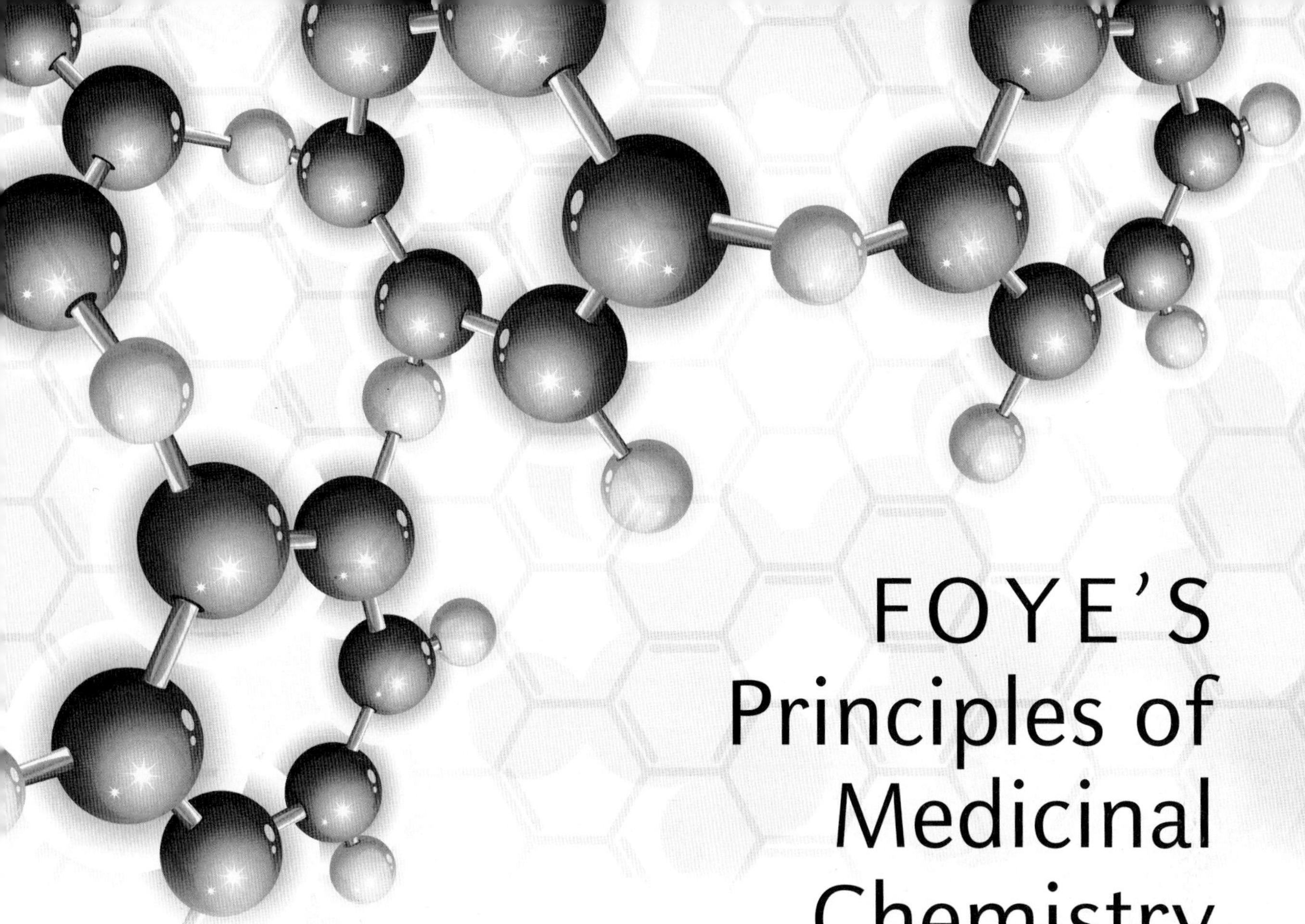

FOYE'S
Principles of Medicinal Chemistry

SEVENTH EDITION

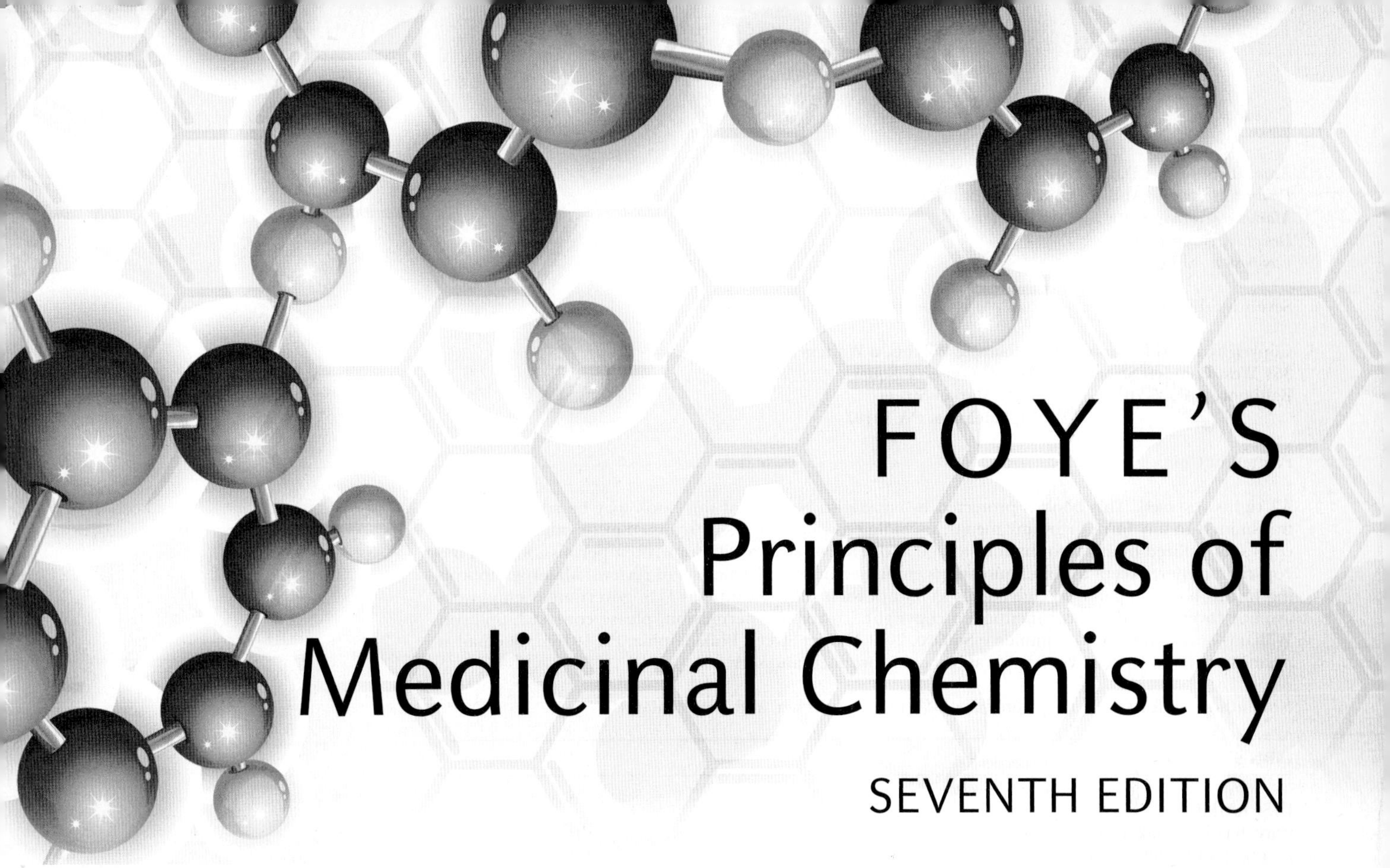

FOYE'S
Principles of Medicinal Chemistry

SEVENTH EDITION

Edited By

THOMAS L. LEMKE, PhD
Professor Emeritus
College of Pharmacy
University of Houston
Houston, Texas

DAVID A. WILLIAMS, PhD
Professor Emeritus of Chemistry
Massachusetts College of Pharmacy and Health Sciences
Boston, Massachusetts

Associate Editors

VICTORIA F. ROCHE, PhD
Professor of Pharmacy Sciences
School of Pharmacy and Health Professions
Creighton University
Omaha, Nebraska

S. WILLIAM ZITO, PhD
Professor Pharmaceutical Sciences
College of Pharmacy and Allied Health Professions
St. John's University
Jamaica, New York

Wolters Kluwer Health | Lippincott Williams & Wilkins

Philadelphia • Baltimore • New York • London
Buenos Aires • Hong Kong • Sydney • Tokyo

Acquisitions Editor: David Troy
Product Managers: Andrea M. Klingler and Paula C. Williams
Marketing Manager: Joy Fischer-Williams
Designer: Doug Smock
Compositor: SPi Global

Seventh Edition

351 West Camden Street
Baltimore, MD 21201

Two Commerce Square
2001 Market Street
Philadelphia, PA 19103

Printed in China

ISBN 978-1-4511-7572-1

DISCLAIMER
Care has been taken to confirm the accuracy of the information present and to describe generally accepted practices. However, the authors, editors, and publisher are not responsible for errors or omissions or for any consequences from application of the information in this book and make no warranty, expressed or implied, with respect to the currency, completeness, or accuracy of the contents of the publication. Application of this information in a particular situation remains the professional responsibility of the practitioner; the clinical treatments described and recommended may not be considered absolute and universal recommendations.

The authors, editors, and publisher have exerted every effort to ensure that drug selection and dosage set forth in this text are in accordance with the current recommendations and practice at the time of publication. However, in view of ongoing research, changes in government regulations, and the constant flow of information relating to drug therapy and drug reactions, the reader is urged to check the package insert for each drug for any change in indications and dosage and for added warnings and precautions. This is particularly important when the recommended agent is a new or infrequently employed drug.

Some drugs and medical devices presented in this publication have Food and Drug Administration (FDA) clearance for limited use in restricted research settings. It is the responsibility of the health care provider to ascertain the FDA status of each drug or device planned for use in their clinical practice.

To purchase additional copies of this book, call our customer service department at (800) 638-3030 or fax orders to (301) 223-2320. International customers should call (301) 223-2300.

Visit Lippincott Williams & Wilkins on the Internet: http://www.lww.com. Lippincott Williams & Wilkins customer service representatives are available from 8:30 am to 6:00 pm, EST.

9 8 7 6 5 4 3 2 1

RRS1112

This textbook is dedicated to our students and to our academic colleagues who mentor these students in the principles and applications of medicinal chemistry. The challenge for the student is to master the chemical, pharmacological, pharmaceutical and therapeutic aspects of the drug and utilize the knowledge of medicinal chemistry to effectively communicate with prescribing clinicians, nurses and other members of the health care team, as well as in discussing drug therapy with patients.

Thomas L. Lemke
David A. Williams
Victoria F. Roche
S. William Zito

Preface

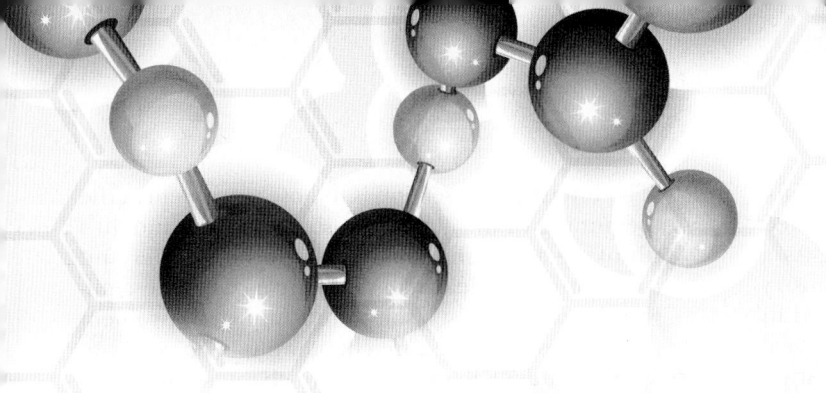

As defined by IUPAC, medicinal chemistry is a chemistry-based discipline, involving aspects of the biological, medical and pharmaceutical sciences. It is concerned with the invention, discovery, design, identification and preparation of biologically active compounds, the study of their metabolism, the interpretation of their mode of action at the molecular level and the construction of structure-activity relationships (SAR), which is the relationship between chemical structure and pharmacological activity for a series of compounds.

As we look back 38 years to the first edition of *Foye's Principles of Medicinal Chemistry* and nearly 63 years to the first edition of Wilson and Gisvold's textbook, *Organic Chemistry in Pharmacy* (later renamed *Textbook of Organic Medicinal and Pharmaceutical Chemistry*), we can examine how the teaching of medicinal chemistry has evolved over the last half of the 20th century. Sixty years ago the approach to teaching drug classification was based on chemical functional groups; in the 1970s it was the relationship between chemical structure and pharmacological activity for a series of compounds, and today medicinal chemistry involves the integration of these principles with pharmacology, pharmaceutics, and therapeutics into a single multi-semester course called pharmacodynamics, pharmacotherapeutics, or another similar name. Drug discovery and development will always maintain its role in traditional drug therapy, but its application to pharmacogenomics may well become the treatment modality of the future. In drug discovery, toxicogenomics is used to improve the safety of drugs mandated by U.S. Food and Drug administration by studying the adverse/toxic effects of drugs in order to draw conclusions on the toxic and safety risk to patients. The scope of knowledge in organic chemistry, biochemistry, pharmacology, and therapeutics allows students to make generalizations connecting the physicochemical properties of small organic molecules and peptides to the receptor and biochemical properties of living systems.

Creating new drugs to combat disease is a complex process. The shape of a drug must be right to allow it to bind to a specific disease-related protein (i.e., receptor) and to work effectively. This shape is determined by the core framework of the molecule and the relative orientation of functional groups in three dimensional space. As a consequence, these generalizations, validated by repetitive examples, emerge in time as principles of drug discovery and drug mechanisms, principles that describe the structural relationships between diverse organic molecules and the biomolecular functions that predict their mechanisms toward controlling diseases.

Medicinal chemistry is central to modern drug discovery and development. For most of the 20th century, the majority of drugs were discovered either by identifying the active ingredient in traditional natural remedies, by rational drug design, or by serendipity. As we have moved into the 21st century, drug discovery has focused on drug targets and high-throughput screening of drug hits and computer-assessed drug design to fill its drug pipeline. Medicinal chemistry has advanced during the past several decades from not only synthesizing new compounds but to understanding the molecular basis of a disease and its control, identifying biomolecular targets implicated as disease-causing, and ultimately inventing specific compounds (called "hits") that block the biomolecules from progressing to an illness or stop the disease in its tracks. Medicinal chemists use structure-activity relationships to improve the "hits" into "lead candidates" by optimizing their selectivity against the specific target, reducing drug activity against non-targets, and ensuring appropriate pharmacokinetic properties involving drug distribution and clearance.

These are tough times for the drug industry, as companies are looking at diminishing pipelines of potential new drugs, growing competition from generic versions of their drugs and increasing pressure from regulatory agencies to ensure that products are both safe and more effective than existing drugs. With the completion of sequencing of the human genome there are now greater challenges facing the drug industry for applications of new technologies in discovery and development. The number of drug targets once considered to be less than 500, has doubled and is expected to increase tenfold. Diseases that were once thought to be caused by a single pathology are now known to have differing etiologies requiring highly specific medications. In order to maintain its pipeline of new drugs, the drug industry is integrating biopharmaceuticals, such as therapeutic antibodies (e.g., in the treatment of arthritis), along with small-molecule drugs. As the drug industry undergoes reform, drug companies are developing collaborations with academia for new sources of drug molecules.

The editors of this textbook are all medicinal chemists, and our approaches to editing this seventh edition of *Foye's Principles of Medicinal Chemistry* are influenced by our respective academic backgrounds. We believe that our collaboration on this textbook represents a melding of our perspectives that will provide new dimensions of appreciation and understanding for all students. In addition we recognize the benefits of medicinal chemistry can only be valuable if the science can be translated into improving the quality of life of our patients. As a result it is essential that the student apply the chemistry of the drugs to their patients and we have attempted to bridge the gap between the science of drugs and the real life situations through the use of scenarios and case studies. Finally in editing this multi-authored book we have tried to promote a consistent style in the organization of the respective chapters.

ORGANIZATIONAL PHILOSOPHY

The organizational approach taken in this textbook builds from the principles of drug discovery, physicochemical properties of drug molecules, and ADMET (absorption-distribution-metabolism-excretion-toxicity) to their integration into therapeutic substances with application to patient care. Our challenge has been to provide a comprehensive description of drug discovery and pharmacodynamic agents in an introductory textbook. To address the increasing emphasis in U.S. pharmacy schools on integrating medicinal chemistry with pharmacology and clinical pharmacy and the creation of one-semester principle courses, we organized the book into four parts: Part I: Principles of Drug Discovery; Part II: Drug Receptors Affecting Neurotransmission and Enzymes as Catalytic Receptors; Part III: Pharmacodynamic Agents (with further subdivision into drugs affecting different physiologic systems); and Part IV: Disease State Management. Parts I and II are designed for a course focused on principles of drug discovery and Parts II through IV are relevant to integrated courses in medicinal chemistry/pharmacodynamics/pharmacotherapeutics.

WHAT IS NEW IN THIS EDITION

The pharmacist sits at the interface between the health-care system and the patient. The pharmacist has the responsibility for improving the quality of life of the patient by assuring the appropriate use of pharmaceuticals. To do this appropriately, the pharmacist must bring together the basic sciences of chemistry, biology, biopharmaceutics and pharmacology with the clinical sciences. In an attempt to relate the importance of medicinal chemistry to the clinical sciences, each of the chapters in Part II, Pharmacodynamic Agents, through Part IV, Disease State Management, includes the following:

- **A clinical significance section:** At the beginning of most chapters, a practicing clinician has provided a statement of the clinical significance of medicinal chemistry to the particular therapeutic class of drugs.
- **A clinical scenario section:** At the beginning of the chapters in Part III and IV the clinician has provided a brief clinical scenario (mini-case) or real-life therapeutic problem related to the disease state under consideration. A solution to the case or problem appears at the end of the chapter along with the medicinal chemist's analysis of the solution. The intent of this section is to pose a problem at the beginning of the chapter to stimulate the student's thinking as he/she reads through the chapter and then bring the learning "full circle" with the clinician's and chemist's solution to the case/problem revealed once the entire chapter has been read.
- **A case study:** Each of the above chapters ends with a case study (see the "Introduction to Medicinal Chemistry Case Studies" section of this preface). As with previous editions of Foye's Principles of Medicinal Chemistry these cases are meant help the student evaluate their comprehension of the therapeutically relevant chemistry presented in the chapter and apply their understanding in a standardized format to solving the posed problem. All cases presented in this text underwent review by a practicing pharmacist to ensure clinical accuracy and relevance to contemporary practice.

In addition, the reader will find at the beginning of most chapters a list of drugs (presented by generic or chemical names) discussed in that chapter. Additionally, at the beginning of each chapter, one will find a list of the commonly used abbreviations in the chapter.

Several new chapters appear in the seventh edition, including Chapter 5, Membrane Drug Transporters; Chapter 16, Anesthetics: General and Local Anesthetics; Chapter 19, CNS Stimulants and Drugs of Abuse; and Chapter 42, Obesity and Nutrition. Lastly, a second color has been added to this edition to help emphasize particular points in the chapters. In most figures where drug metabolism occurs the point of metabolism is highlighted in red with coloration of the functionality which has been changed.

STUDENT AND INSTRUCTOR RESOURCES

Student Resources

A Student Resource Center at http://thePoint.lww.com/Lemke7e includes the following materials:

- Full Text Online
- Additional Case Studies
- Answers to Additional Case Studies
- Practice Quiz Questions
- Drug Updates
- U.S. Drug Regulation: An Overview

Instructor Resources

We understand the demand on an instructor's time. To facilitate and support your educational efforts, you will have access to Instructor Resources upon adoption of *Foye's Principles of Medicinal Chemistry, 7th edition.* An Instructor's Resource Center at http://thePoint.lww.com/Lemke7e includes the following:

- Full Text Online
- Image Bank
- Answers to In-Text Case Studies
- Angel/Blackboard/WebCT Course Cartridges
- U.S. Drug Regulation: An Overview

ACKNOWLEDGEMENTS

We are indebted to our talented and conscientious contributors, for without them this book would not exist. This includes chapter authors, clinicians who wrote both the clinical significance sections and scenarios, and to Victoria Roche and Sandy Zito for creation of the exciting and educational case studies. We also thank our respective academic institutions for the use of institutional resources and for the freedom to exercise the creative juices needed to bring new ideas to a textbook in medicinal chemistry.

We are grateful for the many people at Lippincott Williams & Wilkins who were there to answer questions, make corrections, and support us through their encouraging words. Many of those who shepherded this book through the complex process of publication worked behind the scene and are not known to us, but we specifically acknowledge Andrea M. Klingler and Paula Williams (Product Managers), and David Troy (Acquisitions Editor) for their kind and gentle prodding.

Finally, we want to acknowledge our respective spouses, Pat and Gail, who were supportive of this time-consuming labor of love. Untold hours were spent away from the family sitting in front of our computers in order to bring this project to fruition.

Thomas L. Lemke, PhD
David A. Williams, PhD

INTRODUCTION TO MEDICINAL CHEMISTRY CASE STUDIES

We are pleased to share our newest medicinal chemistry case studies with student and faculty users of *Foye's Principles of Medicinal Chemistry*. One case study is provided at the end of most chapters. This preface is written to explain their scope and purpose, and to help those who are unfamiliar with our technique of illustrating the therapeutic relevance of chemistry get the most out of the exercise.

Like the more familiar therapeutic case studies, medicinal chemistry case studies are clinical scenarios that present a patient in need of a pharmacist's expert intervention. The learner, most commonly in the role of the pharmacist, evaluates the patient's clinical and personal situation and makes a drug product selection from a limited number of therapeutic choices. However, in a medicinal chemistry case study, only the structures of the potential therapeutic candidates are given. To make their professional recommendation, students must conduct a thorough analysis of *key structure activity relationships (SAR)* in order to predict such things as relative potency, receptor selectivity, duration of action and potential for adverse reactions, and then apply the knowledge gained to meet the patient's therapeutic needs.

The therapeutic choices we offer in each case have been purposefully selected to allow students to review the therapeutically relevant chemistry of different classes of drugs used to treat a particular disease. We recognize that this approach might occasionally omit some compounds viewed by practitioners as drugs of choice within a class or the formulary entry at their practice sites. Faculty employing the cases as in-class or take-home assignments might alter the structural choices provided to meet their teaching and learning goals, and this is certainly acceptable. Regardless of how they are used, students working thoughtfully and scientifically through the cases will not only master chemical concepts and principles and reinforce basic SAR, but also learn how to actively use their unique knowledge of drug chemistry when thinking critically about patient care. This skill will be invaluable when, as practitioners, they are faced with a full gamut of therapeutic options to analyze in order to ensure the best therapeutic outcomes for their patients.

In short, here's what we hope students will gain by working our cases.

- Mastery of the important concepts needed to be successful in the medicinal chemistry component of the pharmacy curriculum;
- An ability to identify the relevance of drug chemistry to pharmacological action and therapeutic utility, and to discriminate between therapeutic options based on that understanding;
- An enhanced ability to think critically and scientifically about drug use;
- A commitment to caring about the impact of professional decisions on patients' quality of life;
- The ability to demonstrate the unique role of the pharmacist as the chemist of the health care team.

We hope you find these case studies both challenging and enjoyable, and we encourage you to use them as a springboard to more in-depth discussions with your faculty and/or colleagues about the role of chemistry in rational therapeutic decision-making.

Victoria F. Roche, PhD
S. William Zito, PhD

Contributors

Ali R. Banijamali, PhD
Ironwood Pharmaceuticals
Cambridge, MA

Raymond G. Booth, PhD
University of Florida
College of Pharmacy
Gainsville, FL

Ronald Borne, PhD
The University of Mississippi
School of Pharmacy
University, MS

Robert W. Brueggemeier, PhD
The Ohio State University
College of Pharmacy
Columbus, OH

James T. Dalton, PhD
The Ohio State University
College of Pharmacy
Columbus, OH

Małgorzata Dukat, PhD
Virginia Commonwealth University
School of Pharmacy
Richmond, VA

E. Kim Fifer, PhD
University of Arkansas for Medical Sciences
College of Pharmacy
Little Rock, AR

Elmer J. Gentry, PhD
Chicago State University
College of Pharmacy
Chicago, IL

Marc Gillespie, PhD
St. John's University
College of Pharmacy and Allied Health Professions
Queens, NY

Richard A. Glennon, PhD
Virginia Commonwealth University
School of Pharmacy
Richmond, VA

Robert K. Griffith, PhD
West Virginia University
School of Pharmacy
Morgantown, WV

Marc Harrold, PhD
Duquesne University
Mylan School of Pharmacy
Pittsburgh, PA

Peter J. Harvison, PhD
University of the Sciences in Philadelphia
Philadelphia College of Pharmacy
Philadelphia, PA

Sunil S. Jambhekar, PhD
Lake Erie College of Osteopathic Medicine
Bradenton, FL

David A. Johnson, PhD
Duquesne University
Mylan School of Pharmacy
Pittsburgh, PA

Stephen Kerr, PhD
Massachusetts College of Pharmacy and Health
School of Pharmacy
Boston, MA

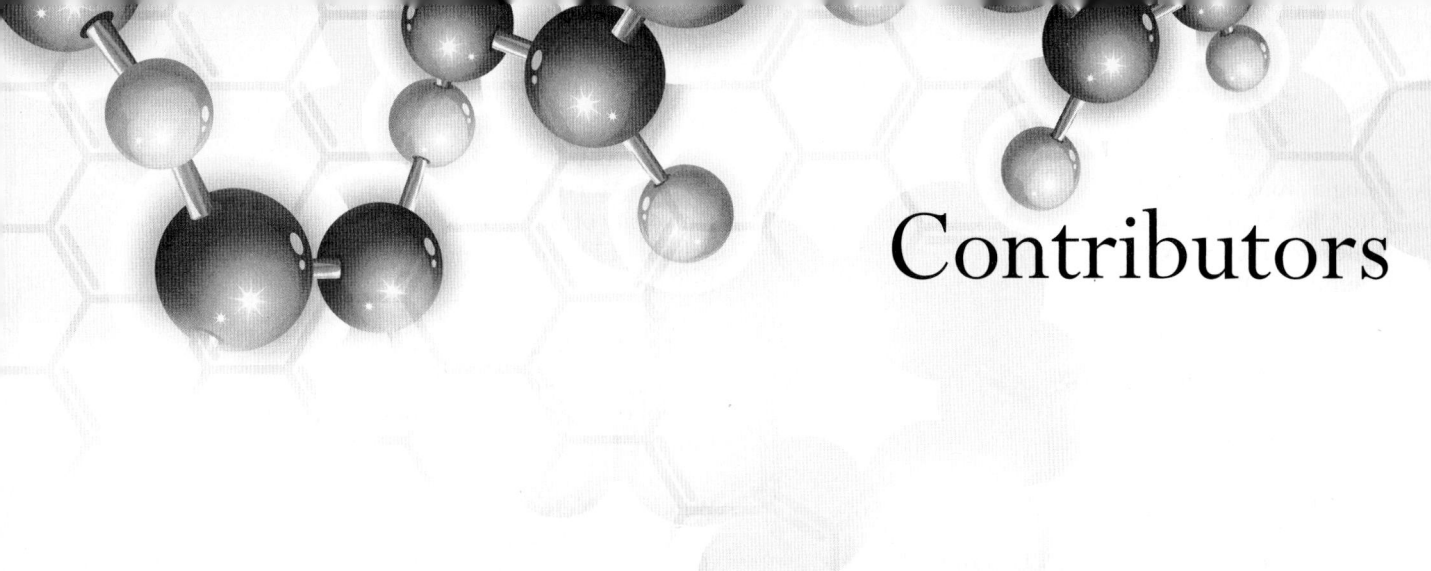

Douglas Kinghorn, PhD
The Ohio State University
College of Pharmacy
Columbus, OH

James J. Knittel, PhD
Western New England College
School of Pharmacy
Springfield, MA

Vijaya L. Korlipara, PhD
St. John's University
College of Pharmacy and Allied Health Professions
Queens, NY

Barbara LeDuc, PhD
Massachusetts College of Pharmacy and Health
School of Pharmacy
Boston, MA

Thomas L. Lemke, PhD
University of Houston
College of Pharmacy
Houston, TX

Mark Levi, PhD
US Food & Drug Administration
National Center for Toxicological Research
Division of Neurotoxicology
Jefferson, AR

Matthias C. Lu, PhD
University of Illinois at Chicago
College of Pharmacy
Chicago, IL

Timothy Maher, PhD
Massachusetts College of Pharmacy and Health Sciences
School of Pharmacy
Boston, MA

Ahmed S. Mehanna, PhD
Massachusetts College of Pharmacy and Health Sciences
School of Pharmacy
Boston, MA

Duane D. Miller, PhD
The University of Tennessee
College of Pharmacy
Memphis, TN

Nader H. Moniri
Mercer University
College of Pharmacy and Health Sciences
Atlanta, GA

Marilyn Morris, PhD
University of Buffalo - SUNY
School of Pharmacy and Pharmaceutical Sciences
Buffalo, NY

Bridget L. Morse
University of Buffalo - SUNY
School of Pharmacy and Pharmaceutical Sciences
Buffalo, NY

Wendel L. Nelson, PhD
University of Washington
School of Pharmacy
Seattle, WA

John L. Neumeyer, PhD
Harvard Medical School
McLean Hospital
Belmont, MA

Gary O. Rankin, PhD
Marshall University
School of Medicine
Huntington, WV

Edward B. Roche, PhD
University of Nebraska
College of Pharmacy
Omaha, NE

Victoria F. Roche, PhD
Creighton University
School of Pharmacy and Health Professions
Omaha, NE

David A. Williams, PhD
Massachusetts College of Pharmacy and Health Sciences
School of Pharmacy
Boston, MA

Norman Wilson, BSc, PhD, CChem, FRSC
University of Edinburgh
Edinburgh, Scotland

Patrick M. Woster, PhD
Medical University of South Carolina
College of Pharmacy
Charleston, SC

Tanaji T. Talele, PhD
St. John's University
College of Pharmacy and Allied Health Professions
Queens, NY

Robin Zavod, PhD
Midwestern University, Chicago
College of Pharmacy
Chicago, IL

S. William Zito, PhD
St. John's University
College of Pharmacy and Allied Health Professios
Queens, NY

Clinical Scenario and Clinical Significance

Paul Arpino, RPh
Harvard Medical School
Department of Pharmacy
Massachusetts General Hospital
Boston, MA

Kim K. Birtcher, MS, PharmD, BCPS, CDE, CLS
University of Houston
College of Pharmacy
Houston, TX

Jennifer Campbell, PharmD
Creighton University
School of Pharmacy and Health Professions
Omaha, NE

Judy Cheng, PharmD
Massachusetts College of Pharmacy and Health Sciences
School of Pharmacy
Boston, MA

Elizabeth Coyle, PharmD
University of Houston
College of Pharmacy
Houston, TX

Joseph V. Etzel, PharmD
St. John's University
College of Pharmacy and Allied Health Professions
Queens, NY

Marc Gillepspie, PhD
St. John's University
College of Pharmacy and Allied Health Professions
Queens, NY

Michael Gonyeau, PharmD, BCPS
Northeastern University
School of Pharmacy
Boston, MA

David Hayes, PharmD
University of Houston
College of Pharmacy
Houston, TX

Elizabeth B. Hirsch, PharmD, BCPS
Northeastern University
School of Pharmacy
Boston, MA

Jill T. Johnson, PharmD, BCPS
University of Arkansas for Medical Sciences
College of Pharmacy
Little Rock, AR

Vijaya L. Korlipara, PhD
St. John's University
College of Pharmacy and Allied Health Professions
Queens, NY

Beverly Lukawski, PharmD
Creighton University
School of Pharmacy and Health Professions
Omaha, NE

Timothy Maher, PhD
Massachusetts College of Pharmacy and Health Sciences
School of Pharmacy
Boston, MA

Susan W. Miller, PharmD
Mercer University
College of Pharmacy and Health Sciences
Atlanta, GA

Kathryn Neill, PharmD
University of Arkansas for Medical Sciences
College of Pharmacy
Little Rock, AR

Kelly Nystrom, PharmD, BCOP
Creighton University
School of Pharmacy and Health Professions
Omaha, NE

Nancy Ordonez, PharmD
University of Houston
College of Pharmacy
Houston, TX

Anne Pace, PharmD
University of Arkansas for Medical Sciences
College of Pharmacy
Little Rock, AR

Nathan A. Painter, PharmD, CDE
University of California, San Diego
Skaggs School of Pharmacy and Pharmaceutical Science
La Jolla, CA

Thomas L. Rihn, PharmD
Duquesne University
School of Pharmacy
Pittsburgh, PA

Jeffrey T. Sherer, PharmD, MPH, BCPS, CGP
University of Houston
College of Pharmacy
Houston, TX

Douglas Slain, PharmD, BCPS
West Virginia University
College of Pharmacy
Morgantown, WV

Autumn Stewart, PharmD
Duquesne University
School of Pharmacy
Pittsburgh, PA

Tanaji T. Talele, PhD
St. John's University
College of Pharmacy and Allied Health Professions
Queens, NY

Mark D. Watanabe, PharmD, PhD, BCPP
Northeastern University
School of Pharmacy
Boston, MA

Reviewers

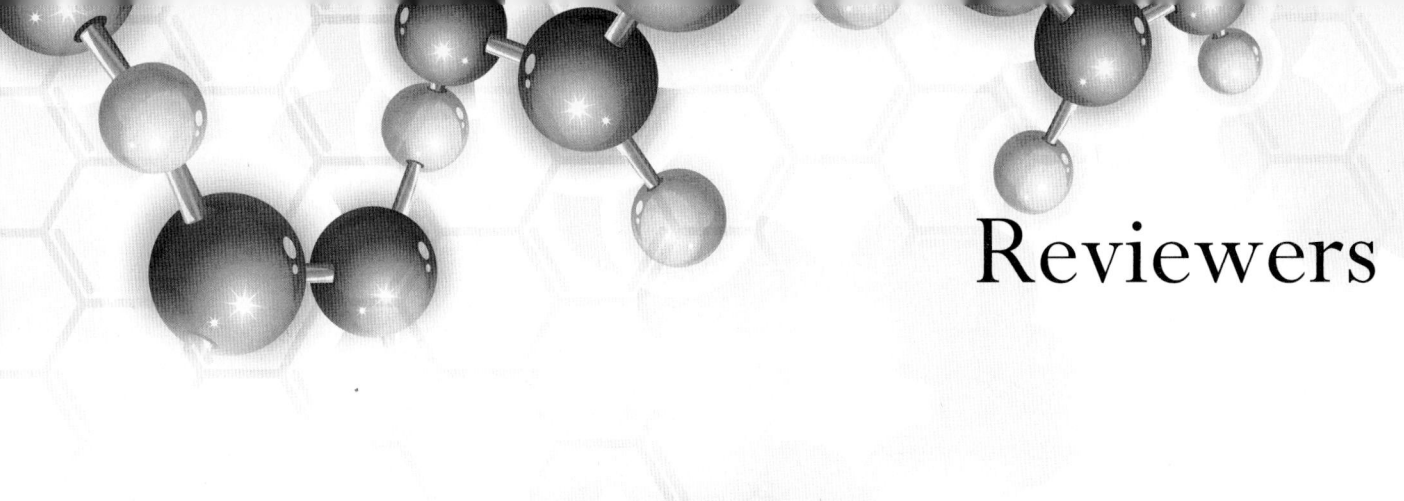

Michael Adams, PharmD, PhD
Assistant Professor
Pharmaceutical Sciences
Campbell University School of Pharmacy
Buies Creek, NC

Zhe-Sheng Chen, MD, PhD
Associate Professor
Pharmaceutical Science
St. John's University
Queens, NY

John Cooperwood, PhD
Associate Professor
Pharmaceutical Sciences
Florida Agricultural and Mechanical University College of Pharmacy
Tallahassee, FL

Matthew J. DellaVecchia, PhD
Assistant Professor of Pharmaceutical Sciences
Gregory School of Pharmacy
Palm Beach Atlantic University
Palm Beach, FL

Marc Harrold, PhD
Professor of Medicinal Chemistry
Mylan School of Pharmacy
Duquesne University
Pittsburgh, PA

Kennerly Patrick, PhD Med Chem
Professor
Pharmaceutical Sciences
Medical University of South Carolina
College of Pharmacy
Charleston, SC

Tanaji Talele, PhD
Associate Professor of Medicinal Chemistry
Department of Pharmaceutical Sciences
College of Pharmacy & Allied Health Professions
St. John's University
Queens, NY

Ganeshsingh Thakur, PhD
Center for Drug Discovery
Assistant Professor
Pharmaceutical Sciences
Northeastern University
Boston, MA

Constance Vance, PhD
Adjunct Assistant Professor
University of North Carolina at Chapel Hill
Chapel Hill, NC

Contents

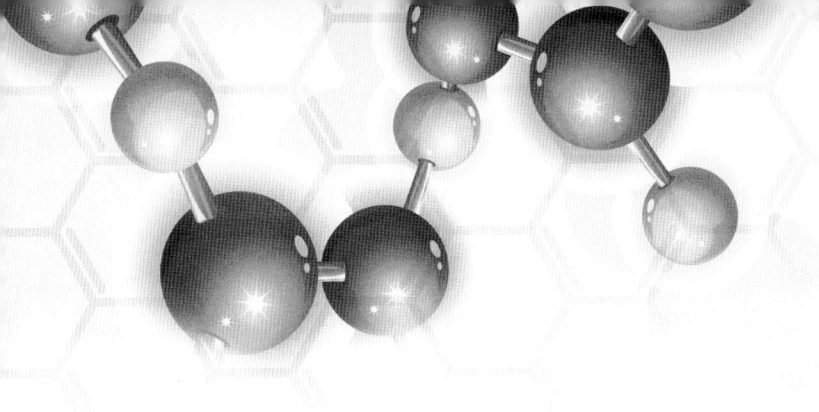

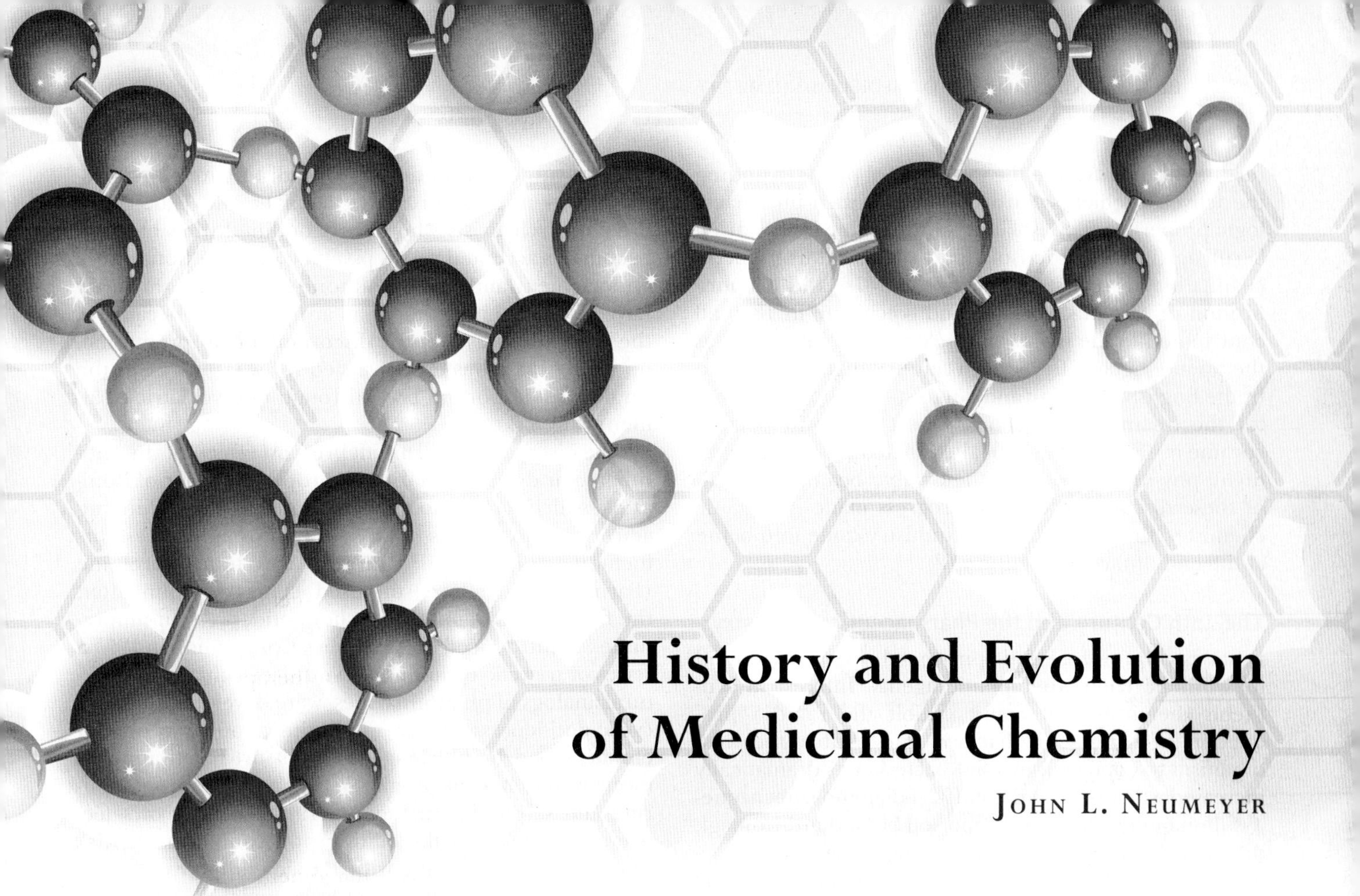

History and Evolution of Medicinal Chemistry

John L. Neumeyer

The unprecedented increase in human life expectancy, which has almost doubled in a hundred years, is mainly due to drugs and to those who discovered them (1).

The history of all fields of science is comprised of the ideas, knowledge, and available tools that have advanced contemporary knowledge. The spectacular advances in medicinal chemistry over the years are no exception. Alfred Burger (1) stated that "...the great advances of medicinal chemistry have been achieved by two types of investigators: those with the genius of prophetic logic, who have opened a new field by interpreting correctly a few well-placed experiments, whether they pertained to the design or the mechanism of action of drugs; and those who have varied patiently the chemical structures of physiologically active compounds until a useful drug could be evolved as a tool in medicine." To place the development of medicinal chemical research into its proper perspective, one needs to examine the evolution of the ideas and concepts that have led to our present knowledge.

Drugs of Antiquity

The oldest records of the use of therapeutic plants and minerals are derived from the ancient civilizations of the Chinese, the Hindus, the Mayans of Central America, and the Mediterranean peoples of antiquity. The Emperor Shen Nung (2735 BC) compiled what may be called a pharmacopeia including *ch'ang shang*, an antimalarial alkaloid, and *ma huang*, from which ephedrine was isolated. Chaulmoogra fruit was known to the indigenous American Indians, and the ipecacuanha root containing emetine was used in Brazil for the treatment of dysentery and is still used for the treatment of amebiasis. The early explorers found that the South American Indians also chewed coca leaves (containing cocaine) and used mushrooms (containing methylated tryptamine) as hallucinogens. In ancient Greek apothecary shops, herbs such as opium, squill, and *Hyoscyamus*, viper toxin, and metallic drugs such as copper and zinc ores, iron sulfate, and cadmium oxide could be found.

The Middle Ages

The basic studies of chemistry and physics shifted from the Greco-Roman to the Arabian alchemists between the 13th and 16th centuries. Paracelsus (1493–1541) glorified antimony and its salts in elixirs as cure-alls in the belief that chemicals could cure disease.

The 19th Century: Age of Innovation and Chemistry

The 19th century saw a great expansion in the knowledge of chemistry, which greatly extended the herbal pharmacopeia that had previously been established. Building on the work of Antoine Lavoisier, chemists throughout Europe refined and extended the techniques of chemical analysis. The synthesis of acetic acid by Adolph Kolbe in 1845 and of methane by Pierre Berthelot in 1856 set the stage for organic chemistry. Pharmacognosy, the science that deals with medicinal products of plant, animal, or mineral origin in their crude state, was replaced by physiologic chemistry. The emphasis was shifted from finding new medicaments from the vast world of plants to finding the active ingredients that accounted for their pharmacologic properties. The isolation of morphine by Friedrich Sertürner in 1803, the isolation of emetine from ipecacuanha by Pierre-Joseph Pelletier in 1816, and his purification of caffeine, quinine, and colchicine in 1820 all contributed to the increased use of "pure" substances as therapeutic agents. In the 19th century, digitalis was used by the English physician and botanist, William Withering, for the treatment of edema. Albert Niemann isolated cocaine in 1860, and in 1864, he isolated the active ingredient, physostigmine, from the Calabar bean. As a result of these discoveries and the progress made in organic chemistry, the pharmaceutical industry came into being at the end of the 19th century (2).

The 20th Century and the Pharmaceutical Industry

Diseases of protozoal and spirochetal origin responded to synthetic chemotherapeutic agents. Interest in synthetic chemicals that could inhibit the rapid reproduction of pathogenic bacteria and enable the host organism to cope with invasive bacteria was dramatically increased when the red dyestuff 2,4-diaminoazobenzene-4′-sulfonamide (Prontosil) reported by Gerhard Domagk dramatically cured dangerous systemic gram-positive bacterial infections in man and animals. The observation by Woods and Fildes in 1940 that the bacteriostatic action of sulfonamide-like drugs is antagonized by *p*-aminobenzoic acid is one of the early examples in which a balance of stimulatory and inhibitory properties depends on the structural analogies of chemicals.

That, together with the discovery of penicillin by Alexander Fleming in 1929 and its subsequent examination by Howard Florey and Ernst Chain in 1941, led to a water-soluble powder of much higher antibacterial potency and lower toxicity than that of previously known synthetic chemotherapeutic agents. With the discovery of a variety of highly potent anti-infective agents, a significant change was introduced into medical practice.

DEVELOPMENTS LEADING TO VARIOUS MEDICINAL CLASSES OF DRUGS

Psychopharmacologic Agents and the Era of Brain Research

Psychiatrists have been using agents active in the central nervous system for hundreds of years. Stimulants and depressants were used to modify the mood and mental states of psychiatric patients. Amphetamine, sedatives, and hypnotics were used to stimulate or depress the mental states of patients. Was it the synthesis of chlorpromazine by Paul Charpentier that caused a revolution in the treatment of schizophrenia? Who really discovered chlorpromazine? Was it Charpentier, who first synthesized the molecule in 1950 at Rhone-Poulenc's research laboratory; Simone Courvoisier, who reported distinctive effects on animal behavior; Henri Laborit, a French military surgeon who first noticed distinctive psychotropic effects in man; or Pierre Deniker and Jean Delay, French psychiatrists who clearly outlined what has now become its accepted use in psychiatry and without whose endorsement and prestige Rhone-Poulenc might never have developed it further as an antipsychotic? Because of the bitter disputes over the discovery of chlorpromazine, no Nobel Prize was ever awarded for what has been the single most important breakthrough in psychiatric treatment (Fig. 1).

The discovery of the antidepressant effects of the antitubercular drug iproniazid (isopropyl congener of isoniazid), which has monoamine oxidase (MAO)–inhibiting activity, led to a series of MAO inhibitor antidepressants including phenelzine (Nardil) and tranylcypromine (Parnate), which are still used clinically. Soon after, the first dibenzazepine (tricyclic) antidepressant imipramine was introduced by Ciba-Geigy Corporation in 1957 a series of tricyclic compounds synthsized initially as structural analogs of phenothiazines, were developed. The tricyclic antidepressants are not antipsychotic, but instead elevate mood by blocking the transport inactivation of monoamine neurotransmitters including norepinephrine and serotonin. In the late 1980s, a series of selective serotonin reuptake or transport inhibitors (SSRIs) were developed, starting with *R,S*-zimelidine from Astra Pharmaceutica (which proved to be toxic) and then *R,S*-fluoxetine (Prozac) from Eli Lilly and Company, the first commercially successful SSRI and the first psychotropic agent to attain an annual market above $1 billion.

The antianxiety agents, including a large series of benzodiazepines (including chlordiazepoxide [Librium] and diazepam [Valium] and the carbamate meprobamate [Miltown]), are examples of the serendipitous discovery of new drugs based on random screening of newly synthesized chemicals (Fig. 1). The discovery of these drugs was based on observations of effects on the behavior of animals used in screening bioassays. In 1946, Frank M. Berger observed unusual and characteristic paralysis and relaxation of voluntary muscles in laboratory animals for different series of compounds. At this point, the treatment of ambulatory anxious patients with meprobamate and psychotic patients with one of the aminoalkylphenothiazine drugs was possible.

There was a need for drugs of greater selectivity in the treatment of anxiety because of the side effects often

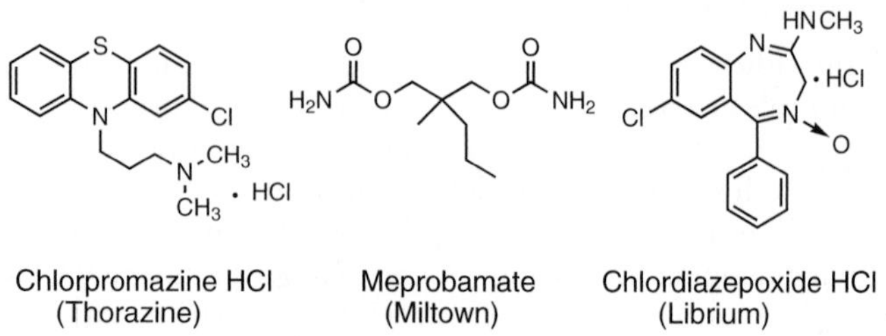

FIGURE 1 Psychopharmacologic agents.

encountered with phenothiazines. Leo Sternback, a chemist working in the research laboratory of Hoffman-La Roche in New Jersey, decided to reinvestigate a relatively unexplored class of compounds that he had studied in the 1930s when he was a postdoctoral fellow at the University of Cracow in Poland. He synthesized about 40 compounds in this series, all of which were disappointing in pharmacologic tests, so the project was abandoned. In 1957, during a cleanup of the laboratory, one compound synthesized 2 years earlier had crystallized and was submitted for testing to L.O. Randall, a pharmacologist. Shortly thereafter, Randall reported that this compound was hypnotic and sedative and had antistrychnine effects similar to those of meprobamate. The compound was named chlordiazepoxide and marketed as Librium in 1960, just 3 years after the first pharmacologic observations by Randall. Structural modifications of benzodiazepine derivatives were undertaken, and a compound 5 to 10 times more potent than chlordiazepoxide was synthesized in 1959 and marketed as diazepam (Valium) in 1963. The synthesis of many other experimental analogs soon followed, and by 1983, about 35 benzodiazepine drugs were available for therapy (see Chapter 15). Benzodiazepines are used in the pharmacotherapy of anxiety and related emotional disorders and in the treatment of sleep disorders, status epilepticus, and other convulsive states. They are used as centrally acting muscle relaxants, for premedication, and as inducing agents in anesthesiology.

Endocrine Therapy and Steroids

The first pure hormone to be isolated from the endocrine gland was epinephrine, which led to further molecular modifications in the area of sympathomimetic amines. Subsequently, norepinephrine was also identified from sympathetic nerves. The development of chromatographic techniques allowed the isolation and characterization of a multitude of hormones from a single gland. In 1914, biochemist Edward Kendall isolated thyroxine from the thyroid gland. He subsequently won the Nobel Prize in Physiology or Medicine in 1950 for his discovery of the activity of cortisone. Two of the hormones of the thyroid gland, thyroxine (T_4) and liothyronine (T_3), have similar effects in the body regulating metabolism, whereas the two hormones from the posterior pituitary gland—vasopressin, which exerts pressor and antidiuretic activity, and oxytocin, which stimulates lactation and uterine motility—differ considerably both in their chemical structure and physiologic activity. (Fig. 2)

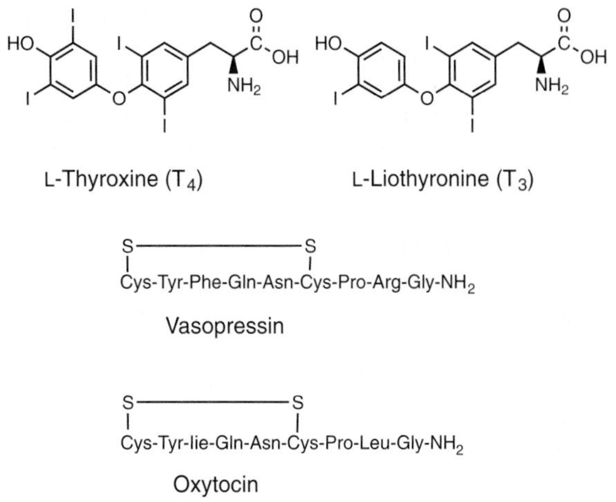

FIGURE 2 Hormones from the endocrine glands.

Less than 50 years after the discovery of oxytocin by Henry Dale in 1904, who found that an extract from the human pituitary gland contracted the uterus of a pregnant cat, the biochemist Vincent du Vigneud synthesized the cyclic peptide hormone. His work resulted in the Nobel Prize in Chemistry in 1955.

A major achievement in drug discovery and development was the discovery of insulin in 1921 from animal sources. Frederick G. Banting and Charles H. Best, working in the laboratory of John J.R. McLeod at the University of Toronto, isolated the peptide hormone and began testing it in dogs. By 1922, researchers, with the help of James B. Collip and the pharmaceutical industry, purified and produced animal-based insulin in large quantities. Insulin soon became a major product for Eli Lilly & Co. and Novo Nordisk, a Danish pharmaceutical company. In 1923, McLeod and Bunting were awarded the Nobel Prize in Medicine or Physiology, and after much controversy, they shared the prize with Collip and Best. For the next 60 years, cattle and pigs were the major sources of insulin. With the development of genetic engineering in the 1970s, new opportunities arose for making synthetic insulin that is chemically identical to human insulin. In 1978, the biotech company Genentech and the City of Hope National Medical Center produced human insulin in the laboratory using recombinant DNA technology. By 1982, Lilly's Humulin became the first genetically engineered drug approved by the U.S. Food and Drug Administration (FDA). At about the same time, Novo Nordisk began selling the first semisynthetic human insulin made by enzymatically converting porcine insulin. Novo Nordisk was also using recombinant technology to produce insulin. Recombinant insulin was a significant milestone in the development of genetically engineered drugs and combined the technologies of the biotech companies with the know-how and resources of the major pharmaceutical industries. Inhaled insulin was approved by the FDA in 2006. Many drugs are now available (see Chapter 27) to treat the more common type 2 diabetes in which insulin production needs to be increased. Insulin had been the only treatment for type 1 diabetes until 2005 when the FDA approved Amylin Pharmaceuticals' Symlin to control blood sugar levels in combination with the peptide hormone. The isolation and purification of several peptide hormones of the anterior pituitary and hypothalamic-releasing hormones now make it possible to produce synthetic peptide agonists and antagonists that have important diagnostic and therapeutic applications.

Extensive and remarkable advances in the endocrine field have been made in the group of steroid hormones. The isolation and characterization of minute amounts of the active principles of the sex glands and from the adrenal cortex eventually led to their total synthesis. Male and female sex hormones are used in the treatment of a variety of disorders associated with sexual development and the sexual cycles of males and females, as well as in the selective therapy of malignant tumors of the breast and prostate gland. Synthetic modifications of the structure of the male and female hormones have furnished improved hormonal compounds such as the anabolic agents (see Chapter 40). Since early days, women have ingested every manner of substance as birth control agents. In the early 1930s, Russell Marker found that, for hundreds of years, Mexican women had been eating wild yams of the *Dioscorea* genus for contraception, with apparent success. Marker determined that diosgenin is abundant in yams and has a structure similar to progesterone. Marker was able to convert diosgenin into progesterone, a substance known to stop ovulation in rabbits. However, progesterone is destroyed by the digestive system when ingested. In 1950, Carl Djerassi, a chemist working at the Syntex Laboratories in Mexico City, synthesized norethindrone, the first orally active contraceptive steroid, by a subtle modification of the structure of progesterone. Gregory Pincus, a biologist working at the Worcester Foundation for Experimental Biology in Massachusetts studied Djerassi's new steroid together with its double bond isomer norethynodrel (Fig. 3).

By 1956, clinical studies led by John Rock, a gynecologist, showed that progesterone, in combination with norethindrone, was an effective oral contraceptive. G.D. Searle was the first on the market with Enovid, a combination of mestranol and norethynodrel. In 2005, it was estimated that 11 million American women and about 100 million women worldwide were using oral contraceptive pills. In 1993, the British weekly *The Economist* considered the pill to be one of the seven wonders of the modern world, bringing about major changes in the economic and social structure of women globally.

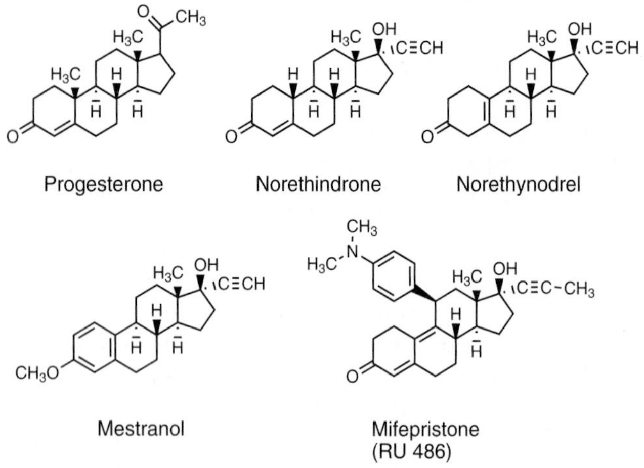

FIGURE 3 Steroidal agents.

In the early 1930s, chemists recognized the similarity of a large number of natural products including the adrenocortical steroids such as hydrocortisone. The medicinal value of Kendall's Compound F and Reichstein's Compound M was quickly recognized. The 1950 Nobel Prize in Physiology or Medicine was awarded to Phillip S. Hench, Edward C. Kendall, and Tadeus Reichstein "...for their discovery relating to the hormones of the adrenal cortex, their structure and biological effects."

An interesting development in the study of glucocorticoids led in 1980 to the synthesis of the "abortion pill," Ru-486, synthesized by Etienne-Emile Beaulieu, a consultant to the French pharmaceutical company, Rousel-Uclaf. Researchers at that time were investigating glucocorticoid antagonists for the treatment of breast cancer, glaucoma, and Cushing syndrome. In screening RU-486, researchers at Rousel-Uclaf found that it had both antiglucocorticoid activity as well as high affinity for progesterone receptors where it could be used for fertility control. RU-486, also known as mifepristone (Mifeprex), entered the French market in 1988, but sales were suspended by Rousel-Uclaf when antiabortion groups threatened to boycott the company. In 1994, the company donated the United States rights to the New York City–based Population Council, a nonprofit reproductive and population control research institution. Mifepristone is now administered in doctors' offices as a tablet in combination with misoprostol, a prostaglandin that causes uterine contractions to help expel the embryo. The combination of mifepristone and misoprostol is more than 90% effective. Plan B, also known as the "morning after pill," has been referred to as an emergency contraceptive. It contains levonorgestrel, the same progestin that is in "the pill," and should be taken within 3 days of unprotected sex and can reduce the risk of pregnancy by 89%.

Anesthetics and Analgesics

The first use of synthetic organic chemicals for the modulation of life processes occurred when nitrous oxide, ether, and chloroform were introduced in anesthesia during the 1840s. Horace Wells, a dentist in Hartford, Connecticut, administered nitrous oxide during a tooth extraction while Crawford Long, a Georgia physician, used ether as an anesthetic for excising a growth on a patient's neck. It was William Morton, a 27-year-old dentist, however, who gave the first successful public demonstration of surgical anesthesia on October 16, 1846, at the surgical amphitheater that is now called the Ether Dome at Massachusetts General Hospital. Morton attempted to patent his discovery but was unsuccessful, and he died penniless in 1868. Chloroform had also been used as an anesthetic at St. Bartholomew's Hospital in London. In

Paris, France, Pierre Fluorens tested both chloroform and ethyl chloride as anesthetics in animals.

The potent and euphoric properties of the extract of the opium poppy have been known for thousands of years. In the 16th century, the Swiss physician and alchemist, Paracelsus (1493–1541) popularized the use of opium in Europe. At that time, an alcoholic solution of opium, known as laudanum, was the method of administration. Morphine was first isolated in pure crystalline form from opium by the German apothecary, Fredrick W. Sertürner, in 1805 who named the compound "morphium" after Morpheus, the Greek god of dreams. It took another 120 years before the structure of morphine was elucidated by Sir Robert Robinson at the University of Oxford. The chemistry of morphine and the other opium alkaloids obtained from *Papaver somniferum* has fascinated and occupied chemists for over 200 years, resulting in many synthetic analgesics available today (see Chapter 20). (−)-Morphine was first synthesized by Marshall Gates at the University of Rochester in 1952. Although a number of highly effective stereoselective synthetic pathways have been developed, it is unlikely that a commercial process can compete with its isolation from the poppy. Diacetylmorphine, known as heroin, is highly addictive and induces tolerance. The illicit worldwide production of opium now exceeds the pharmaceutical production by almost 10-fold. In the United States, some 800,000 people are chemically addicted to heroin, and a growing number are becoming addicted to OxyContin, a synthetic opiate also known as oxycodone. Another synthetic opiate, methadone, relaxes the craving for heroin or morphine. A series of studies in the 1960s at Rockefeller University by Vincent Dole and his wife, Marie Nyswander, found that methadone could also be a viable maintenance treatment to keep addicts from heroin. It is estimated that there are about 250,000 addicts taking methadone in the United States. It has not been widely recognized in the United States that opiate addiction is a medical condition for which there is no known cure. More than 80% of United States heroin addicts still lack access to methadone treatment facilities, primarily due to the stigma against drug users and the medical distribution of methadone.

It has been only within the last 40 years that scientists have begun to understand the effects of opioid analgesics at the molecular level. Beckett and Casey at the University of London proposed in 1954 that opiate effects were receptor mediated, but it was not until the early 1970s that the stereospecific binding of opiates to specific receptors was demonstrated. The characterization and classification of three different types of opioid receptors, *mu*, *kappa*, and *delta*, by William Martin formed the basis of our current understanding of opioid pharmacology. The demonstration of stereospecific binding of radiolabeled ligands to opioid receptors led to the development of radioreceptor binding assays for each of the opioid receptor types, a technique that has been of major importance in the identification of selective opioids as well as many other receptors. In 1973, Avram Goldstein, Solomon Snyder, Ernst Simon, and Lars Terenius independently described saturable, stereospecific binding sites for opiate drugs in the mammalian nervous system. Shortly thereafter, John Hughes and Hans Kosterlitz, working at the University of Aberdeen in Scotland, described the isolation from pig brains of two pentapeptides that exhibited morphine-like actions on the guinea pig ileum. At about the same time, Goldstein reported the presence of peptide-like substances in the pituitary gland showing opiate-like activity. Subsequent research revealed that there are three distinct families of opiate peptides: the enkephalins, the endorphins, and the dynorphins.

Hypnotics and Anticonvulsants

Since antiquity, alcoholic beverages and potions containing laudanum, an alcoholic extract of opium, and various other plant products have been used to induce sleep. Bromides were used in the middle of the 19th century as sedative-hypnotics, as were chloral hydrate, paraldehyde, urethane, and sulfenal. Joseph von Merring, on the assumption that a structure having a carbon atom carrying two ethyl groups would have hypnotic properties, investigated diethyl acetyl urea, which proved to be a potent hypnotic. Further investigations led to 5,5-diethylbarbituric acid, a compound synthesized 20 years earlier in 1864 by Adolph von Beyer. Phenobarbital (5-ethyl-5-phenylbarbituric acid) (Fig. 4) was synthesized by the Bayer Pharmaceutical Company and introduced to the market under the name Luminol. The compound was effective as a hypnotic, but also exhibited properties as an anticonvulsant. The success of phenobarbital led to the testing of more than 2,500 barbiturates, of which about 50 were used clinically, many of which are still in clinical use. Modification of the barbituric acid molecule also led to the development of the hydantoins. Phenytoin (also known as diphenylhydantoin or Dilantin) (Fig. 4) was first synthesized in 1908, but its anticonvulsant properties were not discovered until 1938. Because phenytoin was not a sedative at ordinary doses, it established that antiseizure drugs need not induce drowsiness and encouraged the search for drugs with selective antiseizure action.

Local Anesthetics

The local anesthetics can be traced back to the naturally occurring alkaloid cocaine isolated from *Erythroxylon coca*. A Viennese ophthalmologist, Carl Koller, had

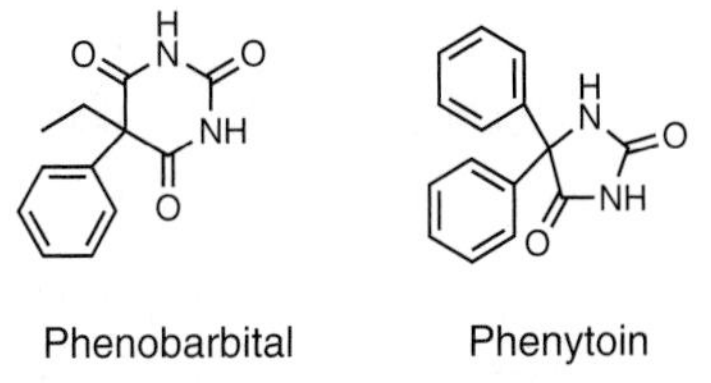

FIGURE 4 Examples of an early hypnotic and anticonvulsant.

experimented with several hypnotics and analgesics for use as a local anesthetic in the eye. His friend, Sigmund Freud, suggested that they attempt to establish how the South American Indians allayed fatigue by chewing leaves of the coca bush. Cocaine had been isolated from the plant by the Swedish chemist Albert Niemann at Gothenburg University in 1860. Koller found that cocaine numbed the tongue, and thus, he discovered a local anesthetic. He quickly realized that cocaine was an effective, nonirritating anesthetic for the eye, leading to the widespread use of cocaine in both Europe and the United States. (Carl Koller's nickname among Viennese medical students was "Coca Koller"). Richard Willstatter in Munich determined the structure of both cocaine and atropine in 1898 and succeeded in synthesizing cocaine 3 years later. Although today cocaine is of greater historic than medicinal importance and is widely abused, few developments in the chemistry of local anesthetics can disclaim a structural relationship to cocaine (Fig. 5). Benzocaine, procaine, tetracaine, and lidocaine all can be considered structural analogs of cocaine, a classic example of how structural modification of a natural product can lead to useful therapeutic agents.

Drugs Affecting Renal and Cardiovascular Function

Included in this category are drugs used in the treatment of myocardial ischemia, congestive heart failure, various arrhythmias, and hypercholesterolemia. Only two examples of drug development will be highlighted. Use of the cardiac drug digoxin dates back to the folk remedy foxglove attributed to William Withering who, in 1775, discovered that the foxglove plant, *Digitalis purpurea*, was beneficial to those suffering from abnormal fluid buildup. The active principles of digitalis were isolated in 1841 by E. Humolle and T. Quevenne in Paris. They consisted mainly of digitoxin. The other glycosides of digitalis were subsequently isolated in 1869 by Claude A. Nativelle and in 1875 by Oswald Schmiedberg. The correct structure of digitoxin was established more than 50 years later by Adolf Windaus at Gothenburg University. In 1929, Sydney Smith at Burroughs Wellcome isolated and separated a new glycoside from *D. purpurea*, known as digoxin. This is now the most widely used cardiac glycoside. Today, dried foxglove leaves are processed to yield digoxin much like the procedure used by Withering. It takes about 1,000 kg of dried foxglove leaves to make 1 kg of pure digitalis.

It is the group of drugs used in the therapy of hypercholesterolemia that has received the greatest success and financial reward for the pharmaceutical industry during the last two decades. Cholesterol-lowering drugs, known as statins, are one of the cornerstones in the prevention of both primary and secondary heart diseases. Drugs such as Merck's lovastatin (Mevacor) and Pfizer's atorvastatin (Lipitor) are a huge success (Fig. 6). In 2004, Lipitor was the world's top selling drug, with sales of more than \$10 billion. As a class, cholesterol- and triglyceride-lowering drugs were the world's top selling category, with sales exceeding \$30 billion. The discovery of the statins can be credited to Akira Endo, a research scientist at Sankyo Pharmaceuticals in Japan (3). Endo's 1973 discovery of the first anticholesterol drug has almost been relegated to obscurity. The story of his research and the discovery of lovastatin are not typical but often escape attention. When Endo joined Sankyo after his university studies to investigate food ingredients, he searched for a fungus that produced an enzyme to make fruit juice less pulpy. The search was a success, and Endo's next assignment was to find a drug which would block the enzyme hydroxymethylglutaryl-coenzyme A (HMG-CoA) a key enzyme essential to the production of cholesterol. With Endo's interest and background, he searched for fungi that would block this enzyme. In 1973, after testing 6,000 fungal broths Endo found a substance made by the mold *Penicillium citrinum* that was a potent inhibitor on the enzyme needed to make cholesterol; it was named compactin (mevastatin) (Fig. 6). However, the substance did not work in rats but did work in hens and dogs. Endo's bosses were unenthusiastic about his discovery and discouraged further research with this compound. With the collaboration of Akira Yamamoto, a physician treating patients with extremely high cholesterol due to a genetic defect, Endo prepared samples of his drug, and it was administered to an 18-year-old

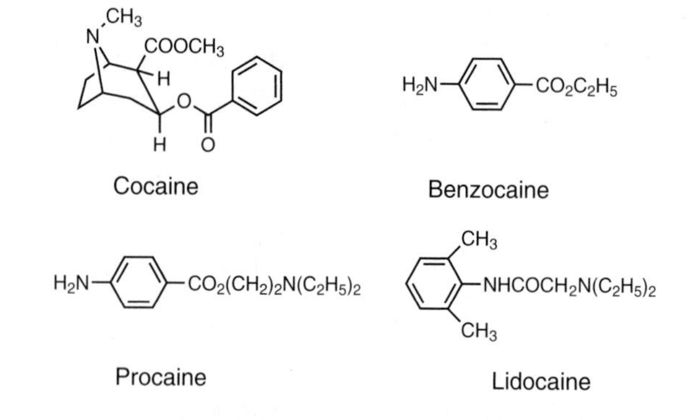

FIGURE 5 Synthetic local anesthetics development based on the structure of cocaine.

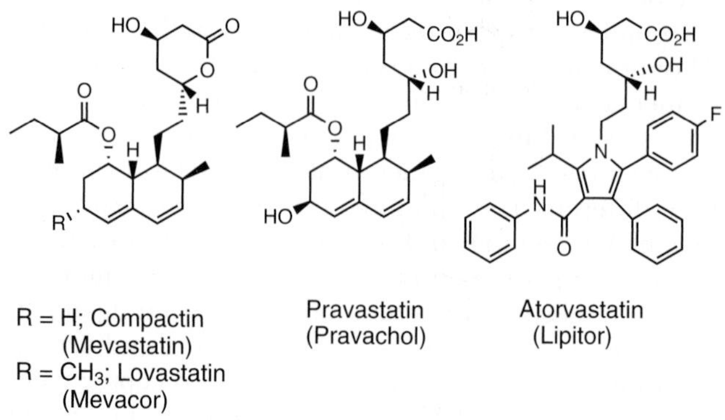

FIGURE 6 The first statins.

woman by Yamamoto. Further testing in nine patients led to an average of 27% lowering of cholesterol. In 1978, using a different fungus, Merck discovered a substance that was nearly identical to Endo's; this one was named lovastatin (Mevacor). Merck held the patent rights in the United States and, in 1987, started marketing it as Mevacor, the first FDA-approved statin. Sankyo eventually gave up compactin and pursued another statin that they licensed to Bristol-Myers Squibb Co., which was sold as Pravachol. In 1985, Michael S. Brown and Joseph Goldstein won the Nobel Prize in Physiology or Medicine for their work in cholesterol metabolism. It was only in January of 2006 that Endo received the Japan Prize, considered by many to be equivalent to the Nobel Prize. There is no doubt that millions of people whose lives have been and will be extended through statin therapy owe it to Akira Endo.

Anticancer Agents

Sulfur mustard gas was used as an offensive weapon by the Germans during World War I, and the related nitrogen mustards were manufactured by both sides in World War II. Later, investigations showed that the toxic gases had destroyed the blood's white cells, which subsequently led to the discovery of drugs used in leukemia therapy. These compounds, although effective antitumor agents, were very toxic. 6-Mercaptopurine (Fig. 7) was really the first effective leukemia drug developed by George Hitchings and his technician, Gertrude Elion, who, working together at Burroughs Wellcome Research Laboratories, shared the Nobel Prize in 1988. By a process now termed "rational drug design," Hitchings hypothesized that it might be possible to use antagonists to stop bacterial or tumor cell growth by interfering with nucleic acid biosynthesis in a similar way that sulfonamides blocked cell growth.

Unlike many cancer drugs available today, cisplatin is an inorganic molecule with a simple structure (Fig. 7). Cisplatin interferes with the growth of cancer cells by binding to DNA and interfering with the cells' repair mechanism and eventually causes cell death. It is used to treat many types of cancer, primarily testicular, ovarian, bladder, lung, and stomach cancers. Cisplatin is now the gold standard against which new medicines are compared. It was first synthesized in 1845, and its structure was elucidated by Alfred Werner in 1893. It was not until the early 1960s when Barnett Rosenberg, a professor of biophysics and chemistry at Michigan State University, observed the compound's effect in cell division, which prompted him to test cisplatin against tumors in mice. The compound was found to be effective and entered clinical trials in 1971. There is an important lesson to be learned from Rosenberg's development of cisplatin. As a biophysicist and chemist, Rosenberg realized that when he was confronted with interesting results for which he could not find explanations, he enlisted the help and expertise of researchers in microbiology, inorganic chemistry, molecular biology, biochemistry, biophysics, physiology, and pharmacology. Such a multidisciplinary approach is the key to the discovery of modern medicines today. Although cisplatin is still an effective drug, researchers have found second-generation compounds such as carboplatin that have less toxicity and fewer side effects.

A third compound in the class of anticancer agents is paclitaxel (Taxol), discovered in 1963 by Monroe E. Wall and Masukh C. Wani at Research Triangle Park in North Carolina (Fig. 7). Taxol was isolated from extracts of the bark of the Pacific yew tree, *Taxus brevifolia*. The extracts showed potent anticancer activity, and by 1967, Wall and his coworkers had isolated the active ingredients; in 1971, they established the structure of the compound. Susan Horwitz, working at the Albert Einstein College of Medicine in New York, studied the mechanism of how Taxol kills cancer cells. She discovered that Taxol works by stimulating growth of microtubules and stabilizing the cell structures so that the killer cells are unable to divide and multiply. It was not until 1993 that Taxol was brought to the market by Bristol-Myers Squibb and soon became an effective drug for treating ovarian, breast, and certain forms of lung cancers. The product became a huge commercial success, with annual sales of approximately $1.6 billion in 2000.

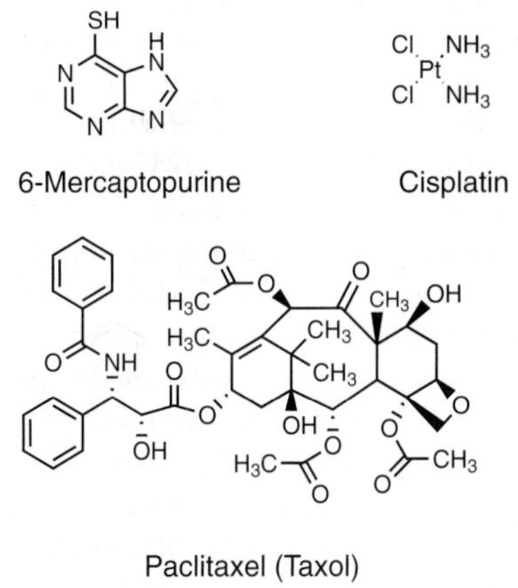

FIGURE 7 Anticancer drugs.

Old Drugs as Targets for New Drugs

Cannabis is used throughout the world for diverse purposes and has a long history characterized by usefulness, euphoria or evil, depending on one's point of view. To the agriculturist cannabis is a fiber crop; to the physician of a century ago it was a valuable medicine; to the physician of today it is an enigma; to the user, a euphoriant; to the police, a menace; to the trafficker, a source of profitable danger; to the convict or parolee and his family, a source of sorrow (4).

The plant, *Cannabis sativa*, the source of marijuana, has a long history in folk medicine, where it has been used for ills such as menstrual pain and the muscle spasms that affect multiple sclerosis sufferers. As in so many other areas of drug research, progress was achieved in the understanding of the pharmacology and biogenesis of a naturally occurring drug only when the chemistry had been well established and the researcher had at his disposal pure compounds of known composition and stereochemistry. Cannabis is no exception in this respect, with the last 60 years producing the necessary know-how in the chemistry of the cannabis constituents so that chemists could devise practical and novel synthetic schemes to provide the pharmacologists with pure substances. The isolation and determination of the structure of tetrahydrocannabinol (Δ^9-THC), the principal active ingredient, were performed in 1964 by Rafael Mechoulam at Hebrew University in Israel. Although cannabis and some of its structural analogs have been and are still used in medicine, in the last few years, research has focused on the endocannabinoids and their receptors as targets for drug development. It was shown that THC exerts its effects by binding to receptors that are targets of naturally occurring molecules termed endocannabinoids that have been involved in controlling learning, memory, appetite, metabolism, blood pressure, emotions such as fear and anxiety, inflammation, bone growth, and cancer. It is no surprise, then, that drug researchers are focusing on developing compounds that either act as agonists or antagonists of the endocannabinoids. In 1990, Lisa Matsuda and Tom Bonner at the National Institutes of Health cloned a THC receptor now called CB_1 from a rat brain. Shortly thereafter, Mechoulam and his coworkers identified the first of these endogenous cannabinoids called anandamide and, a few years later, identified 2-arachidonylgyclerol (2-AG). In 1993, the second cannabinoid receptor, CB_2, was cloned by Muna Abu-Shaar at the Medical Research Council in Cambridge, United Kingdom. The drug rimonabant was an endocannabinoid antagonist developed by the French pharmaceutical company Sanofi-Aventis, and although it was approved initially for promoting weight loss, it has subsequently been removed from the market. The drug binds to CB_1 but not CB_2 receptors, resulting in the weight loss effect. Efforts to develop other endocannabinoids as therapeutic agents are in full swing in many laboratories and include preclinical testing for epilepsy, pain, anxiety, and diarrhea. Thus, a new series of drugs is being developed that are not centered on marijuana itself, but inspired by its active ingredient Δ^9-THC, mimicking the endogenous substances acting in the brain or the periphery.

Molecular Imaging

The clinician now has at his or her disposal a variety of diagnostic tools to help obtain information about the pathophysiologic status of internal organs. The most widely used methods for noninvasive imaging are scintigraphy, radiography (x-ray and computed tomography [CT]), ultrasonography, positron emission tomography (PET), single photon emission computed tomography (SPECT), and magnetic resonance imaging (MRI). Chemists continue to make important contributions to the preparation of radiopharmaceuticals and contrast agents. These optical, nuclear, and magnetic methods are increasingly being empowered by new types of imaging agents. The effectiveness of new and old drugs to treat disease and to monitor the response to therapies is now being routinely used in the drug discovery process.

The expanded use of the cyclotron in the late 1930s and the nuclear reactor in the early 1940s made available a variety of radionuclides for potential applications in medicine. The field of nuclear medicine was founded with reactor-produced radioiodine for the diagnosis of thyroid dysfunction. Soon other radioactive tracers, such as ^{18}F, ^{123}I, ^{131}I, ^{99m}Tc, and ^{11}C, became available. This, together with more sensitive radiation detection instruments and cameras, made it possible to study many organs of the body such as the liver, kidney, lung, and brain. The diagnostic value of these noninvasive techniques served to establish nuclear medicine and radiopharmaceutical chemistry as distinct specialties. A radiopharmaceutical is defined as any pharmaceutical that contains a radionuclide (5).

Historically, radioiodine has a special place in nuclear medicine. In 1938, Hertz, Roberts, and Evans first demonstrated the uptake of ^{128}I by the thyroid gland. ^{131}I, with a longer half-life ($t_{1/2}$; 8 days), became available later and is now widely used. Although iodine has 24 known isotopes, ^{123}I, ^{131}I, and ^{125}I are the only iodine isotopes currently used in medicine. At present, the most widely used PET radiopharmaceutical is the glucose analog ^{18}F-FDG (2-fluoro-2-deoxy-D-glucose; ^{18}F $t_{1/2}$ = 1.8 hrs), which is routinely used for functional studies of brain, heart, and tumor growth. The process is derived from the earlier animal studies quantifying regional glucose metabolism with [^{14}C]-2-deoxyglucose, which passes through the blood–brain barrier by the same carrier-facilitated transport system used for glucose. With the advancement in the development of highly selective PET and SPECT ligands, the potential of the noninvasive imaging procedures will achieve wider application both in pharmacologic research and diagnosis of CNS disorders.

The Next Wave in Drug Discovery: Genomics

Imatinib (Gleevec) was discovered through the combined use of high-throughput screening and medicinal chemistry that resulted in the successful treatment of chronic myeloid leukemia. Through rational molecular modifications based on an understanding of the structure of logical alternative tyrosine kinase targets, improved activity against the platelet-derived growth factor receptor (PDGFR), epidermal growth factor receptor (EGFR) and vascular endothelial growth factor receptor (VEGFR) have been obtained. As a result of the success of imatinib, scientists are modifying their drug discovery and development strategies to one that considers the patient's genes, without abandoning the more traditional drugs. It has been known for many years that genetics plays an important role in an individual's well-being. Attention is now being paid to manipulating the proteins that are produced in response to malfunctioning genes by inhibiting the out-of-control tyrosine kinase enzymes in the body that play such an important role in cell signaling events in growth and cell division. Using the human genome, scientists with knowledge of the sequencing of DNA and genes of various species have shown that some cancers are caused by genetic errors that direct the biosynthesis of dysfunctional proteins. Because proteins carry out the instructions from the genes located on the DNA, dysfunctional proteins such as the kinases deliver the wrong message to the cells, making them cancerous. The emphasis is now to inhibit the proteins in order to slow the progression of the cancerous growth.

An emphasis in the pharmaceutical industry and in academia is to develop drug formulations that guarantee that therapies will reach specific targets in the body. Vaccines based on a proprietary plasmid DNA that will activate skeletal muscles to manufacture desired proteins and antigens are being developed. Plasmid DNA vaccine technology represents a fundamentally new means of treatment that is of great importance for the future of drug targeting. There is currently an increase in the number of products coming out of biotechnology companies. Biotechnology drug discovery and drug development tools are used to create the more traditional small molecules. The promise of pharmacogenetics lies in the potential to identify sources of interindividual variability in drug responses that affect drug delivery and safety. Recent success stories in oncology demonstrate that the field of pharmacogenetics has progressed substantially. The knowledge created through pharmacogenetic trials can contribute to the development of patient-specific medicines as well as to improved decision making along the research and development value chain (6).

Combinatorial Chemistry and High-Throughput Screening

No discussion of the history and evolution of medicinal chemistry would be complete without briefly mentioning combinatorial chemistry and high-throughput screening. Combinatorial chemistry is one of the new technologies developed by academics and researchers in the pharmaceutical and biotechnology industries to reduce the time and cost associated with producing effective, marketable, and competitive new drugs. Chemists use combinatorial chemistry to create large populations of molecules that can be screened efficiently, generally using high-throughput screening. Thus, instead of synthesizing a single compound, combinatorial chemistry exploits automation and miniaturization to synthesize large libraries of compounds. Combinatorial organic synthesis is not random, but systematic and repetitive, using sets of chemical "building blocks" to form a diverse set of molecular entities.

Random screening has been a source of new drugs for several decades. Many of the drugs currently on the market were developed from leads identified through screening of natural products or compounds synthesized in the laboratory. However, in the late 1970s and 1980s, screening fell out of favor in the industry. Using traditional methods, the number of novel selective leads generated did not make this approach cost effective. The last 25 years have seen an enormous advance in the understanding of critical cellular processes, leading to a more rationally designed approach in drug discovery. The availability of cloned genes for use in high-throughput screening to identify new molecules has led to a reexamination of the screening process. Targets are now often recombinant proteins (i.e., receptors) produced from cloned genes that are heterologously expressed in a number of ways. Combinatorial libraries complement the enormous numbers of synthetic libraries available from new and old synthetic programs. The development and use of robotics and automation have made it possible to screen large numbers of compounds in a short period of time. It should also be emphasized that computerized data systems and the analysis of the data have facilitated the handling of the information being generated, leading to the identification of new leads.

SUMMARY

It is fair to say that more than 50% of the drugs in use today had their origin in a plant, animal, or mineral that had been used as a cure for alleviating disease occurring in man. Examples of a number of discoveries of important drugs in use today are recounted as "case studies" in the drug discovery process and are described in more detail in the following chapters. The discoveries briefly described are in large measure due to the increased sophistication brought to bear in the isolation, identification, structure determination, and synthesis of the active ingredients of the drugs used empirically hundreds of years ago.

The emergence of the pharmaceutical industry took place in conjunction with the advances in organic/medicinal/pharmaceutical chemistry, pharmacology, bacteriology, biochemistry, and medicine as distinct fields of science in the late 19th century. Current research efforts are now focused not only on discovering new biologically active compounds using ever increasingly sophisticated technology, but also on gaining a better understanding of how and where drugs exert their effects at the molecular level. One should not underestimate, however, that the discoveries in the 20th and 21st centuries and earlier represent an amazing amount of insight, determination, and luck by researchers in chemistry, pharmacology, biology, and medicine. We owe gratitude and admiration to those earlier scientists who had the imagination and inspiration to develop drugs to cure so many illnesses.

References

1. Burger A. The practice of medicinal chemistry. In: Burger A, ed. Medicinal Chemistry. New York: Wiley, 1970:4–9.
2. Daemmrich A, Bowden ME. A rising drug industry. Chem Eng News Am Chem Soc 2005;83:28–42.
3. Landers P. Stalking cholesterol: how one scientist intrigued by molds found first statin. The Wall Street Journal (Eastern edition), January 9, 2006:A.1.
4. Mikuriya TH. Marijuana in medicine: past present and future. Calif Med 1969;110:34–40.
5. Counsel RE, Weichert JP. Agents for organ imaging. In Foye WO, Lemke TL, Williams DA, eds. Principles of Medicinal Chemistry, 4th Ed. Baltimore, MD: Williams & Wilkins, 1995:927–947.
6. Mullin R. The next wave in biopharmaceuticals. Chem Eng News Am Chem Soc 2005;83:16–19.

Suggested Readings

Djerassi C. The Politics of Contraception. New York: Norton, 1970.

Healy D. The Antidepressant Era. Cambridge, MA: Harvard University Press, 1998.

Marx J. Drugs inspired by a drug. Science 2006;311:322–325.

Podolsky ML. Cures Out of Chaos. Williston, VT: Harwood Academic, 1997.

Sheehan JC. The Enchanted Ring: The Untold Story of Penicillin. Cambridge, MA: MIT Press, 1982.

Triggle DJ. The chemist as astronaut: searching for biologically useful space in the chemical universe. Biochem Pharmacol 2009;78:217–223.

Part I

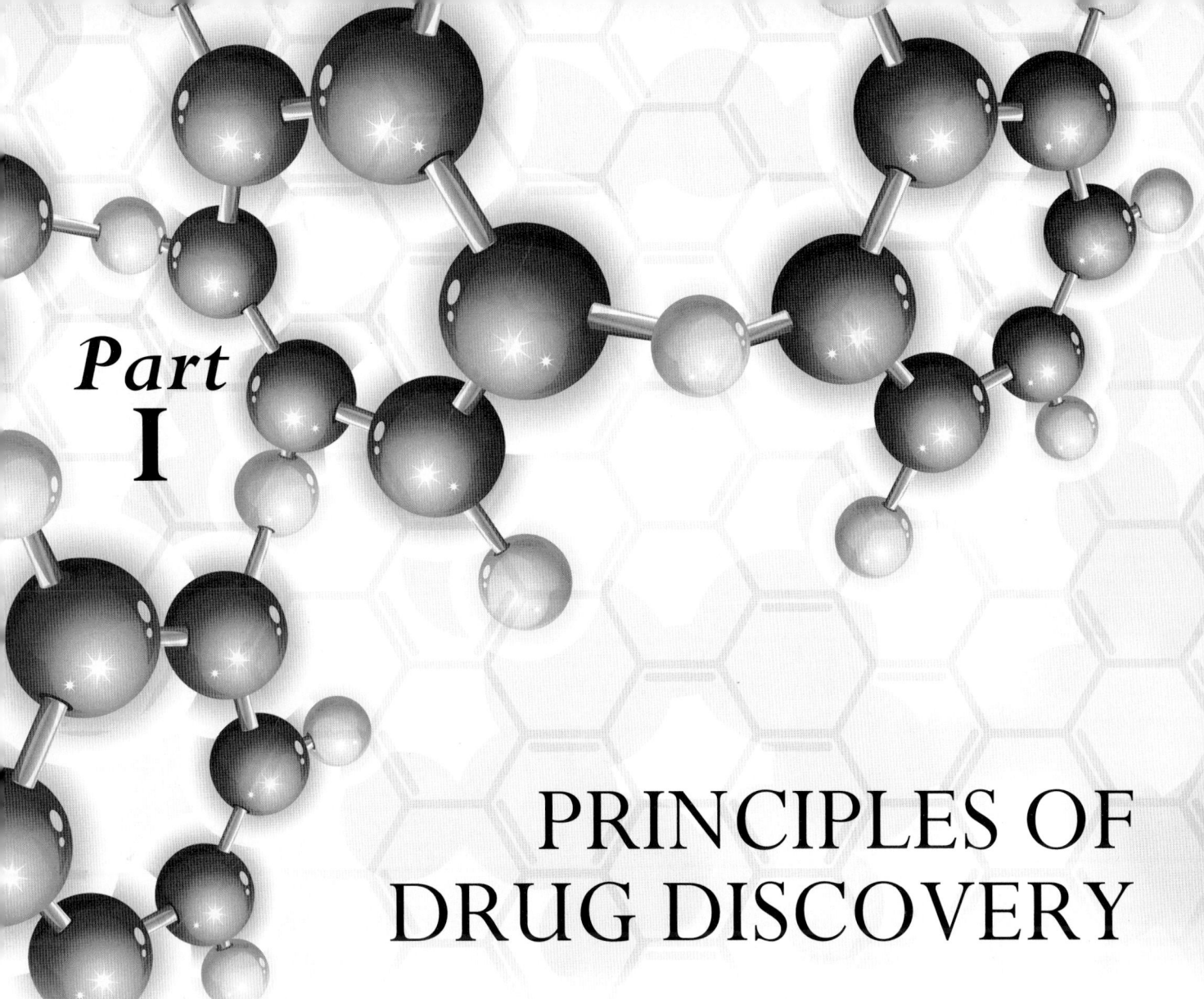

PRINCIPLES OF DRUG DISCOVERY

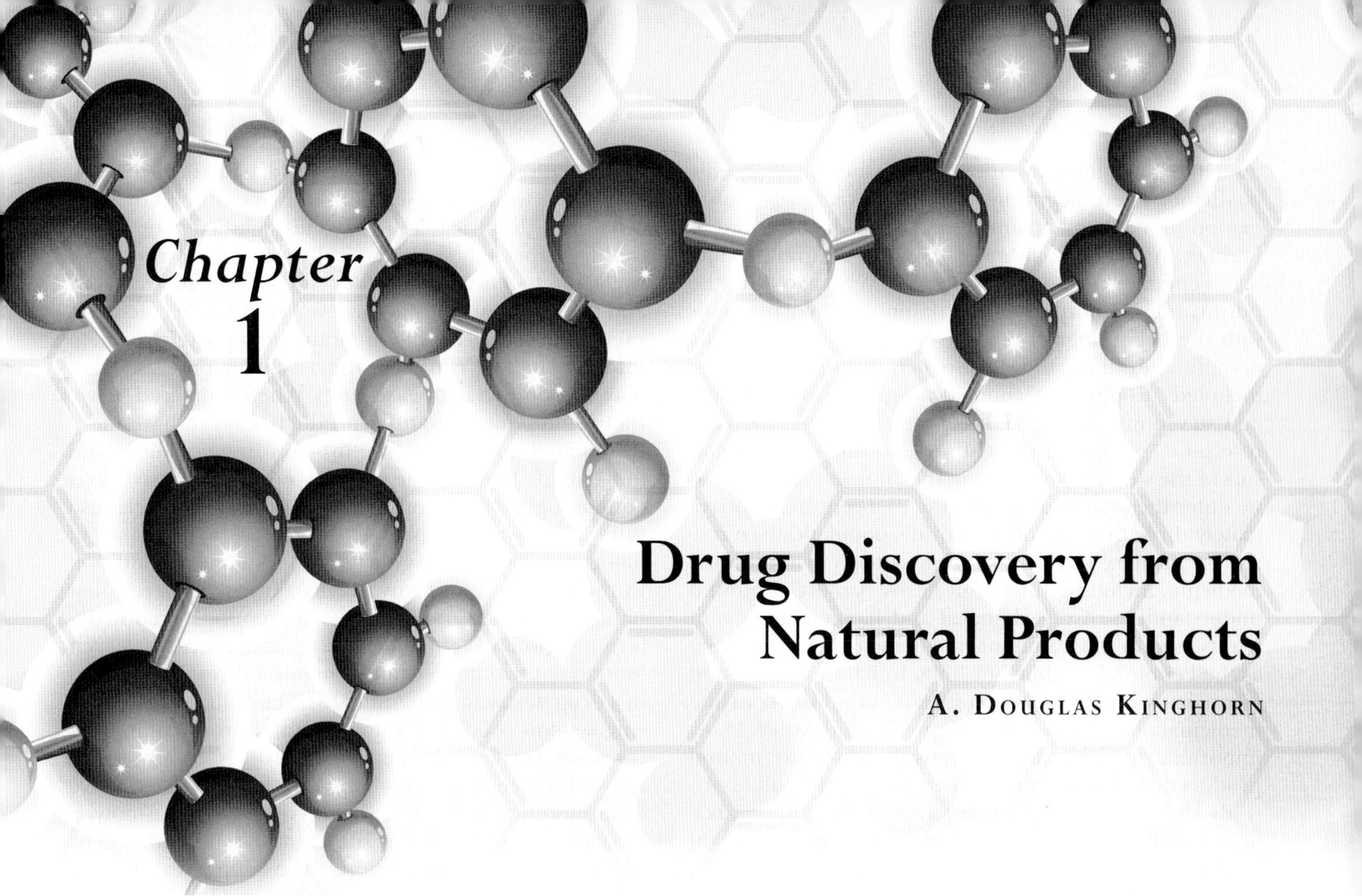

Chapter 1

Drug Discovery from Natural Products

A. Douglas Kinghorn

Abbreviations

CAM, complementary and alternative medicine
CNS, central nervous system
COPD, chronic obstructive pulmonary disease
DSHEA, Dietary Supplement Health and Education Act
GLP-1, glucagon-like peptide-1
HMG-CoA, 5-hydroxy-3-methylglutaryl–coenzyme A
HPLC, high-performance liquid chromatography
HTS, high-throughput screening
LC, liquid chromatography
M6G, morphine-6-glucuronide
MOA, memorandum of agreement
MS, mass spectrometry
NCE, new chemical entity
NMR, nuclear magnetic resonance
PVP, polyvinylpyrrolidone
SCE, single chemical entity
SPE, solid-phase extraction
THC, tetrahydrocannabinol
UNCLOS, United Nations Convention on the Law of the Sea

INTRODUCTION

"Pharmacognosy" is one of the oldest established pharmaceutical sciences, and the term has been used for nearly two centuries. Initially, this term referred to the investigation of medicinal substances of plant, animal, or mineral origin in their crude or unprepared state, used in the form of teas, tinctures, poultices, and other types of formulation (1–4). However, by the middle of the 20th century, the chemical components of such crude drugs began to be studied in more detail. Today, the subject of pharmacognosy is highly interdisciplinary, and incorporates aspects of analytical chemistry, biochemistry, biosynthesis, biotechnology, ecology, ethnobotany, microbiology, molecular biology, organic chemistry, and taxonomy, among others (5). The term "pharmacognosy" is defined on the Web site of the American Society of Pharmacognosy (www.phcog.org) as "the study of the physical, chemical, biochemical, and biological properties of drugs, drug substances, or potential drugs or drug substances of natural origin, as well as the search for new drugs from natural sources."

There seems little doubt that humans have used natural drugs since before the advent of written history. In addition to their use as drugs, the constituents of plants have afforded poisons for darts and arrows used in hunting and euphoriants with psychoactive properties used in rituals. The actual documentation of drugs derived from natural products in the Western world appears to date as far back to the Sumerians and Akkadians in the third century BCE, as well as the Egyptian *Ebers Papyrus* (about 1600 BCE). Other important contributions on the uses of drugs of natural origin were documented by Dioscorides (*De Materia Medica*) and Pliny the Elder in the first century CE and by Galen in the second century. Written records also exist from about the same time period on plants used in both Chinese traditional medicine and Ayurvedic medicine. Then, beginning about 500 years ago, information on medicinal plants began to be documented in herbals. In turn, the laboratory study of natural product drugs commenced approximately 200 years ago, with the purification of morphine from opium. This corresponds with the beginnings of organic chemistry as a scientific discipline. Additional drugs isolated from plant sources included atropine, caffeine, cocaine, nicotine, quinine, and strychnine in the 19th century, and then digoxin, reserpine, paclitaxel, vincristine, and chemical precursors of the steroid hormones in the 20th century. Even as we enter the second decade of the 21st century, approximately three quarters of the world's population are reliant on primary health care from systems of traditional medicine, including the use of herbs. A more profound understanding of the chemical and biologic aspects of plants used in the traditional medicine of countries such as the People's Republic of China, India, Indonesia, and Japan has occurred in recent years, in addition to the medicinal plants used in Latin America and Africa. Many important scientific observations germane to natural product drug discovery have been made as a result (1–4).

By the mid-20th century, therapeutically useful alkaloids had been purified and derivatized from the ergot fungus, as uterotonic and sympatholytic agents. Then, the penicillins were isolated along with further major structural classes of effective and potent antibacterials from terrestrial microbes, and these and later antibiotics revolutionized the treatment of infectious diseases. Of the types of organisms producing natural products, terrestrial microorganisms have been found to afford the largest number of compounds currently used as drugs for a wide range of human diseases, and these include antifungal agents, the "statin" cholesterol-lowering agents, immunosuppressive agents, and several anticancer agents (6,7).

At present, there remains much interest also in the discovery and development of drugs from marine animals and plants. However, to date, marine organisms have had a relatively brief history in serving as sources of drugs, with only a few examples approved for therapeutic use thus far. Although the oceans occupy 70% of the surface of the earth, an intense effort to investigate the chemical structures and biologic activities of the marine fauna and flora has only been ongoing for about 40 years (8).

The term "natural product" is generally taken to mean a compound that has no known primary biochemical role in the producing organism. Such low molecular weight organic molecules may also be referred to as "secondary metabolites" and tend to be biosynthesized by the producing organism in a biologically active chiral form to increase the chances of survival, such as by repelling predators or serving as insect pollination attractants, in the case of plants (9). There have been a number of studies to investigate the physicochemical parameters of natural products in recent years, and it has been concluded that "libraries" or collections of these substances tend to afford a higher degree of "drug-likeness," when compared with compounds in either synthetic or combinatorial "libraries" (10,11). This characteristic might well be expected, since natural products are produced by living systems, where they are subject to transport and diffusion at the cellular level. Small-molecule natural products are capable of modulating protein–protein interactions and can thus affect cellular processes that may be modified in disease states. When compared to synthetic compounds, natural products tend to have more protonated amine and free hydroxy functionalities and more single bonds, with a greater number of fused rings containing more chiral centers. Natural products also differ from synthetic products in the average number of halogen, nitrogen, oxygen, and sulfur atoms, in addition to their steric complexity (12,13). It is considered that natural products and synthetic compounds occupy different regions of "chemical space," and hence, they each tend to contribute to overall chemical diversity required in a drug discovery program (13). Fewer than 20% of the ring systems produced among natural products are represented in currently used drugs (10). Naturally occurring substances may serve either as drugs in their native or unmodified form or as "lead" compounds (prototype bioactive molecules) for subsequent semisynthetic or totally synthetic modification, for example, to improve biologic efficacy or to enhance solubility (1–4,6,8,10,11).

In the present era of efficient drug design by chemical synthesis aided by computational and combinatorial techniques, and with other new drugs obtained increasingly by biotechnologic processes, it might be expected that traditional natural products no longer have a significant role to play in this regard. Indeed, in the past two decades, there has been a decreased emphasis on the screening of natural products for new drugs by pharmaceutical companies, with greater reliance placed on screening large libraries of synthetic compounds (10,11,14,15). However, in a major review article, Newman and Cragg from the U.S. National Cancer Institute pointed out that for the period from 1981 to 2006, about 28% of the new chemical entities (NCEs) in Western medicine were either natural products per se or semisynthetic derivatives of natural products. Thus, of a total of 1,184 NCEs for all disease conditions introduced into therapy in North America, Western Europe, and Japan over the 25.5-year period covered, 5% were unmodified natural products and 23% were semisynthetic agents based on natural product lead compounds. An additional 14% of the synthetic compounds were designed based on knowledge of a natural product "pharmacophore" (the region of the molecule containing the essential organic functional groups that directly interact with the receptor active site and, therefore, confers the biologic activity of interest) (16). The launch of new natural product drugs in Western countries and Japan has continued in the first decade of 21st century, and such compounds introduced to the market recently have been documented (14,16–18).

Thus, it is generally recognized that the secondary metabolites of organisms afford a source of small organic molecules of outstanding chemical diversity that are highly relevant to the contemporary drug discovery process. Potent and selective leads are obtained from more exotic organisms than before, as collection efforts venture into increasingly inhospitable locales throughout the world, such as deep caves in terrestrial areas and thermal vents on the ocean floor. On occasion, a natural lead compound may help elucidate a new mechanism of interaction with a biologic target for a disease state under investigation. Natural products may serve to provide molecular inspiration in certain therapeutic areas for which there are only a limited number of synthetic lead compounds. A valuable approach is the large-scale screening of libraries of partially purified extracts from organisms (11). However, there is a widespread perception that the resupply of the source organism of a secondary metabolite of interest may prove problematic and will consequently hinder the timely, more detailed, biologic evaluation of a compound available perhaps only in milligram quantities initially. In addition, natural product extracts have been regarded as incompatible with the modern rapid screening techniques used in the pharmaceutical industry, and some believe that the successful market development of a natural product–derived drug is too time consuming (10,11,14,15). A further consideration of the factors involved in the discovery of drugs from natural products will be presented in the next section of this chapter. This will be followed by examples of natural products currently used in various therapeutic categories, as well as a few selected representatives with present clinical use or future potential in this regard.

NATURAL PRODUCTS AND DRUG DISCOVERY

Collection of Source Organisms

There are at least five recognized approaches to the choice of plants and other organisms for the laboratory investigation of their biologic components, namely, random screening; selection of specific taxonomic groups, such as families or genera; a chemotaxonomic approach where restricted classes of secondary metabolites such as alkaloids are sought; an information-managed approach, involving the target collection of species selected by database surveillance; and selection by an ethnomedical approach (e.g., by investigating remedies being used in traditional medicine by "shamans" or medicine men or women) (19). In fact, if plant-derived natural products are taken specifically, it has been estimated that of 122 drugs of this type used worldwide from a total of 94 species, 72% can be traced to the original ethnobotanical uses that have been documented for their plant of origin (19). The need for increased natural products discovery research involving ethnobotany should be regarded as urgent, due to the accelerating loss in developing countries of indigenous cultures and languages, inclusive of knowledge of traditional medical practice (20). However, it is common for a given medicinal plant to be used ethnomedically in more than one disease context, which may sometimes obscure its therapeutic utility for a specific disease condition. Another manner in which drugs have been developed from terrestrial plants and fungi is through following up on observations of the causes of livestock poisoning, leading to new drugs and molecular tools for biomedical investigation (21). When the origin of plants with demonstrated inhibitory effects in experimental tumor systems was considered at the U.S. National Cancer Institute, medicinal or poisonous plants with uses as either anthelmintics or arrow and homicidal poisons were three to four times more likely to be active in this regard than species screened at random (22).

Although some shallow water marine specimens may be collected simply by wading or snorkeling down to 20 feet below the water surface, scuba diving permits the collection of organisms to depths of 120 feet. Deep-water collections of marine animals and plants have been made by dredging and trawling and through the use of manned and unmanned submersible vessels. Collection strategies for specimens from the ocean must take into account marine macroorganism–microorganism associations that may be involved in the biosynthesis of a particular secondary metabolite of interest (8). Thus, there seems to be a complex interplay between many marine host invertebrate animals and symbiotic microbes that inhabit them, and it has been realized that several bioactive compounds previously thought to be of animal origin may be produced by their associated microorganisms instead (23).

The process of collecting or surveying a large set of flora (or fauna) for the purpose of the biologic evaluation and isolation of lead compounds is called "biodiversity prospecting" (24). Many natural products collection programs are focused on tropical rain forests, in order to take advantage of the inherent biologic diversity (or "biodiversity") evident there, with the hope of harnessing as broad a profile of chemical classes as possible among the secondary metabolites produced by the species to be obtained. To exemplify this, there may be more tree species in a relatively small area of a tropical rainforest than in the whole of the temperate regions of North America. A generally accepted explanation for the high biodiversity of secondary metabolites in humid forests in the tropics is that these molecules are biosynthesized (a process of chemical synthesis by the host organism) for ecologic roles, in response to a continuous growing season under elevated temperatures, high humidity, and great competition due to the high species density present. Maximal biodiversity in the marine environment is found on the fringes of the ocean or sea bordering land, where there is intense competition among sessile (nonmoving) organisms, such as algae, corals, sponges, and some other invertebrate animals, for attachment space (25).

Great concern should be expressed about the continuing erosion of tropical rain forest species, which is accelerating as the 21st century develops (26). Approximately 25 "hot spots" of especially high biodiversity have been proposed that represent 44% of all vascular plant species and 35% of all species of vertebrates in about 1.4% of the earth's surface (27). At present, many of the endemic (or native) species to these biodiversity "hot spot" areas have been reported to be undergoing massive habitat loss and are threatened with extinction, especially in tropical regions (26,27).

After the United Nations Convention on Biological Diversity, passed in Rio de Janeiro in 1992, biologic or genetic materials are owned by the country of origin (24,28). A major current-day component of being able to gain access to the genetic resources of a given country for the purposes of drug discovery and other scientific study is the formulation of a memorandum of agreement (MOA), which itemizes access, prior informed consent (involving human subjects in cases where ethnomedical knowledge is divulged), intellectual property related to drug discovery, and the equitable sharing of financial benefits that may accrue from the project, such as patent royalties and licensing fees (24,28). When access to marine organisms is desired, the United Nations Convention on the Law of the Sea (UNCLOS) must also be considered (29).

Once a formal "benefit sharing" agreement is on hand, the organism collection process can begin. It is usual to initially collect 0.3 to 1 kg of each dried plant sample and about 1 kg wet weight of a marine organism for preliminary screening studies (30). In the case of a large plant (tree or shrub), it is typical to collect up to about four different organs or plant parts, since it is known that the secondary metabolite composition may vary considerably between the leaves, where photosynthesis occurs, and storage or translocation organs such as the roots and bark (31). There is increasing evidence that considerable variation in the profile of secondary metabolites occurs in the same plant organ when collected from different habitats, depending on local environmental conditions, and thus it may be worth reinvestigating even well-studied species in drug discovery projects. Taxa endemic (native) to a particular country or region are generally of higher priority than the collection of pandemic weeds. It is very important never to remove all quantities of a desired species at the site of collection, in order to conserve the native germplasm encountered. Also, rare or endangered species should not be collected; a listing of the latter is maintained by the *Red List of Threatened Species* of the International Union for Conservation of Nature and Natural Resources (www.redlist.org), covering terrestrial, marine, and freshwater organisms.

A crucial aspect of the organism collection process is to deposit voucher specimens representative of the species collected in a central repository such as a herbarium or a museum, so that this material can be accessed by other scientists, in case of need. It is advisable to deposit specimens in more than one repository, including regional and national institutions in the country in which the organisms were collected. Collaboration with general and specialist taxonomists is very important, because without an accurate identification of a source organism, the value of subsequent isolation, structure elucidation, and biologic evaluation studies will be greatly reduced (31).

Organisms for natural products drug discovery work may be classified into the following kingdoms: Eubacteria (bacteria, cyanobacteria [or "blue-green algae"]), Archaea (halobacterians, methanogens), Protoctista (e.g., protozoa, diatoms, "algae" [including red algae, green algae]), Plantae (land plants [including mosses and liverworts, ferns, and seed plants]), Fungi (e.g., molds, yeasts, mushrooms), and Animalia (mesozoa [wormlike invertebrate marine parasites], sponges, jellyfish, corals, flatworms, roundworms, sea urchins, mollusks [snails, squid], segmented worms, arthropods [crabs, spiders, insects], fish, amphibians, birds, mammals) (24). Of these, the largest numbers of organisms are found for arthropods, inclusive of insects (~950,000 species), with only a relatively small proportion (5%) of the estimated 1.5 million fungi in the world having been identified. At present, with 300,000 to 500,000 known species, plants are the second largest group of classified organisms, representing about 15% of our biodiversity. Of the 28 major animal phyla, 26 are found in the sea, with eight of these exclusively so. There have been more than 200,000 species of invertebrate animals and algal species found in the sea (24). A basic premise inherent in natural products drug discovery work is that the greater the degree of phylogenetic (taxonomic) diversity of the organisms sampled, the greater the resultant chemical diversity that is evident.

Interest in investigating plants as sources of new biologically active molecules remains strong, in part because of a need to better understand the efficacy of herbal components of traditional systems of medicine (32). In the last decade, many new natural product molecules have been isolated from fungal sources (6,7). An area of investigation of great potential expansion in the future will be on other microbes, particularly of actinomycetes and cyanobacteria of marine origin, especially if techniques can continue to be developed for their isolation and culturing in the laboratory (33). Because as many as 99% of known microorganisms are not able to be cultivated under laboratory conditions, the technique of "genome mining" isolates their DNA and enables new secondary metabolite biochemical pathways to be exploited, leading to the possibility of producing new natural products (34). The endophytic fungi that reside in the tissue of living plants have been found to produce an array of biologically interesting new compounds and are worthy of more intensive investigation (35). It is of interest to note that in a survey of the origin of 30,000 structurally assigned lead compounds of natural origin, the compounds were derived from animals (13%), bacteria (33%), fungi (26%), and plants (27%) (12). For the year 2008, it was reported that 24 animal-, 25 bacterial-, 7 fungal-, and

108 plant-derived natural products were undergoing at least phase I clinical trials leading to drug development (36). Therefore, while natural product researchers tend to specialize in the major types of organism on which they work, it is reasonable to expect that the future investigation of all of their major groups mentioned earlier will provide dividends in terms of affording new prototype biologically active compounds of use in drug discovery.

Preparation of Initial Extracts and Preliminary Biologic Screening

Although different laboratories tend to adopt different procedures for initial extraction of the source organisms being investigated, it is typical to extract initially terrestrial plants with a polar solvent like methanol or ethanol, and then subject this to a defatting (lipid-removing) partition with a nonpolar solvent like hexane or petroleum ether, and then partition the residue between a semipolar organic solvent, such as chloroform or dichloromethane, and a polar aqueous solvent (31). Marine and aquatic organisms are commonly extracted fresh into methanol or a mixture of methanol–dichloromethane (30). A peculiarity of working on plant extracts is the need to remove a class of compounds known as "vegetable tannins" or "plant polyphenols" before subsequent biologic evaluation because these compounds act as interfering substances in enzyme inhibition assays, as a result of precipitating proteins in a nonspecific manner. Several methods to remove plant polyphenols have been proposed, such as passage over polyvinylpyrrolidone (PVP) and polyamide, on which they are retained. Alternatively, partial removal of these interfering substances may be effected by washing the final semipolar organic layer with an aqueous sodium chloride solution (31). However, it should be pointed out that there remains an active interest in pursuing purified and structurally characterized vegetable tannins for their potential medicinal value (37). Caution also needs to be expressed in regard to common saturated and unsaturated fatty acids that might be present in natural product extracts, because these may interfere with various enzyme inhibition and receptor binding assays. Fatty acids and other lipids may largely be removed from more polar natural product extracts, using the defatting solvent partition stage mentioned earlier (38).

Drug discovery from organisms is a "biology-driven" process, and as such, biologic activity evaluation is at the heart of the drug discovery process from crude extracts prepared from organisms. So-called high-throughput screening (HTS) assays have become widely used for affording new leads. In this process, large numbers of crude extracts from organisms can be simultaneously evaluated in a cell-based or non-cell-based format, usually using multiwell microtiter plates (39). Cell-based in vitro bioassays allow for a considerable degree of biologic relevance, and manipulation may take place so that a selected cell line may involve a genetically altered organism (40) or incorporate a reporter gene (41). In noncellular (cell-free) assays, natural products extracts and their purified constituents may be investigated for their effects on enzyme activity (42) or on receptor binding (43). Other homogenous and separation-based assays suitable for the screening of natural products have been reviewed (44). For maximum efficiency and speed, HTS may be automated through the use of robotics and may be rendered as a more effective process through miniaturization.

Methods for Compound Purification and Structure Elucidation and Identification

Bioassay-directed fractionation is the process of isolating pure active constituents from some type of biomass (e.g., plants, microbes, marine invertebrates) using a decision tree that is dictated solely by bioactivity. A variety of chromatographic separation techniques are available for these purposes, including those based on adsorption on sorbents, such as silica gel, alumina, Sephadex, and more specialized solid phases, and methods involving partition chromatography inclusive of counter-current chromatography (45). Recent improvements have been made in column technology, automation of high-performance liquid chromatography (HPLC; a technique often used for final compound purification), and compatibility with HTS methodology (46). Routine structure elucidation is performed using combinations of spectroscopic procedures, with particular emphasis on ^{1}H- and ^{13}C-nuclear magnetic resonance (NMR) spectroscopy and mass spectrometry (MS). Considerable progress has been made in the development of cryogenic and capillary NMR probe technology, for the determination of structures of submilligram amounts of natural products (47). In addition, the automated processing of spectroscopic data for the structure elucidation of natural products is a practical proposition (48). Another significant advance is the use of "hyphenated" analytical techniques for the rapid structure determination of natural products without the need for a separate isolation step, such as liquid chromatography (LC)-NMR and LC-NMR-MS (11,46). The inclusion of an online solid-phase extraction (SPE) cartridge is advantageous in the identification of natural product molecules in crude extracts using LC-NMR, coupled with MS and circular dichroism spectroscopy (49).

Dereplication is a process of determining whether an observed biologic effect of an extract or specimen is due to a known substance. This is applied in natural product drug discovery programs in an attempt to avoid the re-isolation of compounds of previously determined structure. A step like this is essential to prioritize the resources available to a research program, so that the costly stage of bioassay-directed fractionation on a promising lead crude extract can be devoted to the discovery of biologically active agents representing new chemotypes (46,50). This has been particularly necessary for many years in studies on anti-infective agents from actinomycetes and bacteria and is also routinely applied to extracts from marine invertebrates and higher plants. Methods for dereplication must be sensitive, rapid, and reproducible, and the analytical methods used generally contain a mass spectrometric component (50). For example, the eluant (effluent) from an HPLC separation of a crude natural product extract may be split into two portions, so that the major part is plated out into a microtiter plate, with the wells then evaluated in an in vitro bioassay of interest. The fractions from the minor portion of the column eluant are introduced to a mass spectrometer, and the molecular weights of compounds present in active fractions can be determined. This information may then be introduced into an appropriate natural products database, and tentative identities of the active compounds present in the active wells can be determined (50).

Metabolomics is a recently developed approach in which the entire or "global" profile of secondary metabolites in a system (cell, tissue, or organism) is catalogued under a given set of conditions. Secondary metabolites may be investigated by a detection step such as MS after a separation step such as gas chromatography, HPLC, or capillary electrophoresis (51). This type of technology has particular utility in systematic biology, genomics research, and biotechnology and should have value in future natural products drug discovery (51,52).

Compound Development

A major challenge in the overall natural products drug discovery process is to obtain larger amounts of a biologically active compound of interest for additional laboratory investigation and potential preclinical development. One strategy that can be adopted when a plant-derived active compound is of interest is to obtain a recollection of the species of origin. To maximize the likelihood that the recollected sample will contain the bioactive compound of previous interest, the plant recollection should be carried out in the same location as the initial collection, on the same plant part, at the same time of the year (31). Some success has been met with the production of terrestrial plant metabolites via plant tissue culture (53). For microbes of terrestrial origin, compound scale up usually may be carried out through cultivation and large-scale fermentation (6,7).

Although evaluation of crude extracts of organisms is not routinely performed in animal models because of limitations of either test material or other project resources, it is of great value to test in vitro–active natural products in a pertinent in vivo method to obtain a preliminary indication of the worthiness of a lead compound for preclinical development. There are also a variety of "secondary discriminator" bioassays that provide an assessment of whether or not a given in vitro–active compound is likely to be active in vivo, and these require quite small amounts of test material. For example, the in vivo hollow fiber assay was developed at the U.S. National Cancer Institute for the preliminary evaluation of potential anticancer agents and uses confluent cells of a tumor model of interest deposited in polyvinylidene fluoride fibers that are implanted in nude mice (31,54). It is also important for pure bioactive compounds to be evaluated mechanistically for their effects on a particular biologic target, such as on a given stage of the life cycle of a pathogenic organism or cancer cell. Needless to say, a pure natural product of novel structure with in vitro and in vivo activity against a particular biologic target relevant to human disease acting through a previously unknown mechanism of action is of great value in the drug discovery process.

Once a bioactive natural product lead is obtained in gram quantities, it is treated in the same manner as a synthetic drug lead and is thus subjected to pharmaceutical development, leading to preclinical and clinical trials. This includes lead optimization via medicinal chemistry, combinatorial chemistry, and computational chemistry, as well as formulation, pharmacokinetics, and drug metabolism studies, as described elsewhere in this volume. Often, a lead natural product is obtained from its organism of origin along with several naturally occurring structural analogs, permitting a preliminary structure–activity relationship study to be conducted. This information may be supplemented with data obtained by microbial biotransformation or the production of semisynthetic analogs, to allow researchers to glean some initial information about the pharmacophoric site(s) of the naturally occurring molecule (10,11). Combinatorial biosynthesis is a contemporary approach with the ability to produce new natural product analogs, or so-called "unnatural" natural products, and these may be used to afford new drug candidates. This methodology involves the engineering of biosynthetic gene clusters in microorganisms and has been applied to the generation of polyketides, peptides, terpenoids, and other compounds. New advances in the biochemical and protein engineering aspects of this technique have led to a greater applicability than previously possible (55).

SELECTED EXAMPLES OF NATURAL PRODUCT–DERIVED DRUGS

In the following sections, examples are provided of both naturally occurring substances and synthetically modified compounds based on natural products with drug use. It is evident that many of the examples shown reflect considerable structural complexity and that the compounds introduced to the market have been obtained from organisms of very wide diversity. More detailed treatises with many more examples of natural product drugs are available (e.g., see references 1–4). Several recent reviews have summarized natural product drugs introduced to the market in recent years and substances on which clinical trials are being conducted (16–18,36).

Drugs for Cardiovascular and Metabolic Diseases

There is a close relationship between natural product drugs and the treatment of cardiovascular and metabolic diseases. The powdered leaves of *Digitalis purpurea* have been used in Western medicine for more than 200 years, with the major active constituent being the cardiac (steroidal) glycoside digitoxin, which is still used now for the treatment of congestive heart failure and atrial fibrillation. A more widely used drug used today is digoxin, a constituent of *Digitalis lanata*, which has a rapid action and is more rapidly eliminated from the body than digitoxin. Deslanoside (deacetyllanatoside C) is a hydrolysis product of the *D. lanata* constituent lanatoside C and is used for rapid digitalization (1–4). The "statin" drugs used for lowering blood cholesterol levels are based on the lead compound mevastatin (formerly known as compactin), produced by cultures of *Penicillium citrinum*, and were discovered using a 5-hydroxy-3-methylglutaryl–coenzyme A (HMG-CoA) reductase assay. Because hypercholesterolemia is regarded as one of the major risk factors for coronary heart disease, several semisynthetic and synthetic compounds modeled on the mevastatin structure (inclusive of the dihydroxycarboxylic acid side chain) now have extremely wide therapeutic use, including atorvastatin, fluvastatin, pravastatin, and simvastatin. Lovastatin is a natural product drug of this type, isolated from *Penicillium brevecompactin* and other organisms (3). There is also a past history of the successful production of cardiovascular agents from a terrestrial vertebrate, namely, the angiotensin-converting enzyme inhibitors captopril and enalapril, which were derived from tetrotide, a nonapeptide isolated from the pit viper, *Bothrops jararaca* (56).

Two further new drugs derived from an invertebrate and a vertebrate source, respectively, are bivalirudin and exenatide. Bivalirudin is a specific and reversible direct thrombin inhibitor that is administered by injection and is used to reduce the incidence of blood clotting in patients undergoing coronary angioplasty. This compound is a synthetic, 20-amino acid peptide and was modeled on hirudin, a substance present in the saliva of the leech, *Haementeria officinalis* (57,58). Exenatide is a synthetic version of a 39-amino acid peptide (exenatide-4), produced by a lizard native to the southwest United States and northern Mexico, called the Gila monster, *Heloderma suspectum*, and acts in the same manner as glucagon-like peptide-1 (GLP-1), a naturally occurring hormone. This drug is also administered by injection and enables improved glycemic control in patients with type 2 diabetes (18,59).

Central and Peripheral Nervous System Drugs

A comprehensive review has appeared on natural products (mostly of experimental value) that affect the central nervous system (CNS), inclusive of potential analgesics, antipsychotics, anti-Alzheimer disease agents, antitussives, anxiolytics, and muscle relaxants, among other categories. The authors point out that apart from the extensive past literature on plants and their constituents as hallucinogenic agents, this area of research inquiry on natural products is not well developed but is likely to be productive in the future (60). Natural products also have the potential to treat drug abuse (61).

The morphinan isoquinoline alkaloid, (−)-morphine, is the most abundant and important constituent of the dried latex (milky exudate) of *Papaver somniferum* (opium poppy) and the prototype of the synthetic opioid analgesics, being selective for μ-opioid receptors (Fig. 1.1). This compound may be considered the paramount natural product lead compound, with many thousands of analogs synthesized in an attempt to obtain derivatives with strong analgesic potency but without any addictive tendencies (1–4). One derivative now in late clinical trials as a pain treatment is morphine-6-glucuronide (M6G), the major active metabolite of morphine, with fewer side effects than the parent compound (18,62). The pyridine alkaloid epibatidine, isolated from a dendrobatid frog (*Epipedobates tricolor*) found in Ecuador, activates nicotinic receptors and has a 200-fold more potent analgesic activity than morphine. The drug potential of epibatidine is limited by its concomitant toxicity, but it is an important lead compound for the development of future new analgesic agents with less addictive liability than the opiate analgesics (63). A nonopioid analgesic for the amelioration of chronic pain has been introduced to the market recently, namely, ziconotide, which is a synthetic version of the peptide, ω-conotoxin MVIIA. The conotoxin class is produced by the cone snail, *Conus magus*, and these compounds are peptides with 24- to 27-amino acid residues. Ziconotide selectively binds to N-type voltage-sensitive neuronal channels, causing a blockage of neurotransmission and a potent analgesic effect (18,64). This is one of the first examples of a new natural product drug from a marine source.

(−)-Δ^9-*trans*-Tetrahydrocannabinol (tetrahydrocannabinol [THC]) is the major psychoactive (euphoriant) constituent of marijuana (*Cannabis sativa*). The synthetic form of THC (dronabinol) was approved more than 25 years ago to treat nausea and vomiting associated with cancer chemotherapy and has been used for a lesser amount

D-Phe-L-Pro-L-Arg-L-Pro-Gly-Gly-Gly-Gly-L-Asn-Gly-L-Asp-L-Phe-L-Glu-L-Glu-
L-Ile-L-Pro-L-Glu-L-Glu-L-Tyr-L-Leu

Bivalirudin

L-His-Gly-L-Glu-Gly-L-Thr-L-Phe-L-Thr-L-Ser-L-Asp-L-Leu-L-Ser-L-Lys-
L-Gln-L-Met-L-Glu-L-Glu-L-Glu-L-Ala-L-Val-L-Arg-L-Leu-L-Phe-L-Ile-L-Glu-L-Trp-
L-Leu-L-Lys-L-Asn-Gly-Gly-L-Pro-L-Ser-L-Ser-Gly-L-Ala-L-Pro-L-Pro-L-Pro-L-Ser-NH_2

Exenatide

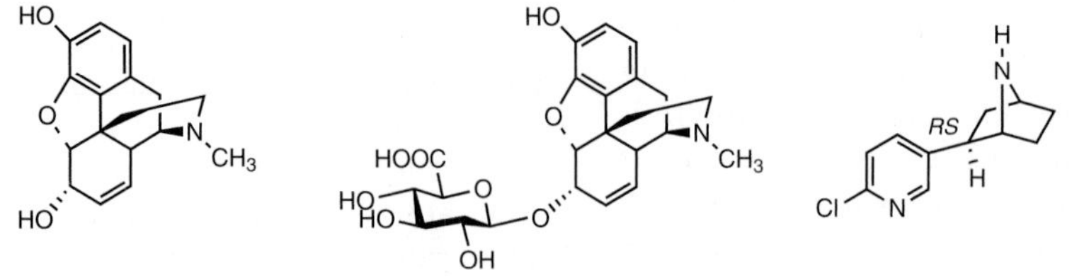

Morphine Morphine-6-O-glucuronide (M6G) Epibatidine

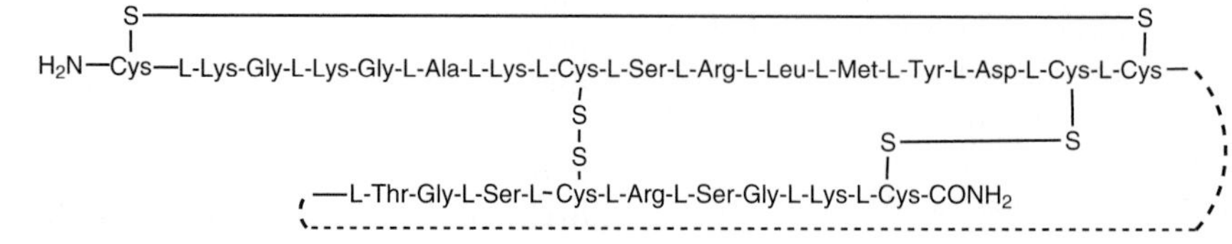

Ziconotide

FIGURE 1.1 Analgesic compounds of natural origin or derived from naturally occurring analgesics.

of time to treat appetite loss in HIV/AIDS patients (3). More recently, an approximately 1:1 mixture of THC and the structurally related marijuana constituent cannabidiol (CBD) has been approved in Canada and the United Kingdom for the alleviation of neuropathic pain and spasticity for multiple sclerosis patients and is administered in low doses as a buccal spray (18,65). There is considerable interest in using cannabinoid derivatives based on THC for medicinal purposes, but it is necessary to minimize the CNS effects of these compounds.

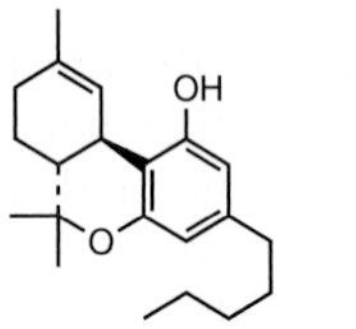

Tetrahydrocannabinol (THC)

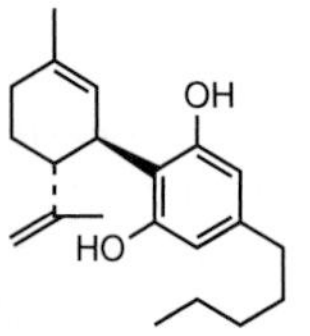

Cannabidiol (CBD)

Another important natural product lead compound is the tropane alkaloid ester atropine [(±)-hyoscyamine], from the plant *Atropa belladonna* (deadly nightshade). Atropine has served as a prototype molecule for several anticholinergic and antispasmodic drugs. One recently introduced example of an anticholinergic compound modeled on atropine is tiotropium bromide, which is used for the maintenance treatment of bronchospasm associated with chronic obstructive pulmonary disease (COPD) (66).

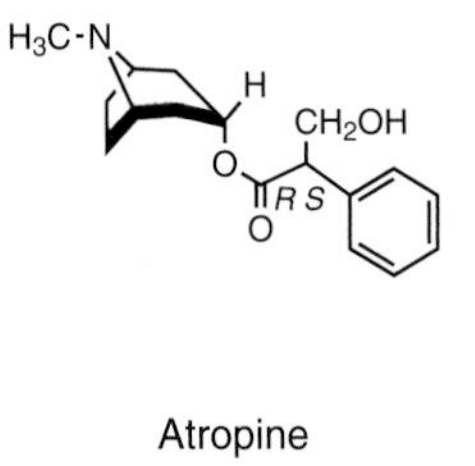

Atropine

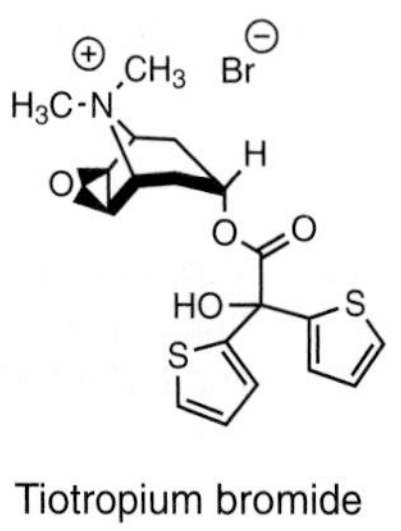

Tiotropium bromide

In the category of anti-Alzheimer disease agents, galantamine hydrobromide is a selective acetylcholinesterase inhibitor that slows down neurologic degeneration by inhibiting this enzyme and by interacting with the nicotinic receptor (67). Galantamine (also known as "galanthamine") is classified as an Amaryllidaceae alkaloid and has been obtained from several species in this family. Because commercial synthesis is not economical, it is obtained from the bulbs of *Leucojum aestivum* (snowflake) and *Galanthus* species (snowdrop) (1–4). There is some evidence that there is an ethnomedical basis for the current use of galantamine (68).

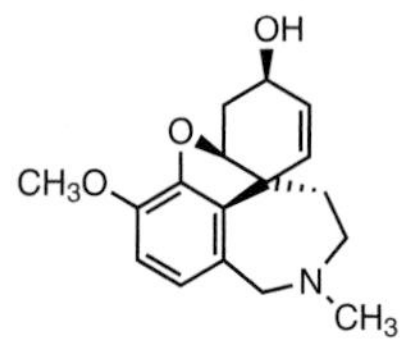

Galantamine

Anti-infective Agents

Since the introduction of penicillin G (benzylpenicillin) to chemotherapy as an antibacterial agent in the 1940s, natural products have contributed greatly to the field of anti-infective agents. In addition to the penicillins, other classes of antibacterials that have been developed from natural product sources are the aminoglycosides, cephalosporins, glycopeptides, macrolides, rifamycins, and tetracyclines. Antifungals, such as griseofulvin and the polyenes, and avermectins, such as the antiparasitic drug ivermectin, are also of microbial origin (1–4). Of the approximately 90 drugs in this category that were introduced in Western countries, including Japan, in the period from 1981 to 2002, almost 80% can be related to a microbial origin (16). Despite this, relatively few major pharmaceutical companies are currently working on the discovery of new anti-infective agents from natural sources, due to possible bacterial resistance against new agents and concerns regarding regulation (17). Higher plants have also afforded important anti-infective agents, perhaps most significantly the quinoline alkaloid quinine, obtained from the bark of several *Cinchona* species found in South America, including *Cinchona ledgeriana* and *Cinchona succirubra.* Quinine continues to be used for the treatment of multidrug-resistant malaria and was the template molecule for the synthetic antimalarials chloroquine, primaquine, and mefloquine (1–4).

The following examples have been chosen to represent an array of different structural types of antibacterial agents recently introduced into therapy (Fig. 1.2) (6,14,17,18). Meropenem is a carbapenem (a group of β-lactam antibiotics in which the sulfur atom in the thiazolidine ring is replaced by a carbon) and is based on thienamycin (Fig. 1.2), isolated from *Streptomyces cattleya.* It is a broad-spectrum antibacterial that was introduced into therapy in the last decade as a stable analog of the initially discovered thienamycin (69). Tigecycline (Fig. 1.2) is member of the glycylcycline class of tetracycline antibacterials and is the 9-*tert*-butylglycylamido derivative of minocycline, a semisynthetic derivative of chlortetracycline from *Streptomyces aureofaciens.* This is a broad-spectrum antibiotic with activity against methicillin-resistant *Staphylococcus aureus* (70). Daptomycin (Fig. 1.2) is the prototype member of the cyclic lipopeptide class of antibiotics and, although isolated initially from *Streptomyces roseosporus,* is produced by semisynthesis. This compound binds to bacterial cell membranes, disrupting the membrane potential, and blocks the synthesis of DNA, RNA, and proteins. Daptomycin is bactericidal against gram-positive organisms including vancomycin-resistant *Enterococcus faecalis* and *Enterococcus faecium* and is approved for the treatment of complicated skin and dermal infections (71). Telithromycin (Fig. 1.2) is a semisynthetic derivative of the 14-membered macrolide erythromycin A from *Saccharopolyspora erthraea* and is a macrolide of the ketolide class that lacks a cladinose sugar but has an extended alkyl-aryl unit attached to a cyclic carbamate unit. It binds to domains II and V of the 23S rRNA unit of the bacterial 50S ribosomal unit, leading to inhibition of the ribosome assembly and protein synthesis. This macrolide antibiotic is used to treat bacteria that infect the lungs and sinuses, including community-acquired pneumonia due to *Streptococcus pneumoniae* (72).

Natural products have been a fruitful source of antifungal agents in the past, with the echinocandins being a new group of lipopeptides introduced recently (73). Of these, three compounds are now approved drugs, including the acetate of caspofungin, which is a semisynthetic derivative of pneumocandin B_0, a fermentation product of *Glarea lozoyensis.* Caspofungin inhibits the synthesis of the fungal cell wall β(1,3)-D-glucan, by noncompetitive inhibition of the enzyme β(1,3)-D-glucan synthase, producing both a fungistatic and a fungicidal effect (73). The compound is administered by slow intravenous infusion and is useful in treating infections by *Candida* species (74).

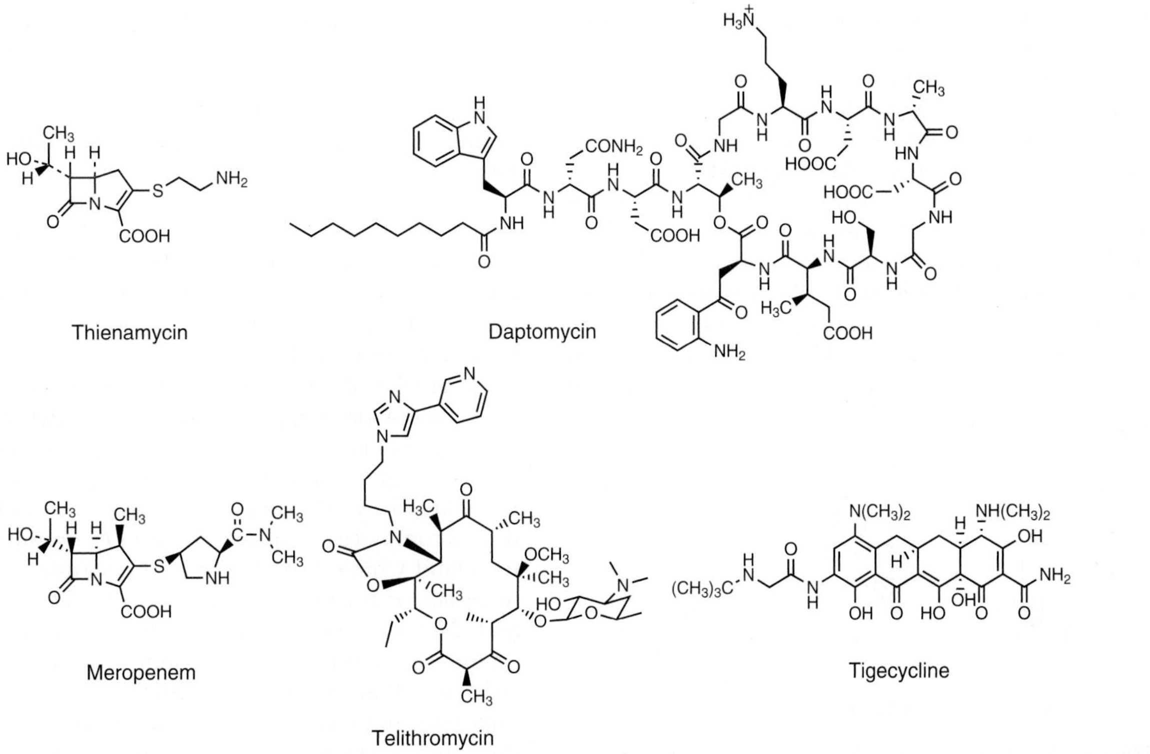

FIGURE 1.2 Examples of Natural and Semisynthetic Anti-infective Agents.

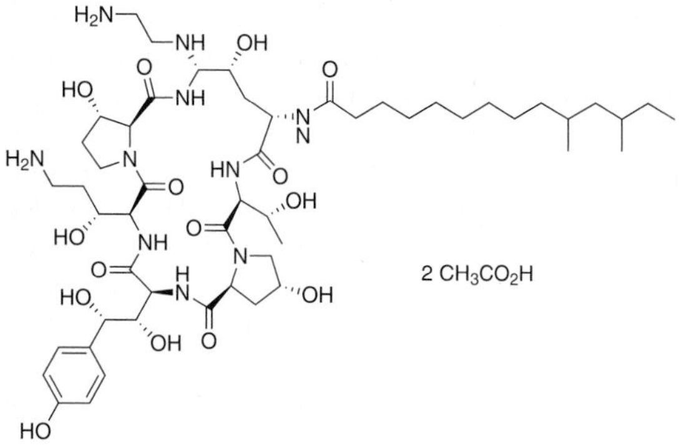

Caspofungin

Malaria remains a parasitic scourge that is still extending in incidence. In 1972, the active principle from *Artemisia annua*, a plant used for centuries in Chinese traditional medicine to treat fevers and malaria, was established as a novel antimalarial chemotype. This compound, artemisinin (*qinghaosu* in Chinese), is a sesquiterpene lactone with an endoperoxide group that is essential for activity, and it reacts with the iron in haem in the malarial parasite, *Plasmodium falciparum* (Fig. 1.3). Because this compound is poorly soluble in water, a number of derivatives have been produced with improved formulation, including arteether and artemether. Although animal experiments have suggested that artemisinin derivatives are neurotoxic, this may not be the case in malaria patients (1–4). Artemisinin-based combination treatments such as coartemether (artemether and lumefantrine) are now widely used for treating drug-resistant *P. falciparum* malaria (75). Coartemether is also known as artemisinin combination therapy and is registered in a large number of countries. A second ether derivative of artemisinin has also been developed, namely, arteether, and is registered in the Netherlands (76).

There are now about 30 approved drugs or drug combinations used to treat HIV/AIDS infections, with most of these being targeted toward the viral enzymes reverse transcriptase or protease. Bevirimat is a semisynthetic 3′,3′-dimethylsuccinyl derivative of the oleanane-type triterpenoid betulinic acid, which is found widely in the plant kingdom, including several species used in traditional Chinese medicine. This compound is now undergoing clinical trials as a potential HIV maturation inhibitor (77,78).

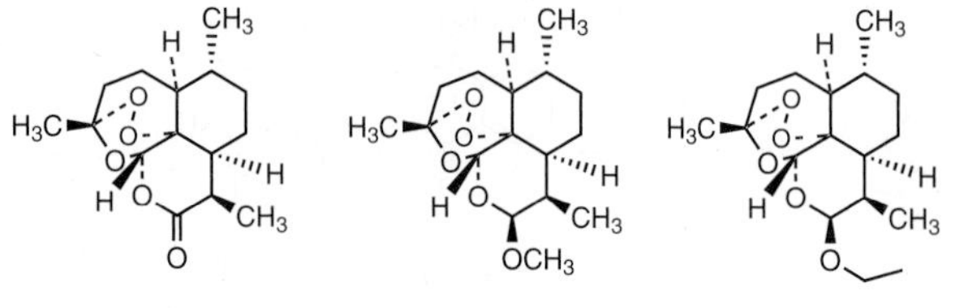

Artemisinin Artemether Arteether

FIGURE 1.3 Artemisinin and two derivatives used for the treatment of malaria.

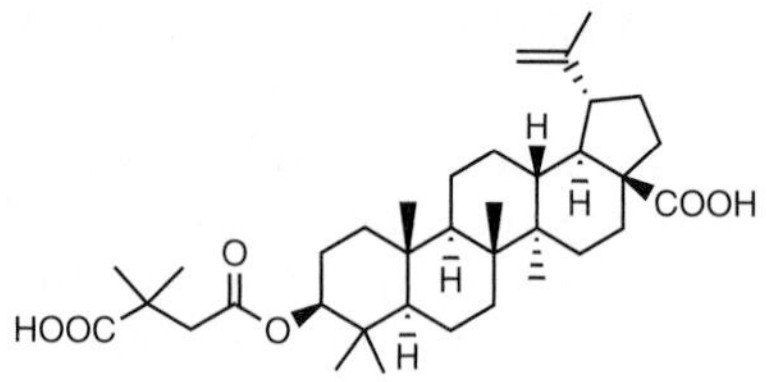

Bevirimat

Anticancer Agents

For several decades, natural products have served as a useful group of structurally diverse cancer chemotherapeutic agents, and many of our most important anticancer agents are of microbial or plant origin. Thus, the antitumor antibiotics include the anthracyclines (daunorubicin, doxorubicin, epirubicin, idarubicin, and valrubicin), bleomycin, dactinomycin (actinomycin D), mitomycin C, and mitoxantrone. Four main classes of plant-derived antitumor agents are used: vinca (*Catharanthus*) bisindole alkaloids (vinblastine, vincristine, and vinorelbine); the semisynthetic epipodophyllotoxin derivatives (etoposide, teniposide, and etoposide phosphate); the taxanes (paclitaxel and docetaxel); and the camptothecin analogs (irinotecan and topotecan) (Fig. 1.4) (1–4,79).

The parent compounds paclitaxel (originally called "taxol") and camptothecin were both discovered in the laboratory of the late Monroe E. Wall and of Mansukh Wani at Research Triangle Institute in North Carolina (Fig. 1.4). Like some other natural product drugs, several years elapsed from the initial discovery of these substances until their ultimate clinical approval in either a chemically unmodified or modified form. One of the factors that served to delay the introduction of paclitaxel to the market was the need for the large-scale acquisition of this compound from a source other than from the bark of its original plant of origin, the Pacific yew (*Taxus brevifolia*), because this would involve destroying this slow-growing tree. Paclitaxel and its semisynthetic analog docetaxel may be produced by partial synthesis. To enable this, the diterpenoid "building block," 10-deacetylbaccatin III, is used as a starting material, which can be isolated from the needles of the ornamental yew, *Taxus baccata*, a renewable botanical resource that can be cultivated in greenhouses (80). A major pharmaceutical company now manufactures paclitaxel by plant tissue culture. The initial source plant of camptothecin, *Camptotheca acuminata*, is a rare species found in regions south of the Yangtze region of the People's Republic of China. Today, camptothecin is not only produced commercially from cultivated *C. acuminata* trees in mainland China, but also from the roots of *Nothapodytes nimmoniana* (formerly known as both *Nothapodytes foetida* and *Mappia foetida*), which is found in the southern regions of the Indian subcontinent (81). It is of interest to note that these two antineoplastic agents are particularly important not only because of the clinical effectiveness of their derivatives as cancer chemotherapeutic agents, having a significant proportion of the market share (80), but

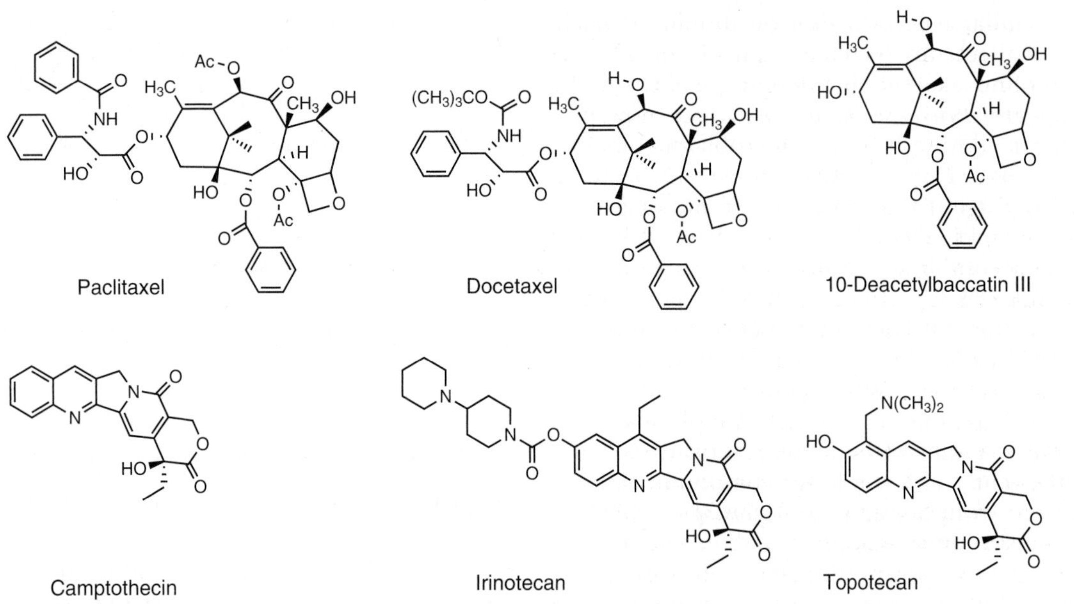

FIGURE 1.4 Lead anticancer compounds paclitaxel, camptothecin, and their respective derivatives.

also because they are prominent lead compounds for synthetic optimization. There are several taxanes and camptothecin derivatives in clinical trial (17,18). Interestingly, endophytic fungi have been reported to produce paclitaxel (82) and camptothecin (83), so it may be possible in the future to produce these important compounds by fermentation rather than by cultivation or other existing methods. Paclitaxel and camptothecin were each found to exhibit a unique mechanism of action for the inhibition of cancer cell growth, with paclitaxel shown to promote the polymerization of tubulin and the stabilization of microtubules and with camptothecin demonstrated as the first inhibitor of the enzyme DNA topoisomerase I (84).

Several other natural product molecules or their derivatives have been introduced to therapy recently (Fig. 1.5) (17,18,85). Ixabepilone, a semisynthetic derivative of epothilone B, is now marketed in the United States for the treatment of locally advanced and metastatic breast cancer (86). The epothilones are derived from the terrestrial myxobacterium *Sorangium cellulosum*

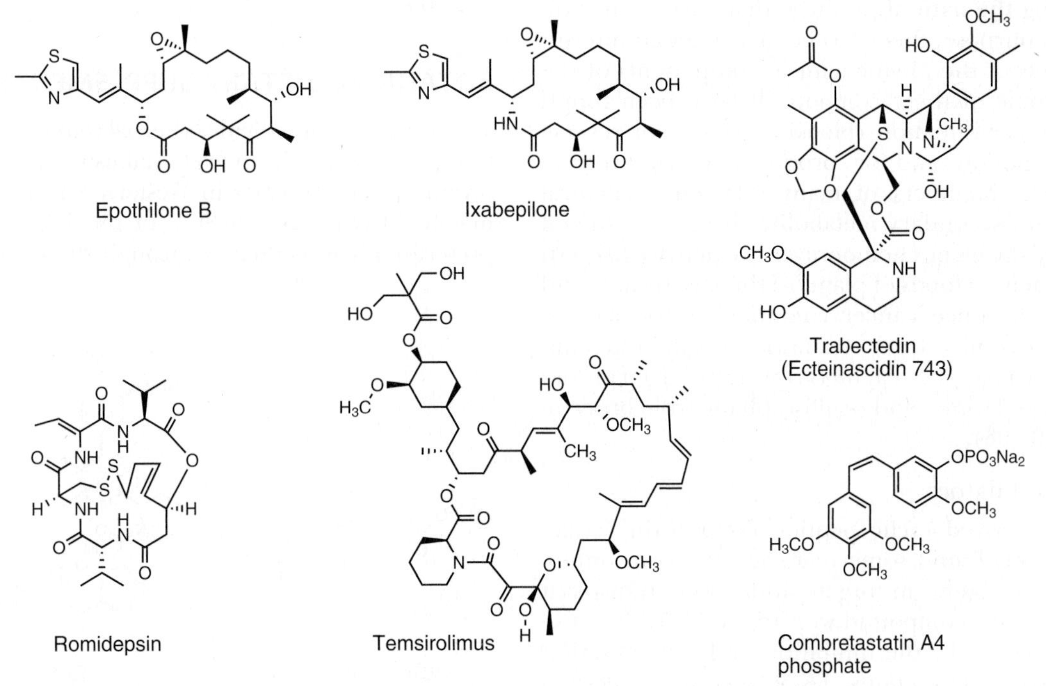

FIGURE 1.5 Potential cancer chemotherapeutic agents from marine, bacterial, plant, and fungal origin.

and have a similar type of action on tubulin as paclitaxel (87). Trabectedin (ecteinascidin-743 or ET-743) is an isoquinoline alkaloid obtained originally from the marine tunicate, *Ecteinascidia turbinata*, but now produced by partial synthesis from a microbial metabolite, cyanosafracin B, of *Pseudomonas fluorescens*. Trabectedin is an alkylating agent that binds to the minor groove of DNA and blocks cells in the G_2-M phase; it is used in Europe as second-line therapy for patients with soft tissue sarcoma (88,89). Romidepsin is a depsipeptide isolated from the soil bacterium, *Chromobacterium violaceum*, in 1994 (90). This compound is an inhibitor of histone deacetylase and was approved in the United States for the treatment of T-cell lymphoma (91). Temsirolimus is a semisynthetic ester derivative of sirolimus (rapamycin), with the latter compound isolated some time ago from *Streptococcus hygroscopicus* (92,93). Recently, temsirolimus was approved in the United States for treating advanced renal cell carcinoma, and mechanistically, this compound is an inhibitor of the mammalian target of rapamycin kinase (92,93). A promising new anticancer agent still in advanced clinical trials is combretastatin A4 phosphate, a water-soluble prodrug of combretastatin A4 from the South African plant, *Combretum caffrum* (94). Combretastatin A4 phosphate binds to tubulin and also affects tumor blood flow as a vascular disrupting agent (94,95).

Cancer chemoprevention is regarded as the use of synthetic or natural agents to inhibit, delay, or reverse the process of carcinogenesis through intervention before the appearance of invasive disease. This relatively new approach toward the management of cancer has involved gaining a better understanding of the mechanism of action of cancer chemopreventive agents (96). Among the natural products that have been studied for this purpose, there has been a renewed interest in the effects of the phytochemical components of the diet, and some of these compounds have been found to block cancer initiation (blocking agents) or reverse tumor promotion and/or progression (suppressing agents) (97). Members of many different structural types of plant secondary metabolites have been linked with potential cancer chemopreventive activity (97,98). Approximately 35 foods of plant origin have been found recently to produce cancer chemopreventive agents, such as curcumin from turmeric, epigallocatechin 3-*O*-gallate from green tea, *trans*-resveratrol from grapes and certain red wines, and *d*-sulforaphane from broccoli (Fig. 1.6) (97,98).

Immunomodulators

The fungal-derived cyclic peptide cyclosporin (cyclosporine A) was found some years ago to be an immunosuppressive agent in organ and tissue transplant surgery. Another compound with this same type of use and that also acts by the inhibition of T-cell activation is the macrolide tacrolimus (FK-506) from *Streptomyces tsukubaensis* (3).

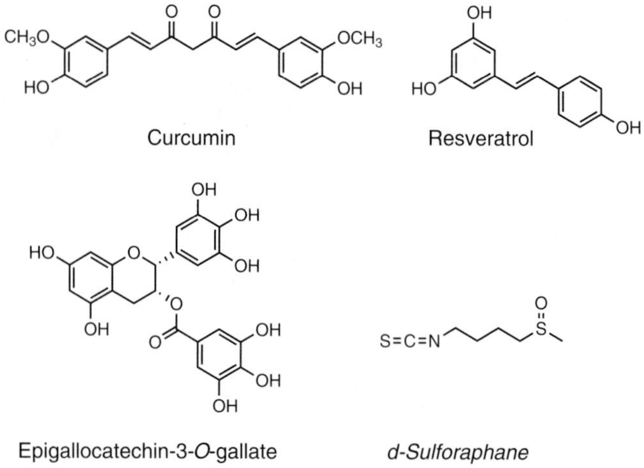

FIGURE 1.6 Naturally occurring cancer chemopreventive agents.

Two additional natural product–derived immunosuppressants are clinically available as mycophenolate sodium and everolimus (Fig. 1.7) (17,18). The active principle of both mycophenolate sodium and an earlier introduced form mycophenolate mofetil (a morpholinoethyl derivative) is mycophenolic acid, obtained from several *Penicillium* species. This compound is a reversible inhibitor of inosine monophosphate dehydrogenase, which is involved in guanosine nucleotide synthesis (17,99). Everolimus is an orally active semisynthetic 40-*O*-(2-hydroxyethyl) derivative of rapamycin (also known as sirolimus) and was originally obtained from *Streptomyces hygroscopicus*. Everolimus is a proliferation inhibitor that blocks growth factor-mediated transduction signals and prevents organ rejection through a different mechanism than mycophenolate mofetil (17,100).

BOTANICAL DIETARY SUPPLEMENTS

The use of phytomedicines (herbal remedies) as prescription products has been well established in Germany and several other countries in Western Europe for approximately 30 years. About 80% of physicians in Germany prescribe phytomedicines through the orthodox health

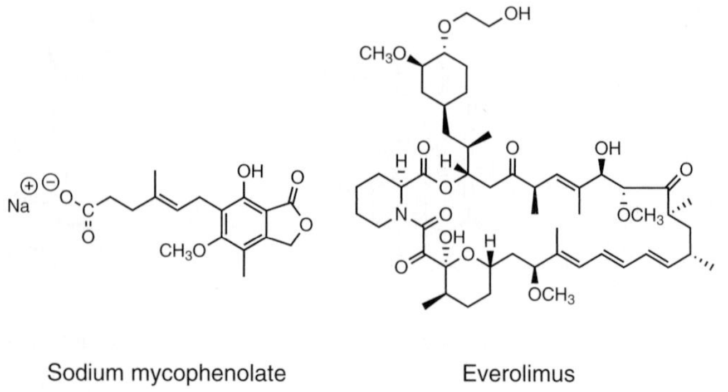

FIGURE 1.7 Naturally occurring immunosuppressants.

care system. Over the last 15 years, there has been a large influx of botanical products into community pharmacy practice and health food stores in the United States as a result of the passage of the Dietary Supplement Health and Education Act (DSHEA) in 1994. Such products are regulated by the U.S. Food and Drug Administration as foods rather than drugs and must adhere to requirements regarding product labeling and acceptable health claims (101). Currently, among the most popular botanical products used in the United States are those containing black cohosh, cranberry, echinacea, evening primrose, garlic, ginkgo, ginger, ginseng, green tea, milk thistle, saw palmetto, soy, St. John's wort, and valerian. These are purchased as either the crude powdered form in compressed tablets or capsules or as galenical preparations, such as extracts or tinctures, and are frequently ingested in the form of a tea (101). In addition to the United States, a parallel increased interest in herbal remedies has occurred in all countries in Western Europe, Canada, and Australia, in part because of a greater awareness of complementary and alternative medicine (CAM). Many clinical trials on these products have been conducted in Europe, and some are occurring in the United States under the sponsorship of the National Institutes of Health.

The recent widespread introduction of a large number of botanical dietary supplements has opened a new door in terms of research inquiry for natural product scientists in the United States. Not all of these products have a well-documented efficacy, however. Three important needs in the scientific investigation of herbal remedies are the characterization of active principles (where these are not known), the development of rigorous and validated analytical methods for quality control procedures, and the determination of their potential toxicity and interactions with prescription medications (102). Unlike compounds approved as single chemical entity (SCE) drugs, it is accepted that combinations of plant secondary metabolites may be responsible for the physiologic effects of herbal medicines. For example, both the terpene lactone (e.g., ginkgolide B; Fig. 1.8) and the flavonoid glycoside constituents of ginkgo (*Ginkgo biloba*) leaves are regarded as being necessary for allevation of the symptoms of peripheral vascular disease for which this phytomedicine is used in Europe (101). Moreover, an acetone-soluble extract of *G. biloba* containing standardized amounts of flavone glycosides (24%) and terpene lactones (6%) has been used in many clinical trials on this herb (101). If the "active principles" of an herbal remedy are known or can be discovered, these substances can act as reference standards, and their specified concentration levels can be quantified in chemical quality control procedures, which are predominantly performed by HPLC. A number of official monographs for the standardization of botanical dietary supplements have been developed over the last decade in the United States (103). Other scientific challenges on herbal remedies are to establish more completely their dissolution, bioavailability, and shelf life. For

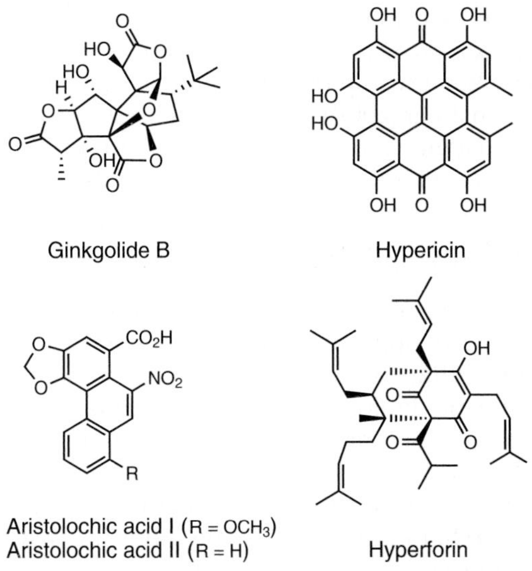

FIGURE 1.8 Chemicals found in various botanical dietary supplements.

example, it has been found that co-effectors such as certain procyanidins present in St. John's wort (*Hypericum perforatum*) can increase the bioavailability of hypericin (Fig. 1.8), one of the constituents of this plant known to exert antidepressant activity (104). These herbal products should be free of adulteration (the deliberate addition of nonauthentic plant material or of biologically active or inactive compounds), as well as free of other additives such as herbicides, pesticides, heavy metals, solvent residues, and microbial and biologic contaminants (101,102).

Unfortunately, many herbal remedies may pose toxicity risks or may be involved in harmful drug interactions. A drastic example of toxicity was caused by the herbal Chinese medicinal plant, *Aristolochia fangchi,* which was substituted in error for another Chinese plant in a weight-reducing regimen taken by a number of women in Belgium several decades ago. Years later, this was linked to the generation of severe renal disease characterized as interstitial fibrosis with atrophy of the tubules, as well as the development of tumors. These toxic symptoms, also known as "Chinese herb nephropathy," were attributed to the presence of the phenanthrene derivatives aristolochic acids I and II (Fig. 1.8) produced by *A. fangchi,* which have been found experimentally to intercalate with DNA (105). The presence of high levels of the phloroglucinol derivative hyperforin (Fig. 1.8) in St. John's wort (*Hypericum perforatum*) products has been found to induce cytochrome P450 enzymes (in particular CYP34A), leading to decreased plasma concentrations of prescription drugs that may be coadministered, such as alprazolam, cyclosporin, digoxin, indinavir, irinotecan, simvastatin, and warfarin, as well as oral contraceptives (106).

In 2006, the first example of a new class of natural product prescription drugs was approved by the U.S. Food and Drug Administration, namely, a mixture of sinecatechins present in a standardized extract of the leaves of green tea (*Camellia sinensis*). This product is approved for the topical treatment of external genital and perianal warts. Stringent criteria must be followed in the manufacture and quality control of this product, and it was subjected to rigorous clinical trials (107).

FUTURE PROSPECTS

The beginning of the second decade of the 21st century seems to be an opportune time for renewed efforts to be made regarding the discovery of new secondary metabolite prototype, biologically active compounds from animals, fungi, microorganisms, and plants of terrestrial and marine origin. Although many pharmaceutical companies have reduced their investment in natural products research, in favor of screening libraries of synthetic compounds and combinatorial chemistry, this has coincided with disappointing numbers of SCE drugs being introduced in recent years (11,14–16). Fortunately, many smaller "biotech" companies have actively taken up the challenge of contemporary natural products drug discovery from organisms. There continues to be a steady stream of new natural product–derived drugs introduced into therapy for the treatment of many common human diseases (e.g., cancer, cardiovascular diseases, neurologic conditions) (17,18). However, there is ample potential for much greater utilization of natural product–derived compounds in the treatment or prophylaxis of such major worldwide scourges as HIV/AIDS, tuberculosis, hepatitis C, and tropical diseases (e.g., lymphatic filariasis, leishmaniasis, schistosomiasis). The search for such agents should be enhanced by the availability of extensive libraries of taxonomically authenticated crude extracts of terrestrial and marine origin, as well as of pure secondary metabolites from microorganisms, plants, and animals. In addition, this will be facilitated by recently developed techniques such as biocatalysis, combinatorial biosynthesis, combinatorial and computational chemistry, metabolic engineering, and tissue culture. The high "drug-like" quality of natural product molecules stands as a constant, and it only remains for natural product chemists and biologists to investigate these substances in the most technically ingenious and expedient ways possible.

It should not be thought that after approximately 200 years of investigation, the prospects of finding new drugs of natural origin are nearing exhaustion; there is still a large scope for success in this type of endeavor. For example, if plants are taken specifically, less than 20% have been evaluated chemically or biologically. The urgency to perform this type of work cannot be understated in view of the increasing erosion of natural resources that will accelerate as the 21st century progresses.

References

1. Heinrich M, Barnes J, Gibbons S, et al. Fundamentals of Pharmacognosy and Phytotherapy. Edinburgh, UK: Churchill Livingstone, 2004.
2. Evans WC. Trease and Evans Pharmacognosy, 16th Ed. New York: Saunders-Elsevier, 2009.
3. Dewick PM. Medicinal Natural Products: A Biosynthetic Approach, 3rd Ed. New York: John Wiley & Sons, 2009.
4. Samuelsson G, Bohlin L. Drugs of Natural Origin. A Treatise of Pharmacognosy, 6th Rev. Ed. Stockholm, Sweden: Swedish Pharmaceutical Press, 2009.
5. Kinghorn AD. Pharmacognosy in the 21st century. J Pharm Pharmacol 2001;53:135–148.
6. Demain AL, Sanchez S. Microbial drug discovery: 80 years of progress. J Antibiot 2009;62:5–16.
7. Pearce C, Eckard P, Gruen-Wollny I, et al. Microorganisms: their role in the discovery and development of medicines. In: Buss AD, Butler MS, eds. Natural Product Chemistry for Drug Discovery. Cambridge, UK: RSC Publishing, 2010:215–241.
8. Molinski TF, Dalisay DS, Lievens SL, et al. Drug development from marine natural products. Nat Rev Drug Discov 2009;8:69–85.
9. Williams DH, Stone MJ, Hauck PR, et al. Why are secondary metabolites (natural products) biosynthesized? J Nat Prod 1989;52:1189–1208.
10. Clardy J, Walsh C. Lessons from natural molecules. Nature 2004;432:829–837.
11. Koehn FE, Carter GT. The evolving role of natural products in drug discovery. Nat Rev Drug Discov 2005;4:206–220.
12. Henkel T, Brunne RM, Muller H, et al. Statistical investigation into the structural complementarity of natural products and synthetic compounds. Angew Chem Int Ed 1999;38:643–647.
13. Feher M, Schmidt JM. Property distributions: differences between drugs, natural products, and molecules from combinatorial chemistry. J Chem Inf Comput Sci 2003;43:218–227.
14. Lam KS. New aspects of natural products in drug discovery. Trends Microbiol 2007;15:279–289.
15. Li JW-H, Vederas JC. Drug discovery and natural products: end of an era or an endless frontier? Science 2009;325:161–165.
16. Newman DJ, Cragg GM. Natural products as sources of new drugs over the last 25 years. J Nat Prod 2007;70:461–477.
17. Butler MS. Natural products to drugs: natural product-derived compounds in clinical trials. Nat Prod Rep 2008;25:475–516.
18. Butler MS. A snapshot of natural product-derived compounds in later stage clinical development at the end of 2008. In: Buss AD, Butler MS, eds. Natural Product Chemistry for Drug Discovery. Cambridge, UK: RSC Publishing, 2010:321–354.
19. Fabricant DS, Farnsworth NR. The value of plants used in traditional medicine for drug discovery. Environ Health Perspect 2001;109:69–75.
20. Lewis WH. Pharmaceutical discoveries based on ethnomedicinal plants: 1985 to 2000 and beyond. Economic Botany 2003;57:126–134.
21. James LF, Panter KE, Gaffield W, et al. Biomedical applications of poisonous plant research. J Agric Food Chem 2004;52:3211–3230.
22. Spjut RW. Relationships between folklore and antitumor activity: an historical review. Sida 2005;21:2205–2241.
23. Piel J. Metabolites from symbiotic bacteria. Nat Prod Rep 2004;21:519–538.
24. Tan GT, Gyllenhaal C, Soejarto DD. Biodiversity as a source of anticancer agents. Curr Drug Targets 2006;7:265–277.
25. Simmons TL, Andrianosolo E, McPhail K, et al. Marine natural products as anticancer drugs. Mol Cancer Ther 2005;4:333–342.
26. Pitman NCA, Jørgensen PM. Estimating the size of the world's threatened flora. Science 2002;298:989.
27. Myers N, Mittermeier RA, Mittermeier CG, et al. Biodiversity hotspots for conservation priorities. Nature 2000;403:853–858.
28. Cordell GA. The Convention on Biological Diversity and its impact on natural products research. In: Buss AD, Butler MS, eds. Natural Product Chemistry for Drug Discovery. Cambridge, UK: RSC Publishing, 2010:81–139.
29. Farrier D, Tucker L. Access to marine bioresources: hitching the conservation car to the bioprospecting horse. Ocean Dev Int Law 2001;32:213–239.
30. Hallock YF, Cragg GM. National Cooperative Drug Discovery Groups (NCDDGs): a successful model for public private partnerships in cancer drug discovery. Pharm Biol 2003;41(Suppl):78–91.
31. Kinghorn AD, Carcache-Blanco EJ, Chai H-B, et al. Discovery of anticancer agents of diverse natural origin. Pure Appl Chem 2009;81:1051–1063.
32. Itokawa H, Morris-Natschke SL, Akiyama T, et al. Plant-derived natural product research aimed at new drug discovery. J Nat Med 2008;62:263–280.
33. Fenical W, Jensen PR, Palladino MA, et al. Discovery and development of the anticancer agent salinosporamide A (NPI-0052). Bioorg Med Chem 2009;17:2175–2180.
34. Challis GL. Genome mining for novel natural product discovery. J Med Chem 2008;51:2618–2628.
35. Gunitalaka AAL. Natural products from plant-associated microorganisms: distribution, structural diversity, and implications of their occurrence. J Nat Prod 2006;69:509–526.
36. Harvey AL. Natural products in drug discovery. Drug Discov Today 2008;13:894–901.
37. Haslam E. Natural polyphenols (vegetable tannins) as drugs: possible modes of action. J Nat Prod 1996;59:205–215.
38. Balunas MJ, Su B, Landini S, et al. Interference by naturally occurring fatty acids in a non-cellular enzyme based aromatase bioassay. J Nat Prod 2006;69:700–703.

39. Parker CH, Ottl J, Gabriel D, et al. Advances in biological screening for lead discovery. In: Buss AD, Butler MS, eds. Natural Product Chemistry for Drug Discovery. Cambridge, UK: RSC Publishing, 2010:245–271.
40. Jacob MR, Walker LA. Natural products and antifungal drug discovery. In: Ernst EJ, Rogers P, eds. Methods in Molecular Medicine, Vol. 118, Antifungal Agents: Methods and Protocols. Totowa, NJ: Humana Press Inc., 2005:83–109.
41. New DC, Miller-Martini DM, Wong YH. Reporter gene assays and their applications to bioassays of natural products. Phytother Res 2003;17:439–448.
42. Nakao Y, Fusetani N. Enzyme inhibitors from marine invertebrates. J Nat Prod 2007;70:689–710.
43. Mora FD, Jones DK, Desai PV, et al. Bioassay for the identification of natural product-based activators of peroxisome proliferator-activated receptor-γ (PPARγ): the marine sponge metabolite psammaplin A activates PPARγ and induces apoptosis in human breast cancer cells. J Nat Prod 2006;69:547–522.
44. Walters WP, Namchuk M. Designing screens: how to make your hits a hit. Nat Rev Drug Discov 2003;2:259–266.
45. Sticher O. Natural product isolation. Nat Prod Rep 2008;25:517–544.
46. Koehn FE. High impact technologies for natural products screening. In: Petersen F, Amstutz R, eds. Progress in Drug Research, Vol. 65; Natural Compounds as Drugs, Vol. 1. Basel, Switzerland: Birkhäuser Verlag, 2008:175–210.
47. Molinski TF. NMR of natural products at the nanomolar scale. Nat Prod Rep 2010;27;321–329.
48. Steinbeck C. Recent developments in automated structure elucidation of natural products. Nat Prod Rep 2004;21:512–518.
49. Spogøe K, Stærk D, Ziegler HL, et al. Combining HPLC-PDA-MS-SFE-NMR with circular dichroism for complete natural product characterization in crude extracts: levorotatory gossypol in *Thespesia danis*. J Nat Prod 2008;71:516–519.
50. Dinan L. Dereplication and partial identification of compounds. In: Sarker SD, Latif Z, Gray AI, eds. Methods in Biotechnology, Vol. 20: Natural Products Isolation, 2nd Ed. Totowa, NJ: Humana Press Inc., 2005:297–321.
51. Sumner LW, Mendes P, Dixon RA. Plant metabolomics: large-scale phytochemistry in the functional genomics era. Phytochemistry 2003;62:817–836.
52. Rochfort S. Metabolomics revisited: a new "omics" platform technology for systems biology and implications for natural products research. J Nat Prod 2005;68:1813–1820.
53. Kolewe ME, Gaurav V, Roberts SC. Pharmaceutically active natural product synthesis and supply via plant cell culture technology. Mol Pharmaceutics 2008;5:243–256.
54. Mi Q, Pezzuto JM, Farnsworth NR, et al. Use of the in vivo hollow fiber assay in natural products anticancer drug discovery. J Nat Prod 2009;72:573–580.
55. Zhang W, Tang Y. Combinatorial biosynthesis of natural products. J Med Chem 2008;51:2629–2633.
56. Sneader W. Drug Discovery: A History. Hoboken, NJ: John Wiley & Sons, 2005.
57. Ledizet M, Harrison LM, Koski RA, et al. Discovery and pre-clinical development of antithrombotics from hematophagous invertebrates. Curr Med Chem Cardiovasc Hematol Agents 2005;3:1–10.
58. Curran MP. Bivalirudin: in patients with ST-segment elevation myocardial infarction. Drugs 2010;70:909–918.
59. Tahrani AA, Piya MK, Barnett AH. Exenatide: incretin therapy for patients with type-2 diabetes. Exp Rev Endocrinol Metab 2008;6:671–690.
60. Clement JA, Yoder BJ, Kingston DGI. Natural products as a source of CNS-active agents. Mini-Rev Organic Chem 2004;1:183–208.
61. Prisinzano TE. Natural products as tools for neuroscience: discovery and development of novel agents to treat drug abuse. J Nat Prod 2009;72:581–587.
62. van Dorp EL, Morariu A, Dahan A. Morphine-6-glucuronide: potency and safety compared to morphine. Expert Opin Pharmacother 2008;9:1955–1961.
63. Daly JW, Spande TF, Garraffo HM. Alkaloids from amphibian skin: a tabulation of over 800 compounds. J Nat Prod 2005;68:1556–1575.
64. Schmidtko A, Lötsch J, Freynhagen R, et al. Ziconotide for treatment of severe chronic pain. Lancet 2010;375:1569–1577.
65. Wade DT, Collin C, Stott C, et al. Meta-analysis of the efficacy and safety of Sativex (nabiximols), on spasticity in people with multiple sclerosis. Mult Scler 2010;16:707–714.
66. Mundy C, Kirkpatrick P. Fresh from the pipeline. Tiotropium bromide. Nat Rev Drug Discov 2004;3:643–644.
67. Suh WH, Suslick KS, Suh Y-H. Therapeutic agents for Alzheimer's disease. Curr Med Chem Central Nerv Syst Agents 2005;5:259–269.
68. Heinrich M, Teoh HL. Galanthamine from snowdrop: the development of a modern drug against Alzheimer's disease from local Caucasian knowledge. J Ethnopharmacol 2004;92:147–162.
69. Zhanel GG, Wiebe R, Dilay L, et al. Comparative review of the carbapenems. Drugs 2007;67:1027–1052.
70. Peterson CM. A review of tigecycline—the first glycylglycine. Int J Antimicrob Agents 2008;32(Suppl 4):S215–S222.
71. Baltz RH. Daptomycin. In: Buss AD, Butler MS, eds. Natural Product Chemistry for Drug Discovery. Cambridge, UK: RSC Publishing, 2010:395–409.
72. Spiers KM, Zervos MJ. Telithromycin. Expert Rev Anti Infect Ther 2004;2:685–693.
73. Renslo AR. The echinocandidins: total and semi-synthetic approaches to antifungal drug discovery. Anti Infect Agents Med Chem 2007;6:201–212.
74. Columbo AL, Ngai AL, Bourque M, et al. Caspofungin use in patients with invasive candidiasis caused by common non-albicans *Candida* species: review of the caspofungin database. Antimicrob Agents Chemother 2010;54:1864–1871.
75. Wernsdorfer WH. Coartemether (artemether and lumefantrine): an oral antimalarial drug. Expert Rev Anti Infect Ther 2004;2:181–196.
76. Yeates RA. Artemotil (Artecef). Curr Opin Investig Drugs 2002;3:545–549.
77. Martin DE, Salzwedel K, Allaway GP. Bevirimat: a novel maturation inhibitor for the treatment of HIV-1 infection. Antivir Chem Chemother 2008;19:107–113.
78. Qian K, Nitz TJ, Yu D, et al. From natural product to clinical trials: bevirimat, a plant-derived anti-AIDS drug. In: Buss AD, Butler MS, eds. Natural Product Chemistry for Drug Discovery. Cambridge, UK: RSC Publishing, 2010:374–391.
79. Cragg GM, Kingston DGI, Newman DJ, eds. Anticancer Agents from Natural Products. Boca Raton, FL: Taylor & Francis/CRC Press, 2005.
80. Oberlies NH, Kroll DJ. Camptothecin and taxol: historic achievements in natural products research. J Nat Prod 2004;67:129–135.
81. Padmanabha BV, Chandrashekar M, Ramesha BT, et al. Patterns of accumulation of camptothecin, an anti-cancer alkaloid, in *Nothapodytes nimmoniana* Graham, in the Western Ghats, India: implications for identifying high-yielding sources of the alkaloid. Curr Sci 2006;90:95–100.
82. Stierle A, Strobel G, Stierle D. Taxol and taxane production by *Taxomyces andreanae*, an endophytic fungus of Pacific yew. Science 1993;260:214–217.
83. Kusari S, Zühlke S, Spiteller M. An endophytic fungus from *Camptotheca acuminata* that produces camptothecin and analogues. J Nat Prod 2009;72:2–7.
84. Cragg GM, Grothaus PG, Newman DJ. Impact of natural products on developing new anti-cancer agents. Chem Rev 2009;109:3012–3043.
85. Bailly C. Commentary. Ready for a comeback of natural products in oncology. Biochem Pharmacol 2009;77:1447–1457.
86. Borzelli RM, Vite GD. Case history: discovery of ixabepilone (IXEMPRA™), a first-in-class epothilone analog for treatment of metastatic breast cancer. In: Macor JE, ed. Annual Reports in Medicinal Chemistry, Vol. 44. San Diego, CA: Academic Press/Elsevier, 2009:301–322.
87. Altmann K-H, Höfle G, Müller R, et al. The epothilones: an outstanding family of anti-tumor agents. In: Kinghorn AD, Falk H, Kobayashi J, eds. Progress in the Chemistry of Organic Natural Products, Vol. 90. Vienna, Austria: Springer-Verlag, 2009:1–260.
88. Henriquez R, Faircloth G, Cuervas C. Ecteinascidin 743 (ET-743; Yondelis™), aplidin, and kahalalide F. In: Cragg GM, Kingston DGI, Newman DJ, eds. Anticancer Agents from Natural Products. Boca Raton, FL: Taylor & Francis/ CRC Press, 2005:215–240.
89. D'Incalci M, Galmarini CM. A review of trabectedin (ET-743): a unique mechanism of action. Mol Cancer Ther 2010;9:2157–2163.
90. Ueda H, Nakajima H, Hori Y, et al. FR901228, a novel antitumor bicyclic depsipeptide produced by *Chromobacterium violaceum* no. 968. I. Taxonomy, fermentation, isolation, physico-chemical and biological properties, and antitumor activity. J Antibiot 1994;47:301–310.
91. Grant C, Rahman F, Piekarz R, et al. Romidepsin: a new therapy for cutaneous T-cell lymphoma and a potential therapy for solid tumors. Expert Rev Anticancer Ther 2010;10:997–1008.
92. Rini B, Kar S, Kirkpatrick P. Fresh from the pipeline. Temsirolimus. Nat Rev Drug Discov 2007;6:599–600.
93. Vezina C, Kudelski A, Sehgal SN. Rapamycin (AY-22,989), a new antifungal antibiotic. I. Taxonomy of the producing streptomycete and isolation of the active principle. J Antibiot 1975;28:721–726.
94. Pinney KC, Jelinek C, Edvarsden K, et al. The discovery and development of the combretastatins. In: Cragg GM, Kingston DGI, Newman DJ, eds. Anticancer Agents from Natural Products. Boca Raton, FL: Taylor & Francis/CRC Press, 2005:23–46.
95. Siemann DW, Chaplin DJ, Walicke PA. A review and update of the current status of the vasculature-disabling agent combretastatin-A4 phosphate (CA4P). Expert Opin Investig Drugs 2009;18:189–197.
96. Kelloff GJ, Hawk ET, Sigman CC, eds. Cancer Chemoprevention. Vol. 1, Promising Cancer Chemopreventive Agents. Totowa, NJ: Humana Press, 2004.
97. Surh Y-J. Cancer chemoprevention with dietary phytochemicals. Nat Rev Cancer 2003;3;768–779.
98. Mehta RG, Murillo G, Naithani R, et al. Cancer chemoprevention by natural products: how far have we come? Pharm Res 2010;27:950–961.
99. Curran MP, Keating GM. Mycophenolate delayed release: prevention of renal transplant rejection. Drugs 2005;65:799–805.
100. Chapman TM, Perry CM. Everolimus. Drugs 2004;64:861–872.
101. Robbers JC, Tyler VE. Tyler's Herbs of Choice. The Therapeutic Use of Phytomedicinals. New York: The Haworth Herbal Press, 1999.

102. Cardellina JH. Challenges and opportunities confronting the botanical dietary supplement industry. J Nat Prod 2002;65:1073–1081.
103. Schiff PL Jr, Srinivasan VS, Giancaspro GI, et al. The development of USP botanical dietary supplement monographs, 1995-2005. J Nat Prod 2006;69:464–472.
104. Nahrstedt A, Butterweck V. Lessons learned from herbal medicinal products: the example of St. John's wort. J Nat Prod 2010;73:1015–1021.
105. Arlt VM, Stiborova M, Schmieser HH. Aristolochic acid as a probable human cancer hazard in herbal remedies: a review. Mutagenesis 2002;17: 265–277.
106. Madabushi R, Frank B, Drewelow B, et al. Hyperforin in St. John's wort drug interactions. Eur J Clin Pharmacol 2006;62:225–233.
107. Chen ST, Dou J, Temple R, et al. New therapies from old medicines. Nat Biotechnol 2008;26:1077–1083.

Chapter 2

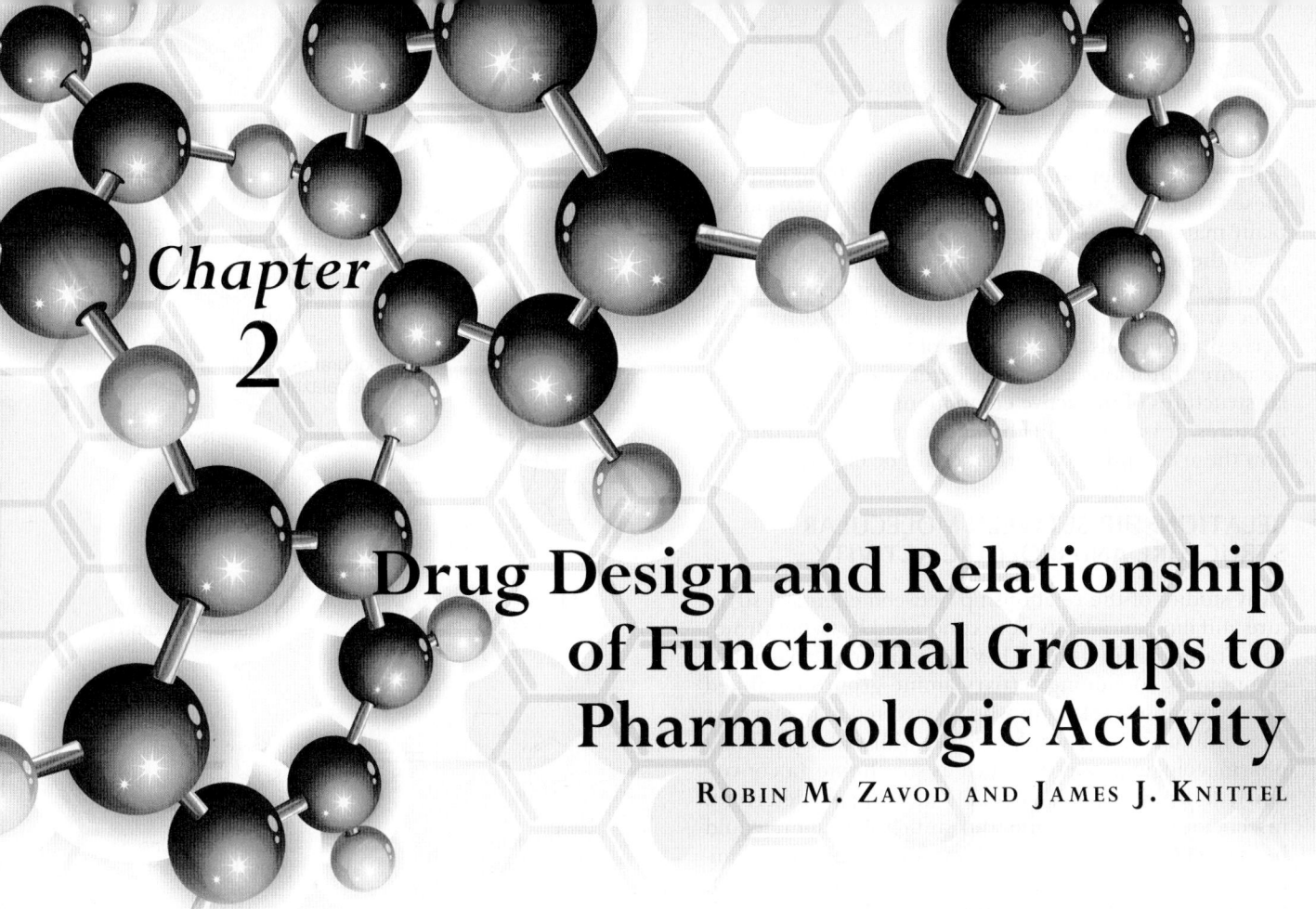

Drug Design and Relationship of Functional Groups to Pharmacologic Activity

ROBIN M. ZAVOD AND JAMES J. KNITTEL

Abbreviations

HCl, hydrochloric acid
IV, intravenous
MW, molecular weight
NaOH, sodium hydroxide
PABA, *p*-aminobenzoic acid
QSAR, quantitative structure–activity relationship
SAR, structure–activity relationship
USP, U.S. Pharmacopeia

Medicinal chemistry is an interdisciplinary science at the intersection of organic chemistry, biochemistry (bioorganic chemistry), computational chemistry, pharmacology, pharmacognosy, molecular biology, and physical chemistry. This branch of chemistry is involved with the identification, design, synthesis, and development of new drugs that are safe and suitable for therapeutic use in humans and pets. It also includes the study of marketed drugs, their biologic properties, and their quantitative structure–activity relationships (QSARs).

Medicinal chemistry studies how chemical structure influences biologic activity. As such, it is necessary to understand not only the mechanism by which a drug exerts its effect, but also how the molecular and physicochemical properties of the molecule influence the drug's pharmacokinetics (absorption, distribution, metabolism, toxicity, and elimination) and pharmacodynamics (what the drug does to the body). The term "physicochemical properties" refers to how the functional groups present within a molecule influence its acid–base properties, water solubility, partition coefficient, crystal structure, stereochemistry, and ability to interact with biologic systems, such as enzyme active sites (Chapter 8) and receptor sites (Chapter 3). To design better medicinal agents, the relative contribution that each functional group (i.e., pharmacophore) makes to the overall physicochemical properties of the molecule must be evaluated. Studies of this type involve modification of the molecule in a systematic fashion followed by a determination of how these changes affect biologic activity. Such studies are referred to as structure–activity relationships (SARs)—that is, the relationship of how structural features of the molecule contribute to, or take away from, the desired biologic activity.

Because of the foundational nature of the content of this chapter, there are numerous case studies presented throughout the chapter (as boxes), as well as at the end. In addition, a list of study questions at the conclusion of—and unique to—this chapter provides further self-study material related to the subject of medicinal chemistry/drug design.

INTRODUCTION

Chemical compounds, usually derived from plants and other natural sources, have been used by humans for thousands of years to alleviate pain, diarrhea, infection, and various other maladies. Until the 19th century, these "remedies" were primarily crude preparations of plant material of unknown constitution. The revolution in synthetic organic chemistry during the 19th century produced a concerted effort toward identification of the structures of the active constituents of these naturally derived medicinals and synthesis of what were hoped to be more efficacious agents. By determining the molecular structures of the active components of these complex mixtures, it was thought that a better understanding of how these components worked could be elucidated.

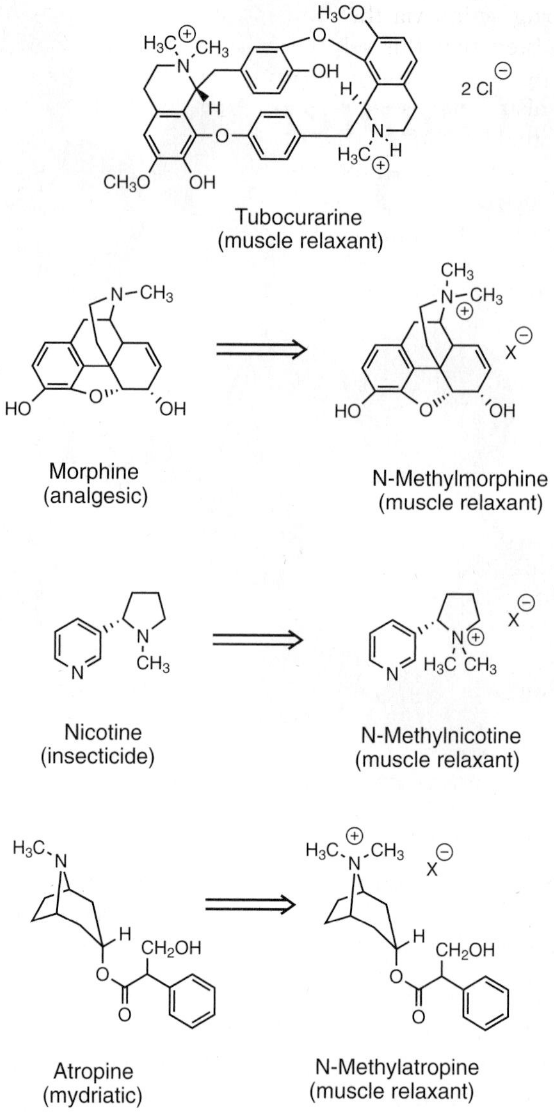

FIGURE 2.1 Effects of methylation on biologic activity.

RELATIONSHIP BETWEEN MOLECULAR STRUCTURE AND BIOLOGIC ACTIVITY

Early studies of the relationship between chemical structure and biologic activity were conducted by Crum-Brown and Fraser (1) in 1869. They demonstrated that many compounds containing tertiary amine groups exhibited activity as muscle relaxants when converted to quaternary ammonium compounds. Molecules with widely differing pharmacologic properties, such as strychnine (a convulsant), morphine (an analgesic), nicotine (a deterrent, insecticide), and atropine (an anticholinergic), could be converted to muscle relaxants with properties similar to those of tubocurarine when methylated (Fig. 2.1). Crum-Brown and Fraser therefore concluded that muscle relaxant activity required the presence of a quaternary ammonium group within the structure. This initial hypothesis was later disproven by the discovery of the natural neurotransmitter and activator of muscle contraction, acetylcholine (Fig. 2.2). Even though Crum-Brown and Fraser's initial hypothesis that related chemical structure with action as a muscle relaxant was incorrect, it demonstrated the concept that molecular structure influences the biologic activity of chemical entities and that alterations in structure produce changes in biologic action.

With the discovery by Crum-Brown and Fraser that quaternary ammonium groups could produce molecules with muscle relaxant properties, scientists began to look for other functional groups that produce specific biologic responses. At this time, it was thought that specific chemical groups, or nuclei (rings), were responsible for specific biologic effects. This led to the postulate, that took some time to disprove, that "one chemical group gives one biological action" (2). Even after the discovery of acetylcholine by Loewi and Navrati (3), which effectively dispensed with Crum-Brown and Fraser's concept of all quaternary ammonium compounds being muscle relaxants, this was still considered to be dogma and took a long time to refute.

SELECTIVITY OF DRUG ACTION AND DRUG RECEPTORS

Although the structures of many drugs or xenobiotics, or at least their functional group composition, were known at the start of the 20th century, how these compounds exerted their effects was still a mystery. Using his observations with regard to the staining behavior of microorganisms, Ehrlich (4) developed the concept of drug receptors. He postulated that certain "side chains" on the surfaces of cells were "complementary" to the dyes (or drug) and suggested that the two could therefore interact with one another. In the case of antimicrobial compounds, interaction of the chemical with the cell surface "side chains" produced a toxic effect. This concept was the first description of what later became known as the receptor hypothesis for explaining the biologic action of chemical entities. Ehrlich also discussed selectivity

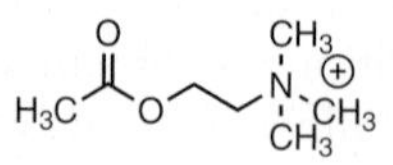

FIGURE 2.2 Acetylcholine, a neurotransmitter and muscle relaxant.

of drug action via the concept of a "magic bullet." He suggested that this selectivity permitted eradication of disease states without significant harm coming to the organism being treated (i.e., the patient). This was later modified by Albert (5) and today is referred to as "selective toxicity." An example of poor selectivity was demonstrated when Ehrlich developed organic arsenicals that were toxic to trypanosomes as a result of their irreversible reaction with thiol groups (-SH) on vital proteins. The formation of As–S bonds resulted in death to the target organism. Unfortunately these compounds were toxic not only to the target organism, but also to the host once certain blood levels of arsenic were achieved.

The "paradox" that resulted after the discovery of acetylcholine—how one chemical group can produce two different biologic effects (i.e., muscle relaxation and muscle contraction)—was explained by Ing (6) using the actions of acetylcholine and tubocurarine as his examples (see also Chapter 9). Ing hypothesized that both acetylcholine and tubocurarine act at the same receptor, but that one molecule fits to the receptor in a more complementary manner and "activates" it, causing muscle contraction. (Ing did not elaborate just how this activation occurred.) The blocking effect of the larger molecule, tubocurarine, could be explained by its occupation of part of the receptor, thereby preventing acetylcholine, the smaller molecule, from interacting with the receptor. With both molecules, the quaternary ammonium functional group is a common structural feature and interacts with the same region of the receptor. If one closely examines the structures of other molecules with opposing effects on the same pharmacologic system, this appears to be a common theme: Molecules that block the effects of natural neurotransmitters, such as norepinephrine, histamine, dopamine, or serotonin for example are called antagonists and, are usually larger in size than the native compound, which is not the case for antagonists of peptide neurotransmitters and hormones such as cholecystokinin, melanocortin, or substance P. Antagonists to these peptide molecules are usually smaller in size. However, regardless of the type of neurotransmitter (biogenic amine or peptide), both agonists and antagonists share common structural features with the neurotransmitter that they influence. This provides support to the concept that the structure of a molecule, its composition and arrangement of functional groups, determines the type of pharmacologic effect that it possesses (i.e., SAR). For example, compounds that are muscle relaxants that act via the cholinergic nervous system possess a quaternary ammonium or protonated tertiary ammonium group and are larger than acetylcholine (compare acetylcholine in Fig. 2.2 with tubocurarine in Fig. 2.1).

SARs are the underlying principle of medicinal chemistry. Similar molecules exert similar biologic actions in a qualitative sense. A corollary to this is that structural elements (functional groups) within a molecule most often contribute in an additive manner to the physicochemical properties of a molecule and, therefore, to its biologic action. One need only peruse the structures of drug molecules in a particular pharmacologic class to become convinced (e.g., histamine H_1 antagonists, histamine H_2 antagonists, β-adrenergic antagonists). In the quest for better medicinal agents (drugs), it must be determined which functional groups within a specific structure are important for its pharmacologic activity and how these groups can be modified to produce more potent, more selective, and safer compounds.

An example of how different functional groups can yield chemical entities with similar physicochemical properties is demonstrated by the sulfanilamide antibiotics. In Figure 2.3, the structures of sulfanilamide and *p*-aminobenzoic acid (PABA) are shown. In 1940, Woods (7) demonstrated that PABA reverses the antibacterial action of sulfanilamide (and other sulfonamide-based antibacterials) and that both PABA and sulfanilamide have similar steric and electronic properties. Both molecules contain acidic functional groups, with PABA containing an aromatic carboxylic acid and sulfanilamide an aromatic sulfonamide. When ionized at physiologic pH, both compounds have a similar electronic configuration, and the distance between the ionized acid and the weakly basic amino group is also very similar. It should be no surprise that sulfanilamide acts as an antagonist to PABA metabolism in bacteria.

Biologic Targets for Drug Action

In order for drug molecules to exhibit their pharmacologic activity, they must interact with a biologic target, typically a receptor, enzyme, nucleic acid, or excitable membrane or other biopolymer. These interactions occur between the functional groups found in the drug molecule and those found within each biologic target. The relative fit of each drug molecule with its target is a function of a number of physicochemical properties including acid–base chemistry and related ionization, functional group shape and size, and three-dimensional spatial orientation. The quality of this "fit" has a direct impact on the biologic response produced. In this chapter, functional group characteristics are discussed as a means to better understand overall drug molecule absorption, distribution, metabolism, and excretion, as well as potential interaction with a biologic target.

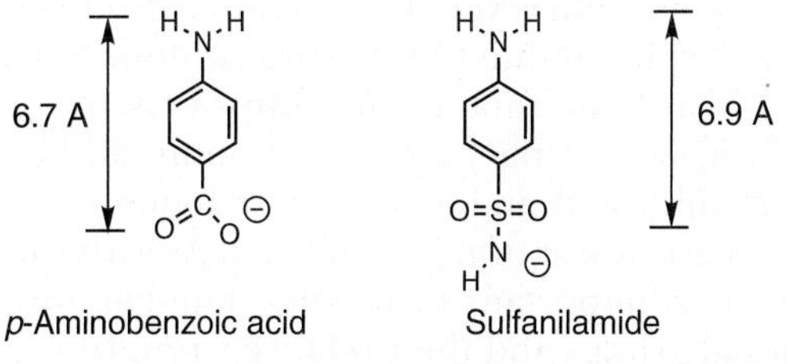

FIGURE 2.3 Ionized forms of *p*-aminobenzoic acid (PABA) and sulfanilamide, with comparison of the distance between amine and ionized acids of each compound. Note how closely sulfanilamide resembles PABA.

PHYSICOCHEMICAL PROPERTIES OF DRUGS

Acid–Base Properties

The human body is 70 to 75% water, which amounts to approximately 51 to 55 L of water for a 160-lb (73-kg) individual. For an average drug molecule with a molecular weight of 200 g/mol and a dose of 20 mg, this leads to a solution concentration of approximately 2×10^{-6} M (2 μM). When considering the solution behavior of a drug within the body, we are dealing with a dilute solution, for which the Brönsted-Lowry (8) acid–base theory is most appropriate to explain and predict acid–base behavior. This is a very important concept in medicinal chemistry, because the acid–base properties of drug molecules have a direct effect on absorption, excretion, and compatibility with other drugs in solution. According to the Brönsted-Lowry Theory, an "acid" is any substance capable of yielding a proton (H^+), and a "base" is any substance capable of accepting a proton. When an acid gives up a proton to a base, it is converted to its "conjugate base." Similarly, when a base accepts a proton, it is converted to its "conjugate acid" (Eqs. 2.1 and 2.2):

Eq. 2.1

$$CH_3COOH + H_2O \rightleftharpoons CH_3COO^{\ominus} + H_3O^{\oplus}$$

Acid (acetic acid)	Base (water)	Conjugate Base (acetate)	Conjugate Acid (hydronium ion)

Eq. 2.2

$$CH_3NH_2 + H_2O \rightleftharpoons CH_3NH_3^{\oplus} + {}^{\ominus}OH$$

Base (methylamine)	Acid (water)	Conjugate Acid (methylammionium ion)	Conjugate Base (hydroxide ion)

Note that when an acidic functional group loses its proton (often referred to as having undergone "dissociation"), it is left with an extra electron and becomes negatively charged. This is the "ionized" form of the acid. The ability of the ionized functional group to participate in an ion-dipole interaction with water (see the Water Solubility of Drugs section) enhances its water solubility. Many functional groups behave as acids (Table 2.1). The ability to recognize these functional groups and their relative acid strengths helps to predict absorption, distribution, excretion, and potential incompatibilities between drugs.

When a basic functional group is converted to the corresponding conjugate acid, it too becomes ionized. In this instance, however, the functional group becomes positively charged due to the extra proton. Most drugs that contain basic functional groups contain primary, secondary, and tertiary amines or imino amines, such as guanidines and amidines. Other functional groups that are basic are shown in Table 2.2. As with the acidic groups, it is important to become familiar with these functional groups and their relative strengths.

Functional groups that cannot give up or accept a proton are considered to be "neutral" (or "nonelectrolytes") with respect to their acid–base properties. Common neutral functional groups are shown in Table 2.3. Quaternary ammonium compounds are neither acidic nor basic and are not electrically neutral. Additional information about the acid–base properties of the functional groups listed in Tables 2.1 through 2.3 can be found in Gennaro (9) and Lemke (10). Review of functional groups and their acid–base properties can also be found at www.duq.edu/pharmacy/faculty/harrold/basic-concepts-in-medicinal-chemistry.cfm.

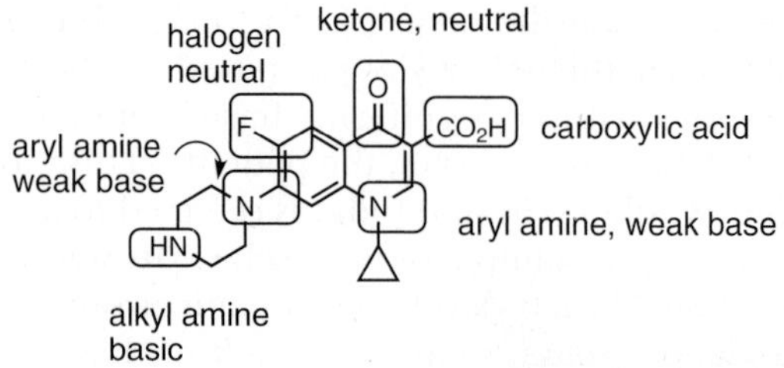

FIGURE 2.4 Chemical structure of ciprofloxacin showing the various organic functional groups.

A molecule can contain multiple functional groups with acid–base properties and, therefore, can possess both acidic and basic character. For example, ciprofloxacin (Fig. 2.4), a fluoroquinolone antibacterial agent, contains a secondary alkylamine, two tertiary arylamines (aniline-like amines), and a carboxylic acid. The two arylamines are weakly basic and, therefore, do not contribute significantly to the acid–base properties of ciprofloxacin under physiologic conditions. Depending on the pH of the physiologic environment, this molecule will either accept a proton (secondary alkylamine), donate a proton (carboxylic acid), or both. Thus, it is described as amphoteric (both acidic and basic) in nature. Figure 2.5 shows the acid–base behavior of ciprofloxacin in two different environments. Note that at a given pH (e.g., pH 1.0 to 3.5), only one of the functional groups (the alkylamine) is significantly ionized. To be able to make this prediction, an appreciation for the relative acid–base strength of both the acidic and basic functional groups is required. Thus, one needs to know which acidic or basic functional group within a molecule containing multiple functional groups is the strongest and which acidic or basic functional group is the weakest. The concept of pK_a not only describes relative acid–base strength of functional groups,

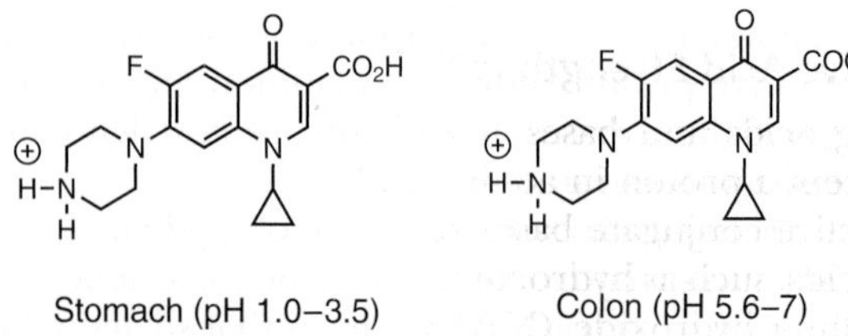

FIGURE 2.5 Predominate forms of ciprofloxacin at two different locations within the gastrointestinal tract.

TABLE 2.1 Common Acidic Organic Functional Groups and Their Ionized (Conjugate Base) Forms

Acids (pKa)			Conjugate Base
Phenol (9-11)	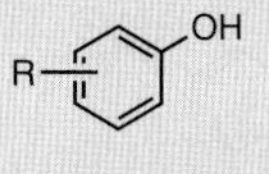	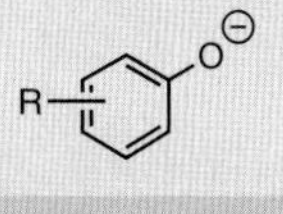	Phenolate
Sulfonamide (9-10)	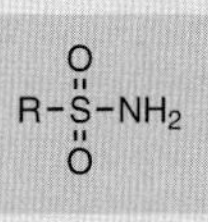	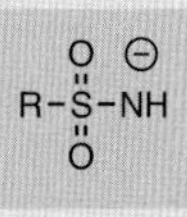	Sulfonamidate
Imide (9-10)	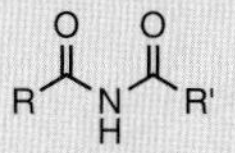	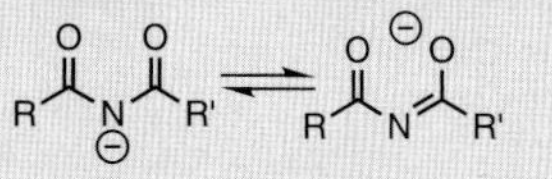	Imidate
Alkylthiol (10-11)	R–SH	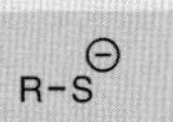	Thiolate
Thiophenol (9-10)	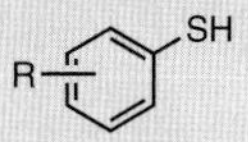	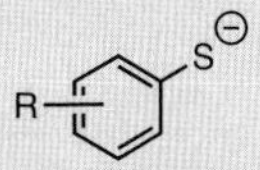	Thiophenolate
N-Arylsulfonamide (6-7)	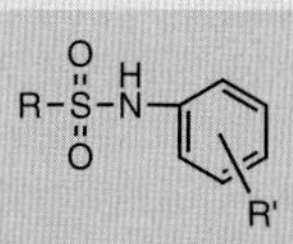	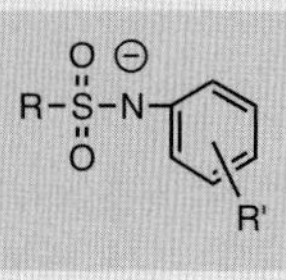	N-Arylsulfonamidate
Sulfonimide (5-6)	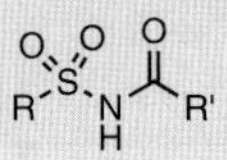	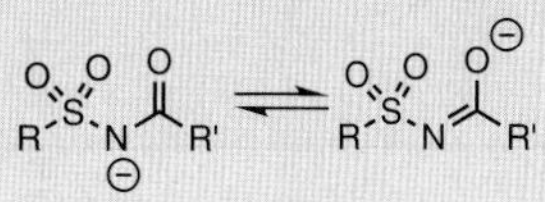	Sulfonimidate
Alkylcarboxylic acid (5-6)	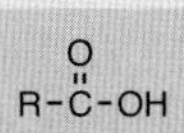	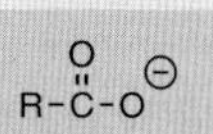	Alkylcarboxylate
Arylcarboxylic acid (4-5)	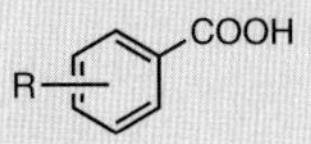	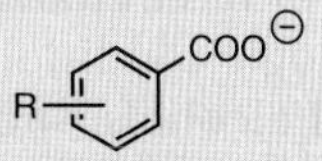	Arylcarboxylate
Sulfonic acid (0-1)	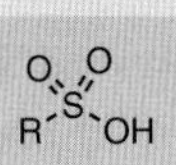	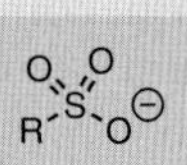	Sulfonate

Acid strength increases as one moves down the table.

but also allows one to calculate, for a given pH, the relative percentages of the ionized and un-ionized forms of the drug. As stated earlier, this helps to predict relative water solubility, absorption, and excretion for a given compound.

Relative Acid Strength (pK_a)

Strong acids and bases completely donate (dissociate) or accept a proton in aqueous solution to produce their respective conjugate bases and acids. For example, mineral acids, such as hydrochloric acid (HCl), or bases, such as sodium hydroxide (NaOH), undergo 100% dissociation in water, with the equilibrium between the ionized and un-ionized forms shifted completely to the right (ionized), as shown in Equations 2.3 and 2.4:

Eq. 2.3 $$HCl + H_2O \rightleftharpoons Cl^{\ominus} + H_3O^{\oplus}$$

Eq. 2.4 $$NaOH + H_2O \rightleftharpoons Na^{\oplus} + OH^{\ominus} + H_2O$$

Acids and bases of intermediate or weak strength, however, incompletely donate (dissociate) or accept a proton, and the equilibrium between the ionized and un-ionized forms lies somewhere in the middle, such that all possible species can exist at any given time. Note that in Equations 2.3 and 2.4, water acts as a base in one instance and as an acid in the other. Water is therefore *amphoteric*—that is, it can act as an acid or a base, depending on the prevailing pH of the solution. From a physiologic perspective, drug molecules are always present as a dilute aqueous solution. The strongest base

TABLE 2.2 Common Basic Organic Functional Groups and Their Ionized (Conjugate Acid) Forms

Base (pKa)			Conjugate Acid
Arylamine (9-11)	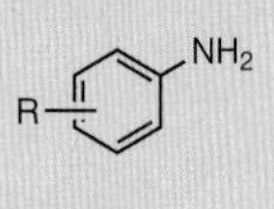	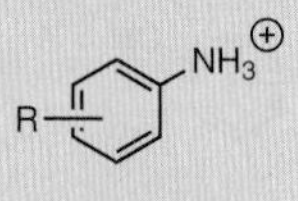	Arylammonium
Aromatic amine (5-6)	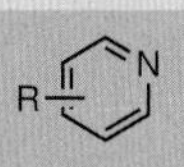	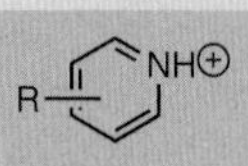	Aromatic ammonium
Imine (3-4)	R-C(H)=NH	R-C(H)=NH ⊕	Iminium
Alkylamines (2° - 10-11) (1° - 9-10)	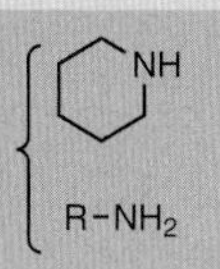	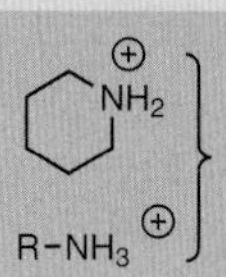	Alkylammonium
Amidine (10-11)	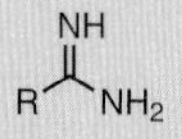	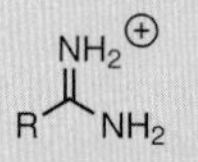	Amidinium
Guanidine (12-13)	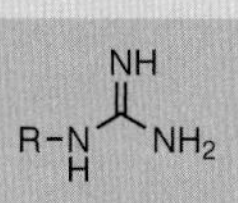	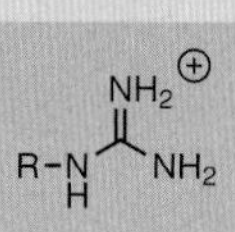	Guanidinium

that is present is OH^-, and the strongest acid is H_3O^+. This is known as the "leveling effect" of water. Thus, some functional groups that have acidic or basic character do not behave as such under physiologic conditions in aqueous solution. For example, alkyl alcohols, such as ethyl alcohol, are not sufficiently acidic to become significantly ionized in an aqueous solution at a physiologically pH. Water is not sufficiently basic to remove the proton from ethyl alcohol to form the ethoxide ion (Eq. 2.5). Therefore, under physiologic conditions, alcohols are neutral with respect to acid–base properties:

Eq. 2.5 $$CH_3CH_2OH + H_2 \not\rightleftharpoons CH_3CH_2O^- + H_3O^{\oplus}$$

Predicting the Degree of Ionization of a Molecule

By knowing if there are acidic and/or basic functional groups present in a molecule, one can predict

TABLE 2.3 Common Organic Functional Groups That are Considered Neutral Under Physiologic Conditions

$R\text{–}CH_2\text{–}OH$	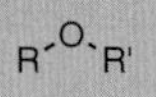	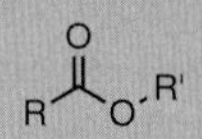	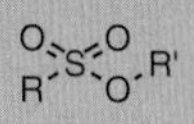
Alkyl alcohol	Ether	Ester	Sulfonic acid ester
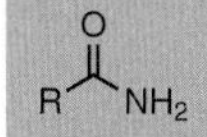	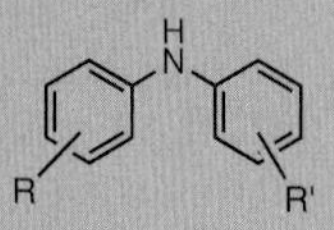	R–C≡N	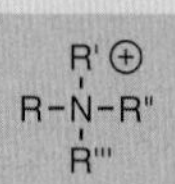
Amide	Diarylamine	Nitrile	Quaternary ammonium
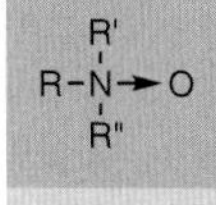	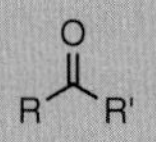	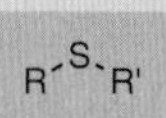	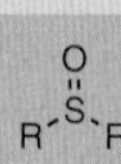 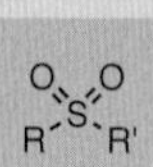
Amine oxide	Ketone & Aldehyde	Thioether	Sulfoxide Sulfone

whether a molecule is going to be predominantly ionized or un-ionized at a given pH. To be able to quantitatively predict the degree of ionization of a molecule, the pK_a values of each of the acidic and basic functional groups present and the pH of the environment in which the molecule will be located must be known. The magnitude of the pK_a value is a measure of relative acid or base strength, and the Henderson-Hasselbalch equation (Eq. 2.6) can be used to calculate the percent ionization of a compound at a given pH (this equation was used to calculate the major forms of ciprofloxacin in Fig. 2.5):

Eq. 2.6
$$pK_a = pH + \log \frac{[\text{acid form}]}{[\text{base form}]}$$

The key to understanding the use of the Henderson-Hasselbalch equation for calculating percent ionization is to realize that this equation relates a constant, pK_a, to the ratio of the acidic form of a functional group to its conjugate base form (and conversely, the conjugate acid form to its base). Because pK_a is a constant for any given functional group, the ratio of acid to conjugate base (or conjugate acid to base) will determine the pH of the solution. A sample calculation is shown in Figure 2.6 for the sedative hypnotic amobarbital.

When dealing with a basic functional group, one must recognize the conjugate acid represents the ionized form of the functional group. Figure 2.7 shows the calculated percent ionization for the decongestant phenylpropanolamine. It is very important to understand that for a base, the pK_a refers to the conjugate acid or ionized form of the compound. To thoroughly comprehend this relationship, calculate the percent ionization of an acidic functional group and a basic functional group at different pH values and carefully observe the trend.

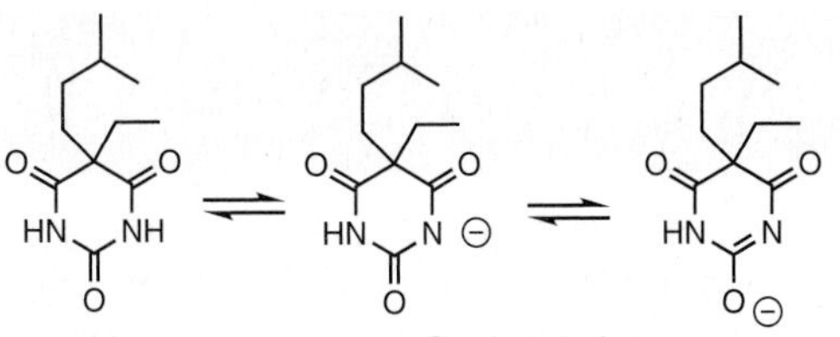

Acid form
pK_a 8.0

Conjugate base

Question: At a pH of 7.4, what is the percent ionization of amobarbital?

Answer:
$$8.0 = 7.4 + \log \frac{[\text{acid}]}{[\text{base}]}$$
$$0.6 = \log \frac{[\text{acid}]}{[\text{base}]}$$
$$10^{0.6} = \frac{[\text{acid}]}{[\text{base}]} = \frac{3.98}{1}$$
$$\%\ \text{acid form} = \frac{3.98 \times 100}{4.98} = 79.9\%$$

FIGURE 2.6 Calculation of percent ionization of amobarbital. Calculation indicates that 80% of the molecules are in the acid (or protonated) form, leaving 20% in the conjugate base (ionized) form.

Water Solubility of Drugs

The solubility of a drug molecule in water greatly affects the routes of administration that are available, as well as its absorption, distribution, and elimination. Two key concepts to keep in mind when considering the water (or fat) solubility of a molecule are the potential for hydrogen bond formation and ionization of one or more functional groups within the molecule.

Hydrogen Bonds

Each functional group capable of donating or accepting a hydrogen bond contributes to the overall water solubility of the compound and increases the hydrophilic (water-loving) nature of the molecule. Conversely, functional groups that cannot form hydrogen bonds do not enhance hydrophilicity and will contribute to the hydrophobic (water-fearing) nature of the molecule. Hydrogen bonds are a special case of what are usually referred to as dipole–dipole interactions. A permanent dipole occurs as a result of an unequal sharing of electrons between the two atoms within a covalent bond. This unequal sharing of electrons only occurs when these two atoms have significantly different electronegativities. When a permanent dipole is present, a partial charge is associated

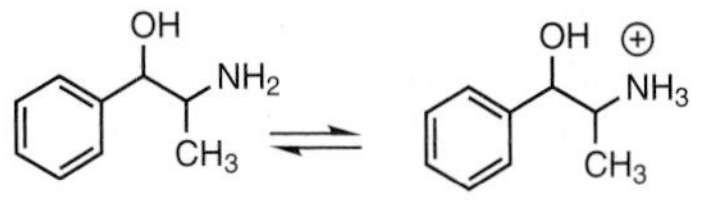

Base form

Conjugate acid form
pK_a 9.4

Question: What is the % ionization of phenylpropanolamine at pH 7.4?

Answer:
$$9.4 = 7.4 + \log \frac{[\text{acid}]}{[\text{base}]}$$
$$2.0 = \log \frac{[\text{acid}]}{[\text{base}]}$$
$$10^{2} = \frac{[\text{acid}]}{[\text{base}]} = \frac{100}{1}$$
$$\%\ \text{ionization} = \frac{100 \times 100}{101} = 99\%$$

FIGURE 2.7 Calculation of percent ionization of phenylpropanolamine. Calculation indicates that 99% of the molecules are in the acid form, which is the same as the percent ionization.

ABSORPTION/ACID–BASE CASE

A long-distance truck driver comes into the pharmacy complaining of seasonal allergies. He asks you to recommend an agent that will act as an antihistamine but that will not cause drowsiness. He regularly takes TUMS for indigestion due to the bad food that he eats while on the road.

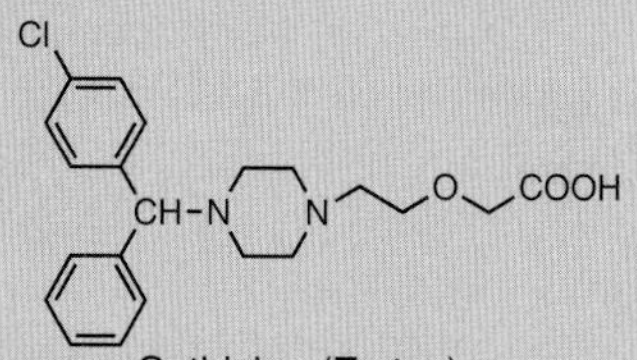

Cetirizine (Zyrtec)

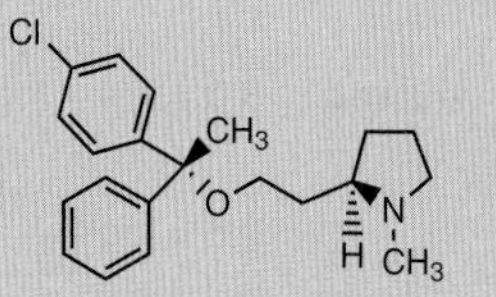

Clemastine (Tavist)

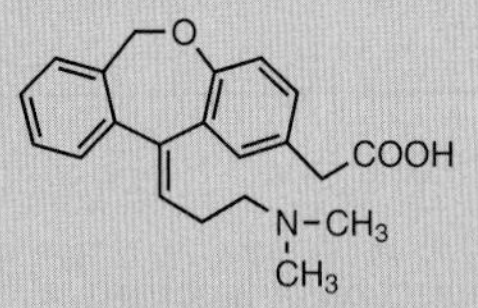

Olopatadine (Patanol)

1. Identify the functional groups present in Zyrtec and Tavist, and evaluate the effect of each functional group on the ability of the drug to cross lipophilic membranes (e.g., blood–brain barrier). Based on your assessment of each agent's ability to cross the blood–brain barrier (and, therefore, potentially cause drowsiness), provide a rationale for whether the truck driver should be taking Zyrtec or Tavist.
2. Patanol is sold as an aqueous solution of the hydrochloride salt. Modify the structure present in the box to show the appropriate salt form of this agent. This agent is applied to the eye to relieve itching associated with allergies. Describe why this agent is soluble in water and what properties make it able to be absorbed into the membranes that surround the eye.
3. Consider the structural features of Zyrtec and Tavist. In which compartment (stomach [pH 1] or intestine [pH 6 to 7]) will each of these two drugs be best absorbed?
4. TUMS neutralizes stomach acid to pH 3.5. Based on your answer to question 3, determine whether the truck driver will get the full antihistaminergic effect if he takes his antihistamine at the same time that he takes his TUMS. Provide a rationale for your answer.

ACID–BASE CHEMISTRY/COMPATIBILITY CASES

The intravenous (IV) technician in the hospital pharmacy gets an order for a patient that includes the two drugs drawn below. She is unsure if she can mix the two drugs together in the same IV bag and is not certain how water soluble the agents are.

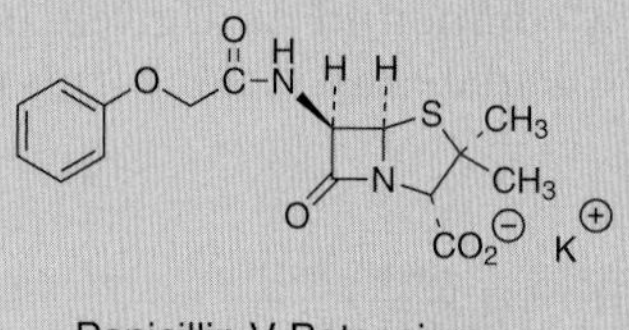

Penicillin V Potassium

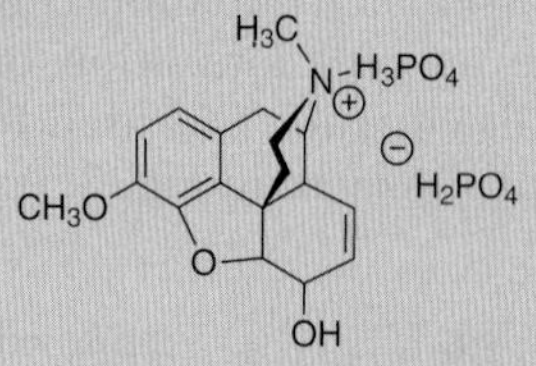

Codine phosphate

1. Penicillin V potassium is drawn in its salt form, whereas codeine phosphate is not. Modify the structure above to show the salt form of codeine phosphate. Determine the acid–base character of the functional groups in the two molecules drawn above as well as the salt form of codeine phosphate.
2. As originally drawn above, which of these two agents is more water soluble? Provide a rationale for your selection that includes appropriate structural properties. Is the salt form of codeine phosphate more or less water soluble than the free base form of the drug? Provide a rationale for your answer based on the structural properties of the salt form of codeine phosphate.
3. What is the chemical consequence of mixing aqueous solutions of each drug in the same IV bag? Provide a rationale that includes an acid–base assessment.

with each of these atoms along a single bond (one atom has a partial negative charge, and one atom has a partial positive charge). The atom with a partial negative charge has higher electron density than the other atom. When two functional groups that contain one or more permanent dipoles approach one another, they align such that the negative end of one dipole is electrostatically attracted to the positive end of the other. When the positive end of the dipole is a hydrogen atom, this interaction is referred to as a "hydrogen bond" (or H-bond). Thus, for a hydrogen bonding interaction to occur, at least one functional group must contain a dipole with an electropositive hydrogen. The hydrogen atom must be covalently bound to an electronegative atom, such as oxygen (O), nitrogen (N), sulfur (S), or selenium (Se). Of these four elements, only oxygen and nitrogen atoms contribute significantly to the dipole, and we will therefore concern ourselves only with the hydrogen-bonding capability (specifically as hydrogen bond donors) of functional groups that contain a bond between oxygen and hydrogen atoms (e.g., alcohols) and functional groups that contain a bond between nitrogen and hydrogen atoms (e.g., primary and secondary amines and amides) (e.g., NH and CONH groups).

Even though the energy associated with each hydrogen bond is small (1 to 10 kcal/mol/bond), it is the additive nature of multiple hydrogen bonds that contributes to the overall water solubility of a given drug molecule. This type of interaction is also important in the interaction between a drug and its biologic target (e.g., receptor). Figure 2.8 shows several types of hydrogen bonding interactions that can occur with a couple of functional groups and water. As a general rule, the more hydrogen

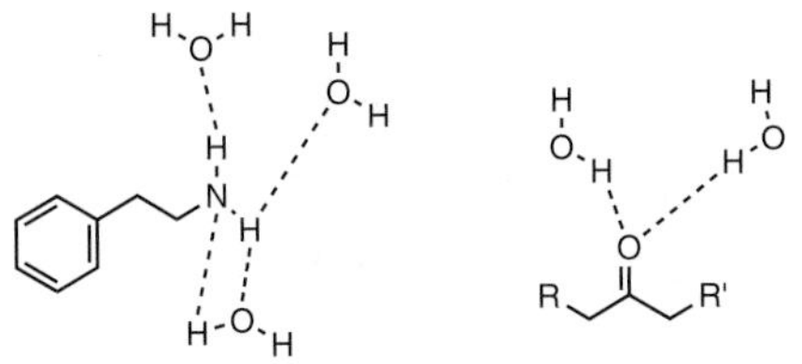

FIGURE 2.8 Examples of hydrogen bonding between water and hypothetical drug molecules.

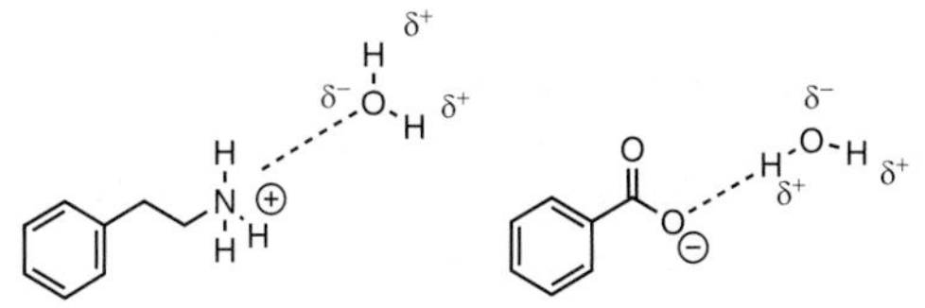

FIGURE 2.9 Examples of ion–dipole interactions.

bonds that are possible between a drug molecule and water, the greater the water solubility of the molecule. Table 2.4 lists several common functional groups and the number of hydrogen bonds in which they can potentially participate. Note that this table does not take into account the possibility of intramolecular hydrogen bond formation. Each intramolecular hydrogen bond decreases water solubility (and increases lipid solubility) because there is one less interaction possible with water.

Ionization

In addition to the hydrogen-bonding capacity of a molecule, another type of interaction plays an important role in determining water solubility: the ion–dipole interaction. This type of interaction can occur with organic salts. Ion–dipole interactions occur between either a cation and the partially negatively charged atom found in a permanent dipole (e.g., the oxygen atom in water) or an anion and the partially positively charged atom found in a permanent dipole (e.g., the hydrogen atoms in water) (Fig. 2.9).

Organic salts are composed of a drug molecule in its ionized form and an oppositely charged counterion. For example, the salt of a carboxylic acid is composed of the carboxylate anion (ionized form of the functional group) and a positively charged ion (e.g., Na^+) and the salt of a secondary amine is composed of the ammonium cation (ionized form of the functional group and a negatively charged ion; e.g., Cl^-). Not all organic salts are very water soluble. To associate with enough water molecules to become soluble, the salt must be highly dissociable; in other words, the cation and anion must be able to separate and interact independently with water molecules. Highly dissociable salts are those formed from strong acids with strong bases (e.g., sodium chloride), weak acids with strong bases (e.g., sodium phenobarbital), or strong acids with weak bases (e.g., atropine sulfate). Examples of strong acids (strong acids are 100% ionized in water [i.e., no ionization constants or pK_a values of <1]) include the hydrohalic (hydrochloric, hydrobromic, and hydrofluoric), sulfuric, nitric, and perchloric acids. All other acids (e.g., phosphoric, tartaric, acetic, and other organic acids, and phenols) are partially ionized with pK_a values from 1 to 14 and are, therefore, considered to be moderate or weak acids. Hydroxides of sodium, potassium, and

ABSORPTION/BINDING INTERACTIONS CASE

A 24-year-old man comes into the pharmacy and asks you to recommend a treatment for the itching and burning he has recently noticed on both feet. He indicates that he would prefer a cream rather than a spray or a powder. Your recommendation to this patient is to use Lamisil (terbinafine), a very effective topical antifungal agent that is sold over the counter.

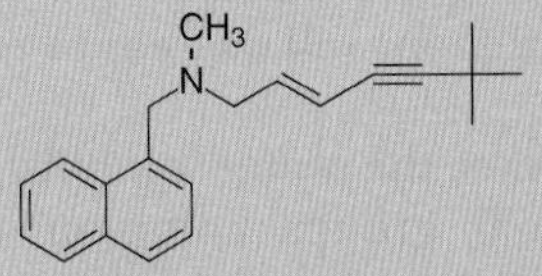

Terbinafine (Lamisil)

1. Identify the structural characteristics and the corresponding properties that make terbinafine an agent that can be used topically.
2. The biologic target of drug action for terbinafine is squalene epoxidase. Consider each of the structural features of this antifungal agent and describe the type of interactions that the drug will have with the target for drug action. Which amino acids are likely to be present in the active site of this enzyme?

TABLE 2.4 Common Organic Functional Groups and Their Hydrogen-Bonding Potential

Functional Groups	Number of Potential H-bonds
R–OH	3
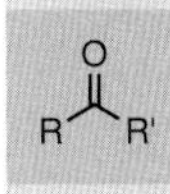	2
$R–NH_2$	3
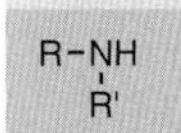	2
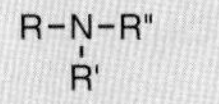	1
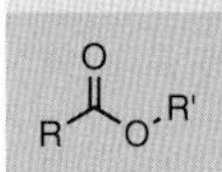	2

calcium are strong bases because they are 100% ionized, whereas other bases, such as amines, are of moderate or weak strength. The salt formed by a carboxylic acid with an alkylamine is the salt of a weak acid and weak base, respectively. This salt does not dissociate appreciably and cannot significantly contribute to the overall water solubility of a given drug molecule. In general, low molecular weight salts are water soluble, and high molecular weight salts are water insoluble. Examples of common organic salts used in pharmaceutical preparations are provided in Figure 2.10.

The extent to which ionized molecules are soluble in water is also dependent on the presence of intramolecular ionic interactions. Molecules with ionizable functional groups of opposite charges have the potential to interact with each other rather than with water molecules. When this occurs, these molecules often become water insoluble. A classic example is the amino acid tyrosine (Fig. 2.11). Tyrosine contains three very polar functional groups, two of which are ionizable (the alkylamine and carboxylic acid) depending on the pH of the environment.

The phenolic hydroxyl group is also ionizable (pK_a 9 to 10); however, it does not contribute significantly to the ionization of tyrosine under pharmaceutically or physiologically relevant conditions (<1% ionized at pH 7). Because of the presence of three very polar functional groups (two of them being ionizable), one would expect tyrosine to be very soluble in water, yet its solubility is only 0.45 g/1,000 mL. The basic alkylamine (pK_a 9.1 for the conjugate acid) and the carboxylic acid (pK_a 2.2) are both ionized at physiologic pH, and a zwitterionic molecule results. These two charged groups are sufficiently close that a strong ion–ion interaction occurs, thereby keeping each group from participating in ion–dipole interactions with surrounding water molecules. This lack of interaction between the ions and the dipoles found in water results in a molecule that is very water insoluble (Fig. 2.12). Not all zwitterions or multiply charged molecules demonstrate this behavior; only those that contain ionized functional groups close enough for an ionic interaction to occur will be poorly soluble. Generally, the greater the separation between charges, the more highly water soluble one anticipates the molecule will be. This is only true, however, up to a certain number of carbon atoms. This will be discussed in more detail later.

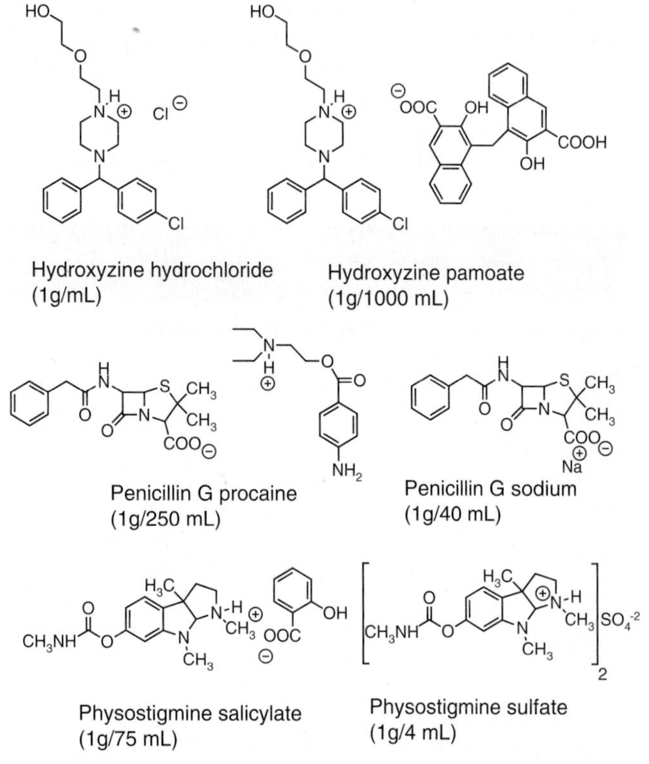

FIGURE 2.10 Water solubilities of different salt forms of selective drugs.

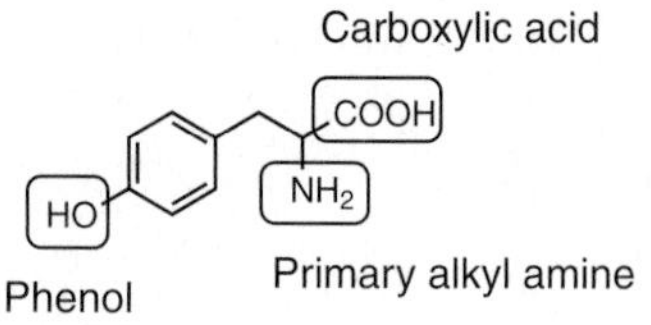

FIGURE 2.11 Organic functional groups in tyrosine (see text for pK_a values).

Predicting Water Solubility: The Empirical Approach

Lemke (10) developed an empiric approach to predicting the water solubility of molecules based on the carbon-solubilizing potential of several functional groups. In his approach, if the solubilizing potential of the functional groups exceeds the total number of carbon atoms present, then the molecule is considered to be water soluble. Otherwise, it is considered to be water insoluble. Participation in intramolecular hydrogen bonding or ionic interactions decreases the solubilizing potential of a given functional group. It is difficult to quantitate how much such interactions will decrease a molecule's overall water solubility.

Table 2.5 shows the water-solubilizing potential for several functional groups common to many drugs. Because most drug molecules contain more than one functional group (i.e., are polyfunctional), the second column in the table will be of more utility. To demonstrate Lemke's method, consider the structure of anileridine. Anileridine (Fig. 2.13) is an opioid analgesic that contains three functional groups that contribute to water

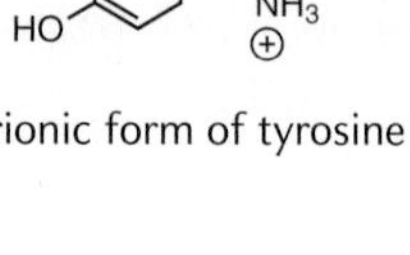

FIGURE 2.12 Zwitterionic form of tyrosine showing ion–ion bond.

BINDING INTERACTIONS CASE

Each of these drug molecules interacts with a different biologic target and elicits a unique pharmacologic response. For each of the three molecules, list the types of interactions that are possible with a biologic target. For each type of interaction, provide one example of an amino acid that could participate in that interaction.

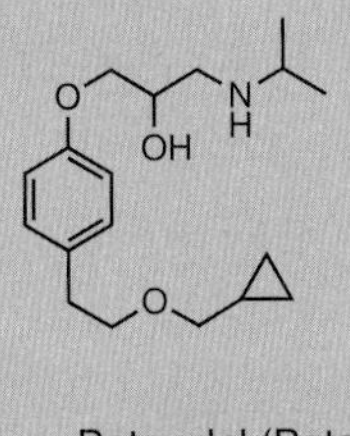

Betaxolol (Betoptic)

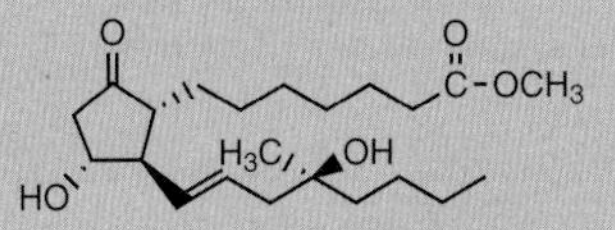

Misoprostol (Cytotec)

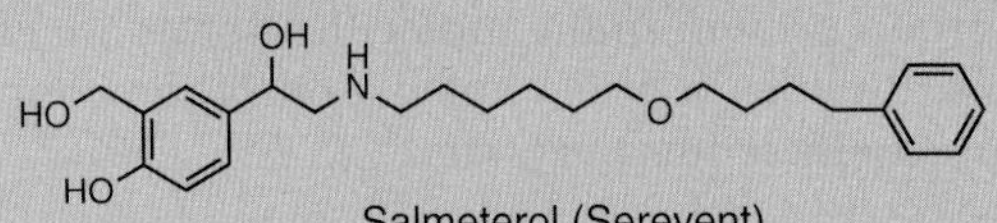

Salmeterol (Serevent)

Example: Binding interaction: Van der Waals
Amino acid: Leucine

WATER/LIPID SOLUBILITY CASE

When you look at any drug molecule, there are a number of functional groups present that contribute to the properties of that drug molecule. Identify the types of functional groups in each molecule and to which physical properties (water/lipid solubility) each contributes.

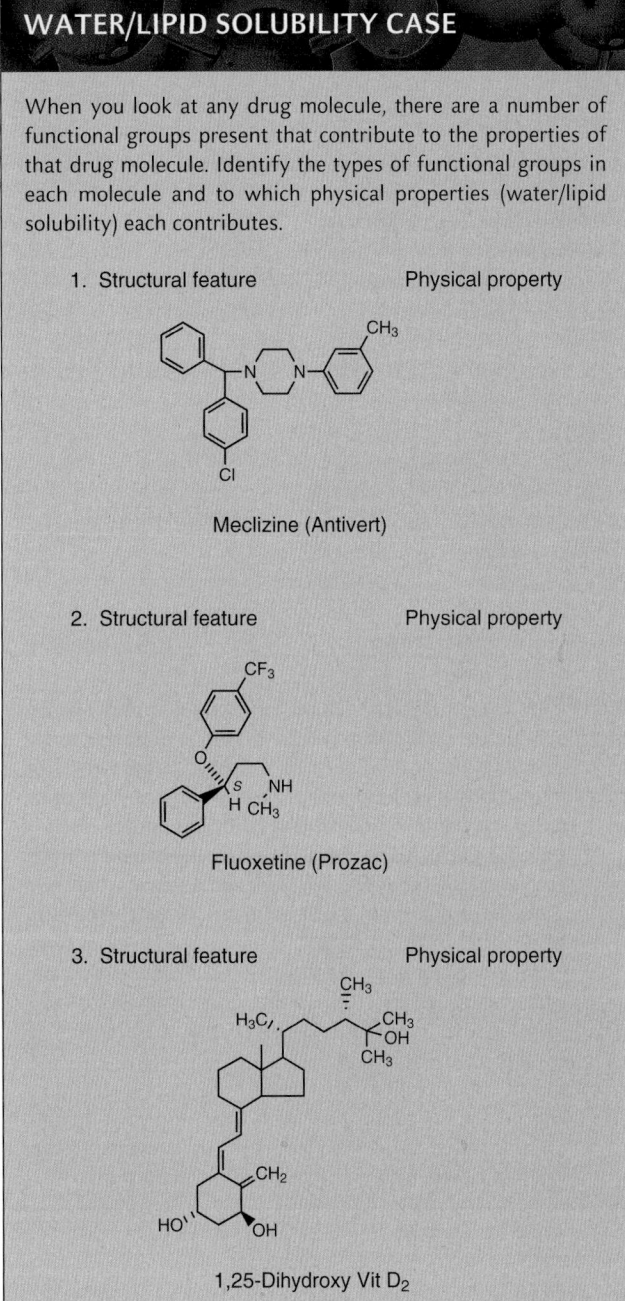

1. Structural feature — Physical property

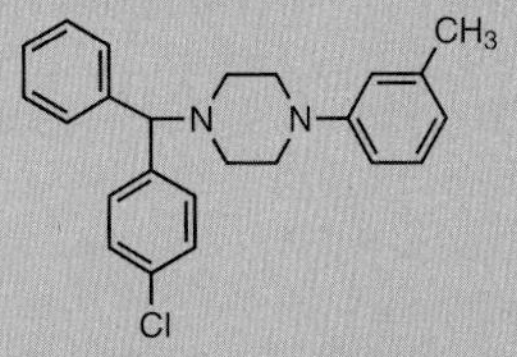

Meclizine (Antivert)

2. Structural feature — Physical property

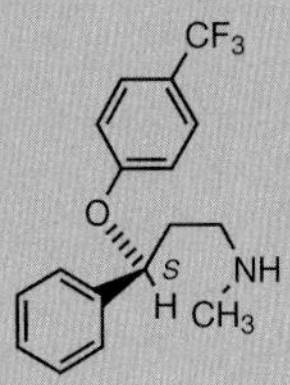

Fluoxetine (Prozac)

3. Structural feature — Physical property

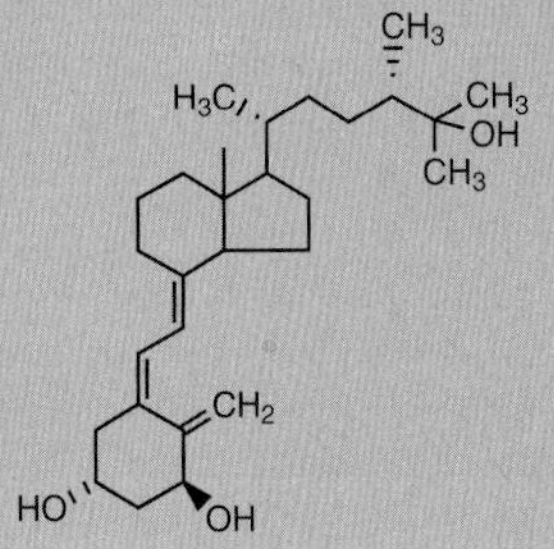

1,25-Dihydroxy Vit D_2

solubility: an aromatic amine (very weak base), a tertiary alkylamine (weak base), and an ester (neutral). There are a total of 21 carbon atoms in the molecule and a solubilizing potential from the three functional groups of nine carbon atoms. Since the solubilizing potential of the functional groups is less than the total number of carbons that are present, it is predicted that anileridine is insoluble in water. This is, indeed, the case: The solubility of anileridine is reported in the U.S. Pharmacopeia (USP) as 1 g/10,000 mL, or 0.01%. Now consider the

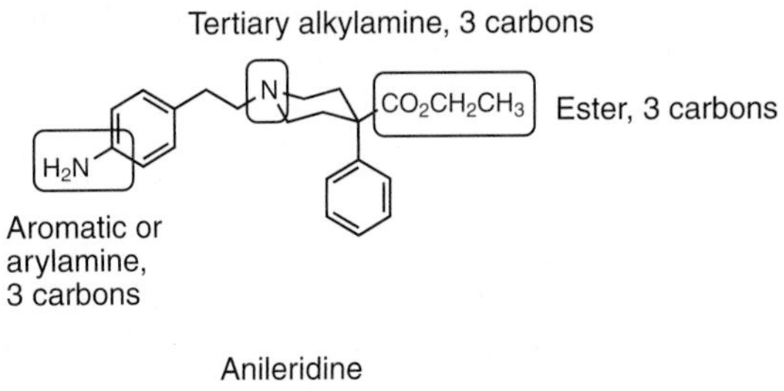

FIGURE 2.13 Identification of functional groups in anileridine.

hydrochloride salt of anileridine. Not only do the three functional groups contribute a solubilizing potential of nine carbon atoms, the positive charge of the alkylammonium contributes also to its water solubility. Lemke (10) estimates that each ionized functional group (cationic or anionic) found within a drug molecule contributes a solubilizing potential of 20 to 30 carbon atoms. Thus, the solubilizing potential for all of the functional groups in anileridine hydrochloride is 29 to 39 carbon atoms, which is more than the total number of carbon atoms in the molecule. This salt should therefore be soluble in water, and it is (to the extent of 0.2 g/mL, or 20%).

INTERACTIONS/SOLUBILITY CASE

J.K. presents a prescription for her 6-month-old daughter for Donatussin Drops. She wants to know if this medication will have an effect on her daughter's alertness.

Components of Donatussin:
Phenylephrine (decongestant)
Chlorpheniramine (antihistamine)
Guaifenesin (expectorant)

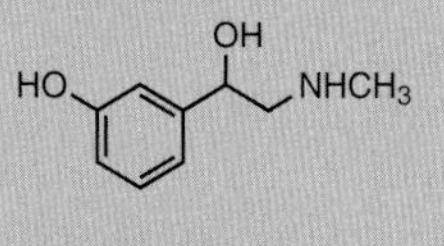

Phenylephrine

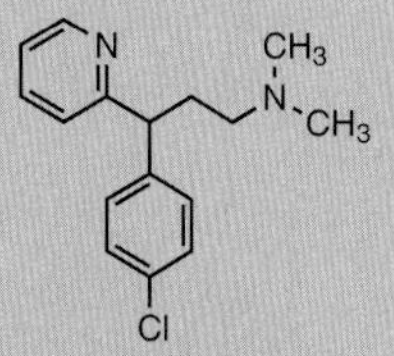

Chlorpheniramine

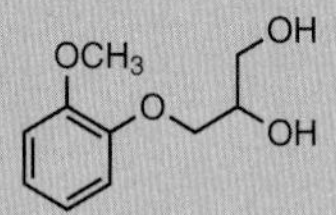

Guaifenesin

1. Identify the structural features/functional groups of phenylephrine and guaifenesin that contribute to improved water solubility (medication given as drops). List the type(s) of interactions that these groups have with water, and draw an example of these interactions (with appropriate labels).
2. Evaluate each of the three molecules, and determine if each molecule contains any functional groups that will allow the drug to cross the blood–brain barrier and have an effect on this child's alertness (create a list of relevant functional groups for each molecule). Based on your evaluation, which agent is likely to have the most significant effect? Identify what property is necessary for these agents to cross this biologic membrane.
3. Identify the binding interactions that chlorpheniramine and guaifenesin could have with their respective targets for drug action. Be sure to identify which functional groups will participate in each of these binding interactions.

Problem 6, found at the end of the chapter, provides an additional opportunity to use this approach to predict water solubility. Solubility data for these drug molecules can be found in the USP. In most instances, discrepancies between approximate and actual water solubilities can be rationalized by careful inspection of the chemical structure.

Predicting Water Solubility: Analytical/Quantitative Approach

Another method for predicting water solubility involves calculation of an approximate logP, or log of the partition coefficient for a molecule. This approach is based on an approximation method developed by Cates (11) and discussed in Lemke (10). In this approach, one sums

TABLE 2.5 Water-solubilizing Potential of Organic Functional Groups in a Mono- or Polyfunctional Molecule

Functional Group	Monofunction Molecule	Polyfunctional Molecule
Alcohol	5 to 6 carbons	3 to 4 carbons
Phenol	6 to 7 carbons	3 to 4 carbons
Ether	4 to 5 carbons	2 carbons
Aldehyde	4 to 5 carbons	2 carbons
Ketone	5 to 6 carbons	2 carbons
Amine	6 to 7 carbons	3 carbons
Carboxylic acid	5 to 6 carbons	3 carbons
Ester	6 carbons	3 carbons
Amide	6 carbons	2 to 3 carbons
Urea, carbonate, carbamate		2 carbons

Water solubility is defined as greater than 1% solubility (9).

the hydrophobic or hydrophilic properties of each functional group present in the molecule. Before we can calculate logP values, a brief explanation of the concept of partition coefficient is necessary.

Eq. 2.7 $$P = C_{oct}/C_{water}$$

In its simplest form, the partition coefficient, P, refers to the ratio of drug concentration in octanol (C_{oct}) to that in water (C_{water}) (Eq. 2.7). Octanol is used to mimic the amphiphilic nature of lipid, because it has a polar head group (primary alcohol) and a long hydrocarbon chain, or tail, similar to the fatty acid tail that makes up part of a lipid membrane. Because P is logarithmically related to free energy (12), P is generally expressed as logP and is, therefore, the sum of the hydrophobic and hydrophilic characteristics of the functional groups that make up the structure of the molecule. Thus, logP is a measure of the lipid/water solubility characteristics of the entire molecule. Because each functional group contained within the molecule contributes to the overall hydrophilic/hydrophobic character of the molecule, a hydrophilic/hydrophobic value (the hydrophobic substituent constant, π) can be assigned to each functional group. Equation 2.8 defines this relationship:

Eq. 2.8 $$\text{LogP} = \Sigma\pi \text{ (fragments)}$$

When calculating logP from hydrophobic substituent constants, the sum is usually referred to as logP_{calc} or ClogP [for software sources to calculate ClogP, see (16)] to distinguish it from an experimentally determined value (MlogP or logP_{meas}). Over the years, extensive tables of π values have been compiled for organic functional groups and molecular fragments (12–15). Table 2.6 is a highly abbreviated summary of π values from Lemke (10), based largely on the manuscript by Cates (11). Using the values in this table, a fairly reasonable estimate for the water solubility of many organic compounds (shown as logP) can be determined.

Again we will consider the structure of the opioid analgesic anileridine to demonstrate the calculation of logP (Fig. 2.13). This compound has a total of 22 carbon atoms, some aliphatic and some aromatic. We need to distinguish between the aliphatic and aromatic carbon atoms because the delocalized π orbitals for the sp^2 hybridized aromatic carbon atoms make them more polar than aliphatic carbons. The compound also contains one tertiary alkylamine, one aromatic or aryl amine, and one ester. Evaluation of esters and amides requires that the oxygen, nitrogen, and ester/amide carbon atoms are counted in this π value. The remaining aliphatic carbons are then counted. Figure 2.14 summarizes the logP calculation for anileridine. The calculation gives a ClogP value for anileridine of +4.8. Water solubility as defined by the USP is solubility greater than 3.3%, which equates to an approximate logP of +0.5. LogP values less than +0.5 are therefore considered to be water soluble, and those greater than +0.5 are considered to be water insoluble. According to our calculation, anileridine would be predicted to be insoluble in water. This calculation agrees with the more empiric procedure discussed earlier.

Other sample calculations are shown in Figure 2.15, and several problems are provided at the end of this chapter. In Figure 2.15, MlogP values (when available) and ClogP values (16) are included for comparison purposes (see Appendix A for additional ClogP values). Even though the π values from Table 2.6 are not as extensive as those in the computer program, there is good general agreement with most of these compounds with respect to their solubility (or insolubility) in water. In addition, other programs besides ClogP are available to predict logP values; some of these programs are available on the Internet. One must keep in mind that due to the assumptions made in these programs, they cannot produce results that are in total agreement with measured values or other prediction programs. ClogP values calculated from ACDLogP (16) are generally more accurate. Other programs for calculating logP values, such as Molinspiration (17) and Interactive Analysis (18), use different methods and assumptions and, therefore, do not always agree with ClogP predictions or experimentally determined values. This is not to say that the latter two programs do not give accurate results. Often, one or all of the programs will have reasonable agreement with measured values, but greater disagreement tends to occur as the number of functional groups in the molecule that participate as hydrogen-bond acceptor and/or hydrogen-bond donor groups increases. This increases the likelihood that intramolecular interactions will occur—something that is not always taken into account with these programs.

TABLE 2.6 Hydrophilic-lipophilic Values (πV) for Organic Fragments (10)

Functional Group	π value (aliphatic)	π value (aromatic)
H		0.00
Alkane	0.50	0.56 (CH_3); 1.02 (CH_2CH_3)
Alkene		0.82
C_6H_5 (phenyl)	2.15	1.96
Br, Cl, F, I	0.60; 0.39; −0.17; 1.00	0.86; 0.71; 0.14; 1.12
NO_2	−0.85	−0.28
NH_2 (primary amine)	−1.19	−1.23
NHR (secondary amine)	−0.67	0.47
NR_2 (tertiary amine)	−0.30	0.18
-NHC=OR (amide)	−0.97	
SC_6H_5	2.32	
OH	−1.12	−0.67
OCH_3		−0.02
-OC=OR (ester)	−0.27	−0.64
CHO (aldehyde)		−0.65
C=OCH_3 (ketone)		−0.55
CO_2H		−0.32
SO_2NH_2 (sulfonamide)		−1.82

The ability to predict the percent ionization or water solubility of a molecule should not be viewed as an exercise in arithmetic, but rather as a way to understand the solution behavior of molecules, especially as it relates to admixtures and the pharmacokinetic differences among molecules. The ionization state of a molecule not only influences its water solubility, but also its ability to traverse

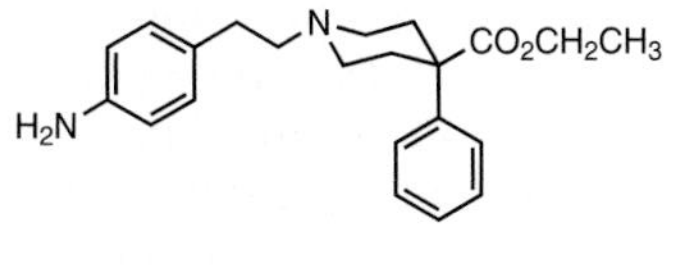

Fragments	π
1 primary alkylamine	-1.23
1 teriary alkylamine	-0.30
9 aliphatic carbons	+4.5
2 phenyl rings	+4.30
1 ester	-0.27
logP	+7.0

FIGURE 2.14 Calculation of logP for anileridine.

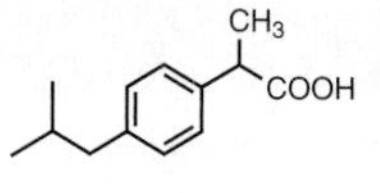

Ibuprofen

Fragments	π
6 carbons	+3.0
1 phenyl	+2.15
1 carboxyl	-0.32
logP	+4.83

MlogP +3.5; ClogP +3.68

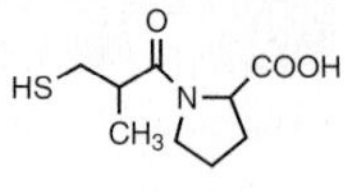

Captopril

Fragments	π
7 carbons	+3.5
1 sulfur	0.0
1 carboxyl	-0.32
1 amide	-0.97
logP	+2.21

ClogP +1.16

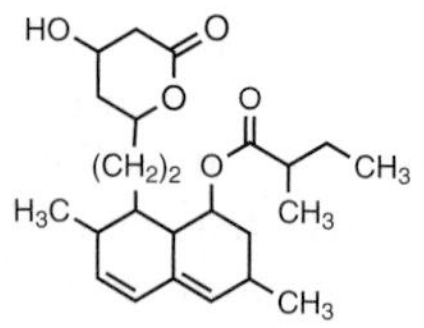

Lovastatin

Fragments	π
22 carbons	+11.0
1 alcohol	-1.12
2 carboxyls	-0.64
logP	+ 9.24

MlogP +4.26; ClogP +4.08

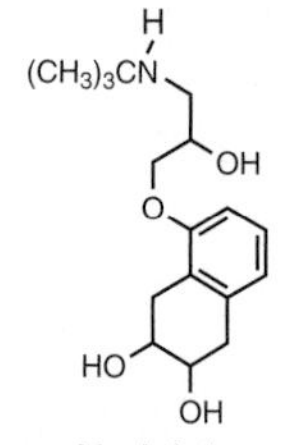

Nadolol

Fragments	π
11 carbons	+5.5
1 phenyl	+2.15
2 IMHB	+1.3
1 secondary amine	-0.67
1 ether	-0.02
3 alcohols	-3.36
logP	+4.90

MlogP +0.71; ClogP +0.23

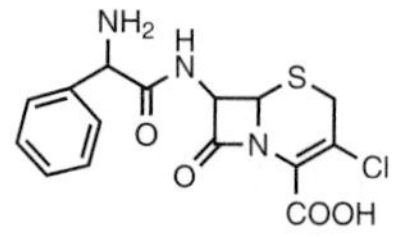

Cefaclor

Fragments	π
6 carbons	+3.0
1 phenyl	+2.15
1 chloride	+0.39
1 primary amine	-1.19
1 sulfur	0.0
2 amides	-1.94
1 carboxyl	-0.32
logP	+2.09

MlogP -1.69; ClogP -1.79

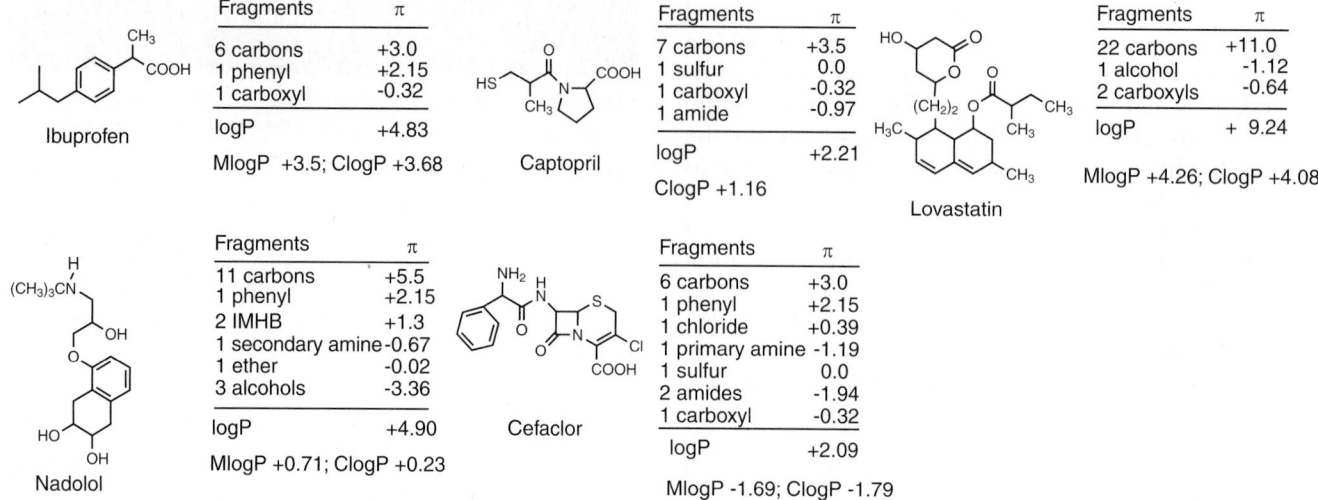

FIGURE 2.15 ClogP calculations for selected compounds.

membranes and, therefore, its ability to be absorbed. The distribution of the drug and its ability to bind to proteins other than its target are also greatly influenced by the ionization state and the hydrophilic/hydrophobic nature of the molecule.

STEREOCHEMISTRY AND DRUG ACTION

Stereoisomers are molecules that contain the same number and kinds of atoms, the same arrangement of bonds, but different three-dimensional structures; in other words, they only differ in the three-dimensional arrangement of atoms in space. There are two types of stereoisomers: enantiomers and diastereoisomers. Enantiomers are pairs of molecules for which the three-dimensional arrangement of atoms represents nonsuperimposable mirror images. Diastereoisomers represent all of the other stereoisomeric compounds that are not enantiomers. Thus, the term "diastereoisomer" includes compounds that contain double bonds (geometric isomers) and ring systems. Unlike enantiomers, diastereoisomers exhibit different physicochemical properties, including, but not limited to, melting point, boiling point, solubility, and chromatographic behavior. These differences in physicochemical properties allow the separation of individual diastereoisomers from mixtures with the use of standard chemical separation techniques, such as column chromatography or crystallization. Enantiomers cannot be separated using such techniques unless a chiral environment is provided or if they are first converted to diastereoisomers (e.g., salt formation with another enantiomer). Examples of enantiomers and diastereoisomers are provided in Figure 2.16.

The physicochemical properties of a drug molecule are dependent not only on what functional groups are present in the molecule but also on the spatial arrangement of these groups. This becomes an especially important factor when the environment that a molecule is in is asymmetric, such as the human body. Proteins and other biologic targets are asymmetric in nature. How a particular drug molecule interacts with these macromolecules is determined by the three-dimensional orientation of the functional groups present. If critical functional groups in the drug molecule do not occupy the proper spatial region, then productive interactions with the biologic target will not be possible. As a result, it is possible that the desired pharmacologic activity will not be achieved. If, however, the functional groups within a drug molecule are located in the proper three-dimensional orientation, then the drug can participate in multiple key interactions with its biologic target. It is important to understand not only which functional groups contribute to the pharmacologic activity of a drug, but also the importance of the three-dimensional nature of these functional groups in predicting drug potency and potential side effects.

Approximately one in every four drugs currently on the market is some type of isomeric mixture. For many of these drugs, the biologic activity can only reside in one isomer (or at least predominate in one isomer). The majority of these isomeric mixtures are termed "racemic mixtures" (or "racemates"). A racemic mixture is comprised of equal amounts of both of the possible drug enantiomers. As mentioned earlier in this chapter, when enantiomers are introduced into an asymmetric, or chiral, environment, such as the human body, they display different physicochemical properties. This can lead to significant differences in their pharmacokinetic and pharmacodynamic behavior, resulting in adverse side effects or toxicity. For example, the individual isomers in a racemic mixture can exhibit significant differences in absorption (especially active transport), serum protein binding, and metabolism. As it relates to drug metabolism, it is certainly possible that only one of the

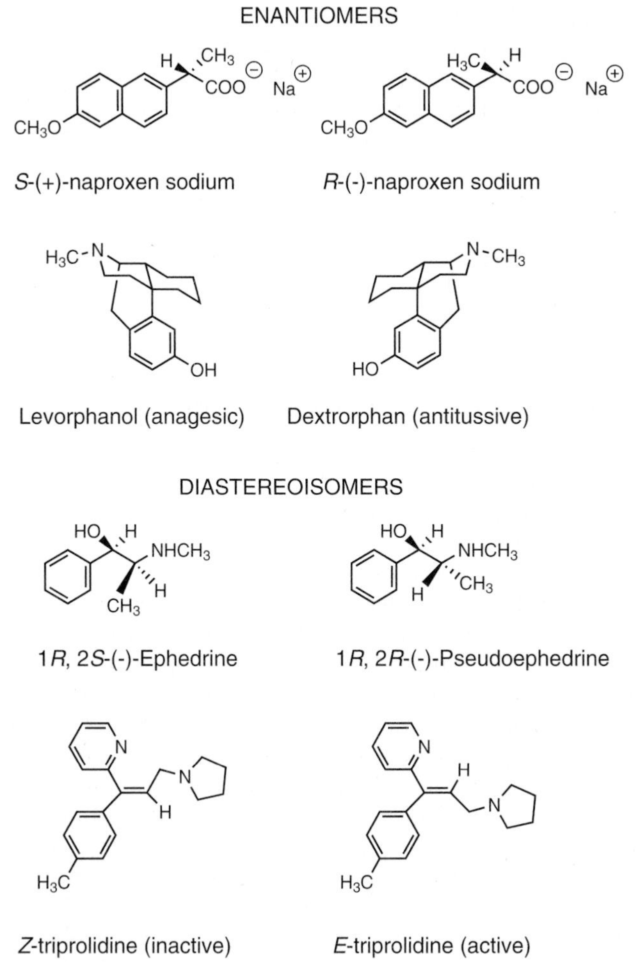

FIGURE 2.16 Examples of stereoisomers.

isomers can be converted into a toxic substance or can influence the metabolism of another drug (Chapter 4). Since stereochemistry can have a profound effect on both the pharmacokinetic and pharmacodynamic properties of a drug, it is important to review the foundational concepts

Stereochemical Definitions

Designation of Absolute Configuration

At first, enantiomers were distinguished by their ability to rotate the plane of polarized light. Isomers that rotate the plane of polarized light to the right, or in a clockwise direction, were designated as dextrorotatory, indicated by a (+)- sign before the chemical name [e.g., (+)-amphetamine or dextroamphetamine]. The opposite designation, levorotatory or (−)-, was assigned to molecules that rotate the plane of polarized light to the left, or in a counterclockwise direction. The letters *d*- and *l*- were formerly used to indicate (+)- and (−)-, respectively. A racemate (racemic mixture)—that is, a 1:1 mixture of enantiomers—is indicated by placement of a (±)- before the compound name. This nomenclature is based on a physical property of the molecule and does not describe the absolute configuration or three-dimensional arrangement of atoms around the chiral center.

In the late 19th century, Fisher and Rosanoff developed a system of nomenclature based on the structure of glyceraldehyde (Fig. 2.17). Since there were no methods at that time to determine the absolute three-dimensional arrangement of atoms in space, the two isomers of glyceraldehyde were arbitrarily assigned the designation of D-(+)- and L-(−). It was not until the 1950s that the absolute configurations of these molecules were determined (Fisher had fortuitously guessed correctly). The configurations of other molecules were then assigned based on their relationship to D- or L-glyceraldehyde via synthetic methods or chemical degradation. Thus, via chemical degradation, it was possible to determine that (+)-glucose, (−)-2–deoxyribose, and (−)-fructose had the same terminal configuration as D-(+)-glyceraldehyde and, therefore, were assigned the D-absolute configuration. Amino acid configurations were assigned based on their relationship to D-(+)- and L-(−)-serine (Fig. 2.17). Unfortunately, this system becomes very cumbersome with molecules that contain more than one chiral center.

QUESTIONS WE CAN NOW ANSWER ABOUT ANY DRUG MOLECULE

Based on your knowledge of acid–base chemistry, from where will this drug primarily be absorbed?
What is the solubility of the drug in the stomach, plasma, or an aqueous IV?
What are the possible interactions that the drug could have with its respective target for drug action?
What is the compatibility of the drug if mixed with other drugs?
How should this drug be delivered? Is it stable in stomach acid?

LEARNING THE LINGO: DRUG MOLECULE EVALUATION

Analysis of Individual Functional Groups:
Name of functional group
Shape of functional group
Hydrophobic vs. hydrophilic character
Polar vs. nonpolar character
Acidic vs. basic (pK_a) character
Binding interactions
Chemical/enzymatic stability

Analysis of the Whole Drug Molecule:
Looking for functional group balance: water solubility and absorption
Ionization issues: effect on solubility and absorption
Drug combinations: acid–base interactions
Drug interactions with biologic target: good fit or not?
Stability and bioavailability: route of administration

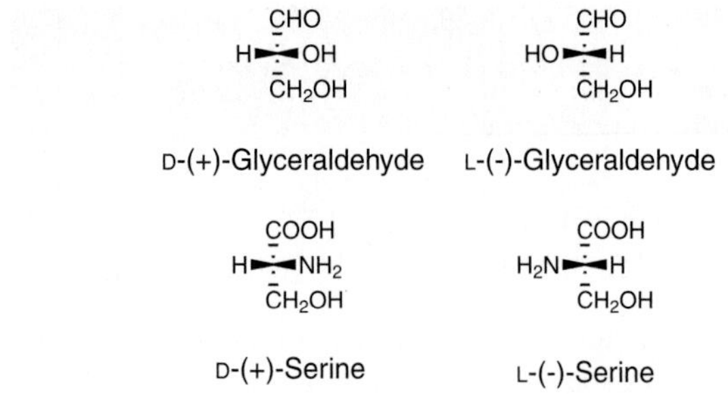

FIGURE 2.17 Relationship of optical isomers of serine to D- and L-glyceraldehyde.

In 1956, a new system of stereochemical nomenclature was introduced by Cahn et al. (19) and is known as the Sequence Rule or CIP system. With this system, atoms attached to a chiral center are ranked based on their atomic number. Highest priority is given to the atom with the highest atomic number, and subsequent atoms are ranked accordingly, from highest to lowest. When a decision cannot be made in the assignment of priority—for example, two atoms with the same atomic number attached to the chiral center—this evaluation extends to the next atom until a priority can be established. When the molecule is then viewed from the side opposite to the lowest-priority atom, the priority sequence from highest to lowest can then be determined. If the priority sequence proceeds to the right, or in a clockwise direction, the chiral center is designated with an *R*-absolute configuration. The designation is *S* when the priority sequence proceeds to the left, or in a counterclockwise direction. An example of this is seen in the neurotransmitter norepinephrine.

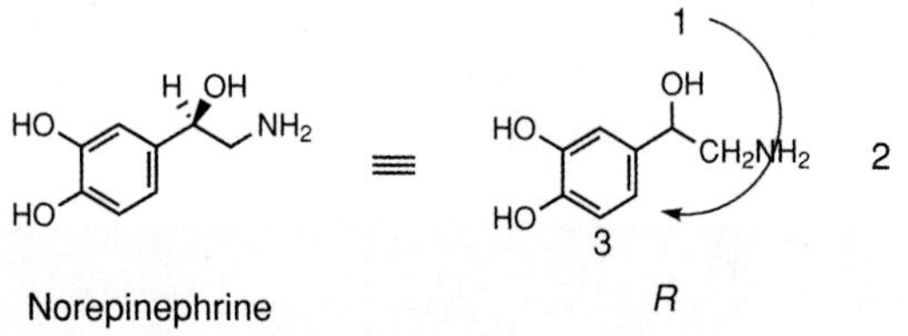

Degradation studies demonstrate that (−)-norepinephrine is related to D-(−)-mandelic acid; therefore, it was given the D-designation using the Fisher system. With the CIP system, norepinephrine is assigned the *R*-absolute configuration.

It should be noted that the CIP nomenclature system uses a set of arbitrary rules and, therefore, should be viewed as a system that tracks absolute configuration only. In many instances, two molecules can have different absolute configurations as designated by the CIP system, but the same relative orientation of the functional groups relevant for biologic activity. An example of this is demonstrated when the absolute configuration of the nonselective β-adrenergic antagonist propranolol is compared to norepinephrine. Because of the presence of the ether oxygen atom, the priority sequence of the functional groups about the chiral center results in the assignment of the *S*-absolute configuration for the more active enantiomer of propranolol. Close inspection of both *R*-norepinephrine and *S*-propranolol, however, shows that the hydroxy group, basic amine, and aromatic rings of both compounds occupy the same regions in three-dimensional space.

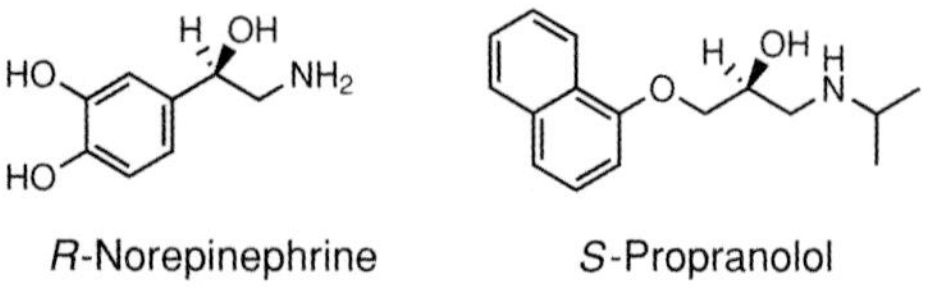

Stereochemistry and Biologic Activity

Easson-Stedman Hypothesis

In 1886, Piutti (20) reported different physiologic actions for the enantiomers of asparagine, with (+)-asparagine having a sweet taste and (−)-asparagine a bland one. This was one of the earliest observations that enantiomers can exhibit differences in biologic action. In 1933, Easson and Stedman (21) reasoned that differences in biologic activity between enantiomers resulted from selective reactivity of one enantiomer with its receptor. They postulated that such interactions require a minimum of a three-point fit to the receptor. This is demonstrated in Figure 2.18 for two hypothetical enantiomers. In Figure 2.18, the letters A, B, and C represent hypothetical functional groups that can interact with complementary sites on the hypothetical receptor surface, represented by A′, B′, and C′. Only

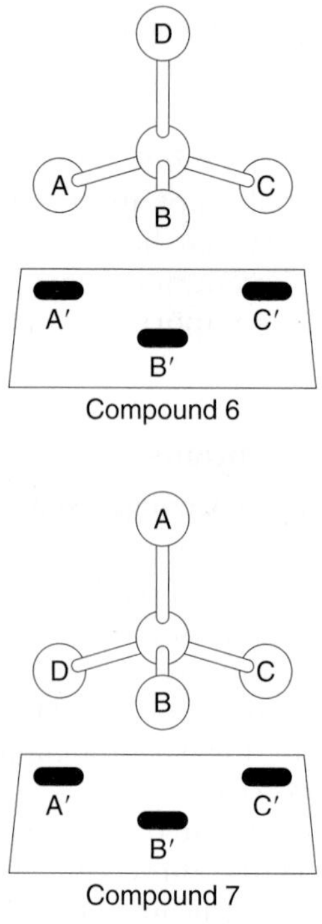

FIGURE 2.18 Optical isomers. Only in compound 6 do the functional groups A, B, and C align with the corresponding sites of binding on the asymmetric surface.

one enantiomer is capable of attaining the correct special orientation to enable all three functional groups to interact with their respective sites on the receptor surface. The inability of the other enantiomer to achieve the same number of interactions with the hypothetical receptor surface explains its reduced biologic activity. The Easson-Stedman Hypothesis states that the more potent enantiomer must be involved in a minimum of three intermolecular interactions with the surface of the biologic target and that the less potent enantiomer only interacts with two sites. This can be illustrated by looking at the differences in vasopressor activity of *R*-(−)-epinephrine, *S*-(+)-epinephrine, and the achiral *N*-methyldopamine (Fig. 2.19). With *R*-(−)-epinephrine, the three points of interaction with the receptor site are the substituted aromatic ring, β-hydroxyl group, and the protonated secondary ammonium group. All three functional groups interact with their complementary sites on the receptor surface, resulting in receptor stimulation (in this case). With *S*-(+)-epinephrine, only two interactions are possible (the protonated secondary ammonium and the substituted aromatic ring). The β-hydroxyl group is located in the wrong place in space and, therefore, cannot interact properly with the receptor. *N*-methyldopamine can achieve the same interactions with the receptor as *S*-(+)-epinephrine; therefore, it is not surprising that its vasopressor response is the same as that of *S*-(+)-epinephrine and less than that of *R*-(−)-epinephrine.

Not all stereoselectivity seen with enantiomers can be attributed to differences in the ability of the drug molecule to interact with its biologic target. Differences in biologic activity can also result from differences in the ability of each enantiomer to reach the biologic target. Because the biologic system encountered by the drug is asymmetric, each enantiomer can experience selective penetration into membranes, metabolism, absorption at sites of loss (e.g., adipose tissue), and/or excretion. Figure 2.20 shows various phases that enantiomers can encounter before reaching the biologic target. An enantiomer cannot encounter stereoselective environments at each of these points; however, enantioselectivity at any

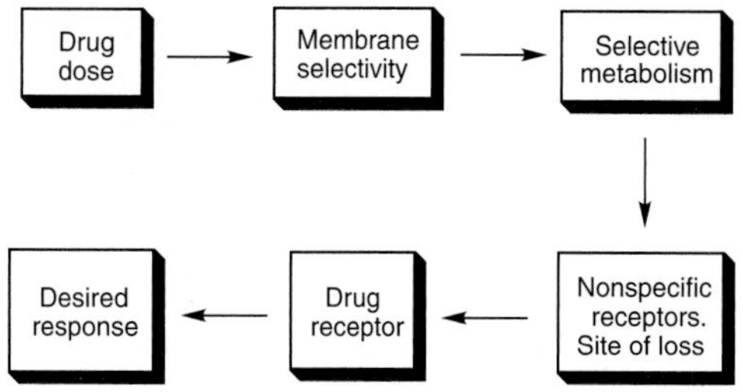

FIGURE 2.20 Selective phases to which optical isomers can be subjected before biologic response.

point can provide enough of an influence to cause one enantiomer to produce a significantly better pharmacologic effect than the other. Conversely, such processes can also contribute to untoward effects of a particular enantiomer. Differences in pharmacologic action among stereoisomers provides an excellent example of how not all pharmacologic effects of a drug are necessarily beneficial to the patient. Although there is no regulatory prohibition on the development of racemic agents, it is reasonable that single enantiomer drugs will become the overwhelming therapeutic choice in the future.

Diastereomers

As mentioned earlier, diastereoisomers are molecules that are nonsuperimposable, non–mirror images. This type of isomer can result from the presence of more than one chiral center in the molecule, double bonds, or ring systems. These isomers have different physicochemical properties, and as a result, it is possible that they can have differences in biologic activity.

Molecules that contain more than one chiral center probably are the most common type of drug-based diastereoisomers. Classic examples are the diastereoisomers ephedrine and pseudoephedrine (Fig. 2.21). When a molecule contains two chiral centers, there can be as

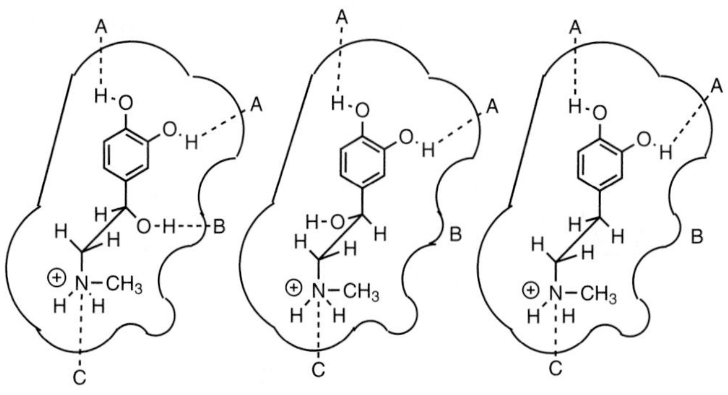

R-(-)-Epinephrine *S*-(+)-Epinephrine *N*-Methyldopamine

FIGURE 2.19 Drug receptor interaction of *R*-(−)-epinephrine, *S*-(+)-epinephrine, and *N*-methyldopamine.

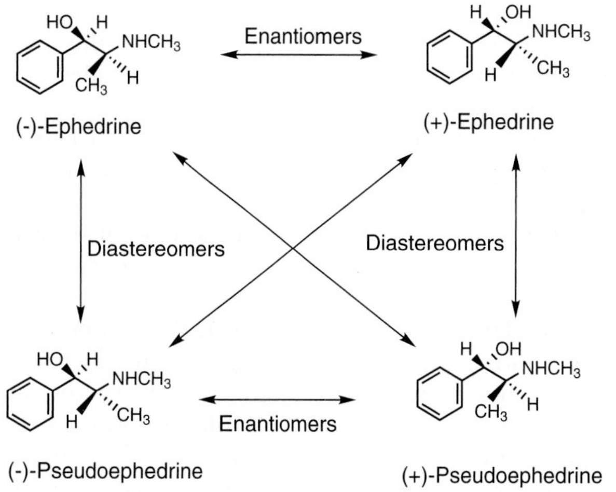

FIGURE 2.21 Relationship between the diastereomers of ephedrine and pseudoephedrine.

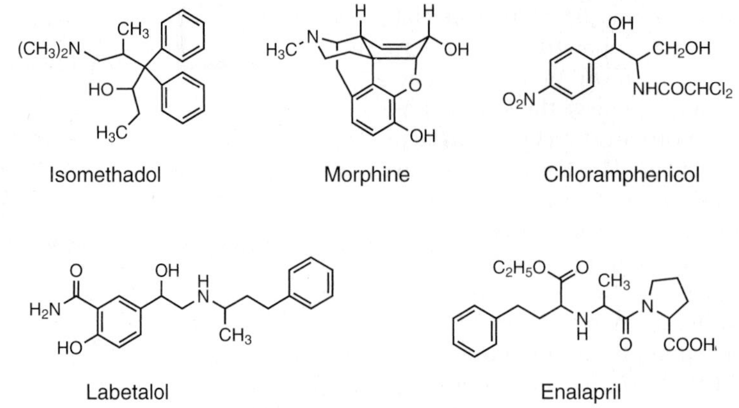

FIGURE 2.22 Examples of chiral drugs with two or more asymmetric centers.

many as four possible stereoisomers consisting of two sets of enantiomeric pairs. When considering an enantiomeric pair of molecules, there is inversion of both chiral centers. In diastereomers, there is inversion of only one chiral center. (Problem 9 at the end of this chapter helps to illustrate this point.) Figure 2.22 shows several examples that contain two or more chiral centers and, therefore, are diastereoisomeric (see Problem 10 at the end of this chapter).

Restricted bond rotation caused by carbon–carbon double bonds (alkenes or olefins) and similar systems, such as imines (C=N), can produce stereoisomers. These are also referred to as geometric isomers, although they more properly are classified as diastereoisomers. In this situation, substituents can be oriented on the same side or on opposite sides of the double bond. The alkene 2-butene is a simple example.

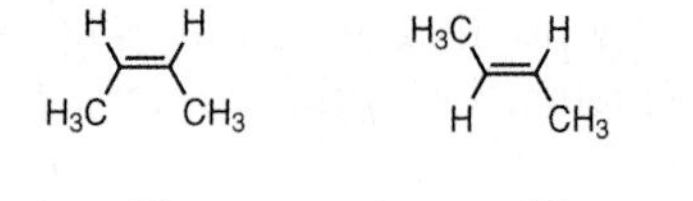

cis or *Z* isomer   *trans* or *E* isomer

With 2-butene, it is readily apparent that the methyl groups can be on the same or on opposite sides of the double bond. When they are on the same side, the molecule is defined as the *cis*- or *Z*-isomer (from the German *zusammen*, meaning "together"); when they are on opposite sides, the designation is *trans*- or *E*- (from the German *entgegen*, meaning "opposite"). With simple compounds, such as 2-butene, it is easy to determine which groups in the molecule are *cis* or *trans* to one another. This becomes more difficult to determine, however, with more complex structures, where it is less obvious which substituents should be referred to when naming the compound. In 1968, Blackwood et al. (22) proposed a system for the assignment of "absolute" configuration with respect to double bonds. Using the CIP sequence rules, each of the two substituents attached to the carbon atoms comprising the double bond are assigned a priority of 1 or 2, depending on the atomic number of the atom attached to the double bond. When two substituents of higher priority are on the same side of the double bond, this isomer is given the designation of *cis* or *Z*. When the substituents are on opposite sides, the designation is *trans* or *E*. The histamine H_1-receptor antagonist triprolidine (Fig. 2.23) is a good example for demonstrating how this nomenclature system works. The *E*-isomer of triprolidine is more active both in vitro and in vivo, indicating that the distance between the pyridine and pyrrolidine rings is critical for binding to the receptor.

Diastereoisomers (as well as enantiomers) can also be found in cyclic molecules. For example, the cyclic alkane 1,2-dimethylcyclohexane can exist as *cis/trans*-diastereoisomers, and the *trans* isomer can also exist as an enantiomeric pair. In Figure 2.24, each of the *trans*-enantiomorphs is depicted in the two possible chair conformations for the cyclohexane ring. Since cyclohexane rings can exhibit significant conformational freedom, this allows for the possibility of conformational isomers. Isomers of this type will be discussed in the next section. When two or more rings share a common bond (e.g., decalin), rotation around the bonds is even more restricted. This prevents ring "flipping" from occurring, and as a result, diastereoisomers and enantiomers are generated.

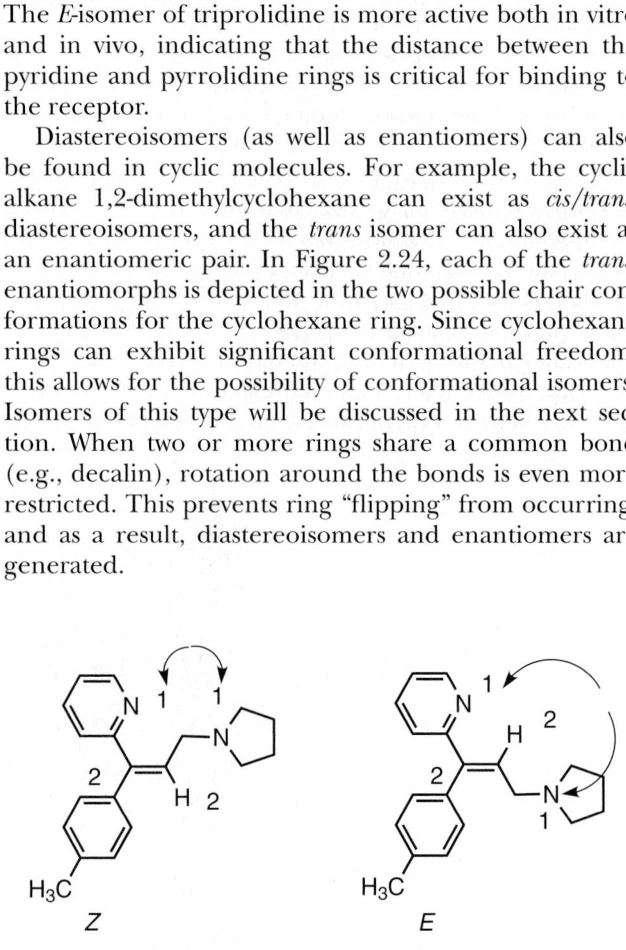

FIGURE 2.23 Geometric isomers of triprolidine.

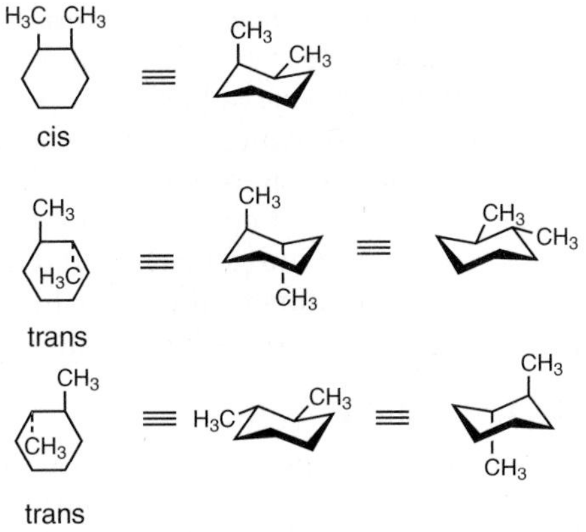

FIGURE 2.24 Diastereomers of 1,2-dimethylcyclohexane.

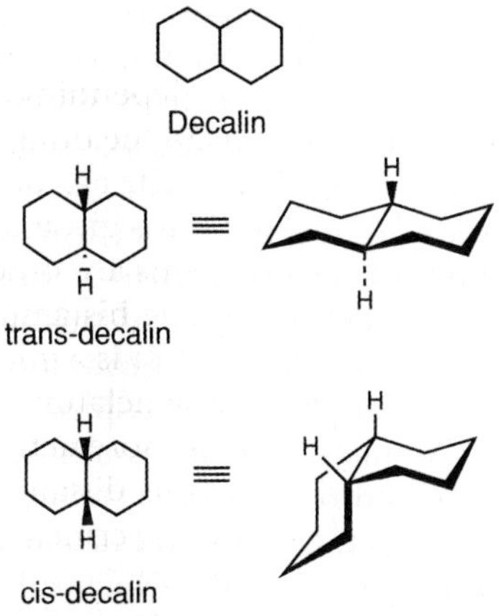

In the case of decalin, a two-ring system, the rings are fused together via a common bond in either the *trans* or *cis* configuration as shown. Steroids, a class of medicinally important compounds that consist of four fused rings (three cyclohexanes and one cyclopentane), exhibit significantly different biologic activity when the first two cyclohexane rings are fused into different configurations, referred to as the 5α- or 5β-isomers (Fig. 2.25). The α-designation indicates that the hydrogen atom in the 5-position is below the "plane" of the ring system; the β-designation refers to the hydrogen atom being above this plane. What appears to be a very minor change in orientation for the substituent results in a very drastic change in the three-dimensional shape of the molecule and in its biologic activity. Figure 2.25 shows the diastereoisomers 5α-cholestane and 5β-cholestane as examples. The chemistry and pharmacology of steroids will be discussed in more detail in Chapters 28 (Adrenocorticoids), 40 (Men's Health: Androgens), and 41 (Women's Health: Estrogens and Progestins).

Conformational Isomerism

Conformational isomerism takes place via rotation about one or more single bonds. Such bond rotation results in nonidentical spatial arrangement of atoms in a molecule. This type of isomerism does not require much energy because no bonds are broken. In the conversion of one enantiomer into another (or diastereoisomer), bonds are broken, which requires significantly more energy. The neurotransmitter acetylcholine can be used to demonstrate the concept of conformational isomers.

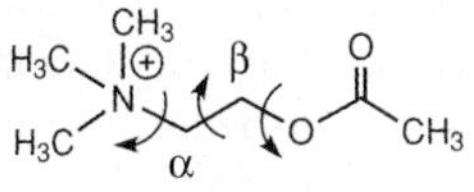

Acetylcholine

Each single bond within the acetylcholine molecule is capable of undergoing rotation, and at room temperature, such rotations readily occur. Rotation around single bonds Cα–Cβ bond of acetylcholine was shown by Kemp and Pitzer (23) in 1936 not to be free but, rather, to have an energy barrier, which is sufficiently low that at room temperature acetylcholine exists in many interconvertible conformations (see Chapter 9). Rotation around the central Cα–Cβ bond produces the greatest spatial rearrangement of atoms compared to rotation around any other bond. Since the atoms at the end of some of the bonds within acetylcholine are identical, rotation about several of these bonds produces redundant structures when viewed along the Cα–Cβ bond, and acetylcholine can be depicted in

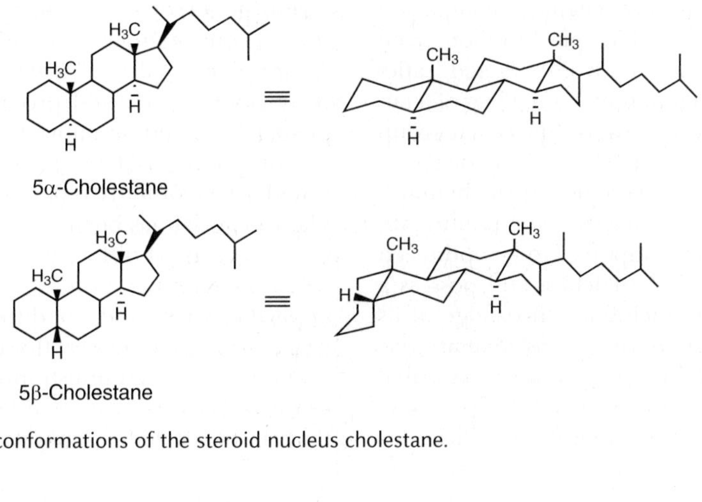

FIGURE 2.25 The 5α and 5β conformations of the steroid nucleus cholestane.

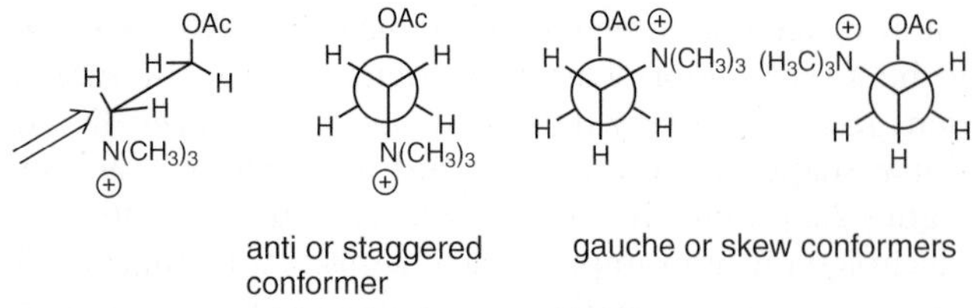

FIGURE 2.26 Anti and gauche conformations of acetylcholine.

the sawhorse or Newman projections, as shown in Figure 2.26. When the ester and trimethylammonium groups are 180° apart, the molecule is said to be in the anti, or staggered, conformation (or conformer or rotamer). This conformation allows maximum separation of the functional groups and is the most stable conformation energetically. It is possible that other conformations are more stable if factors other than steric interactions are considered (e.g., intramolecular hydrogen bonds). Rotation of one end of the Cα–Cβ bond by 120° or 240° results in the two gauche, or skew, conformations shown in Figure 2.26. These are less stable than the anti conformer, although some studies suggest that an electrostatic attraction between the electron-poor trimethylammonium and electron-rich ester oxygen atom stabilizes this conformation. Rotation by 60°, 180°, and 240° produces the least stable conformations in which all of the atoms overlap, what are referred to as eclipsed conformations.

DRUG DESIGN: DISCOVERY AND STRUCTURAL MODIFICATION OF LEAD COMPOUNDS

Process of Drug Discovery

The process of drug discovery begins with the identification of new, previously undiscovered, biologically active compounds, often called "hits," which are typically found by screening many compounds for the desired biologic properties. We will next explore the various approaches used to identify "hits" and to convert these "hits" into "lead" compounds and, subsequently, into drug candidates suitable for clinical trials. Sources of "hits" can originate from natural sources, such as plants, animals, or fungi; from synthetic chemical libraries, such as those created through combinatorial chemistry or historic chemical compound collections; from chemical and biologic intuition from years of chemical–biologic training; from targeted/rational drug design; or from computational modeling of a target site such as an enzyme. Chemical or functional group modifications of the "hits" are performed in order to improve the pharmacologic, toxicologic, physiochemical, and pharmacokinetic properties of a "hit" compound into a "lead" compound. The lead compound to be optimized should be of a known chemical structure and possess a known mechanism of action, including knowledge of its functional groups (pharmacophoric groups) that are recognized by the receptor/active site and are responsible for that molecule's affinity at the targeted receptor site. "Lead optimization" is the process whereby modifications of the functional groups of the lead compound are carried out in order to improve its recognition, affinity, and binding geometries of the pharmacophoric groups for the targeted site (a receptor or enzyme); its pharmacokinetics; or its reactivity and stability toward metabolic degradation. The final step of the drug discovery process involves rendering the lead compound into a drug candidate that is safe and suitable for use in human clinical trials, including the preparation of a suitable drug formulation.

Natural Product Screening

Perhaps the most difficult aspect of drug discovery is that of lead discovery. Until the late 19th century, the development of new chemical entities for medicinal purposes was achieved primarily through the use of natural products, generally derived from plant sources (see Chapter 1). As the colonial powers of Europe discovered new lands in the Western Hemisphere and colonized Asia, the Europeans learned from the indigenous peoples of the newly discovered lands of remedies for many ailments derived from herbs. Salicylic acid was isolated from the bark of willow trees after learning that Native Americans brewed the bark to treat inflammatory ailments. Structural optimization of this lead compound (salicylic acid) by the Bayer Corporation of Germany resulted in acetylsalicylic acid, or aspirin, the first nonsteroidal anti-inflammatory agent. South American natives used a tea obtained by brewing Cinchona bark to treat chills and fever. Further study in Europe led to the isolation of quinine and quinidine, which subsequently were used to treat malaria and cardiac arrhythmias, respectively. Following "leads" from folklore medicine, chemists of the late 19th and early 20th centuries began to seek new medicinals from plant sources and to assay them for many types of pharmacologic actions. This approach to drug discovery is often referred to as "natural product screening." Before the mid-1970s, this was one of the major approaches to obtaining new chemical entities as "leads" for new drugs. Unfortunately, this approach fell out of favor and was replaced with the rational approaches to drug design developed during that period (see next section). Heightened awareness of the fragility of ecosystems, especially the rainforests, has fueled a resurgence of screening products from plants before they become extinct. A new field of pharmacology, called "ethnopharmacology," which is the discipline of identifying potential natural product sources with medicinal properties based on native lore, has emerged as a result.

Compounds isolated from natural sources are usually tested in one or more bioassays for the ailment(s) that the plant material has been purported to treat. Interestingly, the treatment of different ailments can require different methods of preparation (e.g., brewing, chewing, or direct application to wounds) or different parts of the same plant (e.g., roots, stem, leaves, flowers, or sap). As it turns out, each method of administration or part of the plant used can produce one or more different chemical compounds that are necessary to generate the desired outcome.

Drug Discovery via Random Screening of Synthetic Organic Compounds

The random screening of synthetic organic compounds approach to the discovery of new chemical entities for a particular biologic action began in the 1930s, after the discovery of the sulfonamide class of antibacterials. All compounds available to the investigator (natural products, synthetic molecules), regardless of structure, were tested in the pharmacologic assays available at the time. This random screening approach was also applied in the 1960s and 1970s in an effort to find agents that were effective against cancer. Some groups did not limit their assays to identify a particular type of biologic activity but, rather, tested compounds in a wide variety of assays. This large-scale screening approach of drug "leads" is referred to as high-throughput screening, which involves the simultaneous bioassay of thousands of compounds in hundreds to thousands of bioassays. These types of bioassays became possible with the advent of computer-controlled robotic systems for the assays and combinatorial chemistry techniques for the synthesis of large numbers of compounds in small (milligram) quantities. This type of random screening eventually gave way to targeted dedicated screening and rational design techniques.

Drug Discovery from Targeted Dedicated Screening and Rational Drug Design

Rational drug design is a more focused approach that uses greater knowledge (structural information) about the drug receptor (targets) or one of its natural ligands as a basis to design, identify, or create drug "leads." Testing is usually done with one or two models (e.g., specific receptor systems or enzymes) based on the therapeutic target. The drug design component often involves molecular modeling and the use of quantitative structure–activity relationships (QSARs) to better define the physicochemical properties and the pharmacophoric groups that are essential for biologic activity. The development of QSARs relies on the ability to examine multiple relationships between physical properties and biologic activities. In classic QSAR (e.g., Hansch-type analysis), an equation defines biologic activity as a linear free-energy relationship between physicochemical and/or structural properties. It permits evaluation of the nature of interaction forces between a drug and its biological target, as well as the ability to predict activity in molecules. These approaches are better for the development of a lead compound into a drug candidate than for the discovery of a lead compound.

Drug Discovery via Drug Metabolism Studies

New drug entities have been "discovered" as drug leads through investigation of the metabolism of drug molecules that already are clinical candidates or, in some instances, are already on the market. In this method, metabolites of known drug entities are isolated and assayed for biologic activity using either the same target system or broader screen target systems. The broader screening systems are more useful if the metabolite under evaluation is a chemical structure that was radically altered from the parent molecule through some unusual metabolic rearrangement reaction. In most cases, the metabolite is not radically different from the parent molecule and, therefore, would be expected to exhibit similar pharmacologic effects. One advantage of evaluating this type of drug candidate is that a metabolite can possess better pharmacokinetic properties, such as a longer duration of action, better oral absorption, or less toxicity with fewer side effects (e.g., terfenadine and its antihistaminic hydroxylated metabolite, fexofenadine). As it turns out, the sulfonamide antibacterial agents were discovered in this way. The azo dye Prontosil was found to have only antibacterial action in vivo. It was soon discovered that this compound required metabolic activation via reduction of the diazo group to produce the active metabolite 4-aminobenzene sulfonamide (Fig. 2.27). The sulfonamide mimics the physicochemical properties of PABA, a crucial component in microbial metabolism. It is no surprise that the sulfonamide acts as a competitive inhibitor of the enzyme for which PABA is a substrate.

Drug Discovery from the Observation of Side Effects

An astute clinician or pharmacologist can detect a side effect in a patient or animal model that could lead, on further development, to a new therapeutic use for a particular chemical entity. Discovery of new lead compounds via exploitation of side-effect profiles of existing agents is discussed below.

One of the more interesting drug development scenarios is that of the phenothiazine antipsychotics (see Chapter 14). Molecules with this type of biologic activity can be traced back to the first histamine H_1-receptor antagonists developed in the 1930s. In 1937, Bovet and Staub (24) were the first to recognize that it should be possible to antagonize the effects of histamine and, thereby, treat allergic reactions. They tested compounds that were known to act on the autonomic nervous system and, eventually, discovered that benzodioxanes (Fig. 2.28) significantly antagonized the effects of histamine. During an attempt

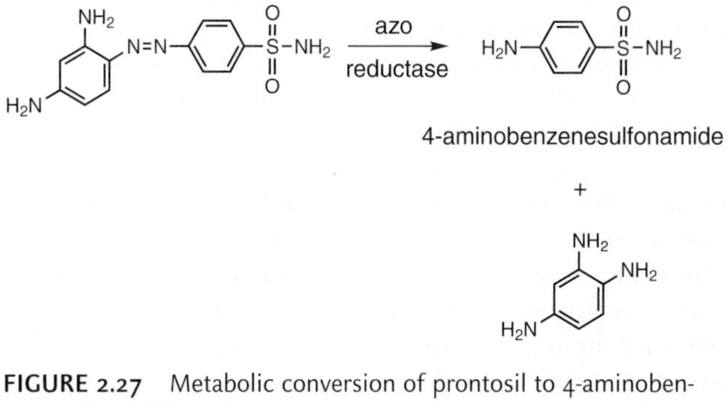

FIGURE 2.27 Metabolic conversion of prontosil to 4-aminobenzenesulfonamide.

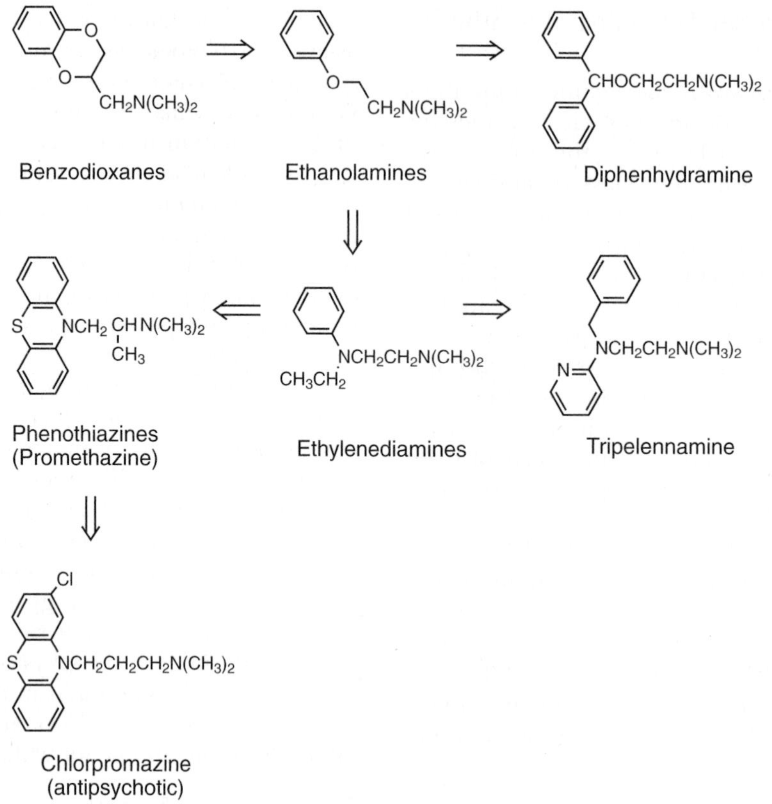

FIGURE 2.28 Development of phenothiazine-type antipsychotic drugs.

to improve the antihistaminergic action of the benzodioxanes, it was discovered that phenyl substituted ethanolamines also demonstrated significant antihistaminergic activity. Further development of this class generated two different classes of antihistamines, the diphenhydramine class of antihistamines represented by diphenhydramine (Fig. 2.28) and the ethylenediamine class, represented by tripelennamine (Fig. 2.28) (see also Chapter 32).

Incorporation of the aromatic rings of the ethylenediamines into the rigid and planar tricyclic phenothiazine structure produced molecules (e.g., promethazine) with good antihistaminergic action and relatively strong sedative properties (see also Chapter 32). At first, these compounds were found to be useful as antihistamines, but their very strong sedative properties led to their use as potentiating agents for anesthesia (25). Further development to increase the sedative properties of the phenothiazines resulted in the development of chlorpromazine in 1950 (26).

Chlorpromazine was found to produce a tendency for sleep, but unlike the antihistamine phenothiazines, it also produced a disinterest in patients with regard to their surroundings (i.e., tranquilizing effects). In patients with psychiatric disorders, an ameliorative effect on the psychosis and a relief of anxiety and agitation were noted. These observations suggested that chlorpromazine had potential for the treatment of psychiatric disorders. Thus, what started out as an attempt to improve antihistaminergic activity ultimately resulted in an entirely new class of chemical entities useful in the treatment of an unrelated disorder (27).

Another example of how new chemical entities can be derived from biologically unrelated molecules is illustrated by the development of the potassium channel agonist diazoxide (Fig. 2.29). This molecule was developed as a result of the observation that the thiazide diuretics, such as chlorothiazide, not only exhibited diuretic activity, due to inhibition of sodium absorption in the distal convoluted tubule, but also demonstrated a direct effect on the renal vasculature. Structural modification to enhance this direct effect led to the development of diazoxide and related potassium channel agonists for the treatment of hypertension (see Chapter 28).

Refinement of the Lead Structure

Determination of the Pharmacophore

Once a "hit" compound has been discovered for a particular therapeutic use, the next step is to identify the pharmacophoric groups. The pharmacophore of a drug molecule

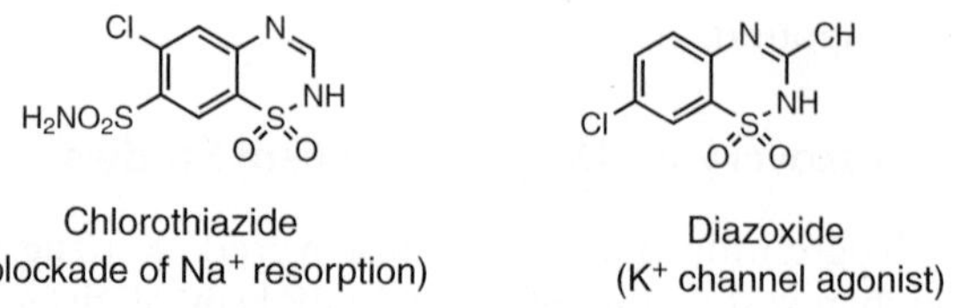

FIGURE 2.29 Structural similarity of chlorothiazide (a diuretic) and diazoxide (an antihypertensive that acts via opening of K^+ channels).

is that portion of the molecule that contains the essential functional group(s) that directly bind with the active site of the biologic target to produce the desired biologic activity. Because drug–target interactions can be very specific (think of a lock [receptor] and key [drug] relationship), the pharmacophore can constitute a small portion of the molecule. In many cases, a very structurally complex molecule can be "stripped down" to a simpler structure with retention of the pharmacophoric groups while maintaining the desired biologic action. An example of this is the opioid analgesic morphine, a tetracyclic compound with five chiral centers. Not only would structure simplification possibly provide molecules with fewer side effects, but a reduction in the number of chiral centers would greatly simplify the synthesis of morphine derivatives. Figure 2.30 shows how the morphine structure has been simplified in the search for molecules with fewer deleterious side effects, such as respiratory depression and addiction potential. Within each class are analogues that are less potent, equipotent, and many times more potent than morphine. As shown in the figure, the pharmacophore of morphine consists of a tertiary alkylamine that is at least four atoms away from an aromatic ring. A more detailed discussion of the chemistry and pharmacology of morphine can be found in Chapter 20.

Alterations in Alkyl Chains: Chain Length, Branching, and Rings

An increase or decrease in the length of an alkyl chain (homologation), branching, and alteration of ring size can have a profound effect on the potency and pharmacologic activity of the molecule. A change in the length of an alkyl chain by one CH_2 unit or branch alters the lipophilic character of the molecule and, therefore, its properties of absorption, distribution, and excretion. If the alkyl chain is directly involved in an interaction with the biologic target, then this type of alteration can influence the quality of those interactions. Molecules that are conformationally flexible can become less flexible if branching is introduced at a key position of an alkyl chain or the alkyl chain is incorporated into a ring equivalent. Changes in conformation can alter the spatial relationship between the pharmacophoric (functional) groups in the molecule and thereby influence interactions with the biologic target. Small structural changes are important to consider in the design of structural analogues.

An example that demonstrates how an increase in hydrocarbon chain length has significant effects not only on potency, but also on drug action (agonist vs. antagonist) is provided by a series of *N*-alkyl morphine analogues (Fig. 2.31). In this series, homologation of R = CH_3 (morphine) to R = $CH_2CH_2CH_3$ (*N*-propylnormorphine) produces a pronounced decrease in agonist activity and an increase in antagonist activity. When further homologated by one methylene unit R = $CH_2CH_2CH_2CH_3$ (*N*-butylnormorphine), the resulting analog is totally devoid of agonist or antagonist activity (i.e., the compound is inactive). Additional increases in chain length (R = $CH_2CH_2CH_2CH_2CH_3$ and R = $CH_2CH_2CH_2CH_2CH_2CH_3$) produce compounds with increasing potency as agonists. When R is β-phenylethyl, the compound is a full agonist, with a potency approximately 14-fold that of morphine (28,29).

Branching of alkyl chains can also produce drastic changes in potency and pharmacologic activity. If the mechanism of action is closely related to the lipophilicity of the molecule, then hydrocarbon chain branching will result in a less lipophilic compound and a significant alteration in

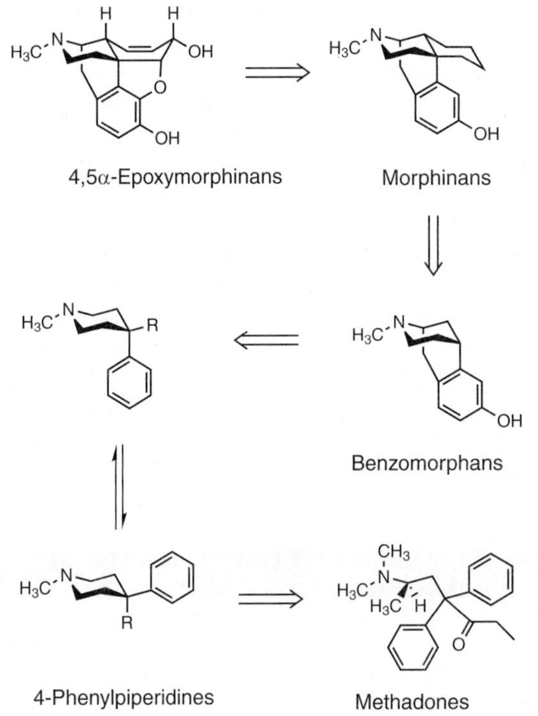

FIGURE 2.30 Morphine pharmacophore and its relationship to analgesic derivatives.

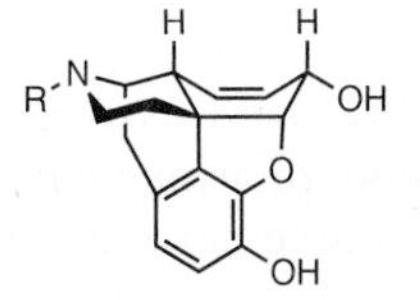

R	Pharmacological activity
$-CH_3$	Analgesic (morphine)
$-CH_2CH_3$	Opioid agonist activity decreased
$-CH_2CH_2CH_3$	Opioid antagonist activity increased
$-CH_2CH_2CH_2CH_3$	Inactive as opioid agonist or antagonist
$-CH_2CH_2CH_2CH_2CH_3$ $-CH_2CH_2CH_2CH_2CH_2CH_3$	Opioid antagonist activity increased
$-CH_2CH_2-C_6H_5$	14X potency of morphine

FIGURE 2.31 Effect of alkyl chain length on activity of morphine.

biologic effect. This decrease in lipophilicity is a result of the alkyl chain becoming more compact and causes less disruption of the hydrogen-bonding network of water. If the hydrocarbon chain is directly involved in interactions with its biologic target, then branching can produce major changes in pharmacologic activity. For example, consider the phenothiazines promethazine and promazine:

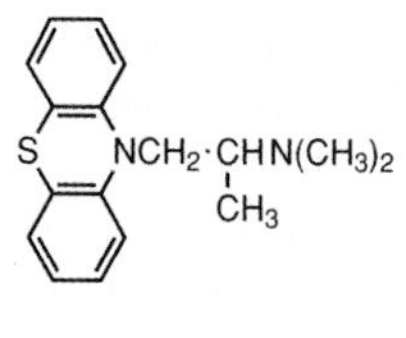

Promethazine

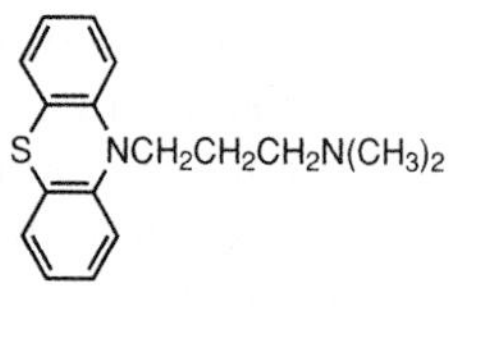

Promazine

The primary pharmacologic activity of promethazine is that of an antihistamine, whereas promazine is an antipsychotic. The only difference between the two molecules is the alkylamine side chain. In the case of promethazine, there is an isopropylamine side chain, whereas promazine contains an *n*-propylamine. In this case, simple modification of one carbon atom from a branched to a linear hydrocarbon radically alters the pharmacologic activity.

Positional isomers of aromatic ring substituents can also possess different pharmacologic properties. Substituents on aromatic rings can alter the electron distribution throughout the ring, which, in turn, can influence how the ring interacts with the biologic target. Aromatic ring substituents can also influence the conformation of the flexible portion of a molecule, especially if the substituents are located ortho to the same carbon attached to the flexible side chain. Ring substituents influence the conformations of adjacent substituents via steric interactions and can significantly alter interactions with the biologic target.

Functional Group Modification: Bioisosterism

Bioisosterism

When a lead compound is first discovered, it often lacks the required potency and pharmacokinetic properties suitable for making it a viable clinical candidate. These can include undesirable side effects, physicochemical properties, other factors that affect oral bioavailability (see also Chapter 3), and adverse metabolic or excretion properties. These undesirable properties are often the result of the presence of specific pharmacophoric (functional) groups in the molecule. Successful modification of the compound to reduce or eliminate these undesirable features without losing the desired biologic activity is the goal. Replacement or modification of specific pharmacophoric (functional) groups with other groups having similar properties is known as "isosteric replacement" or "bioisosteric replacement."

In 1919, Langmuir (30,31) first developed the concept of chemical isosterism to describe the similarities in physical properties among atoms, functional groups, radicals,

TABLE 2.7 Comparison of Physical Properties of N_2O and CO_2

Property	N_2O	CO_2
Viscosity at 20°C	148×10^{-6}	148×10^{-6}
Density of liquid at 10°C	0.856	0.858
Refractive index of liquid, D line 16°C	1.193	1.190
Dielectric constant of liquid at 0°C	1.593	1.582
Solubility in alcohol at 15°C	3.250	3.130

and molecules. The similarities among atoms described by Langmuir resulted primarily from the fact that these atoms contained the same number of valence electrons and came from the same columns within the periodic table. This concept of isosterism was limited to elements in adjacent rows and columns, inorganic molecules, ions, and small organic molecules, such as diazomethane and ketene. Table 2.7 shows a comparison of the physical properties of N_2O and CO_2 to illustrate Langmuir's concept.

To account for similarities between functional groups with the same number of valence electrons but different numbers of atoms, Grimm (32) developed his hydride displacement law. This is not a "law" in the strict sense but, rather, more an illustration of similar physical properties among closely related functional groups. Table 2.8 presents an example of Grimm's hydride displacement. Descending diagonally from left to right in the table, hydrogen atoms are progressively added to maintain the same number of valence electrons for each group of atoms within a column (thus the term "hydride"). Within each column, the groups are considered to be "pseudoatoms" with respect to each another. Thus, NH_2 is considered to be isosteric to OH, and so on. This early view of isosterism did not consider the actual location, motion, and resonance of electrons within the orbitals of these functional group replacements. Careful observation of this table reveals that some groups do share similar physicochemical properties, but others have very different properties, despite having the same number of valence electrons. For example, OH and NH_2 share similar hydrogen-bonding properties and, therefore, should be interchangeable if that is the only important criterion. The NH_2 group is basic, whereas the OH is neutral. Hence, at physiologic pH, the NH_2 group exists in

TABLE 2.8 Grimm's Hydride Displacement "Law"

C	N	O	F	Ne
	CH	NH	OH	FH
		CH_2	NH_2	OH_2
			CH_3	NH_3

its protonated or conjugate acid form and the molecule becomes positively charged. If OH is being replaced by NH_2, the additional positive charge could have a significant effect on the overall physicochemical properties of the molecule in which it is being introduced. The difference in physicochemical properties of the CH_3 group relative to the OH and NH_2 groups is even greater. In addition to acid–base character, this "law" fails to take into account other important physicochemical parameters, such as electronegativity, polarizability, bond angles, size, shape of molecular orbitals, electron density, and partition coefficients, all of which contribute significantly to the overall physicochemical properties of a molecule.

Instead of considering only partial structures, Hinsberg (33) applied the concept of isosterism to entire molecules. He developed the concept of "ring equivalents"—that is, functional groups that can be exchanged for one another in aromatic ring systems without drastic changes in physicochemical properties relative to the parent structure. Benzene, thiophene, and pyridine illustrate this concept (Fig. 2.32). A –CH=CH- group in benzene is replaced by the divalent sulfur, -S-, in thiophene, and a –CH= is replaced by the trivalent –N= to give pyridine. The physical properties of benzene and thiophene are very similar. For example, the boiling point of benzene is 81.1°C, and that of thiophene is 84.4°C (at 760 mm Hg). Pyridine, however, deviates, with a boiling point of 115 to 116°C. Hinsberg therefore concluded that divalent sulfur (-S- or thioether) must resemble –C=C- in shape, and these groups were considered to be isosteric. Note that hydrogen atoms are ignored in this comparison. Today, this isosteric relationship is seen in many drugs e.g., H_1-receptor antagonists (Fig. 2.32).

It is difficult to relate biologic properties to physicochemical properties of individual atoms, functional groups, or entire molecules, because many physicochemical parameters are involved simultaneously and, therefore, are difficult to quantitate. Simple relationships as described earlier often do not hold up across the many types of biologic systems seen with medicinal agents. That is, what can work as an isosteric replacement in one biologic system can not work in another. Because of this, it was necessary to introduce the term "bioisosterism" to describe functional groups related in structure that have similar biologic effects. Friedman (34) introduced the term bioisosterism and defined it as follows: "Bioisosteres are (functional) groups or molecules that have chemical and physical similarities producing broadly similar biological properties."

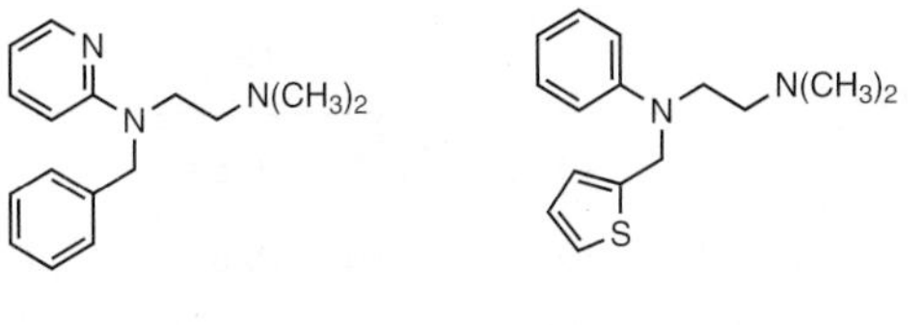

Tripelennamine Methaphenilene

FIGURE 2.32 Isosteric substitution of thiophene for benzene and benzene for pyridine.

Burger (35) expanded this definition to take into account biochemical views of biological activity: "Bioisosteres are compounds or groups that possess near equal molecular shapes and volumes, approximately the same distribution of electrons, and which exhibit similar physical properties such as hydrophobicity. Bioisosteric compounds affect the same biochemically associated systems as agonist or antagonists and thereby produce biological properties that are related to each other."

Classical and Nonclassical Bioisosteres

Bioisosteric groups can be subdivided into two categories: classical and nonclassical bioisosteres. Functional groups that satisfy the original conditions of Langmuir and Grimm are referred to as classical bioisosteres. Nonclassical bioisosteres do not obey steric and electronic definitions of classical bioisosteres and do not necessarily have the same number of atoms as the functional group that they replace. A wider set of compounds and functional groups are encompassed by nonclassical bioisosteres that produce, at the molecular level, qualitatively similar agonist or antagonist action. In animals, many hormones and neurotransmitters with very similar structures and biologic actions can be classified as bioisosteres. An example is the insulins isolated from various mammalian species. Even though these insulins can differ by several amino acid residues, they still produce the same biologic effects. (If this did not occur, the use of insulin to treat diabetes would have had to wait another 60 years for recombinant DNA technology to allow production of human insulin.)

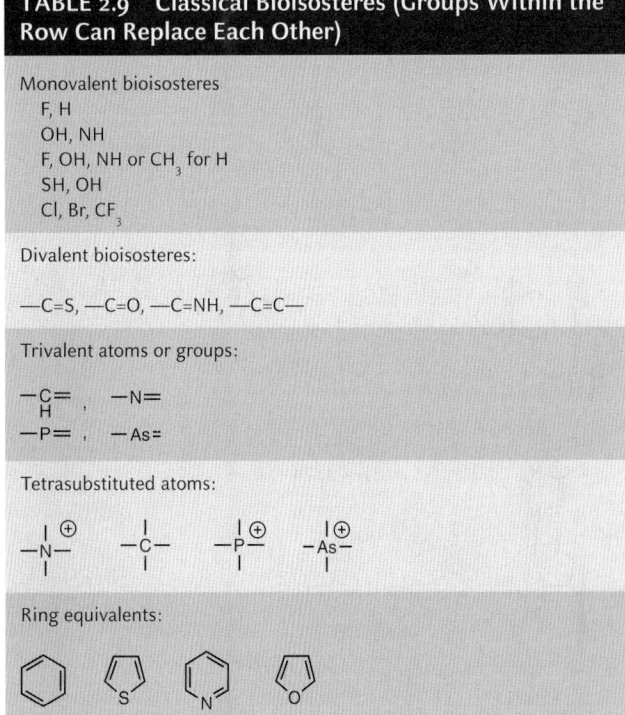

TABLE 2.9 Classical Bioisosteres (Groups Within the Row Can Replace Each Other)

Monovalent bioisosteres
F, H
OH, NH
F, OH, NH or CH_3 for H
SH, OH
Cl, Br, CF_3
Divalent bioisosteres:
—C=S, —C=O, —C=NH, —C=C—
Trivalent atoms or groups:
—CH= , —N=
—P= , —As=
Tetrasubstituted atoms:
$-N^{\oplus}-$ $-C-$ $-P^{\oplus}-$ $-As^{\oplus}-$
Ring equivalents:
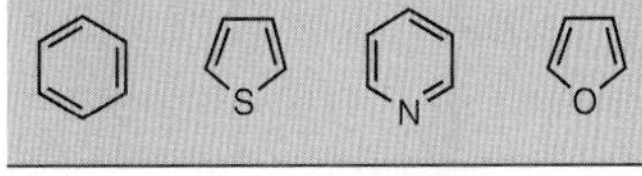

What can be a successful bioisosteric replacement for a given molecule that interacts with a particular biologic target quite has often no effect or abolishes biologic activity in another. Thus, the use of bioisosteric replacement (classical or nonclassical) in the design of new chemical entities (drug discovery) is highly dependent on the biologic system under investigation. No hard-and-fast rules exist to determine which bioisosteric replacement is going to work with a given molecule, although as the following tables and examples demonstrate, some generalizations are possible. Each category of bioisostere can be further subdivided as shown below, and examples are provided in Tables 2.9 and 2.10:

I. Classical bioisosteres
  A. Monovalent atoms and groups
  B. Divalent atoms and groups
  C. Trivalent atoms and groups
  D. Tetrasubstituted atoms
  E. Ring equivalents

II. Nonclassical bioisosteres
  A. Exchangeable groups
  B. Rings versus noncyclic structure

TABLE 2.10 Nonclassical Bioisosteric Replacements

Compounds	Bioisosteric Replacement	References
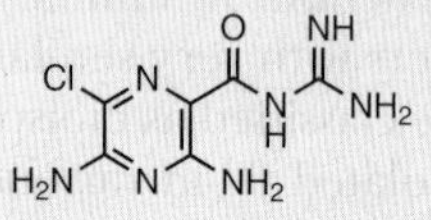	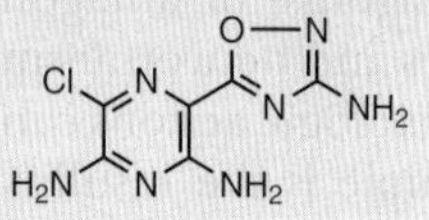	40
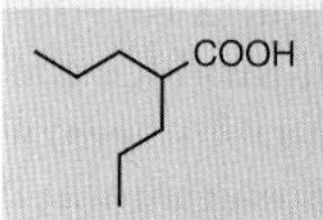	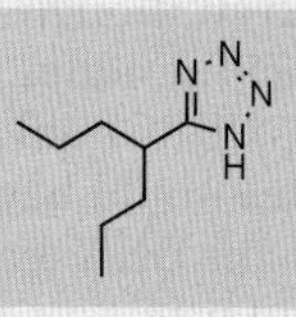	41
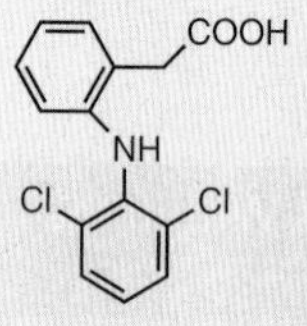	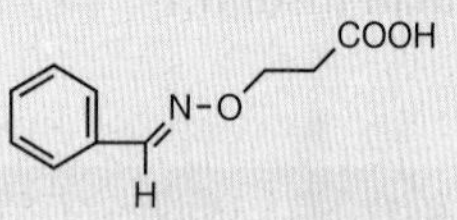	42
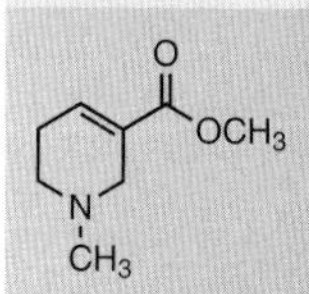	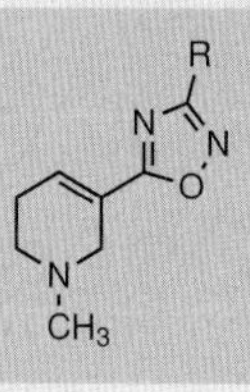	43
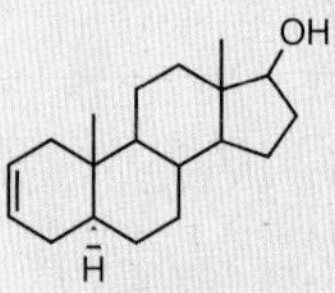	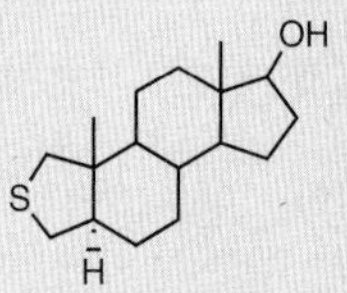	44
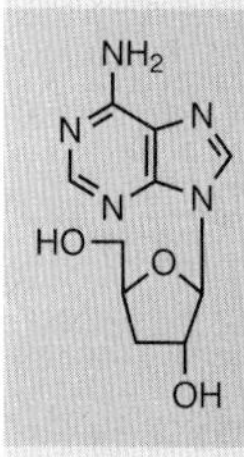	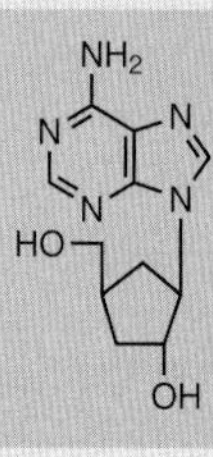	45
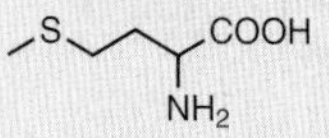	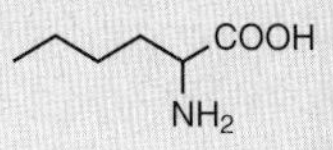	46

Classical Bioisosteres Substitution of hydrogen with fluorine is a common monovalent isosteric replacement. Sterically, hydrogen and fluorine are quite similar, with their van der Waals' radii measuring 1.2 and 1.35 Å, respectively. Because fluorine is the most electronegative element in the periodic table, any differences in biologic activity resulting from replacement of hydrogen with fluorine can be attributed to this property.

A classic example of hydrogen replacement by fluorine is development of the antineoplastic agent 5-fluorouracil from uracil. Another example is shown in Figure 2.33, in which the chlorine of chlorothiazide has been replaced with bromine or a trifluoromethyl group. For each of the substitutions, the electronic (σ, where σ^+ is electron withdrawing and σ^- is electron donating) and hydrophobic (π) properties of each group are maintained relatively constant, but the size of each group varies significantly, as indicated by the Taft steric parameter (E_s).

Figure 2.34 shows an example of classical isosteric substitution of an amino group for a hydroxyl group in folic acid. The amino group is capable of mimicking the tautomeric forms of folic acid and providing the appropriate hydrogen bonds to the enzyme active site.

A tetravalent bioisosteric replacement study was done by Grisar et al. (36) with a series of α-tocopherol analogues (Fig. 2.35). α-Tocopherol has been shown to scavenge lipoperoxyl and superoxide radicals and to accumulate in heart tissue. This is thought to be part of its mechanism of action to reduce cardiac damage resulting from myocardial infarction. All of the bioisosteric analogues were found to produce similar biologic activity.

Nonclassical Bioisosteres As mentioned earlier, nonclassical bioisosteres are replacements of functional groups

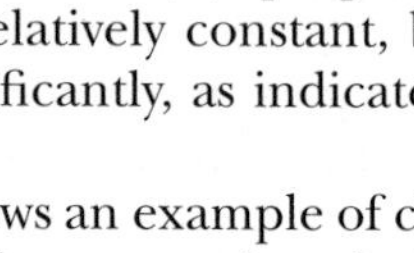

R =	Cl	Br	CF_3
σ	+0.23	+0.23	+0.54
π	+0.71	+0.86	+0.88
E_s	-0.97	-1.16	-2.40

FIGURE 2.33 Isosteric replacement of chlorine in thiazide diuretics. Comparison of physicochemical properties of the substituents.

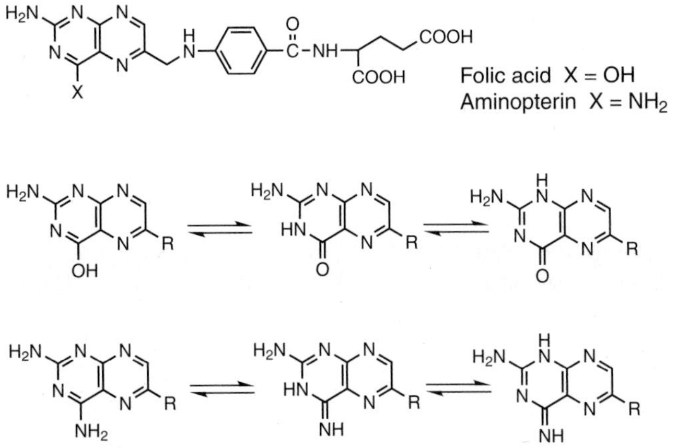

FIGURE 2.34 Isosteric replacement of OH by NH_2 in folic acid and possible tautomers of folic acid and aminopterin.

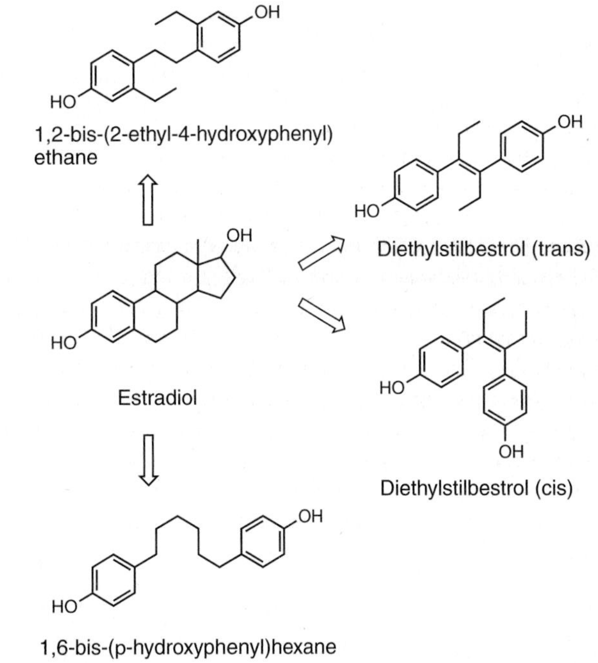

FIGURE 2.36 Noncyclic analogs of estradiol.

not defined by classical definitions. Some of these groups, however, mimic spatial arrangements, electronic properties, or some other physicochemical property of the molecule or functional group critical for biologic activity. One example is the use of a double bond to position essential functional groups into a particular spatial configuration critical for activity. This is shown in Figure 2.36 with the naturally occurring hormone estradiol and the synthetic analogue diethylstilbestrol. The *trans* isomer of diethylstilbestrol has approximately the same potency as estradiol, whereas the *cis* isomer is only one fourteenth as active. In the *trans* configuration, the phenolic hydroxy groups mimic the correct orientation of the phenol and alcohol in estradiol (37,38). This is not possible with the *cis* isomer, and more flexible analogues (Fig. 2.36) have little or no activity (39,40).

Another example of a nonclassical replacement is that of a sulfonamide group for a phenol in catecholamines (Fig. 2.37). With this example, steric factors appear to have less influence on receptor binding than acidity and hydrogen-bonding potential of the functional group on the aromatic ring. Both the phenolic hydroxyl of isoproterenol and the acidic proton of the arylsulfonamide have nearly the same pK_a (~10) (41). Both groups are weakly acidic and capable of losing a proton and interacting with the biologic target as anions (Fig. 2.37). Because the replacement is not susceptible to metabolism by catechol *O*-methyltransferase, it has also the added advantage of increasing the duration of action and making the compound orally active. Other examples of successful bioisosteric replacements are shown in Table 2.10, and a more detailed description of the role of bioisosterism can be found in the review by Patani and LaVoie (42).

PEPTIDE AND PROTEIN DRUGS

Not all drugs are small molecules as described thus far. Some very important therapeutic agents are peptidic in nature (e.g., insulin, calcitonin) and, due to their physical chemical properties, generally cannot be delivered orally and must be administered parenterally. Peptides and proteins are very similar in that they are made up of units, or residues, of amino acids that are linked by amide bonds, also referred to as peptide bonds. There is no definitive number of amino acid residues that delineates a peptide from a protein. However, the term peptide refers generally to molecules that contain 15 to

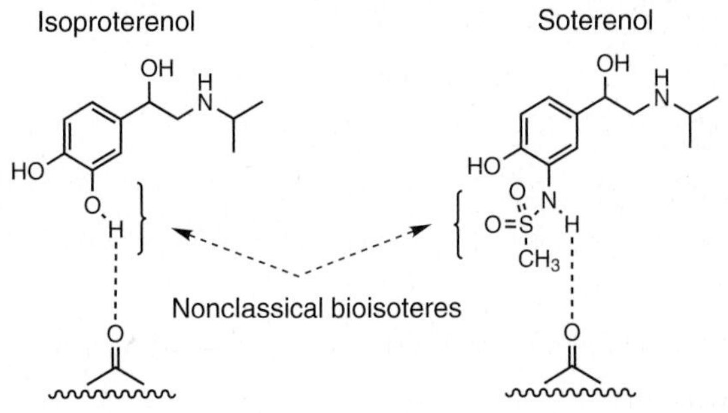

FIGURE 2.37 Bioisosteric replacement of m-OH of isoproterenol with a sulfonamido group and similar hydrogen-bonding capacity to a possible drug receptor.

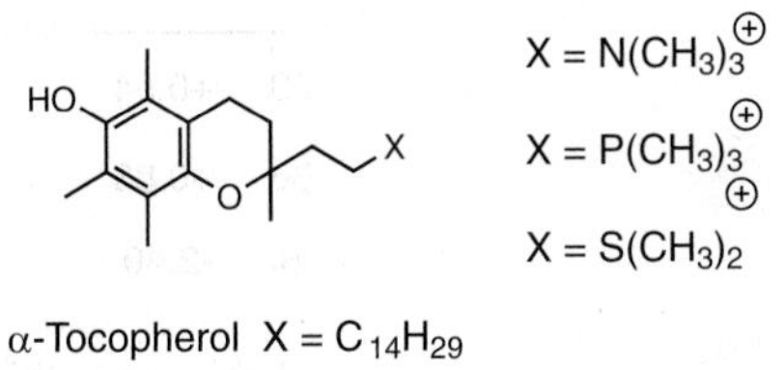

FIGURE 2.35 Tetravalent bioisosteres of α-tocopherol.

50 amino acids. Molecules composed of more than 50 residues are generally referred to as proteins.

There are 20 naturally occurring amino acids that serve as the building blocks for both peptide and protein drugs (Table 2.11). Each amino acid contains a common functional group "backbone" that includes a basic amine attached to the α-carbon of an acidic carboxylic acid. The α-carbon for each amino acid is substituted with a unique side chain. The amino acid side chains contribute significantly to the physical chemical properties of

TABLE 2.11 The Twenty Natural Occurring Amino Acids

Name	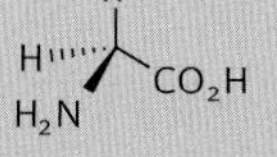 3 Letter code	General Structure Single Letter code	Structure R =	pKa of side chain
Glycine	Gly	G	-H	none
Alanine	Ala	A	$-CH_3$	none
Valine	Val	V	$-CH(CH_3)_2$	none
Isoleucine	Ile	I	$-CH(CH_3)CH_2CH_3$	none
Leucine	Leu	L	$-CH_2CH(CH_3)_2$	none
Proline	Pro	P	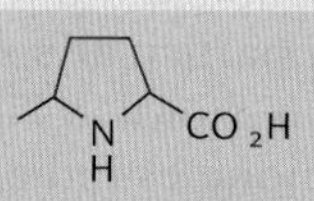 (side chain highligted)	none
Phenylalanine	Phe	F	$-CH_2-C_6H_5$	none
Tryptophan	Trp	W	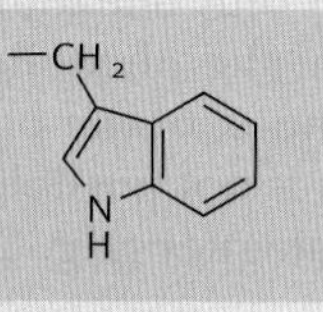	none
Methionine	Met	M	$-CH_2CH_2SCH_3$	none
Cysteine	Cys	C	$-CH_2SH$	(acidic) ~8
Serine	Ser	S	$-CH_2OH$	none
Threonine	Thr	T	$-CH(CH_3)OH$	none
Tyrosine	Tyr	Y	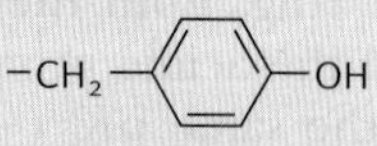	(acidic) ~10
Arginine	Arg	R	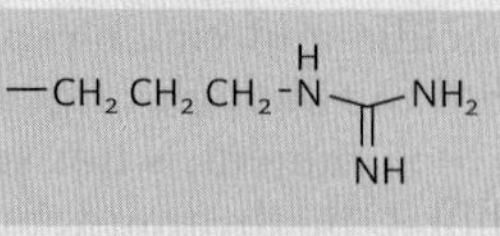	(basic) ~12.5
Lysine	Lys	K	$-CH_2CH_2CH_2NH_2$	(basic) ~10.5
Histidine	His	H	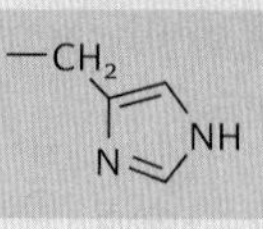	(basic) ~6
Asparagine	Asn	N	$-CH_2CONH_2$	none
Glutamine	Gln	Q	$-CH_2CH_2CONH_2$	none
Aspartic Acid	Asp	D	$-CH_2COOH$	(acidic) ~3.8
Glutamic Acid	Glu	E	$-CH_2CH_2COOH$	(acidic) ~4

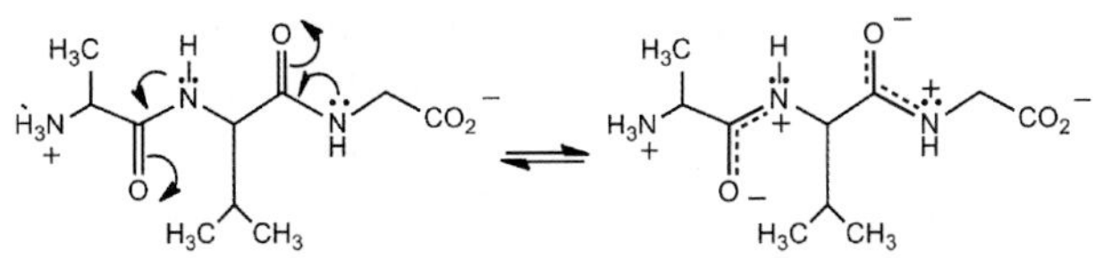

FIGURE 2.38 A tripeptide, Ala-Val-Gly, indicating the planarity of the peptide bonds caused by the restricted rotation around the amide bond.

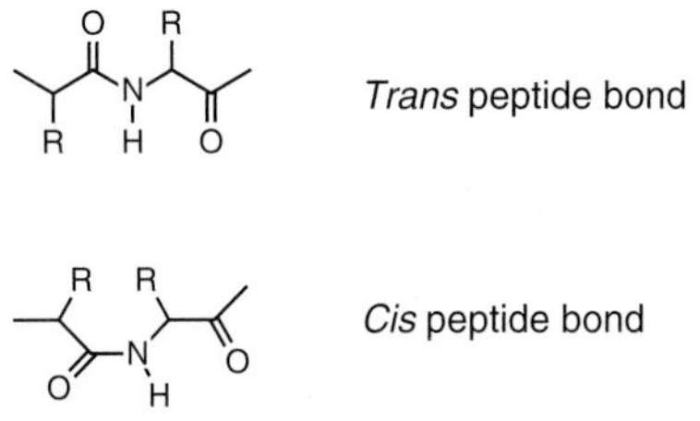

FIGURE 2.39 *Cis/trans* peptide bond configuration.

the peptide that is formed from a unique sequence of amino acids.

As previously mentioned, the amino acid residues are linked by amide bonds, as shown in Figure 2.38. Each carboxylic acid forms an amide bond with the amine group of the next amino acid in the sequence. As with other amide bonds, conjugation between the lone pair of electrons on the nitrogen atom and the adjacent carbonyl group results in the amide bond having partial double-bond character due to a resonance structure as shown in Figure 2.38. This property has two major consequences: 1) the amide bond is therefore co-planar; and 2) there is restricted rotation around the C–N bond (Fig. 2.38). Because of this restricted rotation, there are two conformations possible, *cis* and *trans* (Fig 2.39). The *trans*-conformation is lower in energy due to fewer steric interactions (similar to that found with a carbon–carbon double bond) and is favored. When proline is one of the amino acid residues, the *cis*-conformation can be favored as a result of the amine group being part of a pyrrolidine ring. For this reason, the presence of proline in peptides and proteins is associated with a "kink" or bend in the overall conformation of the peptide chain.

Physical Chemical Properties of Peptides

Since the α-amine and α-carboxylic acid of each amino acid are involved in the peptide backbone (except at each terminus of the chain), the basic and acidic nature of these functional groups does not contribute to the overall physical chemical properties of the molecule. The functional groups found within the amino acid side chains are what are integral to the physicochemical properties of the peptide or protein and represent important points of interaction with the corresponding biologic target. Examination of Table 2.11 shows that the functional groups found within the amino acid side chains can be basic (e.g., amine, guanidine, imidazole), acidic (e.g., carboxylic acid, phenol, thiol), neutral (e.g., thioether, amide), or hydrocarbon (e.g., alkyl, aromatic rings) in nature. All of the functional groups found in amino acid side chains were discussed previously as components of small-molecule drugs. The primary differences in physical chemical properties between peptides and small molecules are due to their large size (molecular weight [MW]) and, as a result, the sheer number of different side chains (i.e., functional groups) present in a given structure. As might be expected, the types and number of functional groups present in the side chains dictate how much more or less polar the peptide is compared to a small-molecule drug. It is certainly plausible that peptide-based drugs will not have optimal logP values for passive absorption across membranes and, given their large MW, will not readily cross membranes (see also Chapter 3).

Metabolism/Degradation of Peptide and Protein Drugs

Peptides and proteins are metabolized extensively by enzymes in the gastrointestinal tract, blood, interstitial fluid, vascular bed, and cell membranes, which results in very poor oral absorption and a short half-life for these molecules. The primary route of metabolism of peptides and proteins involves hydrolysis of the peptide bonds that link the amino acids by enzymes called peptidases. Some of these peptidases exhibit specificity for certain amino acid sequences or have specificity for either the amino or carboxyl terminus of the peptide (exopeptidase). For example, carboxypeptidases cleave off one C-terminal residue, dipeptidyl carboxypeptidases cleave dipeptides from the C terminus, aminopeptidases cleave off one N-terminal residue, and amidases (endopeptidases) cleave internal peptide bonds. There are also peptidase subclasses that exhibit specificity for certain amino acid sequences within the peptide or at either of the termini. Some peptidases (e.g., dipeptidyl peptidase IV) have been found to catalyze the degradation of naturally occurring peptides (e.g., GLP-1) (Fig. 2.40) (see also Chapter 37).

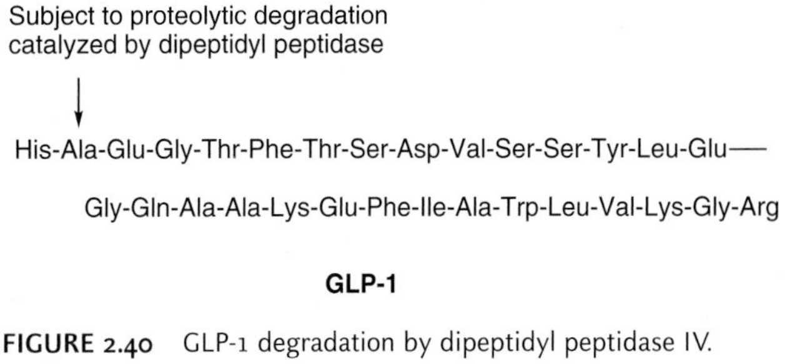

FIGURE 2.40 GLP-1 degradation by dipeptidyl peptidase IV.

SUMMARY

Medicinal chemistry involves the discovery of new chemical entities and the systematic study of the SARs of these compounds for disease state management. Such studies provide the basis for development of better and therapeutically safer medicinal agents from lead compounds found from natural sources, random screening, systematic screening, and focused rational design. Drug design goals include increasing the potency and duration of action of newly discovered compounds and decreasing adverse side effects.

For the pharmacist, it is also important to understand how the physicochemical properties influence the pharmacokinetic properties of the medicinal agents being dispensed. Such knowledge will help the pharmacist not only to better understand the clinical properties of these compounds but also to anticipate the properties of newly marketed agents. An understanding of the chemical properties of the molecule will allow the pharmacist to anticipate formulation problems (especially IV admixtures), as well as potential adverse interactions with other drugs as the result of serum protein binding and metabolism.

PROBLEMS

The following problems are provided for additional study:

1. Calculate the percent ionization of amobarbital at pH 2.0, 5.5, and 8.0. What trend is seen?
2. Calculate the percent ionization of phenylpropanolamine at pH 2.0, 5.5, and 8.0. Compare these results with those obtained in Problem 1.
3. Calculate the percent ionization of sulfacetamide in the stomach, duodenum, and ileum. Draw the structure of the predominate form of the drug in each tissue.
4. Referring to Figure 2.15, redraw each compound in its ionized form.
5. For the organic functional groups listed in Table 2.4, name each functional group, and redraw them, showing all potential hydrogen bonds with water.
6. Using the empiric method of Lemke, predict the water solubility for each of the following molecules (*Note:* Water solubility is defined as >1% solubility):

Aspirin	Carphenazine maleate
Chlordiazepoxide	Codeine
Codeine phosphate	Cyproheptadine hydrochloride
Haloperidol	Phenytoin

7. Calculate the logP value for each of the following:

Aspirin	Carphenazine
Codeine	Cyproheptadine
Haloperidol	Chlordiazepoxide
Phenytoin	

8. Using the Merck Index or other source, find the chemical structures for the following empirical formulae. List as many physicochemical properties as possible for each compound, and compare them within each group of isomers:

$C_4H_{10}O_2$ C_5H_8O

$C_5H_{11}O_2$ $C_7H_7NO_2$ $C_8H_8O_2$

$C_{12}H_{17}NO_3$

$C_{20}H_{30}O_2$

9. Using the Cahn-Ingold-Prelog rules, assign the absolute configuration to each chiral center of ephedrine and pseudoephedrine (Fig. 2.21).
10. For the compounds shown in Figure 2.22, indicate, using an*, where the chiral centers are in each molecule.
11. Draw each possible stereoisomer for chloramphenicol and enalapril. Assign the absolute stereochemistry to each chiral center.
12. I. Draw the Newman projection along the CH_3–N bond of acetylcholine in the staggered conformation. Rotate the bond 120° and 240°. Are these rotameters conformational isomers? Explain why or why not.
    II. Repeat the above exercise with the N1–C2 bond of acetylcholine.
13. Draw the three most stable rotameters of norepinephrine. Of these rotameters, is there the possibility of an intramolecular interaction that would stabilize what normally would be considered an unstable rotameter? Explain.

TABLE 2.12 Drug Structures not Included in Text for Problems at End of Chapter 2

Problem #	Drug Name	Drug structure
3	Sulfacetamide	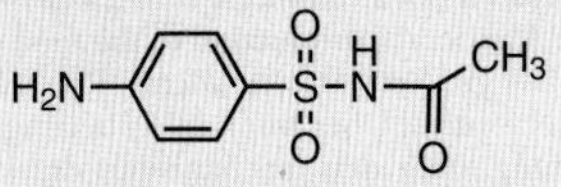
6 + 7	Aspirin	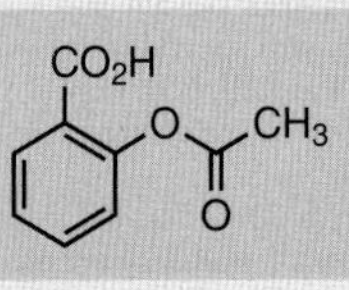
6 + 7	Chlordiazepoxide	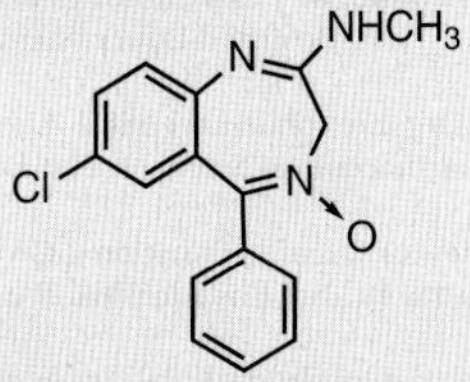
6 + 7	Carphenazine maleate	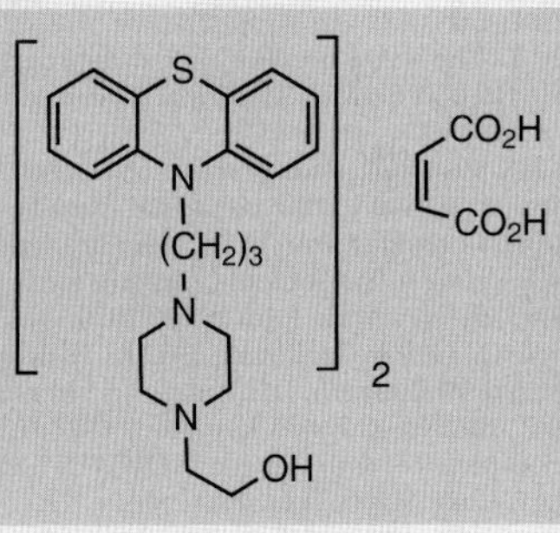
6 + 7	Codeine	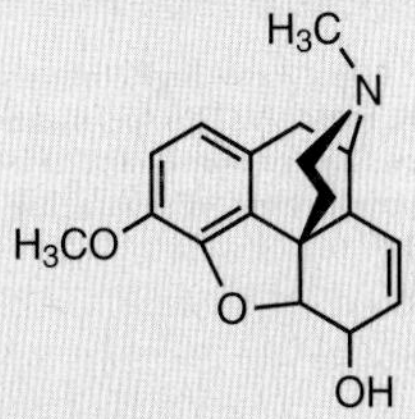
6 + 7	Cyproheptadine	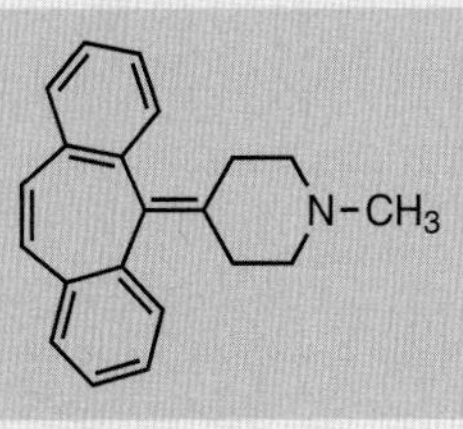
6 + 7	Phenytoin	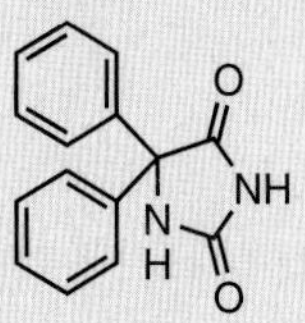
6 + 7	Haloperidol	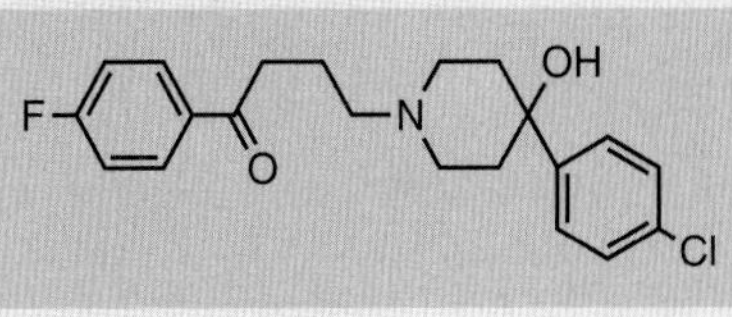
11	Chloramphenicol	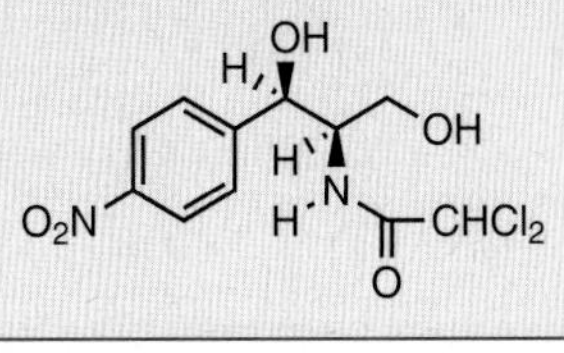

References

1. Crum-Brown A, Fraser TR. On the connection between chemical constitution and physiological action. Part 1: on the physiological action of the ammonium bases derived from Strychia, Brucia, Thebia, Codeia, Morphia, and Nicotia. Trans R Soc Edinburgh 1869;25:257–274.
2. Ariëns EJ. A general introduction to the field of drug discovery. In: Ariëns EJ, ed. Drug Design. New York: Academic Press, 1971:689–696.
3. Loewi O, Navrati E. Über humorale übertragbarkeit der herznervenwirkung XI mitteilung. über den mechanismus der vaguswirkung von physostigmin und ergotamine. Plugers Arch Ges Physiol Menshen Tiere 1926;214:689–696.
4. Ehrlich P. On immunity with special reference to cell life. In: Himmelweit F, ed. Collected Papers of Paul Ehrlich. London: Pergamon, 1957:178–195.
5. Albert A. The long search for valid structure–action relationships in drugs. J Med Chem 1982;25:1–5.
6. Ing HR. The curariform action of onium salts. Physiol Rev 1936;16:527–544.
7. Woods DD. The relation of *p*-aminobenzoic acid to the mechanism of the action of sulfanilamide. Br J Exp Pathol 1940;21:74–90.
8. Kauffman GB. The Brönsted-Lowry acid-base concept. J Chem Ed 1988;85:28–31.
9. Gennaro AR. Organic pharmaceutical chemistry. In: Gennaro AR, ed. Remington's Pharmaceutical Sciences, 21st Ed. Easton, PA: Mack Publishing, 2006:386–409.
10. Lemke TL. Review of Organic Functional Groups: Introduction to Medicinal Organic Chemistry, 4th Ed. Philadelphia, PA: Lippincott Williams & Wilkins, 2003.
11. Cates LA. Calculation of drug solubilities by pharmacy students. Am J Pharm Ed 1981;45:11–13.
12. Fujita T. The extrathermodynamic approach to drug design. In: Hansch C, ed. Comprehensive Medicinal Chemistry. New York: Pergamon Press, 1990;4:497–560.
13. Tute MS. Principles and practice of Hansch analysis: a guide to structure–activity correlation for the medicinal chemist. In: Harper NJ, Simons AB, eds. Advances in Drug Research. London: Academic Press, 1971:1–77.
14. Hansch C, Leo A. Substituent Constants for Correlation Analysis in Chemistry and Biology. New York: John Wiley, 1979.
15. Hansch C, Leo A. Exploring QSAR: Hydrophobic, Electronic, and Steric Constants. Washington, DC: American Chemical Society, 1995.
16. ClogP®, BioByte Corp., Claremont, CA; ACDLogP®, Advanced Chemistry Development Toronto Canada; KOWWIN®, Chemaxon, Budapest, Hungary; CSLogP, ChemSilico, Tewksbury, MA.
17. Molinspiration Chemoinformatics. http://www.molinspiration.com, accessed March 6, 2010.
18. Interactive Analysis. http://www.logP.com, accessed March 6, 2007.
19. Cahn RS, Ingold CK, Prelog V. The specification of asymmetric configuration in organic chemistry. Experientia 1956;12:81–94.
20. Piutti A. Su rune nouvelle espec d'asparagine. Compt Red 1886;103:134–138.
21. Easson LH, Stedman E. Studies on the relationship between chemical constitution and physiological action. V. Molecular dissymmetry and physiological activity. Biochem J 1933;27:1257–1266.
22. Blackwood JE, Gladys CL, Loening KL, et al. Unambiguous specification of stereoisomerism about a double bond. J Am Chem Soc 1968;90:509–510.
23. Kemp JD, Pitzer KS. Hindered rotation of the methyl groups in ethane. J Chem Phys 1936;4:749.
24. Bovet D, Staub A. Action protectice des ethers phenoliques au cours de l'intoxication histaminique. C R Soc Biol (Paris) 1937;124:547–549.
25. Laborit H, Huguenard P, Alluaume R. Un nouveau stabilisateur vegetatif, le 4560 RP. Presse Med 1952;60:206–208.
26. Charpentier P, Gaillot P, Jacob R, et al. Recherches sur les dimethylaminopropyl N-phenothiazines. C R Acad Sci (Paris) 1952;325:59–60.
27. Delay J, Deniker P, Hurl JM. Utilisation en thirapeutique psychiatrique d'une phenothiazine d'action centrale elective. Ann Med Psychol (Paris) 1952;110:112–117.
28. McCawley EL, Hart ER, Marsh DF. The preparation of *N*-allylnormorphine. J Am Chem Soc 1941;63:314.
29. Clark RL, Pessolano AA, Weijlard J, et al. *N*-substituted epoxymorphinans. J Am Chem Soc 1953;75:4964–4967.
30. Langmuir I. The arrangement of electrons in atoms and molecules. J Am Chem Soc 1919;41:868–934.
31. Langmuir I. Isomorphism, isosterism, and covalence. J Am Chem Soc 1919;41:1543–1559.
32. Grimm HG. Über ban und grösse der nichtmetallhydride. Z Elekrochemie 1925;31:474–480.
33. Hinsberg O. The sulfur atom. J Prakt Chem 1916;93:302–311.
34. Friedman HL. Influence of isosteric replacements upon biological activity. In: Symposium on Chemical–Biological Correlation. Publication 206. Washington, DC: National Academy of Science, 1951:206:295–358.
35. Burger A. Isosterism and bioisosterism in drug design. Prog Drug Res 1991;37:288–371.
36. Grisar JM, Marciniak G, Bolkenius FN, et al. Cardioselective ammonium, phosphonium, and sulfonium analogues of α-tocopherol and ascorbic acid that inhibit in vitro and ex vivo lipid peroxidation and scavenge superoxide radicals. J Med Chem 1995;38:2880–2886.
37. Dodds EC, Goldberg L, Lawson W, et al. Estrogenic activity of certain synthetic compounds. Nature 1938;141:247–248.
38. Walton E, Brownlee G. Isomers of stilbestrol and its esters. Nature 1943;151:305–306.
39. Blanchard EW, Stuart AH, Tallman RC. Studies on a new series of synthetic estrogenic substances. Endocrinology 1943;32:307–309.
40. Baker BR. Some analogues of hexestrol. J Am Chem Soc 1943;65:1572–1579.
41. Larsen AA, Gould WA, Roth HR, et al. Sulfonanilides. II. Analogues of catecholamines. J Med Chem 1967;10:462–472.
42. Patani GA, LaVoie EJ. Bioisosterism: a rational approach in drug design. Chem Rev 1996;96:3147–3176.

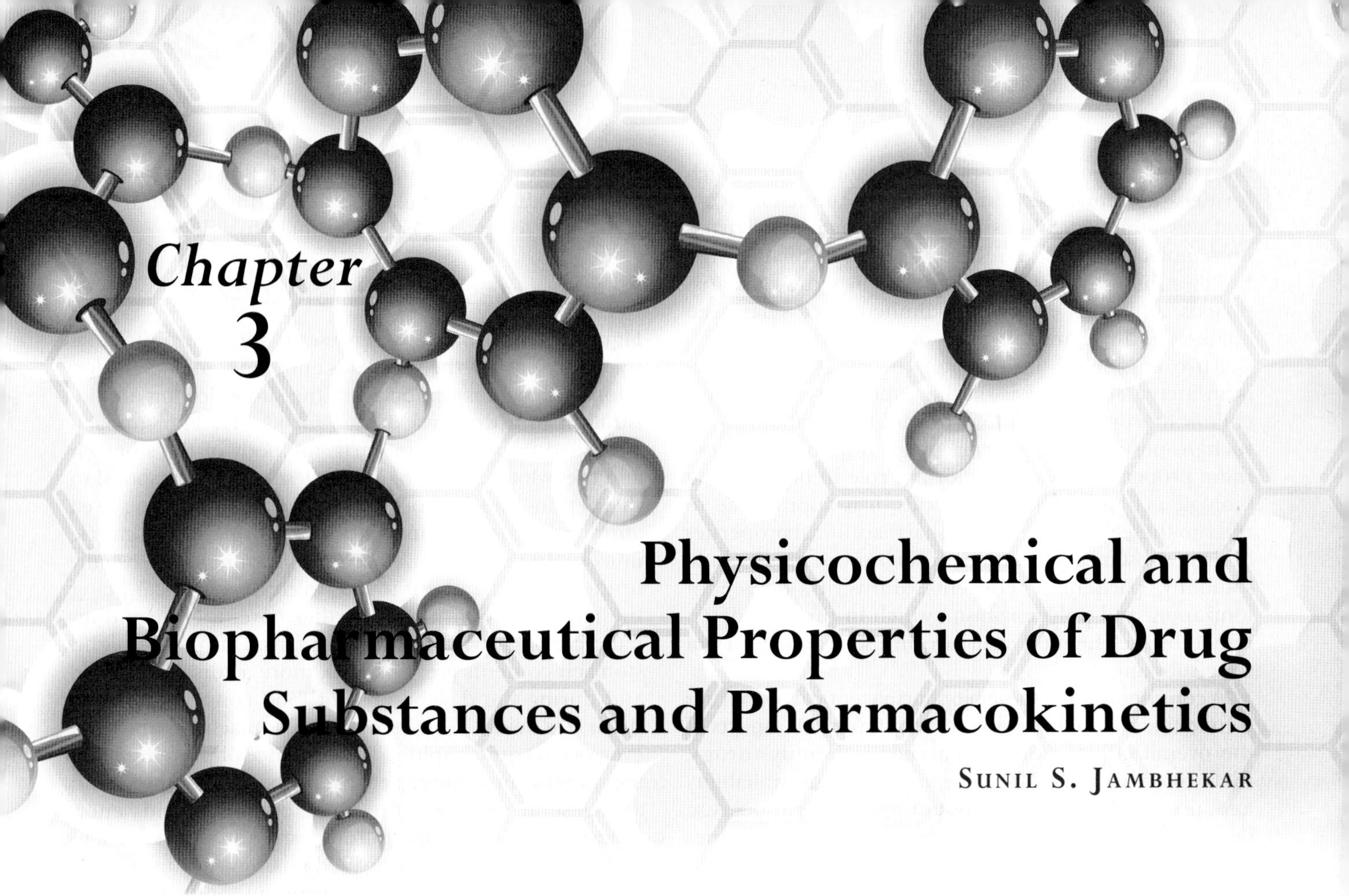

Chapter 3

Physicochemical and Biopharmaceutical Properties of Drug Substances and Pharmacokinetics

Sunil S. Jambhekar

Abbreviations

ADME, absorption, distribution, metabolism, and excretion
AP, absorption potential
ATP, adenosine 5′-triphosphate
ANDA, Abbreviated New Drug Application
AUC, area under the plasma concentration–time curve
$(AUC)_0^\infty$, total area under the plasma concentration–time curve
AUMC, area under the first-moment curve
Cl, clearance
C_o, concentration of drug in the organic or oil phase
$(C_p)_{max}$, plasma peak concentration
C_s, solubility
dC, concentration gradient
ER, extraction ratio
f, bioavailability
F, absolute bioavailability
FDA, U.S. Food and Drug Administration
F_{uni}, fraction of un-ionized form
HCl, hydrochloric acid
IM, intramuscular
IV, intravenous
K, elimination rate constant
K_m, the concentration of drug at half the V_{max}
MAD, maximum absorbable dose
MAT, mean absorption time
MDCK, Madin-Darby canine kidney
MRT, mean residence time
NDA, New Drug Application
P* or log *P, partition coefficient
P_{aq}, aqueous permeability
P-gp, P-glycoprotein
pK_a, the negative logarithm of a dissociation constant, K_a
pK_w, negative logarithm of dissociation constant of water
PSA, polar surface area
PSAd, dynamic polar surface area
P_w, permeability of a drug in the gut wall
Q, blood flow rate
SC, subcutaneous
SITT, small intestinal transit time
SIV, small intestinal volume
S_o, intrinsic solubility
$t_{1/2}$, half-life
t_{max}, peak time
V, volume of distribution
V_1, volume of the luminal content
V_{max}, maximum theoretical transfer rate

Throughout its history, the pharmacy profession has been concerned primarily with the manner in which drugs produce their pharmacologic effects and the dosage forms through which drugs are administered. Since the early 20th century, efforts have been directed to determining, understanding, and providing rational explanations of drug effects on biologic systems, but we have been limited by our ability to correlate the observed physiologic events with a reasonable hypothesis or concept. Pharmacists, at one time, were closely involved in formulating a prescription written by a physician for a patient. Today, most of the formulating is done by the pharmaceutical manufacturer.

Early descriptions of drug action were confined to their reference as tonic or toxic effects. This approach was followed by the concept of receptor theory, which for decades remained primarily an operational concept that was useful for discussing the new actions of drugs on a molecular level (1). Research in receptor theories, however, has provided evidence that the drug receptors do exist as distinct entities, and limited success has been attained in the characterization of receptors (2,3).

An extension of the receptor theory of drug action is an increased emphasis on the importance of physicochemical properties of the drug and the relationship of such properties to the pharmacologic responses. Because these properties have an important role in determining biologic action of pharmaceuticals, it is appropriate to refer to these properties as biopharmaceutical properties of drug substances. Examples of such properties include solubility, partition coefficients, diffusivity, degree of ionization, and polymorphism, which in turn are determined by the chemical structure and stereochemistry of drug substances.

A consideration of these biopharmaceutical properties is fundamental to discussing several important aspects of the overall effects. For a given chemical entity (drug), there often will be a difference in physiologic availability and, presumably, in clinical responses, primarily because drug molecules must cross various biologic membranes and interact with intercellular and intracellular fluids before reaching the elusive region termed the "site of action." Under these conditions, the biopharmaceutical properties of the drug must contribute favorably to facilitate absorption and distribution processes to augment the drug concentration at various active sites. Furthermore, equally important is the fact that these biopharmaceutical properties of a drug must ensure a specific orientation on the receptor surface so that a sequence of events is initiated that leads to the observed pharmacologic effects. Drug molecules that are deficient in the required biopharmaceutical properties can display generally marginal pharmacologic action or be totally ineffective.

Biopharmaceutics is the study of the influence of formulation factors on the therapeutic activity of a drug product or dosage forms. It involves the study of the relationship between some of the physicochemical properties of a drug and the biologic effects observed after the administration of a drug via various dosage forms or drug delivery systems. Almost any alteration in a drug delivery system is likely to alter the drug delivery rate and the amount of the drug delivered to the desired place in the body. This includes the chemical nature of the drug (e.g., ester, salts, complexes), the particle size and surface area of the drug, the type of dosage forms (e.g., solution, suspension, capsule, tablet), and the excipients and processes used in the manufacturing of the drug delivery systems.

Drugs, via drug delivery systems, are most often administered to human subjects by the oral route. Compared to other routes of drug administration, especially the intravenous route, the oral route is unusually complex with respect to the physicochemical conditions existing at the absorption site. Therefore, before we discuss how the biopharmaceutical properties of a drug in a dosage form can affect the availability and action of that drug, it is prudent to review gastrointestinal physiology.

GASTROINTESTINAL PHYSIOLOGY

Figure 3.1 schematically represents the gastrointestinal tract and some of the problems encountered in consideration of drug absorption from the site following administration of a drug via dosage forms (4). The stomach is divided into two main parts: the body of the stomach and the pylorus. Histologically, these parts correspond to the pepsin- and hydrochloric acid (HCl)-secreting area and the mucus-secreting area, respectively, of the gastric mucosa. In the human, the stomach contents are usually in the pH range of 1.0 to 3.5, with pH 1.0 to 2.5 being the most common range. Furthermore, there is a diurnal cycle of gastric acidity in humans. During the night, stomach contents are, as a rule, more acidic (pH, ~1.3), and during the day, because of food consumption, the pH is less acidic. The recovery of stomach acidity, however, occurs quite rapidly. The presence of protein, being amphoteric in nature, acts as an excellent buffer, and as digestion proceeds, the liberated amino acids enormously increase the neutralizing capacity of the stomach.

The small intestine is divided anatomically into three sections: the duodenum, the jejunum, and the ileum. All three areas are involved in the digestion and absorption of food. The available absorbing area is increased by surface folds in the intestinal lining. The surface of these folds possesses villi and microvilli, which are tiny, finger-like projections that protrude from the epithelial lining of the intestinal wall as shown in Figure 3.2. The pH of the duodenal contents in the human is usually in the range of 5 to 7. There is a gradual decrease in acidity along the length of the gastrointestinal tract, with the ultimate pH being 7 to 8 in the lower ileum. It has been estimated that approximately 8 L of fluid enter the upper intestine per day, with approximately 7 L of this arising from digestive juices and fluids and approximately 1 L arising from oral intake. Over the entire length of the large and small intestine and the stomach is the brush border, which consists of a uniform coating (thickness, 3 mm) of mucopolysaccharide. This coating layer serves as a mechanical barrier to bacteria or food particles.

When a dosage form containing a drug or drug molecules moves from the stomach through the pylorus into the duodenum, the dosage form encounters a rapidly changing environment with respect to pH. Furthermore, digestive juices secreted into the small bowel contain many enzymes not found in the gastric juices. Digestion and absorption of foodstuff occur simultaneously in the small intestine. Intestinal digestion is the terminal phase of preparing foodstuff for absorption and consists of two processes: completion of the hydrolysis of large molecules to smaller ones, which are absorbed, and converting the finished product of hydrolysis into an aqueous solution or emulsion.

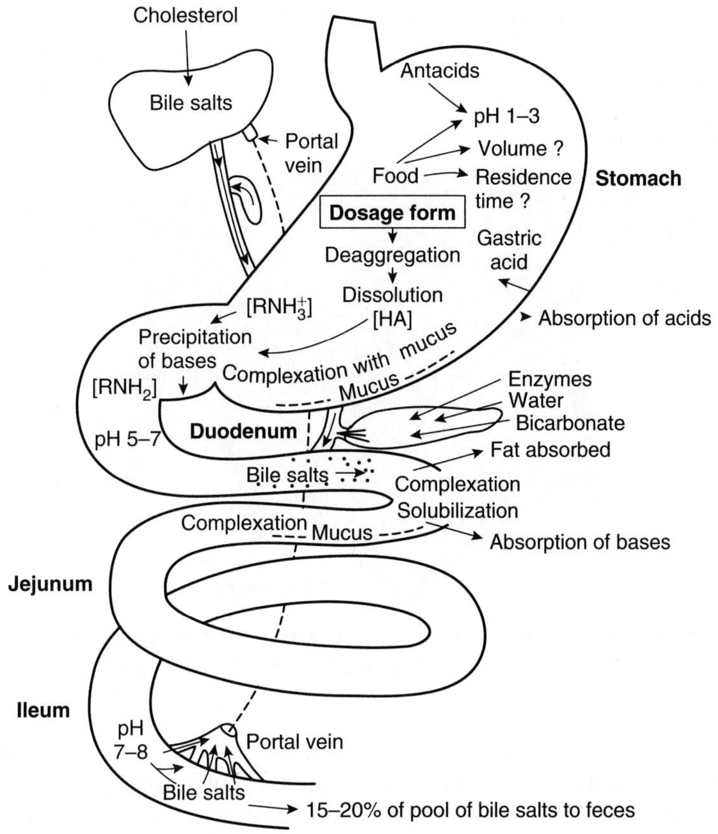

FIGURE 3.1 Processes occurring along with drug absorption when drug molecules travel down the gastrointestinal tract and the factors that affect drug absorption. (From Florence AT, Attwood D. Physiochemical Principles of Pharmacy, 2nd Ed. New York: Chapman and Hall, 1988, with permission.) (21).

Drug absorption, whether from the gastrointestinal tract or from other sites, requires the passage of the drug in a molecular form across the barrier membrane. Most drugs are presented to the body as solid or semisolid dosage forms, and the drug particles must first be released from these dosage forms. These drug particles must dissolve, and if they possess the desirable biopharmaceutical properties, they will pass from a region of high concentration to a region of low concentration across the membrane into the blood or general circulation (Fig. 3.3). Knowledge of biologic membrane structure and its general properties is pivotal in understanding absorption processes and the role of the biopharmaceutical properties of drug substances.

Biologic Membrane

The prevalent view of the gastrointestinal membrane is that it consists of a bimolecular lipoid layer covered on each side by protein, with the lipid molecule oriented perpendicular to the cell surface as shown in Figure 3.4. The lipid layer is interrupted by small, water-filled pores with a radius of approximately 4 Å. A molecule with a radius of 4 Å or less can easily pass through these water-filled pores. Thus, membranes have a specialized transport system to assist the passage of water-soluble material and ions through the lipid interior, a process sometimes termed "convective absorption." The rate of permeation of such

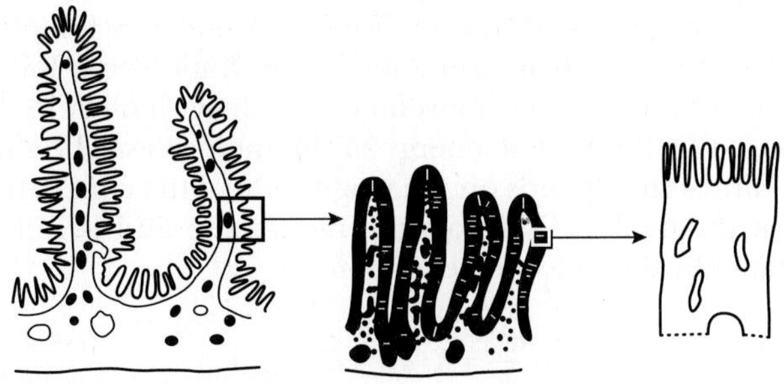

FIGURE 3.2 The epithelium of the small intestine at different levels of magnification. From left to right: the intestinal villi and microvilli that constitute the brush border.

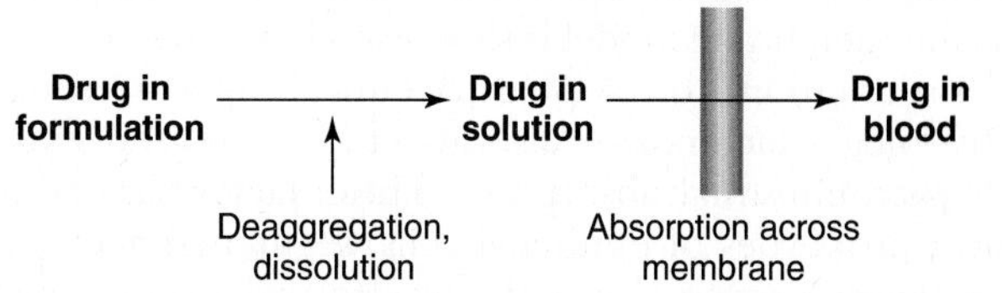

FIGURE 3.3 Sequence of events in drug absorption from formulations of solid dosage forms.

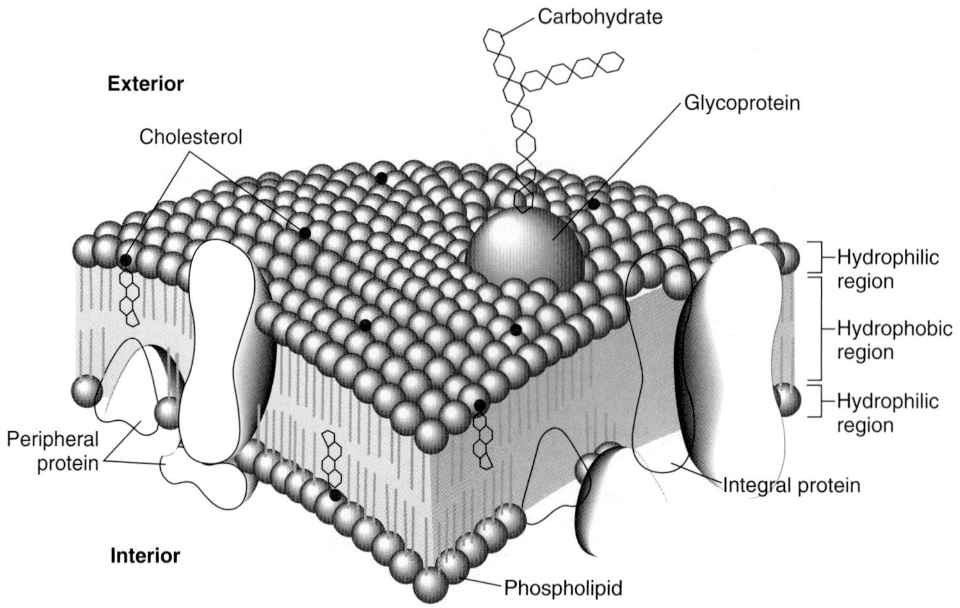

FIGURE 3.4 Basic structure of an animal cell membrane. (From Smith C, Marks A, Lieberman M, eds. Basic Medical Biochemistry. Baltimore: Lippincott Williams & Wilkins, 2004:159–163, with permission.)

small molecules through the pore is affected not only by the relative sizes of the holes and the molecules, but also by the interaction between permeating molecules and the membrane. When permeation through the membrane occurs, the permeating substance is considered to have transferred from solution in the luminal aqueous phase to the lipid membrane phase, then to the aqueous phase on the other side of the membrane. Biologic membranes differ from a polymeric membrane in that they are composed of small amphipathic molecules, phospholipids, and cholesterol. The protein layer associated with membranes is hydrophobic in nature. Therefore, biologic membranes have a hydrophilic exterior and a hydrophobic interior. Cholesterol is a major component of most mammalian biologic membranes, and its removal renders the membrane highly permeable. Cholesterol complexes with phospholipids, and its presence reduces the permeability of the membrane to water, cations, glycerides, and glucose. The shape of the cholesterol molecule allows it to fit closely with the hydrocarbon chains of unsaturated fatty acids in the bilayer. It is the general opinion that the cholesterol makes the membrane more rigid. The flexibility of the biologic membrane to reform and adapt to a changing environment is its important feature. The details of membrane structure are still widely debated, and a more recent membrane model is shown in Figure 3.4.

In addition to biopharmaceutical factors, several physiologic factors can also affect the rate and extent of gastrointestinal absorption. These factors are as follows: properties of epithelial cells, segmental activity of the bowel, degree of vascularity, effective absorbing surface area per unit length of gut, surface and interfacial tensions, electrolyte content and their concentration in luminal fluid, enzymatic activity in the luminal contents, and gastric emptying rate of the drug from stomach.

Mechanisms of Drug Absorption

Drug transfer is often viewed as the movement of a drug molecule across a series of membranes and spaces (Fig. 3.5), which, in aggregate, serve as a macroscopic membrane. The cells and interstitial spaces lying between the gastric lumen and the capillary blood or structure between the sinusoidal space and the bile canaliculi are examples. Each of the cellular membranes and spaces can impede drug transport to varying degrees; therefore, any one of them is a rate-limiting step to the overall process of drug transport. This complexity of structure makes quantitative prediction of drug transport difficult. A qualitative description of the processes of drug transport across functional membranes follows.

Passive Diffusion

The transfer of most drugs across a biologic membrane occurs by passive diffusion, a natural tendency for molecules to move from a higher concentration to a lower concentration. This movement of drug molecules is caused by the kinetic energy of the molecules. The rate of diffusion depends on the magnitude of the concentration gradient (dC) across the membrane and is represented by the following equation:

3.1
$$-\frac{dC}{dt} = K \cdot dC = K(C_{\text{abs}} - C_{\text{b}})$$

where $-dC/dt$ is the rate of diffusion across a membrane; K is a complex proportionality constant that includes the

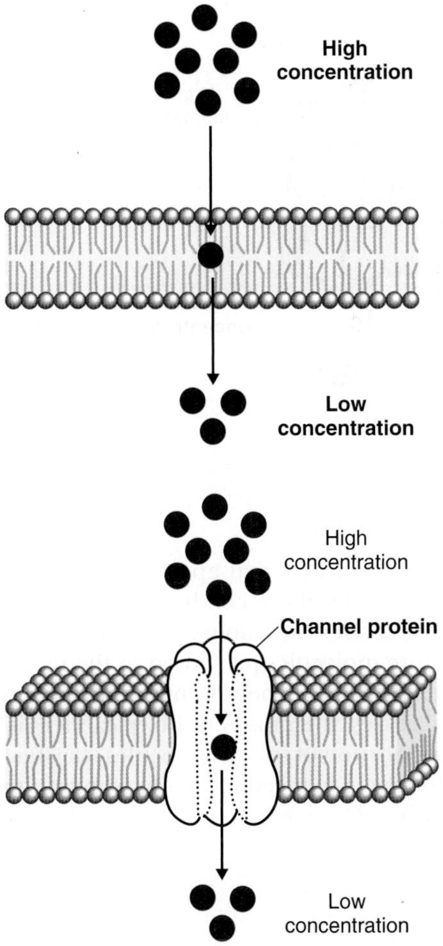

FIGURE 3.5 (A) Simple diffusion. (B). Membrane channels. (From Smith C, Marks A, Lieberman M, eds. Basic Medical Biochemistry. Baltimore: Lippincott Williams & Wilkins, 2004:159–163, with permission.)

area of membrane, the thickness of the membrane, the partition coefficient of the drug molecule between the lipophilic membrane and the aqueous phase on each side of the membrane, and the diffusion coefficient of the drug; C_{abs} is the drug concentration at the absorption site; and C_b is the drug concentration in the blood.

The gastrointestinal absorption of a drug from an aqueous solution requires transfer from the lumen to the gut wall followed by penetration of the epithelial membrane by a drug molecule to the capillaries of the systemic circulation. On entering the blood, the drug distributes itself rapidly in the blood. Because of the volume differences at absorption and distribution sites, the drug concentration in blood (C_b) will be much lower than the concentration at the absorption site (C_{abs}). This concentration gradient is maintained throughout the absorption process—that is, ($C_{abs} - C_b$). As a result, the concentration gradient (dC in Eq. 3.1), is approximately equal to C_{abs}, so Equation 3.1 is written as:

3.2 $$-\frac{dC}{dt} = K \cdot C_1$$

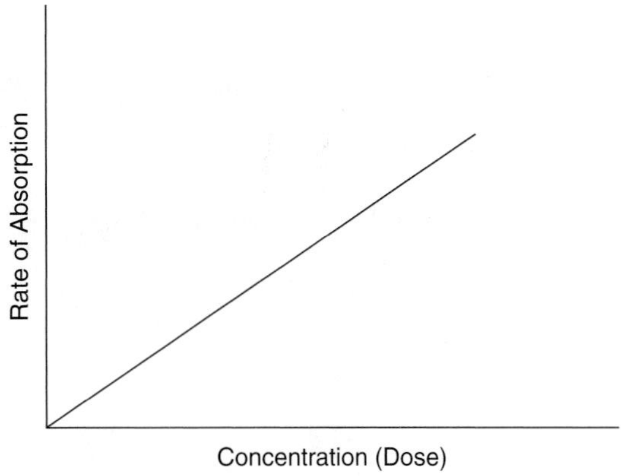

FIGURE 3.6 Effect of drug concentration on the rate of absorption when passive diffusion is operative.

Because absorption by passive diffusion is a first-order process, the rate of absorption (dC/dt in Eq. 3.2) is directly proportional to the concentration at the site of absorption (C_1). The greater the concentration of drug at the absorption site, the faster is the rate of absorption (Fig. 3.6). The percentage of dose absorbed at any time, however, remains unchanged.

A major source of variation is membrane permeability, which depends on the lipophilicity of the drug molecule. This is often characterized by its partition between oil and water. The lipid solubility of a drug, therefore, is a very important physicochemical property governing the rate of transfer through a variety of biologic membrane barriers. Figure 3.7 illustrates the role of partition coefficients in the

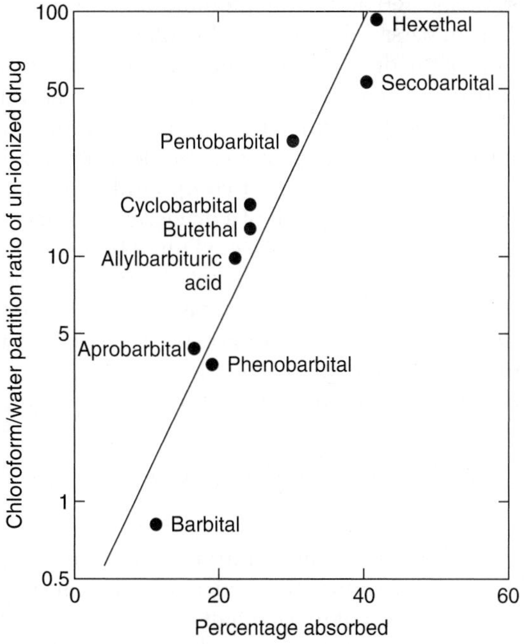

FIGURE 3.7 Comparison between colonic absorption of barbiturates in the rat and lipid-to-water partition coefficient of the un-ionized form of the barbiturates. (From Schanker LS. Absorption of drugs from the colon. J Pharmacol Exp Ther 1959;126:283–294, with permission.) (6).

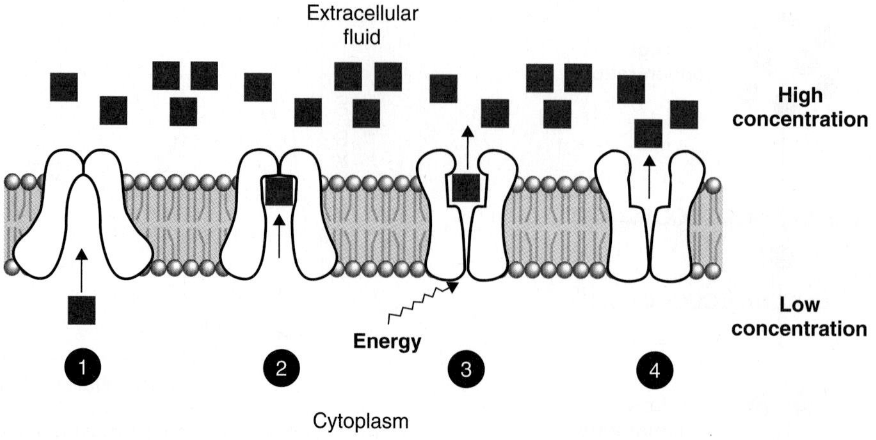

FIGURE 3.8 Active transport. (From Smith C, Marks A, Lieberman M, eds. Basic Medical Biochemistry. Baltimore: Lippincott Williams & Wilkins, 2004:159–163, with permission.)

drug absorption process from the colon and that a good correlation exists between the percentage of drug absorption and the partition coefficient of an un-ionized drug.

Carrier-Mediated or Active Transport

Although most drugs are absorbed from the gastrointestinal tract by passive diffusion, some drugs of therapeutic interest and some chemicals of nutritional value, such as amino acids, dipeptides and tripeptides, glucose, and folic acid, are absorbed by the action of transporter proteins (i.e., a carrier-mediated transport mechanism) (Fig. 3.8). In this type of transport, membranes have a specialized role. The usual requirement for active transport is structural similarities between the drug and the substrate normally transported across the membrane. Active transport differs from passive diffusion in the following ways: 1) The transport of the drug occurs against a concentration gradient; 2) the transport mechanism can become saturated at high drug concentration; and 3) a specificity for a certain molecular structure can promote competition in the presence of a similarly structured compound. This, in turn, can decrease the absorption of a drug. Active or facilitated absorption of a drug is usually explained by assuming that transporter proteins (i.e., carriers in membranes) are responsible for shuttling these solutes in mucosal or serosal direction. The number of apparent carriers in membranes, however, is limited. Therefore, the rate of transfer or absorption is described by the following equation:

3.3 $$\text{Absorption rate} = \frac{dC}{dt} = V_{\max} \cdot C/K_{\mathrm{m}} + C$$

where C is the solute concentration at the absorption site, and $V_{\max}$ (the maximum theoretical transfer rate) and K_{m} (the concentration of drug at half the $V_{\max}$) are constants. Low doses or concentrations, when $K_{\mathrm{m}} >>> C$, reduce Equation 3.3 to:

3.4 $$\frac{dC}{dt} = \frac{V_{\max}}{K_{\mathrm{m}} \cdot C} = K_m \cdot C$$

Equation 3.4 indicates that apparent first-order kinetics is observed. Under these conditions, there are sufficient numbers of carriers available so that a constant proportion of solute molecules presented to the membrane are transported across the membranes. As the solute concentration increases, the number of free carriers is reduced, and the proportion of solute molecules transferred across the membrane is reduced until a maximum saturation is reached, when $C >>> K_{\mathrm{m}}$:

3.5 $$\text{Absorption rate} = \frac{dC}{dt} = V_{\max}$$

Equation 3.5 indicates that a further increase in solute concentration will not result in any further increase in the rate of absorption (Fig. 3.9). The capacity-limited characteristics of carrier-mediated processes suggest that the bioavailability of drugs absorbed in this manner should decrease nonlinearly with increasing doses.

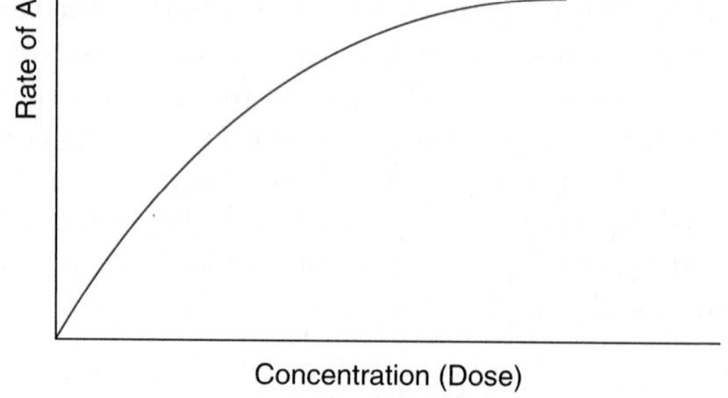

FIGURE 3.9 Relationship between drug concentration and rate of absorption when an active transport process is operative.

Therefore, the use of a large, single oral dose of these drugs is irrational, and if larger daily doses are necessary, one should use divided doses. Examples of substances that are actively transported include amino acids, methyldopa, fluorouracil, penicillamine, and levodopa.

Convective Absorption

The absorption of small molecules (molecular radii less than ~4 Å) through water-filled pores of biologic membrane is referred to as convective absorption. The rate of absorption because of this mechanism is equated to the product of a sieving coefficient, the rate of fluid or water absorption, and the concentration of solute in the luminal content. The sieving coefficient is indirectly related to the relative sizes of the pores and the molecules.

Ion-Pair Absorption In 1967, Higuchi suggested that highly ionized compounds, such as quaternary ammonium compounds, can possibly be absorbed by an ion-pair mechanism (5). In vitro, a relatively large organic anion can combine with a relatively large cation to form an ion pair of neutral properties, which will then cross a water–organic solvent interface and transfer to an organic phase.

PHYSICOCHEMICAL FACTORS AFFECTING DRUG ABSORPTION

The pH-Partition Hypothesis on Drug Absorption

Drug absorption is influenced by many physiologic factors. Additionally, it also depends on many physicochemical properties of the drug itself. Some investigators (6–12) concluded from their research that most drugs are absorbed from the gastrointestinal tract by a process of passive diffusion of the un-ionized moiety across a lipid membrane. Furthermore, the dissociation constant, lipid solubility, and pH of the fluid at the absorption site determine the extent of absorption from a solution. The interrelationship among these parameters is known as the pH-partition theory. This theory provides a basic framework for the understanding of drug absorption from the gastrointestinal tract and drug transport across the biologic membrane. The principle points of this theory are as follows:

1. The gastrointestinal and other biologic membranes act like lipid barriers.
2. The un-ionized form of the acidic or basic drug is preferentially absorbed.
3. Most drugs are absorbed by passive diffusion.
4. The rate of drug absorption and amount of drug absorbed are related to the drug's oil–water partition coefficient (i.e., the more lipophilic the drug, the faster is its absorption).
5. Weak acidic and neutral drugs are absorbed from the stomach, but basic drugs are not.

When a drug is administered intravenously, it is immediately available to body fluids for distribution to the site of action. However, all extravascular routes, such as oral, intramuscular, sublingual, buccal, subcutaneous, dermal, rectal, and nasal routes, can influence the overall therapeutic activity of the drug, primarily because of its dissolution rate, a step that is necessary for a drug to be available in a solution form. When a drug is administered orally in a dosage form such as a tablet, capsule, or suspension, the rate of absorption across the biologic membrane frequently is controlled by the slowest step in the following sequence:

$$\text{Dosage form} \xrightarrow{\text{dissolution}} \text{Drug in solution} \xrightarrow{\text{absorption}} \text{Drug in general circulation}$$

In many instances, the slowest step, or the rate-limiting step, in the sequence is the dissolution of the drug. When dissolution is the controlling step, any factors that affect the rate of dissolution must also influence the rate of absorption. This, in turn, affects the extent and duration of action. Several factors can influence the dissolution rate of drug from solid dosage forms and, therefore, the therapeutic activity. These factors include solubility of a drug, particle size and surface area of drug particles, crystalline and salt form of a drug, and rate of disintegration.

The absorption rate of drugs is also affected by interaction or formation of complexes in the gastrointestinal tract. Generally, such complex formation reduces the concentration of free drug at the absorption site. Because the complexed drug is absorbed either slowly or not at all, the net effect is the reduction of concentration of drug at the absorption site and slower rate of absorption.

Ionization and pH at Absorption Site

The fraction of the drug existing in its un-ionized form in a solution is a function of both the dissociation constant of a drug and the pH of the solution at the absorption site. The dissociation constant, for both weak acids and bases, is often expressed as the pK_a (the negative logarithm of a dissociation constant, K_a). The Henderson-Hasselbalch equation (Eq. 3.6) for the ionization of a weak acid, HA, is presented below.

3.6 $$\text{pH} - \text{p}K_a = \log \frac{[\text{Ionized}]}{[\text{Un-ionized}]}$$

Assuming that α is the fraction of ionized species and that 1 − α is the fraction remaining as the un-ionized form, Equation 3.6 is written as

3.7 $$\text{pH} - \text{p}K_a = \log \frac{\alpha}{1-\alpha}$$

or

3.8 $$\frac{\alpha}{1-\alpha} = \text{antilog}\,(\text{pH} - \text{p}K_a)$$

From Equation 3.8, the fraction or percentage of the absorbable and nonabsorbable forms of a weak acid can be calculated if the pH condition at the site of administration is known. Analogously, the dissociation or basicity constant for a weak base is derived as follows:

3.9 $$pK_a + pK_b = pK_w$$

where pK_w is the negative logarithm of dissociation constant of water. Although the dissociation constant of a weak base is described by the term K_b, it is conventionally expressed in terms of K_a, because of the relationship expressed in Equation 3.9.

3.10 $$pK_a - \mathrm{pH} = \log\frac{[\text{Ionized}]}{[\text{Un-ionized}]}$$

Again, assuming that α is the fraction of ionized species and that 1 − α is the fraction of un-ionized species, Equation 3.10 becomes

3.11 $$pK_a - \mathrm{pH} = \log\frac{\alpha}{1-\alpha}$$

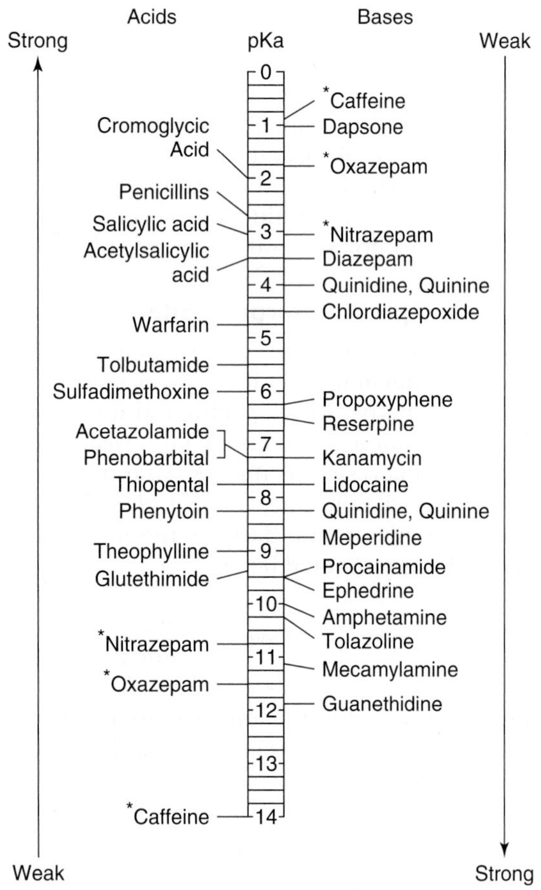

FIGURE 3.10 The pK_a values of certain acidic and basic drugs. Drugs denoted with an asterisk are amphoteric (13). (From Rowland M, Tozer T. Clinical Pharmacokinetics: Concepts and Application, 2nd Ed. Philadelphia: Lea and Febiger, 1989, with permission.)

or

3.12 $$\frac{\alpha}{1-\alpha} = \text{antilog}\,(pK_a - \mathrm{pH})$$

From Equation 3.12, one can calculate the fraction or percentage of absorbable and nonabsorbable form of a weak base if the pH condition at the site of drug absorption is known. Figure 3.10 shows the pK_a values of several drugs and the relative acid or base strength of these compounds.

The relationship between pH and pK_a and the extent of ionization is given by Equations 3.8 and 3.12 for weak acids and weak bases, respectively. Accordingly, most weak acidic drugs are predominantly in the un-ionized form at lower pH of the gastric fluid and, therefore, are absorbed from the stomach as well as from the intestine. Some very weak acidic drugs, such as phenytoin and many barbiturates, the pK_a values of which are greater than 8.0, are essentially un-ionized at all pH values. Therefore, for these weak acidic drugs, transport is more rapid and independent of pH, provided that the un-ionized form is lipophilic or nonpolar. Furthermore, it is important to note that the fraction un-ionized changes dramatically only for weak acids with pK_a values between 3 and 7. Therefore, for the weak acids, a change in the rate of transport with pH is expected, as shown in Figure 3.11 (13). Although the transport of weak acids with pK_a values less than 3.0 should theoretically depend on pH, the fraction un-ionized is so low that transport across the gut membrane is slow even under the most acidic conditions.

Most weak bases are poorly absorbed, if at all, in the stomach, because they are present largely in the ionized form at pH 1 to 2. Codeine, a weak base with a pK_a of approximately 8, will have about 1 in every 1 million

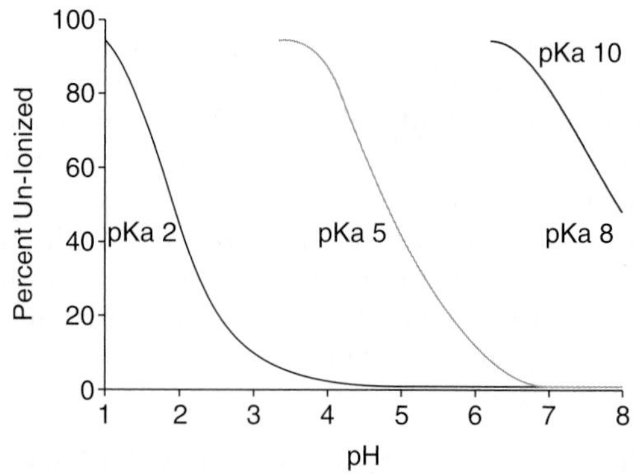

FIGURE 3.11 For very weak acids, pK_a values greater than 8.0 are predominantly un-ionized at all pH values between 1.0 and 8.0. Profound changes in the un-ionized fraction occur with pH for an acid with a pK_a value that lies within the range of 2.0 to 8.0. Although the fraction un-ionized of even strong acids increases with hydrogen ion concentration, the absolute value remains low at most pH values shown. (From Rowland M, Tozer T. Clinical Pharmacokinetics: Concepts and Application, 2nd Ed. Philadelphia: Lea and Febiger, 1989, with permission.) (13).

molecules in its un-ionized form at gastric pH 1.0. Weakly basic drugs with a pK_a of less than 4, such as dapsone, diazepam, and chlordiazepoxide, are essentially un-ionized through the intestine. Strong bases, which are those with pK_a values between 5 and 11, show pH-dependent absorption. Stronger bases, such as guanethidine ($pK_a > 11$) are ionized throughout the gastrointestinal tract and tend to be poorly absorbed.

The evidence of the importance of dissociation in drug absorption is found in the result of studies in which pH at the absorption site is changed (Tables 3.1 and 3.2). Table 3.2 clearly shows the decreased absorption of a weak acid at pH 8.0 compared to pH 1.0 (13). However, an increase to pH 8.0 promotes the absorption of a weak base with practically nothing absorbed at pH 1.0. The data in Table 3.2 also permit a comparison of intestinal absorption of acidic and basic drugs from buffered solutions ranging from pH 4.0 to 8.0 (14). These results are in agreement with the pH-partition hypothesis.

The pH-partition theory provides a basic framework for the understanding of drug absorption and, sometimes, is an oversimplification of a more complex process. For example, experimentally observed pH–absorption curves are less steep (Fig. 3.12) than those expected theoretically and are shifted to higher pH values for bases and lower pH values for acids. This deviation, observed experimentally, has been attributed by several investigators to factors such as limited absorption of ionized species of drugs, the presence of an unstirred diffusion layer adjacent to the cell membrane, and a difference between luminal pH and cell membrane surface pH.

Lipid Solubility

Partition Coefficient Some drugs are poorly absorbed after oral administration even though they are available predominantly in the un-ionized form in the gastrointestinal tract. This is attributed to the low lipid solubility of the un-ionized molecule. A guide to lipid solubility or lipophilic nature of a drug is provided by a property called the partition coefficient (P). Therefore, this parameter influences the transport and absorption processes of drugs, and it is one of the most widely used properties in quantitative structure–activity relationships (15) (see also Chapter 2).

TABLE 3.1 Comparison of Gastric Absorption of Acids and Bases at pH 1 and 8 in the Rat (13,44)

	pK_a	% Absorbed at pH 1	% Absorbed at pH 8
Acids			
5-Sulfosalicylic acid	<2.0	0	0
5-Nitrosalicylic acid	2.3	52	16
Salicylic acid	3.0	61	13
Thiopental	7.6	46	34
Bases			
Aniline	4.6	6	56
p-Toluidine	5.3	0	47
Quinine	8.4	0	18
Dextromethorphan	9.2	0	16

TABLE 3.2 Comparison of Intestinal Absorption of Acids and Bases in the Rat at Several pH Values (13,44)

		% Absorbed from Rat Intestine			
	pK_a	pH 4	pH 5	pH 7	pH 8
Acids					
5-Nitrosalicylic acid	2.3	40	27	0	0
Salicylic acid	3.0	64	35	30	10
Acetylsalicylic acid	3.5	41	27	—	—
Benzoic acid	4.2	62	36	35	5
Bases					
Aniline	4.6	40	48	58	61
Aminopyrine	5.0	21	35	48	52
p-Toluidine	5.3	30	42	65	64
Quinine	8.4	9	11	41	54

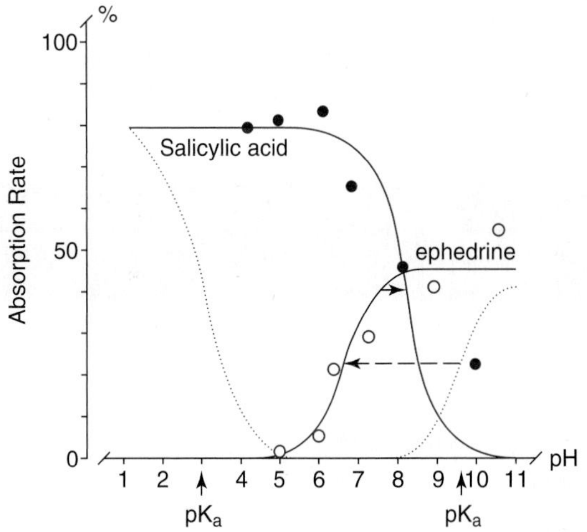

FIGURE 3.12 Relationship between absorption rates of salicylic acid and ephedrine and bulk phase pH in the rat small intestine in vivo. Dashed lines represent curves predicted by the pH-partition theory in the absence of an unstirred layer. (From Winne D. The influence of unstirred layers on intestinal absorption in intestinal permeation. In: Kramer M, Lauterbach F, eds. Workshop Conference Hoechest, Vol 4. Amsterdam: Excerpta Medica, 1977:58–64, with permission.) (16).

The movement of molecules from one phase to another is called partitioning. Drugs partition themselves between the aqueous phase and lipophilic membrane. Preservative emulsions partition between the water and oil phases; antibiotics partition from body fluids to microorganisms; and drug and other adjuvants can partition into the plastic and rubber stoppers of containers. Therefore, it is important that this process is understood.

If two immiscible phases are placed adjacent to each other, with one containing a solute soluble in both phases, the solute will distribute itself between two immiscible phases until equilibrium is attained; therefore, no further transfer of solute occurs. If we consider an aqueous (w) and an organic (o) phase, we write according to theory.

If the solute under consideration forms an ideal solution in either phases or in solvent, the activity coefficient can be replaced by the concentration term to yield Equation 3.13:

3.13 $$P = \frac{C_o}{C_w}$$

Equation 3.13 is used conventionally to calculate the partition coefficient of a drug. In Equation 3.13, C_o, the concentration of drug in the organic or oil phase, is divided by the concentration in the aqueous phase. The greater the value of P, the higher is the lipid solubility of the solute. It has been demonstrated for several systems that the partition coefficient can be approximated by the solubility of the solute in the organic phase divided by the solubility in the aqueous phase. Therefore, the partition coefficient is a measure of the relative affinities of the solute for an aqueous or nonaqueous or oil phase. The effect of lipid solubility and, hence, the partition coefficient on the absorption of a series of barbituric acid derivatives is shown in Table 3.3. The term partition coefficient is more commonly expressed exponentially as log P.

TABLE 3.3 Comparison of Barbiturate Absorption in Rat Colon and Partition Coefficient (Chloroform/Water) of Undissociated Drug (5,45)

Barbiturate	Partition Coefficient	% Absorbed
Barbital	0.7	12
Apobarbital	4.9	17
Phenobarbital	4.8	20
Allylbarbital	10.5	23
Butethal	11.7	24
Cyclobarbital	13.9	24
Pentobarbital	28.0	30
Secobarbital	50.7	40
Hexethal	>100	44

It must be clearly understood that even though drugs with greater lipophilicity and, therefore, partition coefficient are better absorbed, it is imperative that drugs exhibit some degree of aqueous solubility. This is essential, because the availability of the drug molecule in a solution form is a prerequisite for drug absorption and the biologic fluids at the site of absorption are aqueous in nature. Therefore, from a practical viewpoint, drugs must exhibit a balance between hydrophilicity and lipophilicity. This factor is always taken into account while a chemical modification is being considered as a way of improving the efficacy of a therapeutic agent.

Examples of polar or hydrophilic molecules that are poorly absorbed following oral administration and, therefore, must be administered parenterally include gentamicin, ceftriaxone, and streptokinase. Lipid-soluble drugs with favorable partition coefficients generally are well absorbed after oral administration. Often, the selection of a compound with higher partition coefficient from a series of research compounds provides improved pharmacologic activity. Occasionally, the structure of an existing drug is modified to develop a similar pharmacologic activity with improved absorption. Chlortetracycline, which differs from tetracycline by the substitution of a chlorine at C-7, substitution of an n-hexyl (hexethal) for a phenyl ring in phenobarbital, or replacement of the 2-carbonyl of pentobarbital with a 2-thio group (thiopental) are examples of enhanced lipophilicity (Fig. 3.13).

It is important to note that even a minor molecular modification of a drug can also promote the risk of altering the efficacy and safety profile of a drug. For this reason, medicinal chemists prefer the development of a lipid-soluble prodrug of a drug with poor oral absorption characteristics.

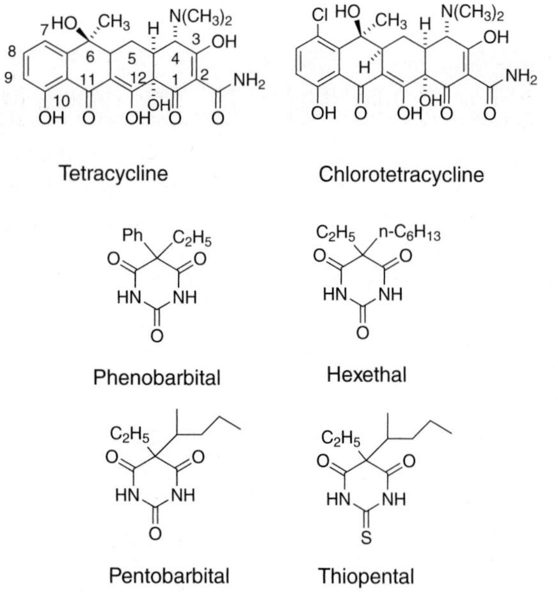

FIGURE 3.13 Drug pairs in which chemical modification enhances lipophilicity.

Estimation of Drug Absorption

When different chemical entities are being investigated for their potential as drug candidates, dosage form performance is one of the possible contributing factors to poor bioavailability. Historically, the concept of bioavailability is closely, if not solely, associated with dosage form performance. Because poor bioavailability in particular is increasingly an issue in the drug discovery and development process, application of the bioavailability principles and techniques has been extended to include animal studies in the selection of potential drug candidates for their full development (17,18).

As the drug travels down the gastrointestinal tract following its oral administration, part of the dose cannot be available for absorption for a number of reasons. These include its chemical degradation, physical inactivation because of binding and complexation with substances in the intestinal tract, incomplete dissolution of the dosage form, microbial metabolism, insufficient contact time in the gastrointestinal tract, poor solubility and poor permeability across the gastrointestinal mucosa, and metabolism within the gut wall. Of the absorbed dose, some of the drug is metabolized in transit during its first passage through the gut wall and the liver. Unchanged drug that reaches the hepatic portal vein can be extracted by the liver via metabolism or biliary excretion. Thus, the bioavailability (f) of an orally administered dose of a drug comprises the individual fractions that survive several barriers encountered by the drug during its first passage from gut lumen to the sampling site, and it is described (19), in general, by the following relationship:

3.14 $$f = F_a F_g F_b$$

where F_a, F_g, and F_b are the fractions of intact drug absorbed (F_a) that escape irreversible elimination as the drug passes sequentially from the gastrointestinal tract across the gut wall (F_g) and traverses the liver (F_b) into systemic circulation. Thus, bioavailability of a drug is equal to or less than the fraction absorbed, depending on the extent of metabolism and loss during the absorption process. Therefore, poor blood levels of a drug can be a consequence of poor absorption or of good absorption accompanied by extensive metabolism.

There appear to be several common misconceptions (20) regarding the nature of absorption. Among these misconceptions are that intestinal absorption, permeability, fraction of drug absorbed, and in some cases, even bioavailability are equivalent properties and, consequently, are used interchangeably. Another common misconception is that absorption and permeability are discrete fundamental properties of a drug molecule and can be predicted solely from its chemical structure. In reality, however, drug absorption is quite a complex process dependent on drug properties such as solubility and permeability, formulation factors, and physiologic variables such as regional permeability differences, pH, luminal and mucosal enzymology, and intestinal motility, among others.

Publication of the so-called "Rule of Five" (21) has generated widespread interest regarding applying calculated physicochemical properties in the drug discovery process to separate out poor drug candidates before better drug candidates go into clinical trials. According to the Rule of Five, poor intestinal absorption is associated with and attributed to the molecule possessing any two of the following properties: molecular weight greater than 750 daltons, number of hydrogen bond donors greater than 5, number of hydrogen bond acceptors greater than 10, and calculated log P greater than 5. These guidelines have been proven to be very useful for approximate predictions of intestinal drug absorption. The critical role of lipid solubility in drug absorption is a major guiding principle in the drug discovery and development process. Because the lipid solubility of a drug molecule is the sum of the individual partition coefficients for each of its functional groups (see Chapter 2), the prediction of lipid solubility (calculated CLog P; see Appendix A for tables of CLog P values) can be estimated.

A recent examination (22) of the relationship of molecular surface properties with biologic performance of a molecule has been revealing. Most notably, it has been demonstrated that polar surface area (PSA) of a drug molecule has a strong correlation predicting drug transport from human intestine and across the drug membrane. The PSA is defined as the sum of the Van der Waals surface areas for the polar atoms, oxygens, nitrogens, and attached hydrogen atom (or the number of H-bond donors and H-bond acceptors). (See www.molinspiration.com for calculating the PSA.) The PSA is a major determinant for oral absorption and brain penetration of drugs that are transported by the transcellular route (movement across cell membranes). This property should be considered in the early phase of drug screening. Another related parameter, dynamic PSA (PSAd), has surfaced (23) as a parameter of value in predicting membrane permeability and oral absorption in humans. Interpolation of the sigmoidal plot for 20 selected compounds suggests that when the PSAd is greater than 140 Å^2, incomplete absorption (< 10%) results, and when the PSAd value is less than 60 Å^2, drug absorption will be in excess of 90%.

A drug's absorption, as reflected in its bioavailability, is a fairly complex process, and although it is related to the drug structure, it is related in a complex manner. Failure to appreciate and understand these complexities, in an attempt to build models, can provide a prediction of marginal and low confidence. Both fraction absorbed and bioavailability are measures of the extent of absorption. Permeability, on the other hand, is related to the rate of absorption (20):

3.15 $$J = P_e \cdot SA \cdot dC$$

where J is the absorptive flux and is equal to the permeability (P_e) of intestinal mucosa to the drug, the surface area available (SA), and the drug concentration gradient (dC) across the mucosa. Factors that can influence permeability include structural characteristics of a drug, including size, shape, solubility, charge, and surface area.

It has been argued (24), on a theoretical basis, that a fundamental relationship exists between the rate measured as a permeability coefficient and the extent of absorption. This has led to the greater interest and increasing use of the in vitro permeability model to serve as an experimental surrogate for predicting oral absorption potential of drug candidates in drug discovery programs. Additionally, although in some instances (24,25) it has been possible to directly correlate absorption with permeability, more often poor correlation exists (20,26), as illustrated in Figure 3.14. At times, good absorption is observed for poorly permeable compounds. These poorly permeable but well-absorbed compounds exhibit high aqueous solubility, generally exceeding 2.5 mg/mL (20,22). This suggests that aqueous solubility can help to compensate for the poor in vitro permeability observed.

Estimating the extent of oral drug absorption and variation in drug absorption, therefore, can be of great value in the selection of a potential therapeutic agent and in identifying ways to optimize the oral drug delivery in patients. This can be facilitated by developing the predictive oral drug delivery models. In turn, these models permit the estimation of drug absorption without performing in vivo studies in humans and impart better understanding of the rate-limiting processes affecting drug absorption, which can assist in developing strategies for the development of oral drug delivery. There are three physical barriers to drug absorption: the dissolution resistance, the aqueous boundary layer resistance, and the membrane resistance (27–29).

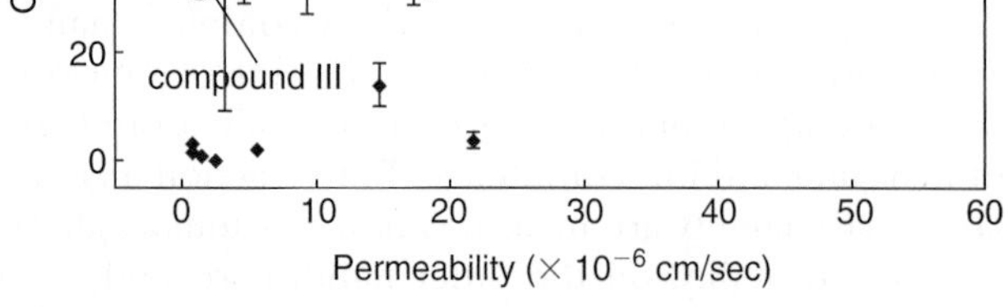

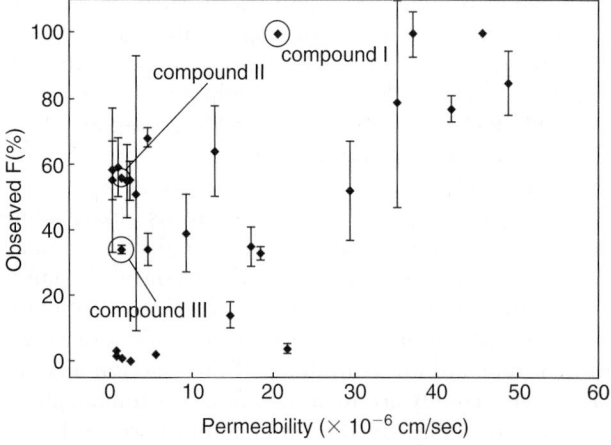

FIGURE 3.14 Poor correlation between oral bioavailability and permeability as measured using Caco-2 cells for three compounds. (From Burton P, Goodwin J, Vidamas T, et al. Predicting drug absorption: how nature made it a difficult problem. J Pharm Exp Ther 2002;303:889–895; and from Hilgers AR, Smith DP, Biermacher JJ, et al. Predicting oral absorption of drugs: a case study with novel class of antimicrobial agents. Pharm Res 2003;20:1149–1155, with permission.) (19).

Although physicochemical properties, such as solubility and permeability, and other properties, such as metabolic stability and toxicity, are important individually, the interrelationship of these properties is what eventually determines the in vivo performance of a drug. In particular, the role of solubility is dependent on the potency, which will determine the dose. In other words, low solubility is problematic for a high-dose drug; however, it can be more acceptable for a low-dose drug.

Measurement of Permeability

Although a variety of models (subcellular fraction, cell monolayer model, isolated intestinal tissue, and intestinal perfusion) are available to predict the permeability of a drug, the cell monolayer model and rat intestinal perfusion techniques are the most commonly used techniques.

Cell Monolayer

These models consist of cells grown on permeable inserts. Transport of compounds across the cell monolayer is used to quantitate the permeability of a new chemical entity in a rapid manner. One of the most popular cell lines is Caco-2, derived from human colon adenocarcinoma cells. The monolayer exhibits ion conductance and possesses transepithelial electrical resistance indicative of fully formed tight junctions that restrict the paracellular transport of a chemical entity. Although Caco-2 cells are the most commonly used cells, Madin-Darby canine kidney (MDCK) cells are becoming more widespread in use, in part because of the shorter culture time (4 to 7 days vs. 21 to 30 days for Caco-2 cells) needed for their use in permeability experiments.

Excellent correlation for permeability coefficient between MDCK and Caco-2 cells was observed for 55 compounds with known human intestinal absorption. Regardless of the type of cells used in determining permeability measurement, establishing the correlation between the permeability coefficient and the fraction of drug absorbed in vivo validates this approach.

Several clones of HT 29 cells have been used (30) to study different aspect of intestinal drug absorption. An enterocytic HT 29 clone, HT 29-18-C1, was proposed as a model to study intestinal permeability. The limitation of the cells is that these cells grow very slowly, and a large number of cultures failed to develop acceptable barrier characteristics.

Biopharmaceutical Drug Classification

It is clear from the discussion thus far that the physicochemical properties, such as drug solubility and drug permeability, have a critical role in the drug absorption process. The following biopharmaceutical drug classification system (30–32) has been developed to optimize the development of an oral dosage form taking into consideration two rate-limiting factors, drug permeability and drug dissolution, the latter of which is related to drug solubility.

Class I Drugs (High Solubility and High Permeability) Class I drugs provide both rapid dissolution and high membrane permeation. This class includes small-molecule hydrophilic drugs that are not ionized in the gastrointestinal tract. Examples include acetaminophen, valproic acid, ketoprofen, disopyramide, verapamil, propranolol, fluconazole, and metoprolol. Class I drugs are well absorbed and are affected by a limited set of interactions that alter drug absorption. Because gastric emptying frequently will control the rate of absorption for this class of drugs, interactions that delay gastric emptying will delay drug absorption. This is important for class I analgesic drugs, for which a rapid rate of absorption and quick rise in the plasma level to within the therapeutic range is needed to alleviate pain quickly.

Class II Drugs (Low Solubility and High Permeability) For immediate-release formulations of many poorly water-soluble drugs, the dissolution rate limits drug absorption. Along with this limitation, a greater impact on drug absorption will be observed with high oral doses. For example, the antifungal drug griseofulvin and the cardiac glycoside drug digoxin are both poorly water soluble and possess similar dissolution profiles, which limit the rate of drug absorption. The extent of griseofulvin absorption, however, is incomplete for a typical dose of 500 mg, whereas a normal, 0.25-mg oral dose of digoxin usually provides a fairly complete absorption. Other examples are diazepam and nifedipine.

Any interactions that increase drug solubility and dissolution rate in the gastrointestinal tract will exert a positive effect on the gastrointestinal absorption of this class of drugs. The absorption of this class of drugs is often enhanced in proportion to the fat content of the coadministered meal. This is attributed to the increased gastrointestinal fluid volume from a coadministered meal, stimulated gastrointestinal secretions, and biliary solubilization effects that increase the dissolution rate. Furthermore, increased gastric residence time as a function of the caloric density permits greater time for drug dissolution.

Class III Drugs (High Solubility and Low Permeability) For drugs possessing high water solubility, the intestinal membrane permeation rate is often the rate-limiting step in drug absorption from immediate-release dosage forms. Many drugs in this class (e.g., acyclovir and chloramphenicol) also show region-dependent absorption with better absorption in the upper small intestine. Therefore, any interactions that compromise upper intestinal absorption can result in a significant decrease in oral bioavailability. Consequently, these drugs show a sharp decrease in absorption with a coadministered meal that is independent of fat content. Meals tend to decrease the absorption of some drugs in this category as a result of simple physical barrier that compromises the availability of drug molecules to the upper intestinal membrane.

Class IV Drugs (Low Solubility and Low Permeability) Poor aqueous solubility cannot necessarily impart high lipophilicity and, therefore, high membrane permeation for a drug. Class IV drugs possess both low solubility and low permeability, both of which are undesirable for good drug absorption. Examples include furosemide and paclitaxel. Drugs in this class, however, still are administered orally if the plasma concentrations obtained are sufficient to produce the desired therapeutic effect and the drugs do not possess a narrow therapeutic index.

Role of Transporters in Drug Absorption

The oral route of drug administration remains the most popular and convenient route of administration, despite its many shortcomings and challenges. Although the advantages associated with oral administration far outweigh the limitations, a major limitation for oral absorption relates to the interactions of drugs with intestinal membrane transporters and metabolizing enzymes (33). The rapidly growing awareness of transporters affecting the rate and extent of intestinal drug absorption has attracted attention in drug discovery and development (Chapter 5). Intestinal membrane transporters affecting the rate of oral absorption are the influx peptide transporters (PepT1, PHTs, and HPT-1), bile salt transporter, phosphate transporter, nucleoside transporters, organic cation/anion transporters (OATP and OCTP), and fatty acid transporters. Transporters affecting drug efflux into the intestinal lumen include P-glycoprotein (P-gp), MRP2, BCRP, and MRP3. The primary intestinal enzyme affecting the absorption of drugs is CYP3A4, as well as the phase II enzymes, glutathione transferase, glucuronyltransferases, and sulfotransferases. Thus, inhibition of these membrane transporters and/or metabolizing enzymes and modulation of the expression of these membrane transporters and/or metabolizing enzymes are key factors affecting the rate and extent of drug absorption. Drug molecules recognized by OATP-B include bile acids, bilirubin and bilirubin glucuronides, estrogen and androgen sulfate conjugates, digoxin, pravastatin, fexofenadine, thyroid hormones, and other lipophilic organic anions. The PepT1 will transport peptide-like drugs, such as β-lactam antibiotics (penicillins and cephalosporins), angiotensin-converting enzyme inhibitors, rennin inhibitors, thrombin inhibitors, and di-/tripeptide prodrugs of antivirals (valacyclovir).

Efflux Transporters

More recently (33–37), the role of efflux transporters in influencing the permeability and the overall bioavailability of drugs has emerged and gained considerable attention. Among these transporters is P-gp, which is expressed on the luminal surface of normal intestinal mucosa. Unlike absorptive transporters that increase the uptake of a substrate from intestinal lumen, P-gp impedes uptake by returning the portion of drug entering the mucosa back to the lumen in a concentration-dependent manner. Two types of P-gp have been observed in mammals: drug-transporting P-gp and phospholipid-transporting P-gp.

The localization suggests that P-gp functionally can protect the body against toxic xenobiotics by excreting these compounds into bile, urine, and the intestinal lumen and by preventing their accumulation in brain and testes. Thus, P-gp can have a significant role in drug absorption and disposition in human and animals. An increasing number of drugs have been shown to be substrate for P-gp, including HIV protease inhibitors and verapamil, which is also an inhibitor of P-gp and, thus, can increase the intestinal permeability of other drugs

P-gp is a cell membrane–associated protein that transports a variety of substances. It has been studied extensively as a mediator of multidrug resistance in cancer, but only recently has the role of P-gp expressed in normal tissue as a determinant of drug pharmacokinetics and pharmacodynamics been investigated.

P-gp is a 170 kDa protein product of the *MDR1* gene. It is a dimer consisting of 1,280 amino acids, with 12 transmembrane segments and 2 adenosine 5′-triphosphate (ATP)-binding domains. P-gp requires binding of ATP to both ATP-binding domains for the transport function. A proposed mechanism by which P-gp secretes substrates is illustrated in Figure 3.15.

Unlike most other transport proteins that recognize a few structurally similar substrates, P-gp recognizes a broad range of pharmacologically and structurally diverse compounds. In general, P-gp substrates are large, lipophilic compounds that tend to be cationic at physiologic pH. An evaluation of 100 structurally diverse compounds revealed that P-gp substrates have a relatively high number of electron-donating groups (i.e., O, N, S, F, Cl, or groups with a π-electron orbital of an unsaturated system).

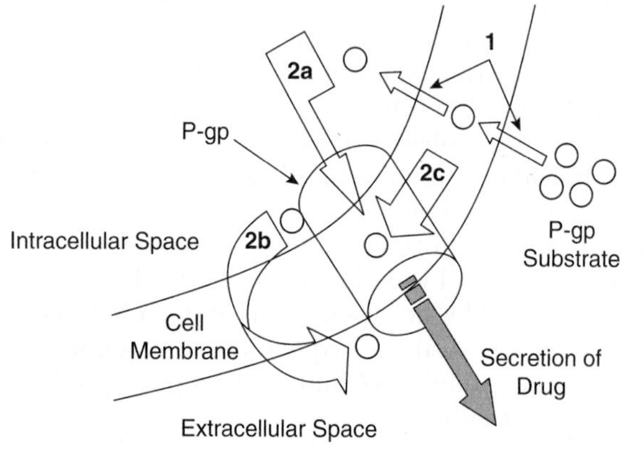

FIGURE 3.15 Proposed mechanism by which P-glycoprotein (P-gp) secretes substrates. (1) Passive drug uptake across cell membrane. (2a) Formation of hydrophobic channel (pore) between the intracellular and extracellular space. (2b) Flippase activity, whereby the drug is flipped from the inner leaflet to the outer leaflet of the cell membrane. (2c) "Vacuum cleaner model," in which the drug interacts with P-gp in the lipid bilayer and is subsequently secreted back into the extracellular space. (From Matheney C, Lamb M, Brouwer K, et al. Pharmacokinetics and pharmacodynamic implications of P-glycoprotein modulation. Rev Ther 2001;21:778–796, with permission.)

In recent years, the role of drug transporters in the intestinal epithelium as major determinants of drug absorption has been recognized, and P-gp and other transporters have been implicated in modulating the absorption and/or intestinal elimination of drugs. Reduction in the small intestinal transit time (SITT) of a drug can decrease the peak plasma concentration and area under the plasma concentration–time curve, the rate and extent of absorption, and, therefore, the bioavailability of a drug. Another potential consequence of increased transit has been proposed for digoxin and, possibly, other drugs that are substrate for P-gp in the small intestine. Because intestinal permeability of such compounds can depend on the relative activity of P-gp in the intestine, factors affecting this activity can also affect absorption. One determinant is drug concentration, which will influence the degree of saturation of the transporters. Another consideration is the specific activity of the transporters with the intestine itself. Evidence suggests that P-gp is not homogenously distributed throughout the intestinal tract but, rather, increases in abundance from the proximal to the distal small intestine. Therefore, drugs that can be substrate for P-gp but that are partly permeable can be well absorbed in the duodenum and proximal jejunum, which have little P-gp. Drugs that inhibit P-gp can alter the absorption, disposition, and elimination of coadministered drugs and can enhance bioavailability or cause unwanted drug–drug interactions.

Prodrugs

Prodrugs are bioreversible derivatives of drug molecules that undergo an enzymatic and/or chemical transformation in vivo to release the active parent drug, which can then exert the desired pharmacologic effect. In both drug discovery and development, prodrugs have become an established tool for improving physiochemical, biopharmaceutical, or pharmacokinetic properties of pharmacologically active agents. The rationale behind the use of a prodrug is generally to optimize absorption, distribution, metabolism, and excretion (ADME) processes. Prodrugs are usually designed to improve oral bioavailability due to poor absorption from the gastrointestinal tract. Prodrugs are now an established concept to overcome barriers to a drug's usefulness. About 5% to 7% of drugs approved worldwide can be classified as prodrugs, and the implementation of a prodrug approach in the early stages of drug discovery is a growing trend. A few examples of noteworthy blockbuster prodrugs are omeprazole, simvastatin, lovastatin, enalapril, clopidogrel, valacyclovir, acyclovir, and oseltamivir (Fig. 3.16).

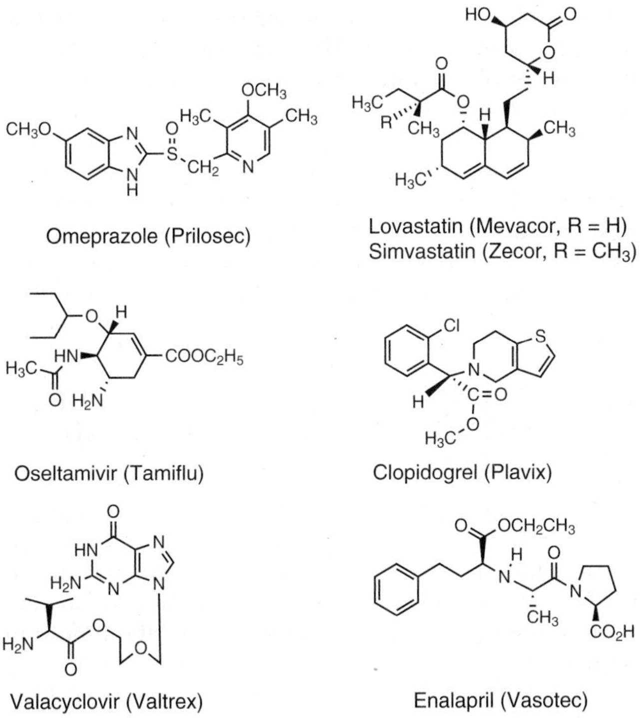

FIGURE 3.16 Commercially available blockbuster prodrugs and their structures.

The term "prodrug" or "proagent" was first introduced by Albert (38) to signify pharmacologically inactive chemical derivatives that could be used to alter the physicochemical properties of drugs, in a temporary manner, to increase their usefulness and/or to decrease associated toxicity. Since Albert discussed the concept of prodrugs in the late 1950s, such compounds have also been called "latentiated drugs," "bioreversible derivatives," and "congeners," but "prodrug" is now the most commonly accepted term (39–41). Usually, "prodrug" implies a metabolizable covalent link between a drug and a chemical moiety, although some authors also use it to characterize some forms of salts of the active drug molecule. Approximately 49% of all marketed prodrugs are activated by hydrolysis, and 23% are bioprecursors (i.e., lacking a promoiety) activated by a biosynthetic reaction (42).

The prodrug approach gained attention as a technique for improving drug therapy in the early 1970s. Numerous prodrugs have been designed and developed since then to overcome pharmaceutical and pharmacokinetic barriers in clinical drug application such as low oral drug absorption, lack of site specificity, chemical instability, toxicity, and poor patient acceptance (e.g., bad taste, odor, pain at injection site) (42).

Prodrugs provide a rationale and opportunities to reach target physiochemical, pharmacokinetic, and pharmacodynamic properties. They are designed to overcome barriers such as insufficient chemical stability, poor solubility, unacceptable taste or odor, irritation or pain, insufficient oral absorption, inadequate blood–brain barrier permeability, marked presystemic metabolism, and toxicity (39).

Strategic Considerations

Beaumont et al. (43), in a recent review on the design of ester prodrugs, conclude with the recommendations that the prodrug strategy should only be considered as a last resort to improve the oral bioavailability of important therapeutic agents. It can be considered in parallel with classical analoging as soon as a problem becomes apparent.

One prodrug strategy that is often applied to improve the solubility of drug candidates is to introduce a promoiety containing phosphate, sulfate, or succinate groups, which can ionize in relevant biologic media. Strategies to improve the permeability by prodrug formulation can be used to develop prodrugs that have increased passive diffusional permeability properties across the enterocytic membrane compared with the parent compound or to develop prodrugs as substrates for absorptive intestinal membrane transporters such as the peptide transporter PepT1.

Regardless of the strategy used, however, a prerequisite is that the drug candidates contain functional group(s) such as carboxylic acid, alcohol, thiol, or amine functionalities that can be applied in the formation of bioreversible linkages between the promoiety and the drug candidate. The most frequently applied prodrug linkage is the ester linkage; however, many other linkages can also be used.

Thus, drug candidates that are alcohols, amines, thiols, or carboxylic acids are formulated as the corresponding ester, amide, thioester, and ester prodrugs, respectively. Conventional ester linkages are, in general, rapidly cleaved in the gastrointestinal fluids and thus characterized by very short half-lives in vivo due to esterase-catalyzed hydrolysis. In cases where the prodrug linkage is hydrolyzed in gastrointestinal fluids, the prodrug formulation does not necessarily increase the oral bioavailability of the parent drug candidate.

Type of Prodrugs

Hard Prodrug: A hard prodrug is a biologically active compound with a high lipid solubility or high water solubility having a long biologic half-life. Examples include cocaine and heroin.

Soft Prodrug: A soft drug is a biologically active compound that is biotransformed in vivo in a rapid and predictable manner into nontoxic moieties. Examples include insulin and adrenaline.

Carrier-Linked Prodrug: A carrier-linked prodrug is a compound that contains an active drug linked to a carrier group that can be removed enzymatically. These prodrugs are generally esters or amides, and such a prodrug would have greatly modified lipophilicity due to the attached carrier. The active drug is realized by hydrolytic cleavage either chemically or enzymatically. The prodrug should be biologically inactive. The chemical linkage between the parent drug and its promoiety must be bioreversible; the prodrug should be sufficiently stable to allow its formulation into an appropriate dosage form. The carrier-linked prodrug is subdivided into a bipartite prodrug that is comprised of one carrier attached to drug. A tripartite prodrug is carrier connected to a linker that is connected to a drug.

Bioprecursors: Bioprecursors are inert molecules obtained by chemical modification of the active drug but do not contain a carrier. Such a moiety has almost the same lipophilicity as the parent drug and is bioactivated generally by enzymatic redox metabolism.

Mutual Prodrug: Two, usually synergistic, drugs are attached to each other. A bipartite or tripartite prodrug is one in which the carrier is a synergistic drug with the drug to which it is linked.

Major Objectives of Prodrug Design

IMPROVED BIOAVAILABILITY Aqueous solubility, drug instability, passive intestinal absorption, targeted active absorption, formulation problems, taste palatability, and metabolic switching are well-established factors limiting bioavailability that need to be circumvented.

IMPROVED AQUEOUS SOLUBILITY Inadequate aqueous solubility is an important factor limiting parenteral, percutaneous, and oral bioavailability. In such cases, a prodrug strategy can bring great pharmaceutical and pharmacokinetic benefit. Charged promoieties (e.g., esters such as phosphates, hemisuccinates, aminoacyl conjugates, dimethylamino acetates) and neutral promoieties (e.g., polyethylene glycols) can be used (e.g., celecoxib and valdecoxib). One of the potential problems in this approach is that solubilizing groups can sometimes generate toxic effects.

IMPROVED PASSIVE INTESTINAL ABSORPTION Providing enhanced lipophilicity for increased passive intestinal absorption is the most frequent rationale when adopting a prodrug strategy (approximately 49% of all marked prodrugs are activated by hydrolysis).

Other pharmaceutical applications of prodrugs include protection against fast metabolism (slow-release prodrugs), improvement of taste, improvement of odor, change of physical form for preparation of solid dosage forms (4), reduction of gastrointestinal irritation, and reduction of pain on injection

Because prodrugs are designed to improve the permeability and oral absorption of the parent drug, they are more lipid soluble than the parent drug and should be rapidly converted to the parent compound during absorption from the gut wall, liver, or site of action. Examples of prodrugs include pivampicillin, the pivalate ester prodrug of ampicillin that is more lipid soluble and, therefore, more efficiently absorbed than the parent compound (35); valacyclovir, an L-valyl ester prodrug of acyclovir; lisdexamfetamine, an L-lysinylamide prodrug of amphetamine that is slowly hydrolyzed to amphetamine; and methyldopa, a prodrug of methyldopamine that is decarboxylated in the brain to methyldopamine. The recognition that di- and tripeptides are transported from the intestine by their PepT1 transporter has led to the development of prodrugs designed as di- or tripeptide analogues (36). For example, the dipeptidyl analogue of methyldopa increased the intestinal absorption of methyldopa by more than 20-fold.

FACTORS AFFECTING THE ABSORPTION OF DRUGS FROM SOLID DOSAGE FORMS AND SUSPENSIONS

When a drug is administered orally via tablet, capsule, or suspension, the rate of absorption is often controlled by how fast the drug particles dissolve in the fluid at the site of administration. Hence, the dissolution rate is often the rate-limiting (slowest) step in the following sequence:

$$\text{Solid drug} \xrightarrow[\text{Step I}]{\text{Dissolution}} \text{Drug in solution} \xrightarrow[\text{Step II}]{\text{Absorption}} \text{Drug in systemic circulation}$$

If the dissolution of the drug is slow or controlling the rate of absorption (Step I), then dissolution is the rate-determining step. Factors controlling dissolution, such as solubility, ionization, or surface area, will then control the overall dissolution process. Figure 3.17 describes the absorption of aspirin from solution and from two different types of tablets.

It is clear from Figure 3.17 that aspirin absorption is more rapid from solution than from tablet formulations. This rapid absorption of aspirin is an indication that the rate of absorption is dissolution rate limited. A general

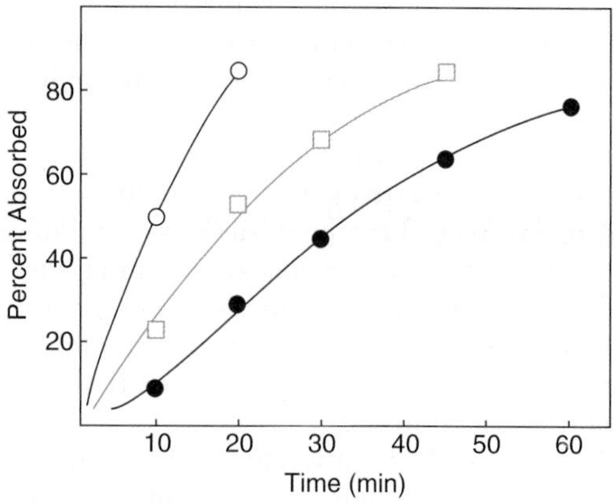

FIGURE 3.17 Absorption of aspirin after oral administration of a 650-mg dose in solution (○), in buffered tablets (□), or in regular tablets (●). (From Kwan KC. Oral bioavailability and first-pass effects. Drug Metab Drug Dispos 1997;25:1329–1336, with permission.) (18).

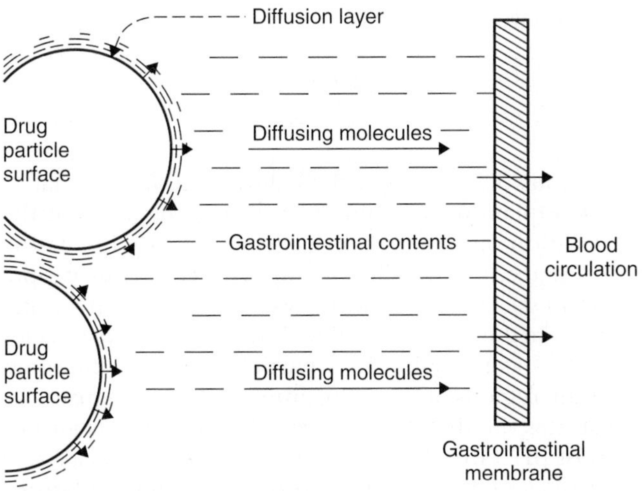

FIGURE 3.18 Dissolution from a solid surface.

relationship describing the dissolution of a drug was first reported by Noyes and Whitney (44). The equation derived by those authors is as follows:

3.16
$$\frac{dc}{dt} = KS(C_s - C_t)$$

where dc/dt is the dissolution rate, K is a constant, S is the surface area of the dissolution solid, C_s is the equilibrium solubility of drug in the solvent, and C is the concentration of drug in the solvent at time t.

The constant K in Equation 3.16 has been shown to be equal to D/h, where D is the coefficient of the dissolving material of the drug and h is the thickness of the diffusion layer surrounding the dissolving solid particles. This diffusion layer is a thin, stationary film of a solution adjacent to the surface of a solid particle (Fig. 3.17) and is saturated with drug (4); in other words, the drug concentration in the diffusion layer is equal to C_s, the equilibrium solubility. The term $(C_s - C_t)$ in Equation 3.16 represents the concentration gradient for the drug between the diffusion layer and the bulk solution. If dissolution is the rate-limiting step in the absorption process, the term C_t in Equation 3.16 is negligible compared to C_s. Under this condition, Equation 3.16 is reduced to:

3.17
$$\frac{dc}{dt} = \frac{DSC_s}{h}$$

Equation 3.17 describes a diffusion-controlled dissolution process (4), which can be visualized as shown in Figure 3.18; when solid drug particles are introduced to the fluids at the absorption sites, the drug promptly saturates the diffusion layer. This is followed by the diffusion of drug molecules from the diffusion layer into the bulk solution, which is instantly replaced in the diffusion layer by molecules from the solid crystal or particle. This is a continuous process. Although it oversimplifies the dynamics of the dissolution process, Equation 3.17 is a qualitatively useful equation and clearly indicates the effects of some important factors on the dissolution and, therefore, the absorption rate of drugs. When dissolution is the rate-limiting factor in the absorption, then bioavailability is affected. These factors are listed in Table 3.4.

The Noyes-Whitney equations (Eqs. 3.16 and 3.17) demonstrate that the equilibrium solubility (C_s) is one of the major factors determining the rate of dissolution. Changes in the characteristics of solvents, such as pH, affecting the solubility of the drug, affect its dissolution rate. Similarly, the use of a different salt or other physicochemical form of a drug, which exhibits a solubility different from the parent drug, usually affects the dissolution rate. Increasing the surface area of a drug exposed to the dissolution medium, by reducing the particle size, usually increases the dissolution rate. In the discussion to follow, some of the more important factors affecting dissolution and, therefore, absorption are presented in greater detail.

Dissolution

pH and Solubility of Weak Acids and Bases

Solubility is another factor determining the rate of dissolution. As solubility increases, so does the dissolution rate. One way of increasing solubility is to use salts. Salts of weak acids and weak bases generally have much higher aqueous solubility than the free acid or base; therefore, if the drug is given as a salt, the solubility can be increased,

TABLE 3.4 The Effect of Changing Parameters from the Dissolution Equation on the Rate of Solution (4)

Equation Parameter	Comments	Effect on Rate of Solution
D (diffusion coefficient of drug)	May be decreased in the presence of substances that increase viscosity of the medium	(−)
A (area exposed to solvent)	Increased by micronization and in "amorphous drugs"	(+)
δ (thickness of diffusion layer)	Decreased by increased agitation in gut or flask	(+)
C_s (solubility in diffusion layer)	That of weak electrolytes altered by change in pH by use of appropriate drug salt or buffer ingredient	(−) (+)
C (concentration in bulk)	Decreased by intake of fluid in stomach, by removal of drug by partition or absorption	(+)

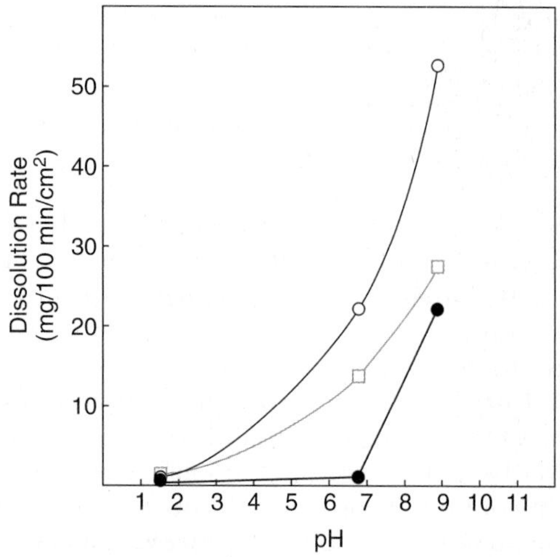

FIGURE 3.19 The pH-dependent dissolution of salicylic acid (o), benzoic acid (□), and phenobarbital (●). (From Gibaldi M. Biopharmaceutics and Clinical Pharmacokinetics, 4th Ed. Philadelphia: Lea and Febiger, 1991, with permission.) (45).

and we should have improved dissolution (Fig. 3.19). This factor can lead to quite different peak plasma concentrations after oral administration.

The solubility of weak acids and bases is a function of the pH of the medium. Therefore, differences in the dissolution rate are expected to occur in different regions of the gastrointestinal tract. The solubility of weak acid is obtained by

3.18 $$C_s = [HA] + [A^-]$$

where [HA] is the intrinsic solubility of the un-ionized acid (i.e., C_o) and $[A^-]$ is the concentration of its anion, which can be expressed in terms of its dissociation constant, K_a, and C_o; that is,

3.19 $$C_s = C_o + \frac{K_a C_o}{[H^+]}$$

In a similar manner, the solubility of a weak base is obtained by

3.20 $$C_s = C_o + \frac{C_o[H^+]}{K_a}$$

By substituting Equations 3.18 and 3.19 into Equation 3.20 for the term C_s, the following dissolution rate equations are obtained:

For weak acids:

3.21 $$\frac{dc}{dt} = \frac{K'(C_o + K_a C_o)}{[H^+]}$$

or

3.22 $$\frac{dc}{dt} = \frac{K'C_o(1 + K_a)}{[H^+]}$$

and for a weak base:

3.23 $$\frac{dc}{dt} = \frac{K'C_o(1 + [H^+])}{K_a}$$

Equations 3.21 through 3.23 show that K' is equal to DS/h. Equations 3.22 and 3.23 clearly suggest that the dissolution rate of weak bases decreases with increasing pH. Hence, the dissolution rate of weak bases is optimum in gastric fluid, but for weak acids, it is at a minimum. Furthermore, the dissolution rate of weak acids increases as the solid drug particles move to the more alkaline regions of the gastrointestinal tract. Figure 3.18 illustrates the dissolution rates of weak acids as a function of pH (45). The absorption of a salt of weak acid or base can be explained by using the following figure:

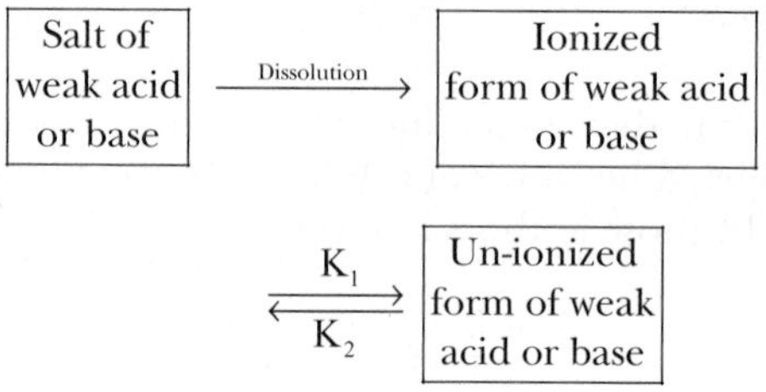

where K_1 and K_2 represent the rate constants associated with the formation of un-ionized and ionized species of a compound, respectively. The ratio of these two rate constants represents the dissociation constant of a compound. The absorption of the un-ionized species of a molecule disturbs the equilibrium of the process. To regain the equilibrium, some of the ionized species, therefore, are converted into un-ionized species, which are then absorbed through the membrane. This process, being a continuous one, permits the absorption of the un-ionized species to take place. Therefore, a drug molecule will eventually be absorbed.

The relatively poor dissolution of weak acids at the pH of gastric fluid further diminishes the importance of the stomach as a drug absorption site. Although gastric absorption of weak acids can occur from solution, it is unlikely that much of the drug dissolves and is absorbed during the short residence time as a solid dosage form in the stomach. A study by Ogata et al. (46) proposed that the critical value of solubility that separates acidic drugs from the absorption sites (stomach or intestine) is approximately 30 mg/mL in 0.1 N HCl when 1 g of drug is administered orally. Those authors found that if the solubility of a drug is less than 3 mg/mL, practically no absorption occurs in the stomach. Changes in the gastric pH also alter the solubility of certain drugs and can affect the dissolution and absorption rates. A patient with achlorhydria has a higher gastric pH and absorbs aspirin more rapidly than a normal subject. On the other hand, similar differences were not observed with respect to the absorption rates of acetaminophen, a much weaker acid, the solubility of which would be unaffected by changes in pH (47).

The relationships between dissolution rate and hydrogen ion concentration, described in Equations 3.22 and 3.23, are approximations and tend to overpredict the dissolution rate of both weak acids in the small intestine and weak bases in the stomach. In reality, the hydrogen ion concentration of the bulk is not equal to the hydrogen ion concentration of the diffusion layer.

Salts

The objective of drug discovery is to identify substances that are highly active in biologic systems. Screening for potential drug candidates is performed in solution at micromolar and nanomolar concentration levels.

Drug substances can be administered by various routes, including oral, which is the most frequently chosen route; parenteral by several modes of injection (intramuscular [IM], intravenous [IV], subcutaneous [SC], and others); intranasal inhalation; and topical to the various areas of the body surface, to name just a few more important routes. Various pharmaceutical dosage forms are formulated to administer drug substances by these routes. Each dosage form requires that a typical set of relevant parameters of the drug substance lie within a certain range, beyond which the development of said dosage form becomes increasingly difficult and eventually impossible. Also, in a mutual interdependence, the selection of dosage form and the applicable technology depend on the physical chemical properties profile of the chosen salt.

Approximately two thirds of the drug substances are weakly acidic or basic entities, and therefore, salt formation provides a significant opportunity to alter the physiochemical properties of drugs in the solid state without altering chemical integrity. The decision whether to pursue a salt form is usually made early in the development process on the basis of known properties of the uncharged molecules. Salt formation will often be considered when the drug has one or more unfavorable properties, including poor dissolution, low aqueous solubility (< 10 μg/mL), poor chemical stability, hygroscopicity, low melting point (< 80°C), poor crystallization (forms oil or amorphous solid on crystallization attempts), or displays multiple polymorphs. A significant number of counterions are suitable for pharmaceutical salt selection studies of weakly acidic or basic drugs, and therefore, there is a broad range of opportunity to obtain different salts with improved and desired physical chemical properties.

The selection of suitable counterions for inclusion in a salt selection search is dependent on safety considerations. For example, chloride and sodium ions are regarded as safe to administer and well tolerated. Counterion selection often uses pK_a values of the acid and base involved to estimate the likelihood of successful salt formation.

Based on the pK_a values, a series of salt formers can then be selected from those frequently used pharmaceutically (Table 3.5), whereas others must be rejected. From experience, to form a stable salt, the pK_a values of an acid–base pair should differ by at least two pK_a units

TABLE 3.5 Most Frequently Used Acids and Bases as Salt Formers

Acids (Anions)	Bases (Cations)
Hydrobromic	Sodium
Hydrochloric	Potassium
Hydroiodic	Zinc
Sulfuric	Choline
Nitric	Calcium
Methanesulfonic	Magnesium
Maleic	Diethylamine
Phosphoric	Tromethamine
Fumaric	Silver
Citric	Ammonium
Succinic	
Acetic	
Tartaric	

(i.e., the pK_a of the acid should be at least two units lower than that of the base). This corresponds to a situation in which both compounds, brought together in water, are ionized to a degree of at least 90%. Strong mineral acids such as HCl ($pK_a \approx -6$) or H_2SO_4 ($pK_a = -3$) can form solid salts with the weak base atazanavir, having a pK_a as low as 4.25, whereas attempts to isolate a salt with either acetic acid ($pK_a = 4.76$) or benzoic acid ($pK_a = 4.19$) would fail with such a weak base.

The final decision on the selection of a salt of a drug substance is based on data collected from analytical and physical characterization of a certain number of prepared salts. The data are evaluated primarily against the requirements set by biopharmaceutical and therapeutic considerations for the use of the drug, pharmaceutical and chemical–technologic aspects in view of the development and manufacturing of dosage forms, and the synthesis and isolation of the drug substance. The most frequently encountered issues while selecting a suitable salt are discussed below.

For injectable solutions, high solubility of a drug under the conditions close to physiologic pH of 7.4 is essential. For a small-volume injectable such as IM and SC, the solubility should be as high as possible to accommodate the dose to be administered in 0.5 to 2 mL for SC or up to 5 mL for IM administration. The solubility requirement for IV injections is less stringent because volumes up to 20 mL can be administered. With lower solubility drugs, one has to resort to infusions of volumes of up to 1,000 mL. Injectable solutions of drugs require particularly high chemical stability. Ideally, a drug substance must withstand heat sterilization in solution and subsequent storage for up to 5 years. For those drug substances lacking such optimum stability, it is possible to circumvent heat stress by sterile filtration. Naturally, for injectables, solid-state drug properties are of minor importance as long as they do not hamper processing or the dissolution of a lyophilizate.

For solid dosage forms, the most critical step, after swallowing a unit dose, is the release of the drug substance. Solubility and, therefore, dissolution can control or limit, respectively, this important process. Therefore, a solubility that is reasonably high in relation to the drug dose is desirable.

In selecting a salt form for a product that is applied topically, it is a prerequisite that it (salt of the drug) must not cause local irritation, whether the target of treatment is the skin surface, dermal tissue, or underlying organs (e.g., joints, muscles, tendons) or even if systemic effects are intended. Weakly acidic to neutral pH values (~5 to 7.5) are tolerated best, and deviations from this range should be avoided. Choosing the right salt form of a drug can offer the following advantages: Annoying polymorphism problems can be circumvented; high hygroscopicity resulting in deliquescence can be avoided; amorphous material can be turned to a crystalline salt; taste and smell problems can be minimized; the melting point can be raised to improve mechanical properties (e.g., for milling), to the extent that liquid bases or acids are turned into solids; and local irritation can be avoided (e.g., for inhalation)

With drug candidates exhibiting absorption difficulties, investigations can even include in vivo studies in animals (e.g., rat, dog) with experimental formulations to identify the most suitable salt form or solid-state form. Sometimes such a search can address the state of distribution of the active substance in an experimental formulation (e.g., micronized, nano-sized, amorphous, suspension, emulsion, microemulsion), and so the borderlines between chemical technical operations and pharmaceutical formulation and processing techniques can become quite diffuse.

Solubility and Dissolution Rate

Chemical stability includes potential interaction between drug entity and counterions and stability in the presence of pharmaceutical excipients (drug/excipient compatibility); stability of the morphic state in bulk form; stability in solid and suspension dosage forms; hydrate formation and stability during storage and processing; chemical stability of hydrated versus anhydrous forms (influence of released hydrate water during storage); and uptake of water of hydration by anhydrates in solid dosage forms with consequences for mechanical properties.

Regarding molecular weight, large counterions can surmount the tolerable drug amount to be packed into a solid dose unit; in contrast, for extremely low–dose drugs, a larger molecular weight can improve handling and content uniformity.

The dissolution rate of a particular salt is usually different from that of a parent compound. Sodium or potassium salts of weak acids dissolve more rapidly than the free acid. The same is true with HCl or other salts of weak bases. Table 3.6 illustrates the dissolution rate differences between some weak acids and their sodium salts (45). The differences in the dissolution rates of salt and parent compound are explained by taking into consideration the pH of the diffusion layer. At a given pH, regardless of salt or free acids/bases, a drug will have a fixed solubility. The classical dissolution equation predicts a slower dissolution of a salt of a drug, and the concept of a diffusion layer becomes useful.

TABLE 3.6 Dissolution Rate of Weak Acids and Their Sodium Salts (44)

Compound	pK_a	Dissolution Rate (mg/100 min/cm^2)		
		0.1 N HCl pH 1.5	0.1 M Phosphate pH 6.8	0.1 M Borate pH 9.0
Benzoic acid	4.2	2.1	14	28
Sodium salt		980	1,770	1,600
Phenobarbital	7.4	0.24	1.2	22
Sodium salt		~200	820	1,430
Salicylic acid	3.0	1.7	27	53
Sodium salt		1,870	2,500	2,420
Sulfathiazole	7.3	<0.1	~0.5	8.5
Sodium salt		550	810	1,300

For sodium or potassium salts of weak acids, the pH of the solution in a diffusion layer is greater than the pH of the diffusion layer for the corresponding weak acid. However, the pH of the solution in the diffusion layer for hydrochloride salts of weak bases is always smaller than the diffusion layer of the corresponding free base. Therefore, effective solubility and dissolution rate of soluble salts on drug absorption are available in the literature. The potassium salt of penicillin V yields a higher peak plasma concentration of antibiotic than the corresponding free acid (48). Sodium salts of barbiturates are reported by Anderson (49) to provide a rapid onset of sedation. Some salts have a lower solubility and dissolution rate than their parent compounds. Examples include aluminum salts of weak acids and pamoate salts of weak bases. In these particular examples, insoluble films of either weak acids or pamoic acid appear to form in the dissolving solids and further retard the dissolution rate.

Surface Area and Particle Size

The surface area per gram (or per dose) of a solid drug is changed by altering the particle size. For example, a cube that is 1 cm on each side has a surface area of 6 cm^2. If this cube is broken into cubes with sides of 0.1 cm, the total surface area is 60 cm^2. If the particles are broken up by grinding, then irregular shapes with even larger surface areas are created. Generally, as the surface area increases, the drug will dissolve more rapidly. Therefore, many poorly soluble and slowly dissolving drugs currently are marketed in a micronized or microcrystalline form. The problems of low water solubility and particle size were not fully appreciated, but they have resulted in reducing the therapeutic dose of some drugs without sacrificing therapeutic efficacy. For example, since the original marketing of spironolactone, its dose has been reduced from 500 to 25 mg as a result of a reformulation that includes micronization. The bioavailability of digoxin increased from 40% to approximately 80% to 97% by reducing the particle size from 100 to approximately 10 nm. A similar result has been obtained for griseofulvin.

Polymorphism

Many pharmaceutical solids can exist in two or more crystalline forms called polymorphs (50,51). Polymorphism is the ability of the same drug molecule to crystallize into more than one different crystal structure that has a different arrangement and/or conformation of molecules in the crystal lattice. However, once they are in the solution phase, polymorphs share a common form. The different arrangements of atoms within the crystal unit cell can have a profound effect on physical and chemical properties of the final crystallized compound and on the final drug product. Amorphous solids consist of disordered arrangements of molecules that do not possess a distinguishable crystal lattice. Solvates are crystalline solid adducts containing either stoichiometric or nonstoichiometric amounts of a solvent incorporated within the crystal structure (50,51). If the incorporated solvent is water, the solvates are commonly known as hydrates. Polymorphs and/or solvates of a pharmaceutical solid or pharmaceutical excipients (e.g., lactose) can have different physical and chemical properties, such as melting point, chemical reactivity, apparent solubility, and dissolution rate. These properties of a drug substance can affect the intended shelf life (stability), rate of dissolution, and bioavailability/bioequivalence of the drug product. A metastable (amorphous) pharmaceutical solid form can change crystalline structure or solvate/desolvate in response to changes in environmental conditions or shelf-life storage. When such differences in physical properties are sufficiently large, bioavailability is altered, and it is often difficult to formulate a bioequivalent drug product using a different polymorph. The Biopharmaceutics Classification System criteria of high solubility and rapid dissolution should be considered in product development decisions when polymorphism exists. Drug substances with different physical form include warfarin sodium, famotidine, and ranitidine, and those with solvation or hydration state include terazosin hydrochloride, ampicillin, and cefadroxil.

Some drugs that exist as polymorphs can have different solubility properties and, thus, different dissolution characteristics. Chloramphenicol palmitate and ritonavir provide good examples of how polymorphism can influence drug dissolution and, thus, drug bioavailability. Chloramphenicol palmitate is a broad-spectrum antibiotic known to crystallize in at least three polymorphic forms and one amorphous (metastable) form, B. The most stable form, known as form A, is the polymorph that is marketed, whereas the metastable form B is approximately eight times more soluble than form A, thus providing an eightfold difference in bioavailability. This large difference in bioavailability creates the danger of fatal dosages when the unwanted polymorph is unwittingly administered because of alterations in process and/or storage conditions. The HIV protease inhibitor ritonavir (Norvir) was withdrawn from the market because an undesirable polymorph of ritonavir had been produced during its shelf life. Ritonavir was found to exist in only one monoclinic form during development and early manufacturing. This form, called "form I," was not sufficiently bioavailable in the solid state by the oral route, requiring the initial product (Norvir) to be formulated as a capsule filled with a hydroalcoholic solution containing the dissolved drug. Two years after the product launch, several lots of Norvir capsules started failing dissolution specifications. Evaluation of the failed lots revealed that a second crystal form of ritonavir, "form II," had precipitated from the formulation during its shelf life. "Form II" was 50% less soluble compared to "form I," resulting in failure of batches in the dissolution test, affecting its bioavailability and causing the eventual withdrawal of the product from the market. Substantial time and effort went into identifying and correcting the problem. To ensure a continuous supply of this life-saving drug, a liquid formulation had to be introduced in the market until the issue of the polymorphic form was resolved. Hence, an inadvertent production of the "wrong" polymorph at the crystallization stage or any transformations of one dosage form to another during processing (e.g., drying, milling, granulation, compression, spray drying, or freeze-drying), storage, and scale-up can result in pharmaceutical dosage forms that are either ineffective or toxic. This highlights that identification of different solid forms of a drug substance and determination of their physical and chemical properties, thermodynamic stabilities, and conditions or kinetics of interconversion are essential for ensuring reproducible behavior of drug products.

Estimate of Dose Absorbed

Johnson and Swindell (52) proposed a simple predictive model that relates the aqueous solubility and absorption rate constant (K_a) to determine the maximum absorbable dose (MAD):

3.24 $$\text{MAD} = K_a C_s V t$$

where K_a is the first-order absorption rate constant; $C_s V$ is a constant, and t is the time.

Hilgers et al. (26) argued that Equation 3.24, proposed by Johnson and Swindell (52), assumes that the drug absorption occurs under highly unrealistic conditions, such as the intestine is exposed to a saturated solution of a drug of interest for a time equal to the normal SITT. For interrelating permeability and solubility of a drug to estimate the absorption potential (30) as MAD by using the predictive model, Hilgers et al. (26) proposed a modified equation:

3.25 $$\text{MAD} = S \cdot K_a \cdot \text{SIV} \cdot \text{SITT}$$

where S is solubility and SIV is the small intestinal volume.

Briefly, the MAD calculates the total mass of drug that could theoretically be absorbed if a saturated solution of a compound with solubility S in the SIV were absorbed with a first-order absorption rate constant (K_a) for a time equivalent to SITT.

The absorption rate constant (K_a) was determined from Caco-2 permeability value with the assumption that the value of K_a and rat ileum permeability values are approximately equal and, consequently, that the estimated rat permeability (P_e) was converted to an absorption rate constant (K_a) from the following relationship:

3.26 $$K_a = P_e\,(A/V)$$

where V is the volume of the intestinal lumen and A is the surface area. For the rats used in this study (26), A/V was equal to 10 cm^{-1}.

Using Equations 3.24 and 3.25 for estimating the oral absorption of oxazolidinone antibiotics data obtained in rat and comparing the predicted MAD to the actually administered dose, Burton et al. (19) and Hilgers et al. (26) reported the relationship illustrated in Figure 3.20.

It is clear from Figure 3.20 that better prediction of MAD is achieved when solubility, permeability, and dose are taken into consideration. Despite this, drug permeability is an important determinant of drug absorption; therefore, it is informative to explore mechanisms contributing to permeability in the light of structure-based models for absorption prediction.

The relationship between the estimate of MAD and the fraction absorbed is hyperbolic (28), analogous to the relationship between drug permeability and fraction absorbed. Incorporating the solubility term in Equation 3.24 yields a more realistic value of estimate of MAD for poorly to moderately soluble compounds. Therefore, the concept of MAD serves to combine two major determinants of oral drug absorption (i.e., intestinal permeability and solubility). In turn, the value of MAD can provide a practical guideline in the early drug discovery program.

If the dose of a potential drug candidate is projected to be greater than the calculated estimated dose absorbed, this serves a cautionary notice that the following should be examined: the potential for solubilization in the gastrointestinal tract, and the formulation variables that could ultimately result in an increased solubility or drug

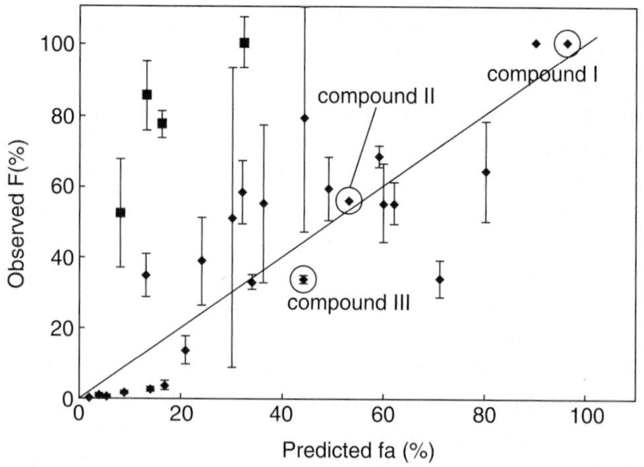

FIGURE 3.20 A better correlation between observed bioavailability and predicted bioavailability when both aqueous solubility and permeability parameters of drugs are used to predict the fraction absorbed for three compounds. (From Burton P, Goodwin J, Vidamas T, et al. Predicting drug absorption: how nature made it a difficult problem. J Pharm Exp Ther 2002;303:889–895; and adapted from Hilgers AR, Smith DP, Biermacher JJ, et al. Predicting oral absorption of drugs: a case study with novel class of antimicrobial agents. Pharm Res 2003;20:1149–1155, with permission.)

dissolution during the gastrointestinal transit to increase the fraction absorbed.

To reach the systemic circulation, a drug must move from the intestinal lumen through an unstirred water layer and mucous coat adjacent to the epithelial cell structure. Movement across the epithelial layers takes place by two independent routes, transcellular flux (i.e., movement across the cells) and paracellular flux (i.e., movement between adjacent epithelial cells). The solute molecules then encounter a basement membrane, interstitial space, and mesenteric capillary wall to access the mesenteric circulation. Any and all of these microenvironments can be considered a resistance to solute molecule movement, each with an associated permeability coefficient. Therefore, the overall process consists of a number of resistances (i.e., reciprocal of permeability) in series. Furthermore, the influence of drug structure with permeability in these different domains is different. For example, permeability in an unstirred water layer is inversely related to solute size, whereas paracellular permeability is a function of both size and charge. Furthermore, cations exhibit greater permeability than neutral species, which in turn manifest greater permeability than anions.

With respect to transcellular permeability, the relationship of solute structure with permeability depends on the mechanism. Historically, a passive diffusion pathway is assumed for most solutes. Nevertheless, a great number of solutes are identified as being associated with active absorption and secretary processes in intestinal epithelial cells. Additionally, although active transport involves specific interactions between a solute and transporter, passive diffusion is dependent on solute partitioning into the cellular plasma membrane and the diffusion coefficient within the membrane. Both processes, however, are influenced by the physicochemical and structural characteristics of the drug. Factors influencing plasma membrane partitioning are solute size, lipophilicity, hydrogen-bonding potential, and charge characteristics, whereas the diffusion coefficient is dependent on size or total molecular surface area. In general, a non-PSA favors partitioning.

For solutes that exhibit marginal (or a lack of) membrane affinity, permeability is low, resulting primarily from paracellular diffusion of the solute. As the propensity of the solute to partition into cell membrane increases, so does the permeability, as a result of the significant increase in surface area of the transcellular pathway relative to the paracellular route. This increase in permeability will approach a plateau, the so-called "aqueous boundary layer–limited situation," in which diffusion across the cell is very rapid relative to diffusion of the solute through the unstirred water/mucous layer.

In the case of ionizable solutes, permeability is also pH dependent. A neutral, uncharged species is capable of transcellular diffusion, whereas a charged species is restricted to the paracellular pathway. Thus, the observed permeability of such molecules is dependent on the relative concentrations of charged and neutral species.

Dressman et al. (53) developed an equation to determine the absorption potential (AP) of a drug by taking into consideration several of its physicochemical properties, including intrinsic solubility (S_o) of the un-ionized species of a drug, fraction of un-ionized form (F_{uni}) of a drug at a specific pH, volume of the luminal content (V_l), permeability of a drug in the gut wall (P_w), and the aqueous permeability (P_{aq}) of a drug. The equation is:

3.27 $$F_{abs} = \left(\frac{P_w}{P_{aq}}\right)(F_{uni})\left(\frac{S_o V_l}{X_o}\right)$$

where F_{abs} is the fraction absorbed and X_o is the administered dose. With the assumption that, in many cases, the permeability ratio (i.e., P_w/P_{aq}) of a drug is proportional to its membrane-water coefficient (P), which can be correlated to the 1-octanol–water partition coefficient (P), Equation 3.27 was simplified to:

3.28 $$AP = \log\left(P \cdot F_{uni} \cdot \frac{S_o V_l}{X_o}\right)$$

where AP is a dimensionless parameter.

Using Equation 3.28 and selecting drugs that represent a wide range of absorption characteristics, from poorly absorbed compounds to those that are virtually completely absorbed, the utility of the AP parameter as a predictor of the fraction absorbed was assessed (53). The physicochemical properties, such as the partition coefficient, solubility, fraction available in un-ionized form, dissociation constant, fraction of dose absorbed, and calculated dimensionless parameter AP for drugs selected in this study (53), are reported in Table 3.7. The observed correlation between the fractions absorbed and the AP is illustrated graphically in Figure 3.21.

From Table 3.7 and Figure 3.21, it is quite apparent that for the compounds selected in this study (53), the dimensionless parameter AP manifests a strong correlation to the fraction absorbed. Negative AP values correspond to poor drug absorption. For the range of AP values between 0 and 1, an increase in AP value correlates with an increase in fraction absorbed, whereas AP values greater than 1 indicate complete drug absorption.

SUMMARY

At one time, it was common to assume that the biologic response to a drug was simply a function of the intrinsic pharmacologic activity of the drug molecule. Today, when assessing the potency of most drugs, consideration is given to plasma drug concentration–response rather than dose–response relationships. The concentration of

TABLE 3.7 Physicochemical Properties and Calculated Absorption Potential (AP) for Representative Drugs (53)

Drug	P	S (mg/mL)	Dose (mg)	pK_a	F_{non} (pH 6.5)	AP	%ABS (range)
Acyclovir	0.018	1.3	200	9.5	1	−1.5	17 (12–23)
Chlorothiazide	0.54	0.4	250	6.7	0.6	−0.89	25 (10–40)
Griseofulvin	151	0.015	250	—	1	0.36	43 (35–51)
Hydrochlorothiazide	0.85	0.6	25	8.8	0.95	0.7	67 (50–90)
Phenytoin	295	0.014	100	9.2	0.99	1.0	90 (80–100)
Prednisone	26	0.235	20	—	1	1.9	99
Digoxin	56	0.024	0.25	—	1	3.13	>90

ABS, % absorbed.

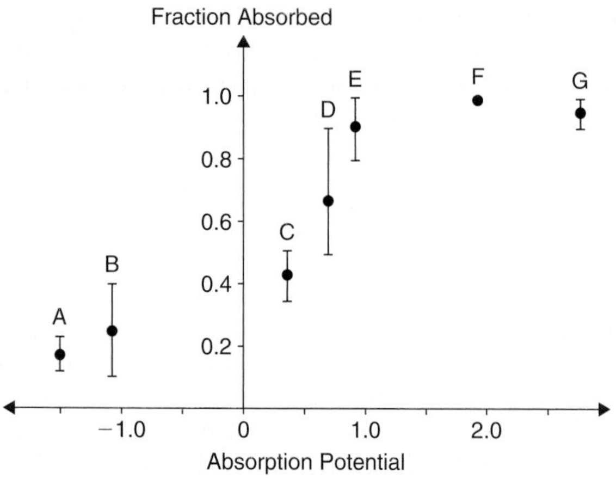

FIGURE 3.21 The relationship between absorption potential (AP) and fraction absorbed for seven representative drugs (see Table 3.7). A, acyclovir; B, chlorothiazide; C, micronized griseofulvin; D, hydrochlorothiazide; E, phenytoin; F, prednisolone; G, digoxin (Lanoxicap). (From Dressman JB, Amidon GL, Fleisher D. Absorption potential: estimating the fraction absorbed for orally administered compounds. J Pharm Sci 1985;74:588–589, with permission.)

a drug in the plasma is dependent on the rate and extent of absorption, which in turn is influenced by the physicochemical properties of drug substances. Drug absorption can markedly affect the onset and intensity of a biologic response to a drug. Clinically significant differences in the absorption of closely related drugs, such as lincomycin and clindamycin, penicillin and pivampicillin, or secobarbital and sodium secobarbital, are invariably the result of significant differences in their physicochemical properties.

Dissolution is simply a process by which a solid substance goes into solution. The determination of dissolution rates of pharmaceutical substances from dosage forms does not predict their bioavailability or their in vivo performance; rather, it indicates the potential availability of drug substance for absorption. Therefore, it is essential for pharmacists and pharmaceutical scientists to know and understand the importance of dissolution and its potential influence on the rate and extent of absorption and availability for drugs.

Factors affecting the dissolution rate of a drug from a dosage form can be related to the physicochemical properties of a drug, formulation of a dosage form, and dissolution apparatus and test parameters. Additionally, a brief introduction of the role of intestinal transporters and metabolizing enzymes (CYP3A4) in drug absorption was provided. The role of intestinal permeability in drug absorption process, techniques of measuring intestinal permeability, and methods that permit the estimation of fraction of dose absorbed by considering the physicochemical properties of a drug also were discussed. Additionally, the biopharmaceutical drug classification based on the two physicochemical properties of drugs, solubility and permeability, and the implications of these properties on drug absorption were covered.

PHARMACOKINETICS

Introduction

The events following drug administration are divided into two phases: a pharmacokinetic phase, in which the ability to adjust a dose, alter the dosage form, and alter the frequency and route of administration are related to the drug concentration–time relationship in the body; and a pharmacodynamic phase, in which the drug concentration at the sites of action is related to the magnitude of effects produced. Once both of these phases have been defined for a drug, a dosage regimen for a drug can be established to achieve the optimum therapeutic goals in individual patients and to predict what can happen when a dosage regimen is changed.

The sites into which drugs are routinely administered are broadly classified as intravascular and extravascular. Intravascular administration refers to the placement of a drug directly into blood, either IV or intra-arterially. Because the drug is placed directly into blood, it is imperative that a drug administered intravascularly be given as a solution. The extravascular routes of administration include oral, IM, sublingual, buccal, SC, dermal, rectal, and nasal routes. To enter the blood, a drug administered extravascularly must be absorbed from the site of administration. In addition, if a drug is orally administered through solid dosage forms, such as tablets or capsules, then the drug must first dissolve at the site of administration. Therefore, the dissolution of a drug is essential before absorption occurs. However, no such absorption step is required when a drug is administered IV.

Pharmacokinetics is the scientific discipline that deals with the mathematical description of biologic processes affecting drugs and affected by drugs. In addition to signifying the relationship of ADME processes to the intensity and time course of pharmacologic effects of drugs, pharmacokinetics describes the time course of a drug's ADME processes, which take place following the administration of a drug. Therefore, it is necessary to describe and analyze these processes and their effects in relation to their rates, rate constants, or time course. A qualitative description of these processes is quite insufficient and seldom leads to adequate and accurate characterizations of the effects of drugs on the body and effects of the body on the drugs. Pharmacokinetics is a quantitative study whose purposes are:

1. To develop mathematical expressions that permit one to describe the temporal changes of the drug concentration;
2. To determine constraints that describes ADME processes succinctly;
3. To make predictions and extrapolations based on the mathematical expressions; and

4. To help establish a dosage regimen that, in turn, will result in improved drug utilization in patients.

At a fundamental level, pharmacokinetics is a useful tool for pharmacists and physicians when optimizing the dosage regimen of drugs for individuals who can differ in their therapeutic response and their ability to absorb and eliminate drugs. Adjustment of dosage regimen to account for individual differences and disease states is, in essence, an exercise in clinical pharmacokinetics and clinical pharmacy practice.

A basic tenet of pharmacokinetics is that the magnitudes of both the desired response and toxicity are functions of drug concentration in the blood. Furthermore, it is not only the efficacy of a drug at the site of action that determines the intensity and duration of its pharmacologic or therapeutic effects, but also the amount of a drug and the rate at which the drug gets to the site of action. The vital processes of the body can delay the transport of drug molecules across membranes, convert drug molecules into metabolites, and remove them from the body as metabolites and/or the unchanged form. In turn, this can result in therapeutic failure, as a result of drug concentrations being too low, or unacceptable toxicity, as a result of the drug concentration being too high. Between these concentrations limits lies a region associated with therapeutic success. This region is regarded as a therapeutic range, or "therapeutic window." Each drug can possess its own therapeutic window, and because the drug concentration is rarely measured at the site of drug action, the drug concentration is measured at alternative and more accessible sites, such as plasma or serum and urine.

Figure 3.22 illustrates the concentration or therapeutic window for a drug. The terms "minimum toxic concentration" and "minimum effective concentration" describe the limits of the therapeutic range for a drug. If the administered dose of a drug produces the plasma concentration within this range, the drug will likely produce its therapeutic effect. The term "onset of action" is defined as the time at which the drug enters the therapeutic range (i.e., above the minimum effect concentration), and "termination of action" is defined as when the plasma concentration of a drug falls below the therapeutic range. The time span between the termination and the onset of action is described as the duration of action.

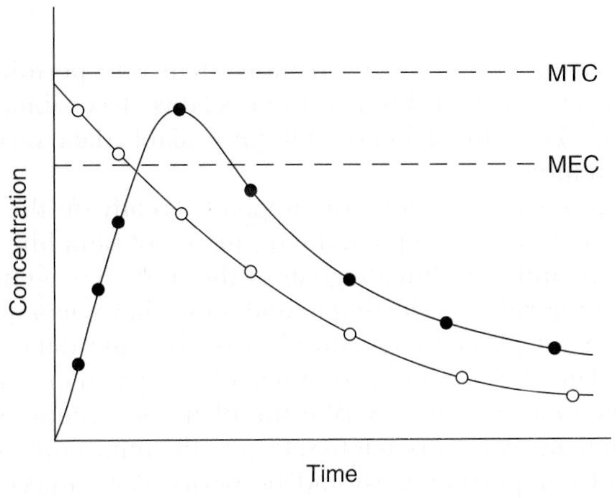

FIGURE 3.22 Typical plasma concentration versus time profile following administration of a dose of a drug by intravascular (o) and extravascular routes (●).

It is clear from Figure 3.22 and the previous definitions that an optimum dosage regimen might be defined as one that maintains the plasma concentration of a drug within the therapeutic range. Furthermore, it can be obvious from the previous discussion that the success of a drug in providing the desired drug concentration depends on factors such as how rapidly the drug reaches the general circulation from the site of administration, particularly following the oral and other extravascular routes; whether the drug is reaching the general circulation in sufficient amounts to provide plasma concentration within the therapeutic range; and the pharmacokinetic properties of a drug.

The purpose of this section is to provide students with a brief overview and the functional understanding of basic pharmacokinetics and its application to how physicochemical properties of drug molecules affect pharmacokinetic properties. Emphasis is placed on how to carry out pharmacokinetic analysis of the data and on how to use the pharmacokinetic parameters for predictive purposes. The mathematical equations presented have been chosen because of their general utility for predicting the plasma concentrations following administration of a drug by intravascular and extravascular routes. Furthermore, this discussion attempts to review and illustrate how the chemical modification of a drug through molecular modifications can alter selected pharmacokinetic parameters of drugs and, therefore, possibly the pharmacologic response in the drug discovery and development process.

Table 3.8 describes the dimensions of various pharmacokinetics parameters and provides examples of the corresponding typical dimensions reported in the literature.

Compartmental Concepts

The most commonly used approach to pharmacokinetic characterization of a drug is to depict the body as a system of compartments, even though these compartments often do not have any apparent physiologic reality. These frequently used compartmental models are illustrated in Figure 3.23.

The one-compartment model considers the body as a single homogenous unit (central compartment). This simplest model is particularly useful for pharmacokinetic analysis of plasma concentration versus time for drugs that are very rapidly distributed in the body. The two-compartment model consists of a central component, which includes the plasma and other highly perfused organs, connected to a peripheral or tissue compartment.

TABLE 3.8 Dimensions of Measurement and Typical Dimensions for Important Pharmacokinetics Parameters

Pharmacokinetics Parameter	Dimension of Measurement	Examples of Typical Dimensions
Mass of drug (e.g., mass of drug in blood, mass of drug at the site of administration, mass of drug in urine, and mass of metabolite in urine)	Amount	mg, μg, etc.
Plasma and/or serum concentration	Amount per unit volume	$mg{\cdot}L^{-1}$, $\mu g{\cdot}mL^{-1}$, mg/L, μg/mL, etc.
Elimination half-life	Time	hr, min, etc.
All first-order rate constants (e.g., elimination, distribution, disposition, absorption, and intercompartmental transfer rate constants)	Reciprocal of time	hr^{-1}, min^{-1}, etc.
All the apparent volumes of drug distribution (e.g., V for one compartment model, and V_c and V_b for two-compartment model)	Volume or volume per unit weight of a subject	L, mL, etc. or $L{\cdot}kg^{-1}$, $mL{\cdot}kg^{-1}$, L/kg, mL/kg, etc.
Zero-order rate constant	Amount, concentration, or percentage per unit time	$mg{\cdot}hr^{-1}$, $\mu g{\cdot}mL{\cdot}hr^{-1}$, $\%{\cdot}hr^{-1}$, mg/hr, μg/hr, %hr, etc.
All rates (zero as well as first order; e.g., absorption rate, elimination rate, and excretion rate)	Amount per time or concentration per time	$mg{\cdot}hr^{-1}$, $\mu g{\cdot}hr^{-1}$, $\mu g{\cdot}mL^{-1}{\cdot}hr^{-1}$, mg/hr, μg/hr, μg/mL/hr, etc.
All clearances (e.g., systemic, renal, metabolic, and creatinine clearance)	Volume per unit time or volume per unit time per unit weight	$mL{\cdot}hr^{-1}$, $L.hr^{-1}$, $mL{\cdot}hr^{-1}{\cdot}kg^{-1}$, $L{\cdot}hr^{-1}{\cdot}kg^{-1}$, mL/hr, L/hr, mL/hr/kg, etc.
Peak time	Time	hr, min, etc.
Dose administered (e.g., single intravenous or oral dose, loading dose, and maintenance dose)	Amount or amount per unit weight	mg, μg, $mg{\cdot}kg^{-1}$, mg/kg etc.
Peak concentration (e.g., for a single dose or multiple doses) etc.	Mass per unit volume	$mg{\cdot}L^{-1}$, $ng{\cdot}mL^{-1}$, mg/L, ng/mL
Area under the plasma concentration–time curve (AUC)	Mass per volume × time	$mg{\cdot}L^{-1}{\cdot}hr$, $ng{\cdot}mL^{-1}{\cdot}hr$, mg/L/hr, ng/mL/hr, etc.
Dosing interval	Time	hr, min., etc.
Absolute or relative bioavailability	Dimensionless	
Blood flow rate	Volume per unit time	$L{\cdot}hr^{-1}$, $mL{\cdot}hr^{-1}$, L/hr, mL/hr, etc.
Extraction ratios	Dimensionless	
Infusion rate	Mass per unit time or mass per unit time per unit weight	$mg{\cdot}kg^{-1}$, $\mu g{\cdot}kg^{-1}$, $\mu g{\cdot}kg^{-1}{\cdot}hr^{-1}$, mg/kg, μg/kg, μg/kg/hr, etc.

Each compartment can be considered to include a group of tissues, fluids, or parts of organs. A somewhat more complex model, illustrated in Figure 3.24, is the three-compartment model, which consists of a central

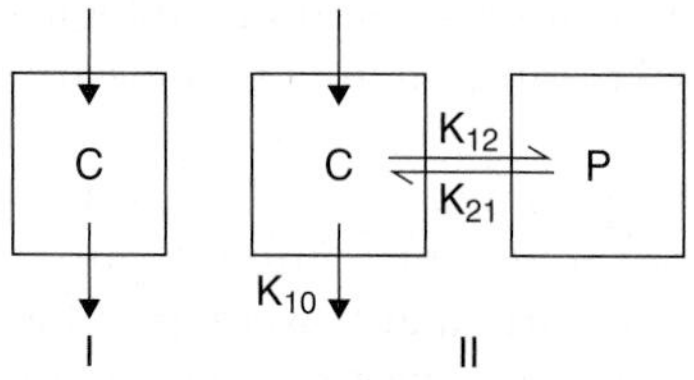

FIGURE 3.23 Schematic representation of the one-compartment (I) and two-compartment (II) models commonly used in pharmacokinetics. Arrows represent transfer of a drug because of the first-order process. C, central compartment (plasma, highly perfused organs); P, peripheral (tissue) compartment.

compartment connected to more than one peripheral compartment that differ in their relative accessibility to a drug. This model is chosen if the available data warrant such a model.

The selection of a model depends greatly on the site and tissue being sampled, the frequency of sampling collection, and the ultimate goals of the study. The general operating rule in selecting a model for pharmacokinetic analysis of plasma concentration versus time data is to postulate the minimum number of compartments necessary to accurately describe the pharmacokinetics of a given drug. An approach to selecting the minimum number of compartments should be performed, unless the experimental evidence dictates that such limited selection can lead to errors in estimating the pharmacokinetic parameters of drugs and in the use of equations to predict blood levels of drugs.

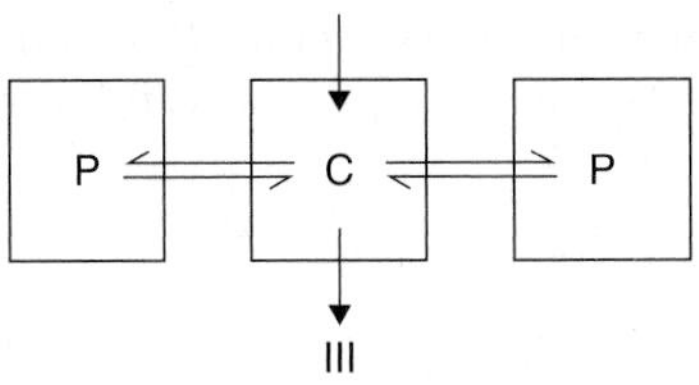

FIGURE 3.24 Schematic representation of a three-compartment (III) model commonly used in pharmacokinetics. Arrows represent transfer of a drug because of the first-order process. C, central compartment; P, peripheral compartment.

Linear and Nonlinear Pharmacokinetics

Linear Pharmacokinetics

Many processes in pharmacokinetics can be accurately described by a first-order process. This means that the rate of drug metabolism, the rate of transfer of a drug between compartments, and the rate of absorption and elimination of drugs from the body are directly proportional to the size of the dose administered. It is also true that passive diffusion is responsible for the transfer of a drug in the body and that a directly proportional relationship exists between the administered dose and the resulting drug concentration in the body. This dose proportionality is often used as an indicator of linear pharmacokinetics. It is important, however, to recognize that the pharmacokinetic parameters, such as elimination half-life and elimination rate constant, are independent of the size of the administered dose. Therefore, linear pharmacokinetics is regarded as dose-independent kinetics.

Nonlinear Pharmacokinetics

The rate of elimination of drugs (e.g., ethanol, salicylate, phenytoin) by metabolism and by other transfer processes, such as protein carrier systems, is not removed from the body by a first-order process, which means that the elimination rate is not proportional to the concentration of drug or to the dose administered, but follows zero-order kinetics—that is, the rate of change of drug concentration is independent of the drug concentration. A constant amount of a drug, rather than the constant percentage of the remaining amount of drug, is eliminated per unit time (i.e., mg/min or µg/mL/min).

The most frequently reported reason for the use of nonlinear kinetics is that metabolism and transfer processes require protein carrier systems. These systems are specific with respect to substrates that have finite capacities. The kinetics of these processes are described by the Michaelis-Menten equation (Eqs. 3.3–3.5).

Nonlinear, or dose-dependent, elimination kinetics can also be the result of effects other than the limited capacity of metabolism or elimination processes. If a drug is partly reabsorbed from the renal tubules by a recycling process with limited capacity, then the elimination of large doses proceeds relatively more rapidly than the elimination of smaller doses. Similarly, lesser binding of drugs to plasma constituents or tissues at higher dosing can result in relatively more rapid drug elimination than is observed at lower drug concentrations.

Evidence suggests that some drug metabolites can inhibit their own formation. This process of product inhibition can also cause dose-dependent effects, with large doses being eliminated relatively more slowly than small doses. The rate of decline of a drug concentration in the postdistribution phase, at any given level of a drug in the body, will be independent of the dose in the case of simple Michaelis-Menten kinetics. In cases of product inhibition, this rate tends to decrease with increasing doses.

Intravascular Administration

IV Bolus Administration and One-Compartment Model After the administration by IV injection, if a drug distributes very rapidly in the body, this confers on the body the characteristics of a one-compartment model, and if the drug elimination from the body can be described by a first-order process, then a plot of the logarithm of plasma drug concentration as a function of time yields a straight line, as shown in Figure 3.25.

The equation responsible for describing plasma drug concentration against time is as follows:

3.29 $$C_p = (C_p)_0 e^{-Kt}$$

where C_p is the plasma drug concentration at time t; $(C_p)_0$ is the initial plasma drug concentration (i.e., t = 0) immediately after the injection; K is the first-order

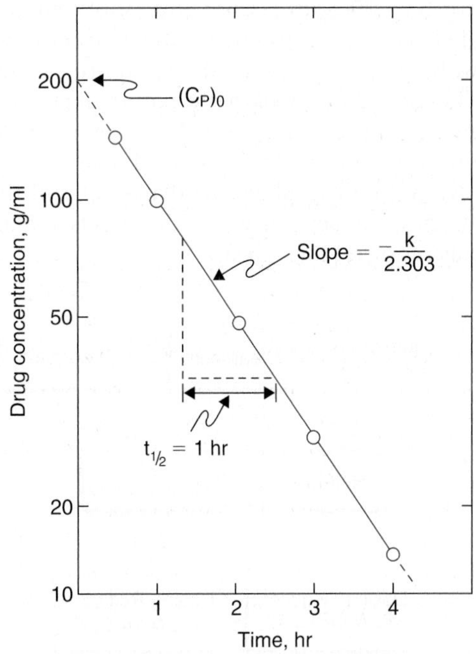

FIGURE 3.25 Schematic representation of plasma concentration of drug in the body as a function of time following rapid intravenous injection.

elimination rate constant; and t represents time. Equation 3.29 is also written as follows:

3.30 $$\ln C_p = \ln (C_p)_0 - Kt$$

or

3.31 $$\log C_p = \log (C_p)_0 - \frac{Kt}{2.303}$$

The initial plasma drug concentration, $(C_p)_0$, can be obtained by extrapolation of the line (Fig. 3.24) to $t = 0$ or the y-intercept of plasma drug concentration versus time plot. Figure 3.24 shows that a plot of the log of plasma drug concentration versus time will be linear under the stated condition.

Three primary factors determine the plasma concentration of the administered drug: 1) the route of administration; 2) the uptake of drug by body tissues; and 3) the elimination of the drug from the body. In the case of IV administration, because the drug is introduced directly into the blood, there is no delay as a result of the absence of the drug absorption process. The drug plasma level, however, depends on the size of the dose, and the maximum plasma drug concentration occurs immediately after completion of the dose administration.

Elimination Rate Constant and Half-Life

The half-life of a drug is a major factor in determining the dosing frequency, which is a function of the drug's clearance (Cl) and apparent volume of distribution (V). The relationship of a drug's half-life to the prediction of human pharmacokinetics and dosing regimen is shown in Figure 3.26 (54–56). Drugs with short half-lives are more likely to require frequent administration, whereas those with long half-lives tend to require dosing once daily. The two pharmacokinetic parameters that determine the half-life of a drug are clearance and volume of distribution. Dosing regimen is also linked to other factors, such as the drug pharmacodynamics and the drug concentrations associated with side effects versus those minimally required for efficacy.

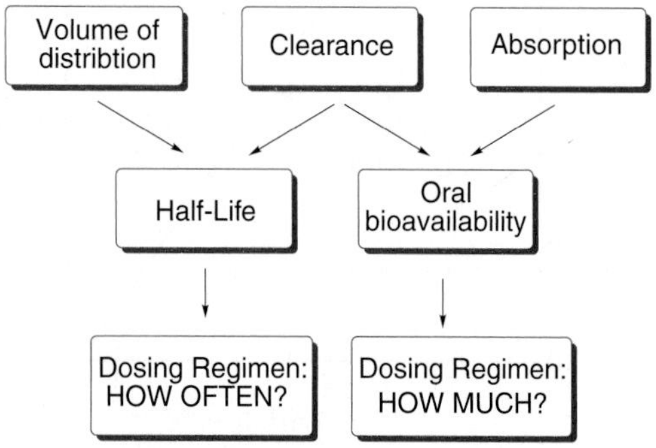

FIGURE 3.26 The relationship of volume of distribution to the prediction of human kinetics.

The elimination rate constant (K) can be determined from the slope of the straight line as follows:

3.32 $$(\text{slope})\ (2.303) = -K$$

However, it is much easier to determine the elimination rate constant by making use of the following relationship:

3.33 $$K = \frac{0.693}{t_{1/2}}$$

where $t_{1/2}$ is the time required for any drug concentration to decrease by half (i.e., 50%) and is also known as the biologic or elimination half-life. The elimination half-life is a pharmacokinetic property of a drug, and it is independent of the size of the administered dose when the administered drug exhibits the characteristics of a first-order process.

The elimination half-life ($t_{1/2}$) and the elimination rate constant (K) of a drug also have an important role in determining the plasma concentration of a drug at a given time. For instance, a drug with a short elimination half-life will be eliminated from the body much more quickly than a drug with a longer elimination half-life. These two parameters of a drug, therefore, become important in maintaining the desired drug blood levels in the body. In essence, these two parameters provide a quantifiable index of the presence of a drug in the body.

The process of drug elimination includes metabolism and excretion, which begin almost immediately when blood circulation distributes some of the drug to organs capable of metabolizing the drug or excreting it from the body. Among the organs of drug elimination, the liver is the principal site of metabolism, and the kidney is primarily responsible for the excretion of unmetabolized drugs and their metabolites. Other organs, however, can also participate in the elimination of selected drugs.

The consequence of metabolism of the drug to metabolite depends on the pharmacologic activity of the individual metabolite(s). Metabolites can be active or completely inactive. Active metabolites can be more or less potent than the parent drug, and they can exhibit similar or dissimilar action. The kinetics of distribution and elimination of metabolites can differ from those of the parent drug, because each metabolite differs from the parent drug in its physicochemical properties as a result of functional group additions or changes.

The elimination rate constant (K) is the sum of the individual rate constants that characterize the elimination of a drug from the body and the form of metabolite or unchanged drug. Thus:

3.34 $$K = K_u + K_m$$

where K_u and K_m represent the first-order rate constants associated with excretion and the form of metabolite or unchanged drug, respectively, removed from the blood.

Apparent Volume of Distribution

Plasma or serum samples, collected immediately following the administration of equal doses (i.e., X_0) of two different drugs, can exhibit large differences in the plasma drug concentration. This is because drug distribution in the body is largely a function of the drug's physicochemical properties and, therefore, of the chemical structure of a drug. The sole purpose of this parameter (V *or* V_d) is to relate the amount (mg) and the concentration (L^{-1}) of drug in the body at a given time. Therefore, it is important to recognize that knowledge of this parameter is essential for the determination of the dose of a drug required to attain the desired initial plasma concentration. The relationship of V to the prediction of human pharmacokinetics and dosing regimen is shown in Figure 3.26. Because it is not a true physical volume but, rather, a mathematical term that describes the behavior of a drug in the body with regard to its degree of partitioning between the plasma compartment and the remainder of the body, V is called "apparent." Drug partitioning into tissues represents a complex combination of physicochemical (lipophilicity, pK_a, plasma protein binding) and physiologic parameters. Drugs that are equally bound to plasma proteins can yield different V values, because the drug with the greater tissue binding will yield the larger V. However, drugs with equal tissue binding can differ in V, with the compounds having the greater plasma protein binding yielding the smaller volume of distribution.

This relationship is shown in Equation 3.35:

3.35 $$(X)_t = V(C_p)_t$$

where $(X)_t$ and $(C_p)_t$ are the amount of the drug and its plasma concentration, respectively, at a given time. V is determined by rearranging Equation 3.35 as follows:

3.36 $$V = \frac{(X)_0}{(C_p)_t} = \frac{\text{Dose}\,(X_0)}{(C_p)_0}$$

where $(X)_0$ is the administered dose of the drug and $(C_p)_0$ is its initial plasma concentration.

V of a drug is a property of the drug rather than of the biologic system and describes the extent to which a particular drug is distributed in the body tissues. The magnitude of V as a rule does not correspond to plasma, extracellular, or total body volume space but can vary from a few liters (7 to 10 L) to several hundred liters (≥ 200 L) in a 70-kg subject. The higher the value of V, the greater is the extent to which the drug is distributed in the body tissues, organs, or both. Furthermore, because body tissues, biologic membranes, and organs are lipophilic in nature, the value of V is correlated with the lipophilicity of a drug, which in turn is influenced by the drug's chemical structure, pK_a, and protein binding. The more lipophilic the drug, the greater is the value of V and the smaller is the initial plasma concentration (assuming the administered doses of drugs are identical). Conversely, if the drug is hydrophilic, the drug will penetrate to a lesser extent into tissue; consequently, the aqueous plasma concentration will be higher and V will be smaller. Therefore, the value of V is influenced by the lipophilicity of the drug molecule.

In most situations, V is independent of the drug concentration, because doubling the amount of a drug in the body usually results in doubling of its plasma concentration (linear pharmacokinetics). V is constant for a drug and remains independent of the dose administered and disease state. Other factors that can influence the blood composition, total body fluid, and the permeability characteristic of tissue, can bring about changes in the value of V. Furthermore, because V reflects the extent to which a drug will penetrate into tissue, alteration in the permeability characteristics of tissue will alter V. In addition, V of a drug can vary in infants, adults, and the geriatric population.

Many acidic drugs, including salicylates, sulfonamides, penicillins, and anticoagulants, are either highly bound to plasma proteins or are too water soluble to enter intracellular fluid and cannot penetrate tissues in a significant amount. Therefore, these drugs have low volumes of distribution and low tissue-to-plasma concentration ratios. A given dose of these drugs will yield relatively higher plasma concentrations. It can be implied that analytical problems in the determination of drug concentration are minimized or do not exist. Basic drugs, including tricyclic antidepressants and antihistamines, are extensively bound to extracellular tissues and are absorbed by adipose tissues. The V for these drugs is large—often larger than the total body space. For example, the value of V for amphetamine is approximately 200 L (3 L/kg). The relatively small doses and V for amphetamine produce a low plasma concentration, which makes its quantitative detection in plasma a difficult task.

Theoretical limits for V could be as low as 5 to 7 L (equivalent to the volume of the body fluid if the drug totally fails to penetrate the tissues or is extremely hydrophilic) or as high 200 L or greater. Because of differences in the magnitude of the V of a drug, a given dose of a drug with a relatively high V will provide low initial drug concentrations, and vice a versa (Eq. 3.35).

Clearance

One of the most important pharmacokinetic properties of a drug is clearance (Cl). In pharmacokinetic terms, clearance refers to the hypothetical volume of distribution from which the drug is entirely removed or cleared in unit time (mL/min or mL min^{-1}). In other words, Cl is an index of drug elimination. Cl is a function both of the intrinsic ability of certain organs, such as kidneys and liver, to excrete or metabolize a drug and of the blood flow rate to these organs. The concept of Cl is illustrated by assuming elimination in a single organ as depicted in Figure 3.27.

Under the conditions described in Figure 4.27, the venous concentration of drug (C_V) will always be less than the arterial concentration (C_A) because of the drug being eliminated or excreted during the passage of blood through the organ. The rate at which the drug enters the organ is the product of blood flow rate (Q) and the arterial concentration. The rate at which the drug leaves the

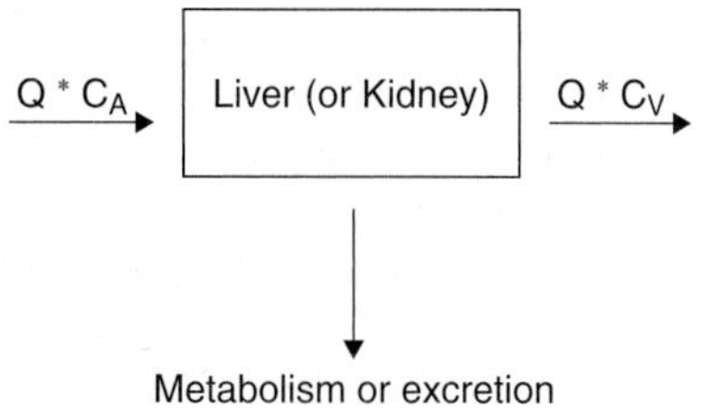

FIGURE 3.27 Schematic representation of drug elimination by the liver (or kidney). $Q \cdot C_A$ is the rate at which the drug enters the liver (or kidney), and $Q \cdot C_V$ is the rate at which the drug leaves the liver (or kidney). The venous drug concentration (C_V) is less than the arterial drug concentration (C_A).

organ, however, is equal to the product of blood flow rate and venous concentration:

3.37 $$\text{The rate in} = Q^{*}C_A$$

3.38 $$\text{The rate out} = Q^{*}C_V$$

The difference between the rate in and rate out is the rate of elimination of a drug by the organ:

3.39 $$\text{rate of elimination} = Q(C_A - C_V)$$

The dimensionless ratio of elimination rate (K) to the rate at which a drug enters the organ (QC_A) is defined as the extraction ratio (ER) and is obtained as follows:

3.40 $$\text{ER} = \frac{Q(C_A - C_V)}{QC_A} = \frac{(C_A - C_V)}{C_A}$$

ER of a drug ranges from 0 to 1 depending on how well the organ eliminates or excretes the drug from the blood flowing through it. If an organ does not eliminate the drug, then $C_A = C_V$, and the ER is 0 (low extraction ratio). If, however, the organ avidly removes the drug so that $C_V \cong 0$, then ER is 1 (high extraction ratio). If liver is the organ responsible for metabolizing the drug, then the extraction ratio is described by using the notation, E_H.

Using the extraction ratio number (i.e., ER of E_H), the drugs have been classified as having a low (ER < 0.3), intermediate (ER = 0.3 to 0.7), or high (ER > 0.7) ER. Table 3.9 lists the representative drugs with their hepatic or extraction ratios. The influence of blood flow and intrinsic clearance of an organ on the clearance of a drug is determined by the ER of the drug.

Cl can also be viewed as a proportionality constant relating the elimination rate of a drug to its plasma concentrations at a given time and is expressed as:

3.41 $$(Cl) = \frac{\text{rate of elimination}}{\bar{C}_p}$$

where $\bar{C}_p$ is the average plasma concentration of a drug at a time that corresponds to the rate of elimination. It follows from an earlier equation (Eq. 3.41) that:

3.42 $$(Cl) = Q^{*}\text{ER}$$

where Q and ER have been previously defined and, because the drug elimination follows a first-order process, *Cl* is independent of the drug concentrations or the dose administered.

The total-body clearance of a drug from the blood is equal to the ratio of the overall elimination rate to drug concentration (Eq. 3.41), where the overall elimination rate is comprised of the sum of the elimination processes occurring in all organs and the removal of a drug in all its forms. Therefore, the overall clearance, $(Cl)_s$, represents the renal clearance (i.e., unchanged form of a drug) and

TABLE 3.9 Hepatic and Renal Extraction Ratios of Selected Drugs and Metabolites

Low (< 0.3)	Intermediate (0.3–0.7)	High (> 0.7)
Hepatic extraction[a]		
Carbamazepine	Aspirin	Alprenolol
Diazepam	Quinidine	Arabinosyl-cytosine
Digitoxin	Codeine	Desipramine
Indomethacin	Nortriptyline	Doxepin
Phenobarbital		Isoproterenol
Phenytoin		Lidocaine
Procainamide		Meperidine
Salicylic Acid		Morphine
Theophylline		Nitroglycerin
Tolbutamide		Pentazocine
Valproic Acid		Propoxyphene
Warfarin		Propranolol
Renal extraction[a]		
Atenolol	Cimetidine	(Many) Glucuronides
Cefazolin	Cephalothin	Hippurates
Chlorpropamide	Procainamide	(Some) Penicillins
Digoxin	(Some) Penicillins	(Many) Sulfates
Furosemide		
Gentamicin		
Lithium		
Phenobarbital		
Sulfisoxazole		
Tetracycline		

[a]At least 30% of the drug is eliminated by this route.

the metabolic clearance (i.e., removal of a drug as metabolic by kidney). It is also useful to keep in mind that the *Cl* can be expressed as the product of the apparent volume of distribution (*V*) and the elimination rate constant (*K*) for drugs that exhibit characteristics of a one-compartment model. Thus:

3.43 $$(Cl)_s = VK$$

Hepatic Clearance

Although metabolism can take place in many organs, the liver frequently has the greater metabolic capacity and, therefore, has been the most thoroughly studied. The most direct quantitative measure of the liver's ability to eliminate a drug is hepatic clearance, $(Cl)_H$, which includes biliary excretion clearance and hepatic metabolic clearance:

3.44 $$(Cl)_H = Q_H E_H$$

where Q_H is the sum of the hepatic portal and hepatic arterial blood flow rates, the values of which are 1,050 and 300 mL/min, respectively.

Under conditions of normal body functions, the pharmacokinetic behavior of most drugs can be established within reasonable limits, and optimal dosage regimens can be designed using the observed values of the pharmacokinetic parameters of the drug. However, when renal function is compromised as a result of acute or chronic renal diseases or the patient's age, drugs that are predominantly eliminated through the kidneys are likely to be retained in the body for a longer duration and accumulate to the extent of providing toxic drug levels with repeated dosing. If the drug is converted to a metabolite, the accumulation of active metabolite can also lead to a toxic effect, and although most metabolites are inactive, their accumulation with repeated dosing can produce toxic reactions by displacement of the parent drug from plasma protein and by inhibiting further drug metabolism.

Renal failure can result from a variety of pathologic conditions. If renal impairment is rapid in onset and short in duration, then renal failure is described as acute. The primary cause of acute renal failure can be prerenal (i.e., acute congestive heart failure or shock), intrarenal (i.e., acute tubular necrosis), or postrenal (i.e., hypercalcemia). Although renal failure is generally reversible, complete restoration of renal function can take 6 to 12 months.

Chronic renal failure is almost always caused by intrinsic renal diseases and is characterized by slow, progressive development. Unlike the acute condition, chronic renal impairment is generally irreversible. The degree or loss of kidney functional capacity in the chronic condition is best described in terms of the intact "nephron" hypothesis, in which the diseased kidney is comprised of nephrons that are essentially nonfunctional because of pathologic conditions along with normal nephrons. Progressive renal impairment is the result of an increasing fraction of nonfunctional nephrons.

The prolonged and progressive nature of chronic renal failure is of particular concern in older patients, who can require a variety of medications, both for their renal condition and for other unrelated conditions. The inability of these patients to adequately excrete drugs and drug metabolites and the influence of their uremic conditions on the functions of other physiologic systems require careful adjustments of drug dosage to obtain accurate and adequate blood levels without increased toxicity.

Drugs are cleared by kidneys as a result of passive filtration through the glomeruli or by active transport in the kidney tubule. Once in the nephrons, drugs (and their unconjugated metabolites) can also be reabsorbed into the circulation. The glomerular filtration rate is measured using any compound that is filtered by glomeruli and not reabsorbed. Although exogenous compounds, such as urea and inulin, are used for this purpose, the relative ease of using endogenous creatinine has made this the method of universal choice. In principle, the following equation determines the relationship between the creatine clearance, $(Cl)_{cr}$, the serum creatinine concentration, $(\bar{C}_s)_{cr}$ and creatinine excretion rate, $(dX_\mu/dt)_{\bar{t}} \cdot cr$:

3.45 $$(Cl)_{cr} = \frac{(dX_\mu/dt)_{\bar{t}} \cdot cr}{(\bar{C}_s)_{cr}}$$

Serum creatinine concentration is constant unless there is a change in the rate of production of creatinine in the body or creatinine clearance. The creatinine clearance in normal kidneys is approximately 110 to 130 mL/min. This value declines with progressive renal impairment, and it drops to zero with severe renal impairment. Creatinine clearance values of 20 to 30 mL/min signify moderate renal impairment; values of less than 10 mL/min signify several renal impairment. Creatinine is poorly secreted and not subject to tubular reabsorption; therefore, its clearance is a useful measure of the glomerular filtration rate. Although creatinine clearance tells us about only one aspect of renal function (i.e., filtration), it is an excellent indicator for assessing the severity of renal impairment.

The extent to which decreased renal function influences drug elimination is a function of the percentage of circulating drug being cleared by the kidneys. From the literature, the influence of renal impairment on the elimination half-life of a drug will clearly be a direct function of the percentage of the drug cleared through the kidneys. If the elimination half-life of a drug that is cleared essentially unchanged via the kidneys is plotted against the endogenous creatinine clearance (Fig. 3.28), the result will be a hyperbola.

IV Bolus Administration (Two-Compartment Model)

After the administration of a drug IV, a finite amount of time has to pass before distribution equilibrium is attained

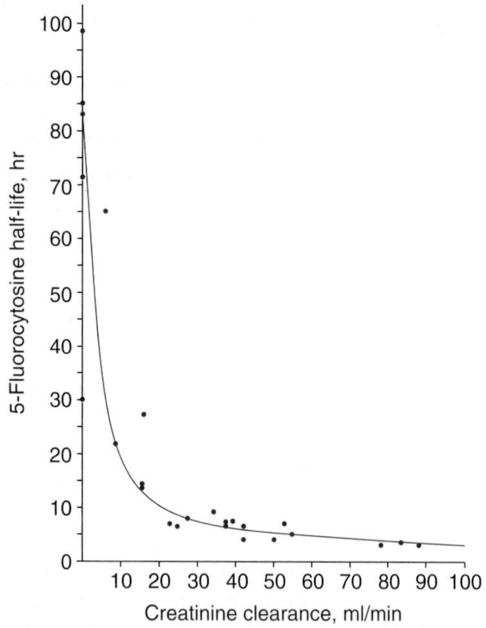

FIGURE 3.28 Curvilinear relationship between the elimination half-life of 5-fluorocytosine and renal function (creatinine clearance). (45).

in the body. During this distribution phase, the plasma drug concentration will decline more rapidly than during the postdistribution phase, as shown in Figure 3.29. There are three possible types of two-compartment models, which differ between whether the elimination of the drug occurs from the central compartment, the peripheral compartment, or both. The three types of two-compartment models are, mathematically, indistinguishable on the basis of available concentration data. The type of two-compartment model illustrated in Figure 3.23 is most

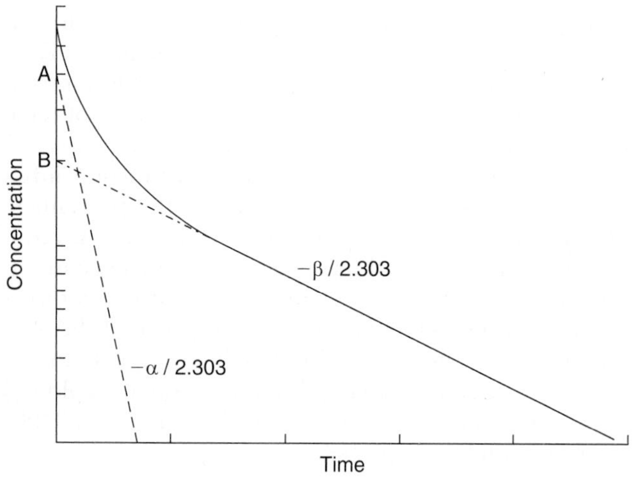

FIGURE 3.29 Semilogarithmic plot of drug concentration in the plasma against time following administration of a rapid intravenous injection when the body can be represented as a two-compartment open model. The dashed line is obtained by "feathering" the curve.

often used to describe the pharmacokinetics of drugs. In this model, it is assumed that drug elimination from a two-compartment model occurs exclusively from the central compartment, because the sites of metabolism and excretion (i.e., liver and kidney) are well perfused with blood and, therefore, presumably rapidly accessible to drug in the systemic circulation. Whether this distribution phase is apparent depends on the early collection of blood samples. A distribution phase can last for only a few minutes or for several hours.

A semilogarithmic plot of plasma drug concentration as a function of time (Fig. 3.29) after rapid IV injection of a drug can often be resolved into two linear components, which can be done graphically by using the residual, or "feathering," method, as shown in Figure 3.29, in which the slopes of rapid and slow disposition phases will permit the determination of α and β, respectively, in Equation 3.46. The intercepts on the concentration axis are designated A and B. The entire plasma concentration–time curve can be described by the following equation:

3.46 $$C_p = Ae^{-at} + Be^{-bt}$$

where α and β are the first-order distribution and disposition rate constants, respectively. A biexponential decline in the plasma drug concentration justifies, mathematically, the representation of the body as a two-compartment model.

Extravascular Route of Administration

When a drug is administered by extravascular routes (such as orally), absorption is requisite for a drug to reach the general circulation. Absorption is defined as a process whereby a drug proceeds from the site of administration to the site of measurement within the body, generally blood, plasma, or serum. Figure 3.30 represents the passage of a drug through the gastrointestinal tract into the general circulation.

When a drug is orally administered, there are several possible sites for drug loss. One such site is the gastrointestinal lumen, where drug decomposition can occur. If it is assumed that the drug survives destruction in the gut lumen and is metabolized by enzymes as it passes through the membrane of the gastrointestinal tract, then even though the drug leaves the site of administration, it is considered not to be systemically absorbed. Indeed, loss at any site in the gastrointestinal tract before reaching the site of measurement can contribute to a decrease in the systemic absorption of the drug. The requirement for an orally administered drug to pass through the gastrointestinal tract makes the extent of absorption not always complete. The loss of a drug as it passes for the first time through gastrointestinal membrane and the lining, during absorption, is known as the first-pass effect. Figure 3.31 represents the time course of a drug and metabolite at each site in the body.

The rate or the change in the amount of drug in the body (dX/dt) following administration of a drug by an

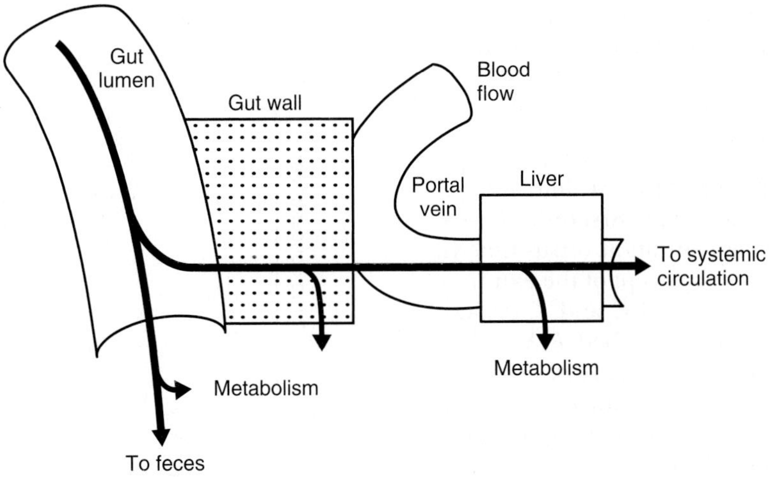

FIGURE 3.30 After oral administration, a drug must pass sequentially through the gut lumen, the gut wall, and then the liver before reaching the general circulation. Metabolism can occur in the lumen before absorption, in the gut wall during absorption, or in the liver after absorption and before reaching the systemic circulation. (From Rowland M, Tozer T. Clinical Pharmacokinetics: Concepts and Application, 2nd Ed. Philadelphia: Lea and Febiger, 1989, with permission.)

extravascular route is a function of both the absorption rate (K_aX_a) and the elimination rate (KX):

3.47 $$\frac{dX}{dt} = K_aX_a - KX$$

where K_aX_a is the first-order absorption rate, KX is the first-order elimination rate, and K_a and K are the first-order absorption and elimination rate constants, respectively.

When the absorption rate is greater than the elimination rate (i.e., $K_aX_a > KX$), the amount of drug in the body and plasma drug concentration increase with time. Conversely, when the amount of drug remaining at the absorption site (X_a) is sufficiently small, the elimination rate exceeds the absorption rate (i.e., $KX > K_aX_a$); therefore, the amount of drug in the body and the drug concentration in the plasma decrease with time.

The peak plasma concentration [$(C_p)_{max}$] after drug administration occurs at the moment when the absorption rate equals the elimination rate (i.e., $K_aX_a = KX$). The faster the drug is absorbed, the higher the $(C_p)_{max}$ and the shorter the time required following administration of a dose to observe the $(C_p)_{max}$. Integration of Equation 3.47 from $t = 0$ to $t = t^*$ and converting the amount to the concentration results in the following equation:

3.48 $$C_p = \frac{K_aF(X_a)_0}{V(K_a - K)}(e^{-Kt} - e^{-K_at})$$

where $(X_a)_0$ is the administered dose and F is the fraction of the administered dose that is absorbed and available to reach the general circulation. Equation 3.48 is often used to determine plasma concentration after administration of a drug by an extravascular route when the administered drug manifests the characteristics of a one-compartment model.

The absorption rate constant (K_a) of a drug frequently is larger than the elimination rate constant (K). Under such a condition, at some time after drug administration, the value of the term e^{-Kt} in Equation 3.48 approaches zero, indicating that no more drug is available for absorption, and Equation 3.48 simplifies to:

3.49 $$C_p = \frac{K_aF(X_a)_0}{V(K_a - K)}(e^{-Kt})$$

3.50 $$C_p = \text{Intercept}(e^{-Kt})$$

3.51 $$\log C_p = \log \text{Intercept} - \frac{Kt}{2.303}$$

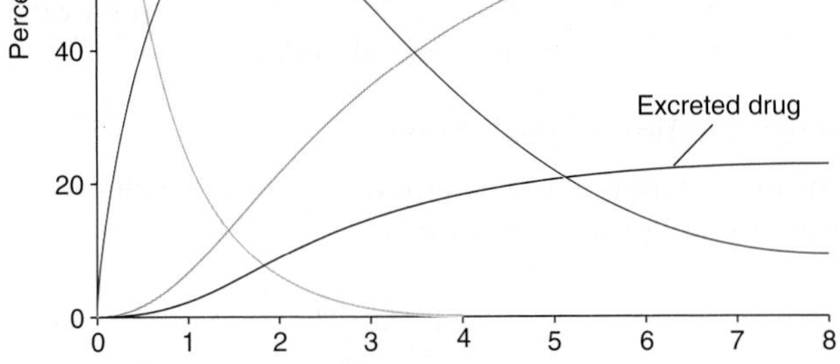

FIGURE 3.31 Time course of a drug at each site following an extravascular administration.

When the absorption is complete, the term $X_a K_a$ disappears from Equation 3.47 and the equation is reduced to:

3.52 $$-\frac{dX}{dt} = KX$$

During the postabsorption phase, the decline in the plasma concentration with time follows first-order kinetics. A typical plot of plasma concentration versus time is shown in Figure 3.32, where the intercept of the extrapolated line (I*) is a complex function of K_a and K, respectively, as well as the dose or amount absorbed, $F(X_a)_0$, and the apparent volume of distribution (V). It is, however, incorrect to assume that the intercept approximates the ratio of dose over the V unless the drug is rapidly and completely absorbed, which rarely occurs.

Importance of Absorption Rate

The influence of absorption on the drug concentration time profile is shown in Figure 3.33. The administration of an equal dose of a drug in three different dosage forms or by three different extravascular routes or three different formulations results in threefold the drug concentration in the plasma. The faster the drug is absorbed (i.e., $K_a >>> K$), the greater is $(C_p)_{max}$ and the shorter the time required to achieve peak plasma drug concentration.

Many drugs do not exhibit demonstrable pharmacologic effects or do not elicit a desired degree of pharmacologic response unless a minimum concentration is reached at the site of an action and, therefore, a minimum therapeutic concentration in the plasma. Thus, the absorption rate of a drug can affect the clinical response if it fails to yield the minimum effective concentration. As evident in Figure 3.33, the more rapid the absorption of a drug is, the faster its onset of response (i.e., curve A). When the drug is absorbed rather slowly (curve C), the minimum effective concentration is just barely attained. The intensity of maximum pharmacologic effects is a function of the drug concentration. The data presented in Figure 3.33 suggest that the administered dose of a drug in curve A can produce a more intense response than observed in curves B and C.

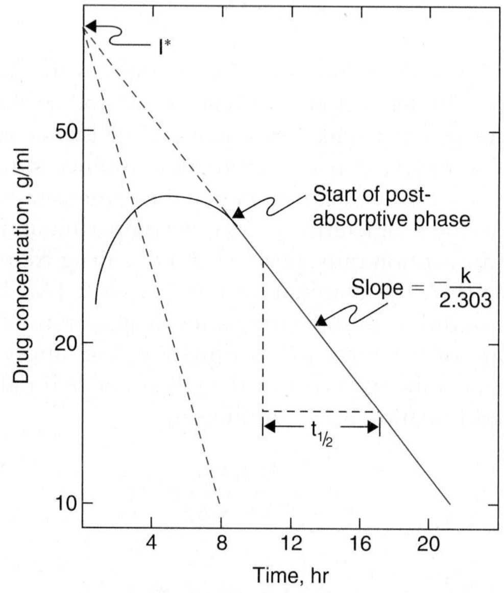

FIGURE 3.32 Typical semilogarithmic plot of drug concentration versus time profile in plasma following the administration of a drug by an extravascular route. The dashed line represents the "feathered line" used to obtain the absorption rate constant (K_a).

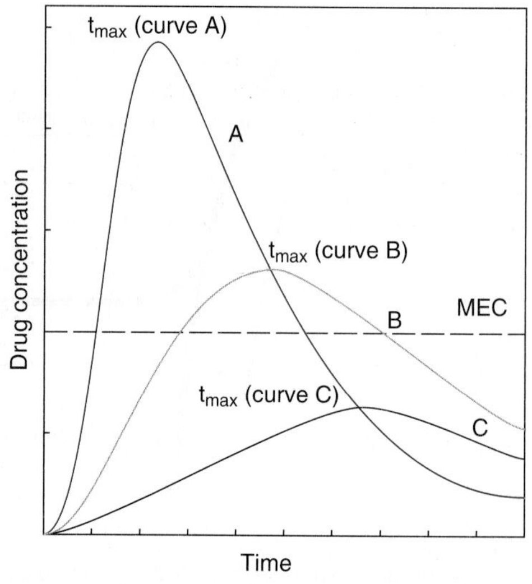

FIGURE 3.33 A plasma concentration versus time profile illustrating the influence of absorption rate constant (K_a) on the rate of absorption as reflected in the peak time (t_{max}) and peak plasma concentration $(C_p)_{max}$.

The peak plasma drug concentration is always lower following administration of a drug by the extravascular route compared with its initial plasma concentration following administration of an identical dose by IV solution. In the former, at peak time, some drugs can still remain at the absorption site and some has been eliminated, whereas the entire dose is in the body immediately following the IV administration.

The delay between drug administration and a drug reaching the general circulation can be of particular importance when a rapid onset of effect is desired. This delay is termed "lag time," and it is anywhere between a few minutes to many hours. Lag time generally is attributed to the slow and poor absorption of the drug, either because of slow disintegration and dissolution of the drug from the dosage form or because of slow removal of the coating material from coated tablets.

Determination of Peak Time

The determination of peak time (t_{max}) can be achieved by using the following equation:

3.53 $$t_{max} = \frac{\ln (K_a/K)}{(K_a - K)}$$

where K_a and K are the first-order absorption and elimination rate constants, respectively. Equation 3.53 shows that the t_{max} is a function only of the relative magnitude of the absorption and elimination rate constants. As the rate of absorption decreases (i.e., smaller K_a value), the t_{max} will be higher, as shown in Figure 3.33, progressing from curve C to curve A.

The rate of drug absorption varies when the extravascular route is changed, when the formulation of a drug is changed, or when the dosage form is changed. These changes will be reflected in different t_{max} for the same dose of a drug. However, t_{max} will be unaffected by a mere change in the size of the administered dose. In many disease states, the impairment in the renal function can affect the elimination rate constant, thereby producing a change in the t_{max}.

Determination of Peak Plasma Concentrations

The maximum peak plasma drug concentration, $(C_p)_{max}$, in the body occurs at time t_{max}, which is described by substituting t_{max} for time t in Equation 3.48:

3.54 $$(C_p)_{max} = \frac{K_a F(X_a)_0}{V(K_a - K)}(e^{-Kt_{max}} - e^{-K_a t_{max}})$$

Equation 3.54 is further simplified into:

3.55 $$(C_p)_{max} = \text{Intercept}\,(e^{-Kt_{max}} - e^{-K_a t_{max}})$$

where the intercept of the plasma drug concentration versus time is equal to $K_a F(X_a)_0 / V(K_a - K)$, as previously described in Equations 3.49 through 3.51.

Peak Time and Peak Plasma Concentration

The most important property of any oral dosage form, intended for a systemic therapeutic effect, is the ability of the oral dosage form to deliver the active ingredient to the bloodstream in an amount and at a rate sufficient to produce the desired therapeutic effect. This property of a dosage form is described as bioavailability.

Bioavailability, essentially, captures two features: how fast the drug enters the systemic circulation (rate of absorption) and how much of the administered dose of a drug enters the systemic circulation (extent of absorption). Assuming that the therapeutic effect of a drug is directly related to the drug concentration in a patient's blood, these two properties of an oral dosage form are, in principle, important in correlating the therapeutic response to a drug's dose. The onset of response is directly linked to the rate of absorption, whereas the time-dependent extent of response is connected to the extent of adsorption.

The bioavailability of a drug, following the administration of an oral dose, can vary because of either patient-related or dosage form–related factors. Patient-related factors can include the nature and timing of meals, age, disease, and gastrointestinal physiology. The dosage form– or drug-related factors can include the chemical form of the drug (such as salt vs. free drug), its physical properties (such as crystal structure and particle size), and an array of formulation (excipients) and manufacturing (processing) variables.

Therefore, the bioavailability of a drug is of clinical, academic, and regulatory interest. The regulatory interest includes agencies such as the U.S. Food and Drug Administration (FDA) and its global partners, which approve safe and effective drug products. Applications from manufacturers seeking regulatory approval of a new drug (New Drug Application [NDA]) must provide exhaustive information about the drug's pharmacokinetics (ADME). The more pertinent interests in the bioavailability of a drug relate to questions about the absolute extent of absorption (absolute bioavailability), the importance of product formulation changes during the drug development process, the comparability of different oral dosage forms, and whether the products can be administered with meals.

Manufacturers seeking regulatory approval of generic drug products by filing an Abbreviated New Drug Application (ANDA) must provide detailed bioavailability evidence showing comparative performance of their product against the innovator's branded product with respect to the rate of absorption and the extent of absorption. To declare product equivalence, while assessing and evaluating the bioequivalence of two or more chemically or pharmaceutically equivalent drug products, both the rate and extent of absorption of the products are expected to be the same within the statistical tolerance of ±80%. In the United States, the FDA has the responsibility to determine how the rate and extent are to be assessed and set standards for what is meant by "significant differences," "same," and "similar." The underlying principle is that generic products should be bioequivalent for the drug or its active metabolite or both to be considered by the FDA for therapeutic equivalence. Therefore, the measurements of the rate and extent of absorption are indicators of therapeutic outcomes or, at least, markers to assess drug product performance

The extent of drug absorption is generally evaluated by measuring the area under the plasma concentration–time curve (AUC), a well-accepted criterion to assess the extent of absorption. In linear pharmacokinetics, all observed plasma drug concentrations rise and decline in proportion to changes in the extent of absorption. The rate of absorption, however, is assessed by measuring peak time (t_{max}) and peak plasma concentration [$(C_p)_{max}$]. The rate of absorption is turning out to be the nemesis of bioequivalence testing because there is disagreement among scientists on how best to assess the rate of absorption. $(C_p)_{max}$ and the time of its occurrence (t_{max}) are considered as universal measures of absorption rate. $(C_p)_{max}$ depends on the extent of absorption and, for this reason, is often not a reliable measure of rate. Moreover, $(C_p)_{max}$ is relatively insensitive to the changes in the absorption rate. The measure of t_{max} has been found to be a relatively sensitive measure of absorption rate. It is, however, a discrete measure that depends on the frequency of the blood sampling in the absorption and elimination phases. Because rate is not a single number and varies with time, it is often difficult to measure absorption rate precisely.

With limitations and debates on assessing the rate of absorption accurately, $(C_p)_{max}$ and t_{max} have an important role characterizing the absorption of a drug following its oral administration. Collectively, both parameters can be used to draw some inferences from the AUC data following the oral administration of a drug. As previously stated, both t_{max} and $(C_p)_{max}$ are used by the FDA to assess the comparative bioavailability and bioequivalence for a drug product. t_{max} can be used to assess the onset of action following oral administration of an identical dose of drug via a different dosage form, different route of administration, or different formulation of the same dosage form. t_{max} is a reflection of the onset of action of a drug. The shorter the t_{max}, the quicker the onset of action of a drug is likely to be. Differences in onset of action and t_{max} are routinely observed when the same dose of a drug is administered by different routes or different dosage forms to a subject.

$(C_p)_{max}$ also has an important role in assessing comparative bioavailability or bioequivalence. Assuming that plasma concentration is a reflection of the pharmacologic effects of a drug, the higher the drug $(C_p)_{max}$ (within the therapeutic range), the better will be the pharmacologic effect or the intensity of the pharmacologic effect. Therefore, $(C_p)_{max}$ is also used to determine the route of drug administration and the selection of a formulation.

Bioavailability

The bioavailability of a drug is defined as the rate and extent to which the administered dose of a drug reaches the general circulation. As a rule, rapid and complete absorption of a drug is desirable if it is used for pain, allergy response, insomnia, and other conditions for which a quick onset of action is desired. As previously indicated in Figure 3.33, the more rapid the absorption is, the shorter the onset of action and the greater the intensity of a pharmacologic response. Bioavailability determines the amount of administered dose that reaches the circulation, which is also related to rate of drug clearance, as shown in Figure 3.26.

The efficacy of a single dose is a function of both the rate and the extent of absorption. Thus, for two dosage forms or two oral routes to be comparable with regard to the bioavailability following the administration of a drug, the absorption rate of a drug and the extent to which a drug reaches the general circulation from each dosage form or oral route of administration must be comparable.

The useful estimate of relative absorption rates of a drug from different products, through different routes of administration or different conditions (i.e., with or without food or in the presence of other drugs, etc.), can be made by comparing the magnitude of time of occurrence of t_{max}, $(C_p)_{max}$, and total area under the plasma concentration–time curve $[\text{AUC}_0^\infty]$. The peak time and peak plasma concentration can be determined by using Equations 3.53 and 3.54 or 3.55, respectively, and the extent of absorption can be determined as described in the following section.

Estimating the Extent of Absorption

The extent of absorption is estimated by determining the total area under the plasma drug concentration–time curve, AUC_0^∞, or the total amount of an unchanged drug excreted in urine, $(X_u)_{\infty}$, following the administration of a drug. AUC_0^∞ can be estimated by several methods, such as by using a planimeter, which is an instrument for measuring the area of a planar irregular figure, and by using the cut-and-weight method, which weighs the paper of plasma concentration–time curve. The weight is converted to weight per unit area. The most common method, however, is the application of the trapezoidal rule and equation, when possible. In a single-dose study, we cannot determine the area under the plasma concentration–time curve by using the trapezoidal rule alone. In this case, a widely used practice is to determine the area under the plasma concentration–time curve from $t = 0$ to $t = t^*$ (the last sampling time) by means of trapezoidal rule and estimate the remaining area by using the following equation:

3.56 $$(\text{AUC})_{t^*}^{\infty} = C_p{}^* / K$$

where $(\text{AUC})_{t^*}^{\infty}$ is the area under the plasma concentration–time curve from the last sampling time to time ∞, $C_p{}^*$ is the last observed plasma concentration, and K is the first-order elimination rate constant. This $(\text{AUC})_{t^*}^{\infty}$ will be added to the area under the curve obtained from $t = 0$ to $t = t^*$ to calculate the total area under the plasma concentration–time curve:

3.57 $$(\text{AUC})_0^{\infty} = (\text{AUC})_0^{t\otimes} + (\text{AUC})_t^{\infty\otimes}$$

When an IV administration of a drug exhibits the characteristics of a one-compartment model, the total area under the plasma concentration–time curve is estimated by the following equation:

3.58 $$(\text{AUC})_0^{\infty} = \frac{\text{dose}}{VK}$$

where VK is the systemic clearance of a drug.

Following the administration of a drug by an IV injection, if it is necessary to use a two-compartment model, the area under the plasma concentration–time curve from $t = 0$ to $t = t^*$ (the last sampling time) is estimated by using trapezoidal rules, as previously mentioned. The area under the plasma concentration–time curve from $t = t^*$ to $t = \infty$ can then be computed using the following equation:

3.59 $$(\text{AUC})_t^{*\infty} = C_p{}^* / \beta$$

where $C_p{}^*$ is the last observed plasma concentration and β is the first-order disposition rate constant.

When a drug is administered by an oral route, one can use the following equation to determine AUC_0^∞:

3.60 $$(AUC)_0^\infty = \frac{F(\text{dose})}{VK}$$

If it is desired to assess the relative extent of drug absorption from a product, AUC_0^∞ of the product is compared to the AUC_0^∞ obtained for a reference drug standard. The reference standard can be an IV injection, an orally administered aqueous or water-miscible solution, or another product accepted as a standard.

When it is desired to assess the absolute bioavailability (F), the reference drug standard becomes an IV injection, and when it is desired to judge the bioequivalence, the reference standard is an innovator product. If the AUC_0^∞ values are identical following the administration of equal doses of a test product and the reference IV solution, we conclude that the test product is completely absorbed and not subject to presystemic metabolism.

Frequently, however, the standard is an innovator product or another established product. If the AUC_0^∞ values are identical following the administration of equal doses of the test and reference products, we conclude that the test product is completely bioavailable relative to the standard. It is essential to use the term "relative to the standard" because we do not know if the standard is completely absorbed or available. Additionally, when two products produce comparable $(C_p)_{max}$ and t_{max} and the reference standard is an innovator product, then the products are judged to be bioequivalent.

By using the ratio of AUC_0^∞ for extravascular to IV routes, one can determine the F of a drug from a test product as follows:

3.61 $$F = \frac{(AUC)_0^\infty \text{ oral}}{(AUC)_0^\infty \text{ IV solution}}$$

where F is the absolute bioavailability of a drug or the fraction of the administered dose that reaches the general circulation following the administration of equal dose of a drug. If the administered doses of a drug are different than the AUC_0^∞, then estimates can be scaled approximately to permit comparison under identical conditions or equivalent doses—assuming, of course, that AUC_0^∞ is directly proportional to the administered dose. The relative bioavailability (F_{rel}) of a drug from a test product is determined by using the following expression:

3.62 $$F_{rel} = \frac{(AUC)_0^\infty \text{ test product}}{(AUC)_0^\infty \text{ reference standard}}$$

Equation 3.62 assumes that the doses administered from each product are identical, and if not, the AUC_0^∞ values should be scaled for the dose differences.

Therefore, the bioavailability of a drug following its extravascular administration can be expressed as:

3.63 $$F = \frac{(X_u)_\infty \text{ extravascular}}{(X_u)_\infty \text{ intravascular}}$$

To determine the assessment of relative bioavailability (F_{rel}), Equation 3.63 becomes:

3.64 $$F_{ref} = \frac{(X_u)_\infty \text{ test product}}{(X_u)_\infty \text{ standard product}}$$

In addition, Equations 3.63 and 3.64 are applicable under the condition that the administered doses are identical. The utility of these equations depends on how much of the drug is eliminated by urinary excretion, the sensitivity of the analytical procedure, and the variability in urinary output of the drug. Many drugs are extensively metabolized, with little, if any, drug appearing in an unchanged form in the urine. In such cases, the bioavailability is estimated from the plasma concentration–time data.

Presystemic or First-Pass Metabolism

After oral administration, a drug must pass sequentially from the gastrointestinal lumen, through the gut wall, and through the liver before reaching the general circulation (Fig. 3.30). Because the gut wall and liver are the sites of drug metabolism, a fraction of the amount of drug absorbed can be eliminated or metabolized before reaching the general circulation. Therefore, an oral dose of a drug can be completely absorbed yet incompletely available to reach the general circulation because of presystemic or first-pass effect (metabolism) in the gut wall or liver. If such is the case, it will be reflected in the values of AUC_0^∞ for the administered dose.

Criteria have been developed to identify and quantify the extent of presystemic metabolism and to indicate when it is occurring. The determination of presystemic metabolism requires only that the systemic availability of a drug is less than the fraction of the dose absorbed. The fraction absorbed can be determined from the urinary excretion of a drug and metabolite after oral administration of a drug relative to that after IV administration. Many drugs undergoing presystemic metabolism in humans have been identified on the basis of this type of information. Differentiation between the gut wall and the liver as the site of presystemic metabolism is more difficult in humans, although relatively easy in animals.

The liver is the most important site of presystemic elimination because of high levels of drug-metabolizing enzymes, its ability to rapidly metabolize different types of drugs, and its unique anatomic location. The following are selected examples of drugs that are subject to considerable hepatic first-pass metabolism: the β-blockers propranolol and metoprolol; the analgesics propoxyphene, meperidine, and pentazocine; the antidepressants imipramine and nortriptyline; and the antiarrhythmic lidocaine.

Hepatic presystemic metabolism is most easily understood when liver is the sole organ of drug elimination. Under these conditions, the clearance of the drug, as determined following IV administration of the drug, is equal to:

3.65 $$(Cl)_H = \frac{\text{dose}}{(\text{AUC})_0^\infty}$$

Hepatic clearance, however, is also equal to:

3.66 $$(Cl)_H = Q_H \cdot E_H$$

where $(Cl)_H$ is the hepatic clearance, Q_H is the hepatic blood flow rate, and E_H is the dimensionless hepatic extraction ratio of the drug. Hepatic blood flow rate (Q_H) has a mean range from approximately 1.1 to 1.8 L/min, with an average of approximately 1.5 L/min. The hepatic extraction ratio (E_H) of a drug can range from 0 to 1, depending on the liver's ability to metabolize the drug. The maximum hepatic clearance of a drug, excluding hepatic metabolism, is equal to hepatic blood flow; this occurs when $E_H = 1.0$. The fraction of a drug eliminated from portal blood (Fig. 3.30) during the absorption phase is given by the hepatic extraction ratio (E_H); the remainder of the drug (i.e., $1 - E_H$) escapes into the systemic circulation and then is cleared from the circulation by the liver according to Equation 3.66.

If the fraction of the oral dose is absorbed and then subjected to hepatic presystemic metabolism, the AUC_0^∞ following oral administration of a drug is given by:

3.67 $$(\text{AUC})_0^\infty = \frac{F(X_a)_0(1 - E_H)}{Q_H \cdot E_H}$$

Because $Q_H \cdot E_H$ is equal to hepatic clearance (Eq. 3.66), which under these conditions is given by the ratio of an IV dose to an area under the concentration–time curve, AUC_0^∞ IV, Equation 3.67 is rewritten as:

3.68 $$\frac{(\text{AUC})_0^\infty \text{ oral}}{(\text{AUC})_0^\infty \text{ IV}} = \frac{F(X_a)_0(1 - E_H)}{(X_a)\text{IV}}$$

The ratio of AUC_0^∞ after oral and IV administration of equal doses of drugs is the systemic availability (i.e., the fraction absorbed). If it is assumed that the drug is completely absorbed (i.e., $F = 1$), then Equation 3.68 reduces to:

3.69 $$F = (1 - E_H)$$

Equation 3.69 shows that the systemic availability of the drug depends on the E_H of the drug, and those drugs with low E_H, such as antipyrine, tolbutamide, and warfarin, undergo little presystemic metabolism.

An estimate of E_H is made from determination of the clearance of a drug following IV administration and comparing this value to the mean value of liver blood flow according to Equation 3.66, when rearranged:

3.70 $$E_H = \frac{(Cl)_H}{Q_H}$$

The IV clearance of propranolol is approximately 1.05 L/min. Assuming that the average liver blood flow is approximately 1.5 L/min, we can determine that the hepatic extraction for propranolol (E_H) is 0.7 and that the fraction absorbed (F) is 0.3. This means that even though propranolol is well absorbed, only 30% of the oral dose is available for systemic circulation.

This type of information, in conjunction with the value of the fraction absorbed (F), has been used to substantiate the predominantly hepatic presystemic elimination of several drugs, including propranolol, lidocaine, and pentazocine. The plasma concentrations for pentazocine, following the oral administration of a 100-mg dose and IV administration of a 30-mg dose, are shown in Figure 3.34, which shows that even though the IV dose is smaller, this route of administration provides higher plasma concentration than an oral dose. The systemic availability (F) of pentazocine after oral administration was reported to be 11% to 32%, with a mean of 18%. This low systemic availability is consistent with its high hepatic clearance.

Repetitive Drug Administration (Multiple Dosing)

If a fixed IV dose of a drug is administered repeatedly at a constant time interval (τ), the plasma concentration of a drug at any time can be calculated using the following expression:

3.71 $$(C_p)_t = \frac{X_0}{V}\left(\frac{1 - e^{-nK\tau}}{1 - e^{-K\tau}}\right)e^{-Kt}$$

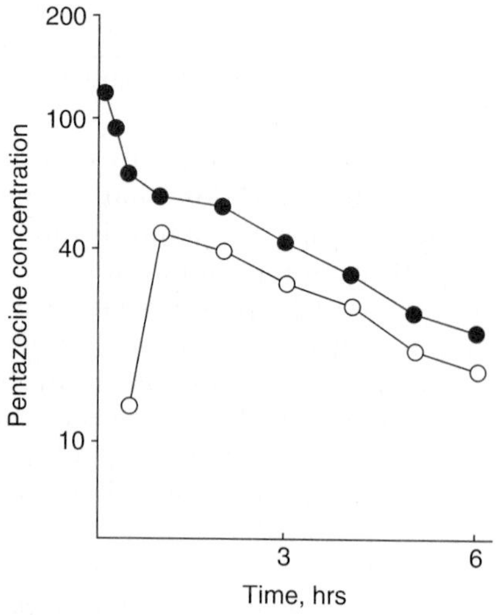

FIGURE 3.34 Pentazocine concentration in plasma (ng/mL) after administration of 100 mg orally (o) or 30 mg intravenously (●). (From Ehrnebo M, Boreus L, Lonroth U. Bioavailability and first-pass metabolism of oral pentazocine in man. Clin Pharmacol Ther 1977;22:888–892, with permission.) (57).

where n is the number of doses that have been administered, t is the time between $t = 0$ and $t = \tau$, τ is the dosing interval, X_0 is the dose administered, V is the apparent volume of distribution of the drug, and K is the elimination rate constant. At the plateau, Equation 3.71 reduces to:

3.72 $$(C_p)_\infty = \frac{X_0}{V}\left(\frac{e^{-Kt}}{1-e^{-K\tau}}\right)$$

where $(C_p)_\infty$ is the steady-state plasma concentration.

The maximum plasma concentration of a drug (Fig. 3.35) at steady-state, $(C_p)_\infty$ max, and its minimum plasma concentration at steady-state, $(C_p)_\infty$ min, is determined by setting $t = 0$ and $t = \infty$, respectively. Equation 3.71 then becomes:

3.73 $$(C_p)_\infty \max = \frac{X_0}{V}\left(\frac{1}{1-e^{-K\tau}}\right)$$

and

3.74 $$(C_p)_\infty \min = \frac{X_0}{V}\left(\frac{1}{1-e^{-K\tau}}\right)e^{-K\tau}$$

When drugs are administered as repetitive doses (multiple doses), it is often of practical use to determine the "average" plasma concentration at the plateau or steady-state, $(\bar{C}_p)_{ss}$ average. This is obtained by:

3.75 $$(\bar{C}_p)_{ss} \text{ average} = \frac{X_0}{VK\tau}$$

where τ is the dosing interval, X_0 is the administered dose, and VK is its systemic clearance. Equation 3.75 clearly indicates that by knowing the V and the K, obtained from the administration of a single IV bolus dose, the average plasma concentration of a drug can be predicted for the IV bolus administration of a fixed dose (X_0) at a constant dosing interval (τ). Equation 3.75 also clearly indicates that only the size of the dose (X_0) and the dosing interval (τ) can be adjusted to obtain the desired average steady-state plasma drug concentration.

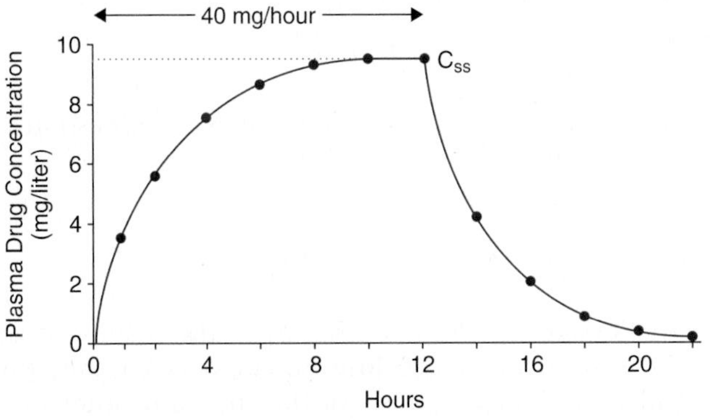

FIGURE 3.35 A typical plasma concentration versus time profile for a drug administered intravenously as a fixed dose (X_0) at a fixed dosing interval (τ).

It is important to recognize that the average steady-state plasma drug concentration, $(\bar{C}_p)_{ss}$ average, is neither the arithmetic nor geometric mean of $(C_p)_\infty$ max and $(C_p)_\infty$ min but, rather, the ratio of the AUC_0^∞ curve during the dosing interval (τ) at the plateau over the dosing interval (τ).

When the drug is administered by the oral route (Fig. 3.36), the mathematical expressions are more complex than the analogous equations for IV administration:

3.76 $$(C_p)_\infty = \frac{K_a F(X_a)_0}{V(K_a - K)}\left(\frac{e^{-Kt}}{1-e^{-K\tau}} - \frac{e^{-K_a t}}{1-e^{-K_a\tau}}\right)$$

where $(X_a)_0$ is the dose administered; F is the fraction absorbed; K_a and K are the first-order absorption and the elimination rate constants, respectively; V is the apparent volume of distribution; and t and τ are time and dosing intervals, respectively. Following the administration of each successive dose in the postabsorption period, Equation 3.76 reduces to:

3.77 $$(C_p)_\infty \min = \frac{K_a F(X_a)_0}{V(K_a - K)}\left(\frac{e^{-K\tau}}{1-e^{-K\tau}}\right)$$

The average steady-state plasma concentration of a drug when administered by an extravascular route is obtained using the following equation:

3.78 $$(C_p)_{ss} \text{ average} = \frac{F(X_a)_0}{VK\tau}$$

Or by substituting Equation 3.60 into Equation 3.78:

3.79 $$(C_p)_{ss} \text{ average} = \frac{(AUC)_0^\infty}{\tau}$$

where F is the fraction absorbed or absolute bioavailability of a drug. Taking the ratio of Equation 3.78 over Equation 3.75 after the attainment of the steady-state condition permits one to determine the bioavailability of a drug; of course, this assumes that the administered doses are identical.

Repeated administration of a fixed dose at a constant dosing interval (τ) produces a gradual increase of drug levels in the body until the steady-state condition is attained. This increase is the result of drug accumulation factor (τ) because of the sequential dosing of the drug. Therefore, predicting the degree of accumulation of a drug under defined conditions becomes important. Multiplying each side of Equation 3.75 by V and dividing by the administered dose, Equation 3.80 is obtained:

3.80 $$\frac{X_{ss} \text{ average}}{X_0} = \frac{1}{K\tau} = \frac{1.44t_{1/2}}{\tau}$$

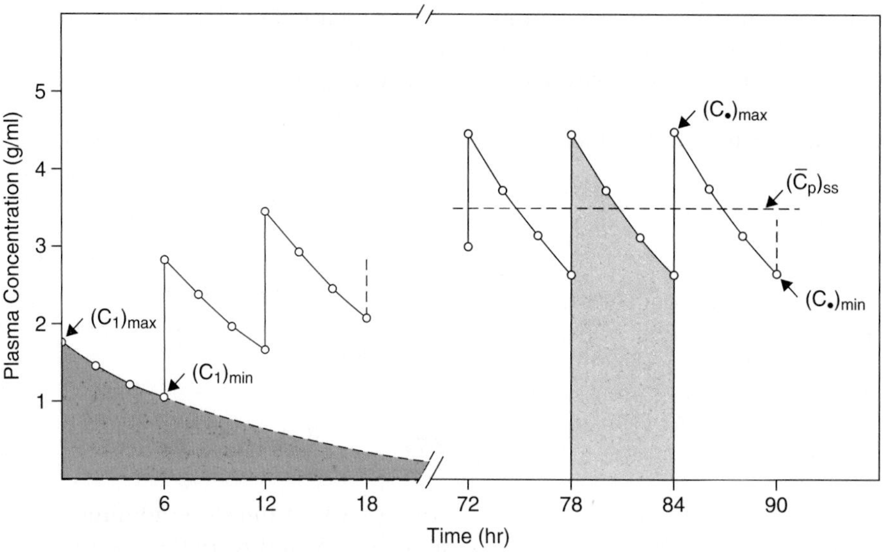

FIGURE 3.36 A typical plasma concentration versus time profile for a drug administered orally as a fixed dose $(X_a)_o$ at a fixed dosing interval (τ).

Where X_{ss} average/X_0 = R = drug accumulation factor and X_{ss} average is the "average" amount of drug in the body at the steady-state condition.

The ratio of the average amount of a drug at its steady-state and the administered dose is defined as drug accumulation (R). Equation 3.80 describes that the magnitude of drug accumulation is a function of the elimination half-life of a drug and the chosen dosing interval. For example, if a drug with an elimination half-life of 12 hours (i.e., $K = 0.0577\ h^{-1}$) is administered every 6 hours (τ), the ratio of X_{ss} average over dose is 2.9. This means that repeated administration of a fixed dose of a drug in the body is approximately 2.9-fold the amount administered in a single dose. It is also clear from Equation 3.80 that the drug accumulation ratio (R) is directly proportional to the elimination half-life of the drug ($t_{1/2}$) and inversely proportional to the dosing interval (τ); however, R is independent of the size of the administered dose.

Because considerable time can elapse before a steady-state condition is attained as a result of repeated drug administration, it is often desirable to administer a large dose initially (i.e., loading dose) to achieve the desired drug levels immediately. Equation 3.29, which describes the time course of drug concentration after a single IV bolus dose, is written as:

3.81 $$(C_p)_1 \min = \frac{X_0}{V}(e^{-K\tau})$$

where $(C_p)_1$ min is the drug concentration immediately before administration of the second dose of the same size as the first one (i.e., the minimum concentration occurs at $t = \tau$ following administration of the first dose). The minimum steady-state plasma concentration, $(C_p)_\infty$ min, is given by Equation 4.74. Thus, the ratio of $(C_p)_\infty$ min to $(C_p)_1$ min (i.e., Eqs. 3.74 and 3.81) is another way to measure the drug accumulation (R), which can be calculated by means of the following expression:

3.82 $$R = \frac{(C_p)_\infty \min}{(C_p)_1 \min} = \frac{1}{1-e^{-K\tau}}$$

This ratio of minimum drug concentrations, numerically, is not equal to the ratio of the "average" dose of a drug at steady-state and the dose administered (Eq. 3.80).

If one wished to administer a loading dose (D_L) that produces the minimum concentration equal to $(C_p)_\infty$ min:

3.83 $$(C_p)_1 \min = (C_p)_\infty \min = \frac{D_L}{V}e^{-K\tau}$$

Dividing Equation 3.74 by Equation 3.83 will result in:

3.84 $$1 = \frac{D}{D_L(1-e^{-K\tau})}$$

Equation 3.84, on rearrangement, yields an expression to determine the loading dose (D_L):

3.85 $$\frac{D_L}{D} = \frac{1}{(1-e^{-K\tau})}$$

In Equations 3.84 and 3.85, D_L is the loading dose and D is the maintenance dose. Equation 3.85 permits the calculation of loading dose for the chosen maintenance dose and dosing interval (τ) and is applicable for the administration of a drug not only by an IV bolus but also by the extravascular route. When a drug is administered by the extravascular route, however, it is essential that each maintenance dose be administered following the complete absorption of a drug from the previous dose. Conversely, Equation 3.85 also permits the determination of the maintenance dose required to maintain the minimum drug level produced by the administration of the initial dose for any chosen dosing interval.

Plasma Protein Binding in Pharmacokinetics

Drug binding to plasma proteins affects drug distribution and elimination as well as the pharmacologic effect of a drug. The high molecular weight of plasma proteins restricts their passage across capillaries, and their low lipid solubility prevents them from crossing the cell membrane. Analogously, binding of drugs to plasma protein restricts their passage across cell membranes. Only that fraction of the drug concentration that is freely circulating or unbound can penetrate the cell membrane and be subject to glomerular filtration. Hepatic metabolism of most drugs is also limited by the availability of free fraction of drug in the blood. Because the interaction of drugs with plasma protein is a rapidly reversible process, one can view the plasma protein-binding phenomenon as being temporary storage of a drug, subject to instant recall.

Drug binding to plasma protein can be attributed to ionic, Van der Waals, and hydrogen bonding. The most important contribution to drug binding in the plasma is made by albumin, which comprises approximately 50% of the total plasma protein. In healthy subjects, albumin concentration in the plasma is approximately 4 g/100 mL. During pregnancy and other diseases, however, low levels of plasma protein are observed. Although albumin binds a wide variety of drug molecules, it has a particularly important role in the binding of weak acidic and neutral drugs.

α_1-Acid glycoprotein is another important binding protein with an affinity for basic drugs. α_1-Acid glycoprotein is a low molecular weight protein. It is an acute-phase reactant, and its concentration in plasma rises in inflammation, malignant diseases, and stress. Conversely, its plasma concentration falls in hepatic diseases and nephrotic syndrome. The average concentration of α_1-acid glycoprotein is approximately 40 to 100 mg/100 mL. Other plasma proteins have a limited role in drug binding. The drug–protein interactions can be described by applying the law of mass action:

3.86 $$D_F + \text{free sites} \underset{K_2}{\overset{K_1}{\rightleftharpoons}} D_B$$

where D_F and D_B represent the free and bound drug, respectively, and K_1 and K_2 are the association and dissociation rate constants, respectively. Thus:

3.87 $$K = \frac{K_1}{K_2} = \frac{[D_B]}{[D_F][\text{free sites}]}$$

3.88 $$K = \frac{K_1}{K_2} = \frac{[D_B]}{[D_F][nP - D_B]}$$

where K is the equilibrium association constant, K_1 and K_2 are binding rate constants, n is the number of available binding sites per mole of protein, and $[D_F]$, $[D_B]$, and P are the molar concentration of free drug, bound drug, and protein, respectively.

The binding rate constants K_1 and K_2 appear to be large, because the equilibrium is established almost immediately. The value of the equilibrium constant (K) varies from zero, at which essentially no drug is bound, to greater than 10^6, at which almost all drug is bound to the protein. The fraction of drug in the plasma that is free or unbound (f_p) is then obtained as follows:

3.89 $$f_p = \frac{[D_F]}{[D_F]+[D_B]}$$

3.90 $$f_p = \frac{[D_F]}{[D_T]}$$

where $[D_T]$ is the total drug concentration in the plasma. In most cases, for a given amount of drug in the body, the greater the binding of drug to plasma protein, the larger is the total drug concentration of drug in the plasma. Changes in drug binding as a rule affect the blood level of total drug and have a role in pharmacokinetic variability.

The free fraction of drug in the plasma (f_p) depends on the magnitude of the equilibrium constant (K), the total drug concentration, $[D_T]$, and the protein concentration, $[P]$. In theory, there are limited numbers of binding sites on the protein. As the plasma drug concentration increases, the number of available free sites decreases, and therefore, the fraction of available free drug increases. In reality, however, the fraction of unbound drug in the plasma for most drugs, when administered in therapeutic doses, is essentially constant over the entire drug concentration range. Concentration-dependent changes in the fraction of free drug in the plasma are most likely to occur with drugs exhibiting a high association constant (K= 10^5 to 10^6) administered in large doses.

The relationship between bioavailability and area under the plasma concentration–time curve is nonlinear and absorption rate dependent when the plasma protein binding of a drug is concentration dependent. Two drug products from which a drug is equally well absorbed will produce different values for the area under the plasma concentration–time curve if a difference exists in the absorption rate. Generally, such a comparison will overestimate the extent of drug absorption of the more slowly absorbed product.

The clearance of many drugs from the blood is directly proportional to the free drug fraction in the plasma (f_p). The steady-state concentration of these drugs is inversely proportional to the free fraction in the plasma. However, clearance of some drugs is largely independent of plasma protein binding. The direction and magnitude of the effect of plasma protein binding on the elimination half-life of a drug depends on the size of the drug's *V* and whether the drug exhibits restrictive clearance (i.e., has an intrinsic clearance less than the liver blood flow). The half-life of a restrictively cleared drug with relatively small *V* (i.e., $V <$ 0.25 L/kg) can show a small decrease in elimination half-life when there is decrease in plasma protein binding (i.e., an increase in the free fraction in plasma. Conversely, the half-life of a nonrestrictively cleared drug with a small apparent volume of distribution can show a small increase in half-life when the free fraction is increased. Drugs with a large value for *V* (i.e., $V >$ 0.5 L/ kg) either will be essentially independent of the changes in plasma protein binding (restrictive clearance) or will show an increase in half-life that is directly proportional to the increase in free fraction (nonrestrictive clearance).

The classical methods of studying protein binding of drugs include equilibrium dialysis and ultrafiltration. Ultrafiltration provides quick measurements but is not as accurate as the equilibrium dialysis method. Detailed discussions for studying protein binding can be found in textbooks listed in the Suggested Readings.

STATISTICAL MOMENT ANALYSIS

Statistical moment analysis is a noncompartmental method, based on statistical moment theory, for calculation of the absorption, distribution, and elimination parameters of a drug. This approach to estimating pharmacokinetic parameters has gained considerable attention in recent years.

The zero moment in the drug plasma concentration–time curve is the total area under the plasma concentration–time curve from $t = 0$ to $t = \infty$, AUC_0^∞. Estimates of the area under this curve are useful in calculating bioavailability as well as drug clearance, which is the ratio of dose over area under the concentration–time curve for an IV dose.

The first moment of the plasma concentration–time profile is the total area under the concentration–time curve resulting from plot of the product of plasma concentration and time (i.e., $C_p t$) versus time, as illustrated in Table 3.10 and Figure 3.37 (45).

Column 2 of Table 3.10 shows the concentration versus time data obtained following a 1-hour constant-rate infusion, and column 3 also includes concentration–time values for the product of concentration × time. These values are plotted against time in Figure 3.34. The area under the curve for the concentration–time plot is obtained by using the trapezoidal rule. The total area under the curve for the product of concentration × time is termed the "area under the first-moment curve" (AUMC).

The ratio of the AUMC over the area under the concentration–time curve for any drug, according to the theory, is the assessment of the mean residence time (MRT). The MRT provides a quantitative estimate of the persistence of a drug in the body, and like the half-life of a drug, MRT or persistence is a function of distribution and elimination of a drug. Comparison of MRTs following administration of a drug as an IV bolus or via any other extravascular route provides information regarding the mean absorption time (MAT).

One of the most useful properties of statistical moment analysis is that it permits estimation of the apparent volume of distribution that is independent of drug elimination (i.e., regardless of the model chosen to describe the concentration–time data).

TABLE 3.10 Drug Concentration and Drug Concentration–Time Data During and After a 1-Hour, Constant-Rate Infusion (45)

Time (hours)	Concentration (µg/mL)	Concentration–Time (µg/mL/h)
0.5	3.2	1.6
1.0	5.9	5.9
2.0	4.2	8.4
3.0	3.0	9.0
4.0	2.1	8.4
5.0	1.5	7.5
6.0	1.1	6.6
8.0	0.5	4.0

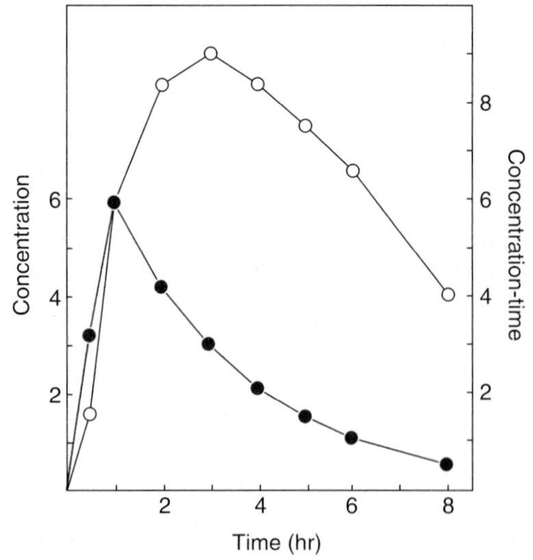

FIGURE 3.37 Plots of drug concentration (µg/mL; ●) and drug concentration × time (µg/mL/h; o) versus time during and after 1 hour of a constant-rate infusion. The area under the concentration versus time plot to infinity is AUC; the area under the concentration × time versus time plot to infinity is AUMC. (45).

Mean Residence Time (MRT)

The MRT of a drug after administration of a single dose is provided by the following equation:

3.91 $$MRT = \frac{AUMC}{AUC}$$

The MRT for a drug administered IV provides a useful estimate of the persistence time in the body. Therefore, in this sense, it is related to the half-life of a drug. When applied to a drug that distributes rapidly (i.e., one-compartment model), it has been shown that:

3.92 $$MRT = \frac{1}{K}$$

where K is the elimination rate constant.

Because the half-life of a drug is equal to $0.693/K$, half-life is a measurement of the time required to eliminate 50% of the administered dose. The MRT, however, indicates the time required to eliminate 63.2% of the administered dose.

When a drug is administered by an extravascular route, statistical moment analysis theory can also be used for estimating the rate of absorption. This approach, however, requires the calculation of MRT for IV as well as extravascular routes, because the method is based on the differences in MRT for different modes of administration. In general:

3.93 $$MAT = (MRT)_{EV} - (MRT)_{IV}$$

where $(MRT)_{EV}$ is the MRT following administration of a drug by an extravascular route and $(MRT)_{IV}$ is the MRT for the IV bolus dose. When the administered drug follows the first-order process:

3.94 $$(MRT)_{EV} = \frac{1}{K_a}$$

where K_a is the first-order absorption rate constant. Under these conditions:

3.95 $$K_a = \frac{1}{MAT}$$

and the absorption half-life is obtained by $0.693/MAT$.

The statistical moment theory offers an attractive alternative for the evaluation and estimation of the absorption data, and even in the absence of intravenous data, this method permits the ranking of several dosage forms, with respect to drug release and absorption, from the available MRT values.

SUMMARY

From this discussion, the efficacy of a drug is not determined by its pharmacodynamic characteristics alone, but efficacy also depends, to a large extent, on the pharmacokinetic parameters of the drug, because ADME processes control the rate and extent to which an administered dose of a drug reaches its site of action.

Because of the high degree of structural variability of drugs, multiplicity of kinetics, and metabolite kinetics, the task of establishing a clear correlation between the structured chemistry of substituents and their pharmacokinetic properties appears somewhat daunting. The pharmacokinetic fate of a drug molecule, however, appears to be a consequence of its physicochemical properties and, therefore, can, to some extent, be predicted from its chemical structure.

Although the drug in the formulation has received considerable attention, many of the alterations in the formulation can be considered as chemical changes. Most of what has been reported applies primarily to the gastrointestinal absorption of drugs and can be viewed as attempts to:

1. Maximize the rate of absorption by increasing the rate of dissolution (i.e., micronization, salt of acid or bases, amorphous form and metastable polymorph, etc.)
2. Decrease the loss of a drug because of its degradation in the stomach (i.e., acid, insoluble esters or salt, and chemically stable derivatives of a drug)
3. Extend the duration of action by reducing the rate of a drug's release from a dosage form (e.g., timed release, depot-forming injectable, macrocrystals, and slowly dissolving salts)
4. Decrease the loss of a drug by reducing the complex formation

These examples for enhancing gastrointestinal absorption represent the response to a particular problem with the parent compound and, therefore, can be viewed as "corrective" research. It is of considerable interest to see this aspect of research become "predictive and preventive," in which the pharmacokinetic parameters of drugs are required in the early phases of drug discovery to optimize the effectiveness of drugs.

An immediate problem facing those who would consider optimizing all factors of a drug is physically locating the receptor site and defining the ideal time course for the drug–receptor interaction and sustained effects. An ideal drug molecule should reach the site of action, arrive rapidly in sufficient quantity, remain at the site of action for sufficient time, be excluded from other sites, and be removed from the site, when appropriate. Although such an ideal drug molecule rarely exists, alternate approaches are chosen to optimize the effectiveness of a drug. Furthermore, if a correlation exists between a biologic response and the plasma blood levels of a drug, then the pharmacokinetic parameters (ADME) have an important role in influencing the biologic response, because these parameters influence the magnitude of the blood level of a drug in the body. The task of examining the examples of drugs illustrating the connection between biologic response and pharmacokinetics study is not an easy one, but the results do convey the important facts that:

1. Pharmacokinetic parameters influence the biologic responses, which are critical in drug design.
2. Pharmacokinetic parameters can be modified by subtle structural changes, which in turn can influence the desired blood level.

The ultimate goal is to design a drug molecule that exhibits the desired pharmacologic effect as a result of the proper balance of ADME processes. Figure 3.37 illustrates how modification of a parent structure can influence the availability of a drug to the receptor site (58).

The following are some of the processes shown in Figure 3.38 that are altered by changing a substituent group on the drug molecule:

- **I.** Supply and loss
  - **A)** Rate of transfer from the dosage form
  - **B)** Binding of a drug in the depot
  - **C)** Stability of a drug in the depot
- **II.** Distribution in the body
  - **A)** Binding of a drug in the central and peripheral compartments
  - **B)** Apparent volume of distribution
  - **C)** Transfer of a drug to the receptor sites
- **III.** Drug–receptor interaction

Consider the following well-known example for the design of a urinary tract anti-infective. The site of infection is the urinary tract. The example selected is the prodrug methenamine. In acidic pH, methenamine is converted to formaldehyde, which acts as an antibacterial agent (Fig. 3.39). Tablets of methenamine are often enteric coated to prevent conversion to formaldehyde in the stomach. Methenamine is cleared intact from the kidney into the urine, where it is hydrolyzed to formaldehyde if the pH is less than 6.5. The rate of hydrolysis is controlled by the urinary pH.

The influence of structural effects on pharmacokinetic parameters can be illustrated using the following examples. The steady-state levels of the antibiotic carbenicillin

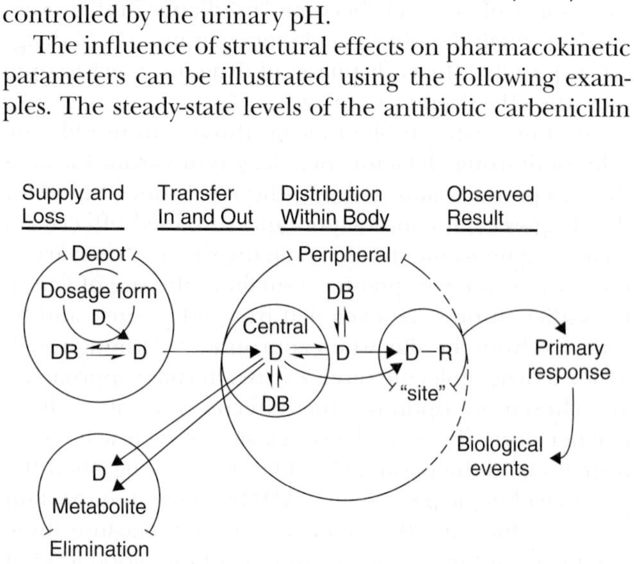

FIGURE 3.38 How some of the processes can be altered by changing a substituent group on a drug molecule.

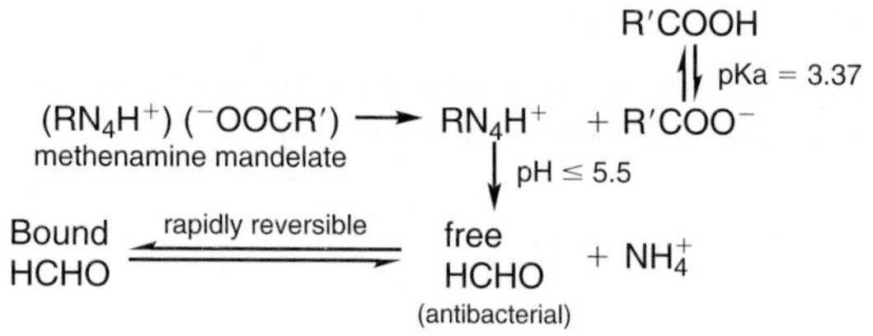

FIGURE 3.39 Conversion of methenamine to formaldehyde in acidic pH.

are twice those of ampicillin. These higher blood levels of carbenicillin following IV administration have been attributed to its efficacy in the treatment of relatively resistant infections, such as *Pseudomonas* species. The reason for these differences in the higher steady-state plasma concentration is the larger apparent volume of distribution for ampicillin, because the elimination rate constants are similar. If all the factors were equal, one can argue that an increased value for the apparent volume of distribution is a clinical advantage, because bacteria germinate more frequently in the tissue than in the blood. The effectiveness of an antibiotic depends on its penetration into tissues, particularly inflamed tissue. Thus, if plasma protein binding is equal for both antibiotics, the antibiotic with a larger volume of distribution would appear to be reaching the site of action with better efficacy, but this is by no means unequivocal. Therefore, the spectrum of research activity in the area of antibiotics would imply that the following goals for molecular modifications are generally pursued:

1. Increased tissue distribution
2. Longer half-life to maintain a higher blood level and decrease the frequency of dose administration
3. Decreased binding capacity to foods and plasma protein

ACKNOWLEDGMENT

The author would like to acknowledge Dr. Philip Breen, Associate Professor of Pharmaceutics, School of Pharmacy and the University of Arkansas for Medical Sciences, for helpful discussions and suggestions in preparing this chapter.

References

1. Ariens EJ. Intrinsic activity: partial agonists and partial antagonists. J Cardiovasc Pharmacol 1983;5:S8–S15.
2. Venter JC, Fraser CM. Mechanism of action and regulation. In: Kito S, Segawa T, Kuriyama K, eds. Neurotransmitter Receptors. New York: Plenum Press, 1984.
3. Lefkowitz RJ, Stadel JM, Caron MG. Adenylate cyclase–coupled β-adrenergic receptors: structure and mechanisms of activation and desensitization. Annu Rev Biochem 1983;52:159–186.
4. Florence AT, Attwood D. Physiochemical Principles of Pharmacy, 2nd Ed. New York: Chapman and Hall, 1988.
5. Wagner JG. Biopharmaceutics and Relevant Pharmacokinetics. Hamilton, IL: The Hamilton Press, 1971.
6. Schanker LS. Absorption of drugs from the rat colon. J Pharmacol Exp Ther 1959;126:283–294.
7. Shore PA, Brodie, BB, Hogben CAM. The gastric of drugs: a pH partition hypothesis. J Pharmacol Exp Ther 1957;119:361–369.
8. Hogben CAM, Tocco DJ, Brodie BB, et al. On the mechanism of intestinal absorption of drugs. J Pharmacol Exp Ther 1959;125:275–282.

9. Schanker LS. On the mechanism of absorption of drugs from the gastrointestinal tract. J Med Pharm Chem 1960;2;343–359.
10. Schanker LS. Mechanism of drug absorption and distribution. Annu Rev Pharmacol 1961;1:29–44.
11. Schanker LS. Passage of drugs across the gastrointestinal epithelium in drugs and membrane. In: Hogben CAM, ed. Proceedings of the First International Pharmacology Meeting, Vol. 4. New York: McMillan Company, 1963.
12. Schanker LS. Physiological transport of drugs. In: Harper NJ, Simon AB, eds. Advances in Drug Research. London: Academic Press, 1966:71–106.
13. Rowland M, Tozer T. Clinical Pharmacokinetics: Concepts and Applications, 2nd Ed. Philadelphia: Lea and Febiger, 1989.
14. Schanker LS. Absorption of drugs from the rat small intestine. J Pharmacol Exp Ther 1958;128:81–87.
15. Zimmerman JJ, Feldman S. Physical–chemical properties and biologic activity. In: Foye WO, ed. Principles of Medicinal Chemistry, 3rd Ed. Philadelphia: Lea and Febiger, 1988:7–38.
16. Winne D. The influence of unstirred layers on intestinal absorption in intestinal permeation. In: Kramer M, Lauterbach F, eds. Workshop Conference Hoechest, Vol. 4. Amsterdam: Excerpta Medica, 1977:58–64.
17. Levy G, Leonard JR, Procknal JA. Development of in vitro dissolution tests which correlate quantitatively with dissolution rate limited absorption. J Pharm Sci 1965;54:1319–1325.
18. Kwan KC. Oral bioavailability and first-pass effects. Drug Metab Drug Dispos 1997;25:1329–1336.
19. Burton P, Goodwin J, Vidamas T, et al. Predicting drug absorption: how nature made it a difficult problem. J Pharmacol Exp Ther 2002;303: 889–895.
20. Lipinsky CA, Lombordo F, Dominy W, et al. Experimental and computational approaches to estimate solubility and permeability in drug discovery and development settings. Adv Drug Deliv Rev 1997;23:3–25.
21. Stewart B, Wang Y, Surendran N. Ex vivo approaches to predicting oral pharmacokinetics in humans. Ann Repts Med Chem 2000;35:299–307.
22. Ertl P, Rohde B, Selzer P. Fast calculation of molecular polar surface area as a sum of fragment-based contributions and its application to the prediction of drug transport properties. J Med Chem 2000;43:3714–3717.
23. Sinko PJ, Leesman GD, Amidon GL. Predicting fraction of dose absorbed in humans using a macroscopic mass-balance approach. Pharm Res 1991;8:979–988.
24. Avdeef A. Absorption and Drug Development: Solubility, Permeability, and Charge State. New York: Wiley-Interscience, 2003.
25. Artusson P, Karlsson J. Correlation between oral drug absorption in humans and the apparent drug permeability coefficient in human intestinal epithelia (Caco-2) cells. Biochem Biophys Res Commun 1991;14:880–885.
26. Hilgers AR, Smith DP, Biermacher JJ, et al. Predicting oral absorption of drugs: a case study with novel class of antimicrobial agents. Pharm Res 2003;20:1149–1155.
27. Amidon GL, Sinko PJ, Fleisher D. Estimating human oral fraction dose absorbed: a correlation using rat intestinal permeability for passive and carrier-mediated compounds. Pharm Res 1988;5:651–654.
28. Dressman JB, Fleisher D. Mixing-tank model for predicting dissolution rate control oral absorption. J Pharm Sci 1986;75:109–116.
29. Johnson DA, Amidon GL. Determination of intrinsic transport parameters from perfused intestine experiments: a boundary layer approach to estimating the aqueous and unbiased membrane permeability. J Theor Biol 1988;131:93–106.
30. Hidalgo I. Assessing the absorption of new pharmaceuticals. Curr Top Med Chem 2001;1:385–401.
31. Fleisher D, Cheng L, Zhou Y, et al. Drug, meal, and formulation interactions influencing drug absorption after oral administration: clinical implications. Clin Pharmacokinet 1999;36:233–254.
32. Amidon G, Lenncranas H, Shah V, et al. A theoretical basis for a biopharmaceutics drug classification: the correlation of in vitro drug product and in vivo bioavailability. Pharm Res 1995;12:413–420.
33. Kunta JR, Sinko PJ. Intestinal drug transporters: in vivo function and clinical importance. Curr Drug Metab 2004;5:109–124.
34. Matheney C, Lamb M, Brouwer K, et al. Pharmacokinetics and pharmacodynamic implications of P-glycoprotein modulation. Pharmacotherapy 2001;21:778–796.
35. Foltz EL. Clinical pharmacology of pivampicillin. Antimicrob Agents Chemother 1970;10:442–454.
36. Surendran N, Covits KMY, Han HK, et al. Evidence for overlapping substrate specificity between large neutral amino acid (LNAA) and dipeptide (hPEPT1) transporters for PD 158473, an NMDT antagonist. Pharm Res 1999;16: 391–395.
37. Lin J, Chiba M, Baillie T. Is the role of the small intestine in first-pass metabolism overemphasized? Pharmacol Rev 1999;51:135–157.
38. Albert A. Chemical aspects of selective toxicity. Nature 1958;182:421–423.
39. Roche EB. Design of Biopharmaceutical Properties through Pro-drugs and Analogs. Washington, DC: American Pharmaceutical Association, 1977.
40. Sinkula AA, Yalkowsky SH. Rationale for design of biologically reversible drug derivatives: pro-drugs. J Pharm Sci 1975;64:181–210.
41. Stella VJ, Charman WN, Naringrekar VH. Prodrugs. Do they have advantages in clinical practice? Drugs 1985;29:455–473.
42. Stella V. Pro-drugs: an overview and definition. In: Higuchi T, Stella V, eds. Pro-drugs as Novel Drug Delivery Systems. ACS Symposium Series. Washington, DC: American Chemical Society, 1975:1–115.
43. Beaumont K, Webster R, Gardner I, et al. Design of ester pro-drugs to enhance oral absorption of poorly permeable compounds: challenges to the discovery scientist. Curr Drug Metab 2003;4:461–485.
44. Noyes NA, Whitney WR. The rate of solution of solid substances in their own solution. J Am Chem Soc 1897;19:930–942.
45. Gibaldi M. Biopharmaceutics and Clinical Pharmacokinetics, 4th Ed. Philadelphia: Lea and Febiger, 1991.
46. Ogata H, Shibazoki T, Inoue T, et al. Studies on dissolution tests of solid dosage forms. IV. Relation of absorption sites of sulfonamides administered orally in solid dosage forms to their solubilities and dissolution rates. Chem Pharm Bull 1979;27:1281–1286.
47. Pottage A, Nimmo J, Prescott LF. The absorption of aspirin and paracetamol in patients with achlorhydria. J Pharm Pharmacol 1974;26:144–145.
48. Juncher H, Raaschou F. Solubility of oral preparation of penicillin V. Antibiotic Med 1957;4:497–507.
49. Anderson KW. Oral absorption of quinalbarbitone and its sodium salt. Arch Int Pharmacodyn Ther 1964;147:171–177.
50. Grant DJW. Theory and origin of polymorphism. In: Brittain HG, ed. Polymorphism in Pharmaceutical Solids. New York: Marcel Dekker, 1999:1–34.
51. Brittain HG, Grant DJW. Effect of polymorphism and solid-state solvation on solubility and dissolution rate. In: Brittain HG, ed. Polymorphism in Pharmaceutical Solids. New York: Marcel Dekker, 1999:34–66.
52. Johnson KC, Swindell AC. Guidance in the setting of drug particle size specifications to minimize variability in drug absorption. Pharm Res 1996;13:1795–1798.
53. Dressman JB, Amidon GL, Fleisher D. Absorption potential: estimating the fraction absorbed for orally administered compounds. J Pharm Sci 1985;74:588–589.
54. Lombardo F, Obach RS, Dicapua FM, et al. A hybrid mixture discriminant analysis–random forest computational model for the prediction of volume of distribution of drugs in human. J Med Chem. 2006;49:2262–2267.
55. Lombardo F, Obach RS, Shalaeva MY, et al. Prediction of volume of distribution values in humans for neutral and basic drugs using physicochemical measurements and plasma protein binding data. J Med Chem 2002;45:2867–2876.
56. Lombardo F, Obach RS, Shalaeva MY, et al. Prediction of human volume of distribution values for neutral and basic drugs. 2. Extended data set and leave-class-out statistics. J Med Chem 2004;47:1242–1250.
57. Ehrnebo M, Boreus L, Lonroth U. Bioavailability and first-pass metabolism of oral pentazocine in man. Clin Pharmacol Ther 1977;22:888–892.
58. Notari R. Pharmacokinetics and molecular modification: implications in drug design and evaluation. J Pharm Sci 1973;62:865–881.

Suggested Readings

Avdeef A. Absorption and Drug Development: Solubility, Permeability, and Charge State. New York: Wiley-Interscience, 2003.
Florence A, Siepman J, eds. Modern Pharmaceutics, 5th Ed. New York: Informa Healthcare, 2009.
Ganellin C, Roberts S, eds. Medicinal Chemistry: The Role of Organic Chemistry in Drug Research, 2nd Ed. New York: Academic Press, 1993.
Garrett E. Classical pharmacokinetics to frontiers. J Pharmacokinet Biopharm 1973;1:341–361.
Gibaldi M. Biopharmaceutics and Clinical Pharmacokinetics, 4th Ed. Philadelphia: Lea and Febiger, 1991.
Gibaldi M, Perrier D. Pharmacokinetics, 2nd Ed., Vol. 15: Drugs and the Pharmaceutical Sciences. New York: Marcel Dekker, 1982.
Hilfiker R, ed. Polymorphism. Weinheim, Germany: Wiley-VCH Verlag, 2006.
Horter D, Dressman JB. Influence of physiochemical properties on dissolution of drugs in the gastrointestinal tract. Adv Drug Deliv Rev 2001;46:75–87.
Hug C. Pharmacokinetics of drugs administered intravenously. Anesth Analg 1978;57:704–723.
Jambhekar S, Breen P. Basic Pharmacokinetics, 1st Ed. London: Pharmaceutical Press, 2009.
Rowland M, Tozer T. Clinical Pharmacokinetics: Concepts and Application, 3rd Ed. Philadelphia: Lea and Febiger, 1994.
Steffansen B, Brodin B, Nielsen U, eds. Molecular Biopharmaceutics. London: Pharmaceutical Press, 2010.
Taylor J, Kennewell P. Modern Medicinal Chemistry: Ellis Horwood Series in Pharmaceutical Technology. New York: Ellis Horwood, 1993.
Wagner J. A modern view of pharmacokinetics. J Pharmacokinet Biopharm 1973;1:363–401.
Wagner J. Do you need a pharmacokinetic model, and, if so, which one? J Pharmacokinet Biopharm 1975;3:457–478.
Welling P. Pharmacokinetics: Processes and Mathematics. Monograph 185. Washington, DC: American Chemical Society, 1986.
Wermuth C, Koga N, Konig H, et al. Medicinal Chemistry for the 21st Century. Boston: Blackwell Scientific Publications, 1992.

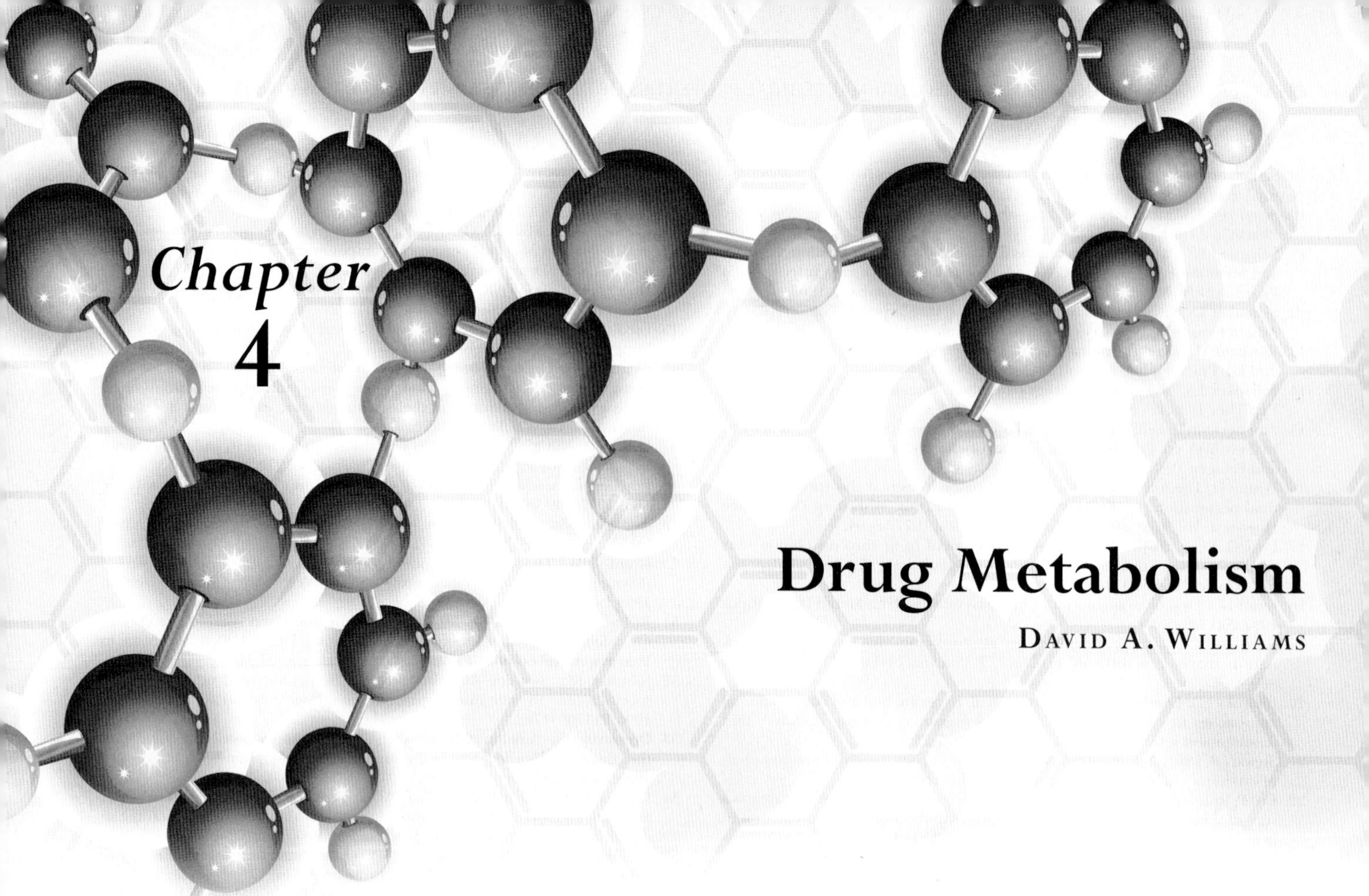

Chapter 4

Drug Metabolism

DAVID A. WILLIAMS

Abbreviations

ADH, alcohol dehydrogenases
AhR, aromatic hydrocarbon receptor
ALHD, aldehyde dehydrogenases
ALT, alanine aminotransferase
AST, aspartate aminotransferase
Ah, aromatic hormone
AKR, aldo-keto reductase
ATP, adenosine triphosphate
CAR, constitutive androstane receptor
CoA, coenzyme A
COMT, catechol-*O*-methyltransferase
COX, cyclooxygenase
DHEA, dehydroepiandrosterone
DIH, drug-induced hepatotoxicity
EHC, enterohepatic cycle
EM, fast or extensive metabolizers
ER, endoplasmic reticulum
FAD, flavin dinucleotide
$FADH_2$, reduced form of flavin dinucleotide
FDA, U.S. Food and Drug Administration
FMN, flavin mononucleotide
$FMNH_2$, reduced form of flavin mononucleotide
FMO, flavin-containing monooxygenase
GSH, glutathione
GSSG, oxidized glutathione
GST, glutathione *S*-transferases
HOCl, hypochlorous acid
HSAB, hard-soft acid-bases
IDR, idiosyncratic drug reaction
kDa, unit of molecular weight
LDL, low-density lipoprotein
MAO, monoamine oxidase
MAOI, monoamine oxidase inhibitors
MDMA, 4-methylenedioxy-methamphetamine
MIC, metabolite-intermediate complex
MPO, myeloperoxidase
MPP^+, 1-methyl-4-phenylpyridinium ion
MPTP, 1-methyl-4-phenyl-1,2,3,6-tetrahydropyridine
NAD^+, nicotinamide adenine dinucleotide
NADH, the reduced form of nicotinamide adenine dinucleotide
$NADP^+$, nicotinamide adenine dinucleotide phosphate
NADPH, the reduced form of nicotinamide adenine dinucleotide phosphate
NAT, *N*-acetyltransferase
NSAID, nonsteroidal anti-inflammatory drug
OATP, organic anion transporter polypeptide
P450, cytochrome P450 monooxygenase
PAH, polycyclic aromatic hydrocarbon
PAPS, 3′-phosphoadenosine-5′-phosphosulfate
PGG_2, prostaglandin G_2
PGI_2, prostacyclin
P-gp, P-glycoprotein
PM, poor metabolizers
PON, paraoxonase
PPAR, peroxisome proliferator-activated receptor
PXR, pregnane X receptor
ROS, reactive oxygen species
SULT, sulfotransferase
TPMT, thiopurine *S*-methyltransferase
UGT, UDP–glucuronosyl transferase
UDP, uridine diphosphate
UDPGA, UDP–glucuronic acid
UM, ultrarapid metabolizers

Scenario

Mark D. Watanabe, PharmD, PhD, BCPP

Y.H., a 32-year-old female with a history of chronic schizophrenia, presented for a routine follow-up visit to the behavioral health clinic. Her psychotic symptoms had been well controlled on risperidone 3 mg daily. At her previous appointment 1 month ago, Y.H. had reported being depressed, so her psychiatrist initiated a trial of paroxetine 20 mg daily as treatment. As the pharmacist was interviewing Y.H. for a medication history, he noticed that there was a resting tremor in her left hand. Y.H. acknowledged that it had first appeared within the last few weeks. She also stated that she was just starting to feel less depressed.

(The reader is directed to the clinical solution and chemical analysis of this case at the end of the chapter).

What is a poison?
All substances are poisons;
There is none that is not a poison.
The right dose differentiates a poison from a drug.

—*Paracelsus (1493–1541)*

Humans are exposed throughout their lives to a large variety of drugs and nonessential exogenous (foreign) compounds (collectively termed "xenobiotics") that can pose health hazards. Drugs taken for therapeutic purposes as well as occupational or private exposures to vapors of volatile chemicals or solvents pose possible health risks; smoking and drinking lead to the absorption of large amounts of substances with potentially adverse health effects. Furthermore, ingestion of natural toxins in vegetables and fruits, pesticide residues in food, as well as carcinogenic pyrolysis products from fats and protein formed during the charbroiling of meat have to be considered as additional health risks. Most of these xenobiotics undergo enzymatic biotransformations by xenobiotic-metabolizing enzymes in the liver and extrahepatic tissues and are eliminated by excretion as hydrophilic metabolites. In some cases, especially during oxidative metabolism, numerous chemical procarcinogens form reactive metabolites capable of covalent binding to biopolymers, such as proteins or nucleic acids—critical components that can lead to mutagenicity, cytotoxicity, and carcinogenicity. Therefore, insight into the biotransformation and bioactivation of xenobiotics becomes an indisputable prerequisite to assess drug safety and estimate risks associated with chemicals and drugs.

Detoxication and toxic effects of drugs and other xenobiotics have been studied extensively in various mammalian species. Frequently, differences in sensitivity to these toxic effects were observed and can now be attributed to genetic differences between species in the isoenzyme/isoforms of cytochrome P450 monooxygenases (P450). The level of expression of the P450 enzymes is regulated by genetics and by a variety of endogenous factors such as hormones, gender, age, and disease, as well as the presence of environmental factors, such as inducing agents. Drugs were developed and prescribed under the old paradigm that "one dose fits all," which largely ignored the fact that humans (both adults and children) are genetically and metabolically different, resulting in variable responses to drugs.

Drugs can no longer be regarded as chemically stable entities that elicit the desired pharmacologic responses, after which they are excreted from the body. Drugs undergo a variety of chemical changes in humans brought about by enzymes of the liver, intestine, kidney, lung, and other tissues, with subsequent alterations in the nature of their pharmacologic activities, durations of activity, and toxicities. Thus, the pharmacologic and toxicologic activities of a drug (or xenobiotic) are, in many ways, consequences of its metabolism.

Drug therapy is becoming more oriented toward control of metabolic, genetic, and environmental illnesses (e.g., cardiovascular disease, mental illness, cancer, and diabetes) than toward short-term therapies. In most cases, drug therapies last for months or even years, and the problem of drug toxicities resulting from long-term therapy has become increasingly important.

The practice of simultaneous prescriptions of several drugs has become common. Thus, an awareness of possible drug–drug interactions is essential to avoid catastrophic synergistic effects and chemical, enzymic, and pharmacokinetic interactions that can produce toxic side effects.

The study of xenobiotic metabolism has developed rapidly during the past few decades (1–9). These studies have been fundamental in the assessment of drug efficacy and safety and in the design of dosage regimens; in the development of food additives and the assessment of potential hazards of contaminants; in the evaluation of toxic chemicals; and in the development of pesticides and herbicides and the assessment of their metabolic fates in insects, other animals, and plants. The metabolism of drugs and other xenobiotics is fundamental to many toxic processes, such as carcinogenesis, teratogenesis, and tissue necrosis. Often, the same enzymes involved in drug metabolism also carry out the regulation and metabolism of endogenous substances such as steroids, vitamin D, prostaglandins, and lipids. Consequently, the inhibition and induction of these enzymes by drugs and xenobiotics can have a profound effect on the normal processes of intermediary metabolism, such as tissue growth and development, hematopoiesis, calcification, and lipid metabolism.

Familiarity with the mechanisms of drug metabolism can often aid the prediction of the consequences of drug–drug interactions, drug–food interactions, and herbal drug–drug interactions, and help to explain patients' adverse responses to drug regimens. Incorporating pharmacogenomics into the selection of drug regimens will change the way in which drugs are prescribed for patients. Selection based on a patient's individual genetic makeup could eliminate previously unpredictable responses to drug treatment caused by genetic polymorphisms that effect metabolism, clearance, and tolerance. Pharmacogenomic testing to determine a patient's phenotype (i.e., poor metabolizer) and, thus, his or her ability to metabolize drugs will become common in the future. Such knowledge will assure improved selection of proper drug regimens and doses before therapy begins.

The increased knowledge of drug metabolism, fed by the need for better safety evaluations of drugs and chemicals, has resulted in a proliferation of publications (e.g., *Drug Metabolism Reviews, Drug Metabolism and Disposition*, and *Xenobiotica*) and a series of monographs that present the current state of knowledge of foreign compound metabolism from biochemical and pharmacologic viewpoints (3–9).

PATHWAYS OF METABOLISM

Drugs, plant toxins, food additives, environmental chemicals, insecticides, and other chemicals foreign to the body undergo enzymic transformations that results frequently in the loss of pharmacologic activity. The term "detoxication" describes the result of such metabolic changes. Although drug metabolism leads as a rule to detoxication, the processes of oxidation, reduction, glucuronidation, sulfonation (sulfo-conjugation), and other enzyme-catalyzed reactions can lead to the formation of metabolites having therapeutic or toxic effects. This process is often referred to as "bioactivation." One of the earliest discoveries of an example of bioactivation was the reduction of Prontosil to the antibacterial agent sulfanilamide. Other examples of drug metabolism that lead to therapeutically active drugs include the hydroxylation of acetanilide to acetaminophen, the *N*-demethylation of the antidepressant imipramine to form desipramine, and conversion of the anxiolytic diazepam to form desmethyldiazepam. The insecticide parathion is desulfurized by both insects and mammals to form paraoxon.

Most drugs and other xenobiotics are metabolized by enzymes normally associated with the metabolism of endogenous constituents (e.g., steroids and biogenic amines). The liver is the primary site of drug metabolism, although other xenobiotic-metabolizing enzymes are found in nervous tissue, kidney, lung, plasma, and the gastrointestinal tract (digestive secretions, bacterial flora, and the intestinal wall).

CLINICAL SIGNIFICANCE

The basic principles of drug metabolism may inform a wide variety of clinical decisions regarding pharmacotherapy. For example, a thorough understanding enables a careful assessment for drug–drug interactions in particular patient cases. Drugs, as chemical entities, can be substrates, inhibitors, or inducers of metabolic enzymes. The interplay of these roles potentially influences serum drug concentrations in ways that may directly affect the desired outcome (i.e., decreases in levels that may prevent therapeutic efficacy or increases that may enhance risks of toxicity). There are certainly many more theoretical pharmacokinetic interactions that invoke these mechanisms than are actually seen in clinical practice. Through careful observation and analysis of unexpected and possibly concentration-dependent events, one could more readily identify and document which interactions are of greater clinical significance by virtue of their actual occurrence in patients. The clinician would then be poised to recommend appropriate dosage adjustments or medication changes based on the actual outcomes of these interactions.

In addition, the biotransformation of drugs may produce reactive metabolites which, through basic chemical reactions, can interact with the components of cellular membranes and proteins in a manner that disrupts normal structure and function. A working knowledge of those functional groups within drug molecules that may be more susceptible to reactive metabolite formation could help explain toxic sequelae when they emerge during a medication trial. This could be useful information whenever alternative therapeutic agents within a given chemical class are being considered.

Ongoing discoveries from studies in the pharmacogenetics field are expanding the drug metabolism literature in directions that hint at the future prospect of truly individualized drug regimens. The need to keep abreast of these new developments is both compelling and exciting, and their application builds upon the principles presented in this chapter.

Mark D. Watanabe, PharmD, PhD, BCPP
Assistant Clinical Specialist
Department of Pharmacy Practice
Northeastern University
Boston, MA

Although hepatic metabolism continues to be the most important route of metabolism for xenobiotics and drugs, other biotransformation pathways have a significant role in the metabolism of these substances. Among the more active extrahepatic tissues capable of metabolizing drugs are the intestinal mucosa, kidney, and lung (see the discussion of extrahepatic metabolism). The ability of the liver and extrahepatic tissues to metabolize substances to either pharmacologically inactive or bioactive metabolites before they achieve systemic blood levels is termed "first-pass metabolism" or the "presystemic first-pass effect." Other metabolite reactions occurring in the gastrointestinal tract are associated with bacteria and other microflora in the tract. The bacterial flora can affect metabolism through: 1) production of toxic metabolites, 2) formation of carcinogens from inactive precursors, 3) detoxication, 4) exhibition of species differences in drug metabolism, 5) exhibition of individual differences in drug metabolism, 6) production of pharmacologically active metabolites from inactive precursors, and 7) production of metabolites not formed by animal tissues.

Phase 1 Reactions

The pathways of xenobiotic metabolism are divided into two major categories. Phase 1 reactions (biotransformations) include oxidation, hydroxylation, reduction, and hydrolysis. In each of these enzymatic reactions, a new functional group is introduced into the substrate molecule, an existing functional group is modified, or a functional group or acceptor site for Phase 2 transfer reactions is exposed, thus making the xenobiotic more polar and, therefore, more readily excreted.

Phase 2 Reactions

Phase 2 reactions (conjugation) are enzymatic syntheses whereby a functional group, such as alcohol, phenol, or amine, is masked by the addition of a new group, such as acetyl, sulfate, glucuronic acid, or certain amino acids, which usually increases the polarity of the drug or xenobiotic. Most substances undergo both Phase 1 and Phase 2 reactions sequentially.

Those xenobiotics that are resistant to metabolizing enzymes or are already hydrophilic are excreted largely unchanged. This basic pattern of xenobiotic metabolism is common to all animal species, including humans, but species can differ in details of the reaction and enzyme control.

FACTORS AFFECTING METABOLISM

As indicated earlier, drug therapy is becoming oriented more toward controlling metabolic, genetic, and environmental illnesses rather than short-term therapy associated with infectious diseases. In most cases, drug therapy lasts for months or even years, and the problems of drug–drug interactions and chronic toxicity from long-term drug therapy have become more serious. Therefore, a greater knowledge of drug metabolism is essential. Several factors influencing xenobiotic metabolism include:

1. *Genetic factors.* Individual differences in drug effectiveness (drug sensitivity or drug resistance), drug–drug interactions, and drug toxicity can depend on racial and ethnic characteristics with the population frequencies of the many polymorphic genes and the expression of the metabolizing enzymes. Pharmacogenetics focuses primarily on genetic polymorphisms (mutations) responsible for interindividual differences in drug metabolism and disposition (10). Genotype–phenotype correlation studies have validated that inherited mutations result in two or more distinct phenotypes causing very different responses following drug administration. The genes encoding for CYP2A6, CYP2C9, CYP2C19, and CYP2D6 are functionally polymorphic; therefore, at least 30% of P450-dependent metabolism is performed by polymorphic enzymes. For example, mutations in the *CYP2D6* gene result in poor, intermediate, or ultrarapid metabolizers of more than 30 cardiovascular and central nervous system drugs. Thus, each of these phenotypic subgroups experiences different responses to drugs extensively metabolized by the CYP2D6 pathway ranging from severe toxicity to complete lack of efficacy. For example, ethnic specificity has been observed with the sensitivity of the Japanese and Chinese to ethanol as compared to Caucasians, CYP2C19 polymorphism (affects ~20% of Asians and ~3% of Caucasians) and the variable metabolism of omeprazole (proton pump inhibitor) and antiseizure drugs, and the polymorphic paraoxonase–catalyzed hydrolysis of the neurotoxic organophosphates and lipid peroxides (atherosclerosis) (see the discussion of genetic polymorphism).

   Incorporating pharmacogenomics, the study of heritable traits affecting patient response to drug treatment, into drug therapy will alter the way in which drug regimens are chosen for patients based on their individual genetic makeup (10), thus eliminating the unpredictable response of drug treatment as a result of genetic polymorphisms that affect metabolism, clearance, and tolerance. Understanding how individuals are genetically predisposed to differences in metabolism risk could facilitate development of new classes of drugs that are metabolized by nonpolymorphic P450 enzymes.
2. *Physiologic factors.* Age is a factor as both very young and old have impaired metabolism. Hormones

(including those induced by stress), sex differences, pregnancy, changes in intestinal microflora, diseases (especially those involving the liver), and nutritional status can also influence drug and xenobiotic metabolism.

Because the liver is the principal site for xenobiotic and drug metabolism, liver disease can modify the pharmacokinetics of drugs metabolized by the liver (11–13). Several factors identified as major determinants of the metabolism of a drug in the diseased liver are the nature and extent of liver damage, hepatic blood flow, the drug involved, the dosage regimen, and the degree of participation of the liver in the pharmacokinetics of the drug. Liver disease affects the elimination half-life of some drugs but not of others, although all undergo hepatic biotransformation (Table 4.1). Some results have shown that the capacity for drug metabolism is impaired in chronic liver disease, which could lead to drug overdosage. Consequently, as a result of the unpredictability of drug effects in the presence of liver disorders, drug therapy in these circumstances is complex, and more than usual caution is needed (13).

Substances influencing drug and xenobiotic metabolism (other than enzyme inducers) include lipids, proteins, vitamins, and metals. Dietary lipid and protein deficiencies diminish microsomal drug-metabolizing activity. Protein deficiency leads to reduced hepatic microsomal protein and lipid metabolism; oxidative metabolism is decreased due to an alteration in endoplasmic reticulum (ER) membrane permeability affecting electron transfer. In terms of toxicity, protein deficiency would increase the toxicity of drugs and xenobiotics by reducing their oxidative microsomal metabolism and clearance from the body.

3. *Pharmacodynamic factors.* Dose, frequency, and route of administration, plus tissue distribution and protein binding of a drug, affect its metabolism.
4. *Environmental factors.* Competition of ingested environmental substances with other drugs and xenobiotics for metabolizing enzymes, and poisoning of enzymes by toxic chemicals such as carbon monoxide or pesticide synergists alter metabolism. Induction of enzyme expression (in which the number of enzyme molecules is increased, while the activity is constant) by other drugs and xenobiotics is another consideration.

Such factors can change not only the kinetics of an enzyme reaction but also the whole pattern of metabolism, thereby altering bioavailability, pharmacokinetics, pharmacologic activity, or toxicity of a xenobiotic. Species differences of responses to xenobiotics must be considered in the extrapolation of pharmacologic and toxicologic data from animal experiments to predict effects in humans. The primary factors in these species differences probably are the rates and patterns of drug and xenobiotic metabolism.

TABLE 4.1 The Effect of Liver Disease in Humans on the Elimination Half-Life of Various Drugs[a]

Difference Reported	No Difference Reported
Acetaminophen	Chlorpromazine
Amylbarbital	Dicoumarol
Carbenicillin	Phenytoin
Chloramphenicol	Phenylbutazone
Clindamycin	Salicylic acid
Diazepam	Tolbutamide
Hexobarbital	
Isoniazid	
Lidocaine	
Meperidine	
Meprobamate	
Pentobarbital	
Phenobarbital	
Prednisone	
Rifamycin	
Tolbutamide	
Theophylline	

[a]Clearance is disputable but can be increased.

DRUG BIOTRANSFORMATION PATHWAY (PHASE 1)

Human Hepatic Cytochrome P450 Enzyme System

Oxidation is probably the most common reaction in xenobiotic metabolism. This reaction is catalyzed by a group of membrane-bound monooxygenases found in the smooth ER of the liver and other extrahepatic tissues, termed the "cytochrome P450 monooxygenase enzyme system" (14) (hereafter, the abbreviation P450 will be used for this enzyme system). Additionally, P450 has been called a mixed-function oxidase or microsomal hydroxylase. The tissue homogenate fraction containing the smooth ER is called the microsomal fraction. P450 functions as a multicomponent electron-transport system, responsible for the oxidative metabolism of a variety of endogenous substrates (e.g., steroids, fatty acids, prostaglandins, and bile acids) and exogenous substances (xenobiotics) including drugs, carcinogens, insecticides, plant toxins, environmental pollutants, and other foreign chemicals. Central to the functioning of this unique superfamily of heme proteins is an iron protoporphyrin. The iron protoporphyrin is coordinated to the sulfur of cysteine and has the ability to form a complex with carbon monoxide, resulting in a complex that has its primary absorption maximum at 450 nm (thus the title of these metabolizing P450 enzymes). P450 has an absolute requirement for NADPH (the reduced form of nicotinamide adenine dinucleotide phosphate) and molecular oxygen (dioxygen). The rate at which various compounds are metabolized by this system depends on the animal species, strain, nutritional status, type of tissue, age, and pretreatment of animals. The variety of reactions catalyzed by P450 (Table 4.2) include the oxidation of alkanes and aromatic compounds; the epoxidation of alkenes, polycyclic hydrocarbons, and halogenated benzenes; the dealkylation of secondary and tertiary amines and ethers; the deamination of primary amines; the conversion of amines to *N*-oxides, hydroxylamine, and nitroso derivatives; and the dehalogenation of halogenated hydrocarbons. It also catalyzes the oxidative cleavage of organic thiophosphate esters, the sulfoxidation of some thioethers, the conversion of phosphothionates to phosphate derivatives, and the reduction of azo and nitro compounds to primary aromatic amines.

The most important function of P450 is to "activate" molecular oxygen (dioxygen), permitting the incorporation of one atom of oxygen into an organic substrate molecule concomitant with the reduction of the other atom of oxygen to water. The introduction of a hydroxyl group into the hydrophobic substrate molecule provides a site for subsequent conjugation with hydrophilic compounds (Phase 2), thereby increasing the aqueous solubility of the product for transport and excretion from the organism. This enzyme system not only catalyzes xenobiotic transformations in ways that typically lead to detoxication but also, in some cases, in ways that lead to products having greater cytotoxic, mutagenic, or carcinogenic properties. A nonheme, microsomal flavoprotein monooxygenase is responsible for the oxidation of certain nitrogen- and sulfur-containing organic compounds.

Components of P450

P450 consists of at least two protein components: a heme protein called P450 and a flavoprotein called NADPH-P450 reductase, containing both flavin mononucleotide (FMN) and flavin dinucleotide (FAD). P450 is the substrate- and oxygen-binding site of the enzyme system, whereas the reductase serves as an electron carrier, shuttling electrons from NADPH to P450. A third component essential for electron transport

TABLE 4.2 Hydroxylation Mechanisms Catalyzed by Cytochrome P450

Mechanism	Reaction
Aromatic hydroxylation	$CH_3CO-\overset{H}{N}-C_6H_5 \xrightarrow{[OH]} CH_3CO-\overset{H}{N}-C_6H_4\text{-}OH$
Aliphatic hydroxylation	$R-CH_3 \xrightarrow{[OH]} R-CH_2\text{-}OH$
Deamination	$R-CH(NH_2)\text{-}CH_3 \xrightarrow{[OH]} (R-C(OH)(NH_2)\text{-}CH_3) \longrightarrow R-CO^{-}CH_3 + NH_3$
O-Dealkylation	$R-O\text{-}CH_3 \xrightarrow{[OH]} (R-O\text{-}CH_2\text{-}OH) \longrightarrow R-OH + CH_2O$
N-Dealkylation	$R-N(CH_3)_2 \xrightarrow{[OH]} (R-N(CH_2OH)(CH_3)) \longrightarrow R-\overset{H}{N}-CH_3 + CH_2O$ $R-NH\text{-}CH_3 \xrightarrow{[OH]} (R-NH\text{-}CH_2OH) \longrightarrow R-NH_2 + CH_2O$
N-Oxidation	$(CH_3)_3-N \xrightarrow{[OH]} ((CH_3)_3-NOH) \longrightarrow (CH_3)_3-NO + H^{\oplus}$
Sulfoxidation	$R-S-R' \xrightarrow{[OH]} (R-\underset{OH}{S}-R') \longrightarrow R-\underset{O}{\overset{\|}{S}}-R' + H^{\oplus}$

from NADPH to P450 is a phospholipid, phosphatidylcholine, which facilitates the transfer of electrons from NADPH-P450 reductase to P450 (14). Although the phospholipid does not function in the system as an electron carrier, it has great influence on the P450 monooxygenase system. The phospholipid constitutes approximately one-third of the hepatic ER and contributes to a negatively charged environment at neutral pH.

Of the three components involved in microsomal oxidative xenobiotic metabolism, P450 is important due to its vital role in oxygen activation and substrate binding. P450 is an integral membrane protein deeply imbedded in the membrane matrix. The environment surrounding the enzyme is negatively charged at neutral pH by of the phospholipids. The electron components of P450 are located on the cytoplasmic side of the ER and the hydrophobic active site toward the lumen of the ER (15). The active site of P450 consists of a hydrophobic substrate-binding domain in which is imbedded an iron protoporphyrin (heme) prosthetic group. This group is exactly like that of hemoglobin, peroxidase, and the b-type cytochromes. The iron in the iron protoporphyrin is coordinated with four nitrogens via a tetradentate link to the porphyrin ring. X-ray studies reveal that in the ferric state, the two nonporphyrin ligands are water and cysteine (Fig. 4.1). The cysteine thiolate ligand (proximal) is present in all states of the enzyme and is absolutely essential for the formation of the reactive oxenoid intermediate. The sixth (distal) coordination position is occupied by an easily exchangeable ligand, most likely water, which is labile and readily exchanged for stronger ligands such as cyanide, amines, imidazoles, and pyridines. The ferrous form loses the water ligand completely, leaving the sixth position open for binding ligands such as oxygen and carbon monoxide.

The vast array of xenobiotics presents a unique challenge to the human body, to metabolize these many lipophilic foreign compounds; this makes it impractical to have one enzyme to metabolize each compound or each class of compounds. Therefore, whereas most cellular functions are in general very specific, oxidation of xenobiotics necessitates P450s with diverse substrate specificities and regioselectivities (multiple sites of oxidation). Several types of P450 enzymes can be found in a single animal species. Humans have 57 genes and more than 59 pseudogenes divided among 18 families of P450 genes and 43 subfamilies, each coding for a different version of the enzyme (isoform), so that together the P450s can metabolize almost any lipophilic compound to which the human is exposed.

Classification of the P450 Multigene Family

Nebert et al. (16) and Gonzalez and Gelboin (17) classified the P450 supergene family on the basis of structural (evolutionary) relationships. P450 monooxygenases resulting from this supergene family have been subdivided into families that possess greater than 40% amino acid homology with subfamilies of greater than 55% homology (16,17). The P450s are named with the root symbol CYP followed by an Arabic numeral designating the family member (e.g., CYP1, CYP2, or CYP3), a letter denoting the subfamily (e.g., CYP1A, CYP2C, CYP2D, or CYP2E), and another Arabic numeral representing the individual gene. Names of genes are written in italics. The nomenclature system is based solely on sequence similarity among the P450s and does not indicate the properties or functions of individual P450s. Of the more than 17 P450 isoforms that have been identified so far, the primary isoforms responsible for drug metabolism in the liver are presented in Figure 4.2 (18). It is evident that the CYP3A and CYP2C families are the isoforms most involved in the metabolism of clinically relevant drugs, whereas the CYP1A2 isoform is predominantly involved in the bioactivation of environmental substances.

In all probability P4540s evolved for the regulation of endogenous substances, such as metabolism of cholesterol to maintain membrane integrity, and for steroid

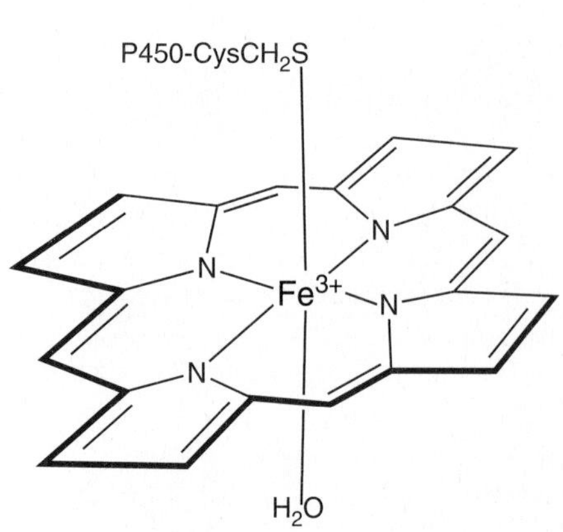

FIGURE 4.1 Ferric heme thiolate catalytic center of P450. The porphyrin side chains are deleted for clarity.

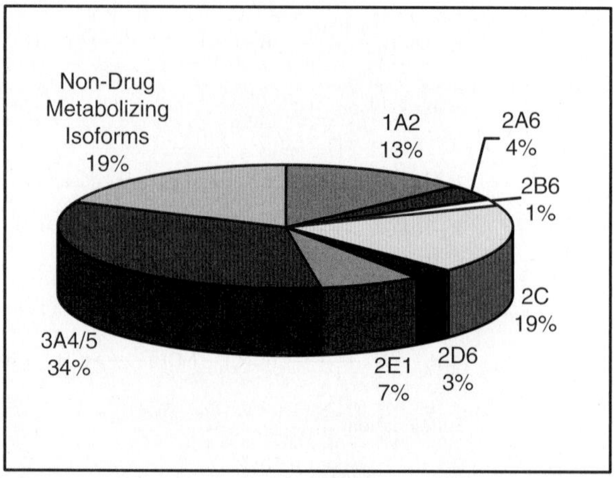

FIGURE 4.2 Total human P450 isoforms expressed in the liver that metabolize drugs.

biosynthesis and metabolism, rather than for metabolizing foreign compounds. P450s are either located in the inner mitochondrial membrane and involved in highly specific steroid hydroxylations or are bound to the ER of the cell and have broad substrate specificity. In evolutionary terms, P450s evolved from a common ancestor, and only more recently (during the last 100 million years), P450 genes have taken on the role of producing enzymes to metabolize a vast array of lipophilic foreign compounds. The xenobiotic P450 genes probably emerged from the steroidogenic P450s to enhance animal survival by synthesizing new P450s to metabolize plant toxins concentrated in the food chain. It is not surprising that animals and humans possess a vast array of P450 enzymes capable of handling a multitude of xenobiotics. Interindividual variation in the expression of xenobiotic P450 genes (genetic polymorphism) or in their inducibility can be associated with differences such as individual susceptibilities to cigarette smoke carcinogenesis. Certain P450 isoforms that clearly exhibit genetic polymorphisms are known to metabolize and as a rule inactivate therapeutic agents. The extent of P450 polymorphism in humans is being investigated to determine the risks of protection against cancers. Food mutagens are typically carcinogens in tissues, but they are activated by CYP1A2 and CYP3A in the liver. Specific forms of P450 in hepatic microsomes are regulated by hormones (e.g., the CYP3A subfamily) and are induced or inhibited by drugs, food toxins, or other environmental xenobiotics (see section on induction and inhibition of P450 isoforms). Identification of a specific P450 isoform as the primary form responsible for metabolism of a specific drug in humans permits reconciliation of the drug's toxicity or other pharmacologic effects.

Substrate Specificity

No evidence exists that the active oxygenating species differ among P450s, suggesting that the substrate specificities, substrate affinities, regioselectivities, and rates of reaction are probably consequences of topographic features of the active site of apoproteins (14,15,19–21). Because a primary function of these enzymes is the metabolism of hydrophobic substrates, it is likely that hydrophobic forces are important in the binding of many substrates to the apoproteins. Nonspecific binding is consistent with the multiple substrate orientations at the active site necessary for the broad regioselectivities observed. A specific binding requirement would decrease the diversity of substrates. Some P450 isoforms have constrained binding sites, and thus, they metabolize small organic molecules (e.g., CYP2E1); CYP1A1/2 isoforms have planar binding sites and metabolize only aromatic planar compounds (i.e., polycyclic aromatic hydrocarbons [PAHs]); CYP2D6 exhibits high affinities for specific apoprotein interactions (hydrogen bonds, ion-pair formation) for specific substrates such as lipophilic amines; and CYP3A4 has broader affinities for a variety of lipophilic substrates (with molecular weights of 200 to 1,200 daltons). If P450 isoforms are tightly membrane bound, substrate access to the active sites is limited to compounds that can diffuse through the membranes, whereas different P450 isoforms that are less tightly bound will metabolize hydrophilic compounds.

In the past, the P450s were often referred to as having broad and overlapping specificities, but it became apparent that the broad substrate specificity could be attributed to multiple isoenzymic forms of P450. The phenotype of an individual with respect to the forms and amounts of individual P450s expressed in the liver can determine the rate and pathway of the metabolic clearance of a compound (see the discussion of genetic polymorphism). Significant differences exist between humans and other animal species with respect to the catalytic activities and regulation of expression of hepatic drug-metabolizing P450s. These differences often make it difficult to extrapolate results of P450-mediated metabolism studies performed experimentally in animal species to humans. Caution is warranted in the extrapolation of rodent data to humans, as some isoforms are similar between species (e.g., CYP1A and CYP3A subfamilies) whereas others are different (e.g., CYP2A, CYP2B, CYP2C, and CYP2D subfamilies).

The unique and diverse characteristics of the P450 ensure that predicting the metabolism of xenobiotics will be difficult. To date, no crystal structure for a mammalian membrane-bound P450 isoform has been described.

Other P450 Isoforms

A large number of other P450 isoforms catalyzing the oxidation of steroids, bile acids, fat-soluble vitamins, and other endogenous substances are shown in Table 4.3. Included are the following: CYP4, an ω-hydroxylase that hydroxylates the ω-methyl group of C20 to C22 fatty acids; CYP5, which causes platelet aggregation through synthesis of thromboxane A_2; CYP7A, which catalyzes the rate-determining step in the biosynthesis of bile acids from cholesterol; CYP7B, a brain-specific form of 7α-hydroxylase that produces several neurosteroids; CYP8A, which regulates hemostasis through prostacyclin (PGI_2) synthesis and opposes the action of CYP5; CYP8B, which catalyzes bile acid biosynthesis; CYP11A1, which has steroid 20α-hydroxylase and steroid 22-hydroxylase activity, the first steps in mitochondrial steroid biosynthesis that oxidatively cleave the 17-side chain of cholesterol to pregnenolone so that defects in this enzyme lead to a lack of glucocorticoids, feminization, and hypertension; CYP11B1, which is found in the inner mitochondrial membrane of the adrenal cortex and catalyzes the 11β-hydroxylation of 11-deoxycortisol to hydrocortisone or 11-deoxycorticosterone to corticosterone; CYP11B2, which hydroxylates corticosterone at the 18-position to aldosterone; CYP17A1,

TABLE 4.3 Other Cytochromes with Indicated Specificities and Actions

CYP450s	Activity	Location	Action
CYP4	ω-hydroxylases		ω-Hydroxylation of fatty acids, leukotrienes, eicosanic acids
CYP5	thromboxane A_2 synthase		Arachidonic acid to thromboxane A_2 effecting platelet aggregation
CYP7A	7α-hydroxylase		Cholesterol to bile acids formation
CYP7B	7α-hydroxylase	Brain	Neurosteroids formation: 7α-hydroxydehydroepiandrosterone and 7α-hydroxypregnenolone
CYP8A	prostacyclin synthase		Synthesis of prostaglandin I_2 regulating hemostasis
CYP8B	12α-hydroxylase		Catalyzes bile acid biosynthesis
CYP11A1	steroid 20α-/22-hydroxylase	Adrenal mitochondria	Catalyze mitochondrial steroid biosynthesis via 17-side chain cleavage of cholesterol to pregnenolone -lack of leads to feminization and hypertension
CYP11B1	11β- hydroxylase	Adrenal cortex	Catalyzes 11-deoxycortisol to hydrocortisone or 11-deoxycorticosterone to corticosterone
CYP11B2	18-hydrolyase	Adrenal zona glomerulosa	Hydroxylates corticosterone at the 18-position leading to aldosterone
CYP17A1	17α-hydroxylase and 17,20-lyase	ER of adrenal cortex	Production of testosterone and estrogen- lack of affects sexual development
CYP19A	Aromatase	ER of gonads, brain, adipose tissue	Aromatization of ring A of testosterone leading to estrogen-lack of causes estrogen deficiency
CYP21A1	C21 steroid hydroxylase	Adrenal cortex	17-hydroxyprogesterone to cortisol
CYP24	24-hydroxylase	Mitochondria	Catalyzes the degradation/inactivation of vitamin D metabolites
CYP26A1	*trans*-retinoic acid hydroxylase		Terminates retinoic acid signal
CYP26B1	retinoic acid hydroxylase		Catalyzes the hydroxylation of *cis*-retinoic acids
CYP26C	retinoic acid hydroxylase		Unknown
CYP27A1	27-hydroxylase		Catalyzes the oxidation of the cholesterol in bile acid biosynthesis
CYP27B1	vitamin D_3 1-α-hydroxylase	Mitochondria	Activates vitamin D_3
CYP27C1			Unknown
CYP39			Catalyzes the 7-hydroxylation of 24-hydroxy cholesterol
CYP46	cholesterol 24-hydroxylase		Unknown
CYP51	lanosterol 14α-demethylase		Converts lanosterol into cholesterol

which exhibits 17α-hydroxylase and 17,20-lyase activities (two enzymes in one), which are required for production of testosterone and estrogen (lack of this enzyme affects sexual development at puberty); and CYP19A, an aromatase, which is found in the ER of gonads, brain, and adipose tissue and is a key steroidogenic enzyme that catalyzes ring A of testosterone aromatization to estrogen (lack of this enzyme causes estrogen deficiency and failure of females to develop at puberty). Aromatase inhibitors target estrogen-sensitive breast cancers, and a number of environmental contaminants can act as aromatase inhibitors, thereby disrupting endocrine function in humans and wildlife through suppression of circulating estrogen levels. CYP21A1 has C21 steroid hydroxylase activity, and a lack of this enzyme prevents cortisol synthesis, thereby diverting excess 17-hydroxyprogesterone into overproduction of testosterone biosynthesis. CYP24 (mitochondrial 25-hydroxyvitamin D_3 24-hydroxylase) catalyzes the degradation/inactivation of vitamin D metabolites; CYP26A1 is involved in terminating the retinoic acid signal and thus turning off a developmental switch. CYP26B1 catalyzes the hydroxylation of *cis*-retinoic acids, which are not recognized by the CYP26A1. CYP26C, a retinoic acid hydroxylase, has an unknown function. CYP27A1, a 27-hydroxylase, catalyzes the oxidation of the cholesterol 17-side chain as the first step in bile acid biosynthesis to the feedback inhibitors cholic acid and chenodeoxycholic acid and 25-hydroxyvitamin D_3. CYP27B1 (mitochondrial vitamin D_3 1-α-hydroxylase) activates vitamin D_3. CYP27C1 has an unknown function. CYP39 catalyzes the 7-hydroxylation of 24-hydroxy cholesterol with unknown function. CYP46 (cholesterol 24-hydroxylase) has an unknown function. CYP51 (lanosterol 14α-demethylase) converts lanosterol into cholesterol, which is the enzyme inhibited by ketoconazole.

Cytochrome P450 Isoforms Metabolizing Drugs/Xenobiotics (18–20)

Figure 4.3 shows the participation (%) of hepatic P450 isoforms in the metabolism of drugs and xenobiotics (19–21). P450s are the most important enzymes responsible for Phase 1 drug metabolism. The polymorphic nature of the P450s influences individual drug responses and drug–drug interactions and induces adverse drug reactions. The crystal structures of eight mammalian P450s (CYP1A2, CYP2B4, CYP2C5, CYP2A6, CYP2D6 CYP2C8, CYP2C9, and CYP3A4) have been published. Outstanding is the fact that approximately two-thirds of all drugs are metabolized by one isoform, CYP3A4, increasing the potential for drug–drug interactions. When two drugs are metabolized by the same isoform, only one drug can serve as a substrate at a time, increasing the likelihood of a drug–drug interaction, especially if one drug has a low therapeutic threshold.

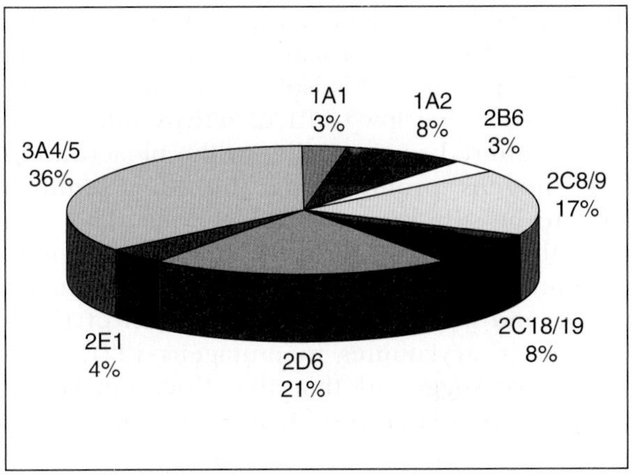

FIGURE 4.3 Percentage of clinically important drugs metabolized by human P450 isoforms.

Family 1

Family 1 consists of three subfamilies (CYP1A1, CYP1A2, and CYP1B1), three genes, and one pseudogene. The human CYP1A subfamily has an integral role in the metabolism of estrogens and two important classes of environmental carcinogens, polycyclic aromatic hydrocarbons (PAHs) and arylamines (Tables 4.4 and 4.5) (22). The PAHs are commonly present in the environment from industrial combustion processes and tobacco products. Several potent carcinogenic arylamines result from the pyrolysis of amino acids in cooked meats and cause colon cancer in rats. Environmental and genetic factors can alter the expression of this subfamily of enzymes.

CYP1A1 The CYP1A1 subfamily (also called aromatic hydrocarbon hydroxylase) is expressed primarily in extrahepatic tissues, small intestine, placenta, skin, and lung as well as in the liver in response to the presence of

TABLE 4.4 Some Substrates and Reaction Type for Human Subfamily CYP1A2[a]

Acetaminophen (imino quinone)
Amitriptyline (*N*-demethylation)
Caffeine (N^1- and N^3-demethylation)
Chlordiazepoxide
Cinacalcet
Clomipramine (*N*-demethylation)
Clopidogrel
Clozapine
Cyclobenzaprine
Desipramine (*N*-demethylation)
Diazepam
Duloxetine
Erlotinib
Estradiol (2- and 4-hydroxylation)
Fluoroquinolones (3′-hydroxylation of piperazine ring)
Flutamide
Fluvoxamine
Haloperidol
Imipramine (*N*-demethylation)
Levobupivacaine
Mexiletine
Mirtazapine
Naproxen
Nortriptyline
Olanzapine
Ondansetron
Propafenone
Propranolol
Ramelteon
Riluzole
Ropinirole
Ropivacaine
Tacrine
Theophylline
Tizanidine
Verapamil
R-warfarin
Zileuton
Zolmitriptan

[a]Drugs in bold italic have been reported to cause drug–drug interactions.

TABLE 4.5 Some Procarcinogens and Other Toxins Activated by Human Cytochrome P450s

CYP1A1	CYP1A2	CYP2E1	CYP3A4
Benzo[a]pyrene and other polycyclic aromatic hydrocarbons	4-Aminobiphenyl	Benzene	Aflatoxin B1
	2-Naphthylamine	Styrene	Aflatoxin G1
	2-Aminofluorene	Acrylonitrile	Estradiol
	2-Acetylaminofluorene	Vinyl bromide	6-Aminochrysene
	2-Aminoanthracene	Trichloroethylene	Polycyclic hydrocarbon
	Heteropolycyclic amines (2-aminoquinolines)	Carbon tetrachloride	Dihydrodiols
	Aflatoxin B1	Chloroform	
	Ipomeanol	Methylene chloride	
		N-nitrosodimethylamine	
		1,2-Dichloropropane	
		Ethyl carbamate	

CYP1A1 inducers such as PAHs (i.e., in cigarette smoke and the carcinogen 3-methylcholanthrene), α-naphthoflavone (a noncarcinogenic inducer related to dietary flavones), and indole-3-carbinol (found in Brussels sprouts and related vegetables). CYP1A1 metabolizes a range of PAHs, including a large number of procarcinogens and promutagens (Table 4.5). Diethylstilbestrol and 2- and 4-hydroxyestradiol (catecholestrogens) are oxidized by CYP1A1 to their quinone analogues, which are normally reduced to inactive metabolites (23). In the absence of a detoxifying reduction step, however, the quinones can accumulate and initiate carcinogenic processes or cell death by covalently damaging DNA or cellular proteins. Interindividual variations in the inducible expression of CYP1A1 might be related to genetic differences in aromatic hormone (Ah) receptor expression, which could explain differences in individual susceptibilities to cigarette smoke–induced lung cancer. Therefore, genetic factors appear to be important in the expression of the *CYP1A1* gene in humans and its involvement in human carcinogenesis. Women who smoke are at greater risk than men to develop lung cancer (adenocarcinoma) and chronic obstructive pulmonary diseases. The mechanism for induction of the *CYP1A1* gene begins with binding of the inducing agents to a cytosolic receptor protein, the Ah receptor, which is then translocated to the nucleus where it binds to the DNA of the *CYP1A1* gene, thus enhancing the rate of transcription. The presence of the Ah receptor in hepatic and intestinal tissues can have implications beyond xenobiotic metabolism and can have a role in the induction of other genes for the control of cellular growth and differentiation. On the other hand, CYP1A1 can metabolize procarcinogens to hydroxylated inactive compounds that are not mutagenic. The question of how the bowel protects itself from ingested compounds known to be activated by CYP1A1 (i.e., PAH) remains unanswered (22).

CYP1A2 The CYP1A2 subfamily (also known as phenacetin *O*-deethylase, caffeine demethylase, or antipyrine *N*-demethylase) is one of the major P450s in human liver that catalyzes the oxidation (and in some cases the bioactivation) of arylamines, nitrosamines, and aromatic hydrocarbons and the bioactivation of promutagens and procarcinogens, caffeine, clozapine, tacrine, theophylline, estrogens, and other substances (Tables 4.4 and 4.5). CYP1A2 is expressed in the liver (13% to 40%), intestine, and stomach and is induced by smoking, PAHs, and isosafrole (a noncarcinogenic dietary compound). CYP1A2 is primarily responsible for activation of the carcinogen aflatoxin B1 in ordinary human exposure and of the pneumotoxin ipomeanol. CYP1A2 is subject to reversible and/or irreversible inhibition by a number of drugs, natural substances, and other compounds. *CYP1A2* gene expresses a 515-residue protein with a molecular mass of 58.3 kDa. The CYP1A2 structure exhibits a relatively compact, planar active site cavity that is highly adapted for the size and shape of its substrates. A large interindividual variability in the expression and activity of CYP1A2 has been observed, which is largely caused by genetic, epigenetic, and environmental factors (e.g., smoking). CYP1A2 is primarily regulated by the aromatic hydrocarbon receptor (AhR). Induction or inhibition of CYP1A2 may provide partial explanation for some clinical drug interactions. More than 15 variant alleles of the *CYP1A2* gene have been identified, and some of them have been associated with altered drug clearance and response and disease susceptibility. Evidence for polymorphism of this isoform has been reported, and it is likely that low CYP1A2 activity will be associated with altered susceptibility to the bioactivation of procarcinogens, promutagens, and other xenobiotics known to be substrates for this enzyme. The expression of the *CYP1A2* gene in the stomach becomes an important issue for gastric carcinogenesis induced by smoking and by the metabolic activation of the procarcinogenic arylamines to mutagens (22). Clinical studies have suggested that the *N*-demethylation of imipramine is greater in smokers than in nonsmokers.

Family 2

The human CYP2A family comprises 16 subfamilies (CYP2A6, CYP2A7, CYP2A13, CYP2B6, CYP2C8, CYP2C9,

CYP2C18, CYP2C19, CYP2D6, CYP2E1, CYP2F1, CYP2J2, CYP2R1, CYP2S1, CYP2U1, CYP2W1), 16 genes, and 16 pseudogenes. CYP2A7 is nonfunctional. CYP2A13 is highly active in the metabolic activation of a major tobacco-specific carcinogen, 4-(methylnitrosamino)-1-(3-pyridyl)-1-butanone, in the human respiratory tract, with a catalytic efficiency much greater than that of other CYP2A. Expressed CYP2A13 is more active than CYP2A6 in the metabolic activation of hexamethylphosphoramide, *N,N*-dimethylaniline, 2'-methoxyacetophenone, and *N*-nitrosomethylphenylamine, but is much less active than CYP2A6 in coumarin 7-hydroxylation.

CYP2A6 CYP2A6 has a low level of hepatic expression and represents only approximately 4% of the total of hepatic P450 isoforms (Fig. 4.2). It is also expressed at low levels in lung and nasal epithelium and exhibits high interindividual variability (polymorphism). Lung CYP2A6 bioactivates many tobacco smoke–specific carcinogens, procarcinogens, and nitrosamines. Mutant alleles of this isoenzyme have been associated with an elevated risk for small-cell lung cancer. Hepatically, CYP2A6 is the major enzyme catalyzing the 7-hydroxylation of coumarin (coumarin 7-hydroxylase) and C5 oxidation of nicotine to cotinine (nicotine C-poxidase) (Table 4.6). Other substrates include the hydroxylation of aflatoxin B1, naproxen, tacrine, clozapine, mexiletine, and cyclobenzaprine. In in vitro studies with human microsomes and expressed human CYP2A6, selegiline and its desmethyl metabolite are mechanism-based CYP2A6 inhibitors of nicotine metabolism. Thus, inhibition of nicotine metabolism by selegiline could increase plasma nicotine in vivo. There is overlapping substrate specificity with CYP2A13. CYP2A6 exhibits polymorphism, with an incidence of 2% in the Caucasian population. This population is characterized as poor metabolizers. Smokers with a defective *CYP2A6* gene smoke fewer cigarettes, implicating a genetic factor in nicotine dependence.

CYP2A13 CYP2A13 is expressed highest in nasal epithelium, followed by lung and trachea, with high interindividual variability. CYP2A13 activates tobacco smoke–specific carcinogens, procarcinogens, and nitrosamines into DNA-altering compounds that cause lung cancer. Individuals with a high level of CYP2A13 expression could likely have an increased risk of developing tobacco smoking–related lung cancers. Although CYP2A13 and CYP2A6 are 93.5% identical in amino acid sequences, CYP2A13 exhibits higher affinity for metabolizing tobacco smoke carcinogens than does CYP2A6. A comparison of the crystal structures of CYP2A13 and CYP2A6 has shown them to be very similar, and like CYP2A6, the CYP2A13 active site cavity is small and highly hydrophobic with a cluster of phenylalanine residues in the active site. Amino acid differences

TABLE 4.6 Some Substrates for CYP2A6

Acetaminophen	Ifosfamide
Aminopyrine	Methoxsalen
Caffeine	Nicotine
Cinnarizine	Omeprazole
Cisapride	Phenacetin
Clomethiazole	Pilocarpine
Cyclophosphamide	Promazine
Disulfiram	Propofol
Efavirenz	Tamoxifen
Etodolac	Tretinoin
Fenchone	Verbenone
Flunarizine	Zidovudine
Halothane	

Adapted from Di YM, Chow VD, Yang LP, et al. Structure, function, regulation and polymorphism of human cytochrome CYP2A6. Curr Drug Metab. 2009;10:754–780.

between CYP2A6 and CYP2A13 at key positions could be the cause of the significant variations observed in ligand binding and catalysis.

CYP2B6 The human CYP2B6 subfamily has not been as fully characterized at the molecular level as have other members of the human P450 family. This family represents less than 1% of the total of hepatic P450 isoforms, and its level of expression mainly in the liver is low and may be co-regulated with CYP3A4. CYP2B6 has been thought to have an insignificant role in human drug metabolism. This enzyme exhibits polymorphic and ethnic differences in CYP2B6 expression and therefore could be important in drug–drug interactions. CYP2B6 can metabolize approximately 8% of clinically used drugs including cyclophosphamide, ifosfamide, tamoxifen, ketamine, artemisinin, nevirapine, efavirenz, bupropion, sibutramine, nicotine, sertraline, and propofol (Table 4.7). CYP2B6 also metabolizes arachidonic acid, lauric acid, 17β-estradiol, estrone, ethinylestradiol, and testosterone and can also bioactivate several procarcinogens and toxicants. The crystal structure of CYP2B6 has not been resolved, whereas several pharmacophore and homology models of human CYP2B6 have been reported. CYP2B6 is closely regulated by the androstane receptor, which can activate CYP2B6 expression upon ligand binding. Pregnane X receptor and glucocorticoid receptor also have a role in the regulation of CYP2B6. Induction of CYP2B6 may partially explain some clinical drug interactions observed. For example, coadministered carbamazepine decreases the blood levels of bupropion. There is a wide interindividual variability in the expression and activity of CYP2B6. Such a large variability is probably a result of the effects of genetic polymorphisms and exposure to drugs that are inducers or inhibitors of CYP2B6. CYP2B6 substrates are by and large small nonplanar molecules, neutral or weakly basic, highly lipophilic with one or two hydrogen-bond acceptors, and frequently active in the CNS. Phenobarbital appears to induce its formation.

TABLE 4.7 Some Substrates for Human Subfamily CYP2B6

Amitriptyline	Diclofenac	Meperidine	Sevoflurane
Artemisinin	Diphenhydramine	Methadone	Sibutramine
Bupropion	Disulfiram	Methoxyflurane	*S*-mephenytoin
Carbamazepine	Efavirenz	Mianserin	*S*-mephobarbital
Carbaryl	Ethylbenzene	Nevirapine	Tamoxifen
Cinnarizine	Fenchone	Nicotine	Temazepam
Cisapride	Fluoxetine	Nor-LAAM	Thiotepa
Clomethiazole	Haloperidol	Prasugrel	Tramadol
Clopidogrel	Ifosfamide	Promazine	Tretinoin
Cyclophosphamide	Imipramine	Propofol	Valproic acid
Desmethylselegiline	Ketamine	Selegiline	Verapamil
Diazepam	l-Acetyl-α-methadol	Sertraline	

Adapted from Mo SL, Liu YH, Duan W, et al. Substrate specificity, regulation, and polymorphism of human cytochrome CYP2B6. Curr Drug Metab. 2009;10:730–53.

CYP2C The CYP2C subfamily is the most complex family, consisting of three subfamilies (CYP2C8, CYP2C9, and CYP2C19), metabolizing approximately 25% of the clinically important drugs (Fig. 4.3), including *S*-warfarin, *S*-mephenytoin, and tolbutamide (Table 4.8). The CYP2C subfamily represents approximately 20% of the total of P450 isoforms in the liver (Fig. 4.2). CYP2C8 is expressed primarily in extrahepatic tissues (kidney, adrenal, brain, uterus, breast, ovary, and intestine) and metabolizes the tricyclic antidepressants, diazepam and verapamil. Its level of expression is less than that of the other CYP2C9 and CYP2C19 subfamilies.

CYP2C9 metabolizes approximately 15% of clinical drugs, including the methyl hydroxylation of tolbutamide and glyburide; 4′-hydroxylation of diclofenac, celecoxib, and phenytoin; oxidation of the hydroxymethyl group of losartan to a carboxylic acid; and 7-hydroxylation of *S*-warfarin and many nonsteroidal anti-inflammatory drugs (NSAIDs) (Table 4.8). CYP2C9 is highly polymorphic. Some natural and herbal compounds are also metabolized by CYP2C9, probably leading to the formation of toxic metabolites. CYP2C9 also metabolizes endogenous compounds such as steroids, melatonin, retinoids, and arachidonic acid. Many CYP2C9 substrates are weak acids, but CYP2C9 has also the capacity to metabolize neutral, highly lipophilic compounds. Ligand-based and homology models of CYP2C9 have been reported, which have provided insight into how its substrates are bound to the active site of CYP2C9. The resolved crystal structure of CYP2C9 has confirmed the importance in substrate specificity and ligand orientation. For example, CYP2C9 is activated by dapsone and its analogues and *R*-lansoprazole in a stereospecific and substrate-dependent manner, probably through binding to the active site and inducing positive cooperativity. CYP2C9 is subject to induction by rifampin, phenobarbital, and dexamethasone, indicating the involvement of pregnane X receptor, the androstane receptor, and the glucocorticoid receptor in the regulation of CYP2C9. A number of compounds inhibit CYP2C9, which could provide an explanation for some clinically important drug interactions. Tienilic acid, suprofen, and silybin are mechanism-based inhibitors of CYP2C9. Given the importance of CYP2C9 in drug metabolism and the presence of polymorphisms, it is important to identify drugs as potential substrates, inducer, or inhibitors of CYP2C9 in drug–drug interactions.

CYP2C19 is found primarily in the liver and intestine. The expression of CYP2C19 in the liver is less than that of CYP2C9 and also exhibits polymorphism (differences in the DNA sequence for the *CYP2C* gene), which changes the enzyme's ability to metabolize these substrates (i.e., poor metabolizer phenotype). Because of this genetic difference in expressing CYP2C isoforms, it is important to be aware of a person's race when prescribing drugs that are metabolized differently by different racial populations (see the section concerning genetic polymorphism). CYP2C19 (*S*-mephenytoin hydroxylase) is the isoform associated with the 4′-hydroxylation of *S*-mephenytoin. The CYP2C subfamily is apparently not inducible in humans.

CYP2D6 CYP2D6 polymorphism is, perhaps, the most studied P450 (see the section on genetic polymorphism). This enzyme is responsible for at least 30 different drug oxidations, representing approximately 21% of clinically important drugs (Fig. 4.3). CYP2D6 is only 3% expressed in the liver and minimally expressed in the intestine, and it does not appear to be inducible (Fig. 4.2). Because there might not be any other way to clear drugs metabolized by CYP2D6 from the system, poor metabolizers of CYP2D6 substrates can be at severe risk for adverse drug reactions or drug overdoses. The metabolism of debrisoquine by CYP2D6 is one of the most studied examples of metabolic polymorphism, with the molecular basis for defective metabolism well understood (Table 4.9) (see the section on genetic polymorphism). This isoform metabolizes a wide variety of lipophilic amines and is probably the only P450 for which a charged or ion-pair interaction is important for substrate binding. It appears

TABLE 4.8 Some Substrates and Reaction Type for Human Subfamily CYP2C[a]

CYP2C8	CYP2C9	CYP2C9 (con't)	CYP2C219
Amiodarone	Amitriptyline	Losartan (hydroxymethyl to carboxylic)	Amitriptyline
Amodiaquine	Bosentan	Mefenamic acid	Carisoprodol
Benzphetamine	Buprenorphine	Meloxicam	Cilostazol
Carbamzepine	Carvedilol	(*R*)-Mephenytoin	Citalopram
Cerivastatin	Celecoxib	Mestranol	Clomipramine
Docetaxel	Chlorpheniramine	Montelukast	***Clopidogrel***
Fluvastatin	Chloramphenicol	Naproxen	Cyclophosphamide
Isotretinoin	Clomipramine	Nateglinide	Desipramine
Paclitaxel	Chlorpropamide	Omeprazole	***Diazepam*** (*N*-demethylation)
Phenytoin	Clopidogrel	Phenobarbital	Escitalopram
Pioglitazone	Dapsone	***Phenytoin*** (4′-hydroxylation)	Esomeprazole
Repaglinide	Desogestrel	Phenylbutazone (4-hydroxylation)	Formoterol
Retinol	Diclofenac (4′-hydroxylation)	Piroxicam	Hexobarbital
Rosiglitazone	***Diazepam***	Prasugrel	Imipramine (*N*-demethylation)
Tolbutamide	Diphenhydramine	***Ramelteon***	Indomethacin
Torsemide	Donepezil	Rosiglitazone	Lansoprazole
Verapamil	Dorzolamide	Rosuvastatin	Loratidine (*N*-decarboethoxylation)
Zopliclone	Dronabinol	Sildenafil	(*S*)-Mephenytoin (4′-hydroxylation)
	Eletriptan	Sulfamethoxazole	(*R*)-Mephenytoin (*N*-demethylation)
	Etodolac	Sulfinpyrazone (aromatic hydroxylation)	(*R*)-Mephobarbital
	Fluoxetine	Suprofen	Moclobemide
	Flurbiprofen (4′-hydroxylation)	Tamoxifen	Nelfinavir
	Fluvastatin	Tenoxicam	Nilutamide
	Formoterol	Terbinafine	Omeprazole (hydroxylation)
	Glibenclamide	Tienilic acid (thiophene ring hydroxylation)	Pantoprazole
	Gliclazide	Tolbutamide (*p*-methylhydroxylation)	Pentamidine
	Glyburide	Tolterodine	Phenobarbital
	Glimepiride	Torsemide	***Phenytoin*** (ring hydroxylation)
	Glipizide	Δ^1-THC (7-hydroxylation)	Progesterone
	Glyburide	Testosterone (16α-hydroxylation)	Proguanil (cyclization)
	Halothane	Trimethadione	Propranolol (side chain hydroxylation)
	Hexobarbital (3′-hydroxylation)	Valdecoxib	Rabeprazole
	Ibuprofen (*i*-butylmethyl-hydroxylation)	Vardenafil	Teniposide
	Imipramine	Valproic acid	***Thioridazine***
	Indomethacin	Valsartan	Progesterone
	Irbesartan	Voriconazole	Tolbutamide
	Irinotecan	*S*-Warfarin (7′-hydroxylation)	***Voriconazole***
	Ketamine	Zafirlukast	*R*-Warfarin
	Lomoxicam	Zileuton	
		Zopiclone	

[a]Drugs in bold italic have been reported to cause drug-drug interactions.

also to preferentially catalyze the hydroxylation of a single enantiomer (stereoselectivity) in the presence of enantiomeric mixtures. Quinidine is an inhibitor of CYP2D6, and concurrent administration with CYP2D6 substrates results in increased blood levels and toxicities for these substrates. If the pharmacologic action of the CYP2D6 substrate depends on the formation of active metabolites, quinidine inhibition results in a lack of a therapeutic response. The interaction of two substrates for CYP2D6 can prompt a number of clinical responses. For example, when substrates have unequal affinities for CYP2D6, the first-pass hepatic metabolism of a substrate (drug) with high affinity for CYP2D6 will inhibit binding of a second substrate that has a lower affinity for this enzyme. The result of this will be a rapid absorption of the second unmetabolized substrate, leading to a higher plasma concentration and to the increased potential for adverse reaction or toxicity.

CYP2E1 Few drugs are metabolized by CYP2E1; however, this isoform has a major role in the metabolism of numerous halogenated hydrocarbons (including volatile general anesthetics) and of a range of low molecular weight organic compounds including dimethylformamide, acetonitrile, acetone, ethanol, and benzene, as well as in the activation of acetaminophen to its reactive metabolite, *N*-acetyl-*p*-benzoquinoneimine (Table 4.10) (24,25). CYP2E1 is of most interest as a result of the oxidation of ethanol into its reactive products, acetaldehyde and 1-hydroxyethyl radicals, and its ability to activate small molecular weight products into electrophilic reactive metabolites, which result in toxicity and carcinogenicity. This enzyme then oxidizes acetaldehyde produced from ethanol to acetic acid. This isoform is only 7% expressed in the liver and is also expressed in the kidney, intestine, and lung. CYP2E1 is inducible under diverse pathophysiologic conditions including

TABLE 4.9 Some Substrates and Reaction Type for Human CYP2D6 Isoform[a]

- Alprenolol (4-hydroxylation)
- ***Amitriptyline*** (10-hydroxylation)
- Amphetamine
- Aripiprazole
- ***Atomoxetine***
- Bifuralol (1′-hydroxylation)
- Bisoprolol
- Captopril
- Carvedilol
- Cevimeline
- Chlorpheniramine (*N*-demethylation, ring hydroxylation, deamination)
- Chlorpromazine
- Chlorpropamide
- Cinacalcet
- Clemastine
- Clomipramine (hydroxylation)
- Clozapine (aromatic hydroxylation)
- ***Codeine*** (O-demethylation)
- Cyclobenzaprine
- Darifenacin
- Debrisoquine (4-hydroxylation)
- ***Desipramine***
- Dexfenfluramine
- ***Dextromethorphan*** (*O*-demethylation)
- Diphenhydramine (*N*-demethylation, ring hydroxylation, cleavage ether bond)
- Dolasetron (hydroxylation of indole ring)
- ***Donepezil***
- ***Doxepin***
- ***Duloxetine***
- Encainide (*N*-demethylation, *O*-demethylation)
- Fenfluramine
- Fluphenazine
- ***Fentanyl***
- ***Flecainide*** (*O*-dealkylation)
- Fluoxetine (*N*-dealkylation)
- Fluvoxamine
- Formoterol
- Galantamine
- Guanoxan (6- and 7-hydroxylation)
- ***Haloperidol***
- ***Hydrocodone***
- Hydroxyzine (ring hydroxylation)
- ***Imipramine*** (2-hydroxylation)
- Indoramin (6-hydroxylation)
- Lidocaine (3-hydroxylation)
- Maprotiline
- ***Meperidine***
- ***Methadone***
- Methamphetamine
- Methoxyamphetamine (4-hydroxylation, *N*-demethylation)
- Metoclopramide
- Metoprolol (*O*-demethylation)
- ***Mexiletine*** (4-hydroxylation and methyl hydroxylation)
- Minaprine
- Mirtazapine
- Morphine
- Nebivolol
- ***Nortriptyline*** (10-hydroxylation)
- Olanzapine
- Ondansetron (hydroxylation of indole ring)
- ***Oxycodone*** (*O*-demethylation)
- Paroxetine
- Perhexiline (4′-hydroxylation)
- Perphenazine (aromatic hydroxylation)
- Phenacetin
- Phenformin (4-hydroxylation)
- Pindolol
- Promethazine (ring hydroxylation, *S*-oxidation, *N*-demethylation)
- ***Propafenone*** (4-hydroxylation)
- ***Propoxyphene***
- Propranolol (4′-hydroxylation)
- Quetiapine
- Quinidine (hydroxylation)
- Ranolazine
- Risperidone
- Ritonavir
- Sertraline
- *S*-Metoprolol
- Sparteine (*N*-oxidation)
- Tamoxifen
- **Thioridazine** (aromatic hydroxylation)
- Timolol (*O*-dealkylation)
- Tolterodine (2-hydroxylation)
- ***Tramadol***
- ***Trazodone***
- Tripelennamine
- Tropisetron (hydroxylation of indole ring)
- Venlafaxine

[a]Drugs in bold italic have been reported to cause drug–drug interactions.

diabetes, obesity, fasting, cancer, alcoholic liver disease, and nonalcoholic liver disease, as well as by the chemical substances ethanol, isoniazid, 4-methylpyrazole, and other chemicals (see Table 4.14). Mitochondrial CYP2E1 induces the formation of reactive oxygen species (ROS), which is associated with oxidative stress and lipid peroxidation and augments ethanol-induced hepatocellular injury. CYP2E1 is also known as the microsomal ethanol-oxidizing system, benzene hydroxylase, or aniline hydroxylase. CYP2E1 is induced in alcoholics, and there is a polymorphism associated with this isoform, which is most common in Chinese people. This isoform also appears to be involved in smoking-induced cancer (c.f., CYP1A2). Most of the compounds that induce CYP2E1 are also substrates for this enzyme. The induction of this enzyme in humans can cause enhanced susceptibility to the toxicity and carcinogenesis of CYP2E1 substrates. Some evidence shows interindividual variation in the in vitro liver expression of this isoform. Ketogenic diets (increased serum ketone levels), including those deficient in carbohydrates or high in fat, are known to enhance the metabolism of halogenated hydrocarbons in rats (25). The mechanism of induction appears to be a combination of an increase in CYP2E1 transcription, mRNA translation efficiency, and stabilization of CYP2E1 against proteolytic degradation. The induction of CYP2E1 resulting from ketosis (i.e., due to starvation, a high-fat diet, uncontrolled diabetes, or obesity) or from exposure to alcoholic beverages or other xenobiotics can be detrimental to individuals simultaneously exposed to halogenated hydrocarbons (increased hepatotoxicity as a result of exposure to halothane or chloroform). Chronic

TABLE 4.10 Some Substrates and Reaction Type for Human CYP2E1 Isoform[a]

Acetaminophen (*p*-benzoquinone imine)
Styrene (epoxidation)
Theophylline (C-8 oxidation)
Disulfiram
Halogenated Hydrocarbons
Dehalogenation of chloroform, methylene chloride
Volatile Anesthetics (fluorinated hydrocarbons)
Enflurane, halothane, methoxyflurane, sevoflurane, desflurane
Miscellaneous Organic Solvents
Ethanol (to acetaldehyde)
Glycerin
Dimethylformamide (*N*-demethylation)
Acetone
Diethylether
Benzene (hydroxylation)
Aniline (hydroxylation)
Acetonitrile (hydroxylation to cyanohydrin)
Pyridine (hydroxylation)

[a]Drugs in bold italics have been reported to cause drug–drug interactions.

alcohol intake is known to enhance the hepatotoxicity of halogenated hydrocarbons. Testosterone appears to regulate CYP2E1 levels in the kidney, and pituitary growth hormone regulates hepatic levels of CYP2E1. Kidney damage in response to halocarbon exposure was greater in male rats than in female rats. This finding could have implications for sexual differences in the nephrotoxicity of CYP2E1 substrates in humans.

Family 3

The human CYP3 family comprises four subfamilies CYP3A4, CYP3A5, CYP3A7, CYP3A43, four genes, and two pseudogenes.

CYP3A4 The CYP3A4 subfamily includes the most abundantly expressed P450s in the human liver and intestine (extrahepatic metabolism). Although CYP3A4 is responsible for approximately two-thirds of CYP3A-mediated drug metabolism, the other minor isoforms (CYP3A5, CYP3A7, and CYP3A43) also contribute. CYP3A5 is the best studied of the minor CYP3A isoforms, with 85% sequence identity with CYP3A4. Approximately 20% of human livers express CYP3A5. The expression of CYP3A5 shows ethnic differences, with the wild-type CYP3A5*1 allele more common in Africans than in Caucasians or Asians. In individuals who express CYP3A5, 17% to 50% of the total hepatic CYP3A is this isoform. Additionally, CYP3A5 is also expressed in a range of extrahepatic tissues (kidney, small intestine, lung, adrenal glands) and is inducible via the pregnane X receptor. Both CYP3A4 and CYP3A5 exhibit significant overlap in substrate specificity but can differ in catalytic activity and regioselectivity. Results from a comparison of CYP3A4 and CYP3A5 enzyme kinetics indicate that CYP3A5 has different enzymic characteristics than CYP3A4 in some CYP3A-catalyzed reactions. The enzyme kinetics of CYP3A5 suggest faster substrate turnover than that observed with CYP3A4.

Approximately one-third of the total P450 in the liver and two-thirds in the intestine is CYP3A4. This isoform is responsible for the metabolism of testosterone and more than one-third of the clinically important drugs. CYP3A4 is expressed in the intestine, lung, placenta, kidney, uterus, and brain and is glucocorticoid-inducible. CYP3A7 is predominantly expressed in fetal liver (~50% of total fetal P450 enzymes) but is also found in some adult livers and extrahepatically. CYP3A7 has a specific role in the hydroxylation of retinoic acid, 16α-hydroxylation of steroids, and hydroxylation of allylic and benzylic carbons, and therefore, it is relevant in both normal development and in carcinogenesis. The most recently discovered CYP3A isoform is CYP3A3. In addition to a low level of liver expression, it is expressed in prostate and testis. Its substrate specificity is currently unclear. Polymorphisms that predict the absence of active enzyme have been identified.

The CYP3A4 subfamily metabolizes approximately 50% to 60% of clinically important drugs (Table 4.11) and is inhibited by a number of xenobiotics (Table 4.12). CYP3A4 also appears to activate aflatoxin B1 and, possibly, to metabolize benzo[a]pyrene. The interindividual differences reported for metabolism of nifedipine, cyclosporine, triazolam, and midazolam are probably related to changes in induction and not to polymorphism. Binding of CYP3A is predominantly lipophilic (14). Drugs known to be substrates for CYP3A4 have low and variable oral bioavailabilities that might be explained by prehepatic metabolism by a combination of intestinal CYP3A4 and P-glycoprotein in the enterocytes of the intestinal wall (see the section on oral bioavailability). Therefore, it is the expression and function of CYP3A4 that governs the rate and extent of metabolism of the substrates for the CYP3A subfamily. The induction of the CYP3A subfamily by phenobarbital in humans could ultimately be responsible for many of the well-documented interactions between barbiturates and other drugs (19,20).

Family 4

The human CYP4 family consists of 6 subfamilies and 13 CYP4 proteins, of which the CYP4A, CYP4B, and CYP4F subfamilies have been most studied. The CYP4A subfamily (fatty acid hydroxylases) catalyzes the hydroxylation of the terminal ω-carbon and, to a lesser extent, the ω-1 position of saturated and unsaturated fatty acids, as well as the ω-hydroxylation of various prostaglandins. The *CYP4A1*, *CYP4A2*, and *CYP4A3* genes are expressed mostly in liver and kidney, and their expression is induced by a class of chemicals known as peroxisome proliferators, which includes the hypolipidemic drug, clofibrate. Induction of CYP4A expression by clofibrate is due to transcriptional activation, mediated possibly via a peroxisome proliferator-activated receptor (PPAR). *CYP4A* gene expression is hormonally regulated. There is a close association between CYP4A1 induction, peroxisome proliferation, and induction of the peroxisomal fatty acid metabolizing

TABLE 4.11 Substrates for Human CYP3A4 Isoform[a]

Alfentanyl	Citopram	Efavirenz	Lansoprazole	Prasugrel	***Prednisone***	***Zileuton***
Alfuzosin	Clarithromycin	***Eplerenone***	Letrozole	Propranolol	***Prednisolone***	***Ziprasidone***
Almotriptan	Clindamycin	***Ergotamine***	Lercanidipine	***Quetiapine***	Dexamethasone	Zolpidem
Alprazolam	Clomipramine	***Erlotinib***	***Lidocaine***	***Quinidine***	***Sunitinib***	***Zonisamide***
Amitriptyline	Clonazepam	***Erythromycin***	Lopinavir	Quinine	***Tacrolimus***	
Amiodarone	***Clopidogrel***	Esomeprazole	Loratidine	Rabeprazole	***Tadalafil***	
Amlodipine	Clozapine	***Eszopiclone***	***Lovastatin***	***Ramelteon***	***Tamoxifen***	
Amprenavir	Cocaine	***Ethinylestradiol***	***Methadone***	***Ranolazine***	***Telithromycin***	
Aprepitant	Codeine	***Ethosuximide***	***Midazolam***	Repaglinide	Temazepam	
Aripiprazole	***Colchicine***	Etonogestrel	***Mifepristone***	Rifampin	Δ^1-THC	
Astemizole	Cyclophosphamide	***Etoposide***	***Mirtazepine***	***Rifabutin***- related	Theophylline	
Atazanavir	***Cyclosporine***	Exemestane	***Modafinil***	compounds	***Tiagabine***	
Atorvastatin	Dapsone	***Felodipine***	***Mometasone***	***Ritonavir***	Tinidazole	
Azole antifungals	***Darifenacin***	***Fentanyl***	***Montelukast***	Salmeterol	***Tipranavir***	
Bepridil	Delavirdine	Fexofenadine	Nateglinide	***Saquinavir***	***Tolterodine***	
Bexarotene	Desogestrel	Finasteride	***Nelfinavir***	***Sertraline***	Toremifene	
Bromocriptine	Dextromethorphan	Flutamide	Nevirapine	Sibuttramine	Tramadol	
Budesonide	Diazepam	***Fluticasone***	***Nicardipine***	***Sildenafil***	***Trazodone***	
Buprenorphine	***Dihydroergotamine***	Galantamine	***Nifedipine***	***Simvastatin***	***Triazolam***	
Buspirone	***Diisopyramide***	Gleevec	***Nisoldipine***	***Sirolimus***	Trimetrexate	
Cafergot	Diltiazem	Haloperidol	Nitrendipine	***Solifenacin***	Valdecoxib	
Caffeine	Docetaxel	Hydrocodone	Norethindrone	Sorafenib	Valproic acid	
Cannabinoids	Dofetilide	Imatinib	***Omeprazole***	Steroids	***Vardenafil***	
Carbamzepine	Dolasetron	Imipramine	***Ondanestron***	Testosterone	***Verapamil***	
Cerivastatin	Domperidone	***Indinavir***	***Oral contraceptives/***	Progesterone	***Vinblastine***	
Cevimeline	Donepezil	Irinotecan	***progestins***	***Estradiol***	***Vincristine***	
Chlorpheniramine	Doxorubicin	***Isradipine***	Oxybutynin	***17α-Ethynylestradiol***	***Voriconazole***	
Cilostazol	Dronabinol	***Itraconazole***	***Paclitaxel***	***Norethisterone***	***R-Warfarin***	
Cinacalcet	Duasteride	***Keotconazole***	Pantoprazole	Hydrocortisone	Zaleplon	
			Pioglitazone	Methylprednisolone		

[a]Drugs in bold italic have been reported to cause drug–drug interactions.

system. The CYP4A subfamily is involved in the metabolism of eicosanoic acids (e.g., arachidonic acid), leading to the formation of physiologically important metabolites involved in such processes as blood flow in the kidney, and brain. CYP4B1 is a major bioactivating factor catalyzing the formation of reactive metabolites, such as the pneumotoxin, 4-ipomeanol. The CYP4F subfamily consists of seven proteins and are ω-hydroxylases, which function as eicosanoid regulators. This family is responsible for inactivating the vascular effects of leukotrienes, ω-3 fatty acids, and tocopherols (vitamin E analogs).

Clearly, no one animal model or combination of animal models represents the metabolic capabilities of humans. By having a complete understanding of the factors (e.g., inducers, inhibitors, and effects of disease states) that alter the expression and activity of an enzyme responsible for the metabolism of a particular compound and by a determination of responsible isoforms and patient phenotyping, it might be possible to predict drug–drug interactions and metabolic clearance.

An alphabetical listing of the clinically important drugs and the CYP450 isoforms catalyzing their oxidative metabolism is presented in Table 4.13.

Catalytic Cycle of Cytochrome P450: Steps of the Catalytic Cycle

The many variant P450 isoforms that have been isolated show a remarkable uniformity for the catalytic mechanism (14,21,26,27). The current view illustrating the cyclic mechanism for reduction and oxygenation of P450 with stepwise interactions with substrate molecules, electron donors, and oxygen is shown in Figure 4.4 and can be summarized as follows (26,27):

Step A. The Fe^{+3}–P450 complex binds reversibly to a molecule of the substrate (RH), resulting in a complex analogous to an enzyme–substrate complex. Binding of the substrate facilitates the first one-electron reduction step.

Step B. The substrate complex of Fe^{+3}–P450 undergoes reduction to a Fe^{+2}–P450 substrate complex by an electron originating from NADPH and transferred by the flavoprotein (NADPH-P450 reductase) from the $FMNH_2$/FADH complex.

Step C. The reduced Fe^{+2}–P450 complex readily binds dioxygen as the sixth ligand of Fe^{+2} to form a dioxygen–Fe^{+2}–P450 complex.

Step D. The dioxygen–Fe^{+2}–P450 complex rearranges by resonance, as a result of the strong electronegativity of oxygen, to an Fe^{+3}–P450–superoxide substrate complex.

Step E. The Fe^{+3}–P450–superoxide substrate complex undergoes further reduction by accepting the rapid delivery of a second electron from the flavoprotein (or possibly cytochrome b_5) to form the equivalent of a two-electron–reduced peroxy–Fe^{+3}–P450 complex. If the electron is not delivered rapidly, the

TABLE 4.12 Cytochrome P450 Inhibitors[a]

CYP1A2	CYP2B6	CYP2C8	CYP2C19	CYP2C9	CYP2D6	CYP2E1	CYP3A4/5/7
Amiodarone	Amiodarone	Anastrozole	Cimetidine	***Amiodarone***	***Amiodarone***	Diethyl dithio-carbamate	***Amiodarone***
Atazanavir	Amlodipine	***Gemfibrozil***	Citalopram	Atazanavir	Bupropion	Disulfiram	***Amprenavir***
Cimetidine	Azelastine	Glitazones	Delavirdine	***Cimetidine***	Celecoxib		***Aprepitant***
Ciprofloxacin	Citalopram	Montelukast	Efavirenz	Clopidogrel	Chloroquine		***Atazanavir***
Citalopram	Clotrimazole	Nicardipine	Felbamate	Cotrimoxazole	Chlorpheniramine		***Cimetidine***
Clarithromycin	Desipramine	Sulfinpyrazone	Fluconazole	Delavirdine	Chlorpromazine		Ciprofloxacin
Diltiazem	Disulfiram	Trimethoprim	***Fluoxetine***	Disulfiram	***Cimetidine***		***Clarithromycin***
Enoxacin	Doxorubicin		Fluvastatin	Efavirenz	***Cinacalcet***		***Cyclosporine***
Erythromycin	Ethinyl estradiol		***Fluvoxamine***	Fenofibrate	Citalopram		Danazol
Ethinyl Estradiol	Fluoxetine		Indomethacin	***Fluconazole***	Clemastine		***Delavirdine***
Fluoroquinolones	Fluvoxamine		Isoniazid	Fluorouracil	Clomipramine		Diethyl dithio-carbamate
Fluvoxamine	Isoflurane		Ketoconazole	***Fluoxetine***	Cocaine		***Diltiazem***
Interferon	Ketoconazole		Lansoprazole	Fluvastatin	***Darifenacin***		***Efavirenz***
Isoniazid	Mestranol		Modafinil	Fluvoxamine	Desipramine		***Erythromycin***
Ketoconazole	Methimazole		Omeprazole	Gemfibrozil	Diphenhydramine		Ethinyl Estradiol
Methoxsalen	Miconazole		Oxcarbazepine	Imatinib	Doxepin		***Fluconazole***
Mibefradil	Nelfinavir		Probenicid	***Isoniazid***	Doxorubicin		Fluoxetine
	Orphenadrine		Ticlopidine	Itraconazole	***Duloxetine***		***Fluvoxamine***
	Paroxetine		Topiramate	Ketoconazole	Escitalopram		Gestodene
	Sertraline			Leflunomide	***Fluoxetine***		Imatinib
	Sorafenib			Lovastatin	Fluphenazine		***Indinavir***
	Tamoxifen			Methoxsalen	Halofantrine		***Isoniazid***
	Ticlopidine			***Metronidazole***	Haloperidol		***Itraconazole***
	Thiotepa			Mexiletine	Hydroxychloroquine		***Ketoconazole***
	Venlafaxine			Modafinil	Hydroxyzine		Methylprednisolne
				Nalidixic acid	Imatinib		***Metronidazole***
				Norethindrone	Levomepromazine		Mibefradil
				Norfloxacin	Methadone		***Miconazole***
				Omeprazole	Metoclopramide		Mifepristone
				Oral Contraceptives	Mibefradil		***Nelfinavir***
				Paroxetine	Midodrine		Nicardipine
				Phenylbutazone	Moclobemide		***Nifedipine***
				Probenicid	Norfluoxetine		Norethindrone
				Sertraline	***Paroxetine***		***Norfloxacin***
				Sulfamethoxazole	Perphenazine		Norfluoxetine
				Sulfaphenazole	Propafenone		Oxiconazole
				Sulfonamides	Propoxyphene		Prednisone
				Tacrine	***Propranolol***		***Quinine***
				Teniposide	Quinacrine		***Ranolazine***
				Ticlopidine	***Quinidine***		***Ritonavir***
				Tipranavir	Ranitidine		***Roxithromycin***
				Troleandomycin	Ranolazine		***Saquinavir***
				Voriconazole	***Ritonavir***		***Sertraline***
				Zafirlukast	***Sertraline***		***Telithromycin***
				Zileuton	Terbinafine		***Troleandomycin***
					Thioridazine		***Verapamil***
					Ticlopidine		***Voriconazole***
					Tipranavir		***Zafirlukast***
					Tripelennamine		***Zileuton***
							Zolpidem

[a]P450 isoform inhibitors presented in bold italics have been associated with drug–drug interactions of clinical relevance or with drug–drug interaction warnings that can require dosage adjustment.
Data from *Stockley's Drug Interactions: A Source Book of Interactions, Their Mechanisms, Clinical Importance and Management.* London and Chicago: Pharmaceutical Press, 2010.

TABLE 4.13 Substrates for the P450 Isoforms Catalyzing Their Metabolism

Acetaminophen	1A2, 2E1, 3A4, 2C9	Efavirenz	2B6
Albendazole	3A4, 1A2	Eletriptan	2C9
Alfentanil	3A4	Enalapril	3A4
Alprazolam	3A4	Encainide	2D6
Amiodarone	3A4, 2C9	Enflurane	2E1
Amitriptyline	1A2, 2C9, 2D6, 3A4, 2C19	Ergot alkaloids	3A4
Amlodipine	3A4	Erythromycin	3A4
Amphetamine	2D6	Esomeprazole	2C19
Aripipraole	2D6, 3A4	Estradiol	1A2
Anastrozole	3A4	Estrogens, oral	3A4
Astemizole	3A4	Ethanol	2E1
Atomoxetine	2D6	Ethinyl estradiol	3A4
Atorvastatin	3A4	Ethosuximide	3A4
Bepridil	3A4	Etodolac	2C9
Bisoprolol	2D6	Etoposide	3A4
Bosentan	2C9	Felodipine	3A4
Bupropion	2C9, 2B6, 2A6, 1A2	Fenfluramine	2D6
Busulfan	3A4	Fentanyl	2D6, 3A4
Caffeine	1A2	Fexofenadine	3A4
Cannabinoids	3A4	Finasteride	3A4
Carbamazepine	2C8, 3A4, 2B6	Flecainide	2D6
Carisoprodol	2C19	Fluconazole	3A4
Carvedilol	2C9, 2D6	Flurbiprofen	2C9
Celecoxib	2C9	Fluoxetine	2C9, 2D6, 2B6
Cerivastatin	3A4	Fluvastatin	2C8, 2C9
Cevimeline	2D6	Fluphenazine	2D6
Chlordiazepoxide	1A2	Flutamide	1A2, 3A4
Chloroquine	3A4	Fluvoxamine	1A2, 2D6
Chlorpromazine	2D6, 3A4	Formoterol	2C9, 2C19, 2D6
Chlorzoxazone	2E1	Galantamine	2D6
Cilostazol	2C19	Glimepiride	2C9
Cimetidine	3A4	Glipizide	2C9
Cisapride	3A4	Glyburide	2C9, 3A4
Citalopram	2C19, 3A4	Granisetron	3A4
Clarithromycin	3A4	Halofantrine	3A4
Clindamycin	3A4	Haloperidol	1A2, 2D6
Clomipramine	1A2, 2C9, 2C19, 2D6, 3A4	Halothane	2E1, 2C9
Clopidogrel	2C19, 2C9,1A2, 3A4/5	Hexobarbital	2C19, 2C9
Clonazepam	3A4	Hydrocodone	2D6, 3A4
Clozapine	1A2, 2D6, 2C19, 3A4	Hydrocortisone	2D6, 3A4
Cocaine	3A4	Ibuprofen	2C9
Codeine	2D6, 3A4	Ifosfamide	2B6, 3A4
Cyclobenzaprine	1A2, 2A6, 2D6, 3A4	Imipramine	1A2, 2C19, 2C9, 2D6, 3A4
Cyclophosphamide	2B6, 2C19, 3A4	Indinavir	2D6, 3A4
Cyclosporine	3A4	Indomethacin	2C9, 2C19
Dapsone	2C9, 3A4	Irbesartan	2C9
Delavirdine	3A4	Isoflurane	2E1, 2B6
Desipramine	1A2, 2C19, 2D6	Isoniazid	2E1
Desogestrel	2C9	Isotretinoin(retinoids)	1A2, 2C8, 3A4
Dexamethasone	3A4	Isradipine	3A4
Dexfenfluramine	2D6	Itraconazole	3A4
Dextromethorphan	2D6, 3A4	Ketamine	2B6, 2C9
Diazepam	1A2, 2C19, 2C9, 3A4	Ketoconazole	3A4
Diclofenac	2C8, 2C9	Labetalol	2D6
Diltiazem	3A4	Lansoprazole	2C19, 3A4
Diphenhydramine	2C9	Lidocaine	2D6, 3A4
Disopyramide	3A4	Leflunomide	1A2, 2C9, 2C19
Divalproex sodium	2C19	Losartan	2C9, 3A4
Docetaxel	2C8, 3A4	Lovastatin	3A4
Dolasetron	2D6, 3A4	Maprotiline	2D6
Donepezil	2D6, 3A4, 2C9	Meclobemide	2C19
Dorazolamide	2D6	Mefenamic acid	2C9
Doxepin	3A4	Mefloquine	3A4
Doxorubicin	2C9	Meloxicam	2C9
Dronabinol	2C9	Meperidine	2D6, 2B6

TABLE 4.13 Substrates for the P450 Isoforms Catalyzing Their Metabolism (*Continued*)

Mephenytoin	2C19
Mephobarbital	2C9, 2B6
Mestranol	2C9
Methadone	1A2, 2D6, 2B6
L-α-Methadol	2B6
Methamphetamine	2D6
Metoprolol	2D6
Mexiletine	1A6, 2D6, 2A6
Mibefradil	3A4
Miconazole	3A4
Midazolam	3A4
Mirtazapine	1A2, 2D6, 3A4
Modafinil	3A4
Montelukast	2C9
Morphine	2D6
Naproxen	1A2, 2C18, 2C9, 2A6
Nateglinide	2C9
Navelbine	3A4
Nefazodone	3A4
Nelfinavir	2B6, 3A4
Nevirapine	3A4
Nicardipine	3A4
Nicotine	2A6, 2B6, 2A13
Nifedipine	3A4/5
Nilutamide	2C19
Nimodipine	3A4
Nisoldpine	3A4
Nitrendipine	3A4
Nortriptyline	1A2, 2D6
Olanzapine	1A2, 2D6, 3A4
Omeprazole	2C19, 2C9, 3A4
Ondansetron	1A2, 2D6, 2E1, 3A4
Oral contraceptives	3A4
Oxycodone	2D6
Paclitaxel	2C8, 3A4
Pantoprazole	2C19
Paroxetine	2D6
Perphenazine	2D6
Phenacetin	1A2
Phenformin	2D6
Phenol	2E1
Phenobarbital	2B6, 2C9
Phenytoin	3A4
Pimozide	2D6, 3A4
Pindolol	2C8, 3A4
Pioglitazone	2C18, 2C9
Piroxicam	2C18, 2C9
Prasugrel	3A4, 2B6, 2C9
Pravastatin	3A4
Praziqantel	2B6, 3A4
Prednisone	3A4
Progesterone	3A4, 2C19
Proguanil	2C18, 2C19
Propafenone	1A2, 2D6, 3A4
Propofol	2B6, 2C9
Propoxyphene	2D6
Propranolol	1A2, 2C18, 2C19, 2D6
Quetiapine	3A4
Quinidine	3A4
Quinine	3A4
Rabeprazole	2C19
Rapaglinide	2C8
Retinoic acid	2C8
Rifabutin	3A4
Rifampin	3A4
Riluzole	1A2
Risperidone	2D6, 3A4
Ritonavir	2A6, 2C19/9, 2D6, 2E1, 3A4
Ropinirole	1A2
Ropivacaine	1A2, 2D6
Rosiglitazone	2C8, 2C9
Rosuvasatain	2C8, 2C9
Salmeterol	3A4
Saquinavir	3A4
Selegiline	2D6, 2B6, 2A6
Sertindole	2D6
Sertraline	2D6, 2C19, 3A4, 2B6
Sevoflurane	2E1
Sibutramine	2B6
Sildenafil	2C9, 3A4
Simvastatin	3A4
Sufentanil	3A4
Sulfamethoxazole	2C9
Suprofen	2C9
Tacrine	1A2, 2A6
Tacrolimus	3A4
Tamoxifen	1A2, 2A6, 2B6, 2D6, 2E1, 3A4
Terfenadine	3A4
Testosterone	3A4
Δ^9-THC	2C9
Theophylline	1A2, 2E1, 3A4
Thiabendazole	1A2
Thioridazine	2C19, 2D6
Tiagabine	3A4
Timolol	2D6
Tolbutamide	2C8,2C9, 2C19
Tolteridine	2D6, 2C9
Torsemide	2C9
Tramadol	2D6
Trazodone	2D6
Valproic acid	2C9, 2A6, 2B6
Valdecoxib	2C9
Vardenafil	3A4
Venlafaxine	2D6
Verapamil	1A2, 3A4, 2C8
Vinblastine	3A4
Vinca alkaloids	3A4
Vincristine	3A4
Voriconazole	2C9
Warfarin	2C18, 2C9
R-warfarin	1A2
S-warfarin	2C9, 2C18
Yohimbine	2D6
Zafirlukast	2C9
Zaleplon	3A4
Zileuton	1A2, 2C9, 3A4
Zolpidem	3A4
Zoplicone	3A4

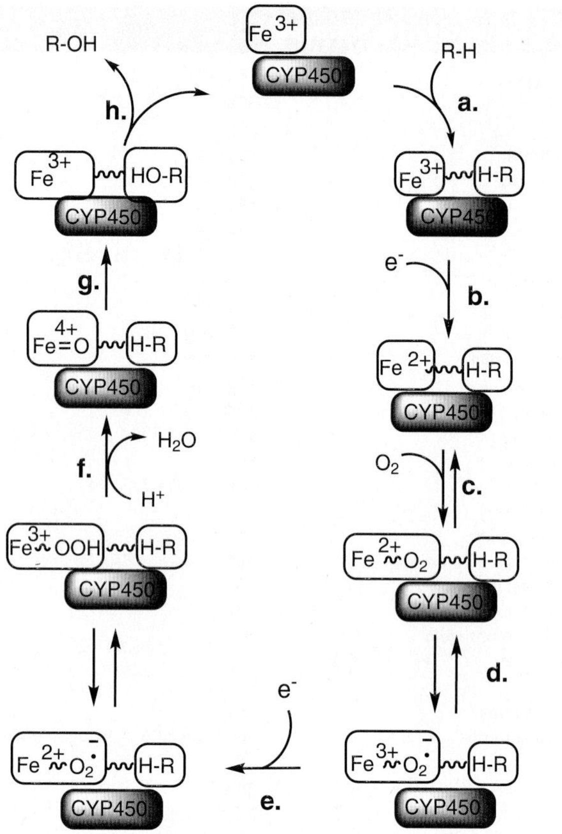

FIGURE 4.4 Cyclic mechanism for P450. The substrate is RH, and the valence state of the heme iron in P450 is indicated.

complex dissociates and is aborted (uncoupled) from subsequent substrate hydroxylation at this step by xenobiotics, which can cause release of the superoxide anion, which decomposes to hydrogen peroxide and dioxygen, with regeneration of the starting point of the cycle, the Fe^{+3}–P450 complex (step A).

Step F. The peroxy–Fe^{+3}–P450 complex undergoes heterolytic cleavage of peroxide anion to form water and a highly electrophilic perferryl oxenoid intermediate (Fe^{+5}=O) or a ferryl (Fe^{+4}=O) oxygen–cysteine–porphyrin resonance-stabilized complex (the more favorable complex). The ferryl oxenoid species represents the catalytically active oxygenation species.

Step G. Abstraction of a hydrogen atom from the substrate by the ferryl oxenoid species produces a carbon-centered radical–ferryl-hydroxide complex; radical addition to a π-bond; or electron abstraction from a heteroatom to form a heteroatom-centered radical–cation-ferryl intermediate.

Step H. Subsequent radical recombination (oxygen rebound) or electron transfer (deprotonation) yields the hydroxylated product and regeneration of the Fe^{+3}–P450 complex (step A).

Until the final step, the oxidizable substrate has been an inactive spectator in the chemical events of oxygen activation. None of the preceding oxygenated intermediates has been sufficiently reactive to abstract hydrogen from the substrate. The ferryl–iron oxenoid complex (step G), however, is a competent hydrogen abstractor, even for relatively inert terminal methyl groups on hydrocarbon chains. Thus, this is evidence that the oxidant exhibits regioselectivity in its choice of hydrogen atoms, balancing stability of the resulting carbon radical with stereochemical constraints (Fig. 4.5). Because the inert aliphatic region of the substrate has been converted to a highly reactive radical, the process is described as substrate activation. Various studies have shown that hydroxylation or alkene formation proceeds not by a direct one-step insertion of an oxygen atom but rather by a two-step two-electron process that involves radical or cationic substrate intermediates with subsequent hydroxyl radical recombination (oxygen rebound) to form products (Fig. 4.6) (28).

Despite considerable experimental evidence, the proposed mechanism and intermediates of the monooxygenation of unsaturated substrates (alkenes, alkynes, and aromatics) remain controversial (19,20,29–31). The proposed mechanism for the oxidation of π-bonds in alkenes is a stepwise sequence of one-electron transfers between the radical complex and the ferryl oxygen intermediate [Fe^{+4}=O], leading to alkene oxidation (Fig. 4.6). After the initial formation of an unsaturated P450 π-complex, the one-electron transfer either yields a radical σ-complex, which can either collapse to an arene or to an alkene epoxide (steps A or D, Fig. 4.6); undergoes a 1,2-group migration to form a carbonyl product (steps A and B, Fig. 4.6); or produces a vinyl hydroxylated product (step C, Fig. 4.6)

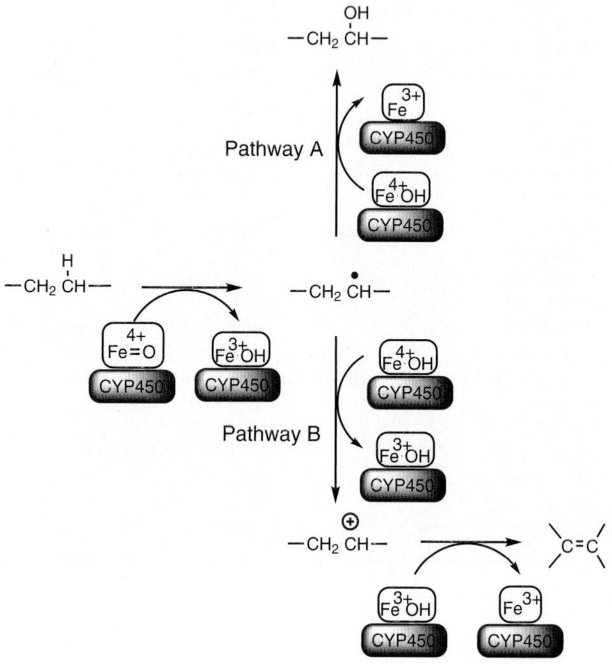

FIGURE 4.5 Proposed mechanisms for the hydroxylation and dehydrogenation of alkanes.

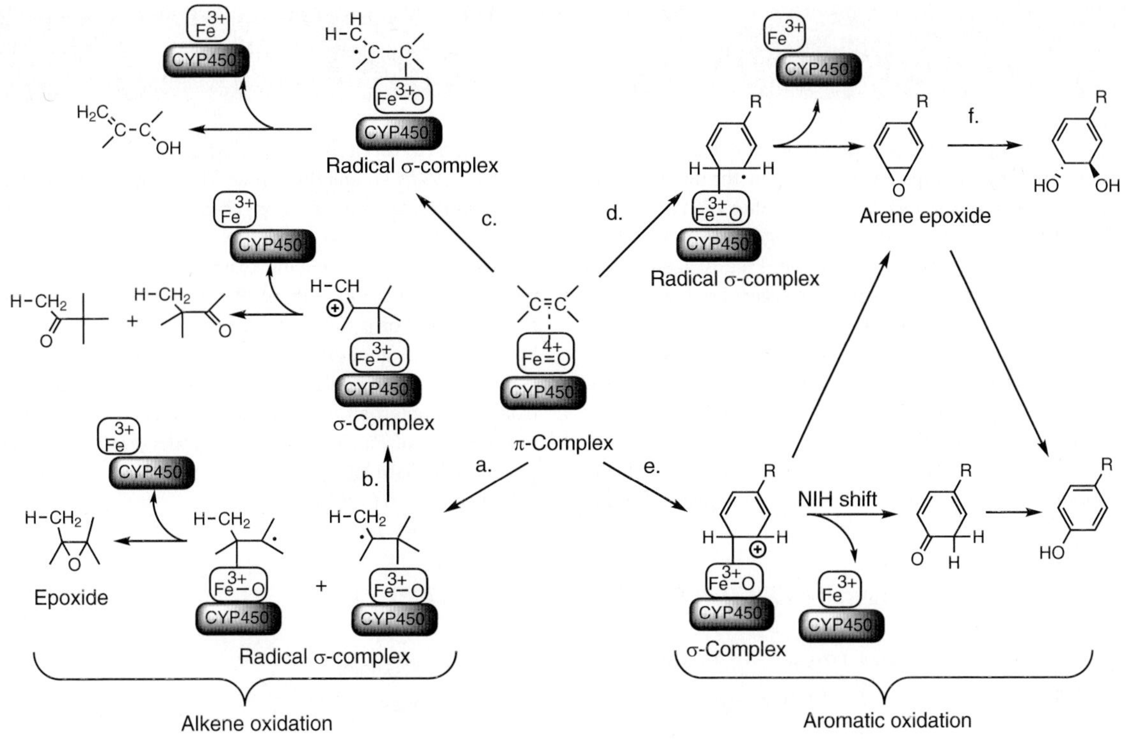

FIGURE 4.6 Proposed mechanisms for the oxidation of alkene and aromatic compounds.

or a σ-complex, which can break down to a phenol (step E, Fig. 4.6). The presence of a hydroxyl radical in the porphyrin ring allows some substrate radicals to covalently bond by *N*-alkylation of a pyrrole nitrogen rather than recombination with $(Fe–OH)^{+3}$ radical. This deviation from the normal course of reaction explains the suicide inhibition exhibited by some xenobiotics, such as the oral contraceptives, erythromycin, and paroxetine (32,33).

In the case of aromatic oxidations (Fig. 4.6), following the initial formation of an arene P450 π-complex, one-electron transfer yields either a π-complex or a radical σ-complex. The radical σ-complex can collapse to the arene epoxide (Fig. 4.6, step D), or the π-complex can proceed to a σ-complex followed by an NIH shift (1,2-group migration) to a phenolic product (Fig. 4.6, step E). Arene oxides are highly unstable entities and rearrange (NIH shift) nonenzymatically to phenols or hydrolyze enzymatically with epoxide hydrolase to 1,2-dihydrodiols (*trans* configuration) (Fig. 4.6, step F), which subsequently are dehydrogenated to 1,2-diphenols. The oxidation of aromatic compounds can be highly specific to individual P450 isoforms, suggesting that substrate binding and orientation at the active site can dominate the mechanism of oxidative catalysis.

The exact mechanism of oxidative *N*-, *O*-, and *S*-dealkylations is unclear. There are two competing mechanisms: single electron transfer or hydrogen atom abstraction (Fig. 4.7). Heteroatom-containing substrates most commonly undergo hydroxylation adjacent (α) to the heteroatom, as compared to other positions. Reactions of this type include *N*-, *O*-, and *S*-dealkylations, as well as dehydrohalogenations and oxidative deamination (dealkylation) reactions. The single electron transfer pathway is abstraction of an electron from the heteroatom to produce a radical cation, followed by the loss of the α-proton from the more labile α-carbon to generate a carbon radical that can recombine with the ferric-bound hydroxyl radical intermediate (oxygen rebound) to generate an unstable geminal hydroxy heteroatom-substituted intermediate (e.g., carbinolamine, halohydrin, hemiacetal, hemiketal, or hemithioketal) that breaks down, releasing the heteroatom and

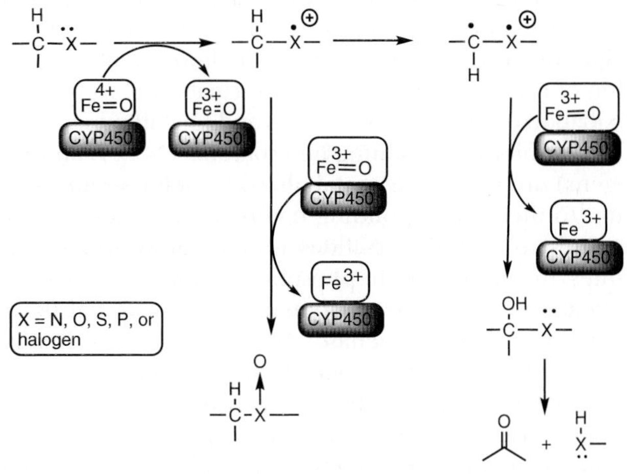

FIGURE 4.7 Proposed mechanism for heteroatom-compound oxidation, dealkylation and dehalogenation.

OXYGEN ACTIVATION

Elemental oxygen (dioxygen) is a relatively unreactive form of oxygen that exists as an unpaired diradical in the triplet form. Alternatively, singlet oxygen is a form of dioxygen in which the diradical electrons are paired. In the singlet form, oxygen is too reactive for biologic systems to handle. Free oxygen atoms (oxenes), which are formed by splitting dioxygen, are highly reactive but are not known to exist in biochemical processes. The solution to the problem of a reactive form of oxygen lies in the suggestion that the reduction of dioxygen occurs to a reactive oxygen species (ROS), such as superoxide radical anion, peroxide, hydroxyl radical, or oxygen atom.

Any of these ROS could oxidize an organic substrate with the net insertion of an oxygen atom. In each case, reductive reactions are required for activation of dioxygen to one of the ROS from electrons supplied by NADPH. The generation of a carbon-centered radical and a hydroxyl radical with triplet oxygen atom has been found to be relevant to a number of enzymatic and chemical reactions involving oxenoids (oxygen rebound mechanism) (28). The function of P450 monooxygenases is mostly hydroxylation of a substrate. A reactive radical-like iron oxenoid intermediate is generated that is reactive enough to split aliphatic C-H bonds, add to bonds α to heteroatoms, or remove single electrons from heteroatoms to produce radical-cations. Although the mechanisms of P450 are not fully understood, the reactive oxygen intermediate has not been isolated or even spectroscopically observed.

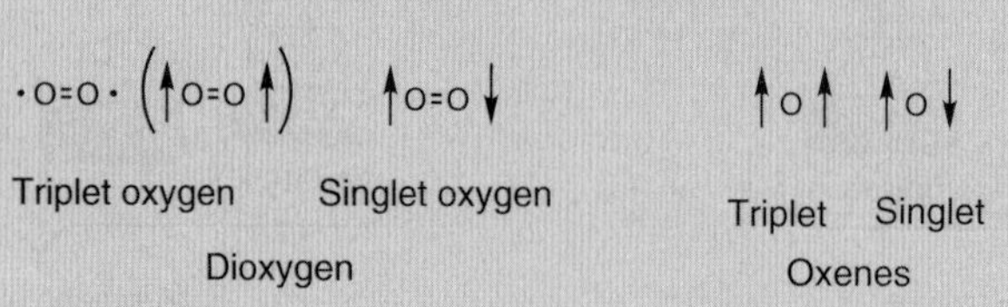

$O_2 + e^- \longrightarrow$:O=O· (⊖)	Superoxide radical anion	Reactive oxygen species (ROS)
$O_2 + 2e^- + 2H^+ \longrightarrow H_2O_2$	Peroxide	
$O_2 + 2e^- + 2H^+ \longrightarrow 2\,HO\cdot + H_2O$	Hydroxyl radical	
$O_2 + 2e^- + 2H^+ \longrightarrow O + H_2O$	Oxygen atom	

forming a carbonyl compound (29–31). The resultant carbon radical is stabilized by the heteroatom. This pathway is feasible for nitrogen, which is easily oxidized and electron rich. However, if the recombination reaction with the ferric-bound hydroxyl radical intermediate (oxygen rebound) is faster than the deprotonation of the α-proton from the adjacent α-carbon, the oxidation will simply result in oxidation of the heteroatom, as in the formation of *N*-oxides or oxidation of sulfides to sulfoxides and/or sulfones.

Xenobiotics containing heteroatoms (N, S, P, and halogens) are frequently metabolized by heteroatom oxidation to their corresponding heteroatom oxides (tertiary amines to *N*-oxides, sulfides to sulfoxides and/or sulfones, or phosphines to phosphine oxides). Heteroatom oxidation can also be attributed to a microsomal flavin-containing monooxygenase. As is the case with heteroatom α-hydroxylation, one-electron oxidation of the heteroatom occurs as the first step to form the heteroatom ferric-hydroxide radical intermediate, which collapses to generate the heteroatom oxide. This reaction is favored by the absence of α-hydrogens and by the stability of the heteroatom radical-cation (29–31).

All known oxidative reactions catalyzed by P450 monooxygenases can be described in the context of a mechanistic scheme that involves the ability of a high-valent iron oxenoid species to bring about the stepwise one-electron oxidation through the abstraction of hydrogen atoms, abstraction of electrons from heteroatoms, or addition to π-bonds. A series of radical recombination reactions completes the oxidation process.

Induction and Inhibition of Cytochrome P450 Isoforms

Induction

Many of the enzymes involved in drug metabolism can be upregulated by exposure to drugs and environmental chemicals or by other coingested/inhaled compounds leading to increased rates of metabolism, thereby altering their pharmacologic and toxicologic effects (34–36). Prolonged administration of a drug or xenobiotic can enhance the metabolism of itself and a wide variety of other compounds. This phenomenon is known as enzyme induction, a dose-dependent phenomenon.

Drugs and xenobiotics exert this effect by inducing transcription of P450 mRNA and synthesis of xenobiotic-metabolizing enzymes in the smooth ER of the liver and other extrahepatic tissues (34,35). Enzyme induction is an adaptive response associated with increases in liver weight, induction of gene expression, and morphologic changes in hepatocytes. Induction is the process whereby the rate of enzyme synthesis is increased relative to the rate of enzyme synthesis in the uninduced organism. In many older studies of mammalian systems, the term "induction" was inferred from the increase in enzyme activity, but the amount of enzyme protein had not been determined. Enzyme induction is important to interpret the results of chronic toxicities, mutagenicities, or carcinogenesis and to explain certain unexpected drug–drug interactions in patients. Enzyme inducers trigger pathways involving the constitutive androstane receptor (CAR), PPAR, AhR, and pregnane X receptor (PXR) (34). CAR is a member of the nuclear receptor superfamily and, along with PXR, upregulates the expression of P450 proteins responsible for the metabolism and excretion of these xenobiotics, and thus is a key regulator of xenobiotic CYP450 metabolism.

Many drugs and xenobiotics stimulate the upregulation of P450 isoforms, as shown in Table 4.14. These stimulators have nothing in common so far as their pharmacologic activities or chemical structures are concerned, but they are all metabolized by one or more of the P450 isoforms. Most are lipid soluble at physiologic pH. PAHs in cigarette smoke, xanthines and flavones in foods, halogenated hydrocarbons in insecticides, polychlorinated biphenyls, and food additives are but a few of the environmental chemicals that alter the activities of P450 enzymes (37).

Enzyme induction, which can last as long as 1 to 3 weeks as drug blood levels decrease, can alter the pharmacokinetics and pharmacodynamics of a drug, with clinical implications for the therapeutic actions of the drug as well as increased potential for drug–drug interactions. As a result of induction, a drug can be metabolized more rapidly to metabolites that are more potent, more toxic, or less active than the parent drug. Induction can also enhance the activation of procarcinogens or promutagens. Not all inducing agents enhance their own metabolism; for example, phenytoin induces CYP3A4 but is hydroxylated by CYP2C9. Some of the more common enzyme inducers of P450 subfamilies, which can also be substrates for the same P450 isoforms, include phenobarbital (CYP2B6, CYP2C, and CYP3A4), rifampicin (CYP3A4), and cigarette smoke (CYP1A1/2) (Table 4.14). The broad range of drugs metabolized by these CYP450 subfamilies (Table 4.13) and that are also affected by these enzyme inducers raises the issue of clinically significant drug–drug interactions and their clinical implications. Examples of a clinically significant P450 drug–drug interaction and an herbal drug–drug interaction are rifampin and oral contraceptives and St. John's wort and oral contraceptives, respectively. Both rifampin and St. John's wort induce the expression of CYP3A4, thereby reducing the serum levels of the oral contraceptive due to increased oxidative metabolism of the oral contraceptives by CYP3A4 to form less active metabolites, thereby increasing the risk for pregnancy. Drugs poorly metabolized by P450 enzymes are less affected by enzyme induction. Inducers of P450 isoforms also stimulate oxidative metabolism and synthesis of endogenous substances: for example, the hydroxylation of androgens, estrogens, progestational steroids (synthetic oral contraceptives), glucocorticoids, vitamin D, and bilirubin, which decreases their biologic activity. These enzyme inducers might also be implicated in deficiencies associated with these steroids. For example, the induction of C-2 hydroxylation of estradiol and synthetic estrogens by phenobarbital,

TABLE 4.14 Drugs That Induce the Expression of P450 Isoforms[a]

Amprenavir	3A4	4-Methylpyrazole	2E1
Aprepitant	2C9	Modafinil	1A2, 2B6, 3A4
Barbiturates	3A4, 2C9, 2C19, 2B6	Nevirapine	3A4, 2B6
Carbamazepine	1A2, 3A4, 2C8, 2C9, 2D6, 2B6	Norethindrone	2C19
Charbroiled meats	1A1/2,	Omeprazole	1A1/2, 3A4
Cigarette smoke	1A1/2	Oxcarbazepine	3A4
Clotrimazole	1A1/2, 3A4	***Phenobarbital***	3A4, 2C, 2B6, 2D6, 1A2
Ethanol	2D6, 2E1	***Phenytoin***	3A4, 1A2, 2B6, 2C8, 2C19, 2D6
Efavirenz	3A4	Primidone	3A4, 2C9, 1A2, 2B6, 2D6
Erythromycin	3A4	Psoralen	1A1/2
Glucocorticoids	3A4, 2A6	***Ethosuximide***	3A4
(Dexamethasone, prednisone)	2C19	Polycyclic aromatic hydrocarbons	1A1/2
Griseofulvin	3A4	Rifampin	2C8, 2C9,2C19, 2D6, 3A4, 2B6
Isoniazid	2E1	Rifampicin	2C8
Lansoprazole	1A1/2, 3A4	Rifabutin	2C8, 3A4
Mephenytoin	2B6	Rifapentine	3A4
		Ritonavir	2D6, 3A4
		St. John's Wort	1A2, 2C9, 3A4
		Troglitazone	3A4
		Topiramate	3A4

[a]Drugs in bold italic have been reported to cause drug–drug interactions.

dexamethasone, or cigarette smoking in women results in the increased formation of the principal and less active metabolite of these estrogenic substances, reducing their effectiveness (38). Thus, cigarette smoking in premenopausal women could result in an estrogen deficiency, increasing the risks of osteoporosis and early menopause. Postmenopausal women who smoke and take estrogen replacement therapy can lose the effectiveness of the estrogen.

In addition to enhancing metabolism of other drugs, many compounds, when chronically administered, stimulate their own metabolism, thereby decreasing their therapeutic activities and producing a state of apparent tolerance. This self-induction can explain some of the changes in drug toxicity observed during prolonged treatments. The duration of the sedative action of phenobarbital, for example, becomes shorter with repeated doses and can be explained in part on the basis of increased metabolism.

The time course of induction varies with different inducing agents and with different P450 isoforms. CYP1A induction always involves AhR. Increased transcription of P450 mRNA has been detected as early as 1 hour after administration of phenobarbital, with maximum induction occurring after 48 to 72 hours. After administration of PAH such as 3-methylcholanthrene and benzo[a]pyrene, maximum induction of the CYP1A subfamily is reached within 24 hours. Less potent inducers of hepatic drug metabolism can take as long as 6 to 10 days to produce maximum induction (34,35). Exposures to a variety of different xenobiotics can increase the hepatic content of specific isoforms of P450 (34–36). Therefore, the process of enzyme induction involves the adaptive increase in the content of specific enzymes in response to the enzyme-inducing agent. Other inducible metabolizing enzymes include uridine diphosphate (UDP)–glucuronosyl transferase and glutathione transferase.

Specific Inducers

Phenobarbital and Rifampin Phenobarbital and rifampin are probably the enzyme inducers that have been studied most extensively. These drugs could alter the pharmacokinetics and pharmacodynamics of many concurrently administered drugs listed in Tables 4.8 (CYP2C) and 4.11 (CYP3A4), which raises the issue of clinically significant drug–drug interactions.

Cigarette Smoke Cigarette smoke has been shown to increase the hydrocarbon-inducible isoforms CYP1A1 and CYP1A2 in the lungs, liver, small intestine, and placenta of cigarette smokers. A decrease in the pharmacologic action and stimulation of the CYP1A1/2 metabolism of several drugs is the end result. Cigarette smoking has been reported to lower blood levels of drugs metabolized by CYP1A1/2, including theophylline, imipramine, estradiol, pentazocine, and propoxyphene; to decrease the urinary excretion of nicotine; and to decrease drowsiness caused by chlorpromazine, diazepam, and chlordiazepoxide.

Dietary Substances A diet containing Brussels sprouts, cabbage, and cauliflower (cruciferous vegetables) was found to stimulate P450 activity in rat intestine (39). It was subsequently determined that indole-3-carbinol in the plants is released from the breakdown of glucobrassicin, a thioglucoside also called a glucosinolate, during gastrointestinal digestion, which was responsible for the enzyme induction. Other examples of chemicals found naturally in foods that are released during digestion that enhance metabolism in animals are flavones, safrole, eucalyptol, xanthines, β-ionone, and organic peroxides. Volatile oils in soft woods (e.g., cedar) have been shown to be enzyme inducers.

Alcohol Sober alcoholics show an increase in CYP2E1 enzyme activity, leading to more rapid clearance of drugs and xenobiotics that are substrates for this isoform from the body. As discussed previously, hepatic CYP2E1 oxidizes ethanol, and chronic ethanol intake increases the activity of CYP2E1 through enzyme induction (24). When intoxicated, alcoholics are more susceptible to the actions of various drugs due to inhibition of drug metabolism as a result of an excessive quantity of alcohol in the liver and an additive or synergistic effect in the central nervous system. The basis for this inhibition is unknown. Furthermore, moderate ethanol consumption reduces the clearance of some drugs, presumably due to competition between ethanol and the other drugs for hepatic biotransformation. The changes in drug metabolism in alcoholics can also be attributed to other factors, such as malnutrition, other drugs, and the trace chemicals that are sources of flavors and odors of particular alcoholic beverages. Heavy drinkers metabolize phenobarbital, tolbutamide, and phenytoin more rapidly than nonalcoholics, which can be clinically important when this leads to problems in adjusting drug therapies for alcoholics.

Inhibition

Another method to alter in vivo effects of xenobiotics metabolized by P450s is the use of inhibitors (Table 4.12). The P450 inhibitors can be divided into three categories according to their mechanisms of action: reversible inhibition, metabolite intermediate complexation of P450, or mechanism-based inactivation of P450 (36,40,41). The polysubstrate nature of P450 is responsible for the large number of documented interactions associated with the inhibition of drug oxidation and drug biotransformation.

Reversible Inhibition Reversible inhibition of P450 is the result of reversible interactions at the heme–iron active center of P450, the lipophilic sites on the apoprotein, or both. The interaction occurs before the oxidation steps of the catalytic cycle, and the effects dissipate quickly when the inhibitor is discontinued. The most effective reversible inhibitors are those that interact strongly with both the apoprotein and the heme iron. It is widely accepted that inhibition has an important impact on the oxidative metabolism and pharmacokinetics of drugs that have a metabolism that cosegregates with that of an inhibitor (Tables 4.4 and 4.8 to 4.11) (40,41). Drugs interacting reversibly with P450 include the fluoroquinolone antimicrobials, cimetidine, the azole antifungals, quinidine (specific for CYP2D isoforms), and diltiazem. Cimetidine is the only H_2 antagonist that inhibits P450 by interacting directly with the P450 heme–iron through one of its imidazole ring nitrogen atoms. Cimetidine is not a universal inhibitor of P450 oxidative metabolism, but it does bind differentially to several P450 isoforms (Table 4.12). Cimetidine inhibits the oxidation of theophylline (CYP1A2), chlordiazepoxide (CYP3A4), diazepam (CYP2C), propranolol (CYP2C18/19 and CYP2D6), warfarin (CYP2C9), and antipyrine (CYP1A2), but not that of ibuprofen (CYP2C9), tolbutamide (CYP2C8/9), mexiletine (CYP2D6), the 6-hydroxylation of steroids (CYP3A4/5), and carbamazepine (CYP3A4/5) (36). The imidazole-based azole antifungals are potent inhibitors of CYP3A4 and of the P450-mediated biosynthesis of endogenous steroid hormones. The azole antifungals exert their fungiostatic effects through inhibition of fungal P450, inhibiting the oxidative biosynthesis of lanosterol to ergosterol, thereby affecting the integrity and permeability of the fungal membranes.

P450 Complexation Inhibition Noninhibitory alkylamine drugs have the ability to undergo P450-mediated oxidation to nitrosoalkane metabolites (Fig. 4.8), which have high affinities to form stable complexes with the reduced (ferrous) heme-P450 intermediates of the CYP2B, CYP2C, and CYP3A subfamilies. This process is termed "metabolite intermediate complexation" (40,41). Thus the P450 isoform is unavailable for further oxidation, and synthesis of the new enzyme is required to restore P450 activity. The process relies on at least one cycle of the P450 catalytic cycle to generate the required heme intermediate. The macrolide antibiotics troleandomycin, erythromycin, and clarithromycin, as well as their analogues, are selective inhibitors of CYP3A4 that are capable of inducing expression of hepatic and extrahepatic CYP3A4 mRNA and of induction of their own biotransformation into nitrosoalkane metabolites. The clinical significance of this inhibition with CYP3A4 is the long-lived impairment of metabolism of a large number of coadministered substrates of this isoform, and the potential for drug–drug interactions and time-dependent nonlinearities in their pharmacokinetics upon long-term administration

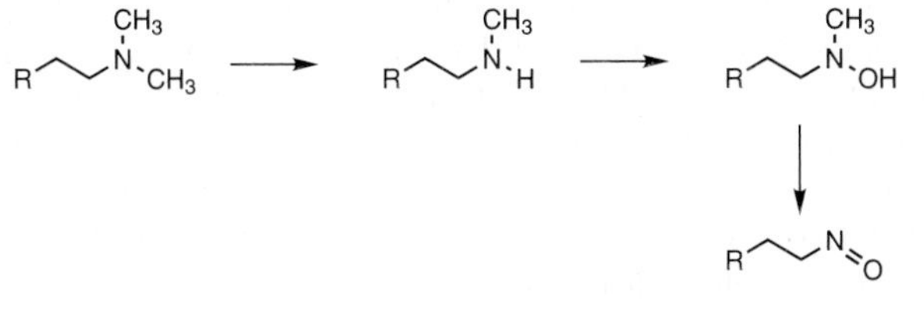

FIGURE 4.8 Sequence of oxidation of dialkylamine to nitroso metabolite intermediate.

(Tables 4.11 and 4.12). For macrolides to be so metabolized, they must possess an unhindered dimethylamino sugar, and the compound itself must be lipophilic. Other alkylamine-based drugs that demonstrate this type of inhibition include orphenadrine (antiparkinson drug), the antiprogestin mifepristone (CYP3A4), and SKF525A (the original P450 inhibitor). Methylenedioxyphenyl compounds (i.e., the insecticide synergist piperonyl butoxide and the flavoring agent isosafrole) generate metabolite intermediates that form stable complexes with both the ferric and ferrous state of P450.

Mechanism-based Inhibition Certain drugs that are not inhibitors of P450 contain functional groups that, when oxidized by P450, generate metabolites that irreversibly bind to the enzyme. This process is termed "mechanism-based inhibition" ("suicide inhibition") and requires at least one catalytic P450 cycle either during or subsequent to the oxygen-transfer step, when the drug is activated to the inhibitory species. Alkenes and alkynes were the first functionalities found to inactivate P450 by generation of a radical intermediate that alkylates the heme structure (see the section on alkene and alkyne hydroxylation) (32,33,40,41). Iron is lost from the heme, and abnormal *N*-alkylated porphyrins are produced. Drugs that are mechanism-based inhibitors of P450 include the 17α-acetylenic estrogen, 17α-ethinyl estradiol, the 17α-acetylenic progestin, norethindrone (norethisterone), and their radical intermediates that *N*-alkylate the heme of CYP3A4 (see Fig. 4.11 and later discussion); chloramphenicol and its oxidative dechlorinated acyl metabolite that alkylates P450 apoprotein; cyclophosphamide and its generated acrolein and phosphoramide mustard that alkylates CYP2B6 apoprotein; spironolactone and its 7-thio metabolite that alkylates heme; 8-methoxypsoralen (a furocoumarin) and its epoxide metabolite that alkylates the P450 apoprotein of CYP2A6; nicotine (CYP1A6 and CYP1A13 isoforms); isoniazid that alkylates CYP1A2, CYP2A6, CYP2C19, and CYP3A4 isoforms; 21-halosteroids; halocarbons; and secobarbital. The selectivity of P450 isoform destruction by several of these inhibitors indicates involvement of this isoform in its bioactivation of such drugs.

Oxidations Catalyzed by Cytochrome P450 Isoforms

Aliphatic and Alicyclic Hydroxylations The accepted mechanism of hydroxylation of alkane C-H bonds is shown in Figure 4.6 and has been reviewed in detail elsewhere (29–31). The principal metabolic pathway of the methyl group is oxidation to the hydroxymethyl derivative followed by P450 oxidation to the carboxylic acid (e.g., tolbutamide) (Fig. 4.9). On the other hand, some methyl groups are oxidized only to the hydroxymethyl derivative, without further oxidation to the acid. Where there are several equivalent methyl groups, as a rule only one methyl group is oxidized. In the case of aromatic methyl groups, the para methyl is the most vulnerable because it is less sterically hindered.

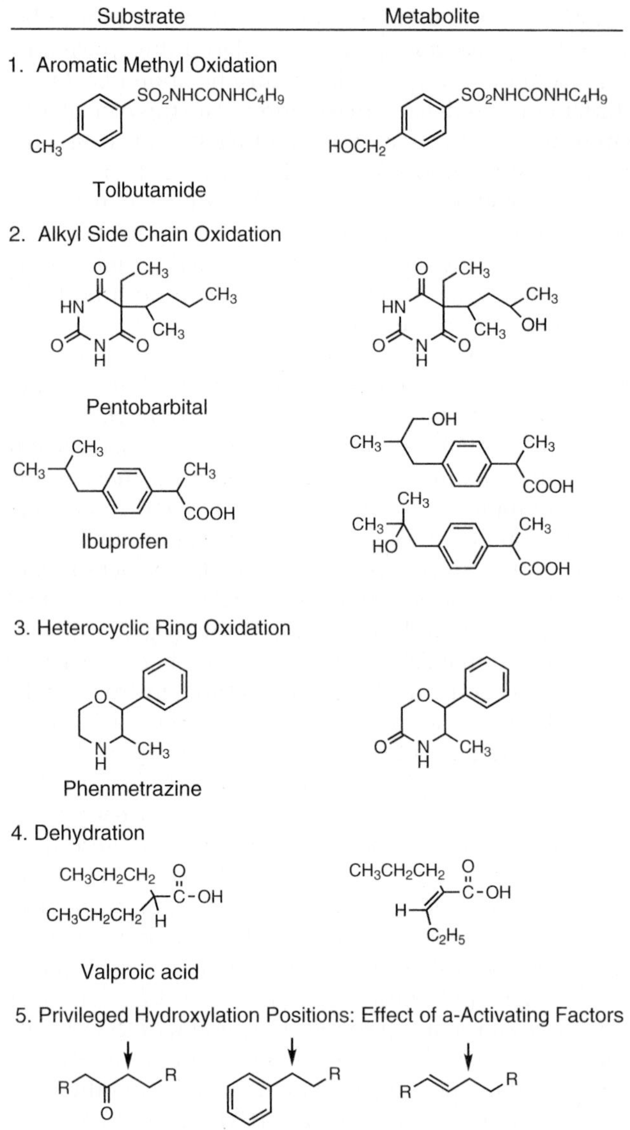

FIGURE 4.9 Examples of oxidative metabolism of aliphatic and alicyclic hydrocarbons catalyzed by CY P450.

Alkyl side chains are often hydroxylated on the terminal or penultimate carbon atoms (e.g., pentobarbital) (Fig. 4.9). The isopropyl group is an interesting side chain that is hydroxylated at the secondary carbon and at either of the equivalent methyl groups (e.g., ibuprofen) (Fig. 4.9). Hydroxylation of alkyl side chains attached to an aromatic ring does not follow the general rules for alkyl side chains, because the aromatic ring activates the α-position of hydroxylation (Fig. 4.9). In general, oxidation occurs preferentially on the benzylic methylene group and, to a lesser extent, at other positions on the side chain.

The methylene groups of an alicycle are readily hydroxylated, usually at the least hindered position, or at an activated position—for example, α to a carbonyl (cyclohexanone), α to a double bond (cyclohexene), or α to a phenyl ring (tetralin). The products of hydroxylation often show regioselectivity and stereoisomerism. Nonaromatic heterocycles normally undergo oxidation at the α-carbon adjacent to the heteroatom (e.g., phenmetrazine) (Fig. 4.9).

In addition to hydroxylation reactions, P450s can catalyze the dehydrogenation of an alkane to an alkene (olefin). The reaction is thought to involve formation of a carbon radical and electron transfer to the ferryl complex of P450, which produces a carbocation that is deprotonated to a dehydrogenated product alkene (Fig. 4.5) (29–31). An example of the ability of P450 to function as both a dehydrogenase and a monooxygenase has been demonstrated with the antiseizure drug valproic acid. Whereas the major metabolic products in humans are formed by β-oxidation and acyl glucuronidation, several alkenes are also formed, including (*E*)2-ene isomer (Fig. 4.9) (42). Presumably, the CYP3A subfamily catalyzes these reactions. The factors that determine whether P450 catalyzes hydroxylation (oxygen rebound/recombination) or dehydrogenation (electron transfer) remain unknown, but hydroxylation is usually favored. In some instances, the product of dehydrogenation can be the primary product (i.e., 6,7-dehydrogenation of testosterone).

Alkene and Alkyne Hydroxylation The oxidation of alkenes yields primarily epoxides and a series of products derived from 1,2-migration (see previous discussion) (Fig. 4.6). The stereochemical configuration of the alkene is retained during epoxidation. The epoxides can differ in reactivity. Those that are highly reactive either undergo pH-catalyzed hydrolyses to excretable vicinal dihydrodiols or covalent reactions (alkylation) with macromolecules such as proteins or nucleic acids, which lead to tissue necrosis or carcinogenicity. Moreover, the ubiquitous epoxide hydrolase can catalyze the rapid hydrolysis of epoxides to nontoxic vicinal dihydrodiols. Several drugs (carbamazepine, cyproheptadine, and protriptyline), however, were found to form stable epoxides at the 10,11-position during biotransformation (Fig. 4.10). The fact that these epoxides could be detected in the urine indicates that these oxides are not particularly reactive and should not readily react covalently with macromolecules.

The epoxidation of terminal alkenes is accompanied by the mechanism-based ("suicide") *N*-alkylation of the heme–porphyrin ring. If the π-complex attaches to the alkene at the internal carbon, the terminal carbon of the double bond can irreversibly *N*-alkylate the pyrrole nitrogen of the porphyrin ring (32,33). The heme adduct formation is observed mostly with monosubstituted, unconjugated alkenes (i.e., 17α-ethylenic steroids and 4-ene metabolite of valproic acid).

In addition to the formation of epoxides, heme adducts, and hydroxylated products, carbonyl products are also created. These latter products result from the migration of atoms to adjacent carbons (i.e., 1,2-group migration). For example, during the P450-catalyzed oxidation of trichloroethylene, a 1,2-shift of chloride occurs to yield chloral (Fig. 4.10).

Like the alkenes, alkynes (acetylenes) are more readily oxidized, but usually faster. Depending on which of the

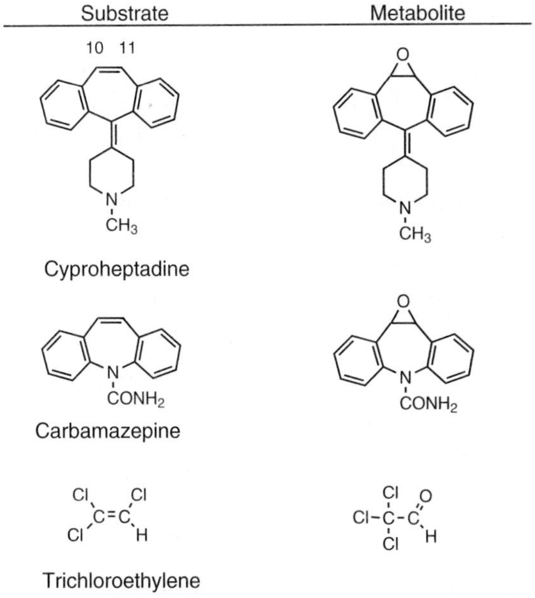

FIGURE 4.10 Examples of oxidative metabolism of alkenes catalyzed by P450.

two alkyne carbons are attacked, different products are obtained (32,33). If attachment of P450 occurs on the terminal alkyne carbon, a hydrogen atom migrates, forming a ketene intermediate that readily hydrolyzes with water to form an acid or that alkylates nucleophilic protein side chains (i.e., lysinyl or cysteinyl) to form a protein adduct (Fig. 4.11). The effect of attaching the ferryl oxygen at the internal alkenyl carbon is *N*-alkylation of a pyrrole nitrogen in the porphyrin ring by the terminal acetylene carbon, with the formation of a keto heme adduct (Fig. 4.11). The latter mechanism has been proposed for the irreversible inactivation of CYP3A4 with 17α-alkenyl steroids (i.e., 17α-ethinyl estradiol).

Aromatic Hydroxylation The metabolic oxidation of aromatic carbon atoms by P450 depends on both the isoform catalyzing the oxidation and the oxidation potential of the aromatic compound. The products are typically phenolic products, and the position of hydroxylation can be activated/deactivated by the type of substituents on the ring, according to the theories of aromatic electrophilic substitution (Fig. 4.12). For example, electron-donating substituents enhance *o*- and *p*-hydroxylation, whereas electron-withdrawing substituents reduce or prevent *o*- or *p*-hydroxylation. Moreover, steric factors must also be considered, since oxidation occurs mostly at the least hindered position. For monosubstituted benzene compounds, *p*-hydroxylation frequently predominates, with some ortho product also formed (Fig. 4.12). When more than one phenyl ring is present, only one ring is typically hydroxylated (e.g., phenytoin).

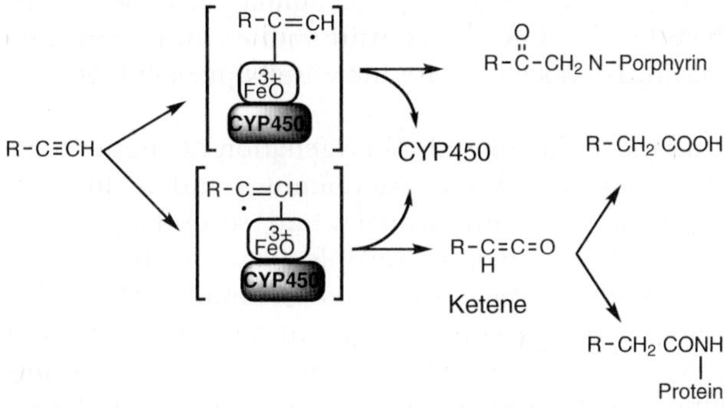

FIGURE 4.11 Alkyne oxidation catalyzed by P450.

Traditionally, hydroxylation of aromatic compounds by P450 has been thought to be mediated by an arene oxide (epoxide) intermediate, followed by the "NIH shift," as discussed previously (29–31) (Fig. 4.6). The formation of phenols and the isolation of urinary dihydrodiols, catechols, and glutathione conjugates (mercapturic acid derivatives) implicate arene oxides as intermediates in the metabolism of both benzene and substituted benzenes. Arene oxides are also prone to conjugate with glutathione to form premercapturic acids (see section on glutathione conjugation).

The CYP1A2 and CYP3A subfamilies are important contributors to 2- and 4-hydroxylation of estradiol, and CYP3A4 is an important contributor to 2-hydroxylation of the synthetic estrogens (e.g., 17α-ethinyl estradiol) (38). The principal metabolite (as much as 50%) for estradiol is 2-hydroxyestradiol, with 4-hydroxy and 16α-hydroxyestradiol as minor metabolites (Fig. 4.12). The 2-hydroxy metabolite of both estradiol and ethinyl estradiol have limited or no estrogenic activity, whereas the C-4 and

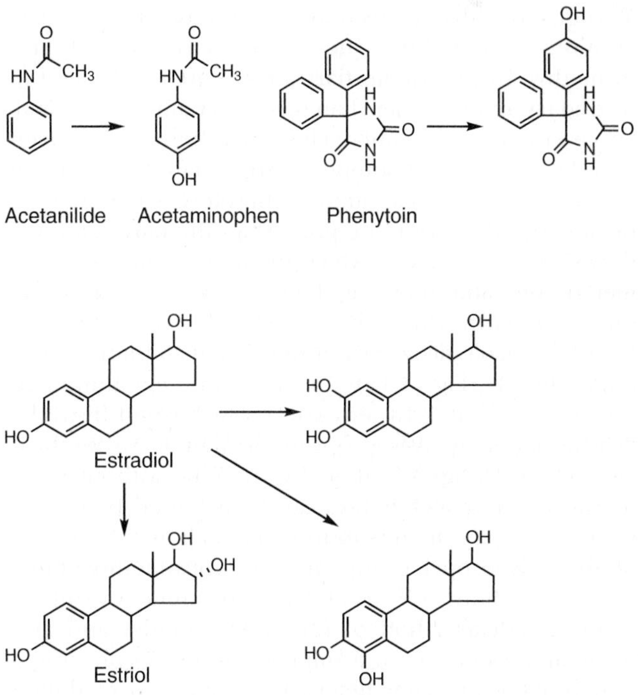

FIGURE 4.12 Examples of oxidative metabolism of aryl compounds catalyzed by P450.

C-16 α-hydroxy metabolites have a potency similar to that of estradiol. In humans, 16α-hydroxyestradiol is the primary estrogen metabolite both in pregnancy and in breast cancer. The metabolites 16α-hydroxyestrone and 4-hydroxyestrone can be carcinogenic in specific cells since they are capable of damaging cellular proteins and DNA after their activation to quinone intermediates.

Xenobiotic-metabolizing enzymes not only detoxify xenobiotics but also cause the formation of active intermediates (bioactivation), which in certain circumstances can elicit a diversity of toxicities, including mutagenesis, carcinogenesis, and hepatic necrosis (37). In addition to glutathione, some nucleophiles, such as other sulfhydryl compounds (most effective), alcohols, and phosphates, can react with arene oxides. Many of these nucleophiles are found in proteins and nucleic acids. The covalent binding of these bioactive epoxides to intracellular macromolecules provides a molecular basis of these toxic effects (see the discussion of toxicity due to oxidative metabolism).

N-Dealkylation, Oxidative Deamination, and *N*-Oxidation

N-dealkylation Dealkylation of secondary and tertiary amines to yield primary and secondary amines, respectively, is one of the most important and frequently encountered reactions in drug metabolism. The proposed mechanism of oxidative *N*-dealkylation involves α-hydrogen abstraction or an electron abstraction from the nitrogen by the ferryl oxygen and has been previously discussed (29–31) (Fig. 4.7).

Typical *N*-substituents removed by oxidative dealkylation are methyl, ethyl, *n*-propyl, isopropyl, *n*-butyl, allyl, and benzyl. Dealkylation occurs mostly with a smaller alkyl group. Substituents that are more resistant to dealkylation include *t*-butyl (no α-hydrogen) and cyclopropylmethyl. In general, tertiary amines are dealkylated to secondary amines faster than secondary amines are dealkylated to primary amines. This rate difference has been correlated with lipid solubility. Appreciable amounts of secondary and primary amines therefore accumulate as metabolites that are more polar than the parent amine, thus slowing the rate at which the amines diffuse across membranes and reducing their accessibility to receptors. Frequently, these amine metabolites contribute to the pharmacologic activity of the parent substance (e.g., imipramine) (Fig. 4.13), or they produce unwanted side effects, such as hypertension, which result from the *N*-dealkylation of *N*-isopropylmethoxamine to methoxamine. The design of an analogous drug without these unwanted drug metabolites can be achieved by proper choice of replacement substituents, such as substitution of the *N*-isopropyl group in *N*-isopropylmethoxamine with a tert-butyl (*N*-tert-butylmethoxamine or butoxamine). *N*-dealkylation of substituted amides and aromatic amines occurs in a similar manner. *N*-substituted nonaromatic nitrogen heterocycles undergo oxidation on the α-carbon to a lactam (nicotine to cotinine) as well as *N*-dealkylation (nicotine to nornicotine, cotinine, and norcotinine) (Fig. 4.13).

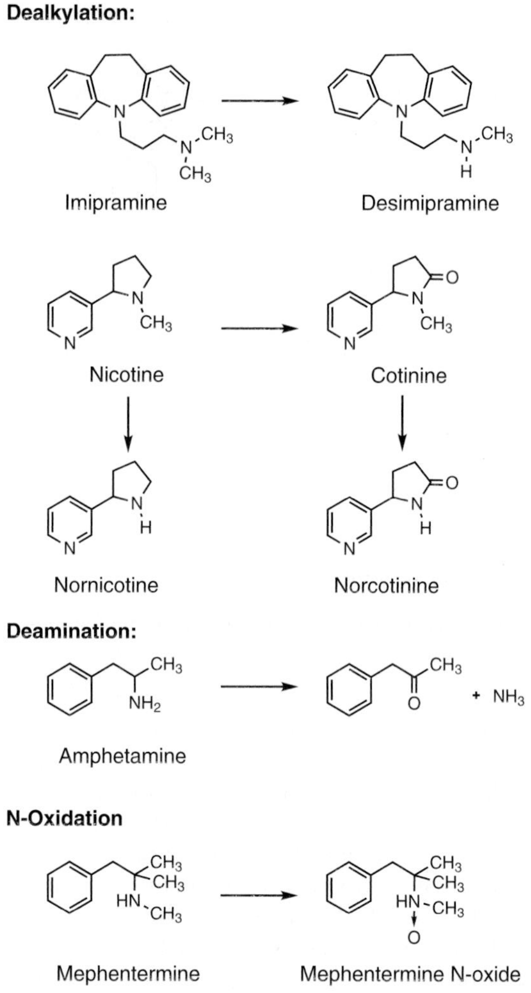

FIGURE 4.13 Examples of *N*-dealkylation, oxidative deamination, and *N*-oxidation reactions catalyzed by P450.

Oxidative Deamination The mechanism of oxidative deamination follows a pathway similar to that of *N*-dealkylation. Initially, oxidation to the iminium ion occurs, followed by decomposition to the carbonyl metabolite and ammonia. Oxidative deamination can occur with α-substituted amines, exemplified by amphetamine (Fig. 4.13). Disubstitution of the α-carbon inhibits its deamination (e.g., phentermine). Some secondary and tertiary amines, as well as amines substituted with bulky groups, can undergo deamination directly, without *N*-dealkylation (e.g., fenfluramine). Apparently, this behavior is associated with increased lipid solubility.

N-oxidation In general, *N*-oxygenation of amines forms stable *N*-oxides with tertiary amines and amides and hydroxylamines with primary and secondary amines, when no α-protons are available (e.g., mephentermine and arylamines) (Fig. 4.13). Tertiary amines having one or more hydrogens on the adjacent carbon dealkylate via the *N*-oxide. Rearrangement of the *N*-oxide to a carbinolamine, which subsequently collapses, produces the secondary amine. Amine metabolites can be *N*-conjugated, increasing their excretion.

O- AND S-DEALKYLATION Oxidative *O*-dealkylation of ethers is a common metabolic reaction with a mechanism of dealkylation analogous to that of *N*-dealkylation: oxidation of the α-carbon and subsequent decomposition of the unstable hemiacetal to an alcohol (or phenol) and a carbonyl product (29–31). *S*-Dealkylation of thioethers to hemithioacetals is a minor pathway in comparison to the major direct P450 oxidation of sulfur to sulfoxides and/or sulfones. The majority of ether groups in drug molecules are aromatic ethers (e.g., codeine, prazosin, and verapamil). For example, codeine is *O*-demethylated to morphine (Fig. 4.14). The rate of *O*-dealkylation is a function of chain length (i.e., increasing chain length or branching reduces the rate of dealkylation). Steric factors and ring substituents influence the rate of dealkylation but are complicated by electronic effects. Some drug molecules contain more than one ether group, in which case only one ether is dealkylated. The methylenedioxy group undergoes variable rates of dealkylation to the 1,2-diphenolic metabolite. Metabolism of such a group is also capable of forming a stable complex with and inhibiting P450.

By analogy to *O*- and *N*-dealkylations, esters and amides can also be P450 oxidized by attaching the α-carbon to the ether oxygen of the ester (or α-carbon to the amide nitrogen). This reaction has not been usually recognized because of it is obscured by the competing, more common hydrolysis of esters and amides.

Aliphatic and aromatic methyl thioethers undergo *S*-dealkylation to thiols and carbonyl compounds. For example, 6-methylthiopurine is demethylated to give the active anticancer drug 6-mercaptopurine (Fig. 4.14). Other thioethers are oxidized to sulfoxides or sulfones (see *N*- and *S*-oxidations).

DEHALOGENATION Many halogenated hydrocarbons, such as insecticides, pesticides, general anesthetics, plasticizers, flame retardants, and commercial solvents, undergo a variety of different dehalogenation biotransformations (24,25). Because of our potential exposure to these halogenated compounds as drugs and environmental pollutants in air, soil, water, or food, it is important to understand the interactions between metabolism and toxicity. Some halogenated hydrocarbons form glutathione or mercapturic acid conjugates, whereas others undergo dehydrohalogenation and reductive dehalogenation catalyzed by

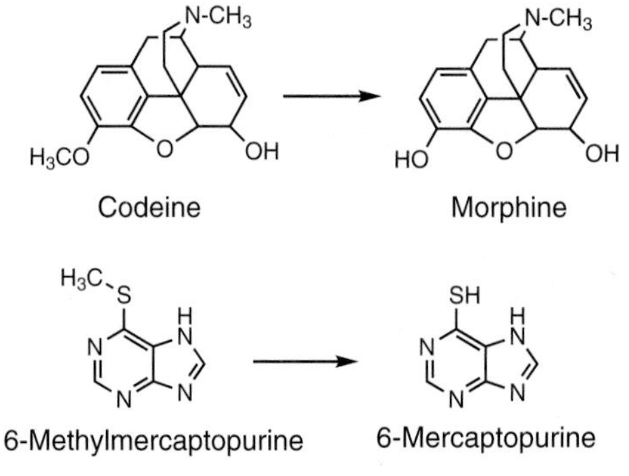

FIGURE 4.14 Examples of *O*- and *S*-dealkylations catalyzed by P450.

CYP2E1. In many cases, reactive intermediates, including radicals, anions, and cations, are produced that can react with a variety of tissue molecules.

Halogenated hydrocarbons differ in their chemical reactivity as a result of the electron-withdrawing properties of the halogens on adjacent carbon atoms, resulting in the α-carbon developing electrophilic character. The halogen atoms have also the ability to stabilize α-carbon cations, free radicals, carbanions, and carbenes.

Oxidative dehydrohalogenation is a common metabolic pathway of many halogenated hydrocarbons (25,29–31). P450-catalyzed oxidation generates the transient gem-halohydrin (analogous to alkane hydroxylation) that can eliminate the hydrohalic acid to form carbonyl derivatives (aldehydes, ketones, acyl halides, and carbonyl halides) (Fig. 4.7). This reaction requires the presence of at least one halogen and one α-hydrogen. gem-Trihalogenated hydrocarbons are more readily oxidized than are the gem-dihalogenated and monohalogenated compounds. The acyl and carbonyl halides formed are reactive metabolites that can react either with water to form carboxylic acids or nonenzymatically with tissue molecules (with a potential for eliciting increased toxicity). Chloramphenicol ($RNHCOCHCl_2$) is biotransformed into an acyl halide (RNHCOCOCl) that selectively acylates the apoprotein of P450 (40,41).

An excellent example of oxidative dehydrohalogenation leading to significant hepatotoxicity and nephrotoxicity is seen with the fluorinated inhalation anesthetics (Fig. 4.15). The toxicity of halothane and the fluranes is related to their metabolism to either an acid chloride (or fluoride) or a trifluoroacetate intermediate. The CYP2E1 has been identified as the isoform catalyzing the biotransformation of the fluranes (25,43,44). The hydroxylated intermediate decomposes spontaneously to reactive intermediates, an acid chloride (or fluoride) or trifluoroacetate, that can either react with water to form halide anions and a fluorinated carboxylic acid or bind covalently to tissue proteins to produce an acylated protein. The acylated protein becomes a "hapten," stimulating an immune response and a hypersensitivity reaction. Halothane has received the most attention as a result of its ability to cause "halothane-associated" hepatitis. This immunologic reaction occurs after repeated exposure in surgical patients to trifluoroacetylate protein. The patient is sensitized to future exposures of the volatile anesthetic. After subsequent exposure to a fluorinated anesthetic, the antigenic trifluoroacetylate protein stimulates an immune response, producing halothane-like hepatitis. Because of the common metabolic pathway involving CYP2E1 for enflurane, isoflurane, desflurane, and methoxyflurane, halothane-exposed patients who have halothane hepatitis can show cross-sensitization to one of the other fluranes, triggering an idiosyncratic hepatic necrosis. The formation of antigenic protein is related to the amount of CYP2E1-catalyzed metabolism of each agent: halothane (20% to 40%) > enflurane (2% to 8%) > isoflurane (0.2% to 1.0%) > desflurane (<0.1%). Enough fluoride ion is generated from oxidative dehalogenation during flurane anesthesia to produce subclinical nephrotoxicity. Interestingly, female rats metabolize halothane more slowly than do male

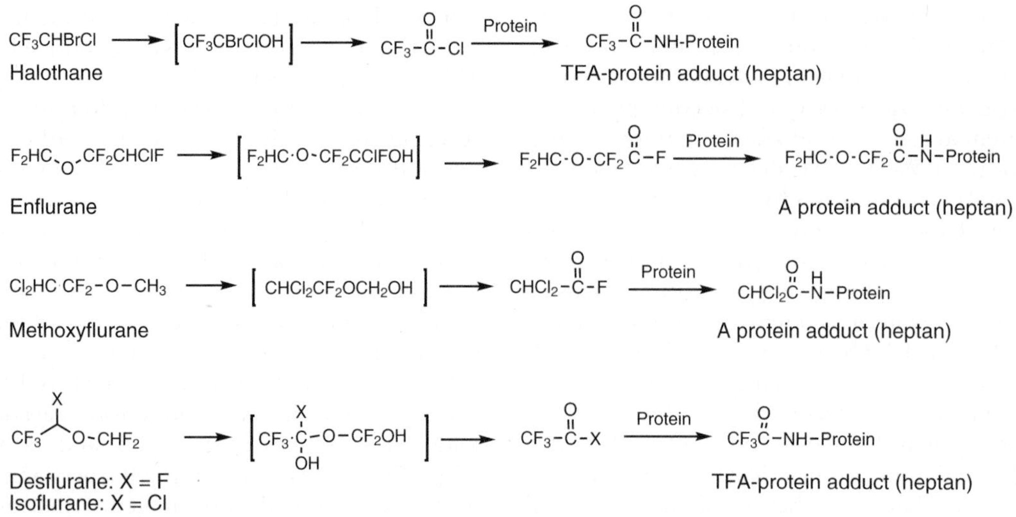

FIGURE 4.15 CYP2E1-catalyzed metabolism of fluorinated volatile anesthetics to antigenic proteins.

rats and are less susceptible to hepatotoxicity than males are. For patients with preexisting liver dysfunction, isoflurane or desflurane can be a better choice of general anesthetic.

In today's environment, most humans have been exposed to many CYP2E1-inducing agents (including recreational, industrial, and agricultural chemicals and alcohol), having an unknown effect on hepatic toxicity from volatile anesthetics. Enhanced activity of CYP2E1 has been observed in obesity, isoniazid therapy, ketogenic diets, and alcoholism.

Azo and Nitro Reduction In addition to the oxidative systems, liver microsomes also contain enzyme systems that catalyze the reduction of azo and nitro compounds to primary amines. A number of azo compounds, such as Prontosil and sulfasalazine (Fig. 4.16), are converted to aromatic primary amines by azoreductase, an NADPH-dependent enzyme system in the liver microsomes. Evidence exists for the participation of P450 in some reductions. Nitro compounds (e.g., chloramphenicol and nitrobenzene) are reduced to aromatic primary amines by a nitroreductase, presumably through nitrosamine and hydroxylamine intermediates. These reductases are not solely responsible of reduction of azo and nitro compounds; reduction by the bacterial flora in the anaerobic environment of the intestine can also occur.

Oxidations Catalyzed by Flavin Monooxygenase

Flavin-containing monooxygenase (FMO) oxidizes drugs, xenobiotics, and environmental chemicals containing a "soft nucleophile," usually nitrogen or sulfur. FMO, unlike P450, is a monooxygenase, utilizing the two-electron reducing equivalents of NADPH (hydride anion) to reduce one atom of molecular oxygen to water while the other oxygen atom is used to oxidize the substrate. Because oxygen activation occurs before substrate addition, any compound binding to 4α-hydroperoxyflavin, the enzyme-bound monooxygenating FMO intermediate, is a potential substrate. The products formed from FMO-catalyzed oxidation are consistent with a two-electron oxidation of the heteroatom. Unlike P450, FMO does not catalyze epoxidation reactions or hydroxylation at unactivated carbon atoms of xenobiotics. FMO and P450 also exhibit similar tissue and cellular location, molecular weight, and substrate specificity, and exist as multiple enzymes under developmental control.

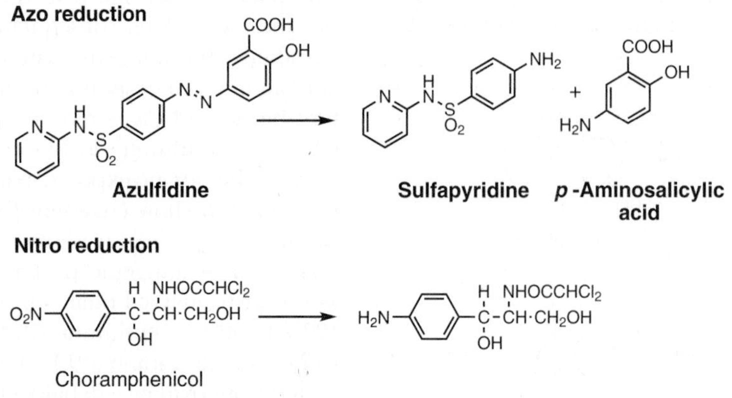

FIGURE 4.16 P450-catalyzed reduction of azo and nitro compounds.

Humans express five different FMOs (FMO1, FMO2, FMO3, FMO4, and FMO5) in a tissue-specific manner, with different substrate specificities. The human FMO functional gene family consists of five families each expressing a single protein unlike P450. Three of the five expressed human FMO genes, *FMO1, FMO2,* and *FMO3,* exhibit genetic polymorphisms. FMO3 is the prominent form in adult human liver that is likely to be associated with the bulk of FMO-mediated metabolism and contributes to the disease known as trimethylaminuria. FMO2 is largely found in the lung. Because of their low expression, less is known about the substrate specificity for FMO4 and FMO5. Thus, these enzymes do not contribute significantly to human drug metabolism. FMO does not require a reductase to transfer electrons from NADPH. The catalytic cycles of FMO and P450 are very different. Another distinction is the lack of induction of FMOs by xenobiotics. In general, P450 is the major contributor to oxidative xenobiotic metabolism. However, FMO activity may be of significance in a number of cases and should not be overlooked. FMO and P450 have overlapping substrate specificities, but often yield different metabolites with potentially diverse toxicologic/pharmacologic consequences. The physiologic functions of FMO are poorly understood (45). Unlike P450, which exhibits interindividual variation in expression to both genetic and environmental factors, FMO is not regulated by environmental factors, and interindividual variability in FMO enzyme expression would be predominately genetic in origin.

N- and *S*-Oxidations

FMO constitutes an alternative biotransformation pathway for converting *N*- and *S*-containing lipophilic drugs and xenobiotics to more polar materials that are more efficiently excreted in the urine. Typically, FMO catalyzes oxygenation of the *N*- and *S*-heteroatoms ("soft nucleophiles") (Fig. 4.17) but not heteroatom dealkylation

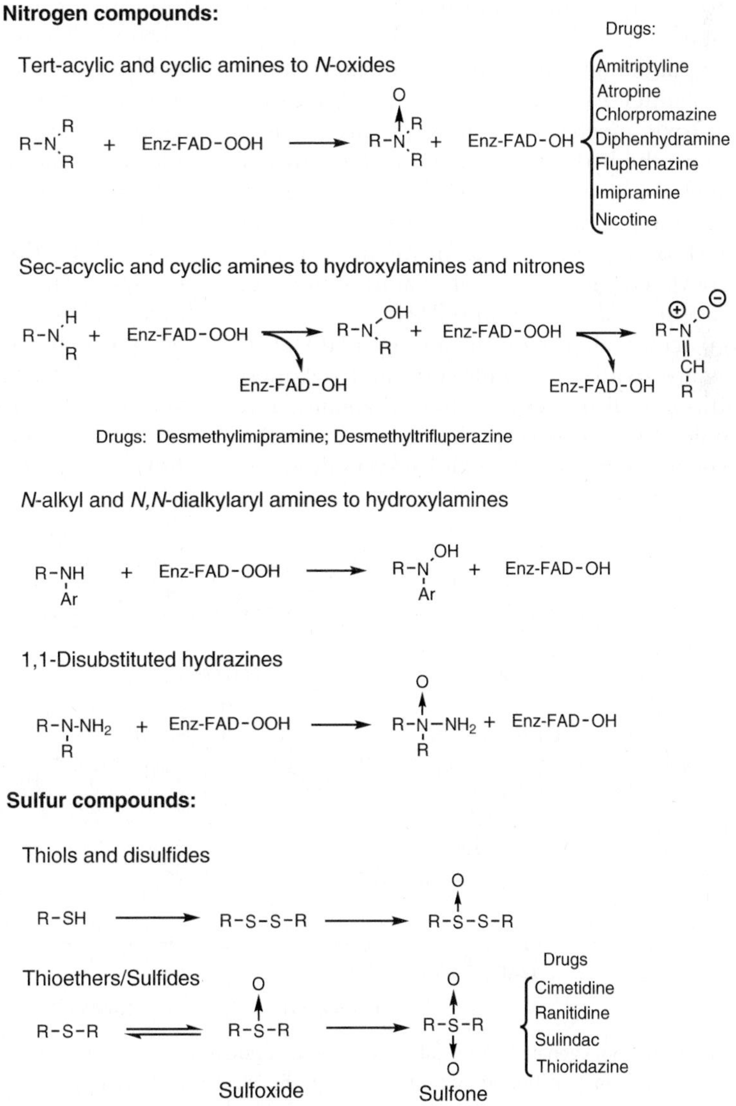

FIGURE 4.17 Examples of flavin monooxygenase (FMO) oxidations.

reactions. Normally, FMO is not inducible by phenobarbital, nor is it affected by P450 inhibitors. With few exceptions, however, xenobiotic substrates of FMO are also substrates of the isoforms of P450, producing similar oxidation products. Which monooxygenase is responsible for the oxidation can be readily determined, because FMO is thermally labile in the absence of NADPH, whereas P450 is stable.

Of the many nitrogen functional groups in xenobiotics, only secondary and tertiary acyclic, cyclic, and arylamines as well as hydroxylamines and hydrazines are oxidized by FMO and excreted in the urine (Fig. 4.17). The tertiary amines form stable amine oxides (*N*-oxides), which are highly polarized, hydrophilic, and less basic compounds that are reduced back to the parent tertiary amine in the gastrointestinal tract. On the other hand, secondary amines are sequentially oxidized to hydroxylamines, nitrones, and a complex mixture of products. Secondary *N*-alkylarylamines can be *N*-oxygenated to reactive *N*-hydroxylated metabolites, which are responsible for the toxic, mutagenic, and carcinogenic activity of these aromatic amines. For example, the chemically unstable hydroxylamine intermediates of aromatic amines degrade into bladder carcinogens (see the discussion of this type of toxic mechanism under glucuronic acid conjugation), and the hydroxamic acid intermediates of *N*-arylacetamides are bioactivated into liver carcinogens. Hepatic FMO, however, will not catalyze the oxidation of primary alkyl- or arylamines, except for the carcinogenic *N*-hydroxylated derivatives of 2-aminofluorene, 2-aminoanthracene, and other amino PAHs.

S-Oxidation occurs almost exclusively by FMO (Fig. 4.17). Sulfides are oxidized to sulfoxides and sulfones; thiols are oxidized to disulfides and thiocarbamates; and mercaptopyrimidines and mercaptoimidazoles (i.e., the antithyroid drug methimazole) are oxidized via sulfenates (RSOH) to sulfinates (R-SO-OH), all of which are eliminated in the urine. FMO *S*-oxygenates a number of sulfur-containing substrates and, in some cases, with great stereoselectivity. The hepatotoxicity of thioureas (e.g., the antimycobacterial drug ethionamide) is the result of metabolic bioactivation of thioureas due to FMO3-dependent *S*-oxidation to produce toxic sulfinic acid metabolites. Metabolic bioactivation of ethionamide by bacterial FMOs may be its antimycobacterial mechanism of action.

Primary aromatic amines and amides, aromatic heterocyclic amines and imines, and the aliphatic primary amine phentermine are *N*-oxidized by P450 to hydroxylamines. P450 oxidizes carbon disulfide to carbon dioxide and hydrogen sulfide and the antipsychotic phenothiazines to sulfoxides.

Catalytic Cycle for Flavin Monooxygenase

The major steps in the catalytic cycle for FMO are shown in Figure 4.18 (45,46). Like most of the other monooxygenases, FMO requires NADPH and oxygen as cosubstrates to catalyze the oxidation of the xenobiotic substrate. Unlike P450, however, the xenobiotic being oxidized does not need to be bound to the 4α-hydroperoxyflavin intermediate (FAD-OOH) for oxygen activation to occur. Apparently, FMO is present within the cell in its enzyme-bound activated hydroperoxide (Enz-FAD-OOH) state ready to oxidize any suitable lipophilic substrate that binds to it. The FMO uses a nonradical, nucleophilic displacement type of mechanism binding dioxygen with a reduced flavin. The reactive oxygen intermediate is a reactive derivative of hydrogen peroxide, flavin-4α-hydroperoxide (Fig. 4.18, insert), which is reactive enough to successfully attack a lone electron pair on a heteroatom, such as nitrogen or sulfur, but not reactive enough to attack a typical C-H bond. These studies suggest the xenobiotic substrate interacts with

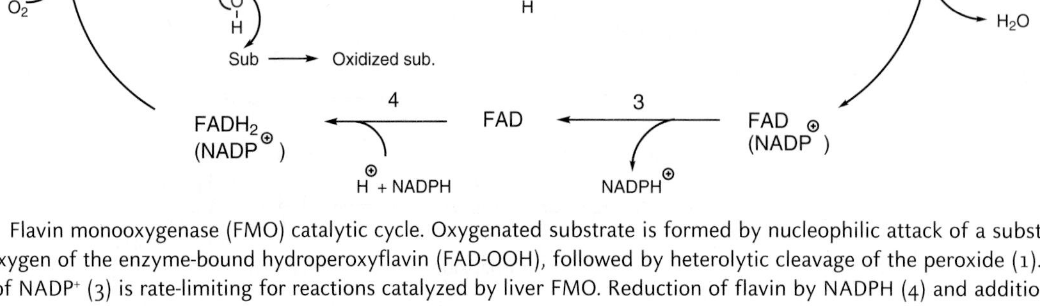

FIGURE 4.18 Flavin monooxygenase (FMO) catalytic cycle. Oxygenated substrate is formed by nucleophilic attack of a substrate (Sub.) by the terminal oxygen of the enzyme-bound hydroperoxyflavin (FAD-OOH), followed by heterolytic cleavage of the peroxide (1). The release of H_2O (2) or of $NADP^+$ (3) is rate-limiting for reactions catalyzed by liver FMO. Reduction of flavin by NADPH (4) and addition of oxygen (5) complete the cycle by regeneration of the oxygenated FAD-OOH.

the 4α-hydroperoxyflavin form of FMO and is oxidized by oxygen transfer from Enz-FAD-OOH to form the oxidized product. Neither the substrate nor the oxidized substrate is essential for any other steps in the cycle. Steps 2 to 5 simply regenerate the oxygenating agent Enz-FAD-OOH from Enz-FAD-OH, NADPH, oxygen, and a proton. Any compound readily crossing cell membranes by passive diffusion and penetrating to the FMO-bound hydroperoxyflavin intermediate is a potential substrate, thus explaining the broad substrate specificity exhibited for FMO. The fact that the xenobiotic substrate is not required for activation of the FMO-hydroperoxyflavin state distinguishes FMO from P450 monooxygenases, in which substrate binding initiates the P450 catalytic cycle and activation of oxygen to the ferryl oxygenating agent. It is not unusual for FMO oxidation products to undergo reduction to the parent xenobiotic, which can enter into repeated redox reactions (termed "metabolic cycling").

Results of substrate specificity studies suggest that the number of ionic groups on endogenous substrate is an important factor enabling FMO to distinguish between xenobiotic and endogenous substrates, preventing the indiscriminate oxidation of physiologically important amine and sulfur compounds (47). Without exception, FMO readily catalyzes the oxidation of uncharged amines or sulfur compounds (in equilibrium with its respective monocation or monoanion; for sulfur compounds, the charge is on sulfur atom). The FMO will not catalyze the oxidation of dianions (e.g., thiamine pyrophosphate), dications (e.g., polyamines), dipolar ions (e.g., amino acids and peptides), or other polyionic compounds with one or more anionic groups (i.e., COO^-) distal to the heteroatom (e.g., coenzyme A).

Unlike the P450 system, only three isoforms of hepatic FMO have been characterized in the adult human liver (48,49): FMO1, the major form in fetal tissue; FMO2; and FMO3. The availability of different forms of FMO can be of clinical importance in the pharmacologic and toxicologic properties of FMO-dependent drug oxidations.

The substrate specificity for FMO3 is distinct from that of FMO1. FMO3 *N*-oxygenates primary, secondary, and tertiary amines, whereas FMO1 is only efficient at *N*-oxygenating tertiary amines. FMO3 is sensitive to steric features of the substrate, and aliphatic amines with linkages between the nitrogen atom and a large aromatic group such as a phenothiazine of at least five carbons are *N*-oxygenated significantly more efficiently than those substrates with two or three carbons. Amines with smaller aromatic substituents, such as phenethylamines, are often efficiently *N*-oxygenated by FMO3. Interindividual variation in FMO3-dependent metabolism of drugs, xenobiotics, and environmental chemicals is therefore more likely to be a result of genetic and not environmental effects. Certain mutations of the *FMO3* gene have been associated with deficient *N*-oxygenation of trimethylamine, which results in an inherited genetic condition called trimethylaminuria. Allelic variations of FMO3 might cause abnormal metabolism of drugs, which has clinical implications for human drug metabolism. For example, (*S*)-nicotine *N*-1′-oxide formation is a highly stereoselective product of FMO3 for adult humans who smoke cigarettes. Thus, *FMO3* genetic polymorphism and poor metabolism phenotype in certain human populations could contribute to adverse drug reactions or exaggerated clinical response to certain medications. *FMO3* may be another example of an environmental gene that participates in a protective mechanism to help shield humans from potentially toxic exposure to chemicals.

Peroxidases and Other Monooxygenases

Peroxidases are hemoproteins and are closely related enzymes to P450 monooxygenase (50,51). The differences between peroxidase and P450 is that the cysteine axial ligand of P450 has been replaced by a histidine residue as well as the inclusion of polar amino acids within proximity of the heme-active site. These polar amino acid differences in the peroxidase heme-active site allow the peroxidase to rapidly catalyze the reduction of hydroperoxides to alcohol (water in the case of hydrogen peroxide) and the simultaneous reoxidation of peroxidase. The normal course of peroxide (ROOH)-catalyzed oxidation involves the formation of the ferryl-oxo intermediate, analogous to the ferryl complex in P450. Thus, the catalytic cycle of peroxidases is simpler than that of P450. Unlike P450, which is capable of oxidizing almost any type of substrate, peroxidase-catalyzed oxidation of drugs and xenobiotics is limited to electron-rich substrates that are easily oxidized (e.g., heteroatom oxygenation, aromatization [oxidation] of 1,4-dihydropyridines [calcium channel blockers] and arylamines).

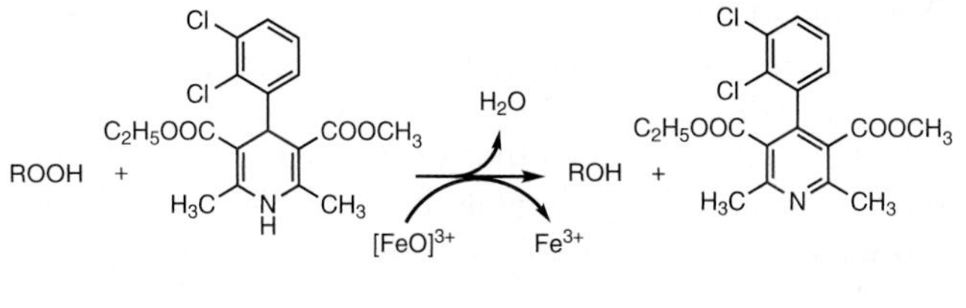

Cyclooxygenase (COX; also known as prostaglandin synthase or prostaglandin endoperoxide synthetase) is a widely distributed heme-peroxidase enzyme responsible for the formation of important biologic mediators called prostanoids, including prostaglandins, prostacyclin, and thromboxane from arachidonic acid (see also Chapter 31). COX catalyzes the heme-peroxidation of arachidonic acid by means of hydrogen atom abstraction from arachidonic acid by a tyrosine radical generated by a ferryl-oxo-heme intermediate to hydroperoxy endoperoxide prostaglandin G_2 (PGG_2), which is then reduced to prostaglandin H_2, regenerating the COX. Two oxygen molecules then react with the arachidonic acid radical to produce PGG_2. During the reduction of PGG_2 to prostaglandin H_2, drug substrates can be oxidized. Three COX isoenzymes are known: COX-1, COX-2, and COX-3. Inhibitors of COX are the NSAIDs.

Myeloperoxidase (MPO) is a heme-peroxidase enzyme most abundantly present in neutrophil granulocytes (a subtype of white blood cells). MPO differs from P450 and other peroxidases in that the substrates are hydrogen peroxide and chloride anion. The chloride anion is oxidized to hypochlorous acid (HOCl) in the granulocyte, which is cytotoxic and very effective in killing bacteria, virus, and other pathogens—the natural function of neutrophils. HOCl is also used to disinfect drinking water. HOCl can also oxidize drugs to reactive intermediates (e.g., nitrenium ions), which can be responsible for causing agranulocytosis. Examples of HOCl-generated reactive intermediates associated with agranulocytosis are the atypical antipsychotic clozapine, the antimalarial amodiaquine, the antipyretic aminopyrine, and the phosphodiesterase cardiotonic vesnarinone.

Other peroxidases include horseradish peroxidase (found in plants), lactoperoxidase found in breast milk, and thyroid peroxidase found in the thyroid gland to produce thyroid hormones from iodide.

Other monooxygenases catalyzing oxidation reactions similar to P450 include dopamine β-monooxygenase, a mammalian copper-containing enzyme catalyzing carbon hydroxylation, epoxidation, *S*-oxygenation, and *N*-dealkylation reactions, and nonheme iron–containing enzymes from bacteria and plants.

Nonmicrosomal Oxidations

In addition to the microsomal monooxygenases, other oxidases and dehydrogenases that catalyze oxidation reactions are present in the mitochondrial and soluble fractions of tissue homogenates.

Oxidation of Alcohols

Alcohol dehydrogenases (ADH) are a family of nicotinamide adenine dinucleotide (NAD)-specific enzyme dehydrogenase enzymes that occur in many organisms and are responsible for catalyzing oxidation of primary and secondary alcohols to aldehydes and ketones, respectively, with reduction of NAD^+ to NADH. ADHs can also catalyze the reverse reaction, reducing NADH to NAD^+. In humans and many other animals, genetic evidence suggests that early on in evolution, ADHs were effective for metabolizing endogenous and exogenous formaldehyde and metabolizing naturally occurring toxic alcohols contained in foods or produced by bacteria in the digestive tract. Another evolutionary purpose may be metabolism of the endogenous alcohol vitamin A (retinol) to generate the hormone retinoic acid. In yeast, plants, and many bacteria, some ADHs catalyze the opposite reaction as part of fermentation to ensure a constant energy supply of NAD^+ for the host organism.

In humans, ADH exists as a dimer with a mass of 80 kDa and is encoded by at least seven different genes. There are five classes (I to V) of ADHs, but the hepatic form that is primarily present in humans is class I. Class I consists of A, B, and C subunits that are encoded by the genes ADH1A, ADH1B, and ADH1C. The human genes that encode class II, III, IV, and V ADHs are ADH4, ADH5, ADH7, and ADH6, respectively. The large number of ADH classes gives the body the capability to metabolize/detoxify a variety of primary and secondary alcohols. Human ADH is present at high levels in the liver and the lining of the stomach and exhibits a broad specificity for alcohols. Most primary alcohols are readily oxidized to their corresponding aldehydes. Some secondary alcohols are oxidized to the ketones, whereas other secondary and tertiary alcohols are excreted either unchanged or as their conjugate metabolite. Some secondary alcohols also show mixed activity due to steric factors and a lack of substrate affinity for the enzyme. The mechanism of dehydrogenation involves abstraction by the enzyme and transfer of a hydride anion from the alcohol to NAD+, reducing NAD+ to NADH, and subsequent formation of an aldehyde. ADH contains a two Zn+2 ions in each subunit. One of those Zn ions is located at the catalytic site and binds the hydroxyl group of the alcohol in place for dehydrogenation to occur. ADH is located in the soluble fraction of tissue homogenates.

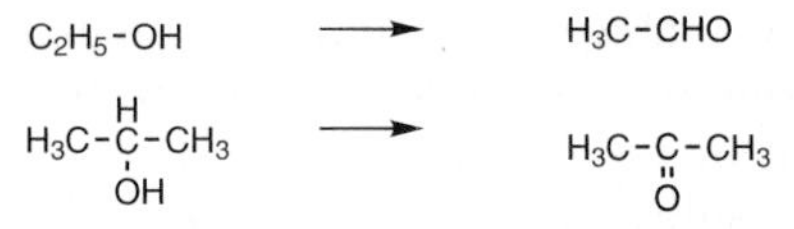

Oxidation by ADH is the principal pathway for ethanol metabolism, but the CYP2E1 isoform has also a significant role in ethanol metabolism and tolerance. Two-thirds of ingested ethanol is oxidized by ADH and the remainder by CYP2E1; during intoxication, however, ethanol induces the expression of CYP2E1. The induction of CYP2E1 contributes to the activation of other drugs and xenobiotics, increasing the vulnerability of heavy drinkers to anesthetic drugs, over-the-counter analgesics, prescription drugs, and chemical carcinogens. In turn, the excessive amounts of acetaldehyde generated cause hepatotoxicity, lipid peroxidation of membranes, formation of protein adducts, and other hepatocellular changes.

The toxicity of methanol and ethylene glycol in humans has long been recognized, but frequent reports of such toxicity are not surprising given the number of consumer products containing methanol and ethylene glycol (automotive antifreeze). Methanol (wood alcohol or methyl alcohol) is commonly used as a solvent in organic synthetic procedures and is available to consumers in a variety of products, including solid fuels (Sterno), paint removers, motor fuels, antifreeze, and alcoholic beverages (an adulterant in wines or an unintentional ingredient). Oral methanol toxicity in humans is characterized by its rapid absorption from the gut, followed by a latent period of many hours before metabolic acidosis (lowered blood pH and bicarbonate levels) and ocular toxicity are evident. The metabolic acidosis and blindness result from the excessive accumulation of formic acid and the inability of the hepatic tetrahydrofolate pathway to oxidize formate to carbon dioxide. The rate of elimination of methanol from the blood is relatively slow compared to the rapid rate for ethanol, accounting for its long latency period. Its half-life ranges from 2 to 3 hours at low blood concentration to 27 hours at high blood concentration. Evidence supports the singular role of liver ADH in the metabolism of methanol to formaldehyde, although it is oxidized slowly by ADH (approximately one-sixth the rate of ethanol). The demonstration that methanol is a substrate for ADH provides a rational basis for the use of ethanol in the treatment of methanol toxicity. Ethanol depresses the rate of methanol oxidation by acting as a competitive substrate for ADH, reducing the formation of formaldehyde. On the other hand, formaldehyde is not customarily detected in the blood as a result of its rapid metabolism by ADH to formate. Although human exposure to methanol vapor is less prevalent, methanol is rapidly absorbed through the skin or by inhalation, and depending on the severity of exposure, this can result in methanol poisoning. Ethylene glycol is oxidized to hydroxyacealdehyde and glyoxal and, subsequently, to oxalate by ADH. When eliminated into the urine, oxalate forms calcium oxalate crystals that can block the kidney tubules. 4-Methylpyrazole (fomepizole) is an alcohol dehydrogenase inhibitor that is used as an antidote for the treatment of methanol or ethylene glycol poisoning. 1,4-Butanediol is a solvent that has became popular as a date-rape drug and drug of abuse due to its metabolism to γ-hydroxybutyrate (see Chapter 13), which binds to the γ-hydroxybutyrate receptor, which in turn produces central nervous system sedation with amnesia.

ADH also functions as a reductase when it catalyzes the reduction of an aldehyde or ketone to an alcohol. In addition, other NADP- or NAD-dependent dehydrogenases in the cytosol are capable of reducing a variety of ketones. Ketones are stable to further oxidation and, consequently, yield reduction products as major metabolites. Examples of reduction include the sedative-hypnotic chloral hydrate to trichloroethanol, the opioid antagonist naltrexone to 6-β-hydroxynaltrexol, the opioid analgesic methadone to α-methadol, the antipsychotic haloperidol to hydroxyhaloperidol, and the antiemetic dolasetron to dihydrodolasetron. These alcohol metabolites are all pharmacologically active.

Aldehyde Dehydrogenase

Aldehyde dehydrogenases (ALHDs) (not to be confused with aldehyde oxidase) are a family of polymorphic NAD^+-specific enzymes that catalyze the NAD^+-dependent oxidation (dehydrogenation) of aldehydes to carboxylic acids, to be subsequently metabolized by the body's muscle and heart. There are three mammalian classes of these enzymes: class 1 (low K_m, cytosolic, ALDH1), class 2 (low K_m, mitochondrial, ALDH2), and class 3 (high K_m, such as those expressed in tumors, stomach, and cornea). In all three classes, constitutive (an enzyme whose activity is constant and active) and inducible forms exist. ALDH1 and ALDH2 are the most important enzymes for aldehyde oxidation, and both are tetrameric enzymes composed of 5-kDa subunits. These enzymes are found in many tissues of the body but are at the highest concentration in the liver. ALDH1 and ADH are responsible for the metabolism of retinol to retinoic acid. ALDH2 has a major role in the hepatic detoxication of acetaldehyde and other aldehydes produced from oxidation of ethanol and other primary alcohols and oxidation of endogenous aldehydes, such as those produced by the oxidation of biogenic amines (norepinephrine, serotonin, dopamine). These aldehydes can be toxic, and health problems arise when the aldehyde cannot be cleared. The accumulation of unmetabolized acetaldehyde in the blood has been shown to be a carcinogen in lab animals. For example, when high levels of acetaldehyde occur in the blood, facial flushing, light headedness, palpitations, nausea, and general "hangover" symptoms occur. These symptoms are indicative of a disease known as "Asian flush" or "Oriental flushing syndrome," due to a mutant form of ALDH2, termed *ALDH2*2*, where a lysine residue replaces a glutamate in the active site. These individuals have about 8% of the wild-type (normal) *ADH2* allele. The mutant allele shows a higher K_m for NAD^+ than the wild-type allele. This mutation is common in Japan, where 41% of a nonalcoholic control group were ALDH2 deficient and where only 2% to 5% of an alcoholic group were ALDH2 deficient. In Taiwan, the numbers are similar, with 30% of the control group showing the deficiency and 6% of alcoholics displaying the deficiency. The deficiency is manifested by slow acetaldehyde removal and low alcohol tolerance, which perhaps leads to a lower frequency of alcoholism. These symptoms are also the same as those observed in people who drink ethanol while being treated with the drug disulfiram (Antabuse), which is why it is used to treat alcoholism. These patients show higher blood levels of acetaldehyde and become violently ill upon consumption of even small amounts of alcohol. Several other drugs (e.g., metronidazole) cause a similar reaction known as "disulfiram-like reaction."

$$H_3C\text{-}CHO \longrightarrow H_3C\text{-}COOH$$

Aldo-Keto Reductases

Aldo-keto reductases (AKRs) are a superfamily of enzymes that are typically monomeric, cytosolic, NAD(P)H-dependent oxidoreductases that share high sequence identity (<40%) and similar three-dimensional structures and are involved in the formation of hyperosmotic sugars, which can contribute to diabetic complications. They also metabolize reactive aldehydes, prostaglandins, steroid hormones, chemical carcinogens, and drugs.

AKRs detoxify endogenous toxicants (e.g., cytotoxic/ mutagenic bifunctional electrophiles derived from the decomposition of lipid hydroperoxides), detoxify nicotine-derived nitrosamino ketone carcinogens in tobacco, and activate polycyclic aromatic trans-dihydrodiols to yield reactive ortho-quinones. AKRs also detoxify mycotoxin metabolites (e.g., aflatoxin dialdehyde), protecting against hepatocellular carcinomas. AKRs could have a central role in the cellular response to osmotic, electrophilic, and oxidative stress.

Molybdenum Hydroxylases

Molybdenum hydroxylases are non-P450 enzymes capable of catalyzing the oxidation of drugs. The molybdenum hydroxylases, which include aldehyde oxidase, xanthine oxidase, and xanthine dehydrogenase, are more commonly found in the cytosol of mammalian liver and carry out the oxidation and detoxification of a number of structurally different azaheterocycles (52). The efficient oxidation of endogenous purine nucleosides suggests that their metabolism and detoxification might be an important physiologic role of the molybdenum hydroxylases. Among the azaheterocycles metabolized are derivatives of pyridine, quinoline, pyrimidine, purine, quinazoline, and pteridines. These hydroxylases, as a rule, oxidize the α-carbon to the nitrogen of the azaheterocycle to oxo metabolites (also known as lactams). The molybdenum hydroxylases are cytosolic homodimeric enzymes (two identical monomers) with a common electron-transfer system in each enzyme subunit: a molybdopterin (a pyranopteridine ligand) cofactor that binds the single molybdenum ion, two iron-sulfur centers, and FAD molecule. The molybdenum hydroxylases catalyze their reactions differently than P450 and other hydroxylase enzymes, requiring water rather than molecular oxygen as the source of the oxygen atom incorporated into the metabolite and with the concomitant reduction of molecular oxygen to superoxide (53,54). The active sites possess a catalytically labile Mo^{5+}-OH (or, possibly, Mo^{6+}-OH_2) group that is transferred to the substrate during the course of the hydroxylation reaction.

Aldehyde Oxidase Aldehyde oxidase is a molybdenum cofactor–specific enzyme that generates carboxylic acids and hydrogen peroxide from aldehydes in the presence of oxygen. The enzyme is a homodimer and requires FAD in addition to molybdenum as cofactors. In addition to metabolizing some aldehydes, aldehyde oxidase also oxidizes a variety of azaheterocycles but not thia- or oxaheterocycles. Of the various purine nucleosides metabolized by aldehyde oxidase, the 2-hydroxy and 2-amino derivatives are more efficiently metabolized, and for the N^9-substituents, the typical order of preference of the acyclic nucleosides is as follows: 9-[(hydroxy-alkyloxy)methyl]-purines) > 2′-arabinofuranosyl > H. The kinetic rate constants for purine analogues reveal that the pyrimidine portion of the purine ring system is more important for substrate affinity than the imidazole portion. Aldehyde oxidase is inhibited by potassium cyanide and menadione (synthetic vitamin K).

Aldehyde oxidase metabolizes an assortment of azaheterocycles including the short-acting sedative-hypnotic drug zaleplon (a pyrazolo[1,5α] pyrimidine derivative) to its 5-oxo metabolite; the anticancer drug thioguanine to 8-oxothioguanine; the α_2-adrenergic agonist brimonidine (a pyrimidine derivative) to its 2-oxo-, 3-oxo-, and 2,3-dioxo- metabolites; quinine and quinidine to their 2-quinolone metabolites; the proantiviral drug famciclovir (a purine derivative) to its active 6-oxo metabolite (penciclovir); O^6-benzylguanine to its 8-oxo metabolite (also formed primarily from CYP3A4); the metabolism of the anticancer drug DACA (an acridine-4-carboxamide derivative) to its 9-acridone metabolite; and the antiseizure drug zonisamide (a 1,2-benzisoxazole derivative) primarily by reductive cleavage of the 1,2-benzisoxazole ring to 2-sulfamoylacetylphenol. Although the azaheterocycles thiazole and oxazole are not metabolized by aldehyde oxidase, their carbocyclic analogues, benzothiazole, benzoxazole and 1,2-benzisoxazole, are metabolized. On the other hand, the heterocycles, benzothiophene and benzofuran, which do not contain a nitrogen atom, are not metabolized by or inhibited by aldehyde oxidase. The hepatotoxic and neurotoxic 1-methyl-4-phenyl-1,2,3,6-tetrahydropyridine (MPTP) is metabolized by aldehyde oxidase to its nontoxic MP-2-pyridone metabolite (MPTP lactam). Both aldehyde oxidase and xanthine oxidase contribute to the first-pass hepatic metabolism of orally administered methotrexate (a 2,4-diaminopteridine) to its 7-hydroxymethotrexate metabolite.

Potent inhibitors of aldehyde oxidase include the selective estrogen receptor modulator raloxifene, tamoxifen, estradiol, and ethinyl estradiol. Other classes of drugs that demonstrate inhibition of aldehyde oxidase included phenothiazines, tricyclic antidepressants, tricyclic atypical antipsychotic agents, dihydropyridine calcium channel blockers, loratadine, cyclobenzaprine, amodiaquine, maprotiline, ondansetron, propafenone, domperidone, quinacrine, ketoconazole, verapamil, tacrine, and salmeterol. Thus, the possibility of clinical drug interactions mediated by inhibition of this aldehyde oxidase could be observed between these drugs and drugs for which aldehyde oxidase is the primary route of metabolism.

Xanthine Oxidase and Xanthine Dehydrogenase Xanthine oxidase and xanthine dehydrogenase represent different forms of the same gene product and are involved in the oxidative metabolism of purines with the formation of the uric acids. Xanthine dehydrogenase can be converted to xanthine oxidase by reversible sulfhydryl oxidation; xanthine dehydrogenase and xanthine oxidase are interconvertible.

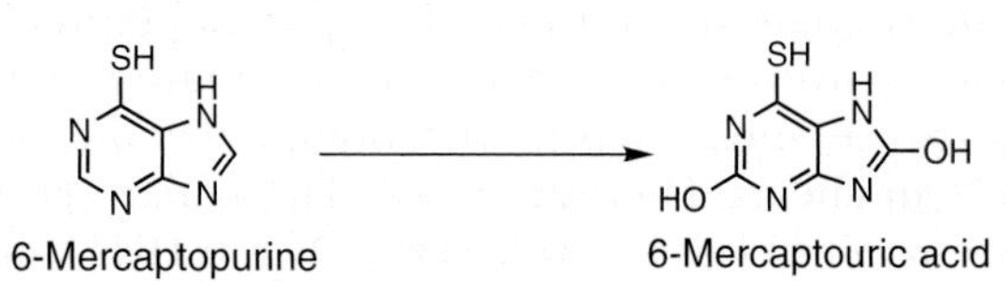

These two enzyme forms and their reactions often are referred to as xanthine oxidoreductase. Xanthine oxidase is the rate-limiting enzyme in human purine catabolism of hypoxanthine to uric acid and can also generate ROS. Xanthine oxidase is a cytosolic 370-kDa molybdoflavoenzyme that requires a molybdopterin cofactor, two iron-sulfur centers, and FAD. Both xanthine oxidase and xanthine dehydrogenase have important roles in the metabolism of a number of purine anticancer drugs to their active and inactive metabolites. Although xanthine oxidase is strongly inhibited by the antigout drug allopurinol, aldehyde oxidase also oxidizes it to oxypurinol. Only xanthine dehydrogenase requires NAD^+ as an electron acceptor for the oxidation of azaheterocycles. 6-Mercaptopurine is metabolized by xanthine oxidase to 6-mercapturic acid. In humans, xanthine oxidase is normally found in the liver and not free in the blood. Xanthinuria is a rare genetic disorder where the lack of xanthine oxidase leads to high concentration of xanthine in blood and can cause health problems such as renal failure. There is no specific treatment for this disorder except to avoid foods high in purine and to maintain a high fluid intake.

Oxidative Deamination of Amines

Monoamine oxidase (MAO) and diamine oxidase catalyze oxidative deamination of amines to the aldehydes in the presence of oxygen. The aldehyde products can be metabolized further to the corresponding alcohol or acid by aldehyde oxidase or dehydrogenase.

Monoamine Oxidase

MAO is a mitochondrial membrane flavin-containing enzyme that catalyzes the oxidative deamination of monoamines where oxygen is used to remove an amine group from a monoamine substrate, resulting in the formation of the corresponding aldehyde and ammonia according to the following equation:

$$R\text{–}CH_2\text{–}NH_2 + O_2 \rightarrow [R\text{–}CH{=}NH] \rightarrow R\text{–}CHO + NH_4$$

Substrates for this enzyme include monoamines and secondary and tertiary amines in which the amine substrates are methyl groups. The amine must be attached to an unsubstituted methylene group, and compounds having substitution at the α-carbon atom are poor substrates for MAO (e.g., aniline, amphetamine, and ephedrine) but are oxidized by the P450 enzymes rather than by MAO (Fig. 4.13). For secondary and tertiary amines, alkyl groups larger than a methyl and branched alkyl groups (i.e., isopropyl, *t*-butyl, or β-phenylisopropyl) inhibit MAO oxidation, but such substrates can function as reversible inhibitors of MAO. Nonselective irreversible inhibitors of MAO include hydrazides (phenelzine) and tranylcypromine and the MAO-B selective inhibitors pargyline and selegiline. MAO is important in regulating the metabolic degradation of catecholamines and serotonin in neural tissues, and hepatic MAO has a crucial defensive role in inactivating circulating monoamines or those that originated in the gastrointestinal tract and were absorbed into the systemic circulation (e.g., tyramine).

There are two types of MAO: MAO-A and MAO-B. They show dissimilar substrate preferences and different sensitivities to inhibitors. MAO-A is found mainly in peripheral adrenergic nerve terminals and shows substrate preference for 5-hydroxytryptamine, norepinephrine, and epinephrine, and is also found in the liver, gastrointestinal tract, and placenta. MAO-B is found principally in platelets and shows selectivity for nonphenolic, lipophilic β-phenethylamines. Common substrates to both MAO-A and MAO-B are dopamine, tyramine, and other monophenolic phenylethylamines.

A contaminant in the synthesis of reversed esters of meperidine, MPTP, was discovered to be a highly selective neurotoxin for dopaminergic cells, producing parkinsonism (see also Chapter 13) (47). The neurotoxicity of MPTP is associated with cellular destruction in the substantia nigra along with severe reductions in the concentration of dopamine, norepinephrine, and serotonin. The neurotoxic action for MPTP involves a sequence of events beginning with the metabolic activation of MPTP to the toxic metabolite MPP^+ (1-methyl-4-phenylpyridinium ion) by MAO-B, specific uptake and accumulation of MPP^+ in the nigrostriatal dopaminergic neurons, and ending with the inhibition of oxidative phosphorylation (of NADH dehydrogenase in complex I). This inhibition results in mitochondrial injury, depriving the sensitive nigrostriatal cells of oxidative phosphorylation with their eventual cell death (neurotoxic actions of MPP^+). The MAO-B inhibitors (e.g., deprenyl) blocked this biotransformation.

MPTP　　　MPP^+

Because of the vital role that MAOs have in the inactivation of neurotransmitters, MAO dysfunction (too much or too little MAO activity) is thought to be responsible for a number of neurologic disorders. For example, unusually high or low levels of MAOs in the body have been associated with depression, schizophrenia, substance abuse, attention deficit disorder, and migraines. Monoamine oxidase inhibitors (MAOIs) are one of the major classes of drugs prescribed for the treatment of depression, although they are last-line treatment due to risk of the drugs interacting with diet or other drugs. Excessive levels of catecholamines (epinephrine, norepinephrine, and dopamine) may lead to a hypertensive crisis, and excessive levels of serotonin may lead to serotonin syndrome.

Diamines, such as $H_2N\text{-}(CH_2)_n\text{-}NH_2$, in which n is less than six, are not attacked and show little affinity for MAO. If the intermolecular distance between the amine groups is increased, the rate of oxidation by MAO increases.

Evidently, the second amine group interferes with attachment of the amine to the enzyme.

Diamine Oxidase

Diamine oxidase, a flavin-containing enzyme, catalyzes the aerobic oxidation of diamines and histamine in much the same way that MAO attacks monoamines, forming aldehydes. This enzyme is inhibited by carbonyl-blocking reagents and produces hydrogen peroxide, supporting the role of pyridoxal phosphate and the flavin prosthetic groups in the catalytic action of the enzyme. Diamine oxidase is found in the cytosolic fraction, kidneys, intestines, liver, lung, and nervous tissue. It limits the biologic effects of histamine and the polymethylene amines putrescine and cadaverine. It also attacks monoamines, but at a higher substrate concentration.

$H_2N\text{-}(CH_2)_4\text{-}NH_2$ — Putrescine

$H_2N\text{-}(CH_2)_5\text{-}NH_2$ — Cadaverine

Plasma amine oxidases are in blood plasma of mammals and include spermine oxidase, which deaminates spermine and other polyamines.

Miscellaneous Reductions

Disulfides (e.g., disulfiram), sulfoxides (e.g., dimethylsulfoxide), *N*-oxides, double bonds such as those in progestational steroids, and dehydroxylation of aromatic and aliphatic hydroxyl derivatives are examples of reductions occurring in microsomal or nonmicrosomal (cytosol enzymes) fractions.

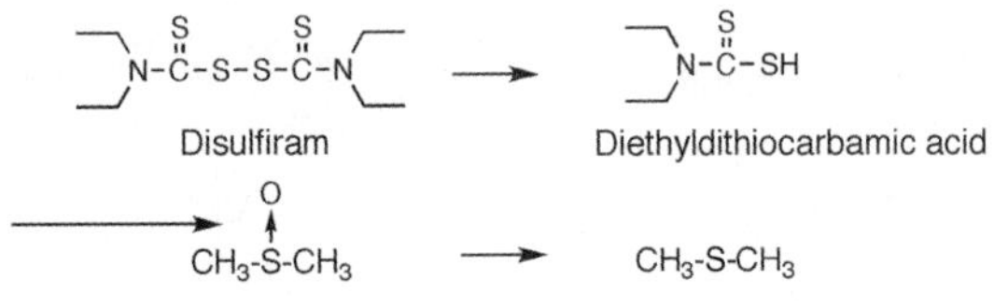

Various studies regarding the biotransformation of xenobiotic ketones have established that ketone reduction is an important metabolic pathway in mammalian tissue. Because carbonyl compounds are lipophilic and can be retained in tissues, their reduction to the hydrophilic alcohols and subsequent conjugation are critical to their elimination. Although ketone reductases (carbonyl reductases) can be closely related to the alcohol dehydrogenases, they have distinctly different properties and use NADPH as the cofactor. Carbonyl reductase participates in arachidonic acid metabolism. The metabolism of xenobiotic ketones to free alcohols or conjugated alcohols has been demonstrated for aromatic, aliphatic, alicyclic, and unsaturated ketones (e.g., naltrexone, naloxone, hydromorphone, and daunorubicin). The carbonyl reductases are distinguished by the stereospecificity of their alcohol metabolites.

β-Oxidation

Alkyl carboxylic acids, as their coenzyme A (CoA) thioesters, are metabolized by oxidation at the β-carbon to the carboxylic carbon (β-oxidation). This pathway involves the oxidative cleavage of two carbon units at a time (as acetate), beginning at the carboxyl terminus and continuing until no more acetate units can be removed. The reaction is terminated when a branch (e.g., valproic acid) or aromatic group is encountered. The metabolism of even and odd phenylalkyl acids can serve as an example:

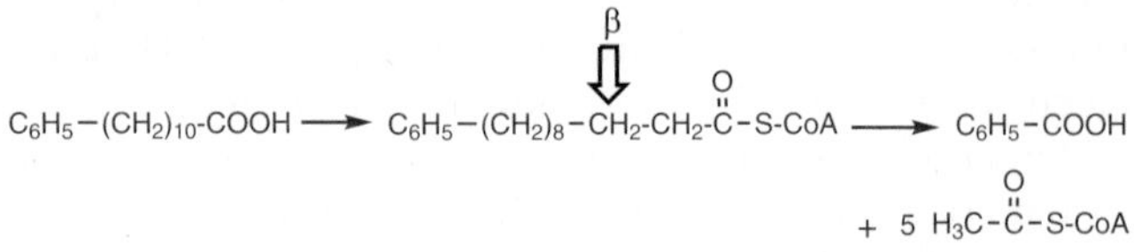

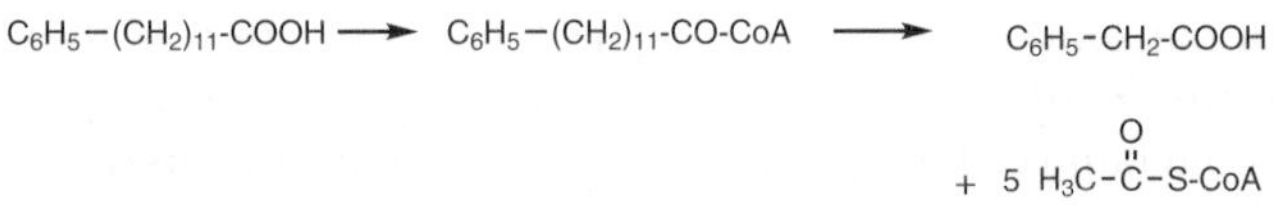

Hydrolysis

In general, esters and amides are hydrolyzed by enzymes in the blood, liver microsomes, intestine, kidneys, and other tissues. Esters and certain amides are rapidly hydrolyzed by a group of enzymes termed "carboxylesterases." The more lipophilic the amide, the more favorable it is as a substrate for this enzyme. In most cases, the hydrolysis of an ester or amide bond in a toxic substance results in bioinactivation to hydrophilic metabolites that are readily excreted. Some of these metabolites can yield conjugated metabolites (i.e., glucuronides). Amides are very common in food as proteins and peptides we eat. Not surprisingly, there are a large number of proteolytic enzymes in the gastrointestinal tract called amino endopeptidases and amino exopeptidases that hydrolyze ingested proteins into amino acids.

Carboxylesterases include cholinesterase (pseudocholinesterase), arylcarboxyesterases, liver microsomal carboxylesterases, and other unclassified liver carboxylesterases. Cholinesterase hydrolyzes choline-like esters (e.g., acetylcholine, succinylcholine) and procaine as well as acetylsalicylic acid. Genetic variant forms of cholinesterase have been identified in human serum (e.g., succinylcholine toxicity when administered as a ganglionic blocker for muscle relaxation). Meperidine is hydrolyzed only by liver microsomal carboxylesterases (Fig. 4.19). Diphenoxylate is hydrolyzed to its active metabolite diphenoxylic acid within 1 hour (Fig. 4.19). Presumably, the lack of a central pharmacologic action of diphenoxylate is attributed to the formation of a zwitterionic diphenoxylic acid, which is readily eliminated in the urine.

A distinct type of esterase is the enzyme serum paraoxonase (PON), which appears to act as an important guardian against the neurotoxicity of organophosphates and functions as an antioxidant by preventing the oxidation

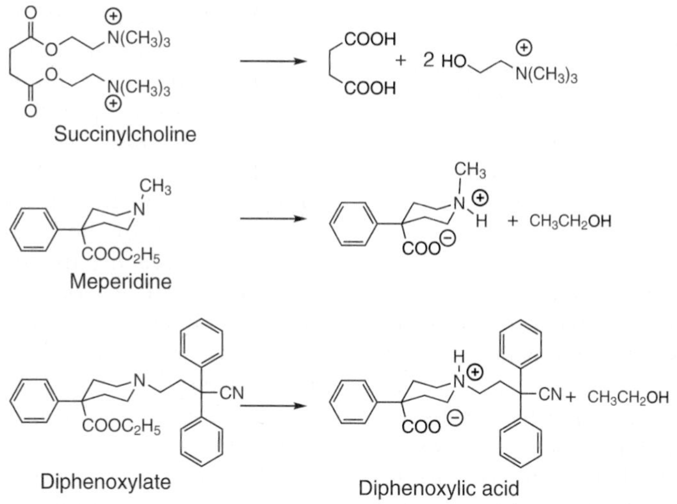

FIGURE 4.19 Examples of hydrolysis reactions.

of low-density lipoprotein (LDL), lowering the risk of developing coronary artery disease and atherosclerosis (55). The PON1 (A-esterase) is similar to an arylesterase in that it catalyzes the hydrolysis of phenyl acetate and other aryl esters. Without PON1, the organophosphate is free to react with and irreversibly inhibit acetylcholinesterase (see Chapter 9). Additionally, PON1 exhibits a substrate-dependent polymorphism. Individuals who are susceptible to the toxic effects of organophosphates such as paraoxon and chlorpyrifos (Dursban) are deficient in this isoenzyme. PON2 is an intracellular protein found in a variety of cell that protects cells against oxidative damage, and PON3 is similar to PON1 in activity but differs from it in substrate specificity.

Esters that are sterically hindered are hydrolyzed more slowly and can appear unchanged in the urine. For example, approximately 50% of a dose of atropine appears unchanged in the urine of humans, and the remainder of atropine appears to consist of unhydrolyzed biotransformed products.

As a rule, amides are more stable to esterase hydrolysis than are esters, and it is not surprising to find amides of drugs excreted largely unchanged. This fact has been exploited in developing the antiarrhythmic drug procainamide. Procaine is not useful as a result of its rapid esterase hydrolysis, but 60% of a dose of procainamide was recovered unchanged from the urine of humans, with the remainder being mostly *N*-acetylprocainamide. On the other hand, the deacylated metabolite of indomethacin (a tertiary amide) is one of the major metabolites detected in human urine. Amide hydrolysis of phthalylsulfathiazole and succinylsulfathiazole by bacterial enzymes in the colon releases the antibacterial agent sulfathiazole.

SUMMARY

Phase 1 metabolic transformations introduce new and polar functional groups into the molecule, which can produce one or more of the following changes:

1. Decreased pharmacologic activity (deactivation)
2. Increased pharmacologic activity (activation)
3. Increased toxicity (carcinogenesis, mutagenesis, cytotoxicity)
4. Altered pharmacologic activity

Drugs exhibiting increased activity or activity different from the parent drug usually undergo further metabolism and conjugation resulting in deactivation and excretion of the inactive conjugates.

DRUG CONJUGATION PATHWAYS (PHASE 2)

Conjugation reactions represent probably the most important xenobiotic biotransformation reaction (7,56–58). Xenobiotics are as a rule lipophilic, well absorbed from the blood, but excreted slowly in the urine. Only after conjugation (Phase 2) reactions have added an ionic hydrophilic moiety, such as glucuronic acid, sulfate ester, or glycine, to the xenobiotic is water solubility increased and lipid solubility decreased enough to make urinary elimination possible. The major proportion of the administered drug dose is excreted as conjugates into the urine and bile. Conjugation reactions can be preceded by Phase 1 reactions. For xenobiotics with a functional group available for conjugation, conjugation can be its fate.

The major conjugation reactions (glucuronidation and sulfonation) were traditionally thought to terminate pharmacologic activity by transforming the parent drug or Phase 1 metabolites into readily excreted ionic polar products (7,56). Moreover, these terminal metabolites would have no significant pharmacologic activity (i.e., poor cellular diffusion and affinity for the active drug's receptor). This long-established view has changed with the discoveries that morphine 6-glucuronide has more analgesic activity than morphine in humans and that minoxidil sulfate is the active metabolite for the antihypertensive minoxidil. For most xenobiotics, conjugation

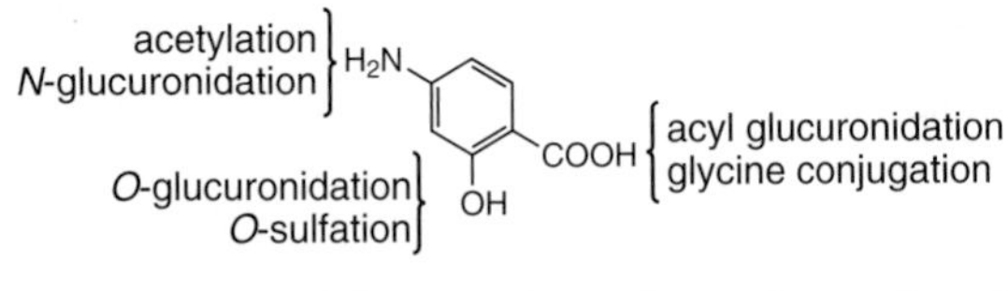

FIGURE 4.20 Sequential conjugation pathways for *p*-aminosalicylic acid.

is a detoxification mechanism. However, some compounds could form reactive intermediates that have been implicated in carcinogenesis, allergic reactions, and tissue damage.

Sequential conjugation of the same drug substance produces multiple conjugated products, for example *p*-aminosalicylic acid in Figure 4.20. Thus, the drug or xenobiotic can be a substrate for more than one metabolizing enzyme. Different conjugation pathways could compete for the same functional group with the outcome being an array of metabolites excreted in the urine or feces. Factors determining the outcome of this interplay include availability of cosubstrates, enzyme kinetics (V_{max}), affinity of the drug/xenobiotic (K_m) for the metabolizing enzyme, and type of tissues (e.g., hepatic, kidney, lung). When a cosubstrate is low or depleted, the competing conjugation reactions can take control. The reactivity of the functional group is also determined by all subsequent conjugation reactions. For example, major conjugation reactions are sulfonation, ether glucuronidation, and methylation for the phenolic hydroxyl groups; acetylation, sulfonation, and glucuronidation for amine groups; and amino acid conjugation, CoA conjugation, and ester glucuronidation for carboxyl groups.

Conjugation enzymes can show stereospecificity toward enantiomers when a racemic drug is administered. The metabolite pattern of the same drug when administered orally can be different when administered intravenously as a result of presystemic intestinal conjugation.

Glucuronic Acid Conjugation

Glucuronide formation is probably the major and most common route for Phase 2 metabolism to water-soluble metabolites, which accounts for the major share of the conjugated metabolites found in the urine and bile (7,56). The significance of glucuronidation lies in the available supply of glucuronic acid in the liver and in the many functional groups forming glucuronide conjugates (e.g., phenols, alcohols, carboxylic acids, and amines).

Mechanism of Glucuronide Conjugation

Glucuronide conjugation involves the direct condensation of the xenobiotic (or its Phase 1 product) with the activated form of glucuronic acid, UDP–glucuronic acid (UDPGA). The overall scheme of the glucuronide conjugation reaction is shown in Figure 4.21. The reaction between UDPGA and acceptor compound is catalyzed by a family of UDP–glucuronosyl transferases (UGT), a multigene family of isozymes located along the ER of liver, epithelial cells of the intestine, and other extrahepatic tissues. Its unique location in the ER along with the P450 isoforms has important physiologic effects in the neutralization of reactive metabolites generated by the P450 isoforms and in controlling the levels of reactive metabolites present in these tissues (Fig. 4.22).This cartoon depicts the spatial orientation and the interrelationship of the ER membrane–bound enzymes such as P450, UGTs, and membrane-bound transporters (57). The transporters carry the UDPGA and xenobiotics (D) from the cytosol into the ER lumen and then transport the glucuronide metabolite from the ER lumen into the cytosol. The presence of the active site for UGT toward the ER lumen catalyzes the reaction between the substrate and UDPGA. Glucuronidation is a low-affinity and high-capacity Phase 2 reaction. The resultant glucuronide has the β-configuration about carbon 1 of glucuronic acid. With the attachment of the hydrophilic carbohydrate moiety containing an easily ionizable carboxyl group (pK_a = 3–4), a lipid-soluble substance is converted into a conjugate that is reabsorbed poorly by the renal tubules from the urine and excreted more readily into the urine or, in some cases, into the bile. Endogenous substances conjugated with glucuronic acid include catecholamines, steroids, bilirubin, and thyroxine. Not all glucuronides are excreted by the kidneys. Some are excreted into the intestinal tract with bile (enterohepatic cycling), where β-glucuronidase in the intestinal flora hydrolyzes the C^1-*O*-glucuronide to the aglycone (xenobiotic or their metabolites) for reabsorption into the portal circulation (see section on enterohepatic cycling).

UGT Families

UGTs have been classified into families according to similarities in amino acid sequences, analogous to the P450 family. The human UGT family is divided into two subfamilies, UGT1 (UGT1A1, 1A2, 1A3, 1A4, 1A5, 1A6, 1A7, 1A8, 1A9, and 1A10) and UGT2 (UGT2B4, 2B7, 2B10, 2B11, 2B15, 2B17, and 2B28) (7,58). Considerable overlap in substrate specificities exists between the two families. UGT1A1 isoform is primarily responsible for the glucuronidation of bilirubin, estradiol, and other estrogenic steroids; UGT1A3 and UGT1A4 catalyze the glucuronidation of drugs with tertiary amines to form quaternary glucuronides and hydroxylated xenobiotics; UGT1A6 exhibits limited substrate specificity for planar phenolic substances; UGT1A9 has a wide range of substrate specificity and can glucuronidate nonplanar phenols, plant substances (e.g., anthraquinones and flavones), steroids, other phenolic drugs, and C-glucuronidate phenylbutazone; and UGT1A10 glucuronidates mycophenolic acid an inhibitor of inosine monophosphate dehydrogenase. Human family 2 isoform UGT2B4 is homologous to UGT2B7 and catalyzes

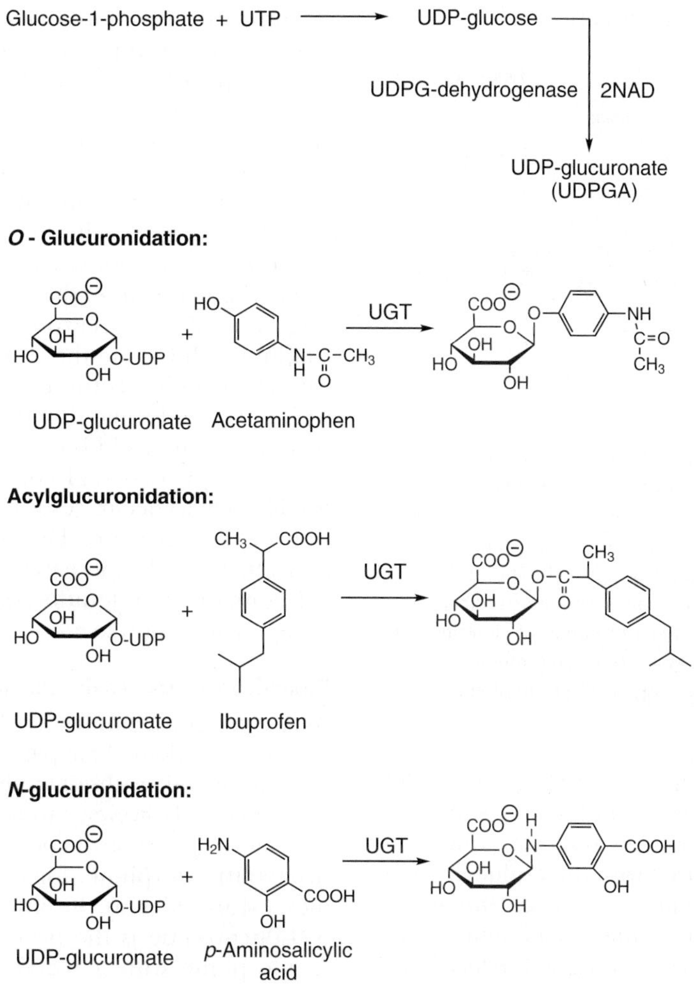

FIGURE 4.21 Glucuronidation pathway catalyzed by UDP-glucuronosyl transferases (UGTs).

the glucuronidation of the 6α-hydroxyl group of bile acids; UGT2B7 glucuronidates the largest number of substrates including the 3- and 6-glucuronidation of morphine and 6-glucuronidation of codeine; UGT2B11 glucuronidates a wide range of planar phenols, bulky alcohols, and polyhydroxylated estradiol metabolites; and UGT2B15 catalyzes the glucuronidation of the 17α-hydroxyl group of dihydrotestosterone and other steroidal compounds as well as phenolphthalein. UGT1A isoforms are inducible with 3-methylcholanthrene and cigarette smoking, and the UGT2B family is inducible by barbiturates. Approximately 40% of the glucuronides are produced by UGT2B7, 20% by UGT1A4, and 15% by UGT1A1.

UGT Distribution

The human liver has been established as the most important tissue for all routes of metabolism, including glucuronidation. Studies have shown that the rate of glucuronidation is not uniform in the different sections of the liver: UGT1A6 content was greatest in the middle section of the liver but can also be found in the bile duct epithelium and in the endothelium of the hepatic artery and portal vein; UGT2B2 was uniformly distributed throughout the liver. The UGTs expressed in the intestine include UGT1A1 (bilirubin-glucuronidating isoform), UGT1A3, UGT1A4, UGT1A6, UGT1A8, UGT1A9, and UGT1A5. Substrate specificities of intestinal UGT isoforms are comparable to those in the liver. The UGT isoforms in the intestine can glucuronidate orally administered drugs, such as morphine, acetaminophen, α- and β-adrenergic agonists, and other phenolic phenethanolamines, as well as other dietary xenobiotics, reducing their oral bioavailability (first-pass metabolism). Although UGT isoforms are found in kidney, brain, nasal epithelia, and lung, they are not uniformly distributed, with UGT1A6 being the isoform that is ubiquitous in extrahepatic tissue.

O-, N-, and S-Glucuronides

The xenobiotics forming glucuronides with alcohols and phenols are ether *O*-glucuronides. Aromatic and some

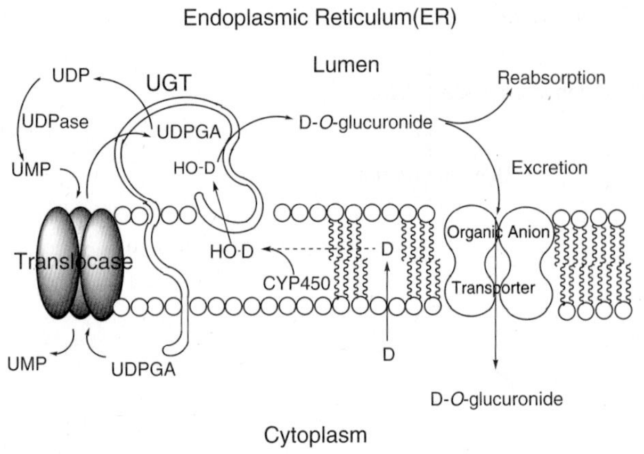

FIGURE 4.22 Proposed topologic model of UGT. A lipophilic drug (D) reaches the active site of P450 from the membrane or cytoplasm and is hydroxylated (HO-D). The hydroxylated metabolite is transferred to UGT, where glucuronidation occurs, followed by release into the lumen and excretion from the cell. The UDPGA is synthesized in the cytoplasm and transported via translocase. (Adapted from Oesch F. Metabolic transformation of clinically used drugs to epoxides: new perspectives in drug–drug interactions. Biochem Pharmacol 1976;25:1935–1937, with permission.)

aliphatic carboxylic acids form ester (acyl) glucuronides. Aromatic amines form *N*-glucuronides and sulfhydryl compounds form *S*-glucuronides, both of which are more labile to acid as compared with the *O*-glucuronides (Fig. 4.21). Some tertiary amines (e.g., tripelennamine) have been reported to form quaternary ammonium *N*-glucuronides. Substances containing a 1,3-dicarbonyl structure (e.g., phenylbutazone) can undergo formation of *C*-glucuronides by direct conjugation without previous metabolism. The acidity of the methylene carbon of the 1,3-dicarbonyl group determines the degree of *C*-glucuronide formation.

Acyl Glucuronides

Drug–acyl glucuronides are reactive conjugates at physiologic pH. The acyl group of the C^1-acyl glucuronide can migrate via transesterification from the original C-1 position of the glucuronic acid to the C-2, C-3, or C-4 positions (Fig. 4.21). The resulting positional isomers are not hydrolyzed by β-glucuronidase, giving the appearance of a new unknown conjugate. However, under physiologic or weakly alkaline conditions, the C^1-acyl glucuronide can hydrolyze in the urine to produce the parent substance (aglycone) or undergo acyl migration to an acceptor macromolecule, forming an immunoreactive hapten. The pH-catalyzed migration of the acyl group from the drug C^1-*O*-acyl glucuronide to a protein or other cellular constituent occurs with the formation of a covalent bond to the protein (59). The acylated protein becomes a "hapten" and could stimulate an immune response against the drug, resulting in the expression of a hypersensitivity reaction or other forms of immunotoxicity. A high incidence of anaphylactic reactions has been reported for several NSAIDs, for example, benoxaprofen, zomepirac, indoprofen, alclofenac, ticrynafen, and ibufenac, which have been removed from the market. All of these NSAIDs are metabolized by humans to acyl glucuronides. Similar reactions have been reported for other NSAIDs, including tolmetin, sulindac, ibuprofen, ketoprofen, and acetylsalicylic acid. The frequency of the immunotoxic response can be related to the stability of the acyl glucuronide, the chemical rate kinetics for the migration of the acyl group, and the concentration and stability/half-life of the antigenic protein. When the acyl glucuronide is the primary metabolite in patients with decreased renal function (i.e., elderly individuals) or when probenecid is coadministered, renal cycling of the unconjugated (aglycone) parent drug or metabolite is likely to occur, resulting in the plasma accumulation of the aglycone. The reduced elimination of the acyl glucuronide increases its hydrolysis to either the aglycone or the migration of the C^1-*O*-acyl group to an acceptor macromolecule.

Bioactivation and Toxic Glucuronides

As a rule, glucuronides are biologically and chemically less reactive than their parent molecules and are readily eliminated without interaction with intracellular substances. However, some glucuronide conjugates are more pharmacologically active than the parent drug (60). Morphine, for example, forms the 3-*O*- and 6-*O*-glucuronides in the intestine and in the liver. The 3-*O*-glucuronide is the primary glucuronide metabolite of morphine with a blood concentration 20-fold that of morphine. Pharmacologically, it is an opiate antagonist. On the other hand, 6-*O*-glucuronide, with a blood concentration twice that of morphine, is a more potent μ-receptor agonist and, whether administered orally or parentally, is 650-fold more analgesic than morphine in humans. Thus, the analgesic effects of morphine are the result of a complex interaction of the drug and its two glucuronide metabolites with the opiate receptor. The 6-*O*-glucuronide is transported into the brain via an anion-transport system.

Glucuronidation is also capable of promoting cellular injury (e.g., hepatotoxicity and carcinogenesis) by facilitating the formation of reactive electrophilic (electron-deficient) intermediates and their transport into target tissues (37). The induction of bladder carcinogenesis by aromatic amines can result from the *O*-glucuronidation of the *N*-hydroxylarylamine. These *O*-glucuronides become concentrated in the urine where they are either hydrolyzed by the acid pH of the urine to produce *N*-hydroxylarylamines or eliminate water from the *N*-hydroxylarylamine under these acidic conditions to yield the formation of an electrophilic arylnitrenium species (see Fig. 4.26, metabolite 5). This reactive species binds covalently with endogenous cellular constituents (e.g., nucleic acids and proteins), initiating carcinogenesis.

Sulfonation and glucuronidation occur side by side, often competing for the same substrate (most commonly phenols, i.e., acetaminophen). The balance between sulfonation and glucuronidation is influenced by such factors as animal species, dose, availability of cosubstrates, and inhibition and induction of the respective transferases.

Sulfonation (Sulfo-Conjugation)

Sulfonation (sulfo-conjugation) is an important conjugation reaction in the biotransformation of steroid hormones, catecholamine neurotransmitters, thyroxine, bile acids, phenolic drugs, and other xenobiotics (7,61,62). The major physiologic consequence of sulfonation of a drug or xenobiotic is its increased aqueous solubility and excretion, because the pK_a of the sulfate group is approximately 1 to 2. Sulfate esters are almost totally ionized in physiologic solution and possess a smaller volume of distribution than unconjugated steroids and drugs. For some drugs, sulfonation can result in their bioactivation to reactive electrophiles or therapeutically active conjugates (e.g., minoxidil sulfate). Cytosolic sulfotransferases are, in general, associated with the sulfonation of phenolic steroids, neurotransmitters, and xenobiotics. Membrane-bound sulfotransferases are localized in the Golgi apparatus of most cells and are responsible for the sulfonation of glycosaminoglycans, glycoproteins, and the tyrosinyl group of peptides and protein but are usually not associated with xenobiotic metabolism.

Mechanism of Sulfonation

Xenobiotics are sulfonated by the transfer of a sulfonic group (-SO_3^-) from 3′-phosphoadenosine-5′-phosphosulfate (PAPS) to the acceptor molecule, a cytosolic reaction catalyzed by a family of multigene sulfotransferases (Fig. 4.23); PAPS is formed enzymatically from adenosine triphosphate (ATP) and inorganic sulfate. Sulfonation is a reaction principally of phenols and, to a lesser extent, of alcohols to form highly ionic and hydrophilic sulfate esters (R-O-SO_2H). The availability of PAPS and its precursor inorganic sulfate determines the sulfonation reaction rate.

The total pool of sulfate is frequently limited and can be readily exhausted due to the large number of substrates. Sulfonation is a high-affinity and low-capacity Phase 2 reaction that works in conjunction with glucuronidation on overlapping substrates. Thus, sulfonation predominates at low substrate concentrations, and glucuronidation predominates at high substrate concentrations (62). Thus, when sulfonation becomes saturated from increasing doses of a drug, sulfonation becomes a less predominant pathway, and the rate of glucuronidation increases until it reaches saturation and the drug is either excreted unchanged or other metabolism pathways become activated. For example, at high doses of acetaminophen, glucuronidation more often than not predominates over that of sulfonation, which prevails at low doses. Other precursors for sulfate include L-methionine and L-cysteine. When PAPS, inorganic sulfate, or the sulfur amino acids are low or depleted or when a substrate for sulfonation is given in high doses, competing reactions with glucuronidation can take control. Additionally, *O*-methylation is a competing reaction for a catecholamine.

Sulfotransferase Family

In humans, sulfotransferases are divided into two families, SULT1 and SULT2 (61). SULT1A1, SULT1A2, and SULT1A3 catalyze the sulfonation of many phenolic drugs, catecholamine, hormones, aromatic amines, and other xenobiotics (62). SULT1A1/2 (formerly known as phenol sulfotransferase thermally stable) preferentially sulfonates small planar phenols in the micromolar concentration range, estradiol and synthetic estrogens, phytoestrogens, acetaminophen, the *N*-oxide of minoxidil, and *N*-hydroxyaromatic and heterocyclic amines. The crystal structure for SULT1A1 has provided insights into this enzyme's substrate specificity and catalytic function, including its role in the sulfonation of endogenous substrates such as estrogens. SULT1A3 (formerly known as phenol sulfotransferase thermally labile) selectively sulfonates the catecholamines dopamine, norepinephrine, and epinephrine, as well as the *N*-oxide of minoxidil and thyroid hormones, but not estrogenic steroids and other hydroxy

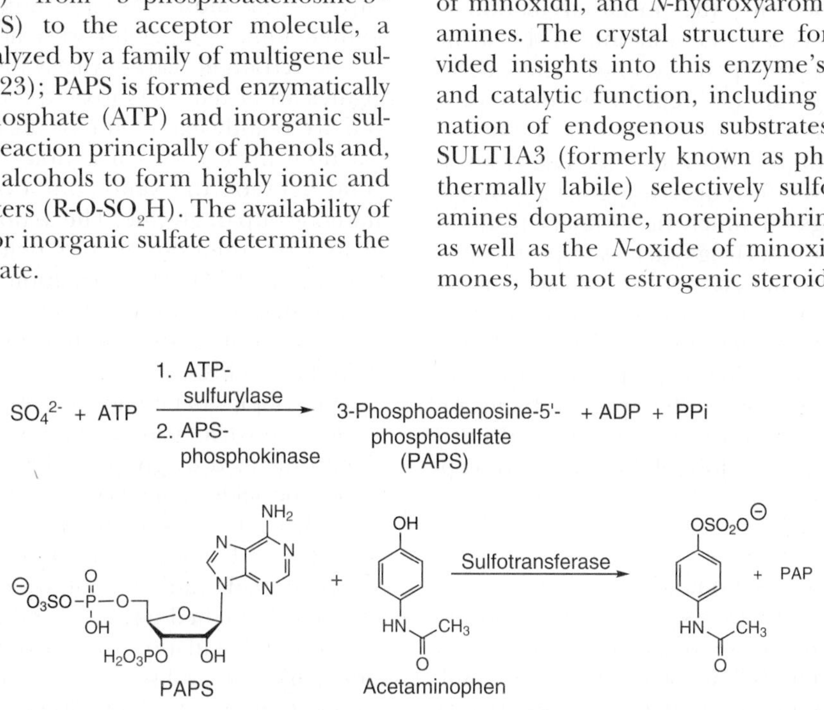

FIGURE 4.23 Sulfonation pathways.

steroids; SULT1B1 catalyzes the sulfonation of the thyroid hormones; SULT1C1 is involved with the bioactivation of procarcinogens via sulfonation; SULT1E1 (formerly known as estrogen sulfotransferase) preferentially sulfonates estradiol in the nanomolar range; SULT2A1 (formerly known as dehydroepiandrosterone [DHEA] sulfotransferase) conjugates DHEA, estradiol (micromolar range), the synthetic estrogens, and other estrogen metabolites; and SULT2B1 (formerly known as hydroxysteroid sulfotransferase) sulfonates DHEA and pregnenolone.

Sulfonation is an important reaction in the transport and metabolism of steroids. Sulfonation decreases the biologic activity of the steroid because the steroid sulfate esters are not capable of binding to their receptors. It provides for the transport of an inactive form of the steroid to its target tissue, where the active steroid is regenerated by sulfatases at the target tissue.

Sulfotransferase Distribution

The SULT1A families are abundantly expressed in the liver, small intestine, brain, kidneys, and platelets (61). For example, phenol is sulfonated by a sulfotransferase in the liver, kidneys, and intestines, whereas steroids are sulfonated only in the liver. The broad diversity of compounds sulfonated in human tissues results, in part, from the multi-isoforms of the cytosolic sulfotransferases and their overlapping substrate specificities. Sulfate esters are almost totally ionized and, therefore, are excreted mostly in the urine, but biliary elimination is common for steroids. When biliary sulfate esters are hydrolyzed in the intestine by sulfatases, the parent drug (or xenobiotic) or its metabolites can be reabsorbed into the portal circulation to be resulfonated for eventual elimination in the urine as a sulfate ester (enterohepatic cycling). The rate of sulfonation appears to be age dependent, decreasing with age. An important site of sulfonation, especially after oral administration, is the intestine. The result is a presystemic first-pass effect, decreasing drug bioavailability of several drugs for which the primary route of conjugation is sulfonation. Drugs such as isoproterenol, albuterol, steroid hormones, α-methyldopa, acetaminophen, and fenoldopam are sulfonated. Competition for intestinal sulfonation between coadministered substrates can influence their bioavailability with either an enhancement of or a decrease in therapeutic effects. An example would be coadministration of a 500-mg dose of acetaminophen and 0.03-mg dose of the oral contraceptive ethinyl estradiol.

Bioactivation and Toxicity

As with glucuronidation, sulfonation is a detoxication reaction, although sulfate esters have been reported to be pharmacologically active (e.g., minoxidil sulfate, dehydroepiandrosterone sulfate, and morphine 6-sulfate) or to be converted into unstable sulfate esters that form reactive intermediates implicated in carcinogenesis and tissue damage (62). SULT1A1 can also sulfonate procarcinogens such as hydroxymethyl polycyclic aromatic hydrocarbons producing reactive intermediates capable of forming DNA adducts, potentially resulting in mutagenesis. Sulfonation of an alcohol generates a good leaving group and can be an activation process for alcohols to produce a reactive electrophilic species (37). However, like the *N*-glucuronides, *N*-sulfates are capable of promoting cytotoxicity by facilitating the formation of reactive electrophilic intermediates. Sulfonation of *N*-oxygenated aromatic amines is an activation process for some arylamines that can eliminate sulfate to produce an electrophilic species capable of reacting with proteins or DNA (e.g., 2-acetylaminofluorene). *N*-sulfonation of arylamines to arylsulfamic acids (R-$NHSO_3H$) is a minor pathway.

Stereoselectivity

SULT1A3 displays stereoselectivity in the sulfonation of chiral phenolic phenethanolamines. This isoform can be responsible, in part, for the enantiomer-specific metabolism observed for the β-adrenergic agonists. For example, the (+)-enantiomers of terbutaline and isoproterenol and the (−)-enantiomer of albuterol are selectively sulfonated.

Conjugation with Amino Acids

Conjugation with amino acids is an important metabolic route in the metabolism of drug or xenobiotic carboxylic acids before elimination (56). This pathway is low in the newborn and could contribute to the toxicity of administered benzoic acid derivatives (e.g., the bacterial preservative benzyl alcohol in intravenous fluids). Glycine, the most common amino acid, forms water-soluble ionic conjugates with aromatic, arylaliphatic, and heterocyclic carboxylic acids. These glycine conjugates are usually less toxic than their precursor acids and are readily excreted into the urine and bile. These reactions involve the formation of an amide or peptide bond between the xenobiotic carboxylic acid and the amino group of glycine. The xenobiotic is first activated to its CoA thioester before reacting with the amino group (Fig. 4.24). The formation of the xenobiotic acyl CoA thioester is of critical importance in intermediary metabolism of lipids as well as intermediate- and long-chain fatty acids.

The major metabolic biotransformations for xenobiotic carboxylic acids include conjugation with either glucuronic acid or glycine. The metabolic fate of these carboxylic acids depends on the size and type of substituents adjacent to the carboxyl group. Most unbranched aliphatic acids are completely oxidized by β-oxidation to acetic acids and do not typically form conjugates, although branched aliphatic and arylaliphatic acids are resistant to β-oxidation and form glycine or acyl glucuronide conjugates: substitution of the α-carbon favors glucuronidation rather than glycine conjugation. Benzoic and heterocyclic aromatic acids are mostly conjugated

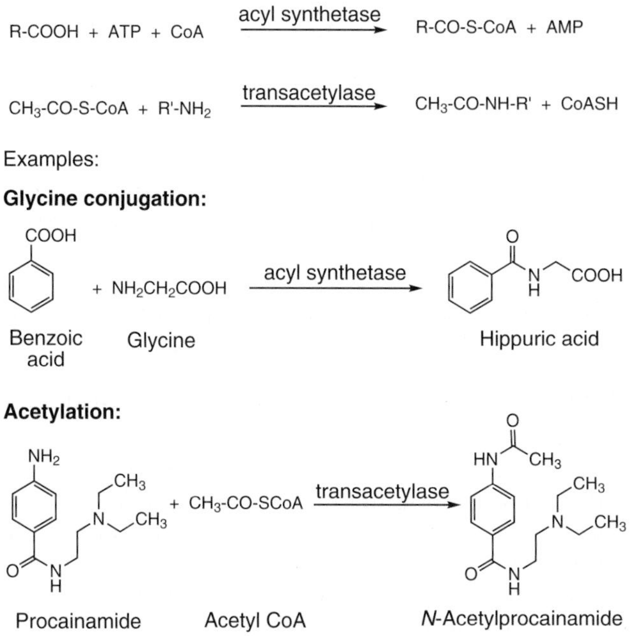

FIGURE 4.24 Amino acid conjugation pathways of carboxylic acids with glycine and acetylation pathways.

with glycine. Glycine conjugation is preferred for xenobiotic carboxylic acids at low doses, and glucuronidation is preferred at high doses with broad substrate selectivity. In humans, glutamine can also form a conjugate with phenylacetic acids and related arylacetic acids. Bile acids form conjugates with glycine and taurine by the action of enzymes in the microsomal fraction rather than in the mitochondria.

In contrast to the enhanced reactivity and toxicity of the various glucuronide, sulfate ester, acetyl, and glutathione conjugates, amino acid conjugates have not proven to be toxic. It has been proposed that amino acid conjugation is a detoxication pathway for reactive acyl CoA thioesters.

Conjugation with CoA

Several carboxylic acid–containing drugs (e.g., zomiperac and benzoxaprofen) have been implicated in rare but serious adverse reactions. These carboxylic acids were withdrawn from the market in the late 1980s as a result of unpredictable idiosyncratic reactions that could have been caused by carboxylic acid–protein adducts formed by reaction of their reactive acyl glucuronide or acyl CoA thioesters with endogenous proteins. Carboxylic acids can be bioactivated via two distinct pathways: UGT-catalyzed conjugation with glucuronic acid to acyl glucuronides, or acyl CoA synthetase–catalyzed formation of acyl CoA thioesters. The reactive CoA thioester intermediates of carboxylic acids are electrophilic and, therefore, can contribute to the acylation of target proteins (see Reactive Metabolites Resulting from Bioactivation and Fig. 4.30-1). Acyl CoA thioester serves as an obligatory intermediate in the formation of glycine conjugates and carnitine esters, which are involved in mitochondrial acyl transfer or elimination of acyl groups into urine. Therefore, their appearance in metabolism studies and urine is of significance, because they serve as biomarkers for the formation of acyl CoA thioesters, which can provide the link between protein-reactive acyl CoA thioesters and the rare and unpredictable idiosyncratic drug reactions in humans.

A nontoxic reaction involving acyl CoA thioesters includes chiral inversions of the 2-arylpropionic acids ("profens"), a major group of NSAIDs that exist in two enantiomeric forms (59). The anti-inflammatory activity (inhibition of cyclooxygenase) for the NSAIDs resides with the *S*-(+)-enantiomer. The intriguing aspect for the metabolism of the NSAIDs is their unidirectional chiral inversion from the *R*-(−)- to the *S*-(+)-enantiomer (Fig. 4.25). The NSAID acyl CoA thioester is the critical intermediate for this chiral inversion of the 2-arylpropionic acids, and the formation of the thioester is stereospecific for the pharmacologically inactive *R*-enantiomer (61). Racemic ibuprofen and related anti-inflammatory 2-arylpropionic acids (e.g., benoxaprofen, carprofen, cicliprofen, clidanac, fenoprofen, indoprofen, ketoprofen, loxoprofen, and naproxen) undergo in vivo metabolic inversion to the more active *S*-enantiomer via the formation, epimerization, and hydrolysis of their respective acyl CoA thioesters (63). The unidirectional *R*- to *S*-inversion of ibuprofen is attributed to the stereoselective thioester formation of *R*-ibuprofen CoA, not to the stereoselectivity of either the epimerization or hydrolysis steps (64). *S*-(+)-ibuprofen does not form its CoA thioester in vivo. Because the formation of 2-arylpropionyl CoA thioester is analogous to the activation and metabolism of medium and long-chain fatty acids, it seems possible that conditions either elevating (e.g., diabetes or fasting)

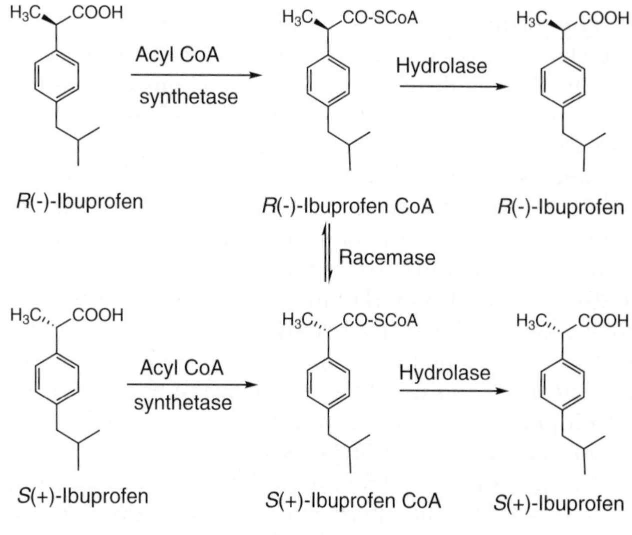

FIGURE 4.25 Coenzyme A (CoA) conjugation pathway: Stereospecific inversion of *R*(−)- to *S*(+)-ibuprofen.

or depleting CoA can alter CoA thioester formation of the 2-arylpropionic acids and their in vivo metabolic inversion. Amino acid conjugation (i.e., CoA activation) is more sensitive to steric hindrance than is glucuronidation (e.g., arylacetic acids).

Acetylation

Acetylation is principally a reaction of amino groups involving the transfer of acetyl CoA to primary aliphatic and aromatic amines, amino acids, hydrazines, or sulfonamide groups (56). The liver is the primary site of acetylation, although extrahepatic sites have been identified. Sulfonamides, being difunctional, can form either N^1 or N^4 acetyl derivatives and in some instances, the diacetylated derivative has been identified. Secondary amines are not acetylated. Acetylation can produce conjugates that retain the pharmacologic activity of the parent drug (e.g., *N*-acetylprocainamide) (Fig. 4.24).

The existence of genetic polymorphism in the rate of acetylation has important consequences for drug therapy and tumorigenicity of xenobiotics. Acetylation polymorphism has been associated with differences in human drug toxicity between the two acetylator phenotypes, slow and fast acetylators. Slow acetylators are more prone to drug-induced toxicities and accumulate higher blood concentrations of the unacetylated drug (e.g., hydralazine and procainamide-induced lupus erythematous, isoniazid-induced peripheral nerve damage, and sulfasalazine-induced hematologic disorders) than do fast acetylators. Fast acetylators eliminate the drug more rapidly by conversion to its relatively nontoxic *N*-acetyl metabolite. However, for some drug substances, fast acetylators can pose a greater risk of liver toxicity than slow acetylators because fast acetylators produce toxic metabolites more rapidly (e.g., isoniazid forms the hepatotoxic monoacetylhydrazine metabolite). Thus, differences in acetylator phenotype can influence adverse drug reactions.

The possibility arises that genetic differences in acetylating capacity can confer differences in susceptibility to chemical carcinogenicity from arylamines. The tumorigenic activity of arylamines (1 in Fig. 4.26) can be the result of a complex series of sequential metabolic reactions commencing with *N*-acetylation (2 in Fig. 4.26), subsequent oxidation to arylhydroxamic acids (3 in Fig. 4.26), and metabolic transformation to acetoxyarylamines by *N*, *O*-acyltransferase (4 in Fig. 4.26). The acetoxyarylamine can eliminate the acetoxy group to form the reactive arylnitrenium ion (5 in Fig. 4.26), which is capable of covalently binding to nucleic acids and proteins, thus increasing the risk for development of bladder and liver tumors (65). The rapid acetylator phenotype is expected to form the acetoxyarylamine metabolite at a greater rate than the slow acetylator and, thereby, to present a greater risk for development of tumors compared with the slow acetylator.

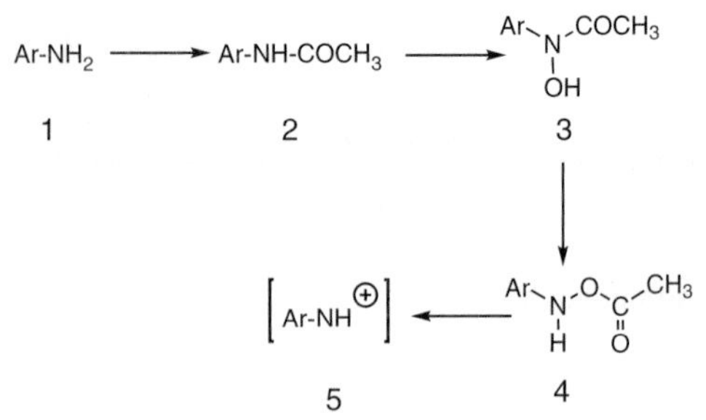

FIGURE 4.26 Bioactivation of acetylated arylamines.

Glutathione Conjugation and Mercapturic Acid Synthesis

Mercapturic acids are *S*-derivatives of *N*-acetylcysteine synthesized from glutathione (GSH) (53,54). The mercapturic acid pathway appears to have evolved as a protective mechanism against xenobiotic-induced hepatotoxicity or carcinogenicity, serving to detoxify a large number of noxious substances that we inhale or ingest or that are produced daily in the human body. Most xenobiotics that are metabolized to mercapturic acids first undergo conjugation with GSH catalyzed by the enzyme glutathione *S*-transferase (GST), a multigene isoenzyme family that is abundant in the soluble supernatant liver fractions. In humans, the GST family consists of cytosolic dimeric isoenzymes of 45 to 55 kDa size that have been assigned to at least eight classes: alpha (five members), kappa (one member), mu (six members), omega (two members), pi (one member), theta (two members), zeta (one member), and microsomal (three members). The principal drug substrates for the mu family are the nitrosourea and mustard-type anticancer drugs. The theta isoform metabolizes small organic molecules, such as solvents, halocarbons, and electrophilic compounds (e.g., α,β-unsaturated carbonyl compounds). The GSH conjugation reaction to mercapturic acid metabolites is depicted in Figure 4.27.

GST increases the ionization of the thiol group of GSH, increasing its nucleophilicity toward electrophiles and thereby increasing the rate of conjugation with these potentially harmful electrophiles, thereby protecting other vital nucleophilic centers in the cell, such as nucleic acids and proteins from these electrophiles. Glutathione is also capable of reacting nonenzymatically with nucleophilic sites on neighboring macromolecules (Fig. 4.27) (see also subsequent section on metabolic activation). Once conjugated with GSH, the electrophiles are, as a rule, excreted in the bile and urine.

A range of functional groups yields thioether conjugates of GSH as well as products other than thioethers (Fig. 4.27). The nucleophilic attack by GSH occurs on electrophilic carbons with leaving groups (e.g., halogen [alkyl, alkenyl, aryl, or aralkyl halides], sulfonates [alkylmethanesulfonates], and nitro [alkyl nitrates]

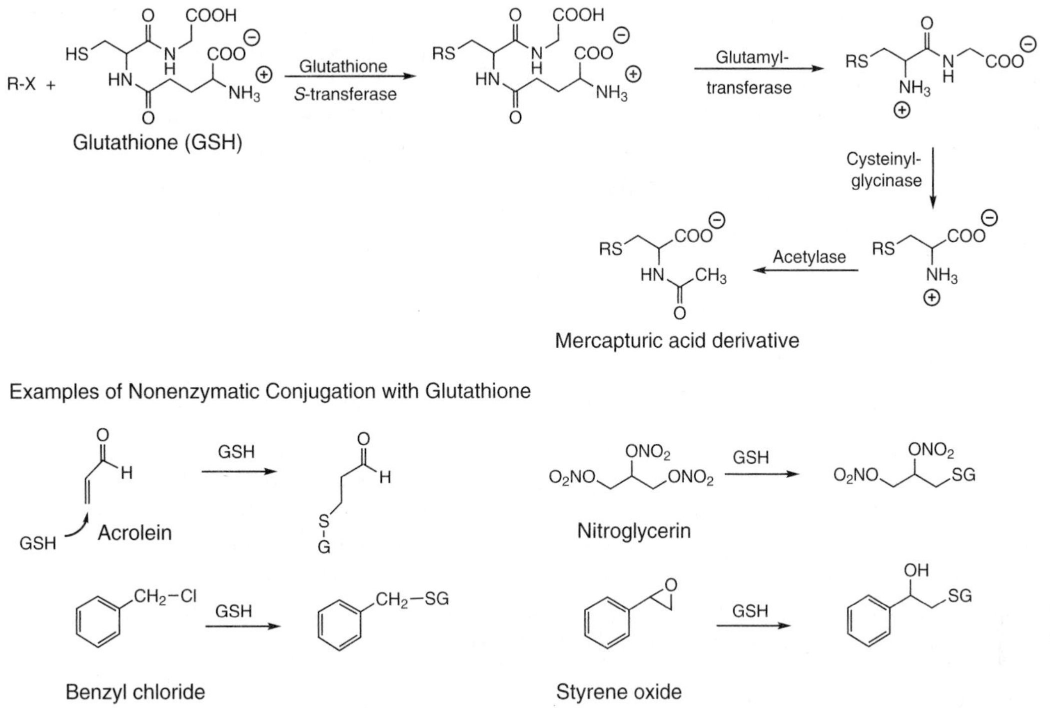

FIGURE 4.27 Glutathione and mercapturic acid conjugation pathways.

groups), ring opening of small ring ethers (epoxides and β-lactones, e.g., β-propiolactone), and the Michael-type addition to the activated β-carbon of an α,β-unsaturated carbonyl compound (e.g., acrolein) (see Reactive Metabolites Resulting from Bioactivation and Fig. 4.32A). Organic nitrate esters (e.g., the coronary vasodilator nitroglycerin) undergo a redox reaction that results in the concurrent oxidation of GSH to GSSG (through formation of the labile *S*-nitrate conjugation product) and reduction of the nitrate ester to an alcohol and inorganic nitrite. The lack of substrate specificity gives argument to the fact that glutathione transferase has undergone adaptive changes to accommodate the variety of xenobiotics to which it is exposed. The conjugation of an electrophilic compound with GSH is usually a reaction of detoxication, but in some cases, carcinogens have been activated through conjugation with GSH (29–31).

The enzymatic conjugation of GSH with epoxides provides a mechanism for protecting the liver from injury caused by certain bioactivated intermediates (see the subsequent Metabolic Bioactivation section). Not all epoxides are substrates for this enzyme, but the more chemically reactive epoxides appear to be better substrates. Important among the epoxides that are substrates for this enzyme are those produced from halobenzenes and PAHs through the action of a P450 monooxygenase. Epoxide formation represents bioactivation, because the epoxides are reactive and potentially toxic, whereas their GSH conjugates are inactive. Conjugation of GSH with the epoxides of aryl hydrocarbons eventually results in the formation of hydroxymercapturic acids (premercapturic acids), which undergo acid-catalyzed dehydration to the mercapturic acids. The halobenzenes are typically conjugated in the para position.

Monohalogenated, gem-dihalogenated, and vicinal dihalogenated alkanes undergo glutathione transferase–catalyzed conjugation reactions to produce *S*-substituted glutathione derivatives that are metabolically transformed into the more stable and less toxic mercapturic acids. This common route of metabolism occurs through nucleophilic displacement of a halide ion by the thiolate anion of glutathione (see the discussion on glutathione conjugation). The mutagenicity of the 1,2-dihaloethanes (e.g,. the pesticide and fumigant ethylene dibromide) has been attributed to GSH displacing bromide with the formation of the *S*-(2-haloethyl) glutathione, which subsequently rearranges to a reactive episulfonium ion electrophile that, in turn, alkylates DNA. Many of the halogenated hydrocarbons exhibiting nephrotoxicity undergo the formation of similar *S*-substituted cysteine derivatives.

A correlation exists between the hepatotoxicity of acetaminophen and levels of GSH in the liver. The probable mechanism of toxicity that has emerged from animal studies is that acetaminophen is CYP1A2 and CYP2E1 oxidized to the *N*-acetyl-*p*-benzoquinonimine intermediate, which conjugates with and depletes hepatic GSH levels (Fig. 4.28). This action allows the benzoquinonimine to bind covalently to tissue macromolecules. The mercapturic acid derivative of acetaminophen represents approximately 2% of the administered dose of acetaminophen. Thus, the possibility exists that those toxic metabolites

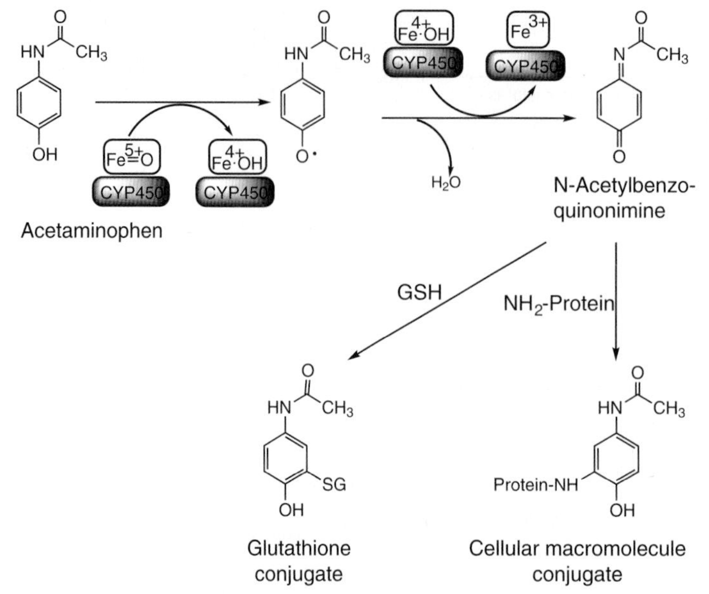

FIGURE 4.28 Proposed mechanism for the P450-catalyzed oxidation of acetaminophen to its *N*-acetyl-*p*-benzoquinoneimine intermediate, which can further react with either glutathione (GSH) or cellular macromolecules (NH_2-protein).

that are mostly detoxified by conjugating with GSH exhibit their hepatotoxicity (or, perhaps, carcinogenicity) because the liver has been depleted of GSH and is incapable of inactivating them. Pretreatment of animals with phenobarbital often hastens the depletion of GSH by increasing the formation of epoxides or other reactive intermediates.

Methylation

Methylation is a common biochemical reaction but appears to be of greater significance in the metabolism of endogenous compounds than for drugs and other xenobiotics (56). Methylation differs from other conjugation processes in that the *O*-methyl metabolites formed can, in some cases, have as great or greater pharmacologic activity and lipophilicity than the parent molecule (e.g., the conversion of norepinephrine to epinephrine). Methionine is involved in the methylation of endogenous and exogenous substrates, because it transfers its methyl group via the activated intermediate *S*-adenosylmethionine to the substrate under the influence of methyl transferases (Fig. 4.29).Methylation results principally in the formation of *O*-methylated, *N*-methylated, and *S*-methylated products.

O-Methylation

O-Methylation is catalyzed by the magnesium-dependent enzyme catechol-*O*-methyltransferase (COMT) transferring a methyl group primarily to the *m*- or 3-hydroxy group of the catechol moiety (3,4-dihydroxylphenyl moiety) of norepinephrine, epinephrine, or dopamine, or, less frequently, to the *p*- or 4-hydroxy group of these catecholamines (regioselectivity), as well as by their deaminated metabolites. COMT does not methylate monophenols or other dihydroxy noncatechol phenols. The meta:para product ratio depends greatly on the type of substituent attached to the catechol ring. Substrates specific for COMT include the catecholamines norepinephrine, epinephrine, and dopamine; the catechol amino acids L-DOPA and α-methyl-DOPA; and 2- and 4-hydroxyestradiol (catechol-like) metabolites of estradiol. The enzyme is thought to function in the biologic inactivation of the adrenergic neurotransmitter norepinephrine as well as other endogenous and exogenous catechol-like substances. It is found in liver, kidneys, nervous tissue, and other tissues.

Hydroxyindole-*O*-methyltransferase, which *O*-methylates *N*-acetylserotonin, serotonin, and other hydroxyindoles, is found in the pineal gland and is involved in the formation of melatonin, a hormone associated with the dark–light diurnal cycle in humans. This enzyme differs from COMT in that it does not methylate catecholamines and has no requirement for magnesium iron.

N-Methylation

N-Methylation of various amines is among several conjugate pathways for metabolizing amines. Specific *N*-methyltransferases catalyze the transfer of active methyl groups from *S*-adenosylmethionine to the acceptor substance. Phenylethanolamine-*N*-methyltransferase methylates a number of endogenous and exogenous phenylethanolamines (e.g., normetanephrine, norepinephrine, and norephedrine) but does not methylate phenylethylamines. Histamine-*N*-methyl transferase methylates specifically histamine, producing the inactive metabolite N^1-methylhistamine. Amine-*N*-methyltransferase will *N*-methylate a variety of primary and secondary amines from a number of sources,

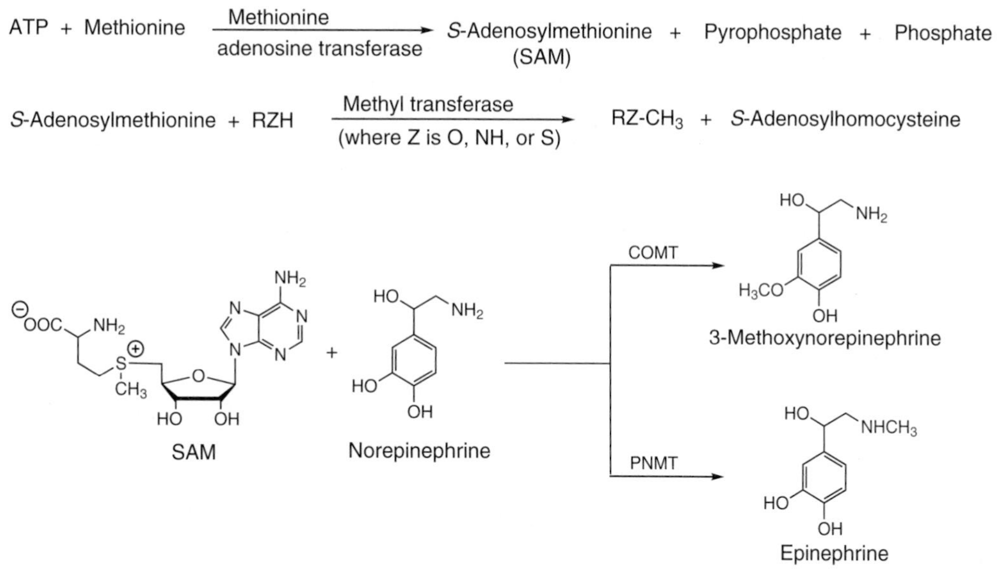

FIGURE 4.29 Methylation pathways.

including endogenous biogenic amines (serotonin, tryptamine, tyramine, and dopamine) and drugs (desmethylimipramine, amphetamine, and normorphine). Amine-*N*-methyl transferases seem to have a role in recycling *N*-demethylated drugs.

S-Methylation

Thiols are, as a rule, toxic, and the role of thiol *S*-methyl transferases is a nonoxidative detoxification pathway of these compounds. *S*-Methylation of sulfhydryl compounds also involves a microsomal enzyme requiring *S*-adenosylmethionine. Although a wide range of exogenous sulfhydryl compounds are *S*-methylated by this microsomal enzyme, none of the endogenous sulfhydryl compounds (e.g., cysteine and GSH) can function as substrates. Clearly, *S*-methylation represents a detoxication step for thiols. Dialkyldithiocarbamates (e.g., disulfiram) and the antithyroid drugs (e.g., 6-propyl-2-thiouracil), mercaptans, and hydrogen sulfide (from thioglycosides as natural constituents of foods, mineral sulfides in water, fermented beverages, and bacterial digestion) are *S*-methylated. Other drugs undergoing *S*-methylation include captopril, thiopurine, azaprine, penicillamine, and 6-mercaptopurine.

Thiopurine methyltransferase or thiopurine *S*-methyltransferase (TPMT) catlyzes the *S*-methylation of thiopurine drugs, such as azathioprine, 6-mercaptopurine, and 6-thioguanine. Interindividual variations in sensitivity and toxicity to thiopurine are correlated with TPMT genetic polymorphisms. Defects in the TPMT gene lead to decreased methylation and decreased inactivation of the thiopurine drugs, leading to enhanced bone marrow toxicity that may cause myelosuppression, anemia, bleeding tendency, leukopenia, and infection. Approximately 5% of all thiopurine therapies will fail due to toxicity as a result of TPMT polymorphism.

Conjugation of Cyanide

The toxicity of hydrogen cyanide is the result of its ionization to cyanide ion in biologic tissues. Cyanide anion is a powerful metabolic inhibitor that arrests cellular respiration by inactivating cytochrome enzymes that are fundamental to the respiratory process as well as combining with hemoglobin to form cyanomethemoglobin, which is incapable of transporting oxygen to tissues. With the wide prevalence of cyanoglycosides in plant-food materials, the ability to detoxify cyanide is a vital function of the liver, erythrocytes, and other tissues. Rhodanase, a mitochondrial enzyme in liver and other tissues, catalyzes the formation of thiocyanate from cyanide rapidly in the presence of thiosulfate and colloidal sulfur, but cysteine and GSH are poor sulfur donors. The detoxification of cyanide depends on the availability of a physiologic pool of thiosulfate, the origin of which is not known. A possible source for thiosulfate is the transamination of cysteine to β-mercaptopyruvate and transfer of the mercapto group by a sulfur transferase to sulfite-producing thiosulfate. Depletion of the thiocyanate pool increases cyanide toxicity. However, in the presence of excess cyanide, minor pathways for cyanide metabolism can occur, including oxidation to cyanate (NCO^-), reaction with cobalamin (vitamin B_{12}) to form cyanocobalamin, and the formation of 2-iminothiazolidine-4-carboxylic acid from the nonenzymatic reaction between cysteine and cyanide (66).

$$S_2O_3^{2-} + CN^{\ominus} \longrightarrow CNS^{\ominus} + SO_3^{2-}$$

ELIMINATION PATHWAYS

Most xenobiotics are lipid-soluble and are altered chemically by the metabolizing enzymes, usually into less toxic and more water-soluble substances, before being excreted into the urine (or, in some cases, bile). The formation of conjugates with sulfonate, amino acids, and glucuronic acid is particularly effective in increasing the polarity of drug molecules. The principal route of excretion of drugs and their metabolites is in the urine. If drugs and other compounds foreign to the body are not metabolized in this manner, substances with a high lipid–water partition coefficient could be reabsorbed readily from the urine through the renal tubular membranes and into the plasma. Therefore, such substances would continue to be recirculated, and their pharmacologic or toxic effects would be prolonged. Very polar or highly ionized drug molecules often are excreted in the urine unchanged.

Urine

Tubular reabsorption is greatly reduced by conversion of a drug into a more hydrophilic substance with a lower partition coefficient. In general, the more resistant a drug is to the metabolizing enzymes, the greater the therapeutic action and the smaller the dose needed to achieve a particular therapeutic goal.

Urine is not the only route for excreting drugs and their metabolites from the animal body. Other routes include bile, saliva, lungs, sweat, and milk. The bile has been recognized as a major route of excretion for many endogenous and exogenous compounds.

Enterohepatic Cycling of Drugs

The liver is the principal organ for the metabolism and eventual elimination of xenobiotics from the human body in either the urine or the bile. When eliminated in the bile, steroid hormones, bile acids, drugs, and their respective conjugated metabolites are available for reabsorption from the duodenal–intestinal tract into the portal circulation, undergoing the process of enterohepatic cycling (EHC) (67). Nearly all drugs are excreted in the bile, but only a few are concentrated in the bile. For example, the bile salts are so efficiently concentrated in the bile and reabsorbed from the gastrointestinal tract that the entire body pool of bile acids/salts are recycled multiple times per day. Therefore, EHC is responsible for the conservation of bile acids, steroid hormones, thyroid hormones, and other endogenous substances. In humans, compounds excreted into the bile typically have a molecular weight greater than 500 daltons, whereas with rats, the critical molecular weight is 325 daltons. Consequently, biliary excretion is more common in rats than in humans. In humans, compounds with a molecular weight between 300 and 500 daltons are excreted in both urine and bile. Some compounds would not be expected to be excreted in the bile as a result of a molecular weight of less than 300 daltons and a relatively nonpolar structure. Compounds excreted into bile are, as a rule, hydrophilic substances that can be either charged (anionic; e.g., dyes) or uncharged (e.g., cardiac glycosides and steroid hormones). Biotransformation of this type of compound by means of Phase 1 and Phase 2 reactions would produce a conjugated metabolite that is anionic and hydrophilic with a molecular weight greater than that of the parent compound. The conjugated metabolites are most often present as their glucuronide conjugates, because glucuronidation adds 176 daltons to the molecular weight of the parent compound. Unchanged drug in the bile is either excreted with the feces, metabolized by the bacterial flora in the intestinal tract, or reabsorbed into the portal circulation via EHC.

The bacterial intestinal flora is directly involved in EHC and the recycling of drugs through the portal circulation (see the discussion of extrahepatic metabolism). A conjugated drug and metabolites excreted via the bile can be hydrolyzed by enzymes of the bacterial flora, releasing the parent drug or its Phase 1 metabolite for reabsorption into the portal circulation (68). Among the numerous compounds metabolized in the enterohepatic circulation are the estrogenic and progestational steroids, digitoxin, indomethacin, diazepam, pentaerythritol tetranitrate, mercurials, arsenicals, and morphine. The oral ingestion of xenobiotics inhibiting the gut flora (i.e., nonabsorbable antibiotics) can affect the pharmacokinetics of the initial drug.

The impact of EHC on the pharmacokinetics and pharmacodynamics of a drug depends on the importance of biliary excretion of the drug relative to renal clearance and on the efficiency of gastrointestinal absorption. The EHC becomes dominant when biliary excretion is the major clearance mechanism for the drug. Because the majority of the bile is stored in the gallbladder and released on the ingestion of food, intermittent spikes in the plasma drug concentration are observed following reentry of the drug from the bile via EHC. From a pharmacodynamic point of view, the net effect of EHC is to increase the duration of a drug in the body and to prolong its pharmacologic action.

Chronic treatment with the enzyme inducer phenobarbital enhances the biliary excretion of drug molecules and their metabolites by increasing liver size, bile flow, and more efficient transport into the bile. This behavior is not shared by all inducers of the P450 monooxygenases. The route of administration can also influence excretion pathways. Direct administration into the portal circulation might be expected to result in more biliary excretion than could be expected via the systemic route.

DRUG METABOLISM AND AGE

Approximately 40% of the population is older than 65 years of age and is responsible for more than 50% of the national drug expenditures. People older than 85 years represent approximately 2% of the population; they are the most medicated and account for more than one-third of all prescription drugs dispensed. The average elderly patient in a health care facility could receive as many as 10 medications daily, which results in the potential

TABLE 4.15 Effect of Age on the Clearance of Some Drugs

No Change	Decrease
Acetaminophen*	Alprazolam
Aspirin	Amitriptyline
Diclofenac	Carbenoxolone
Digitoxin	Chlordiazepoxide
Diphenhydramine	Chlormethiazole
Ethanol	Clobazam
Flunitrazepam	Desmethyldiazepam
Heparin	Diazepam
Lormetazepam	Labetalol
Midazolam	Lidocaine
Nitrazepam	Lorazepam
Oxazepam	Morphine
Phenytoin*	Meperidine
Prazosin	Nifedipine and other dihydropyridines
Propylthiouracil	Norepinephrine
Temazepam	Nortriptyline
Thiopental*	Phenytoin
Tolbutamide*	Piroxicam
Warfarin	Propranolol
	Quinidine
	Quinine
	Theophylline
	Verapamil

*Drugs for which clearance is disputable but can be increased.

for a greater incidence of adverse drug reactions. The widespread use of medications in the elderly increases the potential for an increased incidence of drug-related interactions, which can be related to changes in drug v (Table 4.15). The interpretation of the age-related alteration in drug response must consider the contributions of absorption, distribution, metabolism, and excretion (69). Drug therapy in the elderly is expected to become one of the more significant problems for clinical medicine. It has been well documented that the metabolism of many drugs and their elimination is impaired in the elderly.

Metabolism in the Elderly

The decline in drug metabolism due to old age is associated with physiologic changes that have pharmacokinetic implications affecting the steady-state plasma concentrations and renal clearance for the parent drug and its metabolites (70,71). Those changes relevant to the bioavailability of drugs in the elderly are decreases in hepatic blood flow, glomerular filtration rate, hepatic P450 enzyme activity, plasma protein binding, and body mass. Because the rate of a drug's elimination from the blood through hepatic metabolism is determined by hepatic blood flow, protein binding, and intrinsic renal clearance, a reduction in hepatic blood flow can lead to an increase in drug bioavailability and decreased renal clearance, with the symptoms of drug overdose and toxicity as the outcome (e.g., warfarin in patients with congestive heart failure). Drugs for which renal elimination is dependent on hepatic blood flow have a high extraction ratio and undergo extensive first-pass metabolism when administered orally. Available evidence suggests that age is associated with a reduction in first-pass metabolism of some, but certainly not all, drugs. Those orally administered drugs exhibiting a reduction in first-pass metabolism in the elderly include the dihydropyridine calcium antagonists, chlormethiazole, diazepam, lorazepam, chlordiazepoxide, alprazolam, propranolol, verapamil, labetalol, theophylline, morphine, amitriptyline, and nortriptyline. The bioavailability of drugs with low extraction ratios depends on the percentage of drug–protein binding and not on first-pass hepatic metabolism. Inasmuch as drug binding to plasma proteins is an important factor in the rate of drug metabolism, it appears not to be a significant factor in the elderly.

Age-related changes in drug metabolism are a complicated interplay between age-related physiologic changes, genetics, environmental influences (diet and nutritional status, smoking, and enzyme induction), concomitant diseases states, and drug intake. In most studies, the elderly appear just as responsive to drug-metabolizing enzyme activity (Phase 1 and Phase 2) as young individuals. All the common pathways of drug conjugation, including glucuronidation, sulfonation, and glycine conjugation, are variably affected by aging. Given the number of factors that determine the rate of drug metabolism, it is not surprising that the effects of aging on drug elimination by metabolism have yielded variable results even for the same drug. Therefore, the bioavailability of a drug in the elderly and the potential for drug toxicity is dependant largely on its extraction ratio and mode of administration. The fact that drug renal elimination can be altered in old age suggests that initial doses of metabolized drugs should be reduced in older patients and then modified according to the clinical response (70,71). A decrease in hepatic drug metabolism coupled with age-related alterations in clearance, volume of distribution, and receptor sensitivity can lead to prolonged plasma half-life and increased drug toxicity (Table 4.15).

Drug–Drug Interactions

Although drug–drug interactions constitute only a small proportion of adverse drug reactions in the elderly, they are important, because they are often predictable and, therefore, avoidable or manageable. Their frequency is related to the age of the patient, the number of drugs prescribed, the number of physicians involved in the patient's care, and the presence of increasing frailty. The most important mechanisms for drug–drug interactions are the inhibition or induction of drug metabolism. Interactions involving a loss of action of one of the drugs are at least as frequent as those involving an increased effect. Although only approximately 10% of potential interactions result in clinically significant adverse events, death or serious clinical consequences are rare, but low-grade, clinical morbidity in the elderly can be much more common. Nonspecific complaints (e.g., confusion, lethargy, weakness, dizziness, incontinence, depression, and falling) should all prompt a closer look at the patient's drug list. A number of strategies can be adopted to decrease the risk of potential clinical problems. The number of drugs prescribed for each individual should be limited to as few as necessary. The use of drugs should be reviewed regularly, and unnecessary agents should be withdrawn if possible, with subsequent monitoring. Patients should be encouraged to engage in a "prescribing partnership" by alerting physicians, pharmacists, and other health care professionals to symptoms that occur when new drugs are introduced. Health care professionals should develop a strategy for monitoring their drug treatment, looking for the drug–drug interactions that have been encountered.

Those P450 substrates reported to cause drug–drug interactions are shown in Tables 4.4 through 4.14 in bold italics.

Fetal Metabolism

The ability of the human placenta to metabolize xenobiotics is well established. Drug-metabolizing enzymes expressed in the placenta include CYP1A1, CYP2E1, CYP3A4/5, CYP3A7, CYP4B1, epoxide hydrase, alcohol dehydrogenase, glutathione transferase, UGTs, sulfotransferases, and *N*-acetyltransferase. A 1973 clinical study reported that women ingest an average of 10 drugs during pregnancy, not including general anesthetics, intravenous fluids, vitamins, iron, nicotine, cosmetic products, artificial sweeteners, or exposure to environmental contaminants. The majority of these drugs readily cross the placenta, thus exposing the fetus to a large number of xenobiotic agents. The knowledge regarding the effects of prenatal exposure to drugs, environmental pollutants (e.g., smoking), and other xenobiotics (e.g., ethanol) on the fetus has led to a decrease in the exposure to these substances during pregnancy. The human fetus is at special risk from these xenobiotics due to low or negligible levels of the P450 monooxygenase system. Placentas of tobacco smokers have shown a significant increase in the rate of placental CYP1A activity. Concern for this CYP1A activity is increasing, because this enzyme system is known to catalyze the formation of reactive metabolites capable of covalently binding to macromolecules producing permanent effects (e.g., teratogenicity, hepatotoxicity, or carcinogenicity) in the fetus and newborn. A more disturbing fact is that the conjugation enzymes (i.e., glucuronosyl transferases, epoxide hydrase, glutathione transferase, and sulfotransferase), which are important for the formation of Phase 2 conjugates of these reactive metabolites, are also found in low to negligible levels in the fetus and newborn, increasing the exposure of these infants to these potentially toxic metabolites.

The placenta is not a barrier protecting the fetus from xenobiotics; because most every drug present in the maternal circulation will cross the placenta and reach the fetus. For some drugs, however, the placental efflux transport protein, P-glycoprotein (P-gp; discussed later and in Chapter 7), functions as a maternofetal barrier, pumping drugs and P-gp substrates out of the fetal circulation back into the maternal circulation (72) and protecting the fetus from exposure to potentially harmful teratogenic xenobiotics/drugs and endogenous substances that have been absorbed through the placenta. The P-gp inhibitors should be carefully evaluated for their potential to increase fetal susceptibility to drug or chemical-induced teratogenesis. On the other hand, selective inhibition of P-gp could be used clinically to improve pharmacotherapy of the unborn child. Depending on the pharmacologic activity of the parent substance or its metabolites, adult maternal drug metabolism can be viewed as complimentary yet contradictory. Because metabolites are usually more water soluble than the parent substance, drug metabolites when formed by maternal drug metabolism can be trapped and accumulate on the fetal side of the placenta. Such accumulation can result in drug-induced toxicities or developmental defects. However, the difference between fetal and adult metabolism can be used advantageously and constitutes the rational for transplacental therapy (e.g., the administration of betamethasone several days before delivery can increase the production of surfactant in the fetal lung and prevent respiratory distress syndrome in the neonate).

Neonatal Metabolism

From the day of birth, the neonate is exposed to drugs and other foreign compounds persisting from pregnancy as well as those transferred via breast milk. Many of the drug-metabolizing enzymes operative in the neonate are developed during the first year of life. The routine use of therapeutic agents during labor and delivery, as well as during pregnancy, is widespread, and consideration must be given to the fact that potentially harmful metabolites can be generated by the newborn. Consequently, the use of drugs capable of forming reactive metabolic intermediates (e.g., isotretinoin [Accutane]) should be avoided during pregnancy, delivery, and the neonatal period. The activity of Phase 1 and Phase 2 drug-metabolizing enzymes is high at birth but decreases to normal levels with increasing age. Evidence suggests increased activity of drug-metabolizing enzymes in liver microsomes of neonates resulting from treatment of the mother during the pregnancy with enzyme inducers (e.g., phenobarbital).

GENETIC POLYMORPHISM

The reality of drug therapy is that many drugs do not work in all patients. By current estimates, the percentage of patients who will react favorably to a specific drug ranges from 20% to 80%. Drugs have been developed and dosage regimens prescribed under the old paradigm that "one dose fits all," which ignores largely the fact that humans are genetically different, resulting in interindividual differences in drug metabolism and disposition (10). It is widely accepted that genetic factors have an important impact on the oxidative metabolism and pharmacokinetics of drugs. Genotype–phenotype correlation studies (pharmacogenetics) have shown that inherited mutations in P450 genes (alleles) result in distinct phenotypic subgroups. For example, mutations in the *CYP2D6* gene result in poor (PM), intermediate (or extensive [EM]), and ultrarapid (UM) metabolizers of CYP2D6 substrates (73) (Table 4.9). Each of these phenotypic subgroups experience different responses to drugs extensively metabolized by the CYP2D6 pathway, ranging from severe toxicity to complete lack of efficacy. Genetic studies confirm that "one dose does not fit all," leaving the question of why we would continue to develop and prescribe drugs under the old paradigm. As early as 1997, the U.S. Food and Drug Administration (FDA) recognized that identifying genetic polymorphisms might allow the safe dosing, marketing, and approval of drugs that would otherwise not be approved and advised pharmaceutical companies to incorporate the knowledge of genetic polymorphisms into drug development (see sidebar). Importantly, pharmacogenomic testing (the study of heritable traits affecting patient response to drug treatment) can significantly increase the likelihood of developing drug regimens that benefit most patients without severe adverse events.

Polymorphisms are expressed for a number of metabolizing enzymes, but the polymorphic P450 isoforms that are most important for drug metabolism include CYP2A6, CYP2A13, CYP2B6, CYP2C9, CYP2C19, and CYP2D6. These isoforms have been studied extensively, and despite their low abundance in the liver, they have been found to catalyze the metabolism of many drugs. Most gene variants are expressed into inactive, truncated proteins or fail to express any protein. There is, as yet, no clear information about CYP1A1 and CYP3A4/5 polymorphism. These polymorphic isoforms give rise to phenotypic subgroups in the population differing in their ability to perform clinically significant biotransformation reactions with obvious clinical ramifications (73). Metabolic polymorphism can have several consequences; for example, when enzymes that metabolize drugs used either therapeutically or socially are deficient, adverse or toxic drug reactions can occur in these individuals. The discovery of genetic polymorphism resulted from the observation of increased frequency of adverse effects or no drug effects after normal doses of drugs to some patients (e.g., hyper–central nervous system response from the administration of the antihistamine doxylamine or no analgesic response with codeine). Polymorphism is a difference in DNA sequence found at 1% or greater in a population and expressed as an amino acid substitution in the protein sequence of an enzyme resulting in changes in its rate of activity (V_{max}) or affinity (K_m). Thus, mutant DNA sequences can lead to interindividual differences in drug metabolism. Furthermore, the polymorphisms do not occur with equivalent frequency in all racial or ethnic groups. As a result of these differences, it is important to be aware of a person's race and ethnicity when giving drugs that are metabolized differently by different populations (73–76). Because no other way exists to adequately clear these drugs from the body, PMs can be at greater risk for adverse drug reactions or toxic overdoses. The signs and symptoms of these overdoses are primarily extensions of the drug's common adverse effects or pharmacologic effects (Table 4.16) (73). The level of adverse reactions or overdosage depends very much on the overall contribution of the mutant isoform to the drug's metabolism. Perhaps the most interesting explanation for the various mutant isoforms is that they evolved as protective mechanisms against alkaloids and other common substances in the food chain for the different ethnicities. Although much effort has gone into finding polymorphisms of *CYP3A4* and *CYP1A2* genes, none has yet to be discovered.

FDA ADVISORY ON GENETIC POLYMORPHISM

"When a genetic polymorphism affects an important metabolic route of elimination, large dosing adjustments can be necessary to achieve the safe and effective use of the drug...indeed in some cases understanding how to adjust the dose to avoid toxicity can allow the marketing of a drug that would have an unacceptable level of toxicity were its toxicity unpredictable and unpreventable."
—FDA, *Guidance of Industry, Drug Metabolism/Drug Interaction Studies in the Drug Development Process: Studies in Vitro,* April 1997.

Occasionally, one derives benefit from an unusual P450 phenotype. For example, cure rates for peptic ulcer treated with omeprazole are substantially greater in individuals with defective CYP2C19 due to the sustained high plasma levels achieved.

CYP2A6

CYP2A6 is of particular importance, because it activates a number of procarcinogens to carcinogens and is the major isoform metabolizing the anticoagulant warfarin and nicotine (74). Approximately 15% of Asians express the *CYP2A6*4del* allele, and 2% of Caucasians express the other *CYP2AD6*2* allele. Both of these alleles express zero enzymes or a nonfunctional enzyme; these individuals are referred to as having the PM phenotype. A benefit from being a PM of CYP2A6 substrates might be

TABLE 4.16 Impact of Human P450 Polymorphisms on Drug Treatment in Poor Metabolizers

Polymorphic Enzyme	Decreased Clearance	Adverse Effects (overdosage)	Reduced Activation of Prodrug
CYP2C9	*S*-Warfarin	Bleeding	Losartan
	Phenytoin	Ataxia	
	Losartan		
	Tolbutamide	Hypoglycemia	
	NSAIDs	GI bleeding?	
CYP2C19	Omeprazole		Proguanil
	Diazepam	Sedation	
CYP2D6	Tricyclic antidepressants	Cardiotoxicity	Tramadol
	SSRIs	Serotonin syndrome	Codeine
	Antiarrhythmic drugs	Arrhythmias	Ethylmorphine
	Perhexiline	Neuropathy	
	Haloperidol	Parkinsonism?	
	Perphenazine		
	Zuclopenthixol		
	S-Mianserin		
	Tolterodine		
CYP2A6	Nicotine		

the protection from some carcinogens and smoking as a result of the high plasma levels of nicotine achieved with fewer cigarettes.

CYP2B6

CYP2B6 is of particular interest due to its wide interindividual variability in the expression and enzyme activity (75). Such a large variability for an enzyme that is not highly expressed is probably a result of effects of genetic polymorphisms and exposure to drugs that are inducers or inhibitors of CYP2B6. Variant alleles resulting from splicing defects or gene deletions have been identified in individuals with altered metabolic activity or impaired enzyme function as PMs. At least 28 allelic variants and some subvariants of *CYP2B6* have been shown to have an effect on drug clearance and drug response. For example, HIV-infected African-American individuals with a defective variant of *CYP2B6* are PMs of efavirenz, with plasma levels approximately threefold higher than individuals with the normal *CYP2B6* gene. A different variant of *CYP2B6* is associated with approximately twofold greater plasma levels of nevirapine in HIV-infected patients. A benefit from being a PM of CYP2B6 antiviral drugs might be enhanced HIV protection as a result of the higher plasma levels of the antiviral drugs achieved with low dosages. Smokers with another variant of *CYP2B6* may be more vulnerable to abstinence symptoms and relapse following treatment with bupropion as a smoking cessation agent.

CYP2C9 and CYP2C19

CYP2C9 and CYP2C19 metabolize approximately 15% of clinical drugs such as phenytoin, *S*-warfarin, tolbutamide, losartan, and many NSAIDs (76). Although CYP2C19 metabolizes fewer drugs than CYP2D6 does, the drugs that CYP2C19 does metabolize are clinically important (Table 4.8). A deficit of CYP2C19 is found in the PM phenotype, which is seen in 8% to 13% of Caucasians, 20% to 30% of the Asian population (11% to 23% of Japanese and 5% to 37% of Chinese), up to 20% of the black African-American population, 14% to 15% of Saudi Arabians and Ethiopians, and up to 70% of Pacific Islanders (76). The more common mutant allele in these individuals is *CYP2C19*2*, which expresses an inactive enzyme. The large interindividual variability observed in the therapeutic response to the antiseizure drug mephenytoin is attributed to CYP2C19 polymorphism, which catalyzes the *p*-hydroxylation of its *S*-stereoisomer (76). The *R*-enantiomer is *N*-demethylated by CYP2C8 with no difference in its metabolism between PMs and EMs.

CYP2C9 is highly polymorphic, with at least 33 variants of CYP2C9 being identified so far. *CYP2C9*2* is frequent among Caucasians, with approximately 1% of the population being homozygous carriers and 22% being heterozygous. The corresponding figures for the *CYP2C9*3* allele are 0.4% and 15%, respectively. Clinical studies have addressed the importance of the *CYP2C9*2* and **3* alleles as a determining factor for drug clearance and drug response. CYP2C9 polymorphisms are relevant for the efficacy and adverse effects of numerous NSAIDs, sulfonylurea antidiabetic drugs, and, most critically, oral anticoagulants belonging to the class of vitamin K epoxide reductase inhibitors (e.g., warfarin) (76). A deficiency of this isoform, however, is seen in 8% to 13% of Caucasians, 2% to 3% of African Americans, and 1% of Asians. Individuals with the PM phenotype who possess this deficient isoform variant are ineffective in clearing *S*-warfarin (so much so that they can be fully anticoagulated on just 0.5 mg of warfarin per day) and in clearing phenytoin, which has a potentially very toxic narrow therapeutic range. On the other hand, the prodrug losartan will be poorly activated and ineffective.

CYP2D6

CYP2D6 is of particular importance, because it metabolizes a wide range of commonly prescribed drugs, including antidepressants, antipsychotics, β-adrenergic blockers, and antiarrhythmics (Table 4.9). CYP2D6 deficiency is a clinically important genetic variation of drug metabolism characterized by three phenotypes: UM, EM, and PM. The PM phenotype is inherited as an autosomal recessive trait, with 5 of 30 of the known *CYP2D6* gene mutations leading to either zero expression or the expression of a nonfunctional enzyme (73). Approximately 12% to 20% of Caucasians express the *CYP2D6*4* allele, and 5% express the other *CYP2D6* alleles. Up to 34% of African Americans express the *CYP2D6*17* allele, and 5% express the other *CYP2D6* alleles. Up to 50% of Chinese express the *CYP2D6*10* allele, and 5% express the other *CYP2D6* alleles (these individuals are referred to as PM) (73,75). Conversely, the 20% to 30% of Saudi Arabians and Ethiopians who express the *CYP2D6*2XN* allele are known as UMs of CYP2D6 substrates, because they express excess enzyme as a result of having multiple copies of the gene (73). Inasmuch as CYP2D6 is not inducible, individuals of Ethiopian and Saudi Arabian descent have developed genetically a different strategy to cope with the (presumed) high load of alkaloids and other substances in their diet; thus, the high expression of CYP2D6 using multiple copies of the gene. Those individuals who are deficient in CYP2D6 will be predisposed to adverse effects or drug toxicity from antidepressants or neuroleptics caused by inadequate metabolism or long half-lives, but the metabolism of prodrugs in these patients will be ineffective due to lack of activation (e.g., codeine, which must be metabolized by *O*-demethylation to morphine). Those with the UM phenotype will require a dose that is much higher than normal to attain therapeutic drug plasma concentrations (e.g., one patient required a daily dose of ~300 mg of nortriptyline to achieve therapeutic plasma levels) or a lower dose for prodrugs that require metabolic activation. Individuals with the PM phenotype are also characterized by loss of CYP2D6 stereoselectivity in hydroxylation reactions. It can be anticipated that large differences in steady-state concentration for CYP2D6 substrates will occur between individuals with the different phenotypes when they receive the same dose. Depending on the drug and reaction type, a 10- to 30-fold difference in blood concentrations can be observed in the PM-phenotype debrisoquine polymorphism (76).

Acetylation

Acetylation, a nonmicrosomal form of metabolism, also exhibits polymorphisms and was first demonstrated in the acetylation of isoniazid. Several forms of *N*-acetyl transferase (NAT1 and NAT2) occur in humans. NAT1 (arylamine *N*-acetyltransferase) is widely distributed and catalyzes the *N*-acetylation of acidic arylamines, such as *p*-aminobenzoic acid and *p*-aminosalicylic acid, and so its expression levels in the body have toxicologic importance with regard to drug toxicity and cancer risk, for example bladder cancer and colorectal cancer. NAT2 is found predominately in the liver. Some clinically used drugs undergoing NAT2-catalyzed *N*-acetylation include isoniazid, procainamide, hydralazine, phenelzine, dapsone, caffeine, some benzodiazepines, and the carcinogenic secondary *N*-alkylarylamines (2-aminofluorene, benzidine, and 4-aminobiphenyl). Both NAT1 and NAT2 have a cysteine group at the active site, which is acetylated by acetyl CoA. The *S*-acetyl group is then transferred to the substrate. *o*-Substituents to the amino group sterically block acetylation. Polymorphisms in *NAT2* gene in human populations can be segregated into fast, intermediate, and slow acetylator phenotypes. Polymorphisms in NAT2 are also associated with higher incidences of cancer and drug toxicity. Intestinal *N*-acetyl transferase appears not to be polymorphic (i.e., 5-aminosalicylic acid). The proportion of the fast acetylation phenotype is approximately 30% to 45% in Caucasians, 89% to 90% in Asians, and 100% in Canadian Eskimos. Drug-induced systemic lupus erythematosus from chronic procainamide therapy is more likely to appear in slow acetylators.

The antituberculosis drugs isoniazid and rifampicin in combination are known to cause drug-induced hepatotoxicity (DIH). A higher risk of DIH during antituberculosis treatment has been reported in India compared with the Western populations. The occurrence of DIH in India was approximately 19%, with a higher prevalence of NAT2 slow acetylator genotypes in DIH (~70%) compared with non-DIH (~45%). The frequency of *NAT2*5/*7* and *NAT2*6/*7* genotypes was higher in DIH than non-DIH (20% vs. 7% and 20% vs. 5%, respectively). Thus, genotyping of the *NAT2* gene could possibly identify the high-risk group for developing antituberculosis treatment–induced hepatitis prior to medication

Other Polymorphic Metabolizing Enzymes

The polymorphism for CYP2E1 is expressed more in Chinese than in Caucasians. Those with the CYP2E1 PM phenotype exhibit tolerance to alcohol and less toxicity from halohydrocarbon solvents.

Individuals with a defective variant of *FMO3* are poor metabolizers of trimethylamine to its *N*-oxide metabolite, and therefore exhibit trimethylaminuria, in which affected individuals excrete diet-derived free trimethylamine in the urine. This disease has probably been around since 1400 BC, when a young woman was described as being rejected by society because she smelled like rotting fish. Even Shakespeare likely was referring to a person with trimethylaminuria in a scene from *The Tempest*, Act I, scene II, line 26: "What have we here? A man or a fish? Dead or alive? A fish! He smells like a fish; a very ancient and fishlike smell."

In human populations, serum PON1 exhibits a substrate-dependent polymorphism to the neurotoxic effects of organophosphates in those susceptible individuals who are deficient in PON1 (i.e., PM phenotype) (55). The PON1 catalyzes the hydrolysis of paraoxon, chlorpyrifos (Dursban), and other organophosphates.

Polymorphism has been associated with serum cholinesterases (particularly succinyl cholinesterase, causing skeletal muscle paralysis), alcohol dehydrogenases, aldehyde dehydrogenases, epoxide hydrolase, and xanthine oxidase (74). Approximately 50% of the Asian population lack aldehyde dehydrogenase, resulting in high levels of acetaldehyde following ethanol ingestion and causing nausea and flushing. People with genetic variants of cholinesterase respond abnormally to succinylcholine, procaine, and other related choline esters. The clinical consequence of reduced enzymic activity of cholinesterase is that succinylcholine and procaine are not hydrolyzed in the blood, resulting in prolongation of their respective pharmacologic activities.

A suggestion has been made that those with EM phenotypes can be more prone than those with PM phenotypes to develop cancers, because they are better able to activate procarcinogens. Such interindividual variations can have a major influence in determining the risk of cancer. The activity of a particular P450 isoform can be a rationale for predicting the individual risk from exposure to carcinogenic compounds.

Our increasing knowledge of genetic polymorphism has contributed a great deal to our understanding about interindividual variation in the metabolism of drugs, including how to change dose regimens accordingly to minimize drug toxicity and improve therapeutic efficacy. In humans, drugs not subject to polymorphic metabolism also exhibit substantial interindividual variation in their disposition, which is attributed to a great extent to environmental factors (e.g., inducing agents, smoking, and alcohol ingestion).

For many of these drugs, clear gene–dose and gene–effect relationships have been observed in patients. In this regard, the normal and mutant alleles can be considered as useful biomarkers in monitoring drug response and adverse effects. Genetic testing of mutant alleles is expected to have a role in predicting drug clearance and conducting individualized pharmacotherapy. However, clinical studies with large samples are warranted to establish gene–dose and gene–effect relationships for those enzymes exhibiting polymorphisms and their substrate drugs.

ORAL BIOAVAILABILITY

Oral bioavailability (see Chapter 3) is the fraction of the total dose of a drug that reaches the systemic circulation. The low oral bioavailability for a drug can be the result of disintegration and dissolution properties of the drug formulation, solubility of the drug molecule in the gastrointestinal environment, membrane permeability, presystemic intestinal metabolism, hepatic first-pass metabolism, or susceptibility to membrane transporters, such as P-gp efflux. Other routes of administration (e.g., subcutaneous, intravenous, inhalation, and nasal) for susceptible drugs have been investigated in an attempt to overcome the pronounced presystemic metabolism. The extent of first-pass metabolism depends on the drug delivery system because a formulation can increase or decrease the rate of dissolution, the residence time of a drug in the gastrointestinal tract, and the dose. The more prolonged the residence time, the greater the efficiency of first-pass metabolism. The drug form and delivery system should yield optimal bioavailability and pharmacokinetic profiles, resulting in a reproducible clinical response.

Studies are being performed to determine the effect of presystemic and hepatic first-pass metabolism on the toxicity and carcinogenicity of xenobiotics. For a nontherapeutic toxic substance, the existence of a first-pass effect is desirable, because the liver can bioinactivate the substance, preventing its distribution to other parts of the body. On the other hand, first-pass metabolism can increase a drug's toxicity by biotransforming the toxicant to a more toxic metabolite, which can reenter the blood and exert its toxic effect.

Presystemic First-Pass Metabolism

Although hepatic metabolism continues to be the most important route of metabolism for xenobiotics, the ability of the liver and intestine to metabolize substances to either pharmacologically inactive or bioactive metabolites before reaching systemic blood levels is called prehepatic or presystemic first-pass metabolism, which results in the low systemic availability for susceptible drugs. Sulfonation and glucuronidation are major pathways of presystemic intestinal first-pass metabolism in humans for acetaminophen, phenylephrine, terbutaline, albuterol, fenoterol, and isoproterenol.

The discovery that CYP3A4 is found in the mucosal enterocytes of the intestinal villi signifies its role as key determinant in the oral bioavailability of its numerous drug substrates (Table 4.11) (77). Drugs known to be substrates for CYP3A have a low and variable oral bioavailability that can be explained by presystemic first-pass metabolism by the small intestine P450 isoforms. The concentration of functional intestinal CYP3A is influenced by genetic disposition, induction, and inhibition, which to a great extent determines drug blood levels and therapeutic response. Xenobiotics, when ingested orally, can modify the activity of intestinal CYP3A enzymes by induction, inhibition, and stimulation. By modulation of the isoform pattern in the intestine, a xenobiotic could alter its own metabolism and that of others in a time- and dose-dependent manner. The concentration of CYP3A in the intestine is comparable to that of the liver. The oral administration of dexamethasone induces the formation of CYP3A and erythromycin inhibits it. The glucocorticoid inducibility of CYP3A4 can also be a factor in differences of metabolism between males and females. Studies have suggested that intestinal CYP3A4 C-2 hydroxylation of estradiol contributes to the oxidative metabolism of endogenous estrogens circulating with the enterohepatic recycling pool (38). Norethisterone has a low oral bioavailability of 42% due to oxidative first-pass metabolism (CYP3A), but levonorgestrel is completely available in women with no conjugated metabolites.

Several clinically relevant drug–drug interactions between orally coadministered drugs and CYP3A4 can be explained by a modification of drug metabolism at the P450 level. If a drug has high presystemic elimination (low bioavailability) and is metabolized primarily by CYP3A4, then coadministration with a CYP3A4 inhibitor can be expected to alter the drug's pharmacokinetics by reducing its metabolism, thus increasing its plasma concentration. Drugs and some foods (e.g., grapefruit juice) that are known inhibitors, inducers, or substrates for intestinal CYP3A4 can potentially interact with the metabolism of a coadministered drug, affecting its area under the curve and rate of clearance (Tables 4.12 and 4.14) (78). Inducers can reduce absorption and oral bioavailability, whereas these same factors are increased by inhibitors. For example, erythromycin can enhance the oral absorption of another drug by inhibiting its metabolism in the small intestine by CYP3A4. By virtue of being competitive substrates for CYP3A4, prednisone, prednisolone, and methylprednisolone (but not dexamethasone) are competitive inhibitors of synthetic glucocorticoid metabolism. This is because a major metabolic pathway for synthetic glucocorticoids involves CYP3A4. In addition to coadministered drugs, metabolic interactions with exogenous CYP3A4 substrates secreted in the bile are possible. The poor oral bioavailability for cyclosporine is attributed to a combination of intestinal metabolism by CYP3A4 and efflux by P-gp (79).

Because the intestinal mucosa is enriched with glucuronosyltransferases, sulfotransferases, and glutathione transferases, presystemic first-pass metabolism for orally administered drugs susceptible to these conjugation reactions results in their low oral bioavailability (65). Presystemic metabolism often exceeds liver metabolism for some drugs. For example, more than 80% of intravenously administered albuterol is excreted unchanged in urine, with the balance as glucuronide conjugates, whereas when albuterol is administered orally, less than 5% is systemically absorbed as a result of intestinal sulfonation and glucuronidation. Presystemic metabolism is a major pathway in humans for most β-adrenergic agonists, such as glucuronides or sulfate esters for terbutaline, fenoterol, albuterol, and isoproterenol, morphine (3–*O*-glucuronide), acetaminophen (*O*-sulfate), and estradiol (3–*O*-sulfate). The bioavailability of orally administered estradiol or ethinyl estradiol in females is approximately 50%. Mestranol (3-methoxyethinyl estradiol) has greater bioavailability, however, because it is not significantly conjugated. Levodopa has a low oral bioavailability as a result of its metabolism by intestinal L-aromatic amino acid decarboxylase. The activity of this enzyme depends on the percentage bound of its cofactor pyridoxine (vitamin B_6). Tyramine, which occurs in fermented foods such as cheeses and red wines, ripe bananas, and yeast extracts, is metabolized by both MAO-A and MAO-B in the gut wall.

The extensive presystemic first-pass sulfonation of phenolic drugs, for example, can lead to increased bioavailability of other drugs by competing for the available sulfate pool, resulting in the possibility of drug toxicity (56). Concurrent oral administration of acetaminophen with ethinyl estradiol resulted in a 48% increase in ethinyl estradiol blood levels. Ascorbic acid, which is sulfonated, also increases the bioavailability of concurrently administered ethinyl estradiol. Sulfonation and glucuronidation occur side by side, often competing for the same substrate, and the balance between sulfonation and glucuronidation is influenced by several factors, such as species, doses, availability of cosubstrates, inhibition, and induction of the respective transferases.

First-Pass Metabolism

Several orally administered drugs are known to undergo liver first-pass metabolism during their transport to the systemic circulation from the gastrointestinal tract

TABLE 4.17 Examples of Drugs Exhibiting First-Pass Metabolism

Acetaminophen	Isoproterenol	Oxprenolol
Albuterol	Lidocaine	Pentazocine
Alprenolol	Meperidine	Propoxyphene
Aspirin	Methyltestosterone	Propranolol
Cyclosporin	Metoprolol	Salicylamide
Desmethylimipramine	Dihydropyridines	Terbutaline
Fluorouracil	(Nifedipine)	Verapamil
Hydrocortisone	Nortriptyline	
Imipramine	Organic nitrates	

(e.g., metoprolol). Thus, the liver can remove substances from the blood after their absorption from the gastrointestinal tract, thereby preventing distribution to other parts of the body. This effect can seriously impair the bioavailability of an orally administered drug, reducing the amount of the drug that reaches the systemic circulation and, ultimately, its receptor to produce its pharmacologic effect. Drugs subject to first-pass metabolism are included in Table 4.17.

P-Glycoprotein

Another factor that must be considered in the oral bioavailability of many CYP3A4 substrates is intestinal P-gp (80). Originally discovered as a transmembrane transporter protein associated with the resistance (elimination) of anticancer drugs, P-gp can also have a role in how a drug is absorbed, distributed, metabolized, and eliminated from the body (see Chapter 5) (79–81). Considering its role as a transporter protein (efflux pump), it is logical that it should exhibit saturable (nonlinear) kinetics. P-gp exhibits a broad specificity for a large number of substrates, inhibitors, and inducers (Table 4.18). The common link between P-gp substrates is that most of the same compounds are also substrates for CYP3A4. The close physical location of P-gp and CYP3A4 in the endothelial cells of the intestinal mucosa allows these proteins to work in concert with each other to decrease drug plasma concentrations of CYP3A4 substrates, suggesting a complementary protective mechanism for these two proteins, forming a barrier to the intestinal absorption of CYP3A4 substrates. Hepatic and renal P-gp also appears to function in a complementary manner, promoting the elimination of substrates into the bile and urine, respectively. For example, if a drug is a substrate for intestinal P-gp, its oral absorption will be incomplete and this same drug will be actively transported by the renal tubules into the urine, enhancing its elimination. On the other hand, inhibiting P-gp would be expected to improve the oral bioavailability of P-gp substrates, but if the inhibitor is also a substrate for CYP3A4, increased metabolism (presystemic) would occur. Drugs with low oral bioavailability or high first-pass metabolism can be particularly susceptible to alterations in the transport kinetics of P-gp. Because P-gp exhibits saturation (nonlinear) kinetics, drugs

TABLE 4.18 Some Substrates, Inhibitors, and Inducers for P-Glycoprotein

Substrate	Lidocaine*	**Inhibitors**	Lovastatin*	**Foods**
Acetolol	Loperamide*	Amiodarone*	Maprotiline	Daidzein
Amiodarone*	Methotrexate	Amitriptyline*	Mefloquine*	Genistein
Atorvastatin*	Mibefradil	Astemizole*	Mibefradil*	Grapefruit juice*
Celiprolol	Nadolol	Atorvastatin*	Midazolam*	Orange juice
Cimetidine*	Nelfinavir*	Carvedilol	Mifepristone*	Isoflavones
Ciprofloxacin	Nicardipine*	Chlorpromazine*	Nelfinavir*	**Inducers**
Colchicine	Ondansetron*	Clarithromycin*	Nicardipine*	Dexamethasone*
Cyclosporin*	Paclitaxel*	Cyclosporin*	Nifedipine*	Prazosin
Daunorubicin*	Pravastatin*	Desipramine	Nitrendipine*	Progesterone*
Debrisoquine	Quinidine*	Dexverapamil*	Ofloxacin	Quercetin
Dexamethasone*	Quinolones	Diltiazem*	Prochlorperazine	Rifampin
DHEA	Ranitidine	Dipyridamole	Progesterone*	St. John's Wort*
Digoxin*	Rifampin*	Disulfiram	Propranolol	
Diltiazem*	Ritonavir*	Doxepin	Propafenone*	
Docetaxel*	Saquinavir*	Erythromycin*	Quinidine*	
Domperidone*	Tacrolimus*	Flupentixol	Quinine*	
Doxorubicin*	Taxol*	Felodipine*	Reserpine	
Enoxacin	Teniposide*	Fluphenazine	Rifampin*	
Erythromycin*	Terfenadine*	Glibenclamide	Ritonavir*	
Estradiol*	Timolol	Haloperidol*	Saquinavir*	
Etoposide*	Verapamil*	Hydrocortisone*	Tacrolimus*	
Fexofenadine*	Vinblastine*	Imipramine*	Testosterone*	
Hydrocortisone*	Vincristine *	Itraconazole*	Tamoxifen*	
Idarubicin	Vindesine*	Ivermectin	Trimipramine	
Indinavir*		Ketoconazole*	Verapamil*	
Ivermectin		Lidocaine*		

*CYP3A4 substrate, inhibitor, or inducer.

with low dosages can have their oral bioavailability enhanced by increasing its oral dosage, thus saturating the P-gp pump. As with CYP3A4, there is significant interindividual variation (4- to 10-fold) in the intestinal expression of P-gp, which could explain the variance observed in the pharmacokinetics for CYP3A4 substrates. The interactive nature of CYP3A4 and P-gp will be of importance in controlling and improving the oral bioavailability of CYP3A4 substrates and drug regimens. The presence of inhibitors of P-gp in grapefruit juice (e.g., 6,7-dihydroxybergamottin and other furanocoumarins) has confirmed that the inhibition of efflux transport of drugs and of drug metabolism by CYP3A4 could be an important cause of drug–grapefruit juice interaction (82).

In summary, oral bioavailability for xenobiotics is dependent on a combination of factors, including physical properties of the drugs and formulation and biologic factors such as metabolizing enzymes, membrane permeability, and the membrane efflux pump, P-gp.

EXTRAHEPATIC METABOLISM

Because the liver is the primary tissue for xenobiotic metabolism, it is not surprising that our understanding of mammalian P450 monooxygenase is based chiefly on hepatic studies. Although the tissue content of P450s is highest in the liver, P450 enzymes are ubiquitous, and their role in extrahepatic tissues remains unclear. P450 pattern in these tissues differs considerably from that in the human liver (83). In addition to liver tissue, P450 enzymes are found in lung, nasal epithelium, intestinal tract, kidney, and adrenal tissues and brain. It is possible that the expression of the polymorphic genes and induction of the isoforms in the extrahepatic tissues can affect the activity of the P450 isoforms in the metabolism of drugs, endogenous steroids, and xenobiotics. Therefore, characterization of P450, UGT, SULT, and other polymorphic drug-metabolizing enzymes in extrahepatic tissues is important to our overall understanding about the biologic importance of these isoform families to improved drug therapy, design of new drugs and dosages forms, toxicity, and carcinogenicity.

The mucosal surfaces of the gastrointestinal tract, the nasal passages, and the lungs are major portals of entry for xenobiotics into the body and, as such, are continuously exposed to a variety of orally ingested or inhaled airborne xenobiotics, including drugs, plant toxins, environmental pollutants, and other chemical substances. As a consequence of this exposure, these tissues represent a major target for necrosis, tumorigenesis, and other chemically induced toxicities. Many of these toxins and chemical carcinogens are relatively inert substances that must be bioactivated to exert their cytotoxicity and tumorigenicity. The epithelial cells of these tissues are capable of metabolizing a wide variety of exogenous and endogenous substances, and these cells provide the principal and initial source of biotransformation for these xenobiotics during the absorptive phase. The consequences of such presystemic biotransformation is either a decrease in the amount of xenobiotics available for systemic absorption by facilitating the elimination of polar metabolites or toxification by activation to carcinogens, which can be one determinant of tissue susceptibility for the development of intestinal cancer. The risk of colon cancer can depend on dietary constituents that contain either procarcinogens or compounds modulating the response to carcinogens.

Intestinal Metabolism

Many of the clinically relevant aspects of P450 can, in fact, occur at the level of the intestinal mucosa and could account for differences among patients in dosing requirements. The intestinal mucosa is enriched especially with CYP3A4 isoform, glucuronosyl transferases, sulfotransferases, and GSTs, making it particularly important for orally administered drugs susceptible to oxidation (77), glucuronidation, or sulfonation conjugation pathways (56), or glutathione conjugation pathways. The highest concentrations of P450s occur in the duodenum, with gradual tapering into the ileum. In the human intestine, CYP2E, CYP3A, CYP2C8, CYP2C9, CYP2C19, and CYP2D6 have been identified. Therefore, intestinal P450 isoforms provide potential presystemic first-pass metabolism of ingested xenobiotics affecting their oral bioavailability (e.g., hydroxylation of naloxone) or bioactivation of carcinogens or mutagens. It is not surprising that dietary factors can affect the intestinal P450 isoforms. For example, a 2-day dietary exposure to cooked Brussels sprouts significantly decreased the 2α-hydroxylation of testosterone yet induced CYP1A2 activity for PAH. An 8-oz glass of grapefruit juice inhibited the sulfoxidation metabolism of omeprazole (CYP3A4) but not its hydroxylation (CYP2C19), thus increasing its systemic blood concentration. These types of interactions between a drug and a dietary inhibitor could result in a clinically significant drug interaction.

Intestinal UGT isoforms can glucuronidate orally administered drugs, such as morphine, acetaminophen, α- and β-adrenergic agonists, and other phenolic phenethanolamines and other dietary xenobiotics, resulting in a reduction of their oral bioavailability (increasing first-pass metabolism), thus altering their pharmacokinetics and pharmacodynamics. The UGTs expressed in the intestine include UGT1A1 (bilirubin-glucuronidating isoform), UGT1A3, UGT1A4, UGT1A6, UGT1A8, UGT1A9, and UGT1A5. Substrate specificities of intestinal UGT isoforms are comparable to those in the liver. Glucuronidase hydrolysis of biliary glucuronide conjugates in the intestine can contribute to EHC of the parent drug.

Likewise, the sulfotransferases in the small intestine can sulfonate orally administered drugs and xenobiotics for which the primary route of conjugation is sulfonation (e.g., isoproterenol, albuterol, steroid hormones, α-methyldopa, acetaminophen, and fenoldopam), decreasing their oral bioavailability and, thus, altering their pharmacokinetics and pharmacodynamics. Competition for intestinal sulfonation between coadministered substrates can influence their bioavailability with either an enhancement or a decrease of therapeutic effects. Sulfatase hydrolysis of biliary sulfate esters in the intestine can contribute to EHC of the parent drug.

The occurrence of intestinal P450 enzymes and bacterial enzymes in the microflora allows the metabolism of relatively stable environmental pollutants and food-derived xenobiotics (i.e., plants contain a variety of protoxins, promutagens, and procarcinogens) into mutagens and carcinogens (68). For example, cruciferous vegetables (Brussels sprouts, cabbage, broccoli, cauliflower, and spinach) are all rich in indole compounds (e.g., indole 3-carbinol), which with regular and chronic ingestion are capable of inducing some intestinal P450s (CYP1A subfamily) and inhibiting others (CYP3A subfamily). It is likely that these vegetables would also alter the metabolism of food-derived mutagens (e.g., heterocyclic amines produced during charbroiling of meat are P450 *N*-hydroxylated and become carcinogenic in a manner similar to arylamines) and carcinogens.

The extent of a drug's metabolism in the small bowel and its role in clinically relevant drug interaction remain to be evaluated and must be taken into account during oral pharmacokinetics analysis of future drug interaction studies. Clinically significant interaction will not always occur when a drug is combined with other isoform subfamily substrates. Oral coadministration of a drug with drugs that interact with its metabolism need not be avoided. The blood concentration of the drug must be monitored closely, however, and the dose should be adapted to avoid adverse drug reactions.

Intestinal Microflora

When drugs are orally ingested or there is considerable biliary excretion of a drug or its metabolites into the gastrointestinal tract, such as with a parentally administered drug (EHC or recirculation), the intestinal bacterial microflora can have a role in the metabolism of these drugs. The microflora has an important role in the enterohepatic recirculation of xenobiotics via their conjugated metabolites (e.g., digoxin, the oral contraceptives norethisterone and ethinyl estradiol, and chloramphenicol) and endogenous substances (steroid hormones, bile acids, folic acid, and cholesterol), which reenter the gut via the bile (68). Compounds eliminated in the bile are conjugated with glucuronic acid, glycine, sulfate, and glutathione, and once secreted into the small intestine, the bacterial β-glucuronidase, sulfatase, nitroreductases, and various glycosidases catalyze the hydrolysis of the conjugates. The activity of orally administered conjugated estrogens (e.g., Premarin) involves the hydrolysis of the sulfate esters by sulfatases, releasing estrogens to be reabsorbed from the intestine into the portal circulation. The clinical use of oral antibiotics (e.g., erythromycin, penicillin, clindamycin, and aminoglycosides) has a profound effect on the gut microflora and the enzymes responsible for the hydrolysis of drug conjugates undergoing EHC. Bacterial reduction includes nitro reduction of nitroimidazole, azo reduction of azides (sulfasalazine to 5-aminosalicylic acid and sulfapyridine), and reduction of the sulfoxide to its sulfide. The sulfoxide of sulindac is reduced by both gut microflora and hepatic P450s. Other ways in which bacterial flora can affect metabolism include the following: 1) production of toxic metabolites, 2) formation of carcinogens from inactive precursors, 3) detoxication, 4) exhibition of species differences in drug metabolism, 5) exhibition of individual differences in drug metabolism, 6) production of pharmacologically active metabolites from inactive precursors, and 7) production of metabolites not formed by animal tissues. In contrast to the predominantly hepatic oxidative and conjugative metabolism of the liver, gut microflora is largely degradative, hydrolytic, and reductive, with a potential for both metabolic activation and detoxication of xenobiotics.

Lung Metabolism

Some of the hepatic xenobiotic biotransformation pathways are also operative in the lung (84,85). Because of the differences in organ sizes, the total content of the pulmonary xenobiotic-metabolizing enzyme systems is usually lower than in the liver, creating the impression of a minor role for the lung in xenobiotic elimination. CYP2E1 is expressed in the lung to the greatest extent. The expression of other P450s, FMO, epoxide hydrolase, and the Phase 2 conjugation pathways are comparable to those in the liver. Thus, the lungs can have a significant role in the metabolic elimination or activation of small molecular weight inhaled xenobiotics. When drugs are injected intravenously, intramuscularly, or subcutaneously, or after skin absorption, the drug initially enters the pulmonary circulation, after which the lung becomes the organ of first-pass metabolism for the drug. The blood levels and therapeutic response of the drug are influenced by genetic disposition, induction, and inhibition of the pulmonary metabolizing enzymes. By modulation of the P450 isoform pattern in the lung, a xenobiotic could alter its own metabolism and that of others in a time- and dose-dependent manner. Because of its position in the circulation, the lung provides a second-pass metabolism for xenobiotics and their metabolites exiting from the liver, but it is also susceptible to the cytotoxicity or carcinogenicity of hepatic activated metabolites. Antihistamines, β-blockers, opioids, and tricyclic antidepressants are among the basic amines known to accumulate in the lungs as a result of their binding to surfactant phospholipids in lung tissue. The significance of this relationship to potential pneumotoxicity remains to be seen.

Nasal Metabolism

The nasal olfactory mucosa is recognized as a first line of defense for the lung against airborne environmental xenobiotics, because the mucosa is constantly exposed to the airborne external environment (86). Drug metabolism in the olfactory nasal epithelium represents a major metabolic pathway for protecting the brain against the entry of drugs, inhaled environmental pollutants, or other volatile chemicals into the CNS and brain. In some instances, these enzymes can biotransform drugs, environmental pollutants, or airborne xenobiotics into more reactive and potentially toxic metabolites, increasing the risk of carcinogenesis in the nasopharynx and lung (e.g., procarcinogens and nitrosamines in cigarette smoke). P450 activity is high in olfactory tissue, and olfactory-specific isoforms have been identified, including CYP1A2, CYP2A6, CYP2A13, CYP2E1, CYP3A4, and CYP2G1, as well as several isoforms of the flavin-dependent monooxygenases. Phase 2 enzymes found in the olfactory mucosa include UGTs, glutathione-*S*-transferases, carboxylesterases, aldehyde oxidases, and epoxide hydrolases. The most striking feature of the nasal epithelium is that P450 catalytic activity is higher than in any other extrahepatic tissue, including the liver. Nasal decongestants, essences, anesthetics, alcohols, nicotine, and cocaine have been shown to be metabolized in vitro by P450 enzymes from the nasal epithelium. Because the P450s in the nasal mucosa are active, first-pass metabolism should be considered when delivering susceptible drugs to the nasal tissues.

The nasal mucosa is also exposed to a wide range of odorants. Odorants, which are mostly small lipophilic molecules, enter the mucosa and reach the odorant receptors on sensory neurons by a transient process requiring signal termination, which could be provided by biotransformation of the odorant in the epithelial supporting cells. Thus metabolism of odorants could be involved in both the termination and initiation of olfactory stimuli.

Metabolism in Other Tissues

The isoforms of P450s and their regulation in the brain are of interest in defining the possible involvement of P450s in central nervous system toxicity and carcinogenicity. P450s in the kidney and adrenal tissues include isoforms primarily involved in the hydroxylation of steroids, arachidonic acid, and 25-hydroxycholcalciferol.

STEREOCHEMICAL ASPECTS OF DRUG METABOLISM

In addition to the physicochemical factors that affect xenobiotic metabolism, stereochemical factors have an important role in the biotransformation of drugs. This involvement is not unexpected, because the xenobiotic-metabolizing enzymes are also the same enzymes that metabolize certain endogenous substrates, which for the most part are chiral molecules. Most of these enzymes show stereoselectivity but not stereospecificity; in other words, one stereoisomer enters into biotransformation pathways preferentially but not exclusively. Metabolic stereochemical reactions can be categorized as follows: substrate stereoselectivity, in which two enantiomers of a chiral substrate are metabolized at different rates; product stereoselectivity, in which a new chiral center is created in a symmetric molecule and one enantiomer is metabolized preferentially; and substrate-product stereoselectivity, in which a new chiral center of a chiral molecule is metabolized preferentially to one of two possible diastereomers (87). An example of substrate stereoselectivity is the preferred decarboxylation of *S*-α-methyldopa to *S*-α-methyldopamine, with almost no reaction for *R*-α-methyldopa. The reduction of ketones to stereoisomeric alcohols and the hydroxylation of enantiotropic protons or phenyl rings by monooxygenases are examples of product stereoselectivity. For example, phenytoin undergoes aromatic *p*-hydroxylation of only one of its two phenyl rings to create a chiral center at C-5 of the hydantoin ring, methadone is reduced preferentially to its α-diastereometric alcohol, and naltrexone is reduced to its 6-β-alcohol. An example of substrate-product stereoselectivity is the reduction of the enantiomers of warfarin and the β-hydroxylation of *S*-α-methyldopamine to (1*R*,2*S*)-α-methylnorepinephrine, whereas *R*-α-methyldopamine is hydroxylated only to a negligible extent. In vivo studies of this type often can be confused by the further biotransformation of one stereoisomer, giving the false impression that only one stereoisomer was formed preferentially. Moreover, some compounds show stereoselective absorption, distribution, and excretion, which proves the importance of performing in vitro studies. Although studies regarding the stereoselective biotransformation of drug molecules are not yet extensive, those that have been done indicate that stereochemical factors have an important role in drug metabolism and, in some cases, could account for the differences in pharmacologic activity and duration of action between enantiomers (see the discussion of chiral inversion of the NSAIDs).

METABOLIC BIOACTIVATION: ROLE IN HEPATOTOXICITY, IDIOSYNCRATIC REACTIONS, AND CHEMICAL CARCINOGENESIS

Drug-Induced Hepatotoxicity

Drug-induced hepatotoxicity is the leading cause of hepatic injury, accounting for approximately half of all cases of acute liver failure in the United States (88,89). Recent studies have shown that drug-induced hepatotoxicity represents a larger percentage of adverse drug reactions than reported previously and that the incidence and severity of drug-induced liver injury is underestimated among the general population.

Acetaminophen overdose is the leading cause for calls to Poison Control Centers (>100,000 calls/year) and accounts for more than 56,000 emergency room visits, 2,600 hospitalizations, and an estimated 458 deaths from acute liver failure each year. Among the listed drugs in Table 4.19, acetaminophen is the most frequent hepatotoxic agent and can cause extensive hepatic necrosis with as little as 10 to 12 g (30 to 40 tablets). Chronic alcohol intake enhances acetaminophen hepatotoxicity by more than five times as compared to acute alcohol intake, yet acetaminophen is heavily marketed for its safety as compared to nonsteroidal analgesics. United States drug manufacturers continue to market and promote extra-strength acetaminophen products (500 to 750 mg/tablet) and a variety of extra-strength acetaminophen–drug combination products. Self-poisoning with acetaminophen (paracetamol) is also a common cause of hepatotoxicity in the Western world. To reduce the number of acetaminophen poisonings in the United Kingdom, over-the-counter (nonprescription) sales of acetaminophen are limited to 16 tablets per packet.

Drug-induced hepatic damage is also the most frequent reason that new therapeutic agents are not approved by the FDA (e.g., ximelagatran in 2004) and the most common adverse drug reaction leading to withdrawal of a drug from the market (Table 4.19). Hepatotoxicity almost always involves metabolism with P450 enzymes rather than Phase 2 enzymes. More than 600 drugs, chemicals, and herbal remedies can cause hepatotoxicity, of which more than 30 drugs have either been withdrawn from the United States market as a result of hepatotoxicity or have carried a black box warning for hepatotoxicity since 1990. Table 4.19 includes some of the more common drugs that have exhibited drug-induced hepatotoxicity ranging from severe, requiring the drug's regulatory withdrawal from the market (bold in Table 4.19); moderate to severe, requiring black box warning restrictions (italics in Table 4.19); or mild to moderate, requiring frequent liver function monitoring.

SOME DRUGS EXHIBITING DRUG-INDUCED HEPATOTOXICITY NOT APPROVED FOR USE IN UNITED STATES

Drugs with reactive metabolites that were used in other countries but never approved in the United States include: alpidem, amineptine, amodiaquine, cinchophen, dihydralazine, dilevalol, ebrotidine, glafenine, ibufenac, isoxicam, niperotidine, perhexiline, pirprofen, and tilbroquinol.

However, Watkins et al. (90) reported in the *Journal of the American Medical Association* that one-third of 106 patients taking a maximum daily acetaminophen dose of 4 g for 8 days, either alone or in combination with hydrocodone, exhibited a threefold increase in liver enzymes associated with acetaminophen-induced liver injury. This threefold increase in transaminase levels is a signal for potential liver safety concerns in those individuals who are at risk of acetaminophen-induced liver toxicity. Drug-induced injury is most common and includes hepatic necrosis and steatosis, which can affect significant portions of the liver (88). Drugs reported to cause hepatocellular necrosis include acetaminophen, methyldopa, valproic acid, trazodone,

TABLE 4.19 Some Drugs Causing Hepatic Injury[a]

Acarbose	Fenofibrate	Methotrexate	Rosiglitazone
Acetaminophen	*Fluconazole*	Methsuximide	Rosuvastatin
Allopurinol	*Flutamide*	Methyldopa	*Saquinavir*
Amiodarone	Fluvastatin	Nabumetone	Simvastatin
Amprenavir	Gemfibrozil	Naproxen	Sulindac
Anagrelide	Gemtuzumab	**Nefazodone (2005)**	*Tacrine*
Atomoxetine	Griseofulvin	*Nevirapine*	Tamoxifen
Atorvastatin	*Halothane*	Niacin (SR)	**Tasosartan (1998)**
Azathioprine	Imatinib	Nitrofurantoin	*Terbinafine*
Bicalutamide	Indinavir	Olanzapine	Testosterone
Bosentan	*Infliximab*	Oxaprozin	Thioguanine
Bromfenac (1998)	*Interferon-β_{1a}*	Peg-interferon-α_{2a}	Tizanidine
Carbamazepine	Interferon-β_{1b}	**Pemoline (2005)**	*Tolcapone*
Celecoxib	Isoflurane	Pentamidine	**Troglitizone (2000)**
Dapsone	*Isoniazid*	Pioglitazone	*Trovafloxacin*
Deferasirox	Fenofibrate	Piroxicam	*Valproic acid*
Diclofenac	Isotretinoin	Pravastatin	Voriconazole
Disulfiram	Itraconazole	*Pyrazinamide*	**Ximelagatran** *(2004)*
Duloxetine	*Ketoconazole*	Ribavirin	*Zileuton*
Efavirenz	*Ketorolac*	Rifabutin	*Zifirlukast*
Ethotoin	Lamivudine	*Rifampin*	
Ethosuximide	*Leflunomide*	Riluzole	
Felbamate	Lovastatin	Ritonavir	

[a]Drugs in **bold** have exhibited severe drug-induced hepatotoxicity and were withdrawn either voluntarily or by a regulatory agency (year given). Drugs in *italics* have exhibited moderate–severe drug-induced hepatotoxicity requiring a black box warning restricting their use. The other drugs have exhibited mild to moderate drug-induced hepatotoxicity that can need frequent liver transaminase testing for those at risk (see Table 4.20).

nefazodone, venlafaxine, and lovastatin. Drug-induced liver damage occurs after a prolonged period of drug administration.

The most commonly used indicators of hepatotoxicity (i.e., liver injury) are increased levels of the liver transaminases, aspartate aminotransferase (AST) and alanine aminotransferase (ALT) (88,89). Drug-induced hepatotoxicity can develop rapidly, often before abnormal laboratory tests are noticed, which are characterized by rapid elevations in ALT and AST of 8 to 500 times the upper normal limit, with variable elevations in bilirubin. Drugs causing acute liver injury (hepatocellular necrosis) exhibit elevations in hepatic transaminases ranging from 50 to 100 times higher than the normal level. On the other hand, the elevations of ALT and AST in alcoholic liver disease are two to three times higher than normal. Some hepatotoxins, however, do not elevate transaminases, whereas nonhepatic toxins can elevate ALT.

Most drug-induced hepatotoxicity is of an idiosyncratic nature, occurring in a small percentage of patients (1 in 5,000) who ingest the drug (88,89). These reactions tend to be of two distinct types: 1) hypersensitivity reactions that are immune mediated, occurring within the first 4 to 6 weeks, and are associated with fever, rash, eosinophilia, and a hepatitis-like picture (e.g., phenytoin, sulindac, and allopurinol); and 2) metabolic idiosyncratic reactions that tend to occur at almost any time during the first year of treatment (e.g., troglitazone and isoniazid). The incidence of overt idiosyncratic liver diseases varies with the drug, ranging from approximately 1 in 100 with isoniazid to 1 in 1,000 with phenytoin, to 1 in 10,000 or more with sulindac and troglitazone, and 1 in 100,000 with diclofenac. To detect a single case of drug-induced hepatotoxicity with 95% confidence requires the number of patients studied to be threefold the incidence of the reaction. For one adverse drug reaction in 10,000 patients, at least 30,000 patients need to be evaluated. Thus, many drugs are approved before liver toxicity is observed. It is the responsibility of postmarketing surveillance and monitoring of liver transaminases to identify potential cases of liver-adverse drug reactions.

Risk factors (Table 4.20) for drug-induced liver injury, such as age, gender, genetic predisposition, multiple drugs or dietary supplements, and degree of alcohol consumption, appear to increase the susceptibility to drug-induced hepatotoxicity (88,89). Patients with mild to moderate chronic liver disease do not appear to be at increased risk for idiosyncratic hepatic injury from drugs. However, the drugs in Table 4.19 should be used with caution in these patients, because such patients can have altered metabolism of these drugs and, therefore, can be at increased risk for liver injury. The coadministration of drugs in Table 4.19 with enzyme inducers, such as phenobarbital, phenytoin, ethanol, and/or cigarette smoke, can induce hepatic enzymes, resulting in the enhancement of hepatotoxicity.

Most hepatic adverse effects associated with drugs occur in adults rather than children. Drug-induced liver injury occurs at a higher rate in patients older than 50

TABLE 4.20 Risk Factors for Drug-Induced Liver Injury

Race	Some drugs exhibit different toxicities based on race as a result of individual P450 polymorphism. For example, blacks and Hispanics can be more susceptible to isoniazid (INH) toxicity.
Age	Elderly persons are at increased risk of hepatic injury due to decreased clearance, drug-to-drug interactions, reduced hepatic blood flow, variation in drug binding, and lower hepatic volume. In addition, poor diet, infections, and multiple hospitalizations are important reasons for drug-induced hepatotoxicity. Hepatic drug reactions are rare in children (e.g., acetaminophen, halogenated general anesthetics).
Gender	Although the reasons are unknown, hepatic drug reactions are more common in females. Females are more susceptible to acetaminophen, halothane, nitrofurantoin, diclofenac, and sulindac.
Alcohol	Alcoholics are susceptible to drug toxicity, because alcohol induces liver injury and cirrhotic changes that alter drug metabolism. Alcohol causes depletion of glutathione (hepatoprotective) stores, making the person more susceptible to toxicity by drugs (e.g., acetaminophen, statins).
Liver disease	Patients with chronic liver disease are not uniformly at increased risk of hepatic injury. Although the total P450 level is reduced, some patients can be affected more than others. The modification of doses in persons with liver disease should be based on knowledge of the specific P450 isoform involved in the metabolism. Patients with HIV infection who are coinfected with hepatitis B or C virus are at increased risk for hepatotoxic effects. Similarly, patients with cirrhosis are at increased risk to hepatotoxic drugs (e.g., methotrexate, methyldopa, valproic acid).
Genetic factors	Genetic (polymorphic) differences in the formation of P450 isoforms (2C family and 2D6) can result in abnormal reactions to drugs, including idiosyncratic reactions (see Table 4.18).
Other comorbidities	Patients with AIDS, renal disease, or diabetes mellitus; persons who are malnourished; and persons who are fasting can be susceptible to drug reactions as a result of low glutathione stores.
Pharmacokinetics	Long-acting drugs can cause more injury than shorter-acting drugs, as well as sustained-release drug product formulations.
Drug adulterants	Contaminants are often found in noncertified herbal supplements (e.g., hepatitis C).

years, and drug-associated jaundice occurs also more frequently in the geriatric population (88,89). This age-related risk can be the result of increased frequency of drug exposure, multidrug therapy, and age-related changes in drug metabolism.

For reasons that are unclear, drug-induced liver injury affects females more than males: Females accounted for approximately 79% of all reactions to acetaminophen and 73% of all idiosyncratic drug-induced reactions (88). Females exhibit increased risk of hepatic injury from drugs such as atorvastatin, nitrofurantoin, methyldopa, and diclofenac.

Genetic factors as a result of enzyme polymorphism in affected individuals can decrease the ability to metabolize or eliminate drugs, thus increasing their duration of action and the drug exposure and/or decreasing the ability to modulate the immune response to drugs or metabolites. Chronic ingestion of alcohol can also predispose many patients to increased hepatotoxicity from drugs by lowering the store of glutathione (a detoxifying mechanism), which prevents trapping of the toxic metabolites as mercapturate conjugates that are excreted in the urine.

Other factors include the effect of drug formulation (sustained vs. rapid release; increased exposure) on pharmacokinetics, for example, elimination half-life of the drug or adulterants (e.g., enzyme inducers) in dietary supplements.

Drug-induced hepatotoxicity can be categorized as an intrinsic (predictable) or idiosyncratic (unpredictable) drug reaction (89). Most drugs involved in hepatotoxicity belong to the idiosyncratic group. Intrinsic hepatotoxins produce liver injury in a dose-related manner when the toxic amount of drug is ingested without bioactivation, such as these toxins found in the *Amanita* mushroom. Fortunately, few drugs are intrinsic hepatotoxins. Idiosyncratic hepatotoxicity is the result of the toxic effects of a drug's metabolites.

The common trigger for both mild and severe forms of hepatotoxicity is bioactivation of relatively inert functional groups to reactive electrophilic intermediates, which is considered to be an obligatory event in the etiology of many drug-induced idiosyncratic hepatotoxicities (91,92). A great deal of evidence now shows that reactive metabolites are formed from drugs known to cause idiosyncratic hepatotoxicity, but how these toxic species initiate and propagate tissue damage remains poorly understood. However, the relationship between bioactivation and the occurrence of hepatic injury is not simple. For example, many drugs at therapeutic doses undergo bioactivation in the liver but are not hepatotoxic. The tight coupling of bioactivation with bioinactivation pathways can be one reason for the lack of hepatotoxicity with these drugs. Examples of bioinactivation (detoxification) pathways include glutathione conjugation of quinones by GSTs and hydration of arene oxides to dihydrodiols by epoxide hydrolases. When reactive metabolites are poor substrates for such detoxifying enzymes, they can escape bioinactivation and, thereby, damage proteins and nucleic acids, prompting hepatotoxicity.

Most drugs, however, are not directly chemically reactive but, through the normal process of drug metabolism, can form electrophilic, chemically reactive metabolites (90–92). Formation of chemically reactive metabolites is mainly catalyzed by P450 enzymes, but products of Phase 2 metabolism (e.g., acylglucuronides, acyl CoA thioesters, or *N*-sulfates) can also lead to toxicity. However, if P450 drug bioactivation is closely coupled with Phase 2 bioinactivation (e.g., glutathione conjugation to mercapturates), then the net chemical process is one of detoxification if the final product is rapidly cleared. Toxicity can accrue when accumulation occurs of a chemically reactive metabolite that, if not detoxified, can lead to covalent modification of biologic macromolecules. The identity of the target macromolecule and the functional consequence of its modification will dictate the resulting toxicologic response. P450 enzymes are present in many organs, mainly the liver but also the kidney and lung, and thus can bioactivate chemicals to cause organ-specific toxicity. Evidence for the formation of reactive metabolites was found for 5 of the 6 drugs that have been withdrawn from the market since 1995 and for 8 of the 15 drugs that have black box warnings. Evidence for reactive metabolite formation has been found for acetaminophen, bromfenac, diclofenac, clozapine, and troglitazone (91–93). Acetaminophen is the most studied hepatotoxin. The current hypothesis of how reactive metabolites lead to liver injury suggests that hepatic (target) proteins can be modified by reactive metabolites. Much more important can be the identification of the target proteins modified by these toxic metabolites and how this reaction alters the function of the target proteins. Additionally, it is important to note that the toxicity of reactive metabolites can also be mediated by noncovalent binding mechanisms, which can have profound effects on normal liver physiology. Technologic developments in the wake of the genomic revolution now provide unprecedented power to characterize and quantify covalent modification of individual target proteins and their functional consequences (93). Such information should dramatically improve our understanding of drug-induced hepatotoxic reactions. Moreover, covalent binding per se does not necessarily lead to drug hepatotoxicity. The regioisomer of acetaminophen, 3-hydroxyacetanilide, becomes covalently bound to hepatic proteins in rodents without inducing hepatotoxicity (94).

Therefore, it is necessary to identify targets for these reactive metabolites (i.e., covalently modified macromolecules) that are critical to the toxicologic process. Hard electrophiles react as a rule with hard nucleophiles, such as the basic groups in DNA and lysine ω-amino residues in proteins. Soft electrophiles react with soft nucleophiles, which include cysteine residues in proteins and in

HARD/SOFT ACIDS/BASES

The nonenzymatic reaction of an electrophilic metabolite with a nucleophilic molecule occurs usually via a substitution or addition mechanism involving the donation of an electron pair by the nucleophile to an acceptor molecule, an electrophile, with subsequent formation of a covalent bond and an adduct product (Coles B. Effects of modifying structure on electrophilic reactions with biological nucleophiles. Drug Metab Rev 1984–1985;15:1307–1334). The most accepted concept classifies electrophiles and nucleophiles according to Pearson's "hard-soft acid-bases" (HSAB) model. Thus, hard electrophiles have a formal positive charge at the electrophilic center, and the valence electrons are not easily delocalized or polarized (e.g., acylonium ions, carbocations, nitrenium ions; see Figs. 4.30 and 4.33), whereas soft electrophiles have a partial positive charge density and valence electrons that are delocalized (polarized), such as activated double bonds of α,β-unsaturated carbonyl compounds as shown in Fig. 4.32. Hard nucleophiles have high electronegativity (oxygen and nitrogen groups) and low polarization of valence electrons, whereas soft nucleophiles have low electronegativity and are more polarizable. The softest biologic nucleophilic sites are cysteine thiol groups on proteins and GSH. The primary and secondary amino groups of lysine and histidine or the hydroxyl groups of serine or threonine on proteins are hard nucleophiles, whereas the hardest nucleophiles are the oxygen atoms of purines and pyrimidines on DNA and RNA.

Based on the HSAB theory, the reaction rates and selectivities of electrophiles and nucleophiles are dependent upon comparable states of "hardness." Specifically a soft electrophile such as quinoneimine will react predominantly with a soft nucleophile such as the thiol group of cysteine. A hard electrophile such as the acylonium ion formed from acyl glucuronide will react with hard nucleophiles such as the hydroxyl group of serine. This preferential nonenzymatic reactivity is due primarily to the high-energy transition state that acts as a barrier to the reaction of a hard electrophile with a soft nucleophile such as the delocalized double bonds of *p*-benzoquinoneimines, *p*-benzoquinonemethides, and other α,β-unsaturated carbonyl intermediates that react by Michael-type addition of the nucleophile to the polarized (partial positive charge) located on the β-carbon.

Adduct formation is dependent not only on the physiochemical nature of the electrophilic but also on the microenvironment of the nucleophilic center, which can vary significantly even among centers of the same elemental type (e.g., sulfur or amino groups). Thus, nucleophilic reactivity among free sulfhydryl groups on proteins can be diverse, and consequently, soft electrophilic metabolites will form adducts with the more reactive thiol groups on a given protein or free thiols on glutathione. This diversity in nucleophilic reactivity is a function of both steric and electronic factors mediated primarily by the tertiary structure of a protein. For example, adjacent acidic and basic amino acids on a protein significantly influence the reactivity of the target nucleophilic group. Depending on the physiochemical nature of the electrophile, the resulting electrophilic metabolite can produce toxicity by reacting with either soft thiol nucleophilic sites on proteins and free thiols such as GSH or harder nucleophilic centers on DNA and RNA to produce adducts.

For example, metabolic epoxidation of an aromatic ring produces an epoxide, a relatively hard electrophilic metabolite that will form a ring-opened hydroxyl adduct primarily with hard nucleophilic centers on guanine and adenine on DNA and not with soft thiol nucleophiles. On the other hand, a soft electrophile, such as the *N*-acetyl *p*-benzoquinone imine metabolite of acetaminophen, will form adducts with thiol groups on proteins and free thiols on GSH, but not with hard nucleophilic groups on lysine or serine on proteins or with those on guanine and adenine on DNA. Glutathione offers little protection against carcinogens, most of which are hard nucleophiles. These examples show that the bioactivated metabolite can exhibit distinct electrophilic characteristics and different nucleophilic target molecules. Thus, soft electrophiles are associated with organ-specific toxicities (e.g., hepatotoxicity, renal toxicity), and hard electrophiles are associated with carcinogenicity.

glutathione. Unfortunately, no simple rules predict the target macromolecules for a particular chemically reactive metabolite or the biologic consequences of a particular modification. Furthermore, noncovalent interactions have also a role, because covalent binding of hepatotoxins is not indiscriminate with respect to proteins. Even within a single protein, there can be selective modification of an amino acid side chain found repeatedly in the primary structure. Thus, the microenvironment (e.g., pK_a and hydrophobicity) of the amino acid in the tertiary structure appears to be the crucial determinant of selective binding and, therefore, the impact of covalent binding on protein function. In turn, the extent of binding and the biochemical role of the protein will determine the toxicologic insult of drug bioactivation. The resulting pathologic consequences will be a balance between the rates of protein damage and the rates of protein replacement and cellular repair.

Drug-Induced Idiosyncratic Reactions

Idiosyncratic drug reactions (IDR; type B adverse drug reactions) occur in from 1 in 1,000 to 1 in 50,000 patients, are not predictable from the known pharmacology or toxicology of the drug, are not produced experimentally in vitro and in vivo, and are dose independent. The occurrence of IDRs during late clinical trials or after a drug has been released can lead to severe restriction of its use and even its withdrawal. The IDRs do not, as a rule, result from the drug itself because most people can tolerate the drug, but rather from a unique set of patient characteristics, including gender, age, genetic predisposition, and a lack of drug-metabolizing enzymes, that can increase the risk of these adverse drug reactions. Most IDRs are caused by hypersensitivity reactions and can result in hepatocellular injury. The hepatic injury occurs within 1 week to 12 months after initiation of drug therapy and often is accompanied by systemic characteristics of allergic drug reactions, such as rash and fever. Signs of hepatic injury reappear with subsequent administration of the same drug with only one or two doses. Hypersensitivity reactions can be severe and associated with fatal reactions as a multiorgan clinical syndrome characterized by the following: 1) fever; 2) rash; 3) gastrointestinal symptoms (e.g., nausea, vomiting, diarrhea, or abdominal pain); 4) generalized malaise, fatigue, or achiness; and 5) respiratory symptoms (e.g., dyspnea, cough, or pharyngitis). Examples of drugs causing IDRs through a hypersensitivity mechanism include penicillin, methyldopa, chlorpromazine, erythromycin, azathioprine toxicity in thiopurine methyltransferase–deficient individuals, sulfonamide and acetaminophen hepatotoxicity in alcoholics and in UGT1A6-deficient cats, ivermectin neurotoxicity in Collie dogs deficient in P-gp, perhexilene hepatotoxicity in CYP2D6-deficient individuals, phenytoin toxicity in CYP2C9-deficient individuals, and valproic acid hepatotoxicity.

The clinical features of some cases of drug-induced idiosyncratic hepatotoxicity strongly suggest an involvement of the immune system (95). These clinical characteristics include the following: 1) concurrence of rash, fever, and eosinophilia; 2) delay of the initial reaction (1 to 8 weeks) or requirement of repeated exposure to the culprit drug; 3) rapid recurrence of toxicity on reexposure to the drug; and 4) presence of antibodies specific for native or drug-modified hepatic proteins. Our current understanding of drug-induced adaptive immune responses is largely based on the hapten hypothesis.

Idiosyncratic drug reactions that are connected with hepatotoxicity involve the formation of reactive metabolites (91,92). Such reactions are not predictable, but current bioanalytical technology has enabled the in vivo identification of the formation of reactive metabolites, as evidenced by the detection of biomarkers (i.e., mercapturate or cysteine adducts) in urine, drug-specific antibodies, or antibodies to P450 isoforms (93). As a result, some drugs known to cause hepatic injury continue to be used, because the drug's benefit outweighs its risk and no alternative efficacious drug exists. For example, isoniazid, a drug commonly used to treat tuberculosis, is implicated in approximately 15% to 20% of the individuals who show increased serum transaminases after receiving the drug as a single agent for tuberculosis prophylaxis. Of these individuals, an estimated 1 in 1,000 patients can develop severe hepatic necrosis. Additionally, NSAIDs, including cyclooxygenase-2 inhibitors, commonly are associated with idiosyncratic liver injury. Most of the idiosyncratic toxins listed in Table 4.21 that have been studied to date produce reactive metabolites.

Current hypotheses regarding IDRs suggest that metabolic activation of a drug to a reactive metabolite is a necessary yet insufficient step in the generation of an idiosyncratic reaction (91,92). Evidence for this hypothesis comes from drugs that are associated with hepatotoxicity (Table 4.21) and the detection of drug metabolite–specific antibodies in affected patients.

For the other drugs that have been associated with idiosyncratic hepatotoxicity but that do not have black box warnings, either evidence for hepatotoxicity was not available or suitable studies had not been carried out. High doses increase the risk for an IDR (e.g., clozapine at 300 mg/d vs. olanzapine at 20 mg/d). Strong evidence also exists that T cells have an important role in immune-mediated IDR and can trigger cell death. In patients exhibiting IDR, pretreatment with immunosuppressants prevented the IDR (rash). The incidence of IDRs also appears to be lower in patients with low T-cell counts.

The hapten hypothesis proposes that the reactive metabolites of the drugs act as haptens and bind covalently to endogenous proteins to form immunogenic drug–protein adducts triggering either antibody or cytotoxic T-cell responses (92,96). The hapten hypothesis is supported by the detection of antibodies that recognize drug-modified hepatic proteins in the sera of drug-induced liver injury patients. For example, antibodies that recognize trifluoroacetate-altered hepatic proteins have been detected in the sera of patients with halothane-induced hepatitis. Such drug-specific antibodies or autoantibodies that recognize native liver proteins

TABLE 4.21 Some Examples of Idiosyncratic Toxins

Abacavir	Hypersensitivity
Acetaminophen	Hepatotoxicity
Amiodarone	Hepatotoxicity
Aromatic anticonvulsants	Hypersensitivity
Cefaclor	Hepatotoxicity
Clozapine	Agranulocytosis
Diclofenac	Hepatotoxicity
Felbamate	Aplastic anemia
Fibrates	Hepatotoxicity
Halothane	Hepatotoxicity
Indomethacin	Hepatotoxicity
Isoniazid	Hepatotoxicity
Levamisole	Hepatotoxicity
Nefazodone	Hepatotoxicity
Nevirapine	Agranulocytosis
Oral contraceptives	Hepatotoxicity
Paroxetine	Hepatotoxicity
Phenytoin	Hepatotoxicity
Statins	Hepatotoxicity
Sulfonamides	Stevens-Johnson syndrome
Tamoxifen	Hepatotoxicity
Tacrine	Hepatotoxicity
Tienilic acid	Hypersensitivity
Ticlopidine	Agranulocytosis
Troglitazone	Hepatotoxicity
Valproic acid	Hepatotoxicity
Vesnarinone	Agranulocytosis
Penicillinamine[a]	Hypersensitivity

[a]Does not produce reactive metabolites.

have also been found in patients with liver injury caused by other drugs, such as diclofenac. In patients who developed IDRs of the liver and other organs, drug-specific T cells have been detected, and in some cases, T-cell clones were generated. Most drugs are small molecules and are unlikely to form haptens. Electrophilic acylators (hard electrophiles) can react with the lysine ω-amino residues (hard nucleophiles) of the target protein or guanosine residues of DNA. How much chemical modification is required to trigger an IDR remains unknown. Halothane is the most studied molecule for supporting this hypothesis regarding IDRs (91). Therefore, it is not surprising that irreversible chemical modification of a protein, which has a profound effect on function, is a mechanism of idiosyncratic hepatotoxicity. However, it is important to note that a number of drugs (e.g., penicillins, aspirin, and omeprazole) rely on covalent binding to proteins for their efficacy; thus, prevention of their covalent binding through chemical modification of the compound can also, inadvertently, lead to loss of efficacy.

Drug-induced stress and/or damage of hepatocytes can trigger activation and inflammatory responses of the immune system within the liver (95,96). Evidence to support this idea has been obtained mainly from studies of liver injury induced by overdoses of acetaminophen, which is one of the few drugs that provide an experimental animal model of drug-induced liver injury. Evidence is growing that the initial benzoquinoneimine-induced hepatocyte damage can lead to activation of immune cells within the liver, thereby stimulating hepatic infiltration by inflammatory cells. Activated T cells of the immune system produce a range of inflammatory mediators, including cytokines, chemokines, and reactive oxygen and nitrogen species, that contribute to the progression of liver injury. On the other hand, the immune cells also represent a major source of hepatoprotective factors.

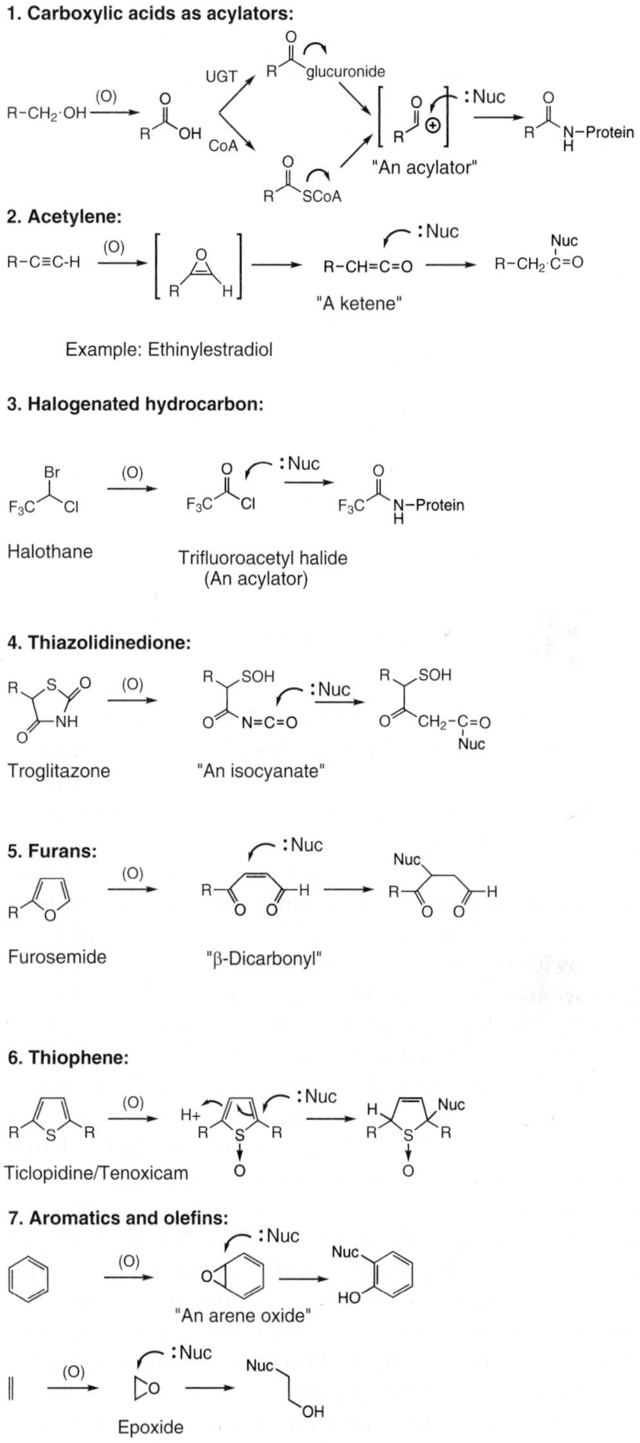

FIGURE 4.30 Some examples of electrophilic intermediates resulting from bioactivation. NUC, nucleophiles.

Reactive Metabolites Resulting from Bioactivation

Electrophiles

The concept that small organic molecules can undergo bioactivation to electrophiles and free radicals and elicit toxicity by chemical modification of cellular macromolecules has its basis in chemical carcinogenicity and the pioneering work of Miller and Miller (97) and Gillette et al. (98–100). A number of different types of reactive metabolites exist; however, they can be broadly classified as either electrophiles (Fig. 4.30) or free radicals (Fig. 4.31) (93,101). These reactive metabolites are short-lived, with half-lives of usually less than 1 minute, and are not normally detectable in plasma or urine except as Phase 2 conjugates or other biomarkers. Electrophiles are reactive because they possess electron-deficient centers (polarization-activated double bonds or positive-charge acylators) (Figs. 4.30 and 4.32) and can form covalent bonds with electron-rich biologic nucleophiles. They are either soft electrophiles that react directly with soft nucleophiles (:Nuc), such as the thiol groups in either glutathione or cysteine residues within proteins, or hard electrophiles that react with hard nucleophiles, such as basic groups in DNA and lysine ω-amino residues in proteins, or are mediated by bioinactivation enzymes, such as glutathione transferase

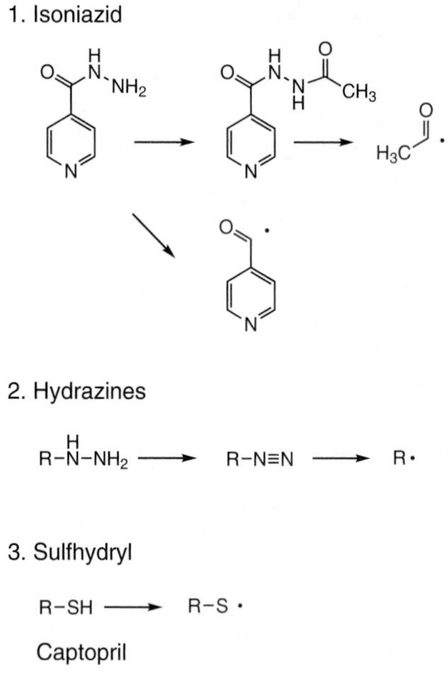

FIGURE 4.31 Drug bioactivation to free radicals.

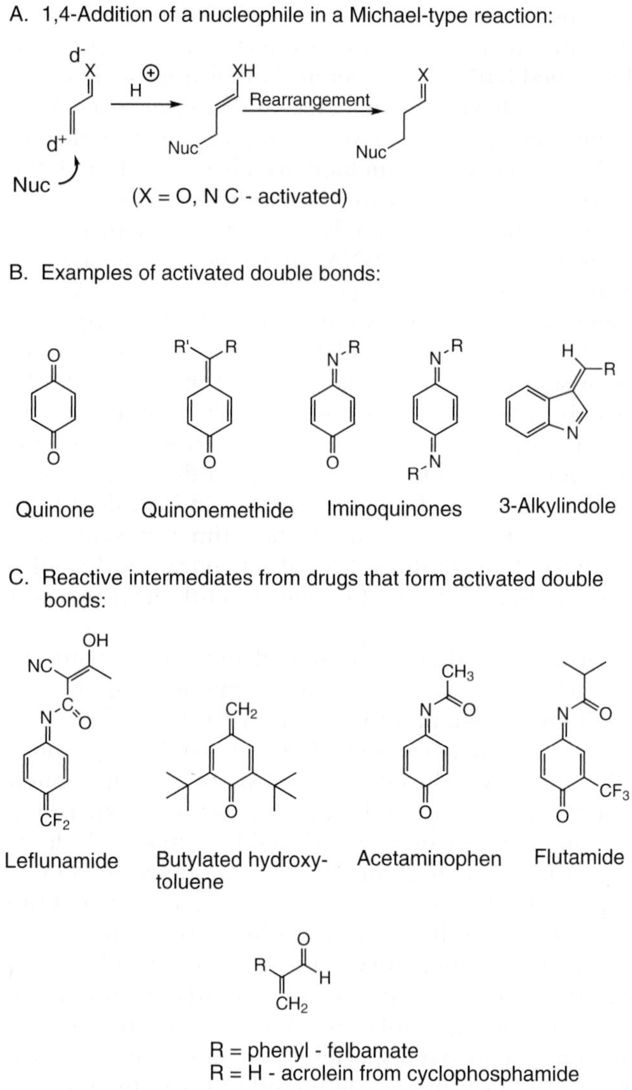

FIGURE 4.32 Some examples of activated double bonds as electrophilic reactive intermediates.

or epoxide hydrase. Softness and hardness are associated with the polarizability of the electrophilic/nucleophilic species (see Hard/Soft Acids/Bases). Activated double bonds are soft electrophilic intermediates as shown in Figure 4.32.

Examples of activated double bond electrophiles include α,β-unsaturated carbonyl compounds, quinones, quinoneimines, quinonemethides, and diiminoquinones, as shown in Figure 4.32B. These electrophilic intermediates are highly polarized and can react with nucleophiles in a 1,4-Michael-type addition at the more electrophilic or β-carbon of the activated double bond intermediate to the addition product (Fig. 4.32A). Specific examples of activated double bond electrophiles that have been proposed for the anticancer drug leflunamide, the food antioxidant butylated hydroxytoluene, acetaminophen, the antiandrogen flutamide, the anticonvulsant felbamate, and the cytotoxic cyclophosphamide are shown in Figure 4.32C. The bioinactivation pathways for these electrophilic intermediates can involve either direct addition, with or without transferases, depending on the degree of polarization and reactivity of the electrophilic intermediate (hard vs. soft electrophiles).

Other commonly found electrophilic intermediates for drug molecules in Figure 4.30 include the formation of ketenes from the bioactivation of acetylenic groups (e.g., ethinylestradiol) (Fig. 4.30-2); isocyanates from thiazolidinediones (e.g., the "glitazones") (Fig. 4.30-4) (93); acylonium ions from halogenated hydrocarbons (e.g., halothane) (Fig. 4.30-3) (93) and carboxylic acids; β-dicarbonyl from furans (e.g., furosemide) (Fig. 4.30-5) (93); activated thiophene-*S*-oxide from thiophenes, such as ticlopidine; tenoxicam, which cause the IDR of agranulocytosis (Fig. 4.30-6) (93); and epoxides and arene oxides from olefins and aromatic compounds (Fig. 4.30-7) (93). Drugs possessing structural features prone to metabolic epoxidations are abundant. Therefore the incidence of epoxide metabolites in mediating adverse biologic effects has aroused concern about clinically used drugs known to be metabolized to epoxides. Metabolically produced epoxides have been reported for allobarbital, secobarbital, protriptyline, carbamazepine, and cyproheptadine and are implicated with 8-methoxypsoralen and other furanocoumarins (6,7-dihydroxybergamottin in grapefruit juice), phenytoin, phensuximide, phenobarbital, mephobarbital, lorazepam, and imipramine (81). The alarming biologic effects of some epoxides, however, do not imply that all epoxides have similar effects. Epoxides vary greatly in molecular geometry, stability, electrophilic reactivity, and relative activity as substrates for epoxide-transforming enzymes (e.g., epoxide hydrolase, glutathione *S*-transferase, and others).

Some carboxylic acid–containing drugs have been implicated in rare IDRs, which was the basis for the market withdrawal of the NSAIDs zomiperac and benzoxaprofen. These drugs (e.g., NSAIDs, fibrates, "statins," and valproic acid) can be bioactivated to acyl glucuronides or acyl CoA thioesters (Fig. 4.30-1). These products are electrophilic acylators that can acylate target proteins if they escape inactivation by *S*-glutathione–thioester formation. A crucial factor is the concentration of acyl glucuronides in hepatocytes due to their transport by conjugate export pumps, where acylglucuronides can selectively acylate canalicular membrane proteins. Acyl CoA esters can be either rapidly hydrolyzed or further metabolized in hepatocytes. Evidence is accumulating that acyl glucuronides can alter cellular function by haptenation of peptides, target protein acylation or glycation, or direct stimulation of neutrophils and macrophages. The role of acyl CoA reactive metabolites is less clear. It should be noted that some noncarboxylic acid drugs can be biotransformed by oxidative metabolism in the liver to the respective carboxylic acids.

Free Radicals

P450 activates molecular dioxygen to generate ROS, such as singlet oxygen ($^1O_2$) or superoxide (see Oxygen Activation, p. 118). Reactive metabolites that possess unpaired electrons are free radicals (molecular species that contain an odd unpaired electron), which can react with molecular oxygen (ground state triplet) to generate intracellular oxidative stress damage (93,98–100). Free radicals abstract a hydrogen atom from other molecules rather than becoming covalently bound. Free radical reactions can be self-propagating by abstracting a hydrogen atom from the double bond of a lipid that initiates a chain reaction leading to lipid peroxidation, oxidative stress, or other types of modification of biologic molecules.

Some examples of free radicals generated by the bioactivation of drug molecules are shown in Figure 4.31. Isoniazid is acetylated to its major metabolite acetylisoniazid, which is hydrolyzed to acetylhydrazine and isonicotinic acid (Fig. 4.31-1). Acetylhydrazine is further metabolized by the CYP2E1 to an *N*-hydroxy intermediate that hydrates into an acetyl radical, which can then initiate the process that leads to hepatic necrosis. Other carbon-centered radicals are formed from hydrazines such as the antihypertensive hydralazine and thio-radicals from the angiotensin-converting enzyme inhibitor captopril (Fig. 4.31-2 and -3).

Bioinactivation Mechanisms

Several enzyme systems exist as cellular defense (detoxification) pathways against the chemically reactive metabolites generated by P450 metabolism (91,92,102,103). These include GST, epoxide hydrolase, and quinone reductase, as well as catalase, glutathione peroxidase, and superoxide dismutase, which detoxify the peroxide and superoxide byproducts of metabolism. The efficiency of the bioinactivation process is dependent on the inherent chemical reactivity of the electrophilic intermediate, its affinity and selectivity of the reactive metabolite for the bioinactivation enzymes, the tissue expression of these enzymes, and the rapid upregulation of these enzymes and cofactors mediated by the cellular sensors of chemical stress. The reactive metabolites that can evade these defense systems can damage target proteins and nucleic acids by either oxidation or covalent modification.

The most abundant agents of cellular defense are thiols. Glutathione is a soft electrophile and, therefore, will only react noncatalytically with soft electrophiles, such as activated double bonds (Fig. 4.32). Glutathione conjugation to mercapturates is one of the most important defenses against hepatocellular injury. Glutathione protects cellular enzymes and membranes from toxic metabolites, and its inadequate stores can compromise efficient detoxification of the reactive metabolites. The subsequent inability to detoxify the reactive metabolites can result in hepatocellular injury. The rate-limiting factor for glutathione synthesis is the intracellular concentration of cysteine. *N*-acetylcysteine is often used as an alternative to glutathione to trap the iminoquinone intermediate in the treatment of acute acetaminophen toxicity. Glutathione has a protective role in the hepatic tissue injury produced by acetaminophen but not by furosemide.

The relationship between bioactivation, bioinactivation, and DNA adduct formation has been well established for a number of hepatocarcinogens. Glutathione conjugation of hard electrophiles becomes more efficient when catalyzed by GSTs, an important example being the detoxication of the hepatocarcinogen aflatoxin. Aflatoxin, a hepatocarcinogen and a hepatotoxin found in mold growing on peanuts, is converted into aflatoxin B1 epoxide in rodents, which is more readily detoxified by GST enzymes than by epoxide hydrolase. The balance between these transferase reactions explains the greater DNA damage in humans compared with rodents, because human forms of GST are less able to catalyze the conjugation of aflatoxin epoxide compared with the rodent forms. Transgenic knockout mice have been used to establish the role of bioactivation by P450 and bioinactivation by GSTs for a number of carcinogenic PAHs.

Substances that detoxify free radicals include the antioxidants vitamin C, vitamin E, and carotene, which scavenge free radicals, including reactive metabolites and ROS generated as a consequence of chemical stress.

Specific Examples

Some examples of bioactivation to hepatotoxic or IDR electrophilic intermediates are shown in Figure 4.33. Bioactivation can occur by both oxidation and

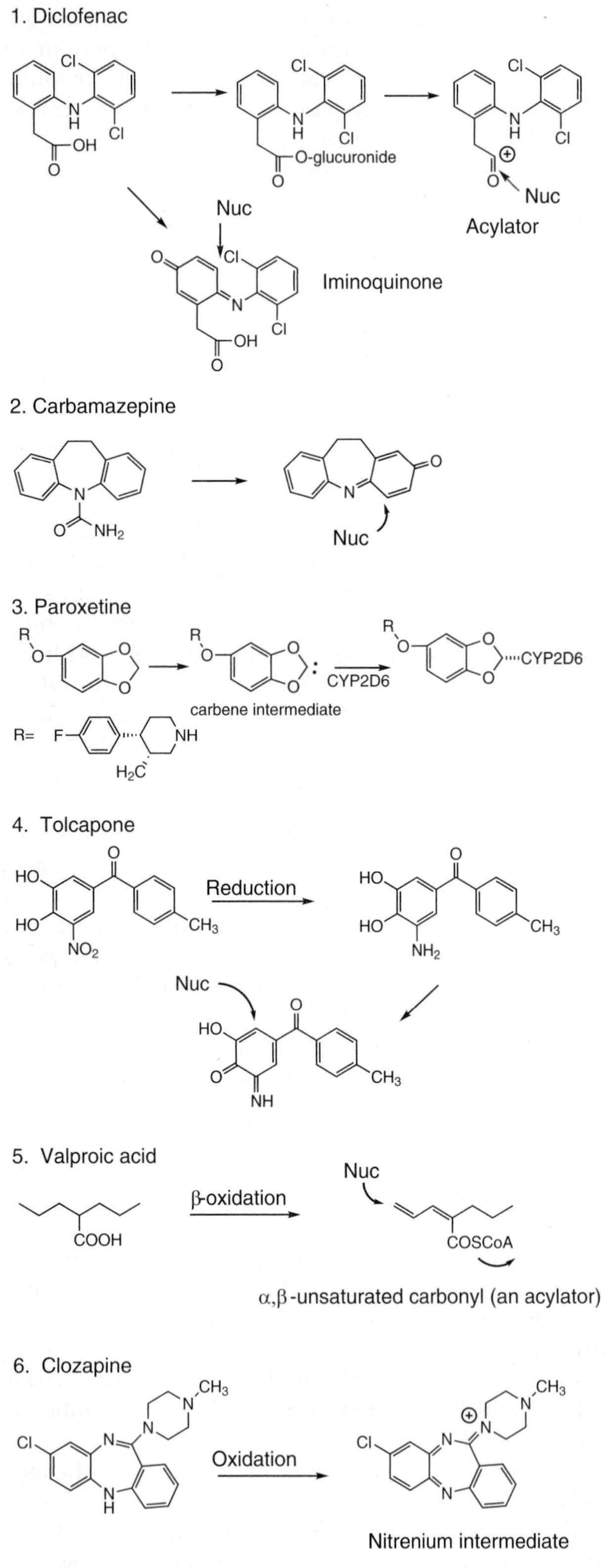

FIGURE 4.33 Some examples of drug bioactivation to their hepatotoxic intermediates.

conjugation reactions, such as those with diclofenac, which undergoes the formation of an acyl glucuronide and/or acyl CoA (acylator intermediates), or to produce iminoquinones via formation of a phenol intermediator (Fig. 4.33-1) (92). The anticonvulsant carbamazepine is 2-hydroxylated, and the elimination of the amide group yields the reactive quinoneimine intermediate (Fig. 4.33-2); and the antidepressant paroxetine and other xenobiotics with the common methylenedioxyphenyl nucleus undergo methylene oxidation to a carbene intermediate (Fig. 4.33-3). In the COMT inhibitor used in the treatment of parkinsonism, tolcapone, the nitro group is first reduced to an amine and then oxidized to a *o*-quinoneimine (Fig. 4.33-4). The mitochondrial/hepatotoxicity of the anticonvulsant valproic acid results from the formation of an activated α,β-unsaturated CoA thioester via mitochondrial β-oxidation, most commonly associated with the oxidation of fatty acids (Fig. 4.33-5). The agranulocytosis resulting from the ingestion of the antipsychotic clozapine is bioactivated by its oxidation by hypochlorous acid in neutrophils to a nitrenium intermediate (Fig. 4.33-6) (93). The effect of structure modification for troglitazone that reduced its hepatotoxicity is shown in Figure 4.34. The *p*-dihydroxy elements of the chroman ring nucleus (outlined in red in Fig. 4.34) of troglitazone is bioactivated to an activated double bond (*p*-quinone) and has been replaced with a pyridine ring that is not bioactivated, although the thiazolidone ring can be bioactivated to an isocyanate (Fig. 4.30) (92).

The oxidation of acetaminophen to the chemically reactive *N*-acetyl-*p*-benzoquinoneimine (Fig. 4.32) is catalyzed by the isoforms CYP1A2 and CYP2E1, which can either react covalently with glutathione to form an inactive product or with cellular macromolecules, initiating the processes leading to hepatic necrosis (Fig. 4.28) (93). The usual route for acetaminophen metabolism is glucuronidation. If insufficient UDP-glucuronic acid is present, then bioactivation will dominate.

Furosemide, a frequently used diuretic drug, is reportedly a human hepatocarcinogen. The hepatic toxicity apparently results from metabolic activation of the furan ring to a β-dicarbonyl intermediate (Fig. 4.30-5) (93). Ticlopidine and tenoxicam, reported to cause agranulocytosis, do so via metabolic activation of the thiophene ring to an *S*-oxide (Fig. 4.30-6) (93). The agranulocytosis resulting from the ingestion of clozapine is via its bioactivation to a nitrenium ion intermediate (Fig. 4.33-6) (96–101).

Drug-Induced Chemical Carcinogenesis

The mechanism whereby xenobiotics are transformed into chemical carcinogens is usually accepted as bioactivation to reactive metabolites, which are responsible for initiating carcinogenicity (98–100). Many carcinogens elicit their cytotoxicity through a covalent linkage to DNA. This process can lead to mutations and, potentially, to cancer. Most chemical carcinogens of concern are chemically inert but require activation by the xenobiotic-metabolizing enzymes before they can undergo

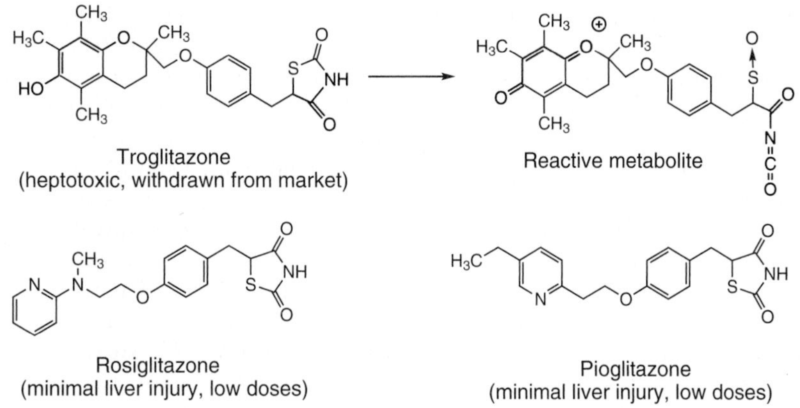

FIGURE 4.34 The effect of structure modification on the drug-induced hepatotoxicity of troglitazone.

reaction with DNA or proteins (cytotoxicity). There are many ways to bioactivate procarcinogens, promutagens, plant toxins, drugs, and other xenobiotics (37) (Fig. 4.35). Oxidative bioactivation reactions are by far the most studied and common. Conjugation reactions (Phase 2), however, are also capable of activating these xenobiotics to produce electrophiles, in which the conjugating derivative acts as a leaving group. These reactive metabolites are mostly electrophiles, such as epoxides, quinones, or free radicals formed by the P450 enzymes or FMO. The reactive metabolites tend to be oxygenated in sterically hindered positions, making them poor substrates for subsequent bioinactivation transferases, such as epoxide hydrolase and GST. Therefore, their principal fate is formation of covalent linkage to intracellular macromolecules, including enzyme proteins and DNA. Experimental studies indicate that the CYP1A subfamily can oxygenate aromatic hydrocarbons (e.g., PAHs) in sterically hindered positions to arene oxides. Activation by *N*-hydroxylation of polycyclic aromatic amines (e.g., aryl *N*-acetamides) appears to depend on either FMO

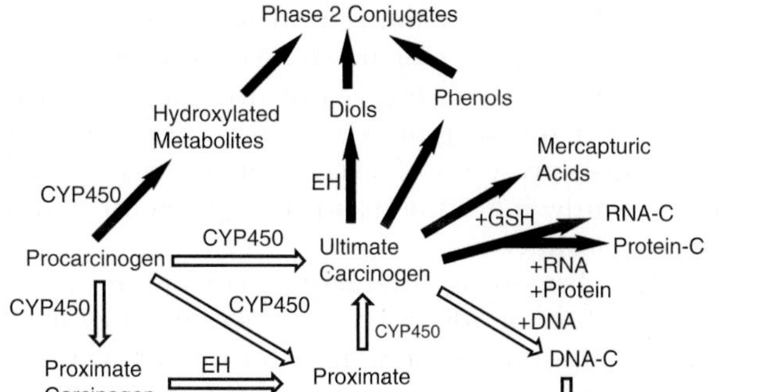

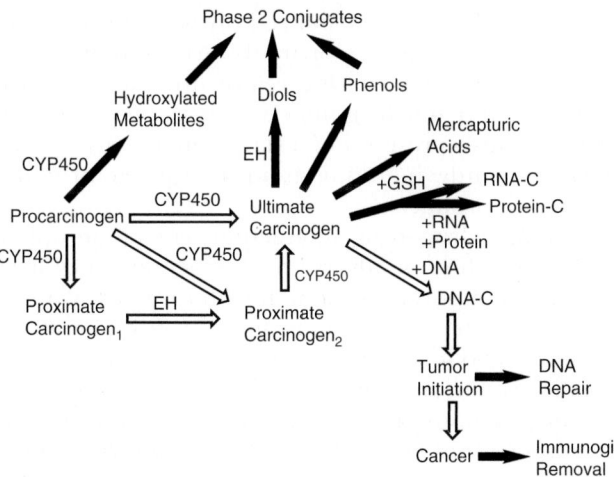

FIGURE 4.35 The bioactivation of procarcinogens and a proposed mechanism of chemical carcinogenesis.

or P450 isoforms. The formation of chemically reactive metabolites is important, because they frequently cause a number of different toxicities, including tumorigenesis, mutagenesis, tissue necrosis, and hypersensitivity reactions.

Our understanding of these reactions was advanced by the studies of Miller and Miller (97) and Gillette et al. (98–100). They proposed that the proportion of the dose that binds covalently to critical macromolecules could depend on the quantity of the reactive metabolite that is formed.

A scheme illustrating the complexities of drug-induced chemical carcinogenesis is shown in Figure 4.35. Reactions that proceed via the open arrows eventually lead to neoplasia. Some carcinogens can form the "ultimate carcinogen" directly through P450 isoform bioactivation; others, like the PAHs (e.g., benzo[a]pyrene), appear to involve a multistep reaction sequence forming an epoxide, reduction to a diol by epoxide hydrase, and perhaps, the formation of a second epoxide group on another part of the molecule. Other procarcinogens form the *N*-hydroxy intermediate that requires transferase-catalyzed conjugation (e.g., *O*-glucuronide and *O*-sulfate) to form the "ultimate carcinogen." The quantity of "ultimate carcinogen" formed should relate directly to the proportion of the dose that binds or alkylates DNA.

The solid-arrow reaction sequences in Figure 4.35 are intended to show detoxification mechanisms, which involve several steps. First, the original chemical can form less active products (phenols, diols, mercapturic acids, and other conjugates). Second, the "ultimate carcinogen" can rearrange so as to be prevented from its reaction with DNA (or whatever the critical macromolecule is). Third, the covalently bound DNA can be repaired. Fourth, immunologic removal of the tumor cells can occur. Several mechanisms within this scheme could regulate the quantity of covalently bound carcinogen: 1) The activity of the rate-limiting enzyme, such as epoxide hydrolase, P450 isoform, or one of the transferases, could be involved; 2) the availability of cosubstrates, such as glutathione, UDP-glucuronic acid, or PAPS, can be rate-limiting; 3) relative P450 activities for detoxification and activation must be considered; 4) availability of alternate reaction sites for the ultimate carcinogen (e.g., RNA and protein can be involved); 5) and possible specific transport mechanisms that deliver either the procarcinogen or its ultimate carcinogen to selected molecular or subcellular sites.

It is now well established that numerous organic compounds that are essentially nontoxic as long as their structure is preserved can be converted into cytotoxic, teratogenic, mutagenic, or carcinogenic compounds by normal biotransformation pathways in both animals and humans (37). The reactive electrophilic intermediate (hard acids) involves its reaction with cellular constituents (hard bases) forming either detoxified products or binding covalently with essential macromolecules, initiating processes that eventually lead to the toxic effect. A better understanding of the mechanisms underlying these reactions can lead to more rational approaches to the development of nontoxic therapeutic drugs. For the present, it seems that new advances in drug therapy cannot occur without some risk of causing structural tissue lesions. Special attention to risk factors is required for drugs that will be used for long periods in the same patient.

Some toxic chemicals exert their toxic action by lethal injury or biologic auto-oxidation (radical lipid peroxidation). Lethal injury involves the disruption of cellular energy metabolism by inhibition of oxidative phosphorylation or adenosine triphosphatase, resulting in disruption of subcellular organelles, cell death, and tissue necrosis. Because the early stages of lethal injury are reversible, complete recovery can occur. Auto-oxidation is the process whereby cellular components are irreversibly oxidized and damaged by free radicals or free radical–generating systems. This results in the oxidation and depletion of glutathione, various thiol enzymes, or lipid peroxidation, which in turn leads to the disruption of cellular membranes and to cell death, tissue necrosis, and death of the organism. When cell death does not occur, nonlethal changes, such as mutations and malignant transformations, are likely.

DRUG–DRUG INTERACTIONS

Drug–drug interactions represent a common clinical problem, which has been compounded by the introduction of many new drugs and the expanded use of herbal medicines. Between 1999 and 2005, approximately 100 drug–drug interactions were reported, of which approximately 50% involved P450 inhibition. Drug–drug interactions occur when the efficacy or toxicity of a medication is changed by coadministration of another substance, drug, food (e.g., grapefruit), or herbal product (103,104). Pharmacokinetic interactions often occur as a result of a change in drug metabolism. For example, CYP3A4 oxidizes more than 60% of the clinically used drugs with a broad spectrum of structural features, and its location in the small intestine and liver permits an effect on both presystemic and systemic drug disposition. Some drug–drug interactions with CYP3A4 substrates/inhibitors can also involve inhibition of P-gp. Other clinically important drug–drug interactions resulting from coadministration of CYP3A4 substrates or inhibitors include rhabdomyolysis with the coadministration of some 3-hydroxy-3-methylglutaryl–CoA reductase inhibitors ("statins"), symptomatic hypotension with some dihydropyridine calcium antagonists, excessive sedation from benzodiazepine or nonbenzodiazepine hypnosedatives, ataxia with carbamazepine, and ergotism with ergot alkaloids.

The clinical importance of any drug–drug interaction depends on factors that are drug-, patient-, and administration-related. Drugs with low oral bioavailability or high first-pass metabolism are particularly susceptible to drug–drug interactions as a result of coadministration of inhibitors that alter absorption, distribution, and elimination. In general, a doubling or more in the plasma drug concentration has the potential for enhanced adverse or beneficial drug response. Less pronounced pharmacokinetic drug interactions can still be clinically important for drugs with a steep concentration–response relationship or narrow therapeutic index. In most cases, the extent of drug interaction varies markedly among individuals; this is likely to be dependent on interindividual differences in P450 content (polymorphism), preexisting medical conditions, and possibly, age. Drug–drug interactions can occur under single-dose conditions or only at steady-state. The pharmacodynamic consequences can or cannot closely follow pharmacokinetic changes. Drug–drug interactions can be most apparent when patients are stabilized on the affected drug and the P450 substrates or inhibitors are then added to the regimen (103). One reason for the increased incidence of drug–drug interactions is the practice of simultaneously prescribing several potent drugs as well as concurrently ingesting nonprescription products and herbal products.

Although drug–drug interactions constitute only a small proportion of adverse drug reactions, they have become an important issue in health care. Many of the drug–drug interactions can be explained by alterations in the metabolic enzymes in the liver and other extrahepatic tissues, and many of the major pharmacokinetic interactions between drugs are caused by hepatic P450 isoenzymes being affected by coadministration of other drugs. Some drugs act as potent enzyme inducers, whereas others are inhibitors. Drug–drug interactions involving enzyme inhibition, however, are much more common. Understanding these mechanisms of enzyme inhibition or induction is extremely important to give appropriate multidrug therapies. In the future, individuals at greatest risk for drug–drug interactions and adverse events need to be identified. P450s have a dominant role in the metabolism and elimination of drugs from the body, and their substrates are shown in Tables 4.4 and 4.8 through 4.11. Drugs in bold italics have been associated with drug–drug interactions (103). Inhibitors of P450 are shown in Table 4.12. Pharmacokinetic interactions can arise when the biotransformation and elimination of a drug are impaired by coadministered drugs. Thus, drugs can compete for biotransformation by a common P450. Adverse drug reactions, including toxicity, can occur if elimination is dependent on a P450 that exhibits defective gene variants. Thus, the genetic makeup of the individual (see the section on genetic polymorphism) has a major influence on the duration of drug action as well as on drug efficacy and safety. P450 pharmacogenetics affects the tendency for certain drug–drug interactions to occur. Thus, the future safe use of drug combinations in patients can require genotyping and phenotyping of individuals before the commencement of therapy. Identification of subjects who metabolize drugs in a different fashion from the general population should minimize the impact of pharmacogenetic variation on drug pharmacokinetics.

Metabolism-Based Enzyme Inhibition

Many drug–drug interactions are the result of inhibition or induction of P450 enzymes. Metabolism-based enzyme inhibition involves mostly competition between two drugs for the enzyme-active site. Metabolic drug–drug interactions occur when drug A (or its metabolite) alters the pharmacokinetics of a coadministered drug B by inhibiting, activating, or inducing the activity of the enzymes that metabolize drug B. Inhibitory drug–drug interactions could result in serious adverse effects, including fatalities in patients receiving multiple medications. This process is competitive and begins with the first dose of the inhibitor, and the extent of inhibition correlates with the relative affinities for the enzymes and the metabolic half-lives of the drugs involved. However, mechanism-based (irreversible) inhibition results from a metabolite that binds irreversibly with a covalent bond to the enzyme, rendering the enzyme inactive. Enzyme-specific P450 inhibitors, including metabolism- and mechanism-based inhibitors, are metabolized by specific P450 isoforms and are by and large excluded from further consideration for new drug development. Not only is CYP3A4 the most abundant isoform in human liver, but it also metabolizes more than 60% of the drugs in clinical use, which renders CYP3A4 highly susceptible to both metabolism- (reversible) and mechanism-based inhibition. The CYP3A subfamily is involved in many clinically significant drug–drug interactions, and therefore metabolism-based inhibition of CYP3A can cause clinically significant drug–drug interactions, such as those involving nonsedating antihistamines and cisapride, which can result in cardiac dysrhythmias. For example, inhibitors of CYP1A2 can increase the risk of toxicity from clozapine or theophylline. Inhibitors of CYP2C9 can increase the risk of toxicity from phenytoin, tolbutamide, and oral anticoagulants (e.g., warfarin). Inhibitors of CYP3A4 can increase the risk of toxicity from many drugs, including carbamazepine, cyclosporine, ergot alkaloids, lovastatin, protease inhibitors, rifabutin, simvastatin, tacrolimus, and vinca alkaloids. Inhibitors of CYP2D6 can increase risk of toxicity of many antidepressants, opiate analgesics, and psychotherapeutic agents. An excellent example of a metabolism-based inhibition drug–drug interaction that resulted in a life-threatening ventricular arrhythmia associated with QT prolongation (torsades de pointes) occurred when CYP3A4 substrates or inhibitors were coadministered with terfenadine, astemizole, cisapride, or pimozide. This potentially lethal drug interaction led to the withdrawal of terfenadine and cisapride from clinical use and to the approved marketing of fexofenadine, the active metabolite of terfenadine, which does not have this interaction. Examples of enzyme inducers include barbiturates, carbamazepine, glutethimide, griseofulvin, phenytoin, primidone, rifabutin, and rifampin. Some drugs, such as ritonavir, can act as either an enzyme inhibitor or an enzyme inducer, depending on the situation. Drugs metabolized by CYP3A4 or CYP2C9 are particularly susceptible to enzyme induction.

Mechanism-Based Enzyme Inhibition

Mechanism-based inhibition differs from reversible inhibition in that the inhibitors require enzymatic activation by the target enzyme prior to exerting their inhibitory effect. This initial activation step leads to the formation of an active inhibitor, often referred to as the metabolite-intermediate complex (MIC). The MIC can then exert its inhibitory effect by either forming a direct covalent link with the enzyme or forming a noncovalent tight binding complex. Mechanism-based inhibition is characterized by NADPH-, time-, and concentration-dependent enzyme inactivation, occurring when some drugs are converted by P450s to reactive metabolites (103). Mechanism-based inactivation of CYP3A4 by drugs can be the result of chemical modification of the heme, the apoprotein, or both, as a result of covalent binding of the modified heme to the protein. The clinical pharmacokinetic effect of a mechanism-based CYP3A4 inhibitor is a function of its enzyme kinetics (i.e., K_m and V_{max}) and the rate of synthesis of new or replacement enzyme. Predicting drug–drug interactions involving CYP3A4 inactivation is possible when pharmacokinetic principles are followed. Such prediction can become difficult, however, because the clinical outcomes of CYP3A4 inactivation depend on many factors associated with the enzyme, the drugs, and the patients.

Some of the clinically important drugs that have been identified to be mechanism-based CYP3A4 inhibitors include antibacterials (e.g., clarithromycin, erythromycin, isoniazid), anticancer drugs (e.g., irinotecan, tamoxifen, raloxifene), antidepressants (e.g., fluoxetine, paroxetine), anti-HIV agents (e.g., ritonavir, delavirdine), antihypertensives (e.g., dihydralazine, verapamil), steroids and their receptor modulators (e.g., ethinyl estradiol, gestodene, raloxifene), dihydrotestosterone reductase inhibitors (e.g., finasteride), and some herbal constituents (e.g., bergamottin, glabridin). Drugs inactivating CYP3A4 often possess several common moieties such as a tertiary amine, furan ring, or an acetylene group. The chemical properties of a drug critical to CYP3A4 inactivation include formation of reactive metabolites by P450 isoenzymes, P450 inducers, and P-gp substrate and the occurrence of clinically significant pharmacokinetic interactions with coadministered drugs.

Compared to the more common metabolism-based (reversible) inhibition, mechanism-based inhibitors of CYP3A4 more frequently cause pharmacokinetic–pharmacodynamic drug–drug interactions and are frequently the cause of unfavorable drug–drug interactions, because the inactivated CYP3A4 must be replaced by newly synthesized CYP3A4 protein. The resultant drug interactions may lead to adverse drug effects, including some fatal events. Also, raloxifene, a drug approved for the treatment of osteoporosis and chemoprevention of breast cancer in postmenopausal women at high risk for invasive breast cancer, has demonstrated the ability to act as a mechanism-based inhibitor of CYP3A4 by forming adducts with the apoprotein. It has been established that 3′-hydroxyraloxifene is produced exclusively via CYP3A4-mediated oxygenation to produce a reactive diquinone methide excluding the alternative arene oxide pathway.

However, predicting drug–drug interactions involving CYP3A4 inactivation is difficult because the clinical outcomes depend on a number of factors that are associated with drugs and patients. The apparent pharmacokinetic effect of a mechanism-based inhibitor of CYP3A4 would be a function of its enzyme kinetics and the synthesis rate of new or replacement enzyme. Most CYP3A4 inhibitors are also P-gp substrates/inhibitors, confounding the in vitro to in vivo extrapolation. The clinical significance of CYP3A inhibition for drug safety and efficacy warrants closer understanding of the mechanisms for each inhibitor. Furthermore, such inactivation may be exploited for therapeutic gain in certain circumstances. Clinicians should have good knowledge about these CYP3A4 inhibitors and avoid their combination use.

Although CYP2D6 constitutes a relatively minor fraction of the total hepatic P450 content (Fig. 4.2), the contribution of this isoform is significant as a result of its role in the metabolism and clearance of many therapeutic agents that target the cardiovascular and central nervous system (Fig. 4.3) (Table 4.9). In addition, clinically significant polymorphisms in the *CYP2D6* gene have been identified in a variety of populations with altered metabolic activity as PMs or individuals with impaired enzyme function resulting from splicing defects or gene deletions. On the other hand, EMs or individuals with normal enzyme function are heterozygous or homozygous for the wild-type allele. In vivo clearance of CYP2D6 substrates in PMs is usually much lower than in EMs, leading to higher plasma concentrations and the potential for clinical toxicities with therapeutic doses. For example, paroxetine is a selective serotonin reuptake inhibitor that is both a substrate for and an inhibitor of CYP2D6 (also see Chapter 19). Paroxetine is metabolized by CYP2D6 via the formation of a carbene intermediate of the methylenedioxy group yielding an irreversible complex with CYP2D6 (Fig. 4.33) (105). Also, an in vitro study of 3,4-methylenedioxy-methamphetamine (MDMA, ecstasy) suggested that a typical recreational MDMA dose could inactivate most hepatic CYP2D6 within an hour, and the return to a basal level of CYP2D6 could take at least 10 days, impacting its pharmacokinetics.

Because of the pivotal role of P450 isoenzymes in drug metabolism, significant inactivation of these isoforms and particularly the major human hepatic and intestinal CYP3A4 and hepatic CYP2D6 could result in drug–drug interactions and adverse drug reactions. Compared with the reversible inhibition of CYP3A4 and CYP2D6, mechanism-based inhibitors of these isoenzymes more frequently cause pharmacokinetic/pharmacodynamic drug–drug interactions, as the inactivated isoenzyme has to be replaced by newly synthesized P450 protein. Pharmacokinetic interactions often occur as a result of a change in drug metabolism. For example, the macrolides increased the plasma concentrations of a number of therapeutic agents that are substrates of CYP3A4 (Table 4.11). Diltiazem has been shown to inhibit the metabolism of a variety of coadministered drugs including carbamazepine, quinidine, midazolam, and lovastatin (Table 4.11). Inhibition of CYP3A by ritonavir explains, in part, the remarkable elevation of blood concentrations and area under the plasma concentration-time curve of other concomitantly administered drugs that are extensively metabolized by CYP3A4 and have significant first-pass metabolism. These drugs include rifabutin (400%), clarithromycin (77%), ketoconazole, saquinavir (5,000%), amprenavir (210%), nelfinavir (152%), lopinavir (7,700%), and indinavir (380%) (103). Furthermore, such inactivation can be exploited for therapeutic gain in certain circumstances (e.g., the protease inhibitors ritonavir/indinavir).

Beneficial Drug–Drug Interactions

By understanding the unique functions and characteristics of these P450 isoenzymes, health care practitioners can better anticipate and manage drug–drug interactions. They can also predict or explain an individual's response to a particular therapeutic regimen. A beneficial drug interaction, for example, is the coadministration of a CYP3A4 inhibitor with cyclosporine. By inhibiting CYP3A4, the plasma concentrations of cyclosporine (a CYP3A4 substrate) are increased, which allows a reduction of the cyclosporine dosage, thereby improving clinical efficacy and reducing its cost. Similarly, certain HIV protease inhibitors, such as saquinavir, have a low oral bioavailability due to intestinal CYP3A4 metabolism. The oral bioavailability of saquinavir can be profoundly increased by the addition of a low dose of the mechanism-based CYP3A4 inhibitor, ritonavir. This concept of altering drug pharmacokinetics by adding a low, subtherapeutic dose of a mechanism-based CYP3A4 inhibitor (ritonavir) to increase the oral bioavailability of another protease inhibitor, lopinavir (CYP3A4 substrate), led to the marketing of Kaletra, a new drug combination of lopinavir and ritonavir.

Another beneficial mechanism-based inhibition is of the P2Y12 receptor (a protein found on the surface of blood platelet cells and that is an important regulator in blood clotting) by the antiaggregating platelet prodrugs, clopidogrel and prasugrel. Clopidogrel is bioactivated to its reactive metabolite by CYP2C19, CYP1A2, and CYP3A4, whereas prasugrel is bioactivated by CYP3A4 and CYP2B6. The bioactivated metabolites can then react with the P2Y12 receptor protein.

Grapefruit Juice–Drug Interactions

The discovery that grapefruit juice can markedly increase the oral bioavailability of CYP3A4 metabolized drugs was based on an unexpected observation from an interaction study between the dihydropyridine calcium channel antagonist felodipine and ethanol in which grapefruit juice was used to mask the taste of the ethanol. Subsequent investigations confirmed that grapefruit juice significantly increased the oral bioavailability of felodipine by reducing presystemic felodipine metabolism through selective inhibition of CYP3A4 expression in the intestinal wall (106).

Grapefruit juice is a beverage often consumed at breakfast for its health benefits and to mask the taste of drugs or foods. Unlike other citrus fruit juices, however, grapefruit juice can significantly increase the oral bioavailability of drugs that are metabolized primarily by intestinal CYP3A4, causing an elevation in their serum concentrations (Table 4.22). Those drugs with high oral bioavailabilities (>60%), however, are all likely safe to take with grapefruit juice, because their high oral bioavailability leaves little room for elevation by grapefruit juice. The importance of the interaction appears to be influenced by individual patient susceptibility, type and amount of grapefruit juice, and administration-related factors.

Grapefruit juice can alter oral drug pharmacokinetics by different mechanisms. Irreversible inactivation of intestinal CYP3A4, which can persist up to 24 hours, is produced by grapefruit juice given as a single, normal, 200- to 300-mL drink or by whole fresh fruit segments (Table 4.22). As a result, presystemic metabolism is reduced, and oral drug bioavailability is increased. Enhanced oral drug bioavailability can occur up to 24 hours after juice consumption. Inhibition of P-gp is a possible mechanism that increases oral drug bioavailability by reducing intestinal and/or hepatic efflux transport. Inhibition of organic anion–transporting polypeptides by grapefruit juice and apple juice has been observed; intestinal uptake transport appeared to be decreased as oral drug bioavailability was reduced. Numerous medications used in the prevention or

TABLE 4.22 Some CYP3A4 Substrates and Interactions with Grapefruit Juice (78)

Drug	Interaction[a]	Drug	Interaction[a]	Drug	Interaction[a]
Calcium channel blocker		HIV protease inhibitors		CNS Drugs	
Amlodipine	Y	Indinavir	N?	Buspirone	Y
Felodipine	Y	Nelfinavir	N?	Carbamazepine	Y
Nifedipine	Y	Ritonavir	N?	Diazepam	Y
Nimodipine	Y	Saquinavir	Y	Midazolam	Y
Nisoldipine	Y	Macrolides		Triazolam	Y
Nitrendipine	Y	Clarithromycin	N	Immunosuppressants	
Pranidipine	Y	HMG-CoA reductase inhibitors		Cyclosporine	Y
Antiarrhythmics		Atorvastatin	Y	Tacrolimus	Y?
Diltiazem	N	Cerivastatin	Y?	Other	
Verapamil	N	Fluvastatin	N?	Methadone	Y
Antihistamines		Lovastatin	Y	Sildenafil	Y
Ebastine	Y?	Pravastatin	N?		
Loratidine	Y?	Simvasta	Y		

[a]Y (yes) and N (no) indicate published evidence of the presence or absence of an interaction with grapefruit juice. Y? and N? indicate expected findings based on available data. Those drugs with Y or Y? should not be consumed with grapefruit juice in an unsupervised manner.

treatment of coronary artery disease and its complications have been observed or predicted to interact with grapefruit juice. Such drug–drug interactions can increase the risk of rhabdomyolysis when dyslipidemia is treated with the HMG-CoA reductase inhibitors ("statins"). Such drug–drug interactions could also cause excessive vasodilatation when hypertension is managed with the dihydropyridines felodipine, nicardipine, nifedipine, nisoldipine, or nitrendipine. An alternative agent could be amlodipine. The therapeutic effect of the angiotensin II type I receptor antagonist losartan can be reduced by grapefruit juice. Grapefruit juice interacting with the antidiabetic agent repaglinide can cause hypoglycemia, and interaction with the appetite suppressant sibutramine can cause elevated blood pressure and heart rate. In angina pectoris, administration of grapefruit juice could result in atrioventricular conduction disorders with verapamil or attenuated antiplatelet activity with clopidogrel. Grapefruit juice can enhance the drug toxicity for antiarrhythmic agents, such as amiodarone, quinidine, disopyramide, or propafenone and for the congestive heart failure drug carvedilol. Some drugs for the treatment of peripheral or central vascular disease also have the potential to interact with grapefruit juice. Interaction with sildenafil, tadalafil, or vardenafil for erectile dysfunction can cause serious systemic vasodilatation, especially when combined with a nitrate. In stroke, interaction with nimodipine can cause systemic hypotension.

If a drug has low inherent oral bioavailability from presystemic metabolism by CYP3A4 or efflux transport by P-gp and the potential to produce serious overdose toxicity, avoidance of grapefruit juice entirely during pharmacotherapy appears mandatory. Although altered drug response is variable among individuals, the outcome is difficult to predict, and avoiding the combination will guarantee that toxicity is prevented. The elderly are at particular risk, because they often are prescribed medications and frequently consume grapefruit juice.

The mechanism by which grapefruit juice produces its effect is through inhibition of the enzymatic activity and a decrease in the intestinal expression of CYP3A4. The P-gp efflux pump also transports many CYP3A4 substrates; thus, the presence of inhibitors of P-gp in grapefruit juice (e.g., 6′,7′-dihydroxybergamottin and other furanocoumarins) could be a related factor for drug–grapefruit juice interactions (82). Numerous studies have shown that grapefruit juice acts on intestinal CYP3A4, not at the hepatic level.

Does the quantity of juice matter? The majority of the presystemic CYP3A4 inhibition is obtained following ingestion of one glass of grapefruit juice; however, 24 hours after ingestion of a glass of grapefruit juice, 30% of its effect is still present (78). The reduction in intestinal CYP3A4 concentration is rapid: A 47% decrease occurred in a healthy volunteer within 4 hours after consuming grapefruit juice. Daily ingestion of grapefruit juice results in a loss of CYP3A4 from the small intestinal epithelium. Consumption of very large quantities of grapefruit juice (six to eight glasses/day) can lead to inhibition of hepatic CYP3A4.

The active constituents found in grapefruit juice responsible for its effects on CYP3A4 include flavonoids (e.g., naringenin and naringin) and furanocoumarins (e.g., bergamottin and 6′,7′-dihydroxybergamottin) (82). Of particular interest are the effects of naringin and 6′,7′-dihydroxybergamottin on the activity of intestinal CYP3A4.

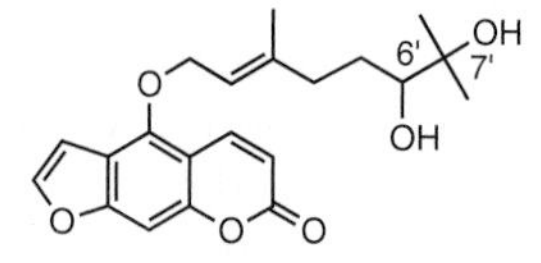

6',7'-Dihydroxybergamottin

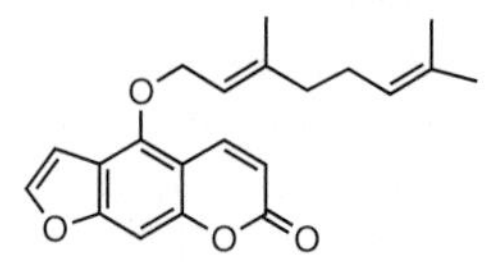

Bergamottin

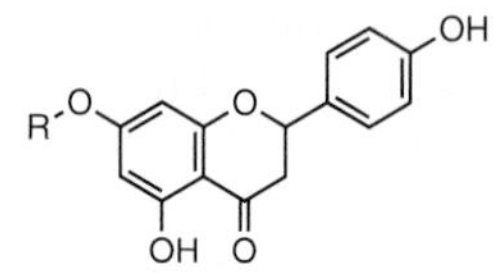

Naringin R: rhamnose-glucoside-
Naringinin R: H-

The majority of studies to date have used either freshly squeezed grapefruit juice, reconstituted frozen juice, commercial grapefruit juice, grapefruit segments, or grapefruit extract; all are capable of causing drug–drug interactions with CYP3A4 substrates (blended grapefruit juices have not yet been investigated). The active constituents in grapefruit juice are present not just in the juice but also in the pulp, peel, and core of the fruit and are responsible for its flavor. Bergamottin and 6′,7′-dihydroxybergamottin are potent mechanism-based inhibitors of CYP3A4, and naringenin isomers are competitive inhibitors of CYP3A4 (82). Higher concentrations of 6′,7′-dihydroxybergamottin and naringin are present in grapefruit segments. Thus, any therapeutic concern for a drug interaction with grapefruit juice should now be extended to include whole fruit and other products derived from the grapefruit peel. The difference in the in vitro CYP3A4 inhibition between grapefruit juice and orange juice is that orange juice contained no measurable amounts of 6′,7′-dihydroxybergamottin.

If a patient has been taking medication with grapefruit juice for some time without ill effects, is it safe to continue to do so? Much of this unpredictability results from the inconsistency of the juice concentrations and the sporadic manner in which grapefruit juice is consumed, suggesting that this approach cannot be entirely safe (106). Given the unpredictability of the effect of grapefruit juice on the oral bioavailability of the drugs in Table 4.22, patients should be advised to avoid this combination, thus preventing the onset of potential adverse effects. Each patient's situation should be considered, and advice should be based on consumption history and the specific medications involved. The benefits of increased and controlled drug bioavailability by grapefruit juice can, in the future, be achieved through either standardizing the constituents or coadministration of the isolated active ingredients. This would then lead to a safe, effective, and cost-saving means to enhance the absorption of many therapeutic agents.

P-Glycoprotein–Drug Interactions

From the earlier discussion regarding P-gp, it is obvious that P-gp–mediated transport has an important role in pharmacokinetic-mediated drug–drug interactions (79). Thus, inhibition of P-gp–mediated transport could dramatically increase the systemic bioavailability of an otherwise poorly absorbed drug. Similar consequences could be expected with a reduction in renal or biliary clearances (e.g., digoxin). Numerous investigations with drugs such as digoxin, etoposide, cyclosporine, vinblastine, paclitaxel, loperamide, domperidone, and ondansetron demonstrate that P-gp has an important role in determining the pharmacokinetics of substrate drugs (79). For example, if drug A is a substrate for both P-gp and *only* for CYP3A4 and if a second drug B is added that is an inhibitor for both P-gp and CYP3A4 (Table 4.18), then the plasma drug concentration for unmetabolized drug A will be elevated, with increased potential for drug–drug interactions as adverse effects or for causing a drug overdose. If drug A is a substrate for multiple P450 isoforms, however, then drug A will be metabolized by these other isoforms, with minimal effect on plasma drug concentrations. On the other hand, if the second drug B is only an inhibitor for P-gp, then drug A will be subject to CYP3A4 metabolism, thus decreasing the plasma concentration for drug A to subtherapeutic levels. The effect of P-gp inhibition is to increase the oral bioavailability so that the later actions of CYP3A4 inhibition will be increased. One of the best examples is the interaction between digoxin and quinidine. Quinidine blocks P-gp in the intestinal mucosa and in the proximal renal tubule; thus, digoxin elimination into the intestine and urine is inhibited, increasing the plasma digoxin concentration to toxic levels. Another example is loperamide, which is an opiate antidiarrheal normally kept out of the brain by the P-gp pump; however, inhibition of P-gp allows accumulation of loperamide in the brain, leading to respiratory depression. Increasingly, the relevant clinical data for drug–drug interactions can be found on the World Wide Web.

The components of grapefruit juice reportedly inhibit P-gp, and this can be one of the mechanisms for the increase in bioavailability of drugs that are substrates for P-gp (Table 4.18). Although fexofenadine is a P-gp substrate, rather than a decrease in its plasma levels when it is coadministered with grapefruit juice, the blood levels are increased as a result of fexofenadine being a substrate of the organic anion transporter polypeptide (OATP) in the intestine. Studies have shown that apple and other fruit juices are more potent inhibitors of OATP than of P-gp.

Food–Drug Interactions

Drug pharmacokinetics can be altered by the fat content of food through changes in drug solubility as well as the nutritional status of a patient (107). The fact that grapefruit juice can increase the bioavailability of certain drugs by reducing their presystemic intestinal metabolism has led to renewed interest in the area of "food–drug interactions," with particular interest regarding the effects of grapefruit constituents. Specific naturally occurring chemicals in food have been associated with drug–drug interactions. For example, severe hypertensive reactions have occurred when patients treated with antidepressant MAO inhibitors have ingested cheeses and other foods rich in the biogenic amine tyramine (see Chapter 18).

Drug–Dietary Supplement Interactions

The increasing use of dietary supplements presents a special challenge in health care; thus, there is an increasing need to predict and avoid these potential adverse drug–dietary supplement interactions. The present interest and widespread use of herbal remedies has created the possibility of interaction between them and over-the-counter or prescription drugs if they are used simultaneously. As herbal medicines become more popular, herbal hepatotoxicity is being increasingly recognized. Females appear to be predisposed to hepatotoxicity, and coadministered agents that induce P450 enzymes (e.g., St. John's wort) can also increase individual susceptibility to some dietary supplements. Currently, nearly one in five adults taking prescription medicines is also taking at least one dietary supplement. The mechanisms for drug–dietary supplement interactions are similar to those for drug–drug interactions affecting the pharmacokinetics of the respective drug. Little is known regarding the pharmacokinetic properties of many of the substances in dietary supplements. Therefore, the potential for drug–dietary supplement interactions has greatly increased.

St. John's Wort

A commonly reported drug–dietary supplement interaction is between St. John's wort and HIV protease inhibitors, leading to drug resistance and treatment failure. St. John's wort is a popular dietary supplement often used for depression. Of the two substances found in St. John's wort, hypericin and hyperforin, hyperforin appears to be the main constituent, with in vitro selective serotonin reuptake inhibitor activity (also see Chapter 18).

Hyperforin appears also to be the more potent inducer of CYP3A enzymes based on in vitro and in vivo studies.

The FDA has issued a statement that "concomitant use of St. John's wort with protease inhibitors or nonnucleoside reverse transcriptase inhibitors is not recommended." St. John's wort appeared to have minimal effects on the CYP3A4 enzymes after acute administration; however, chronic administration (≥2 weeks) of St. John's wort selectively induced CYP3A4, with a greater effect in the small intestine than in the liver. Administration of St. John's wort for 8 weeks decreased the plasma levels of norethindrone, a low-dose oral contraceptive; reduced the half-life of ethinyl estradiol, consistent with increased CYP3A activity; increased breakthrough bleeding; and reduced contraceptive efficacy. Based on these in vivo and in vitro studies, the efficacy of drugs that are substrates for the CYP3A family or P-gp can be reduced with coadministration of St. John's wort. St. John's wort should be listed along with other known CYP3A inducers (e.g., rifampin and rifabutin) as possibly decreasing plasma levels of CYP3A substrates. The drug products Kaletra (lopinavir and ritonavir), Mifeprex (mifepristone, RU-486), Nuvaring (etonogestrel/ethinyl estradiol), Gleevec (imatinib), Neoral (cyclosporine), Rapamune (sirolimus), and Prograf (tacrolimus) include information about drug interactions with St. John's wort in their labeling. Thus, patients ingesting St. John's wort products should be advised that St. John's wort can have potentially dangerous drug–drug interactions with some prescription drugs and to consult a physician before taking St. John's wort if currently taking anticoagulants, oral contraceptives, antidepressants, antiseizure medications, drugs to treat HIV or prevent transplant rejections, or any other prescription drug.

St. John's wort also decreases the absorption of digoxin and fexofenadine, apparently by inducing P-gp in the intestinal and renal endothelium, increasing their elimination in the intestine and urine, respectively, and their plasma concentrations.

Echinacea

In vitro or in vivo chronic administration studies of echinacea, an herbal product used for the treatment of colds and viral infections, inhibited hepatic CYP1A2 and intestinal CYP3A activities and induced hepatic CYP3A. Based on these preliminary findings, the effect of echinacea on various CYP3A substrates can vary depending on the relative contribution to a given drug's overall clearance by intestinal CYP3A versus hepatic CYP3A in the individual substrate's clearance pathway.

Ginkgo Biloba

In vitro studies with ginkgo biloba, often used for memory improvement, exhibited induction of CYP2C19. The extent of induction appears to be CYP2C19 genotype dependent.

Kava

Reports of hepatotoxicity have been associated with the use of kava, a popular drug in Europe and North America. Hepatotoxicity was not observed when kava was prepared as a water infusion but was observed with solvent-extracted products available in stores and on the Internet. The three kava lactones (methysticin, desmethoxyyangonin, and yangonin; active principles) are potent inhibitors of CYP1A2, CYP2C9, CYP2C19, CYP2E1, and CYP3A4, with methysticin being the most potent enzyme inhibitor as well as the most cytotoxic. The potent inhibition of P450 enzymes suggests a high potential for drug–drug interactions with drugs and other herbs that are metabolized by the same P450 enzymes. Long-term use or use in individuals with liver disorders should be avoided, and liver function transaminases need to be checked frequently.

Other Dietary Supplements Exhibiting Drug-Induced Hepatotoxicity

DHEA and androstenedione are testosterone precursors that have been associated with hepatic toxicity and should be avoided in those with hepatic disease or coingestion with other potentially hepatotoxic products or enzyme inducers that might increase the risk of liver damage. Liver enzymes should be monitored once or twice a year. Boldo, an herbal medicine, can cause hepatotoxicity and exacerbate existing liver disease. Because chaparral, comfrey, germander, skullcap, and valerian root can cause acute and chronic liver injury, these products should be considered unsafe. Pennyroyal oil can cause acute hepatotoxic liver injury, which has been attributed to the bioactivation of the terpine, *R*-(+)-pulegone, resulting in depletion of hepatic glutathione. In some cases, unknown adulterants found in these herbal products can be responsible for the hepatotoxicity. Black cohosh, commonly used by women for menopausal symptoms, including hot flashes and sleep disorders, formed quinone metabolites in vitro, but no mercapturate conjugates were detected in urine samples from women who consumed multiple oral doses of up to 256 mg of a standardized black cohosh extract. At moderate doses of black cohosh, the risk of liver injury is minimal (108).

Silybum marianum (milk thistle) is used in the treatment of chronic or acute liver disease as well as in protecting the liver against toxicity (109). Silybum is cited as one of the oldest known herbal medicines. The active constituents of milk thistle are flavonolignans, which are known collectively as silymarin. The most remarkable use of silymarin is in the treatment of *Amanita* mushroom poisoning. *Amanita* mushrooms possess two extremely powerful hepatotoxins, amanitin and phalloidin (the median lethal dose of amanitin is 0.1 mg/kg body weight). Severe liver damage (and death) is avoided if silymarin is administered within 24 hours following ingestion of *Amanita*. It is also a hepatoprotective for chronic exposure to ethanol and acetaminophen toxicity.

Miscellaneous Drug–Drug Interactions

The ability of drugs and other foreign substances to stimulate (induction) metabolism of other drugs has already been discussed. Phenobarbital, for example, stimulates metabolism of a variety of drugs (e.g., phenytoin and coumarin anticoagulants). Stimulation of bishydroxycoumarin metabolism can create a problem in patients undergoing anticoagulant therapy. If phenobarbital administration is stopped, the rate of metabolism of the anticoagulant decreases, resulting in greater plasma concentrations of bishydroxycoumarin and enhanced anticoagulant activity, increasing the possibility of hemorrhage. Serious side effects have resulted from this type of interaction. These observations indicate that combined therapy of a potent drug (e.g., bishydroxycoumarin) and an inducer of drug metabolism (e.g., phenobarbital) can create a hazardous situation if the enzyme inducer is withdrawn and therapy with the potent drug is continued without an appropriate decrease in dose.

Some drugs are competitive inhibitors of nonmicrosomal metabolic pathways. Serious reactions have been reported in patients treated with an MAO inhibitor, such as tranylcypromine or iproniazid, because they are, as a rule, sensitive to a subsequent dose of a sympathomimetic amine (e.g., amphetamine) or a tricyclic antidepressant (e.g., amitriptyline), which is metabolized by MAO.

Allopurinol, a xanthine oxidase inhibitor used for the treatment of gout, inhibits metabolism of 6-mercaptopurine and other drugs metabolized by this enzyme. A serious drug interaction results from the concurrent use of allopurinol for gout and 6-mercaptopurine to block the immune response from a tissue transplant or as antimetabolite in neoplastic diseases. In some cases, however, allopurinol is used in conjunction with 6-mercaptopurine to control the increase in uric acid elimination from 6-mercaptopurine metabolism. The patient should be supervised closely, because when given in large doses, allopurinol, an inhibitor of purine metabolism, can have serious effects on bone marrow.

GENDER DIFFERENCES IN DRUG METABOLISM

The role of gender as a contributor to variability in xenobiotic metabolism and IDRs, which are more common in women than in men, is not clear, but increasing numbers of reports show differences in metabolism between men and women, raising the intriguing possibility that endogenous sex hormones, hydrocortisone, or their synthetic equivalents can influence the activity of inducible CYP3A. For example, *N*-demethylation of erythromycin was significantly higher in females than males. Nevertheless, the *N*-demethylation was persistent throughout adulthood. In contrast, males exhibited unchanged *N*-demethylation values.

Gender-dependent differences of metabolic rates have been detected for some drugs. Side-chain oxidation of propranolol was 50% faster in males than in females, but no differences between genders were noted in aromatic ring hydroxylation. *N*-demethylation of meperidine was depressed during pregnancy and for women taking oral contraceptives. Other examples of drugs cleared by oxidative drug metabolism more rapidly in men than in women included chlordiazepoxide and lidocaine. Diazepam, prednisolone, caffeine, and acetaminophen are metabolized slightly faster by women than by men. No gender differences have been observed in the clearance of phenytoin, nitrazepam, and trazodone, which interestingly are not substrates for the CYP3A subfamily. Gender differences in the rate of glucuronidation have been noted.

More investigation is warranted, and future pharmacokinetic studies examining the alteration in drug metabolism in one gender need to be reexamined with respect to the other gender. Even in postmenopausal women, CYP3A function can be altered and influenced by the lack of estrogen or the presence of androgens.

MAJOR PATHWAYS OF METABOLISM

Table 4.12 contains an extensive list of commonly used drugs and the P450 isoforms that catalyze their metabolism. In addition, Phase 1 and Phase 2 metabolic pathways for some common drugs are listed in Table 4.23.

TABLE 4.23 Metabolic Pathways of Common Drugs

Drug	Pathway	Drug	Pathway
Amphetamines 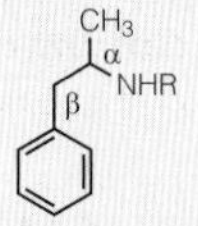	Deamination (followed by oxidation and reduction of the ketone formed) *N*-oxidation *N*-dealkylation Hydroxylation of the aromatic ring Hydroxylation of the β-carbon atom Conjugation with glucuronic acid of the acid and alcohol products from the ketone formed by deamination	Barbiturates 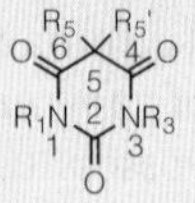	Oxidation and complete removal of substituents at carbon 5 *N*-dealkylation at N^1 and N^3 Desulfuration at carbon 2 (thiobarbiturates) Scission of the barbiturate ring at the 1:6 bond to give substituted malonylureas
Phenothiazines 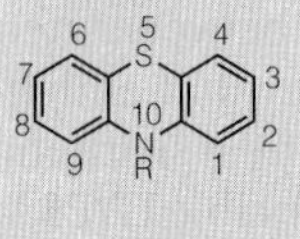	*N*-dealkylation in the N^{10} side chain *N*-oxidation in the N^{10} side chain Oxidation of the heterocyclic S atom to sulfoxide or sulfone Hydroxylation of one or both aromatic rings Conjugation of phenolic metabolites with glucuronic acid or sulfate Scission of the N^{10} side chain	Sulfonamides 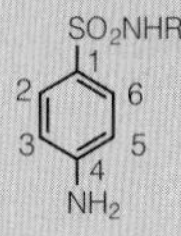	Acetylation at the N^4 amino group Conjugation with glucuronic acid or sulfate at the N^4 amino group Acetylation or conjugation with glucuronic acid at the N^1 amino group Hydroxylation and conjugation in the heterocyclic ring, R
Phenytoin 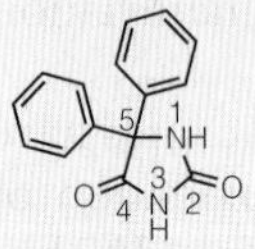	Hydroxylation of one aromatic ring Conjugation of phenolic products with glucuronic acid or sulfate Hydrolytic scission of the hydantoin ring at the bond between carbons 3 and 4 to give 5,5-diphenylhydantoic acid	Meperidine 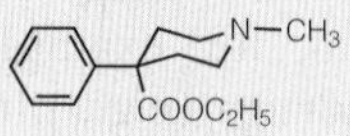	Hydrolysis of ester to acid *N*-dealkylation Hydroxylation of aromatic ring *N*-oxidation Both *N*-dealkylation and hydrolysis Conjugation of phenolic products
Pentazocine 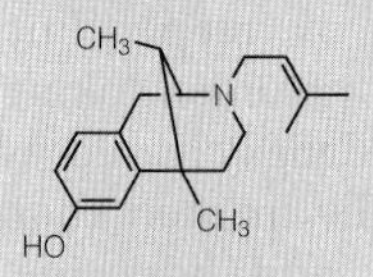	Hydroxylation of terminal methyl groups of the alkenyl side chain to give cis and trans (major) alcohols Oxidation of hydroxymethyl product of the alkenyl side chain to carboxylic acids Reduction of alkenyl side chain and oxidation of terminal methyl group	Cocaine 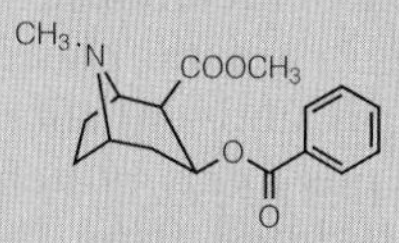	Hydrolysis of methyl ester Hydrolysis of benzoate ester *N*-dealkylation Both hydrolysis and *N*-dealkylation
Phenmetrazine 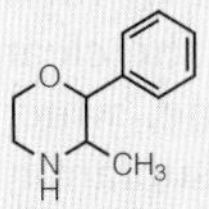	Oxidation to lactam Aromatic hydroxylation *N*-oxidation Conjugation of phenolic products	Ephedrine 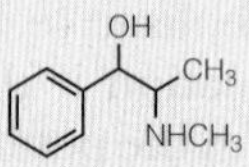	*N*-dealkylation Oxidative deamination Oxidation of deaminated product to benzoic acid Reduction of deaminated product to 1,2-diol
Propranolol 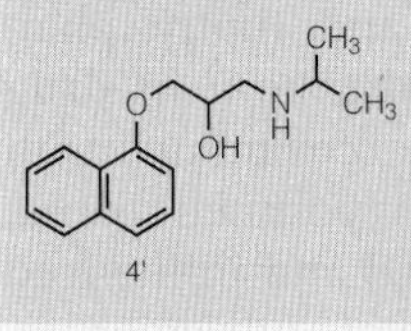	Aromatic hydroxylation at C-4′ *N*-dealkylation Oxidative deamination Oxidation of deaminated product to naphthoxylactic acid Conjugation with glucuronic acid *O*-dealkylation	Indomethacin 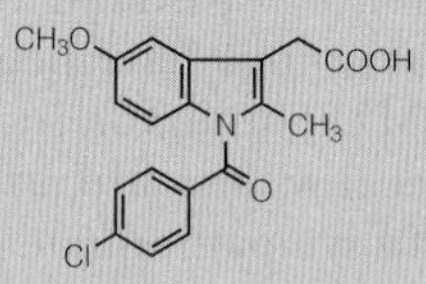	*O*-demethylation *N*-deacylation of *p*-chlorobenzoyl group Both *O*-dealkylation and *N*-deacylation Conjugation of phenolic products with glucuronic acid Other conjugation products
Diphenoxylate 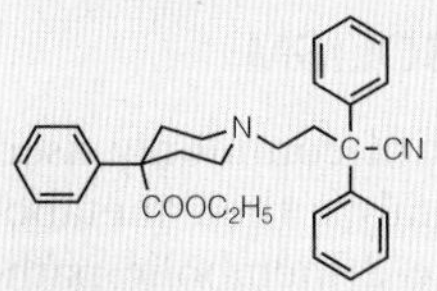	Hydrolysis of ester to acid Hydroxylation of one aromatic ring attached to the *N*-alkyl side chain	Diazepam 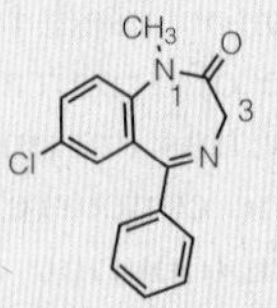	*N*-dealkylation at N^1 Hydroxylation at carbon 3 Conjugation with glucuronic acid Both *N*-dealkylation of N^1 and hydroxylation at carbon 3
Prostaglandins 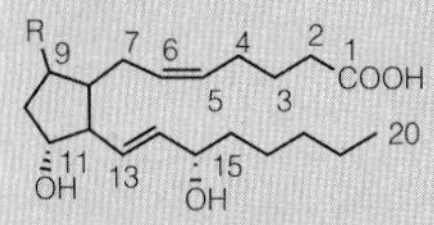	Reduction of double bonds at carbons 5 and 6 and 13 and 14 Oxidation of 15-hydroxyl to ketone β-Oxidation of carbons 3, 5, and 7 ω-Oxidation of carbon 20 to acid	Cyproheptadine 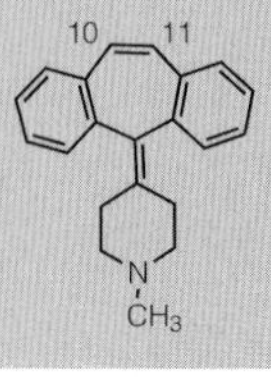	*N*-dealkylation 10,11-Epoxide formation Both *N*-dealkylation and 10,11-epoxidation

TABLE 4.23 Metabolic Pathways of Common Drugs *(Continued)*

Drug	Pathway	Drug	Pathway
Hydralazine 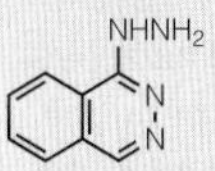	*N*-acetylation with cyclization to a methyl-s-triazolophthalazine *N*-formylation with cyclization to an s-triazolophthalazine Aromatic hydroxylation of benzene ring Oxidative loss of hydrazinyl group to 1-hydroxy Hydroxylation of methyl of methyl-s-triazolophthalazine Conjugation with glucuronic acid	Methadone 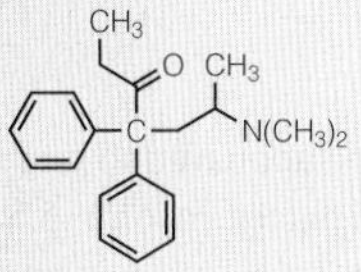	Reduction of ketone to hydroxyl Aromatic hydroxylation of one aromatic ring *N*-dealkylation of alcohol product *N*-dealkylation with cyclization to pyrrolidine
Lidocaine 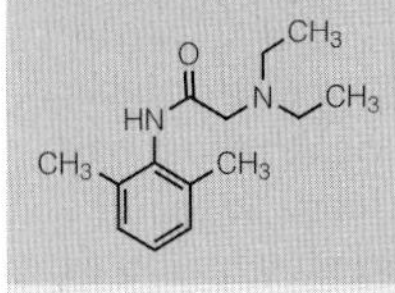	*N*-dealkylation Oxidative cyclization to a 4-imidazolidone *N*-oxidation of amide N Aromatic hydroxylation ortho to methyl Hydrolysis of amide	Imipramine 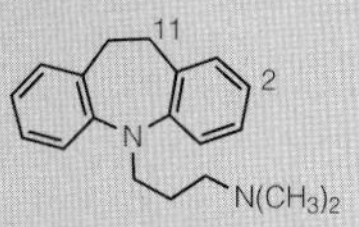	*N*-dealkylation Hydroxylation at C-11 Aromatic hydroxylation (C-2) *N*-oxidation Both *N*-dealkylation and hydroxylation
Cimetidine 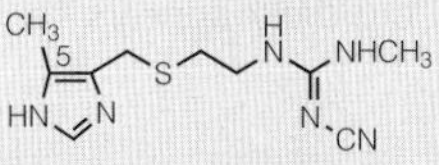	*S*-oxidation Hydroxylation of 5-methyl	Valproic acid 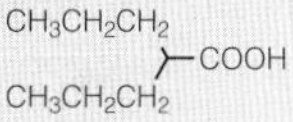	CoA thioester Dehydrogenation to (E) 2-ene Dehydrogenation to (E) 2,4-diene Dehydrogenation to 4-ene 3-Hydroxylation
Piroxicam 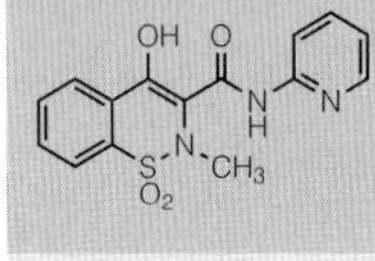	Pyridine 3′-hydroxylation Hydrolysis of amide Decarboxylation	Caffeine 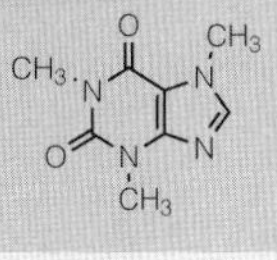	N^3-demethylation N^1-demethylation N^7-demethylation to theophylline C-8 oxidation to uric acids Imidazole ring opened
Theophylline 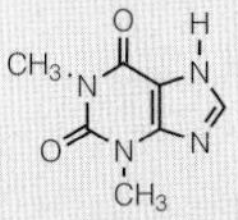	N^3-demethylation N^1-demethylation C-8 oxidation to uric acids Imidazole ring opened 1-Me xanthine to 1-Me uric acid–xanthine oxidase	Nicotine 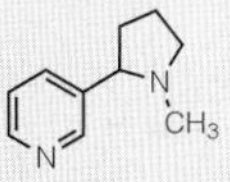	Pyrrolidine 5′-hydroxylation to cotinine Pyrrolidine *N*-oxidation (FMO) *N*-demethylation (nornicotine and norcotinine) Pyridine *N*-methylation 3′-Hydroxylation of cotinine
Ibuprofen 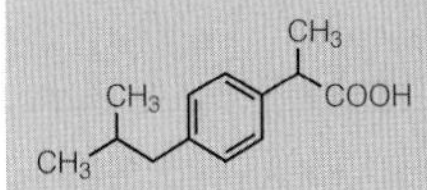	CoA thioester and epimerization of R− to S+ enantiomer Methyl hydroxylation to CH$_2$OH CH$_2$OH to COOH Acylglucuronide	Tamoxifen 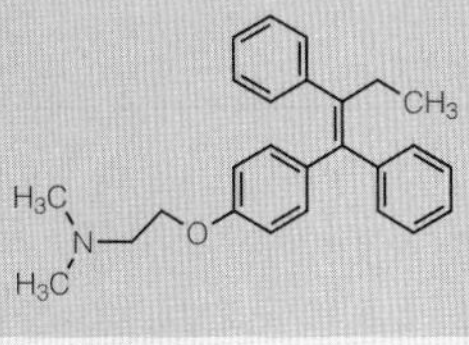	*N*-demethylation 4′-Hydroxylation *N*-oxidation (FMO) 4′-*O*-sulfate 4′-*O*-glucuronide
Lovastatin 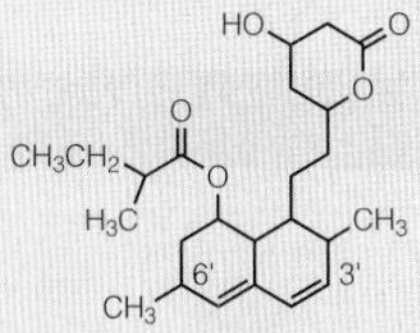	6′-Hydroxylation 3′-Side chain hydroxylation 3′-Hydroxylation β-oxidation of lactone *O*-glucuronides	Ciprofloxacin 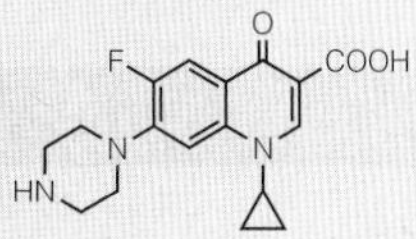	Piperazine 3′-hydroxylation *N*-sulfonation
Labetalol 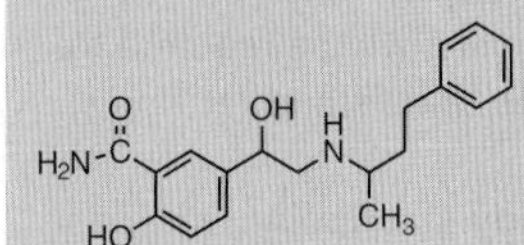	*O*-sulfate (major) *O*-glucuronide	Acetaminophen 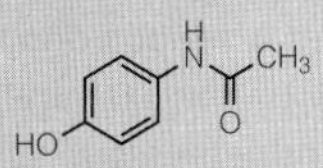	*O*-glucuronide *O*-sulfate Oxidation to *N*-acetyl-*p*-benzoquinoneimine Conjugation of *N*-acetyl-*p*-benzoquinoneimine with glutathione
Tripelennamine 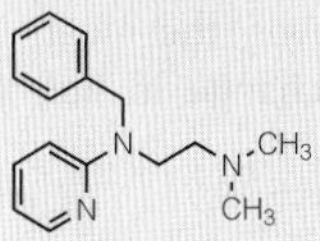	*p*-Hydroxylation Benzylic *C*-hydroxylation *N*-depyridinylation *N*-debenzylation	Felodipine 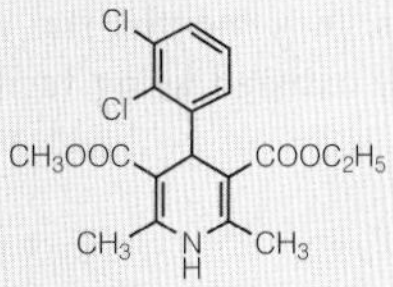	Aromatization Ester hydrolysis Methyl hydroxylation

SCENARIO: OUTCOME AND ANALYSIS

Outcome

Mark D. Watanabe, PharmD, PhD, BCPP

Because both the risperidone and paroxetine appeared to demonstrate a therapeutic effect for Y.H., the pharmacist recommended that the dose of risperidone be decreased to 2 mg daily while continuing paroxetine 20 mg daily. At her next appointment the following month, Y.H. stated that her mood was "getting back on an even keel" and her left hand was no longer shaking.

Chemical Analysis

Victoria Roche and S. William Zito

Risperidone is an antipsychotic agent that acts through the inhibition of dopamine D_2 and serotonin 5-HT_2 receptors. If serum levels exceed those associated with safe therapeutic use, adverse effects associated with excessive D_2 receptor antagonism, including tremor, can commonly manifest. Like many psychotropic agents, risperidone is metabolized by CYP2D6. The active metabolite generated by this isoform is 9-hydroxyrisperidone. Paroxetine is an antidepressant that works by inhibiting the reuptake of 5-HT. It too is metabolized by CYP2D6, yielding an inactive catechol metabolite that can further oxidize to an orthoquinone.

Coadministration of paroxetine and risperidone would result in competition for limited quantities of CYP2D6. As risperidone serum levels increase, the side effects of tremor, dystonia, and akathisia could reasonably be anticipated. Maintaining these two CYP2D6 substrates in Y.H.'s mental health drug regimen demands a reduction in the dose of risperidone so that the metabolism-mediated increase in serum concentration keeps blood levels within the therapeutic range and out of the toxic range. The reduction in dose from 3 to 2 mg daily appears to have accomplished this goal.

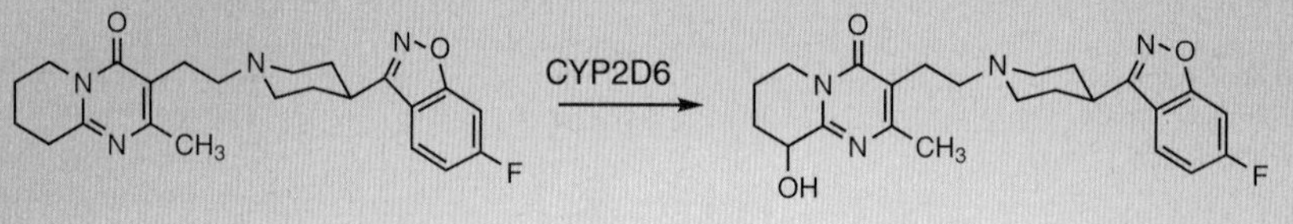

Risperidone 9-Hydroxyrisperidone

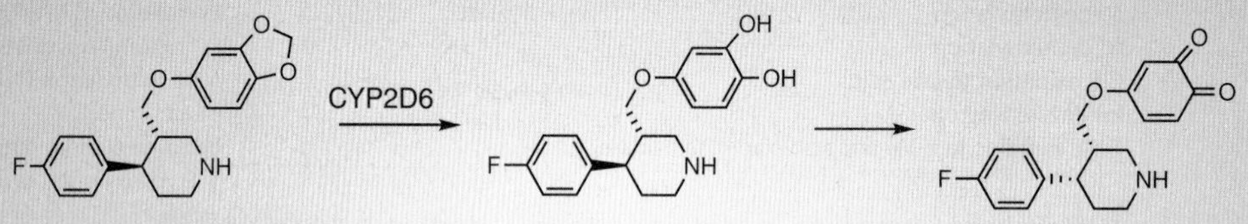

Paroxetine Catechol metabolite *o*-Quinone metabolite

CASE STUDY

Victoria Roche and S. William Zito

NH is a 79-year-old widow who has been in a slow cognitive decline for the past 3 years. Always fiercely independent, her progressive mental impairment has prompted a serious depression that has been fairly well controlled with fluvoxamine, a serotonin reuptake transporter inhibitor antidepressant drug metabolized by CYP1A2 and 2D6. Recently, NH became lost and disoriented while driving to the local supermarket. In a panic, she caused a car accident that resulted in significant property damage but, thankfully, no personal injuries. In 3 months she will be moving into Brookside Manor, a new assisted living facility known for its high-quality care of Alzheimer's patients. NH is a pack-a-day smoker, but Brookside is totally smoke free. NH is dreading the smoking cessation program she will be required to complete before she moves in, but does understand (at times) that she has no choice.

From a cognitive impairment therapy standpoint, NH was doing well on the NMDA receptor antagonist memantine (Namenda), which is minimally metabolized by CYP isoforms and predominantly excreted unchanged. However, the most recent upheaval in her life and the pending change in her living situation have prompted a worsening of her cognitive dysfunction symptoms. Her physician is now trying tacrine (Cognex), a centrally acting acetylcholinesterase inhibitor, in place of Namenda. After a week on this medication NH had initially complained of diarrhea and "feeling hot and sweaty" (symptoms of tacrine toxicity). Now that she's quitting smoking, these symptoms have intensified, she's experiencing urinary incontinence, and her hepatic transaminase enzymes are significantly elevated. As the consultant pharmacist for Brookside, how would you advise this patient and her current providers?

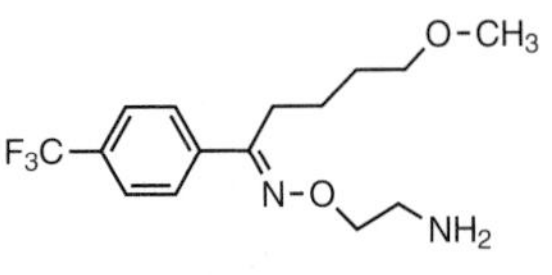

Fluvoxamine

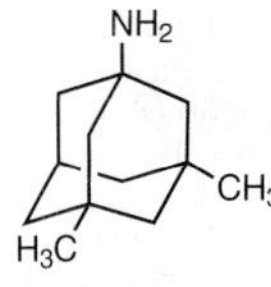

Memantine

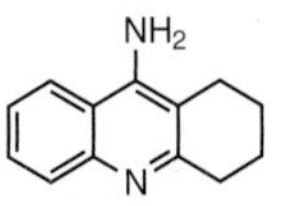

Tacrine

1. Conduct a thorough metabolic analysis of the therapeutic options in the case.
2. Apply the chemical understanding gained from the metabolic analysis to this patient's specific needs to make a therapeutic recommendation.

References

1. Williams RT. Detoxication Mechanisms, 2nd Ed. New York: John Wiley and Sons, 1959.
2. Anders M, ed. Bioactivation of Foreign Compounds. New York: Academic Press, 1985.
3. Jakoby W, ed. Enzymatic Basis of Detoxication, vols I and II. New York: Academic Press, 1980.
4. Jakoby W, Bend JR, Caldwell J, eds. Metabolic Basis of Detoxication—Metabolism of Functional Groups. New York: Academic Press, 1982.
5. Mulder GJ, ed. Conjugation Reactions in Drug Metabolism: An Integrated Approach. London: Taylor and Francis, 1990.
6. Ortiz de Montellano PR, ed. Cytochrome P450: Structure Mechanism and Biochemistry, 2nd Ed. New York: Plenum Press, 1995.
7. Testa B, Krämer SD. The Biochemistry of Drug Metabolism. Volume 1: Principles, Redox Reactions, Hydrolyses and Volume 2: Conjugations, Consequences of Metabolism, Influencing Factors. New York: Wiley-VCH, 2005.
8. Rodrigues AD. Drug-Drug Interactions, 2nd Ed (Drugs and the Pharmaceutical Sciences Volume 179). New York: Informa Healthcare, 2008.
9. Pearson PG, Wienkers LC. Handbook of Drug Metabolism, 2nd Ed (Drugs and the Pharmaceutical Sciences Volume 186). New York: Informa Healthcare, 2008.
10. Murphy MP. Pharmacogenomics: a new paradigm for drug development. Drug Discov World 2000;1:23–32.
11. Wilkinson GR, Schenker S. Drug disposition and liver disease. Drug Metab Rev 1975;4:139–175.
12. McLean AJ, Morgan DJ. Clinical pharmacokinetics in patients with liver disease. Clin Pharmacokinet 1991;21:42–69.
13. Rodighiero V. Effects of liver disease on pharmacokinetics. An update. Clin Pharmacokinet 1999;37:399–443.
14. Groves JT. Models and mechanisms of cytochrome P450. In: Ortiz de Montellano PR, ed. Cytochrome P450: Structure Mechanism and Biochemistry, 3rd Ed. New York: Plenum Press, 2005:1–44.
15. Nielson KA, Moller BL. Cytochrome P450 in plants. In: Ortiz de Montellano PR, ed. Cytochrome P450: Structure Mechanism and Biochemistry, 3rd Ed. New York: Plenum Press, 2005:553.
16. Nebert DW, Nelson DR, Coon MJ, et al. The P450 superfamily: update on new sequences, gene mapping and recommended nomenclature. DNA Cell Biol 1991;10:1–14.
17. Gonzalez FJ, Gelboin HV. Human cytochromes P450: evolution and cDNA-directed expression. Environ Health Perspect 1992;98:810–885.
18. Rendic S, DiCarlo FJ. Human cytochrome P450 enzymes: a status report summarizing their reactions substrates inducers and inhibitors. Drug Metab 1997;29:413–580.
19. Guengerich FP. Enzymatic oxidation of xenobiotic chemicals. Crit Rev Biochem Mol Biol 1990;25:97–153.
20. Meunier B, de Visser SP, Shaik S. Mechanism of oxidation reactions catalyzed by cytochrome P450 enzymes. Chem Rev 2004;104:3947–3980.
21. Guengerich FP. Human cytochrome P450 enzymes. In: Ortiz de Montellano PR, ed. Cytochrome P450: Structure Mechanism and Biochemistry, 3rd Ed. New York: Plenum Press, 2005:377–530.
22. Traber PG, McDonnell WM, Wang R. Expression and regulation of cytochrome P450I genes (CYP1A1 and CYP1A2) in the rat alimentary tract. Biochim Biophys Acta 1992;1171:167–175.
23. Roy D, Bernhardt A, Strobel H, et al. Catalysis of the oxidation of steroid and stilbene estrogens to estrogen quinone metabolites by the β-naphthoflavone–inducible cytochrome CYP1A family. Arch Biochem Biophys 1992;296:450–456.
24. Koop DR. Oxidative and reductive metabolism of cytochrome P4502E1. FASEB J 1992;6:724–730.
25. Raucy JL, Kraner JC, Lasker JM. Bioactivation of halogenated hydrocarbons by cytochrome P4502E1. Crit Rev Toxicol 1993;23:1–20.
26. White RE, Coon MJ. Oxygen activation by cytochrome P450. Ann Rev Biochem 1980;49:315–356.
27. Makris TM, Denisov L, Schlichting L, et al. Activation of molecular oxygen by cytochrome P450 enzymes. In: Ortiz de Montellano PR, ed. Cytochrome P450: Structure Mechanism and Biochemistry, 3rd Ed. New York: Plenum Press, 2005:149–182.
28. Groves JT. Key elements of the chemistry of cytochrome P450. The oxygen rebound mechanism. J Chem Educ 1985;62:928–931.
29. Ortiz de Montellano PR, DeVoss JJ. Substrate oxidation by cytochrome P450 enzymes. In: Ortiz de Montellano PR, ed. Cytochrome P450: Structure Mechanism and Biochemistry, 3rd Ed. New York: Plenum Press, 2005:193–198.
30. Guengerich FP, MacDonald TL. Mechanisms of cytochrome P450 catalysis. FASEB J 1990;4:2453–2459.
31. Ortiz de Montellano PR. Cytochrome P-450 catalysis: radical intermediates and dehydrogenation reactions. Trends Pharmacol Sci 1989;10:354–359.
32. Correia MA, Ortiz de Montellano PR. Inhibition of cytochrome P450 enzymes. In: Ortiz de Montellano PR, ed. Cytochrome P450: Structure Mechanism and Biochemistry, 3rd Ed. New York: Plenum Press, 2005:247–322.
33. Ortiz de Montellano PR. Alkenes and alkynes. In: Anders M, ed. Bioactivation of Foreign Compounds. New York: Academic Press, 1985:121–155.
34. Williams SN, Dunkan E, Bradfield CA. Induction of cytochrome P450 enzymes. In: Ortiz de Montellano PR, ed. Cytochrome P450: Structure Mechanism and Biochemistry, 3rd Ed. New York: Plenum Press, 2005:323–346.
35. Okey AB. Enzyme induction in the cytochrome P450 system. Pharmacol Ther 1990;45:241–298.
36. Barry M, Feely J. Enzyme induction and inhibition. Pharmacol Ther 1992;48:71–94.
37. Guengerich FP. Metabolic activation of carcinogens. Pharmacol Ther 1992;54:17–61.
38. Martucci CP, Fishman J. P450 enzymes of estrogen metabolism. Pharmacol Ther 1993;57:237–257.
39. Conney AH, Pantuck EJ, Kuntzman R, et al. Nutrition and chemical biotransformations in man. Clin Pharmacol Ther 1977;22:707–711.
40. Murray M, Reidy GF. Selectivity in the inhibition of mammalian cytochromes P-450 by chemical agents. Pharmacol Rev 1990;42:85–101.
41. Murray M. P450 enzymes. Clin Pharmacokinet 1992;23:132–146.
42. Ballie TA. Metabolism of valproate to hepatotoxic intermediates. Pharm Weekbl Sci 1992;14:122–125.
43. Thummel KE, Kharasch ED, Podoll T, et al. Human liver microsomal enflurane defluorination catalyzed by cytochrome P-450 2E1. Drug Metab Dispos 1993;21:350–356.
44. Elliot RH, Strunun L. Hepatotoxicity of volatile anesthetics. Br J Anaesth 1993;70:339–348.
45. Zeigler DM. Flavin-containing monooxygenases. Drug Metab Rev 1988;19:1–32.
46. Zeigler DM. Flavin-containing monooxygenases: enzymes adapted for multisubstrate specificity. Trends Pharmacol Sci 1990;11:321–324.
47. Singer TP, Ramsay RR. Mechanism of neurotoxicity of MPTP. FEBS Lett 1990;274:1–8.
48. Krueger SK, Williams DE. Mammalian flavin-containing monooxygenases: structure/function, genetic polymorphisms and role in drug metabolism. Pharmacol Ther 2005;106:357–387.
49. Cashman JR, Wang Z, Yang L, et al. Stereo- and regioselective N- and S-oxidation of tertiary amines and sulfides in the presence of adult liver microsomes. Drug Metab Dispos 1993;21:492–501.
50. Hollenberg PF. Mechanism of cytochrome P450 and peroxide-catalyzed xenobiotic metabolism. FASEB J 1992;6:686–694.
51. Marnett LJ, Kenned TY. Comparison of the peroxidase activity of hemeproteins and cytochrome P450. In: Ortiz de Montellano PR, ed. Cytochrome P450: Structure Mechanism and Biochemistry, 3rd Ed. New York: Plenum Press, 2005:49–80.

52. Hille R. Molybdenum enzymes. Essays Biochem 1999;34:125–137.
53. Kitamura S, Sugihara K, Ohta S. Drug-metabolizing ability of molybdenum hydroxylases. Drug Metab Pharmacokinet 2006;21:83–98.
54. Lang D, Kalgutkar AS. Non-P450 mediated oxidative metabolism of xenobiotics. In: Lee JS, Obach RS, Fisher MB, eds. Drug Metabolizing Enzymes: Cytochrome P450 and Other Enzymes in Drug Discovery and Development. New York: FontisMedia-Marcel Dekker, 2003:483–539.
55. Costa LG, Li WF, Richter RJ, et al. The role of paraoxonase (PON1) in the detoxication of organophosphates and its human polymorphism. Chem Biol Interact 1999;119–120:429–439.
56. Mulder GJ, ed. Conjugation Reactions in Drug Metabolism: An Integrated Approach. New York: Taylor and Francis, 1990.
57. Jansen PLM, Mulder PJ, Burchell B, et al. New developments in glucuronidation research: report of a workshop on "glucuronidation, its role in health and disease." Hepatology 1992;15:532–544.
58. Burchell B, Mcgurk K, Brierly CH, et al. UDP-glucuronosyltransferases. In: Guengerich FP, ed. Comprehensive Toxicology, Vol 3. New York: Pergamon–Elsevier Science, 1997:449–473.
59. Spahn-Langguth H, Benet LZ. Acylglucuronides revisited: is the glucuronidation process a toxification as well as a detoxication mechanism. Drug Metab Rev 1992;24:5–48.
60. Mulder GJ. Pharmacological effects of drug conjugates: is morphine 6-glucuronide an exception. Trends Pharmacol Sci 1992;13:302–304.
61. Falani CN. Enzymology of human cytosolic sulfotransferases. FASEB J 1997;11:206–216.
62. Lindsay J, Wang LL, Li Y, et al. Structure, function and polymorphism of human cytosolic sulfotransferases. Curr Drug Metab 2008;9:99–105.
63. Caldwell J, Hutt AJ, Fournel-Gigleux S. The metabolic chiral inversion and dispositional enantioselectivity of the 2-arylpropionic acids and their biological activity. Biochem Pharmacol 1988;37:105–115.
64. Tracy TS, Wirthwein DP, Hall SD. Metabolic inversion of R-ibuprofen. Drug Metab Dispos 1993;21:114–119.
65. Nelson SD. Arylamines and arylamide: oxidation mechanisms. In: Anders M, ed. Bioactivation of Foreign Compounds. New York: Academic Press, 1985:349–375.
66. Ahmed AE. Nitriles. In: Anders M, ed. Bioactivation of Foreign Compounds. New York: Academic Press, 1985:485–489.
67. Dobrinska MR. Enterohepatic circulation of drugs. J Clin Pharmacol 1989;29:577–580.
68. Ilett KF, Tee LBG, Reeves PT, et al. Metabolism of drugs and other xenobiotics in the gut lumen and wall. Pharmacol Ther 1990;46:67–93.
69. Schmucker DL. Aging and drug disposition: an update. Pharmacol Rev 1985;37:133–145.
70. Durnas C, Loi CM, Cusack BJ. Hepatic drug metabolism and aging. Clin Pharmacokinet 1990;19:359–389.
71. Woodhouse K, Wynne HA. Age-related changes in hepatic function: implications for drug therapy. Drugs Aging 1992;2:243–246.
72. Smit JW, Huisman MT, van Tellingen O, et al. Absence or pharmacological blocking of placental P-glycoprotein profoundly increases fetal drug exposure. J Clin Invest 1999;104:1441–1447.
73. Ingelmann-Sundberg M, Oscarson M, McLellan RA. Polymorphic human cytochrome P450 enzymes: an opportunity for individualized drug treatment. Trends Pharmacol Sci 1999;20:342–349.
74. Di YM, Chow VD, Yang LP, et al. Structure, function, regulation and polymorphism of human cytochrome CYP2A6. Curr Drug Metab 2009;10:754–780.
75. Mo SL, Liu YH, Duan W, et al. Substrate specificity, regulation, and polymorphism of human cytochrome CYP2B6. Curr Drug Metab 2009;10:730–753.
76. Zhou SF, Zhou ZW, Huang M. Polymorphisms of human cytochrome CYP2C9 and the functional relevance. Toxicology 2010;278:165–188.
77. Kaminsky LS, Fasco MJ. Small intestinal cytochromes P450. Crit Rev Toxicol 1991;21:407–422.
78. Kane GC, Lipsky JJ. Drug–grapefruit juice interactions. Mayo Clin Proc 2000;75:933–942.
79. Yu Dk. The contribution of P-glycoprotein to the pharmacokinetics of drug–drug interactions. J Clin Pharmacol 1999;39:1203–1211.
80. Silverman JA. Multidrug resistance transporters. Pharm Biotechnol 1999;12:353–386.
81. Oesch F. Metabolic transformation of clinically used drugs to epoxides: new perspectives in drug–drug interactions. Biochem Pharmacol 1976;25:1935–1937.
82. Ohnishi A, Matsuo H, Yamada S, et al. Effect of furanocoumarin derivatives in grapefruit juice on the uptake of vinblastine by Caco-2 cells and on the activity of cytochrome CYP3A4. Br J Pharmacol 2000;130:1369–1377.
83. Watkins PB. Role of cytochrome P450 in drug metabolism and hepatotoxicity. Semin Liver Dis 1990;10:235–250.
84. Roth RA, Vinegar A. Action by the lungs on circulating xenobiotic agents, with a case study of physiologically based pharmacokinetic modeling of benzo[a]pyrene disposition. Pharmacol Ther 1990;48:143–155.
85. Reed CJ. Drug metabolism in the nasal cavity. Drug Metab Rev 1993;25:173–205.
86. Sarkar MA. Drug metabolism in the nasal mucosa. Pharmacol Res 1992;9:1–8.
87. Testa B, Jenner P, eds. Drug Metabolism: Chemical and Biological Aspects. New York: Marcel Dekker, 1976.
88. Lee WM. Drug-induced hepatotoxicity. N Engl J Med 2003;349:474–485.
89. Navarro VJ, Senior JR. Drug-related hepatotoxicity. N Engl J Med 2006;354:731–739.
90. Watkins PB, Kaplowitz N, Slattery JT, et al. Aminotransferase elevations in healthy adults receiving 4 grams of acetaminophen daily. JAMA 2006;296:87–93.
91. Park BK, Kitteringham NR, Maggs JL, et al. The role of metabolic activation in drug-induced hepatotoxicity. Annu Rev Pharmacol Toxicol 2005;45:177–202.
92. Williams DP, Kitteringham NR, Naisbitt DJ, et al. Are chemically reactive metabolites responsible for adverse reactions to drugs? Curr Drug Metab 2002;3:351–366.
93. Kalgutkar AS, Gardner I, Obach RS, et al. A comprehensive listing of bioactivation pathways of organic functional groups. Curr Drug Metab 2005;6:161–225.
94. Myers TG, Dietz EC, Anderson N, et al. A comparative study of mouse liver proteins arylated by reactive metabolites of acetaminophen and its nonhepatotoxic regioisomer, 3'-hydroxyacetanilide. Chem Res Toxicol 1995;8:403–413.
95. Holt MP, Ju C. Mechanisms of drug-induced liver injury. AAPS J 2006;8:E48–E54.
96. Ju C, Uetrecht JP. Mechanism of idiosyncratic drug reactions: reactive metabolite formation, protein binding and the regulation of the immune system. Curr Drug Metab 2002;3:367–377.
97. Miller EC, Miller JA. Mechanisms of chemical carcinogenesis. Cancer 1981;47:1055–1064.
98. Gillette JR. The problem of chemically reactive metabolites. Drug Metab Rev 1982;13:941–961.
99. Reed DJ. Cellular defense mechanisms against reactive metabolites. In: Anders M, ed. Bioactivation of Foreign Compounds. New York: Academic Press, 1985:71–108.
100. Nelson SD, et al. Role of metabolic activation in chemical-induced tissue injury. In: Jerina DM, ed. Drug Metabolism Concepts. ACS Symposium Series 44. Washington, DC: American Chemical Society, 1977:155–185.
101. Uetrecht J. Bioactivation. In: Lee JS, Obach RS, Fisher M, eds. Drug-Metabolizing Enzymes: Cytochrome P450 and Other Enzymes in Drug Discovery and Development. Weimar, TX: Culinary and Hospitality Industry Publications Services, 2003:87–145.
102. Boelsterli UA. Xenobiotic acyl glucuronides and acyl CoA thioesters as protein-reactive metabolites with the potential to cause idiosyncratic drug reactions. Curr Drug Metab 2002;3:439–450.
103. Zhou S, Yung Chan S, Cher Goh B, et al. Mechanism-based inhibition of cytochrome CYP3A4 by therapeutic drugs. Clin Pharmacokinet 2005;44:279–304.
104. Dressor GK, Spence JD, Bailey DG. Pharmacokinetic–pharmacodynamic consequences and clinical relevance of cytochrome CYP3A4 inhibition. Clin Pharmacokinet 2000;38:41–57.
105. Murray M. Mechanisms of inhibitory and regulatory effects of methylenedioxyphenyl compounds on cytochrome P450-dependent drug oxidation. Curr Drug Metab 2000;1:67–84.
106. Bailey DG, Dresser GK, Kreeft JH, et al. Grapefruit–felodipine interaction: effect of unprocessed fruit and probable active ingredients. Clin Pharmacol Ther 2000;68:468–477.
107. Evans AM. Influence of dietary components on the gastrointestinal metabolism and transport of drugs. Ther Drug Monit 2000;22:131–136.
108. Johnson BM, Van Breemen RB. In vitro formation of quinoid metabolites of the dietary supplement cimicifuga racemosa (black cohosh). Chem Res Toxicol 2003;16:838–846.
109. Saller R, Meier R, Brignoli R. The use of silymarin in the treatment of liver diseases. Drugs 2001;61:2035–2063.

Suggested Readings

Anders M, ed. Bioactivation of Foreign Compounds. New York: Academic Press, 1985.

Caldwell J, Jakoby W, eds. Biological Basis of Detoxication. New York: Academic Press, 1983.

Jakoby W, ed. Enzymatic Basis of Detoxication, Vols I and II. New York: Academic Press, 1980.

Jakoby W, Bend JR, Caldwell J, eds. Metabolic Basis of Detoxication—Metabolism of Functional Groups. New York: Academic Press, 1982.

Lee JS, Obach RS, Fisher M, eds. Drug-Metabolizing Enzymes: Cytochrome P450 and Other Enzymes in Drug Discovery and Development. Weimer, TX: Culinary and Hospitality Industry Publications Services, 2003.

Mulder GJ, ed. Conjugation Reactions in Drug Metabolism: An Integrated Approach. London: Taylor and Francis, 1990.

Ortiz de Montellano PR, ed. Cytochrome P450: Structure Mechanism and Biochemistry, 3rd Ed. New York: Plenum Press, 2005.

Testa B, Jenner P, eds. Concepts in Drug Metabolism. New York: Marcel Dekker, 1981.

Testa B, Jenner P, eds. Drug Metabolism: Chemical and Biochemical Aspects. New York: Marcel Dekker, 1976.

Williams RT, ed. Detoxication Mechanisms, 2nd Ed. New York: John Wiley and Sons, 1959.

Wolf TF, ed. Handbook of Drug Metabolism. New York: Marcel Dekker, 1999.

Chapter
5

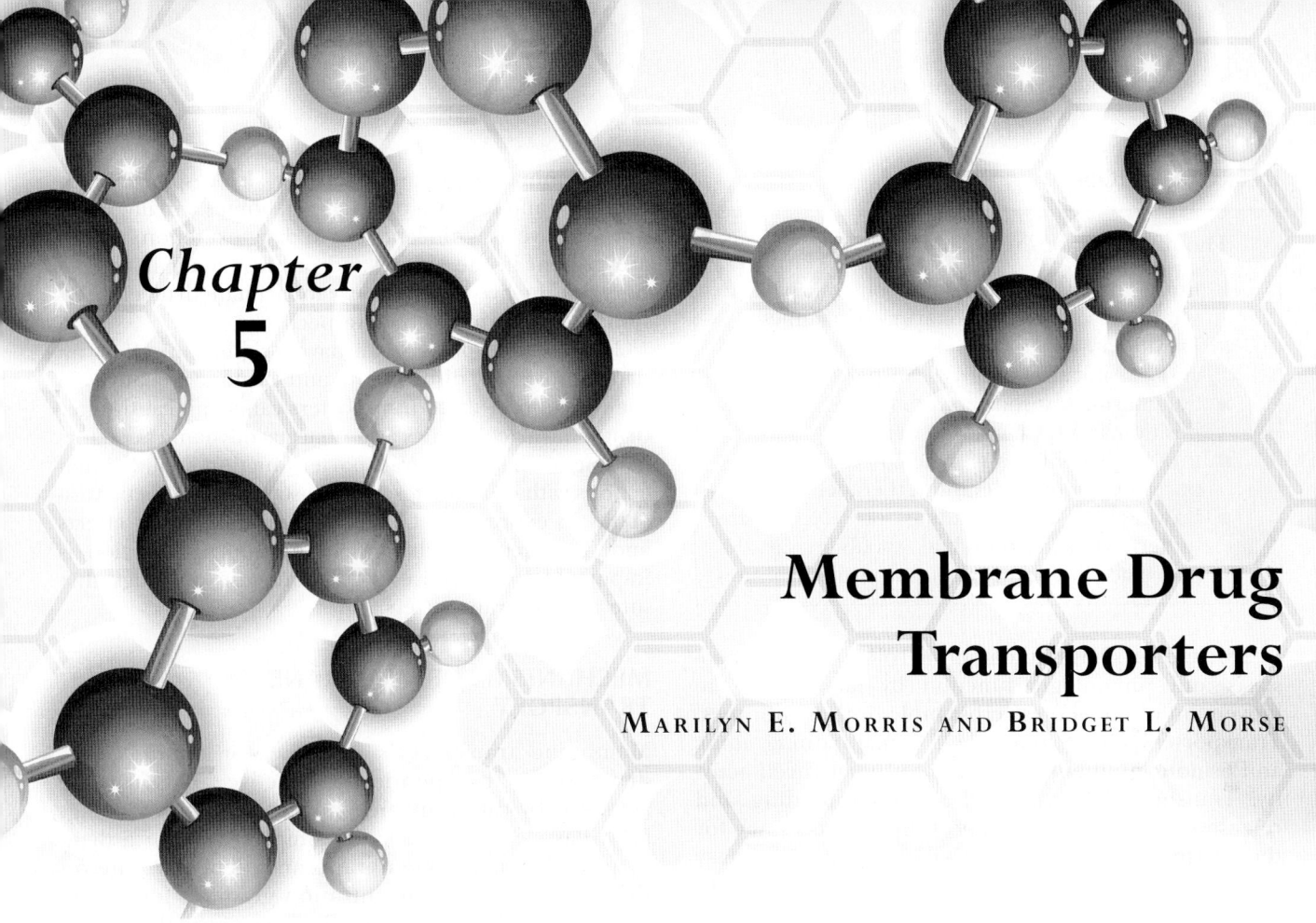

Membrane Drug Transporters

MARILYN E. MORRIS AND BRIDGET L. MORSE

Drugs Covered in This Chapter

- Acyclovir
- Adefovir
- Atorvastatin
- Cerivastatin
- Cidofovir
- Cisplatin
- Cyclosporine
- Digoxin
- Doxorubicin
- Fexofenadine
- Furosemide
- Gabapentin
- Gabapentin enacarbil
- Gemfibrozil
- Lamivudine
- Methotrexate
- Nitrofurantoin
- Olmesartan
- Oxaliplatin
- Paclitaxel
- Penicillin
- Pravastatin
- Probenecid
- Repaglinide
- Rifampin
- Rosuvastatin
- Simvastatin
- Tenofovir
- Topotecan
- Valacyclovir
- Valsartan

Abbreviations

ABC, ATP-binding cassette
ACE, angiotensin-converting enzyme
ATP, adenosine triphosphate
AUC, area under the curve
BBB, blood–brain barrier
BCRP, breast cancer resistance protein
BSEP, bile salt export pump
CNT, concentrative nucleoside transporter
ENT, equilibrative nucleoside transporter
FXR, farnesoid X receptor
GI, gastrointestinal
GHB, γ-hydroxybutyrate
HMG-CoA, 3-hydroxy-3-methyl-glutaryl–coenzyme A
LAT, L-type amino acid transporter
MATE, multidrug and toxin extrusion transporter
MCT, monocarboxylate transporter
MDR, multidrug resistance
MRP, multidrug resistance–associated protein
OAT, organic anion transporter
OATP, organic anion transporting polypeptide
OCT, organic cation transporter
OCTN, organic cation/carnitine transporter
P-gp, P-glycoprotein
PEPT, peptide transporter
PHT, peptide/histidine transporter
PXR, pregnane X receptor
SLC, solute carrier
SMCT, sodium-coupled monocarboxylate transporter
SNP, single nucleotide polymorphism

INTRODUCTION

The objectives of the chapter are:

- Emphasize the significance of transport in pharmacokinetics and pharmacodynamics
- Provide an overview of transport mechanisms and classification of drug transporters
- Summarize transporters relevant to drug disposition and their relevant drug substrates
- Provide evidence and mechanisms for transport interactions relevant to therapeutics
- Provide an understanding of mechanisms underlying interindividual variability in the pharmacokinetics of drug transporter substrates

Transporters have fundamental roles in cell homeostasis and physiologic function by facilitating the movement of molecules across biological membranes. Transporters are responsible for maintaining ionic and osmotic gradients necessary for normal cell activity. Transporters facilitate the oxygen binding and release in red blood cells, and they are necessary for the transport of nutrients to vital organs. The primary function of transporters is to transport endogenous substances, such as hormones, glucose, and amino acids; however, many of these transporters also transport xenobiotics. It is these drug transporters that are of importance when considering drug disposition and drug response.

Drug transporters are localized to barrier membranes of the body responsible for xenobiotic entry and exit. They are expressed in organs of absorption, such as the intestine, and clearance organs including the liver and kidney. Transporters are also expressed on membranes that separate particularly susceptible organs from the rest of the body, including the blood–brain and blood–placenta barriers, where they facilitate the influx of nutrients and efflux of potentially harmful xenobiotics. Because of their location on barrier membranes, transporters have an important role in drug pharmacokinetics and pharmacodynamics. Transporters can have a role in drug absorption and can facilitate or prevent drug entry into the body. Also, transporters have a role in drug distribution, as they facilitate the movement of drugs between the blood and peripheral tissues. The role of transporters in drug distribution can also affect drug response by allowing or preventing drug access to the site of action. One of the most interesting roles of drug transporters is their indirect effects on drug metabolism. Transporters can restrict or allow a drug's distribution into organs that contain drug-metabolizing enzymes, particularly the liver and the intestine. In this regard, there can be extensive transport-metabolism interplay, and transport or metabolism can be the rate-limiting process controlling drug elimination. Transporters are also responsible for transport and removal of drug metabolites. Finally, transporters have a significant role in drug excretion, as they are present in the kidney and on the canalicular membrane of the liver where they can facilitate drug elimination into the urine or bile, respectively.

Because transporters can have a significant effect on drug absorption, distribution, and clearance, changes in the function of these transporters can significantly alter drug pharmacokinetics and pharmacodynamics. Factors leading to changes in transporter function include interactions with other drugs, disease states, and genetic variability in expression. Understanding transporter effects and the effects of changes in transporter function is important for effective therapeutic use of drugs that interact with transporters.

MECHANISMS OF MEMBRANE TRANSPORT

Membrane transport is essential for almost every drug to be therapeutically effective. This can be achieved by different mechanisms of transport (Fig. 5.1). Passive diffusion is the simplest way for a drug to pass through a membrane and depends only on the existence of a concentration gradient for a molecule across the membrane. Because of the lipophilicity of biologic membranes, diffusion is energetically unfavorable for drugs that are relatively hydrophilic, particularly for drugs that are predominantly ionized at physiologic pH, and these molecules require facilitated transport. Facilitated transport refers to any transport aided by a facilitating protein. Similar

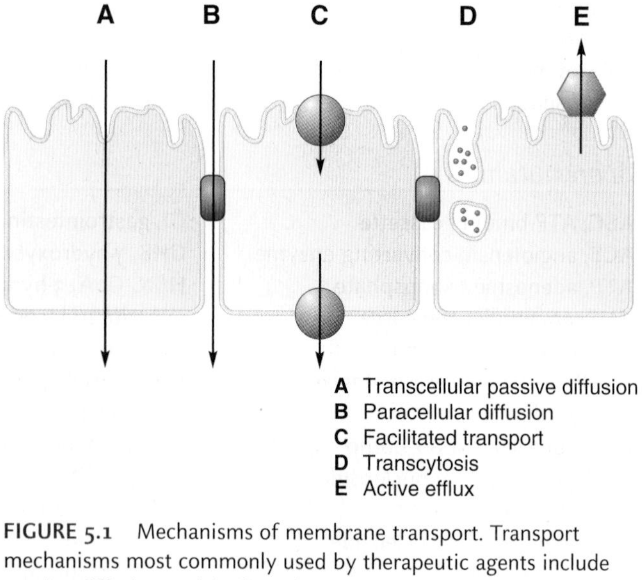

FIGURE 5.1 Mechanisms of membrane transport. Transport mechanisms most commonly used by therapeutic agents include passive diffusion and facilitated transport.

to diffusion, passive facilitated transport depends only on the existence of a concentration gradient and involves movement of molecules down this gradient. Active transport uses a separate energy source to move molecules against their concentration gradient. Drug transporters can use either passive or active transport mechanisms. Paracellular transport (transfer of substances between cells of an epithelial cell layer) and transcytosis (vesicular transfer of substances across the interior of a cell) are less commonly used mechanisms of membrane transport. Mannitol can pass through membranes via paracellular transport and can be used as a probe for this type of transport. Transcytosis is often receptor mediated and is a mechanism of transport for endogenous substances such as insulin and transferrin.

Molecules can use one or more of these mechanisms to cross biological membranes. Transporter substrates can be lipophilic and also capable of passive diffusion; therefore, drug transport can often be described with the following equation:

$$J = \frac{V_{max} \times C}{K_m + C} + P \times C$$

where J is the rate of total drug transport, V_{max} is the maximum rate of the saturable transporter system, K_m reflects the affinity of a drug substrate for the transporter system, P is the rate of nonsaturable transport or passive diffusion, and C is the drug concentration. The importance of a transporter depends on to what extent transporter-mediated transport (V_{max}/K_m) is responsible for membrane passage of a drug compared to other mechanisms like passive diffusion (P). Transporter-mediated transport becomes particularly important when the need is present to move a molecule against its concentration gradient, as this type of transport can only be achieved by active transporters and P due to passive diffusion is negligible.

When considering drug transport, it is important to consider the polarization of biological membranes, in that different membranes can have different properties relating to their function as a barrier, including the expression of different transporters. The membrane facing the systemic circulation is referred to as the basolateral membrane, or the sinusoidal membrane in the liver. The membrane facing the exterior, such as the gut lumen, is referred to as the apical membrane. The apical membrane is also called the brush border membrane in the kidney or intestine and the canalicular membrane in the liver. Transport is actually a two-step process in which molecules must be transported across the apical then basolateral membrane or vice versa. Drug transport is a concerted action between transporters expressed on both membranes.

CLASSIFICATION OF TRANSPORTERS

Facilitative Versus Active Transporters

Although all transporters are facilitating proteins, the terms facilitative and active transporters refer to transporters that transport substrates down and against their concentration gradients, respectively. Transporters that are classified as facilitative transporters only move molecules down their concentration gradient, without the use of a separate energy source. The transporters of this type should not be confused with channels. Channels also facilitate the movement of ions and hydrophilic molecules across membranes and down their concentration gradient; however, channels control transport or flow of substrates by gating mechanisms, whereas transporters bind to their substrates and undergo a conformational change to transport the substrate across a membrane.

Primary Versus Secondary Active Transporters

Most drug transporters are active transporters that use an energy source other than the drug's concentration gradient to transport substrates across membranes from a region of lower concentration to a region of higher concentration (i.e., against its concentration gradient). Active transporters are further classified as primary or secondary active transporters. Primary active transporters most commonly use adenosine triphosphate (ATP) as an energy source for substrate transport. Secondary active transporters use the concentration gradient of another substance, such as protons or sodium ions, but also other ionic endogenous substances as energy sources to drive transport. The concentration gradients that drive secondary active transport are generally created by primary active transporters; an example of interplay between the two types of transporters is depicted in Figure 5.2. As shown, primary active transport by the Na^+/K^+ ATPase results in a concentration gradient of Na^+ ions. This concentration gradient drives secondary active transport by the Na^+/H^+ exchanger, and the resulting proton gradient drives transport of the drug substrate against its concentration gradient. The Na^+/K^+ ATPase and Na^+/H^+ exchanger do not transport drug substrate, but are involved in drug transport by producing the sodium and proton gradients used as driving forces. Molecules used to drive secondary active transport are also substrates for the secondary active transporter and are simultaneously transported across the membrane. This simultaneous transport may be in the same direction, referred to as *symport,* or in opposite directions, referred to as *antiport.*

Influx Versus Efflux Transporters

Influx transporters transport substrates from extracellular spaces into cells. Efflux transporters transport

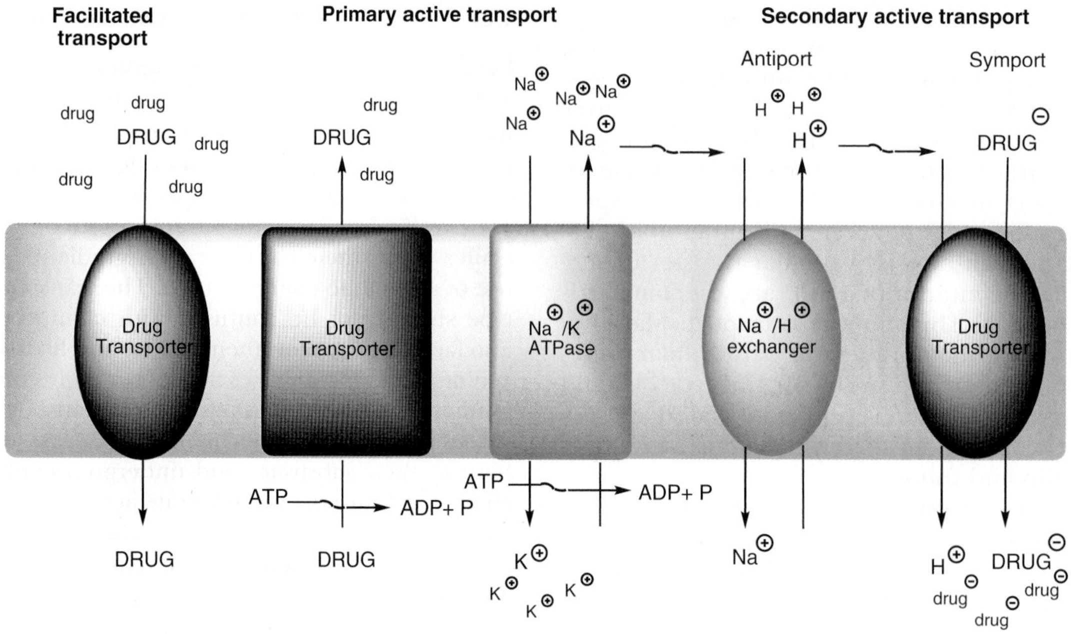

FIGURE 5.2 Types of drug transporters. Primary active transporters use ATP and have the ability to transport substrates against their concentration gradient. Secondary active transporters used gradients created by primary active transport to transport drug substrates. Facilitated transporters only transport substrates down their concentration gradient. Transporters that transport drug substrates are shown in *red,* whereas those shown in *gray* provide driving forces for drug transport.

substrates out of cells. Transporters are usually responsible for either drug influx or drug efflux, but in some cases facilitate both types of transport.

Secretory Versus Absorptive Transporters

Secretory transporters facilitate drug clearance and are responsible for transport of drugs from the blood, such as excretion into the urine. Absorptive transporters allow a drug access into the blood, such as those facilitating absorption in the gut or reabsorption in the kidney. A transporter can be both secretory and absorptive depending on its physiologic locations. The same transporter is often expressed at both the site responsible for drug absorption and that responsible for drug clearance; hence, the transporter would serve both secretory and absorptive functions. When considering transport across membranes of the brain and placenta, the terms secretion and absorption are applied differently. With respect to these sites, absorptive transporters allow access into the sites and out of the circulation, and secretory transporters efflux drugs out of these sites and back into the blood circulation.

ABC Versus SLC Transporters

Drug transporters have been classified into two families, namely the ABC (ATP-binding cassette) and SLC (solute carrier) families. Members of the ABC family are primary active transporters that use ATP as an energy source. Most SLC transporters are secondary active transporters, using the concentration gradients of several different molecules as a driving force for transport. The SLC family also includes a handful of facilitative transporters. Many members of each family have a role in drug disposition, and these transporters are summarized in Table 5.1.

ABC Transporters

ABC transporters are efflux transporters, many of which are located on the apical side of biological membranes, facilitating drug secretion. ABC transporters are primary active transporters and use ATP as an energy source. The widespread physiologic expression of ABC transporters and their extensive range of substrates make it inevitable for these transporters to have effects on drug pharmacokinetics and elicit clinically significant drug interactions. Substrates and inhibitors for ABC transporters are given in Table 5.2.

Multidrug Resistance (MDR) Proteins *(ABCB)*

MDR1 (ABCB1) MDR1, more commonly known as P-glycoprotein (P-gp), is the most extensively researched of all the transporters. The structure of P-gp consists of two homologous halves each with six transmembrane-spanning domains and one ATP binding site (Fig. 5.3). Transport by P-gp has been discovered to be notably complicated, with at least two binding sites and three different proposed mechanisms by which it transports substrates (1).

TABLE 5.1 Drug Transporters

Transporter Family	Family Member	Gene Name	Location	Role in Drug Disposition
MDR	MDR1	*ABCB1*	Intestine, liver, kidneys, brain, heart, placenta	• Role in oral absorption, biliary clearance, renal secretion, and drug penetration of blood–brain barrier • Drug–drug interactions • Relevant polymorphisms • Role in multidrug resistance
MRP	MRP1	*ABCC1*	Liver, intestine, brain	• Role in multidrug resistance • Facilitates basolateral drug efflux
	MRP2	*ABCC2*	Intestine, liver, kidney	• Role in oral absorption, biliary clearance, and renal secretion of drugs and drug conjugates
	MRP3	*ABCC3*	Liver, brain	• Facilitates sinusoidal efflux of drugs and drug conjugates
	MRP4	*ABCC4*	Kidney, liver, brain	• Facilitates renal secretion and sinusoidal efflux of drugs and drug conjugates
BCRP	BCRP1	*ABCG2*	Intestine, liver, kidney, brain, heart, placenta	• Role in oral absorption, biliary secretion, and drug penetration of blood–brain barrier • Drug–drug interactions • Relevant polymorphisms • Role in multidrug resistance
OCT	OCT1	*SLC22A1*	Liver	• Facilitates sinusoidal uptake • Drug–drug interactions • Relevant polymorphisms
	OCT2	*SLC22A2*	Kidney	• Facilitates renal secretion • Drug–drug interactions • Relevant polymorphisms
OCTN	OCTN1	*SLC22A4*	Kidney, intestine	• Role in oral absorption and renal secretion
	OCTN2	*SLC22A5*	Kidney, intestine	• Role in oral absorption and renal secretion
OAT	OAT1	*SLC22A6*	Kidney	• Facilitates renal secretion • Drug–drug interactions
	OAT2	*SLC22A7*	Liver	• Facilitates sinusoidal uptake
	OAT3	*SLC22A8*	Kidney	• Facilitates renal secretion • Drug–drug interactions
	OAT4	*SLC22A11*	Kidney	• Facilitates renal reabsorption
OATP	OATP1A2	*SLCO1A2*	Brain, intestine	• Role in oral absorption and brain uptake
	OATP1B1	*SLCO1B1*	Liver	• Facilitates sinusoidal uptake • Drug–drug interactions • Relevant polymorphisms
	OATP1B3	*SLCO1B3*	Liver	• Facilitates sinusoidal uptake • Relevant polymorphisms
	OATP2A1	*SLCO2A1*	Intestine, liver	• Role in oral absorption and sinusoidal uptake
	OATP2B1	*SLCO2B1*	Intestine, liver	• Role in oral absorption and sinusoidal uptake
	OATP4C1	*SLCO4C1*	Kidney	• Facilitates renal secretion
MATE	MATE1	*SLC47A1*	Kidney, liver	• Role in renal and biliary secretion • Drug–drug interactions
	MATE2-K	*SLC47A2*	Kidney	• Facilitates renal secretion
MCT	MCT1	*SLC16A7*	Ubiquitous	• Role in oral absorption and renal reabsorption • Overexpression in tumor cells
PEPT	PEPT1	*SLC15A1*	Intestine, kidney	• Facilitates oral absorption • Drug–drug interactions
	PEPT2	*SLC15A2*	Kidney	• Facilitates renal reabsorption
CNT	CNT1	*SLC28A1*	Intestine, kidney, liver	• Role in absorption and disposition of nucleoside analogs
	CNT2	*SLC28A2*	Intestine, Kidney, liver	• Role in absorption and disposition of nucleoside analogs
	CNT3	*SLC28A3*	Kidney, brain, placenta	• Role in distribution and renal reabsorption of nucleoside analogs
ENT	ENT1	*SLC29A1*	Ubiquitous	• Role in absorption and disposition of nucleoside analogs
	ENT2	*SLC29A2*	Ubiquitous	• Role in absorption and disposition of nucleoside analogs

TABLE 5.2 Relevant Drug Substrates and Inhibitors of ABC Transporters

Transporter	Substrates	Inhibitors
MDR1	Amphotericin B, cyclosporine, daunorubicin, dexamethasone, digoxin, diltiazem, docetaxel, doxorubicin, erythromycin, etoposide, fexofenadine, hydrocortisone, ketoconazole, methadone, mitoxantrone, morphine, paclitaxel, phenytoin, rifampin, ritonavir, saquinavir, tacrolimus, verapamil, vinblastine, vincristine	Clarithromycin, cyclosporine, elacridar, quinidine, verapamil
MRP2	Ampicillin, ceftriaxone, cisplatin, daunomycin, doxorubicin, etoposide, fluorouracil, glucuronide conjugates, glutathione conjugates, irinotecan, methotrexate, mitoxantrone, olmesartan, pravastatin, ritonavir, rosuvastatin, saquinavir, SN-38-glucuronide, valsartan, vinblastine, vincristine	Cyclosporine, probenecid, efavirenz, emtricitabine
MRP3	Fexofenadine, glucuronide conjugates, methotrexate	Efavirenz, emtricitabine
MRP4	Adefovir, furosemide, methotrexate, tenofovir, topotecan	Diclofenac
BCRP	Ciprofloxacin, imatinib, irinotecan, methotrexate, mitoxantrone, nitrofurantoin, rosuvastatin, sorafenib, topotecan	Elacridar

P-gp is expressed in most tissues and is involved in drug transport in the intestine, liver, kidney, brain, and placenta, and in tumor cells. This is one reason P-gp has been and remains a transporter of clinical interest. The ability of P-gp to transport a wide range of substrates is another remarkable feature. These substrates span many therapeutic areas and drug classes, making it difficult to determine the structure–activity relationship for P-gp–mediated transport. Digoxin serves as a probe for P-gp in both in vitro and in vivo studies (2). Other substrates include many chemotherapeutic drugs and HIV protease inhibitors. One common feature of P-gp substrates is that they are generally lipophilic, commonly containing aromatic rings (Fig. 5.4). The relative lipophilicity of these substrates implies that most P-gp substrates are also capable of passive diffusion. This means that P-gp transport must be efficient to have an effect on the passage of its substrates across membranes, and P-gp transport does not always result in clinically relevant effects. P-gp substrates are rarely specific and are also often substrates of other transporters and drug-metabolizing enzymes, particularly CYP3A4, making it difficult to attribute in vivo pharmacokinetic effects or interactions entirely to P-gp alone. Intestinal efflux by P-gp has been demonstrated to contribute to the low bioavailability of many compounds (3). Significant drug interactions have also been demonstrated to involve P-gp in the intestine, as well as in the kidneys (4,5). P-gp is also likely important in pregnancy in that it protects the fetus from xenobiotics by effluxing them back into the maternal blood circulation (6). In addition, as the original name "multidrug resistance protein" (MDR) implies, P-gp is also recognized as an important factor for chemotherapeutic drug resistance due to its overexpression in tumor cells, and P-gp inhibitors have recently gained interest as concurrent treatment with chemotherapy (7).

Multidrug Resistance–Associated Proteins *(ABCC)*

MRP2 (ABCC2) Multidrug resistance–associated protein 2 (MRP2) is primarily localized to three apical membrane barriers, the liver canalicular membrane, the brush border membrane in the kidney, and the

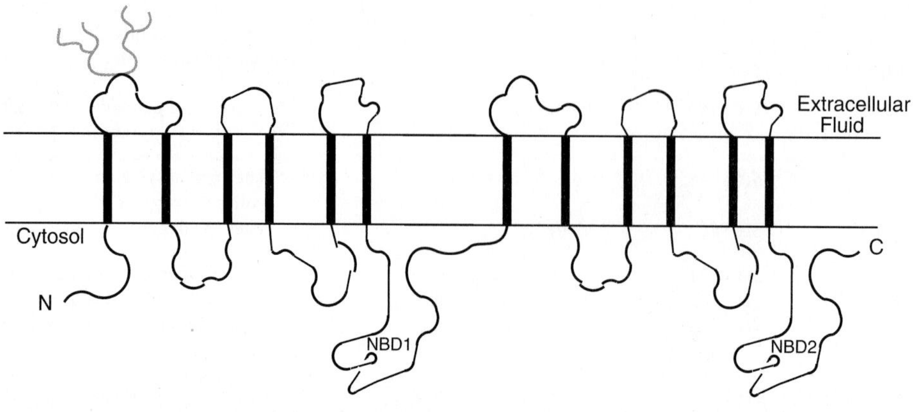

FIGURE 5.3 Structure of P-glycoprotein including 12 transmembrane-spanning domains and 2 nucleotide-binding domains (NBDs).

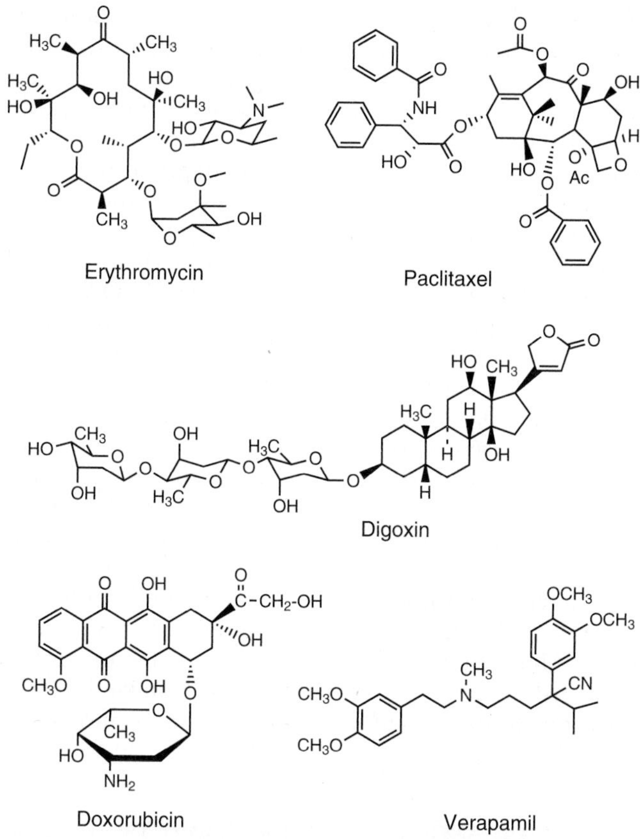

FIGURE 5.4 Examples of P-gp substrates.

apical membrane of the gut, where it serves to excrete substrates into the bile, urine, and back into the gut lumen, respectively. The major substrates of MRP2 are conjugates, including glucuronide, glutathione, and sulfate conjugates, and the primary function of MRP2 is the secretion of bile acid conjugates across the canalicular membrane into the bile. MRP2 substrates also include phase 2 drug metabolites and many unconjugated therapeutic drugs including vinca alkaloids. Glutathione symport is often required for transport of unconjugated substances (8). MRP2 can contribute to the renal secretion of some drug substrates; however, the main role of MRP2 in drug disposition appears to be hepatobiliary transport (1,9). Due to transport of drug conjugates, MRP2 has an important role in enterohepatic cycling. MRP2 transports conjugates into the bile, which empties into the gut lumen. Bacteria in the gut metabolize the conjugate back to the parent drug, which can then be reabsorbed back into the systemic blood circulation. In this way, MRP2 can be responsible for maintaining plasma concentrations of drugs that are not substrates, due to transport of their conjugated metabolites. P-gp is also expressed on the canalicular membrane, although it does not appear to have a role in biliary secretion of drug conjugates.

Other MRPs

In contrast to the apical expression of MRP2, MRPs 1, 3, 4, 5, and 6 are basolateral efflux transporters. MRP1 is another ABC transporter that can be overexpressed in cancer cells, resulting in resistance to chemotherapy (8). MRP3 has an important role in the transport of conjugated drug metabolites in the liver, particularly glucuronide conjugates. Located on the sinusoidal membrane, MRP3 serves to efflux metabolites out of hepatocytes into the plasma, resulting in conjugate excretion into the urine. MRP3 also transports conjugated bile acids and can be induced in cholestatic conditions (10). This also occurs with MRP4, which is located on the sinusoidal membrane as well. MRP4 is also expressed on the brush border membrane of the kidney and has a role in anionic drug secretion into the urine (9).

Breast Cancer Resistance Protein

BCRP (ABCG2) Breast cancer resistance protein (BCRP) is actually a "half" transporter, in that it consists of only six transmembrane-spanning domains and one ATP binding site (Fig. 5.5). Like P-gp, BCRP expression is widespread. Its highest expression is in the placenta, and it is present in the intestine, liver, kidney, brain, heart, and ovaries (11). As its name implies, BCRP has also been attributed with causing chemotherapeutic drug resistance due to overexpression in tumor cells, and among its substrates are several chemotherapeutic agents. BCRP shares many substrates with P-gp and is commonly localized with P-gp, making it difficult to attribute drug transport or inhibition to BCRP. However, the use of BCRP inhibitors and knockout animals has demonstrated the importance of BCRP in drug disposition. Significant effects of BCRP transport have been demonstrated with drug absorption, with biliary clearance, and interestingly on drug transport in the mammary gland, mediating the transport of some drugs into breast milk (12–14). BCRP has a similar role to P-gp in pregnancy, as it is highly expressed at the

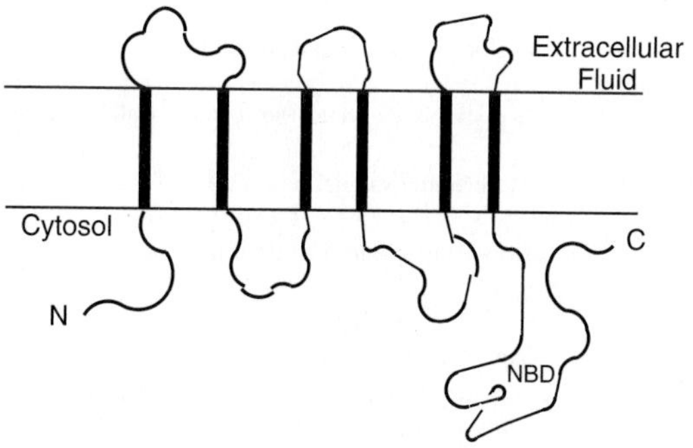

FIGURE 5.5 Structure of BCRP. BCRP is regarded as a half transporter due to its structure including only six transmembrane-spanning domains and one nucleotide-binding domain (NBD).

blood–placenta barrier, where it also serves a protective function to efflux potentially harmful xenobiotics (6).

SLC Transporters

Members of the SLC transporter family are secondary active transporters and, as such, use the concentration gradients of many other substances to transport drug substrates. The concentration gradients of these other substances generally facilitate drug influx, although in some physiologic locations, they can facilitate efflux, and some transporters can be capable of transport in both directions. Like the ABC transporters, SLC transporters are physiologically expressed throughout the body. They transport many different xenobiotics along with many endogenous substances, leading to effects on drug disposition and drug interactions. Substrates and inhibitors of SLC transporters are given in Table 5.3.

Organic Anion Transporting Polypeptides *(SLCO)*

OATP1B1 (SLCO1B1) This transporter is one of the most clinically relevant transporters in that its substrates include drugs such as the 3-hydroxy-3-methylglutaryl–coenzyme A (HMG-CoA) reductase inhibitors, or statins, which are widely prescribed. This transporter is localized specifically on the sinusoidal membrane of the liver, where it serves to influx substrates into hepatocytes, where they can be metabolized or transported into bile. Organic anion transporter polypeptide (OATP) 1B1 and other OATPs are antiporters, using the high intracellular concentration of glutathione as a driving force. Although the name implies anion transport, OATPs are also capable of transporting cationic and neutral compounds, with OATP1B1 displaying the broadest substrate specificity overall. OATP1B1 transports many endogenous substrates including bilirubin and estrogen conjugates. Common drug substrates of OATP1B1 and other OATPs are given in Figure 5.6. Inhibitors of this transporter are also commonly used in the clinic for similar or concomitant disease states and include drugs like gemfibrozil. Rifampin functions as an inhibitor as well as being a substrate. This transporter has also gained attention due to the recognition that it is highly polymorphic, with a large number of single nucleotide polymorphisms (SNPs) having been identified in the *SLCO1B1* gene. Many of these SNPs have been demonstrated to translate into decreased hepatic uptake in vivo, resulting in decreased clearance of statins and other OATP1B1 substrates (15).

TABLE 5.3 Relevant Drug Substrates and Inhibitors of SLC Transporters

Transporter	Substrates	Inhibitors
OATP1B1	Atorvastatin, bosentan, caspofungin, cerivastatin, enalapril, fexofenadine, fluvastatin, methotrexate, olmesartan, pravastatin, repaglinide, rifampin, rosuvastatin, simvastatin, SN-38, valsartan	Atorvastatin, clarithromycin, cyclosporine, erythromycin, gemfibrozil, paclitaxel, rifampin, ritonavir, saquinavir, tacrolimus, telmisartan
OATP1B3	Digoxin, docetaxel, fexofenadine, olmesartan, paclitaxel, rifampin	Clarithromycin, cyclosporine, erythromycin, rifampin, ritonavir
OATP1A2	Digoxin, erythromycin, fexofenadine, imatinib, levofloxacin, methotrexate, pitavastatin, rocuronium, rosuvastatin, saquinavir	Grapefruit juice, rifampin, ritonavir, saquinavir, verapamil
OATP2B1	Atorvastatin, bosentan, fexofenadine, pravastatin, rosuvastatin	Cyclosporine, gemfibrozil, rifampin
OAT1	Acyclovir, adefovir, cidofovir, ciprofloxacin, lamivudine, methotrexate, penicillins, tenofovir, zidovudine	Probenecid
OAT3	Bumetanide, cefaclor, ceftizoxime, furosemide, NSAIDs, penicillins	Probenecid
OCT1	Metformin, lamivudine, oxaliplatin	Disopyramide, quinidine
OCT2	Cisplatin, lamivudine, metformin, oxaliplatin, procainamide	Cetirizine, cimetidine, quinidine
MATE1	Metformin, oxaliplatin	Cimetidine, quinidine, procainamide
MCT1	Atorvastatin, salicylic acid, pravastatin, valproic acid, γ-hydroxybutyric acid	Dietary flavonoids
PEPT1	Captopril, cefadroxil, cephalexin, enalapril, valacyclovir	Glycyl-proline, zinc
PEPT2	Captopril, cefadroxil, cephalexin, enalapril, valacyclovir	Fosinopril
CNT/ENT	Clofarabine, gemcitabine, ribavirin, other nucleoside analogs	Dipyridamole

NSAIDs, nonsteroidal anti-inflammatory drugs.

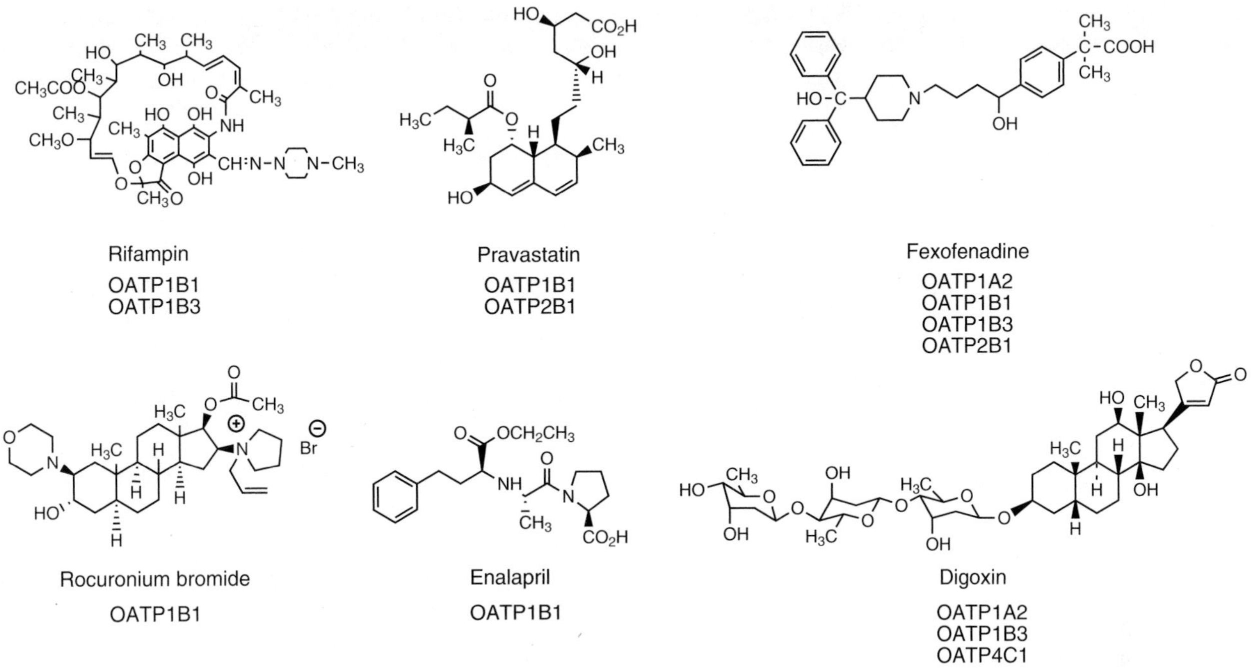

FIGURE 5.6 Common OATP substrates.

Other OATPs

OATP1B3 is expressed like OATP1B1 exclusively on the sinusoidal membrane of the liver. The substrates for OATP1B3 are generally shared by OATP1B1, with the exceptions of digoxin, docetaxel, and paclitaxel (15). OATP1B3 can act as a compensatory transport mechanism when transport by OATP1B1 is deficient due to inhibition or genetic polymorphisms. The other OATPs with identified drug substrates and effects on drug disposition include OATP1A2, 2B1, and 4C1. OATP1A2 is expressed in the intestine and expressed highly in the brain and is responsible for both oral absorption and blood–brain barrier transport of drugs and endogenous substances. OATP2B1 is also expressed on the sinusoidal membrane of the liver with OATP1B1 and 1B3; however, unlike these transporters, it is also expressed in other tissues including the kidney and intestine. OATP4C1 is expressed on the basolateral membrane of the kidney. Among its substrates are digoxin and the antidiabetic drug sitagliptin, and this transporter can have a role in the renal secretion of these drugs (16,17).

Organic Anion Transporters *(SLC22A)*

The organic anion transporters (OATs) are highly expressed in the kidney where they have a significant role in the renal clearance of many anionic drugs. The driving forces and polarized renal expression of OATs support renal secretion of drug substrates from the blood circulation into the urine. OAT1 is expressed exclusively in the kidney, on the basolateral membrane of renal tubule cells, along with OAT3. These transporters facilitate anion transport into renal tubule cells through antiport with intracellular dicarboxylates like α-ketoglutarate. Located on the apical membrane, OAT4 can transport drugs from the tubule cells into the urine, but it is likely primarily responsible for renal reabsorption (18). OATs transport an expansive range of drugs, and the importance of OAT expression in the kidney has been demonstrated with numerous clinically relevant drug interactions. Coadministration of OAT inhibitors can lead to decreased renal secretion of OAT substrates including penicillin antibiotics and diuretic agents (Tables 5.3 and 5.4) (9). Along with renal transport, OATs also mediate hepatic anion transport. The primary location of OAT2 is on the liver sinusoidal membrane, where it facilitates anion uptake into hepatocytes. OATs are also present on the choroid plexus (a structure in the brain where cerebrospinal fluid is produced), where they can have a role in transfer of drugs between the blood and cerebrospinal fluid.

Organic Cation/Carnitine Transporters *(SLC22)*

Organic cation transporters (OCTs) are electrogenic uniporters, which use only the cation concentration as a driving force. They require no cosubstrate, resulting in unequal distribution of ionic charges across the membrane. OCT1 is expressed in the liver and OCT2 in the kidney, both on the basolateral membrane. Although they are named cation transporters, these transporters are also capable of transporting some anionic and neutral compounds. Drug interactions and drug toxicity have been attributed to OCT-mediated

TABLE 5.4 Clinically Relevant Transporter-Mediated Drug Interactions[a]

Transporter	Substrate	Inhibitor(s)	Effect on Substrate Pharmacokinetics
MDR1	Digoxin	Clarithromycin (4), cyclosporine (95), ritonavir (5)	↑ plasma AUC, ↓ Cl_R and/or ↑ F
	Paclitaxel	Cyclosporine (43)	↑ F
BCRP	Topotecan	Elacridar (13)	↑ F
	Rosuvastatin	Atazanavir/ritonavir (44)	↑ plasma AUC and C_{max}
OATP1B1/1B3	Statins	Gemfibrozil (54),[b] cyclosporine (58),[b] lopinavir/ritonavir (96)	↑ plasma AUC, ↓ Cl
	Bosentan	Lopinavir/ritonavir (97)	↑ AUC and C_{max}
OAT1/3	Acyclovir, cidofovir, furosemide, penicillins	Probenecid (9,74)	↑ plasma AUC, ↓ Cl_R
OCT2/MATE1	Metformin	Cimetidine (19)	↑ plasma AUC, ↓ Cl_R

AUC, area under the curve; Cl, clearance; Cl_R, renal clearance; F, bioavailability; C_{max}, peak plasma concentration.
[a] Interactions that have been demonstrated in humans to elicit clinically significant effects on substrate pharmacokinetics or pharmacodynamics in vivo.
[b] Also involves enzyme inhibition.

transport, due to their substrate range that includes commonly prescribed therapeutic agents, such as metformin (Table 5.3). Coadministration of OCT inhibitors (e.g., cimetidine) and genetic variation in OCT2 have been demonstrated to increase plasma concentrations of the antidiabetic drug metformin due to its decreased renal secretion (Tables 5.4) (19,20). Renal transport of cisplatin by OCT2 has also been identified as a significant factor in cisplatin-induced nephrotoxicity (21). OCT3 transports monoamines and is primarily located in the brain and placenta, where its primary role can be to eliminate catecholamines from the fetal blood circulation (22). Decreased OCT3 transport has also been suggested to be related to cases of preeclampsia (23).

Organic cation/carnitine transporter (OCTN) 1 and OCTN2 are proton antiporters and are primarily expressed in the kidney, where they are localized on the apical membrane. Expression of human OCTN1/2 mRNA has also been detected in the intestine (24). These transporters share substrates with OCTs, and their apical expression allows for the concerted movement of these substrates across membranes. These transporters are of particular importance in the placenta, as they are responsible for transporting carnitine to the fetus (22). Some antiepileptics, like valproate, inhibit OCTNs, and it has been suggested that inhibition of carnitine transport can be partly responsible for teratogenicity and other adverse effects associated with valproate use (25). Mutations in OCTN2 lead to systemic carnitine deficiency syndrome, causing early-onset cardiomyopathy, including congestive heart failure (26). The anticholinergic drugs ipratropium and tiotropium are transported primarily by OCTN2 and, to a lesser extent, by OCTN1, by bronchial epithelial cells. These findings are consistent with the pharmacologic activity of the drugs after administration via inhalation.

Multidrug and Toxin Extrusion Transporters (*SLC47A*)

Multidrug and toxin extrusion transporter (MATE) 1 and MATE2-K are cation transporters that use proton antiport as a driving force. MATE1 is located primarily on the apical membrane of the kidney and canalicular membrane of the liver, where it acts in concert with OCTs expressed on

TABLE 5.5 Nuclear Receptors Involved in Transporter Regulation

Nuclear Receptor or Transcription Factor	Agents That Act on Receptor	Transporters Affected
Pregnane X receptor (PXR)	Rifampin, cytokines	MDR1, MRP2, OATP1A2
Constitutive androstane receptor (CAR)	Phenobarbital	MDR1, MRP2, MRP4
Farnesoid X receptor (FXR)	Bile acids	MRP2, MRP3, MRP1, OATP1B3
Peroxisome proliferator-activated receptor γ (PPARγ)	Thiazolidinediones	BCRP

the basolateral membranes of these organs to transport cationic substrates, including therapeutic agents. MATE2-K is kidney specific. The significance of MATE1 transport in metformin pharmacokinetics was characterized in Mate1 knockout mice, in which the renal clearance of metformin was decreased to less than 20% that of controls, indicating the importance of this transporter for metformin renal secretion (27). It has also been demonstrated that MATE1 has a role in the nephrotoxicity of platinum agents, where MATE1 secretion appears protective due to the prevention of renal cell accumulation (28,29). Many drug substrates and inhibitors of these transporters have been identified, and the therapeutic relevance of these transporters is expected to increase as their transport and effects on in vivo drug disposition are further characterized (Table 5.3) (30).

Monocarboxylate Transporters (*SLC16A* and *SLC5A*)

The first discovered monocarboxylate transporters (MCTs) were proton coupled, transporting monocarboxylates via symport. Because the transport of substrates by MCTs is driven by the proton gradient, these transporters can influx or efflux substrates depending on this gradient. The MCTs are ubiquitously expressed, and their role in the transport of endogenous substances, including lactate and pyruvate, has been extensively characterized (31). Many therapeutic agents have also been identified as substrates; however, the clinical relevance of MCT transport of these agents is unclear (Table 5.3). A relevant therapeutic aspect of MCT1 is its high expression in the intestine, making this transporter a target as a means for oral drug absorption (32). MCT1 has also been identified to be overexpressed in tumor cells, and inhibition of this transporter represents a possible therapeutic strategy for some cancers (33). The drug of abuse γ-hydroxybutyrate (GHB) has been identified as an MCT substrate, and the relevance of MCT transport of this drug has been established. Inhibition of the MCT-mediated renal reabsorption of GHB has been demonstrated to increase its renal and total clearance, making MCT inhibition a possible strategy for the treatment of GHB overdose (34).

Another subset of MCTs has been identified that use sodium for monocarboxylate symport and are referred to as sodium-coupled MCTs (SMCTs). Expression of SMCTs is also widely distributed, including the apical membranes of the intestine and kidney, where they likely act in conjunction with proton-coupled MCTs to transport monocarboxylates across membranes.

Peptide Transporters (*SLC15A*)

Peptide transporters (PEPTs) mediate the transport of di- and tripeptides via proton symport. PEPT1 has very high expression on the apical membrane of the intestine and, as such, is used for drug delivery. Transport mediated by PEPT1 facilitates sufficient oral absorption to allow oral administration for many therapeutic drugs and prodrugs structurally designed to target this transporter (Fig. 5.7 and Table 5.3) (32). PEPT1 is also present at lower levels on the brush border membrane of the kidney; however, PEPT2 is the major peptide transporter at this site. PEPT2 is also localized to the apical membrane where it serves mainly to reabsorb peptides from the urine in renal tubule cells. It also facilitates transport of drug substrates similar to PEPT1 including β-lactam antibiotics and angiotensin-converting enzyme (ACE) inhibitors (Table 5.3) (35). Two peptide/histidine transporters (PHTs) were recently identified, PHT1 and PHT2. Expression of these transporters has been demonstrated in the intestine, and they likely have a role in peptide absorption, along with PEPT1. Expression of mRNA for these transporters has also been identified in several other human tissues (36). The role of the PHTs in drug disposition has yet to be elucidated.

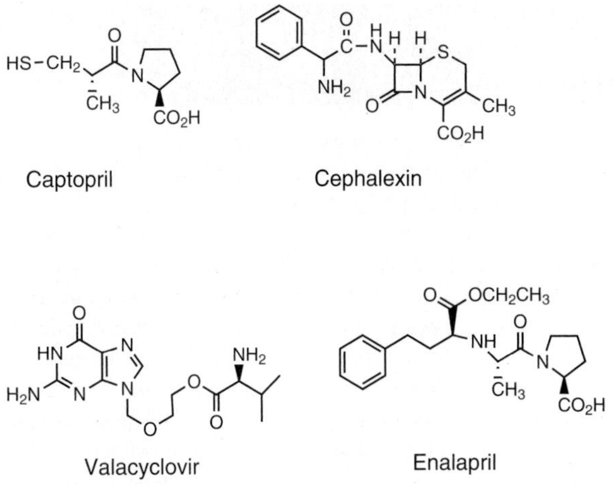

FIGURE 5.7 Drug substrates of peptide transporters.

Nucleoside Transporters (*SLC28* and *SLC29*)

Two nucleoside transporter groups exist, the concentrative nucleoside transporters (CNTs) and the equilibrative

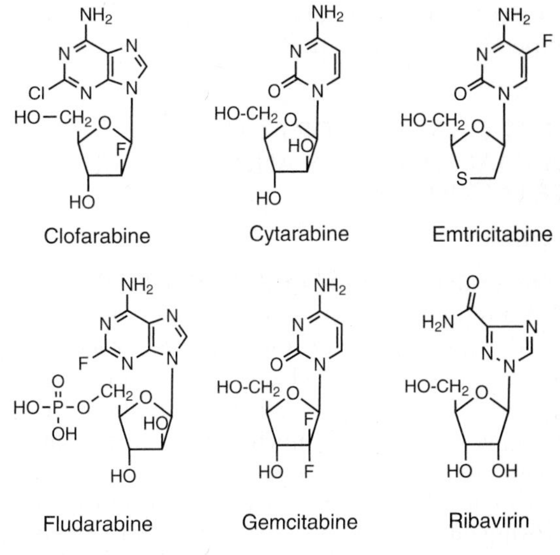

FIGURE 5.8 Drug substrates of nucleoside transporters.

EVALUATING TRANSPORTER EFFECTS IN VIVO

Many transporters share substrates with other transporters and with drug-metabolizing enzymes, making it difficult to attribute in vivo effects to a specific transporter. The use of probe substrates and specific inhibitors makes this identification easier, but these are not available for all transporters or may not be suitable for in vivo use. Knockout animals can be used to assess the effects of a specific transporter in vivo, whereas transfected cell lines or oocytes and specific silencing of a transporter using small interfering, double-stranded RNA can be useful to assess effects in vitro. When evaluating the effects of drug transport on bioavailability, it can be difficult to attribute effects to transport in the intestine alone, as changes in both bioavailability and clearance can affect plasma concentrations after oral administration. It is necessary to assess administration of substrates and inhibitors both orally and intravenously to determine if transport primarily affects substrate bioavailability or systemic clearance. Often both parameters are affected by changes in transport because the same transporters are responsible for both processes. Significant effects on absorption cannot always be demonstrated with efflux transporter substrates in vivo. This can be due to the very high luminal concentrations of substrate causing transporter saturation and to the passive membrane permeability of these compounds. A lack of effect can also be due to shared transporter substrates, allowing compensatory transport by one transporter when another is inhibited.

nucleoside transporters (ENTs). CNTs are present on the apical membrane of cells and are sodium dependent, whereas ENTs are facilitative and located primarily on basolateral membranes (37). These two groups of transporters work together to achieve vectorial transport of purines and pyrimidines. The expression of both groups of transporters is widespread, and although their primary function is to facilitate cellular uptake of nucleosides, they also transport many nucleoside analogs (Fig. 5.8), and these transporters are associated with toxicity and therapeutic response to these drugs (Table 5.3) (37,38).

EFFECT OF TRANSPORT ON DRUG PHARMACOKINETICS AND DRUG–DRUG INTERACTIONS

Intestinal Transport

The importance of transporter-mediated influx or efflux in the intestine depends primarily on two factors. The first is the contribution of transporter-mediated transport compared to the other mechanisms of drug passage across the gut wall. The second is drug concentration. Drug concentrations are generally much higher in the gut lumen compared to the systemic blood circulation due to a lower volume of distribution. This causes the concentration gradient driving diffusion to be very large but, more importantly, can lead to transporter saturation. This can lead to low

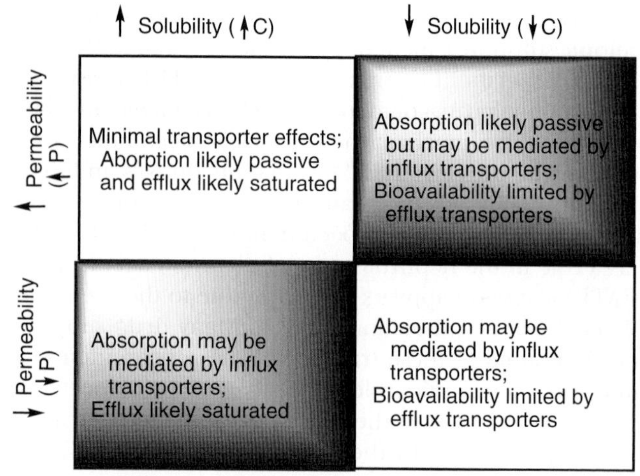

FIGURE 5.9 Role of transporters in drug absorption. High aqueous drug solubility will result in high luminal drug concentrations, allowing for possible transporter saturation. High permeability results in high nonsaturable transport, allowing these drugs to be orally absorbed without dependence on transporters. (Adapted from Shugarts S, Benet LZ. The role of transporters in the pharmacokinetics of orally administered drugs. Pharm Res 2009;26:2039–2054.)

bioavailability due to saturation of influx transporters and nonlinearity in drug absorption. Transporter saturation can also aid in drug absorption in that high drug concentrations in the enterocyte can saturate efflux transporters. High drug concentrations in the gut can also result in drug interactions affecting oral absorption. The U.S. Food and Drug Administration–recommended Biopharmaceutics Classification System names solubility and permeability as determining factors of oral absorption (39), factors which can be translated into effects on drug concentration (C) and nonsaturable transport (P) in the intestine. Considering these factors, the predicted effects of drug transporters on oral absorption are given in Figure 5.9 (40).

The polarized expression of relevant drug transporters in the intestine is illustrated in Figure 5.10. Clinical relevance of drug transport is determined not only by the presence of transporters on a biologic membrane, but also by their relative expression. The transporters with highest intestinal expression include BCRP, PEPT1, P-gp, and MCT1 (41). High expression of influx transporters, like PEPT1 and MCT1, allows the use of these high-capacity transporters as a drug delivery mechanism. High expression of efflux transporters makes these transporters important in limiting drug bioavailability.

Along with drug transporters, present in the enterocytes forming the gut wall are drug-metabolizing enzymes, including phase 1 and phase 2 enzymes. First-pass metabolism in the gut can be a reason for low oral bioavailability. Transporters often share substrates with drug-metabolizing enzymes, and the intestine is one site in which substantial transport–metabolism interplay has been recognized. In particular, it has been noted that P-gp shares many substrates with the enzyme CYP3A4, and it is proposed that P-gp can prevent oral absorption through drug efflux

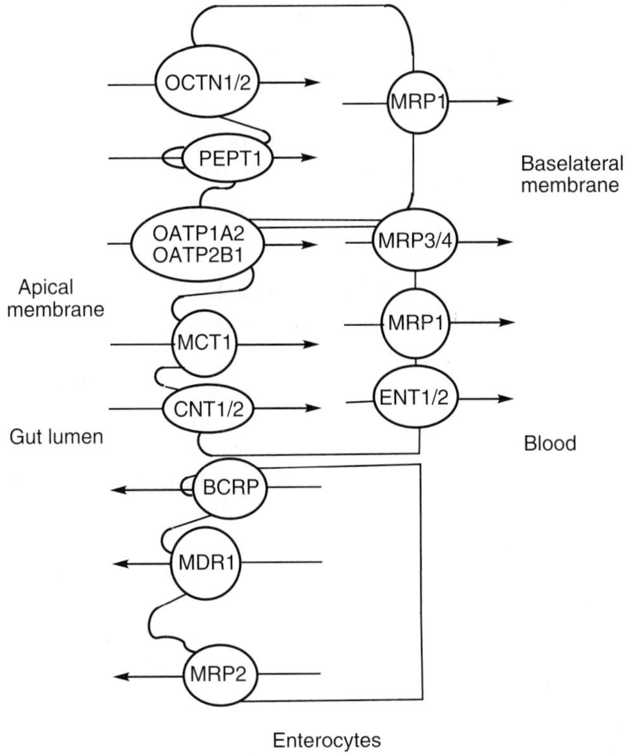

FIGURE 5.10 Polarized expression of drug transporters in the intestine.

and by facilitating drug metabolism by CYP3A4 (42). This is achieved by the cycling of substrates through the gut lumen and enterocytes, allowing enzymes such as CYP3A4

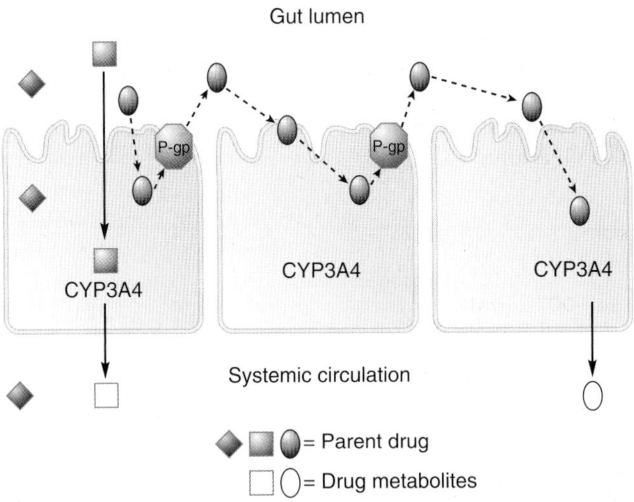

FIGURE 5.11 Transport–metabolism interplay in the intestine. Drugs may be orally absorbed without undergoing metabolic conversion. Drugs may undergo metabolism in the gut, and this may occur upon initial entry into the enterocyte or after cycling between the gut lumen and the enterocyte. P-gp facilitates CYP3A4 metabolism by allowing the enzyme multiple opportunities for drug metabolism, as demonstrated by the molecule shown in red. (Adapted from Benet LZ. The drug transporter-metabolism alliance: uncovering and defining the interplay. Mol Pharm 2009;6:1631–1643.)

multiple opportunities to metabolize their substrates. This interplay is depicted in Figure 5.11.

Efflux Transporters and Drug Bioavailability

Studies using specific P-gp inhibitors and Mdr1 knockout animals have demonstrated the importance of P-gp in the oral bioavailability of drugs including HIV protease inhibitors, β-receptor antagonists, morphine, and many other therapeutic agents (3). Many of the drug interactions in the intestine involve P-gp or other efflux transporters, usually involving inhibition of transport, resulting in increased bioavailability of the transporter substrate. Administration of P-gp inhibitors and inducers has demonstrated clinically significant effects on the bioavailability of P-gp substrates, including digoxin and paclitaxel (4,43).

Drug bioavailability can also be limited by BCRP. Administration of the P-gp/BCRP inhibitor elacridar increased the bioavailability of topotecan sixfold in Mdr1 knockout mice, and oral coadministration with elacridar has been shown to increase the bioavailability of topotecan in humans to almost 100% (12,13). Similarly, oral coadministration of the statin rosuvastatin, a BCRP substrate, and the antivirals atazanavir/ritonavir, known to inhibit BCRP, significantly increased rosuvastatin exposure in humans, most likely due to inhibition of BCRP-mediated intestinal efflux and biliary secretion (44).

Influx Transporters and Drug Bioavailability

Select influx transporters in the intestine can be used to facilitate oral absorption. The high expression of PEPT1

P-GP AND DIGOXIN: CLINICAL SIGNIFICANCE

Digoxin undergoes little metabolism in humans, and transport by P-gp is the primary determinant of digoxin pharmacokinetics. One of the first drug interactions noted with digoxin was that with cyclosporine, leading to decreased digoxin clearance and digoxin-associated arrhythmias (45). It was later discovered that cyclosporine and other therapeutic agents decrease digoxin clearance due to inhibition of P-gp–mediated renal secretion (46). Nonrenal clearance of digoxin is minimal; however, P-gp inhibitors have similarly been demonstrated to decrease digoxin biliary excretion (47). P-gp function also affects digoxin absorption, and concomitant oral administration of clarithromycin was demonstrated to increase digoxin bioavailability along with decreasing digoxin renal clearance (4). Because in vivo P-gp inhibition can affect both absorption and clearance, there exists substantial risk of elevated digoxin plasma concentrations and digoxin-associated toxicity with concomitant inhibitor administration.

P-gp induction can also affect digoxin pharmacokinetics. In a study of human volunteers, chronic rifampin administration resulted in a 3.5-fold increase in duodenal P-gp expression leading to a decrease in digoxin bioavailability (48). P-gp expression correlated well with digoxin area under the curve (AUC) in this study, emphasizing the significance of intestinal P-gp on digoxin exposure.

MCT1 AND ORAL DRUG DELIVERY

The antiepileptic agent, gabapentin, has unfavorable oral pharmacokinetics, with low, dose-dependent bioavailability and poor rates of clinical response. In an effort to improve the oral delivery of gabapentin, a prodrug, gabapentin enacarbil, was designed to target absorption by MCT1. In a pilot study comparing the pharmacokinetics of gabapentin to the prodrug, gabapentin displayed dose-dependent bioavailability ranging from 27% to 65%, whereas gabapentin enacarbil displayed bioavailability above 68% for all doses and dose-proportional oral exposure (52). Gabapentin enacarbil resulted in higher plasma concentrations of gabapentin at similar doses compared to gabapentin itself. This case emphasizes the utility of high-capacity transporters like MCT1 for facilitating oral drug delivery and achieving clinically desirable drug pharmacokinetics.

has made it a target for oral drug delivery, and among its substrates are ACE inhibitors, β-lactam antibiotics, and the antiviral drug valacyclovir. Nonlinearity in the oral pharmacokinetics of valacyclovir can be attributed to saturable PEPT1-mediated absorption (49). Other transporters involved in oral drug delivery include OATP1A2 and 2B1, OCTN1/2, and MCT1 (32).

Influx transporters can also be responsible for drug interactions in the intestine, although fewer drug interactions have been noted than for efflux transporters. Plasma concentrations of fexofenadine, an OATP1A2 substrate, are decreased with concomitant ingestion of grapefruit juice (50). This is most likely due to transporter inhibition by the furanocoumarins in grapefruit juice, to which drug interactions with intestinal P-gp have also been attributed (51).

Hepatic Transport

As a clearance organ, the liver can eliminate drug through two pathways, metabolism and biliary excretion. Uptake into the liver is necessary for both of these processes, and for hydrophilic or ionic drugs, this is often a transporter-mediated process. Active transporters are also necessary for biliary excretion, as diffusion of drugs into the bile is unlikely due to the low volume of the bile canaliculus resulting in high drug concentrations. The transporters facilitating both drug uptake and drug excretion in the liver are depicted in Figure 5.12.

Role of Transporters in Drug Metabolism and Drug Interactions at the Sinusoidal Membrane

As with the intestine, there exists transporter–metabolism interplay in the liver because transporters regulate the distribution of drug substrates into the liver and therefore their access to drug-metabolizing enzymes. Just as the significance of a transporter on a drug's membrane permeability is determined by the contribution of that transport process to overall transport, uptake by transporters needs to be a rate-limiting process for uptake to be a significant factor in drug elimination. Uptake by OATP1B1 located on the sinusoidal membrane appears to be the rate-limiting process for elimination of many of its substrates, and changes in OATP1B1 transport have been demonstrated to affect drug clearance. The relevance of OATP transport has been demonstrated with the HMG-CoA reductase inhibitors, several of which are OATP1B1 substrates. Drug interactions resulting in OATP1B1 inhibition and numerous polymorphisms in the *SLCO1B1* gene demonstrate decreased clearance of statins and other OATP substrates, including repaglinide, olmesartan, and the active metabolite of irinotecan, SN-38 (15,53). Polymorphisms in the other sinusoidal uptake transporters have also been identified, and effects on their drug substrates emphasize their role in hepatic uptake. Polymorphism in *SLCO1B3* has been correlated with increased myelosuppresssion associated with docetaxel, and polymorphisms in *SLC22A1* have been demonstrated to be related to decreased metformin clearance (53).

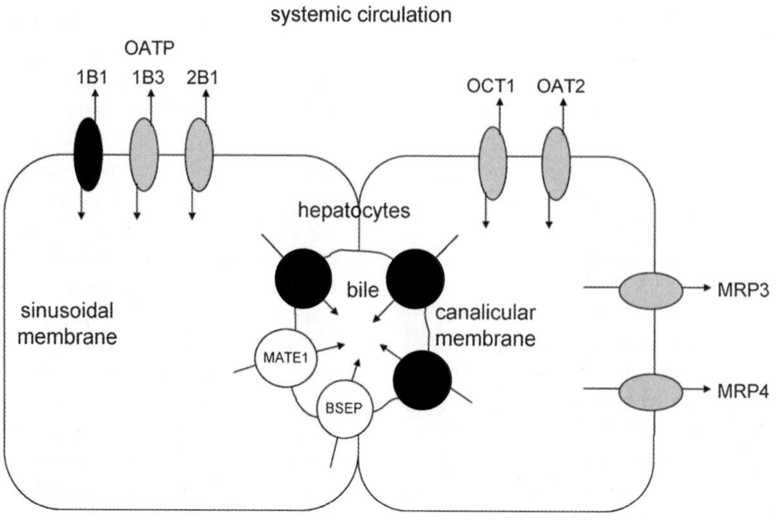

FIGURE 5.12 Drug transporter expression in hepatocytes. Transporters most relevant to drug disposition are shown in *red*.

OATP1B1 AND STATIN DISPOSITION

Although the metabolism and disposition of statin drugs can involve many drug-metabolizing enzymes and drug transporters, OATP1B1 has emerged as a protein of significance, with increasing clinical evidence supporting its involvement in the clearance, response, and toxicity of these drugs. One of the first interactions noted was the several-fold increase in cerivastatin plasma concentrations following gemfibrozil administration, resulting in severe cases of rhabdomyolysis (54). This drug interaction was determined to be due to inhibition of OATP1B1 and CYP2C8 by gemfibrozil (55). Gemfibrozil has been shown to increase the plasma AUC of other statins, which undergo little metabolism, indicating the significance of OATP-mediated transport (15,55,56). Similar effects on statin pharmacokinetics have also been demonstrated with other OATP1B1 inhibitors, including cyclosporine and rifampin (57–59). The effect of OATP1B1 polymorphisms on statin pharmacokinetics and response further emphasizes the significance of OATP-mediated uptake. Studies of subjects with the common SLCO1B1 c.521CC genotype have reported increases in plasma AUC from 65% with rosuvastatin to 221% with simvastatin compared to subjects carrying the wild-type allele (15). Polymorphisms in SLCO1B1 have also been correlated with increased rates of myopathy, along with decreased lipid-lowering effects (60,61). Alterations in the function of this transporter can significantly affect the safe and effective use of statins, and the use of OATP inhibitors with statin therapy can require dosage adjustment. SLCO1B1 genotyping may become useful for individualizing statin therapy.

Role of Transporters in Biliary Drug Excretion and the Effect of Drugs on Canalicular Membrane Transport

Some of the first drug interactions discovered to affect biliary clearance of drugs in humans involved the ABC transporter P-gp. It was demonstrated that quinidine and verapamil, known P-gp inhibitors, significantly decreased the biliary clearance of digoxin, resulting in increased digoxin plasma concentrations (47,62). P-gp efflux also has a role in the biliary excretion of doxorubicin, as demonstrated by an 80% to 90% decrease in doxorubicin biliary clearance in Mdr1 knockout mice (63,64). MRP2 also mediates biliary excretion of doxorubicin, along with that of other therapeutic agents including pravastatin and valsartan (Table 5.2) (64–66). MRP2 has a significant role in the biliary excretion of drug conjugates and in enterohepatic circulation, but it appears that BCRP has a more significant role in the excretion of sulfate conjugates, along with its role in secreting unconjugated drugs. Decreased biliary excretion of acetaminophen sulfate and other sulfate conjugates has been reported to be decreased in mice lacking Bcrp but not in those lacking Mdr2 (67,68). BCRP knockout or inhibition results in decreased biliary clearance of therapeutic agents including topotecan, nitrofurantoin, and ciprofloxacin (12,14,69). In addition, polymorphisms in the *ABCG2* gene have been shown to correlate with increased response to rosuvastatin, which can be explained by increased concentrations in the liver, the site of action, due to decreased biliary excretion by BCRP (70). Drugs have also been demonstrated to interact with the bile salt export pump (BSEP), which is expressed at the canalicular membrane and is responsible for bile acid secretion. Drugs with significant hepatotoxicity, such as cyclosporine, rifampin, and troglitazone, have been demonstrated to inhibit BSEP, leading to liver injury presumably due to inhibition of bile acid transport (71,72). The primary metabolite of troglitazone, troglitazone sulfate, has been demonstrated to inhibit BSEP and likely contributes to troglitazone-induced hepatotoxicity (71).

Renal Transport

Renal clearance is mediated by three primary pathways: glomerular filtration, tubular secretion, and renal reabsorption. Small-molecule drugs that are not protein bound will be filtered at the glomerulus. Drugs that undergo glomerular filtration can have negligible renal clearance if they are sufficiently lipophilic to be passively reabsorbed from the tubular lumen back into systemic circulation. Drugs that are hydrophilic or ionized will usually be passively excreted into the urine unless they are actively reabsorbed by transporters. Drugs can have extensive renal clearance, sometimes much greater than the glomerular filtration rate, if they undergo renal secretion. Renal secretion of drugs from the blood into urine requires active transport because drug concentrations in the tubular lumen are generally higher than those in the blood. The following equation can be used to determine renal clearance considering the possibility of all three processes:

$$Clr = (GFR * f_{up} + Cl_{rs})(1 - FR)$$

where *GFR* is the glomerular filtration rate; f_{up} is the fraction unbound in the plasma; Cl_{rs} is the clearance by renal secretion; and *FR* is the fraction of unchanged drug that is filtered and secreted in the urine, which is reabsorbed. Transporters are involved in both active secretion and active reabsorption. Secretion and reabsorption require transport of drug across both apical and basolateral membranes, and the polarized expression of organic anion and organic cation transporters on both membranes allows directional transport of ionized substrates. The transporters responsible for active secretion and active reabsorption and their polarized expression in the kidney are illustrated in Figure 5.13.

Renal Clearance of Anions

Tubular secretion of anions across the basolateral membrane is mediated primarily by OAT1 and OAT3. Substrates of these transporters include β-lactam antibiotics, nonsteroidal anti-inflammatory drugs, and many other anionic therapeutic agents (Table 5.3). Probenecid is a known inhibitor of OATs, and coadministration with OAT substrates leads to decreased renal clearance of

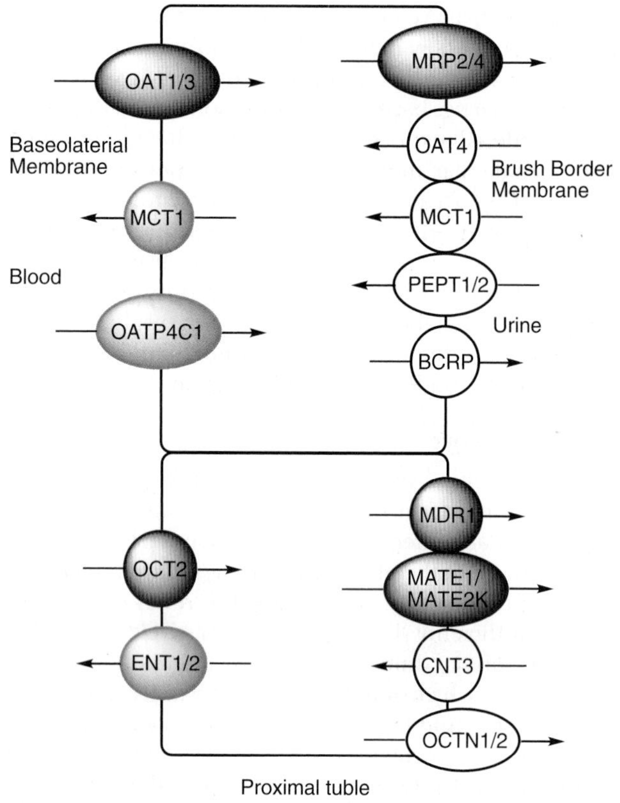

FIGURE 5.13 Drug transporter expression in the proximal renal tubule. Transporters most relevant to drug disposition are shown in *red*.

RENAL CLEARANCE BY OCT2/MATE: CISPLATIN TOXICITY

The platinum agents are used clinically for treatment of a variety of cancers. Treatment with cisplatin has been limited by its adverse effects, including nephrotoxicity, ototoxicity, and neurotoxicity (78). Transport by OCT2 has been attributed with facilitating cisplatin toxicity in the kidney, demonstrated by decreased nephrotoxicity with coadministration of OCT2 inhibitors and in Oct2 knockout animals (79,80). Genetic polymorphism in OCT2 has also been correlated with decreased serum creatinine concentrations in patients undergoing cisplatin treatment (21). Oxaliplatin, another OCT2 substrate, is not associated with severe nephrotoxicity. Oxaliplatin is efficiently transported by MATE1 and MATE2-K, allowing for secretion of this drug from tubule cells into the urine (29). Cisplatin is a poor MATE substrate, and cisplatin has been demonstrated to accumulate in renal tubule cells (81). Carboplatin, another platinum-based agent, is a substrate for neither OCT2 or MATE transporters and, similarly to oxaliplatin, does not display nephrotoxicity (29). It is apparent that the effects of cisplatin in the kidney can be attributed to OCT2-mediated influx followed by inefficient apical efflux, resulting in renal cell accumulation and toxicity. Recently, OCT2 was also found to be present in the cochlea, and Oct2 knockout prevented cisplatin-induced ototoxicity, along with reducing nephrotoxicity (80). OCT2 inhibition represents a potentially clinically relevant therapy for the prevention of both toxicities during cisplatin therapy.

these substrates. One of the most highly recognized transporter interactions is that between probenecid and penicillin derivatives, and coadministration of probenecid has been demonstrated to decrease the renal clearance of numerous drugs of this class including piperacillin, nafcillin, ticarcillin, and others (9). Inhibition of OAT transport by probenecid also causes decreased renal clearance of diuretics like furosemide and results in diminished diuretic effect due to decreased tubular drug concentrations (73,74). OAT-mediated drug interactions affect renal secretion of many other OAT substrates including methotrexate, acyclovir, and zidovudine (9). Secretion of anions across the renal brush border membrane is primarily mediated by MRP2 and MRP4. Probenecid is also an MRP2 inhibitor, and some of its effects on renal clearance can be due to combined inhibition of OATs and MRP2. The role of MRP4 in renal anion secretion has recently been elucidated, and it can be of greater importance at this site than MRP2 because MRP4 expression was reported to be five times that of MRP2 in human renal cortex (75). Mrp4 knockout mice display significant renal cell accumulation of the nucleotide phosphonates adefovir and tenofovir (76). Interestingly, cidofovir does not appear to be transported by MRP4, and this may be a reason for the significant nephrotoxicity associated with this drug. These drugs are also OAT substrates, and OAT inhibition can have therapeutic potential for preventing renal accumulation and toxicity with these agents (76).

Renal Clearance of Cations

Renal secretion of cations involves transport across the basolateral membrane by OCT2 followed by transport across the brush border membrane by MATE1, OCTNs, or possibly P-gp. Metformin is a substrate of both OCT2 and MATE1, and inhibition or knockout of either of these transporters results in significant decreases in metformin renal clearance (19,27). Genetic variants of both OCT2 and MATE1 have also been correlated with decreased metformin clearance and/or increased glucose-lowering effects with metformin treatment (20,77). Platinum-based chemotherapeutic agents also use the OCT2/MATE transport system, and this transport is a factor in toxicity of these agents (23).

Blood–Brain Barrier Transport

The blood–brain barrier (BBB) serves an important protective function for the CNS and presents both structural and metabolic barriers for xenobiotic penetration into the brain. The endothelial cells of the BBB form tight junctions with minimal fenestrations, limiting BBB penetration to drug molecules that are capable of transcellular diffusion. For entry of polar or charged essential nutrients such as amino acids and glucose, transport processes are necessary. Transporters present on the BBB for this function have been exploited to facilitate brain penetration of agents like levodopa, one of the most commonly used agents in Parkinson disease, which is transported into the brain by the L-type amino acid transporter (LAT) 1 (82). Influx transporters including LAT1 remain important for brain delivery of select drugs; however, attention has recently shifted to the efflux transporters expressed at the BBB, including P-gp, BCRP, and MRPs. Secretion of drug into the blood by these transporters has been recognized as another important barrier for drug penetration into the brain. Mdr1 knockout mice display substantially higher brain/plasma ratios for many P-gp substrates, with over 10-fold increases exhibited for digoxin, paclitaxel, and protease inhibitors compared to wild-type animals (83–85). Inhibition of P-gp has been used as a strategy to increase BBB penetration and has been demonstrated to be effective in animal models (43,84). The use of P-gp inhibitors in studies with human subjects shows similar but much more modest effects on brain penetration. This decreased effect is due in part to the lower inhibitor concentrations reached at doses used in human subjects, and evaluating the effects of these inhibitors at relevant concentrations is a priority for determining the utility of this strategy (85). Bcrp knockout animals have demonstrated the ability of this efflux transporter to limit brain penetration of drugs such as sorafenib (86). Many anticancer drugs are cosubstrates for P-gp and BCRP, and knockout of both transporters has demonstrated synergistic effects on brain accumulation of these drugs (86–88). The use of coinhibitors represents a potential strategy for improving treatment of brain tumors with these agents (43).

Regulation of Transporters and Interindividual Variability

Transcriptional regulation of transporters, effects mediated by nuclear receptors, can contribute to interindividual variability. The nuclear receptors that affect transporter expression are summarized in Table 5.5. Rifampin, an agonist of the nuclear receptor pregnane X (PXR), induces the expression of several enzymes and transporters including CYP3A4 and MDR1. During rifampin treatment, decreased drug exposure is observed with CYP3A4/MDR1 cosubstrates such as cyclosporine, calcium channel blockers, and chemotherapeutic agents, leading to a complete loss of response for some of these substrates (89,90). Interesting effects on transporter and enzyme regulation also occur in the presence of disease states. During cholestasis, hepatic transporter expression changes to facilitate bile acid secretion into the plasma by MRP3 and MRP4 and decrease secretion into the bile by MRP2 and BSEP (10). This change in transporter function has been attributed to the effect of bile acids on the farnesoid X receptor (FXR), causing upregulation of sinusoidal efflux transporters and downregulation of those at the canalicular membrane (91). Changes in enzyme and transporter expression have also been demonstrated in other disease states, including cancer, chronic renal failure, inflammation, and epilepsy, which display considerable interindividual variability (92–94). Current literature supports the involvement of select nuclear receptors in the regulation of affected proteins in some of these conditions (93). Understanding regulatory effects with these diseases and the mechanisms by which enzyme and transporter functions are altered will aid in accurate dosing of these patient populations.

CONCLUSIONS

Transporters have important roles in the pharmacokinetics of their drug substrates. Transport can result in drug–drug interactions, nonlinear pharmacokinetics, and interindividual variability. Changes in transporter function can translate into drug toxicity, although transporter interactions also have the potential to be beneficial for drug therapy. Application of transport principles and understanding the effects of transport on drug substrate concentrations promote the safe and effective use of these agents. Further investigation of transporter effects in vivo is expected to reveal additional significant effects of drug transporters on drug disposition.

ACKNOWLEDGMENT

Supported in part by National Institutes of Health Grant DA 023223. B.L.M. is supported in part by a fellowship from Pfizer.

References

1. Hoffmann U, Kroemer HK. The ABC transporters MDR1 and MRP2: multiple functions in disposition of xenobiotics and drug resistance. Drug Metab Rev 2004;36:669–701.
2. Giacomini KM, Huang SM, Tweedie DJ, et al. Membrane transporters in drug development. Nat Rev Drug Discov 2010;9:215–236.
3. Mealey KL. Therapeutic implications of the MDR-1 gene. J Vet Pharmacol Ther 2004;27:257–264.
4. Rengelshausen J, Goggelmann C, Burhenne J, et al. Contribution of increased oral bioavailability and reduced nonglomerular renal clearance of digoxin to the digoxin-clarithromycin interaction 2003. Br J Clin Pharmacol 2003;56:32–38.
5. Ding R, Tayrouz Y, Riedel KD, et al. Substantial pharmacokinetic interaction between digoxin and ritonavir in healthy volunteers. Clin Pharmacol Ther 2004;76:73–84.
6. Hutson JR, Koren G, Matthews SG. Placental P-glycoprotein and breast cancer resistance protein: influence of polymorphisms on fetal drug exposure and physiology. Placenta 2010;31:351–357.
7. Zhou SF. Structure, function and regulation of P-glycoprotein and its clinical relevance in drug disposition. Xenobiotica 2008;38:802–832.
8. Schinkel AH, Jonker JW. Mammalian drug efflux transporters of the ATP binding cassette (ABC) family: an overview. Adv Drug Deliv Rev 2003;55:3–29.
9. Masereeuw R, Russel FG. Therapeutic implications of renal anionic drug transporters. Pharmacol Ther 2010;126:200–216.
10. Zamek-Gliszczynski MJ, Hoffmaster A, Nezasa K, et al. Integration of hepatic drug transporters and phase II metabolizing enzymes: mechanisms of hepatic excretion of sulfate, glucuronide, and glutathione metabolites. Eur J Pharm Sci 2006;27:447–486.
11. Takano M, Yumoto R, Murakami T. Expression and function of efflux drug transporters in the intestine. Pharmacol Ther 2006;109:137–161.
12. Jonker JW, Smit JW, Brinkhuis RF, et al. Role of breast cancer resistance protein in the bioavailability and fetal penetration of topotecan. J Natl Cancer Inst 2000;92:1651–1656.
13. Kruijtzer CM, Beijnen JH, Rosing H, et al. Increased oral bioavailability of topotecan in combination with the breast cancer resistance protein and P-glycoprotein inhibitor GF120918. J Clin Oncol 2002;20:2943–2950.
14. Merino G, Jonker JW, Wagenaar E, et al. The breast cancer resistance protein (BCRP/ABCG2) affects pharmacokinetics, hepatobiliary excretion, and milk secretion of the antibiotic nitrofurantoin. Mol Pharmacol 2005;67:1758–1764.
15. Kalliokoski A, Niemi M. Impact of OATP transporters on pharmacokinetics. Br J Pharmacol 2009;158:693–705.

16. Chu XY, Bleasby K, Yabut J, et al. Transport of the dipeptidyl peptidase-4 inhibitor sitagliptin by human organic anion transporter 3, organic anion transporting polypeptide 4C1, and multidrug resistance P-glycoprotein. J Pharmacol Exp Ther 2007;321:673–683.
17. Mikkaichi T, Suzuki T, Onogawa T, et al. Isolation and characterization of a digoxin transporter and its rat homologue expressed in the kidney. Proc Natl Acad Sci U S A 2004;101:3569–3574.
18. Ekaratanawong S, Anzai N, Jutabha P, et al. Human organic anion transporter 4 is a renal apical organic anion/dicarboxylate exchanger in the proximal tubules. J Pharmacol Sci 2004;94:297–304.
19. Somogyi A, Stockley C, Keal J, et al. Reduction of metformin renal tubular secretion by cimetidine in man. Br J Clin Pharmacol 1987;23:545–551.
20. Chen Y, Li S, Brown C, et al. Effect of genetic variation in the organic cation transporter 2 on the renal elimination of metformin. Pharmacogenet Genomics 2009;19:497–504.
21. Filipski KK, Mathijssen RH, Mikkelsen TS, et al. Contribution of organic cation transporter 2 (OCT2) to cisplatin-induced nephrotoxicity. Clin Pharmacol Ther 2009;86:396–402.
22. Ganapathy V, Prasad PD. Role of transporters in placental transfer of drugs. Toxicol Appl Pharmacol 2005;207(2 Suppl):381–387.
23. Ciarimboli G. Organic cation transporters. Xenobiotica 2008;38:936–971.
24. Koepsell H, Lips K, Volk C. Polyspecific organic cation transporters: structure, function, physiological roles, and biopharmaceutical implications. Pharm Res 2007;24:1227–1251.
25. Wu SP, Shyu MK, Liou HH, et al. Interaction between anticonvulsants and human placental carnitine transporter. Epilepsia 2004;45:204–210.
26. Tein I. Carnitine transport: pathophysiology and metabolism of known molecular defects. J Inherit Metab Dis 2003;26:147–169.
27. Tsuda M, Terada T, Mizuno T, et al. Targeted disruption of the multidrug and toxin extrusion 1 (mate1) gene in mice reduces renal secretion of metformin. Mol Pharmacol 2009;75:1280–1286.
28. Nies AT, Koepsell H, Damme K, et al. Organic cation transporters (OCTs, MATEs), in vitro and in vivo evidence for the importance in drug therapy. Handb Exp Pharmacol 2011;201:105–167.
29. Yonezawa A, Inui KI. Organic cation transporter OCT/SLC22A and H(+)/organic cation antiporter MATE/SLC47A are key molecules for nephrotoxicity of platinum agents. Biochem Pharmacol 2011;581:563–568.
30. Tanihara Y, Masuda S, Sato T, et al. Substrate specificity of MATE1 and MATE2-K, human multidrug and toxin extrusions/H(+)-organic cation antiporters. Biochem Pharmacol 2007;74:359–371.
31. Merezhinskaya N, Fishbein WN. Monocarboxylate transporters: past, present, and future. Histol Histopathol 2009;24:243–264.
32. Varma M, Ambler C, Ullah M, et al. Targeting intestinal transporters for optimizing oral drug absorption. Curr Drug Metab 2010;11:730–742.
33. Kennedy KM, Dewhirst MW. Tumor metabolism of lactate: the influence and therapeutic potential for MCT and CD147 regulation. Future Oncol 2010;6:127–148.
34. Morris ME, Hu K, Wang Q. Renal clearance of gamma-hydroxybutyric acid in rats: increasing renal elimination as a detoxification strategy. J Pharmacol Exp Ther 2005;313:1194–1202.
35. Rubio-Aliaga I, Daniel H. Peptide transporters and their roles in physiological processes and drug disposition. Xenobiotica 2008;38:1022–1042.
36. Herrera-Ruiz D, Wang Q, Gudmundsson OS, et al. Spatial expression patterns of peptide transporters in the human and rat gastrointestinal tracts, Caco-2 in vitro cell culture model, and multiple human tissues. AAPS PharmSci 2001;3:E9.
37. Huber-Ruano I, Pastor-Anglada M. Transport of nucleoside analogs across the plasma membrane: a clue to understanding drug-induced cytotoxicity. Curr Drug Metab 2009;10:347–358.
38. Endres CJ, Moss AM, Govindarajan R, et al. The role of nucleoside transporters in the erythrocyte disposition and oral absorption of ribavirin in the wild-type and equilibrative nucleoside transporter 1-/- mice. J Pharmacol Exp Ther 2009;331:287–296.
39. Amidon GL, Lennernas H, Shah VP, et al. A theoretical basis for a biopharmaceutic drug classification: the correlation of in vitro drug product dissolution and in vivo bioavailability. Pharm Res 1995;12:413–420.
40. Shugarts S, Benet LZ. The role of transporters in the pharmacokinetics of orally administered drugs. Pharm Res 2009;26:2039–2054.
41. Englund G, Rorsman F, Ronnblom A, et al. Regional levels of drug transporters along the human intestinal tract: co-expression of ABC and SLC transporters and comparison with Caco-2 cells. Eur J Pharm Sci 2006;29:269–277.
42. Benet LZ. The drug transporter-metabolism alliance: uncovering and defining the interplay. Mol Pharm 2009;6:1631–1643.
43. Breedveld P, Beijnen JH, Schellens JH. Use of P-glycoprotein and BCRP inhibitors to improve oral bioavailability and CNS penetration of anticancer drugs. Trends Pharmacol Sci 2006;27:17–24.
44. Busti AJ, Bain AM, Hall RG, et al. Effects of atazanavir/ritonavir or fosamprenavir/ritonavir on the pharmacokinetics of rosuvastatin. J Cardiovasc Pharmacol 2008;51:605–610.
45. Dorian P, Strauss M, Cardella C, et al. Digoxin-cyclosporine interaction: severe digitalis toxicity after cyclosporine treatment. Clin Invest Med 1988;11:108–112.
46. Koren G, Woodland C, Ito S. Toxic digoxin-drug interactions: the major role of renal P-glycoprotein. Vet Hum Toxicol 1998;40:45–46.
47. Hedman A, Angelin B, Arvidsson A, et al. Digoxin-verapamil interaction: reduction of biliary but not renal digoxin clearance in humans. Clin Pharmacol Ther 1991;49:256–262.
48. Greiner B, Eichelbaum M, Fritz P, et al. The role of intestinal P-glycoprotein in the interaction of digoxin and rifampin. J Clin Invest 1999;104:147–153.
49. Bolger MB, Lukacova V, Woltosz WS. Simulations of the nonlinear dose dependence for substrates of influx and efflux transporters in the human intestine. AAPS J 2009;11:353–363.
50. Dresser GK, Kim RB, Bailey DG. Effect of grapefruit juice volume on the reduction of fexofenadine bioavailability: possible role of organic anion transporting polypeptides. Clin Pharmacol Ther 2005;77:170–177.
51. Won CS, Oberlies NH, Paine MF. Influence of dietary substances on intestinal drug metabolism and transport. Curr Drug Metab 2010;11:778–792.
52. Cundy KC, Sastry S, Luo W, et al. Clinical pharmacokinetics of XP13512, a novel transported prodrug of gabapentin. J Clin Pharmacol 2008;48:1378–1388.
53. Fahrcanr C, Fromm MF, Konig J. Hepatic OATP and OCT uptake transporters: their role for drug-drug interactions and pharmacogenetic aspects. Drug Metab Rev 2010;42:380–401.
54. Backman JT, Kyrklund C, Neuvonen M, et al. Gemfibrozil greatly increases plasma concentrations of cerivastatin. Clin Pharmacol Ther 2002;72:685–691.
55. Shitara Y, Hirano M, Sato H, et al. Gemfibrozil and its glucuronide inhibit the organic anion transporting polypeptide 2 (OATP2/OATP1B1:SLC21A6)-mediated hepatic uptake and CYP2C8-mediated metabolism of cerivastatin: analysis of the mechanism of the clinically relevant drug-drug interaction between cerivastatin and gemfibrozil. J Pharmacol Exp Ther 2004;311:228–236.
56. Schneck DW, Birmingham BK, Zalikowski JA, et al. The effect of gemfibrozil on the pharmacokinetics of rosuvastatin. Clin Pharmacol Ther 2004;75:455–463.
57. Kostapanos MS, Milionis HJ, Elisaf MS. Rosuvastatin-associated adverse effects and drug-drug interactions in the clinical setting of dyslipidemia. Am J Cardiovasc Drugs 2010;10:11–28.
58. Neuvonen PJ, Niemi M, Backman JT. Drug interactions with lipid-lowering drugs: mechanisms and clinical relevance. Clin Pharmacol Ther 2006;80:565–581.
59. Lau YY, Huang Y, Frassetto L, et al. Effect of OATP1B transporter inhibition on the pharmacokinetics of atorvastatin in healthy volunteers. Clin Pharmacol Ther 2007;81:194–204.
60. Link E, Parish S, Armitage J, et al. SLCO1B1 variants and statin-induced myopathy—a genomewide study. N Engl J Med 2008;359:789–799.
61. Romaine SP, Bailey KM, Hall A, et al. The influence of SLCO1B1 (OATP1B1) gene polymorphisms on response to statin therapy. Pharmacogenomics J 2010;10:1–11.
62. Angelin B, Arvidsson A, Dahlqvist R, et al. Quinidine reduces biliary clearance of digoxin in man. Eur J Clin Invest 1987;17:262–265.
63. van Asperen J, van Tellingen O, Beijnen JH. The role of mdr1a P-glycoprotein in the biliary and intestinal secretion of doxorubicin and vinblastine in mice. Drug Metab Dispos 2000;28:264–267.
64. Vlaming ML, Mohrmann K, Wagenaar E, et al. Carcinogen and anticancer drug transport by Mrp2 in vivo: studies using Mrp2 (Abcc2) knockout mice. J Pharmacol Exp Ther 2006;318:319–327.
65. Yamazaki M, Akiyama S, Ni'inuma K, et al. Biliary excretion of pravastatin in rats: contribution of the excretion pathway mediated by canalicular multispecific organic anion transporter. Drug Metab Dispos 1997;25:1123–1129.
66. Yamashiro W, Maeda K, Hirouchi M, et al. Involvement of transporters in the hepatic uptake and biliary excretion of valsartan, a selective antagonist of the angiotensin II AT1-receptor, in humans. Drug Metab Dispos 2006;34:1247–1254.
67. Chen C, Hennig GE, Manautou JE. Hepatobiliary excretion of acetaminophen glutathione conjugate and its derivatives in transport-deficient (TR-) hyperbilirubinemic rats. Drug Metab Dispos 2003;31:798–804.
68. Zamek-Gliszczynski MJ, Nezasa K, Tian X, et al. The important role of Bcrp (Abcg2) in the biliary excretion of sulfate and glucuronide metabolites of acetaminophen, 4-methylumbelliferone, and harmol in mice. Mol Pharmacol 2006;70:2127–2133.
69. Ando T, Kusuhara H, Merino G, et al. Involvement of breast cancer resistance protein (ABCG2) in the biliary excretion mechanism of fluoroquinolones. Drug Metab Dispos 2007;35:1873–1879.
70. Hu M, To KK, Mak VW, et al. The ABCG2 transporter and its relations with the pharmacokinetics, drug interaction and lipid-lowering effects of statins. Expert Opin Drug Metab Toxicol 2011;7:49–62.
71. Funk C, Ponelle C, Scheuermann G, et al. Cholestatic potential of troglitazone as a possible factor contributing to troglitazone-induced hepatotoxicity: in vivo and in vitro interaction at the canalicular bile salt export pump (Bsep) in the rat. Mol Pharmacol 2001;59:627–635.
72. Mita S, Suzuki H, Akita H, et al. Inhibition of bile acid transport across Na+/taurocholate cotransporting polypeptide (SLC10A1) and bile salt export pump (ABCB 11)-coexpressing LLC-PK1 cells by cholestasis-inducing drugs. Drug Metab Dispos 2006;34:1575–1581.
73. Walshaw PE, McCauley FA, Wilson TW. Diuretic and non-diuretic actions of furosemide: effects of probenecid. Clin Invest Med 1992;15:82–87.

74. Honari J, Blair AD, Cutler RE. Effects of probenecid on furosemide kinetics and natriuresis in man. Clin Pharmacol Ther 1977;22:395–401.
75. Smeets PH, van Aubel RA, Wouterse AC, et al. Contribution of multidrug resistance protein 2 (MRP2/ABCC2) to the renal excretion of p-aminohippurate (PAH) and identification of MRP4 (ABCC4) as a novel PAH transporter. J Am Soc Nephrol 2004;15:2828–2835.
76. Imaoka T, Kusuhara H, Adachi M, et al. Functional involvement of multidrug resistance-associated protein 4 (MRP4/ABCC4) in the renal elimination of the antiviral drugs adefovir and tenofovir. Mol Pharmacol 2007;71:619–627.
77. Becker ML, Visser LE, van Schaik RH, et al. Genetic variation in the multidrug and toxin extrusion 1 transporter protein influences the glucose-lowering effect of metformin in patients with diabetes: a preliminary study. Diabetes 2009;l58:745–749.
78. de Jongh FE, van Veen RN, Veltman SJ, et al. Weekly high-dose cisplatin is a feasible treatment option: analysis on prognostic factors for toxicity in 400 patients. Br J Cancer 2003;88:1199–1206.
79. Katsuda H, Yamashita M, Katsura H, et al. Protecting cisplatin-induced nephrotoxicity with cimetidine does not affect antitumor activity. Biol Pharm Bull 2010;33:1867–1871.
80. Ciarimboli G, Deuster D, Knief A, et al. Organic cation transporter 2 mediates cisplatin-induced oto- and nephrotoxicity and is a target for protective interventions. Am J Pathol 2010;176:1169–1180.
81. Yokoo S, Yonezawa A, Masuda S, et al. Differential contribution of organic cation transporters, OCT2 and MATE1, in platinum agent-induced nephrotoxicity. Biochem Pharmacol 2007;74:477–487.
82. Pinho MJ, Serrao MP, Gomes P, et al. Over-expression of renal LAT1 and LAT2 and enhanced L-DOPA uptake in SHR immortalized renal proximal tubular cells. Kidney Int 2004;66:216–226.
83. Schinkel AH, Wagenaar E, van Deemter L, et al. Absence of the mdr1a P-glycoprotein in mice affects tissue distribution and pharmacokinetics of dexamethasone, digoxin, and cyclosporin A. J Clin Invest 1995;96:1698–1705.
84. Kemper EM, van Zandbergen AE, Cleypool C, et al. Increased penetration of paclitaxel into the brain by inhibition of P-glycoprotein. Clin Cancer Res 2003;9:2849–2855.
85. Eyal S, Ke B, Muzi M, et al. Regional P-glycoprotein activity and inhibition at the human blood-brain barrier as imaged by positron emission tomography. Clin Pharmacol Ther 2010;87:579–585.
86. Agarwal S, Sane R, Ohlfest JR. The role of the breast cancer resistance protein (ABCG2) in the distribution of sorafenib to the brain. J Pharmacol Exp Ther 2011;336:223–233.
87. Kodaira H, Kusuhara H, Ushiki J, et al. Kinetic analysis of the cooperation of P-glycoprotein (P-gp/Abcb1) and breast cancer resistance protein (Bcrp/Abcg2) in limiting the brain and testis penetration of erlotinib, flavopiridol, and mitoxantrone. J Pharmacol Exp Ther 2010;333:788–796.
88. Zhou L, Schmidt K, Nelson FR, et al. The effect of breast cancer resistance protein and P-glycoprotein on the brain penetration of flavopiridol, imatinib mesylate (Gleevec), prazosin, and 2-methoxy-3-(4-(2-(5-methyl-2-phenyloxazol-4-yl)ethoxy)phenyl)propanoic acid (PF-407288) in mice. Drug Metab Dispos 2009;37:946–955.
89. Harmsen S, Meijerman I, Beijnen JH, et al. The role of nuclear receptors in pharmacokinetic drug-drug interactions in oncology. Cancer Treat Rev 2007;33:369–380.
90. Niemi M, Backman JT, Fromm MF, et al. Pharmacokinetic interactions with rifampicin: clinical relevance. Clin Pharmacokinet 2003;42:819–850.
91. Huang L, Zhao A, Lew JL, et al. Farnesoid X receptor activates transcription of the phospholipid pump MDR3. J Biol Chem 2003;278:51085–51090.
92. Dreisbach AW. The influence of chronic renal failure on drug metabolism and transport. Clin Pharmacol Ther 2009;86:553–556.
93. Morgan ET, Goralski KB, Piquette-Miller M, et al. Regulation of drug-metabolizing enzymes and transporters in infection, inflammation, and cancer. Drug Metab Dispos 2008;36:205–216.
94. Potschka H. Modulating P-glycoprotein regulation: future perspectives for pharmacoresistant epilepsies? Epilepsia 2010;51:1333–1347.
95. Robieux I, Dorian P, Klein J, et al. The effects of cardiac transplantation and cyclosporine therapy on digoxin pharmacokinetics. J Clin Pharmacol 1992;32:338–343.
96. Kiser JJ, Gerber JG, Predhomme JA, et al. Drug/drug interaction between lopinavir/ritonavir and rosuvastatin in healthy volunteers. J Acquir Immune Defic Syndr 2008;47:570–578.
97. Dingemanse J, van Giersbergen PL, Patat A, et al. Mutual pharmacokinetic interactions between bosentan and lopinavir/ritonavir in healthy participants. Antivir Ther 2010;15:157–163.

Chapter 6

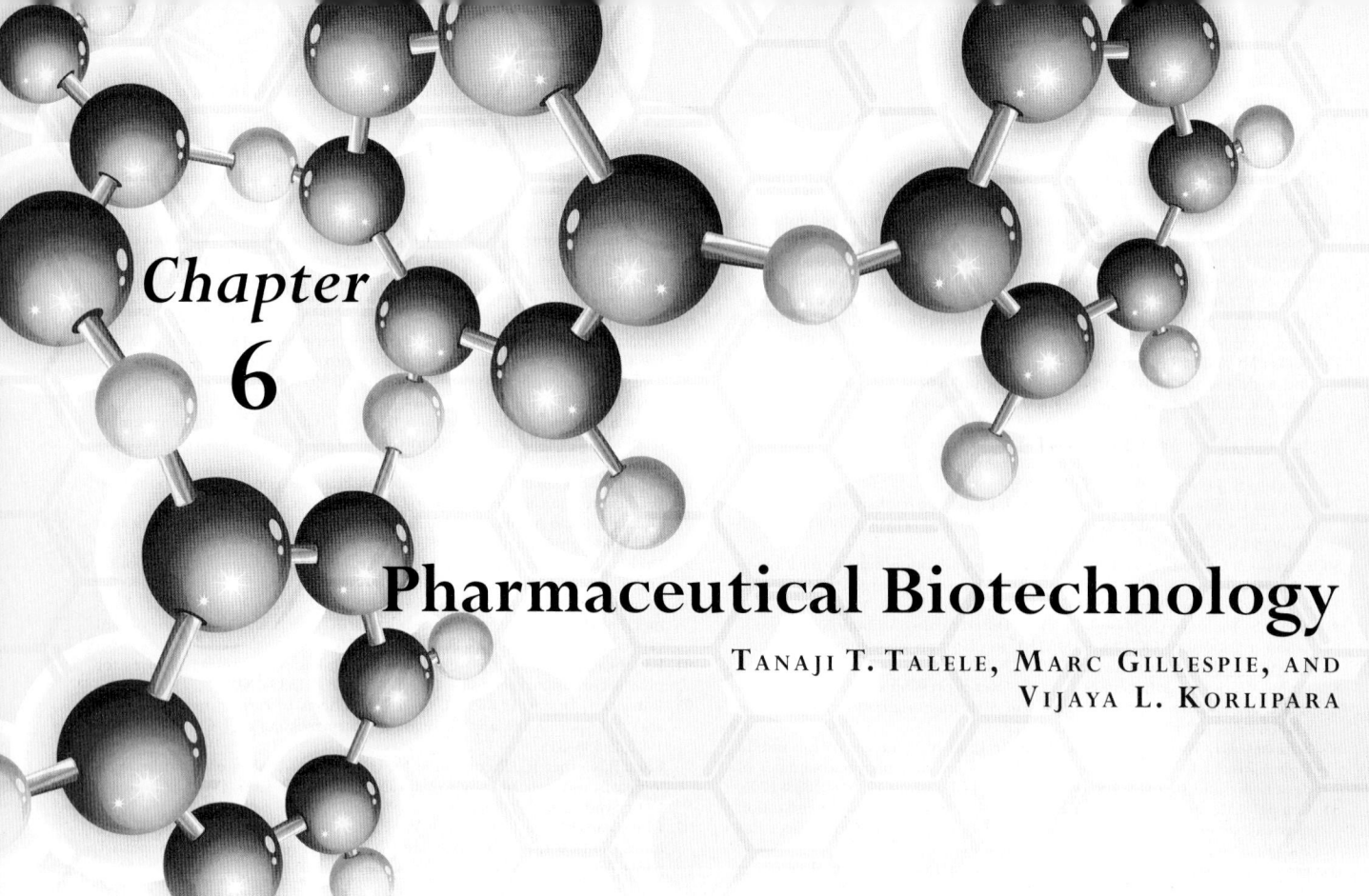

Pharmaceutical Biotechnology

Tanaji T. Talele, Marc Gillespie, and Vijaya L. Korlipara

Drugs Covered in This Chapter

Adrenocorticotropin hormones
- Adrenocorticotropin hormone
- Cosyntropin

Corticotropin-releasing factor
- Corticorelin ovine triflutate

Cytokines
- Anakinra
- Consensus interferon
- Denileukin diftitox
- Interferon α
- Interferon β
- Interferon γ
- Interleukin-1
- Interleukin-2/aldesleukin
- Interleukin-2 fusion protein
- Interleukin-11/oprelvekin
- Rilonacept

Enzymes
- Tissue plasminogen activators
    - Alteplase
    - Dornase alfa
    - Reteplase
    - Tenecteplase

Enzyme replacement therapy
- Alglucosidase alfa
- Idursulfase
- Imiglucerase

Gonadotropins
- Follitropin alfa
- Follitropin beta
- Lutropin alfa
- Menotropins
- Urofollitropin

Gonadotropin-releasing hormones
- Abarelix
- Cetrorelix acetate
- Ganirelix acetate
- Gonadotropin-releasing hormone
- Goserelin acetate
- Histrelin acetate
- Leuprolide acetate
- Nafarelin acetate
- Triptorelin pamoate

Growth hormones
- Pegvisomant
- Somatropin

Hematopoietic growth factors
- Erythropoietin (epoetin alfa)
- Filgrastim
- Sargramostim

Monoclonal antibodies
- Alemtuzumab
- Bevacizumab
- Canakinumab
- Catumaxomab
- Certolizumab pegol
- Cetuximab
- Denosumab
- Eculizumab
- Golimumab
- Ibritumomab tiuxetan
- Ofatumumab
- Panitumumab
- Ranibizumab
- Tositumomab
- Trastuzumab
- Ustekinumab

Pancreatic hormones
- *Amylin*
- Glucagon
- Insulin
- Pramlintide acetate

Parathyroid hormones
- Teriparatide

Pituitary hormones
- Desmopressin acetate
- Oxytocin
- Vasopressin

Placental hormones
- Choriogonadotropin alfa
- Human chorionic gonadotropin

Somatostatins
- Indium pentetreotide
- Octreotide acetate

Thyrotropin

Thyroid hormones
- Calcitonin salmon

- **Tumor necrosis factors**
- Abatacept
- Etanercept

Other growth factors

- Clotting factor VIII, factor IX, and anticoagulants

Vaccines

Abbreviations

ACTH, adrenocorticotropin hormone
ART, assisted reproductive therapy
ATP, adenosine triphosphate
bp, base pair
cDNA, complementary DNA
CDR, complementarity-determining region
CF, cystic fibrosis
CHO, Chinese hamster ovary
CLL, chronic lymphocytic leukemia
CRF, corticotropin-releasing factor
CSF, colony-stimulating factor
CT, calcitonin
CTCL, cutaneous T-cell lymphoma
CTLA-4, cytotoxic T-lymphocyte–associated antigen-4
CTP, cytidine triphosphate
ddNTP, 2′,3′-dideoxynucleotide triphosphate
DM, diabetes mellitus
DMARD, disease-modifying antirheumatic drug
DTPA, diethylenetriaminepentaacetic acid
EGF, epidermal growth factor
EGFR, epidermal growth factor receptor
EpCAM, epithelial cell adhesion molecule
EPO, erythropoietin
ERT, enzyme replacement therapy
Fab, functional human antibody
FDA, U.S. Food and Drug Administration
FSH, follicle-stimulating hormone
GAG, glycosaminoglycan
G-CSF, granulocyte colony-stimulating factor
gDNA, genomic DNA
GH, growth hormone
GM-CSF, granulocyte-macrophage colony-stimulating factor
GnRH, gonadotropin-releasing hormone
GTP, guanosine triphosphate
HAMA, human anti-mouse antibody
hCG, human chorionic gonadotropin
hGH, human growth hormone
5-HM, 5-hydroxymethyl metabolite
IL, interleukin
IFN, interferon
IgG, immunoglobulin G
^{111}In, indium-111
IRR, infusion-related reaction
IVF, in vitro fertilization
LH, luteinizing hormone
MAb, monoclonal antibody
MAPK, mitogen-activated protein kinase
M-CSF, macrophage colony-stimulating factor
MPS, mucopolysaccharidosis
mRNA, messenger RNA
MS, multiple sclerosis
MTX, methotrexate
MW, molecular weight
NHL, non-Hodgkin lymphoma
oCRF, sheep corticotropin-releasing factor
4OH-TAM, 4-hydroxy tamoxifen
PCR, polymerase chain reaction
PDGF, platelet-derived growth factor
PEG, polyethylene glycol
PI3K, phosphatidylinositol 3-kinase
PTH, parathyroid hormone
RA, rheumatoid arthritis
RANK, receptor activator of nuclear factor-κB
RANKL, receptor activator of nuclear factor-κB ligand
rDNA, recombinant DNA
rh, recombinant human
rRNA, ribosomal RNA
SC, subcutaneous
SNP, single nucleotide polymorphism
TNF, tumor necrosis factor
t-PA, tissue-type plasminogen activator
tRNA, transfer RNA
UGT1A1, UDP-glucuronosyl transferase 1A1
UTP, uridine triphosphate
VEGF, vascular endothelial growth factor
VEGFR, vascular endothelial growth factor receptor
VIP, vasoactive intestinal peptide

INTRODUCTION

Pharmaceutical biotechnology generates basic scientific knowledge, useful therapeutic and diagnostic products, and promising methodologies for future research and clinical applications. The techniques of biotechnology lead to the development of novel therapeutics, improved methods of manufacturing pharmaceuticals, and significant contributions to our understanding of disease etiology, pathophysiology, and biochemistry. Genomics, transcriptomics, proteomics, pharmacogenomics, and metabolomics, the core approaches to pharmaceutical biotechnology, are making major contributions in three areas:

1. Identification of new genes
2. Identification of drug targets
3. Development of "personalized medicine"

Although many of the first biotechnology-derived therapeutics were initially used in acutely ill, hospitalized patients, the products of today's pharmaceutical biotechnology have an impact on chronic disease patient populations constituting much of ambulatory care practice.

PHARMACOGENETICS

The application of genetic information from the Human Genome Project to disease diagnosis and drug therapy is a major development that is bringing about a wealth of change. The main benefits of pharmacogenetic screening are a reduction in the health care costs arising from drug toxicity and lack of efficacy in drug therapy.

Mutations are the result of heritable, permanent changes in DNA base sequence. These usually come about by one of three mechanisms: substitution, addition, or deletion. The number of base pairs involved in a single gene mutation can vary from a single base pair change or single nucleotide polymorphism (SNP), to a large number of gross changes in the gene structure

CLINICAL SIGNIFICANCE

The biotechnology industry has grown explosively over the past 30 years, with U.S. health care biotech revenues of publicly traded biotech industry companies rising from $8 billion in 1992 to $56.6 billion in 2009 (1). Fifteen new biopharmaceutical products were approved by the U.S. Food and Drug Administration in 2009.

Improved manufacturing of pharmaceuticals was the first major contribution of biotechnology to pharmaceutical care in the 1980s. Biotechnology-produced human insulin, growth hormone, and erythropoietin—all replacements of highly specific, endogenous molecules—were major advances in therapy. Since the late 1980s, however, pharmaceutical biotechnology also has helped to identify new compounds with new mechanisms of action. Significant contributions to our understanding about the mechanism of disease at the molecular level continue to be made by biotechnology researchers and will translate into newer, better pharmaceuticals. The impact of biotechnology on pharmaceutical care is expected to increase exponentially as advances in technology continue to yield novel medicinal agents, such as the colony-stimulating factors, tissue-type plasminogen activator, new vaccines, DNase, fusion protein drugs, and specific monoclonal antibodies. Products of biotechnology are playing a critical role in the discovery and design, as well as in the production, of treatments for life-threatening diseases including genetic disorders, cancer, and AIDS.

Pharmaceutical care using biotechnology-derived products requires:

1. An understanding of how the handling and stability of biopharmaceuticals differ from those of other drugs that pharmacists dispense.
2. A preparation of the product for patient use, including reconstitution or compounding, if required.
3. Patient education regarding their disease, benefits of the prescribed biopharmaceutical, potential side effects or drug interactions to be aware of, and the techniques to self-administer the biotechnology drug.
4. Patient counseling about the reimbursement issues involving an expensive product.
5. Monitoring of the patient for compliance.

Key areas of biotechnology growth include pharmacogenomics/pharmacogenetics; recombinant-based therapies, such as vaccines delivered by novel administrative routes; genetic modification of the patient; and cloning of human tissues and organs. The field has matured sufficiently with the generic-like versions of original biotech drugs, called "biogenerics," "biosimilars," or "follow-on biologics" (2,3).

Tanaji T. Talele, Marc Gillespie, and Vijaya L. Korlipara
Department of Pharmaceutical Sciences
St. John's University College of Pharmacy and Allied Health Professions
Queens, New York

involving insertion, deletion, or rearrangements of a very large number of base pairs.

Mutations result in a variety of changes to the gene product. If the base change occurs within the reading frame of the gene product, it may alter the amino acid sequence of the gene product (protein). SNPs have been defined as single base mutations that occur in 1% or more of the population (4). Many of these SNPs may be responsible for the production of a malfunctioning gene product that, in turn, is responsible for a serious disease. The well-used example is the A → T mutation in the β-globin gene, in which the GAG glutamic acid codon is changed to the GTG valine codon, resulting in abnormal aggregation of the hemoglobin molecules and causing sickle cell anemia. Another example is one form of β-thalassemia that results from a mutation of a CAG glutamine codon to the TAG stop codon early in the DNA sequence, resulting in premature termination of the translation process and total loss of the β subunit of the adult hemoglobin molecule.

In principle, one is able to manipulate the therapeutic outcome of a patient population by separating patients who will not respond normally to a particular drug therapy from those who will, based on an analysis of established genetic biomarkers related to the drug's metabolic profile (Fig. 6.1). Patients who are homozygous for the genetic biomarkers indicating poor metabolism of the recommended therapeutic agent may, depending on the therapeutic window of the drug, exhibit a response resembling an overdose to the normal drug dose and require a reduced dose to achieve therapeutic levels (patient A in Fig. 6.2), whereas patients carrying the biomarkers indicating extensive metabolism may exhibit a lack of efficacy at normal doses and require an increased dose of the drug to achieve therapeutic activity (patient D in Fig. 6.2). The patients who are homozygous or heterozygous for the normal (wild-type) genetic biomarker (patients B and C, respectively, in Fig. 6.2) may require no alteration of the "normal" dose of the drug for adequate therapeutic outcome.

The application of genetic variation to drug therapy centered on the variations seen in a number of drug metabolism enzymes and much of the pharmacogenetic research has developed with the phase I (oxidative) and phase II (conjugative) metabolic enzymes. Currently, considerable data relate SNPs in the coding and regulatory regions of these genes to poor metabolism of particular drugs that have the potential to result in drug overdoses in patients carrying the genetic variations and given the "normal" dose of drug (Fig. 6.3).

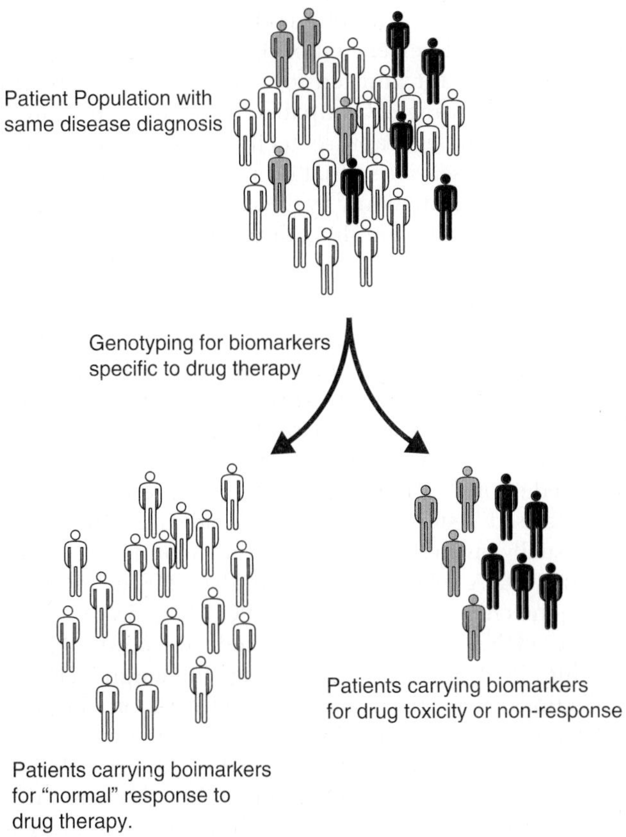

FIGURE 6.1 Manipulating therapeutic outcomes: manipulating therapeutic outcomes through pharmacogenetic analysis of a population with the same disease diagnosis to eliminate patients with genetic biomarkers indicating an adverse response to a particular drug therapy.

The action of a drug on the body is a complex interaction involving the metabolism of drugs, the transport of drugs throughout the body, and the interaction of the drug with its target. The parameters that describe this interaction are the pharmacokinetic (absorption, distribution, metabolism, and excretion) and pharmacodynamic (drug–target interaction) features of drug therapy. The biologic or pharmacodynamic targets of drug therapy are often candidate genes for biotechnology research (Fig. 6.4).

Transport proteins that move drugs through membrane barriers are critical in the absorption, distribution, and excretion of drugs and drug metabolites, whereas enzymes are critical in the metabolism of drugs in the body (Fig. 6.4). The pharmacodynamic pathway is represented most abundantly by the drug receptor pathway of drug response. This involves drug receptors as well as the numerous biochemical events that occur subsequent to drug–receptor interaction and before the measurement of the pharmacologic response. The complexity of the pharmacodynamic pathway can be simplified if one takes the modular biology approach and considers the many biochemical pathways between the drug–receptor interaction and the drug response to be linked modules of biochemical systems.

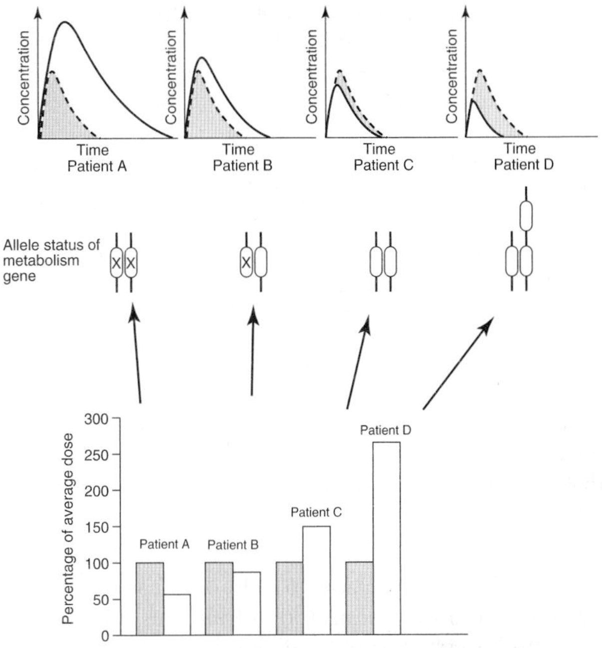

FIGURE 6.2 Dose–genotype relationship. A schematic representation of the potential benefit of adjusting drug dose to patient genotype. The theoretical "normal" drug concentration/time curve is depicted by the dashed line in the concentration/time curves of Patients A to D at the top of the figure, whereas the theoretical "genetic" drug concentration/time curve for each patient is expressed by the solid line. The allele status for each patient is shown below the theoretical plots. The oval containing the "X" indicates the presence of the detrimental allelic variation. The extra oval in Patient D indicates duplication of one of the normal alleles. The bar graph at the bottom of the figure indicates the normal doses (shaded) compared to the dose adjustments that should be made based on the patient's allele status (Kirchheiner J, Brockmoller J. Clinical consequences of cytochrome P450 2C9 polymorphisms. Clin Pharmacol Ther 2005;77:1–16.)

Thus, the candidate genes for the therapeutic drug pathway include the genes for drug metabolism, drug transport, and drug response (Table 6.1).

Genomics

Genomics is the study of the full complement of genetic information, both coding and noncoding, in an organism's genome. The main genomics technique is the use of SNPs as biomarkers to inform clinicians about subtypes of disease that require differential treatments and provide pharmacists with information for selection of the best therapeutic methodology to effectively manage the disease as well as provide an indication of the patients at risk of experiencing adverse reactions or those who will not respond to a given drug dose.

The general genotyping procedure for detecting known SNPs consists of polymerase chain reaction (PCR) amplification of the region of interest in the genome, discrimination of the alleles in that region, and detection of the discrimination products. Many genotyping

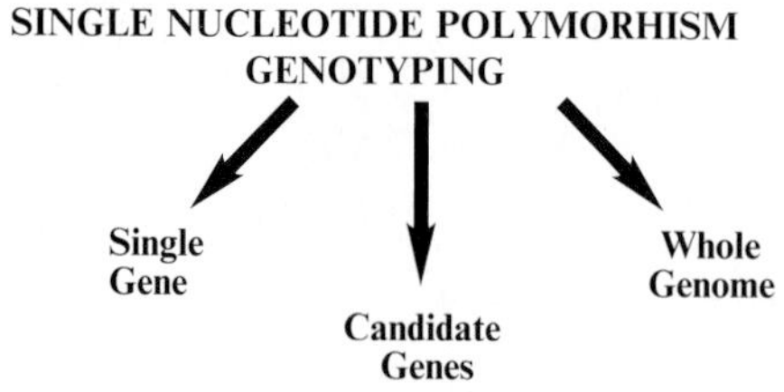

FIGURE 6.3 Single-nucleotide polymorphism (SNP) genotyping: approaches to genotyping for drug therapy. The single-gene approach has been used successfully in pharmacogenetic studies of a number of phase I and phase II metabolic enzymes. The candidate gene approach involves the selection of the genes for proteins that are demonstrated to be involved in a particular drug action, including metabolic enzymes, transport proteins, drug targets, and proteins involved in modular drug response pathways. The whole-genome approach uses SNPs evenly spaced throughout the genome.

technologies are available to choose from, and each has their advantages and disadvantages (Table 6.2). Discriminating between the alleles in the genomic region being examined is generally done by one of the five techniques illustrated in Figure 6.5.

The technique of choice for high-throughput genotyping is the minisequencing/primer extension technique augmented with the 5′-tag technology to permit the purification of the extended products via specific tags (Fig. 6.6). The genomic region of interest is PCR amplified, and the amplified DNA is exposed to allele-specific primers with 5′-tags that are complementary to oligonucleotides immobilized at specific locations in the wells of microtiter plates or on specific colored beads. Single base extension using DNA polymerase and fluorescently labeled 2′,3′-dideoxynucleotide triphosphates (ddNTPs) in solution is used to detect the SNP. The resulting fluorescently labeled and tagged DNA fragments are captured by complementary tags

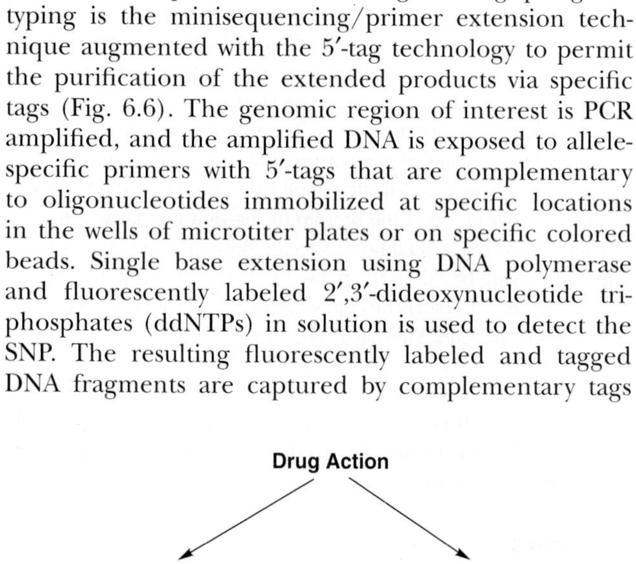

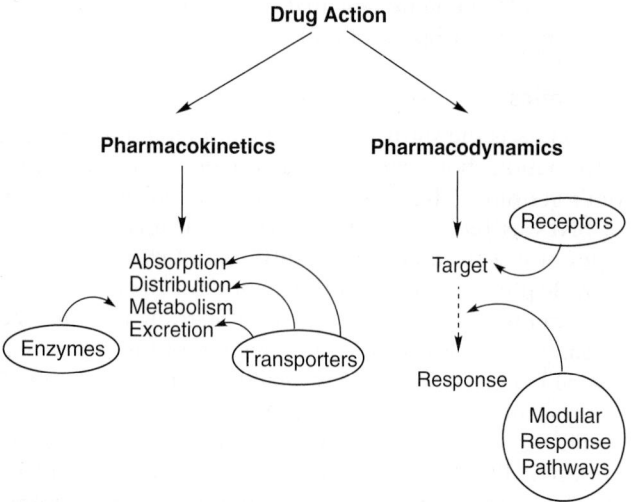

FIGURE 6.4 Schematic representation of the multigenic therapeutic drug pathway.

on microtiter plates or color-coded beads. Fluorescence resulting from laser excitation of the plates or beads is read by a detector and fed to a computer database for analysis and storage. Companies providing the single-base-extension tag–capture technology also provide a primer design service so that users can take advantage of multiplexing limited only by the capacity to design effective primers for the amplification and detection steps.

Transcriptomics

Transcriptomics is the technology behind the study of the full complement of mRNA transcripts in the cell's transcriptome and also is known as expression profiling. Methods of expression profiling are either "open" or "closed." Open systems do not require any advance knowledge of the sequence of the genome being examined; closed systems require some advance knowledge and usually involve the use of oligonucleotide or complementary DNA (cDNA) array hybridization technologies (the gene chip) and quantitative PCR (Fig. 6.7).

The cDNA arrays are prepared by spotting gene-specific PCR products, including full-length cDNAs, collections of partially sequenced cDNAs, or randomly chosen cDNAs from any library of interest onto a glass, silicon, gel, or bead matrix or a nylon or nitrocellulose membrane. The matrix (most often glass) is coated with polylysine, amino silanes, or amino-reactive silanes to assist in the attachment of the cDNA probes. The PCR products of the clones are purified and spotted onto the matrix by robots through contact printing or noncontact piezo or ink-jet devices. After cross-linking the probe to the matrix by ultraviolet irradiation, the probe is made single stranded by heat or alkali treatment. The mRNA target is prepared from both a test and reference sample by reverse transcription to produce cDNA, which is then labeled with fluorescent probes (one for the test and another for the reference). The fluorescent targets are pooled and hybridized to the probe array under very stringent conditions. Laser excitation of the hybridized samples on the matrix and comparison of the fluorescence intensity of the reference sample with the fluorescence intensity of the test sample using computer algorithms yield an emission characteristic of the increase or decrease of mRNA expression under test conditions.

Proteomics

Proteomics is the technology behind the study of the total protein complement of a genome, or the complete set of proteins expressed by a cell, tissue, or organism. The presence of an open reading frame in a DNA sequence indicates the presence of a gene, but it does not indicate gene transcription, RNA editing, translation, or posttranslational modification and the presence of isoforms. Analysis of the transcriptome does not indicate alteration of protein levels by proteolysis, recycling, and sequestration. Therefore, it is important to determine protein levels, protein expression, and protein–protein interactions directly.

TABLE 6.1 Specific Examples of the Application of Allelic Variation in Drug Therapy

Protein	Action	Drug	Therapy	Efficacy/Toxicity
CYP450 2D6	Drug metabolism	Codeine	Pain	Efficacy
CYP450 2C9	Drug metabolism	Warfarin	Coagulation	Toxicity (hemorrhage)
Thiopurine *S*-methyltransferase	Drug metabolism	Mercaptopurine	Acute lymphoblastic leukemia	Toxicity (myelotoxic)
HER2/neu	Drug target	Herceptin	Breast cancer	Efficacy
bcr/abl	Drug target	Gleevec	Chronic myelogenous leukemia	Efficacy
EGFR	Drug target	Erbitux	Colon cancer	Efficacy
Apolipoprotein E4	Marker	Tacrine	Alzheimer disease	Efficacy
Cholesteryl ester transferase	Marker	Statins	Atherosclerosis	Efficacy
ATP-binding cassette B1	Drug transport	Saquinavir	HIV	Efficacy
		Indinavir	Leukemia	
		Ritonavir		
		Daunorubicin		
		Etoposide		
UDP-glucuronosyl-transferase 1A1	Drug metabolism	Irinotecan	Cancer	Toxicity (myelotoxic)
N-Acetyltransferase 2	Drug metabolism	Isoniazid	Tuberculosis	Toxicity (hepatotoxic)
Pseudocholinesterase	Drug metabolism	Suxamethonium	Muscle relaxation during surgery	Toxicity (prolonged apnea)

Proteomics is divided into three main areas (5):

1. Microcharacterization for large-scale identification of proteins and posttranslational modifications (5).
2. Differential gel electrophoresis for comparison of protein levels (6).
3. Protein–protein interaction studies using protein chips (7), mass spectrometry isotope-coded affinity tag technology (8), and the yeast two-hybrid system (9).

Metabolomics

Metabolomics is the technology behind the measurement of metabolite concentrations, fluxes, and secretions in cells and tissues (metabolome). Metabolomics is at the cross-roads of genotype/phenotype interactions, where the interrelationship of metabolic pathways is considered to be the fundamental component of an organism's phenotype. Metabolomics is distinguished by the fact that metabolites are not directly linked to the genetic code but actually are products of a concerted action of many enzyme networks and other regulatory proteins (10). Metabolites also are more complex than nucleic acids, which are composed of four nucleotides, or proteins, which in turn are composed of 20 different amino acids. As a result, metabolites cannot be sequenced like genes and proteins so that their characterization requires that the structure of each metabolite be determined individually through description of elemental composition and stereochemical orientation of functional groups.

Metabolites are more than just products of enzyme-catalyzed reactions. They also are sensors and regulators of complex molecular interactions in the organism, and as a result, the composition of the metabolome can be altered by changes in the individual's environment. Therefore, a study of the metabolome is complicated not only by the uniqueness of the individual's genome but also by the uniqueness of the individual's environment. On the other side of the coin, however, one could consider the metabolome to be a very sensitive indicator of the individual's phenotype (11,12).

Metabolomics can be approached by using several different but related strategies:

1. Target analysis investigates the primary metabolic effect of a genetic variation, in which the analysis usually is limited to the substrate and/or product of the protein expressed by the altered gene.
2. Metabolic profiling limits the investigation to a number of predefined metabolites, usually in a specific metabolic pathway.
3. Metabolomics is a comprehensive analysis (both identification and quantification) of metabolites in a biologic system, which investigates the effect of multiple genetic variations on many different biochemical pathways.
4. Metabolic fingerprinting is a strategy to screen a large number of metabolites for biologic relevance in diagnostic or other analytical procedures in which it is important to rapidly distinguish

TABLE 6.2 Genotyping Technologies

Technique[a]	Mechanism of Allele Discrimination	Reaction Formate	Detection Mechanism[b]
Reverse dot blot	Hybridization	Solid support	Colorimetric
Microarray	Hybridization	Solid support	Fluorescence
DASH	Hybridization	Solid support	Fluorescence
Molecular beacons	Hybridization	Homogeneous reaction	FRET
5′-Nuclease cleavage (TaqMan)	Hybridization	Homogeneous reaction	FRET or FP
Cleavase (Invader Assay)	Hybridization	Homogeneous reaction	FRET, FP, MS
Biosensor microchip	Hybridization	Solid support	Electrochemical and fluorescence
AS-PCR	Primer extension	Homogeneous reaction	Fluorescence or FRET
AS-PE	Primer extension	Solid support	Fluorescence
APEX	Primer extension	Solid support	Fluorescence
FP-TDI	Primer extension	Homogeneous reaction	FRET or FP
MALDI-TOF MS	Primer extension	Homogeneous reaction	MS
Pyrosequencing	Primer extension	Homogeneous reaction or solid support	Luminescence
BioBeads and TagArrays	Primer extension	Homogeneous reaction and solid support capture	Fluorescence
OLA	Ligation	Homogeneous and solid support	Colorimetric and fluorescence
RCA	Ligation	Solid support	Fluorescence
Closed tube	Ligation	Homogeneous reaction	FRET
Microsphere/microarray ligation	Ligation	Homogeneous reaction	Fluorescence

[a]DASH, dynamic allele-specific hybridization; AS-PCR, allele-specific polymerase chain reaction; AS-PE, allele-specific primer extension; APEX, arrayed primer extension; FP-TDI, fluorescence polarization template directed dye terminator incorporation; MALDI-TOF-MS, matrix-assisted laser desorption/ionization time-of-flight mass spectrometry; OLA, oligonucleotide ligation assay; RCA, rolling circle amplification.
[b]FRET, fluorescence resonance energy transfer; FP, fluorescence polarization; MS, mass spectrometry.

between individuals in a population. Metabolic fingerprinting is the ultimate characterization of an individual's phenotype for disease diagnosis and drug therapy. Once the technologic problems of high-throughput metabolic analysis are developed in this area, it will be a major competitor of SNP analysis in pharmacogenomics.

The analytical technologies used in metabolomic investigations are nuclear magnetic resonance and mass spectrometry alone or in combination with liquid or gas chromatographic separation of metabolites. Other techniques include thin-layer chromatography, Fourier-transform infrared spectrometry, metabolite arrays, and Raman spectroscopy.

PHARMACEUTICAL BIOTECHNOLOGY METHODS

Pharmaceutical biotechnology is defined, at its most basic level, as the manipulation of nucleic acids in the production of therapeutic and diagnostic agents. In order to understand both DNA and RNA, the fundamental genetic material, it is important to understand the basic process that moves information from DNA to RNA. This process starts with transcription.

Transcription

The genetic information in DNA is transcribed to the intermediate RNA molecule that moves to the cytoplasm, where it directs the synthesis of the gene product it encodes using ribosomes. RNA differs chemically from DNA in that the sugar molecule is ribose and thymine in DNA is replaced by uracil in RNA. Structurally, RNA contains both single-stranded runs and short, double helical regions.

There are several types of RNA molecules in the cell, three of which are highlighted here. Messenger RNA (mRNA) is transcribed from a particular DNA sequence. Transfer RNAs (tRNAs) are covalently linked to specific amino acids and carry the anticodon triplet that recognizes a complementary trinucleotide sequence of mRNA specific for the amino acid that it carries. The ribosome contains both ribosomal RNA (rRNA) and proteins.

Several differences exist in the mechanism of transcription between prokaryotes and eukaryotes. These differences are important when evaluating if recombinant

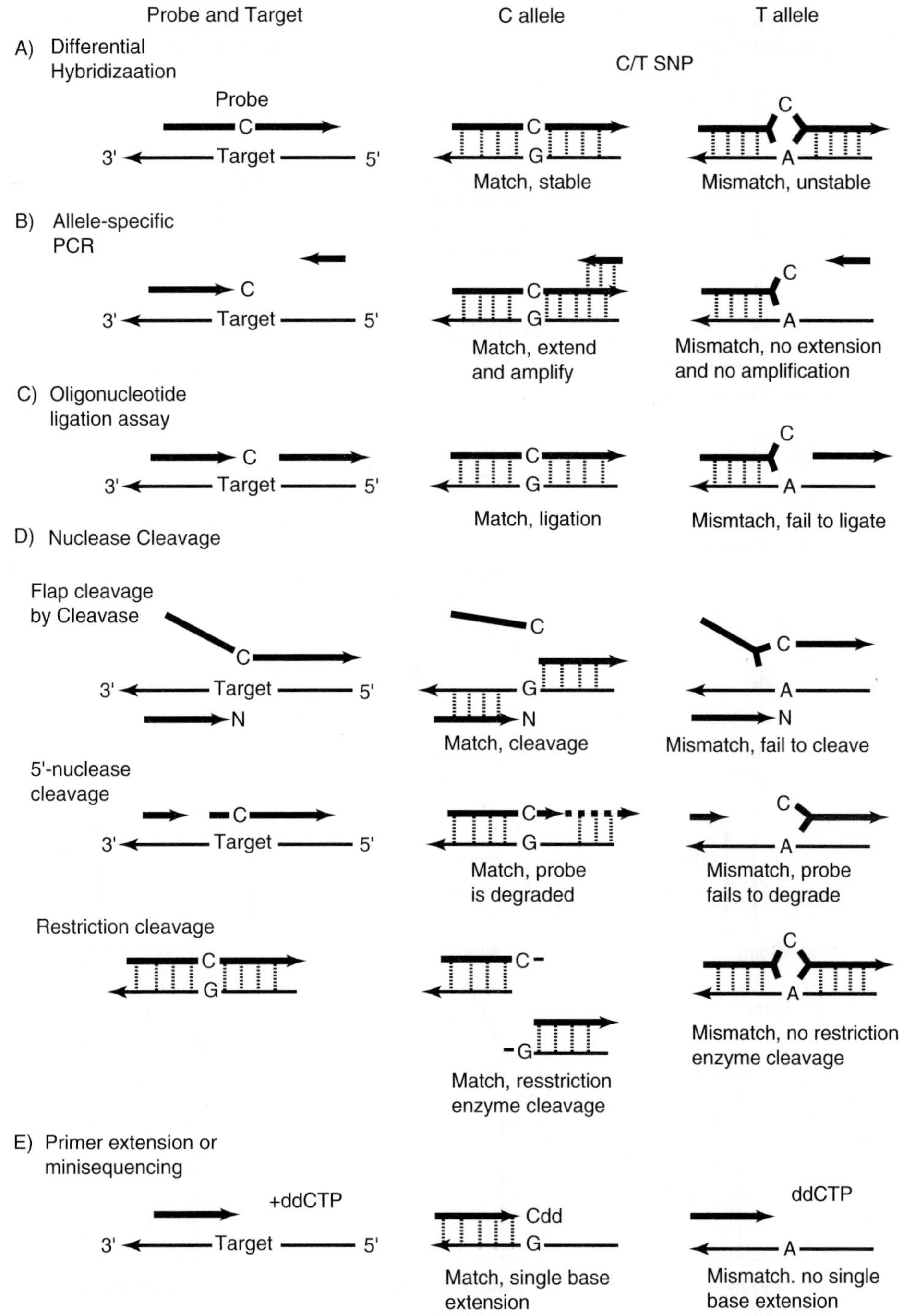

FIGURE 6.5 Allele discrimination strategies for the detection of the C allele of a C/T transition. Figure summarizes the five main biochemical reaction principles that underlie the single nucleotide polymorphism (SNP) genotyping technologies. Bold arrows indicate the probes; thinner arrows indicate the target. (From Syvanen AG. Accessing genetic variation: genotyping single-nucleotide polymorphisms. Nat Rev Genet 2001;2:930–942; Carlson CS, Newman TL, Nickerson DA. SNPing in the human genome. Curr Opin Chem Biol 2001;5:78–85, with permission.)

expression of a protein should be carried out in a eukaryotic or prokaryotic system. For our purposes, we describe transcription in a eukaryotic system.

Transcription is carried out by RNA polymerases, of which there are three types in the eukaryote. RNA pol I catalyzes the synthesis of rRNAs, RNA pol II is responsible for the synthesis of mRNA, and RNA pol III synthesizes tRNA. All three polymerases are large enzymes containing 12 or more subunits.

Each eukaryotic RNA polymerase copies DNA from the 3′ end, thus catalyzing mRNA formation in the 5′⇒ 3′ direction and synthesizing RNA complementary to the antisense DNA template strand. The reaction requires the precursor nucleotides adenosine triphosphate

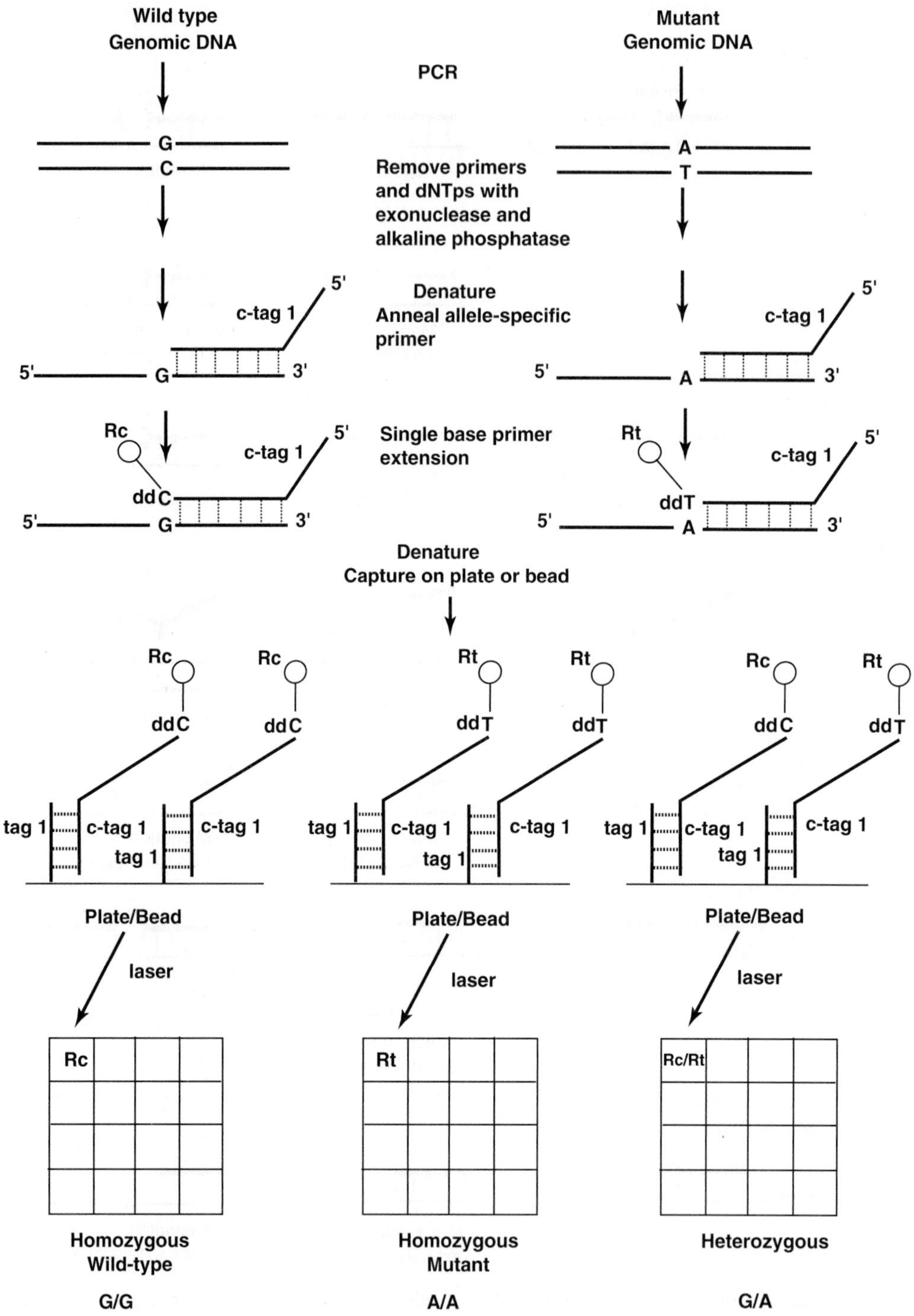

FIGURE 6.6. Tag-array and bead technology. Tag 1 is specific for the G/A mutation at a particular position in the gene under investigation. Other tags can be designed for other single nucleotide polymorphisms (SNPs) to permit multiplexing in the same well of the microtiter plate to produce an "array of arrays." R, reporter fluorescent label.

(ATP), guanosine triphosphate (GTP), cytidine triphosphate (CTP), and uridine triphosphate (UTP) and does not require a primer for initiation of transcription. The five stages of eukaryotic transcription include initiation, elongation and termination, capping, polyadenylation, and splicing.

Initiation

Eukaryotes have different RNA polymerase–binding promoter sequences than prokaryotes. The TATA consensus sequence of the eukaryotic promoter region is located 25 to 35 base pairs (bp) upstream from the transcription start site (Fig. 6.8). The low activity of

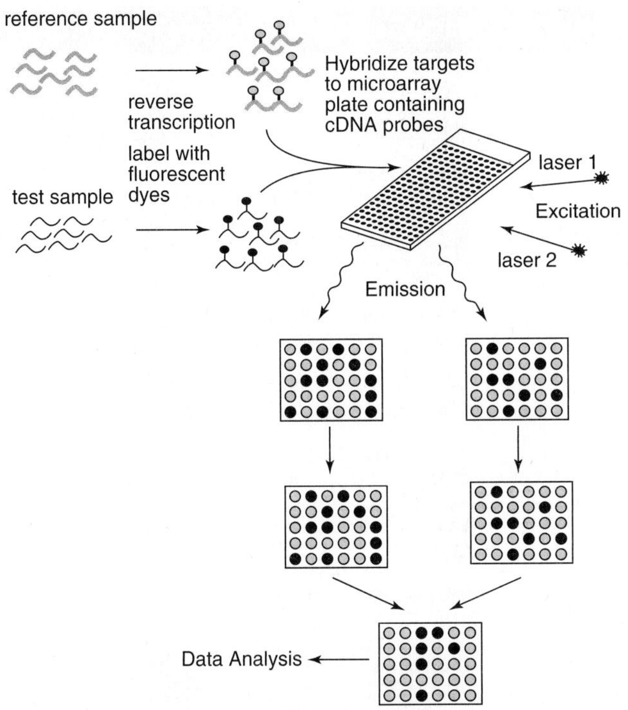

FIGURE 6.7 Schematic representation of a cDNA microarray chip. Probes of interest are obtained from DNA clones and printed on coated glass microscope slides. Analysis of mRNA expression is carried out by taking total mRNA from both a test and control sample, fluorescently labeling the samples with either Cy3- or Cy5-dUTP during a single round of reverse transcription, pooling the fluorescent targets, and hybridizing to the immobilized probes on the array under very stringent conditions. Laser excitation of the incorporated targets yields an emission with a characteristic spectrum, which is measured using a scanning confocal laser microscope and analyzed using a computer program. (From Duggan DJ, Bittner M, Chen Y, et al. Expression profiling using cDNA microarrays. Nat Genet 1999;21[Suppl 1]:10–14.)

basal promoters is greatly increased by the presence of upstream regulatory elements located 40 to 200 bp upstream of the promoter sequence and includes the SP1 box, the CCAAT box, and the hormone response elements. Transcription from many eukaryotic promoters can be stimulated by control elements, called enhancers, located many thousands of base pairs away from the transcription start site.

Elongation and Termination

RNA polymerase moves along the DNA template until a terminator sequence is reached. The RNA molecule made from a protein-coding gene by RNA pol II in eukaryotes is called pre-mRNA. The pre-mRNA from a eukaryotic protein-coding gene is extensively processed within the nucleus before export to the cytoplasm.

Capping

At the end of polymerization, the 5′ end of the pre-mRNA molecule is modified by addition of an *N*-7-methyl guanine molecule (Fig. 6.9).

Polyadenylation

The 3′ end of the pre-mRNA is generated by nucleases catalyzed cleavage followed by the addition of a run, or tail, of 100 to 200 adenosine nucleotides, resulting in what is called the poly(A) tail. Cleavage and polyadenylation require specific sequences in the DNA and its pre-mRNA transcript that are part of the transcription termination signal. The poly(A) tail helps stabilize the mRNA molecule, reducing its sensitivity to 3′-nuclease activity.

RNA Splicing

Splicing is the precise excision of the intron sequences and joining of exons to produce a functional mRNA molecule.

Translation

Once the fully processed mRNA has been transported from the nucleus to the cytoplasm, protein synthesis occurs. The triplet genetic code carried on the mRNA is translated into a protein sequence by the ribosome. Amino acids are delivered to the ribosome by tRNAs that carry specific amino acids attached to their 3′-terminus based on the tRNA anticodon sequence. The anticodon complements the triplet codon sequence in mRNA, and

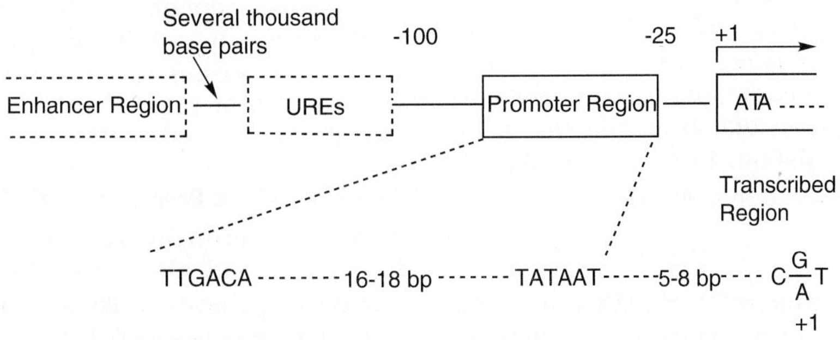

FIGURE 6.8 Schematic representation of the eukaryotic transcription unit showing the relationship between the promoter, upstream regulatory elements, and enhancer region. Note that transcription usually starts with a purine base in the 1 position. (Reproduced from Turner et al. BIOS Instant Notes in Molecular Biology. Garland Science/Taylor & Francis Books, Inc., 1997, with permission.)

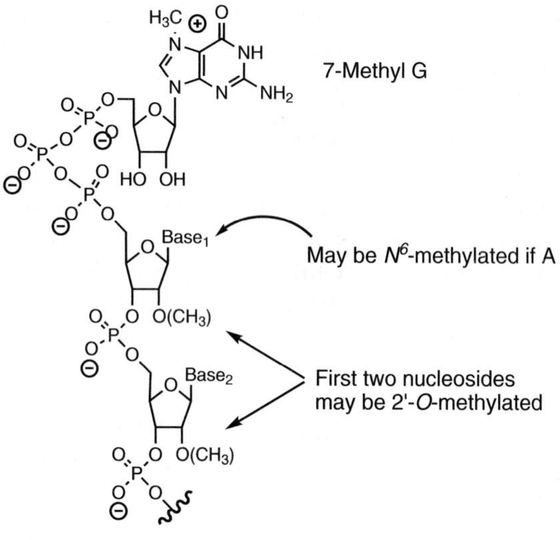

FIGURE 6.9 Chemical structure of the 5′-cap of mRNA. Cap 0 consists of the 7-methylguanosine triphosphate attached to the 5′ end of the mRNA. Cap 1 consists of the 7-methylguanosine and 2′-*O*-methylation of the 5′ base. Cap 2 consists of the 7-methylguanosine and the 2′-*O*-methylation of the first two bases in the sequence.

61 triplet sequences code for 20 amino acids (Table 6.3). Three codons are nonsense or stop codons that terminate translation. The code is degenerate with 18 of the 20 common amino acids coded for by more than one codon. Two amino acids, Met (AUG) and Trp (UGG), each have one unique codon. From a fixed start point on the mRNA (start codon, AUG), which establishes the open reading frame, each group of three bases in the coding region of the mRNA represents a codon that is recognized by a complementary triplet on the tRNA molecule.

There are four stages in the protein synthesis in both prokaryotes and eukaryotes:

1. *Initiation*—assembly of the ribosome on an mRNA molecule.
2. *Elongation*—repeated cycles of amino acid addition.
3. *Termination*—recognition of the stop codon, release of the new protein chain, and breakdown of the synthetic complex.
4. *Posttranslational modification*—usually includes protein cleavage by carboxy or amino peptidases, and chemical modification such as acetylation, sulfonylation, phosphorylation, hydroxylation, lipidation, and/or addition of polysaccharides.

Genes

A gene is the segment of genomic DNA (gDNA) involved in producing a polypeptide chain. The mRNA assembled from the gene includes regions preceding (the leader or 5′-untranslated region) and following (the trailer or 3′-untranslated region) the coding region as well as intervening sequences such as introns that are removed in the processing of the pre-mRNA. With the discovery of other processes that contribute to the penultimate sequence of the mature mRNA, the definition of a gene is evolving (13).

TABLE 6.3 The Genetic Code

First Position	Second Position				Third Position
	U	C	A	G	
U	Phe UUU	Ser UCU	Tyr UAU	Cys UGU	U
	Phe UUC	Ser UCC	Tyr UAC	Cys UGC	C
	Leu UUA	Ser UCA	Stop UAA	Stop UGA	A
	Leu UUG	Ser UCG	Stop UAG	Trp UGG	G
C	Leu CUU	Pro CCU	His CAU	Arg CGU	U
	Leu CUC	Pro CCC	His CAC	Arg CGC	C
	Leu CUA	Pro CCA	Gln CAA	Arg CGA	A
	Leu CUG	Pro CCG	Gln CAG	Arg CGG	G
A	Ile AUU	Thr ACU	Asn AAU	Ser AGU	U
	Ile AUC	Thr ACC	Asn AAC	Ser AGC	C
	Ile AUA	Thr ACA	Lys AAA	Arg AGA	A
	Met AUG	Thr ACG	Lys AAG	Arg AGG	G
G	Val GUU	Ala GCU	Asp GAU	Gly GGU	U
	Val GUC	Ala GCC	Asp GAC	Gly GGC	C
	Val GUA	Ala GCA	Glu GAA	Gly GGA	A
	Val GUG	Ala GCG	Glu GAG	Gly GGG	G

Cloning and the Preparation of DNA Libraries

Two discoveries in the early 1970s provided breakthroughs in nucleic acid chemistry: the discovery of bacterial enzymes capable of cleaving nucleic acids at specific, palindromic (symmetrical) base sequences (Figs. 6.10 and 6.11) and the discovery of bacterial plasmids as vehicles (vectors) to amplify and carry the gene fragments produced by those restriction enzymes. Plasmids are small,

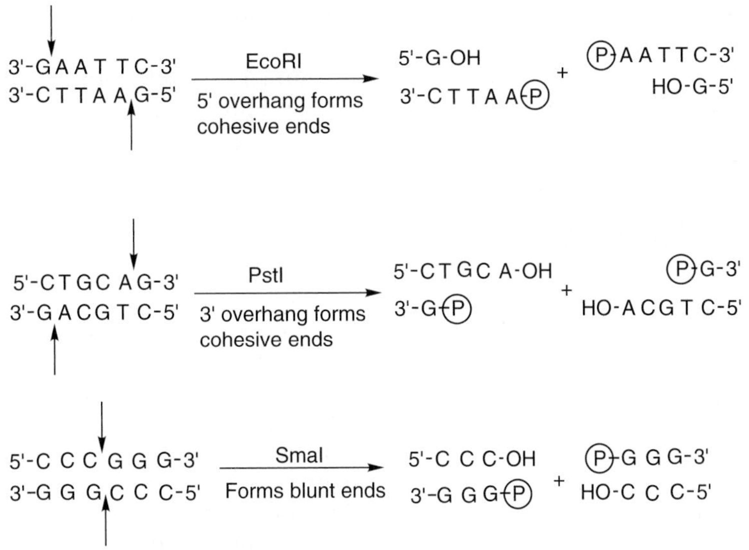

FIGURE 6.10 Actions of restriction endonucleases *EcoRI*, *PstI*, and *SmaI* at their recognition sequences. Note that *EcoRI* and *PstI* enzymes produce "sticky ends," with overlapping sequences, whereas *SmaI* produces "blunt ends," or nonoverlapping sequences.

circular, extrachromosomal nucleic acid molecules in bacteria that replicate independently within the bacterial cell. Restriction enzymes (and now PCR) are used to produce relatively small DNA fragments that are inserted into bacterial plasmid vectors, forming recombinant DNA (rDNA) molecules. The rDNA vectors are inserted into bacterial hosts, where the plasmid replicates with the bacteria, producing a large number of identical rDNA molecules known as clones, thus completing the process known as DNA cloning.

Sequencing DNA Fragments The two previous methods of nucleic acid sequencing, the Maxam and Gilbert method (chemical method) (14) and Sanger's dideoxy method (15), have been superseded by the far faster massive parallel sequencing methods. In short, high-throughput sequencing involves breaking up gDNA into fragments and placing the individual fragments onto specially designed microbeads where the many copies of each fragment have been amplified. The amplified fragments are then loaded into the small wells of a substrate. As the wells are loaded with sample, reagents are pumped across the plate. The addition of the reagents results in an enzymatic reaction between complimentary bases in the DNA fragments, and a fluorescent signal is released and read by a computational sequence analyzer (16).

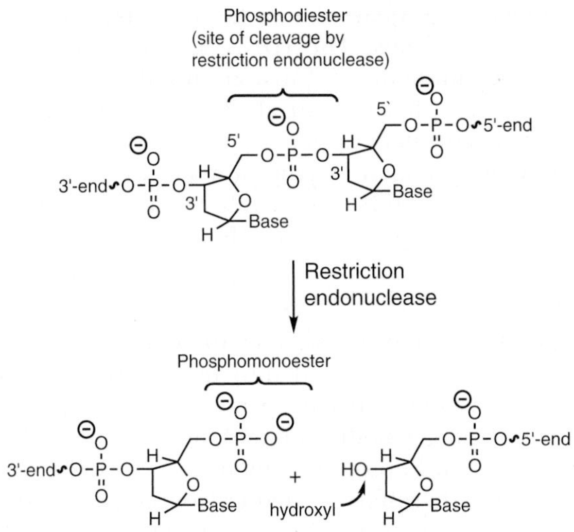

FIGURE 6.11 Cleavage by restriction endonuclease.

Synthesizing Oligonucleotides The need for short oligonucleotides of known sequence has grown tremendously with the need for radiolabeled and fluorescently labeled probes to isolate and characterize nucleic acids. The phosphite triester (17) and the phosphotriester methods (18) are convenient solid-phase automated techniques for the synthesis of oligonucleotides (Fig. 6.12).

Polymerase Chain Reaction Working with small quantities of nucleic acids isolated from cell and tissue sources is difficult, and there is often a need to amplify these sequences. PCR is used to amplify fragments of DNA without the need for cloning (19). The process can amplify samples that contain as little as a single nucleotide fragment used as template. There is a requirement for the sequences flanking the boundaries of the fragment to be amplified so that oligonucleotide primers can be prepared.

Protein Synthesis Through Recombinant DNA Once the gene coding for the desired protein has been identified and isolated (Fig. 6.13), the genetic material is

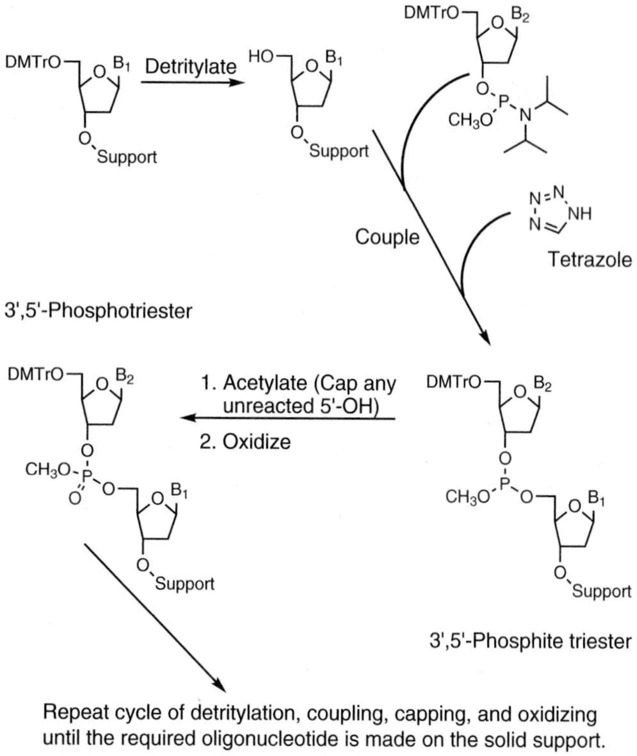

FIGURE 6.12 Solid-phase phosphate triester method of oligonucleotide synthesis.

introduced into cells on a vector capable of DNA replication and initiation of transcription. A cloning vector is a carrier molecule, the vehicle that is used to insert foreign DNA into a host cell. Typically, vectors are genetic elements that can be replicated in a host cell separately from that cell's chromosomes. Bacterial plasmids are circular DNA of only a few thousand base pairs that replicate freely within the cells and are ideal for carrying the gene into the host organism. DNA fragments coding for the desired protein can be cloned from gDNA or cDNA and inserted into the vector that carries the code to synthesize the protein in the host.

The vector containing the code for the target protein is then inserted into the host. Host cells are typically bacteria (e.g., *Escherichia coli*), eukaryotic yeast (e.g., *Saccharomyces cerevisiae* [baker's yeast]), or mammalian cell lines. The choice of host system is influenced primarily by the type of protein to be expressed and by the key differences among the various host cells (20). Overall protein yields generally are much lower in mammalian cells, but in some cases, this may be the only system that produces the specific protein of interest. It should be noted that recombinant proteins produced in gram-negative bacteria may contain endotoxins.

The host cells containing the vector are grown under selection to identify a clone that contains the desired gene and is able to produce the best protein (21). The selected cloned cells are used as inoculum first for a small-scale cell culture/fermentation, which is then followed by larger fermentations in bioreactors. The medium is carefully controlled to enhance cell reproduction and protein synthesis. The host produces its natural proteins along with the desired protein, which may be secreted into the growth medium. The protein of interest can then be isolated from the fermentation, purified, and formulated to give a potential rDNA-produced pharmaceutical.

Protein Isolation and Purification The isolation and purification of the final protein product from the complex mixture of cells, cellular debris, medium nutrients, and other host metabolites is a challenging task (20,21). The structure, purity, potency, and stability of the recombinant protein must be considered. Often, sophisticated filtrations, phase separations, precipitation, and complex multiple-column chromatographic procedures are required to obtain the desired protein. Although isolation of the recombinant protein, produced in culture in relatively large amounts, generally is easier than isolating the native protein, ensuring the stability and retention of the bioactive three-dimensional structure (correct protein folding) of any biopharmaceutical is a more arduous task. In addition, recombinant proteins from bacterial hosts require removal of endotoxins, whereas viral particles may need to be removed from mammalian cell culture products (22). A discussion of these techniques is beyond the scope of this chapter; however, useful reviews on the extraction and purification (20,21,23) and the analysis and chromatography (24–28) of biotechnology products are available as a resource for further information.

GENERAL PROPERTIES OF BIOTECHNOLOGY-PRODUCED MEDICINAL AGENTS

rDNA and hybridoma technologies have made it possible to produce large quantities of highly pure, therapeutically useful proteins. The rDNA-derived proteins and monoclonal antibodies (MAbs) are not dissimilar to the other protein pharmaceuticals or biopharmaceuticals that pharmacists have dispensed in the past. As polymers of amino acids joined by peptide bonds, the properties of these proteins differ generally from those of small organic molecule pharmaceuticals.

Stability of Biotech Pharmaceuticals

The instability of proteins, including protein pharmaceuticals, can be separated into three distinct classes. Chemical instability results from bond formation or cleavage yielding a modification of the protein and a new chemical entity. Photoinstability of protein drugs upon exposure to light results in chemical and physical instability. Physical instability involves a change to the secondary

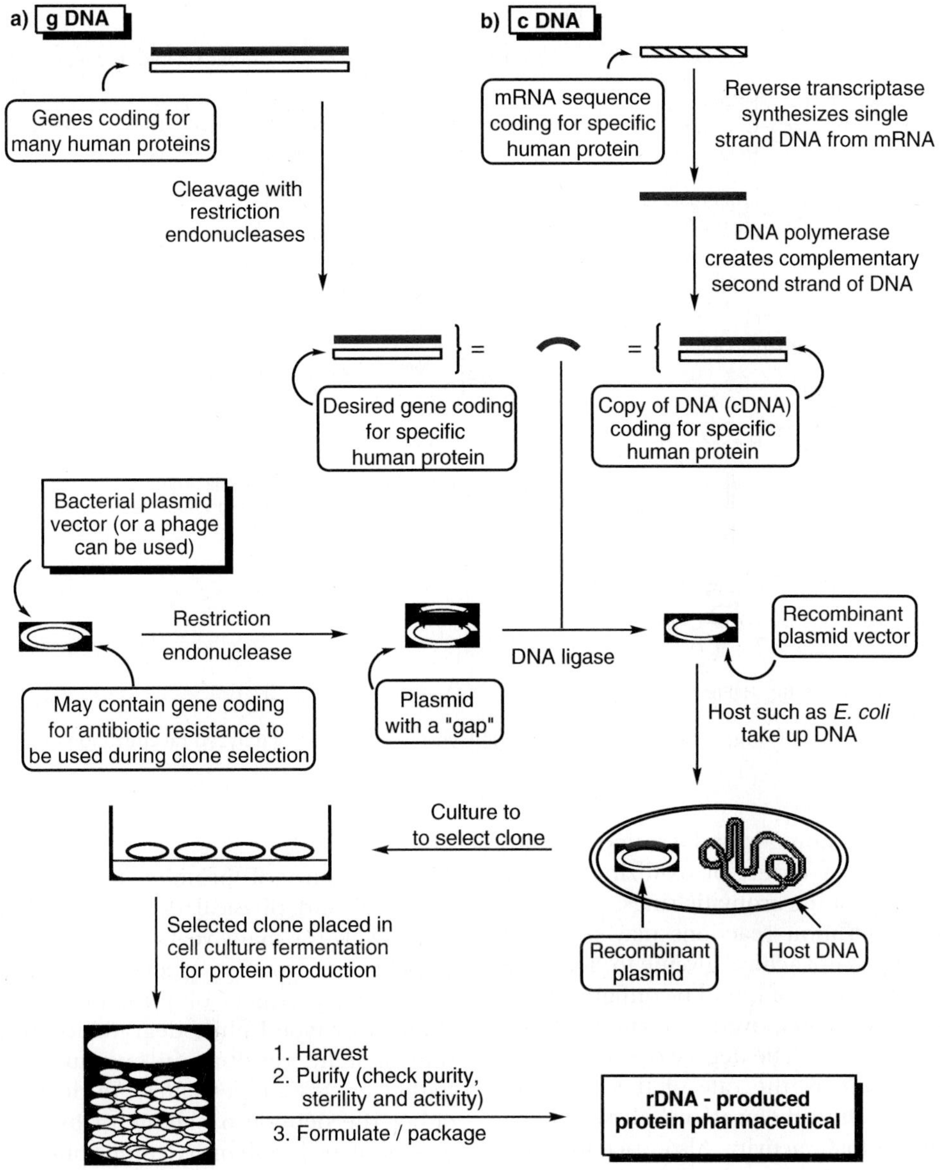

FIGURE 6.13 Summary of typical rDNA production of a protein from either (a) genomic DNA or (b) cDNA.

or higher-order structure of the protein rather than a covalent bond-breaking modification (29–36).

Chemical Instability

A variety of reactions give rise to the chemical instability of proteins, including hydrolysis, oxidation, racemization, β-elimination, and disulfide exchange (Fig. 6.14). Each of these changes may cause a loss of biologic activity. Proteolytic hydrolysis of peptide bonds results in fragmentation of the protein chain. It is well established that in dilute acids, aspartic acid residues in proteins are hydrolyzed at a rate at least 100-fold faster than that of other peptide bonds because of the mechanism of the reaction. An additional hydrolysis reaction is the deamidation of the neutral residue of asparagine and glutamine side-chain linkages, forming the ionizable carboxylic acid residues aspartic acid and glutamic acid (Fig. 6.14a). This conversion may be considered primary sequence isomerization.

Oxidative degradative reactions can occur to the side chains of sulfur-containing methionine and cysteine residues and the aromatic amino acid residues histidine, tryptophan, and tyrosine in proteins during their isolation and storage. The weakly nucleophilic thioether group of methionine ($R\text{-}S\text{-}CH_3$) can be oxidized at low pH by hydrogen peroxide as well as by oxygen in the air to the sulfoxide ($R\text{-}SO\text{-}CH_3$) and the sulfone ($R\text{-}SO_2\text{-}CH_3$). The thiol (sulfhydryl, R-SH) group of cysteine can be successively oxidized to the corresponding sulfenic acid (R-SOH), disulfide (R-SS-R), sulfinic acid ($R\text{-}SO_2H$), and finally, sulfonic acid ($R\text{-}SO_3H$). A number of factors, including pH, influence the rate of this oxidation.

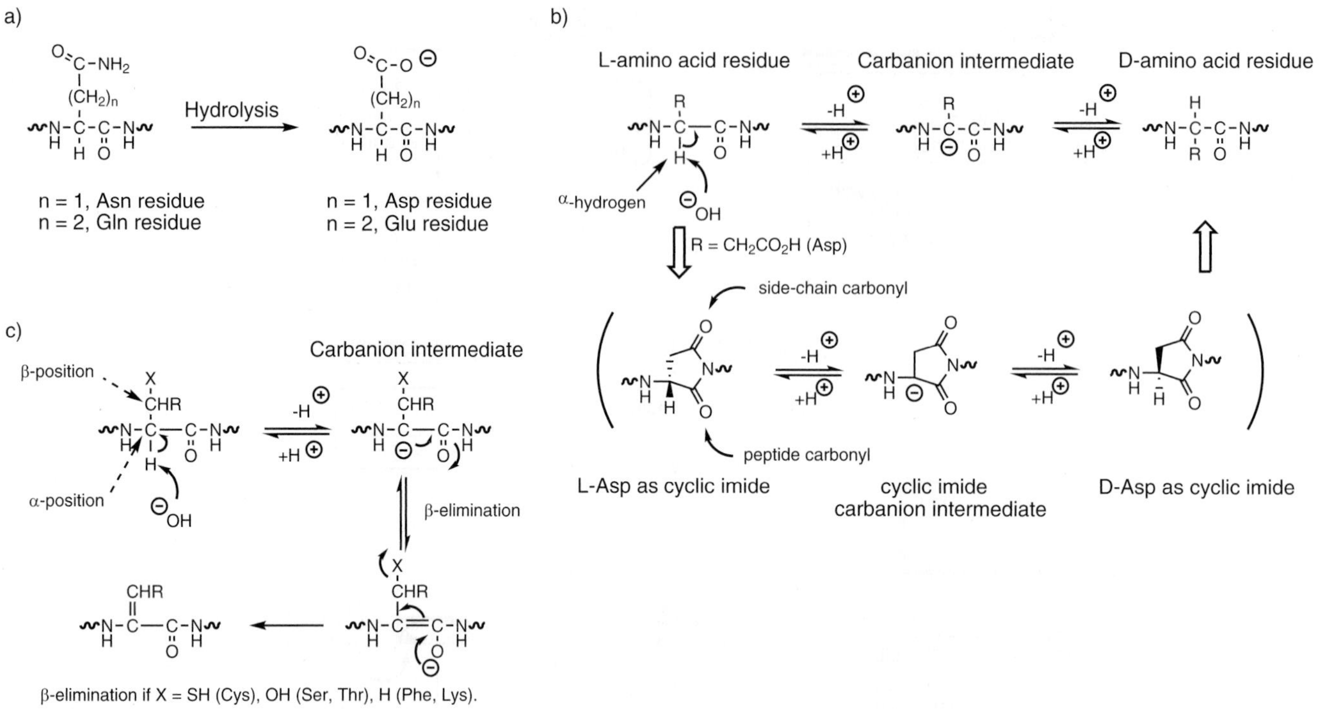

FIGURE 6.14 Chemical instability of protein biopharmaceuticals. (a) Hydrolysis. (b) Base-catalyzed racemization. (c) β-Elimination.

Oxidation of histidine, tryptophan, and tyrosine residues is believed to occur with a variety of oxidizing agents, resulting in the cleavage of the aromatic rings.

Base-catalyzed racemization reactions may occur in any of the amino acids except achiral glycine to yield residues in proteins with mixtures of L- and D-configurations. The α-methine hydrogen is removed to form a carbanion intermediate (Fig. 6.14b). The degree of stabilization of this intermediate controls the rate of this reaction. Racemization generally alters the proteins' physicochemical properties and biologic activity. Also, racemization generates nonmetabolizable D-configuration forms of the amino acids. Aspartate residues in proteins racemize at a 10^5-fold faster rate than when free, in contrast to the 2- to 4-fold increase for the other residues. The facilitated rate of racemization for aspartic acid residues is believed to result from the formation of a stabilized cyclic imide.

Proteins containing cysteine, serine, threonine, phenylalanine, and lysine are prone to β-elimination reactions under alkaline conditions (Fig. 6.14c). The reaction proceeds through the same carbanion intermediate as racemization. The reaction is influenced by a number of additional factors, including temperature and the presence of metal ions.

The interrelationships of disulfide bonds and free sulfhydryl groups in proteins are important factors influencing the chemical and biologic properties of protein pharmaceuticals. Disulfide exchange can result in incorrect pairings and major changes in the higher-order structure (secondary and above) of proteins. The exchange may occur in neutral, acidic, and alkaline media.

Photoinstability

The exposure of proteins to light and the ensuing chemical and physical degradation have been studied extensively for many years (36). The peptide backbone, tryptophan, tyrosine, phenylalanine, and cysteine are the primary targets of photodegradation in proteins. Primary or type I photodegradation begins with absorption of light, resulting in excitation of an electron to higher energy singlet states. Absorption occurs through either the peptide backbone or by the amino acid side chains of tryptophan, tyrosine, phenylalanine, and cysteine. In aqueous solution, the absorption wavelengths are 180 to 230 nm for the peptide backbone, 280 to 305 nm for tryptophan, 260 to 290 nm for tyrosine, 240 to 270 nm for phenylalanine, and 250 to 300 nm for cysteine. Although tryptophan is present in relatively low abundance in proteins, it has the highest molar absorption coefficients and is therefore a major player in the photodegradation of protein drugs.

The major photolytic pathways of tryptophan in proteins are shown in Figure 6.15. Following absorption of light, the excited state tryptophan will either relax to the lowest energy singlet state followed by fluorescence, undergo intersystem crossing to the triplet state (^{3}tryptophan), or eject an electron with formation of a tryptophan radical cation that will rapidly deprotonate to form the neutral tryptophan radical. The tryptophan radical may extract a hydrogen from a nearby tyrosine, repairing the tryptophan and forming a tyrosine phenoxy radical; react with oxygen, if present, forming a peroxy radical on the Trp; or react with nearby amino acids.

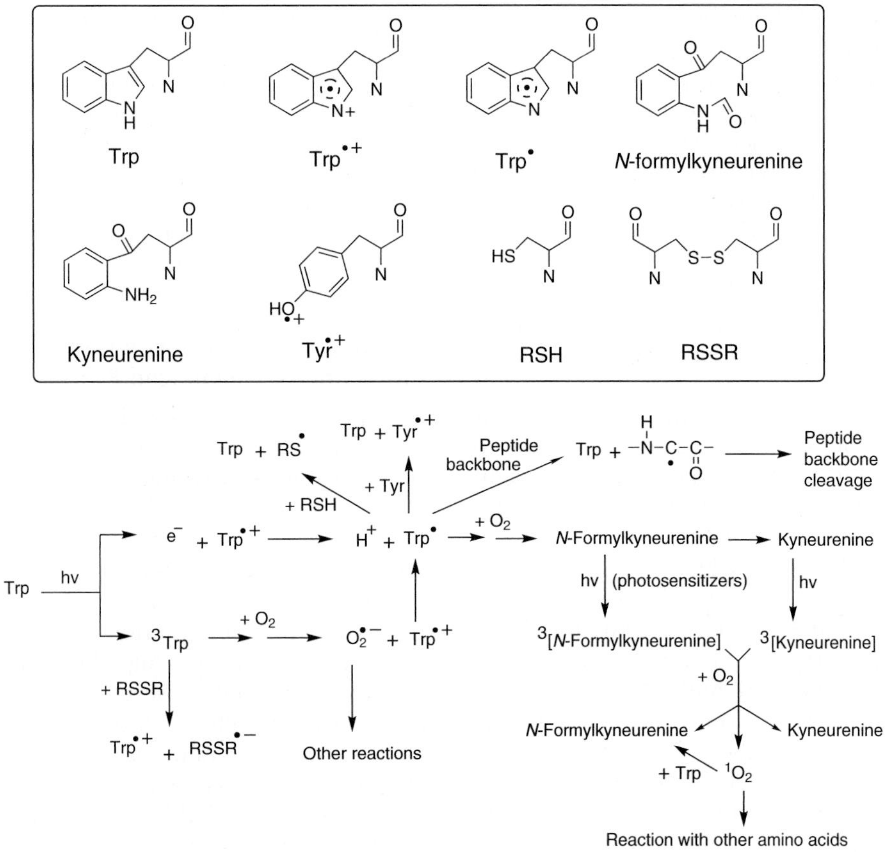

FIGURE 6.15 Structure of tryptophan (Trp) and common photolytic pathways.

The ejected electron can become solvated forming an e^-_{aq} or migrate along the peptide backbone and react with cystine residues, forming a disulfide radical anion as discussed below. Under anaerobic conditions, the tryptophan triplet state generally either relaxes back to the ground state with formation of light at 420 to 500 nm or electron transfers to a nearby cystine with subsequent reactions as discussed earlier. In the presence of oxygen, formation of the tryptophan-based peroxy radical can undergo further reaction to produce *N*-formylkyneurenine and kyneurenine. Interestingly, the *N*-formylkyneurenine and kyneurenine absorb light at longer wavelengths than Trp, thereby acting as photosensitizers to visible light, causing additional damage to the protein. Likewise, photodegradation of tyrosine, phenylalanine, cysteine, and histidine residues in proteins can occur.

Changes in the primary structure of the protein can result in changes in the secondary and tertiary structures impacting long-term stability, bioactivity, and immunogenicity of the peptide and protein drugs. Complete protection of the proteins from light is the only method to prevent photodegradation. This is achieved with primary and secondary packaging containers such as cardboard boxes that block incoming light to the protein. Addition of excipients such as methionine is also used to further reduce the protein aggregation as in the case of darbepoetin alfa formulation. Methionine is known to react with peroxide to form methionine sulfoxide and likely reduces protein aggregation through its effect as a peroxide scavenger. Because photodegradation reactions occur through generation of singlet oxygen species, which are generated during the photolytic process by reaction of molecular dioxygen, some biopharmaceutical products, both liquid and lyophilized, are packaged in inert atmospheres.

Physical Instability

Generally not encountered in most small organic molecules, physical instability is a consequence of the polymeric nature of proteins. Proteins adopt secondary, tertiary, and quaternary structures, which influence their three-dimensional shape and, therefore, their biologic activity. Any change to the higher order structure of a protein may alter both. Physical instability includes denaturation, adsorption to surfaces, and noncovalent self-aggregation (soluble and precipitation). The most widely studied aspect of protein instability is denaturation. Noncovalent aggregation, however, is one of the primary mechanisms of protein degradation (29).

A protein, in principle, can be folded into a virtually infinite number of conformations. Denaturation occurs by disrupting the weaker noncovalent interactions that hold a protein together in its secondary and tertiary structures. Temperature, pH, and the addition of organic solvents and solutes may cause denaturation. The process can be reversible or irreversible. In general, denaturation affects the protein by decreasing aqueous solubility, altering three-dimensional molecular shape, increasing susceptibility to enzymatic hydrolysis, and causing the loss of the native protein's biologic activity.

Handling and Storage of Biotechnology-Produced Products

The preparation and administration of protein drugs of synthetic, recombinant, or hybridoma origin are dissimilar to the nonprotein pharmaceuticals. Proteins generally have more limited shelf stability. The average shelf life for a biotechnology product is 12 to 18 months, compared with more than 36 months for a small-molecule weight drug. Although each individual biotechnology drug may be different, several generalizations can be made.

Proper storage of the lyophilized and the reconstituted drug is essential. Most of these drugs are expensive, so special care must be taken not to inactivate the therapeutic protein during storage and handling. The human proteins have limited chemical and physical stability, which is shortened on reconstitution. Expiration dating ranges from 2 hours to 30 days. The self-association of either native state or misfolded protein subunits may readily occur under certain conditions. This can lead to aggregation and precipitation and results in a loss of biologic activity. Self-association mechanisms depend on the conditions of formulation and may occur as a result of hydrophobic interactions.

Many of the biotechnology-produced drugs are stored refrigerated, but not frozen (2°C to 8°C). In general, temperature extremes must be avoided. One example is the rDNA-produced, blood clot–dissolving drug alteplase. A recombinant version of a naturally occurring human tissue-type plasminogen activator, lyophilized alteplase is stable at room temperature for several years if protected from light (37). Freezing or exposure to excessive heat decreases the physical stability of the protein. Anything that causes denaturation or self-aggregation, even though labile peptide bonds are not broken, may inactivate the protein. Some pharmacy facilities may need to increase cold storage capacity to accommodate biotech storage needs. If the patient must travel any distance home after receiving the medication, the pharmacist should help package the biotechnology product according to the manufacturer's directions. This may mean supplying a reusable cooler for the patient's use. Because the protein drug should not be frozen, the cooler should contain an ice pack rather than dry ice.

Some rDNA-derived pharmaceuticals, particularly the cytokines (e.g., the interferons, interleukin-2, and colony-stimulating factors), require human serum albumin in their formulation to prevent adhesion of the protein drug to the glass surface of the vial, which results in loss of protein (37–39). The amount of human serum albumin added varies with the biotech product. The vials should not be shaken to prevent foaming of the albumin, which causes protein loss or inactivation of the biotechnology-derived proteins. Care must be exercised in reconstituting protein pharmaceuticals. The diluent used for reconstitution of biotechnology drugs varies with the product and is specified by the manufacturer. Diluents can include normal saline, bacteriostatic water, and 5% dextrose. Several reviews of biotechnology drugs written for pharmacists contain additional information on the subjects of handling and storage (40–45).

Pharmacokinetic Considerations of Biotechnology-Produced Proteins

The processes of absorption into, distribution within, metabolism by, and excretion from the body (i.e., ADME) of biotechnology-produced pharmaceuticals are important factors affecting the time course of their pharmacologic effect. To deliver quality pharmaceutical care with biotech products, a pharmacist must be able to apply pharmacokinetic principles to establish and maintain a nontoxic, therapeutic effect. The pharmacokinetics of protein and peptide drugs differ in some pharmacokinetic aspects from those of the small-molecule organic agents with which we are most familiar. Although a lengthy discussion of this topic is beyond the scope of this chapter, a brief overview of metabolism follows. Useful reviews also are available for further information (46,47).

The plasma half-life of most administered proteins and peptides is relatively short, because they are susceptible to a wide variety of metabolic reactions. The enzymes involved in peptide bond hydrolysis and, thus, the degradation of peptides and proteins are known as peptidases and can be found in the blood, in the vascular bed, in the interstitial fluid, on cell membranes, and within cells. These enzymes include carboxypeptidases (cleaves C-terminal residues), dipeptidyl carboxypeptidases (cleaves dipeptides from the C-terminus), aminopeptidases (cleaves N-terminal residues), and amidases (cleaves internal peptide bonds). For the most part, these enzymes are all specific for the natural amino acids of the L-configuration. Overall, the metabolic products of most proteins and peptides are not considered to be a safety issue. They generally are broken down into amino acids and reincorporated into new, endogenously biosynthesized proteins.

Metabolic oxidation reactions may occur to the side chains of sulfur-containing residues, similar to that observed for in vitro chemical instability. Methionine can be oxidized to the sulfoxide, whereas metabolic oxidation of cysteine residues forms a disulfide. Metabolic reductive cleavage of disulfide bridges in proteins may occur, yielding free sulfhydryl groups.

Biotechnology Drug Delivery

Protein-based pharmaceuticals, whether produced by biotechnology or isolated from traditional sources, present challenges to drug delivery because of the unique demands imposed by their physicochemical and biologic properties. Although a detailed discussion of this topic is beyond the scope of this chapter, a brief overview follows. Useful reviews also are available for further information (31,48–52).

Delivery of large molecular weight, biotechnology-produced drugs into the body is difficult because of the poor absorption of these drugs, the acid lability of peptide bonds, and the rapid enzymatic degradation of these drugs in the body. In addition, protein pharmaceuticals are susceptible to physical instability, complex feedback control mechanisms, and peculiar dose–response relationships.

Given the limitations of today's technology, the strongly acidic environment of the stomach, the peptidases in the gastrointestinal tract, and the barrier to absorption presented by gastrointestinal mucosal cells preclude successful oral administration of most protein and peptide drugs. Therefore, administration of all the biotechnology-produced protein drugs and some natural or synthetic peptides currently is parenteral (by intravenous, subcutaneous, or intramuscular injections) to provide a better therapeutic profile. Manufacturers supply most of these drugs as sterile solutions without a preservative. In such cases, it is recommended that only one dose be prepared from each vial to prevent bacterial contamination.

Novel solutions to overcome delivery problems associated with biotechnology protein products and natural or synthetic peptide drugs are being explored. Oral drug delivery approaches in development for proteins and peptide drugs include conjugated systems (e.g., PEGylation with polyethylene glycol), amino acid substitution, liposomes, microspheres, erythrocytes as carriers, and viruses as drug carriers (30).

PEGylation is frequently used to improve the pharmacokinetic properties of biotechnology-produced drugs (53). This method involves the attachment of a flexible strand or strands of polyethylene glycol (PEG) to a protein. PEG is a simple, water-soluble, nontoxic polymer that is nonimmunogenic, is readily cleared from the body, and has been approved for human administration by mouth, injection, and topical application. The most common process used for PEGylation of protein is to activate the PEG with functional groups suitable for reaction with lysine and N-terminal amino groups. PEGylated proteins are less rapidly broken down by the body's enzymes than are unmodified proteins. PEG can extend the duration of action of proteins and peptides in the body from minutes, to hours, to days, depending on the PEG molecule used. By increasing the biologic half-life and improving the efficacy of proteins in the body, these modifications can reduce the frequency of injections a patient requires. They also reduce the rapidity and intensity of the body's immune reaction against molecules such as interferon. Several PEGylated protein products (e.g., pegvisomant, certolizumab pegol, peginterferon α2a) are currently marketed, and many are under development.

When metabolism studies indicate a predominant cleavage site, attempts can be made to replace that residue with another that retains the receptor-binding activity of the protein/peptide drug while yielding enhanced resistance to peptidase activity. Often, this can be accomplished by replacing the offending L-residue with its enantiomer, the D-amino acid, or another D-residue. Many peptidases are unable to cleave peptide bonds consisting of a "fraudulent" D-amino acid, and peptides containing such changes are designed as a means to increase their half-life. Also, the replacement of an L-amino acid with L-proline or *N*-methylation of the amide nitrogen offers the possibility of generating a peptide that is more resistant to enzymatic hydrolysis. The introduction of pseudopeptide bonds (54) and the design of retro-inverso peptides (55) are two examples of strategies that can afford peptidase resistance to peptide drugs.

Adverse Effects

An important consideration in the pharmaceutical care of a patient being administered a biotechnology-produced medicinal agent is the potential for adverse reactions. Many of the protein drugs are biotechnology-derived versions of endogenous human proteins normally present, on stimulus, in minute quantities near their specific site of action. Therefore, the same protein administered in much larger quantities may cause adverse effects not commonly observed at normal physiologic concentrations (46,47,56). Careful monitoring of patients administered biotechnology-produced drugs is critical for the health care team.

Immunogenicity

The immune system may respond to an antigen, such as a protein pharmaceutical, by triggering the production of antibodies. Biotechnology-derived proteins may possess a different set of antigenic determinants (i.e., regions of a protein recognized by an antibody) because of structural differences between the recombinant protein and the natural human protein (29,46,52). Factors that can contribute to this immunogenicity include lack of or incorrect glycosylation, amino acid modifications, and amino acid additions and deletions. A number of recombinant proteins produced with bacterial vectors contain an N-terminal methionine in addition to the natural human amino acid sequence. Bacterial vector-derived recombinant protein preparations also may contain small amounts of immunoreactive bacterial polypeptides as possible contaminants. Additionally, immunogenicity may result from proteins that are misfolded, denatured, or aggregated.

THERAPEUTIC PEPTIDE AND PROTEIN DRUGS

The following sections introduce a variety of peptide and protein hormones, both natural and synthetic, and their recombinant analogs that are commercially available for the treatment of various diseases or are used for diagnostic purposes. These hormones are obtained synthetically, from natural sources, or via genetic engineering. They are listed, for the most part, according to their endocrine organ of origin. Space does not allow us to discuss other biologically significant peptides and proteins. Table 6.4, however, summarizes some of the interesting peptides and proteins used in medicine. Recombinant DNA technology provides a powerful tool for new pharmaceutical product development and production. Biotechnology-produced medicinal agents discussed in this chapter include hormones, enzymes, cytokines, hematopoietic growth factors, other growth factors, blood clotting factors and anticoagulants, vaccines, and monoclonal antibodies.

Production of Peptide and Protein Drugs

The production of many of important peptides and proteins, via synthetic procedures as well as through biotechnology, involves the pharmaceutical industry. Of necessity, peptides of low to moderate molecular weight, chemically modified peptides, and those containing pseudopeptide bonds or fraudulent amino acids will continue to be made by synthetic procedures rather than through biotechnology. Many of these hormones are available as chemical analogs, and these also are discussed, particularly the chemical changes made and the implications of these changes to the resulting biologic action.

Peptide and Protein Hormones and Analogs

Hormones of Hypothalamic Origin

The hypothalamus, a relatively small organ that is located in the brain and is responsible for thermoregulation, among other functions, is the secretory source for a number of peptide hormones that are transported to the pituitary gland situated immediately below it. These hormones regulate the synthesis of other peptide hormones produced by the anterior pituitary (adenohypophysis) and are thus called releasing hormones, releasing factors, or inhibitory factors, as the case may be. The release of these hypothalamic hormones is regulated via cholinergic and dopaminergic stimuli from higher brain centers, and their synthesis and release are controlled by feedback mechanisms from their target organs.

Gonadotropin-Releasing Hormone

Gonadotropin-releasing hormone (GnRH) is a decapeptide (Fig. 6.16) that causes the release of the gonadotropins, luteinizing hormone (LH) and follicle-stimulating hormone (FSH), from the anterior pituitary gland, but

TABLE 6.4 Additional Significant Peptides and Proteins of Biologic Interest

Generic Name	Trade Name	General Use or Action
Exenatide	Byetta	39-Peptide known as an incretin mimetic; an agonist of glucagon-like peptide-1, used adjunctively in type 2 diabetes mellitus
Liraglutide	Victoza	Analog of human glucagon-like peptide-1 of rDNA origin used adjunctively in type 2 diabetes mellitus
Insulin-like growth factor-1 (human)		Protein of rDNA origin that has orphan drug status and is used in treating major burns requiring hospitalization
Secretin, synthetic human	Chirhostim	27-peptide used to evaluate exocrine pancreas function and in diagnosis of gastrinoma (Zollinger-Ellison syndrome)
Thymopentin	Timunox	Synthetic 5-peptide consisting of residues 32–36 of thymopoietin, an immunologically active polypeptide. It is an investigational drug used for its immunomodulating properties.
Thyrotropin alfa	Thyrogen	Recombinant form of human thyroid-stimulating hormone (rhTSH); used diagnostically for serum thyroglobulin testing
Carfilzomib		Multiple myeloma
Nesiritide	Natrecor	Acute decompensated congestive heart failure
Enfuvirtide	Fuzeon	HIV-1 infection
Ziconotide	Prialt	Chronic pain
Lanreotide	Somatuline	Acromegaly
Romiplostim	Nplate	Chronic idiopathic thrombocytopenic purpura
Degarelix	Firmagon	Advanced prostate cancer
Botulinum toxin A	Dysport	Inhibits release of acetylcholine, leading to its utility in diseases characterized by excessive efferent activity in motor nerves
Ecallantide	Kalbitor	Acute attacks of hereditary angioedema
Tesamorelin acetate	Egrifta	Analog of growth hormone-releasing hormone for HIV-associated lipodystrophy

not in equal amounts. Therefore, GnRH is intimately involved in the control of both male and female reproduction. Medicinal chemists have capitalized on the relatively simple decapeptide structure of GnRH by preparing many analogs as potential fertility and antifertility agents, several of which are commercially available, especially those that are referred to as superagonists. It is known that GnRH can be degraded by enzymatic cleavage between Tyr 5–Gly 6 and Pro 9–Gly 10 (57). Structure–activity relationship studies of GnRH analogs have shown that when Gly 6 is replaced with certain D-amino acids, as well as with changes in the peptide C-terminus, they generally are less susceptible to proteolytic enzymes, resulting in a longer-lasting action. For that reason, they are referred to as superagonists. Furthermore, half-life of GnRH analogs is enhanced by substituting hydrophobic D-amino acids at position 6 (Fig. 6.16).

In physiologic doses, GnRH agonists are able to induce ovulation and spermatogenesis by increasing LH and FSH levels and the resulting sex steroid levels, as does the normal hormone. In larger pharmacologic (therapeutic) doses, however, GnRH agonists, especially the superagonists, block implantation of the fertilized egg, cause luteolysis of the corpus luteum, and can act as postcoital contraceptive agents (although not approved for this latter use). This "paradoxical" antifertility effect seen with the superagonists has been attributed to the fact that GnRH must be administered in a low-dose, pulsatile manner for it to be therapeutically effective as a fertility agent. Natural GnRH release from the hypothalamus occurs in a pulsatile manner. When GnRH or, especially, a superagonist is administered in pharmacologic doses each day, LH and FSH levels will initially rise but then begin to fall after a few days because of target tissue desensitization/downregulation of pituitary GnRH receptors. The continued use of these agents in a nonpulsatile manner will result in a drastic drop of the gonadal steroid levels to near castrate levels in both males and females, thereby giving rise to their use in such conditions as precocious puberty, endometriosis, and advanced metastatic breast and prostate carcinoma. Typically, however, the GnRH superagonists take approximately 2 weeks to finally desensitize the GnRH receptors, and during this time, there is a transient rise in LH and FSH levels, which often results in an initial "flare-up" of the original symptoms. The following discussion concerns the medicinal chemistry and medical use of the commercially available GnRH analogs (58).

Specific Drugs

Leuprolide Acetate Leuprolide acetate, a synthetic nonapeptide analog of GnRH that possesses greater potency than the natural hormone, is a superagonist that is commercially available. Leuprolide acetate contains substitutions that hinder enzymatic degradation, D-Leu and NH-Et in place of glycine 6 and glycine 10 -NH_2, respectively (Fig. 6.16). Leuprolide acetate exhibits 15-fold higher potency than natural GnRH. When given continuously and in therapeutic doses, leuprolide acetate inhibits LH and FSH secretion by desensitizing/downregulating the GnRH receptors, as discussed previously. After an initial stimulation, chronic administration of leuprolide acetate results in suppression of ovarian and testicular steroidogenesis. In premenopausal females, estrogens are reduced to postmenopausal levels; in males, testosterone is reduced to castrate levels.

Leuprolide acetate is administered by daily injections or as depot injections every month, every 3 months, every 4 months, or every 6 months as a palliative treatment in advanced prostatic carcinoma (as an alternative to orchiectomy). An implant version (Viadur) also is available for long-term palliative therapy; after implantation of the device into the upper arm, leuprolide acetate is continuously released over a 12-month period. Because dihydrotestosterone, a metabolite of testosterone, is able to stimulate the growth of prostate cancer, the ability of leuprolide acetate to bring testosterone to near castrate levels is why this drug finds use as a palliative in the advanced disease. The addition of a nonpeptidyl antiandrogen, such as flutamide or bicalutamide, to the leuprolide acetate regimen inhibits adrenal and testicular synthesized androgens from binding to or being taken up by target prostate cancer tissue. This combination therapy helps to control the initial flare-up, by blocking all sources of androgen, and is referred to as maximal androgen blockade.

Leuprolide acetate, in monthly and every-3-month depot formulations, is useful in treating women diagnosed with endometriosis, but not for longer than 6 months because of the chance of developing osteoporosis. Because estrogens stimulate the growth of endometrial tissue, the ability of this drug to drastically reduce estrogen levels suggests why leuprolide acetate is useful in treating endometriosis.

Central precocious puberty that is idiopathic, or gonadotropin dependent, can cause the development of secondary sexual characteristics in girls before the age of 8 years and in boys before the age of 9 years. In addition to the psychological and physiologic changes that occur because of entering puberty too early, there is the risk of the child failing to reach his or her full adult height. Therefore, leuprolide acetate's ability to suppress LH and sex steroid levels (testosterone and estradiol) to prepubertal levels is the reason that leuprolide acetate is approved for treating children with this disease. Use of this drug in a child with precocious puberty will slow or stop that child's secondary sexual development, slow linear growth and skeletal maturation, and in girls, bring about the cessation of menstruation.

Uterine leiomyomas (fibroids), which are benign neoplasms derived from smooth muscle, can cause, among other problems, excessive vaginal bleeding that may progress to anemia. Leuprolide acetate, concomitant with iron therapy, is used in treating the anemia that arises from uterine leiomyoma. The decrease in the formation of the steroid sex hormones reduces fibroid and uterine volume, produces a relief in the clinical symptoms (pelvic pain), and stops the excessive vaginal bleeding, thus correcting the anemia.

Goserelin Acetate Goserelin acetate, like leuprolide acetate, is a synthetic superagonist nonapeptide analog of GnRH that possesses greater potency than the natural hormone. It contains D-Serine (Bu^t) and $NH\text{-}NHCONH_2$ in place of glycine 6 and glycine 10 $\text{-}NH_2$, respectively (Fig. 6.16). That is, the C-terminal modification simply has an NH substituting for the CH_2 of glycine, and like the C-terminal change in leuprolide acetate, this inhibits enzymatic degradation of the peptide by the postproline carboxyamide peptidase.

Goserelin acetate is available in the form of a small, solid pellet that is administered as subcutaneous (SC) implant for the palliative treatment of advanced, metastatic breast cancer in pre- and perimenopausal women or, similarly, as a palliative in advanced prostatic cancer. The rationale for this drug's use is, as described earlier, its ability as a superagonist to bring the levels of estradiol or testosterone to near castrate levels, thus slowing the progression of breast or prostate carcinoma, respectively. Additionally, goserelin acetate is approved for use in treating endometriosis for up to 6 months.

Goserelin acetate also is used in combination with the antiandrogen flutamide for shrinking prostate carcinoma before radiation therapy. This maximal androgen blockade combination is used when the prostate carcinoma has been staged as locally confined to the prostate gland, with one or both lobes as well as the seminal vesicles involved. The treatment should start 8 weeks before radiation treatment begins and be continued throughout the radiation therapy.

Furthermore, women who are to undergo hysterectomy for menorrhagia can benefit from previous treatment with goserelin acetate, because it is able to induce endometrial thinning. This thinning of the endometrium improves the operating environment by causing less intrauterine bleeding, increased postoperative amenorrhea, and decreased dysmenorrhea following surgery, which is why goserelin acetate is approved for inducing endometrial thinning prior to a patient undergoing a hysterectomy for heavy menstrual bleeding.

Nafarelin Acetate Nafarelin acetate, another synthetic superagonist decapeptide analog of GnRH, contains D-Nal(2) 6 [Nal = 3-(2-naphthyl)-Ala] in place of glycine 6, but the C-terminus, glycine 10 $\text{-}NH_2$, is identical with natural GnRH (Fig. 6.16). Nafarelin acetate is available as a 0.2% nasal spray for the relief of endometriosis. Estrogen, of course, is needed for the growth of endometrial tissue; thus, decreased estrogen leads to shrinkage of errant endometrial tissue. The observed side effects of nafarelin acetate are related to falling estrogen levels and include decreased libido, amenorrhea, hot flashes, and vaginal dryness. When used consistently, nafarelin acetate will inhibit ovulation and stop menstruation.

Nafarelin acetate also is used in children, male and female, for the treatment of central precocious puberty. By suppressing the release of LH, the estradiol or testosterone levels fall to prepubertal levels; early secondary sexual development is arrested, linear growth and skeletal maturation are slowed, and in girls, menstruation stops.

Histrelin Acetate Histrelin acetate, a superagonist analog of GnRH, contains D-histidine (N^1-Bzl) 6 in place of glycine 6, and the C-terminus is identical with leuprolide acetate—namely, NH-Et in place of glycine 10 $\text{-}NH_2$ (Fig. 6.16). This GnRH analog is commercially available in the form of an implantable device (SC in the upper arm) that slowly releases the drug over a 12-month period, resulting in decreased testicular steroidogenesis, for the palliative treatment of advanced prostate cancer.

Triptorelin Pamoate Triptorelin pamoate is another superagonist of GnRH, which like nafarelin acetate contains only a single amino acid substitution (D-tryptophan 6 for glycine 6) when compared to the natural hormone

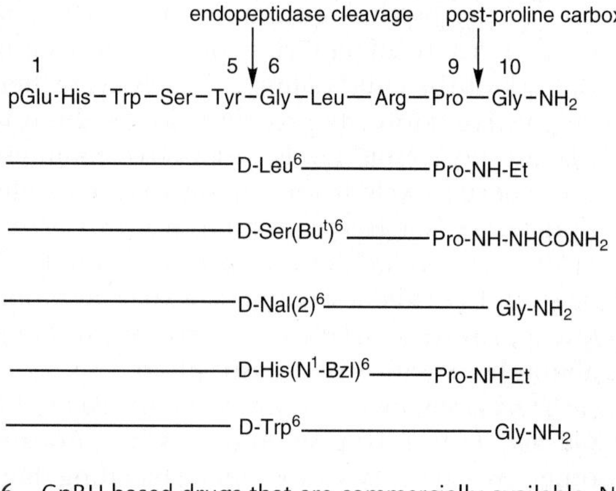

Drug	Trade Name
GnRH	
Leuprolide acetate	Eligard, Lupron, Viadur
Goserelin acetate	Zoladex
Nafarelin acetate	Synarel
Histrelin acetate	Vantas
Triptorelin pamoate	Trelstar LA and Depot

FIGURE 6.16 GnRH-based drugs that are commercially available. Note that leuprolide, goserelin, nafarelin, histrelin, and triptorelin are all superagonists and contain a D-amino acid in place of Gly^6, and that three of the five are missing the C-terminal Gly (the line indicates an identical sequence of amino acids). Note: pGlu = pryoglutamic acid = Bu^t = *t*-butyl; D-Nal(2) = D-3-(2-naphthyl)alanine; N^1-Bzl = 1-benzyl-D-histamine.

(Fig. 6.16). In the treatment of advanced prostate cancer, it is important to reduce serum testosterone levels to very low levels, which can be achieved surgically by orchiectomy. When this surgical method is unacceptable to the patient, an alternative approach is "chemical castration," which can be achieved by use of estrogen therapy, leuprolide, goserelin or histrelin acetates, and triptorelin pamoate. This product is available for intramuscular depot injection (monthly or every 3 months), wherein serum testosterone concentration drops to a level generally seen in surgically castrated men.

Ganirelix Acetate Ganirelix acetate is an analog of GnRH with substitutions at residues 1, 2, 3, 6, 8, and 10 (Fig. 6.17). It is not a superagonist but, rather, is a synthetic decapeptide with high antagonist activity and the first GnRH antagonist to be marketed. It is approved for the suppression of LH surges in women who are undergoing ovarian hyperstimulation fertility treatment; LH surges normally promote ovulation. The goal of this drug is to significantly reduce the number of medication days necessary to suppress the LH surge, thereby maintaining eggs in the ovaries. In vitro fertilization (IVF) treatment cycles were historically initiated by the administration of leuprolide acetate to suppress the premature release of LH. This inhibits ovulation so that the eggs remain available for retrieval by a fertility specialist. For this purpose, leuprolide acetate usually is injected for as many as 26 days. Clinical studies have shown that ganirelix acetate can shut down the LH surge in only 5 days of treatment, that the suppression of LH is more pronounced than that of FSH, and that the shorter treatment time minimizes unpleasant side effects, such as hot flashes and headaches.

Cetrorelix Acetate Cetrorelix acetate is an analog of GnRH with amino acid substitutions at residues 1, 2, 3, 6, and 10 and differing from ganirelix at amino acids 1, 6, and 8 (Fig. 6.17). These substitutions are synthetic, non–DNA-directed amino acids and, like ganirelix acetate, impart GnRH antagonist activity to cetrorelix acetate. This drug also is marketed for use in women undergoing assisted reproductive therapy (ART) procedures, in which it is necessary to control their LH surge. This allows the follicles to develop to a size, as determined by ultrasound, that increases the success of timed insemination and oocyte retrieval for IVF. Like ganirelix acetate, cetrorelix acetate has an advantage over GnRH agonists, such as leuprolide acetate, because it reduces the fertility therapy cycle to days rather than weeks.

Abarelix Abarelix is another GnRH receptor antagonist with substitutions or alterations of the natural hormone at seven residues; the amino acids at positions 4, 7, and 9 are identical with those in GnRH. Abarelix differs from ganirelix at amino acids 1, 5, 6, and 8 (Fig. 6.17). Unlike ganirelix and cetrorelix, however, abarelix is not used in women undergoing ART but, rather, as a palliative in men with advanced prostate cancer. Like the superagonists, abarelix affords a drop in testosterone to castrate levels. Abarelix does not, however, causes the initial rise in testosterone levels and resulting flare-up of symptoms often seen with the superagonists. Still, because of the risk of life-threatening allergic reactions associated with its use, this drug is specifically relegated to a select group of men with advanced symptomatic prostate cancer who are not candidates for other hormone therapies and who choose not to undergo orchiectomy. Abarelix is available only from health care providers who have participated in a special education program that allows them to identify allergic reactions associated with its use.

Somatostatins

Somatostatin is a cyclic 14-peptide that was first isolated by Guillemin in 1973 and is probably the most thoroughly investigated and most important of the inhibitory factors produced by the hypothalamus (Fig. 6.18). The principal activity of somatostatin is inhibition of the release of growth hormone (GH) from the anterior pituitary. Too much GH, as in pituitary tumors, causes acromegaly, a form of gigantism. However, too little GH leads to dwarfism. Somatostatin also has been found in the pancreas and the gastrointestinal tract, where it inhibits the secretion of both insulin and glucagon from the pancreas as well as the secretion of a variety of intestinal peptides (e.g., gastrin, secretin, pepsin, and renin). The short half-life of somatostatin, which is less than 3 minutes, has precluded its use as a therapeutic agent. Many derivatives of somatostatin have been prepared to increase its duration

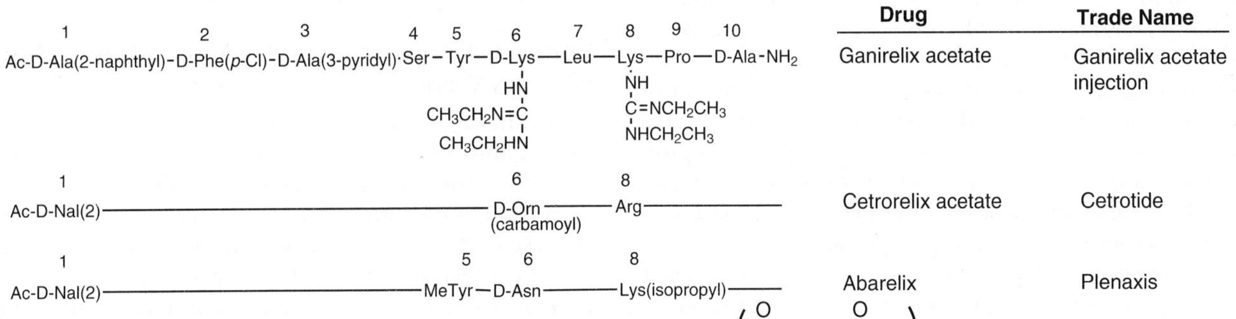

FIGURE 6.17 GnRH receptor antagonists. Note: D-Orn(carbamoyl) = D-ornithine 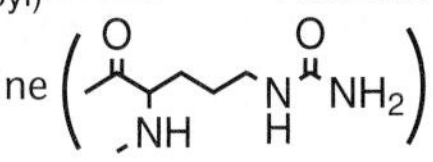

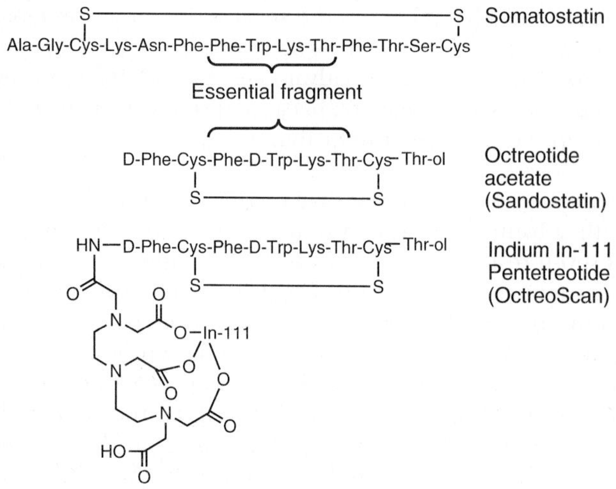

FIGURE 6.18 Somatostatin and its analog octreotide.

of action and/or to enhance its selectivity of action. The culmination of these structure–activity studies was the development of octreotide acetate.

SPECIFIC DRUGS

Octreotide Acetate Octreotide acetate, a long-acting octapeptide analog of somatostatin, has a half-life of approximately 100 minutes. A comparison of the primary structures of octreotide and somatostatin suggests little similarity, but studies suggested that the essential fragment for its activity was the tetrapeptide phenylalanine7-tryptophan8-lysine9-threonine10 (Fig. 6.18). These studies helped in the design of the potent drug now known as octreotide acetate (59). This drug suppresses the secretion of gastroenteropancreatic peptides, such as gastrin, vasoactive intestinal peptide (VIP), insulin, and glucagon, as well as pituitary GH. Furthermore, it is more potent than natural somatostatin in inhibiting the release of glucagon, insulin, and GH.

Octreotide acetate is used by SC injection in the palliative treatment of patients with metastatic carcinoid tumors, which are tumors of the endocrine system, gastrointestinal tract, and lung. It is also used in the palliative management of VIP-secreting tumors (VIPomas, usually pancreatic tumors). Patients with VIPomas suffer a profuse, watery diarrhea syndrome, and octreotide acetate is able to help by decreasing the release of damaging intestinal tumor cell secretions. Octreotide also helps to reduce hypokalemia by correcting electrolyte imbalances.

Octreotide acetate is able to decrease the secretion of GH from the pituitary and is used in treating patients with acromegaly who are unresponsive to previous pituitary radiation therapy or surgery. It is used in the treatment of acromegaly, because it reduces the blood levels of both GH and insulin-like growth factor-1. The long-acting repository form of octreotide acetate also is used in treating acromegaly, carcinoid tumors, and VIPomas, but in monthly depot injections.

Octreotide for intravenous injection is used in the treatment of acute bleeding from esophageal varices. Variceal bleeding occurs in about half the patients with cirrhosis of the liver and is responsible for about one-third of deaths in these patients. Octreotide is a potent vasoconstrictor that reduces portal and collateral blood flow by constricting visceral vessels, which leads to reduced portal blood pressure and decreases the bleeding.

Indium-111 Pentetreotide (OctreoScan) Somatostatin receptors have a broad distribution in normal tissue as well as in a variety of human malignancies (e.g., small-cell lung, brain, breast, pituitary, and endocrine pancreatic cancers). For this reason, octreotide, which binds to somatostatin receptors, was converted to a radionuclide-containing peptide by reacting the amino terminus with an active ester of diethylenetriaminepentaacetic acid (DTPA) to give DTPA-octreotide and then chelated to the radionuclide indium-111 (111In) (Fig. 6.18). This radiopharmaceutical is used as a diagnostic agent for the early detection and localization of small tumors and their metastases in the body, especially tumors that originate from neuroendocrine cells.

Corticotropin-Releasing Factor

The primary function of corticotropin-releasing factor (CRF), a hypothalamic 41-peptide, is the regulation of the release of adrenocorticotropin hormone (ACTH) from the anterior pituitary gland, which then stimulates the release of hydrocortisone from the adrenal gland. Human CRF, which was previously commercially available, has been replaced by the sheep CRF (oCRF).

Corticorelin Ovine Triflutate (Acthrel) The ovine form of the hormone oCRF, which shares 83% homology with the human form, has a longer half-life and greater potency (60). Usually, ACTH deficiency in humans is associated with a pituitary disorder rather than with a deficiency of CRF, and oCRF can be used to distinguish between pituitary hypersecretion of ACTH (Cushing disease) and ectopic ACTH secretion, both of which are conditions that cause a hypersecretion of hydrocortisone. In the case of ectopic ACTH secretion, the administration of oCRF will elicit little to no response in the production of ACTH and hydrocortisone. Therefore, synthetic oCRF trifluoroacetate salt is marketed as a diagnostic agent for patients with ACTH-dependent Cushing syndrome.

Hormones Originating in the Anterior Lobe of the Pituitary Gland

The pituitary, lying just below the hypothalamus, is a small gland that can be divided into an anterior and a posterior lobe. This gland is responsible for the secretion of several important peptide hormones, two of which are released by the posterior lobe. The anterior pituitary peptide hormones control important functions such as growth, reproduction, metabolic and ion balance, as well as a number of other functions.

Growth Hormone

Human GH, a 191–amino acid protein with a molecular weight (MW) of 22 kDa is roughly spherical with a hydrophobic interior. GH is secreted by the anterior pituitary in response to the liberation of GH-releasing factor from the hypothalamus. This contrasts with somatostatin, which inhibits the release of GH. The primary function of GH in the body is to promote skeletal growth. When GH is absent during childhood, or if there is an inadequate supply, dwarfism results. Before 1985, children of short stature were sometimes treated with human GH (hGH) of pituitary origin, which was obtained from cadavers, but hGH of natural origin was discontinued by the U.S. Food and Drug Administration (FDA) when several young adults who had received hGH died. Their deaths were attributed to contaminated hGH, and the contaminant was later found to be an infective agent, known as a prion, that causes Creutzfeldt-Jakob disease, a rare and fatal neurodegenerative disease (61). Naturally occurring hGH has been replaced with material that is prepared by rDNA methodology (62).

Specific Drugs

Somatropin (Genotropin, Humatrope, Norditropin, Nutropin, Saizen, Serostim, Zorbtive) Somatropin, which is an hGH that is prepared by rDNA procedures, contains exactly the same sequence of 191 amino acids as the natural hormone. Several of these products are indicated for the long-term treatment of children who fail to grow because of inadequate secretion of the body's normal endogenous GH and for growth problems associated with chronic renal failure (63). Even adults who are diagnosed with GH deficiency, which can arise as a result of pituitary or hypothalamic disease, surgery, radiation therapy, or other reasons, can benefit from hGH replacement therapy. Turner syndrome, a genetic disease in which there is a complete or partial absence of one of the two X chromosomes in females, causes short stature as one of its many symptoms. Girls suffering from Turner syndrome can benefit from the use of Humatrope, Norditropin, or Nutropin during their growth years. A long-acting dosage form of somatotropin is approved for use in children with Prader-Willi syndrome, a rare genetic disorder that causes short stature; an involuntary, continuous urge to eat that is life-long and may be life-threatening; low muscle tone; and cognitive disorders. The formulation was designed to reduce the frequency of injections to once or twice a month by encapsulating the agent in biodegradable microspheres.

The anabolic properties of hGH are the basis for the orphan drug uses of several of these recombinant products. hGH is used in AIDS-associated catabolism or weight loss, in cachexia resulting from AIDS, and as an anabolic agent in patients with severe burns. In addition, the anabolic property of recombinant hGH is the reason for the use of Zorbtive, along with specialized nutritional support, in the treatment of short bowel syndrome.

Pegvisomant (Somavert) This product contains 191 amino acid residues (of recombinant origin), the same number as in GH, but there are substitutions at residues 18, 21, 120, 167, 168, 171, 172, 174, and 179. This product is then covalently linked to several PEG molecules, and this PEGylated protein is a GH receptor antagonist. Thus, pegvisomant binds to the GH receptor and blocks endogenous GH from binding. The result is a blocking of the GH-stimulated overproduction of insulin-like growth factor-1 that contributes to the disabling symptoms and long-term health problems associated with acromegaly.

Gonadotropins

The gonadotropins, FSH and LH, are large glycoproteins released by the anterior pituitary on stimulation from GnRH produced by the hypothalamus. Both FSH and LH consist of two noncovalently associated α and β subunits. The α subunits contain 92 amino acids and are identical in both hormones, whereas the β subunit consists of 121 amino acids in LH and 111 amino acids in FSH, with the β subunits being dissimilar (64). Thus, the β subunit gives each hormone its specific function.

Both LH and FSH are referred to as gonadotropins, because they act on the male and female gonads, which results in the production of the sex steroids testosterone and estradiol, respectively. In the female, FSH and LH act in concert in regulating ovarian function: egg maturation, ovulation, and transformation of the ruptured follicle into the corpus luteum. In males, spermatogenesis is dependent on these two hormones. FSH is a 34 kDa glycoprotein (~14% carbohydrate) that, in females, facilitates the maturation of ovarian follicle cells and their secretion of estradiol, whereas in males, it stimulates the maturation of sperm in the testes. In females, LH promotes ovulation, formation of the corpus luteum, and progesterone secretion; in males, it enables the secretion of testosterone from the testes.

Male infertility is generally caused by the quality and/or quantity of the sperm produced. In the case of female infertility, however, it may be caused by several factors, such as the inability to produce an egg, to ovulate, for fertilization to occur, and for implantation of the fertilized ovum in the uterus. Several of the commercially available gonadotropins can help in enhancing both male and female fertility and are discussed below.

Specific Drugs

Menotropins (Menopur, Repronex) Menotropins are natural products that are obtained from the urine of postmenopausal women and then biologically standardized (international units) for FSH and LH activities in an approximate ratio of 1:1. Menotropins are used in males with primary (hypothalamic) or secondary (pituitary) hypogonadism to stimulate spermatogenesis, provided they have been treated previously with human chorionic gonadotropin (hCG; a peptide hormone of placental origin that has activity very similar to LH; discussed below) to effect masculinization (increased testosterone production). In females, menotropins and hCG are given sequentially for the purposes of inducing ovulation in women who are having difficulty ovulating as a result of either hypothalamic or pituitary hormonal dysfunction. The menotropins are given for 7 to 12 days, and after clinical evaluation (via ultrasound) indicates the presence of a mature follicle, a single dose of hCG is given to simulate the typical LH surge that normally triggers ovulation. Also, women use the combination of menotropins and hCG to promote the development of multiple follicles when they are participating in an IVF program requiring the recruitment of follicles.

Follitropins Follitropins are hormonal products that consist entirely of FSH and are used to stimulate ovarian follicle growth in women who do not have primary ovarian failure. In the absence of an adequate endogenous LH surge, however, hCG must be given following the use of follitropins to stimulate ovulation.

Urofollitropins (Bravelle) Urofollitropin, a natural product like the menotropins, is obtained from the urine of postmenopausal women and then highly purified so as to contain only FSH, reportedly with only minute amounts of LH. Urofollitropin is used for its ability to stimulate follicle development, such as in women undergoing drug-induced pituitary suppression (GnRH antagonist or superagonist) for purposes of IVF (i.e., multiple follicle development or egg donation). When the number and size of the ovarian follicles are correct, as determined by ultrasound, hCG is administered so as to effect ovulation, and the oocytes are retrieved for IVF.

This drug also is indicated for women who have infertility caused by polycystic ovary syndrome, which generally is observed clinically as enlarged, cystic ovaries containing relatively small follicles. These patients often develop hirsutism, their androgen and LH levels appear elevated while their FSH levels are low, and the early exposure to these improper hormone levels may be causing the follicular atresia (65).

Lately, it has become desirable to have a nonnatural source of pure FSH. It is believed that exposure to increased amounts of LH early in follicular development, as would be the case with menotropins, is detrimental to fertility. Also, urofollitropin is derived from menopausal urine, and the supply of this natural product is limited and, in addition, contains variable levels of urine-derived contaminant proteins (66). These problems have given rise to recombinant forms of FSH.

Follitropin alfa and follitropin beta are human FSH preparations produced by rDNA technology (67). The production of rhFSH in a Chinese hamster ovary (CHO) cell line has proved to be particularly challenging. Follitropin alfa was the first heterodimeric glycoprotein to be produced by rDNA technology. Before the product of rDNA origin was available for infertility treatment, FSH was isolated from urine at less than 5% purity.

Follitropin Alfa (Gonal-F, Gonal-F RFF, Gonal-F RFF Pen) Follitropin alfa is a human FSH preparation of rDNA origin. Because FSH is a glycoprotein, alterations in the carbohydrate side-chain attachments afford different isoforms, which leads to different pharmacokinetic and pharmacodynamic properties. Because it is of recombinant origin and not isolated from urine, it is free of any additional substances, such as urinary proteins and LH.

Like urofollitropin, it is marketed for enhancing the development of multiple follicles that can then be induced to ovulate, via hCG administration, so that the oocytes can be collected for IVF. It also is used in treating women who wish to become pregnant and are anovulatory because of polycystic ovary syndrome, in whom it can enhance follicle maturation before hCG administration for final ovulation.

Men with infertility also can benefit from therapy with follitropin alfa if their infertility is related to hypothalamic or pituitary hormonal dysfunction and not primary testicular failure, because it induces spermatogenesis. Just as with therapy using menotropins, pretreatment with hCG is performed for 3 months to achieve serum testosterone levels within the normal range, before hCG and follitropin alfa therapy.

Follitropin Beta (Follistim AQ) Follitropin beta is a human FSH preparation of rDNA origin that differs chemically from natural FSH and follitropin alfa only by slight variances in the composition of the carbohydrate side chains. In fact, the primary and tertiary structures of both follitropins alfa and beta are indistinguishable from those of human FSH of natural origin. Furthermore, bioassays and physiochemical studies indicate that follitropins alfa and beta are indistinguishable from each other. Therefore, follitropin beta is approved for the same medical uses as follitropin alpha.

Lutropin Alfa (Luveris) Lutropin alfa is the first pure human LH preparation and is of rDNA origin. According to physicochemical and biologic assays, it is indistinguishable from human LH of natural origin. It is indicated for use in infertile women who are undergoing ART, specifically those with severe LH deficiency. It is meant to be coadministered with follitropin alfa so as to stimulate follicular growth in these women. When the follicles are of correct size, as determined by ultrasound examination, hCG is administered to stimulate ovulation.

Anterior Pituitary Hormones

Adrenocorticotropin hormone (H.P. Acthar Gel) The anterior pituitary, under the influence of the hypothalamic hormone hCRF, releases ACTH, a single-chain peptide of 39 amino acids (also known as corticotropin). The sequence of 24–amino acid residues beginning from the amino terminus contains all the biologic activity of the parent. The remaining 15 C-terminal residues confer species specificity as well as enhance the stability of ACTH toward proteolytic cleavage. Amino acids 1 through 24, which are critical for ACTH activity, are identical in humans, pigs, sheep, and beef, whereas the species differ only slightly from each other in the final 15 amino acids. The main action of ACTH on the adrenal cortex involves the release of the glucocorticoid hormone hydrocortisone and the mineralocorticoid hormone aldosterone.

Commercial ACTH is obtained from natural sources and is available in 16% gelatin (repository gel) to prolong its release after SC or intramuscular injection. ACTH has both anti-inflammatory and immunosuppressant properties, which contributes to its use in the treatment of acute exacerbations of multiple sclerosis.

Cosyntropin (Cortrosyn) Cosyntropin is a synthetic polypeptide that consists of amino acids 1 through 24 of human ACTH, but that has the full biologic activity of its parent. Because it is of synthetic origin, it is less allergenic than ACTH of natural origin. Cosyntropin is used as a diagnostic agent in the screening of patients suspected of having adrenocortical insufficiency. Normally, parenteral administration of cosyntropin acts rapidly on the adrenal cortex to effect release of plasma hydrocortisone; when performing the test, the hydrocortisone levels are compared to a control blood sample taken earlier.

Thyrotropin (Thyrogen)

Thyroid-stimulating hormone (thyrotropin) is a 28 to 30 kDa glycoprotein secreted by the anterior lobe of the pituitary gland that is necessary for the growth and function of the thyroid. A recombinant thyrotropin α useful for the detection and treatment of cancer was approved by the FDA in 1998.

Hormones Released from the Posterior Lobe of the Pituitary Gland

As previously discussed, the pituitary gland is responsible for the secretion of several peptide hormones, only two of which are released by the posterior lobe. In fact, these two hormones, oxytocin and vasopressin, are synthesized in neurons originating in the hypothalamus and are transported to the posterior pituitary for storage until release is required.

Oxytocin Oxytocin is a cyclic nonapeptide that, like somatostatin, contains a ring that encompasses a disulfide bridge (Fig. 6.19). Oxytocin has uterotonic action, contracting the muscles of the uterus during gestation, and plays an important role in milk ejection. Exogenous oxytocin most commonly is used for induction of labor, wherein it improves uterine contractions to achieve early vaginal delivery for fetal or maternal reasons (e.g., preeclampsia, Rh factor problems, pregnancy that has exceeded 42 weeks). It also finds use following delivery of the placenta, because it promotes contraction and vasoconstriction and helps to control postpartum bleeding.

Vasopressin Human vasopressin, or Arg-vasopressin, is chemically very similar to oxytocin and therefore sometimes is referred to as [phenylalanine 3, arginine 8] oxytocin (Fig. 6.19). The physiologic role of vasopressin is the regulation of water reabsorption in the renal tubules, and thus, it is often referred to as the antidiuretic hormone. In high doses, vasopressin promotes the contraction of arterioles and capillaries, resulting in an increase in blood pressure, thus the name vasopressin. An inadequate output of pituitary antidiuretic hormone can cause diabetes insipidus, which is characterized by the chronic excretion of large amounts of pale urine and results in dehydration and extreme thirst.

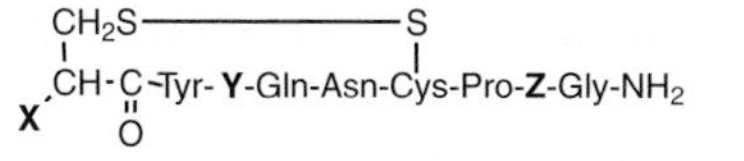

Drug	Trade name
Oxytocin (**X** = NH_2 ; **Y** = Ile; **Z**= Leu)	Pitocin
Vasopressin (**X** = NH_2 ; **Y** = Phe; **Z**= Arg)	
Desmopressin acetate (**X** = H ; **Y** = Phe; **Z**= D-Arg)	DDAVP Stimate

FIGURE 6.19 Structural relationship between oxytocin, vasopressin, and its analog.

Desmopressin Acetate Desmopressin, as its acetate salt, is a synthetic analog of vasopressin in which the N-terminal cysteine is devoid of its α-amino function (1-deamino) and where arginine 8 is present as its D-isomer (D-arginine 8), thus the commercial acronym DDAVP (Fig. 6.19). The presence of D-Arg and the absence of the N-terminal amine in the desmopressin structure have increased its half-life such that it is available for oral, parenteral, or nasal use. It is used by all three of these routes of administration to prevent or control polydipsia (excessive thirst), polyuria, and dehydration of patients with diabetes insipidus caused by a deficiency of vasopressin. It also has been approved for the treatment of nocturnal enuresis (bed-wetting), which is believed to be caused by an absence of the normal nighttime rise in vasopressin levels.

Desmopressin is known to cause an increase in both plasma factor VIII (antihemophilic factor) and plasminogen activator. Therefore, it is approved by the FDA for use, parenterally and nasally, in reducing spontaneous or trauma-induced bleeding episodes in patients with hemophilia A and type I von Willebrand disease, provided that their plasma factor VIII activity is greater than 5%. Stimate, the nasal spray used in treating patients with hemophilia A and type I von Willebrand disease, is 15-fold the concentration of DDAVP nasal spray; the latter is used in treating diabetes insipidus.

Hormones of Placental Origin

If, after ovulation occurs in females, the liberated ovum is fertilized and then implants in the endometrium, the resulting placenta that forms between mother and fetus begins to release a hormone, hCG, the function of which is to maintain and prolong the life of the ovarian corpus luteum. The corpus luteum is important for the continued production of progesterone. Progesterone is especially important because it prepares the uterus for pregnancy and helps in the maintenance of the placenta. hCG begins to appear in the maternal bloodstream and urine shortly after conception and implantation of the fertilized ovum. As a result of this early release of hCG, its detection in the urine forms the basis for the home pregnancy kits that have become so popular in the early prediction of pregnancy.

Human Chorionic Gonadotropin (hCG, Pregnyl) Placental hCG is a complex protein that consists of an α and β subunit. The α subunit consists of 92 amino acids that are identical in sequence with those found in both LH and FSH, whereas the β subunit contains 145 amino acids and is responsible for its biologic specificity. The biologic actions of hCG closely resemble those of LH, but the former has a longer half-life than the latter and has minimal FSH activity.

Like LH, hCG stimulates the production of testosterone by the testes; therefore, it is used in treating male hypogonadism and prepubertal cryptorchidism in young males (age, 4 to 9 years), in whom it stimulates testicular descent. In treating infertility caused by pituitary dysfunction, hCG, in combination with menotropins (as discussed previously) or clomiphene, can induce ovulation and pregnancy in anovulatory females. This hCG, which is of natural origin, is purified from the urine of pregnant women.

Choriogonadotropin Alfa (Ovidrel) Choriogonadotropin alfa is obtained by rDNA technology and is biologically and chemically identical to hCG of natural origin. It is used, like hCG of natural origin, for inducing ovulation in women with anovulatory infertility. Following proper pretreatment with a GnRH antagonist or superagonist to desensitize the pituitary, women participating in ART are treated with a follicle-stimulating agent (e.g., menotropins) to effect the final maturation of the follicles within the ovaries. Ultrasonograms are used to determine proper follicle maturation before the administration of choriogonadotropin alfa to induce ovulation. A distinct advantage of this product is that it can be self-administered by the patient via SC injection.

Hormone of Parathyroid Origin

The parathyroid glands (four) exist as two pairs, one pair of which is embedded on the back surface of each lobe (two) of the thyroid gland. These very small glands are responsible for the secretion of parathyroid hormone (PTH), the action of which is the regulation of both calcium and phosphate metabolism within bone and kidney. In humans, the Ca^{2+} concentration is carefully regulated, and when it falls below a normal level, the parathyroid glands secrete PTH, an 84–amino acid, single-chain protein (see Chapter 30 and Fig. 30.2). Depending on whether PTH is administered intermittently or continuously, it can either stimulate bone formation or breakdown (resorption), respectively.

Teriparatide (Forteo) Teriparatide, a polypeptide prepared by rDNA techniques, consists of the first 34 amino acids from the N-terminal end of PTH (see Chapter 30 and Fig. 30.2). It has been shown to contain all the structural requirements for the full biologic activity of PTH. When teriparatide is administered daily by SC injection, it stimulates osteoblastic activity at the expense of osteoclastic activity, and this enhances bone formation. This is the basis for teriparatide's use in treating high-risk patients in danger of bone fracture resulting from osteoporosis, men with primary or hypogonadal osteoporosis, and women with postmenopausal osteoporosis.

Hormone Secreted by the Parafollicular C Cells of the Thyroid Gland

The majority of the thyroid gland contains follicular cells responsible for the production of the thyroid hormones. A second population of endocrine cells within the thyroid known as C (clear) cells, or parafollicular cells, produce the hormone calcitonin (CT), which has an opposing action to that of PTH in that it decreases the Ca^{2+} concentration in body fluids. It accomplishes this by inhibiting the activity of osteoclasts (i.e., decreasing Ca^{2+} release from bone by inhibiting bone resorption). The actual biosynthesis and release of CT is regulated by the concentration of Ca^{2+} in plasma (i.e., when it is high, CT secretion increases).

Salmon Calcitonin (Fortical, Miacalcin) Calcitonin is a single-chain polypeptide consisting of 32 amino acids (Fig. 6.20). Calcitonins as obtained from different species are identical at seven of the first nine amino acids, contain glycine at position 28, and all terminate with proline-NH_2. The C-terminal proline amide (proline-NH_2) is very important for the biologic function of CT, as is the disulfide bridge between cysteine amino acids at positions 1 and 7. In contrast, the amino acids from 10 through 27 can be varied and seem to influence CT's potency as well as its duration of action. Salmon CT differs from human CT at 16 amino acids.

Only salmon CT is commercially available for medical use, because on a weight basis, it is approximately 45-fold more potent than human CT. Salmon CT, in parenteral form, is approved for treating Paget disease of bone (generally seen in older persons; involves increased bone resorption and softening of bones), postmenopausal osteoporosis, and hypercalcemia of malignancy (multiple myeloma or advanced breast carcinoma). Salmon CT also is available in a nasal spray formulation, which is used exclusively in the treatment of postmenopausal osteoporosis.

S—S (Cys1–Cys7)
Cys-Ser-Asn-Leu-Ser-Thr-Cys-Val-Leu-Gly-Lys-Leu-Ser-Gln-Glu-Leu-His-Lys-Leu-Gln-
1 5 10 15 20
Thr-Tyr-Pro-Arg-Thr-Asn-Thr-Gly-Ser-Gly-Thr-Pro-NH_2 Salmon CT
25 30

S—S (Cys1–Cys7)
Cys-Gly-Asn-Leu-Ser-Thr-Cys-Met-Leu-Gly-Thr-Tyr-Thr-Gln-Asp-Phe-Asn-Lys-Phe-His-
1 5 10 15 20
Thr-Phe-Pro-Gln-Thr-Ala-Ile-Gly-Val-Gly-Ala-Pro-NH_2 Human CT
25 30

FIGURE 6.20 Primary structures of salmon and human calcitonin (CT). Similarities are highlighted in *red*.

Hormones of Endocrine Pancreatic Origin

The exocrine pancreas consists mostly (~99%) of gland cells known as pancreatic acini, which are responsible for secreting several digestive enzymes. The endocrine pancreas, or the remaining 1% of the gland, consists of a group of cells known as pancreatic islets or islets of Langerhans. Each of these islets consists of four distinct cell types, designated as α, β, γ, and δ cells. The α cells secrete glucagon, the β cells insulin and amylin, the δ cells a peptide that is identical with somatostatin of hypothalamic origin, and the γ cells pancreatic polypeptide, of which little concerning its physiologic action is known. Insulin, glucagon, and somatostatin are essential in regulating carbohydrate, lipid, and amino acid metabolism. Insulin is responsible for promoting the storage of glucose as glycogen and effecting hypoglycemia, whereas glucagon mobilizes glucose from its glycogen stores and causes hyperglycemia. The primary action of somatostatin of hypothalamic origin is to inhibit the release of GH from the pituitary, but pancreatic somatostatin suppresses the production of both insulin and glucagon. Amylin, which is cosecreted with insulin from the β cells, has physiologic actions that include slowing of gastric emptying, suppression of postprandial glucagon secretion, reduction of food intake, and inhibition in the secretion of both stomach acid and pancreatic digestive enzymes (see Chapter 27).

Specific Drugs

Insulin Insulin has anabolic properties that include the stimulation of both skeletal muscle and liver cells to incorporate glucose and convert it to glycogen, to synthesize proteins from amino acids in the blood, and to act on fat cells to enhance their uptake of glucose and the synthesis of fat. In short, insulin encourages anabolism rather than catabolism, because it promotes the synthesis of glycogen, proteins, and lipids. A deficiency of insulin, which characterizes the disease diabetes mellitus (DM), causes extreme changes in the entire metabolic pattern of individuals with DM. Patients with DM often demonstrate elevated blood glucose levels, excess glucose in the urine, and failure to properly use carbohydrate and lipids. Untreated DM can be fatal. Even when treated, however, there can be numerous circulatory and renal complications, and some metabolic abnormalities may lead to blindness (diabetic retinopathy).

The human insulin molecule, consisting of 51 amino acids, has the structural characteristics of a large protein, yet is only the size of a polypeptide. Two disulfide bonds (cysteine [Cys] A7 to Cys B7 and Cys A20 to Cys B19) link two polypeptide chains, with the A-chain consisting of 21 amino acids and the B-chain consisting of 30 amino acids. An additional disulfide loop is found in the A-chain between Cys A6 and Cys A11 (Fig. 6.21).

The primary sequences of insulin from several species are known, and porcine insulin is the closest to that

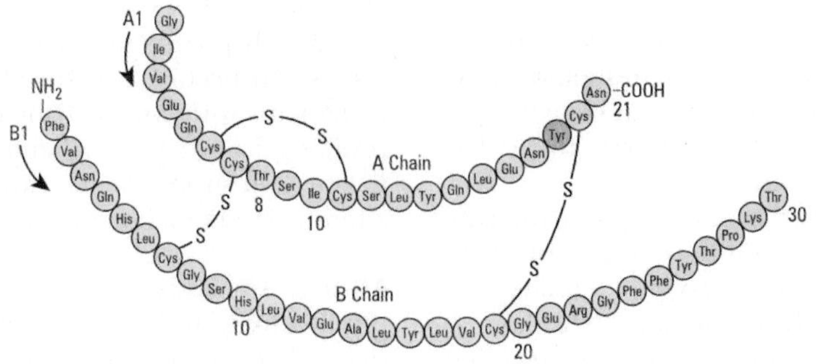

FIGURE 6.21 Primary structure of human insulin chains A and B, including the interchain disulfide bonds A7-B7 and A20-B19 and intrachain disulfide bond A6-A11.

of humans. Their A-chains are identical, and they differ only in their B-chains, with alanine 30 (porcine) in place of threonine 30 (human). Human and bovine insulin differ in each chain, with alanine 8 and valine 10 in the A-chain (bovine) and alanine 30 in the B-chain (bovine). Nearly all human insulin is produced by rDNA technology, and insulin obtained from porcine sources is being phased out. Recombinant insulin approved in 1982 for the treatment of insulin-dependent diabetes, is the first FDA-approved rDNA drug. The biotechnology solution has several advantages over insulin derived from animal sources:

1. It should have potentially fewer serious immune reactions.
2. It is pyrogen-free.
3. It is not contaminated with other peptide hormones, such as glucagon, somatostatin, and proinsulin, as found in isolated products.
4. It can be produced in larger amounts.

The first successful attempt to tailor a protein hormone for therapy by rDNA techniques has yielded interesting insulin analogs (68–70).

Human insulin of rDNA origin is available commercially as Humulin, Novolin, and several analogs. The Humulin and Novolin products are produced using genetically modified strains of two different microorganisms. Humulin is prepared using recombinant *E. coli* bacteria. The pharmaceutical preparation is reported to contain less than 4 ppm of immunoreactive bacterial polypeptides that act as possible contaminants. Baker's yeast (*S. cerevisiae*) serves as the recombinant organism for the production of Novolin. Before 1986, Humulin was produced by chemically joining together the separately rDNA-derived A-chain and B-chain. Today, the product is prepared by enzymatically cleaving the connecting peptide in recombinant proinsulin.

Studies in animals, healthy adults, and patients with type 1 DM have shown human insulin to have pharmacologic effects identical to those of purified porcine insulin. A comparable pharmacokinetic profile also has been shown. Human insulin, however, administered intramuscularly or intravenously, may have a slightly faster onset and slightly shorter duration of action when compared with purified porcine insulin in patients with diabetes. The usual precautions concerning toxic potentials observed with insulin of animal origin should be followed with rDNA human insulin. As would be expected, the recombinant product has been shown to be less immunogenic than animal insulins.

Insulin remains the only treatment option for type 1 diabetes and is still widely used to treat patients with type 2 diabetes who do not respond adequately to other pharmacotherapies. Recombinant DNA technology has led to the development of insulin analogs that have greater utility in certain situations and may more closely resemble the normal diurnal pattern of insulin secretion (Table 27.6). The newly engineered analogs have specific amino acid sequence modifications that improve absorption properties and biologic profiles (71). Insulin lispro (Humalog) has a more rapid onset and shorter duration of action than regular human insulin. Unlike regular insulin that must be injected 30 to 60 minutes before a meal, recombinant insulin lispro is effective when injected 15 minutes before a meal. The analog differs from natural human insulin, because the B-chain amino acids B28 proline and B29 lysine are exchanged. Insulin aspart (Novolog), which is homologous with human insulin except for the single amino acid substitution of aspartic acid for proline at B28, is effective when injected 5 to 10 minutes before a meal. Insulin glargine (Lantus) is the newest rDNA-derived human insulin analog. An ultra-long-acting agent, insulin glargine differs from human insulin in that the amino acid asparagine at residue A21 is replaced by glycine, and two arginines are added to the C-terminus of the B chain. When administered subcutaneously, insulin glargine has a duration of action up to 24 to 48 hours. This change in action profile resulted from structural modifications that enhanced the product's basicity, thus causing the product to precipitate at neutral pH postinjection and, therefore, increasing its duration of action.

Glucagon (GlucaGen)

1 5 10 15
His-Ser-Gln-Gly-Thr-Phe-Thr-Ser-Asp-Tyr-Ser-Lys-Tyr-Leu-Asp-Ser
Thr-Asn-Met-Leu-Trp-Gln-Val-Phe-Asp-Gln-Ala-Arg–Arg
25 20

Glucagon, a 29–amino acid, straight-chain polypeptide of α-cell pancreatic origin, triggers liver glycogenolysis and gluconeogenesis, thereby elevating glucose levels. The principal action of glucagon is the liver-mediated release into the blood of abnormally high concentrations of glucose, which causes hyperglycemia. This means that glucagon has an effect on blood glucose levels that is opposite to what occurs with insulin.

Glucagon of rDNA origin is now available (69). Replacing the bovine product with the rDNA-derived drug would eliminate the risk of acquiring bovine spongiform encephalopathy from glucagon therapy. Human glucagon of rDNA origin is marketed for the treatment of severe hypoglycemic reactions in patients with diabetes, as can occur when there is an overdose of insulin. In patients with type 1 diabetes, the increase in glucose resulting from glucagon administration may not be sufficient, and supplemental carbohydrates may need to be administered quickly, especially in children.

AMYLIN Amylin is a 37–amino acid peptide that is structurally similar to CT. Amylin works together with insulin to regulate glucose concentrations after a meal. When in solution, amylin is viscous, unstable, and tends to aggregate; therefore, it cannot be used parenterally and is not commercially available.

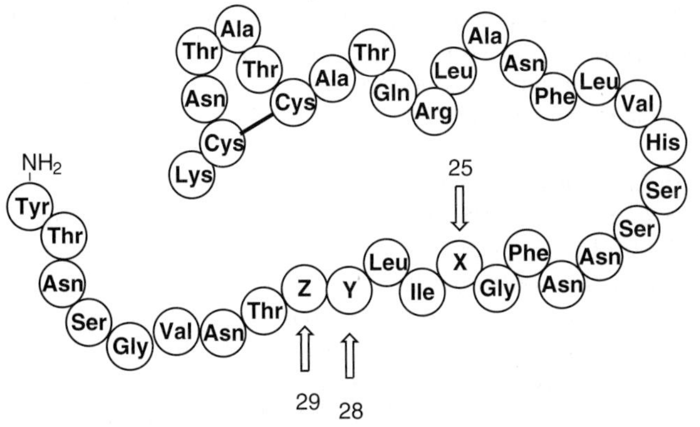

Amylin (human) X = Ala, Y = Z = Ser

Pramlintide (Symlin) X = Y = Z = Pro

Pramlintide acetate (Symlin) Pramlintide acetate is a synthetic analog of amylin (a 37–amino acid peptide) with proline substitutions at amino acids 25, 28, and 29. These substitutions change its physical properties such that it is commercially available for SC injection. When pramlintide is used in combination with insulin, it slows gastric emptying, lowers blood glucose levels after meals, and affords a feeling of fullness that leads to decreased caloric intake and the potential for weight loss. Pramlintide has been approved for use in adults with type 1 or type 2 diabetes as an adjunct along with insulin.

ENZYMES

Tissue-Type Plasminogen Activator

The fibrinolytic system is activated in response to the presence of an intracellular thrombus or clot. The process of clot dissolution is initiated by the conversion of plasminogen to plasmin. Plasminogen activation is catalyzed by two endogenous highly specific serine proteases, urokinase-type plasminogen activator and tissue-type plasminogen activator (t-PA).

The mature human t-PA is a glycoprotein consisting of a single chain of 527 amino acids. Its MW is approximately 70 kDa. Human t-PA contains 35 cysteines assigned to 17 disulfide bonds (Fig. 26.24). A serine protease domain of approximately 260 amino acids is located at the carboxy-terminal end of this protein. A fibronectin "finger" domain, two kringle domains, and an epidermal growth factor domain also are present. The t-PA protease domain is approximately 35% to 40% homologous with typical serine protease, such as bovine trypsin and chymotrypsin.

Mammalian cells produce two t-PA variants of *N*-linked glycosylation, type 1 (at asparagines 117, 184, and 448) and type 2 (only at asparagines 117 and 448). The rate of fibrin-dependent plasminogen activation is two- to threefold faster for type 2 compared with type 1. The cDNA obtained from a human melanoma cell line was expressed in CHO cells to achieve glycosylation and a protein identical to the natural protein. Protein engineering studies have produced variant t-PA molecules with modified pharmacokinetics, affinity for fibrin, catalytic activity, and side effects.

Three rDNA thrombolytic agents are approved in the United States (20,72–74) (Fig. 26.24). The first is alteplase, an enzyme equivalent to human t-PA. It is indicated for the treatment of acute myocardial infarction (administered as a bolus), acute massive pulmonary embolism (administered by intravenous infusion), and ischemic stroke. It is the first fibrin-selective thrombolytic agent preferentially activating fibrinogen bound to fibrin. Thus, the thrombolytic effect is localized to a blood clot and avoids systemic activation of fibrinogen, preventing bleeding elsewhere in the body. Plasma t-PA concentrations are proportional to the rate of infusion. Alteplase is rapidly cleared from circulating plasma, with 50% cleared within 5 minutes after termination of infusion. The mechanisms for clearance of t-PA from the blood are poorly understood. Detectable levels of antibody against alteplase have been found in patients receiving the drug, although 12 days to 10 months later, antibody determinations have been negative.

The second, reteplase, a recombinant, is a nonglycosylated deletion mutation of human t-PA containing 355 of 527 amino acids of native t-PA. The drug is indicated for acute myocardial infarction and is given as a 10 U + 10 U double bolus.

The most recent addition to the marketed rDNA-derived t-PAs is tenecteplase. This recombinant protein contains three modifications from natural human t-PA. In the kringle 1 domain of natural t-PA, threonine 103 is replaced by arginine; the kringle 1 domain asparagine 117 is replaced by glutamine; and in the protease domain, four amino acids (lysine, histidine, and two arginines) are replaced by four alanines. The drug is indicated for acute myocardial infarction. Bleeding at the injection site is similar to that with alteplase, but there is a reduction in the noncerebral bleeding complications. It is administered as a single, 5-second bolus.

DNase—Dornase Alfa (Pulmozyme) According to the Cystic Fibrosis Foundation, cystic fibrosis (CF) is the most common fatal genetic disorder, afflicting approximately 30,000 patients, most of whom die before the age of 30 years. They develop thick mucous secretions and suffer from severe, frequent lung infections. Studies during the 1950s and 1960s determined that CF-related secretions in the lungs contained large amounts of DNA. Mucous-thickening DNA release resulted from an inflammatory response and ensuing white blood cell death. The enzyme DNase I specifically cleaves extracellular DNA, such as that found in the mucous secretion of CF patients, and has no effect on the DNA of intact cells. The FDA has approved a recombinant human DNase (75).

The enzyme DNase I is a glycoprotein containing 260 amino acids with an approximate MW of 37 kDa.

The recombinant protein is expressed by genetically engineered CHO cells encoding for the native enzyme, although DNase I was not purified or sequenced from human sources at the time. A degenerate sequence, based on the sequence of bovine DNase (263 amino acids), was used to synthesize probes and screen a human pancreatic DNA library. The primary amino acid sequence of rhDNase is identical to native human DNase I.

The only FDA-approved DNase product, dornase alfa (inhalation solution), has been developed as a therapeutic agent for the management of CF. It is administered by nebulizer aerosol delivery systems.

Dornase alfa is indicated for daily administration in conjunction with standard CF therapies to reduce the frequency of respiratory infections requiring parenteral antibiotics to improve pulmonary function. The breakdown of DNA in infected sputum results in improved airflow in the lung and reduced risk of bacterial infection. Although effective for the management of the respiratory symptoms of CF, dornase alfa is not a replacement for antibiotics, bronchodilators, and daily physical therapy. This product also finds application in treating chronic bronchitis.

Enzyme Replacement Therapy

Enzyme replacement therapy (ERT) is available for many of the lysosomal storage diseases, including Gaucher disease, Fabry disease, Pompe disease, mucopolysaccharidosis (MPS) type I (Hurler, Scheie, and Hurler/Scheie syndromes), MPS II (Hunter syndrome), and MPS VI (Maroteaux-Lamy syndrome) (76). The most frequent drug-related adverse events of ERT are infusion-related reactions. Antibodies formed against infused enzymes are usually of the immunoglobulin G (IgG) serotype. Signs and symptoms of infusion-related reactions (IRRs) can include cutaneous reactions, pyrexia, headache, and hypertension. Precise relationship between antibody formation and occurrence of IRRs is unclear. Not all IRRs are antibody mediated, and not all patients who develop antibodies develop IRRs (76).

Imiglucerase (Cerezyme) Type 1 Gaucher disease, the most common form, is an inherited disorder. Fewer than 1 in 40,000 people in the general population have Gaucher disease. Patients with the disease lack the normal form of the enzyme glucocerebrosidase. They cannot break down glucocerebroside, leading to accumulation of glucocerebroside within the lysosomes. This leads to the poor functioning of macrophages and an accumulation of "Gaucher cells" in the spleen, liver, and bone marrow. Imiglucerase is an analog of glucocerebrosidase produced by rDNA technology using mammalian cell culture system. The drug is a monomeric glycoprotein consisting of 497 amino acids (approximate MW = 60 kDa), with four *N*-linked glycosylation sites, and differs from the human placental glucocerebrosidase by one amino acid (histidine 495 replaces arginine). Imiglucerase carries out the normal function of the missing enzyme and has been shown to be safe in long-term safety studies (77).

Alglucosidase Alfa (Myozyme, Lumizyme) Pompe disease, a rare genetic disorder affecting nearly 1 in every 40,000 births, is caused by the mutation in a gene that makes the α-glucosidase enzyme (78). It was the first disease to be identified as a lysosomal storage disorder. α-Glucosidase enzyme is responsible for the breakdown of glycogen to glucose. The lack of degradation results in the accumulation of glycogen in lysosomes in all tissues, most notably in skeletal and cardiac muscles. The disease is characterized as early onset or late onset Pompe disease based on the age of onset of disease. Severe α-glucosidase deficiency manifests during infancy with rapidly progressing muscle weakness, hypotonia, and cardiomyopathy and eventually lethal muscle disorder. As with other lysosomal storage disorders, ERT is the patient's only hope. Alglucosidase alfa was developed and launched in 2006 for the treatment of infants and children with Pompe disease (79). Another alglucosidase alfa drug (Lumizyme) was approved by the FDA in 2010 for patients age 8 years and older with late-onset (noninfantile) Pompe disease. Alglucosidase alfa is a recombinant human enzyme produced by transfected CHO cells as a 110 kDa precursor that targets lysosomes via the mannose-6-phosphate receptor. Following endocytosis, the enzyme is transformed to its mature 76 kDa form that restores glycogen processing and reverses accumulation. Alglucosidase alfa therapy has been shown to improve cardiac and muscle function.

Idursulfase (Elaprase) MPS II (Hunter syndrome), a disease with an incidence of approximately 1 in 162,000 births, is caused by the deficiency of the lysosomal enzyme iduronate-2-sulfatase. This enzyme is responsible for a crucial step in degradation of two glycosaminoglycans (GAGs), dermatan sulfate and heparin sulfate, in the lysosomes of various cells. Iduronate-2-sulfatase deficiency causes an accumulation of GAGs in tissue, and the patient's only recourse is ERT. The clinical manifestations of this deficiency are short stature, joint stiffness, harsh facial features, hepatosplenomegaly, and progressive mental retardation. Recombinant iduronate-2-sulfatase has been available in the United States since 2006 and is produced from HT-1080 cells for proper translational attachment of *N*-linked oligosaccharides and the crucial mannose-6-phosphate groups as the targeting phosphate into lysosomes (80). In addition to being fully glycosylated with eight mannose-6-phosphate groups, the enzyme possesses sialylated moieties that improve its stability in circulation. For full activity, cysteine 59 must undergo modification to formylglycine. Idursulfase has been designated as an orphan product by the FDA.

Cytokines

Cytokines communicate in a dynamic cellular network during an immune/inflammatory response to an antigen (75,81–83). Lymphokine and monokine are the terms used for a cytokine derived from lymphocytes and macrophages, respectively. Chemokines are a group of at least 25 structurally homologous, low molecular weight cytokines that stimulate leukocyte movement and regulate the migration of leukocytes from the blood to tissues. Cytokines, usually released and targeted to produce a localized effect, regulate the growth, differentiation, and activation of the hematopoietic cells responsible for the maintenance of the immune response. A wide array of glycoproteins, including interferons, interleukins, hematopoietic growth factors, and tumor necrosis factors (TNFs), are cytokines. Cytokines can only act on target cells that express receptors for that cytokine. There are five families of cytokine receptor proteins: class I cytokine receptors, class II cytokine receptors, TNF receptors, chemokine receptors, and immunoglobulin superfamily receptors (Table 6.5) (20,84–90).

INTERFERONS The interferons (20,85) are a family of cytokines discovered in the late 1950s with broad-spectrum antiviral and potential anticancer activity, making them biologic response modifiers. Biotherapy (the therapeutic use of any substance of biologic origin) of cancer is different than standard chemotherapy. That is, biotherapeutic agents belong to a group of compounds that enhance normal immune interactions (therefore, they also are immunomodulators) with cells in a specific or nonspecific fashion. Chemotherapeutics interact directly with the cancer cells themselves. Three types of naturally occurring interferons have been found in small quantities: leukocyte interferon (IFN-α), produced by lymphocytes and macrophages; fibroblast interferon (IFN-β), produced by fibroblasts, epithelial cells, and macrophages; and immune interferon (IFN-γ), synthesized by $CD4^+$, $CD8^+$, and natural killer lymphocytes. Both IFN-α and IFN-β, also known as type I interferons, exhibit approximately 30% primary sequence homology but no structural similarity to IFN-γ, a type II interferon. All three are glycoproteins. Previously only available in low yields by chemical synthesis or isolation, several rDNA interferon pharmaceuticals now have been marketed in the United States, including three IFN-α products, two IFN-β agents, and an IFN-γ drug.

TABLE 6.5 The Five Families of Cytokine Receptors and Some Ligands

Receptor Families	Ligands
Class I cytokine receptors	IL-2, IL-7, IL-9, IL-11, IL-13, IL-15, GM-CSF, G-CSF
Class II cytokine receptors	INF-α, INF-β, INF-γ
Tumor necrosis factor receptors	TNF-α, TNF-β, CD30, CD40, FAS
Chemokine receptors	IL-8, RANTES, MIP-1, PF-4, MCAF
Immunoglobin superfamily receptors	IL-1, M-CSF

Interferon-α At least 24 different human genes producing 16 distinct mature IFN-α molecules with slight structural variations are known (20,85,91). Human IFN-α proteins generally are composed of either 165 or 166 amino acids. The two primary subtypes, IFN-α2a (Roferon-A) and IFN-α2b (Intron A), both contain 165 amino acids, differing only at position 23, with IFN-α2a containing a lysine residue and IFN-α2b an arginine residue at this position. They have MWs of approximately 19 kDa. Although cultures of genetically modified *E. coli* produce two recombinant FDA-approved IFN-α products, IFN-α2a and IFN-α2b, their method of purification differs. Purification of IFN-α2a includes affinity chromatography using a murine MAb, whereas that of IFN-α2b does not.

Interferon-α possesses complex antiviral, antineoplastic, and immunomodulating activities. Although the precise mechanism of action of IFN-α is not known, it is believed to interact with cell surface receptors to produce the biologic effects. The actions appear to result from a complex cascade of biologic modulation and pharmacologic effects that include the modulation of host immune responses; cellular antiproliferative effects; cell differentiation, transcription, and translation processes; and reduction of oncogene expression. Interferon-α is filtered through the glomeruli in the kidney and undergoes rapid proteolytic degradation during tubular reabsorption.

Consensus Interferon (IFN Alfacon-1) Hepatitis C infection results in a chronic disease state in 50% to 70% of cases and is now the most important known cause of chronic liver disease (92). Following the acute phase, as many as 80% of patients may progress to the chronic phase of the infectious disease. An estimated 20% of patients with a chronic form of the disease progress to cirrhosis. The only agents shown to be effective in the treatment of hepatitis C are the interferons. A unique recombinant molecule, a consensus IFN, known as IFN alfacon-1, has been approved for the treatment of chronic hepatitis C infection. It is a 19.5 kDa recombinant protein produced in *E. coli* and contains 166 amino acids in a relationship in which each amino acid position in the molecule contains the most commonly occurring amino acid among all the natural IFN-α subtypes. IFN alfacon-1 exhibits 5- to 10-fold higher biologic activity when compared to either IFN-α2a or IFN-α2b.

Interferon-β Normally produced by fibroblasts, human IFN-β (20,85,91) was first cloned and expressed in 1980; however, its instability made it unsuitable for clinical use.

The more stable recombinant IFN-β1b (Betaseron), a 165–amino acid analog of human IFN-β, differs from the native protein with a serine residue substituted for cysteine at position 17. The highly purified rDNA technology-derived product has a MW of 18.5 kDa. It is produced in a recombinant *E. coli*. Approved in 1993 by the FDA, IFN-β1b is indicated for the treatment of patients with exacerbating-remitting multiple sclerosis (MS). The National MS Society says that 250,000 to 300,000 Americans have this disease, with more than 60% of patients falling into the exacerbating-remitting category. A vial of recombinant IFN-β1b contains 0.3 mg of protein with dextrose and human albumin as stabilizers. The exact mechanism of action of IFN-β1b is not known. Its immunomodulating effects, however, may benefit patients with MS by decreasing the levels of endogenous IFN-γ. Levels of IFN-γ are believed to rise before and during acute attacks in patients with MS.

Whereas IFN-β1b of rDNA origin was the first to the market, IFN-β1a (Avonex) also is now available. IFN-β1a is produced in mammalian cells and has the same amino acid sequence and carbohydrate side chain as natural IFN-β. Recombinant IFN-β1a is administered to patients once weekly by intramuscular injection. This differs from the SC administration every other day of rDNA-produced IFN-β1b.

Interferon-γ Human IFN-γ (20,85,91,93) is a single-chain glycoprotein with a MW of approximately 15.5 kDa. The cytokine mainly exists as a noncovalent dimer of differentially glycosylated chains in solution in vivo. Glycosylation does not appear to be necessary for biologic activity. The 140–amino acid IFN-γ1b (Actimmune) is produced by fermentation of a recombinant *E. coli*. IFN-γ1b was approved in 1990 by the FDA.

IFN-γ1b possesses biologic activity identical to the natural human IFN-γ derived from lymphoid cells. Although all the IFNs share certain biologic effects, IFN-γ differs distinctly from IFN-α and IFN-β by its potent capacity to activate phagocytes involved in host defense. These activating effects include the ability to enhance the production of toxic oxygen metabolites within phagocytes, resulting in a more efficient killing of various microorganisms. This activity is the basis for the use of IFN-γ1b in the management of chronic granulomatous disease. Chronic granulomatous disease is a group of rare X-linked or autosomal genetic disorders of the phagocytic oxygen metabolite–generating system, leaving patients susceptible to severe infections. The drug extends the time that patients spend without being hospitalized for infectious episodes. Investigational applications of IFN-γ include the treatment of renal cell carcinoma, small-cell lung cancer, infectious disease, trauma, atopic dermatitis, asthma, allergies, rheumatoid arthritis, and venereal warts.

INTERLEUKINS Interleukins are cytokines involved in immune cell communication. Synthesized by monocytes, macrophages, and lymphocytes, interleukins serve as soluble messengers between leukocytes. Currently, at least 18 interleukins have been observed. One of the most studied cytokines is interleukin (IL)-2, originally called T-cell growth factor because of its ability to stimulate growth of T lymphocytes.

Interleukin-1 IL-1 is a major inflammatory mediator and exists in two forms: IL-1α and IL-1β. Each form is a product of two separate genes, but is related to each other structurally at a three-dimensional level. IL-1β is a systemic, hormone-like mediator intended to be released from cells, whereas IL-1α is primarily a regulator of intracellular events and mediator of local inflammation. The recombinant protein anakinra, which is an IL-1 receptor antagonist, and the fusion protein rilonacept, which blocks the excessive IL-1β signaling are commercially available and described below (94,95).

Anakinra (Kineret) Rheumatoid arthritis (RA) is a chronic, inflammatory disease affecting synovial joints. Patients with persistent, active disease are traditionally treated with disease-modifying antirheumatic drugs (DMARDs). IL-1 receptor antagonist is an endogenous cytokine that blocks the binding of proinflammatory cytokine IL-1 to its receptor, thereby balancing the cartilage destruction and bone resorption mediated by IL-1. Anakinra is the first recombinant human IL-1 receptor antagonist and differs from the native human protein in that it is not glycosylated and has an additional N-terminal methionine (rmetHuIL-1 receptor antagonist). Anakinra, a 17.3 kDa recombinant protein expressed in *E. coli*, was approved in 2001 for treating the signs and symptoms and the joint-destructive components of RA (94–96). However, the challenge for anakinra for occupying the large number of IL-1 receptors is formidable, as these receptors are expressed on all cells except red blood cells; moreover, anakinra is rapidly excreted by the kidney, and blood levels are low after 24 hours. IL-1 receptors are also readily generated each day, necessitating a daily SC injection.

Rilonacept (Arcalyst) Cryopyrin-associated periodic syndromes are inherited disorders caused by mutations in the nucleotide-binding domain, leucine-rich family, pyrin domain containing-3 (*NLRP-3*) gene, which encodes the protein cryopyrin. Cryopyrin regulates the protease caspase-1 and controls activation of IL-1β. Mutations in the *NLRP-3* gene can cause an overactive inflammasome, resulting in excessive levels of activated IL-1β, which causes inflammation, joint pain, rash or skin lesions, fever and chills, eye redness or pain, and fatigue. Rilonacept is a 252 kDa recombinant fusion protein produced by the CHO cells and approved by the FDA in 2008 for the long-term treatment of familial cold autoinflammatory syndrome and Muckle-Wells syndrome, two cryopyrin-associated periodic syndromes that are extremely rare, affecting approximately 300 people in the United States. Rilonacept's mechanism of intervention involves blockade of excessive IL-1β signaling (94,95,97). Rilonacept combines the extracellular binding domains of the human IL-1 receptor component and IL-1 receptor accessory protein in a single chain, with two of these chains joined to the fragment crystallizable (Fc) portion of human IgG creating a dimeric molecule. Rilonacept serves as an effective soluble IL-1β sink or trap since the coupled receptor components bind IL-1β with higher affinity than either individual receptor. It exerts its effects through multicomponent receptor system and is more effective than drugs that target only one of the components such as the IL-1 receptor antagonist anakinra. With its weekly subcutaneous dosing regimen, it may have better patient compliance than anakinra. Concomitant administration of other IL-1 blockers and anti-TNF-α agents has been associated with an increased risk of serious infection and neutropenia. Because IL-1 blockade may interfere with the immune response to infections, patients should not initiate rilonacept with an existing infection. Patients with chronic inflammation tend to have suppressed formation of CYP450 enzymes. Treatment with rilonacept is expected to normalize CYP450 distribution, so plasma levels of coadministered drugs that are CYP450 substrates with narrow therapeutic indexes should be carefully monitored for potential dose modification.

Interleukin-2 Human IL-2 is a 133–amino acid, 15.4 kDa protein that is *O*-glycosylated at a threonine in position 3. An intramolecular disulfide bond between cysteine 58 and cysteine 105 is essential for biologic activity. A recombinant version of IL-2 is marketed as aldesleukin (Proleukin) (20,85,91,98–101). Aldesleukin differs from the native protein by the absence of glycosylation, a lack of the N-terminal alanine residue at position 1 (132 amino acids), and the replacement of cysteine with serine at position 125 of the primary sequence. Sequence changes were accomplished by site-directed mutagenesis to the IL-2 gene before cloning and expression. Aldesleukin exists as noncovalent microaggregates with an average size of 27 recombinant IL-2 molecules. The recombinant drug does possess the biologic activity of the native protein.

Aldesleukin is used in cancer biotherapy as a biologic response modifier for the treatment of metastatic renal cell carcinoma and metastatic melanoma. Side effects are the major dose-limiting factor, because aldesleukin is an extremely toxic drug. The manufacturer's labeling should be consulted for full details. Careful patient selection and thorough patient monitoring are essential. The incidence of nonneutralizing anti–IL-2 antibodies in patients treated on an every-8-hour regimen is quite high (76% in one clinical study).

Interleukin-2 Fusion Protein Using ligation chemistry approaches during the preparation of recombinant proteins, researchers have created biologically active molecules that combine the activities of two individual proteins into "fusion molecules." These fusion technologies hold promise for developing custom molecules expressing a wide variety of dual activities.

Denileukin Diftitox (Ontak). The FDA approved the fusion protein denileukin diftitox in 1999 for the treatment of patients with persistent or recurrent cutaneous T-cell lymphoma (CTCL) whose malignant cells express the CD25 component of the IL-2 receptor (102–105). CTCL is a general term for a group of low-grade, non-Hodgkin lymphomas (NHLs) affecting approximately 1,000 new patients per year. Malignant T cells manifest initially in the skin. Over time, there is systemic involvement. For many patients, CTCL is a persistent, disfiguring, and debilitating disease that requires multiple treatments. Malignant CTCL cells express one or more of the components of the IL-2 receptor. Thus, the IL-2 receptor may be a homing device to attract a "killer drug." The incidence of CTCL in the United States is approximately 1,500 cases per year. Men are twice as likely as women to have the disease.

Denileukin diftitox is a rDNA-derived, cytotoxic IL-2 fusion protein that is composed of two different components: the first 389 amino acids of diphtheria toxin fused to amino acids 2 to 133 of human IL-2. Thus, the fusion protein binds to IL-2 receptors on neoplastic T cells and gets internalized via receptor-mediated endocytosis, bringing diphtheria toxin directly to kill the CTCL target. Interestingly, although denileukin diftitox was originally thought to act primarily by binding to CD25, now that the components of IL-2 receptor are better delineated, it appears that clinical activity of denileukin diftitox is associated with the presence of CD122.

Interleukin-11 IL-11 is a thrombopoietic growth factor that directly stimulates the proliferation of hematopoietic stem cells and megakaryocyte progenitor cells (106). This induces megakaryocyte maturation, resulting in increased platelet production. IL-11 is a 178–amino acid glycosylated cytokine produced by bone marrow stromal cells. Primary osteoblasts and mature osteoclasts express mRNAs for an IL-11 receptor (IL-11Rα). Thus, bone-forming cells and bone-resorbing cells are potential targets of IL-11. In 1997, the FDA approved an rDNA-derived version of IL-11 produced in *E. coli.* Oprelvekin (Neumega) contains only 177 amino acids, lacking the amino terminal proline of the native IL-11. Produced in *E. coli*, the cytokine analog is nonglycosylated. Oprelvekin has potent thrombopoietic activity in animal models of compromised hematopoiesis. It is indicated for the prevention of thrombocytopenia following myelosuppressive chemotherapy. Pharmacists should monitor for possible fluid retention and electrolyte states when it is used with chronic diuretic therapy.

TUMOR NECROSIS FACTOR TNFs, a family of cytokines produced mainly by activated mononuclear phagocytes, have both beneficial and potentially harmful effects, mediating cytotoxic and inflammatory reactions (20). The TNFs are endogenous pyrogens capable of inducing chills, fever, and other flu-like symptoms. TNF-α, also called cachectin (and commonly referred to as TNF), and TNF-β, also called lymphotoxin, both bind to the same receptor and induce similar biologic activities. Biologic effects of TNF-α include selective toxicity against a range of tumor cells, mediation of septic shock, activation of elements of the immune system in response to gram-negative bacteria, and induction/regulation of inflammation. The TNF-α of rDNA origin has been studied extensively, but it has not been developed into a useful drug.

Etanercept is a rDNA-produced fusion protein that binds specifically to TNF and blocks its interaction with cell surface TNF receptors (107,108). It is indicated for the treatment of moderate to severe active RA in adults and for juvenile RA in patients who have had an inadequate response to one or more DMARDs. It is a genetically engineered protein that includes two components. The extracellular, ligand-binding portion (p75) of the human TNF receptor is linked as a fusion protein to the Fc portion of the human IgG1 antibody. Each etanercept molecule binds specifically to two TNF molecules found in the synovial fluid of patients with RA, blocking the interaction of TNF with the TNF receptor. The drug inhibits both TNF-α and TNF-β. The Fc portion of the fusion protein helps to clear the etanercept–TNF complex from the body.

Abatacept (Orencia) With the recognition that T cells play a central role in the pathogenesis of RA, abatacept has been developed as a novel, rational approach to interfere with the upstream effector of the inflammation to meet the needs of patients who fail to respond adequately to existing therapy using traditional DMARDs such as methotrexate (MTX) or TNF-blocking agents. Abatacept is a soluble 92 kDa human fusion protein approved for the treatment of RA as a new class of DMARDs (109). Structurally, abatacept consists of a fusion between the extracellular domain of human cytotoxic T-lymphocyte–associated antigen-4 (CTLA-4) linked to the modified Fc portion of human IgG1. Abatacept selectively modulates the CD80/CD86:CD28 costimulatory signal required for full T-cell activation. By targeting the activation of T cells, an upstream event in the immune cascade that underlies RA, abatacept has the potential to impact multiple downstream aspects of RA immunogenesis, such as the production of cytokines, autoantibodies, and inflammatory proteins. The immunoglobulin portion of the abatacept serves as a handle to facilitate purification of the protein that is produced by rDNA technology in a mammalian cell expression system. It also enhances the solubility and serum half-life of the fusion protein. Serum half-life of 14.7 days is independent of dose, and rate of elimination remains constant, supporting the lack of antidrug antibody generation. Abatacept was found to be well tolerated for up to 7 years of exposure in patients with RA who had an inadequate response to MTX or other traditional DMARDs or who failed to respond to treatment with anti-TNF agents (110). The potential for increased risk of infection is an important safety concern in patients with RA receiving biologic therapies. During abatacept treatment, live vaccinations should be avoided because the drug may diminish the effectiveness of some immunizations, and anti-TNF agents should be avoided due to risk of infections.

Hematopoietic Growth Factors Hematopoiesis is the complex series of events involved in the formation, proliferation, differentiation, and activation of red blood cells, white blood cells, and platelets. Hematopoietic growth factors are cytokines that regulate these events (20,111–114). Investigators have identified and cloned at least 20 factors, including IL-3 (or multi–colony-stimulating factor [CSF]), IL-4, IL-5, IL-6, IL-7, erythropoietin (EPO), granulocyte-macrophage colony-stimulating factor (GM-CSF), granulocyte colony-stimulating factor (G-CSF), macrophage colony-stimulating factor (M-CSF), and stem cell factor. Figure 6.22 summarizes the elaborate hematopoietic cascade. All blood cells originate within the bone marrow from a single class of pluripotent stem cells. In response to various external and internal stimuli, regulated by hematopoietic growth factors, stem cells give rise to additional new stem cells (self-renewal) and differentiate into mature, specialized blood cells.

Erythropoietin–Epoetin Afa (Epogen, Procrit) EPO (20,111,115–119), a glycoprotein with a MW of 30 to 34 kDa produced by the kidney, stimulates the division and differentiation of erythroid progenitors in the bone marrow, increasing the production of red blood cells. Epoetin alfa (sometimes called rHuEPO-α), a recombinant EPO prepared from cultures of genetically engineered mammalian CHO cells, consists of the identical 165–amino acid sequence of endogenous EPO. The MW is approximately 30.4 kDa. The protein contains two disulfide bonds (linking cysteine 7 with 161 and 29 with 33) and four sites of glycosylation (one *O*-site and three *N*-sites); the disulfide bonds and glycosylation are necessary for the hormone's biologic activity. Deglycosylated natural EPO and bacterial-derived EPO (without glycosylation) have greatly decreased in vivo activity, although in vitro activity is largely conserved. The sugars may play a role in thermal stability or the prevention of aggregation in vivo.

The marketed products are formulated as a sterile, colorless, preservative-free liquid for intravenous or SC administration. Epoetin alfa is indicated for the treatment of various anemias. Epoetin alfa represents a major scientific advance in the treatment of patients with chronic renal failure, serving as a replacement therapy for inadequate production of endogenous EPO by failing kidneys. Epoetin alfa may decrease the need for infusions in dialysis patients. By several mechanisms related to elevating the erythroid progenitor cell pool, epoetin alfa increases the production of red blood cells.

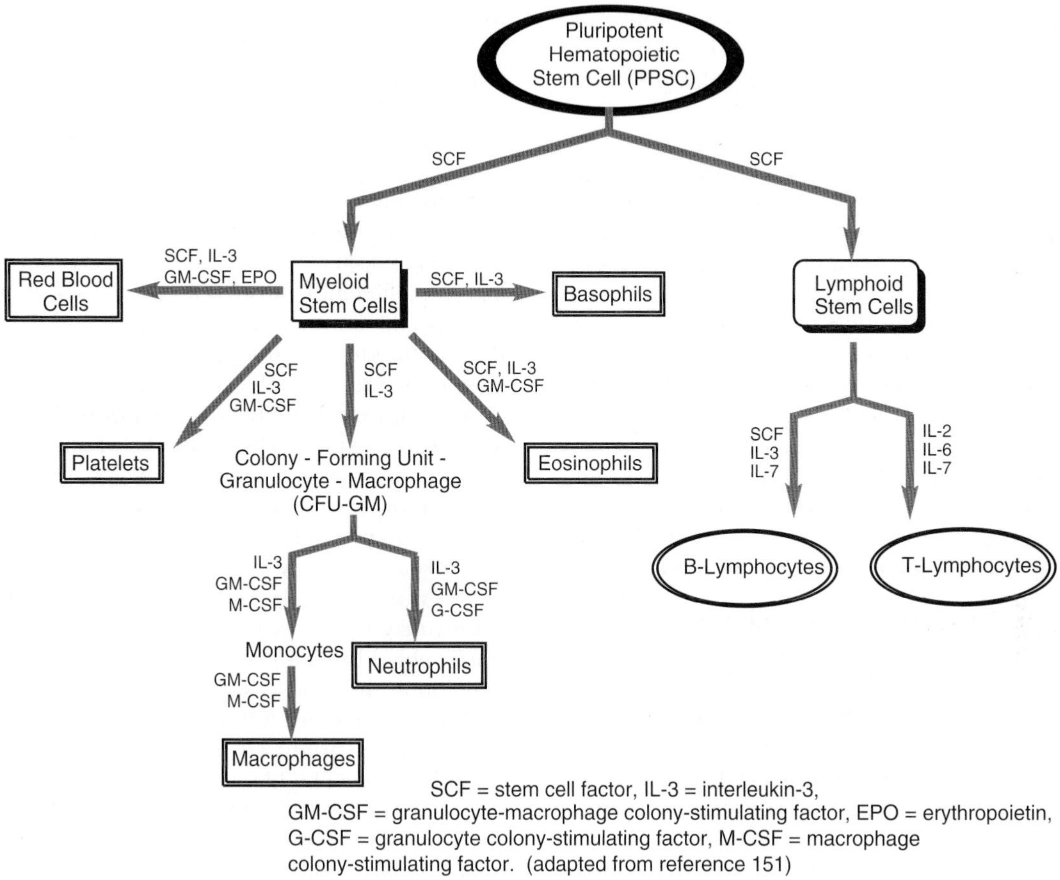

FIGURE 6.22 Schematic overview of hematopoiesis.

The manufacturer's full prescribing information should be consulted for dosing regimens, because the dose is titrated individually to maintain the patient's target hematocrit. The circulating half-life is 4 to 13 hours in patients with chronic renal failure. Peak serum levels are achieved within 5 to 24 hours following subcutaneous administration.

Colony-Stimulating Factors The CSFs are glycoprotein cytokines that promote progenitor proliferation, differentiation, and some functional activation. The name "colony-stimulating factor" results from the fact that these proteins often are assayed by their ability to stimulate the formation of cell colonies in bone marrow cultures. The names added to "CSF" reflect the types of cell colonies that arise in these assays.

Granulocyte Colony-Stimulating Factor—Filgrastim (Neuprogen). Recombinant DNA–derived G-CSF (20,111,120–124), or filgrastim, was approved by the FDA in 1991 to decrease the incidence of infection in patients with nonmyeloid malignancies who are receiving myelosuppressive anticancer drugs. Filgrastim is a 175–amino acid, single-chain protein with a MW of 18.8 kDa. Filgrastim, produced by a recombinant bacteria, differs from the endogenous human protein by the addition of a methionine at the N-terminus (recombinant methionyl G-CSF is sometimes called r-metHuG-CSF) and the lack of glycosylation. Glycosylation, however, does not appear to be necessary for the biologic activity.

It is administered by intravenous infusion or by SC injection or infusion. The drug is rapidly absorbed, with peak serum concentrations in 4 to 5 hours. Elimination half-life is approximately 3.5 hours.

Filgrastim is lineage selective for the neutrophil lineage type of white blood cells, whereas GM-CSF is multilineage, stimulating progenitors of neutrophils, monocytes, basophils, and eosinophils. The drug reduces the period of neutropenia, the number of infections, and the number of days the patient is on antibiotics. Filgrastim generally is well tolerated, with medullary bone pain being the most frequently encountered side effect.

Granulocyte-Macrophage Colony-Stimulating Factor—Sargramostim (Leukine). GM-CSF (20,111,120–124) has been produced by rDNA technology in the yeast *S. cerevisiae*. Sargramostim is a glycoprotein of 127 amino acids, differing from the endogenous human GM-CSF by substituting leucine at position 23. Also, the glycosylation pattern may differ from that of the native protein.

Cellular division, maturation, and activation are induced through the binding of GM-CSF to specific receptors expressed on the surface of target cells. On 2-hour intravenous infusion, the alpha half-life is 12 to 17 minutes, followed by a slower decrease (beta half-life) of 2 hours.

Other Growth Factors Growth factors are cytokines responsible for regulating cell proliferation, differentiation, and function (20). They act as intercellular signals. Each cell type's response is specific for each particular growth factor and differs from growth factor to growth factor. Platelet-derived growth factor (PDGF) is an endogenous growth-promoting protein that is released from cells involved in the healing process and is evident at the cell proliferation stage of a healing open wound. A recombinant human (rH) PDGF B homodimer has been produced from genetically engineered *S. cerevisiae* cells (125). Becaplermin is the B-chain of the PDGF B protein. Thus, becaplermin is also referred to as rHPDGF-BB. The 25 kDa protein is formulated into a gel that mimics natural PDGF when applied to diabetic foot ulcers.

Clotting Factor VIII, Factor IX, and Anticoagulants

Antihemophiliac factor, or factor VIII, is required for the transformation of prothrombin (factor II) to thrombin by the intrinsic clotting pathway (20,74,126). Hemophilia A, a lifelong bleeding disorder, results from a deficiency of factor VIII. Conventional biotherapy for the treatment of hemophilia A includes protein concentrates from human plasma collected by transfusion services or commercial organizations. Therefore, the concentrates may contain other native human proteins and microorganisms, such as viruses (e.g., HIV and hepatitis), derived from infected blood. Four versions of recombinant factor VIII (antihemophiliac factor), highly purified, microorganism-free proteins are now available. All four therapeutic proteins are produced by the insertion of cDNA encoding for the entire factor VIII protein into mammalian cells. The mature, heavily glycosylated protein is composed of 2,332 amino acids (1 to 2 million daltons) and contains sulfate groups. Stability of the large protein is a concern. The products have proved to be safe and effective for reducing bleeding time in patients. There is the possibility, however, of induction of inhibitors in previously untreated patients.

Hemophilia B results when a patient is deficient in specific clotting factor IX (20). It affects males primarily and makes up approximately 15% of all hemophilia cases. A recombinant human factor IX is now available.

Surgeons have used medicinal leeches (*Hirudo medicinalis)* for years to prevent thrombosis in fine vessels of reattached digits. Hirudin is the potent, specific thrombin inhibitor isolated from the leech. Lepirudin is a rDNA-derived (recombinant yeast) polypeptide that differs from the natural polypeptide, having a terminal leucine instead of isoleucine and missing the sulfate group at Tyr 63 (127).

Vaccines

There are two types of immunization: active immunization and passive immunization. Active immunization is the induction of an immune response either through exposure to an infectious agent or by deliberate immunization with a vaccine (vaccination) made from the microorganism or its products to develop protective immunity. Passive immunization involves the transfer of products produced by an immune animal or human (preformed antibody or sensitized lymphoid cells) to a previously nonimmune recipient host, usually by injection. Sufficient active immunity may take days, several weeks, or even months to induce (possibly including booster vaccinations), but it generally is long lasting (even lifelong) through the clonal selection of genetically specific immunologic memory B and T lymphocytes. Passive immunity, although often providing effective protection against some infection, is relatively brief, lasting only until the injected immunoglobulin or lymphoid cells have disappeared (a few weeks or months). Thus, vaccines enable the body to resist infection by diseases. In response to an injection of vaccine, the immune system makes antibodies, which recognize surface antigens found in the vaccine. If the subject is later exposed to a virulent form of the virus, the immune system is primed and ready to eliminate it. Many viral vaccines are produced from the antigens isolated from pooled human plasma of virus carriers. Vaccinations are among the most cost-effective and widely used public health interventions. Although generally safe, the minimal risk of vaccine-produced infections can be eliminated by administration of highly purified vaccine antigens of recombinant origin (20,127–129). The different types of vaccines are described below, and the vaccines currently available in the Unites States are listed in Table 6.6.

Live, Attenuated Vaccines

To make a live, attenuated vaccine, the disease-causing organism is grown under special laboratory conditions that cause it to lose its virulence, or disease-causing properties.

Inactivated Vaccines

Inactivated vaccines are produced by killing the disease-causing microorganism with chemicals or heat.

Subunit Vaccines

Sometimes vaccines developed from antigenic fragments are able to evoke an immune response, often with fewer side effects than might be caused by a vaccine made from the whole organism.

Toxoid or Inactivated Vaccines

A toxoid is an inactivated toxin, the harmful substance produced by a microbe. Many of the microbes that infect people are not themselves harmful. It is the powerful toxins they produce that can cause illness. To inactivate such powerful toxins, vaccine manufacturers treat them by chemical means (formalin solution) and irradiation to completely cripple any disease-causing ability.

Conjugate Vaccines

The bacteria that cause some diseases, such as pneumococcal pneumonia and certain types of meningitis, have special outer coats. These coats disguise antigens so that

TABLE 6.6 Some FDA-Approved Vaccines

Generic Name	Trade Name	Vaccine Type	Protection Against
Anthrax	BioThrax	Inactivated	Anthrax
Chicken pox	Varivax	Live attenuated	Chicken pox
Diphtheria	Pediarix	Toxoid	Diphtheria
Haemophilus influenza type b (Hib)	ActHib, PedvaxHib	Conjugate	*H. influenza*
Hepatitis A	Havrix, Vaqta	Inactivated	Hepatitis A
Hepatitis B	Engerix-B, Recombivax	Recombinant subunit	Hepatitis B
HepA-HepB	Twinrix	Inactivated-recombinant	Hepatitis A and B
Herpes zoster	Zostavax	Live attenuated	Herpes zoster
Human papilloma virus	Gardasil, Cervarix	Recombinant	Cervical cancer
Influenza	Fluarix, Fluvirin, Fluzone, Flulaval, Afluria, Agriflu, FluMist	Inactivated Live attenuated	Influenza
Japanese encephalitis	Ixiaro, JE-Vax	Inactivated	Japanese encephalitis
Measles	Attenuvax	Live attenuated	Measles
Meningococcal conjugate	Menactra, Menomune, Menveo	Inactivated	Meningococcal
Mumps	Mumpsvax	Live attenuated	Mumps
Pertussis	Boostrix	Subunit	Pertussis
Pneumococcal	Prevnar, PCV13, Pneumovax23	Conjugate	Pneumococcal
Polio	Ipol	Inactivated	Polio
Sipuleucel-T	Provenge	Autologous	Prostate cancer
Rabies	Imovax, Rabavert	Inactivated	Rabies
Rotavirus	Rotarix, RotaTeq	Live attenuated	Rotavirus
Rubella	Meruvax	Live attenuated	Measles
Tetanus toxoid (TT)		Toxoid	Tetanus
Typhoid	Typherix, Vivotif Berna, Typhim Vi	Inactivated	Typhoid
Varicella	Varivax	Live attenuated	Varicella
Vaccinia (smallpox)	ACAM2000	Live attenuated	Smallpox
Yellow fever	YF-Vax	Live attenuated	Yellow fever

the immature immune systems of infants and younger children are unable to recognize these harmful bacteria. In a conjugate vaccine, proteins or toxins from a second type of organism, one that an immature immune system can recognize, are linked to the outer coats of the disease-causing bacteria. This enables a young immune system to respond and defend against the disease agent.

DNA Vaccines or Naked Vaccine

Genes encoding antigens of an infectious organism are expressed by the host's own cells. Genes are inserted into a bacterial plasmid under the control of a mammalian promoter. The chimeric plasmid is either directly injected into muscle or the DNA is conjugated to a solid matrix such as gold particles.

Recombinant Vector Vaccines

A vaccine vector, or carrier, is a weakened virus or bacterium into which harmless genetic material from another disease-causing organism can be inserted.

MONOCLONAL ANTIBODIES

Introduction to Antibodies

The cell-mediated branch of the immune system includes the antibody-secreting B cells or plasma cells (81–83).

Antibodies or immunoglobulins are soluble proteins that are produced in response to an antigenic stimulus. As part of the normal immune system, each B cell produces as many as 100 million antibody proteins (polyclonal antibodies) directed against bacteria, viruses, and other foreign invaders. Antibodies act by binding to a particular antigen, thereby "tagging" it for removal or destruction by other immune system components.

The production of antigen-"neutralizing" antibodies or immunoglobulins and the detection of a sufficient antibody titer are important concepts for an understanding of vaccinations and exposure to antigens. The humoral response to an antigen involves the creation of memory B cells and the transformation of B lymphocyte into plasma cells that serve as factories for the production of secreted antibodies. Approximately 4 days after initial contact with an antigen (immunization), immunoglobulin M antibodies (one of five types of immunoglobulin structure) appear and then peak approximately 4 hours later. Approximately 7 days after exposure, IgG, the major class of circulating immunoglobulin, appears. The antibodies bind to the antigen and effect additional immune system–mediated events, "neutralizing" the antigen and leading to its elimination. The concentration of an immunoglobulin specific for a given antigen at a given time is referred to as the antibody titer and may be a measure of the effectiveness of the initial antigen exposure/vaccination to elicit immunologic memory.

Antibody Structure

Antibodies are glycoproteins. The simplest structure of an immunoglobulin molecule consists of two identical long peptide chains (the heavy chains) and two identical short polypeptide chains (the light chains) interconnected by several disulfide bonds. The selectivity of any immunoglobulin for a particular antigen is determined by its structure and, specifically, by the variable or antigen-binding regions (Fig. 6.23). Enzymatic digestion of the antibody with papain yields the functional human antibody (Fab) fragment, which contains the antigen-binding sites, and the Fc fragment, which specifies the other biologic activities of the molecule.

Hybridoma Technology

MAbs are ultrasensitive, hybrid immune system–derived proteins designed to recognize specific antigens. Nobel Laureates Kohler and Milstein first reported MAbs in 1975 (130). MAbs have been used in laboratory diagnostics, site-directed drugs, and home test kits (85,128,131–134). The B lymphocyte produces a wide range of structurally diverse antibody proteins with varying degrees of specificity in response to a single antigen stimulus. Because of their structural diversity, these antibodies would be called polyclonal antibodies. MAbs are homogeneous hybrid proteins produced by a selected, single clone of an engineered B lymphocyte. They are designed to recognize specific sites or epitopes on antigens.

Hybridoma technology (the technology used to produce MAbs) consists of combining or fusing two different cell lines: a myeloma cell (generally from a mouse) and a plasma spleen cell (B lymphocyte) capable of producing an antibody that recognizes a specific antigen (Fig. 6.24). The resulting fused cell, or hybridoma, possesses some of the characteristics of both original cells: the myeloma cell's ability to survive and reproduce in culture (immortality), and the plasma spleen cell's ability to produce antibodies to a specific antigen.

Monoclonal antibodies are more attractive than polyclonal antibodies for diagnostic and therapeutic applications because of their increased specificity of antigen recognition. Thus, they can serve as target-directed "homing devices" to find and attach to the targeted antigen. Developments in hybridoma technology have led to highly specific diagnostic agents for home use in

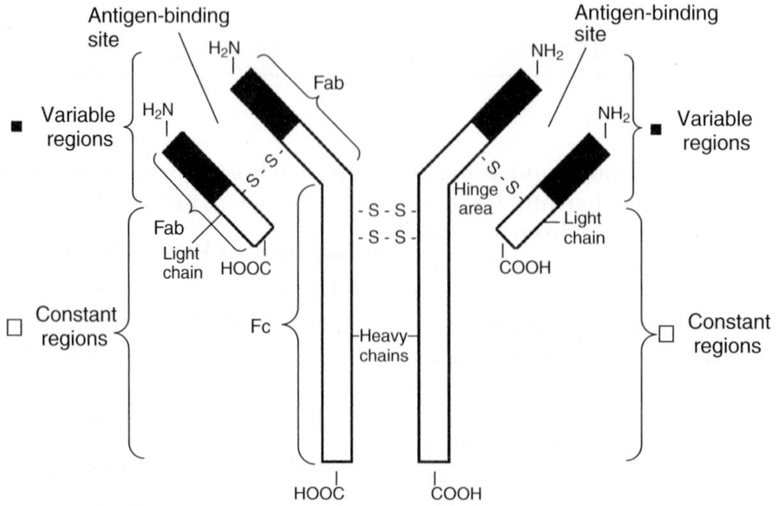

FIGURE 6.23 Schematic model of an antibody molecule.

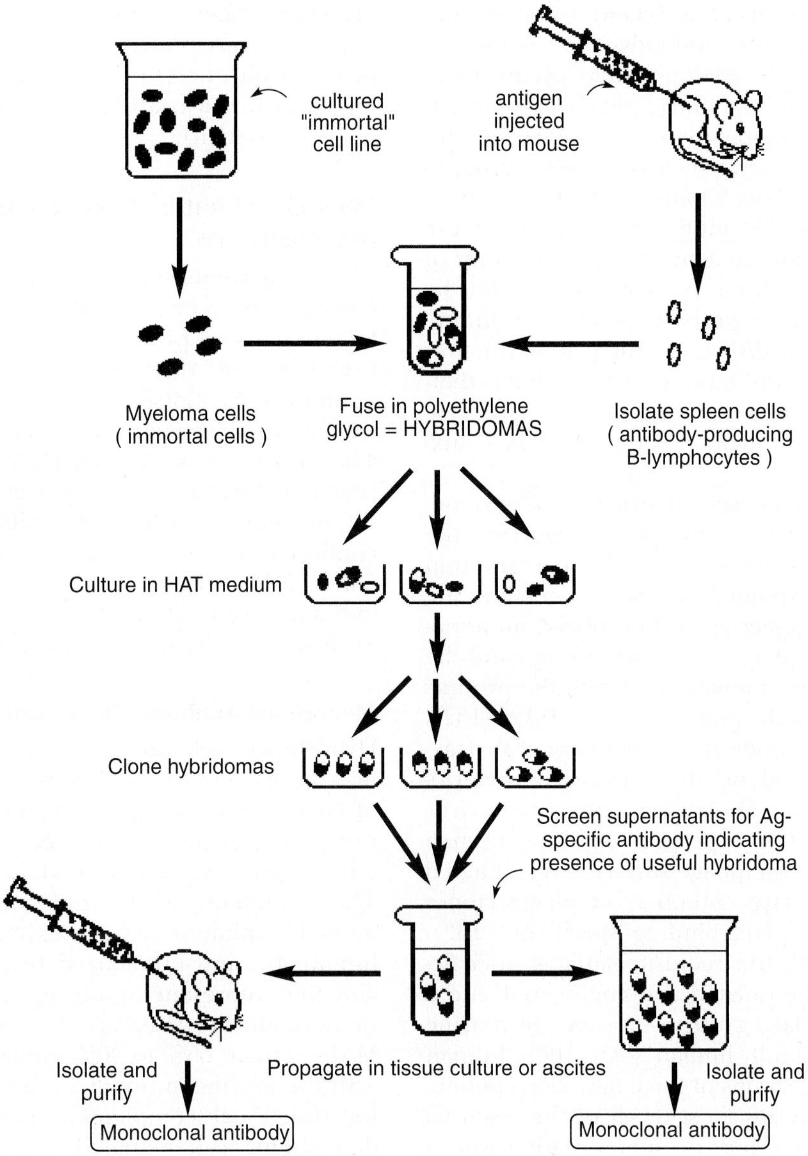

FIGURE 6.24 Outline of hybridoma creation and monoclonal antibody (MAb) production.

pregnancy testing and ovulation prediction kits; laboratory use in detection of colorectal cancer, ovarian cancer, and others; and design of site-directed therapeutic agents, such as trastuzumab to combat metastatic breast cancer and abciximab as an adjunct for the prevention of cardiac ischemic complications.

Monoclonal Antibody Immunogenicity

Nearly 25 years after the pioneering work of Kohler and Milstein, MAbs began to realize their therapeutic potential. Until recently, most MAbs were murine proteins based on their production. Initial clinical trials of murine MAbs showed that these mouse proteins were highly immunogenic in patients after just a single dose (135). Human patients formed antibodies to combat the foreign MAb that was administered. The human anti-mouse antibody response is known as HAMA. So, far from being the "magic bullets" that were proposed, immunogenic murine MAbs were useless in chronic therapy. Thus, a different approach was needed to eliminate the unwanted immune response (HAMA) in patients.

The variable regions of an immunoglobulin must be of a specific chemical structure with the ability to bind to the antigen they "recognize." The part within the variable region that forms the intermolecular interactions with the antigen is the complementarity-determining region (CDR). The variable domains of antibody light and heavy chains each contain three CDRs.

It was determined that immune responses against the mouse-produced MAbs were directed against both the variable and the constant regions of the antibody. Human and murine antibodies are very homologous in chemical structure. Thus, an MAb should be engineered to decrease the immunogenicity of an MAb by replacing the mouse constant regions of an IgG with human constant regions, making the antibody less mouse-like (131,136–139). In practice, what generally occurs is the variable heavy-chain and variable light-chain domains (CDRs) of human immunoglobulins are replaced with those of a murine antibody, which possesses the requisite antigen specificity. This "chimeric" MAb will retain its ability to recognize the antigen (a property of the murine MAb) and retain the many effector functions of an immunoglobulin (both murine and human), but be much less immunogenic (a property of a human immunoglobulin). A chimeric MAb, containing approximately 70% human sequence, will have a longer half-life than its murine counterpart in a human patient. Therapeutic MAbs that are chimeric include catumaxomab, cetuximab, and infliximab.

The discovery of the conserved structure of antibodies, particular IgGs, across many species suggested the possibility of chimeric antibodies, and the realization that the homology extended to the antigen-binding site facilitated the engineering of humanized immunoglobulins. Advances in phage display technology and the production of transgenic animals has led to the production of humanized or fully human MAbs (119,129–132). Functional human antibody fragments (e.g., Fab fragments) can be displayed on the surface of bacteriophages. A bacteriophage, also called a phage, is a virus that infects bacteria. The expression of these human antibody fragments on the phage surface has facilitated efficient screening of large numbers of phage clones (phage display) for antigen-binding specificity (133). Once a fragment with the requisite antigen specificity is selected, it can be isolated and engineered into a humanized MAb (replacing up to 95% of the murine protein sequence) or a fully human MAb (100% human sequence). Transgenic strains of mice have been genetically engineered to possess most or all of the essential human antibody genes. Thus, on immunization with a foreign antigen, the transgenic mice will develop humanized or fully human antibodies in response. Both of these techniques, although very complex and expensive, have yielded FDA-approved, humanized antibody pharmaceuticals, such as alemtuzumab, bevacizumab, eculizumab, and trastuzumab. The half-life of humanized antibodies is dramatically enhanced (from hours to weeks), and immunogenicity is drastically reduced.

Monoclonal Antibody Diagnostic Agents

Several ultrasensitive diagnostic MAb-based products have enjoyed great success; these include a variety of imaging agents for the detection of blood clots and cancer cells. A monoclonal Fab fragment, technetium-99m–arcitumomab (CEA-Scan), can detect the presence and indicate the location of recurrent and metastatic colorectal cancer. Colorectal cancer and ovarian cancer can be detected with satumomab pendetide (OncoScint CR/OV). Capromab pendetide (ProstaScint) is used for detection, staging, and follow-up of patients with prostate adenocarcinoma. Small-cell lung cancer can be detected with nofetumomab (Verluma). The first imaging MAb for myocardial infarction is imiciromab pentetate (MyoScint).

Monoclonal Antibody–Based, In-Home Diagnostic Kits

The strong trend toward self-care, coupled with a heightened awareness by the public of available technology and an emphasis on preventive medicine, has increased the use of in-home diagnostics (140–142). MAb specifically minimizes the possibilities of interference from other substances that might yield false-positive test results. The antigen being selectively detected by MAb-based pregnancy test kits is human chorionic gonadotropin, the hormone produced if fertilization occurs and that continues to increase in concentration during the pregnancy. Table 6.7 lists some examples of MAb-containing in-home pregnancy test kits as well as some examples of MAb-based, in-home ovulation prediction kits.

Monoclonal Antibody Therapeutic Agents

Hybridoma technology and advanced antibody engineering has led to the design of an increasing number of site-directed therapeutic agents for the treatment and prevention of transplant rejection, therapy in rheumatoid arthritis, treatment of NHL, and other indications. These products are examples of murine (e.g., tositumomab), chimeric (e.g., cetuximab), human (e.g., panitumumab), and humanized (e.g., trastuzumab) MAbs, and they represent significant advances in pharmacotherapy. Murine MAbs are derived from mice. Chimeric MAbs contain 65% to 90% human protein that is fused with the murine antibody variable region, which allows for functional complement activation and antibody-dependent cell-mediated cytotoxicity in humans. Variations of chimeric MAbs, such as partially humanized and de-immunized MAbs, are 95% human protein and are composed of a few critical residues involved in the antigen binding site from the murine antibody or modified murine variable domains containing nonimmunogenic amino acid sequences, respectively. As described earlier, to prevent any HAMA response, fully humanized MAbs containing only human protein sequences have been developed from mice that have had human immunoglobulin genes placed in their genome. Therapeutic MAbs (Table 6.8) can be divided into three main classes based on their mechanism of action: 1) MAbs as directed targeted therapy: these MAbs either block or stimulate a particular cell membrane molecule (e.g., growth factor signal receptor) or ligand (vascular endothelial growth factor [VEGF]) and thereby inhibit tumor growth or activate effector cells; 2) cytotoxicity by chaperoning cytotoxic molecules (immunoconjugates): these MAbs are conjugated to various cytotoxic molecules/atoms including chemotherapy or radioisotopes such as

TABLE 6.7 Some MAb-Based In-Home Test Kits[a]

Manufacturer	Product Distributor	Positive End Point
Pregnancy		
Answer Plus	Carter Products	Plus in test window = +
Answer Quick & Simple	Carter Products	Plus in test window = +
Clear Blue Easy	Unipath	Blue line in large window = +
Clear Blue Easy One Min.	Unipath	Blue line in large window = +
Conceive	Quidel	Pink to purple test line = +
1 Step E.P.T.	Warner Lambert	Pink color in test and control = +
Clear Blue Easy	Unipath	Blue line in large window = +
Clear Blue Easy One Min.	Unipath	Blue line in large window = +
Conceive	Quidel	Pink to purple test line = +
1 Step E.P.T.	Warner Lambert	Pink color in test and control = +
Clear Blue Easy	Unipath	Blue line in large window = +
Clear Blue Easy One Min.	Unipath	Blue line in large window = +
Ovulation		
Answer Quick & Simple	Carter Products	Purple stick line darker than reference = +
Conceive 1 Step	Quidel	Pink to purple test line darker than reference = +
First Response 1 Step	Carter Products	Purple test line darker than reference = +
ClearPlan Easy	Unipath	Blue test line in large window similar or darker than line in small window = +
Ovukit Self Test	Quidel	White to shades of blue compared to LH surge guide = +
OvuQuick	Quidel	Test spot appears darker than reference = +
Q Test	Quidel	Purple test line darker than reference = +

[a]Information from Pray W. Nonprescription Product Therapeutics, 2nd Ed. Philadelphia: Lippincott Williams & Wilkins, 2006:778–780; Quattrocchi E, Hove I. Ovulation & pregnancy home testing products. U.S. Pharmacist 1998;23:54–63; and Rosenthal WM, Briggs GC. Home testing and monitoring devices. In: Allen LV Jr, Berardi RR, DeSimone EM II, et al., eds. Handbook of Nonprescription Drugs. Washington, DC: American Pharmaceutical Association, 2000:917–942.

yttrium-90, which is in clinical use, cellular toxins such as diphtheria toxin, or biologic agents such as IFN; and 3) modulating an immunologic mechanism: in this case, MAbs exert their cytotoxic effects by antibody-dependent cell-mediated cytotoxicity or complement-dependent cytotoxicity.

Specific Drugs

Catumaxomab (Removab) Catumaxomab is a 180 kDa, chimeric murine IgG2a/rat IgG2b anti-EpCAM/anti-CD3, trifunctional MAb produced in the rat/mouse quadroma cell line (143). The human epithelial cell adhesion molecule (EpCAM) protein is overexpressed on a variety of carcinomas, and its inhibition has emerged as a viable approach for the immunotherapy of cancer. In addition to targeting EpCAM, catumaxomab has anti-CD3 arm that targets the T-cell antigen CD3; binding to the CD3 receptor activates T cells to release cytotoxic cytokines and to promote T-cell–mediated lysis. The trifunctionality comes from an intact Fc region that selectively binds to FCg receptor–positive accessory cells, such as macrophages, dendritic cells, and natural killer cells that promote phagocytosis and antibody-dependent cell cytotoxicity. Catumaxomab was generated using a hybrid hybridoma or quadroma, where two hybridoma cells producing different MAbs are fused together to form a new hybrid cell that contains sets of genes encoding the two parent antibodies. Catumaxomab is used for the intraperitoneal treatment of malignant ascites in patients with EpCAM-positive carcinomas where standard therapy is not available or no longer feasible.

Trastuzumab (Herceptin) One of the major advances in breast cancer treatment in the last decade has been the development of MAbs targeting growth factor receptors. Advances in the understanding of tumor pathobiology and molecular biology have facilitated the development of these targeted therapies, in particular in breast cancer.

TABLE 6.8 FDA-Approved MAb Therapeutic Agents

Generic Name	Trade Name	MAb Type	Indication
Abciximab	ReoPro	Chimeric	Adjunct to percutaneous transluminal coronary angioplasty for prevention of acute cardiac complications
Adalimumab	Humira	Fully human	Rheumatoid arthritis
Alemtuzumab	Campath	Humanized	B-cell chronic lymphocytic leukemia
Basiliximab	Simulect	Chimeric	Prevention of transplant rejection
Belimumab	Benlysta	Fully human	Systemic lupus erythematosus plus standard therapy
Bevacizumab	Avastin	Humanized	Metastatic colorectal cancer
Canakinumab	Ilaris	Fully human	Cryopyrin-associated periodic syndromes and Muckle-Wells syndrome
Catumaxomab	Removab	Chimeric	Malignant ascites
Certolizumab pegol	Cimzia	Humanized	Crohn disease
Cetuximab	Erbitux	Chimeric	Colorectal cancer
Daclizumab	Zenapax	Humanized	Prevention of transplant rejection
Denosumab	Prolia	Fully human	Postmenopausal osteoporosis in women
Eculizumab	Soliris	Fully human	Paroxysmal nocturnal hemoglobinuria
Efalizumab	Raptiva	Humanized	Psoriasis
Etanercept	Embrel	Fusion MAb	Rheumatoid and psoriatic arthritis and ankylosing spondylitis
Gemtuzumab	Mylotarg	Fusion MAb	Treatment of CD33-positive acute myeloid leukemia
Golimumab	Simponi	Fully human	Rheumatoid and psoriatic arthritis and ankylosing spondylitis
Ibritumomab tiuxetan	Zevalin	Murine	Non-Hodgkin lymphoma
Infliximab	Remicade	Chimeric	Crohn disease
Ipilimumab	Yervoy	Fully human	Late-stage melanoma
Muromonab-CD3	Orthoclone-OKT3	Murine	Reversal of transplant rejection
Natalizumab	Tysabri	Humanized	Multiple sclerosis
Ofatumumab	Arzerra	Fully human	Chronic lymphocytic leukemia
Omalizumab	Xolair	Humanized	Asthma
Palivizumab	Synagis	Humanized	Respiratory syncytial virus prophylaxis
Panitumumab	Vectibix	Fully human	First- or second-line treatment of metastatic colorectal cancer
Ranibizumab	Lucentis	Fully human	Neovascular age-related macular degeneration
Rituximab	Rituxan	Chimeric	Treatment of B-cell non-Hodgkin lymphoma
Tositumomab	Bexxar	Murine	Non-Hodgkin lymphoma
Trastuzumab	Herceptin	Humanized	Refractory breast cancer
Ustekinumab	Stelara	Fully human	Moderate to severe psoriasis

HER2 (or erbB2) is a transmembrane tyrosine kinase receptor that belongs to the family of the epidermal growth factor receptor (EGFR). HER2 protein overexpression is observed in 25% to 30% of primary breast cancers. Activated erbBs stimulate many intracellular signaling pathways, mainly the mitogen-activated protein kinase (MAPK) and the phosphatidylinositol 3-kinase (PI3K)-Akt pathways. In 1998, trastuzumab was approved by the FDA for clinical use largely based on a randomized clinical trial that compared chemotherapy with chemotherapy plus trastuzumab as a front-line treatment for patients with erbB2-overexpressing metastatic breast cancer (144).

Trastuzumab is a recombinant humanized anti-erbB2 MAb that binds the extracellular domain of the receptor and blocks intracellular signaling. Both cytostatic and cytotoxic mechanisms of action of trastuzumab were identified in preclinical studies. In vitro, downregulation of erbB2 disrupts receptor dimerization and signaling through the downstream PI3K cascade. It effectively prevents cell proliferation of the erbB2-overexpressing breast cancer SK-BR-3 cell line.

Trastuzumab, administered as single-agent, first-line therapy in women with erbB2-overexpressing metastatic breast cancer and in women with erbB2-overexpressing metastatic breast cancer that has progressed after chemotherapy, produces durable objective responses with a median duration of response of 9.1 months (144).

Bevacizumab (Avastin) Angiogenesis, the process of developing new blood vessels from existing ones, is critical for tumor cell growth, survival, invasion, and metastasis. Numerous growth factors work in the tumor microenvironment to promote angiogenesis. Of these, VEGF may be among the most important factors implicated in angiogenesis, based on its specificity as an endothelial cell mitogen and the ability of many tumor types to produce it in physiologically relevant quantities. Oncogenic activation, loss of tumor suppressor factors, and tumor hypoxia lead to upregulation of VEGF production. There are four isoforms of the VEGF (A, B, C, and D) and three types of VEGF receptors (VEGFRs). Once produced, VEGF-A binds to two tyrosine kinase receptors, termed VEGFR-1 and VEGFR-2, which are predominantly located on the surface of vascular endothelial cells. VEGFR-2 appears to be the more important of the two receptors for mediating the angiogenic effects of VEGF, whereas VEGFR-1 may be a decoy receptor that modulates the amount of VEGF available for binding to VEGFR-2. VEGF and its receptors have emerged as anticancer targets based on their central and specific role in angiogenesis. In principle, VEGF-targeted therapy may inhibit tumor growth by blocking new vessel growth. Bevacizumab was approved in 2004 for the treatment of metastatic colorectal cancer in combination with fluorouracil-based chemotherapy (145).

Bevacizumab, a 149 kDa recombinant humanized monoclonal IgG1 antibody (93% human, 7% murine sequences) directed against VEGF-A, is believed to globally prevent the binding of all VEGF isoforms to all VEGFRs. Bevacizumab is composed of two identical light chains (214 amino acids) and two heavy chains (453 amino acids) and is produced in a CHO cell expression system (145).

Panitumumab (Vectibix) EGFR, a transmembrane cell surface glycoprotein belonging to the subfamily of type I tyrosine kinase receptors, is overexpressed in certain human cancers including colon and rectum cancers. The binding of ligands such as EGF and transforming growth factor-alpha to EGFR triggers autophosphorylation and internalization of EGFR, thereby activating various signaling pathways involved in proliferation, angiogenesis, inhibition of apoptosis, and metastasis.

Panitumumab is a 147 kDa recombinant, fully human IgG2 anti-EGFR MAb produced in genetically engineered mammalian CHO cells. Panitumumab was discovered using Abgenix's XenoMouse technology and was approved by the FDA in 2006 (146). Proposed mechanisms explaining the antitumor activity of panitumumab include downregulation of EGFR expression resulting from receptor internalization, induction of apoptosis via inhibition of EGFR signaling pathways and induction of cell cycle arrest, induction of autophagy, and inhibition of angiogenesis. Panitumumab is used in combination with chemotherapy for the first- or second-line treatment of metastatic colorectal cancer or as monotherapy for the treatment of chemotherapy-refractory metastatic colorectal cancer in patients with wild-type rather than mutant K-*ras* tumors. K-*ras* protein is a membrane bound G protein and is activated by receptor tyrosine kinases and is found to be mutated in 30% to 40% of colorectal cancer patients (147,148). Panitumumab has an acceptable tolerability profile when administered as monotherapy or in combination with chemotherapy. It is associated with skin-related toxicities, which is a characteristic of EGFR inhibitors.

Cetuximab (Erbitux) As discussed previously, EGFR overexpression is detected in many human cancers, including colorectal cancer. Cetuximab was approved in 2004 for the second-line treatment of colorectal cancer either alone or in combination with chemotherapy (149). Cetuximab, a recombinant human/mouse chimeric MAb with an approximate MW of 152 kDa, is produced in mammalian murine myeloma cell culture. It binds specifically to the extracellular domain of the human EGFR on normal and tumor cells and competitively inhibits the binding of the EGF and other ligands, such as transforming growth factor-alpha. Binding of cetuximab to the EGFR blocks phosphorylation and activation of receptor-associated kinases, resulting in inhibition of cell growth, induction of apoptosis, decreased matrix metalloproteinase, and VEGF reduction. Cetuximab is eliminated by binding to EGFRs in various tissues, followed by internalization of the antibody–EGFR complex.

Ofatumumab (Arzerra) Chronic lymphocytic leukemia (CLL) is the most common adult leukemia and one of the most common malignant lymphoid diseases. Based on 2007 worldwide estimates, leukemia accounted for more than 330,000 new cases and more than 245,000 deaths (150). CLL cells are malignant B cells that have low surface expression levels of CD20 molecules. B cells normally protect the body from invading pathogens by developing into plasma cells, which make antibodies.

These antibodies directly inactivate pathogens or attach to pathogens to prepare them for destruction by other white blood cells. Ofatumumab received accelerated approval in 2009 for the treatment of patients with CLL refractory to fludarabine and alemtuzumab.

Ofatumumab is a fully human 149 kDa IgG1κ anti-CD20 MAb generated via transgenic mouse and hybridoma technology and is produced in a recombinant murine cell line (NS0) using standard mammalian cell cultivation and purification technologies (151). Ofatumumab binds specifically to both the small and large extracellular loops of the CD20 molecule. Ofatumumab is highly potent in lysing B cells, which is presumably due to its binding to the membrane-proximal, small extracellular loop of the target CD20 protein and its slow release from the target molecule (152). As with other human monoclonal antibodies, ofatumumab induces both antibody-dependent cell-mediated cytotoxicity and complement-dependent cytotoxicity.

Alemtuzumab (Campath-1H) Alemtuzumab was introduced in 2001 for the treatment of patients with B-cell CLL who had been treated with alkylating agents and failed fludarabine therapy. Alemtuzumab is an rDNA-derived humanized IgG1κ MAb specific for the cell surface glycoprotein CD52 expressed on normal and malignant human peripheral-blood B and T lymphocytes as well as natural killer cells, monocytes, macrophages, and tissues of the male reproductive system. It is produced in CHO cells and has an approximate MW of 150 kDa. The mechanism of action is not completely understood but involves a number of effects, including complement-mediated cell lysis, antibody-dependent cellular toxicity, and the induction of apoptosis (153,154).

Ibritumomab Tiuxetan (Zevalin) Radioimmunotherapy is an innovative form of cancer therapy, combining a MAb against a specific target antigen with a source of radiation such as a radioisotope. Technical advances have made it possible to link radionuclides such as yttrium-90 (^{90}Y) to MAbs specifically to target radiation to lymphoma cells. Yttrium-90 is a beta-emitting radionuclide that delivers 90% of its radiation (2.3 MeV) over a mean path length of 5 mm and has a half-life of 64 hours. These characteristics are particularly advantageous for treating bulky, poorly vascularized tumors and tumors with heterogeneous antigen expression. Ibritumomab tiuxetan therapeutic regimen became the first radioimmunotherapy approved by the FDA in 2002 for the treatment of NHL, the fifth leading type of cancer in the United States, with approximately 300,000 people affected by this cancer at present.

Ibritumomab tiuxetan, a 148 kDa radioimmunoconjugate, is a short-course therapy that uses immunobiologic and radiolytic mechanisms of action to destroy both dividing and nondividing tumor cells. Ibritumomab is a murine IgG1κ MAb produced in CHO cells. It is directed against the CD20 antigen found on the surface of malignant B lymphocytes in patients with B-cell NHL as well as on normal mature B lymphocytes. Tiuxetan, [*N*-[2-bis(carboxymethyl)amino]-3-(*p*-isothiocyanatophenyl)propyl]-[*N*-[bis(carboxy-methyl) amino-2-(methyl)-ethyl]glycine forms a stable covalent thiourea-type linkage with the lysine and arginine residues of the antibody and can chelate a radionuclide via its carboxyl groups (Fig. 6.25). Ibritumomab tiuxetan can chelate indium-111 (^{111}In) for imaging or ^{90}Y for therapy. Thus, the antibody specifically targets radiation to CD20-positive cells while sparing normal nonlymphoid cells. Ibritumomab tiuxetan is indicated for the treatment of patients with relapsed or refractory, low-grade, follicular or transformed B-cell NHL, including patients with rituximab-refractory follicular NHL. After ^{90}Y Zevalin enters the bloodstream, the MAb ibritumomab recognizes and attaches to the CD20 antigen, allowing beta radiation emitted by the ^{90}Y isotope to penetrate and damage the B cell as well as neighboring cells (155).

Tositumomab (Bexxar) Tositumomab was introduced in 2003 as a novel radioimmunotherapeutic antibody for the treatment of B-cell NHL. Therapeutic regimen of the drug is composed of tositumomab and iodine-131 (^{131}I)-tositumomab. Tositumomab is a murine IgG2a lambda monoclonal antibody directed against the CD20 antigen, which is found on the surface of normal and malignant B lymphocytes. Tositumomab is produced in an antibiotic-free culture of mammalian cells and is composed of two murine gamma 2a heavy chains of 451 amino acids each and two lambda light chains of 220 amino acids each. The approximate MW of tositumomab is 150 kDa. ^{131}I-tositumomab is a radio-iodinated derivative of tositumomab that has been covalently linked to ^{131}I through tyrosine residues.

Tositumomab actions include induction of apoptosis, complement-dependent cytotoxicity, and antibody-dependent cellular cytotoxicity. Additionally, cell death is associated with ionizing radiation from the radioisotope. ^{131}I has a half-life of 8 days and emits β and γ rays. The antitumor

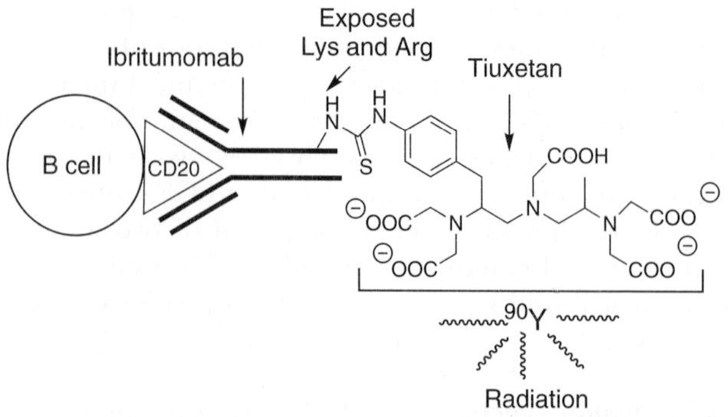

FIGURE 6.25 Structure of ibritumomab tiuxetan radioimmunoconjugate monoclonal antibody (MAb) and its binding to the target CD20 on the surface of the B cell.

activity results from the β-particles. Thus the mechanisms of action of this radioimmunotherapeutic drug involve combining tumor-targeting ability of the cytotoxic MAb with patient-specific delivery of radiation dose directly to the tumor cells. The therapeutic regimen of the radioimmunotherapeutic antibody is indicated for the treatment of patients with CD20 antigen–expressing relapsed or refractory, low-grade, follicular, or transformed NHL, including patients with rituximab-refractory NHL (155).

Storage of the radioimmunotherapeutic drug requires special considerations. The lead pot containing ^{131}I-tositumomab must be stored in a freezer at a temperature of −20°C or below until it is removed for thawing prior to administration to the patient. Thawed dosimetric and therapeutic doses of ^{131}I-tositumomab are stable for up to 8 hours at 2°C to 8°C or at room temperature. Any unused portion must be discarded according to federal and state laws.

Canakinumab (Ilaris) Canakinumab was approved in 2009 for the treatment of cryopyrin-associated periodic syndromes known as familial cold autoinflammatory syndrome and Muckle-Wells syndrome in patients 4 years of age or older. The two syndromes are serious inherited autoimmune inflammatory disorders that are believed to result from cryopyrin-activated overproduction of IL-1β. Canakinumab is a 150 kDa, fully human, IgG1 anti–IL-1β MAb produced in mouse hybridoma Sp2/0-Ag14 cell line by rDNA technology (156). Compared to other drugs targeting IL-1β, such as anakinra and rilonacept, canakinumab possesses a less frequent dosing regimen and instigates fewer injection site reactions. Because IL-1β suppression can hinder the immune response, the labeling recommends that patients receive all recommended vaccinations before starting canakinumab therapy. No live vaccines should be administered during treatment with canakinumab, and patients should be tested for latent tuberculosis before receiving canakinumab. Similar to rilonacept, the labeling warns against the concomitant administration of canakinumab and TNF inhibitors, and therapeutic monitoring is recommended with concurrent administration of drugs that interact with the CYP450 system.

Certolizumab Pegol (Cimzia) Crohn disease is an immunologically mediated chronic relapsing inflammatory bowel disease of the gastrointestinal tract that can potentially affect the entire gastrointestinal tract, but most commonly occurs in the terminal ileum and colon. Active Crohn disease is associated with excessive levels of proinflammatory cytokines including TNF-α. It is growing in incidence in both developing and developed countries. The incidence rate in North America is among the highest with 1 to 15 cases per 100,000 person-years. Certolizumab pegol is a TNF-α blocker approved for the treatment of moderate to severe Crohn disease (157,158). It is specifically indicated for reducing signs and symptoms and maintaining clinical response in adult patients who have had an inadequate response to conventional therapy. Certolizumab pegol is a 91 kDa humanized antibody fragment Fab′ that is manufactured in *E. coli*, purified, and conjugated to PEG. The addition of PEG moiety significantly enhances the plasma half-life of the antibody, allowing for less frequent dosing. Certolizumab is the third anti–TNF-α biologic to be marketed for Crohn disease behind infliximab and adalimumab and has higher affinity than both of these drugs for TNF-α. Unlike the full-length antibodies infliximab and adalimumab, certolizumab pegol does not contain an Fc region and, therefore, does not induce complement activation, antibody-dependent cellular cytotoxicity, or apoptosis in vitro. As with other TNF-α inhibitors, the drug is associated with an increased risk of opportunistic infections and malignancy, and it carries a warning of the risk of serious infections such as histoplasmosis.

Golimumab (Simponi) The proinflammatory cytokine TNF-α has been implicated as the primary mediator of articular inflammation in diseases such as RA, psoriatic arthritis, and ankylosing spondylitis. Targeting TNF-α has been a successful strategy in the intervention of a range of immunoinflammatory disorders. Golimumab is a 150 kDa, fully human, IgG1 anti-TNF MAb produced in murine Sp2/0 cell line. It was approved by the FDA in 2009 (159). Drugs previously introduced include infliximab (chimeric MAb), etanercept (fusion protein comprised of the ligand-binding segment of the soluble TNF receptor) in the late 1990s, and adalimumab (fully human) and certolizumab pegol (PEGylated humanized) in more recent years. Golimumab binds to both soluble and transmembrane forms of TNF-α, is the first once-monthly SC agent to enter the market, and is currently approved for the treatment of RA and psoriatic arthritis in combination with MTX and for treatment of ankylosing spondylitis. The drug is administered as an SC injection once a month. Live vaccines should not be administered while being treated with golimumab. The drug carries a boxed warning regarding the risk of serious infections including tuberculosis and invasive fungal infections, such as histoplasmosis. Furthermore, patients are also warned that lymphoma and other malignancies, some fatal, have been reported in children and adolescent patients treated with TNF blockers, of which golimumab is a member.

Ustekinumab (Stelara) Psoriasis is a chronic inflammatory disease that affects approximately 2% to 3% of the world population. The most common form of the disease is plaque psoriasis. Conventional treatment options for psoriasis include topical corticosteroids, phototherapy, and systemic drugs, but all of these drugs have limitations. Ustekinumab is a fully human 149 kDa IgG1κ MAb developed in transgenic mouse and expressed in unspecified recombinant cell line. Ustekinumab inhibits IL-12 and IL-23 signaling by blocking p40 binding to IL-12/23 receptors. It was approved by the FDA in 2009 for the treatment of moderate to severe psoriasis in patients who cannot tolerate other treatment modalities with ease or in whom these modalities have failed (160). As a human IgG1κ MAb, ustekinumab is expected to be degraded into small peptides and amino acids via catabolic pathways in the same manner as endogenous IgG. The mean half-life of ustekinumab ranges from 15 to 46 days across all psoriasis studies following intravenous and SC administration.

Eculizumab (Soliris) Paroxysmal nocturnal hemoglobinuria is a clonal hematopoietic stem cell disorder that is characterized by the production of abnormal red blood cells. Eculizumab, a fully humanized anti-CD5 MAb with an approximate MW of 148 kDa, is used for the treatment of patients with paroxysmal nocturnal hemoglobinuria to reduce hemolysis (161,162). It is the first therapy to be introduced for this rare and life-threatening form of hemolytic anemia. Eculizumab is effective in controlling serum hemolytic activity. Eculizumab has been granted orphan drug status from both the FDA and European regulatory agencies. The drug carries a black box warning for the potential increased risk of meningococcal infections and requires patients to receive meningococcal vaccine at least 2 weeks prior to receiving the first dose of eculizumab.

Ranibizumab (Lucentis) Ranibizumab is a recombinant, fully humanized IgG1 MAb fragment produced by the *E. coli* expression system. It neutralizes all active forms of VEGF-A and is indicated for the treatment of neovascular age-related macular degeneration (163,164). The full-length anti-VEGF-A MAb, bevacizumab, is approved for the treatment of colorectal cancer. The Fab domain of ranibizumab differs from the Fab domain of bevacizumab by six amino acids. The smaller size of ranibizumab (~48 kDa) is expected to facilitate retinal penetration and hence is more suitable for intraocular use. The binding of ranibizumab to VEGF-A prevents the interaction with its receptors (VEGFR-1 and VEGFR-2) on the surface of endothelial cells, thereby reducing endothelial cell proliferation, vascular leakage, and new blood vessel formation. Ranibizumab is administered once a month by intravitreal injection.

Denosumab (Prolia) Osteoporosis is a chronic, debilitating disease in which the bones become porous and break easily. Approximately 10 million people in the United States are estimated to have osteoporosis, and almost 34 million Americans are estimated to have low bone mass, placing them at increased risk for osteoporosis. Receptor activator of nuclear factor-κB ligand (RANKL) is a protein expressed by osteoblasts and bone-lining cells that binds to receptor activator of nuclear factor-κB (RANK) receptors on osteoclast and osteoclast precursors. The RANKL/RANK complex stimulates osteoclast precursors to mature to osteoclasts and increases osteoclast activity on bone resorption. After menopause, as estrogen levels drop, RANKL levels increase. Denosumab, a 147 kDa fully human MAb produced in genetically engineered mammalian CHO cells, is specific for RANKL and was approved by the FDA in 2010 for the treatment of postmenopausal osteoporosis in women (also see Chapter 30). By inhibiting RANKL, denosumab inhibits osteoclast function and bone resorption. Denosumab has been shown to increase bone mineral density and decrease fracture risk in postmenopausal women with osteoporosis (165).

PHARMACOGENOMICS AND PERSONALIZED MEDICINE

Personalized medicine is defined as the utilization of molecular biomarkers from an individual's genome, transcriptome, proteome, and metabolome under the influence of the individual's envirome in the assessment of predisposition to disease, screening and early diagnosis of disease, assessment of prognosis, pharmacogenomic prediction of therapeutic drug efficacy and risk of toxicity, and monitoring of illness until the final therapeutic outcome is determined (Fig. 6.26) (166).

The concept of personalized medicine was anticipated by Sir William Osler (1849–1919), a well-known Canadian physician during his time. He recognized that "variability is the law of life, and as no two faces are the same, so no two bodies are alike, and no two individuals react alike and behave alike under the abnormal conditions we know as disease." Personalized medicine has rapidly advanced the prediction of disease incidence as well as the prevention of incorrect drug prescription based on a person's clinical, genetic, and environmental information. The goal of personalized medicine is optimizing the medical care and outcomes for each patient (167).

Pharmacogenomics uses genomic tools to understand the genotype effects of relevant genes on the behavior of a drug, as well as the effects of a drug on gene expression. The best examples of successful pharmacogenomic applications are presented below.

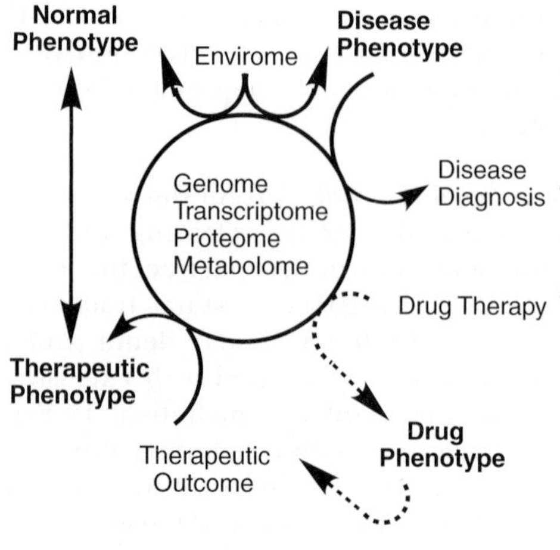

FIGURE 6.26 Schematic representation of the concept of molecular profiling for personalized medicine. Dashed arrows indicate the critical components of pharmacogenomics: disease diagnosis, drug therapy, drug phenotype, and therapeutic outcome.

The oral anticoagulant warfarin is prescribed for the long-term treatment and prevention of thromboembolic events. An investigation of the pharmacokinetic and pharmacodynamic drug properties of warfarin indicated the additive involvement of two genes when determining the dosage. One of these genes encodes CYP2C9, which is responsible for the metabolic clearance (~80%) of the pharmacologically potent *S*-enantiomer of warfarin. There are three allele types, CYP2C9*1, *2, and *3, and both CYP2C9*2 and *3 cause a reduction in warfarin clearance. A 10-fold difference in warfarin clearance was observed between groups of individuals having the genotype of the highest metabolizer (CYP2C9*1 homozygote) and lowest metabolizer (CYP2C9*3 homozygote) (168).

Trastuzumab is a MAb that specifically targets breast cancers overexpressing the *HER2/neu* gene and thus is marketed solely for the subset of breast cancer patients (~10%) overexpressing the *HER2/neu* gene. Because trastuzumab was developed for marker-positive individuals who comprise a rather low proportion of breast cancer patients, trastuzumab therapy may be one of the best examples of a genomic technology paving the way for personalized medical treatment (169).

Tamoxifen is a prodrug that is metabolized by members of the CYP450 family into two active metabolites: 4-hydroxy tamoxifen (4OH-TAM) and 4-hydroxyl-*N*-desmethyltamoxifen (endoxifen) (Fig. 6.27). CYP3A4/5 is responsible for the conversion of tamoxifen into *N*-desmethyltamoxifen, which is then converted into its active metabolite, endoxifen, by CYP2D6. CYP2D6 is also responsible for the conversion of tamoxifen into 4OH-TAM. In a recent study of steady-state levels of tamoxifen and active tamoxifen metabolites, there was interpatient variability for all three metabolites. A recent study investigating the CYP2D6*4 allele (inactive enzyme), a poor metabolizer that is common in Caucasians, in patients being treated with tamoxifen found that individuals who were homozygous for CYP2D6*4 had significantly lower endoxifen levels than patients who had the wild-type gene. This study clearly indicates that genotyping of patients with impaired CYP2D6 function may be beneficial in a clinical setting to determine which patients will derive the most benefit from tamoxifen therapy (170).

Tolterodine [(*R*)-*N*,*N*-diisopropyl-3-(2-hydroxy-5-methylphenyl)-phenylpropanamine] is a new antimuscarinic drug for the treatment of urinary urge incontinence and other symptoms associated with an overactive bladder. Two different oxidative metabolic pathways, hydroxylation and *N*-dealkylation, have been identified in humans (Fig. 6.28). Hydroxylation to the pharmacologically active 5-hydroxymethyl metabolite (5-HM) is catalyzed by CYP2D6, whereas the *N*-dealkylation pathway is catalyzed by CYP3A4. Further oxidation of 5-HM catalyzed by alcohol and aldehyde dehydrogenases yields the carboxylic acid of tolterodine and its *N*-dealkylated form, along with *N*-dealkylated 5-HM. As described previously, CYP2D6 is subject to genetic polymorphism, with important implications for drugs that are metabolized by this enzyme such as tolterodine. Clinical studies have demonstrated that individuals with reduced CYP2D6-mediated metabolism represent a high-risk group in the population, with a propensity to develop adverse drug effects. In fast metabolizers, the mean systemic clearance of tolterodine was found to be 44 L/hour, yielding a half-life of 2 to 3 hours. In contrast, poor metabolizers have a fivefold lower clearance and a mean half-life of 9 hours, which results in a sevenfold higher maximum serum concentration of tolterodine at steady-state (171).

Irinotecan (also known as CPT-11 or Camptosar) is an approved topoisomerase I inhibitor used to treat patients with metastatic colon cancer. Acute and delayed diarrhea and neutropenia often occur after treatment with irinotecan. Diarrhea following treatment with irinotecan occurs due to the excretion of an active metabolite (SN-38,10-hydroxy-7-ethylcamptothecin) initially into the bile and subsequently

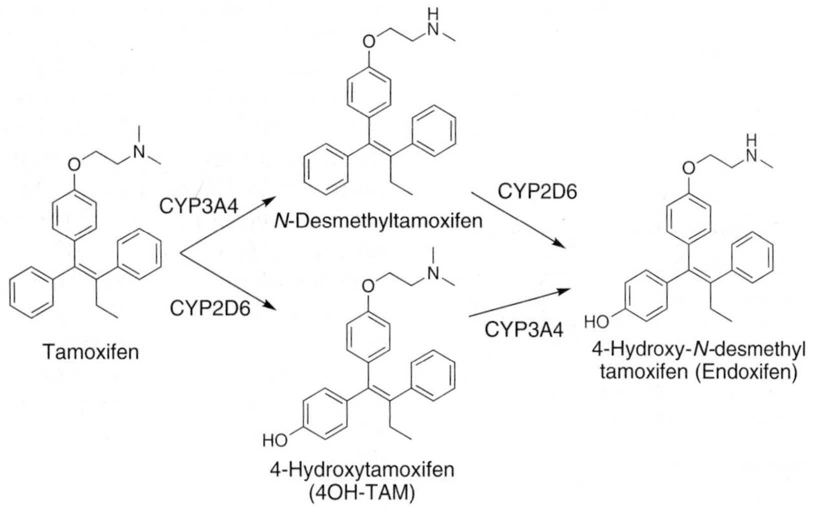

FIGURE 6.27 Tamoxifen metabolic pathway.

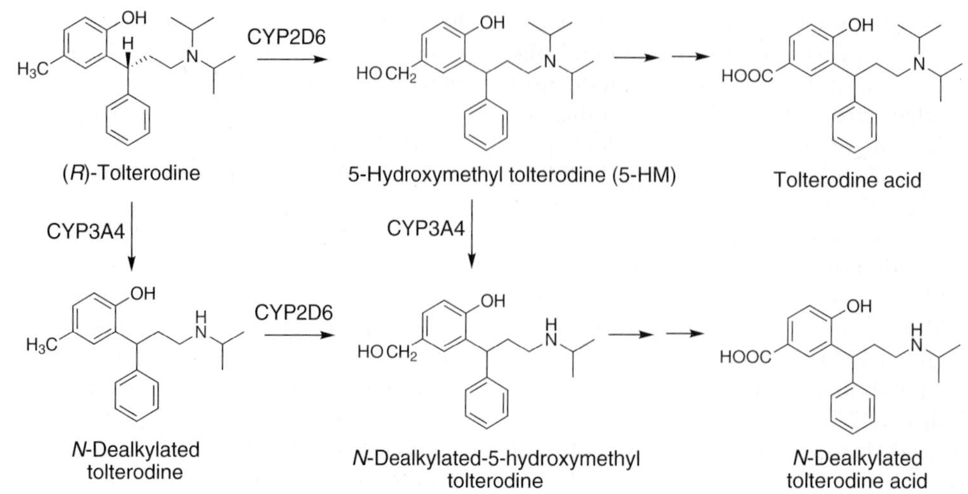

FIGURE 6.28 Tolterodine metabolic pathway.

the colon (Fig. 6.29; for more details, see Chapter 37 and Fig. 37.18). Irinotecan treatment is associated with an increased frequency of severe and potentially life-threatening toxicity among patients with genetic polymorphisms that markedly reduce glucuronidation of SN-38. Patients with decreased capacity to glucuronidate SN-38 (e.g., patients homozygous for specific UDP-glucuronosyl transferase 1A1 [UGT1A1] genotypes such as UGT1A1*28 [TA7]) are at increased risk for severe neutropenia after treatment with irinotecan or SN-38 than patients with wild-type sequence (172).

GENE THERAPY

The premise of gene therapy is that genes can (173) be used as pharmaceutical products to cause in vivo

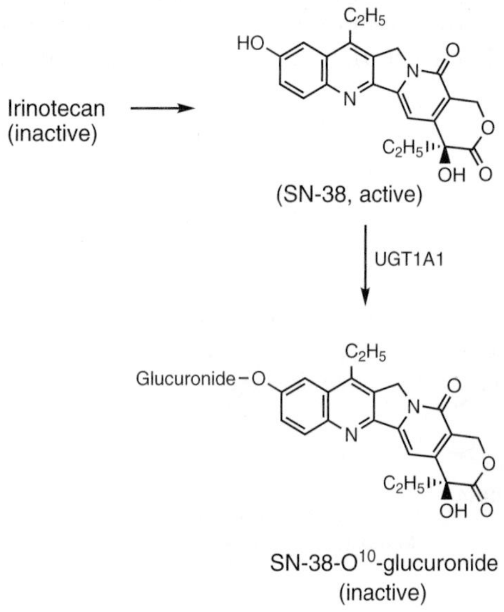

FIGURE 6.29 Metabolic activation of irinotecan.

production of therapeutic proteins. There is considerable confidence that gene therapy, as a therapeutic paradigm, will provide a number of novel pharmaceutical products, diagnostics, and therapeutic approaches in the years to come (173). A major problem in gene therapy is similar to the problem encountered in all forms of drug therapy—the assurance of drug efficacy through efficient delivery of the therapeutic agent to its biologic target in a fully functional form. Gene therapy is unique in the sense that it is the product of gene expression, the protein, and not the gene itself that is the therapeutic agent. Hence, we must not only deliver the gene to its proper target but also assure that when the gene reaches its target, it will arrive in a form that will produce the therapeutic agent in such a form that it, too, will be assured of reaching its specified target (174–176). A number of gene therapy products are under various phases of clinical investigation for different disease conditions including a severe combined immunodeficiency disease due to adenosine deaminase deficiency ($CD34^+$ cells transduced with adenosine deaminase gene), glioblastoma (Toca511, a retroviral replicating vector), age-related macular degeneration (AAV2-sFLT01), Parkinson disease (CERE-120: adeno-associated virus delivery of neurturin), advanced osteocarcinoma (Her2 chimeric antigen receptor expressing T cells), CLL (autologous T lymphocytes engrafted with a chimeric antigen receptor targeting the kappa light chain), and Alzheimer disease (CERE-110: adeno-associated virus delivery of nerve growth factor). The steps (administration, delivery, and expression) involved in the delivery of the therapeutic gene are shown in Figure 6.30 (177). Because gene therapy has yet to reach the market, a detailed discussion on gene therapy and the ethical challenges it presents is beyond the scope of this chapter.

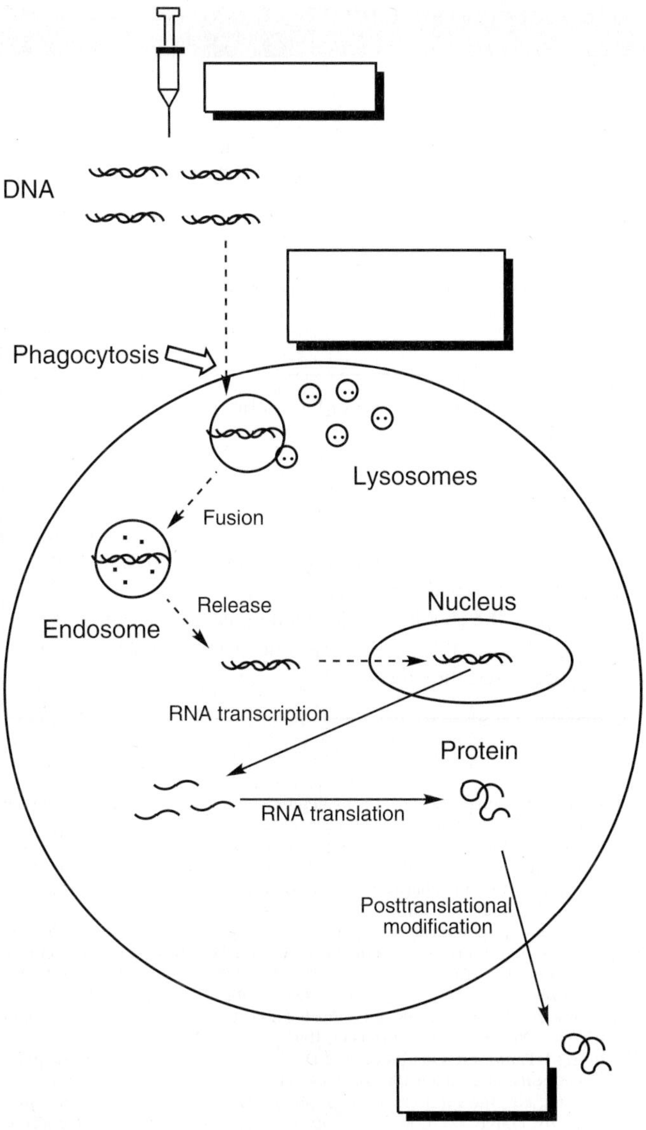

FIGURE 6.30 Steps in gene therapy. Gene therapy involves the steps of administration, delivery, and expression. (Note: dashed arrow represents uptake and transport).

SUMMARY

Completion of the Human Genome Project in 2003 resulted in the elucidation of the entire sequence of the 3 billion base pairs in the human genome, estimated to contain some 25,000 genes. The full impact that this scientific advance will have on our lives has yet to be determined, but the social, legal, ethical, and economic issues are certain to be extensive and complex. The manipulation and analysis of the genomic information obtained from the Human Genome Project is paving the path for transformative biomedical developments. DNA-based tests are among the first commercial medical applications. Gene tests can be used to diagnose and confirm disease, provide prognostic information about the course of disease, and predict the risk of future disease in healthy individuals.

Knowledge of genes involved in diseases, disease pathways, and drug-response sites will result in the discovery of novel therapeutic targets beyond the 500 or so that were known prior to the completion of the Human Genome Project, providing a tremendous opportunity for the discovery of drugs that work through previously unexplored mechanisms.

Discovery of genomic biomarkers can help determine the type of drug therapy. For example, one of the most commonly used predictive biomarkers in cancer is immunohistochemical staining for the presence of the estrogen receptor in breast cancer. Only estrogen receptor–positive breast tumors are likely to respond to antihormonal therapy. Identification of biomarkers for various diseases can help in the selection of patients most likely to benefit from a potential drug, which in turn will speed the design of clinical trials that are more efficient and have the potential to reduce drug approval time and associated costs. Predicting toxicity is another important outcome of the availability of the genomic information. For example, patients who have mutations in the thiopurine *S*-methyltransferase gene will metabolize the chemotherapeutic mercaptopurine drugs at a reduced rate and can be overdosed on their treatment. Similarly, an SNP in the coding region of genes expressing drug-metabolizing CYP450 enzymes results in either poor (overdose) or fast (subtherapeutic dose) metabolism of drugs.

The future will see an altered form of health care using a genetic information infrastructure to contain costs and predict outcomes, create advanced personalized therapies, and develop a predict-and-manage paradigm of health care. The recent years have witnessed the introduction of a steady stream of biotechnology-derived drugs. The trend is expected to continue for the foreseeable future. The expiration of patents on biotechnology-derived drugs will introduce an era of more affordable biosimilars or follow-on biologics.

CASE STUDY

S. William Zito and Victoria Roche

TS is a 24-year-old white woman who is 8 months postpartum. She complains of excruciating back pain in the sacral area as well as left lower quadrant pain. The pain worsens about 1.5 weeks before her periods and continues during her menses. She gets only mild relief with nonsteroidal anti-inflammatory drugs. Since the delivery TS has been taking oral contraceptive pills; the pills regulate her cycles but do not seem to alleviate the pain. TS recounts that during her pregnancy she was pain-free for the first time in 5 years. The menstrual pain began when she was approximately 19 years old. On further questioning she notes occasional painful intercourse, especially just before menses. A pelvic examination reveals a retroverted uterus, which is tender to palpation. Cervix and vaginal mucosa are unremarkable. The Papanicolau, *Neisseria gonorrheae,* and chlamydia tests were negative.

Because oral contraceptive pills do not alleviate the symptoms, TS's gynecologist suspects endometriosis and wants to prescribe a gonadotropin-releasing hormone superagonist to help control the symptoms while awaiting laparoscopy and biopsy for diagnostic confirmation. Which of the following peptides do you recommend?

5 6 9 10
pGlu-His-Trp-Ser-Tyr-Gly-Leu-Arg-Pro-Gly-NH_2

1

5 6 9 10
pGlu-His-Trp-Ser-Tyr-D-Nal(2)-Leu-Arg-Pro-Gly-NH_2

2

S———S
D-Phe-Cys-Phe-D-Trp-Lys-Thr-Cys-Thr-ol

3

1. Conduct a thorough and mechanistic SAR analysis of the three therapeutic options in the case.
2. Apply the chemical understanding gained from the SAR analysis to this patient's specific needs to make a therapeutic recommendation.

References

1. Ernst & Young. Beyond Borders Global Biotechnology Report 2010. Available at: http://www.ey.com/FR/fr/Newsroom/News-releases/Communique-de-presse—Beyond-Borders-Global-Biotechnology-Report-2010.
2. Kresse GB. Biosimilars: science, status, and strategic perspective. Eur J Pharm Bipharm 2009;72:479–486.
3. Zuniga L, Calvo B. Biosimilars approval process. Regul Toxicol Pharmacol 2010;56:374–377.
4. Wang DG, Fan JB, Siao CJ, et al. Large-scale identification, mapping, and genotyping of single-nucleotide polymorphisms in the human genome. Science 1998;280:1077–1082.
5. Pandey A, Mann M. Proteomics to study genes and genomes. Nature 2000;405:837–846.
6. Tonge R, Shaw J, Middleton B, et al. Validation and development of fluorescence two-dimensional differential gel electrophoresis proteomics technology. Proteomics 2001;1:377–396.
7. Zhu H, Snyder M. Protein arrays and microarrays. Curr Opin Chem Biol 2001;5:40–45.
8. Smolka MB, Zhou H, Purkayastha S, et al. Optimization of the isotope-coded affinity tag-labeling procedure for quantitative proteome analysis. Anal Biochem 2001;297:25–31.
9. Uetz P, Giot L, Cagney G, et al. A comprehensive analysis of protein–protein interactions in *Saccharomyces cerevisiae.* Nature 2000;403:623–627.
10. Saghatelian A, Cravatt BF. Global strategies to integrate the proteome and metabolome. Curr Opin Chem Biol 2005;9:62–68.
11. Bino RJ, Hall RD, Fiehn O, et al. Potential of metabolomics as a functional genomics tool. Trends Plant Sci 2004;9:418–425.
12. Fiehn O. Metabolomics—the link between genotypes and phenotypes. Plant Mol Biol 2002;48:155–171.
13. Gerstein MB, Bruce C, Rozowsky JS, et al. What is a gene, post-ENCODE? History and updated definition. Genome Res 2007;17:669–681.
14. Maxam AM, Gilbert W. A new method of sequencing DNA. Proc Natl Acad Sci U S A 1977;74:560–564.
15. Sanger F, Nicklen S, Coulson AR. DNA sequencing with chain-terminating inhibitors. Proc Natl Acad Sci U S A 1977;74:5463–5467.
16. Tucker T, Marra M, Friedman JM. Massively parallel sequencing: the next big thing in genetic medicine. Am J Hum Genet 2009;85:142–154.
17. Atkinson A, Smith M. Solid-phase synthesis of oligodeoxyribonucleotides by the phosphite-triester method. In: Gait MJ, ed. Oligonucleotide Synthesis: A Practical Approach. Oxford, UK: IRL Press Ltd., 1984:35–82.
18. Sproat BS, Gait MJ. Solid-phase synthesis of oligodeoxyribonucleotides by the phosphotriester method. In: Gait MJ, ed. Oligonucleotide Synthesis: A Practical Approach. Oxford, UK: IRL Press Ltd., 1984:83–115.
19. Newton CR, Graham A. Introduction to biotechniques-PCR. In: Billington D, ed. PCR, 2nd Ed. New York: Springer-Verlag, 1997.
20. Walsh G. Biopharmaceutical: Biochemistry and Biotechnology. Chichester, UK: John Wiley & Sons Ltd., 1998:293–336.
21. Kadir F. Production of biotech compounds—cultivation and downstream processing. In: Crommelin DJA, Sindelar RD, eds. Pharmaceutical Biotechnology: An Introduction for Pharmacists and Pharmaceutical Scientists. Amsterdam: Harwood Academic Publishers, 1997:53–70.
22. Crommelin D. Formulation of biotech products, including biopharmaceutical considerations. In: Crommelin DJA, Sindelar RD, eds. Pharmaceutical Biotechnology: An Introduction for Pharmacists and Pharmaceutical Scientists. Amsterdam: Harwood Academic Publishers, 1997:71–99.
23. Seetharam R, Sharma SK, eds. Purification and Analysis of Recombinant Proteins. New York: Marcel Dekker, 1991.
24. Briggs J, Panfili PR. Quantitation of DNA and protein impurities in biopharmaceuticals. Anal Chem 1991;63:850–859.
25. Dwyer J, ed. Analytical chromatography of amino acids, peptides, and proteins. In: Franks F, ed. Protein Biotechnology. Totowa, NJ: Humana Press, 1993:49–90.
26. Hancock W, Willis B. The future of analytical chemistry in the characterization of biopharmaceuticals. Am Lab 1996:31–34.
27. Horvath C, Ettre LS, eds. Chromatography in Biotechnology. Washington, DC: American Chemical Society, 1993.
28. Prankerd R, Schulman SG. Analytical methods in biotechnology. In: Pezzuto JM, Johnson ME, Manasse HR, eds. Biotechnology and Pharmacy. New York: Chapman & Hall, 1993:71–96.
29. Oeswein J, Shire SJ. Physical biochemistry of protein drugs. In: Peptide and Protein Drug Delivery. New York: Marcel Dekker, 1991:167–202.
30. Wang Y, Pearlman R, eds. Stability and Characterization of Protein and Peptide Drugs: Case Histories. New York: Plenum Press, 1993.
31. Burgess D. Drug delivery aspects of biotechnology products. In: Pezzuto JM, Johnson ME, Manasse HR, eds. Biotechnology and Pharmacy. New York: Chapman & Hall, 1993:116–151.
32. Lemke T. Review of Organic Functional Groups: Introduction to Medicinal Organic Chemistry, 5th Ed. Philadelphia: Lippincott Williams & Wilkins, 2012.
33. Li S, Schoneich C, Borchardt RT. Chemical instability of proteins. Pharm News 1995:12–16.
34. Frokjaer S, Otzen DE. Protein drug stability: a formulation challenge. Nat Rev Drug Discov 2005;4:298–306.
35. Powell M. Peptide stability in drug development: in vitro peptide degradation in plasma and serum. Annu Rep Med Chem 1993;28:285–294.
36. Kerwin BA, Remmele RL Jr. Protect from light: photodegradation and protein biologics. J Pharm Sci 2007;96:1468–1479.
37. Genentech. Written Information on storage, reconstitution, compatibility, stability, and administration on file. South San Francisco: Genentech, Inc., 1995.
38. Banga A, Reddy IK. Biotechnology drug: pharmaceutical issues. Pharm Times 1994;March:68–76.

39. Koeller J, Fields S. Biologic response modifiers. Contemp Pharm Issues 1991:4.
40. Sindelar R. The pharmacy of the future—biotechnology and your practice. Drug Topics 1993;137:66–78.
41. Hall P. Pharmaceutical Biotechnology. New York: Global Medical Communications, 1992.
42. Evens R, Louie SG, Sindelar R, et al. Biotech Rx: Biotechnology in Pharmacy Practice: Science, Clinical Applications, and Pharmaceutical Care—Opportunities in Therapy Management. Washington, DC: American Pharmaceutical Association, 1997.
43. Fields S. Dispensing biotechnology products. Am Pharm 1993;NS33:28–29.
44. Kane B, Kuhn JG. Biotechnology: new roles and challenges for the pharmacist in ambulatory care. Drug Topics 1992:3–13.
45. Piascik P, Smith GH. Dispensing biotechnology products: handling professional education and product information. In: Crommelin, D, Sindelar RD, eds. Pharmaceutical Biotechnology: An Introduction for Pharmacists and Pharmaceutical Scientists, 2nd Ed. London: Taylor and Francis, 2002:356–381.
46. Braeckman R. Pharmacokinetics and pharmacodynamics of peptide and proteins and drugs. In: Crommelin DJA, Sindelar RD, eds. Pharmaceutical Biotechnology: An Introduction for Pharmacists and Pharmaceutical Scientists. Amsterdam: Harwood Academic Publishers, 1997:101–121.
47. Reddy I, Belmonte AA. Pharmacokinetics of protein and peptide drugs. In: Zito SW, ed. Pharmaceutical Biotechnology: A Programmed Text. Lancaster, PA: Technomic Publishing, 1997:183–203.
48. Goldberg M, Gomezz-Orellana I. Challenges for the oral delivery of macromolecules. Nat Rev Drug Discov 2003;2:289–295.
49. Crommelin DJA, Storm G. Drug targeting. In: Sammes G, Taylor JD, eds. Comprehensive Medicinal Chemistry. New York: Oxford Press, 1990:661–701.
50. Bayley H. Protein therapy—delivery guaranteed. Nat Biotech 1999;17:1066–1067.
51. Lee V. Peptide and Protein Drug Delivery. New York: Marcel Dekker, 1991.
52. Reddy I. Protein and peptide drug delivery. In: Zito SW, ed. Pharmaceutical Biotechnology: A Programmed Text. Lancaster, PA: Technomic Publishing, 1997:159–182.
53. Shantha Kumar TR, Soppimath K, Nachaegari SK. Novel delivery technologies for protein and peptide therapeutics. Curr Pharm Biotech 2006;7: 261–276.
54. Spatola AF. Peptide backbone modifications: a structure–activity analysis of peptides containing amide bond surrogates, conformational constraints, and replacement. In: Weinstein B, ed. Chemistry and Biochemistry of Amino Acids, Peptides, and Proteins. New York: Marcel Dekker, 1983.
55. Goodman M, Chorev M. On the concept of linear modified retro-peptide structures. Acc Chem Res 1979;12:1–7.
56. Stewart C, Fleming RA. Biotechnology products: new opportunities and responsibilities for the pharmacist. Am J Hosp Pharm 1989;46(Suppl 2):S4–S8.
57. Crowley WF Jr, Conn PM. Modes of Action of GnRH and GnRH Analogues. New York: Springer-Verlag, 1991.
58. Chengalvala MV, Pelletier JC, Kopf GS. GnRH agonists and antagonists in cancer therapy. Curr Med Chem 2003;3:399–410.
59. Bauer W, Briner U, Doepfner W, et al. SMS 201-995: a very potent and selective analogue of somatostatin with a prolonged action. Life Sci 1982;31:1133–1140.
60. Emeric-Sauval E. Corticotropin-releasing factor. Psychoneuroendocrinology 1986;11:277–294.
61. Hintz RL. Untoward events in patients treated with growth hormone in the USA. Horm Res 1992;38(Suppl):44–49.
62. Marian M. Growth hormones. In: Crommelin DJA, Sindelar RD, eds. Pharmaceutical Biotechnology: An Introduction for Pharmacists and Pharmaceutical Scientists. Amsterdam: Harwood Academic Publishers, 1997:241–253.
63. Cázares-Delgadillo J, Ganem-Rondero A, Kalia YN. Human growth hormone: new delivery systems, alternative routes of administration, and their pharmacological relevance. Eur J Pharm Biopharm 2011;78:278–288.
64. Combarnous Y. Molecular basis of the specificity of binding of glycoprotein hormones to their receptors. Endocr Rev 1992;13:670–691.
65. Homburg R, Giudice LC, Chang RJ. Polycystic ovary syndrome. Hum Reprod 1996;11:465–466.
66. Lispi M, Bassett R, Crisci C, et al. Comparative assessment of the consistency and quality of a highly purified FSH extracted from human urine (urofollitropin) and a recombinant human FSH (follitropin α). Reprod Biomed Online 2006;13:179–193.
67. Sam T, De Boer W. Follicle-stimulating hormone (FSH). In: Crommelin DJA, Sindelar RD, eds. Pharmaceutical Biotechnology: An Introduction for Pharmacists and Pharmaceutical Scientists. Amsterdam: Harwood Academic Publishers, 1997:315–320.
68. AHFS drug information. Am Soc Hospital Pharmacists 1999:2714–2728.
69. Facts and Comparisons. St. Louis, MO: Wolters Kluwer, 2000:287–290.
70. Beals J, Kovach PM. Insulin. In: Crommelin DJA, Sindelar RD, eds. Pharmaceutical Biotechnology: An introduction for Pharmacists and Pharmaceutical Scientists. Amsterdam: Harwood Academic Publishers, 1997:229–239.
71. Riley T, DeRuiter J. How effective are the new insulin analogs in regulating glucose metabolism? US Pharmacist 2000;25:56–64.
72. Brixner D. Biotechnology products: an overview. In: Pezzuto JM, Johnson ME, Manasse HR, eds. Biotechnology and Pharmacy. New York: Chapman & Hall, 1993:392–395.
73. Higgins DL, Bennett WF. Tissue plasminogen activator: the biochemistry and pharmacology of variants produced by mutagenesis. Annu Rev Pharmacol Toxicol 1990;30:91–121.
74. Modi N. Recombinant tissue-type plasminogen activator and factor VIII. In: Crommelin DJA, Sindelar RD, eds. Pharmaceutical Biotechnology: An Introduction for Pharmacists and Pharmaceutical Scientists. Amsterdam: Harwood Academic Publishers, 1997:297–306.
75. Marian M, Sinicropi D. Recombinant human deoxyribonuclease. In: Crommelin DJA, Sindelar RD, eds. Pharmaceutical Biotechnology: An Introduction for Pharmacists and Pharmaceutical Scientists. Amsterdam: Harwood Academic Publishers, 2002:349–358.
76. Burton BK, Whiteman DAH. Incidence and timing of infusion-related reactions in patients with mucopolysaccharidosis type II (Hunter syndrome) on idursulfase therapy in the real-world setting: a perspective from the Hunter Outcome Survey (HOS). Mol Genet Metab 2011;103:113–120.
77. Starzyk K, Richards S, Yee J, et al. The long-term international safety experience of imiglucerase therapy for Gaucher disease. Mol Genet Metab 2007;90:157–163.
78. National Institute of Neurological Disorders and Stroke. Pompe disease. Available at: http://www.ninds.nih.gov/disorders/pompe/pompe.htm. Accessed on April 18, 2011.
79. Hegde S, Schmidt M. Alglucosidase alfa. Ann Rep Med Chem 2007;42:511–512.
80. Hegde S, Schmidt M. Idursulfase. Ann Rep Med Chem 2007;42:520–522.
81. Abbas AK, Pober JS. Cellular and Molecular Immunology, 4th Ed. Philadelphia: WB Saunders, 2000:235–269.
82. Janeway CA, Walport M, Travers P. Immunobiology: The Immune System in Health and Disease, 4th Ed. New York: Elsevier Science Ltd/Garland Publishing, 1999:288–292.
83. Roitt I, Brostoff J, Male D. Immunology, 5th Ed. London: Mosby International, 1998:121–125.
84. Arai KI, Lee F, Miyajima A, et al. Cytokines: coordinators of immune and inflammatory responses. Annu Rev Biochem 1990;59:783–836.
85. Klegerman ME. Lymphokines and monokines. In: Pezzuto JM, Johnson ME, Manasse HR, eds. Biotechnology and Pharmacy. New York: Chapman & Hall, 1993:53–70.
86. Louie SG, Jung B. Clinical effects of biologic response modifiers. Am J Hosp Pharm 1993;50(Suppl 3):S10–S18.
87. Pestka S, Krause CD, Walter MR. Interferons, interferon-like cytokines and their receptors. Immunol Rev 2004;202:8–32.
88. Rodriguez FH, Nelson S, Kolls JK. Cytokine therapeutics for infectious diseases. Curr Pharm Des 2000;6:665–680.
89. Urdal D. Cytokine receptors. Ann Rep Med Chem 1991;26:221–228.
90. Xing Z, Wang J. Consideration of cytokines as therapeutic targets. Curr Pharm Des 2000;6:599–611.
91. Tami J. Interleukins and interferons. In: Crommelin, DJA, Sindelar RD, eds. Pharmaceutical Biotechnology: An Introduction for Pharmacists and Pharmaceutical Scientists. Amsterdam: Harwood Academic Publishers, 1997:215–227.
92. Ebert S, De Muth JE. Hepatitis C: From Pathogenesis to Prognosis. Thousand Oaks, CA: Amgen, 1997.
93. Todd AV, Fuery CJ, Impey HL, et al. DzyNA-PCR: use of DNAzymes to detect and quantify nucleic acid sequences in a real-time fluorescent format. Clin Chem 2000;46:625–630.
94. Molto A, Olivé A. Anti-IL-1 molecules: new comers and new indications. Joint Bone Spine 2010;77:102–107.
95. Hoffman HM. Therapy of autoinflammatory syndromes. J Allerg Clin Immunol 2009;124:1129–1138.
96. Bernardelli P, Gaudilliere B, Vergne F. Anakinra. Ann Rep Med Chem 2002;37:261.
97. Hegde S, Schmidt M. Rilonacept (genetic autoinflammatory syndromes). Ann Rep Med Chem 2009;44:615–616.
98. Romanelli F. Interleukin-2 for the management of HIV infection. J Am Pharm Assoc (Wash) 1999;39:867–868.
99. Rosenberg SA, Lotze M, Mule JJ. New approaches to the immunotherapy of cancer using interleukin-2. Ann Intern Med 1988;108:853–864.
100. Siegel JP, Puri RK. Interleukin-2 toxicity. J Clin Oncol 1991;9:694–704.
101. Solimando JD, Hanna WJ. Aldesleukin and levamisole. AMJ Hosp Pharm 1998;33:1172–1177.
102. Hussan D. New drugs of 1999. J Am Pharm Assoc 2000;40:181–221.
103. Piascik P. FDA approves fusion protein for treatment of lymphoma. J Am Pharm Assoc (Wash) 1999;39:571–572.
104. Manoukian G, Hagemeister F. Denileukin diftitox: a novel immunotoxin. Expert Opin Biol Ther 2009;9:1445–1451.
105. Vose JM. Denileukin diftitox use in relapsed and refractory NHL. Clin Adv Hematol Oncol 2006;4:1–7.
106. Vu K, Solimando DA Jr. Oprelvekin. AMJ Hosp Pharm 1998;33:387–389.
107. Hoy SM, Scott LJ. Etanercept a review of its use in the management of ankylosing spondylitis and psoriatic arthritis. Drugs 2007;67:2609–2633.
108. Newton RC, Decicco CP. Therapeutic potential and strategies for inhibiting tumor necrosis factor-alpha. J Med Chem 1999;42:2295–2314.

109. Kaine JL. Abatacept for the treatment of rheumatoid arthritis: a review. Curr Ther Res 2007;68:379–399.
110. Khraishi M, Russell A, Olszynski WP. Safety profile of abatacept in rheumatoid arthritis: a review. Clin Ther 2010;32:1855–1870.
111. Flynn J, Rosman AW. Interleukins and interferons. In: Crommelin DJA, Sindelar RD, eds. Pharmaceutical Biotechnology: An Introduction for Pharmacists and Pharmaceutical Scientists. Amsterdam: Harwood Academic Publishers, 1997:185–214.
112. Huber SL, Yee G, Michau D. New Product Bulletin: Filgrastim. Washington, DC: American Pharmaceutical Association, 1993.
113. Kouides PA. The hematopoietic growth factors. In: Haskell CM, ed. Cancer Treatment. Philadelphia: WB Saunders, 1995:69–77.
114. Summerhayes M. Myeloid hematopoietic growth factors in clinical practice—a comparative review. Eur Hosp Pharm 1995;Parts 1 and II:1, 30–36, 67–74.
115. Faulds D, Sorkin EM. Epoetin (recombinant human erythropoietin). Drugs 1989;38:863–899.
116. Graber SE, Krantz SB. Erythropoietin: biology and clinical use. Hematol Oncol Clin North Am 1989;3:369–400.
117. Jensen JD, Madsen JK, Jensen LW, et al. Pharmacokinetics of epoetin in dialysis patients before and after correction of the anemia. Drug Invest 1994;8:278–287.
118. Johnson C. Epoetin alfa: a therapeutic achievement from pharmaceutical biotechnology. US Pharmacist 1989(Nov):1–11.
119. Mertelsmann R. Hematopoietins: biology, pathophysiology, and potentials therapeutic agents. Ann Oncol 1991;2:251–263.
120. Blackwell S, Crawford J. Colony-stimulating factors: clinical applications. Pharmacotherapy 1992;12(2 Pt 2):20S–31S.
121. Lieschke GJ, Burgess AW. Granulocyte colony-stimulating factor and granulocyte-macrophage colony-stimulating factor. N Engl J Med 1992;327:28–35.
122. Louie S, Rho J. Pharmacotherapeutics of biotechnology-produced drugs. In: Zito SW, ed. Pharmaceutical Biotechnology: A Programmed Text. Lancaster, PA: Technomic Publishing, 1997:224–231.
123. Petros WP. Pharmacokinetics and administration of colony-stimulating factors. Pharmacotherapy 1992;12(2 Pt 2):32S–38S.
124. Smith SP, Yee GC. Hematopoiesis. Pharmacotherapy 1992;12(2 Pt 2):11S–19S.
125. Becaplermin. Drugs Fut 1999;24:123–127.
126. Piascik P. Use of Regranex gel for diabetic foot ulcers. J Am Pharm Assoc (Wash) 1998;38:628–630.
127. Jiskoot W, Kersten GFA, Beuvery EC. Vaccines. In: Crommelin DJA, Sindelar RD, eds. Pharmaceutical Biotechnology: An Introduction for Pharmacists and Pharmaceutical Scientists. Amsterdam: Harwood Academic Publishers, 1997:255–278.
128. Glick BR, Pasternak J, eds. Molecular biotechnology. In: Principles and Applications of Recombinant DNA. Washington, DC: ASM Press, 1994:207–233.
129. Hikal AH, Hikal EM. The ABCs of hepatitis. Drug Topics 1998;146:60–69.
130. Hoogenboom HR. Selecting and screening recombinant antibody libraries. Nat Biotechnol 2005;23:1105–1116.
131. Adair F. Immunogenicity: the last hurdle for clinically successful therapeutic antibodies. Pharm Tech 2000;24:50–56.
132. Adams VR, Karlix JL. Monoclonal antibodies. In: Concepts in Immunology and Immunotherapeutics. Bethesda, MD: American Society of Health-System Pharmacists, 1997:269–299.
133. Chamow SM, Ashkenazi A. Overview. In: Chamow SM, Ashkenazi A, eds. Antibody Fusion Proteins. New York: Wiley-Liss, 1999:1–12.
134. Shen W-C, Louie SG. Immunology for Pharmacy Students. Amsterdam: Harwood Academic Publishers, 1999:45–58.
135. Hakimi J, Mould D, Waldmann TA. Development of Zenapax: a humanized anti-Tac antibody. In: Harris WJ, Adair JR, eds. Antibody Therapeutics. Boca Raton, FL: CRC Press, 1997:277–300.
136. Van Dijk MA, Vidarsson G. Monoclonal antibody-based pharmaceuticals. In: Crommelin D, Sindelar RD, eds. Pharmaceutical Biotechnology: An Introduction for Pharmacists and Pharmaceutical Scientists, 2nd Ed. London: Taylor and Francis, 2002:283–199.
137. Glover D. Fully human monoclonal antibodies come to fruition. Scrip Mag 1999:16–19.
138. Holliger P, Hoogenboom H. Antibodies come back from the brink. Nat Biotechnol 1998;16:1015–1016.
139. Vaughan TJ, Osbourn JK, Tempest PR. Human antibodies by design. Nat Biotechnol 1998;16:535–539.
140. Pray W. Nonprescription Product Therapeutics, 2nd Ed. Philadelphia: Lippincott Williams & Wilkins, 2006:778–799.
141. Quattrocchi E, Hove I. Ovulation & pregnancy home testing products. US Pharmacist 1998;23:54–63.
142. Rosenthal WM, Briggs GC. Home testing and monitoring devices. In: Allen LV Jr, Berardi RR, DeSimone EM II, et al., eds. Handbook of Nonprescription Drugs. Washington, DC: American Pharmaceutical Association, 2000:917–942.
143. Hegde S, Schmidt M. Catumaxomab. Ann Rep Med Chem 2010;45:486–488.
144. Bernard-Marty C, Lebrun F, Awada A, et al. Monoclonal antibody-based targeted therapy in breast cancer: current status and future directions. Drugs 2006;66:1577–1591.
145. Press MF, Lenz H-J. EGFR, HER2 and VEGF pathways: validated targets for cancer treatment. Drugs 2007;67:2045–2075.
146. Keating GM. Panitumumab: a review of its use in metastatic colorectal cancer. Drugs 2010;70:1059–1078.
147. Gaedcke J, Grade M, Jung K, et al. KRAS and BRAF mutations in patients with rectal cancer treated with preoperative chemoradiotherapy. Radiother Oncol 2010;94:76–81.
148. Castagnola P, Giaretti W. Mutant KRAS, chromosomal instability and prognosis in colorectal cancer. Biochim Biophys Acta 2005;1756:115–125.
149. Drug Facts and Comparisons. Philadelphia: Wolters Kluwer Health, Inc., April 2004.
150. American Cancer Society. Global Cancer Facts and Figures 2007. Atlanta, GA: American Cancer Society, 2007.
151. Cheson BD. Ofatumumab, a novel anti-CD20 monoclonal antibody for the treatment of B-cell malignancies. J Clin Oncol 2010;28:3525–3530.
152. Sanford M, McCormack PL. Ofatumumab. Drugs 2010;70:1013–1019.
153. Gawronski KM, Rainka MM, Patel MJ, et al. Treatment options for multiple sclerosis: current and emerging therapies. Pharmacotherapy 2010;30:916–927.
154. Minagar A, Alexander JS, Sahraian MA, et al. Alemtuzumab and multiple sclerosis: therapeutic application. Expert Opin Biol Ther 2010;10:421–429.
155. Dillman RO. Radiolabeled anti-CD20 monoclonal antibodies for the treatment of B-cell lymphoma. J Clin Oncol 2002;20:3545–3557.
156. Hegde S, Schmidt M. Canakinumab. Ann Rep Med Chem 2010;45:484–485.
157. Panés J, Gomollon F, Taxonera C, et al. Crohn's disease: a review of current treatment with a focus on biologics. Drugs 2007;67:2511–2537.
158. Rivkin A. Certolizumab pegol for the management of Crohn's disease in adults. Clin Ther 2009;31:1158–1176.
159. Hegde S, Schmidt M. Golimumab. Ann Rep Med Chem 2010;45:503–505.
160. Chien AL, Elder JT, Ellis CN. Ustekinumab: a new option in psoriasis therapy. Drugs 2009;69:1141–1152.
161. Hegde S, Schmidt M. Eculizumab. Ann Rep Med Chem 2008;43:468–469.
162. Charneski L, Patel PN. Eculizumab in paroxysmal nocturnal haemoglobinuria. Drugs 2008;68:1341–1346.
163. Blick SKA, Keating GM, Wagstaff AJ. Ranibizumab. Drugs 2007;67:1199–1206.
164. Chappelow AV, Kaiser PK. Neovascular age-related macular degeneration potential therapies. Drugs 2008;68:1029–1036.
165. Abraham J. Denosumab: a new alternative for metastases. Commun Oncol 2008;5:291–294.
166. Group BDW. Biomarkers and surrogate endpoints: preferred definitions and conceptual framework. Clin Pharmacol Ther 2001;69:89–95.
167. Hong KW, Oh B. Overview of personalized medicine in the disease genomic era. BMB Rep 2010;43:643–648.
168. Voora D, McLeod HL, Eby C, et al. The pharmacogenetics of coumarin therapy. Pharmacogenomics 2005;6:503–513.
169. Ross JS, Schenkein DP, Pietrusko R, et al. Targeted therapies for cancer 2004. Am J Clin Pathol 2004;122:598–609.
170. Rofaiel S, Muo EN, Mousa SA. Pharmacogenetics in breast cancer: steps toward personalized medicine in breast cancer management. Pharmacogen Personalized Med 2010;3:129–143.
171. Postlind H, Danielson A, Lindgren A, et al. Tolterodine, a new muscarinic receptor antagonist, is metabolized by cytochromes P450 2D6 and 3A in human liver microsomes. Drug Metab Dispos 1998;26:289–293.
172. Gagne JF, Montminy V, Belanger P, et al. Common human *UGT1A* polymorphisms and the altered metabolism of irinotecan active metabolite 7-ethyl-10-hydroxycamptothecin (SN-38). Mol Pharmacol 2002;62:608–617.
173. Kohn DB, Candotti F. Gene therapy fulfilling its promise. N Engl J Med 2009;360:447–458.
174. Terazaki Y, Yano S, Yuge K, et al. An optimal therapeutic expression level is crucial for suicide gene therapy for hepatic metastatic cancer in mice. Hepatology 2003;37:155–163.
175. Goverdhana S, Puntel M, Xiong W, et al. Regulatable gene expression systems for gene therapy applications: progress and future challenges. Mol Ther 2005;12:189–211.
176. Chen P, Tian J, Kovesdi I, et al. Promoters influence the kinetics of transgene expression following adenovector gene delivery. J Gene Med 2008;10:123–131.
177. Ledley FD. Nonviral gene therapy: the promise of genes as pharmaceutical products. Hum Gene Ther 1995;6:1129–1144.

Chapter 7

Receptors as Targets for Drug Discovery

David A. Johnson and Timothy J. Maher

Abbreviations

ATP, adenosine triphosphate
cAMP, cyclic adenosine monophosphate
cGMP, cyclic guanosine monophosphate
DAG, diacylglycerol
DAT, dopamine transporter
ERK, extracellular signal-regulated kinase
GDP, guanosine diphosphate
GPCR, G protein–coupled receptors
Grb2, growth factor receptor-bound protein 2
GSK-3, glycogen synthase kinase 3
GTP, guanosine triphosphate
HTS, high-throughput screening
IP_3, inositol 1,4,5-triphosphate
JAK, Janus kinase
LGIC, ligand-gated ion channel
MAPK, mitogen-activated protein kinase
MEK, MAPK kinase
PLC, phospholipase C
STAT, signal transducer and activator of transcription

INTRODUCTION

The human body is an example of an exquisitely designed, extremely complex machine that functions day-in and day-out to allow for survival of the organism in response to a never-ending onslaught of external challenges. When one considers the enormous variety of environmental stressors to which the body is continually subjected, it is not surprising to anticipate the existence of a multitude of checks and balances associated with its physiologic and biochemical systems. These systems, including endocrine, nervous, and enzymatic, typically function in concert to adapt to changing environmental conditions. Such systems are designed to respond quickly (i.e., within milliseconds) and for a short time; others are designed to act more slowly but usually have significantly longer durations ranging from minutes to hours to days and, in some case, even months to years. Together, these systems support the organism's survival. Malfunctioning of the control of such systems often leads to disease and, potentially, the eventual demise of the individual.

The use of specific chemical compounds to treat disease dates back to early humans. Many primitive cultures used plants and other natural sources in an attempt to mitigate the influences of evil spirits and other factors rooted in superstition, which were believed to be the foundations of such illnesses. Over the centuries, a number of serendipitous observations involving the ability of largely botanical preparations to alter disease processes laid the foundation for the modern, more systematic approach to the discovery of medicinals for therapeutic use. The collaboration of chemical and biological scientists continues this quest for the "magic bullet" to treat those diseases that challenge the individual's well-being.

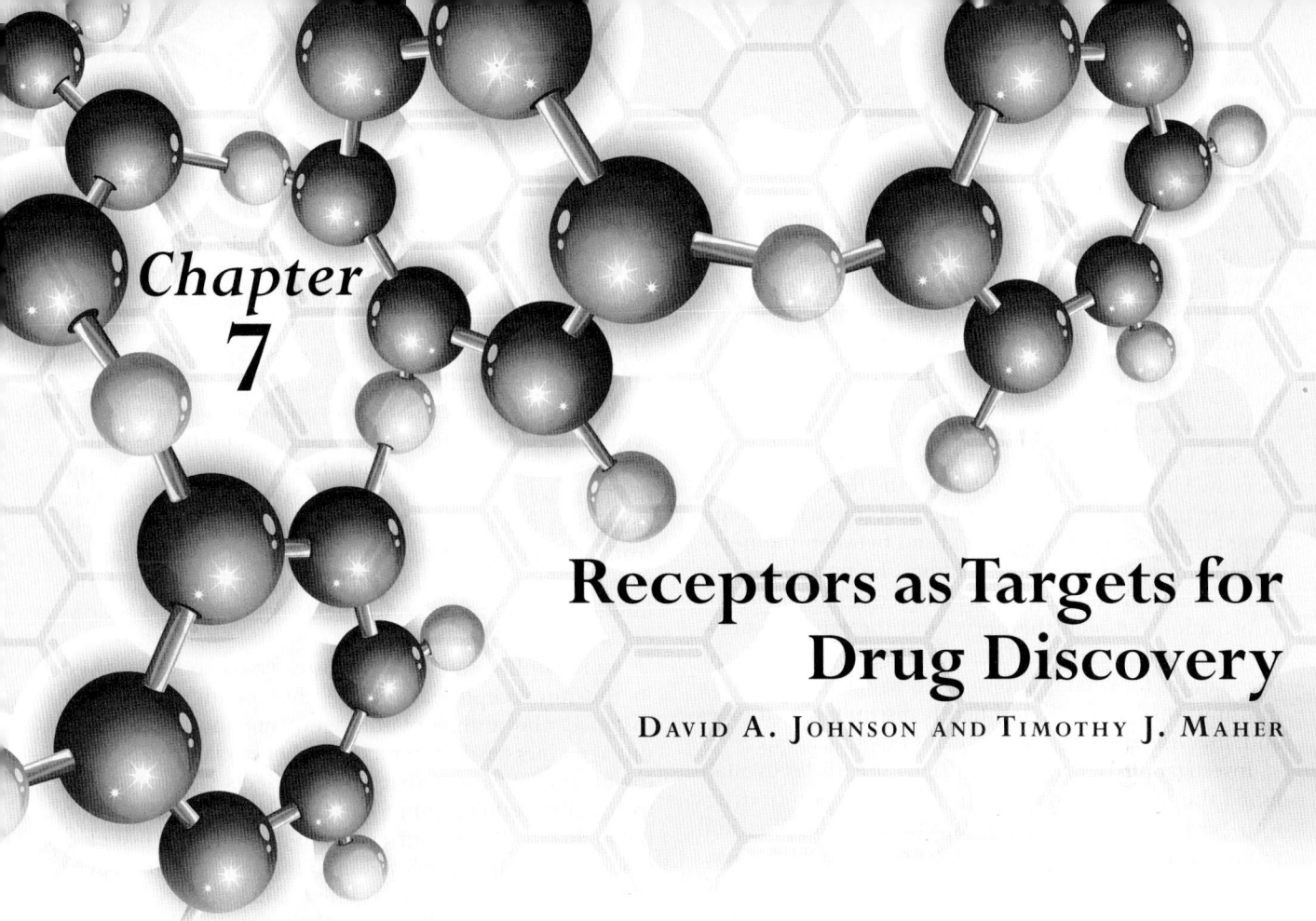

HISTORICAL PERSPECTIVES

For years, it had been known that some drugs were capable of producing their effects by acting at specific sites within the body. Claude Bernard was the first to demonstrate this in the mid-1800s, with his classical experiments involving curare (1). He showed that this neuromuscular blocking agent, which was used as an arrow poison by the South American natives, was capable of preventing skeletal muscle contraction following nerve stimulation, but was without effect when the muscle was stimulated directly. This work demonstrated for the first time a localized site of action for a drug and, most importantly, suggested that a gap, or synapse, existed between the nerve and the muscle. From these findings, he postulated that some chemical substance normally communicated the information between the nerve and the target tissue—in this case, the muscle. These findings established the foundations for what is known today as "chemical neurotransmission," a process frequently disrupted by diseases and, likewise, the target of many therapeutic agents.

Investigations by J.N. Langley (2) in the early 1900s established the initial foundations for the interaction of drugs with specific cellular components, later to be identified and termed "receptors." Before this time, many leading experts believed that most drugs acted nonselectively on virtually all the cells in the body to produce their biologic responses, with a response resulting from their general physical characteristics (e.g., lipid solubility) and not related to specific structural features of the compound. Langley noted that the natural product pilocarpine, which act to mimic the parasympathetic division of the autonomic nervous system, were very selective and also extremely potent. Additionally, the natural product atropine was capable of blocking, in a rather selective fashion, the effects of pilocarpine and parasympathetic nervous system stimulation. Importantly, he concluded that these two compounds interacted with the same component of the cell.

Paul Ehrlich (3), a noted microbiologist during the late 19th and early 20th centuries, is credited with coining the term "receptive substance," or "receptor." His observations that various organic compounds appeared to produce their antimicrobial effects with a high degree of selectivity led him to speculate that drugs produced their effects by binding to such a receptive substance. The interaction or binding of the drug with the receptor was analogous to a "lock" (the receptor) and a "key" (the drug), which gave rise to the lock and key fit theory for drug receptors. Thus, certain organic compounds would properly fit into the receptor and activate it, leading to a high degree of specificity. Although such a situation might be considered to be ideal for drug therapy, few drugs actually interact only with their intended receptors. The frequency of side effects is not associated with a simple extension of their desired pharmacologic actions; instead, drug molecules can also bind with other receptors or nonreceptor entities on or within cells to produce a host of other—and often undesirable—effects.

Some drugs produce their desired therapeutic effects without interaction with a specific receptor. For instance, osmotic diuretics produce their pharmacologic effects simply by creating an osmotic gradient in the renal tubules and, thereby, promoting the elimination of water in the urine. This is purely the result of a physical characteristic of the drug. Similarly, antacids produce their beneficial effects by chemically neutralizing the hydrochloric acid found in the stomach. No absorption of the drug is even required for its effects to be realized. Often, the failure of a drug to be absorbed and, thus, only act locally at the desired biologic site constitutes a tremendous advantage regarding the safety of that compound. Unfortunately, from a practical standpoint, most pharmacologic agents require absorption following administration to reach the intended target; thus, side effects typically are a serious consideration.

More sophisticated mechanisms can also be involved in the nonreceptor actions of therapeutic agents. For instance, the antineoplastic agent mechlorethamine, a nitrogen mustard, produces its beneficial (pharmacologic) and adverse (toxicologic) effects via interaction with many cellular components in both cancerous and normal cells. Via its conversion to a highly reactive electrophilic ethyleniminium ion intermediate, this agent reacts with nucleophilic cellular components, such as amino, hydroxyl, sulfhydryl, phosphate, carboxyl, and imidazole groups. In particular, by alkylating the N-8 position of guanine in DNA, this agent produces miscoding (cytosine normally base pairs with guanine in DNA; however, thymine now substitutes for cytosine) and the eventual death of the cell (4). When one realizes that all replicating cells contain an N-8 nitrogen in guanine in their DNA, it is easy to see why mechlorethamine produces nonselective destruction of cells throughout the body. Thus, no specific receptor is involved in the actions of this class of pharmacologic agent.

DRUG DISCOVERY

The discovery of pharmacologic agents by modern pharmaceutical companies and universities often involves the use of receptor–ligand binding techniques. Following the synthesis of a series of new chemically related compounds, which can constitute hundreds to thousands of compounds, the determination of the desired biologic activity was once a rather daunting task. Before the advent of receptor–ligand binding techniques, the initial screening of these compounds involved injecting each agent individually into experimental animals or incubating each agent with isolated tissues (e.g., intestine, heart, and skeletal muscle), which are techniques that require a large investment of resources, including personnel, time, animals, and money. Today, receptor–ligand binding techniques, such as high-throughput screening (HTS), are used to narrow large numbers of compounds down to those that display the greatest affinity for a receptor, thereby significantly decreasing the time and cost associated with identifying "lead" compounds (5). Initial *in silico* analytical techniques use molecular modeling software to "virtually screen" trillions of candidate structures found in "chemical libraries" for the potential to bind to target proteins or other molecules of interest. Once the structural features of candidate molecules are identified, HTS techniques are employed that combine computer-controlled robotics, detectors, and data processing to identify compounds that interact with target molecules or biochemical pathways. Typically, HTS uses microtiter plates that contain from 96 to 3,456 wells that hold volumes of liquid as small as nanoliters (Fig. 7.1). The liquid in the wells contains substrates or cells of interest to which the chemical entities are added. Automated analytical machines then detect reactions and identify "hits" that represent compounds that will undergo further testing. The most current HTS processes can screen 100 million reactions in 10 hours. "Hits" are confirmed by retesting initially using identical assay conditions. Once confirmed, dose–response curves are generated using a range of concentrations of the compound. Next, the compounds undergo further testing using alternative assays and experimental conditions. The original "hit" compound can be structurally modified to optimize activity, potency, and stability using approaches such as combinatorial chemistry to create a "lead" or drug candidate. Converting a "hit" to a "lead" is the most important and difficult part of drug discovery. However, a danger associated with this initial screening approach is the failure to recognize potentially useful compounds that might require biotransformation before exerting a biologic effect, such as a prodrug. It should be remembered that ligand binding based on the affinity of a drug for its receptor does not differentiate agonists from antagonists. Despite these potential pitfalls associated with receptor–ligand binding techniques, modern drug discovery relies heavily on these approaches.

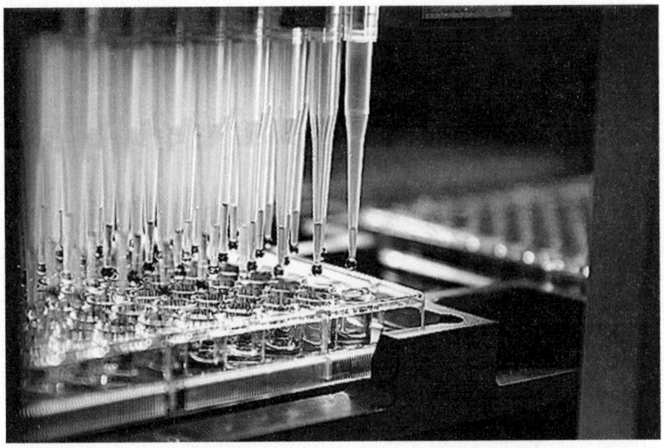

FIGURE 7.1 A pipetting robot system for fully automated high-throughput screening arrays.

Another contemporary approach to drug development is "rational drug design," which is a process for discovering new drug entities through detailed knowledge of the structure of the biologic target. For example, the elucidation of the three-dimensional crystal structure of the bacterial leucine transporter (Fig. 7.2) provided a template to serve as a model for analogous mammalian monoamine transporters such as the dopamine transporter (DAT) (6). With knowledge of the amino acid sequences for both the leucine transporter and DAT, it was possible using computer modeling and site-directed mutagenesis techniques to discover chemical bonding interactions between key amino acids in the binding site of DAT and substrates such as dopamine and amphetamine. With this information, it becomes possible to design "leads" for ligands that could serve as either substrates or inhibitors of DAT. Drugs developed through this process can then be effective in treating a number of diseases such as Parkinson disease, attention-deficit disorders, and drug addiction.

AFFINITY: THE ROLE OF CHEMICAL BONDING

During the early 1900s, A.V. Hill used the natural products nicotine and curare in isolated muscle preparations and noted the effects of temperature in his experiments (1). He concluded that the ability of a drug to produce an effect must result from specific chemical interactions between the drug and specific sites. He also noted that the effects of many drugs were reversible, because washing the isolated tissue often restored the sensitivity of the tissue to nerve stimulation. These studies set the foundation for our understanding of the chemical interactions between drugs and receptors.

When a drug interacts with a receptor, multiple chemical interactive forces, both weak and strong, between two molecules (a drug and its receptor) are believed to be responsible for the initial interaction. Such forces having a role in ligand–receptor binding include covalent, ionic, and hydrogen bonds and hydrophobic interactions as shown in Fig. 7.3. Compounds attracted to a receptor macromolecule are said to have affinity for that receptor and can be classified as agonists or antagonists. Compounds with affinity for a receptor are referred to as ligands. An agonist is a compound that has affinity for its receptor and thus is capable of producing a positive biologic response as a result of its interaction with its receptor (7). The ability to produce a response is termed "efficacy" or "intrinsic activity." On the other hand, antagonists are compounds with "affinity" for a receptor but do not activate the receptor to produce a biologic response. Antagonists are said to have affinity, but lack intrinsic activity. The affinity of a compound for a receptor is dependent on its correct three-dimensional characteristics, such as its size, stereochemical orientation of its functional groups, and its physical and electrochemical properties (e.g., ionic and dipole interactions).

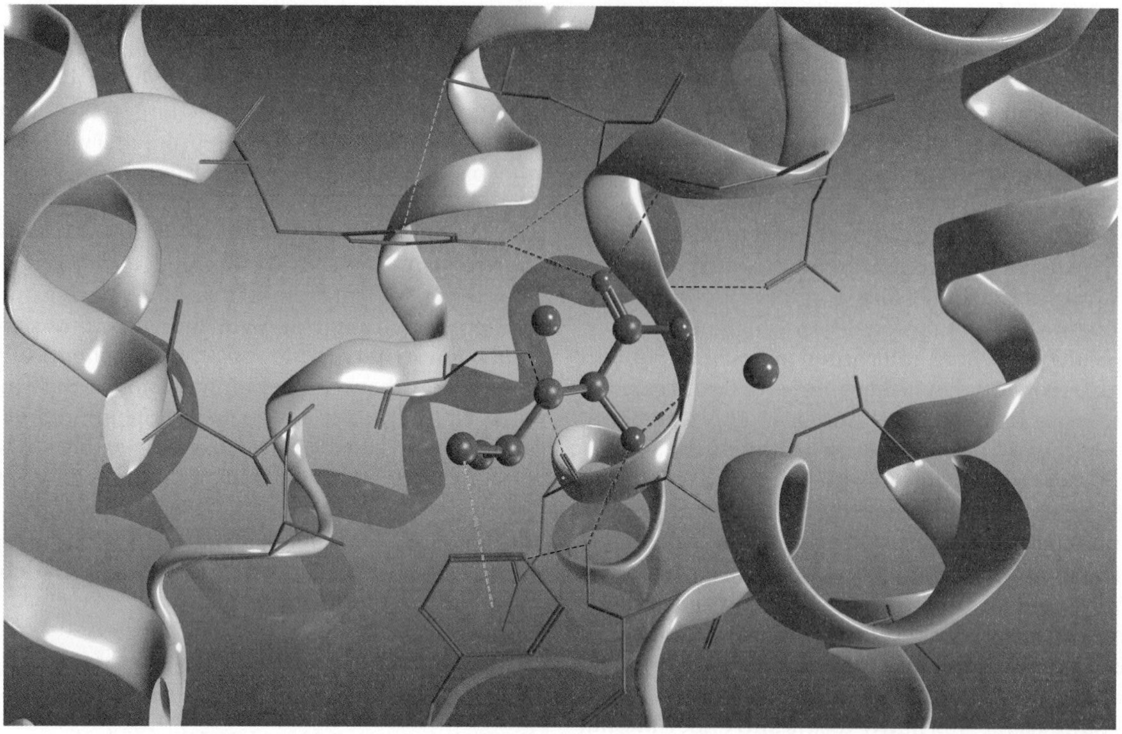

FIGURE 7.2 Molecular recognition of the bacterial leucine transporter (LeuT, pdb:3GWW) with co-crystallized leucine substrate (shown as ball-and-stick). Side-chain residues within 4.5 Å (line rendering) of the leucine molecule are shown, along with two Na^+ ions (black spheres), which are required for transport. Hydrogen bonding and hydrophobic interactions between LeuT and substrate are shown as dotted lines, respectively. Figure rendered using Molecular Operating Environment (MOE) software (CCG, Montreal, Quebec, Canada). (From Zhou Z, Zhen J, Karpowich NK, et al. Antidepressant specificity of serotonin transporter suggested by three LeuT-SSRI structures. Nat Struct Mol Biol 2009;16:652–657.)

Assuming that a compound has been distributed to the general vicinity of a receptor, based on its physical characteristics, the binding of the drug to the receptor will then initially depend on the types of chemical bonds that can be established between the drug and its receptor. The overall strengths of these bonds will vary (Fig. 7.3) and will determine the degree of affinity between the drug and its receptor.

Covalent Bond

The strongest of bonds involved in drug–receptor interactions is the covalent bond, in which two atoms, one from the ligand and one from the receptor, share a pair of electrons to form a covalent bond. Because of the significant strength of the covalent bond (50 to 150 kcal/mol), covalent bonding often produces a situation in which the ligand is irreversibly bound by the receptor and, thus, leads to the receptor's eventual destruction via endocytosis and chemical destruction. Full recovery of cellular function therefore requires the synthesis of new receptors.

An example of an irreversible covalent bond formation between drug and its receptor involves the long-lasting blockade of α-adrenoceptors by phenoxybenzamine (a haloalkylamine) (see Chapter 10). Phenoxybenzamine under physiologic pH forms a highly reactive carbonium ion intermediate that covalently links by reaction (alkylation) with amino, sulfhydryl, or carboxyl groups to the α-adrenoceptor. The receptor is thus rendered irreversibly nonfunctional and, eventually, destroyed. The synthesis of a new receptor requires a number of days, thus accounting for the extremely prolonged duration of the inhibition associated with this agent. This property of phenoxybenzamine to irreversibly bind the α-adrenoceptor by a covalent bond is critical for the

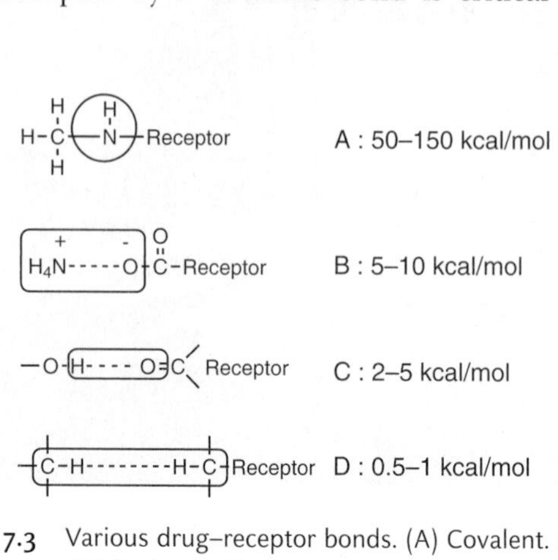

FIGURE 7.3 Various drug–receptor bonds. (A) Covalent. (B) Ionic. (C) Hydrogen. (D) Hydrophobic.

demonstration of spare receptors (8,9). Because other receptors and cellular components also contain molecular groups that are capable of reacting with the bioactivated (reactive) phenoxybenzamine intermediate, it is not surprising to find that receptors that mediate the actions of other neurotransmitters (such as acetylcholine, serotonin, or histamine) are also subject to alkylation and inhibition, demonstrating the lack of selectivity of phenoxybenzamine.

Another important example of a class of compounds that produces its effects via a covalent bond to its receptor is the organophosphate acetylcholinesterase inhibitors (see also Chapter 9). Examples of such agents include the insecticides parathion and malathion and the nerve-gas agents sarin, soman, and tabun. These type of inhibitors are capable of reacting (phosphorylating or forming a covalent phosphate bond) with the active site of acetylcholinesterase, which normally is responsible for metabolizing acetylcholine, the neurotransmitter found at the neuromuscular junction and within many sites of the autonomic and central nervous systems. Reaction of the enzyme with its normal substrate acetylcholine leads to a readily hydrolyzable acetylated enzyme, which rapidly regenerates to the active enzyme. Covalent bonding by the organophosphates results in phosphorylation of a serine residue within the active site of the enzyme, which is extremely stable and essentially irreversible. Recovery of enzymatic function in the tissue requires the synthesis of new enzyme molecules.

Ionic Bond

When two ions of opposite charge are attracted to each other through electrostatic forces, an ionic bond is formed. The strength of this type of bond varies between 5 and 10 kcal/mol, and it decreases proportionally to the square of the distance between the two atoms. The ability of a drug to bind to a receptor via ionic interactions therefore increases significantly as the drug molecule diffuses closer to the receptor. Additionally, the strength associated with the ionic bond is strong enough to support an initial transient interaction between the receptor and the drug, but unlike the covalent bond, the ionic bond is not so strong as to prevent dissociation of the drug–receptor complex.

The tendency of an atom to participate in ionic bonding is determined by its degree of electronegativity. Hydrogen, as a standard, has an electronegativity value of 2.2; fluorine is 4.2, chlorine 2.9 and nitrogen 3.1 (Linus Pauling units). Fluorine and chlorine atoms, as well as hydroxyl, sulfhydryl, and carboxyl groups, form strong ionic bonds because of a stronger attraction for electrons compared with that of hydrogen. On the other hand, alkyl groups do not participate in ionic bonds because of a weaker tendency to attract electrons compared with that of hydrogen.

Hydrogen Bond

A hydrogen bond (or hydrogen bonding) is a strong electrostatic dipole–dipole interaction between a hydrogen atom and an electronegative atom, such as oxygen, nitrogen, or fluorine. The hydrogen bond is extremely strong because oxygen, nitrogen, and fluorine are extremely good at attracting the relative positive charge of hydrogen, resulting in an extreme dipole situation. This type of bond can occur between molecules (intermolecular hydrogen bonds) or within the same molecule (intramolecular hydrogen bonds). At 2 to 5 kcal/mol, a single hydrogen bond is stronger than a van der Waals interaction, but weaker than covalent or ionic bonds, and thus would not be expected to support a drug–receptor interaction alone. However, when multiple intermolecular hydrogen bonds are formed between drugs and receptors, as typically is the case, a substantial amount of stability is conferred on the drug–receptor interaction, an essential requirement for drug–receptor interactions. For example, a water molecule behaves as an electronic dipole and can easily form intermolecular hydrogen bonds with other water molecules, which gives water its high boiling point of 100°C. Intramolecular hydrogen bonding is partly responsible for the secondary, tertiary, and quaternary structures of proteins and nucleic acids.

Hydrophobic Interactions

Hydrophobic interactions (hydrophobic effect; fear of water) are intermolecular interactions or dispersion forces that occur between nonpolar organic molecules and contribute to the binding forces that attract a ligand to its receptor, other than ionic, covalent, or hydrogen bonds. These interactions are often referred to as van der Waals forces or London forces, which require two nonpolar molecules to come in close range to one another, or between groups within the same molecule. Dispersion forces (or London dispersion forces) are induced dipole–dipole electrostatic interactions between atoms/molecules at close distances and occur over a large surface area (i.e., at the interface of the ligand and binding site) and thus contribute to receptor binding. London forces are weaker than van der Waals forces. These forces tend to align the atoms/molecules in order to increase their interaction, thereby reducing their potential energy. Theorists have suggested that for these forces to operate, a momentary dipolar structure needs to exist to allow such association. This induced dipolar interaction results from a temporary imbalance of charge distribution between or within molecules. These forces are very weak (0.5 to 1 kcal/mol) and decrease proportionally to the seventh power of the interatomic distance. The hydrophobic effect is the ability of polar water molecules to exclude (repel) nonpolar hydrocarbon-like molecules.

AFFINITY: THE ROLE OF CONFORMATION

Most therapeutically useful drugs bind only transiently and reversibly to their intended receptor. The combination of a variety of bonds, including ionic, hydrogen, and van der Waals attractive forces, collectively contributes to the strength of drug binding to the receptor. The functional groups (critical portion of the structure) of the drug that bind to the receptor are termed "pharmacophores" or "pharmacophoric groups." Once the drug has bound, a biologic response may result (e.g., especially if the drug is an agonist). Either following or during the process of binding to the receptor, a conformational change can occur in the receptor that initiates the activation of the biologic response and increases the affinity/binding between the drug and its receptor. This conformational change in the receptor can also contribute to the dissociation of the drug–receptor complex. This simple explanation of the interaction between a drug and its receptor producing a biologic response is commonly referred to as the "occupancy theory," which predicts that the biologic response is directly related to the number of receptors bound by an agonist.

Another theory of drug–receptor interactions is the "rate theory," which suggests that the number of drug–receptor interactions per unit time determines the intensity of the response. Thus, drugs that associate with and then rapidly dissociate from the receptor, thus allowing other drug molecules to subsequently interact with the receptor, would be expected to produce the most robust responses. The "induced-fit theory" suggests that as the drug (agonist) approaches the inactive state of the receptor (conformation A), the agonist induces a specific conformational change (perturbation) in the inactive receptor, which allows for effective drug–receptor binding or formation of the drug–receptor complex (conformation B) and the desired biologic response (Fig. 7.4). According to this theory, the receptor exists in an inactive state/configuration (conformation A) without the proper conformation to form the drug–receptor complex. Following dissociation of the drug–receptor complex (conformation B), the receptor then reverts to its original or inactive state (conformation A). According to this theory, an antagonist, on the other hand, induces a nonspecific conformational change in the receptor (conformation C), which fails to produce the desired drug–receptor complex; thus, no biologic response is elicited. Combining the induced-fit and rate theories yields the "macromolecular perturbation theory," which suggests that two types of conformational changes exist and that the rate of their existence determines the observed biologic response. This theory can partially account for the activity of partial agonists. Finally, the "activation-aggregation theory" indicates that receptors are always in a dynamic equilibrium between active and inactive states. Agonists function by shifting the equilibrium toward the activated state, whereas antagonists prevent the activated state. This theory can account for the activity of inverse agonists, which produce neither a typical agonist response nor an antagonist response (i.e., blocking the receptor) but, rather, produce biologic responses opposite to those of the agonist.

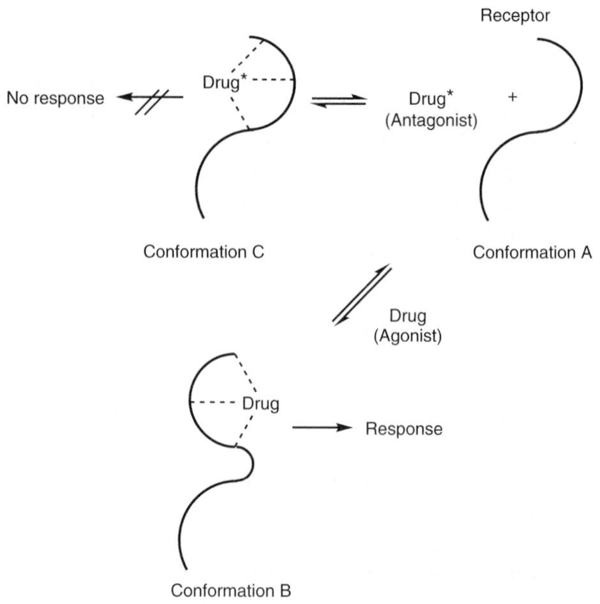

FIGURE 7.4 Diagrammatic representation of drug-induced fit theory, in which an agonist (Drug) or antagonist (Drug*) interacts with three different conformations of the receptor.

AFFINITY: THE ROLE OF STEREOCHEMISTRY

Very specific three-dimensional requirements must be satisfied for a compound to effectively act as an agonist. To elegantly demonstrate the specificity of a drug for its receptor, the unique three-dimensional characteristics of chiral compounds can be used as an example. As early as 1901, Pasteur (10) noted the significance of asymmetric compounds in biologic systems. Since that time, much has been learned from chiral compounds regarding three-dimensional binding requirements of receptors. For instance, although the individual enantiomers (i.e., nonsuperimposable mirror images) of norephedrine (2-amino-3-phenyl-1-propanol) (Fig. 7.5) have identical molecular weights, melting points, lipid solubility, and empirical formulae, these compounds have significantly different α-adrenoceptor agonistic activities. The 1*R*,2*S* enantiomer (levo) is approximately 100-fold more potent than the 1*S*,2*R* enantiomer (dextro) both in vivo and

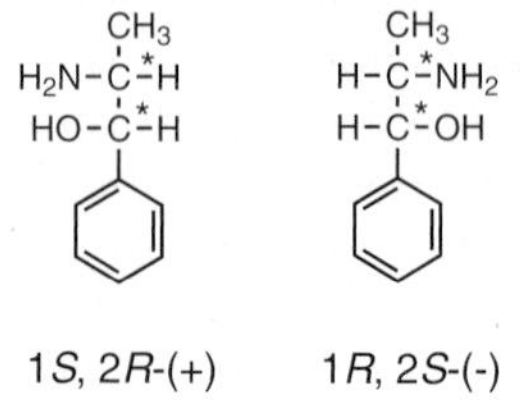

FIGURE 7.5 Projection formulae of 2-amino-3-phenyl-1-propanol stereoisomers. (From Maher TJ, Johnson DA. Review of chirality and its importance in pharmacology. Drug Dev Res 1991;24:149–156, with permission.)

in vitro (11,12). (Because there are two chiral centers, there is also another set of stereoisomers called diastereomers, 1*S*,2*S* and 1*R*,2*R*, that have an even different pharmacologic profile.) Thus, the greater efficacy of the 1*R*,2*S* enantiomer most likely is dependent on its ability to bind and activate the receptor as a result of its preferential fit into the receptor.

Labetalol, an adrenoceptor-blocking agent structurally related to epinephrine, has two asymmetric centers, and therefore, four diastereomers exist (Fig. 7.6). The formulation available for use as a mixed α- and β-adrenoceptor blocker contains equal amounts of each diastereomer. The *R,R*-isomer accounts for much of the β-adrenoceptor blocking activity, whereas the *S,R*-isomer has the greatest effect on α-adrenoceptors. The *S,S*-isomer has some α-adrenoceptor blocking activity but no activity at β-adrenoceptors. The *R,S*-isomer is essentially devoid of activity at both α- and β-adrenoceptors.

Many synthetically prepared therapeutic agents are a mixture of two enantiomers (racemates), with one enantiomer, termed the "eutomer," being largely responsible for the desired pharmacologic effect (13). The other enantiomer, termed the "distomer," can be inactive or even contribute more significantly to the toxicity of the therapeutic agent. For example, the bronchodilator albuterol is available as equimolar mixtures of *R*- and *S*-enantiomers. *R*-Albuterol binds to the β_2-adrenergic receptor with high affinity to produce bronchodilation, whereas its *S*- enantiomer exhibits weak binding to the β_2-adrenergic receptor and induces airway bronchoconstriction (toxicity).

Thus, knowledge of chirality and stereochemistry of drug action has a significant role in drug development due to the advances gained in receptor theory as well as in therapeutics. It has been generally accepted in drug discovery that the development of enantiomerically pure drugs could provide safer and more efficacious alternatives to the racemate, when the beneficial effects are attributable to receptor selectivity by one of the enantiomers. An understanding of the role of chirality in the properties of the drug molecule is important to the rational process of developing chiral drugs as well as the clinical use of chiral drugs. The pharmacokinetic properties of a racemate can be very different from the single enantiomer, with differences in bioavailability as a result of stereoselective metabolism, transport, or elimination. Stereochemical aspects of drug action have been known for many decades; however, only within the last couple of decades has emphasis been placed on stereochemistry of drug disposition.

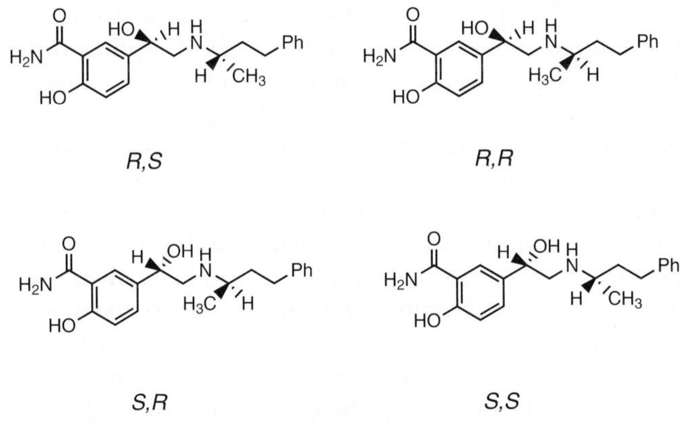

FIGURE 7.6 Diastereomers of labetalol.

DOSE–RESPONSE RELATIONSHIPS

A.J. Clark is generally given credit for being the first to apply the law of mass action principles to the concept of drug–receptor interactions, thus providing further evidence for the dose–effect phenomenon (14). This concept, as applied by Clark, states that the greater the number of agonist molecules at the site of the receptors, the greater the response (i.e., a direct relationship); however, these principles of the law of mass action in drug–receptor interactions have been questioned. The law of mass action applies to compounds dissolved in fluids that are allowed to freely diffuse. Since much is known about the anchoring of most receptors to, or within, cell membranes where drug–receptor interactions are thought to occur, this environment would actually constitute a solid–liquid interface. Thus, the law of mass action as applied to compounds dissolved in fluids where they are allowed to freely diffuse might not be completely applicable.

Equation 7.1 illustrates the interaction of a drug ([D]) with a receptor ([R]), which results in a drug–receptor complex ([DR]) and a biologic response. The interaction between most therapeutically useful drugs and their receptors is generally reversible:

7.1 $$[D] + [R] \rightleftarrows [DR] \rightarrow \text{Biologic Response}$$

After administration of a drug, one can monitor the biologic responses produced. Plotting the dose or concentration of the drug versus the effect produced (% response) yields a rectangular hyperbolic function, as illustrated in Figure 7.7A. This type of function is mathematically difficult from which to accurately extrapolate quantitative information due to the constantly changing slope of the curve. When the effect produced is plotted against the log of the drug concentration or the dose administered, however, a sigmoidal function results, as illustrated in Figure 7.7B. This function possesses a relatively linear portion of the curve about its central point, thereby making quantitative extrapolations more accurate.

Dose–response curves are typically plotted to determine both quantitative and qualitative parameters of potency and efficacy. Potency is inversely related to the dose required to produce a given response (typically half-maximum), and efficacy is the ability of a drug to produce a full response (100% maximum). In Figure 7.8, drug X is equally efficacious to drug Y, but drug X is

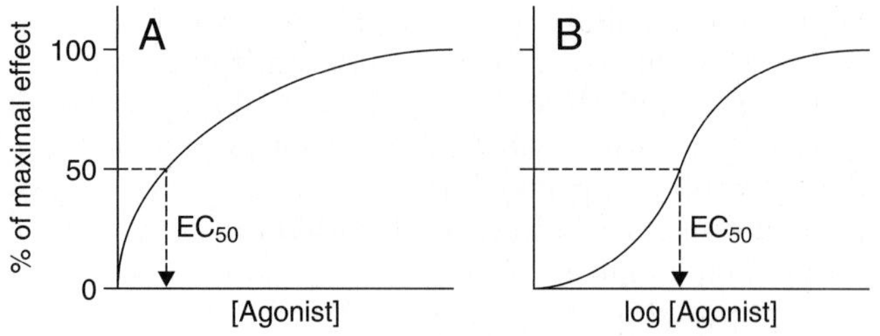

FIGURE 7.7 Plot of (A) dose or concentration and (B) log of the dose or concentration of a drug versus the effect produced.

more potent than drug Y. That is to say, both drug X and drug Y produce a 100% response, but drug X reaches that response at a lower dose. Visual inspection of such dose–response curves allows easy qualitative interpretations (e.g., in a series of curves). Those curves positioned to the left are more potent than those positioned to the right, as illustrated in Figure 7.8, drug Z is more potent than drug Y, and drug Z is equipotent to drug X. However, comparisons of efficacy are visually apparent, because the greater the maximum response (i.e., efficacy), the higher the maximum point on the dose–response curve. Thus, in Figure 7.8, drug X and drug Y are of equal efficacy, and drug X and drug Y are of greater efficacy than drug Z.

The potency of an agonist is decreased in situations where the agonist must compete with an antagonist for binding at the same site (competitive antagonism). The potency of the agonist is decreased as the concentration of antagonist is increased. Graphically, this is demonstrated as a parallel shift to the right in the dose–response curve with no decrease in maximal response (Fig. 7.9A). An antagonist can also inhibit activation of a receptor by binding to a separate allosteric site (noncompetitive antagonism). In this case, by binding to the allosteric site, the antagonist prevents the conformational change in receptor tertiary structure to the active state even with agonist binding to the primary site. Graphically, in the presence of a noncompetitive binding, the dose–response curve is shifted to the right, and the maximal response is reduced (Fig. 7.9B).

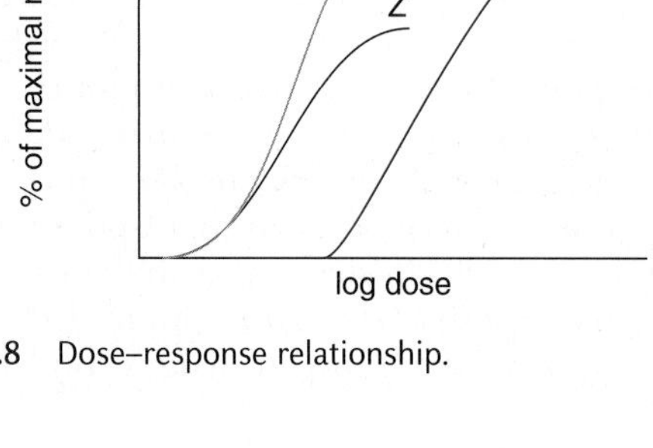

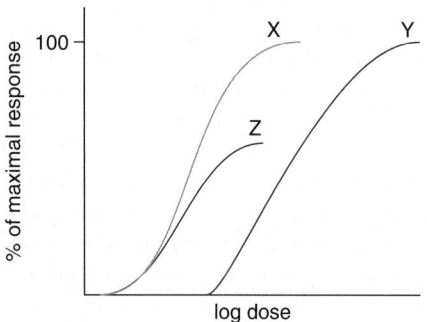

FIGURE 7.8 Dose–response relationship.

PRESYNAPTIC AND POSTSYNAPTIC RECEPTOR LOCATIONS

When an action potential arrives at the nerve cell's axon, a depolarization-induced exocytosis of the neurotransmitter from its storage sites in the presynaptic terminal occurs. Through this process, the action potential continues the flow of information to the target site, the postsynaptic cell. The neurotransmitter diffuses across the extracellular fluid-filled space known as the synapse to interact with its postsynaptic receptors. The released neurotransmitter, however, is also capable of interacting with presynaptic receptors located on the neurons that just released the neurotransmitter. The function of these receptors typically involves the regulation of nerve transmission, and they are are termed "autoreceptors," because the neurotransmitters that activate them function to control their own release.

An exquisite example of both receptor locations and the action of autoreceptors in the control of neurotransmission is observed in norepinephrine-containing postganglionic neurons of the sympathetic nervous system (Fig. 7.10) (15). Norepinephrine, which is capable of stimulating both α- and β-adrenoceptors, is initially released from the presynaptic neuron and is present at low concentration in the synapse. Low concentrations of norepinephrine are capable of preferentially stimulating β-adrenoceptors located presynaptically, which function to increase the release of more neurotransmitter and, thereby, magnify the intended response. The epinephrine released from the adrenal medulla during sympathetic stimulation is also thought to have an important role in facilitating neuronal norepinephrine release. This is an example of a positive-feedback system, which allows a rapid rise in the concentration of the neurotransmitter and, thus, the intended signal. Following this initial period of robust norepinephrine release, very high norepinephrine concentrations result in the synaptic cleft, which is then capable of stimulating other presynaptic autoreceptors, this time terminating the additional release of neurotransmitter. This negative-feedback system allows the signal to be terminated very quickly.

Together, the presynaptic facilitatory β-adrenoceptor–mediated mechanism and the presynaptic inhibitory α-adrenoceptor–mediated mechanism allow a rapid, robust, and well-controlled signal to be delivered. If one were to design a system that was to respond quickly to stressors, such as the sympathetic nervous system is believed to be designed to do, then a system that turns on rapidly and can be terminated quickly would be ideal and, presumably, an evolutionary advantage. Many other neurotransmitter autoreceptors have been identified, such as in the serotoninergic, dopaminergic, and histaminergic transmitter systems. Examples exist whereby a neurotransmitter can interact with a presynaptic receptor to influence the release of a

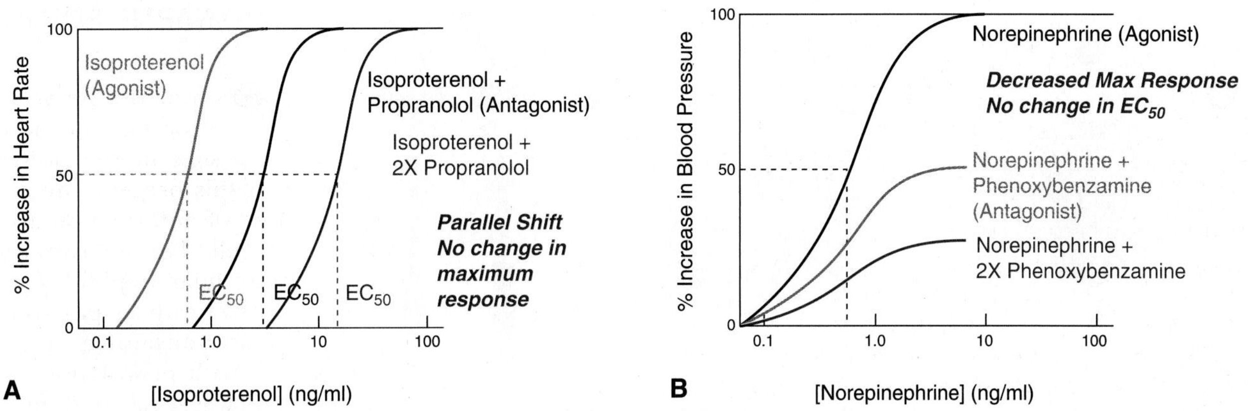

FIGURE 7.9 Dose–response curves for the effect of the agonist isoproterenol on heart rate in: (A) the presence of two concentrations of the competitive antagonist propranolol. Note the rightward shift of the dose–response curve with no change in maximum effect; and dose-response curves for the effect of the agonist norepinephrine on blood pressure (B) in the presence of two concentrations of the noncompetitive antagonist phenoxybenzamine. Note the decrease in maximum response and the absence of a rightward shift of the dose–response curves. (From Clarkson CW. Basic principles of pharmacology. Available at: http://tmedweb.tulane.edu/pharmwiki/doku.php/drug_receptor_theory.)

different neurotransmitter. For instance, norepinephrine released from neurons in the gastrointestinal tract can function to decrease acetylcholine release. This is termed a heteroreceptor.

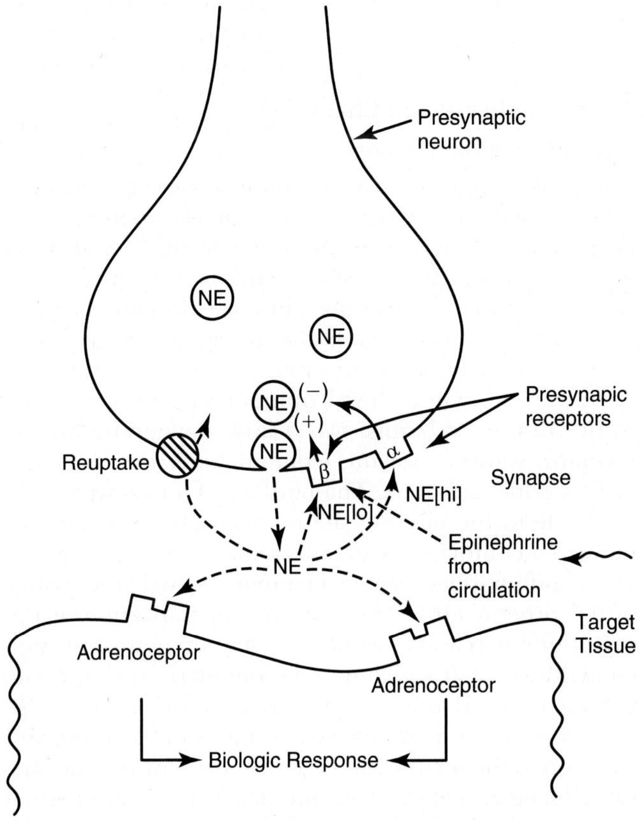

FIGURE 7.10 Autoreceptor control of neurotransmission as observed in norepinephrine-containing postganglionic neurons of the sympathetic nervous system. NE, norepinephrine; NE[lo], low norepinephrine concentration; NE[hi], high norepinephrine concentration; α, α-adrenoceptor; β, β-adrenoceptor; (–), inhibit; (+), stimulate.

DRUG RECEPTORS AND THE BIOLOGIC RESPONSE

There are four major families of receptors that drugs, which mimic, modify, or antagonize endogenous neurotransmitters, hormones, or autocoids, are capable of interacting with in the body (Fig. 7.11). Some receptors allow a rapid response to a released neurotransmitter/hormone or an administered drug. These responses are generally important for the immediate response to a significant homeostatic challenge to the individual. Both ion channel and G protein–coupled receptors tend to be rapid responders, with some catalytic receptors also characterized this way. These responses tend to be short-lived. On the other hand, many catalytic and just about all cytoplasmic/nuclear receptors are likely to respond much more slowly, on the order of hours to days, and these responses are much longer in duration than the rapid-responding receptors.

Signal Transduction

Signal transduction is a communication process by which a cell converts an extracellular signal or stimulus by transmitting this signal across the cell membrane to the interior of the cell. Proteins on the cell's extracellular surface function as receptors for specific molecules, ligands, or agonists (first messengers). The binding of the ligand to the receptor initiates an interlinked series of processes, termed "signal transduction," that involve a sequence of biochemical reactions inside the cell, which are carried out by enzymes, proteins, and ions (especially calcium) that are linked through second messengers, such as cyclic adenosine monophosphate (cAMP) or inositol 1,4,5-trisphosphate (IP_3). This signal is relayed via a second messenger that results in specific cellular responses or changes in gene expression in the nucleus as shown in Figure 7.12. Such processes take place in as little as a millisecond or as long as a few

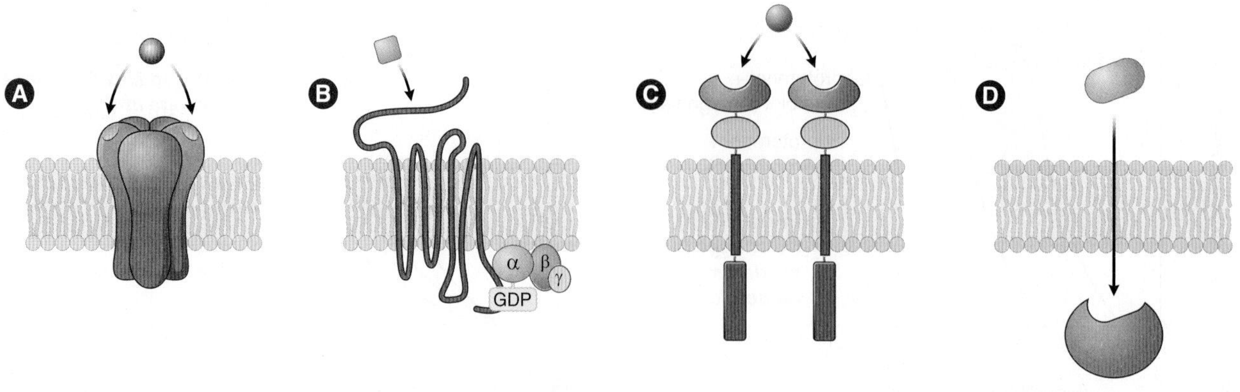

FIGURE 7.11 Major classes of drug receptors. (A) Transmembrane ligand-gated ion channel receptor. (B) Transmembrane G protein–coupled receptor (GPCR). (C) Transmembrane catalytic receptor or enzyme-coupled receptors. (D) Intracellular cytoplasmic/nuclear receptor. (From Simon JB, Golan DE, Tashjian A, et al., eds. Chapter 1: drug–receptor interactions. In: Principles of Pharmacology: The Pathophysiologic Basis of Drug Therapy. Baltimore: Lippincott Williams & Wilkins, 2008:3–16, with permission.)

seconds. Slower processes are rarely referred to as signal transduction.

The process of signal transduction serves several critical roles. First, it enables extracellular molecules to affect cellular function without entering the intracellular environment. This "long distance" communication is accomplished by the binding of a ligand (agonist) to the receptor protein and stabilizing the receptor structure in an active conformation. The active receptor conformation can then facilitate the flow of ions through a membrane channel by the removal of steric or electronic hindrances (opening of channel gates). For those receptors that produce signals via activation of intracellular metabolic pathways, the active state or conformation of the receptors changes the intracellular molecular environment in such a way as to activate, directly or indirectly, intracellular regulatory enzymes. Second, several different signals can affect one another by facilitating or inhibiting the activation of regulatory enzymatic proteins via common or opposing metabolic pathways. Thus, signal transduction mechanisms can interact in such a way as to yield an integrated response to multiple stimuli. Third, via the activation of enzymes and the production of second messengers (e.g., cAMP, diacylglycerol [DAG], and IP_3), an initially weak signal can be amplified many times, and its duration prolonged, to produce a robust cellular response. This amplification occurs through several mechanisms. The kinetic time frame for enzyme activation and the presence of key metabolites can be much longer than the time of receptor activation itself. Thus, a brief activation of a small number of receptors can result in a magnified response by the cell. Amplification can also occur via a molecular "cascade," in which one initial signal can trigger a multitude of intracellular reactions that lead to an enhanced cellular response. Outcomes of signal transduction can include one or more of the following: 1) a change in cell membrane polarity in electrically excitable tissues, such as nerves and muscles, which then results in the facilitation or inhibition of an action potential, thus affecting the excitability of the tissue; 2) the activation of cytosolic metabolic cascades, resulting in alterations of cellular morphology or function; and 3) gene activation, leading to the synthesis of new proteins that can then modify cellular structures and physiology.

Transmembrane Ion Channels

Ligand-Gated Ion Channels

The most rapid cellular responses to receptor activation are mediated via ligand-gated ion channels (LGICs) (Fig. 7.11A). The main component of this signal transduction pathway is a plasma membrane–spanning protein composed of multiple peptide subunits, each of which contains four membrane-spanning domains. The nicotinic acetylcholine receptor is, perhaps, the best characterized LGIC. The nicotinic receptor is composed of five distinct subunits, two α and, depending on the receptor subtype, various combinations of additional α, β, γ, and δ subunits. The binding of an acetylcholine molecule to the binding site on each of two α subunits induces a conformational change in the receptor, opening a sodium-selective ion channel through the center of the protein (16). The result is depolarization of the surrounding plasma membrane. Other neurotransmitter-activated LGICs include γ-aminobutyric acid, glycine, glutamate, and some serotonin receptors (17). These receptors share a similar structural conformation and function to the nicotinic receptor, except for the specificity of the ligand-binding site and selectivity of the channel for particular ions. The primary reason for the rapidity (milliseconds) of the cellular response with LGICs is that the transduction of the signal requires the activation of a single molecule. Therefore, this transduction mechanism is especially suited for physiologic processes necessitating

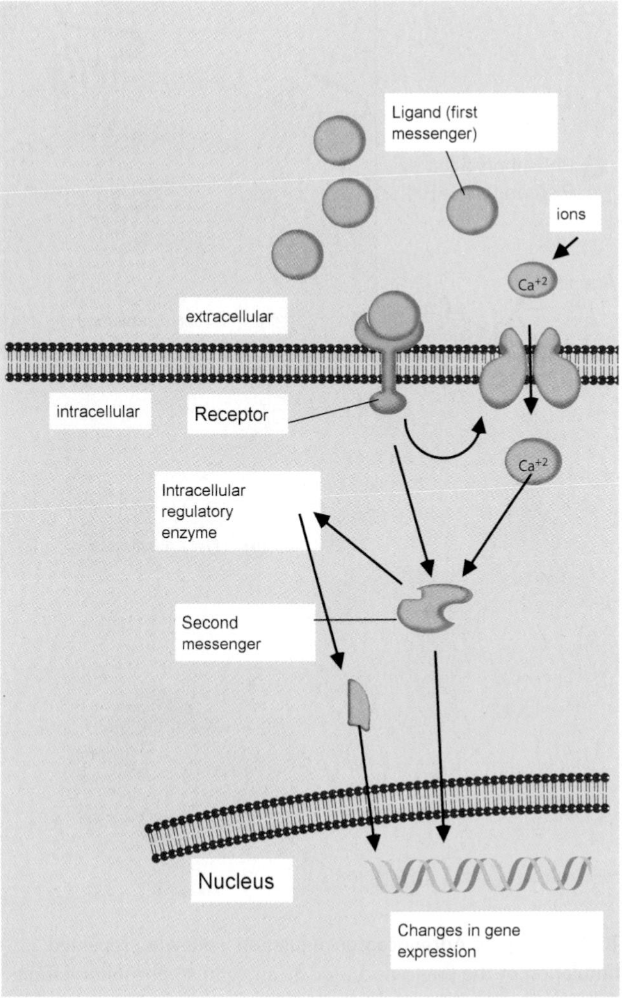

FIGURE 7.12 Overview of signal transduction in cellular regulation and gene expression via second messengers.

an immediate response, such as the stimulation of nerves and muscles.

Voltage-Gated and Second Messenger–Gated Channels

Other ion channels are controlled by either voltage changes or second messenger molecules. An example of a voltage-gated channel includes the sodium channels responsible for impulse conduction in sensory nerve fibers that transmit information about pain and temperature. Following administration, the local anesthetic lidocaine enters the nerve cell via diffusion in its unprotonated form. Once inside the nerve cell, lidocaine is protonated and, in this charged form, is capable of blocking the sodium channel from the intracellular side. Some second messenger molecules (e.g., cAMP and IP_3) generated following the activation of G protein–coupled receptors can influence the degree of channel opening or closing. The most common channels influenced by these second messengers include those for calcium and potassium.

Transmembrane G Protein–Coupled Receptors

The G protein–coupled receptors (GPCRs) are a class of large membrane-bound proteins that share a well-conserved structure and transduce their signal via the activation of an intracellular guanine nucleotide–binding protein (G protein). This family of proteins has seven hydrophobic (heptahelical) domains that span the plasma membrane; therefore, it is sometimes referred to as having a serpentine structure (Fig. 7.11B). The extracellular region of the protein is composed of the amino terminus and several loops, which comprise the ligand-binding site. Smaller ligands tend to bind deep within the extracellular loops, close to the plasma membrane, whereas larger molecules have binding sites that are more superficial. The carboxy end of the receptor is located in the area of the protein that protrudes into the cytoplasm. The intracellular side of the receptor also includes the binding site for the G protein, which usually binds to the third loop between the sixth and seventh transmembrane regions of the protein. Close to the carboxy terminus are serine and threonine residues, which are targets for adenosine triphosphate (ATP)-dependent phosphorylation. Following prolonged activation, phosphorylation of these residues is hypothesized to occur via a negative-feedback regulatory metabolic pathway, which facilitates the binding of modulating molecules that subsequently impair the coupling of G proteins to the receptor. The result is receptor desensitization.

More than 100 different GPCRs bind to a variety of ligands encompassing biogenic amines, such as acetylcholine, norepinephrine, and serotonin; amino acid neurotransmitters, such as glutamate and glycine; and peptide hormones, such as angiotensin II and somatostatin. There are multiple GPCR types for a single ligand. The result is the possibility that a single ligand can activate a variety of transduction pathways and produce a multiplicity of cellular responses. Thus, a receptor is defined not just by which ligand binds to it but also by how the signal is transduced and the resultant physiologic response. As an example, at least nine different adrenergic receptor subtypes exist (18). Norepinephrine can bind to the β_1 receptor, which is coupled to a G protein (designated G_s). Following receptor stimulation of G_s, there is activation of the enzyme adenylyl cyclase, thus leading ultimately to an increase in heart rate and force of contraction. Norepinephrine binding to α_1-receptors, on the other hand, results in the binding to a different G protein (G_q), which activates the production of the second messengers IP_3 and DAG, which then initiate a cascade of intracellular events leading to smooth muscle contraction. Therefore, a single ligand can induce a wide range of responses as a consequence of coupling to different G proteins. Which G protein is activated depends on factors such as the presence and availability of individual G proteins within a particular cell type, kinetic issues (e.g., the binding affinity of the G protein for the receptor protein), and finally, the affinity of the activated G protein subunits for signal transduction enzymes.

G Proteins

G proteins are heterotrimeric in structure with the subunits (in decreasing size) designated as α, β, and γ. At least 13 types of G proteins have been identified, which are divided among four families, G_s, G_i, G_q, and G_{12}. Individual G proteins transduce the receptor activation signal via one of a number of second messenger systems discussed below. The best-understood second messenger systems associated with each G protein family are summarized in Table 7.1.

The characteristics of the α subunit are what determine the designation of the G protein. Receptor activation leads to a conformational change in the associated G protein, triggering the release of bound guanosine diphosphate (GDP) from the α subunit, which is then replaced by a molecule of guanosine triphosphate (GTP). With the binding of GTP, the α-subunit GTP complex dissociates from the αβ subunits and binds to a particular target enzyme, resulting in its activation or inhibition. Within a short period of time, the α subunit catalyzes the dephosphorylation of the associated GTP molecule to GDP, resulting in the reassociation of the α subunit with the αβ subunits and, thus, the return of the G protein to the inactivated state (Fig. 7.13). Variations on this scheme include the activation of proteins such as G protein–gated ion channels by dissociated αβ subunits and the ability of receptor proteins to activate more than a single G protein. The simultaneous activation of more than one type of GPCR results in the initiation of multiple signals, which can then interact with one another (a phenomenon commonly referred to as cross-talk). This interaction can be of several types: If both receptors use a common signal transduction pathway, the activation can result in an additive response by the cell. Conversely, if simultaneous receptor activation triggers opposing signal transduction pathways, the outcome will be an attenuated cellular response. Other types of interactions can include the desensitization or activation of other receptor proteins or second messenger pathways. The final outcome of the activation of multiple signals is an integrated response by the cell.

TABLE 7.1 G-Protein Transducers and Second Messengers

G Protein Transducer Family	Second Messenger System
G_s	Stimulates adenylyl cyclase activity and Ca^{2+} channels
G_i	Inhibits adenylyl cyclase activity and activates K^+ channels
G_q	Stimulates phospholipase C activity
G_{12}	Modulates sodium/hydrogen ion exchanger

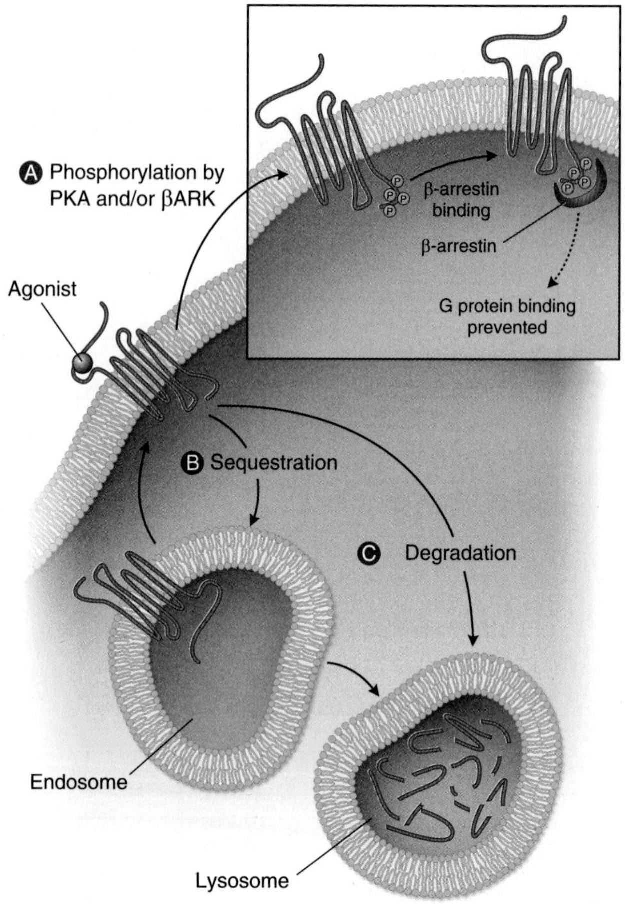

FIGURE 7.13 β-Adrenoceptor regulation. Following repeated stimulation of the β-adrenoceptor by an agonist, phosphorylation of amino acids on the intracellular C-terminal domain by protein kinase A (PKA) and/or β-adrenergic receptor kinase (βARK) can (A) prevent subsequent G protein binding, (B) enhance removal of the receptor from the membrane via sequestration into endosomes, or (C) enhance degradation via lysosomal internalization and cleavage. (From Simon JB, Golan DE, Tashjian A, et al., eds. Chapter 1: drug–receptor interactions. In: Principles of Pharmacology: The Pathophysiologic Basis of Drug Therapy. Baltimore: Lippincott Williams & Wilkins, 2008:16, with permission.)

Second Messenger Pathways

As previously discussed, in response to receptor activation, G proteins activate plasma membrane-bound enzymes, which then trigger a metabolic cascade that results in a cellular response (19). The products of these enzymatic actions are termed "second messengers," because they mobilize other enzymatic and structural proteins, which then produce the cellular response. The enzymes catalyzing the synthesis of second messengers fall generally into two categories: those that convert the purine triphosphates ATP and GTP into their respective cyclic monophosphates (e.g., cAMP, cyclic guanosine monophosphate [cGMP]), and enzymes that synthesize second messengers from plasma membrane phospholipids (e.g., DAG and IP_3). The most thoroughly studied second messenger system is controlled by a family of 10 plasma membrane-bound isoenzymes of adenylyl cyclase*, which catalyze the conversion of ATP to cAMP (Fig. 7.14). Adenylyl cyclase is activated by the G_s family of G proteins and inhibited by the G_i family. Following synthesis, cAMP activates cAMP-dependent protein kinases by triggering the dissociation of regulatory subunits from catalytic subunits. The catalytic subunits then activate other target proteins via phosphorylation, which then trigger the cellular response. The magnitude of the cellular response is proportional to the concentration of cAMP. Degradation of cAMP occurs via phosphodiesterases or by reducing cAMP concentration via active transport out of the cell. The result is termination of the signal.

A similar, although less ubiquitous, second messenger pathway is associated with guanylyl cyclase**. Guanylyl cyclase is activated in response to catalytic receptors selective for ligands including atrial natriuretic factor and nitric oxide. When stimulated, guanylyl cyclase then catalyzes the synthesis of cGMP from GTP. cGMP subsequently activates cGMP-dependent protein kinases, which then activate other proteins. The actions of cGMP are terminated by enzymatic degradation of the second messenger or the dephosphorylation of substrates. One effect of this second messenger pathway is relaxation of smooth muscle via the dephosphorylation of myosin light chains.

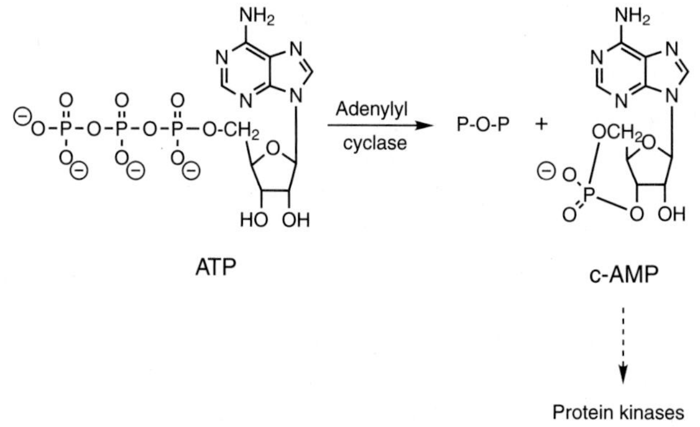

FIGURE 7.14 Conversion of adenosine triphosphate (ATP) to cyclic adenosine monophosphate (cAMP) catalyzed by adenylyl cyclase.

*This enzyme is known by two names, *adenylate cyclase* (EC 4.6.1.1), its official name from the International Union of Biochemistry and Molecular Biology Nomenclature Committee, or its alternative name, adenylyl cyclase.

**This enzyme is known by two names, *guanylate cyclase* (EC 4.6.1.2), its official name from the International Union of Biochemistry and Molecular Biology Nomenclature Committee, or its alternative name, guanylyl cyclase.

The generation of second messengers from plasma membrane phospholipids is mediated primarily by G protein activation of phospholipase C (PLC) (20). There are three families of PLC, designated PLC-β, PLC-γ, and PLC-δ. PLC-β can be activated by the α subunit of the G_q family of G proteins or the βγ subunits of other G proteins. PLC-γ is activated via tyrosine kinase receptors, but the mechanism for PLC-δ is not yet understood. On activation, PLC hydrolyzes phosphatidyl inositol-4,5-bisphosphate to DAG and IP_3 (Fig. 7.15). The water-soluble IP_3 diffuses into the cytoplasm, where it triggers the release of calcium from intracellular stores. Intracellular calcium then binds to the protein calmodulin and also to protein kinase C, both of which then stimulate, via protein phosphorylation, a broad range of enzymes and other proteins, including specific kinases. The other product of PLC, DAG, is lipid soluble and remains in the plasma membrane, where it facilitates the activation of protein kinase C by calcium. The signal is terminated via inactivation of IP_3 by dephosphorylation, whereas DAG is inactivated by phosphorylation to phosphatidic acid or deacetylation to fatty acids. The

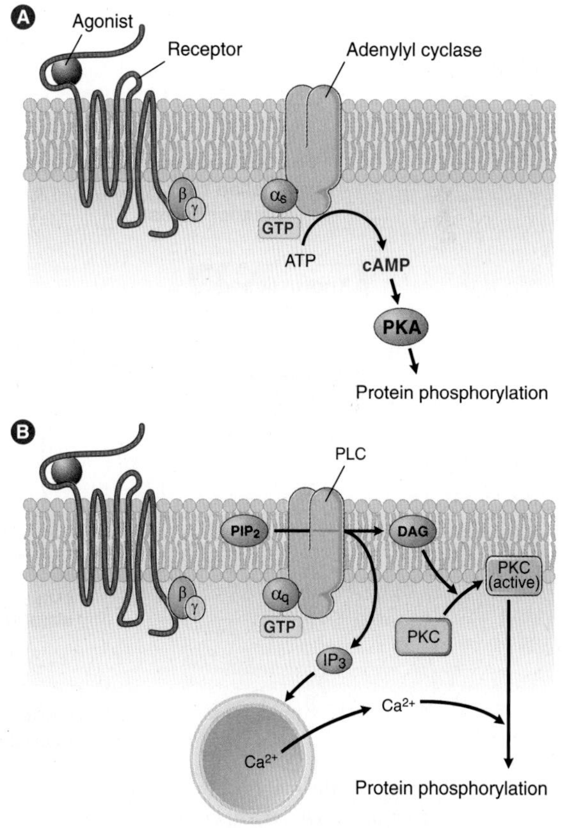

FIGURE 7.15 Second messenger mechanisms for cyclic adenosine monophosphate (cAMP) and inositol trisphosphate. (From Simon JB, Golan DE, Tashjian A, et al., eds. Chapter 1: drug– receptor interactions. In: Principles of Pharmacology: The Pathophysiologic Basis of Drug Therapy. Baltimore: Lippincott Williams & Wilkins, 2008:3–16, with permission.)

concentration of intracellular calcium is reduced by sequestration within cytoplasmic organelles or transport out of the cell. Activation of phospholipase D hydrolyzes phosphatidylcholine to phosphatidic acid, which can then be metabolized to DAG via phosphatidate phosphohydrolase. This pathway prolongs the duration of elevated levels of DAG. Phospholipase A_2 is activated by increased concentrations of intracellular calcium and metabolizes phosphatidylcholine to arachidonic acid. Arachidonic acid then functions as a substrate for the synthesis of autocoids, including prostaglandins, thromboxane A_2, and leukotrienes.

Frizzled is another family of GPCR proteins that regulate functions such as embryonic development, the formation of neural synapses, and cell polarity via a signal transduction cascade composed of protein kinases such as glycogen synthase kinase 3 (GSK-3), phosphatases, and proteolytic enzymes. A target molecule for this cascade is β-catenin, which promotes specific gene expression.

With the development of screening assays of cDNA libraries, a number of GPCRs have been identified for which there is no known endogenous ligand. These receptors are termed "orphan receptors." When the endogenous ligand is identified, the receptor is said to be "adopted." Strategies for identifying the ligand of orphan receptors include: 1) expression of the GPCR in a recombinant assay system; 2) screening candidate ligands against the receptor; 3) detecting active ligands by activation of signal transduction cascades; and 4) further testing of the ligand against other GPCRs to determine selectivity. An example of an adopted orphan GPCR is Axor 35, which was ultimately characterized as the histamine H_4 receptor (Fig. 7.16) (21).

Transmembrane Catalytic Receptors

Catalytic receptors are a class of plasma membrane-bound receptors characterized by a monomer with a ligand-binding site in the extracellular domain, a single membrane-spanning domain, and an intracellular domain with enzymatic activity (Fig. 7.11C). This family of receptors is activated predominately by peptide hormones, such as insulin, epidermal growth factor,

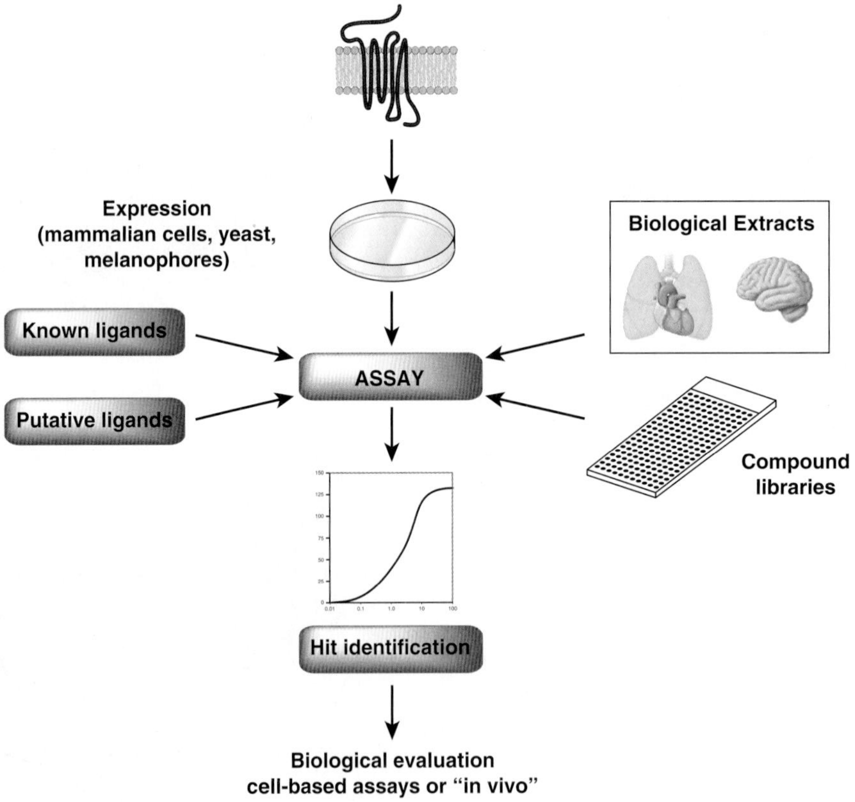

FIGURE 7.16 Strategy for the identification of ligands for orphan GPCRs. Orphan GPCRs are expressed in a recombinant expression system, such as mammalian cells, yeast, or *Xenopus* melanophores. Following expression, it is usual to generate an assay amenable to the screening of candidate ligands in microtiter plate formats. The identification of an activating ligand is detected according to the activation of an intracellular signaling cascade. An activating ligand is identified according to its ability to cause a concentration-dependent increase in the activity of a signaling cascade. Once identified, the ligand can be further characterized against other GPCRs to determine its activity and selectivity profile prior to being used in cell-based, tissue, and, in some cases, whole-animal experiments in order to study the physiologic role of the newly liganded receptor.

platelet-derived growth factor, and atrial natriuretic factor. The catalytic portion of the receptor functions as a protein kinase, targeting primarily tyrosine residues; however, the receptor for atrial natriuretic factor, rather than having kinase activity, activates guanylyl cyclase and metabolizes GTP to cGMP (22). Receptor activation occurs by ligand binding, which then triggers dimerization of receptor proteins via the cross-phosphorylation of tyrosine residues. The dimeric protein is the active form of the catalytic receptor. One consequence of activation via dimerization is that the intracellular signal can be maintained even after the ligand has dissociated from the binding site. The phosphorylation of intracellular proteins by this receptor type results in effects such as the opening of ion channels, changes in cytoplasmic function, or initiation of genomic expression. Other catalytic receptors, activated by transforming growth factor-β, use serine/threonine kinases in regulating cellular growth and differentiation. Major signal transduction pathways activated by receptor tyrosine kinases include the mitogen-activated protein kinase (MAPK) cascade.

The MAPK Cascade

The MAPK cascade is comprised of a series of proteins that activate enzymatic substrates via phosphorylation (Fig. 7.17). Once a tyrosine hydroxylase receptor is activated by a ligand (most commonly hormones that affect gene expression), an adaptor protein, growth factor receptor-bound protein 2 (Grb2), binds to the receptor and the complex then activates a small GTPase called Ras. Ras then binds to and activates the serine/threonine-specific protein kinase c-Raf. c-Raf then phosphorylates a MAPK kinase (MEK), which phosphorylates MAPK (MAPKs are also referred to as extracellular signal-regulated kinases [ERKs]). Activated MAPK can then activate transcription factors that bind to DNA sequences that control the transfer of genetic information from DNA to messenger RNA. Ultimately, activation of catalytic receptors results in the stimulation of gene

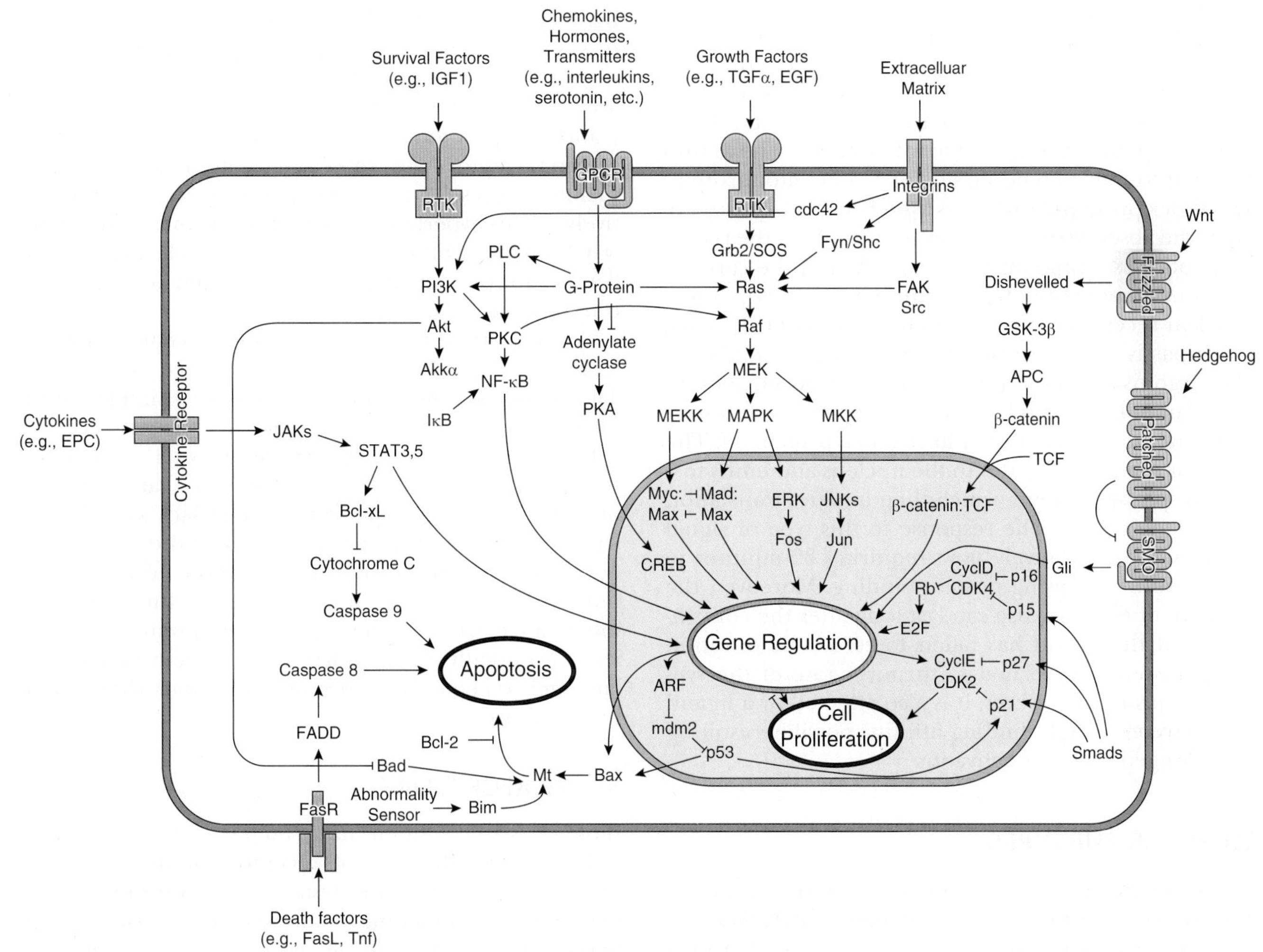

FIGURE 7.17 Signal transduction cascades that regulate gene expression and apoptosis. (From Wikipedia. Mitogen-activated protein kinase. Available at: http://en.wikipedia.org/wiki/Mitogen-activated_protein_kinase.)

expression, cell growth and division, differentiation, and apoptosis.

Enzyme-Coupled Receptors

Enzyme-coupled receptors are similar in their function to catalytic receptors, except rather than inherent catalytic activity, enzyme-coupled receptors bind to separate enzymatic proteins (Fig. 7.11C). This class of receptor binds cytokines, including growth hormone, erythropoietin, and interferon. Like catalytic receptors, enzyme-coupled receptors are activated via dimerization following ligand binding. Kinase activity is accomplished by separate, noncovalently bound protein kinases of the Janus kinase (JAK) family. After dimerization, JAKs are activated and phosphorylate receptor tyrosine residues. The phosphorylated receptor then binds other molecules, termed "signal transducers and activators of transcription" (STATs), which are phosphorylated by the JAKs and, subsequently, dissociate into the cytoplasm. The STATs then translocate to the nucleus, where they initiate gene transcription.

Intracellular Cytoplasmic/Nuclear Receptors

Cytoplasmic/nuclear receptors differ from those described earlier in that they are not associated with the plasma membrane but, rather, are located within the cytoplasm or are bound to the surface of the nucleus (Fig. 7.11D). These receptors are composed of a single polypeptide with three functional domains. The amino terminal contains a binding site for a modulator protein, heat shock protein-90, which is associated with the receptor in the absence of agonist. In the middle of the receptor peptide is a binding site for DNA, and the carboxy terminus contains the ligand-binding site. Cytoplasmic/nuclear receptors are activated by lipid-soluble ligands, which passively diffuse through the plasma membrane (23). Agonists include nitric oxide, steroid hormones, and vitamin D. Ligand binding activates the receptor by inducing the dissociation of heat shock protein-90. The receptor then translocates to the nucleus and binds to a DNA response element, which then initiates translation of the target gene. The response to this type of signal transduction is relatively slow, requiring 30 minutes to several hours following protein binding. Moreover, the duration of the response can last long after the concentration of the ligand has fallen to zero. The duration of the response is related to turnover rate of the synthesized protein; however, it is also affected by a ligand with extremely high binding affinity, possibly resulting in prolonged receptor activation.

RECEPTOR SUBTYPES

Careful examination of the effects of a series of sympathomimetics by Ahlquist (24) led him to postulate the existence of at least two types of adrenoceptors, which he termed α and β. Realizing that adrenoceptor agonists were capable of causing either relaxation or contraction of isolated smooth muscles, he noted that although a compound like norepinephrine had potent excitatory actions but weak inhibitory actions, another catecholamine, isoproterenol, had potent inhibitory actions but weak excitatory actions. When a series of related compounds were tested for potency in various tissues, it was demonstrated that for the α-adrenoceptor, the order of potency was epinephrine ≥ norepinephrine >>> isoproterenol, and for the β-adrenoceptor, the order of potency was isoproterenol > epinephrine ≥ norepinephrine. Following the findings of Ahlquist, others used specific antagonists that had become available to further support this designation of receptor subtypes. With the development of highly selective antagonists and procedures for cloning and determining the amino acid sequence of proteins, the classification of receptors into subtypes has expanded at a tremendous rate (25). For example, the α-adrenoceptor noted earlier can be subclassed as α_{1A}, α_{1B}, α_{1C}, α_{1D}, α_{2A}, α_{2B}, and α_{2C} based on cloning experiments (Table 7.2).

The therapeutic significance of such distinctions is not yet known, however, due to a lack of selective agonists or antagonists. Some therapeutic distinction can be made between α_1 and α_2 adrenoceptors in a general way, in that α_1 vasoconstriction antagonism by prazosin and central nervous system α_2-adrenoceptor stimulation by clonidine are useful in the treatment of hypertension. Similarly, β-adrenoceptor antagonists are available that antagonize β_1-adrenoceptors with some selectivity. Thus, the use of metoprolol, a selective β_1-antagonist, is effective and relatively safe in hypertensive patients with compromised airway function, whereas the use of a nonselective (β_1 and β_2) antagonist, such as propranolol, would be clearly contraindicated in such a patient.

A summary of the most important receptor subtypes from a therapeutic standpoint is presented in Table 7.3. The reader should realize that this is a simplification of what is currently known about the various receptor subtypes. For instance, within the general category of serotonin receptors, at least 13 subtypes can be identified from cloning experiments. The lack of selective agonists and antagonists to characterize the pharmacology of each of these subtypes, however, has hindered our understanding of their individual functions and importance from a therapeutic standpoint. Our ability to eventually develop drugs that selectively manipulate such receptor subtypes has enormous therapeutic implications.

SPARE RECEPTORS

Biologic systems often have built-in safety factors to enhance the efficiency of receptor–stimulus coupling and, thereby, assure the desired neurotransmission. In many tissues containing α-adrenoceptors, only a small percentage of the available receptors need to be occupied to produce a maximum response. This depends on the particular tissue being studied and the agonist used.

TABLE 7.2 Adrenoreceptor Families

Receptor Type	Subtype	Transduction Mechanism	Tissue Function
α_1	1A	Activates $G_{q/11}$	Smooth muscle and myocardial contraction
α_1	1B	Activates $G_{q/11}$	Smooth muscle contraction
α_1	1D	Activates $G_{q/11}$	Smooth muscle contraction
α_2	2A	Activates $G_{i/o}$	Hypotension, sedation, analgesia, anesthesia
α_2	2B	Activates $G_{i/o}$	Vasoconstriction
α_2	2C	Activates $G_{i/o}$	Not established
β_1	—	Activates G_s	Increases heart rate and force of contraction
β_2	—	Activates G_s	Smooth muscle relaxation
β_3	—	Activates or inhibits adenylyl cyclase	Lipolysis, cardioinhibition

Therefore, 100% occupancy of the available receptors is not always required, because spare receptors (or a receptor reserve) are present. Studies using phenoxybenzamine, which alkylates the α-adrenoceptor and, therefore, irreversibly inactivates the receptor, indicate that only 5% to 10% of the available receptors need to be activated to elicit a maximum response to a full, or strong, agonist, such as norepinephrine or phenylephrine (8,9,26). To obtain a maximum response to a partial agonist like ephedrine, however, nearly 100% of the receptors need to be occupied. The explanation behind this difference can involve a less than ideal receptor–drug interaction for partial agonists. A partial agonist can function as an antagonist if it interferes with the ability of a full agonist to bind to its receptor and produce a response. In the absence of a full agonist, however, the partial agonist only displays agonistic activity.

DYNAMIC NATURE OF RECEPTORS

As is characteristic of most individual components of living systems, receptors are not static but, rather, are constantly in a state of dynamic adaptation. One could envision these protein molecules floating within the fluid mosaic of the biologic membrane awaiting interaction with normal physiologic signals. The function of such receptors, once stimulated, involves attempts to respond to perturbations of the normal physiology of the cell or organism. The role in maintaining homeostasis within the organism requires constant adaptation of receptor number and/or sensitivity in response to the changing environment in the vicinity of the receptor. One approach to controlling receptor activation is by regulating the concentration of neurotransmitter at the receptor binding site. This is accomplished by the modulation of release via activation of presynaptic receptors, as described earlier. Altering the rate of synthesis, degradation, or efficiency of the enzymes that create or degrade neurotransmitter molecules is also used to regulate neurotransmitter concentrations at the receptor.

A second mechanism for modulating the cellular response to receptor activation is to alter receptor number and/or sensitivity. The process is best understood for GPCRs but has also been characterized for ion channel receptors, such as the nicotinic receptor. The alteration in the availability or functional capacity of a given receptor constitutes an adaptive mechanism whereby the cell or organism is protected from agonist overload. For example, the chronic administration of a β-adrenoceptor agonist, such as isoproterenol, is known to produce a desensitization of the β-adrenoceptors in the heart (27). During the period of overstimulation, the receptor becomes desensitized to further activation via phosphorylation by G protein–coupled kinases, such as protein kinase A or β-adrenoceptor kinase, at serine and threonine residues on the C-terminal domain that interferes with G_S binding (Fig. 7.13). Desensitization can also occur at other receptors with analogous phosphorylation sites (heterologous desensitization). A more prolonged or powerful overstimulation typically results in a decrease in receptor number and is termed "downregulation." In these GPCRs, downregulation initiated by phosphorylation of amino acids near the intracellular C-terminal domain results in binding to β-arrestins that facilitate their internalization via a clathrin-dependent pathway. Following internalization, the receptor can either be recycled back into the plasma membrane via endosomes or degraded by lysosomes. Reduced receptor numbers can also be accomplished via changes in the transcription and/or translation of genes that code for the receptor. Changes in receptor number or efficiency of receptors that lead to diminished responses and, thus, diminished efficacy of a drug with repeated or long-term use are examples of pharmacodynamic tolerance. As a

TABLE 7.3 Survey of Receptor Subtypes

Receptor Class	Subtype	Selective Selective Agonist	Antagonist	Effector	Cloned
Adrenoceptors	α_1	Phenylephrine	Prazosin	IP_3/DAG	Yes
	α_2	Clonidine	Yohimbine	↓cAMP	Yes
	β_1	Dobutamine	Atenolol	↑cAMP	Yes
	β_2	Terbutaline	Butoxamine	↑cAMP	Yes
Dopamine receptors	D_1	Fenoldopam	Dihydroxidine	↑cAMP	Yes
	D_2	Bromocriptine	(–)Sulpiride	↓cAMP	Yes
Excitatory amino acid receptors	NMDA	NMDA	D-AP5	↓Na^+/Ca^{2+}	Yes
	AMPA	AMPA	CNQX	↑Na^+	Yes
	Kainate	Kainate	?	↑Na^+/K^+	Yes
GABA receptors	$GABA_A$	Muscimol	Bicuculline	↑Cl^-	Yes
	$GABA_B$	Baclofen	Saclofen	↓cAMP	Yes
Histamine receptors	H_1	2-(*m*-Fluorophenyl) Histamine	Mepyramine	IP_3/DAG	Yes
	H_2	Dimapril	Ranitidine	↑cAMP	Yes
Muscarinic receptors	M_1	Oxotremorine	Pirenzepine	IP_3/DAG	Yes
	M_2	Oxotremorine	AF-DX116	↓cAMP	Yes
Nicotinic receptors	N_{muscle}	?	Decamethonium	↑Na^+/Ca^{2+}	Yes
	$N_{neuronal}$	?	Hexamethonium	↑Na^+/Ca^{2+}	Yes
Opioid receptors	Mu	Sufentanil	CTAP	↓cAMP	Yes
	Delta	[D-Ala²] deltorphin	Naltrindole	↓cAMP	Yes
	Kappa	Dynorphin	Nor-binaltorphimine	↓cAMP	Yes
Serotonin receptors (5-HT)	$5\text{-}HT_{1A}$	8-OH-DPAT	Spiperone	↓cAMP	Yes
	$5\text{-}HT_{2A}$	α-Methyl-5-HT	Ketanserin	IP_3/DAG	Yes

?, no known selective compounds available; cloned, receptor subtype has been cloned and the amino acid structure is known. Chemical abbreviations used: AF-DX116, 11-([2-[(diethylamino)methyl]-1-piperidinyl]acetyl)-5-11-dihydro-6H-pyridol[2,3-b] [1,4]benzodiazepine-6-one; AMPA, D,L-α-amino-3-hydroxy-5-methyl-4-isoxalone propionic acid; cAMP, cyclic adenosine 3′,5′-monophosphate; CNQX, 6-cyano-7-nitroquinoxaline-2,3-dione; CTAP, D-Phe-Cys-Tyr-DTrp-Arg-Thr-Pen-Thr-NH2; DAG, diacyl glycerol; D-AP5, D-amino-5-phosphonopentanoate; GABA, γ-aminobutyric acid; 5-HT, 5-hydroxytryptamine, serotonin; IP_3, inositol 1,4,5-triphosphate; NMDA, N-methyl-D-aspartate; 8-OH-DPAT, 8-hydroxy-2-(di-n-propylamino)tetralin.

general principle, the body will always attempt to maintain homeostasis, whether perturbed by environmental challenges, disease processes, or even the administration of drugs. Actually, the body sees the administration of drugs as a perturbation of homeostasis and, usually, attempts to overcome the effects of the drug by invoking receptor adaptations. Often, however, with appropriate dosing schedules, drugs can be used with little observed receptor adaptation such that the desired pharmacologic effect continues to be observed.

In a similar fashion to the example described earlier, chronic administration of the β-adrenoceptor antagonist propranolol leads to a state of receptor supersensitivity or upregulation. The cells within the tissue, such as the heart, sense an alteration in the normal rate of basal β-adrenoceptor stimulation and, thus, respond by either increasing the number or the affinity of the receptors for their natural agonists, norepinephrine and epinephrine. An enhanced efficiency of the interaction between the receptor and its transducing systems can also account for a portion of the observed supersensitivity. The knowledge that such a receptor adaptation occurs has paramount practical therapeutic implications, because abrupt withdrawal of this class of agents can precipitate acute myocardial infarction. Thus, this practice should be scrupulously avoided.

Some pathophysiologic states are characterized by perturbations in receptor dynamics. Prinzmetal angina is thought to be characterized by an imbalance between vasodilatory β_2-adrenoceptor function and vasoconstrictor α_1-adrenoceptor function. In this disease state, the excessive alpha vasoconstriction of coronary arteries leads to myocardial ischemia and pain. The inadvertent use of a β-adrenoceptor antagonist, which is safely employed in typical angina pectoris to prevent β-adrenoceptor vasodilation, can leave unopposed alpha vasoconstrictor inputs and actually precipitate anginal pain. Thus, an understanding of the role that receptors have in physiology, pathophysiology, and pharmacology is essential for optimal therapeutic interventions.

FUTURE DIRECTIONS

Our understanding about the nature and role of receptors has increased tremendously since the early work of Langley and Ehrlich. Today, with the advances made in the field of molecular biology, it is possible to clone individual receptor subtypes (Table 7.3) and determine their function in cell culture. By modifying the amino acid structure at those sites believed to be involved in agonist binding, a better appreciation for the interaction of drugs currently available—and the rational design of those awaiting discovery—can be realized. Additionally, as we begin to be able to determine the structure of receptor subtypes through cloning techniques, we hopefully will better understand those disease processes that result from, or lead to, receptor adaptations or dysfunction.

Promising therapeutic approaches that exploit ligand receptor interactions include gene therapy and pharmacogenomics. Gene therapy uses knowledge about genetic defects in receptors, enzymes, and other proteins to treat inherited diseases. The approach of gene therapy is to administer genetically engineered viruses as vectors that contain normal genes for proteins that can function in place of defective gene products. One target of gene therapy research is cystic fibrosis, a genetic disorder that affects the protein transmembrane conductance regulator, a cAMP-regulated chloride channel. The goal of gene therapy in this case is to introduce functional transmembrane conductance regulator genes into affected tissues and ultimately decrease the thick mucus that is the primary pathologic manifestation of the disease. Pharmacogenomics is based on drug therapy targeting particular isoforms of receptors and enzymes expressed as a consequence of the individual genotype of the patient. The expectation of the pharmacogenomic approach is to optimize drug therapy by selecting drugs and doses that have the best potency and efficacy for the expressed protein.

References

1. Leake CD. A Historical Account of Pharmacology in the 20th Century. Springfield, IL: Charles C. Thomas, 1975.
2. Langley JN. On the reaction of cells and nerve endings to certain poisons. J Physiol 1905;33:374–413.
3. Ehrlich P. In: Himmelweit F, ed. Collected Papers of Paul Ehrlich, Vol III. London: Pergammon, 1957.
4. Price CC. Chemistry of alkylation. In: Sartorelli AC, Johns DG, eds. Antineoplastic and Immunosuppressive Agents, Part II—Handbuch der Experimentellen Pharmakologie, Vol 38. Berlin: Springer-Verlag, 1975:1–5.
5. Persidis A. High-throughput screening. Nat Biotechnol 1998;16:488–489.
6. Gedeon PC, Indarte M, Surratt CK, et al. Molecular dynamics of leucine and dopamine transporter proteins in a model cell membrane lipid bilayer. Proteins 2010;78:797–811.
7. Nickerson M. Receptor occupancy and tissue response. Nature 1956;178:697–698.
8. Minneman KP, Abel PW. Relationship between α_1-adrenoceptor density and functional response of rat vas deferens. Studies with phenoxybenzamine. Naunyn Schmiedebergs Arch Pharmacol 1984;327:238–246.
9. Besse JC, Furchgott RF. Dissociation constants and relative efficacies of agonists acting on α-adrenergic receptors in rabbit aorta. J Pharmacol Exp Ther 1976;197:66–78.
10. Pasteur L. On the asymmetry of naturally occurring organic compounds, the foundations of stereochemistry. In: Richardson GM, ed. Memoirs by Pasteur, Van't Hoff Le Bel, and Wislicenus. Stuttgart: Birkhauser, 1901:3–33.
11. Moya-Huff FA, Maher TJ. β-Adrenoceptor influences on the α_1- and α_2-mediated vasoconstriction induced by phenylpropanolamine and its two component isomers in the pithed rat. J Pharm Pharmacol 1988;40:876–878.
12. Johnson DA, Maher TJ. Vasoactive properties of phenylpropanolamine and its enantiomers in isolated rat caudal artery. Drug Dev Res 1991;23:159–169.
13. Maher TJ, Johnson DA. Review of chirality and its importance in pharmacology. Drug Dev Res 1991;24:149–156.
14. Parascandola J, Clark AJ. Quantitative pharmacology and the receptor theory. Trends Pharamcol Sci 1982;4:421–423.
15. Starke K. Presynaptic α-autoreceptors. Rev Physiol Biochem Pharmacol 1987;107:73–146.
16. Brisson A, Unwin PNT. Quaternary structure of the acetylcholine receptor. Nature 1985;315:474–477.
17. Kemp JA, Leeson PD. The glycine site of the NMDA receptor—five years on. Trends Pharmacol Sci 1993;14:20–25.
18. Kobilka BK. Adrenergic receptors as models for G protein–coupled receptors. Annu Rev Neurosci 1992;15:87–114.
19. Gilman AG. G proteins: transducers of receptor-generated signals. Annu Rev Biochem 1987;56:615–649.
20. Berridge MJ. Inositol triphosphate and diacylglycerol: two interacting second messengers. Ann Rev Biochem 1987;56:159–193.
21. Wise A, Jupe SC, Rees S. The identification of ligands at orphan G-protein coupled receptors. Annu Rev Pharmacol Toxicol 2004;44:43–66.
22. Chinkers M, Garbers DL, Chang MS, et al. A membrane form of guanylate cyclase is an atrial natriuretic peptide receptor. Nature 1989;338:78–83.
23. Evans RM. The steroid and thyroid hormone receptor superfamily. Science 1988;240:889–895.
24. Ahlquist RP. A study of the adrenotropic receptors. Am J Physiol 1948;153:586–600.
25. Minneman KP, Esbenshade TA. α_1-Adrenergic receptor subtypes. Annu Rev Pharmacol Toxicol 1994;34:117–133.
26. Furchgott RF. The use of β-haloalkylamines in the differentiation of receptors and in the determination of dissociation constants of receptor-agonist complexes. In: Harper NJ, Simmonds AB, eds. Advances in Drug Research, Vol 3. New York: Academic Press, 1966:21–55.
27. Tattersfield AE. Tolerance to β-agonists. Bull Eur Physiopathol Respir 1985;21:1S–5S.

Suggested Readings

Aranda A, Pascual A. Nuclear hormone receptors and gene expression. Physiol Rev 2001;8:1269–1304.

Ariens EJ. Affinity and intrinsic activity in the theory of competitive inhibition: problems and theory. Arch Int Pharmacodynam 1954;99:32–49.

Black JW, Leff P. Operational models of pharmacological agonists. Proc R Soc Lond Biol 1983;220:141–162.

Bylund DB. Subtypes of α_1- and α_2-adrenergic receptors. FASEB J 1992;6:832–839.

Kebabian JW, Neumeyer JL. The RBI Handbook of Receptor Classification. Natick, MA: Research Biochemicals International, 1998.
Kenakin T. Pharmacologic Analysis of Drug-Receptor Interaction, 2nd Ed. New York: Raven, 1993.
Liebmann C. G protein–coupled receptors and their signaling pathways: classical therapeutical targets susceptible to novel therapeutic concepts. Curr Pharm Design 2004;10:1937–1958.
Tallarida RJ, Jacobs LS. The Dose–Response Relation in Pharmacology. New York: Springer-Verlag, 1979.
Trends in Pharmacological Sciences. 2000 Receptor & Ion Channel Nomenclature Supplement. Oxford: Elsevier Science Ltd, 2000.

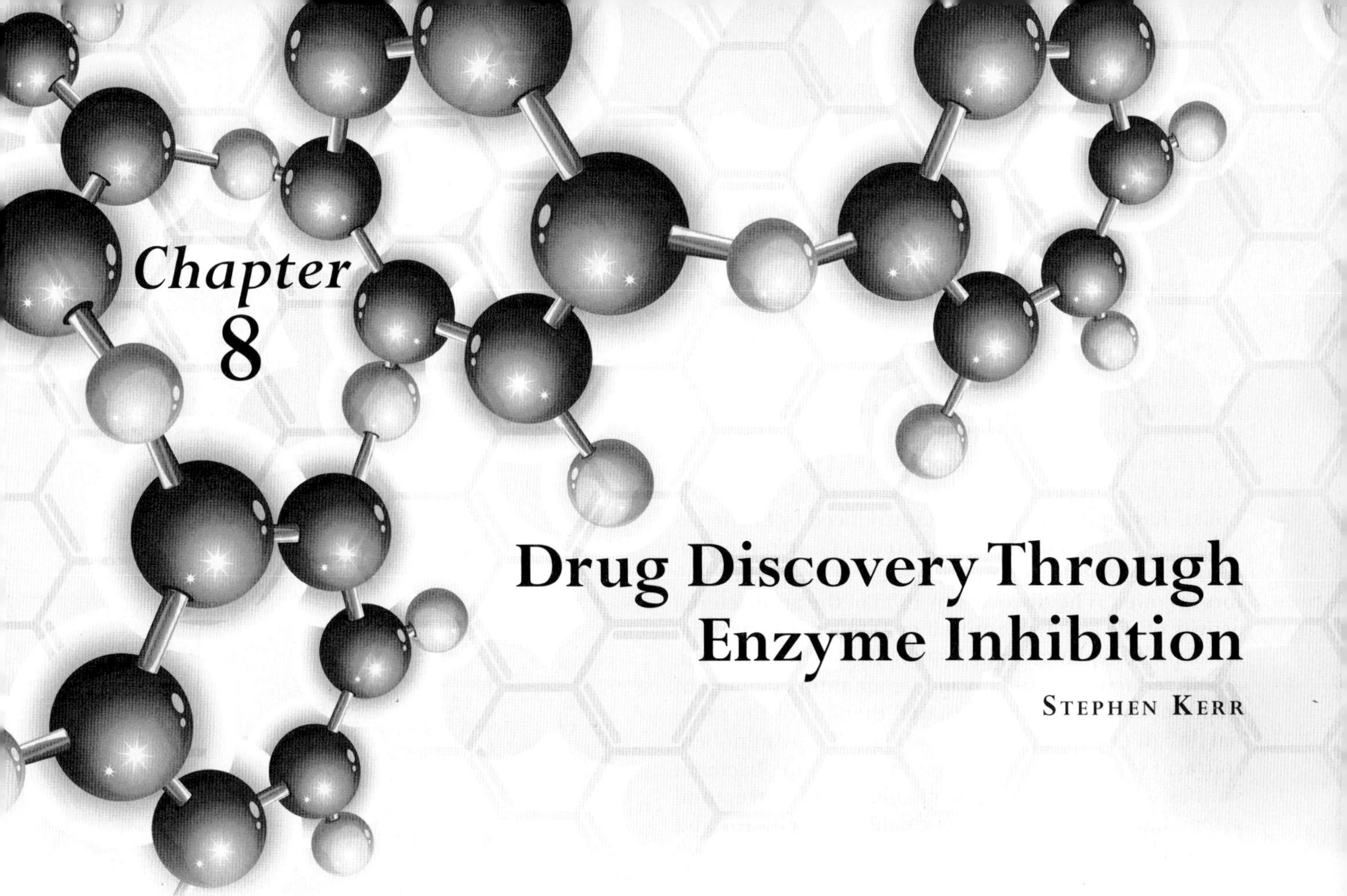

Chapter 8

Drug Discovery Through Enzyme Inhibition

Stephen Kerr

Abbreviations

ACE, angiotensin-converting enzyme
AChE, acetylcholinesterase
AMP, adenosine monophosphate
ANP, atrial natriuretic peptide
Ara-C, cytosine arabinoside
ATP, adenosine triphosphate
AZT, azidothymidine
cAMP, cyclic adenosine monophosphate
cGMP, cyclic guanosine monophosphate
CML, chronic myelogenous leukemia
dC, deoxycytidine
ddC, 2,′3′-dideoxycytidine
DHFR, dihydrofolate reductase
dNTP, deoxynucleotide triphosphate
EC, Enzyme Commission
FdUMP, 5-fluorodeoxyuridine monophosphate
5-FU, 5-flurouracil
GABA-T, γ-aminobutyric acid transaminase
GTP, guanosine triphosphate
k_{cat}, catalytic or first-order rate constant
K_d, enzyme–substrate dissociation constant
K_i, inhibition constant
K_m, Michaelis-Menten constant or apparent substrate–enzyme dissociation constant
M, moles/L
mTOR, mammalian target of rapamycin
PAP, 2-phenylamionopyrimidine
PDE, phosphodiesterase
PLP, pyridoxal phosphate
RT, reverse transcriptase
SAR, structure–activity relationship
3-TC, 3-thiacytidine
TKI, tyrosine kinase inhibitor
TLCK, tosyl-lysyl-chloromethyl-ketone
TPCK, tosyl-phenylalanyl-chloromethyl-ketone
v, velocity or rate of enzyme reaction
V_{max}, maximum velocity or rate of enzyme reaction

OVERVIEW OF ENZYMES AS CATALYTIC RECEPTORS

A Perspective

The concept of using small molecules that specifically target one or more enzymatic systems in the body is not new. Historically, compounds that were extracted from natural products have been used as medicinal agents (see Chapter 1). Subsequently, they have been shown to have their therapeutic effect by targeting certain systemic enzymes (1). A classic example is the bark of the willow tree, known since ancient days to have antipyretic and analgesic effects. Its active ingredient, salicin, a glycoside, is metabolized in vivo to salicylic acid, which is a known inhibitor of cyclooxygenase, a key enzyme in the formation of prostaglandins, which are mediators of pain and fever. Similarly, physostigmine, isolated from the West African Calabar bean, was used as a treatment for glaucoma in the mid-1800s.

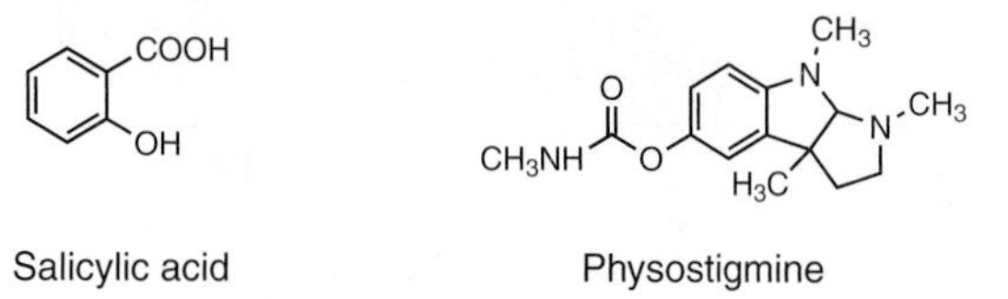

Physostigmine's mechanism of action was only later determined to be inhibition of acetylcholinesterase (1). Inhibition of acetylcholinesterase in the eye leads to improved drainage and, thus, a decrease in the intraocular pressure giving relief to glaucoma patients. It was only in the 20th century, with the concept of the "magic bullet" having selective toxicity, introduced by Ehrlich as a rational approach to chemotherapy (1), that the concept of rational design and discovery of enzyme inhibitors followed. The discovery in 1935 of the antibacterial activity of the azo dye prontosil by Domagk (2), and the subsequent explanation in 1940 by Woods (3) of its metabolic reduction to sulfanilamide, an antimetabolite of *p*-aminobenzoic acid, finally paved the way for the rational design of enzyme inhibitors (Fig. 8.1). *p*-Aminobenzoic acid is an essential metabolite used in the bacterial synthesis of folic acid. Sulfanilamide, by its structural resemblance to *p*-aminobenzoic acid, competes for and selectively inhibits the bacterial enzyme dihydropteroate synthase (Fig. 8.2). In the absence of dihydropteroic acid, the bacteria are unable to synthesize tetrahydrofolic acid, an essential cofactor in one-carbon transfers that is involved in the de novo synthesis of purines and in the synthesis of thymidylate. This concept of designing drugs as antimetabolites, or structural analogs of essential metabolites, became the hallmark for the development of enzyme inhibitors. This was especially important in cancer therapy during the early days of rational drug design (4). As mechanisms of enzymes became better understood, the inhibitor design strategy grew more sophisticated, resulting in more potent and selective inhibitors being developed. The present-day focus on drug design through enzyme inhibition makes use of the antimetabolite theory as well as detailed kinetic and mechanistic information about the enzymatic pathways. These strategies use sophisticated assays, enzyme crystal structures and active site environments, site-directed mutagenesis experiments of catalytic groups of enzymes, and molecular docking experiments employing computers equipped with modeling or docking software. However, it must be mentioned that in the drug design

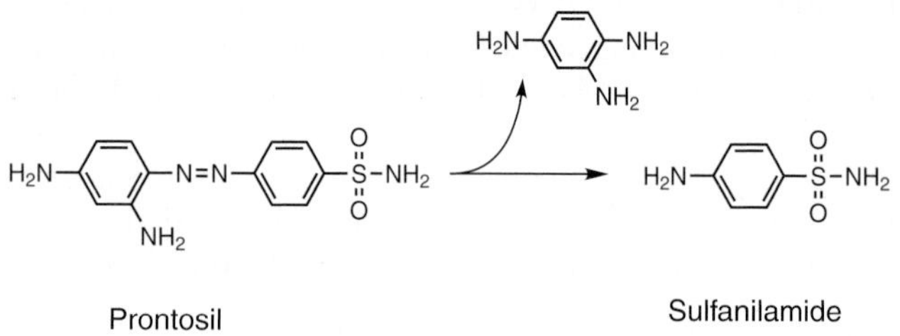

FIGURE 8.1 Metabolic reduction of prontosil to sulfanilamide.

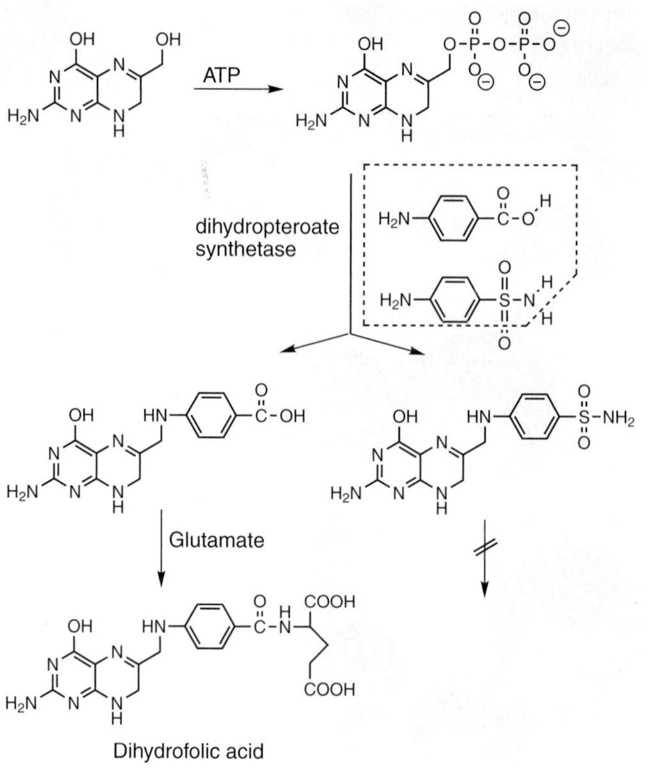

FIGURE 8.2 Metabolic pathway leading to dihydrofolic acid and its inhibition by sulfanilamide. This figure shows the structural resemblance to *p*-aminobenzoic acid.

process, designing a potent inhibitor of an enzyme is only the first step in the long and difficult process of drug development. Other factors, including pharmacokinetic profile of the inhibitor, toxicities and side effects, and animal and preclinical studies, must all be satisfactorily completed or addressed before the inhibitor can even enter clinical studies as a new drug candidate. Hence, even though an enormous amount of data exist regarding enzyme inhibitors, only a selected few turn out to be marketable drugs (Table 8.1). In the following sections, an overview of enzymes as catalytic proteins and general concepts of enzyme inhibitors and their rational design into drugs will be discussed with selected examples.

Overview

Enzymes are specialized proteins that function as catalysts to increase the rate of biochemical reactions. By interacting with substrates (reactant molecules upon which an enzyme acts), enzymes catalyze chemical reactions involved in the biosynthesis of many cellular products. Enzymes derive their name from Greek, in which the term *enzyme* means "in yeast" and was mainly used to distinguish the whole microorganism, such as yeast ("organized ferments"), from that of extracts of the whole microorganisms ("unorganized ferments"). The implication was that enzymes were unorganized ferments in yeast. Although the vast majority of enzymes are proteins, certain nucleic acids (RNAs) also possess

TABLE 8.1 A Partial Listing of Enzyme Inhibitor Drugs Presently Used as Drugs

Inhibitor (Drug)	Enzyme Inhibited	Use	Organism
Caspofungin	1,3-β-Glucan synthase	Antifungal	Fungal
Trilostane	3 (or 17)β-Hydroxysteroid dehydrogenase	Breast cancer	Human
Sildenafil	3′,5′-Cyclic GMP phosphodiesterase	Erectile dysfunction	Human
Theophylline	3′,5′-Cyclic nucleotide phosphodiesterase	Asthma	Human
Nitisinone	4-Hydroxyphenylpyruvate dioxygenase	Tyrosinemia	Human
Finasteride	Steroid 5α-reductase	Benign prostatic hyperplasia	Human
Pyridostigmine	Acetylcholinesterase	Myasthenia gravis	Human
Pentostatin	Adenosine deaminase	Cancer	Human
Cycloserine	Alanine racemase	Tuberculosis	Bacterial
Fomepizole	Alcohol dehydrogenase	Alcoholism	Human
Disulfiram	Aldehyde dehydrogenase	Alcoholism	Human
Acarbose	α-Amylase	Diabetes	Human
Miglitol	α-Glucosidase	Diabetes	Human
Ethambutol	Arabinosyltransferase	Tuberculosis	Bacterial
Zileuton	Arachidonate 5-lipoxygenase	Inflammation	Human
Carbidopa	Aromatic L-amino acid decarboxylase	Parkinson disease	Human
Clavulanic acid	β-Lactamase	In combination with penicillins	Bacterial
Acetazolamide	Carbonate dehydratase (carbonic anhydrase)	Glaucoma	Human
Entacapone	Catechol *O*-methyltransferase	Parkinson disease	Human
Miglustat	Ceramide glucosyltransferase	Gaucher disease	Human
Methotrexate	Dihydrofolate reductase	Cancer	Human
Trimethoprim	Dihydrofolate reductase	Antibacterial	Bacterial
Sulfamethoxazole	Dihydropteroate synthase	Antibacterial	Bacterial
Topotecan	DNA topoisomerase	Cancer	Human
Ciprofloxacin	DNA gyrase	Antibacterial	Bacterial
Acyclovir	DNA-directed DNA polymerase	Antiviral (anti-HSV)	Viral
Rifampin	DNA-directed RNA polymerase	Antibacterial	Bacterial
Bacitracin	Dolichyl phosphatase	Antibacterial	Bacterial
Isoniazid	Fatty acid enoyl reductase	Tuberculosis	Bacterial
Oseltamivir	Viral neuraminidase	Anti-influenza	Viral
Fondaparinux	Factor Xa	Thrombosis	Human
Alendronate	Farnesyl-diphosphate farnesyltransferase	Osteoporosis	Human
Pyrazinamide	Mycobacterial fatty acid synthase	Tuberculosis	Bacterial
Valproic acid	Histone acetyltransferase	Seizures	Human
Nelfinavir	HIV protease	AIDS (anti-HIV)	Viral
Esomeprazole	H^+/K^+-ATPase	Gastroesophageal reflux disease	Human

(*Continued*)

TABLE 8.1 A Partial Listing of Enzyme Inhibitor Drugs Presently Used as Drugs (*Continued*)

Inhibitor (Drug)	Enzyme Inhibited	Use	Organism
Atorvastatin	HMG-CoA reductase	Hyperlipidemia	Human
Mycophenolate	IMP dehydrogenase	Immune suppression	Human
Propylthiouracil	Iodide peroxidase	Hyperthyroid	Human
Cilastatin	Renal dehydropeptidase	In combination with imipenem	Human
Eflornithine	Ornithine decarboxylase	Trypanosomes	Parasitic
Allopurinol	Xanthine oxidase	Gout	Human
Captopril	Peptidyl-dipeptidase A (angiotensin-converting enzyme)	Hypertension	Human
Pemetrexed	Phosphoribosylglycinamide formyltransferase	Cancer	Human
Aprotinin	Plasma kallikrein	Thrombosis	Human
Aminocaproic acid	Plasmin	Thrombosis	Human
Etodolac	Prostaglandin-endoperoxide synthase (cyclooxygenase)	Inflammation	Human
Bortezomib	Proteasome endopeptidase complex	Myeloma	Human
Imatinib	Protein-tyrosine kinase	Cancer	Human
Gemcitabine	Ribonuleoside-diphosphate reductase	Cancer	Human
Ribavirin	IMP dehydrogenase	Anti-viral (broad spectrum)	Viral
Azidothymidine	HIV reverse transcriptase	AIDS (anti-HIV)	Viral
Lamivudine	Reverse transcriptase	AIDS, hepatitis B	Viral
Penicillin	Serine-type D-Ala—Ala carboxypeptidase	Antibiotic	Bacterial
Digitoxin	Na^+/K^+-ATPase	Congestive heart failure	Human
Terbinafine	Squalene monooxygenase	Antifungal	Fungal
Itraconazole	Sterol 14 α-demethylase	Antifungal	Fungal
Lepirudin	Thrombin	Thrombosis	Human
Floxuridine	Thymidylate synthase	Cancer	Human
Orlistat	Triacylglycerol lipase	Obesity	Human
Metyrosine	Tyrosine 3-monooxygenase	Pheochromocytoma	Human
Fosfomycin	UDP-*N*-acetylglucosamine 1-carboxyvinyltransferase	Antibacterial	Bacterial
Aminoglutethimide	Monooxygenase	Breast cancer	Human
Acetohydroxamic acid	Urease	Gastritis	Bacterial
Dicumarol	Vitamin K–epoxide reductase	Thrombosis	Human

(Adapted from Robertson J. Mechanistic basis of enzyme-targeted drugs. Biochemistry 2005;44:5561–5771, with permission.)

enzymatic activity (i.e., ribozymes). Enzymes are the most efficient catalysts known in nature, because they have the ability to increase reaction rates by enormous factors. Like all catalysts, enzymes have the ability to lower the activation energy of reactions, and the tremendous catalytic power they possess results from their inherent ability to provide stabilization to the reacting molecules at their activated complex states. A preliminary enquiry shows that enzymatic rates for reactions in aqueous solutions are limited by the diffusion rate constant so that the second-order rate constant of an enzyme (k_{cat}/K_m) is approximately 10^9 M s^{-1} (diffusion rate constant of water) (5). This implies that every collision of a reactant molecule (substrate) with the enzyme leads to product formation. Because for many enzymes, K_m (the Michaelis-Menten or apparent substrate–enzyme dissociation constant) values are in the micromolar or submicromolar range (10^{-4} M), one can compute the k_{cat} (the catalytic or first-order rate constant or the number of molecules of substrate converted to product per unit time per enzyme) value to be approximately 10^5. Estimates (6) for uncatalyzed reactions in water have ranged from 10^{-1} to 10^{-20}; thus, the rate enhancements for enzyme-catalyzed reactions over the noncatalyzed reaction (also referred to as the proficiency of an enzyme) can range from 10^6- to over 10^{25}-fold—truly remarkable proficiencies. Moreover, enzymes display great specificity toward particular chemical bonds (bond specificity; e.g., peptidases for peptide bonds) or functional groups (group specificity; e.g., esterases for esters), or they display absolute specificity toward a single molecule (e.g., carbonic anhydrase, which catalyzes the hydration of carbon dioxide). Furthermore, this specificity and catalytic proficiency are carried out, in most cases, at ambient temperatures and normal pressures in aqueous solutions. It is no wonder that enzymes have intrigued scientists for centuries.

Enzymes have been classified on the type of reaction catalyzed, and six major classes (families) of enzymes, numbered from 1 to 6, have been assigned by the Enzyme Commission (EC) of the International Union of Biochemistry and Molecular Biology (7). These classes are as follows: 1) oxidoreductases (e.g., dehydrogenases); 2) transferases (group transfer enzymes; e.g., kinases); 3) hydrolases (hydrolytic reactions; e.g., esterases); 4) lyases (formation or removal of double bonds; e.g., hydratase—addition of water across a double bond); 5) isomerases (e.g., mutarotation of glucose by mutases); and 6) ligases (joining of two substrates at the expense of energy, also referred to as synthetases). All discovered enzymes are identified by the prefix EC followed by an Arabic numeral based on the major class of reaction catalyzed, as indicated earlier. Furthermore, this is followed by a series of three more Arabic numerals, which indicate the subclass (functionality), sub-sub class (specific bond type), and serial number of the enzyme in that class, respectively. For example, the enzyme acetylcholinesterase has been given the following assignment: EC 3.1.1.7. As can been seen in this example, the numeral 3 indicates that this enzyme belongs to the family of hydrolases, the first 1 indicates that the nature of the bond being hydrolyzed is an ester, the second 1 indicates that specific ester bond is a carboxylic acid ester, and the last number is the serial number of this enzyme in this sub-subclass.

Many enzymes require cofactors, which enable them to carry out the catalysis. These small molecules (including ions) are intimately bound to the enzyme and are essential to the functioning of the enzyme. As macromolecular proteins, enzymes have the inherent ability to bind substrates. In effecting the transformation of these substrates to products (catalyzing the chemical reaction), enzymes use all the necessary tools in the chemical bonding arsenal to hold these substrates extremely tight in the active site as the reaction occurs. Because all chemical reactions require covalent bond breakage and formation, the substrate must go through a transition state, or an "activated complex," which is a destabilizing event, because bonds are being polarized and there is development of a partial charge. It is the inherent capability of the enzyme to greatly stabilize such activated complexes that give them their role in nature and allows their phenomenal catalytic power.

Pauling (8) first proposed the stabilization theory of the activated complex by enzymes. He concluded that the active site of the enzyme is complementary to the structure of the activated complex so that the binding of the enzyme to the activated complex is extremely tight. The ability to stabilize such complexes and correspondingly reduce the activation energy of the reaction and, thus, enhance the reaction rate is caused by many factors, both noncovalent as well as covalent (9). Noncovalent influences include entropic effects, such as proximity and orientation; restricted motion, where enzymes, by their evolvement, have the inherent ability to bring reacting molecules closer together and in the correct orientation for bonds to form; desolvation effects, to strip solvent (water) molecules from the reactants; transition state electrostatic stabilization, to stabilize the partial charges being developed in the activated complex; induced-fit effects, in which the flexibility of the enzyme can accommodate the substrate, intermediate, and/or product; strain and distortion effects, to increase the reactivity of compounds; and many other such ancillary effects. Moreover, covalent effects also play a vital role in the enzyme's catalytic role. Covalent effects imply a covalent bond being made by the enzyme (or its cofactor) to the substrate being transformed. These covalent effects would include general acid-base catalysis, in which amino acid side-chain groups partake in the overall biochemical reaction through proton donation (general acid) or proton abstraction (general base), as well as nucleophilic and electrophilic catalysis, in which there is bond formation with an amino acid side-chain group (or cofactor) to the substrate.

It should be mentioned that "covalent catalysis" has traditionally implied a group transfer reaction between one substrate and another being facilitated through an enzyme-group intermediate (e.g., the enzyme sucrose phosphorylase transfers a glucose moiety from sucrose to phosphate giving the products glucose-1-phosphate and fructose through an enzyme-glucosyl intermediate). Many amino acid side-chain groups (i.e., acidic and basic amino acids, e.g., aspartate, glutamate, histidine, lysine, arginine, tyrosine, and cysteine) as well as nucleophilic amino acid groups, such as cysteine, allow such covalent effects. Recent analysis of enzyme rate enhancements has postulated that noncovalent effects allow an increase of as much as 11-fold over the noncatalyzed reaction, whereas for those enzymes with rate enhancements greater than 11-fold over noncatalyzed reactions, covalent catalysis in the transition state accounts for this exceptional increase in rate enhancement (10).

Noncovalent effects like proximity and orientation may be explained on the basis that enzymes have the inherent ability to affect the order of reactions by the "effective concentration" principle—for example, to change a second-order reaction to a first-order one by bringing the reacting molecules closer to each other so that there is a lower amount of entropic loss (restriction of molecular motion) for the reacting substrates. In the example shown in Figure 8.3, which is taken from physical-organic chemical studies (11), one can consider the hydrolysis of a nitrophenyl ester by an amine in two scenarios: reaction (i), with two individual molecules reacting (i.e., amine and ester), versus reaction (ii), with a single molecule having an "inbuilt" amine on the ester molecule. If the reaction rate constants are compared [one needs to keep in mind that we are comparing a first-order rate constant for (ii), with a second-order rate constant for (i), which may not be a true comparison, because mechanisms are likely to be different], however, one finds that the first-order rate reaction [reaction (ii)] has a rate enhancement over reaction (i) by a factor of approximately 5,000 M attributed to the fact that reaction (i) needs to give up more degrees of freedom (entropy) [as compared to reaction (ii)] to react (i.e., form productive collision complexes, leading to product formation). This proximity effect indicates that by using such a system (bringing the reacting centers closer to each other), one can effectively increase the concentration of the reactants by this factor, resulting in a faster reaction. This enhancement factor of 5,000 M (i.e., effectively changing a second-order reaction to that of a first-order one) has been termed the "effective concentration," because this is an unrealistic increase in the concentration of the reactants, which gives rise to the higher rate constant (i.e., it is impossible to make a solution of 5,000 M of the reactants).

The next example, which is shown in Figure 8.4, illustrates that besides the proximity factor, one also can use "orientation" effects to bring about an increase in the reaction rate constant (12). For example, as shown in Figure 8.4, one may use alkyl groups to sterically hinder rotation about single bonds, effectively freezing the molecule in a particular conformation to provide maximum orbital overlap for bonding. Thus, using a "dimethyl lock" system in molecule II, which restricts rotation, ensures that lactonization for molecule II is faster by a factor of 4×10^4 than molecule I. Both of these effects, proximity and orientation, are thought to be part of an enzyme's arsenal of tools in allowing enzymes to lower the activation energy for reactions. Other noncovalent effects, such as desolvation of the reactant molecules, can also be effectively achieved by enzymes. Enzymes have the capacity, by lining their exterior and/or interior surfaces with appropriately situated hydrophobic amino acids (e.g., phenylalanine, valine, tryptophan, leucine), to effectively strip away water molecules from substrates as they enter into the active site of the enzyme through such channels. Thus, no further expense of energy is required to desolvate the substrate before the reaction.

As previously mentioned, enzymes also use covalent chemistry as a means to effect catalysis. Indeed, it has been postulated that covalent chemistry plays a far greater role in enzyme catalysis than previously thought (10). Nucleophilic catalysis by hydrolytic enzymes, such as the serine proteases or esterases, are classic examples of covalent effects in enzyme catalysis. In such systems, for example, as in the case of the serine protease chymotrypsin, which hydrolyzes peptide bonds containing aromatic amino acids (e.g., phenylalanine and tyrosine), the covalent effects occur at the level of general acid, general base, and nucleophilic covalent catalysis.

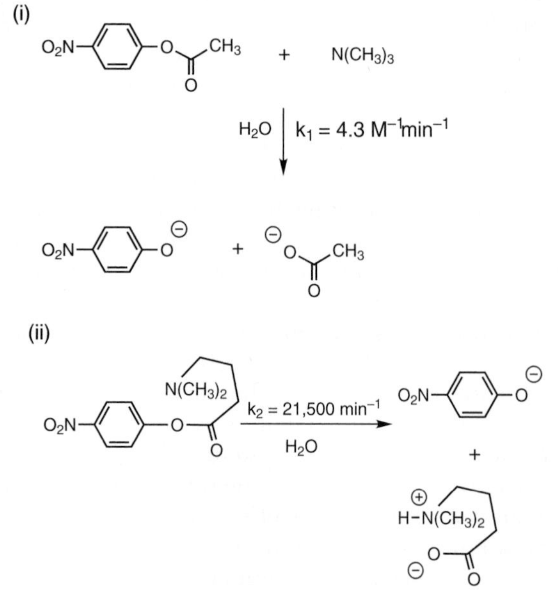

Effective concentration = k_2/k_1 = 5,000 M (approx.)

FIGURE 8.3 Concept of proximity and effective concentration.

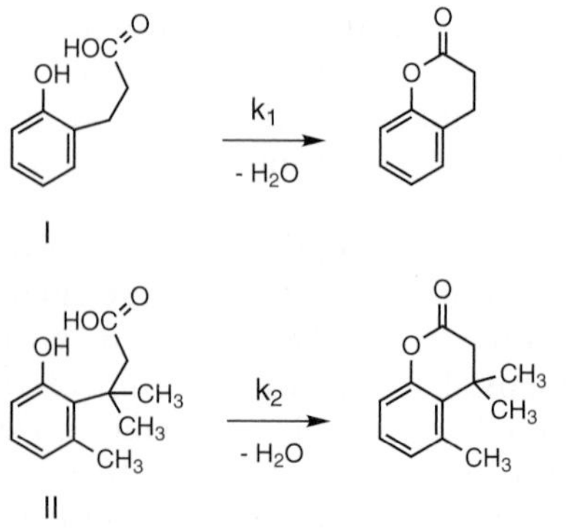

Relative rate, $k_2/k_1 = 4 \times 10^4$

FIGURE 8.4 Concept of orientation.

Figure 8.5 illustrates an accepted mechanism for such enzymes. It should be noted that all serine proteases contain a "catalytic triad" (a set of three amino acid groups in the active site that function together and are directly involved in catalysis), designated as Ser-195, His-57, and Asp-102 (numerals represent the amino acid position in the protein primary structure), which are present in the active sites of these proteases. The catalysis is effected by making the hydroxyl group of the Ser more nucleophilic for attack at the carbonyl center of the peptide bond. One should recall that, in general, hydroxyl groups have pK_a values in the range of greater than 14 and, as such, are not acidic and unable to ionize at physiologic pH. However, because of the catalytic triad of amino acids, the proton from the Ser-OH group is transferred to the Asp moiety through the His group in a "charge relay system" such that the Ser-OH group is made into the highly nucleophilic alkoxide ion. This is achieved by the Asp group acting as a general base to pick up the proton from His, which can also abstract a proton from the Ser-OH group (see I in Fig. 8.5). Thus, His behaves as a tautomeric catalyst in this enzyme (i.e., acts as both a general acid and a general base) and, in essence, relays the proton from Ser to Asp. The Ser (as its alkoxide) is now a much more powerful nucleophile and can attack the peptidyl carbonyl group to generate a "tetrahedral oxyanion intermediate" (see II in Fig. 8.5), which collapses to liberate a new amino terminus of the peptide and the acylated Ser enzyme (see III in Fig. 8.5). The next part of the reaction involves a water molecule (which also is made more nucleophilic by a similar mechanism; see III in Fig. 8.5) that goes on to hydrolyze, through a tetrahedral intermediate (see IV in Fig. 8.5), the Ser-acyl bond to liberate the new carboxyl terminus of the peptide (R_1COOH) and the free enzyme, which can be recycled for another round of catalysis.

Knowledge of the mechanisms and interactions, both noncovalent and covalent, that allow enzymes to function as such efficient catalysts provides the medicinal chemist with insights to design molecules that achieve selective inhibition of the enzyme. Such knowledge also paves the way to the design and discovery of drugs.

GENERAL CONCEPTS OF ENZYME INHIBITION

The body is composed of thousands of different enzymes, many of them acting in concert to maintain homeostasis. Although disease states may arise from the malfunctioning of a particular enzyme, or the introduction of a foreign enzyme through infection by microorganisms, inhibiting a specific enzyme to alleviate a disease state is a challenging process. Most bodily functions occur through a cascade of enzymatic systems, and it becomes extremely difficult to design a drug molecule that can selectively inhibit an enzyme and result in a therapeutic benefit. However, to address this problem, the basic mechanism of enzyme action needs to be understood. Once knowledge of a particular enzymatic pathway is determined and the mechanism and kinetics are worked out, the challenge is then to design a suitable inhibitor that is selectively used by the enzyme causing its inhibition.

As outlined earlier, enzymes (E) represent the best-known biochemical catalysts, because they are uniquely designed to carry out specific biochemical reactions in a highly efficient manner (5). They initially act by binding a substrate (S) to form an enzyme–substrate complex [E·S],

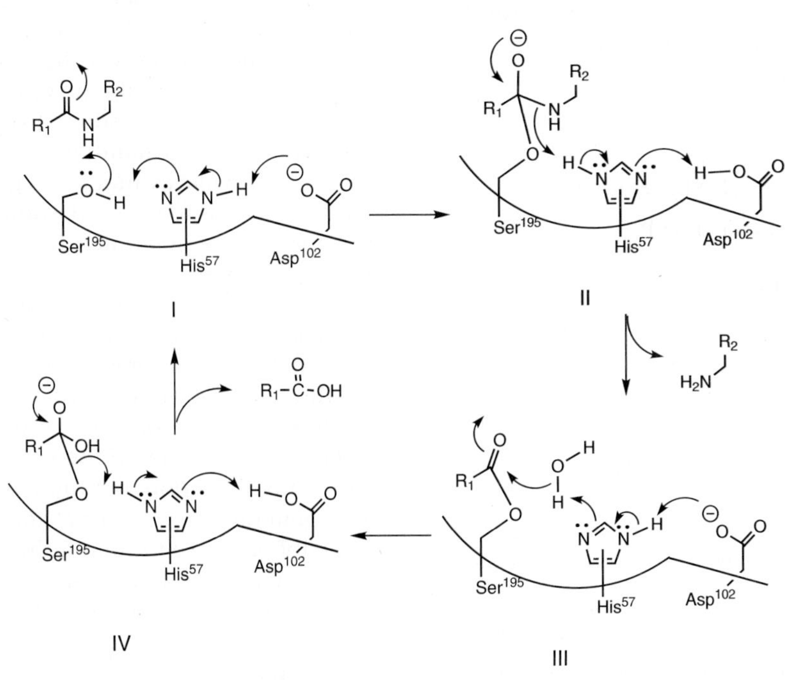

FIGURE 8.5 Acid, base, and nucleophilic covalent catalysis by chymotrypsin.

which undergoes specific chemistry (catalysis) to give the enzyme–product complex [E·P], followed by dissociation of product (P) and liberating the free enzyme (E). Equation 8.8.1 represents a simplified version of this scenario:

8.1 $$E + S \underset{}{\overset{K_d(\text{or } K_m)}{\rightleftharpoons}} [E \cdot S] \overset{k_{cat}}{\rightleftharpoons} [E \cdot P] \rightleftharpoons E + P$$

where K_d is the enzyme–substrate dissociation constant and k_{cat} represents the rate constant for the catalytic step (chemical modification step or slowest step in the overall pathway). If the binding step of E + S to form [E·S] is relatively fast as compared to the catalytic step and one assumes steady-state conditions, then K_m [the substrate concentration at half-maximum velocity ($V_{max}/2$)], may be equated to the K_d, as shown in Equation 8.2: where v = velocity/rate of the reaction

8.2
$$\text{Michaelis-Menten equation}: v = \frac{V_{max}[S]}{K_m + [S]}$$
$$\text{Lineweaver-Burk equation}: \frac{1}{v} = \frac{K_m}{V_{max}} \cdot \frac{1}{[S]} + \frac{1}{V_{max}}$$

The rate of the reaction can then be derived in terms of K_m and V_{max} (or $k_{cat} = V_{max}/[E]$). From the knowledge of the dissociation constant ($K_{m(d)}$) and the rate constant for catalysis (k_{cat}), it is then possible to compare inhibitors and the dissociation constant for the inhibitors, K_i, in relation to the natural substrates and the effect on the catalytic rates. These kinetic parameters, k_{cat} and $K_{m(d)}$ (or K_i) can then give an indication as to the affinity (K_i versus $K_{m(d)}$) and specificity (k_{cat}/K_i or $k_{cat}/K_{m(d)}$) of the inhibitor for a particular enzyme. Equations 8.3 and 8.4 represent the general scheme of reversible inhibition, and Figure 8.6 illustrates graphically and mathematically the relationship of the velocity of the enzyme reaction to the substrate [S] and inhibitor [I] concentration as well as the kinetic parameters K_m, K_i, and V_{max} (or $k_{cat} = V_{max}/[E]$):

Competitive Inhibition

8.3
$$E + S \overset{K_m}{\rightleftharpoons} [E \cdot S] \rightleftharpoons E + P$$
$$E + I \overset{K_i}{\rightleftharpoons} [E \cdot I] \rightarrow P$$

Noncompetitive Inhibition

8.4
$$\begin{array}{lcc} E + S \overset{K_m}{\rightleftharpoons} [E \cdot S] & \searrow\!\!\!\nwarrow & +I \\ & [E.S.I] & \\ E + S \overset{K_i}{\rightleftharpoons} [E \cdot S] & \nearrow\!\!\!\swarrow & +S \end{array}$$

Inhibition of enzymes may be broadly classified under two categories—reversible and irreversible inhibitors—as shown in Equation 8.5:

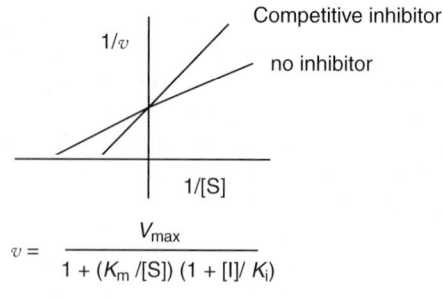

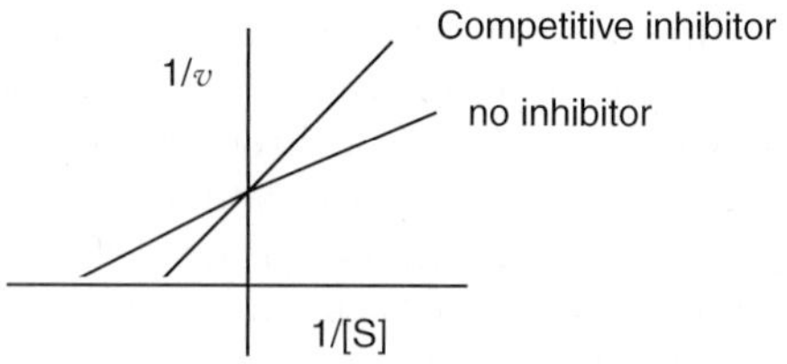

$$v = \frac{V_{max}}{1 + (K_m/[S])\,(1 + [I]/K_i)}$$

(K_m increases, V_{max} unchanged)

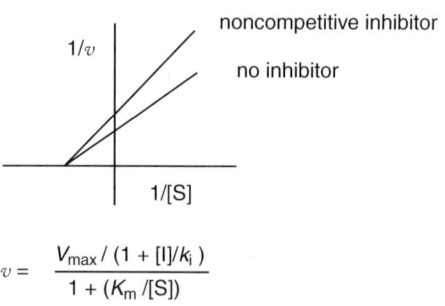

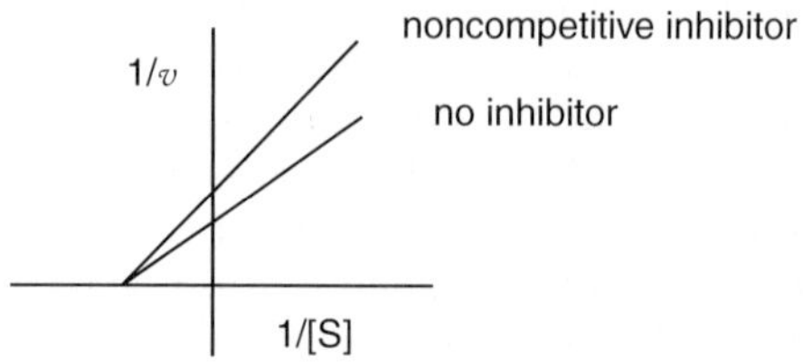

$$v = \frac{V_{max}/(1 + [I]/k_i)}{1 + (K_m/[S])}$$

(K_m unchanged, V_{max} decreases)

FIGURE 8.6 Graphic representation of competitive and noncompetitive enzyme inhibition.

8.5
$$E + I \overset{K_i}{\rightleftharpoons} [E \cdot I]\,(\text{reversible inhibition})$$
$$E + I \overset{K_i}{\rightleftharpoons} [E - I]\,(\text{irreversible inhibition}$$

In the presence of inhibitor, the enzyme–substrate complex, [E·S], is replaced by the enzyme–inhibitor complex, [E·I], which may block or retard the formation of product. In the presence of a reversible inhibitor, the enzyme is tied up and the reaction retarded or stopped; however, the enzyme can be subsequently regenerated from the enzyme–inhibitor complex, [E·I], to react again with substrate and produce product (see Eqs. 8.3 and 8.4). On the other hand, irreversible inhibition implies that the enzyme cannot be regenerated, and the only way for catalysis to proceed would be if new molecules of the enzyme are generated from gene transcription and translation. Irreversible inhibition is commonly associated with covalent bond formation between inhibitor and enzyme [E—I], which *cannot* be easily broken and is often defined as a time-dependent loss of enzyme activity. Reversible inhibition, on the other hand, does not necessarily imply noncovalent bond formation. In many instances, reversible inhibition can occur through covalent bond formation, but these bonds can be hydrolyzed to regenerate free enzyme and inhibitor. Thus, for a reversible enzyme inhibitor, there is no time-dependent loss of activity, and enzyme activity can always be recovered. There are instances when reversible inhibition tends to look kinetically like irreversible inhibition. This scenario results whenever there is a tight binding of a reversible inhibitor to the enzyme; consequently, the dissociation of the enzyme from this enzyme–inhibitor complex is extremely slow. Kinetically, it is extremely difficult to distinguish this type of inhibition from an irreversible inhibitor, because over time, the enzyme does tend to look like it loses its activity and, for all practical purposes, the enzyme behaves as if it were irreversibly tied up. To differentiate between tight-binding reversible and irreversible inhibitors, one can dialyze the enzyme–inhibitor complex. In case of the reversible inhibitor, on dialysis, the inhibitor will be removed from the enzyme, resulting in recovery of the enzyme activity; however, this does not occur with the irreversible inhibitor.

Reversible Enzyme Inhibition

Reversible enzyme inhibition may be classified under two main headings, competitive and noncompetitive, with both following Michaelis-Menten kinetics. Competitive inhibition, by definition, requires that the inhibitor competes with the substrate for binding to the enzyme at the active site, and this binding is mutually exclusive. That is, if the inhibitor binds to the enzyme, the substrate will not be able to bind, and vice versa. However, competitive inhibition also suggests that the inhibition can be reversed in the presence of saturating amounts of substrate, because in this case, all enzyme active sites will be occupied by substrate-displacing inhibitor. In contrast, noncompetitive inhibition implies independent binding (i.e., both inhibitor and substrate may bind to the enzyme at different sites). Because binding of the inhibitor to the enzyme is at a site other than the active site, noncompetitive inhibition cannot be reversed by increasing the concentration of substrate. Graphing the kinetics of inhibition as shown in Figure 8.6, the Lineweaver-Burk plot of $1/V$ versus $1/[S]$ shows distinguishing characteristics between the two types of inhibition. In competitive inhibition, there is no change in the V_{max} of the reaction (the intercept on the *y*-axis remains constant in the presence of inhibitor). However, the slope of the curve (K_m/V_{max}) is different with the inhibitor present, and K_m changes because of the presence of the competitive inhibitor (Fig. 8.6, competitive inhibition). In the case of noncompetitive inhibition, only the V_{max} of the reaction decreases, while the K_m remains unchanged (intercept on the *x*-axis unchanged with inhibitor; Fig. 8.6, noncompetitive inhibition).

Most of the rationally designed and clinically useful reversible inhibitors are competitive inhibitors. Table 8.1 lists several currently approved drugs that act as enzyme inhibitors. The majority of enzyme inhibitors generally bear some structural resemblance to the natural substrate of the enzyme. The design of such inhibitors would thus seem to be a logical and rational task that is uniquely suited to the medicinal chemist who can use the principles of bioisosteric modification of natural enzyme substrates and metabolites, or modification of "lead" structures and structure–activity relationships (SARs), to create selective and potent inhibitors (see Chapter 2). However, there are pitfalls in this endeavor because even the most rationally designed drug must still overcome transport and other cellular barriers before exerting its effects. In the case of the noncompetitive inhibitors, the design is not as straightforward. These inhibitors can have widely differing structures, which in many instances bear no resemblance to the natural substrate. In general, inhibitors of the noncompetitive type have been obtained primarily through random screening of chemically novel molecules followed by further synthetic manipulation of the pharmacophore to optimize their inhibitory effects.

Examples of Reversible Inhibitors

The design of enzyme inhibitors has included random screening of synthetic chemical agents, natural products, and combinatorial libraries followed by molecular optimization or SARs of so-called "lead" structures as well as bioisosteric analogs of the enzyme substrates themselves. Drugs (e.g., finasteride) also have been developed for one indication but, based on observed side effects, have led to other uses.

The rational approach in the design of enzyme inhibitors is greatly aided if the enzymatic reaction is characterized in terms of its kinetic mechanism. Such a characterization would include the knowledge of the kinetic parameters (rate constants and dissociation constants) of individual steps in the overall reaction pathway as well as the characterization of (any) intermediates involved in these individual steps. Examples of such "rational" inhibitors include both reversible and irreversible inhibitors of enzymes.

ANTIMETABOLITES Antimetabolites are agents that interfere with the functioning of an essential metabolite and that most often are designed as structural analogs of the natural metabolite. As described earlier, the mechanism of action of sulfanilamide is that of a competitive inhibitor of *p*-aminobenzoic acid. However, in the case of the sulfanilamide, the mechanism was only determined after the bacterial inhibitory action was noted. This is often the case when a drug is discovered to have a certain therapeutic effect and, later, this effect is "rationalized" as being caused by an enzyme-inhibitory action (1). Other classic examples of a competitive inhibitor acting as an antimetabolite include a number of nucleoside analogs used as antiviral and anticancer agents. These agents bear

USE OF FINASTERIDE

Finasteride (Proscar) an inhibitor of steroid 5α-reductase, an enzyme involved in the catalytic reduction of testosterone to dihydrotestosterone, was originally developed as an agent to treat prostate hyperplasia. In addition to this original use, finasteride is also indicated as an agent (Propecia) to stimulate hair growth for treatment of male pattern baldness. This benefit was recognized as a useful side effect during clinical trials of finasteride as an antiprostate agent.

structural resemblance to natural nucleosides, which in their triphosphate form are substrates for nucleic acid polymerases involved in the synthesis of nucleic acids. Nucleic acid polymerases catalyze the condensation of the free 3′-hydroxy end of a nucleic acid with an incoming 5′-triphosphate derivative of a nucleoside (deoxynucleotide triphosphate [dNTP]), resulting in a 3′,5′-phosphodiester linkage. Hence, nucleoside analogs, to compete with the natural substrate in the synthesis of nucleic acid, must be converted intracellularly to their mono-, di-, and finally, triphosphate derivative before exerting their inhibitory effects on nucleic acid synthesis. Certain drug design strategies incorporate a "masked" phosphate group on the nucleoside such that once absorbed, they enter into the systemic circulation as the monophosphate (13). The majority of these analogs are designed such that they lack the 3′-hydroxy group and are dideoxy derivatives of the natural substrate. Thus, these analogs ensure that once they are incorporated into a nucleic acid, further extension of the nucleic acid is prevented because of the lack of a 3′-hydroxy group.

Inhibition of HIV-reverse Transcriptase

Azidothymidine (AZT). The advent of AIDS stimulated a great interest in designing inhibitors against the essential viral polymerase—HIV-reverse transcriptase (HIV-RT). AZT is a potent inhibitor of HIV-RT (14), the retroviral polymerase that catalyzes the formation of proviral DNA from viral RNA. Structurally, AZT is similar to the natural nucleoside thymidine but has an azide group ($-N_3$) rather than a hydroxy group (–OH) at the 3′-position of the sugar deoxyribose (Fig. 8.7). AZT is activated intracellularly to its triphosphate and competes with thymidine triphosphate for uptake by HIV-RT into DNA (15). Once incorporated, further chain extension of the DNA is prevented, because there is no 3′-hydroxyl group to continue the DNA synthesis. In this fashion, AZT is an effective chain terminator of viral DNA synthesis.

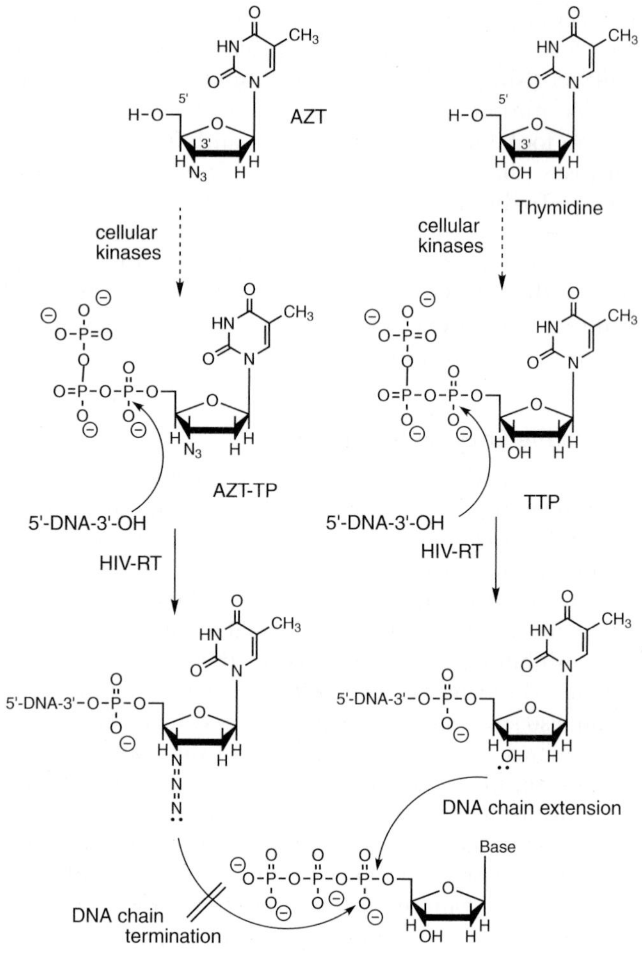

FIGURE 8.7 Activation, incorporation, and chain-terminating action of azidothymidine (AZT), a thymidine analog, as a reversible inhibitor of human immunodeficiency virus–reverse transcriptase (HIV-RT).

Dideoxycytidine (Zalcitabine) and 3-thiacytidine (Lamivudine). 2′,3′-Dideoxycytidine (ddC) is another antiretroviral agent used against HIV-RT. In this case, ddC resembles the natural metabolite, deoxycytidine (dC), and as in the case of AZT, it is a 3′-deoxy analog of dC, where the 3′-OH group of dC is replaced by a hydrogen atom. Similarly, 3-thiacytidine (3-TC) is another anti-HIV agent that resembles dC. However, in this example, rather than replacing the 3′-hydroxyl functionality as in ddC, the 3′-carbon position of the sugar has been substituted by a sulfur atom.

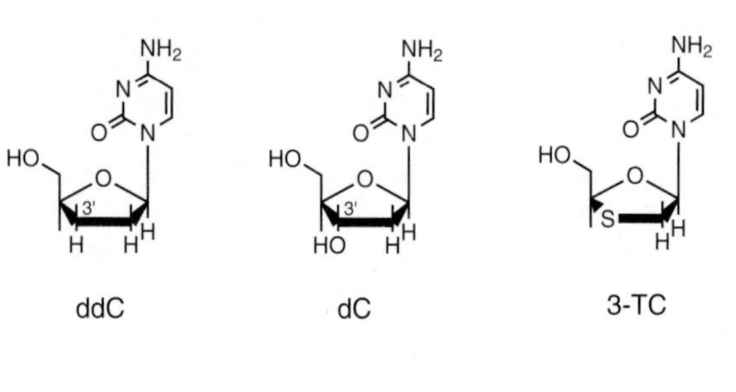

Nevirapine. An example of a potent noncompetitive inhibitor of HIV-RT is the drug nevirapine, a benzodiazepine analog (16), which is extremely tight-binding to the enzyme, having a K_i in the nanomolar range.

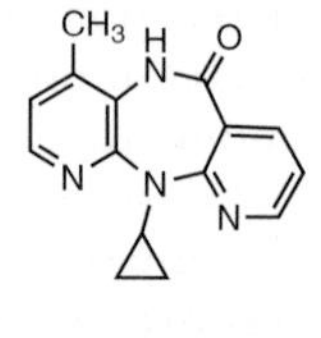

Nevirapine

As can be seen in the structure of nevirapine, the drug bears no resemblance to any of the natural nucleotide substrates and was discovered through a random screening program. X-ray crystallographic studies of HIV-RT complexed with nevirapine have shown it binding in a hydrophobic pocket at a site adjacent to and slightly overlapping the nucleotide-binding site of HIV-RT (17). Kinetic studies with the enzyme have revealed an

HISTORIC DEVELOPMENT OF AZT

Interestingly, AZT was originally synthesized as an anticancer agent to inhibit cellular DNA synthesis, but it was found to be too toxic. Subsequently, in the mid-1980s, during a random screening of nucleoside agents for potential inhibitory effects against HIV-RT, AZT was found to have selectivity for the HIV-RT (14). As such, its effects on host cell polymerases result in its dose-limiting bone marrow toxicity.

extremely slow binding rate for the drug; however, once bound, the polymerization rate for the reaction is effectively reduced (18).

However, a drawback for nevirapine is that the virus can develop resistance very rapidly, through mutation of the amino acid groups in the binding pocket (19). Thus, its usefulness is limited to combination therapy with other antiretroviral agents rather than single-drug therapy.

Reversible Inhibitors Used in Cancer Therapy. The design of several anticancer agents have been based on the antimetabolite theory. Because cancer results in overproliferation and uncontrolled cell growth, antimetabolite drugs designed against cancer have been based on inhibiting DNA synthesis in the cell (see Chapter 37). Thus, these drugs have been targeted against those enzymes, including the nucleic acid polymerases, thymidylate synthase and dihydrofolate reductase (DHFR), which have a role in DNA synthesis. Examples of drugs that have been designed against nucleic acid polymerases include cytosine arabinoside (Ara-C) and 5-fluorouracil (5-FU) (Fig. 8.8). Ara-C is first converted to its triphosphate, and as such, it functions as an antimetabolite of deoxycytidine triphosphate to inhibit DNA polymerase. As can be seen from its structure, Ara-C is the arabino isomer of cytidine, where the 2′-hydroxyl group in Ara-C is in the arabino configuration rather than the ribo configuration of cytidine. Because of this stereochemical change in the placement of the 2′-hydroxyl group, Ara-C resembles more dC rather than cytidine. In this way, Ara-C inhibits DNA polymerases by competing with dC. 5-FU is an analog of the pyrimidine base uracil, where the hydrogen at the 5-position in uracil has been substituted by the bioisosteric fluorine (F) atom. This makes 5-FU look very similar to uracil. 5-FU, after conversion to 5-fluorodeoxyuridine monophosphate (FdUMP), becomes an inhibitor of thymidylate synthase, the enzyme involved in the de novo synthesis of thymidylate. In this case, FdUMP is an antimetabolite of deoxyuridine monophosphate.

Methotrexate is a potent inhibitor of DHFR, the enzyme responsible for the reduction of folic acid to dihydro- and tetrahydrofolic acid, precursors to one-carbon donation in purine and pyrimidine de novo synthesis. Methotrexate is an analog of folic acid where the 4-hydroxyl group (–OH) on the pteridine ring of

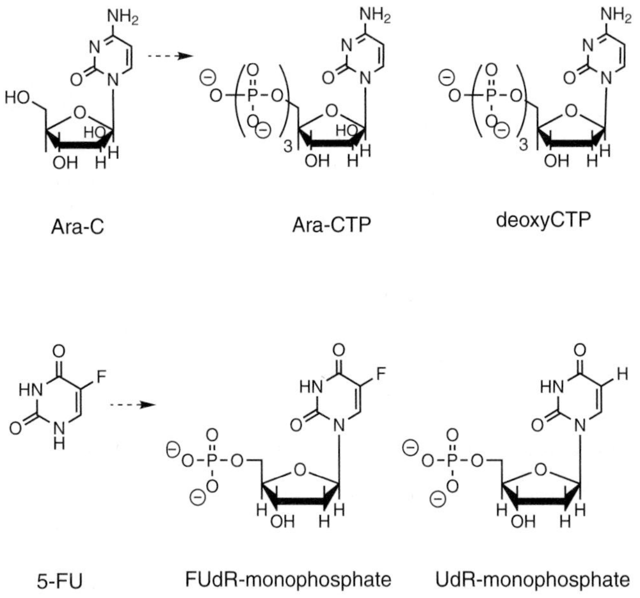

FIGURE 8.8 Structures of pyrimidine antimetabolites used in cancer chemotherapy.

folic acid has been replaced by an amino ($-NH_2$) group and the nitrogen atom at the 10-position is methylated (Fig. 8.9). These substitutions led to methotrexate having an affinity for DHFR orders of magnitude greater than that for the natural metabolite, folic acid, and allows it to be an extremely potent inhibitor of DHFR.

Inhibition of Acetylcholinesterase Acetylcholinesterase (AChE) is the enzyme that catalyzes the catabolism of the neurotransmitter acetylcholine to acetate and choline (see Chapter 9). Thus, inhibition of AChE would lead to increased concentrations of acetylcholine in both of the cholinergic muscarinic and nicotinic synapses resulting in a prolonged cholinergic action. Inhibitors of AChE have found use in cases of myasthenia gravis, glaucoma, and Alzheimer disease. To appreciate the design of these inhibitors, it is useful to first understand the mechanism

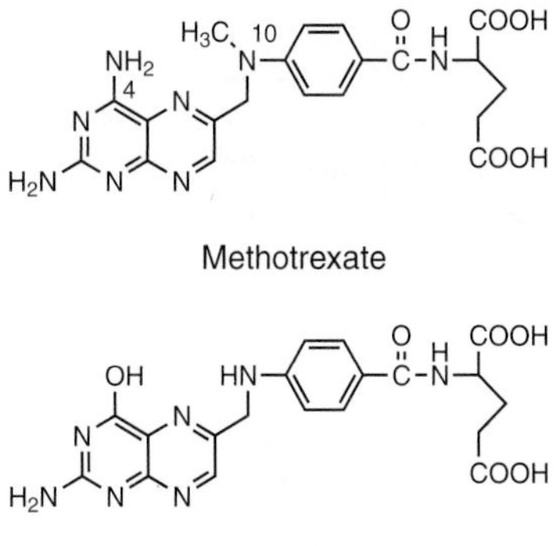

FIGURE 8.9 Methotrexate, the antimetabolite of folic acid.

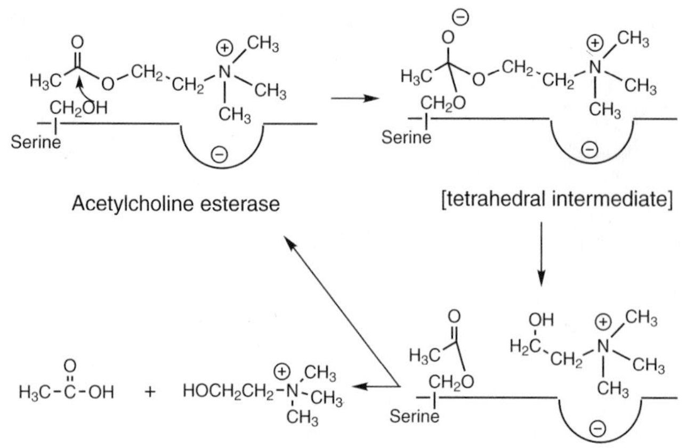

FIGURE 8.10 Mechanism of hydrolysis of acetylcholine by acetylcholine esterase.

of action of AChE. AChE has an anionic active site that can bind the positively charged quaternary ammonium group of the choline functionality and an active esteratic site that contains a nucleophilic Ser-CH_2-OH group that is involved in the hydrolysis of the ester bond as shown in Figure 8.10. The hydrolysis mechanism involves attack of the nucleophilic Ser-CH_2-OH group on the ester carbonyl group of acetylcholine to form a tetrahedral intermediate that collapses, releasing choline and forming an acetylated Ser-CH_2-O-AChE complex, which subsequently hydrolyzes with water to release AChE, acetic acid (as acetate ion), and choline.

Physostigmine has been used in the treatment of glaucoma. It is an alkaloid with a carbamate moiety that resembles the ester linkage of acetylcholine. Being an alkaloid, it is protonated at physiologic pH and, thus, can bind to the anionic site of AChE. Similar to the mechanism for the hydrolysis of acetylcholine by AChE, the Ser-CH_2-OH group of AChE can attack the carbamate carbonyl group of physostigmine, and in the process, the Ser-CH_2OH group is carbamylated as shown in Figure 8.11. This carbamyl Ser-CH_2O-AChE intermediate is more stable to

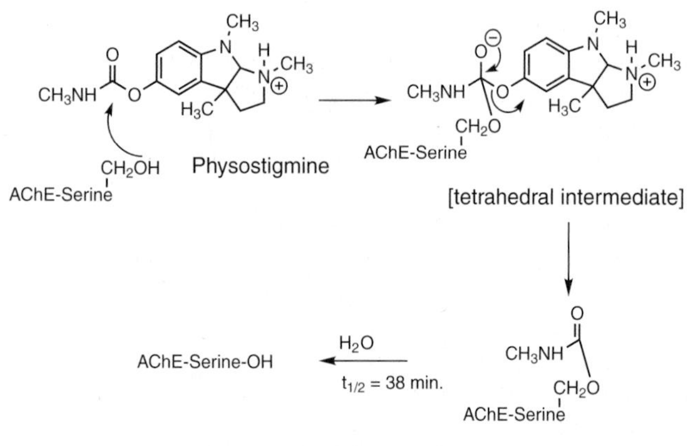

FIGURE 8.11 Mechanism of inhibition of acetylcholine esterase by physostigmine.

enzymatic hydrolysis than is acetylated Ser-CH_2-O-AChE, and its subsequent hydrolysis by water occurs extremely slowly. The carbamylated AChE intermediate is slowly regenerated with a half-life of 38 minutes—more than 10 million-fold (10^7) slower than that for AChE's natural substrate, acetylcholine. This is an example of a reversible inhibitor involved in covalent bond formation with the enzyme that ultimately gets hydrolyzed.

Inhibitors of Angiotensin-Converting Enzyme Angiotensin-converting enzyme (ACE) is a carboxypeptidase having a zinc ion as a cofactor and is involved in the renin–angiotensin cascade of blood pressure control (20). The design of the antihypertensive drug captopril, a clinically important and potent reversible inhibitor of ACE, is an example of one of the early successes of a rationally designed enzyme inhibitor (21) (see Chapter 23). The design of captopril was based on several factors. These included knowledge that ACE was similar in its enzymatic mechanism to carboxypeptidase A, except that ACE cleaved off a dipeptide whereas carboxypeptidase A cleaved single amino acid groups from the carboxyl end of the protein. The discovery of benzylsuccinic acid as a potent inhibitor of carboxypeptidase A and studies of a potent pentapeptide inhibitor of ACE, $BPP_{5\alpha}$ (Glu-Lys-Trp-Ala-Pro), from the venom of the Brazilian viper (*Bothrops jararaca*) showed that the N-terminal peptide fragments, including tetra-, tri-, and dipeptide fragments (Ala-Pro) of $BPP_{5\alpha}$, retained some inhibitory activity. Benzylsuccinic acid has been described as a bi-product inhibitor of carboxypeptidase A, wherein its design was based on the combination of the products of the peptidase reaction (i.e., the two peptide fragments, one with a free carboxyl end that coordinates the zinc ion of carboxypeptidase A and the other with a free amino terminus) (Fig. 8.12) (22). In the case of benzylsuccinic acid, the amino (–NH_2) functionality is replaced by the bioisosteric methylene (–CH_2–) group. Using the above concepts, it was rationalized that succinyl amino acids could behave similarly as bi-product inhibitors of ACE. Starting with a succinyl-proline moiety, the SAR developmental effort finally resulted in captopril with the substitution of the stronger zinc coordinating mercapto functionality in place of the carboxylic acid moiety of succinic acid and a stereospecific R methyl group on the succinyl moiety to represent the methyl group on the natural L-Ala group in L-Ala-Pro (the dipeptide fragment that had previously shown inhibitory activity). Captopril soon became clinically successful as an antihypertensive agent and, especially in combination with diuretics, in controlling hypertension.

Following on the heels of captopril was another bi-product ACE inhibitor, enalaprilat (Fig. 8.12). Enalaprilat incorporated a phenylethyl moiety with the *S*-configuration and made use of a hydrophobic binding pocket in ACE that was overlooked during the design of captopril (23). Recalling that the tripeptide fragment of $BPP_{5\alpha}$ (L-Trp-L-Ala-L-Pro) contained the aromatic tryptophan (Trp) group and

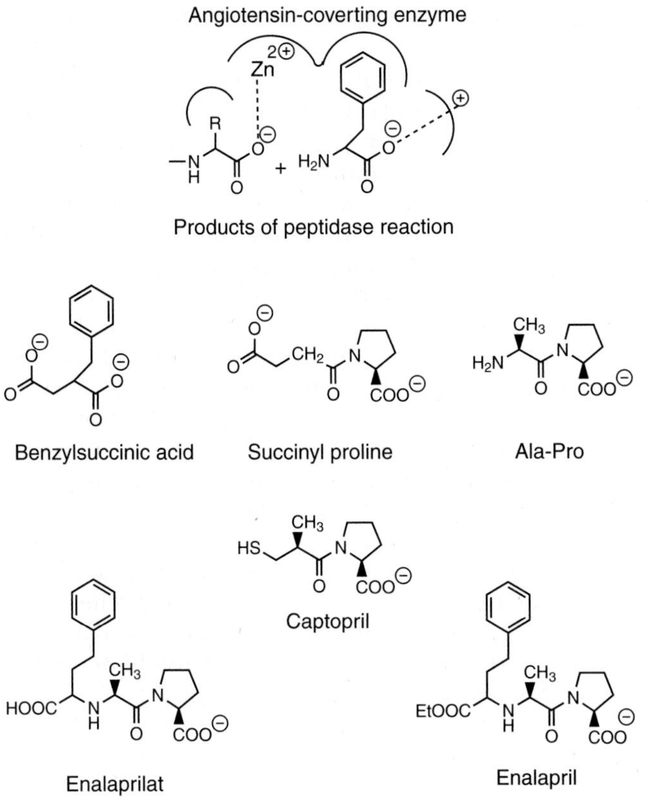

FIGURE 8.12 Angiotensin-converting enzyme (ACE) inhibitors and efforts that led to their development.

showed weak inhibitory properties suggested the benefit of an aromatic binding site. Substituting the tryptophan moiety with a phenyl group allowed the design of enalaprilat, which retained the carboxylic group as the coordinating ligand for zinc, which resulted in a 20-fold increase in antihypertensive potency over captopril. However, the diacid enalaprilat as its dianion was poorly absorbed from the gastrointestinal tract; thus, a prodrug monoethyl ester of enalaprilat, called enalapril, was developed. Enalapril had superior pharmacokinetics to enalaprilat and was rapidly metabolized to the active drug.

Transition-State Analogs

Transition-state analogs are compounds that resemble the substrate portion of the hypothetical transition state of an enzymatic reaction. All chemical reactions progressing from substrate to product must cross an energy barrier and proceed through a transition state or activated high-energy complex. This energy barrier is described as the activation energy. In the case of enzyme-catalyzed reactions, it is accepted that the enzyme reduces this energy barrier as compared to the nonenzyme-catalyzed reaction. Factors contributing to this reduced energy barrier are several and include stabilization of the transition state and intermediate forms of the reaction during the course of transition from substrate to product as well as conformational effects of distortion of the substrate while traversing toward the product (5). In 1948, Pauling (8) initially suggested that compounds resembling the transition state of an enzyme-catalyzed reaction would be effective inhibitors of the enzyme, because the substrate transition state should have the greatest affinity for the enzyme. Later, Wolfenden (24) proposed that thermodynamically, it is possible to relate the hypothetical equilibrium dissociation constants between substrate and its transition state of an enzyme-catalyzed reaction with that of the nonenzyme-catalyzed one. Using such an analysis, he showed that the ratio of the hypothetical transition-state dissociation constants of the nonenzyme-catalyzed reaction to that of the enzyme-catalyzed one is equal to the ratio of the first-order rate constants of formation of transition state for enzyme-catalyzed reaction to noncatalyzed reaction. Because the ratio of the enzyme-catalyzed rate constant to that of the noncatalyzed one ranges from 10^7 to 10^{10}, it follows that the substrate transition state would bind the enzyme 10^7- to 10^{10}-fold more tightly than the substrate itself (25). Hence, transition-state analogs that resemble the substrate would be extremely tight-binding compounds. To design a transition-state inhibitor, knowledge of the enzyme chemistry and its mechanism is a basic requirement. However, it must be understood that these substrate transition states are, by nature, unstable transient species existing for no longer than a few picoseconds. Nevertheless, experimental evidence has shown that even crudely designed transition-state inhibitors resembling the substrate are extremely potent inhibitors (25).

Transition-State Inhibitor of Adenosine Deaminase Adenosine deaminase hydrolyzes adenosine (or deoxyadenosine) to inosine (or deoxyinosine) and is important for purine metabolism (Fig. 8.13). High levels of adenosine are toxic to B cells of the immune system and can result in an immunocompromised state. People who also lack the gene for adenosine deaminase have the genetic condition of severe combined immunodeficiency and are extremely susceptible to opportunistic infections. Many cancer and antiviral agents are also degraded by this enzyme; hence, there is a role for the development of inhibitors of this enzyme (26). The mechanism proposed for adenosine deaminase is nucleophilic attack of water at the 6-position of adenosine to form a tetrahedral intermediate (Fig. 8.13). The transition state presumably resembles this intermediate.

During the course of the deaminase reaction, the hybridization of the 6-carbon changes from an sp^2-hybridized state to an sp^3 state. Subsequently, there is a loss of ammonia to form the product inosine. To develop a transition-state inhibitor for this enzyme, one would have to factor in this change in the hybridization of the substrate molecule; thus, molecules having an sp^3-hybridized carbon at this position and resembling the substrate would potentially be candidates for transition-state inhibitors. The compound 1,6-dihydro-6-hydroxymethylpurine has such geometry, and its potent

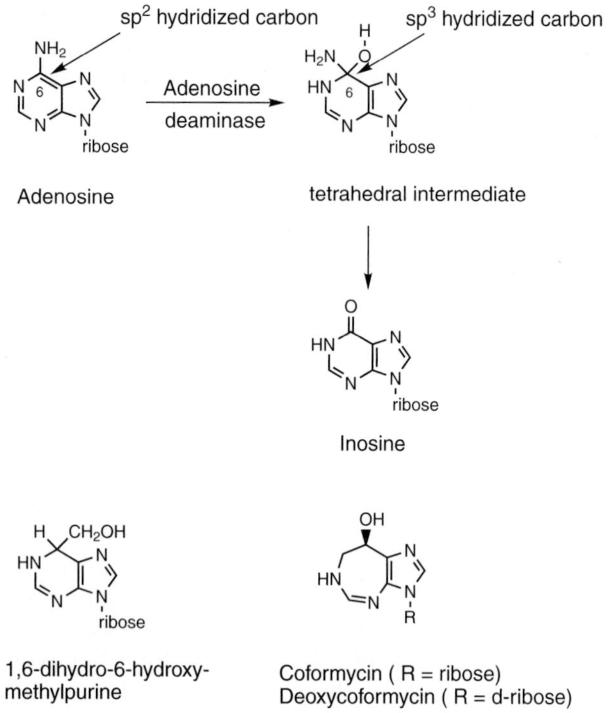

FIGURE 8.13 Mechanism and transition-state inhibitors of adenosine deaminase.

inhibitory properties of adenosine deaminase ($K_i < 1$ μM, as compared to a K_m for adenosine of 31 M) have been rationalized as being transition-state inhibitors (27). Two compounds that nature has provided, coformycin and its deoxyribose analog, deoxycoformycin (Fig. 8.13), are extremely potent inhibitors of adenosine deaminase (K_i = 2 pM). Both of these compounds contain a seven-member ring structure, which through its flexibility is presumed to resemble the hypothesized distorted sp^2–sp^3 transition state that forms during the addition of water to adenosine (28).

Irreversible Enzyme Inhibition

As previously described, irreversible enzyme inhibition is defined as "time-dependent inactivation of the enzyme," which implies that the enzyme has been permanently modified, because it can no longer carry out its catalytic function. This modification is the result of a covalent bond being formed between the inhibitor and an amino acid group in the protein. Furthermore, the covalent bond is extremely stable and, for all practical purposes, is not hydrolyzed to give back the enzyme in its original state or structure. In most examples of irreversible inhibition, a new enzyme must be generated through gene transcription and translation for the enzyme to continue its normal catalytic action. Basically, there are two types of irreversible enzyme inhibitors, the affinity labels or active site–directed irreversible inhibitors and the mechanism-based irreversible enzyme inactivators.

Affinity Labels and Active Site–Directed Irreversible Inhibitors

The affinity labels are those chemical entities that are inherently reactive and can target any nucleophilic group in the enzyme, especially those residing in and around the catalytic center of the protein. These agents generally resemble the substrate so that they can bind in the active site of the enzyme. In most examples, these agents also contain an electrophilic group, which includes groups such as halo-methyl ketones ($X\text{-}CH_2C{=}O$, where X = halide), sulfonyl fluorides (SO_2F), nitrogen mustards [$(ClCH_2CH_2)_2NH$], diazoketones ($COCHN_2$), and other such reactive groups, that can "label," or alkylate, a nucleophilic amino acid group in the enzyme. They generally tend to be indiscriminate in their action and have little therapeutic value, because they are nonselective and, thus, inherently toxic. They have been mainly used as biochemical tools to probe active sites of enzyme to differentiate the types of amino acid groups both in and around the catalytic center of an enzyme. The classic example of an affinity label is TPCK (tosyl-phenylalanyl-chloromethyl-ketone), an irreversible inhibitor of the serine protease chymotrypsin (29).

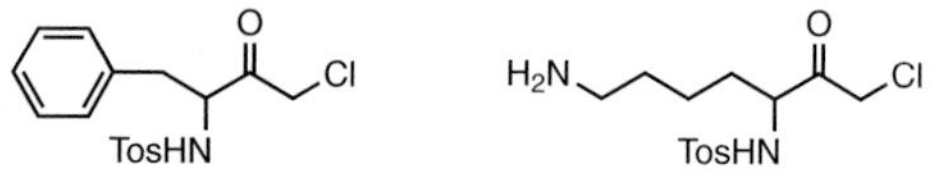

TPCK TLCK

Because TPCK resembles the amino acid phenylalanine, it can bind to the active site of the chymotrypsin, the selectivity of which is for such hydrophobic amino acid groups (Phe and Tyr). During the course of normal peptide hydrolysis, the reactive chloromethyl-ketone labels the nucleophilic histidine group present as part of the catalytic triad (Ser-His-Asp) in the active site of the protease (Fig. 8.14). Another similarly designed affinity

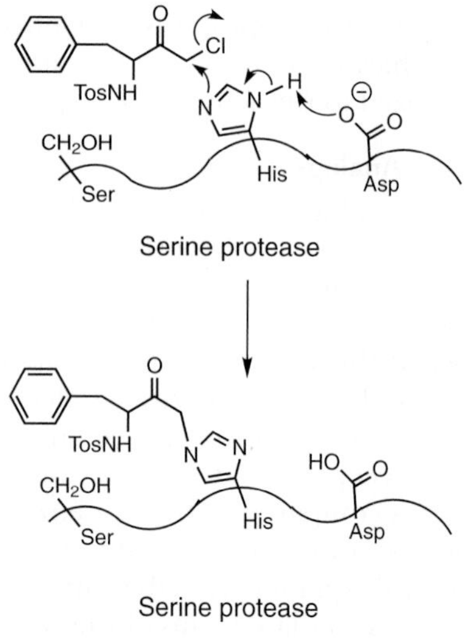

FIGURE 8.14 Mechanism of affinity label of serine protease with TPCK (tosyl-phenylalanyl-chloromethyl-ketone).

label is TLCK (tosyl-lysyl-chloromethyl-ketone), the specificity of which is for the protease trypsin. Trypsin cleaves peptide bonds adjacent to the basic amino acids, lysine and arginine. It was found that TLCK was a specific inhibitor of trypsin but had no activity for chymotrypsin. On the other hand, TPCK, although extremely specific for chymotrypsin, showed no activity for trypsin.

Because of the inherent reactivity and nonselectivity of these affinity labels and their limited utility in drug therapy, the late B.R. Baker (30) extended this concept to design inhibitors that would have greater selectivity and specificity and, thus, be potential drug candidates. He designed several analogs, termed active site–directed irreversible inhibitors, targeted toward thymidylate synthase, a key enzyme involved in the de novo metabolism of thymidylate. These analogs contained a substrate-binding region linked to a reactive group, such as a halomethyl ketone, by a tether whose chain length could be manipulated. The substrate portion of the analog ensures both affinity and rapid binding to the enzyme active site. Once the substrate is bound, areas in and around the binding site and on the surface of the enzyme could be probed for nucleophilic amino acid groups. By manipulating the length of the tether, ideal inhibitors could then be designed such that any suitably located, sufficiently nucleophilic amino acid group on the surface of the enzyme could potentially be alkylated by the halomethyl ketone (Fig. 8.15). Once alkylated, the tether "bridges" the active site with the labeled amino acid group, thus "tying up" and preventing further catalysis by the enzyme.

Mechanism-Based Irreversible Enzyme Inhibitors

OVERVIEW The mechanism-based irreversible inhibitors have also been termed "suicide substrates," "k_{cat} inhibitors," "Trojan horse inhibitors," or "latent alkylating agents." These inhibitors are inherently unreactive but, on normal catalytic processing by the enzyme, are activated into highly reactive moieties (31–33). These reactive groups can irreversibly alkylate a nucleophilic amino acid group or cofactor in the enzyme and, in essence, cause the enzyme's death ("suicide"). Basically, these inhibitors have a latent reactive group that only becomes apparent after binding and acted on by the normal catalytic machinery of the enzyme. This type of inhibitor design differs from the active site–directed inhibitors in that these inhibitors have one more level of built-in selectivity. The kinetic scheme for such inhibition is shown in Equation 8.6, in which enzyme, E, binds with substrate (inhibitor), S, to give an [E–S] complex with dissociation constant of K_i:

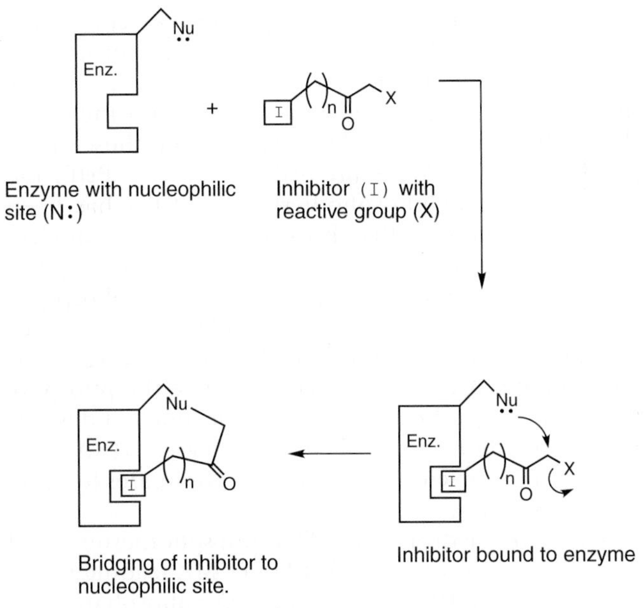

FIGURE 8.15 Model showing Baker's (30) active site–directed irreversible inhibitors.

8.6
$$\begin{array}{c} E + S \underset{}{\overset{K_i}{\rightleftharpoons}} [E{\cdot}S] \overset{k_{cat}}{\rightarrow} [E{\cdot}S^*] \overset{k_{inact}}{\rightarrow} [E-S] \\ \downarrow k_{diff} \\ E + S^* + Nu{:} \rightarrow [Nu\text{-}S] \end{array}$$

Next, the [E–S] complex is converted into a highly activated complex [E–S*] by the catalytic machinery (k_{cat}) of the enzyme, which can then go on to alkylate the enzyme, [E–S]. Note that it is possible for the reactive species [S*] to diffuse (k_{diff} dissociate) from the enzyme and react with some other target (nucleophilic species)—that is, the system is "leaky." However, if this happens, the inhibitor cannot be classified as a "true" suicide substrate, because specificity is lost.

Several requirements need to be met by these inhibitors in order for them to be classified as suicide substrates. These include the following: 1) inactivation should be time dependent (reaction is irreversible); 2) kinetics should be first order; 3) the enzyme should show saturation kinetics; 4) the substrate should be able to protect the enzyme; and 5) stoichiometry of the reaction should be 1:1 (one active site to one inhibitor).

EXAMPLES OF MECHANISM-BASED IRREVERSIBLE INHIBITORS During the past three decades, besides the rational design of hundreds of molecules that have been synthesized and tested as mechanism-based irreversible inhibitors, it has also come to light that nature itself has known about this mechanistic mode of enzyme inhibition and provided us with several extremely potent mechanism-based irreversible inhibitors. Below are a few selected examples to demonstrate the mode of action of these inhibitors.

Halo Enol Lactones Halo enol lactones are examples of irreversible inhibitors for serine proteases. These analogs were developed by Katzenellenbogen and coworkers at the University of Illinois (34). On normal catalytic processing by the Ser-CH_2-OH group, the analogs produce a reactive halo-methyl ketone, which subsequently alkylates a nearby nucleophilic group on the enzyme (Fig. 8.16). Other inhibitors for

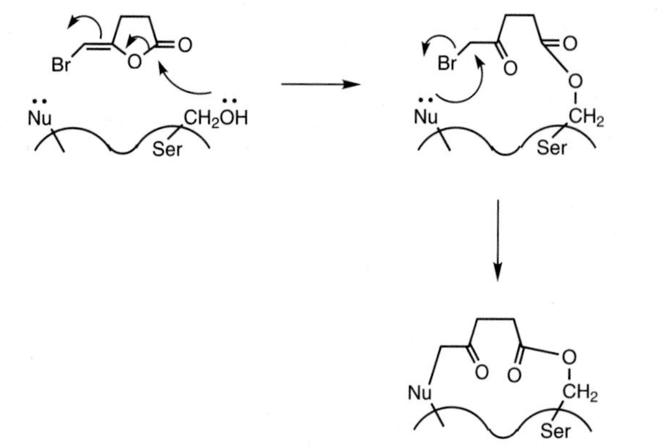

FIGURE 8.16 Mechanism-based inhibition of serine proteases by Katzenellenbogen's halo enol lactone.

the serine proteases have been designed by various researchers (32).

Clavulanic Acid Clavulanic acid is a potent inhibitor of bacterial β-lactamase (35). This enzyme is a serine protease and can hydrolyze β-lactams, such as the penicillin antibiotics. It is the principal enzyme responsible for penicillin-resistant bacteria. Clavulanic acid is a β-lactam and, when given in combination with penicillin, is preferentially taken up by β-lactamase and hydrolyzed. However, during the process of hydrolysis, the clavulanic acid undergoes a cleavage, leading to the formation of a "Michael acceptor," which subsequently alkylates a nucleophilic group on β-lactamase, causing irreversible inhibition as shown in Figure 8.17. Such combinations of a β-lactamase inhibitor and a penicillin have resulted in clinically useful agents, for example clavulanic acid plus amoxicillin (Augmentin).

Gabaculin Gabaculin, a naturally occurring neurotoxin, is a potent mechanism-based inhibitor of the enzyme γ-aminobutyric acid transaminase (GABA-T) with an interesting mechanism of action (36). GABA-T is a pyridoxal phosphate (PLP)–dependent enzyme

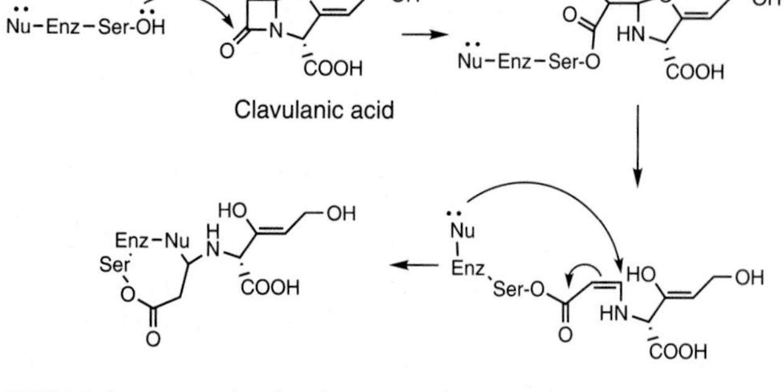

FIGURE 8.17 Mechanism-based inhibition of β-lactamases by clavulanic acid.

(PLP is a cofactor) involved in the catabolism (transamination) of the excitatory neurotransmitter, GABA, to succinate semialdehyde and pyridoxamine as shown in Figure 8.18. As part of the normal catalytic mechanism of PLP-dependent enzymes, the *m*-amino group of gabaculin initially reacts with the aldehyde group of PLP to form an adduct, which subsequently undergoes an aromatization reaction, resulting in an extremely stable covalent bond with PLP. Hence, in this case, rather than an enzymatic nucleophilic group being alkylated, the cofactor is unavailable, resulting in the inhibition.

Finasteride Finasteride is a clinically useful agent in the treatment of prostate hyperplasia and male pattern baldness. It is a potent inhibitor that targets human steroid-5α-reductase, the enzyme responsible for the reduction of testosterone to more potent dihydrotestosterone (Fig. 8.19) (see Chapter 40). The inhibitory action of finasteride has been attributed both to its similarity in structure to testosterone, which allows the drug to bind to the enzyme and be reduced to dihydrofinasteride in place of testosterone, as well as to its ability to act as a mechanism-based inhibitor, during which it makes the cofactor NADPH unavailable by forming a covalent NADP-dihydrofinasteride adduct as shown in Figure 8.19 (see Chapter 40). This adduct very slowly releases dihydrofinasteride with a half-life of 1 month (37).

Recent Inhibitors of Clinically Important Enzymes

Cyclic Nucleotide Phosphodiesterase Inhibitors

Phosphodiesterases (PDEs) belong to a large family of enzymes that hydrolyze phosphate ester bonds, linking two hydroxyl groups with phosphoric acid. In nature, there are numerous biomolecules containing such phosphodiester bonds including glycerol phosphates (phospholipids), sugar phosphates, inositol phosphates, nucleic acids, and nucleotides including the cyclic nucleotides. Although, all of these phosphodiesters are essentially hydrolyzed by a PDE, the specific name of phosphodiesterase (PDE) has been applied to enzymes that hydrolyze the cyclic nucleotide monophosphates, cyclic adenosine monophosphate (cAMP) and cyclic guanosine monophosphate (cGMP), both of which are involved in signal transduction and second messenger cell signaling (Fig. 8.20) (see Chapter 3). Enzymes that hydrolyze the phosphodiester bonds other than the cyclic nucleotides are known by other names, such as nucleases (DNAses or RNAses, for nucleic acids) and phospholipases for glycerol phosphates.

The PDEs hydrolyze the 3′-5′ phosphodiester bond of its primary substrates, cAMP or cGMP, leading to the formation of AMP (5′-adenosine monophosphate) and GMP (5′-guanosine monophosphate), respectively. The PDEs can bind either cyclic nucleotide with selectivity

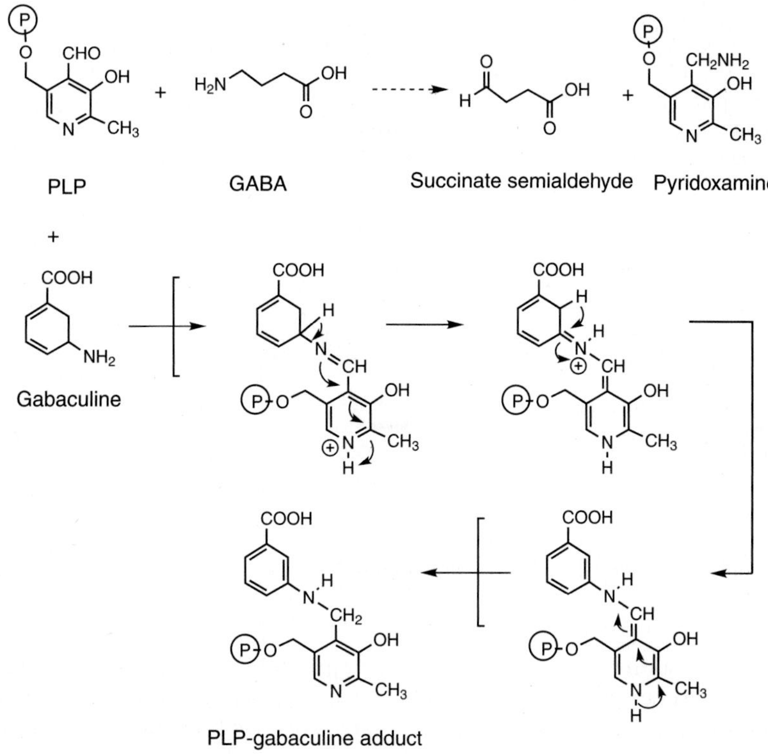

FIGURE 8.18 Pyridoxal phosphate–dependent γ-aminobutyric acid transaminase (GABA-T) reaction and the mechanism of suicide inhibition by gabaculin.

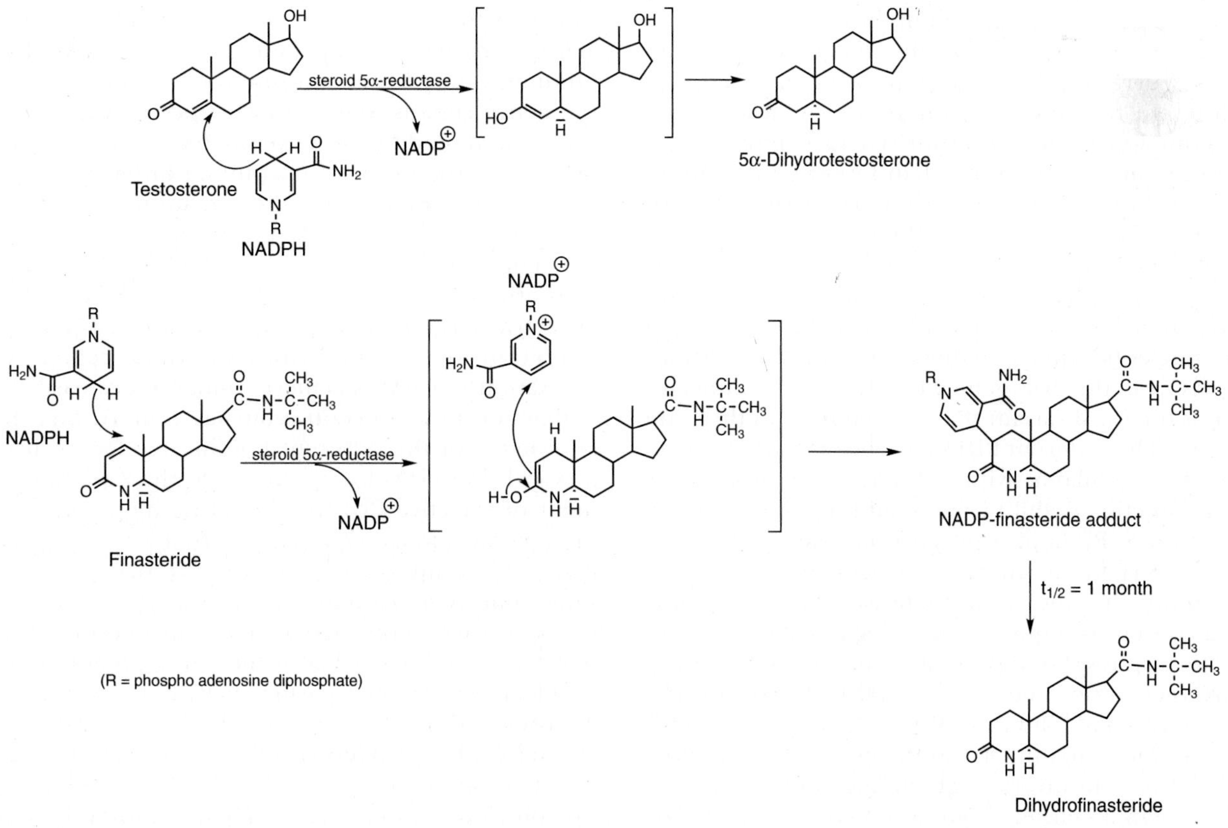

FIGURE 8.19 Mechanism of steroid reductase reduction on finasteride and testosterone and the structure of hypothesized NADPH-dihydrofinasteride adduct (37).

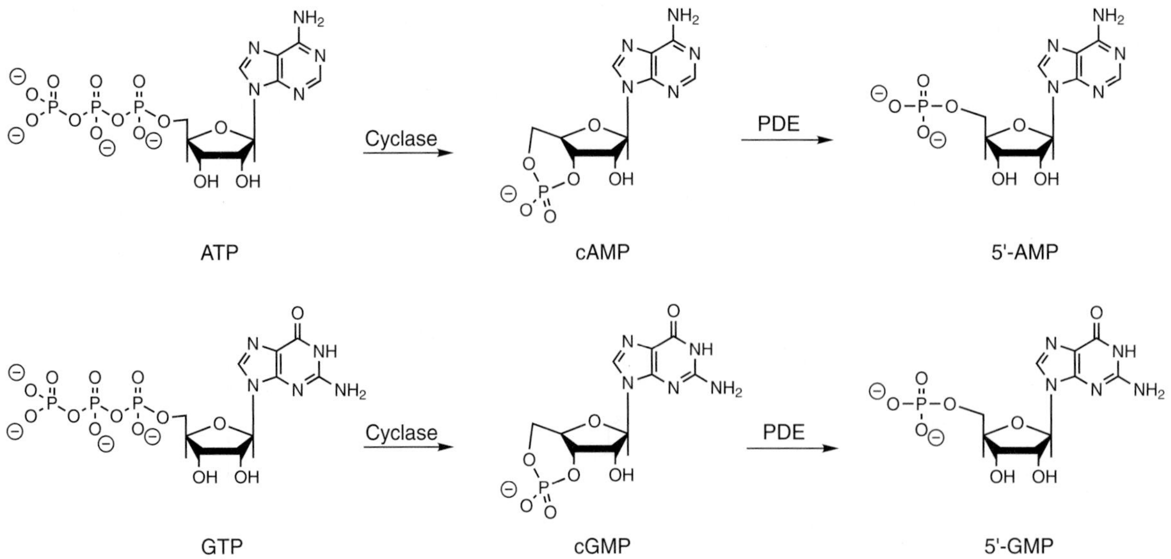

FIGURE 8.20 Enzymatic interconversions of cyclic and linear nucleotides.

depending on the particular isoenzyme. cAMP and cGMP are formed from their precursor nucleotide triphosphates, adenosine triphosphate (ATP) and guanosine triphosphate (GTP), respectively (Fig. 8.20). There are many different isoforms of the PDEs present in cells, which allows for great diversity in substrate specificity and cell regulation. This diversity further governs specific roles for each of these PDEs in various cellular locales and physiologic and pathologic conditions. Currently, the PDEs have been classified into 11 different families based on gene products (amino acid homology) and are estimated to comprise over 100 different mRNAs from 21 different genes due to alternative splicing and transcription start sites (38,39). The nomenclature of these PDE families is based on the species of origin, the gene, and the variant discovered. For example, HsPDE2A3 signifies that the origin is from homo sapiens (Hs), PDE denotes that it is a cyclic nucleotide phosphodiesterase, the 2A indicates that it is from the PDE gene 2 family A, and 3 indicates that it is the third variant that was reported in the gene database. The different PDEs have been shown to regulate various cellular activities, and hence because of this diverse functional ability, one could develop drugs to control these PDEs in a selective manner (Table 8.2) (40–42). Structural studies of several of these PDEs have shown that they all contain a "catalytic domain" with a consensus sequence denoting a metal ion binding site (a phosphorylase sequence, containing a signature recognition sequence for all PDEs) of two His and two Asps that bind Zn^{2+}/Mg^{2+}; a "glutamine switch," which accounts for the substrate specificity (cAMP or cGMP) where an invariant glutamine amino acid moiety can rotate to either H-bond with cAMP or cGMP or is constrained from binding to either cAMP or cGMP, thus favoring binding to the other nucleotide; and a "regulatory domain" based on the specific PDE family (e.g., Ca^{2+}-calmodulin binding site for PDE1) as well as an allosteric binding site for cGMP (38,39).

X-ray crystallographic studies with inhibitors bound with the enzyme have indicated that there are several binding modes for inhibition and the active site architecture is often unique for different PDEs. Inhibitors can bind to the enzyme through H-bonds with amino acid groups that make up the active site for cAMP/cGMP binding, with groups that line the channel leading to the active site, as well as by H-bonding with water to groups that bind to the active site metal ions. Moreover, because of the order of magnitude differences in cellular concentrations of the cyclic nucleotides (as compared to its precursor, nucleotide triphosphate molecule, <1 to 10 μM for cAMP/cGMP vs. mM concentrations for ATP/GTP) (38), these PDEs become attractive targets to design drugs. (Since competitive inhibition for a natural substrate whose cellular concentration is 1 μM is achieved much more easily than if the substrate concentration was 1 mM). Structural knowledge of the different binding modes for inhibitors with the PDEs has given rise to the rapid development of selective PDE inhibitors to allow for specific interactions along regulatory pathways involving such PDEs. While inhibitors of PDEs have been known for some time (e.g., caffeine and theophylline have been in use as therapeutic agents for many decades as nonselective inhibitors of PDE), the development of drugs to selectively inhibit a particular PDE is a more recent discovery. Moreover, selective PDE inhibitors would also have a better safety profile, as one would expect a decreased amount of side/adverse effects. For example, theophylline, a nonselective PDE inhibitor, is known to have a narrow therapeutic index because of its interaction with multiple PDEs.

TABLE 8.2 Specificity and Potency of PDE Inhibitors

PDE	Specificity	Inhibitor	IC$_{50}$[a] (nM)	PDE	Specificity	Inhibitor	IC$_{50}$[a] (nM)
PDE1B	Duel	Rolipram	>200,000	PDE6	cGMP	Sildenafil	50[b]
		Cilomilast	87,000			Vardenafil	11[c]
		Roflumilast	>200,000			Tadalafil	2,000[b]
		Sildenafil	1,500	PDE7B	cAMP	Rolipram	>2,000,000
		Vardenafil	300			Cilomilast	44,000
		Tadalafil	50,000			Roflumilast	>200,000
PDE2A	Duel	Rolipram	>200,000			Sildenafil	78,000
		Cilomilast	160,000			Vardenafil	1,900
		Roflumilast	>200,000			Tadalafil	74,000
		Sildenafil	35,000	PDE8A	cAMP	Rolipram	>200,000
		Vardenafil	3,100			Cilomilast	7,000
		Tadalafil	130,000			Roflumilast	>200,000
PDE3B	cAMP > cGMP	Rolipram	>200,000			Sildenafil	>200,000
		Cilomilast	87,000			Vardenafil	57,000
		Roflumilast	>200,000			Tadalafil	>200,000
		Sildenafil	15,000	PDE9A	cGMP	Rolipram	>200,000
		Vardenafil	580			Cilomilast	>200,000
		Tadalafil	280,000			Roflumilast	>200,000
PDE4B	cAMP	Rolipram	570			Sildenafil	5,600
		Cilomilast	25			Vardenafil	680
		Roflumilast	0.84			Tadalafil	150,000
		Sildenafil	20,000	PDE10A	cAMP<cGMP	Rolipram	140,000
		Vardenafil	3,800			Cilomilast	73,000
		Tadalafil	9,200			Roflumilast	>200,000
PDE4D	cAMP	Rolipram	1,100			Sildenafil	6,800
		Cilomilast	11			Vardenafil	880
		Roflumilast	0.68			Tadalafil	19,000
		Sildenafil	14,000	PDE11A	Duel	Rolipram	>200,000
		Vardenafil	3,900			Cilomilast	21,000
		Tadalafil	19,000			Roflumilast	25,000
PDE5A	cGMP	Rolipram	>200,000			Sildenafil	6,100
		Cilomilast	53,000			Vardenafil	240
		Roflumilast	17,000			Tadalafil	10
		Sildenafil	2.2				
		Vardenafil	1.0				
		Tadalafil	1.2				

[a] Data are from Sutherland and Rall (40) unless stated otherwise. The numbers shown in the table are the 50% inhibition concentration (IC50). The cAMP and cGV; concentrations used were far below the K_m of all the PDEs assayed except for PDE9A, in which case it was close to the K_m. The IC50s obtained are good approximations of the inhibition constant K_i. Selectivities of an inhibitor may be determined by taking ratios of the numbers given in the table.

[b] K_i values are from Card et al. (41).

[c] Value from Hatzelmann and Schudt (42).

PDE5 Selective Inhibitors The impetus for the development of PDE inhibitors arose from the knowledge that vasodilation (for treatment of high blood pressure) could be achieved through the stimulation of atrial natriuretic peptide (ANP), an endogenous peptide that allows for renal excretion of sodium/water. Furthermore it was also known that ANP stimulated the synthesis of cGMP through its activation of guanyl cyclase. Thus, inhibition of cGMP hydrolysis was a rational target for the development of PDE inhibitors as vasodilators. Since ANP worked in the kidney, the idea was to target the specific PDE in the kidney. The lead compound for the development of these PDE inhibitors was a xanthine derivative, zaprinast (Fig. 8.21), previously shown to demonstrate weak PDE inhibition (43). Analysis of the heterocyclic ring of zaprinast and comparison with the purine heterocycle of cGMP led to the development of a number of derivatives displaying PDE5 inhibitory activity, including the design of one containing a pyrazolopyrimidinone, which ultimately resulted in the development of the potent PDE5 inhibitor sildenafil (44). During clinical trials of sildenafil as an antihypertensive and vasodilator, it was discovered to have a (beneficial) side effect regarding erectile dysfunction. This pharmacologic effect was recognized, appreciated, and commercialized into a new line of therapeutic agents to treat erectile dysfunction. Inhibition of cGMP hydrolysis by PDE5 in the corpus cavernosum in the penis results in elevated levels of cGMP, leading to increased smooth muscle relaxation and increased blood flow and maintenance of an erection. Presently, PDE5 selective inhibitors include the drugs sildenafil (Viagra), vardenafil (Levitra). and tadalafil (Cialis) (Fig. 8.21) (see Chapter 40). They have been some of the most widely marketed and commercially successful drugs in recent years to treat erectile dysfunction in males and also more recently have been approved to treat pulmonary hypertension (see Chapter 24). These drugs have high selectivity to inhibit PDE5 over the other PDE classes. PDE5 is a PDE that specifically hydrolyzes cGMP to GMP at low substrate levels and also has a high affinity binding site for cGMP on its regulatory domain. PDE5, originally isolated from platelets, was later found to be a regulator in vascular smooth muscle contraction present in the lungs and brains. The drugs are all reversible inhibitors of PDE5 where they bind in the active site of PDE5, the heterocyclic nucleus of the inhibitors binding in the space reserved for the guanosine ring (of cGMP). A side effect is hypotension, and also, because the active site structures of PDE5 and PDE6 are similar in architecture, some cross inhibition of PDE6 enzymes has been observed. PDE6 enzymes regulate the phototransduction cascade where PDE6 rapidly reduces the steady-state concentration of cGMP in response to light stimuli. Thus, a side effect of PDE5 inhibitors involves decreased vision in some patient populations. The drug tadalafil, however, is approximately 1,000-fold more selective for PDE5 than for PDE6. Several other selective competitive PDE inhibitors are approved for use, and these include the PDE4 inhibitors cilomilast and roflumilast for treatment of chronic obstructive pulmonary disease (Fig. 8.22) as well as the PDE3 inhibitors dipyridamole and cilostazol, as antiplatelet drugs (Fig. 8.23), and inamrinone and milrinone, as positive inotropic agents (Fig. 8.24).

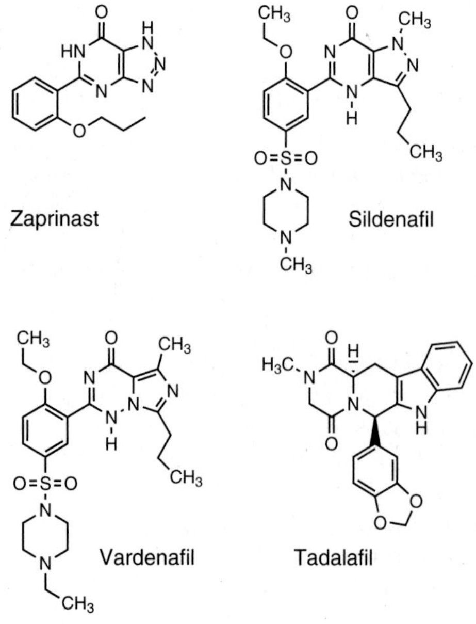

FIGURE 8.21 Inhibitors of PDE5.

Protein Kinase Inhibitors

Protein kinases belong to the family of group transfer phosphorylating enzymes that transfer a phosphate group from ATP onto amino acid groups of proteins. It is estimated that there are over 500 of these kinases encoded by the human genome, and this reaction, when coupled with a phosphatase (i.e., reversible phosphorylation of proteins), offers cells a precise regulatory mechanism to control their differentiation, maturation,

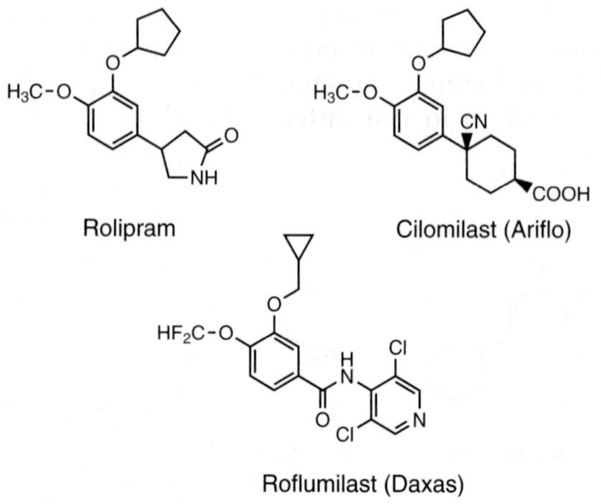

FIGURE 8.22 Competitive inhibitors of PDE4.

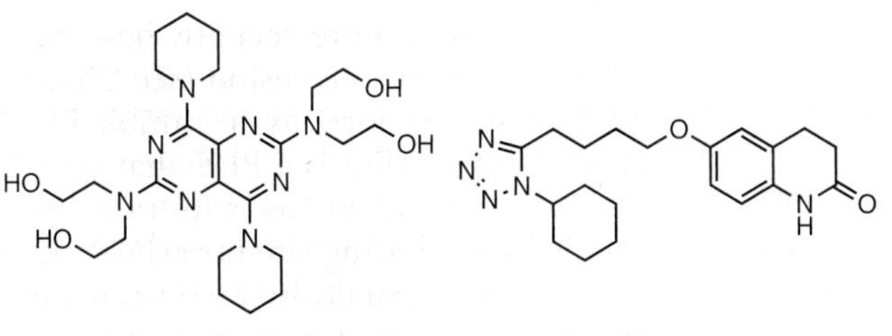

Dipyridamole Cilostazol

FIGURE 8.23 Antiplatelet inhibitors of PDE3.

proliferation, apoptosis, and other cellular functions (45). The substrate amino acid groups on proteins that are phosphorylated belong largely to the hydroxyl-bearing amino acids, such as serine, threonine, and tyrosine. Therefore, these kinases are referred to as either serine/threonine kinases or tyrosine kinases. Because these proteins are involved in regulatory functions of the cell, it becomes apparent that mutations or aberrations of expression of these proteins can lead to dysregulation of cellular functions, giving rise to tumors and cancers. Indeed, research has shown that of the 518 kinase genes present in the human genome, 244 map to disease loci and cancer (45). Moreover, targeting these enzymes with inhibitors would be a way to selectively target cancers without the noxious side effects seen with conventional anticancer drugs such as the alkylating agents or antitumor antibiotics (see Chapter 37). Research over the last decade for kinase inhibitors has provided a rationale to develop targeted anticancer therapy where such kinases that manifest themselves in certain cancers have been specifically targeted for inhibition, resulting in dramatic decreases of cancer cells and greater survival times for the patient (46). Examples of such targeted anticancer drugs have involved primarily the development of the tyrosine kinase inhibitors (TKIs), several of which are U.S. Food and Drug Administration approved (see Chapter 37); however, more recently, inhibitors of serine/threonine kinases are also being developed and are in clinical trials.

Tyrosine Kinase Inhibitors The tyrosine kinases are a group of enzymes responsible for signal transduction and intracellular signaling functions, many of which are involved in cell differentiation and proliferation. They can be divided into two major types depending on where they act in the cell: receptor tyrosine kinases, membrane-spanning proteins having an extracellular ligand binding domain and an intracellular catalytic (kinase) domain involved in the transduction of extracellular signals from the membrane to the cytoplasm, or the non–receptor tyrosine kinases involved in cytosolic signaling events. Inhibitors for both of these kinases have been developed and have shown excellent and selective activity in cancers manifested by aberrant expression of these enzymes. The development of a TKI to selectively treat chronic myelogenous leukemia (CML) was the impetus leading to the large number of presently available TKIs. CML in the majority of patients is due to a reciprocal translocation of chromosomes 9 and 22, resulting in a fusion of the *abl* (Abelson leukemia virus) gene of chromosome 9 to the *bcr* (break point cluster) gene of chromosome 22, leading to the *bcr-abl* fusion gene (the Philadelphia chromosome). Although the *abl* gene normally produces a non–receptor tyrosine kinase whose activity is highly regulated, the *bcr-abl* fusion gene produces a tyrosine kinase that is constitutively active and whose activity is required for the transformation of cells to become malignant (47). The knowledge of this direct correlation between expression of the abnormal fusion protein and CML allowed for the development of specific inhibitors for this enzyme and other such dysregulated kinases that are overexpressed in many cancers. Using a high-throughput screening program to develop inhibitors for receptor tyrosine kinases as a possible treatment for such cancers, 2-phenylamionopyrimidine (PAP) became a lead compound. Further SAR optimization and refinement of this lead led to imatinib (Gleevec) (Fig. 8.25), the first targeted drug for treatment of CML (48,49). Note that the SAR to imatinib included addition of a pyridine, a methyl, and a benzamide to enhance the potency of the basic PAP nucleus. The piperazinyl functionality helped to increase water solubility, allowing for better "drug-like" properties. Imatinib also proved to be inhibitory in many other cancers with overexpressed kinases, such as gastrointestinal stromal tumors (which overexpress *c-kit*), myelodysplastic diseases associated with platelet-derived growth factor receptor, and Philadelphia chromosome–positive adult lymphoblastic leukemia (50). X-ray

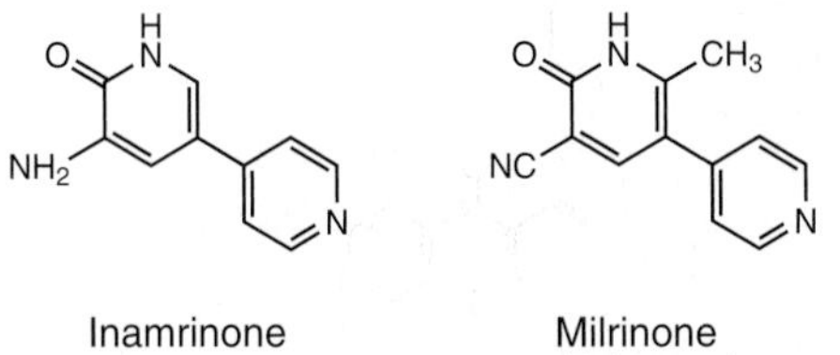

Inamrinone Milrinone (Primacor)

FIGURE 8.24 PDE3 inhibitors with cardiac and pulmonary effects.

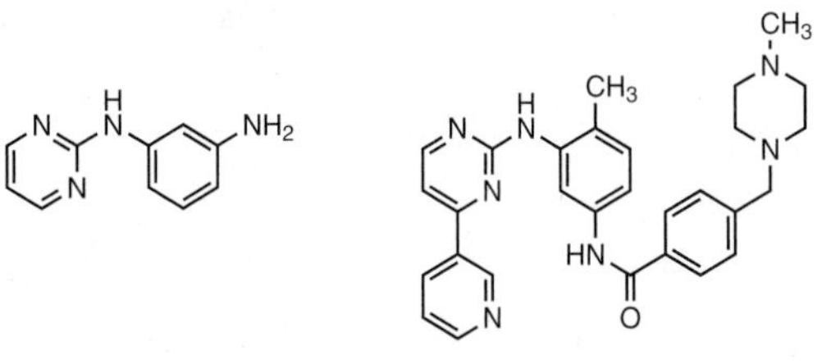

2-Phenylaminopyrimidine Imatinib

FIGURE 8.25 Structures of 2-phenylaminopyrimidine and imatinib.

crystallographic studies with imatinib co-crystallized with the tyrosine kinase expressed from *abl* showed that imatinib binds to the ATP binding site of the enzyme in its inactive conformation (off state) and this binding prevented the kinase from achieving its productive binding conformation with ATP (51,52). These kinases all have an "activation loop," which contains a tyrosine phenolic group (Tyr 393), the major phosphorylated group, that allows switching the kinase from inactive to active forms and allows for ATP binding. Studies showed that with the enzyme-bound imatinib, the phenolic group of Tyr 393 was not phosphorylated and the conformation of this activation loop in the nonphosphorylated enzyme changed to that resembling substrate (ATP) being bound to the kinase. In this way, the altered geometry brought about by imatinib binding to the active site of the enzyme prevented the enzyme from binding its true substrate, ATP. Resistance develops to imatinib due to mutations in the hydrophobic pocket that prevent access of imatinib to the enzyme in the off state, thus allowing for the kinase to bind ATP and cancer to progress. TKIs have also been developed to bind the kinase in its "on state" (active conformation), where the drugs can access hydrophobic regions in the ATP binding pocket, and to bind both "on" and "off" forms (dual-mode inhibitors that are more potent than imatinib) (52).

Since the introduction of imatinib, many other TKI drugs have been developed for related tyrosine kinases such as epidermal growth factor receptor, platelet-derived growth factor receptor, and vascular endothelial growth factor receptor. All of these inhibitors make use of a heterocyclic functionality (resembling the adenine of ATP) and bind in the putative binding site of ATP (a highly conserved nucleotide binding region in the catalytic domain of the kinase). The inhibitors make use of differences in the variable region of the enzyme surrounding the ATP binding pocket, which allows for specific binding interactions with the various groups present on the individual inhibitors. Resistance to these inhibitors manifests due to mutations to these variable regions on the enzyme as well as to cellular efflux pumps being activated. Examples of some of these inhibitors such as dasatinib (for imatinib resistance), sunitinib (inhibitor of vascular endothelial growth factor receptor), and gefitinib (inhibitor of epidermal growth factor receptor) are shown in Figure 8.26.

Serine/Threonine Kinase Inhibitors The serine/threonine kinases are a family of enzymes that phosphorylate the hydroxyl groups of serine and threonine present on enzymes. One of the most studied of these enzymes is protein kinase C, an intracellular kinase that is activated by Ca^{2+} ions or diacylglycerol, leading to various signal transduction events in the cell through its activation of the mitogen-activated protein kinase family (53). Examples of other serine/threonine kinases include mammalian target of rapamycin (mTOR), a protein involved in the activation of immune B and T cells, and the Aurora kinases, which are involved in cell cycle regulation during mitosis. Inhibitors of mTOR include rapamycin (sirolimus) a macrolide originally isolated from a microbe on Easter Island and used as an immunosuppressant drug. The Aurora kinase inhibitors encompass inhibitors for Aurora A and Aurora B kinases, both of which are overexpressed in cancer cells leading to dysregulation during mitosis and chromosomal destabilization (54). Generally, mitosis is a highly regulated process with multiple checkpoints to regulate chromosomal segregation. One of these regulatory mechanisms involves phosphorylation of proteins by serine/threonine kinases (mitotic kinases). The Aurora kinases are one such mitotic kinase where they interact with many proteins, including tumor suppressors and activators from the mitotic entry stage all the way to cytokinesis. It is not surprising then that they are overexpressed in many tumors (breast, colon, gastric, ovarian, and pancreatic) and thus have become an

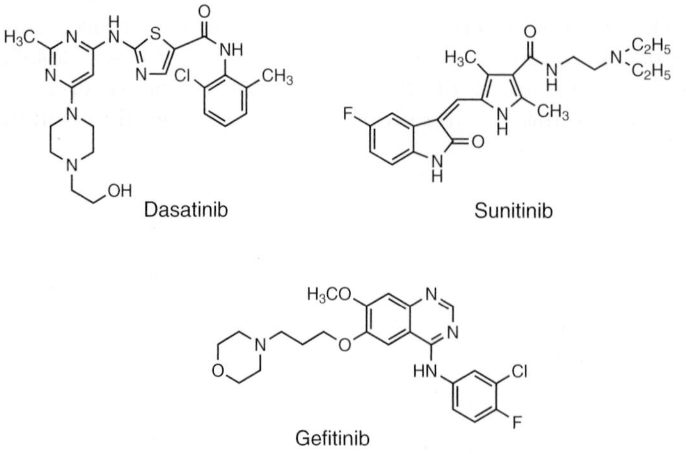

FIGURE 8.26 Structures of the tyrosine kinase inhibitors, dasatinib, sunitinib, and gefitinib.

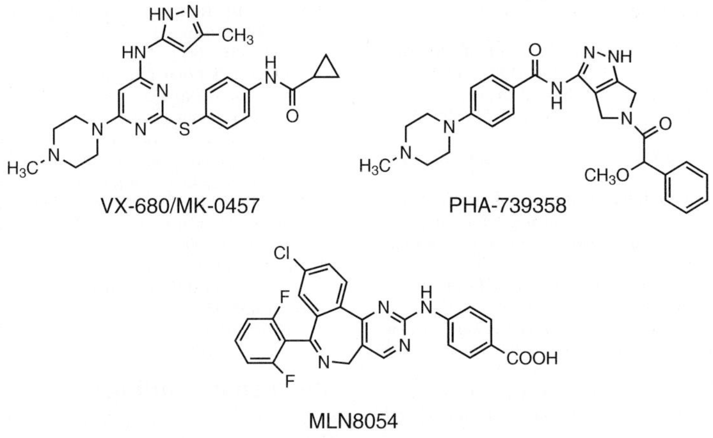

FIGURE 8.27 Structures of the Aurora kinase inhibitors undergoing clinical trials.

attractive target for anticancer drug development (55). Examples of some of these Aurora kinase inhibitors in clinical trials include VK680/MK-0457, PHA-739358, and MLN8054 (Fig. 8.27).

SUMMARY

This chapter has attempted to give the reader an overview of enzyme catalysis and the various ways in which enzymes can act as catalytic proteins. Based on these properties and mechanisms of enzyme action, the essentials of drug design and discovery through enzyme inhibition with a few choice examples have been outlined. The reader is referred to the Suggested Reading material for more detailed explanations and insights regarding the rationale and design strategies of enzyme inhibitors. In conclusion, drug design by enzyme inhibition is a continually developing enterprise. There will always be the need to discover more selective and more potent inhibitors in an effort to increase the therapeutic benefit to patients. This chapter has tried to give a brief insight into this fascinating area of medicinal chemistry and the various types of enzyme inhibitors that can be rationally designed.

References

1. Albert A. Selective Toxicity—The Physicochemical Basis of Therapy, 7th Ed. New York: Chapman & Hall, 1985.
2. Domagk G. Ein beitrag zur chemotherapie der bakteriellen infektionen. Dtsch Med Wochenschr 1935;61:250–253.
3. Woods DD. Relation of *p*-aminobenzoic acid to mechanism of action of sulfanilamide. Br J Exp Pathol 1940;21:74–90.
4. Albert A. Chapter 9. In: Selective Toxicity—The Physicochemical Basis of Therapy, 7th Ed. New York: Chapman & Hall, 1985.
5 Fersht A. Structure and Mechanism in Protein Science: A Guide to Enzyme Catalysis and Protein Folding, 3rd Ed. New York: W.H. Freeman, 2000.
6. Lad C, Williams H, Wolfenden, R. The rate of hydrolysis of phosphomonoester dianions and the exceptional catalytic proficiencies of protein and inositol phosphatases. Proc Natl Acad Sci U S A 2003;100:5607–5610.
7. Nomenclature Committee of the International Union of Biochemistry and Molecular Biology. Enzyme nomenclature. Available at: http://www.chem.qmul.ac.uk/iubmb/enzyme/. Accessed April 4, 2006.
8. Pauling L. The nature of forces between large molecules of biological interest. Nature 1948;161:707–709.
9. Garcia-Viloca M, Gao J, Karplus M, et al. How enzymes work: analysis by modern rate theory and computer simulations. Science 2004;303:186–195.
10. Zhang X, Houk KN. Why enzymes are proficient catalysts: beyond the Pauling paradigm. Acc Chem Res 2005;38:379–385.
11. Bruice TC, Benkovic SJ. A comparison of the bimolecular and intramolecular nucleophilic catalysis of the hydrolysis of substituted phenyl acylates by the dimethylamino group. J Am Chem Soc 1963;85:1–8.
12. Michael C, Gaston S. Formation and hydrolysis of lactones of phenolic acids. J Am Chem Soc 1980;102:4815–4821.
13. Sastry JK, Nehete PN, Khan S, et al. Membrane-permeable dideoxyuridine 5′-monophosphate analog inhibits human immunodeficiency virus infection. Mol Pharmacol 1992;41:441–445.
14. Mitsuya H, Weinhold KJ, Furman PA, et al. 3′-Azido-3′-deoxythymidine (BW A509U): an antiviral agent that inhibits the infectivity and cytopathic effect of human T-lymphotropic virus type III/lymphadenopathy-associated virus in vitro. Proc Natl Acad Sci U S A 1985;82:7096–7100.
15 Furman PA, Fyfe JA, St. Clair MH, et al. Phosphorylation of 3″-azido-3′-deoxythymidine and selective interaction of the 5′-triphosphate with human immunodeficiency virus reverse transcriptase. Proc Natl Acad Sci U S A 1986;83:8333–8337.
16. Grob PM, Wu JC, Cohen KA, et al. Nonnucleoside inhibitors of HIV-1 reverse transcriptase: nevirapine as a prototype drug. AIDS Res Hum Retrovir 1992;8:145–152.
17. Kohlstaedt LA, Wang J, Friedman JM, et al. Crystal structure at 3.5 A resolution of HIV-1 reverse transcriptase complexed with an inhibitor. Science 1992;256:1783–1790.
18. Spence RA, Kati WM, Anderson KS, et al. Mechanism of inhibition of HIV-1 reverse transcriptase by nonnucleoside inhibitors. Science 1995;267:988–993.
19. Mellors JW, Dutschman GE, Im GJ, et al. In vitro selection and molecular characterization of human immunodeficiency virus-1 resistant to nonnucleoside inhibitors of reverse transcriptase. Mol Pharmacol 1992;41:446–451.
20. Harrold M. Angiotensin-converting enzyme inhibitors, angiotensin antagonists and calcium blockers. In: Lemke T, Williams DA eds. Foye's Principles of Medicinal Chemistry, 6th Ed. Philadelphia, PA: Williams & Wilkins, 2007:738–768.
21. Cushman DW, Cheung HS, Sabo EF, et al. Design of potent competitive inhibitors of angiotensin-converting enzyme. Carboxyalkanoyl and mercaptoalkanoyl amino acids. Biochemistry 1977;16:5484–5491.
22. Byers LD, Wolfenden R. Binding of the by-product analog benzylsuccinic acid by carboxypeptidase A. Biochemistry 1973;12:2070–2078.
23. Patchett AA, Harris E, Tristram EW, et al. A new class of angiotensin-converting enzyme inhibitors. Nature 1980;288:280–283.
24. Wolfenden R. Transition-state analogs for enzyme catalysis. Nature 1969;223:704–705.
25. Wolfenden R. Transition-state analogs as potential affinity labeling agents. Methods Enzymol 1977;46:15–28.
26. Shannon WM, Schabel FM Jr. Antiviral agents as adjuncts in cancer chemotherapy. Pharmacol Ther 1980;11:263–390.
27. Evans BE, Wolfenden RJ. A potential transition-state analog for adenosine deaminase. J Am Chem Soc 1970;92:4751–4752.
28. Nakamura H, Koyama G, Iitaka Y, et al. Structure of coformycin, an unusual nucleoside of microbial origin. J Am Chem Soc 1974;96:4327–4328.
29. Walpole CSJ, Wrigglesworth R. Enzyme inhibitors in medicine. Nat Prod Rep 1989;63:311–346.
30. Baker BR. Design of Active Site Directed Irreversible Enzyme Inhibitors. New York: Wiley, 1967.
31. Walsh C. Recent developments in suicide substrates and other active site–directed inactivating agents of specific target enzymes. Horiz Biochem Biophys 1977;3:36–81.
32. Abeless RH. Suicide enzyme inactivators. Chem Eng News 1983;61:48–55.

33. Rando RR. Mechanism based irreversible enzyme inhibitors. Methods Enzymol 1977;46:28–41.
34. Kraft GA, Katzenellenbogen JA. Synthesis of halo enol lactones. Mechanism-based inactivators of serine proteases. J Am Chem Soc 1981;103:5459–5466.
35. Charnas RL, Knowles JR. Inactivation of RTEM β-lactamase from *Escherichia coli* by clavulanic acid and 9-deoxyclavulanic acid. Biochemistry 1981;20:3214–3219.
36. Rando RR. Mechanisms of naturally occurring irreversible enzyme inhibitors. Acc Chem Res 1975;8:281–288.
37. Bull HG, Garcia-Calvo M, Andersson S, et al. Mechanism-based inhibition of human steroid 5α-reductase by finasteride: enzyme-catalyzed formation of NADP-dihydrofinasteride, a potent bisubstrate analog inhibitor. J Am Chem Soc 1996;118:2359–2365.
38. Bender AT, Beavo JA. Cyclic nucleotide phosphodiesterases: molecular regulation to clinical use. Pharmacol Rev 2006;58:488–520.
39. Lugnier C. Cyclic nucleotide phosphodiesterase (PDE) superfamily: a new target for the development of specific therapeutic agents. Pharmacol Ther 2006;109:366–398.
40. Sutherland EW, Rall TW. Fractionation and characterization of a cyclic adenine ribonucleotide formed by tissue particles. J Biol Chem 1958;232:1077–1091.
41. Card GI, England BP, Suzuki Y, et al. Structural basis for the activity of drugs that inhibit phosphodiesterases. Structure (Camb) 2004;12:2233–2247.
42. Hatzelmann A, Schudt C. Anti-inflammatory and immunomodulatory potential of the novel PDE4 inhibitor roflumilast in vitro. J Pharmacol Exp Ther 2001;297:267–279.
43. Emmons PR, Harrison MJG, Honour AJ, et al. Effect of dipyridamole on human platelet behavior. Lancet 1965;2:603–606.
44. Terrett NK, Bell AS, Brown P, et al. Sildenafil (Viagra), a potent and selective inhibitor of type 5 cGMP phosphodiesterase with utility for the treatment of male erectile dysfunction. Bioorg Med Chem Lett 1996;6:1819–1824.
45. Manning G, Whyte DB, Martinez R, et al. The protein complement of the human genome. Science 2002;298:1912–1934.
46. Noble MEM, Endicott JA, Johnson LN. Protein kinase inhibitors: insights into drug design from structure. Science 2004;303:1800–1805.
47. Sawyers C. Chronic myeloid leukemia. N Eng J Med 1999;340:1330–1340.
48. Zimmermann J, Buchdunger E, Mett H, et al. Phenylamino-pyrimidine (PAP) derivatives: a new class of potent and highly selective PDGF-receptor autophosphorylation inhibitors. Bioorg Med Chem Lett 1996;6:1221–1226.
49. Druker BJ, Tamura J, Buchdunger E, et al. Effects of a selective inhibitor of the ABL tyrosine kinase on the growth of the Bcr-Abl positive cells. Nat Med 1996;2:561–566.
50. Aurora A, Scholar EM. Role of tyrosine kinase inhibitors in cancer therapy. J Pharmacol Exp Ther 2005;315:971–979.
51. Schindler T, Bornmann W, Pellicena P, et al. Structural mechanism for STI-571 inhibition of Abelson tyrosine kinase. Science 2000;289:1938–1942.
52. Nagar B, Bornmann WG, Pellicena P, et al. Crystal structures of the kinases domain of c-Abl in complex with the small molecule inhibitors PD173955 and imatinib (STI-571). Can Res 2002;62:4236–4243.
53. Spitaler M, Cantrell DA. Protein kinase C and beyond. Nat Immunol 2004;5:785–790.
54. Vader G, Lens SMA. The Aurora family in cell division and cancer. Biochem Biophys Acta 2008;1786:60–72.
55. Katayama H, Sen S. Aurora kinase inhibitors as anticancer molecules. Biochem Biophys Acta 2010;1799:829–839.

Suggested Readings

Abeless RH. Suicide enzyme inactivators. Chem Eng News 1983;61:48–55.

Albert A. Selective Toxicity—The physicochemical Basis of Therapy, 7th Ed. New York: Chapman & Hall, 1985.

Baker BR. Design of Active Site Directed Irreversible Enzyme Inhibitors. New York: Wiley, 1967.

Kalman TI, ed. Drug Action & Design—Mechanism-Based Enzyme Inhibitors. New York: Elsevier Science, 1979.

Seiler N, Jung MJ, Kock-Weser J, eds. Enzyme-Activated Irreversible Inhibitors. New York: Elsevier North Holland, 1978.

Silverman RB. The Organic Chemistry of Drug Design and Drug Action, 2nd Ed. New York: Elsevier–Academic Press, 2004.

Silverman RB. The Organic Chemistry of Enzyme Catalyzed Reactions, Revised Ed. London: Academic Press, 2002.

Smith JS, ed. Smith and Williams' Introduction to the Principles of Drug Design and Action, 3rd Ed. Amsterdam: Harwood Academic Press, 1998.

Sneader W. Drug Discovery: A History. New York: John Wiley & Sons, 2005.

Walpole CSJ, Wrigglesworth R. Enzyme inhibitors in medicine. Nat Prod Rep 1989;63:311–346.

Wolfenden R. Transition-state analogs as potential affinity labeling agents. Methods Enzymol 1977;46:15–28.

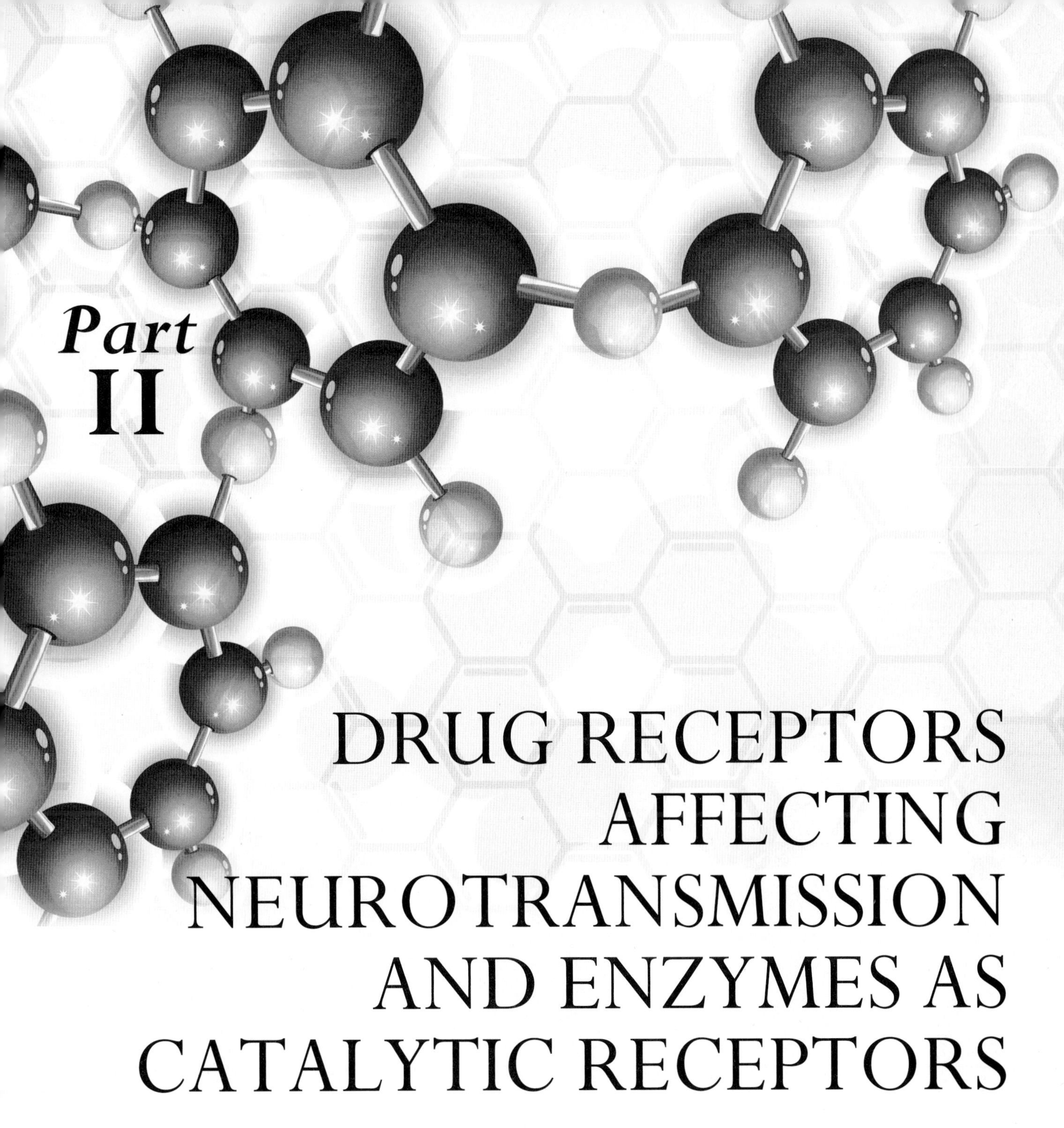

Part II

DRUG RECEPTORS AFFECTING NEUROTRANSMISSION AND ENZYMES AS CATALYTIC RECEPTORS

Chapter 9

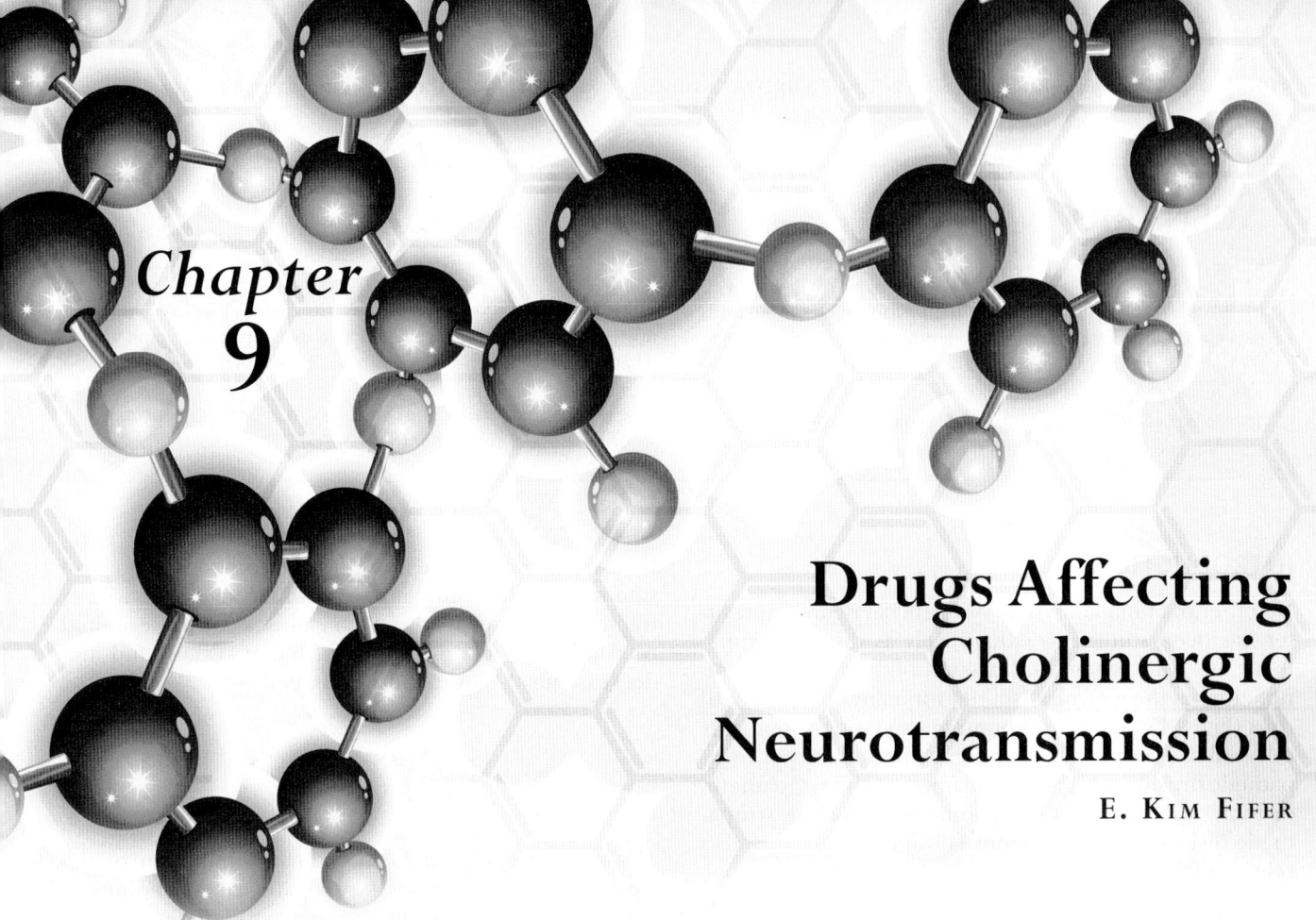

Drugs Affecting Cholinergic Neurotransmission

E. KIM FIFER

Drugs Covered in This Chapter

ACETYLCHOLINE MIMETICS—MUSCARINIC AGONIST
- Methacholine chloride
- Carbachol chloride
- Bethanechol chloride
- Pilocarpine
- Cevimeline

ACETYLCHOLINESTERASE INHIBITORS (ANTICHOLINESTERASES)
- Physostigmine
- Neostigmine
- Pyridostigmine
- Carbaryl
- Edrophonium
- Echothiophate iodide

ACETYLCHOLINESTERASE INHIBITORS FOR THE TREATMENT OF ALZHEIMER DISEASE
- Tacrine
- Donepezil
- Rivastigmine
- Galantamine

INSECTICIDAL ACETYLCHOLINESTERASE INHIBITORS
- Parathion
- Malathion
- Paraoxin
- Schradan
- Dichlofenthion
- Chlorpyrifos

CHOLINESTERASE REACTIVATOR—TREATMENT OF ACETYLCHOLINESTERASE INHIBITOR POISONING
- Pralidoxime chloride

ACETYLCHOLINE ANTAGONISTS—MUSCARINIC ANTAGONISTS
- Atropine
- Scopolamine
- Homatropine
- Tiotropium
- Trospium
- Ipratropium
- Glycopyrrolate
- Procyclidine
- Trihexyphenidyl
- Tolterodine
- Orphenadrine
- Benztropine
- Flavoxate
- Propantheline
- Oxybutynin
- Solifenacin
- Darifenacin
- Fesoterodine

NICOTINIC ANTAGONISTS—NEUROMUSCULAR BLOCKING AGENTS
- Decamethonium bromide
- Succinylcholine chloride
- d-Tubocurarine
- Metocurine
- Pancuronium bromide
- Vecuronium bromide
- Pipecuronium bromide
- Rocuronium bromide
- Atracurium besylate
- Mivacurium chloride
- Doxacurium chloride

Abbreviations

acetyl-S-CoA, acetyl coenzyme A
AChE, acetylcholinesterase
AChEI, acetylcholinesterase inhibitor
AD, Alzheimer disease
ATP, adenosine triphosphate
CNS, central nervous system
CoA, coenzyme A
GABA, γ-aminobutyric acid
GDP, guanosine diphosphate
GPCR, G protein–coupled receptor
GTP, guanosine triphosphate
IP_3, inositol-1,4,5-triphosphate
M, moles/L
mAChR, muscarinic acetylcholinergic receptor
nAChR, nicotinic acetylcholinergic receptor
NM, Neuromuscular (somatic) nAChR
NN, Neuronal Ganglionic nAChR
NMR, nuclear magnetic resonance
2-PAM, 2-pyridine aldoxime methyl chloride
SAR, structure–activity relationship

SCENARIO

Kathryn Neill, PharmD

LT is a 62-year-old man who calls the pharmacy after taking his new medication inappropriately. He brought in a new prescription for tiotropium (Spiriva) 2 days ago. A 1-month supply of capsules was dispensed with the Handihaler inhalation device. LT was counseled regarding proper use and demonstrated good understanding and technique. LT says this morning he "just popped the Spiriva in my mouth with my blood pressure pill and swallowed it." He wants to know if he should take ipecac or try to vomit and whether to take another dose with the inhaler for his lungs.

(The reader is directed to the clinical solution and chemical analysis of this case at the end of the chapter).

INTRODUCTION

No other mammalian system or chemical neurotransmitter has been studied as exhaustively as the parasympathetic nervous system and acetylcholine. Acetylcholine functions as the neurotransmitter for many different neurons (Fig. 9.1) (1). In the autonomic nervous system, it is released by pre- and postganglionic fibers of the parasympathetic division, preganglionic fibers of the sympathetic division, and a few postganglionic fibers of the sympathetic division (e.g., sweat and salivary glands). It is also released by neurons of the somatic (voluntary) nervous system and by some neurons in the CNS. Neurons that release acetylcholine are referred to as cholinergic, as are the receptors on which these neurons synapse. These receptors are further classified as either muscarinic or nicotinic, depending on their ability to bind the naturally occurring alkaloids muscarine or nicotine, respectively.

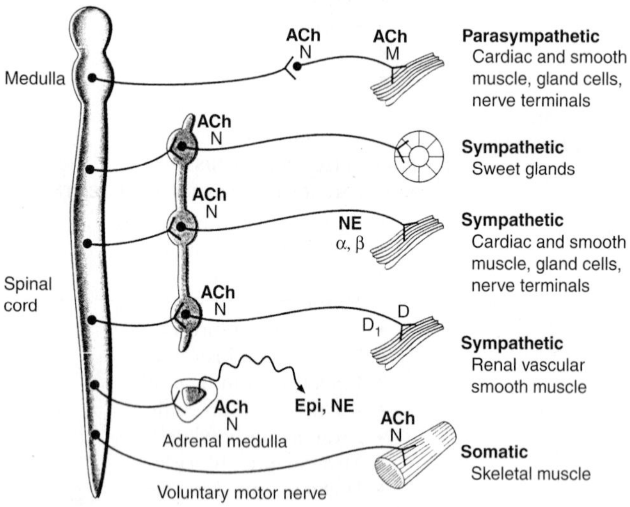

FIGURE 9.1 Schematic representation of autonomic and somatic motor nerves. The sites of action of acetylcholine (ACh), norepinephrine (NE), epinephrine (Epi), and dopamine (D) are indicated. Cholinergic receptors are designated as nicotinic (N) or muscarinic (M). (From Katzung BG. Introduction to autonomic pharmacology. In: Katzung BG, Masters SB, Trevor AJ, eds. Basic and Clinical Pharmacology, 11th Ed. New York: McGraw-Hill, 2009:78, with permission.)

Parasympathetic nerve impulses stimulate contraction of smooth muscle in the gastrointestinal tract and urinary tract, contraction of the ciliary muscle of the eye, and relaxation of smooth muscle of blood vessels, and also decrease heart contractility and rate.

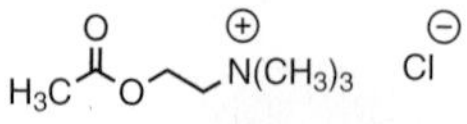

Acetylcholine chloride

Chemical compounds that cause stimulation of the parasympathetic nervous system are called cholinomimetic or, more specifically, parasympathomimetic agents. Cholinomimetic agents are 1) agonists that act directly on cholinergic receptors or 2) function as inhibitors of acetylcholinesterase (AChE), the enzyme responsible for hydrolysis of acetylcholine. Those compounds that possess affinity for cholinergic receptors but exhibit no intrinsic activity are called cholinergic antagonists, cholinolytic, or parasympatholytic agents. This chapter is devoted to the discussion of cholinergic agonists and antagonists and to the biochemistry of cholinergic neurotransmission.

Studies of the parasympathetic nervous system and cholinergic agents led to the concept of neurochemical transmission and were instrumental in the development of early drug receptor hypotheses and our understanding of the stereochemical influence on drug action. An excellent summary of this history is presented by Holmstedt (2).

In 1914, Dale defined two subdivisions of the parasympathetic nervous system when he observed that ethers and esters (including acetylcholine) of choline produced effects similar to those of either muscarine (muscarinic effects) or nicotine (nicotinic effects) (Fig 9.2) (2). The initial experiments were performed using an ergot extract contaminated with acetylcholine, although Dale was unaware of this contamination. Ewins, a chemist who collaborated with Dale, isolated acetylcholine from the ergot extract and subsequently synthesized acetylcholine, thus allowing Dale to show that the unexpected muscarinic effects observed with the ergot preparation were the result of acetylcholine. He proposed the term "parasympathomimetic" to describe the ability of acetylcholine to produce the same effects as electrical stimulation of parasympathetic nerves, and he suggested that

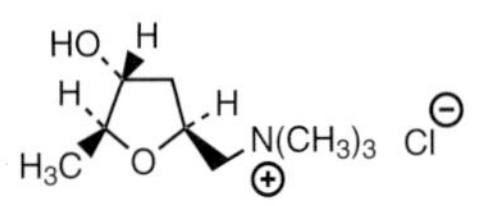

L(+)-Muscarine chloride

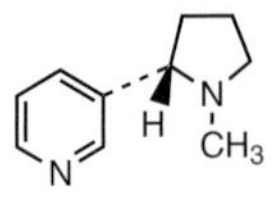

S(-)-Nicotine

FIGURE 9.2 Structures of *L*-(+)-muscarine chloride and (-)-nicotine.

acetylcholine was a chemical neurotransmitter in the parasympathetic nervous system. Dale also observed that the action of acetylcholine was short-lived, and he proposed that tissues contained an esterase that hydrolyzed acetylcholine. In 1921, Loewi (3) demonstrated that a chemical compound mediated impulses between nerves; he referred to the chemical substance in his preparation as *vagusstoff*. In 1926, Loewi and Navratil (4) provided experimental evidence suggesting that vagusstoff was acetylcholine.

These classic studies are the foundation of our current understanding of the role of acetylcholine in cholinergic nerve transmission and our recognition of muscarinic acetylcholinergic receptors (mAChR) and nicotinic acetylcholinergic receptors (nAChRs). These classic studies provided the stimulus for subsequent studies of acetylcholine biochemistry, synthesis of new organic compounds (e.g., cholinergic and anticholinergic drugs), and purification of cholinergic receptors.

The concept that mAChRs and nAChRs can explain the different physiologic responses produced by acetylcholine was derived from this early research of Dale and Loewi. Although it is now recognized that there are multiple subclasses of both mAChRs and nAChRs, the general classification of these two types of cholinergic receptors continues to effectively explain the different physiologic responses produced by acetylcholine.

Because of the important role of acetylcholine as a chemical neurotransmitter in the autonomic nervous system, an imbalance in parasympathetic tone can lead to serious consequences. Conceptually, deficiencies in acetylcholine could be treated by administering the neurotransmitter itself, but acetylcholine is a poor therapeutic agent. Its actions are nonselective, producing effects at all cholinergic receptor sites, which could result in serious consequences for the patient. Because acetylcholine is a quaternary ammonium salt, it is poorly absorbed across biologic membranes, resulting in poor bioavailability regardless of the route of administration. Furthermore, its ester functional group is rapidly hydrolyzed in the acidic conditions of the gastrointestinal tract and by esterases in plasma.

Muscarinic cholinergic agents are used postsurgically to reestablish smooth muscle tone of the gastrointestinal and urinary tracts inorder to relieve abdominal distention and urinary retention. These agents are also used to

CLINICAL SIGNIFICANCE

Agents affecting cholinergic neurotransmission are some of the most widely studied agents to date. They are also one of the most intriguing classes of study in that the clinical utility of these compounds runs the gamut from the life-saving potential of atropine given to patients undergoing cardiac life support to the life-threatening capacity of chemical warfare agents, such as sarin. Advancements in our understanding of muscarinic and nicotinic receptor activity and compounds that modulate these effects have led to decreased morbidity and mortality and enhanced quality of life for millions of individuals throughout the world. In addition, those agents employed as insecticides or pesticides have had tremendous economic impact. Agents affecting cholinergic neurotransmission are used to treat a variety of clinical conditions, including impaired or excessive gastric motility/secretion, glaucoma, bradycardia, Alzheimer's disease, Parkinson's disease, and myasthenia gravis. Nicotinic antagonists are used to facilitate surgical procedures by reducing the amount of anesthetic or sedative agent required, thus reducing risk to the patient. A thorough understanding of the structure–activity relationships of these compounds has led to an ability to enhance their desired pharmacodynamic effects while minimizing unwanted or harmful adverse effects.

For the clinician, the impact of the application of this knowledge is multifaceted. Examples include the synthesis of newer chemical compounds used to treat Alzheimer's disease that provide greater affinity for acetylcholinesterase in the brain than in the periphery, decrease the frequency of dosing required, and alleviate the risk of hepatotoxicity associated with the first Alzheimer's agent, tacrine. These advances have increased the utility of these agents and given hope to countless individuals and families affected by this devastating disease. Modifications to neuromuscular blocking agents have resulted in differences in onset and length of activity, reduction in adverse effects (e.g., hypotension), and alternate routes of elimination, which increase their utility for patients with certain comorbid conditions (e.g., cardiac disease or renal dysfunction). Finally, it is important for the clinician to recognize the capacity of certain chemical configurations to be allergenic or more prone to producing adverse effects so the best agent for a particular patient can be selected.

Kathryn Neill, Pharm.D.
Hospital Experiential Director
Assistant Professor
Critical Care Specialist
Department of Pharmacy Practice
College of Pharmacy
University of Arkansas for Medical Sciences
Little Rock, AR

treat some forms of glaucoma by enhancing the outflow of aqueous humor, thereby reducing intraocular pressure. Cholinomimetic compounds with central nervous system (CNS) activity are used for the treatment of cognitive disorders (e.g., Alzheimer disease). Those that exhibit nicotinic effects are commonly used to treat myasthenia gravis.

Cholinergic muscarinic antagonists (anticholinergic drugs) are sometimes referred to as antispasmodics due to their ability to reduce smooth muscle spasms resulting from overstimulation of the gastrointestinal smooth muscles. Newer drugs in this class have found use in the treatment of overactive bladder.

Many synthetic cholinergic agonists have been designed using structure–activity relationships (SARs) based on the structure of acetylcholine. To design cholinergic agents that are selective for specific cholinergic receptors, it is necessary to have a thorough understanding of acetylcholine neurochemistry as well as the chemical nature and role of cholinergic receptors.

CHOLINERGIC RECEPTORS

History

Knowledge of the structure and function of cholinergic receptors has increased substantially since the concept of distinct mAChRs and nAChRs was first postulated. Early efforts to describe these receptors were hindered in that receptors were only a concept. Indeed, the existence of receptors was not established until 1973, when Pert and Snyder (5) provided demonstrable evidence for the existence of opiate receptors.

Early attempts to characterize cholinergic receptors were based on SAR and stereochemical studies of cholinergic agonists and antagonists. This led to synthesis of agonists and antagonists with exceptionally high affinity and selectivity for cholinergic receptors as well as to synthesis of radiolabeled cholinergic ligands with high specific radioactivity. Parallel advances in biochemistry, molecular pharmacology, and molecular biology made possible purification and sequencing of small quantities of protein, measurement of ligand binding to cell membranes and subcellular components, and cloning and sequencing of genes. This led to isolation, purification, and amino acid sequencing of one of the nAChRs—the first acetylcholine receptor and the first neurotransmitter receptor to be fully characterized (6,7). Subsequently, mAChRs were isolated, purified, and sequenced using these techniques.

Current research in pharmacology and molecular biology indicates that multiple mAChR and nAChR subtypes exist (8,9). However, the traditional classification of mAChRs and nAChRs adequately describes the actions of most cholinergic medicinal agents and is used throughout this chapter. Furthermore, most of the current therapeutic agents acting at mAChRs exhibit little selectivity for the receptor subtypes, with the exception of a few recently introduced anticholinergic agents for treatment of overactive bladder.

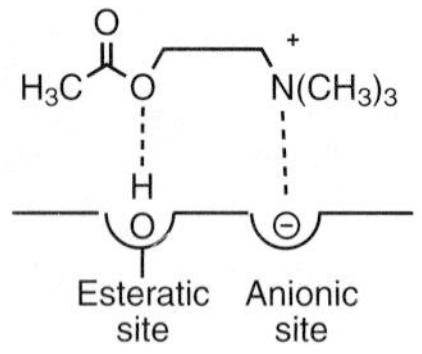

FIGURE 9.3 Original representation of the mAChR.

Muscarinic Receptors

The SAR regarding affinity and efficacy of cholinergic agonists provided the basis for early models of mAChR structure. An early model of the mAChR, depicted in Figure 9.3, illustrates the importance of muscarinic agonists having an ester functional group and a quaternary ammonium group separated by two carbons. This model depicts ionic bonding between the positively charged quaternary nitrogen of acetylcholine and a negative charge at the anionic site of the receptor. The negative charge was suggested to result from a carboxylate ion from the free carboxyl group of a dicarboxylic amino acid (e.g., aspartate or glutamate) at the binding site on the receptor protein. This model also involved a hydrogen bond between the ester oxygen of acetylcholine and a hydroxyl group contributed by the esteratic site of the receptor.

Although this early mAChR model accounted for two important SAR requirements for muscarinic agonists, it failed to explain the following: 1) at least two of the alkyl groups bonded to the quaternary nitrogen must be methyl groups; 2) the known stereochemical requirements for agonist binding to the receptor; and 3) the fact that all potent cholinergic agonists have only five atoms between the quaternary nitrogen and the terminal hydrogen atom. This last point is known as Ing's "Rule of Five" (10).

Subsequent models of the mAChR have depicted the receptor as a binding site on a protein molecule and explained more completely the structural and stereochemical requirements for cholinergic agonist activity. Interestingly, it was once proposed that the mAChR and AChE were the same entity, but this proposal was dispelled by experiments demonstrating that interaction of cholinergic ligands with the mAChR did not lead to hydrolysis of the ligand. None of these models, however, completely explained the diverse pharmacologic effects produced by all muscarinic agonists and antagonists.

Subsequent developments suggested that mAChR stimulation results in at least two important events: 1) inhibition of adenylyl cyclase*, and 2) activation of phospholipase C and subsequent biosynthesis of second messengers. Both involve a guanosine triphosphate (GTP)-dependent mechanism. Two other important developments that helped characterize mAChRs were the synthesis of radiolabeled muscarinic ligands and the utilization of molecular biology techniques.

*This enzyme is known by two names, *adenylate cyclase (EC 4.6.1.1)*, its official name from the International Union of Biochemistry and Molecular Biology Nomenclature Committee, or its alternative name, *adenylyl cyclase*.

Heterogeneity in the mAChR population was first suggested in the late 1970s during pharmacologic studies using the muscarinic antagonist pirenzepine. At the time, pirenzepine was the only muscarinic antagonist to block gastric acid secretion at concentrations that did not block the effects of muscarinic agonists. This observation initiated research that ultimately led to discovery of mAChR subtypes, designated as M_1, M_2, and M_3 based on their pharmacologic responses to various ligands. Rapid advances in molecular biology led to cloning of cDNAs that encoded for five mAChRs, designated as m1 through m5; m1, m2, and m3 correspond to the respective M_1 through M_3 receptors identified by their pharmacologic specificity. The International Union of Pharmacology Committee on Receptor Nomenclature and Drug Classification has recommended that the uppercase nomenclature M_1 through M_5 be used to designate both pharmacologic and molecular subtypes (8).

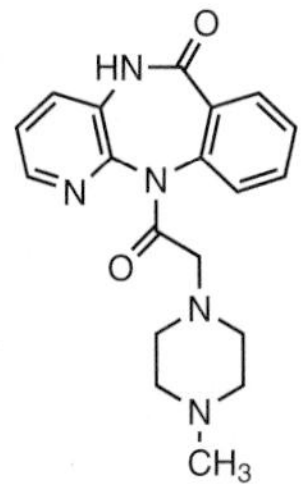

Pirenzepine

All mAChR subtypes (M_1 to M_5) are found in the CNS, whereas other tissues can contain more than one. These receptors are summarized in Table 9.1 (11). As more mAChR subtypes have been discovered, it has become apparent that there is a lack of known antagonists exhibiting "very high subtype selectivity" and that there "are no muscarinic agonists with high selectivity" (8). Thus, proof for involvement of any one receptor subtype in a given system currently requires use of more than one antagonist. Additionally, if the selectivity of a novel muscarinic antagonist or putative agonist is to be assessed, it should be through use of recombinant mAChRs expressed in cell lines rather than with native receptors.

Cloning and sequencing of genes encoding mAChRs have led to major advances in understanding of their chemical nature and function (8,12–14). These experiments demonstrated that mAChRs are coupled to guanine nucleotide–binding proteins and are referred to as G protein–coupled receptors (GPCR) (8,15,16). The guanine nucleotide regulatory protein to which the receptors are coupled has three subunits (α, β, and γ) that link the receptor to effectors that produce second messenger molecules within the cell. Binding of muscarinic agonists to GPCRs leads to a variety of effector responses (see below). The ultimate observable response is a function of the tissue where the receptor is located.

Amino acid sequences of mAChR proteins expressed by cloned genes for the GPCRs have been deduced from the base sequence of the respective genes. These GPCRs are components of the cell membrane and consist of seven hydrophobic transmembrane helical domains as well as hydrophilic extracellular and intracellular domains (17). The N-terminus of the GPCR protein is extracellular, and the C-terminus is intracellular. This proposed arrangement and the deduced amino acid sequence for the human type M_1 mAChR has been reported (12). Computer-assisted molecular modeling has made it possible to obtain three-dimensional models of the mAChR (17); a proposed top-view model of the M_1 mAChR is shown in Figure 9.4 (18). This model suggests that the quaternary nitrogen of acetylcholine participates in an ionic bond with the free carboxylate group of an aspartate residue (ASP105 in transmembrane domain 3)—one of the receptor functional groups that was originally hypothesized to be involved in receptor binding of acetylcholine.

A current model for mAChRs that better describes signal transduction is illustrated in Figure 9.5 (14). In this model, acetylcholine binds to the mAChR located in the cell membrane, and this ligand–receptor interaction is translated, presumably by a conformational perturbation, through the receptor protein to the receptor-coupled guanine nucleotide regulatory protein (G protein). A relationship between the guanine nucleotide regulatory protein and the effector is illustrated in Figure 9.6. In this scheme, the G protein is in the inactive state, with guanosine diphosphate (GDP) bound to its α subunit. Upon interaction of an agonist with the mAChR, the α subunit releases GDP and binds GTP. The α subunit–GTP complex then dissociates from the βγ subunits. Both the α subunit–GTP complex and the βγ subunits interact with membrane-bound effectors (phospholipase C or adenylate cyclase) or ion channels (K^+ and Ca^{2+}), either independently or in a parallel manner. The α subunit possesses GTPase activity and quickly hydrolyzes the GTP to GDP to terminate signal transmission, at which time the α, β, and γ subunits reassociate and migrate back to the receptor protein. Characteristics of the α subunit determine the classification of the particular G protein:

G_s increases adenylyl cyclase activity and increases Ca^{2+} currents;
G_i decreases adenylyl cyclase activity and increases K^+ currents;
G_o decreases Ca^{2+} currents; and
G_q increases phospholipase C activity.

The βγ subunits are involved with receptor-operated K^+ currents and with activity of adenylyl cyclase and phospholipase C.

Signal transduction at the stimulatory "odd-numbered" mAChRs (i.e., M_1, M_3, and M_5) is via coupling with a $G_{q/11}$ protein that is involved with mobilization of intracellular calcium. Agonist binding to these receptors results in activation of phospholipase C, with subsequent production of the second messengers, diacylglycerol and inositol-1,4,5-triphosphate (IP_3). Stimulation of IP_3 ion channel receptors leads to release of intracellular calcium from the endoplasmic reticulum. The diacylglycerol

TABLE 9.1 Muscarinic Acetylcholine receptor Subtypes[a]

Receptor	G Protein	Tissue Location	Cellular Response	Function
M_1	$G_{q/11}$	CNS, gastric and salivary glands, autonomic ganglia, enteric nerves	PLC activation (↑IP_3 & ↑DAG → ↑Ca^{2+} & PKC); depolarization and excitation (↑sEPSP); PLA_2 and PLD_2 activation; ↑AA	↑ Cognitive function ↑ Seizure activity ↑ Secretions ↑ Autonomic ganglia depolarization ↓ DA release and locomotion
M_2	G_i/G_o	Autonomic nerve terminals; CNS; heart; smooth muscle	Inhibition of adenylyl cyclase (↓cAMP) & voltage-gated Ca^{2+} channels; activation of inwardly rectifying K^+ channels	↓ Heart rate ↑ Smooth muscle contraction Neural inhibition in periphery via autoreceptors and heteroreceptor ↓ Ganglionic transmission Neural inhibition in CNS ↑ Tremors, hypothermi,a & analgesia
M_3	$G_{q/11}$	CNS (less than other mAChRs), smooth muscle, glands, heart	Same as M_1	↑ Smooth muscle contraction (e.g., bladder) ↑ Salivary gland secretion ↑ Food intake, body fat deposits Inhibits dopamine release Synthesis of nitric oxide
M_4	G_i/G_o	CNS	Same as M_2	Inhibition of autoreceptor- and heteroreceptor-mediated transmitter release in CNS Analgesia Cataleptic activity Facilitates dopamine release
M_5	$G_{q/11}$	Low levels in CNS & periphery; predominate mAChRs in dopaminergic neurons of substantia nigra & ventral tegmentum area	Same as M_1	Mediates dilation of cerebral arteries Facilitates dopamine release Augments drug-seeking behavior and reward

[a]CNS, central nervous system; PLC, Phospholipase C; IP_3 inositol-1, 4, 5-triphosphate; DAG, diacylglycerol; PLD_2 phospholipase D; AA, arachidonic acid; PKC, protein kinase C; sEPSP, slow excitatory postsynaptic potential; mAChRs, muscarinic acetylcholine receptor subtypes; PLA, phospholipase A; cAMP, cyclic adenosine monophosphate; VTA, ventral tegmentum area.
Adapted from Westfall TC, Westfall DP, Neurotransmission: the autonomic and somatic motor nervous systems. In: Brunton LL, Lazo JS. Parker KL, eds. Goodman and Gilman's The Pharmacological Basis of Therapeutics, 11th Ed. New York: McGraw-Hill, 2006, pp. 137-181; with permission.

produced, along with calcium, activates protein kinase C, which phosphorylates proteins to afford various physiologic responses. The M_1, M_3, and M_5 receptors also stimulate phospholipase A_2 and phospholipase D. Activation of phospholipase A_2 results in release of arachidonic acid, with subsequent synthesis of eicosanoids (C_{20} fatty acids).

The "even-numbered" mAChR subtypes (i.e., M_2 and M_4) are coupled to G_i/G_o proteins, whose activation inhibits adenylyl cyclase. This results in a decrease in cyclic adenosine monophosphate, inhibition of voltage-gated calcium channels, and activation of inwardly rectifying potassium channels (19). The result is hyperpolarization and inhibition of these excitable membranes.

The M_1 receptors are sometimes described as "neural" due to their abundance in the cerebral cortex, hippocampus, and striatum. M_1 receptors have been implicated in Alzheimer disease and are thought to be involved with memory and learning. Early studies suggested that the agonist McN-A-343 was selective for the M_1 receptor, but more recent evidence indicates otherwise. It can show moderate selectivity for M_4 receptors. Additionally, M_1 receptors are found at autonomic ganglia, enteric nerves, and salivary and gastric glands. Agonists at M_1 receptors show the greatest promise for treatment of the cholinergic deficit associated with Alzheimer disease.

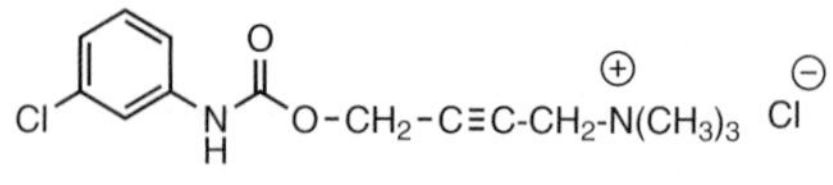

McN-A-343

M_2 receptors are found in abundance in the heart, where activation exerts both negative chronotropic and inotropic actions, and stimulate contraction of smooth muscle. Activation of M_2 autoreceptors located on nerve

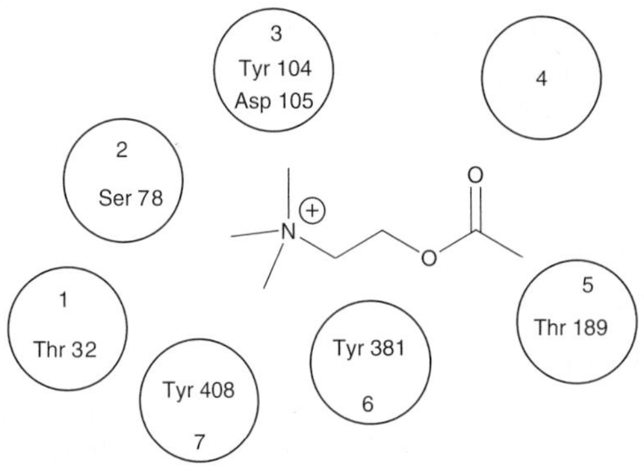

FIGURE 9.4 Model of acetylcholine interaction with muscarinic M_1 receptor. Circles represent seven transmembrane domains (18).

terminals affords neural inhibition by decreasing acetylcholine release.

M_3 receptors are found in abundance in smooth muscle and glands, where their stimulation leads to contraction and secretion, respectively. Knowledge of this effect on smooth muscle of the bladder has led to development and subsequent approval of several M_3 receptor antagonists for treatment of overactive bladder (see below). Although widely distributed in the CNS, their concentration in the CNS is lower than those of other mAChRs. M_3 mAChRs function to decrease neurotransmitter release.

M_4 receptors are found in the striatum and basal forebrain, where they decrease transmitter release in both the CNS and periphery. Their activation in smooth muscle and secretary glands leads to inhibition of potassium and calcium channels.

M_5 receptors are the least characterized of the mAChRs, and there is evidence for their existence in the CNS and periphery, whereby they can regulate dopamine release in the CNS.

Nicotinic Receptors

nAChRs are found at the skeletal neuromuscular junction, adrenal medulla, and autonomic ganglia. nAChRs have been the focus of intensive research interest, even though the majority of clinically effective cholinergic medicinal agents are either muscarinic agonists or antagonists (20). The best known nicotinic agonist is nicotine, which is an alkaloid obtained from *Nicotiana tabacum* plant. (Fig. 9.2). Interest in nAChRs stems from the availability of the receptor protein from the electric organs of the electric eel (*Electrophorus electricus*) and the marine ray (*Torpedo californica*) and the important role they play in myasthenia gravis, an autoimmune disease.

The multiplicity of nAChRs is based on different structural requirements for agonists and antagonists acting at the autonomic ganglia and the skeletal neuromuscular junction and is supported by molecular biology research (20). Both ganglionic neuronal (NN) and neuromuscular (somatic muscle) (NM) nAChRs are classified as ligand-gated ion channel receptors that are structurally and functionally related to other ligand-gated ion channel receptors, such as those for γ-aminobutyric acid (GABA), 5-hydroxytryptamine (serotonin), and glycine (21). The nAChR creates a transmembrane ion channel (the gate), and acetylcholine (the ligand) serves as a gatekeeper by binding with the nAChR to modulate passage of ions, principally K^+ and Na^+, through the channel.

The nAChR was the first neurotransmitter receptor to be isolated and purified in the active form using the same molecular biologic techniques described earlier for isolation and purification of mAChRs. The primary sequence of nAChRs has been deduced from cloning and sequencing of genes that encode their receptor proteins (22,23). nAChRs are pentameric transmembrane proteins made up of subunits designated as α, β, γ (or ε), and δ (24).

The nAChR of skeleton (somatic) muscle tissue is a transmembrane glycoprotein consisting of four types of subunits—α, β, γ (or ε), and δ. Only the α_1 subtype of the α subunit is present in muscle. In a mature muscle end plate, the γ subunit is replaced by an ε subunit. This change in gene expression encoding the γ and ε subunits affects ligand selectivity along with receptor turnover and/or tissue location.

One class of neuronal nAChRs exists as a heteromeric pentamer composed of α (α_2 to α_6) and β (β_2 to β_4) subunits (25–27)—for example, $\alpha_4\beta_3$ with a stoichiometry of two α_4 and three β_3 subunits. Another class of functional homomeric nAChRs is composed of α_7 through α_{10} subunits. The diversity of the subunits and the pentameric structure suggest that a large number of nAChR subtypes can exist.

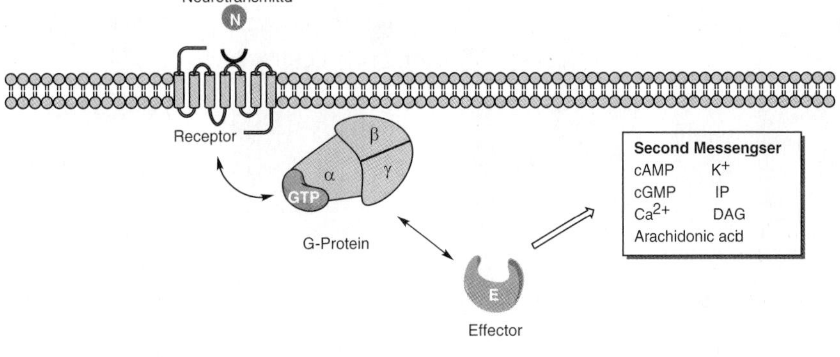

FIGURE 9.5 Model of signal transduction by a G protein–coupled receptor. This illustrates a proposed relationship between receptor, G protein, effector, and various second messengers.

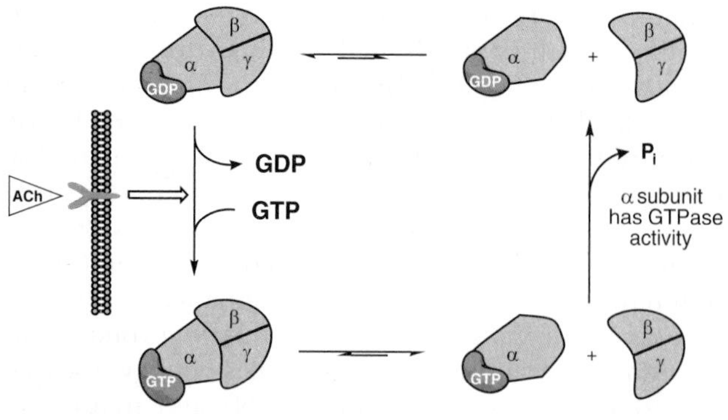

FIGURE 9.6 Diagram of a GTPase cycle and subunit association/dissociation proposed to control signal transduction between muscarinic G protein–coupled receptors and the effector. The acetylcholine (ACh)–receptor interaction facilitates GTP binding and activates the α subunit. The α subunit–GTP complex then dissociates from the βγ subunit, and each is free to activate effector proteins. The duration of separation is determined by the rate of α subunit–mediated GTP hydrolysis.

The five subunits of each nAChR protein in muscle tissue are arranged around a central pore that serves as the ion channel. Based on molecular modeling of the deduced primary structure of the individual subunits, it has been proposed that each subunit [α, β, γ (or ε), and δ] possesses a hydrophilic extracellular N-terminus, a hydrophilic intracellular C-terminus, and four α helical hydrophobic transmembrane domains (M_1 to M_4) (Fig. 9.7) (26,28). (Note: Do not confuse these transmembrane domains of the nAChRs with the domains of the mAChRs.) A pentameric arrangement of these five amphipathic subunits makes up the walls of the ion channel. Two acetylcholine binding sites exist on the extracellular domain of each nAChR molecule. In Figure 9.7, one binding site is located on each α subunit at the αγ and αδ interfaces (28). The binding sites show a positive cooperativity, even though the binding sites are not adjacent to each other in the pentameric receptor. Some central and peripheral nAChR subtypes are summarized in Table 9.2 (11).

Our knowledge and understanding of mAChR and nAChRs have advanced tremendously from the time when these receptors were only ethereal concepts. This understanding provides the basis for the rational design of new selective therapeutic agents to treat diseases associated with cholinergic neurons.

DRUGS AFFECTING CHOLINERGIC NEUROTRANSMISSION

Acetylcholine Neurochemistry

The neurochemistry of acetylcholine includes its biosynthesis, storage, release, and metabolism. These are illustrated in Figure 9.8.

Biosynthesis

Acetylcholine is biosynthesized in cholinergic neurons by the enzyme-catalyzed transfer of the acetyl group from acetyl coenzyme A (acetyl-*S*-CoA) to choline, a quaternary ammonium alcohol (Fig. 9.9) (29). The enzyme catalyzing this reaction, choline acetyltransferase, is also biosynthesized in the cholinergic neuron. Choline used for biosynthesis of acetylcholine in the CNS comes from several sources. About 35% to 50% of the choline produced by AChE-catalyzed hydrolysis of acetylcholine in the synaptic space is transported into the neuron (see below). This accounts for about half of the choline required for acetylcholine synthesis (30). Two stores of choline are the lipid phosphatidylcholine, found in the plasma, and phosphorylcholine, stored in lipid. Although, choline will not cross the blood–brain barrier, phosphatidylcholine and phosphorylcholine will. Once in the CNS, these phosphatidylcholine esters can be hydrolyzed to afford choline (30). Choline can be biosynthesized from the amino acid serine (Fig. 9.9), but most of the choline used to form acetylcholine is recycled after AChE-catalyzed hydrolysis of acetylcholine in the synaptic space. The choline acetyltransferase-catalyzed reaction is not the rate-limiting step in acetylcholine biosynthesis. Active uptake of choline into the neuron is rate-determining. Choline is taken up into cells by both low-affinity and high-affinity transport sites. The low-affinity (K_m = 10 to 100 μM) transporter is found

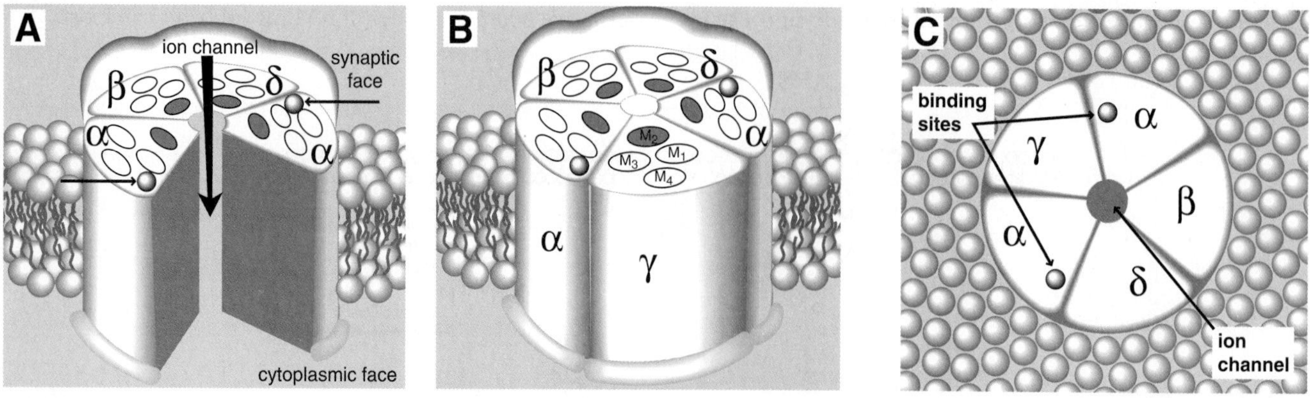

FIGURE 9.7 nAChR: (A) Longitudinal view (γ subunit removed) showing the internal ion channel. Acetylcholine binding sites on the α subunits are indicated by the arrows. These are located at the αγ and αγ interfaces. (B) Each of the five transmembrane subunits (α, α, β, δ, and γ) are composed of four hydrophobic membrane spanning segments (M_1 to M_4). (C) Top view of the nAChR showing the subunits surrounding the ion channel.

TABLE 9.2 Nicotinic Acetylcholine Receptor Subtypes

Receptor	Location	Membrane Response	Molecular Mechanism	Agonists	Antagonists
Neuromuscular (N_M) $(\alpha_1)_2\beta_1\epsilon\delta$ $(\alpha_1)_2\beta_1\gamma\delta$	Skeletal (somatic) neuro-muscular junction (postjunctional)	Excitatory; end plate depolarization; contraction (skeletal muscle)	Increased Na^+ & K^+ permeability	ACh; nicotine; succinylcholine	Atracurium; Vecuronium; *d*-tubocurarine; pancuronium; α-conotoxin; α-bungarotoxin
Ganglionic neuronal (N_N) $(\alpha_3)_2(\beta_4)_3$	Autonomic ganglia; adrenal medulla	Excitatory; depolarization firing of postganglionic neuron; depolarization & secretion of catecholamines	Increased Na^+ & K^+ permeability	ACh; nicotine; epibatidine; dimethylphenyl-piperazinium	Trimethaphan; mecamylamine; dihydro-β erythrodine; erysodine lophotoxin
Central neuronal $(\alpha_4)_2(\beta_4)_3$ (α-bungarotoxin insensitive)	CNS; pre- & postjunctional	Pre- & postsynaptic excitation; prejunctinal control of transmitter release	Increased Na^+ & K^+ permeability	Cytisine; epibatidine; Anatoxin A	
$(\alpha_7)_5$ (α-bungarotoxin sensitive)	CNS; pre- and postsynaptic	Same as central neuronal	Increased Ca^{2+} permeability	Anatoxin A	Methyllycaconities α-conotoxin; α-bungarotoxin

Adapted from Westfall TC, Westfall DP. Neurotransmission: the autonomic and somatic motor nervous systems. In: Brunton LL, Lazo JS. Parker KL, eds. Goodman and Gilman's The Pharmacological Basis of Therapeutics, 11th Ed. New York: McGraw-Hill, 2006. pp. 137–181; with permission.

in cells that synthesize choline-containing phospholipids (e.g., corneal epithelium). The high-affinity (K_m = 1 to 5 μM) transporter is a sodium-choline cotransporter and is found in cholinergic nerve endings, where it is responsible for uptake of most of the choline recycled from the synapse (30). Because this high-affinity uptake site is saturable at greater than 10 μM, the rate of choline uptake by the neuron is limited. Thus, choline uptake is considered to be the rate-determining step in biosynthesis of acetylcholine. Hemicholinium-3 is a research tool that inhibits reuptake of choline at high-affinity uptake sites.

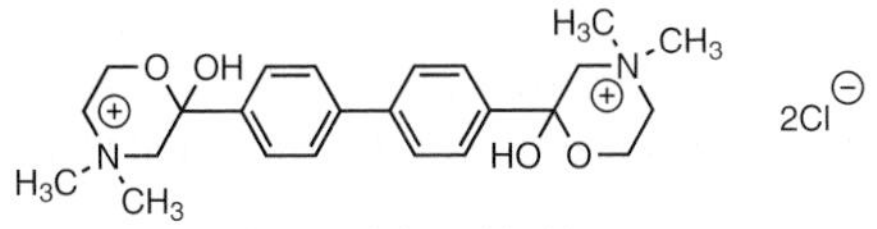

Hemicholinium chloride

Storage

Most newly biosynthesized acetylcholine is actively transported into cytosolic storage vesicles located in presynaptic nerve endings, where it is maintained with adenosine triphosphate (ATP) (10:1 ratio) along with calcium and magnesium ions until it is released. Some acetylcholine remains in the cytosol and eventually is hydrolyzed. Only the stored form serves as the functional neurotransmitter.

EFFORTS TO MODULATE ACETYLCHOLINE BIOSYNTHESIS

Efforts to develop therapeutic agents based on regulation of acetylcholine biosynthesis have not been successful. Dexpanthenol, the dextrorotatory enantiomer of the alcohol derived from pantothenic acid (a vitamin), was once used as a cholinomimetic agent to help reestablish normal smooth muscle tone in the gastrointestinal tract following surgery. Pantothenic acid is essential for the biosynthesis of coenzyme A (CoA). The apparent rationale for the therapeutic use of dexpanthenol was that it would be biotransformed to pantothenic acid, which would be incorporated into CoA. This would lead to increased intracellular levels of acetyl CoA, which would facilitate increased biosynthesis of acetylcholine. The limited therapeutic success of dexpanthenol, difficulty with administration, and effectiveness of synthetic cholinergic agonists led to its discontinuation. The quaternary pyridinium salt, *trans*-*N*-methyl-4-(1-naphthylvinyl)pyridinium iodide, is an effective inhibitor of choline acetyltransferase in vitro, but it has proven to be a poor inhibitor in whole animal experiments.

Although efforts have been made to design cholinergic agents based on the mechanism of biosynthesis of acetylcholine, such agents would be expected to have nonselective effects, because it currently is thought that acetylcholine is biosynthesized by the same mechanism in all cholinergic neurons.

Release

Release of acetylcholine from the storage vesicles is initiated by an action potential that has traveled down the axon to the presynaptic nerve membrane. This action potential leads to opening of voltage-dependent calcium channels, affording an influx of Ca^{2+} and exocytotic release of acetylcholine into the synapse. The increase in intracellular Ca^{2+} can induce fusion of acetylcholine storage vesicles with the presynaptic membrane before release of the neurotransmitter. Each synaptic vesicle contains a quantum of acetylcholine; one quantum represents between 12,000 and 60,000 molecules of

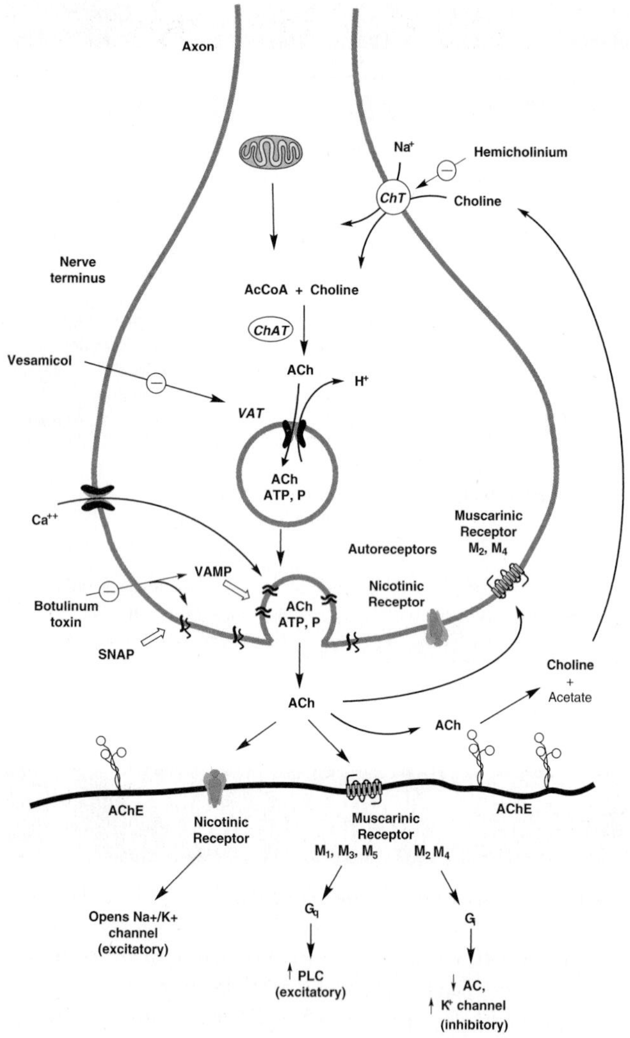

FIGURE 9.8 General cholinergic nerve junction showing location of receptor sites and biosynthesis, storage, release, and hydrolysis of acetylcholine.

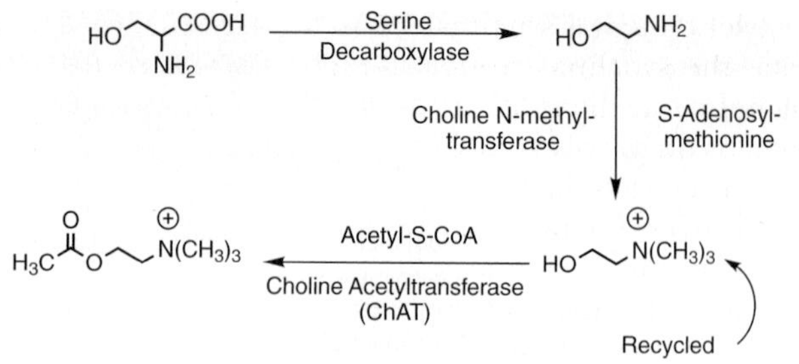

FIGURE 9.9 Biosynthesis of acetylcholine.

Stereochemistry

One shortcoming of early models for cholinergic receptors was that they did not account for the observed stereoselectivity of the receptors for agonist and antagonist ligands. Even though acetylcholine is achiral, many synthetic and naturally occurring agonists and antagonists possess chirality; usually, one enantiomer is many times more active than the other. It was apparent to early receptor investigators that the stereochemistry of cholinergic ligands was important for receptor binding. In this regard, the stereochemical–activity relationships of cholinergic ligands have been studied extensively to provide a rational basis for design of cholinergic drugs as well as to describe the properties and functions of cholinergic receptors.

The stereochemistry of acetylcholine resides in the different arrangements in space of its atoms by virtue of rotation about σ bonds (i.e., conformational isomerism). Because of relatively unrestricted rotation about these single covalent bonds, acetylcholine can exist in an infinite number of conformations. Most studies of the conformational isomerism of acetylcholine have focused on torsion angles between the ester oxygen atom and the quaternary nitrogen resulting from rotation about the Cα–Cβ bond. Four of these conformations are illustrated by Newman projections in Figure 9.10.

Nuclear magnetic resonance (NMR) studies in aqueous solution revealed that the preferred conformation between the ester oxygen and the quaternary nitrogen of

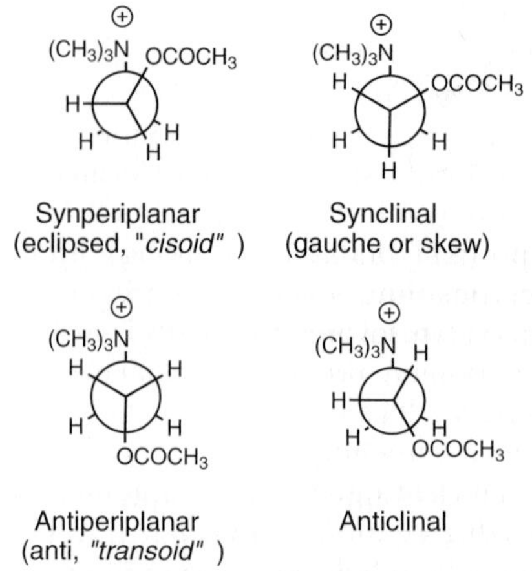

FIGURE 9.10 Conformational isomers of acetylcholine.

acetylcholine. A single action potential causes release of several hundred quanta of acetylcholine into the synapse.

Metabolism

Acetylcholine in the synapse can bind with cholinergic receptors on postsynaptic or presynaptic membranes to produce a response. Free acetylcholine that is not bound to a receptor is hydrolyzed by AChE. Hydrolysis is the physiologic mechanism for terminating the action of acetylcholine. Enough AChE is present in the synapse to hydrolyze approximately 3×10^8 molecules of acetylcholine in 1 millisecond; thus, adequate enzyme activity exists to hydrolyze all the acetylcholine (~3×10^6 molecules) released by one action potential. A number of useful therapeutic cholinomimetic agents have been developed based on the ability of the compounds to inhibit AChE; these agents are addressed later in this chapter.

acetylcholine was synclinal (gauche or skew). Using x-ray data, the synclinal conformation was observed for acetylcholine in the solid crystalline state as well. The same conclusion was also obtained for the preferred conformation of acetylcholine using molecular orbital calculations. These experimental and theoretical determinations of the acetylcholine conformation differ from the antiperiplanar conformation that might be expected when using molecular models to visualize minimum steric interactions. The synclinal conformation would be stabilized by intramolecular electrostatic interactions between the quaternary nitrogen and the carbonyl oxygen.

It must be emphasized that the experimentally determined synclinal conformation of acetylcholine is only that measured in aqueous solution (NMR) or the crystalline state (x-ray). This might not be the conformation preferred by the receptors. Indeed, the conformation of receptor-bound acetylcholine could be much different and might not be a thermodynamically preferred conformation.

In recognition of this possibility, conformationally restricted acetylcholine analogs have been synthesized and pharmacologically evaluated in an effort to determine the conformation of acetylcholine when it binds to cholinergic receptors. The most significant study in this regard is that of Armstrong et al. (31), who synthesized and evaluated the muscarinic and nicotinic activity of *cis*- and *trans*-isomers of a conformationally rigid model of acetylcholine, *cis*- and *trans*-2-acetoxycyclopropyl-1-trimethylammonium iodide (ACTM). Because this model is based on the cyclopropane ring, the ester and quaternary ammonium functional groups cannot change their relative positions by bond rotation. The *cis*- and *trans*-isomers are rigidly constrained to the conformations shown. The *cis*-isomer is similar to the synperiplanar conformation of acetylcholine, and the *trans*-isomer approximates the anticlinal conformation. The (+)-*trans*-enantiomer was observed to be equally as or more potent, depending on the pharmacologic test used, than acetylcholine at mAChRs; it was much more potent than the (−)-*trans*-enantiomer. The racemic *cis*-compound had almost no activity in the same mAChR test system, and all compounds were very weak nicotinic agonists.

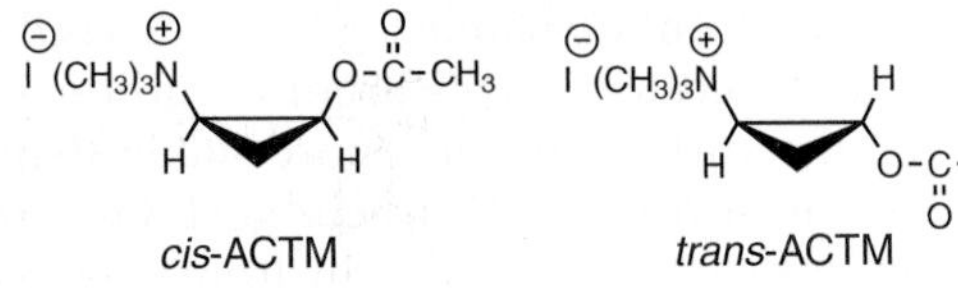

cis-ACTM *trans*-ACTM

The important conclusion drawn from this study (31) was that acetylcholine would most probably interact with mAChRs in its less favored anticlinal conformation. The most active isomer, the (+)-*trans*-enantiomer, of these cyclopropane analogs was found to have a torsion angle of 137 degrees (anticlinal) between the ester oxygen and the quaternary nitrogen. This is significantly different from the 60-degree torsion angle in the synclinal conformation found by NMR and x-ray determinations to be the preferred conformation.

Stereochemistry of cholinergic ligands and stereoselectivity of receptors has played an important role in design of cholinergic ligands as therapeutic agents. This role becomes apparent in subsequent sections.

Acetylcholine Mimetics—Muscarinic Agonists

Interaction of cholinergic agonists with mAChRs leads to well-defined pharmacologic responses depending on the tissue or organ in which the receptor is located. These responses include contractions of smooth muscle, vasodilation, increased secretion from exocrine glands, miosis, and decreased heart rate and force of contraction.

Acetylcholine

Acetylcholine is the prototypical muscarinic and nicotinic agonist, because it is the physiologic chemical neurotransmitter for the cholinergic nervous system. However, it is a poor therapeutic agent due to its lack of specificity for nAChRs or mAChRs and due to the chemical and physicochemical properties associated with its ester and quaternary ammonium salt functional groups. It is quite stable in the solid crystalline form but undergoes rapid hydrolysis in aqueous solution. This hydrolysis is accelerated in the presence of catalytic amounts of either acid or base. For this reason, acetylcholine cannot be administered orally due to rapid hydrolysis in the gastrointestinal tract. Even when administered parenterally, its pharmacologic action is fleeting as a result of hydrolysis by butyrylcholinesterase (also known as pseudocholinesterase or plasma cholinesterase) in serum. The quaternary ammonium functional group of acetylcholine imparts excellent water solubility, but quaternary ammonium salts are poorly absorbed across lipid membranes due to their high hydrophilic and ionic character. Thus, even if acetylcholine were stable enough to be administered orally, it would be poorly absorbed. When used during ocular surgery to produce complete miosis within seconds, acetylcholine must be directly instilled into the anterior chamber. It cannot be administered topically, because it is not lipophilic enough to penetrate the cornea, and it must be reconstitution immediately before instillation due to its hydrolytic lability.

Structure–Activity Relationship for Muscarinic Activity

The necessity to design compounds that would serve as therapeutic muscarinic alternatives to acetylcholine and as probes to study the role of acetylcholine in muscarinic neurotransmission led to an exhaustive study of the structural features required for the muscarinic action of acetylcholine. SARs that developed from these studies have provided the basis for the design of all muscarinic agonists currently used as therapeutic agents.

To review the SAR, it is logical to divide the structure of acetylcholine into the three components shown below to examine the effects of chemical modification of each group.

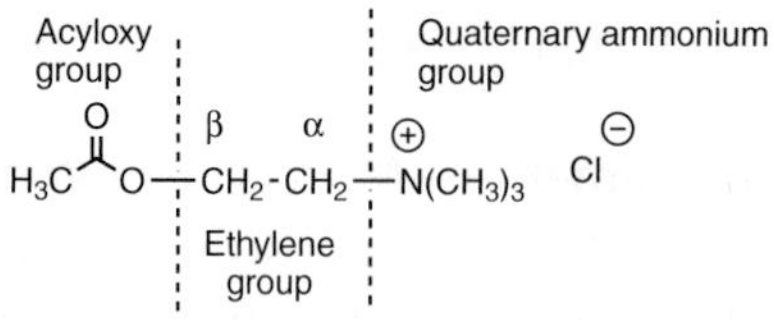

Modification of the Quaternary Ammonium Group Analogs of acetylcholine in which the nitrogen atom was replaced by arsenic, phosphorus, sulfur, or selenium have been synthesized (10,32,33). Although these analogs exhibited some of the activity of acetylcholine, these compounds are less active and are not used clinically. It was concluded that only compounds possessing a positive charge on the atom in the position of the nitrogen had appreciable muscarinic activity.

Compounds in which all three methyl groups on the nitrogen are replaced by larger alkyl groups are inactive as agonists. When the methyl groups are replaced by three ethyl groups, the resulting compound is a cholinergic antagonist. Replacement of only one methyl group by an ethyl or propyl group affords a compound that is active, but much less so than acetylcholine (32). Furthermore, successive replacement of one, two, or three of the methyl groups with hydrogen atoms to afford a tertiary, secondary, or primary amine, respectively, leads to successively diminishing muscarinic activity (34,35).

Modification of the Ethylene Bridge Synthesis of acetic acid esters of quaternary ammonium alcohols of greater length than choline led to a series of compounds with activity that was rapidly reduced as the chain length increased. This observation led Ing (10) to postulate his Rule of Five. This rule suggests that there should be no more than five atoms between the nitrogen and the terminal hydrogen atom for maximal muscarinic potency. Present concepts suggest that the mAChR cannot successfully accommodate molecules larger than acetylcholine and still produce its physiologic effect. Although larger analogs of acetylcholine can bind to the receptor, they lack efficacy and demonstrate antagonist properties.

Replacement of the hydrogen atoms of the ethylene bridge by alkyl groups larger than methyl affords compounds that are much less active than acetylcholine. Introduction of a methyl group on the carbon β to the quaternary nitrogen affords acetyl-β-methylcholine (methacholine), which has muscarinic potency almost equivalent to that of acetylcholine and much greater muscarinic than nicotinic selectivity.

A methyl group on the carbon α to the quaternary nitrogen affords acetyl-α-methylcholine. Although activity relative to acetylcholine is reduced at both mAChRs and nAChRs, it exhibits greater nicotinic than muscarinic potency. This compound is not currently used as a therapeutic agent.

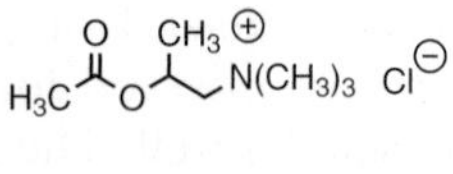

Acetyl-β-methylcholine chloride (Methacholine)

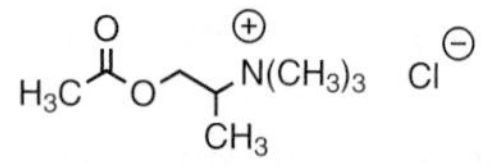

Acetyl-α-methylcholine chloride

Addition of methyl groups to either one or both of the ethylene carbons results in chiral molecules. mAChRs display stereoselectivity for the enantiomers of methacholine. Thus, *S*-(+)-methacholine (see Fig. 9.11) is equipotent with acetylcholine, whereas the *R*-(−)-enantiomer is approximately 20-fold less potent. Acetylcholinesterase hydrolyzes the *S*-(+)-isomer much slower (approximately half the rate) than acetylcholine. The *R*-(−)-isomer is not hydrolyzed by AChE and even acts as a weak competitive inhibitor of the enzyme. This stability toward AChE hydrolysis as well as the AChE inhibitory effect of the *R*-(−)-enantiomer can explain why racemic *R,S*-methacholine produces a longer duration of action than acetylcholine. The mAChR and AChE exhibit little stereoselectivity for the optical isomers of acetyl-α-methylcholine.

Modification of the Acyloxy Group As would be predicted by the Rule of Five (10), when the acetyl group is replaced by higher homologs (i.e., the propionyl or butyryl groups), the resulting esters are less potent than acetylcholine. Choline esters of aromatic or higher molecular weight acids possess cholinergic antagonist activity.

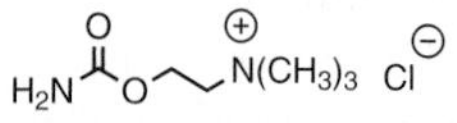

Carbachol

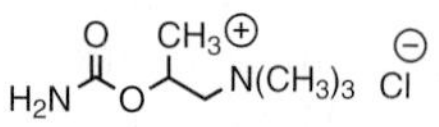

Bethanechol

Because the fleeting pharmacologic action and chemical instability of acetylcholine result from its rapid hydrolysis, a logical approach to the development of better muscarinic therapeutic agents was to replace the acetyloxy functional group with a functional group more resistant to hydrolysis. This led to synthesis of the carbamic acid ester of choline (carbachol), a potent cholinergic agonist possessing both muscarinic and nicotinic activity. Esters derived from carbamic acid are referred to as carbamates, and because their carbonyl carbon is less electrophilic, the carbamates are more stable than carboxylate esters to hydrolysis. Carbachol exhibits greater stability than acetylcholine toward hydrolysis by gastric acid, AChE, or butyrylcholinesterase and therefore is administered orally.

This same chemical logic was extended to methacholine and led to synthesis of its carbamate ester, bethanechol, an orally effective potent muscarinic agonist with almost no nicotinic activity at therapeutic doses. mAChRs exhibit stereoselectivity for the two optical isomers of bethanechol, and similar to methacholine, the *S*-(+)-enantiomer exhibits greater binding affinity at mAChRs than does the *R*-(−)-enantiomer in isolated receptor preparations.

The profound muscarinic activity of the alkaloid muscarine provided substantial rationale for synthesizing ethers of choline. Muscarine, which is obtained from the red variety of mushroom (*Amanita muscaria*) as well as other mushrooms, is one of the oldest known cholinergic agonists and is the compound for which mAChRs were named (see Fig. 9.2). Muscarine was used in many pharmacologic experiments during the latter 19th century and the early part of the 20th century, and its use preceded the discovery and chemical characterization of acetylcholine (2). The chemical structure of muscarine (see Fig. 9.11), however, was not completely characterized until 1957. Muscarine possesses three chiral centers (C2, C3, and C5). Thus, eight optical isomers (four enantiomeric pairs) are possible. Of these, only the naturally occurring alkaloid, 2*S*,3*R*,5*S*-(+)-muscarine [also called *L*-(+)-muscarine], is correctly referred to as muscarine. The C5 carbon of (+)-muscarine has the same absolute configuration as the analogous chiral β carbon in *S*-(+)-methacholine. Thus, acetylcholine and methacholine can adopt three-dimensional structures through molecular flexibility, similar to *L*-(+)-muscarine (see Fig. 9.11).

Other choline ethers and alkylaminoketones have been synthesized and evaluated for muscarinic activity. Choline ethyl ether exhibits significant muscarinic activity and is chemically stable, but it has not been used clinically. The most potent ketone derivatives possess the carbonyl on the carbon δ to the quaternary nitrogen; this is the same relative position as the carbonyl in acetylcholine. This suggests that these carbonyl groups bind by either a hydrogen bond or other dipole–dipole interaction with an appropriate group on the mAChR. Furthermore, the activity of these ethers and ketones demonstrates that neither the ester functional group nor a carbonyl is required for muscarinic agonist activity.

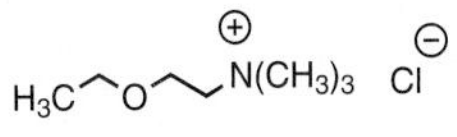

Choline ethyl ether

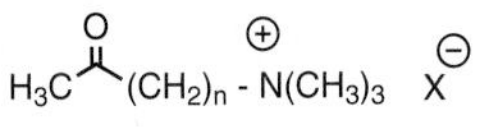

Alkylaminoketones

The classic SAR for muscarinic agonist activity can be summarized as follows:

- The molecule must possess a nitrogen atom capable of bearing a positive charge, preferably a quaternary ammonium salt.

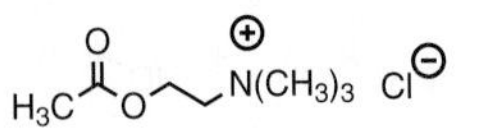

Acetylcholine chloride

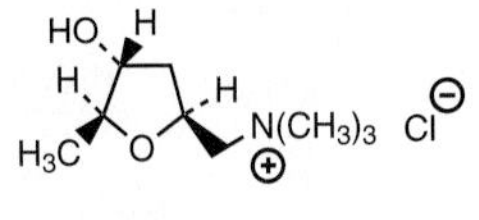

L(+) - Muscarine chloride

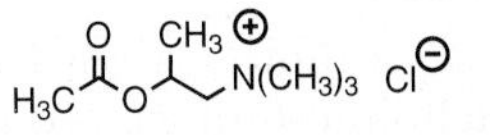

S-(+)Acetyl-β-methylcholine chloride
S-(+)Methacholine)

FIGURE 9.11 Structural relationships between acetylcholine, *L*-(+)-muscarine, and (*S*)-(+)-methacholine.

- For maximum potency, the size of the alkyl groups substituted on the nitrogen should not exceed the size of a methyl group.
- The molecule should have an oxygen atom, preferably an ester-like oxygen, capable of participating in a hydrogen bond.
- There should be a two-carbon unit between the oxygen atom and the nitrogen atom.

It is important to note that this SAR was based on in vitro and in vivo pharmacologic evaluations performed over a 60-year period without the luxury of modern, highly refined biologic testing systems (i.e., protein-binding assays, cell membrane–binding assays, and single-cell models) that are considered to be state-of-the-art today for pharmacologic evaluation of new medicinal agents. This is why some classic muscarinic agonists and many of the more modern agents do not adhere to this SAR. Indeed, SAR rules are not static; they should change as new experimental data refine the structural and stereochemical requirements for muscarinic agonist activity.

Specific Muscarinic Agonists

Methacholine Chloride (Provocholine) Methacholine, acetyl β-methylcholine, (see previous structure p. 12 and SAR discussion) is marketed as the racemic mixture. It is a selective muscarinic agonist with very little activity at nAChRs. Although methacholine chloride is marketed as the racemic mixture, the *S*-(+)-enantiomer is 240-fold more potent than the *R*-(−)-isomer at mAChRs. In addition, AChE hydrolyzes *S*-(+)–methacholine at approximately 54% the rate of acetylcholine, whereas the *R*-(−)–enantiomer is a weak inhibitor. Methacholine chloride is used via inhalation for the diagnosis of asthma. The resulting bronchospasm can be relieved with bronchodilators. Methacholine chloride is available as a powder that is reconstituted for inhalation.

Carbachol Chloride (Isopto Carbachol) Carbachol (see structure p. 12), the carbamate analog of acetylcholine, exhibits affinity for both mAChRs and nAChRs. Because it is a carbamate ester, carbachol is more resistant toward acid-, base-, or enzyme (AChE)-catalyzed hydrolysis than acetylcholine. It is also reported to exhibit weak anticholinesterase activity. Both of these actions work to prolong the duration of action of carbachol. Because of erratic absorption and its actions at nAChRs, use of carbachol has been limited to the treatment of glaucoma and for the induction of miosis in ocular surgery. Carbachol is available as an intraocular solution and an ophthalmic solution.

Bethanechol Chloride (Urecholine) Bethanechol (see structure p. 12), the carbamate analog of methacholine, is selective for mAChRs and exhibits almost no affinity for nAChRs. It is used to treat postsurgical and postpartum urinary retention and abdominal distention. Bethanechol is administered orally, because there is danger of a cholinergic crisis if it is given by intravenous or intramuscular injection.

Pilocarpine Hydrochloride (Isopto Carpine) Pilocarpine hydrochloride, the salt of an alkaloid obtained from *Pilocarpus jaborandi,* is an example of a muscarinic agonist with affinity for the M_3 mAChR that does not adhere to the traditional SAR of muscarinic agonists. In 1876, Langley reported that extracts containing the alkaloid stimulated the end organs of parasympathetic neurons. The structure of pilocarpine was reported in 1901. It possesses two chiral centers at C3 and C4. Thus, four optical isomers (two enantiomeric pairs) are possible, and of these, the naturally occurring alkaloid is 3*S*,4*R*-(+)-pilocarpine, with a pK_a of 6.8 and a logD at pH 7.4 of 1.03.

Pilocarpine is marketed as tablets (Salogen), an ophthalmic solution, and gel. It penetrates the eye well and is the miotic of choice for open-angle glaucoma and to terminate acute angle closure attacks. It is also used for the treatment of xerostomia (dryness of the mouth) caused by radiation therapy of the head and neck, Sjögren syndrome, and mucositis following chemotherapy. Because pilocarpine is a lactone, its solutions are subject to 1) hydrolysis to afford the pharmacologically inactive pilocarpic acid, and 2) base-catalyzed epimerization at C3 in the lactone to give isopilocarpine, an inactive stereoisomer of pilocarpine. Epimerization is not believed to be a serious problem if the drug is properly stored. Its solutions can be stored at room temperature, but the gel should be refrigerated and labeled with a 2-week expiration date when dispensed.

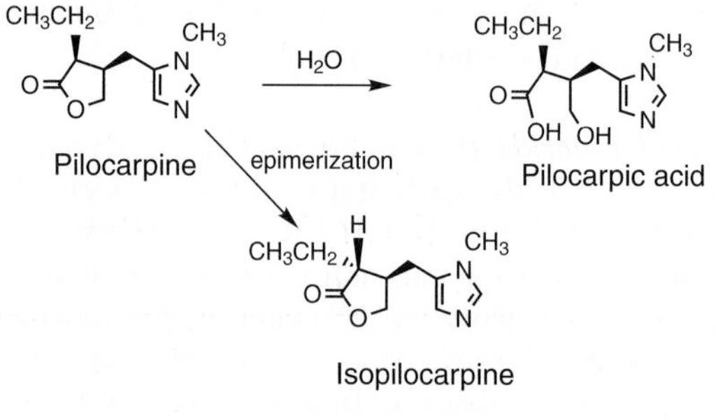

Cevimeline Hydrochloride (Evoxac) Cevimeline is a nonclassical muscarinic agonist. It is a quinuclidine derivative that exhibits partial direct M_1 receptor agonist activity in the CNS and affinity for M_3 receptors in epithelial tissue of lacrimal and salivary glands. Its elimination half-life is 3 to 5 hours. It is metabolized by CYP2D6, CYP3A3, and CYP3A4 to inactive metabolites, the *cis*- and *trans*-sulfoxide, *N*-oxide, and glucuronide. Cevimeline hydrochloride is available as an oral capsule for the treatment of xerostomia (dry mouth) associated with Sjögren syndrome. Before its approval, pilocarpine was the only drug for this condition.

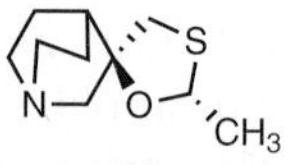

Cevimeline

FUTURE MUSCARINIC AGONISTS Current research interest in the design and synthesis of new muscarinic agonists is focused on discovering agents that might be effective in the treatment of Alzheimer disease and other cognitive disorders. Investigators are searching actively for muscarinic agonists that exhibit selectivity for mAChRs in the brain. Among these compounds are analogs of arecoline, oxotremorine, and McN-A-343 (see above) as well as many other novel chemical structures possessing muscarinic agonist activity.

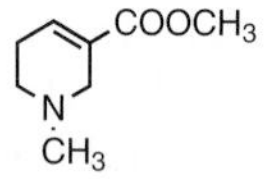

Arecoline

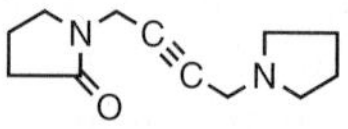

Oxotremorine

Arecoline is of historical interest because its structure, like those of many other early medicinal agents, was determined and confirmed by a 19th century German pharmacist, E. Jahns (2). Xanomeline can be viewed as a nonclassical bioisostere of the ester moiety of arecoline. It is a muscarinic M_1/M_4 agonist that is showing promise in clinical trials for the treatment of Alzheimer disease (36). Although it is not tolerated at orally effective doses, transdermal delivery systems are showing promise.

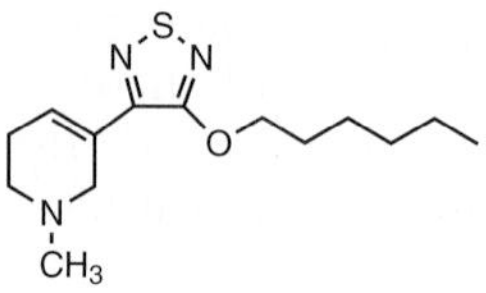

Xanomeline

Acetylcholinesterase Inhibitors

Another means of producing a cholinergic response is to interfere with the mechanism by which the action of acetylcholine is terminated. Thus, inhibition of its rapid hydrolysis by AChE increases the concentration of acetylcholine in the synapse and results in production of both muscarinic and nicotinic effects.

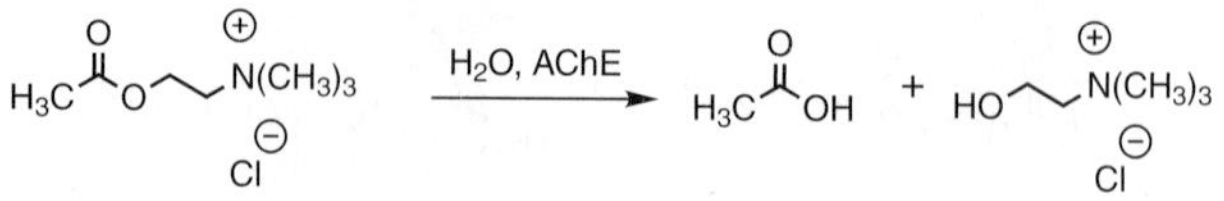

Therapeutic Application

Acetylcholinesterase inhibitors (AChEIs), sometimes referred to as anticholinesterases, are classified as indirect cholinomimetics, because their principle mechanism of action does not involve binding to cholinergic receptors, but indirectly increasing the synaptic concentration of acetylcholine. These agents are used therapeutically to improve muscle strength in myasthenia gravis. They are also used in open-angle glaucoma to decrease intraocular pressure by stimulating contraction of the ciliary muscle and sphincter of the iris. This facilitates outflow of aqueous humor via the canal of Schlemm. Recently, AChEIs have found use in the treatment of symptoms of Alzheimer disease and similar cognitive disorders (37,38), which are conditions characterized by a cholinergic deficiency in the cortex and basal forebrain. They are used extensively as insecticides and are in military arsenals as chemical warfare agents.

Mechanism of Acetylcholinesterase-Catalyzed Hydrolysis of Acetylcholine

Extensive studies of AChE have resulted in purification and amino acid sequencing of the enzyme from several sources, as well as the description of its quaternary structure from x-ray crystallographic and molecular modeling studies (39). The active site of AChE consists of the esteratic site at which hydrolysis of the ester occurs and an "anionic-binding site" where the cationic portion of acetylcholine binds (Fig. 9.12). Using *Torpedo californica*, Sussman et al. (39) showed that the active site lies at the bottom of a deep, narrow gorge that is 18 to 20 Å deep and is lined with aromatic amino acids (39). The amino acids composing the gorge in AChEs from a number of species are highly conserved (40).

Describing AChE as possessing an "anionic site" is a misnomer. This site was originally proposed to be the free carboxylate group of a glutamate residue, but Sussman et al. (39), using AChE from *Torpedo californica,* showed that it is actually uncharged and lipophilic. Rather than an ionic bond being responsible for binding of the quaternary ammonium group, the quaternary nitrogen binds to the π-electrons of a tryptophan residue forming a cation-π bonding interaction. This is supported by mutagenesis studies using human

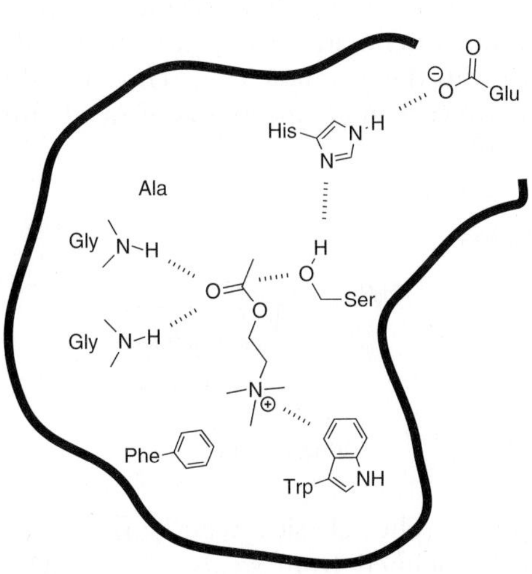

FIGURE 9.12 Binding of acetylcholine to catalytic site of acetylcholinesterase; role of serine and histidine residues is illustrated.

AChE (41). The aromatic residues found in the gorge can act as low-affinity sites that guide the substrate to the active site while the strong cation-π interaction is responsible for binding the choline portion of acetylcholine (40) (see Fig. 9.12).

Like other serine hydrolases, the functional catalytic unit of AChE is composed of a catalytic triad of glutamate, histidine, and serine at the esteratic site (42,43). The serine hydroxyl group serves as the nucleophile, while the histidine residue increases the nucleophilicity by serving as a general acid–base catalyst. The glutamic acid residue is believed to provide stabilization to the transition state (43,44). Also found at the esteratic site is an "oxyanion hole" formed by hydrogen bonding between *NH* groups of two glycine residues and an alanine (43,45). These hydrogen bonds with the carbonyl oxygen stabilize the transition state.

The proposed mechanism of hydrolysis is illustrated in Figure 9.13. Transition state B is unstable and collapses to form choline and acetylated AChE (C); this form of the enzyme is referred to as the acylated enzyme. As long as the enzyme is acylated, it cannot bind another molecule of acetylcholine; the enzyme is in an inactive state. The acylated enzyme then undergoes rapid hydrolysis (D) to regenerate the active form of AChE and a molecule of acetic acid (E) (43).

Hydrolysis of the acylated enzyme (deacylation) is important in the development of AChEIs. If the enzyme becomes acylated by a functional group (i.e., carbamyl or phosphate) that is more stable toward hydrolysis than a carboxylate ester, the enzyme remains inactive for a longer period of time. Application of this chemical principle regarding rates of hydrolysis led to discovery and design of two classes of AChEIs, the reversible inhibitors and the irreversible inhibitors.

Reversible Inhibitors of Acetylcholinesterase

MECHANISM OF ACTION Reversible AChEIs are 1) those compounds that are substrates for and react with AChE to form an acylated enzyme, which is more stable than the acetylated enzyme but still capable of undergoing hydrolytic regeneration or 2) those that bind to AChE with greater affinity than acetylcholine but do not react with the enzyme as a substrate. Both types of inhibitors have found clinical applications. Those that acylate AChE include the aryl carbamates, such as esters of carbamic acid and phenols (e.g., physostigmine). Alkyl carbamates (esters of carbamic acid and alcohols), such as carbachol and bethanechol, which are structurally related to acetylcholine, are also substrates for and competitively inhibit AChE because they are hydrolyzed very slowly by AChE. For reasons previously discussed, carbachol and bethanechol are more resistant than acetylcholine to AChE-catalyzed hydrolysis.

When aryl carbamate AChEIs, such as physostigmine and its analogs, bind to the catalytic site of AChE, hydrolysis of the carbamate occurs by transesterification by the carbamoyl group to the serine residue, forming what

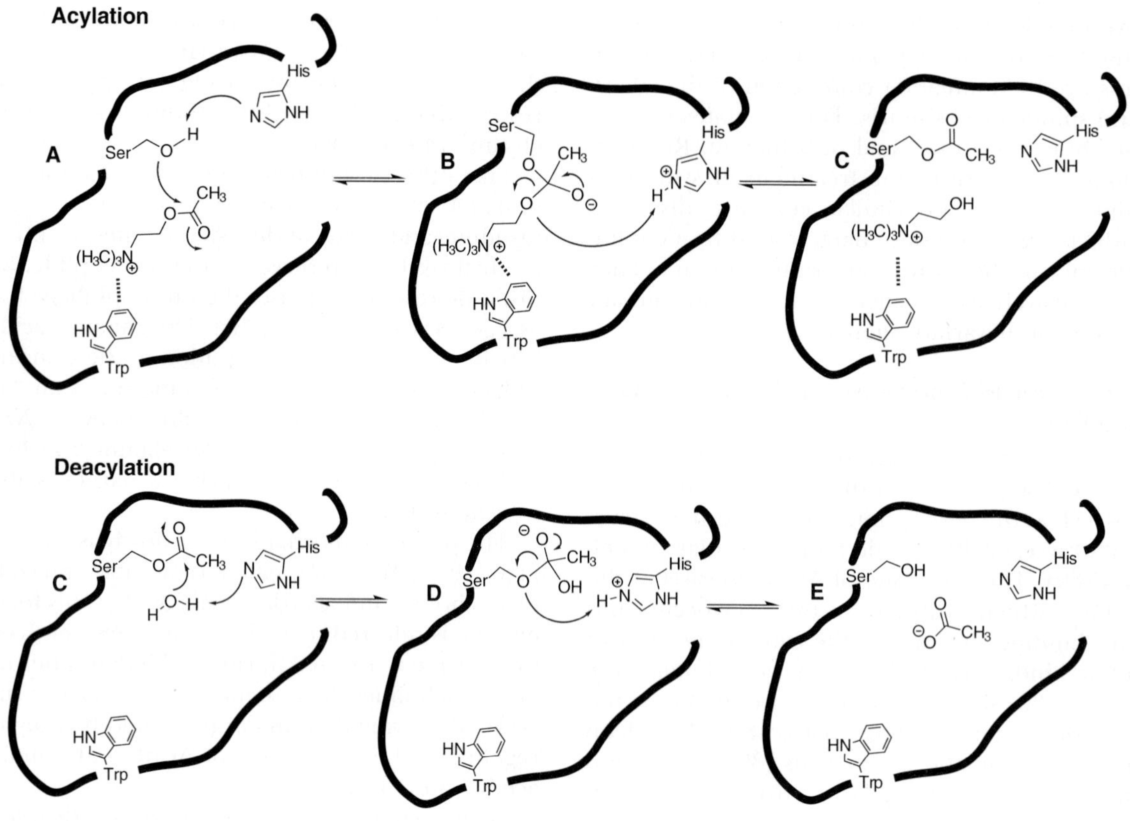

FIGURE 9.13 Mechanistic steps in the hydrolysis of acetylcholine (Ach).

is termed a "carbamylated enzyme." The rate of carbamylation follows this order: unsubstituted carbamic acid esters > methylcarbamic acid esters > dimethylcarbamic acid esters (46).

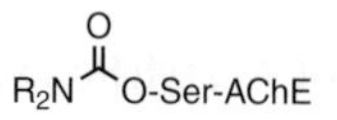

Carbamylated AChE

Regeneration of active AChE by hydrolysis of the carbamylated enzyme is much slower than hydrolysis of the acetylated enzyme. The rate for hydrolytic regeneration of the carbamylated AChE is measured in minutes (e.g., the half-life for methyl carbamylated enzyme is ~15 minutes); the rate of hydrolytic regeneration of acetylated AChE is measured in a fraction of a millisecond (e.g., the half-life for acetylated enzyme is ~0.2 milliseconds). Despite the longer time required to regenerate the carbamylated enzyme, the active form of AChE eventually is regenerated. Therefore, these inhibitors are considered to be reversible.

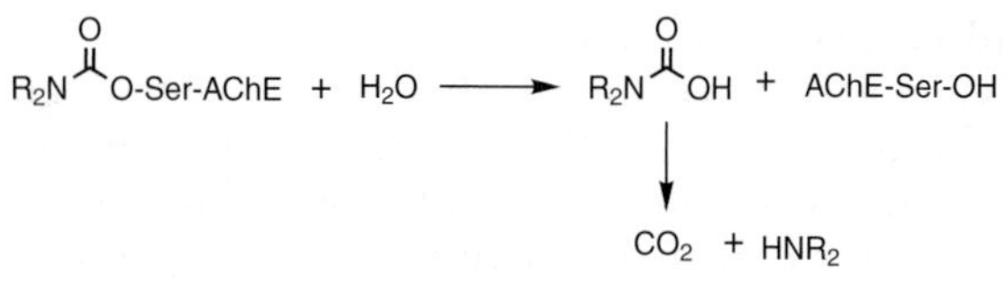

Aryl carbamates are superior to alkyl carbamates as AChEIs, because they have better affinity for AChE and, therefore, carbamylate AChE more efficiently. Physostigmine and other aryl carbamates exhibit inhibition constants (K_i) on the order of 10^{-9} to 10^{-8} M and are three to four orders of magnitude more effective than alkyl carbamates, such as carbachol ($K_i \sim 10^{-5}$ M). This is to be expected because phenoxide anions are more stable and, hence, are better leaving groups than alkoxide anions. Phenoxide anions are stabilized through resonance with the aromatic ring. Thus, the therapeutically effective carbamate inhibitors of AChE are derived from phenols.

Specific Agents

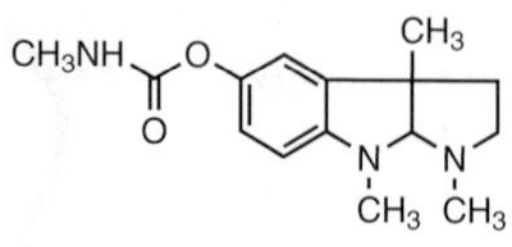

Physostigmine

Physostigmine The classic AChEI, physostigmine, is an alkaloid obtained from seeds of the Calabar bean (*Physostigma venenosum*) (38). Its parasympathomimetic effects were recognized long before its structure was elucidated in 1923. In 1929, Stedman found that the mechanism of the parasympathomimetic effects of physostigmine was inhibition of AChE; it inhibits AChE by acting as a substrate and carbamylating the enzyme. Acetylcholinesterase is carbamylated at a slow rate, but physostigmine has exceptionally high affinity ($K_i \sim 10^{-9}$ M) for the catalytic site of the enzyme. By comparison, the K_s for acetylcholine is on the order of 10^{-4} M. Thus, physostigmine is classified as a reversible AChEI that carbamylates the enzyme at a slow rate; the carbamylated AChE is also regenerated quite slowly. Because physostigmine is a tertiary amine with a pK_a of 8.2 (BH^+) rather than a quaternary ammonium salt, it is more lipophilic than many other AChEIs and can diffuse across the blood–brain barrier. The tertiary amine also imparts pH dependence to its ability to inhibit AChE, because its affinity for AChE is greater when the amine is protonated. Physostigmine is metabolized in vivo by esterases to the phenol and has an elimination half-life of 1 to 2 hours. Its aqueous solutions are subject to hydrolytic decomposition to form eseroline, which undergoes light-catalyzed oxidation to form rubreserine, a red-colored compound (Fig. 9.14). Both degradation products are inactive as AChEIs.

Physostigmine has been used for many years in ophthalmology for the treatment of glaucoma. More recently, the salicylate salt has been used in hospital emergency rooms to treat overdoses of compounds possessing significant anticholinergic CNS effects, such as atropine and tricyclic antidepressants. Physostigmine's ability to cross the blood–brain barrier has led to renewed interest in this molecule, and it is also one of a number of centrally active AChEIs being investigated as indirect cholinomimetics for use in the treatment of Alzheimer disease and other cognitive disorders.

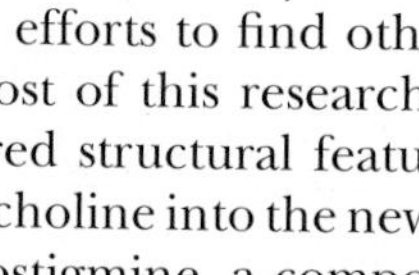

Neostigmine bromide

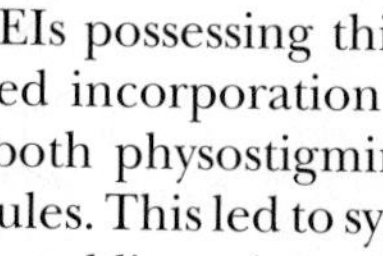

Pyridostigmine bromide

Neostigmine (Prostigmin) The discovery that physostigmine and other aryl carbamates inhibit AChE reversibly led to efforts to find other AChEIs possessing this activity. Most of this research involved incorporation of the required structural features of both physostigmine and acetylcholine into the new molecules. This led to synthesis of neostigmine, a compound resembling physostigmine but having a much simpler structure. Neostigmine retains the substituted carbamate group, the benzene ring, and the nitrogen atom of the first heterocyclic ring of physostigmine. The distance between the ester and the quaternary ammonium group is approximately the same as that found in acetylcholine and physostigmine. Because of its quaternary ammonium group, it lacks central activity. Neostigmine is metabolized by plasma cholinesterases, in liver, and in skeletal muscle to 3-hydroxyphenyltrimethylammonium chloride, 3-hydroxyphenyldimethylamine, and their *O*-glucuronide conjugates (Fig. 9.15). It has an elimination half-life of 15 to 90 minutes. Neostigmine is indicated for prophylaxis of postoperative abdominal distension and urinary retention, myasthenia gravis, and reversal of neuromuscular blockade.

Pyridostigmine (Mestinon) Pyridostigmine, a closely related structure to neostigmine that incorporates the charged nitrogen into a pyridine ring, acts by the same mechanism as physostigmine, and, like neostigmine, it lacks CNS activity. It is orally effective and, compared to neostigmine, has a longer duration of action and a lower incidence of side effects. Thus, it is a better choice for oral therapy of myasthenia gravis. It is approved for U.S. military use as an adjunct for prophylaxis of soman nerve gas exposure. It is also administered parenterally to reverse the effects of nondepolarizing neuromuscular blocking agents. Its elimination half-life is 1 to 2 hours. Its metabolism pathway and metabolites are similar to those for neostigmine.

Carbaryl (Sevin) Carbaryl is a reversible, carbamate-derived AChEI that has tremendous economic impact as an insecticide for use on houseplants and vegetables as well as for control of fleas and ticks on pets. Its structural relationship to physostigmine and neostigmine is readily apparent. A number of other carbamate AChEIs are also commercially available for this use.

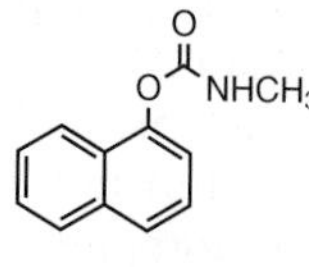

Carbaryl

Edrophonium Chloride (Enlon, Reversol) Edrophonium is a quaternary ammonium-substituted phenol. Because it is a phenol rather than a carbamate ester of a phenol, it does not carbamylate AChE. It does, however, inhibit AChE in a reversible manner, and also exhibits a direct cholinomimetic effect at skeletal muscle. Edrophonium

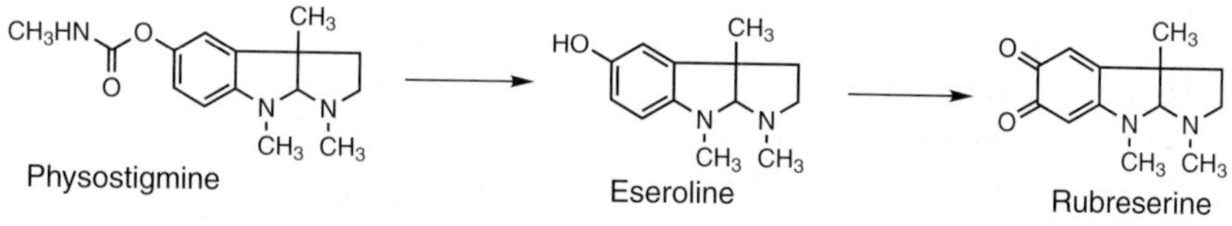

FIGURE 9.14 In vitro degradation of physostigmine.

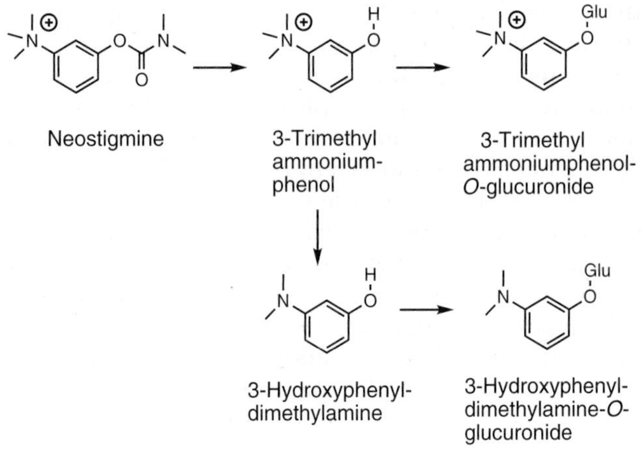

FIGURE 9.15 Metabolism of neostigmine bromide.

is used intravenously for the diagnosis of myasthenia gravis, where it acts rapidly to increase muscle strength. It is also administered intramuscularly to rapidly reverse the effects of nondepolarizing neuromuscular blocking agents like *d*-tubocurarine and gallamine. It is not effective, however, at reversing the effects of the depolarizing blockers such as succinylcholine and decamethonium. Its elimination half-life is 1.3 to 2.4 hours.

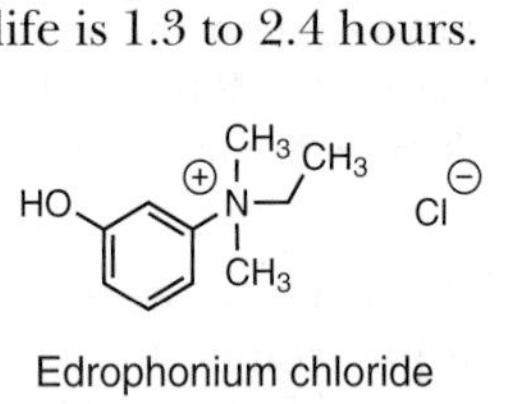

Reversible Acetylcholinesterase Inhibitors for Treatment of Alzheimer Disease Of all the age-related disorders in which dementia is a component, Alzheimer disease (AD) is probably the best known. Much effort has been expended to discover the cause of AD. Autopsy examination of the brains of patients who had AD has revealed microscopic structural changes characteristic of the disease. In addition, neurotransmitter dysfunction involving reduction in acetylcholine, serotonin, norepinephrine, dopamine, and glutamate levels has been reported. For a review of AD and the search for therapies, see Rzeszotarski (47). It is known that in AD patients, there is widespread atrophy in the primary motor and sensory cortices and cerebellum. There is a disruption in cholinergic innervation in these areas of the brain, along with decreases in choline acetyltransferase, high-affinity nicotinic acetylcholine receptor binding, and choline transporter sites (48–51). Impairment of short-term memory is the first observable symptom of the disease, and progressive memory impairment, severe mood changes, and depression coupled with loss of judgment and reasoning ability follow. The U.S. Food and Drug Administration has approved four AChEIs for the treatment of AD: tacrine, donepezil, rivastigmine, and galantamine. Although these four AChEIs are not without problems, they do provide some benefit in early to mild AD. Their clinical effectiveness in advanced AD has yet to be shown.

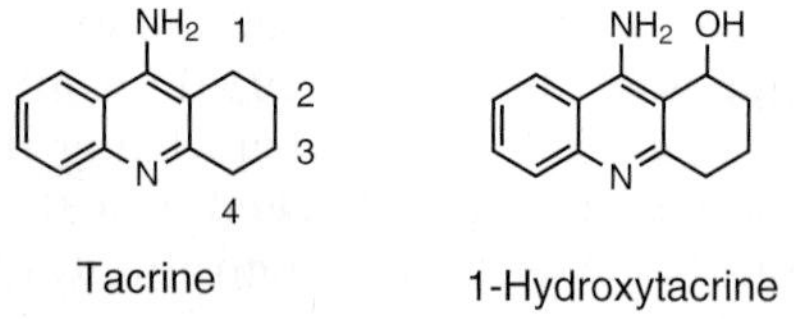

Tacrine Hydrochloride (Cognex) Tacrine, an aminoacridine synthesized in the 1930s, is a nonclassical cholinesterase inhibitor that binds to both AChE and butyrylcholinesterase (52). It was approved in 1993 for treatment of AD. Approximately 20% of tacrine-treated patients show improvement. However, its use is limited due to hepatotoxicity and development of safer AChEIs. Tacrine is extensively metabolized by CYP1A2 to the 2-, 3-, and 4-hydroxy metabolites. All show reduced AChEI activity relative to tacrine, with the major metabolite, 1-hydroxytacrine, being the most active. Its elimination half-life is between 1.5 and 4 hours, with metabolites being are excreted via the urine.

Donepezil (Aricept) Donepezil is another "nonclassical," centrally acting, reversible, noncompetitive AChEI that was approved in 1997 for treatment of mild-to-moderate AD and dementia. Its selectivity for AChE is 570 to 1,250-fold than for butyrylcholinesterase, and it also exhibits greater affinity for brain AChE than for peripheral AChE (53). When compared to tacrine, donepezil exhibits greater CNS AChE selectivity, longer elimination half-life (70 to 104 hours in subjects older than 55 years), and little or no potential for hepatotoxicity. Donepezil is metabolized by CYP2D6 and CYP3A4 via O-demethylation, N-debenzylation, oxidation to the *cis*-*N*-oxide, and O-glucuronidation (Fig. 9.16). Donepezil is hepatically metabolized, and the predominant route for the elimination of both parent drug and its metabolites is renal. The major plasma metabolites of donepezil include O-dealkylation to M1 and M2 metabolites and

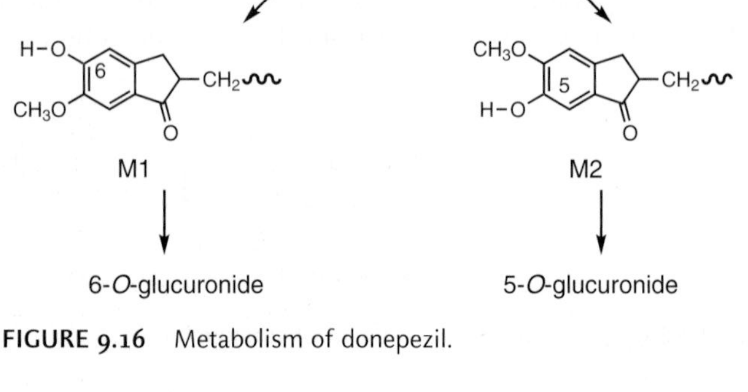

FIGURE 9.16 Metabolism of donepezil.

N-oxidation (M6) (Fig. 9.16). Unchanged donepezil accounted for approximately 25% of the dose and 17% in urine. Urinary metabolites included the *O*-glucuronides of M1 and M2, but also M4 the *N*-debenzylated metabolite. The 6-*O*-desmethyl metabolite (M1) accounted for 11% of the dose, and it exhibits AChE inhibitory activity comparable to that of the parent compound.

Rivastigmine Tartrate (Exelon) Rivastigmine is a centrally selective, arylcarbamate AChEI that was approved in 2000 for oral administration in the treatment of AD. It has an elimination half-life of 1.4 to 1.7 hours. Rivastigmine inhibits both plasma cholinesterase and acetylcholinesterase (unlike donepezil, which selectively inhibits acetylcholinesterase). It is thought that rivastigmine works by inhibiting these cholinesterase enzymes, which would otherwise break down acetylcholine. However, it inhibits AChE for up to 10 hours due to the slow hydrolysis of the carbamylated enzyme. Thus, it has been referred to as a pseudo-irreversible AChEI (53). When given orally, rivastigmine is well absorbed with a bioavailability of about 40%. Peak plasma concentrations are seen in about 1 hour, and peak spinal fluid is seen at 1.4 to 3.8 hours. When given by once-daily transdermal patch, the pharmacokinetic profile of rivastigmine is much smoother as compared with capsules, with lower peak plasma concentrations and reduced plasma concentration fluctuations. The 9.5 mg/24 hours rivastigmine patch provides comparable exposure to 12 mg/day capsules (the highest recommended oral dose). The drug crosses the blood–brain barrier. It is rapidly and extensively hydrolyzed by plasma and CNS cholinesterases with minimal involvement of hepatic CYP450 enzymes. The phenolic metabolite is excreted primarily via the kidneys. Like donepezil, rivastigmine exhibits a low potential of hepatotoxicity and drug–drug interactions due to lack of hepatic metabolism by CYP450 enzymes.

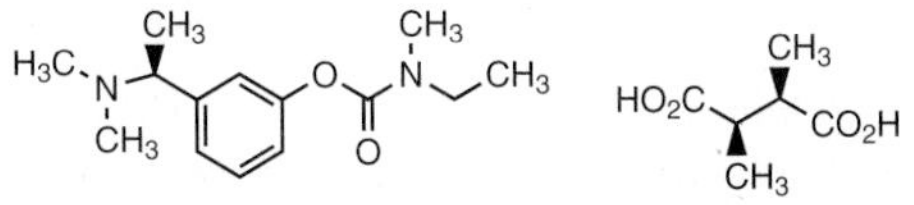

Rivastigmine tartrate

Galantamine Hydrobromide (Razadyne) Galantamine, introduced in 2001, is an alkaloid found in plants of the family Amaryllidaceae, which includes the daffodil (*Narcissus pseudonarcissus*) and snowflake (*Leucojum aestivum*). It is a reversible inhibitor of AChE, but it does not appear to inhibit butyrylcholinesterase. Because it is a tertiary amine and can cross the blood–brain barrier, it is indicated for treatment of mild-to-moderate AD and dementia. It has been used outside the United States for more than 30 years as an anticurare agent in anesthesia. Galantamine differs from other cholinesterase inhibitors, because it allosterically binds to nAChRs, giving it a dual cholinergic action. It is primarily metabolized (75%) by CYP2D6 to *O*-desmethyl and *O*-desmethylnormethyl metabolites and by CYP3A4 to the normethyl metabolite, along with other minor metabolites (Fig. 9.17). Unlike tacrine, galantamine is not associated with hepatotoxicity. Its elimination half-life is 5.7 hours.

Irreversible Inhibitors of Acetylcholinesterase

MECHANISM OF ACTION The chemical logic involved in the development of effective AChEIs was to synthesize compounds that would be substrates for AChE and result in an acylated enzyme more stable to hydrolysis than a carboxylate ester. Phosphate esters are very stable to hydrolysis, being even more stable than many amides. Application of this chemical property to the design of AChEI compounds led to derivatives of phosphoric, pyrophosphoric, and phosphonic acids that are effective inhibitors of AChE. These act as inhibitors by the same mechanism as the carbamate inhibitors, except that they form phosphate esters with the enzyme. The rate of hydrolysis of the phosphorylated enzyme is much slower than that of the carbamylated enzyme, and its rate is measured in hours (e.g., the half-lives for diethyl phosphates are ~8 hours). Because the duration of action of these compounds is much longer than that of carbamate esters, they are referred to as irreversible inhibitors of AChE.

An important difference between irreversible phosphoester-derived AChEIs and reversible (carbamate-derived) AChEIs is that the phosphorylated AChE can undergo a process known as aging (Fig. 9.18). Aging plays an important role in the toxicity of these irreversible AChEIs. It is the result of hydrolysis of one or more of the phosphoester bonds while leaving the AChE phosphorylated. This reaction affords an anionic phosphate in which the phosphorus atom is much less electrophilic and, therefore, much less likely to undergo hydrolytic regeneration than the original phosphoester. Aging occurs over a period of time and depends on the rate of the P–O bond cleavage reaction. Prior to aging of the

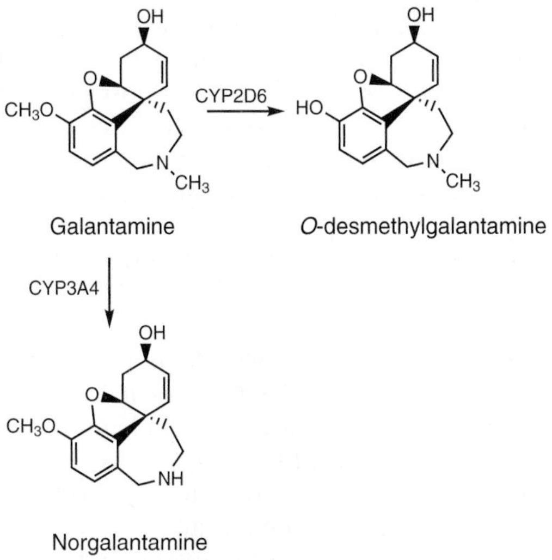

FIGURE 9.17 Metabolism of galantamine.

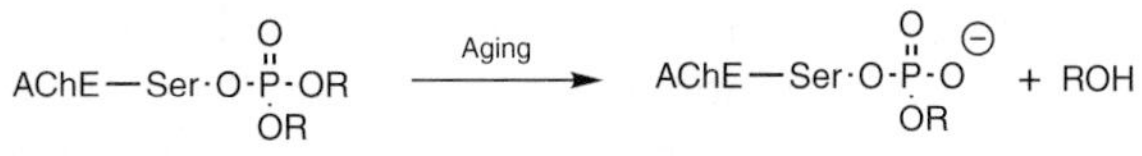

FIGURE 9.18 Aging of phosphorylated AChE.

enzyme, the antidotes to phosphate ester poisoning can be effective.

Only those phosphorus-derived AChEIs that have at least one phosphoester group undergo the aging process. Knowledge of the chemical mechanisms associated with irreversible inhibition of AChE and the aging process led to development of deadly phosphorus-derived chemical warfare "nerve agents," one of which is sarin (GB is the two-letter North Atlantic Treaty Organization designation for this nerve agent). When sarin phosphorylates AChE, only one aging reaction takes place, and then the enzyme becomes refractory to regeneration by the currently available antidotal agents. Other organophosphate nerve agents include tauban (GA), soman (GD), GF, and VX.

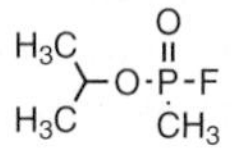

Sarin

SPECIFIC AGENTS

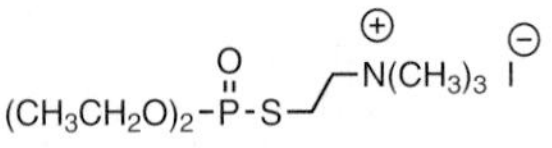

Echothiophate iodide

Echothiophate Iodide (Phospholine Iodide) Echothiophate iodide has found therapeutic application for the treatment of glaucoma and strabismus. Echothiophate is applied topically as a solution and is the only irreversible AChEI for the treatment of glaucoma. The decrease in intraocular pressure observed can last up to 4 weeks. Phosphoester AChEIs exhibit cataractogenic properties; thus, their use should be reserved for patients who are refractory to other forms of treatment (i.e., short-acting miotics, β-blockers, epinephrine, and possibly, carbonic anhydrase inhibitors). Because of its toxicity, echothiophate is not used for its systemic action. Selectivity of echothiophate for the AChE catalytic site was enhanced by incorporation of a quaternary ammonium salt functional group two carbons removed from the phosphoryl group.

Insecticidal AChEIs A number of lipophilic phosphoester AChEIs have been designed as insecticides; the structures of some of these are shown in Figure 9.19. This group of irreversible AChEI insecticides is beneficial to agricultural production throughout the world. In addition to being extremely lipophilic, another physicochemical property common to these compounds is a high vapor pressure. This combination of physicochemical

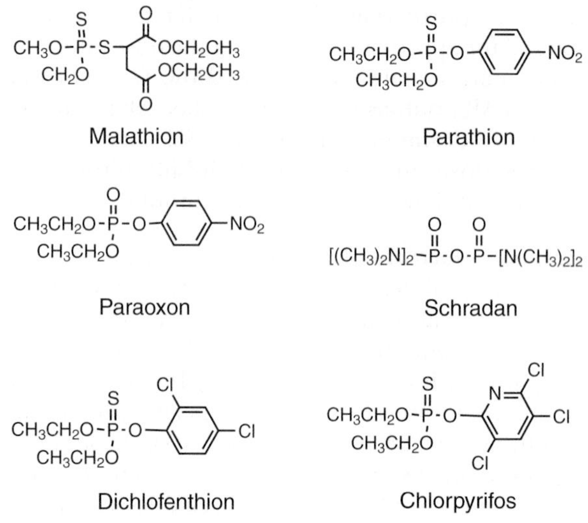

FIGURE 9.19 Irreversible acetylcholinesterase inhibitors used as insecticides.

properties makes it imperative that these compounds be used with extreme caution in the presence of humans and other mammals to prevent inhalation of the vapors and their absorption through the skin. Both routes of exposure cause a number of poisoning accidents every year, some of which are fatal.

Some of these irreversible AChEI insecticides have a sulfur atom bonded to the phosphorus atom with a coordinate-covalent bond. These compounds exhibit little AChEI activity, but they are rapidly bioactivated via desulfurization by microsomal oxidation in insects to afford the corresponding oxo-derivatives (phosphate esters), which are quite potent. A good example of this bioactivation phenomenon is illustrated by the commercially available insecticide parathion and its bioactivation to a toxic metabolite paraoxon.

Malathion (Ovide). Malathion (Fig. 9.19) is a dithiophosphate ester that has found use both as an aerial insecticide and clinically as a mitocide for topical treatment of lice infestations of the hair and scalp. It will kill both hatched lice and their eggs (nits) within 3 seconds after application. Compared to other organophosphate AChEIs, malathion exhibits lower transdermal absorption. On intact skin, less than 10% of a topical dose is systemically absorbed. Similar to parathion, malathion is bioactivated in insects to its toxic phosphate ester metabolite. It is much less toxic in humans, mammals, and birds than in insects. This selectivity toward insects is achieved because, in humans, plasma esterases hydrolyze the carboxylate esters to less toxic carboxylic acid metabolites that are rapidly eliminated in urine as carboxylate anions. This does not occur in insects. Acute toxicity with malathion is rare and usually occurs only after oral ingestion. The lethal dose in mammals is approximately 1 g/kg.

ANTIDOTES FOR IRREVERSIBLE ACHEIS

Background The marked toxicity of phosphate ester irreversible AChEIs, their widespread use as insecticides, and their proliferation as chemical warfare agents posed serious problems that stimulated research to develop antidotes for these agents. This required rational use of reaction kinetics, organic reaction mechanisms, and synthetic organic chemistry. Water is a nucleophile capable of rapidly hydrolyzing acetylated AChE and regenerating the active enzyme. Phosphorylated AChE (irreversibly inhibited), however, was known to involve a phosphate ester of serine. It is well established from reaction kinetic studies that the rate of hydrolysis is much slower for organic phosphate esters than for carboxylate esters and that a significantly stronger nucleophile than water would be required for efficient cleavage of phosphate esters. The problem required the design of reagents capable of efficiently catalyzing phosphate ester cleavage to regenerate active AChE while being safe enough for use as therapeutic agents. The resolution of this problem is an elegant example of application of chemical principles to the solution of a therapeutic problem (54–56).

Hydroxylamine (NH_2OH) is a strong nucleophilic compound that efficiently cleaves phosphate esters and significantly increases the rate of reactivation of phosphorylated AChE, but only at toxic concentrations (57). The nucleophilicity of hydroxylamine prompted the development of a number of structurally related hydroxylamines in the hope of eliminating its toxicity. The toxicity inherent in hydroxylamine would most probably be present in any structurally related compound, but this toxicity might be minimized if sufficiently small doses could be used. It would be logical to design a compound that would have a high degree of selectivity and strong binding affinity for AChE and also carries a hydroxylamine-like nucleophile into close proximity to the phosphorylated serine residue. This design was achieved by the synthesis of hydroxylamine derivatives of organic compounds possessing a functional group bearing a positive charge.

Reaction of hydroxylamine with aldehydes or ketones affords oximes, which possess the desired nucleophilic oxygen atom. A pyridine ring was considered an attractive carrier for the oxime function, because such groups are common in a number of biochemical systems (e.g., NAD^+ and $NADP^+$), indicating a possible low order of toxicity. Furthermore, three readily available positional isomers of pyridine aldehyde can be easily converted to oximes. Finally, the nitrogen atom of the pyridine ring can be converted to a quaternary ammonium salt by treatment with methyl iodide. This cationic charge would be expected to increase affinity of the compound for the anionic-binding site of the phosphorylated AChE.

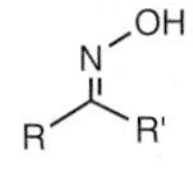

Oxime

The three isomeric pyridine aldoxime methiodides were synthesized and biologically evaluated. Of these, the most effective is the isomer derived from 2-pyridinylaldehyde. This compound, known as pralidoxime chloride (2-PAM, or 2-pyridine aldoxime methyl chloride) currently is the only available agent proven to be clinically effective as an antidote for poisoning by phosphate ester AChEIs. The proposed mechanism for regeneration of AChE by 2-PAM is illustrated in Figure 9.20. The initial step involves binding of the quaternary ammonium nitrogen of 2-PAM to the anionic-binding site of phosphorylated AChE. This places the nucleophilic oxygen of 2-PAM in close proximity to the electrophilic phosphorus atom. Nucleophilic attack of the oxime oxygen results in breaking of the ester bond between the serine oxygen atom and the phosphorus atom. The final products of the reaction are the regenerated active form of AChE and phosphorylated 2-PAM.

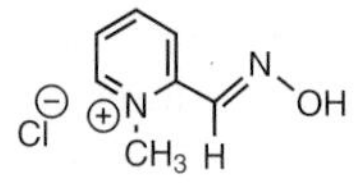

Pralidoxime chloride (2-PAM)

Pralidoxime is administered subcutaneously, intramuscularly, or intravenously, and it must be given within a short period of time after enzyme phosphorylation, generally a few hours after exposure, for it to be effective due to the aging process of the phosphorylated enzyme. Little reactivation is likely if given 36 hours after exposure. If the phosphorylated AChE has aged, 2-PAM will not regenerate the enzyme. For this reason, as well as because new phosphate ester AChEIs capable of aging rapidly are being developed as insecticides and chemical warfare agents, there is a continuing effort to discover new and better substitutes for 2-PAM. This research is focused on finding substitutes for 2-PAM that are better nucleophiles and, therefore, more effective generators of active AChE, as well as compounds that cross the blood–brain barrier to regenerate phosphorylated AChE in the brain.

Acetylcholine Antagonists—Muscarinic Antagonists

Muscarinic antagonists are compounds that have high binding affinity for mAChRs but exhibit no intrinsic activity. When the antagonist binds to the receptor, it is

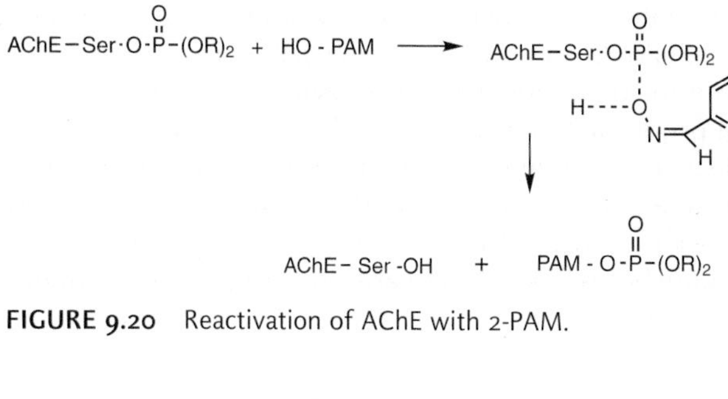

FIGURE 9.20 Reactivation of AChE with 2-PAM.

proposed that the receptor protein undergoes a conformational perturbation that is different from that produced by an agonist. Therefore, antagonist binding to the receptor produces no response. Muscarinic antagonists are often referred to as anticholinergics, antimuscarinics, cholinergic blockers, antispasmodics, or parasympatholytics. The term "anticholinergic" refers, in a pure sense, to medicinal agents that are antagonists at both mAChRs and nAChRs. Common usage of the term, however, has become synonymous with muscarinic antagonist, and it is used as such in this section.

Therapeutic Application

Muscarinic antagonists are employed as both prescription drugs and over-the-counter medications. Because they act as competitive (reversible) antagonists of acetylcholine, these compounds have pharmacologic effects that are opposite those of muscarinic agonists. Responses of muscarinic antagonists include decreased contractions of smooth muscle of the gastrointestinal and urinary tracts, dilation of the pupils, and reduced gastric, mucociliary, and salivary secretions. It follows that these compounds have therapeutic value in treating smooth muscle spasms associated with increased tone of the gastrointestinal tract or with overactive bladder, in ophthalmologic examinations, and in treatment of gastric ulcers. Compounds possessing muscarinic antagonist activity are common components of cold and flu remedies that act to reduce nasal and upper respiratory tract secretions.

In addition to reducing gastric motility, anticholinergic agents decrease gastric acid secretion and were once widely used to manage peptic ulcers. Histamine H_2 antagonists and, more recently, the proton pump inhibitors have largely replaced them for this use. When used systemically, they tend to produce undesirable side effects, such as blurred vision, photophobia, dry mouth, and difficulty in urination. These side effects tend to reduce patient compliance.

Anticholinergic agents exhibit a mydriatic action and, thus, must be used with caution due to their effect on intraocular pressure. Drainage of the canal of Schlemm is restricted by the iris when the pupil is dilated, and this can cause an increase in intraocular pressure. Hence, muscarinic antagonists are contraindicated in patients with glaucoma.

The aforementioned side effect of causing difficulty in urination has been used as an indication for several anticholinergic agents—darifenacin, trospium, solifenacin, tolterodine, and oxybutynin—for the treatment of overactive bladder.

Centrally acting belladonna alkaloids, such as scopolamine, have been used in transdermal delivery systems for prevention of motion sickness. They are most effective when used prophylactically; they have less effect when used after nausea and vomiting have begun. Several synthetic muscarinic antagonists have been used to treat parkinsonism and to block the extrapyramidal effects of antipsychotic agents. The anticholinergic alkaloid atropine is used for treatment of central and peripheral symptoms associated with poisoning by organophosphorous anticholinesterase agents.

Specific Agents—Solanaceous Alkaloids

The earliest known anticholinergic agents were alkaloids found in the family Solanaceae, a large family of plants that includes potatoes. *Atropa belladonna* (deadly nightshade), *Hyoscyamus niger* (black henbane), and *Datura stramonium* (jimsonweed, thorn apple) are plants that have significant historical importance to our understanding of the parasympathetic nervous system. Pharmacologic effects of extracts from these plants have been recognized since the Middle Ages, although these effects were not associated with the autonomic nervous system until the latter part of the 19th century. (−)-Hyoscyamine, isolated as atropine, and scopolamine are the two alkaloids that have found the widespread clinical applications.

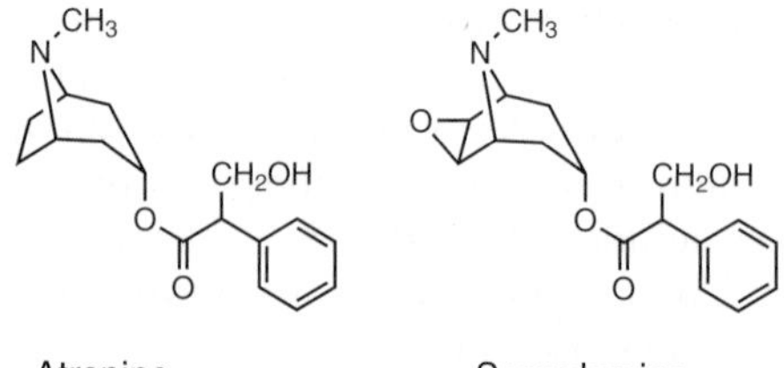

Atropine

Atropine is the tropic acid ester of tropine and is marketed as the sulfate salt. The naturally occurring alkaloid, (−)-hyoscyamine, undergoes base-catalyzed racemization during isolation from plants of the Solanaceae to give (±)-hyoscyamine or atropine. It was the first compound shown to block the effects of muscarine and electrical stimulation of the parasympathetic nervous system. Atropine sulfate has a number of clinical uses; two of the most common are treatment of bradycardia and as a preoperative agent to reduce secretions before surgery. Its use for management of parkinsonism has been supplanted by newer agents with fewer peripheral side effects. It has been used in ophthalmology as a cycloplegic agent to paralyze the iris and ciliary muscle in treatment of iritis and uveitis and as a cycloplegic/mydriatic agent. Atropine is contraindicated in glaucoma due to its ability to increase intraocular pressure during mydriasis. Its prolonged duration of mydriasis makes other drugs more attractive for this purpose. In poisoning by organophosphate nerve agents and insecticides, atropine decreases muscarinic cholinergic actions (e.g., lacrimation, salivation, sweating, bradycardia, and breathing problems) associated with this poisoning. It only treats the symptoms and does not reverse the underlying AChE inhibition. Approximately 50% of an oral dose of atropine is eliminated in the urine unchanged, 24% is eliminated as noratropine, 15% is eliminated as *N*-oxide, and less than 5% undergoes nonenzymatic ester hydrolysis. Its elimination half-life is 4 hours in adults and 6.5 hours in children.

SCOPOLAMINE Scopolamine, another Solanaceous alkaloid, is chemically and pharmacologically similar to atropine. Scopolamine is the generic name given to (−)-hyoscine, the naturally occurring alkaloid. The racemic compound, isolated during extraction of the alkaloid from plants, is atroscine. Scopolamine is marketed as the hydrobromide salt, because it is less deliquescent than some of its other salts. Interestingly, scopolamine is a CNS depressant at usual therapeutic doses, whereas atropine and other antimuscarinic agents are CNS stimulants. It has been used for the treatment of uveitis, iritis, and parkinsonism, but its most widespread use is for the treatment of motion sickness. For this indication, scopolamine is used in a transdermal patch applied to the skin behind the ear and is well-absorbed percutaneously following application. Plasma levels are observed within 4 hours and peak levels within 24 hours. It crosses the placenta and the blood–brain barrier. Although not well characterized, scopolamine is extensively metabolized in the liver and conjugated with less than 5% of the total dose appearing unchanged in the urine. Following patch removal, plasma levels decline linearly with an observed half-life of 9.5 hours.

Structure–activity Relationship Atropine, the prototype anticholinergic agent, provided the structural model that guided the design of synthetic muscarinic antagonists for almost 70 years. The circled portion of the atropine molecule depicts the segment resembling acetylcholine.

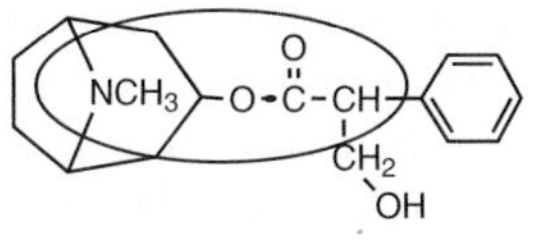

Although the amine functional group is separated from the ester oxygen by more than two carbons, the conformation assumed by the tropine ring orients these two atoms such that the intervening distance is similar to that in acetylcholine. One important structural difference between atropine and acetylcholine, both of which are esters of amino alcohols, is the size of the acyl portion of the molecules. Based on the assumption that size was a major factor in blocking action, many substituted acetic acid esters of amino alcohols were prepared and evaluated for biologic activity.

It became apparent that the most potent antagonists were those that possessed two lipophilic ring substituents on the carbon α to the carbonyl of the ester moiety. This is the first of the classic SARs for muscarinic antagonist activity, and this SAR became defined more precisely as research on these antagonists continued. The SAR for muscarinic antagonists can be summarized as follows:

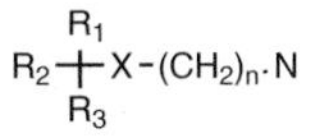

1. Substituents R_1 and R_2 should be carbocyclic or heterocyclic rings for maximal antagonist potency. The rings can be identical, but the more potent compounds have different rings. Generally, one ring is aromatic and the other saturated or possessing only one olefinic bond. Substituents R_1 and R_2, however, can be combined into a fused aromatic tricyclic ring system, such as that found in propantheline (Fig. 9.22). The size of these substituents is limited. For example, substitution of naphthalene rings for R_1 and R_2 affords compounds that are inactive, apparently due to steric hindrance of the binding of these compounds to the mAChR.
2. The R_3 substituent can be a hydrogen atom, a hydroxyl group, a hydroxymethyl group, or a carboxamide, or it can be a component of one of the R_1 and R_2 ring systems. When this substituent is either a hydroxyl group or a hydroxymethyl group, the antagonist is usually more potent than the same compound without this group. The hydroxyl group presumably increases binding strength by participating in a hydrogen bond interaction at the receptor.
3. The X substituent in the most potent anticholinergic agents is an ester, but an ester functional group is not an absolute necessity for muscarinic antagonist activity. This substituent can be an ether oxygen, or it can be absent completely.
4. The N substituent is a quaternary ammonium salt in the most potent anticholinergic agents. This

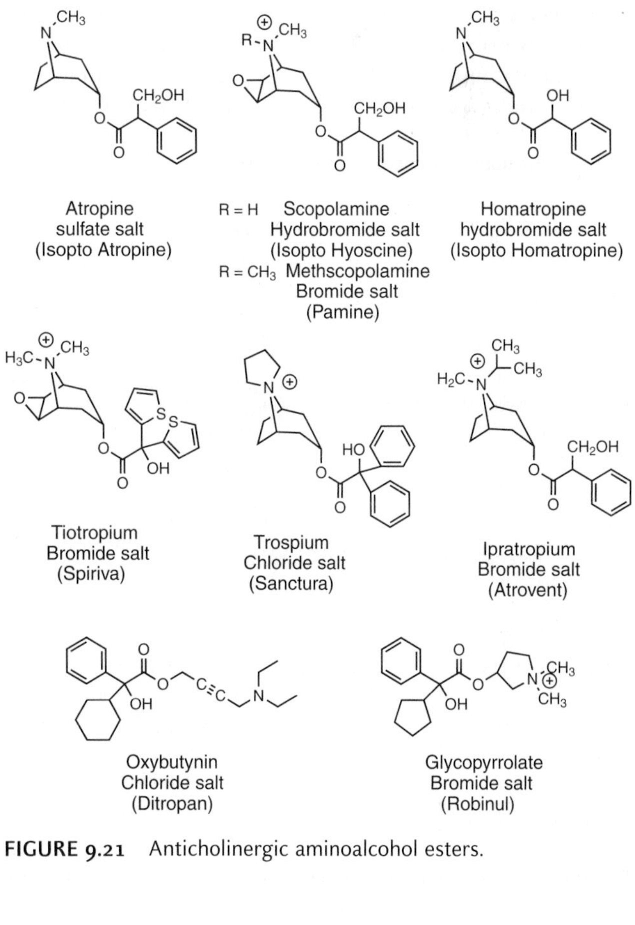

FIGURE 9.21 Anticholinergic aminoalcohol esters.

is not a requirement, however, because tertiary amines also possess antagonist activity, presumably by binding to the receptor in the cationic (conjugate acid) form. The alkyl substituents are usually methyl, ethyl, propyl, or isopropyl.

5. The distance between the ring-substituted carbon and the amine nitrogen apparently is not critical; the length of the alkyl chain connecting these can be from two to four carbons. The most potent anticholinergic agents have two methylene units in this chain.

Muscarinic antagonists must compete with agonists for a common receptor. Their ability to do this effectively is because the large groups R_1 and R_2 enhance binding to the receptor. Because antagonists are larger than agonists, this suggests that groups R_1 and R_2 bind outside the binding site of acetylcholine. It has been suggested that the area surrounding the binding site of acetylcholine is hydrophobic in nature (58). This accounts for the fact that in potent cholinergic antagonists, groups R_1 and R_2 must be hydrophobic (usually phenyl, cyclohexyl, or cyclopentyl). This concept is also supported by the current models for mAChRs.

Figures 9.21 and 9.22 and Table 9.3 include structures and pharmacologic properties of some of the anticholinergic agents that have found clinical application. These compounds reflect the SAR features that have been described. All these compounds are effective when administered orally or parenterally. Anticholinergic agents possessing a quaternary ammonium functional group are generally not well absorbed from the gastrointestinal tract due to their ionic character. These drugs are useful primarily in the treatment of ulcers or other conditions for which a reduction in gastric secretions and reduced motility of the gastrointestinal tract are desired. Those antagonists having a tertiary nitrogen are much better absorbed and distributed following all routes of administration and are especially useful when systemic distribution is desired. The tertiary amino-derived anticholinergic agents readily cross the blood–brain barrier. These have proven to be particularly beneficial in the treatment of Parkinson disease and other diseases requiring a central anticholinergic effect.

All these drugs display pronounced selectivity for mAChRs; however, some of those possessing the quaternary ammonium functional group exhibit nicotinic antagonist activity at high doses. With the exception of the M_3 antagonists, solifenacin and darifenacin, these agents display no marked selectivity for other mAChR subtypes.

Recent Muscarinic Antagonists More recently discovered muscarinic antagonists display a higher affinity for the receptors compared with the older agents, as exemplified by quinuclidinylbenzilate, which has structural features common to the classic anticholinergic agents. Radiolabeled quinuclidinylbenzilate was instrumental in the development of mAChR labeling techniques as well as the discovery of subtypes of mAChRs. This latter research depended also on the M_1-selective antagonist pirenzepine, a compound having a novel structure for muscarinic antagonist activity. A number of compounds structurally related to pirenzepine have demonstrated a similar M_1 selectivity; among these is telenzepine (59). Because of their selectivity for muscarinic M_1 receptors, pirenzepine and telenzepine have been evaluated in clinical trials for the treatment of duodenal ulcers. It is of interest to note that AFDX-116, structurally similar to pirenzepine, is a

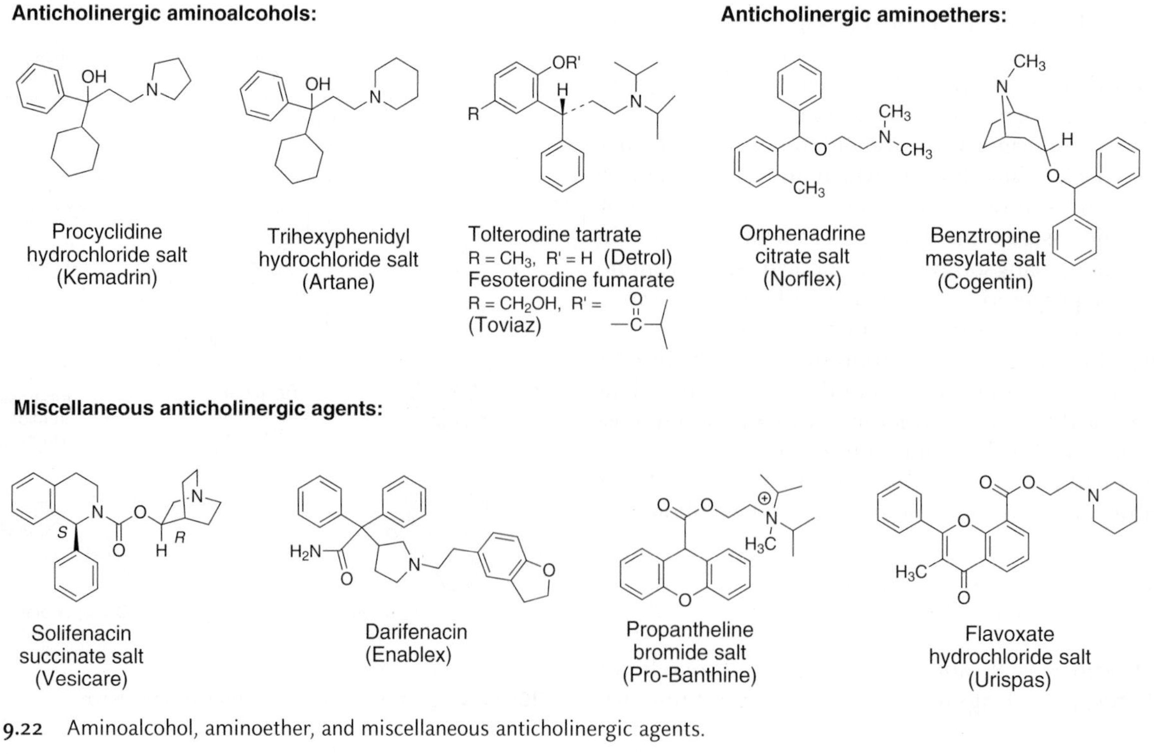

FIGURE 9.22 Aminoalcohol, aminoether, and miscellaneous anticholinergic agents.

TABLE 9.3 Anticholinergic Agents

Name	Calculated[a] LogP and LogD (pH 7)	Half-Life	Metabolism	Indications	Comments
Atropine	1.53 −1.21	3.5 ± 1.5 h	Hydrolysis; N-dealkylation; *N*-oxide	Bradycardia; parkinsonism; cycloplegic/mydriatic	Nonselective muscarinic antagonist; stimulates the CNS
Scopolamine	0.76 0.29	8 h	Almost completely metabolized (liver)	Uveitis; iritis; parkinsonism; motion sickness	Nonselective muscarinic antagonist; CNS depressant
Homatropine (Isopto Homatropine)	1.57 −1.17	—	—	Cycloplegic/mydriatic	Nonselective muscarinic antagonist; less potent and shorter duration than atropine
Ipratropium bromide (Atrovent)	—	2 h	Hydrolysis	Bronchodilator (oral inhalation); seasonal rhinitis (nasal spray)	Nonselective muscarinic antagonist; slow onset after inhalation
Tiotropium bromide (Spiriva)	—	5–6 d	CYP2D6 and CYP3A4; hydrolysis; N-dealkylation; glucuronide conjugation	Chronic obstructive pulmonary disease (oral inhalation)	Equal affinity for M_1, M_2, and M_3 receptors
Trospium chloride (Sanctura)	—	20 h	Hydrolysis; conjugation	Urinary and gastrointestinal antispasmodic	High affinity for M_1 and M_3 receptors; lesser affinity for M_2
Oxybutynin (oral: Ditropan and Ditropan XL; transdermal: Oxytrol)	5.19 3.93	2–5 h	CYP3A4; hydrolysis; N-dealkylation	Overactive bladder	Nonselective muscarinic antagonist
Solifenacin (Vesicare)	3.70 1.70	55 h	4-(*R*)-Hydroxy (active); *N*-glucuronide; *N*-oxide; 4*R*-hydroxy-*N*-oxide	Overactive bladder	Selective M_3 antagonist
Tolterodine (Detrol)	5.77 2.79	2–4 h (extensive metabolizers); 9.6 h (poor metabolizers)	Primary pathway: CYP2D6 (primary); 7% of Caucasians and 2% of African Americans lack CYP2D6; CYP3A4 is the primary pathway in the latter. Metabolites: 5-hydroxymethyl (active), 5-carboxylic acid, *N*-dealkylated-5-carboxylic acid	Overactive bladder	Nonselective muscarinic antagonist
Fesoterodine fumarate (Toviaz)	5.08 ± 0.28 2.09	7	Hydrolysis to 5-hydroxymethyl tolterodine, followed by CYP2D6 and CYP3A4 to give carboxy, carboxy-*N*-desisopropy, *N*-desisopropyl metabolites	Overactive bladder	Prodrug of 5-hydroxymethyl tolterodine, a nonselective muscarinic agonist
Darifenacin (Enablex)	4.50 2.25	—	CYP2D6 (primary; see tolterodine above); hydroxylation of the dihydrobenzofuran; ring opening (dihydrobenzofuran); N-dealkylation	Overactive bladder	Selective M_3 antagonist

[a] Values calculated using ACD Lab Solarius, Chemical Abstracts Service, 2006, Columbus, OH (values for quaternary compounds are not listed).

muscarinic antagonist exhibiting selectivity for cardiac M_2 receptors.

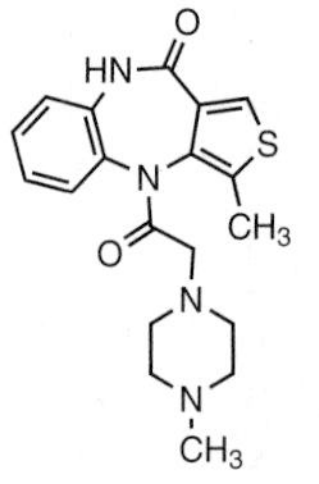
Telenzepine

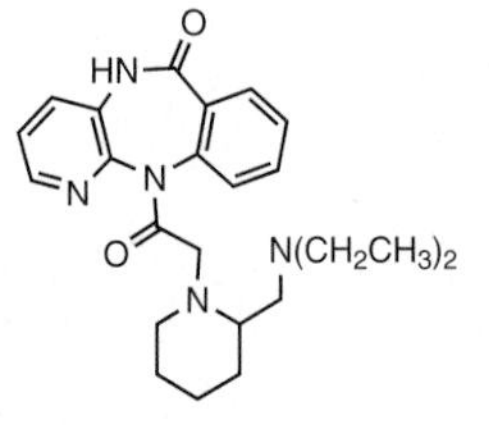
AFDX - 116

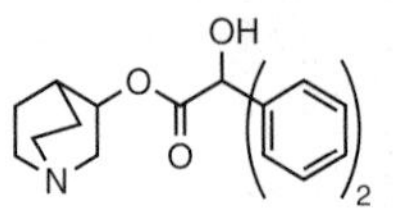
3-Quinuclidinylbenzilate (QNB)

NICOTINIC ANTAGONISTS—NEUROMUSCULAR BLOCKING AGENTS

Nicotinic antagonists are chemical compounds that bind to nAChRs but have no efficacy. All therapeutically useful nicotinic antagonists are competitive antagonists; in other words, the effects are reversible with acetylcholine. There are two subclasses of nicotinic antagonists—skeletal neuromuscular blocking agents and ganglionic blocking agents—classified according to the two populations of nAChRs, NM and NN, respectively. This section emphasizes nicotinic antagonists used clinically as neuromuscular blocking agents. These medicinal agents should not be confused with those skeletal muscle relaxant compounds that produce their effects through the CNS.

History

In terms of the historical perspective, tubocurarine, the first known neuromuscular blocking drug, was as important to the understanding of nicotinic antagonists as atropine was to that of muscarinic antagonists. The neuromuscular blocking effects of extracts of curare were first reported as early as 1510, when explorers of the Amazon River region of South America found natives using these plant extracts as arrow poisons. Early research with these crude plant extracts indicated that the active components caused muscle paralysis by effects on either the nerve or the muscle (remember that the concept of neurochemical transmission was not introduced until the late 19th century). In 1856, however, Bernard described the results of his experiments, which demonstrated unequivocally that curare extracts prevented skeletal muscle contractions by an effect at the neuromuscular junction, rather than the nerve innervating the muscle or the muscle itself (60).

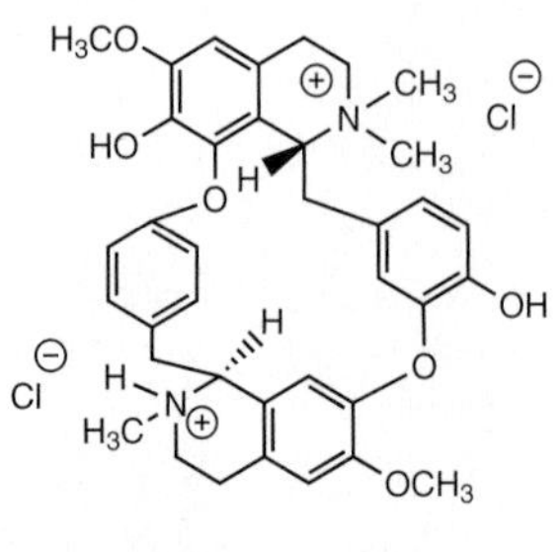
d-Tubocurarine chloride

Much of the early literature concerning the effects of curare is confusing and difficult to interpret. This is not at all surprising considering that this research was performed using crude extracts, many of which came from different plants. It was not until the late 1800s that scientists recognized that curare extracts contained quaternary ammonium salts. This knowledge prompted the use of other quaternary ammonium compounds to explore the neuromuscular junction. In the meantime, curare extracts continued to be used to block the effects of nicotine and acetylcholine at skeletal neuromuscular junctions and to explore the nAChRs.

In 1935, King (61) isolated a pure alkaloid, which he named *d*-tubocurarine, from a tube curare of unknown botanical origin. The word "tube" refers to the container in which the South American natives transported their plant extract. It was almost 10 years later that the botanical source for *d*-tubocurarine was clearly identified as *Chondodendron tomentosum*. The structure that King assigned to tubocurarine possessed two nitrogen atoms, both of which were quaternary ammonium salts (e.g., a *bis*-quaternary ammonium compound). It was not until 1970 that the correct structure was reported by Everett et al. (62). The correct structure, shown here, has only one quaternary ammonium nitrogen; the other nitrogen is a tertiary amine salt. Nevertheless, the incorrect structure of tubocurarine served as the model for the synthesis of all the neuromuscular blocking agents in use today. These compounds have been of immense therapeutic value for surgical and orthopedic procedures and have been essential to research that led to the isolation and purification of nAChRs.

The potential therapeutic benefits of the neuromuscular blocking effects of tubocurarine as well as the difficulty in obtaining pure samples of the alkaloid encouraged medicinal chemists to design structurally related compounds possessing nicotinic antagonist activity. Using the incorrectly assigned *bis*-quaternary ammonium structure of tubocurarine, as reported by King (61), as a guide, a large number of compounds were synthesized and evaluated. It became apparent that a *bis*-quaternary ammonium compound having two quaternary ammonium salts separated by 10 to 12 carbon atoms (similar to the distance between the nitrogen atoms in tubocurarine) was a requirement for neuromuscular blocking activity. The rationale for this structural requirement was that in contrast to mAChRs, nAChRs possessed two anionic-binding sites, both of which had to be occupied for a neuromuscular blocking effect. It is important to observe that the current transmembrane model for the nAChR protein has two anionic sites in the extracellular domain.

Some of the new *bis*-quaternary ammonium agents produced depolarization of the postjunctional membrane at the neuromuscular junction before causing blockade; other compounds, such as tubocurarine, did not produce this depolarization. Thus, the structural features of the remainder of the molecule determined whether the nicotinic antagonist was a depolarizing or a nondepolarizing neuromuscular blocker.

Therapeutic Application

Neuromuscular blocking agents are used primarily as an adjunct to general anesthesia. Their pharmacokinetics are shown in Table 9.4. They produce skeletal muscle relaxation that facilitates operative procedures such as abdominal surgery. Furthermore, they reduce the depth requirement for general anesthetics; this decreases the overall risk of a surgical procedure and shortens the postanesthetic recovery time. Muscles producing rapid movements are the first to be affected by neuromuscular blocking agents. These include muscles of the face, eyes, and neck. Muscles of the limbs, chest, and abdomen are affected next, with the diaphragm (respiration) being affected last. Recovery generally is in the reverse order.

Neuromuscular blocking agents have also been used in the correction of dislocations and the realignment of fractures. Short-acting neuromuscular blocking agents, such as succinylcholine, are routinely used to assist in tracheal intubation. When choosing a neuromuscular blocking agent, four questions must be considered:

1. Will the compound produce the desired neuromuscular blockade?
2. What is its duration of action?
3. What are its adverse effects?
4. What is its relative cost?

Side Effects

Adverse reactions to most, but not all, of the neuromuscular blocking agents can include hypotension, bronchospasm, and cardiac disturbances. The depolarizing agents also cause an initial muscle fasciculation before relaxation. Many of these agents cause release of histamine and subsequent cutaneous (flushing, erythema, urticaria, and pruritus), pulmonary (bronchospasm and wheezing), and cardiovascular (hypotension) effects.

Specific Depolarizing Neuromuscular Blocking Agents

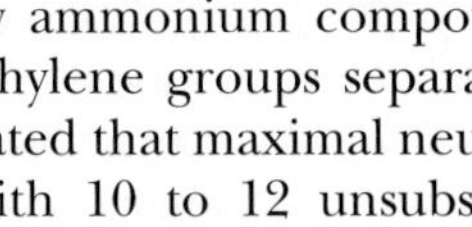

Decamethonium bromide

Decamethonium Bromide

Decamethonium was one of the first neuromuscular blocking agents synthesized. An SAR study on a series of *bis*-quaternary ammonium compounds with varying numbers of methylene groups separating the nitrogen atoms demonstrated that maximal neuromuscular blockade occurred with 10 to 12 unsubstituted methylene groups. Activity diminished as the number of carbons was either decreased or increased. The compound with six methylene groups, hexamethonium, is a nicotinic antagonist at autonomic ganglia (ganglionic blocking agent). All compounds in this series that possessed neuromuscular blocking activity also caused depolarization of the postjunctional membrane.

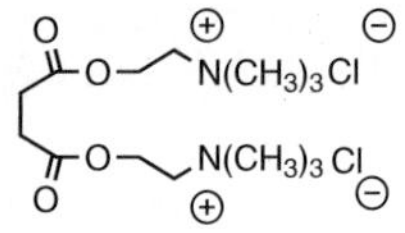

Succinylcholine chloride

Succinylcholine Chloride (*Anectine*)

Succinylcholine is a depolarizing neuromuscular blocking agent that represents a dimer of acetylcholine bonded through the α-carbon atom of each. The molecule can exist in an extended conformation (antiperiplanar). This would account for the appropriate separation of the quaternary nitrogens. Succinylcholine is rapidly hydrolyzed and rendered inactive both in aqueous solution and by plasma esterases; this chemical instability must be considered when preparing solutions for parenteral administration. This same chemical property, however, gives the compound a brief duration of action. As a result, succinylcholine is frequently used for rapid induction of neuromuscular blockade and when blockade of short duration is desired (Table 9.4). As such, it is used primarily to produce muscle relaxation during endotracheal intubation or endoscopic procedures. The depolarizing property is undesirable in neuromuscular blockers, so most research efforts have been directed toward the design of nondepolarizing agents.

Specific Nondepolarizing Neuromuscular Blocking Agents

Compounds in this class have one or two quaternary ammonium groups. Those with only one quaternary ammonium group, however, exist as *bis*-cations in vivo due to the second positive charge being on a protonated tertiary amine. The various structures of these compounds serve primarily as a "scaffold" to position two positive charges in the correct three-dimensional orientation for interaction with the transmembrane nAChRs.

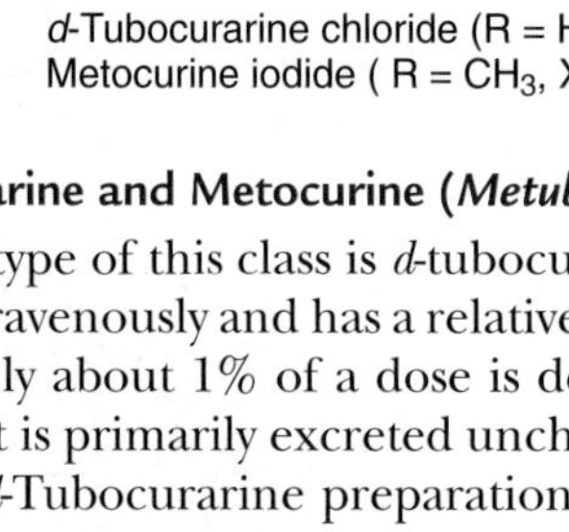

d-Tubocurarine chloride (R = H, X = Cl)
Metocurine iodide (R = CH_3, X = I)

d-Tubocurarine and Metocurine (*Metubine Iodide*)

The prototype of this class is *d*-tubocurarine. It is administered intravenously and has a relatively long duration of action. Only about 1% of a dose is demethylated in the liver, and it is primarily excreted unchanged in the urine and bile. *d*-Tubocurarine preparations contain bisulfites and, thus, can potentiate allergic reactions in patients with bisulfate allergy. It is the most potent inducer of

TABLE 9.4 Properties of Clinically Useful Neuromuscular Blocking Agents

Agent	Time of Onset (min)	Duration of Action (min)	Half-life (min)	Mode of Elimination
Succinylcholine	1–1.5	6–8	<1	Hydrolysis by plasma chclinesterases
d-Tubocurarine	4–6	80–120	173	Renal elimination, liver clearance
Vecuronium	2–4	30–40	65–80	Liver metabclism and clearance renal relimination
Pancuronium	4–6	120–180	89–140	Renal elimination, liver metabolism and clearance
Pipecuronium	2–4	80–100	137–161	Renal elimination, liver metabolism and clearance
Rocuronium	1–2	30–40	84–131	Liver metabolism and clearance
Atracurium	2–4	30–40	16–20	Hofmann degradation, hydrolysis by plasma cholinesterases
Mivacurium	2–4	12–18	1.8–2.0	Hydrolysis by plasma cholinesterases
Doxacurium	4–6	90–120	72–96	Renal elimination, liver metabolism and clearance

Adapted from Taylor P. Agents acting at the neuromuscular junction and autonomic ganglia. In: Brunton LL, Lazo JS, Parker KL, eds. Goodman and Gilman's The pharmacological Basis of Therapeutics, 11th Ed. New York: McGraw-Hill, 2006:217–236; with permission.

histamine release of all the nondepolarizing neuromuscular blockers.

Reaction of *d*-tubocurarine with methyl iodide affords metocurine iodide (see above), in which the two phenolic hydroxyl groups of *d*-tubocurarine are changed to the methyl ethers and the tertiary amine becomes quaternary. This agent is approximately fourfold more potent than *d*-tubocurarine in neuromuscular blocking activity. Like *d*-tubocurarine, it has a long duration of action and is eliminated (predominantly unchanged) via the kidney.

Steroid-Based Neuromuscular Blocking Agents

An ideal neuromuscular blocking agent would be a nondepolarizing compound that is metabolically inactivated and rapidly eliminated. Efforts to design such a neuromuscular blocker have resulted in the development of several synthetic neuromuscular agents. Those that have found clinical use are either aminosteroids derived from (+)-malouetine (an aminosteroid found in the rain forest of central Africa) (Fig. 9.23) or tetrahydroisoquinoline derivatives (Fig. 9.24).

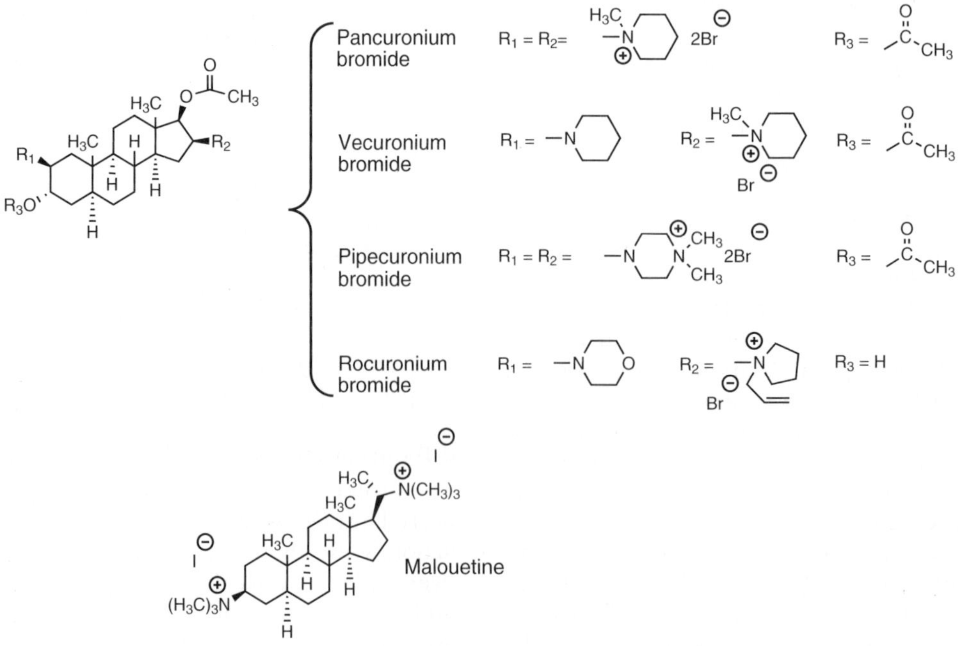

FIGURE 9.23 Aminosteroid–based neuromuscular blocking agents.

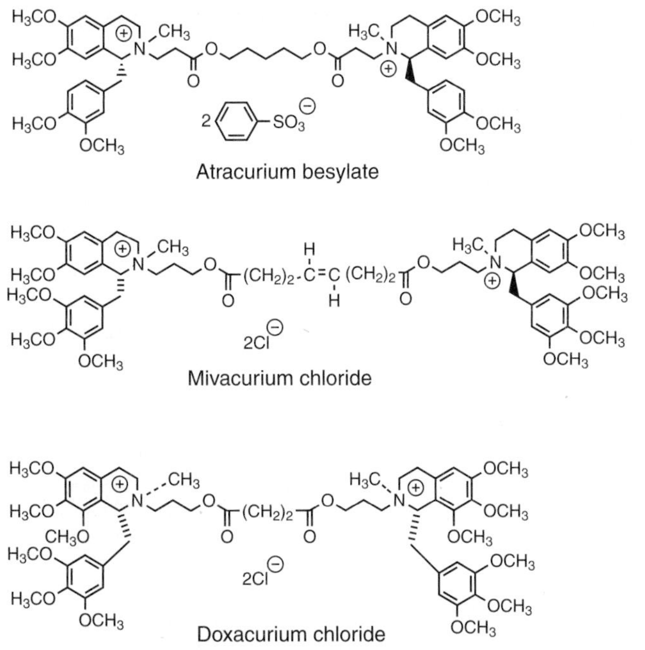

FIGURE 9.24 Tetrahydroisoquinoline-based neuromuscular blocking agents.

Pancuronium Bromide (*Pavulon*) Pancuronium, a long-acting agent, is more active than tubocurarine. It can cause increases in heart rate and blood pressure and should not be used in patients with coronary artery disease. Pancuronium undergoes hydrolysis in the liver to the active 3-hydroxy metabolite and the inactive 17-hydroxy and 3,17-dihydroxy metabolites; it is excreted primarily in the urine, with small amounts in the bile.

Vecuronium Bromide (*Norcuron*) Removal of the methyl group from the quaternary piperidinium group at position 3 of pancuronium affords vecuronium, an intermediate-acting agent. Vecuronium has the advantage of not inducing histamine release at normal doses and of not exhibiting significant cardiovascular effects. One-third of an administered dose of vecuronium is hydrolyzed to the 3-hydroxy, 17-hydroxy, and 3,17-dihydroxy metabolites, all of which are active. Accumulation of the 3,17-dihydroxy metabolite is responsible for prolonged neuromuscular blockade in patients receiving long-term therapy with vecuronium.

Pipecuronium Bromide (*Arduan*) Pipecuronium bromide, a long-acting neuromuscular blocking agent, exhibits minimal cardiovascular effects. Like pancuronium and vecuronium, pipecuronium undergoes some hydrolysis but is excreted primarily unchanged in the urine with very small amounts in the bile. Pipecuronium can be used in patients with coronary artery disease, but neuromuscular blockade is prolonged in patients with renal failure.

Rocuronium Bromide (*Zemuron*) Rocuronium bromide is an intermediate-acting agent with a duration of action similar to vecuronium and atracurium but with a more rapid onset. It does not appear to cause significant histamine release.

Tetrahydroisoquinoline-Based Neuromuscular Blocking Agents

Atracurium Besylate (*Tracrium*) Atracurium besylate is a nondepolarizing neuromuscular blocker in which the quaternary ammonium groups are located in two substituted tetrahydroisoquinoline rings separated by an aliphatic diester. Its duration of action is slightly longer than that of succinylcholine. Atracurium is not metabolized in the liver; rather, it undergoes hydrolysis of the

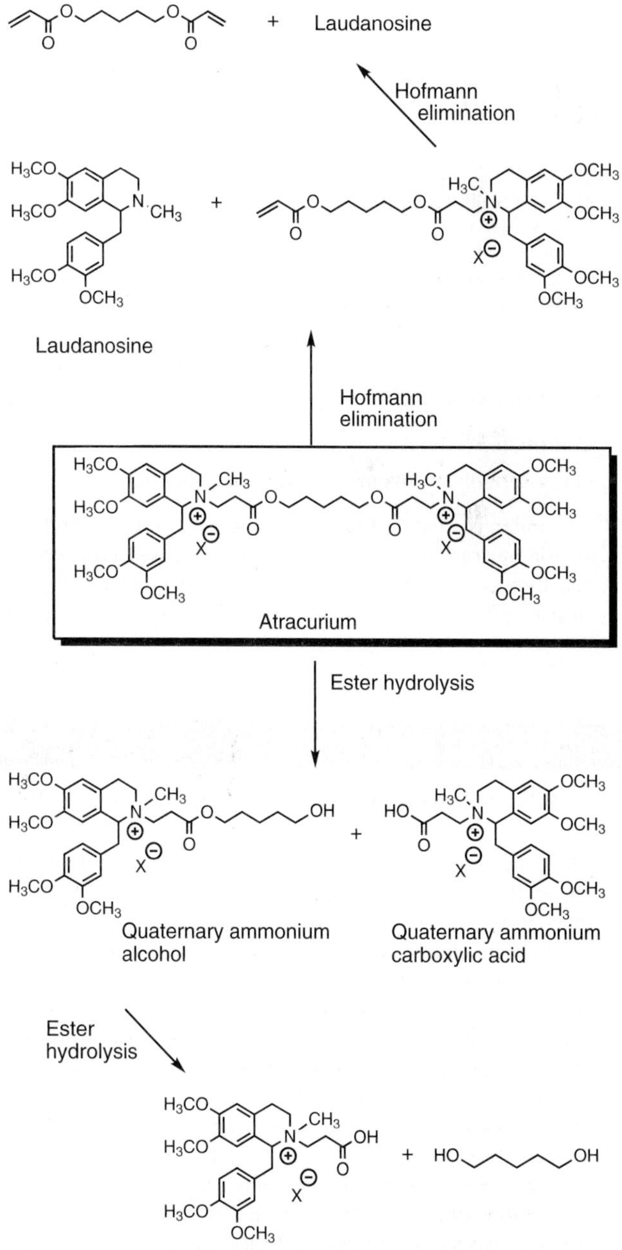

FIGURE 9.25 Inactivation of atracurium by Hofmann elimination and hydrolysis.

ester functional groups that connect the two quaternary nitrogens. It also undergoes Hofmann elimination, a nonenzymatic, base-catalyzed decomposition, to yield laudanosine, which is inactive (Fig. 9.25) (63,64). Thus, termination of the effects of atracurium is independent of renal elimination. Because of this unusual metabolic profile, it is useful in patients with hepatic or renal disease.

Mivacurium Chloride (*Mivacron*) Mivacurium chloride is a mixture of three stereoisomers, with the *trans-trans* (92% to 96%) and the *cis–trans* diesters being equipotent. The *cis–cis* diester produces only minimal (<5%) neuromuscular blockade. It is hydrophilic, has a small volume of distribution, and is distributed primarily to extracellular fluids. Mivacurium is short acting (Table 9.4), with mean elimination half-lives for the *trans–trans* and *cis–trans* stereoisomers of 2.0 and 1.8 minutes, respectively, in adults receiving opioid/nitrous oxide/oxygen anesthesia. It is rapidly hydrolyzed and does not undergo Hofmann elimination like atracurium.

Doxacurium Chloride (*Nuromax*) Doxacurium is a mixture of three *trans-trans* stereoisomers, a *dl* pair [1*R*,1′*R*,2*S*,2′*S* and 1*S*,1′*S*,2*R*,2′*R*] and a *meso* form 1*R*,1′*S*,2*S*,2′*R*. Doxacurium is hydrophilic, has a small volume of distribution, and is distributed primarily to extracellular fluids. It is not metabolized by plasma cholinesterase or hepatic enzymes and does not undergo Hofmann elimination.

Scenario: Outcome and Analysis

Outcome

Kathryn Neill, PharmD

The pharmacist reviews the package insert and tells LT that he does not need to take ipecac or try to make himself expel the medication. There is little chance he will experience any symptoms, but the main symptom he may experience is dry mouth. The pharmacist also recommends LT take a regular daily dose of tiotropium using the inhalation device.

Chemical Analysis

Kathryn Neill, S. William Zito, and Victoria Roche

Tiotropium is a long-acting anticholinergic agent with an affinity for muscarinic receptors M1–M5. It causes bronchodilation through inhibition of M3 receptors in bronchial smooth muscle; effects can last more than 24 hours. Tiotropium is the dithienyl derivative of *N*-methyl scopolamine, a quaternary ammonium analog of naturally occurring scopolamine in *Atropa belladonna.*

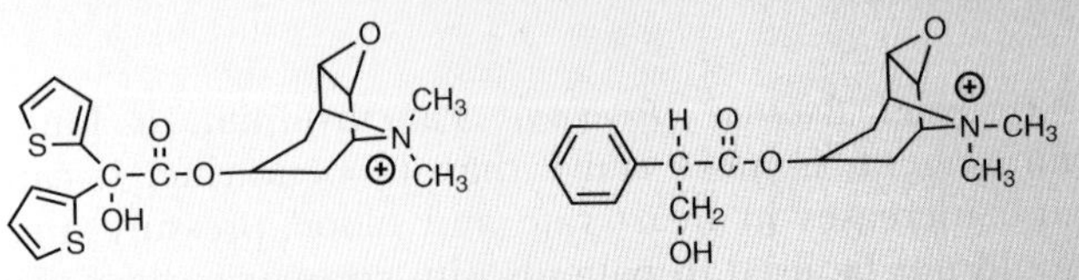

Tiotropium bromide N-Methyl scopolamine

The bioavailability of inhaled tiotropium is approximately 19% in healthy volunteers, and therapeutic bronchodilation is predominantly a site-specific effect. Gastrointestinal absorption is minimal, with an oral solution resulting in bioavailability of only about 2%.

Case Study

S. William Zito and Victoria Roche

NM is a 43-year-old man of East Indian heritage. He presents to the ophthalmology department of the hospital where you are on rotation. He explains to the ophthalmologist that he has been experiencing blurred vision in his left eye. He is a senior executive in a software company and his work involves a lot of reading and computer work. He has been having this problem for the last 3 to 4 months, and it is becoming increasingly difficult for him to work at the computer. On examination he had a visual acuity of 20/20 in the right eye and 20/40 in the left eye. The lens in the left eye showed a small central cataract whereas the right eye was normal. Anterior segment examination showed normal anterior chambers with normal pupils. Fundus examination showed no abnormality and intraocular pressure was 14 mm Hg in the left eye and 16 mm Hg in the right. Retinal examination also was normal in both the eyes. It was decided to conduct cataract surgery in the left eye via phacoemulsification. The ophthalmologist wants to use a cholinergic agonist for the induction of meiosis. Your preceptor shows you the following structures and asks you which one you would recommend for this surgery.

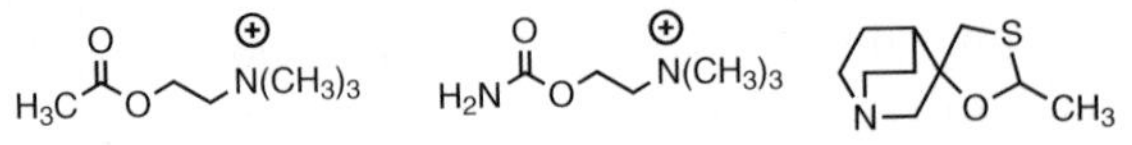

1 2 3

1. Conduct a thorough and mechanistic SAR analysis of the three therapeutic options in the case.
2. Apply the chemical understanding gained from the SAR analysis to this patient's specific needs to make a therapeutic recommendation.

References

1. Katzung BG. Introduction to autonomic pharmacology. In: Katzung BG, ed. Basic and Clinical Pharmacology, 11th Ed. New York: McGraw-Hill, 2009:77–94.
2. Holmstedt G. Pages from the history of research on cholinergic mechanisms. In: Waser PG, ed. Cholinergic Mechanisms. New York: Raven Press, 1975:1–21.
3. Loewi O. Humoral transfer of heart action. Arch Ges Physiol 1921;189:237–242.
4. Loewi O, Navratil E. Mechanism of the action of physostigmine and of ergotamine on vagus action. Arch Ges Physiol 1926;214:689–696.
5. Pert CB, Snyder SH. Opiate receptor: demonstration in nervous tissue. Science 1973;179:1011–1114.
6. Changeaux JP, Devillers-Thiery A, Chemouilli P. Acetylcholine receptor: an allosteric protein. Science 1984;225:1335–1345.
7. Mishina M, Kurodaki T, Tobimatsu T, et al. Expression of functional acetylcholine receptor from cloned cDNAs. Nature 1984;307:604–608.
8. Caulfield JP, Birdsall NJM. International Union of Pharmacology. XVII. Classification of muscarinic acetylcholine receptors. Pharmacol Rev 1998;50:279–290.
9. Lukas RJ, Bencherif M. Heterogeneity and regulation of nicotinic acetylcholine receptors. Int Rev Neurobiol 1992;34:25–131.
10. Ing HR. The structure–action relationships of the choline group. Science 1949;109:264–266.
11. Westfall TC, Westfall DP. Neurotransmission: the autonomic and somatic motor nervous systems. In: Brunton LL, Lazo JS, Parker KL, eds. Goodman and Gilman's The Pharmacological Basis of Therapeutics, 11th Ed. New York: McGraw-Hill, 2006:137–181.
12. Lameh J, Cone RI, Maeda S, et al. Structure and function of G protein coupled receptors. Pharm Res 1990;7:1213–1221.
13. Drubbisch V, Drubbisch V, Lameh J, et al. Mapping the ligand binding pocket of the human muscarinic cholinergic receptor Hm1: contribution of tyrosine-82. Pharm Res 1992;9:1644–1647.
14. Dixon RAF, Strader CD, Sigal IS. Structure and function of G protein–coupled receptors. Annu Rep Med Chem 1988;23:221–233.
15. Linder ME, Gilman AG. G proteins. Sci Am 1992;267:56–65.
16. Ehlert FJ, Ostrom RS, Sawyer GW. Subtypes of the muscarinic receptor in smooth muscle. Life Sci 1997;61:1729–1740.
17. Nordvall G, Hacksell U. Binding-site modeling of the muscarinic m_1 receptor: a combination of homology-based and indirect approaches. J Med Chem 1993;36:967–976.
18. Humblet C, Mirzadegan T. Three-dimensional models of G protein–coupled receptors. Annu Rep Med Chem 1992;27:291–300.
19. van Koppen CJ, Kaiser B. Regulation of muscarinic acetylcholine signaling. Pharmacol Ther 2003;98:197–220.
20. Lindstrom J, Anand R, Peng X, et al. Neuronal nicotinic receptor subtypes. Ann N Y Acad Sci 1995;757:100–116.
21. Le Novere N, Changeux JP. Molecular evolution of the nicotinic acetylcholine receptor: an example of multigene family in excitable cell. J Mol Evol 1995;40:155–172.
22. Changeux JP. The nicotinic acetylcholine receptor: an allosteric protein prototype if ligand-gated ion channels. Trends Pharmacol Sci 1990;11:485–492.
23. Luyten WHML, Heinemann SG. Molecular cloning of the nicotinic acetylcholine receptor: new opportunities in drug design. Annu Rep Med Chem 1987;22:281–291.
24. Arias HR. Localization of agonist and competitive antagonist binding sites on nicotinic acetylcholine receptors. Neurochem Int 2000;36:595–645.
25. Picciotto MR, Caldarone BJ, Brunzell DH, et al. Neuronal nicotinic acetylcholine receptor subunit knockout mice: physiological and behavioral phenotypes and possible clinical implications. Pharmacol Ther 2001;92:89–108.
26. Taylor P. Agents acting at the neuromuscular junction and autonomic ganglia. In: Brunton LL, Lazo JS, Parker KL, eds. Goodman and Gilman's The Pharmacological Basis of Therapeutics, 11th Ed. New York: McGraw-Hill, 2006:217–236.
27. Holladay MW, Dart MJ, Lynch JK. Neuronal nicotinic receptors as targets for drug discovery. J Med Chem 1997;40:4170–4194.
28. Changeux JP. Chemical signaling in the brain. Sci Am 1993;269:58–62.
29. Tucek S. Choline acetyltransferase and synthesis of acetylcholine. In: Wittaker VP, ed. The Cholinergic Synapse: Handbook of Experimental Pharmacology. Berlin: Springer-Verlag, 1988:125–165.
30. Atri A, Chang MS, Strichartz GR. Cholinergic pharmacology. In: Golan DE, Tashjian, AH Jr, Armstrong EJ, et al., eds. Principles of Pharmacology, 2nd Ed. Philadelphia, PA: Wolters Kluwer–Lippincott Williams & Wilkins, 2008:109–128.
31. Armstrong PD, Cannon JG, Long JP. Conformationally rigid analogues of acetylcholine. Nature 1968;220:65–66.
32. Ing HR, Kordik P, Williams DPHT. Studies on the structure–action relationships of the choline group. Br J Pharmacol 1952;7:103–116.
33. Welch AD, Roepke MH. A comparative study of choline and certain of its analogues. I. The pharmacological activity of acetylphosphocholine and acetylarsenocholine relative to acetylcholine. J Pharmacol Exp Ther 1935;55:118–126.
34. Hotlon P, Ing HR. The specificity of the trimethylammonium group in acetylcholine. Br J Pharmacol 1949;4:190–196.
35. Stehle RL, Melville KI, Oldham FK. Choline as a factor in the elaboration of adrenaline. J Pharmacol Exp Ther 1936;56:473–481.
36. Bocick NC, Offen WW, Levey AI, et al. Effects of xanomeline, a selective muscarinic receptor agonist, on cognitive function and behavioral symptoms in Alzheimer's disease. Arch Neurol 1997;54:465–473.
37. John V, Lieberburg I, Thorsett ED. Alzheimer's disease: current therapeutic approaches. Annu Rep Med Chem 1993;28:197–206.
38. Karczmar AG. Anticholinesterase agents: In: Raduoco-Thomas C, ed. International Encyclopedia of Pharmacology and Therapeutics, Section 13, Vol 1. New York: Pergamon Press, 1970:1–44.
39. Sussman JL, Harel M, Frolow F, et al. Atomic structure of acetylcholinesterase from *Torpedo californica*: a prototypic acetylcholine-binding protein. Science 1991;253:872–879.
40. Scrutton NS, Raine ARC. Cation-π bonding and amino-aromatic interactions in the biomolecular recognition of substituted ammonium ligands. Biochem J 1996;319:1–8.
41. Ordentlich A, Barak D, Kronman C, et al. Dissection of the human acetylcholinesterase active center determinants of substrate specificity. Identification of residues constituting the anionic site, the hydrophobic site, and the acyl pocket. J Biol Chem 1993;268:17083–17095.
42. Shafferman A, Kronman C, Flashner Y. Mutagenesis of human acetylcholinesterase. J Biol Chem 1992;267:17640–17648.
43. Zhang Y, Kua J, McCammon JA. Role of catalytic triad and oxyanion hole in acetylcholinesterase catalysis: an abinitio QM/MM study. J Am Chem Soc 2002;124:10572–10577.
44. Taylor P, Brown JH. Acetylcholine: In: Siegel GJ, Agranoff BW, Alders RW, et al., eds. Basic Neurochemistry, Molecular, Cellular and Medical Aspects, 6th Ed. Philadelphia, PA: Lippincott-Raven, 1999:213–242.
45. Harel M, Quinn DM, Nair HK, et al. The X-ray structure of a transition state analog complex reveals the molecular origins of the catalytic power and substrate specificity of acetylcholinesterase. J Am Chem Soc 1996;118:2340–2346.
46. Wilson IB, Harrison MA, Ginsberg S. Carbamyl derivatives of acetylcholinesterase. J Biol Chem 1961;236:1498–1500.
47. Rzeszotarski WJ. Alzheimer's disease: search for therapeutics. In: Abraham DJ, ed. Burger's Medicinal Chemistry & Drug Discovery, Vol 6, 6th Ed. Hoboken, NJ: John Wiley & Sons, 2003:743–777.
48. Schroder H, Giacobini E, Strubble RG, et al. Nicotinic cholinoceptive neurons of the frontal cortex are reduced in Alzheimer's disease. Neurobiol Aging 1991;12:259–262.
49. Nordberg A, Winblad B. Reduced number of [H³]nicotine and [H³] acetylcholine binding sites in the frontal cortex of Alzheimer brains. Neurosci Lett 1986;72:115–119.
50. Sugaya K, Giacobini E, Chiappinelli VA. Nicotinic acetylcholine receptor subtypes in human frontal cortex: changes in Alzheimer's disease. J Neurosci Res 1990;27:349–359.
51. Whitehouse PJ, Martino AM, Antuono PG, et al. Nicotinic acetylcholine binding sites in Alzheimer's disease. Brain Res 1986;371:146–151.
52. Shutske GM, Pierrat FA, Kapples KJ, et al. 9-Amino-1,2,3,4-tetrahydroacridin-1-ols: synthesis and evaluation as potential Alzheimer's disease therapeutics. J Med Chem 1989;32:1805–1813.
53. Galatsis P. Market to market—1997. Annu Rep Med Chem 1998;33:327–353.
54. Wilson IB, Ginsburg S. A powerful reactivator of alkylphosphate-inhibited acetylcholinesterase. Biochim Biophys Acta 1955;18:168–170.
55. Wilson IB. Molecular complementarity and antidotes for alkyl phosphate poisoning. Fed Proc 1959;18:752–758.
56. Wilson IB. Acetylcholinesterase. XI. Reversibility of tetraethylpyrophosphate inhibition. J Biol Chem 1951;190:111–117.
57. Hestrin S. Acetylation reactions mediated by purified acetylcholine esterase. J Biol Chem 1949;180:879–881.
58. Ariens EJ. Receptor theory and structure–activity relationships. Adv Drug Res 1966;3:235–285.
59. Mihm G, Wetzel B. Peripheral actions of selective muscarinic agonists and antagonists. Annu Rep Med Chem 1988;23:81–90.
60. McIntyre AR. History of curare. In: Cheymol J, ed. International Encyclopedia of Pharmacology and Therapeutics, Section 14, Vol 1. Oxford: Pergamon Press, 1972:187–203.
61. King H. Curarie alkaloids. I. Tubocurarine. J Chem Soc 1935:1381–1389.
62. Everett AJ, Lowe AJ, Wilkinson S. Revision of the structures of (+)-tubocurarine chloride and (+)-chondrocurine. J Chem Soc 1970;16:1020–1021.
63. Stenlake JB, Waigh RD, Urwin J, et al. Atracurium: conception and inception. Br J Anaesth 1983;55:3S–10S.
64. Basta SJ, Ali HH, Savarese JJ, et al. Clinical pharmacology of atracurium besylate (BW33A): a new nondepolarizing muscle relaxant. Anesth Analg 1983;61:723–729.

Suggested Readings

Belleau B. Conformational perturbation in relation to the regulation of enzyme and receptor behaviour. In: Harper NJ, Simmons AR, eds. Advances in Drug Research, Vol 2. New York: Academic Press, 1965:89–126.

Cannon JG. Cholinergics. In: Abraham, DJ, ed. Burger's Medicinal Chemistry & Drug Discovery, Vol 6, 6th Ed. New York: John Wiley & Sons, 2003:39–108.

Rama Sastry BV. Anticholinergic drugs. In: Abraham, DJ, ed. Burger's Medicinal Chemistry & Drug Discovery, Vol 6, 6th Ed. New York: John Wiley & Sons, 2003:109–165.

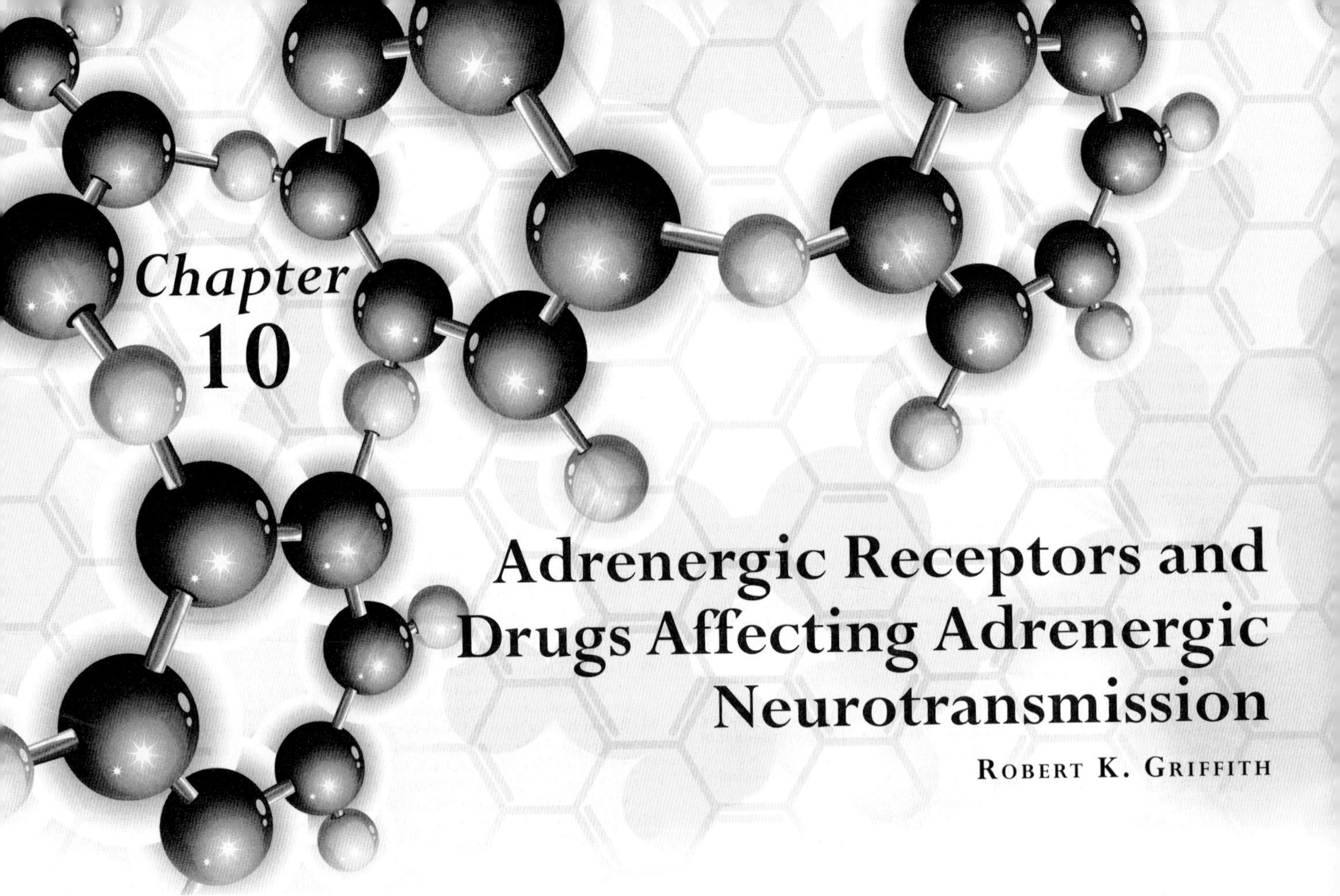

Chapter 10

Adrenergic Receptors and Drugs Affecting Adrenergic Neurotransmission

ROBERT K. GRIFFITH

Drugs Covered in This Chapter

β_2-ADRENERGIC AGONISTS
- Albuterol
- Bitolterol
- Formoterol, arformoterol (*R,R*-formoterol)
- Indacaterol
- Isoproterenol
- Pirbuterol
- Ritodrine
- Salmeterol
- Terbutaline

β_1-ADRENERGIC AGONISTS
- Dopamine
- Dobutamine

β-ADRENERGIC ANTAGONISTS (ALSO CHAPTER 24)

MIXED α/β-ADRENERGIC ANTAGONISTS (ALSO CHAPTER 24)

MIXED-ACTING SYMPATHOMIMETICS
- Phenylpropanolamines
  - (−)-Ephedrine
  - (+)-Pseudoephedrine
  - (+)-Phenylpropanolamine
- Phenylisopropylamines
  - Amphetamine
  - Methamphetamine

NONSELECTIVE ADRENERGIC AGONISTS
- Epinephrine
- Norepinephrine

NONSELECTIVE α-ADRENERGIC ANTAGONISTS
- Phenoxybenzamine
- Phentolamine
- Tolazoline

SELECTIVE α_1-ADRENERGIC AGONISTS
- Metaraminol
- Methoxamine
- Oxymetazoline
- Phenylephrine
- Tetrahydrozoline

SELECTIVE α_2-ADRENERGIC AGONISTS
- Apraclonidine
- Brimonidine
- Clonidine
- Guanfacine
- Guanabenz
- Methyldopa
- Tizanidine

SELECTIVE α_2-ADRENERGIC ANTAGONISTS (SEE ALSO CHAPTER 40)
- Alfuzosin
- Alfuzosin
- Doxazosin
- Prazosin
- Silodosin
- Terazosin
- Tamsulosin

Abbreviations

ATP, adenosine triphosphate
BPH, benign prostatic hyperplasia
cAMP, cyclic adenosine monophosphate
CNS, central nervous system
COMT, catechol-*O*-methyltransferase
DAG, 1,2-diacylglycerol
DOPGAL, 3,4-dihydroxyphenylglycolaldehyde
L-DOPA, L-dihydroxyphenylalanine
GPCR, G protein–coupled receptor
IP_3, inositol-1,4,5-triphosphate
MAO, monoamine oxidase
SAR, structure–activity relationship
TMD, transmembrane domain

SCENARIO

SJ is a 28-year-old white woman with pneumonia and acute psychosis. She has used illicit drugs extensively. Upon arrival to the emergency department, SJ was disoriented and combative and was sedated. She was started on intravenous antibiotics, fluids, and dopamine 800 mg in 250 mL of D5W at 5 mcg/kg/min. Hours later the patient remained combative and believed the hospital staff were trying to poison her. When the nurse went to retrieve another dose of sedation, SJ disconnected the intravenous tubing and drank the remaining dopamine infusion. Upon finding the bag empty, the nurse called the pharmacy for recommendations.

(The reader is directed to the clinical solution and chemical analysis of this case at the end of the chapter).

INTRODUCTION

Adrenergic drugs are a broad class of agents employed in the treatment of disorders of widely varying severity. Adrenergic drugs include popular prescription drugs, such as albuterol for asthma and atenolol for hypertension, as well as many common over-the-counter cold remedies, such as the nasal decongestant pseudoephedrine.

Adrenergic drugs act on effector cells through adrenoceptors that normally are activated by the neurotransmitter norepinephrine (noradrenaline), or they can act on the neurons that release the neurotransmitter. The term "adrenergic" stems from the discovery early in the 20th century that administration of the hormone adrenaline (epinephrine) had specific effects on selected organs and tissues similar to the effects produced by stimulation of the sympathetic (adrenergic) nervous system. For a number of years, adrenaline was thought to be the neurotransmitter in the sympathetic nervous system, but it was also recognized that the effects of administered epinephrine were not quite identical to those of sympathetic stimulation. Finally, in the 1940s, norepinephrine was identified as the true neurotransmitter at the terminus of the sympathetic nervous system (1,2). Adrenoceptors are widely located in various organs and tissues as well as on neurons of both the peripheral nervous system and central nervous system (CNS).

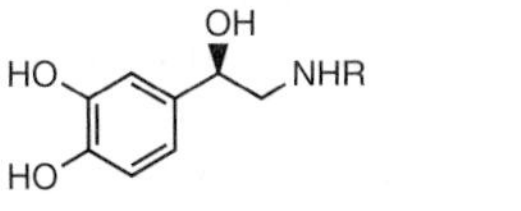

Norepinephrine, R = H
Epinephrine, R = CH_3

Norepinephrine and epinephrine are members of a class of pharmacologically active substances known as catecholamines, because they contain within their structures both an amine and an *ortho*-dihydroxybenzene moiety, which is known by the common chemical name of catechol. Many adrenergic drugs are also catecholamines, and their structure–activity relationships (SARs) will be discussed.

Neurons at the terminus of an adrenergic neuron fiber release norepinephrine to influence the target tissue through binding to receptors on cells of the tissue or organ. The cells bearing the receptors are called effector cells, because they produce the effect seen by adrenergic stimulation.

In general, stimulation of the sympathetic nervous system causes what is known as a "fight-or-flight" response. These effects include an increased rate and force of heart contraction, a rise in blood pressure, a shift of blood flow to skeletal muscles, dilation of bronchioles and pupils, and an increase in blood glucose levels through gluconeogenesis and glycogenolysis. These responses are what one might predict in a mammal that is enraged and preparing to fight or in one that is frightened and preparing to flee. Drugs can influence adrenergic responses through a variety of mechanisms, and an understanding of these mechanisms requires knowledge regarding the details of norepinephrine biosynthesis, storage, release, and fate after release.

BIOSYNTHESIS, STORAGE, AND RELEASE OF NOREPINEPHRINE

Biosynthesis of norepinephrine takes place within adrenergic neurons near the terminus of the axon and junction with the effector cell. The biosynthetic pathway (Fig. 10.1) begins with the active transport of the amino acid L-tyrosine into the adrenergic neuron cell (1). In the first step within the cytoplasm, the enzyme tyrosine hydroxylase (tyrosine-3-monooxygenase) oxidizes the 3′ position of tyrosine to form the catechol amino acid L-dihydroxyphenylalanine (L-DOPA). This is the rate-limiting step in norepinephrine biosynthesis, and the activity of tyrosine hydroxylase is carefully controlled (3). The enzyme is under feedback inhibition control by product catecholamines and is controlled through a complex pattern of phosphorylation/dephosphorylation, in which phosphorylation by protein kinases activates the enzyme and dephosphorylation by phosphatases decreases activity.

In the second step, L-DOPA is decarboxylated to dopamine by aromatic L-amino acid decarboxylase, another cytoplasmic enzyme. Aromatic L-amino acid decarboxylase was discovered in the 1930s and originally

CLINICAL SIGNIFICANCE

Through the years, an increased understanding of adrenergic receptors and compounds that modulate their activity has led to decreased morbidity and mortality as well as increased quality of life for millions of patients worldwide; multiple drugs in this category are on the Top 200 list of prescriptions dispensed. Agents affecting adrenergic neurotransmission are used to treat a variety of clinical conditions, including hypertension, hypotension, angina, heart failure, arrhythmias, and asthma. In fact, our understanding of structure-activity relationships led to an ability to alter the pharmacodynamic effects of various agents even before the specific receptor types were identified.

A thorough understanding of the structure–activity relationships of these compounds and application of the principles of medicinal chemistry to alter their pharmacodynamic effects has enhanced the desired properties and diminished the incidence and/or severity of associated unwanted adverse effects. Furthermore, therapeutic utility and patient compliance has been improved with the advent of orally active agents with longer elimination times and decreased frequency of dosing. For clinicians, a thorough understanding of the resultant pharmacodynamic properties of these agents is necessary to substantiate therapeutic decision making for an individual patient. For example, a patient with hypotension resulting in shock is treated with an adrenergic agonist that will increase blood pressure. If the patient's hypotension results from distributive shock, an agent with α_1-stimulant properties is necessary. If hypotension results from cardiogenic shock, however, a β_1-agonist drug would be most effective, and, in actuality, an α_1 stimulant agent may cause the patient to further decompensate by increasing cardiac workload without lending support to the failing heart. Manipulation of three sites on the basic phenylethanolamine structure alter these receptor specificities, which allows a clinician to tailor drug selection for an individual patient based on the specific desired pharmacological effects of each compound.

A second example would be selection of a β_1-selective receptor blocking agent like metoprolol, as opposed to a nonspecific β-antagonist like propranolol, to treat a patient with asthma who has experienced a myocardial infarction. This allows the patient to benefit from the potential mortality reduction associated with the β-blocking agent while minimizing the risk of decreasing β_2-agonist utility for bronchospasm. These are only a couple of simple illustrations of altering the structure–activity relationship of adrenergic compounds to increase their utility for specific disease processes, outlining the importance of understanding the pharmacodynamic impact of these alterations.

Kathryn Neill, PharmD
Hospital Experiential Director
Assistant Professor
Critical Care Specialist
Department of Pharmacy Practice
College of Pharmacy
University of Arkansas for Medical Sciences

named DOPA decarboxylase. Researchers discovered subsequently that DOPA decarboxylase is not specific for L-DOPA and decarboxylates other aromatic L-amino acids having the L (or *S*) absolute configuration, such as 5-hydroxy-L-tryptophan, L-tryptophan, and L-tyrosine. Nevertheless, the enzyme is often referred to by the older name.

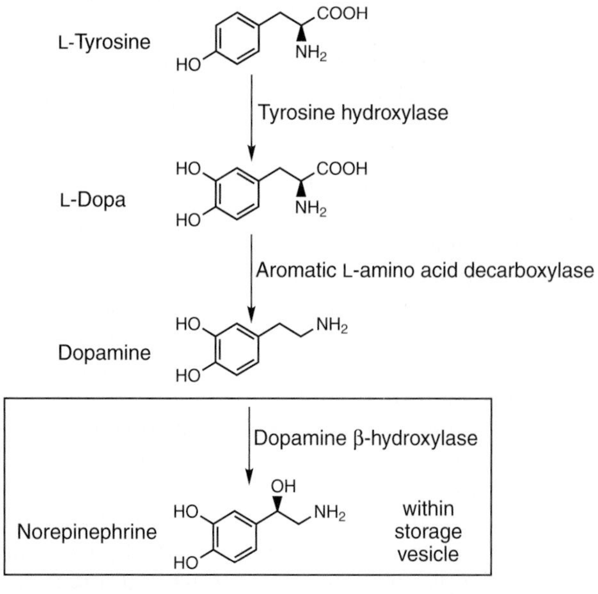

FIGURE 10.1 Biosynthesis of norepinephrine.

The dopamine formed in the cytoplasm by decarboxylation of L-DOPA is then taken up by active transport into storage vesicles or granules located near the terminus of the adrenergic neuron. Within these vesicles, the enzyme dopamine β-hydroxylase stereospecifically introduces a hydroxyl group in the (*R*) absolute configuration on the carbon atom β to the amino group to generate the neurotransmitter norepinephrine. Norepinephrine is stored in the vesicles in a 4:1 complex with adenosine triphosphate (ATP) in such quantities that each vesicle in a peripheral adrenergic neuron contains between 6,000 and 15,000 molecules of norepinephrine (4). The norepinephrine remains in the vesicles until released into the synapse during signal transduction. When a wave of depolarization reaches the terminus of an adrenergic neuron, it triggers the transient opening of voltage-dependent calcium channels, causing an influx of calcium ions. This influx of calcium ions triggers fusion of the storage vesicles with the neuronal cell membrane, spilling the norepinephrine and other contents of the vesicles into the synapse through exocytosis (Fig. 10.2). The pathway for epinephrine biosynthesis in the adrenal medulla is the same as for norepinephrine with the additional step of conversion of norepinephrine to epinephrine by the enzyme phenylethanolamine-*N*-methyltransferase.

REUPTAKE AND METABOLISM OF NOREPINEPHRINE FOLLOWING RELEASE

After its release, norepinephrine diffuses through the intercellular space to bind reversibly to α- or β-adrenoceptors on the effector cell, inducing a conformational change in the receptor. This conformational change triggers a biochemical cascade that results in a physiologic response by the effector cell. As well as the receptors on effector cells, there are also α_2-adrenoreceptors that respond to norepinephrine on the presynaptic neuron, which, when stimulated by norepinephrine, inhibit the release of additional norepinephrine into the synapse. It must be noted that there are also postsynaptic α_2-receptors, particularly in the CNS. Once it has been released and is stimulating its various receptors, there must be mechanisms for removing the norepinephrine from the synapse and terminating the adrenergic impulse. The most important of these mechanisms for removing the norepinephrine is transmitter recycling through active transport reuptake into the presynaptic neuron. This process, called uptake-1, is efficient, and in some tissues, up to 95% of released norepinephrine is likely removed from the synapse by this mechanism (5). Part of the norepinephrine taken into the presynaptic neuron by uptake-1 is metabolized to 3,4-dihydroxyphenylglycolaldehyde (DOPGAL) by mitochondrial monoamine oxidase (MAO) (Fig. 10.3), and part of it is sequestered in the storage vesicles to be used again as a neurotransmitter. A less efficient uptake process, called uptake-2, operates in a variety of other cell types but only in the presence of high concentrations of norepinephrine. That portion of released norepinephrine that escapes uptake-1 diffuses out of the synapse and is metabolized in extraneuronal sites by catechol-*O*-methyltransferase (COMT), which methylates the *meta* hydroxyl group of norepinephrine. Norepinephrine is also metabolized to DOPGAL by MAO at extraneuronal sites, principally the liver and blood platelets. Both DOPGAL and normetanephrine are subject to further metabolism, as outlined in Figure 10.3 (6). These pathways are also important to drugs that are structural analogs of norepinephrine. In particular, drugs that are catechols (a 1,2-diphenolic moiety) are subject to metabolism by COMT, and drugs with unsubstituted aliphatic amino groups are often substrates for MAO.

As summarized in Figure. 11.3, following biosynthesis and storage in a vesicle, norepinephrine release into the synapse is triggered by depolarization-induced calcium influx. The norepinephrine in the synapse interacts with postsynaptic G protein–linked α- or β-receptors on the effector cell, triggering effector cell response, or with presynaptic α_2-receptors on the neuron, which inhibit release of more norepinephrine. Most of the synaptic neurotransmitter is transported back into the presynaptic neuron by uptake-1 active transport. Some of the norepinephrine is metabolized by MAO, and the remainder is stored in a vesicle to be used again. That portion of norepinephrine not captured by uptake-1 diffuses out of the synapse and is metabolized by COMT and MAO.

CHARACTERIZATION OF ADRENERGIC RECEPTOR SUBTYPES

The discovery of subclasses of adrenergic receptors and the ability of relatively small-molecule drugs to stimulate differentially or block these receptors represented

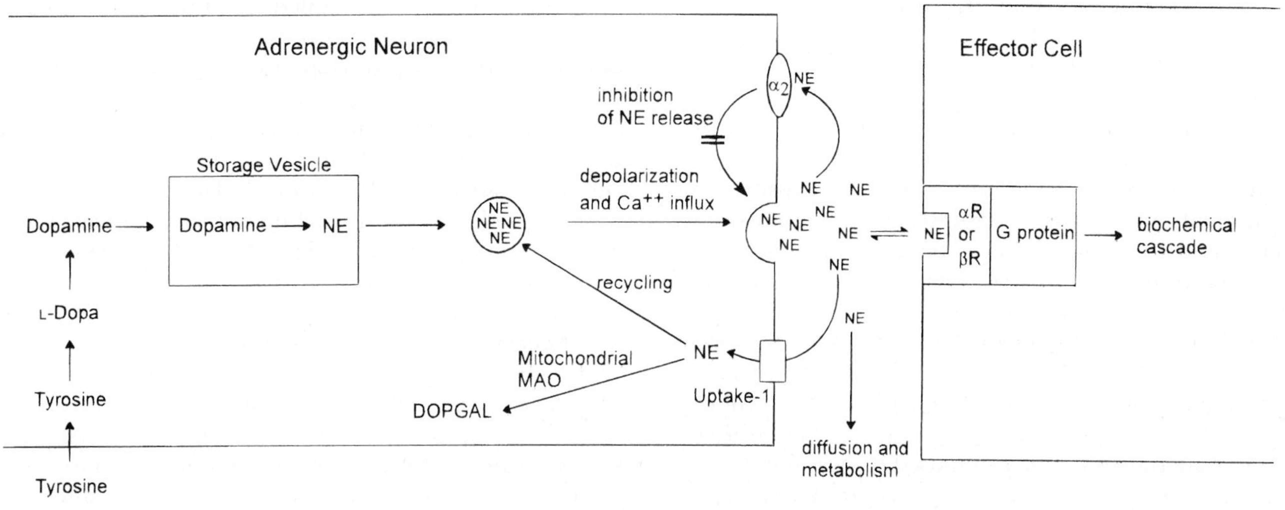

FIGURE 10.2 Neurotransmission events in an adrenergic neuron and effector cell. DOPGAL, 3,4-dihydroxyphenylglycolaldehyde; MAO, monoamine oxidase; NE, norepinephrine; αR, α-adrenoceptor; βR, β-adrenoceptor.

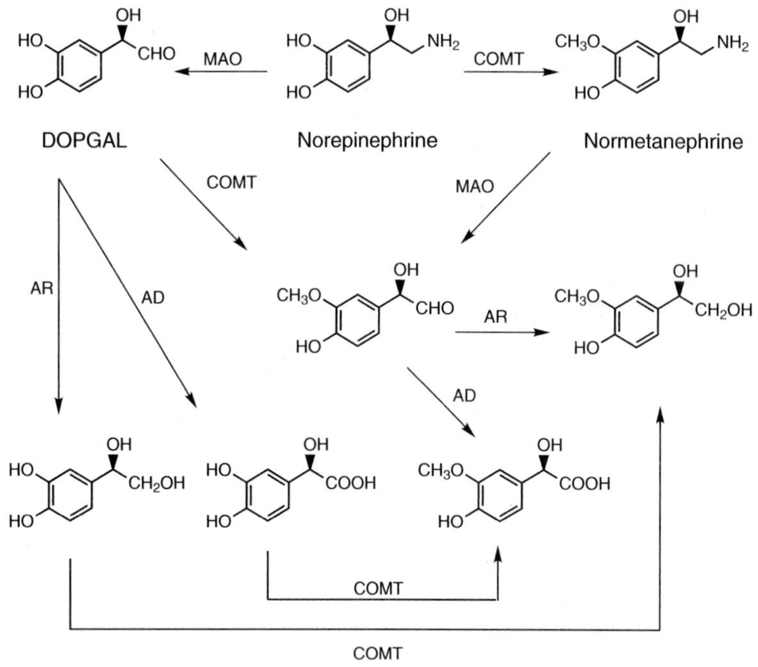

FIGURE 10.3 Metabolism of norepinephrine. AD, aldehyde dehydrogenase; AR, aldehyde reductase; COMT, catechol-*O*-methyltransferase; MAO, monoamine oxidase.

a major advance in several areas of pharmacotherapeutics. Adrenergic receptors were subclassified by Ahlquist (7) in 1948 into α- and β-adrenoreceptor classes according to their responses to different adrenergic receptor agonists, principally norepinephrine, epinephrine, and isoproterenol. These catecholamines are able to stimulate α-adrenoceptors in the following descending order of potency: epinephrine > norepinephrine > isoproterenol. In contrast, β-adrenoceptors are stimulated in the following descending order of potency: isoproterenol > epinephrine > norepinephrine.

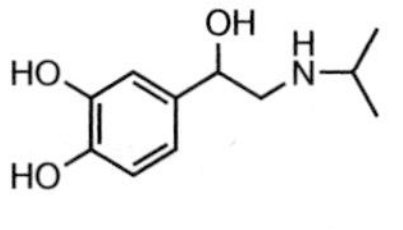

Isoproterenol

In the years since Ahlquist's original classification, additional small-molecule agonists and antagonists have been used to allow further subclassification of α- and β-receptors into the α_1 and α_2 subtypes of α-receptors and the β_1, β_2, and β_3 subtypes of β-adrenoceptors. The powerful tools of molecular biology have been used to clone, sequence, and identify even more subtypes of α-receptors for a total of six. Currently, three types of α_1-adrenoceptors, called α_{1A}, α_{1B}, and α_{1D}, are known. (There is no α_{1C} because identification of a supposed α_{1C} was found to be incorrect.) Currently, three subtypes of α_2, known as α_{2A}, α_{2B}, and α_{2C}, are also known (8). The data derived from molecular biology provide a wealth of information on the structures and biochemical properties of both α- and β-receptors. Intensive research continues in this area, and the coming years can provide evidence of additional subtypes of both α- and β-receptors. At this time, however, only the α_1-, α_2-, β_1-, and β_2-receptor subtypes are sufficiently well differentiated by their small-molecule binding characteristics to be clinically significant in pharmacotherapeutics, although therapeutic agents acting selectively on β_3-adrenoceptors to induce fat catabolism could become available in the near future (9).

The adrenoceptors, both α and β, are members of a receptor superfamily of membrane-spanning proteins, including muscarinic, serotonin, and dopamine receptors, which are coupled to intracellular guanosine triphosphate–binding proteins (G proteins), which determine the cellular response to receptor activation (10). All these receptors exhibit a common motif of a single polypeptide chain that is looped back and forth through the cell membrane seven times with an extracellular N-terminus and intracellular C-terminus. The human β_2-adrenoceptor was one of the first to be cloned and thoroughly studied (Fig. 10.4) (11). The seven transmembrane domains, TMD1 through TMD7, are composed primarily of lipophilic amino acids arranged in α-helices connected by regions of hydrophilic amino acids. The hydrophilic regions form loops on the intracellular and extracellular faces of the membrane. In all the adrenoceptors, the agonist/antagonist recognition site is located within the membrane-bound portion of the receptor. This binding site is within a pocket formed by the membrane-spanning regions of the peptide, as illustrated in Figure 10.5 for epinephrine bound to the

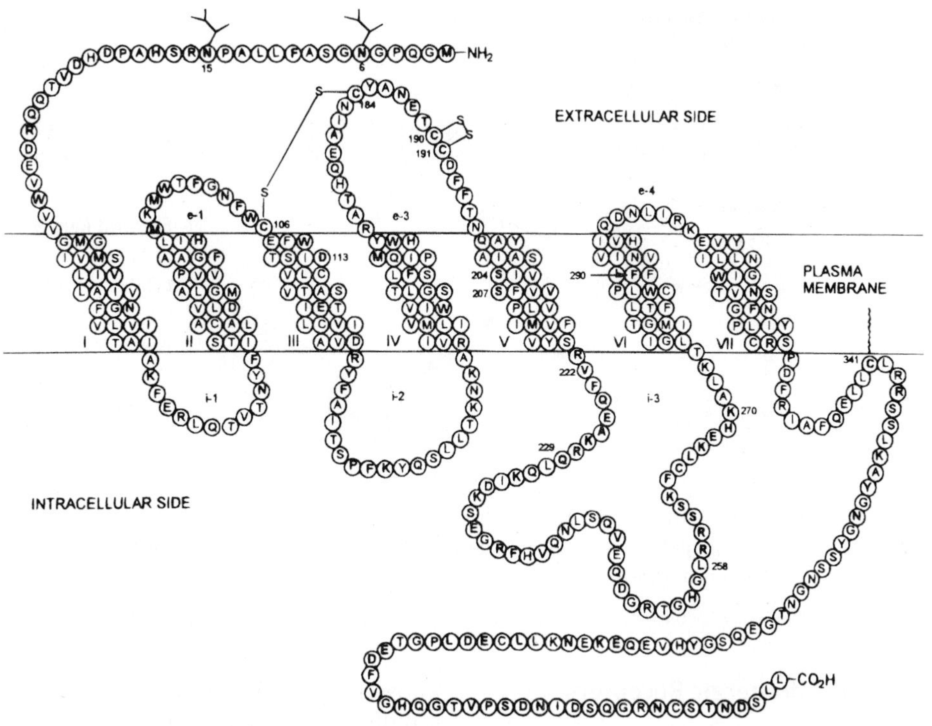

FIGURE 10.4 Human β_2-adrenergic receptor: amino acid sequence of the human β_2-receptor showing the seven transmembrane domains (I–VII), the connecting intracellular and extracellular loops, extracellular glycosylation sites at asparagines 6 and 15, and intrachain disulfide bonds between cysteines 106 to 184 and 190 to 191. Also indicated are the amino acids identified as participating in neurotransmitter binding—aspartate 113 in transmembrane domain III, which binds the positively charged amine of the neurotransmitter, and serines 204 and 207 of transmembrane domain V, which form hydrogen-bonds with the catechol hydroxyls. Phenylalanine 290 can participate in agonist binding as well. Amino acids 222 to 229 and 258 to 270 of the third intracellular loop are critical for G protein coupling, and palmitoylated cysteine 341 is critical for proper adenylyl cyclase activation. (Reprinted with permission from the Annual Review of Pharmacology and Toxicology, Volume 32 © 1992 by Annual Reviews, http://www.annualreviews.org.)

human β_2-receptor. All the adrenoceptors are coupled to their effector systems through a G protein, which is linked through reversible binding interactions with the third intracellular loop of the receptor protein.

Salient features of the extensively studied β_2-adrenoreceptor are indicated in Figure 10.4. Binding studies with selectively mutated β_2-receptors have provided strong evidence for binding interactions between agonist functional groups and specific residues in the transmembrane domains of adrenoceptors. Such studies indicate that Asp113 in transmembrane domain 3 (TMD3) of the β_2-receptor is the acidic residue that forms a bond, presumably ionic or a salt bridge, with the positively charged amino group of catecholamine agonists. An aspartic acid residue is also found in a comparable position in all the other adrenoceptors as well as other known G protein–coupled receptors (GPCRs) that bind substrates having positively charged nitrogens in their structures. Elegant studies with mutated receptors and analogs of isoproterenol demonstrated that serines at 204 and 207 of TMD5 are the residues that form hydrogen bonds with the catechol hydroxyls of β_2-agonists (12). Furthermore, the evidence indicates that Ser204 interacts with the *meta* hydroxyl group of the ligand, whereas Ser207 interacts specifically with the *para* hydroxyl group. Serine residues are found in corresponding positions in TMD5 of the other known adrenoceptors. Evidence indicates that the phenylalanine residue of TMD6 is also involved in ligand-receptor bonding with the catechol ring. Studies such as these and others that indicated the presence of specific disulfide bridges between cysteine residues of the β_2-receptor led to the binding scheme shown in Figure 10.5.

Structural differences exist among the various adrenoceptors with regard to their primary structure, including the actual peptide sequence and length. Each of the adrenoceptors is encoded on a distinct gene, and this information was crucial to the proof that each adrenoreceptor is, indeed, distinct although related. The amino acids that make up the seven transmembrane regions are highly conserved among the various adrenoreceptors, but the hydrophilic portions are quite variable. The largest differences occur in the third intracellular loop connecting TMD5 and TMD6, which is the site of linkage between the receptor and its associated G protein. Compare the diagram of the β_2-receptor in Figure 10.4 with that of the α_2-receptor in Figure 10.6 (13).

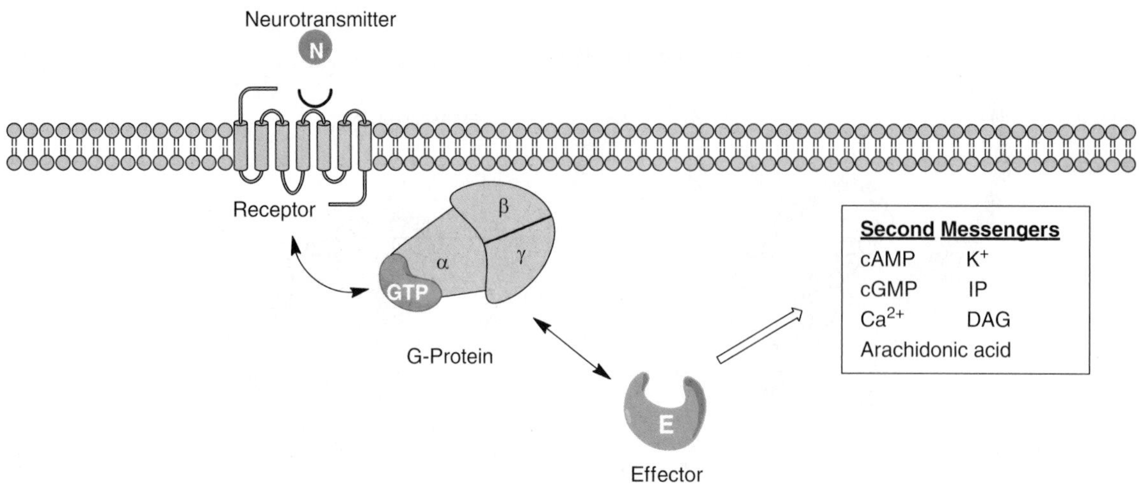

FIGURE 10.5 Proposed arrangement for the transmembrane helices of the β_2-adrenergic receptor depicting the binding site for epinephrine as viewed from the extracellular side. (Reprinted with permission from the Annual Review of Pharmacology and Toxicology, Volume 32 © 1992 by Annual Reviews, http://www.annualreviews.org.)

Effector Mechanisms of Adrenergic Receptors

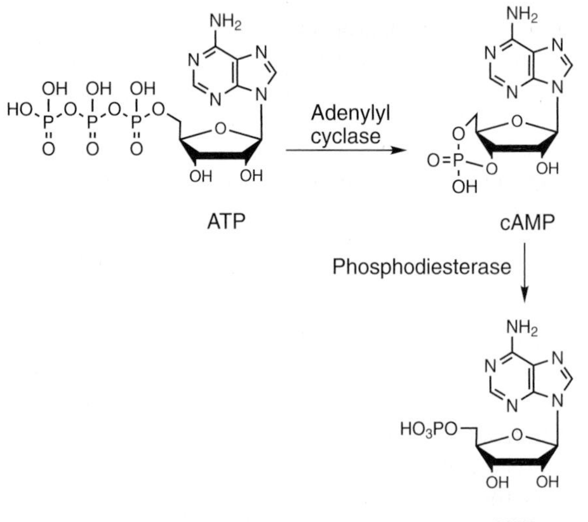

Each adrenoceptor is coupled through a G protein to an effector mechanism. Effector mechanisms are proteins that are able to translate the conformational change caused by activation of the receptor into a biochemical event within the cell. All the β-adrenoceptors are coupled via specific G proteins (G_S) to the activation of adenylate cyclase (14). Thus, when the receptor is stimulated by an agonist, adenylate cyclase is activated to catalyze the formation of cyclic adenosine monophosphate (cAMP) from ATP. Called a second messenger for the β-adrenoceptors, cAMP is known to function as a second messenger for a number of other receptor types. cAMP is considered to be a messenger because it can diffuse through the cell for at least short distances to modulate biochemical events remote from the synaptic cleft. Modulation of biochemical events by cAMP includes a phosphorylation cascade of other proteins. cAMP is also rapidly deactivated by hydrolysis of the phosphodiester bond by the enzyme phosphodiesterase. The α_2-receptor can use more than one effector system depending on the location of the receptor. To date, however, the best-understood effector system of the α_2-receptor appears to be similar to that of the β-receptors, except that linkage via a G protein (G_i) leads to inhibition of adenylyl cyclase instead of activation.

α_1-Adrenoreceptor is linked through yet another G protein to a complex series of events involving hydrolysis of polyphosphatidylinositol (15). The first event set in motion by activation of the α_1-receptor is activation of the enzyme phospholipase C. Phospholipase C catalyzes the hydrolysis of phosphatidylinositol-4,5-biphosphate. This hydrolysis yields two products, each of which has biologic activity as second messengers of the α_1-receptor (see Chapter 7). These two products are 1,2-diacylglycerol (DAG) and inositol-1,4,5-triphosphate (IP_3). The latter, IP_3, causes the release of calcium ions from intracellular storage sites in the endoplasmic reticulum, resulting in an increase in free intracellular calcium levels. Increased free intracellular calcium is correlated with smooth muscle contraction. The other product, DAG, is thought to activate cytosolic protein kinase C, which can induce slowly developing contractions of vascular smooth muscle. The end result of a complex series of protein interactions triggered by agonist binding to the α_1-receptor includes increased intracellular free calcium, which leads to smooth muscle contraction. When the smooth muscle innervated by α_1-receptors is in vascular walls, stimulation leads to vascular constriction.

Receptor Localization

The generalization made in the past about synaptic locations of adrenoreceptor subtypes was that all

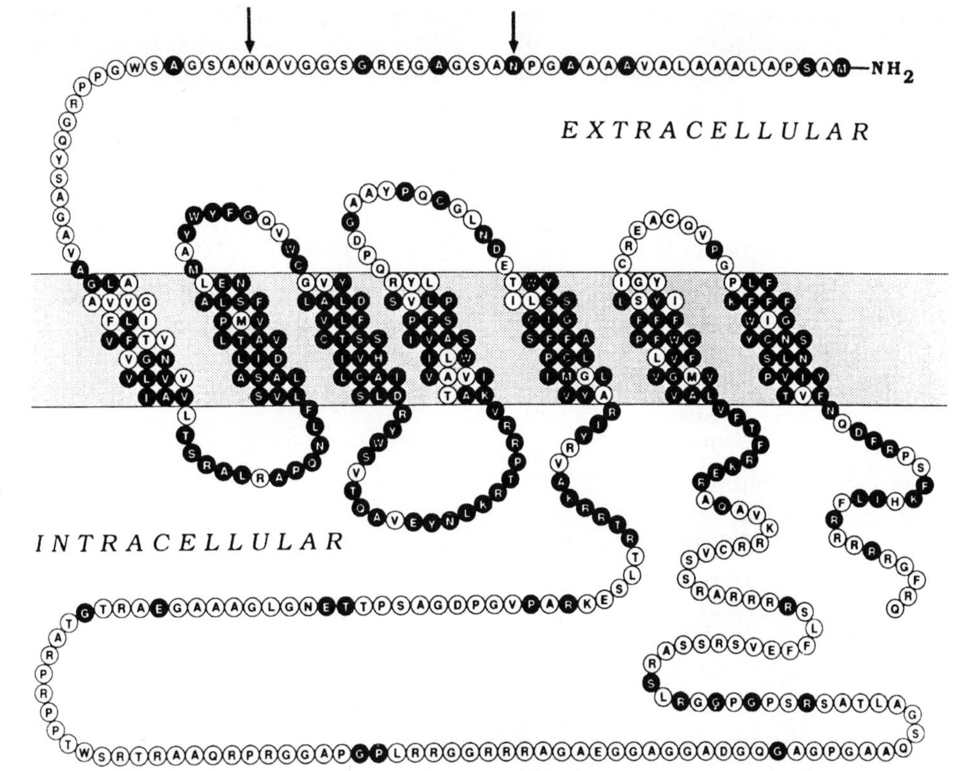

FIGURE 10.6 Human kidney α_2-adrenergic receptor: amino acid sequence of the human kidney α_2-receptor showing the seven transmembrane domains and the connecting intracellular and extracellular loops. Note particularly the large third intracellular loop, which is the G protein–binding site. The arrows point to the sites of glycosylation. Amino acids in black circles are those identical to the amino acids in the human platelet α_2-receptor. (From Regan JW, Kobilka TS, Yang-Feng TL, et al. Cloning and expression of a human kidney cDNA for an α_2-adrenergic receptor subtype. Proc Natl Acad Sci U S A 1988;85:6301–6305, with permission.)

α_1-, β_1-, β_2-, and β_3-receptors are postsynaptic receptors that are linked to stimulation of biochemical processes in the postsynaptic cell. Presynaptic β-receptors, however, are known to occur, although their function is unclear. Traditionally, the α_2-receptor has been viewed as a presynaptic receptor that resides on the outer membrane of the nerve terminus or presynaptic cell and reacts with released neurotransmitter. The α_2-receptor serves as a sensor and modulator of the quantity of neurotransmitter present in the synapse at any given moment. Thus, during periods of rapid nerve firing and neurotransmitter release, the α_2-receptor is stimulated and causes an inhibition of further release of neurotransmitter. This is a well-characterized mechanism for modulation of neurotransmission. Not all α_2-receptors are presynaptic, but the physiologic significance of postsynaptic α_2-receptors is less well understood (16).

Therapeutic Relevance of Adrenergic Receptor Subtypes

The clinical utility of receptor-selective drugs becomes obvious when one considers the adrenoreceptor subtypes and effector responses of only a few organs and tissues innervated by the sympathetic nervous system. The major adrenoceptor subtypes are listed in Table 10.1. For example, the predominant response to adrenergic stimulation of smooth muscle of the peripheral vasculature is constriction causing a rise in blood pressure. Because this response is mediated through α_1-receptors, an α_1-antagonist would be expected to cause relaxation of the blood vessels and a drop in blood pressure with clear implications for treating hypertension. The presence of α_1-adrenoceptors in the prostate gland also leads to the use of α_1-antagonists in treating benign prostatic hyperplasia. The principal therapeutic uses of adrenergic agonists and antagonists are shown in Table 10.2. A smaller number of β_2-receptors on vascular smooth muscle mediate arterial dilation, particularly to skeletal muscle, and a few antihypertensives act through stimulation of these β_2-receptors. (Adrenergic antihypertensives are discussed more thoroughly in Chapter 24.) Adrenergic stimulation of the lungs causes smooth muscle relaxation and bronchodilation mediated through β_2-receptors. Drugs acting as β_2-agonists are useful for alleviating respiratory distress in persons with asthma or other obstructive pulmonary diseases (see Chapter 39). Activation of β_2-receptors in the uterus also causes muscle relaxation, and so some β_2-agonists are used to inhibit uterine contractions in premature labor. Adrenergic stimulation of the heart causes an increase in rate and force of contraction,

TABLE 10.1 Selected Tissue Responses to Stimulation of Adrenoceptor Subtypes

Organ or Tissue	Major Receptor Type	Response
Arterioles, vascular bed	α_1, α_2	Constriction
Skeletal muscle	β_2	Dilation
Eye (radial muscle)	α_1	Contraction (papillary dilation)
Heart	β_1	Increased rate and force
Lungs	β_2	Relaxation (bronchodilation)
Liver	α_1, β_2	Increased gluconeogenesis and glycogenolysis
Fat cells	α_1, β_3	Lipolysis
Uterus (pregnant)	α_1	Contraction
	β_2	Relaxation
Intestine	α_1, β_2	Decreased motility

TABLE 10.2 Principal Therapeutic Uses of Adrenergic Agonists and Antagonists

Adrenoceptor	Drug Action	Therapeutic Uses
α_1	Agonists	Shock, hypotension (to raise blood pressure)
		Nasal decongestants
	Antagonists	Antihypertensives
		Benign prostatic hyperplasia
α_2	Agonists	Antihypertensives
		Glaucoma
		Analgesia
		Sedatives
β_1	Antagonists	Antihypertensives
		Antiarrhythmics
β_2	Agonists	Bronchodilators (asthma and chronic obstructive pulmonary disorder)
		Glaucoma
β_3	Agonists	Weight loss (investigational drugs)

which is mediated primarily by β_1-receptors. Drugs with β_1-blocking activity slow the heart rate and decrease the force of contraction. These drugs have utility in treating hypertension, angina, and certain cardiac arrhythmias (see Chapters 21 and 24).

From the preceding discussions of the biosynthesis, storage, release, and fate of norepinephrine, one can readily conceive of a number of possible sites of drug action for adrenergic drugs. As mentioned, there are drugs that act directly on the receptors as agonists and antagonists, drugs that affect storage and release from vesicles, drugs that affect neurotransmitter biosynthesis, and drugs that affect uptake and catabolism of norepinephrine and epinephrine. These categories are discussed in turn. Most adrenergic drugs fit into well-defined classes with readily defined SARs, but a few adrenergic drugs do not permit such straightforward structural definition of their activity. We begin with a discussion of phenylethanolamine (or phenethanolamine) agonists, which do have reasonably clear SARs. Although many of these drugs directly stimulate adrenoceptors, others exhibit what is termed "indirect activity." Indirect agonists do not directly bind to and activate adrenergic receptors; rather, they are taken up into the presynaptic neuron, where they cause the release of norepinephrine, which can diffuse into the receptor causing the observed response. Mixed-acting drugs have both a direct and an indirect component to their action, and the relative amount of direct versus indirect activity for a given drug varies considerably with its chemical structure, the tissue preparation examined, and the experimental animal species.

STRUCTURE–ACTIVITY RELATIONSHIPS OF ADRENERGIC AGONISTS

Phenylethanolamine Agonists

The structures of many clinically useful phenylethanolamine-type adrenergic agonists are summarized in Table 10.3. Agents of this type have been extensively studied over the years since discovery of the naturally occurring prototypes, epinephrine and norepinephrine, and the structural requirements and tolerances for substitutions at each of the indicated positions have been established (2). In general, a primary or secondary aliphatic amine separated by two carbons from a substituted benzene ring is minimally required for high agonist activity in this class. Because of the basic amino groups (pK_a range, ~8.5 to 10), all these agents are highly positively charged at physiologic pH. By definition, agents in this class have a hydroxyl group on C1 of the side chain, β to the amine, as in epinephrine and norepinephrine. This hydroxyl-substituted carbon must be in the (*R*) absolute configuration for maximal direct activity as in the natural neurotransmitter, although most drugs currently are sold as mixtures of both (*R*) and (*S*) stereoisomers at this position (racemates). Given these features in common, the nature of the other substituents determines receptor selectivity and duration of action. In the following discussions, keep in mind that saying a drug is selective for a given receptor does not mean it has no activity at other

TABLE 10.3 Phenylethanolamine Adrenergic Agonists

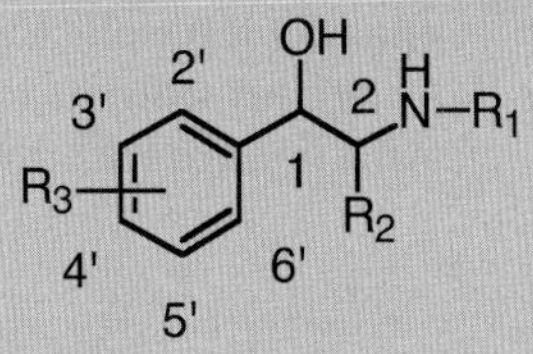

Drug	R^1	R^2	R^3	Receptor Activity
Norepinephrine	H	H	3',4'-diOH	$\alpha + \beta$
Epinephrine	CH_3	H	3',4'-diOH	$\beta \geq \alpha$
α-Methylnorepinephrine	H	CH_3	3',4'-diOH	$\alpha + \beta$
Ethylnorepinephrine	H	CH_2CH_3	3',4'-diOH	$\beta > \alpha$
Isoproterenol	$CH(CH_3)_2$	H	3',4'-diOH	General β
Isoetharine	$CH(CH_3)_2$	CH_2CH_3	3',4'-diOH	selective β_2
Colterol	$C(CH_3)_3$	H	3',4'-diOH	Selective β_2
Metaproterenol	$CH(CH_3)_2$	H	3',5'-diOH	Selective β_2
Terbutaline	$C(CH_3)_3$	H	3',5'-diOH	Selective β_2
Albuterol	$C(CH_3)_3$	H	3'-CH_2OH, 4'-OH	Selective β_2
Phenylephrine	CH_3	H	3'-OH	α
Metaraminol	H	CH_3	3'-OH	α
Methoxamine	H	CH_3	2',5'-diOCH_3	α
Ephedrine, pseudoephedrine	CH_3	CH_3	H	$\alpha + \beta$
Phenylpropanolamine	H	CH_3	H	$\alpha + \beta$
Salmeterol	$-(CH_2)_6-O-(CH_2)_4-C_6H_5$	H	3'-CH_2OH, 4'-OH	$\beta_2 > \beta_1$
Formoterol	$-CH(CH_3)CH_2-C_6H_4-4-OCH_3$	H	3'-NH-COH, 4'-OH	$\beta_2 > \beta_1$
Arformoterol (*R,R*-formoterol)	$-CH(CH_3)CH_2-C_6H_4-4-OCH_3$	H	3'-NH-COH, 4'-OH	$\beta_2 > \beta_1$

receptors and that the clinically observed degree of selectivity is frequently dose-dependent.

R^1, Substitution on the Amino Nitrogen

We have already seen that as R^1 is increased in size from hydrogen in norepinephrine to methyl in epinephrine to isopropyl in isoproterenol, that activity at α-receptors decreases, and that activity at β-receptors increases. These compounds were used to define α- and β-activity long before receptor proteins could be isolated and characterized. The activity at both α- and β-receptors is maximal when R^1 is methyl as in epinephrine, but α-agonist activity is dramatically decreased when R^1 is larger than methyl and is negligible when R^1 is isopropyl, as in isoproterenol, leaving only β-activity. In fact, the β-activity of isoproterenol actually is enhanced over norepinephrine and epinephrine. Presumably, the β-receptor has a large lipophilic binding pocket adjacent to the amine-binding aspartic acid residue, which is absent in the α-receptor. As R^1 becomes larger than *t*-butyl into aryl-α-methylalkyl groups, affinity for α_1-receptors, but not intrinsic activity, returns, which means large lipophilic groups can afford compounds with α_1-blocking activity (e.g., labetalol, a mixed α/β-antagonist). The *N*-substituent can also provide selectivity for different β-receptors, with a *t*-butyl group affording selectivity for β_2-receptors. For example, with all other features of the molecules being constant, colterol is a selective β_2-agonist, whereas isoproterenol is a nonselective β-agonist. When considering use as a bronchodilator, a nonselective β-agonist, such as isoproterenol, has undesirable cardiac stimulatory properties because of its β_1-activity, which is greatly diminished in a selective β_2-agonist, such as albuterol. Also, an arylalkyl group (where the alkyl chain ranges from 2 to 11 carbon/oxygen atoms) can provide β-selectivity with increased lipophilicity and cell penetration for longer duration of action.

R^2, Substitution α to the Basic Nitrogen, Carbon-2

Small alkyl groups, methyl or ethyl, can be present on the carbon adjacent to the amino nitrogen, carbon-2 in Table 10.3. Such substitution slows metabolism by MAO but has little overall effect on duration of action in catecholamines, because they remain substrates for COMT. Resistance to MAO activity is more important in noncatechol, indirect-acting phenylethylamines. An ethyl group in this position diminishes α-activity far more than β-activity, affording compounds with β-selectivity, such as ethylnorepinephrine. Substitution on this carbon also introduces another asymmetric center into these molecules producing pairs of diastereomers, which can have significantly different biologic and chemical properties. For example, maximal direct activity in the stereoisomers of α-methylnorepinephrine resides with the *erythro* stereoisomer with the 1*R*,2*S* absolute configuration (17). The configuration of C2 has a great influence on receptor binding, because the 1*R*,2*R* diastereomer of α-methylnorepinephrine has primarily indirect activity, even though the absolute configuration of the hydroxyl-bearing C1 is the same as in norepinephrine. With respect to α-activity, this additional methyl group also makes the direct-acting 1*R*,2*S* stereoisomer of α-methylnorepinephrine more selective for α_2-adrenoceptors than for α_1-adrenoceptors. This has important consequences in the antihypertensive activity of α-methyldopa, which is discussed later and in Chapter 24. The same stereochemical relationships hold for metaraminol and other phenylethanolamines, in which stereochemical properties have been investigated.

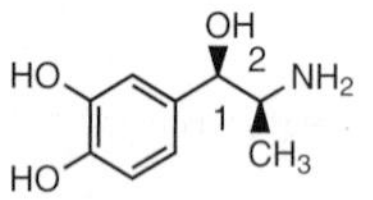

α-Methylnorepinephrine
direct acting stereoisomer

R^3, Substitution on the Aromatic Ring

The natural 3′,4′-dihydroxy–substituted benzene ring in norepinephrine provides excellent receptor activity for both α- and β-sites. Such catechol-containing compounds have poor oral activity, however, because they are rapidly metabolized by COMT. Alternative substitutions have been found that retain good activity but are more resistant to COMT metabolism. 3′,5′-Dihydroxy compounds are not good substrates for COMT but provide selectivity for β_2-receptors. Thus, because of its 3′,5′-dihydroxy ring substitution pattern, metaproterenol is an orally active bronchodilator with little of the β_1 cardiac stimulatory properties possessed by 3′,4′-dihydroxy ring substitution pattern for isoproterenol.

Other substitutions are possible that enhance oral activity and provide selective β_2-activity, such as the 3′-hydroxymethyl and 4′-hydroxy substitution pattern of albuterol, the 3′-amino or 3′-formylamino, which are also resistant to COMT. At least one of the groups must be capable of forming hydrogen bonds, and if there is only one, it should be at the 4′ position to retain β-activity. For example, ritodrine has only a 4′-OH for R^3 yet retains good β-activity, with the large substituent on the nitrogen making it β_2-selective. Ritodrine has been administered to pregnant women to prevent premature labor, consistent with β_2-adrenoceptor stimulation relaxing the uterus.

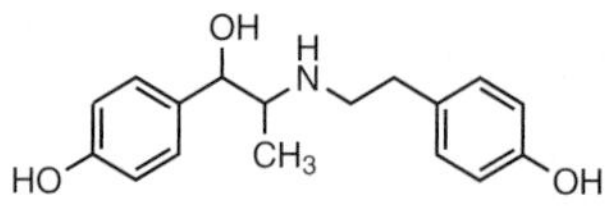

Ritodrine

If R^3 is only a 3′-OH or 3′-sulfonamide, however, activity is reduced at α_1 sites but almost eliminated at β sites, thus affording selective α_1-agonists, such as phenylephrine and metaraminol. Further indication that α_1 sites have a wider range of substituent tolerance for agonist activity is shown by the 2′,5′-dimethoxy substitution of methoxamine, which is a selective α_1-agonist as a result of 5′-*O*-demethylation to 5′-hydroxy metabolite, which also has β-blocking activity at high concentrations. In keeping with the presence of α_1-adrenoceptors in the peripheral vasculature, all three of these agents cause vasoconstriction.

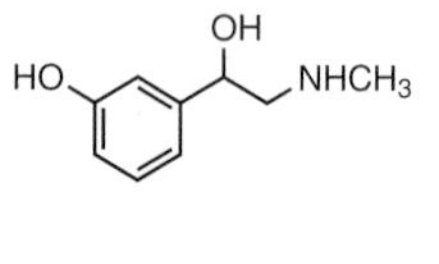

Phenylephrine

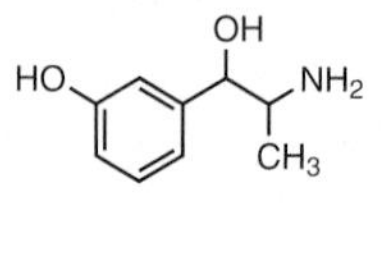

Metaraminol

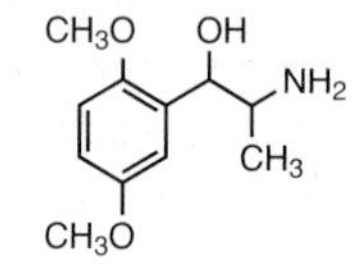

Methoxamine

When the phenyl ring has no phenolic substituents (i.e., R^3 = H), these phenylethanolamines can have both direct and indirect activity. Direct activity (i.e., agonist) is the stimulation of an adrenoceptor by the drug itself; indirect activity is the result of displacement of norepinephrine from its storage granules or reuptake inhibition, resulting in nonselective stimulation of the adrenoceptors by the displaced norepinephrine. Because norepinephrine stimulates both α- and β-adrenoceptors, indirect activity cannot be selective. Stereochemistry of the various substituents can also have a role in determining the extent of direct/indirect activity.

For example, ephedrine and pseudoephedrine have the same substitution pattern, but substitution of both carbons 1 and 2 means four stereoisomers are possible. Racemic (±)-ephedrine is a mixture of the erythro enantiomers 1*R*,2*S* and 1*S*,2*R*, whereas the threo pair of enantiomers, 1*R*,2*R* and 1*S*,2*S*, are known as racemic pseudoephedrine (ψ-ephedrine). As discussed for α-methylnorepinephrine, (−)-ephedrine is the naturally occurring stereoisomer and has the 1*R*,2*S* absolute configuration with a mixed direct activity on both α- and β-receptors and some indirect activity. Its 1*S*,2*R*-(+)-enantiomer exhibits primarily indirect activity. 1*S*,2*S*-(+)-Pseudoephedrine has virtually no direct receptor activity and is mostly indirect acting.

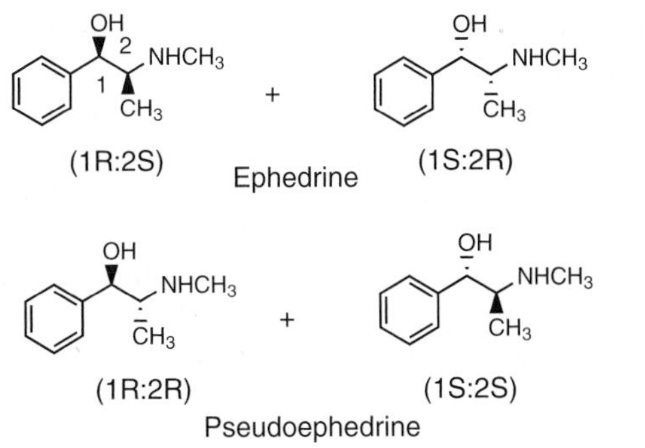

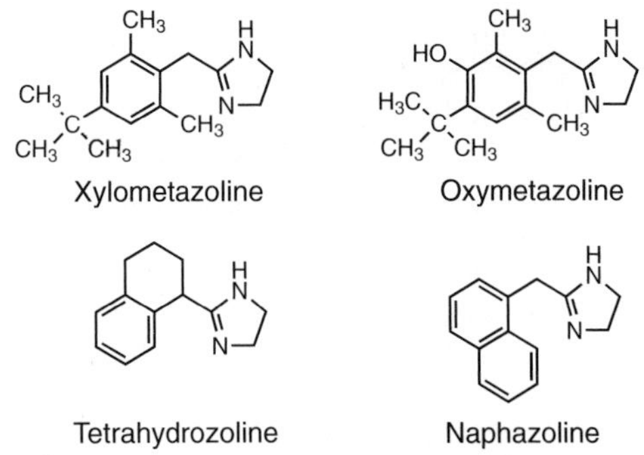

FIGURE 10.7 Imidazoline α_1-adrenergic agonists.

Norepinephrine and Epinephrine

Norepinephrine has limited clinical application because of the nonselective nature of its action, which causes both vasoconstriction and cardiac stimulation. In addition, it must be given intravenously, because it has no oral activity (poor oral bioavailability) as a result of its rapid metabolism by intestinal and liver COMT and MAO, 3′-*O*-glucuronidation/sulfation in the intestine, and low lipophilicity. Rapid metabolism by MAO and COMT limits its duration of action to only 1 or 2 minutes, even when given by infusion. The drug is used to counteract various hypotensive crises, because its α-activity raises blood pressure, and as an adjunct treatment in cardiac arrest, where its β-activity stimulates the heart.

Epinephrine is far more widely used clinically than norepinephrine, although it also lacks oral activity for the same reasons as norepinephrine. Epinephrine, similar to norepinephrine, is used to treat hypotensive crises and, because of its greater β-activity, to stimulate the heart in cardiac arrest. The β_2-activity of epinephrine leads to its administration intravenously and in inhalers to relieve bronchoconstriction in asthma and to application in inhibiting uterine contractions. Because it has significant α-activity, epinephrine has been used in nasal decongestants. Constriction of dilated blood vessels in mucous membranes shrinks the membranes and reduces nasal congestion, although significant rebound congestion can limit its utility.

Selective α-Adrenergic Agonists

α_1-Agonist Phenylethanolamines: Metaraminol, Methoxamine, and Phenylephrine

Metaraminol, methoxamine, and phenylephrine are selective for α_1-receptors and have minimal cardiac stimulatory properties. Because they are not substrates for COMT, their duration of action is significantly longer than that of norepinephrine. Their α_1-agonist activity makes them strong vasoconstrictors, however, and their primary systemic use is limited to treating hypotension during surgery or severe hypotension accompanying shock. Methoxamine is bioactivated by 5′-*O*-demethylation to an active 5′-phenolic metabolite. The β-blocking activity of methoxamine, which is seen at high concentrations, affords some use in treating tachycardia. Phenylephrine, which is also a selective α_1-agonist, is used similarly to metaraminol and methoxamine for hypotension. It also has widespread use as a nonprescription nasal decongestant in both oral and topical preparations. However, its oral bioavailability is less than 10% because of its hydrophilic properties and intestinal 3′-*O*-glucuronidation/sulfation. Phenylephrine preparations applied topically to the eye constrict the dilated blood vessels of bloodshot eyes and, in higher concentrations, are used to dilate the pupil during eye surgery.

2-Arylimidazoline α_1-Agonists

In addition to phenylethanolamine derivatives, α-adrenoceptors accommodate a very diverse assortment of structures. The imidazoline derivatives in Figure 10.7 are also selective α_1-agonists and, therefore, are called vasoconstrictors/vasopressors. They all contain a one-carbon bridge between C2 of the imidazoline ring (pK_a range, 10 to 11) and a phenyl substituent; therefore, the general skeleton of a phenylethylamine is contained within the structures. Lipophilic substitution on the phenyl ring *ortho* to the methylene bridge appears to be required for agonist activity at α_1- and α_2-receptors (15). Presumably, the bulky lipophilic groups attached to the phenyl ring at the *meta* or *para* positions provide selectivity for the α_1-receptor by diminishing affinity for α_2-receptors. These highly ionic compounds are widely used only in topical preparations as nasal decongestants and eye drops (Table 10.4). Systemically, they are potent vasoconstrictors.

α_2-Adrenergic Agonists: 2-Aminoimidazolines and Other α_2-Agonists

Three subtypes of α_2-adrenoceptors, α_{2A}, α_{2B}, and α_{2C}, are recognized. Each has a role in the different clinical

TABLE 10.4 Imidazoline α_1-Agonists in Over-the-Counter Vasoconstrictors

Drug	Nasal Decongestant	Eye Drops
Xylometazoline	Otrivin, Inspire	—
Oxymetazoline	Afrin, Duration, Neo-Synephrine, Vicks Sinex	Visine L.R. Ocu Clear
Tetrahydrozoline	—	Murine, Visine, Soothe
Naphazoline	4-Way Fast Acting, Privine	Naphcon, Clear Eyes

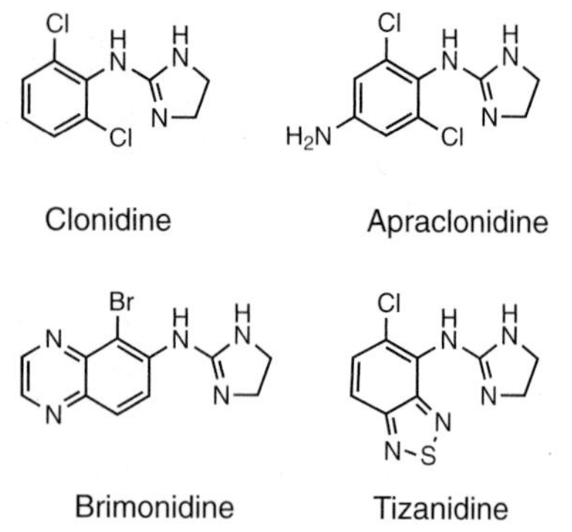

FIGURE 10.8 Imidazoline α_2-adrenergic agonists.

applications of α_2-agonists, which include use as antihypertensives (see Chapter 24), antiglaucoma drugs, and analgesics. The first of these drugs, clonidine, was introduced as an antihypertensive, an effect attributed to central α_{2A}-adrenoceptors in cardiovascular control areas of the brain (18).

Clonidine (Catapres) Closely related structurally to the imidazoline nasal decongestants is clonidine and other developed analogs (Fig. 10.8). Clonidine was originally synthesized as a vasoconstricting nasal decongestant but, in early clinical trials, was found to have dramatic hypotensive effects—in contrast to all expectations for a vasoconstrictor (19). Subsequent pharmacologic investigations showed that clonidine not only has some α_1-agonist (vasoconstrictive) properties in the periphery but also is a powerful α_2-adrenergic agonist and exhibits specific binding to nonadrenergic imidazoline binding sites in the CNS (mainly in the medulla oblongata), causing inhibition of sympathetic output (sympathoinhibition) (see Chapter 24). Because of its peripheral activity on extraneuronal vascular postsynaptic α_{2B}-receptors (18), initial doses of clonidine can produce a transient vasoconstriction and an increase in blood pressure that is soon overcome by vasodilation as clonidine penetrates the blood–brain barrier and interacts with CNS α_{2A}-receptors.

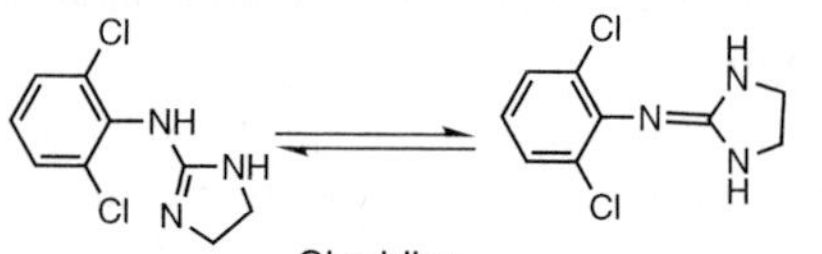

Clonidine

Similar to the imidazoline α_1-agonists, clonidine has lipophilic *ortho*-dichloro substituents on the phenyl ring, but the most readily apparent difference between clonidine and the α_1-agonists in Figure 10.7 is the replacement of the CH_2 bridge on C1 of the imidazoline by an amine NH. This makes the imidazoline ring part of a guanidino group, and the uncharged form of clonidine exists as a pair of tautomers as shown.

Clonidine has a pK_a of 8.3 and is approximately 80% ionized at physiologic pH. Its experimental logD$_{pH\ 7.4}$ = 1.03. The positive charge is shared through resonance by all three nitrogens of the guanidino group. Steric crowding by the bulky *ortho*-chlorine groups does not permit a coplanar conformation of the two rings, as illustrated in Figure 10.9.

In addition to its use as an antihypertensive, clonidine has been proven useful in a wide variety of conditions. Clonidine has sedative properties and has been used to treat attention-deficit hyperactivity disorder, nicotine and opiate withdrawal, and glaucoma, among other uses. Epidural anesthesia has been found to be enhanced by α_2-agonists (20), and clonidine is available in an injectable form for epidural administration.

Tizanidine (Zanaflex) Tizanidine (Fig. 10.8) is a centrally active muscle relaxant analog of clonidine that is approved for use in reducing spasticity associated with cerebral or spinal cord injury. Tizanidine has a pK_a of 7.4 and is approximately 50% ionized at physiologic pH. Its logD$_{pH\ 7.4}$ = 1.8. Its mechanism of action for reducing spasticity suggests presynaptic inhibition of motor neurons at the α_2-adrenergic receptor sites, reducing the release of excitatory amino acids and inhibiting facilitatory ceruleospinal pathways, thus resulting in a reduction in spasticity. Tizanidine only has a small fraction of the antihypertensive action of clonidine, presumably because of action at a selective subgroup of α_{2C}-adrenoceptors, which appear to be responsible for the analgesic and antispasmodic activity of imidazoline α_2-agonists (20).

Apraclonidine (Iopidine) and Brimonidine (Alphagan) The other imidazoline α_2-agonists in Figure 10.8 that are clinically used for treatment of glaucoma are apraclonidine (pK_a = 9.22, logD$_{pH7.4}$=0.01) and brimonidine (pK_a=7.4, logD$_{pH7.4}$=0.49). Stimulation of α_2-receptors in the eye reduces production of aqueous humor and enhances outflow of aqueous humor, thus reducing intraocular pressure, and also has a neuroprotective effect apparently through α_{2A}-receptors located in the retina (21,22). Animal and human studies suggest that apraclonidine's primary mechanism of action can be related to a vreduction of aqueous humor formation, whereas brimonidine lowers intraocular pressure by reducing aqueous humor production and increasing uveoscleral outflow. Brimonidine is approximately 1,000-fold more selective for α_2-receptors than are clonidine or apraclonidine and is a first-line agent for treating glaucoma. It exhibits minimal effect on blood pressure and heart rate. Although both are applied topically to the eye, measurable quantities of these drugs are detectable in plasma, so caution must be employed when cardiovascular agents are also being coadministered to the patient. Plasma brimonidine levels peaked within 1 to 4 hours and declined with a systemic half-life of approximately 3 hours. Brimonidine has been reported to enter the brain and can potentially cause fatigue and/or drowsiness in some patients. Brimonidine is primarily metabolized by aldehyde oxidase.

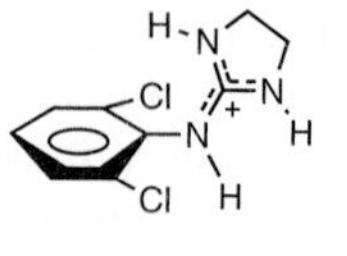

FIGURE 10.9 Protonated clonidine.

GUANFACINE (TENEX) AND GUANABENZ (WYTENSIN) After the discovery of clonidine, extensive research into the SAR of central α_2-agonists showed that the imidazoline ring was not necessary for activity in this class but that the phenyl ring required at least one *ortho* chlorine or methyl group. Two clinically useful antihypertensive agents resulting from this effort are guanfacine and guanabenz (see Chapter 24). These are ring-opened analogs of clonidine, and their mechanism of action is the same as that of clonidine.

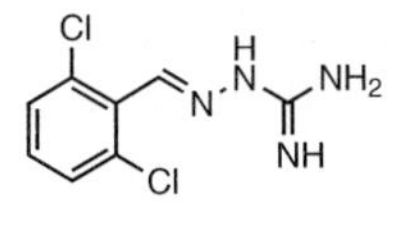

Guanabenz

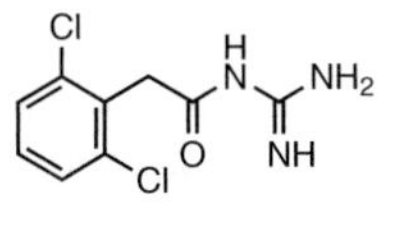

Guanfacine

METHYLDOPA (ALDOMET) Although structurally unrelated to the aminoimidazolines or the guanidines, the prodrug L-α-methyldopa (methyldopa) is an α_2-agonist acting in the CNS via its active metabolite, α-methylnorepinephrine (Fig. 10.10). Methyldopa is transported across the blood–brain barrier, where it is decarboxylated by aromatic L-amino acid decarboxylase in the brain to α-methyldopamine, which is then stereospecifically hydroxylated to 1*R*,2*S*-α-methylnorepinephrine. This stereoisomer is a selective α_2-agonist and acts as an antihypertensive agent much like clonidine to inhibit sympathetic neural output from the CNS, thus lowering blood pressure. α-Methylnorepinephrine and α-methyldopamine do not cross the blood–brain barrier because of their hydrophilicity. Originally synthesized as a norepinephrine biosynthesis inhibitor, methyldopa was thought to act through a combination of inhibition of norepinephrine biosynthesis through DOPA decarboxylase inhibition and metabolic decarboxylation to generate α-methylnorepinephrine. The latter was thought to replace norepinephrine in the nerve terminal and, when released, to have less intrinsic activity than the natural neurotransmitter. This latter mechanism is an example of the concept of a false neurotransmitter. (The antihypertensive properties for methyldopa are further described in Chapter 24.)

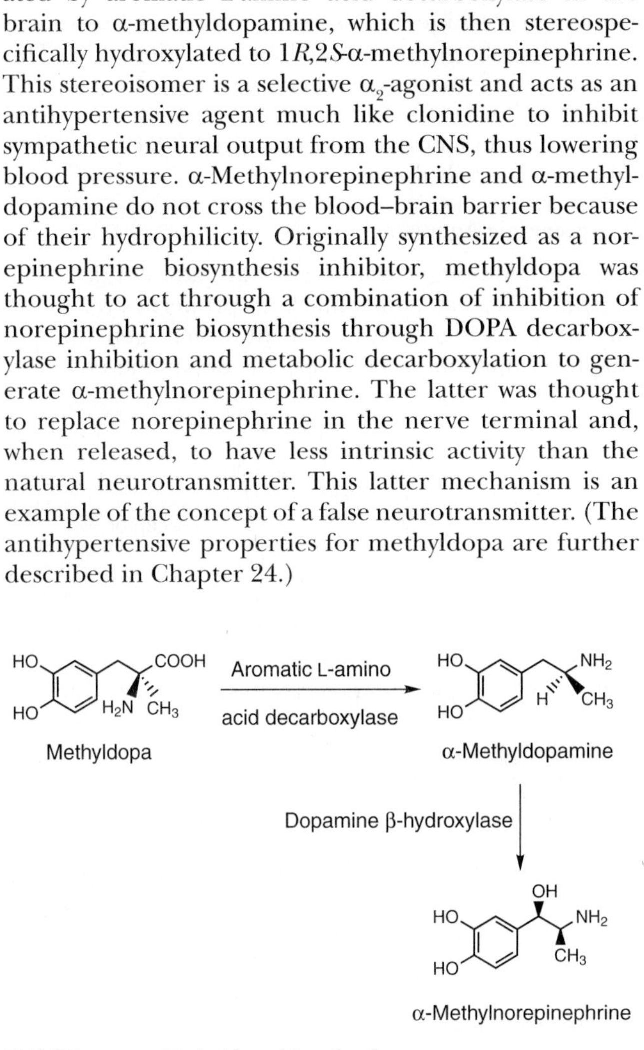

FIGURE 10.10 Methyldopa bioactivation.

b-Adrenergic Agonists

β_2-Agonist Phenylethanolamines

Most of the β_2-selective adrenergic agonists listed in Table 10.3 are used primarily as bronchodilators in asthma and other constrictive pulmonary conditions (see Chapter 39 for pharmacokinetic details about these drugs). Isoproterenol is a nonselective β-agonist (β_2/β_1 = 1), and the cardiac stimulation caused by its β_1-activity and its lack of oral activity have led to its diminished use in favor of more selective β_2-agonists.

SHORT-ACTING β_2-ADRENERGIC AGONISTS

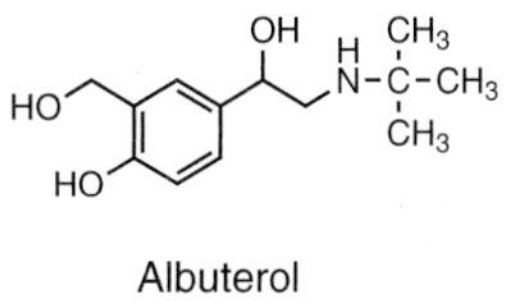

Albuterol

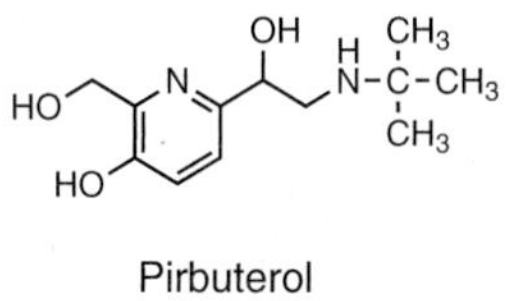

Pirbuterol

Albuterol (Ventolin, Proventil), Pirbuterol, (Maxair) Terbutaline (Bricanyl, Brethine) The noncatechol, selective b2-agonists, such as racemic albuterol (b2/b1 = 60), metaproterenol, and terbutaline, are available in oral dosage forms as well as in inhalers. All have similar activities and durations of action. Pirbuterol is an interesting analog of albuterol in which the benzene ring has been replaced by a pyridine ring, altering its pharmacokinetic properties. Similar to albuterol, pirbuterol is a selective b2-agonist currently available only for administration by inhalation.

Studies with the *R/S* enantiomers of albuterol have shown that the *S*-enantiomer can be proinflammatory, exacerbating airway reactivity to a variety of spasmogens and, thereby, enhancing bronchial muscle contraction, thus opposing the bronchodilation effects of the *R*-enantiomer levoalbuterol. Moreover, racemic albuterol exhibits enantioselective presystemic metabolism. Levalbuterol undergoes more rapid metabolism (sulfation) than the *S*-(+)-isomer, resulting in a lower oral bioavailability and rapid elimination. Because of its slower metabolism, *S*-albuterol has a higher and more prolonged tissue concentration than levalbuterol, increasing airway reactivity. These adverse effects of *S*-albuterol are completely avoided by using the *R*-enantiomer, levalbuterol (Xopenex). Thus, the removal of *S*-albuterol from racemic albuterol increases the clinical potency of levalbuterol, such that bronchodilator efficacy is achieved at one-fourth the dose of racemic albuterol along with a marked reduction in side effects.

LONG-ACTING B2-ADRENERGIC AGONISTS The mechanisms behind the long duration of the bronchodilating effect of the b2-adrenoceptor agonists formoterol, arformoterol, salmeterol, and indicaterol are only partially understood. Their long duration is attributed to their higher lipophilicity and greater receptor affinity compared to those of the short-acting agonists at the b2-adrenoceptor. Lipophilicity determines the amount of drug entering into the cell membrane of the b2-adrenoceptor and how much b2-adrenoceptor agonist must remain at the receptor for maximal sustained activity.

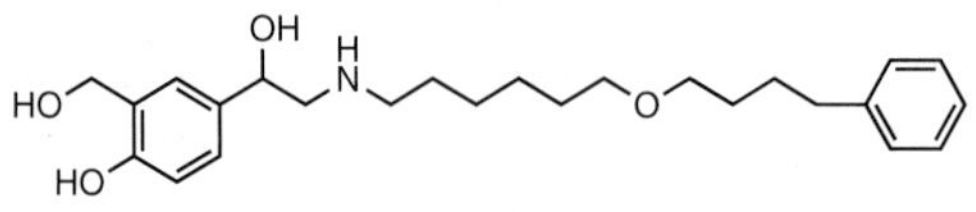

Salmeterol

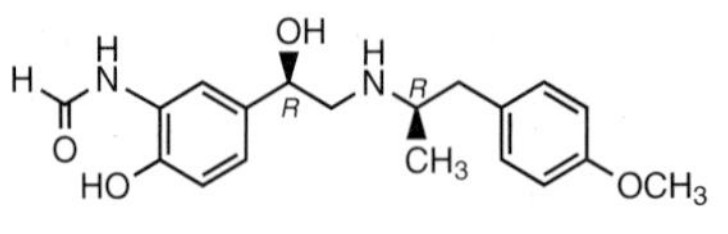

Formoterol
R,R-Arformoterol

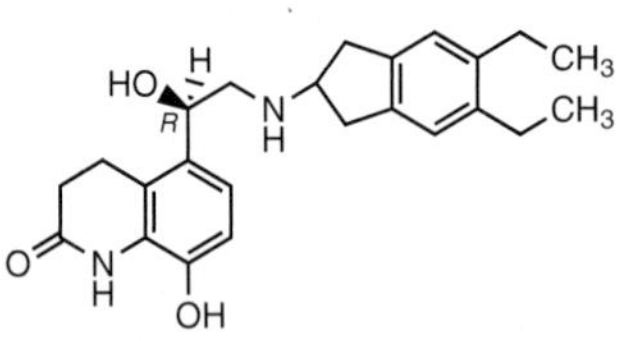

Indacaterol

Salmeterol (Serevent) A β_2-agonist with a slow onset and extended duration of action is salmeterol. Salmeterol has the same phenyl ring substitution R^3 as albuterol but also an unusually long and lipophilic group R^1 on the nitrogen. The octanol–water partition coefficient, logP, for salmeterol is 3.88, compared with 0.66 for albuterol. Salmeterol is approximately 50-fold more selective than albuterol for the β_2-receptor. Substantial evidence indicates that its long duration of action results from a specific binding interaction ("anchoring") of the phenyl group at the end of the extended lipophilic side chain with a specific region of the β_2-receptor, affording salmeterol a unique binding mechanism (Fig. 10.11).

Salmeterol is usually prescribed for severe persistent asthma following previous treatment with a short-acting β-agonist, such as albuterol. The noticeable differences between salmeterol and albuterol are the onset of action and their duration of action (see Chapter 39 for pharmacokinetic details). When used regularly every day as prescribed, inhaled salmeterol decreases the number and severity of asthma attacks. It is not used, however, for relieving an acute asthma attack that has already started.

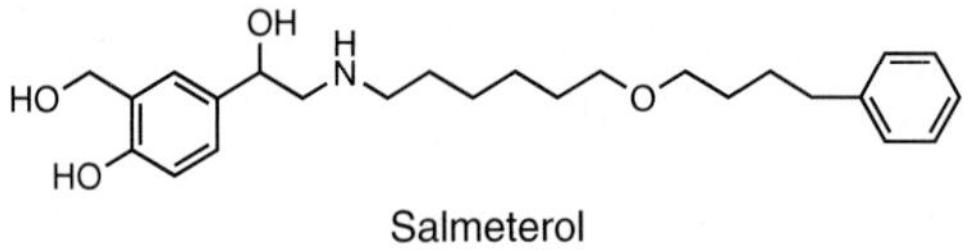

Salmeterol

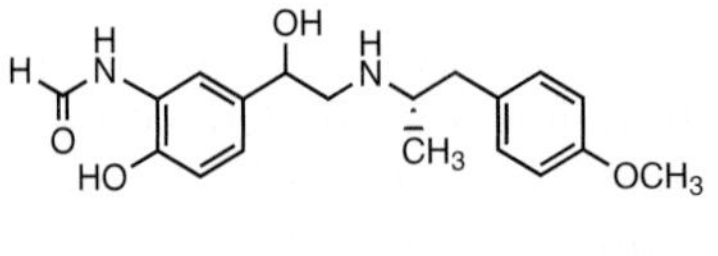

Formoterol

Formoterol (Foradil) and Arformoterol (Brovana) Formoterol has 3′-formylamino and 4′-hydroxy ring R^3 substitution pattern but also an alkoxyphenylethyl lipophilic group R^1 on the nitrogen, similar to ritodrine. Although it is less lipophilic (logP = 1.6) than salmeterol, it has a 12-hour duration of action similar to that for salmeterol. It is administered as an inhaled dry powder, because it is unstable to heat and moisture. Formoterol is a mixture of *R,R*-(−)- and *S,S*-(+)-stereoisomers, with the *R,R*-isomer having approximately 1,000-fold more affinity for the β_2-receptor than the *S,S*-isomer. Arformoterol is the single *R,R* active stereoisomer. Formoterol and arformoterol have a faster onset of action than salmeterol as a result of lower lipophilicity.

Indacaterol (Arcapta, Neohaler) Indacaterol is the newest bronchodilator, which is U.S. Food and Drug Administration approved for use in chronic obstructive pulmonary disease. Although the calculated logP for indacaterol is the same as salmeterol (logP = 3.88), the pK_a of the phenolic OH of indacaterol (pK_a = 6.7) is significantly lower than that of salmeterol (pK_a = 10.2), leading to a significant amount of indacaterol existing in solution at physiologic pH (7.4) as the zwitterion (protonated amine/phenoxide), whereas salmeterol is predominately the protonated amine cation (23). This difference in ionization has been shown to affect interactions with lipid membranes (24). As a result, indicaterol has a much longer duration of action of 24 hours, permitting once-daily dosing (25).

β_1-Adrenergic Agonists

Dopamine Although not strictly an adrenergic drug, dopamine is a catecholamine with properties related to the cardiovascular activities of the other agents in this chapter. Dopamine acts on specific dopamine receptors

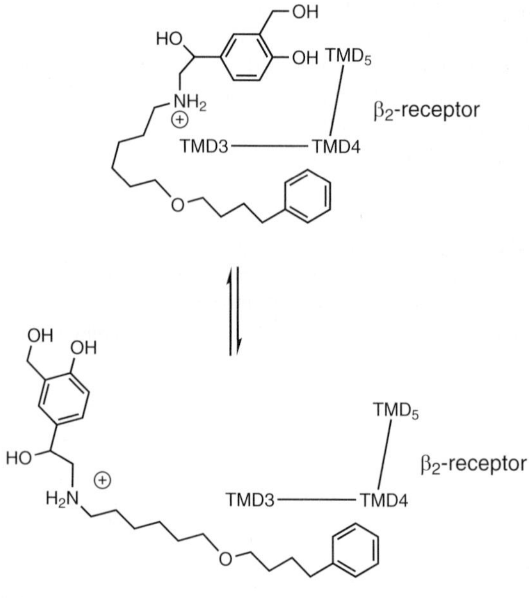

FIGURE 10.11 Mechanism of action for salmeterol.

to dilate renal vessels, increasing renal blood flow. Dopamine also stimulates cardiac β_1-receptors through both direct and indirect mechanisms. It is used to correct hemodynamic imbalances induced by conditions such as shock, myocardial infarction, trauma, or congestive heart failure. As a catechol and primary amine, dopamine is rapidly metabolized by COMT and MAO and, similar to dobutamine, has a short duration of action with no oral activity. It is administered as an intravenous infusion.

DOBUTAMINE (DOBUTREX) Not all the adrenergic agonists with direct activity have an aliphatic β-hydroxyl group such as the agents discussed so far. One of these is the catechol dobutamine. Dobutamine is a dopamine analog with a bulky arylalkyl group on the nitrogen and one chiral (asymmetric) center. Racemic (±)-dobutamine has direct activity on both α_1- and both β-receptors, but because of some unusual properties of its two enantiomers, the overall pharmacologic response looks similar to that of a selective β_1-agonist. The *S*-(−)-enantiomer of dobutamine exhibits β_1-agonist activity and is also an α_1-agonist and vasopressor. The *R*-(+)-isomer is an α_1-antagonist and general $\beta_1\beta_2$-agonist; thus, when the racemate is used clinically, the α-effects of the enantiomers cancel each other, leaving primarily the β_1-effects (26,27). The stereochemistry of the methyl substituent does not affect the ability of the drug to bind to the α_1-receptor but does affect the ability of the molecule to activate the receptor. That is, the stereochemistry of the methyl group affects intrinsic activity but not affinity. Because both stereoisomers are β_1-agonists, with the (−)-isomer having approximately one-tenth the potency of the (+)-isomer, the net effect is β_1 stimulation. Dobutamine is used as a cardiac stimulant after surgery or congestive heart failure. As a catechol, dobutamine is readily metabolized by COMT and has a short duration of action with no oral activity.

Mixed-Acting Sympathomimetics

PHENYLPROPANOLAMINES

(−)-Ephedrine As previously discussed, ephedrine is a natural product isolated from several species of ephedra plants, which have been used for centuries in folk medicines in a variety of cultures worldwide (28). Its occurrence in ephedra is approximately 80% to 90% of the alkaloid content. Other substances also found include (+)-pseudoephedrine (10% to 15%) and *N*-methylephedrine (2% to 5%). Pure ephedrine was first isolated and crystallized in 1887 from a Chinese herbal medicine called Ma Huang. Its sympathomimetic activity was not recognized until 1917, and the pure drug was used clinically even before epinephrine and norepinephrine were isolated and characterized. Ephedrine does not have any phenolic substituents on the phenyl ring, giving it a mixed-acting response and good oral activity, because it is not a substrate for COMT. Lacking hydrogen-bonding phenolic substituents, ephedrine is less polar than the other compounds discussed thus far and crosses the blood–brain barrier far better than the catechols do. Because of its ability to penetrate the CNS, ephedrine has been used as a stimulant and exhibits side effects related to its action in the brain. Ephedrine is widely used for many of the same indications as epinephrine, including use as a bronchodilator, vasopressor, cardiac stimulant, and nasal decongestant.

(+)-Pseudoephedrine Pseudoephedrine, as previously discussed, is the threo diastereomer of ephedrine, with virtually no direct activity and fewer CNS side effects than ephedrine. (+)-Pseudoephedrine is widely used as a nasal decongestant but is also used in the illicit manufacture of the widely abused drug methamphetamine. For this reason, sale of pseudoephedrine over-the-counter products is becoming increasingly restricted.

(+)-Phenylpropanolamine Phenylpropanolamine (Table 10.3) is the *N*-desmethyl analog of ephedrine, also known as stereoisomers of norephedrine and norpseudoephedrine, which is as a stimulant, nasal decongestant, and anorectic agent. Lacking the *N*-methyl group, however, phenylpropanolamine has none of the β_2-agonist activity of ephedrine, is slightly less lipophilic, and therefore, does not enter the CNS as well as ephedrine. Phenylpropanolamine, similar to ephedrine, is a mixture of *erythro* enantiomers with mixed direct and mostly indirect activity. In the United States, phenylpropanolamine is no longer sold without a prescription due to a proposed increased risk of stroke in younger women. In Europe, however, it is still available both by prescription and over the counter. In Canada, it was withdrawn from the market, and in the United Kingdom, it is available in many "all-in-one" cough and cold medications, which also contain acetaminophen (paracetamol) or another analgesic and caffeine. It is still available for veterinary use in dogs as a treatment for urinary incontinence.

PHENYLISOPROPYLAMINES

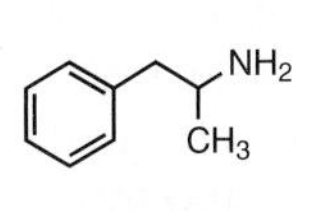

Amphetamine

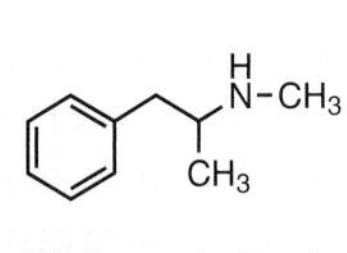

Methamphetamine

Amphetamine and Methamphetamine Other methyl-substituted phenylethylamines (phenylisopropylamines), such as *S*-(+)-amphetamine and *S*-(+)-methamphetamine, which lack both ring substituents and a side-chain hydroxyl, are sufficiently lipophilic to cross the blood–brain barrier readily and cause dramatic CNS stimulation, which gives them serious abuse potential. The clinical utility of *S*-(+)-amphetamine and its derivatives is entirely based on CNS stimulant and central appetite suppressant effects. The only amphetamine product available that is used for the treatment of attention-deficit disorder combines the sulfate, saccharate, and aspartate salts of dextroamphetamine and amphetamine (total amphetamine base, 3.1 mg; Adderall). (These agents and the methoxylated amphetamines are discussed in Chapter 19.)

STRUCTURE–ACTIVITY RELATIONSHIPS OF ADRENERGIC ANTAGONISTS

Nonselective α-Antagonists

Phenoxybenzamine

Because α-agonists cause vasoconstriction and raise blood pressure, one would expect α-antagonists to be therapeutically used as antihypertensive agents. An old but powerful drug in this class is phenoxybenzamine (dibenzyline), a β-haloalkylamine that alkylates α-receptors. β-Haloalkylamines are present in nitrogen mustard anticancer agents and are highly reactive alkylating agents. The acid salt of phenoxybenzamine is stable, but at physiologic pH, equilibrium exists between the protonated drug and free base. The unshared electrons of the unprotonated amino group are nucleophilic and displace the β-chlorine atom in an intramolecular reaction to form a highly reactive aziridinium ion (Fig. 10.12). If this occurs in the vicinity of an α-receptor, a nucleophile group X on the receptor can open the aziridinium ion in a nucleophilic reaction to form a covalent bond between the receptor and the drug. The substituents attached to the haloalkylamine provide selectivity for binding to α-adrenoceptors so that the nucleophile generally is part of the target receptor. The nucleophile X is presumably part of an amino acid side chain, such as a cysteine thiol, serine hydroxyl, or lysine amino group, but the specific site of covalent attachment to the α-receptor has not been determined. Because the reaction in which phenoxybenzamine forms covalent bonds with the receptors is irreversible, new receptors must be synthesized before the effects can be overcome. Therefore, the α-blockade is long-lasting.

Unfortunately, other biomolecules besides the target α-receptor are also alkylated. Because of its receptor nonselectivity and toxicity, the use of phenoxybenzamine largely is limited to alleviating the sympathetic effects of pheochromocytoma. This tumor of chromaffin cells of the adrenal medulla produces large amounts of epinephrine and norepinephrine, which are released into the bloodstream, producing hypertension and generalized sympathetic stimulation.

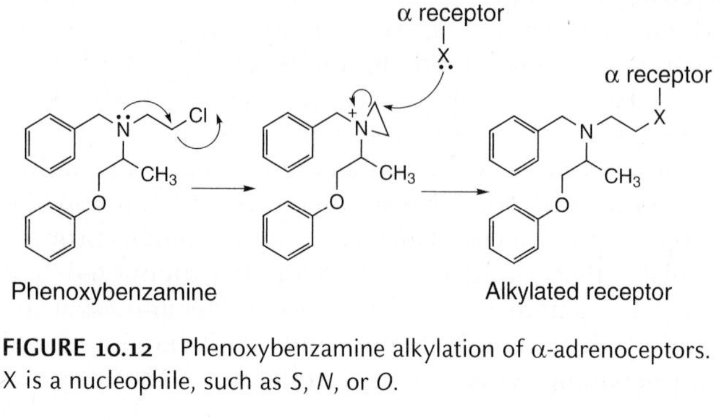

FIGURE 10.12 Phenoxybenzamine alkylation of α-adrenoceptors. X is a nucleophile, such as *S*, *N*, or *O*.

Tolazoline and Phentolamine

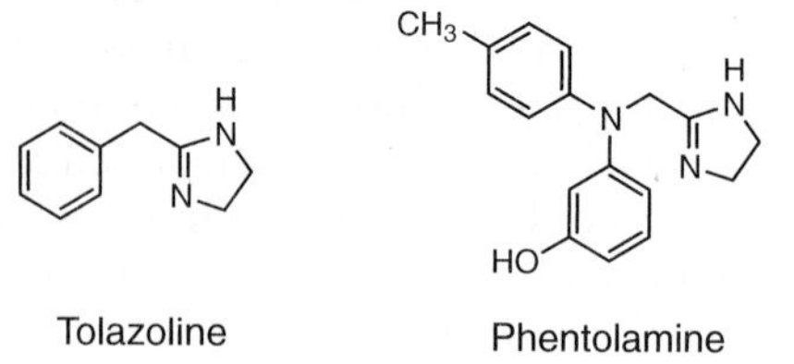

Tolazoline and phentolamine are two imidazoline nonselective α-antagonists that also have antihypertensive activity, although they have been replaced in general clinical use by far better agents. Tolazoline has clear structural similarities to the imidazoline α_1-agonists, such as naphazoline and xylometazoline (Fig. 10.7), but does not have the lipophilic substituents required for agonist activity. The resemblance of phentolamine is not as readily apparent, but extensive molecular modeling studies have provided a topologic scheme for α_1-antagonist SAR (19). This pattern, however, cannot be readily visualized without computer graphics and is beyond the scope of this chapter.

Both phentolamine and tolazoline are potent but rather nonspecific α-antagonists. Both drugs stimulate gastrointestinal smooth muscle, an action blocked by atropine, which would indicate cholinergic activity, and they both stimulate gastric secretion, possibly through release of histamine. Because of these and other side effects, the clinical applications of tolazoline and phentolamine are also limited to treating the symptoms of pheochromocytoma and hypertensive crises induced by certain illicit drugs.

Selective α_1-Antagonists

Prazosin, Doxazosin, Terazosin, Tamsulosin, Alfuzosin, and Silodosin

Prazosin, the first known selective α_1-blocker, was discovered in the late 1960s (29) and is now one of a small group of selective α_1-antagonists that includes three other quinoxaline antihypertensives terazosin, doxazosin, and alfuzosin and the nonquinazoline benzensulfonamides tamsulosin and silodosin (Fig. 10.13). Prazosin, doxazosin, and terazosin contain a 4-amino-6,7-dimethoxyquinazoline ring system attached to a piperazine ring, whereas alfuzosin has a rotatable propylenediamine group (an open piperazine ring). The other structural differences are the heterocyclic acyl groups attached to the second nitrogen of the piperazine or the propyl chain. The differences in these groups afford dramatic differences in some of the pharmacokinetic properties of these agents (Table 10.5). For example, reduction of the furan ring for prazosin to the tetrahydrofuran ring of terazosin increases its duration of action by altering its rate of metabolism. Some of the important clinical parameters of the quinazolines are shown in Table 10.5. The long half-lives and durations of action for terazosin, doxazosin, tamsulosin, and silodosin permit once-a-day dosing and generally lead to increased patient compliance.

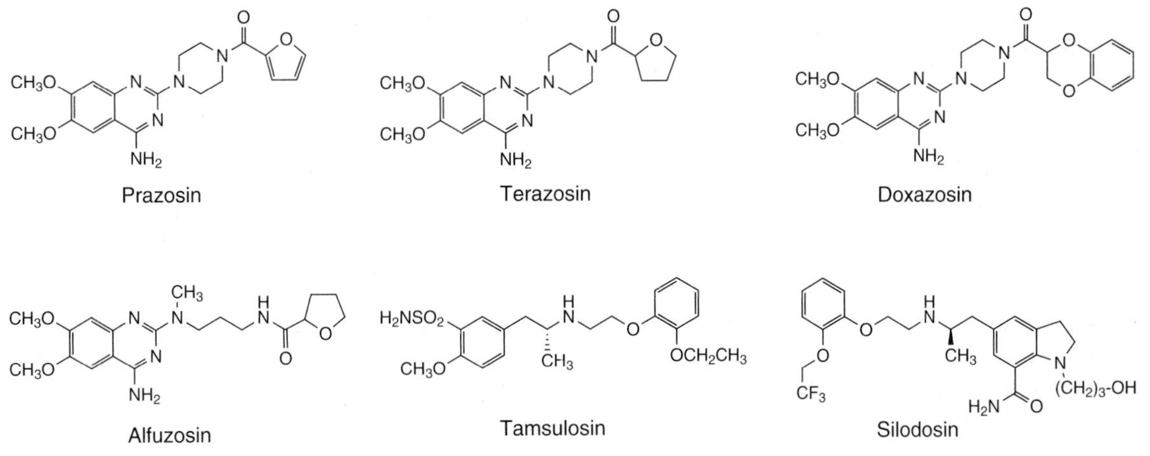

FIGURE 10.13 Selective α_1-adrenergic antagonists.

Prazosin is an antihypertensive agent, as are terazosin and doxazosin. The latter two were subsequently discovered to block α_1-receptors in the prostate gland and alleviate the symptoms of benign prostatic hyperplasia (BPH) (see Chapter 40). The subsequently developed tamsulosin and alfuzosin are more selective for the subtype of α_1-adrenoceptor found in the prostate gland, α_{1A}, over those found in vascular tissue. The most recently developed drug, silodosin, is the most selective of the group for α_{1A}-receptors found in the prostate (30). Thus, tamsulosin, alfuzosin, and silodosin are first-line drugs for the treatment of BPH and have no utility in treating hypertension. They have fewer cardiovascular side effects than terazosin and doxazosin in treating BPH. (Details on the use and pharmacokinetics of α_1-antagonists in treating hypertension and BPH are provided in Chapters 24 and 40, respectively.)

β-Adrenergic Antagonists

In the 1950s, dichloroisoproterenol, a derivative of isoproterenol in which the catechol hydroxyls had been replaced by chlorines, was discovered to be a β-antagonist that blocked the effects of sympathomimetic amines on bronchodilation, uterine relaxation, and heart stimulation (31). Although dichloroisoproterenol had no clinical utility, replacement of the 3,4-dichloro substituents with a carbon bridge to form a naphthylethanolamine derivative did afford a clinical candidate, pronethalol, which was introduced in 1962 only to be withdrawn in 1963 because of tumor induction in animal tests.

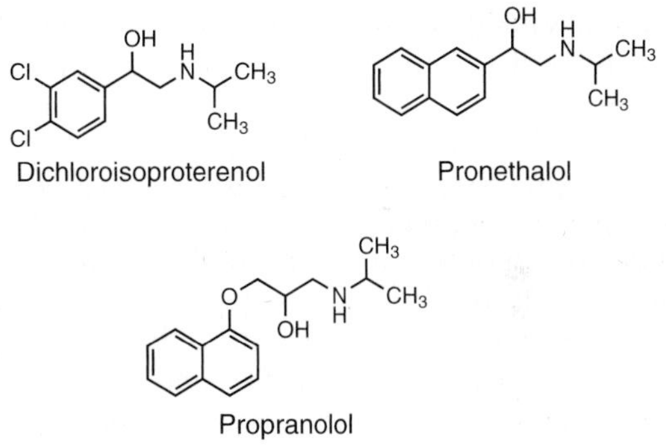

Structure–Activity Relationships

Shortly thereafter, a major innovation in drug development for the β-adrenergic antagonists was introduced when it was discovered that an oxymethylene bridge,

TABLE 10.5 Selected Clinical Parameters of α_1-Adrenergic Antagonists

Drug	Trade Name	cLogP/logD$_{pH\ 7.0}$	Half-Life (hours)	Duration of Action (hours)	Bioavailability (%)
Prazosin	Minipres	−1.1/−1.3	2–3	4–6	45–65
Terazosin	Hytrin	−1.0/−1.0	12	>18	90
Doxazosin	Cardura	0.7/0.5	22	18–36	65
Tamsulosin	Flomax	2.2/0.5	14–15	>24	<50 with food 50–90 fasting
Alfuzosin	Uroxatral	−1.0/−2.7	3–5	>48	65
Silodosin	Rapaflo	2.33/0.48	13	>24	18-43 with food

[a] Chemical Abstracts, American Chemical Society, calculated using Advanced Chemistry Development (ACD/Labs) Software V8.19 for Solaris (1994–2011 ACD/Labs).

OCH_2, could be inserted into the arylethanolamine structure of pronethalol to afford propranolol, an aryloxypropanolamine and the first clinically successful β-blocker. Note that along with the introduction of the oxymethylene bridge, the side chain has been moved from C2 of the naphthyl group to the C1 position. In general, the aryloxypropanolamines are more potent β-blockers than the corresponding arylethanolamines, and most of the β-blockers currently being used clinically are aryloxypropanolamines. β-Blockers have found wide use in treating hypertension (Chapter 24) and certain types of glaucoma.

Initially, it might appear that lengthening the side chain would prevent appropriate binding of the required functional groups to the same receptor site. Molecular models, however, show that the side chains of aryloxypropanolamines can adopt a conformation that places the hydroxyl and amine groups into approximately the same position in space (Fig. 10.14). Although the simple two-dimensional drawing in Figure 10.14 exaggerates the true degree of overlap, elaborate molecular modeling studies confirm that the aryloxypropanolamine side chain can adopt a low-energy conformation that permits close overlap with the arylethanolamine side chain (32).

Stereochemistry of the β-Adrenergic Antagonists

A factor that sometimes causes confusion when comparing the structures of arylethanolamines with aryloxypropanolamines is the stereochemical nomenclature of the side-chain carbon bearing the hydroxyl group. For maximum effectiveness in receptor binding, the hydroxy group must occupy the same region in space as it does for the phenylethanolamine agonists in the *R* absolute configuration. Because of the insertion of an oxygen atom in the side chain of the aryloxypropanolamines, the Cahn-Ingold-Prelog priority of the substituents around the asymmetric carbon changes, and the isomer with the required special arrangement now has the *S* absolute configuration. This is an effect of the nomenclature rules; the groups still have the same spatial arrangements (Fig. 10.15).

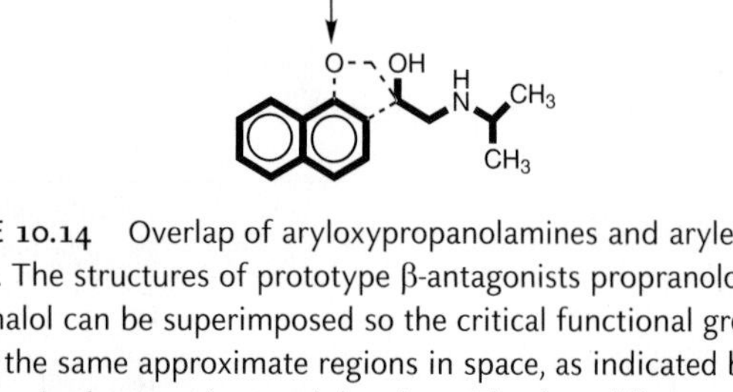

FIGURE 10.14 Overlap of aryloxypropanolamines and arylethanolamines. The structures of prototype β-antagonists propranolol and pronethalol can be superimposed so the critical functional groups occupy the same approximate regions in space, as indicated by the bold lines in the superimposed drawings. The dotted lines are those parts that do not overlap but are not necessary to receptor binding.

Propranolol and Other β-Blockers Propranolol was initially introduced for the treatment of angina pectoris and later underwent trials as an antiarrhythmic. During clinical trials as an antianginal, propranolol was discovered to have antihypertensive properties, and it has been widely employed for that purpose for decades (33). Propranolol rapidly became widely used for a variety of cardiac arrhythmias as well. In addition, because of its high lipophilicity and ability to penetrate the CNS, propranolol has found use in treating disorders of the CNS, such as anxiety.

At approximately this same time, a new series of 4-substituted phenyloxypropanololamines emerged that selectively inhibited sympathetic cardiac stimulation. These observations led to the recognition that not all β-receptors were the same, which in turn led to the introduction of β_1 and β_2 nomenclature to differentiate cardiac β_1-receptors from others. Development of β-blockers proceeded rapidly, and today, a large number of additional drugs, both nonselective β-antagonists and selective β_1-antagonists, are available on the world market. (Clinical use of β-blockers as antihypertensives is covered in Chapter 24.) Of those antagonists that are selective for the cardiac β_1-receptor, most have also some β_2-antagonist properties at the higher levels of therapeutic dosing (dose dependent). With the exception of sotalol, all the drugs shown in Figures 10.16 and 10.17 are aryloxypropanolamines. Metipranolol (Fig. 10.16) is an exception to the general rule that 4-substituted aryloxypropanolamines are selective β_1-blockers.

Other than β_1-selectivity of 4-substituted aryloxypropanolamines, little obvious structural pattern relates β-blockers to specific clinical applications, with the exception of esmolol. Esmolol is the methyl ester of a carboxylic acid, which makes it susceptible to hydrolysis by serum esterases. The acid metabolite generated by hydrolysis is essentially inactive and readily excreted as its zwitterion. For this reason, esmolol has a half-life of only approximately 8 minutes and is used to control supraventricular tachycardia during surgery when a short-acting β_1-adrenergic antagonist is desirable. Nebivolol (Fig. 10.17) is also unique in this group of selective β_1-blockers in that it has

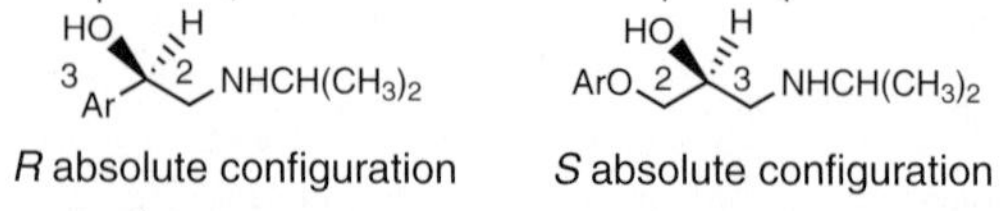

FIGURE 10.15 Stereochemical nomenclature for arylethanolamines versus aryloxypropanolamines. The relative positions in space of the four functional groups are the same in the two structures; however, one is designated *R* and the other *S*. This is because the introduction of an oxygen atom into the side chain of the aryloxypropanolamine changes the priority of two of the groups used in the nomenclature assignment.

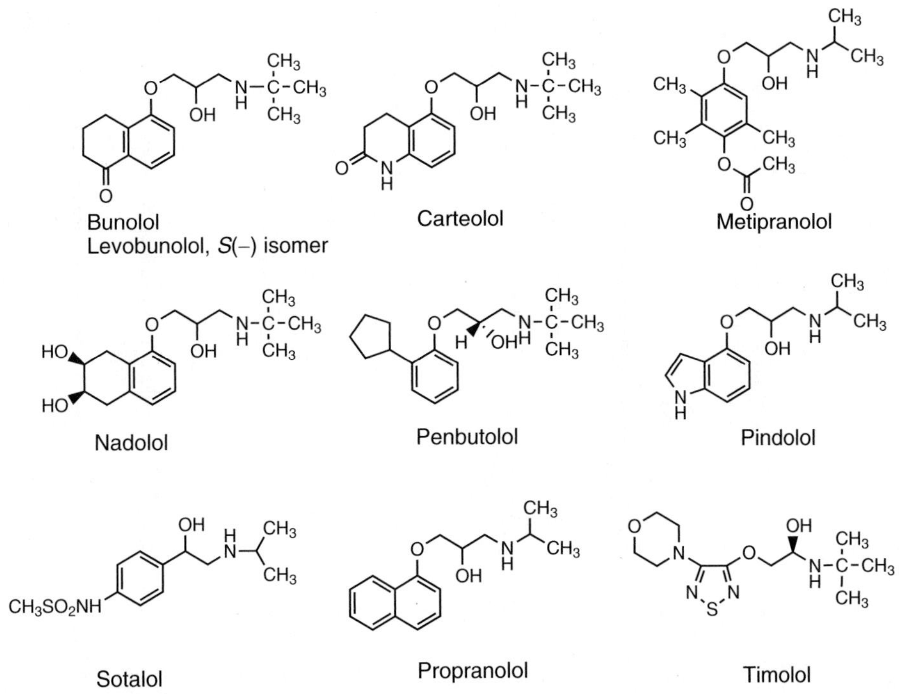

FIGURE 10.16 Nonselective β-adrenergic antagonists.

a nitric oxide potentiating effect (34). This gives the drug vasodilating effects in addition to its β-effects on the heart.

Another physicochemical parameter with some clinical correlation is the relative lipophilicity of different agents. Propranolol is by far the most lipophilic of the available β-blockers, and it enters the CNS far better than the less lipophilic agents, such as atenolol or nadolol. Lipophilicity as measured by octanol–water partitioning also correlates with the primary site of clearance, as seen in Table 10.6. The more lipophilic drugs are primarily cleared by the liver, whereas the more hydrophilic agents are cleared by the kidney. This could influence the choice of agents in cases of renal failure or liver disease. Several of the β-blockers must be dose adjusted in patients with impaired renal function, as indicated in Table 10.6.

β-Blockers have also found extensive use in treating glaucoma, although the mechanism of action in treating glaucoma is more difficult to explain. The

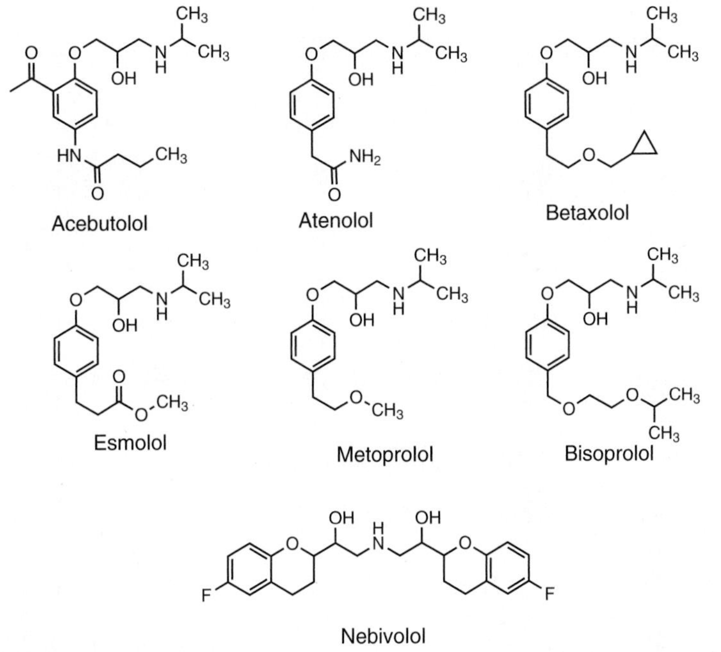

FIGURE 10.17 Selective β_1-adrenergic antagonists.

TABLE 10.6 Pharmacologic/Pharmacokinetic Properties of β-Adrenergic Blocking Agents

Drug	Adrenergic Receptor Blocking Activity	Membrane Stabilizing Activity	Intrinsic Sympathomimetic Activity	cLogP/ $logD_{pH 7.4}$ [a]	Extent of Absorption (%)	Absolute Oral Bioavailability (%)	Half-Life (h)	Protein Binding (%)	Metabolism/Excretion
Acebutolol (Sectral)	β_1 [b]	+	+	2.67/0.52	90	20–60	3–4	26	Hepatic; renal excretion, 30%–40%; nonrenal excretion, 50%–60% (bile)
Atenolol (Tenormin)	β_1 [b]	0	0	0.1/–2.0	50	50–60	6–9	16–16	~50% excreted unchanged in feces
Betaxolol (Kerlone, Betoptic)	β_1 [b]	+	0	2.7/0.6	~100	89	14–22	~50	Hepatic; >80% recovered in urine, 15% unchanged
Bisoprolol (Zebeta)	β_1 [b]	0	0	2.2/0.1	≥90	80	9–12	~30	~50% excreted unchanged in urine, remainder as inactive metabolites; <2% excreted in feces
Esmolol (Brevibloc)	β_1 [b]	0	0	1.9/–0.22	na[f]	na[f]	0.15	55	Rapid metabolism by esterases in cytosol of red blood cells
Metoprolol Lopressor) Metoprolol, LA	β_1 [b]	0[c]	0	1.8/–0.34	95	40–50 77	3–7	12	Hepatic; renal excretion, <5% unchanged
Carteolol (Cartrol, Ocupress)	β_1 β_2	0	++	1.7/–0.4	80	85	6	23–30	50%–70% excreted unchanged in urine
Nadolol (Corgard)	β_1 β_2	0	0	1.3/0.84	30	30–50	20–24	30	Urine, unchanged
Nebivolol (Bystolic)	β_1 [b]	0	0	3.7/2.3	nd[g]	12% EM[h] 96% PM[h]	10 EM 30–50 PM	98	38%–67% in urine; 44%–13% in feces
Penbutolol (Levatol)	β_1 β_2	0	+	4.2/2.1	~100	~100	5	80–98	Hepatic (conjugation, oxidation); renal excretion of metabolites (17% as conjugate)
Pindolol (Visken)	β_1 β_2	+	+++	1.97/–0.2	95	~100	3–4[d]	40	Urinary excretion of metabolites (60%–65%) and unchanged drug (35%–40%)
Propranolol (Inderal) Propranolol, LA	β_1 β_2	++	0	3.1/1	90	30 9–18	3–5 8–11	90	Hepatic; <1% excreted unchanged in urine
Sotalol (Betapace)	β_1 β_2	0	0	0.3/–1.8	nd[g]	90–100	12	0	Not metabolized; excreted unchanged in urine
Timolol (Blocadren, Timoptic)	β_1 β_2	0	0	–4.3/–2	90	75	4	10	Hepatic; urinary excretion of metabolites and unchanged drug
Labetalol[e] (Normodyne)	β_1 β_2 α_1	0	0	2.9/0.99	100	30–40	5.5–8	50	55%–60% excreted in urine as conjugates or unchanged drug
Carvedilol (Coreg)	β_1 β_2 α_1	0	0	4.2/3.2	>90	25–35	7–10	98	

[a] cLogP and LogD calculated using Advanced Chemistry Development (ACD/Labs) Software V8.19 for Solaris (1994–2011 Chemical Abstracts, American Chemical Society.
[b] Inhibits β_2-receptors (bronchial and vascular) at higher doses.
[c] Detectable only at doses much greater than required for β-blockade.
[d] In elderly hypertensive patients with normal renal function, half-life is variable (7–15 hours).
[e] Not labetalol monograph.
[f] Not applicable (available intravenously only).
[g] No data.
[h] EM, extensive metabolizers in CYP2D6; PM, poor metabolizers in CYP2D6.
0 = none; + = low; ++ = moderate; +++ = high.

β-blockers lower intraocular pressure by decreasing the amount of aqueous humor fluid produced in the eye by the ciliary body, and β_2-receptors have been found in that tissue. Observations have shown, however, that the ciliary body has no adrenergic innervation, that the effect is not stereoselective, and that a correlation of activity exists with decreased ciliary blood flow and decreased dopamine levels, indicating that the mechanism of action of β-blockers in treating glaucoma is unusual (35).

Mixed α/β-Adrenergic Antagonists

Labetalol and carvedilol are antihypertensives with α_1-, β_1-, and β_2-blocking activity (Fig. 10.18) (see Chapter 24). In terms of SAR, recall from the earlier discussion of phenylethanolamine agonists that the type of *N*-substituents, such as *N*-isopropyl and *N*-*t*-butyl, eliminated α_1-receptor activity; however, arylalkyl groups with α-methyl substituent returned α_1-affinity but not intrinsic activity (c.f., dobutamine). Thus, these two drugs have structural features that permit binding to the α_1-receptor and nonselectively to both β-receptors. The β-blocking activity of labetalol is approximately 1.5-fold that of its α_1-blocking activity. Carvedilol has an estimated β-blocking activity 10- to 100-fold its α_1-blocking activity. Carvedilol also has unique properties that make it particularly good for treating heart failure. In addition to both α_1- and β-blocking activity, the carbazole portion of the molecule also has antioxidant properties that provide further protection to the heart by scavenging free radicals (36,37).

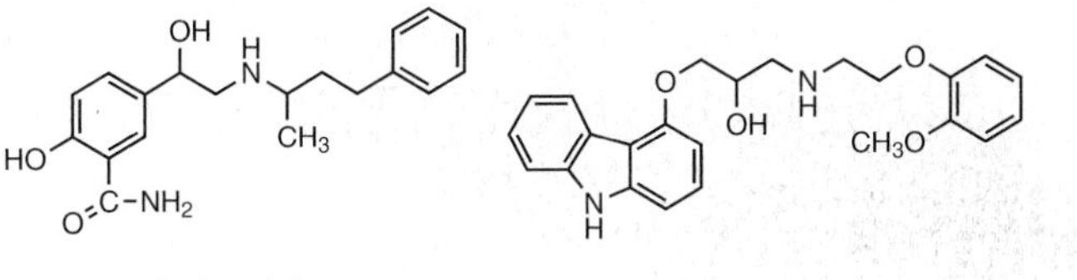

FIGURE 10.18 Mixed α/β-adrenergic antagonists.

DRUGS AFFECTING NOREPINEPHRINE/ EPINEPHRINE BIOSYNTHESIS

Hypothetically, inhibitors of any of the three enzymes involved in the conversion of tyrosine to norepinephrine could be used as drugs to moderate adrenergic transmission. Inhibitors of the rate-limiting enzyme tyrosine hydroxylase would be the most logical choice. One inhibitor of tyrosine hydroxylase, metyrosine or α-methyl-L-tyrosine, is in limited clinical use to help control hypertensive episodes and other symptoms of catecholamine overproduction in patients with the rare adrenal tumor pheochromocytoma (38). Metyrosine, a competitive inhibitor of tyrosine hydroxylase, inhibits the production of catecholamines by the tumor. Although metyrosine is useful in treating hypertension caused by excess catecholamine biosynthesis in pheochromocytoma tumors, it is not useful for treating essential hypertension. The drug metyrosine is the (*S*)-stereoisomer of α-methyltyrosine. The enantiomer, (*R*)-α-methyltyrosine, does not bind to the active site of tyrosine hydroxylase and, thus, has no useful pharmacologic activity.

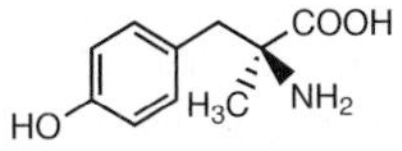

Metyrosine

Powerful inhibitors of the next enzyme in the pathway, aromatic L-amino acid decarboxylase (e.g., carbidopa), have proven clinically useful, but not as modulators of peripheral adrenergic transmission. Rather, these agents are used to inhibit the metabolism of exogenous L-DOPA administered in the treatment of Parkinson disease (see Chapter 13).

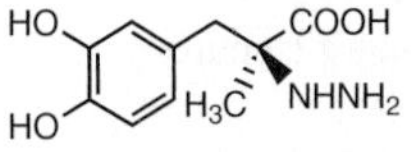

Carbidopa

The next enzyme in the biosynthetic pathway to norepinephrine and epinephrine, dopamine β-hydroxylase, has been the subject of extensive research into its chemical mechanism and the subject of many enzyme inhibition studies. The inhibitors known to date, however, are primarily of basic biochemical research interest and have no therapeutic relevance. The same is true of phenylethanolamine-*N*-methyltransferase, the last enzyme in the biosynthesis of epinephrine in the adrenal medulla.

SCENARIO: OUTCOME AND ANALYSIS

Outcome

Kathryn Neill, PharmD

Based on the infusion record, SJ ingested approximately 200 mL of dopamine solution. After reviewing the administration and solubility information for dopamine, the pharmacist recommended no intervention for the ingested dopamine. In addition, the pharmacist instructed the nurse that the dopamine infusion could be restarted if needed for continued treatment of hypotension with vigilant monitoring based on the patient's mental status.

Chemical Analysis

Victoria Roche, S. William Zito, and Kathryn Neill

Dopamine is a catechol-containing primary phenethylamine manufactured as a water-soluble hydrochloride salt. It is a precursor molecule in the biosynthesis of the adrenergic neurotransmitter norepinephrine and the neurohormone epinephrine. It lacks the β-OH group found on the true endogenous adrenergic agonists and, as a result, has a lower affinity for α and β adrenoceptors than norepinephrine or epinephrine. However, dopamine's close structural similarity with norepinephrine allows it to compete with its "sister" neurotransmitter for access to catacholaminergic reuptake sites, which leaves more norepinephrine in adrenergic synapses to act on postsynaptic receptors. Because it promotes the action of the true adrenergic neurotransmitter at its receptors, dopamine can be viewed as an indirect-acting adrenergic agonist. Another mechanism through which dopamine can act indirectly as an adrenergic agonist is by stimulating the release of the adrenergic neurotransmitter from vesicles in the presynaptic terminals of adrenergic neurons.

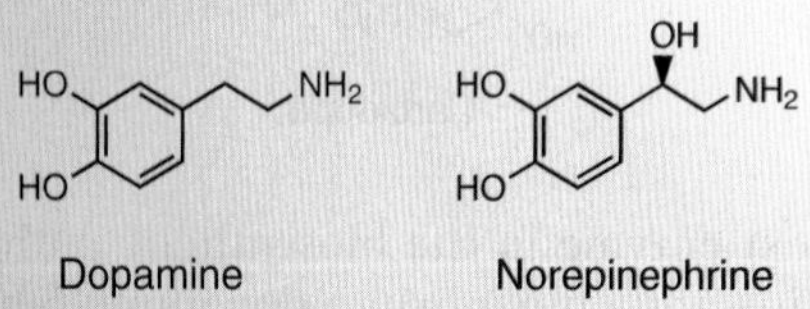

Dopamine increases renal blood flow through the stimulation of specific renal dopamine receptors and exerts dose-dependent pharmacodynamic effects through the direct and indirect stimulation of adrenergic receptors, as described above. By directly stimulating β receptors and causing release of norepinephrine from sympathetic storage sites, dopamine produces increases in myocardial inotropy and chronotropy. Stimulation of α receptors increases at higher doses and results in vasoconstriction.

Dopamine is administered intravenously because it is unstable in the gastrointestinal tract. The lack of substituents (e.g., CH_3) on the α-carbon makes dopamine exceptionally vulnerable to prehepatic (gut) and first pass (liver) deamination by monoamine oxidase, which would yield the inactive 3,4-dihydroxyphenylacetaldehyde. This short-lived aldehyde intermediately would be rapidly biotransformed to 3,4-dihydroxyphenylacetic acid by cytosolic aldehyde dehydrogenase. The catechol nucleus also would be vulnerable to rapid, inactivating COMT methylation to 3-methoxytyramine, using S-adenosylmethionine as the methyl-donating cofactor. As a result of these inactivating biotransformations, there would essentially be no active drug delivered to SJ's bloodstream after oral ingestion of an aqueous dopamine solution, so the patient is not at risk for dopamine toxicity as a result of her misadventure.

It should also be noted that dopamine, like all catechols, is unstable to base and can also auto-oxidize on exposure to light (hυ) and oxygen in the air. The decomposition product generated by any of these conditions is the inactive orthoquinone. If the dopamine infusion is restarted, care should be taken to not co-administer bicarbonate or any other intravenous solution with an alkaline pH and to protect the catecholic solution from light and air.

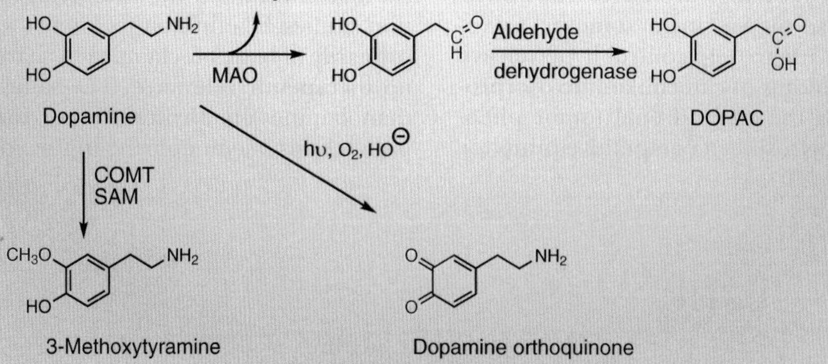

CASE STUDY

Victoria Roche and S. William Zito

It is a hot and humid Saturday afternoon, and you are chatting casually with a patient in the full-service neighborhood apothecary you've established in your hometown. Things were relatively quiet until BW, a 49-year-old woman who lives right around the corner from your pharmacy, phones in a panic. Her husband, LW, had been doing some yard work when he disturbed a nest of wasps with his weed whacker. He suffered several stings on his hands and arms before he was able to make it back to the house. His limbs immediately began to swell and, as BW was putting ice packs on them, LW lost color in his face and began to breathe in a labored manner. You tell her to phone 911 ask your pharmacist coworker to call LW's physician for the needed prescription, grab the life-saving medication, and run to assist. You find LW clearly hypotensive and in the beginning stages of respiratory crisis.

One of the three structures drawn below needs to be administered stat. Which one did you bring with you to save the day?

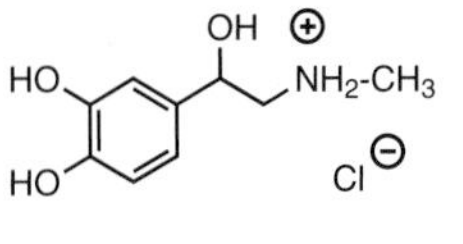

1

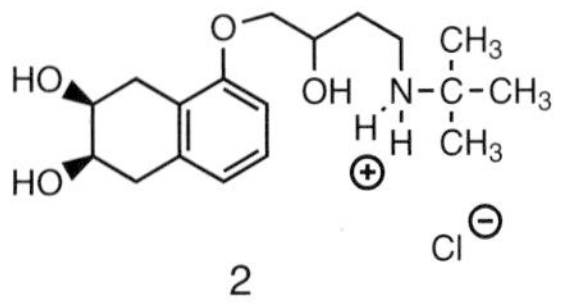

2

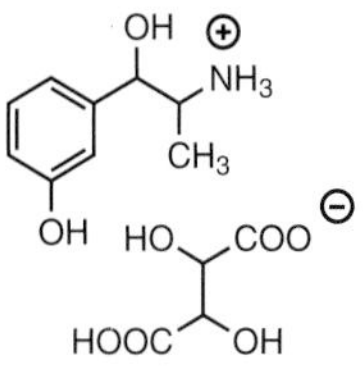

3

1. Conduct a thorough and mechanistic SAR analysis of the three therapeutic options in the case.
2. Apply the chemical understanding gained from the SAR analysis to this patient's specific needs to make a therapeutic recommendation.

References

1. Von Euler US. Synthesis, uptake, and storage of catecholamines in adrenergic nerves: the effect of drugs. In: Blaschko H, Marshall E, ed. Catecholamines. New York: Springer, 1972:186–230.
2. Griffith RK. Adrenergics and adrenergic-blocking drugs. In: Abraham DJ, ed. Burger's Medicinal Chemistry and Drug Discovery. Hoboken, NJ: John Wiley and Sons, 2003:1–37.
3. Kaufman S, Nelson TJ. Studies on the regulation of tyrosine hydroxylase activity by phosphorylation and dephosphorylation. In: Dahlstrom A, Belmaker RH, Sandler M, eds. Progress in Catecholamine Research. Part A: Basic Aspects and Peripheral Mechanisms. New York: Alan R Liss, 1988:57–60.
4. Philippu A, Matthaei H. Transport and storage of catecholamines in vesicles. In: Trendelenburg U, Weiner N, eds. Catecholamines I. New York: Springer, 1988:1–42.
5. Trendelenburg U. Factors influencing the concentration of catecholamines at the receptors. In: Blaschko H, Marshall E, eds. Catecholamines. New York: Springer, 1972:726–761.
6. Kopin IJ. Metabolic degradation of catecholamines. In: Blaschko H, Marshall E, eds. Catecholamines. New York: Springer, 1972:270–282.
7. Ahlquist RP. A study of the adrenotropic receptors. Am J Physiol 1948;153:586–600.
8. Harrison JK, Pearson WR, Lynch KR. Molecular characterization of α_1- and α_2-adrenoceptors. Trends Pharmacol Sci 1991;12:62–67.
9. De Souza CJ, Burkey BF. β_3-Adrenoceptor agonists as antidiabetic and antiobesity drugs in humans. Curr Pharm Des 2001;7:1433–1449.
10. Trumpp-Kallmeyer S, Hoflack J, Bruinvels A, et al. Modeling of G protein–coupled receptors: application to dopamine, adrenaline, serotonin, acetylcholine, and mammalian opsin receptors. J Med Chem 1992;35:3448–3462.
11. Ostrowski J, Kjelsberg MA, Caron MG, et al. Mutagenesis of the β_2-adrenergic receptor: how structure elucidates function. Annu Rev Pharmacol Toxicol 1992;32:167–183.
12. Strader CD, Candelore MR, Hill WS, et al. Identification of two serine residues involved in agonist activation and the β-adrenergic receptor. J Biol Chem 1989;264:13572–13578.
13. Regan JW, Kobilka TS, Yang-Feng TL, et al. Cloning and expression of a human kidney cDNA for an α_2-adrenergic receptor subtype. Proc Natl Acad Sci U S A 1988;85:6301–6305.
14. Kobilka B. Adrenergic receptors as models for G protein–coupled receptors. Annu Rev Neurosci 1992;15:87–114.
15. Nichols AJ, Ruffolo RR Jr. Structure–activity relationships for α-adrenoceptor agonists and antagonists. In: Ruffolo RR Jr, ed. α-Adrenoceptors: Molecular Biology, Biochemistry, and Pharmacology. New York: Karger, 1991:75–114.
16. Timmermans PB, van Zwieten PA. α_2-Adrenoceptors: classification, localization, mechanisms, and targets for drugs. J Med Chem 1982;25:1389–1401.
17. Patil PN, Jacobowitz D. Steric aspects of adrenergic drugs. IX. Pharmacologic and histochemical studies on isomers of cobefrin (α-methylnorepinephrine). J Pharmacol Exp Ther 1968;161:279–295.
18. Kanagy NL. α_2-Adrenergic receptor signaling in hypertension. Clin Sci (Lond) 2005;109:431–437.
19. Kobinger W. Central α-adrenergic systems as targets for hypotensive drugs. Rev Physiol Biochem Pharmacol 1978;81:39–100.
20. Fairbanks CA, Stone LS, Kitto KF, et al. α_{2C}-Adrenergic receptors mediate spinal analgesia and adrenergic-opioid synergy. J Pharmacol Exp Ther 2002;300:282–290.
21. Wheeler LA, Woldemussie E. α_2-Adrenergic receptor agonists are neuroprotective in experimental models of glaucoma. Eur J Ophthalmol 2001;11(Suppl 2):S30–S35.
22. Wheeler L, WoldeMussie E, Lai R. Role of α_2-agonists in neuroprotection. Surv Ophthalmol 2003;48(Suppl 1):S47–S51.
23. Baur F, Beattie D, Beer D, et al. The identification of indacaterol as an ultralong-acting inhaled β_2-adrenoceptor agonist. J Med Chem 2010;53:3675–3684.
24. Lombardi D, Cuenoud B, Kramer SD. Lipid membrane interactions of indacaterol and salmeterol: do they influence their pharmacological properties? Eur J Pharm Sci 2009;38:533–547.
25. Beeh KM, Derom E, Kanniess R, et al. Indacaterol, a novel inhaled β_2-agonist, provides sustained 24-h bronchodilation in asthma. Eur Resp J 2007;29:871–878.
26. Ruffolo RR, Spradlin TA, Pollock GD, et al. Alpha and beta adrenergic effects of the stereoisomers of dobutamine. J Pharmacol Exp Ther 1981;219:447–452.
27. Pollock GD, Bowling N, Tuttle RR, et al. Effects of (S)-dobutamine on ischemic myocardium caused by coronary artery narrowing. J Cardiovasc Pharmacol 1994;24:64–73.
28. Chen KK, Schmidt CF. Ephedrine and related substances. Medicine 1930;9:1–117.
29. Scriabine A, Constantine JW, Hess HJ, et al. Pharmacological studies with some new antihypertensive aminoquinazolines. Experientia 1968;24:1150–1151.
30. Rossi M, Roumeguere T. Silodosin in the treatment of benign prostatic hyperplasia. Drug Des Dev Ther 2010;4:291–297.
31. Moran NC. New adrenergic blocking drugs: their pharmacological, biochemical, and clinical actions. Ann N Y Acad Sci 1967;139:545–548.
32. Jen T, Frazee JS, Schwartz MS, et al. Adrenergic agents. 8.1. Synthesis and β-adrenergic agonist activity of some 3-*tert*-butylamino-2-(substituted phenyl)-1-propanols. J Med Chem 1977;20:1263–1268.
33. Evans DB, Fox R, Hauck FP. β-Adrenergic receptor blockers as therapeutic agents. Ann Rep Med Chem 1979;14:81–90.

34. Weiss R. Nebivolol: a novel beta-blocker with nitric oxide-induced vasodilation. Vasc Health Risk Manag 2006;2:303–308.
35. Lesar TS. Comparison of ophthalmic β-blocking agents. Clin Pharm 1987;6:451–463.
36. Ruffolo RR, Gellai M, Hieble JP, et al. The pharmacology of carvedilol. Eur J Clin Pharmacol 1990;38:S82–S88.
37. Ruffolo RR, Feuerstein GZ, Neurohormonal activation: oxygen free radicals, and apoptosis in the pathogenesis of congestive heart failure. J Cardiovasc Pharmacol 1998;32:S22–S30.
38. Brogden RN, Heel RC, Speight TM, et al. α-Methyl-*p*-tyrosine: a review of its pharmacology and clinical use. Drugs 1981;21:81–89.

Suggested Reading

Westfall TC, Westfall DP. Adrenergic agonists and antagonists. In: Brunton LL, Lazo JS, Parker KL, eds. Goodman and Gilman's The Pharmacological Basis of Therapeutics, 11th Ed. New York: McGraw-Hill, 2006:237–295.

Chapter 11

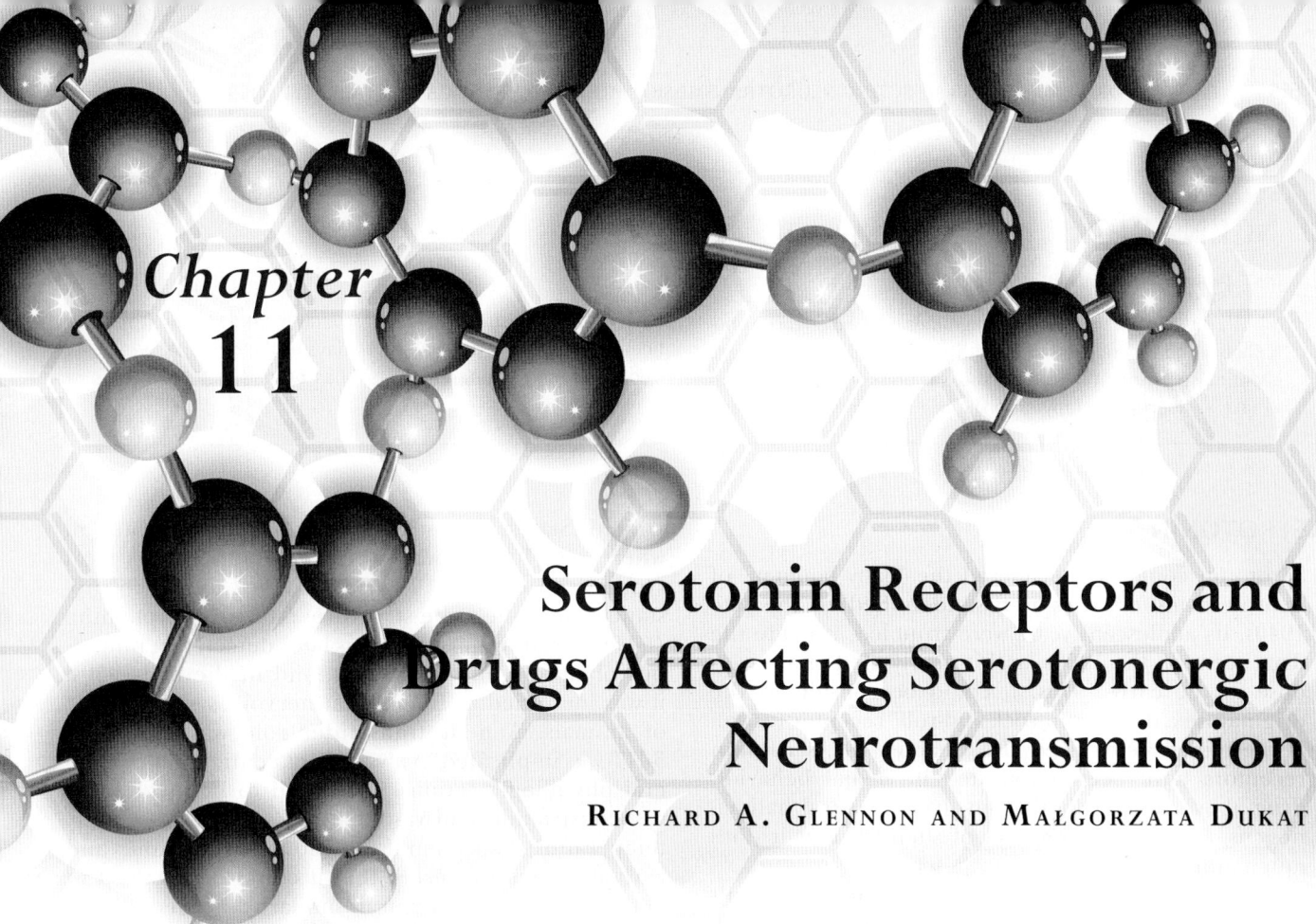

Serotonin Receptors and Drugs Affecting Serotonergic Neurotransmission

Richard A. Glennon and Małgorzata Dukat

Drugs Covered in This Chapter*

Antiemetic drugs (5-HT_3 receptor antagonists)
- Alosetron
- Dolasetron
- Granisetron
- Ondansetron
- Palonosetron
- *Tropisetron*

Drugs for the treatment of migraine (5-$HT_{1D/1F}$ receptor agonists)
- Almotriptan
- Eletriptan
- Frovatriptan
- Naratriptan
- Rizatriptan
- Sumatriptan
- Zolmitriptan

Drug for the treatment of irritable bowel syndrome (5-HT_4 agonists)
- Tegaserod

Drugs for the treatment of neuropsychiatric disorders
- Buspirone
- Citalopram
- Clozapine
- Desipramine
- Fluoxetine
- Imipramine
- Olanzapine
- Propranolol
- Quetiapine
- Risperidone
- Tranylcypromine
- Trazodone
- Ziprasidone
- *Zotepine*

Hallucinogenic agents
- Lysergic acid diethylamide
- 2,5-dimethyl-4-bromoamphetamine
- 2,5-dimethoxy-4-iodoamphetamine

Abbreviations

cAMP, cyclic adenosine monophosphate
CNS, central nervous system
5-CT, 5-carboxamidotryptamine
DOB, 2,5-dimethyl-4-bromoamphetamine
DOI, 2,5-dimethoxy-4-iodoamphetamine
EMDT, 2-ethyl-5-methoxy-*N,N*-dimethyltryptamine
GABA, γ-aminobutyric acid
5-HT, serotonin
5-HTP, 5-hydroxytryptophan
IBS, irritable bowel syndrome
IBS-C, irritable bowel syndrome with constipation
IBS-D, irritable bowel syndrome with diarrhea
LCAP, long-chain arylpiperazine
L-DOPA, L-dihydroxyphenylalanine
LSD, lysergic acid diethylamide
MAO, monomaine oxidase
MAOI, monoamine oxidase inhibitor
***m*CPBG**, *m*-chlorophenylbiguanide
***m*CPG**, *m*-chlorophenylguanidine
***m*CPP**, *m*-chlorophenylpiperazine
nM, nanomoles/L
MT, melatonin
MTR, melatonin receptor
NET, norepinephrine reuptake transporter
8-OH DPAT, 8-hydroxy-2-(di-n-propylamino)tetralin
PMDT, 2-phenyl-5-methoxy-*N,N*-dimethyltryptamine
SAFIR, structure–affinity relationship
SAR, structure–activity relationship
SERT, serotonin transporter
SSRI, selective serotonin reuptake inhibitor

*Drugs available outside the U.S. are shown in italics.

SCENARIO

Jill T. Johnson, PharmD, BCPS

MB is a 34-year-old woman with migraines. She experiences photophobia and severe headaches with nausea and vision changes about twice per month. Recently she was prescribed sumatriptan to take as abortive therapy once she begins to feel the migraine aura. After using sumatriptan for several months, taking it routinely up to 300 mg per day for 15 days of the month, she realized it was not working as well as it had been.

SEROTONIN

Serotonin could be considered the "baby boomer" of neurotransmitters: It was first identified in the late 1940s, its adolescent years were troubled, it made the drug scene in the 1960s, and it nearly died of an overdose in the early 1970s. It could be considered the original "sex, drugs, and rock-and-roll" receptor (as will be described below [see also Chapter 19], serotonin receptors have been implicated in sexual behavior, drug abuse [especially that involving classical hallucinogens], and the perception of sound)—but, it does much more.

At one time, it was remarked that "serotonin doesn't do anything" (1). On reaching its middle years, serotonin matured and became an important topic of study, a household name, and more complicated than ever. Serotonin has been associated with, among other things, anxiety, depression, schizophrenia, drug abuse, sleep, dreaming, hallucinogenic activity, headache, cardiovascular disorders, sexual behavior, and appetite control. Television ads now routinely refer to serotonin and serotonin receptor antagonists. This, subsequently, prompted the comment that "it almost appears that serotonin is involved in everything" (1). A review of the current patent literature provides an indication of some of the claims being made for serotonergic agents (Table 11.1). Tens of thousands of papers have been published on serotonin. Much is known—but an incredible amount remains to be learned.

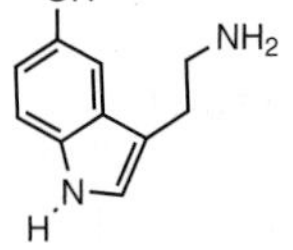

Serotonin (5-HT)

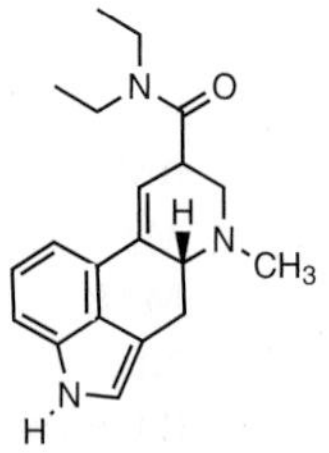

(+)-Lysergic acid diethylamide (LSD)

A hormonal substance was independently identified in the late 1940s by two groups of investigators, one in the United States and the other in Italy. In the United States, the substance was called serotonin, whereas in Italy, it was termed enteramine. Its total synthesis in the early 1950s confirmed that both substances were the same structure: 5-hydroxytryptamine (5-HT). Serotonin (5-HT) was later detected in numerous plant and animal species, and in the mid-1950s, it was identified in the central nervous system (CNS) of animals. A neurotransmitter role was proposed. 5-HT was implicated in a variety of central and peripheral physiologic actions. It seemed to be involved in vasoconstriction and vasodilation, regulation of body temperature, sleep, and hormonal regulation, and early evidence suggested that it could be involved in depression. The structural similarity between 5-HT

TABLE 11.1 Some Indications and Treatment Claims for Novel Serotonergic Agents in the Patent Literature

Aggression disorders	Esophagitis	Obsessive-compulsive
Alcoholism	Gastric motility	Pain
Alzheimer's disease	Head injury	Panic disorders
Amnesia	Headache	Parkinson's disease
Anorexia	Hypertension	Psychosis
Bulimia	Impotence	Raynaud's disease
Cardiac failure syndrome	Irritable bowel	Schizophrenia
Cardiovascular disorders	Ischemia	Sedation
Cerebrovascular disorders	Migraine	Sexual dysfunction
Cognition disorders	Movement	Sleep disorders
Depression	Nausea	Substance abuse
Drug abuse	Neurodegenerative disease	Substance dependence
Emesis	Obesity	Thromboembolism

CLINICAL SIGNIFICANCE

Discovery of the different types of serotonin receptors during the past few years has created the potential to target these receptors. Altering the chemical structures may improve tolerability, reduce the risk of side effects, improve efficacy, enhance compliance, or simply provide an alternative drug should another in the class fail to provide relief for a given patient.

The clinical effects of serotonin receptors are multifaceted. At this time, only a few of the identified receptors have drugs that are currently marketed for use in humans. Buspirone stimulates the 5-HT1A receptor to cause antianxiety effects. The 5-HT1D agonists, or the "triptans," vary by side chains on essentially the same core structure to create compounds with different affinities for the 5-HT1D receptors and, likely, for other serotonin receptors as well. The varying affinities of each triptan for receptors change the profiles of their effectiveness and adverse or complimentary effects. As a rule, the triptans work to treat migraine headaches by causing vasoconstriction.

Unfortunately, they also may cause coronary vasoconstriction, making them contraindicated in patients with underlying coronary artery disease. Antagonists of the 5-HT3 receptor, ondansetron, and granisetron, work to lessen emesis in chemotherapy-induced and radiation-associated emesis as well as postoperative nausea and vomiting. A variety of drugs work to inhibit selective serotonin reuptake without acting on any specific serotonin receptor. Drugs such as fluoxetine, paroxetine, sertraline, and fluvoxamine have been effective in the treatment of depression, obsessive-compulsive disorder, and panic disorder with varying degrees of side effects like weight gain, weight loss, and drowsiness.

Jill T. Johnson, Pharm.D., BCPS
Associate Professor
Department of Pharmacy Practice
College of Pharmacy
University of Arkansas for Medical Science
Little Rock, AR

and the then recently discovered hallucinogenic agent (+)-lysergic acid diethylamide (LSD) intrigued investigators. The observation led to speculation that 5-HT could be involved in the mechanism of action of this psychoactive substances and could also have a role in certain mental disorders. LSD was shown to behave as a potent 5-HT receptor agonist in certain peripheral receptor assays and as a potent antagonist in others. The late 1960s and early 1970s, however, witnessed a decline in 5-HT research as the result of three factors: 1) sophisticated experimental techniques were still lacking for the investigation of the central actions of 5-HT; 2) apart from ergolines (LSD-related agents), only a few potent 5-HT agonists or antagonists had been developed; and 3) it was becoming increasingly difficult to understand how a single putative neurotransmitter substance could be involved in so many different central and peripheral actions. As a consequence, research interest in 5-HT entered the "doldrums." Subsequent development of histochemical fluorescence techniques and 5-HT radioligand binding methodology led to the mapping of serotonergic pathways, identifying binding sites in the brain, and measuring the affinity (i.e., K_i values) of serotonergic agents for 5-HT receptors. This rekindled interest in 5-HT receptors—big time. Much of the early work on serotonin receptors and their ligands has been reviewed (2–4); as a result, a substantial amount of the older literature is not cited here, and the interested readers are urged to consult these reviews for references to the primary literature.

Serotonin Biosynthesis, Catabolism, and Function as Targets for Drug Manipulation

5-HT is biosynthesized from its dietary precursor L-tryptophan (5) (Fig. 11.1). Serotonergic neurons contain tryptophan hydroxylase (L-tryptophan-5-monooxygenase) that converts tryptophan to 5-hydroxytryptophan (5-HTP), in what is the rate-limiting step in 5-HT biosynthesis, and aromatic L-amino acid decarboxylase (a nonselective decarboxylase previously called 5-HTP decarboxylase) that decarboxylates 5-HTP to 5-HT. This latter enzyme is also responsible for the conversion of L-dihydroxyphenylalanine (L-DOPA) to dopamine (see Chapter 13). The major route of metabolism of 5-HT is oxidative deamination by monoamine oxidase (MAO; specifically, by MAO-A) to the unstable 5-hydroxyindole-3-acetaldehyde, which is either reduced to 5-hydroxytryptophol (~15%) or to the oxidized product 5-hydroxyindole-3-acetic acid (~85%) under normal physiologic conditions. In the pineal gland, 5-HT is acetylated by 5-HT *N*-acetyltransferase to *N*-acetylserotonin, which undergoes *O*-methylation by 5-hydroxyindole-*O*-methyltransferase to melatonin.

RADIOLIGANDS

Radioligand binding techniques measure the affinity of agonists and antagonists for their respective receptors (i.e., K_i values). Radioligands are receptor agonists or antagonists to which a radioactive atom (label) is covalently attached.

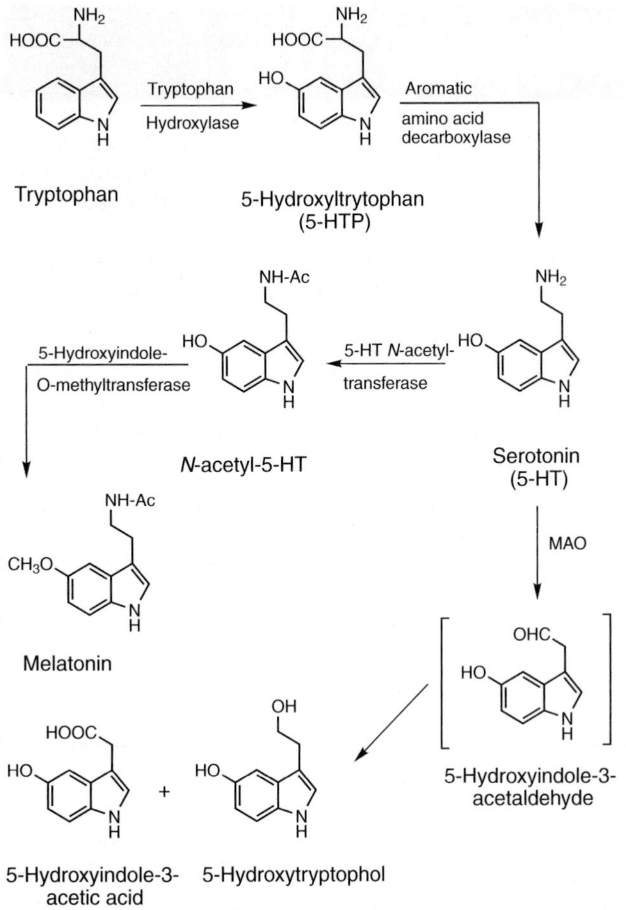

FIGURE 11.1 Biosynthesis and catabolism of serotonin. In the pineal, serotonin is converted to melatonin. Melatonin is an agonist at melatonin (MT), not 5-HT, receptors. Ac, acetyl.

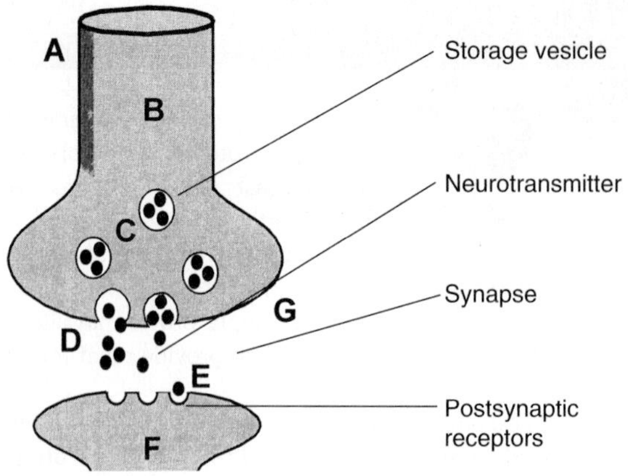

FIGURE 11.2 Steps involved in serotonergic neurotransmission. The serotonin precursor tryptophan is taken up into the neuron (A) and converted to 5-HT (B). Synthesized 5-HT is stored in synaptic vesicles (C). Under the appropriate conditions, the synaptic vesicles migrate to and fuse with the cell membrane, releasing their store of 5-HT (D). Released neurotransmitter interacts with postsynaptic receptors (E) and, in the case of G protein–coupled receptors, activates second messenger systems (F). The action of 5-HT is terminated (G) either by diffusion of 5-HT away from the synapse, with subsequent metabolism, or by the 5-HT being taken back up by 5-HT transporters into the presynaptic neuron (i.e., reuptake), where it can be re-stored in synaptic vesicles or is metabolized (by MAO).

Distinct types of melatonin receptors (MTRs; MTR_1/MTR_2) have been identified.

Each step in 5-HT biosynthesis, metabolism, and function is a hypothetical target for drug manipulation (Fig. 11.2). Tryptophan depletion, by reducing or restricting dietary tryptophan consumption, results in decreased 5-HT biosynthesis; conversely, tryptophan "loading," by increasing dietary tryptophan, results in the overproduction of 5-HT. The latter effect also can occur in nonserotonergic neurons, such as in dopaminergic neurons, because of the nonselective nature of aromatic amino acid decarboxylase. Inhibitors of tryptophan hydroxylase, such as *para*-chlorophenylalanine, are used as pharmacologic tools; they are not used therapeutically.

Therapeutically exploited serotonergic targets include presynaptic receptors, postsynaptic receptors, the reuptake mechanism (i.e., the serotonin transporter [SERT]), second messenger systems, and 5-HT metabolism. MAO inhibitors (MAOI) effectively interfere with the oxidative deamination of 5-HT to increase synaptic concentrations of 5-HT. The MAOI tranylcypromine, for example, has been employed since the 1960s as an antidepressant agent.

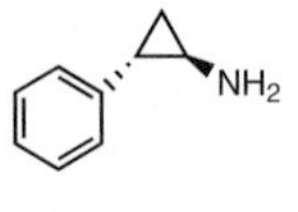

Tranylcypromine

A problem associated with many MAOIs is that they are notoriously nonselective and can interfere with the metabolism of other neurotransmitters, amines found in certain foods, and exogenously administered amine-containing therapeutic agents. Serotonin receptors and SERT are discussed below.

SEROTONIN RECEPTORS

Initially, 5-HT was thought to interact with what were termed 5-HT receptors. Today, seven distinct families or populations of serotonergic receptors have been identified, 5-HT_1 through 5-HT_7, and several are divided into subpopulations (Table 11.2). The discovery of the individual populations and subpopulations of 5-HT receptors follows the approximate order of their numbering and, as a consequence, more is known about 5-HT_1 and 5-HT_2 receptors than about 5-HT_6 and 5-HT_7 receptors. Factors contributing to our current lack of understanding about

TABLE 11.2 Classification and Nomenclature for the Various Populations of 5-HT Receptors

Populations and Subpopulations	Second Messenger System[a]	Currently Accepted Name[b]	Comments
5-HT_1			
5-HT_{1A}	AC(−)	5-HT_{1A}	Cloned and pharmacologic 5-HT_{1A} receptors
5-HT_{1B}	AC(−)	5-HT_{1B}	Rodent homolog of 5-HT_{1B} receptors
$5\text{-HT}_{1B\beta}$			A mouse homolog of $h5\text{-HT}_{1B}$ receptors
5-HT_{1D}			Sites identified in binding studies using human and calf brain homogenates
$5\text{-HT}_{1D\alpha}$	AC(−)	$h5\text{-HT}_{1D}$	A cloned human 5-HT_{1D} subpopulation
$5\text{-HT}_{1D\beta}$	AC(−)	$h5\text{-HT}_{1B}$	A second cloned human 5-HT_{1D} subpopulation; human counterpart of rat 5-HT_{1B}
5-HT_{1E}	AC(−)	5-HT_{1E}	Sites identified in binding studies using brain homogenates and cloned receptors
$5\text{-HT}_{1E\alpha}$			An alternate name that has been used for cloned human 5-HT_{1E} receptors
$5\text{-HT}_{1E\beta}$	AC(−)	5-ht_{1F}	A cloned mouse homolog of 5-HT_{1F} receptors
5-HT_{1F}			A cloned human 5-HT_1 receptor population
5-HT_2			
5-HT_2	PI	5-HT_{2A}	Original "5-HT_2" (sometimes called $5\text{-HT}_{2\alpha}$) receptors
5-HT_{2F}	PI	5-HT_{2B}	5-HT_2-like receptors originally found in rat fundus
5-HT_{1C}	PI	5-HT_{2C}	Originally described as 5-HT_{1C} ($5\text{-HT}_{2\beta}$) receptors
5-HT_3			
5-HT_3	Ion channel	5-HT_3	An ion channel receptor
5-HT_4	AC(+)	5-HT_4	5-HT_4 population originally described in functional studies
5-HT_{4S}			Short form of cloned 5-HT_4 receptors
5-HT_{4L}			Long form of cloned 5-HT_4 receptors
$5\text{-HT}_{4(b)-4(d)}$			Recently identified human 5-HT_4 receptor isoforms
5-HT_5			
5-HT_{5A}	?	5-HT_{5A}	Cloned mouse, rat, and human 5-HT_5 receptors
5-HT_{5B}	?	5-HT_{5A}	Cloned mouse and rat 5-HT_{5A}–like receptor
5-HT_6			
5-HT_6	AC(+)	5-HT_6	Cloned rat and human 5-HT receptor
5-HT_7			
5-HT_7	AC(+)	5-HT_7	Cloned rat, mouse, guinea pig, and human 5-HT receptors

[a] AC = adenylate cyclase; (−) = negatively coupled; (+) = positively coupled; PI = phospholipase coupled.

[b] Currently accepted names are taken from Hoyer et al. (9).

the function of certain 5-HT receptor populations (e.g., 5-HT_{1E} or 5-HT_5 receptors) is the absence of agonists and/or antagonists with selectivity for these receptors.

History

Tritiated LSD ([^{3}H]LSD), the first radioligand used to identify a brain 5-HT binding site, suggested it could be a "hallucinogen receptor." Tritiated 5-HT ([^{3}H]5-HT)–labeled serotonergic sites displayed high affinity for LSD. Thus, not only did 5-HT and LSD share structural similarity, there was now evidence that these agents could be acting via a common receptor type. According to the *interconvertible receptor conformation hypothesis* that was popular at the time, 5-HT (known to be an agonist) interacted with the agonist conformation of the receptor, whereas [^{3}H]LSD (LSD being known to be a partial agonist) labeled both the agonist and antagonist conformations. A search was initiated for 5-HT receptor antagonists that could serve to label the antagonist conformation of 5-HT receptors. After the serendipitous discovery that a tritiated version of the dopamine antagonist spiperone not only labeled dopaminergic receptors but also labeled nondopaminergic receptors in other brain regions, it was shown that 5-HT displayed modest affinity for some of these sites, indicating they could represent 5-HT receptors.

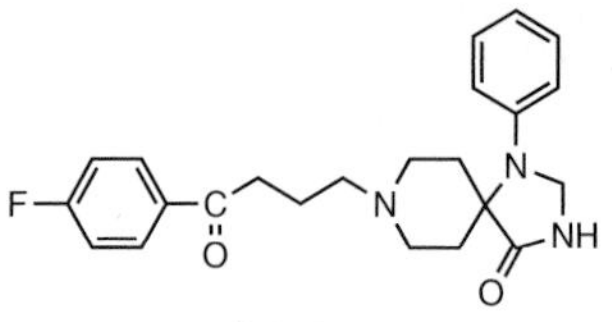

Spiperone

Spiperone was also shown to antagonize some of the pharmacologic effects of 5-HT in functional assays. These data, coupled with the additional observation that 5-HT receptor agonists tended to display higher affinity for [^{3}H]5-HT–labeled sites, whereas 5-HT antagonists displayed higher affinity for [^{3}H]spiperone-labeled sites, led to the conclusion that [^{3}H]5-HT and [^{3}H]spiperone label two distinct populations (not conformations) of sites, termed 5-HT_1 and 5-HT_2 receptors, respectively (6). Soon thereafter, 5-HT_1 receptors were found to consist of 5-HT_{1A} and 5-HT_{1B} subpopulations. Earlier, during the 1950s, Gaddum and Picarelli had demonstrated the existence of two populations of serotonergic receptors in isolated guinea pig ileum and termed these receptors 5-HT-D (because phenoxybenzamine or dibenzyline blocked the actions of 5-HT at this receptor) and 5-HT-M (because morphine and cocaine blocked the actions of 5-HT at the second population). Later, 5-HT-D receptors were found to be similar to 5-HT_2 receptors, and 5-HT-M receptors were eventually renamed 5-HT_3 receptors. By the early 1980s, 5-HT_{1A}, 5-HT_{1B}, 5-HT_2, and 5-HT_3 receptors had been identified, and interest in 5-HT research exploded. Molecular biology intervened in the late 1980s and early 1990s; new populations of serotonergic receptors were cloned and expressed. Perhaps the multitude of actions of 5-HT, previously thought impossible to understand, are mediated by multiple subtypes of 5-HT receptors. This led to attempts to develop selective agonists and antagonists for each subpopulation (2,7).

Table 11.2 lists the receptor classification and nomenclatures that have been employed for serotonergic receptors. Care should be used when reading the older primary literature because 5-HT receptor nomenclature has changed so dramatically and, often, can be confusing and very frustrating to comprehend.

All of the seven serotonergic receptor populations (and subpopulations) have been cloned and, together with the cloning of other neurotransmitter receptors, has led to generalizations regarding amino acid sequence homology (8). Any two receptors with amino acid sequences that are approximately 70% to 80% identical in their transmembrane-spanning segments are called the *intermediate-homology group*. This group of receptors could be members of the same subfamily and have highly similar to nearly indistinguishable pharmacologic profiles or second messenger systems. A *low-homology group* (~35% to 55% transmembrane homology) consists of distantly related receptor subtypes from the same neurotransmitter family, and a *high-homology group* (~95% to 99% transmembrane homology) consists of species homologs from the same gene in different species (8). Species homologs of the same gene reveal high sequence conservation in regions outside the transmembrane domains, whereas intraspecies receptor subtypes usually are quite different (8). Current 5-HT receptor classification and nomenclature require that several criteria be met before a receptor population can be adequately characterized. Receptor populations must be identified on the basis of drug binding characteristics (*operational* or *recognitory criteria*), receptor–effector coupling (*transductional criteria*), and gene and receptor structure sequences for the nucleotide and amino acid components, respectively (*structural criteria*) (7–9).

5-HT_1 Receptor Family

5-HT_1 receptors were one of the first two populations of 5-HT receptors to be identified (6), and 5-HT_{1A}, 5-HT_{1B}, 5-HT_{1D}, 5-HT_{1E}, and 5-HT_{1F} receptor subpopulations have since been defined. 5-HT_{1C} receptors were initially described, but subsequent classification (employing the previously mentioned criteria) resulted in their being moved to the 5-HT_2 receptor family and being renamed 5-HT_{2C} receptors. With the exception of 5-HT_{1E} receptors, all 5-HT_1 receptors exhibit high affinity for 5-carboxamidotryptamine (5-CT).

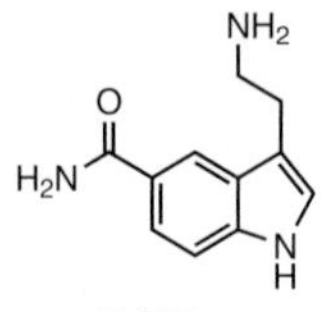

5-CT

5-HT_{1A} Receptors and Agents

5-HT_{1A} receptors are, as are all 5-HT receptors except for 5-HT_3 receptors, G protein–coupled receptors that consist of seven transmembrane-spanning helices connected

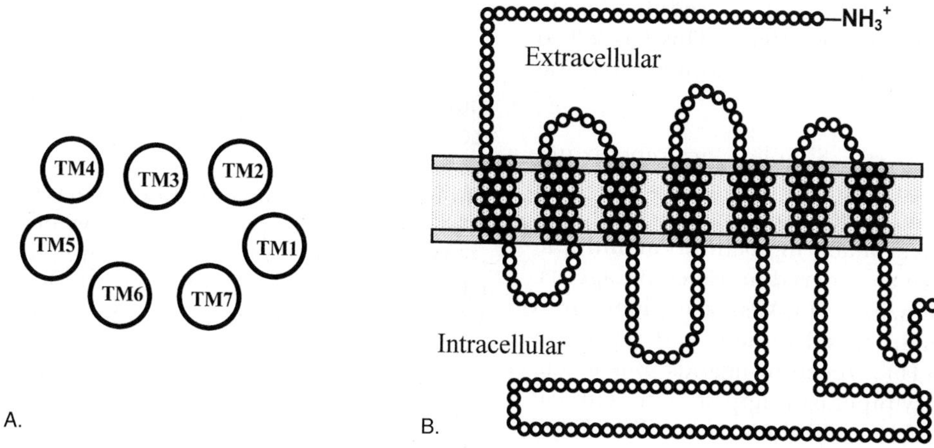

FIGURE 11.3 Top (A) and side (B) views of a schematic representation of a typical G protein–coupled receptor (GPCR). In B, the transmembrane-spanning helical portions are numbered, from left to right, as TM1 to TM7. The seven helices are connected by extracellular and intracellular loops. The large intracellular loop between TM5 and TM6 is believed to be associated with coupling to a second messenger system. The helices are arranged in such a manner that TM1 is adjacent to TM7, as shown in A. Molecular graphics studies suggest that agonists could bind in a manner that utilizes an aspartate residue in TM3 (common to all G protein–coupled 5-HT receptors) and residues in the TM4, TM5, and TM6 regions, whereas antagonists likely utilize the aspartate moiety but residues in the TM6, TM7, and TM1 regions.

by intracellular and extracellular loops (see Fig. 11.3 for a schematic representation of a generalized G protein receptor structure). The receptors are negatively coupled to an adenylate cyclase*[1] second messenger system, and the 5-HT_{1A} receptors located in the raphe nuclei correspond to somatodendritic autoreceptors (Fig. 11.4). 5-HT_{1A} receptors differ significantly in structure from most other 5-HT receptors and exhibit a substantial similarity to adrenergic receptors, which likely explains why a number of adrenoceptor agents bind at 5-HT_{1A} receptors with high affinity (see below). Cloned 5-HT_{1A} receptors and 5-HT_{1A} receptor ligands have been reviewed (9,10–18).

Structure–Activity Relationship of 5-HT_{1A} Receptor Agonists

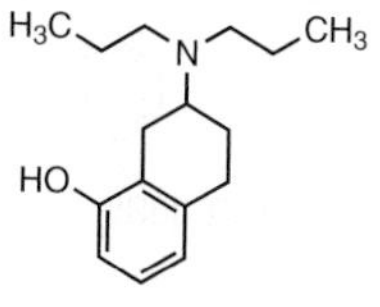

8-OH DPAT

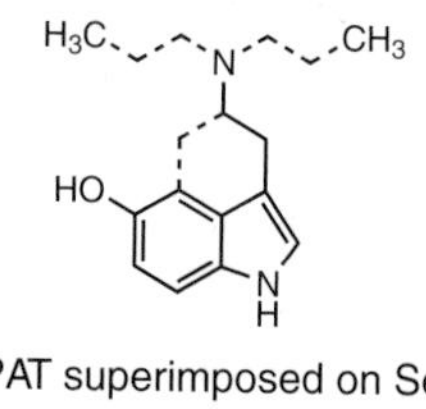

8-OH DPAT superimposed on Serotonin

Numerous 5-HT–related tryptamines bind with high affinity at 5-HT_{1A} receptors, but most are notoriously nonselective. One of the most selective 5-HT_{1A} receptor agonists is the aminotetralin derivative 8-hydroxy-2-(di-n-propylamino)tetralin (8-OH DPAT), and its early discovery was significant in advancing understanding of 5-HT_{1A} receptors. Furthermore, because the structure of 8-OH DPAT is similar to that of 5-HT (see 8-OH DPAT/5-HT superimposition), its activity indicated that an intact indole nucleus was not required for 5-HT_{1A} receptor action. Although numerous 8-OH DPAT

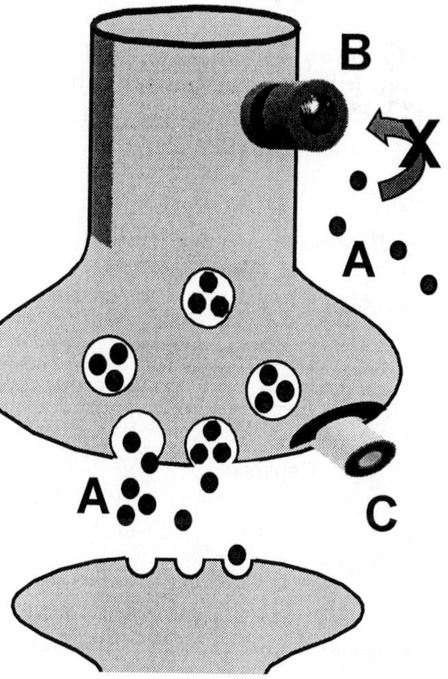

FIGURE 11.4 Typical nerve ending showing the cell body (i.e., somatodendritic) autoreceptors (B) and the terminal autoreceptors (C). Neurotransmitter molecules are also shown (A). 5-HT can interact with cell body autoreceptors (B) to regulate synthesis, and with terminal autoreceptors (C) to regulate release. Shown above is a drug molecule blocking the cell body autoreceptor and preventing an interaction with the neurotransmitter.

*This enzyme is known by two names, *adenylate cyclase (EC 4.6.1.1)*, its official name from the International Union of Biochemistry and Molecular Biology Nomenclature Committee, or its alternative name, adenylyl cyclase.

derivatives have been reported, none is used therapeutically because of low oral bioavailability. This has led to efforts to develop novel aminotetralins with greater oral bioavailability.

Long-Chain Arylpiperazines Simple arylpiperazines (i.e., those bearing no N_4-substituent or only a small N_4-substituent), such as 1-(phenyl)piperazine (Fig. 11.5), bind with modest to reasonably high affinity at multiple receptor types and are considered nonselective agents. Long-chain arylpiperazines (LCAPs) are piperazines possessing a long-chain N_4 substituent and represent the largest class of 5-HT_{1A} receptor ligands. Buspirone (Fig. 11.5), the first arylpiperazine approved for clinical use as an anxiolytic agent, and the structurally related gepirone and ipsapirone bind at 5-HT_{1A} receptors and behave as agonists or partial agonists. Structure–activity relationships (SARs) and structure–affinity relationships (SAFIRs) have been formulated, and this has led to LCAPs with enhanced 5-HT_{1A} receptor affinity and selectivity (12–15). With the LCAPs, there is substantial structural latitude for 5-HT_{1A} receptor binding (14,15).

The aryl portion of these agents (Fig. 11.6) typically is a phenyl, substituted phenyl, or heteroaryl group (such as 2-pyrimidinyl). The intact piperazine ring seems to be optimal for binding to 5-HT_{1A} receptors. A spacer or linker separates the N_4-nitrogen atom of the piperazine and the terminus or terminal structural moiety. There has been controversy as to whether the spacer participates in binding to the receptor or whether it acts simply as a "connector"; in any event, a chain of two to five atoms is common. The terminus typically is an amide or imide, but it has been shown that neither is required for binding. Alternatively, the terminus can be a phenyl or some other aryl or heteroaryl substituent (14). With respect to spacer length, when the spacer is -$(CH_2)_n$–, 2 to 4 methylene groups appear optimal. Chain length (n) can influence affinity and selectivity. When the terminus contains a heteroarylamide, $n = 4$ seems to be optimal, whereas when the terminus is an alkylamide, optimal affinity is associated with $n = 2$. A region of bulk tolerance is associated with the terminus, or at least a portion thereof, and very bulky groups have been introduced into this part of the molecule (12–15). Some LCAPs are nonselective and variously bind at other populations of 5-HT receptors, dopamine receptors, or adrenoceptors.

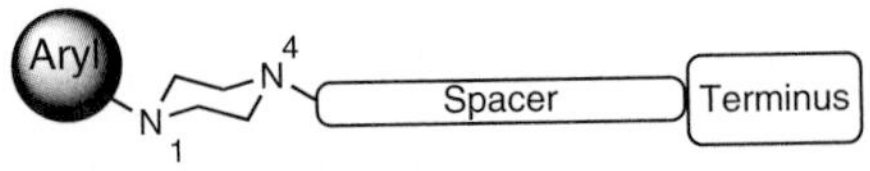

FIGURE 11.6 General structure of long-chain arylpiperazines (LCAPs).

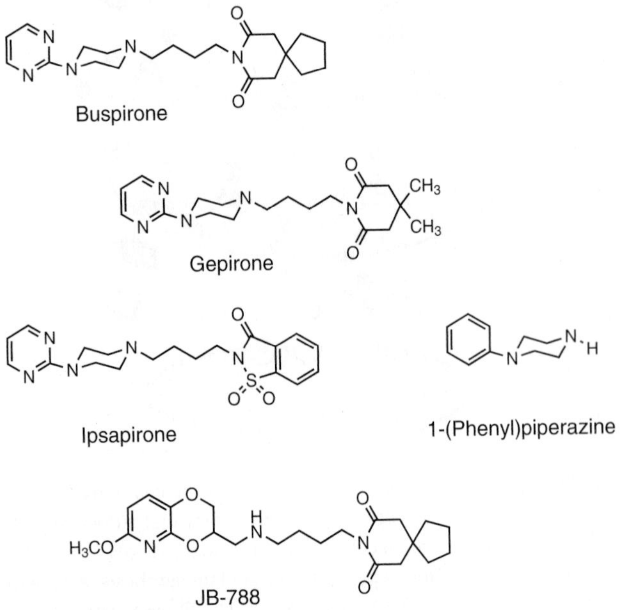

FIGURE 11.5 5-HT_{1A} receptor agonists (arylpiperazines).

Structure–activity Relationships of 5-HT_{1A} Receptor Antagonists

Many 5-HT_{1A} receptor antagonists possess a 2-methoxyphenyl group with structural similarity to buspirone. BMY 7378 and NAN-190 were among the first agents shown to be very low-efficacy partial agonists at 5-HT_{1A} receptors and were used as antagonists for many years (Fig. 11.7). Certain aminotetralins [e.g., S(–)UH-301] and arylpiperazines (e.g., WAY 100135 and WAY 100635) represent

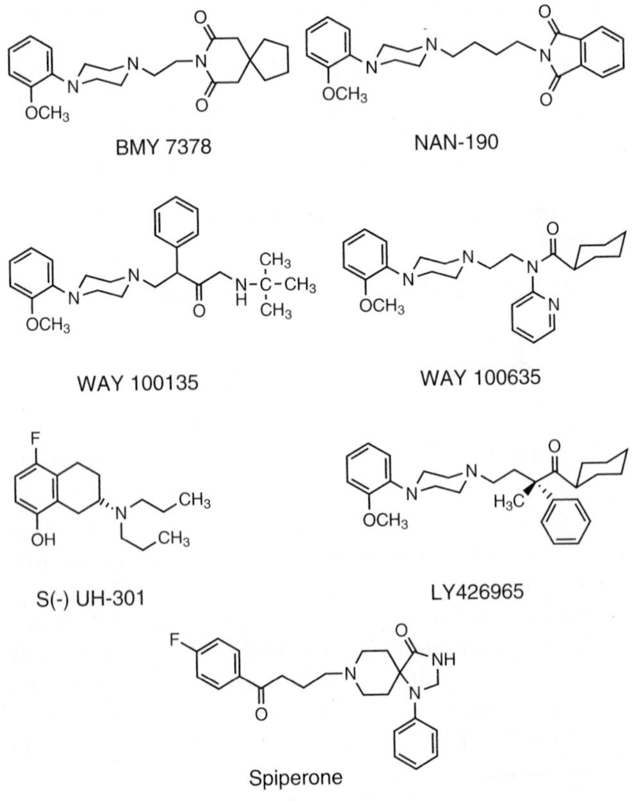

FIGURE 11.7 5-HT_{1A} receptor antagonists.

new classes of 5-HT$_{1A}$ receptor antagonists, termed "silent antagonists," because they are "seemingly" without any 5-HT$_{1A}$ agonist action. The alkylpiperidine spiperone is a 5-HT$_{1A}$ antagonist, but spiperone displays high affinity for D$_2$-dopamine receptors and 5-HT$_{2A}$ receptors.

Molecular graphics studies suggest that 5-HT and 5-HT$_{1A}$ receptor agonists interact with amino acid residues associated with helices 4, 5, and 6 (Site 1), whereas 5-HT$_{1A}$ receptor antagonists likely interact with amino acid residues in helices 1, 2, 7, and, perhaps, 6 (Site 2) (16). The basic amine for both types of agents is thought to bind at a common aspartate residue found in TM helix 3 (Fig. 11.3). The 5-hydroxy group of 5-HT is thought to form a hydrogen bond with the threonine residue in TM5 (16).

5-HT$_{1A}$ Receptor Agonists: Clinical Significance

In preclinical studies, 5-HT$_{1A}$ receptor agonists have demonstrated antianxiety, antidepressant, antiaggressive, and perhaps, anticraving, anticataleptic, antiemetic, and neuroprotective properties (15,17). Evidence also exists indicating that 5-HT$_{1A}$ receptors could be involved in sleep, impulsivity, alcoholism, sexual behavior, appetite control, thermoregulation, and cardiovascular function (17,19,20). The main focus of drug development for 5-HT$_{1A}$ receptors is their therapeutic potential for the treatment of anxiety and depression (15,19). Buspirone (Buspar) was the first LCAP to become clinically available as an anxiolytic agent. A number of structurally related agents hold promise as novel anxiolytics (11,12,21); one of the newest is JB-788 (22). 5-HT$_{1A}$ receptor agents could also be useful in the treatment of depression (15), and there seems to be a relationship between 5-HT metabolism, depression, and violent behavior. The antianxiety actions of 5-HT$_{1A}$ receptor (partial) agonists could involve, primarily, presynaptic somatodendritic 5-HT$_{1A}$ receptors, whereas the antidepressant actions of 5-HT$_{1A}$ receptor agents could primarily involve postsynaptic 5-HT$_{1A}$ receptors (17). Gepirone produced marked improvement in depressed patients, and buspirone was effective in the treatment of mixed anxious-depressive patients. 5-HT$_1$ and, possibly, 5-HT$_{1A}$ receptors have been implicated in obsessive-compulsive disorders.

5-HT$_{1A}$ Receptor Antagonists: Clinical Significance

A new direction in 5-HT$_{1A}$ receptor research targets the development of 5-HT$_{1A}$ receptor antagonists (15,23). Agents such as the acknowledged dopaminergic antagonist spiperone and the β-adrenoceptor antagonist propranolol were among the first to see application as 5-HT$_{1A}$ receptor antagonists. These agents are, obviously, nonselective; they bind at other populations of neurotransmitter receptors with comparable or higher affinities than they display at 5-HT$_{1A}$ receptors. The next generation of 5-HT$_{1A}$ receptor antagonists, the LCAPs BMY 7378 and NAN-190, possessed postsynaptic antagonist character but also behaved as low-efficacy partial agonists (14,23) (Fig. 11.7). A third generation of agents—"silent" 5-HT$_{1A}$ receptor antagonists—has been developed and includes WAY 100635, WAY 100135 (a structural relative of BMY 7378 and NAN-190), and S(−)UH-301 (a derivative of the 5-HT$_{1A}$ agonist 8-OH DPAT); these are both presynaptic and postsynaptic 5-HT$_{1A}$ receptor antagonists (23,24). Silent 5-HT$_{1A}$ receptor antagonists, such as WAY 100135 and S(−) UH-301, are not intrinsically inactive and can indirectly produce non–5-HT$_{1A}$ serotonin-mediated actions (25,26). These antagonists presumably block presynaptic 5-HT$_{1A}$ autoreceptors, increasing the synaptic concentration of 5-HT, which results in the activation of other 5-HT receptor populations. Human evaluation of "so-called" silent and selective 5-HT$_{1A}$ receptor antagonists should prove interesting and could open new vistas in 5-HT$_{1A}$ research and therapeutics. For example, pretreatment of patients with 5-HT$_{1A}$ receptor antagonists accelerates the effects of selective serotonin reuptake inhibitors (SSRIs) and enhance their clinical efficacy as antidepressants (27). The 5-HT$_{1A}$ receptor antagonist WAY 100635 enhances the anorectic effect of citalopram in animals (28) and, thus, may be of benefit in weight reduction. Combination therapy using an SSRI plus a 5-HT$_{1A}$ receptor antagonist, including the β-blocker pindolol, which binds at 5-HT$_{1A}$ receptors, has been reported (29). A new LCAP, LY426965, is more metabolically stable than WAY 100635 and is orally bioavailable. In combination with fluoxetine, LY426965 increase extracellular levels of 5-HT beyond that achievable by fluoxetine alone, and it is being examined for the treatment of depression and as a smoking cessation agent (30). The therapeutic potential of 5-HT$_{1A}$ receptor antagonists is quite intriguing.

5-HT$_{1B}$ Receptors and Agents

Early studies identified 5-HT$_{1B}$ receptors in rodent brain homogenates using radioligand binding techniques but failed to find them in human brain. 5-HT$_{1B}$ receptors are located both presynaptically, where they regulate the release of 5-HT (Fig. 11.4), and postsynaptically (31). Like 5-HT$_{1A}$ receptors, they are negatively coupled to adenylate cyclase. (See 5-HT$_{1D}$ Receptors for further related discussion.)

5-HT$_{1B}$ Receptors: Clinical Significance

Rodent 5-HT$_{1B}$ receptors have been implicated as having a role in thermoregulation, respiration, appetite control, sexual behavior, aggression, locomotor activity, sleep regulation, sensorimotor inhibition, and anxiety (32).

5-HT$_{1D}$ Receptors

5-HT$_{1D}$ receptors were first identified by radioligand binding techniques, and they are widely distributed throughout the CNS (33). They are G protein–linked and are coupled to inhibition of adenylate cyclase. Two human subpopulations of 5-HT$_{1D}$ receptors, 5-HT$_{1D\alpha}$ and 5-HT$_{1D\beta}$ receptors, display approximately 77% sequence homology, and their pharmacologic properties are nearly indistinguishable. Because of the high degree of species homology with rat and mouse 5-HT$_{1B}$ receptors, human 5-HT$_{1D\beta}$ receptors have been renamed h5-HT$_{1B}$ receptors. Human 5-HT$_{1D\alpha}$ receptors have been renamed h5-HT$_{1D}$. Most agents that bind at 5-HT$_{1B}$ receptors bind at 5-HT$_{1D}$ receptors.

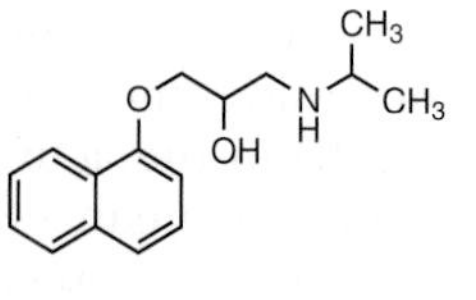

Propranolol

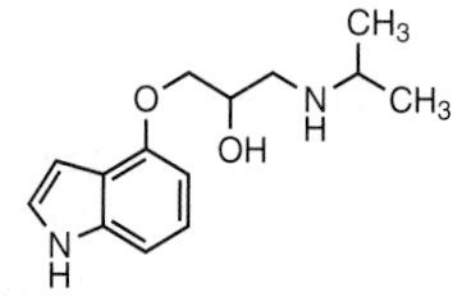

Pindolol

Curious exceptions have been noted with certain aryloxyalkylamines, however, such as the β-blockers, propranolol and pindolol, which exhibit very low affinity (K_i ~ 5,000 nM) for human (h) 5-HT$_{1D}$ receptors (34,35). The major functional difference between rat 5-HT$_{1B}$ receptors and h5-HT$_{1B}$ receptors has been attributed to both the presence of a threonine residue at position 355 (i.e., Thr^{355}) in TM7 of the latter and the presence of an asparagine residue at the corresponding position in 5-HT$_{1B}$ receptors; site-directed mutagenesis studies have demonstrated that conversion of Thr^{355} to an asparagine (i.e., a T355N mutant) accounts for the binding differences of certain ligands (e.g., aryloxyalkylamines such as propranolol). Combined ligand SAR, site-directed mutagenesis, and molecular modeling studies have led to the conclusion that although most typical serotonergic agonists bind in the central cavity formed by TM3, TM4, TM5, and TM6 (Site 1) (Fig. 11.3), propranolol most likely occupies the region defined by TM1, TM2, TM3, and TM7 (Site 2). The higher affinity of propranolol for T355N mutant 5-HT$_{1B}$ receptors relative to the wild-type receptors was specifically attributed to the formation of two hydrogen bonds between the receptor asparagine and the ether and hydroxyl oxygen atoms of propranolol (35).

5-HT$_{1D}$ Agonists and Antagonists

There are few 5-HT$_{1D}$–selective agonists, but one agent commonly referred to as a prototypical 5-HT$_{1D}$ receptor agonist is sumatriptan (Imitrex). Sumatriptan, however, exhibits only 2- to 20-fold greater selectivity for the 5-HT$_{1D}$ receptors than for certain other populations of 5-HT$_1$ (especially 5-HT$_{1A}$) receptors, binds at h5-HT$_{1D}$ and h5-HT$_{1B}$ receptors with nearly identical affinity and also binds at 5-HT$_{1F}$ receptors (36). SARs for 5-HT$_{1D}$ receptor agonists have been reported for many indolealkylamines or tryptamine derivatives, which bind with high affinity but with little selectivity. Newer agents displaying high affinity and reasonable selectivity for h5-HT$_{1D}$/h5-HT$_{1B}$ receptors over other populations of 5-HT receptors (37) include, for example, zolmitriptan (Zomig), naratriptan (Amerge), rizatriptan (Maxalt), and alniditan. Of these, all are tryptamine derivatives or sumatriptan-related structures except for the benzopyran alniditan. Many of these are commercially available or currently undergoing clinical trials. Other investigational agonists are shown in Figure 11.8.

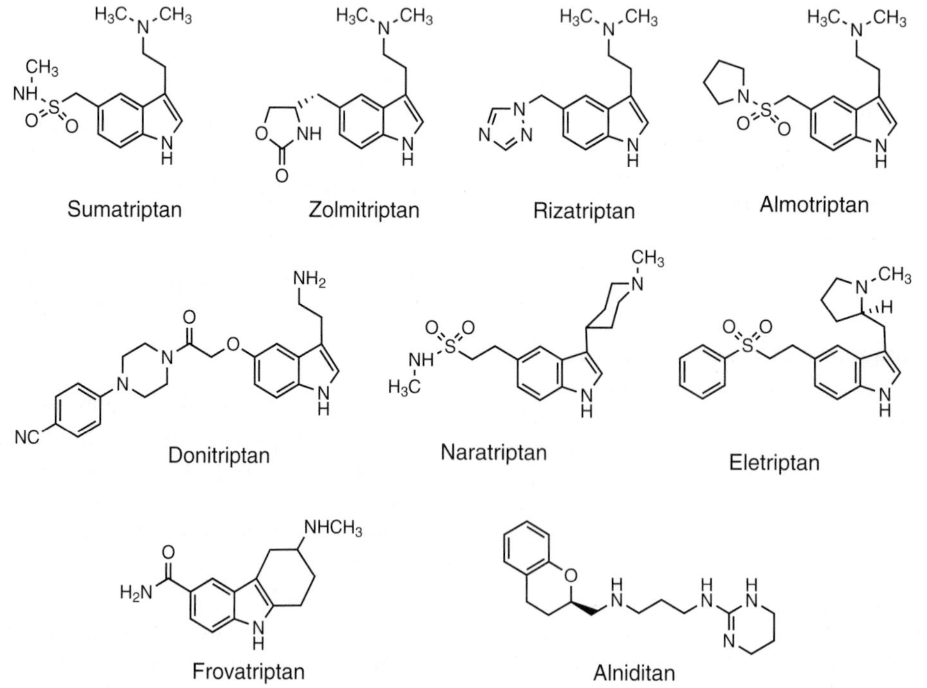

FIGURE 11.8 5-HT$_{1D}$ receptor agonists.

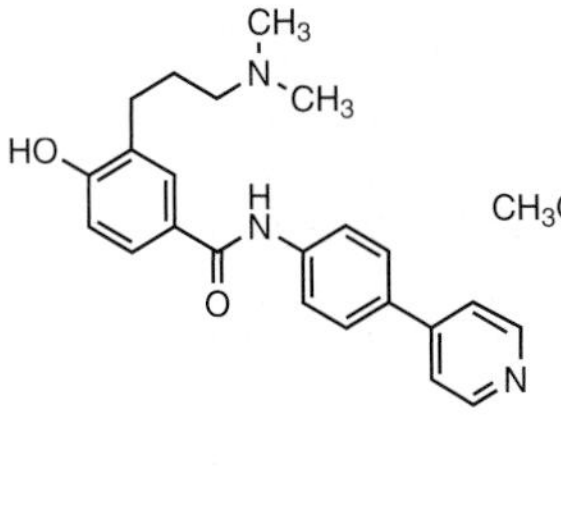

GR 55562

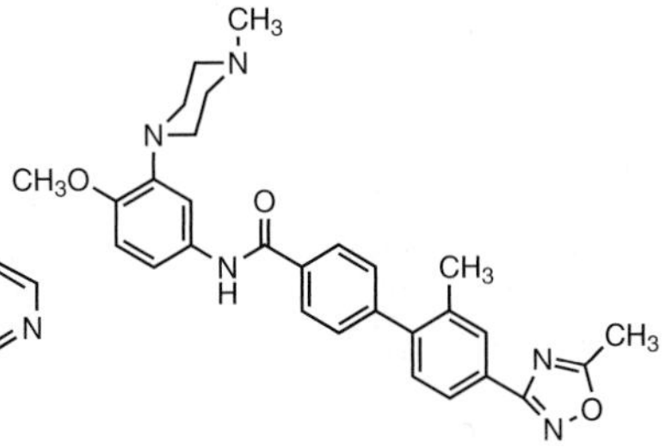

GR 127935

Several 5-HT_{1D} receptor antagonists have been developed, including GR127935 (high affinity for h5-HT_{1D}/h5-HT_{1B} receptors but possibly a low-efficacy partial agonist) and GR55562. Both of these agents antagonize many of the effects of sumatriptan.

5-HT_{1D} Receptors: Clinical Significance

The clinical significance of 5-HT_{1D} receptors remains largely unknown. These receptors are speculated to be involved in anxiety, depression, and other neuropsychiatric disorders, but this remains to be substantiated. However, recent studies show that 5-HT_{1D} receptors are the dominant species in human cerebral blood vessels. Sumatriptan and several closely related agents are clinically effective in the treatment of migraine, and logical extrapolation implies a role for 5-HT_{1D} receptors in this disorder. Agents with 5-HT_{1D} receptor agonist activity that have found application in the treatment of migraine are, as a group, termed *triptans,* because the first agent introduced was suma*triptan.* As efficacious as the triptans may be however, it is unknown if their activity involves action only in the periphery or in the CNS as well (38). Sumatriptan is an h5-HT_{1B} and h5-HT_{1D} receptor agonist. It is also an agonist at 5-HT_{1F} receptors. Most triptans share a similar binding profile. The vasoconstrictor properties of sumatriptan probably are mediated by its action on arterial smooth muscle. The triptans are also believed to inhibit the activation of peripheral nociceptors (38), and this could be related to the localization of 5-HT_{1D} receptors on peptide nociceptors.

Relatively little sumatriptan normally penetrates the blood–brain barrier. Although it has been speculated that transient changes in blood–brain barrier permeability could occur during migraine attacks (38), agents with greater lipophilicity (and, hence, enhanced ability to penetrate the blood–brain barrier) have been introduced, including zolmitriptan and rizatriptan (Table 11.3). Their greater lipophilicity, however, does not seem to correlate with significantly improved clinical efficacy over sumatriptan (38). Other triptans (Fig. 11.8) currently being examined include eletriptan, almotriptan, donatriptan, and frovatriptan (37).

In general, the newer triptans (e.g., zolmitriptan, rizatriptan, and naratriptan) have a higher oral bioavailability and a longer plasma half-life than sumatriptan (39,40) (Table 11.3). Most triptans also bind at 5-HT_{1F} receptors, and 5-HT_{1F} receptor agonists have demonstrated efficacy in the treatment of migraine (41). The 5-HT receptor binding characteristics of various triptans have been compared (37).

The safety of the triptans has been established; more than 8 million patients have been treated for more than 340 million attacks with sumatriptan alone. All triptans narrow coronary arteries by 10% to 20% at clinical doses and should not be administered to patients with coronary or cerebrovascular disease. Triptans with potential for significant drug–drug interactions include sumatriptan, naratriptan, rizatriptan, almotriptan, and MAOIs; rizatriptan and propranolol; zolmitriptan and cimetidine; zolmitriptan, naratriptan, and eletriptan; CYP3A4-metabolized drugs; and P-glycoprotein pump inhibitors.

The rational employment of triptans should be governed by the use of these medications for patients with disability associated with migraine. Patients with greater than 10 days of at least 50% disability during 3 months have benefited from treatment with triptans as their first-line treatment for acute attacks. When the decision has been made to treat with a triptan, the patient should be instructed to treat early in the attack, when the pain is at a mild phase. This approach increases the likelihood of achieving a pain-free response, with fewer adverse events and with lower likelihood of the headache recurring.

5-HT_{1E} Receptors and Agents

In early binding experiments using [^{3}H]5-HT as radioligand, masking of brain 5-HT_{1A} and 5-HT_{1B} receptors resulted in biphasic competition curves providing evidence for additional 5-HT_1-like receptor populations. One of these was the 5-HT_{1D} receptors; the other was termed 5-HT_{1E} receptors.

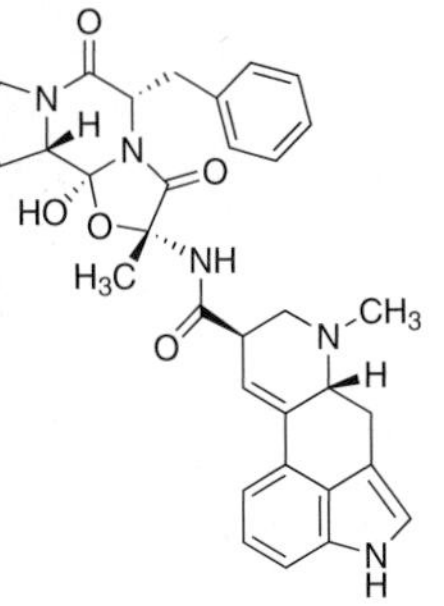

Ergotamine

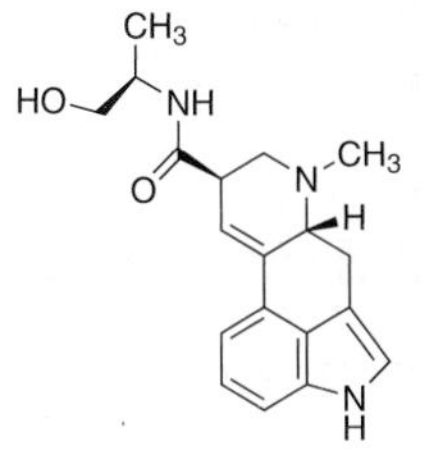

Ergonovine

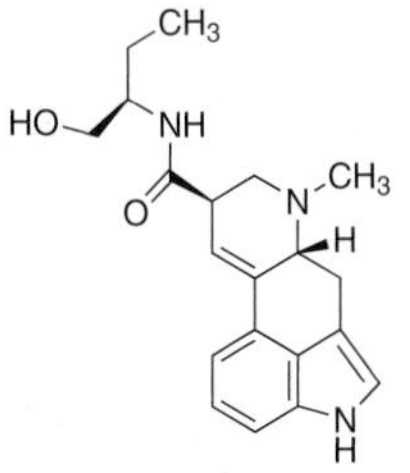

Methylergonovine

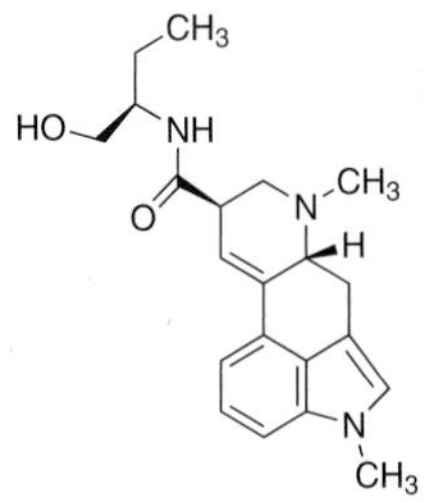

Methysergide

The low affinity of 5-CT and ergotamine for 5-HT_{1E} receptors allowed their differentiation from 5-HT_{1D}

TABLE 11.3 Pharmacokinetics of the 5-HT_1 Agonists (the Triptans)

Parameters	Sumatriptan	Zolmitriptan	Naratriptan	Rizatriptan	Almotriptan	Frovatriptan	Eletriptan
Trade name	Imitrex	Zomig	Amerge	Maxalt	Axert	Frova	Relpax
LogP (calc)[a]	0.7 ± 0.6	1.6 ± 0.4	1.4 ± 0.6	0.9 ± 0.6	1.9 ± 0.6	0.9 ± 0.4	3.1 ± 0.6
LogD (pH 7) (calc)[a]	−1.7	−0.8	−1.2	−1.4	−0.5	−2.1	0.18
Bioavailability (%)							
Oral (PO)	14–15[b]	40–50[b]	70[c]	40–50[b]	70–80	20–30[b]	50[cd]
Nasal	17	102	—	—	—	—	—
Subcutaneous (SC)	97		—	—	—	—	—
Protein binding (%)	14–20	25	28–30	14	35	15	85
Volume of distribution (L/kg)	PO: 50	PO: 7	PO: 170	PO: 110–140	PO: 180–200	PO: 3–4	PO: 138
		Nasal: 9					
Elimination half-life (h)	PO: 2.5	PO: 2–3	PO: 5–6	PO: 2–3	PO: 3–4	PO: 25	PO: 4–5
	SC: 2.5	Nasal: 3–4					PO Elderly: 6
Major metabolites (%)	Indoleacetic acid	*N*-Demethyl (act)[e]: 4	Hepatic: 50%	Indolacetate	Indolacetate	*N*-Demethyl (act)	*N*-Demethyl (act)
	Glucuronides	Indoleacetate: 31		*N*-Demethyl (act)	GABA	*N*-Ac demethyl	
	Hepatic: 60%			6-OH	*N*-demethyl		
					Hepatic: 60%		
Metabolizing enzymes	MAO-A	CYP3A4	CYP3A4	MAO-A	CYP3A4/CYP2D6: 12%	CYP1A2	CYP3A4
			MAO-A	CYP3A4	MAO-A: 27%		
Excretion (%)	Urine metab: ~60	Urine metab: 60	Urine metab: 30	Urine metab: 80	Urine metab: 75	Urine metab: 10–30	Urine metab: ~90%
	Feces metab: ~40	Feces metab: 30	Feces metab: ~15	Feces metab: 12	Feces metab: 10	Feces metab: 60	Unchanged: <10
	Unchanged: 3–22	Unchanged: <10	Unchanged: 50	Unchanged: 14	Unchanged: 40–50		
Time to peak concentration (min)	SC: 12 (5–20)	PO: 120–240	PO: 60–180	PO: 60–90	PO: 60–240	PO: 120–240	PO: 60–90
	Nasal: 60–90	Nasal: 180–240			SC: <30		
	PO: 60–120						
Onset (min)	SC: <10	PO: 60	PO: 60–180	PO: 30–120	PO: 60–120	PO: 120	PO: <60
	Nasal: <15				SC: 60–120		
	PO: <30						
Dosage range (mg)	SC: 6	PO: 1.25–5.00	PO: 1.0–2.5	PO: 5–10	PO: 6.25–12.5	PO: 2.5–5.0	PO: 20–40
	Nasal: 5–20	Max PO: 10/24 h	Max PO: 5/24 h	Max PO: 25/24 h	Max PO: 25/24 h	Max PO: 7.5/24 h	Max PO: 80/24 h
	PO: 25–100		Duration PO: <24 h	Duration PO: 14–16 h		Duration PO: <24 h	Duration PO: 18 h
	Max PO: 200/24 h						
	Duration PO: 2–4 h						

[a] Chemical Abstracts, American Chemical Society, calculated using Advanced Chemistry Development (ACD/Labs) Software V8.14 for Solaris (1994-2006 ACD/Labs).
[b] First-pass metabolism.
[c] Delayed by food.
[d] Slower onset during migraine attack.
[e] act= active metabolite

receptors. No tryptamine analog binds at 5-HT$_{1E}$ receptors with substantially higher affinity than 5-HT (K_i ~ 10 nM), and even simple *O*-methylation of 5-HT reduces its affinity for this receptor by approximately 100-fold (42). Ergolines, such as ergonovine (Ergotrate), methylergonovine (Methergine), and methysergide (Sansert), bind to 5-HT$_{1E}$ receptors with K_i values in the 50 to 150 nM range (42). Studies indicate that these receptors are negatively coupled to adenylate cyclase. No 5-HT$_{1E}$–selective receptor agonists or antagonists have yet been reported (43); this has created a problem for investigating this receptor subpopulation. One problem stalling development of selective agents is the lack of 5-HT$_{1E}$ receptors in rodent (i.e., mouse, rat) brain, the animal species commonly employed in preclinical drug development; however, the recent discovery of this receptor type in guinea pig brain bodes well for future studies.

5-HT$_{1F}$ Receptors

The newest 5-HT$_1$ receptor subpopulation to be cloned is the human 5-HT$_{1F}$ receptor (44), which exhibits intermediate (~50% to 70%) amino acid sequence homology with other 5-HT$_1$ receptor subpopulations. The receptors are coupled to inhibition of adenylate cyclase. Detection of these receptors in the uterus and mesentery suggests a possible role in vascular contraction. Although their distribution in the brain appears to be limited, distributional similarities with h5-HT$_{1B}$ receptors have been observed. A 4-(3-indolyl)piperidine, LY-334370, and an aminocarbazole, LY-344864, were identified as the first 5-HT$_{1F}$–selective agonists (45) with potential for the treatment of migraine. A more selective (nearly 300-fold more selective over 5-HT$_{1E}$) agent, lasmiditan, has been recently identified (46). Preliminary evidence suggests that lasmiditan, unlike most of the triptans, will not constrict the coronary artery (46). The nonselective 5-HT$_1$ receptor antagonist methiothepin has been shown to act as a 5-HT$_{1F}$ receptor antagonist. The SAFIR for the binding of tryptamines at 5-HT$_{1F}$ receptors has been reported (43). Interestingly, there is a statistically significant correlation between the affinities of several dozen tryptamine derivatives at 5-HT$_{1E}$ and 5-HT$_{1F}$ receptors (43), indicating common or similar binding requirements; interestingly, 5-HT$_{1F}$, but not 5-HT$_{1E}$ (vide supra), receptors allow substitution at the tryptamine 5-position. This opens the door for the development of additional 5-HT$_{1F}$– versus 5-HT$_{1E}$–selective agents. Many agents that bind at 5-HT$_{1E}$ receptors typically bind as well at 5-HT$_{1F}$ receptors; however, not all 5-HT$_{1F}$ receptor ligands bind at 5-HT$_{1E}$ receptors (see below).

5-HT$_{1F}$ Receptors: Clinical Significance

The clinical significance of 5-HT$_{1F}$ receptors is unknown at this time. The binding of sumatriptan to this receptor population suggests a relationship between 5-HT$_{1F}$ receptor binding and antimigraine activity. Other antimigraine agents, including naratriptan, rizatriptan, and zolmitriptan, also bind at 5-HT$_{1F}$ receptors (37). Studies show that 5-HT$_{1D}$ receptors are the dominant species in human cerebral blood vessels but that 5-HT$_{1F}$ receptors are also expressed both in neural and vascular tissue; however, 5-HT$_{1F}$ receptor agents could have a role in migraine as well (41). Indeed, lasmiditan could represent a prototype for a new generation of antimigraine agents that, because they do not bind at 5-HT$_{1B/1D}$ receptors, are likely to display reduced coronary vasoconstrictor action associated with the triptans.

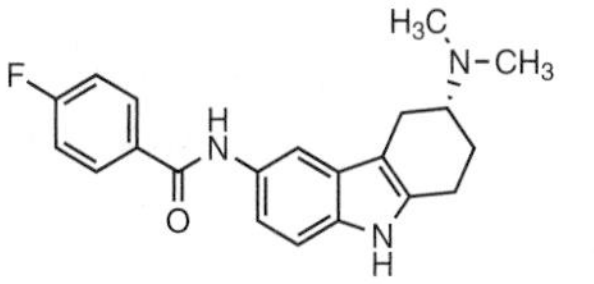

LY-344864

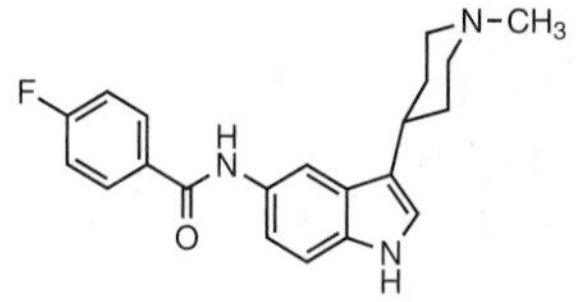

LY-334370

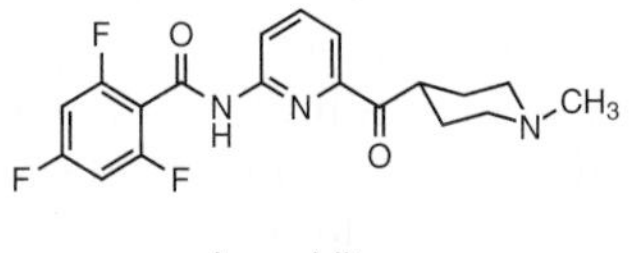

Lasmiditan

5-HT$_2$ Receptor Family

Serotonin receptors were first divided into 5-HT$_1$ and 5-HT$_2$ receptor families in 1979 (6), and the latter was subsequently divided into the subfamilies 5-HT$_{2A}$, 5-HT$_{2B}$, and 5-HT$_{2C}$ (formerly 5-HT$_{1C}$) receptors. Now, the term "5-HT$_2$" refers to a receptor family, not to an individual population of receptors. Ketanserin (Fig. 11.9) was

ERGOLINES

Ergolines, a large group of indole alkaloids with varied effects known for more than 2,000 years, are isolated from the ergot fungus, Claviceps purpurea, a plant parasite principally infecting rye. Eating rye grain contaminated with ergot caused a severely debilitating and painful disease during the Middle Ages called St. Anthony's Fire (ergotism), but in small doses, ergot was known to midwives for centuries for its ability to stimulate uterine contractions. Gangrene with burning pain in the extremities was one of two common presentations of ergot poisoning, which also could produce convulsions, hallucinations, severe psychosis, and death. St. Anthony was the patron saint of those who were stricken, and the Order of St. Anthony provided care for these patients. Outbreaks of "dancing mania," which occurred between the 13th and 16th centuries, sometimes have been attributed to ergotism, and one appealing—if unprovable—theory proposes that the women accused of witchcraft in the Salem trials of 1692 were suffering from ergot-induced psychosis and convulsions. The pharmacology of the various ergolines is complex, and they exhibit affinity for α-adrenergic, dopaminergic, and serotonergic receptor systems. The ergolines have been largely displaced by other more selective and effective drugs.

identified early on as a 5-HT_2 receptor antagonist with no affinity for 5-HT_1 receptors, and [^{3}H]ketanserin was introduced as a radioligand to label 5-HT_2 receptors. 1-(2,5-Dimethoxy-4X-phenyl)-2-aminopropane, where X = -Br and -I (DOB and DOI, respectively), was introduced as a 5-HT_2 receptor agonist. A significant amount of pharmacology was published, and structure–activity studies led to the development of many novel agents. Many of the original agents thought to be 5-HT_2 selective, including standard antagonists such as ketanserin and the agonists DOB and DOI, were later shown to bind nonselectively both to 5-HT_{2A} and 5-HT_{2C} receptors. Consequently, pharmacologic actions originally thought to be 5-HT_2 mediated could actually involve 5-HT_{2A} receptors, 5-HT_{2C} receptors, or a combination of 5-HT_{2A} and 5-HT_{2C} receptors. The structures of the three 5-HT_2 receptor subpopulations were found to be consistent with those of transmembrane-spanning G protein–coupled receptors, and the receptors all use a phospholipase C second messenger system. Approximately 70% to 80% sequence homology is found among the three receptor subtypes (10). Only relatively recently have novel agents with subpopulation selectivity been reported.

5-HT_{2A} Receptors

5-HT_{2A} receptors, formerly termed 5-HT_2 receptors, have been extensively reviewed (47–51). 5-HT_{2A} receptors have been cloned from various species, including human, and exhibit a high degree (>90%) of species homology. Significant (78%) amino acid sequence homology is found between the transmembrane portions of cloned 5-HT_{2A} receptors and 5-HT_{2C} receptors; this could explain the observed similarities in the binding of various ligands at the two receptor subpopulations. Evidence was provided that 5-HT_{2A} receptors exist in a high-affinity state and a low-affinity state (sometimes referred to as 5-HT_{2H} and 5-HT_{2L} states, respectively); under normal conditions, the low-affinity state predominates. The tritiated antagonist, [^{3}H]ketanserin, displays comparable affinity for both states, whereas agonists display higher affinity for the high-affinity state (e.g., when a tritiated agonist is employed as radioligand).

5-HT_{2A} Agonists The SAFIRs for 5-HT_{2A} receptor binding have been reviewed (47,51). Most indolealkylamines are nonselective 5-HT_{2A} receptor ligands, and typically bind with high affinity at the tritiated agonist-labeled high-affinity state. Investigations suggest that all indolealkylamines could not bind in the same manner at 5-HT_{2A} receptors (52). Phenylalkylamines, such as DOB and DOI, act as 5-HT_{2A} receptor agonists or high-efficacy partial agonists (see Chapter 19) and are significantly more selective than the indolealkylamines because of the low affinity of the former for non–5-HT_{2A} sites, but they do not differentiate between 5-HT_2 receptor subpopulations. [^{3}H]DOB and [^{125}I]DOI have been introduced as agonist radioligands (53). Interestingly, although *N*-alkylation of DOB-type compounds typically results in decreased affinity, it was found that *N*-benzyl-α-desmethyl DOB is a very high-affinity compound and, furthermore, that it behaves as a 5-$HT_{2A/2C}$ agonist (54). The structurally related INBMeO has been introduced as a radioligand to label 5-$HT_{2A/2C}$ receptors (55). Another 5-$HT_{2A/2C}$ agonist with DOB-like effects is the 1*R*,2*R*-isomer of β-hydroxy DOB (β-OH DOB) (56,57).

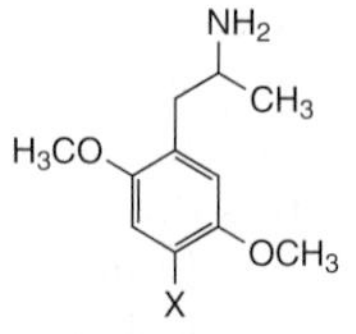

DOB X = Br
DOI X = I

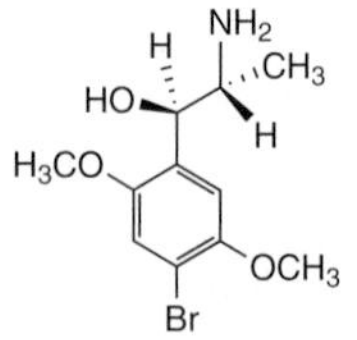

1*R*,2*R*-β-OH DOB

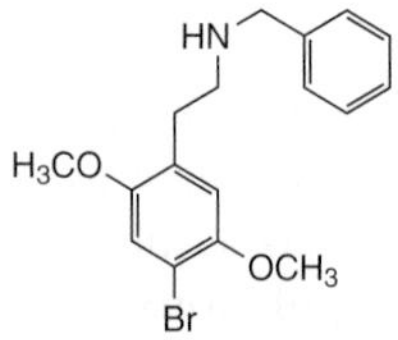

N-Benzyl-α-desmethyl DOB

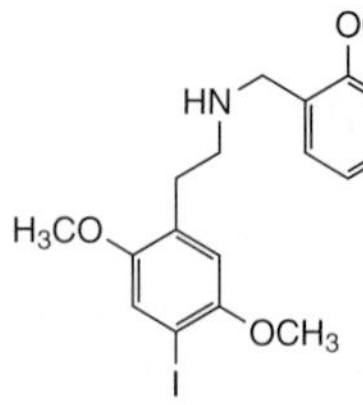

INBMeO

5-HT_{2A} Antagonists One of the largest and more selective classes of 5-HT_{2A} receptor antagonists is the *N*-alkylpiperidines. The best-known examples are ketanserin and ritanserin. Although numerous ketanserin-related derivatives have been reported, their SAR still has not been completely defined. Nevertheless, far less than the entire structure of ketanserin is required for high affinity. Some 5-HT_{2A} receptor antagonists, although fairly selective for 5-$HT_{2A/2C}$ receptors versus most other populations of 5-HT receptors, bind with modest to high affinity at dopaminergic, histaminergic, and/or adrenergic receptors. The tricyclic antipsychotics, atypical antipsychotics (risperidone, clozapine, and olanzapine) (Fig. 11.9), and tricyclic antidepressants also bind at 5-HT_{2A} receptors. Spiperone (Fig. 11.7) has been employed as a 5-HT_{2A} receptor antagonist with 1,000-fold selectivity for 5-HT_{2A} versus 5-HT_{2C} receptors, but spiperone is also a potent dopamine receptor antagonist, a 5-HT_{1A} receptor antagonist, and a 5-HT_7 receptor antagonist. Spiperone, volinanserin (MDL 100,907 or M100907), and AMI-193 were the first 5-HT_{2A}– versus 5-HT_{2C}–selective antagonists available (58,59) (Fig. 11.10). The binding selectivity of various antagonists (and agonists) at 5-HT_{2A}, 5-HT_{2B}, and 5-HT_{2C} receptors has been compared (60). Spiperone and AMI-193 bind at 5-HT_{2A} receptors with 1,000- to 3,000-fold selectivity relative to 5-HT_{2C} receptors but display high affinity for 5-HT_{1A} and D_2 dopamine receptors. A newer member of this series, KML-010, is a spiperone-related derivative that lacks affinity for 5-HT_{2C} and 5-HT_{1A} receptors and binds with low affinity at D_2-dopamine receptors (59).

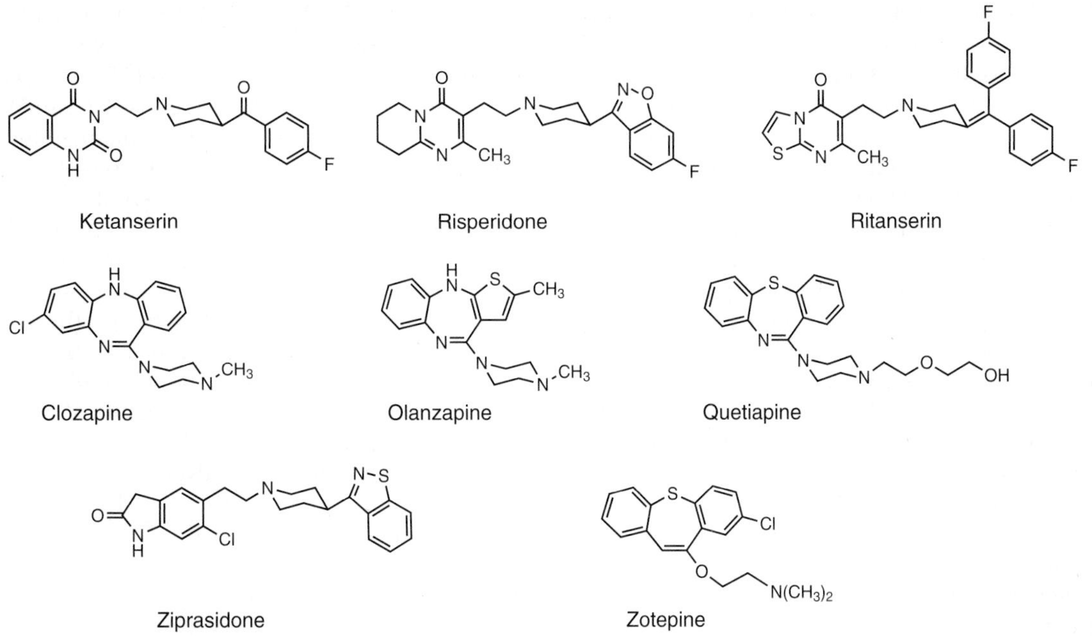

FIGURE 11.9 5-HT_2 receptor antagonists.

Volinanserin is a widely used pharmacologic tool with greater than 100-fold selectivity over most other receptor types (58). Pimavanserin and nelotanserin (ADP-125) display 10-fold and 250-fold selectivity, respectively, for 5-HT_{2A} versus 5-HT_{2C} receptors; one of the most selective antagonists is pruvanserin (EMD-281,014) with about 4,000-fold selectivity (Fig. 11.10).

5-HT_{2A} RECEPTORS: CLINICAL IMPLICATIONS The potential therapeutic roles of 5-HT_{2A} ligands and the possible involvement of 5-HT_{2A} receptors in modulating normal physiologic functions and various pathologic and psychopathologic conditions have been extensively reviewed (3,11,20). 5-HT_{2A} receptors appear to have a role in thermoregulation and sleep, and they could be involved in appetite control, learning, and, along with various other serotonergic receptor populations, cardiovascular function and muscle contraction. Many of the clinical implications of 5-HT_{2A} receptors could actually involve 5-HT_{2C} receptors or a combination of 5-HT_{2A} and 5-HT_{2C} receptors, due to the high homology between the two receptor populations resulting in many antagonists that bind to both with relatively little selectivity. For example, 5-HT_{2A} (and/or 5-HT_{2C}) antagonists could be useful for the treatment of anxiety (particularly posttraumatic stress disorder) and sleep, cognitive, and mood disorders (61,62). With the recent development of subpopulation-selective agents, this is currently an important area of research. For example, nelotanserin, pimavanserin, pruvanserin, and volinanserin are being examined for their effectiveness in treating insomnia, schizophrenia, depression, and anxiety.

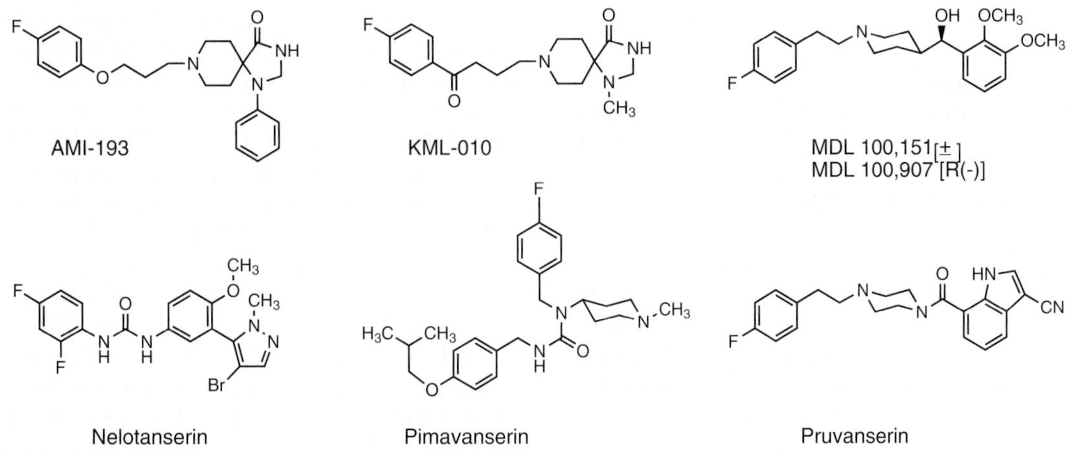

FIGURE 11.10 Examples of 5-HT_{2A} subpopulation selective agents.

Antipsychotic Agents and Antidepressants Various typical and atypical antipsychotic agents (see Chapter 14) and antidepressants (see Chapter 18) bind with relatively high affinity at 5-HT_{2A} receptors as antagonists (15,63). Although no direct correlation exists between their receptor affinities and clinically effective doses, evidence suggests that these disorders involve, at least to some extent, 5-HT_{2A} receptors. For example, chronic administration of 5-HT_{2A} antagonists results in a paradoxical downregulation of 5-HT_{2A} receptors. Such a downregulation would be of benefit in the treatment of depression. Several agents with 5-HT_{2A} antagonist action possess antipsychotic activity; an example is the atypical antipsychotic risperidone. Some 5-HT_{2A} antagonists also bind at dopamine receptors. Indeed, the atypical antipsychotics clozapine, olanzapine, quetiapine, risperidone, ziprasidone, and zotepine, bind both at 5-HT_{2A} and dopamine D_2 receptors (63,64) and often at other serotonergic and nonserotonergic receptors. Although this can obfuscate the role of 5-HT_{2A} antagonism as being important for (atypical) antipsychotic activity, it has been suggested that certain types of schizophrenia could actually be more responsive to the combined effect. That is, D_2-dopaminergic antagonist antipsychotics have been claimed to be more effective for treating the positive symptoms of schizophrenia, whereas the 5-HT_{2A} antagonists could be more effective in treating the negative symptoms; this has led to the development of the serotonin–dopamine antagonists. This theory also suggests that increasing the 5-HT_{2A} component of binding could be related to a decrease in extrapyramidal side effects associated with these types of agents. However, a recent study has found that whereas certain atypical antipsychotics (e.g., clozapine, olanzapine, risperidone) are more efficacious than typical antipsychotics agents against overall positive and negative symptoms of schizophrenia, this was not true for certain others (e.g., quetiapine, ziprasidone, zotepine) (65). Nevertheless, all agents produced decreased extrapyramidal stimulation as an undesirable side effect. From preclinical studies, there are indications that certain 5-HT_{2A} receptor antagonists also possess anxiolytic properties; for example, ritanserin (Fig. 11.9) has been demonstrated to produce both antipsychotic and antianxiety effects in humans.

Classical Hallucinogens 5-HT_{2A} receptors can be involved in the actions of the classical hallucinogens (66) (see Chapter 19). Although indolealkylamine (e.g., 5-methoxy-*N*,*N*-dimethyltryptamine) and ergoline-related (e.g., LSD) classical hallucinogens are fairly nonselective agents that bind to multiple populations of serotonergic receptors, the phenylalkylamine hallucinogens (e.g., DOB, and DOI) are much more 5-HT_2–selective agonists. Furthermore, a significant correlation exists between the human hallucinogenic potencies of classical hallucinogens and their 5-HT_{2A} receptor affinities (66). Interestingly, phenylalkylamine hallucinogens also bind at 5-HT_{2B} and 5-HT_{2C} receptors, and here, too, a significant correlation is found between human potency and receptor affinity for 17 different agents (67). Recent studies suggest that 5-HT_{2A} receptors can have a more prominent role than 5-HT_{2B} or 5-HT_{2C} receptors for the behavioral actions of hallucinogens (67), and differences may exist in the manner in which hallucinogens activate the different receptor populations (68,69).

An interesting twist, with potential therapeutic ramifications, was the development of the 1*R*,2*R* isomer of β-OH DOB (56). 5-HT_{2A} receptors are found in the eye, and activation of these receptors can reduce intraocular pressure and could be of benefit for the treatment of glaucoma. However, 5-HT_{2A} agonists such as DOB are hallucinogenic. A DOB analog, β-OH DOB, was developed as a less lipid-soluble version of DOB. With its reduced lipophilicity, and because of its route of administration (ocular installation), the adverse effects of this agent should be minimized. Other 5-HT_2 agonists are now being examined in this regard (57).

5-HT_{2B} Receptors

The rat fundus preparation is a peripheral tissue assay that has been used as a functional assay for serotonergic action for more than 50 years. Long-standing questions concerning the pharmacologic similarity of serotonergic fundus receptors (now called 5-HT_{2B} receptors) to the 5-HT_2 family of receptors were answered once they were cloned (70). The 5-HT_{2B} receptors exhibit approximately 70% homology to 5-HT_{2A} and 5-HT_{2C} receptors, and like 5-HT_{2A} receptors, they appear to couple functionally to phosphoinositol hydrolysis. Nevertheless, rat and human 5-HT_{2B} receptors display more than 90% transmembrane sequence homology. Therefore, most agents that bind at rat 5-HT_{2B} receptors also bind with similar affinity at human 5-HT_{2B} receptors. There are, however, some exceptions (71). The standard 5-HT_{2A} receptor antagonist ketanserin and the 5-HT_{2A} receptor agonists DOI and DOB display higher affinity for 5-HT_{2A} and 5-HT_{2C} receptors than for 5-HT_{2B} receptors (67). Evidence suggests that human 5-HT_{2B} receptors, like human 5-HT_{2A} receptors, also exist in high-affinity and low-affinity states (71). 5-HT_{2B} receptors are found on cardiovascular tissue. Activation of such receptors by agents with a 5-HT_{2B} agonist character could result in cardiac valvulopathy; valvular heart disease associated with the anorectic agent fenfluramine could involve its metabolism to norfenfluramine—a high-affinity 5-HT_{2B} agonist (72). The designer drug 3,4-methylenedioxymethamphetamine (MDMA; Ecstasy) and its *N*-desmethyl analog MDA also show a 5-HT_{2B} agonist character (73). A series of 1-substituted β-carbolines (e.g., LY-23728, LY-287375, and LY-266097) have been reported to be the first 5-HT_{2B}–selective antagonists (74).

In the periphery, 5-HT_{2B} receptors seem to be involved in muscle contraction; however, their function in the CNS (if any) is still a matter of speculation. On the basis of some preliminary studies, and considering their central distribution in brain, 5-HT_{2B} receptors could be involved, at least in rodents, in anxiety, cognition, food intake, neuroendocrine regulation, locomotor coordination, and balance (75).

5-HT_{2C} Receptors

The 5-HT_{2C} receptors, formerly called 5-HT_{1C} receptors, originally were identified in various regions of the brain using autoradiographic and radioligand binding techniques. Cloned human 5-HT_{2C} receptors display a high amino acid sequence homology with 5-HT_{2A} receptors, and like 5-HT_{2A} receptors, they are coupled to phosphoinositol hydrolysis. As previously mentioned, some pharmacologic functions once attributed to "5-HT_2" receptors actually could involve a 5-HT_{2C} receptor mechanism. For example, the hyperthermic activity of a series of phenylisopropylamines is significantly correlated not only with 5-HT_{2A} but also with their 5-HT_{2C} receptor affinity. Numerous atypical antipsychotic agents bind at 5-HT_{2C} receptors as well as at 5-HT_{2A} receptors; however, no significant correlation exists between their atypical properties and binding affinity. 5-HT_{2C} receptors can have a greater role than 5-HT_{2A} receptors in migraine. Other studies suggest that 5-HT_{2C} receptor modulators could be useful in the treatment of obesity, schizophrenia, depression, anxiety, drug abuse, erectile dysfunction, urinary incontinence, and Parkinson disease (76). Several selective agents are now available.

A series of isotryptamine derivatives, including Ro 60-0175 (ORG-35030), has been shown to display high selectivity for 5-HT_{2C} versus 5-HT_{2A} receptors and to possess 5-HT agonist activity (77); however, some of the results could not be replicated (78). Structurally related tricyclic analogs, such as Ro 60-0332 (ORG-35035), also have been examined and display more than 100-fold selectivity (79). 10-Methoxy-9-methylpyrazino[1,2-a] indole, Ro 60-0175, and Ro 60-0332 all were active in animal models predictive of therapeutic utility for obsessive-compulsive disorders, panic disorders, and depression (79). WAY-163909 (Fig. 11.11), a full agonist at 5-HT_{2C} receptors with weak partial agonist action at 5-HT_{2B} receptors and inactive at 5-HT_{2A} receptors, was effective in animal models of obesity, psychotic-like behavior, and depression (80). Lorcaserin (APD-356) (Fig. 11.11) is a 5-HT_{2C} receptor agonist developed for the treatment of obesity (81); although it has completed phase III clinical trials, it has not yet been approved by the U.S. Food and Drug Administration. 1*R*,3*S*(−) *trans*-1-Phenyl-3-dimethylamino-1,2,3,4-tetrahydronaphthalene, or 1*R*,3*S*(−) *trans*-PAT (Fig. 11.11), a full agonist at 5-HT_{2C} receptors, is an inverse agonist and competitive antagonist at 5-HT_{2A} and 5-HT_{2B} receptors and produced anorexia in animals (82).

Interestingly, selective 5-HT_{2C} receptor antagonists appear to target some of the same actions as 5-HT_{2C} receptor agonists. Perhaps the first 5-$HT_{2C/2B}$–selective antagonist was SB-206553, which was identified in the 1990s; continued work with this molecule ultimately resulted in SB-243213—actually, an inverse agonist (83,84). The latter displays greater than 100-fold selectivity over the other two populations of 5-HT_2 receptors and is being

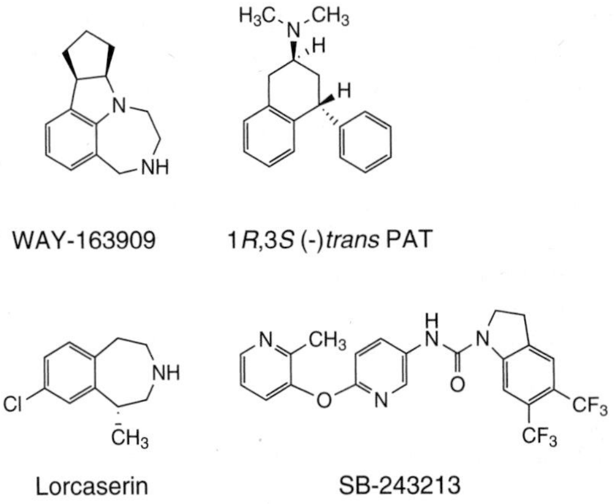

FIGURE 11.11 5-HT_{2C} receptor–selective agonists and antagonists.

examined for its potential use in the treatment of anxiety, depression, and schizophrenia. SB-243213 is claimed to possess an improved anxiolytic profile relative to the benzodiazepines and could have utility in the treatment of schizophrenia and motor disorders (83). It should be noted that agomelatine (Valdoxan), although not strictly a 5-HT_{2C}–selective receptor antagonist, has been found more effective than fluoxetine in a randomized double-blind study in patients with severe major depressive disorder (85), and is currently in clinical trials in the United States. Initially developed as a melatonin (MT) receptor agonist, agomelatine is a nonselective MT_1/MT_2 receptor agonist with 5-HT_{2C} receptor antagonist character (Chapter 18).

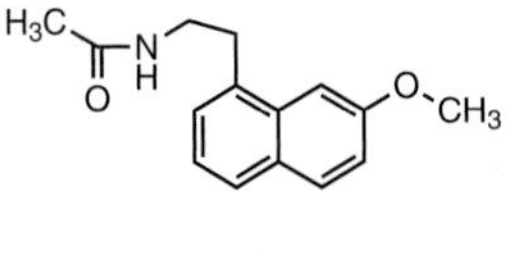

Agomelatine

It is still not known with confidence specifically what pharmacologic effects are related to what 5-HT_2 receptor subpopulation. However, with the availability of subtype-selective agents, the problem comes closer to being solved.

5-HT_3 Receptor Family

Unlike with most 5-HT receptor populations, early 5-HT_3 pharmacologic studies relied almost exclusively on functional (i.e., peripheral tissue) assays. It was a number of years before radioligands were available to identify 5-HT_3 receptors in brain. 5-HT_3 receptors, ligand-gated ion channel receptors, are members of the Cys-loop family that includes nicotinic acetylcholine, γ-aminobutyric acid $(GABA)_A$ and glycine receptors, and a Zn^{2+}-activated cation channel (86,87). They consist of five subunits surrounding a cation-permeable (Na^+, Ca^{2+}, K^+), water-filled pore. Each subunit is composed of four transmembrane-spanning helices (TM1 to TM4) with the TM2 domains of each forming the channel pore (Fig. 11.12). Both, a large N-terminus with a Cys-loop and a short C-terminus are located extracellularly (86,87). Approximately 70% to 80% of 5-HT_3 receptors in brain are located presynaptically (87). Evidence indicates that 5-HT_3 receptors modulate release of other neurotransmitters, including dopamine, acetylcholine, GABA, and 5-HT (88).

Five 5-HT_3 subunits have been cloned. 5-HT_{3A}, 5-HT_{3B}, 5-HT_{3C}, and 5-HT_{3E} subunits are similar in their topology, whereas the 5-HT_{3D} subunit lacks most of the N-terminus including the Cys-loop. The 5-HT_{3A} subunit is the only one that forms functional homomeric receptors when expressed in *Xenopus* oocytes. The other subunits are unable to form functional homomeric receptors in vitro, but they can assemble to functional heteromeric receptors with the 5-HT_{3A} subunit (87). This could be explained by lack of a tryptophan residue in the N-terminus of all four subunits (5-HT_{3B}, 5-HT_C, 5-HT_D, and 5-HT_E) shown to be essential for binding. Conversely, the latest reports indicate that subunits 5-HT_{3C}, 5-HT_{3D}, and 5-HT_{3E} could be present on the cell surface when expressed alone in CHO cells (89). 5-HT_{3A}- and 5-HT_{3AB} receptors are the most studied to date. 5-HT_{3AB} receptors differ from 5-HT_{3A} in that they have higher single-channel conductance, a lower Ca^{2+} permeability, faster activation and deactivation, and a lower potency for 5-HT. The subunit composition of recombinant 5-HT_{3AB} receptors in HEK293 cells has been shown to be B-B-A-B-A, but this could not be the case for native 5-HT_3 receptors (87). The orthosteric ligand binding site is believed to be located at the interface of two adjacent subunits where it is formed by three loops (A to C) of the "principal" and three loops (D to F) of the "complementary" subunit as shown for acetylcholine binding protein and adapted for 5-HT_3 receptors. To fully activate the ion channel of homomeric 5-HT_{3A} receptors, three molecules of agonist are necessary, whereas in the case of heteromeric 5-HT_{3AB} receptors, with presumed stoichiometry of 5-$HT_{3(A)2(B)3}$, only two agonist molecules are necessary (87).

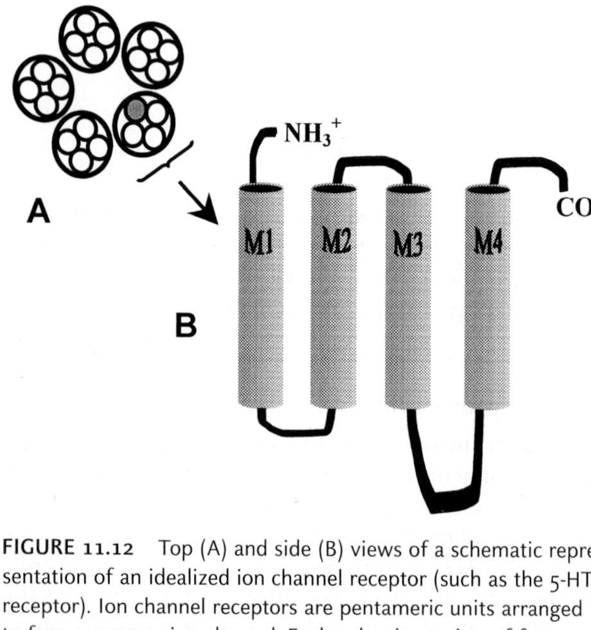

FIGURE 11.12 Top (A) and side (B) views of a schematic representation of an idealized ion channel receptor (such as the 5-HT_3 receptor). Ion channel receptors are pentameric units arranged to form a pore or ion channel. Each subunit consists of four transmembrane-spanning amino acid chains (M_1–M_4) constructed such that the M_2 chain faces the channel. The transmembrane portions are connected by extracellular and intracellular loops. In the serotonin family, only 5-HT_3 receptors have been identified as ion channel receptors.

Structure–Activity Relationships of 5-HT_3 Agonists

Only a few 5-HT_3 receptor agonists have been identified (Fig 12.13), and the topic has been comprehensively reviewed (90). Many tryptamine analogs bind at 5-HT_3 receptors in a nonselective manner. Simple *O*-methylation of 5-HT significantly decreases its affinity for 5-HT_3 receptors. Ergolines either do not bind or bind only with very low affinity. 5-HT is a nonselective 5-HT_3 receptor agonist that binds only with modest affinity (K_i ~ 500 to 1,000 nM). Its 2-methyl analog, 2-methyl 5-HT (K_i = 1,200 nM) (Fig. 11.13), is somewhat more selective but binds with slightly lower affinity than 5-HT. Although 2-methyl 5-HT may be only a partial agonist, it has found widespread application in 5-HT_3 research due to its greater selectivity over 5-HT. Recently, however, 2-methyl 5-HT was shown to bind with high affinity at 5-HT_6 receptors (see below). The *N,N,N*-trimethyl quaternary amine analog of 5-HT, 5-HTQ, binds with approximately 10-fold greater affinity and is much more selective than 5-HT; however, because of its quaternary nature, it could not readily penetrate the blood–brain barrier when administered systemically. Using cloned mouse 5-HT_3 receptors, 5-HT and 5-HTQ act as full agonists, suggesting that the quaternary nature of 5-HTQ has little effect on efficacy, whereas 2-methyl 5-HT and tryptamine act as partial agonists. Another example of a low-affinity (K_i ~ 1,000 nM) 5-HT_3 agonist is phenylbiguanide. *m*-Chlorophenylbiguanide (*m*CPBG), which binds in the low nanomolar range (K_i ~ 20 to 50 nM) and retains agonist character, has largely replaced phenylbiguanide. Because of its polar nature, *m*CPBG does not readily penetrate the blood–brain barrier. *m*-Chlorophenylguanidine (MD-354; *m*CPG) shows that the entire biguanide moiety is not required for serotonergic activity. Adding multiple chloro groups to *m*CPBG or *m*CPG increases their lipophilicity and affinity (90).

Simple arylpiperazines were among the first serotonergic agents investigated at 5-HT_3 receptors (Fig 12.13). Many are nonselective 5-HT_3 ligands (see previous discussion of 5-HT_{1A} receptors). Depending on the particular substitution pattern, they can behave as 5-HT_3 agonists, partial agonists, or antagonists (90). This nonselectivity probably accounts for the initial lack of interest in arylpiperazines as 5-HT_3 ligands, but today, there is renewed interest in these

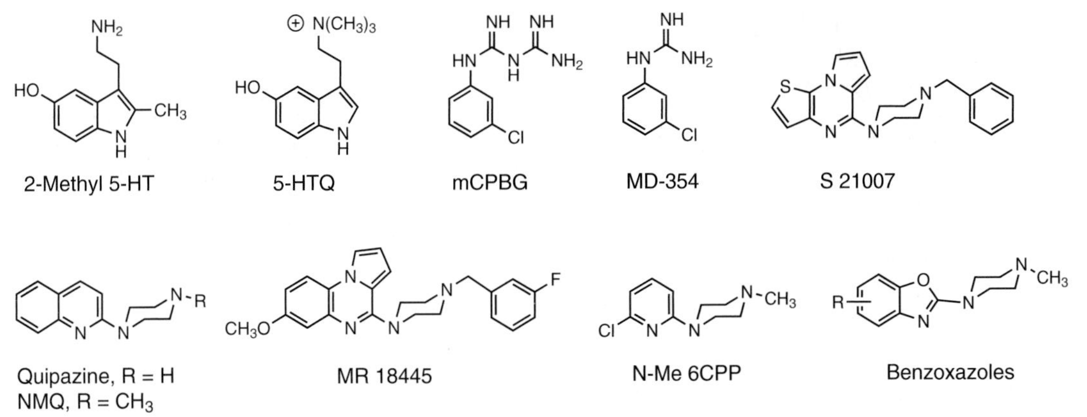

FIGURE 11.13 5-HT$_3$ receptor agonists or partial agonists.

types of agents. Quipazine was the first arylpiperazine shown to bind at 5-HT$_3$ receptors, even though it is also a 5-HT$_{2A}$ agonist. It binds with much higher affinity than 5-HT at 5-HT$_3$ receptors (K_i ~ 1 nM) and was subsequently shown to act as an agonist in certain assays and as an antagonist in others. Interestingly, its structure was quite different from that of other 5-HT$_3$ antagonists known at that time. Early structure–affinity studies showed that its fused pyridine ring attached to N_4-piperazine nitrogen distance (~5.5 Å) was similar to that of 5-HT. Other findings indicated that 1) the N_4-piperazine nitrogen atom, but not the N_1-piperazine nitrogen atom, was important for binding; 2) the quinoline ring nitrogen atom was a major contributor to binding; 3) the benzene ring portion of the quinoline nucleus was not required for binding, but its presence was optimal for high affinity; and 4) N_4-methylation (*N*-methylquipazine) enhances 5-HT$_3$ receptor selectivity (Fig. 11.13) (90). With the availability of newer arylpiperazines, it has been possible to conduct more comprehensive structure–activity studies. A summary of quipazine SAR is shown in Figure 11.14; results of other SAR studies and several pharmacophoric models have been described (90). Appropriate structural modification of arylpiperazines can result in rather selective 5-HT$_3$ agonists (Fig. 11.13). For example, ring-fused quipazine-related analogs, such as the pyrrolo[1,2-*a*]quinoxalines, represent novel 5-HT$_3$ receptor agonists. Some are full agonists, whereas others (e.g., MR 18445) are partial agonists (90–93).

Structure–Activity Relationship of 5-HT$_3$ Antagonists

Bemesetron (MDL-72222) was the first selective 5-HT$_3$ receptor antagonist (Fig. 11.15). Its development stems from the structural modification of cocaine, an agent that had been previously shown to be a weak 5-HT$_3$ antagonist. Since then, many hundreds of 5-HT$_3$ antagonists have been identified as antiemetics (93,94). Many of these agents belong to the structural class of compounds broadly referred to as keto compounds and contain an amide, reverse amide, ester, reverse ester, carbamoyl, or ketone function. Typical of these 5-HT$_3$ antagonists is retention of the bulky tropane or tropane-like amine group. Some of the more widely used or newer antiemetic agents include dolasetron (Anzemet), granisetron (Kytril), itasetron, renzapride, ricasetron, tropisetron, WAY-100289, zacopride, and zatosetron. It should be noted that some of these keto compounds also bind at 5-HT$_4$ receptors.

A related group of antagonists that possess an imidazole or related heterocyclic terminal amine include ondansetron (Zofran), alosetron (Lotronex), fabesetron, and ramosetron (Fig. 11.16). Many others have been described (93,94). The SARs of 5-HT$_3$ antagonists have been reviewed in detail (93–95).

Studies have identified pharmacophoric features (Fig. 11.17) that are common to many 5-HT$_3$ receptor antagonists.

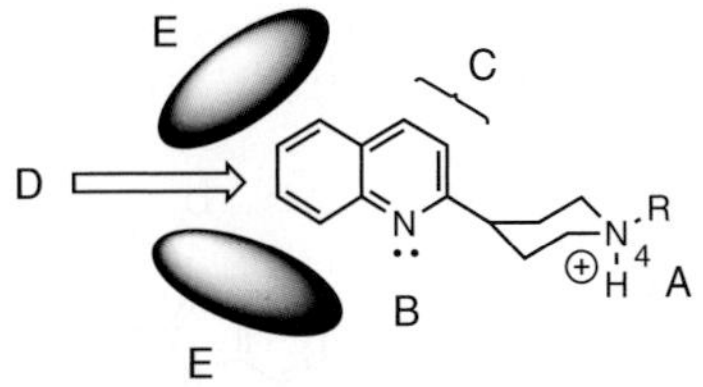

FIGURE 11.14 Structure–activity composite for quipazine analogs binding at 5-HT$_3$ receptors. (A) The N_4-piperazine nitrogen atom, but not the N_1-piperazine nitrogen atom, is important for binding; a 5-position-CH$_3$ is tolerated and results in somewhat greater 5-HT$_3$ selectivity. (B) The quinoline nitrogen atom is required for high affinity, and its replacement by an sp^2-hybridized carbon atom results in a more than 100-fold decrease in affinity. (C) Substituents in this region are tolerated and can influence intrinsic activity. (D) An aromatic moiety (e.g., benzene ring or isosteric structure), although not required for binding, results in optimal affinity. (E) Regions of limited bulk tolerance.

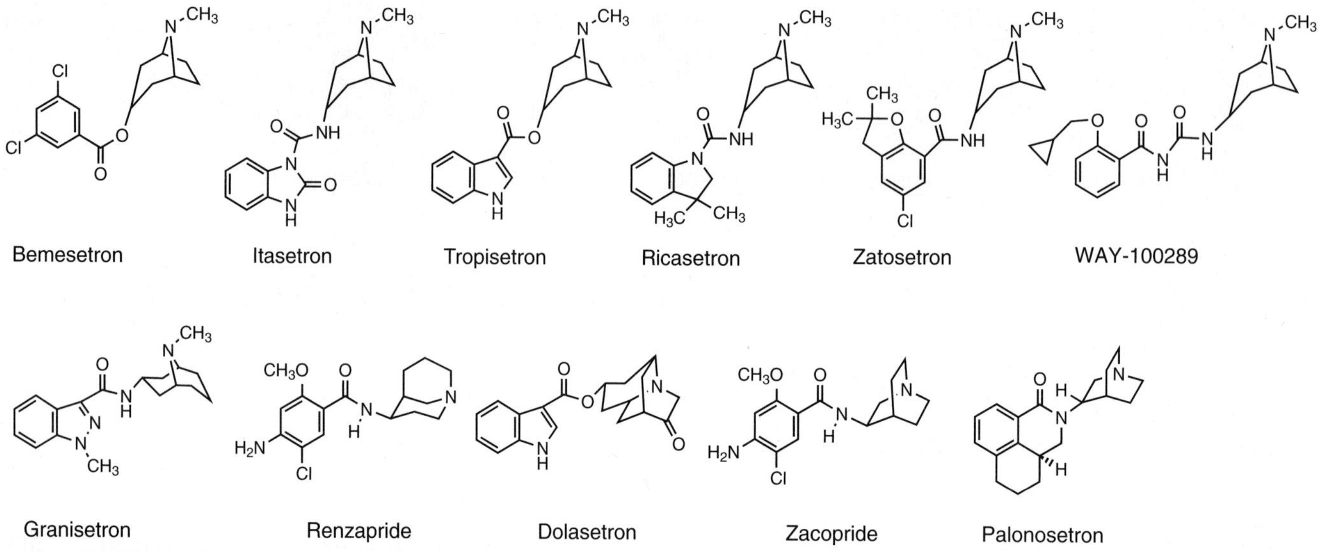

FIGURE 11.15 5-HT_3 receptor antagonists.

5-HT_3 Receptors: Clinical Implications

One of the most noteworthy clinical success stories in 5-HT research relates to the antiemetic properties of 5-HT_3 receptor antagonists. Ondansetron was introduced as an antiemetic in the 1990s, and 5-HT_3 receptor antagonists are now the "gold standard" for treatment of chemotherapy- and radiation-induced nausea and vomiting (96). Twenty or so years ago, nausea and vomiting were inevitable side effects that forced many patients to delay or avoid chemotherapy (97). With the current antiemetic therapy, nausea and vomiting can be prevented in nearly 80% of patients (97). The most commonly employed 5-HT_3 receptor antagonists are ondansetron, granisetron, dolasetron and, in Europe, tropisetron; a newer 5-HT_3 antagonist in clinical use in the United States is palonosetron (98). The various 5-HT_3 antagonists are commonly perceived as being of comparable efficacy and safety (99); however, they vary widely in their pharmacologic and pharmacokinetic properties (96–99) (Table 11.4). For example, their duration of action and elimination half-lives differ considerably. Ondansetron displays the shortest half-life (~4 hours), whereas the half-life of palonosetron has been reported to be up to 128 hours (99). Another difference in their pharmacology is that ondansetron is a competitive 5-HT_3 antagonist, whereas granisetron and tropisetron (and, perhaps, palonosetron) produce an insurmountable antagonism (98,99). Selection of a particular 5-HT_3 antiemetic follows specific guidelines that are related, at least in part, to such factors as the emeticity of the chemotherapeutic regimen, side effect tolerability, patient history, and financial considerations. Patients who are refractory to the effect of a particular antiemetic may benefit by switching antiemetic agents—improvement could be related to different routes of metabolism (96) (Table 11.4).

Preclinical and limited clinical studies suggest that 5-HT_3 receptor antagonists could potentially be of benefit for the treatment of alcohol and substance abuse, anxiety, autism, bipolar disorder, cognitive impairment,

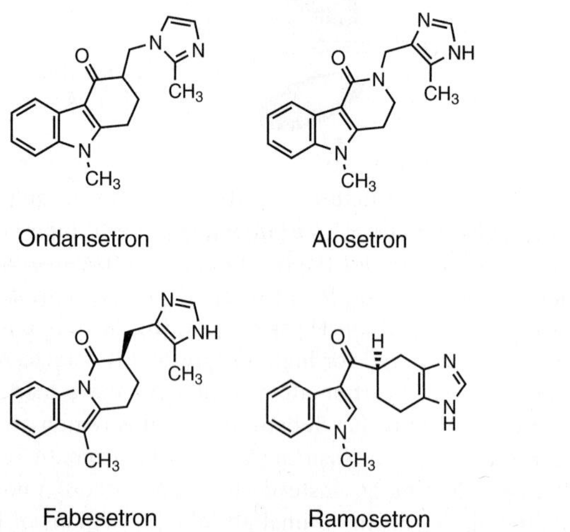

FIGURE 11.16 Imidazole-containing 5-HT_3 receptor antagonists.

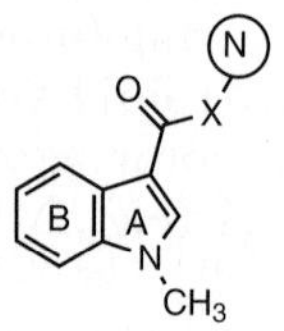

FIGURE 11.17 A composite pharmacophore model for 5-HT_3 receptor antagonists. An aromatic centroid (A) to oxygen (O) distance of 3.3 to 3.5 Å is thought to be optimal. Distances calculated from the terminal amine (N) to the oxygen atom (O) and from the terminal amine N to centroid A are from 5.1 to 5.2 and from 6.7 to 7.2 Å, respectively. It has been speculated that ring A is not required for binding and acts as a spacer. Ring B can be more important for binding, and associated hydrophobic binding regions have been proposed.

TABLE 11.4 Pharmacokinetics of the 5-HT3 Antagonists (Setrons)

Parameters	Ondansetron	Dolasetron	Granisetron	Alosetron	Palonosetron	Tropisetron
Trade name	Zofran	Anzemet	Kytril	Lotronex	Aloxi	Navoban
CLogP (calc)[a]	2.1 ± 0.5	2.8 ± 0.5	1.5 ± 0.5	0.88 ± 0.8	2.6 ± 0.5	3.6 ± 0.3
LogD (pH 7) (calc)[a]	1.5	2.8	−1.5	0.4	0.01	0.8
Bioavailability (%)	56–70[d]	Hydrodolasetron: 60–80	60[d]	50–60[bc]	IV	60 (60–100)
Protein binding (%)	70–76	Hydrodolasetron: 70–80	65	82	62	71
Volume of distribution (L/kg)	PO: 2.2–2.5	Hydrodolasetron: PO: 5.8–10	PO: 3.9	PO: 70 (65–95)	IV: 6.8–12.5	IV: 500
		PO: 6-7				
Elimination half-life (h)	PO: 3–6	PO: <10 min	IV: 4–5	PO: 1.5–2.0	PO: 30–40	EM: PO: 6–8
	Elderly: PO: 11	Hydrodolasetron: PO: 4–9	PO: ~6			PM: PO: 30
Major metabolites (%)	Hydroxylation	Hydrodolasetron	*N*-Demethyl	6-Hydroxylation	*N*-oxide	Hydrolyzation
	Glucuronidation	Hydroxylation	Hepatic	*N*-Demethyl	6S-Hydroxy	Glucuronides
	Hepatic	*N*-Demethyl			Hepatic: 50%	
Metabolizing enzyme (%)	CYP3A4	Carbonyl reductase	CYP3A4	CYP2C9: 30	CYP2D6	CYP2D6
	CYP2D6	CYP2D6		CYP3A4: 20	CYP3A4	
		CYP3A4 (*N*-oxide)		CYP1A2: 10	CYP1A2	
Time to peak plasma concentration (h)	PO: 1–2	Hydrodolasetron IV: <0.5	PO: 2–3	PO: 0.5–2	IV: 30 s	EM: PO: 3
		Hydrodolasetron PO: <1				PM: PO: 4
Excretion (%)	Urine metab: 40–60	Urine metab: 45	Urine metab: 48	Urine metab: 70	Urine metab: 80	Urine metab: ~70
	Feces metab: 25	Feces: 30	Feces metab: 38	Feces metab: 25		Feces metab: ~15
	Unchanged: <10	Unchanged hydrodolasetron: 60	Unchanged: <10	Unchanged: <10	Unchanged: 40	Unchanged: <10
Duration (h)	——	——	8–24	1–10	>24	——

IM, intramuscular; IV, intravenous; PO, oral.
[a] Chemical Abstracts, American Chemical Society, calculated using Advanced Chemistry Development (ACD/Labs) Software V8.14 for Solaris (1994–2006 ACD/Labs).
[b] First-pass metabolism.
[c] Food delays absorption and peak plasma concentrations.
[d] Food increase extent of absorption.

depression, eating disorders, gastrointestinal disorders, pain, and schizophrenia (87).

Very little is known about the potential therapeutic utility of 5-HT$_3$ receptor agonists (90).

5-HT$_4$ Receptors and Agents

A novel population of serotonergic receptors, originally identified in primary cell cultures of mouse embryo colliculi neurons and later termed 5-HT$_4$ receptors, have broad tissue distribution and are positively coupled to adenylate cyclase (100). In the brain, 5-HT$_4$ receptors appear to be localized on neurons and can mediate the slow excitatory responses to 5-HT. Peripherally, these receptors facilitate acetylcholine release in guinea pig ileum and can have a role in peristalsis. The uniqueness of this receptor type and its potential therapeutic utility spurred initial interest in drug development. Human 5-HT$_4$ receptors have been cloned and display low transmembrane sequence homology (<50%) with other 5-HT receptors. In fact, two 5-HT$_4$ isoforms have been isolated, a long form (5-HT$_{4L}$) and a short form (5-HT$_{4S}$). These isoforms are splice variants and differ only in their C-terminus ends, with identical transmembrane regions

(101). In general, the potency of agonists to stimulate cyclic adenosine monophosphate (cAMP) was greater for the 5-HT_{4S} receptor than for the 5-HT_{4L} receptor. A mouse 5-HT_{4L} receptor has been cloned, and a human pseudogene has been identified that codes for a 5-HT_4-like receptor. Indeed, several new human 5-HT_4 receptor isoforms have been cloned and expressed (102). The new 5-HT_4 receptors have been termed 5-$HT_{4(b)}$, 5-$HT_{4(c)}$, and 5-$HT_{4(d)}$; the stimulatory pattern of cAMP formation in response to the 5-HT_4 agonist renzapride was found to be different for the various isoforms, suggesting that the splice variants could differ in the manner by which they trigger signal transduction following receptor activation (102). In the rat gastrointestinal tract, both 5-HT_{4L} and 5-HT_{4S} receptors are expressed, whereas only 5-HT_{4S} receptors are found in the heart, with localization almost exclusively in the atrium. The 5-HT_{4a} receptors have been cloned from human atrium and appear to correspond to the rodent 5-HT_{4S} isoform. It has been proposed that the cardiac effects of 5-HT are mediated by this short splice variant, whereas 5-HT_{4L} determines the neuronal effects of 5-HT (102).

Although 5-HT_3 receptors are ion channel receptors and 5-HT_4 receptors represent G protein–coupled receptors (Table 11.2), a number of 5-HT_3 receptor ligands are active at 5-HT_4 receptors. Even more interesting is that a number of 5-HT_3 antagonists, or what were considered at one time to be 5-HT_3–selective antagonists (e.g., renzapride and zacopride), actually exhibited 5-HT_4 agonist activity. Even today, there is considerable structural similarity among various 5-HT_3 and 5-HT_4 receptor ligands. In addition to their lack of selectivity for 5-HT_4 versus other 5-HT receptors, many early 5-HT_4 receptor ligands suffered from several other disadvantages, such as their affinity for other receptor types, inability or difficulty in penetrating the blood–brain barrier, and hydrolytic instability (103).

Structure–Activity Relationships of 5-HT_4 Agonists

In general terms, 5-HT_4 agonists can be divided into several different categories (Fig. 11.18) (90): tryptamines (e.g., 5-HT and 5-CT, with 2-methyl 5-HT and 5-methoxy-*N,N*-dimethyltryptamine being nearly inactive), benzamides (particularly those bearing a 2-methoxy-4-amino-5-chloro substitution pattern, e.g., SC 53116, renzapride, zacopride, and cisapride), benzimidazolones (e.g., BIMU 8), quinolines (e.g., SDZ 216,908), naphthalimides (e.g., *S*-RS 56532), benzoates (ML-10302), and ketones (e.g., RS 67333).

Structure–Activity Relationships of 5-HT_4 Antagonists

The 5-HT_3 antagonist tropisetron was the first agent to see application as a 5-HT_4 antagonist, and its low affinity for 5-HT_4 receptors prompted a search for higher affinity agents. Various agents have been identified (94,104,105), and 5-HT_4 antagonists are derived from structural classes similar to those from which the 5-HT_4 agonists are derived. These include indole esters and amides (e.g., GR 113,808), benzoates (e.g., SB 204070), benzimidazolones (e.g., DAU 6285), imidazoles (e.g., SC 53606), and ketones (e.g., RS 100235) (Fig. 11.19). These are just a few representative examples of the many agents that have been examined as 5-HT_4 antagonists. Structure–activity details for several different receptor preparations have been reviewed (94,104,105). It is worth noting that apart from 5-HT_3 receptors, 5-HT_4 receptors are the only other population of serotonergic sites that seem to accommodate quaternary amines.

5-HT_4 Receptors: Clinical Implications

Selective 5-HT_4 agents have been recently developed, and studies regarding their clinical potential are still in their infancy. Peripheral actions currently being examined include irritable bowel syndrome (IBS), gastrointestinal tract motility, bladder contraction, gastroesophageal reflux, corticosteroid secretion, and atrial contractility. Cisapride is available as a prokinetic drug that enhances gastrointestinal activity. With respect to their central effects, it has been suggested that 5-HT_4 agonists can restore deficits in cognitive function and that 5-HT_4 antagonists could be useful as anxiolytics or in the treatment of dopamine-related disorders. It is further speculated that 5-HT_4 receptors may be involved in memory and learning, and it has been noted that 5-HT_4 receptors

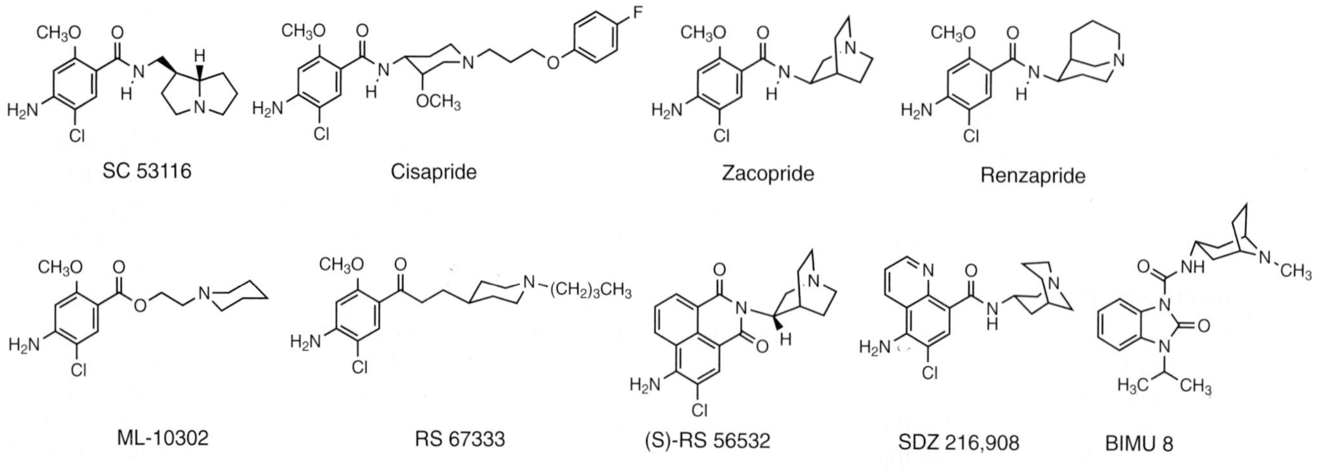

FIGURE 11.18 5-HT_4 receptor agonists.

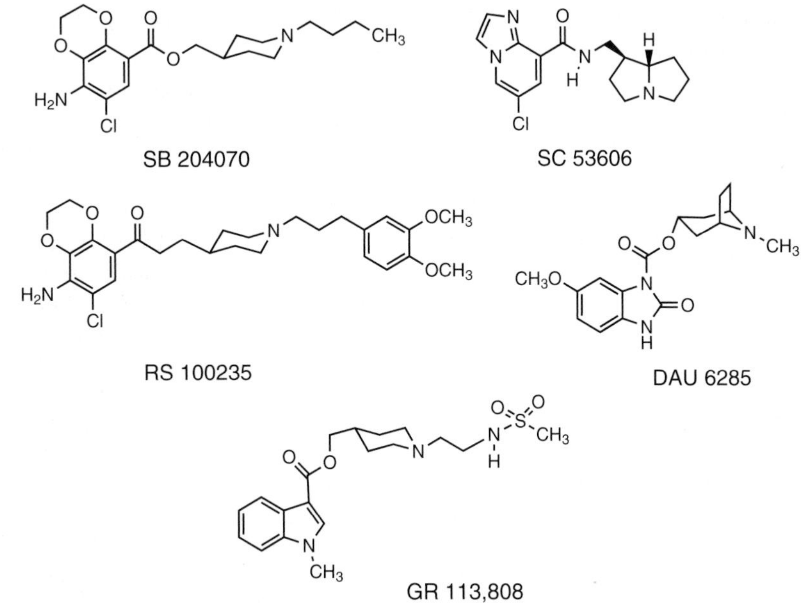

FIGURE 11.19 5-HT_4 receptor antagonists.

are markedly decreased in patients with Alzheimer disease (106,107). A high density of 5-HT_4 receptors in the nucleus accumbens has led some to speculate that these receptors may be involved in the reward system and that they could influence drug self-administration behavior. Other central roles are also beginning to emerge; for example, repeated administration of antidepressants decreases the responsiveness of central 5-HT_4 receptors to activation (108). It would appear that therapeutic roles exist for both 5-HT_4 antagonists and 5-HT_4 agonists. However, it has been cautioned that the use of highly potent and selective 5-HT_4 agonists could result in cardiovascular side effects (107). If different 5-HT_4 receptor isoforms can be shown to mediate the various effects for which 5-HT_4 receptors have been implicated, the potential exists for the development of selective agents. Another problem associated with 5-HT_4 agents is their lack of oral bioavailability (109).

IBS is one of the most common gastrointestinal disorders in the United States, accounting for more than 3.5 million doctor visits per year (110). IBS is characterized by abdominal discomfort or pain associated with altered bowel function (i.e., constipation [IBS-C]), diarrhea (IBS-D), or alternating constipation and diarrhea. Until recently, treatment has been limited by the poor efficacy or side effects of available agents. Agents commonly used to treat IBS include laxatives, antispasmodics and smooth muscle relaxants (e.g., dicyclomine and hyoscyamine), and tricyclic antidepressants, but only 40% of patients are satisfied with these medications (110). Because more than 95% of all 5-HT in the body is found in the gut, it would seem logical that serotonergic agents should be of benefit in the treatment of IBS.

In general, peristaltic and secretory reflexes are initiated by 5-HT acting at 5-HT_{1P} receptors (111)—that is, a population of 5-HT receptors found only in the gut. 5-HT_3 receptors are associated with excitation of the gastrointestinal tract, resulting in increased motility, secretion, and excitation (110) as well as signaling to the CNS (111); 5-HT_3 antagonists reduce colonic transit and improve fluid absorption (110). The 5-HT_3 antagonists tend to be constipating (111). The 5-HT_4 receptors mediate both excitatory and inhibitory effects on gut function (110).

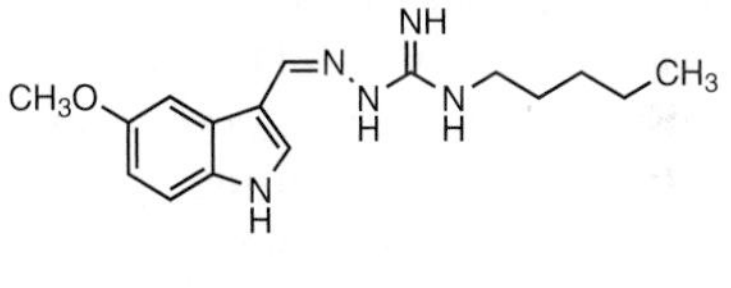

Tegaserod

Alosetron (Fig. 11.16), a 5-HT_3 antagonist, and tegaserod (Zelnorm), a 5-HT_4 agonist, are two of the most recent entries for the treatment of IBS. Recent clinical trials have found that both agents are more effective than placebo for the treatment of IBS-C and IBS-D (110). Tegaserod acts by accelerating small bowel and colonic transit in patients with IBS. It is rapidly absorbed following oral administration, with a bioavailability of approximately 10%, except that food reduces the bioavailability by 40% to 65%. Peak plasma concentrations are reached in approximately 1 hour. Tegaserod is approximately 98% bound to plasma proteins, primarily to α_1-acid glycoprotein. Its volume of distribution is approximately 368 L/kg. Tegaserod undergoes presystemic acid-catalyzed hydrolysis in the stomach, followed by hepatic oxidation to its principal inactive metabolite (5-methoxyindole-3-carboxylic acid), its acyl glucuronide, and three isomeric *N*-glucuronides. The terminal half-life is approximately 11 hours following intravenous administration. Approximately two-thirds of the orally administered dose of tegaserod is excreted unchanged in feces, with the remainder excreted in urine, primarily as glucuronide. Tegaserod exhibits dose-proportional kinetics when given twice daily at therapeutic doses for 5 days, with no relevant accumulation. No dosage adjustment is required in elderly patients or those with mild to moderate hepatic or renal impairment. No clinically relevant drug–drug interactions have been identified with tegaserod. However, in 2007, tegaserod was removed from the U.S. market due increased risks of heart attack or stroke and was made available only through a restricted distribution program. As of 2008, tegaserod is available only in emergency life-threatening situations.

5-HT$_5$ Receptors and Agents

Two 5-HT$_5$ receptors, expressed primarily in the mouse CNS, have been identified as 5-HT$_{5A}$ and 5-HT$_{5B}$ receptors (112). The two 5-HT$_5$ receptors exhibit 77% amino acid sequence homology but less than 50% homology with other cloned serotonergic receptors. To some extent, 5-HT$_5$ receptors appear to resemble 5-HT$_1$ receptors (e.g., high affinity for 5-HT and 5-CT); however, their low homology with other 5-HT$_1$ receptors suggests that they represent a distinct family of receptors. Only 5-HT$_{5A}$ receptors have been identified in humans (112). Human 5-HT$_{5A}$ receptors are G protein–coupled receptors with a complex second messenger system (113).

Radiolabeled LSD binds to both 5-HT$_{5A}$ and 5-HT$_{5B}$ receptors, with 5-CT having 10-fold greater affinity for human 5-HT$_{5A}$ receptors than 5-HT, which binds with modest affinity (K_i = 100 to 250 nM). The SAR for the binding of various ligands at 5-HT$_{5A}$ receptors has been reviewed elsewhere (114). Ergotamine and methiothepin bind with high affinity at human 5-HT$_{5A}$ receptors, whereas agents such as spiperone, sumatriptan, yohimbine, ketanserin, propranolol, zacopride, and clozapine bind with much lower affinity (K_i > 1,000 nM). To date, no 5-HT$_{5A}$–selective agonists or antagonists have been reported.

5-HT$_5$ Receptors: Clinical Implications

Pharmacologic functions of 5-HT$_5$ receptors are currently unknown. It has been speculated, on the basis of their localization, that they could be involved in motor control, feeding, anxiety, depression, learning, memory consolidation, adaptive behavior, and brain development (112). 5-HT$_{5A}$ receptors also could be involved in a neuronally driven mechanism for regulating astrocyte physiology with relevance to gliosis; disruption of 5-HT neuronal–glial interactions can be involved in the development of certain CNS pathologies, including Alzheimer disease, Down syndrome, and some drug-induced developmental deficits. Recent evidence indicates that genes that encode for the human 5-HT$_{5A}$ receptor could be involved in schizophrenia (115) and that spinal 5-HT$_{5A}$ receptors could have a role in nociception and control of pelvic floor musculature (116).

5-HT$_6$ Receptors and Agents

A novel G protein–coupled serotonergic receptor that appears to be localized exclusively in the CNS was cloned from rat brain and named 5-HT$_6$. This receptor exhibits only 40% transmembrane homology with 5-HT$_{1A}$, 5-HT$_{1B}$, 5-HT$_{1D}$, 5-HT$_{1E}$, 5-HT$_{2A}$, and 5-HT$_{2C}$ receptors. Both LSD and 5-HT display modest affinity for 5-HT$_6$ receptors (K_i ~ 50 to 150 nM). Of interest is that a number of typical and atypical antipsychotic agents and tricyclic antidepressants bind with K_i values in the nanomolar range.

The human 5-HT$_6$ receptor was cloned, and its gene structure, distribution, and pharmacology were found to be similar to those of the rat receptor (117). Like the rat receptor, the human receptor is positively coupled to adenylate cyclase. 5-HT binds at human 5-HT$_6$ receptors with moderate affinity (K_i = 65 nM), and one of the highest affinity, albeit nonselective, agents is the antipsychotic methiothepin (K_i = 0.4 nM). Agents that bind at human 5-HT$_6$ receptors with K_i less than 50 nM include 5-methoxytryptamine, bromocriptine, octoclothepin, the atypical antipsychotic agents clozapine and olanzapine, and the typical antipsychotics chlorpromazine, loxapine, and fluphenazine (118). Agents with K_i greater than 500 nM include 5-CT, sumatriptan, quipazine, ketanserin, 8-OH DPAT, haloperidol, risperidone, and mesulergine (118). A number of other antipsychotic agents, both typical and atypical, as well as antidepressants bind with low nanomolar affinity (114,117,118).

5-HT$_6$ Agonists and Antagonists

2-Ethyl-5-methoxy-*N*,*N*-dimethyltryptamine (EMDT) represented the first reasonably selective 5-HT$_6$ agonist (119), and Ro 04-6790 and Ro 63-0563 represented the first 5-HT$_6$–selective antagonists (120) (Fig. 11.20). These were soon followed by the antagonists SB-271046 (121), MS-245 (119,122), and PMDT (2-phenyl-5-methoxy-*N*,*N*-dimethyltryptamine, also known as BGC20-761) (119). Since then, work has continued on related structure types, leading to agents with greater metabolic stability and bioavailability (114). It should be noted that most of the early 5-HT$_6$ antagonists contained an arylsulfonamide moiety. Interestingly, the importance of this functionality was an independent discovery from several different laboratories, and this structural feature is now commonplace among many 5-HT$_6$ agents. In some cases, the sulfonamido moiety can be replaced by a sulfone (e.g., naphthylsulfones) (Fig. 11.20). Numerous structural modifications have now been reported, and one of the interesting findings is that the basic side chain of MS-245–type compounds can be moved to the indole 4-position (Fig. 11.20) (123,124) or removed altogether (e.g., amino-BSS) (114) with retention of antagonist action. 5-Sulfonamidotryptamines also bind with high affinity at 5-HT$_6$ receptors and, depending on the nature of their pendent substituents, act as 5-HT$_6$ agonists, partial agonists, or antagonists (125,126). A comprehensive review of 5-HT$_6$–related agents and their SARs has been published (127).

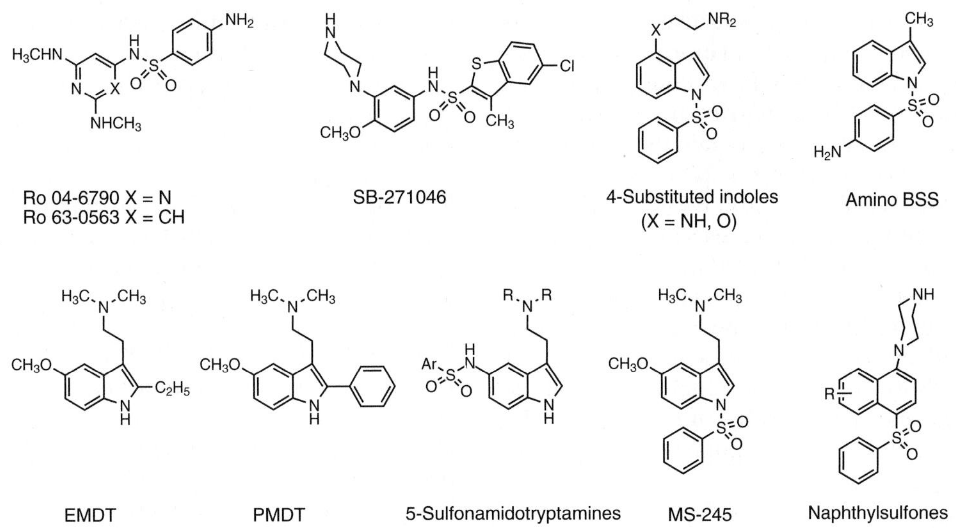

FIGURE 11.20 5-HT_6 receptor agonists and antagonists.

5-HT_6 Receptors: Clinical Implications

The exact clinical significance of 5-HT_6 receptors is unknown at this time. The high affinity of various antipsychotics, particularly atypical antipsychotics (see Chapter 14), and antidepressants suggests a possible connection between 5-HT_6 receptors and certain psychiatric disorders (128). The different binding profiles of atypical antipsychotics can be responsible for their atypical nature (e.g., D_2:5-HT_{2A} ratio); for example, certain agents, such as clozapine, can be classified as atypical on the basis of their binding with higher affinity at 5-HT_{2A} than at D_2 receptors. However, antipsychotics that produce the fewest extrapyramidal side effects in humans (e.g., clozapine, olanzapine, and fluperlapine) also possess high affinity for 5-HT_6 receptors (118). The atypical antipsychotic agent risperidone, which produces some extrapyramidal symptoms, binds with 1,000-fold higher affinity at 5-HT_{2A} than at 5-HT_6 receptors; thus, affinity of agents for 5-HT_6 receptors can contribute to the difference between typical and certain atypical antipsychotics (118). Furthermore, preclinical studies indicate that combinations of a 5-HT_6 antagonist and a 5-HT_{2A} antagonist were effective in models of psychosis and cognition (129). PMDT differs from most other 5-HT_6 antagonists in that it combines both types of antagonist action in the same molecule (114). In 5-HT_6 knockout mice, a behavioral syndrome is produced that seems to involve an increase in cholinergic function. Blocking the receptors in rats with 5-HT_6 antagonists produces a similar effect. This has led to speculation that one of the roles of 5-HT_6 receptors may be to control cholinergic neurotransmission and that 5-HT_6–selective antagonists could be useful in the treatment of anxiety and memory deficits. Other studies have shown that although 5-HT_6 antagonists could not influence basal levels of dopamine by themselves, they apparently increase amphetamine-induced increases in brain dopamine and can potentiate certain dopamine-mediated behavioral effects (130,131). The exact mechanisms underlying this process are not understood, but 5-HT_6 receptors have a role in neuronal plasticity (132) and can influence the actions of dopaminergic agents. Evidence also suggests that 5-HT_6 receptors could be involved in motor function, mood-dependent behavior, anxiety disorders, appetite control, anticonvulsant activity, and early growth processes involving 5-HT (117,119,123). With the newly identified 5-HT_6 agonists and antagonists, interest in the therapeutic potential of such agents is on the upswing.

5-HT_7 Receptors and Agents

Like 5-HT_5 receptors, 5-HT_7 receptors were once considered to be orphan receptors. Rat, mouse, guinea pig, and human 5-HT_7 receptors have now been cloned and are expressed mainly in the CNS (114,133). Structural analysis of the 5-HT_7 receptor suggests a seven transmembrane-spanning G protein–coupled receptor. These receptors are positively coupled to adenylate cyclase, and several splice variants have been identified. Alternative splicing in rat and human receptors results in four 5-HT_7 receptor isoforms that vary with respect to the length of their C-terminus chains (114,134). In rat, the isoforms are named 5-HT_{7a}, 5-HT_{7b}, and 5-HT_{7c}. Two of the isoforms are homologous in rat and human (5-HT_{7a} and 5-HT_{7b}). The third human isoform is named 5-HT_{7d}. These different isoforms could have important functional consequences, such as different distribution or G protein–coupling efficiency or different susceptibility to desensitization (134,135). Apparently, the three human isoforms are pharmacologically indistinguishable and show similar affinity for various ligands. Evidence suggests that 5-HT_7 receptors are constitutively active and that the degree of constitutive activity could vary among the isoforms. Nonselective agents with K_i values at 5-HT_7 receptors of 10 nM or less include 5-HT, 5-methoxytryptamine, LSD, methiothepin, and mesulergine; those with K_i values in the range of 10 to 100 nM include 8-OH

DPAT (long considered a 5-HT$_{1A}$–selective agonist!), spiperone, ritanserin, metergoline, mianserin, and chlorpromazine; those with K_i values in the range of 100 to 1,000 nM include NAN-190, sumatriptan, and haloperidol; and those with K_i values of greater than 1,000 nM include 2-methyl 5-HT, tropisetron, pindolol, and ketanserin. Reportedly, 5-HT, 5-CT, and 8-OH DPAT act as agonists, whereas methiothepin, mianserin, mesulergine, ritanserin, spiperone (a 5-HT$_{1A}$, 2-HT$_{2A}$, and D$_2$ antagonist), NAN-190 (a 5-HT$_{1A}$ antagonist), and clozapine act as antagonists. Numerous antidepressants and antipsychotic agents bind at 5-HT$_7$ receptors with nanomolar or subnanomolar affinity ($K_i \leq 10$ nM), including fluphenazine, acetophenazine, chlorprothixene, zotepine, clorotepine, clozapine, fluperlapine, pimozide, tiospirone, and risperidone (114,135).

5-HT$_7$ Antagonists

Several reasonably selective 5-HT$_7$ agents have been identified. The first reported 5-HT$_7$ antagonist was SB-258719 ($K_i \sim 30$ nM) (136), and attempts to optimize binding affinity and selectivity led to SB-269970 (*S*-isomer, K_i = 1.3 nM) (Fig. 11.21). Both compounds displayed some inverse agonist action. The high in vivo blood clearance of SB-269970 resulted in further structural modification, leading to compounds such as SB-656104 (*S*-isomer, K_i = 2 nM) (114). Another early series of 5-HT$_7$ antagonists was the DR compounds: DR4004 was the first of these to show activity as a competitive antagonist; structural modification resulted in others, including DR4365 (K_i = 4 nM) (137). Other antagonists Fig. 11 include phenylpyrrole-containing LCAPs (Fig. 11.21), which because of their structural similarity to other 5-HT$_{1A}$ ligands could have been expected to—and do—bind at 5-HT$_{1A}$ receptors (138); arylpiperazinosulfonamides; and tetrahydroisoquinolinylsulfonamides (139). Actually, the latter two types of compounds have been demonstrated to act as inverse agonists (139).

5-HT$_7$ Agonists

N-Arylaminoimidazolines (Fig. 11.22) were identified as the first 5-HT$_7$ agonists (140); however, they have not been pursued because of their profound effects on blood pressure and heart rate, which are probably a consequence of their affinity for α-adrenoceptors. Several new 5-HT$_7$ agonists have been recently reported, including the piperazinylhexanones (141) and 2-aminotetralins (142) (Fig. 11.22); the latter can function either as agonists (e.g., R = *n*Pr) or antagonists (e.g., R = Me), depending on the nature of the R group. Pharmacophore models have been proposed for 5-HT$_7$ agonists (143), antagonists (144), and inverse agonists (139).

5-HT$_7$ Receptors: Clinical Implications

Because of the previous unavailability of 5-HT$_7$–selective agents, the pharmacology of the 5-HT$_7$ system is still relatively unexplored. Nevertheless, studies with nonselective agents, 5-HT$_7$ receptor knockout animals, and some of the first few selective agents that were identified have provided some tantalizing clues (114,135,145–147). The 5-HT$_7$ receptors could be involved in mood and learning as well as in neuroendocrine and vegetative behaviors. The 5-HT$_2$ ligand ritanserin, certain tricyclic antidepressants (e.g., amitriptyline), classical antipsychotic agents (e.g., chlorpromazine), and nonclassical antipsychotic agents (e.g., clozapine) bind with K_i values of less than 100 nM (128). On this basis, it has been speculated that 5-HT$_7$ receptors may have a role in certain neuropsychiatric disorders. Consistent with these suggestions, 5-HT$_7$ receptors are sensitive to antidepressant treatment (148). The 5-HT$_7$ receptors have been implicated in serotonergic regulation of circadian rhythm, leading to suggestions that 5-HT$_7$–selective agents could be effective in the treatment of jet lag or sleep disorders of a circadian nature (149). 5-HT$_7$ receptors could also be involved in sleep disorders, anxiety, memory and cognition, epilepsy, pain, migraine, and thermoregulation. In the periphery, 5-HT produces both contraction and relaxation of coronary artery from various species (150). It has been proposed that relaxation of coronary artery may be mediated by 5-HT$_7$ receptors. Agents active at 5-HT$_7$ receptors could thus be effective in the treatment of coronary heart disease. Now that newer, more selective agents are finally available, many of these hypotheses can be further tested.

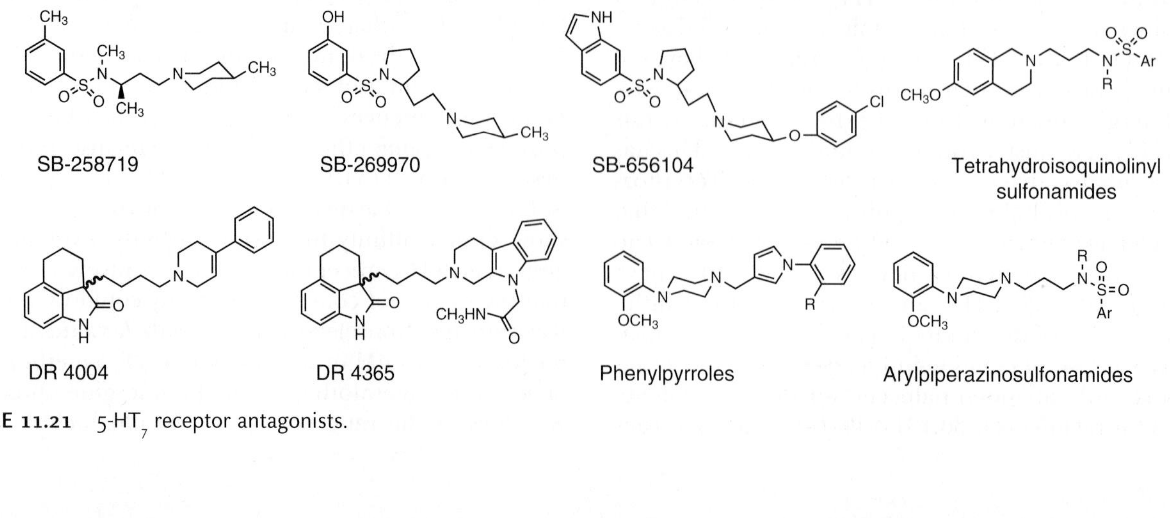

FIGURE 11.21 5-HT$_7$ receptor antagonists.

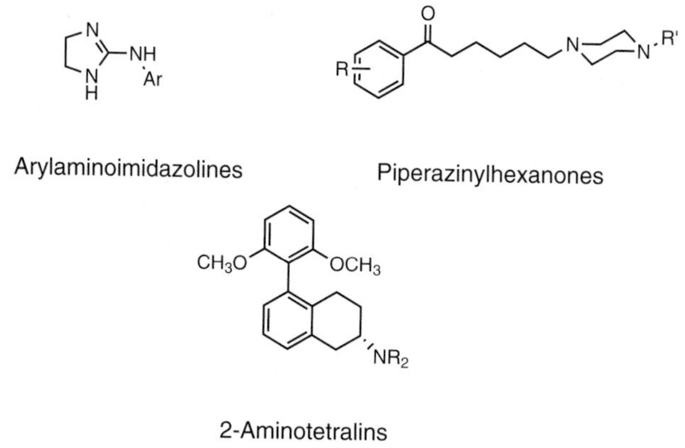

FIGURE 11.22 5-HT_7 receptor agonists.

THE SEROTONIN TRANSPORTER

The actions of 5-HT are terminated by its diffusion away from the synapse, by enzymatic degradation, and by reuptake into the presynaptic terminal (see Chapter 18 for further discussion). After reuptake, once 5-HT is inside the neuron, it can be re-stored in storage vesicles or metabolized. The 5-HT reuptake process involves a high-affinity transporter protein that is localized in the presynaptic terminal membrane. The 5-HT reuptake transporter (SERT) regulates the duration and magnitude of postsynaptic response to 5-HT. A different transporter is associated with different neurotransmitters (e.g., norepinephrine reuptake transporter [NET] transports norepinephrine). SERT has been cloned and expressed (138), and its putative structure is roughly similar to the general receptor structure shown in Figure 11.3 except that 1) it consists of 12 membrane-spanning helices, 2) both the amino terminus and the carboxy terminus are located on the intracellular side, and 3) it has an exaggerated extracellular loop between TM3 and TM4 (Fig. 11.23). SERT possesses approximately 50% homology with the NET and the dopamine transporter. For 5-HT transport, a ternary complex of protonated 5-HT, Na^+, and Cl^- binds to the transporter protein to form a quaternary complex; the transporter undergoes a conformational change to release 5-HT into the cytoplasm of the neuron (151).

The 5-HT transporter has been implicated as having a role in affective disorders (Chapter 18). Agents that block the transporter and, thereby, increase synaptic levels of 5-HT are useful for the treatment of depression, obsessive-compulsive behavior, and panic disorders. Tricyclic antidepressants (e.g., imipramine, desipramine) block the 5-HT transporter and the NET to varying degrees. Some display a preference for one transporter over the other, but most are nonselective (152). SSRIs display greater selectivity for SERT than for NET. The first SSRI to be used clinically was fluoxetine; several other agents have since become available. The SARs of SSRIs have been reviewed elsewhere (153); see Chapter 18 for further discussion of antidepressants and examples. Certain drugs of abuse (e.g., cocaine) also block the 5-HT transporter, although cocaine's primary mechanism of action likely involves the dopamine transporter.

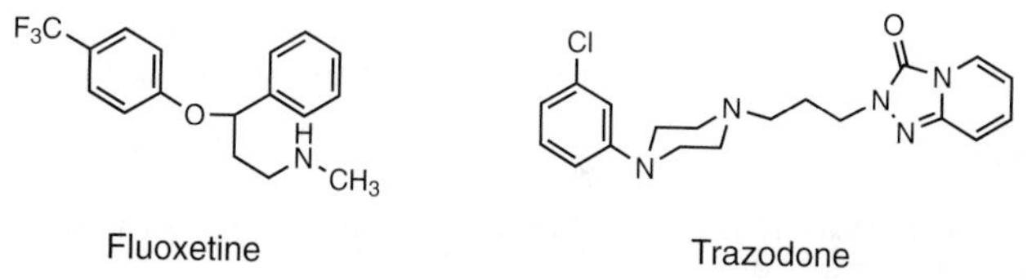

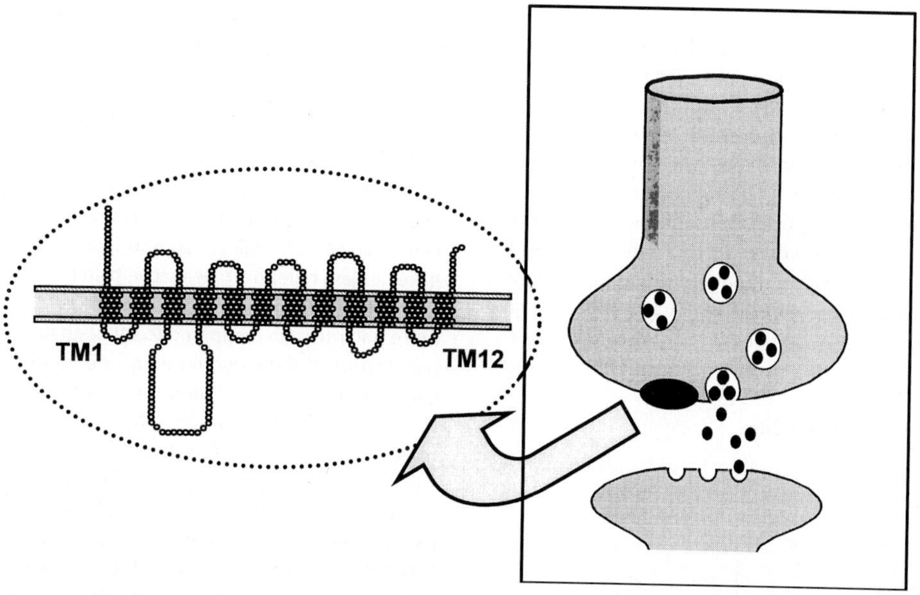

FIGURE 11.23 Schematic of a neuron showing the general location and basic structure (inset) of a serotonin transporter (SERT). Note that the transporter possesses 12 transmembrane-spanning helices (TM1–TM12). Both the amine terminus (attached to TM1) and the carboxy terminus (attached to TM12) are on the intracellular side.

Various tricyclic antidepressants and SSRIs, including fluoxetine, also bind at 5-HT_{2A} and 5-HT_{2C} receptors (154,155). The role, if any, derived from a direct interaction of these agents with 5-HT_2 receptors versus their interaction at SERT remains to be determined. 5-HT_2 antagonists typically downregulate 5-HT_2 receptors. The antidepressant trazodone, for example, is a weak SSRI but binds at 5-HT_2 receptors and is also a 5-HT_2 antagonist (155). The 5-HT_{2C} agonist *m*-chlorophenylpiperazine (*m*CPP) induces panic attacks in patients with panic disorder and increases obsessive compulsions in patients with obsessive-compulsive disorder (156), implicating a role for this specific 5-HT_{2C} subpopulation. The 5-HT_{2C} receptor antagonists could be useful targets for the development of novel agents to treat these disorders. This issue is complicated, however, by findings that trazodone is metabolized to *m*CPP and that, in some instances, trazodone possesses 5-HT_{2C} agonist properties (157). In any event, long-term treatment with tricyclic antidepressants (and MAOIs) leads to a downregulation in the number of 5-HT_2 receptors, the time course for which approximates the clinical response in depressed patients (152). Some SSRIs produce adaptive changes involving decreased responsiveness of 5-HT_2 receptors, whereas electroconvulsive therapy increases the number of 5-HT_2 receptors (152). Several 5-HT receptor populations have been implicated in the actions of antidepressants (e.g., 5-HT_1, 5-HT_2, 5-HT_6, and 5-HT_7), but SERT remains an attractive target for the development of novel psychotherapeutic agents.

SUMMARY

5-HT is a major neurotransmitter in the brain and is also involved in a number of peripheral actions. Seven families or populations of 5-HT receptors have been identified (5-HT_1 to 5-HT_7), and several are divided into distinct subpopulations (Table 11.2). Excluding splice variants, 14 different populations and subpopulations of 5-HT receptors have been cloned. Over the past 30 years, selective agonists and antagonists have been developed and identified for many of the subpopulations, but subpopulations remain for which selective agents have yet to be developed. The availability of such agents is important, because it aids functional investigations of the different 5-HT receptors. In addition to acting directly on 5-HT receptors, therapeutic agents with other mechanisms are available for influencing serotonergic transmission, including SSRIs and MAO inhibitors. Studies with 5-HT receptors have led to the introduction of agents useful for treating anxiety (e.g., buspirone), migraine (e.g., sumatriptan), irritable bowel syndrome (e.g. tegaserod), and chemotherapy-induced emesis (e.g., ondansetron); numerous other agents are currently in clinical trials for the treatment of depression, schizophrenia, and obsessive-compulsive and other disorders. Investigations also have led to a greater understanding of cardiovascular pharmacology, obesity, neurodegenerative disorders, aggression, sexual behavior, and drug abuse, just to mention a few examples. To reiterate a phrase from the introduction, "[I]t almost appears that 5-HT is involved in everything" (1).

SCENARIO: OUTCOME AND ANALYSIS

Outcome

Jill T. Johnson, PharmD, BCPS

The pharmacist referred her back to her physician to seek a different "triptan." The pharmacist also counseled the patient about using the drug for aborting migraines, not as prophylaxis. The pharmacist described medication overuse headaches that one can experience from taking triptans too often. Because the maximum dose of sumatriptan for migraines is 200 mg per day, the patient likely was experiencing overuse headaches. She was prescribed rizatriptan, which has worked to abort her migraines for many months. She takes rizatriptan only for aborting migraines and limits its use to not more than 15 mg in 24 hours. She now has fewer than 3 migraines in a month.

Chemical Analysis

Victoria Roche and S. William Zito

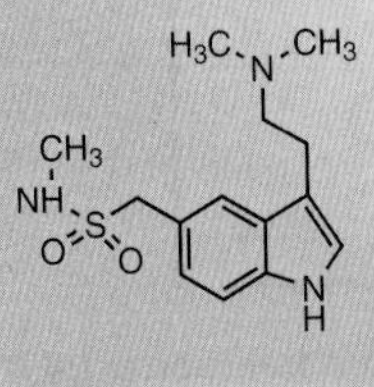

Sumatriptan

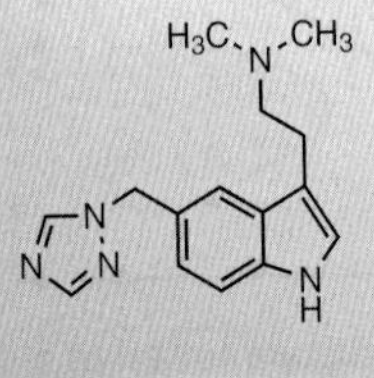

Rizatriptan

Both of the triptans associated with this scenario are indoleethylamines (tryptamines) that abort migraine headaches through their agonist action at 5-HT1D receptors. Sumatriptan was the first molecule in this class to be developed, and its selectivity for this receptor subtype, while acceptable, is not absolute. Other serotonergic receptors stimulated by sumatriptan include the 1B (formerly classified as a 1D receptor), 1A, and 1F subtypes, the latter of which also may be beneficial in treating migraines. Triptans work by constricting central vessels that dilate during migraine headaches. Overuse of vasoconstrictors results in rebound vasodilation, which could explain why MB's inappropriate (daily) use of sumatriptan gave her less relief from headache pain than expected.

The sulfonamide sidechain of sumatriptan produces a more polar triptan compared to other analogs that followed, and penetration of the blood–brain barrier under normal physiological conditions is low. Though rizatriptan's triazole substituent is certainly not the most lipophilic of rings, the drug's log P is higher than that of sumatripan (1.4 vs. 0.8). The more lipophilic structure confers a higher oral bioavailability on rizatriptan and allows a more facile penetration of the blood–brain barrier to reach central sites of action. The actual therapeutic impact of this enhanced distribution profile is, however, uncertain. The triazole ring of rizatriptan also confers a higher level of 5-HT1D selectivity than the methylsulfonamide moiety of sumatriptan.

SCENARIO: OUTCOME AND ANALYSIS *(Continued)*

As ethylamines, both sumatriptan and rizatriptan are vulnerable to oxidative deamination by MAO-A, and this is the major biotransformation route for both drugs. The *N*-dealkylated metabolite of rizatriptan (which forms before deamination) is known to be equally active with the parent structure, although it is generated to a minor (14%) extent.

Either triptan should be effective to abort MB's headaches if taken as directed, which is during the very early phase of a migraine when the pain level is low. Likewise, either triptan, if taken on a chronic basis rather than as needed, will promote rebound vasodilation and undermine therapeutic efficacy when it's needed most.

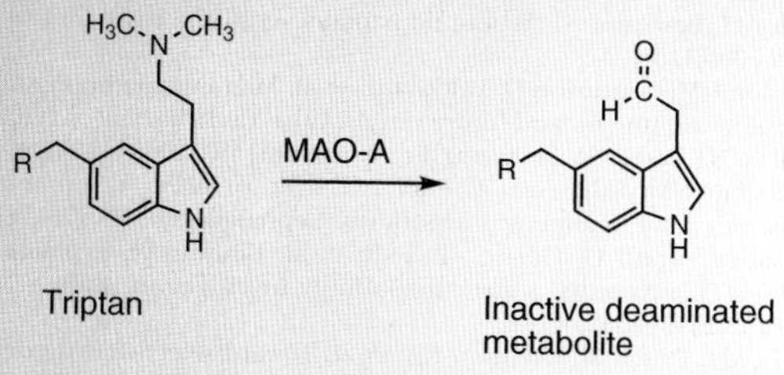

CASE STUDY

Victoria Roche and S. William Zito

Sr. MT is a 61-year-old woman with newly diagnosed ovarian cancer, and is a member of the Sisters of St. Agnes. The mission of this order of nuns includes community outreach related to social justice and health care, and Sr. MT is beloved by all those whom she has served over the years, including members of your family. Sr. MT will soon begin cisplatin/doxorubicin chemotherapy known as the AP regimen. She has been told that these two drugs induce severe nausea and vomiting that, in addition to occurring during or shortly after therapy, can also be delayed for several days after drug administration. Sr. MT has moderate coronary artery disease, and she is currently taking rosuvastatin to lower serum lipids and is taking propranolol (β-blocker)/hydrochlorothiazide (diuretic) antihypertensive therapy. Though she believes the propranolol in her blood pressure medication is helping her feel less anxious about the discomforting side effects of her chemotherapy, she also wants to minimize the disabling nausea and vomiting so she can continue serving her community for as long as possible.

Recognizing the value of serotonergic receptor antagonists in the treatment of chemotherapy-induced nausea, you recall the structures of three serotonin-related agents you studied in Medicinal Chemistry class, and contemplate their value in easing your friend's way in the days ahead.

1. Conduct a thorough and mechanistic SAR analysis of the three therapeutic options in the case.
2. Apply the chemical understanding gained from the SAR analysis to this patient's specific needs to make a therapeutic recommendation.

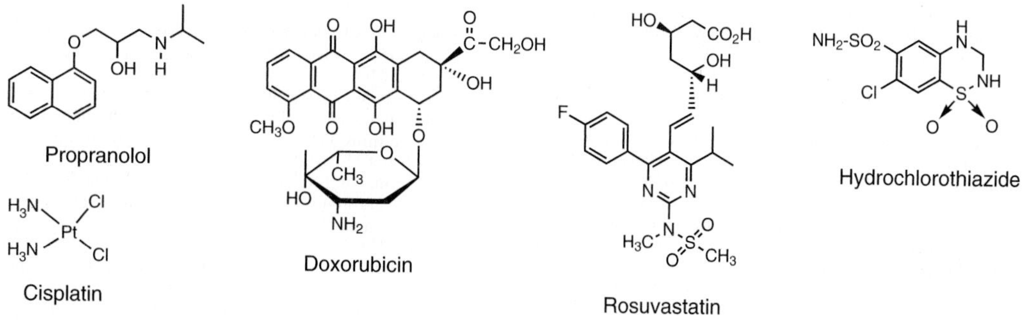

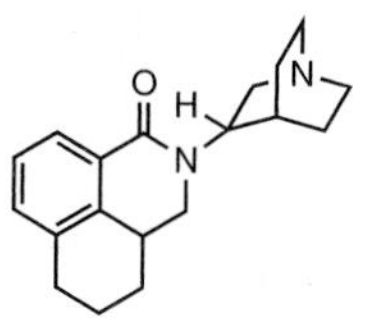

1

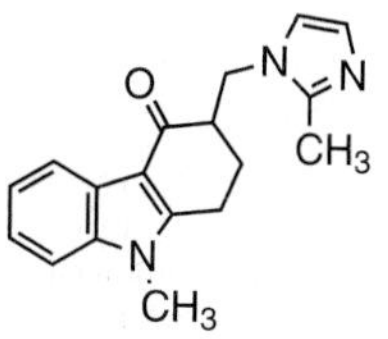

2

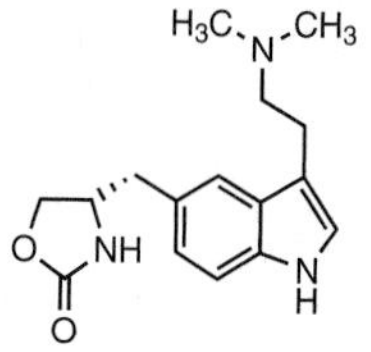

3

References

1. Rapport MR. The discovery of serotonin. Perspect Biol Med 1997;40:260–273.
2. Glennon RA, Dukat M. Serotonin receptors and drugs affecting serotonergic neurotransmission. In: Lemke TL, Williams DA, Roche VF, et al., eds. Foye's Principles of Medicinal Chemistry, 6th Ed. Philadelphia, PA: Lippincott Williams & Wilkins, 2008:415–443.
3. Roth BL, ed. The Serotonin Receptors: From Molecular Pharmacology to Human Therapeutics. Totowa, NJ: Humana Press, 2006.
4. Nichols DE, Nichols CD. Serotonin receptors. Chem Rev 2008;108:1614–1641.
5. Frazer A, Hensler JG. Serotonin. In: Siegel GJ, Agranoff BW, Albers RW, et al., eds. Basic Neurochemistry. New York: Raven Press, 1993:283–308.
6. Peroutka SJ, Snyder SH. Multiple serotonin receptors: differential binding of [^{3}H]5-hydroxytryptamine, [^{3}H]lysergic acid diethylamide and [^{3}H]spiroperidol. Mol Pharmacol 1979;16:687–699.
7. Hoyer D, Hannon JP, Martin GR. Molecular, pharmacological, and functional diversity of 5-HT receptors. Pharmacol Biochem Behav 2002;71:533–534.
8. Hartig PR, Branchek TA, Weinshank RL. A subfamily of 5-HT$_{1D}$ receptor genes. Trends Pharmacol Sci 1992;3:152–159.
9. Hoyer D, Clarke DE, Fozard JR, et al. International Union of Pharmacology Nomenclature and Classification of receptors for 5-hydroxytryptamine (serotonin). Pharmacol Rev 1994;46:157–203.
10. Westkaemper RB, Roth BL. Structure and function reveal insights into the pharmacology of 5-HT receptors. In: Roth BL, ed. The Serotonin Receptors: From Molecular Pharmacology to Human Therapeutics. Totowa, NJ: Humana Press, 2006:39–58.
11. van Wijngaarden I, Soudijn W, Tulp MTM. 5-HT$_{1A}$ receptor ligands. In: Olivier B, van Wijngaarden I, Soudin W, eds. Serotonin Receptors and Their Ligands. Amsterdam: Elsevier, 1997:17–43.
12. Glennon RA, Dukat M. 5-HT$_1$ receptor ligands: update 1997. Invest Drugs Res Alerts 1997;2:351–372.
13. Glennon RA. Strategies for the development of selective serotonergic agents. In: Roth BL, ed. The Serotonin Receptors: From Molecular Pharmacology to Human Therapeutics. Totowa, NJ: Humana Press, 2006.
14. Glennon RA. Concepts for the design of 5-HT$_{1A}$ serotonin agonists and antagonists. Drug Dev Res 1992;6:251–274.
15. Glennon RA, Iversen L. Antidepressants. In: Abraham DJ, Rotella DP, eds. Burger's Medicinal Chemistry and Drug Discovery, 7th Ed, Vol 8, CNS Disorders. New York: Wiley, 2010:219–264.
16. Kuipers W. Structural characteristics of 5-HT$_{1A}$ receptors and their ligands. In: Olivier B, van Wijngaarden I, Soudin W, eds. Serotonin Receptors and Their Ligands. Amsterdam: Elsevier, 1997:45–64.
17. De Vry J. 5-HT$_{1A}$ receptor agonists: recent developments and controversial issues. Psychopharmacology 1995;121:1–26.
18. Caliendo G, Santagada V, Perissutti E, et al. Derivatives as 5-HT$_{1A}$ receptor ligands—past and present. Curr Med Chem 2005;12:1721–1753.
19. File SE. Recent developments in anxiety, stress, and depression. Pharmacol Biochem Behav 1996;54:3–12.
20. Jones BJ, Blackburn TP. The medical benefit of 5-HT research. Pharmacol Biochem Behav 2002;71:555–568.
21. Chessick CA, Allen MH, Thase M, et al. Azapirones for generalized anxiety disorder. Cochrane Database Syst Rev 2006;3:CD006115.
22. Picard M, Morisset S, Cloix JF, et al. Pharmacological, neurochemical, and behavioral profile of JB-788, a new 5-HT$_{1A}$ agonist. Neuroscience 2010;169:1337–1347.
23. Fletcher A, Cliffe I, Dourish CT. Silent 5-HT$_{1A}$ receptor antagonists: utility as research tools and therapeutic agents. Trends Pharmacol Sci 1993;14:441–448.
24. Assie M-B, Koek W. Effects of 5-HT$_{1A}$ receptor antagonists on hippocampal 5-hydroxytryptamine levels: (S)-WAY100135, but not WAY100635, has partial agonist properties. Eur J Pharmacol 1996;304:15–21.
25. Darmani NA, Reeves SL. The mechanism by which the selective 5-HT$_{1A}$ receptor antagonist S-(–)-UH-301 produces head-twitches in mice. Pharmacol Biochem Behav 1996;55:1–10.
26. Mundey MK, Fletcher A, Marsden CA. Effects of 8-OH DPAT and 5-HT$_{1A}$ antagonists WAY 100135 and WAY 100635 on guinea pig behavior and dorsal raphe 5-HT neuron firing. Br J Pharmacol 1996;117:750–756.
27. Arborelius L, Nomikos GG, Hertel P, et al. The 5-HT$_{1A}$ receptor antagonist (S)-UH-301 augments the increase in extracellular concentrations of 5-HT in the frontal cortex produced by both acute and chronic treatment with citalopram. Naunyn-Schmiedeberg Arch Pharmacol 1996;353:630–640.
28. Grignaschi G, Invernizzi RW, Fanelli E, et al. Citalopram-induced hypophagia is enhanced by blockade of 5-HT$_{1A}$ receptors: role of 5-HT$_{2C}$ receptors. Br J Pharmacol 1998;124:1781–1787.
29. Segrave R, Nathan PJ. Pindolol augmentation of selective serotonin reuptake inhibitors: accounting for the variability of results of placebo-controlled double-blind studies in patients with major depression. Human Psychopharmacol 2005;20:163–174.
30. Rasmussen K, Calligaro DO, Czachura JF, et al. The novel 5-hydroxytryptamine$_{1A}$ antagonist LY426965: effects on nicotine withdrawal and interactions with fluoxetine. J Pharmacol Exp Ther 2000;294:688–700.
31. Schoeffter P, Hoyer D. Interaction of arylpiperazines with 5-HT$_{1A}$, 5-HT$_{1B}$, 5-HT$_{1C}$, and 5-HT$_{1D}$ receptors. Do discriminatory 5-HT$_{1B}$ receptor ligands exist? Naunyn-Schmiedeberg Arch Pharmacol 1989;339:675–683.
32. Glennon RA, Westkaemper RB. 5-HT$_{1D}$ receptors: a serotonin receptor population for the 1990s. Drug News Perspect 1993;6:390–405.
33. Middlemiss DN, Beer MS, Matassa VG. 5-HT1D receptors. In: Olivier B, van Wijngaarden I, Soudin W, eds. Serotonin Receptors and Their Ligands. Amsterdam: Elsevier, 1997:101–138.
34. Adham N, Tamm JA, Salon JA, et al. A single point mutation increases the affinity of serotonin 5-HT$_{1D\alpha}$, 5-HT$_{1D\beta}$, 5-HT$_{1E}$, and 5-HT$_{1F}$ receptors for β-adrenergic antagonists. Neuropharmacology 1994;33:387–391.
35. Glennon RA, Dukat M, Westkaemper RB, et al. The binding of propranolol at 5-hydroxytryptamine$_{1D\beta}$ T355N mutant receptors may involve formation of two hydrogen bonds to asparagine. Mol Pharmacol 1996;49:198–206.
36. Hamel E. 5-HT$_{1D}$ receptors: pharmacology and therapeutic potential. Serotonin 1996;1:19–29.
37. Saxena PR, Tfelt-Hansen P. Success and failure of triptans. J Headache Pain 2001;2:3–11.
38. Ahn AH, Basbaum AI. Where do triptans act in the treatment of migraine? Pain 2005;115:1–4.
39. Villalon CM, Centurion D, Valdivia IF, et al. Migraine: pathophysiology, pharmacology treatment, and future trends. Curr Vasc Pharmacol 2003;1:71–84.
40. Mathew NT, Loder EW. Evaluating the triptans. Am J Med 2005;118(Suppl 1):28S–35S.
41. Ramadan NM, Skljarevski V, Phebus LA, et al. 5-HT$_{1F}$ receptor agonists in acute migraine treatment: a hypothesis. Cephalgia 2003;23:778–785.
42. Dukat M, Smith C, Herrick-Davis K, et al. Binding of tryptamine analogs at h5-HT$_{1E}$ receptors: a structure–affinity investigation. Bioorg Med Chem 2004;12:2545–2552.
43. Klein MT, Dukat M, Glennon RA, et al. Toward selective drug development for the human 5-HT$_{1E}$ receptor: a comparison of 5-HT$_{1E}$ and 5-HT$_{1F}$ receptor structure-affinity relationships. J Pharmacol Exp Ther 2011;337:860–867.
44. McAllister G, Castro JL. 5-HT$_{1E}$ and 5-HT$_{1F}$ receptors. In: Olivier B, van Wijngaarden I, Soudin W, eds. Serotonin Receptors and Their Ligands. Amsterdam: Elsevier, 1997:141–157.
45. Phebus LA, Johnson KW, Zgombick JM, et al. Characterization of LY344864 as a pharmacological tool to study 5-HT$_{1F}$ receptors: binding affinities, brain penetration, and activity in the neurogenic dural inflammation model of migraine. Life Sci 1997;61:2117–2126.
46. Nelson DL, Phebus LA, Johnson KW, et al. Preclinical pharmacological profile of the selective 5-HT$_{1F}$ receptor agonist lasmiditan. Cephalalgia 2010;30:1159–1169.
47. Sanders-Bush E, Fentress H, Hazelwood L. Serotonin 5-HT$_2$ receptors: molecular and genomic diversity. Mol Interventions 2003;3:319–330.
48. Leysen JE. 5-HT$_2$ receptors. Curr Drug Targets CNS Neurol Disord 2004;3:11–26.
49. Gavarini S, Becamel C, Chanrion B, et al. Molecular and functional characterization of proteins interacting with the C-terminal domains of 5-HT$_2$ receptors: emergence of 5-HT$_2$ "receptorsomes." Biol Cell 2004;96:373–381.
50. Roth B, Willins DL, Kristiansen K, et al. 5-hydroxytryptamine2-family receptors (5-hydroxytryptamine$_{2A}$, 5-hydroxytryptamine$_{2B}$, 5-hydroxytryptamine$_{2C}$): where structure meets function. Pharmacol Ther 1998;79:231–257.
51. van Wijngaarden I, Soudijn W. 5-HT$_{2A}$, 5-HT$_{2B}$, and 5-HT$_{2C}$ receptor ligands. In: Olivier B, van Wijngaarden I, Soudin W, eds. Serotonin Receptors and Their Ligands. Amsterdam: Elsevier, 1997:161–197.
52. Johnson MP, Wainscott DB, Lucaites VL, et al. Mutations of transmembrane IV and V serines indicate that all tryptamines do not bind to rat 5-HT$_{2A}$ receptors in the same manner. Mol Brain Res 1997;49:1–6.
53. Glennon RA, Seggel MR, Soine WH, et al. [^{125}I]-1-(2,5-Dimethoxy-4-iodophenyl)-2-aminopropane: an iodinated radioligand that specifically labels the agonist high-affinity state of 5-HT$_2$ serotonin receptors. J Med Chem 1988;31:5–7.
54. Glennon RA, Dukat M, El-Bermawy M, et al. Influence of amine substituents on 5-HT$_{2A}$ versus 5-HT$_{2C}$ binding of phenylalkyl- and indolylalkylamines. J Med Chem 1994;37:1929–1935.
55. Nichols DE, Frescas SP, Chemel BR, et al. High specific activity tritium-labeled N-(2-methoxybenzyl)-2,5-dimethoxy-4-iodophenethylamine (INBMeO): a high-affinity 5-HT$_{2A}$ receptor-selective agonist radioligand. Bioorg Med Chem 2008;16:6116–6123.
56. Glennon RA, Bondarev ML, Khorana N, et al. β-Oxygenated analogues of the 5-HT$_{2A}$ serotonin agonist 1-(4-bromo-2,5-dimethoxyphenyl)-2-aminopropane. J Med Chem 2004;47:6034–6041.
57. Sharif NA. Serotonin-2 receptor agonists as novel ocular hypotensive agents and their cellular and molecular mechanisms of action. Curr Drug Targets 2010;11:978–993.
58. Kehne JH, Baron BM, Carr AA, et al. Preclinical characterization of the potential of the putative atypical antipsychotic MDL 100,907 as a potent 5-HT$_{2A}$ antagonist with a favorable CNS safety profile. J Pharmacol Exp Ther 1996;277:968–981.
59. Metwally KA, Dukat M, Egan CT, et al. Spiperone: influence of spiro ring substituents on 5-HT$_{2A}$ serotonin receptor binding. J Med Chem 1998;41:5084–5093.
60. Knight AR, Misra A, Quirk K, et al. Pharmacological characterisation of the agonist radioligand binding site of 5-HT$_{2A}$, 5-HT$_{2B}$ and 5-HT$_{2C}$ receptors. Naunyn Schmiedeberg Arch Pharmacol 2004;370:114–123.
61. Monti JM. Serotonin 5-HT$_{2A}$ receptor antagonists in the treatment of insomnia: present status and future prospects. Drugs Today 2010;46:183–193.

62. Landolt HP, Wehrle R. Antagonism of serotonergic 5-HT$_{2A/2C}$ receptors: mutual improvement of sleep, cognition and mood? Eur J Neurosci 2009;29:1795–1809.
63. Meltzer HY, Li Z, Kaneda Y, et al. Serotonin receptors: their key role in drugs to treat schizophrenia. Prog Neuropsychopharmacol Biol Psychiatry 2003;27:1159–1172.
64. Reynolds GP. Receptor mechanisms in the treatment of schizophrenia. J Psychopharmacol 2004;18:340–345.
65. Leucht S, Corves C, Arbter D, et al. Second-generation versus first-generation antipsychotic drugs for schizophrenia: a meta-analysis. Lancet 2009;373:31–41.
66. Glennon RA. Do hallucinogens act as 5-HT$_2$ agonists or antagonists? Neuropsychopharmacology 1990;56:509–517.
67. Nelson DL, Lucaites VL, Wainscott DB, et al. Comparison of hallucinogenic phenylisopropylamine binding affinities at cloned human 5-HT$_{2A}$, 5-HT$_{2B}$, and 5-HT$_{2C}$ receptors. Naunyn-Schmiedeberg Arch Pharmacol 1999;359:1–6.
68. Smith RL, Canton H, Barrett RJ, et al. Agonist properties of N,N-dimethyltryptamine at serotonin 5-HT$_{2A}$ and 5-HT$_{2C}$ receptors. Pharmacol Biochem Behav 1998;61:323–330.
69. Newton RA, Phipps SL, Flanigan TP, et al. Characterisation of human 5-hydroxytryptamine$_{2A}$ and 5-hydroxytryptamine$_{2C}$ receptors expressed in the human neuroblastoma cell line SH-SY5Y: comparative stimulation by hallucinogenic drugs. J Neurochem 1996;67:2521–2531.
70. Nelson DL. The serotonin2 (5-HT$_2$) subfamily of receptors: pharmacological challenges. Med Chem Res 1993;3:306–316.
71. Wainscott DB, Sasso DA, Kursar JD, et al. [^{3}H]Rauwolscine: an antagonist radioligand for the cloned human 5-hydroxytryptamine$_{2B}$ (5-HT$_{2B}$) receptor. Naunyn-Schmiedeberg Arch Pharmacol 1998;375:17–24.
72. Rothman RB, Baumann MH, Savage JE, et al. Evidence for possible involvement of 5-HT$_{2B}$ receptors in the cardiac valvulopathy associated with fenfluramine and other serotonergic medications. Circulation 2000;102:2836–2841.
73. SetolaV,HufeisenSJ,Grande-AllenKJ,etal.3,4-Methylenedioxymethamphetamine (MDMA, "Ecstasy") induces fenfluramine-like proliferative actions on human cardiac valvular interstitial cells in vitro. Mol Pharmacol 2003;63:1223–1229.
74. Auclair AL, Cathala A, Sarrazin F, et al. The central serotonin 2B receptor: a new pharmacological target to modulate the mesoaccumbens dopaminergic pathway activity. J Neurochem 2010;114:1323–1332.
75. Duxon MS, Flanigan TP, Reavley AC, et al. Evidence for expression of the 5-hydroxytryptamine-2B receptor system in the rat central nervous system. Neuroscience 1997;76:323–329.
76. Lee J, Jung ME, Lee J. 5-HT$_{2C}$ receptor modulators: a patent survey. Expert Opin Ther Pat 2010;20:1429–1455.
77. Bős M, Jenck F, Martin JR, et al. Novel agonists of 5-HT$_{2C}$ receptors. Synthesis and biological evaluation of 2-(indol-1-yl)-1-methylethylamines and 2-(indeno[1,2-b]pyrrol-1-yl)-1-methylethylamines. Improved therapeutics for obsessive compulsive disorder. J Med Chem 1997;40:2762–2769.
78. Chang-Fong J, Addo J, Dukat M, et al. Evaluation of isotryptamine derivatives at 5-HT$_2$ serotonin receptors. Bioorg Med Chem Lett 2002;12:155–158.
79. Martin JR, Bos M, Jenck F, et al. 5-HT$_{2C}$ receptor agonists: pharmacological characteristics and therapeutic potential. J Pharmacol Exp Ther 1998;286:913–924.
80. Dunlop J, Marquis KL, Lim HK, et al. Pharmacological profile of the 5-HT2C receptor agonist WAY-163909; therapeutic potential in multiple indications. CNS Drug Rev 2006;12:167–177.
81. Smith BM, Smith JM, Tsai JH, et al. Discovery and structure-activity relationship of (1*R*)-8-chloro-2,3,4,5-tetrahydro-1-methyl-1*H*-3-benzazepine (lorcaserin), a selective 5-HT$_{2C}$ receptor agonist for the treatment of obesity. J Med Chem 2008;51:305–313.
82. Booth RG, Fang L, Huang Y, et al. (1*R*,3*S*)-(-)-*trans*-PAT: a novel full-efficacy serotonin 5-HT$_{2C}$ receptor agonist with 5-HT$_{2A}$ and 5-HT$_{2B}$ receptor inverse agonist/antagonist activity. Eur J Pharmacol 2009;61:1–9.
83. Wood MD, Reavill C, Trail B, et al. SB-243213; a selective 5-HT$_{2C}$ receptor inverse agonist with improved anxiolytic profile: lack of tolerance and withdrawal anxiety. Neuropharmacology 2001;41:186–199.
84. Bromidge SM, Dabbs S, Davies DT, et al. Biarylcarbamoylindolines are novel and selective 5-HT$_{2C}$ receptor inverse agonists: identification of 5-methyl-1-[[2-[(2-methyl-3-pyridyl)oxy]-5-pyridyl]carbamoyl]-6-trifluoromethylindoline (SB-243213) as a potential antidepressant/ anxiolytic agent. J Med Chem 2000;43:1123–1134.
85. Hale A, Corral RM, Mencacci C, et al. Superior antidepressant efficacy results of agomelatine versus fluoxetine in severe MDD patients: a randomized, double-blind study. Int Clin Psychopharmacol 2010;25:305–314.
86. Lummis SC. The transmembrane domain of the 5-HT$_3$ receptors: its role in selectivity and gating. Biochem Soc Trans 2004;32(Part 3):535–539.
87. Walstab J, Rappold G, Niesler B. 5-HT$_3$ receptors: role in disease and target of drugs. Pharmacol Ther 2010;128:146–169.
88. Farber L, Haus U, Spath M, et al. Physiology and pathophysiology of the 5-HT$_3$ receptor. Scand J Rheumatol Suppl 2004;119:2–8.
89. Holbrook JD, Gill CH, Zebda N, et al. Characterisation of 5-HT$_{3C}$, 5-HT$_{3D}$ and 5-HT$_{3E}$ receptor subunits: evolution, distribution and function. J Neurochem 2009;108:384–396.
90. Dukat M. 5-HT$_3$ serotonin receptor agonists: a pharmacophoric journey. Curr Med Chem 2004;4:77–94.
91. Campiani G, Cappelli A, Nacci V, et al. Novel and highly potent 5-HT$_3$ receptor agonists based on a pyrroloquinozaline structure. J Med Chem 1997;40:3670–3678.
92. Katounina T, Besret L, Dhilly M, et al. Synthesis and biological investigations of [^{18}F]MR 18445, a 5-HT$_3$ receptor partial agonist. Bioorg Med Chem 1998;6:789–795.
93. Gozlan H. 5-HT$_3$ receptors. In: Olivier B, van Wijngaarden I, Soudin W, eds. Serotonin Receptors and Their Ligands. Amsterdam: Elsevier, 1997:221–258.
94. Gaster LM, King FD. Serotonin 5-HT$_3$ and 5-HT$_4$ receptor antagonists. Med Res Rev 1997;17:163–214.
95. Heidempergher F, Pillan A, Pinciroli V, et al. Phenylimidazolidin-2-one derivatives as selective 5-HT$_3$ receptor antagonists and refinement of the pharmacophore model for 5-HT$_3$ receptor binding. J Med Chem 1997;40:3369–3380.
96. De Wit R, Aapro M, Blower PR. Is there a pharmacological basis for differences in 5-HT$_3$-receptor antagonist efficacy in refractory patients? Cancer Chemother Pharmacol 2005;56:231–238.
97. Jordin K, Kasper C, Schmoll H-J. Chemotherapy-induced nausea and vomiting: current and new standards in antiemetic prophylaxis and treatment. Eur J Cancer 2005;41:199–205.
98. Aapro M, Blower P. 5-Hydroxytryptamine type-3 antagonists for chemotherapy-induced and radiotherapy-induced nausea and vomiting. Cancer 2005;104:1–13.
99. Aapro M. Optimizing antiemetic therapy: what are the problems and how can they be overcome? Curr Med Res Opin 2005;21:885–897.
100. Bockaert J, Claeysen S, Compau V, et al. 5-HT$_4$ receptors. Curr Drug Targets CNS Neurol Disord 2004;3:39–51.
101. Gerald C, Adham N, Kao H-T, et al. The 5-HT$_4$ receptor: molecular cloning and pharmacological classification of two splice variants. EMBO J 1995;14:2806–2815.
102. Blondel O, Gastineau M, Dahmoune Y, et al. Cloning, expression, and pharmacology of four human 5-hydroxytryptamine$_4$ receptor isoforms produced by alternative splicing in the carboxyl terminus. J Neurochem 1998;70:2252–2261.
103. Eglen RM, Bonhaus DW, Clark RD, et al. (R) and (S) RS 56532: mixed 5-HT$_3$ and 5-HT$_4$ receptor ligands with opposing enantiomeric selectivity. Neuropharmacology 1994;33:515–526.
104. Langlois M, Fischmeister R. 5-HT$_4$ receptor ligands: applications and new prospects. J Med Chem 2003;30:319–344.
105. Lopez-Rodriguez ML, Benhamu B, Morcillo MJ, et al. 5-HT$_4$ receptor antagonists: structure–affinity relationships and ligand receptor interactions. Curr Top Med Chem 2002;2:625–641.
106. Maillet M, Robert SJ, Lezoualch F. New insights into serotonin 5-HT$_4$ receptors: a novel therapeutic target for Alzheimer's disease? Curr Alzheimer Res 2004;1:79–85.
107. Eglen RM, Wong EHF, Dumuis A, et al. Central 5-HT$_4$ receptors. Trends Pharmacol Sci 1995;16:391–398.
108. Bijak M, Tokarski K, Maj J. Repeated treatment with antidepressant drugs induces subsensitivity to the excitatory effect of 5-HT$_4$ receptor activation in the rat hippocampus. Naunyn-Schmiedeberg Arch Pharmacol 1997;355:14–19.
109. Schaus JM, Thompson DC, Bloomquist WE, et al. Synthesis and structure–activity relationships of potent and orally active 5-HT$_4$ receptor antagonists: indazole and benzimidazolone derivatives. J Med Chem 1998;41: 1943–1955.
110. Johanson JF. Options for patients with irritable bowel syndrome: contrasting traditional; and novel serotonergic therapies. Neurogastroenterol Motil 2004;16:701–711.
111. Gershon MD. Review article: serotonin receptors and transporters—roles in normal and abnormal gastrointestinal motility. Aliment Pharmacol Ther 2004;20(Suppl 7):3–14.
112. Nelson DL. 5-HT$_5$ receptors. Curr Drug Targets CNS Neurol Disord 2004;3:53–58.
113. Raymond JR, Turner JH, Gelasca AK, et al. 5-HT receptor signal transduction pathways. In: Roth BL, ed. The Serotonin Receptors: From Molecular Pharmacology to Human Therapeutics. Totowa, NJ: Humana Press, 2006:143–206.
114. Glennon RA. Higher-end serotonin receptors: 5-HT$_5$, 5-HT$_6$, and 5-HT$_7$. J Med Chem 2003;46:2795–2812.
115. Dubertret C, Hanoun N, Ades J, et al. Family-based association studies between 5-HT$_{5A}$ receptor gene and schizophrenia. J Psychiat Res 2004;38:371–376.
116. Doly S, Fischer J, Brisorgueh M-J, et al. 5-HT$_{5A}$ receptor localization in the rat spinal cord suggests a role in nociception and control of pelvic floor musculature. J Comp Neurol 2004;476:316–329.
117. Woolley ML, Marsden CA, Fone KC. 5-HT$_6$ receptors. Curr Drug Targets CNS Neurol Disord 2004;3:59–79.
118. Kohen R, Metcalf MA, Khan N, et al. Cloning, characterization, and chromosomal localization of a human 5-HT6 serotonin receptor. J Neurochem 1996;66:47–56.

119. Glennon RA, Lee M, Rangisetty JB, et al. 2-Substituted tryptamines: agents with selectivity for 5-HT_6 serotonin receptors. J Med Chem 2000;43:1011–1018.
120. Sleight AJ, Boess FG, Bos M, et al. Characterization of Ro 04-6790 and Ro 63-0563; potent and selective antagonists at human and rat 5-HT_6 receptors. Br J Pharmacol 1998;124:556–562.
121. Bromidge SM, Brown AM, Clarke SE, et al. 5-Chloro-*N*-(4-methoxy-3-piperazin-1-yl-phenyl)-3-methyl-2-benzothiophenesulfonamide (SB-271046): a potent, selective, and orally bioavailable 5-HT_6 receptor antagonist. J Med Chem 1999;42:202–205.
122. Tsai Y, Dukat M, Slassi A, et al. *N*1-(Benzenesulfonyl)tryptamines as novel 5-HT_6 antagonists. Bioorg Med Chem Lett 2000;10:2295–2299.
123. Russell MGN, Baker RJ, Barden L, et al. *N*-Arylsulfonylindole derivatives as serotonin 5-HT_6 receptor ligands. J Med Chem 2001;44:3881–3895.
124. Zhou P, Yan Y, Bernotas R, et al. 4-(2-Aminoethoxy)-*N*-(phenylsulfonyl) indoles as novel 5-HT_6 receptor ligands. Bioorg Med Chem Lett 2005;15:1393–1396.
125. Holenz J, Merce R, Diaz JL, et al. Medicinal chemistry driven approaches toward novel and selective 5-HT_6 receptor ligands. J Med Chem 2005;48:1781–1795.
126. Cole DC, Lennox WJ, Lombardi S, et al. Discovery of 5-arylsulfonamido-3-(pyrrolidin-2-ylmethyl)-1*H*-indole derivatives as potent, selective 5-HT_6 receptor agonists and antagonists. J Med Chem 2005;48:353–356.
127. Glennon RA, Siripurapu U, Roth BL, et al. The medicinal chemistry of 5-HT_6 receptor ligands with a focus on arylsulfonyltryptamines. Curr Topics Med Chem 2010;10:579–595.
128. Roth BL, Craigo SC, Choudhary MS, et al. Binding of typical and atypical antipsychotic agents to 5-hydroxytryptamine-6 and 5-hydroxytryptamine-7 receptors. J Pharmacol Exp Ther 1994;268:1403–1410.
129. Hedley L, Kamphuis S, Secchi R, et al. The combined effects of the 5-HT_{2A} antagonist MDL 100,907 and the selective 5-HT_6 receptor antagonist Ro 4368554 in rat models of psychosis and cognition. Behav Pharmacol 2005;16(Suppl 1):S23.
130. Frantz KJ, Hannson KJ, Stouffer DG, et al. 5-HT_6 receptor antagonism potentiates the behavioral and neurochemical effects of amphetamine but not cocaine. Neuropharmacology 2002;42:170–180.
131. Dawson LA, Nguyen HQ, Li P. Potentiation of amphetamine-induced changes in dopamine and 5-HT by a 5-HT_6 receptor antagonist. Brain Res Bull 2003;59:513–521.
132. Svenningsson P, Tzavara ET, Liu F, et al. DARPP-32 mediates serotonergic neurotransmission in the forebrain. Proc Nat Acad Sci USA 2002;99:3188–3193.
133. Eglen RM, Jasper JR, Chang DJ, et al. The 5-HT_7 receptor: orphan found. Trends Pharmacol Sci 1997;18:104–107.
134. Heidmann DE, Metcalf MA, Kohen R, et al. Four 5-hydroxytryptamine$_7$ (5-HT_7) receptor isoforms in human and rat produced by alternative splicing. Species differences due to altered intron–exon organization. J Neurochem 1997;68:1372–1381.
135. Vanhoenacker P, Haegeman G, Leysen JE. 5-HT_7 receptors: current knowledge and future prospects. Trends Pharmacol Sci 2000;21:70–77.
136. Forbes IT, Dabbs S, Duckworth DM, et al. *R*-3,*N*-Dimethyl-*N*-[1-methyl-3-(4-methylpiperidin-1-yl)propyl]benzenesulfonamide: the first selective 5-HT_7 receptor antagonist. J Med Chem 1998;41:655–657.
137. Kikuchi C, Ando T, Watanabe T, et al. 2α-[4-(Tetrahydropyrodoindol-2-yl) butyl]tetrahydrobenzindole derivatives: new, selective, antagonists of the 5-hydroxytryptamine$_7$ receptor. J Med Chem 2002;45:2197–2206.
138. Paillet-Loilier M, Fabis F, Lepailleur A, et al. Phenylpyrroles, a new chemolibrary virtual screening class of 5-HT_7 receptor ligands. Bioorg Med Chem Lett 2005;15:3753–3757.
139. Vermeulen ES, van Smeden M, Schmidt AW, et al. Novel 5-HT7 receptor inverse agonists. Synthesis and molecular modeling of arylpiperazine- and 1,2,3,4-tetrahydroisoquinolin-based arylsulfonamides. J Med Chem 2004;47:5451–5466.
140. Parikh V, Welch WM, Schmidt AW. Discovery of a series of (4,5-dihydroimidazol-2-yl)biphenylamine 5-HT_7 agonists. Bioorg Med Chem Lett 2003;13:269–271.
141. Perrone R, Berardi F, Colabufo NA, et al. Synthesis and structure–affinity relationships of 1-[ω-(4-aryl-1-piperazinyl)alkyl]-1-aryl ketones as 5-HT_7 receptor ligands. J Med Chem 2003;46:646–649.
142. Holmberg P, Sohn D, Leideborg R, et al. Novel 2-aminotetralin and 3-aminochroman derivatives as selective serotonin 5-HT_7 receptor agonists and antagonists. J Med Chem 2004;47:3927–3930.
143. Vermeulen ES, Schmidt AW, Sprouse JS, et al. Characterization of the 5-HT_7 receptor. Determination of the pharmacophore for 5-HT_7 receptor agonism and CoMFA-based modeling of the agonist binding site. J Med Chem 2003;46:5365–5374.
144. Lopez-Rodriguez ML, Porras E, Morcillo MJ, et al. Optimization of the pharmacophore model for 5-HT_7R antagonism. Design and synthesis of new naphtholoactam and naphthosultam derivatives. J Med Chem 2003;46:5638–5650.
145. Pouzet B. SB-258741: a 5-HT_7 receptor antagonist of potential clinical interest. CNS Drug Rev 2002;8:90–100.
146. Thomas DR, Hagan JJ. 5-HT_7 receptors. Curr Drug Targets CNS Neurol Disord 2004;3:81–90.
147. Hedlund PB, Sutcliffe JG. Functional, molecular and pharmacological advances in 5-HT_7 receptor research. Trends Pharmacol Sci 2004;25: 481–486.
148. Sleight AJ, Carolo C, Petit N, et al. Identification of 5-hydroxytryptamine$_7$ receptor binding sites in rat hypothalamus: sensitivity to chronic antidepressant treatment. Mol Pharmacol 1995;47:99–103.
149. Lovenberg TW, Baron BM, de Lecea L, et al. A novel adenylyl cyclase–activating serotonin receptor (5-HT_7) implicated in the regulation of mammalian circadian rhythms. Neuron 1993;11:449–458.
150. Cushing DJ, Zgombick JM, Nelson DL, et al. LY215840, a high-affinity 5-HT_7 receptor ligand blocks serotonin-induced relaxation in canine coronary artery. J Pharmacol Exp Ther 1996;277:1560–1566.
151. Barker EL, Blakely RD. Norepinephrine and serotonin transporters. In: Bloom FE, Kupfer DJ, eds. Psychopharmacology: The Fourth Generation of Progress. New York: Raven Press, 1995:321–333.
152. Maes M, Meltzer HY. The serotonin hypothesis of major depression. In: Bloom FE, Kupfer DJ, eds. Psychopharmacology: The Fourth Generation of Progress. New York: Raven Press, 1995:933–944.
153. Soudjin W, van Wijngaarden I. 5-HT transporter. In: Olivier B, van Wijngaarden I, Soudin W, eds. Serotonin Receptors and Their Ligands. Amsterdam: Elsevier, 1997:327–361.
154. Stanford SC. Prozac: panacea or puzzle? Trends Pharmacol Sci 1996;17:150–154.
155. Jenck F, Moreau JL, Mutel V, et al. Brain 5-HT_{1C} receptors and antidepressants. Prog Neuropsychopharmacol Biol Psychiatry 1994;18:563–574.
156. Broekkamp CLE, Leysen D, Peeters BWMM, et al. Prospects for improved antidepressants. J Med Chem 1995;38:4615–4633.
157. Marcoli M, Maura G, Tortarolo M, et al. Trazodone is a potent agonist at 5-HT_{2C} receptors mediating inhibition of the *N*-methyl-D-aspartate/nitric oxide/cyclic GMP pathway in rat cerebellum. J Pharmacol Exp Ther 1998;285:983–986.

Chapter 12

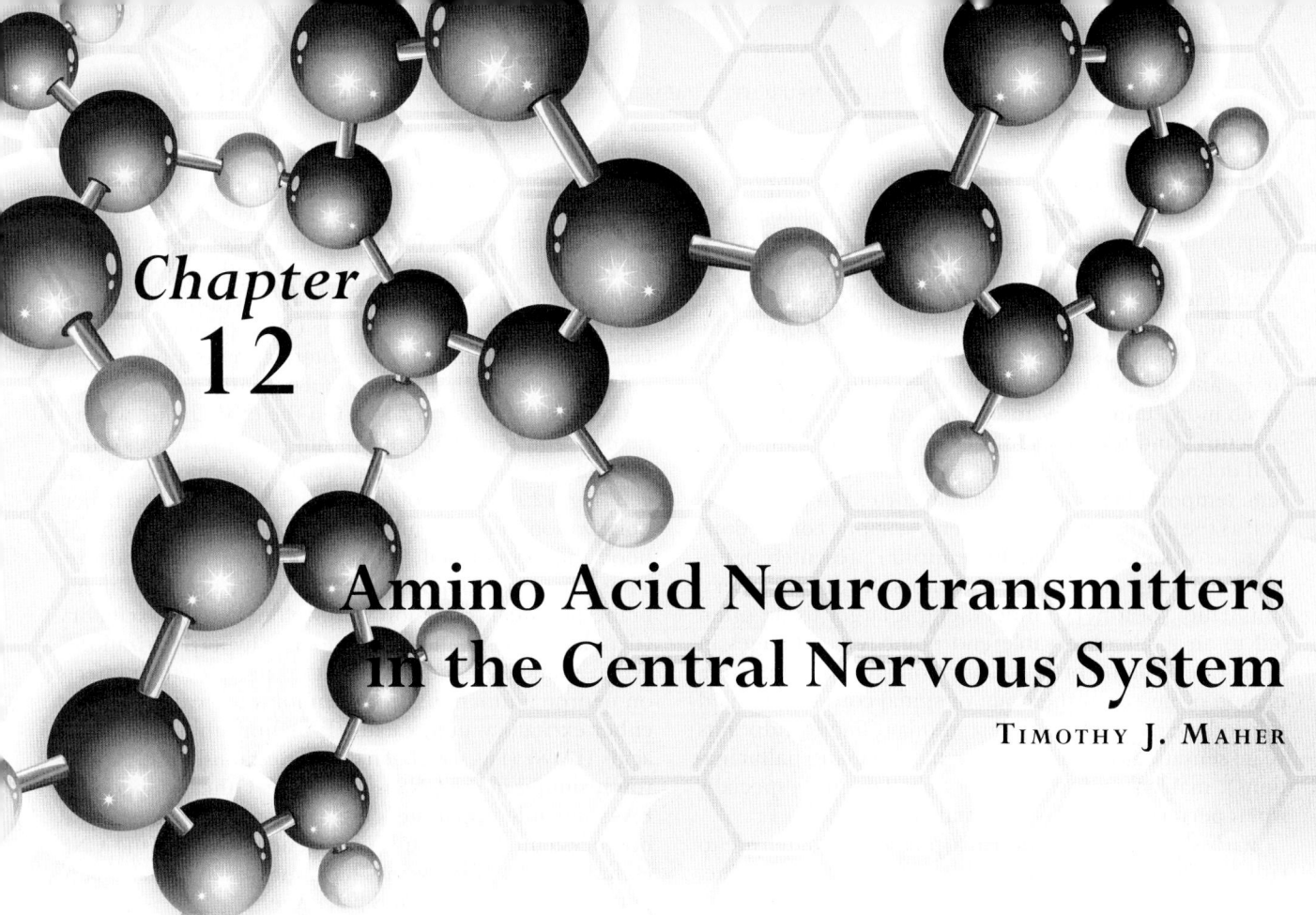

Amino Acid Neurotransmitters in the Central Nervous System

TIMOTHY J. MAHER

Abbreviations

ALS, amyotrophic lateral sclerosis
AMPA, α-amino-3-hydroxy-5-methyl-4-isoxazole propionic acid
ATP, adenosine triphosphate
CNS, central nervous system
EAA, excitatory amino acids
EAAT, excitatory amino acid transporter
EDTA, ethylenediamine tetra-acetic acid
GABA, γ-aminobutyric acid
GABA-T, GABA transaminase
GAD, glutamic acid decarboxylase
GHB, γ-hydroxybutyrate
GPCR, G protein–coupled receptor
IAA, inhibitory amino acids
MSG, monosodium glutamate
NMDA, *N*-methyl-D-aspartate
PLC, phospholipase C
SHMT, serine hydroxymethyltransferase
SSA, succinic semialdehyde
SSADH, SSA dehydrogenase
VGAT, vesicular GABA transporter
VGLUT1, vesicular glutamate transporter 1

HISTORICAL BACKGROUND

Scientists in the late 1800s and early 1900s studying the physiology of the body began to postulate that the medicinals available at that time produced their responses by interacting with a special group of structures termed "receptive substances." This suggestion was based on the observation that seemingly very minor changes in the chemical structures of a series of compounds could greatly alter the biologic responses observed following administration of these compounds to animals or people. Later, it was recognized that many of these drugs typically were acting as mimics or antagonists of endogenous compounds and that their responses were caused by interactions with what we today term "receptors." Thus the era of chemical neurotransmission was born, which challenged the long-accepted dogma that communication between cells was simply the result of electrical transmission.

Acetylcholine released from the parasympathetic nerves innervating the heart and termed "vagustuff" was the first neurotransmitter to be recognized. Drugs that acted similarly to the then-unknown acetylcholine molecule, including muscarine and nicotine, led to the eventual characterization of muscarinic cholinergic and nicotinic cholinergic receptors, respectively. Epinephrine found in adrenal gland extracts and termed "adrenaline" was also described in those early days of discovery in the field of neurotransmitter pharmacology. Each of these substances could produce very powerful responses when released from nerves or tissues or when applied exogenously to isolated tissues or intact animals. Today, we know that these compounds serving as neurotransmitters, neuromodulators, and/or hormones are the normal endogenous mediators of information transfer throughout the body.

The earliest characterizations of chemical compounds as neurotransmitters involved studies of physiologic systems in the periphery and used both chemical and physiologic techniques. Later, investigators started to apply some of the same techniques used in characterizing these peripheral neurotransmitters and their receptors to the central nervous system (CNS), which is comprised of the brain and spinal cord. These investigations were often much more difficult because of the greater complexity of structures and functions in the CNS. The seemingly less well defined and more ambiguous areas (e.g., limbic system, temporal lobe, and prefrontal cortex) in the CNS as well as the smaller and more diverse synaptic connections (e.g., axo-axonal and somato-dendritic) presented significant challenges to early investigators. In the periphery, stimulation of a nerve innervating a target tissue often led to an easily observable end point (e.g., changes in heart rate or blood pressure, hormone release), but stimulation of nerves in the brain or spinal cord often failed to produce easily observable and quantifiable endpoints (e.g., sensations of warmth, fear, memory, and hallucinations), making such studies very challenging, especially when performed in experimental animals.

Early studies by Falk and Hillarp used formaldehyde to visualize neurons containing the monoamines dopamine, norepinephrine, and epinephrine (fluoresces green) as well as serotonin (fluoresces yellow) in brain slices. With improvements in the chemical techniques for measuring these classical monoamines and acetylcholine and, eventually, the enzymes involved with their synthesis and degradation, investigators began to map the neurons in the CNS that used these neurotransmitters and began to appreciate the neurochemical basis of drug action in the brain and spinal cord. In the late 1950s and early 1960s, however, investigators began to observe the neuronal effects of simple amino acids in these brain tissues. The suggestion that simple amino acids could function as sophisticated neurotransmitters was met with considerable resistance and skepticism. Amino acids are typically reserved for protein synthesis and serve many metabolic functions, and they did not appear to have the same unique functional characteristics of the classical monoamine neurotransmitters and acetylcholine. As studies continued to support the neurotransmitter role of amino acids such as γ-aminobutyric acid (GABA), glutamic acid (glutamate), and glycine, however, overwhelming evidence has led to their nearly universal acceptance as the major neurotransmitters in the CNS. Quantitatively, the amino acids are the most prevalent neurotransmitters in the CNS. For example, it has been estimated that more than 40% of all neurons in the CNS use GABA as a neurotransmitter substance and that less than 10% use one of the other classical monoamines, such as norepinephrine and serotonin, or acetylcholine.

Although overall neuronal functioning is rather complex, a simplistic view of the two major effects of neurotransmitters involves changes in membrane potential toward states of either depolarization or hyperpolarization (Fig. 12.1). Such changes in membrane potential usually result from alterations in membrane conductance to ions such as Na^+, K^+, Ca^{2+}, and Cl^-, which typically flow down their electrochemical gradients when a selective ion channel is opened. Ion channels need only open for 0.1 to 100 milliseconds to effect this change. Thus, when a neuron is to be depolarized, Na^+ or Ca^{2+} typically enters the cell, making the membrane potential more positive and more likely to reach the threshold potential and lead to an action potential (Fig. 12.1A). On the other hand, when a neuron is hyperpolarized, typically either K^+ moves out of the cell into the extracellular space or Cl^- moves into the cell (Fig. 12.1B). Both of these ion fluxes result in a hyperpolarization of the membrane, which decreases the likelihood that a neuronal cell will become excited and fire. Thus, these two opposing alterations in neuronal membrane potentials commonly are referred to as excitatory (depolarization) and inhibitory (hyperpolarization). When amino acid neurotransmitters produce their effects on neuronal function, they commonly are categorized as either excitatory amino acids (EAAs) or inhibitory amino acids (IAAs) (Fig. 12.2). The major established EAA neurotransmitter in the CNS is glutamate. Other endogenous EAAs include aspartate (aspartic acid), cysteine, and homocysteine. The major endogenous IAAs in the CNS include GABA and glycine, but much evidence also supports a role for taurine and β-alanine.

NEUROTRANSMITTER CRITERIA

For a compound to be classified as a neurotransmitter, a number of criteria must be satisfied. First, the neurotransmitter must be present. As a rule, the concentrations of the neurotransmitter in various parts of the CNS will vary such that a unique and unequal distribution can be demonstrated. For some amino acids, this unequal distribution is difficult to demonstrate, because most of these amino acids are also used to support protein synthesis and for intermediary metabolism, unlike the monoamine neurotransmitters, for which an unequal distribution is relatively easy to demonstrate. Although substances such as glucose and sodium are present in the CNS, their regional distribution is rather uniform, and few would consider either of these to be a classical neurotransmitter. Besides determining the concentration of the neurotransmitter itself, evidence that can also be used to support this criterion includes the distribution of specific receptors, reuptake systems, and enzymes involved with synthesis and/or degradation of the particular amino acid neurotransmitter. Today, with the aid of molecular biologic techniques (e.g., mRNA, cloning techniques, and in situ hybridization), the location and quantification of proteins that serve as receptors, transporters, or metabolizing enzyme are more easily achieved. Second, the neurotransmitter must be released when the nerve cell is stimulated. To date, the vast majority of amino acid neurotransmitter release, like that of the monoamines and acetylcholine, has been found to be Ca^{2+} dependent and originating from presynaptic storage vesicles. Release

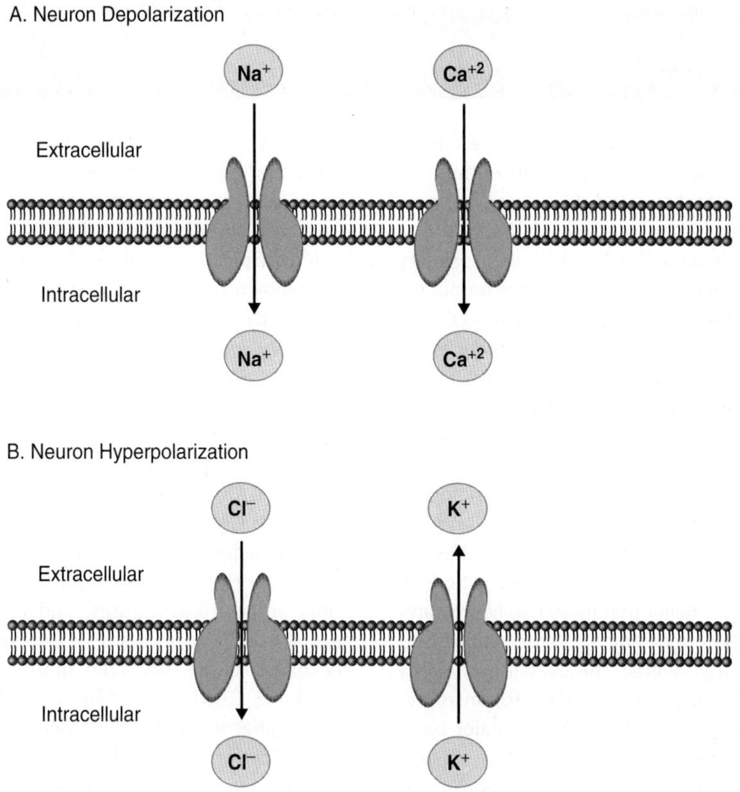

FIGURE 12.1 Electrophysiology of excitatory and inhibitory neurotransmitters. The tendency of an ion to move across the membrane depends on the difference in its electrochemical gradient on either side of the membrane. The electrochemical gradient depends on the difference in the concentration of the ion between the two sides of the membrane, the charge of the ion, and the transmembrane potential (the difference in voltage between the two sides of the membrane).

can be determined using brain slices prelabeled with radioactive neurotransmitter or with in vivo microdialysis, in which the extracellular fluid surrounding neurons is continuously sampled. Furthermore, there should be a mechanism in place that terminates the action of the neurotransmitter (e.g., reuptake, removal into astroglia or other cells, metabolism, or some other form of inactivation). And finally, for a substance to be considered a neurotransmitter, the exogenous administration or application of the suspected neurotransmitter must mimic the

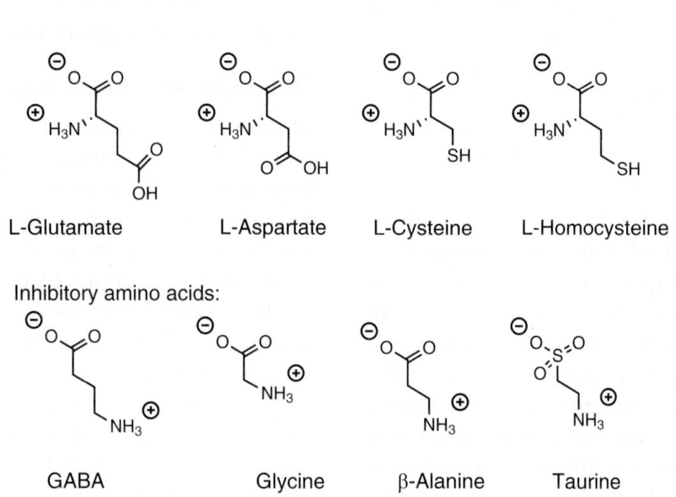

FIGURE 12.2 Endogenous excitatory and inhibitory amino acid neurotransmitters.

CLINICAL SIGNIFICANCE

Amino acids are the most abundant neurotransmitters in the CNS, and the majority of neurons in the mammalian brain utilize either glutamate or GABA as their primary neurotransmitters. These amino acids are responsible for almost all of the fast signaling between neurons, with a modulatory role for many of the other neurotransmitters. Glutamate is the most abundant excitatory neurotransmitter and GABA is the most abundant inhibitory neurotransmitter in the human CNS. Thus, these amino acids serve to regulate reciprocally the level of excitability of most neurons in the CNS and therefore have been implicated as important mediators of many critical physiological processes as well as pathophysiological conditions that underlie brain function and/or dysfunction. Pharmacological studies utilizing drugs that selectively inhibit/block or mimic the actions of GABA or glutamate support the belief that these two neurotransmitters, because of their often opposing excitatory and inhibitory actions, control, to a large degree, the overall excitability of the CNS. Glutamate is the major excitatory neurotransmitter and is distributed in all regions of the brain. Three major types of glutamate receptors have been identified: *N*-methyl- D-aspartate (NMDA), α-amino-3-hydroxy-5-methylisoxazole-4-propionic acid (AMPA), and kainate (KA) receptors. GABA, metabolically derived from glutamate, is the major inhibitory neurotransmitter in the brain. Glycine is an inhibitory neurotransmitter found mostly in the brain stem and spinal cord but which has also a role as a co-agonist on certain glutamate receptors.

Glutamate is involved in cognitive functions in the brain such as learning and memory, and it has been implicated in epileptic seizures. GABA and glycine are the most important inhibitory amino acid neurotransmitters in the brain and brainstem/spinal cord, respectively. These inhibitory amino acids are of particular interest because many therapeutically useful drugs act by selectively affecting these two neurotransmitter systems. Specific inhibitors of GABA reuptake transporters have been shown to have antiseizure and/or antinociceptive properties in laboratory animals. Receptors for both inhibitory and excitatory amino acid neurotransmitters are either ionotropic (i.e., their activation results in enhanced membrane ion conductance) or metabotropic (i.e., their activation results in increased intracellular levels of a second messenger). $GABA_A$ receptors are ionotropic receptors that lead to increased Cl^- ion conductance, whereas $GABA_B$ receptors are metabotropic receptors that are coupled to G proteins and thereby alter neuronal excitability.

Subsequent chapters will describe the mechanisms of action of the sedative-hypnotic benzodiazepines, nonbenzodiazepines, barbiturates, and anesthetic agents at $GABA_A$ receptors; baclofen and γ-hydroxybutyric acid at $GABA_B$ receptors; GABA reuptake inhibitors as antiseizure agents, tiagabine; GABA-transaminase inhibitors, gabaculine, valproate, vigabatrin; and GABA analogs as antiseizure drugs and analgesics for neuropathic pain, pregabalin, gabapentin. The hallucinogenic drug phencyclidine (more commonly known as PCP) antagonizes glutamate noncompetitively at the NMDA receptor.

Timothy Maher
Professor
Department of Pharmaceutical Sciences
Massachusetts College of Pharmacy and Health Sciences
Boston, MA

effects (e.g., depolarization, hyperpolarization, activation of protein kinase C, inhibition of adenylyl cyclase, etc.) that are observed when the neurotransmitter is released endogenously following presynaptic nerve cell stimulation.

EXCITATORY AMINO ACID NEUROTRANSMITTERS

Glutamate

The major EAA neurotransmitter in the CNS is L-glutamate. (Note that all amino acids with the exception of glycine mentioned in this chapter are considered to be in the "L" configuration; thus, the "L" will be omitted, unless specifically indicated as "D"). Early studies in invertebrates demonstrated the potent actions of the acidic amino acid glutamate, as well as another acidic amino acid, aspartate. Acceptance of glutamate as a neurotransmitter in the CNS was delayed for many years as neuroscientists attempted to distinguish its role as a component of protein and peptides (e.g., glutathione), an important intermediate in numerous metabolic processes, and a precursor to the inhibitory neurotransmitter GABA. Whereas glutamate is found in all cells within the CNS, an unequal distribution of this amino acid and of aspartate has been demonstrated.

Glutamate Synthesis, Storage, and Release

Glutamate is synthesized in the CNS via the transamination of α-ketoglutarate (Fig. 12.3), which is produced from glucose in the Krebs cycle. Glutamate can also be synthesized from glutamine via glutaminase. Once produced, glutamate can be stored in neuronal vesicles. With the vast number of compounds that can feed into the Krebs cycle and the various sources of glucose, it is not surprising that the control of glutamate synthesis in the CNS is still poorly understood.

The oral ingestion of glutamate in protein, as the individual amino acid in the form of a dietary supplement or in the form of the flavor enhancer monosodium glutamate (MSG), fails to significantly increase CNS levels of this amino acid neurotransmitter. Following

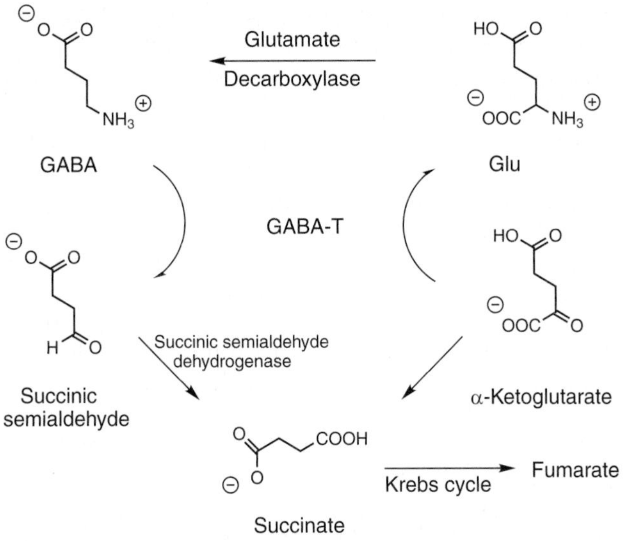

FIGURE 12.3 Glutamate and GABA biosynthesis.

Similar concerns have been voiced regarding the safety of the acidic amino acid aspartate in the artificial sweetener aspartame (L-aspartyl-L-phenylalanine methylester). As with MSG, however, the homeostatic mechanisms regulating plasma aspartate levels following aspartate consumption do not allow for large increases in plasma aspartate that could alter CNS function. In fact, the concern regarding the safety of aspartame results from the other amino acid present, phenylalanine, which much more readily crosses the blood–brain barrier and can alter CNS function. This is especially important for people who unknowingly are heterozygous for the genetic metabolic disorder of phenylketonuria (2).

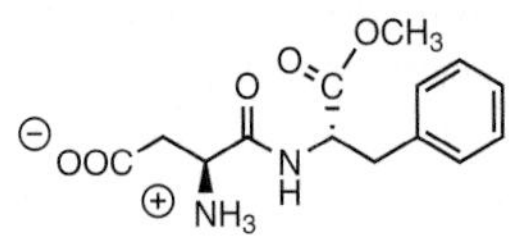

Aspartame

its ingestion, blood glutamate levels do increase transiently, but largely because of the ability of the blood–brain barrier to regulate the entry of glutamate into the CNS, no significant changes in brain glutamate are observed. This ability to regulate synaptic glutamate levels in brain despite fluctuations in peripheral levels is very important, because uncontrolled variations in CNS glutamate would lead to serious consequences, including seizures and coma for increases and decreases of glutamate, respectively. Within the blood–brain barrier, there exist transport proteins that are responsible for controlling the influx of amino acids into the CNS. Of the three major types—acidic, basic, and neutral amino acid transporters—it is the acidic amino acid transporter that carries glutamate. These transporters function by facilitated diffusion and cannot operate against a concentration gradient (as seen with active transport). In actuality, the acidic amino acid transporter normally functions to move glutamate out of the CNS. There have been studies in which glutamate, often in the form of MSG, has been injected subcutaneously into neonatal mice or nonhuman primates and hypothalamic lesions noted. The lesions are mostly restricted to the circumventricular organs (those near the fourth ventricle in the brain), where the blood–brain barrier is significantly diminished. Moreover, when MSG is directly injected into the brains of laboratory animals, cellular necrosis is observed. However, when MSG is given orally in very high doses, the homeostatic processes in liver and other tissues help to regulate plasma glutamate concentrations, and large fluctuations are not observed. The blood–brain barrier also functions to keep CNS glutamate at appropriate levels. The studies in which glutamate in the form of MSG is parenterally injected do not reflect the chemical fluctuations that occur following oral ingestion and should not be interpreted as an indicator of toxicity of MSG (1).

The vesicular glutamate transporter 1 (VGLUT1) transports glutamate into storage vesicles in preparation for the Ca^{2+}-mediated release of this neurotransmitter that uses adenosine triphosphate (ATP) to concentrate glutamate against its concentration gradient (ATP-dependent transporter). Unrelated to any of the other families of neurotransmitter vesicle transporters, VGLUT1 originally was thought to be an inorganic phosphate membrane transporter. Today, it is known that VGLUT1 uses a vacuolar ATPase to cleave ATP to provide the energy required to generate and maintain an electrochemical proton gradient that allows the concentration of glutamate to remain extremely high in synaptic vesicles compared to that in the cytoplasm—and especially compared to that in the synapse. Although probably not the basis of their main pharmacologic actions, known inhibitors of VGLUT1 include the ergot bromocriptine (a dopamine agonist used in the treatment of Parkinson disease and hyperprolactinemia) and some of the azo-dyes, including Evans Blue (3). Recently, a family of endogenous inhibitory proteins has been identified that not only blocks glutamate vesicular transport but also GABA vesicular transport. The significance of the role that these proteins, known as IPFα, IPFβ, and IPFγ, have in regulating glutamatergic neurotransmission is still poorly understood (4). As more is learned about such proteins and other yet unknown regulatory mechanism, a better appreciation regarding the pathology of various disease states can be realized, and therapeutic interventions can be designed based on this knowledge.

Like most other recognized neurotransmitter substances, vesicular release of glutamate occurs in a Ca^{2+}-dependent manner following depolarization of the presynaptic terminal. In cell culture or isolated tissue studies, agents that bind Ca^{2+}, such as ethylenediamine tetra-acetic acid (EDTA) or the use of Ca^{2+}-free perfusion solutions, the vesicular release of glutamate can be diminished or prevented. Thus, this is one of the techniques that can be employed to distinguish, in part, between the neurotransmitter and metabolic roles of glutamate in a particular biologic system.

Glutamate Reuptake and Metabolism

Transporter proteins that regulate the synaptic concentrations of glutamate are essential in keeping the basal levels of this EAA neurotransmitter low and in helping to terminate the responses to neuronally released glutamate. These high-affinity, sodium-dependent transporters are so efficient at sequestering glutamate from the synaptic cleft that the concentration of glutamate inside the presynaptic terminal is most often several thousandfold greater than that found in the synapse (5).

These EAA transporters (EAATs) have been identified and categorized into five major subtypes: EAAT1, EAAT2, EAAT3, EAAT4, and EAAT5 (Table 12.1 and Fig. 12.4). Their distribution tends to be primarily cellular, and relative anatomic distribution of the subtypes in brain for each subtype is such that EAAT1 and EAAT2 are mostly found in astroglial cells in the cerebellum and forebrain, respectively. The astroglial reuptake of neuronally released glutamate is believed to be very important in terminating the glutamate-mediated synaptic signal. The EAAT3 and EAAT4 subtypes are highly concentrated in the cortical and cerebellar Purkinje neurons, respectively, whereas EAAT5 is most abundant in the retina. The reuptake of glutamate or aspartate via any of the EAAT subtypes is coupled to the cotransport of H^+ and $3Na^+$ into astroglia or neurons, with the extrusion of K^+, as shown in Figure 12.4.

The EAATs are capable of transporting D-aspartate, aspartate, and glutamate but do not transport D-glutamate. The known inhibitors of glutamate reuptake transport are classified as either competitive (these, as a rule, act as substrates and are transported) or noncompetitive (these are nontransported), but no therapeutically useful agents have yet been discovered. The actions of glutamate are terminated via its reuptake into the presynaptic neuron, from where it originally was released, into the surrounding glia and into the postsynaptic neuron that houses the various target EAA receptors (6). Following its release, glutamate that is taken up via EAATs into neurons or astroglial cells can be recycled, in part, directly into vesicles for subsequent release or, more likely, is converted to glutamine via glutamine synthetase and is available for eventual recycling to glutamate via the activity of the enzyme glutaminase, as shown in Figure 12.4.

TABLE 12.1 Excitatory Amino Acid Transporters

Subtype	Predominant Brain Distribution
EAAT1	Cerebellar glia
EAAT2	Forebrain glia
EAAT3	Cortical neurons
EAAT4	Cerebellar Purkinje neurons
EAAT5	Retina

Ischemic brain injury has been shown to upregulate EAAT2, which can provide some neuroprotection by increasing the removal of glutamate from the extracellular space where it can be in contact with excitatory receptors and further the ischemic insult (7). Recently, two endogenous inflammatory mediators, tumor necrosis factor-α and nuclear factor-κB, have been shown to upregulate EAAT2, suggesting that selectively modulating this transporter might be a pharmacologic approach to reducing ischemic brain damage in the future. Similarly, the β-lactam antibiotic ceftriaxone, which enhances the activity of some EAATs, has been effective in attenuating neurodegeneration in an animal model of amyotrophic lateral sclerosis (ALS; also known as Lou Gehrig disease) (8). The EAATs continue to be a promising target for therapeutic interventions involving diseases of the CNS, which involve excessive excitatory amino acid neurotransmission.

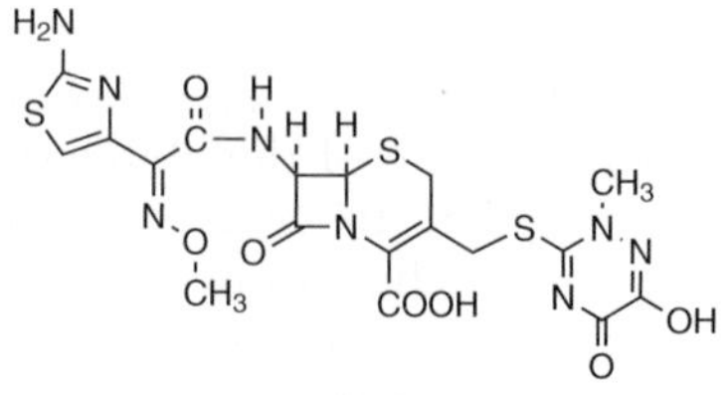

Ceftriazone

EAA Receptors

The receptors for glutamate and the other EAAs are categorized into major two groups: ionotropic and metabotropic (Fig. 12.4). The three ionotropic receptor types are classified based on their selective affinity for the EAA ligands: *N*-methyl-D-aspartate (NMDA), α-amino-3-hydroxy-5-methyl-4-isoxazole propionic acid (AMPA), and kainite (Table 12.2). AMPA is a homologue of the neurotoxin ibotenic acid found in *Amanita* mushrooms, whereas kainate is a neurotoxin isolated from red algae.

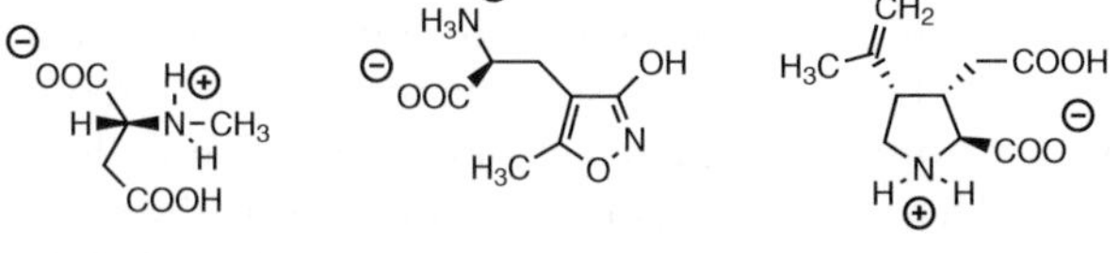

NMDA L-AMPA Kainate

These ligand-gated ion channel receptors are composed of homo- or heterotetramers of individual subunits that confer cation selectivity. Each subunit has an extracellular N-terminus with three transmembrane domains, an intramembrane reentrant "p-loop" between the first and third transmembrane domains, and an intracellular C-terminus (Fig. 12.5) (9). The metabotropic glutamate receptors belong to the larger family of G protein–coupled receptors (GPCRs). When activated, these metabotropic receptors can alter the activity of effector proteins, such as adenylyl cyclase and phospholipase C (PLC).

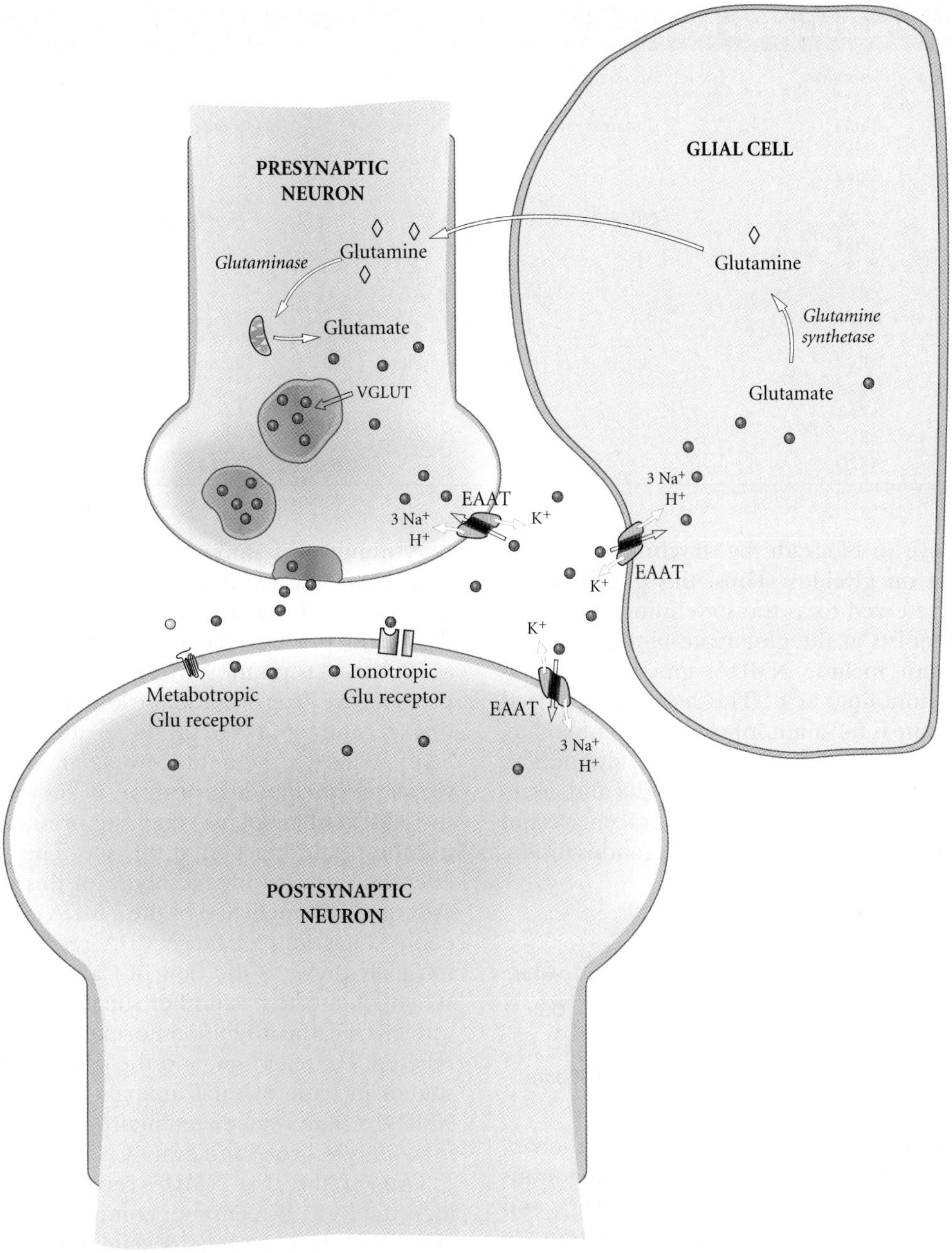

FIGURE 12.4 The glutamate neuron showing the formation of glutamate (o) from glutamine (◊), ionotropic and metabotropic receptors, storage vesicles, and reuptake transporters.

To date, at least eight distinct EAA metabotropic receptor subtypes appear to exist. The EAA receptors, in balance with the receptors for the IAAs, likely are crucial for the regulation of neuronal plasticity involving dynamic changes in neurons as a response to environmental stimuli. Neuronal plasticity accounts for the ability of an organism to learn and adapt, which includes both long-term potentiation and long-term depression.

Ionotropic Receptors

NMDA Receptor The NMDA receptor is a heterotetramer comprised of a number of subunit forms—GLU_{N1}, GLU_{N2A}, GLU_{N2B}, GLU_{N2C}, GLU_{N2D}, GLU_{N3A}, and GLU_{N3B}—that can confer unique pharmacology to individual receptors (Table 12.2). Splice variants can also lead to a number of isoforms of the above subunits with the potential of changing the binding characteristics and functions on the receptor. Activation of the NMDA receptor requires the binding of two agonists: glutamate to the GLU_{N2} subunit, and glycine to a binding site on the GLU_{N1} subunit (10). Glycine appears to act as an important co-agonist positive modulator at a unique recognition site on the GLU_{N1} subunit, and unlike the actions of glycine as an IAA neurotransmitter, this recognition

TABLE 12.2 Ionotropic Glutamate Receptor Subtypes

Subtype	Subunits	Agonists	Actions
AMPA	GluR1 GluR2 GluR4	Glutamate or AMPA	Increases Na^+ influx, increases K^+ efflux
Kainate	GluR5 GluR6 GluR7 KA1 KA2	Glutamate or kainate	Increases Na^+ influx, increases K^+ efflux
NMDA	NR1 NR2A NR2B NR2C NR2D	Glutamate or NMDA with glycine	Increases Na^{2+} and Ca^{2+} influx, increases K^+ efflux

site is not sensitive to blockade by strychnine (see the following section on glycine). Thus, this glycine binding site is often referred to as the strychnine-insensitive receptor site. Agonists at the glutamate binding site on the GLU_{N2} subunit include NMDA, glutamate, aspartate, and homoquinolinic acid. The best-characterized antagonist at this site is D-2-aminophosphonopentanoate. D-Serine is a well-known agonist at the GLU_{N1} glycine site. D-Serine, which normally is found only in glia and astrocytes, is synthesized from L-serine via serine racemase and is thought to be one of the important endogenous modulators of NMDA receptor activity.

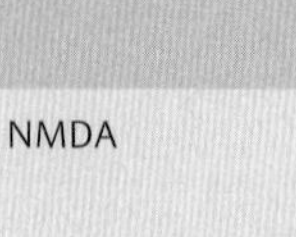
Homoquinolinate

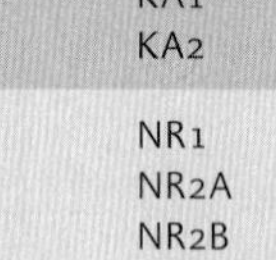
D-AP5

L-Serine

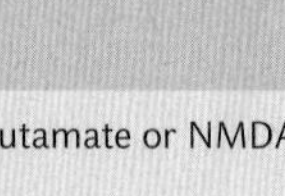
D-Serine

The NMDA receptor has also many sites for channel modulation by pharmacologic agents. Endogenous inhibitory channel modulators include Mg^{2+}, Zn^{2+}, and protons. Neurosteroids can either inhibit or potentiate NMDA receptor channel function depending on how the subunits comprising the tetrameric structure are assembled. For instance, the neurosteroid pregnenolone sulfate inhibits NMDA receptors that are assembled as GLU_{N1}/GLU_{N2C} but potentiates those assembled as GLU_{N1}/GLU_{N2A} and GLU_{N1}/GLU_{N2B} (11). Polyamines, such as spermine and spermidine, are known to be positive channel modulators.

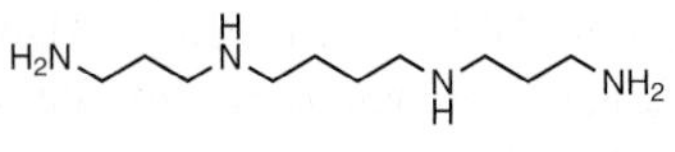
Spermine

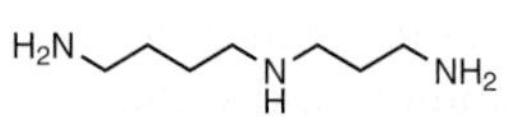
Spermidine

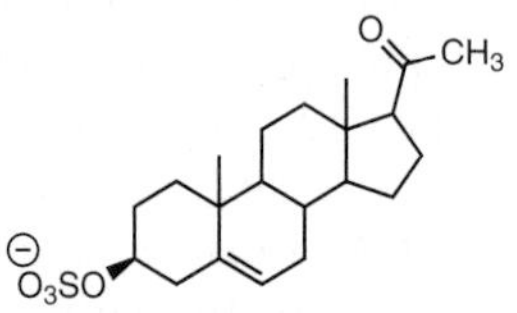
Pregnenolone sulfate

A number of important NMDA channel antagonists (Fig. 12.6) also exist, and these include amantadine (an antiviral agent that also releases dopamine and is used in Parkinson disease), ketamine (a dissociative anesthetic agent that acts via the NMDA receptor), phencyclidine (a psychoactive drug of abuse also known as PCP), and memantine (recently approved for the treatment of Alzheimer disease). Whereas the antitussive agent dextromethorphan, via its metabolite dextrorphan, is known to block within the NMDA channel, its cough-suppressant activity likely is not the result of action at this site. The psychotomimetic effects observed with the abuse of this compound, however, are likely mediated by the NMDA receptor. An endogenous antagonist of the NMDA receptor is Mg^{2+}, which normally prevents the flow of Ca^{2+} through the channel. When glutamate or another suitable agonist binds, along with glycine, the inhibition normally maintained by Mg^{2+} is relieved, Ca^{2+} can flow, and the cell can depolarize. Some studies in experimental animals have demonstrated the NMDA receptor–mediated neuroprotective effects of Mg^{2+} in models of stroke and other CNS insults.

One of the first NMDA receptor antagonists to be identified was dizocilpine, commonly known as MK-801 (Fig. 12.6). Initially, much excitement was generated with the discovery of MK-801, because the ability to block the excessive intracellular cation flow (Ca^{2+}, Na^+) that follows neuronal hypoxic insults, as are seen following cerebral vascular accidents (stroke) or head trauma, might lead to effective treatments for such pathologic conditions. Whereas MK-801 was very effective in decreasing infarct size in various rodent models of stroke, poor clinical efficacy was noted in humans. The generation of severe psychotic behaviors was also deemed to be unacceptable.

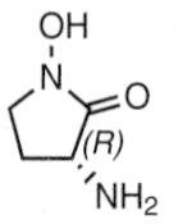
(R)-HA-966

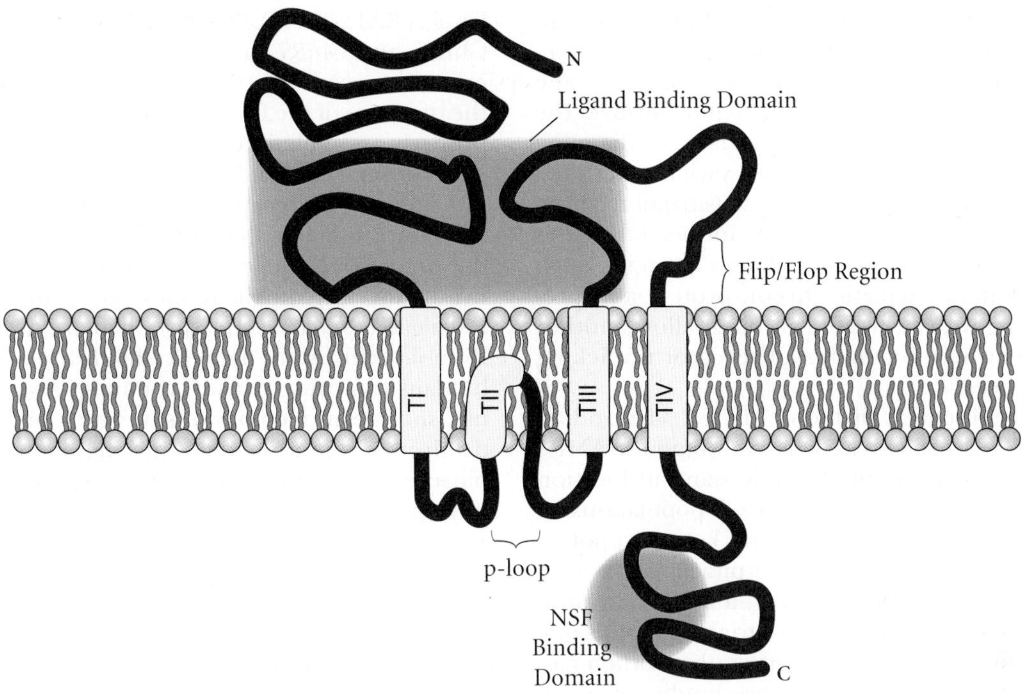

FIGURE 12.5 The ionotropic glutamate receptor showing the p-loop, ligand binding domain, *N*-ethylmaleimide–sensitive fusion protein (NSF) binding domain (shaded area), flip-flop region, and the N- and C-terminal regions.

The strychnine-insensitive binding site on the NMDA receptor has also been a target for researchers, because an agent that would antagonize this binding site might be useful in preventing the neuronal damage that occurs following hypoxic insults that lead to excessive glutamate release or in controlling electrical neuronal dysfunction associated with epilepsy. One agent, *R*-(+)-3-amino-1-hydroxypyrrolidin-2-one [(*R*)-HA-966], is an antagonist at the strychnine-insensitive binding site on the NMDA receptor that, unfortunately, has not been used therapeutically because of its hepatotoxic properties unrelated to the NMDA receptor. However, the dicarbamate anticonvulsant felbamate (see Chapter 17) produces part of its activity by inducing conformational (allosteric) changes in the receptor (allosterism) that alters the binding of glycine at the NMDA glycine binding site. Felbamate also has interactions at the AMPA and kainate receptors that contribute to its anticonvulsant activity (12,13).

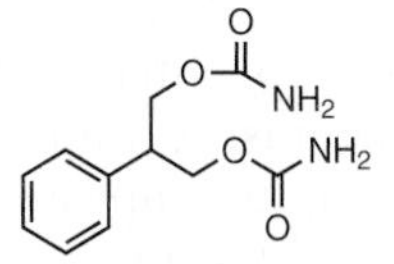

Felbamate

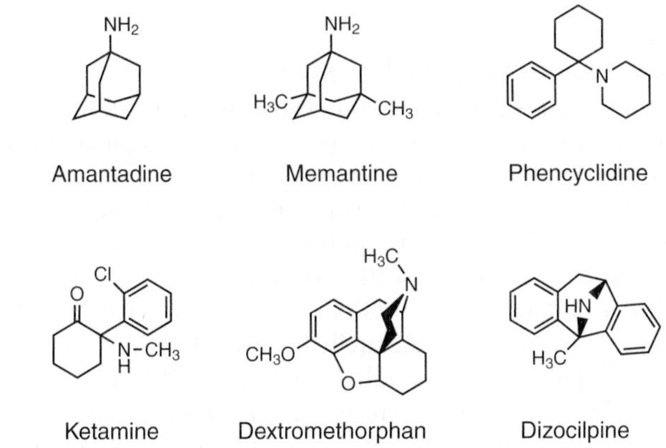

FIGURE 12.6 NMDA channel antagonists.

AMPA Receptors Another ionotropic EAA receptor is preferentially activated by AMPA. Although at one time, this receptor was referred to as the quisqualate receptor, the AMPA receptor mediates fast synaptic activity via the influx of Na^+ and, in some neurons, K^+ efflux (Table 12.2). The AMPA receptor, which is found in high abundance in the cerebral cortex and hippocampus, is comprised of four subunits: GluR1, GluR2, GluR3, and GluR4. One of these subunits, GluR2, when present prevents the formation of an ionophore that can efficiently conduct Ca^{2+}. However, when the

AMPA receptor does not contain a GluR2 subunit, Ca^{2+} is capable of being conducted through the ion channel. On the extracellular loop between transmembrane segments III and IV there exists a region termed the "flip-flop" that is sensitive to splice variants of the gene coding for each subunit. Such splice variants can lead to significant differences in the desensitization kinetics of the receptor (14). Moreover, intracellular sites on the C-terminus, where modulatory proteins such as *N*-ethylmaleimide–sensitive fusion protein and protein interacting with C kinase can bind, allow another important site where regulation of receptor trafficking can be influenced.

Recently, the discovery that some of the 2,3-benzodiazepines (e.g., GYKl 53655) can selectively bind the AMPA receptor has aided in studies to understand its location and functions, especially where mixed populations of EAA receptors are present (15). Agents known to potentiate AMPA receptor activity include piracetam (a drug for improving mental performance), a cyclic derivative of GABA, and the benzothiazide diuretic, cyclothiazide (Fig. 12.7). Some evidence also suggests that certain barbiturates and volatile anesthetics have binding sites on the AMPA receptor. Riluzole (2-amino-6-fluoromethoxy benzothiazole), approved for the treatment of ALS and which acts partly by reducing glutamate release and altering AMPA receptor expression, has been found to have potential utility in treatment-resistant unipolar depression, bipolar depression, and generalized anxiety disorders (16).

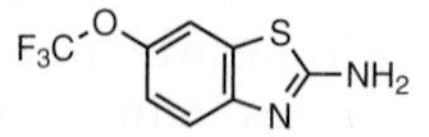

Riluzole

Agents that act to cause conformational changes that positively modulate the AMPA receptor have been termed "ampakines" and have been suggested to improve memory, to enhance the activity of certain antipsychotic agents, to improve attention-deficit hyperactivity disorder, to improve Parkinson disease symptoms, and to provide neuroprotection following CNS ischemic insults (17).

Kainate Receptors The ionotropic kainate receptor is a heterotetramer comprised of subunits GluR5, GluR6, GluR7, KA1, and KA2 (Table 12.2). The subunits GluR5, GluR6, and GluR7 can form functional homo- and heteromeric receptors; the KA1 and KA2 subunits require the presence of the GluR5, GluR6, and GluR7 subunits to properly assemble into functional receptors. Similarities exist between the binding characteristics of AMPA receptors and kainite receptors such that few pharmacologic agents are available that effectively differentiate between the two (18). Kainate receptors tend to be more sensitive to the phycotoxin domoic acid, an EAA found in red algae (*Pseudonitzschia* sp.), than are AMPA receptors. Domoic acid causes amnesic shellfish poisoning that in humans can cause nausea, vomiting, abdominal cramping, short-term memory loss, seizures, arrhythmias, and death in severe cases following ingestion. Domoic acid bioaccumulates in shellfish that feed on the red algae phytoplankton.

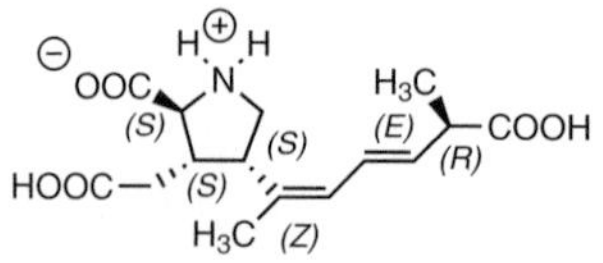

Domoic acid

Kainate receptors are located postsynaptically and mediate neuronal excitation, as do NMDA and AMPA receptors, but kainate receptors have also been found to be located presynaptically. Such presynaptic receptors appear to regulate the release of GABA in the hippocampus and glutamate in some other brain regions. Some kainate receptors have also been shown to be linked to a pertussis toxin–sensitive G protein, which via interaction with PLC can in turn act to influence nearby voltage-dependent Ca^{2+} channels (19). This dual signaling capability of kainate receptors appears to be unique for an EAA ionotropic receptor and can facilitate the role of this receptor subtype in influencing both short- and long-term synaptic plasticity (adaptive changes to the synapse affecting the efficacy of neurotransmission) in the CNS.

Metabotropic Glutamate Receptors

Another class of EAA receptors are the G protein–coupled metabotropic receptors (m), which are categorized into one of three groups based on their pharmacology, sequence similarity, and intracellular effector signaling systems. Group I, which includes mGlu1 and mGlu5, are positively coupled to PLC via $G_{q/11}$. Group II, which includes mGlu2 and mGlu3, and group III, which includes mGlu4, mGlu6, mGlu7, and mGlu8, are negatively coupled via $G_{i/o}$ to adenylyl cyclase (20). The term "metabotropic" is used to indicate that activation of these receptors results in alterations in metabolic processes within the cell. All of the metabotropic receptors are

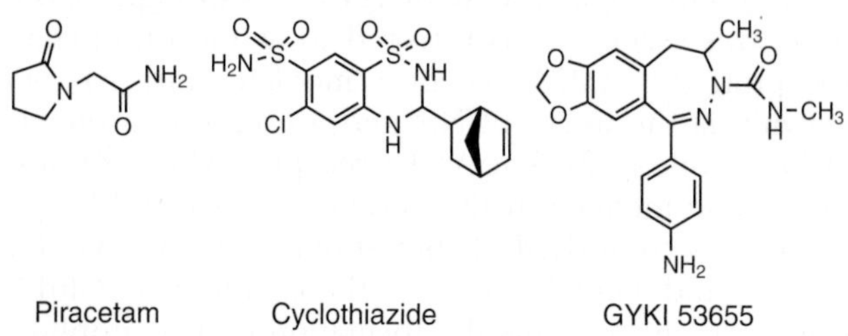

Piracetam Cyclothiazide GYKI 53655

FIGURE 12.7 AMPA agonists.

activated by glutamate and ibotenate, but none is activated by NMDA, AMPA, or kainate.

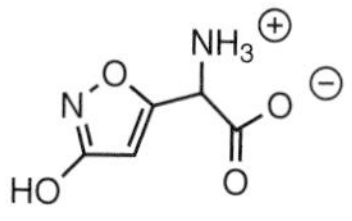

Ibotenate

Few useful selective agonists or antagonists are available for these receptors subtypes, but some researchers have used knockout mice to explore the role of a particular metabotropic receptor. For instance, mice lacking the mGlu5 receptor fail to display the reinforcing and locomotor stimulant effects of cocaine, suggesting that an agent that is selective at antagonizing the mGlu5 receptor might find utility in treating patients dependent on cocaine (21). Because the mGlu5 receptor is located in areas of the brain thought to be involved with anxiety, compounds that negatively modulate this receptor subtype have been shown to be anxiolytic in animal studies. The group II mGlu receptors are also highly concentrated in areas involved with anxiety, such that agents that are selective positive modulators for this receptor subtype are found to act as anxiolytics. Finally, positive modulators of the mGlu4 receptor subtype have been suggested as an approach for treating Parkinson disease (22). As more information is revealed about the distribution, function, binding characteristics, and trafficking of the metabotropic receptor subtypes in the CNS, advances in the therapy of disease states such as Parkinson disease, schizophrenia, chronic pain, epilepsy, depression, and drug dependence can be realized (23).

A steady accumulation of evidence supports a role for glutamate and its mGlu1 and mGlu5 receptors in depression and antidepressant activity. Furthermore, evidence also implicates glutamate release, which can result in activation of NMDA and mGlu1 and mGlu5 receptors, an underlying cause for depression and anxiety. Studies with NMDA receptor antagonists of mGlu1 and mGlu5 receptors as well as positive modulators of AMPA receptors have demonstrated antidepressant-like activity in a variety of preclinical models. The concept of NMDA antagonists as antidepressants has generated considerable interest in the NMDA receptor as a target for new antidepressant therapies (see Chapter 18). Several studies have shown that chronic antidepressant treatment can modulate NMDA receptor expression and function. Preclinical studies with NMDA receptor antagonists have demonstrated their potential antidepressant properties. Other studies, which have demonstrated that NMDA receptors have a role in the development and maintenance of alcohol dependence, suggest that NMDA receptors that are upregulated by alcohol could be a target for therapeutic interventions (24).

INHIBITORY AMINO ACID NEUROTRANSMITTERS

γ-Aminobutyric Acid

The major IAA neurotransmitter in the mammalian CNS is GABA (Fig. 12.2). Initially found to be involved with neuromuscular transmission in the lobster, GABA has since been well characterized as a neurotransmitter in the brain and spinal cord of mammals. In the periphery, in tissues such as the liver, spleen, sympathetic ganglia, and splenic nerve, GABA and its receptors are also found. The levels are very low, however, and their function in these non-CNS tissues is poorly understood. While levels of GABA in the CNS are very high (millimoles per gram of tissue) compared to those of the classical monoamine neurotransmitters (nanomoles per gram of tissue), the distribution of GABA in the CNS is unique, with an unequal distribution, thus supporting a neurotransmitter role. Unlike many of the other putative amino acid neurotransmitters that are also components of CNS proteins, GABA is not known to be incorporated into proteins, thus making it easier to support a role for GABA as a neurotransmitter.

The synthesis of GABA uses glutamate and the enzyme glutamic acid decarboxylase (GAD), the levels of which closely parallel those of GABA (Fig. 12.3). Although glutamate itself functions as an important neurotransmitter, the control of GABA synthesis appears to be dependent on the activity of GAD and its cofactor, pyridoxal phosphate. Glutamate can be synthesized from α-oxoglutaric acid, α-ketoglutarate, and glutamine (25) (Fig. 12.3). Glucose and pyruvate can also be converted to glutamate via metabolism involving the Krebs cycle. Two isoforms of GAD derived from different genes have been characterized: GAD-65 and GAD-67. The lower molecular weight GAD-65 has a much higher affinity for its pyridoxal cofactor than does the larger GAD-67. There also appears to be different cellular and subcellular distribution patterns between the two GAD isoforms, but the significance of their unique roles in GABAergic neurotransmission is not fully understood (26).

In a similar manner to most other classical neurotransmitters, GABA, once synthesized, is stored in vesicles located in the presynaptic nerve terminals, as shown in Figure 12.8. A specific vesicular GABA transporter protein (VGAT) has been identified that transports largely GABA into the storage vesicles (27). The VGAT lacks complete selectivity, because the other major IAA neurotransmitter glycine is also a substrate for VGAT, which has been shown to be present in glycinergic terminals. Unlike the well-defined vesicular transporters for the monoamine neurotransmitters, which are characterized by 12 transmembrane-spanning segments, VGAT only contains 10 such transmembrane-spanning segments. However, similar to the monoamine vesicular transporters, VGAT appears to be driven by an H^+ electrochemical gradient generated by an ATP-dependent H^+ pump in the vesicle plasma membrane. Whereas vigabatrin potently

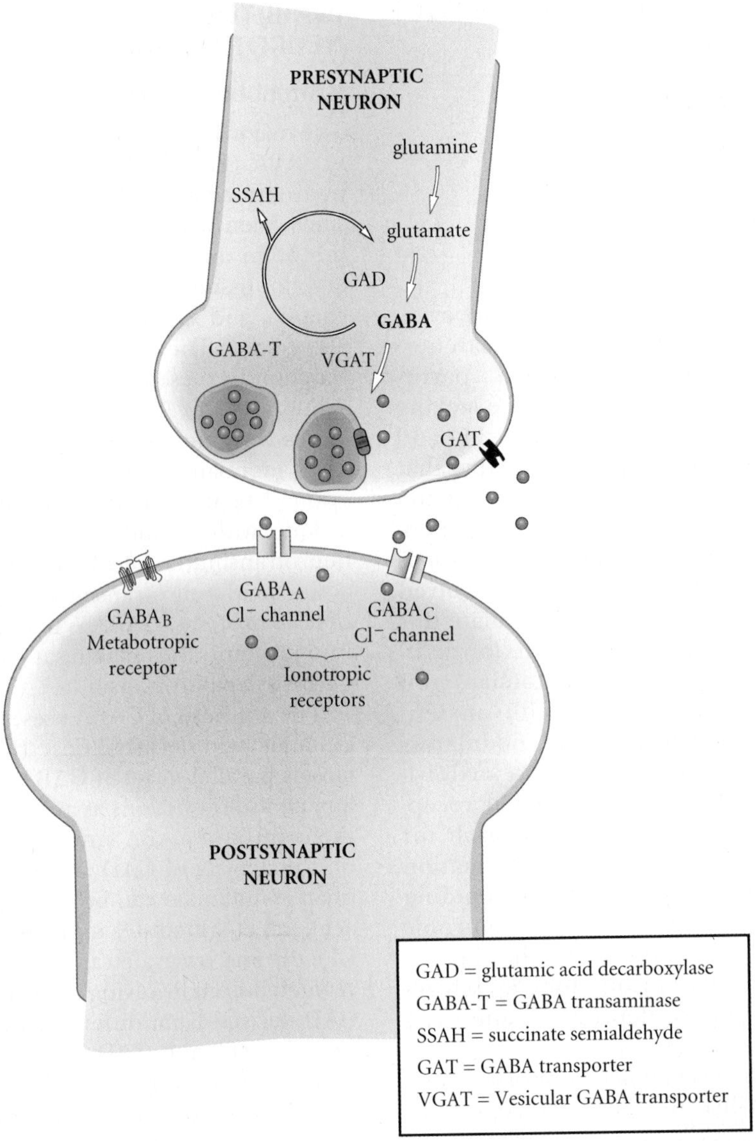

FIGURE 12.8 The GABA neuron, showing the formation of GABA, ionotropic and metabotropic receptors, and reuptake transporters.

inhibits VGAT and nipecotic acid weakly inhibits VGAT, the role of VGAT inhibition in the overall pharmacologic actions of these agents is not well understood, because both agents probably act largely via non–GABA-mediated mechanisms.

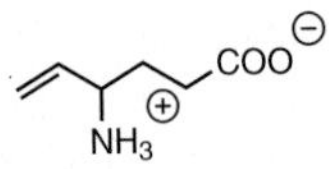

Vigabatrin

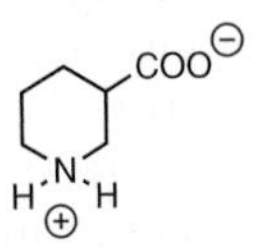

Nipecotate

Nerve stimulation leading to depolarization of GABAergic presynaptic terminals causes the Ca^{2+}-mediated exocytosis of vesicles containing GABA. Once released, GABA diffuses across the synapse to the postsynaptic side, where interaction with GABA receptors takes place, leading to hyperpolarization of the postsynaptic neuron, as shown in Figure 12.8 (these receptor subtypes are described in detail below). Some regulation of GABA release occurs via presynaptic $GABA_B$ autoreceptors that decrease subsequent neurotransmitter release. The termination of the GABA-mediated signal takes place as a result of reuptake transporter systems that transport GABA back into the presynaptic neuron or into surrounding glial cells and astrocytes. This dual neuronal–glial reuptake process is distinct from that observed with the classical monoamines, for which neuronal reuptake largely predominates. Four transporters with 12 transmembrane-spanning segments have been identified and cloned: GAT-1, GAT-2, GAT-3, and BGT-1 (28). All four are capable of transporting GABA, but they can also transport other IAAs, particularly glycine, β-alanine, and taurine (Fig. 12.2). One of the transporters, BGT-1, is capable of transporting the dimethylated glycine derivative betaine and thus is also known as the betaine transporter.

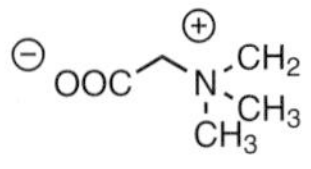

Betaine

A number of inhibitors of these transporters are known, but only one currently is available for therapeutic use. Tiagabine, by selectively inhibiting GAT-1, which can be the major GABA neuronal reuptake transporter, is an approved agent for the treatment of partial seizures (see Chapter 17). Clinical trials are under way for its use in the treatment of anxiety, neuropathic pain, and insomnia (29). Two GABA analogues that have been shown to interact with GAT-1 are gabapentin and pregabalin. The concentrations required to inhibit GAT, however, are very high, and a GABAergic mechanism of action most likely does not explain their anticonvulsant activity (30). Despite their close structural similarity to GABA, inhibition of a voltage-gated calcium channel containing the $\alpha_2\delta_1$ subunit is believed to be responsible for their anticonvulsant actions.

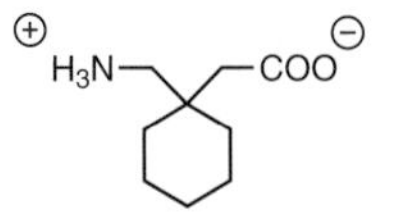

Gabapentin

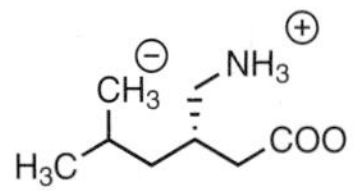

Pregabalin

Metabolism of GABA occurs via a series of enzymatic steps starting with GABA transaminase (GABA-T), as shown in Figure 12.3. This reversible mitochondrial enzyme uses pyridoxal phosphate as a cofactor and is widely distributed throughout the CNS. Transamination results in the formation of succinic semialdehyde (SSA), which can be further metabolized to succinate via SSA dehydrogenase (SSADH) or, alternatively, reduced to γ-hydroxybutyrate (GHB) (see Fig 12.12). Other metabolites of unknown significance include carnitine, homoanserine, homopantothenic acid, and a number of γ-butyryl derivatives, including γ-butyryllysine, γ-butyrylhistidine, and γ-butyrylcholine. Vigabatrin (γ-vinyl-GABA), an irreversible inhibitor of GABA-T, increases the levels of GABA by inhibiting its metabolism and is used for the treatment of seizure disorders in some countries. Other inhibitors of GABA-T include gabaculline and acetylenic GABA. These agents display anticonvulsant activity in experimental animal models of epilepsy.

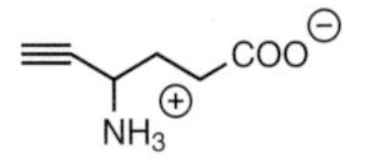

Acetylenic GABA

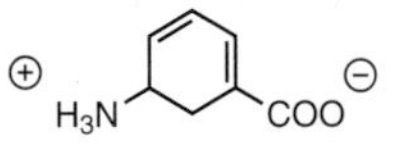

Gabaculine

GABA$_A$ Receptors

The initial observations that application of GABA was capable of hyperpolarizing neurons, as well as the lack of activity of structurally related amino acids and other compounds, suggested that a receptor likely mediated this response. At least three different families of GABA receptors have been identified to date: GABA$_A$, GABA$_B$, and GABA$_C$ (Fig. 12.9). The GABA$_A$ receptor was the first to be identified and was found to be a neurotransmitter-gated ion channel (ionotropic) that, when activated, allows the entry of chloride ion into the cell, thereby hyperpolarizing the neuron and making cell firing less likely to occur. The GABA$_A$ receptor (Fig. 12.9) is a member of the Cys-loop (cysteine–cysteine loop located on the N-terminal region) family of receptors that also include the strychnine-sensitive glycine, nicotinic acetylcholine, and serotonin 5-HT$_3$ receptors. The pentameric GABA$_A$ receptor is composed of various combinations of subunits (α, β, γ, δ, ε, π, ρ, and θ). Various subunit isoforms have been identified with 6α, 3β, 3γ, and 3ρ subunits (some have suggested that the ρ subunits are found only in the GABA$_C$ receptor). Each subunit is a four

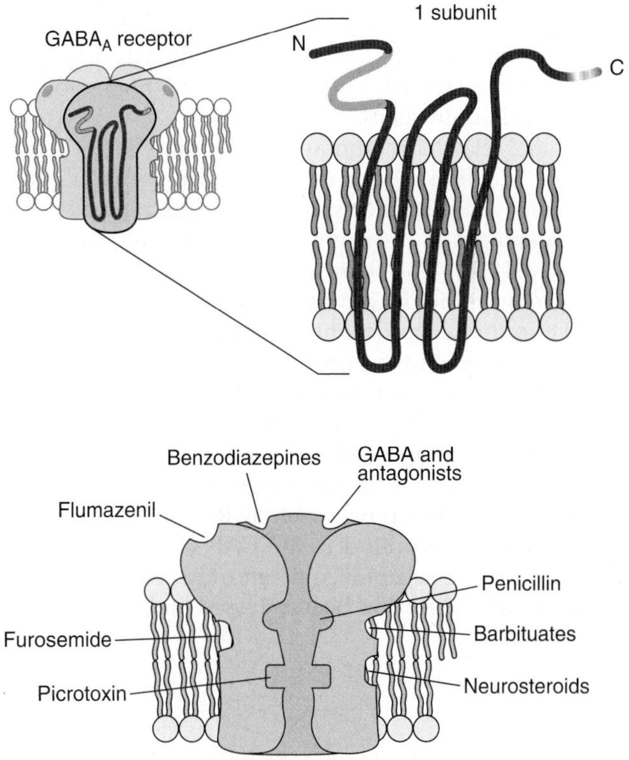

FIGURE 12.9 GABA$_A$ receptor. (A) The structure of the GABA$_A$ receptor, showing the N- and C-terminal regions of the four membrane-spanning regions for each of the five subunits. (B) The major binding sites on the GABA$_A$ receptor. (From Chou J, Strichartz GR, Lo EH. Pharmacology of excitatory and inhibitory neurotransmitters, Chapter 10. In: Golan DE, Tashjian A, Tashjian A, et al., eds. Principles of Pharmacology: The Pathophysiologic Basis of Drug Therapy. Baltimore, MD: Lippincott Williams & Wilkins, 2004:139–160, with permission.)

transmembrane-spanning protein that, when arranged in a circle, forms the ion channel with a diameter of approximately 8 nm that remains closed until GABA binds to its ligand recognition site. One of the most common $GABA_A$ receptor conformations in the mammalian CNS consists of a pair of α_1 subunits, a pair of β subunits, and a single γ_2 subunit, as shown in Figure 12.10. Other commonly identified receptors contain α_1, α_2, α_3, and α_5 as well as forms of the β subunit and, typically, the γ_2 subunit, and always in a 2:2:1 stoichiometry (31). The binding of two molecules of GABA, as shown in Figure 12.10, probably to the individual β subunits near the α–β interface, is believed to be required for normal receptor activation. In fact, among $GABA_A$ receptors, 17 different combinations of subunits have been identified. Having a family of receptors that all share the same basic structure but that differ in specific subunit composition allows greater levels of functional diversity. Each of the receptor varieties varies in binding affinity, channel activity, and the degree to which GABA binding is affected by different endogenous modulators. As a result, inhibitory neurotransmission can be more finely controlled. Such receptor heterogeneity also allows more control at the genomic level, in turn allowing postsynaptic cells to respond to changing environmental needs or variable activity at the synapse (plasticity). In contrast, altered subunit compositions could also be partly responsible for an increased susceptibility to pathophysiologic conditions in individuals.

A major class of compounds that modulate $GABA_A$ receptor function is that of the benzodiazepines (e.g., diazepam). The binding site for benzodiazepines likely is the α subunit in proximity to the β subunit, as shown in Figure 12.10. The form of the γ subunit appears to help to determine the affinity of the individual benzodiazepine to the receptor. The benzodiazepines appear to bind more efficiently to receptors containing γ_2 than to the γ_1 subunit, as shown in Table 12.3. Similarly, very low-affinity binding is observed if a receptor contains the α_6 subunit. In fact, the α_6 subunit seems to confer binding preference to inverse agonists (agents that stabilize the inactive/resting receptor), such as Ro194603. The benzodiazepines do not bind to the GABA (ligand-recognition) site on the receptor and can only produce effects if presynaptic GABA has been released and is present at the receptors.

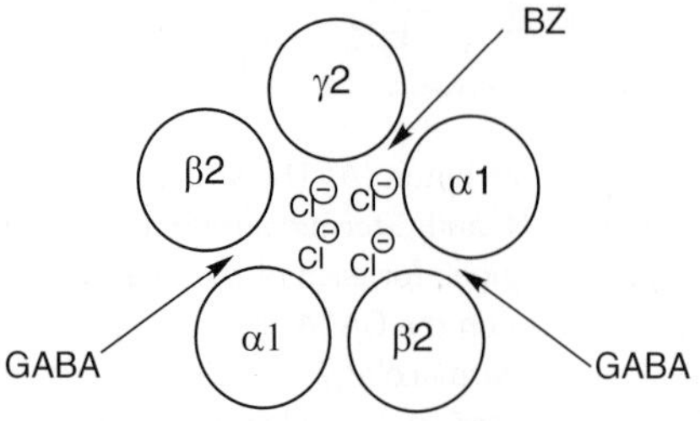

FIGURE 12.10 Extracellular view of the $GABA_A$ receptor showing the location of benzodiazepine (BZ) and low-affinity GABA binding sites.

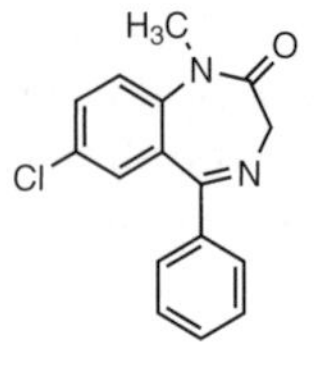

Diazepam

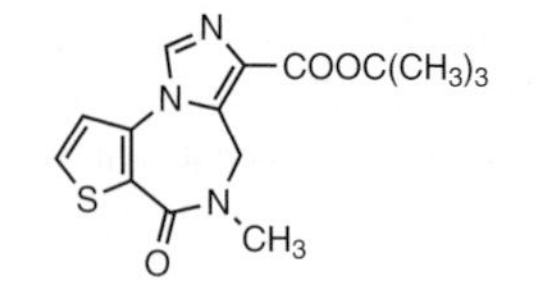

Ro-19-4603

Benzodiazepines are allosteric modulators, or ligands that bind at a secondary binding site on a receptor that is distinct from the primary ligand binding site, resulting in conformational changes in the structure of the receptor that either activates or, sometimes, inhibits the receptor. Thus, the benzodiazepines allosterically modulate the $GABA_A$ receptor, increasing the frequency of the chloride channel opening when GABA is bound, thus potentiating the response of exogenously released GABA. Clinically the benzodiazepines are very safe when used alone in the absence of CNS depressants, because they are not active on GABA receptors alone. This is in contrast to the barbiturates that can directly activate the $GABA_A$ receptor when present at higher concentration and, thus, have a much lower therapeutic index. Flumazenil, a benzodiazepine receptor antagonist, is used for the treatment of severe overdoses of benzodiazepines. Flumazenil competitively antagonizes the binding and allosteric effects of benzodiazepine agonists as well as benzodiazepine inverse agonists, such as the β-carbolines.

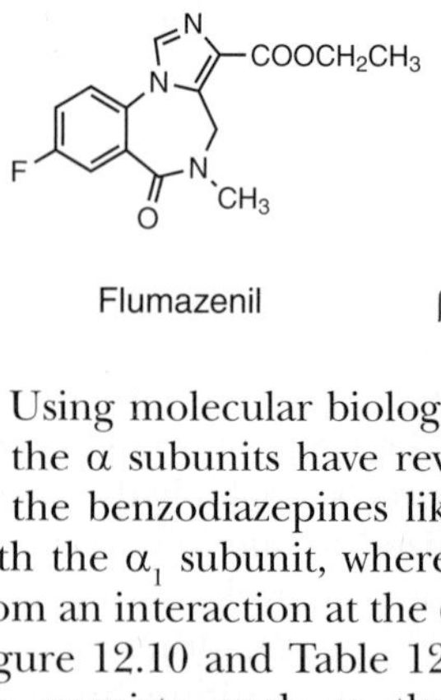

Flumazenil

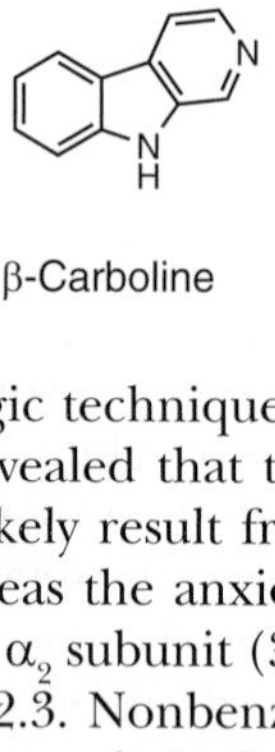

β-Carboline

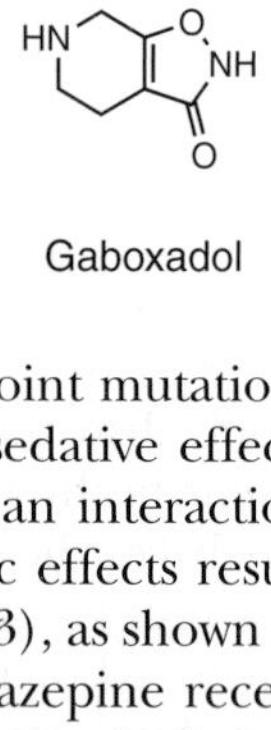

Gaboxadol

Using molecular biologic techniques, point mutations of the α subunits have revealed that the sedative effects of the benzodiazepines likely result from an interaction with the α_1 subunit, whereas the anxiolytic effects result from an interaction at the α_2 subunit (32,33), as shown in Figure 12.10 and Table 12.3. Nonbenzodiazepine receptor agonists, such as the sedative-hypnotics indiplon, zaleplon, zopiclone, and zolpidem (see Chapter 16), are α_1 subunit–preferring ligands, as shown in Table 12.3 (34).

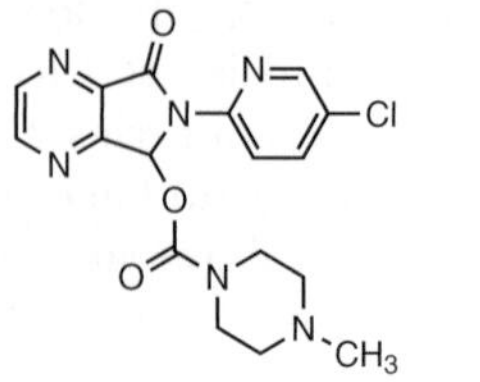

Zopiclone

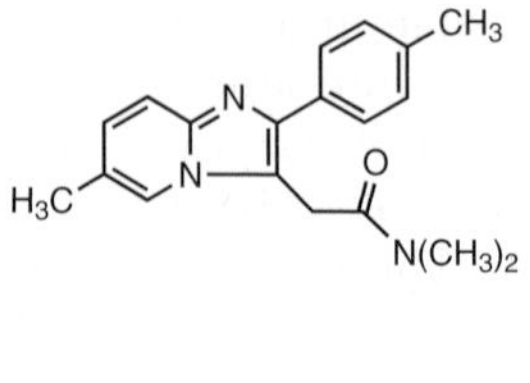

Zolpidem

An agent that acts on the $GABA_A$ receptor that does not interact with the benzodiazepine binding site is gaboxadol (previously called THIP). This sedative-hypnotic

TABLE 12.3 A Comparison of the Binding Affinities (nm) of Benzodiazepine and Nonbenzodiazepine Ligands for $GABA_A$ Receptor Subtypes (45)

Compound	$GABA_A$ Receptor Subtypes					
	$\alpha_1\beta\gamma_2$	$\alpha_2\beta\gamma_2$	$\alpha_3\beta\gamma_2$	$\alpha_4\beta\gamma_2$	$\alpha_5\beta\gamma_2$	$\alpha_6\beta\gamma_2$
Benzodiazepines						
Diazepam	16	17	17	>10,000	15	>10,000
Clonazepam	1.3	1.7	2.0	—	—	>10,000
Triazolam	1.8	1.2	3.0	—	1.2	—
Flumazenil	1.0	1.1	1.5	107	2.4	90
Nonbenzodiazepines						
Zaleplon	130	1,820	1,530	>10,000	490	>10,000
Zolpidem	17	290	357	—	>15,000	—
Zopiclone	19	33	—	—	—	—

binds with high affinity to the extrasynaptic $\alpha_4\beta_x\delta$ $GABA_A$ receptor and does not alter sleep onset or REM sleep as do the benzodiazepines. On the other hand, gaboxadol increases slow-wave sleep (35).

The barbiturates bind to a different portion of the $GABA_A$ receptor and, similar to the benzodiazepines, enhance the activity of GABA. The binding of a barbiturate leads to an increase in the duration of ion channel opening. Higher concentrations of the barbiturates can directly open the chloride channel; thus, overdoses of barbiturates can lead to life-threatening, CNS-mediated respiratory and cardiovascular depression.

A number of compounds are known to directly activate the $GABA_A$ receptor. Of these compounds, muscimol, the decarboxylated metabolite of ibotenate, and isoguvacine are the most well known. Unlike GABA, which does not cross the blood–brain barrier, these agents do cross the blood–brain barrier and display GABA-mimetic activity following peripheral administration. A number of compounds can also bind to the $GABA_A$ receptor and antagonize the actions of GABA. Bicuculline, by binding to the GABA recognition site and preventing GABA from binding, produces convulsions in experimental animals. Picrotoxin, via its active metabolite picrotoxinin, binds in the chloride channel to prevent ion flow when the receptor is activated by GABA. Picrotoxin does not alter GABA binding but, instead, prevents ions from flowing and is a potent convulsant.

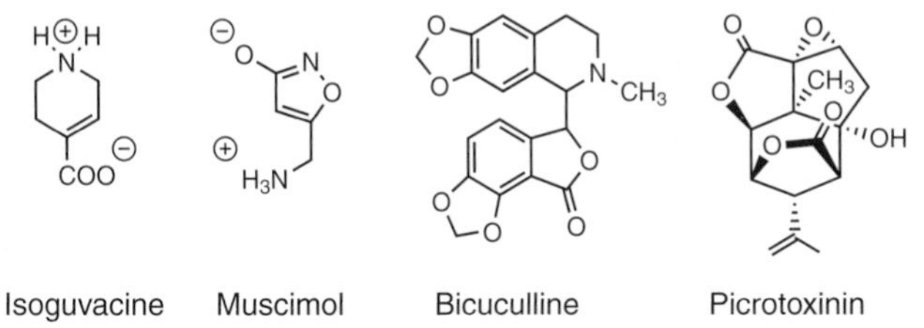

Isoguvacine Muscimol Bicuculline Picrotoxinin

With the many possible subunit assembly sequences of $GABA_A$ receptors, advances in medicinal chemistry can someday lead to the design of compounds that target specific pentameric subunit assemblies to preferentially produce specific effects (36). For instance, located on the base of the dendritic spines of hippocampal pyramidal cells are $GABA_A$ receptors with an α_5 subunit composition. These receptors are thought to counteract the excitatory input because of glutamatergic NMDA receptor activation involved in learning and memory. Activation of $GABA_A$ receptors in this area disrupts learning and memory, whereas NMDA receptor activation improves learning and memory. Administration of an inverse agonist of the $GABA_A$ receptor with selectivity for the α_5 subunit improves memory performance in experimental animals (37). Furthermore, α_3-selective agonists can be useful in treating schizophrenia, because this subtype of $GABA_A$ receptor appears to have a role in decreasing the release of dopamine from overactive neurons in the mesolimbic system (38).

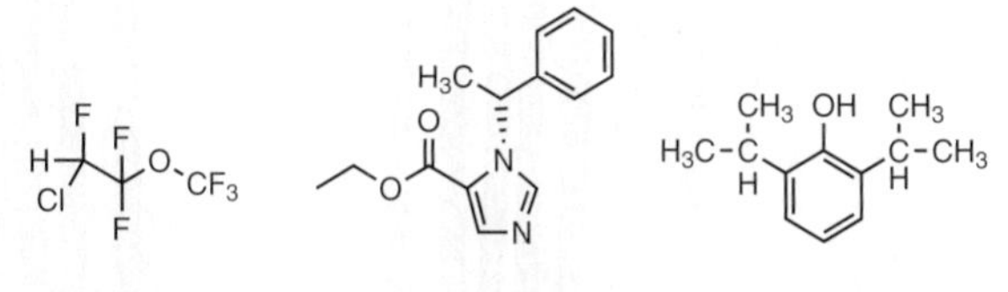

Enflurane Etomidate Propofol

General anesthetics (see Chapter 14) also appear to have interactions with the $GABA_A$ receptor in producing their various anesthetic effects, including immobilization, respiratory depression, and hypnosis via binding to hydrophobic pockets within the receptor. Using point-mutated knock-in mice, general anesthetic agents, such as enflurane, etomidate, and propofol, have been found to interact with the β_3 subunit of the $GABA_A$ receptor to produce immobilization and hypnosis (38). The heart rate and body temperature depressant effects of etomidate and propofol, however, do not appear to be mediated by the sub-β_3 subunit. Studies are under way to improve our understanding of the molecular mechanisms of this chemically varied group of agents used as general anesthetics.

Neurosteroids are also capable of modulating the activity of GABA at the $GABA_A$ receptor by binding to a site distinct from that used by GABA, benzodiazepines, and barbiturates. These steroids, including the progesterone metabolites pregnenolone, allopregnenolone, and allotetrahydrodeoxycorticosterone, enhance GABA-mediated inhibitory activity. The presence of the δ subunit in the pentameric $GABA_A$ receptor greatly increases the affinity of steroid binding and efficacy. High concentrations of these steroids can also result in direct activation of the receptor.

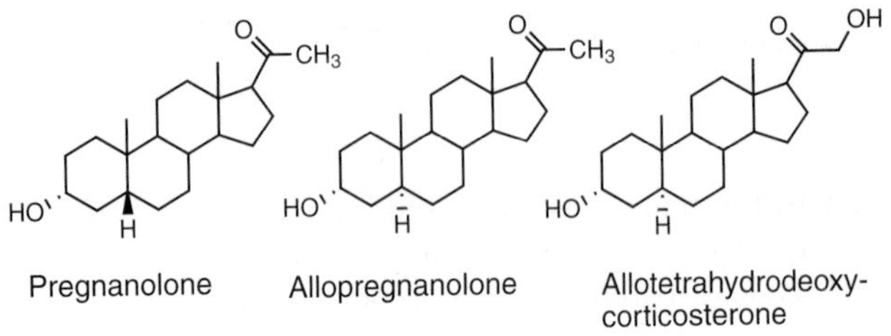

Thus, it can be possible in the future to selectively target the various modulatory sites on the $GABA_A$ receptor to produce preferential pharmacologic effects—for example, benzodiazepines that are anxiolytic without sedative effects, antischizophrenic agents that lack sedation and extrapyramidal side effects, and general anesthetics that do not alter respiratory and/or heart rates.

$GABA_B$ Receptors

As studies continued, the application of GABA to cells occasionally was found to produce effects that were not blocked by the standard GABA receptor antagonist bicuculline. Standard GABA agonists, such as muscimol and isoguvacine, were also ineffective as agonists in such systems. This led to the suggestion that a different subtype of GABA receptor mediated these observed effects. In 1998, the structure of the $GABA_B$ receptor was elucidated and found to be a GPCR heterodimer comprised of $GABA_{B1}$ and $GABA_{B2}$ subunits (Fig. 12.11). Each subunit had a seven membrane-spanning segment, which allowed their intracellular C-termini to connect in a 1:1 stoichiometric fashion (39). The $GABA_{B1}$ subunit was also found to exist in two isoforms, $GABA_{B1a}$ and $GABA_{B1b}$. Some have suggested that the $GABA_{B1a}$ subunit is preferentially located presynaptically, whereas the $GABA_{B1b}$ subunit is located postsynaptically. Within this metabotropic receptor, the $GABA_{B1}$ subunits contain the GABA binding domain extracellularly, whereas the $GABA_{B2}$ subunit couples to the G-protein mechanism intracellularly. Both subunits are required for normal receptor function, as shown in Figure 12.11. Knockout mice lacking either of these subunits typically display epileptiform seizures, hyperalgesia, hyperlocomotion, and impaired memory function (40). Besides the normal endogenous agonist GABA, a structural analogue, (−)-baclofen, acts stereoselectively as an agonist at the $GABA_B$ receptor.

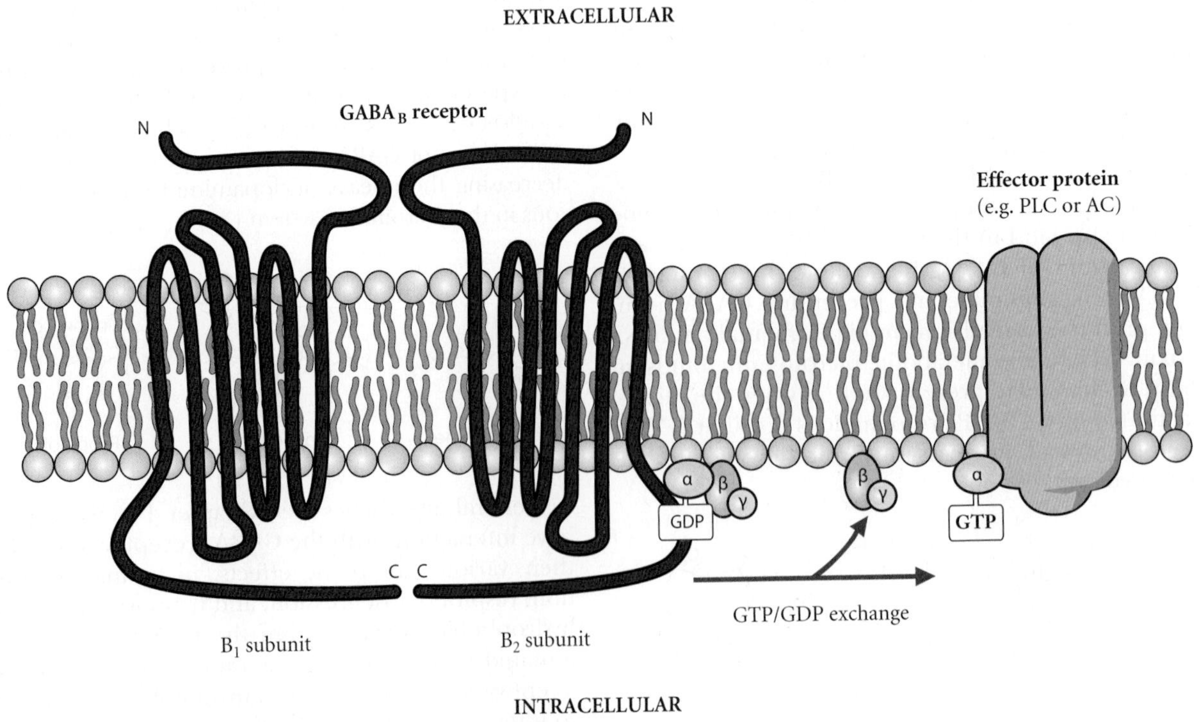

FIGURE 12.11 The $GABA_B$ receptor, showing its B_1 and B_2 subunits and its mechanism of signal transduction.

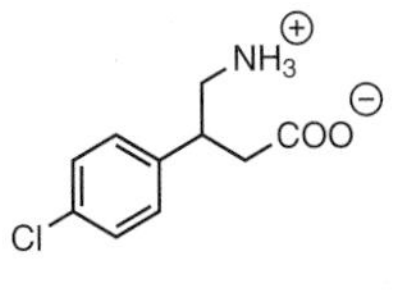

Baclofen

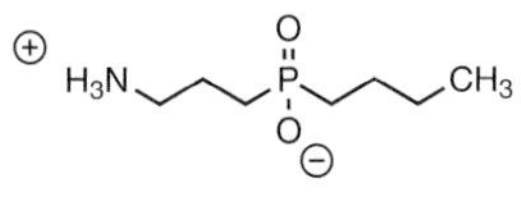

CGP 36742

(±)-Baclofen, which enters the brain via a selective transporter, has been approved for therapeutic use since 1972 for the treatment of spasticity as a muscle relaxant (41). Besides relaxing skeletal muscles, baclofen is capable of exacerbating absence seizures, decreasing cognitive function, increasing food intake, and decreasing drug-seeking behaviors. Drug development of selective $GABA_B$ receptor antagonists can someday lead to therapeutically useful agents for the treatment of absence seizures, depression, anxiety, and cognitive impairments. One such compound currently undergoing clinical trials is the orally bioavailable $GABA_B$ receptor antagonist CGP-36742, which is in clinical trials for the treatment of mild cognitive impairment and Alzheimer disease. The inhibition of $GABA_B$ receptors is believed to cause disinhibition of somatostatin (a peptide neurotransmitter in the CNS) release, which then allows activation of NMDA receptors in the hippocampus that normally are required for memory and cognitive functions (42).

γ-Hydroxybutyrate

Another endogenous compound that binds to and weakly activates the $GABA_B$ receptor is GHB (43). This compound, which can be formed as a result of the metabolism of GABA, has a unique distribution in the CNS, but it does not parallel closely that of GABA, as shown in Figure 12.12. Levels of GHB are increased significantly in patients and knockout mice lacking the enzyme SSADH, which is responsible for the conversion of SSA to succinic acid, with eventual entry into the citric acid cycle. A deficiency of this enzyme in patients is caused by a rare, autosomal recessive inheritance and is termed "GHB aciduria" (44).

Endogenous GHB likely interacts with a recently discovered GHB receptor, but the function of GHB in the CNS is not completely understood. A specific GHB receptor was reportedly cloned in 2003 and found to have no sequence homology with the $GABA_B$ receptor—or with any other known GPCR (45). This putative receptor is a member of the GPCR family and is distributed in most brain regions known to bind GHB. The association is not perfect, however, because high levels of mRNA for the GHB receptor are found in the cerebellum even though little GHB normally binds here.

In the United States, GHB is approved for the treatment of cataplexy associated with the sleeping disorder narcolepsy (46). Narcolepsy is most often characterized by a lack of the CNS 11-amino acid polypeptide orexin (also known as hypocretin) or, possibly, its receptors. Patients with narcolepsy experience excessive bouts of sudden-onset daytime sleepiness and have been treated in the past with

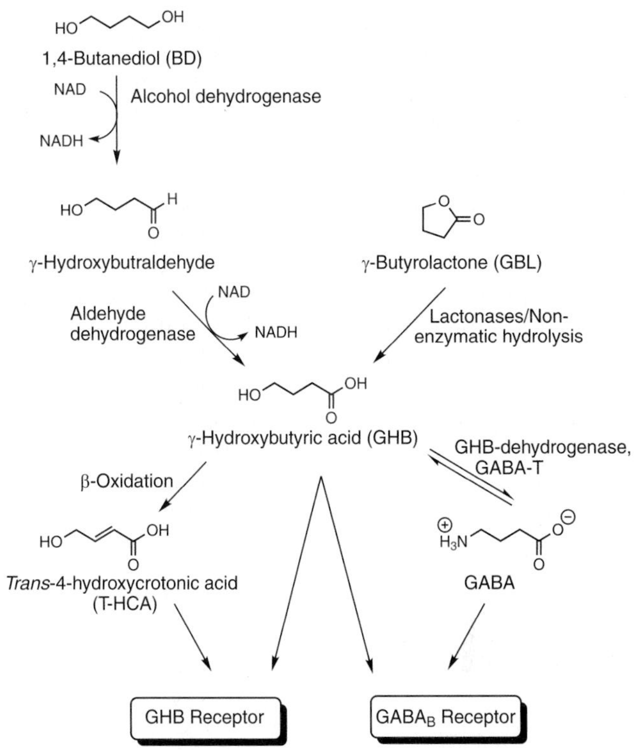

FIGURE 12.12 Biotransformation of 1,4-butanediol (BD) and γ-butyrolactone (GBL) and the receptor sites for their metabolites, γ-hydroxybutyrate (GHB), GABA, and trans-4-hydroxycrotonic acid (T-HCA).

stimulants, such as methylphenidate and amphetamine, or with modafinil (see Chapter 22) or antidepressants. The use of GHB in narcolepsy takes a different approach in that dosing is at bedtime and, being a CNS depressant, it acts to enhance sleep quality. Patients then awake the following morning and experience a rebound insomnia, which counteracts any propensity for daytime sleepiness. Although not a U.S. Food and Drug Administration–approved use, GHB is being investigated for its efficacy in treating fibromyalgia. Exogenously administered GHB appears to produce its clinical and toxic effects via interaction with $GABA_B$ receptors, because most studies have been able to block its effects with $GABA_B$ receptor antagonists but not with the GHB receptor antagonist NCS-382 (although NCS-382 is not an ideal antagonist because it can function as a partial agonist).

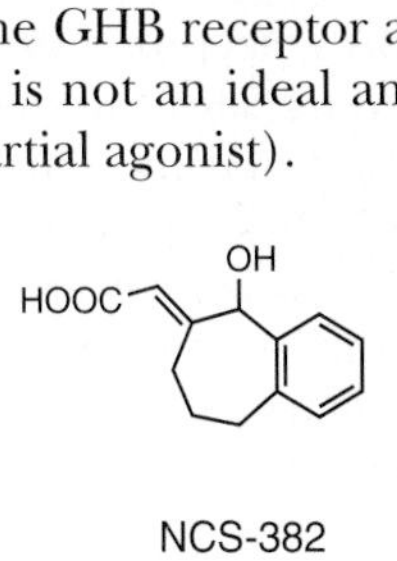

NCS-382

In addition, GHB has been used for illicit purposes. Because GHB produces CNS sedation with amnesia, some have used this compound for drug-facilitated sexual assault (e.g., "date rape"). As governmental regulations on the availability of GHB became tighter, the use of GHB precursors, such as γ-butyrolactone and 1,4-butanediol, became popular (47). Figure 12.12 diagrams the biotransformation of γ-butyrolactone and 1,4-butanediol to GHB and GABA, explaining their relationship to GHB and $GABA_B$ receptors. The popularity of these compounds as drugs of abuse is facilitated by their ready availability as industrial solvents. Furthermore, GHB can be further metabolized by β-oxidation to *trans*-4-hydroxycrotonic acid, which can also bind to the GHB receptor. Body builders use GHB and its precursor compounds as well in an attempt to enhance the release of growth hormone, which actually increases due to their ability to produce sleep. Most often, however, chronic abuse leads to tolerance, with a need to increase dosing and a propensity to produce physical dependence (48). A serious and difficult-to-treat withdrawal syndrome from GHB abuse has been documented.

$GABA_C$ Receptor

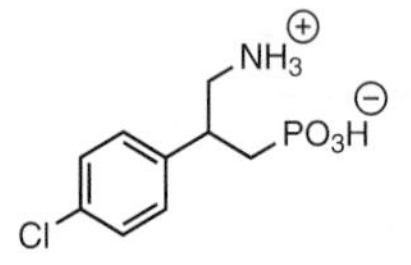

Phaclofen

Another receptor that binds GABA but is not antagonized by bicuculline ($GABA_A$) or phaclofen ($GABA_B$) and is not influenced by either the benzodiazepines or barbiturates is known as the $GABA_C$ receptor. The endogenous neurotransmitter GABA is an order of magnitude more potent on the $GABA_C$ receptor as compared with the $GABA_A$ receptor, and the responses to activation of the $GABA_C$ receptor are much slower and sustained as compared with the rapid and brief responses following $GABA_A$ receptor activation. The $GABA_C$ receptor is most abundant in the retina, with significant levels in the spinal cord and pituitary gland. This ligand-gated ion chloride channel is a pentamer of subunits that form the ion channel. Some have suggested that the ρ subunit is unique to the $GABA_C$ receptor (49). On the extracellular domain are binding sites for zinc, which is a potent modulator of receptor activity. The most well-described antagonist is TPMPA. Interestingly, isoguvacine, an agonist at the $GABA_A$ receptors, acts as an antagonist at the $GABA_C$ receptor. Much information regarding the location, function, and pharmacology of the $GABA_C$ receptor is needed to begin to take advantage of this receptor for therapeutic purposes.

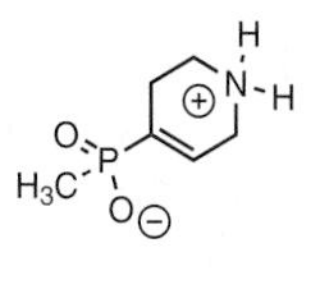

TPMPA

GLYCINE

The simplest of all amino acids, glycine, which classically causes hyperpolarization of neurons in the CNS, satisfies all the required criteria for neurotransmitter candidacy (50). Glycine in the CNS is unevenly distributed, with the highest concentrations found in the ventral gray areas of the spinal cord and in the medulla oblongata in the brainstem (51). The retina is also a structure with high concentrations of glycine (52). The synthesis of glycine in glycinergic neurons appears to be from L-serine and to be regulated by the enzyme serine hydroxymethyltransferase (SHMT), the concentrations of which in the CNS parallel those of glycine. Another substrate of SHMT, however, is L-threonine, which can also serve as a precursor of glycine. Administration of large doses of L-serine to animals fails to alter CNS glycine levels, but administration of L-threonine, which passes the blood–brain barrier more readily than L-serine does, increases CNS glycine levels (53). L-Threonine has been used as an orphan drug to treat a rare form of spasticity, familial spastic paraparesis, in humans (54). The synthesis of glycine could also occur via a transamination reaction involving glutamate in which glycine and α-ketoglutarate are produced. The understanding of the synthesis of glycine in the CNS for its neurotransmitter functions has been a difficult hurdle to overcome, likely because of the varied roles of glycine in the synthesis of protein, porphyrin, bile salts, and nucleic acids in addition to intermediary metabolic processes involving one-carbon fragments.

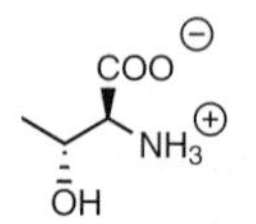

L-Threonine

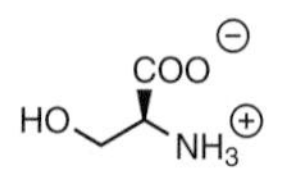

L-Serine

Glycine is stored in vesicles, and its uptake is mediated via VGAT, which is also capable of transporting GABA. Release of glycine occurs from presynaptic terminals in a Ca^{2+}-dependent fashion and, similarly, is taken back up into these terminals and, possibly, nearby glial cells (55,56). Endocannabinoids released from the postsynaptic membrane can act retrogradely at presynaptic glycinergic terminals via the cannabinoid-1 receptor to inhibit the release of glycine (57). Reuptake is via Na^+/Cl^--dependent neurotransmitter transporters known as GLYT-1 and GLYT-2. These 12 transmembrane-spanning transporters are located in areas where glycine is believed to act as a neurotransmitter or coagonist at NMDA receptors. The GLYT-1 transporters are largely found on glial cells and at glutamatergic neurons, whereas the GLYT-2 transporter is found mostly on presynaptic glycinergic neurons (58). Few pharmacologic tools are available to examine the role of either form of the membrane transporters.

The glycine receptor mediating the inhibitory actions of glycine is similar to the $GABA_A$ receptor and other members of the Cys-loop family in being a pentameric, circular ion channel that allows the conduction of chloride (59). Unlike the GABA receptor, however, the inhibitory glycine receptor can be a homopentamer of α subunits or a heteropentamer comprised of two α subunits and three β subunits. Four isoforms of the α subunits have been identified, whereas only one β subunit is known. The neurotransmitter glycine, in addition to taurine, D-alanine, L-alanine, β-alanine, hypotaurine, serine, and β-aminobutyric acid, can bind to any of three sites on the receptor to lead to activation. Positive modulators of the inhibitory glycine receptor include zinc, neurosteroids, propofol, ethanol, and volatile anesthetics, such as isoflurane (60,61).

The best-described antagonist of the inhibitory glycine receptor is the convulsant strychnine. Strychnine binds to a different site than that which recognizes glycine. Sometimes, the inhibitory glycine receptor is referred to as the "strychnine-sensitive" glycine receptor to distinguish it from the glycine modulatory site on the glutamatergic NMDA receptor. The $GABA_A$ receptor antagonist picrotoxin can also inhibit the IAA glycine receptor. More recently, the endocannabinoids, such as anandamide and 2-arachidonylglycerol, have also been shown to antagonize the activity of IAA glycine at this receptor (57). Ginkgolide B has similarly been shown to act as an antagonist at the IAA glycine receptor. Agents that act as agonists at the IAA glycine receptor can find utility as anticonvulsants, muscle relaxants, sedatives, and general anesthetics.

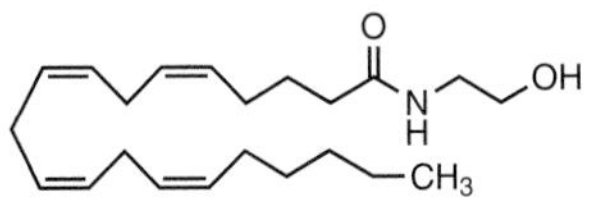

Anandamide

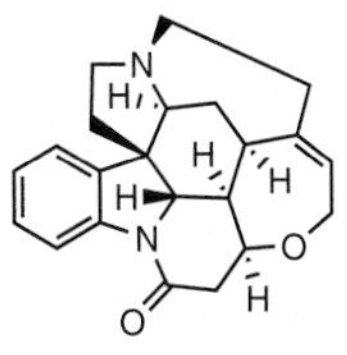

Strychnine

As more information regarding the control of the synthesis of the neurotransmitter pool of glycine becomes available and more compounds with selectivity for the IAA glycine receptor are discovered or developed, useful therapeutic agents that take advantage of modulating glycinergic neurotransmission can be realized.

FUTURE DIRECTIONS

The amino acids have an essential role in the normal control of neurotransmission in the CNS, but during disease, these same amino acids can mediate a number of the pathologic consequences that are observed. Currently there are many therapeutic agents available that take advantage of one or more aspects of amino acidergic neurotransmission to produce their pharmacologic effects. As agents are developed that are more specific for a particular isoform configuration of an amino acid receptor or transporter, or other aspect of amino acid neurotransmitter function, the treatment of various diseases likely will become more effective. Associations between disease states and receptor isoform configurations, transporter density, and activity of enzymes involved in the synthesis and degradation of amino acid neurotransmitters can help to improve our understanding of the pathology of these diseases and lead to improved therapies.

CASE STUDY

S. William Zito and Victoria Roche

SW is a 67-year-old white man who was recently in a car accident and sustained minor soft tissue bruising and shoulder and neck muscle spasms. SW is an academic and spends most of his day working at his computer. The neck and shoulder muscle spasms are severe enough to make it difficult to work for more than 20 minutes at a time before having to take a break. SW visits his primary care physician (PCP) seeking relief from his muscle spasms so he can complete a writing commitment on time. A review of SW's current medication includes Lipitor for hyperlipidemia (10 mg daily) and Uloric for gout (40 mg daily). Clinical laboratory tests indicate that both conditions are under control. His PCP knows that SW is a health care educator who likes chemistry and presents him with the following three structure choices and asks him for his opinion.

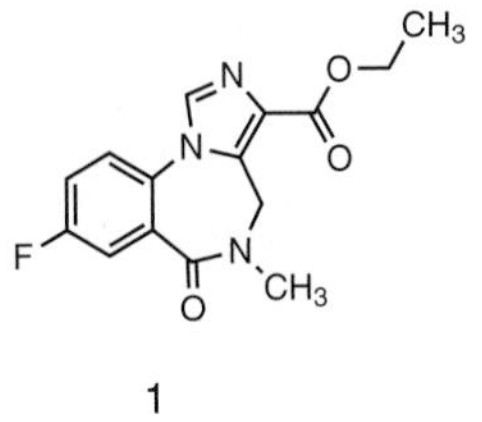

1

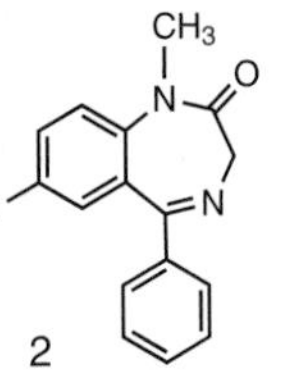

2

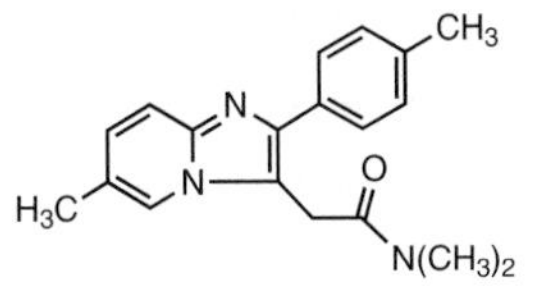

3

1. Conduct a thorough and mechanistic SAR analysis of the three therapeutic options in the case.
2. Apply the chemical understanding gained from the SAR analysis to this patient's specific needs to make a therapeutic recommendation.

References

1. Raiten DJ, Talbot JM, Fisher KD, eds. Analysis of adverse reactions to monosodium glutamate (MSG). Report prepared for Center for Food Safety and Applied Nutrition, Food and Drug Administration. Bethesda, MD: Life Sciences Research Office, Federation of American Societies for Experimental Biology, 1995.
2. Maher TJ. Effects of phenylalanine or aspartame on catecholamine synthesis and catecholamine-mediated behaviors. In: Belmaker R, Sandler M, Dahlstrom A, eds. Progress in Catecholamine Research. Part C: Clinical Aspects. New York: Liss, 1988:55–60.
3. Carlson MD, Kish PE, Ueda T. Glutamate uptake into synaptic vesicles: competitive inhibition by bromocriptine. J Neurochem 1989;53:1889–1894.
4. Ozkan ED, Lee FS, Ueda T. A protein factor that inhibits ATP-dependent glutamate and GABA accumulation into synaptic vesicles: purification and initial characterization. Proc Natl Acad Sci U S A 1997;94:4137–4142.
5. Zerangue N, Kavanaugh MP. Flux coupling in a neuronal glutamate transporter. Nature 1996;383:634–637.
6. Dunlop J. Glutamate-based therapeutic approaches: targeting the glutamate transport system. Curr Opin Pharmacol 2006;6:103–107.
7. Chao X-D, Fei F, Fei Z. The role of excitatory amino acid transporters in cerebral ischemia. Neurochem Res 2010;35:1224–1230.
8. Bunch L, Erichsen MN, Jensen AA. Excitatory amino acid transporters as potential drug targets. Expert Opin Ther Targets 2009;13:719–731.
9. Dingdledine R, Borges K, Bowie D, et al. The glutamate receptor ion channels. Pharmacol Rev 1999;51:7–61.
10. Erreger K, Chen PE, Wyllie DJ, et al. Glutamate receptor gating. Crit Rev Neurobiol 2004;16:187–224.
11. Malejev A, Gibbs TT, Farb DH. Inhibition of the NMDA response by pregnenolone sulfate revels subtype selective modulation of NMDA receptors by sulfated steroids. Br J Pharmacol 2002;135:901–909.
12. Subramaniam S, Rho JM, Penix L, et al. Felbamate block of the *N*-methyl-D-aspartate receptor. J Pharmacol Exp Ther 1995;273:878–886.
13. De Sarro G, Ongini E, Bertorelli R, et al. Excitatory amino acid neurotransmission through both NMDA and non-NMDA receptors is involved in the anticonvulsant activity of felbamate in DBA/2 mice. Eur J Pharmacol 1994;262:11–19.
14. Brorson JR, Li D, Suzuki T. Selective expression of heteromeric AMPA receptors driven by flip-flop differences. J Neurosci 2004;24:3461–3470.
15. Paternain AV, Morales M, Lerma J. Selective antagonism of AMPA receptors unmasks lainate receptor–mediated responses in hippocampal neurons. Neuron 1995;14:185–189.
16. Mathew SJ, Manji HK, Charney DS. Novel drugs and therapeutic targets for severe mood disorders. Neuropsychopharmacology 2008;33:2080–2092.
17. Lynch G. Glutamate-based therapeutic approaches: ampakines. Curr Opin Pharmacol 2006;6:82–88.
18. Lerma J, Paternain AV, Rodriguez-Moreno A, et al. Molecular physiology of kainate receptors. Physiol Rev 2001;81:971–998.
19. Lerna J. Kainate receptor physiology. Curr Opin Pharmacol 2006;6:89–97.
20. Foster AC, Kemp JA. Glutamate- and GABA-based CNS therapeutics. Curr Opin Pharmacol 2006;6:7–17.
21. Chiamulera C, Epping-Jordan MP, Zocchi A. Reinforcing and locomotor stimulant effects of cocaine are absent in mGluR5 null mutant mice. Nature Neurosci 2001;4:873–874.
22. Valenti O, Marino MJ, Wittmann M, et al. Group II metabotropic glutamate receptor–mediated modulation of the striatopallidal synapse. J Neurosci 2003;23:7218–7226.
23. Marino MJ, Conn PJ. Glutamate-based therapeutic approaches: allosteric modulators of metabotropic glutamate receptors. Curr Opin Pharmacol 2006;6:98–102.
24. Heinz A, Beck A, Wrase J, et al. Neurotransmitter systems in alcohol dependence. Pharmacopsychiatry 2009;42(Suppl 1):S95–S101.
25. Wang L, Maher TJ, Wurtman RJ. Oral L-glutamine increases GABA levels in striatal tissue and extracellular fluid. FASEB J 2007;21:1227–1232.
26. Sheikh SN, Martin SB, Martin DL. Regional distribution and relative amounts of glutamate decarboxylase isoforms in rat and mouse brain. Neurochem Int 1999;35:73–80.
27. McIntire SL, Reimer RJ, Schuske K, et al. Identification and characterization of the vesicular GABA transporter. Nature 1997;389:870–876.
28. Soudijin W, Van Wijingaarden I. The GABA transporter and its inhibitors. Curr Med Chem 2000;7:1063–1079.
29. Foster AC, Kemp JA. Glutamate- and GABA-based CNS therapeutics. Curr Opin Pharmacol 2006;6:7–17.
30. Sills GJ. The mechanisms of action of gabapentin and pregabalin. Curr Opin Pharmacol 2006;6:108–113.
31. Rudolph U, Mohler H. GABA-based therapeutic approaches: $GABA_A$ receptor subtype functions. Curr Opin Pharmacol 2006;6:18–23.
32. Rudolph U, Crestani F, Benke D, et al. Benzodiazepine actions mediated by specific γ-aminobutyric acid(A) receptor subtypes. Nature 1999;401:796–800.
33. Low K, Crestani F, Keist R, et al. Molecular and neuronal substrates for the selective attenuation of anxiety. Science 2000;290:131–134.
34. Foster AC, Pelleymounter MA, Cullen MJ, et al. In vivo pharmacological characterization of indipion, a novel pyrazolopyrimidine sedative-hypnotic. J Pharmacol Exp Ther 2004;311:547–559.
35. Lancel M, Langebartels A. γ-Aminobutyric acid(A) agonist 4,5,6,7-tetrahydroisoxazolo[4,5-*c*]pyridine-3-ol persistently increases sleep maintenance and intensity during chronic administration to rats. J Pharmacol Exp Ther 2000;293:1084–1090.
36. Whiting PJ. GABA-A receptors: a viable target for novel anxiolytics? Curr Opin Pharmacol 2006;6:24–29.
37. Sternfeld F, Carling RW, Jelly RA, et al. Selective, orally active γ-aminobutyric acid(A) α_5 receptor inverse agonists as cognition enhancers. J Med Chem 2004;47:2176–2179.
38. Yee BK, Keist R, von Boehmer L, et al. A schizophrenia-related sensorimotor deficit links α_3-containing $GABA_A$ receptors to a dopamine hyperfunction. Proc Natl Acad Sci U S A 2005;102:17154–17159.
39. Jurd R, Arras M, Lambert S, et al. General anesthetic actions in vivo strongly attenuated by point mutation in the GABA(A) receptor β_3 subunit. FASEB J 2003;17:250–252.
40. White JH, Wise A, Main M, et al. Heterodimerization is required for the formation of a functional $GABA_B$ receptor. Nature 1998;396:679–682.
41. Bowery NG. $GABA_B$ receptor: a site of therapeutic benefit. Curr Opin Pharmacol 2006;6:37–43.
42. Van Bree JB, Heijligers-Feijen CD, de Boer AG, et al. Stereoselective transport of baclofen across the blood-brain barrier in rats as determined by the unit impulse response methodology. Pharm Res 1991;8:259–262.
43. Malcangio M, Bowery NG. Possible therapeutic application of GABAB receptor agonists and antagonists. Clin Neuropharmacol 1995;18:285–305.
44. Crunelli V, Emri Z, Leresche N. Unravelling the brain targets of γ-hydroxybutyric acid. Curr Opin Pharmacol 2006;6:44–52.
45. Gibson KM. γ-Hydroxybutyric aciduria: a biochemist's education from a heritable disorder of GABA metabolism. J Inherit Metab Dis 2005;28:247–265.
46. Andrianmampandry C, Taleb O, Viry S, et al. Cloning and characterization of a rat brain receptor that binds the endogenous neuromodulator γ-hydroxybutyrate (GHB). FASEB J 2003;17:1691–1693.
47. Lemon MD, Strain JD, Farver DK. Sodium oxybate for cataplexy. Ann Pharmacother 2006;40:433–440.
48. Quang LS, Desai MC, Shannon MW, et al. Pretreatment of CD-1 mice with 4-methylpyrazole blocks toxicity from the γ-hydroxybutyrate precursor, 1,4-butanediol. Life Sci 2002;71:771–778.
49. Carai MAM, Quang LS, Atzeri S, et al. Withdrawal syndrome from γ-hydroxybutyric acid (GHB) and 1,4-butanediol (1,4-BD) in Sardinian alcohol-preferring rats. Brain Res Brain Res Protoc 2005;15:75–78.
50. Seighart W, Sperk G. Subunit composition, distribution, and function of GABA(A) receptor subtypes. Curr Topics Med Chem 2002;2:795–816.
51. Werman R, Davidoff RA, Aprison MH. Inhibitory action of glycine on spinal neurons in the cat. J Neurochem 1968;31:81–95.
52. Boehme DH, Fordice MW, Marks N, et al. Distribution of glycine in human spinal cord and selected regions of the brain. Brain Res 1973;50:353–359.
53. Berger SJ, McDaniel ML, Carter JC, et al. Distribution of four potential transmitter amino acids in the monkey retina. J Neurochem 1977;28:149–163.
54. Maher TJ, Wurtman RJ. L-Threonine administration increases glycine concentrations in the rat central nervous system. Life Sci 1980;26:1283–1286.
55. Nader TM, Gowdeu JH, Maher TS, et al. L-Threonine administration increases CSF glycine levels and suppresses spasticity. Neurology 1987;375(Suppl 1):125.
56. Shank RP, Aprison MH. Method for multiple analysis of concentration and specific radioactivity of individual amino acids in nervous tissue extracts. Anal Biochem 1970;35:136–145.
57. Xu T-L, Gong N. Glycine and glycine receptor signaling in hippocampal neurons: diversity, function and regulation. Prog Neurobiol 2010;91:349–361.
58. Keck T, White JA. Glycinergic inhibition in the hippocampus. Rev Neurosci 2009;20:13–22.
59. Neal MJ, Pickles H. Uptake of ^{14}C-glycine by spinal cord. Nature (Lond) 1969;222:679–680.
60. Breitinger HG, Becker CM. The inhibitory glycine receptor—simple views of a complicated channel. Chem Bio Chem 2003;3:1042–1052.
61. Lobo IA, Harris RA. Sites of alcohol and volatile anesthetic action on glycine receptors. Int Rev Neurobiol 2005;65:53–87.

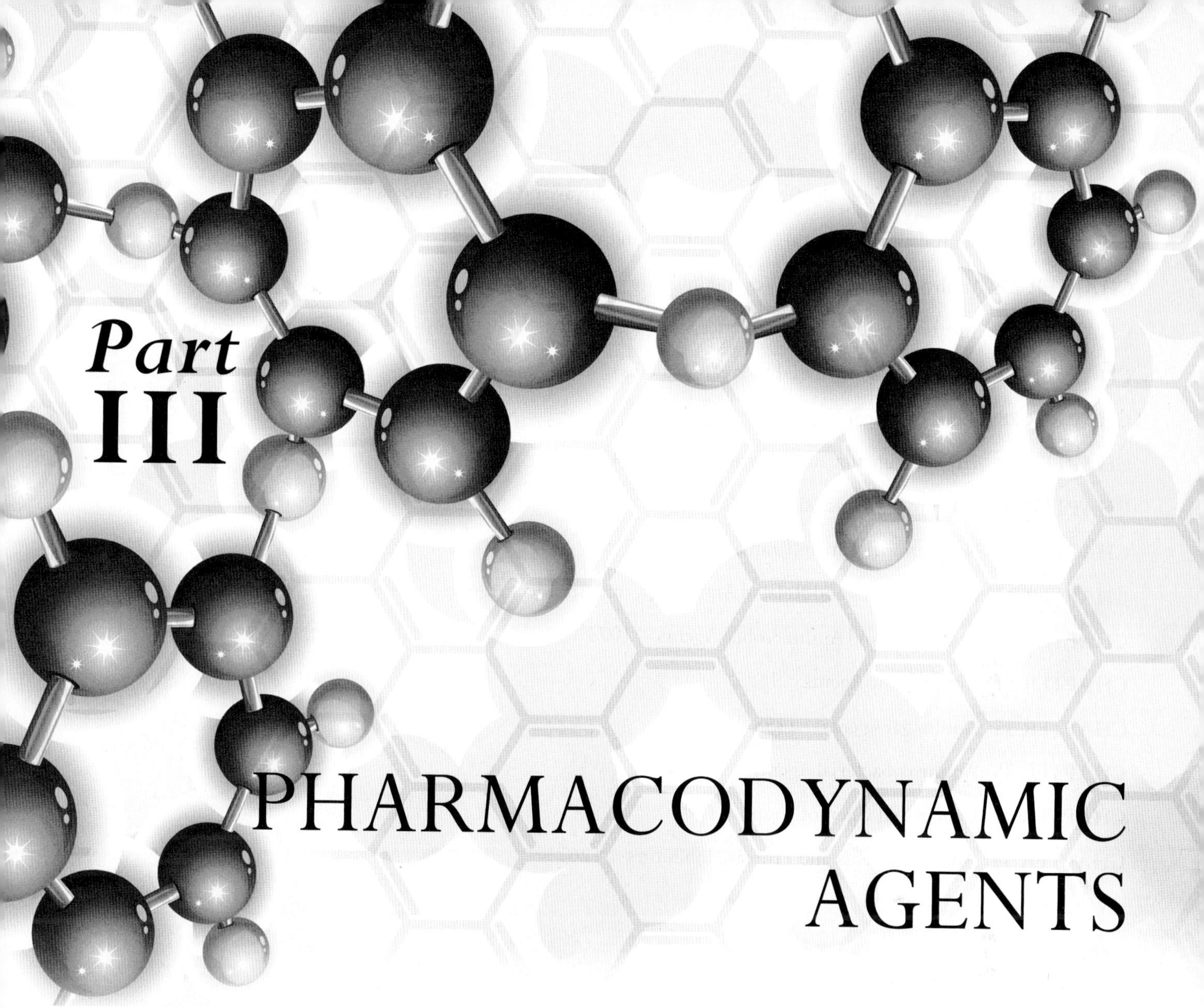

Part III

PHARMACODYNAMIC AGENTS

Chapter 13

Drugs Used to Treat Neuromuscular Disorders: Antiparkinsonian and Spasmolytic Agents

RAYMOND G. BOOTH

Drugs Covered in This Chapter[*]

- Amantadine
- Apomorphine
- Baclofen
- Botulinum toxin-type A
- Bromocriptine
- Cabergoline
- Dantrolene
- Diazepam
- Entacapone
- *Istradefylline*
- L-DOPA
- Memantine
- *Pergolide*
- Pramipexole
- Rasagiline
- Ropinirole
- Rotigotine
- Safinamide
- *Sarizotan*
- Selegiline
- Tizanidine
- Tolcapone

Abbreviations

A-5,6-DTN, 2-amino-5,6-dihydroxy-1,2,3,4-tetrahydronaphthalene
ATP, adenosine triphosphate
CNS, central nervous system
COMT, catechol-*O*-methyltransferase
DA, dopamine
DAT, DA transporter
DOPAC, 3,4-dihydroxyphenylacetic acid
DOPAL, 3,4-dihydroxyphenylacetaldehyde
FDA, U.S. Food and Drug Administration
Gα, G protein α-subunit
GABA, γ-aminobutyric acid
GDP, guanosine diphosphate
GPCR, G protein–coupled receptor
GTP, guanosine triphosphate
5-HT, 5-hydroxytryptamine
HVA, homovanillic acid
l-DOPA/levodopa, L-dihydroxyphenylalanine
MAO, monoamine oxidase
MPDP⁺, 1-methyl-4-phenyl-2,3-dihydropyridinium
MPP⁺, 1-methyl-4-phenylpyridinium
MPPP, 1-methyl-4-propionoxy-4-phenylpiperidine
MPTP, 1-methyl-4-phenyl-1,2,3,6-tetrahydropyridine
NMDA, *N*-methyl-D-aspartate
PD, Parkinson disease
PET, positron emission tomography
SAMe, *S*-adenosyl-L-methionine
SPECT, single photon emission computed tomography
UPS, ubiquitin–proteasome system
VMAT2, vesicular monoamine transporter 2

[*] Drugs listed include those available in the United States; those available outside the United States are shown in italics.

SCENARIO

David Hayes, PharmD

A 56-year-old man is referred to a neurology clinic by his primary care physician secondary to a 6-month unilateral intermittent tremor in his left arm that is triggered by stress. His evaluation at the clinic reveals normal cognition, absence of oculomotor dysfunction, mild left arm rigidity and resting tremor, with normal gait and postural reflexes. The neurologist's impression is early stage of Parkinson disease. His medications include HCTZ 25 mg daily, lovastatin 20 mg at bedtime, and a daily multivitamin. His medical history is significant for hypertension and hyperlipidemia. Should pharmacotherapy be started for this patient, and which would be best suited to his condition?

(The reader is directed to the clinical solution and chemical analysis of this case at the end of the chapter).

OVERVIEW OF NEUROMUSCULAR DISORDERS

Neuromuscular disorders covered in this chapter include the neurodegenerative movement disorder, Parkinson disease (PD), and various spasticity disorders. PD is characterized by debilitating tremor, rigidity, and bradykinesia. The neuropathology (but not the etiology) of PD, with resulting dopamine (DA) neurotransmitter deficit, has been well defined for decades; however, pharmacotherapy of the disorder remains far from satisfactory. The development of prophylactic and, perhaps, curative pharmacotherapy of PD requires advances in understanding of the causes and pathogenesis of the disease, and this chapter reviews some current research in these areas in addition to available pharmacotherapy. Considered are genetic, maturational, metabolic, and environmental contributors to risk for the disease.

Spasticity disorders covered here are characterized by a general increase in tonic stretch reflexes and flexor muscle spasms together with muscle weakness. Muscle spasticity may accompany a number of different disorders but mostly is associated with cerebral palsy, multiple sclerosis, spinal cord injury, and stroke. These disorders do not share a similar pathophysiology with neurodegenerative diseases, such as parkinsonism. Accordingly, drugs used to treat spastic neuromuscular disorders have mechanisms of action that differ from those used to treat PD. Nevertheless, most drugs described in this chapter to treat neurodegenerative or spastic neuromuscular disorders have in common the ability to reduce muscle tone by virtue of their action on the central nervous system (CNS).

PARKINSON DISEASE

Clinical Features and Neuropathology

PD, first described by James Parkinson (1) in 1817, typically presents after age 55 and affects approximately 1% to 2% of the population over age 65; after age 84, incidence increases to 3% to 5% per year (2). Clinically, PD presents as a classic triad of signs: 1) resting tremor that improves with voluntary activity; 2) bradykinesia or slow initiation and paucity of voluntary movements; and 3) rigidity of muscle and joint motility that includes postural disturbances. Dementia is about six times more common among elderly patients with PD, and there can be other spontaneous or treatment-associated neuropsychiatric disturbances, including hallucinations and depression (3). Although L-dihydroxyphenylalanine (L-DOPA or levodopa) pharmacotherapy has decreased morbidity and mortality, mortality among PD patients still is approximately 60% greater than in age-matched controls (4).

Neuropathologically, PD is a slowly progressive, neurodegenerative disorder of the extrapyramidal dopaminergic pathway that has cell bodies in the A9 substantia nigra region and nerve terminals in the corpus striatum (Fig. 13.1). The disease is characterized by gradual destruction of DA-containing neurons in the pars compacta component of the pigmented midbrain substantia nigra, leading to a deficiency of the neurotransmitter in DA nerve terminals of the corpus striatum (3). Degenerative changes in the pigmented nuclei of the noradrenergic locus ceruleus region also are typical, as is the appearance of intraneuronal inclusions called Lewy bodies (5). Neurochemically, the striatal DA deficiency accounts for the major motor symptoms of the disease, but loss of noradrenergic nerve terminals with concomitant reductions in norepinephrine may account for several of the nonmotor features seen in PD, including fatigue and abnormalities of blood pressure regulation. The mainstay of pharmacologic treatment (3), developed in the mid-1960s, continues to be replacement therapy with the α-amino acid L-dihydroxyphenylalanine, the biochemical precursor to the catecholamine neurotransmitters DA and norepinephrine (Fig. 13.2).

Pathophysiology

PD primarily affects the nigrostriatal pathway in the part of the brain known as the basal ganglia, which consists of five interconnected, subcortical nuclei that span the telencephalon (forebrain), diencephalon, and mesencephalon (midbrain). These nuclei include the striatum (caudate and putamen), globus pallidus, subthalamic nucleus, substantia nigra pars compacta, and substantia nigra pars reticulata. Medium-sized spiny neurons that produce the inhibitory amino acid transmitter

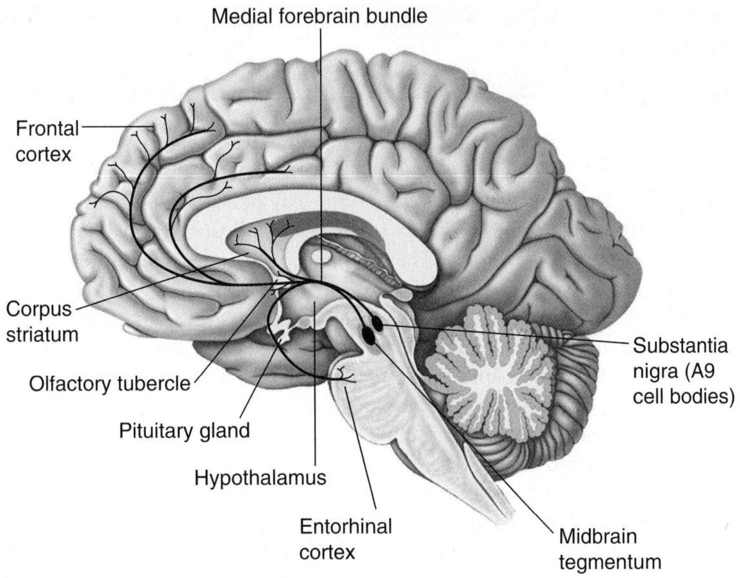

FIGURE 13.1 Some dopaminergic pathways in the brain. The nigrostriated pathway (A9 cell bodies in substantia nigra; nerve terminals in striatum) is degenerated in PD.

γ-aminobutyric acid (GABA) are the principal neurons in the striatum. They receive input from descending corticostriatal projections mediated by the excitatory amino acid neurotransmitter L-glutamic acid, as well as dopaminergic input from the substantia nigra. There are also acetylcholine-producing interneurons in the striatum. Both GABA-producing and acetylcholine-producing neurons in the striatum respond to DA through several DA receptor types.

Dopamine Receptors

DA receptors are grouped into excitatory D_1 types (D_1 and much less prevalent D_5 receptors), and inhibitory D_2 types (D_2 with long and short splice variants, and less abundant D_3 and D_4 types) (6). All are members of the G protein–coupled receptor (GPCR) superfamily and consist of 387 to 477 amino acids. GPCRs are thermodynamically flexible, which manifests as thermal instability when attempts are made to extract the protein from lipid membranes with a detergent, making crystal generation difficult (7). Currently, the only human GPCR x-ray crystal structures solved are for the β_2-adrenergic (8) and adenosine A_{2A} (9) receptors. DA receptors, putatively, are structurally similar to these other GPCRs, consisting of seven relatively hydrophobic transmembrane regions, linked by four extracellular and four intracellular loop segments, with an extracellular amino terminus and cytoplasmic carboxy terminus; a schematic representation based on crystal structure of the human β_2-adrenergic GPCR (8) is shown in Figure 13.3 (10).

The third intracellular loop segment varies most among the DA receptor subtypes, and this is likely where the specific α-subunit of the heterotrimeric (α, β, γ) guanine nucleotide–binding (G) protein binds. The inherent structural flexibility of GPCRs translates to numerous thermodynamic conformations (7). Certain GPCR conformations are constitutively active; that is, the GPCR is able to activate the associated G protein α-subunit (Gα) in the absence of a ligand. In other cases, agonist ligands bind and stabilize GPCR conformations that lead to Gα activation. Upon receptor activation, the Gα subunit releases guanosine diphosphate (GDP) in exchange for binding guanosine triphosphate (GTP) and the β/γ-dimer dissociates. The Gα and Gβ/γ subunits then activate various intracellular effector systems, including adenylyl cyclase (stimulated by D_1-like and inhibited by D_2-like receptors) and phospholipase C (stimulated by D_2/D_4 and inhibited by D_3 receptors), to result in physiologic and/or psychological effects (and side effects, where drug therapy is concerned). It is now realized that the same GPCR can couple to different Gα proteins to result in "multifunctional" signaling that provides a mechanistic basis for "functional selectivity" with regard to design of drugs targeting DA receptors (11–14); this concept is discussed in Chapter 14 relative to antipsychotic drugs; there are no known functionally selective drugs used to treat PD.

Neural Mechanisms in Parkinson Disease

The neuroanatomic connections of the basal ganglia, cerebral cortex, and motor neurons of the spinal cord are complex, and current understanding is incomplete. Figure 13.4 shows a schematic representation of basal ganglia anatomic connections (3,15–18) that can be used as a framework to understand pharmacologic management of the disease. In this model, DA released from nerve terminals of dopaminergic neuron cell bodies originating in the substantia nigra modulates activity of

CLINICAL SIGNIFICANCE

There is some degree of debate as to when to begin therapy, and many clinicians believe that early treatment of PD could lead to a decrease in the progression of disease. The approach to initial treatment should take into consideration the patient-specific factors (e.g., age, comorbid conditions); treatment specific factors (augmentation of the synthesis of brain DA, stimulation of dopamine release from presynaptic sites, direct stimulation of dopamine receptors, decreasing re-uptake of dopamine at presynaptic sites, or decreasing metabolism of DA or its precursor L-dopa); and disease-related factors (rate of progression, presenting phenomenology, related physical disability) to result in a decreased rate of progression and preservation of functionality. Current guidelines and consensus agree that levodopa/carbidopa, second-generation dopamine agonist, and monoamine oxidase-B (MAO-B) can be considered for initial therapy. Attention to the chemistry of these agents may provide an understanding of their benefit and potential detriment for specific patients. Though levodopa/carbidopa therapy is the most effective therapy to treat motor symptoms, there is the potential for dyskinesia and motor fluctuations, which may occur for some as early as within 5 years but for the majority within 15 years. There also is concern that this approach may result in increased oxidative pressure and disease progression. Therefore, it is generally accepted that levodopa/carbidopa therapy should be reserved for those with disability. Second-generation dopamine agonists may hold value as initial therapy but may be limited by nausea and vomiting, psychiatric disturbances, and postural hypotension; interestingly, these agents may convey some neuroprotective qualities. MAO-B inhibitors can be considered, but the lack of evidence supporting selegiline as monotherapy, along with it having an amphetamine metabolite that holds potential for benefit (L-dopa potentiating) and detriment (vasoactive properties), may persuade some to consider rasagline, an agent for which sufficient clinical evidence exists for efficacy as initial monotherapy. Furthermore, some preliminary clinical data has demonstrated a neuroprotective effect at the lower dose range for this agent. Therefore, in a younger patient population the clinician should be mindful of the chemistry of dopamine agonists as they relate to improvement in motor function, but acknowledge that motor fluctuation may occur and recognize the need to reserve these agents for patients who exhibit disability. Clearly, the utility of rasagline or second-generation dopamine agonist potentially exhibiting neuroprotective effects to address early-stage PD without disability should be recognized.

David Hayes, PharmD
Clinical Assistant Professor
Department of Clinical Sciences & Administration
University of Houston College of Pharmacy

inhibitory GABA neurons in the striatum. In turn, striatal GABA neurons, through a series of "direct" and "indirect" neuronal pathways, modulate neuronal outflow to the thalamus that provides excitatory (glutamatergic) input to the motor cortex.

In the direct pathway are two sequential inhibitory GABAergic links that provide input directly to the thalamus. The first set of GABAergic neurons in striatum contains a predominance of excitatory DA D_1-type receptors. Thus, the net effect of DA D_1-mediated stimulation of striatal GABA neurons in the direct pathway is increased excitatory outflow from the thalamus to the motor cortex.

The indirect pathway uses two sequential GABAergic links, like the direct pathway, that are followed by an excitatory glutamatergic link and another inhibitory GABAergic input to the thalamus. The first set of striatal GABAergic neurons in the indirect pathway contains a predominance of inhibitory D_2-type receptors. Thus, the net effect of DA D_2-mediated modulation of striatal GABAergic neurons in the indirect pathway is to reduce excitatory outflow from the thalamus to the motor cortex.

In the normal condition, the direct pathway is dominant, but in PD, reduced levels of striatal DA negates this preference, and the indirect pathway becomes more apparent, with a net effect of decreased excitatory input to the motor cortex. The clinical result is that the striatal DA deficiency accounts for the major motor symptoms of PD, particularly bradykinesia. The mainstay of pharmacologic treatment (3) continues to be replacement therapy with the immediate biochemical precursor of DA, L-DOPA, (see Fig. 13.2), in an effort to produce nearly physiologic agonism of both D_1 and D_2 DA receptors.

Etiology

Genetic Component

Although the neuropathology is well defined, the cause of PD is unknown. The development of effective pharmacotherapeutic and prophylactic therapy will require advances in understanding the etiology of the disease. Currently, there are several, convergent theories regarding the cause of PD: "proteolytic stress," which recently has been characterized in connection with rare PD genetic mutations as well as environmental and/or endogenous neurotoxicants; mitochondrial dysfunction; and oxidative metabolism—any and all of which may lead to "oxidative stress." This section describes these and some alternative proposals regarding the etiology of PD.

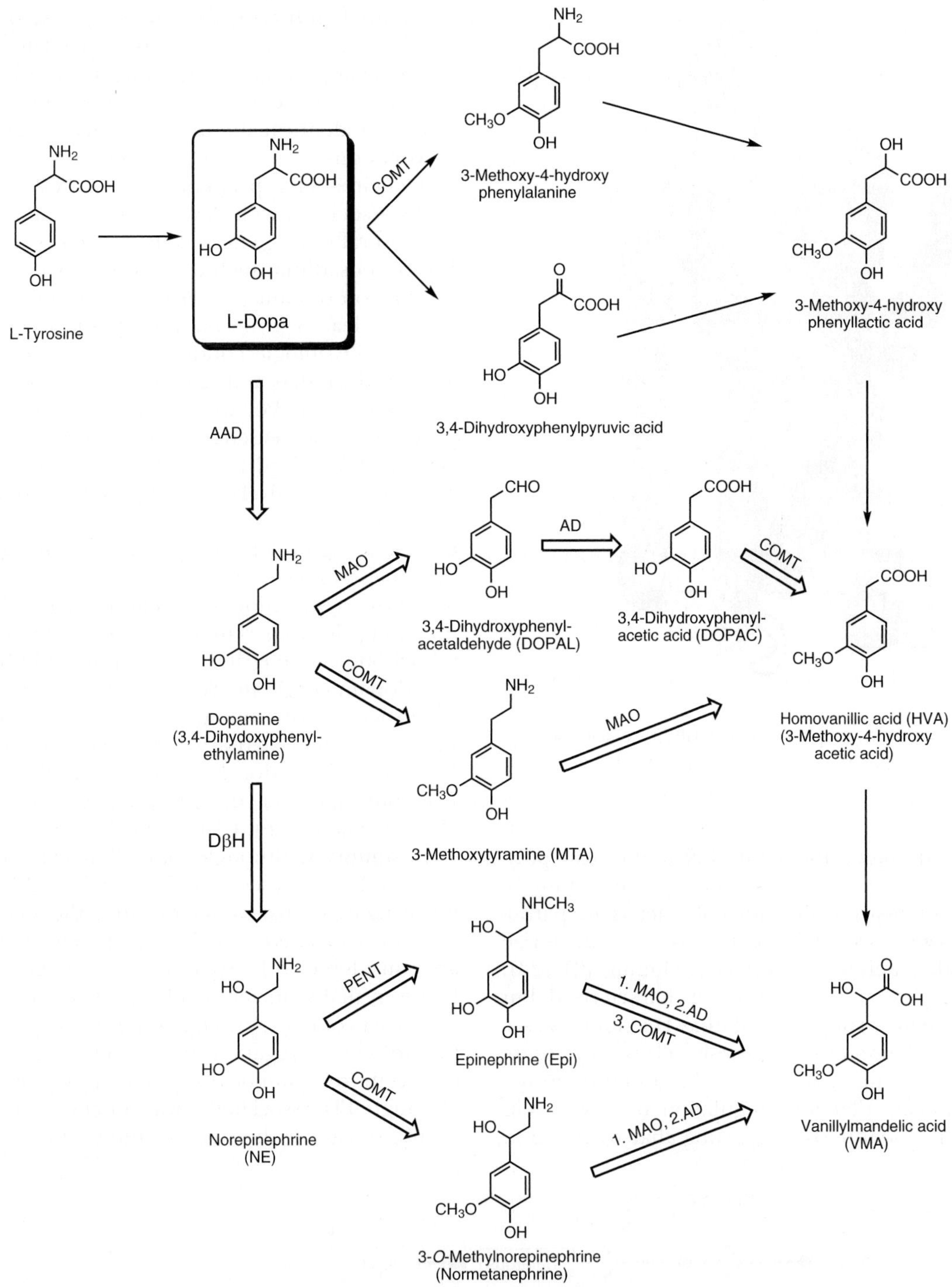

FIGURE 13.2 Pathways in the biosynthesis and catabolism of L-DOPA and DA. Heavy and light arrows indicate major or minor reactions. AAD, aromatic L-amino acid decarboxylase; AD, aldehyde dehydrogenase; COMT, catechol-*O*-methyltransferase; DH, DA β-hydroxylase; MAO, monoamine oxidase; PENT, phenylethanolamine-*N*-methyltransferase.

Several neurodegenerative disorders (including the movement disorder Huntington disease) are genetically determined; thus, researchers have investigated a possible genetic influence in PD. Epidemiologic studies have found that apart from age, a family history of PD is the strongest predictor of an increased risk of the disorder (19,20); however, the role of shared environmental exposure in families must be considered.

One familial form of PD is characterized by mutations in the α-synuclein gene, originally reported in a single large Italian family, three smaller Greek families, and a German pedigree (21,22). The protein α-synuclein

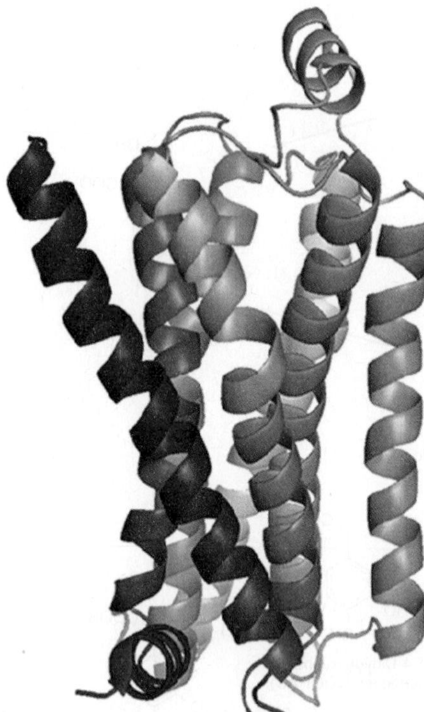

FIGURE 13.3 G protein–coupled receptor (GPCR) secondary structure model based on the crystal structure of the human β_2-adrenergic GPCR.

is a highly conserved, abundant, 140-amino acid polypeptide expressed mainly in cerebral nerve terminals. Aggregation of α-synuclein molecules leads to pathologic inclusions (synucleinopathy) that characterize many neurodegenerative disorders, including PD (23). The function of α-synuclein is not well-characterized, but it appears to play a role in regulating DA homeostasis, including modulation of DA synthesis, release, and reuptake at nerve terminals. In vitro studies using neuronal cells (24) indicate that downregulation of α-synuclein enhances DA biosynthesis, suggesting that dysfunction of α-synuclein may lead to increased intraneuronal levels of DA that become neurotoxic (see later discussion). Nevertheless, several studies failed to detect mutations in the α-synuclein gene in large family samples (25,26) or in studies of identical and heterozygous twins (27,28).

Mutations in four other genes—*DJ-1*, *PINK1*, *parkin*, and leucine-rich repeat kinase 2 (*LRRK-2*)—are unequivocally associated with development of familial PD (29), and several other genetic mutations also are implicated. It is proposed that such mutations may lead to excessive production of damaged proteins and/or dysfunction of protein clearance mechanisms in the brain (30,31). In normal physiologic conditions, damaged proteins usually are degraded and cleared by the ubiquitin–proteasome system (UPS). Increased production of damaged proteins or decreased UPS-mediated degradation and clearance may lead to protein aggregation and proteolytic stress, negatively affecting cellular structures and processes (32,33). For example, the UPS protein parkin mediates engulfment of dysfunctional mitochondria by autophagosomes (34), and dysfunctional parkin may fail to remove dysfunctional mitochondria. PINK1 appears to function prior to parkin in the same pathway to maintain mitochondrial integrity and functioning in both muscles and dopaminergic neurons (35,36). In cases of familial PD associated with mutations of *LRRK-2* (a kinase encoding the protein dardarin), protein accumulation and Lewy body formation have been identified postmortem (37), but such data currently are unavailable for the parkin (a UPS enzyme), DJ-1, and PINK-1 mutations.

In summary, although compelling evidence exists for apparently rare cases of genetically linked PD, primarily involving early onset of the disorder, the majority of cases are not associated with known genetic mutations and are considered to be sporadic (38). It should be noted, however, that synucleinopathy has been detected in sporadic cases of PD (39), suggesting that hypotheses involving protein aggregation may be relevant to the etiology of the more common forms of the disease. Moreover, although PD associated with genetic mutation is rare (<10% of cases), the study of these cases has facilitated

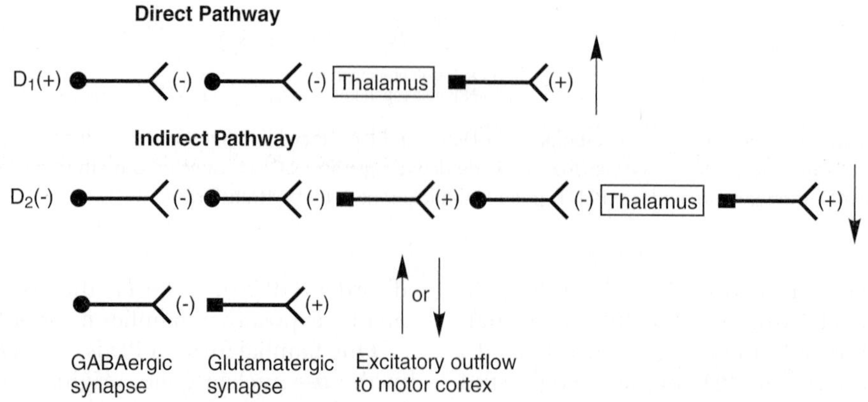

FIGURE 13.4 Striatal dopaminergic stimulation of the direct and indirect pathways modulates the thalamus excitatory outflow to the motor cortex.

understanding of the molecular pathways that lead to neurodegeneration, especially involving dopaminergic neurons.

In contrast to PD forms that are associated with genetic mutations, little evidence suggests that the disorder is autoimmune related (40). Likewise, although a form of parkinsonism associated with influenza virus–induced encephalitis did occur in a 1918 epidemic, recent studies indicate no evidence for a communicable infectious etiology of PD (41).

Oxidative Metabolism Component

Analysis of postmortem brain tissue from PD patients has revealed decreased levels of glutathione (42), increased lipid peroxidation (43), and increased oxidation of DNA (44) and proteins (45). Accordingly, oxidative metabolism involving the synthesis and catabolism of DA has been implicated in the PD disease process (46) through production of chemically reactive products, including epoxides (47,48), free radicals (49), and quinones (50,51).

Synthesis of DA, as well as the catecholamine neurotransmitters norepinephrine and epinephrine, proceeds by initial aromatic oxidation (*meta*-position) of the precursor amino acid L-tyrosine to L-DOPA, in a rate-limiting step catalyzed by tyrosine hydroxylase (L-tyrosine-3-mono-oxygenase; see Fig. 13.2). The mechanism of this hydroxylation may involve direct insertion of an oxygen atom into L-tyrosine to form L-DOPA, or through an intermediate arene epoxide (48) (Fig. 13.5), as is case for metabolic conversion of benzene to phenol (52) and of estradiol to catechol-estrogens (47,53). It is hypothesized that an analogous epoxide intermediate, formed during the conversion of tyrosine to L-DOPA, may alkylate nucleophilic functionalities on proteins, RNA, or DNA to produce neurotoxicity (47).

Once formed, DA can auto-oxidize to the corresponding electrophilic semiquinone and quinone (Fig. 13.5) species that can alkylate protein sulfhydryl groups, including glutathione (50,54). Manganese ion can catalyze this oxidation of DA, and the resulting semiquinone and quinone species have been implicated (51) in a PD-like syndrome among South American manganese miners (55). The auto-oxidation of DA also leads to the formation of the polymeric black pigment neuromelanin (54). The pigment is increasingly deposited in catecholaminergic neurons with advancing age, however, and it has been suggested that its accumulation in nigral neuronal cells eventually causes cell death (5).

In addition to neurotoxic metabolites derived from the auto-oxidation of DA, the monoamine oxidase (MAO)-catalyzed oxidation of DA may be relevant to PD. During MAO catalysis of DA and the other monoamine neurotransmitters (norepinephrine and serotonin), hydrogen peroxide is generated (see Equation 1 in Fig. 13.5) that can undergo a redox reaction with superoxide, according to the Haber-Weiss reaction (56), to form the extremely cytotoxic hydroxy radical (see Equation 2 in Fig. 13.5).

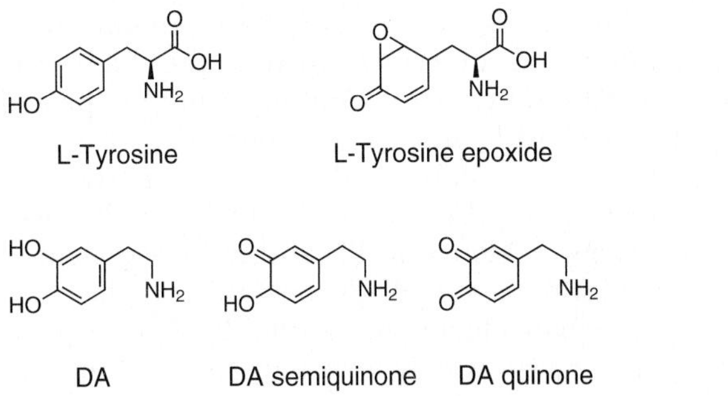

Equation 1:

$$RCH_2CH_2NH_2 + O_2 + H_2O \longrightarrow RCH_2CHO + NH_3 + H_2O_2$$

Equation 2:

$$H_2O_2 + O_2^{\bullet\ominus} \longrightarrow O_2 + {}^{\ominus}OH + {}^{\bullet}OH$$

FIGURE 13.5 Putative and known compounds involved in DA synthesis and catabolism, some of which may cause DA neuronal cell death.

Dysfunction of mitochondrial redox processes also is hypothesized to play a role in PD neuronal cell death (57,58). Postmortem samples of brain and peripheral tissue from PD patients indicate selective mitochondrial complex I deficiency, including in the substantia nigra and other sites (59,60). It is hypothesized that resulting decreased adenosine triphosphate (ATP) synthesis and altered homeostasis of reactive species such as hydrogen peroxide, superoxide, and free hydroxyl radicals might contribute to neuronal cell death in PD. In fact, mitochondrial dysfunction and altered oxidative metabolism of DA may converge such that decreased energy production by mitochondria may impede vesicular storage of DA, leading to increased cytoplasmic concentration of DA that can undergo MAO-catalyzed oxidation to hydroxyl radicals, as well as auto-oxidize to quinones and semiquinones (61).

In summary, toxic products from normal oxidative metabolism and/or altered mitochondrial function may contribute to the progressive loss of DA neurons that occurs normally with maturation and aging at a rate of approximately of 13% per decade after age 45 (62–64). Clinical symptoms of PD emerge as losses of DA neurons exceed 65% (65). Conceivably, the symptoms of parkinsonism could be produced by two processes, a specific disease-related insult combined with pathologic changes resulting from normal aging. This two-pronged pathophysiology may explain why PD is a progressive disorder of late onset (66). Hypotheses concerning the initial pathologic event have centered on environmental neurotoxicants.

Environmental Neurotoxicants Component

There has been accumulated compelling evidence to suggest that environmental toxicants play an important role in the etiology (and perhaps treatment) of PD. For example, as described earlier, the high prevalence of PD among South American miners probably is associated with manganese neurotoxicity. There is also evidence linking herbicides and pesticides to PD. For example, there is a remarkably high correlation between incidence of PD and use of pesticides in an agricultural region of Québec (67). In fact, *N,N'*-dimethyl-4,4'-bipyridinium dichloride (Paraquat, Fig. 13.6) is one of the most widely used herbicides in the world (68) and is structurally similar to the selective DA neurotoxicant 1-methyl-4-phenylpyridinium (MPP^+; Fig. 13.6), which was marketed as the herbicide Cyperquat (69,70). Paraquat, like MPP^+ and the pesticide rotenone (see later discussion), inhibits mitochondrial complex I and cellular respiration, although only at concentrations (~10 mmol/L) considerably higher than are required for MPP^+ (~10 μmol/L) or rotenone (~10 nmol/L) (69). Some investigators have reported Paraquat-induced postmortem losses of nigral DA neurons and degeneration of striatal DA nerve terminals, as well as decreased locomotor activity (71). Others, however, have found no evidence of neurotoxic changes after exposure to Paraquat (72), and Paraquat neurotoxicity, unlike MPP^+-associated parkinsonism, probably is not highly selective for DA neurons (69). Finally, the ability of Paraquat itself to gain entry to the brain remains uncertain (70) because it is a (double) quaternary ammonium compound, unlike the much more lipophilic molecule rotenone, discussed in the following paragraph.

Rotenone is an isoflavone, many of which are found in roots and stems of several plants; this association allows rotenone to be labeled as "natural" and to be used in organic food farming (68). Rotenone is a lipophilic molecule that crosses the blood–brain barrier and neuronal cell membranes where it is proposed to inhibit mitochondrial complex I to cause degeneration of nigrostriatal DA neurons (69,70), producing hypokinesia and rigidity, as well as accumulation of fibrillar cytoplasmic inclusions that contain ubiquitin and α-synuclein (73).

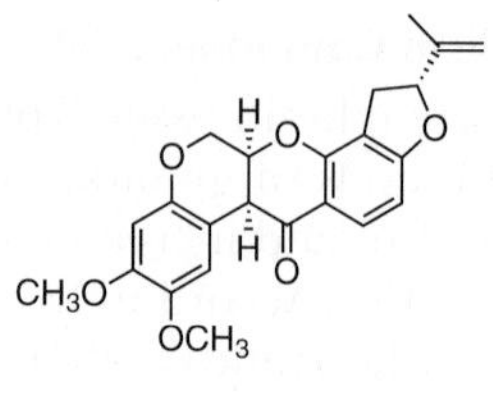

Rotenone

Another environmental link to PD is the lower incidence of the disease in cigarette smokers than in nonsmokers (74,75). It has been proposed that something in cigarette smoke may protect against a toxicant (environmental or endogenous) relevant to parkinsonian neuropathology. Several mechanisms might account for this inverse correlation, which might enhance understanding of neuroprotective or even curative pharmacotherapy in neurodegenerative disorders. For example, several constituents in tobacco smoke are MAO inhibitors, including farnesylacetone, a selective inhibitor of MAO-B (76,77), which is thought to be the predominant MAO isoform

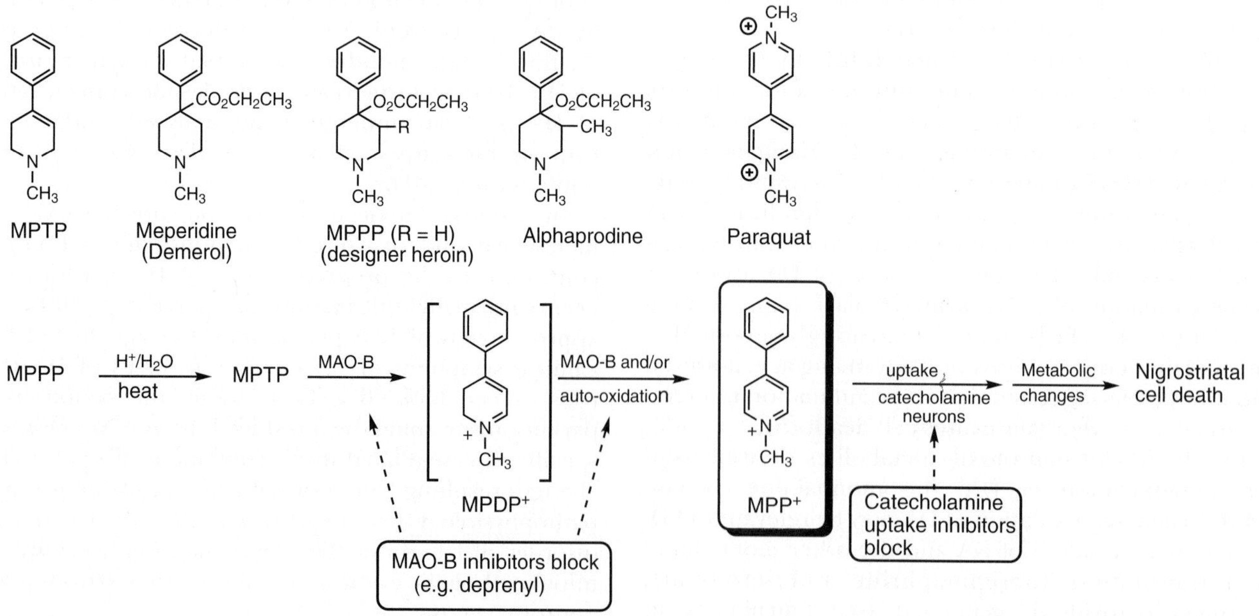

FIGURE 13.6 Phenylpiperidine analgesics and metabolic activation of MPTP. In the presence of acid and heat, MPPP forms MPTP that undergoes an MAO-B–catalyzed two-electron oxidation to $MPDP^+$. $MDPP^+$ undergoes a two-electron auto-oxidation (also can be catalyzed by MAO-B) to MPP^+ that is accumulated into DA neurons by the DA transporter and subsequently into mitochondria where it disrupts cellular respiration, producing neuronal cell death.

responsible for metabolism of DA in brain (glial cells). Moreover, prolonged nicotine exposure can increase activity of the UPS system (78), discussed earlier.

There also is an inverse correlation between risk of developing PD and coffee and caffeine consumption (79). Caffeine is a nonselective adenosine A_1/A_2 receptor antagonist that reduces parkinsonism-like tremor in rodent models of PD (80). The adenosine A_{2A} receptor subtype is expressed abundantly on medium spiny neurons. Aberrant interneuronal signaling associated with A_{2A}-linked intracellular kinase activation is proposed to account for parkinsonism-like signs and the dyskinetic motor response produced by DA agonist therapy in rodent and primate models of PD (81). Accordingly, adenosine A_{2A} receptor antagonists, such as istradefylline (see later discussion, Fig. 13.13), have been proposed as pharmacotherapy for PD (82). Antagonism of adenosine A_1 receptors also may reduce parkinsonism-like tremor in rodents (80), but no clinical candidate anti-A_1 drugs have emerged.

In conclusion, there are several potential links between the environment and the etiology and pathophysiology of PD, including exposure to pesticides, herbicides, well water, wood pulp mills, and rural living (83,84). Pathologic mechanisms involving environmental neurotoxicants may converge with dysfunctional oxidative metabolism. A particularly well-studied example of such convergence involves the discovery that 1-methyl-4-phenyl-1,2,3,6-tetrahydropyridine (MPTP, Fig. 13.6) produces a severe parkinsonism syndrome in humans and some laboratory animals that is remarkably similar to the idiopathic disease. As such, MPTP has been a useful tool to study the etiology and pharmacotherapy of PD.

Parkinsonism Caused by MPTP

The cyclic tertiary amine MPTP (Fig. 13.6) induces a form of parkinsonism in humans and monkeys similar in neuropathology and motor abnormalities to idiopathic PD (85–87). The role of MPTP in parkinsonian disorders was revealed by a serendipitous series of events. In 1977, a 23-year-old college student suddenly developed parkinsonian symptoms, with severe rigidity, bradykinesia, and mutism. The abrupt and early onset of symptoms was so atypical that the patient initially was thought to have catatonic schizophrenia. The subsequent diagnosis of parkinsonism was substantiated by a therapeutic response to L-DOPA, whereupon the patient was referred to the National Institute of Mental Health in Bethesda, Maryland. The patient admitted having synthesized and used several illicit drugs, after which the psychiatrist who had elicited the patient's history visited his home and collected glassware that had been used for chemical syntheses. Chemical analysis revealed several pyridines, including MPTP, formed as by-products during synthesis of the target molecule, 1-methyl-4-propionoxy-4-phenylpiperidine (MPPP, Fig. 13.6). MPPP, known as "designer heroin" or "synthetic heroin," is the reverse ester of the narcotic analgesic meperidine (Fig. 13.6) and lacks only the 3-methyl moiety of the analgesic α-1,3-dimethyl-4-phenyl-4-propionoxypiperidine or alphaprodine (Nisentil, Fig. 13.6). Initially, it was unclear whether MPTP or other constituents of the injected mixture accounted for the neurotoxicity that produced parkinsonism.

After the patient returned home, he continued to abuse drugs and died of an overdose; autopsy revealed degeneration of the substantia nigra—the hallmark neuropathologic feature of PD. Subsequently, other patients were identified with virtually identical parkinsonian symptoms who had also been receiving intravenous injections of MPPP preparations containing varying amounts of MPTP. In several patients, MPTP was the principal or sole constituent injected, providing the first definitive evidence that MPTP is a parkinsonism-producing neurotoxicant. Both the clinical and neuropathologic features of MPTP-induced parkinsonism resemble idiopathic PD more closely than any previous animal or human disorder elicited by toxins, metals, viruses, or other means. Accordingly, understanding the molecular pathophysiology of MPTP neurotoxicity has shed light on the neurodegenerative mechanisms in idiopathic parkinsonism.

Mechanisms of Neuronal Cell Death in MPTP-Induced Parkinsonism

Consideration of the chemical structure of MPTP would suggest that the compound is relatively chemically inert, because no highly reactive functional group is present. Almost immediately, it was recognized that MPTP might undergo some type of metabolic activation to a more reactive metabolite. Researchers soon discovered that brain MAO-B catalyzes the two-electron oxidation of MPTP at the allylic α-carbon to give the unstable intermediate product 1-methyl-4-phenyl-2,3-dihydropyridinium ($MPDP^+$), which subsequently undergoes a further two-electron oxidation to the stable 1-methyl-4-phenylpyridinium species (MPP^+) via auto-oxidation, disproportionation, and enzyme-catalyzed mechanisms (Fig. 13.6) (88–90). Inhibitors of MAO-B subsequently were shown to prevent MPTP-induced parkinsonism in primates (91), and it currently is accepted that MPP^+ is the major metabolite of MPTP responsible for the destruction of DA neurons, although a role for the unstable dihydropyridinium species $MPDP^+$ has not been ruled out.

The relationship of MAO and MPTP has neurobiologic relevance beyond MPTP neurotoxicity. MAO catalyzes the α-carbon oxidation of the monoamine neurotransmitters (e.g., DA, norepinephrine, and serotonin) (Fig. 13.2). Oxidation of a heterocyclic tertiary amine (i.e., MPTP) by MAO suggests a novel physiologic role for this enzyme. For example, MAO could be important in regulating the oxidation state of pyridine systems, such as those involving NADH, which is relevant to mitochondrial function (see later discussion) (92). Interestingly, biochemical and epidemiologic evidence suggests that cigarette smokers have depressed MAO-B activity (93), which may be relevant to the lower incidence of PD seen in smokers (74,75). Nicotine is not a particularly potent inhibitor of MAO, and in fact, nicotine increases the neurotoxicity of MPTP (94). As mentioned earlier, however, other components of cigarette smoke do inhibit MAO (76,77), and cigarette smoke protects against MPTP-induced depletion of striatal DA in mice (95).

Although extensive metabolic, biochemical, and toxicologic investigations have established that the nigrostriatal neurodegenerative properties of MPTP are mediated by the MAO-B–derived metabolite, MPP^+, this bioactivation reaction must proceed outside of the target nigrostriatal DA neurons because they apparently do not contain MAO-B (96). It is thought that MPTP is oxidized to MPDP in MAO-B–rich glial cells near striatal nerve terminals and nigral cell bodies; the conjugate base MPDP presumably diffuses out of glial cells and is subsequently oxidized to the MPP^+ metabolite. The MPP^+ is sequestered into striatal dopaminergic nerve terminals via the DA neurotransporter, which accepts MPP^+ as a substrate (Fig. 13.6) (97). Intraneuronally, MPP^+ is concentrated into mitochondria, where it selectively inhibits complex I of the electron-transport chain, inhibiting NADH oxidation and, eventually, depleting the nigrostriatal neuronal cell of ATP (98,99). Thus, it is proposed that the mechanism of nigrostriatal cell death induced by MPTP (via MPP^+) is energy failure at the level of the mitochondrial respiratory chain (100,101).

Several sequential factors may account for the selective damage of nigrostriatal DA neurons by MPTP (Fig. 13.6). First, MPTP binds selectively to MAO-B, which is highly concentrated in glial cells in human substantia nigra and corpus striatum. Then, the MPP^+ produced from MPTP is selectively accumulated by DA neurotransporters into nigral DA cells and striatal DA nerve terminals. Finally, within nigral cell bodies, MPP^+ binds to neuromelanin and may be gradually released in a depot-like fashion, maintaining a toxic intracellular concentration of MPP^+ that inhibits mitochondrial respiration.

The serendipitous discovery and subsequent scientific investigation of the mechanism of parkinsonism produced by MPTP refocused study of the etiology and pathogenesis of idiopathic PD. For example, discovery of the selective ability of MPTP to induce nigral cell death has stimulated broad interest in identifying potential environmental or endogenous toxicants that may be causative agents in PD, as discussed earlier. Likewise, the mechanism of MPP^+ to cause DA cell death via inhibition of mitochondrial respiration provides support for theories involving mitochondrial dysfunction and oxidative metabolism in general (oxidative stress) in the etiology of idiopathic PD. Specifically, it has been documented that there is a 30% to 40% reduction in mitochondrial complex I activity in the substantia nigra of patients with PD (102,103). In general, mitochondrial dysfunction and disorders of oxidative metabolism, which can include a genetic component (29), now are considered to be critical components of most theories of nigral cell degeneration in PD. Delineation of the neurobiochemical mechanism of MPTP-induced parkinsonism also has led to new pharmacotherapeutic approaches aimed at slowing neurodegeneration in PD, focusing, notably, on MAO-B and oxidative stress. Clinical studies to evaluate the effectiveness of coadministration of an MAO-B inhibitor plus the antioxidant vitamin E to slow progression of neurodegeneration in PD, however, have not yielded encouraging results (104–106). In fact, as indicated in the next section, despite progress toward understanding the etiology and pathophysiology of PD summarized earlier, no treatment has conclusively been proven to stop or even reliably slow the progressive neurodegeneration in the disease (3).

Pharmacotherapy of PD

Due to the failure of various neuroprotection strategies to provide unequivocal disease-modifying benefit for PD patients, the mainstay of PD pharmacotherapy continues to be palliative or symptomatic, involving replacement of the DA deficiency in striatum. This is accomplished currently by one or more of the following means: 1) augmentation of the synthesis of brain DA; 2) stimulation of DA release from presynaptic sites; 3) direct stimulation of DA receptors; 4) decreasing reuptake of DA at presynaptic sites; or 5) decreasing metabolism of DA or its precursor L-DOPA. Some of these treatments, notably DA receptor agonists and MAO-B inhibitors (decrease DA metabolism), might also provide putative neuroprotective benefit (3).

L-DOPA Therapy

More than 40 years after its introduction, L-DOPA (Fig. 13.2) remains the most effective symptomatic pharmacotherapy for PD (3). Despite controversy regarding long-term efficacy, adverse effects, and even potential neurotoxicity, most PD patients derive a substantial benefit from L-DOPA over the entire course of their illness. Moreover, L-DOPA increases life expectancy among patients with PD, and survival is significantly reduced if the initiation of L-DOPA therapy is delayed (107).

In 1960, Ehringer and Hornykiewicz (108) assayed DA in the brains of patients dying with PD and found that tissue concentrations of DA in the corpora striata of many of these patients averaged only 20% of normal. Signs of PD in patients resembled behavioral changes in rats treated with reserpine or other amine-depleting agents. These findings led Birkmayer and Hornykiewicz (109) to administer high oral doses of racemic DOPA to PD patients in Vienna in 1960. Subsequent clinical trials led by Barbeau in Montréal in the early 1960s (110) and by Cotzias in New York in the late 1960s (112) confirmed this effect of racemic DOPA. Barbeau and Cotzias also demonstrated the greater potency and safety of the physiologic enantiomer L-DOPA (111,112).

Development of L-DOPA as a therapeutic agent in PD is a rare example of a rationally predicted and logically pursued clinical treatment in a neuropsychiatric disorder, based on neurochemical pathology and basic pharmacologic theory (113). The effectiveness of L-DOPA treatment requires its penetration into the CNS and local decarboxylation to

DA. DA does not cross the blood–brain diffusion barrier because its amino moiety is protonated under physiologic conditions (pK_a = 10.6 [NH_2]), making it relatively hydrophilic (114). However, the precursor amino acid to DA, L-DOPA, is less basic (pK_a = 8.72 [NH_2]) and polar at physiologic pH, and thus more able to penetrate the CNS, in part facilitated by transport into brain with other aromatic and neutral aliphatic amino acids (114–116).

Biosynthesis and Metabolism L-DOPA is normally a trace intermediary metabolite in the biosynthesis of catecholamines. L-DOPA is readily decarboxylated by the cytoplasmic enzyme L-aromatic amino acid decarboxylase ("DOPA decarboxylase") to form DA (see Fig 13.2). The main by-products of DA are 3,4-dihydroxyphenylacetic acid (DOPAC) and homovanillic acid (HVA; 3-methoxy-4-hydroxyphenylacetic acid; Fig. 13.2). The effects observed after systemic administration of L-DOPA have been attributed to its peripheral and cerebral metabolites, mainly DA, with much less conversion to norepinephrine by β-hydroxylation, or epinephrine formed by *N*-methylation of norepinephrine by phenylethanolamine-*N*-methyltransferase (Fig. 13.2). A small amount of L-DOPA is *O*-methylated by catechol-*O*-methyltransferase (COMT) to L-3-*O*-methyldopa (L-3-methoxytyrosine or 3-methoxy-4-hydroxyphenylalanine, Fig 13.2), which accumulates in the CNS because of its long half-life. Most exogenous L-DOPA, however, is rapidly decarboxylated to DA in peripheral tissues, including liver, heart, lung, and kidney (Fig 13.7). In fact, only about 1% of an orally administered dose of L-DOPA reaches the brain; thus, L-DOPA, by itself, has very limited dose effectiveness (117). In humans, appreciable quantities of L-DOPA enter the brain only when administered alone in doses (3 to 6 g daily) high enough to compensate for losses caused by peripheral metabolism.

L-DOPA peripheral decarboxylation can be competitively inhibited (118) by coadministration of carbidopa (combined with L-DOPA in Sinemet) or benserazide (combined with L-DOPA in Prolopa in countries other than the United States) (Fig. 13.8). Such polar decarboxylase inhibitors do not appreciably penetrate the brain to inhibit cerebral decarboxylase, thus markedly increasing the proportion of L-DOPA that reaches the brain for conversion to DA (Fig 13.7), allowing for a 2.5- to 30-fold lower dose (0.2 to 1.2 g/d) of L-DOPA (17). Patients with PD are typically started on a combination product, either alone or with other adjunctive agents discussed later. Products containing extended-release preparations of decarboxylase inhibitors should provide more sustained benefits with less "wearing off" of benefit after several hours, but the bioavailability and performance of these products is variable. In general, tissue uptake of L-DOPA is highly dependent on competition with other aromatic and neutral aliphatic amino acids and can be decreased substantially by a protein meal.

Pyridoxine (vitamin B_6) is the cofactor for L-aromatic amino acid decarboxylase. In high doses, vitamin B_6 can reverse the therapeutic effects of L-DOPA by increasing

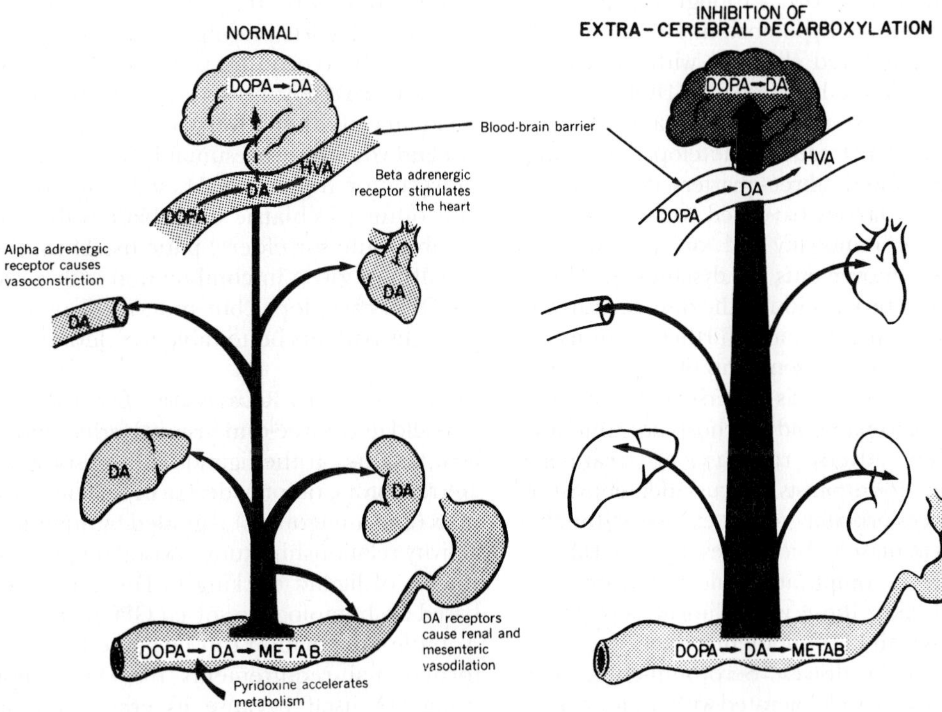

FIGURE 13.7 Diagrammatic representation of the peripheral decarboxylation of levodopa to form dopamine (DA) and the mode of action of extracerebral decarboxylase on levodopa metabolism and distribution in vivo. The concurrent administration of levodopa and a decarboxylase inhibitor decreases the amount of levodopa required to elicit a therapeutic response in parkinsonism. HVA, homovanillic acid.

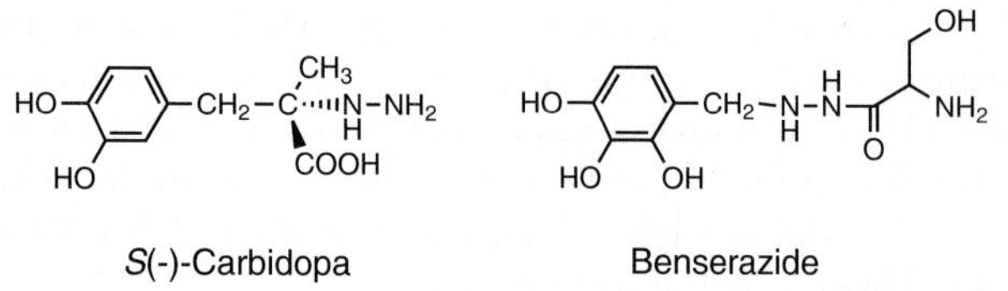

FIGURE 13.8 Drugs that inhibit peripheral L-aromatic amino acid decarboxylase

peripheral decarboxylase activity. Competitive blockade of peripheral decarboxylation with carbidopa or benserazide, however, minimizes this potential effect of pyridoxine.

SIDE EFFECTS Common adverse effects of L-DOPA therapy are nausea and vomiting, likely due to direct gastrointestinal irritation as well as stimulation by DA of the chemoreceptor trigger zone in the area postrema of the brainstem, an emesis-inducing center that is largely unprotected by the blood–brain diffusion barrier. An important advantage of combining L-DOPA with a peripheral decarboxylase inhibitor is a marked reduction of required L-DOPA dose; thus, there is less risk of emesis or other adverse effects associated with formation of excess DA. These can include activation of peripheral adrenergic and DA receptors, in part by releasing endogenous adrenergic catecholamines (119), as summarized in Figure 13.7. Theoretically, vasoconstriction and hypertension might occur by stimulation of peripheral α-adrenoceptors, tachycardia by stimulation of cardiac β-adrenoceptors, and direct renal and mesenteric vasodilatation by DA, although DA agonists and L-DOPA usually induce hypotension. However, such effects are rarely encountered clinically with the use of a peripheral decarboxylase inhibitor with L-DOPA (17).

After about 5 years of continuous treatment with L-DOPA, at least half of PD patients develop fluctuating motor responses, and nearly three-quarters do so by 15 years (120). These fluctuations (so-called "on-off" effects) include "off" periods of immobility and "on" periods with abnormal involuntary movements or dyskinesias. These phenomena may reflect progression of the disease with striatal nerve terminal degeneration and further lowering of DA levels, and possibly increased sensitivity of DA receptors.

Psychiatric disturbances such as hypersexuality, mania, visual hallucinations, and paranoid psychosis are common and sometimes severe adverse responses to treatment with L-DOPA or direct DA agonists (discussed later). Such behavioral disturbances probably reflect excessive stimulation of DA receptors in mesolimbic or mesocortical DA systems. These side effects complicate clinical management of PD patients, including those with clinical depression commonly associated with PD or dementia that sometimes arises in late stages of the disease. Serotonin-enhancing antidepressants usually are well tolerated with minor risk of worsening bradykinesia (120). Use of antipsychotic drugs, however, is limited to those with minimal risk of worsening bradykinesia and other aspects of extrapyramidal motor dysfunction (121,122). Clozapine, although potentially toxic and relatively expensive, is best tolerated and may have particular efficacy for visual hallucinations in PD patients. Moderate doses of quetiapine and ziprasidone are tolerated, but their efficacy is not established, and other second-generation antipsychotic agents including olanzapine, risperidone, paliperidone, and even the DA partial agonist aripiprazole usually are poorly tolerated by PD patients due to increased bradykinesia (121–124).

Dopamine Receptor Agonists

MECHANISM OF ACTION The nigrostriatal neurodegeneration that proceeds over the course of PD limits the number of striatal nerve terminals that are available to decarboxylate L-DOPA to DA. Drugs that act directly to stimulate DA receptors, however, do not require functioning dopaminergic nerve terminals and can be useful in the management of late-stage disease problems during L-DOPA therapy. DA receptor agonists currently available are nonselective, and without balanced activity at D_1-type and D_2-type receptors, for example, clinically used agents are full or partial agonists primarily at D_2-type receptors. Use of DA agonist monotherapy (i.e., without L-DOPA) has been suggested as initial therapy for PD based on the hypothesis that oxidative metabolites of DA (formed from exogenous and endogenous L-DOPA) may be neurotoxic. At present, however, no substantial evidence supports an indirect neuroprotective effect of DA receptor agonists (3). Meanwhile, DA receptor agonists have a longer duration of action (8 to 24 hours) compared to L-DOPA (6 to 8 hours) and may be less likely than L-DOPA to induce on/off effects and dyskinesias. In fact, the DA receptor agonists pramipexole and ropinirole (see later discussion) do produce reduced motor fluctuations compared to L-DOPA; however, they also produce increased incidence of other adverse effects (125,126), such as nausea and vomiting (presumably from activation of the chemoreceptor trigger zone), sedation, and hallucinations and other psychiatric disturbances that are particularly troublesome for elderly patients. Thus, the DA agonists usually are given in combination with a reduced dose of L-DOPA/carbidopa, but monotherapy may be used for younger patients better able to tolerate side effects (3).

STRUCTURE–ACTIVITY RELATIONSHIP Because there is currently no validated three-dimensional orientation of the amino acid residues at the ligand-binding site for D_1- or D_2-type DA receptors, rational design of selective DA receptor agonists (and antagonists) is guided by quantitative structure–activity relationship studies based on probe molecules and studies of ligand docking to DA molecular models built based on homology to solved GPCR crystal structures.

Little information can be gained concerning the conformational requirements for DA receptor activation using DA itself because its ethylamine side chain has unlimited flexibility, with unrestricted rotation about the β-carbon–phenyl bond (Fig. 13.9). Accordingly, compounds in which the catechol ring and the amino-ethyl moiety of DA are held in rigid conformation have been synthesized to probe molecular determinants for receptor binding and activation. Such rigid analogs include aporphines, notably starting with the morphine acid-rearrangement product, *R*-(−)-apomorphine (Fig. 13.9).

The alkaloid apomorphine has been employed in experimental neuropharmacology since the late nineteenth century (127,128). The *trans*-α-rotamer conformation of DA (Fig. 13.9) most closely aligns with apomorphine, as confirmed by the x-ray crystal structure of apomorphine (129). In contrast, *R*-(−)-isoapomorphine (Fig. 13.9) mimics the structure of DA in the *trans*-β-rotameric conformation and has less activity than apomorphine as a DA receptor agonist. The analog *R*-(−)-1,2-dihydroxyaporphine (Fig. 13.9) mimics the *cis*-α-rotamer conformation of DA and is inactive as a DA receptor agonist (130). In addition to the aporphines, the semi-rigid aminotetralin, 2-amino-5,6-dihydroxy-1,2,3,4-tetrahydronaphthalene (A-5,6-DTN, Fig. 13.9), that has its benzene ring and amino side chain in a *trans*-α-rotamer conformation, is a more potent DA agonist than its 6,7-dihydroxy congener (A-6,7-DTN, Fig. 13.9) with a *trans*-β-rotamer conformation (131). Studies of these rigid dopaminomimetic compounds suggest that the preferred conformation of DA is the extended *trans* conformation (α- or β-rotamer). Results from mutagenesis, molecular modeling, and computational chemistry indicate that ligand activity at D_1 versus D_2 receptors is critically dependent on the position of protonated nitrogen moieties of candidate ligands (as in the *trans* conformation of DA) that can support high-affinity ionic bonding at a proposed anionic aspartic acid residue in the third transmembrane α-helix (D3.32), as a preferred docking site of DA receptors (132–134).

Aporphine-Type Dopamine Receptor Agonists

R-(−)-Apomorphine (Fig. 13.9) was reintroduced as a useful adjunct in the therapy of PD (135), following years of neglect after promising early observations (136). Lack of oral bioavailability, short duration of action, and potent central emetic action discouraged its clinical use. Nevertheless, in 1993, *R*-(−)-apomorphine received regulatory approval in the United Kingdom for control of refractory motor dysfunction and wide fluctuations in responses ("on-off" syndrome) to L-DOPA or DA agonists (later approved in the U.S. as Apokyn) (137,138). Improved motility in response to an acute challenge dose of apomorphine also can predict responsiveness to L-DOPA treatment (139,140). *R*-(−)-Apomorphine is an agonist for both D_1- and D_2-type DA receptors. With a pK_a of about 9, it is mostly protonated at physiologic pH, but sufficiently lipophilic to cross the blood–brain barrier readily. Apomorphine can be administered subcutaneously by intermittent self-administration

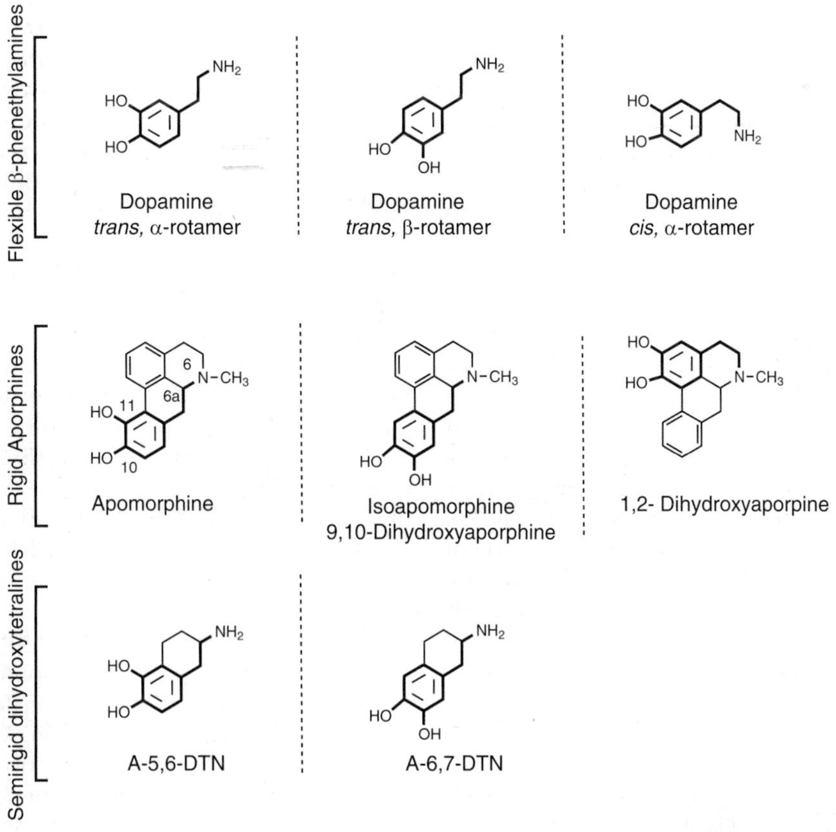

FIGURE 13.9 Conformations of dopamine in the *trans*-α-rotameric, *trans*-β-rotameric, and *cis*-rotameric forms, and their structural relationships to the rigid DA analogs apomorphine, isoapomorphine, and 1,2-dihydroxyaporphine. Also shown are the corresponding semirigid dihydroxyaminotetralin analogs of DA, A-5,6-DTN, and A-6,7-DTN.

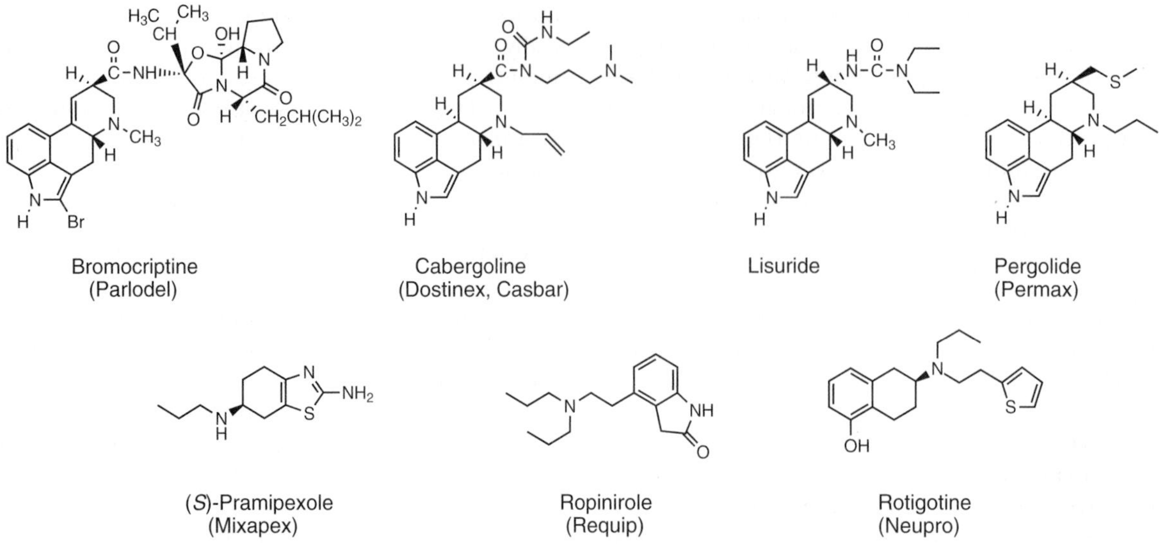

FIGURE 13.10 DA receptor agonist drugs that target primarily D_2-type receptors.

with a small self-injector (Penject) or by continuous infusion with a portable minipump.

Ergot-Type Dopamine Receptor Agonists

Bromocriptine (Fig. 13.10) is an ergot alkaloid peptide that is a partial agonist at D_2 and D_3 DA receptors (141) that lacks appreciable activity at D_1-type or D_4 receptors (142). It was the first direct DA agonist to be used in the treatment of PD, after its development for use at lower doses as a prolactin inhibitor (143). Bromocriptine inhibits prolactin release from anterior pituitary mammotrophic cells that selectively express D_2 DA receptors. These receptors respond to DA produced in the hypothalamus, released into the hypophysioportal blood vessels, and carried to the pituitary to act as a prolactin-inhibitory hormone. Bromocriptine is an effective prolactin inhibitor at daily doses of 1 to 5 mg, for which it is used to treat hyperprolactinemia associated with pituitary adenomas or to suppress prolactin output in prolactin-sensitive metastatic carcinoma of the breast. As a D_2 partial agonist, bromocriptine acts as an agonist at pituitary D_2 receptors that are normally in a high-sensitivity state. At daily doses of 10 to 20 mg, bromocriptine and other D_2 partial agonist ergolines appear to act as D_2 full agonists with antiparkinson effects; this full agonist activity probably reflects the supersensitized status of denervated DA receptors in PD (144,145). Bromocriptine is absorbed after oral administration, but approximately 90% undergoes extensive first-pass hepatic metabolism; the remainder is hydrolyzed in the liver to inactive metabolites eliminated mainly in bile, and the overall elimination half-life is approximately 3 hours.

Another ergoline, cabergoline (Fig. 13.10), is a full agonist at D_2 receptors and a partial agonist at D_3 and D_4 receptors, without appreciable activity at D_1-type receptors (141,142), and with a relatively long half-life of approximately 48 hours (3). Cabergoline is superior to placebo for treating motor signs of PD, but its comparative efficacy versus L-DOPA is poorly documented (146). Lisuride (Fig. 13.10) is an ergoline partial agonist at D_2, D_3, and D_4 receptors with little activity at D_1-type receptors (141,142). This relatively short-acting agent is being evaluated in patients with advanced PD, using either patch or infusion delivery methods (3,147).

The peptide component of bromocriptine evidently is unnecessary for dopaminergic activity. Pergolide (formerly Permax, Fig. 13.10) was the first nonpeptide ergoline used successfully to treat PD, as well to inhibit release of prolactin (143,148). Pergolide shows greater agonist effects at both D_2- and D_1-type DA receptors than does bromocriptine, but it was recently withdrawn from clinical use due to association with valvular heart disease (149,150). This adverse cardiac effect is due to activation of serotonin 5-HT_{2B} receptors by pergolide, as has been hypothesized for other drugs with potent 5-HT_{2B} agonist activity, including cabergoline (Fig. 13.10) (151,152). Moderate cardiac tricuspid valve regurgitation was more frequent in patients taking cabergoline repeatedly in relatively high doses for PD than in newly exposed or untreated controls (153). However, doses of cabergoline used to treat hyperprolactinemia are much lower (154) and may avoid valvular heart disease (154,155). Ergolines such as bromocriptine and lisuride that lack 5-HT_{2B} agonist activity do not appear to induce cardiac valvular damage (150,156,157).

Other Small-Molecule Dopamine Receptor Agonists

Currently, pramipexole and ropinirole (Fig. 13.10) are among the most commonly prescribed direct DA agonists for PD in the United States (17). They were introduced primarily for advanced stages of PD to limit fluctuations in response to L-DOPA therapy and as a "rescue" therapy when L-DOPA became insufficiently effective. These direct D_2 DA agonists are relatively well tolerated. Moreover, in light of concern that L-DOPA might itself cause DA neuronal toxicity through formation of reactive oxidized by-products, pramipexole and ropinirole are sometimes used as first-line treatments. In fact, a study in patients initially treated with pramipexole demonstrated a reduction in loss of striatal nerve terminals (104,105). An additional advantage of these agents is that they have relatively prolonged dopaminergic actions (long half-life), to provide more sustained clinical benefit with less risk of motor fluctuations than with L-DOPA (126).

Rotigotine (Fig. 13.10) is a relatively new, nonergoline, synthetic DA agonist that is administered by transdermal patch and used to treat both early and advanced PD (158). Rotigotine is an agonist at D_1 as well as D_2 and D_3 receptors (159), similar to apomorphine. It is highly lipophilic and undergoes extensive first-pass hepatic clearance when given orally, encouraging use of the long-acting transdermal patch formulation (159). Rotigotine provides benefits in PD both alone and combined with L-DOPA and is better tolerated than other DA agonists (160–162).

The direct DA agonists generally produce similar adverse effects, including initial nausea and vomiting, postural hypotension, and fatigue. These effects are especially likely with the ergolines. Additional risks include psychotic reactions when DA agonists are given alone or with L-DOPA. These reactions include hallucinations, delusions, and confusion, and are most likely in elderly PD patients with symptoms of dementia. Treatment is similar to psychotic reactions encountered during L-DOPA therapy.

Experimental Dopamine D_1 Receptor Agonists

The opposing actions of the direct and indirect pathways in the basal ganglia (Fig. 13.4) suggest that coordinated neurotransmission requires activation of the direct pathway and attenuation of the indirect pathway involving DA neurotransmission in the basal ganglia. Such neuromodulation may require a balance of stimulatory actions at D_1-type receptors and inhibitory actions at D_2-type receptors. Consistent with a role for D_1 receptors in the direct output pathway, their stimulation represents a plausible pharmacotherapeutic approach for PD.

Clinical trials in PD with early, selective D_1 partial agonists (Fig. 13.11) such as the benzergoline CY-208-243 and the *R*-(+)-phenylbenzazepine SKF-38393 found these drugs to be either short acting or ineffective, suggesting that full D_1 agonist activity may be required (163,164). Several analogs of SKF-38393 (Fig. 13.11) are full-efficacy D_1 agonists, including *R*-(+)-SKF-81297 and its 6-halo derivatives, 6-Br-APB and 6-Cl-APB (SKF-82958) (165,166). In MPTP-lesioned monkeys, 6-Cl-APB produced antiparkinson effects (167), but its duration of action was less than 1 hour (168) and it produced severe dyskinetic effects (169). Moreover, *R*-(+)-SKF-81297, as well as the benzophenanthridine dihydrexidine (Fig. 13.11) (168), showed beneficial results only in monkeys with severe parkinsonism. It has been suggested that long-acting D_1 agonists may be most useful in late stages of PD (170).

Dihydrexidine (Fig. 13.11) was the first full-efficacy D_1 agonist to be developed, although it also has some

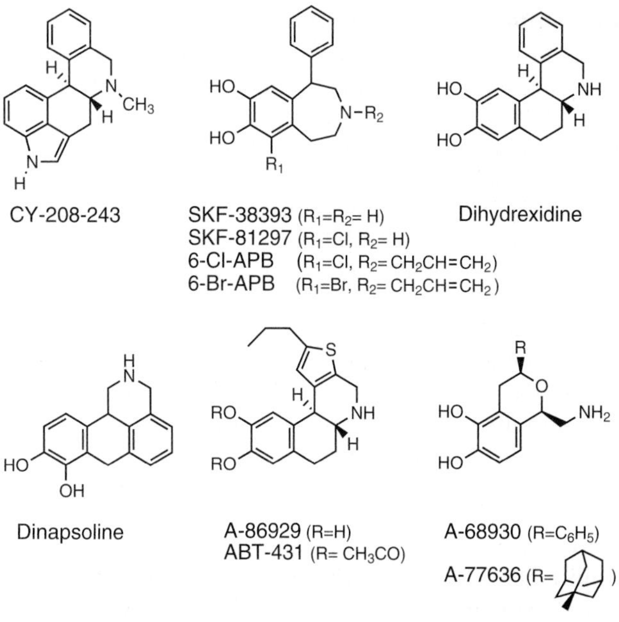

FIGURE 13.11 Experimental DA receptor agonist drugs that target primarily D_1 receptors.

D_2-type activity (171,172). In MPTP-lesioned monkeys, dihydrexidine essentially eliminated all parkinsonian signs, and this effect was fully blocked by a selective D_1 antagonist but not by a selective D_2 antagonist (173). Continuous administration of dihydrexidine to rats for 2 weeks produced very little change in D_1 receptor density or D_1 receptor-mediated DA-stimulated adenylyl cyclase activity, suggesting that tolerance might not develop to its antiparkinson effects. In PD patients, however, dihydrexidine has a narrow therapeutic index, with dose-limiting adverse effects that include flushing, hypotension, and tachycardia after single intravenous doses (174).

A D_1 receptor pharmacophore model developed for dihydrexidine was used to design other novel molecular structures as full-efficacy D_1 agonists (175), including, dinapsoline (Fig. 13.11) (176), the dihydrexidine isostere A-86929, and its diacetyl prodrug ABT-431. These analogs are full-efficacy D_1 agonists with sustained antiparkinson effects in MPTP-lesioned monkeys (177). In PD patients, ABT-431 was highly effective against bradykinesia but produced dyskinesias (178).

Several isochromans also are full D_1 agonists. In primates pretreated with MPTP, A-68930 produced seizures, whereas the analog A-77636 showed antiparkinson effects without inducing seizures (Fig. 13.11) (179). However, A-77636 showed rapid desensitization to its beneficial effects (180), possibly related to its prolonged action that exceeds 20 hours (169). Other conformationally restricted analogs containing the β-phenyldopamine pharmacophore continue to be reported, including some with impressive D_1-type over D_2-type receptor agonist activity (181); however, in vivo studies with D_1 agonists have, so far, given disappointing results.

Monoamine Oxidase Inhibitors

Given the role of MAO in catabolism of DA (Fig. 13.2), leading to neurotoxic oxidation products of both endogenous (Fig. 13.5) and exogenous (Fig. 13.6) substrates, MAO inhibition has the potential to boost levels of brain DA and prevent formation of MAO-derived oxidation products that could cause neurotoxicity. Furthermore, by reducing the oxidation of DA, MAO inhibitors can extend the duration of response to L-DOPA and allow use of lower doses (106).

MAO is expressed as two isoforms, A and B. Histochemical and immunohistochemical studies reveal that in human brain MAO-A is found primarily in noradrenergic neurons, whereas MAO-B is found primarily in serotoninergic and histaminergic neurons as well as in glial cells. There is no consensus on which form may predominate in brain DA neurons (182); thus, there is some uncertainty as to whether to target MAO-A or -B in treatment of PD. Less is known about the structural requirements for highly specific reversible MAO-A inhibitors (183) compared to selective MAO-B inhibitors (see Chapter 18, several of which produce clinical benefits in PD. A compelling link between PD etiology and MAO is that levels of MAO-B are increased in the brains of PD patients as a consequence of gliosis (184). Involvement of MAO-B in age-related neurologic disorders that include PD also is suggested by observations that human and rodent MAO-B levels increase with aging (185,186). Increased MAO-B levels would be expected to not only diminish DA levels, but also to increase levels of potentially neurotoxic oxidation products. Another link between MAO and PD is that 3,4-dihydroxyphenylacetaldehyde (DOPAL), the aldehyde that is the MAO-derived two-electron oxidation product of DA (Equation 1 in Fig 13.5), has been implicated in the aggregation of α-synuclein (187).

Selegiline and Rasagiline

Long-acting, irreversible, nonselective MAO-A/B inhibitors, such as phenelzine and tranylcypromine (Fig. 13.12; also, see Chapter 18) are contraindicated in combination with L-DOPA because of the risk of inducing hypertensive crises and delirium (17,188).

Selegiline (L-deprenyl; *R*-[−]-*N*,2-dimethyl-*N*-2-propynyl-phenethylamine) and rasagiline (Fig. 13.12) are propargylamine-type selective irreversible inhibitors of MAO-B. In addition to potentiating DA actions and allowing for reduction of L-DOPA dose, it has been proposed that MAO-B inhibitors may prevent formation of neurotoxic oxidation products of DA and slow neurodegeneration in PD; however, data from recent clinical studies do not support this attractive "neuroprotective" hypothesis (3,104–106). Nevertheless, MAO-B inhibitors have a beneficial effect on motor fluctuations because of their levodopa-sparing effect (106).

Selegiline and rasagiline undergo extensive hepatic metabolism. Selegiline is *N*-dealkylated via CYP2B6 and CYP2C19 to (−)-methamphetamine and, subsequently, to (−)-amphetamine, which has vasoactive activity similar to (+)-amphetamine (189). The amphetamine metabolites

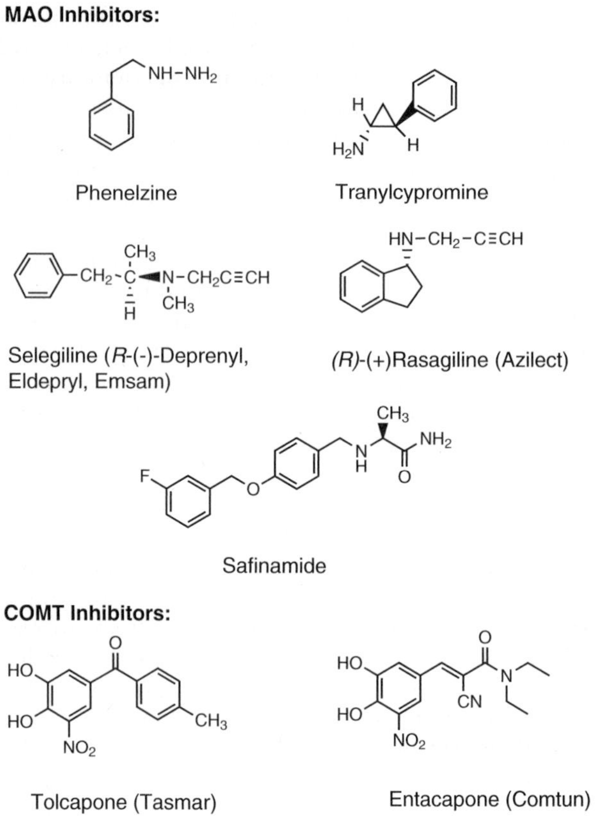

FIGURE 13.12 Drugs that inhibit monoamine oxidase (MAO) or catechol-*O*-methyltransferase (COMT).

of selegiline may contribute to its other pharmacologic property of DA and norepinephrine reuptake inhibition, thus potentiating the pharmacologic effects of L-DOPA. The amphetamine metabolites of selegiline have been associated with cardiovascular (orthostatic hypotension) and psychiatric (hallucinations) side effects.

Rasagiline is *N*-dealkylated primarily by CYP1A2 to (*R*)-1-aminoindan, which does not have vasoactive activity (189). Recently, rasagiline underwent clinical trials to assess its ability to provide neuroprotection (190). Rasagiline at a dose of 1.0 mg/d met endpoints consistent with a disease-modifying (neuroprotective) effect, but rasagiline at 2 mg/d failed; the authors of the study hypothesize that the stronger symptomatic effect of the higher dose masked an underlying disease-modifying effect. Rasaagiline has recently been approved by United States FDA for treatment of PD.

Safinamide (Fig. 13.12) is an α-aminoamide derivative that is a reversible selective MAO-B inhibitor shown to provide benefits in early PD (191,192). In addition to its MAO-B inhibitor properties, safinamide also blocks voltage-dependent sodium and calcium channels and inhibits glutamate release (192). It is currently in phase III trials in the United States and in Europe (3).

Catechol-*O*-Methyltransferase Inhibitors

The peripheral metabolism of L-DOPA given alone leads to very limited access of the amino acid to the CNS. It is rapidly decarboxylated by L-aromatic amino acid decarboxylase and 3-*O*-methylated by COMT (Fig. 13.2). Inactivation of L-DOPA and DA can be slowed by using a COMT inhibitor.

COMT is methyltransferase that uses as its methyl donor the cofactor *S*-adenosyl-L-methionine (SAMe). COMT converts L-DOPA and catecholamines preferentially to their *m*-methoxy derivatives (Fig. 13.2). These include 3-*O*-methyl-DOPA and 3-*O*-methyl-DA (3-methoxytyramine, 3-methoxy-4-hydroxyphenethylamine), as well as the 3-*O*-methylated, deaminated compound HVA, the major final metabolite of DA in humans. Treatment with L-DOPA can reduce tissue concentrations of SAMe (115), with uncertain consequences that should be limited by co-treatment with a COMT inhibitor. COMT acts in both peripheral and cerebral tissues, although the effect of COMT inhibitors to potentiate L-DOPA probably occurs mainly in peripheral tissues (193,194).

Tolcapone and Entacapone

Tolcapone and entacapone (Fig. 13.12) are reversible COMT inhibitors. Examination of their chemical structures reveals obvious similarities, and the molecular mechanisms by which these drugs interact with human COMT are proposed to be similar (195,196). Although the mechanisms of action and pharmacotherapeutic effects are similar for tolcapone and entacapone, they differ with respect to pharmacokinetic properties and adverse effects. Tolcapone has a relatively longer duration of action (8 to 12 hours) and acts both in the brain and periphery, whereas entacapone has a shorter duration of action (2 hours) and acts mostly in the periphery. Some common adverse effects of these agents are predictable and attributable to increased brain DA (e.g., nausea, vivid dreams, confusion, and hallucinations). A potentially fatal adverse effect, however, occurs only with tolcapone; after marketing, three fatal cases of fulminant hepatic failure were observed, leading to its market withdrawal in some countries and restriction in the United States to only those patients who have not responded to other therapies and who have appropriate monitoring for hepatic toxicity. The unforeseen hepatotoxicity associated with tolcapone has left entacapone as the only COMT inhibitor in wide clinical use; however, since the labeling restrictions in 1998, there have been no additional reports of hepatic fatality associated with entacapone (197). The mechanism by which liver damage is induced by tolcapone is believed to involve uncoupling of mitochondria oxidative phosphorylation, significantly reducing cellular generation of ATP (198,199). Additionally, it was shown that tolcapone (but not entacapone) induces cytotoxic pro-oxidant radical formation in hepatocytes (200). Finally, both COMT inhibitors may cause severe diarrhea and produce increased dyskinesias that may require a reduction in the dose of L-DOPA (201).

Approved and Experimental Drugs for PD That Target Nondopaminergic Proteins

Glutamate Antagonists

The dyskinesias associated with L-DOPA therapy may involve overactivity of thalamocortical excitatory glutamatergic input to the motor cerebral cortex (Fig. 13.4). In addition, excessive release of glutamate due to synaptic overactivity is hypothesized to lead to "excitotoxicity," resulting from excess neuronal Ca^{2+} influx due to opening of *N*-methyl-D-aspartate (NMDA) ion channel receptors (202), at which glutamate is a coagonist (along with glycine).

Amantadine and its dimethylated congener memantine (Fig. 13.13) are NMDA glutamate receptor antagonists that might provide neuroprotective effects (203). Both have moderately beneficial effects early in PD, can enhance the effects of L-DOPA, and can perhaps limit the severity of dyskinesias induced by L-DOPA therapy (204). Also, memantine has been used as a spasmolytic agent in the treatment of both PD and dementia (205). Amantadine was originally developed as an antiviral agent, and its use in PD patients with influenza revealed unexpected improvement in PD symptoms (206). The pK_a of this primary amine is 10.8; thus, it exists mainly in the protonated form at physiologic pH. The lipophilic cage-like structure of both amantadine and memantine likely facilitates their entry into brain and may provide resistance to metabolism by oxidative enzymes; both drugs are excreted mostly unchanged in the urine (207,208). In addition, amantadine causes release of DA and norepinephrine from intraneuronal storage sites and blocks reuptake of DA and was initially considered a DA-potentiating agent for use in mild PD (209).

Adenosine Receptor Antagonists

Adenosine is a nucleoside signaling molecule that acts at four GPCR subtypes, A_1, A_{2A}, A_{2B}, and A_3. The mRNA for A_{2A} receptor protein is highly concentrated in the striatum, nucleus accumbens, and olfactory tubercle, and co-localizes with D_2 receptor mRNA in these brain regions (210). Activation of A_{2A} receptors inhibits GABA release in striatum (211). Thus, antagonism of A_{2A} receptors is expected to increase GABA-mediated inhibition of the medium spiny output neurons to help compensate for loss of DA D_1 receptor–stimulated

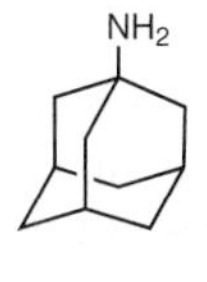

Amantadine (Symmetrel)

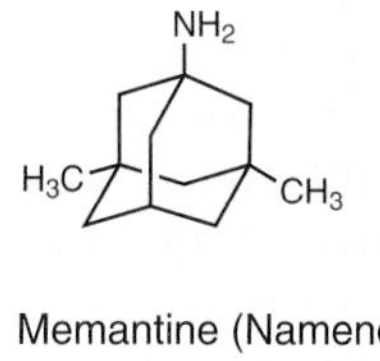

Memantine (Namenda)

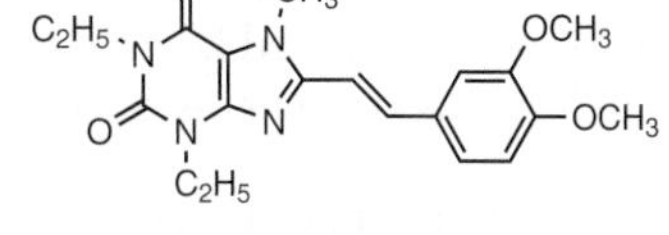

Istradefylline (KW 6002)

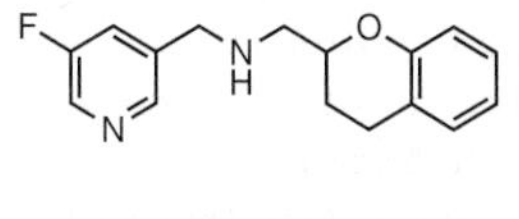

Sarizotan (EMD 128130)

FIGURE 13.13 Approved and experimental drugs for PD that target nondopaminergic proteins.

GABA release and D_2 receptor–mediated inhibition of these neurons in PD (212) (see Fig. 13.4). Adenosine A_{2A} receptors also oppose the actions of D_1 and D_2 receptors on gene expression (213) and second-messenger systems and reduce the binding affinity of DA for D_2 receptors (214). An A_{2A} antagonist presumably would block these A_{2A} receptor–mediated inhibitory effects on DA neurotransmission. Activation of A_{2A} receptors also stimulates release of acetylcholine in striatum (215), and it has long been known that muscarinic receptor antagonists can ameliorate some signs of PD. As mentioned, there is an inverse relationship between the risk of developing PD and consumption of caffeine, a nonselective antagonist at adenosine A_1 and A_2 GPCRs (216,217).

Istradefylline (formerly KW 6002; Fig. 13.13) is a potent and selective antagonist at adenosine A_{2A} receptors that was shown to improve motor disability in primate models of PD (218). A recent double-blind, placebo-controlled clinical trial (219) showed that in patients stabilized on L-DOPA and other PD drug regimens, istradefylline-treated subjects had significant reductions in motor fluctuations and the drug was, in general, well tolerated. In a subsequent study assessing istradefylline as monotherapy for PD, the drug was well tolerated but did not demonstrate efficacy to improve motor symptoms (220). Studies with A_1 receptor antagonists lag behind; however, there is evidence that they reduce parkinsonian-type tremor in rodents (221).

Serotonin 5-HT$_{1A}$ Agonists

Dysfunction of neurotransmission mediated by 5-hydroxytryptamine (5-HT; serotonin) occurs in the basal ganglia of patients with PD, and excessive serotonergic transmission may contribute to dyskinesias associated with dopaminergic treatments (222). The central and peripheral psychological and physiologic effects of 5-HT are mediated by 14 serotonin receptor subtypes grouped into the 5-HT$_1$ to 5-HT$_7$ families. The 5-HT$_1$ family consists of five GPCRs subtypes, 5-HT$_{1A,1B,1D}$, $_{1E}$, and $_{1F}$ (223). The 5-HT$_{1A}$ autoreceptor is expressed presynaptically on 5-HT terminals. When 5-HT$_{1A}$ autoreceptors are activated, serotonin release is decreased (224), and diminished dyskinesias occur in rodent and primate models of PD (225). Activation of 5-HT$_{1A}$ receptors also can reverse parkinsonism-like catalepsy induced by the DA D_2 antagonist haloperidol (221); thus, 5-HT$_{1A}$ receptor activation might also counteract losses of nigrostriatal DA neurotransmission in PD. Moreover, in patients with advanced PD, intact striatal 5-HT terminals are an important site of decarboxylation of exogenous L-DOPA to DA. A 5-HT$_{1A}$ agonist might act at striatal serotonergic terminals to limit release of DA produced by L-DOPA treatment and release from 5-HT terminals as a "false transmitter."

Sarizotan (formerly EMD-128130; Fig. 13.13) is an aminomethylchroman derivative that has high affinity (K_i ~ 0.05 nM) and full-efficacy agonist activity at human 5-HT$_{1A}$ receptors (226). Sarizotan also has appreciable affinity (K_i ~3 nM/L) at human DA D_2-type receptors. It is a partial agonist at D_2 but demonstrates no apparent activation of D_3 and D_4 receptors. Given by itself to MPTP-lesioned monkeys, sarizotan had no effect on the severity of motor deficits or on beneficial responses to L-DOPA, but it reduced L-DOPA–induced choreiform dyskinesias by more than 90% (224). Thus, there appears to be no compelling clinical evidence to support concern that sarizotan might limit release of DA from 5-HT terminals via 5-HT$_{1A}$ activation or from DA nerve terminals via D_2 activation. The beneficial effects of sarizotan in parkinsonian monkeys may be specific to 5-HT$_{1A}$ agonism because effects were reversed by a selective 5-HT$_{1A}$ antagonist. In PD patients with dyskinesias resulting from L-DOPA therapy, adding sarizotan pharmacotherapy produced significant increases in periods of time without dyskinesia and significant reduction in periods of time with troublesome dyskinesias (227). A subsequent clinical study that assessed improvement of dyskinesias gave mixed results, depending on the dyskinesia rating scale that was used; however, the drug proved to be safe and relatively well tolerated (228). A recent study using the MPTP monkey PD model confirmed that sarizotan produces a sustained antidyskinetic effect while maintaining L-DOPA antiparkinsonian effects (229), suggesting the 5-HT$_{1A}$ agonist field may prove fruitful in PD drug discovery.

Adjunct Therapy—Muscarinic and Histamine H1 Antagonist Drugs

Cholinergic interneurons in the striatum exert mainly excitatory effects on GABAergic output from the striatum. Drugs that increase cholinergic neurotransmission (e.g., the cholinesterase inhibitor physostigmine and the direct agonist carbachol) have long been known to aggravate parkinsonism, whereas centrally active muscarinic antagonists (such as the belladonna alkaloids, including atropine) have moderately beneficial effects (17,230). Accordingly, before the discovery of L-DOPA, drug therapy for parkinsonism depended primarily on the limited efficacy of the natural belladonna alkaloids and newer synthetic antimuscarinic alkaloids, as well as histamine H_1 antagonists that also exert central antimuscarinic actions (Table 13.1). Synthetic centrally active muscarinic antagonists include benztropine mesylate, trihexylphenidyl, procyclidine, and biperiden; histamine H_1 antagonists with antimuscarinic activity include diphenhydramine and the phenothiazine ethopropazine.

The muscarinic and histamine H_1 antagonist drugs in Table 13.1 have limited therapeutic benefit in PD. Moreover, they exert a range of undesirable adverse effects associated with blockade of peripheral muscarinic receptors, including, dry mouth, impaired visual accommodation, constipation, urinary retention, and tachycardia. Adverse CNS effects include delirium,

CLINICAL APPLICATIONS: RADIOPHARMACEUTICALS IN DIAGNOSIS OF PD

Even for an experienced clinical neurologist, diagnosis of PD can be difficult to confirm, especially in the early stages of this disease. Signs of PD vary markedly among patients and in the same person over time; disability can fluctuate dramatically, and progression of the disorder is unpredictable. In addition, a number of conditions mimic PD and vary in their responses to antiparkinson drugs. Given these difficulties, brain imaging techniques using positron emission tomography (PET) and single photon emission computed tomography (SPECT) are increasingly used for diagnosis of PD and to assess DA nerve terminal function.

Spatial resolution is greater with PET, but SPECT technology is less expensive and more widely accessible in many clinical settings. In addition, positron-emitting nuclides used in PET imaging have very short half-lives (^{11}C, 20 minutes; ^{18}F, 109 minutes) and usually require an on-site cyclotron for their production. SPECT nuclides have longer half-lives (^{123}I, 13 hours; ^{99m}Tc, 6 hours) and often can be supplied commercially, and [^{99m}Tc]-labeled radioligands can be prepared locally as needed.

Quantitative assessment of nigrostriatal presynaptic DA nerve terminal function by PET using [^{18}F]-labeled 6-fluoro-L-DOPA ([^{18}F]DOPA) has proved useful for the early diagnosis of PD (231). Also, it has been known for some time that cocaine binds to the DA transporter (DAT) protein; however, cocaine also binds to other monoamine transporters and is rapidly hydrolyzed at its benzoyl ester function, making it impractical for use as an imaging agent (232). Linking the phenyl ring of cocaine directly to a tropane system, however, yields nonhydrolyzable, long-acting phenyltropanes that have been developed into clinically useful radiopharmaceuticals.

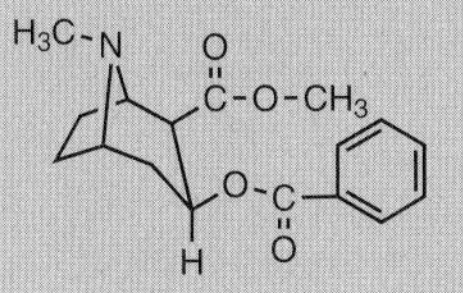

Cocaine

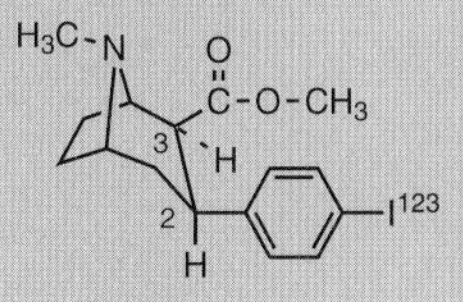

[^{123}I]-β-CIT (DopaScan)

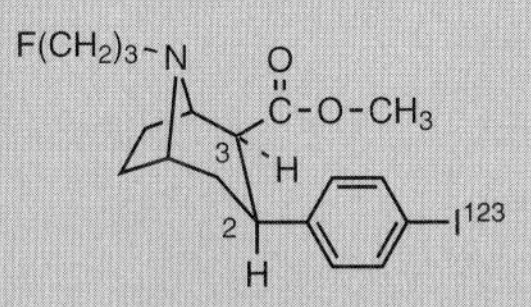

[^{123}I]-FP-CIT (DAT Scan)

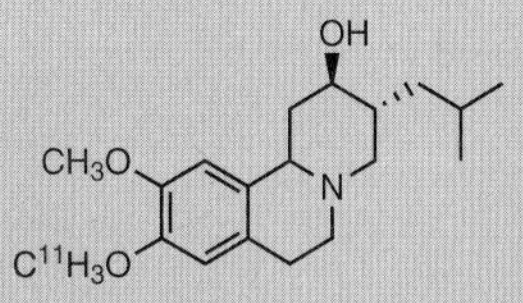

(+)-[^{11}C]-Dihydrotetrabenazine

The first tropane-based imagining to emerge was [^{123}I]2-β-carbomethoxy-3β-(4-iodophenyl)tropane, known as [^{123}I]β-CIT or RTI-55 (233). The radioactive iodine atom in the para position of the phenyl ring provides for the imaging properties of [^{123}I]β-CIT. A limiting factor with [^{123}I]β-CIT, however, is that it must be administered 8 hours before imaging to achieve peak uptake to DA nerve terminal regions. In an effort to improve the pharmacokinetic profile of [^{123}I]β-CIT, Neumeyer et al. (234) developed the *N*-3-fluoropropyl analog of β-CIT, known as [^{123}I]FP-CIT or [^{123}I]ioflupane. This DA nerve terminal imaging agent rapidly reaches its target sites (DA reuptake proteins) so that patients can be imaged 1 to 2 hours after injection of [^{123}I]FP-CIT. A radioligand suitable for PET imaging is obtained by replacing the fluorine atom with [^{18}F] in FP-CIT (235). DAT scan ([^{123}I]FP-CIT) is approved for clinical use, and both [^{123}I]β-CIT and [^{123}I]FP-CIT are used as research tools to assess DA nerve terminal function in neurodegenerative and neuropsychiatric disorders.

An alternative biomarker for assessing DA neuronal loss in PD is the vesicular monoamine transporter 2 (VMAT2) protein. VMAT2 is the transporter that moves nerve terminal cytoplasmic DA into synaptic vesicles for storage and subsequent exocytotic release. Recently, the PET radioligand (+)-[^{11}C]-dihydrotetrabenazine was reported as an investigational imaging agent for VMAT2 (236–238).

confusion, memory impairment, and psychotic symptoms. Despite their relatively unfavorable benefit/risk ratio, these drugs still are used in treatment of PD in combination with L-DOPA, particularly to help control tremor (230). They demonstrate better efficacy to control adverse extrapyramidal neurologic effects of potent D_2-receptor antagonist antipsychotic drugs such as haloperidol (17).

SPASTICITY DISORDERS

Clinical Evaluation

Spasticity is characterized by skeletal muscle spasms and an increase in tonic stretch reflexes, sometimes with accompanying muscle weakness. Spasticity often is associated with cerebral palsy, multiple sclerosis, spinal cord injury, or stroke. The mechanisms that underlie clinical

TABLE 13.1 Muscarinic and Histamine H1 Antagonist Drugs for Parkinson Disease

Class and Generic Name	Trade Name	Chemical Structure	Initial Single Oral Dose
Synthetic anticholinergic agents			
Benztropine mesylate	Cogentin	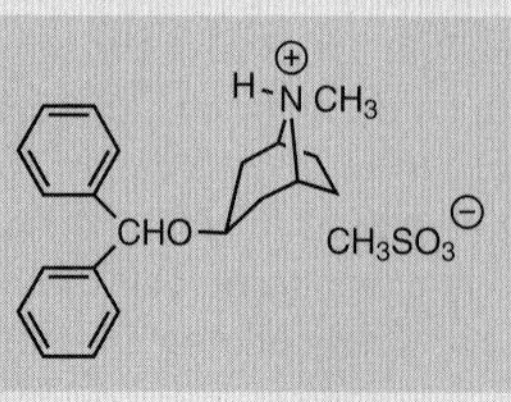	0.5–1.0 mg
Trihexyphenidyl hydrochloride	Artane Pipanol (x = 2) Tremin	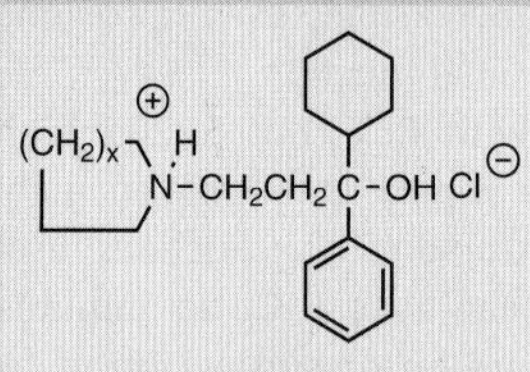	1.0–2.0 mg
Procyclidine hydrochloride	Kemadrin (x= 1)		2.0–5.0 mg
Biperiden hydrochloride	Akineton	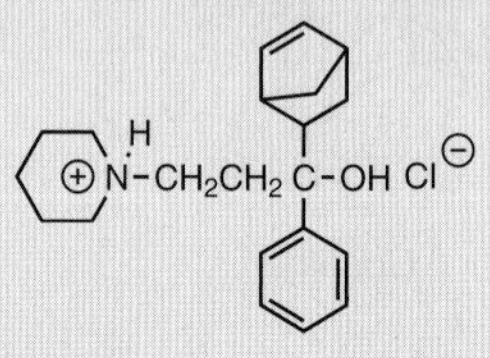	1.0–2.0 mg
Antihistamine			
Diphenhydramine hydrochloride	Benadryl	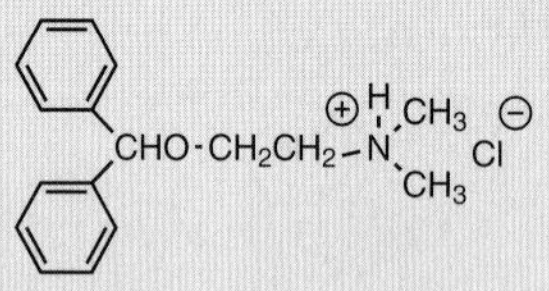	25.0 mg
Phenothiazine (Antihistamine)			
Ethopropazine hydrochloride	Parsidol	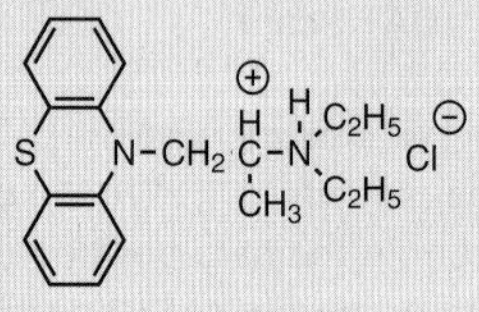	50.0 mg

spasticity appear to involve damage to descending pathways in the spinal cord that results in hyperexcitability of motor neurons (239). In addition to lack of accurate experimental models, a limiting factor in characterizing the pathophysiology of spasticity and effectiveness of antispasmodic drugs continues to be lack of quantitative methodology for assessment of the spasmodic condition (240,241). Simple tests of muscle tone or reflex latency have not been fruitful; however, global clinical assessments, such as the number of painful spasms per day, have been more useful. Even the combined subjective impressions of improvement by the patient, family, and physician, however, may not establish that a particular drug is efficacious. Furthermore, spasm frequently coexists with pain, and spasmolytic drug efficacy may be related to both skeletal muscle relaxation and analgesia (242,243). A straightforward strategy to establish whether a spasmolytic drug produces any benefit is gradual withdrawal of the drug. The diversity of neurologic disorders that culminate in spasticity and the subjectivity of many of the measurements make it difficult to establish efficacy of any one of the spasmolytic drugs. In summary, clinical evidence for efficacy of oral antispasmodic agents is scarce and weak.

Spasmolytic Drugs

Skeletal Muscle Relaxants

Background The drugs used for spasmolytic conditions are diverse in their chemical structures and their sites and mechanisms of action. The first drug recognized to exhibit spasmolytic activity was antodyne or

3-phenoxy-1,2-propanediol. In guinea pigs and rabbits, antodyne produced prolonged paralysis without impairing consciousness. Antodyne was introduced into clinical medicine in 1910 as an analgesic and antipyretic. The duration of its skeletal muscle relaxant effect, however, was too short-lived to be clinically useful. In 1943, structure–activity relationship studies of a series of simple glyceryl ethers related to antodyne led to the development and introduction of mephenesin (Table 13.2) in 1946 (244). Pharmacologic studies revealed that mephenesin selectivity depressed polysynaptic, while sparing monosynaptic, spinal cord reflexes. The relative safety and selective action of mephenesin on the spinal cord led to its use as the first widely prescribed

TABLE 13.2 Skeletal Muscle Relaxants

Class and Generic Name	Trade Name	Chemical Structure	Initial Single Oral Dose
Glycerol monoethers and derivatives			
Mephenesin		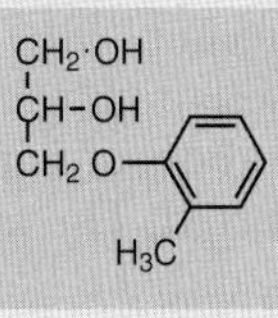	1–2 g (oral)
Chlorphenesin carbamate	Maolate (R_1 = H, R_2 = Cl)	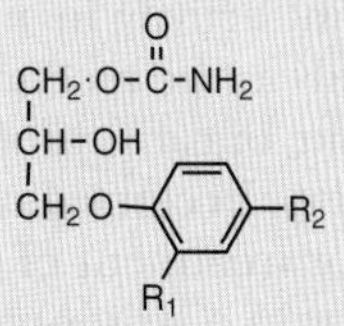	800 mg (oral)
Methocarbamol	Robaxin (R_1 = OCH_3, R_2 = H)		1–2 g (oral) 500 mg IM 1–3 g daily (IV)
Subtituted alkanediols and derivatives			
Meprobamate	Equanil Miltown (R = H)	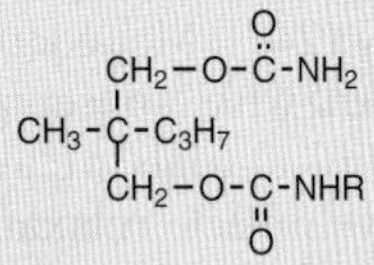	400 mg
Carisoprodol	Rela Soma (R = $CH(CH_3)_2$)		250–350 mg
Metaxalone	Skelaxin	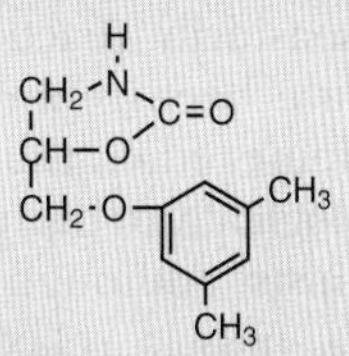	800 mg
Benzazole			
Chlorzoxazone	Paraflex	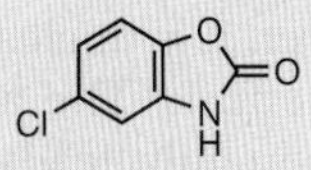	250–750 mg
Miscellaneous			
Orphenadrine citrate	Norflex	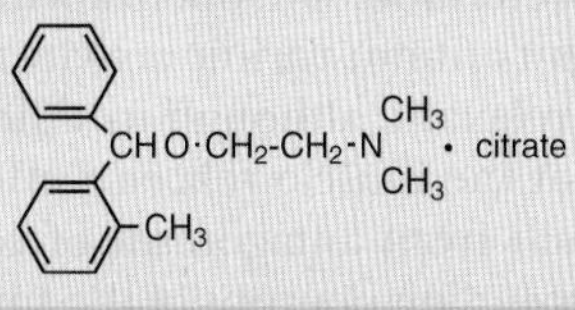	100 mg (oral) 60 mg IM or IV
Cyclobenzaprine	Flexaril	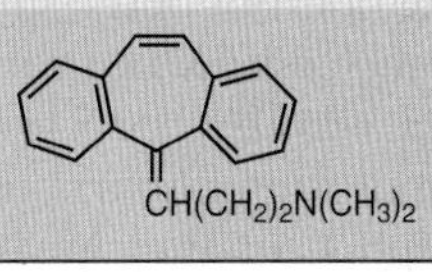	10 mg

centrally acting skeletal muscle relaxant. Accordingly, mephenesin is the prototype of the interneuronal blocking type of muscle relaxant, albeit mephenesin itself no longer is used. In general, the pharmacology of the mephenesin-like muscle relaxants is remarkably similar to that of sedative-hypnotics. Indeed, the only apparent difference is that the spasmolytics have greater selectivity for modulating effects mediated by the spinal cord, thus producing less sedation than general sedative-hypnotics. Both classes produce a reversible, nonspecific depression of the CNS, and sedation, dizziness, and muscle weakness are common side effects.

Table 13.2 shows several compounds with mephenesin-like pharmacologic profiles that have been developed and marketed as antispasmodic muscle relaxants. Chlorphenesin carbamate and methocarbamol are carbamate analogs of mephenesin that are designed to have longer lasting effects; however, their duration of action has not been carefully evaluated and reported. The alcohol carbon of methocarbamol is chiral, and the *R*-(+)-enantiomer has greater muscle relaxant activity in mice (245); however, the drug is available only as the racemate. Meprobamate is the principal metabolite of carisoprodol; thus, the pharmacology of the two overlap. In clinical studies, carisoprodol has modest efficacy for treatment of low back pain associated with sprain or strain. Carisoprodol and meprobamate have sedative and anxiolytic effects similar to benzodiazepines, such as diazepam, and carry a similar liability for abuse and dependency (241). Metaxalone, on the other hand, is not associated with abuse, and although no data from high-quality clinical trials are available, it generally is reported to achieve muscle relaxation without excessive sedation. Chlorzoxazone is another agent marketed as a skeletal muscle relaxant, but with unclear efficacy in spasmodic conditions. A considerable drawback to empirical use of chlorzoxazone is that idiosyncratic hepatotoxicity and several sensitivity reactions (urticaria, erythema, and pruritus) have been reported (241). Orphenadrine is an ethanolamine ether that is related both chemically and pharmacologically to diphenhydramine-type histamine H_1 antagonists. Although its efficacy is not clearly established, any muscle relaxant effects of orphenadrine may be caused by CNS anticholinergic (muscarinic antagonist) activity. Orphenadrine also is an NMDA receptor antagonist; however, it is unclear if this activity may lead to antispasmodic effects. The antimuscarinic activity of orphenadrine certainly leads to unpleasant peripheral side effects, such as dry mouth, blurred vision, and urinary retention. Cyclobenzaprine is another agent with prominent antimuscarinic activity that is used as a skeletal muscle relaxant, although its efficacy is modest. It is proposed that the muscle relaxant effects of cyclobenzaprine may result from antagonism of serotonin 5-HT_2 receptors in descending neurons of the spinal cord (246), but anticholinergic mechanisms cannot be ruled out. Although the presence of a double bond in the cycloheptyl ring of cyclobenzaprine is the only structural difference from the tricyclic antidepressant amitriptyline, cyclobenzaprine is not an efficacious antidepressant. Cyclobenzaprine has a long plasma half-life (1 to 3 days), and accumulation on multiple dosing contributes to its high incidence of sedation.

In summary, it should be noted that there is no clear evidence that so-called skeletal muscle relaxants directly inhibit muscle contraction (as is the case for dantrolene, discussed later) or of whether their effects are related more to sedation and other nonspecific effects. In the United States, the drugs discussed above are approved for treatment of musculoskeletal conditions, whereas the drugs discussed below (baclofen, dantrolene, tizanidine) are approved specifically for muscle spasticity (243).

Diazepam

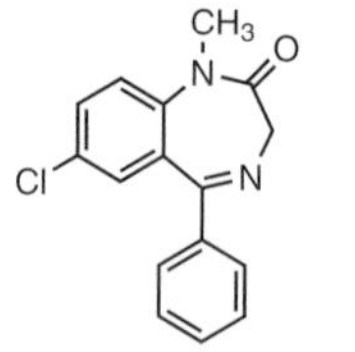

Diazepam (Valium)

Although benzodiazepines, such as diazepam, often are used as skeletal muscle relaxants, they are not approved by the U.S. Food and Drug Administration (FDA) for this purpose (243). Diazepam and other benzodiazepines are proposed to exert skeletal muscle relaxant effects via their binding as agonists at the benzodiazepine receptor of the $GABA_A$ receptor complex, which enhances GABA potency to increase chloride conductance (see Chapter 17). The muscle relaxant properties of classical benzodiazepines, such as diazepam, appear to be mediated mainly by the $GABA_A$ α_2 and α_3 subunits (247,248). The result is neuronal hyperpolarization, probably at both supraspinal and spinal sites for spasmolytic activity. The actions of diazepam are sufficient to relieve spasticity in patients with lesions affecting the spinal cord and in some patients with cerebral palsy (242). Few clinical trials that include appropriate control groups have been conducted to assess diazepam efficacy as a muscle relaxant. It is currently generally accepted that diazepam is no more efficacious than, for example, carisoprodol, cyclobenzaprine, or tizanidine (i.e., efficacy is marginal) (240,241). Moreover, diazepam produces drowsiness and fatigue in most patients at doses required to significantly reduce muscle tone.

Baclofen

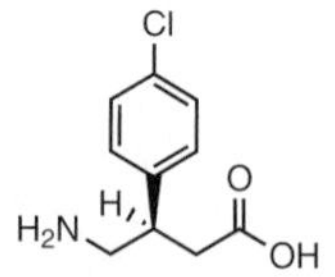

Baclofen
Racemic mixture (Lioresal)

Baclofen (β-*p*-chlorophenyl-GABA) is a $GABA_B$ receptor agonist and is one of the most commonly used antispastic agents (243). The (*R*)-(−)-enantiomer is the active isomer at $GABA_B$ receptors, but the racemate (Lioresal) is approved for use as a spasmolytic agent. The molecular mechanisms of $GABA_B$ receptors in muscle spasticity are not understood any better than other putative receptor-based mechanisms discussed earlier. It is proposed that baclofen inhibits spinal cord monosynaptic and polysynaptic reflexes via $GABA_B$ receptor–mediated opening of neuronal potassium channels that leads to hyperpolarization of primary afferent fiber terminals. In spinal motor neurons, baclofen suppresses excitability by reducing calcium persistent inward currents (239). Adverse effects of oral baclofen include sedation, excessive weakness, vertigo, and psychological disturbances. Baclofen is completely absorbed after oral administration, undergoes minimal hepatic metabolism, and is excreted mainly as the parent compound in urine and feces, with a half-life of approximately 3 to 4 hours. Intrathecal administration via an implanted infusion pump is used to control severe spasticity and pain that is not responsive to medication given by oral or other parenteral routes.

Dantrolene

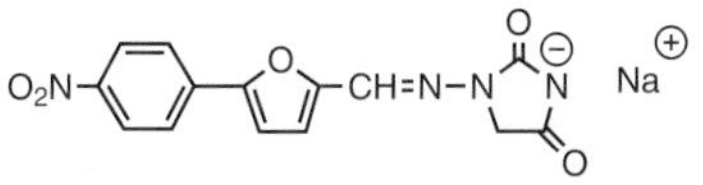

Dantrolene sodium (Dantrium)

Dantrolene is a hydantoin derivative that acts peripherally to reduce spasticity and is indicated for use in spinal cord injury, stroke, cerebral palsy, and multiple sclerosis (249). The site of action of dantrolene is believed to be at the sarcoplasmic reticulum in skeletal muscle cells. Dantrolene binds to a calcium channel protein (ryanodine receptor) on the sarcoplasmic reticulum to close the channel and inhibit the release of calcium; the alkaloid ryanodine activates the same receptor to open the channel. Dantrolene is believed to act directly on the contractile mechanism of skeletal muscle to decrease the force of contraction in the absence of any demonstrated effects on neural pathways, on the neuromuscular junction, or on the excitable properties of the muscle fiber membranes (249). Cardiac muscle and smooth muscle are minimally affected by dantrolene, likely because calcium release from sarcoplasmic reticulum of these muscle cell types occurs via a mechanism that differs from skeletal muscle. The muscle relaxant effect of dantrolene on skeletal muscle, however, is not specific, and generalized muscle weakness occurs as a major adverse side effect. Like other hydantoins, dantrolene is a weak base (pK_a = 7.5) that can cross the blood–brain barrier; thus, CNS depressant side effects (e.g., sedation) are common. Dantrolene sodium salt is slowly absorbed from the gastrointestinal tract. The mean half-life of the drug in adults is approximately 9 hours after a 100-mg dose. It is slowly metabolized by the liver to give the 5-hydroxy and acetamido (nitro reduction and acetylation) metabolites, as well as unchanged drug, excreted in the urine. Interestingly, dantrolene also is valuable in alleviating the signs of malignant hyperthermia. This rare, genetically determined condition, which can be triggered by a variety of stimuli, including inhalation anesthetics and neuromuscular blocking drugs, involves an impaired ability of the sarcoplasmic reticulum to sequester calcium. For treating malignant hyperthermia, dantrolene is administered intravenously.

Tizanidine

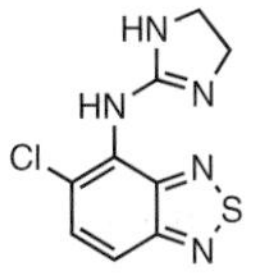

Tizanidine (Zanaflex)

Tizanidine is a centrally acting adrenergic α_2 receptor agonist used to treat chronic muscle spasticity conditions. It is the only antispastic skeletal muscle relaxant to be studied for treatment of low back pain, in which its use is primarily as an adjunctive medication with analgesics (243). Tizanidine is postulated to act presynaptically to produce α_2 receptor–mediated decreased release of the excitatory neurotransmitters glutamate and aspartate from spinal interneurons (239). Tizanidine is structurally related to the α_2-agonist clonidine that is used to treat hypertension; however, the blood pressure–lowering potency of tizanidine is approximately 10% to 20% that of clonidine. Nevertheless, patients may experience hypotension with tizanidine, together with muscle weakness, that may result in dizziness and falls in mobile patients. Tizanidine is rapidly and almost completely absorbed from the gastrointestinal tract; however, the estimated bioavailability is only 10% to 15% because of extensive first-pass metabolism, mainly by CYP1A2 (250), which results in oxidative degradation of the imidazoline ring and hydroxylation of the aromatic system (251). Elevated liver enzyme values are not frequent with tizanidine use. Hepatic injury and death because of liver failure have been reported, however, and this complication should be considered in view of its marginal antispasmodic efficacy (240,241). Other frequently reported side effects of tizanidine are drowsiness and dry mouth. Clonidine also has been used to treat spasticity, having been shown to suppress polysynaptic reflexes in vivo in lab animals (239); however, data from well-controlled clinical trials is not reported.

Botulinum Toxin-Type A Botulinum toxin was identified in 1897 by the microbiologist Emile van Ermengem, who was the first to correlate botulism food poisoning with a bacterium found in raw, salted pork and the postmortem tissue of victims who had consumed the contaminated meat; he later isolated the bacterium that was subsequently named *Clostridium botulinum* (252). There are seven immunologically distinct forms of botulinum neurotoxin, designated as serotypes A, B, C1, D, E, F, and G, all consisting of a 100-kda heavy chain and a 50-kda light chain (253). For all the serotypes, the C-terminal region of the toxin binds with high affinity to synaptic vesicle protein (SV2) receptors expressed on presynaptic acetylcholine motor nerve endings. After binding, botulinum toxin is taken up into the motor neuron via receptor-mediated endocytosis (254). Once in the cytoplasm, the light chain, a zinc-containing protease, targets synaptobrevin proteins (e.g., NSAP-25, VMAP, syntaxin) (255,256) that mediate fusion of acetylcholine-containing synaptic vesicles. The result is inhibition of acetylcholine release at the neuromuscular junction, thereby abolishing the motor end-plate potential (257) and, thus, inducing temporary muscle denervation and relaxation. The major clinical difference between the toxin serotypes is the duration of blockade of acetylcholine release. For type A botulinum toxin, clinical muscle relaxation persists for 4 to 6 months, longer than for the other serotypes. In 1989, the FDA approved type A botulinum toxin (Botox) for treatment of involuntary muscle contraction disorders. There are now several different brands of type A botulinum toxin available, and it should be noted that dosage is measured in "units" that differ for each brand (258).

Administration of botulinum toxin is by injection into target muscles that are believed responsible for the clinical muscle spasticity (258). Despite the relatively high toxicity of botulinum toxin, it has proven safe because the protein does not diffuse beyond 2 cm from the injection site (256). The clinical effect of the toxin is observed about 4 days after injection, is optimal at about 1 month, and lasts about 3 to 4 months (258). The result is a weakening and relaxation of muscle spasticity that facilitates physical stretching and lengthening of the afflicted muscles, as well as allowing for an opportunity to strengthen antagonist muscles to restore the proper balance between the two (256,258). Clinical evidence continues to accumulate that supports the safe use of botulinum toxin to reduce muscle spasticity and improve voluntary muscle movement and active function in certain patients. Injection of botulinum toxin also is used cosmetically to relax facial muscles, the contraction of which results in alteration of the form and structure of the overlying connective tissue (i.e., wrinkles).

SCENARIO: OUTCOME AND ANALYSIS

Outcome

David Hayes, PharmD

After careful consideration, the patient is started on rasagiline secondary to his early-stage PD, lack of disability, and the potential for this agent to provide some neuroprotection. He is seen in the neurology clinic 3 months after starting this treatment and reports that he has not experienced any tremor and has tolerated the medication well.

Chemical Analysis

Victoria Roche and S. William Zito

Rasagiline is an inhibitor of monoamine oxidase B (MAO-B), the enzyme responsible for the inactivating deamination of dopamine.

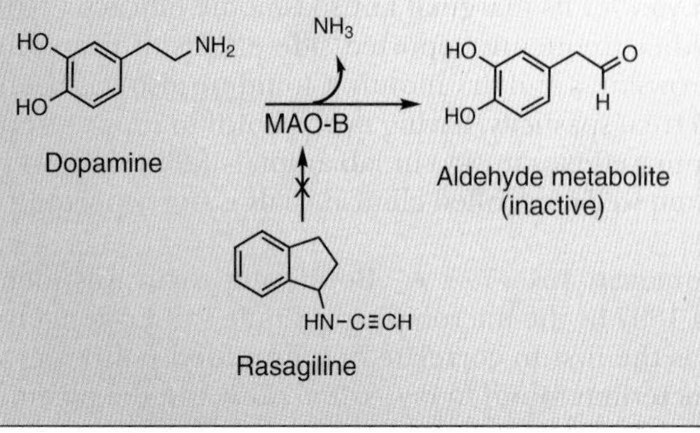

Rasagiline is vulnerable to CYP-mediated *N*-dealkylation but, as an indan-base structure, it does not produce the potent vasoconstricting amphetamine and methamphetamine metabolites that selegiline, a related phenethylamine-based MAO-B inhibitor, does. While these metabolites have some potential benefit in augmenting L-DOPA-mediated dopaminergic action in the CNS, their value may be overridden by the increase in blood pressure that patients will experience. Given that this patient was on a thiazide diuretic to lower elevated blood pressure, the amphetamine metabolites could have been highly problematic. Rasagiline would definitely be the safer MAO-B inhibitor for use in this hypertensive patient.

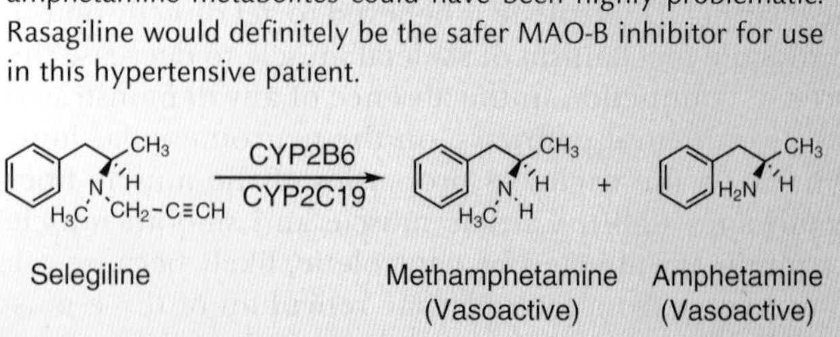

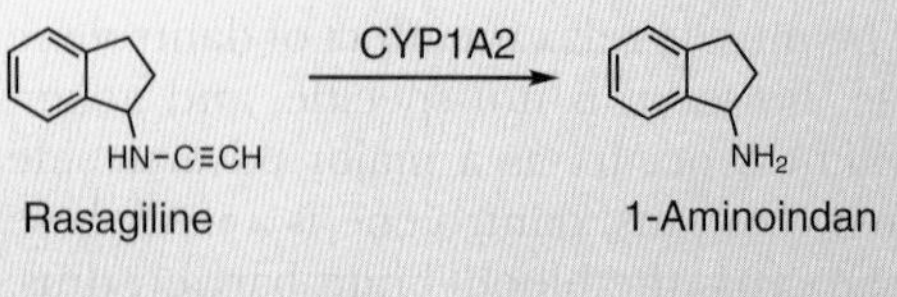

CASE STUDY

FB is a 64-year-old Cultural Studies faculty member at a prestigious university. A beloved teacher and well-respected scholar, he has spent his professional life totally engaged in his work and loving every moment of it. Nine months ago FB began to experience a slight unsteadiness when standing and walking, and these symptoms have now progressed to the point where he must use a power chair to negotiate the campus. Despite repeated attempts to pinpoint a diagnosis, his physicians are uncertain about what's causing his decline, although multiple sclerosis has not been ruled out. FB's job requires a great deal of reading, and he is currently conducting a thorough review of the literature for a new textbook he is writing. For as long as he can, he wants to stand while teaching his courses, rather than deliver his lectures from his chair.

FB has begun to experience painful muscle spasms in his lower limbs that heat and massage do not adequately control, and you are being asked for an opinion related to an appropriate therapeutic agent to relieve them. FB had a myocardial infarction 5 years ago and is currently taking the β-blocker metoprolol to keep his cardiac function and blood pressure in check. Depressive episodes related to his future prompted his physician to start him on the tricyclic antidepressant imipramine. He is continuing this therapy despite occasional dizziness and some problematic drowsiness.

Consider the three potential therapeutic choices drawn below.

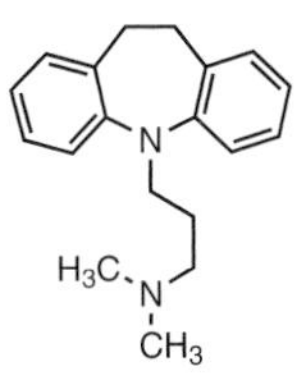

Imipramine

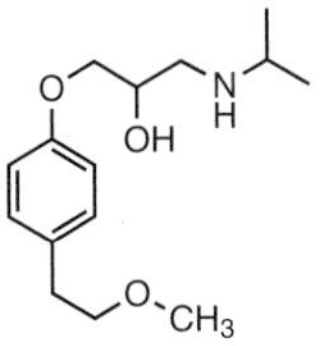

Metoprolol

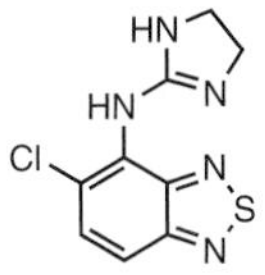

1

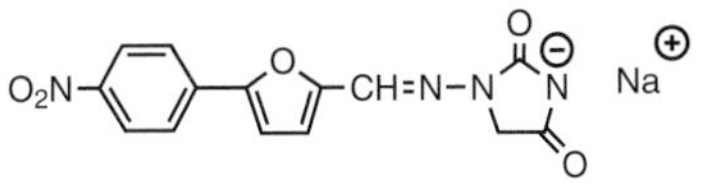

2

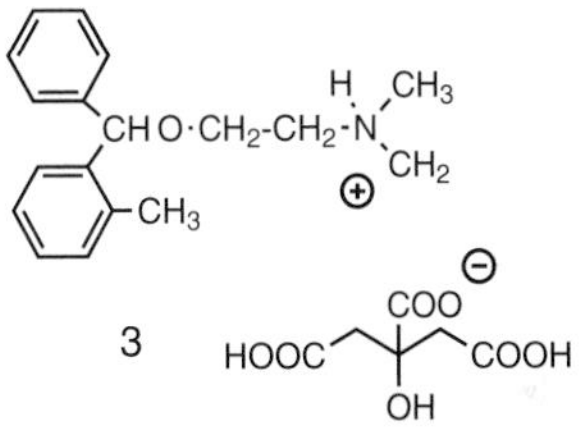

3

1. Conduct a thorough and mechanistic SAR analysis of the three therapeutic options in the case.
2. Apply the chemical understanding gained from the SAR analysis to this patient's specific needs to make a therapeutic recommendation.

References

1. Parkinson J. An Essay on the Shaking Palsy. London: Whittingham and Rowland for Sherwood, Neely and Jones, 1817.
2. Alves G, Forsaa EB, Pedersen KF, et al. Epidemiology of PD. J Neurol 2008;255(Suppl 5):18–32.
3. Olanow CW, Stern MB, Sethi K. The scientific and clinical basis for the treatment of Parkinson disease. Neurology 2009;72(21 Suppl 4):S1–S136.
4. Chen H, Zhang SM, Schwarzschild MA, et al. Survival of PD patients in a large prospective cohort of male health professionals. Mov Disord 2006;21:1002–1007.
5. Forno LS. Neuropathology of PD. J Neuropathol Exp Neurol 1996;55:259–272.
6. Baldessarini RJ, Tarazi FI. Brain DA receptors: a primer on their current status, basic and clinical. Harv Rev Psychiatry 1996;3:301–325.
7. Rosenbaum DM, Rasmussen SG, Kobilka BK. The structure and function of G-protein-coupled receptors. Nature 2009;459:356–363.
8. Rasmussen SG, Choi HJ, Rosenbaum DM, et al. Crystal structure of the human beta2 adrenergic G-protein-coupled receptor. Nature 2007;450:383–387.
9. Jaakola VP, Griffith MT, Hanson MA, et al. The 2.6 angstrom crystal structure of a human A2A adenosine receptor bound to an antagonist. Science 2008;322:1211–1217.
10. Córdova -Sintjago T, Villa N, Canal C, Booth R. Human Serotonin 5-HT2C G Protein-Coupled Receptor Homology Model from the β_2 Adrenoceptor Structure: Ligand Docking and Mutagenesis Studies, International Journal of Quantum Chemistry, in press June 2011, DOI:10.1002/qua.23231.
11. Milligan G. Mechanisms of multifunctional signaling by G protein–linked receptors. Trends Pharmacol Sci 1993;14:239–244.
12. Raymond JR. Multiple mechanisms of receptor–G protein signaling specificity. Am J Physiol 1995;269:F141–F158.
13. Kenakin T. Inverse, protean, and ligand-selective agonism: matters of receptor conformation. FASEB J 2001;15:598–611.
14. Urban JD, Clarke WP, von Zastrow M, et al. Functional selectivity and classical concepts of quantitative pharmacology. J Pharmacol Exp Ther 2007;320:1–13.
15. Parent A, Cicchetti F. The current model of basal ganglia organization under scrutiny. Mov Disord 1998;13:199–202.
16. Carlsson A, Waters N, Carlsson ML. Neurotransmitter interactions in schizophrenia: therapeutic implications. Biol Psychiatry 1999;46:1388–1395.
17. Standaert DG, Young AB. Treatment of central nervous system degenerative disorders. In Brunton LL, Lazo JS, Parker KL, eds. Goodman and Gilman's the Pharmacological Basis of Therapeutics. New York: McGraw-Hill, 2006:527–546.
18. DeLong MR, Wichmann T. Circuits and circuit disorders of the basal ganglia. Arch Neurol 2007;64:20–24.
19. Semchuk KM, Love EJ, Lee RG. PD: a test of the multifactorial etiologic hypothesis. *Neurology* 1993;43:1173–1180.
20. Gwinn-Hardy K. Genetics of parkinsonism. Mov Disord 2002;17:645–656.
21. Polymeropoulos MH, Lavedan C, Leroy E, et al. Mutation in the α-synuclein gene identified in families with PD. Science 1997;276:2045–2047.
22. Kruger R, Kuhn W, Muller T, et al. Ala30Pro mutation in the gene encoding α-synuclein in PD. Nat Genet 1998;18:106–108.
23. Norris EH, Giasson BI, Lee VM. α-Synuclein: normal function and role in neurodegenerative diseases. Curr Top Dev Biol 2004;60:17–54.
24. Liu D, Jin L, Wang H, et al. Silencing alpha-synuclein gene expression enhances tyrosine hydroxylase activity in MN9D cells. Neurochem Res 2008;33:1401–1409.
25. Gasser T, Muller-Myhsok B, Wszolek ZK, et al. Genetic complexity and PD. Science 1997;277:388–389.
26. Scott WK, Staijich JM, Yamaoka LH, et al. Genetic complexity and PD. Deane Laboratory Parkinson Disease Research Group. Science 1997;277:387–388.
27. Ward CD, Duvoisin RC, Ince SE, et al. PD in 65 pairs of twins and in a set of quadruplets. Neurology 1983;33:815–824.
28. Wirdefeldt K, Gatz M, Schalling M, et al. No evidence for heritability of Parkinson disease in Swedish twins. Neurology 2004;63:305–311.
29. Jain S, Wood NW, Healy DG. Molecular genetic pathways in PD: a review. Clin Sci (Lond) 2005;109:355–364.
30. McNaught KS, Olanow CW. Protein aggregation in the pathogenesis of familial and sporadic PD. Neurobiol Aging 2006;27:530–545.

31. Dodson MW, Guo M. Pink1, Parkin, DJ-1 and mitochondrial dysfunction in PD. Curr Opin Neurobiol 2007;17:331–337.
32. Ciechanover A, Brundin P. The ubiquitin–proteasome system in neurodegenerative diseases. Sometimes the chicken, sometimes the egg. Neuron 2003;40:427–446.
33. Goldberg AL. Protein degradation and protection against misfolded or damaged proteins. Nature 2003;426:895–899.,
34. Narendra D, Tanaka A, Suen DF, et al. Parkin is recruited selectively to impaired mitochondria and promotes their autophagy. J Cell Biol 2008;183:795–803.
35. Clark IE, Dodson MW, Jiang C, et al. Drosophila pink1 is required for mitochondrial function and interacts genetically with parkin. Nature 2006;441:1162–1166.
36. Park J, Lee SB, Lee S, et al. Mitochondrial dysfunction in Drosophila PINK1 mutants is complemented by parkin. Nature 2006;441:1157–1161.
37. Biskup S, Mueller JC, Sharma M, et al. Common variants of LRRK2 are not associated with sporadic PD. Ann Neurol 2005;58:905–908.
38. Gasser T. Genetics of PD. Curr Opin Neurol 2005;18:363–369.
39. Baba M, Nakajo S, Tu PH, et al. Aggregation of α-synuclein in Lewy bodies of sporadic PD and dementia with Lewy bodies. Am J Pathol 1998;152:879–884.
40. Duvoisin RC. The cause of PD. In: Marsden CD, Fahn S, eds. Movement Disorders. London: Butterworth Scientific, 1982:8–24.
41. Gajdusek DC, Salazar AM. Amyotrophic lateral sclerosis and parkinsonian syndromes in high incidence among the Auyu and Jakai people of West New Guinea. Neurology 1982;32:107–126.
42. Sian J, Dexter DT, Lees AJ, et al. Alterations in glutathione levels in PD and other neurodegenerative disorders affecting basal ganglia. Ann Neurol 1994;36:348–355.
43. Dexter DT, Holley AE, Flitter WD, et al. Increased levels of lipid hydroperoxides in the parkinsonian substantia nigra: an HPLC and ESR study. Mov Disord 1994;9:92–97.
44. Alam ZI, Jenner A, Daniel SE, et al. Oxidative DNA damage in the parkinsonian brain: an apparent selective increase in 8-hydroxyguanine levels in substantia nigra. J Neurochem 1997;69:1196–1203.
45. Alam ZI, Daniel SE, Lees AJ, et al. A generalised increase in protein carbonyls in the brain in Parkinson's but not incidental Lewy body disease. J Neurochem 1997;69:1326–1329.
46. Langston JW, Irwin I, Ricaurte GA. Neurotoxins, parkinsonism, and PD. Pharmacol Ther 1987;32:19–49.
47. Soloway AH. Potential endogenous epoxides of steroid hormones: initiators of breast and other malignancies? Med Hypoth 2007;69:1225–1229.
48. Soloway AH. Potential endogenous epoxides of tyrosine: causative agents in initiating idiopathic Parkinson's disease? Med Hypotheses Res 2009;5:19–26.
49. Chinta SJ, Andersen JK. Redox imbalance in Parkinson's disease. Biochim Biophys Acta 2008;1780:1362–1367.
50. Graham DG, Tiffany SM, Bell WR Jr, et al. Autoxidation versus covalent binding of quinones as the mechanism of toxicity of dopamine, 6-hydroxydopamine, and related compounds toward C1300 neuroblastoma cells in vitro. Mol Pharmacol 1978;14:644–653.
51. Graham DG. Catecholamine toxicity: a proposal for the molecular pathogenesis of manganese neurotoxicity and Parkinson's disease. Neurotoxicology 1984;5:83–95.
52. Boyd DR, Hamilton JTG, Sharma ND, et al. Isolation of a stable benzene oxide from a fungal biotransformation and evidence for an 'NIH shift' of the carbomethoxy group during hydroxylation of methyl benzoates. Chem Commun 2000;1481–1482.
53. Menberu D, Nguyen PV, Onan KD, et al. Convenient syntheses of stereoisomeric 1,2-epoxyestr-4-en-3-ones, putative intermediates in estradiol metabolism. J Org Chem 1992;57:2065–2072.
54. Jenner P. Oxidative stress in PD. Ann Neurol 2003;53(Suppl 3):S26–S36.
55. Cotzias GC. Manganese in health and disease. Physiol Rev 1958;38:503–532.
56. Haber F, Weiss J. The catalysis of hydrogen peroxide. Naturwissenschaften 1932;20:948–950.
57. Beal MF. Mitochondria take center stage in aging and neurodegeneration. Ann Neurol 2005;58:495–505.
58. Shankar JC, Andersen JK. Redox imbalance in PD. Biochim Biophys Acta 2008;1780:1362–1367.
59. Mizuno Y, Ohta S, Tanaka M, et al. Deficiencies in complex I subunits of the respiratory chain in PD. Biochem Biophys Res Commun 1989;163:1450–1455.
60. Mann VM, Cooper JM, Krige D, et al. Brain, skeletal muscle and platelet homogenate mitochondrial function in PD. Brain. 1992;115(Pt 2):333–342.
61. Dauer W, Przedborski S. PD: mechanisms and models. Neuron 2003; 39:889–909.
62. Knoll J. Deprenyl (selegiline): the history of its development and pharmacological action. Acta Neurol Scand Suppl 1983;95:57–80.
63. Seeman P, Bzowej NH, Guan HC, et al. Human brain DA receptors in children and aging adults. Synapse 1987;1:399–404.
64. Luo Y, Roth GS. The roles of DA oxidative stress and DA receptor signaling in aging and age-related neurodegeneration. Antioxid Redox Signal 2000;2:449–460.
65. Riederer P, Woketich S. Time course of nigrostriatal degeneration in PD. A detailed study of influential factors in human brain amine analysis. J Neural Transm 1976;38:277–301.
66. Calne DB. PD is not one disease. Parkinsonism Rel Disord 2000;7:3–7.
67. Barbeau A, Roy M, Bernier G, et al. Ecogenetics of Parkinson's disease: prevalence and environmental aspects in rural areas. Can J Neurol Sci 1987;14:36–41.
68. Cicchetti F, Drouin-Ouellet J, Gross RE. Environmental toxins and Parkinson's disease: what have we learned from pesticide-induced animal models? Trends Pharmacol Sci 2009;30:475–483.
69. Miller GW. Paraquat: the red herring of Parkinson's disease research. Toxicol Sci 2007;100:1–2.
70. Hatcher JM, Pennell KD, Miller GW. Parkinson's disease and pesticides: a toxicological perspective. Trends Pharmacol Sci 2008;29:322–329.
71. Brooks AI, Chadwick CA, Gelbard HA, et al. Paraquat elicited neurobehavioral syndrome caused by dopaminergic neuron loss. Brain Res 1999;823:1–10.
72. Naylor JL, Widdowson PS, Simpson MG, et al. Further evidence that the blood/brain barrier impedes paraquat entry into the brain. Hum Exp Toxicol 1995;14:587–594.
73. Betarbet R, Sherer TB, MacKenzie G, et al. Chronic systemic pesticide exposure reproduces features of Parkinson's disease. Nat Neurosci 2000;3:1301–1306.
74. Kessler II, Diamond EL. Epidemiologic studies of PD. I. Smoking and PD: a survey and explanatory hypothesis. Am J Epidemiol 1971;94:16–25.
75. Tanner CM, Goldman SM, Aston DA, et al. Smoking and PD in twins. Neurology 2002;58:581–588.
76. Yu PH, Boulton AA. Irreversible inhibition of monoamine oxidase by some components of cigarette smoke. Life Sci 1987;41:675–682.
77. Khalil AA, Davies B, Castagnoli N Jr. Isolation and characterisation of a monoamine oxidase B selective inhibitor from tobacco smoke. Bioorg Med Chem 2006;14:3392–3398.
78. Chapman MA. Does smoking reduce the risk of PD through stimulation of the ubiquitin-proteasome system? Med Hypotheses 2009;73:887–891.
79. Hernan MA, Takkouche B, Caamano-Isorna F, et al. A meta-analysis of coffee drinking, cigarette smoking, and the risk of Parkinson's disease. Ann Neurol 2002;52:276–284.
80. Trevitt J, Kawa K, Jalali A, et al. Differential effects of adenosine antagonists in two models of parkinsonian tremor. Pharmacol Biochem Behav 2009;94:24–29.
81. Chase TN, Bibbiani F, Bara-Jimenez W, et al. Translating A2A antagonist KW6002 from animal models to parkinsonian patients. Neurology 2003;61 (11 Suppl 6):S107–S111.
82. Petzer JP, Castagnoli N Jr, Schwarzschild MA, et al. Dual-target-directed drugs that block monoamine oxidase B and adenosine A(2A) receptors for Parkinson's disease. Neurotherapeutics 2009;6:141–151.
83. Lai BC, Marion SA, Teschke K, et al. Occupational and environmental risk factors for Parkinson's disease. Parkinsonism Relat Disord 2002;8:297–309.
84. Tanner CM, Langston JW. Do environmental toxins cause Parkinson's disease? A critical review. Neurology 1990;40(Suppl 3):17–30.
85. Davis GC, Williams AC, Markey SP, et al. Chronic parkinsonism secondary to intravenous injection of meperidine analogues. Psychiatr Res 1979;1:249–254.
86. Langston JW, Ballard P, Tetrud JW, et al. Chronic parkinsonism in humans due to a product of meperidine-analog synthesis. Science 1983;219:979–980.
87. Burns RS, Chiueh CC, Markey SP, et al. A primate model of parkinsonism: selective destruction of dopaminergic neurons in the pars compacta of the substantia nigra by N-methyl-4-phenyl-1,2,3,6-tetrahydropyridine. Proc Natl Acad Sci U S A 1983;80:4546–4550.
88. Chiba K, Trevor A, Castagnoli N Jr. Metabolism of the neurotoxic tertiary amine, MPTP, by brain monoamine oxidase. Biochem Biophys Res Commun 1984;120:574–578.
89. Salach JI, Singer TP, Castagnoli N Jr, et al. Oxidation of the neurotoxic amine 1-methyl-4-phenyl-1,2,3,6-tetrahydropyridine (MPTP) by monoamine oxidases A and B and suicide inactivation of the enzymes by MPTP. Biochem Biophys Res Commun 1984;125:831–835.
90. Peterson LA, Caldera PS, Trevor A, et al. Studies on the 1-methyl-4-phenyl-2,3-dihydropyridinium species 2,3-MPDP$^+$, the monoamine oxidase catalyzed oxidation product of the nigrostriatal toxin 1-methyl-4-phenyl-1,2,3,6-tetrahydropyridine (MPTP). J Med Chem 1985;28:1432–1436.
91. Langston JW, Irwin I, Langston EB, et al. Pargyline prevents MPTP-induced parkinsonism in primates. Science 1984;225:1480–1482.
92. Snyder SH, D'Amato RJ. MPTP: a neurotoxin relevant to the pathophysiology of PD. The 1985 George C. Cotzias Lecture. Neurology 1986;36:250–258.
93. Yong VW, Perry TL. Monoamine oxidase B, smoking, and PD. J Neurol Sci 1986;72:265–272.
94. Behmand RA, Harik SI. Nicotine enhances 1-methyl-4-phenyl-1,2,36-tetrahydropyridine neurotoxicity. J Neurochem 1992;58:776–779.
95. Shahi GS, Das PN, Moochhala SM. 1-Methyl-4-phenyl-1,2,36-tetrahydropyridine-induced neurotoxicity: partial protection against striatonigral DA depletion in C57BL/6J mice by cigarette smoke exposure and by β-naphthoflavone-pretreatment. Neurosci Lett 1991;127:247–250.
96. Berry MD, Juorio AV, Paterson IA. The functional role of monoamine oxidases A and B in the mammalian central nervous system. Prog Neurobiol 1994;42:375–391.
97. Javitch JA, D'Amato RJ, Strittmatter SM, et al. Parkinsonism-inducing neurotoxin, N-methyl-4-phenyl-1,2,3,6-tetrahydropyridine: uptake of the metabolite N-methyl-4-phenylpyridine by DA neurons explains selective toxicity. Proc Natl Acad Sci U S A 1985;82:2173–2177.

98. Vyas I, Heikkila RE, Nicklas WJ. Studies on the neurotoxicity of 1-methyl-4-phenyl-1,2,3,6-tetrahydropyridine: inhibition of NAD-linked substrate oxidation by its metabolite, 1-methyl-4-phenylpyridinium. J Neurochem 1986;46:1501–1507.
99. Ramsay RR, McKeown KA, Johnson EA, et al. Inhibition of NADH oxidation by pyridine derivatives. Biochem Biophys Res Commun 1987;146:53–60.
100. Castagnoli N Jr, Rimoldi JM, Bloomquist J, et al. Potential metabolic bioactivation pathways involving cyclic tertiary amines and aza-arenes. Chem Res Toxicol 1997;10:924–940.
101. Watanabe H, Muramatsu Y, Kurosaki R et al. Protective effects of neuronal nitric oxide synthase inhibitor in mouse brain against MPTP neurotoxicity: an immunohistological study. Eur Neuropsychopharmacol 2004;14:93–104.
102. Schapira AH, Mann VM, Cooper JM, et al. Mitochondrial function in PD. The Royal Kings and Queens PD Research Group. Ann Neurol 1992;32:S116–S124.
103. Mann VM, Cooper JM, Krige D, et al. Brain, skeletal muscle, and platelet homogenate mitochondrial function in PD. Brain 1992;115:33–42.
104. The Parkinson's Disease Study Group. Impact of tocopherol and deprenyl in DATATOP subjects not requiring levodopa. Ann Neurol 1996;39:29–36.
105. The Parkinson's Disease Study Group. Impact of tocopherol and deprenyl in DATATOP subjects requiring levodopa. Ann Neurol 1996;39:37–45.
106. Macleod AD, Counsell CE, Ives N, et al. Monoamine oxidase B inhibitors for early PD. Cochrane Database Syst Rev 2005;3:CD004898.
107. Rajput AH, Uitti RJ, Offord KO. Timely levodopa administration prolongs survival in PD. Parkinsonism Relat Disord 1997;3:159–165.
108. Ehringer H, Hornykiewicz O. [Distribution of noradrenaline and dopamine (3-hydroxytyramine) in the human brain and their behavior in diseases of the extrapyramidal system.]. Klin Wochenschr 1960;38:1236–1239.
109. Birkmayer W, Hornykiewicz O. [The L-3,4-dioxyphenylalanine (DOPA)-effect in Parkinson-akinesia.] Wien Klin Wochenschr 1961;73:787–788.
110. Barbeau A. Biochemistry of Parkinson's disease. Proceedings of the Seventh International Congress of Neurology 1961;2:925.
111. Barbeau A. L-DOPA therapy in Parkinson's disease: a critical review of nine years' experience. Can Med Assoc J 1969;101:59–68.
112. Cotzias GC, Papavasiliou PS, Gellene R. Modification of Parkinsonism—chronic treatment with L-DOPA. N Engl J Med 1969;280:337–345.
113. Carlsson A. Treatment of Parkinson's disease with L-DOPA. The early discovery phase, and a comment on current problems. J Neural Transm 2002;109:777–787.
114. Nagatssu T. Biochemistry of Catecholamines. Baltimore: University Park Press, 1973:289–651.
115. Chalmers JP, Baldessarini RJ, Wurtman RJ. Effects of L-DOPA on norepinephrine metabolism in the brain. Proc Natl Acad Sci U S A 1971;68:662–666.
116. Baldessarini RJ, Fischer JE. Substitute and alternative neurotransmitters in neuropsychiatric illness. Arch Gen Psychiatry 1977;34:958–964.
117. Vogel WH. Determination and physiological disposition of p-methoxyphenylethylamine in the rat. Biochem Pharmacol 1970;19:2663–2665.
118. Burkard WP, Gey KF, Pletscher A. Inhibition of decarboxylase of aromatic amino acids by 2,3,4-trihydroxybenzylhydrazine and its seryl derivative. Arch Biochem Biophys 1964;107:187–196.
119. Baldessarini RJ, Fischer JE. Substitute and alternative neurotransmitters in neuropsychiatric illness. Arch Gen Psychiatry 1977;34:958–964.
120. Miyawaki E, Lyons K, Pahwa R. Motor complications of chronic levodopa therapy in PD. Clin Neuropharmacol 1997;20:523–530.
121. Tarsy D, Baldessarini RJ, Tarazi FI. Effects of newer antipsychotics on extrapyramidal function. CNS Drugs 2002;16:23–45.
122. Diederich NJ, Fénelon G, Stebbins G, et al. Hallucinations in Parkinson disease. Nat Rev Neurol 2009;5:331–342.
123. Friedman JH, Berman RM, Goetz CG, et al. Open-label flexible-dose pilot study to evaluate the safety and tolerability of aripiprazole in patients with psychosis associated with Parkinson's disease. Mov Disord 2006;21:2078–2081.
124. Zahodne LB, Fernandez HH. Pathophysiology and treatment of psychosis in Parkinson's disease: a review. Drugs Aging 2008;25:665–682.
125. Parkinson Study Group. Pramipexole vs. levodopa as initial treatment for PD: a randomized, controlled trial. JAMA 2000;284:1931–1938.
126. Rascol O, Brooks DJ, Korczyn AD, et al. A five-year study of the incidence of dyskinesia in patients with early PD who were treated with ropinirole or levodopa. 056 Study Group. N Engl J Med 2000;342:1484–1491.
127. Baldessarini RJ, Arana GW, Kula NS, et al. Apomorphine and Other Dopaminomimetics, Basic Pharmacology, Vol. I. New York: Raven Press, 1981:219–228.
128. Neumeyer JL, Baldessarini RJ. Apomorphine: new uses for an old drug. Pharmaceutical News 1997;4:12–16.
129. Giesecke J. The absolute configuration of apomorphine. Acta Cryst 1977;B33:302–303.
130. Neumeyer JL, McCarthy M, Battista S, et al. Aporphines. 9. The synthesis and pharmacological evaluations of (±)-9,10-dihyroxyaporphine, ([±]-isoapomorphine), (±)-, (−)-, and (+)-1,2-dihydroxyaporphine, and (+)-1,2,9,10-tetrahydroxyaprophine. J Med Chem 1973;16:1228–1233.
131. Westerink BHC, Dijkstra D, Feenstra MG, et al. Dopaminergic pro-drugs: brain concentrations and neurochemical effects of 5,6- and 6,7-ADTN after administration as dibenzoyl esters. Eur J Pharmacol 1980;61:7–15.
132. Fu W, Shen J, Luo X, et al. Dopamine D1 receptor agonist and D2 receptor antagonist effects of the natural product (-)-stepholidine: molecular modeling and dynamics simulations. Biophys J 2007;93:1431–1441.
133. Mansour A, Meng F, Meador-Woodruff JH, et al. Site-directed mutagenesis of the human dopamine D2 receptor. Eur J Pharmacol 1992;227:205–214.
134. Wilcox RE, Tseng T, Brusniak MY, et al. CoMFA-based prediction of agonist affinities at recombinant D_1 vs D_2 DA receptors. J Med Chem 1998;41:4385–4399.
135. Stibe CM, Lees AJ, Kempster PA, Stern GM. Subcutaneous apomorphine in parkinsonian on-off oscillations. Lancet 1988;1:403–406
136. Schwab RS, Amador LV, Lettvin JY. Apomorphine in Parkinson's disease. Trans Am Neurol Assoc 1951;56:251–253.
137. Colosimo C, Merello M, Albanese A. Clinical usefulness of apomorphine in movement disorders. Clin Neuropharmacol 1994;17:243–259.
138. Stocchi F. Use of apomorphine in Parkinson's disease. Neurol Sci 2008;(29 Suppl 5):S383–S386.
139. Frankel JP, Lees AJ, Kempster PA, et al. Subcutaneous apomorphine in the treatment of Parkinson's disease. J Neurol Neurosurg Psychiatry 1990;53:96–101.
140. Hughes AJ, Bishop S, Kleedorfer B, et al. Subcutaneous apomorphine in Parkinson's disease: response to chronic administration for up to five years. Mov Disord 1993;8:165–170.
141. Newman-Tancredi A, Cussac D, Audinot V, et al. Differential actions of antiparkinson agents at multiple classes of monoaminergic receptor. II. Agonist and antagonist properties at subtypes of dopamine D(2)-like receptor and alpha(1)/alpha(2)-adrenoceptor. J Pharmacol Exp Ther 2002;303:805–814.
142. Millan MJ, Maiofiss L, Cussac D, et al. Differential actions of antiparkinson agents at multiple classes of monoaminergic receptor. I. A multivariate analysis of the binding profiles of 14 drugs at 21 native and cloned human receptor subtypes. J Pharmacol Exp Ther 2002;303:791–804.
143. Blanchet PJ. Rationale for use of dopamine agonists in Parkinson's disease: review of ergot derivatives. Can J Neurol Sci 1999;26(Suppl 2):S21–S26.
144. Baldessarini RJ, Tarsy D. Dopamine and the pathophysiology of dyskinesias induced by antipsychotic drugs. Annu Rev Neurosci 1980;3:23–41.
145. Brandstädter D, Oertel WH. Treatment of drug-induced psychosis with quetiapine and clozapine in Parkinson's disease. Neurology 2002;58:160–161.
146. Hutton JT, Morris JL, Brewer MA. Controlled study of the antiparkinsonianian activity and tolerability of cabergoline. Neurology 1993;43:613–616.
147. Stocchi F, Ruggieri S, Vacca L, et al. Prospective randomized trial of lisuride infusion versus oral levodopa in patients with Parkinson's disease. Brain 2002;125(Pt 9):2058–2066.
148. Rascol O, Brooks DJ, Korczyn AD, et al. A five-year study of the incidence of dyskinesia in patients with early Parkinson's disease who were treated with ropinirole or levodopa. 056 Study Group. N Engl J Med 2000;342:1484–1491.
149. Horvath J, Fross RD, Kleiner-Fisman G, et al. Severe multivalvular heart disease: a new complication of the ergot derivative dopamine agonists. Mov Disord 2004;19:656–662.
150. Roth BL. Drugs and valvular heart disease. N Engl J Med 2007;356:6–9.
151. Rothman RB, Baumann MH, Savage JE, et al. Evidence for possible involvement of 5-HT(2B) receptors in the cardiac valvulopathy associated with fenfluramine and other serotonergic medications. Circulation 2000;102:2836–2841.
152. Setola V, Hufeisen SJ, Grande-Allen KJ, et al. 3,4-Methylenedioxymethamphetamine (MDMA, "ecstasy") induces fenfluramine-like proliferative actions on human cardiac valvular interstitial cells in vitro. Mol Pharmacol 2003;63:1223–1229.
153. Colao A, Galderisi M, Di Sarno A, et al. Increased prevalence of tricuspid regurgitation in patients with prolactinomas chronically treated with cabergoline. J Clin Endocrinol Metab 2008;93:3777–3784.
154. Wakil A, Rigby AS, Clark AL, et al. Low dose cabergoline for hyperprolactinaemia is not associated with clinically significant valvular heart disease. Eur J Endocrinol 2008;159:R11–R14.
155. Vallette S, Serri K, Rivera J, et al. Long-term cabergoline therapy is not associated with valvular heart disease in patients with prolactinomas. Pituitary 2009;12:153–157.
156. Hofmann C, Penner U, Dorow R, et al. Lisuride, a dopamine receptor agonist with 5-HT2B receptor antagonist properties: absence of cardiac valvulopathy adverse drug reaction reports supports the concept of a crucial role for 5-HT2B receptor agonism in cardiac valvular fibrosis. Clin Neuropharmacol 2006;29:80–86.
157. Berger M, Gray JA, Roth BL. The expanded biology of serotonin. Annu Rev Med 2009;60:355–66.
158. Hutton JT, Metman LV, Chase TN, et al. Transdermal dopaminergic D(2) receptor agonist therapy in Parkinson's disease with N-0923 TDS: a double-blind, placebo-controlled study. Mov Disord 2001;16:459–463.
159. Morgan JC, Sethi KD. Rotigotine for the treatment of Parkinson's disease. Expert Rev Neurother 2006;6:1275–1282.
160. LeWitt PA, Lyons KE, Pahwa R; SP 650 Study Group. Advanced Parkinson disease treated with rotigotine transdermal system: PREFER study. Neurology 2007;68:1262–1267.
161. Poewe WH, Rascol O, Quinn N, et al. Efficacy of pramipexole and transdermal rotigotine in advanced Parkinson's disease: a double-blind, double-dummy, randomized controlled trial. Lancet Neurol 2007;6:513–520.

162. Watts RL, Jankovic J, Waters C, et al. Randomized, blind, controlled trial of transdermal rotigotine in early Parkinson disease. Neurology 2007;68:272–276.
163. Braun A, Fabbrini G, Mouradian MM, et al. Selective D-1 dopamine receptor agonist treatment of Parkinson's disease. J Neural Transm 1987;68:41–50.
164. Emre M, Rinne UK, Rascol A, et al. Effects of a selective partial D1 agonist, CY 208-243, in de novo patients with Parkinson disease. Mov Disord 1992;7:239–243.
165. Neumeyer JL, Baindur N, Niznik HB, et al. (+/-)-3-Allyl-6-bromo-7,8-dihydroxy-1-phenyl-2,3,4,5-tetrahydro-1H-3- benzazepin, a new high-affinity D1 dopamine receptor ligand: synthesis and structure-activity relationship. J Med Chem 1991;34:3366–3371.
166. Neumeyer JL, Kula NS, Baldessarini RJ, et al. Stereoisomeric probes for the D1 dopamine receptor: synthesis and characterization of R-(+) and S-(-) enantiomers of 3-allyl-7,8-dihydroxy-1-phenyl-2,3,4,5-tetrahydro-1H-3-benzazepine and its 6-bromo analogue. J Med Chem 1992;35:1466–1471.
167. Kuno S. Differential therapeutic effects of dopamine D1 and D2 agonists in MPTP-induced parkinsonian monkeys: clinical implications. Eur Neurol 1997;38(Suppl 1):18–22.
168. Grondin R, Bédard PJ, Britton DR, et al. Potential therapeutic use of the selective dopamine D1 receptor agonist, A-86929: an acute study in parkinsonian levodopa-primed monkeys. Neurology 1997;49:421–426.
169. Andringa G, Lubbers L, Drukarch B, et al. The predictive validity of the drug-naive bilaterally MPTP-treated monkey as a model of Parkinson's disease: effects of L-DOPA and the D1 agonist SKF 82958. Behav Pharmacol 1999;10:175–182.
170. Goulet M, Madras BK. D(1) dopamine receptor agonists are more effective in alleviating advanced than mild parkinsonism in 1-methyl-4-phenyl-1,2,3, 6-tetrahydropyridine-treated monkeys. J Pharmacol Exp Ther 2000;292:714–724.
171. Brewster WK, Nichols DE, Riggs RM, et al. Trans-10,11-dihydroxy-5,6,6a,7,8,12b-hexahydrobenzo[a]phenanthridine: a highly potent selective dopamine D1 full agonist. J Med Chem 1990;33:1756–1764.
172. Lovenberg TW, Brewster WK, Mottola DM, et al. Dihydrexidine, a novel selective high potency full dopamine D-1 receptor agonist. Eur J Pharmacol 1989;166:111–113.
173. Taylor JR, Lawrence MS, Redmond DE Jr, et al. Dihydrexidine, a full dopamine D1 agonist, reduces MPTP-induced parkinsonism in monkeys. Eur J Pharmacol 1991;199:389–391.
174. Blanchet PJ, Fang J, Gillespie M, et al. Effects of the full dopamine D1 receptor agonist dihydrexidine in Parkinson's disease. Clin Neuropharmacol 1998;21:339–343.
175. Mottola DM, Laiter S, Watts VJ, et al. Conformational analysis of D1 dopamine receptor agonists: pharmacophore assessment and receptor mapping. J Med Chem 1996;39:285–296.
176. Ghosh D, Snyder SE, Watts VJ, et al. 9-Dihydroxy-2,3,7,11b-tetrahydro-1H-naph[1,2,3-de]isoquinoline: a potent full dopamine D1 agonist containing a rigid-beta-phenyldopamine pharmacophore. J Med Chem 1996;39:549–555.
177. Asin KE, Domino EF, Nikkel A, et al. The selective dopamine D1 receptor agonist A-86929 maintains efficacy with repeated treatment in rodent and primate models of Parkinson's disease. J Pharmacol Exp Ther 1997;281:454–459.
178. Rascol O, Nutt JG, Blin O, et al. Induction by dopamine D1 receptor agonist ABT-431 of dyskinesia similar to levodopa in patients with Parkinson disease. Arch Neurol 2001;58:249–254.
179. Kebabian JW, Britton DR, DeNinno MP, et al. A-77636: a potent and selective dopamine D1 receptor agonist with antiparkinsonian activity in marmosets. Eur J Pharmacol 1992;229:203–209.
180. Lin CW, Bianchi BR, Miller TR, et al. Persistent activation of the dopamine D1 receptor contributes to prolonged receptor desensitization: studies with A-77636. J Pharmacol Exp Ther 1996;276:1022–1029.
181. Cueva JP, Giorgioni G, Grubbs RA, et al. Trans-2,3-dihydroxy-6a,7,8,12b-tetrahydro-6H-chromeno[3,4-c]isoquinoline: synthesis, resolution, and preliminary pharmacological characterization of a new dopamine D1 receptor full agonist. J Med Chem 2006;49:6848–6857.
182. Saura J, Bleuel Z, Ulrich J, et al. Molecular neuroanatomy of human monoamine oxidases A and B revealed by quantitative enzyme radioautography and in situ hybridization histochemistry. Neuroscience 1996;70:755–774.
183. Edmondson DE, Binda C, Wang J, et al. Molecular and mechanistic properties of the membrane-bound mitochondrial monoamine oxidases. Biochemistry 2009;48:4220–4230.
185. Youdim MBH, Edmondson D, Tipton KF. The therapeutic potential of monoamine oxidase inhibitors. Nat Rev 2006;7:295–309.
186. Fowler JS, Logan J, Volkow ND, et al. Monoamine oxidase: radiotracer development and human studies. Methods 2002;27:263–277.
186. Mallajosyula JK, Kaur D, Chinta SJ, et al. MAO B elevation in mouse brain astrocytes results in Parkinson's pathology. PloS One 2008;3:e1616.
187. Burke WJ, Kumar VB, Pandey N, et al. Aggregation of R-synuclein by DOPAL, the monoamine oxidase metabolite of dopamine. Acta Neuropathol 2008;115:193–203.
188. Baldessarini RJ. Drug therapy of depression and anxiety disorders. Pharmacotherapy of psychosis and mania. In: Brunton LL, Lazo JS, Parker KL, eds. Goodman and Gilman's the Pharmacological Basis of Therapeutics. New York: McGraw-Hill, 2006:429–460.
189. Glezer S, Finberg JP. Pharmacological comparison between the actions of methamphetamine and 1-aminoindan stereoisomers on sympathetic nervous function in rat vas deferens. Eur J Pharmacol 2003;472:173–177.
190. Olanow CW, Hauser RA, Jankovic J, et al. A randomized, double-blind, placebo-controlled, delayed start study to assess rasagiline as a disease modifying therapy in Parkinson's disease (the ADAGIO study): rationale, design, and baseline characteristics. Mov Disord 2008;23:2194–2201.
191. Stocchi F, Arnold G, Onofrj M, et al. Improvement of motor function in early Parkinson disease by safinamide. Neurology 2004;63:746–748.
192. Caccia C, Maj R, Calabresi M, et al. Safinamide: from molecular targets to a new anti-Parkinson drug. Neurology 2006;67(7 Suppl 2):S18–S23.
193. Factor SA, Molho ES, Feustel PJ, et al. Long-term comparative experience with tolcapone and entacapone in advanced Parkinson's disease. Clin Neuropharmacol 2001;24:295–299.
194. Teräväinen H, Rinne U, Gordin A. Catechol-O-methyltransferase inhibitors in Parkinson's disease. Adv Neurol 2001;86:311–325.
195. Lautala P, Ulmanen I, Taskinen J. Molecular mechanisms controlling the rate and specificity of catechol O-methylation by human soluble catechol O-methyltransferase. Mol Pharmacol 2001;59:393–402.
196. Gordin A, Kaakkola S, Teravainen H. Clinical advantages of COMT inhibition with entacapone—a review. J Neural Transm 2004;111:1343–1363.
197. Olanow CW, Watkins PB. Tolcapone: an efficacy and safety review. Clin Neuropharmacol 2007;3:287–294.
198. Korlipara LV, Cooper JM, Schapira AH. Differences in toxicity of the catechol-O-methyl transferase inhibitors, tolcapone and entacapone, to cultured human neuroblastoma cells. Neuropharmacology 2004;46:562–569.
199. Haasio K, Nissinen E, Sopanen L, et al. Different toxicological profile of two COMT inhibitors in vivo: the role of uncoupling effects. J Neural Transm 2002;109:1391–1401.
200. Tafazoli S, Spehar DD, O'Brien PJ. Oxidative stress mediated idiosyncratic drug toxicity. Drug Metab Rev 2005;37:311–332.
201. Kurth MC, Adler CH, St. Hilaire MS, et al. Tolcapone improves motor function and reduces levodopa requirement in patients with PD experiencing motor fluctuations: a multicenter, double-blind, randomized, placebo-controlled trial. Neurology 1997;48:81–87.
202. Gardoni F, Di Luca M. New targets for pharmacological intervention in the glutamatergic synapse. Eur J Pharmacol 2006;545:2–10.
203. Merello M, Nouzeilles MI, Cammarota A, et al. Effect of memantine (NMDA antagonist) on Parkinson's disease: a double-blind crossover randomized study. Clin Neuropharmacol 1999;22:273–276.
204. Paci C, Thomas A, Onofrj M. Amantadine for dyskinesia in patients affected by severe Parkinson's disease. Neurol Sci 2001;22:75–76.
205. Moryl E, Danysz W, Quack G. Potential antidepressive properties of amantadine, memantine and bifemelane. Pharmacol Toxicol 1993;72:394–397.
205. Schwab RS, Poskanzer DC, England AC, et al. Amantadine in the treatment of Parkinson's disease. Review of more than two years' experience. JAMA 1972;222:792–795.
207. Geldenhuys WJ, Malan SF, Bloomquist JR, et al. Pharmacology and structure-activity relationships of bioactive polycyclic cage compounds: a focus on pentacycloundecane derivatives. Med Res Rev 2005;25:21148.
208. Geldenhuys WJ, Malan SF, Bloomquist JR, et al. Structure-activity relationships of pentacycloundecylamines at the N-methyl-d-aspartate receptor. Bioorg Med Chem 2007;15:1525–1532.
209. Le DA, Lipton SA. Potential and current use of N-methyl-D-aspartate (NMDA) receptor antagonists in diseases of aging. Drugs Aging 2001;18:717–724.
210. Fink JS, Weaver DR, Rivkees SA, et al. Molecular cloning of the rat A2 adenosine receptor: selective co-expression with D2 dopamine receptors in rat striatum. Brain Res Mol Brain Res 1992;14:186–195.
211. Mori A, Shindou T, Ichimura M, et al. The role of adenosine A2a receptors in regulating GABAergic synaptic transmission in striatal medium spiny neurons. J Neurosci 1996;16:605–611.
212. Richardson PJ, Kase H, Jenner PG. Adenosine A2A receptor antagonists as new agents for the treatment of Parkinson's disease. Trends Pharmacol Sci 1997;18:338–344.
213. Pinna A, di Chiara G, Wardas J, et al. Blockade of A2a adenosine receptors positively modulates turning behaviour and c-Fos expression induced by D1 agonists in dopamine-denervated rats. Eur J Neurosci 1996;8:1176–1181.
214. Ferré S, O'Connor WT, Fuxe K, et al. The striopallidal neuron: a main locus for adenosine-dopamine interactions in the brain. J Neurosci 1993;13:5402–5406.
215. Kurokawa M, Koga K, Kase H, et al. Adenosine A2a receptor-mediated modulation of striatal acetylcholine release in vivo. J Neurochem 1996;66: 1882–1888.
216. Hernan MA, Takkouche B, Caamano-Isorna F, et al. A meta-analysis of coffee drinking, cigarette smoking, and the risk of Parkinson's disease. Ann Neurol 2002;52:276–284.
217. Trevitt J, Kawa K, Jalali A, et al. Differential effects of adenosine antagonists in two models of parkinsonian tremor. Pharmacol Biochem Behav 2009;94:24–29.
218. Kanda T, Jackson MJ, Smith LA, et al. Adenosine A2A antagonist: a novel antiparkinson's agent that does not provoke dyskinesia in parkinsonian monkeys. Ann Neurol 1998;43:507–513.

219. Hauser RA, Shulman LM, Trugman JM, et al. Study of istradefylline in patients with Parkinson's disease on levodopa with motor fluctuations. Mov Disord 2008;23:2177–2185.
220. Fernandez HH, Greeley DR, Zweig RM, et al; 6002-US-051 Study Group. Istradefylline as monotherapy for Parkinson disease: results of the 6002-US-051 trial. Parkinsonism Relat Disord 2010;16:16–20.
221. Christoffersen CL, Meltzer LT. Reversal of haloperidol-induced extrapyramidal side effects in cebus monkeys by 8-hydroxy-2-(di-n-propylamino)tetralin and its enantiomers. Neuropsychopharmacology 1998;18:399–402.
222. Melamed E, Zoldan J, Friedberg G, et al. Involvement of serotonin in clinical features of Parkinson's disease and complications of L-DOPA therapy. Adv Neurol 1996;69:545–550.
223. Sanders-Bush E, Mayer SE. 5-Hydroxytryptamine (serotonin): receptor agonists and antagonists. In: Brunton LL, Lazo JS, Parker KL, eds. Goodman and Gilman's the Pharmacological Basis of Therapeutics. New York: McGraw-Hill, 2006:297–315.
224. Blier P, Piñeyro G, el Mansari M, et al. Role of somatodendritic 5-HT autoreceptors in modulating 5-HT neurotransmission. Ann N Y Acad Sci 1998;861:204–216.
225. Bibbiani F, Oh JD, Chase TN. Serotonin 5-HT1A agonist improves motor complications in rodent and primate parkinsonian models. Neurology 2001;57:1829–1834.
226. Bartoszyk GD, van Amsterdam C, Greiner HE, et al. Sarizotan, a serotonin 5-HT1A receptor agonist and dopamine receptor ligand: 1. Neurochemical profile. J Neural Transm 2004;111:113–126.
227. Olanow CW, Damier P, Goetz CG, et al. Multicenter, open-label trial of sarizotan in Parkinson's disease patients with levodopa-induced dyskinesias (SPLENDID study). Clin Neuropharmacol 2004;27:58–62.
228. Goetz CG, Damier P, Hicking C, et al. Sarizotan as a treatment for dyskinesias in Parkinson's disease: a double-blind placebo-controlled trial. Mov Disord 2007;22:179–186.
229. Grégoire L, Samadi P, Graham J, et al. Low doses of sarizotan reduce dyskinesias and maintain antiparkinsonian efficacy of L-dopa in parkinsonian monkeys. Parkinsonism Relat Disord 2009;15:445–452.
230. Felder CC, Bymaster FP, Ward J, et al. Therapeutic opportunities for muscarinic receptors in the central nervous system. J Med Chem 2000;43:4333–4353.
231. Garnett ES, Firnau G, Chan PK, et al. [18F]Fluoro-DOPA, an analogue of DOPA, and its use in direct external measurements of storage, degradation, and turnover of intracerebral dopamine. Proc Natl Acad Sci U S A 1978;75:464–477.
232. Volkow ND, Fowler JS, Wang GJ, et al. Decreased dopamine transporters with age in health human subjects. Ann Neurol 1994;36:237–239.
233. Neumeyer JL, Wang SY, Milius RA, et al. [123I]-2 Beta-carbomethoxy-3 beta-(4-iodophenyl)tropane: high-affinity SPECT radiotracer of monoamine reuptake sites in brain. J Med Chem 1991;34:3144–3146.
234. Neumeyer JL, Wang S, Gao Y, et al. N-omega-fluoroalkyl analogs of (1R)-2 beta-carbomethoxy-3 beta-(4-iodophenyl)-tropane (beta-CIT): radiotracers for positron emission tomography and single photon emission computed tomography imaging of dopamine transporters. J Med Chem 1994:37:1558–1561.
235. Chaly T, Dhawan V, Kazumata K, et al. Radiosynthesis of [18F] N-3-fluoropropyl-2-beta-carbomethoxy-3-beta-(4-iodophenyl) nortropane and the first human study with positron emission tomography. Nucl Med Biol 1996;23:999–1004.
236. Kilbourn M, Lee L, Vander Borght T, et al. Binding of alpha-dihydrotetrabenazine to the vesicular monoamine transporter is stereospecific. Eur J Pharmacol 1995;278:249–252.
237. Bohnen NI, Albin RL, Koeppe RA, et al. Positron emission tomography of monoaminergic vesicular binding in aging and Parkinson disease. J Cereb Blood Flow Metab 2006;26:1198–1212.
238. Martin WR, Wieler M, Stoessl AJ, et al. Dihydrotetrabenazine positron emission tomography imaging in early, untreated Parkinson's disease. Ann Neurol 2008;63:388–394.
239. Elbasiouny SM, Moroz D, Bakr MM, et al. Management of spasticity after spinal cord injury: current techniques and future directions. Neurorehabil Neural Repair 2010;24:23–33.
240. Montane E, Vallano A, Laporte JR. Oral antispastic drugs in nonprogressive neurologic diseases: a systematic review. Neurology 2004;63:1357–1363.
241. Beebe FA, Barkin RL, Barkin S. A clinical and pharmacologic review of skeletal muscle relaxants for musculoskeletal conditions. Am J Ther 2005;12:151–171.
242. Delgado MR, Hirtz D, Aisen M, et al. Practice parameter: pharmacologic treatment of spasticity in children and adolescents with cerebral palsy (an evidence-based review): report of the Quality Standards Subcommittee of the American Academy of Neurology and the Practice Committee of the Child Neurology Society. Quality Standards Subcommittee of the American Academy of Neurology and the Practice Committee of the Child Neurology Society. Neurology 2010;74:336–343.
243. Chou R. Pharmacological management of low back pain. Drugs 2010;70:387–402.
244. Berger FM, Bradley W. The pharmacological properties of an alpha, beta-dihydroxy-gama-(2-methylphenoxy)-propane (Myanesisn). Br J Pharmacol Chemother 1946;1:265–272.
245. Souri E, Sharifzadeh M, Farsam H, et al. Muscle relaxant activity of methocarbamol enantiomers in mice. J Pharm Pharmacol 1999;51:853–855.
246. Kobayashi H, Hasegawa Y, Ono H. Cyclobenzaprine, a centrally acting muscle relaxant, acts on descending serotonergic systems. Eur J Pharmacol 1996;5:29–35.
247. Crestani F, Low K, Keist R, et al. Molecular targets for the myelorelaxant action of diazepam. Mol Pharmacol 2001;59:442–445.
248. Basile AS, Lippa AS, Skolnick P. Anxioselective anxiolytics: can less be more? Eur J Pharmacol 2004;500:441–451.
249. Zafonte R, Lombard L, Elovic E. Antispasticity medications: uses and limitations of enteral therapy. Am J Phys Med Rehabil 2004;83:S50–S58.
250. Granfors TM, Backman JT, Laitila J, et al. Tizanidine is mainly metabolized by cytochrome P450 1A2 in vitro. Br J Clin Pharmacol 2004;**57**:349–353.
251. Koch P, Hirst DR, von Wartburg BR. Biological fate of sirdalud in animals and man. Xenobiotica 1989;19:1255–1265.
252. Ting PT, Freiman A. The story of Clostridium botulinum: from food poisoning to Botox. Clin Med 2004;4:258–261.
253. Dolly JO, Aoki KR. The structure and mode of action of different botulinum toxins. Eur J Neurol 2006;13(Suppl 4):1–9.
254. Dolly JO, Black J, Williams RS, et al. Acceptors for botulinum neurotoxin reside on motor nerve terminals and mediate its internalization. Nature 1984;307:457–460.
255. Schiavo G, Benfenati F, Poulain B, et al. Tetanus and botulinum-B neurotoxins block neurotransmitter release by proteolytic cleavage of synaptobrevin. Nature 1992;359:832–835.
256. Koussoulakos S. Botulinum neurotoxin: the ugly duckling. Eur Neurol 2009;61:331–342.
257. Dolly JO, Lande S, Wray DW. The effects of in vitro application of purified botulinum neurotoxin at mouse motor nerve terminals. J Physiol 1987;386:475–484.
258. Ward AB. Spasticity treatment with botulinum toxins. J Neural Transm 2008;115:607–616.

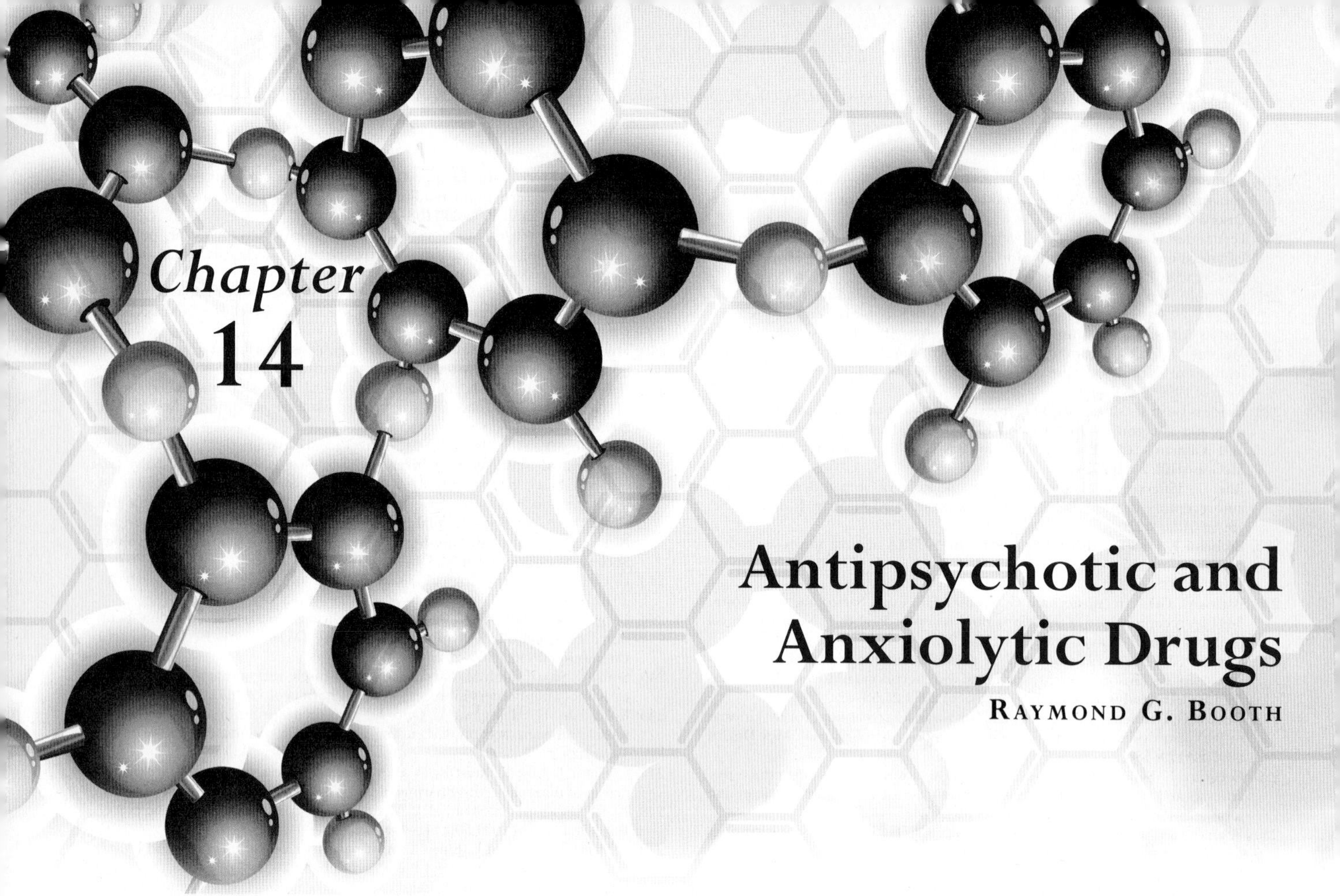

Chapter 14

Antipsychotic and Anxiolytic Drugs

RAYMOND G. BOOTH

*Drugs Covered in This Chapter**

BENZAMIDE CLASS

BENZAZEPINES
- Asenapine
- Clozapine
- Loxapine
- Olanzapine
- Quetiapine

BENZISOXAZOLES AND BENZISOTHIAZOLES
- Iloperidone
- Lurasidone
- Paliperidone
- Risperidone
- Ziprasidone

BENZODIAZEPINES
- Chlordiazepoxide
- Diazepam
- Flurazepam
- Oxazepam

BUTYROPHENONE CLASS
- Droperidol
- Haloperidol
- Pimozide
- *Spiperone*
- *Trifluperidol*

MISCELLANEOUS ANTIPSYCHOTIC AGENTS
- Aripiprazole
- Molindone
- Sertindole

MISCELLANEOUS ANXIOLYTIC AGENTS
- Buspirone

NONBENZODIAZEPINE AGONISTS
- Eszopiclone
- Zaleplon
- Zolpidem

PHENOTHIAZINE CLASS

THIOXANTHENES CLASS
- Thiothixene

Abbreviations

BZR, benzodiazepine receptor
cAMP, cyclic adenosine monophosphate
βCCE, β-carboline-3-carboxylic acid ethyl ester
CNS, central nervous system
DMCM, 6,7-dimethoxy-4-ethyl-β-carboline-3-carboxylic acid methyl ester
DSM-IV-TR, *Diagnostic and Statistical Manual of Mental Disorders, Fourth Edition, Text Revision*
FDA, U.S. Food and Drug Administration
GABA, γ-aminobutyric acid
GPCRs, G protein-coupled receptors
HPTP, haloperidol 1,2,3,6-tetrahydropyridine
HPP^+, haloperidol pyridinium
5-HT, serotonin
MPTP, 1-methyl-4-phenyl-1,2,3,6-tetrahydropyridine
$MPDP^+$, 1-methyl-4-phenyl-2,3-dihydropyridinium
MPP^+, 1-methyl-4-phenylpyridinium
NMDA, *N*-methyl-D-aspartate
7-OH-DPAT, (+)-7-hydroxy-*N*,*N*-di-n-propyl-2-aminotetralin
SSRI, selective serotonin reuptake inhibitor

*Drugs available outside the United States are shown in italics.

SCENARIO

David Hayes, PharmD

Ben is a 25 year old who was diagnosed with paranoid schizophrenia 1 year ago, after having a psychotic episode consisting of auditory hallucinations and delusions of people hiding in his attic. He was encouraged by his mother to see a psychiatrist, at which time he was initiated on olanzapine 5 mg daily. Six months ago he started feeling paranoid and believing that the FBI was following him, so his psychiatrist increased his dose to 10 mg daily; since then Ben has been stable. Ben has no medical history other than schizophrenia and takes no other medications. His family history is significant—his father had type 2 diabetes and obsessive compulsive disorder. Ben recently went to see his primary care physician and it was noted that he had gained 25 lb since his visit 1 year ago. In addition, during this visit he was diagnosed with prediabetes, with a fasting blood glucose level of 119 mg/dL. The clinical question is whether to switch his antipsychotic in favor of one with fewer metabolic effects or to leave the antipsychotic as it is since Ben is stable.

(The reader is directed to the clinical solution and chemical analysis of this case at the end of the chapter).

OVERVIEW OF MENTAL ILLNESSES

Mental illnesses that can be treated with psychotropic drugs are broadly categorized as psychoses, neuroses, and mood (depression, bipolar) disorders. Different classes of psychotropic agents differ in their ability to modify symptoms of these mental illnesses; thus, an appropriate diagnosis is critical to selecting an efficacious psychotropic drug. This chapter is focused on the medicinal chemistry of drugs that are used to treat psychoses (including the manic phase of bipolar illness) and anxiety disorders. The definitive diagnostic criteria for psychiatric disorders in the United States are well described in the *Diagnostic and Statistical Manual of Mental Disorders of the American Psychiatric Association* (DSM-IV-TR) (1). The psychoses (e.g., schizophrenia) are among the most severe mental illnesses and commonly include symptoms of delusions and sensory hallucinations. In anxiety disorders (neuroses), the ability to comprehend reality is retained, but mood changes (anxiety, panic, dysphoria) and thought (obsessions, irrational fears) and behavioral (rituals, compulsions, avoidance) dysfunction can be disabling. Mood and panic disorders often include dysfunction of the autonomic nervous system (e.g., altered patterns of sleep and appetite) in addition to psychic abnormalities. Depression (see Chapter 18) can lead to self-harm and suicide. In general, antipsychotic agents, which can have severe neurologic and metabolic (obesity, type 2 diabetes) side effects, should be used to treat only the most severe mental illnesses (i.e., psychoses such as schizophrenia).

SCHIZOPHRENIA

Definition

An historical definition of schizophrenia began approximately 100 years ago, with the German psychiatrist Emil Kraepelin's description of a type of dementia that was characterized as a severe, chronic mental disorder without known external causation wherein functional deterioration progresses with the symptoms of hallucinations, delusions, thought disorder, incoherence, blunted affect, negativism, stereotyped behavior, and lack of insight (2). The deterioration progresses to catatonia and hebephrenia (illogical, incoherent, and senseless thought processes and actions, delusions, and hallucinations). Meanwhile, the Swiss psychiatrist Eugen Bleuler coined the term "schizophrenia" to take into account the perceived "schism" or splitting in mental functioning (3).

A modern definition of schizophrenia comes from DSM-IV (1). The diagnostic criteria for schizophrenia require two or more of the following characteristic symptoms to be present for a significant proportion of time during a 1-month period: delusions, hallucinations, disorganized speech, or grossly disorganized or catatonic behavior. There is, however, flexibility in the diagnostic criteria that leaves room for professional psychiatric judgment. For example, it is enough if hallucinations consist of a voice maintaining a running commentary on the patient's behavior or there are two or more voices that converse with each other. Also, for a significant proportion of time, one or more areas of social functioning, such as work, interpersonal relationships, or self-care, are markedly below the level achieved before the onset of symptoms. Continuous symptoms must persist for 6 months. Finally, before a diagnosis of schizophrenia is made, affective disorders as well as drug/alcohol abuse or other medical conditions must be ruled out. According to DSM-IV parameters, the common estimate for schizophrenia incidence is about 1% of the population.

Etiology of Schizophrenia

A neurobiologic basis for schizophrenia and related psychotic syndromes remains elusive. Compelling evidence linking genetic factors to the etiology of schizophrenia is not apparent despite enormous progress in the field of molecular genetics and numerous investigations of hereditary factors associated with psychotic illnesses. Current epidemiologic evidence suggests that individual variation in susceptibility to schizophrenia involves alleles of moderate to small effect in multiple genes (4). Investigations of environmental causative factors have

CLINICAL SIGNIFICANCE

As you review the chemistry of the antipsychotics and their receptor affinity and interaction (e.g., agonist, partial agonist, antagonism, and reverse agonist), think about potential for benefit and/or adverse effects. It is believed that those agents with lower affinity to D_2 receptor and higher affinity to 5-HT_{2A} may reduce the probability of extrapyramidal syndromes and provide effective therapy for the symptoms schizophrenia and/or psychosis. It has been determined that antipsychotics exhibit metabolic effects; however, the exact mechanism of metabolic effects such as weight gain has not been fully elucidated. There is some data to support that agents with affinity and antagonistic activity at the 5-HT_{2C} and/or histamine H_1 GPCR receptors have greater metabolic impact. Olanzapine and clozapine both share high to moderate affinity and antagonistic activity at these receptors and both have been determined to have the significant impact on weight gain in their clinical evaluation. Conversely, agents with affinity but that act as a partial agonist, such as aripiprazole, have demonstrated lesser effects on weight gain. Therefore, an understanding of receptor affinity and interaction in relation to the potential for benefit and/or adverse effects tempered with clinic evidence may provide the clinician with support for the choice of an initial therapy or aid in the decision to switch secondary to the occurrence of an adverse effect such as weight gain. This consideration may be most important for those patients who are already overweight and/or at risk for metabolic diseases such as type 2 diabetes.

David Hayes, PharmD
Clinical Associate Professor
Department of Clinical Sciences and Administration
University of Houston College of Pharmacy

focused on prenatal and perinatal risk factors for brain damage. For example, studies have examined the incidence of schizophrenics who were born under conditions of obstetrical complications, influenza epidemics, food shortages, and Rh factor incompatibility. Gene–environment interactions have been linked to the etiology and pathology of schizophrenia, with a role for inflammatory processes most clearly implicated (5). In fact, regulators of inflammatory processes such as cytokines are a common link between the genetic and environmental components of schizophrenia etiology, and it is noteworthy that inflammatory processes involved in maternal infection, obstetric complications, neonatal hypoxia, and brain injury involve cytokines. Gene–environment interactions involving chromosomal abnormalities and obstetric/perinatal complications may converge with precipitating factors such as stress or chemical agents to result in a neurodegenerative component of schizophrenia (6). Neuroanatomic hypotheses include increased ventricular volume; however, neuropathologic changes associated with schizophrenic brains are not obvious as in, for example, Parkinson disease. In contrast, neurochemical abnormalities are well documented. Alterations of brain dopaminergic neurotransmission in psychoses have been studied for more than 30 years, and this field of psychobiologic research generally revolves around the "dopamine hypothesis" of schizophrenia.

The Dopamine Hypothesis

The dopamine hypothesis of schizophrenia arose from observations that the first relatively safe and effective antipsychotic drugs, the phenothiazines, such as chlorpromazine, used in the early 1950s affected brain dopamine metabolism (7). Simply put, the dopamine hypothesis of schizophrenia suggests that the disease results from increased dopaminergic neurotransmission and that approaches that decrease dopaminergic neurotransmission will alleviate psychotic symptoms. Most antipsychotic agents have activity to limit dopaminergic neurotransmission (8–10), providing some indirect evidence to support the dopamine hypothesis of schizophrenia. In a seminal study (11), the average daily dose of an antipsychotic was found to correlate well with affinity for dopamine D_2-type receptors. Moreover, extrapyramidal side effects of antipsychotic drugs correlate with their dopamine D_2 affinity. It should be noted, however, that functional interaction of antipsychotic drugs with the D_2 receptor is complex, involving antagonism, inverse agonism, and partial agonism. For example, recent studies show that essentially all clinically used antipsychotic drugs are D_2 inverse agonists or partial agonists (12), suggesting that biochemical as well as clinical effects may not be explained by simple blockade of endogenous agonist (dopamine) access to the D_2 receptor.

The dopamine hypothesis of schizophrenia and pharmacotherapy involving targeting of dopamine receptors (especially the D_2-type) has dominated research directions, but it should be noted that this approach is somewhat "pharmacocentric." Consideration of potential new drugs as antipsychotic agents usually is limited to compounds that have demonstrated behavioral or biochemical evidence of antidopaminergic actions. In fact, this circular approach may be practical considering the lack of proven alternative neuropharmacologic explanations of antipsychotic drug activity; nevertheless, after about 50 years of research focusing on brain dopaminergic systems, uncontested evidence linking the etiology of psychotic illnesses to the neurobiology of dopaminergic systems remains elusive. Alternative explanations, especially those involving adrenergic and serotonergic receptor systems, probably will gain popularity as more atypical antipsychotic drugs (e.g., clozapine) are introduced and also found to have actions at these receptor systems, perpetuating and expanding a pharmacocentric approach to antipsychotic drug design and development.

Dopamine Receptors in Schizophrenia

As discussed in Chapter 13, there are five different dopamine receptors, D_1, D_2 (with short and long splice variants), D_3, D_4, and D_5—all are G protein–coupled receptors (GPCRs), and as is the case for almost all GPCRs, three-dimensional x-ray crystal structural information is not available. Currently, there are no drugs or even medicinal chemical probes that are specific enough to distinguish between the five subtypes; thus, dopamine receptors often are classified as the D_1-type (includes D_5), which stimulate adenylyl cyclase, or the D_2-type (includes D_3, and D_4), which inhibit adenylyl cyclase.

Several chemical probes are available that can distinguish between the general D_1-type and D_2-type receptor families (Fig. 14.1). The *R*-(+)-isomer of the benzazepine derivative, SKF 38393, is used for research as a selective D_1-type partial agonist. Meanwhile, the structurally related benzazepine derivative, *R*-(+)-SCH 23390, is used as a selective D_2-type receptor antagonist. Although not very selective for D_1-type over D_2-type receptors, the rigid benzophenanthridine derivative (–)-dihydrexidine is a useful research tool, because it is a D_1-type full-efficacy agonist (13,14). Selective D_2-type full agonists, such as the pyrazole derivative (–)-quinpirole, and D_2-type antagonists, such as (–)-sulpiride, also are available to researchers. The dopamine D_3 receptor subtype is of particular neuropharmacologic interest because of its preferential distribution in certain limbic regions of mammalian brain, notably in the nucleus accumbens of the basal forebrain. It is proposed that highly D_3-selective drugs might be developed as antipsychotic agents with preferential limbic antidopaminergic actions while sparing the extrapyramidal basal ganglia, presumably decreasing the neurologic movement disorder side effects associated with antipsychotic drug therapy. The tetrahydronaphthalene, (+)-7-hydroxy-*N*,*N*-di-n-propyl-2-aminotetralin (7-OH-DPAT), and some of its congeners are particularly promising D_3-selective lead agents. The benzazepine clozapine, the prototype of second-generation atypical antipsychotics (see later discussion), shows relatively greater affinity for the D_4 dopamine receptor subtype in addition to its relatively high affinity for serotonin 5-HT_2, adrenergic α_1 and α_2, muscarinic M_1, and histamine H_1 receptors (15).

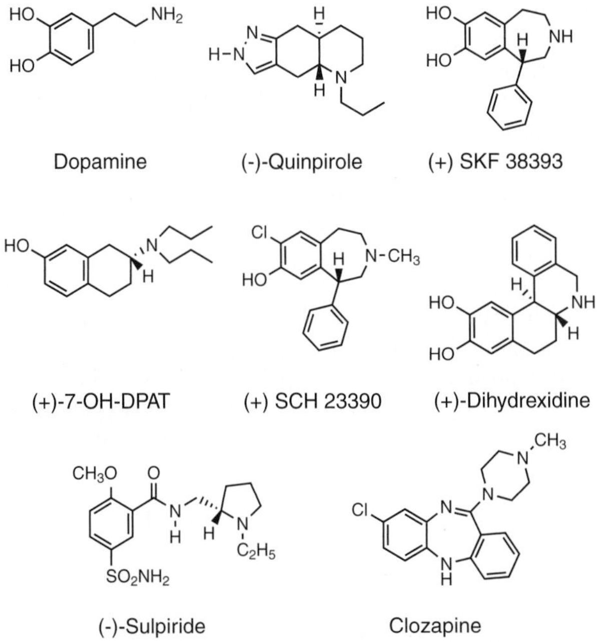

FIGURE 14.1 Structures of compounds useful for characterizing dopamine receptors.

The dopamine D_1-type and D_2-type receptor families are differentially distributed in mammalian forebrain dopaminergic pathways. The extrapyramidal nigrostriatal pathway, which plays a key role in locomotor coordination, consists of neurons with cell bodies in the A9 pars compacta of the substantia nigra in the midbrain. These neurons project to the basal ganglia structures of the caudate nucleus and putamen (collectively referred to as striatum) in the forebrain (Fig. 14.2). Degeneration of neurons in the nigrostriatal pathway is the hallmark pathologic feature of Parkinson disease, clinically manifested as bradykinesia, muscular rigidity, resting tremor, and impairment of postural balance. Blockade of dopamine receptors on cholinergic neurons in striatum is associated with the sometimes severe extrapyramidal, parkinsonian-like side effects (muscular rigidity, bradykinesia, akathisia) that frequently occur with antipsychotic drug treatment.

The mesolimbic and mesocortical pathway, involved in integration of emotions, behaviors, and higher thought processes, consists of neurons with cell bodies in the A10 ventral tegmentum. These neurons project to limbic forebrain structures, including the nucleus accumbens and amygdala, and to higher levels of cerebral function, such as the frontal cortex (Fig. 14.2). According to the dopamine hypothesis, increased dopaminergic neurotransmission in limbic pathways contributes to the "positive" symptoms (e.g., hallucinations and excited delusional behavior that can be reduced with typical antipsychotic drugs) but not necessarily to the "negative" symptoms (e.g., catatonia) observed in the clinical manifestation of schizophrenia.

Typical antipsychotic drugs act in both extrapyramidal and limbic brain regions at D_2-type dopamine receptors that can be located postsynaptically (on cell bodies, dendrites, and nerve terminals of other neurons) as well as presynaptically on dopamine neurons. Dopamine receptors located presynaptically on dopamine cell bodies and nerve terminals are called autoreceptors and act to negatively modulate neuronal firing and dopamine synthesis and release (Fig. 14.3). Low concentrations of certain dopamine agonists can stereospecifically activate dopamine D_2-type autoreceptors to decrease dopamine synthesis (16) and release (17), thus reducing dopaminergic

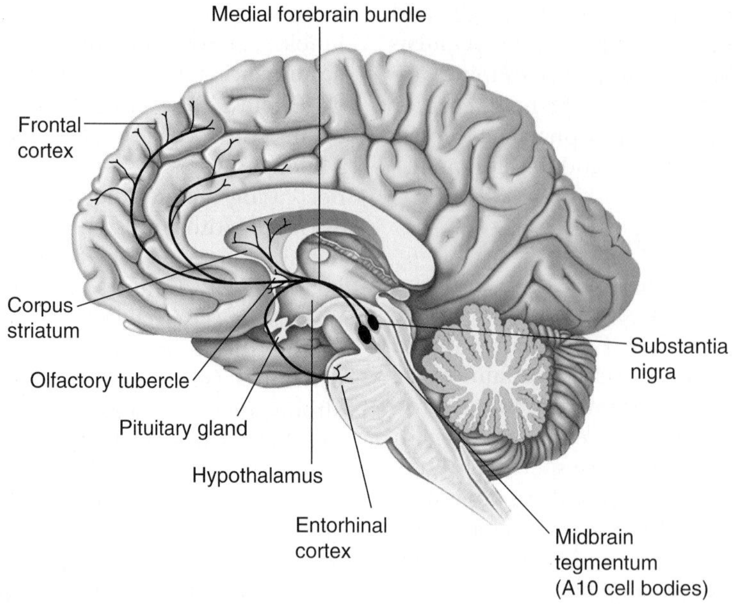

FIGURE 14.2 Some dopamine pathways in human brain.

neurotransmission. Consistent with the dopamine hypothesis of schizophrenia, selective dopamine autoreceptor agonists could, theoretically, be pharmacotherapeutic agents in schizophrenia and related mental illnesses.

GPCR Functional Selectivity

It is now realized that the same GPCR can couple to different Gα proteins to result in "multifunctional" signaling that provides a mechanistic basis for "functional selectivity" with regard to design of drugs targeting DA receptors (18,19). Molecular mechanisms to account for GPCR multifunctional signaling involve the concept of "GPCR permissiveness," which assumes a high degree of flexibility in the interactions between a ligand, receptor, and G protein (20). These interactions occur mainly between the G proteins and the second and third intracellular loops and carboxy-terminal tail of the receptor. Some factors that influence this interaction include receptor:G protein ratios and amounts, alternative GPCR splicing, and conformational changes in the G protein and/or receptor.

A critical assumption of GPCR multifunctional signaling theory is that a heterogeneity of active and inactive receptor conformations exists and that ligands differ in their ability to stabilize different receptor conformations, as described in the "stimulus trafficking" hypothesis (21). Of particular relevance to medicinal chemistry, it follows that upon binding, ligand chemical structural parameters are among the most important determinants of GPCR conformation stabilized. It follows that ligand stereochemistry and other structural parameters influence the type of Gα protein and intracellular signaling pathway activated, resulting in ligand-specific functional outcomes (22–24). Ligands that show such functional selectivity can be exploited for drug design purposes. A clinically relevant example is the second-generation (atypical) antipsychotic drug aripiprazole (25), which interacts with dopamine D_2 receptors to produce agonist, partial agonist, inverse agonist, or neutral antagonist functional effects, depending on the D_2 receptor cellular milieu (e.g., G protein complement and concentration) and particular location (e.g., presynaptic vs. postsynaptic and extrapyramidal vs. limbic brain regions).

Other Brain Neurotransmitter Systems in Schizophrenia

In addition to postsynaptic dopamine receptors and presynaptic dopamine D_2-type autoreceptors, heteroreceptors, such as adenosine (A_2) (26), histamine (H_1) (27), and serotonin (5-HT_{1A}) (28), located on or near presynaptic dopaminergic nerve terminals in the striatum (extrapyramidal) or nucleus accumbens (limbic) regions of brain can modulate dopamine synthesis (and release) by altering the activity of tyrosine hydroxylase, the rate-limiting step in catecholamine biosynthesis. Similarly, activation of adrenergic (α_2) autoreceptors in the limbic structure hippocampus negatively modulates the release of the neurotransmitter norepinephrine (29). It is proposed that atypical antipsychotic drugs, such as clozapine, may interact with these other neurotransmitter receptor systems (i.e., histamine, serotonin, and adrenergic) instead of (or in addition to) dopamine receptor systems. Preceding the introduction of the first clinically successful phenothiazine-type neuroleptic, chlorpromazine, the first phenothiazine to be used to treat psychiatric patients in the 1940s (unsuccessfully) was promethazine, an "antihistamine" H_1 antagonist.

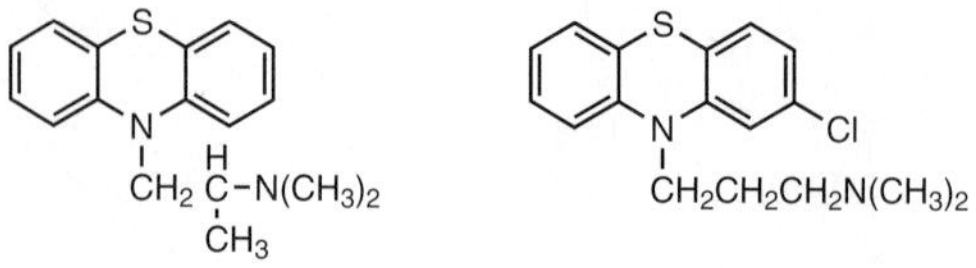

Promethazine　　Chlorpromazine

Serotonin 5-HT_{2A} and 5-HT_{2C} GPCRs that are expressed in the mesolimbic and mesocortical pathways also are

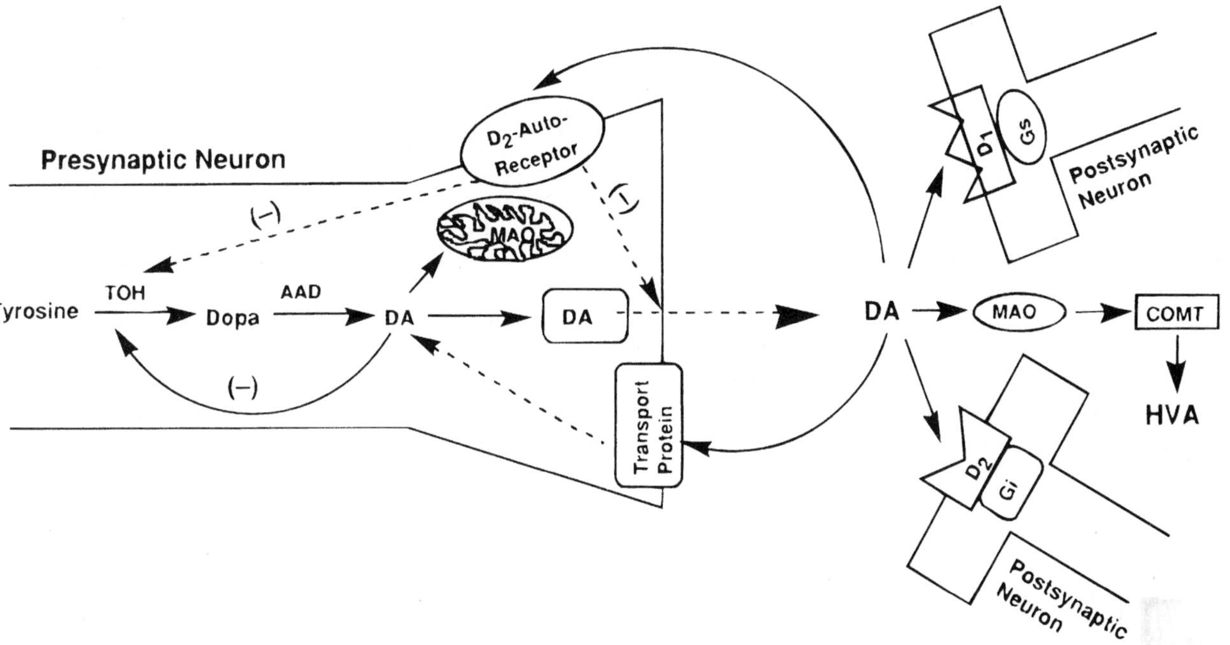

FIGURE 14.3 Tyrosine is hydroxylated in a rate-limiting step by tyrosine hydroxylase (TOH) to form dihydroxyphenylalanine (DOPA), which is decarboxylated by L-aromatic amino acid decarboxylase (AAD) to form dopamine (DA). Newly synthesized DA is stored in vesicles, from which release occurs into the synaptic cleft by depolarization of the presynaptic neuron in the presence of Ca^{2+}. The DA released into the synaptic cleft may go on to stimulate postsynaptic D_1- and D_2-type autoreceptors that negatively modulate DA synthesis (via inhibition of TOH) and release. The action of synaptic DA is inactivated largely via reaccumulation into the presynaptic neuron by high-affinity DA neurotransport proteins located on the nerve terminal membrane. Free cytoplasmic DA negatively modulates DA synthesis via end-product (feedback) inhibition of TOH by competition with biopterin cofactor. Cytoplasmic pools of DA may undergo metabolic deamination by monoamine oxidase (MAO), an enzyme bound to the outer membrane of mitochondria, to form dihydroxyphenylacetaldehyde, which oxides to dihydroxyphenylacetate (DOPAC). The DA or DOPAC may undergo methylation by catechol-*O*-methyltransferase (COMT), ultimately forming homovanillic acid (HVA), a metabolite excreted in urine.

linked to the pathophysiology and treatment of schizophrenia. For example, activation of 5-HT_{2A} receptors mediates psychotomimetic effects of some classes of hallucinogenic drugs (30), activation of 5-HT_{2C} receptors leads to antipsychotic effects in various rodent models of schizophrenia, and some second-generation (atypical) antipsychotic drugs such as clozapine have higher affinity for human serotonin 5-HT_2–type receptors than dopamine D_2-type receptors (15). Moreover, obesity associated with especially atypical antipsychotic drugs (e.g., clozapine) is thought to be due to their antagonist or inverse agonist actions at 5-HT_{2C} receptors (31), whereas selective activation of 5-HT_{2C} receptors reduces food intake (32). The other member of the 5-HT_2 family is the 5-HT_{2B} GPCR, which although also expressed in brain, is best known for its notorious role in the periphery where its activation has been linked to cardiac valvulopathy (33–35). Thus, the desired 5HT_2-type pharmacology for treatment of schizophrenia without propensity for weight gain appears to be 5-HT_{2A} receptor antagonism or inverse agonism and/or 5-HT_{2C} receptor agonism, with no tolerance for activation of 5-HT_{2B} receptors (36). As for dopamine receptors, our understanding of the role of serotonin 5-HT_2 GPCRs (as well as other 5-HT receptor subtypes) in schizophrenia comes mainly from our understanding of drug pharmacology at these receptors; this pharmacocentric approach becomes more complex in light of recent evidence that all three 5-HT_2 subtypes demonstrate multifunctional signaling (37–40); that is, the same drug may be an agonist, partial agonist, inverse agonist, or antagonist at the same receptor, depending on the intracellular milieu.

Pharmacotherapy of Schizophrenia and Related Psychoses

The most widely used class of drugs in the treatment of psychotic disorders is the so-called neuroleptics. This term suggests that such medicines "take hold" (*lepsis*) of the central nervous system (CNS) to suppress movement as well as behavior. Although the connotation has been stretched to include biochemical and clinical antagonism of dopamine D_2 receptors, debilitating extrapyramidal movement side effects are implicit in the clinical definition of neuroleptic antipsychotic drugs. Indeed, the term "neuroleptic" is so synonymous with neurologic side effects that newer antipsychotic drugs, without substantial risk of extrapyramidal effects, are referred to as atypical neuroleptic drugs. Also implied in the term "atypical" is a mechanism of antipsychotic action other than (or in addition to) postsynaptic D_2 receptor blockade. There is currently a trend by researchers and clinicians to refer to typical neuroleptics, with relatively potent dopamine D_2 receptor antagonist activity and high propensity for extrapyramidal side effects, as "first generation," whereas, atypical antipsychotics, which have relatively less affinity for D_2 receptors and less incidence of movement disorder side effects, are called "second generation."

In general, pharmacotherapy with typical first-generation neuroleptics benefits patients with schizophrenia or other psychiatric illnesses marked by agitation, aggressive and impulsive behavior, and impaired reasoning. Positive symptoms respond better to treatment with typical neuroleptics, whereas negative symptoms are not appreciably affected. In general, the first-generation neuroleptics provide calming, mood-stabilizing, and antihallucinatory effects, and their beneficial impact on psychiatric medicine is unquestioned despite their sometimes severe extrapyramidal side effects. Chemical classes of typical neuroleptics include the phenothiazines, thioxanthenes, and butyrophenones. Second-generation antipsychotic drug classes include the dibenzodiazepines and benzisoxazoles, which have less potential for extrapyramidal side effects and have significant activity at brain serotonin 5-HT_2-type, adrenergic α_1/α_2, muscarinic, and/or histamine H_1 receptors, in addition to some activity at dopamine receptors.

First-Generation (Typical) Antipsychotic Drugs

Mechanism of Action Given that the pathogenesis of schizophrenia and related psychiatric disorders is unknown, it is perhaps naïve to suggest how drugs act at the molecular level to relieve the symptoms of these disorders. Nevertheless, it generally is agreed that the antipsychotic mechanism of action of neuroleptics includes modulation of dopamine neurotransmission in the mesolimbic–mesocortical pathways. This is achieved via direct interaction with D_2-type receptors, at which they have very high affinity (K_i < 5 nmol/L) and functional activity spanning the spectrum of inverse agonism, antagonism, and partial agonism. It is noted that phenothiazine neuroleptics (e.g., chlorpromazine) also have appreciable affinity (K_i < 100 nmol/L) at human cloned dopamine D_1-type, serotonin 5-HT_{2A}, 5-HT_{2C}, 5-HT_6, 5-HT_7, adrenergic α_1-type and α_2-type, cholinergic $M_{1\text{-}5}$, and histamine H_1 GPCRs (15) that may account for clinical antipsychotic efficacy and certainly account for their numerous side effects (see later discussion). Likewise, the butyrophenone-type antipsychotic drug haloperidol binds with very high affinity (K_i < 10 nmol/L) at dopamine D_2-type, high affinity (K_i < 20 nmol/L) at adrenergic α_1-type, and moderate affinity (K_i < 100 nmol/L) at dopamine D_1 and serotonin 5-HT_{2A} (but not 5-HT_{2C}) GPCRs (15).

Side Effects Many of the side effects associated with typical antipsychotic agents can be attributed to their interaction with the GPCRs mentioned earlier in both the CNS and periphery. For example, antipsychotic drug side effects such as sedation, hypotension, sexual dysfunction, and other autonomic effects reflect blockade of histamine H_1 and adrenergic α_1/α_2 receptors. Antimuscarinic ($M_{1\text{–}5}$) actions of neuroleptics account for cardiac, ophthalmic, gastrointestinal, and genitourinary side effects. Such untoward antimuscarinic actions also are characteristic of atypical antipsychotics such as clozapine. On the other hand, it has been proposed that anticholinergic activity may be beneficial in controlling negative symptoms in patients with schizophrenia. The parkinsonian-like movement side effects of neuroleptics result from antagonism of dopamine D_2 receptors in the nigrostriatal pathway, and the severity of these extrapyramidal side effects increases with the ratio of their antidopaminergic to anticholinergic potency. Extrapyramidal side effects occur in 30% to 50% of patients receiving standard doses of typical neuroleptics and tend to occur during the first to eighth week of therapy. Extrapyramidal side effects include acute dystonias (e.g., facial grimacing, torticollis, and oculogyric crisis), akathisia (motor restlessness), and parkinsonian-type symptoms, such as bradykinesia, cogwheel rigidity, tremor, masked face, and shuffling gait. The higher the D_2 potency of the neuroleptic is, the worse the side effects, some of which can be reversed using anticholinergic drugs. Tardive dyskinesia occurs in 15% to 25% of patients after prolonged treatment with typical neuroleptics and is characterized by stereotyped, involuntary, repetitive, choreiform movements of the face, eyelids, mouth (grimaces), tongue, extremities, and trunk. There also are metabolic and endocrine side effects of neuroleptics, such as weight gain, hyperprolactinemia, and gynecomastia. Relatively common dermatologic reactions (e.g., urticaria and photosensitivity) also are observed especially with the phenothiazines. Interestingly, anticholinergic and dopaminergic agents worsen tardive dyskinesia, whereas antidopaminergic agents tend to suppress the symptoms. The pathophysiology of tardive dyskinesia is not known, and the disorder essentially is irreversible.

Meanwhile, antagonism of dopamine D_2-type receptors in the chemoreceptor trigger zone in the brainstem is responsible for beneficial antiemetic effects produced by neuroleptics. Several phenothiazines (e.g., promethazine and prochlorperazine) are marketed to exploit this pharmacologic effect.

Development of Phenothiazine and Thioxanthene Neuroleptics

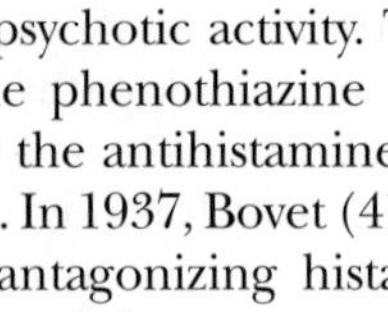

Phenothiazine

Although the phenothiazine nucleus was synthesized in 1883, and although it was used as an anthelmintic for many years, it has no antipsychotic activity. The basic structural type from which the phenothiazine antipsychotic drugs trace their origins is the antihistamines of the benzodioxane type I (Fig. 14.4). In 1937, Bovet (41) hypothesized that specific substances antagonizing histamine should exist, tried various compounds known to act on the autonomic nervous system, and was the first to recognize antihistaminic activity. With the benzodioxanes as a starting point, many molecular modifications were carried out in various laboratories in a search for other types of antihistamines. The benzodioxanes led to ethers of ethanolamine of type II, which after further modifications led to the benzhydryl

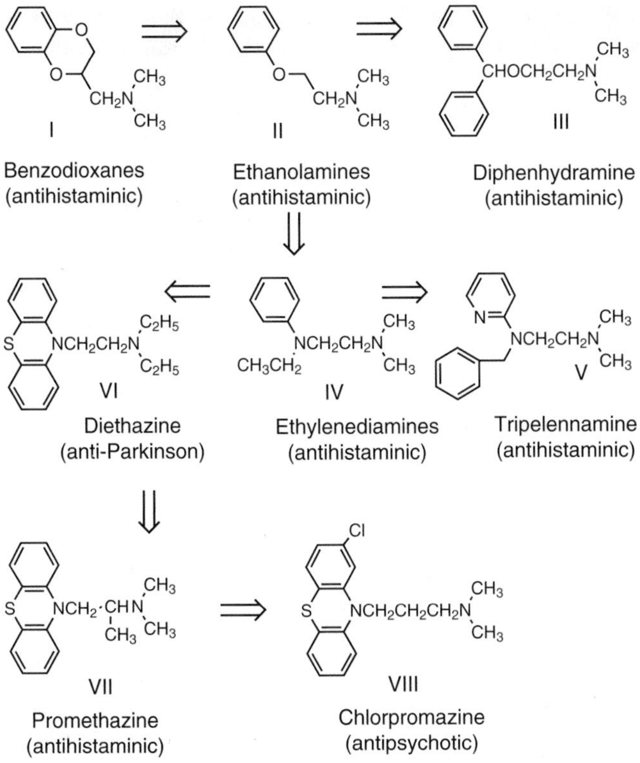

FIGURE 14.4 Development of phenothiazine-type antipsychotic drugs.

ethers (type III), which are characterized by the clinically useful antihistamine diphenhydramine, or to ethylenediamine (type IV), which led to antihistamine drugs, such as tripelennamine (type V). Further modification of the ethylenediamine type of antihistamine resulted in the incorporation of one of the nitrogen atoms into a phenothiazine ring system, which produced phenothiazine (type VI), a compound that was found to have antihistaminic properties and, similar to many other antihistaminic drugs, a strong sedative effect. Diethazine (type VI) is more useful in the treatment of Parkinson disease (because of its potent antimuscarinic action) than in allergies, whereas promethazine (type VII) is clinically used as an antihistaminic. After the ability of promethazine to prolong barbiturate-induced sleep in rodents was discovered, the drug was introduced into clinical anesthesia as a potentiating agent.

To enhance the sedative effects of such phenothiazines, Charpentier and Courvoisier synthesized and evaluated many modifications of promethazine. This research effort eventually led to the synthesis of chlorpromazine (type VIII) in 1950 at the Rhône-Poulenc Laboratories (42). Soon thereafter, the French surgeon Laborit and his coworkers described the ability of this compound to potentiate anesthetics and produce artificial hibernation (43). They noted that chlorpromazine, by itself, did not cause a loss of consciousness but did produce only a tendency to sleep and a marked disinterest in the surroundings. The first attempts to treat mental illness with chlorpromazine alone were made in Paris in 1951 and early 1952 by Paraire and Sigwald. In 1952, Delay and Deniker began their important work with chlorpromazine (44). They were convinced that chlorpromazine achieved more than symptomatic relief of agitation or anxiety and that this drug had an ameliorative effect on psychosis. Thus, what initially involved minor molecular modifications of an antihistamine that produced sedative side effects resulted in the development of a major class of drugs that initiated a new era in the drug therapy for the mentally ill. More than anything else in the history of psychiatry, the phenothiazines and related drugs have positively influenced the lives of schizophrenic patients, enabling them to assume a greatly improved role in society.

More than 24 phenothiazine and the related thioxanthene derivatives are used in medicine, most of them for psychiatric conditions. The structures, generic and trade names, doses, and effects of phenothiazine-type and thioxanthene-type neuroleptics currently in use are listed in Table 14.1.

STRUCTURE–ACTIVITY RELATIONSHIPS It is presumed that phenothiazine and thioxanthene neuroleptics mediate their pharmacologic effects mainly through interactions at D_2-type dopamine receptors. Examination of the x-ray structures of dopamine (in the preferred *trans*-α-rotamer conformation) and chlorpromazine shows that these two structures can be partly superimposed (Fig. 14.5) (45). In the preferred conformation of chlorpromazine, its side chain tilts away from the midline toward the chlorine-substituted ring.

The electronegative chlorine atom on ring "a" is responsible for imparting asymmetry to this molecule, and the attraction of the amine side chain (protonated at physiologic pH) toward the ring containing the chlorine atom indicates an important structural feature of such molecules. Phenothiazine and related compounds lacking a chlorine atom in this position are, in most cases, inactive as neuroleptic drugs. In addition to the ring "a" substituent, another major requirement for therapeutic efficacy of phenothiazines is that the side-chain amine contain three carbons separating the two nitrogen atoms (Fig. 14.5). Phenothiazines with two carbon atoms separating the two nitrogen atoms lack antipsychotic efficacy. Compounds such as promethazine (Fig. 14.4, VII) are primarily antihistaminic and are less likely to assume the preferred conformation.

When thioxanthene derivatives that contain an olefinic double bond between the tricyclic ring and the side chain are examined, it can be seen that such structures can exist in either the *cis* or *trans* isomeric configuration. For example, the *cis* isomer of the neuroleptic thiothixene (marketing was recently discontinued) is several-fold more active than both the *trans* isomer and the compound obtained from saturation of the double bond.

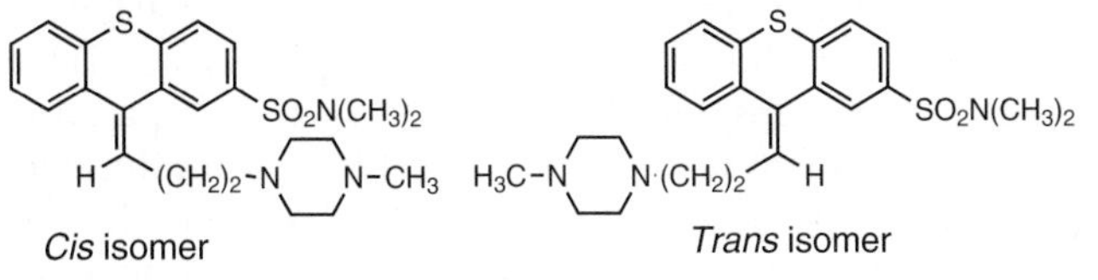

Thiothixene

Structure D in Figure 14.5 shows that the active structure of dopamine does not superimpose with a *trans*-like

TABLE 14.1 Phenothiazine and the Thioxanthene Derivatives Used as Neuroleptics*

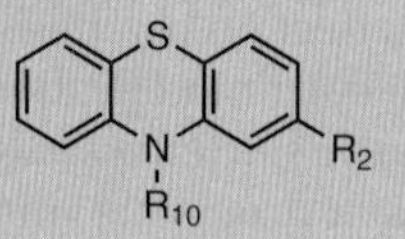

Phenothiazine-Type Generic Name	Trade Name	R_{10}	R_2	Adult Antipsychotic Oral Dose Range (mg/d)	Side Effects** Sedative Effects	Extra-pyramidal Effects	Hypotensive Effects	Other Effects
Chlorpromazine hydrochloride	Thorazine	$(CH_2)_3N(CH_3)_2 \cdot HCl$	Cl	300–800	+++	++	Oral ++ IM +++	Antiemetic dose 10–25 mg every 4–6 h
Thioridazine hydrochloride	Mellaril	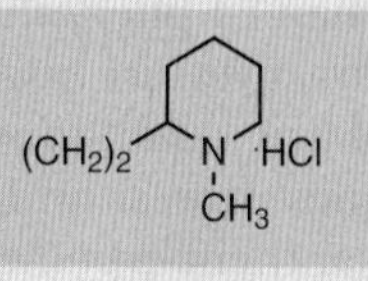	SCH_3	200–600	+++	+	++	
Mesoridazine mesylate	Serentil	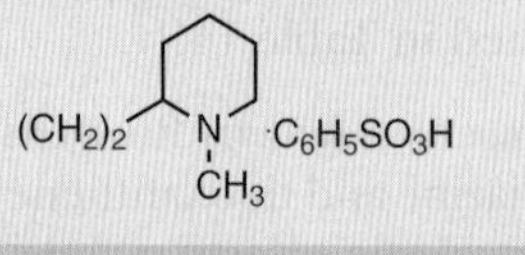	$\overset{O}{\overset{\|}{S}}CH_3$	75–300	+++	+	++	
Perphenazine	Trilafon	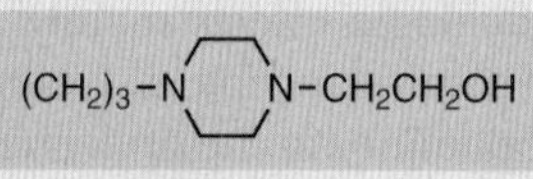	Cl	8–32	++	+++	+	
Prochlorperazine edisylate, maleate	Compazine	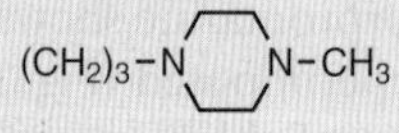	Cl	75–100	++	+++	+	Antiemetic dose 5–10 mg every 4–6 h
Fluphenazine hydrochloride	Permitil, Prolixin	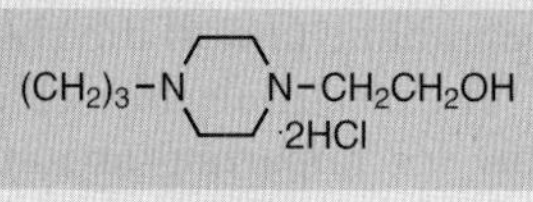	CF_3	1–20	+	+++	+	
Trifluoperazine hydrochloride	Stelazine	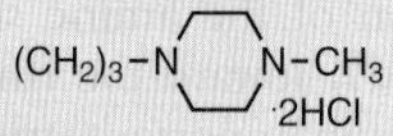	CF_3	6–20	+	+++	+	
Thiethylperazine maleate	Torecan	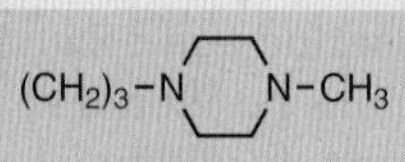	SCH_2CH_3		+	+	+	Antiemetic dose 10–30 mg daily
Thioxanthene-Type								
Thiothixene hydrochloride	Navane	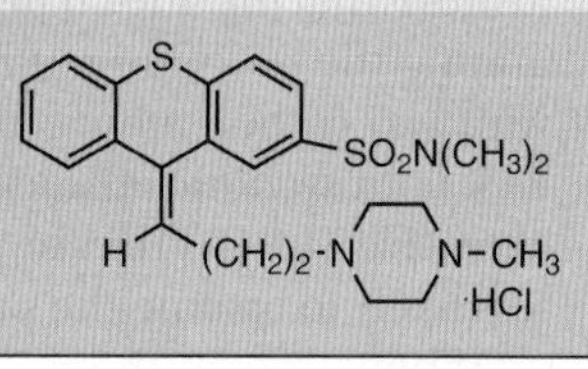		6–30	++	++	++	

*The phenothiazine derivatives that are effective in the treatment of nausea and vomiting are included in this listing. ** +++, high; ++, medium; +, low. IM, intramuscular.

conformer of chlorpromazine that would be predicted to be inactive.

Long-Acting Neuroleptics The duration of action of many of the neuroleptics with a free hydroxyl moiety (OH, as in perphenazine, fluphenazine, and acetophenazine; Table 14.1) can be considerably prolonged by the preparation of long-chain fatty acid esters (Table 14.2). Thus, fluphenazine decanoate and fluphenazine enanthate were the first of these esters to appear in clinical use and are longer acting, with fewer side effects, than the unesterified precursor. The ability to treat patients with a single intramuscular injection every 1 to 2 weeks with the enanthate or every 2 to 3 weeks with the decanoate ester means that problems associated with patient compliance to the drug regimens and with drug malabsorption can be reduced. Table 14.2 lists long-acting forms of phenothiazine-type and thioxanthene-type neuroleptics that are derivatives available in the United States and other countries. Long-acting forms of other typical (haloperidol) and atypical antipsychotics are given in the corresponding sections below.

Metabolism Increasing evidence suggests that the metabolism of neuroleptic drugs is of major significance in the effects of these drugs. Although considerable information about the metabolism of the extensively studied

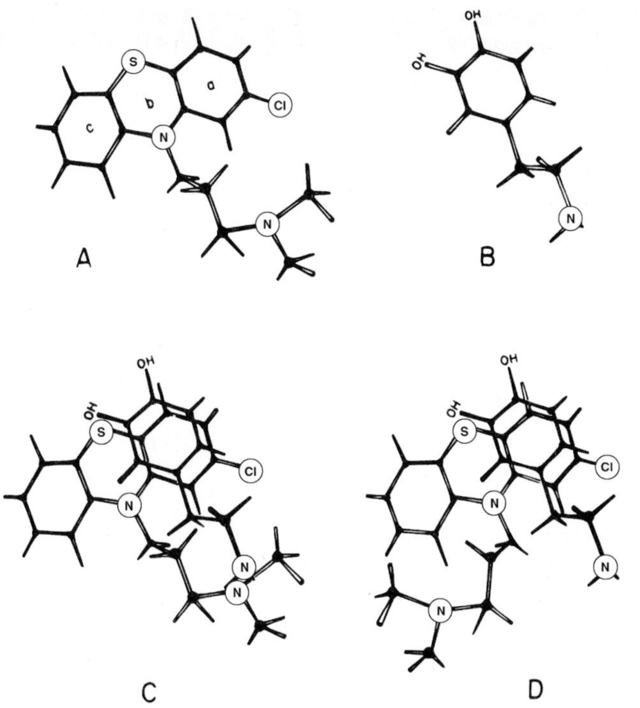

FIGURE 14.5 Conformations of chlorpromazine (A), dopamine (B), and their superposition (C) as determined by x-ray crystallographic analysis. The a, b, and c in (A) designate rings. Also shown (D) is another conformation in which the alkyl side chain of chlorpromazine is in the *trans* conformation (ring a and amino side chain), which is not superimposable onto dopamine. (Adapted from Horn AS, Snyder SH. Chlorpromazine and dopamine: conformational similarities that correlate with the antischizophrenic activity of phenothiazine drugs. Proc Natl Acad Sci USA 1971;68:2325–2328, with permission.)

chlorpromazine is available, information about many of the other drugs administered for prolonged periods is scant. Generally, however, the liver microsomal cytochrome P450–catalyzed metabolic pathways for neuroleptics are similar to those for many other drugs. Some metabolic pathways for chlorpromazine are shown in Figure 14.6. It should be kept in mind that during metabolism, several processes can and do occur for the same molecule. For example, chlorpromazine can be demethylated, sulfoxidized, hydroxylated, and glucuronidated to yield 7-*O*-glu-nor-CPZ-SO. The combination of such processes leads to more than 100 identified metabolites. Evidence indicates that the 7-hydroxylated derivatives and, possibly, other hydroxylated derivatives, as well as the mono- and didesmethylated products (nor_1-CPZ, nor_2-CPZ), are active in vivo and at dopamine D_2 receptors, whereas the sulfoxide (CPZ-SO) is inactive. Although the thioxanthenes are closely related to the phenothiazines in their pharmacologic effects, there seems to be at least one major difference in metabolism: Most of the thioxanthenes do not form ring-hydroxylated derivatives. Metabolic pathways for phenothiazines and thioxanthenes are significantly altered, both quantitatively and qualitatively, by a number of factors, including species, age, gender, interaction with other drugs, and route of administration.

Development of Butyrophenone Neuroleptics

In the late 1950s, Janssen and coworkers synthesized the propiophenone and butyrophenone analogs of meperidine in an effort to increase its analgesic potency (46). Both the propiophenone and butyrophenone analogs had greater analgesic potency than meperidine, but, only the butyrophenone analog also displayed activity resembling that of chlorpromazine.

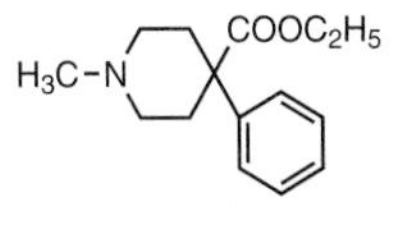

Meperidine

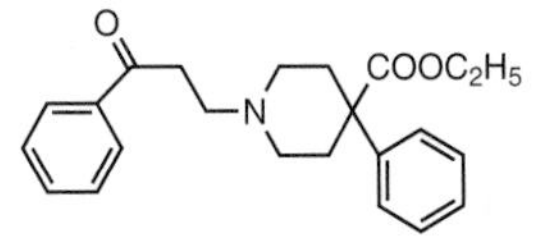

Propiophenone analog

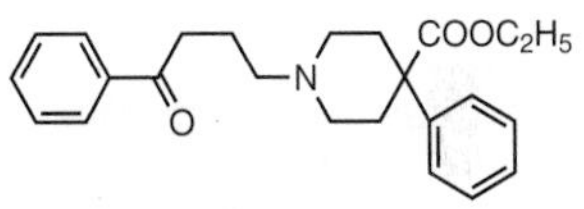

Butyrophenone analog

The structure–activity results of Janssen and coworkers showed that it was possible to eliminate the analgesic activity and, simultaneously, to enhance the chlorpromazine-like neuroleptic activity in the butyrophenone series.

STRUCTURE–ACTIVITY RELATIONSHIPS All butyrophenone derivatives displaying high neuroleptic potency have the following general structure:

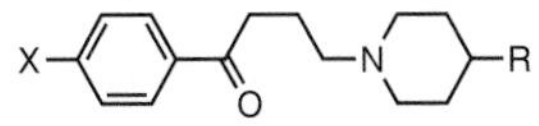

X = F or OCH_3

The attachment of a tertiary amino group to the fourth carbon of the butyrophenone skeleton is essential for neuroleptic activity; lengthening, shortening, or branching of the three-carbon propyl chain decreases neuroleptic potency. Replacement of the keto moiety (e.g., with the thioketone group as in the butyrothienones, with olefinic or phenoxy groups, or reduction of the carbonyl group) decreases neuroleptic potency. In addition, most potent butyrophenone compounds have a fluorine substituent in the para position of the benzene ring. Variations are possible in the tertiary amino group without loss of neuroleptic potency; for example, the basic nitrogen usually is incorporated into a six-membered ring (piperidine, tetrahydropyridine, or piperazine) that is substituted in the para position.

In most respects, the pharmacologic effects of butyrophenones differ in degree, but not in kind, from those of the piperazine phenothiazines. Consistent with its higher affinity for dopamine D_2 receptors (15), haloperidol produces a higher incidence of extrapyramidal reactions than chlorpromazine, but sedative effects in moderate

TABLE 14.2 Long-Acting Neuroleptics for Intramuscular Depot Injection

Phenothiazines Generic Name	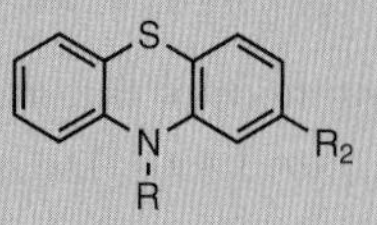 R	R_2	Dosage Range (mg)	Typical Duration of Action (wk)
Fluphenazine enanthate	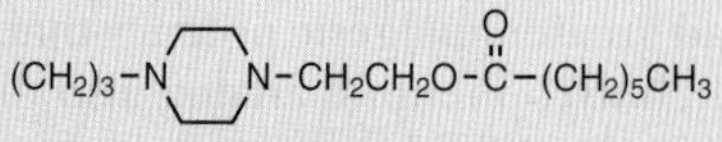	CF_3	25–100	112
Fluphenazine decanoate	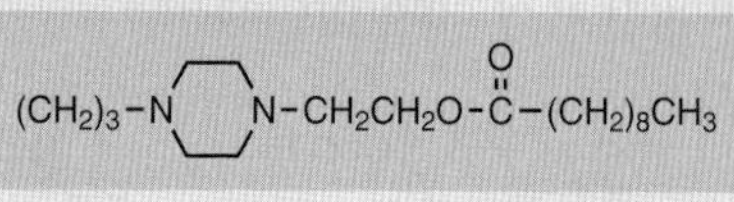	CF_3	25–200	2–3
Perphenazine enanthate	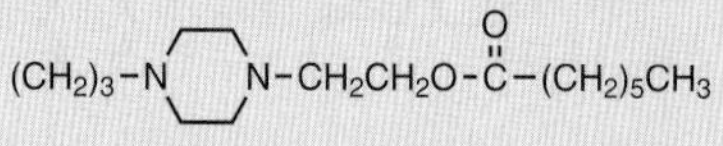	Cl	25–100	1–2
Thioxanthene				
Flupenthixol decanoate	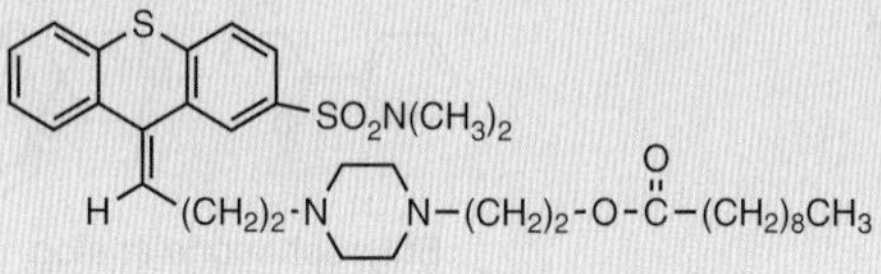		100–200	1–2

Adapted from Simpson and Lee (48) and Baldessarini and Tarsy (9,10).

doses are less than those observed with phenothiazines (47). Butyrophenones have less prominent autonomic effects than the phenothiazine-type antipsychotic drugs, and only mild hypotension occurs. Also, haloperidol has less propensity to induce weight gain than chlorpromazine and most of the second-generation antipsychotic drugs (see later discussion).

Haloperidol was introduced for the treatment of psychoses in Europe in 1958 and in the United States in 1967 (48). It is an effective alternative to more familiar antipsychotic phenothiazine drugs and also is used for the manic phase of bipolar (manic-depressive) disorder. Haloperidol decanoate has been introduced as depot maintenance therapy. When injected every 4 to 6 weeks, the drug appears to be as effective as daily orally administered haloperidol. Other currently available (mostly in Europe) butyrophenones include the very potent spiperone (spiroperidol) as well as trifluperidol and droperidol (Fig. 14.7). Droperidol, a short-acting, sedating butyrophenone, is used in anesthesia for its sedating and antiemetic effects and, sometimes, in psychiatric emergencies as a sedative-neuroleptic. Droperidol often is administered in combination with the potent narcotic analgesic fentanyl for preanesthetic sedation and anesthesia.

Modification of the haloperidol butyrophenone side chain by replacement of the keto function with a di-4-flurophenylmethane moiety results in diphenylbutyl piperidine neuroleptics, such as pimozide, penfluridol, and fluspirilene. The diphenylbutyl piperidine neuroleptics have a longer duration of action than the butyrophenone analogs. All are effective in the control of schizophrenia, and pimozide in particular has been shown to be useful in treating acute exacerbation of schizophrenia and in reducing the rate of relapse in chronic schizophrenic patients (49).

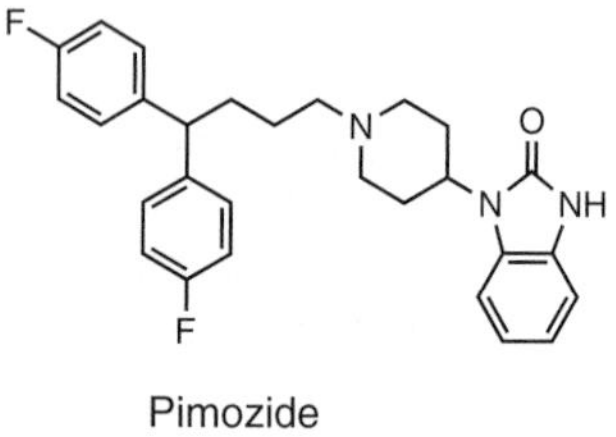

Pimozide

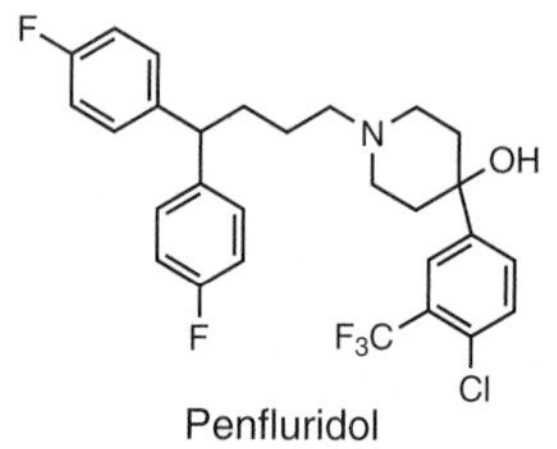

Penfluridol

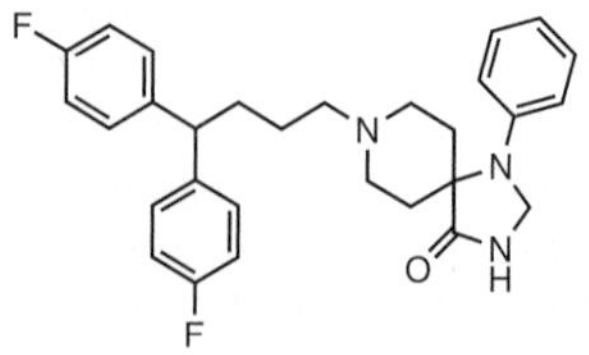

Fluspirilene

Pimozide (Orap) also is used for treatment of Tourette syndrome (49), a movement disorder that is characterized by facial tics, grimaces, strange and uncontrollable sounds, and sometimes, involuntary shouting of obscenities. This disorder may be misdiagnosed by clinicians as schizophrenia. Typically, the onset of Tourette syndrome occurs at age 10, and standard treatment for Tourette syndrome in the past has been the neuroleptics, such as

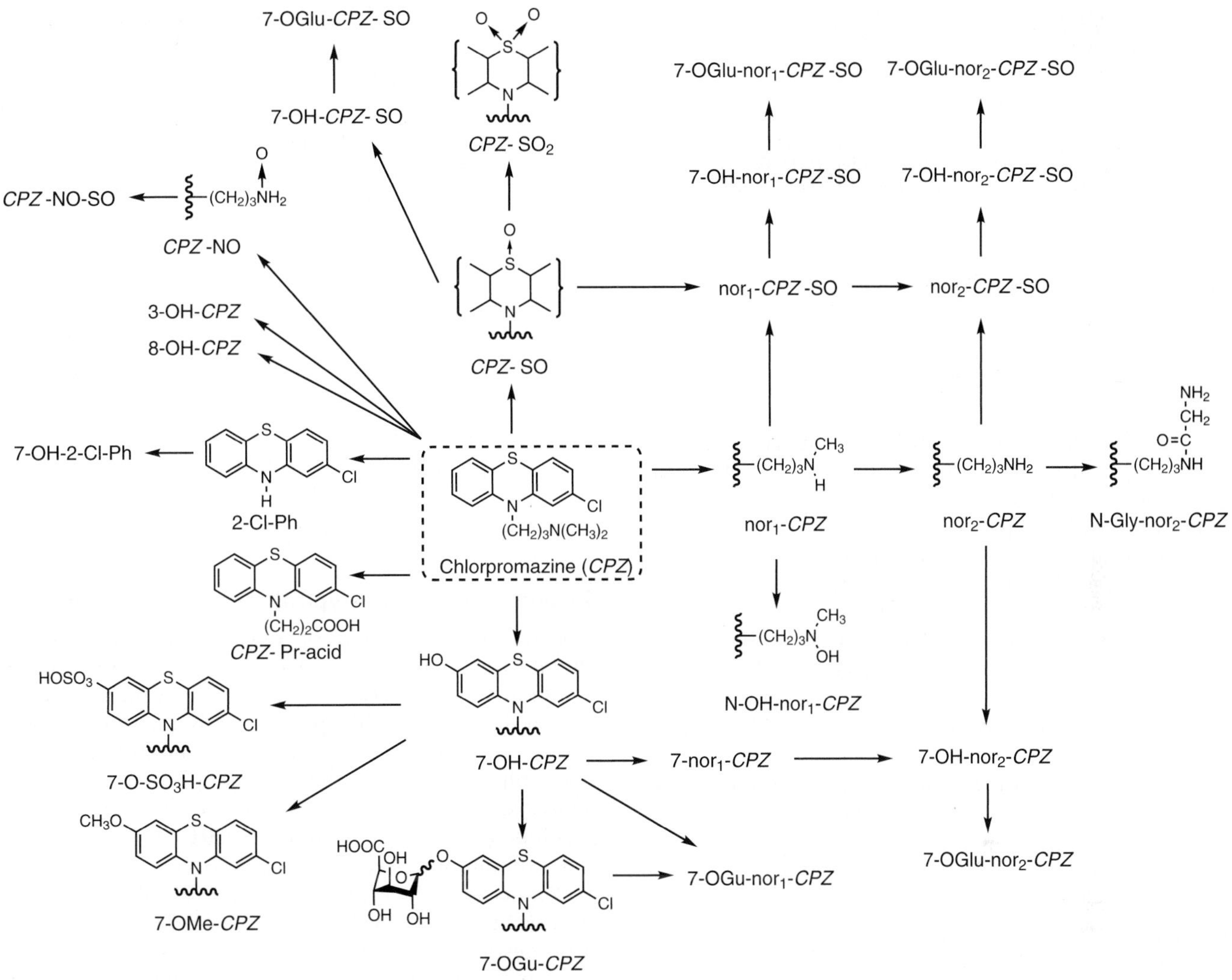

FIGURE 14.6 Metabolism of chlorpromazine. CPZ, chlorpromazine; NO, *N*-oxide; O-Glu, *O*-glucuronide; O-SO_3H, sulfate; Ph, phenothiazine; Pr-acid, propionic acid; SO, sulfoxide; SO_2, sulfone.

haloperidol. Chronic treatment of Tourette syndrome with haloperidol as well as with pimozide carries the risk of producing tardive dyskinesia. Penfluridol and fluspirilene, although not currently available in the United States, are other examples of long-acting neuroleptics in this structure class.

Metabolism Haloperidol is readily absorbed from the gastrointestinal tract. Peak plasma levels occur 2 to 6 hours after ingestion. The drug is concentrated in the liver and CNS. Approximately 15% of a given dose is excreted in the bile, and approximately 40% is eliminated through the kidney. Figure 14.8 shows the typical oxidative metabolic pathway of butyrophenones as exemplified by haloperidol (50,51).

Benzamide Derivatives with Neuroleptic Activity

Similar to the phenothiazine antiemetics (e.g., promethazine), certain benzamide derivatives such as metoclopramide antagonize dopamine D_2-type receptors in the chemoreceptor trigger zone of the brainstem and have neuroleptic activity (52,53). Metoclopramide is an efficacious antiemetic drug that modifies gastric motility, but it is not clinically effective for psychoses. Its antagonism of D_2 receptors in myenteric motor neurons increases acetylcholine release to result in a prokinetic effect on the gastrointestinal tract (54). Metoclopramide also binds to serotonin 5-HT_3 and 5-HT_4 receptors with low affinity (15), and these systems also are proposed to account for its effects to lower esophageal sphincter tone and stimulate antral and small intestine contractions, making it useful to treat gastroesophageal reflux disease and to promote gastric emptying (54).

Several analogs of metoclopramide in which the side chain is incorporated into a pyrrolidine ring include *S*-(−)-sulpiride and *S*-(−)-remoxipride. Both drugs display neuroleptic properties.

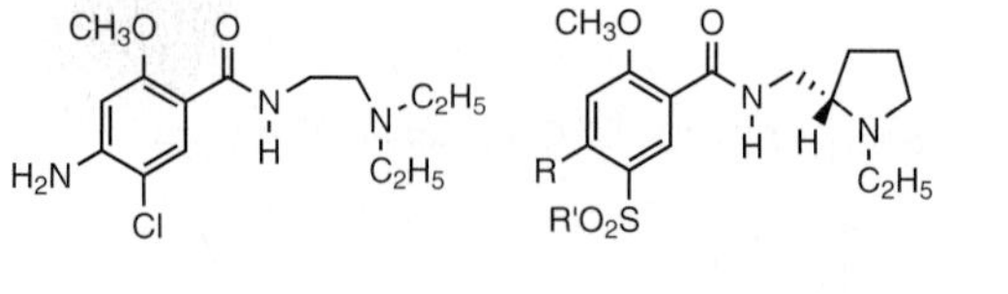

Metoclopramide (Reglan)

S-(-)-Sulpiride, R = H, R' = NH_2
Amisulpride, R = NH_2, R' = Et

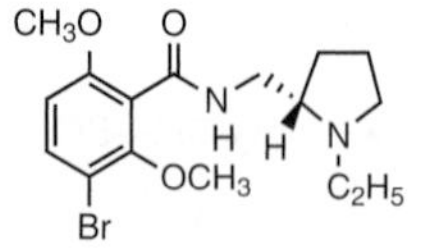

S-(-)-Remoxipride

Sulpiride produces a relatively low incidence of extrapyramidal side effects, putatively because of a preferential effect on limbic versus extrapyramidal (striatum) tissue. The hydrophilic properties of sulpiride may account for its poor oral absorption, limited penetration into the CNS, and resulting low potency. The racemic para-amino congener of sulpiride, amisulpride, is used as an antipsychotic agent outside the United States. Remoxipride was a promising neuroleptic that is comparable to haloperidol in potency and efficacy and has less incidence of extrapyramidal and autonomic side effects. Life-threatening aplastic anemia, however, was reported with remoxipride use, which prompted its withdrawal from the market.

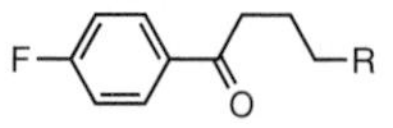

Generic names	Trade names	R
Haloperidol	Haldol	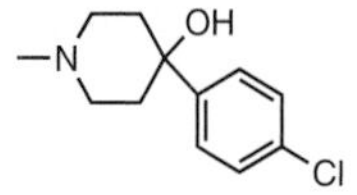
Haloperidol decanoate		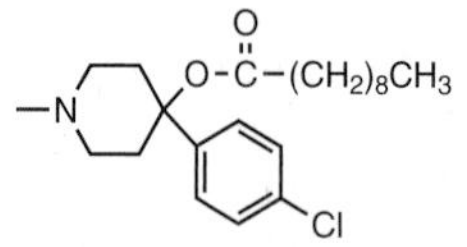
Spiperone		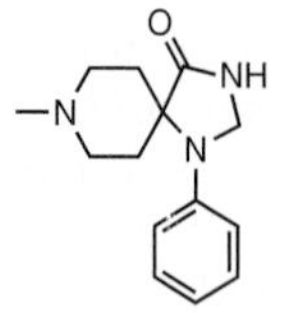
Trifluperidol		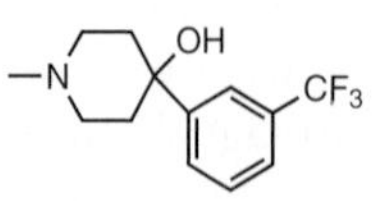
Droperidol	Inapsine	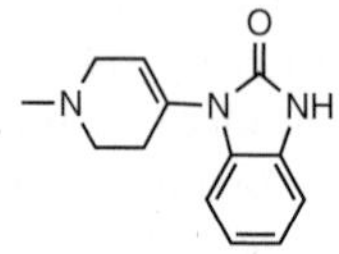

FIGURE 14.7 Haloperidol and it analogs.

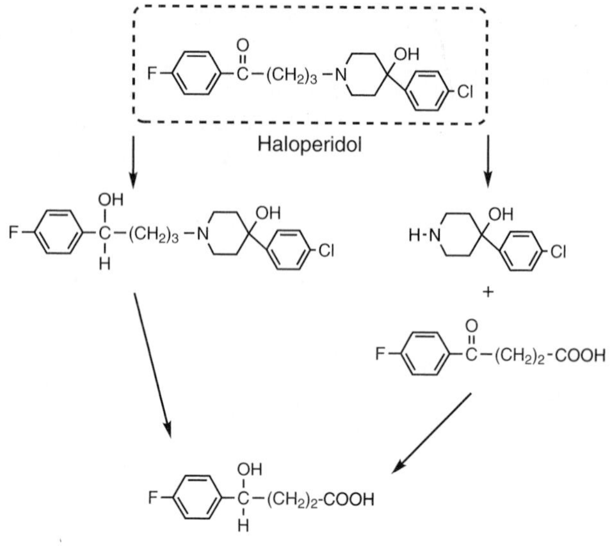

FIGURE 14.8 Metabolism of haloperidol.

Second-Generation (Atypical) Antipsychotic Drugs

The second generation of so-called atypical antipsychotic drugs emerged in 1990 with the introduction of the benzazepine derivative, clozapine, which was initially indicated for schizophrenia resistant to treatment by typical antipsychotics such as the phenothiazines and butyrophones. This was followed by approval of the first benzisoxazole and benzisothiazole derivatives such as risperidone (1994) and ziprasidone (2001). The arylpiperazine quinolinone derivative, aripiprazole (introduced in 2002), occasionally is referred to as a "third-generation" antipsychotic drug because its mechanism of action is hypothesized to involve GPCR functional selectivity; however, its GPCR binding profile is characteristic of other second-generation antipsychotics, and it is classified as such here. It is reiterated that atypical second-generation antipsychotics interact with several aminergic neurotransmitter GPCRs, have a mechanism of antipsychotic action other than (or in addition to) postsynaptic dopamine D_2 receptor blockade, and produce less incidence of extrapyramidal movement disorder side effects.

Mechanism of Action for Antipsychotic Efficacy and Side Effects

Currently, it is generally accepted that the efficacy of second-generation (atypical) antipsychotic drugs involves their actions at both dopamine D_2-type and serotonin 5-HT_{2A} receptors. It is naïve with current understanding to definitively classify such actions as inverse agonism, agonism, partial agonism, or neutral antagonism given that ligands interacting at dopamine and serotonin GPCRs are functionally selective (21–25) (i.e., drug functional activity depends on the neurophysiologic neuroanatomic circumstances). It is likely that activity of atypical antipsychotics at other serotonin GPCRs (5-HT_{1A}, 5-HT_6, and/or 5-HT_7), adrenergic (α_1 and/or α_2) GPCRs, acetylcholine

NEUROTOXICOLOGY OF HALOPERIDOL

As discussed in the section on side effects of neuroleptics, untoward extrapyramidal effects occur in 30% to 50% of patients receiving standard doses of typical neuroleptics. Extrapyramidal side effects include acute dystonias, akathisia, and parkinsonian-type symptoms, such as bradykinesia, cogwheel rigidity, tremor, masked face, and shuffling gait. Tardive dyskinesia, a severe extrapyramidal side effect that occurs in 15% to 25% of patients after prolonged neuroleptic treatment, is characterized by stereotyped, involuntary, repetitive, choreiform movements of the face, eyelids, mouth, tongue, extremities, and trunk. The pathophysiology of tardive dyskinesia is not known, and the disorder essentially is irreversible.

The severe and sometimes irreversible dyskinesias associated with haloperidol pharmacotherapy are hypothesized to result from neurotoxicity involving dopaminergic systems. In fact, the central and peripheral biochemical and resulting pathophysiologic features of haloperidol-induced movement disorders are similar to the potent dopaminergic neurotoxicant and parkinsonian-producing agent, 1-methyl-4-phenyl-1,2,3,6-tetrahydropyridine (MPTP) (see Chapter 13).

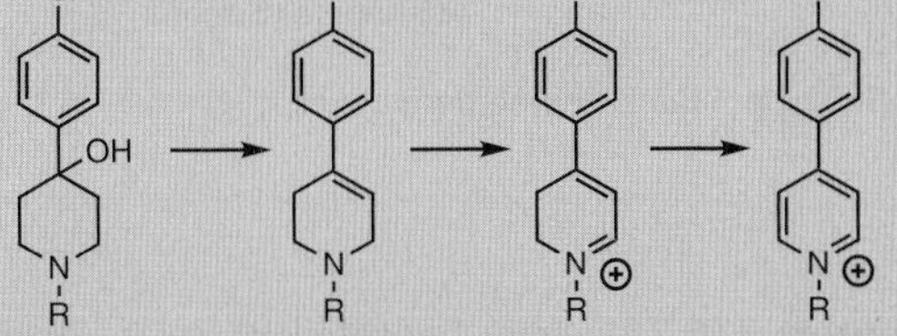

HP HPTP HPP+

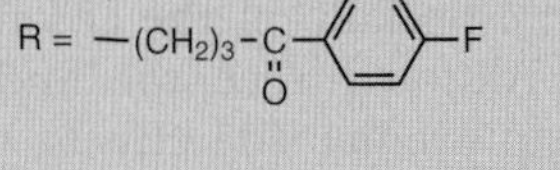

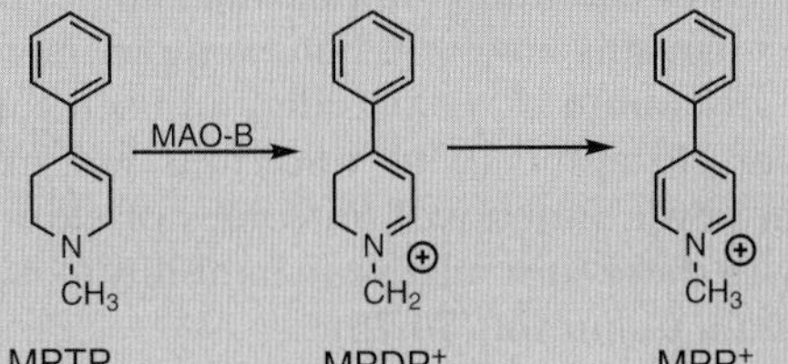

MPTP MPDP+ MPP+

Microsomal-catalyzed dehydration of haloperidol yields the corresponding haloperidol 1,2,3,6-tetrahydropyridine derivative (HPTP) that is a close analog of the parkinsonian-inducing neurotoxicant MPTP. Long-term (58-week) administration of HPTP to nonhuman primates alters both presynaptic and postsynaptic dopaminergic neuronal function, which may contribute to the parkinsonian-type side effects and tardive dyskinesia that are relatively common with haloperidol pharmacotherapy (55). In baboons treated chronically with HPTP, animals developed orofacial dyskinesia, and histopathologic studies revealed volume loss in the basal forebrain and hypothalamus, along with other neuronal cell loss that may be relevant to the pathophysiology of tardive dyskinesia (56). In humans and baboons, HPTP is oxidized in vivo to the corresponding haloperidol pyridinium species (HPP^+) similar to the oxidation of MPTP to its ultimate neurotoxic species MPP^+. HPP^+ is neurotoxic to dopaminergic and, especially, serotonergic neurons in vivo in rats (57), and HPP^+ has been identified in the urine of humans treated with haloperidol (58). Furthermore, in a recent study involving psychiatric patients who were treated chronically with haloperidol, the severity of tardive dyskinesia and parkinsonism was associated with an increased serum concentration ratio of HPP^+ to haloperidol (59), providing compelling clinical evidence for the neurotoxicity of HPP^+. Investigations continue to determine if neuroleptic-induced pathology of the extrapyramidal motor system, such as that associated with tardive dyskinesia, may be related to production of MPP^+/HPP^+-type species in humans.

See Chapter 13 for a related discussion of Parkinson disease caused by MPTP.

muscarinic (M_1, M_5) GPCRs, and/or histamine H_1 GPCRs also accounts for their psychotherapeutic effects, especially modulation of "negative" signs/symptoms (8,9,60). Certainly, antipsychotic drug action at these other neurotransmitter systems in the brain and periphery can contribute to untoward side effects (e.g., sedative, cardiovascular, gastrointestinal, ophthalmic, sexual, urinary).

The high 5-HT_{2A} receptor affinity of second-generation antipsychotics may account for their low propensity to cause extrapyramidal side effects, but reduced affinity for D_2 receptors likely plays a role. Nevertheless, antagonism of presynaptic 5-HT_{2A} receptors that inhibit dopamine release from striatal dopaminergic nerve terminals could increase dopaminergic neurotransmission in the striatum to modulate postsynaptic D_2 blockade and reduce extrapyramidal symptoms.

Weight gain and general metabolic dysregulation that leads to type 2 diabetes and cardiovascular disease is problematic for both first-generation (typical) and second-generation (atypical) antipsychotic drugs; however, this issue previously was obscured for the first-generation drugs due to concern about their much more serious extrapyramidal side effects. The mechanism for antipsychotic-induced weight gain and metabolic syndrome is not known for certain, but likely involves serotonin 5-HT_{2C} and/or histamine H_1 GPCR antagonism or inverse agonism (31,32,36,61,62). Meta-analyses consistently show that clozapine and olanzapine produce the most weight gain in the most patients, whereas quetiapine, risperidone, and chlorpromazine produce intermediate effects, and haloperidol, ziprasidone, and aripiprazole cause smaller changes in weight.

With regard to antipsychotic efficacy between the first-generation (typical) and the second-generation (atypical) drugs, a recent meta-analysis indicates there is no evidence for differences (63–65). Furthermore, there is no evidence for superiority of one second-generation versus another second-generation antipsychotic drug with regard to treatment of positive or negative symptoms of schizophrenia (66–70). Differences between first-generation and second-generation antipsychotic drugs, as well as differences among second-generation antipsychotic drugs, are only in regard to their side effect profile (8–10,60–71).

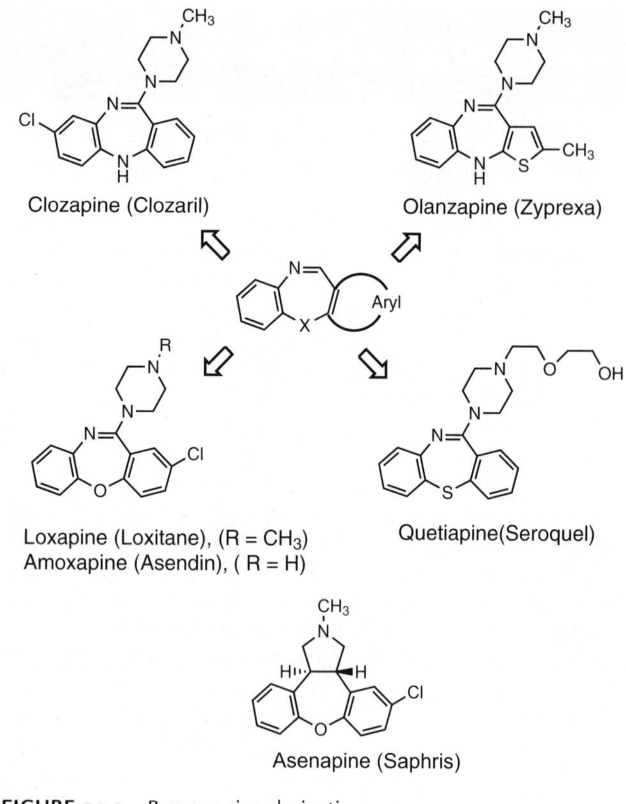

FIGURE 14.9 Benzazepine derivatives.

Benzazepine and Related Analogs

The structures of the benzazepine derivatives, clozapine, olanzapine, loxapine, amoxapine, and quetiapine, and the related dibenzo-oxepine asenapine, are shown in Figure 14.9.

Specific Drugs

Clozapine The dibenzazepine clozapine is the prototype of second-generation atypical antipsychotic drugs that have minimal extrapyramidal side effects and do not produce tardive dyskinesia with long-term use. Clozapine also appears to effectively alleviate the negative symptoms of schizophrenia and has proven to be beneficial in treating patients who do not respond adequately to typical first-generation neuroleptic agents, such as the phenothiazines or butyrophenones. A serious drawback to the use of clozapine, however, is the potentially fatal agranulocytosis that is reported to occur in 1% to 2% of patients; decreased white blood cell count is not common with other second-generation antipsychotics, including drugs from the benzazepine (e.g., olanzapine, quetiapine) and benzisoxazole (e.g., risperidone) chemical classes (66–70,72).

The GPCR profile for clozapine is very well characterized with respect to binding (15) but not with respect to function. According to the literature, most researchers and clinicians seem to assume that clozapine is an antagonist at various GPCRs (8–10,66–70); however, the functional selectivity hypothesis (18–21) suggests this view may be too simplistic. Moreover, neurotransmitter receptor systems for which clozapine has no apparent affinity, such as glutamate *N*-methyl-D-aspartate (NMDA) receptors (15,73), may be relevant to its antipsychotic mechanism of action. Thus, receptor binding profiles can offer only a clue to the mechanism of action for predicting efficacy, especially, in the absence of functional selectivity data. Although receptor binding profiles may be useful to help predict side effects, they fall short to advance understanding of pharmacologic and physiologic mechanisms involved. For example, myriad studies link the histamine H_1 (especially) and serotonin 5-HT_{2C} affinity of clozapine to its notorious weight gain side effect; however, functional outcomes of clozapine interaction with these sites relative to its ability to cause weight gain remain unknown (74,75).

Clozapine has moderate affinity (K_i ~250 to 500 nmol/L) at human dopamine D_1, D_2, and D_3, but moderate affinity (K_i ~50 nmol/L) at D_4 and D_5 GPCRs. It also has moderate affinity (K_i ~25 to 100 nmol/L) at cholinergic muscarinic M_3, M_4, and M_5 GPCRs but high affinity (K_i ~10 nmol/L) at M_1 and M_2 GPCRs. High affinity (K_i ≤10 nmol/L) also is apparent at serotonin 5-HT_{2A}, 5-HT_{2B}, 5-HT_{2C}, 5-HT_6, and 5-HT_7 GPCRs (moderate affinity at 5-HT_{1A}). Clozapine has very high affinity (K_i ≤5 nmol/L) at histamine H_1 and adrenergic α_1-type GPCRs (moderate affinity at α_2). The incidence of clozapine-induced weight gain is the highest among second-generation antipsychotic drugs except olanzapine, and clozapine also produces a higher incidence of sedation and seizures (61,66–70).

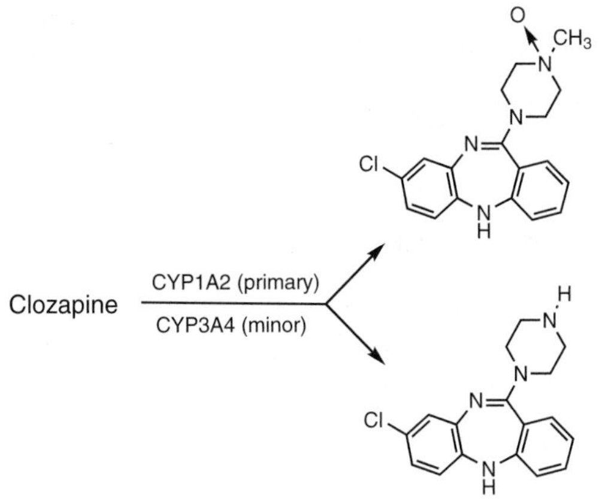

FIGURE 14.10 Metabolism of clozapine.

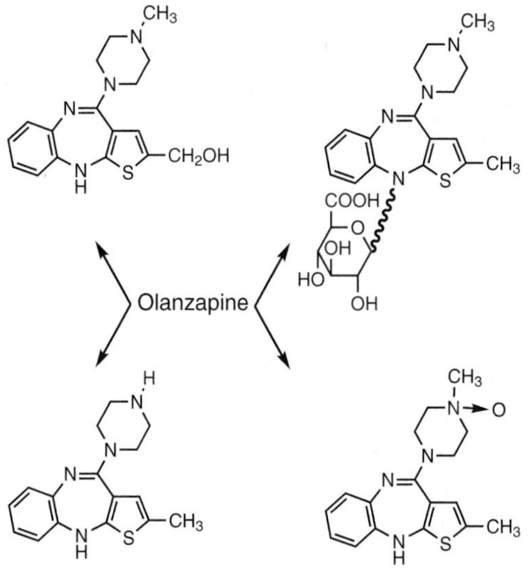

FIGURE 14.11 Metabolism of olanzapine.

Clozapine is orally active and metabolized mainly by CYP1A2 with an important contribution by CYP3A4, although there is a high degree of between-subject and within-subject variability (Fig. 14.10) (76,77). The main products of metabolism are inactive hydroxyl and *N*-oxide derivatives, and the half-life is approximately 12 hours. *N*-Desmethylclozapine is an active metabolite with a receptor binding profile generally similar to clozapine (15), although with higher affinity at 5-HT_{1A} GPCRs. It is noted that caffeine is metabolized primarily by CYP1A2, and it has been observed that some patients who consume caffeine-containing beverages while taking clozapine show signs of increased arousal and extrapyramidal symptoms, and removal of caffeine results in resolution of these problems (78), suggesting a clinically relevant drug interaction. Also, cigarette smoking induces activity of CYP1A2, and patients who smoke while taking clozapine may have significantly lower serum levels of clozapine (79,80).

Olanzapine The thienobenzodiazepine olanzapine (Fig. 14.9) shares close chemical structural resemblance to clozapine and has a similar receptor binding profile, except it has higher affinity at dopamine D_2 and serotonin 5-HT_{2A} receptors (15). The side effect profile is similar to clozapine, with the exception of agranulocytosis that is not usually seen with olanzapine use. Olanzapine is well absorbed after oral administration and is metabolized mainly by CYP1A2 to inactive metabolites similar to those seen with clozapine (*N*-oxide and *N*-demethylation) along with methyl oxidation and phase 2 glucuronidation (77,81) (Fig. 14.11). The drug had a variable half-life of approximately 20 to 50 hours. There is a long-acting injectable formulation of olanzapine pamoate complex available.

Loxapine The dibenzoxazepine loxapine (Fig. 14.9) has equally high affinity for dopamine D_2-type, serotonin 5-HT_2-type, and histamine H_1 GPCRs, but relatively low affinity at muscarinic GPCRs (15). It undergoes phase 1 aromatic hydroxylation to yield several phenolic metabolites that have even higher affinity for D_2-type receptors than the parent. Loxapine also undergoes *N*-desmethylation to form amoxapine (Fig. 14.9), which is used to treat depression, psychotic depression, and depression accompanied by anxiety or agitation. As with loxapine, aromatic hydroxylation of amoxapine produces metabolites that have D_2 antagonist activity similar to haloperidol. Unlike loxapine, amoxapine has moderate affinity (K_i ~25 nmol/L) for norepinephrine and serotonin neurotransporters and blocks reuptake of these neurotransmitters, a correlate of antidepressant activity. Other benzazepine derivatives, as well as other antipsychotic drugs in general, have no appreciable affinity for norepinephrine, serotonin, or dopamine neurotransporters (15).

Quetiapine Quetiapine (Fig. 14.9) is a dibenzothiazepine with a receptor binding profile similar to that of clozapine, binding with high affinity at histamine H_1 GPCRs and with moderate affinity at dopamine D_2/D_3 (but not D_4), serotonergic 5-HT_{2A} (but not 5-HT_{2C}), adrenergic α_1 and α_2, and muscarinic M_1 (but not M_2 to M_5) GPCRs. Thus, the quetiapine GPCR affinity profile differs from clozapine mainly regarding its selective affinity at M_1 versus other muscarinic receptors and its selective affinity for 5-HT_{2A} versus 5-HT_{2C} receptors. Quetiapine is 100% bioavailable, but first-pass metabolism yields at least 20 metabolites, with the major metabolites shown in Figure 14.12. The major products are the sulfoxide (catalyzed by CYP3A4) and the carboxylic acid (76,82). It does not appear that CYP2D6 or CYP1A2 is involved in quetiapine metabolism, and cigarette smoking does not affect the pharmacokinetics of this drug (77). The half-life of quetiapine is approximately 6 hours.

Asenapine The receptor binding profile of asenapine (Fig. 14.9), as reported by its manufacturers

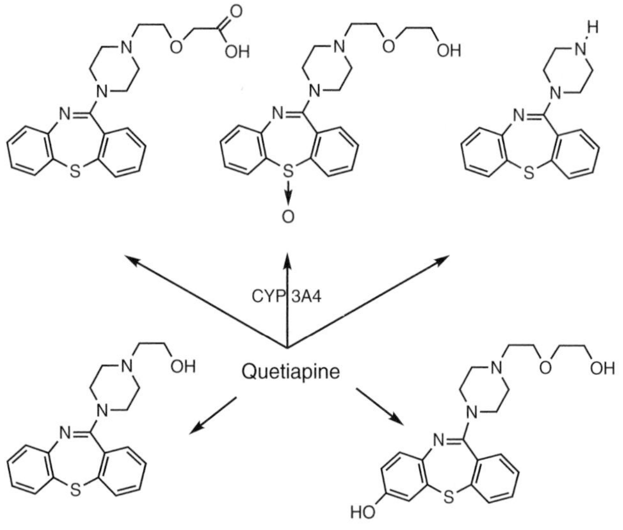

FIGURE 14.12 Major metabolic products of quetiapine.

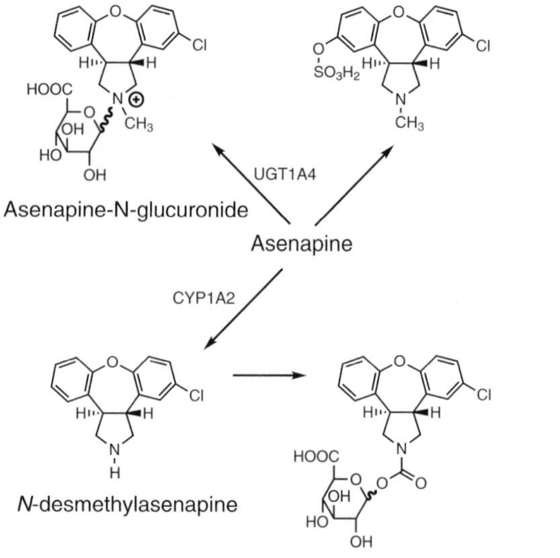

FIGURE 14.13 Major metabolic plasma products for asenapine.

(83), indicates this benzazepine analog significantly differs from clozapine and the other benzazepines in that it has very high affinity (K_i <1 nmol/L) for all of the serotonin 5-HT GPCRs associated with antipsychotic activity (i.e., 5-HT_{1A}, 5-HT_{2A}, 5-HT_{2C}, 5-HT_6, and 5-HT_7). It is reported that asenapine antagonizes the ability of serotonin to activate these receptors (83), but functional selectivity is not reported. Asenapine also antagonizes the ability of dopamine, norepinephrine, and histamine to activate D_2-type, α_2-type, and H_1 receptors, respectively, without regard to functional selectivity (83). Also in contrast to other benzazepines, asenapine has essentially no affinity (K_i >10 μmol/L) for cholinergic muscarinic (M_1 to M_5) GPCRs. Despite some uniqueness regarding its GPCR binding profile, there does not appear to be any efficacy advantages for asenapine over other antipsychotic drugs (first and second generation) for treatment of schizophrenia or bipolar disorder (84,85). Moreover, its side effect profile is similar to other first- and second-generation antipsychotics, except it (expectedly) produces a lower incidence of extrapyramidal effects compared to haloperidol and weight gain is less than with olanzapine (84,85). When given as sublingual tablet, bioavailability is about 35% (<2%, orally) with a half-life of 24 hours. The drug is extensively metabolized to compounds with little or no contributing activity. Direct conjugation by UGT1A4 appears to be a major route of metabolism, giving asenapine-*N*-glucuronide along with *N*-demethylation and aromatic oxidation (primarily by CYP1A2) followed by conjugation (83,84,86) (Fig. 14.13). Approximately 50% of the administered dose is lost via the kidney, and 40% is lost via the fecal route.

Benzisoxazole and Benzisothiazole Derivatives

Neuroanatomic and neurophysiologic interactions between dopaminergic and serotonergic systems, together with evidence that several benzazepine-type antipsychotic agents have high affinity for 5-HT_{2A} receptors, led to the proposal that a combination of D_2/5-HT_{2A} receptor antagonism is required for efficacy in schizophrenia (87,88). Combining the chemical features present in potent benzamide D_2 antagonists (e.g., remoxipride) with those of the benzothiazolyl piperazine 5-HT_{2A} antagonists (e.g., tiospirone) led to the development of the 3-(4-piperidinyl)-1,2-benzisoxazole nucleus present in the 5-HT_{2A}/D_2 antagonists (K_i<5 nmol/L) risperidone and ziprasidone (Fig. 14.14), which also have high affinity (K_i ~5 nmol/L) at histamine H_1 and adrenergic α_1 receptors.

Specific Drugs

Risperidone and Paliperidone Risperidone has very high affinity (K_i ~0.5 nmol/L) for serotonin 5-HT_{2A} and high affinity (K_i ~5 nmol/L) for dopamine D_2 GPCRs (15). It is proposed that the 5-HT_{2A} antagonist activity of risperidone uninhibits dopaminergic neurotransmission in the striatum and cortex, reducing the severity of D_2 antagonist–induced extrapyramidal side effects and alleviating negative symptoms of schizophrenia, while maintaining a blockade of limbic system D_2 receptors (89). In practice, risperidone and its active metabolite marketed as paliperidone (Fig. 14.14) demonstrate a higher incidence of extrapyramidal side effects compared to other second-generation antipsychotics, and they are associated with risk for development of tardive dyskinesia (90,91). Perhaps even more unusual for a second-generation antipsychotic than high D_2-type (including D_3 and D_4) affinity is the essentially zero affinity of risperidone for all five muscarinic GPCRs (15). Other aspects of its GPCR binding profile are unremarkable, including high affinity (K_i <5 nmol/L) for histamine H_1 and adrenergic α_1-type (moderate affinity at α_2-type) receptors. Risperidone is one of the few antipsychotic drugs with very high affinity

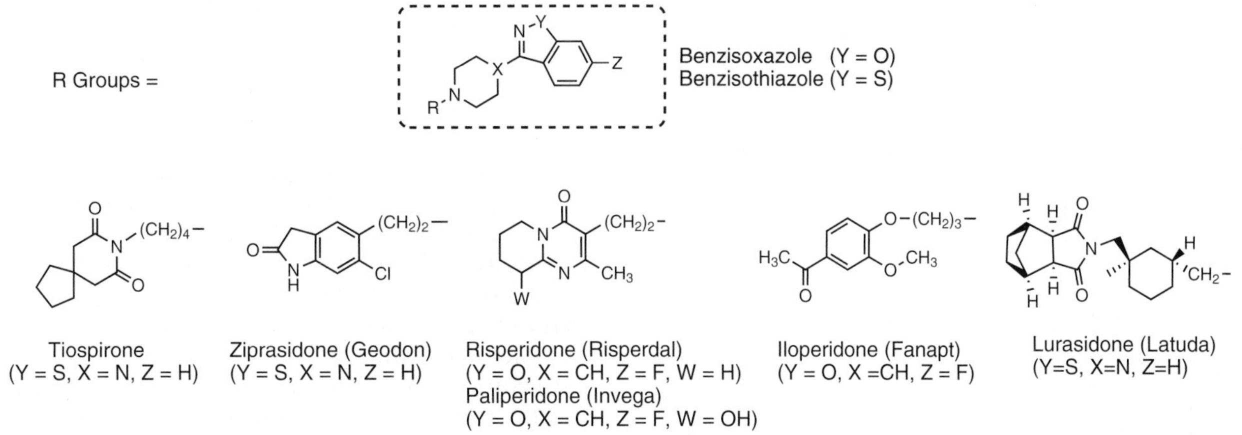

FIGURE 14.14 Benzisoxazole and benzisothiazole antipsychotic agents.

for 5-HT_{2A} receptors that does not also bind tightly to 5-HT_{2C} (K_i ~100 nmol/L) receptors; nevertheless, it produces significant weight gain on par with most other antipsychotics (61).

Risperidone is well absorbed orally and undergoes hepatic CYP2D6- and CYP3A4-catalyzed *N*-dealkylation and 9-hydroxylation; the racemic version of the 9-hydroxy metabolite is marketed separately for schizophrenia as paliperidone (Fig. 14.14). Paliperidone is not extensively metabolized by the liver and is excreted largely unchanged through the kidney. The half-life of risperidone and its 9-hydroxy metabolite (paliperidone) is approximately 22 hours. Patients differ regarding proportions of the (+)- and (−)-enantiomers of paliperidone produced in vivo, with the (+)-enantiomer arising from hydroxylation of risperidone by CYP2D6 and the (−)-enantiomer being formed mainly by action of CYP3A4 (92). There does not appear to be much difference between risperidone and paliperidone regarding pharmacotherapeutic activity or side effect profile (93). Most clinical trials for both drugs were conducted versus placebo, but the limited data available for comparison to other antipsychotics do not show superiority of these agents to other second-generation antipsychotics (94,95). Both drugs are available as long-acting injectable forms—risperidone in a physical complex with carbohydrate microspheres and paliperidone as the palmitate fatty acid ester.

Ziprasidone Ziprasidone is chemically similar to risperidone but with a substitution of piperzinyl and benzisothiazole for piperidinyl and benzisoxazole and with minor aromatic modification (Fig. 14.14). Like risperidone, ziprasidone is a high-affinity antagonist at 5-HT_{2A}, 5-HT_{2C}, and D_2 receptors as well as at adrenergic α_1/α_2 and histamine H_1 receptors. Moreover, ziprasidone can activate 5-HT_{1A} receptors (96) that regulate dopaminergic neurotransmission in brain regions involved in critical cognitive functions, and this activity is thought to be important regarding antipsychotic efficacy (97). It also is suggested that ziprasidone 5-HT_{1A} partial agonist activity contributes to its relatively low incidence of extrapyramidal side effects. Interestingly, ziprasidone has relatively low propensity for inducing weight gain (61) despite its significant affinity at histamine H_1 and serotonin 5-HT_{2C} receptors, which are most often associated with this side effect (31,32,36,61,62). Ziprasidone (half-life, 6 hours) has an oral bioavailability of approximately 60%, which can be enhanced in the presence of fatty foods. It is extensively metabolized (<5% excreted unchanged) by aldehyde oxidase, which results in reductive cleavage of the S–N bond, and then by *S*-methylation. Ziprasidone also can undergo CYP3A4-catalyzed *N*-dealkylation and *S*-oxidation (Fig. 14.15) (98).

Lurasidone Limited data from the manufacturer indicate that lurasidone (Fig. 14.14) is similar to risperidone regarding mainly high affinity (K_i ~2 nmol/L) for serotonin 5-HT_{2A} and dopamine D_2 GPCRs; under the reported assay conditions, lurasidone is an antagonist at these receptors and a partial agonist at 5-HT_{1A} receptors (K_i~7 nmol/L) (99). Lurasidone also is a very high affinity (K_i ~0.5 nmol/L) antagonist at the 5-HT_7 GPCR. There is no significant activity (K_i >10 μmol/L) at muscarinic and histamine H_1 GPCRs.

Currently, there are no rigorous clinical trial data available comparing lurasidone to other antipsychotic drugs; it was approved for treating schizophrenia based on its superiority to placebo only. The most common adverse events reported by the manufacturer are somnolence, akathisia, nausea, parkinsonism, and agitation, along with weight gain (100). Under similar study conditions, lurasidone-induced weight gain was about one-fourth of the olanzapine-induced weight gain. Metabolism is reported (package insert) as oxidative *N*-dealkylation, hydroxylation of the norbornane ring, and *S*-oxidation, mainly by CYP3A4, with a half-life of 18 hours, suitable for once-daily dosing.

Iloperidone This benzisoxazole is very similar to risperidone regarding both its chemical structure and its

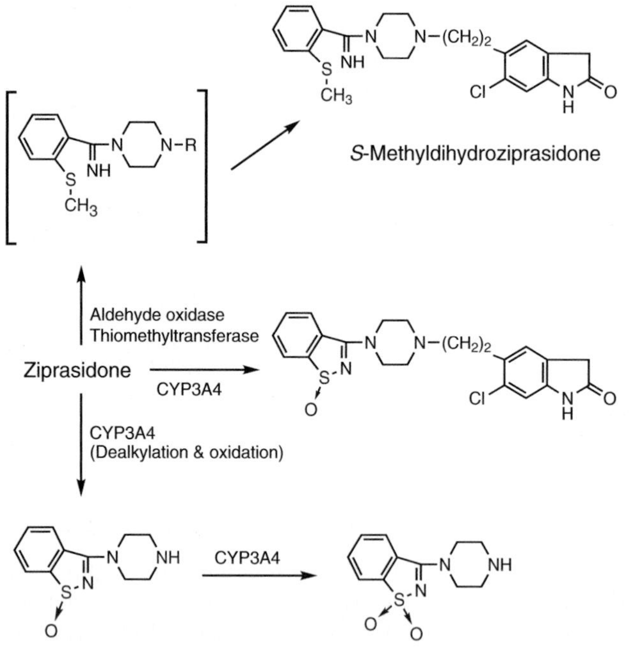

FIGURE 14.15 Metabolism of ziprasidone.

GPCR binding profile (15). Currently, it is not possible to determine with certainty and accuracy how iloperidone may differ from risperidone clinically because clinical trial data currently are available only from industry-sponsored supplemental reports that did not undergo the usual peer-review process (101). In any event, in the few studies where iloperidone was compared to other antipsychotic drugs (haloperidol, risperidone, ziprasidone), there was no difference in antipsychotic efficacy. Not surprisingly, iloperidone produces less severe extrapyramidal side effects than haloperidol, but no comparisons were made with atypical (second-generation) antipsychotics. Iloperidone produces significant weight gain (>7% in acute studies), about the same as haloperidol and much more than risperidone (2.1 vs. 1.8 kg); interestingly, iloperidone and risperidone have about the same affinity at serotonin 5-HT_{2C} and histamine H_1 receptors, which are thought to be responsible for antipsychotic-induced weight gain. As is the case for risperidone, iloperidone is well absorbed orally and undergoes hepatic CYP2D6- and CYP3A4-catalyzed *N*-dealkylation. A majority of iloperidone is recovered unchanged in feces, indicating biliary excretion. Overall, there are currently no comparison data with other atypical antipsychotic drugs that indicate that iloperidone is more efficacious, produces less side effects, or is less expensive; thus, the clinical relevance of iloperidone is not substantiated.

Miscellaneous Chemical Classes of Antipsychotic Drugs

Aripiprazole (Abilify) Aripiprazole (Fig. 14.16) is an arylpiperazine quinolinone derivative that has received relatively extensive attention in the clinical and basic science literature, albeit its efficacy is not superior to other second-generation or even first-generation antipsychotic drugs (including for negative symptoms) (63–71), and its GPCR affinity profile is not very different from other second-generation antipsychotic drugs (15). For example, characteristic of other second-generation antipsychotic drugs, aripiprazole has significant affinity (K_i ~50 nmol/L) at adrenergic α_1-type and α_2-type and histamine H_1 GPCRs, although contribution of these molecular targets to antipsychotic efficacy is unknown. Aripiprazole is similar to risperidone in that it lacks appreciable affinity at cholinergic M_1-M_5 muscarinic receptors, which offers advantages regarding the side effect profile.

The affinity of aripiprazole for dopamine D_2/D_3 receptors is very high (K_i ~1 nmol/L); however, it has a low propensity to cause untoward extrapyramidal

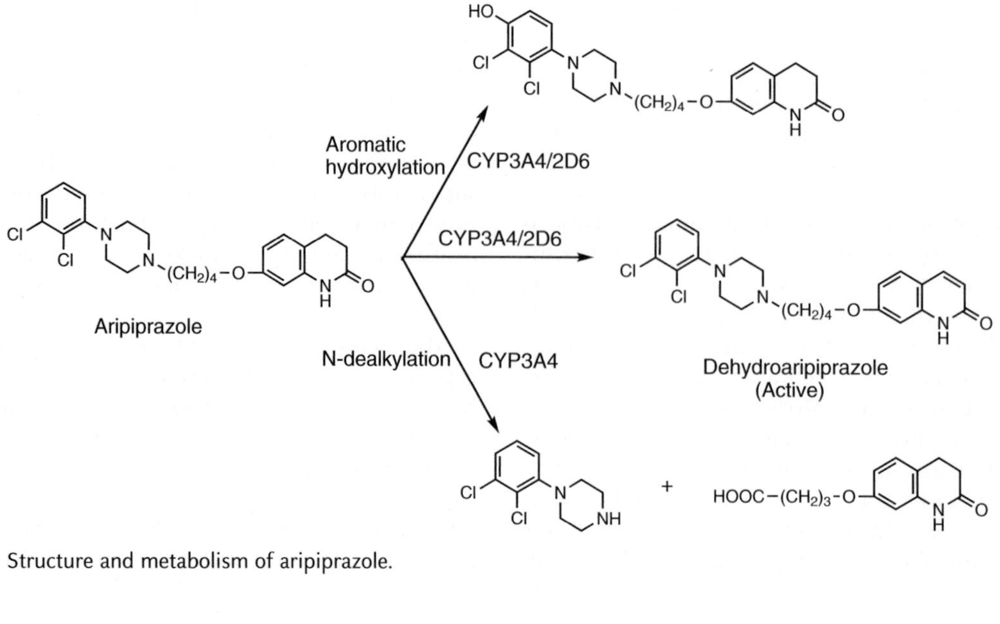

FIGURE 14.16 Structure and metabolism of aripiprazole.

symptoms and hyperprolactinemia (102). Partly, this may be explained by the GPCR functional profile of aripiprazole, which is better characterized than most other second-generation antipsychotic drugs. For example, it is a partial agonist at D_2-type (including D_3/D_4) receptors (103), whereas D_2 antagonism or inverse agonism produces extrapyramidal and hyperprolactinemia side effects. In fact, the D_2-type functional activity of aripiprazole depends on the anatomic location and type of cell type that expresses the D_2-type receptor; that is, aripiprazole is a functionally selective drug (25,103,104). Thus, it is a full agonist that activates brain dopamine D_2 autoreceptors to negatively modulate dopamine synthesis and release (105); according to the dopamine hypothesis, this type of antidopaminergic activity would be beneficial to treat schizophrenia (16,17). Meanwhile, aripiprazole is a partial agonist regarding D_2-mediated inhibition of cyclic adenosine monophosphate (cAMP) second messenger formation, and characteristic of a partial agonist, aripiprazole antagonizes the ability of dopamine to inhibit cAMP formation (106,107).

Aripiprazole also has significant affinity (K_i <10 nmol/L) for serotonin GPCRs, notably 5-HT_{1A}, 5-HT_{2A}, 5-HT_{2C}, and 5-HT_7 (15), all thought to be important in the pathophysiology and pharmacotherapy of schizophrenia (8,9,60). Aripiprazole is a partial agonist at 5-HT_{2A} and 5-HT_{2C} receptors (103); the 5-HT_{2C} partial agonist properties of aripiprazole may reduce its potential for weight gain because 5-HT_{2C} activation is associated with satiety (32,108).

Aripiprazole has good oral bioavailability (90%) with a half-life of approximately 75 hours. It undergoes hepatic CYP3A4- and CYP2D6-catalyzed *N*-dealkylation and hydroxylation as well as dehydrogenation to dehydroaripiprazole (Fig. 14.16), which is an active metabolite with a half-life of about 90 hours (109).

Molindone (Moban)

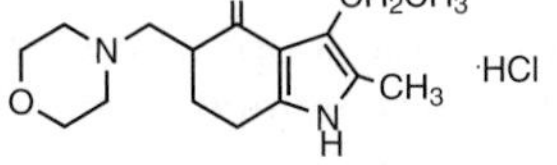

Molindone hydrochloride, a tetrahydro-indolone derivative, is a neuroleptic agent that is structurally unrelated to any of the other marketed neuroleptics. Molindone has no appreciable affinity at serotonin, cholinergic, adrenergic, or histaminergic GPCRs (15). Even at the dopamine D_2 GPCR, its affinity (K_i ~10 nmol/L) is less potent than haloperidol; however, it nonetheless can produce extrapyramidal side effects. Metabolism studies in humans show molindone to be rapidly absorbed and metabolized when given orally. There are 36 recognized metabolites, with less than 2% to 3% unmetabolized molindone being excreted in urine and feces. Clinical studies show that the antipsychotic effects of molindone last more than 24 hours, suggesting that one or more metabolites may contribute to its activity in vivo (110).

Sertindole (Serdolect)

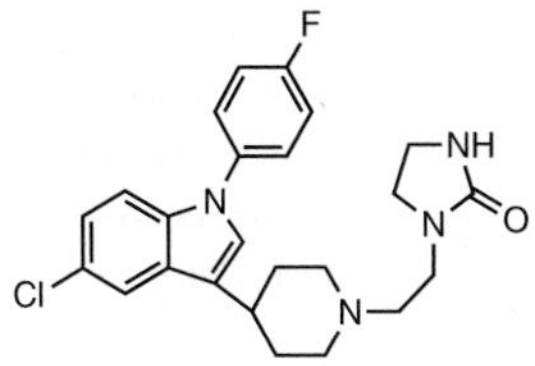

Sertindole is an indole-containing compound with high affinity (K_i <5 nmol/L) at serotonin 5-$HT_{2A/2C}$, dopamine $D_{2/3/4}$, and adrenergic α_{1A} GPCRs. Meanwhile, sertindole has essentially no affinity at cholinergic M_1 to M_5 GPCRs, and this is apparent clinically in that it has low propensity to cause anticholinergic side effects (111), which, in part, gives some justification for its reintroduction in 2002 after being withdrawn in 1998. It is about as effective as haloperidol in the treatment of acute and chronic positive symptoms of schizophrenia, but with much lower incidence of extrapyramidal side effects, and it is more effective at treating negative symptoms (105). Also, compared to other antipsychotics, sertindole is relatively nonsedating (112), perhaps, reflecting its low affinity for histamine H_1 receptors (15) as well as muscarinic receptors. Sertindole has a long plasma half-life of approximately 3 days that offers advantages regarding patient compliance (112).

ANXIETY AND ANXIETY DISORDERS

Definitions

Anxiety can be defined as a sense of apprehensive expectation. In reasonable amounts and at appropriate times, anxiety is helpful (e.g., anxiety before an examination may cause a student to initiate an appropriate study plan). Too much anxiety, however, can be deleterious. Anxiety can be considered pathologic when it is either completely inappropriate to the situation or is in excess of what the situation normally should call for. An example of the former is nocturnal panic attacks—episodes of extreme anxiety that arise out of one of the most physiologically quiet times of the day, stage III/IV sleep (113). An example of the latter is specific phobias—for example, an irrational fear to venture outside of one's home.

According to the DSM-IV (1), abnormal anxiety is that level of anxiety that interferes with normal social or occupational functioning. This definition is helpful to distinguish between normal and pathologic levels of anxiety. To meet general DSM-IV criteria, anxiety symptoms must not be caused by an exogenous factor (e.g., caffeine) or a medical condition (e.g., hyperthyroidism). Examples of anxiety disorders include specific phobias, generalized anxiety disorder (chronic abnormally high level of anxiety), social phobia (e.g., fear of public speaking), obsessive-compulsive disorder, panic disorder with or without agoraphobia (avoidance of situations believed by the patient to precipitate panic attacks), and posttraumatic stress disorder.

Etiology of Anxiety Disorders

Studies of patients with anxiety disorders have not revealed a general gross neuroanatomic lesion. In vivo functional imaging studies, however, show altered blood oxygen levels (as a manifestation of blood flow) or glucose utilization in specific brain areas in patients with anxiety conditions (114,115), including obsessive-compulsive disorder (116,117), panic disorder (118,119), specific phobia (120,121), and posttraumatic stress disorder (122,123), mostly implicating the prefrontal cortex and hippocampus (and other limbic areas) as being involved in the anatomy of pathologic anxiety. It is important to note that there is significant comorbidity for anxiety and major depressive disorders in both children and adults, and it is not clear if one illness has primacy or is part of the other (124,125). Likewise, although there may be genetic predisposition to general distress that can lead to anxiety and/or depression, no clear genetic evidence suggests specific symptoms of either disorder.

A variety of neurotransmitters, neuromodulators (e.g., adenosine), and neuropeptides (e.g., cholecystokinin, corticotropin-releasing factor, and neuropeptide Y) are suggested to be involved in the pathophysiology of anxiety. Currently, abundant evidence exists to document the involvement of the neurotransmitters γ-aminobutyric acid (GABA), norepinephrine, and serotonin in anxiety, and research increasingly is revealing that these neurotransmitter systems have complex anatomic and functional interrelationships.

GABA Receptors

The major inhibitory neurotransmitter in the mammalian CNS, GABA, is widespread, with approximately one-third of all synapses in the CNS using this neurochemical for intercellular communication. The two major classes of GABA receptors (126) are inotropic $GABA_A$ and metabotropic $GABA_B$ receptors. It is currently recommended by the International Union of Pharmacology to not use the term "$GABA_C$" receptor to describe a gene product that was described, precloning, as a GABA receptor–like protein with pharmacology distinct from $GABA_A$ and $GABA_B$ receptors (126). It appears that so-called $GABA_C$ receptors may be a $GABA_A$ subtype that expresses a certain ρ subunit (see later discussion), although the overall subunit makeup of this putative $GABA_A$ subtype is not established.

$GABA_A$ Receptor

The $GABA_A$ receptor is a member of the gene superfamily of ligand-gated ion channels that is known as the "cys-loop" family because of the presence of a cysteine loop in their N-terminal domain (126,127). These receptors exist as heteropentameric subunits arranged around a central ion channel (Fig. 14.17). The five polypeptide subunits are composed of an extracellular region, four membrane-spanning α-helical cylinders, and a large intracellular cytoplasmic loop. The $GABA_A$ ion channel conducts chloride and is defined by the second of the four membrane-spanning α-helical cylinders. The first $GABA_A$ polypeptide subunit was sequenced in 1987 (128), and so far, 19 different subunits have been isolated. These polypeptides are denoted as α_{1-6}, β_{1-3}, γ_{1-3}, δ, ε, π, θ, and ρ_{1-3}. The subunits can combine in varied proportions, and alternatively spliced variants are common. Thus, many possible receptor subtypes may exist. The major (60%) $GABA_A$ receptor isoform in the adult mammalian (rat) brain consists of α_1, β_2, and γ_2 subunits ($GABA_{A1a}$) (129).

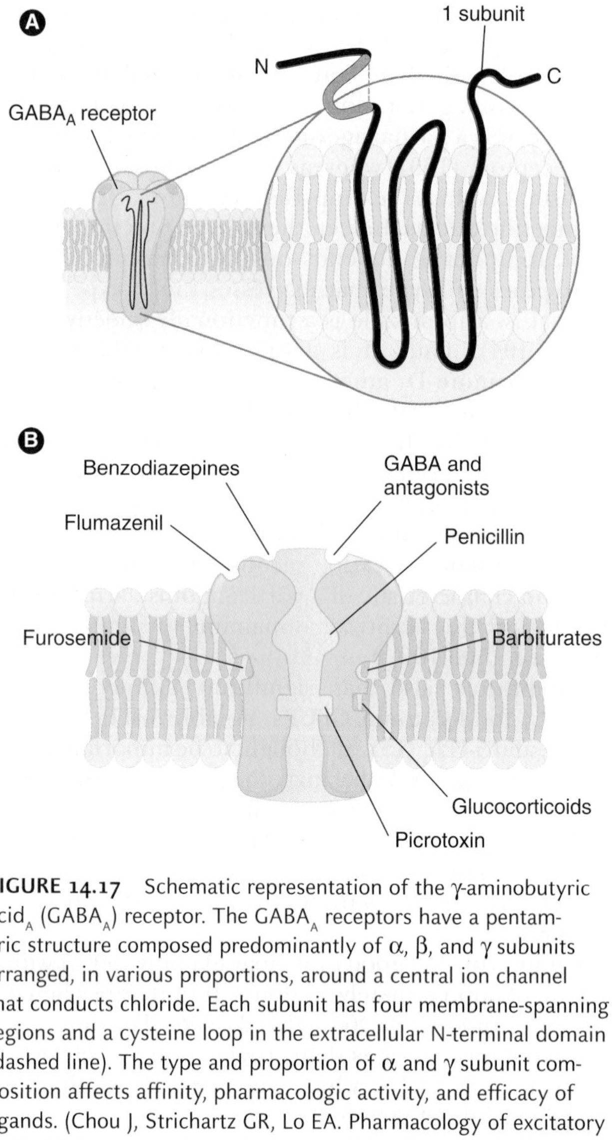

FIGURE 14.17 Schematic representation of the γ-aminobutyric $acid_A$ ($GABA_A$) receptor. The $GABA_A$ receptors have a pentameric structure composed predominantly of α, β, and γ subunits arranged, in various proportions, around a central ion channel that conducts chloride. Each subunit has four membrane-spanning regions and a cysteine loop in the extracellular N-terminal domain (dashed line). The type and proportion of α and γ subunit composition affects affinity, pharmacologic activity, and efficacy of ligands. (Chou J, Strichartz GR, Lo EA. Pharmacology of excitatory and inhibitory neurotransmission. In: Golan DE, ed. Principles of Pharmacology. Philadelphia: Lippincott Williams & Wilkins, 2005:142, with permission.)

The $GABA_A$ extracellular N-terminal region contains a number of distinct binding sites for neuroactive drugs (e.g., barbiturates, benzodiazepines, β-carbolines, and neurosteroids). The benzodiazepines, commonly prescribed as anxiolytic (and sedative) agents, bind to the benzodiazepine receptor (BZR), which is defined mostly by the α and γ subunits (126). The α and γ subunit composition can dramatically affect affinity and efficacy of BZR ligands (130,131). Early research on the BZR gave rise to the pharmacologic concept of inverse agonism in addition to the better known concepts of agonism and antagonism. Inverse agonist compounds bind to the BZR on the $GABA_A$ receptor complex and negatively modulate GABA binding and neurophysiologic activity (i.e., agonists decrease chloride conductance), producing physiologic effects opposite those of GABA (e.g., anxiogenesis and proconvulsant action). The BZR agonist ligands potentiate GABA binding and activity to increase chloride conductance, enhancing physiologic effects of GABA (e.g., sedation and anticonvulsant activity). The BZR antagonists occupy the receptor but have no intrinsic activity to modulate GABA binding and function. A clinical example of a BZR antagonist is the compound flumazenil, which is used to reverse benzodiazepine-induced sedation in overdose. There also have been developed agents that are partial agonists and inverse partial agonists at the BZR/$GABA_A$ receptor complex. The existence of a $GABA_A$ receptor complex that recognizes benzodiazepines has implications for our understanding of both normal and pathologic anxiety states and suggests the existence of endogenous $GABA_A$ receptor ligands. Thus, anxiety could conceivably be either a lack of an endogenous $GABA_A$ receptor agonist or a relative excess of a $GABA_A$ receptor antagonist or inverse agonist.

$GABA_B$ Receptors

The $GABA_B$ receptors are GPCRs that exist as two major subtypes, $GABA_{B(1)}$ and $GABA_{B(2)}$. The $GABA_{B(1)}$ subtype can be expressed as $GABA_{B(1a)}$ and $GABA_{B(1b)}$ isoforms that differ in their extracellular NH_2-terminal domains but are derived from the same gene (126). Interestingly, it was discovered early on that compared to native $GABA_B$ receptors, recombinant $GABA_{B(1a)}$ and $GABA_{B(1b)}$ receptors expressed in heterologous cells display 100- to 150-fold lower affinity for agonist ligands. Likewise, recombinant $GABA_{B(1a)}$ and $GABA_{B(1b)}$ receptors were shown to couple inefficiently to their effector systems (predominantly via $G\alpha_i$ and $G\alpha_o$). These surprising pharmacologic findings were explained by the discovery that recombinant $GABA_{B(1a)}$ and $GABA_{B(1b)}$ receptors expressed in heterologous cells are retained in the endoplasmic reticulum. In fact, it turned out that $GABA_{B(1)}$ receptors do not traffic to the cell membrane surface in the absence of $GABA_{B(2)}$ receptors. This remarkable discovery that the $GABA_{B(2)}$ receptor co-expresses on the cell surface with the $GABA_{B(1a)}$ or $GABA_{B(1b)}$ receptor to form a functional heterodimeric GPCR was reported simultaneously by three industry research groups in 1998 (130–135). The $GABA_B$ receptors were the first GPCR shown to function not as a single protein but, rather, as two distinct subunits, neither of which is functional by itself (Fig. 14.18). Homodimerization and/or heterodimerization (and oligomerization) now are documented for many GPCRs and may account for the diverse signaling functionality for this protein family.

Drugs Used in the Treatment of Anxiety

Benzodiazepines

The benzodiazepines are efficacious drugs for treatment of anxiety disorders (140), putatively, via their interaction with $GABA_A$ receptors (see Chapter 15 for a discussion of benzodiazepines and their sedative-hypnotic utility). Chlordiazepoxide was the first benzodiazepine to be marketed for clinical use in 1960. Its effectiveness and wide margin of safety were major advances over compounds, such as barbiturates, used previously. A variety of new benzodiazepines followed, each with some minor differences from the competition. The major factors considered when selecting an agent include rate and extent of absorption, presence or absence of active metabolites, and degree of lipophilicity. These factors help to determine how a benzodiazepine is marketed and used; for example, an agent that is rapidly absorbed, highly lipid soluble, and without active metabolites would be useful as a sedative but less useful for treatment of a chronic

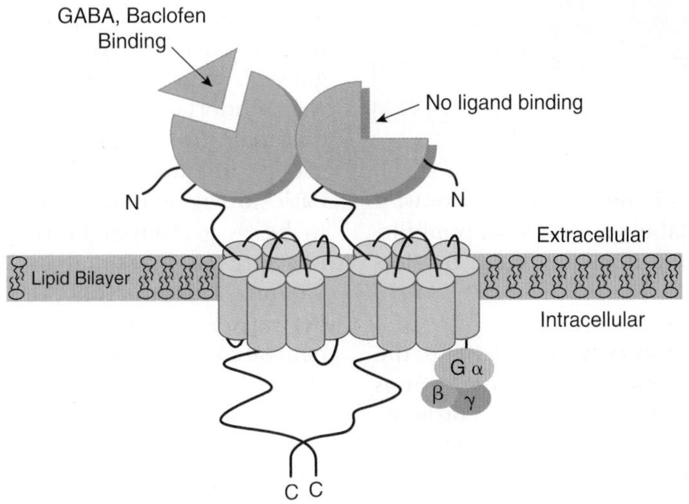

FIGURE 14.18 Schematic representation of the heterodimeric γ-aminobutyric $acid_B$ ($GABA_B$) receptor.

$GABA_B$ RECEPTORS

The structure of functional heterodimeric $GABA_{B(1)}/GABA_{B(2)}$ GPCRs (Fig. 14.18) is assumed to be very different and considerably more complex in comparison to other aminergic GPCRs that are able to function as monomers. Functional $GABA_B$ receptors are proposed to contain a binding pocket that consists of two globular lobes separated by a hinge region. Functional $GABA_B$ receptors are proposed to contain a binding pocket that consists of two globular lobes separated by a hinge region. According to the Venus flytrap model, the two lobes close on ligand binding; however, it is thought that ligands bind in only one of the lobes (136–138). The individual $GABA_{B(1)}$ and $GABA_{B(2)}$ subunits can affect a number of other membrane and cytoplasmic proteins to result in complex signaling and a diverse array of pharmacologic and physiologic effects. For example, $GABA_B$ receptors modulate activity of calcium channels, potassium channels, adenylyl cyclase, and phospholipase C via $G_{\alpha i}$, $G_{\alpha o}$, and $G_{\beta\gamma}$ proteins. Meanwhile, preclinical data suggest that drugs that affect $GABA_B$ receptor function may produce, for example, anxiolytic, anticonvulsant, and antidepressant effects as well as muscle relaxant and analgesic effects (137,138).

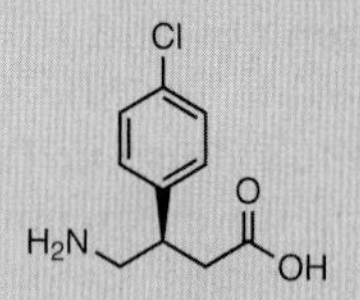

R(-)-Baclofen

The only drug currently in clinical use that selectively interacts with $GABA_B$ receptors is baclofen (β-*p*-chlorophenyl-GABA). Baclofen was first synthesized in 1962 and was shown to have potent muscle relaxant and analgesic activity. In 1972, the racemate was marketed to treat spasticity disorders. In 1980, the *R*-(−)-enantiomer of baclofen was shown to stereoselectively interact (as an agonist) with what is now known as the $GABA_B$ receptor (139). The role of $GABA_B$ receptors in anxiety, however, is not clear, and baclofen (racemate) is approved only for use as a spasmolytic agent (see Chapter 13).

anxiety state. On the other hand, a compound with slower absorption, active metabolites, and low lipophilicity would be a more effective antianxiety agent but less helpful as a soporific.

Development of Benzodiazepine Anxiolytics In the 1950s, the medicinal chemist Sternbach noted that "basic groups frequently impart biological activity," and in accordance with this observation, he synthesized a series of compounds by treating various chloromethylquinazoline N-oxides with amines to produce what he hoped would be products with "tranquilizer" activity at the New Jersey

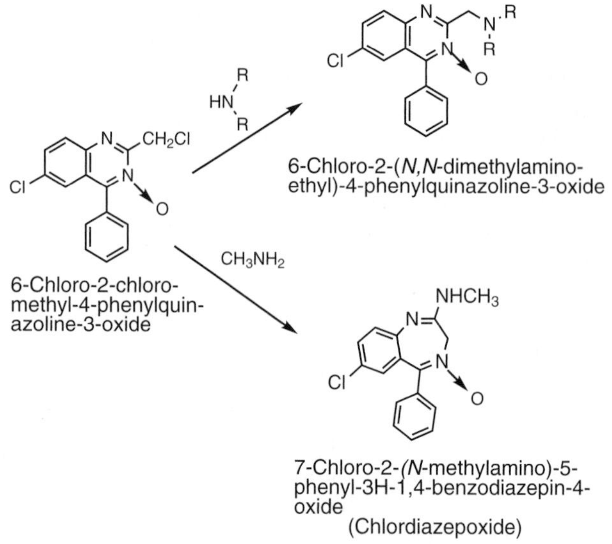

FIGURE 14.19 Synthesis of chlordiazepoxide.

laboratories of Hoffman LaRoche (141,142). Sternbach's studies included the reaction of 6-chloro-2-chloromethyl-4-phenylquinazoline-3-oxide with methylamine, which yielded the unexpected rearrangement product 7-chloro-2-(N-methylamino)-5-phenyl-3H-1,4,-benzodiazepin-4-oxide (Fig. 14.19). This product was given the code name RO 50690 and screened for pharmacologic activity in 1957. Subsequently, Randall et al. (143,144) reported that RO 50690 was hypnotic and sedative and had antistrychnine properties similar to the propanediol meprobamate, a sedative that has tranquilizer (anxiolytic) properties only at intoxicating doses. Renamed chlordiazepoxide, RO 50690 was marketed in 1960 as Librium, a safe and effective anxiolytic agent.

Chlordiazepoxide turned out to have rather remarkable pharmacologic properties and tremendous potential as a pharmacotherapeutic product, but it possessed a number of unacceptable physical chemical properties. In an effort to enhance its "pharmaceutical elegance," structural modifications of chlordiazepoxide were undertaken that eventually led to the synthesis of diazepam in 1959. In contrast to the maxim that basic groups impart biologic activity, diazepam contains no basic nitrogen moiety. Diazepam, however, was found to be 3- to 10-fold more potent than chlordiazepoxide and was marketed in 1963 as the anxiolytic drug Valium. Subsequently, thousands of benzodiazepine derivatives were synthesized, and more than two dozen benzodiazepines are in clinical use in the United States (Fig. 14.20).

A major advance in the BZR field was made in 1981 with the first report that the imidazobenzodiazepinone derivative, flumazenil, binds with high affinity to the BZR and blocks the pharmacologic effects of the classical benzodiazepines in vitro and in vivo (149).

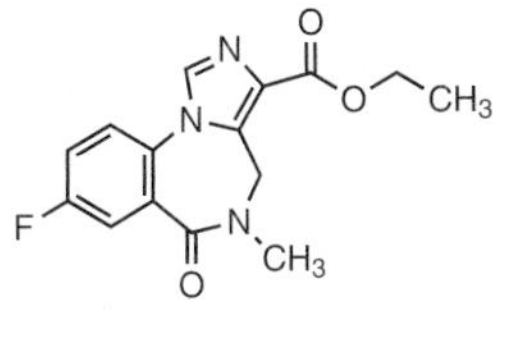

Flumazenil

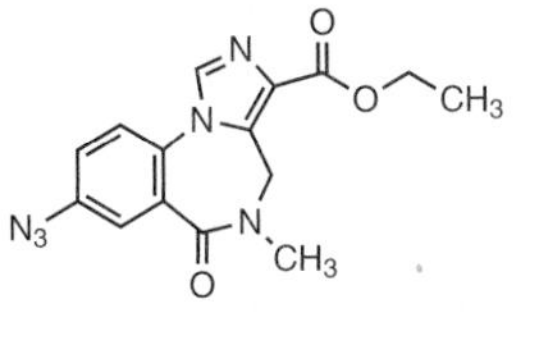

RO 15-4513

Unlike agonists, binding of [^{3}H]flumazenil to the BZR is not affected by modulators such as GABA and several ions that induce changes in receptors (150). The insensitivity of flumazenil to changes in BZR conformation suggests that the ligand does not induce a conformational change in the receptor to trigger a biologic response and is a pure antagonist (148). Such benzodiazepine antagonists have been used to characterize the pharmacologic nature of the BZR, and several of these agents, including flumazenil, are used to treat benzodiazepine overdose. Other imidazobenzodiazepinone derivatives are not true BZR antagonists but, rather, have inverse agonist activity. For example, RO 15-4513 is reported to be a partial inverse agonist that produces anxiogenic-like effects in rats (146), a pharmacologic activity quite different from a true BZR competitive antagonist, such as flumazenil.

Mechanism of Action of Anxiolytic Benzodiazepines The BZR ligands, regardless of intrinsic activity, do not directly alter transmembrane chloride conduction to produce their observed characteristic physiologic anxiolytic or anxiogenic effects. The BZR is an allosteric modulator of GABA binding to the $GABA_A$ receptor complex that, in turn, modulates the transmembrane conductance of chloride. In the presence of BZR agonists or partial agonists, affinity and functional potency of GABA at $GABA_A$ receptors are enhanced maximally or submaximally, respectively, and conductance of chloride is increased. Inverse agonists and partial inverse agonists reduce the effect of GABA, and $GABA_A$ receptor–mediated conductance of chloride is accordingly decreased. The $GABA_A$ receptor–chloride channels thus become either more or less sensitive to GABA in the presence of BZR agonists or inverse agonists, respectively. BZR competitive antagonists block access of agonists to the BZR but have no intrinsic activity to affect GABA-modulated conductance of chloride.

A representation of the relationship between ligand interaction with the BZR and intrinsic activity to modulate $GABA_A$ receptor function is shown in Figure 14.21. The interaction of agonists, competitive antagonists, and inverse agonists with the BZR, as shown in the figure, is a simplistic rendering of the proposed three-state model of the BZR and $GABA_A$ receptor interrelationship (151,152). This model is based on the hypothesis that the BZR and $GABA_A$ receptor exist in three spontaneously oscillating conformational states, functionally described as "active" or agonist, "neutral" or "resting," and "inactive" or inverse agonist. The BZR agonists and partial agonists bind to and stabilize the "active" state, inducing a conformational change in the $GABA_A$ receptor complex that results in chloride channel opening, which may lead to an anticonvulsant or anxiolytic effect. The BZR inverse agonists and partial inverse agonists bind to and stabilize the "inactive" state, resulting in the chloride channel remaining closed, which may lead to a convulsant or anxiogenic effect. The BZR competitive antagonists presumably bind equally well to both states (hence, they bind to a "neutral" state) and affect no change in $GABA_A$ receptor function or chloride conductance, but access of agonists to the BZR is blocked.

The classical BZR is located on the $GABA_A$ receptor complex mainly at the interface of the α and γ subunits (126) that can be rendered benzodiazepine-insensitive by a point mutation in the α subunit, replacing a critical histidine residue for arginine (153). Different α and γ subunit compositions give rise to subtypes of the BZR receptor that are pharmacologically distinct with regard to ligand affinity and intrinsic activity (154–156), providing a

ENDOGENOUS BZR LIGANDS

An endogenous ligand with affinity for the BZR of the $GABA_A$ receptor complex has not been conclusively identified. Several compounds of endogenous origin, however, that inhibit the binding of radiolabeled benzodiazepines to the BZR have been reported. In 1980, Braestrup et al. (145) reported the presence in normal human urine of β-carboline-3-carboxylic acid ethyl ester (βCCE), which has very high affinity for the BZR complex. It was subsequently shown, however, that βCCE formed as an artifact from Braestrup's extraction procedure, during which the urine extract was heated with ethanol at pH 1, a condition favoring formation of the ethyl ester from β-carboline-3-carboxylic acid, a tryptophan metabolite.

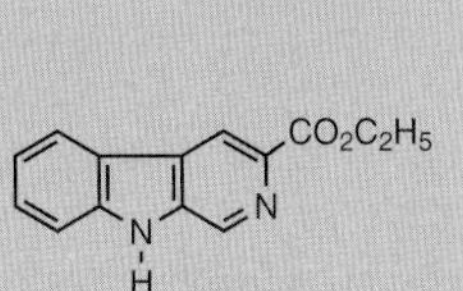

βCCE

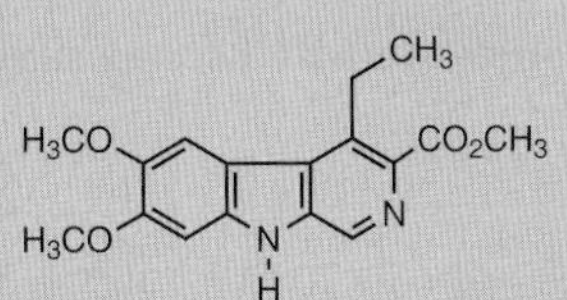

DMCM

Although βCCE actually was shown not to be of endogenous origin, its discovery as a high-affinity BZR ligand stimulated research that led to the synthesis of a series of β-carboline derivatives with a variety of intrinsic activities, presumably mediated through the BZR that is associated with the $GABA_A$ receptor complex. For example, although βCCE is considered to be a partial inverse agonist at this site, 6,7-dimethoxy-4-ethyl-β-carboline-3-carboxylic acid methyl ester (DMCM) appears to be a full inverse agonist (146). In fact, βCCE blocks the convulsions produced by the very potent convulsant DMCM (147). These effects are even more complex and interesting in light of the approximately 10-fold higher affinity that βCCE shows for the BZR labeled by [^{3}H]diazepam when compared to DMCM (148). The β-carbolines currently are important research tools to probe the agonist, competitive antagonist, inverse agonist, and partial agonist/inverse agonist pharmacophores of the BZR/GABA receptor complex.

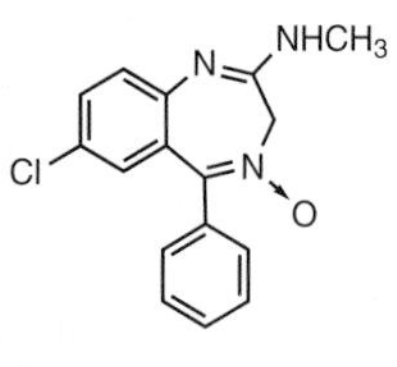

Chlordiazepoxide (Librium)

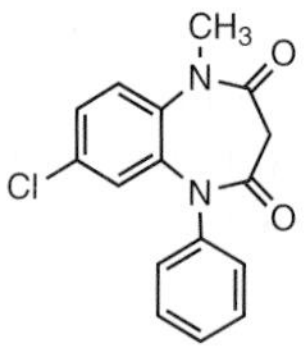

Clobazam (Frisium)

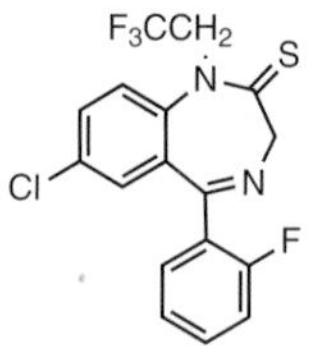

Quazepam (Doral)

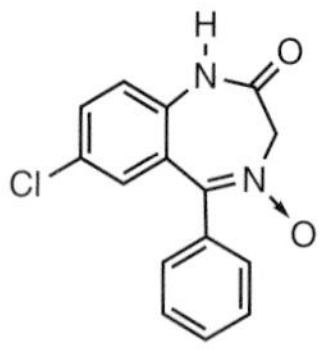

Demoxepam

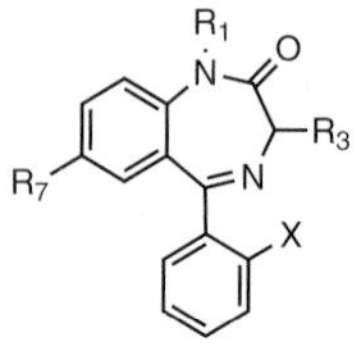

Class A Benzodiazepines

Generic name	Trade name	R_1	R_3	R_7	X
Clonazepam	Klonopin	H	H	NO_2	Cl
Clorazepate	Tranxene	H	COOK	Cl	H
Diazepam	Valium	CH_3	H	Cl	H
Flurazepam	Dalmane	$(CH_2)_2NC_2H_5)_2$	H	Cl	F
Halazepam	Paxipam	CH_2CF_3	H	Cl	H
Lorazepam	Ativan	H	OH	Cl	Cl
Oxazepam	Serax	H	OH	Cl	H
Temazepam	Restoril	CH_3	OH	Cl	H

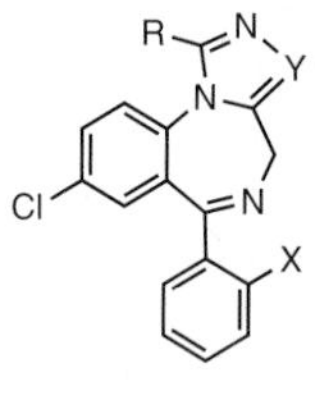

Class B Benzodiazepines

Generic name	Trade name	R	X	Y
Alprazolam	Xanax	CH_3	H	N
Estazolam	ProSom	H	H	N
Midazolam	Versed	CH_3	F	CH
Triazolam	Halcion	CH_3	Cl	N

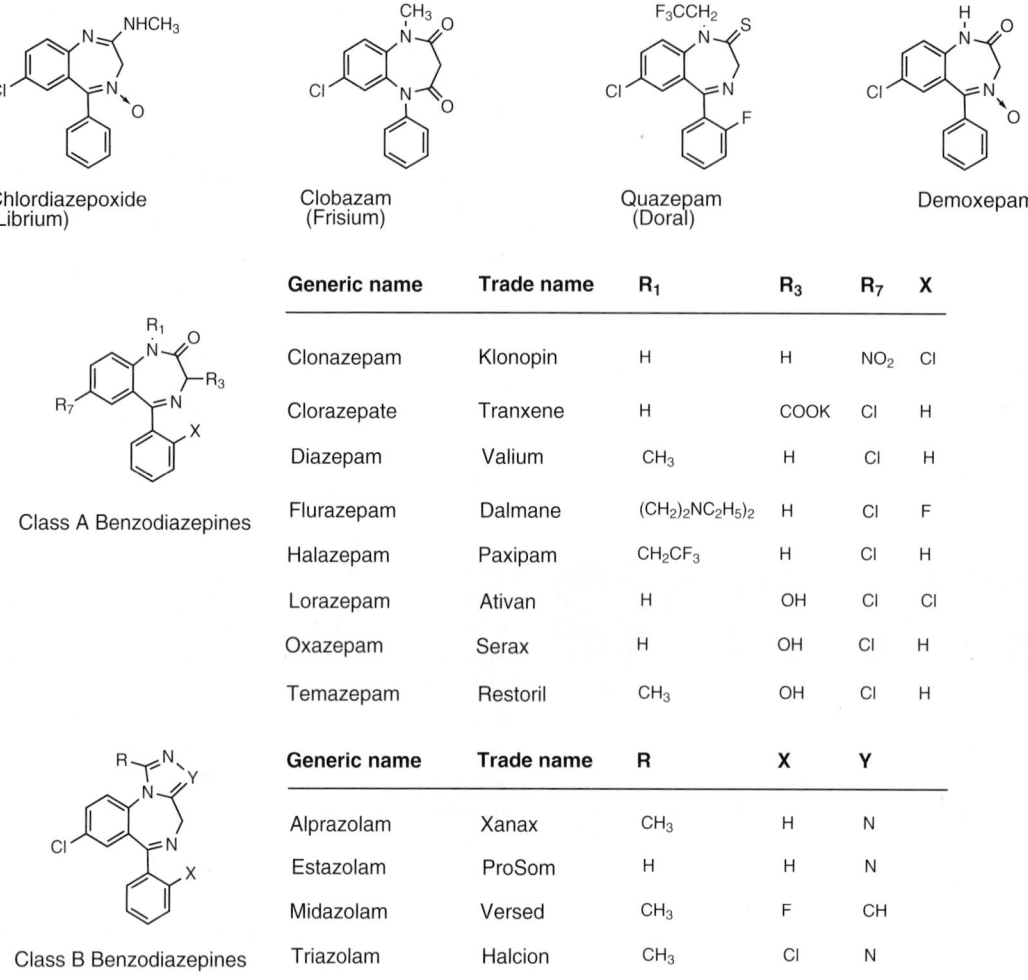

FIGURE 14.20 Some commercially available benzodiazepines.

mechanistic basis for development of ligands that are anxioselective (i.e., anxiolysis in the absence of sedation, muscle relaxation, amnesia, and ataxia). Thus, current drug discovery approaches target specific α and γ molecular subunits of the $GABA_A$ receptor complex in the quest for benzodiazepine and nonbenzodiazepine (see later discussion) drugs that demonstrate anxioselectivity. As a group, currently used benzodiazepines are not α subtype–selective. In studies using nonhuman primates, it has been suggested that $GABA_A$ α_2, α_3, and α_5 subunits mediate anxiolytic and muscle relaxant effects of benzodiazepines, whereas α_1 receptors mediate the sedative effects (157). Several putative anxioselective compounds have reached the clinic; however, they have not exhibited the degree of anxioselectivity predicted from preclinical testing and, usually, have lower efficacy than standard benzodiazepines (131). Of possible clinical importance, "uncoupling" of the BZR/$GABA_A$ receptor complex has been observed in response to chronic benzodiazepine exposure both in vitro (158) and in vivo (159). In the absence of exogenous influences, however, coupling efficiency appears to be determined by the composition and stoichiometry of the α subunits (156), whereas benzodiazepine affinity, intrinsic activity, and efficacy are determined by the nature of both the α and γ subunits (131,155,156).

Structure–Activity Relationships

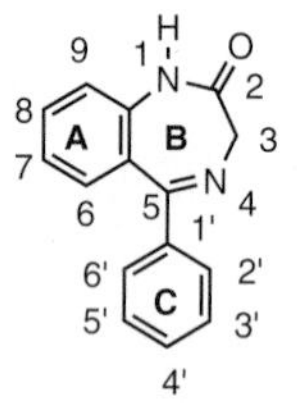

The structure–activity relationship for classical 5-phenyl-1,4-benzodiazepine-2-one anxiolytic agents has been described by Sternbach and other investigators (141,148,151,160). Thousands of benzodiazepine derivatives with a variety of substituents have been synthesized that interact with the BZR; however, classical quantitative structure–activity relationship and molecular modeling techniques have been used to reduce this myriad of structures to the minimal common molecular features necessary for binding (161–164). The pharmacologic activity continuum (agonist, antagonist, inverse agonist) displayed by BZR ligands would seem to suggest that such diverse functional activity be mediated by ligand interaction with different sites on the $GABA_A$ receptor–chloride channel complex. This continuum of activity, however, is

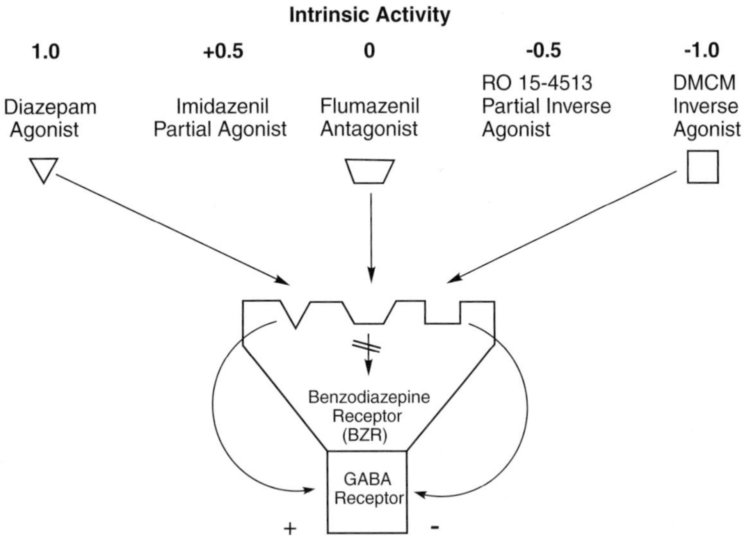

FIGURE 14.21 Ligand interaction with the γ-aminobutyric acid$_A$ (GABA$_A$)/benzodiazepine receptor complex.

displayed by ligands within the same chemical class, and small modifications in the chemical structure of a ligand can shift the intrinsic activity from agonist to antagonist to inverse agonist. Moreover, each functional class of BZR ligands can competitively inhibit the binding of the other two classes as well as functionally antagonize each other. These observations suggest that the binding sites of functionally diverse BZR receptor ligands, at least, overlap. Nevertheless, most BZR pharmacophore models that describe ligand functional activity are based initially on the BZR pharmacophore for ligand binding activity at a single binding domain, and this approach is used here to summarize the structure–activity relationship for benzodiazepine derivatives at the BZR receptor.

Ring A In general, the minimum requirement for binding of 5-phenyl-1,4-benzodiazepin-2-one derivatives to the BZR includes an aromatic or heteroaromatic ring (ring A), which is believed to participate in π-π stacking with aromatic amino acid residues of the receptor. Substituents on ring A have varied effects on binding of benzodiazepines to the BZR, but such effects are not predictable based on electronic or (within reasonable limits) steric properties. It is generally true, however, that an electronegative group (e.g., halogen or nitro) substituted at the 7-position markedly increases functional anxiolytic activity, although effects on binding affinity in vitro are not as dramatic. On the other hand, substituents at positions 6, 8, or 9 generally decrease anxiolytic activity. Other 1,4-diazepine derivatives in which ring A is replaced by a heterocycle generally show weak binding affinity in vitro and even less pharmacologic activity in vivo when compared to phenyl-substituted analogs.

Ring B A proton-accepting group is believed to be a structural requirement of both benzodiazepine and nonbenzodiazepine ligand binding to the GABA$_A$ receptor, putatively for interactions with a histidine residue that serves as a proton source in the GABA$_A$ α_1 subunit (156). For the benzodiazepines, optimal affinity occurs when the proton-accepting group in the 2-position of ring B (i.e., the carbonyl moiety) is in a coplanar spatial orientation with the aromatic ring A. Substitution of sulfur for oxygen at the 2-position may affect selectivity for binding to GABA BZR subpopulations, but anxiolytic activity is maintained. Substitution of the methylene 3-position or the imine nitrogen is sterically unfavorable for antagonist activity but has no effect on agonist (i.e., anxiolytic) activity. Derivatives substituted with a 3-hydroxy moiety have comparable potency to nonhydroxylated analogs and are excreted faster. Esterification of a 3-hydroxy moiety also is possible without loss of potency. Neither the 1-position amide nitrogen nor its substituent is required for in vitro binding to the BZR, and many clinically used analogs are not *N*-alkylated (Fig. 14.20). Although even relatively long *N*-alkyl side chains do not dramatically decrease BZR affinity, sterically large substituents like *tert*-butyl drastically reduce receptor affinity and in vivo activity. Neither the 4,5-double bond nor the 4-position nitrogen (the 4,5-[methyleneimino] group) in ring B is required for in vivo anxiolytic activity, although in vitro BZR affinity is decreased if the C=N bond is reduced to C–N. It is proposed that in vivo activity of such derivatives results from oxidation back to C=N. It follows that the 4-oxide moiety of chlordiazepoxide can be removed without loss of anxiolytic activity.

Ring C The 5-phenyl ring C is not required for binding to the BZR in vitro. This accessory aromatic ring may contribute favorable hydrophobic or steric interactions to receptor binding, however, and its relationship to ring A planarity may be important. Substitution at the 4′-(*para*)-position of an appended 5-phenyl ring is unfavorable for agonist activity, but 2′-(*ortho*)-substituents are not detrimental to agonist activity, suggesting that limitations at the para position are steric, rather than electronic, in nature.

1,2-Annelation

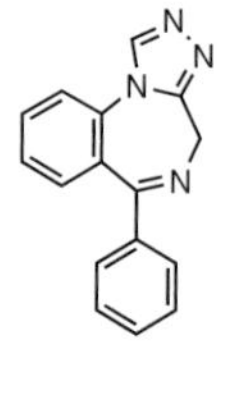

s-Triazolo[4,3a][1,4]benzodiazepine

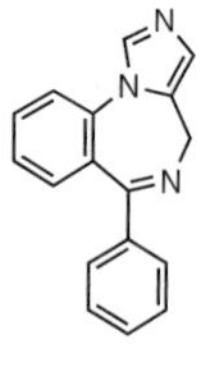

Imidazo[1,5a][1,4]benzodiazepine

Annelating the 1,2-bond of ring B with an additional "electron-rich" (i.e., proton acceptor) ring, such as *s*-triazole or imidazole, also results in pharmacologically active benzodiazepine derivatives with high affinity for the BZR (Fig. 14.21). For example, the *s*-triazolo-benzodiazepines triazolam, alprazolam, and estazolam and the imidazo-benzodiazepine midazolam are clinically effective anxiolytic agents (Fig. 14.20).

Stereochemistry

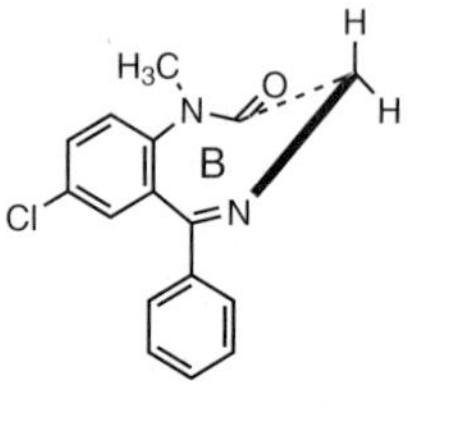

a

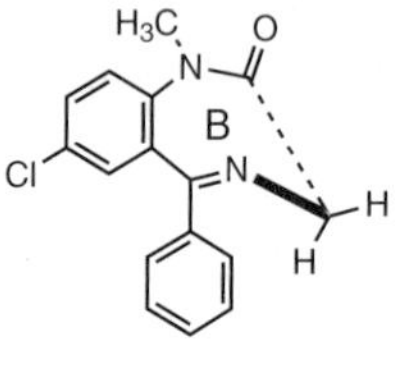

b

Most clinically useful benzodiazepines do not have a chiral center; however, the seven-membered ring B may adopt one of two possible boat conformations, *a* and *b*, that are "enantiomeric" (mirror images) to each other. Nuclear magnetic resonance studies indicate that the two conformations can easily interconvert at room temperature, making it impossible to predict which conformation is active at the BZR a priori. Evidence for stereospecificity for binding to the BZR was provided by introducing a 3-substituent into the benzodiazepine nucleus to provide a chiral center and enantiomeric pairs of derivatives (148). In vitro BZR binding affinity and in vivo anxiolytic activity of several 3-methylated enantiomers was found to reside in the *S*-isomer. Moreover, the *S*-enantiomer of 3-methyldiazepam was shown to stabilize conformation *a* for ring B, whereas the *R*-enantiomer stabilizes conformation *b*. Also, the 3-*S* configuration and *a* conformation for ring B are present in both the crystalline state (165) and in solution (166) for 3-methyldiazepam. Despite the enantioselectivity demonstrated for benzodiazepines, the commonly used 3-hydroxylated derivatives (e.g., lorazepam and oxazepam) are commercially available only as racemic mixtures.

Physiochemical and Pharmacokinetic Properties The physiochemical and pharmacokinetic properties of the various benzodiazepines vary widely, and these properties have clinical implications. For example, depending on the nature of substituents, particularly with regard to electronegative substituents, the lipophilicity of the benzodiazepines may vary by more than three orders of magnitude, which affects absorption, distribution, and metabolism. In general, most benzodiazepines have relatively high lipid:water partition coefficients (logP values) and are completely absorbed after oral administration and rapidly distributed to the brain and other highly perfused organs. A notable exception is clorazepate (Fig. 14.20), which is rapidly decarboxylated at the 3-position to *N*-desmethyldiazepam and, subsequently, quickly absorbed. Overall, the clinical and pharmacokinetic properties of clorazepate are similar to chlordiazepoxide and diazepam (see later discussion).

Most benzodiazepines and their metabolites bind to plasma proteins. The degree of protein binding is dependent on lipophilicity of the compound and varies from approximately 70% for more polar benzodiazepines, such as alprazolam, to 99% for very lipophilic derivatives, such as diazepam. Hepatic microsomal oxidation, including *N*-dealkylation and aliphatic hydroxylation by a wide variety of cytochrome P enzymes, accounts for the major metabolic disposition of most benzodiazepines. Subsequent conjugation of microsomal metabolites by glucuronyl transferases yields polar glucuronides that are excreted in urine. In general, the rate and product of benzodiazepine metabolism vary, depending on route of administration and the individual drug.

Specific Drugs

Chlordiazepoxide Chlordiazepoxide is well absorbed after oral administration, and peak blood concentration usually is reached in approximately 4 hours. Intramuscular absorption of chlordiazepoxide, however, is slower and erratic. The half-life of chlordiazepoxide is variable but usually quite long (6 to 30 hours). Hepatic metabolism is mainly by CYP3A4 to give the initial *N*-desmethylation product, *N*-desmethylchloridiazepoxide, which undergoes deamination to form the demoxepam (Fig. 14.22), which is extensively metabolized, with less than 1% of a dose of chlordiazepoxide excreted as demoxepam. Demoxepam can undergo four different metabolic fates. Removal of the *N*-oxide moiety yields the active metabolite, *N*-desmethyldiazepam (desoxydemoxepam). This product is a metabolite of both chlordiazepoxide and diazepam and can be hydroxylated to yield oxazepam, another active metabolite that is rapidly glucuronidated and excreted in the urine. Another possibility for metabolism of demoxepam is hydrolysis to the "opened lactam," which is inactive (Fig. 14.22). The two other metabolites of demoxepam are the products of ring A hydroxylation (9-hydroxydemoxepam) or ring C hydroxylation (4′-hydroxydemoxepam), both of which are inactive. The majority of a dose of chlordiazepoxide is excreted as glucuronide conjugates of oxazepam and other phenolic (9- or 4′-hydroxylated) metabolites. As with diazepam (see next secton), repeated administration of

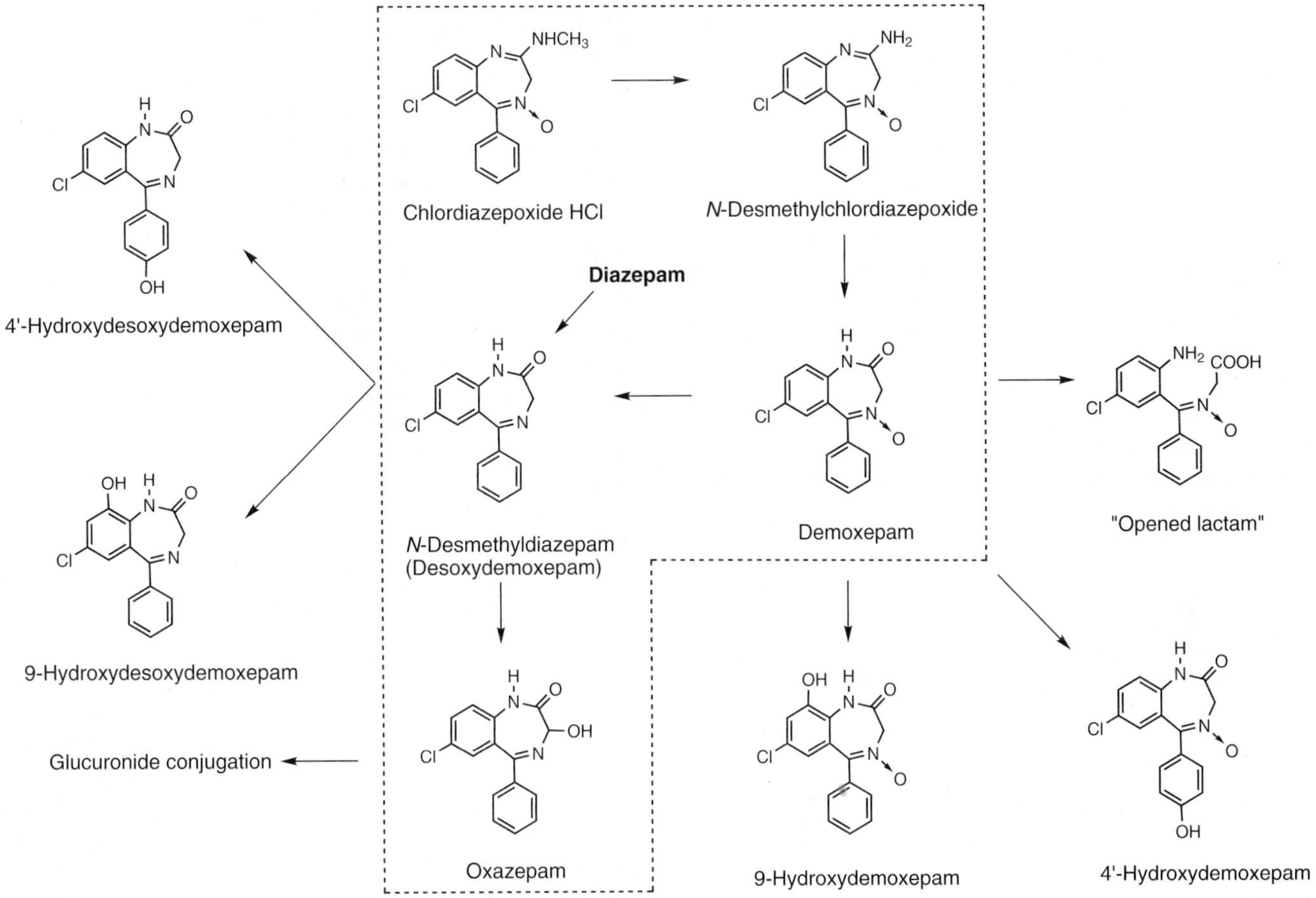

FIGURE 14.22 Metabolism of chlordiazepoxide and related benzodiazepines.

chlordiazepoxide can result in accumulation of parent drug and its active metabolites, which may have important clinical implications, including excessive sedation.

Diazepam Diazepam is rapidly and completely absorbed after oral administration. Maximum peak blood concentration occurs in 2 hours, and elimination is slow, with a half-life of approximately 20 to 50 hours. As with chlordiazepoxide, the major metabolic product of diazepam (by CYP3A4) is *N*-desmethyldiazepam, which is pharmacologically active and undergoes even slower metabolism than its parent compound. Repeated administration of diazepam or chlordiazepoxide leads to accumulation of *N*-desmethyldiazepam, which can be detected in the blood for more than 1 week after discontinuation of the drug. Hydroxylation of *N*-desmethyldiazepam at the 3-position gives the active metabolite oxazepam (Fig. 14.22).

Oxazepam Oxazepam is an active metabolite of both chlordiazepoxide and diazepam and is marketed separately as a short-acting anxiolytic agent. Oxazepam is rapidly inactivated to glucuronidated metabolites that are excreted in the urine (Fig. 14.22). The half-life of oxazepam is approximately 4 to 8 hours, and cumulative effects with chronic therapy are much less than with long-acting benzodiazepines, such as chlordiazepoxide and diazepam. Lorazepam is the 2′-chloro derivative of oxazepam and has a similarly short half-life (2 to 6 hours) and similar pharmacologic activity.

Flurazepam Flurazepam is administered orally as the dihydrochloride salt. It is rapidly ^{1}N-dealkylated (primarily by CYP3A4) to give the 2′-fluoro derivative of *N*-desmethyldiazepam, and it subsequently follows the same metabolic pathways as chlordiazepoxide and diazepam (Fig. 14.22) (also see Fig. 15.7 for metabolism). The half-life of flurazepam is fairly long (~7 hours); consequently, it has the same potential as chlordiazepoxide and diazepam to produce cumulative clinical effects and side effects (e.g., excessive sedation) and residual pharmacologic activity, even after discontinuation.

Midazolam The pK_a of midazolam is 6.2 (see Appendix), making it one of the few benzodiazepines that is highly water soluble (pH<4), as well as highly lipid soluble (pH>4). It is the most commonly used benzodiazepine as a premedication for anesthesia, with a quick onset (1 to 2 minutes) and recovery (20 minutes) after a bolus injection (167). The time to full alertness after midazolam premedication, however, is about 40 minutes, which is much longer than for nonbenzodiazepine agents such as propofol (10 minutes). The intravenously administered preparation is a dihydrochloride salt preparation that is buffered to pH 3; at this pH, acid-catalyzed diazepine ring opening at the 4,5-double bond occurs that assists water solubility but renders the compound inactive. The dihydrochloride salt preparation consists of about 8% to 85% of the ring-opened structure II and 15% to 20% of the ring-closed form Ia (168). The diazepine ring completely reforms to the active midazolam compound (I) upon intravenous injection (i.e., at pH 7.4) (168). Midazolam undergoes hepatic metabolism mainly by CYP3A4 and CYP3A5 to yield primarily hydroxylated derivatives that likely do not contribute to pharmacologic activity at usual doses; these are subsequently excreted as glucuronide conjugates (167).

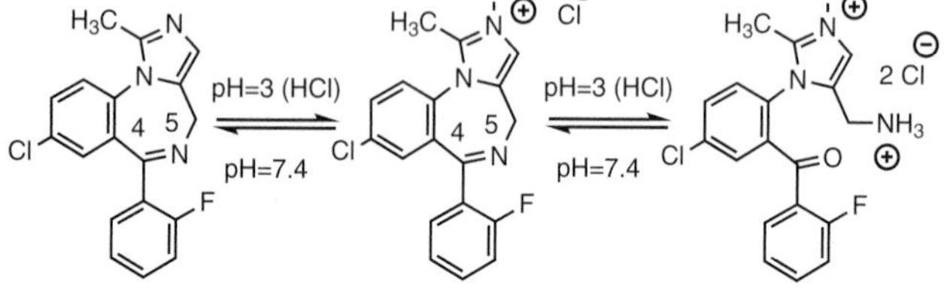

I Ia II

Detailed Pharmacokinetic Analysis Detailed pharmacokinetic analysis for most benzodiazepines is complex. Two-compartment models may be adequate to describe the disposition of most derivatives, but three-compartment models are necessary for highly lipophilic agents, such as diazepam. The distribution of such lipophilic drugs is further complicated by enterohepatic circulation. Thus, the usually stated elimination half-life of benzodiazepines may not adequately account for the pharmacodynamics of the distributive phase of the drug, which can be clinically important. For example, the distributive (α) half-life of diazepam is approximately 1 hour, whereas the elimination (β) half-life is approximately 1.5 days acutely and even longer after chronic dosing that results in accumulation of drug. Furthermore, plasma concentration and clinical effectiveness of benzodiazepines are difficult to correlate, and only a two-fold increase in clinically effective levels produces sedative side effects. Consequently, despite the long half-life of many benzodiazepines, they are not safe or effective when given in one daily dose and usually are divided into two to four doses per day for treatment of daytime anxiety. Both therapeutic and toxic effects may persist several days after discontinuation of chronically administered, long-acting benzodiazepines, such as chlordiazepoxide and diazepam. Thus, short-acting benzodiazepines, such as oxazepam, that are rapidly metabolized to inactive products should be considered in elderly or hepato-compromised patients.

Nonbenzodiazepine Agonists at the Benzodiazepine Receptor

Relatively few structural classes of nonbenzodiazepine compounds have clinically relevant affinity for the BZR and show pharmacologic activity in vivo. Examples of these classes include the β-carbolines, triazolopyridazines, cyclopyrrolones, pyrazolopyrimidines, and imidazopyridines. Representative drugs of these classes in current clinical use are the pyrazolopyrimidine zaleplon, the cyclopyrrolone eszopiclone, and the imidazopyridazine zolpidem (also see Chapter 15). These nonbenzodiazepine BZR ligands show greater selectivity for $GABA_A$ receptors containing the α_1 subunit; however, it should be noted that the α_2, α_3, α_5, and γ subunits may be important in mediating anxiolytic effects of BRZ agonists (131).

β-Carboline

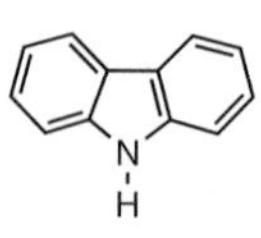

Several β-carbolines have approximately 10-fold higher affinity for the BZR when compared to diazepam. The ethyl ester of βCCE, identified in human urine extracts as an artifact of the extraction procedure, has very high affinity for the BZR. Although βCCE and other β-carbolines are not endogenous BZR ligands (see previous discussion) and are not currently approved for clinical use, they are used to characterize different $GABA_A$/BZR subtypes (based on α and γ subunit composition) and function (e.g., the partial agonist abecarnil) toward the discovery of anxioselective drugs. In this regard, the β-carboline ring system is planar in comparison to the boat conformation of the 1,4-benzodiazepines (see the discussion of stereochemistry); thus, β-carbolines have been useful to extend structure–activity relationship information for the agonist, antagonist, and inverse agonist pharmacophores of the various $GABA_A$/BZR subtypes.

CL 218,872

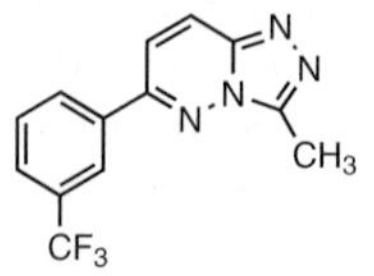

The triazolopyridazine CL 218,872 is another research tool used to probe BZR heterogeneity, because it is known to have selective high affinity at BZR subtypes containing the α_1 subunit, hypothesized to mediate anxioselective actions (131,169). CL 218,872 has lower efficacy than benzodiazepines in potentiating GABA-gated chloride currents, but it produces anxiolytic effects in animal models at substantially lower doses than those required to produce untoward side effects (e.g., sedation, ataxia, and muscle relaxation) (127,169).

Eszopiclone (Lunesta)

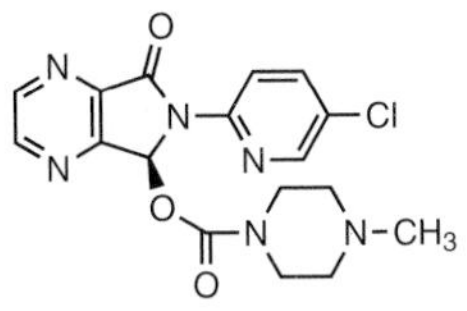

The cyclopyrrolone zopiclone is described as a "superagonist" at BZRs with the subunit composition $\alpha_1\ \beta_2\ \gamma_2$ and $\alpha_1\ \beta_2\ \gamma_3$, because it potentiates the GABA-gated current more than the benzodiazepine (flunitrazepam) reference agonist (170). Racemic zopiclone has been available in Europe since 1992, and the higher affinity *S*-enantiomer (eszopiclone) was marketed in the United States in 2005, primarily to treat insomnia, because of its rapid onset and moderate duration (half-life, ~6 hours) of hypnotic-sedative effect (171). Less than 10% of orally administered eszopiclone is excreted unchanged, because it undergoes extensive CYP3A4- and CYP2E1-catalyzed oxidation and demethylation to metabolites excreted primarily in urine (see Fig. 15.12 and Chapter 15).

Pyrazolopyrimidines

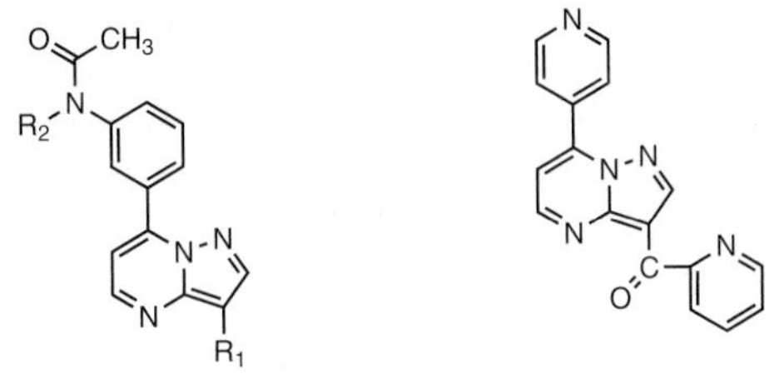

Zaleplon (Sonata) R_1 = CN, R_2 = CH_2CH_3 Ocinaplon

Indiplon R_1 = 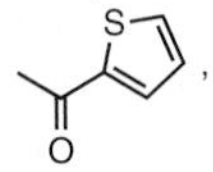 , R_2 = CH_3

The pyrazolopyrimidines zaleplon, indiplon, and ocinaplon have selective high affinity for α_1-containing BZRs but also produce effects at other BZR/$GABA_A$ subtypes. In patients with insomnia, zaleplon is effective to decrease sleep latency and does not appear to induce withdrawal symptoms or rebound insomnia on discontinuation. Indiplon is similar and currently under review by the U.S. Food and Drug Administration (FDA). Zaleplon is absorbed rapidly and reaches peak plasma concentrations in approximately 1 hour, with a half-life of approximately 1 hour as well. Less than 1% of a dose of zaleplon is excreted unchanged, because most is oxidized by aldehyde dehydrogenase and CYP3A4 to inactive metabolites, which are converted to glucuronides and eliminated in urine (see Fig. 15.13).

Indiplon has demonstrated efficacy to improve latency to sleep onset and total sleep time when compared to placebo, with limited rebound insomnia and tolerance (172). Currently, however, the drug is not yet approved by the U.S. FDA.

Ocinaplon was studied primarily for its putative anxioselective activity rather than for its sedative effects. In rats, ocinaplon produced muscle relaxation, ataxia, and sedation only at doses 25-fold higher than the effective anxiolytic dose (169). Likewise, in patients with generalized anxiety disorder, ocinaplon produced anxiolytic effects at doses that do not cause greater incidence of sedation or dizziness than placebo. Development of ocinaplon, however, was discontinued due to liver toxicity.

As a group, the pyrazolopyrimidines may be useful compounds to study discrepancies observed using molecular ($GABA_A$ subunit–selective) approaches versus transgenic animals and other in vivo models in the quest for anxioselective drugs. For example, for some compounds, partial agonism at a particular α subunit may be sufficient to produce a full anxiolytic activity in vivo, whereas other compounds must be full agonists for clinically relevant anxiolysis. Currently, it appears that high relative potency and high relative efficacy at multiple receptor subtypes can account for anxioselective properties of certain compounds, including for ocinaplon.

Imidazopyridines

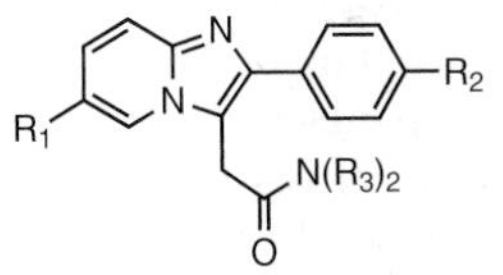

Zolpidem (Ambien) R_1=R_2=R_3 = CH_3
Alpidem R_1=R_2 = Cl, R_3 = $CH_2CH_2CH_3$

The imidazopyridines, zolpidem and alpidem, represent another example of α_1 subunit–selective BZR/$GABA_A$ ligands that have clinical profiles different from those of typical benzodiazepines. For example, although the agonist effects of zolpidem on $GABA_A$ receptors qualitatively resemble those of benzodiazepines, clinically it shows a weaker anticonvulsant effect and a stronger sedative effect, which may mask anxiolytic effects. Zolpidem was marketed as a sedative-hypnotic in the United States in 1993, and it appears to be effective in shortening sleep latency and prolonging total sleep time, without affecting sleep stages, in patients with insomnia (173). Zolpidem is readily absorbed from the gastrointestinal tract and is extensively metabolized by the liver to inactive oxidized products, with a half-life of approximately 2 hours (see Fig. 15.11). Alpidem is similar to zolpidem in that it apparently induces no significant changes in sleep parameters (174) and has no effect on memory or muscle tone (175). Alpidem was

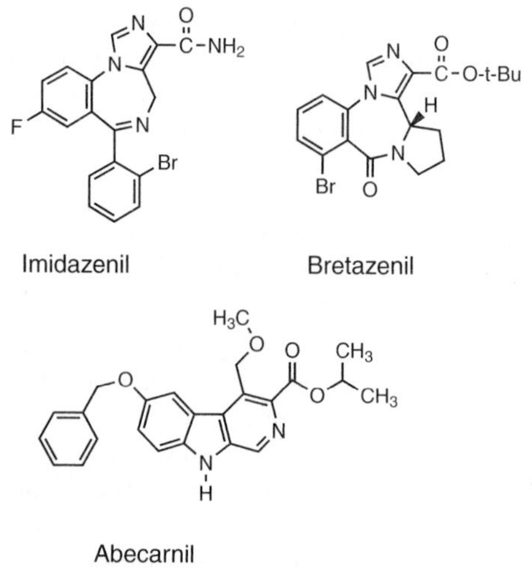

FIGURE 14.23 $GABA_A$ receptor partial agonists.

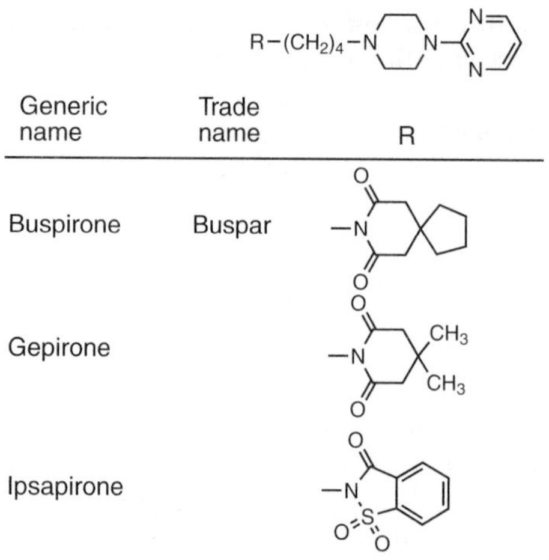

FIGURE 14.24 Azapirone-type $5\text{-}HT_{1A}$ partial agonists.

found to be of at least equal efficacy to lorazepam in the treatment of patients with generalized anxiety disorder (176); however, it was withdrawn because of hepatotoxicity (177).

$GABA_A$ Partial Allosteric Modulators

Partial agonists of the $GABA_A$ receptor complex offer some theoretical and practical advantages over full agonists. For example, compared to the benzodiazepine-type full agonists, partial agonists seem to have lesser side effects, such as sedation, ataxia, and potentiation of alcohol. Also, there may be less abuse potential associated with partial agonists. Three partial agonists of $GABA_A$ receptors were investigated: imidazenil, bretazenil, and abecarnil (Fig. 14.23). Abecarnil is reported by some investigators to have preferential affinity for BZR/$GABA_A$ α_1 subunits, whereas imidazenil and bretazenil are not subtype selective. In any event, abecarnil and bretazenil exhibit anxioselectivity in animal models, but data from clinical trials do not support the anxioselective profile predicted from preclinical results (131).

Imidazenil is an imidazobenzodiazepine carboxamide that has higher BZR affinity than diazepam but is only about half as efficacious at modulating GABA effects on chloride currents. Consistent with the general pharmacologic principle that partial agonists may show antagonist functional effects in competition with a more efficacious agonist, imidazenil blocks the sedative and ataxic effects of diazepam (178). Interestingly, however, imidazenil does not block the anticonvulsant effects of diazepam; accordingly, it has been proposed as an alternative to flumazenil in the alleviation of benzodiazepine-induced withdrawal symptoms (178). Bretazenil has qualitatively similar binding and clinical characteristics as imidazenil (179). Its anxiolytic activity comes with significant sedation, however, and this led to discontinuation of its development. Abecarnil is a β-carboline with anxiolytic properties. Typical of other partial allosteric modulators, abecarnil demonstrates antianxiety and anticonvulsant activities, with little or no development of tolerance to these effects (180). Like bretazenil, however, doses of abecarnil required to produce anxiolysis also produce sedation, and it is unlikely that this drug lead will be developed (97).

Miscellaneous Anxiolytic Agents

Serotonin Receptor–Active Agents

In the development of anxiolytic agents that do not act via the $GABA_A$ receptor complex, serotonin receptors have been the focus of intensive research in recent years, because preclinical and clinical evidence supports the involvement of serotonin in anxiety (181). For example, serotonin $5\text{-}HT_{1A}$ receptors are found in relatively high density in the septohippocampal region of the brain, which is involved in the modulation of anxiety (182). In the structures of the limbic system, $5\text{-}HT_{1A}$ receptors are predominantly postsynaptic, whereas presynaptic $5\text{-}HT_{1A}$ receptors are found in the dorsal and median raphe nuclei. Presynaptic $5\text{-}HT_{1A}$ receptors function as autoreceptors to inhibit serotonergic neurotransmission, and postsynaptic receptor activation also results in decreased neuronal activity.

Azapirones The pyrimidinylbutylpiperazines (azapirones), buspirone, ipsaperone, and gepirone (Fig. 14.24), are partial agonists at brain $5\text{-}HT_{1A}$ receptors and have anxiolytic activity in humans (181,183). Their anxiolytic effects appear only after several days of treatment, and although it is well established that agonistic activity is required, the optimal level of intrinsic activity is still a matter of debate. Thus, it is unclear whether their mechanism of action is to acutely increase serotonergic activity or chronically decrease serotonergic activity (184). Buspirone is the only one of these agents currently marketed in the United States. It also has antidopaminergic activity that complicates interpretation of its interaction with 5-HT_{1A} receptors regarding anxiolytic effects. In any event, buspirone is shown to be effective in the treatment of generalized anxiety disorders that are mild to moderate in severity, although it is not superior in efficacy to benzodiazepines and not as well tolerated (183).

Serotonin Reuptake Inhibitors Several selective serotonin reuptake inhibitors (SSRIs; see Chapter 18), including escitalopram, fluoxetine, fluvoxamine, paroxetine, and sertraline (Fig. 14.25), demonstrate efficacy as first-line treatment of some anxiety disorders, with the purported advantage that they lack the addictive properties of benzodiazepines (181). Specifically, the SSRIs have been shown to be effective in obsessive-compulsive disorder (185), panic disorder (186), and social phobia (187). The mechanism of action of these agents in anxiety may differ with their role in the treatment of depression; however, current understanding centers on functional imaging studies that show SSRI treatment can dampen brain excitability (181). A recent review of the literature (188) that included data on the SSRIs escitalopram, fluoxetine, and paroxetine in comparison to several benzodiazepines, an azapirone (buspirone), a second-generation antipsychotic (olanzapine; see previous section), and other non-SSRI antidepressants (venlafaxine, duloxetine; see Chapter 18) concluded that efficacy of the drug classes and specific drugs is similar.

Atypical Antipsychotic Drugs The second-generation (atypical) antipsychotic drugs olanzapine, quetiapine, and risperidone have been investigated for efficacy as pharmacotherapy for generalized anxiety disorder and social phobia (189,190). Notably, quetiapine was more efficacious than placebo, but study patients were more likely to drop out due to adverse events, including weight gain, sedation, and extrapyramidal side effects. When quetiapine was compared with antidepressants, there was no significant difference in efficacy-related outcomes, but, again, more participants in the quetiapine groups dropped out due to adverse events. The scarce data available for olanzapine and risperidone are inconclusive. Overall, in contrast to antidepressants and benzodiazepines, the long-term risk and benefit of atypical antipsychotic drugs in the treatment of anxiety disorders is not currently established.

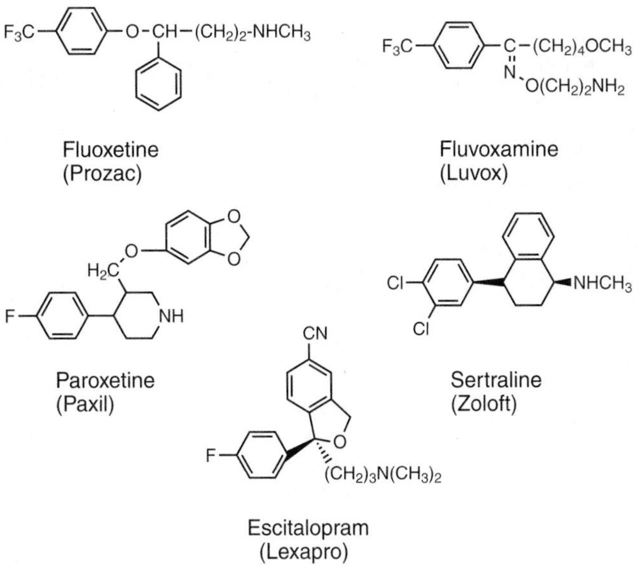

FIGURE 14.25 Structures of some selective serotonin reuptake inhibitors (SSRIs).

SCENARIO: OUTCOME AND ANALYSIS

Outcome

David Hayes, PharmD

The decision is made to switch to aripiprazole because the metabolic effects are generally less often caused by its receptor affinity and interaction, and it has demonstrated good efficacy among patients with schizophrenia. In addition, Ben is encouraged to institute an exercise and diet regimen and an appointment with a dietician is made. Ben returns to his psychiatrist in 3 months after starting his new treatment and reports that he has not experienced any psychotic or delusional episodes. He sees his primary care physician a week later and has lost 21 lb since his last visit and has a fasting blood glucose of 99 mg/dL.

Chemical Analysis

Victoria Roche and S. William Zito

Olanzapine is a thiobenzodiazepine antipsychotic agent that exhibits a high affinity for two main receptor subtypes: dopamine D_2 and serotonin 5-HT_{2A}. The presence of an aromatic moiety and a nitrogen atom capable of becoming cationic at a physiological pH contribute to high affinity at both receptor surfaces. Though 5-HT_{2C} is believed to be the serotonin receptor most closely linked to weight gain, it is known that $5HT_{2A}$ and $5HT_{2C}$ receptors share a strong structural similarity, and ligands of one subtype often bind with comparable affinity to the other. Some authors claim that some therapeutic activities ascribed to antagonism of the 2A subtype might be caused by, at least partially, antagonism of the 2C receptor. Along with its chlorinated dibenzdiazepine analog clozapine, olanzapine prompts some of the most disturbing weight gain of the atypical antipsychotics.

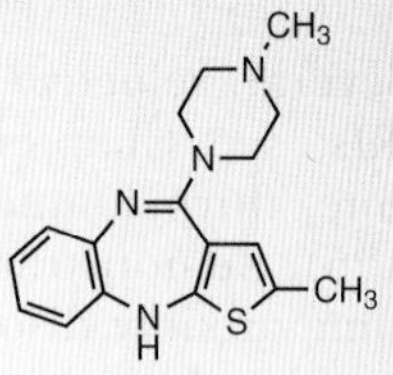

Olanzapine

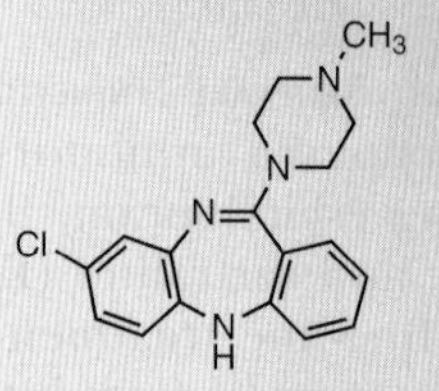

Clozapine

Aripiprazole is a quinolinone-based atypical antipsychotic agent that acts at a wider variety of dopamine and serotonin receptor surfaces than the diazepine-containing molecules. Rather than antagonizing 5-HT_{2C} receptors like olanzapine does, it acts as a partial agonist. That pharmacodynamic action might help Ben feel less hungry and, therefore, consume fewer calories. Weight control and proper nutrition are essential in keeping prediabetic patients from progressing into full-blown disease. Like the other agents that bind to receptors expecting arylethylamine ligands, aripiprazole contains two aromatic nuclei and an ionizable piperazino nitrogen atom.

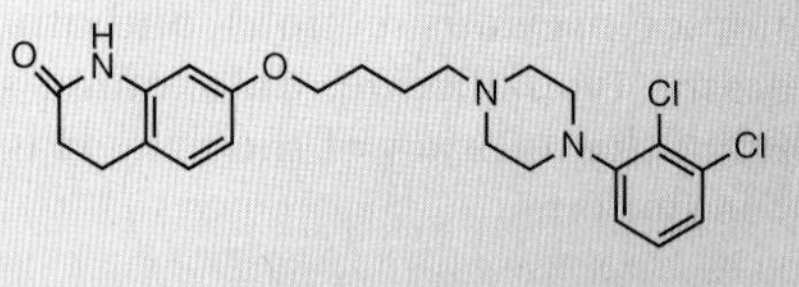

Aripiprazole

CASE STUDY

Victoria Roche and S. William Zito

As a Board-certified psychiatric pharmacist, you have enjoyed a professionally rewarding practice in Hollywood, where the demand for your services seems to be essentially nonstop. You have recently been brought in on a high-profile case involving SN, an actor whose public antics have always been fodder for the tabloids but whose behavior has become increasing aberrant both in public and in private. SN has a history of substance abuse, which has negatively impacted his mental health. His type A personality is exacerbated by the 1 to 2 pots of coffee he drinks daily, particularly after a night of serious partying. He has chain-smoked unfiltered cigarettes for years.

Upon a brief hospitalization after an even shorter stint in a celebrity detoxification center, a diagnosis of schizophrenia is made. SN's medication profile was thoroughly reviewed during his hospitalization and every drug he had been taking was discontinued except for his low-dose diazepam (for anxiety) and diltiazem (for paroxysmal superventricular tachycardia). Your advice about a suitable antipsychotic agent to manage his schizophrenia is now being sought. While interviewing SN you learn that he expects to return to his highly rated daytime soap opera and is already compulsively memorizing his lines. Though he appears physically fit to the casual observer, he is obsessing over the 10 lbs he gained during his days away from his in-home fitness center and personal trainer. He's convinced that, for every pound he's gained, the camera will add five and he'll soon be out of work

Consider the structure of the three antipsychotic agents drawn below and decide which might be the best initial therapeutic choice for this patient.

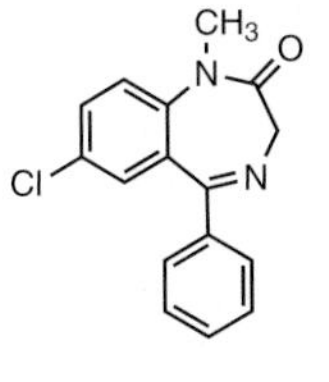

Diazepam

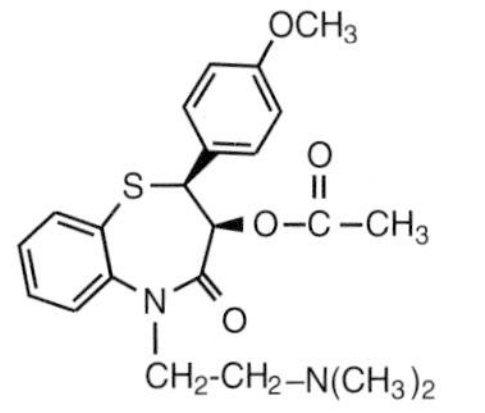

Diltiazem

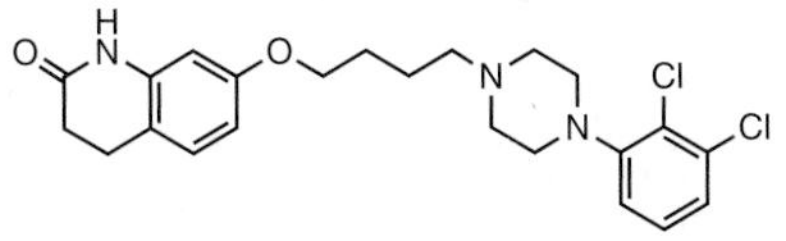

1

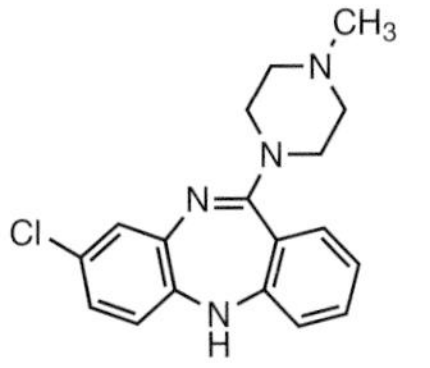

2

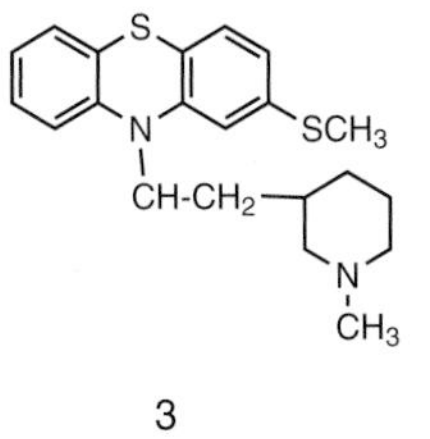

3

1. Conduct a thorough and mechanistic SAR analysis of the three therapeutic options in the case.
2. Apply the chemical understanding gained from the SAR analysis to this patient's specific needs to make a therapeutic recommendation.

References

1. American Psychiatric Association. Diagnostic and Statistical Manual of Mental Disorders, 4th Ed, Revised Text. Washington, DC: APA Press, 2000.
2. Kraepelin E. Dementia Praecox and Paraphrenia (Barclay RM, Roberston GM, trans.). Edinburgh: Livingstone, 1919.
3. Bleuler E. Dimentia Praecox oder Gruppe der Schizophrenien. In: Aschaffenberg G, ed. Handbuch der Psychiatrie (Spezieller Teil, 4. Abteilung). Leipzig, Germany: Denticke, 1911.
4. Owen MJ, Craddock N, O'Donovan MC. Suggestion of roles for both common and rare risk variants in genome-wide studies of schizophrenia. Arch Gen Psychiatry 2010;67:667–773.
5. Watanabe Y, Someya T, Nawa H. Cytokine hypothesis of schizophrenia pathogenesis: evidence from human studies and animal models. Psychiatry Clin Neurosci 2001;64:217–230.
6. Archer T. Neurodegeneration in schizophrenia. Expert Rev Neurother 2010;10:1131–1141.
7. Carlsson A, Lindquist M. Effect of chlorpromazine and haloperidol on formation of 3-methoxytyramine and normetanephrine in mouse brain. Acta Pharmacol Toxicol 1963;20:140–144.
8. Miller R. Mechanisms of action of antipsychotic drugs of different classes, refractoriness to therapeutic effects of classical neuroleptics, and individual variation in sensitivity to their actions: part I. Curr Neuropharmacol 2009;7:302–314.
9. Baldessarini RJ, Tarazi FI. Pharmacotherapy of psychosis and mania. In: Brunton LL, Lazo JS, Parker KL, eds. The Pharmacological Basis of Therapeutics, 11th Ed. New York: McGraw-Hill, 2006:461–500.
10. Baldessarini RJ, Tarazi FI. Chemotherapy in Psychiatry: Principles and Practice, 3rd Ed. Cambridge, MA: Harvard University Press, 1996.
11. Seeman P, Lee T, Chau-Wong M, et al. Antipsychotic drug doses and neuroleptic/dopamine receptors. Nature 1976;261:717–719.
12. Strange PG. Antipsychotic drug action: antagonism, inverse agonism or partial agonism. Trends Pharmacol Sci 2008;29:314–321.
13. Lovenberg TW, Brewster WK, Mottola DM, et al. Dihydrexidine, a novel selective high potency full dopamine D_1 receptor agonist. Eur J Pharmacol 1989;166:111–113.
14. Knoerzer TA, Nichols DE, Brewster WK, et al. Dopaminergic benzo[*a*]phenanthridines: resolution and pharmacological evaluation of the enantiomers of dihydrexidine, the full efficacy D_1 dopamine receptor agonist. J Med Chem 1994;37:2453–2460.
15. Psychoactive Drug Screening Program. BL Roth, Director. NIMH Contract NO2MH80002, University of North Carolina, Chapel Hill, NC. http://pdsp.med.unc.edu/.
16. Booth RG, Baldessarini RJ, Kula NS, et al. Presynaptic inhibition of dopamine synthesis in rat striatal tissue by enantiomeric mono- and dihydroxyaporphines. Mol Pharmacol 1990;38:92–101.
17. Arbilla S, Langer SZ. Stereoselectivity of presynaptic autoreceptors modulating dopamine release. Eur J Pharmacol 1981;76:345–351.
18. Milligan G. Mechanisms of multifunctional signaling by G protein–linked receptors. Trends Pharmacol Sci 1993;14:239–244.
19. Urban JD, Clarke WP, von Zastrow M, et al. Functional selectivity and classical concepts of quantitative pharmacology. J Pharmacol Exp Ther 2007;320:1–13.
20. Raymond JR. Multiple mechanisms of receptor–G protein signaling specificity. Am J Physiol 1995;269:F141–F158.
21. Kenakin T. Inverse, protean, and ligand-selective agonism: matters of receptor conformation. FASEB J 2001;15:598–611.
22. Mottola DM, Kilts JD, Lewis MM, et al. Functional selectivity of dopamine receptor agonists. I. Selective activation of postsynaptic dopamine D_2 receptors linked to adenylate cyclase. J Pharmacol Exp Ther 2002;301:1166–1178.
23. Kilts JD, Connery HS, Arrington EG, et al. Functional selectivity of dopamine receptor agonists. II. Actions of dihydrexidine in D2L receptor-transfected MN9D cells and pituitary lactotrophs. J Pharmacol Exp Ther 2002;301:1179–1189.
24. Moniri NH, Covington-Strachan D, Booth RG. Ligand-directed functional heterogeneity of histamine H_1 receptors: novel dual-function ligands selectively activate and block H_1-mediated phospholipase C and adenylyl cyclase signaling. J Pharmacol Exp Ther 2004;311:274–281.
25. Urban JD, Vargas GA, von Zastrow M, et al. Aripiprazole has functionally selective actions at dopamine D2 receptor-mediated signaling pathways. Neuropsychopharmacology 2007;32:67–77.
26. Booth RG, Baldessarini RJ. Adenosine A_2 stimulation of tyrosine hydroxylase activity in rat striatal minces is reversed by dopamine D_2 autoreceptor activation. Eur J Pharmacol 1990;185:217–221.
27. Choksi NY, Nix William B, Wyrick SD, et al. A novel phenylaminotetralin recognizes histamine H1 receptors and stimulates dopamine synthesis in vivo in rat brain. Brain Res 2000;852:151–160.
28. Johnson EA, Tsai CE, Shahan YH, et al. Serotonin 5-HT_{1A} receptors mediate inhibition of tyrosine hydroxylase in rat striatum. J Pharmacol Exp Ther 1993;266:133–141.
29. El Tamer A, Prokopenko I, Wulfert E, et al. Mivazerol, a novel α_2-agonist and potential anti-ischemic drug, inhibits KC1-stimulated neurotransmitter release in rat nervous tissue preparations. J Neurochemistry 1996;67:636–644.
30. Nichols DE. Hallucinogens. Pharmacol Ther 2004;101:131–181.
31. Kirk SL, Glazebrook J, Grayson B, et al. Olanzapine-induced weight gain in the rat: role of 5-HT2C and histamine H1 receptors. Psychopharmacology (Berl) 2009;207:119–125.
32. Rowland NE, Crump EM, Nguyen N, et al. Effect of (-)-*trans*-PAT, a novel 5-HT2C receptor agonist, on intake of palatable food in mice. Pharmacol Biochem Behav 2008;91:176–180.
33. Rothman RB, Baumann MH, Savage JE, et al. Evidence for possible involvement of 5-HT(2B) receptors in the cardiac valvulopathy associated with fenfluramine and other serotonergic medications. Circulation 2000;102:2836–2841.
34. Fitzgerald LW, Burn TC, Brown BS, et al. Possible role of valvular serotonin 5-HT(2B) receptors in the cardiopathy associated with fenfluramine. Mol Pharmacol 2000;57:75–81.
35. Launay JM, Hervé P, Peoc'h K, et al. Function of the serotonin 5-hydroxytryptamine 2B receptor in pulmonary hypertension. Nat Med 2002;8:1129–1135.
36. Booth RG, Fang L, Huang Y, et al. (1*R*,3*S*)-(-)-*trans*-PAT: a novel full-efficacy serotonin 5-HT2C receptor agonist with 5-HT2A and 5-HT2B receptor inverse agonist/antagonist activity. Eur J Pharmacol 2009;615:1–9.

37. Moya PR, Berg KA, Gutiérrez-Hernandez MA, et al. Functional selectivity of hallucinogenic phenethylamine and phenylisopropylamine derivatives at human 5-hydroxytryptamine (5-HT)2A and 5-HT2C receptors. J Pharmacol Exp Ther 2007;321:1054–1061.
38. González-Maeso J, Weisstaub NV, Zhou M, et al. Hallucinogens recruit specific cortical 5-HT(2A) receptor-mediated signaling pathways to affect behavior. Neuron 2007;53:439–452.
39. Huang XP, Setola V, Yadav PN, et al. Parallel functional activity profiling reveals valvulopathogens are potent 5-hydroxytryptamine(2B) receptor agonists: implications for drug safety assessment. Mol Pharmacol 2009;76:710–722.
40. Canal CE, Morgan D, Booth RG. A functionally-selective serotonin 2 receptor ligand for drug-induced psychoses and schizophrenia. College on Problems of Drug Dependence Abstracts. 73rd Annual Meeting, 2011, http://www.cpdd.vcu.edu/.
41. Bovet D, Staup AM. Action protectrice des éthers phénoliques au cours da l'intoxication histaminique. C R Soc Biol (Paris) 1937;124:547–549.
42. Charpentier P, Gailliot P, Jacob R, et al. Rescherches sur les di methylamino-propyl-N-phenothiazines substituees. C R Acad Sci (Paris) 1952;235:59–60.
43. Laborit H, Huguenard P, Alluaume R. A new vegetative stabilizer. Presse Med 1952;60:206–208.
44. Delay J, Deniker P, Harl J. Utilization therapeutique psychiatrique d'une phenothiazine d'action centrale elective. Ann Med Psychol (Paris) 1952;110:112–117.
45. Horn AS, Snyder SH. Chlorpromazine and dopamine: conformational similarities that correlate with the antischizophrenic activity of phenothiazine drugs. Proc Natl Acad Sci U S A 1971;68:2325–2328.
46. Janssen PA. The butyrophenone story. In: Ayd FI, Blackwell B, eds. Discoveries in Biological Psychiatry. Philadelphia: Lippincott, 1970:165–179.
47. Yang SY, Kao Yang YH, Chong MY, et al. Risk of extrapyramidal syndrome in schizophrenic patients treated with antipsychotics: a population-based study. Clin Pharmacol Ther 2007;81:586–594.
48. Simpson GM, Lee JH. A ten-year review of antipsychotics. In: Lipton MA, ed. Psychopharmacology: A Generation of Progress. New York: Raven Press, 1978:1131–1137.
49. Párraga HC, Harris KM, Párraga KL, et al. An overview of the treatment of Tourette's disorder and tics. J Child Adolesc Psychopharmacol 2010;20:249–462.
50. Janssen PAJ, Van Bever FM. Applications. In: Usdin E, Forrest IS, eds. Psychotherapeutic Drugs. Part II. New York: Marcel Decker, 1977:839–921.
51. Petzer JP, Bergh JJ, Mienie LJ, et al. Metabolic defects caused by 1-methyl-4-phenyl-1,2,3,6-tetrahydropyridine (MPTP) and by HPTP (the tetrahydropyridinyl analog of haloperidol), in rats. Life Sci 2000;66:1949–1954.
52. Augrist BM. The neurobiologically active benzamides and related compounds: some historical aspects. In: Rotrosen J, Stanley M, eds. The Benzamides: Pharmacology, Neurobiology, and Clinical Effects. New York: Raven Press, 1982:1–6.
53. Jenner P, Marsden CD. Neuroleptic agents; acute and chronic receptor actions. In: Horwell DC, ed. Drugs in Central Nervous System Disorders. New York: Marcel Dekker, 1985:149–262.
54. Pasricha PJ, Brunton LL, Lazo JS, Parker KL, eds. The Pharmacological Basis of Therapeutics, 11th Ed. New York: McGraw-Hill, 2006:983–1008.
55. Subramanyam B, Pond S, Eyles D, et al. Identification of a potentially neurotoxic pyridinium metabolite in the urine of schizophrenic patients treated with haloperidol. Biochem Biophys Res Commun 1990;181:573–578.
56. Halliday GM, Pond SM, Cartwright H, et al. Clinical and neuropathological abnormalities in baboons treated with HPTP, the tetrahydropyridine analogue of haloperidol. Exp Neurol 1999;158:155–163.
57. Igarashi K, Matsubara K, Kasuya F, et al. Effect of a pyridinium metabolite derived from haloperidol on the activities of striatal tyrosine hydroxylase in freely moving rats. Neurosci Lett 1996;214:183–186.
58. Rollema H, Skolnick M, D'Engelbronner J, et al. MPP-like neurotoxicity of a pyridinium metabolite derived from haloperidol: in vivo microdialysis and in vitro mitochondrial studies. J Pharmacol Exp Ther 1994;268:380–387.
59. Ulrich S, Sandmann U, Genz A. Serum concentrations of haloperidol pyridinium metabolites and the relationship with tardive dyskinesia and parkinsonism: a cross-section study in psychiatric patients. Pharmacopsychiatry 2005;38:171–177.
60. Wong EH, Tarazi FI, Shahid M. The effectiveness of multi-target agents in schizophrenia and mood disorders: relevance of receptor signature to clinical action. Pharmacol Ther 2010;126:173–185.
61. Reynolds GP, Kirk SL. Metabolic side effects of antipsychotic drug treatment—pharmacological mechanisms. Pharmacol Ther 2010;125:169–179.
62. Kroeze WK, Hufeisen SJ, Popadak BA, et al. H_1-histamine receptor affinity predicts short-term weight gain for typical and atypical antipsychotic drugs. Neuropsychopharmacology 2003;28:519–526.
63. Crossley NA, Constante M, McGuire P, et al. Efficacy of atypical v. typical antipsychotics in the treatment of early psychosis: meta-analysis. Br J Psychiatry 2010;196:434–439.
64. Leucht S, Corves C, Arbter D, et al. Second-generation versus first-generation antipsychotic drugs for schizophrenia: a meta-analysis. Lancet 2009;373:31–41
65. Bhattacharjee J, El-Sayeh HG. Aripiprazole versus typical antipsychotic drugs for schizophrenia. Cochrane Database Syst Rev 2008;3:CD006617.
66. Asenjo Lobos C, Komossa K, Rummel-Kluge C, et al. Clozapine versus other atypical antipsychotics for schizophrenia. Cochrane Database Syst Rev 2010; 11:CD006633.
67. Leucht S, Komossa K, Rummel-Kluge C, et al. A meta-analysis of head-to-head comparisons of second-generation antipsychotics in the treatment of schizophrenia. Am J Psychiatry 2009;166:152–163.
68. Komossa K, Rummel-Kluge C, Schwarz S, et al. Risperidone versus other atypical antipsychotics for schizophrenia. Cochrane Database Syst Rev 2011;1:CD006626.
69. Komossa K, Rummel-Kluge C, Hunger H, et al. Olanzapine versus other atypical antipsychotics for schizophrenia. Cochrane Database Syst Rev 2010;3:CD006654.
70. Komossa K, Rummel-Kluge C, Schmid F, et al. Aripiprazole versus other atypical antipsychotics for schizophrenia. Cochrane Database Syst Rev 2009;4:CD006569.
71. Tandon R, Nasrallah HA, Keshavan MS. Schizophrenia, "just the facts." 5. Treatment and prevention. Past, present, and future. Schizophr Res 2010;122:1–23.
72. Alvir JMJ, Jeffrey PH, Lieberman JA, et al. Clozapine-induced agranulocytosis. Incidence and risk factors in the United States. N Engl J Med 1993;329:162–167.
73. Yadav PN, Abbas AI, Farrell MS, et al. The presynaptic component of the serotonergic system is required for clozapine's efficacy. Neuropsychopharmacology 2011;36:638–651.
74. Kirk SL, Glazebrook J, Grayson B, et al. Olanzapine-induced weight gain in the rat: role of 5-HT2C and histamine H1 receptors. Psychopharmacology (Berl) 2009;207:119–125.
75. Deng C, Weston-Green K, Huang XF. The role of histaminergic H1 and H3 receptors in food intake: a mechanism for atypical antipsychotic-induced weight gain? Prog Neuropsychopharmacol Biol Psychiatry 2010;34:1–4.
76. Raedler TJ, Hinkelmann K, Wiedemann K. Variability of the in vivo metabolism of clozapine. Clin Neuropharmacol 2008;31:347–352.
77. Urichuk L, Prior TI, Dursun S, et al. Metabolism of atypical antipsychotics: involvement of cytochrome p450 enzymes and relevance for drug-drug interactions. Curr Drug Metab 2008;9:410–418.
78. Vainer JL, Chouinard G. Interaction between caffeine and clozapine. J Clin Psychopharmacol 1994;14:284–285.
79. Desai HD, Seabolt J, Jann MW. Smoking in patients receiving psychotropic medications: a pharmacokinetic perspective. CNS Drugs 2001;1:469–494.
80. Haring C, Meise U, Humpel C, et al. Dose-related plasma levels of clozapine: influence of smoking behaviour, sex and age. Psychopharmacology (Berl) 1989;99(Suppl):S38–S40.
81. Kassahun K, Mattiuz E, Nyhart Jr E, et al. Disposition and biotransformation of the antipsychotic agent olanzapine in humans. Drug Met Dispos 1997;25:81–93.
82. DeVane LC, Nemeroff CB. Clinical pharmacokinetics of quetiapine an atypical antipsychotic. Clin Pharmacokin 2001;40:509–522.
83. Shahid M, Walker GB, Zorn SH, Wong EH. Asenapine: a novel psychopharmacologic agent with a unique human receptor signature. J Psychopharmacol 2009;23:65–73.
84. Citrome L. Asenapine for schizophrenia and bipolar disorder: a review of the efficacy and safety profile for this newly approved sublingually absorbed second-generation antipsychotic. Int J Clin Pract 2009;63:1762–1784.
85. McIntyre RS, Cohen M, Zhao J, et al. A 3-week, randomized, placebo-controlled trial of asenapine in the treatment of acute mania in bipolar mania and mixed states. Bipolar Disord 2009;11:673–686.
86. van de Wetering-Krebbers SF, Jacobs PL, Kemperman GJ, et al. Metabolism and excretion of asenapine in healthy male subjects. Drug Metab Dispos 2011;39:580–590.
87. Meltzer HY, Matsubara S, Lee JC. The ratios of $serotonin_2$ and $dopamine_2$ affinities differentiate atypical and typical antipsychotic drugs. Psychopharmacol Bull 1989;25:390–392.
88. Busatto GF, Kerwin RW. Perspectives on the role of serotonergic mechanisms in the pharmacology of schizophrenia. J Psychopharmacol 1997;11:3–12.
89. Kapur S, Remington G. Serotonin–dopamine interaction and its relevance to schizophrenia. Am J Psychiatry 1996;153:466–476.
90. Tarsy D, Baldessarini RJ. Epidemiology of tardive dyskinesia: is risk declining with modern antipsychotics? Mov Disord 2006;21:589–598.
91. Citrome L. Paliperidone: quo vadis? Int J Clin Pract 2007;61:653–662.
92. Yasui-Furukori N, Hidestrand M, Spina E, et al. Different enantioselective 9-hydroxylation of risperidone by the two human CYP2D6 and CYP3A4 enzymes. Drug Metab Dispos 2001;29:1263–1268.
93. Megens AA, Awouters FHL. In vivo pharmacological profile of 9-hydroxyrisperidone, the major metabolite of the novel antipsychotic risperidone. Drug Dev Res 1994;33:399–412.
94. Kramer M, Simpson G, Maciulis V, et al. Paliperidone extended-release tablets for prevention of symptom recurrence in patients with schizophrenia: a randomized, double-blind, placebo-controlled study. J Clin Psychopharm 2007; 27:6–14.
95. Melnik T, Soares BG, Puga ME, et al. Efficacy and safety of atypical antipsychotic drugs (quetiapine, risperidone, aripiprazole and paliperidone) compared with placebo or typical antipsychotic drugs for treating refractory schizophrenia: overview of systematic reviews. Sao Paulo Med J 2010;128:141–166.

96. Newman-Tancredi A, Gavaudan S, Conte C, et al. Agonist and antagonist actions of antipsychotic agents at 5-HT_{1A} receptors: a [^{35}S]GTPγS binding study. Eur J Pharmacol 1998;55:245–256.
97. Meltzer HY, Li Z, Kaneda Y, et al. Serotonin receptors: their key role in drugs to treat schizophrenia. Prog Neuro-Psychopharmacol Biol Psychiatry 2003;27:1159–1172.
98. Beedham C, Miceli JJ, Obach RS. Ziprasidone metabolism, aldehyde oxidase, and clinical implications. J Clin Psychopharmacol 2003;23:229–232.
99. Ishibashi T, Horisawa T, Tokuda K, et al. Pharmacological profile of lurasidone, a novel antipsychotic agent with potent 5-hydroxytryptamine 7 (5-HT7) and 5-HT1A receptor activity. J Pharmacol Exp Ther 2010;334:171–181.
100. lCitrome L. Lurasidone for schizophrenia: a review of the efficacy and safety profile for this newly approved second-generation antipsychotic. Int J Clin Pract 2011;65:189–210.
101. Marino J, Caballero J. Iloperidone for the treatment of schizophrenia. Ann Pharmacother 2010;44:863–780.
102. Potkin SG, Saha AR, Kujawa MJ, et al. Aripiprazole, an antipsychotic with a novel mechanism of action, and risperidone vs placebo in patients with schizophrenia and schizoaffective disorder. Arch Gen Psychiatry 2003;60:681–690.
103. Shapiro DA, Renock S, Arrington E, et al. Aripiprazole, a novel atypical antipsychotic drug with a unique and robust pharmacology. Neuropsychopharmacology 2003;28:1400–1411.
104. Mailman RB, Murthy V. Third generation antipsychotic drugs: partial agonism or receptor functional selectivity? Curr Pharm Des 2010;16:488–501.
105. Kikuchi T, Tottori K, Uwahodo Y, et al. 7-(4-[4-(2,3-Dichlorophenyl)-1-piperazinyl]butyloxy)-3,4-dihydro-2(1H)-quinolinone (OPC-14597), a new putative antipsychotic drug with both presynaptic dopamine autoreceptor agonistic activity and postsynaptic D2 receptor antagonistic activity. J Pharmacol Exp Ther 1995;274:329–336.
106. Lawler CP, Prioleau C, Lewis MM, et al. Interactions of the novel antipsychotic aripiprazole (OPC-14597) with dopamine and serotonin receptor subtypes. Neuropsychopharmacology 1999;20:612–627.
107. Burris KD, Molski TF, Xu C, et al. Aripiprazole, a novel antipsychotic, is a high-affinity partial agonist at human dopamine D2 receptors. J Pharmacol Exp Ther 2002;302:381–389.
108. Vickers SP, Clifton PG, Dourish CT, et al. Reduced satiating effect of D-fenfluramine in serotonin 5-HT_{2C} receptor mutant mice. Psychopharmacology (Berl) 1999;143:309–314.
109. Winans E. Aripiprazole. Am J Health Syst Pharm 2003;60:2437–2445.
110. Owen RR Jr, Cole JO. Molindone hydrochloride: a review of laboratory and clinical findings. J Clin Psychopharmacol 1989;9:268–276.
111. Kasper S. Do we need another atypical antipsychotic? Eur Neuropsychopharmacol 2008;18(Suppl 3):S146–S152.
112. Galatsis P. Market to market. In: Bristol JA, ed. Annual Reports in Medicinal Chemistry, Vol. 32. San Diego: Academic Press, 1997:305–326.
113. Mellman TA, Uhde TW. Electroencephalographic sleep in panic disorder. Arch Gen Psychiatry 1989;46:178–184.
114. Campbell-Sills L, Simmons AN, Lovero KL, et al. Functioning of neural systems supporting emotion regulation in anxiety-prone individuals. Neuroimage 2011;54:689–696.
115. Martin EI, Ressler KJ, Binder E, Nemeroff CB. The neurobiology of anxiety disorders: brain imaging, genetics, and psychoneuroendocrinology. Clin Lab Med 2010;30:865–891.
116. Baxter L. Positron-emission tomography studies of cerebral glucose metabolism in obsessive-compulsive disorder. J Clin Psychiatry 1994;55:54–59.
117. Page LA, Rubia K, Deeley Q, et al. A functional magnetic resonance imaging study of inhibitory control in obsessive-compulsive disorder. Psychiatry Res 2009;174:202–209.
118. Nordahl TE, Semple WE, Gross M, et al. Cerebral glucose metabolic differences in patients with panic disorder. Neuropsychopharmacology 1990;3:261–272.
119. Beutel ME, Stark R, Pan H, et al. Changes of brain activation pre- post short-term psychodynamic inpatient psychotherapy: an fMRI study of panic disorder patients. Psychiatry Res 2010;184:96–104.
120. Rauch S, Savage C, Alpert N, et al. A positron-emission tomographic study of simple phobic symptom provocation. Arch Gen Psychiatry 1995;52:20–28.
121. Caseras X, Mataix-Cols D, Trasovares MV, et al. Dynamics of brain responses to phobic-related stimulation in specific phobia subtypes. Eur J Neurosci 2010;32:1414–1422.
122. Semple WE, Goyer P, McCormick R. Preliminary report: brain blood flow using PET in patients with posttraumatic stress disorder and substance abuse histories. Biol Psychiatry 1993;34:115–118.
123. Roy MJ, Francis J, Friedlander J, et al. Improvement in cerebral function with treatment of posttraumatic stress disorder. Ann N Y Acad Sci 2010;1208:142–149.
124. Gershenfeld HK, Philibert RA, Boehm GW. Looking forward in geriatric anxiety and depression: implications of basic science for the future. Am J Geriatr Psychiatry 2005;13:1027–1040.
125. Cheung A, Mayes T, Levitt A, et al. Anxiety as a predictor of treatment outcome in children and adolescents with depression. J Child Adolesc Psychopharmacol 2010;20:211–216.
126. Olsen RW, Sieghart W. International Union of Pharmacology. LXX. Subtypes of gamma-aminobutyric acid(A) receptors: classification on the basis of subunit composition, pharmacology, and function. Update. Pharmacol Rev 2008;60:243–260.
127. Wafford KA. $GABA_A$ receptor subtypes: any clues to the mechanism of benzodiazepine dependence? Curr Opin Pharmacol 2005;5:47–52.
128. Schofield PR, Darlison MG, Fujita N, et al. Sequence and functional expression of the $GABA_A$ receptor shows a ligand gated ion channel family. Nature 1987;328:221–227.
129. Wisden W, Laurie DJ, Monyer H, et al. The distribution of 13 $GABA_A$ receptor subunit mRNAs in the rat brain: I. Telencephalon, diencephalon, mesencephalon. J Neurosci 1992;12:1040–1062.
130. Sanger DJ, Benavides J, Perrault G, et al. Recent developments in the behavioral pharmacology of benzodiazepine (ω) receptors: evidence for the functional significance of receptor subtypes. Neurosci Biobehav Rev 1994;18:355–372.
131. Basile AS, Lippa AS, Skolnick P. Anxioselective anxiolytics: can less be more? Eur J Pharmacol 2004;500:441–451.
132. Kaupmann K, Malitschek B, Schuler V, et al. GABA-B receptor subtypes assemble into functional heteromeric complexes. Nature 1998;396:683–687.
133. Couve A, Filippov AK, Connolly CN, et al. Intracellular retention of recombinant GABA-B receptors. J Biol Chem 1998;273:26361–26367.
134. Jones KA, Borowsky B, Tamm JA, et al. GABA-B receptors function as a heteromeric assembly of the subunits GABA-BR1 and GABA-BR2. Nature 1998;396:674–679.
135. White JH, Wise A, Main MJ, et al. Heterodimerization is required for the formation of a functional GABA-B receptor. Nature 1998;396:679–682.
136. Quiocho FA, Ledvina PS. Atomic structure and specificity of bacterial periplasmic receptors for active transport and chemotaxis: variation of common themes. Mol Microbiol 1996;20:17–25.
137. Bettler B, Kaupmann K, Mosbacher J, et al. Molecular structure and physiological functions of $GABA_B$ receptors. Physiol Rev 2004;84:835–867.
138. Cryan JF, Kaupmann K. Don't worry 'B' happy!: a role for $GABA_B$ receptors in anxiety and depression. Trends Pharmacol Sci 2005;26:36–43.
139. Bowery NG, Hill DR, Hudson AL, et al. (−)-Baclofen decreases neurotransmitter release in the mammalian CNS by an action at a novel GABA receptor. Nature 1980;238:92–94.
140. Cloos JM, Ferreira V. Current use of benzodiazepines in anxiety disorders. Curr Opin Psychiatry 2009;22:90–95.
141. Sternbach LH. Chemistry of 1,4-benzodiazepines and some aspects of the structure-activity relationship. In: Garattini S, Mussini E, Randall LD, eds. The Benzodiazepines. New York: Raven Press, 1973:1–25.
142. Sternbach LH. The benzodiazepine story. J Med Chem 1979;22:1–7.
143. Randall LO, Schallek W, Heise GA, et al. The psychosedative properties of methaminodiazepoxide. J Pharmacol Exp Ther 1960;129:163–171.
144. Randall LO, Scheckel CL, Banziger RF. Pharmacology of the metabolites of chlordiazepoxide and diazepam. Curr Ther Res Clin Exp 1965;7:590–606.
145. Braestrup C, Nielsen M, Olsen CE. Urinary and brain β-carboline-3-carboxylates as potent inhibitors of brain benzodiazepine receptors. Proc Natl Acad Sci U S A 1980;121:2288–2292.
146. Cole BJ, Hillman M, Seidelmann D, et al. Effects of benzodiazepine receptors partial inverse agonists in the elevated plus maze test of anxiety in the rat. Psychopharmacology 1995;121:118–126.
147. Braestrup C, Schmiechen R, Neef G, et al. Interaction of convulsive ligands with benzodiazepine receptors. Science 1982;216:1241–1243.
148. Haefely W, Kyburz E., Gerecke M, et al. Recent advances in the molecular pharmacology of benzodiazepine receptors and the structure-activity relationships of these agonists and antagonists. In: Advances in Drug Research, Vol. 14. London: Academic Press, 1985:166–322.
149. Hunkeler W, Möhler H, Pieri L, et al. Selective antagonists of benzodiazepines. Nature 1981;290:514–516.
150. Möhler H, Richards JG. Agonist and antagonist benzodiazepine receptor interaction in vitro. Nature 1981;294:763–765.
151. Fryer RI. Ligand interaction at the benzodiazepine receptor. In: Hansch C, ed. Comprehensive Medicinal Chemistry, Vol. 3. New York: Pergamon Press, 1990:539–566.
152. Haefely W. The GABA-benzodiazepine interaction fifteen years later. Neurochemical Res 1990;15:169–174.
153. Wieland HA, Lüddens H, Seeburg PH. A single histidine in $GABA_A$ receptors is essential for benzodiazepine agonist binding. J Biol Chem 1992;267:1426–1429.
154. Huh KH, Delorey TM, Endo S, et al. Pharmacological subtypes of the γ-aminobutyric $acid_A$ receptors defined by a gamma-aminobutyric acid analogue 4,5,6,7-tetrahydroisoxazolo[5,4-*c*] pyridin-3-ol and allosteric coupling: characterization using subunit-specific antibodies. Mol Pharmacol 1995;48:666–675.
155. Pritchett DB, Sontheimer H, Shivers BD, et al. Importance of a novel $GABA_A$ receptor subunit for benzodiazepine pharmacology. Nature 1989;338:582–585.
156. Pritchett DB, Seeburg PH. γ-Aminobutyric $acid_A$ receptor α_5 subunit creates novel type II benzodiazepine receptor pharmacology. J Neurochem 1990;54:1802–1804.

157. Rowlett JK, Platt DM, Lelas S, et al. Different $GABA_A$ receptor subtypes mediate the anxiolytic, abuse-related, and motor effects of benzodiazepine-like drugs in primates. Proc Natl Acad Sci U S A 2005;102:915–920.
158. Wong G, Lyon T, Skolnick P. Chronic exposure to benzodiazepine receptor ligands uncouples the γ-aminobutyric acid type A receptor in WSS-1 cells. Mol Pharmacol 1994;46:1056–1062.
159. Tietz EI, Chiu TH, Rosenberg HC. Regional GABA/benzodiazepine receptor/chloride channel coupling after acute and chronic benzodiazepine treatment. Eur J Pharmacol 1989;167:57–65.
160. Crippen GM. Distance geometry analysis of the benzodiazepine binding site. Mol Pharmacol 1982;22:11–19.
161. Zhang W, Koehler KF, Zhang P, et al. Development of a comprehensive pharmacophore model for the benzodiazepine receptor. Drug Des Discov 1995;12:193–248.
162. Diaz-Arauzo H, Koehler KF, Hagen TJ, et al. Synthetic and computer assisted analysis of the pharmacophore for agonists at benzodiazepine receptors. Life Sci 1991;49:207–216.
163. Villar HO, Davies MF, Loew GH, et al. Molecular models for recognition and activation at the benzodiazepine receptor: a review. Life Sci 1991;48:593–602.
164. Falco JL, Lloveras M, Buira I, et al. Design, synthesis and biological activity of acyl substituted 3-amino-5-methyl-1,4,5,7-tetrahydropyrazolo[3,4-*b*]pyridin-6-ones as potential hypnotic drugs. Eur J Med Chem 2005;40:1179–1187.
165. Blount JF, Fryer RI, Gilman NW, et al. Quinazolines and 1,4-benzodiazepines. 92. Conformational recognition of the receptor by 1,4-benzodiazepines. Mol Pharmacol 1983;24:425–428.
166. Sunjic V, Lisin A, Sega A, et al. Conformation of 7-chloro-5-phenyl-d5-3(s)-methyldihydro-1,4-benzodiazepine-2-one in solution. Heterocyc Chem 1979;16:757–761.
167. Olkkola KT, Ahonen J. Midazolam and other benzodiazepines. Handb Exp Pharmacol 2008;182:335–360.
168. Gerecke M. Chemical structure and properties of midazolam compared with other benzodiazepines. Br J Clin Pharmacol 1983;16(Suppl 1):11S–16S.
169. Lippa A, Czobor P, Stark J, et al. Selective anxiolysis produced by ocinaplon, a $GABA_A$ receptor modulator. Proc Natl Acad Sci U S A 2005;102:7380–7385.
170. Davies M, Newell JG, Derry JM, et al. Characterization of the interaction of zopiclone with γ-aminobutyric acid type A receptors. Mol Pharmacol 2000;58:756–762.
171. Rosenberg R, Caron J, Roth T, et al. An assessment of the efficacy and safety of eszopiclone in the treatment of transient insomnia in healthy adults. Sleep Med 2005;6:15–22.
172. Lemon MD, Strain JD, Hegg AM, et al. Indiplon in the management of insomnia. Drug Des Dev Ther 2009;3:131–142.
173. Herrmann WM, Kubicki ST, Boden S, et al. Pilot controlled double-blind study of the hypnotic effects of zolpidem in patients with chronic "learned" insomnia: psychometric and polysomnographic evaluation. J Int Med Res 1993;21:306–322.
174. Saletu B, Schultes M, Grunberger J. Sleep laboratory study of a new antianxiety drug, alpidem: short-term trial. Curr Ther Res 1986;40:769–779.
175. Bartholini G. Nonbenzodiazepine anxiolytics and hypnotics: concluding remarks. Pharmacol Biochem Behav 1988;29:833–834.
176. Diamond BI, Nguyen H, et al. A comparative study of alpidem, a nonbenzodiazepine, and lorazepam in patients with nonpsychotic anxiety. Psychopharmacol Bull 1991;27:67–71.
177. Berson A, Descatoire V, Sutton A, et al. Toxicity of alpidem, a peripheral benzodiazepine receptor ligand, but not zolpidem, in rat hepatocytes: role of mitochondrial permeability transition and metabolic activation. J Pharmacol Exp Ther 2001;299:793–800.
178. Auta J, Costa E, Davis JM, et al. Imidazenil: an antagonist of the sedative but not the anticonvulsant action of diazepam. Neuropharmacology 2005;49:425–429.
179. Puia G, Ducic I, Vicini S, et al. Molecular mechanisms of the partial allosteric modulatory effects of bretazenil at γ-aminobutyric acid type A receptor. Proc Natl Acad Sci U S A 1992;89:3620–3624.
180. Ozawa M, Sugimachi K, Nakada-Kometani Y, et al. Chronic pharmacological activities of the novel anxiolytic β-carboline abecarnil in rats. J Pharmacol Exp Ther 1994;269:457–462.
181. Gross C, Hen R. The developmental origins of anxiety. Nat Rev Neurosci 2004;5:545–552.
182. Gray JAG. The Neuropsychology of Anxiety: An Enquiry into the Functions of the Septo-Hippocampal System. New York: Oxford University Press, 1982.
183. Chessick CA, Allen MH, Thase M, et al. Azapirones for generalized anxiety disorder. Cochrane Database Syst Rev 2006;3:CD006115.
184. Peroutka SJ. 5-Hydroxytryptamine receptors. J Neurochem 1993;60:408–416.
185. Pigott TA, Pato BT, Bernstein SE, et al. Controlled comparisons of clomipramine and fluoxetine in the treatment of obsessive-compulsive disorder. Arch Gen Psychiatry 1990;47:926–932.
186. Schneirer FR, Liebowitz MR, Davies SO, et al. Fluoxetine in panic disorder. J Clin Psychopharmacol 1990;10:119–121.
187. Black B, Uhde TW, Tancer ME. Fluoxetine for the treatment of social phobia. J Clin Psychopharmacol 1992;12:293–295.
188. Davidson JR, Feltner DE, Dugar A. Management of generalized anxiety disorder in primary care: identifying the challenges and unmet needs. Prim Care Companion J Clin Psychiatry 2010;12:PCC.09r00772.
189. Gao K, Sheehan DV, Calabrese JR. Atypical antipsychotics in primary generalized anxiety disorder or comorbid with mood disorders. Expert Rev Neurother 2009;9:1147–1158.
190. Depping AM, Komossa K, Kissling W, et al. Second-generation antipsychotics for anxiety disorders. Cochrane Database Syst Rev 2010;12:CD008120.

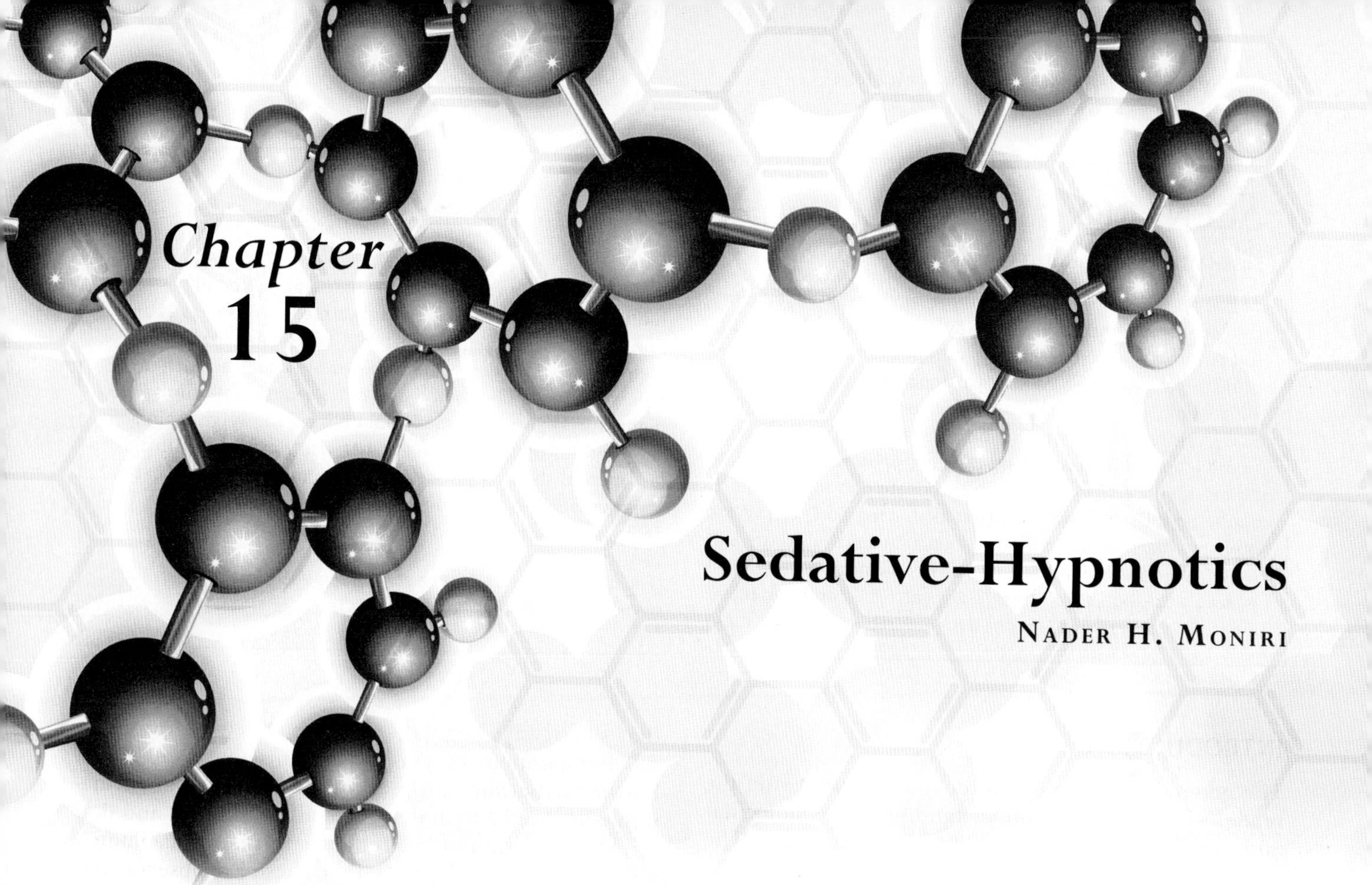

Chapter 15

Sedative-Hypnotics

NADER H. MONIRI

Drugs Covered in This Chapter

BARBITURATES

- Amobarbital
- Butabarbita
- Pentobarbital
- Phenobarbital
- Secobarbital
- Thiamylal
- Thiobarbital

BENZODIAZEPINE SEDATIVE-HYPNOTICS

- Estazolam
- Flurazepam
- Quazepam
- Temazepam
- Triazolam

HISTAMINE H_1 RECEPTOR ANTAGONISTS

- Diphenhydramine
- Doxepin
- Doxylamine

MELATONIN RECEPTOR AGONISTS

- Ramelteon

NONBENZODIAZEPINE SEDATIVE-HYPNOTICS

- Eszopiclone
- Zaleplon
- Zolpidem

Abbreviations

AA-NAT, arylalkylamine *N*-acetyltransferase
AMP, adenosine monophosphate
AMPA, α-amino-3-hydroxy-5-methyl-4-isoxazole propionic acid
APR, antiplanar region
ARAS, ascending reticular activating system
BZ, benzodiazepine
CNS, central nervous system
EEG, electroencephalography
ERR, electron-rich region
FDA, U.S. Food and Drug Administration
FRAR, freely rotating aromatic ring region
$GABA_A$, γ-aminobutyric acid A receptors
GPCR, G protein–coupled receptor
HIOMT, hydroxyindole-*O*-methyltransferase
MT, melatonin
NPS, neuropeptide S
PAR, planar aromatic region
PKA, protein kinase A
REM, rapid eye movement
SAR, structure–activity relationship
SCN, suprachiasmatic nucleus
TMH, transmembrane helix
TMN, tuberomammillary nucleus

SCENARIO

Susan W. Miller, PharmD, CGP, FASCP

WK, a 78-year-old white woman, presents to the ambulatory care clinic for a medication therapy management (MTM) consult before her appointment for a routine examination with her primary care provider. WK is accompanied by her daughter, with whom she lives. WK's medical problems (and medications) are type 2 diabetes (glipizide 5 mg po QD), hypertension (verapamil SR 180 mg po QD), osteoporosis (alendronate 70 mg po once weekly, calcium carbonate 600 mg/vitamin D 200 iu po BID), and insomnia (zolpidem 5 mg po Q HS). WK's problems have been controlled, but at today's visit, an 8-lb weight gain in 6 months is noted. Her hemoglobin A_{1C} level is now 7.6% but it had been stable at 6.8%, and her blood pressure is 126/78 mm Hg. The daughter reports that her mom has begun to wander through the house at night and has been found on several occasions eating warmed-up leftovers at 2 AM. The daughter also reports that WK has begun to experience memory loss. WK denies these behaviors and reports that she falls asleep just fine, but she is not sleeping well during the night. WK is also concerned about her recent weight gain and she confides that, as a result of her visit to the dermatologist last month, she was prescribed a new medicine, itraconazole capsules, for the newly diagnosed fungal infection in the fingernails on her right hand.

(The reader is directed to the clinical solution and chemical analysis of this case at the end of the chapter).

INTRODUCTION

The general objective of this chapter is to provide the reader with an in-depth understanding of the molecular and chemical basis of sedative-hypnotic drug action. The reader is first introduced to neuronal regulation of the sleep/wake cycle and the effects on regulating the stages of sleep. Emphasis is placed on introducing the targets of sedative-hypnotic agents, particularly γ-aminobutyric acid A receptors ($GABA_A$), melatonin (MT) MT1/MT2 receptors, and histamine H_1 receptors. Specific agents that modulate the functions of these receptors to promote sleep will be discussed from the perspectives of structure–activity relationships, as well as physiochemical and pharmacokinetic properties that affect their activity.

NEUROBIOLOGY OF SLEEP

Sleep is a reversible process that is typified by sensory and motor inactivity as well as reduced cortical responses to external stimuli. This process is distinct from complete states of unconsciousness (e.g., coma), in which decreased cortical activity is unresponsive to all external stimuli. In human physiology, sleep/wake cycles are regulated to a large degree by endogenous circadian rhythms as well as homeostatic mechanisms, which in turn are governed by a myriad of neuronal pathways. Critical experiments performed in felines in the late 1940s demonstrated that impairment of the reticular formation within the brainstem triggered behavioral and electroencephalographic (EEG) activity consistent with coma-like states, suggesting that this area of the brain was involved in regulating sleep and wakefulness (1). This was contrary to observations that showed that felines with lesions of ascending sensory neurons distal to the reticular formation displayed no impairment to wakefulness or sleep, indicating that sleep/wake regulation by the reticular formation was independent of sensory neurons that *leave* it (2). Further experiments showed that the reticular formation contained a high density of afferent input and that direct stimulation of the reticular formation facilitated wakefulness (3). Taken together, these key observations suggested that sleep and wakefulness were likely controlled by factors within the reticular formation and that this structure behaves as a relay center that transmits afferent input to the cortex. These and other pioneering studies led to the ascending reticular activating system (ARAS) hypothesis of sleep/wake regulation and subsequent identification of ARAS function as being critical in modification of sleep/wake transitions. Many decades of ensuing research on sleep/wake responses of the ARAS have revealed that projections to and from various nuclei within the brainstem can modulate ARAS activity to facilitate wakefulness and sleep. These include serotonergic neurons of the raphe nucleus within the reticular formation itself; cholinergic neurons of the pedunculopontine tegmentum and noradrenergic neurons of the locus coeruleus, within the pons; as well as dopaminergic neurons of the substantia nigra and ventral tegmental areas of the midbrain. These structures themselves are regulated in a highly orchestrated manner primarily by the excitatory neurotransmitter glutamate and the inhibitory neurotransmitter GABA to regulate their respective activities.

In addition to the cell structures that make up the brainstem ARAS, there are additional populations of highly specialized cells that can modulate sleep/wakefulness either independently or in concert with cells of the ARAS. For example, stimulation of the tuberomammillary nucleus (TMN) within the posterior hypothalamus facilitates wakefulness and arousal, and these cells are predominantly active only during wakeful periods (4). TMN-mediated regulation of wakefulness is dependent on histaminergic neurons that densely project into the cortex as well as other wake-promoting structures within the brainstem (5). The firing rate of these cortical-projecting histaminergic TMN neurons decreases upon sleep and increases upon arousal, whereas lesioning of histaminergic neurons within the TMN promotes sleep (6–8). Biochemically, the release of histamine from these neurons is increased upon and during wakefulness and is under the control of glutaminergic-stimulatory and GABAergic-inhibitory circuits (9,10). Studies with histamine receptor knockout mice and in vivo pharmacologic studies have established that the TMN effects of histamine on wakefulness and sleep are mediated primarily by histamine H_1 receptors.

Whereas the posterior-hypothalamic TMN is involved in regulating arousal, the anterior-hypothalamus, specifically the suprachiasmatic nucleus (SCN), is involved in induction of sleep. This has been demonstrated by studies that show that lesions to the posterior hypothalamus (e.g., TMN) induce sleepfulness, whereas lesions of the anterior hypothalamus are associated with wakefulness (11). Decades of further work have established that the SCN is critical for the maintenance of circadian rhythms, in essence behaving as the brain's endogenous master clock, thereby regulating sleep/wake cycles and synchronizing circadian phase timings with other brain structures. Importantly, the SCN receives visual input from the retina via the retinohypothalamic tract, and this key connection serves to synchronize circadian rhythms to daylight (12). The firing rate of SCN neurons is strongly correlated with day/night cycles, which serve to establish an approximate 24-hour circadian rhythm. Although the SCN is largely under the control of glutaminergic and GABAergic neurons, which originate in the preoptic nucleus, it also works in concert with the pineal gland to regulate circadian rhythms (13). As such, inhibitory GABAergic outflow from SCN neurons to the pineal gland is enhanced during the daylight hours and declines proportionally to decreases in daylight. Light-sensitive neurons from the SCN project to the hypothalamic paraventricular nuclei and through the lateral horn of the spinal cord primarily by way of vasopressin and GABAergic neurons. The signal is then relayed to the pineal gland through noradrenergic ganglionic sympathetic fibers, which directly innervate the pineal gland. Hence, during periods of light, GABA output is elevated, which inhibits the release of norepinephrine at the pineal gland. On the contrary, during periods of darkness, the inhibitory GABAergic outflow from the SCN is reduced, resulting in increased levels of norepinephrine released at the level of the pineal gland (12). Here, norepinephrine acts primarily through pineal β_1- and α_{1B}-adrenergic receptors to stimulate a rapid and profound (~10-fold) synthesis and release of melatonin, another key regulator of circadian rhythms and the sleep/wake cycle, into the bloodstream (14).

The synthesis of melatonin occurs within the pineal gland, where the amino acid L-tryptophan is converted to serotonin, which is subsequently acetylated to yield *N*-acetylserotonin by the enzyme arylalkylamine *N*-acetyltransferase (AA-NAT). *N*-acetylserotonin is converted to melatonin by the

CLINICAL SIGNIFICANCE

Medications from several classes are useful pharmacotherapeutic agents for managing insomnia. The benzodiazepines are safe and effective and are the most commonly prescribed sedative-hypnotic agents. Within the class of benzodiazepines, those with shorter elimination half-lives, such as the triazolobenzodiazepines triazolam and estazolam, provide improved sleep patterns and minimal daytime sedation. Relative duration of action, as well as sedative-hypnotic potency and risk of residual morning depressant effects, can be readily assessed from an evaluation of benzodiazepine structure. The nonbenzodiazepine $GABA_A$ agonists of zolpidem, zaleplon, and eszopiclone have comparable efficacy to the benzodiazepines in improving sleep patterns and can be selectively used to reduce sleep latency, nighttime awakenings, and/or total sleep time. The melatonin receptor agonist ramelteon is a newer alternative as a sedative-hypnotic agent. The antihistamine H_1-receptor antagonists diphenhydramine and doxylamine, members of the highly sedative aminoalkylether class of antihistamines, as well as the antidepressants trazodone and doxepin (a member of the tertiary tricyclics well known for sedative side effects) are useful as sedative-hypnotic agents, but selection of these should be based on the side effect profile of the individual agent. Barbiturates are well established as effective sedative-hypnotic agents and their well-defined structure-activity relationships can help guide clinicians in drug product selection when they are truly indicated; however, their associated toxicities of central nervous system depression, physical dependence, and tolerance as well as their activity as potent hepatic enzyme inducers have limited their use as sedative-hypnotic agents. Identifying the chemical classes and their associated physical chemical properties and metabolic fates will greatly facilitate the understanding and utilization of these useful therapeutic agents.

Susan W. Miller, PharmD
Professor
College of Pharmacy and Health Sciences
Mercer University

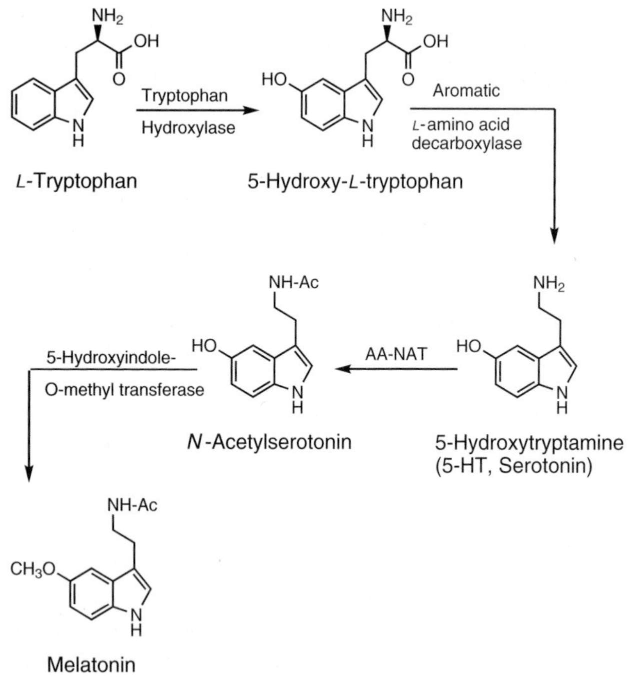

FIGURE 15.1 Biosynthesis of melatonin.

enzyme 5-hydroxyindole-*O*-methyltransferase (HIOMT) (Fig. 15.1). The activity of AA-NAT is greatly influenced by β_1-adrenergic receptors, which are activated upon the release of norepinephrine via the SCN circuit described earlier. β_1-receptor–mediated increases in intracellular cyclic adenosine monophosphate (AMP) stimulate AA-NAT expression and also increase protein kinase A (PKA)–mediated phosphorylation of AA-NAT, which stabilizes and activates the enzyme (15). The rhythm of AA-NAT activity is thus correspondingly coupled to light exposure because increases in light lead to decreases in AA-NAT activity. Activity of AA-NAT can also be effectively abolished by lesions of the SCN, further demonstrating that melatonin synthesis is dependent on retinohypothalamic input (16). Once synthesized, melatonin diffuses into capillary blood vessels and rapidly reaches all tissues of the body, where it can agonize its cognate G protein–coupled receptors (GPCRs), MT1R and MT2R, leading to various physiologic responses. With specific regard to sleep, melatonin has profound effects in the SCN, where it agonizes MT1R to mediate the acute inhibition of SCN neurons, thereby promoting sleep. Additionally, agonism of MT2R in the SCN is associated with the phase-shifting effects on circadian rhythms.

HUMAN SLEEP CYCLES

EEG has afforded researchers the ability to assess the electrical activity of the brain during the course of sleep, and these findings have revealed the presence of distinct EEG activity that correlates to five stages of sleep. These stages, which cycle throughout the night, include four non–rapid eye movement (REM) stages, often referred to as "quiet sleep," as well a single stage of REM sleep, referred to as "active sleep." Non-REM sleep stages correlate to periods of low metabolic rate and low neuronal activity; hence, brain activity and EEG events are "quiet." In non-REM sleep, heart rate and blood pressure are also reduced due to an increase in parasympathetic nervous system activity coupled with a decrease in sympathetic activity. As a result of these autonomic reflexes, non-REM sleep also causes pupillary constriction, which diminishes the amount of light that is allowed to enter the retina (17). The initial period of sleep is stage 1, which lasts only a brief period of time (5 to 15 minutes) and represents the period of transitioning from wakefulness to sleep. Although EEG activity in awake humans mainly consists of high-frequency (15 to 25 Hz) alpha-wave events, the progression to stage 1 sleep results in the emergence of slower theta waves with lower frequency (4 to 10 Hz) as the individual progresses to the light or drowsy sleep characterized by stage 1. In stage 2 sleep, which often lasts 15 to 20 minutes, background theta waves continue but are periodically interrupted by characteristic sleep spindles, which are short bursts of higher frequency (12 to 15 Hz) EEG events. Stage 2 of the sleep cycle is still considered a light sleep; however, skeletal muscle activity is decreased in this stage compared to the transitionary stage 1. Stages 3 and 4, often referred to as slow-wave sleep, are characterized by appearance of higher amplitude, slower frequency (0.5 to 4 Hz) delta waves, which occur less often in stage 3 and more often in stage 4. Both of these stages represent deep sleep because the characteristic delta activity is least similar to arousal-state alpha activity. If awakened in this stage of sleep, an individual will likely be confused and disoriented (18).

The fifth stage of sleep is referred to as REM sleep and is characterized by increases in eye movement, respiration rate, and brain activity. Electroencephalographic changes in REM sleep include high-voltage firing spikes, which seem to originate in the pons, lateral geniculate nucleus, and occipital cortex, and these spikes are correlated with bursts of rapid eye movements associated with this stage of sleep (19). The increased brain activity in REM sleep is consistent with an increase in dreaming and an increase in metabolic rate, thus the naming convention "active sleep"; yet, it is inversely proportional to skeletal muscle tonicity, which effectively paralyzes skeletal movements.

The sleep stages are normally cycled every 90 to 100 minutes throughout the night, and it is important to note that sleep does not necessarily advance sequentially through the five stages. Healthy adults typically enter sleep through a progression through the stages, with the first REM stage occurring after 75 to 90 minutes of non-REM sleep and a typical return to stage 2 or 3 sleep thereafter. As sleep progresses over the course of a night, the amount of time spent in REM sleep increases such that over a typical 8-hour sleep cycle, approximately 55% to 60% of sleep time is spent in stages 1 and 2 (light sleep), 20% in stages 3 and 4 (deep sleep), and 20% to 25% in stage 5 (REM sleep).

PHARMACOLOGIC TARGETS OF SEDATIVE-HYPNOTIC AGENTS

As described earlier in the brief introduction, there are many physiologic and biochemical factors that can influence the various stages of sleep, and as such, numerous targets for pharmacologic intervention have arisen. In fact, nearly every neurotransmitter system in the mammalian brain, including the adenosinergic, serotonergic, dopaminergic, adrenergic, histaminergic, and cholinergic systems, have at one time or another been associated with induction of sleep or wakefulness. Despite this wide breadth of potential biochemical targets, the development of sedative-hypnotic agents has primarily focused on 1) agents that cause CNS depression via agonism of $GABA_A$ receptors, and 2) agents that modulate hypothalamic histamine or melatonin circadian systems that, as described earlier, regulate sleep and arousal. This chapter will focus on structure–activity relationships (SARs) and pharmacodynamics of these agents, including barbiturates, benzodiazepines, nonbenzodiazepine $GABA_A$ agonists, melatonin receptor agonists and histamine H_1 receptor antagonists. Development of agents that modulate the activity of novel protein targets such as orexin and neuropeptide S receptors will also be discussed towards the end of the chapter.

$GABA_A$ Receptors

GABA is the major inhibitory neurotransmitter in the mammalian central nervous system (CNS) and is critical in balancing neuronal excitation. GABA is widely distributed throughout the CNS and can be in found at concentrations up to 1,000-fold (high μmol/L to low mmol/L) greater than that of monoaminergic neurotransmitters in various CNS nuclei. GABA-induced physiologic functions are mediated by at least two distinct classes of membrane-bound receptors, ionotropic $GABA_A$ receptors and metabotropic $GABA_B$ receptors. $GABA_B$ receptors belong to the second messenger–linked GPCR superfamily and share homology with metabotropic glutamate receptors. Meanwhile, $GABA_A$ receptors are ligand-gated ion channels that modulate conductance of chloride ions through the cell membrane upon binding of GABA. The activation of $GABA_A$ receptors on excitable neurons leads to membrane hyperpolarization, which facilitates an increase in the firing threshold potential and consequently reduces the likelihood of generating an action potential. Hence, agonism of GABA receptors leads to neuronal inhibition and CNS depression, and not surprisingly, $GABA_A$ receptors are important targets for treatment of a variety of CNS disorders in which CNS depression provides a therapeutic benefit, including anxiety (see Chapter 14), anesthesia (see Chapter 16), convulsions and seizures (see Chapter 17), and sleep disorders. In this regard, drugs that increase $GABA_A$-mediated chloride flux (e.g., $GABA_A$ agonists) provide anxiolytic, anesthetic, anticonvulsant, and sedative-hypnotic activity, whereas agents that block the chloride channel (e.g., picrotoxin) can lead to convulsions and a heightened state of arousal.

The $GABA_A$ receptor-channel complex is related to the nicotinic acetylcholine receptor superfamily, which also includes the strychnine-sensitive glycine receptors and serotonin $5\text{-}HT_3$ receptors. In the human brain, $GABA_A$ complexes are formed by oligomerization of individual subunits that produce heteropentomeric complexes consisting of α, β, γ, δ, ε, or ρ subunits, which assemble a ligand-gated channel with a central pore that allows for the conductance of chloride (Fig. 15.2) (20). Moreover, the α, β, and γ subunits of $GABA_A$ receptors are expressed as distinct alternatively spliced variants (e.g., $\alpha_{[1\text{-}6]}$, $\beta_{[1\text{-}3]}$, $\gamma_{[1\text{-}3]}$). Functional channels typically require multiple α and β subunits in combination with another subunit, allowing for tremendous diversity in the makeup of the channels (Fig. 15.2). The distribution of various $GABA_A$ receptors varies according to the subtype combinations. The $\alpha_1\beta_2\gamma_2$, $\alpha_2\beta_3\gamma_2$, and $\alpha_3\beta_3\gamma_2$ subtypes are the most abundant receptors, accounting for nearly 80% of $GABA_A$ receptors in the mammalian brain (20). The α_1 subunit is the most widely expressed, whereas α_4, α_5, and α_6 subunits are restricted to localized neuronal populations (20). Two distinct GABA binding sites are formed at the two α and β subunit interfaces, whereas the binding sites for GABA-modulating drugs such as barbiturates and benzodiazepines are at allosteric sites (Fig. 15.2). Upon binding of barbiturates or benzodiazepines to their respective allosteric sites on the $GABA_A$ receptor, alterations in the conductance of Cl^- occur, as described for each class of agent in the following sections.

Barbiturates

Barbiturates are potent CNS depressants with sedative-hypnotic, anesthetic, and anticonvulsant activity and were widely considered sedative-hypnotic agents of choice until the marketing of benzodiazepines in the late 1960s. Barbiturates played a crucial role in our understanding of $GABA_A$ receptor function, and although there are special instances that call for barbiturate use, they have largely been replaced as sedative-hypnotic agents by other agents due to safety concerns, which include tolerance, dependence, potential for abuse, and a relatively low toxicity threshold that can lead to overdosage and poisoning. Currently, there are five barbiturates approved by

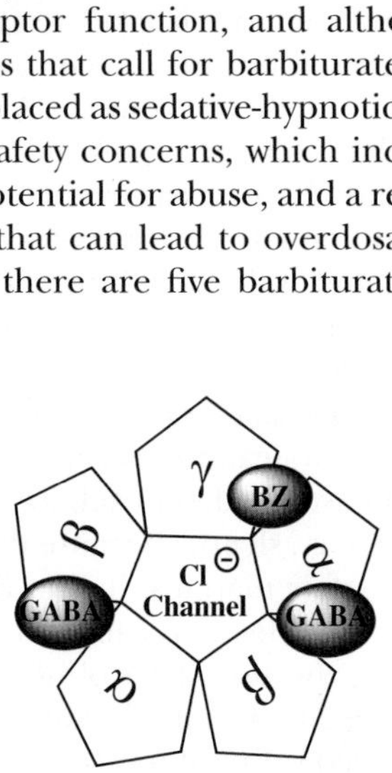

FIGURE 15.2 The pentameric assembly of $GABA_A$ receptors, whose monomers assemble to form the chloride channel at the center. The distinct GABA and benzodiazepine binding sites of this αβγ-type receptor are noted.

the U.S. Food and Drug Administration (FDA) for use as sedative-hypnotics: amobarbital, butabarbital, pentobarbital, phenobarbital, and secobarbital.

Barbiturate Mechanism of Action Upon binding of GABA to the receptor, the chloride ion (Cl^-) conductance channel opens in bursts of approximately 1 millisecond, 5 millisecond, and 10 millisecond of duration, followed by brief periods of closure. Channel opening increases in frequency and duration upon increases in GABA concentrations. Binding of barbiturates to their $GABA_A$ binding site causes an increase in the binding of GABA to the receptor, facilitating an enhancement of the actions of GABA and leading to prolongation of the longest-duration open state (21). Although the exact site of barbiturate binding remains elusive, it is known that this site is distinct from both the GABA and benzodiazepine (BZ) sites and that the barbiturate site likely does not require specific subunits, unlike the BZ site (see later discussion). Higher therapeutic concentrations of barbiturates can also enhance binding of benzodiazepines, whereas supratherapeutic concentrations of barbiturates can cause opening of the channel independently of GABA, although the clinical importance of this response has not been widely studied (22). Notably, in addition to their augmentation of $GABA_A$ responses, the physiologic effects of higher concentrations of barbiturates can also be mediated by kainite-sensitive α-amino-3-hydroxy-5-methyl-4-isoxazole propionic acid (AMPA) glutamate receptors, as well as voltage-gated Na^+ and Ca^{2+} channels.

Pharmacologic Effects of Barbiturates Barbiturates act as reversible inhibitors of virtually all excitable neurons and can produce dose-dependent CNS depression, which ranges in effect from weak sedation to general anesthesia. With regard to their effects on sleep, barbiturates significantly decrease the time it takes to fall asleep (sleep latency), increase the total time of sleep, and also decrease occurrences of nighttime awakenings. As a consequence of these effects, barbiturates significantly impair psychomotor abilities and also decrease memory and cognitive performance. Additionally, barbiturates can cause physical dependence, and sudden withdrawal of these agents can lead to serious neuropsychiatric symptoms and convulsions of excitable tissue, which can facilitate seizures and respiratory spasms. Long-term use of barbiturates has also been shown to lead to tolerance, in which higher doses of the agent are needed to achieve the same therapeutic endpoints (e.g., sleep). Because these agents have relatively narrow safety margins, higher doses that result as a consequence of tolerance can lead to toxicity. Due to these concerns, the use of barbiturates in treatment of insomnia has been virtually discontinued, and when these agents are used for treatment of insomnia, they are used in special cases and/or restricted to only short-term use. Other, older barbiturate-like drugs (e.g., chloral hydrate, glutethimide, and ethylchlorvynol) also act on the $GABA_A$ receptor to produce sedative-hypnotic effects but have fallen out of favor due to numerous untoward effects. These agents have been reviewed in previous editions of this text.

Structure–Activity Relationships of Barbiturates Barbiturates are derivatives of a cycylized ureide of malonic acid, commonly referred to as barbituric acid (2,4,6-trioxyhexahydropyrimidine) (Fig. 15.3), which is itself devoid of sedative-hypnotic, anxiolytic, and anticonvulsant activity. As shown in Figure 15.3, barbituric acid can undergo pH-dependent keto-enol tautomerization through transfer of either imino hydrogen or methylene hydrogen to a keto oxygen. This tautomerization is based on a fairly acidic carbon ($pK_a \sim 4$) at the 2-position, which can be stabilized in either molecular form based on the acidity of the solution. Empirical and computational studies have demonstrated that the tri-keto form is the most stable in aqueous solutions, whereas the 4,6-dialcohol tautomeric forms are the least stable (23,24). Although barbituric acid itself lacks pharmacologic activity, addition of 5,5-disubstituents to the barbituric backbone yields compounds with potent sedative-hypnotic, anxiolytic, and anticonvulsant activity. Termed *barbiturates,* the 5,5-disubstituted barbituric acids all possess a high degree of lipophilicity and, as weak acids, can be easily converted to sodium salts by treatment with sodium hydroxide.

Although thousands of barbiturate-like compounds have been synthesized, the 5,5-disubstituted barbituric acid backbone is the primary pharmacophore required for sedative-hypnotic activity, and efforts to further derivatize this backbone lead to a general loss in activity. These efforts show that esterification of either of the 1,3-diazine nitrogens decreases hypnotic activity. Although substitution of these nitrogens with aliphatic carbons retained anticonvulsant effects, it led to only weak hypnotic activity for *N*-methylated substituents, and this activity was lost upon increases in chain length or bulk (25,26). Likewise, esterification of the 5-position substituents (e.g., 5-phenyl, 5-methylester) yielded agents with analgesic activity but only weak hypnotic effects (27). Although early work on barbiturate derivatization demonstrated the importance of the 5-position substitutions on CNS depressant activity, the inclusion of polar functional groups at the 5-position

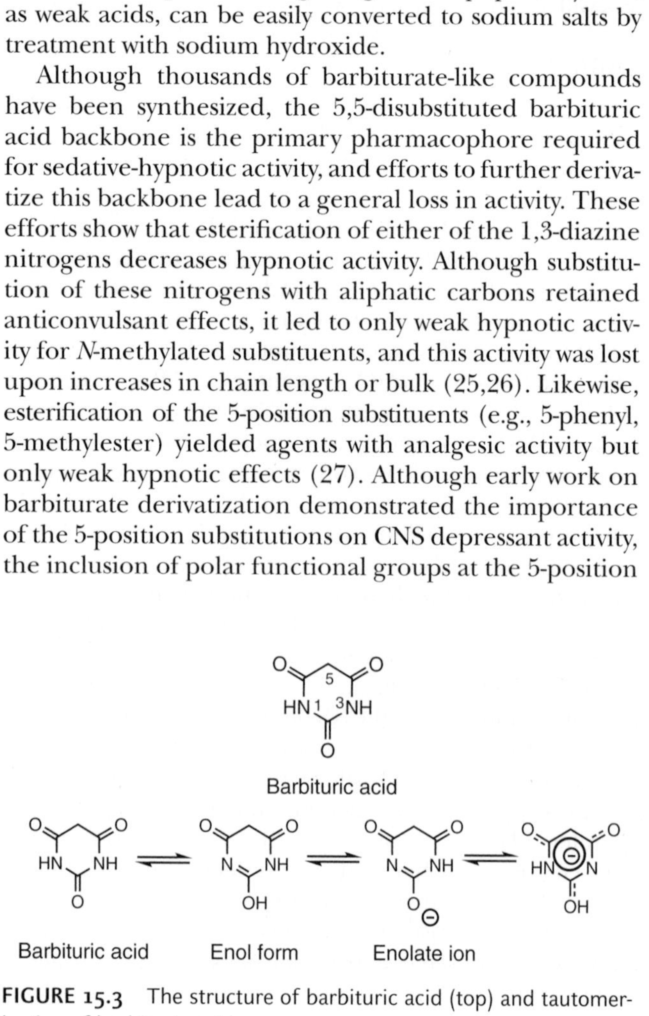

FIGURE 15.3 The structure of barbituric acid (top) and tautomerization of barbituric acid.

resulted in compounds that were fully devoid of sedative-hypnotic or anticonvulsant activity (28).

There are currently five barbiturates approved by the FDA for short-term sedative-hypnotic use and treatment of insomnia (Fig. 15.4). Structurally, pharmacologic activity is imparted to all five compounds due to the lipophilic di-substitutions at the 5-position (e.g., R_1 and R_2; Table 15.1). With the exception of secobarbital, which contains an allylic group at R_1, the remaining agents contain an ethyl substitution at this position (Fig. 15.4). Differences in these sedative-hypnotic barbiturates lie predominately at the R_2 position, where substitutions can affect the potency, rate of onset, and duration of action of the various congeners. The activity of these agents is strongly influenced by the lipophilicity of both substituents at the 5-position. As the number of carbon atoms at the R_2 position increases, the lipophilicity of the barbiturate will also increase such that comparative predictions on activity and time to onset can be made. For example, pentobarbital is more potent and has faster onset compared to butabarbital, which contains one less methylene group and is thus less lipophilic (Fig. 15.4, Table 15.1). Although the lipophilicity of the molecule greatly influences its ability to cross the blood–brain barrier, leading to potency and affecting the time of onset (see later discussion), too high a degree of lipophilicity will offset the required hydrophilicity that is necessary for dissolution and solubility of the compound in aqueous fluids. Hence, a limit to lipophilicity is reached and pharmacologic activity will begin to decrease if this threshold is surpassed.

The first commercially marketed barbiturate, barbital, contained identical 5,5-diethyl substituents, and as such, a plane of symmetry. However, many clinically useful barbiturates contain distinct 5,5-disubstitutions and substituted nitrogens, which form an asymmetric chiral center at the C-5 carbon and/or within one of the 5-position alkyl chains. Although barbiturates are dispensed as racemic mixtures, L-stereoisomers typically have twice the potency of the respective D-stereoisomers, consistent with observations that demonstrate stereoselectivity of $GABA_A$ receptors.

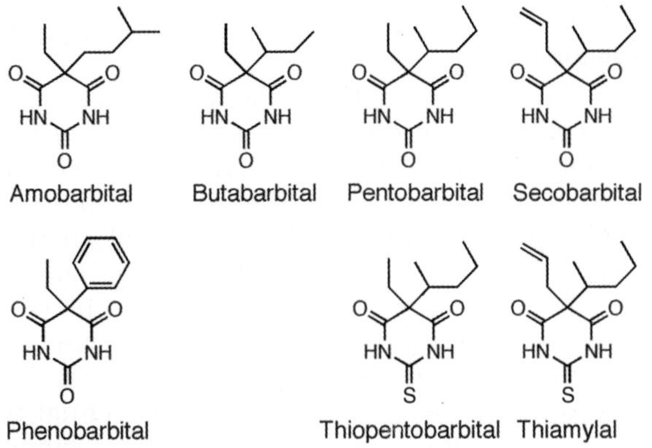

FIGURE 15.4 The barbiturates that are indicated for sedative-hypnotic use and the thiobarbiturates underneath their respective oxybarbiturate congeners.

A final note regarding the SAR of barbiturates is more critical in the role of this class as anesthetic agents and as such is only briefly discussed here. Specifically, modification of the 2-position oxygen of the barbiturate backbone with the larger sulfur atom yields thiobarbiturate derivatives with increased lipophilicity, faster time of onset, and shorter duration of action compared to the oxy-derivatives. For example, thiopentobarbital and thiamylal have much faster onsets and shorter durations than their respective oxy-congeners, pentobarbital and secobarbital, respectively (Fig. 15.4). Because thiobarbiturates have a specialized role as anesthetics, the reader is referred to Chapter 16 for further discussion of these agents.

Pharmacokinetics and Metabolism of Barbiturates Barbiturate salts that are approved for use as sedative-hypnotics are rapidly and completely absorbed following oral ingestion, in contrast to the free acids, which are absorbed at a much slower rate. The time of onset and duration of action are also significantly influenced by the lipophilicity of the individual agent and the route of administration. The five sedative-hypnotic barbiturates described here are all highly lipophilic, with corresponding logP values above 1.5, compared to barbital, which has a logP of 0.65 (Table 15.1) (29). Given the high proportion of cardiac output that is directed toward the brain, more lipophilic barbiturates are more rapidly distributed to the CNS and will have a faster time of onset. As with other CNS-acting agents, the time of onset is also dependent on the route of administration, with intravenous administration being the fastest and having near immediate effects, followed by intramuscular administration, which leads to faster brain distribution than the 10 to 60 minutes typical of orally administered sedative-hypnotics (Table 15.1).

Lipophilicity facilitates the relatively short duration of action of the barbiturates due to redistribution from the brain to other body compartments upon equilibration. This redistribution of barbiturates from the brain to other sites (e.g., adipose tissue) is the major mechanism that contributes to the loss of sedative-hypnotic activity of these agents, leading to durations of 3 to 8 hours for the short- and intermediate-acting agents and 10 to 16 hours for phenobarbital, which has the least lipophilicity and therefore the longest corresponding duration of action (Table 15.1). Because lipophilicity and route of administration can affect both time to onset and duration of action of barbiturates, these factors will influence a particular barbiturate's place in therapy. The anticonvulsant barbiturates are typically less lipophilic (e.g., phenobarbital) and correspondingly have slow onsets and long durations upon oral dosing, whereas the sedative-hypnotic agents described here are typically administered orally to achieve an optimum balance between achievement of sleep onset and duration. On the contrary, anesthesia-inducing barbiturates such as thiamylal are termed ultra-short acting due to their extremely high

TABLE 15.1 Pharmacokinetic Parameters of Barbiturates Approved for Sedative-Hypnotic Use

Barbiturate	R1	R2	LogP	Onset Time (min)[d]	Duration of action (hour)	Classification
Pentobarbital	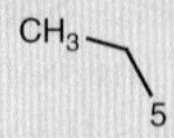	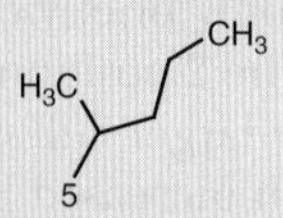	2.10[a]	10–15	3–4	Short-acting
Secobarbital	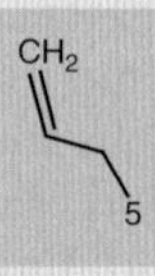	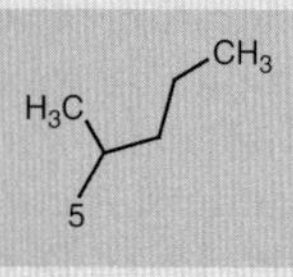	2.36[b]	10–15	3–4	Short-acting
Amobarbital	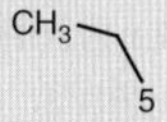	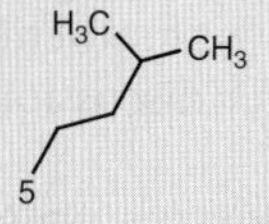	2.07[d]	45–60	6–8	Intermediate acting
Butabarbital	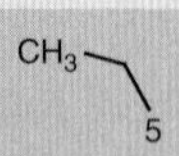	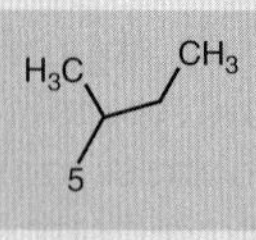	1.60[b]	45–60	6–8	Intermediate acting
Phenobarbital	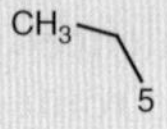	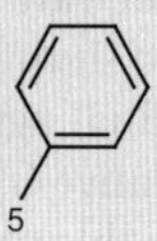	1.46[b]	30–60	10–16	Long-acting

[a] From Freese IE, Levin BC, Pearce R, et al. Correlation between the growth inhibitory effects, partition coefficients and teratogenic effects of lipophilic acids. Teratology. 1979;20:413–440.
[b] Average determinations from Slater B, McCormack, A, Avdeef A, et al. pH-metric log P.4. Comparison of partition coefficients determined by HPLC and potentiometric methods to literature values. J. Pharm. Sci 1994;83:1280–1283
[c] From Kakemi K, Arita T, Hori R, et al. Absorption and excretion of drugs. XXXI. On the relationship between partition coefficients and chemical structures of barbituric acid derivatives. Chem Pharm Bull. 1967;15:1705–17
[d] Upon oral administration.

lipophilicity (logP > 3), which confers immediate onset and very short durations upon intravenous injection.

Although loss of barbiturate sedative-hypnotic activity occurs primarily due to redistribution, the agents are also metabolically transformed. Metabolism of barbiturates is dependent on their individual degrees of lipid solubility—the more lipophilic compounds generally undergo greater metabolic transformations. It is important to understand that metabolism of barbiturates leads to metabolites that lack a high degree of lipophilicity and that, as a result, lack sedative-hypnotic activity. To achieve loss of lipophilicity, barbiturates are typically conjugated with glucuronide or sulfate conjugates that are hydrophilic and will allow for renal excretion of the agents. The most important pathway of barbiturate metabolism is oxidation or removal of the substituents at the 5-position carbon (Fig. 15.5). These phase 1 oxidation transformants are typically alcohols, or phenols in the case of phenobarbital, which can appear in the urine as either free or conjugated metabolites as a result of further phase 2 reactions leading to glucuronides or sulfates. The formed alcohols can also be further oxidized to yield ketones or carboxylic acid metabolites, which can be excreted freely or also conjugated (Fig. 15.5). Although not as significant as the route described earlier, oxidative desulfuration of thiobarbiturates can also occur, leading to more hydrophilic oxybarbiturates. Oxybarbiturate metabolites of thiamylal and thiopentobarbital are subsequently oxidized by the phase 1 and phase 2 reactions described earlier (Fig. 15.5).

Benzodiazepines

As with the barbiturates, benzodiazepines modulate the function of $GABA_A$ receptors, leading to neuronal hyperpolarization and CNS depressant effects. In contrast to the barbiturate binding site of $GABA_A$ receptors, the benzodiazepine binding site has been well characterized and is known to be formed by the interface of α and γ subunits. Not surprisingly, $GABA_A$ receptors that lack the γ subunit (e.g., $\alpha_6\beta\delta$) are completely insensitive to all benzodiazepines. Additionally, it has been shown that isoforms of the α subunit have differential benzodiazepine binding affinities, with the α_1 subunit–containing receptors (often termed BZ_1 receptors) having high benzodiazepine affinity and the α_2, α_3, and α_5 subunit–containing receptors (BZ_2 receptors) having

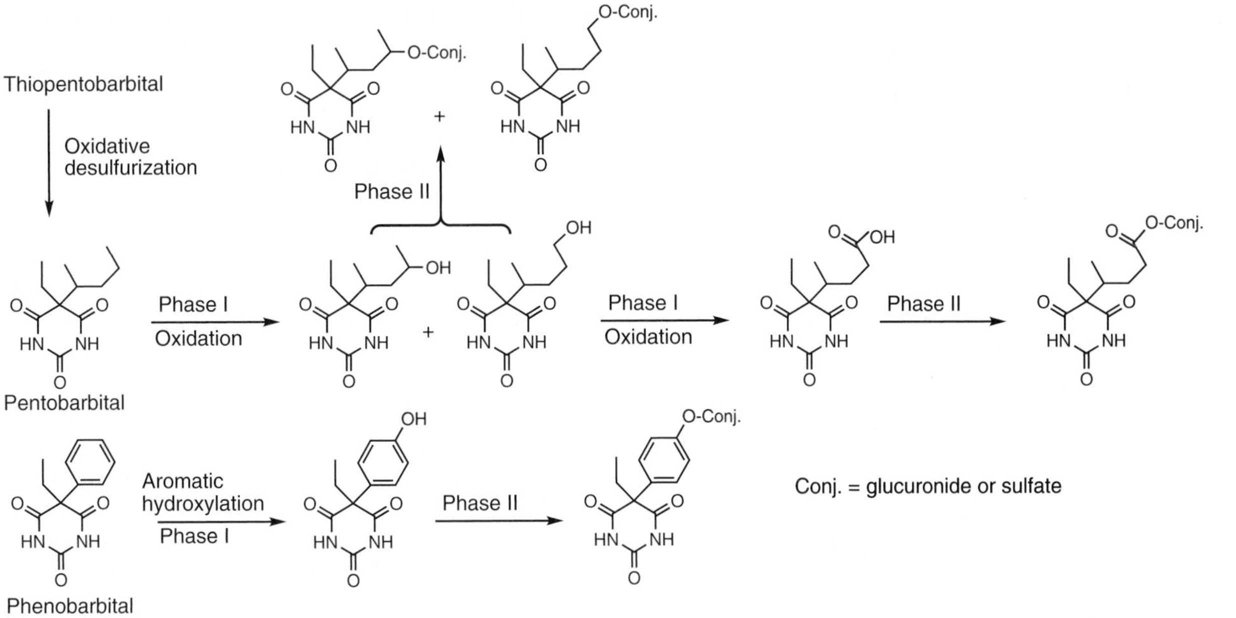

FIGURE 15.5 Major routes of metabolism of barbiturates. Thiopentobarbital and pentobarbital are used as examples to describe metabolism of alkyl thio- and oxybarbiturates, whereas phenobarbital exhibits the metabolism of an aromatic substituent. Coloration indicates site of metabolism.

moderate benzodiazepine affinity. Furthermore, some combinations that include α_4 or α_6 subunits are completely insensitive to benzodiazepine agonists, even in the presence of an appropriate γ subunit (20).

Binding of benzodiazepines to the allosteric BZ binding site can produce agonist, partial agonist, inverse agonist, or antagonist physiologic responses. Benzodiazepine agonists are used clinically as sedative-hypnotic agents as well as for the treatment of anxiety and convulsant disorders, in accordance with their ability to allosterically augment GABA-mediated inhibitory Cl^- conductance through the $GABA_A$ channel. Specifically, binding of benzodiazepines to the BZ site leads to increases in the binding-on rate and affinity of one GABA molecule to the first GABA binding site of the receptor (30–32). The increased affinity and rate of binding of GABA correlate with an increase in the frequency of the open-channel bursts. It is important to distinguish that benzodiazepines increase the frequency of channel opening, whereas barbiturates increase the duration of the open channel, and as such, the two classes of agents have distinct molecular effects on the $GABA_A$ receptor. Furthermore, benzodiazepines lack any effects in the absence of GABA, unlike the barbiturates. The reader is referred to Chapter 14 for more detailed descriptions of benzodiazepine binding and function.

Pharmacologic Effects of Benzodiazepines All benzodiazepines are capable of producing sedative-hypnotic effects; however, currently only five shorter acting benzodiazepine agents are approved by the FDA for use as sedative-hypnotics: estazolam, flurazepam, quazepam, temazepam, and triazolam. Residual hypnosis and psychomotor and cognitive inhibition are common side effects associated with their use. All of these agents are agonists of the BZ site of $GABA_A$ receptors containing α and γ subunits. Physiologically, all of the agents significantly reduce sleep latency and the number and duration of nighttime awakenings, resulting in an increase in total sleep time. The clinical use of these agents as sedative-hypnotics is not free from untoward effects, which are primarily manifested as excessive residual next-day sleepiness, tolerance upon long-term use, and withdrawal upon discontinuation. Another effect that is clinically important is the ability of benzodiazepines to produce a high degree of anterograde amnesia, in which recent events are not transferred to long-term memory (33).

Structure–Activity Relationships of Benzodiazepines The SARs of benzodiazepines are described in detail in Chapter 14, and the reader is referred to that chapter for the particulars of benzodiazepine binding requirements. Regarding the SAR of sedative-hypnotic benzodiazepines, all five agents contain the 5-phenyl-1,4-benzodiazepine-2-one backbone required for $GABA_A$ activity, and all include an electronegative 7-position chloro substitution as required on ring A (see Chapter 14 and Fig. 15.6). Similarly, all contain a pendant 5-phenyl ring (ring C) that is required for in vivo agonism and that can be substituted with ortho-electronegative halogens to increase lipophilicity, as is the case with flurazepam, quazepam, and triazolam. Interestingly, parasubstitution on ring C leads to inactive benzodiazepines, suggesting that steric restrictions are important at this site. Of note, several benzodiazepines, including

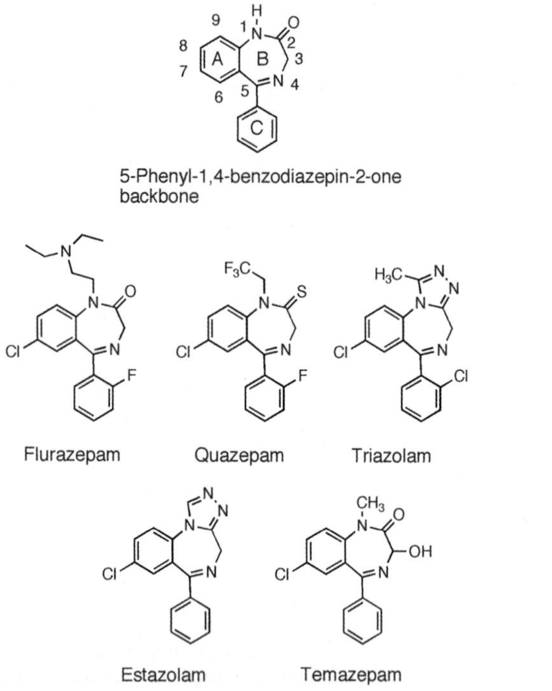

FIGURE 15.6 The benzodiazepine backbone and the benzodiazepines that are indicated for sedative-hypnotic use.

estazolam, are metabolized at the *para-* (4′) position, leading to inactivation of the agent. The major structural differences that impart distinct pharmacokinetic properties to the sedative-hypnotic benzodiazepines are located within ring B, the major site of metabolic transformation of these agents. The structural features of ring B that contribute to metabolism are discussed in the following section.

Pharmacokinetics and Metabolism of Benzodiazepines Benzo diazepine agents, like the barbiturates, are lipophilic and can be easily absorbed upon oral ingestion and rapidly distributed to the brain. Among the oral benzodiazepine formulations specifically indicated for the treatment of insomnia, flurazepam is absorbed most rapidly, achieving mean peak plasma concentrations within 0.5 to 1.0 hour. Temazepam and triazolam reach mean peak plasma concentrations within 0.5 to 2.0 hours, whereas estazolam and quazepam take longer (Table 15.2).

The sedative-hypnotic duration and side effect potential of benzodiazepines is greatly influenced by metabolism of the parent agent and the activity of resulting metabolites. Flurazepam has an elimination half-life of approximately 2 hours and is primarily metabolized by CYP3A4-mediated *N*-dealkylation and hydroxylation yielding active N^1-desalkyl and N^1-hydroxyethyl metabolites with elimination half-lives of 47 to 100 and 2 to 4 hours, respectively (Fig. 15.7, Table 15.2) (34). After a single 30-mg dose, the N^1-hydroxyethyl is undetectable in the plasma after 24 hours. On the contrary, levels of N^1-desalkylflurazepam are five- to sixfold higher after 7 days of administration than they are after 24 hours, suggesting buildup of this active metabolite. Conjugation of N^1-hydroxyethylflurazepam in phase 2 reactions allows for urinary excretion, and this conjugate is the major urinary metabolite accounting for up to 55% of a single dose (Fig. 15.7). The long half-life of these metabolites explains the clinical findings that flurazepam exhibits faster sleep latency and decreases in total wake time following several days of use and also why it is still efficacious for one to two nights following discontinuation of the parent. These observations are especially important in elderly populations, in whom the elimination half-life of *N*1-desethylflurazepam is significantly higher (up to 160 hours).

Quazepam is metabolized by microsomal CYP450 oxidases to yield 2-oxoquazepam, which is subsequently *N*-dealkylated to *N*-desalkyl-2-oxoquazepam (Fig. 15.7) (35). Both of these metabolites are pharmacologically active and have long durations, with mean plasma elimination half-lives of 40 and 73 hours, respectively (Table 15.2) (35). Both 2-oxoquazepam and *N*-desalkyl-2-oxoquazepam can be further hydroxylated at the 3-position, yielding 3-hydroxy-2-oxoquazepam and 3-hydroxy-*N*-desalkyl-2-oxoquazepam, respectively. These hydroxylated metabolites are inactive and can be *O*-glucuronidated and excreted readily in the urine (Fig. 15.7). As a consequence of the slow elimination of multiple active metabolites of both flurazepam and quazepam, residual hypnotic effects, including excessive daytime drowsiness, oversedation, and cognitive decline and confusion, are common and clinically relevant adverse effects.

These problems led to the development of newer triazolobenzodiazepines, such as estazolam and triazolam, with high $GABA_A$ receptor affinity and relatively shorter durations. The 1,4-triazolo ring of these congeners prevents oxidative metabolism typical of the benzodiazepines, which as in the case of flurazepam and quazepam results in formation of active metabolites with long elimination half-lives. The presence of the fused fourth ring of these agents also changes the numbering convention, such that numbering priority proceeds around the triazole ring (Fig. 15.8). Estazolam has a longer elimination half-life (10 to 24 hours) compared to flurazepam, but this agent is primarily metabolized by CYP3A4 yielding 4′-hydroxyestazolam as a major metabolite and 1-oxoestazolam as a minor metabolite (Fig.15.8, Table 15.2). Additionally, a 4-hydroxyestazolam metabolite has been identified in humans and is also detected in the urine at high levels (36). Although these metabolites have weak pharmacologic activity, three important factors prevent them from contributing to any significant sedative-hypnotic effects. The first is the low affinities of the metabolites for the $GABA_A$ receptor. In particular, 4′-hydroxestazolam is sterically hindered from optimal $GABA_A$ binding, consistent with SAR findings that parasubstitutions of ring C lead to decreased potency. The second factor that impedes the activity of estazolam metabolites is their decreased lipophilicity compared to the parent drug. This decrease facilitates the final

TABLE 15.2 Pharmacokinetic Parameters of Benzodiazepines Approved for Sedative-Hypnotic Use

Drugs	Trade name	Log P[a]	Time to peak conc. (hrs)	Parent elimination half-life (hrs)	Major metabolites (t1/2, hrs)	Predominant CYP isoform(s)
Flurazepam	Dalmane	2.35	0.5–1.0	2 ca.	*N*1-desalkyl (47–100, active) *N*1-hydroxyethyl (2-4, active)	3A4
Quazepam	Doral	4.03	2 ca.	39	2-Oxo (40, active) N-desalkyl (73, active)	3A4/2C9
Estazolam	Prosom	3.51	0.5–6.0	10–24	4′-Hydroxy; 4-Hydroxy; 1-Oxo (all inactive)	3A4
Triazolam	Halcion	2.42	<2	1.5–5.5	α-Hydroxy (50-100% active) 4-Hydroxy (inactive)	3A4
Temazepam	Restoril	2.19	1.2–1.6	0.4–0.6	O-glucuronide	–

[a] From Sangster Research Laboratories LOGKOW database

factor, which is that the circulating metabolites are found in low concentrations due to direct excretion of the hydrophilic free metabolites or their rapid *O*-glucuronidation, which readily allows for urinary excretion of the agents (Fig. 15.8).

Triazolam has a short duration of approximately 4 hours and is metabolized in humans to six metabolites, one of which, α-hydroxytriazolam, has been shown to retain 50% to 100% of the potency of the parent compound. Although only small amounts of the parent drug

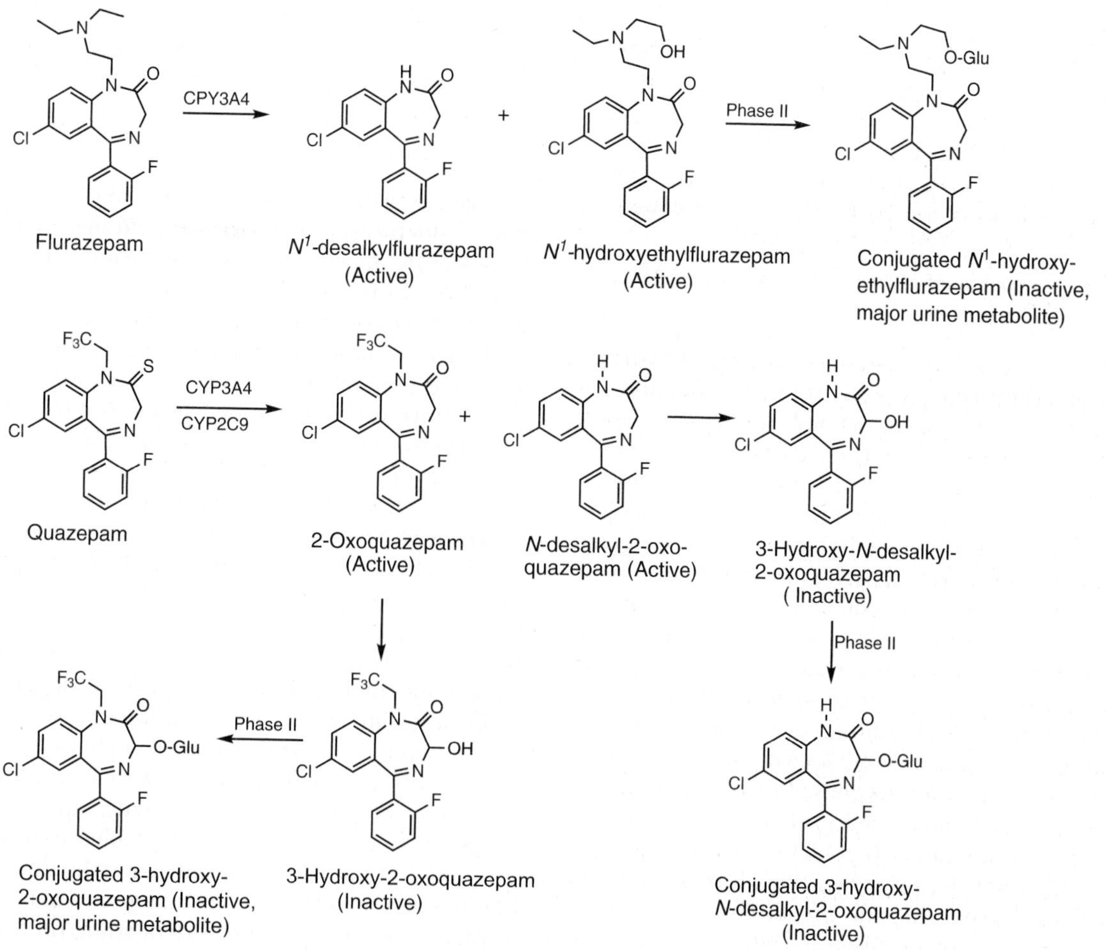

FIGURE 15.7 Metabolism of flurazepam and quazepam leads to formation of multiple long-acting active metabolites. Coloration indicates site of metabolism.

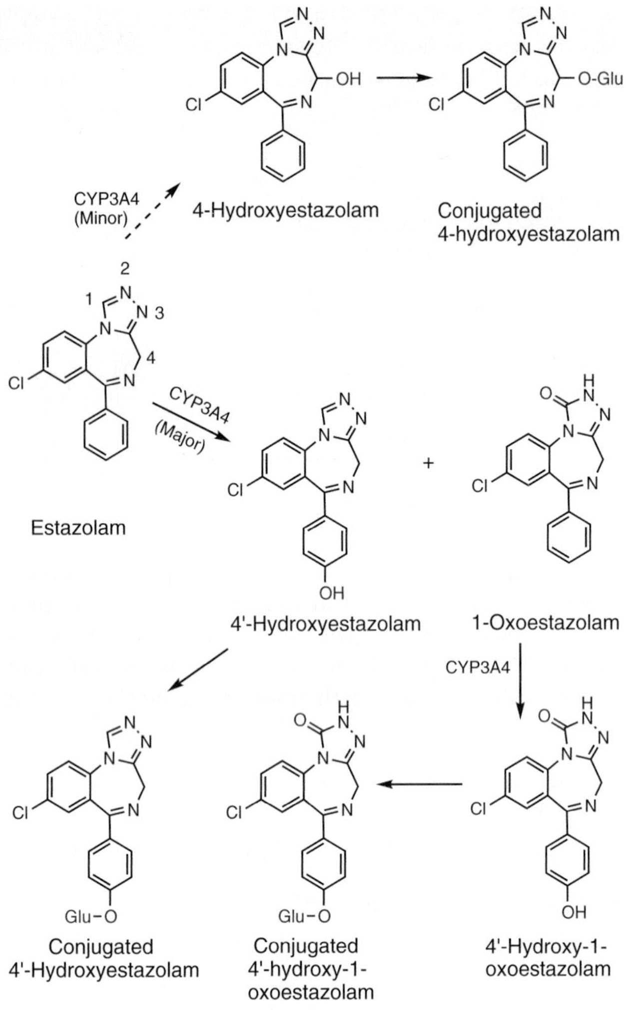

FIGURE 15.8 Metabolism of estazolam. Coloration indicates site of metabolism.

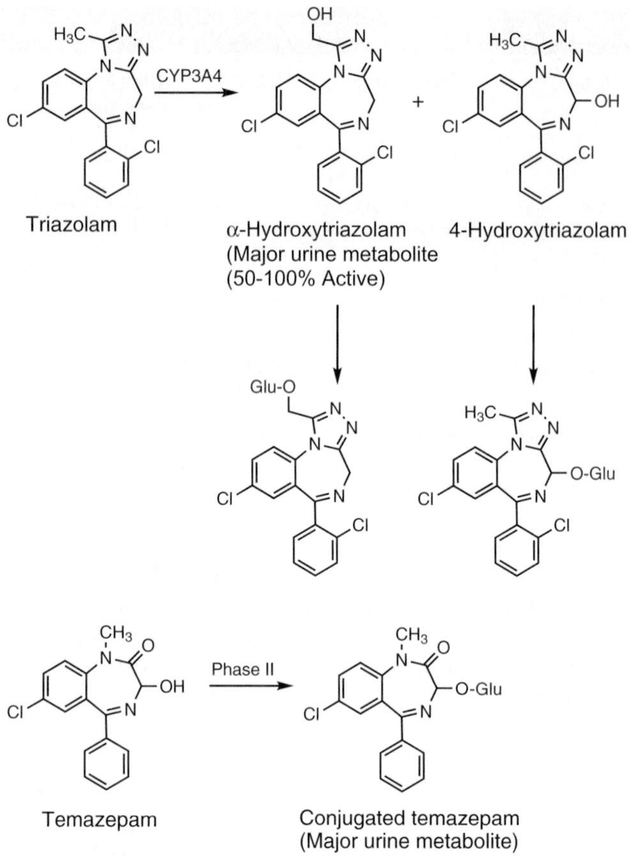

FIGURE 15.9 Metabolism of triazolam and temazepam. Coloration indicates site of metabolism.

are found in the urine, α-hydroxytriazolam and 4-hydroxytriazolam are the principal glucuronidated metabolites found in the urine, and these account for approximately 80% of triazolam excretion (Fig. 15.9) (37). There is no evidence of accumulation of triazolam metabolites, and the clinical effects of the active α-hydroxytriazolam are unclear because this metabolite has been detected in the plasma primarily in its glucuronidated form. Taken together, the relatively short half-life of the parent coupled with the urinary excretion of glucuronidated metabolites afford triazolam a relatively short duration of action compared with other benzodiazepines.

Temazepam is unique among the sedative-hypnotic benzodiazepines in that it contains a 3-hydroxy group, and as such, the agent circumvents phase 1 oxidation reactions prior to conjugation and excretion. This feature affords a 0.4- to 0.6-hour elimination half-life and rapid excretion of the parent, while also providing the additional benefit of bypassing oxidative hepatic metabolism (Fig. 15.9). Based on this route of metabolism, temazepam has no active metabolites. In fact, the only significant metabolites that have been described are the *O*-glucuronide of the parent, which is the major metabolite (>90%), and the *O*-glucuronide of *N*-desmethyltemazepam (<10%). Importantly, these products are formed independently of CYP450 isoforms and are rapidly excreted in the urine with half-lives of approximately 2 hours.

Benzodiazepines are used as sedative-hypnotic agents, as well as general muscle relaxants, anxiolytics, and anticonvulsants, yet as mentioned previously, their use can be confounded by presentation of undesirable side effects. Although death by benzodiazepine overdose is rare and typically only results as a consequence of concomitant use with other CNS depressants, these agents are not free from adverse effects and toxicities. Nearly all benzodiazepines have been reported to cause dose-dependent alterations in behavior, specifically bizarre, uninhibited, and confused behaviors. The propensity of benzodiazepines to cause tolerance and their potential for physical dependence and abuse also limit their use. Additionally, misuse of short-acting hypnotic benzodiazepines such as flunitrazepam (Rohypnol) has had profound social and medicolegal implications due to their use as "date rape" or "robbery" drugs. This elicit use is based on the ability to produce rapid hypnosis in combination with anterograde amnesia. In addition to cognitive effects, benzodiazepines may also exhibit respiratory depressant effects depending on the dose and the duration, and as such, they are contraindicated in patients with pulmonary conditions or sleep apnea. These factors contributed to the development of nonbenzodiazepine sedative-hypnotics, which were devoid of many of the adverse effects induced by classical benzodiazepines.

Nonbenzodiazepine $GABA_A$ Agonists

Due to advances in molecular biology, genetics, and pharmacology in the late 1980s to early 1990s, numerous lines of evidence demonstrated that different $GABA_A$ receptor subtypes may bring about distinct functions depending on their localization in the brain. Future work revealed that α_2, α_3, and α_5 subtype–containing $GABA_A$ receptors (BZ_2) play critical roles in the anxiolytic, anticonvulsant, muscle relaxant, and cognitive impairment properties of classical benzodiazepines, whereas modulation of the α_1-containing $GABA_A$ receptor subtypes (BZ_1) was shown to be the key to benzodiazepine-induced sedation and hypnosis (38–42). Importantly, these findings revealed that it could be feasible to design functionally selective drugs that act as selective agonists at specific $GABA_A$ subtypes to yield the appropriate pharmacotherapeutic outcomes. For example, selective α_2- or α_3-acting agents could have anxiolytic properties while being devoid of sedative effects, whereas selective α_1-acting agents would behave specifically as sedative-hypnotic agents. Although classical benzodiazepines described here and in Chapter 14 are nonselective and demonstrate sedative-hypnotic, anxiolytic, and other effects, the discovery of novel nonbenzodiazepine compounds with a high degree of selectivity for α_1 subtype–expressing $GABA_A$ receptors allowed for the specific use of these agents as sedative-hypnotics. Currently, three structurally distinct nonbenzodiazepines—zolpidem, eszopiclone, and zaleplon, which are often referred to as the Z-drugs—are approved in the United States for treatment of insomnia, and several other investigational agents are in various stages of clinical trials.

ZOLPIDEM

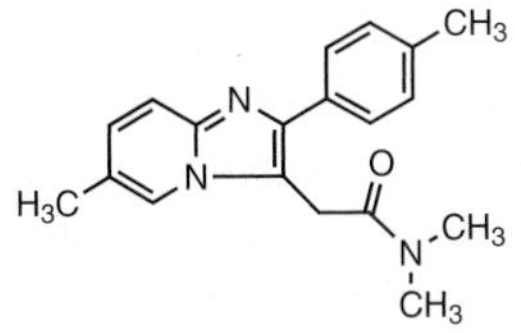

Zolpidem is an imidazopyridine that is a highly selective agonist of the α_1 subunit–expressing $GABA_A$ receptors (BZ_1), demonstrating 5- and 10-fold greater affinity for α_1 versus α_2 and α_3 subtypes, respectively (43). Similar to the benzodiazepines, zolpidem lacks appreciable affinity for α_4 and α_5 receptors (43). Of the three marketed nonbenzodiazepine drugs, zolpidem also has the greatest functional potency at potentiating GABA currents (44). The hypnotic effects of zolpidem parallel those seen for temazepam and triazolam, but based on its selective pharmacologic profile, zolpidem demonstrates weaker anxiolytic, anticonvulsant, and muscle relaxant effects compared to the classical benzodiazepines. Zolpidem has been shown to significantly improve sleep latency and prolong the duration of sleep in healthy volunteers and in patients with insomnia. Studies that compare the sleep outcomes of zolpidem with those of benzodiazepines have generally revealed comparable onset and sleep durations, while also showing that zolpidem leads to significantly fewer nighttime wakenings and, at the same time, does not cause residual morning sedation, confusion, or memory impairment (44–48). Further studies demonstrated that zolpidem exhibits significant improvements with regard to sleep latency, and subjective accounts indicated improved sleep quality compared to benzodiazepines. Extensive review of trial data that compare sleep outcomes of zolpidem to various benzodiazepines shows that zolpidem is comparable or superior to various benzodiazepines (49–51).

Zolpidem is currently available in the United States in two different formulations, immediate or controlled release. Oral administration of both formulations leads to bioavailability of approximately 70% and peak maximal plasma concentrations within 1.6 hours (Table 15.3). Although plasma concentrations of zolpidem begin to decrease at approximately 2 hours following administration of the immediate-release formulation, the extended-release formulation produces a more sustained peak plasma concentration that results in higher plasma concentrations over an 8-hour period. Direct comparison of the two formulations shows that plasma concentration profiles are generally identical for 2 hours following administration, after which decreases in blood levels are seen with the immediate-release formulation. The controlled-release formulation allows for this peak blood level to be extended for approximately 1 to 2 additional hours, affording correspondingly sustained blood levels throughout the night. Administration of the agent with food doubles the time required to reach peak and lowers the peak concentration by 30%. Accumulation of zolpidem does not seem to occur upon repeated exposure, regardless of the formulation. Recently, the FDA has approved a zolpidem oral spray formulation, which is distinguished by the fact that it allows for significantly faster time of onset of approximately 15 minutes (Table 15.3) and, as such, is clinically useful for patients with difficulties in achieving sleep initiation.

Structure–Activity Relationships of Zolpidem There have been many medicinal–chemical efforts that have attempted to define the SARs of zolpidem and to characterize interaction of the agent with the BZ_1 receptor. Anzini et al. (52) have integrated these models using the structurally similar, but non–α_1-selective, imidazopyridine anxiolytic agent alpidem. Based on these results, they have described a freely rotating aromatic ring region (FRAR), an electron-rich region (ERR), an antiplanar region (APR), and a planar aromatic region (PAR) (Fig. 15.10), which contribute to the binding of alpidem to BZ receptors. Studies on each of these regions have demonstrated that the replacement of alpidem's electronegative chloro groups at both the FRAR and PAR with methyl groups, as in zolpidem, does not affect receptor binding affinity, but significantly increases the selectivity for

TABLE 15.3 Pharmacokinetic Parameters of Nonbenzodiazepines Approved for Sedative-Hypnotic Use.

Drugs	Trade name	Log P[a]	Time to peak conc. (hrs)	Parent elimination half-life (mean hrs)	Major metabolites (t1/2, hrs)	Predominant CYP isoform(s)
Zolpidem	Ambien	2.31	Immediate-release 1.6[a]/1.6[b] Control-release 1.5[c] Oral spray 0.25	Immediate-release 2.5[a]/2.6[b] Control-release 2.6[c]	None active	3A4 (major) 2C9, 1A2, and 2D6 (minor)
Eszopiclone	Lunesta	−0.34	1	6.5	*N*-oxide (inactive) *N*-desmethyl (active, lower affinity)	1A2, 3A4
Zaleplon	Sonata	1.23	1	1	None active	3A4 (minor)

[a] 5 mg tablets.
[b] 10 mg tablets.
[c] 12.5 mg tablets.

α_1-subtype receptors (53). Further studies on the ERR have shown that conversion of either of the imidazole nitrogens to hydrogen bond donors leads to complete loss of selectivity for a1 subtype $GABA_A$ receptors (52). These data suggest a role for the imidazole nitrogen's ability to behave as hydrogen bond acceptors within the $GABA_A$ receptor binding site. (52). The importance of the ERR is also demonstrated by studies that convert the imidazole of zolpidem to its azaisostere congener. This simple change does not affect binding to α_1-subtype receptors but decreases binding to α_2 and α_3 such that potency at these subtypes is negligible, similar to that seen for the α_5 subtype (54). The antiplanar group has also been shown to be critical in facilitating binding to $GABA_A$ receptors by allowing for hydrogen bonding interactions. Molecular modeling studies have shown that the antiplanar carbonyl group of zolpidem can hydrogen bond to Ser^{204} or near Thr^{206}/Gly^{207} within the backbone of loop C of α_1 subunits, as well as to Arg^{194} within loop F of γ_2 subunits, which forms $\alpha_1\gamma_2$ complexes (55). Finally, the antiplanar group also contributes to binding selectivity and affinity, as sterically hindered bulky amide nitrogen substitutions show decreased binding to α_1-subtype receptors. This study also identified three additional α_1 and three additional γ_2 residues that are within 5 Å of zolpidem on molecular docking simulations, suggesting that other hydrogen-bonding or salt-bridge interactions can occur within the ligand binding domain.

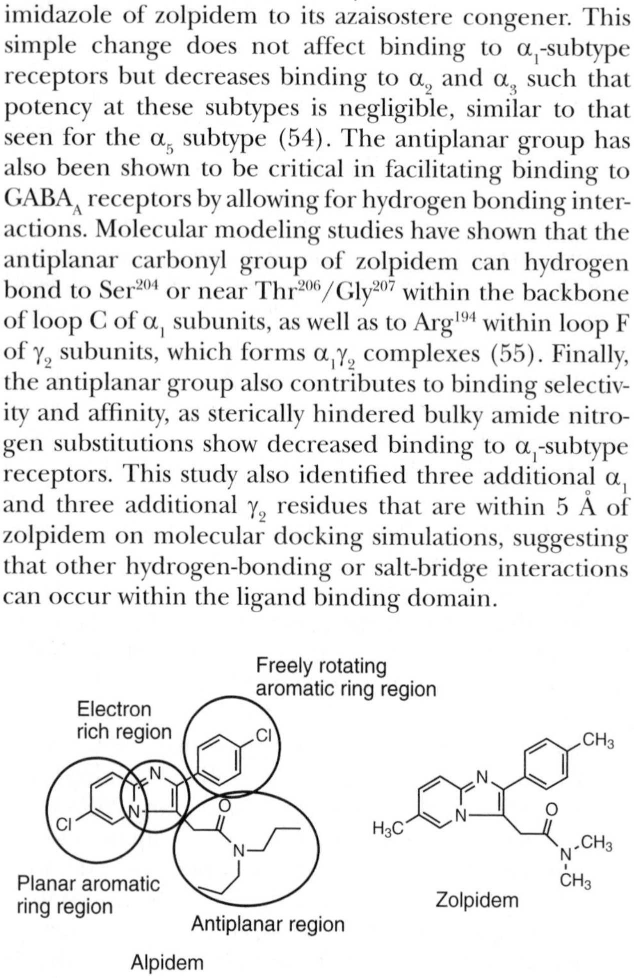

FIGURE 15.10 Structural relationship between of alpidem and zolpidem.

Metabolism of Zolpidem Zolpidem is rapidly eliminated, with a mean half-life of approximately 2.5 hours (Table 15.3). Repeated doses do not seem to accumulate, and elimination of the parent is achieved through extensive metabolism with only trace amounts of unchanged drug being found in urine or feces (56). In humans, zolpidem can be oxidatively metabolized to yield four primary metabolites, M II, M IV, M X, and M XI, all of which lack pharmacologic activity. As shown in Figure 15.11, the major metabolite is formed by CYP3A4-mediated hydroxylation of the *p*-tolyl methyl group yielding M III, which is subsequently oxidized to the corresponding carboxylic acid, M I (57). The M I metabolite is the principal metabolite found in human urine, accounting for approximately 70% to 85% of the administered dose. Microsomal enzyme-mediated hydroxylation of the *p*-methyl substituent on the imidazopyridine backbone can also occur, leading to formation of metabolite M IV, which can be further oxidized to the corresponding carboxylic acid M II, which accounts for approximately 10% of the administered dose. Importantly, M III was also shown to be formed by CYP2D6 and to a lesser degree by CYP1A2, whereas MI V formation by CYP1A2 and CYP3A4 was more modest (57). Because expression of CYP1A2 and CYP2D6 in human liver is generally significantly less than that of CYP3A4, the clinical contribution of these enzymes in transformation of zolpidem is expected to be minor. More recent studies have confirmed these suspicions and demonstrated that the contribution of CYP enzymes to zolpidem metabolism is greatest for CYP3A4 (61%), followed by CYP2C9 (22%), CYP1A2 (14%), and less than 3% for CYP2D6 (58). Because M III and M IV are not detectable in human urine or feces, but the respective carboxylic acids M I and M II are, it was proposed that rapid formation of these secondary metabolites occurs. Indeed, studies in rodents have demonstrated that the conversion of the alcohol metabolites to their corresponding acids occurs very rapidly and requires a nonmicrosomal enzyme, perhaps alcohol dehydrogenase (59). Finally, as shown in Figure 15.11, CYP3A4-mediated oxidation of zolpidem can also lead to formation of the M X and M XI minor metabolites, which are hydroxylated

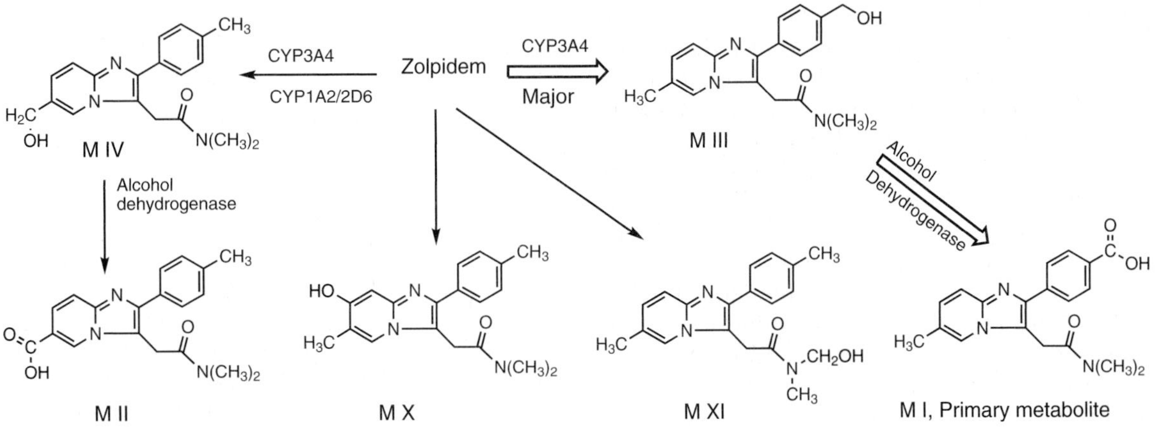

FIGURE 15.11 Metabolism of zolpidem. Coloration indicates site of metabolism.

on the imidazopyridine ring and the substituted amide nitrogen, respectively.

In elderly populations, dose adjustments must be made to account for the 50% increase in elimination half-life of the drug (60). Similarly, in patients with hepatic dysfunction, the plasma concentration of zolpidem doubles, with an increase in elimination half-life to a mean of 10 hours. Interestingly, there has been recent interest in the likelihood of differential gender-based metabolism of zolpidem based on the ability of testosterone to positively contribute to CYP3A4 activity such that higher circulating free testosterone increases CYP3A4 activity (60,61). Given this correlation, women are likely to have higher plasma concentrations of zolpidem and, as such, may be more likely to have higher degrees of zolpidem-mediated adverse effects (62).

Eszopiclone

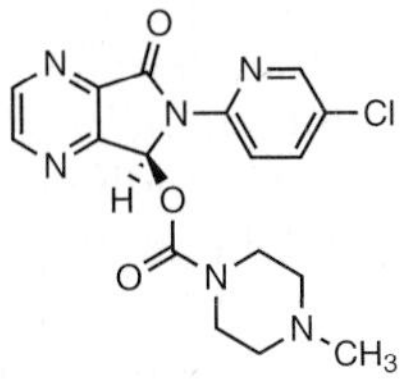

(S)-Zopiclone

Eszopiclone, a pyrrolopyrazine cyclopyrrolone, is the active (*S*)-enantiomer of zopiclone, a racemic mixture that is no longer marketed in the United States. Eszopiclone significantly improves sleep latency and sleep maintenance, increases the time spent in stage III and IV sleep, and is distinguished by the fact that its approval is not limited to short-term utilization and that it has no potential for development of tolerance or abuse. Several trials have demonstrated that hypnotic efficacy is maintained and eszopiclone is well tolerated upon chronic dosing, lasting up to 12 months (63). In contrast to the racemic zopiclone, eszopiclone is devoid of substantial residual next-day sedative and cognitive effects. Unlike zolpidem, eszopiclone is not subtype selective. Yet, despite this lack of selectivity, it does not behave as classical benzodiazepines with respects to its pharmacodynamics and pharmacologic activity (see next section on SAR). Eszopiclone binds with higher affinity to α_1 receptors but also has appreciable affinity for α_3 subunits, and thus has hypnotic and other CNS activities. The affinity of the agent for α_1-subtype receptors is less than the other marketed nonbenzodiazepine agonists.

Eszopiclone is rapidly absorbed following oral administration, and peak plasma concentrations are reached within 1 hour with an elimination half-life of 6.5 hours, the longest of the nonbenzodiazepine hypnotics (Table 15.3). Similar to zolpidem, eszopiclone does not accumulate following repeated administration, and administration after a high-fat meal delays the time to peak plasma concentration by 1 hour and decreases this concentration by more than 20% (64). Eszopiclone dosing in the elderly must also be adjusted to account for 41% greater drug levels and a significantly longer half-life of 9 hours in this population. Similar dose adjustments must be made in patients with liver dysfunction as total exposure to eszopiclone increases twofold at the 2-mg dose, although the time to peak concentration and the concentration itself were unaffected (64).

Structure–Activity Relationships of Eszopiclone Eszop iclone (Fig. 15.12) exhibits 50-fold greater binding affinity for GABAA receptors than does the (R)-enantiomer. This leads to significant improvement in GABA potency, but more importantly, enantiomeric separation of the (S)-enantiomer seems to reduce adverse effects such as residual sedative effects seen with racemic zopiclone, despite the fact that the racemic mixture has a shorter half-life (5.0 vs. 6.5 hours). Racemization of one enantiomer to the other does not occur in mammals in vivo. Although SAR studies for cyclopyrrolones have not been performed to a great degree, it is known that this subclass recognizes a distinct site of the GABAA receptor complex that is allosteric to the recognition site for classical benzodiazepines (65). The regional distribution and specificity of sites labeled by radiolabeled cyclopyrrolones are similar to those labeled by classical benzodiazepine ligands, suggesting that the cyclopyrrolone binding site resides on the BZ site of the GABAA complex (65). However, unlike classical benzodiazepine agonists, binding of cyclopyrrolones is not affected by GABA or barbiturates. Furthermore, radioreceptor displacement binding studies revealed a noncompetitive interaction of cyclopyrrolones at sites labeled by classical benzodiazepines, whereas displacement of radiolabeled cyclopyrrolones by classical benzodiazepines occurred competitively, suggesting that cyclopyrrolones recognize a site on the BZ receptor complex that is allosteric to the recognition site of classical benzodiazepines (65). Others have suggested that perhaps cyclopyrrolones can interact with one of multiple BZ binding sites on the GABAA receptor and, in doing so, cause allosteric changes in the ligand affinity at the remaining sites, potentiating further binding (66). With regard to binding within the ligand recognition site, molecular modeling and mutagenesis studies have shown that eszopiclone is within 4 Å of many amino acid residues within the GABA-BZ complex binding pocket, and such proximity allowed anchoring and stabilization by multiple hydrogen bond interactions with Arg144, Tyr209, Tyr159, and various other residues (55). These studies also revealed that the structural requirements for eszopiclone binding are different than those of zolpidem, and these differences may account for the lack of selectivity of eszopiclone (55).

Metabolism of Eszopiclone Eszopiclone is metabolized extensively by CYP3A4 and CYP1A2 isozymes, which yield the primary metabolites (*S*)-*N*-desmethylzopiclone and (*S*)-*N*-oxidezopiclone, respectively. The oxide metabolite is inactive, whereas *N*-desmethylzopiclone exhibits lower potency and affinity at $GABA_A$ receptors and therefore has only very weak hypnotic activity compared to the parent (Fig. 15.12). Interestingly, due to its lower affinity and lack of subtype selectivity, together with its weak sedative effects, this metabolite has been investigated as a novel anxiolytic agent (67). Only small amounts (<7%) of unchanged eszopiclone are excreted in the urine, and greater than 75% of a dose is excreted via this route as inactive transformants of the two primary metabolites.

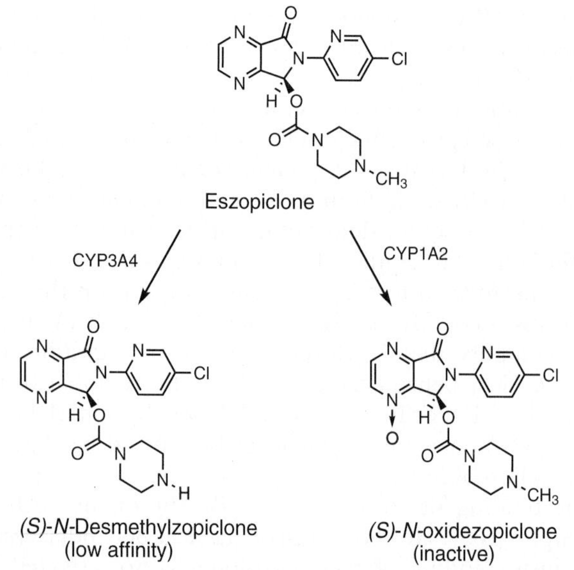

FIGURE 15.12 Metabolism of eszopiclone. Coloration indicates site of metabolism.

ZALEPLON

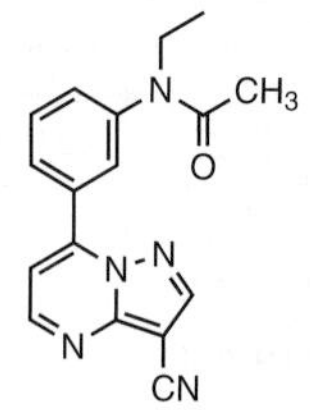

Zaleplon, a pyrazolopyrimidine, is a hypnotic agent that has a pharmacologic profile similar to zolpidem but is primarily distinguished by its extremely rapid onset and short half-life. Similar to zolpidem, zaleplon has greater affinity at the α_1- versus α_2- and α_3-containing receptors, albeit with one-third to one-half the potency of zolpidem (68). Unlike zolpidem, which does not recognize α_5-containing receptors with any appreciable affinity, zaleplon is able to potentiate the effects of GABA at α_5-containing receptors; however, its affinity for α_5-containing receptors is approximately 15-fold less than for α_1-containing receptors (68). Hence, zaleplon is considered an α_1-selective GABA modulator, which lacks the classical benzodiazepine effects on sleep.

The distinguishing features that afford zaleplon a unique place in the therapy of insomnia are its rapid rate of onset combined with its relatively faster rate of excretion. Oral administration of zaleplon leads to a mean peak plasma concentration in less than 1 hour, regardless of dose, the fastest of the nonbenzodiazepines (69). Although zaleplon is completely absorbed following oral administration, it is subject to first-pass metabolism, leading to an absolute bioavailability of 30% (Table 15.3) (69). As with zolpidem and eszopiclone, administration with heavy meals, particularly high-fat foods, delays the time to peak plasma concentration to 3 hours and reduces the peak plasma concentration by 35% (70,71). Following oral administration, zaleplon is rapidly eliminated with a mean elimination half-life of 1 hour, an effect that is delayed significantly in patients with hepatic dysfunction. Taken together, these pharmacokinetic properties facilitate the rapid onset and short duration hypnotic effects (70,71).

Clinically, zaleplon is distinguished by its ability to significantly reduce sleep latency for up to 5 weeks compared to placebo, an effect that can be contributed to its rapid onset (71,72). However, numerous clinical trials have failed to consistently show that a 50 or 10-mg nightly dose of zaleplon significantly improves sleep duration, decreases the number of awakenings, or improves overall sleep quality compared with placebo, likely due to the short half-life of the agent, which precludes hypnotic effects throughout the night. Higher nightly doses of zaleplon (20 mg) do significantly improve either sleep latency or duration, but effects on total sleep quality and number of awakenings compared to placebo have been inconsistent in clinical trials at this dose (71). Tolerance and withdrawal effects have not been reported during short-term treatment (up to 5 weeks), and the agent also seems to be free from rebound insomnia and residual next-day sedative effects, similar to other nonbenzodiazepine hypnotics (72). As a result of these effects, zaleplon is approved only for patients with difficulties falling asleep; however, an extended-release formulation that could improve sleep maintenance and duration has been under development for some time.

Structure–Activity Relationships of Zaleplon Unlike for zolpidem and eszopiclone, extensive studies that examine the SARs of zaleplon have not been performed with regard to binding potency and interaction within the binding pocket. However, there have been numerous studies that compare the binding and function of zaleplon to the closely related compound indiplon (Fig. 15.13), allowing for deduction of SAR from pharmacologic results. These studies show that zaleplon exhibits approximately 7- and 10-fold greater selectivity for α_1- over α_3- and α_5-containing $GABA_A$ receptors, respectively, whereas indiplon demonstrates only 1.6- and 4-fold selectivity (73). Importantly, indiplon has 3-, 12-, and 7-fold higher affinity at α_1-, α_3-, and α_5-containing receptors, respectively, than does zaleplon. Further work has demonstrated that indiplon is greater than 100-fold more potent than zaleplon at potentiating GABA currents through α_1-containing receptors but is also 46- and 25-fold more potent at doing so through α_3- and α_5-containing receptors, respectively (44,73). This work suggests that the thiophene-2-carbonyl moiety of indiplon (Fig. 15.13) drives higher binding affinity and thus potency, but decreases overall selectivity for one subtype over another. Meanwhile, zaleplon contains only a cyano group at this position, suggesting that electronic rather than steric factors influence selectivity.

Metabolism of Zaleplon As described earlier, zaleplon is subjected to significant first-pass metabolism, which accounts for its low oral bioavailability. Following oral administration of the agent in humans, less than 0.1% of the drug is recovered unchanged in the urine. Animal studies have demonstrated distinct interspecies variability in metabolism of orally administered zaleplon due to interspecies differences in activity of hepatic aldehyde oxidase, which is the principle metabolic enzyme responsible for transformation of zaleplon (74). In rodents and canines, which have decreased expression and activity of aldehyde oxidase, zaleplon is predominantly metabolized by CYP3A4 to *N*-desethylzaleplon, with only minor oxidation of zaleplon by aldehyde oxidase to yield 5-oxozaleplon. In humans, these metabolic routes are interchanged due to greater activity of aldehyde oxidase, and as a result, the major metabolite is 5-oxozaleplon, whereas CYP3A4-mediated transformation, yielding *N*-desethylzaleplon, is a minor route (Fig. 15.13). Both primary metabolites are inactive and, once formed, can either be directly eliminated in the urine or oxidized further and excreted as a glucuronide conjugate. In addition, the *N*-desethylzaleplon metabolite can be rapidly converted, presumably also via aldehyde oxidase, to 5-oxo-*N*-desethylzaleplon (Fig. 15.13) (70). Following oral administration of radiolabeled zaleplon to healthy volunteers, 70% of the dose is recovered in the urine within 2 days, almost exclusively as the two primary metabolites or their glucuronide conjugates (70). The 5-oxozaleplon metabolite

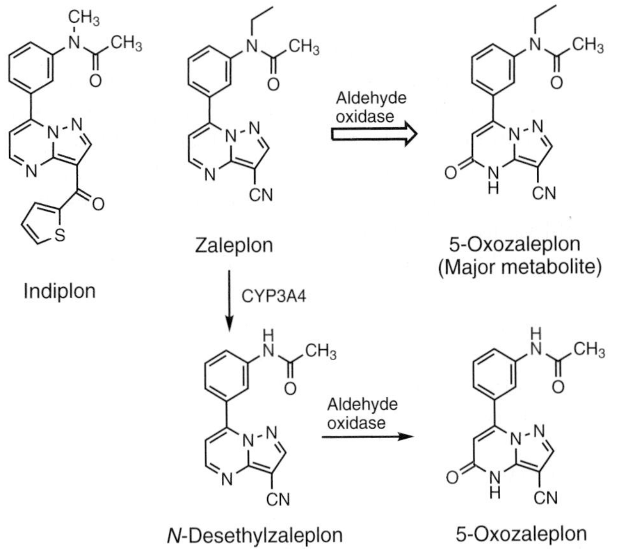

FIGURE 15.13 Structural relationship of zaleplon to indiplon and metabolism of zaleplon. Coloration indicates site of metabolism.

also predominates in the feces, where more than 15% of an administered dose can be found within 6 days.

The nonbenzodiazepines represent major advancements in treatment of insomnia. They are highly effective hypnotic agents with negligible residual daytime drowsiness and are generally free from the psychomotor and cognitive side effects of classical benzodiazepines. Despite their primary use at nighttime and their relatively short half-lives, these agents are also not completely devoid of adverse effects. Recently, there has been an increase in reported occurrences of nonbenzodiazepine-induced sleepwalking and associated amnesic sleep-related complex behaviors such as sleep driving, sleep eating, sleep cooking, sleep talking, and sleep sex (75–83). These effects have been reported at therapeutic and supertherapeutic doses and are potentiated by alcohol consumption. Importantly, patients do not have any recall or memory of these events. Although these unintended effects are rare, they are potentially very serious because they can affect social, emotional, and physical health and pose risks for fatal incidents.

Melatonin Receptor Agonists

As described previously, melatonin is a neurohormone that is primarily synthesized in the pineal gland from its precursor serotonin (Fig. 15.1). Because melatonin synthesis is concurrent with sleep, the increase in endogenous nighttime melatonin levels correlates with the onset of sleepiness. The sleep-promoting and circadian effects of melatonin are due to agonism of both MT1 and MT2 receptors (MT1R, MT2R), both of which are present in very high density (~4 fmol/mg protein) within the SCN (84). Agonism of SCN MT1 receptors directly facilitates inhibition of SCN neuron firing promoting sleep, whereas activation of SCN MT2 receptors affects the circadian rhythm settings related to the central clock (85,86).

Melatonin itself is a poor chemotherapeutic agent due to its poor absorption and low oral bioavailability of less than

10%, as well as its ubiquitous effects on sleep and circadian rhythms. Moreover, because melatonin is a supplement that is not regulated by the FDA, preparations vary in their purity and concentration, and as a result, poor sleep outcomes are often encountered. The significant effects of MT receptor agonism on sleep coupled with the relatively poor nature of melatonin as a drug prompted intense medicinal–chemical efforts to develop novel small-molecule congeners of melatonin that behave as potent agonists of MT receptors. These efforts led to the successful launch of the first in-class melatonin receptor agonist (*S*)-ramelteon, which has an excellent sleep and safety profile. Other investigational MT agonists, such as tasimelteon, are also being developed for treatment of insomnia.

Ramelteon (Rozerem)

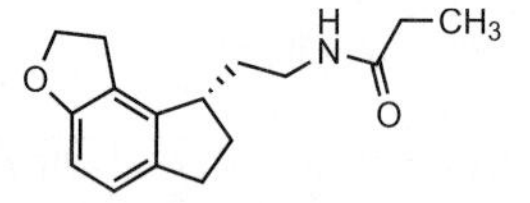

(*S*)-Ramelteon

(*S*)-Ramelteon (TAK-375) selectively binds to both MT1R and MT2R, recognizing the human receptors with extremely high affinity of 14 and 112 pmol/L, respectively, exhibiting 8- to 10-fold greater affinity for MT1R compared to MT2R and 6-fold greater affinity than melatonin for MT1R (87). The high potency and slight preference for MT1R correlate to the ability of the drug to primarily reduce sleep latency as opposed to regulation of phase-circadian rhythms. With regard to functional pharmacology, in Chinese hamster ovary cells ectopically expressing the human MT1R and MT2R, ramelteon was 4- and 17-fold more potent at inhibiting cyclic AMP production compared to melatonin, respectively, consistent with observations that demonstrate coupling of MT receptors to $G\alpha_{i/o}$ proteins (87). Moreover, ramelteon does not have any appreciable affinity for a third physiologically relevant melatonin binding site known as MT3R, which is a melatonin-sensitive quinine reductase that is not involved in the sleep/wake functions (88,89). Taken together, the absence of binding to brain receptors other than MT1R/MT2R and the potent activity of ramelteon at these melatonin receptors make ramelteon an efficacious sleep-inducing agent that is free from many of the CNS side effects common to other sedative-hypnotics.

Animal studies demonstrate that ramelteon significantly decreases wakefulness and increases both short-wave and REM sleep compared with placebo (88,90). In clinical trials, no effects on short-wave sleep have been noted, but the agent leads to significant decreases in sleep latency and increases in total sleep duration over a 5-week period compared to placebo (91–93). Importantly, ramelteon, consistent with its melatonin receptor–related mechanism, which is free of endogenous GABAergic signaling, does not produce residual next-day sedation or decreases in psychomotor function (93). Likewise, due to its unique mechanism, ramelteon does not hinder learning, cognition, and memory like the benzodiazepine agents do, and it also lacks the potential for abuse, does not lead to tolerance, and poses no risk of withdrawal or rebound insomnia upon discontinuation (92–94). One potential adverse effect that can be predicted for melatonin receptor agonists is based on the ability of melatonin to influence prolactin and testosterone levels via agonism of MT1 and MT2 receptors located within endocrine and reproductive tissue. Similarly, ramelteon has been reported to affect mean free and total testosterone levels (88). Further studies are necessary to gauge the clinical consequences, if any, that exogenous melatonin receptor agonists have on endocrine and reproductive function. In summary, from a sleep therapy standpoint, melatonin receptor agonists such as ramelteon have highly efficacious hypnotic effects while being free of many of the cognitive and residual effects common to $GABA_A$ modulating agents.

Structure–Activity Relationships of Ramelteon SARs for melatonin and its congeners have been reviewed at length previously (95–98). Early studies demonstrated that the indole backbone of melatonin was not required for activity so long as it was replaced by an aromatic isostere as in ramelteon (which contains an indane) or as in the investigational MTR agonists tasimelteon and agomelatine, which are currently undergoing clinical trials for treatment of insomnia (Fig. 15.14) (99). It has been proposed that the importance of the aromatic ring system here is to offer optimum distance between the amide side chain at position 3 and the 5-methoxy substitution (100,101). The aromatic moiety has also been suggested to interact with aromatic receptor residues within the binding pocket through *pi–pi* stacking. Although the aromatic portion contributes to spacing and likely *pi–pi* interactions, the 3-position amide and the 5-methoxy side chains are responsible for binding and functional activation of the receptors by interacting with two proposed binding pockets. The amide group is critical for agonist activity at both MT receptors and is thought to interact with key serine (Ser^{110} and Ser^{114}) and asparagine (Asn^{175}) residues in transmembrane helix (TMH) III of MT1 and TMH IV of MT2, respectively (102). Meanwhile, the 5-methoxy moiety is critical for functional effects. It has been proposed that the methoxy oxygen interacts with His^{195} and His^{208} within TMH VI of MT1R and MT2R, respectively (101,103). Movement of the methoxy group to the 4-, 6-, or 7-positions significantly decreases functional activity, suggesting that distance to these conserved histidine residues is critical in maintaining binding affinity and functional activity (97). Additionally, Val^{192}, which is located nearly one turn above His^{195} within the ligand binding domain has been shown to be involved in binding the methyl component of the methoxy group (101). Finally, the binding pocket of MTRs is highly stereoselective, an important feature that must be considered for drug design. As a consequence of the three-dimensional requirements of binding to MT receptors, ramelteon is dispensed as the enantiomerically pure (*S*)-enantiomer, which has 500-fold greater affinity for MT1 than does (*R*)-ramelteon.

Metabolism of Ramelteon (*S*)-Ramelteon is rapidly absorbed after oral administration, and mean peak plasma concentrations are achieved at 0.75 hours. In a study in healthy volunteers who were administered radiolabeled ramelteon, 84% of recovered radioactivity was found in the urine and 4% in the feces, suggesting that at least 84% of the drug was absorbed. However, ramelteon is subject to extensive first-pass metabolism, leading to an absolute oral bioavailability of only approximately 2% (104). Ramelteon has a short elimination half-life of 1 to 2.5 hours, and once-nightly dosing does not lead to accumulation of the drug. The time to peak plasma concentration was delayed by 45 minutes upon administration with food, and the peak plasma concentrations were decreased by 22% in this case (104). Ramelteon is primarily metabolized by oxidation in phase 1 reactions, with secondary metabolites being excreted as glucuronide conjugates (105). Hepatic CYP1A2 is the major isoform responsible for transformation (49%), whereas CYP2C19 (42%) and CYP3A4 (8.6%) isoforms are also contributors to ramelteon metabolism in the liver. On the contrary, in the intestines, only CYP3A4 contributes to transformation (106). The major metabolite of ramelteon in humans is the hydroxylated propionamide M II metabolite (Fig. 15.15), which is active, has a 2- to 5-hour half-life, and has 20- to 100-fold greater systemic exposure than that of the parent, suggesting slower removal from the circulation (104,105). Moreover, this metabolite has one-fifth to one-tenth the binding affinity of the parent for human MT1 and MT2 receptors and shows potent hypnotic effects in animals, suggesting that it may contribute to the sedative-hypnotic effects of ramelteon (88). In addition to the M II metabolite, ramelteon can be oxidized to the ring-opened M I metabolite or transformed to a keto-metabolite, M III (Fig. 15.15), both of which are inactive. Biotransformation of the M II and M III metabolites by sequential oxidation steps can lead to formation of M IV. The rank order of prevalence of the four metabolites in human serum is M II, M IV, M I, and M III, and all three of the hydroxylated metabolites can be excreted as glucuronide conjugates (Fig. 15.15). Importantly, ramelteon is also subject to a significant drug interaction upon coadministration with the antidepressant fluvoxamine, a strong CYP1A2 inhibitor. Coadministration of these agents leads to a greater than 100-fold increase in total systemic exposure of ramelteon and should be avoided.

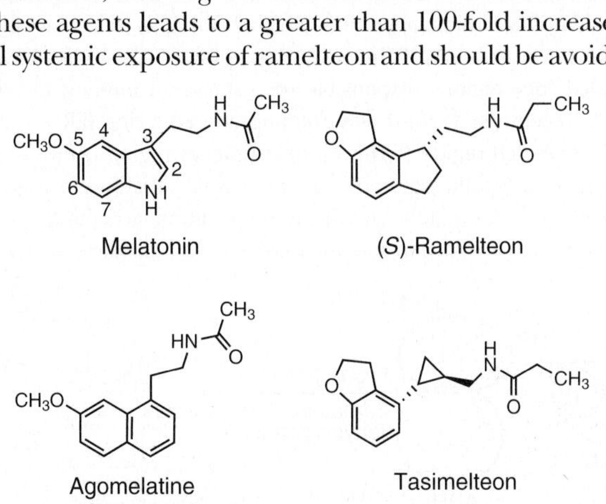

FIGURE 15.14 Structures of melatonin and the melatonin receptor agonists (*S*)-ramelteon, agomelatine, and tasimelteon.

Histamine H_1 Receptor Antagonists

The first generation of ethanolamine ether histamine H_1 receptor antagonists (i.e., antihistamines) that cross the blood–brain barrier are used for acute insomnia due to their sedation-promoting side effects. In particular, diphenhydramine and doxylamine, both high-affinity (low-nanomolar) H_1 receptor antagonists, are sold as over-the-counter sleep aids. Recently, the tricyclic antidepressant doxepin, which is a potent subnanomolar affinity H_1 antagonist, has also been approved for treatment of insomnia at lower doses than those used for depression (Silenor). The benefit of these agents for treatment of insomnia comes from H_1 receptor antagonism within the TMN of the posterior hypothalamus, where the normal release of histamine during the day causes arousal, and its decreased release at night reduces arousal responses. Antagonism of H_1 receptors within the TMN promotes sedation and drowsiness by inhibiting TMN outflow to other brain structures such as the dorsal raphe nucleus, paraventricular nucleus and locus coeruleus. Overall, antihistamines bring about increased drowsiness and sedation with marginal beneficial effects on sleep latency and total sleep time. There is very little in the way of rigorous clinical trial data that support their sedative-hypnotic efficacy, and to the contrary, some results reveal that these agents disrupt sleep architecture by delaying the onset to, and duration of, REM sleep. Regardless, these drugs are used heavily as sedative-hypnotics, and in the case of diphenhydramine and doxylamine, patients are able to readily self-medicate due to the ease in their availability. While diphenhydramine, doxylamine, and doxepin also exhibit antimuscarinic activity, leading to corresponding side effects such as dry mouth, urinary retention, vand blurred vision, a major side effect of these agents is excessive daytime drowsiness and residual next-day sedation, which are not uncommon. These next-day effects can lead to impaired cognition and performance and are attributed to the relatively longer half-lives. Finally, nightly use of first-generation antihistamines as sleep aids has been associated with tolerance to the hypnotic effect over long-term use. These agents are discussed further with respects to their SARs and metabolic transformations in Chapter 32.

FUTURE SEDATIVE-HYPNOTICS

As demonstrated within this chapter, $GABA_A$ receptor–acting hypnotics continue to be the mainstay for the pharmacotherapeutic management of insomnia. Although the pharmaceutical industry has a number of newer nonbenzodiazepine $GABA_A$ agonists such as indiplon under development, these agents are likely to have similar pharmacologic profiles as the currently used Z-drugs. The arrival of ramelteon to the marketplace was a major advance in development of sedative-hypnotics because it represented the first new class to be approved in several decades. Despite this relative paucity of novel sedative-hypnotics, there are several promising new CNS targets that have been exploited for their effects on the sleep/wake cycle, including $5\text{-}HT_{2A}$, orexin, and neuropeptide S (NPS) receptors. As a result, the pharmaceutical industry

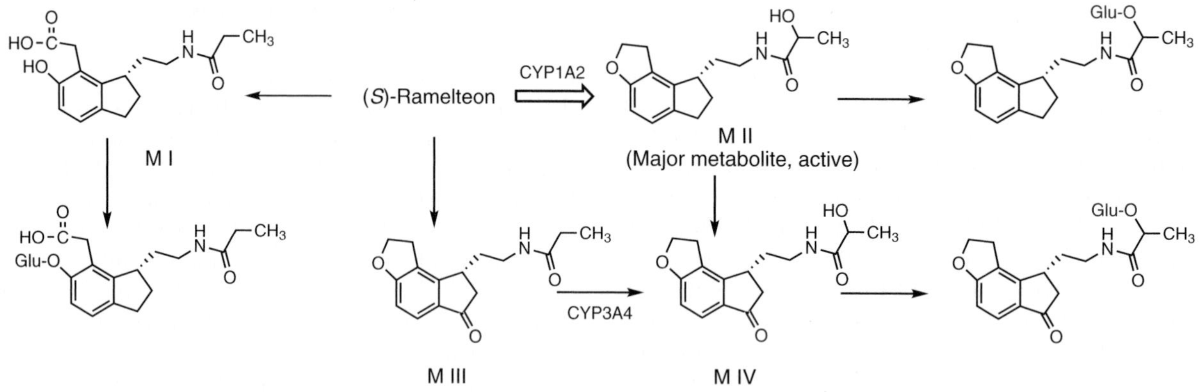

FIGURE 15.15 Metabolism of (*S*)-ramelteon. Coloration indicates site of metabolism.

has developed small-molecule antagonists of these targets with the hope of inducing and promoting sleep. Ritanserin, eplivanserin, and esmirtazapine are all 5-HT_{2A} receptor antagonists that are currently under investigation in various stages of clinical trials for treatment of insomnia. Because the effects of serotonin in the human brain are both broad and profound, further studies with these agents should shed light on the complexities of this system in regard to its regulation of the sleep/wake cycle.

Numerous lines of preclinical evidence support a key role of the orexin neuropeptides in promotion of wakefulness and alertness. Orexin neurons have been shown to extensively innervate key sleep/wake-regulating brain regions, in particular, the histaminergic neurons of the TMN. Binding of orexins to their cognate GPCRs, OX1 and OX2, has been demonstrated to promote wakefulness and alertness, suggesting that orexin receptor antagonism may have opposite effects. Indeed, almorexant is a first-in-class orexin receptor antagonist that is currently in phase III clinical trials for treatment of insomnia. This agent exhibits potent hypnotic effects in animals and humans, including those with insomnia, with minimal adverse effects and tolerability issues, suggesting that orexin receptor antagonism may provide a unique approach to treat insomnia.

Similarly, NPS is another recently described neuropeptide that is expressed in distinct brain regions, most notably in the locus coeruleus. As with the orexins, injection of NPS has been found to significantly increase wakefulness and suppress all stages of sleep. These effects are mediated by the recently discovered NPS receptor, another GPCR, and suggest that antagonism of NPS receptors could lead to a hypnotic effect. Because GPCRs are relatively amicable drug targets—approximately 40% to 50% of all marketed drugs target a GPCR—these novel targets offer promising strategies for the development of new sedative-hypnotic agents.

SCENARIO: OUTCOME AND ANALYSIS

Outcome

Susan W. Miller, PharmD, CGP, FASCP

The pharmacist's review concluded that one of the warnings associated with the use of zolpidem includes new onset of behavioral changes and complex behaviors. Sleep-eating is one of these complex behaviors and the consumption of additional food may account for the weight gain and the elevated hemoglobin A_{1C} level. The pharmacist's recommendations for the MTM were to taper the zolpidem over 4 days to discontinue its use and to initiate therapy with ramelteon dosed at 8 mg po 30 minutes before bedtime on day 5 of the taper. (Use of ramelteon is also associated with the development of complex behaviors.) The pharmacist also recommended discontinuation of the itraconazole because of the potential for drug interaction with the verapamil and zolpidem (now discontinued) and initiation of topical therapy with ciclopirox for treatment of the fingernail onychomycosis. WK should continue to monitor her diabetes and weight and return for a follow-up visit in 3 months. No changes were suggested for the diabetes or hypertension therapies at this time.

Chemical Analysis

S. William Zito and Victoria Roche

Zolpidem is an imidazopyridine, which is a highly selective agonist of the α_1-subunit of the $GABA_A$ receptors. SAR studies have revealed four regions responsible for zolpidem's binding to the $GABA_A$ receptors: 1) the freely rotating aromatic ring (FRAR), 2) an electron-rich region (ERR), 3) an antiplanar region (APR), and 4) a planar aromatic region (PAR). The methyl substituents found on FRAR and PAR regions and the hydrogen-bond–accepting imidazole nitrogen are responsible for zolpidem's α1 selective ability.

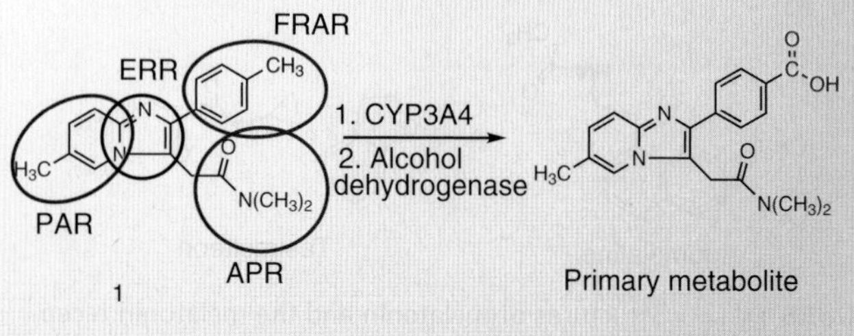

SCENARIO: OUTCOME AND ANALYSIS *(Continued)*

Zolpidem is a short-acting nonbenzodiazepine hypnotic that works like the BZs by binding to the γ-aminobutyric acid receptors. Zolpidem is used for the short-term treatment of insomnia. It works quickly (usually within 15 minutes) and has a short half-life (2 to 3 hours). The onset of zolpidem toxicity (behavioral changes and complex behaviors such as sleep-eating) is most likely caused by the addition of itraconazole, which is a CYP 3A4 inhibitor. Because zolpidem is metabolized by CYP 3A4, its metabolism will be inhibited by itraconazole and lead to behavioral toxicity.

Ramelteon is an analog of melatonin, the biological activity of which is related to circadian rhythm and induction of sleep. There are three melatonin receptors (MT1, MT2, and MT3) found in the CNS. MT1 is associated with induction of sleep and MT2 with setting the body's "biological clock." The role for MT3 has yet to be determined. Ramelteon changes the indole ring of melatonin to an indane ring and constrains the 5-methoxy group into a furan ring to form an indenofuran moiety.

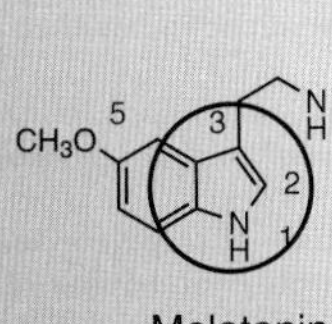

Melatonin

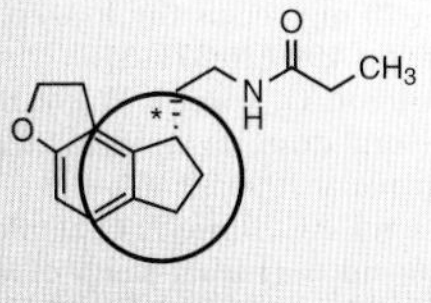

Ramelteon

The amide side chain on position 3 is critical for agonist activity at both MT1 and MT2 receptors. Ramelteon contains a stereochemical center at position 3 and the (*S*)-enantiomer has 500-fold greater affinity for MT1 than does (*R*)-ramelteon.

Ramelteon is primarily metabolized by phase I oxidation followed by excretion of the glucuronide conjugates. CYP1A2 is the major isoform responsible for transformation (49%), whereas CYP2C9 (42%) and CYP3A4 (8.6%) isoforms also contribute. The low percent of metabolism of ramelteon by CYP3A4 would not preclude the use of itraconazole; however, because WK is taking verapamil, which is metabolized by CYP3A4, the decision to discontinue itraconazole is justified.

Ciclopirox is a hydroxylated pyridinone that is used topically to treat superficial dermatophytic infections, primarily onychomycosis. Ciclopirox has a unique mechanism of action through chelation of polyvalent cations, such as Fe^{3+}, which causes inhibition of a number of metal-dependent enzymes within the fungal cell. Ciclopirox is metabolized by phase II glucuronidation and does not inhibit any CYP450 isoforms and would not interfere with the metabolism of the other of WK's medications.

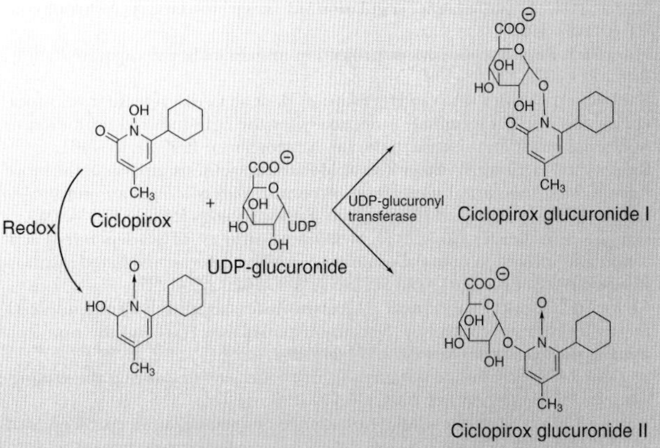

CASE STUDY

S. William Zito and Victoria Roche

BB is a 40-year-old school teacher who suffers from chronic insomnia. She experiences 3 to 5 awakenings every night and then finds it difficult to fall asleep again. She also experiences daytime fatigue and is unable to concentrate on her teaching responsibilities. Upon questioning, BB vaguely remembers being involved in a stressful family inheritance dispute years ago just before the onset of her sleep difficulty. BB also reports anxiety at bedtime because of the prospect of another sleepless night. BB has a history of hypertension, which is under control by treatment with diltiazem HCl (480 mg daily) and enalapril maleate (10 mg daily).

BB has been diagnosed with psychophysiological insomnia, sometimes referred to as "behavioral insomnia." The mainstay of treatment for this type of chronic insomnia is behavioral therapy, which can take 2 to 3 months to learn and provides clinical benefit. BB's physician wants to prescribe a sedative-hypnotic treatment until she experiences the benefits of the behavioral therapy. Evaluate the three choices for use in this case, given below.

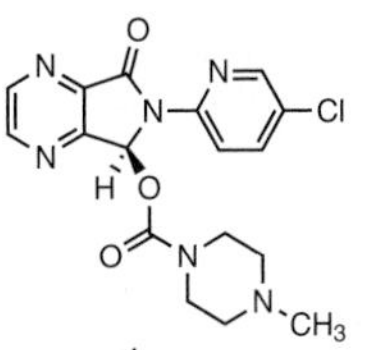

1

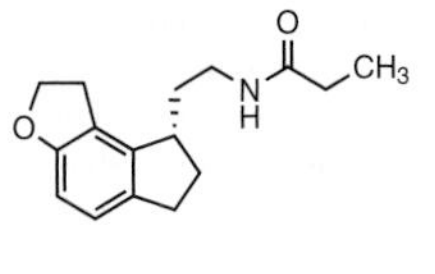

2

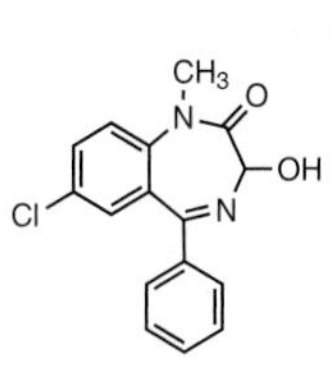

3

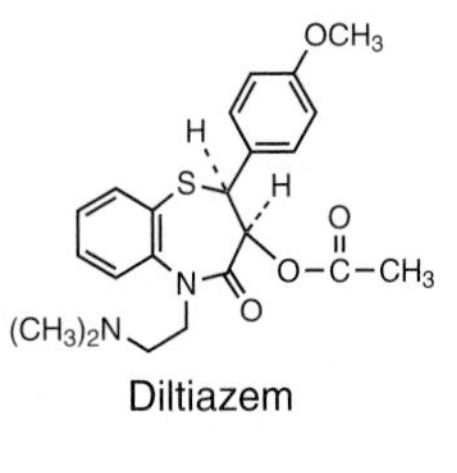

Diltiazem

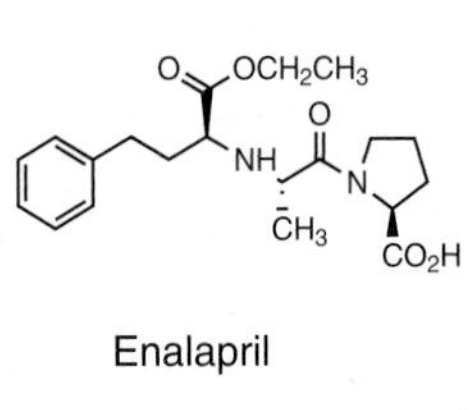

Enalapril

1. Conduct a thorough and mechanistic SAR analysis of the three therapeutic options in the case.
2. Apply the chemical understanding gained from the SAR analysis to this patient's specific needs to make a therapeutic recommendation.

References

1. Moruzzi G, Magoun HW. Brain stem reticular formation and activation of the EEG. Electroencephalogr Clin Neurophysiol 1949;1:455–473.
2. Lindsley DB, Schreiner LH, Knowles WB, et al. Behavioral and EEG changes following chronic brain stem lesions in the cat. Electroencephalogr Clin Neurophysiol 1950;2:483–498.
3. Maghoun HW. Caudal and cephalic influences of the brain stem reticular formation. Physiol Rev 1950;30:459–474.
4. Lu J, Greco MA. Sleep circuitry and the hypnotic mechanism of GABA drugs. J Clin Sleep Med 2006;2:S10–S26.
5. Panula P, Pirvola U, Auvinen S, et al. Histamine immunoreactive nerve fibers in the rat brain. Neuroscience 1989;28:585–610.
6. Takahashi K, Lin JS, Sakai K. Neuronal activity of histaminergic tuberomammillary neurons during wake-sleep states in the mouse. J Neurosci 2006;26:10292–10298.
7. Reiner PB, McGeer EG. Electrophysiological properties of cortically projecting histamine neurons of the rat hypothalamus. Neurosci Lett 1987;73:43–47.
8. Lin JS, Jouvet M. Evidence for histaminergic arousal mechanisms in the hypothalamus of cat. Neuropharmacology 1988;27:111–122.
9. Mochizuki T, Yamatodani A, Okakura K, et al. Circadian rhythm of histamine release from the hypothalamus of freely moving rats. Physiol Behav 1992;51:391–394.
10. Lin JS, Sakai K, Vanni-Mercier G, et al. A critical role of the posterior hypothalamus in the mechanisms of wakefulness determined by microinjection of muscimol in freely moving rats. Brain Res 1989;479:225–240.
11. Nauta WH. Hypothalamic regulation of sleep in rats. J Neurophysiol 1946;9:285–316.
12. Moore RY. Retinohypothalamic projection in mammals: a comparative study. Brain Res 1973;49:403–409.
13. Kalsbeek A, Cutrera RA, Van Heerikhuize JJ, et al. GABA release from suprachiasmatic nucleus terminals is necessary for the light-induced inhibition of nocturnal melatonin release in the rat. Neuroscience 1999;91:453–461.
14. Roseboom PH, Coon SL, Baler R, et al. Melatonin synthesis: analysis of the more than 150-fold nocturnal increase in serotonin *N*-acetyltransferase messenger ribonucleic acid in the rat pineal gland. Endocrinology 1996;13:3033–3045.
15. Ganguly S, Weller JL, Ho A, et al. Melatonin synthesis: 14-3-3-dependent activation and inhibition of arylalkylamine *N*-acetyltransferase mediated by phosphoserine-205. Proc Natl Acad Sci U S A 2005;102:1222–1227.
16. Klein DC, Moore RY. Pineal *N*-acetyltransferase and hydroxyindole-*O*-methyltransferase: control by the retinohypothalamic tract and the suprachiasmatic nucleus. Brain Res 1979;174:245–262.
17. Steriade M. Acetylcholine systems and rhythmic activities during the waking-sleep cycle. Prog Brain Res 2004;145:179–196.
18. Datta S. Cellular and chemical neuroscience of mammalian sleep. Sleep Med 2010;11:431–440.
19. Datta S. Cellular basis of pontine ponto-geniculo-occipital wave generation and modulation. Cell Mol Neurobiol 1997;17:341–365.
20. McKernan RM, Whiting PJ. Which GABAA-receptor subtypes really occur in the brain? Trends Neurosci 1996;19:139–143.
21. Macdonald RL, Rogers CJ, Twyman RE. Barbiturate regulation of kinetic properties of the GABAA receptor channel of mouse spinal neurones in culture. J Physiol 1989;417:483–500.
22. Akaike N, Maruyama T, Tokutomi N. Kinetic properties of the pentobarbitone-gated chloride current in frog sensory neurones. J Physiol 1987;394:85–98.
23. Jeffrey GA, Ghose S, Warwicker JO. The crystal structure of barbituric acid dehydrate. Acta Cryst 1961;14:881–887.
24. Senthilkumar K, Kolandaivel P. Quantum chemical studies on tautomerism of barbituric acid in gas phase and in solution. J Comp Aided Molec Des 2002;16:263–272.
25. Vida JA, Hooker ML. Anticonvulsants. 3. Phenobarbital and mephobarbital derivatives. J Med Chem 1973;16:602–605.
26. Vida JA, Hooker ML, Samour CM. Anticonvulsants. 4. Metharbital and phenobarbital derivatives. J Med Chem 1973;16:1378–1381.
27. Vida JA, Samour CM, O'Dea MH, et al. Analgesics. 2. Selected 5-substituted 5-(1-phenylethyl)barbituric acids. J Med Chem 1974;17:1194–1197.
28. Blicke FH, Cox RH, eds. Medicinal Chemistry, Vol. 4. New York: Wiley, 1959.
29. Basak SC, Harriss DK, Magnuson VR. Comparative study of lipophilicity versus topological molecular descriptors in biological correlations. J Pharm Sci 1984;73:429–437.
30. Lavoie AM, Twyman RE. Direct evidence for diazepam modulation of GABAA receptor microscopic affinity. Neuropharmacology 1996;35:1383–1392.
31. Twyman RE, Rogers CJ, Macdonald RL. Differential regulation of gammaaminobutyric acid receptor channels by diazepam and phenobarbital. Ann Neurol 1989;25:213–220.
32. Windholz M, ed. The Merck Index, 9th Ed. Rahway, NJ: Merck & Co., 1976.
33. Mejo SL. Anterograde amnesia linked to benzodiazepines. Nurse Pract 1992;17:49–50.
34. Clatworthy AJ, Jones LV, Whitehouse MJ. The gas chromatography mass spectrometry of the major metabolites of flurazepam. Biomed Mass Spectrom 1977;4:248–254.
35. Zampaglione N, Hilbert JM, Ning J, et al. Disposition and metabolic fate of 14C-quazepam in man. Drug Metab Dispos 1985;13:25–29.
36. Miura M, Otani K, Ohkubo T. Identification of human cytochrome P450 enzymes involved in the formation of 4-hydroxyestazolam from estazolam. Xenobiotica 2005;35:455–465.
37. Eberts FS Jr, Philopoulos Y, Reineke LM, et al. Triazolam disposition. Clin Pharmacol Ther 1981;29:81–93.
38. Sanger DJ, Benavides J, Perrault G, et al. Recent developments in the behavioral pharmacology of benzodiazepine (omega) receptors: evidence for the functional significance of receptor subtypes. Neurosci Biobehav Rev 1994;18:355–372.
39. McKernan RM, Rosahl TW, Reynolds DS, et al. Sedative but not anxiolytic properties of benzodiazepines are mediated by the GABA(A) receptor alpha1 subtype. Nat Neurosci 2000;3:587–592.
40. Löw K, Crestani F, Keist R, et al. Molecular and neuronal substrate for the selective attenuation of anxiety. Science 2000;290:131–134.
41. Collinson N, Kuenzi FM, Jarolimek W, et al. Enhanced learning and memory and altered GABAergic synaptic transmission in mice lacking the alpha 5 subunit of the GABAA receptor. J Neurosci 2002;22:5572–5580.
42. Crestani F, Keist R, Fritschy JM, et al. Trace fear conditioning involves hippocampal alpha5 GABA(A) receptors. Proc Natl Acad Sci U S A 2002;99:8980–8985.
43. Smith AJ, Alder L, Silk J, et al. Effect of alpha subunit on allosteric modulation of ion channel function in stably expressed human recombinant gamma-aminobutyric acid(A) receptors determined using (36)Cl ion flux. Mol Pharmacol 2001;59:1108–1118.
44. Petroski RE, Pomeroy JE, Das R, et al. Indiplon is a high-affinity positive allosteric modulator with selectivity for alpha1 subunit-containing GABAA receptors. J Pharmacol Exp Ther 2006;317:369–377.
45. Frattola L, Maggioni M, Cesana B, et al. Double blind comparison of zolpidem 20 mg versus flunitrazepam 2 mg in insomniac in-patients. Drugs Exp Clin Res 1990;16:371–376.
46. Bensimon G, Foret J, Warot D, et al. Daytime wakefulness following a bedtime oral dose of zolpidem 20 mg, flunitrazepam 2 mg and placebo. Br J Clin Pharmacol 1990;30:463–469.
47. Declerck AC, Ruwe F, O'Hanlon JF, et al. Effects of zolpidem and flunitrazepam on nocturnal sleep of women subjectively complaining of insomnia. Psychopharmacology 1992;106:497–501.
48. Roger M, Attali P, Coquelin JP. Multicenter, double-blind, controlled comparison of zolpidem and triazolam in elderly patients with insomnia. Clin Ther 1993;15:127–136.
49. Priest R, Terzano M, Parrino L, et al. Efficacy of zolpidem in insomnia. Eur Psychiatry 1997;12S:5–14.
50. Kerkhof G, Van Vianen BG, Kamphuisen HC. A comparison of zolpidem and temazepam in psychophysiological insomniacs. Eur Neuropsychopharmacol 1996;6:155–156.
51. Holm KJ, Goa KL. Zolpidem: an update of its pharmacology, therapeutic efficacy and tolerability in the treatment of insomnia. Drugs 2000;59:865–889.
52. Anzini M, Cappelli A, Vomero S, et al. Molecular basis of peripheral vs central benzodiazepine receptor selectivity in a new class of peripheral benzodiazepine receptor ligands related to alpidem. J Med Chem 1996;39:4275–4284.
53. Trapani G, Franco M, Ricciardi L, et al. Synthesis and binding affinity of 2-phenylimidazo[1,2-alpha]pyridine derivatives for both central and peripheral benzodiazepine receptors. A new series of high-affinity and selective ligands for the peripheral type. J Med Chem 1997;40:3109–3118.
54. Selleri S, Bruni F, Costagli C, et al. A novel selective GABA(A) alpha1 receptor agonist displaying sedative and anxiolytic-like properties in rodents. J Med Chem 2005;48:6756–6760.
55. Hanson SM, Morlock EV, Satyshur KA, et al. Structural requirements for eszopiclone and zolpidem binding to the gamma-aminobutyric acid type-A (GABAA) receptor are different. J Med Chem 2008;51:7243–7252.
56. Sauvantet JP, Langer SZ, Morselli PL, eds. Imidazopyridines in Sleep Disorders. New York: Raven Press, 1988.
57. Pichard L, Gillet G, Bonfils C, et al. Oxidative metabolism of zolpidem by human liver cytochrome P450S. Drug Metab Dispos 1995;23:1253–1262.
58. Von Moltke LL, Greenblatt DJ, Granda BW, et al. Zolpidem metabolism in vitro: responsible cytochromes, chemical inhibitors, and in vivo correlations. Br J Clin Pharmacol 1999;48:89–97.
59. Gillet G, Thénot JP, Morselli PL. In vitro and in vivo metabolism of zolpidem in three animal species and in man. Proc 3rd Intl ISSX Meeting, Amsterdam, the Netherlands, 1991, p. 153.
60. Olubodun JO, Ochs HR, von Moltke LL, et al. Pharmacokinetic properties of zolpidem in elderly and young adults: possible modulation by testosterone in men. Br J Clin Pharmacol 2003;56:297–304.
61. Nakamura H, Nakasa H, Ishii I, et al. Effects of endogenous steroids on CYP3A4-mediated drug metabolism by human liver microsomes. Drug Metab Dispos 2002;30:534–540.
62. Cubała WJ, Landowski J, Wichowicz HM. Zolpidem abuse, dependence and withdrawal syndrome: sex as susceptibility factor for adverse effects. Br J Clin Pharmacol 2008;65:444–445.

63. Hair PI, McCormack PL, Curran MP. Eszopiclone: a review of its use in the treatment of insomnia. Drugs 2008;68:1415–1434.
64. Lunesta (eszopiclone) tablets 1 mg, 2 mg, 3 mg: US prescribing information. Marlborough, MA: Sepracor, Inc., January 2009.
65. Trifiletti RR, Snyder SH. Anxiolytic cyclopyrrolones zopiclone and suriclone bind to a novel site linked allosterically to benzodiazepine receptors. Mol Pharmacol 1984;26:458–469.
66. Sieghart W. Structure and pharmacology of gamma-aminobutyric acid-A receptor subtypes. Pharmacol Rev 1995;47:181–234.
67. Carlson JN, Haskew R, Wacker J, et al. Sedative and anxiolytic effects of zopiclone's enantiomers and metabolite. Eur J Pharmacol 2001;415:181–189.
68. Sanna E, Busonero F, Talani G, et al. Comparison of the effects of zaleplon, zolpidem, and triazolam at various GABA(A) receptor subtypes. Eur J Pharmacol 2002;451:103–110.
69. Rosen AS, Fournié P, Darwish M, et al. Zaleplon pharmacokinetics and absolute bioavailability. Biopharm Drug Dispos 1999;20:171–175.
70. Sonata (zaleplon) capsules 5 mg, 10 mg: US prescribing information. Bristol, TN: King Pharmaceuticals, Inc., March 2006.
71. Dooley M, Plosker GL. Zaleplon: a review of its use in the treatment of insomnia. Drugs 2000;60:413–445.
72. Walsh JK, Vogel GW, Scharf M, et al. A five week, polysomnographic assessment of zaleplon 10 mg for the treatment of primary insomnia. Sleep Med 2000;1:41–49.
73. Wegner F, Deuther-Conrad W, Scheunemann M, et al. GABAA receptor pharmacology of fluorinated derivatives of the novel sedative-hypnotic pyrazolopyrimidine indiplon. Eur J Pharmacol 2008;580:1–11.
74. Kawashima K, Hosoi K, Naruke T, et al. Aldehyde oxidase-dependent marked species difference in hepatic metabolism of the sedative-hypnotic, zaleplon, between monkeys and rats. Drug Metab Dispos 1999;27:422–428.
75. Dolder CR, Nelson MH. Hypnosedative-induced complex behaviours: incidence, mechanisms and management. CNS Drugs 2008;22:1021–1036.
76. Hoque R, Chesson AL Jr. Zolpidem-induced sleepwalking, sleep related eating disorder, and sleep-driving: fluorine-18-flourodeoxyglucose positron emission tomography analysis, and a literature review of other unexpected clinical effects of zolpidem. J Clin Sleep Med 2009;5:471–476.
77. Tsai JH, Yang P, Chen CC, et al. Zolpidem-induced amnesia and somnambulism: rare occurrences? Eur Neuropsychopharmacol 2009;19:74–76.
78. Siddiqui F, Osuna E, Chokroverty S. Writing emails as part of sleepwalking after increase in zolpidem. Sleep Med 2009;10:262–264.
79. Doane JA, Dalpiaz AS. Zolpidem-induced sleep-driving. Am J Med 2008;121:e5.
80. Sansone RA, Sansone LA. Zolpidem, somnambulism, and nocturnal eating. Gen Hosp Psychiatry 2008;30:90–91.
81. Iruela LM. Zolpidem and sleepwalking. J Clin Psychopharmacol 1995;15:223.
82. Ferentinos P, Paparrigopoulos T. Zopiclone and sleepwalking. Int J Neuropsychopharmacol 2009;12:141–142.
83. Liskow B, Pikalov A. Zaleplon overdose associated with sleepwalking and complex behavior. J Am Acad Child Adolesc Psychiatry 2004;43:927–928.
84. Gauer F, Masson-Pevet M, Stehle J, et al. Daily variations in melatonin receptor density of rat pars tuberalis and suprachiasmatic nuclei are distinctly regulated. Brain Res 1994;641:92–98.
85. Liu C, Weaver DR, Jin X, et al. Molecular dissection of two distinct actions of melatonin on the suprachiasmatic circadian clock. Neuron 1997;19:91–102.
86. Dubocovich ML, Yun K, Al-Ghoul WM, et al. Selective MT2 melatonin receptor antagonists block melatonin-mediated phase advances of circadian rhythms. FASEB J 1998;12:1211–1220.
87. Kato K, Hirai K, Nishiyama K, et al. Neurochemical properties of ramelteon (TAK-375), a selective MT1/MT2 receptor agonist. Neuropharmacology 2005;48:301–310.
88. Miyamoto M, Nishikawa H, Doken Y, et al. The sleep-promoting action of ramelteon (TAK-375) in freely moving cats. Sleep 2004;27:1319–1325.
89. Nosjean O, Ferro M, Coge F, et al. Identification of the melatonin-binding site MT3 as the quinone reductase 2. J Biol Chem 2000;275: 31311–31317.
90. Yukuhiro N, Kimura H, Nishikawa H, et al. Effects of ramelteon (TAK-375) on nocturnal sleep in freely moving monkeys. Brain Res 2004;1027:59–66.
91. Mini L, Wang-Weigand S, Zhang J. Ramelteon 8 mg/d versus placebo in patients with chronic insomnia: post hoc analysis of a 5-week trial using 50% or greater reduction in latency to persistent sleep as a measure of treatment effect. Clin Ther 2008;30:1316–1323.
92. Roth T, Stubbs C, Walsh JK. Ramelteon (TAK-375), a selective MT1/MT2-receptor agonist, reduces latency to persistent sleep in a model of transient insomnia related to a novel sleep environment. Sleep 2005;28:303–307.
93. Erman M, Seiden D, Zammit G, et al. An efficacy, safety, and dose-response study of Ramelteon in patients with chronic primary insomnia. Sleep Med 2006;7:17–24.
94. Griffiths RR, Johnson MW. Relative abuse liability of hypnotic drugs: a conceptual framework and algorithm for differentiating among compounds. J Clin Psychiatry 2005;66:31–41.94.
95. Zlotos DP. Recent advances in melatonin receptor ligands. Arch Pharm 2005;338:229–247.
96. Mor M, Plazzi PV, Spadoni G, et al. Melatonin. Curr Med Chem 1999;6:501–518.
97. Spadoni G, Mor M, Tarzia G. Structure-affinity relationships of indole-based melatonin analogs. Biol Signals Recept 1999;8:15–23.
98. Rivara S, Mor M, Bedini A, et al. Melatonin receptor agonists: SAR and applications to the treatment of sleep-wake disorders. Curr Top Med Chem 2008;8:954–968.
99. Yous S, Andrieux J, Howell HE, et al. Novel naphthalenic ligands with high affinity for the melatonin receptor. J Med Chem 1992;35:1484–1486.
100. Sugden D, Davidson K, Hough KA, et al. Melatonin, melatonin receptors and melanophores: a moving story. Pigment Cell Res 2004;17:454–460.
101. Dubocovich ML, Delagrange P, Krause DN, et al. International Union of Basic and Clinical Pharmacology. LXXV. Nomenclature, classification, and pharmacology of G protein-coupled melatonin receptors. Pharmacol Rev 2010;62:343–380.
102. Farce A, Chugunov AO, Logé C, et al. Homology modeling of MT1 and MT2 receptors. Eur J Med Chem 2008;43:1926–1944.
103. Gerdin MJ, Mseeh F, Dubocovich ML. Mutagenesis studies of the human MT2 melatonin receptor. Biochem Pharmacol 2003;66:315–320.
104. Rozarem (ramelteon) tablets 8 mg: US prescribing information. Deerfield, IL: Takeda Pharmaceuticals America, Inc., October 2008.
105. Karim A, Tolbert D, Cao C. Disposition kinetics and tolerance of escalating single doses of ramelteon, a high-affinity MT1 and MT2 melatonin receptor agonist indicated for treatment of insomnia. J Clin Pharmacol 2006;46:140–148.
106. Obach RS, Ryder TF. Metabolism of ramelteon in human liver microsomes and correlation with the effect of fluvoxamine on ramelteon pharmacokinetics. Drug Metab Dispos 2010;38:1381–1391.

Chapter 16

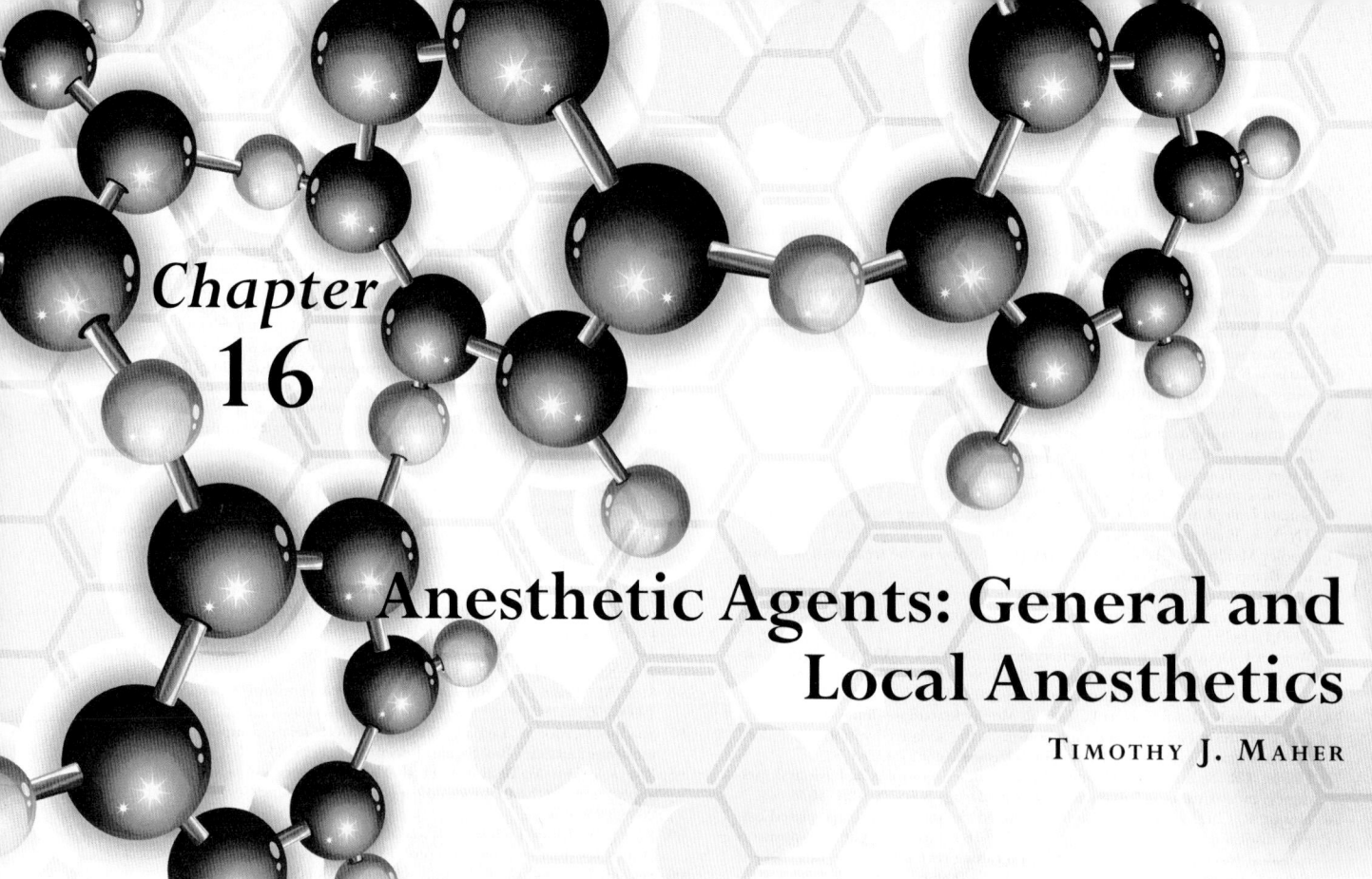

Anesthetic Agents: General and Local Anesthetics

TIMOTHY J. MAHER

Drugs Covered in This Chapter

INHALED GENERAL ANESTHETICS

- Ether
- Halothane
- Desflurane
- Enflurane
- Isoflurane
- Methoxyflurane
- Sevoflurane
- Nitrous oxide

INTRAVENOUS GENERAL ANESTHETICS

- Etomidate
- Ketamine
- Propofol
- Fospropofol
- Thiopental

LOCAL ANESTHETICS

- Articaine
- Benzocaine
- Bupivacaine
- Chloroprocaine
- Cocaine
- Dibucaine
- Dyclonine
- Mepivacaine
- Levobupivacaine
- Lidocaine
- Prilocaine
- Procaine
- Ropivacaine
- Tetracaine

Abbreviations

BTX, batrachotoxin
CNS, central nervous system
$COCl_2$, phosgene
EEG, electroencephalograph
EMLA, Eutectic Mixture of a Local Anesthetic
GABA, γ-aminobutyric acid
HBr, hydrobromic acid
HCl, hydrochloric acid
MAC, minimum alveolar concentration
Na/K-ATPase, sodium-potassium adenosine triphosphatase
NO, nitric oxide
NMDA, *N*-methyl-D-aspartate
PABA, *p*-aminobenzoic acid
PCP, phencyclidine
STX, saxitoxin
TTX, tetrodotoxin

SCENARIO

Paul Arpino, R.Ph.

CDL is a 70-year-old obese man scheduled for carpal tunnel surgery. A review of his medical file indicates a history of obstructive sleep apnea and benign prostatic hypertrophy (BPH). CDL sleeps with a continuous positive pressure airway device and his BPH is treated with tamsulosin, 0.4 mg daily. Given that patients with sleep apnea are at high risk for respiratory depression, the clinical team decides that a peripheral nerve block would be a better alternative to both neuraxial and general anesthesia. During the preoperative assessment before the scheduled day of surgery, the team discovers that CDL has an undefined allergy to procaine (Novocain) and that he experienced severe blistering after a dental procedure many years ago and was told he cannot receive "drugs like Novocain again."

(The reader is directed to the clinical solution and chemical analysis of this case at the end of the chapter).

INTRODUCTION

Anesthesia, defined as a loss of sensation with or without loss of consciousness, can be effectively achieved with a wide range of drugs with very diverse chemical structures. The list of such compounds includes not only the classic anesthetic agents, such as the general and local anesthetics, but also many central nervous system (CNS) depressants, such as analgesics, sedative/hypnotics (barbiturates and benzodiazepines), anticonvulsants, and skeletal muscle relaxants. Although various mechanisms of action are attributed to these agents, ultimately they all produce their anesthetic actions by interfering with conduction in sensory neurons and sometimes also motor neurons. Many of these agents are routinely used today in clinical practice to facilitate surgical and medical procedures. This chapter will focus on those agents typically classified as "general" and "local" anesthetics.

GENERAL ANESTHETICS

Prior to the mid-1800s, pain-producing surgical and dental procedures typically were undertaken without the aid of effective anesthetic agents. Chemical methods available at the time included intoxication with ethanol, hashish (cannabis), or opium, whereas physical methods included packing a limb in ice, creating ischemic conditions with tourniquets, inducing unconsciousness by a blow to the head, or the most common technique, employing strong-armed assistants to hold down the helpless patient during the entire painful surgical procedure. Additionally, at this time, many practicing physicians had been erroneously taught that pain was a requirement for effective healing; therefore, the observation of a patient in terrible pain was viewed as part of the normal healing process. These factors, along with the lack of knowledge regarding aseptic techniques or the availability of suitable infection-fighting agents, made surgical procedures a last resort approach to treating disease.

There have been many accounts of the first demonstration by the Hartford dentist Horace Wells of the use of nitrous oxide as a general anesthetic for surgery in 1844. Wells first observed the anesthetic actions of nitrous oxide at a public demonstration of "laughing gas." One of the volunteers, a pharmacy clerk named Samuel Cooley, injured his leg while under the influence of this gas and appeared to experience no pain. The next day, Wells inhaled the gas himself and, with the aid of a colleague, had one of his own teeth extracted without any sensation of pain. Wells then began routinely using nitrous oxide for dental procedures in his own practice. In 1845, he attempted to demonstrate the anesthetic effects of nitrous oxide at the Massachusetts General Hospital in Boston. This demonstration was considered to be a failure, however, because the patient cried out in the middle of the procedure. Following this unfortunate incident, the use of nitrous oxide was minimal until it resurfaced in dental practice during the mid-1860s, when it was combined with oxygen and made available in steel cylinders. This gas is still commonly used today, especially in combination with other anesthetic and analgesic agents.

The general anesthetic that gained greatest popularity shortly after the failed demonstration of Wells was diethyl ether. William Morton, a Boston dentist, was familiar at the time with the use of nitrous oxide by Wells. He also had heard of the interesting effects of diethyl ether and began to experiment on animals and himself with this volatile liquid. In 1846, he was allowed an opportunity to demonstrate the anesthetic actions of diethyl ether at, again, the Massachusetts General Hospital. In the famed "Ether Dome," which still stands today, Morton administered diethyl ether with a specially designed delivery device to the nervous patient, and the surgical procedure was performed without apparent pain. Following this demonstration, word of its success spread quickly, and soon, dental and medical practices throughout the United States and Europe were employing diethyl ether as a general anesthetic agent. Today, diethyl ether is no longer used in procedures because of its toxicity and dangerous physical properties (e.g., it is flammable and explosive!).

Other general anesthetic agents that enjoyed early popularity were chloroform and cyclopropane. Chloroform vapor depresses the CNS of a patient, allowing a doctor to perform various otherwise painful surgical procedures.

CLINICAL SIGNIFICANCE

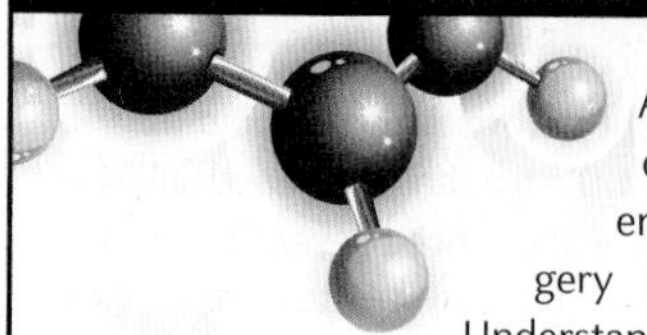

Anesthetics are a structurally diverse class of medications that enable clinicians to perform surgery and other noxious procedures. Understanding the essential components of the anesthetic state (i.e., immobilization, analgesia, and amnesia) as well as the medicinal chemistry of the various anesthetic agents allows the clinician to optimize therapy to meet patient specific needs. The patient undergoing a minimally invasive ambulatory surgical procedure may only require a local anesthetic with adjunctive pain control. Alternatively, patients undergoing a major surgical procedure may require general anesthesia with several different classes of anesthetics as well as several adjunctive medications to counteract deleterious emergence reactions related to the anesthetics. In both cases, a thorough understanding of the basic chemical properties of the drugs and their respective mechanisms of action will prove invaluable to making appropriate clinical decisions.

The practice of anesthesia is typically not considered to be therapeutic; therefore, the practice as well as the development of new agents is aimed at reducing adverse reactions, maintaining optimal physiologic conditions during procedures, and minimizing postoperative complications related to the procedure itself. The study of medicinal chemistry gives us hope for future treatment options, and knowledge of structure-activity relationships fosters the development of new medications and administration techniques. New generations of drugs are being created by modifying the structures of existing compounds to improve the side effect and pharmacokinetic profiles. Clinicians will have to stay up to date with new developments in anesthesia practices, the molecular actions of anesthetics, and the pharmacokinetic properties of the drugs to provide the best therapeutic outcomes for patients.

Paul Arpino, RPh
Harvard Medical School
Department of Pharmacy
Massachusetts General Hospital
Boston, MA

In 1847, the Scottish obstetrician James Young Simpson first used chloroform for general anesthesia during childbirth. The use of chloroform during surgery expanded rapidly thereafter in Europe. In the United States, chloroform replaced diethyl ether as an anesthetic at the beginning of the 20th century; however, it was quickly abandoned due to its cardio and CNS toxicity. Cyclopropane is a hydrocarbon with anesthetic properties like diethyl ether, except it is also explosive and is no longer used. As described later in this chapter, the inhalational general anesthetic agents used today are typically hydrocarbons and halogenated ethers (Cl, Br, or F); nitrous oxide is the exception. Table 16.1 lists the characteristics of the "ideal" general anesthetic agent. Unfortunately, the agent that fulfills all these characteristics is currently unknown.

Stages of General Anesthesia

The ideal general anesthetic state is characterized by a loss of all sensations and includes analgesia and muscle relaxation. Neuronal depression in specific areas of the CNS is believed to be largely responsible for such an anesthetic state. The areas involved include many cortical regions that are represented by excitatory pyramidal cells and inhibitory/excitatory stellate cells. Excitation of the pyramidal cells helps to maintain consciousness, whereas the degree of inhibition or excitation of stellate cells determines the overall activity level of the pyramidal cells with which they synapse. As the concentration of the anesthetic agent increases in the brain, the degree of overall neuronal depression also increases, resulting in progressively deeper stages of anesthesia. Based on observations using diethyl ether, Guedel in 1920 originally described this progression as four distinct stages, and Gillespie subsequently further subdivided these stages (Fig. 16.1), as described in the following sections.

Stage 1: Analgesia

Characterized by a mild depression of higher cortical neurons, this stage is suitable for minor surgical procedures that do not require significant neuromuscular relaxation. Depression of thalamic centers probably accounts for the observed analgesia, because many of the neuronal systems that mediate pain sensation traverse through this anatomic area. Some general anesthetic agents do not possess significant analgesic activity, but they all produce a loss of consciousness that, in turn, can produce some degree of insensitivity to painful stimuli.

TABLE 16.1 Characteristics of the Ideal General Anesthetic Agent

Rapid and pleasant induction of surgical anesthesia
Rapid and pleasant withdrawal from surgical anesthesia
Adequate relaxation of skeletal muscles
Potent enough to permit adequate oxygen supply in mixture
Wide margin of safety
Nontoxic
Absence of adverse effects
Nonflammable/nonexplosive
Chemically compatible with anesthetic devices
Nonreactive
Inexpensive

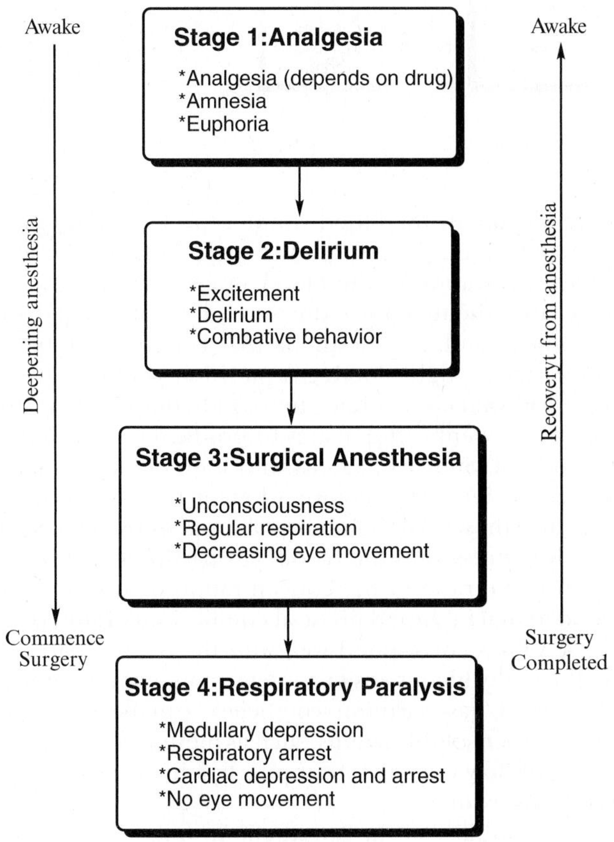

FIGURE 16.1 Stages of general anesthesia.

Stage 2: Delirium

As depression of inhibitory neurons in the CNS progresses, especially in the reticular formation (a network of neurons in the brainstem), a resultant excitation of cortical motor neurons leads to significant involuntary muscle activity, such as urination, delirium, uncontrolled skeletal muscular movements, and increased heart rate, blood pressure, and respiration. These paradoxical responses are caused by suppression of inhibitory neurons that normally function to closely regulate such neuronal activity. Ideally, an anesthetic agent should produce little or no excitatory phase. Together, stages 1 and 2 comprise the induction period, which ideally should be of short duration.

Stage 3: Surgical Anesthesia

This stage is divided into four planes characterized by increasing CNS depression: first, loss of spinal reflexes; second, decreased skeletal muscle reflexes; third, paralysis of intercostal muscles; and fourth, loss of most muscle tone. Stage 3 is also characterized by regular breathing, a loss of many reflexes, and roving eyeball movements.

Stage 4: Respiratory Paralysis

Characterized by respiratory and vasomotor paralysis, this stage represents an overdose or toxic level that should be avoided. Normally, this stage is never reached, because the anesthesiologist is careful to monitor abdominal respiration to prevent apnea, blood pressure to prevent hypotension, and heart rate to prevent asystole (a state of no cardiac electrical activity).

Modern General Anesthetic Agents

Although these stages have been described for diethyl ether, an anesthetic agent no longer used today. Some of today's clinically useful general anesthetic agents fail to follow this described pattern of anesthetic progression. Some attempts have been made to correlate changes in the electroencephalograph (EEG) with the depth of anesthesia. Most of these studies, however, have failed to yield a reliable predictor for anesthesiologists to use. Additionally, concomitant drugs used as preanesthetic agents can alter the EEG while not altering the depth of anesthesia. Rather than describing specific stages or using EEG patterns, a number of useful signs that more accurately reflect the depth of anesthesia for most of the anesthetic agents are currently used. When during the initial period of anesthetic administration a patient has irregular respiratory depth and rate, is still swallowing, and blinks the eyes when the eyelashes are touched, the desired surgical stage of anesthesia likely has not been reached. However, when a loss of the eyelash reflex occurs along with rhythmic breathing, however, a level of adequate surgical anesthesia has generally begun. If a patient at this stage exhibits elevations in blood pressure, increased respiration rate, or increased jaw tension when a surgical incision is attempted, the subject is considered to be "light" and typically requires additional anesthesia to facilitate further surgical manipulations. These responses decrease further—until they are abolished—as the depth of anesthesia progresses. By monitoring reflexes, blood pressure, and respiration rate and depth, today's anesthesiologist is capable of effectively maintaining an appropriate depth of surgical anesthesia without producing unwanted medullary depression.

Pharmacokinetic Principles of Volatile Anesthetics

The production and maintenance of the anesthetic state is believed by most to be dependent on the concentration, or partial pressure, of the anesthetic agent in yet unknown areas of the brain. Obviously, the concentration of the anesthetic agent in the gas mixture administered, as well as the rate and depth of respiration of the patient, will influence the rate of anesthesia induction. The rate at which delivery of anesthetic agents to these sites occurs is dependent on their physicochemical properties, particularly their solubility in lipid and blood (Fig. 16.2).

Administration of Volatile Anesthetics

The administration of gaseous or volatile liquid anesthetics involves a number of sophisticated devices that have been refined over the years to aid the anesthesiologist in carefully controlling the amount of anesthetic delivered to the patient while minimizing the exposure of the

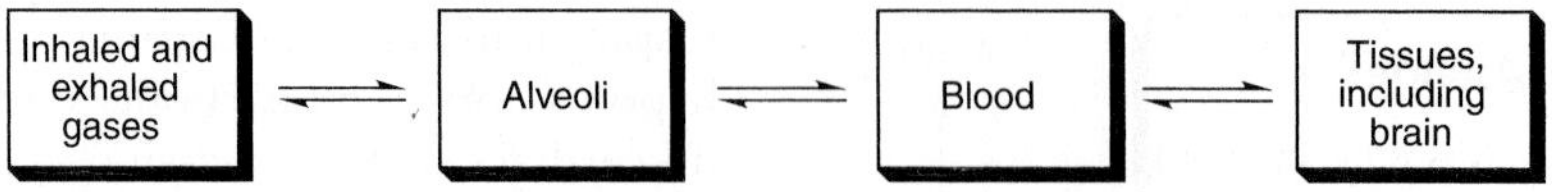

FIGURE 16.2 Dynamic equilibria existing during the state of anesthesia.

surgical personnel to these agents. Early systems used a gauze pad in a mask placed over the nose and mouth of the patient. The anesthesiologist would then put drops of the volatile anesthetic on the gauze pad, and as the patient breathed, the anesthetic was delivered to the lungs. This procedure was somewhat effective, but it allowed little or no control over the amount of anesthetic and oxygen delivered to the patient. Thus, the anesthetic agent not inhaled was allowed to evaporate into the surrounding area in the surgical suite and posed a significant risk to the surgical personnel. Today, flowmeters, vaporizers, and absorber devices are routinely available, allowing precise determination and control of the amount of volatile anesthetic, oxygen, and carbon dioxide administered while preventing significant exposure to workers. Typically, oxygen is bubbled through a volatile anesthetic liquid, and the resultant gas mixture is delivered to the patient for continual inhalation. Many of these devices are described in greater detail elsewhere (1).

The inhaled anesthetic concentration is controlled by the anesthesiologist, who can either increase or decrease this concentration depending on the observed depth of anesthesia. Eventually, with continued administration, the concentration of anesthetic in the bronchiolar alveoli reaches equilibrium with that in the inspired gas mixture (Fig. 16.2). Transfer from the alveolar space to the blood proceeds quickly, and depending on the concentrations of anesthetic used and its physiochemical characteristics, equilibrium with the arterial blood is achieved. However, before appreciable amounts of anesthetic agent dissolved in the blood will enter the brain, the blood must be saturated with the anesthetic. Therefore, anesthetics that are more soluble in the blood (have a low blood/gas partition coefficient, Fig. 16.2) will require a longer time to achieve saturation of the blood–brain compartment. In such cases, the time for induction will be prolonged. On the other hand, an anesthetic that is poorly soluble in blood (has a high blood/gas partition coefficient, Fig. 16.2) will quickly saturate the blood compartment and then rapidly enter the tissues to produce a short induction period. Similarly, agents with high blood/gas partition coefficients will require a longer time for recovery from anesthesia. The solubility of an agent in the blood is usually expressed as the blood/gas partition coefficient, which is the ratio of the concentration of anesthetic in blood to that in the gas phase at equilibrium (Table 16.2). These values correspond well with the oil/gas partition coefficient, which is easier to determine experimentally. The blood/gas partition coefficient can be very high (e.g., 12) for soluble agents, such as methoxyflurane, and extremely low (e.g., 0.47) for poorly soluble agents, such as nitrous oxide.

The solubility of the anesthetic in tissue is expressed as the tissue/blood partition coefficient. Because the concentration of the anesthetic in the brain is probably of most interest, the brain/blood partition coefficient is more useful. Because the solubility of the anesthetic in lean tissues is essentially equal to that in blood, the tissue/blood or brain/blood partition coefficient is typically close to a value of 1. In fatty tissues, however, the partition coefficient can be much larger due to lipid solubility. The rate of blood flow to a particular organ will also influence the rate at which anesthetics reach their sites of action. The brain, liver, and kidneys have relatively high

TABLE 16.2 Partition Coefficients, MACs, and Metabolism of Some General Anesthetics

Anesthetics	Partition Coefficients at 37°C		MAC (vol %)[a]			% Metabolism
	Oil/Gas	Blood/Gas	Without N_2O	With N_2O (%)	MAC-Awake (Vol %)	
Methoxyflurane	970	12	0.16	0.07 (56)	—	50
Halothane	224	2.3	0.77	0.29 (66)	0.4	20
Enflurane	99	1.9	91.7	0.60 (70)	0.4	2.4
Isoflurane	97	1.4	1.15	0.50 (70)	0.4	0.17
Sevoflurane (2)	53	0.60	1.71	0.66 (64)	0.6	4–6
Desflurane (3)	19	0.42	6.0	2.83 (60)	2.4	0.02
Nitrous oxide	1.4	0.47	104	—	60	None

[a]MAC = minimum alveolar concentration, expressed as volume %, that is required to produce immobility in respect to a standard surgical incision in 50% of middle-aged humans.

blood flows, whereas skeletal muscle at rest and fat tissues have relatively poor blood flows and would be expected to accumulate less of the anesthetic agent.

Reversal of the anesthetic state and recovery requires a reduction in the concentration of the anesthetic in the brain. This is achieved by stopping the delivery of the anesthetic through the lungs. As the patient continues to breathe, the anesthetic is continually removed, which favors diffusion from the brain to the blood, to the alveoli, and finally, to the expired air. The rate at which this occurs generally parallels that of induction, because the solubility of an agent in the brain and in the blood determines how quickly these compartments will return to a preanesthetic state. The main route of elimination is via the expired air, which can be mostly captured by gas-scavenging devices with absorbers, but some metabolism of these agents does take place (discussed below).

Minimum Alveolar Concentration

The minimum alveolar concentration (MAC) is defined as the concentration at 1 atmosphere of anesthetic in the alveoli that is required to produce immobility in 50% of adult patients subjected to a standard surgical incision. A further increase to 1.3 MAC will frequently cause immobility in 99% of patients. At equilibrium, the concentration (or partial pressure) of an anesthetic in the alveoli is equal to that in the brain, and it is this concentration in the brain that most closely reflects the concentration at the site responsible for the anesthetic actions. Thus, the MAC is often used as a measure of the potency of individual anesthetic agents. The MAC of many of the volatile and gaseous anesthetics in use today is shown in Table 16.2.

When anesthetic agents are used in combination, the MACs for inhaled anesthetics are simply additive. For instance, the anesthetic depth achieved with 0.5 MAC of enflurane plus 0.5 MAC of nitrous oxide is equivalent to that produced by 1.0 MAC of either agent alone. The combination of two anesthetics is a very common practice, because this technique allows for a reduction in the patient exposure to any one of the individual agents, thereby decreasing the likelihood of adverse reactions.

Many factors influence the MAC via a number of different mechanisms (Table 16.3). Factors that have been shown to increase the MAC for many volatile anesthetics include elevated catecholamines in the CNS following pharmacologic treatments, hypernatremia, and hyperthermia. Factors known to decrease MAC include ethanol ingestion, clonidine, lithium, lidocaine, centrally administered opioids, and drugs that decrease central catecholamine levels. Additionally, hyponatremia, hypotension, hypothermia, hypoxia, increasing age, and pregnancy have also been shown to decrease MAC. Plasma potassium, hypertension, gender, and the duration of anesthesia typically generally have minimal to no effect on the MAC (2).

Another term, the "MAC-Awake," is used to describe the concentration of anesthetic at which appropriate responses to verbal commands are lost in 50% of the patients tested. At this concentration, amnesia and a loss of awareness are evident, and the patient is said to be in a state of hypnosis. The MAC-Awake occurs at concentrations significantly lower (e.g., 50% to 75% lower) than those required for surgical anesthesia.

TABLE 16.3 Factors That May Alter MAC

Increase MAC	Increased catecholamine levels in CNS Hypernatremia Hyperthermia	
Decrease MAC	Decreased catecholamine levels in CNS Alcohol Ingestion Clonidine Lidocaine Lithium Opioids	 Hyponatremia Hypotension Hypothermia Hypoxia Increased age Pregnancy
No effect on MAC	Plasma potassium Gender Hypertension Duration of anesthesia	

Theories About the Mechanisms of Anesthesia

Meyer-Overton Theory

In the early 1900s, Hans Meyer and Charles Overton suggested that the potency of a substance as an anesthetic was directly related to its lipid solubility, or oil/gas partition coefficient (Table 16.2) (3–5). This has commonly been referred to as the "unitary theory of anesthesia." They used olive oil, octanol, and other "membrane-like" lipids to determine the lipid solubility of the agents available at that time. Compounds with high lipid solubility required lower concentrations (i.e., lower MAC) to produce anesthesia. It was later postulated that the interaction of the anesthetic molecules with a hydrophobic portion of the nerve membrane caused a distortion of the nerve membrane near the channels that conducted Na^+, those that mediated the fast action potentials and neuronal cell firing. The presence of this critical volume of anesthetic dissolved within the membrane caused the membrane to "bloat" and cause a "squeezing in" on the Na^+ channel to interfere with Na^+ conductance and normal neuronal depolarization. In support of this theory, it was found that at high pressures (40 to 100 atmospheres), the anesthetic actions of many of these agents could be partially reversed, presumably by compressing membranes back to their original conformation. Arguing against this theory, however, is the finding that not all highly lipid-soluble substances are capable of producing anesthesia. Additionally, more recent work involving protein–drug interactions has seriously challenged this theory. Today, more than 150 years after the first demonstration of the use of a volatile anesthetic agent, most theories about the mechanisms of anesthesia suggest that multiple selective lipid–protein membrane interactions, involving numerous receptor types, are responsible for the anesthesia produced and that no reason exists to believe that all anesthetic agents need to produce their effects via identical actions. Thus, a single molecular target for anesthetic actions is no longer required (6).

Stereochemical Aspects

The volatile anesthetics isoflurane, desflurane, enflurane, and halothane each contain an asymmetric carbon and, thus, can exist as (+)- or (−)-enantiomers. Although all of the commercially available preparations are racemates, some researchers have been able to determine the anesthetic properties of individual enantiomers. The (+)-enantiomer of isoflurane is at least 50% more potent as an anesthetic in the rat than is the (−)-enantiomer (7). In that study, the MAC values were 1.06% and 1.62% for the (+)- and (−)-enantiomers, respectively. In another study, however, the potency of the individual isoflurane enantiomers to depress myocardial activity was not found to be different, suggesting possible involvement of mechanisms dissimilar from those responsible for producing anesthesia (8). These findings argue against the original and simple lipid-solubility theory of anesthesia, and they support a more complex mechanism, probably likely involvement of proteins in the form of receptor–anesthetic interactions (9).

Ion Channel and Protein Receptor Hypotheses

More recently, investigators have determined the effects of anesthetics on a number of protein receptors within the CNS. Features that support the likelihood of an interaction with a protein include 1) the steep dose–response curves observed, 2) the stereochemical requirements of various anesthetics, 3) the finding that increasing the molecular weight and corresponding lipid solubility of an anesthetic can actually decrease or abolish anesthetic activity, and 4) the finding that specific ion channels and neurotransmitter receptor systems are required for most of the observed effects of the anesthetics. What appears to be emerging as a central theme for the mechanism of action of general anesthetics involves the interaction of the anesthetics with receptors that allosterically modulate the activity of ion channels (e.g., chloride and potassium) or with the ion channel directly (e.g., sodium). Many other mechanisms are also emerging to help explain the mechanisms of action of the general anesthetics.

Chloride Channel The ion channel that has received the most investigative attention is that for chloride (Fig. 16.3). Both the γ-aminobutyric acid$_A$ (GABA$_A$) and the glycine$_A$ (strychnine-sensitive) receptors are ligand-gated ion channels and linked to chloride channels that normally mediate inhibitory responses within the CNS. Halothane, isoflurane, and other volatile anesthetics are capable of inhibiting the synaptic destruction of GABA, thereby increasing the GABAergic neurotransmission, which typically is inhibitory in nature (10). Studies have also demonstrated the ability of these anesthetics to enhance the binding of GABA or other allosteric modulators within the GABA receptor complex (11). In one such study, (+)-isoflurane was significantly more potent than the (−)-enantiomer at enhancing GABAergic function (12). The volatile anesthetics, and many of the intravenous general anesthetic agents, bind to discrete cavities within the GABA$_A$

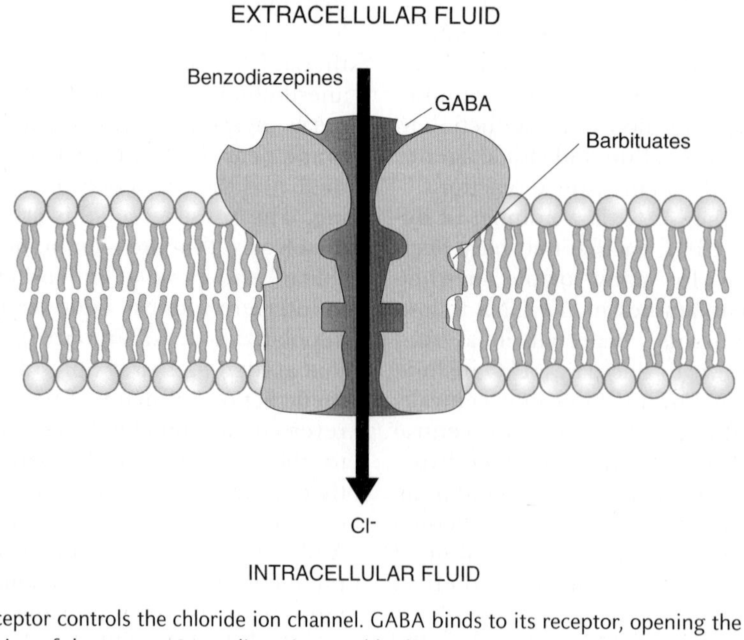

FIGURE 16.3 The GABA$_A$ receptor controls the chloride ion channel. GABA binds to its receptor, opening the chloride ion channel and resulting in hyperpolarization of the neuron. Benzodiazepines and barbiturates can produce anesthesia by allosterically enhancing GABA opening of chloride channels, which are located at inhibitory synapses on pyramidal cells.

receptor complex to enhance GABA neurotransmission (13,14). Studies using mutant chimeric $GABA_A$ receptors have identified a specific binding site for general anesthetics located between transmembrane segments 2 and 3 (15). At therapeutic concentrations, just about all of the inhalational general anesthetics are capable of enhancing GABAergic function, whereas at considerably higher concentrations, many also can act directly as GABA mimetics (16). Recent studies have demonstrated an effect of these agents not only on the synaptic $GABA_A$ receptor function that mediates phasic neuronal responses but also on those extrasynaptic $GABA_A$ receptors that mediate tonic neuronal activity (17). Other specific anesthetic agents can alter $GABA_A$ receptor function via different mechanisms. For instance, propofol, an intravenous general anesthetic, appears to slow the desensitization of the $GABA_A$ receptor during bouts of rapid, repetitive activation at inhibitory synapses (18). Most of these agents also potentiate the actions of glycine, the other important inhibitory amino acid neurotransmitter (16). The combination of GABAergic and glycinergic potentiation by the general anesthetics probably accounts for the vast majority of the observed activity of the inhalational agents as well as that of the barbiturates.

Sodium Channels One channel that has received much attention regarding the mediation of drug-induced anesthetic actions is the ligand-gated Na^+ channel within the *N*-methyl-D-aspartate (NMDA) receptor complex. When activated by the excitatory amino acid neurotransmitter, glutamate, an increase in the conductance to Na^+ occurs that promotes neuronal depolarization (Fig. 16.4) (19). Compounds known to stimulate NMDA receptors are typically capable of increasing alertness and of acting as convulsants, whereas pharmacologic agents that act as antagonists at this site are usually sedatives, anticonvulsants, and dissociative anesthetics (e.g., ketamine). Halothane has been demonstrated to specifically antagonize the glutamate-stimulated depolarization of neurons (20), whereas isoflurane has been shown to decrease glutamate release and enhance its removal from the synaptic cleft (21). Glutamate acting at NMDA and other non-NMDA receptors within the CNS is probably one of the most important excitatory inputs that supports consciousness. It is not surprising that the general anesthetics would act by altering neurotransmission in this system (22). Others have reported an interaction of general anesthetics with the neuronal nicotinic acetylcholine receptor–linked Na^+ channel (23). Voltage-gated Na^+ channels in small, nonmyelinated hippocampal axons also appear to be inhibited by general anesthetics, such as isoflurane (24).

Potassium Channels Potassium ion channels have also been suggested as a site for general anesthetic agents. Increasing K^+ conductance normally functions to maintain the polarized state of neurons and to assist in the

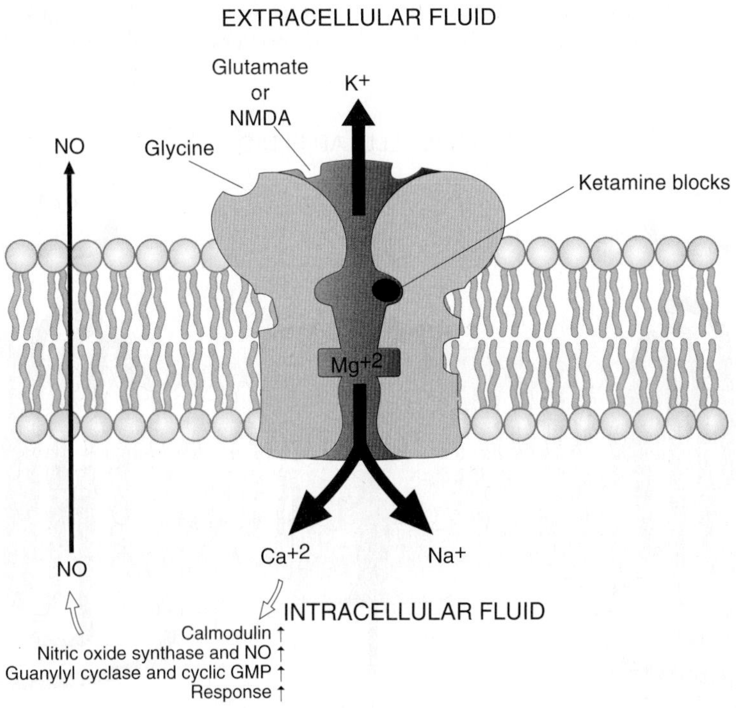

FIGURE 16.4 Glutamate or NMDA receptors in the CNS. Binding of agonists (glutamate or NMDA) opens the channel, allowing K^+ to flow outward to extracellular fluid and sodium and calcium ions to flow into the nerve cells. Increased intracellular fluid calcium ion concentration triggers a cascade that produces a response and liberates the retrograde neuronal messenger nitric oxide (NO). Ketamine can produce anesthesia by blocking these NMDA-controlled channels, which are located at excitatory synapses on pyramidal cells (3). Glycine acts as a positive allosteric modulator at the NMDA receptor.

repolarization of neurons following their stimulation-induced depolarization (Fig. 16.5). Thus, enhancing the activity of certain K^+ channels would be expected to result in a decreased likelihood of neuronal excitation. A novel, anesthetic-sensitive K^+ current [$I_{K(an)}$] has been identified that is stereoselectively activated by isoflurane (25). Mice with a targeted deletion of the TREK-1 two-pore-domain K^+ channel show significantly reduced sensitivity to general anesthetics compared to wild-type controls (26). Additionally, certain α_2-adrenoceptor agonists (e.g., dexmedetomidine) when injected produce an anesthetic state that is mediated by a G protein–coupled receptor that allosterically modulates K^+ channels. These responses can be antagonized by pertussis toxin and 4-aminopyridine, agents that inactivate G proteins and block K^+ channels, respectively, lending further support to the role of this ion channel (27). Similarly, G protein–mediated mechanisms appear to be involved with the action of morphine via the μ-opioid receptor (Fig. 16.5).

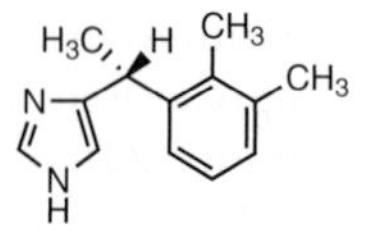

Dexmedetomidine

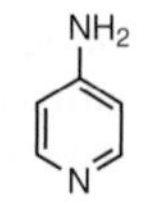

4-Aminopyridine

Halogenated Hydrocarbons and Ethers

Historical Aspects

Ether The useful volatile anesthetics, with the exception of nitrous oxide, are halogenated hydrocarbons and ethers. Diethyl ether (Fig. 16.6), one of the first agents to be introduced as a general anesthetic, has high potency with significant analgesic and neuromuscular relaxing effects. This agent is extremely flammable, and when mixed with air, oxygen, or nitrous oxide, is explosive. Induction with diethyl ether is very slow; significant time is spent progressing through the delirium stage. Irritation of the respiratory tract by diethyl ether can lead to excessive bronchial secretions, complicating adequate ventilation. In addition to its unpleasant induction and adverse effects, recovery is similarly prolonged and can be accompanied by vomiting. These pharmacologic and physical characteristics of diethyl ether have limited the utility of this anesthetic in humans.

Short-Chain Hydrocarbons Many of the short-chain alkanes, alkenes, and alkynes are capable of producing an anesthetic state when administered to patients. Potency generally increases as chain length increases. However, because of their flammability and increased propensity to cause cardiovascular toxicity, these nonsubstituted hydrocarbons are not useful as anesthetic agents.

Chloroform Another of the earlier anesthetic agents to be used was chloroform ($CHCl_3$). This halogenated hydrocarbon was first officially used in the United States in 1847; however, its toxicity seriously limited its utility. The addition of halogens to the hydrocarbon backbone increases potency and volatility, as well as decreases flammability. Similar effects are also observed with such substitutions on ethers. As an anesthetic agent, chloroform is very potent and possesses significant analgesic and neuromuscular

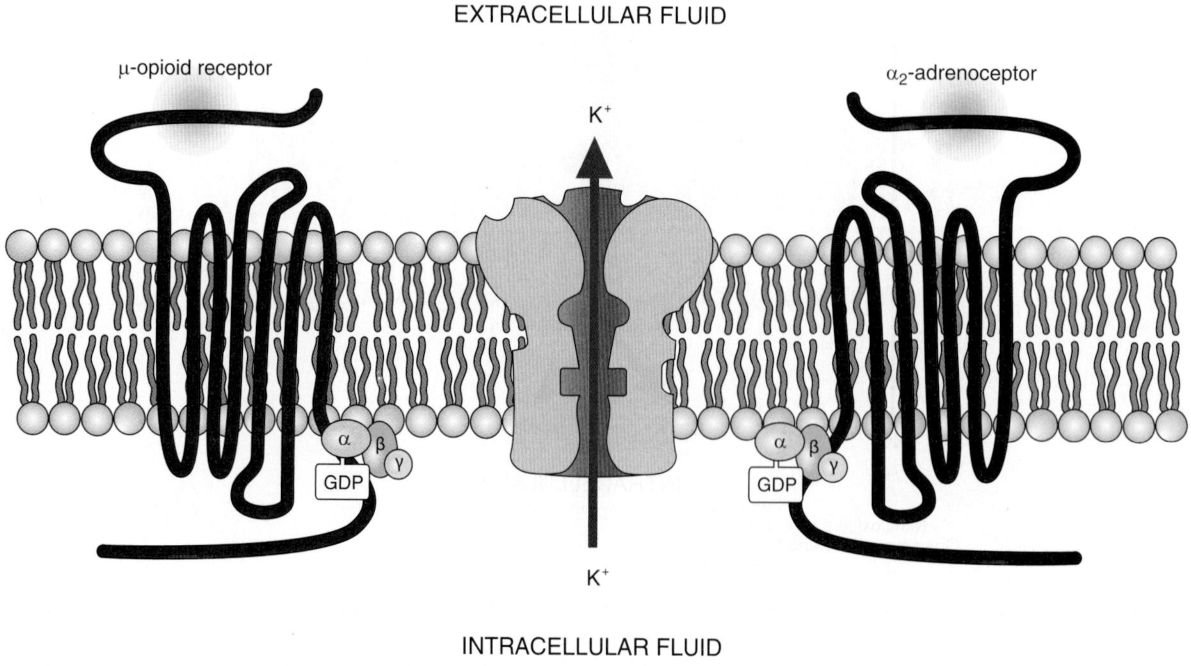

FIGURE 16.5 Morphine and α_2-agonists activate their respective G proteins, which hyperpolarize neurons by lowering intracellular fluid K^+ ion concentration.

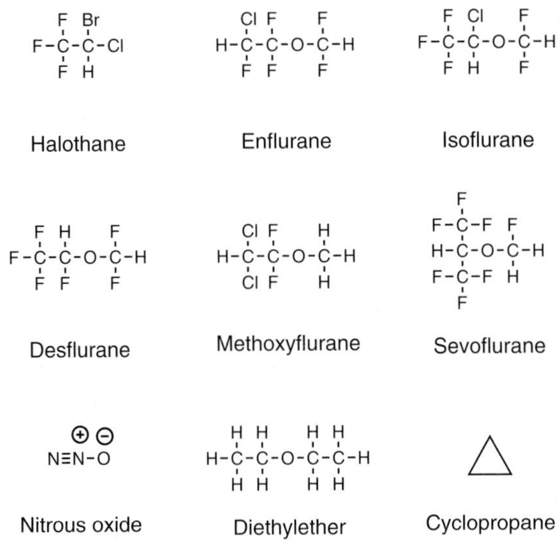

FIGURE 16.6 General anesthetics.

relaxing activity. Chloroform, a known carcinogen, has the disadvantage of being both hepatotoxic and nephrotoxic, in addition to producing adverse cardiovascular effects, such as arrhythmias and severe hypotension. As a result of these toxicities, chloroform has an unacceptable therapeutic index that prohibits its use in anesthesia. Two other halogenated compounds that found limited use in the mid-1900s included trichloroethylene and fluroxene. Neither of these agents is used today. Knowledge regarding the influence of the halogen substitutions on the potency and flammability of hydrocarbons and ethers, however, significantly contributed to our understanding of the structure–activity relationship of volatile anesthetics and the eventual design of substantially improved agents.

Flammability The occurrence of fires in operating rooms is of great concern to all participants in the surgical procedure. Although the introduction of "nonflammable" agents, such as halothane, enflurane, and isoflurane, has substantially decreased this hazard, such fires still occur. Three essential ingredients are required for any combustion: 1) an ignition source (e.g., a laser), 2) a combustible material (e.g., gauze, drapes, or rubber tubes), and 3) an oxidizing agent (e.g., oxygen or nitrous oxide). Many substances are flammable in pure oxygen, nitrous oxide, or mixtures, but not air. Certain substances are flammable in nitrous oxide at concentrations that are too low to permit ignition in pure oxygen (28). The concentrations required for combustion, as indicated in Table 16.4, are higher than those generally encountered, except possibly during induction.

Clinically Useful Inhalation Agents

Fluorinated Hydrocarbons

The structure, physical properties and partition coefficients of the volatile anesthetics are given in Tables 16.2 and 16.5, respectively. Toxic degradation products

TABLE 16.4 Relative Flammability of "Nonflammable" Anesthetics

	Halothane (%)	Enflurane (%)	Isoflurane (%)
MFC of agent in 30% O_2 with remaining atmosphere N_2O	4.75	5.75	7.0
MAC of agent given in above atmosphere	0.28	0.65	0.46
MAC in humans in the absence of N_2O	0.75	.68	1.15
MFC/MAC in N_2O	17	8.9	15.2

MFC, minimum flammable concentration; MAC, minimum effective alveolar concentration

are formed by reaction of the anesthetic agent with the basic substances such as soda lime, used as carbon dioxide absorbents during anesthesia. This reaction results in the conversion of halothane to 2-bromo-2-chloro-1,1-difluoroethylene, sevoflurane to 2-(fluoromethoxy)-1,1,3,3,3-pentafluoro-1-propene (Compound A), and desflurane, isoflurane, and enflurane to carbon monoxide. Compound A forms a glutathione *S*-conjugate, which undergoes hydrolysis to cysteine *S*-conjugates and bioactivation of the cysteine *S*-conjugates by renal cysteine conjugate β-lyase to give nephrotoxic metabolites.

Halothane Halothane (Fig. 16.6) was introduced into medical practice in the United States in 1956 as a nonflammable, nonexplosive, halogenated volatile anesthetic that is usually mixed with air or oxygen. The presence of

TABLE 16.5 Physicochemical Properties of Clinically Useful Volatile Anesthetics

Generic Name (Trade Name) and Structure	Boiling Point (°C)	Chemically Stable[a]
Desflurane (Suprane) $F_2HC–O–CHF–CF_3$	23.5	Yes
Enflurane (Ethrane) $F_2HC–O–CF_2–CHFCl$	56.5	Yes
Halothane (Fluothane) $F_3C–CHBrCl$	50.2	No
Isoflurane (Forane) $F_2HC–O–CHCl-CF_3$	48.5	Yes
Methoxyflurane (Penthrane) $H_3C–O–CF_2–CHCl_2$	104.7	No
Nitrous oxide N_2O	–*8.0	Yes
Sevoflurane (Ultane) $(CF_3)_2CH–O–CH_2F$	58.5	No

[a]Indicates stability to soda lime, ultraviolet light, and common metals.

the carbon–halogen bonds contributes to its nonflammability, volatility, and high lipid solubility (blood/gas partition coefficient = 2.3). This clear liquid with a sweet odor was developed based on predictions that its halogenated structure would provide chemical stability, an intermediate blood solubility, and significant anesthetic potency. Halothane is the only useful volatile anesthetic possessing a bromine atom, which has been suggested to contribute to its potency. Similarly, the addition of fluorine atoms, of which halothane has three, contributes to its increased potency, volatility, and relative chemical stability of the hydrocarbon skeleton (Table 16.5).

Halothane produces rapid onset and recovery from anesthesia with high potency when used alone or in combination with nitrous oxide. Most metals, with the exception of chromium, nickel, and titanium, are easily tarnished by halothane. Although halothane is relatively stable, it is subject to spontaneous oxidative decomposition to hydrochloric acid (HCl), hydrobromic acid (HBr), and phosgene ($COCl_2$). For this reason, it comes in dark, amber glass containers with thymol added as a preservative to minimize decomposition. Halothane can permeate into the rubber components of the anesthetic delivery devices, which might account for some slowing of the induction onset and recovery. Approximately 20% of an administered dose is metabolized, which accounts, in part, for the increased hepatotoxicity observed with this agent (Fig. 16.7).

Enflurane Enflurane (Fig. 16.6) was introduced into medical practice in the United States in 1973 and is a clear, colorless, nonflammable liquid with a mild, sweet odor. Although relatively stable chemically, enflurane does not attack aluminum, copper, iron, or brass and is soluble in rubber, which can prolong induction/recovery times, as seen with halothane (Table 16.5). Enflurane has an intermediate solubility in blood (blood/gas partition coefficient = 1.9) and significant potency. Most of its pharmacologic properties are similar to those of halothane, although there can be slightly less nausea, vomiting, arrhythmias, and postoperative shivering than observed with halothane. High concentrations of enflurane, however, are more likely to produce convulsions and circulatory depression. Enflurane also relaxes the uterus and, thus, should not be used as an anesthetic during labor. Metabolism via CYP2E1 accounts for 2% of an

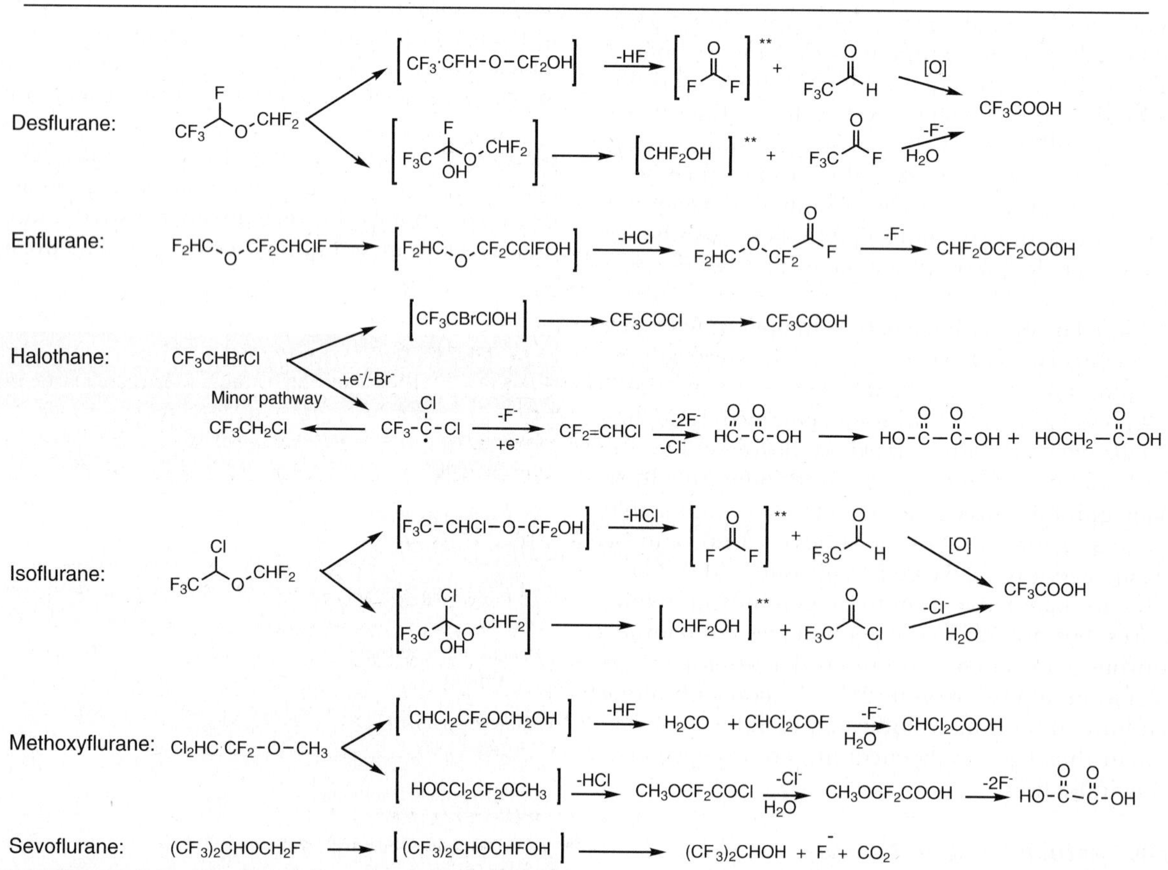

*Data from references 28 and 29.

**Decomposition of unstable intermediates: $CF_2O \longrightarrow 2F^- + CO_2$; $CHF_2OH \longrightarrow 2F^- + HCOOH$;

FIGURE 16.7 Proposed metabolites of fluorinated anesthetics.

inhaled dose and includes metabolism to form a fluoride ion and fluoromethoxydifluoroacetic acid (Fig. 16.7) (30). During recovery, enflurane leaves the fatty tissues rapidly and, therefore, is not available for a prolonged period of time for significant metabolism to proceed.

Isoflurane Isoflurane (Fig. 16.6) was introduced in the United States in 1981 and is a potent anesthetic agent with many similarities to its isomer enflurane (potent, nonflammable, and intermediate blood solubility; with blood/gas partition coefficient = 1.4). However, it does produce significantly fewer cardiovascular effects than enflurane and can be used safely with epinephrine without a concern for arrhythmia production. Isoflurane has a more pungent odor than halothane and, thus, can cause irritation to the throat and respiratory tract, triggering coughing and laryngospasm. To overcome this problem, it is often supplemented with intravenous agents. Less than 0.2% of an administered dose is metabolized, mostly to fluoride and trifluoroacetic acid (Fig. 16.7). As discussed below, some minimal potential for hepatotoxicity is associated with a trifluoroacetyl halide metabolite.

A comparative assessment of the volatile anesthetic properties of enflurane, halothane, and isoflurane is shown in Table 16.6.

Desflurane Desflurane (Fig. 16.6) was introduced in the United States in 1992 and is a pungent, volatile agent that is nonflammable and noncorrosive to metals. With poor blood solubility (blood/gas partition coefficient = 0.42), similar to that of nitrous oxide, desflurane rapidly induces anesthesia. Because the boiling point of desflurane is close to room temperature, a specially designed, heated vaporizer is used to deliver the anesthetic with appropriate concentrations of oxygen either alone or in combination with nitrous oxide. Recovery from the anesthetic state is also rapid, being approximately twice as rapid as that with isoflurane. Because of the rapid induction and recovery associated with desflurane, this anesthetic has gained popularity in outpatient surgical procedures. Desflurane is rather pungent, so patients often are induced with an intravenous anesthetic agent and then maintained with desflurane. Desflurane is not metabolized to any great extent and, therefore, has not been associated with hepatotoxicity or nephrotoxicity (31). Metabolites, mostly trifluoroacetate, account for less than 0.02% of the administered dose (Fig. 16.7). Although desflurane can react with soda lime or Baralyme to form carbon monoxide, no reports of adverse outcomes in patients have appeared.

TABLE 16.6 Comparative Assessment of Enflurane (E), Halothane (H), and Isoflurane (I)

Property	Superior	Intermediate	Inferior
Stability	I = E	—	H
Blood solubility	I	E	H
Pungency	H	I	E
Respiratory depression	H	I	E
Circulatory depression	I	H	E
Induction of arrhythmias	I	E	H
Muscle relaxation	I = E	—	H
Increased intracranial pressure/cerebral blood flow	I	E	H
Seizure activity	H = E	—	E
Metabolism	I	E	H
Toxicity	I	E	H

Adapted from Wade JC, Stevens WC. Isoflurane: an anesthetic for the eighties? Anesth Analg 1981;60:666–682; with permission.

Sevoflurane Sevoflurane (Fig. 16.6) is a nonflammable, nonirritating, pleasant-odored volatile anesthetic available for use in the United States. Similar to desflurane in many of its pharmacologic actions, except sevoflurane which has low blood solubility (blood/gas partition coefficient = 0.60), higher potency, and the advantage of not being irritating to the respiratory tract. Induction and recovery are rapid. Sevoflurane undergoes significantly more metabolism (CYP2E1) than desflurane, however, and as much as 3% of an administered dose can be recovered as hexafluoroisopropanol (Fig. 16.7). Some fluoride ion can also be produced, but the incidence of nephrotoxicity or hepatotoxicity appears low, especially when used infrequently for short periods of time. There have been concerns regarding the reactivity of sevoflurane with soda lime or Baralyme, in which a potentially toxic olefin byproduct termed "Compound A" (2-(fluoromethoxy)-1,1,3,3,3-pentafluoro-1-propene) can be formed. With appropriate precautions, however, sevoflurane can be used safely in both children and adults.

Methoxyflurane Methoxyflurane (Fig. 16.6) is seldom used because of its propensity to cause renal toxicity. It is the most potent of the agents discussed here, and it has high solubility in blood (blood/gas partition coefficient = 12). Induction and recovery would be expected to be slow. Chemically, it is rather unstable, and as much as 50% of an administered dose can be metabolized. Toxic metabolites significantly limit its utility as a general anesthetic (Fig. 16.7).

Toxicity of Fluorinated General Anesthetics Although few signs of toxicity usually are observed during the short-term, infrequent administration of general anesthetics, a few well-defined toxic effects have been noted. For instance, halothane and methoxyflurane are known to produce hepatotoxicity and nephrotoxicity, respectively. Both of these toxic reactions are believed to result from highly reactive metabolites of the parent compound.

Overall, however, the therapeutic ratio for most of the general anesthetics approaches 4:1 (32).

Hepatotoxicity Hepatitis caused by halothane occurs in 1 in 20,000 patients exposed to this anesthetic and is thought to result from the binding of a reactive free radical metabolite to liver tissue (Fig. 16.7). The resultant abnormal molecular product in the liver is viewed by the immune system as a foreign substance (i.e., an antigen), which then sensitizes cells to produce antibodies. Some have suggested that the trifluoroacetyl halide metabolite is responsible for the initiation of halothane hepatitis. Interestingly, both enflurane and isoflurane can be metabolized to the acylated halides and produce a similar immune-mediated syndrome, although to a much lesser extent. Additionally, there appears to be cross-reactivity among these three agents, because the antigen formed is similar enough in structure to elicit the immune system response. Some investigations have suggested that a genetic susceptibility factor could be responsible, in part, for this serious form of hepatitis.

Halothane also can produce another form of hepatotoxicity. This is a self-limiting hepatic dysfunction characterized by elevated liver transaminase enzymes, which probably results from impaired oxygenation of the hepatocytes during exposure to this anesthetic. Isoflurane and enflurane have also been reported to produce a similar elevation of liver enzymes, although to a lesser extent than halothane.

Malignant Hyperthermia This rare (1 in 15,000 anesthetic uses) but potentially fatal complication associated with the use of certain anesthetics (e.g., halothane) is characterized by a rapid rise in core body temperature associated with hypermetabolic reactions in the skeletal muscle of genetically susceptible subjects. Such individuals appear to have an autosomal dominant–mediated defect in the Ca^{2+}-release channel commonly referred to as the ryanodine receptor. The large amounts of heat generated, massive increase in oxygen consumption, and production of carbon dioxide can quickly lead to death or permanent neurologic damage unless appropriate supportive treatment, including rapid cooling, 100% oxygen, and control of acidosis, is promptly initiated. The administration of the skeletal muscle relaxant dantrolene, which blocks release of Ca^{2+} from the sarcoplasmic reticulum, reduces muscle rigidity and heat production, which significantly improves the prognosis of the patient. Besides the fluorinated volatile anesthetics, some depolarizing neuromuscular blocking agents (e.g., succinylcholine) and some neuroleptics (e.g., haloperidol) are also reportedly associated with similar malignant hyperthermic syndromes, although the underlying mechanism mediating these can differ somewhat from those associated with the general anesthetics.

Nephrotoxicity Fluorinated anesthetics that undergo metabolism to form inorganic fluoride ion have the potential to produce damage to the renal tubular cells. Of the fluorinated anesthetics, methoxyflurane is the only agent commonly associated with nephrotoxicity. Methoxyflurane is metabolized (Fig. 16.7) to produce plasma fluoride ion levels in excess of the threshold value for renal damage of 40 μmol/L. Others, such as sevoflurane, have only very rarely been associated with nephrotoxicity—and then usually in patients with severe renal compromise. Plasma levels of fluoride only reach 15 to 20 μmol/L following 2.5 MAC-hour exposure to enflurane (33). The rates of metabolic defluorination of the useful anesthetic agents are as follows: methoxyflurane > enflurane = sevoflurane > isoflurane > desflurane = halothane.

Low-level Chronic Exposure Typically, patients are exposed to greater-than-MAC concentrations of the volatile anesthetics for limited periods of time, such as a number of hours during a surgical procedure, and not for extended periods of time (e.g., days or weeks). Because surgical and dental personnel, however, can be exposed to low levels of the general anesthetics for prolonged periods over many years or even decades, the ability of such agents to produce chronic toxicity is of paramount concern. Although the occupational exposure to these agents has been minimized with improved waste gas–scavenging devices, some epidemiologic studies have demonstrated increased levels of spontaneous abortions, congenital birth defects in offspring, and increased rates of certain cancers in chronically exposed medical personnel (34).

Nitrous Oxide

Commonly called "laughing gas," nitrous oxide (N_2O) is a gas at room temperature, the least potent of the inhalation anesthetics used today and poor blood solubility (blood/gas partition coefficient = 0.47) (Table 16.5). With an MAC value in excess of 105%, this colorless, tasteless, and odorless to slightly sweet-smelling gas is not normally capable of producing surgical anesthesia when administered alone. The MAC for nitrous oxide has been demonstrated to be between 105% and 140% and, thus, cannot achieve surgical anesthesia under conditions at standard barometric pressure. To demonstrate that the MAC was greater than 100%, Bert in 1879 used a mixture of 85% nitrous oxide with oxygen at 1.2 atmospheres in a pressurized chamber. Only at this elevated pressure could an MAC adequate for surgical anesthesia be achieved. Decreasing the oxygen content of a nitrous oxide mixture to values less than 20% to allow an increase in the concentration of nitrous oxide to greater than 80% can be dangerous, because hypoxia would be expected to result. Thus, when administered alone, nitrous oxide finds utility as an anesthetic agent during certain procedures (e.g., dental) in which full surgical anesthesia is not required. Most commonly, however, nitrous oxide is used in combination with other general anesthetics, because it is capable of decreasing the concentration of the added anesthetic required to produce an adequate depth of anesthesia for surgical procedures.

Although no firm underlying mechanisms have been demonstrated, some authors have suggested that irreversible oxidation of the cobalt atom in vitamin B_{12} by nitrous oxide can lead to inactivation of enzymes dependent on this vitamin, with resultant metabolic aberrations. Such examples have included methionine synthetase and thymidylate synthetase, which are essential in the synthetic pathways leading to the production of myelin and thymidine, respectively. Should these enzymes be impaired during the sensitive periods of in utero development, the potential for malformations can unfortunately be realized. To date, no studies have been able to demonstrate conclusively that low-level exposure to nitrous oxide is associated with a meaningful disruption of crucial metabolic functions to produce the above-described toxicity; however, measures including improved waste gas–scavenging systems should be taken to minimize exposure of personnel.

Clinically Useful Intravenous General Anesthetic Agents

Propofol

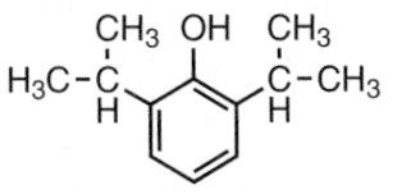

Propofol

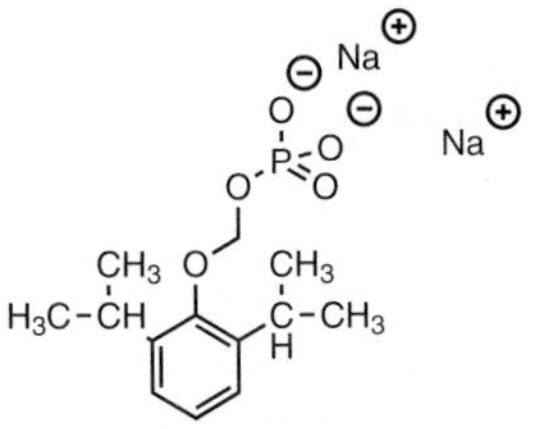

Fospropofol

One of the most commonly used parenteral anesthetics used in the United States is propofol (Diprivan). Used intravenously, propofol is not chemically related to the barbiturates or other intravenous anesthetics. Propofol appears to act via enhancing GABAergic neurotransmission within the CNS. This occurs most likely at the $GABA_A$ receptor complex, but at a site distinct from where the benzodiazepines bind. Because of its poor water solubility (partition coefficient ~6,200), propofol is formulated as a 1% or 2% emulsion with soybean oil, egg lecithin, and glycerol. Sodium metabisulfite (an antioxidant) or ethylenediaminetetraacetic acid (metal chelating agent) is also included in the parenteral dosage form for stability. Because of the likelihood of bacterial contamination of open containers, propofol should be either administered or discarded shortly after sterility seals are broken. Following intravenous administration of a dose of 2.0 to 2.5 mg/kg, a state of hypnosis is achieved within 30 to 60 seconds, which lasts for approximately 5 to 10 minutes. A longer anesthetic state can be achieved by additional propofol dosing or, as typically is the case, maintenance with a volatile anesthetic agent. Blood pressure and heart rate usually are decreased following propofol administration. Propofol is highly bound to plasma proteins (approximately 98%). Metabolism of propofol proceeds rapidly via hepatic conversion to its glucuronide and sulfate conjugates, with less than 0.3% excreted unchanged. Because this agent produces a rapid induction and recovery and is infrequently associated with episodes of vomiting, propofol has found utility as an anesthetic agent in outpatient surgical environments.

Fospropofol

Due to its water solubility, the phosphate ester prodrug of propofol (Lusedra), fospropofol, avoids the emulsion formulation concerns described earlier for propofol. All of the pharmacodynamic effects of fospropofol are attributed to propofol, which is liberated following hydrolytic metabolism by serum alkaline phosphatases. Typical dosing is 6.5 mg/kg, with supplemental doses of 1.6 mg/kg as needed. While formaldehyde and phosphate are also released by this metabolic conversion, the levels of these compounds do not increase to levels beyond those normally found endogenously and thus do not pose any toxicity concerns, except perhaps in overdose situations. Due to its requirement for conversion to the active propofol, the onset of fospropofol is delayed (4 to 10 minutes) when compared to that for propofol (30 to 60 seconds) and has a prolonged duration of anesthetic action.

Ketamine

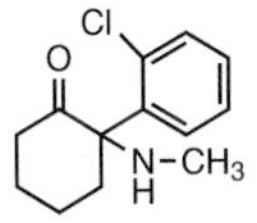

Ketamine

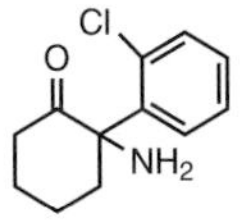

Norketamine

Ketamine hydrochloride is an injectable, very potent, rapidly acting anesthetic agent. As with propofol, its duration of anesthetic activity is also relatively short (10 to 25 minutes). Ketamine does not relax skeletal muscles and, therefore, can only be used alone in procedures of short duration that do not require muscle relaxation. Recovery from anesthesia can be accompanied by "emergence delirium," which is characterized by visual, auditory, and confusional illusions. Disturbing dreams and hallucinations can occur up to 24 hours after the administration of ketamine. Its elimination half-life is 2 to 3 hours, and its volume of distribution is 2 to 3 L/kg. Ketamine has an oral bioavailability of less than 16%. Termination of the acute action of ketamine is largely a result of its redistribution from the brain into other tissue; however, the formation of the glucuronide conjugate and metabolism in the liver to a number of metabolites does occur. One of these metabolites of interest, norketamine, is formed via the action of CYP2B6. This *N*-demethylated derivative retains significant activity at the NMDA receptor and can account for some of the longer-lasting effects of this anesthetic agent. Eventual conversion of norketamine to hydroxylated metabolites and subsequent conjugation leads to metabolites that can be renally eliminated. Less than 4% of a dose is excreted unchanged in the urine.

Ketamine is capable of producing a "dissociative" anesthesia, which is characterized by EEG changes indicating a dissociation between the thalamocortical and limbic systems (35). These neuronal systems, which normally are associated with one another, help to maintain the neuronal connections required for consciousness. When disassociated, the subject will appear to be cataleptic, with the eyes open in a slow, nystagmic gaze (oscillating movement of the eyeball) (1). A potent analgesic and amnesic effect is produced, as is an increase in muscle tone in some areas. Although patients can appear to be awake, they are incapable of communicating and do not remember the event or the people around them. Blood pressure and heart rate usually are increased following ketamine administration.

Ketamine appears to act similarly to phencyclidine (PCP; also known as Angel Dust), which acts as an antagonist within the cationic channel of the NMDA receptor complex (36). By preventing the flow of cations through this channel, ketamine prevents neuronal activation, which normally is required for the conscious state. The analgesic activity of ketamine, however, is more likely the result of an interaction with an opioid receptor or the less well-understood non-opioid sigma receptor. Other studies have suggested a possible involvement of serotonin receptors and muscarinic receptors (37). Ketamine, like PCP, has a significant potential for abuse.

Etomidate

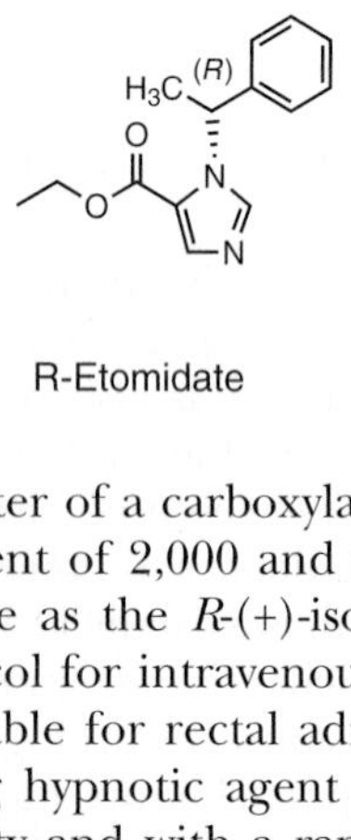

R-Etomidate

Etomidate is the ester of a carboxylated imidazole, with a partition coefficient of 2,000 and a weak base pK_a of 4.5, that is available as the *R*-(+)-isomer solubilized in 35% propylene glycol for intravenous injection in addition to being available for rectal administration. It is a potent, short-acting hypnotic agent (<3 minutes) without analgesic activity and with a rapid onset of action. This agent is useful for the induction of anesthesia in hemodynamically unstable patients prone to hypotension because of hypovolemia, coronary artery disease, or cardiomyopathies. Recovery is similarly rapid following discontinuance of the drug. Etomidate is hydrolyzed by hepatic esterases to the corresponding inactive carboxylic acid, with subsequent renal and biliary excretion terminating its action. Its apparent elimination half-life is approximately 5 to 6 hours, with a volume of distribution of 5 to 7 L/kg. Changes in hepatic blood flow or hepatic metabolism will have only moderate effects on etomidate disposition. Concerns regarding the ability of etomidate to precipitate myoclonic jerks and inhibit adrenal steroid synthesis have been reported.

Ultrashort-Acting Barbiturates

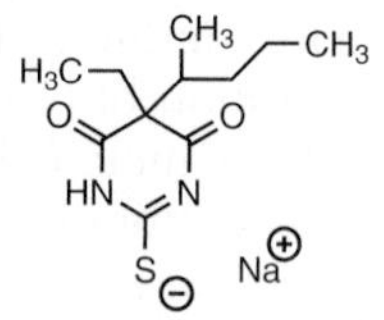

Thiopental

Thiopental, an ultrashort-acting barbiturate (partition coefficient ~390), is used intravenously to produce a rapid unconsciousness for surgical and basal anesthesia. This agent is used initially to induce anesthesia, which then can be maintained during the surgical procedure with a general anesthetic agent. The induction typically is very rapid and pleasant. (The ultrashort-acting barbiturates are discussed in Chapter 15.)

LOCAL ANESTHETICS

Local anesthetic agents are drugs that, when given either topically or administered directly into a localized area, produce a state of local anesthesia by reversibly blocking nerve conductances that transmit the sensations of pain from this localized area to the brain. Unlike the anesthesia produced by general anesthetics, the anesthesia produced by local anesthetics is without loss of consciousness or impairment of vital central cardiorespiratory functions. Local anesthetics block nerve conductance by binding to selective sites on the Na^+ channels in the excitable membranes, thereby reducing Na^+ passage (i.e., conductance) through the pores and, thus, interfere with the generation of action potentials. Although local anesthetics decrease the excitability of nerve membranes, they do not affect the neuron's resting potential. Local anesthetics, in contrast to analgesic compounds, do not interact with the pain receptors or inhibit the release or the biosynthesis of pain mediators.

The Discovery of Local Anesthetics

As with many modern drugs, the initial leads for the design of clinically useful local anesthetics originated from natural sources. As early as 1532, the anesthetic properties of coca leaves (*Erythroxylon coca* Lam) became known to Europeans from the natives of Peru, who chewed the leaves for a general feeling of well-being and to reduce hunger. Saliva from chewing the leaves was often used by the natives to relieve painful wounds. The active principle of the coca leaf, however, was not discovered until 1860 by Niemann, who obtained a crystalline alkaloid from the leaves, to which he gave the name cocaine, and who noted the anesthetic effect on the tongue (see Fig. 16.8 for structure of cocaine). Although Moréno y Maiz in 1868 first asked the question of whether cocaine could be used as a local anesthetic, Von Anrep in 1880, after many animal experiments, recommended that cocaine

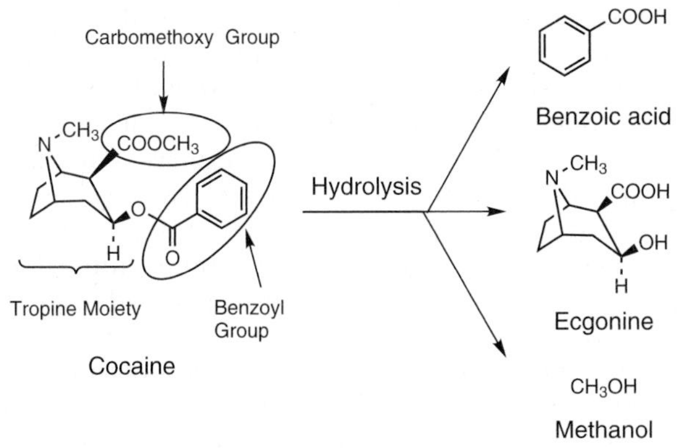

FIGURE 16.8 Structures of cocaine and its hydrolysis products.

be used clinically as a local anesthetic. The first report of successful surgical use of cocaine appeared in 1884 by Koller, an Austrian ophthalmologist. This discovery led to the rapid development of new local anesthetic agents and anesthetic techniques (38).

Cocaine dependence (or addiction) is psychological dependency on the regular use of cocaine. The use of cocaine, depending on the severity, can cause mood swings, paranoia, insomnia, psychosis, high blood pressure, tachycardia, panic attacks, cognitive impairments, and drastic changes in the personality that can lead to aggressive, compulsive, criminal, and/or erratic behaviors. The symptoms of cocaine withdrawal range from moderate to severe: dysphoria, depression, anxiety, psychological and physical weakness, pain, and compulsive craving.

Although the structure of cocaine was not known until 1924, many attempts were made to prepare new analogs of cocaine that lacked its addicting liability and other therapeutic shortcomings, such as allergic reactions, tissue irritations, and poor stability in aqueous solution. Also, cocaine is easily decomposed to hydrolysis products, ecgonine and benzoic acid, when the solution is sterilized (Fig. 16.8).

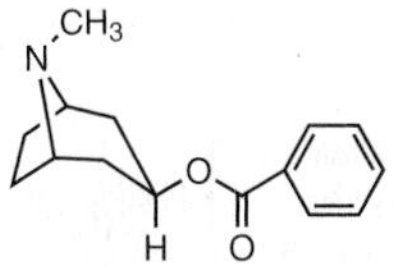

Benzoyltropine

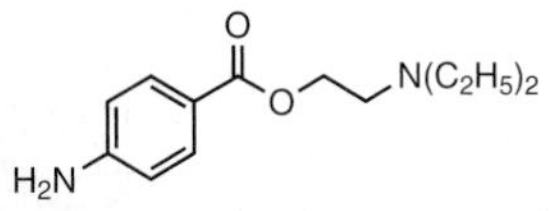

Procaine

When the chemical structure of ecgonine became known, the preparation of active compounds containing the ecgonine nucleus accelerated. It was soon realized that a variety of benzoyl esters of amino alcohols, including benzoyltropine, exhibited strong local anesthetic properties without any of cocaine's addiction liability. Thus, removal of the 2-carbomethoxy group from cocaine also abolished its addiction liability. This discovery eventually led to the synthesis of procaine in 1905 (known as Novocain), which then became the prototype for local anesthetics for nearly half a century, largely because it lacked the severe local and systemic toxicities of cocaine.

Although the intrinsic potency of procaine was low and its duration of action relatively short compared with that of cocaine, it was found that these deficiencies could be remedied when procaine was combined with a vasoconstrictor, such as epinephrine. Vasoconstrictor agents reduce the local blood supply and, thereby, prolong the residence time of the local anesthetic at the injection site.

Following the introduction of procaine, hundreds of structurally related analogs were prepared and their local anesthetic properties examined in an attempt to identify agents with enhanced potency and duration of action compared to the weak and short-acting procaine. Among these compounds, tetracaine remains the most potent, long-acting, ester-type local anesthetic agent, which is used in spinal anesthesia.

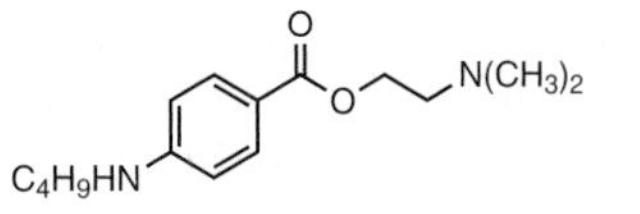

Tetracaine

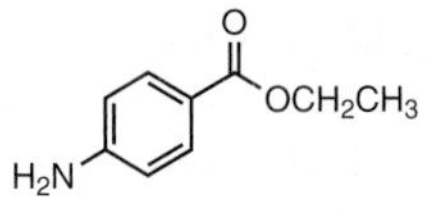

Benzocaine

The topical anesthetic agent benzocaine was synthesized by Ritsert in 1890 and found to have good anesthetizing properties and low toxicity. However, due to its limited water solubility, except at low pH values as a result of the lack of a basic aliphatic amino group, the preparation of pharmaceutically acceptable parenteral solutions could not be achieved.

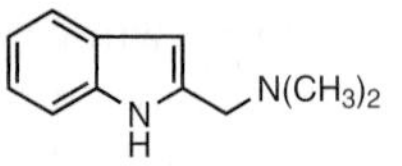

Isogramine

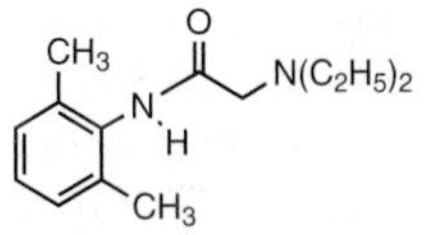

Lidocaine

The serendipitous discovery of the local anesthetic activity of another natural alkaloidal product, isogramine, in 1935 by von Euler and Erdtman was the next major turning point in the development of clinically useful local anesthetic agents. This observation led to the synthesis of lidocaine (Xylocaine) by Löfgren in 1946; lidocaine was the first nonirritating, amide-type local anesthetic agent with good local anesthetic properties yet less prone to allergenic reactions than procaine analogs, and was found to be stabile in aqueous solution due to its more stable amide functionality. Structurally, lidocaine can be viewed as an open-chain analog of isogramine and, thus, is a bioisosteric analog of isogramine.

Since the discovery of lidocaine in the 1940s, much more progress has been achieved in the fields of neurophysiology and neuropharmacology than in the synthesis of local anesthetics by medicinal chemists. Most of this research has significantly increased our understanding of how nerve conduction occurs and how compounds interact with the neuronal membranes to produce local anesthesia. It should be noted, however, that although a number of current clinically useful local anesthetic agents have been introduced into the market, the ideal local anesthetic drug has, unfortunately, not yet been realized.

Characteristics of an Ideal Local Anesthetic

The ideal local anesthetic should produce reversible blockade of sensory neurons with a minimal effect on the motor neurons. It also should possess a rapid onset, have a sufficient duration of action for the completion of major surgical procedures without any systemic toxicity, and be easily sterilized and not inordinately expensive (Table 16.7). Hopefully through further structure–activity relationship studies, particularly with regard to their selective actions on the voltage-gated Na^+ channels, the ideal local anesthetic agent can be realized. Additional leads for the design of ideal local anesthetics could also come from a more systematic metabolic and toxicity study of currently available agents. To understand the chemical aspects of local anesthetics and, thus, to provide a proper background for practical uses of these compounds, it is necessary to have a working knowledge of basic neuroanatomy and electrophysiology of the nervous system.

Neuroanatomy and Electrophysiology of the Nervous System

Neuroanatomy

Sensory neurons (afferent neurons) transmit sensory electrochemical impulses from sensory endings (receptors) in the skin and other sensory organs toward the CNS (i.e., brain and spinal cord) where the information is processed. On the other hand, motor neurons (efferent neurons) transmit electrochemical impulses from the CNS toward motor endings or other target (effector) cells that, when stimulated, produce a response such as contraction of muscle or stimulation/inhibition of sweat glands or exocrine glands. The transmission of a nerve impulse along an axon occurs as a result of electrochemical changes in the Na^+ and K^+ potential across the neuronal membrane. Such neurons are bundled together into a cable-like structure and wrapped in a connective tissue sheath (the perineurium), called a nerve. Within a nerve, each axon is wrapped by a layer of connective tissue called the endoneurium. Finally, the entire nerve is wrapped in a layer of connective tissue called the epineurium (much like an electrical cable of wires wrapped with a plastic casing), as shown in Figure 16.9. (39). A nerve provides a common pathway for the transmission of electrochemical impulses. Thus, each nerve is a cord-like structure that contains groups of neurons in small bundles. The cell bodies of the sensory neurons are found at the point at which the nerve enters the vertebrae and can be seen as enlargements on the nerve bundles (spinal or dorsal root ganglion). The cell bodies (anterior horn cell) of the motor neurons are found within the gray matter of the spinal cord.

Figures 16.9 and 16.10 also illustrate that each axon has its own membranous covering, the endoneurium (often called the nerve membrane), which is tightly surrounded by a myelin sheath of the Schwann cell. The myelin sheath is not continuous along the fiber, with intermittent gaps or interruptions at the nodes of Ranvier, which serve to facilitate neuronal conduction.

TABLE 16.7 Characteristics of the Ideal Local Anesthetic Agent
Produces a reversible blockade
Selective for sensory neurons with no effect on motor neurons
Rapid onset
Sufficient duration of action
Chemically stable when sterilized
No systemic toxicity
Wide margin of safety
Compatible with other coadministered drugs
Absence of adverse effects
Inexpensive

Electrophysiology of Nerve Membrane

Resting Potential Most nerves have a resting membrane potential (unstimulated or polarized state) of approximately −70 to −90 mV as a result of a slight imbalance of electrolyte ions (e.g., sodium, potassium, calcium, magnesium, and chloride) across the nerve membranes, between the intracellular cytoplasm and the extracellular fluid (40). In the polarized state, the nerve membrane is somewhat impermeable to Na^+ as seen by the low intracellular Na^+ concentration, whereas K^+ flows in and out of the cell with greater ease, indicating that the neuronal membrane is highly permeable to K^+. A high K^+ concentration is retained intracellularly by the attractive forces

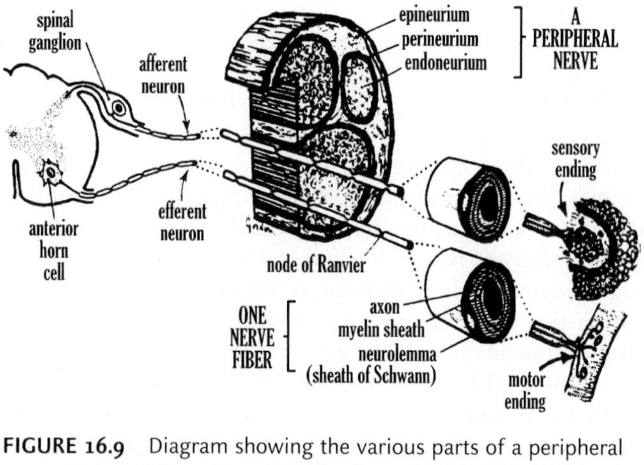

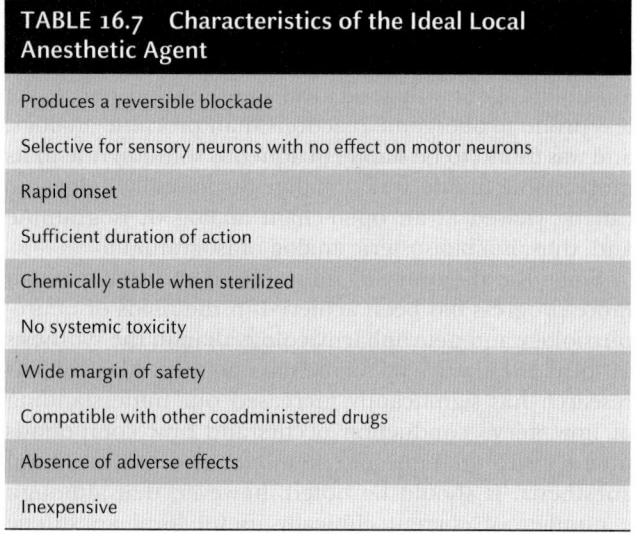

FIGURE 16.9 Diagram showing the various parts of a peripheral nerve. (Adapted from Ham AW. Histology, 6th Ed. Philadelphia: JB Lippincott, 1969:524, with permission.)

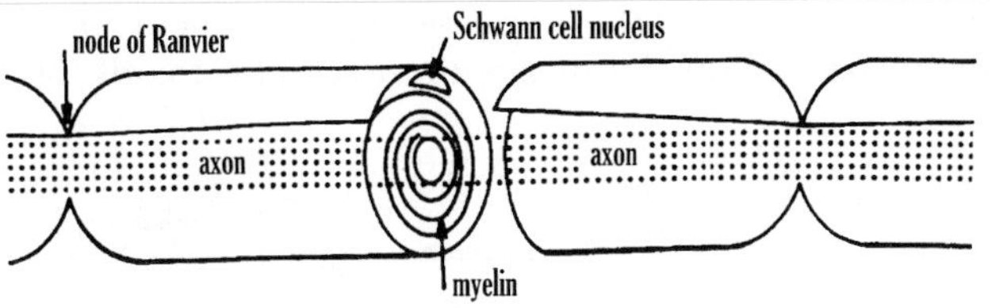

FIGURE 16.10 Single myelinated nerve fiber.

provided by the negatively charged intracellular protein molecules. Thus, the predominant intracellular cations are K^+ (~110 to 170 mmol/L), and the predominant extracellular cations are Na^+ (~140 mmol/L) and chloride (~110 mmol/L).

Because changes in the intracellular or extracellular concentration of K^+ would be expected to markedly alter the resting membrane potential, electrophysiologists modeled the excitable cell as if it were an electrochemical, or Nernst, cell. Thus, the resting potential for K^+ can be determined by the familiar Nernst equation:

$$E = -RT/zF \ln\, [K^+]_i/[K^+]_o$$

in which E = membrane potential, intracellular minus extracellular; R = gas constant; T = temperature; z = ion valence; F = Faraday's constant; $[K^+]_i$ = activity of intracellular K^+; and $[K^+]_o$ = activity of extracellular K^+.

Action Potential In most cells, action potentials are transient transmembrane depolarizations that result from the influx of Na^+ through a brief opening of the voltage-gated Na^+ channels upon excitation of the cell (40). The transmembrane potential during an action potential changes from −70 to approximately +40 mV (a total net change of 110 mV) (depolarized state) and then promptly returns to the resting (polarized state) potential; the entire event typically lasts approximately 1 millisecond (Fig. 16.11). An action potential is capable of traveling long distances along the neuron because open Na^+ gates stimulate neighboring Na^+ gates to open.

The transmembrane potential for Na^+ at the peak of its action potential can be predicted from the Nernst equation by substituting appropriate Na^+ concentrations for those of K^+. Thus, it appears that the excitable nerve membrane can be transformed from a potassium electrode to a sodium electrode during the active process (41).

As the cell approaches its peak action potential, the membrane permeability to Na^+ again decreases (Na^+ inactivation). If no other event occurred, this cell would slowly return to its resting potential, but the cell again becomes highly permeable to K^+, allowing K^+ to flow out into extracellular fluid and quickly restore the membrane potential (repolarization). After an action potential, the cell would therefore be left with a small increase in Na^+ and a decrease in K^+. To explain how the nerve is restored to its original electrolyte composition at the resting potential, it is necessary to postulate a mechanism

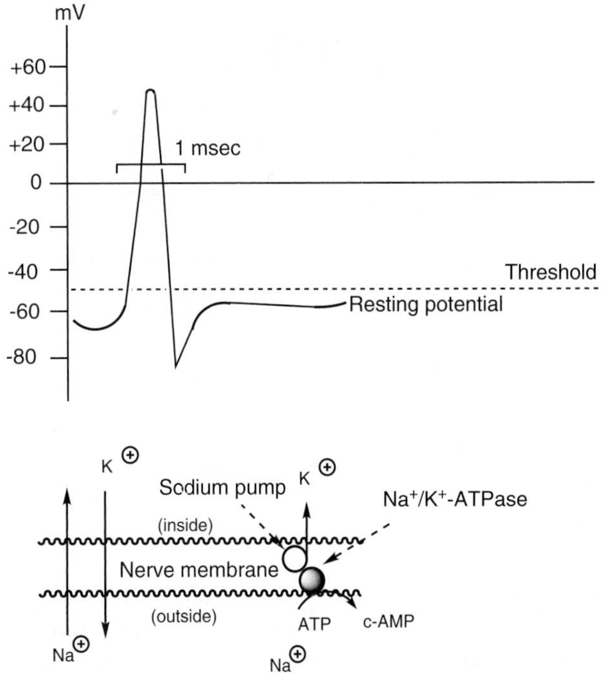

FIGURE 16.11 Relationship between membrane action potential and ionic flux across the nerve membrane.

by which intracellular Na^+ could be rapidly transported (effluxed) from inside the membrane to the outside extracellular fluid and extracellular K^+ could be transported (influxed) from extracellular fluid to inside the membrane. This is accomplished by the "sodium pump," which requires energy from the splitting of adenosine triphosphate by sodium-potassium adenosine triphosphatase (Na/K-ATPase) to adenosine monophosphate. This pump transports three Na^+ to the outside of the membrane for every two K^+ that enter the inside of the membrane.

Threshold The voltage necessary to change localized electrochemical differences into a propagated action potential is called the threshold voltage, which is closely related to the stimulus duration—the longer the stimulus, the lower the threshold voltage. An electrical stimulus of less than a certain voltage can only result in local electrochemical changes and cannot elicit a propagated action potential.

Refractoriness A state of absolute refractoriness (i.e., complete inexcitability) occurs immediately after an impulse has been propagated, and no stimulus, no matter how strong or long, can produce an excited state. Shortly thereafter, the axon becomes relatively refractory; it responds with a propagated impulse only to stimulation that is greater than the normal threshold. The length of the refractory period is affected by the frequency of stimulation and by many drugs (Fig. 16.12).

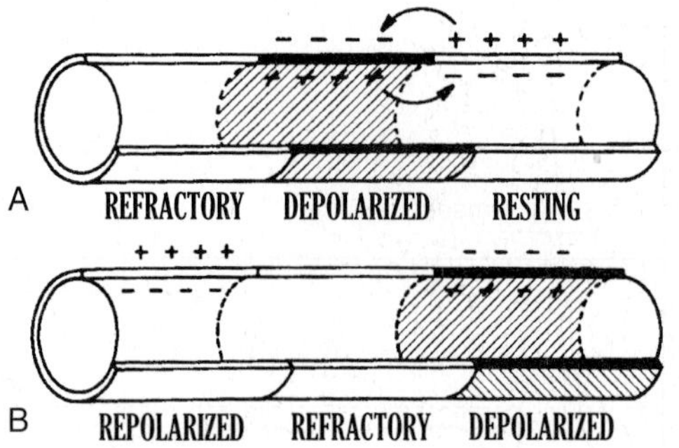

FIGURE 16.12 Impulse propagation. (A) The wave of depolarization passes down the nerve, followed by a wave of refractoriness. (B) The wave of refractoriness is followed by a wave of repolarization. (Adapted from De Jong RH, Freund FG. Physiology of peripheral nerve and local anesthesia. Int Anesthesiol Clin 1970;8:35–53, with permission.)

Conductance Velocity and Nodal Conduction The conductance velocity is the velocity at which an impulse is conducted along the nerve and is proportional to the diameter of the axon. Because longitudinal resistance is inversely proportional to cross-sectional area, impulses are conducted faster in large-diameter axons. The squid giant axon, used in many neurophysiology investigations, is unmyelinated and exceptionally large (~500 to 1,000 μm); therefore, impulses are conducted rapidly along the axon. However, contraction of the mantle of a squid, which this axon controls, is an uncomplicated procedure that does not require a complex sensorimotor feedback system. Perhaps during evolution, vertebrates developed a complicated input–output system of many axons collected in bundles, as shown in Figure 16.9.

Conduction along these neurons would be slow if they were not insulated with a myelin coat of connective tissue, interrupted at intervals by the nodes of Ranvier, where electrical current enters and exits. These ionic fluxes occurring at the nodes allow the electrical impulse to jump along the axon from node to node much faster than could occur in an unmyelinated axon (42).

Sodium Channel The voltage-gated Na^+ channels are discrete, membrane-bound glycoproteins that mediate Na^+ permeability and, thus, are responsible for the generation of action potentials in skeletal muscle, nerve, and cardiac tissues (43–50). Our understanding of the structural domains and binding sites on voltage-gated Na^+ channels has evolved considerably since the first cloning and expression studies of the channel protein by Noda (43). The channel gating kinetics have been extensively studied with the use of selective blockers of Na^+ channels, such as tetrodotoxin (TTX) and saxitoxin (STX), and by site-directed mutagenesis (49). Both TTX and STX bind stoichiometrically to the outer opening of the channels and are detected with patch-clamp electrophysiologic techniques on the cut-open squid giant axon (50). Neher and Sakmann, two German scientists, were awarded the Nobel Prize in 1991 for physiology and medicine for their work on ion channels with these neurotoxins (50).

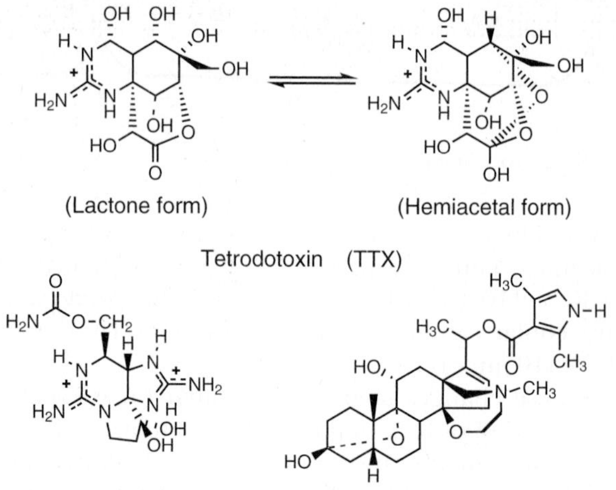

(Lactone form) (Hemiacetal form)

Tetrodotoxin (TTX)

Saxitoxin (STX) Batrachotoxin

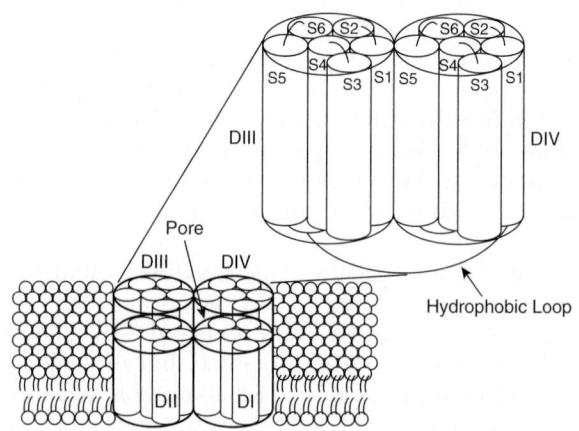

Recent mapping of receptor binding sites within the channel protein for lipid-soluble neurotoxins, such as batrachotoxin (BTX), and for local anesthetics using site-directed mutagenesis has provided further insight regarding these channels (49). For example, mammalian voltage-gated Na^+ channels contain one large α-subunit and one or two smaller β-subunits (15). The primary structure of the α-subunit is composed of four homologous domains (D1 to D4), each with six transmembrane segments (S1 to S6) and a hydrophobic loop thought to dip into the membrane to align the aqueous pore into a pseudotetrameric arrangement (Fig. 16.13) (47–49).

Furthermore, the voltage sensor for activation gating and the structure for fast inactivation gating have been delineated to involve the positively charged S4 segments of each domain (also known as the ion selectivity filter, which contains positively charged amino acid residues).

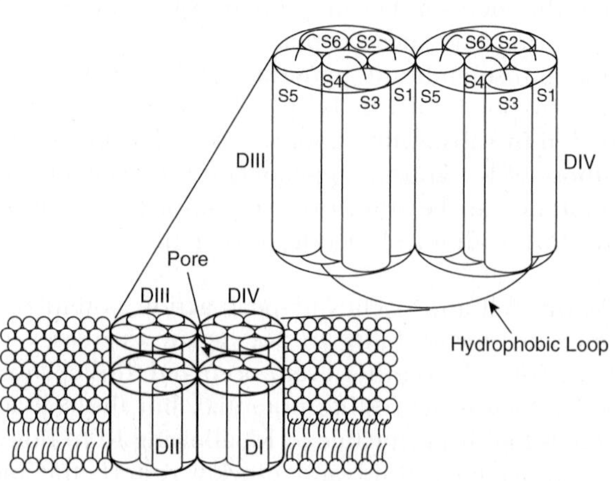

FIGURE 16.13 A schematic representation of the α subunit of the sodium channel and the pore-forming unit. (From Anger T, Madge DJ, Mulla M, et al. Medicinal chemistry of neuronal voltage-gated sodium channel blockers. J Med Chem 2001;44:115–137, with permission.)

The selective filter discriminates Na^+ from other ions (i.e., Na^+ passes through this pore approximately 12-fold faster than does K^+). Sodium channels open and close as they switch between several conformational states: the resting/closed form (polarized nonconducting state), the open channel (depolarized conducting state), and the inactivated form (polarized nonconducting state).

At resting potential, the Na^+ channels are in a resting/closed polarized state and are impermeable to the passage of Na^+. On activation, the channels undergo conformational changes to an open depolarized state, allowing the rapid influx of Na^+ across the neuronal membrane.

Thus, when the threshold potential is exceeded, most of the Na^+ channels are in an open, or conducting, state. At the peak of the action potential, the open channels spontaneously convert to an inactivated polarized state by the "sodium pump" (i.e., nonconducting and nonactivatable), leading to a decrease in Na^+ permeability. When a Na^+ channel is in the inactivated polarized state, it cannot be opened without first being transformed to the normal resting/closed form.

Therapeutic Considerations for Using Local Anesthetic Drugs

Since the discovery of cocaine in 1880 as a surgical local anesthetic, several thousand new compounds have been tested and found to produce anesthesia by blocking nerve conductance. Among these agents, approximately 20 are currently clinically available in the United States as local anesthetic preparations (Table 16.8). Table 16.9 contains chemical structures of the different types of agents in current or recent use.

Pharmaceutical Preparations

Local anesthetic agents generally are prepared in various dosage forms: aqueous solutions for parenteral injection, and creams and ointments for topical applications. Thus, chemical stability and aqueous solubility become primary factors in the preparations of suitable pharmaceutical dosage forms.

WHAT ARE THE SOURCES OF THESE NEUROTOXINS?

TTX is a potent neurotoxin isolated from the ovaries and liver of many marine species of Tetraodontidae, especially the Japanese fugu (or puffer fish). STX, produced by the marine dinoflagellates, *Gonyaulax catenella* or *Gonyaulax tamarensis*, is found concentrated in certain bivalve shellfish (e.g., mussels and clams). Consumption of contaminated mussels or clams causes paralytic shellfish poisoning, which is usually associated with toxic "red tide" environmental episodes in various coastal regions. BTX, a cardiotoxic and neurotoxic steroid isolated originally from the poisonous dart frog, *Phyllobates terribilis*, is a lipid-soluble neurotoxin that is at least 10-fold more toxic than TTX.

In general, compounds containing an amide linkage have greater chemical hydrolytic stability than do the ester types. In this regard, an aqueous solution of an amino ester–type local anesthetic is more likely to hydrolyze under normal conditions and cannot withstand heat sterilization as a result of base-catalyzed hydrolysis of the ester.

Local anesthetic activity usually increases with increasing lipid solubility. Unfortunately, this increase in lipid solubility is often inversely related to water solubility. For this reason, a suitable parenteral dosage form might not be available for these agents because of poor water solubility under acceptable conditions. For example, benzocaine, which lacks a sufficiently basic aliphatic amino group needed for salt formation, is insoluble in water at neutral pH. Protonation of the aromatic amino group in benzocaine results in a salt with a pK_a of 2.78, which is too acidic and, therefore, unsuitable for use as a parenteral dosage form for injection. For this reason, benzocaine and its closely related analog, butamben, are used mostly in creams or ointments to provide topical anesthesia of accessible mucous membranes or skin for burns, cuts, or inflamed mucous surfaces.

Many attempts have been made to substitute oils, fats, or fluid polymers for the aqueous vehicle commonly used in injectable local anesthetics. Unfortunately, the pharmacologic results of these experiments have been quite disappointing, often as a result of the undesirable toxicity of the nonaqueous vehicle.

The only commonly accepted organic additives to local anesthetics are vasoconstrictors, such as epinephrine and levonordefrin (α-methylnorepinephrine). These compounds often increase the frequency of successful anesthesia and, to a limited degree, increase the duration of activity by reducing the rate of drug loss from the injection site, by constricting arterioles that supply blood to the area of the injection. The effect of these vasoconstrictors is less pronounced if the vasoconstrictors are added to a local anesthetic solution that is injected in an area that has profuse venous drainage but is remote from an arterial supply. By slowing the diffusion of the local anesthetic away from the targeted site of injection, the exposure of other tissues in the body is likely minimized such that the local anesthetic never reaches high enough concentrations to produce unwanted toxicities. However, there is a flip slide to the benefit of the use of vasoconstrictors: A prolonged local anesthetic effect long after the surgical procedure is completed can lead to prolonged numbness and inadvertent soft tissue damage due to mechanical irritation (e.g., biting one's lip or tongue following dental procedures) as a result of the continued loss of pain sensations. Soft tissue injury to the lip in children 4 to 7 years of age following mandibular nerve block has been reported to be as high as 16%. Recently, an approach to reverse the vasoconstrictor-induced prolonged anesthetic state has utilized phentolamine, an α-adrenoceptor antagonist. Phentolamine mesylate in doses of 0.4 to 0.8 mg in adults and adolescents and 0.2

TABLE 16.8 Clinically Available Local Anesthetics

Generic Name	Trade Name	Recommended Application
Articaine	Septocaine, Septanest	Parenteral (dental)
Benoxinate	Oxybuprocaine	Mainly in ophthalmology
Benzocaine	Americaine, Anbesol, Benzodent, Orajel, Oratect, Rid-A-Pain, Hurricaine	Topical
Benzyl alcohol		Topical, mainly in combination with pramoxine
Bupivacaine	Marcaine, Sensorcaine	Parenteral
Butamben	Butesin	Topical
Chloroprocaine	Nesacaine	Parenteral
Dibucaine	Nupercainal, Cinchocaine	Topical
Dyclonine	Sucrets	Topical (mucosal only)
Etidocaine	Duranest	Parenteral
Ethyl chloride		Extracutaneous, temperature decreasing
Eugenol		Topical, especially in dentistry
Levobupivacaine	Chirocaine	Parenteral
Lidocaine	Xylocaine, L-Caine, DermaFlex, Dilocaine, Lidoject, Lignocaine, Octocaine,	Parenteral, topical
Mepivacaine	Carbocaine, Polocaine, Isocaine	Parenteral, topical
Menthol	Chloraseptic lozenges, Dermoplast, Pramegel, Pontacaine ointment	Topical, mainly in combination with benzocaine or pramoxine or tetracaine
Phenol	Anbesol	Topical, mainly in combination with benzocaine
Pramoxine	Prax, Tronothane	Topical
Prilocaine	Citanest	Parenteral, topical
Procaine	Novocain	Parenteral
Proparacaine	Alcaine, Ophthaine, Ak-Taine	Mainly in ophthalmology
Propoxycaine	Blockaine, Ravocaine	Parenteral
Ropivacaine	Naropin	Parenteral
Tetracaine	Pontocaine, Amethocaine, Prax	Parenteral, topical

to 0.4 mg in children reverses the vasoconstriction and allows for a more rapid diffusion of the local anesthetic from the injection site and a recovery of sensation (51).

Administration of a local anesthetic in a carbonic acid–carbon dioxide aqueous solution rather than the usual solution of a hydrochloride salt appreciably improves the time of onset and duration of action without causing increased local or systemic toxicity.

Carbon dioxide is believed to potentiate the action of local anesthetics by initial indirect depression of the axon, followed by diffusion trapping of the active form of the local anesthetic within the nerve. Use of the carbonate salt appears to be one pharmaceutical modification of the classic local anesthetic agents that can result in significant clinical advantages.

A Eutectic Mixture of a Local Anesthetic (EMLA) cream containing 2.5% lidocaine and 2.5% prilocaine (or etidocaine) is used for the topical application of local anesthetic through the keratinized layer of the intact skin to provide dermal or epidermal analgesia. This mode of administration allows the use of higher concentrations of local anesthetic with minimal local irritation and lower systemic toxicity. The use of EMLA creams, especially those containing prilocaine, on mucous membranes is not recommended, however, because of the faster absorption of the drugs and, therefore, the increasing

TABLE 16.9 Structures of Local Anesthetics

Amino Esters

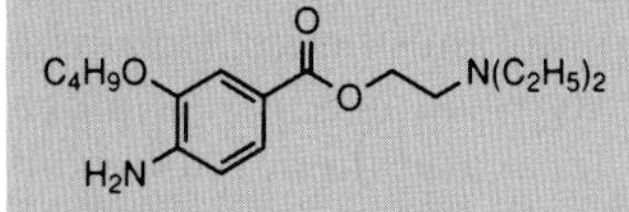

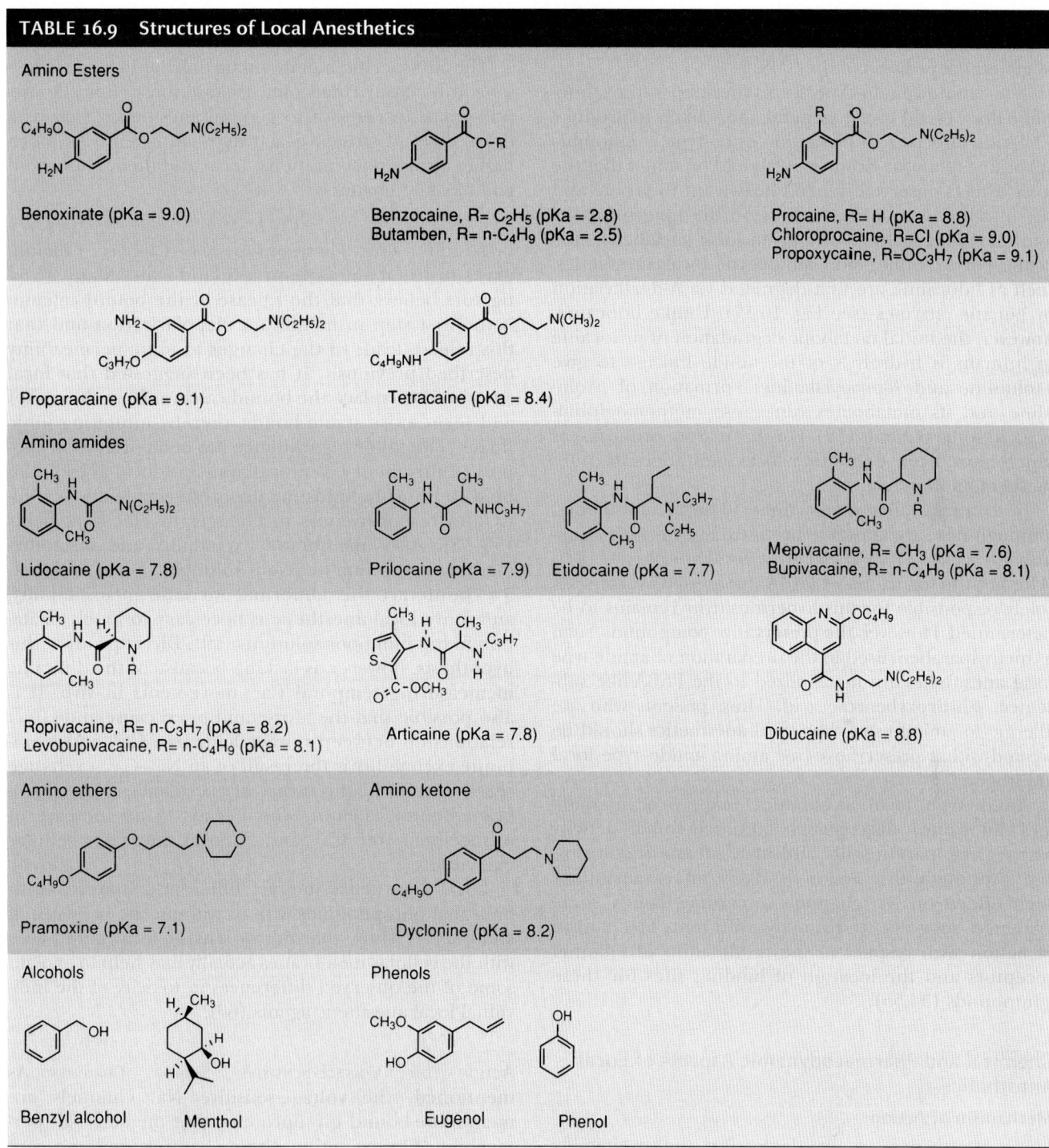

Benoxinate (pKa = 9.0)

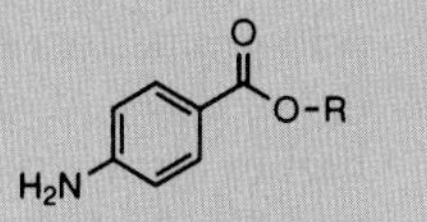

Benzocaine, R= C_2H_5 (pKa = 2.8)
Butamben, R= n-C_4H_9 (pKa = 2.5)

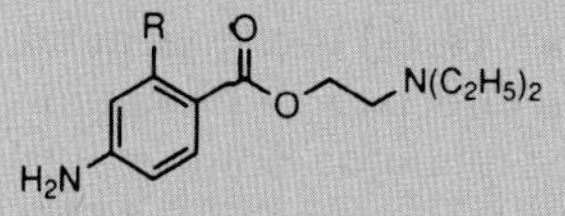

Procaine, R= H (pKa = 8.8)
Chloroprocaine, R=Cl (pKa = 9.0)
Propoxycaine, R=OC_3H_7 (pKa = 9.1)

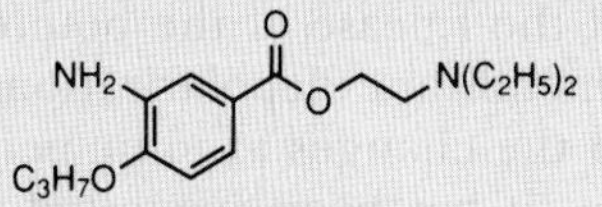

Proparacaine (pKa = 9.1)

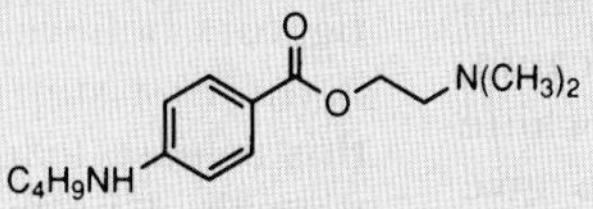

Tetracaine (pKa = 8.4)

Amino amides

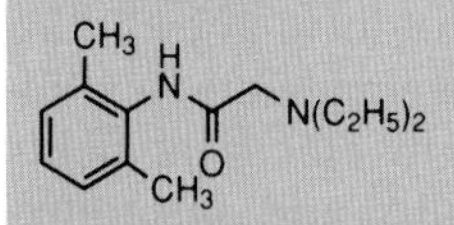

Lidocaine (pKa = 7.8)

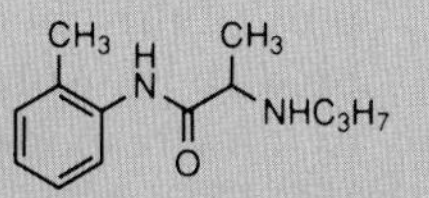

Prilocaine (pKa = 7.9)

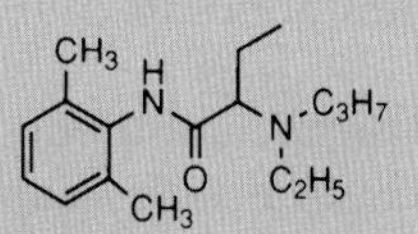

Etidocaine (pKa = 7.7)

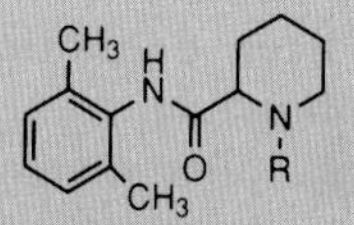

Mepivacaine, R= CH_3 (pKa = 7.6)
Bupivacaine, R= n-C_4H_9 (pKa = 8.1)

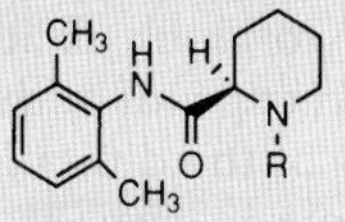

Ropivacaine, R= n-C_3H_7 (pKa = 8.2)
Levobupivacaine, R= n-C_4H_9 (pKa = 8.1)

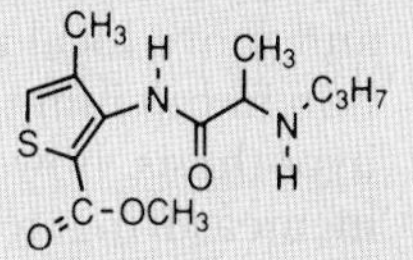

Articaine (pKa = 7.8)

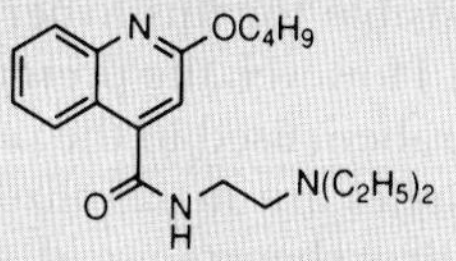

Dibucaine (pKa = 8.8)

Amino ethers

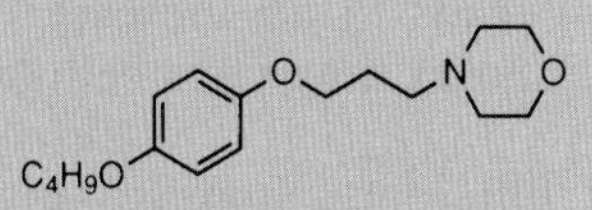

Pramoxine (pKa = 7.1)

Amino ketone

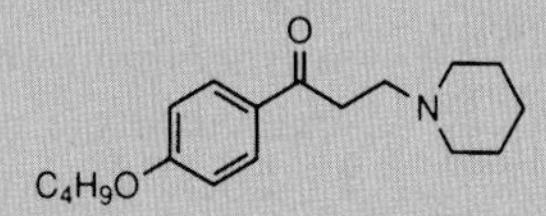

Dyclonine (pKa = 8.2)

Alcohols

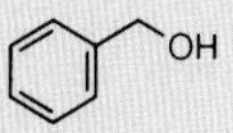

Benzyl alcohol

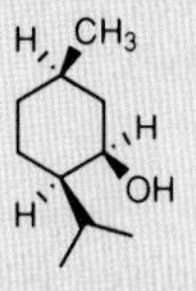

Menthol

Phenols

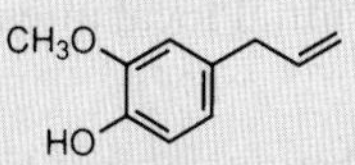

Eugenol

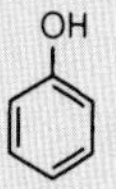

Phenol

risk of systemic toxicity, such as methemoglobinemia, specifically with prilocaine (52).

Toxicity and Side Effects

The side effects and toxicity of local anesthetics seem to be related to their actions on other excitable membrane proteins, such as in the Na^+ and K^+ channels in the heart, the nicotinic acetylcholine receptors in the neuromuscular junctions, and the nerve cells in the CNS. In general, neuromuscular junctions and the CNS are more susceptible than the cardiovascular system to the toxic effects of local anesthetics.

The actions on skeletal muscles tend to be transient and reversible, whereas the CNS side effects can be more deleterious. The primary effect of the toxicity seems to be convulsions, followed by severe CNS depression, particularly of the respiratory and cardiovascular centers. This can be related to an initial depression of inhibitory neurons, such as GABAergic systems, causing convulsions, followed by depression of other neurons, leading to general depression of the CNS.

The amino amide–type local anesthetics (i.e., lidocaine derivatives) are, in general, more likely to produce CNS side effects than the amino ester–type compounds (procaine analog). However, it should be noted that the toxic effects observed depend heavily on the route and site of administration as well as on the lipid solubility and metabolic stability of a given local anesthetic molecule. For example, most amide-type local anesthetics, such as lidocaine, are first degraded via *N*-dealkylation by hepatic enzymes (see Fig. 16.17). Unlike lidocaine, however, the initial metabolic degradation of prilocaine in humans is hydrolysis of the amide linkage to give *o*-toluidine and *N*-propylalanine. Formation of *o*-toluidine and its metabolites can cause methemoglobinemia in some patients (52). For this reason, prilocaine is much more likely than other local anesthetics to cause methemoglobinemia.

In contrast, allergic reactions to local anesthetics, although rare, are known to occur exclusively with *p*-aminobenzoic acid (PABA) ester-type local anesthetics (53). Whether the formation of PABA upon ester hydrolysis is solely responsible for this hypersensitivity remains to be determined. However, the preservative compounds, such as methylparaben, used in the preparation of amide-type local anesthetics are metabolized to the PABA-like substance, *p*-hydroxybenzoic acid. Thus, patients who are allergic to amino ester–type local anesthetics should be treated with a preservative-free amino amide–type local anesthetic.

Amide-type local anesthetics (e.g., procainamide and lidocaine) also possess antiarrhythmic activity when given parenterally and at a subanesthetic dosage. Although this action is likely an extension of their effects on Na^+ channels in cardiac tissues, some evidence suggests a distinctly different mechanism of action with respect to the modulation of channel receptors and the location of binding sites for these compounds (54,55).

Chemical and Pharmacodynamic Aspects of Local Anesthetics

Mechanism of Action

Local anesthetics act by decreasing the excitability of nerve cells without affecting the resting potential. Because the action potential, or the ability of nerve cells to be excited, is associated with the movement of Na^+ across the nerve membranes, anything that interferes with the movement of these ions will interfere with cell excitability. For this reason, many hypotheses have been suggested to explain how local anesthetics regulate the changes in Na^+ permeability that underlie the nerve impulse. These hypotheses include direct action on ionic channels that interfere with ionic fluxes and interaction with phospholipids and calcium that reduces membrane flexibility and responsiveness to changes in electrical fields.

The nonspecific membrane actions of local anesthetics can be easily ruled out, because most clinically useful agents, in contrast to general anesthetics, possess a defined set of structure–activity relationships. At much higher drug concentrations, local anesthetics also bind and block K^+ channels.

Interaction with Phospholipids and Calcium Calcium exists in the membrane in a bound state. Many investigators believe that the release of the bound calcium is the first step in membrane depolarization and that this release leads to the changes in ionic permeability described previously. It has been suggested that local anesthetics displace the bound calcium from these sites and form more stable bonds, thereby inhibiting ionic fluxes. The following evidence has been offered in support of this theory: Both calcium and local anesthetics bind to phospholipids in vitro, reducing their flexibility and responsiveness to changes in electrical fields (56–58). Also, membrane excitability and instability increase in calcium-deficient solutions. Local anesthetics counteract this abnormal increase in excitability, and more local anesthetic is necessary to block excitation in calcium-poor solutions (59). Direct proof of this hypothesis, however, is lacking because of the difficulty in measuring temporal Ca^{2+} movements in vivo. It is also possible that the aforementioned cause-and-effect relationship between intracellular free Ca^{2+} and membrane excitability is the result of an Na^+–Ca^{2+} exchange reaction; that is, the influx of Na^+ displaces the membrane-bound calcium, which leads to an increase of intracellular free Ca^{2+} and, thereby, increases cellular excitability.

Local anesthetics interact differently, however, with neuronal phospholipids with or without the presence of cholesterol. Thus, the interactions of local anesthetics with the cellular membranes actually may help to explain some of the observed differences in toxicity of the individual local anesthetic agents (60).

Action on Voltage-Sensitive Sodium Channels As mentioned, the voltage-sensitive Na^+ channels are membrane-bound glycoproteins that mediate Na^+ permeability. On excitation, these channels undergo conformational changes from a closed to an open state, thus allowing a rapid influx of sodium. The movement of Na^+ is blocked by the neurotoxins TTX and STX and by local anesthetics (61). Most electrophysiologists and neuropharmacologists now agree that the mechanism of action of local anesthetics results primarily from their binding to one or more sites within the Na^+ channels, thus blocking Na^+ conductance (62). However, the exact location of these binding sites and whether all local anesthetics interact with a common site remain matters of dispute.

Action on Sodium Conductance Local anesthetics block Na^+ conductance by two possible modes of action: tonic inhibition and phasic inhibition (63,64). Tonic inhibition results from the binding of local anesthetics to nonactivated closed Na^+ channels and, thus, is independent of channel activation. Phasic inhibition is accomplished when local anesthetics bind to activated, open states (conducting) or to inactivated states (nonconducting) of the Na^+ channels. Thus, it is not surprising that a greater phasic inhibition usually is obtained with repetitive depolarization and is referred to as use-dependent blockade.

Two reasons have been suggested to explain this observation. First, channel inactivation during depolarization increases the number of binding sites that normally are inaccessible to local anesthetics at resting potential. Second, both the open and the inactivated channels possess binding sites with a higher affinity; therefore, local anesthetics bind more tightly and result in a more stable nerve block.

Furthermore, it is generally agreed that most of the clinically useful local anesthetics exert their actions by binding to the inactivated forms of the channels and, thus, prevent their transition to the original resting state (64). Because most of these drugs exhibit both tonic and phasic inhibitions, whether tonic and phasic block results from drug interaction at the same or different sites remains unclear.

Local Anesthetics Binding to Sodium Channels Most of the clinically useful local anesthetics are tertiary amines with a pK_a of 7.0 to 9.0. Thus, under physiologic conditions, both protonated forms (onium ions) and the un-ionized, molecular forms are available for binding to the channel proteins. In fact, the ratio between the onium ions [BH^+] and the un-ionized molecules [B] can be easily calculated based on the pH of the medium and the pK_a of the drug molecule by the Henderson-Hasselbalch equation:

$$pH = pK_a - \log [BH^+]/[B]$$

The effect of pH changes on the potency of local anesthetics has been extensively investigated (65). Based on these studies, it was concluded that local anesthetics block the action potential by first penetrating the nerve membrane in their un-ionized forms and then binding to a site within the channels in their onium forms. Perhaps the most direct support for this hypothesis comes from the experimental results of Narahashi et al. (66,67), who studied the effects of internal and external perfusion of local anesthetics (both tertiary amines and quaternary ammonium compounds), at different pH values, on the Na^+ conductance of the squid giant axon. The observation that both tertiary amines and quaternary ammonium compounds produce greater nerve blockage when applied internally indicates an axoplasmic site of action for these compounds.

Furthermore, only the tertiary amines exhibit a reduction in their local anesthetic activities when the internal pH is raised from 7.0 to 8.0. Because the increase of internal pH to 8.0 favors the existence of the un-ionized forms, this result again suggests that the onium ions are required for binding to the channel receptors. Narahashi and Frazier (68) further estimated that approximately 90% of the blocking actions of lidocaine can be attributed to onium forms of the drug molecule, whereas only approximately 10% can result from un-ionized molecule and, perhaps, at a hydrophobic binding site other than the primary binding site. Benzocaine, because of its lack of a basic amine group (pK_a = 2.78), and other neutral anesthetics, such as benzyl alcohol, have been suggested to bind to this hydrophobic binding site.

In 1984, Hille (69) proposed a unified theory involving a single binding site in the Na^+ channels for both onium ions (protonated tertiary amines and quaternary ammonium compounds) and un-ionized forms of local anesthetics. As depicted in Figure 16.14, a number of pathways are available, depending on the size, pK_a, and lipid solubility of the drug molecules as well as the voltage and frequency-dependent modulation of the channel states, for a drug to reach its binding sites. Protonated anesthetic molecules [BH^+] and quaternary ammonium compounds reach their target sites via the hydrophilic pathway externally (pathway b in Fig. 16.14), which is available only during channel activation.

The lipid-soluble anesthetic molecules, on the other hand, diffuse across the neuronal membrane in their un-ionized forms. They can interact with the same binding sites from either the hydrophilic pathway (pathway b′ in Fig. 16.14) on reprotonation to their onium ions [BH^+] or via the hydrophobic pathway (pathway a in Fig. 16.14) in their un-ionized forms [B]. Benzocaine and other nonbasic local anesthetic molecules use this hydrophobic pathway and, thus, bind in the hydrophobic domain to produce their actions. Site-directed mutagenesis studies (70–73) suggest that local anesthetics bind to the hydrophobic amino acid residues near the center and the intracellular end of the S6 segment in the domain

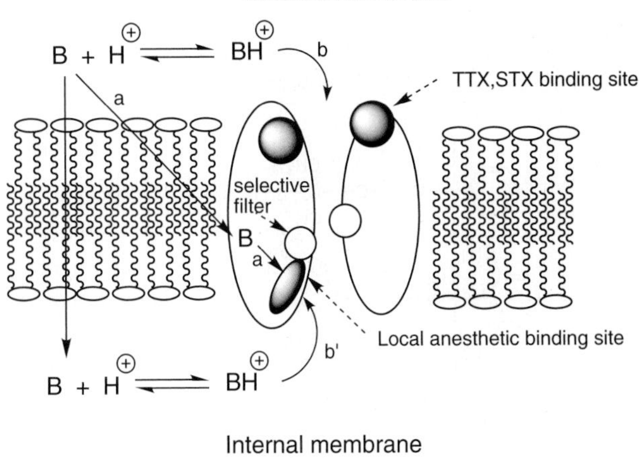

FIGURE 16.14 Model of a sodium channel, as suggested by Hille (69), depicting a hydrophilic pathway (denoted by b and b′) and a hydrophobic pathway (denoted by a) by which local anesthetics can reach their binding sites.

D4, whereas the BTX receptor is within segment S6 in domain D1 of the α subunit of the Na^+ channels (Fig. 16.14) (49).

Structure–Activity Relationships

A quick perusal of Table 16.9 reveals that many diverse chemical structures possess local anesthetic properties: amino esters (procaine analogs), amino amides (lidocaine analogs), amino ethers (pramoxine), amino ketones (dyclonine), alcohols (benzyl alcohol and menthol), and phenols (eugenol and phenol). Although it would seem that there is no obvious structure–activity relationship among these agents, most of the clinically useful local anesthetics are tertiary amines with pK_a values of 7.0 to 9.0. These compounds exhibit their local anesthetic properties by virtue of the interactions of the onium ions with a selective binding site within the Na^+ channels (Fig. 16.14). For this reason, any structural modifications that alter the lipid solubility, pK_a, and metabolic inactivation have a pronounced effect on the ability of a drug molecule to reach or interact with the hypothetical binding sites, thus modifying its local anesthetic properties.

Lipophilic Portion The lipophilic portion of the molecule is essential for local anesthetic activity. For most of the clinically useful local anesthetics, this portion of the molecule consists of either an aromatic group directly attached to a carbonyl function (the amino ester series) or a 2,6-dimethylphenyl group attached to a carbonyl function through an —NH— group (the amino amide series) (Fig. 16.15). Both groups are highly lipophilic

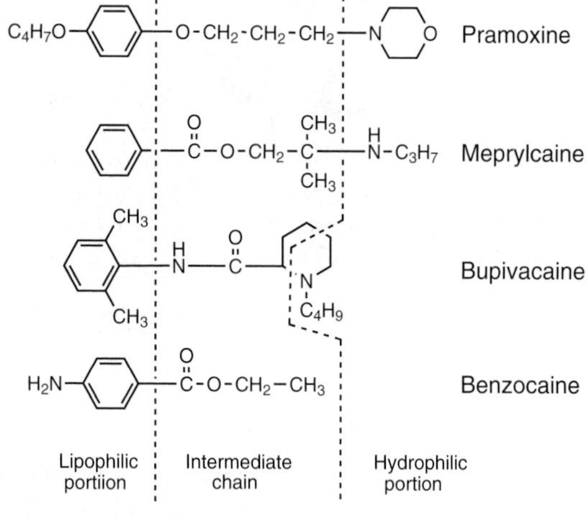

FIGURE 16.15 Structure–activity relationship comparison of local anesthetics.

and appear to play an important role in the binding of local anesthetics to the channel proteins. Structural modification of this portion of the molecule has a profound effect on its physical and chemical properties, which in turn alters its local anesthetic properties.

In the amino ester series, an electron-donating substituent in the *ortho* or *para* (or both) positions increases local anesthetic potency. Such groups as an aromatic amino (procaine, chloroprocaine, and propoxycaine), an alkylamino (tetracaine), or an alkoxy (proparacaine and propoxycaine) group contribute electron density to the aromatic ring by both resonance and inductive effects, thereby enhancing local anesthetic potency over nonsubstituted analogs (e.g., meprylcaine).

As illustrated in Figure 16.16, resonance is expected to give rise to a zwitterionic form (i.e., the electrons from the amino group can be resonance delocalized onto the carbonyl oxygen). Although neither drawn structure of procaine in Figure 16.16 can accurately represent the structure of procaine when it interacts with the local anesthetic binding site, it is reasonable to assume that the greater the resemblance to the zwitterionic form, the greater the affinity for the binding site (i.e., binding from both the hydrophilic pathway b′ and hydrophobic pathway a in Fig. 16.14). This is particularly true for the affinity of benzocaine for its binding site, because it lacks a basic amine group. Therefore, it can only bind from the hydrophobic pathway a. Thus, addition of any aromatic substitution that can enhance the formation of the resonance form through electron donation or inductive effects will produce more potent local anesthetic agents. Electron-withdrawing groups, such as nitro (—NO_2), reduce the local anesthetic activity.

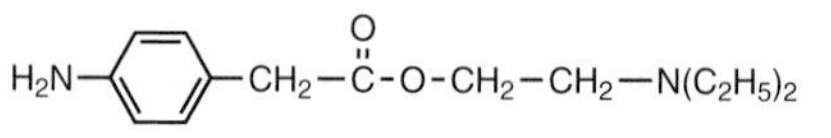

Insertion of a methylene group between the aromatic moiety and the carbonyl function as shown above in the procaine molecule, which prohibits the formation of the zwitterionic form, has led to a procaine analog with greatly reduced anesthetic potency. This observation lends further support for the involvement of the resonance form when an ester-type local anesthetic binds to the binding

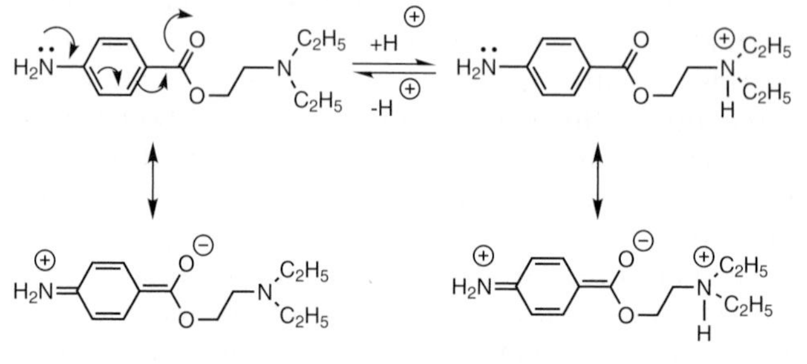

FIGURE 16.16 Possible zwitterionic forms for procaine.

site. When an amino or an alkoxy group is attached to the *meta* position of the aromatic ring, however, no resonance delocalization of their electrons is possible. The addition of this function only increases (alkoxy group) or decreases (amino group) the lipophilicity of the molecule (e.g., benoxinate, $\log D_{pH\ 7.4} = 3.19$; and proparacaine, $\log D_{pH\ 7.4} = 2.05$).

Furthermore, tetracaine is approximately 50-fold more potent than procaine. Experimentally, this increase in potency cannot be correlated solely with the 2,500-fold increase of lipid solubility by the *n*-butyl group ($\log D_{pH\ 7.4} = 2.73$ vs. procaine $\log D_{pH\ 7.4} = -0.32$). Perhaps part of this potentiation of local anesthetic activity can be attributed to the electron-releasing property of the *n*-butyl group via the inductive effect, which indirectly enhances the electron density of the *p*-amino group, which in turn increases the formation of the zwitterionic form available for interaction with the binding site proteins via both the hydrophobic and the hydrophilic pathways of the receptor.

Another important aspect of aromatic substitution has been observed from structure–activity relationship studies. In the amino amides (lidocaine analogs), the *o,o'*-dimethyl groups are required to provide suitable protection from amide hydrolysis to ensure a desirable duration of action. Similar conclusions can be made to rationalize the increase in the duration of action of propoxycaine by the *o*-propoxy group. The shorter duration of action, however, observed with chloroprocaine when compared with that of procaine can only be explained by the inductive effect of the *o*-chloro group, which pulls the electron density away from the carbonyl function, thus making it more susceptible to nucleophilic attack by the plasma cholinesterases.

INTERMEDIATE CHAIN The intermediate chain almost always contains a short alkyl chain of one to three carbons in length linked to the aromatic ring via several possible organic functional groups. The nature of this intermediate chain determines the chemical stability of the drug, which also influences the duration of action and relative toxicity. In general, amino amides are more resistant to metabolic hydrolysis than the amino esters and, thus, have a longer duration of action. The placement of small alkyl groups (i.e., branching), especially around the ester function (e.g., meprylcaine) or the amide function (e.g., bupivacaine, etidocaine, prilocaine, or ropivacaine), also hinders esterase- or amidase-catalyzed hydrolysis, prolonging the duration of action (Fig. 16.15 and Table 16.9). It should be mentioned, however, that prolonging the duration of action of a compound usually increases its systemic toxicities unless it is more selective toward the voltage-gated Na^+ channel, as in the case of levobupivacaine (74,75).

In the lidocaine series, lengthening of the alkyl chain from one to two or three increases the pK_a of the terminal tertiary amino group from 7.7 to 9.0 or 9.5, respectively. Thus, lengthening of the intermediate chain effectively reduces local anesthetic potency as a result of a reduction of onium ions under physiologic conditions. As mentioned earlier, the onium ions are required for effective binding of the amino amide–type local anesthetics to the channel binding sites.

HYDROPHILIC PORTION Most clinically useful local anesthetics have a tertiary alkylamine, which readily forms water-soluble salts with mineral acids, and this portion is commonly considered to be the hydrophilic portion of the molecule (Fig. 16.9). The necessity of this portion of the molecule for amino ester–type local anesthetics remains a matter of debate. The strongest opposition for requiring a basic amino group for local anesthetic action comes from the observation that benzocaine, which lacks the basic aliphatic amine function, has potent local anesthetic activity. For this reason, it is often suggested that the tertiary amine function in procaine analogs is needed only for the formation of water-soluble salts suitable for pharmaceutical preparations. With the understanding of the voltage-activated Na^+ channel and the possible mechanism of action of local anesthetics previously discussed, however, it is quite conceivable that the onium ions produced by protonation of the tertiary amine group are also required for binding in the voltage-gated Na^+ channels (Fig. 16.14).

From Table 16.9, the hydrophilic group in most of the clinically useful drugs can be in the form of a secondary or tertiary alkyl amine or part of a nitrogen heterocycle (e.g., pyrrolidine, piperidine, or morpholine). As mentioned earlier, most of the clinically useful local anesthetics have pK_a values of 7.5 to 9.0. The effects of an alkyl substituent on the pK_a depend on the size, length, and hydrophobicity of the group; and thus, it is difficult to see a clear structure–activity relationship among these structures. It is generally accepted that local anesthetics with higher lipid solubility and lower pK_a values appear to exhibit more rapid onset and lower toxicity.

Stereochemistry

Are there any stereochemical requirements of local anesthetic compounds when they interact with the Na^+ channel binding sites? A number of clinically used local anesthetics do contain a chiral center (i.e., bupivacaine, etidocaine, mepivacaine, and prilocaine) (Table 16.9), but in contrast to other classes of drugs (e.g., cholinergics), the effect of optical isomerism on isolated nerve preparations revealed a lack of stereospecificity. In a few cases (e.g., prilocaine, bupivacaine, and etidocaine), however, small differences in the total pharmacologic profile of optical isomers have been noted when administered in vivo (76–78). Whether these differences result from differences in uptake, distribution, and metabolism or from direct binding to the Na^+ channel have not been determined. When structural rigidity has been imposed on the molecule, however, as in the case of some aminoalkyl spirotetralin succinimides (79), differences in local anesthetic potency of the enantiomers have been observed (range, 1:2 to 1:10). Although these differences in enantiomers clearly are not as pronounced as those with other pharmacologic agents, such as adrenergic antagonists or anticholinergic drugs, steric requirements are necessary for effective interaction between a local anesthetic agent and its proposed channel binding sites.

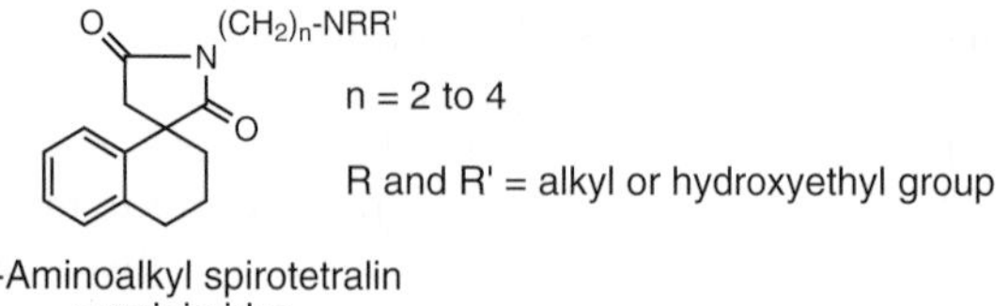

N-Aminoalkyl spirotetralin succinimides

Stereochemistry of the local anesthetics, however, plays an important role in their observed toxicity and pharmacokinetic properties. For example, ropivacaine and levobupivacaine, the only optically active local anesthetics currently being marketed, have considerably lower cardiac toxicities than their close structural analog, bupivacaine (80). Furthermore, the degree of separation between motor and sensory blockade is more apparent with ropivacaine and levobupivacaine relative to bupivacaine at a lower end of the dosage scale (81). Thus, the observed cardiac toxicity of bupivacaine has been attributed to the *R*-(+)-bupivacaine enantiomer (76–78). The exact mechanisms for this enantiomeric difference remain unknown. Longobardo and colleagues observed a stereoselective blockade on the cardiac hKv1.5 channels by the *R*-(+)-enantiomers of bupivacaine, ropivacaine, and mepivacaine (82,83). It should be noted that *S*-(−)-bupivacaine, which is approved by the U.S. Food and Drug Administration and marketed under the name of Chirocaine, has even less CNS toxicity than ropivacaine.

Metabolism of Local Anesthetics

An understanding of the metabolism of local anesthetics is important in clinical practice because the overall toxicity of a drug depends not only on its uptake and tissue distribution but also on how it is deactivated in vivo. The amino ester–type local anesthetics are rapidly hydrolyzed by plasma cholinesterase (also known as pseudocholinesterase), which is widely distributed in body tissues. These compounds can therefore be metabolized in the blood, kidneys, and liver and, to a lesser extent, at the site of administration. For example, both procaine and benzocaine are easily hydrolyzed by cholinesterase into PABA and the corresponding *N,N'*-diethylaminoethyl alcohol.

It is not surprising that potential drug interactions exist between the amino ester–type local anesthetics and other clinically important drugs, such as cholinesterase inhibitors or atropine-like anticholinergic drugs (see Chapter 9). These compounds either inhibit or compete with local anesthetics for cholinesterases, therefore prolonging local anesthetic activity and/or toxicity. Another potential drug interaction with clinical significance can be envisioned between benzocaine and sulfonamides; that is, the hydrolysis of benzocaine to PABA can antagonize the antibacterial activity of sulfonamides.

The amino amide–type local anesthetics, however, are metabolized primarily in the liver, involving CYP1A2 isozymes (84). A general metabolic scheme for lidocaine is shown in Figure 16.17.

Marked species variations occur in the quantitative urinary excretion of these metabolites. For example, rats produce large quantities of the 3-hydroxy derivatives of both lidocaine and monoethylglycinexylidide, which are subsequently conjugated and recycled in the bile. Significant quantities of these two metabolites, however, are not produced by guinea pigs, dogs, or humans. Therefore, it is unlikely that biliary excretion is a major pathway for excretion in humans. Species variability is important primarily when the acute and chronic toxicity of nonester-type local anesthetic agents is being evaluated.

Although the exact mechanism for the CNS toxicity of lidocaine remains unclear, the metabolic studies of lidocaine provide some insight for future studies. Of all the metabolites of lidocaine, only monoethylglycinexylidide (and not glycinexylidide) contributes to some of the CNS side effects of lidocaine. This observation suggests that the toxicities of lidocaine are, perhaps, related to the

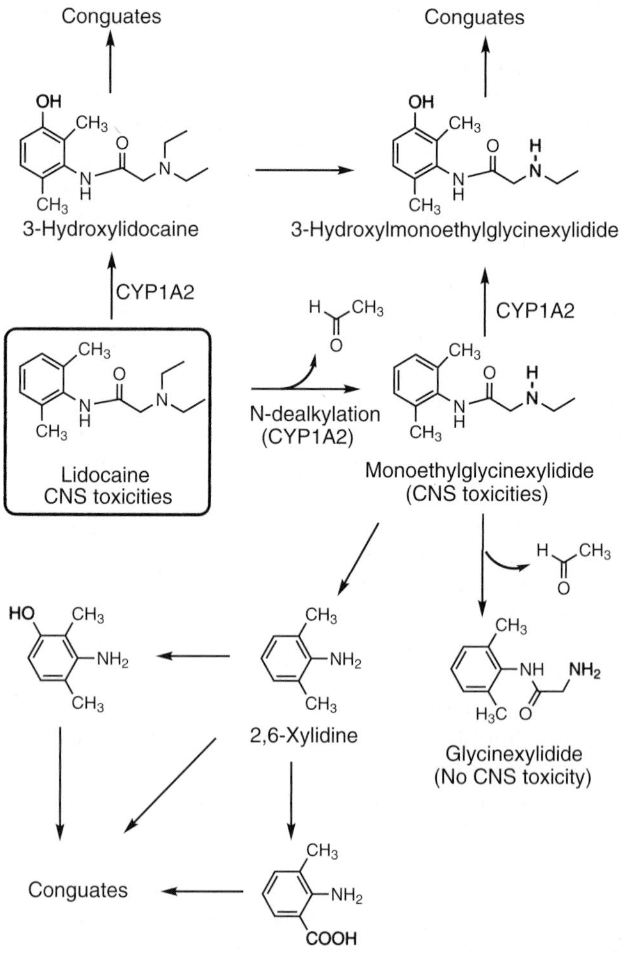

FIGURE 16.17 Metabolic scheme for lidocaine.

removal of the *N*-ethyl groups of lidocaine after crossing the blood–brain barrier. Support for this hypothesis can be obtained from the fact that reaction of a tryptophan derivative with formaldehyde under physiologic conditions gives rise to a β-carboline derivative, which is a CNS convulsant (Fig. 16.18). Advances in the $GABA_A$ receptor–benzodiazepine receptor–chloride ion channels and their role in the mechanism of action of benzodiazepine anticonvulsants lends further support to this hypothesis (i.e., many β-carbolines are inverse agonists at the benzodiazepine binding site).

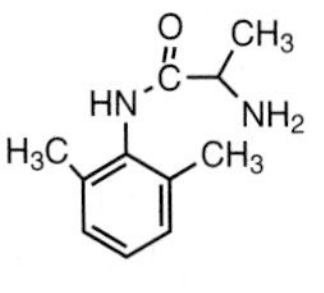

Tocainide

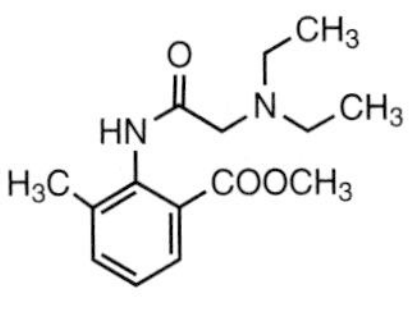

Tolycaine

To minimize these unwanted side effects of lidocaine, tocainide and tolycaine have been prepared and found to possess good local anesthetic activity without any appreciable CNS side effects. Tocainide, which lacks the vulnerable *N*-ethyl group but has an α-methyl group to prevent degradation of the primary amine group from amine oxidase, has desirable local anesthetic properties. Tolycaine has an *o*-carbomethoxy substituted for one of the *o*-methyl groups of lidocaine. The carbomethoxy group is fairly stable in tissues but is rapidly hydrolyzed in the blood to the polar carboxylate group and, thus, is unable to cross the blood–brain barrier.

For this reason, tolycaine lacks any CNS side effects, even though it still contains the *N*-ethyl group. It should be noted, however, that both tocainide and tolycaine are primarily used clinically as antiarrhythmic agents.

Furthermore, the metabolism of nonester-type drugs, especially lidocaine derivatives, is also known to be more prone to being influenced by enzyme induction or inhibition due to other coadministered medications (e.g., cimetidine and barbiturates).

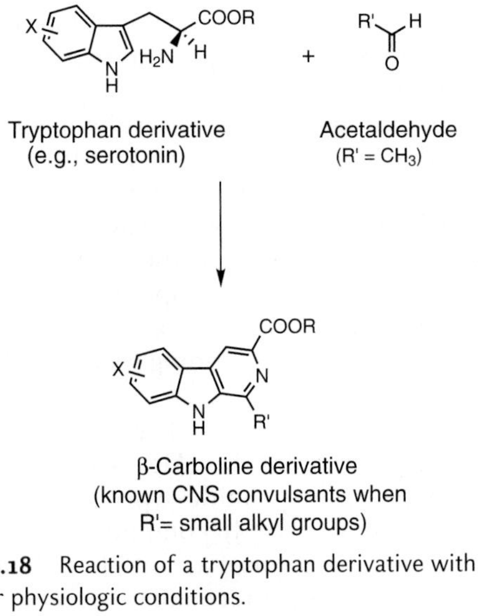

FIGURE 16.18 Reaction of a tryptophan derivative with acetaldehyde under physiologic conditions.

Common Agents Used for Local Anesthesia

Local anesthetics are widely used in many primary care settings. Techniques for their administration in these settings include topical application, local infiltration, field block, and peripheral nerve block. Their use can be maximized by an understanding of their potencies, durations of action, routes of administration, and pharmacokinetic and side effect profiles. The generic name, trade name, and recommended application are given in Table 16.8, and the chemical structures of these agents can be found in Table 16.9.

Articaine

Articaine (Table 16.9) has been widely used in dentistry since its U.S. Food and Drug Administration approval in 2000 due to its quick onset and short duration of action. The structure of articaine differs from the structures of all other amino amide–type local anesthetics in that it contains the bioisosteric thiophene ring instead of a benzene ring and a carbomethoxy group. This renders the molecule more lipophilic and, thus, makes it easier to cross lipoidal membranes.

Its local anesthetic potency is approximately 1.5-fold that of lidocaine, even though it has similar pK_a (7.8) and smaller log $D_{pH\ 7.4}$ (1.65 vs. log$D_{pH\ 7.4}$ of 2.26 for lidocaine) and plasma protein binding (76%) properties. Articaine is metabolized primarily by plasma cholinesterases because of the presence of an ester group and, therefore, has a much shorter duration of action than lidocaine (i.e., only approximately one-fourth that of lidocaine). Articaine undergoes rapid hydrolysis of the carbomethoxy group to give articainic acid, which is eliminated either unchanged (75%) or as its glucuronides (25%). Compared with other short-acting, amino amide–type local anesthetics, such as mepivacaine, lidocaine, or prilocaine, articaine is said to be a much safer drug for regional anesthesia and is the drug of choice for dental procedures.

Benzocaine

Benzocaine (Table 16.9) is used topically by itself or in combination with menthol or phenol in nonprescription dosage forms such as gels, creams, ointments, lotions, aerosols, and lozenges to relieve pain or irritation caused by such conditions as sunburn, insect bites, toothache, teething, cold sores or canker sores in or around the mouth, and fever blisters. Benzocaine is a lipophilic local anesthetic agent with a short duration of action.

Like most amino ester–type local anesthetics, it is easily hydrolyzed by plasma cholinesterase. However, because of its low pK_a, it is un-ionized under most physiologic conditions and, therefore, can only bind to the lipid site in the sodium channel (log$D_{pH\ 7.4}$ = 1.91) (Fig. 16.14). When administered topically to abraded skin, it can easily cross membranes into the systemic circulation to cause systemic toxicities. Furthermore, being a PABA derivative, it has similar allergenic properties to procaine and is contraindicated with sulfonamide antibacterial agents.

Bupivacaine and Levobupivacaine

Bupivacaine hydrochloride (Table 16.8) is a racemic mixture of the *S*-(−)- and *R*-(+)-enantiomers. Bupivacaine has higher lipid solubility ($logD_{pH\ 7.4}$ = 2.54) and a much decreased rate of hepatic degradation compared with lidocaine. For this reason, bupivacaine has significantly greater tendency than lidocaine to produce cardiotoxicity. Because of its greater affinity for voltage-gated Na^+ channels, the *R*-(+)-enantiomer confers greater cardiotoxicity than racemic bupivacaine.

It was not surprising to see the approval of levobupivacaine, the *S*-(-)-enantiomer of (±)-bupivacaine, as the second optically active, amino amide–type local anesthetic for parenteral applications. Like ropivacaine, levobupivacaine has a lower cardiotoxicity than bupivacaine, but it also has a lower CNS toxicity than both ropivacaine and lidocaine.

Possible pathways for metabolism of bupivacaine include CYP1A2 aromatic 3-hydroxylation, CYP3A4 *N*-dealkylation, and to a minor extent, the amide hydrolysis. Only the *N*-dealkylated product, however, has been identified in urine after epidural or spinal anesthesia.

Chloroprocaine

Chloroprocaine (Fig. 16.8) is a very short-acting, amino ester–type local anesthetic used to provide regional anesthesia by infiltration as well as by peripheral and central nerve block, including lumbar and caudal epidural blocks. The presence of a chlorine atom *ortho* to the carbonyl of the ester function increases its lipophilicity ($logD_{pH\ 7.4}$ = 0.95) and its rate of hydrolysis by plasma cholinesterase at least threefold compared to procaine and benzocaine. Thus, chloroprocaine can be used in maternal and neonatal patients with minimal placental passage of chloroprocaine. The lower plasma cholinesterase activity in the maternal epidural space must still have sufficient activity for degrading chloroprocaine and, thus, not allowing it to cross the placental barrier. Like PABA, the hydrolysis product of chloroprocaine, 4-amino-2-chlorobenzoic acid, also inhibits the action of sulfonamides. Therefore, its use with sulfonamides should be avoided.

Lidocaine

Lidocaine (Fig. 16.8) is the most commonly used amino amide–type local anesthetic. Lidocaine is very lipid soluble ($logD_{pH\ 7.4}$ = 2.26) and, thus, has a more rapid onset and a longer duration of action than most amino ester–type local anesthetics, such as procaine and tetracaine. It can be administered parenterally (with or without epinephrine) or topically either by itself or in combination with prilocaine or etidocaine as a eutectic mixture that is very popular with pediatric patients. The use of lidocaine–epinephrine mixtures should be avoided, however, in the areas with limited vascular supply to prevent tissue necrosis. Lidocaine is also frequently used as a class IB antiarrhythmic agent for the treatment of ventricular arrhythmias, both because it binds and inhibits Na^+ channels in the cardiac muscle and because of its longer duration of action than amino ester–type local anesthetics (Chapter 21).

CNS changes are the most frequently observed systemic toxicities of lidocaine. The initial manifestations are restlessness, vertigo, tinnitus, slurred speech, and eventually, seizures. Subsequent manifestations include CNS depression with a cessation of convulsions and the onset of unconsciousness and respiratory depression or cardiac arrest. This biphasic effect occurs because local anesthetics initially block the inhibitory GABAergic pathways, resulting in stimulation, and eventually block both inhibitory and excitatory pathways (i.e., block the Na^+ channels associated with the NMDA receptors, resulting in overall CNS inhibition) (85).

Lidocaine is extensively metabolized in the liver by CYP3A4 *N*-dealkylation and aromatic hydroxylation catalyzed by CYP1A2 (Fig. 16.17). Lidocaine also possesses a weak inhibitory activity toward the CYP1A2 isozymes and, therefore, can interfere with metabolism of other medications (86).

Mepivacaine

Mepivacaine hydrochloride (Fig. 16.8) is an amino amide–type local anesthetic agent widely used to provide regional analgesia and anesthesia by local infiltration, peripheral nerve block, and epidural and caudal blocks. The pharmacologic and toxicologic profile of mepivacaine is quite similar to that of lidocaine, except that mepivacaine is less lipophilic ($logD_{pH\ 7.4}$ = 1.95) and has a slightly longer duration of action but lacks the vasodilator activity of lidocaine. For this reason, it serves as an alternate choice for lidocaine when addition of epinephrine is not recommended in patients with hypertensive vascular disease.

Mepivacaine undergoes extensive hepatic metabolism catalyzed by CYP3A4 and CYP1A2, with only a small percentage of the administered dosage (<10%) being excreted unchanged in the urine. The major metabolic biotransformations of mepivacaine are *N*-dealkylation (to give the *N*-demethylated compound 2′,6′-pipecoloxylidide) and aromatic hydroxylations. These metabolites are excreted as their corresponding glucuronides.

Ropivacaine

S-Ropivacaine hydrochloride (Fig. 16.8) is the first optically active, amino amide–type local anesthetic marketed in recent years. It combines the anesthetic potency and long duration of action of (±)-bupivacaine with a side effect profile intermediate between those of

SCENARIO: OUTCOME AND ANALYSIS

Outcome

Paul Arpino

After consulting with the covering pharmacist and the hospital's allergy specialist, the team decides to proceed with the type of anesthesia and surgery as planned. On the day of the surgery, CDL received the peripheral nerve block with ropivacaine and required minimal adjunctive medications during the procedure. Postoperatively, CDL's pain was well controlled and there was no evidence of an allergic reaction.

Chemical Analysis

S. William Zito and Victoria Roche

Procaine is a local anesthetic developed from the investigation of cocaine analogs that were synthesized in an effort to enhance the local anesthetic properties and reduce cocaine's addiction and acute toxicity liability. Cocaine and procaine are benzoic acid derivatives and both are known to cause allergic reactions.

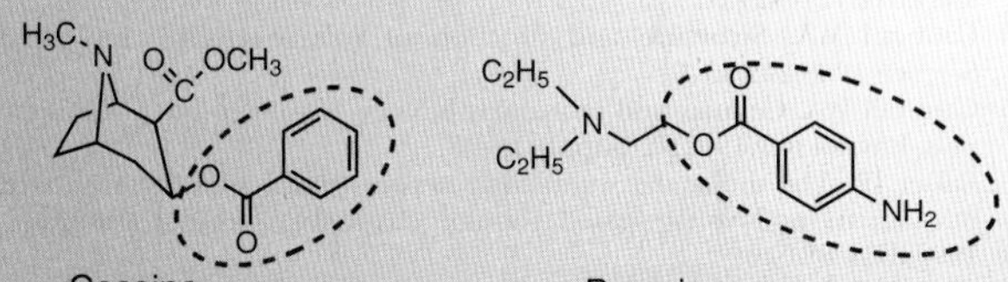

Cocaine Procaine

The aminoalkyl side chain is not necessary for local anesthetic activity but is useful for forming water-soluble salts for parenteral administration. The para-amino phenyl substituent enhances local anesthetic effect by increasing the electron density of the carbonyl oxygen through electron induction.

Ropivacaine is a local anesthetic developed from another natural alkaloid, isogramine. Structure activity studies of isogramine led to the development of the lidocaine class (anilides) of local anesthetics.

The lidocaine types of local anesthetics are bioisosteres of isogramine. The amino alkyl side chain serves to form water-soluble salts for parenteral administration. As anilides, these compounds have a longer duration of action compared with the benzoic acid ester class, and the 2,6-dimethyls of the aromatic ring also serve to increase duration of action.

This class of local anesthetics is less irritating upon injection and, most importantly for this case, have no cross–allergic sensitivity with the benzoic acid class of local anesthetics. General anesthesia must be avoided in this case because it suppresses upper airway muscle activity, and it may impair breathing by allowing the airway to close. General anesthesia thus may increase the number of and duration of sleep apnea episodes of this patient.

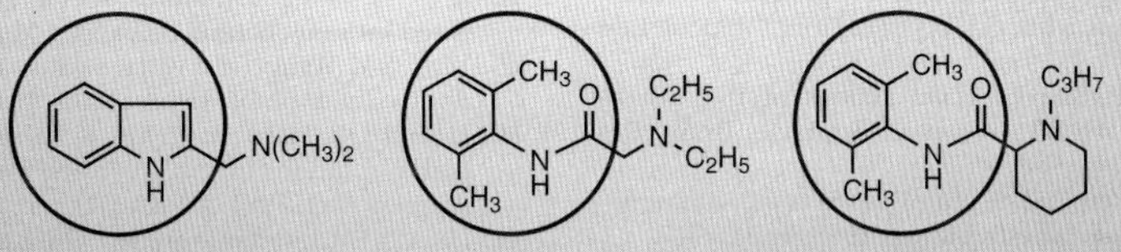

Isogramine Lidocaine Ropivacaine

CASE STUDY

S. William Zito and Victoria Roche

BB is a 19-year-old pregnant woman in her second trimester. Until now she has had an unremarkable pregnancy. However, today she presents to the emergency department complaining of 3 days of right lower quadrant pain, anorexia, and persistent nausea and vomiting. A physical examination of BB revealed vital signs of blood pressure, 127/68 mm Hg; heart rate, 86 beats per minute; respiratory rate, 18 breaths per minute, and a temperature of 97.5 °F. A diagnosis is made of acute appendicitis and surgery is recommended. Preoperative testing showed slight leucocytosis with a white blood cell count of 12,000/mm^3; her hemoglobin was 12.1 gm/dL, with a hematocrit level of 34.9% and platelet count of 306,000/mm^3. BB's medical history was unexceptional; she has had no previous health issues and she is not taking any medications except for prenatal multivitamins, which contain folic acid and iron. She reports no surgical history and that her parents have had operations for which, to her knowledge, there were no anesthetic sequelae. The surgical trauma team expects the operation to take 45 minutes and plans to use general anesthesia using rapid induction and securing her airway with a small cuffed endotracheal tube. The following three general anesthetics are proposed. Which one would you recommend?

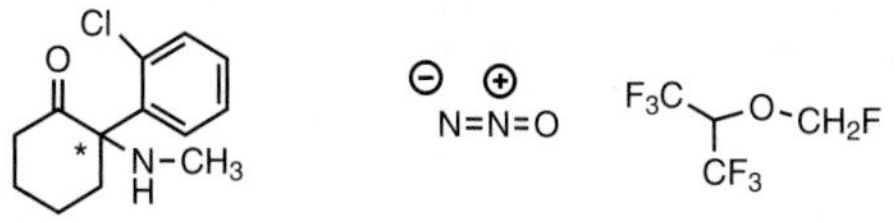

1 2 3

1. Conduct a thorough and mechanistic SAR analysis of the three therapeutic options in the case.
2. Apply the chemical understanding gained from the SAR analysis to this patient's specific needs to make a therapeutic recommendation.

bupivacaine and lidocaine. Although ropivacaine has a pK_a nearly identical to that of bupivacaine, it is two- to threefold less lipid soluble ($logD_{pH\ 7.4}$ = 2.06) and has a smaller volume of distribution, a greater clearance, and a shorter elimination half-life than bupivacaine in humans.

The metabolism of ropivacaine in humans is mediated by hepatic CYP1A2 and, to a minor extent, by CYP3A4 (87). The major metabolite is 3-hydroxyropivacaine, and the minor metabolite is *S*-2′,6′-pipecoloxylidide (an *N*-dealkylated product).

References

1. Stoelting RK, Miller, RD. Basics of Anesthesia, 5th Ed. Philadelphia: Elsevier Health Sciences, 2007.
2. Stevens WC, Kingston HGG. Inhalation anesthesia. In: Barash PG, Cullen BF, Stoelting RK, eds. Clinical Anesthesia, 2nd Ed. Philadelphia: JB Lippincott, 1992:439–465.
3. Harrison NL, Flood P. Molecular mechanisms of general anesthetic action. Sci Med 1998;50:18–27.
4. Meyer HH. The theory of narcosis. JAMA 1906;26:1499–1502.
5. Overton E. Studien ueber die narkose, zugleich ein beitrag zur allgemeinem pharmakologie. Jena, Germany: Gustav Fischer, 1901.
6. Hemming HC, Akabas MH, Goldstein PA, et al. Emerging molecular mechanisms of general anesthetic action. Trends Pharmacol Sci 2005;26: 503–510.
7. Lysco GS, Robinson JL, Casto R, et al. The stereospecific effects of isoflurane isomers in vivo. Eur J Pharmacol 1994;263:25–29.
8. Graf BM, Boban M, Stowe DF, et al. Lack of stereospecific effects of isoflurane and desflurane isomers in isolated guinea pig hearts. Anesthesiology 1994;81:129–136.
9. Sidebotham DA, Schug SA. Stereochemistry in anesthesia. Clin Exp Pharmacol Physiol 1997;24:126–130.
10. Cheng S-C, Brunner EA. Effects of anesthetic agents on synaptosomal GABA disposal. Anesthesiology 1981;55:34–40.
11. Olsen RW. The molecular mechanism of action of general anesthetics: structural aspects of interactions with $GABA_A$ receptors. Toxicol Lett 1998;100–101:193–201.
12. Moody EJ, Harris BD, Skolnick P. Stereospecific actions of the inhalation anesthetic isoflurane at the $GABA_A$ receptor complex. Brain Res 1993;615:101–106.
13. Tomlin SL. Stereoselective effects of etomidate optical isomers on γ-aminobutyric acid type A receptors and animals. Anesthesiology 1998;88:708–717.
14. Krasowski MD, Harrison NL. General anesthetic actions at ligand-gated ion channels. Cell Mol Life Sci 1999;55:1278–1303.
15. Koltchine VV. Agonist gating and isoflurane potentiation in the human $GABA_A$ receptor determined by the volume of a TM2 residue. Mol Pharmacol 1999;56:1087–1093.
16. Belelli D, Pistis M, Peters JA, et al. General anesthetic action at transmitter-gated inhibitory amino acid receptors. Trends Pharmacol Sci 1999;20:496–502.
17. Bai D. Distinct functional and pharmacological properties of tonic and quantal inhibitory postsynaptic currents mediated by γ-aminobutyric acid A receptors in hippocampal neurons. Mol Pharmacol 2001;59:814–824.
18. Bai D. The general anesthetic propofol slows deactivation and desensitization of $GABA_A$ receptors. J Neurosci 1999;19:10635–10646.
19. Flohr H, Glade U, Motzko D. The role of the NMDA synapse in general anesthesia. Toxicol Lett 1998;100–101:23–29.
20. Perouansky M, Kirson ED, Yaari Y. Mechanism of action of volatile anesthetics: effects of halothane on glutamate receptors in vitro. Toxicol Lett 1998;100–101:65–69.
21. Larsen M, Langmoen IA. The effect of volatile anesthetics on synaptic release and uptake of glutamate. Toxicol Lett 1998;100–101:59–64.
22. Hudspith MJ. Glutamate: a role in normal brain function, anesthesia, analgesia and CNS injury. Br J Anaesth 1997;78:731–747.
23. Narahashi T, Aistrup GL, Lindstrom JM, et al. Ion modulation as the basis for general anesthetics. Toxicol Lett 1998;100–101:185–191.
24. Shiraishi M, Harris RA. Effects of alcohol and anesthetics on recombinant voltage-gated Na^+ channels. J Pharmacol Exp Ther 2004;309:987–994.
25. Franks NP, Lieb WR. Stereospecific effects of inhalational general anesthetic optical isomers on nerve ion channels. Science 1991;25:427–430.
26. Heurteaux C. TREK-1, a K^+ channel involved in neuroprotection and general anesthesia. EMBO J 2004;23:2684–2695.
27. Doze VA, Chen BX, Ticklenberg JA, et al. Pertussis toxin and 4-aminopyridine differentially affect the hypnotic-anesthetic action of dexmedetomidine and pentobarbital. Anesthesiology 1990;73:304–307.
28. Perry LB, Gould AB, Leonord PE. Case history number 82: "nonflammable" fires in the operating room. Anesth Analg 1975;54:152–154.
29. Eger EI II. Anesthetic Uptake and Action. Baltimore: Williams & Wilkins, 1974.
30. Christ DD, Kenna JG, Kammerer W, et al. Enflurane metabolism produces covalently bound liver adducts recognized by antibodies from patients with halothane hepatitis. Anesthesiology 1988;69:833–888.
31. Koblin DD. Characteristics and implications of desflurane metabolism and toxicity. Anesth Analg 1992;75:S10–S16.
32. Dodds C. General anesthesia: practical recommendations and recent advances. Drugs 1999;58:453–467.
33. Mazze RI, Calverely RK, Smith NT. Inorganic fluoride nephrotoxicity: prolonged enflurane and halothane anesthesia in volunteers. Anesthesiology 1977;46:265–271.
34. Lane GA Nahrwold ML, Tait AR. Anesthetics as teratogens: nitrous oxide is fetotoxic, xenon is not. Science 1980;210:899–901.
35. Reich DL, Silvay G. Ketamine: an update on the first twenty-five years of clinical experience. Can J Anaesth 1989;36:186–197.
36. Yamamura T, Harada K, Okamura A, et al. Is the site of action of ketamine anesthesia the N-methyl-D-aspartate receptor? Anesthesiology 1990;72:704–710.
37. Toro-Matos A, Redon-Platas AM, Avila-Valdez E, et al. Physostigmine antagonizes ketamine. Anesth Analg 1980;59:764–767.
38. Liljestrand G. The historical development of local anesthesia in local anesthetics. In: Lechat P, ed. International Encyclopedia of Pharmacology and Therapeutics. Oxford: Pergamon Press, 1971:1–38.
39. Arey LB. Developmental Anatomy, 7th Ed. Philadelphia: WB Saunders, 1965.
40. De Jong RH, Freund FG. Physiology of peripheral nerve and local anesthesia. Int Anesthesiol Clin 1979;8:35–53.
41. Hodgkin AL, Huxley AF. The dual effect of membrane potential on sodium conductance in the giant axon of *Loligo*. J Physiol (Lond) 1952;116:497–506.
42. Tasaki I. Nerve Transmission. Springfield, IL: Charles C Thomas, 1953.
43. Noda M, Shimizy S, Tanabe T, et al. Primary structure of *Electrophorus electricus* sodium channel deduced from complimentary DNA sequence. Nature 1984;312:121–127.
44. Catterall WA. Structure and function of voltage-sensitive ion channels. Science 1988;242:50–61.
45. Catterall WA. Cellular and molecular biology of voltage-gated sodium channels. Physiol Rev 1992;72(Suppl):15–48.
46. Balser JR. The molecular interaction between local anesthetic/antiarrhythmic agents and voltage-gated sodium channels. Trends Cardiovasc Med 1998;8:83–88.
47. Clare JJ, Tate SN, Nobbs M, et al. Voltage-gated sodium channels as therapeutic targets. Drug Discov Today 2000;5:506–520.
48. Anger T, Madge DJ, Mulla M, et al. Medicinal chemistry of neuronal voltage-gated sodium channel blockers. J Med Chem 2001;44:115–137.
49. Yang S-Y, Wang GK. Voltage-gated sodium channels as primary targets of diverse lipid-soluble neurotoxins. Cell Signal 2003;15:151–159.
50. Hamill OP, Marty A, Neher E, et al. Improved patch-clamp techniques for high-resolution current recording from cells and cell-free membrane patches. Pflügers Arch 1981;391:85–100.
51. Hersch EV, Lindenmyere RG. Phentolamine mesylate for accelerating recovery from lip and tongue anesthesia. Dent Clin North Am 2010;54:631–642.
52. Arthur GR. Pharmacokinetics of local anesthetics. In: Strichartz GR, ed. Local Anesthetics. Handbook of Experimental Pharmacology. Berlin: Springer, 1987;81:165–186.
53. Eggleston ST, Lush LW. Understanding allergic reactions to local anesthetics. Ann Pharmacother 1996;30:851–857.
54. Bean BP, Cohen CJ, Tsien RW. Lidocaine block of cardiac sodium channels. J Gen Physiol 1983;81:613–642.
55. Makielski JC, Sheets MF, Hanck DA, et al. Sodium current in voltage clamped internally perfused canine Purkinje cells. Biophys J 1987;52:1–11.
56. Welin-Berger K, Neelissen JAM. Engblom J. Physicochemical interaction of local anesthetics with lipid model systems—correlation with in vitro permeation and in vivo efficacy. J Control Release 2002;81:33–43.
57. Feistein MB. Reaction of local anesthetics with phospholipids. A possible chemical basis for anesthesia. J Gen Physiol 1964;48:357–374.
58. Blaustein MP, Goldman DE. Competitive action of calcium and procaine on lobster axon. J Gen Physiol 1966;49:1043–1063.
59. Ritchie JM, Greengard P. On the mode of action of local anesthetics. Annu Rev Pharmacol 1966;6:405–430.
60. Pardo L, Blanck TJJ, Recio-Pinto E. The neuronal lipid membrane permeability was markedly increased by bupivacaine and mildly affected by lidocaine and ropivacaine. Eur J Pharmacol 2002;455:81–90.
61. Tamkun MM, Talvenheimo JA, Catterall WA. The sodium channel from rat brain: reconstitution of neurotoxin-activated ion flux and scorpion toxin binding from purified components. J Biol Chem 1984;259:1676–1688.
62. Butterworth JF IV, Strichartz GR. Molecular mechanisms of local anesthetics: a review. Anesthesiology 1990;72:711–734.
63. Strichartz GR. The inhibition of sodium currents in myelinated nerve by quaternary derivatives of lidocaine. J Gen Physiol 1973;62:37–57.
64. Courtney KR. Mechanism of frequency-dependent inhibition of sodium currents in frog myelinated nerve by the lidocaine derivative GEA 968. J Pharmacol Exp Ther 1975;195:225–236.
65. Narahashi T, Frazier DT. Site of action and active form of local anesthetics. Neurosci Res (NY) 1971;4:65–99.

66. Narahashi T, Yamada M, Frazier DT. Cationic forms of local anesthetics block action potentials from inside the nerve membrane. Nature 1969;223: 748–749.
67. Narahashi T, Frazier DT, Yamada M. The site of action and active form of local anesthetics. I. Theory and pH experiments with tertiary compounds. J Pharmacol Exp Ther 1970;171:32–44.
68. Narahashi T, Frazier DT. Site of action and active form of procaine in squid giant axons. J Pharmacol Exp Ther 1975;194:506–513.
69. Hille B. Mechanisms of blocks. In: Hille B, ed. Ionic Channels of Excitable Membranes. Sunderland, MA: Sinauer Associates, 1984:272–302.
70. Ragsdale DR, McPhee JC, Scheuer T, et al. Molecular determinants of state-dependent block of Na^+ channels by local anesthetics. Science 1994;265:1724–1728.
71. Wang GK, Quan C, Wang SY. Local anesthetic block of batrachotoxin-resistant muscle Na^+ channels. Mol Pharmacol 1998;54:389–396.
72. French RJ, Zamponi GW, Sierralta IE. Molecular and kinetic determinants of local anesthetic action on sodium channels. Toxicol Lett 1998;100–101: 247–254.
73. Scheuer T. A revised view of local anesthetic action: what channel state is really stabilized? J Gen Physiol 1999;113:3–6.
74. Mather LE, Chang DH. Cardiotoxicity with modern local anesthetics. Is there a safer choice? Drugs 2001;61:333–342.
75. Rood JP, Coulthard P, Snowdon AT, et al. Safety and efficacy of levobupivacaine for postoperative pain relief after the surgical removal of impacted third molars: a comparison with lignocaine and adrenaline. Br J Oral Maxillofac Surg 2002;40:491–496.
76. Rutten AJ, Mather LE, McLean CF. Cardiovascular effects and regional clearances of IV bupivacaine in sheep: enantiomeric analysis. Br J Anaesth 1991;67:247–256.
77. Denson DD, Behbehani MM, Gregg RV. Enantiomer-specific effects of an intravenously administered arrhythmogenic dose of bupivacaine on neurons of the nucleus tractus solitarius and the cardiovascular system in the anesthetized rat. Reg Anesth 1992;17:311–316.
78. Rutten AJ, Mather LE, McLean CF, et al. Tissue distribution of bupivacaine enantiomers in sheep. Chirality 1993;5:485–491.
79. Aåkerman SBA, Camougis G, Sandburg RV. Stereoisomerism and differential activity in excitation block by local anesthetics. Eur J Pharmacol 1969;8:337–347.
80. McClure JH. Ropivacaine. Br J Anesth 1996;76:300–307.
81. Markham A, Faulds D. Ropivacaine. A review of its pharmacology and therapeutic use in regional anesthesia. Drugs 1996;52:429–449.
82. Longobardo M, Delpon E, Caballero R, et al. Structural determinants of potency and stereoselective block of hKv1.5 channels induced by local anesthetics. Mol Pharmacol 1998;54:162–169.
83. Franqueza L, Longobardo M, Vicente J, et al. Molecular determinants of stereoselective bupivacaine block of hKv1.5 channels. Circ Res 1997;81:1053–1064.
84. Imaoka S, Enomotl K, Oda Y, et al. Lidocaine metabolism by human cytochrome P-450s purified from hepatic microsomes: comparison of those with rat hepatic cytochrome P-450s. J Pharmacol Exp Ther 1990;255: 1385–1391.
85. Castaneda-Castellanos DR, Nikonorov I, Kallen RG, et al. Lidocaine stabilizes the open state of CNS voltage-dependent sodium channels. Mol Brain Res 2002;99:102–113.
86. Wei X, Dai R, Zhai S, et al. Inhibition of human liver cytochrome P-450 1A2 by the class 1B antiarrhythmics mexiletine, lidocaine, and tocainide. J Pharmacol Exp Ther 1999;289:853–858.
87. Arlander E, Ekstrom G, Alm C, et al. Metabolism of ropivacaine in humans is mediated by CYP1A2 and to a minor extent by CYP3A4: an interaction study with fluvoxamine and ketoconazole as in vivo inhibitors. Clin Pharmacol Ther 1998;64:484–491.

Suggested Readings

Akeson M, Deamer DW. Anesthetics and membranes: a critical review. In: Aloia RC, Curtain CC, Gordon LM, eds. Drug and Anesthetic Effects on Membrane Structure and Function. New York: Wiley-Liss, 1991:71–89.
Arthur GR. Pharmacokinetics of local anesthetics. In: Strichartz GR, ed. Local Anesthetics. Handbook of Experimental Pharmacology. Berlin: Springer, 1987;81:165–186.
Brunton LL, Chabner BA, Knollmann BC. The Pharmacological Basis of Therapeutics, 12th Ed. New York: McGraw Hill, 2011.
Cooper JR, Bloom FE, Roth RH. The Biochemical Basis of Neuropharmacology, 8th Ed. New York: Oxford University Press, 2002.
Courtney KR, Strichartz GR. Structural elements which determine local anesthetic activity. In: Strichartz GR, ed. Local Anesthetics. Handbook of Experimental Pharmacology. Berlin: Springer, 1987;81:53–94.
Covino BG. Local anesthetics. In: Feldman SA, Scurr CF, Paton W, eds. Drugs in Anesthesia: Mechanisms of Action. London: Edward Arnold, 1987:261–291.
Covino BG. Toxicity and systemic effects of local anesthetic agents. In: Strichartz GR, ed. Local Anesthetics. Handbook of Experimental Pharmacology. Berlin: Springer, 1987;81:187–212.
Ezekiel MR. Handbook of Anesthesiology. 2007–2008 Edition. Laguna Hills, CA: CCS Publishing, 2007.
Franks NP. General anaesthesia: from molecular targets to neuronal pathways of sleep and arousal. Nat Rev Neurosci 2008;9:370–386.
Mashour GA, Forman GA, Campagna SA, et al. Mechanisms of general anesthesia: from molecules to mind. Best Pract Res Clin Anesthesiol 2005;19:349–364.
Stoelting RK, Hillier, SC. Pharmacology and Physiology of Anesthetic Practice, 4th Ed. Philadelphia: Lippincott Williams & Wilkins, 2005.
Stoelting RK, Miller RD. Basics of Anesthesia, 5th Ed. Philadelphia: Elsevier Health Sciences, 2007.
Strichartz R, Ritchie JM. The action of local anesthetics on ion channels of excitable tissues. In: Strichartz GR, ed. Local Anesthetics. Handbook of Experimental Pharmacology. Berlin: Springer, 1987;81:21–52.
Tung A. New anesthesia techniques. Thorac Surg Clin 2005;15:27–38.
Vandam LD. Some aspects of the history of local anesthesia. In: Strichartz GR, ed. Local Anesthetics. Handbook of Experimental Pharmacology. Berlin: Springer, 1987;81:1–19.

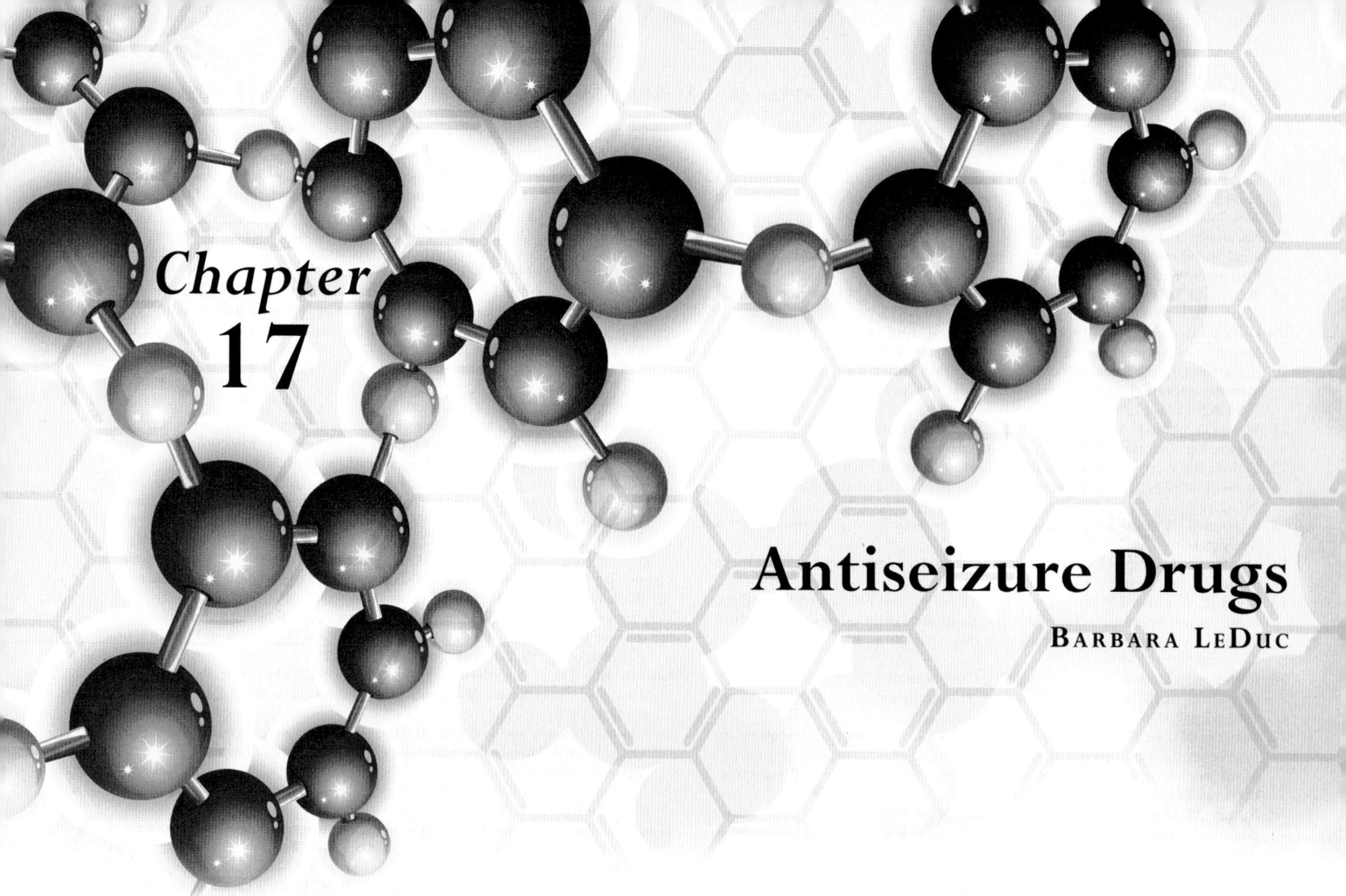

Chapter 17

Antiseizure Drugs

Barbara LeDuc

Drugs Covered in This Chapter

Primary drugs for treatment of seizures
- Carbamazepine
- Clonazepam
- Clorazepate Dipotassium
- Diazepam
- Ethosuximide
- Fosphenytoin
- Lorazepam
- Midazolam
- Phenytoin

Alternative drugs for treatment of seizures
- Ethotoin
- Mephenytoin
- Mephobarbital
- Methsuximide
- Phenobarbital
- Phensuximide
- Primidone

Adjunct drugs for treatment of seizures
- Dimethadione
- Ezogabine
- Felbamate
- Gabapentin
- Lacosamide
- Lamotrigine
- *S*-(−)-Levetiracetam
- Oxcarbazepine
- Pregabalin
- Rufinamide
- Tiagabine
- Topiramate
- Trimethadione
- Valproic acid
- Vigabatrin
- Zonisamide

Abbreviations

ABC, adenosine triphosphate binding cassette
AED, antiepileptic drug
AMPA, L-α-amino-3-hydroxy-5-methyl-4-isoxazole propionate
AUC, area under the curve
CBMA, 3-carbamoyl-2-phenylpropionaldehyde
CBZ, carbamazepine
C_{max}, maximum plasma concentration
CNS, central nervous system
C_{ss}, steady-state plasma concentration
CRMP-2, collapsin-response mediator protein 2
D5W, 5% dextrose in water
EEG, electroencephalography
FDA, U.S. Food and Drug Administration
GABA, γ-aminobutyric acid
GAT1, GABA transporter 1
HPPH, 5-(4′-hydroxyphenyl)-5-phenylhydantoin
IM, intramuscular
IV, intravenous
KA, kainate
MES, maximal electroshock
MHD, 10-monohydroxycarbazepine
NMDA, *N*-methyl-D-aspartate
2-OHIS, 2-hydroxyiminostilbene
PEMA, phenylethylmalonamide
UGT, uridine diphosphoglucuronosyltransferase
V_d, volume of distribution

SCENARIO

Michael Gonyeau, PharmD

BG is a 70-year-old white woman who has been admitted to your hospital after having a tonic clonic seizure at home, which was witnessed by her husband, who states that BG has been complaining of 5 days of nausea and vomiting, has seemed more confused, and has had problems walking (she almost fell down the stairs twice in the past 2 days). Her medical history is significant for seizure disorder, hypertension, end-stage renal disease on hemodialysis, and coronary artery disease. She has no known allergies and currently takes the following medications: phenytoin 300 mg XL po once daily, lisinopril 10 mg po daily, and atorvastatin 20 mg po daily. Notable laboratory data include reduced renal function (creatinine clearance, 39 mL/min), albumin 1.5 mg/dL, and phenytoin level 9 mcg/mL (therapeutic goal, 10–20 mcg/mL). Based on the patient's recent seizure and the subtherapeutic phenytoin level, the admitting physician gives a 500 mg po bolus dose of phenytoin, increases the daily dose to 400 mg XL po daily, asks the pharmacist for any further recommendations.

(The reader is directed to the clinical solution and chemical analysis of this case at the end of the chapter).

INTRODUCTION

As early as 2000 BC, it was recognized that some people suffered from convulsive seizures. The term "epilepsy," based on the Greek word *epilambanein* (meaning "to seize"), was first used by Hippocrates. In the world's first scientific monograph on epilepsy, entitled *On the Sacred Disease* (~400 BC), Hippocrates disputed the myth that the cause of epilepsy is supernatural and the cure magic. He described epilepsy as a disease of the brain, which should be treated by diet. At the same time, Hippocrates provided the first classification of epilepsy, which is still used. He distinguished true (idiopathic) epilepsy (i.e., a disorder for which the cause is unknown) from symptomatic (organic) epilepsy (i.e., a disorder resulting from a physiologic abnormality, e.g., brain injury, tumor, infection, intoxication, or metabolic disturbances).

Two opinions were put forward as to the causes of epilepsy. One was that epilepsy is a single disease entity and all forms of it have a common cause. On the other hand, it was proposed that different types of epilepsy result from different chemical, anatomic, or functional disorders. At the Symposium on Evaluation of Drug Therapy in Neurologic and Sensory Disease, the general opinion was that "epilepsy is a symptom complex characterized by recurrent paroxysmal aberrations of brain functions, usually brief and self-limited" (1).

All forms of epilepsy originate in the brain and appear to be the result of changes in neuronal activity. In turn, these changes, such as an excessive neuronal discharge, can be brought about by a disturbance of physicochemical function and electrical activity of the brain. However, the cause of this abnormality is not clearly understood.

The most important property of the nerve cell is its excitability. It responds to excitation by generating an action potential, which can lead to repeated discharges. All normal neurons can become epileptic if subjected to excessive excitation. DeRobertis et al. (2) list two possible mechanisms for convulsive disorders: a loss of the normal inhibitory control mechanism, and a chemical supersensitivity that increases excitability of neuronal elements.

The origin of the seizures was established as early as the 19th century by Jackson (3). According to him, an intense discharge of gray matter in various regions of the brain initiates the seizures. As a result, it is only a normal reaction of the brain to initiate convulsive seizures. The discharge of excessive electrical (nervous) energy has, indeed, been substantiated by brain-wave studies made possible by electroencephalography (EEG).

Attempts to classify epileptic seizures have been only partially successful, primarily due to limited knowledge regarding the pathologic processes of the brain. At the turn of the century, a classification of seizures had been published (4), and even more attempts appeared during the 1950s and 1960s (5–9). In 1981, the Commission on Classification and Terminology of the International League Against Epilepsy put forward a new proposal (10). The classification outlined in Table 17.1 is a short version of this proposal, which is based on clinical seizure type, ictal (seizure-induced) EEG expression, and interictal (occurring between attacks or paroxysms) EEG expression.

SEIZURE CLASSIFICATION

Seizures result from the sudden, excessive firing of neurons. They are broadly classified as either partial seizures, in which the abnormal firing initially occurs in a small number of neurons but can spread to adjacent areas, or generalized seizures, in which virtually the entire brain is affected simultaneously (11). Seizures can be characterized by clinical symptoms and by EEG patterns. In addition, computed tomography and magnetic resonance imaging of the head are used in virtually all patients with suspected epilepsy to aid in identifying the seizure type.

Partial (Local, Focal) Seizures

Partial seizures are divided into three categories: simple partial, complex partial, and partial progressing to generalized seizures. The key distinction between simple and complex partial seizures is the level of consciousness of the person undergoing the seizure. In partial seizures, the initial

TABLE 17.1 Classification of Epileptic Seizures

Classification	Subtypes
Partial (local, focal) seizures	Simple (consciousness not impaired)
	Complex partial seizures (psychomotor seizures) 1. Beginning as simple partial seizures, progressing to complex seizures 2. With impairment of consciousness at onset
	Partial seizures evolving to secondarily generalized tonic-clonic convulsions
Generalized seizures (convulsive or nonconvulsive)	Absence seizures: typical (petit mal) and atypical
	Myoclonic
	Clonic
	Tonic
	Tonic-clonic (grand mal)
	Atonic
Unclassified epileptic seizures (includes some neonatal seizures)	

neuronal discharge originates from a specific, limited cortical area, which is termed a "focus." Development of the focus is thought to be caused by scarring after head trauma, infection, or oxygen deprivation. The abnormal EEG seizure patterns are restricted to one region of the brain, at least at the onset. These types of seizures are possible at all ages but are most frequent in the elderly. Partial seizures respond fairly well to antiseizure drugs (most commonly referred to as antiepileptic drugs [AEDs]) (Fig. 17.1) (12).

Medications to combat partial seizures are effective against secondary or generalized tonic-clonic seizures as well. These seizures respond well to carbamazepine, hydantoins, and barbiturates, although this latter group unfortunately displays substantial sedative effects. The newer AEDs (gabapentin, lamotrigine, levetiracetam, oxcarbazepine, tiagabine, topiramate, and zonisamide) are useful for either monotherapy or as adjunctive drugs. On the other hand, oxazolidinediones and succinimides are ineffective in the treatment of partial seizures. Valproate is appropriate when tonic-clonic seizures are combined with either myoclonic or absence seizures.

Simple Partial Seizures

The specific symptoms displayed during a simple partial seizure will depend on the area of the brain that is affected, and they will occur on the opposite side of

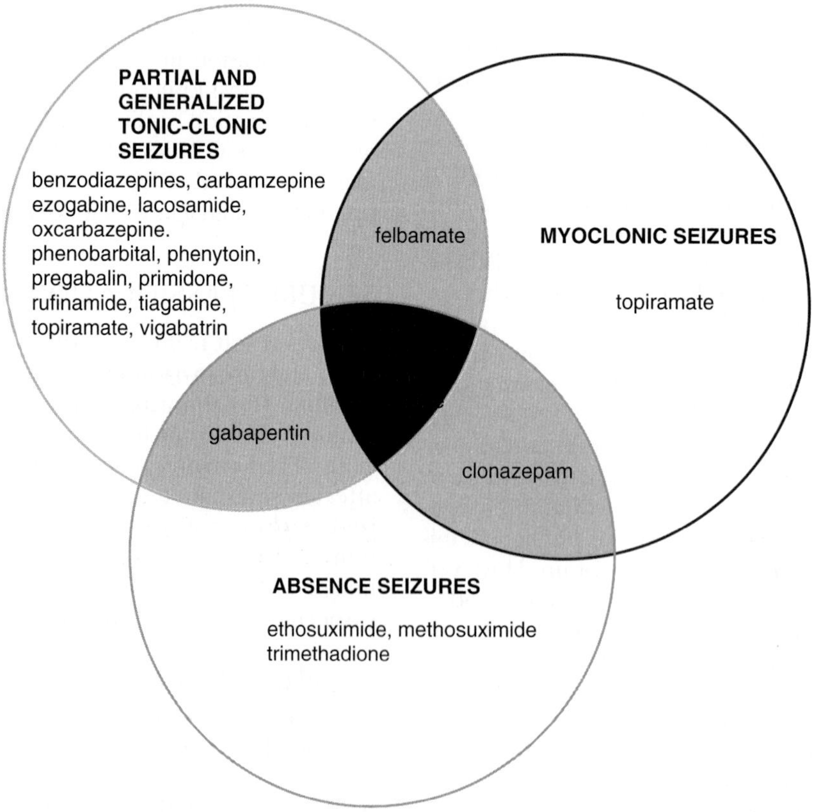

FIGURE 17.1 The antiseizure drugs used in treatment of the various seizures.

CLINICAL SIGNIFICANCE

Seizure disorders can be devastating to a patient's quality of life. Experiencing a seizure is associated with a loss of control of both the body as well as one's control of life events. The unpredictable nature of seizure occurrence and the resultant fear of recurrence can have a significantly negative effect on quality of life. Restrictions placed on patients with epilepsy include revocation of driver's licenses, potential physical limitations, work absenteeism, and various emotional and mental issues related to the disease and to side effects of many antiepileptic medications. Some of these factors may in turn result in poor adherence to antiepileptic medications, which is associated with increased mortality and morbidity; side effects of antiepileptic drugs are attributed to almost half of all recorded treatment failures.

Medicinal chemistry plays a vital role in the understanding of epilepsy, particularly in its treatment. Molecular agents used to treat seizures exert varying effects on neuronal function through their structure-activity relationships and chemical interactions with ion channels (carbamazepine, phenytoin, ethosuximide, zonisamide) and their similarities to naturally occurring neurotransmitters, such as GABAs (benzodiazepines, barbiturates, topiramate, gabapentin, tiagabine). They can directly affect ion channels or indirectly influence synthesis, metabolism, or function of neurotransmitters or receptors that control channel opening and closing.

Many patients cannot be controlled on monotherapy, and a significant number of patients will require drug combinations. Freedom from seizures can be achieved by combining drugs with different or overlapping or similar mechanisms of action to attain synergy in an individual patient. There have been a number of newer antiepileptic drugs approved since 1993, and a solid understanding of basic chemical principles of antiseizure drugs is critical in making appropriate clinical recommendations. The pharmacokinetics of antiseizure medications are very complex and require a strong foundational knowledge base rooted in medicinal chemistry. Monitoring side effects—specifically the multitude of drug interactions associated with these agents—is extremely important to ensure patient safety and efficacy in the clinical setting, with the ultimate goal to keep patients seizure free and maintain their quality of life.

Improved understanding of the medicinal chemistry aspects of antiepileptic drugs, as well as mechanisms of action and pharmacokinetics, will help the clinician make a rational choice of agent based on knowledge about which is most effective against each type of seizure as well as minimize adverse effects and drug interactions and improve patients' quality of life.

Michael Gonyeau PharmD
Associate Clinical Professor
Northeastern University
Department of Pharmacy Practice
Bouvé College of Health Sciences
Boston, Massachusetts

the body from the lesion. Combinations of symptoms are frequent, making accurate diagnosis a challenge. The temporal lobes are the most common origination site for partial seizures. Seizure foci located within the temporal lobe result in psychic symptoms, such as fear, panic, or hallucinations; autonomic signs, such as flushing and sweating; or unpleasant smells or tastes. Frontal lobe foci usually present with motor symptoms. Focal motor attacks most commonly start in one hand, one foot, or one side of the face. Often, however, the onset of focal seizures is not specific. Should the focal motor seizures spread to contiguous cortical areas, there can be an orderly sequence of repeated events (movement of hands, face, and legs) known as an epileptic march. This type of seizure is termed a "jacksonian seizure." If the unilateral movements characteristic of focal motor or jacksonian seizures steadily spread to the other half of the body, a generalized seizure can follow. In contrast, seizures beginning in the parietal lobes are termed "sensory seizures" and present with altered sensations, tingling, numbness, or pain. Foci in the occipital lobes produce nystagmus, blinking, or visual disturbances, such as flashing lights or the appearance of strange colors.

In simple partial seizures, the patient's consciousness is not impaired. Thus, the person remains able to respond to simple commands, perform simple deliberate movements, and recall events that occurred during the seizure.

Complex Partial Seizures

When consciousness is impaired, the seizure is classified as a complex partial seizure. Impaired consciousness will be manifested by the person's staring, inability to respond to simple commands, inaccurate recall, or amnesia of events occurring during the seizure. Clouding of consciousness can be apparent initially or can appear subsequent to the start of a simple partial seizure. With the exception of the mental status, the other symptoms of complex partial seizures are similar to those outlined earlier. Many complex seizures have bilateral hemispheric involvement and frequently are accompanied by automatisms (i.e., repetitive involuntary movements, including chewing, swallowing, or wringing the hands).

Partial Seizures Evolving to Secondarily Generalized Seizures

The abnormal electrical activity responsible for any type of partial seizure can generalize throughout the brain, thus evolving into a secondary generalized tonic-clonic seizure. The diagnosis of partial seizures is therefore difficult to establish. The generalization can occur rapidly, or it can occur slowly enough that the symptoms of the partial seizure are experienced by the patient as an "aura" before the generalized tonic-clonic phase. Auras are comprised of symptoms such as seeing blinking lights or hearing unusual sounds, and they serve as an important warning for the patient. The symptoms of tonic-clonic seizures are described below.

Generalized Seizures (Convulsive or Nonconvulsive)

These disorders are generalized from the outset, and they show simultaneous involvement of both cerebral hemispheres and loss of consciousness. It is not possible to single out one anatomic or functional system in one hemisphere of the brain that is responsible for the clinical symptoms. The initial neuronal discharge spreads quickly into the entire gray matter or at least the greater part of the gray matter. The EEG pattern consists of bilateral, essentially synchronous and symmetric discharges from the start and indicates the widespread nature of neuronal discharge. The cause is rarely known, but it is usually attributed to diffuse lesions, to toxic and metabolic disturbances, or to constitutional genetic factors. People of all ages are affected by generalized convulsions. There are several classes of generalized seizures, and useful drugs are selected according to the seizure type that transpires (Fig. 17.1).

Absence (Petit Mal) Seizures

Both typical and atypical absence seizures bring about brief loss of consciousness. Typical absence seizures have a rapid onset and cessation, which can cause them to be misinterpreted as daydreaming; however, the person cannot be alerted or awakened during the seizures. Absence seizures often begin with a change in facial expression, which is followed by a period of motionless, blank staring. After the brief interruption in consciousness (typically ~10 seconds), the activity that was in progress before the seizure is resumed. The individuals have neither memory of events during the seizure nor postictal confusion. Typical absence seizures (petit mal) are more common in children than in adults. They are particularly disabling because they tend to occur many times daily. Most children will respond to drug treatment, but a small percentage will go on to develop generalized tonic-clonic seizures as adults. Complex typical absence seizures can include additional phenomena, such as clonic or myoclonic motions, automatisms, or more elaborate behaviors. Between 25% and 40% of affected children have a family history of absence seizures.

Atypical absence seizures have a slower onset and cessation, and they last longer (up to several minutes) than typical absence seizures. They can include clonic motions, automatisms, or autonomic symptoms. Differential diagnosis between these types is made on the basis of the EEG. Typical absence seizures display a 3-Hz spike-and-wave EEG pattern, but the pattern of atypical absence seizures is slower, usually in the range of 1.5 to 2.5 Hz.

Both forms of absence seizure often occur as part of one of the recognized epilepsy syndromes. Typical absence seizures respond fairly well to AEDs; ethosuximide and valproate are first-choice drugs. Clonazepam is effective but sedating, and tolerance to the antiabsence effects can develop. Lamotrigine can be useful. Treatment of atypical absence seizures with AEDs is less successful.

Lennox-Gastaut syndrome is a mixed seizure disorder combining the atypical absence seizures with tonic, tonic-clonic, or myoclonic motor patterns. The syndrome begins in childhood and usually includes mental retardation. Although adequate control of the seizures is rarely achieved, valproate, phenytoin, felbamate, lamotrigine, topiramate, and clonazepam have been useful.

Myoclonic Seizures

Myoclonic seizures consist of sudden, very brief, jerking contractions that can involve the entire body or be confined to limited areas, such as the face and neck. The contractions can affect individual muscles or groups, with simultaneous contraction of both extensor and flexor muscles. These seizures occur in all age groups, with symptoms ranging from rapid tremors to falling down. No loss of consciousness is detectable due to the brief duration of the seizure. Myoclonic seizures often occur in combination with other seizure types. Valproate and clonazepam are used most often to treat myoclonic seizures; lamotrigine and topiramate also have shown some efficacy.

Tonic Seizures

Tonic seizures occur mostly in children and are characterized by increased tone in extensor muscles, resulting in falling to the ground. Although brief, the duration of contractions is somewhat longer than in myoclonic seizures. Vocalization can occur as a result of contraction of thoracic muscles, forcing air past the larynx. Brief periods of apnea and postictal tiredness can be associated.

Atonic Seizures

In atonic seizures, a very sudden decrease in muscle tone occurs, leading to a head drop, drooping of a limb, or loss of all muscle tone, resulting in falling. The risk of injury is high in these sudden "drop attacks." Atonic seizures are more common in children.

Attaining good control of tonic or atonic seizures is difficult. Valproate, felbamate, lamotrigine, benzodiazepines, and topiramate have proven to be effective in some individuals.

Clonic Seizures

Clonic seizures nearly always occur in babies or young children. A loss or impairment of consciousness occurs simultaneously with a decrease in muscle tone or with a generalized tonic contraction, and it is followed by period of asymmetric jerking motions.

Tonic-Clonic (Grand Mal) Seizures

Generalized tonic-clonic seizures represent a maximal epileptic response of the brain. These seizures are characterized by the absence of an aura and by tonic stiffening of all muscle groups, causing the patient to fall. The initial contraction can be flexor and is rapidly followed by prolonged extension. Subsequently, there is a period of bilateral symmetric jerking of the extremities. The seizure can be associated with loss of bladder control and biting of the tongue or inside of the mouth. There is a pronounced postictal state (altered state of consciousness lasting from 5–30 minutes) following the seizure, and the person can pass directly into sleep before waking several hours later.

Status Epilepticus

Status epilepticus is a condition in which there is a single prolonged seizure lasting more than 5 minutes or in which there is insufficient time between multiple seizures to permit recovery. Several types exist, depending on the type of seizure involved (i.e., tonic-clonic, simple partial, complex partial, or absence). Tonic-clonic status epilepticus is both the most common and the most life-threatening. Pharmacologic treatment of most forms of status epilepticus can include intravenous (IV) administration of diazepam or lorazepam, fosphenytoin, and phenobarbital. Although lorazepam is not approved by the U.S. Food and Drug Administration (FDA) for this purpose, it sometimes is preferred due to its longer half-life.

Absence status epilepticus is a condition of impaired consciousness, perhaps including mild motor symptoms, that lasts from 30 minutes to 12 hours. It can be distinguished from ongoing seizures as a result of organic or toxic causes by the spike-and-wave EEG pattern that is characteristic of absence seizures. The usual pharmacologic treatment of absence status uses diazepam or lorazepam, followed by ethosuximide.

MECHANISMS OF ACTION FOR THE ANTISEIZURE DRUGS

Seizures result from bursts of abnormal synchronous discharging by a network of neurons. Although the mechanisms of seizure generation are still poorly understood, the causes of abnormal firing appear to involve neuronal ion channels and an imbalance between excitatory and inhibitory synaptic function. Various AEDs exhibit different mechanisms of action on neuronal function, causing them to show selective efficacy against different seizure types (13) (Fig. 17.2).

Ion Channels

Sodium and chloride ions are present at greater concentration outside the cell, whereas potassium, organic cations, and charged proteins are more numerous within the cell. Because the membrane is permeable only to small ions and not large ions or proteins, the neuronal membranes maintain a charge separation, resulting in a "resting potential" in the range of −50 to −80 mV versus the outside of the cell.

An increase in interior negativity, termed "hyperpolarization," decreases the resting potential (e.g., to −90 mV), thus making it more difficult for a neuron to reach threshold and subsequently fire. A reduction in interior negativity, termed "depolarization," can result in generation of an action potential if the depolarization is sufficient to reach threshold (approximately −40 mV). Neuronal firing is initiated by an influx of sodium ions.

After each depolarization, voltage-dependent sodium channels adopt an inactive state and remain refractory to reopening for a period of time. While those channels are unable to open, rapid repetitive firing is diminished, and spread of electrical seizure activity to adjacent brain regions is suppressed (14). Stabilization and prolongation of this inactive state appears to be the primary mechanism of action of phenytoin, carbamazepine, and lamotrigine and can be instrumental in the antiseizure actions of phenobarbital, oxcarbazepine, valproate, topiramate, and zonisamide (Fig. 17.2).

Alterations in the structure or function of an ion channel caused by mutations in a gene encoding one of the channel's subunits are termed "channelopathies." Initially, these abnormalities were associated with cardiac and muscular disorders, but today, it is recognized that channelopathies are responsible for several forms of epilepsy (15,16). Presently, most of the discovered channel mutations appear to be associated with the development of idiopathic generalized epilepsy; most partial seizures are believed to be acquired. Minor alterations in gene structure or expression, however, can predispose a given individual to partial seizures. It is estimated that 40% of adult and childhood epilepsy can result from genetic factors.

Mutations in sodium and potassium channels are most common, because they give rise to hyperexcitability and burst firing. Mutations in the sodium channel subunit gene *SCN2A1* have been associated with benign familial neonatal epilepsy, mutations in *SCN1A* have been associated with severe myoclonic epilepsy of infancy, and mutations in *SCN1A* and *SCN1B* have been associated with generalized epilepsy with febrile seizures. Mutation of the *SCN1B* gene has been shown to reduce the channel's response to phenytoin (17). The potassium channel genes *KCNQ2* and *KCNQ3* are implicated in some cases of benign familial neonatal epilepsy. Chloride channels have been implicated as well. Mutations of the *CLCN2* gene have been found to be altered in several cases of classical idiopathic generalized epilepsy subtypes: childhood and juvenile absence epilepsy, juvenile myoclonic epilepsy, and epilepsy with grand mal on awakening. Mutations of γ-aminobutyric acid (GABA) A receptor ($GABA_A$) subunits also have been detected. The gene encoding the α_1 subunit, *GABRG1*, has been linked to juvenile myoclonic epilepsy; mutated *GABRG2*, encoding an abnormal γ subunit, has been associated with generalized epilepsy with febrile seizures and childhood absence epilepsy. Lastly, mutations of calcium channel subunits have been

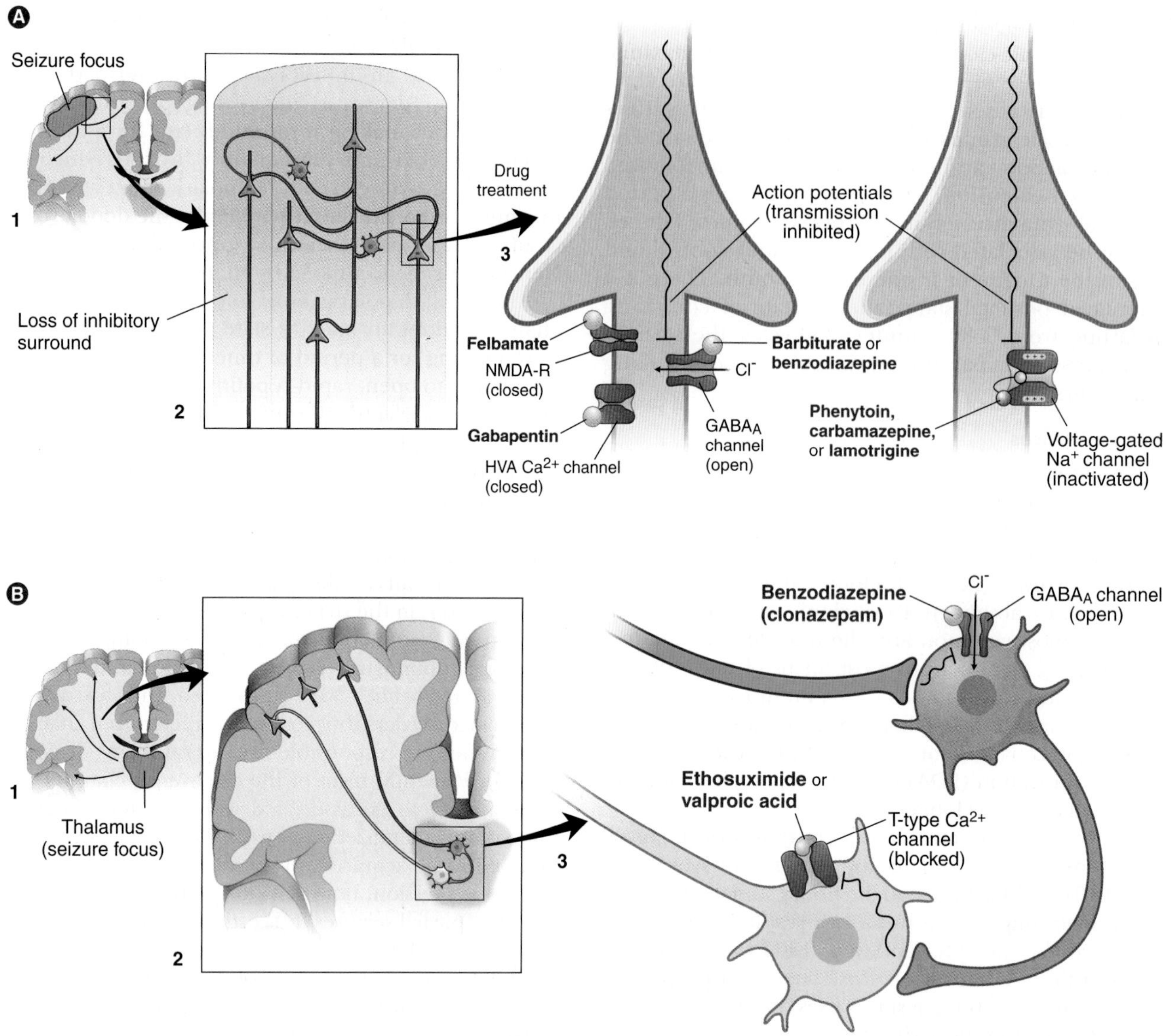

FIGURE 17.2 Mechanisms of antiseizure drugs. (A) Drugs for partial seizures: 1) Seizure activity spreads due to loss of surround inhibition; 2) drugs act in the surrounding region to 3) enhance γ-aminobutyric acid (GABA) inhibition or prolong Na^+ channel inactivation. (B) Drugs for absence seizures: 1) The seizure activity results from cyclic activity between the thalamus and the cortex; 2) drugs prevent synchronization by either 3) deactivating the inhibitory reticular neurons and decreasing hyperpolarization of the thalamic relay neurons or blocking T-type Ca^{2+} channels to prevent burst firing by the thalamic relay neurons. (From Griffin EA Jr, Lowenstein DH. Pharmacology of abnormal electrical neurotransmission in the central nervous system. In: Golan DE, Tashjian A, Armstrong E, et al., eds. Principles of Pharmacology: The Pathophysiologic Basis of Drug Therapy, 2nd Ed. Baltimore: Lippincott Williams & Wilkins, 2008, pp. 225–236, with permission.)

identified in juvenile absence epilepsy (mutation in *CACNB4*; the B4 subunit of the L-type calcium channel) and idiopathic generalized epilepsy (*CACN1A1*) (15,16).

Synaptic Inhibition and Excitation

For a neuron, whether an action potential is generated depends on the balance between excitatory and inhibitory stimulation. The predominant inhibitory neurotransmitter in the brain is GABA. It is synthesized from an amino acid, glutamic acid, by glutamic acid decarboxylase and is inactivated by GABA-transaminase. GABA binds to two receptor types, $GABA_A$ and $GABA_B$. $GABA_A$ receptors occur on chloride ion channels, and the binding of GABA causes chloride influx and neuronal hyperpolarization. $GABA_B$ receptors are linked via G proteins and second messengers to potassium and calcium channel activity, also mediating inhibition in the central nervous system (CNS). $GABA_B$ receptors also can have a role in oscillatory rhythms in some forms of epilepsy (18) (Fig. 17.3).

A number of AEDs augment GABA-mediated inhibition or affect GABA concentration. Benzodiazepines,

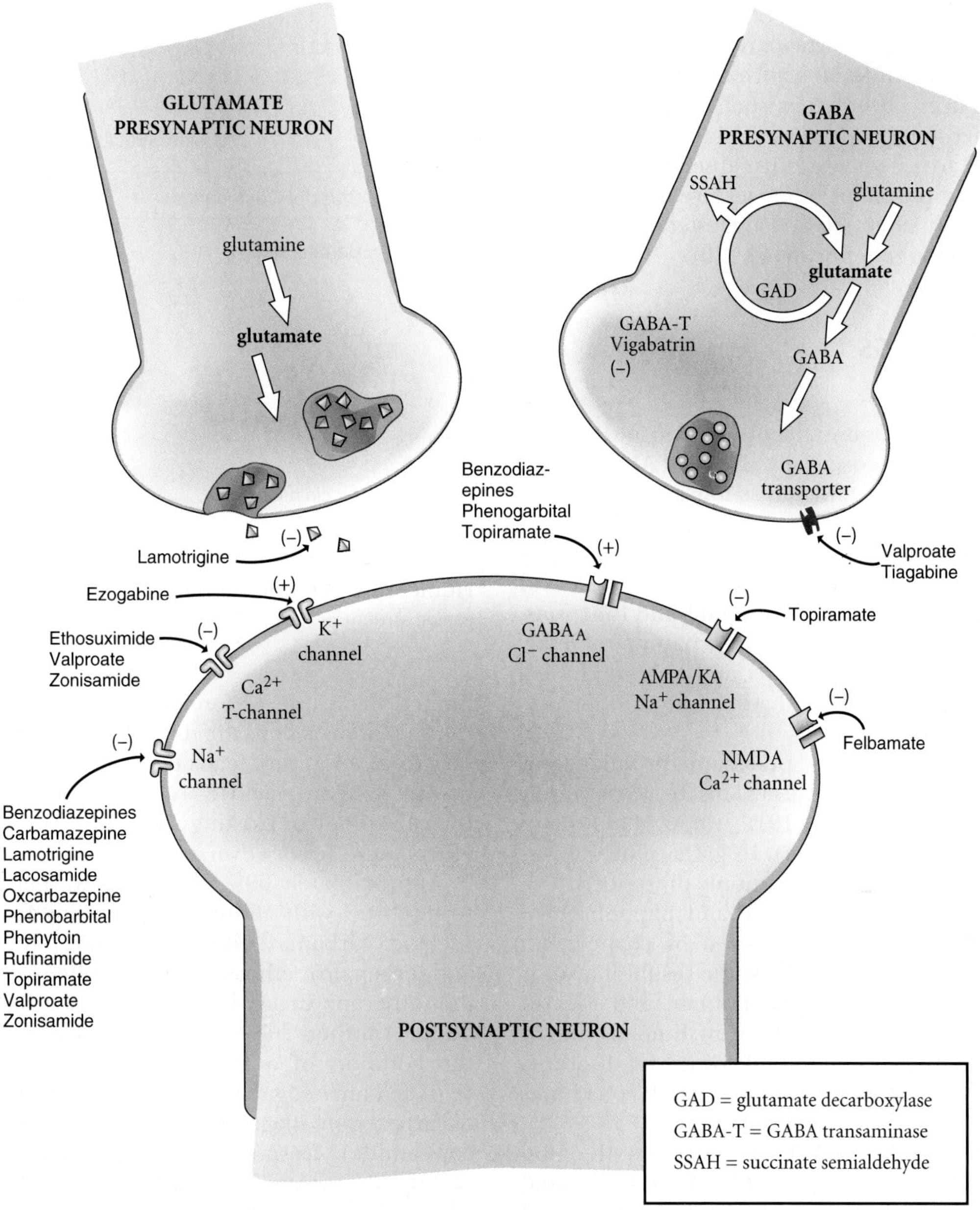

FIGURE 17.3 A summary of the sites of action for the antiepileptic drugs (Adapted from Taylor CP. Mechanisms of new antiepileptic drugs. In: Delgado-Escueta AV, Wilson WA, Olsen RW, et al., eds. Jasper's Basic Mechanisms of the Epilepsies, 3rd Ed. (Advances in Neurology, Vol 79.) Philadelphia: Lippincott Williams & Wilkins, 1999:1012–1027, with permission.)

barbiturates, and perhaps topiramate enhance the action of GABA on the $GABA_A$ chloride channel. Tiagabine decreases the reuptake of GABA, and perhaps, gabapentin decreases its metabolism.

The ionotropic neurotransmitter glutamate provides excitatory neurotransmission via two types of receptors, the *N*-methyl-D-aspartate (NMDA) and L-α-amino-3-hydroxy-5-methyl-4-isoxazole propionate (AMPA) and kainate (KA) receptors (see Chapter 12). NMDA, AMPA, and KA are specific agonists for these receptors that are used in experiments to distinguish the glutamate ionotropic receptors.

Activation of these ligand-gated channels enables sodium and calcium influx and potassium efflux, facilitating depolarization. Blockade of the NMDA receptor by felbamate or of the AMPA/KA receptor by phenobarbital and topiramate inhibits depolarization (Fig. 17.3).

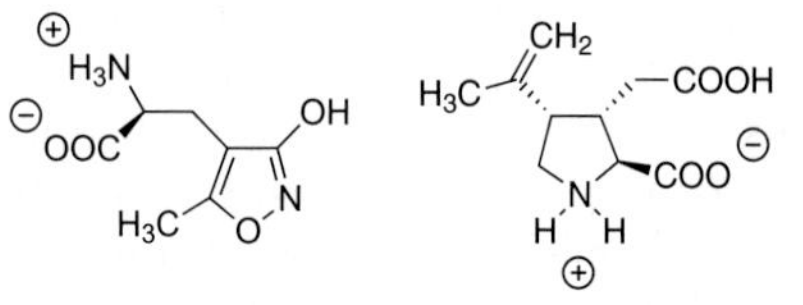

AMPA Kainate

Low-threshold T-type calcium currents act as pacemakers for normal brain activity, particularly the thalamic oscillatory currents thought to be involved in the generation of absence seizures (19). Drugs such as ethosuximide, the oxazolidinediones, and zonisamide, which inhibit T-type currents, are effective against absence seizures but ineffective against partial or other seizure types. In addition, Kv7 potassium channels are suggested as the site of action of certain antiepileptic drugs (20).

ANTISEIZURE DRUGS

Introduction

The primary use of AEDs is in the prevention and control of epileptic seizures. Theoretically, the ideal AED should, among other things, completely suppress seizures in doses that do not cause sedation or other undesired CNS toxicity. The AED should be well tolerated and highly effective against various types of seizures and be devoid of undesirable side effects on vital organs and functions. Its onset of action should be rapid after parenteral injection for control of status epilepticus, and it should have a long duration of effect after oral administration for prevention of recurrent seizures.

The first effective remedy, potassium bromide, was introduced by Locock in 1857 (21). This drug was largely replaced by phenobarbital in 1912, when Hauptmann tried this sedative in epilepsy (22). Its great value was recognized at once, and it is still commonly prescribed.

The usefulness of both bromide and phenobarbital in convulsive disorders was discovered by chance, but phenytoin was developed in 1937 as the result of a study of potential AEDs in animals by Putnam and Merritt (23,24). Bromide is highly effective in humans and is relatively nonsedating. Treatment of convulsive disorders using bromide, phenobarbital, and phenytoin constitutes an important advance in clinical therapy.

Many of the standard AEDs that contain the ureide structure, as shown in Figure 17.4, have been used clinically for more than 30 years without much change in their ureide structures. Small changes in the X substituent of the ureide structure can cause significant changes in the type of seizures controlled, which will be discussed for each of the respective drugs. As a result of rapid developments in molecular biologic techniques for the study of the neurophysiology of epilepsy and in the interactions of AEDs with neurotransmitters at ion channels or brain receptors (AMPA/KA glutamate receptors), a new generation of clinically available AEDs has emerged. These AEDs include felbamate, gabapentin, lamotrigine, levetiracetam, oxcarbazepine, tiagabine, topiramate, and zonisamide. Their mechanisms of action are targeted toward ion channels and brain receptors either by enhancing brain GABA activity (e.g., tiagabine) or by inhibiting excitatory amino acids (L-Glu; e.g., lamotrigine and felbamate) (Fig. 17.2). These new-generation AEDs also exhibit

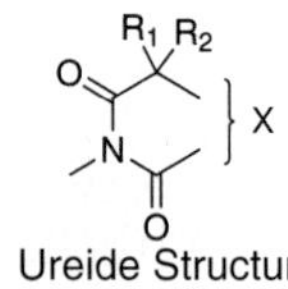

Ureide Structure

Class of Compounds	X
Barbiturates	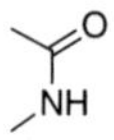
Hydantoins	
Oxazolidinediones	
Succinimides	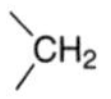

FIGURE 17.4 Structure of anticonvulsant drugs containing the ureide structure.

limited drug interactions with fewer adverse effects. A rational approach to the drug discovery process is necessary to develop new leads to novel effective therapy and to use structure–activity relationships to fine-tune the pharmacology of existing AEDs with the same or better efficacy and fewer adverse effects (25).

Approximately 60% of patients with epilepsy become seizure-free with monotherapy using frontline drugs, such as carbamazepine, benzodiazepine (clonazepam and diazepam), ethosuximide, or phenytoin. Alternative monotherapy drugs include phenobarbital and primidone. Another 20% have their epilepsy controlled by the addition of a second AED called adjunct drugs (e.g., felbamate, gabapentin, lamotrigine, levetiracetam, oxcarbazepine, tiagabine, topiramate, valproic acid, and zonisamide). Despite recent advances in neurobiology and significant insight regarding the molecular dysfunction of epilepsy, the remaining 20% do not completely respond to the current frontline therapeutic drugs and most often are prescribed more than two AEDs without any obvious benefit (11). Recently, much effort has been made to discover new AEDs effective in refractory seizures and partial complex seizures.

Seizure control requires continuous antiseizure action and is not achievable unless plasma concentrations remain relatively consistent at therapeutic levels throughout all 24 hours of the day. Therefore, a knowledge of the therapeutic ranges of plasma concentrations, time to peak serum concentrations, and elimination half-lives helps to guide AED administration to achieve consistent therapeutic serum concentrations that control seizures without causing intolerable toxicity (26). Enzymatic biotransformation is the principal determinant of the pharmacokinetic properties for most AEDs, although some drugs are excreted by the kidneys predominantly as unchanged drug. Most AEDs exhibit linear enzyme kinetics, in which changes in daily dose lead to proportional changes in serum concentration if clearance remains constant. The traditional concept of administering a drug at intervals equal to one elimination half-life, however, does not apply to some drugs, in which the half-life of biologic activity can exceed its elimination half-life. The standard AEDs have the greatest potential to be involved in pharmacokinetic drug interactions when they are coadministered with other AEDs or other drugs (27). These interactions usually involve changes in the rate of biotransformation or in the protein binding of one or both coadministered drugs (26). Drug-induced changes in the pharmacokinetics for many of the AEDs are particularly pronounced in children, requiring a higher oral dose per kilogram body weight than in adults to obtain an effective plasma concentration (28).

This chapter surveys the structure–activity relationship, mechanism of action, metabolism, and pharmacokinetic parameters for the new generation of AEDs (felbamate, gabapentin, lamotrigine, oxcarbazepine, levetiracetam, tiagabine, topiramate, zonisamide, and vigabatrin) and the standard AEDs (phenytoin, carbamazepine, phenobarbital, primidone, valproate, ethosuximide, and the benzodiazepines) as well as for several of the older AEDs that are less commonly used today. The application of AEDs in the treatment of various kinds of epilepsies is shown in Figure 17.1; this illustration is based on AEDs used in clinical therapy. Table 17.2 lists the AEDs, their mechanisms of action, and some of the pharmacokinetic properties.

Drugs Effective against Partial and Generalized Tonic-Clonic Seizures

Hydantoins

The hydantoins have a five-membered ring structure containing two nitrogens in an ureide configuration (Fig. 17.4) and were tested as antiepileptics by Merritt and Putnam (23,24). These drugs suppressed electrically induced convulsions in animals but were ineffective against convulsions induced by pentylenetetrazole, picrotoxin, or bicuculline. The structures for the clinically available hydantoins are listed in Figure 17.5.

PHENYTOIN (DIPHENYLHYDANTOIN) Phenytoin is the prototype and most commonly prescribed member of the hydantoin family of drugs. Bioequivalency is a problem with the hydantoins as a result of their very poor water solubility (~32 mg/L) and low therapeutic ratio. Phenytoin exhibits nonlinear pharmacokinetics that exaggerate the effects of changes in the fraction of dose absorbed. Its apparent pK_a is in the range of 8.06 to 8.33 and, thus, can form a water-soluble sodium salt (~15 mg/mL at solution pH > 11). Aqueous solutions of phenytoin sodium (pH 11 to 12) gradually absorb carbon dioxide, neutralizing the alkalinity of the solution and causing partial hydrolysis and crystallization of free phenytoin resulting in turbid solutions. When phenytoin sodium is administered intramuscularly (IM), its absorption can be erratic as a result of crystallization of insoluble phenytoin at the injection site due to the decrease in pH from 11.5. Phenytoin sodium injection is physically and chemically incompatible in 5% dextrose in water (D5W), normal saline, or with parenteral solutions of many drugs, especially salts of basic drugs. The nature of the incompatibility depends on several factors, including the type of salt, concentrations of the drugs, diluents used, resulting pH of the final admixture (must be pH > 11), and temperature. Phenytoin sodium capsules also will absorb carbon dioxide over time, resulting in the formation of free phenytoin with a different dissolution profile.

Mechanism of Action Phenytoin is indicated for initial monotherapy or adjunct treatment of complex partial or tonic-clonic seizures, convulsive status epilepticus, and prophylaxis. It often is selected for initial monotherapy due to its high efficacy and relatively low incidence of side effects (29). Phenytoin is not used in the treatment of absence seizures, because it can increase their frequency of occurrence (30). Phenytoin binds to and stabilizes the inactivated state of sodium channels, thus producing a use-dependent blockade of repetitive firing and inhibition of the spread of seizure activity to adjacent cortical areas (31).

Pharmacokinetics Phenytoin sodium from immediate-release capsules is rapidly absorbed and generally attains peak serum concentration in 1.5 to 3.0 hours; extended-release phenytoin sodium is absorbed more slowly, attaining peak serum concentration in 4 to 12 hours. The oral bioavailability for sodium phenytoin (70% to 100%) can vary enough among formulations from different manufacturers to result in a subtherapeutic serum concentration, and therefore, it can be ineffective in controlling seizures. Alternatively, switching formulation may result in a toxic blood concentration. Capsules of sodium phenytoin will absorb carbon dioxide, causing dissociation or neutralization to free phenytoin, thus altering its oral bioavailability (gastrointestinal dissolution), pharmacokinetics, and plasma concentrations, which can cause breakthrough seizures. Therapeutic plasma concentrations for phenytoin are usually 7.5 to 20.0 μg/mL, although in some patients, seizure control is not achieved at these plasma concentrations. Phenytoin is highly protein bound (Table 17.2).

Phenytoin is metabolized predominately by CYP2C9 to its primary metabolite, 5-(4′-hydroxyphenyl)-5-phenylhydantoin (HPPH) (Fig. 17.5) (32). Approximately 60% to 75% of an oral dose is excreted as HPPH glucuronide or sulfate metabolites. Approximately 1% is excreted unchanged in urine, and some undergoes enterohepatic circulation. Other minor metabolites also appear in urine. Up to 10% of the oral phenytoin can be excreted unchanged by the kidneys at toxic doses. Phenytoin is notorious for displaying nonlinear pharmacokinetics, because the route of metabolism is a saturable process. Therefore, small

TABLE 17.2 Mechanism(s) of Action and Pharmacokinetics for Antiseizure Drugs

Drug	Mechanism of Action[a]	Elimination Half-Life in Children (hours)	Elimination Half-Life in Adults (hours)	Time to Steady-State Plasma Concentration (hours)	Protein Binding (%)	LogD (pH 7.4)
Carbamazepine (Tegretol)	A	14–27 (children), 8–28 (neonates)	14–27	2–8	66–89	2.2
Clonazepam (Klonopin)	A, B	20–40	20–40	—	95–98	2.3
Diazepam (Diastat)	A, B	17	36	—	40	2.6
Ethosuximide (Zarontin)	C	20–60	20–60	7–10	0	0.38
Ezogabine (Potiga)	F	—	6–10	—	80	0.81[d]
Felbamate (Felbatol)	E	15.9	20–23	—	20–25	1.2[d]
Gabapentin (Neurontin)	D	4	5–7	2–3	<3%	−1.3[d]
Lacosamide (Vimpat)	A	—	13	1–4 days	<15	0.9[d]
Lamotrigine (Lamictal)	A, E	19	25–70	—	55	−0.2[d]
Levetiracetam (Keppra)	I	—	6–8	2 days	<10	−0.67[d]
Oxcarbazepine (Trileptal)	A	—	7–11[b]	2–3	40	1.25[d]
Phenobarbital	A, B	37–73	40–136	12–21	40–60	1.53
Phenytoin (Dilantin)	A	5–14 (children), 10–60 (neonates)	12–36	7–28	69–96	2.39
p-Hydroxyphenytoin (metabolite)						1.72
Pregabalin (Lyrica)	D	—	5–6.5	24–48	0	−1.38[d]
Primidone (Mysoline)	A, B	23	3–7	4–7	20–30	0.91
Rufinamide (Banzel)	A	—	6–10	—	34	0.05[d]
Tiagabine (Gabitril)	A	3–6	7–9	—	96	3.2[d]
Topiramate (Topamax)	A, B	10–15, 6–8[c]	20–30, 12–15[c]	—	15	2.9[d]
Valproic acid (Depakene, Depakote, Depacon)	A, C, G	8–15	6–15	1–4 3–5 (sustained release)	80–95	0.13
Vigabatrin (Sabril)	H	5.7	7.5	—	0	−2.6[d]
Zonisamide (Zonegran)	A, C	—	27–46	10–12	40	−0.10[d]

[a]See the *Mechanism of Action* sections of this chapter for discussion. A, sodium channels; B, γ-aminobutyric acid A receptor currents; C, T-calcium currents; D, P/Q calcium currents; E, glutamate receptor antagonist; F, potassium channel agonist; G, GAT1 antagonist; H, γ-aminobutyric acid–transaminase inhibitor; I, unknown.
[b]Monohydroxy metabolite.
[c]In the presence of enzyme-inducing drugs, such as carbamazepine, phenobarbital, or primidone.
[d]LogD calculated at pH 7.4 using Advanced Chemistry Development (ACD Labs) PhysChem Suite V12, 2010.

increases in dosage can produce substantial increases in plasma phenytoin concentrations; the steady-state plasma concentration (C_{ss}) can double or triple as a result of a 10% or more increase in dosage, possibly resulting in toxicity. Phenytoin also induces CYP3A4 and uridine diphosphoglucuronosyltransferases (UGTs; increased glucuronidation). Therefore, plasma concentrations for drugs metabolized by these isoforms will be affected (see also Chapter 4). Thus, the addition of phenytoin to an AED regimen can reduce their plasma levels by inducing their CYP3A4 metabolism for carbamazepine, felbamate, lamotrigine, oxcarbazepine, tiagabine, valproate, and zonisamide. Other drugs, for which metabolism is induced by phenytoin, include methadone, theophylline, warfarin, and oral contraceptives. On the other hand, plasma phenytoin levels are increased by carbamazepine, felbamate, cimetidine, warfarin, chloramphenicol, isoniazid, and disulfiram. Plasma phenytoin levels are decreased by rifampin, antacids, and valproate (free phenytoin levels remain the same).

The pharmacokinetics of phenytoin are significantly affected by age. Its rate of elimination is strongly dose

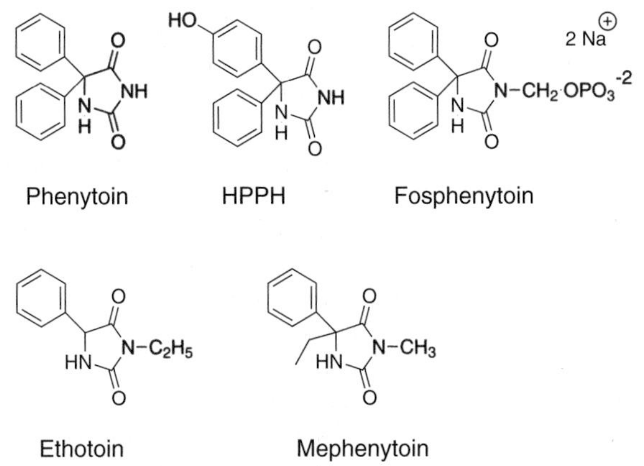

FIGURE 17.5 Hydantoins.

dependent (nonlinear) at all ages. The elimination half-life for phenytoin in children increases with age because of an age-dependent decrease in its rate of metabolism (28). The combination of these factors makes it difficult to predict the phenytoin plasma concentrations following the dose (dose per kilogram) adjustments in neonates and children, particularly when phenytoin is coadministered with other liver enzyme–inducing AEDs, such as phenobarbital and carbamazepine.

Adverse Effects Drug interactions, especially with other AEDs and CYP3A4 substrates, are extensive. Although toxic effects can begin in the upper normal plasma range (>20 μg/mL), serious toxicity is rare. CNS effects are most frequent and include nystagmus, ataxia, dysarthria, and sedation. Gingival hyperplasia, usually reversible, is common. Aromatic anticonvulsants, such as phenytoin, have been associated with a number of toxic effects, including a drug-induced hypersensitivity syndrome that manifests with a triad of reactions, such as rash, agranulocytosis, thrombocytopenia, lymphadenopathy, Stevens-Johnson syndrome, and hepatitis, that have occurred in affected individuals. Although anticonvulsant-induced hypersensitivity reactions are relatively rare events, occurring with an incidence of between 1:1,000 and 1:10,000 exposures, these idiosyncratic reactions can be potentially life-threatening. The hypersensitivity syndrome is consistent with an immune etiology, with symptoms typically appearing within 2 to 8 weeks after the initiation of therapy and generally abating on discontinuation of phenytoin. Dermal metabolism of phenytoin to reactive metabolites can be related to the occurrence of hypersensitivity rashes (33). Although the mechanism by which the aromatic anticonvulsants induce hypersensitivity reactions has not been well characterized, recent studies have suggested that the immune response elicited by phenytoin can be caused, at least in part, by its metabolism into chemically reactive metabolites and can be the critical step in the formation of protein adducts and subsequent immune responses. Identification of the reactive metabolite(s) for phenytoin has been difficult because the rate at which human liver microsomes convert phenytoin to metabolites capable of binding to proteins is quite low. It also is important to note that phenytoin is typically administered in doses ranging from hundreds of milligrams to grams per day, suggesting that substantial amounts of reactive metabolites could be formed on a daily basis. Therefore, it is conceivable that individuals with a low capacity to detoxify reactive metabolites via glucuronidation or other secondary pathways can represent individuals at risk for idiosyncratic toxicity.

The incidence of phenytoin toxicity can be increased in the elderly or in those patients with hepatic or renal impairment, as a result of alterations in its pharmacokinetics. Plasma level determinations can be indicated in these cases. Although a role for P-glycoprotein transporter alleles in the development of phenytoin toxicity remains controversial, phenytoin is a robust substrate for the non–ABC efflux transporter RLIP76. Because RLIP76 has been found to be overexpressed in excised human epileptic foci, its action can account for treatment failures; conversely, inhibition of transport can cause toxicity (34). There is a 2% to 3% increase in the risk of fetal epilepsy syndrome if the mother is taking phenytoin. Phenytoin is contraindicated in cardiac patients with bradyarrhythmias. Induction of CYP2C19 by ginkgo biloba can increase phenytoin clearance and precipitate serious seizures (35).

FOSPHENYTOIN (CEREBYX) Fosphenytoin sodium (Fig. 17.5) is a soluble prodrug disodium phosphate ester of phenytoin (142 mg/mL) that was developed as a replacement for parenteral phenytoin sodium to circumvent the pH and solubility problems associated with parenteral phenytoin sodium formulations (36). Unlike phenytoin, fosphenytoin is freely soluble in aqueous solutions and is rapidly absorbed by the IM route (37). It is rapidly metabolized (conversion half-life, 8 to 15 minutes) to phenytoin by in vivo phosphatases. Therapeutic free (unbound) and total plasma phenytoin concentrations are consistently attained after IM or IV administration of fosphenytoin (26). It is administered IV after benzodiazepines for control of status epilepticus or whenever there is a need to rapidly achieve therapeutic plasma concentrations. Severe bradycardiac adverse events to fosphenytoin, including some fatalities, have been reported (38). A dose reduction in patients who are elderly or have renal or hepatic impairment has been suggested.

ETHOTOIN (PEGANONE) Ethotoin differs from phenytoin in that one phenyl substituent at position 5 has been replaced by hydrogen, and the N-H at position 3 is replaced by an ethyl group (Fig. 17.5). Ethotoin can be used for treatment of tonic-clonic and complex partial (psychomotor) seizures. Because it is considered to be less toxic but also less effective and more sedating than phenytoin, ethotoin usually is reserved for use as an add-on drug (39). Ethotoin does not share phenytoin's profile of antiarrhythmic action. The metabolism of ethotoin, like phenytoin, is saturable and nonlinear. Its administration is contraindicated in patients with hepatic abnormalities and hematologic disorders.

Mephenytoin Mephenytoin is *N*-methylated at position 3 with an ethyl group replacing one of the phenyl substituents at position 5 (Fig. 17.5). It is indicated for focal and jacksonian seizures in patients refractory to less toxic AEDs. Mephenytoin produces more sedation than phenytoin and should be used only when safer drugs have failed, because it is associated with an increased incidence of serious toxicities, such as severe rash, agranulocytosis, and hepatitis (40). Its *N*-desmethyl metabolite, 5-phenyl-5-ethylhydantoin, contributes to both efficacy and toxicity for mephenytoin. The drug is no longer commercially available inside the United States but is still available outside the United States

Iminostilbenes

Carbamazepine Carbamazepine (CBZ; Tegretol) (Fig. 17.6) was approved by the FDA in 1968 and is presently indicated as initial or adjunct therapy for complex partial, tonic-clonic, and mixed-type seizures. It is one of the two safest and most effective older AEDs for these seizure types (phenytoin is the other) and is chosen for monotherapy as a result of its high effectiveness and relatively low incidence of side effects (40). Its tricyclic structure resembles that of the psychoactive drugs imipramine, chlorpromazine, and maprotiline and also shares some structural features with the AEDs phenytoin, clonazepam, and phenobarbital. In addition, CBZ has been found to be effective for treatment of bipolar disorder and trigeminal neuralgia.

Mechanism of Action In animals, the profile of antiseizure properties for CBZ is similar to that of phenytoin. CBZ is effective in the maximal electroshock (MES) test (electrically induced seizure test) but is ineffective against pentylenetetrazole-induced seizures. CBZ is not effective for absence or myoclonic seizures and, indeed, can exacerbate their onset (30,41). Like phenytoin, CBZ acts on voltage-dependent sodium channels to prevent the spread of seizures. CBZ depresses synaptic transmission in the reticular activating system, thalamus, and limbic structures. In a double-blind, crossover study in patients whose seizures were not controlled completely by combinations of AED, CBZ was equal in efficacy to phenobarbital and phenytoin in controlling seizure frequency, and side effects were minimal.

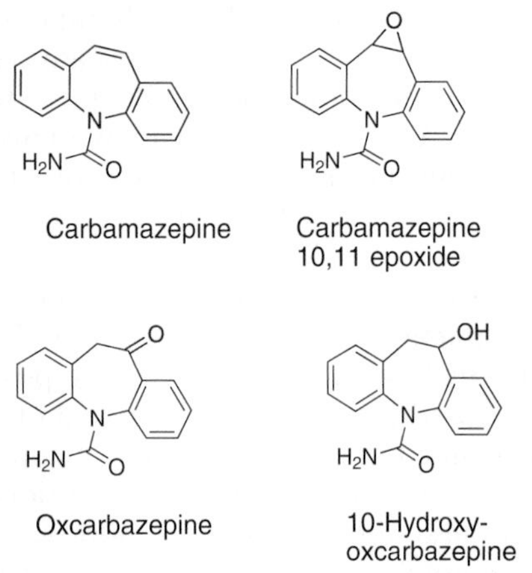

FIGURE 17.6 Iminostilbenes.

Pharmacokinetics After the administration of an oral dose, CBZ is slowly absorbed, with the attainment of peak concentration from immediate-release tablets in 4 to 5 hours and from extended-release tablets in 3 to 12 hours. The normal half-life averages between 12 and 17 hours; however, due to autoinduction, the half-life can range from 8 to 29 hours. The half-life for CBZ-10,11-epoxide is 5 to 8 hours. Therapeutic plasma concentrations range from 4 to 12 μg/mL (in adults) and can require a month to achieve a stable therapeutic concentration for the desired antiseizure effect because of induction of hepatic metabolizing enzymes.

CBZ is principally metabolized by CYP3A4 to its 10,11-epoxide, with CYP2C8 and CYP1A2 having minor roles. CBZ epoxide is hydrolyzed by epoxide hydrase to inactive 10,11-dihydroxy CBZ. CBZ epoxide is active and appears to be more toxic than CBZ (42,43). However, CBZ not only induces CYP3A4 activity but also its own metabolism (an autoinducer) as well as UGT and the increased formation of glucuronide metabolites. Like phenytoin, CBZ has been associated with a number of toxic effects, including a drug-induced hypersensitivity syndrome. Although phenytoin-induced hypersensitivity reactions are relatively rare events, they can be potentially life-threatening. Although the mechanism by which CBZ induces hypersensitivity reactions has not been well characterized, recent studies have suggested that the immune reaction can be caused, at least in part, by its metabolism into chemically reactive metabolites, which can be the critical step in the formation of protein adducts and subsequent immune responses. Identification of the reactive metabolite(s) has been difficult, because the rate at which human liver microsomes convert CBZ to metabolites capable of binding to proteins is quite low. Furthermore, it is also important to note that CBZ is typically administered in doses ranging from hundreds of milligrams to grams per day, suggesting that substantial amounts of reactive metabolites can be formed on a daily basis. Therefore, it is conceivable that individuals with a low capacity to detoxify reactive metabolites via glucuronidation or other pathways can be at risk for idiosyncratic toxicity. Although an arene oxide was originally proposed as the reactive species, either an iminoquinone metabolite derived from the CBZ metabolite (CBZ-IQ) or 2-hydroxyiminostilbene (2-OHIS) are potential candidates for the reactive metabolite, because quinone- and iminoquinone-type metabolites have been implicated in drug-induced hepatotoxicity (see also Chapter 4). CYP3A4-catalyzed secondary metabolism of 2-hydroxycarbamazepine to 2-OHIS or to CBZ-IQ, followed by nonenzymatic reduction to 2-OHIS, can well underlie subsequent development of drug-induced hypersensitivity to CBZ (Fig. 17.7) (44). Based on the formation of glutathione and *N*-acetylcysteine conjugates, it has been suggested that 2-OHIS is the target for the formation of protein adducts, which could lead to localized idiosyncratic toxicities. Like phenytoin, CBZ is highly protein bound (Table 17.2) and is extensively transformed. Approximately 72% of an oral dose is excreted in the urine as metabolites and 3% as unchanged drug. The 28% found in the feces can be the result of incomplete absorption and enterohepatic cycling. As previously mentioned, interindividual variability in apparent plasma half-life and total-body clearance is related to the phenomenon of autoinduction.

Adverse Effects Gastric upset from CBZ can be diminished by taking the drug after meals. Common toxicities include blurred vision, dizziness, drowsiness, and ataxia. Tremor, depression, hyponatremia, and cardiac disturbances are seen at high serum concentrations. Idiosyncratic rashes are common; rarer severe idiosyncratic effects include aplastic anemia, agranulocytosis, thrombocytopenia, and jaundice. Therefore, patients receiving CBZ should have periodic blood count determinations and liver function tests. Both CBZ and oxcarbazepine can reduce plasma 25-hydroxyvitamin D levels (45). CBZ increases levels of phenytoin and decreases levels of felbamate, lamotrigine, oral contraceptives, theophylline, valproate, and zonisamide. CBZ levels are increased by propoxyphene, erythromycin, chloramphenicol, isoniazid, verapamil, and cimetidine. CBZ levels are decreased by phenobarbital, phenytoin, felbamate, and primidone. Lamotrigine and valproic acid can elevate CBZ epoxide levels. Administration of the extended-release form has been associated with fewer side effects and with improved seizure control (46).

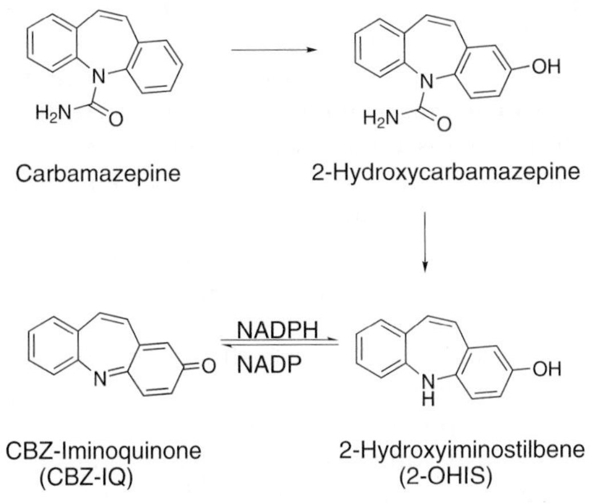

FIGURE 17.7 Bioactivation pathway for carbamazepine.

Macrolide antibiotics inhibit CBZ metabolism, thus increasing CBZ plasma levels and decreasing clearance with the potential for toxicity effects. Drug-induced changes in CBZ pharmacokinetics are particularly pronounced in children (28).

CBZ should be used with caution in patients with a history of congestive heart failure or cardiac arrhythmias (because it can aggravate them) and with a history of hematologic reactions to other drugs or hypersensitivity to tricyclic antidepressants. Blood levels should be monitored in patients with renal or hepatic impairment.

OXCARBAZEPINE Oxcarbazepine (Trileptal) is the 10-keto analog of CBZ (Fig. 17.6). It is indicated as monotherapy or adjunctive therapy for partial seizures in adults with epilepsy, as monotherapy for the treatment of partial seizures in children 4 years of age or older, and as adjunct therapy in children 2 to 4 years of age.

Mechanism of Action Although oxcarbazepine is less potent that CBZ, its mechanism of action is similar (47). The majority of the pharmacologic activity for oxcarbazepine is attributed to its primary metabolite, 10-monohydroxycarbazepine (MHD) (Fig. 17.6), the plasma levels of which can be ninefold higher than those for CBZ. Both oxcarbazepine and MHD produce a blockade of voltage-dependent sodium channels, thus decreasing repetitive firing and spread of electrical activity. An additional action on calcium and potassium channels can contribute to the therapeutic effect. Like carbamazepine, oxcarbazepine can worsen juvenile myoclonic or absence seizures (41).

Pharmacokinetics Oxcarbazepine is completely absorbed, and food has no effect on its absorption. Unlike CBZ, it does not cause autoinduction of its own metabolism. The metabolism of oxcarbazepine is different from that of CBZ. Oxcarbazepine is reduced by cytosolic enzymes to MHD before its *O*-glucuronidation. More than 95% of its oral dose is excreted as conjugated metabolites, with approximately 4% of the drug converted to inactive 10,11-dihydroxy CBZ. Unlike CBZ, no epoxide or aromatic hydroxylation metabolites are formed. The half-life is 2 hours for oxcarbazepine and 9 hours for the active 10-monohydroxy metabolite. In patients with impaired renal function, the half-life for MHD is prolonged to 19 hours, with a doubling in its area under the plasma concentration curve. Peak plasma concentration following an oral dose occurs at approximately 4.5 hours.

Oxcarbazepine induces CYP3A4/5 and UGT and inhibits CYP2C19, producing significant alterations on the plasma concentration of other drugs. Therefore, oxcarbazepine decreases felodipine bioavailability and lowers plasma levels for lamotrigine, CBZ, CBZ epoxide, calcium channel blockers, and oral contraceptives (48). Oxcarbazepine increases plasma levels of phenobarbital and phenytoin. Unlike CBZ, oxcarbazepine has no effect on plasma levels of risperidone or olanzapine (49,50). The plasma levels for oxcarbazepine or MHD are decreased by CBZ, phenobarbital, phenytoin, valproate, and verapamil. Serum MHD can decrease during pregnancy but increase following delivery (51). Oxcarbazepine clearance is decreased in renal impairment and the elderly. In children, a higher dose per kilogram for oxcarbazepine than in adults is required to obtain an effective plasma concentration.

Adverse Effects Patients with hypersensitivity reactions to carbamazepine can be expected to show cross-sensitivity (e.g., rash) or related problems to oxcarbazepine. The improved toxicity profile for oxcarbazepine when compared to CBZ can result from absence of the epoxide or CBZ-iminoquinone metabolites (47). The most common side effects are headache, dizziness, nystagmus, blurred vision, somnolence, nausea, ataxia, and fatigue. The incidence of adverse effects has been related to elevated serum MHD concentrations (52). Adverse effects on cognitive status, hyponatremia, and serious dermatologic reactions have been reported, as has hyponatremia (53).

Barbiturates

The barbiturates are substituted pyrimidine derivatives with an ureide configuration (Fig. 17.4). They are lipophilic weak acids (pK_a = 7 to 8) that are well distributed into brain (see Appendix A for the respective pK_a values). Although many barbiturates display sedative-hypnotic activity (see Chapter 15), only a few have antiseizure properties. Paradoxically, many barbiturates cause convulsions at larger doses. The barbiturates clinically useful as AEDs are phenobarbital, mephobarbital, and primidone (Fig. 17.8). In laboratory animals, phenobarbital is effective by several tests in nontoxic doses. It is active against MES, and it elevates the threshold for pentylenetetrazole stimulation. The mechanism of antiseizure action for the barbiturates is unknown but is thought to involve blockade of sodium channels and enhancement of GABA-mediated inhibitory transmission.

Phenobarbital Phenobarbital is commonly used for convulsive disorders and is the drug of choice for seizures in infants up to 2 months of age. Phenobarbital is indicated for the treatment of partial and generalized tonic-clonic seizures in all age groups, although it is less effective than phenytoin or CBZ in adults (40). Although occasionally used as monotherapy, it usually is combined with another AED. Phenobarbital can be administered parenterally, as its sodium salt, for emergency control of acute convulsive disorders associated with eclampsia (although magnesium sulfate is the standard treatment), meningitis, tetanus, and toxic reactions to strychnine or local anesthetics. Because of its slow onset of action, it is administered after benzodiazepines for the treatment of status epilepticus.

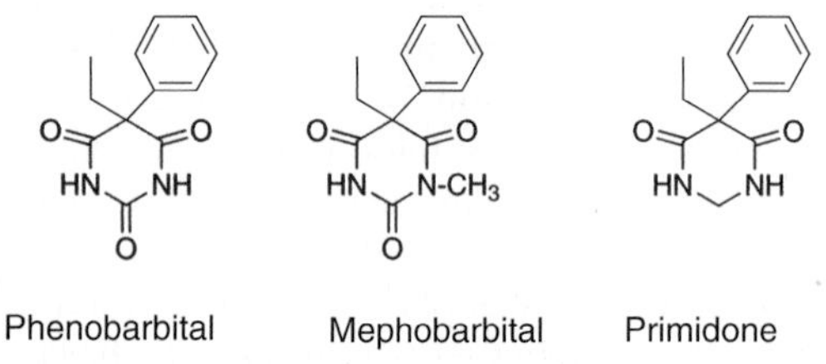

FIGURE 17.8 Barbiturates.

Pharmacokinetics Phenobarbital is a weak acid (pK_a = 7.4; $\log D_{pH\,7.4}$ = 1.53) that is approximately 50% ionized at physiologic pH and is well distributed into the CNS. Its oral absorption is slow but nearly complete, with an oral bioavailability of 80% to 100%, and it shows linear kinetics. Phenobarbital is 40% to 60% protein bound and exhibits a long plasma half-life of 2 to 6 days, which yields an extremely stable plasma concentration. Approximately 25% to 50% of a phenobarbital dose is excreted unchanged in the urine. The remainder is metabolized primarily by hydroxylation to its inactive metabolite, 5-*p*-hydroxyphenyl-5-ethyl-barbituric acid, which is then conjugated as its glucuronide or sulfate and is excreted in the urine. Some of the conjugated metabolites can appear in the feces from enterohepatic cycling. Alkalinizing the urine or increasing the urine flow substantially increases the rate of excretion of unchanged phenobarbital and its metabolites. Phenobarbital is a potent liver enzyme–inducing drug of CYP3A4 and increases the ability of the liver to metabolize many drugs, when taken concurrently, that are normally metabolized by CYP3A4. It also induces UGTs and increased formation of glucuronidation. No conclusive evidence, however, shows that phenobarbital induces its own metabolism (autoinduces), as does CBZ.

Because of its inducing effect on hepatic enzymes, phenobarbital has many drug interactions, decreasing plasma levels of CBZ, valproate, lamotrigine, tiagabine, zonisamide, warfarin, theophylline, cimetidine, and other CYP3A4 substrates. Serum concentrations of phenobarbital are increased by valproate.

Adverse Effects Serious toxicity is rare; however, drowsiness is the most common side effect reported for phenobarbital. Of the barbiturates, only phenobarbital, mephobarbital, and primidone are antiseizure at subhypnotic doses. The sedative effect of phenobarbital limits its use in older children and adults, although tolerance to the sedative effects often develops. When compared to phenytoin or CBZ, phenobarbital shows more sedation, irritability, paradoxical hyperactivity, and impaired intellectual function. This can prove to be particularly troublesome in children, especially those of school age, and in the elderly. Quite rare are idiosyncratic hypersensitivity reactions to phenobarbital that include rash, agranulocytosis, aplastic anemia, and hepatitis. Although the mechanism by which the phenobarbital and other aromatic anticonvulsants induce hypersensitivity reactions has not been well characterized, recent studies have suggested that the immune response elicited can be caused, at least in part, by the metabolism of phenobarbital into chemically reactive metabolites, which can be the critical step in the formation of protein adducts and subsequent immune responses (see discussion for CBZ). Long-term use of phenobarbital can precipitate folate, vitamin K, or vitamin D deficiencies.

Phenobarbital should be used with caution in patients with hepatic impairment; therefore, a dose reduction can be needed. It should be avoided in patients with renal impairment. Barbiturates are known to cause fetal abnormalities and a neonatal coagulation defect responsive to vitamin K.

Mephobarbital (Mebaral) Mephobarbital is a barbiturate-derivative AED with a pK_a of 7.7 ($\log D_{pH\ 7.4}$ = 1.84). Approximately 50% of an oral dose of mephobarbital is absorbed from the gastrointestinal tract. The plasma concentrations required for its therapeutic effects are unknown. The principal route of mephobarbital metabolism is *N*-demethylation by the liver to form phenobarbital, which can be excreted in the urine unchanged and as its *p*-hydroxy metabolite and glucuronide or sulfate conjugates. Conversion to the 4-hydroxy metabolite is stereoselective, being catalyzed by either CYP2C19 (*R*-enantiomer) or CYP2B6 (*S*-enantiomer); individuals who are CYP2C19-poor metabolizers show decreased clearance (54). Approximately 75% of a single oral dose of mephobarbital is converted to phenobarbital. It has not been determined whether mephobarbital contributes to the antiseizure effect or whether it results from its active metabolite, phenobarbital. Similarly, it is unclear whether mephobarbital, like phenobarbital, is a potent inducer of the enzymes involved in the metabolism of other drugs, but because the drug is chemically and pharmacologically similar to phenobarbital and is metabolized to phenobarbital, this possibility is likely.

Mephobarbital is less commonly used in the treatment of generalized and partial seizures. Like phenobarbital, it is classified as a long-acting barbiturate. No evidence exists that it is more effective than phenobarbital in equivalent doses; however, it can be less sedating in children.

Primidone (Mysoline) Primidone is the 2-deoxy derivative of phenobarbital (Fig. 17.8) and is approved by the FDA for initial or adjunctive treatment of simple partial, complex partial, and tonic-clonic seizures. It is less effective against these types of seizures than is phenytoin or CBZ, and it shares the antiseizure and sedative actions of phenobarbital. Although not approved for the purpose, it often is used to treat benign familial tremor (essential tremor).

Pharmacokinetics Approximately 60% to 80% of an oral dose of primidone is absorbed and slowly metabolized by the liver to phenobarbital and phenylethylmalonamide (PEMA) (55,56). All three molecules have antiseizure effects, but PEMA appears to be weaker and to be the more toxic metabolite. During chronic therapy, approximately 15% to 25% of an oral dose of primidone is excreted in the urine unchanged, 15% to 25% is metabolized to phenobarbital, and 50% to 70% is excreted as PEMA (half-life, 24 to 48 hours). The phenobarbital metabolite can be excreted in the urine unchanged, as its *p*-hydroxy metabolite, and as glucuronide or sulfate conjugates. Following an oral dose, the peak plasma levels for primidone are reached in approximately 4 hours, with a reported half-life of 10 to 12 hours. Plasma concentrations in the range of 8 to 12 μg/mL control seizures and minimize adverse effects. Primidone shows antiseizure activity before the phenobarbital levels reach therapeutic range. Only after chronic dosing of primidone are the levels of phenobarbital significant, suggesting autoinduction. Serum levels of chronically administered primidone exceed those of its metabolite, phenobarbital, thus demonstrating that it has antiseizure activity independent of phenobarbital. When primidone is coadministered with enzyme-inducing AEDs, the levels of its phenobarbital metabolite can be two- to threefold higher than those in the noninduced state. Protein binding of primidone and PEMA is negligible, and the phenobarbital metabolite is approximately 50% protein bound.

Primidone use is associated with decreases in CBZ, lamotrigine, valproate, tiagabine, and zonisamide serum levels. Primidone levels are increased by nicotinamide and isoniazid. Hydantoins increase the plasma concentrations of primidone, phenobarbital, and PEMA. CBZ increases levels of phenobarbital derived from primidone. Primidone levels are decreased by succinimides, CBZ, and acetazolamide.

Adverse Effects As with phenobarbital, serious toxicity for primidone is rare, although it can cause disabling sedation, irritability, and decreased mental functioning in a number of persons. Ataxia, dysphoria, idiosyncratic rash, leukopenia, agranulocytosis, lymphadenopathy, hepatitis, and a systemic lupus erythematosus–like syndrome have been reported adverse effects for primidone. Deficiencies of folic acid and of vitamins D and K are possible with long-term therapy of primidone, as is a folate-responsive megaloblastic anemia. Measurement of the complete blood cell count should be performed at 6-month intervals (40).

Benzodiazepines

This class of drugs has been widely used as sedative-hypnotics and antianxiety drugs (see Chapters 15 and 14, respectively). In laboratory animals, benzodiazepines display outstanding antiseizure properties against seizures induced by MES and pentylenetetrazole. The benzodiazepines diazepam, lorazepam, clonazepam, clorazepate dipotassium, and midazolam are effective for seizure control (Table 17.2 and Fig. 17.9). All benzodiazepines enter cerebral tissue rapidly. Although the duration of action is short for diazepam (2 hours) and midazolam

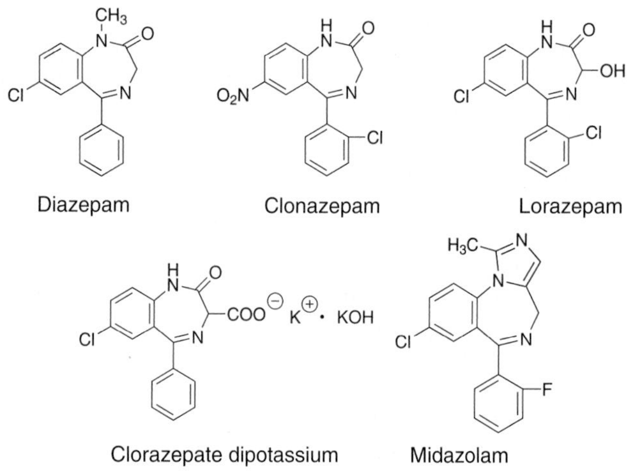

FIGURE 17.9 Benzodiazepines.

(3 to 4 hours), longer for clonazepam (24 hours), and much longer for lorazepam (up to 72 hours), no correlation exists with the plasma concentration–time profiles for these drugs (57,58). Diazepam and lorazepam can be administered either IV or IM for control of status epilepticus; however, absorption is slower from the IM site. Midazolam is particularly useful for treating status epilepticus, because its imidazole ring is open at low pH, allowing it to be dissolved in aqueous solution for IM injection, but is closed at physiologic pH, increasing lipophilicity with rapid IM absorption, brain penetration, and fast onset of action. When administered IM, midazolam has a faster onset of action than diazepam and lorazepam due to its rapid absorption from the injection site, with an efficacy at least equal to that of IV diazepam (57,58). Seizure arrest usually is attained within 5 to 10 minutes. In addition, the use of midazolam by the buccal route for initial treatment of acute seizure activity has been shown to be more effective and without increased respiratory depression as compared to the use of rectal diazepam (59). Midazolam has been used intranasally as well (60,61). Lorazepam, although not approved by the FDA for this purpose, is preferred by some clinicians for the treatment of status epilepticus as a result of its longer duration of action.

Mechanism of Action The benzodiazepines are thought to produce their antiseizure effects primarily by enhancing the effect of the inhibitory neurotransmitter GABA on the $GABA_A$ chloride channel (Figs. 17.1 and 17.2). Additional evidence suggests that the benzodiazepines can diminish voltage-dependent sodium, potassium, and calcium currents in a manner independent of the $GABA_A$/benzodiazepine receptor complex or alter expression of $GABA_A$ receptor subunit expression (62).

Diazepam (Valium) Diazepam is given orally for adjunctive control of convulsive disorders, as a rectal gel (Diastat) for refractory patients with epilepsy on a stable regimen of AEDs who require intermittent use of diazepam to control bouts of increased seizure activity, and parenterally as part of the regimen for the treatment of status epilepticus or other severe, recurrent seizures. Rectal diazepam gel is an effective and well-tolerated therapy for acute repetitive seizures (59).

Pharmacokinetics Orally administered diazepam is less effective as an AED, because tolerance to the antiseizure effects of diazepam develops within a short period. Diazepam gel is rapidly absorbed rectally, having greater than 90% bioavailability. In addition to cluster seizures, it has been proven to be useful to control prolonged febrile seizures in children.

Intravenously administered diazepam is the route of choice for rapid control of status epilepticus. Because of its high lipid solubility, IV diazepam enters the CNS rapidly. However, the initial high brain concentration is reduced quickly as a result of its redistribution; thus, status epilepticus can return. To prevent the return of status epilepticus, the initial dose of diazepam is followed sequentially by parenteral phenytoin (fosphenytoin) and phenobarbital as needed for control of tonic-clonic status epilepticus. For absence status epilepticus, diazepam usually is followed by ethosuximide.

The half-life for diazepam is 46 hours, and diazepam is metabolized by CYP2C19 and CYP3A4 to desmethyldiazepam, an active metabolite with a half-life of 71 hours. Diazepam is 95% protein bound. Cimetidine, by inhibiting CYP3A4, decreases the metabolism and clearance of diazepam. Drugs that affect the activity of CYP2C19 or CYP3A4 can alter diazepam kinetics, and vice versa.

Adverse Effects The most frequent side effect for diazepam is somnolence; dizziness, ataxia, headache, nervousness, euphoria, and rash occur less frequently. Excessive use of rectal diazepam can produce rebound seizures (63). Intravenous administration can produce infrequent respiratory depression and hypotension. Other sedative drugs, such as barbiturates, valproate, narcotics, phenothiazines, monoamine oxidase inhibitors, and antidepressants, can potentiate the effects of diazepam.

Because diazepam clearance is decreased in the elderly and in patients with hepatic insufficiency, a dosage reduction can be warranted. Intravenous diazepam should be used cautiously in patients who are elderly, very ill, or have limited pulmonary reserve, because respiratory depression has occurred. IV Diazepam is rarely given to patients for absence status (typical and atypical) seizures, because it may precipitate tonic status epileptic seizures.

Clonazepam Clonazepam (Klonopin) was approved in 1975 for monotherapy or adjunctive treatment of akinetic (atonic), myoclonic, and absence variant seizures (64). Clonazepam also was found to be effective in controlling absence seizures, but because of its high incidence of side effects, it is rated second to ethosuximide. It can be useful, however, in absence seizures when succinimide therapy has failed. It is considered to be a third-line drug after 1) ethosuximide or valproate and 2) lamotrigine or valproate for the treatment of absence seizures. It is ineffective for treatment of generalized clonic-tonic seizures.

Clonazepam is well absorbed, 95% to 98% protein bound, and extensively metabolized by CYP3A4. Clonazepam displays a wide spectrum of antiseizure activities and is one of the most potent AEDs. Side effects are common, however, and the development of tolerance is more frequent than with ethosuximide or valproate. Sedation is prominent, especially early in treatment. Drowsiness, ataxia, and behavioral changes can be disabling, but slowly increasing its dose over a 2-week period is recommended to minimize adverse effects. Diplopia (double vision), headaches, nystagmus (involuntary eye movement), and other neurologic effects have been reported with the use of clonazepam.

Serum levels of clonazepam are decreased by the enzyme-inducing properties of phenobarbital, phenytoin, and CBZ. Concurrent administration of amphetamines, methylphenidate, ethanol, antianxiety drugs, or antipsychotics can cause CNS depression or altered respiration. The combined administration of clonazepam and valproate can cause absence status, and in patients displaying a mixed seizure pattern, clonazepam can precipitate grand mal seizures.

Clorazepate Dipotassium Clorazepate dipotassium (Tranxene) was approved for use as an AED by the FDA in 1981. It is less commonly used as adjunct therapy for the management of partial seizures in adults and children older than 9 years. Clorazepate is decarboxylated by the acidity of the stomach to desmethyldiazepam, which is also the major active metabolite of diazepam. Therefore, clorazepate exhibits the profile and properties of diazepam.

Lorazepam (Ativan) Lorazepam is a benzodiazepine (Fig. 17.6), with pK_a values of 1.3 and 11.5. Its parenteral solutions are formulated with polyethylene glycol, and dilution with diluents can cause its crystallization from solution. Lorazepam is also used IV or IM for the management of status epilepticus. Although IV diazepam has been used more extensively, some clinicians prefer IV lorazepam due to its more prolonged duration of effect. It has been recommended for initial treatment of generalized convulsive status epilepticus in the elderly (65). A long-acting AED, such as IV phenytoin or fosphenytoin, can be added to IV benzodiazepine therapy for the management of recurring seizures associated with status epilepticus.

Intramuscular lorazepam is slowly absorbed with peak plasma concentrations (C_{max}) reached in approximately 60 to 90 minutes. The half-life for unconjugated lorazepam is approximately 16 hours when given IV or IM, and it is eliminated in the urine as its major metabolite, lorazepam 3-*O*-glucuronide. Lorazepam glucuronide has no demonstrable CNS activity in animals but has a half-life of approximately 18 hours. Lorazepam is 85% bound to plasma proteins. Drugs that inhibit or induce the oxidative metabolism of benzodiazepines (CYP3A4) are less likely to affect lorazepam, because it undergoes only glucuronide conjugation.

Other Benzodiazepines In addition to their anxiolytic and sedative-hypnotic properties, several other benzodiazepines also display antiseizure activity. They include clobazam and nitrazepam, which are used outside the United States; these drugs have not demonstrated any clinical advantage over clonazepam.

Biscarbamates

Felbamate (Felbatol)

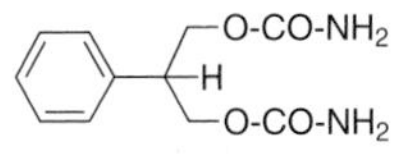

Felbamate

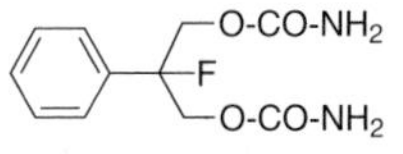

2-Fluorofelbamate

Felbamate is a dicarbamate that is structurally similar to the antianxiety drug meprobamate. It was approved by the FDA for antiseizure use in 1993. Following the occurrence of rare cases of aplastic anemia and of severe hepatotoxicity associated with the use of felbamate during early 1994, however, a black box warning was added to the drug's package insert (53). Despite this, felbamate continues to be used in many patients, although not as a first-line treatment. These toxicity effects can be attributed to the formation of toxic metabolites (66). Although felbamate use is now uncommon, it is used for severe refractory seizures, either partial, myoclonic, or atonic, or in Lennox-Gastaut syndrome.

Mechanism of Action Although its mechanism of action is unknown, felbamate alters the gating behavior of the NMDA receptor by binding to the receptor pore and lowering calcium currents (Fig. 17.2) (67).

Metabolism and Pharmacokinetics Although the metabolism of felbamate has not been fully characterized, felbamate is esterase hydrolyzed to its monocarbamate metabolite, 2-phenyl-1,3-propanediol monocarbamate, which is subsequently oxidized via aldehyde dehydrogenase to its major human metabolite 3-carbamoyl-2-phenylpropionic acid (Fig. 17.10). Other metabolites include the *p*-hydroxy and mercapturic acid metabolites of felbamate, which have been identified in human urine. Felbamate is a substrate for CYP2C19, with minor activity for CYP3A4 and CYP2E1. Thompson et al. (68) have provided evidence for the formation of the reactive metabolite, 3-carbamoyl-2-phenylpropionaldehyde (CBMA), from the alcohol oxidation of 2-phenyl-1,3-propanediol monocarbamate. CBMA then undergoes spontaneous elimination to another reactive intermediate, 2-phenylpropenal (more commonly known as atropaldehyde), which is proposed to have a role in the

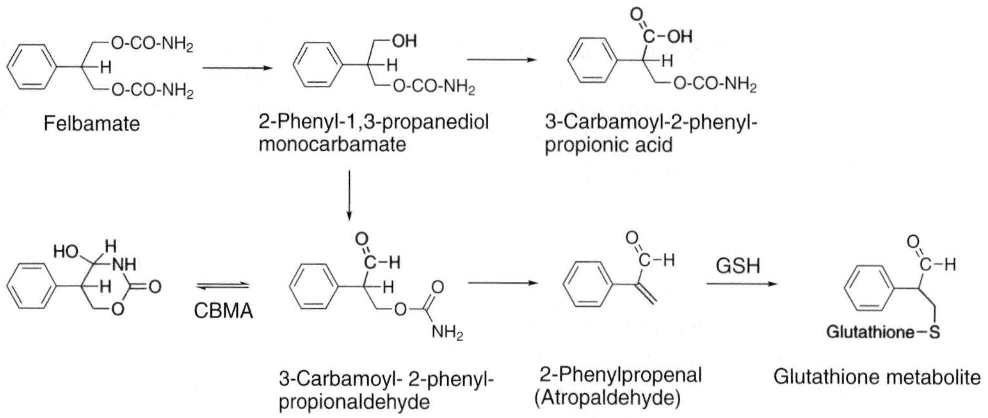

FIGURE 17.10 Metabolism of felbamate.

development of toxicity during felbamate therapy. CBMA or a further product has been shown to provoke an immune response in mice (69). Evidence for in vivo atropaldehyde formation was confirmed with the identification of its mercapturic acid conjugates in human urine after felbamate administration. This is consistent with the hypothesis that atropaldehyde reacts rapidly with thiol nucleophiles, such as glutathione, to form mercapturates (see Chapter 4). More recently, a fluorine analog of felbamate was synthesized in which the benzylic C_2 hydrogen of the propane chain was replaced with a fluorine atom, preventing the formation of atropaldehyde and confirming that the acidic benzylic hydrogen plays a pivotal role in its formation (70). This analog is presently undergoing drug development. Felbamate administration exhibited linear kinetics, with a half-life of 20 to 23 hours in the absence of enzyme-inducing AEDs. Approximately 50% of an oral dose of felbamate is excreted unchanged.

Adverse Effects Felbamate has exhibited the rare occurrence of aplastic anemia and of severe hepatotoxicity, which can be associated with the in vivo formation of reactive metabolites. Felbamate increases phenytoin and valproate serum levels but decreases the level of CBZ. The increase in valproate plasma concentrations by felbamate is through the inhibition of β-oxidation. No clinically relevant pharmacokinetic interactions have been noted between felbamate and lamotrigine, clonazepam, vigabatrin, or the active monohydroxy metabolite of oxcarbazepine. The enzyme inducers phenytoin, phenobarbital, and CBZ decrease felbamate plasma levels by increasing its clearance.

Miscellaneous Antiepileptic Drugs

Ezogabine (Retigabine; Potiga)

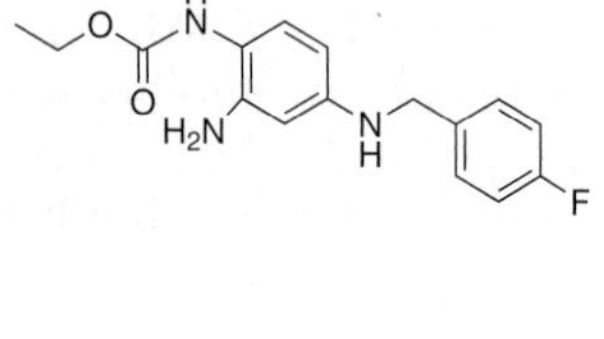

Ezogabine (retigabine in Europe) is an anticonvulsant possessing a new mechanism of action: It affects certain voltage-gated potassium channels known to be expressed in brain. It is indicated for the adjunctive treatment of partial-onset seizures in adults.

Mechanism of Action Ezogabine stabilizes the open state of Kv7.2 to Kv7.5 potassium channels (products of *KCNQ2* to *KCNQ5* genes). Kv7.2 and Kv7.3 are the predominant components of the slow voltage-gated M channel, which regulates neuronal excitability (71). Ezogabine produces a hyperpolarizing shift in their voltage gating, increases the channels' open time, and decreases substantially their closed time, reducing excitability. In addition, it produces faster opening of the channels during depolarization, thus suppressing repetitive firing (72). Kv7.2 and Kv7.3 are present on the axon initial segments of CA1 pyramidal neurons. The drug does not affect cardiac Kv7.1 channels because these lack a requisite tryptophan residue. It is noteworthy that mutations in *KCNQ2* and *KCNQ3* are known to be associated with a form of human epilepsy.

Pharmacokinetics Ezogabine is rapidly absorbed, having a bioavailability of up to 60%. It reaches C_{max} in approximately 1.5 hours, has a half-life of approximately 6.3 hours, and has a volume of distribution (V_d) of 6.2 L/kg. It is not metabolized by CYP450. Ezogabine's predominant metabolites are two *N*-glucuronides formed by UGT1A1, UGT1A4 and UGT1A9, plus lesser acetylated derivatives (73). Ezogabine has been shown to modestly increase the clearance of lamotrigine, whereas lamotrigine increased the AUC of ezogabine by 15%, probably as a result of competition for renal elimination. Phenytoin and CBZ can increase the clearance of ezogabine.

Adverse Effects In clinical studies, urinary retention and dizziness have caused withdrawal of the drug. Weight gain, somnolence, headache, fatigue, confusion, and slurred speech have been noted, although the drug is generally well tolerated (74). Serious adverse events have included nephritis and urinary retention. Monitoring patients for urinary retention can be required.

GABAPENTIN (NEURONTIN)

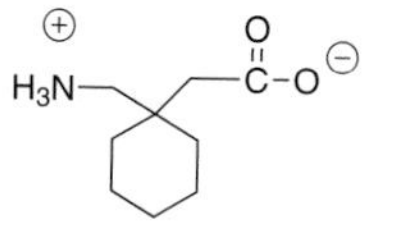

Mechanism of Action Gabapentin is a water-soluble amino acid originally designed to be a GABA-mimetic analog capable of penetrating the CNS. Surprisingly, it has no direct GABA-mimetic activity. As with pregabalin, the mechanism of action involves drug binding to the α-2-δ subunit of the P/Q-type calcium channels, decreasing their activity. In addition, gabapentin raises brain GABA levels in patients with epilepsy (75). Recent studies have demonstrated gabapentin binding to calcium channels in a manner that can be allosterically modulated (76).

Gabapentin is indicated as an adjunct for use against partial seizures with or without secondary generalization, in patients older than 12 years, and as adjunct for the treatment of partial seizures in children 3 to 12 years of age. It also is approved for the treatment of postherpetic neuralgia.

Pharmacokinetics The pharmacokinetic properties for gabapentin are generally favorable, with a bioavailability of 60% when given in low doses and somewhat less when given at higher doses as a result of saturable intestinal uptake by the L-amino acid transporter (77). The L-amino acid transporter is very susceptible to substrate saturation (low K_m value). Its absorption and distribution into the CNS appear to be dependent on this amino acid transporter. Following the administration of an oral dose, gabapentin reaches peak plasma concentration in 2 to 3 hours. Additionally, it exhibits linear pharmacokinetics. Moreover, it is not extensively metabolized and is not an inducer of hepatic metabolizing enzymes. The elimination of unmetabolized gabapentin occurs by the renal route. Although its therapeutic range is not well characterized, gabapentin has a broad therapeutic index. This implies that a wide range of doses can be used, based on individual patient needs, without significant limitation because of dose-dependent side effects. Protein binding is negligible. Its elimination half-life of 5 to 7 hours is not affected by the dose or by other drugs, and its short half-life necessitates multiple daily administration.

Adverse Effects Adverse effects of gabapentin are uncommon and not serious. The CNS effects include mild to moderate sedation, fatigue, ataxia, headache, dizziness, and diplopia. Gabapentin can exacerbate myoclonus, but the effect is mild and does not require discontinuance of the drug (53,78). It has been associated with the development of neuropsychiatric adverse events in children.

Drug interactions are infrequent with gabapentin. It does not induce hepatic metabolizing enzymes, nor do other AEDs affect its metabolism and elimination. Antacids can decrease absorption. Gabapentin dosage can need to be decreased in patients with renal disease or in the elderly.

LACOSAMIDE (VIMPAT)

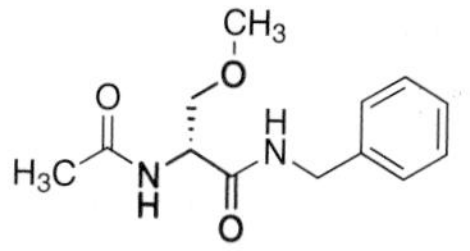

Lacosamide is an amino acid–related compound that was approved by the FDA in 2008 for adjunctive treatment of partial-onset seizures in patients age 17 years or older. Although the drug acts on voltage-gated sodium channels, it has a mechanism of action different from phenytoin and CBZ.

Mechanism of Action Lacosamide is a functionalized amino acid amide, the optical antipode of the natural amino acid L-serine (outlined in color), and enhances sodium channel slow inactivation with no effect on fast inactivation. Following opening, sodium channels adopt a "fast inactivated state" before returning to the resting state. This fast inactivated state is acted on by classical anticonvulsants such as phenytoin, CBZ, or lamotrigine. However, after repetitive firing, sodium channels can adopt a "slow inactivated state" over several seconds. It is this state that is enhanced by lacosamide, thus prolonging depolarization and diminishing rapid repetitive firing (79,80). In addition, lacosamide binds collapsin-response mediator protein 2 (CRMP-2), which is involved in polarization, regulation of gene expression, and growth of axons and dendrites. Whether this contributes to the drug's anticonvulsant antiseizure effects is presently unknown. (79)

Pharmacokinetics Lacosamide's oral bioavailability is complete without any food effect. It displays linear pharmacokinetics, with a half-life of approximately 12 to 13 hours and reaching C_{max} in 1 to 4 hours. It is less than 15% bound by plasma proteins and shows a V_d of 0.6 L/kg. The drug is converted by hepatic CYP2C19 to an inactive *O*-desmethyl metabolite; this metabolite plus 40% of the unchanged drug are excreted renally (80). Although CYP2C19 is polymorphic, no significant differences in lacosamide pharmacokinetics have been reported in poor metabolizers (81). Dosage adjustments can be needed in patients with moderate hepatic or severe renal impairment. Drug interactions are minimal. Lacosamide has no effect on CYP450s and thus does not affect other anticonvulsant levels (79). Only small decreases in lacosamide plasma concentrations are seen with CBZ, phenytoin, or phenobarbital coadministration. Lacosamide does not affect oral contraceptive efficacy (80).

Adverse Effects Because mild PR interval prolongation has been reported, there can be an increased risk of atrial fibrillation in patients with cardiac disease. Dizziness, headache, nausea, vomiting, diplopia (double vision), and blurred vision have occurred. Only one case of severe hypersensitivity reaction was noted in clinical trials.

Lamotrigine (Lamictal)

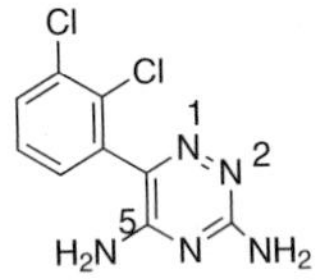

Lamotrigine is a 5-phenyl-1,2,4-triazine derivative indicated as monotherapy or as an adjunct for partial seizures in adults, as adjunct in patients with Lennox-Gastaut syndrome, and as adjunct for partial seizures in children 2 years of age and older. Lamotrigine can have additional benefit in combating myoclonic and typical absence seizures. It is approved for use in the maintenance treatment of bipolar disorder.

Mechanism of Action The most probable explanation for lamotrigine's efficacy is its ability to produce a blockade of sodium channel repetitive firing. In addition, lamotrigine appears to reduce glutaminergic excitatory transmission and inhibit neuronal nicotinic acetylcholine receptors (82,83).

Pharmacokinetics Following oral administration, lamotrigine is absorbed rapidly and completely, exhibiting linear pharmacokinetics and modest protein binding (55%). Lamotrigine is metabolized predominantly by *N*-glucuronidation and subsequent urinary elimination of its major metabolite, the quaternary 2-*N*-glucuronide (80% to 90%), the minor 5-amino-*N*-glucuronide (8% to 10%), and unchanged drug (8% to 10%) (84). Lamotrigine's usual elimination half-life of 24 to 35 hours is reduced to 13 to 15 hours in patients taking enzyme-inducing AEDs. The presence of valproate increases the lamotrigine half-life substantially by inhibiting *N*-glucuronidation, necessitating a reduction in dose to avoid toxicity. Hepatic disease patients can demonstrate a reduced capacity for lamotrigine glucuronidation, thus reducing its rate of clearance.

Adverse Effects The usefulness of lamotrigine is limited by the increased incidence of serious rashes, particularly in children or patients taking valproate (53). This increased incidence, however, can be attenuated by very slow dose escalation, because most rashes appear within the first 8 weeks of treatment. The drug should be discontinued if a rash appears at any time. In 2010, the FDA warned that lamotrigine can cause aseptic meningitis. Furthermore, lamotrigine can be associated with development of myoclonus after 2 to 3 years of drug treatment (85). Additional common side effects associated with lamotrigine therapy include dizziness, diplopia, headache, ataxia, blurred vision, somnolence, and nausea.

S-(−)-Levetiracetam (Keppra)

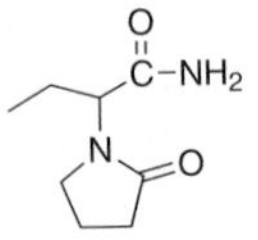

S-(−)-Levetiracetam is a pyrrolidone derivative unrelated to the structures of other AEDs. It is indicated as an adjunct in the treatment of partial-onset seizures in adults, and it has shown some benefit in clinical trials for generalized tonic-clonic seizures and myoclonic seizures in adults and children (86,87).

Mechanism of Action The mechanism of action for *S*-(−)-levetiracetam is unknown. It does not appear to interact with any of the recognized excitatory or inhibitory neural mechanisms. A CNS-specific binding site for *S*-(−)-levetiracetam has been identified as the synaptic vesicle protein (SV2A). Knockout animals without SV2A proteins accumulated presynaptic Ca^{2+} during consecutive action potentials that destabilized synaptic circuits and induced epilepsy. Thus, it appears that SV2A has a major role in the antiepileptic properties of *S*-(−)-levetiracetam, which acts by modulating the functions of SV2A, expression of the associated calcium sensor protein synaptotagmin, and the regulation of Ca^{2+}-mediated synaptic transmission (88). These data support previous indications that *S*-(−)-levetiracetam possesses a mechanism of action distinct from that of other antiepileptic drugs. Three SV2 isoforms (SV2A, SV2B, and SV2C) have been identified, each of which has a unique distribution in brain, suggesting synapse-specific functions as well as antagonism of neuronal synchronization (78,89).

Pharmacokinetics *S*-(−)-Levetiracetam displays rapid and complete absorption, although food slows the rate but not the extent of absorption. It exhibits linear pharmacokinetics and is minimally protein bound (90). Approximately 60% of an oral dose is excreted into the urine unchanged, and 24% to 30% is excreted as its carboxylic acid metabolite, with an elimination half-life in adults of approximately 7 hours. Although *S*-(−)-levetiracetam is not metabolized by hepatic CYP450, UGT, or epoxide hydrolase, it is esterase hydrolyzed to its carboxylic acid metabolite (loss of the amido group), which is not affected by the hepatic metabolizing enzymes.

Adverse Effects The risk of clinically relevant drug interactions is minimal with *S*-(−)-levetiracetam because it does not alter the pharmacokinetics of coadministered drugs by inhibition or induction of hepatic enzymes (91). Toxic effects include mild to moderate somnolence, asthenia, ataxia, and dizziness; these effects seldom require discontinuance. An increase in the incidence of behavioral abnormalities in children and in adults having a previous history of neuropsychiatric problems has been noted (92). Its use in the elderly or in patients with renal impairment will require an individualization of dose, and an additional dose is needed after renal dialysis. Levetiracetam was associated with developmental toxicity in the offspring of pregnant animals.

PREGABALIN (LYRICA)

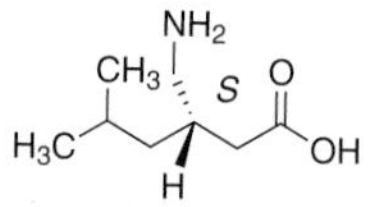

Pregabalin is a GABA analog with similarities in structure and effects to gabapentin; however, it is 3 to 10 times more potent as an AED than is gabapentin. It is the pharmacologically active *S*-enantiomer of 3-isobutyl GABA and is FDA approved for the adjunctive treatment of partial-onset seizures in adults.

Mechanism of Action The drug acts by binding to the α-2-δ subunit of the P/Q-type voltage-sensitive calcium channels present on presynaptic neurons, modulating their activity and decreasing neuronal calcium currents (93).

Pharmacokinetics The absorption of pregabalin is rapid and nearly complete following oral administration. It displays linear pharmacokinetics, with a half-life of 5 to 6.5 hours and reaching C_{max} in approximately 1.5 hours. Although the rate of absorption is decreased by food, there is no clinically detectable decrease in the AUC or half-life; thus it can be administered with or without food. Pregabalin is not bound to plasma proteins and shows only minor metabolism to *N*-methylated (0.9%) and unidentified (0.4%) metabolites. Neither induction nor inhibition of the metabolism of other anticonvulsant agents has been demonstrated; no interaction with oral contraceptives has been reported. However, CBZ and other enzyme-inducing drugs can reduce pregabalin plasma concentrations. Dose adjustments are indicated in renal insufficiency, and supplemental doses are required following renal dialysis.

Adverse Effects Common adverse effects include ataxia, dizziness, somnolence, and confusion. In postmarketing studies, behavioral effects (agitation, irritability, and depression) and weight gain were the most frequent cause of drug discontinuance (93). Instances of severe constipation requiring withdrawal of the drug have been cited. Precautions include withdrawal symptoms of insomnia, nausea, headache, and diarrhea, plus increased seizure occurrence on abrupt discontinuance. Therefore, it is recommended that the drug be tapered off over a minimum of 1 week. In studies, an increase in the cardiac PR interval was seen, but neither this nor heart block has been reported as an adverse effect. Because the medication has been associated with life-threatening rash with respiratory symptoms, caution is indicated for patients with a history of hives. Concomitant use of other angioedema-provoking agents such as the angiotensin-converting enzyme inhibitors can lead to a further increase in risk. The use of pregabalin in patients receiving thiazolidinedione antidiabetic drugs can further increase weight gain and peripheral edema. Infrequent increases in the creatine kinase plasma levels are known, and a few cases of rhabdomyolysis have been reported. Patients should be monitored for creatine kinase elevation; discontinuance is recommended for myopathy symptoms or significant creatine kinase elevation.

RUFINAMIDE (BANZEL)

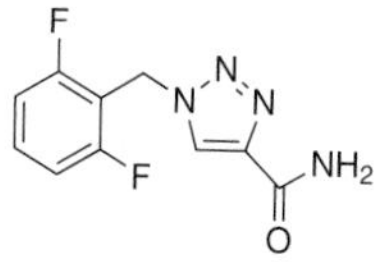

Rufinamide is a triazole derivative that differs structurally from other anticonvulsants.

It is FDA approved as an orphan drug for adjunctive treatment of seizures associated with Lennox-Gastaut syndrome in children 4 years of age of greater and in adults. It was determined to be cost effective for treatment of Lennox-Gastaut syndrome. Additionally, the drug is being evaluated for adjunctive treatment of refractory partial-onset seizures; the European Union brand name is Inovelon.

Mechanism of Action Rufinamide is thought to act by prolonging the inactive state of voltage-gated sodium channels, thereby limiting repetitive firing (94). High plasma concentrations inhibit the mGlu receptor (95).

Pharmacokinetics The bioavailability of rufinamide is approximately 85%. It should be given with food as this further increases absorption. The drug is 34% plasma protein bound, reaches maximum concentrations between 4 and 6 hours after administration, and has a half-life of 8 to 12 hours. It is extensively metabolized: Only 4% is excreted unchanged in urine and feces. The predominant metabolite (78%) is due to carboxylesterase hydrolysis of the carboxamide group, leading to an inactive metabolite; additionally, there is minor non–CYP450-mediated oxidative cleavage at the benzylic carbon. Rufinamide is a weak inhibitor of CYP2E1 and a weak inducer of CYP3A4, but does not affect any other CYPs (94,95). Rufinamide plasma concentrations are affected by several drug interactions (81). Rufinamide concentrations are increased up to 70% by valproic acid, whereas they are decreased by CBZ, phenobarbital, primidone, vigabatrin, and phenytoin. Rufinamide increases plasma concentrations of phenobarbital and phenytoin and decreases concentrations of lamotrigine, CBZ, and triazolam. Additionally, rufinamide lowers the efficacy of oral contraceptives.

Adverse Effects QT interval shortening occurred in up to 65% of patients; thus familial short QT syndrome is an absolute contraindication. There can be an increased risk if combined with other agents known to shorten QT intervals. Multiorgan hypersensitivity syndrome was observed in one patient. Common adverse effects include fatigue, drowsiness, ataxia, somnolence, dizziness, headache, and nausea (95). Abrupt discontinuance can precipitate rebound seizures.

Tiagabine (Gabitril)

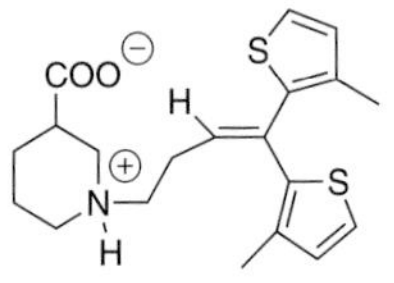

Mechanism of Action Tiagabine is a nipecotic acid derivative with an improved ability to cross the blood–brain barrier. It was rationally designed to be a GABA uptake inhibitor based on the fact that nipecotic acid (piperidine-3-carboxylic acid) inhibits GABA uptake by glial cells. Tiagabine binds to GABA transporter 1 (GAT1), blocking the uptake of GABA into both neurons and glia, thus enhancing GABA-mediated inhibition (Fig. 17.2) (53,96). Tiagabine is presently approved for adjunct use in patients with epilepsy who are older than 12 years and have partial seizures not controlled by first-line drugs.

Pharmacokinetics Tiagabine is well absorbed, with an oral bioavailability of 90% to 95%. It displays linear pharmacokinetics, with a plasma half-life of 5 to 8 hours, necessitating a multiple daily dosing regimen. It also is highly protein bound (96%). The major pathway of metabolism for tiagabine is oxidation by CYP3A4, followed by glucuronidation. Its pharmacokinetics are altered by the coadministration of enzyme-inducing AEDs, even though tiagabine does not appear to induce or inhibit hepatic microsomal metabolizing enzymes.

Adverse Effects Side effects are more common with tiagabine than with other adjunct drugs and most often involve the CNS. They include somnolence, headache, dizziness, tremor, abnormal thinking, depression, and psychosis. Furthermore, recent reports have implicated tiagabine in the development of nonconvulsive status epilepticus (97). There is an increased risk of seizure in patients being treated for off-label psychiatric indications. Tiagabine can interfere with visual color perception (98).

Tiagabine does not affect the hepatic metabolism of other AEDs, but its half-life is decreased by enzyme-inducing AEDs, such as CBZ, phenytoin, and barbiturates. Other CYP3A4-inducing drugs can act similarly. Valproate decreases the protein binding of tiagabine. increasing its plasma concentration in these patients.

Hepatic disease causes decreased clearance of tiagabine, and a dose reduction can be required. Renal disease does not affect elimination.

Topiramate (Topamax)

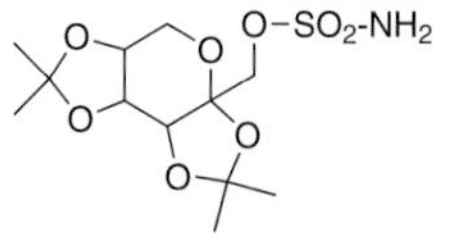

Topiramate is a sulfamate-substituted monosaccharide derived from fructose with a broad spectrum of AED activity. It is FDA approved for monotherapy or as an adjunct drug for partial or primary generalized tonic-clonic seizures in patients older than 10 years, as adjunct therapy in children age 2 to 10 years with partial-onset seizures, and in persons older than 2 years with Lennox-Gastaut syndrome (40,53). Topiramate also is approved for the prophylaxis of migraine headaches.

Mechanism of Action The mechanism of action for topiramate is unknown, but several actions are thought to contribute to its AED activity (99). It blocks repetitive firing by acting on sodium channels, can enhance $GABA_A$-mediated chloride flux, and appears to be an antagonist at the AMPA and KA receptors, thus blocking the effect of glutamate (Fig. 17.2) (100,101).

Pharmacokinetics Topiramate is rapidly absorbed, with at least an 80% to 95% oral bioavailability that is unaffected by food. Following an oral dose of topiramate, peak plasma concentration is reached in 1 to 4 hours exhibiting linear pharmacokinetics (102). Protein binding is minimal (<20%), and the usual elimination half-life is 20 to 30 hours, allowing a twice-daily dosing regimen. In the absence of enzyme-inducing drugs, approximately 70% to 80% of the drug is excreted unchanged in the urine, with the remainder as metabolites resulting from oxidation and hydrolysis. Enzyme-inducing AEDs alter the pharmacokinetics of topiramate by reducing its plasma levels and increasing its rate of elimination.

In children from 4 to 17 years of age, topiramate exhibits linear pharmacokinetics with a 50% increase in clearance rate compared to adults (102). Topiramate can require up to a 50% dose reduction in patients with renal insufficiency, and a replacement dose can be needed after renal dialysis. Topiramate has demonstrated teratogenicity in animal studies.

Adverse Effects Common CNS side effects associated with topiramate therapy include drowsiness, dizziness, impaired concentration and memory, speech and language difficulties, and confusion. These effects develop during the first weeks of therapy and can decline over time. Acute closed-angle glaucoma caused by topiramate requires immediate evaluation (103). Only rare hepatic or bone marrow effects have been noted thus far; however, an increased incidence of renal stones is troublesome and probably related to the drug's activity as a carbonic anhydrase inhibitor, reducing citrate excretion and increasing urinary pH. Use of additional carbonic anhydrase inhibitors, a ketogenic diet, or a family history of nephrolithiasis can be considered as contraindications for using topiramate.

Topiramate is not devoid of potential interaction properties: It induces CYP3A4 and inhibits CYP2C19, thus significantly increasing plasma phenytoin levels. Topiramate can also decrease the effectiveness of oral contraceptives.

Valproic Acid and Its Derivatives

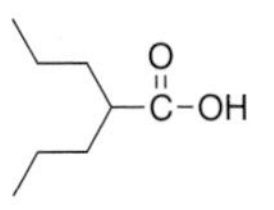

Valproic acid (dipropylacetic acid)

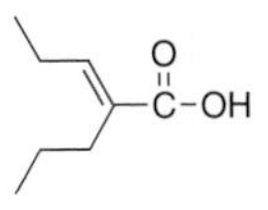

(E)-2-ene-valproic acid

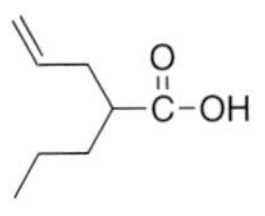

4-ene-valproic acid

Valproate is available as valproic acid (Depakene), divalproex sodium (Depakote), and valproate sodium (Depacon) for IV use. Its AED properties were discovered serendipitously when it was used as a solvent for potential new AEDs undergoing clinical testing. It is effective against both MES test—and pentylenetetrazole-induced seizures in animals and possesses a satisfactory margin of safety. Because the pK_a of valproic acid is 4.7, the drug is completely ionized at physiologic pH; thus, the valproate ion is almost certainly the pharmacologically active species.

Mechanism of Action Although its mechanism of action is not clearly established, valproate appears to increase the inhibitory effect of GABA, possibly by activation of glutamic acid decarboxylase or inhibition of GABA-transaminase (Fig. 17.2). The high drug concentrations required to achieve treatment levels cast doubt on the clinical relevance of this effect. Furthermore, valproate has been shown to decrease the uptake of GABA into cultured astrocytes; this action can contribute to the AED efficacy (104). Valproate is known to produce a blockade of high-frequency repetitive firing by slowing the rate of Na^+ recovery from inactivation, a mechanism consistent with the actions of phenytoin and CBZ. Valproate blocks the low-threshold T-type Ca^{2+} channel. Consequently, the overall therapeutic utility of valproate is likely caused by multiple effects.

Valproate is indicated for initial or adjunct treatment of absence seizures or as an adjunct when absence seizures occur in combination with either tonic-clonic seizures, myoclonic seizures, or both. For patients with unambiguous idiopathic generalized epilepsy, valproate often is the drug of choice, because it controls absence, myoclonic, and generalized tonic-clonic seizures well (105). It also is approved by the FDA for use in complex partial seizures, occurring with or without other seizure types in adults or children 10 years of age or older. In new patients with typical absence seizures, ethosuximide is preferred to valproate due to valproate's risk of producing hepatotoxicity. In a comparative trial, sodium valproate and ethosuximide were equally effective when either drug was given alone or in combination with other AEDs in children with typical absence seizures. In atypical absence seizures (Lennox-Gastaut syndrome), sodium valproate is more effective, whereas in myoclonic seizures, it is less effective than clonazepam. Valproate is approved by the FDA for use in bipolar disorder and as a treatment for migraine headaches.

Pharmacokinetics Valproate undergoes rapid and complete absorption, which is only slightly slowed by food. It is 90% protein bound, and its clearance is dose dependent as a result of an increase in the free fraction of the drug at higher doses. It is metabolized almost entirely by the liver, with 30% to 50% of an orally administered dose being eliminated in the urine as its acyl glucuronide conjugate, 40% from mitochondrial β-oxidation, approximately 15% to 20% by ω-oxidation, and less than 3% is excreted unchanged in urine. Its major active metabolite is (E)-2-ene valproate (*trans*-2-ene valproate). Its 4-ene metabolite has been proposed to be a reactive metabolite responsible for the hepatotoxicity of valproate (see Chapter 4). Other metabolites found in the urine include 3-oxo- and 4-hydroxyvalproate. The elimination half-life for valproate ranged from 9 to 16 hours following oral dosing regimens of 250 to 1,000 mg. Patients who are not taking enzyme-inducing AEDs (CBZ, phenytoin, and phenobarbital) will clear valproate more rapidly; therefore, monitoring of AED plasma concentrations should be intensified whenever concurrent AEDs are introduced or withdrawn.

Adverse Effects The most commonly observed side effects for valproate are gastrointestinal (anorexia, nausea, and indigestion). These effects can be minimized by selecting divalproex sodium, which is enterically coated, and by initiating therapy at a low dose. More importantly, however, valproate is associated with the development of fatal hepatotoxicity, especially in children or when coadministered with other AEDs. Frequent monitoring of liver function tests is mandatory for determining the onset of toxicity, particularly during the first 6 months of treatment. Tremors, hematologic dyscrasias, pancreatitis, stupor, depression, behavioral anomalies, and coma have also been observed with valproate therapy.

Valproate, a substrate for hepatic CYP2C19 and CYP2C9, has an extensive pattern of drug interactions. It increases the plasma concentrations of lamotrigine, CBZ, and phenobarbital and the free fraction of phenytoin by either displacing these drugs from plasma proteins or inhibiting their metabolism. Phenytoin, phenobarbital, and CBZ cause decreased plasma concentrations of valproate, whereas felbamate increases valproate levels.

Because of its propensity for causing liver damage, valproate therapy should be avoided in persons with liver disease. It should be used with caution before surgery because it can produce thrombocytopenia and inhibition of platelet aggregation. During pregnancy, it has been associated with an increased risk of fetal epilepsy syndrome and spina bifida.

Vigabatrin (Sabril)

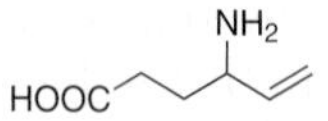

Vigabatrin is γ-vinyl GABA, a synthetic derivative of GABA that was FDA approved in 2009 as monotherapy in the treatment of infantile spasms (West syndrome) in children of 1 month to 2 years of age and as adjunctive treatment of adults with refractory complex partial seizures who are not adequately controlled by other anticonvulsants. Vigabatrin exists as two enantiomers, but only the *S*(+) form is pharmacologically active. The drug is supplied as the racemic mixture (106). Because of the risk of permanent visual field constriction, vigabatrin is available only through a restricted distribution program. The drug should be withdrawn if patients do not show substantial clinical benefit within 3 months.

Mechanism of Action While the exact mechanism for vigabatrin's anticonvulsant effect is unclear, the drug is known to be an irreversible inhibitor of GABA-transaminase, the enzyme responsible for GABA degradation. Although brain GABA concentrations are increased, there is no correlation between the plasma concentration and drug efficacy. Peak antiepileptic response is not seen until 2 to 4 weeks after initiating vigabatrin therapy. Furthermore, drug concentration has no direct relationship to seizure frequency.

Pharmacokinetics Oral bioavailability is up to 80%. The C_{max} is 2.5 hours in infants and 1 hour in children; the half-life is 5.7 hours in infants and 7.5 hours in adults. It does not bind to plasma proteins, is widely distributed (V_d = 1.1 L/kg), and does not undergo significant metabolism. Nevertheless, it has been shown to induce CYP2C9. The drug is excreted unchanged by the kidneys, warranting a dose reduction in renal impairment (106). Coadministration of vigabatrin increases CBZ plasma concentration by 24%, while decreasing phenytoin plasma levels by 16% to 20%.

Adverse Effects Vigabatrin carries a black box warning; up to 30% of patients suffer retinopathy manifesting as irreversible bilateral visual field constriction. Periodic vision testing is required for patients taking vigabatrin; it should not be used in patients at high risk for other types of irreversible vision loss. Gradual tapering of the dose is recommended when discontinuing the drug to avoid increased rebound in seizure frequency.

Zonisamide (Zonegran)

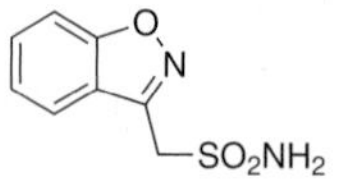

Mechanism of Action Zonisamide is a sulfonamide derivative that is indicated as an adjunct for partial seizures in patients older than 16 years whose seizures are not controlled by first-line drugs. In Japan, it is used for myoclonic seizures as well. Apparently, it has more than one mechanism of action—all of which are, as of yet, unidentified. It is known to produce blockade of both sodium and T-type calcium channels (Fig. 17.2) (107). Because it also affects dopaminergic transmission, bipolar or schizoaffective disorder patients can improve.

Pharmacokinetics The absorption for orally administered zonisamide is slow but nearly complete. Its pharmacokinetics are nonlinear, with a half-life of 50 to 70 hours when administered alone or 27 to 46 hours when administered concurrently with enzyme-inducing AEDs. Protein binding is moderate (<50%). An oral dose of zonisamide is completely absorbed, with peak plasma concentration occurring in 2 to 6 hours. Although the presence of food will delay the attainment of its peak plasma concentration, oral bioavailability does not appear to be altered. More than one-third of each oral dose is excreted in the urine in an unchanged form. The routes of metabolism for zonisamide include acetylation to form its *N*-acetyl metabolite, reduction by CYP3A4/CYP2D6, and the formation of an open-ring metabolite, 2-sulfamoylacetyl phenol. These metabolites subsequently are eliminated unconjugated or glucuronidated in the urine with an elimination half-life of 63 hours. Its coadministration with enzyme-inducing AEDs, such as phenytoin, CBZ, or phenobarbital, and with valproate will alter its pharmacokinetics by reducing its half-life and serum concentration. The half-life for zonisamide is decreased to 27 hours in the presence of phenytoin, to 38 hours in the presence of either CBZ or phenobarbital, and to 46 hours with valproate. Other drugs that inhibit or induce CYP3A4 could affect the metabolism of zonisamide. Zonisamide should be used with caution in patients with hepatic or renal disease. It also has shown to be teratogenic in animal studies.

Adverse Effects Zonisamide is contraindicated in patients with a history of allergy to sulfonamides. The most frequent side effects include somnolence, anorexia, dizziness, agitation, confusion, headache, cognitive impairment, and memory loss. In addition, an incidence of drug-induced psychosis has been noted (108). Reports from both the United States and Europe have indicated that development of renal stones can occur with use of this drug. A family history of nephrolithiasis can be a contraindication, and urinary monitoring for hypercalciuria can be warranted in bedridden patients or those receiving multiple AEDs. Although the incidence of severe rashes attributable to zonisamide is low, sulfonamides are associated with Stevens-Johnson syndrome. Thus, it is recommended to discontinue the drug immediately should a rash occur.

Drugs Effective against Absence Seizures

Drugs that are effective against absence seizures include the five-membered ureides, the oxazolidinediones, and the succinimides (Fig. 17.11); clonazepam and lamotrigine, which have been previously discussed, are also effective. An examination of the structure–activity relationship for the five-membered heterocyclic ureides (Fig. 17.4) reveals that a small substructural difference between ring N (hydantoins), ring O (oxazolidinediones), and ring CH_2 (methylene and succinimides) results in switching from AEDs effective against partial and generalized tonic-clonic seizures to those effective against absence seizures.

Oxazolidinediones

These compounds are some of the oldest AEDs in use, having been introduced into antiseizure therapy between 1946 and 1948. At that time, no effective drugs were available to control absence seizures (petit mal disorders). Therefore, the FDA acceptance of trimethadione in 1946 and of paramethadione in 1948 for the control of absence seizures was rapid. At present, trimethadione (Tridione) (Fig. 17.11) is indicated only for control of absence seizures refractory to treatment with other AEDs. It is ineffective against other seizure types. Trimethadione is a prodrug and is metabolized by *N*-demethylation to dimethadione, which is effective in the pentylenetetrazole test and which acts by decreasing T-type calcium currents. Trimethadione is rapidly absorbed, is not protein bound, and has a half-life of 16 to 24 hours. The half-life of dimethadione, however, is substantially longer (i.e., 6 to 13 days), and dimethadione accumulates to concentrations greater than the parent drug. Because of its potentially fatal side effects, including aplastic anemia, nephrosis, idiosyncratic rashes, and exfoliative dermatitis, trimethadione is rarely used today. It causes malformations or fetal death in up to 87% of pregnancies. Paramethadione is no longer clinically available in the United States.

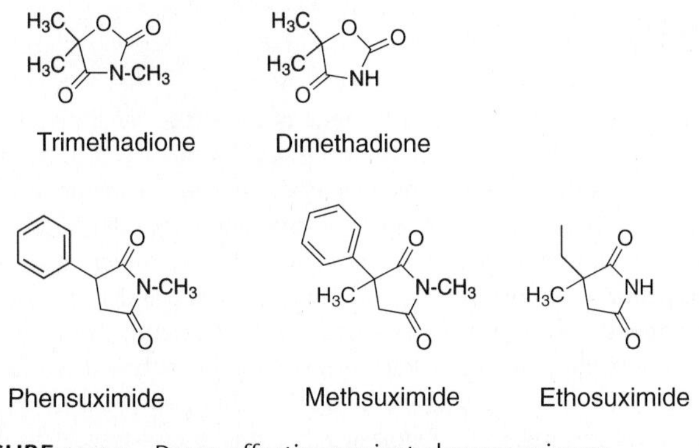

FIGURE 17.11 Drugs effective against absence seizures.

Succinimides

Because oxazolidinediones are toxic, an extensive search was undertaken to replace them with less toxic drugs. Substituting the ring O in the oxazolidinediones with a methylene group gave the antiseizure succinimides. The clinically used succinimides include ethosuximide, methsuximide, and phensuximide, which were introduced between 1951 and 1958 (Fig. 17.11) and widely accepted for the treatment of absence seizures.

Mechanism of Action Succinimides suppress the paroxysmal 3-Hz spike-and-wave activity associated with the lapses of consciousness associated with absence (petite mal) seizures, thus reducing the frequency of seizures and raising the threshold to seizures. The proposed mechanism of action involves a decrease in T-type calcium channel activity (Fig. 17.2).

Succinimides are indicated for the monotherapy of absence seizures or with concomitant therapy when additional forms of seizures occur in combination with absence seizures. These drugs are readily absorbed from the gastrointestinal tract and display very low protein binding. The drug interactions for the succinimides are less extensive than with the oxazolidinediones. They can increase plasma phenytoin levels, decrease plasma primidone levels, and either increase or decrease valproate levels, although the changes might not be clinically significant.

Rena or hepatic disease does not appear to enhance their toxicity. Extreme caution is advised, however, because succinimides can cause morphologic changes to kidneys and liver. Periodic monitoring of the blood count, hepatic function, and urinalysis is recommended with the use of succinimides.

Ethosuximide (Zarontin) Ethosuximide is the drug of choice for treatment of simple absence seizures (109). It is not effective against partial complex or tonic-clonic seizures and can increase the frequency of grand mal attacks. Thus, it must be administered in combination with other AEDs when treating persons with mixed seizure types. Ethosuximide is a substrate for both CYP3A4 and CYP2E1. The major metabolite for ethosuximide is 3-(1-hydroxyethyl) succinimide, which is inactive and excreted unconjugated into the urine. Several additional metabolites have been characterized recently (110). Approximately 20% of an oral dose is excreted unchanged.

Although ethosuximide is thought to be the least toxic of the succinimides, it can cause gastrointestinal disturbances and dose-related CNS effects, such as drowsiness, dizziness, ataxia, sleep disturbances, and depression.

Idiosyncratic hypersensitivity reactions include severe rashes, leukopenia, agranulocytosis (some fatal), systemic lupus erythematosus, and parkinsonian-like symptoms. In addition to being less toxic than trimethadione, ethosuximide offers a wider range of protection against different kinds of absence seizures.

Methsuximide Although methsuximide is less commonly used, it can be indicated for the control of absence seizures refractory to other drugs. Although it does not precipitate tonic-clonic convulsions, it often is combined with phenytoin or phenobarbital when absence seizures coexist with tonic-clonic symptoms. Much of the efficacy of methsuximide is attributed to its desmethyl metabolite. The half-life of methsuximide is between 2.6 and 4.0 hours, but the half-life for *N*-desmethylsuximide is 25 hours, causing it to accumulate substantially. Concentrations of greater than 40 mcg/mL can be associated with toxicity. Methsuximide is considered to be more toxic than ethosuximide.

Phensuximide Phensuximide occasionally is used for the treatment of absence seizures refractory to other drugs, although it is considered to be less effective than ethosuximide. It is excreted in both urine and bile, and it can cause harmless pink to red discoloration of the urine. It should be used with caution in patients with acute intermittent porphyria.

Drugs Effective against Myoclonic Seizures

Clonazepam and valproate commonly are used to control myoclonic seizures. Studies suggest that lamotrigine and topiramate can be effective as well, although neither is approved by the FDA for this indication.

Drugs for Status Epilepticus

Diazepam, administered IV or IM, is a drug of choice for rapid control of status epilepticus. Lorazepam, although not approved by the FDA for the purpose, is preferred by some clinicians for its longer duration of action (40), and midazolam is preferred for its more rapid onset of action (58). Because of its high lipid solubility, IV diazepam enters the CNS rapidly. The initially high brain concentration is quickly reduced, however, due to its redistribution, increasing the chance of recurring status epilepticus. Concomitant IV injection of diazepam and phenobarbital or fosphenytoin has been suggested to overcome this difficulty.

ANTIEPILEPTIC DRUGS IN PHASE III CLINICAL TRIALS

Antiepileptic drugs in phase III clinical trials are shown in Figure 17.12. Brivaracetam is the 4-*n*-propyl analog of levetiracetam (Keppra), which is an SV2A ligand, and thereby can regulate neurotransmitter release. Carisbamate (RWJ 333369) is a monocarbamate derivative of felbamate, which is an antagonist at KA receptors. Clobazam is a benzodiazepine that has long been used in Europe and has U.S. orphan drug status for treatment of Lennox-Gastaut syndrome.

Eslicarbazepine (Stedesa) is a prodrug converted to *S*-licarbazepine, an active metabolite of oxcarbazepine by hepatic esterases. Like carbamazepine, it is a sodium channel antagonist.

Perampanel (E2007) is the first-in-class highly selective noncompetitive AMPA-type glutamate receptor antagonist.

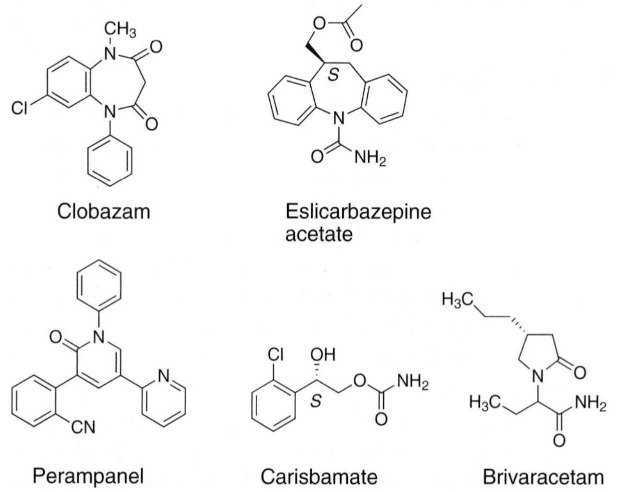

FIGURE 17.12 Antiepileptic drugs in phase III clinical trials.

SCENARIO: OUTCOME AND ANALYSIS

Outcome

Michael Gonyeau, PharmD

Though it may at first appear that the patient experienced a seizure caused by a subtherapeutics phenytoin level, the corrected phenytoin level reveals that the patient experienced the symptoms of nausea and vomiting, ataxia (problems walking), and the seizure that precipitated the hospitalization from phenytoin toxicity. Because of the nature of phenytoin kinetics, namely 90% protein binding, corrected phenytoin levels should be ascertained in any patient with hypoalbuminemia or end-stage renal disease because the free fraction of the drug will be increased in such patients and the potential for toxicity exists even at therapeutic or subtherapeutic observed levels of total phenytoin. The admitting physician only looked at the observed level, which is subtherapeutic (therapeutic range, 10–20 mcg/mL), and increased the patient's dose because she had a recent seizure. However, because of the patient's corrected phenytoin level based on her medical history of end-stage renal disease and her hypoalbuminemia level (36 mcg/mL), increasing her phenytoin dose at this

SCENARIO: OUTCOME AND ANALYSIS *(Continued)*

time will compound the current problem by increasing phenytoin levels even higher in a non–dose-dependent fashion because of its nonlinear kinetics. The end result could be more seizures, increased confusion, coma, or death. The pharmacist in this situation quickly identified the toxic phenytoin level and discussed with the physician, and the phenytoin was held and the patient's symptoms resolved over the next several days with close observation and monitoring in the hospital setting.

Chemical Analysis

S. William Zito and Victoria Roche

Phenytoin is a hydantoin AED. Structurally it is a five-member ring containing two nitrogens in a ureide configuration. Other AEDs containing the ureide moiety are barbiturates (x = –CONH–), oxazolidinediones (x = –O–) and the succinamides (x = $-CH_2-$).

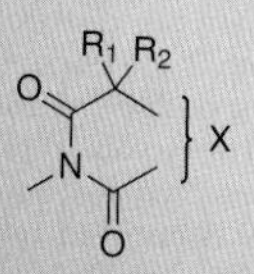

Ureide Structure

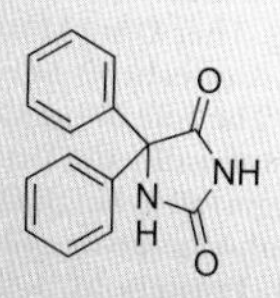

Phenytoin

Seizures result from abnormal synchronous neuronal discharge in the CNS involving ion channels and an excitatory/inhibitory synaptic imbalance. Various structural types of AEDs show selective efficacy versus different seizure types. Phenytoin is effective in the treatment of partial and generalized tonic-clonic seizures. Its mechanism of action is to stabilize the inactive state of the voltage-gated Na^+ channel. When phenytoin binds to the sodium channel it produces a use-dependent blockade of repetitive firing, thus inhibiting the spread of seizure activity.

Phenytoin is metabolized predominately by CYP2C9. Approximately 60 to 75% of an oral dose is excreted as 5-(4′-hydroxyphenyl)-5-phenylhydantoin (HPPH) glucuronide or sulfate (HPPH). Minor amounts are excreted unchanged in the urine, and some undergo enterohepatic circulation. Phenytoin is notorious for displaying nonlinear pharmacokinetics because the route of metabolism is a saturable process, making the therapeutic index very narrow. The steady-state plasma concentration (C_{ss}) can double or triple as a result of a 10% or more increase in dosage, possibly resulting in toxicity. Phenytoin also induces CYP3A4 and uridine diphosphoglucuronosyltransferases (increases glucuronidation); therefore, co-administered drugs metabolized by these isoforms will be affected. In addition, carbamazepine, felbamate, cimetidine, warfarin, chloramphenicol, isoniazid and disulfiram can increase plasma phenytoin levels. The key problem in this case is the pharmacokinetic parameter of plasma binding. Phenytoin is highly protein bound (90%), and because this patient is in the end stage of renal disease and is hypoalbuminemic, the patient was actually suffering from phenytoin toxicity and not subtherapeutic dosing.

CASE STUDY

S. William Zito and Victoria Roche

BJ a 50-year-old woman who reports increased tonic clonic seizures to her neurologist during their most recent visit. She is currently taking oxcarbazepine and gabapentin, and previous trials with phenytoin, phenobarbital, lamotrigine and valproic acid as either monotherapy or adjunct therapy were unsuccessful in seizure control. The physician wants to try adding one of the following three antiepileptic drugs.

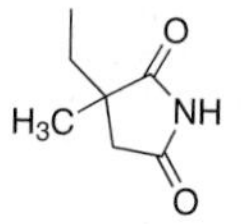

1

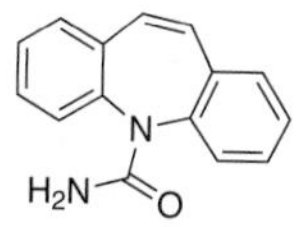

2

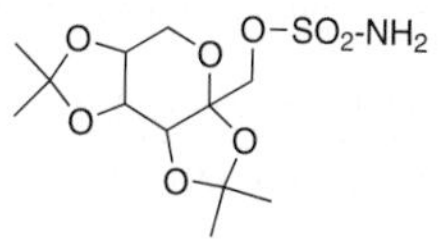

3

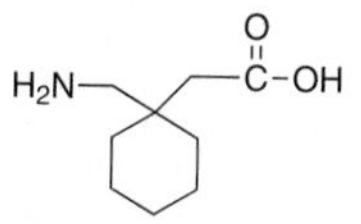

Gabapentin

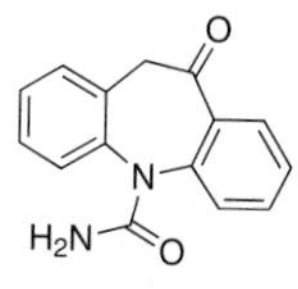

Oxcarbazepine

1. Conduct a thorough and mechanistic SAR analysis of the three therapeutic options in the case.
2. Apply the chemical understanding gained from the SAR analysis to this patient's specific needs to make a therapeutic recommendation.

References

1. Forster FM, ed. Report of the Panel on Epilepsy. Madison, WI: University of Wisconsin Press, 1961:91.
2. DeRobertis E, DeLores-Arnaiz GR, Alberici M. Ultrastructural neurochemistry. In: Jasper HH, Pope A, Ward AA, eds. Basic Mechanisms of the Epilepsies. Boston: Little, Brown and Co., 1969:137–158.
3. Jackson JH. On the anatomical and physiological localization of movements in the brain. In: Taylor J, ed. Selected Writings of John Hughlings Jackson, Vol 1. London: Hodder and Stoughton, 1958:52.
4. Gowers WR. Epilepsy and Other Chronic Convulsive Diseases: Their Causes, Symptoms, and Treatment, 2nd Ed. London: J. and A. Church, 1901.
5. Gastaut H. A proposed international classification of epileptic seizures. Epilepsia (Amst) 1964;5:297–303.
6. Lennox WG. Epilepsy and Related Disorders. Boston: Little, Brown and Co., 1960.
7. Penfield W, Jasper HH. Epilepsy and the Functional Anatomy of the Human Brain. Boston: Little, Brown and Co., 1954:20.
8. Gastaut H. Classification of the epilepsies. Proposal for an international classification. Epilepsia 1969;10(Suppl):14–21.
9. Masland RL. Comments on the classification of epilepsy. Epilepsia 1969;10(Suppl):22–28.
10. Proposal for revised clinical and electroencephalographic classification of epileptic seizures. Epilepsia 1981;22:489–501.
11. Browne TR, Holmes GL. Types of seizures. In: Handbook of Epilepsy, 4th Ed. New York: Lippincott Williams & Wilkins, 2008:24–45.
12. Golan, DE, Tashjian AH, Armstrong EJ, et al., eds. Principles of Pharmacology: The Pathophysiologic Basis of Drug Therapy. Philadelphia: Lippincott Williams & Wilkins, 2005.
13. Taylor CP. Mechanisms of new antiepileptic drugs. In: Delgado-Escueta AV, Wilson WA, Olsen RW, et al., eds. Jasper's Basic Mechanisms of the Epilepsies, 3rd Ed. (Advances in Neurology, Vol 79.) Philadelphia: Lippincott Williams & Wilkins, 1999:1012–1027.
14. MacDonald RI, Meldrum B. Principles of antiepileptic drug action. In: Levy RH, Meldrum BS, eds. Antiepileptic Drugs, 4th Ed. New York: Raven Press, 1995:61–78.
15. Armijo JA, Shushtarian M, Valdizan EM, et al. Ion channels and epilepsy. Curr Pharm Des 2005;11:1975–2003.
16. Lerche H, Weber YG, Jurkat-Rott K, et al. Ion channel defects in idiopathic epilepsies. Curr Pharm Des 2005;11:2737–2752.
17. Lucas PT, Meadows LS, Nicholls J, et al. An epilepsy mutation in the β_1 subunit of the voltage-gated sodium channel results in reduced channel sensitivity to phenytoin. Epilepsy Res 2005;64:77–84.
18. Bal T, Debay D, Destexhe A. Cortical feedback controls the frequency and synchrony of oscillations in the visual thalamus. J Neurosci 2000;20:7478–7488.
19. Browne TR, Holmes GL. Epilepsy: definitions and background. In: Handbook of Epilepsy, 4th Ed. New York: Lippincott Williams & Wilkins, 2008:1–23.
20. Zhaobing G, Tangzhi Z, Meng W, et al. Isoform-specific prolongation of Kv7 (KCNQ) potassium channel opening mediated by new molecular determinants for drug-channel interactions. J Biol Chem 2010;285:28322–28332.
21. Swinyard EA, Woodhead JH, White HS, et al. General principles, experimental selection, quantification, and evaluation of anticonvulsants. In: Levy R, Mattson, RH, Meldrum B, et al., eds. Antiepileptic Drugs, 3rd Ed. New York: Raven Press, 1989:85–102.
22. Vida JA. Central Nervous system depressants: sedative-hypnotics. In: Foye WO, ed. Principles of Medicinal Chemistry, 2nd Ed. Philadelphia: Lea & Febiger, 1981:173–188.
23. Swinyard EA, Brown WC, Goodman LS. Comparative assays of antiepileptic drugs in mice and rats. J Pharmacol Exp Ther 1952;106:319–330.
24. Woodbury LA, Davenport VD. Design and use of a new electroshock seizure apparatus, and analysis of factors altering seizure threshold and pattern. Arch Int Pharmacodyn 1952;92:97–106.
25. Emilien G, Maloteaux JM. Pharmacological management of epilepsy. Mechanism of action, pharmacokinetic drug interactions, and new drug discovery possibilities. Int J Clin Pharmacol Ther 1998;36:181–194.
26. Browne, TR. Pharmacokinetics of antiepileptic drugs. Neurology 1998;51(Suppl 4):S2–S7.
27. Benedetti MS. Enzyme induction and inhibition by new antiseizure drugs: a review of human studies. Fundam Clin Pharmacol 2000;14:301–319.
28. Battino D, Estienne M, Avanzini G. Clinical pharmacokinetics of antiseizure drugs in pediatric patients. Part II. Phenytoin, carbamazepine, sulthiame, lamotrigine, vigabatrin, oxcarbazepine, and felbamate. Clin Pharmacokinet 1995;29:341–369.
29. Mattson RH, Department of Veterans Affairs Epilepsy Cooperative Study No. 118 Group. A comparison of carbamazepine, phenobarbital, phenytoin, and primidone in partial and secondarily generalized tonic-clonic seizures. N Engl J Med 1985;313:145–151.
30. Thomas P, Valton L, Genton P. Absence and myoclonic status epilepticus precipitated by antiepileptic drugs in idiopathic generalized epilepsy. Brain 2006;129:1281–1292.
31. Lipkind GM, Fozzard HA. Molecular model of anticonvulsant drug binding to the voltage-gated sodium channel pore. Mol Pharmacol 2010;78:631–638.
32. Cuttle L, Munns AJ, Hogg NA, et al. Phenytoin metabolism by human cytochrome P450: involvement of P450 3A and 2C forms in secondary metabolism and drug-protein adduct formation. Drug Metab Dispos 2000;28:945–950.
33. Lu W, Uetrecht JP. Peroxidase-mediated bioactivation of hydroxylated metabolites of carbamazepine and phenytoin. Drug Metab Dispos 2008;36:1624–1636.
34. Awasthi S, Hallene KL, Fazio V, et al. RLIP76, a non-ABC transporter, and drug resistance in epilepsy. BMC Neurosci 2005;6:61–76.
35. Kupiec T, Raj V. Fatal seizures due to potential herb–drug interactions with ginkgo biloba. J Anal Toxicol 2005;29:755–758.
36. Browne TR, Kugler AE, Eldon MA. Pharmacology and pharmacokinetics of fosphenytoin. Neurology 1996;46(Suppl1):S3–S7.
37. Aaronson PM, Belgado BS, Spillane JP, et al. Evaluation of intramuscular fosphenytoin vs intravenous phenytoin loading in the ED. Am J Emerg Med 2010, DOI: 10.1016/j.ajem.2010.05.005.
38. Adams BD, Buckley NH, Kim JY, et al. Fosphenytoin can cause hemodynamically unstable bradydysrhythmias. J Emerg Med 2006;30:75–79.
39. Biton V, Gates JR, Ritter FJ, et al. Adjunctive therapy for intractable epilepsy with ethotoin. Epilepsia 1990;31:433–437.
40. Browne TR, Holmes GL. Antiepileptic drugs. In: Handbook of Epilepsy, 4th Ed. New York: Lippincott Williams & Wilkins, 2008:176–222.
41. Gelisse P, Genton P, Kuate C, et al. Worsening of seizures by oxcarbazepine in juvenile idiopathic generalized epilepsies. Epilepsia 2004;45:1282–1286.
42. Bu H, Kang P, Deese AJ, et al. Human in vitro glutathionyl and protein adducts of carbamazepine-10,11-epoxide, a stable and pharmacologically active metabolite of carbamazepine. Drug Metab Dispos 2005;33:1920–1924.
43. Potter JM, Donnelly A. Carbamazepine-10-11 epoxide in therapeutic drug monitoring. Ther Drug Monit 1998;20:652–657.
44. Pearce RE, Uetrecht JP, Leeder JS. Pathways of carbamazepine bioactivation in vitro: II. The role of human cytochrome P450 enzymes in the formation of 2-hydroxyiminostilbene. Drug Metab Dispos 2005;33:1819–1826.
45. Misra A, Aggarwal A, Singh O, et al. Effect of carbamazepine therapy on vitamin D and parathormone in epileptic children. Pediatr Neurol 2010;43:320–324.
46. Ficker DM, Privitera M, Krauss G, et al. Improved tolerability and efficacy in epilepsy patients with extended-release carbamazepine. Neurology 2005;65:593–595.
47. Benes J, Parada A, Figueiredo AA, et al. Anticonvulsant and sodium channel–blocking properties of novel 10,11-dihydro-5H-dibenz[b,f]azepine-5-carboxamide derivatives. J Med Chem 2000;42:2582–2587.
48. Reddy DS. Clinical pharmacokinetic interactions between antiepileptic drugs and hormonal contraceptives. Expert Rev Clin Pharmacol 2010;3:183–192.
49. Muscatello MR, Pacetti M, Cacciola M, et al. Plasma concentrations of risperidone and olanzapine during coadministration with oxcarbazepine. Epilepsia 2005;46:771–774.
50. Besag FMC, Berry D. Interactions between antiepileptic and antipsychotic drugs. Drug Saf 2006;29:95–118.
51. Mazzucchelli I, Onat FY, Ozkara C, et al. Changes in the disposition of oxcarbazepine and its metabolites during pregnancy and the puerperium. Epilepsia 2006;47:504–509.
52. Striano S, Striano P, DiNocera P, et al. Relationship between serum monohydroxy-carbazepine concentrations and adverse effects in patients with epilepsy on high-dose oxcarbazepine therapy. Epilepsy Res 2006;69:170–176.
53. Wong IC, Lhatoo SD. Adverse reactions to new anticonvulsant drugs. Drug Saf 2000;23:35–56.
54. Kobayashi K, Morita J, Chiba K, et al. Pharmacogenetic roles of CYP2C19 and CYP2B6 in the metabolism of R- and S-mephobarbital in humans. Pharmacogenetics 2004;14:549–556.
55. Goodman LS, Swinyard EA, Brown WC, et al. Anticonvulsant properties of 5-phenyl-5-ethyl-hexandropyrimidine-4,6-dione (Mysoline), a new antiepileptic. J Pharmacol Exp Ther 1953;108:428–434.
56. Butler TC, Waddell WJ. Metabolic conversion of pyrimidone (Mysoline) to phenobarbital. Proc Soc Exp Biol Med 1956;93:544–546.
57. Fountain NB, Adams RE. Midazolam treatment of acute and refractory status epilepticus. Clin Neuropharmacol 1999;22:261–267.
58. Towne AR, DeLorenzo RJ. Use of intramuscular midazolam for status epilepticus. J Emerg Med 1999;17:323–328.
59. McIntyre J, Robertson S, Norris E, et al. Safety and efficacy of buccal midazolam versus rectal diazepam for emergency treatment of seizures in children: a randomized controlled trial. Lancet 2005;366:205–210.
60. McMullan J, Sasson C, Pancioli A, et al. Midazolam versus diazepam for the treatment of status epilepticus in children and young adults: a meta-analysis. Acad Emerg Med 2010;17:575–582.
61. Pang T, Hirsch LJ. Treatment of convulsive and nonconvulsive status epilepticus. Curr Treat Options Neurol 2005;7:247–259.
62. Mikko UO, Esa K. Regulation of GABAA receptor subunit expression by pharmacological agents. Pharmacol Rev 2010;62:97–135.
63. Brodtkorb E, Aamo T, Henricksen O, et al. Rectal diazepam: pitfalls of excessive use in refractory epilepsy. Epilepsy Res 1999;35:123–133.
64. Schmidt D, Bourgeois B. A risk–benefit assessment of therapies for Lennox-Gastaut syndrome. Drug Saf 2000;22:467–477.
65. Treiman DM, Walker MC. Treatment of seizure emergencies: convulsive and nonconvulsive status epilepticus. Epilepsy Res 2006;68(Suppl 1):S77–S82.

66. Thompson CD, Barthen MT, Hopper DW, et al. Quantification in patient urine samples of felbamate and three metabolites: acid carbamate and two mercapturic acids. Epilepsia 1999;40:769–776.
67. Chang HR, Kuo CC. Molecular determinants of the anticonvulsant felbamate binding site in the N-methyl-D-aspartate receptor. J Med Chem 2008;51:1534–545.
68. Thompson CD, Gulden PH, Macdonald TL. Identification of modified atropaldehyde mercapturic acids in rat and human urine after felbamate administration. Chem Res Toxicol 1997;10:457–462.
69. Popovic M, Nierkens S, Pieters R, et al. Investigating the role of 2-phenylpropenal in felbamate-induced idiosyncratic drug reactions. Chem Res Toxicol 2004;17:1568–1576.
70. Parker RJ, Hartman NR, Roecklein BA, et al. Stability and comparative metabolism of selected felbamate metabolites and postulated fluorofelbamate metabolites by postmitochondrial suspensions. Chem Res Toxicol 2005;18:1842–1848.
71. Schenzer A, Friedrich T, Pusch M, et al. Molecular determinants of KCNQ (Kv7) K^+ channel sensitivity to the anticonvulsant retigabine. J Neuroscience 2005;25:5051–5060.
72. Brown DA, Passmore GM. Neural KCNQ (Kv7) channels. Br J Pharmacol 2009;156:1185–1195.
73. Borlak J, Gasparic A, Locher M, et al. N-glucuronidation of the antiepileptic drug retigabine: results from studies with human volunteers, heterologously expressed human UGTs, human liver, kidney, and liver microsomal membranes of Crigler-Najjar type II. Metabolism 2006;55:711–721.
74. Brodie MJ, Lerche H, Gil-Nagel A, et al. Efficacy and safety of adjunctive ezogabine (retigabine) in refractory partial epilepsy. Neurology 2010;75:1–8.
75. Petroff OA, Hyder F, Rothman DL, et al. Effects of gabapentin on brain GABA, homocarnosine, and pyrrolidinone in epilepsy patients. Epilepsia 2000;41:675–680.
76. Taylor MT, Bonhaus DW. Allosteric modulation of [^{3}H]gabapentin binding by ruthenium red. Neuropharmacology 2000;39:1267–1273.
77. Luer MS, Hamani C, Dujovny M, et al. Saturable transport of gabapentin at the blood-brain barrier. Neurol Res 1999;21:559–562.
78. Asconape J, Diedrich A, DellaBadia J. Myoclonus associated with the use of gabapentin. Epilepsia 2000;41:479–481.
79. Chung SS. Lacosamide: new adjunctive treatment option for partial-onset seizures. Expert Opin Pharmacother 2010;11:1595–1602.
80. Harris JA, Murphy JA. Lacosamide: an adjunct agent for partial-onset seizures and potential therapy for neuropathic pain. Ann Pharmacother 2009;43:1809–1817.
81. Johannessen-Landmark CJ, Patsalos PN. Drug interactions involving the new second- and third-generation antiepileptic drugs. Expert Rev Neurother 2010;10:119–140.
82. Lingamanemi R, Hemmings HC Jr. Effects of anticonvulsants on veratridine- and KCl-evoked glutamate release from rat cortical synaptosomes. Neurosci Lett 1999;276:127–130.
83. Zheng C, Yang K, Liu Q, et al. The anticonvulsive drug lamotrigine blocks neuronal {alpha}4{beta}2 nicotinic acetylcholine receptors. J Pharmacol Exp Ther 2010;335:401–408.
84. Magdalou J, Herber R, Bidault R, et al. In vitro N-glucuronidation of a novel antiepileptic drug, lamotrigine, by human liver microsomes. J Pharmacol Exp Ther 1992;260:1166–1173.
85. Jansky J, Rasonyi G, Halasz P, et al. Disabling erratic myoclonus during lamotrigine therapy with high serum level—report of two cases. Clin Neuropharmacol 2000;23:86–89.
86. Grunewald R. Levetiracetam in the treatment of idiopathic generalized epilepsies. Epilepsia 2005;46(Suppl 9):154–160.
87. Vigevano F. Levetiracetam in pediatrics. J Child Neurol 2005;20:87–93.
88. Yao J, Nowack A, Kensel-Hammes P, et al. Cotrafficking of SV2 and synaptotagmin at the synapse. J Neurosci 2010;30:5569–5578.
89. Margineanu GD. Inhibition of neuronal hypersynchrony in vitro differentiates levetiracetam from classical antiepileptic drugs. Pharmacol Res 2000;42:281–285.
90. Patsalos PN. Pharmacokinetic profile of levetiracetam: toward ideal characteristics. Pharmacol Ther 2000;85:77–85.
91. Gidal BE, Baltes E, Otoul C, et al. Effect of levetiracetam on the pharmacokinetics of adjunctive antiepileptic drugs: a pooled analysis of data from randomized clinical trials. Epilepsy Res 2005;64:1–11.
92. Briggs DE, French JA. Levetiracetam safety profiles and tolerability in epilepsy. Expert Opin Drug Saf 2004;3:415–424.
93. Arain AM. Pregabalin in the management of partial epilepsy. Neuropsychiatr Dis Treat 2009;5:407–413.
94. Luszczki JJ. Third-generation antiepileptic drugs: mechanisms of action, pharmacokinetics and interactions. Pharmacol Rep 2009;61:197–216.
95. Wisniewski CS. Rufinamide: a new antiepileptic medication for the treatment of seizures associated with Lennox-Gastaut syndrome. Ann Pharmacother 2010;44:658–667.
96. Soudijn W, van Wijngaarden I. The GABA transporter and its inhibitors. Curr Med Chem 2000;7:1063–1079.
97. Koepp MJ, Edwards M, Collins J, et al. Status epilepticus and tiagabine therapy revisited. Epilepsia 2005;46:1625–1632.
98. Sorri I, Kalviainen R, Mantyjarvi M. Color vision and contrast sensitivity in epilepsy patients treated with initial tiagabine monotherapy. Epilepsy Res 2005;67:101–107.
99. Shank RP, Gardocki JF, Streeter AJ, et al. An overview of the preclinical aspects of topiramate: pharmacology, pharmacokinetics, and mechanism of action. Epilepsia 2000;41(Suppl 1):S3–S9.
100. Skradski S, White HS. Topiramate blocks kainate-evoked cobalt influx into cultured neurons. Epilepsia 2000;41(Suppl 1):S45–S47.
101. DeLorenzo RJ, Sombati S, Coulter DA. Effects of topiramate on sustained repetitive firing and spontaneous recurrent seizure discharges in cultured hippocampal neurons. Epilepsia 2000;41(Suppl 1):S40–S44.
102. Garnett WR. Clinical pharmacology of topiramate: a review. Epilepsia 2000;41(Suppl 1):S61–S65.
103. Craig JE, Ong TL, Lousi DL, et al. Mechanism of topiramate-induced acute-onset myopia and angle closure glaucoma. Am J Ophthalmol 2004;137:193–195.
104. Fraser CM, Sills GJ, Butler E, et al. Effects of valproate, vigabatrin, and tiagabine on GABA uptake into human astrocytes cultured from fetal and adult brain tissue. Epileptic Disord 1999;1:153–157.
105. Benbadis SR. Practical management issues for idiopathic generalized epilepsies. Epilepsia 2005;46(Suppl 9):125–132.
106. Krasowski MD, Therapeutic drug monitoring of the newer anti-epilepsy medications. Pharmaceuticals 2010;3:1909–1935.
107. Leppik IE. Zonisamide: chemistry, mechanism of action, and pharmacokinetics. Seizure 2004;13(Suppl 1):S5–S9.
108. Miyamoto T, Kohsaka M, Koyama T. Psychotic episodes during zonisamide treatment. Seizure 2000;9:65–70.
109. Tracy G, Avital C, Shlomo S, et al. Ethosuximide, valproic acid, and lamotrigine in childhood absence epilepsy. N Engl J Med 2010;362:790–799.
110. Millership JS, Mifsud J, Galea D, et al. Chiral aspects of the human metabolism of ethosuximide. Biopharm Drug Dispos 2005;26:225–232.

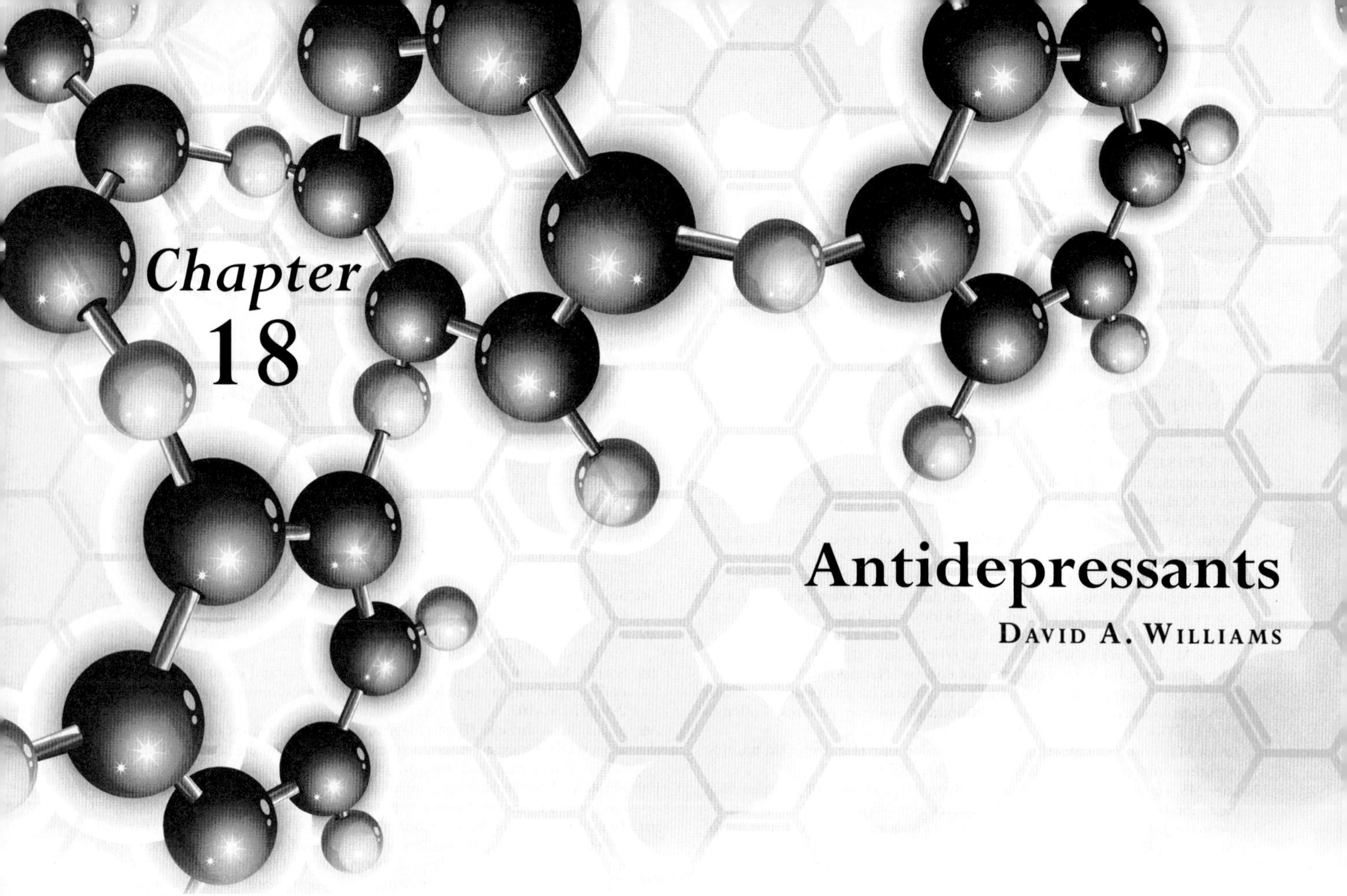

Chapter 18

Antidepressants

DAVID A. WILLIAMS

Drugs Covered in This Chapter*

SELECTIVE NOREPINEPHRINE REUPTAKE INHIBITORS (SNRIs)

- Amoxapine
- Desipramine
- Maprotiline
- Nisoxetine
- Nortriptyline
- Protriptyline
- *Reboxetine*
- R-Atomoxetine

SELECTIVE SEROTONIN REUPTAKE INHIBITORS (SSRIs)

- Citalopram
- Escitalopram (S-citalopram)
- Fluoxetine
- Fluvoxamine
- Paroxetine
- Sertraline

NOREPINEPHRINE AND SEROTONIN REUPTAKE INHIBITORS (NSRIs)

- Amitriptyline
- Clomipramine
- Desvenlafaxine (O-desmethylvenlafaxine)
- Doxepin
- *Dosulepin*
- Duloxetine
- Imipramine
- *Lofepramine*
- Milnacipran
- Trimipramine
- Venlafaxine

DOPAMINE AND NOREPINEPHRINE REUPTAKE INHIBITORS (DNRIs)

- Bupropion

SEROTONIN ANTAGONIST/REUPTAKE INHIBITORS (SARIs)

- Aripiprazole
- Trazodone
- *Vilazodone*

NORADRENERGIC AND SPECIFIC SEROTONERGIC ANTIDEPRESSANTS (NaSSAs)

- Mirtazapine

MONOAMINE OXIDASE INHIBITORS (MAOIs)

- *Moclobemide*
- Phenelzine
- Tranylcypromine

MOOD STABILIZERS

- Lithium carbonate

MELATONERGIC AGONIST/SEROTONIN ANTAGONIST

- *Agomelatine*

Abbreviations

ACh, acetylcholine
ACTH, adrenocorticotropic hormone
ADHD, attention-deficit hyperactivity disorder
ATP, adenosine triphosphate
AUC, area under the curve
BDNF, brain-derived neurotrophic factor
CNS, central nervous system
CRF, corticotropin-releasing factor
CYP, cytochrome P450
DA, dopamine
DAT, dopamine reuptake transporter
DCPP, 2,3-dichlorophenylpiperazine
DSM-IV, *Diagnostic and Statistical Manual of Mental Disorders*
ECT, electroconvulsive therapy
FDA, U.S. Food and Drug Administration
GABA, γ-aminobutyric acid
GI, gastrointestinal
GSK-3, glycogen synthase kinase-3
HPA, hypothalamus-pituitary-adrenal axis

*Drugs listed include those available in the United States. Drugs available outside the United States are shown in italics.

Abbreviations (Continued)

5-HT, serotonin
IC_{50}, half maximal inhibitory concentration
IP, intraperitoneal
MAO, monoamine oxidase
MAOIs, monoamine oxidase inhibitors
***m*-CPP**, *m*-chlorophenylpiperazine
MDD, major depression disorder
MIF-1, melanocyte-stimulating hormone release–inhibiting factor-1
MT, melatonin receptor
nM, nanomoles/L
nAChRs, nicotinic receptors
NaSSAs, noradrenergic and specific serotonergic antidepressants
NE, norepinephrine
NET, norepinephrine reuptake transporter
NK_1, neurokinin-1
NMDA, *N*-methyl-D-aspartate
NSRIs, norepinephrine and serotonin reuptake inhibitors
ODV, *O*-desmethylvenlafaxine
P-gp, P-glycoprotein
RIMAs, reversible inhibitors of MAO-A
SARIs, serotonin antagonist/reuptake inhibitors
SERT, serotonin reuptake transporter
SNRIs, selective norepinephrine reuptake inhibitors
SSRIs, selective serotonin reuptake inhibitors
TCAs, tricyclic antidepressants
TM, transmembrane domain
UV, ultraviolet

SCENARIO

Nancy Ordonez, PharmD

GP is a 45-year-old man who presents to the internal medicine clinic for a follow-up visit for his diabetes and lipids. His medical history is significant for uncontrolled hypertension, type 2 diabetes mellitus, coronary artery disease, and peripheral neuropathy. Six months before this visit he had complained of decreased energy, increased appetite, and loss of interest in his hobbies of golf and running. He was diagnosed with depression at that visit and was started on venlafaxine 37.5 mg twice daily, which was gradually increased to 150 mg twice daily. GP still is not seeing any improvement in his depressive symptoms. His current medications are simvastatin 40 mg, metoprolol 20 mg, amitriptyline 25 mg at bedtime, glyburide 20 mg, and lisinopril 10 mg once daily. He has gained 20 lb in 6 months. His blood pressure readings from today are 160/90 and 165/85, and from his blood pressure log his readings have ranged from 165 to 185 systolic and 75 to 90 diastolic. In addition, GP states that his peripheral neuropathy has worsened significantly even though he is maintaining good glucose control, and he complains that amitriptyline makes him quite drowsy in the morning.

(The reader is directed to the clinical solution and chemical analysis of this case at the end of the chapter).

Canst thou not minister to a mind diseas'd
Pluck from the memory a rooted sorrow,
Raze out the written troubles of the brain
And with some sweet oblivious antidote
Cleanse the stuff'd bosom of that perilous stuff
Which weighs upon the heart?

—*William Shakespeare*

INTRODUCTION

Depression is an ancient and prevalent mental condition that has been referenced throughout history in song, poetry, and literature. In a depressed state, one feels hopeless and experiences an overwhelming sense of despair. Depression immobilizes a person, afflicting men and women, rich and poor, and young and old alike. Depression makes one feel exhausted, worthless, helpless, and hopeless. It is an illness that involves the body, mood, and thoughts and affects the way one eats and sleeps, the way one feels about oneself, and the way one thinks about things. It often interferes with normal functioning, causing pain and suffering not only to those who suffer from depression but also to those around them. Serious depression can destroy family life and the life of the person who is ill. A depressive disorder is not the same as a passing blue mood. Without treatment, symptoms can last for weeks, months, or years. Appropriate treatment, however, can help most people who suffer from depression. Negative thinking fades as treatment begins to take effect. Unfortunately, many people do not recognize that depression is a treatable illness. Much of this suffering is unnecessary because *depression is one of the most treatable mental illnesses.*

"Depression is the flaw in love. The meaninglessness of every enterprise and every emotion, the meaninglessness of life itself, becomes self-evident. The only feeling left in this loveless state is insignificance."

"My depression had grown on me as that vine had conquered the oak; it had been a sucking thing that had wrapped itself around me, ugly and more alive than I. It had a life of its own that bit by bit asphyxiated all of my life out of me. My moods belonged to the depression as surely as the leaves on that oak tree's high branches belonged to the vine."

"Drug therapy hacks through the vine. You can feel it happening, how the medication seems to be poisoning the parasite so that bit by bit it withers away. You feel the weight going, feel the way that the branches can recover much of their natural bent. But even with the vine gone, you may still have a few leaves and shallow roots and the rebuilding of your self cannot be achieved with any drugs that now exist.

Rebuilding of the self in and after depression requires love, insight and most of all, time."

—*Andrew Solomon, The Noonday Demon: An Atlas of Depression*

Depression affects approximately 10% to 12% of the Western population (United States, ~10%; Europe, 9% to 12%; Australia, ~18%), with women outnumbering men 2:1. One in 4 women and 1 in 10 men can expect to develop depression during their lifetime. Thus, depression ranks among the top five diseases in these countries. In the United States alone, approximately 19 million adults will be afflicted yearly with depression, and at least 50% of those with major depression will suffer one or more repeated episodes of depression during their adult lifetime (1,2). Depression affects at least 1 in 50 children under the age of 12 years and 1 in 20 teenagers, mostly girls. The increase in the rate of depression among adolescent girls is related more to physical changes that occur during puberty, suggestive of hormonal changes. Premenstrual syndrome and postpartum depression are additional conditions involving depression that specifically affect women and are suggestive of hormonal involvement in the pathogenesis of depression. About half of all cases of depression go unrecognized and untreated, and approximately 10% to 15% of those with depression will take their own lives yearly.

Depression in the elderly (17% to 35%) often is dismissed as a normal part of aging and may go undiagnosed and untreated, causing needless suffering for the family and for the individual who could otherwise live a fruitful life. Often, the symptoms described usually are physical, and the older person often is reluctant to discuss feelings of hopelessness, sadness, loss of interest in normally pleasurable activities, or extremely prolonged grief after a loss. Some symptoms may be the result of adverse (side) effects of medication that the elderly person is taking for other physical problems, or they may be caused by a concurrent illness. Improved recognition and treatment of depression will make life more enjoyable and fulfilling for the depressed elderly person, the family, and the caretakers.

The economic cost for depressive illnesses in the United States is estimated to be $53 billion per year (2005), but the cost in human suffering cannot be estimated. In 2009, antidepressants drugs (primarily norepinephrine and serotonin reuptake inhibitors [NSRIs] and selective serotonin reuptake inhibitors [SSRIs]) ranked in the top 50 drugs dispensed, third in total prescriptions written, and third in total dollar prescription sales, at approximately $12.5 billion (~5% of total prescription drug sales).

TYPES OF DEPRESSIVE DISORDERS

Why are some people more susceptible to depression than others? Hippocrates, the father of medicine, theorized that we are born into one of four primary temperament styles and that each style has its own unique outlook on life: Choleric (aggressive), Sanguine (emotional), Phlegmatic (passive), and Melancholy (analytical). Of these four styles, the introverted Melancholy is the most perfection driven and depression prone. The analytical Melancholy influence gives one tremendous attention to detail, but it also can create stress, anxiety, and depression. In fact, the term "melancholy" has become synonymous with depression. People with the Melancholy temperament style are by their very nature sensitive, judgmental, and critical. People with this temperament style become depressed primarily because they fail to reach their own incredibly high standards. This depression often leads to suicide, violence against others, or both.

CLINICAL SIGNIFICANCE

The antidepressant class of drugs are well known and widely used today not only for the treatment of mood disorders, such as depression, and bipolar disorders, but also for the treatment of neuropathic pain, smoking cessation, and obsessive-compulsive disorders, among others. The application of medicinal chemistry in the development of newer antidepressants, such as selective serotonin uptake inhibitors (SSRIs), in the past 20 years has significantly affected the treatment of depression. The SSRIs have become first-line therapy in the treatment of major depressive disorder, and they are used as adjunct treatment for patients with other mood disorders. This new generation of antidepressants has more favorable side effect and pharmacokinetic profiles than the older generations of antidepressants, such as tricyclic antidepressants and monoamine oxidase inhibitors. This has resulted in improved patient compliance and therapeutic outcomes for patients with major depressive disorder. Modifications of the structure–activity relationships of the antidepressant drugs have produced medications with multiple indications. For example, both duloxetine and buproprion are indicated for major depressive disorder, but duloxetine also is used for diabetic neuropathic pain and buproprion for smoking cessation. With a growing number of antidepressants on the market, it is more important than ever for the clinician to be knowledgeable about drugs' structure–activity relationships, adverse effects, drug interactions, and pharmacokinetic properties to properly select the optimal drug regimen for the patient.

Nancy Ordonez, PharmD
Clinical Assistant Professor
University of Houston
College of Pharmacy
Houston, Texas

Major Depression Disorder

Major depression disorder (MDD; also called unipolar depression) is the most serious type of depression; it is manifested through a combination of symptoms that interfere with the ability to work, study, sleep, eat, and enjoy once-pleasurable activities. MDD may reoccur several times during a lifetime (3,4). Many people with major depression cannot continue to function normally. Major depression seems to run in families, suggesting that depressive illnesses can be inherited. Early signs (prodromal symptoms) of major depression include changes in brain function among those individuals having low self-esteem, who consistently view themselves and the world with pessimism or who are readily overwhelmed by stress. The treatments for major depression are medication, psychotherapy, and, in extreme cases, electroconvulsive therapy.

Dysthymia

This is a mild, chronic depression that lasts for 2 years (1 year for children and adolescents) or longer and is characterized by chronic symptoms that do not disable but that keep one from functioning well or from feeling good about himself or herself (4). Many of those with dysthymia also experience major depressive episodes at some point in their lives. Most people may not realize that they are depressed and continue to function at work or school, but often with the feeling that they are "just going through the motions." Antidepressants or psychotherapy can help.

Bipolar Disorder (Manic-Depressive Illness)

Bipolar disorders can be divided into bipolar I (episodes of severe mood swings from mania to depression), bipolar II (milder episodes of hypomania that alternate with depression), cyclothymia (milder episodes of bipolar II; low-grade bipolar II), or rapid-cycling bipolar disorder (more than four episodes within a year affecting women more than men) (4). Clinical studies over the years have provided evidence that monoamine signaling and hypothalamic-pituitary-adrenal axis disruption are integral to the pathophysiology of bipolar disorder (5). Bipolar disorders also seem to run in families and affect men and women equally. Not nearly as prevalent as the other forms of depressive disorders, bipolar disorders are characterized by cyclical periods of depression (lows) with periods of abnormal behavior (highs) known as hypomania or mania. Sometimes, the mood switches are dramatic and rapid, but most often, they are gradual. When in the depressed cycle, an individual can exhibit the symptoms of a depressive disorder. When in the hypomanic/manic cycle, the individual may be overactive and overtalkative and have a great deal of energy. The hypomanic/manic cycle often affects thinking, judgment, and social behavior in ways that cause serious problems and embarrassment. For example, the individual in the hypomanic/manic cycle may feel elated and full of grand schemes that might range from unwise business decisions to romantic sprees. Lithium, carbamazepine, topiramate, and valproic acid are effective mood-stabilizing treatments for bipolar disorders. In addition, the atypical antipsychotics, olanzapine and aripiprazole (see Chapter 14), are used as mood stabilizers for acute bipolar mania or in conjunction with antidepressants (e.g., Symbyax, a combination of olanzapine and fluoxetine).

Other Types of Depressive Disorders

Other less common types of depression include seasonal affective disorder, a popular name that describes a type of depression that happens during particular seasons of the year (seasonal pattern) but that it is not a *Diagnostic and Statistical Manual of Mental Disorders* (DSM-IV) (4) diagnosis. This disorder involves symptoms of depression that occur during the fall and winter seasons, when the days are shorter and there is less exposure to natural sunlight. When the spring and summer seasons begin and there is greater exposure to longer hours of daylight, the symptoms of depression disappear. Adjustment disorder with depressed mood is a type of depression that results when a person has something bad happen that depresses them (e.g., loss of one's job can cause this type of depression). It generally fades as time passes and the person gets over whatever it was that happened (4). Additional factors involved in its onset include stresses at home, work, or school, and symptoms may persist for as long as 6 months.

BIOLOGIC BASIS OF DEPRESSION

Existing treatments for MDD usually take weeks to months to achieve their antidepressant effects, and about 25% of these patients do not have adequate improvement even after months of treatment to achieve response and remission, which commonly results in morbidity and disruption in personal, professional, family, and social life. In addition, increased risk of suicide attempts is a major public health concern during the first month of standard antidepressant therapy. Thus, new antidepressant treatment strategies presenting a rapid improvement of depressive symptoms—within hours or even a few days—and whose effects are sustained would have an enormous impact on public health. Thus, improved therapeutics that can exert their antidepressant effects within hours or a few days of their administration are urgently needed.

Current theories regarding the causes of depression support the role of the neurotransmitters serotonin (5-HT) and norepinephrine (NE) in depression and their interrelationships with each other and with dopamine (DA) (Fig. 18.1). Although the precise nature of the depression is not fully understood at the level of the chemistry in the brain, several theories have been proposed to explain the role of NE and 5-HT in the causes of depression (6).

However, evidence for hypercholinergic mechanisms in depression and hypocholinergic mechanisms in mania

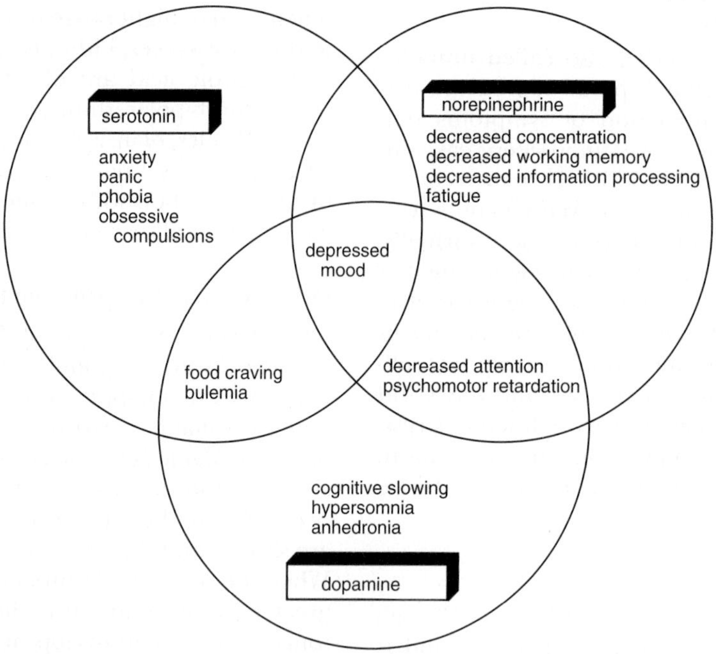

FIGURE 18.1 Neurotransmitter deficiency syndromes and their interactions.

has been building over the last several decades, especially the clinical relationships between tobacco use and depression, which suggest important effects of nicotine in MDD. About 120 years ago, Willoughby (*Lancet*, Pilocarpine in Threatening Mania, Lancet 1889;133:1030–1031.) first reported the use of pilocarpine (a cholinomimetic) to treat acute mania. During the 1970s, Janowsky and Davis (6) and others hypothesized that a cholinergic imbalance (i.e., hypercholinergic tone) was a primary factor in depressive illnesses. Since that time, a number of key findings from both animal and human studies have supported this hypothesis, with focus specifically on central nicotinic cholinergic rather than muscarinic pathways. Further support for this hypothesis is the loss of high-affinity nicotinic cholinergic receptors in Alzheimer patients. Most clinically prescribed antidepressants target NE and 5-HT neurotransmitter systems; however, many of the drugs that target these systems, such as SSRIs or selective norepinephrine reuptake inhibitors (SNRIs) and tricyclic antidepressants (TCAs), also act as potent noncompetitive antagonists of nicotinic acetylcholine receptors (nAChRs) at clinically effective doses for treatment of major depression (6). The rapid monoamine effects of the antidepressants and their delayed therapeutic onset of action have led to reconsideration of alternative hypotheses regarding the mechanism of action of antidepressants.

Animal studies with the *N*-methyl-D-aspartate (NMDA) antagonist ketamine (Chapters 12 and 16) have consistently shown antidepressant effects within a few hours of its administration, and thus, NMDA produces its antidepressant response in a much shorter period of time than existing antidepressant medications. Another alternative approach to improved treatment of depression focuses on the dual-acting melatonin receptor agonists/serotonin receptor antagonists. Melatonin is a neurohormone secreted by the pineal gland in the brain that is an important regulator of the body's circadian (sleep/wake) rhythms, reproduction, and other hormones, which are thrown off balance in depression. Understanding the molecular basis of the NMDA and the dual-acting melatonin receptor agonists/serotonin receptor antagonists can lead to the development of improved antidepressant pharmacotherapy rather than simply furthering our knowledge of current standard antidepressants.

Monoamine Hypothesis

The monoamine hypothesis proposes that depression results from a deficiency in 5-HT and/or NE (7, 9–13) and that antidepressant therapy aims to correct these deficiencies. The role of DA in depression remains unclear. Schildkraut et al. (7) postulated that depression arises as a consequence of a deficiency of NE and that the effects caused by catecholamine depletion can be reversed by TCAs. Depression in animals following reserpine administration can be reversed by TCAs, suggesting that the stimulating effects for desipramine (a secondary amine TCA) and monoamine oxidase (MAO) inhibitors (MAOIs) were NE based.

During the late 1960s, Kielholz, a Swiss psychiatrist, argued that different antidepressants did quite different things and that it was important to select the right antidepressant for the right patient. He differentiated the TCAs based on whether they possessed the ability to sedate (e.g., trimipramine), to stimulate (e.g., desipramine or nortriptyline), or to improve mood (e.g., clomipramine).

By the end of the decade, the broad consensus was that secondary amine TCAs (like desipramine or nortriptyline) inhibited the reuptake of NE into noradrenergic neurons and that blocking 5-HT reuptake by tertiary amine TCAs (such as clomipramine) gave an explanation for the mood elevation of some antidepressants.

The catecholamine hypothesis was then modified to include 5-HT in the etiology of depression (9,10). It should be noted, however, that not all inhibitors of monoamine reuptake are antidepressants, because cocaine, a potent inhibitor of NE and DA reuptake, is not an antidepressant but, rather, an addictive stimulant. Subsequent studies with inhibitors of monoamine biosynthesis appear to confirm Kielholz's opinion and Schildkraut's modified theory that clinical depression is the result of a deficiency in both 5-HT and NE and that the antidepressive mechanism of action most likely affects levels of both.

Inhibition of 5-HT biosynthesis reverses the therapeutic effects of treatment with antidepressants that have predominantly 5-HT reuptake inhibitory activity (e.g., fluoxetine) but less so with those that have predominantly NE reuptake inhibitory activity (e.g., desipramine) (11,12). Also, inhibition of 5-HT biosynthesis produced a relapse in depressed patients who had their depression successfully treated with imipramine or tranylcypromine, whereas inhibitors of DA or NE synthesis had no effect on these depressed patients (13). A depletion of catecholamines reverses the therapeutic effects of desipramine more than that of fluoxetine or sertraline. These studies appear to confirm that the antidepressive action of antidepressants is, indeed, a function of their monoamine activity.

Kielholz further reasoned that because NE reuptake inhibitors (activating antidepressants) were likely to trigger suicide, the greatest hazard of an antidepressant, and 5-HT reuptake inhibitors would be less likely to lead to suicide that it would be worth developing drugs that selectively inhibited the reuptake of 5-HT, producing agents more useful for the treatment of depression.

Changes in NE and 5-HT levels do not affect mood in everyone. Some evidence also suggests that, for a subset of patients, DA plays a role in depression. Dopaminergic substances have been used as antidepressants when other measures have failed. The DA hypothesis of schizophrenia and the emphasis on other neurotransmitters, most notably NE and 5-HT, in the pathogenesis of depression have focused attention away from DA and its role in affective disorders. Recent clinical evidence suggests the involvement of DA in several subtypes of depression, psychomotor retardation, and diminished motivation and in seasonal mood disorder (11). The biochemical evidence in patients with depression indicates diminished DA turnover. In addition, a considerable amount of pharmacologic evidence exists regarding the efficacy of antidepressants with dopaminergic effects in the treatment of depression. However, the role of DA in depression must be understood in the context of existing theories involving other neurotransmitters that may act independently and interact with DA and other neurochemicals to contribute to depression (12).

Thus, the clinical efficacy/toxicity produced by these antidepressants is due to a combination of inhibitory actions on different targets including reuptake transporters for the neurotransmitters 5-HT, NE, DA, muscarinic acetylcholine receptors, nAChRs, histamine H_1 receptors, and α-adrenergic$_1$ receptors (10).

Limitations of the Monoamine Hypothesis

Although the monoamine deficiency hypothesis of depression has been commonly used to explain the mechanism of actions of the antidepressant drugs, a growing body of evidence has been accumulating over the past two decades supporting alternative nonmonoamine mechanisms of action: the hypercholinergic hypothesis of depression (6,8), NMDA antagonists, dual-acting melatonin receptor agonists/serotonin receptor antagonists (14), and neuropeptides.

Almost 40 years ago, the cholinergic theory of depression and mania hypothesized a balance between cholinergic and adrenergic systems, suggesting that hyperactivity of the cholinergic system over the adrenergic system would lead to symptoms of depression, mediated through excessive neuronal nicotinic receptor activation. Thus the therapeutic actions of many antidepressants may be, in part, mediated through inhibition of these nAChRs (6). On the other hand, hypocholinergic activity would lead to the symptoms of mania (6). Consistent with this hypothesis, physostigmine (a cholinesterase inhibitor-hypercholinergic response; Chapter 9), when administered to normal subjects, produces symptoms of depression: anxiety, irritability, aggressiveness, and hostility (6). When physostigmine was administered to patients with MDD, these depressive symptoms were more pronounced and longer lasting in these patients (6); physostigmine also induced depression in patients with acute mania. The hypercholinergic effects of physostigmine are mediated primarily through acetylcholine activation of neuronal nAChRs, not muscarinic receptors. Over the past 20 years, various groups have reported on the nAChR inhibitory actions of classic TCAs, including imipramine, nortriptyline, amitriptyline, and desipramine, and the serotonin reuptake inhibitors, including fluoxetine, sertraline, paroxetine, and citalopram (8). Mecamylamine, a potent ganglionic blocker as a hypotensive agent that is devoid of monoamine reuptake, is a potent nAChR receptor antagonist that is undergoing clinical trials as an antidepressant to reduce symptoms of major depression and bipolar disorders (to be discussed later). nAChRs modulate not only the release of monoamines, but also γ-aminobutyric acid (GABA), glutamate, and various neuropeptides. Perhaps one of the most interesting antidepressants to have nAChR inhibitory activity is the atypical antidepressant, bupropion. Bupropion is unique because it is metabolized to hydroxybupropion, which is an SNRI and a reuptake inhibitor of DA, with little or no direct action on serotoninergic neurotransmission, and is used in nicotine cessation.

In addition, transdermal nicotine administration (patch) has been shown to substantially improve the depressive symptoms of patients with MDD, an effect believed to be due to nicotine's antagonist effects on nAChRs. These effects have been attributed primarily to inhibition of a high-affinity nAChR subtype in the brain, the $\alpha_4\beta_2$ subunit, representing the predominant mammalian brain nAChR subtype. Thus, cigarette smoking may exert antidepressant effects in patients with MDD who were refractory to SSRI treatment (7), supporting the view that depressed smokers self-medicate by smoking.

Thus, there is an increasing amount of evidence supporting a possible role of neuronal nAChRs in depression as well as in the clinical effectiveness of antidepressants and that the therapeutic action of many antidepressants may be mediated, at least partially, through inhibition of excessive neuronal nAChR activity.

Major depression is frequently accompanied by alterations in circadian (light/dark) rhythms of behavior, sleep, reproduction, and the secretion of hydrocortisone and other hormones (14). These circadian disturbances in depression are associated with an abnormal pineal release of melatonin, a key synchronizer of biologic circadian rhythms that is tightly coupled to sleep/wake and seasonal cycles. Melatonin production appears to be lower in depression even though the administration of melatonin itself is ineffective in the treatment of MDD. Aging is also associated with a weakened response of the circadian clock to environmental stimuli. These observations support the resynchronization of sleep/wake rhythms by melatonergic mechanisms as a new strategy for improving the pharmacotherapy of MDD.

Receptor Sensitivity Hypothesis

The receptor sensitivity hypothesis proposes that it is not simply the level of NE or 5-HT in the synapse that matters but, rather, the sensitivity of the postsynaptic receptors to these neurotransmitters. Those with depression, it is speculated, possess postsynaptic receptors that have grown hypersensitive to NE and 5-HT because of their depletion in the synaptic cleft. Thus, a low level of NE and 5-HT at their respective receptors can lead to changes in the receptors themselves, even if there are no clinical signs of depression. Increased receptor sensitivity (hypersensitivity) and an increase in receptor numbers on the neuronal cell membrane are events that may correlate with the start of depression. This theory is an important step toward understanding the long delay between administration of antidepressant drugs and their clinical response. According to this hypothesis, relief from the symptoms of depression following chronic administration of antidepressants comes from a normalization of receptor sensitivity (reducing receptor hypersensitivity) by increasing the concentration of NE and 5-HT in the synaptic cleft. Therefore, the use of reuptake inhibitors and the MAOIs as antidepressants increases the concentration of NE and/or 5-HT in the synaptic cleft and, over time, causes the postsynaptic neuron to compensate by decreasing receptor sensitivity (desensitization) and the number of receptor sites (decrease in the expression of NE and 5-HT receptors: downregulation). Approximately one-third of depressed patients, however, fail to respond to antidepressant therapy. For some unknown reason, the increased concentrations of NE and/or 5-HT fail to desensitize the postsynaptic receptors.

Permissive Hypothesis

The permissive hypothesis (10) emphasizes the importance of the balance between 5-HT and NE in regulating mood, not the absolute levels of these neurotransmitters or their receptors. If 5-HT levels are too low, the balanced control of the NE system is lost, permitting abnormal levels of NE to cause mania, as seen in bipolar disorders. If the NE levels fall, the balanced control of the 5-HT system is lost, allowing abnormal levels of 5-HT to cause the person to exhibit the symptoms of depression.

Hormonal Hypothesis

The hormonal hypothesis suggests that changes in the hypothalamus-pituitary-adrenal axis (HPA) can influence the levels of 5-HT, NE, and acetylcholine (ACh) released by nerve cells in the brain and, subsequently, their function (15). In the event of stress, ACh stimulates the hypothalamus to produce a hormone locally in the brain called corticotrophin-releasing factor (CRF), which in turn stimulates the pituitary gland to secrete adrenocorticotropic hormone (ACTH) into the blood, where it stimulates the adrenal glands to release hydrocortisone (cortisol), which prepares the body for dealing with stress. Stress also directly stimulates the adrenal gland to secrete epinephrine and NE. Hydrocortisone can cause depression, especially when released in higher-than-usual amounts. The release of hydrocortisone may push the individual over the edge into depression or contribute to the component of anxiety, which so often accompanies depressive illnesses. Approximately 50% of those with MDD have elevated hydrocortisone levels as a result of hyper-CRF activity.

Moreover, one of the most replicated findings in biologic psychiatry is that large numbers of unmedicated depressed patients exhibit HPA hyperactivity. The available evidence suggests that nAChRs play important roles in mediating stress-related and possibly depression-inducing neuroendocrine effects of ACh. ACh (hypercholinergic activity), in response to stress, can stimulate the HPA through activation of nAChRs. Thus, antidepressants may reduce symptoms of depression, in part, through blockade of nAChRs involved with stress-induced activation of the HPA (8).

Living organisms operate in a state of imbalance, and the neural (autonomic) and endocrine systems have evolved to modify the rates of biochemical pathways to maintain homeostasis. One of the hallmarks of these regulatory systems is the short-lived nature of the nerve signals produced. The half-life of neurotransmitters is measured in seconds, whereas those of the circulating hormones may be minutes or hours. A rationale for the short-lived nature of the neurotransmitters is to permit these signaling pathways to quickly reset themselves to meet the next challenge. Readjustments (i.e., plasticity) in these systems include uncoupling of receptor responses from signaling events, degradation of receptors, and up- and downregulation of signaling molecules that affect the primary signaling pathway. These hypotheses are not mutually exclusive, and in each, it is assumed that the more extreme the event, the more severe the clinical outcome.

GENERAL APPROACHES TO TREATMENT OF DEPRESSION

Before 1950, there were no antidepressants—at least not as we know them today. The two treatments for depressive illness were either amphetamine stimulants, which often were ineffective and had the general effect of increasing energy and activity (16), or electroconvulsive therapy, which was effective but had the disadvantage of terrifying and often endangering the patient. Not until the late 1950s was the first generation of antidepressants discovered (the TCAs and MAOIs), not by design but by chance. While searching for "chlorpromazine-like" compounds to treat schizophrenia, imipramine was recognized by Kuhn (16) for its antidepressant properties, thus becoming the forerunner for the tricyclic class of monoamine reuptake inhibitor antidepressants (i.e., the TCAs). The second compound to be discovered was the antitubercular drug isoniazid (17), which proved to have powerful mood-enhancing properties, becoming the forerunner of the MAOIs. With the introduction of imipramine and isoniazid, the theory and treatment of depression changed. These early studies still summarize much of our current knowledge regarding the therapeutic effects of antidepressant treatments.

Between 1960 and 1980, TCAs were the major pharmacologic treatment for depression (18). The TCAs, however, have many other actions in addition to blocking monoamine reuptake and nicotinic receptors, including anticholinergic, antihistaminergic, and cardiotoxic side effects that are related to their affinity for muscarinic, histamine, and α_1-adrenergic receptors as well as their action on cardiac and central nervous system (CNS) sodium channels in membranes. The improved safety, tolerability, and reuptake selectivity of the newer antidepressants (i.e., SSRIs, SNRIs, and NSRIs) have resulted in displacement of the TCAs as the first choice for prophylactic treatment of major depression. The TCAs occupy a narrower—but still important—role in the psychopharmacologic therapy.

The early MAOIs irreversibly inhibited the oxidative deamination of the neurotransmitter monoamines, the proposed mechanism of their antidepressant activity. The biggest liability for these MAOIs was their potential to cause life-threatening hypertensive reactions, resulting from the irreversible inhibition of both MAO-A and MAO-B, which decreases the intestinal and hepatic degradation of dietary sources of tyramine. This inhibition of MAO allows excessive amounts of dietary tyramine, a weak sympathomimetic vasoconstrictor, to be absorbed from the food, resulting in increased blood pressure (refer to the section on MAOIs in this chapter for more details). Inhibition of MAOs also can alter the pharmacokinetics of monoamine over-the-counter and prescription drugs, allowing them to accumulate in the blood and, thus, increasing their potential for causing adverse drug effects and drug–drug interactions. Minimizing drug and food interactions of these early MAOIs inspired the development of a new generation of MAOIs that are both reversible and selective for MAO-A. The demise of the early MAOIs allowed the TCAs to become the gold standard for the treatment of depressive disorders.

The discovery that certain antihistaminic agents without the condensed aromatic ring systems are selective inhibitors of 5-HT reuptake with little affinity for the other neuroreceptors and almost devoid of cardiotoxicity questioned the need for the 10,11-ethylene bridge for the TCAs. Thus, the search for inhibitors that selectively blocked 5-HT reuptake without the seven-membered central ring of the TCAs resulted in the synthesis of the diarylpropylamine analogs of the TCAs (Fig. 18.2). Thus, during the late 1960s and early 1970s, antihistamine molecules were structurally manipulated in the search for compounds that selectively inhibited 5-HT reuptake with greater potency. The initial breakthrough came with the synthesis of *Z*-zimeldine (the *cis*-isomer; also known as zimelidine, Zemid, patented in 1971), the first SSRI that selectively inhibited the presynaptic reuptake of 5-HT without the adverse events associated with the multireceptor activities of the TCAs (19,20). Zimelidine was synthesized from the manipulation of the antihistamine pheniramine into a diaryl allylamine, the *cis*-isomer (rigid analog) of the propylamine group (Fig. 18.2).

Other structural changes that enhanced its potency and selectivity for blocking 5-HT reuptake was moving the regional position of the 2-pyridyl ring of pheniramine to the 3-pyridyl position and substitution of a halogen into the 4-position of the phenyl ring (2-substitutions selectively block NE reuptake). The secondary amine and primary metabolite, norzimelidine, was 15 times more potent than zimelidine for blocking 5-HT reuptake. On the other hand, *E*-zimelidine (the *trans*-isomer) is an inhibitor of both 5-HT and NE reuptake, whereas its corresponding secondary amine is a potent and selective inhibitor of NE reuptake. It is not unusual for geometric isomers to differ markedly from each other with regard to their receptor or transporter selectivity, affinity, and pharmacodynamic properties. Thus, zimelidine became the first SSRI to be marketed as an antidepressant, but unfortunately, several cases of Guillain-Barré syndrome (an autoimmune disorder attacking the peripheral nervous system) were associated with the use of this drug and led to its withdrawal from the market in 1983. During postmarketing clinical studies, zimelidine showed an increase in the number of suicide attempts over what had been expected—this adverse event was to become a major issue with the SSRIs 20 years later.

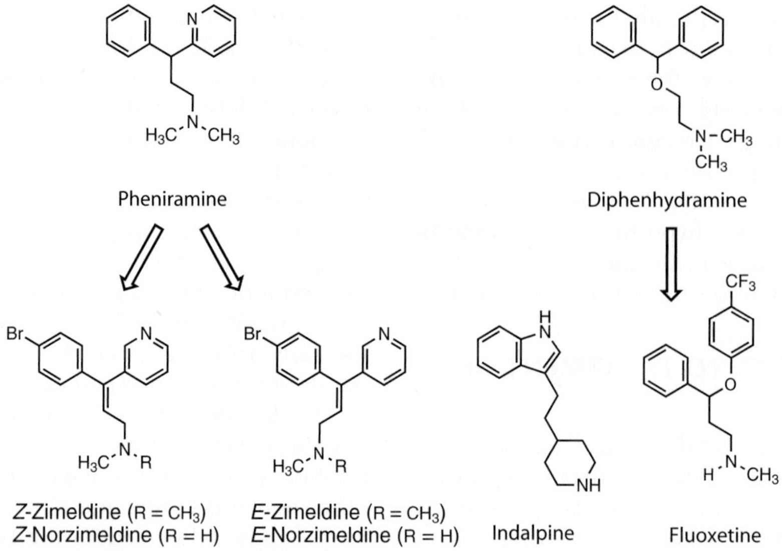

FIGURE 18.2 Structural relationship between antihistamines and antidepressants that block the reuptake of 5-HT.

The success of zimelidine as an SSRI, however, led to the discovery and marketing of several nontricyclic SSRIs from multiple pharmaceutical companies worldwide. Another manipulation of the antihistamines produced indalpine (patented 1977 by Rhône Poulenc) (Fig. 18.2). It produced responses in patients who had not responded to the TCAs or MAOIs but then ran into trouble, because clinical trials suggested that it might cause agranulocytopenia (a lowering of the white blood cell count). For the most part, this is not a serious problem, but in rare cases, if undetected, it can be fatal. It was removed from the European market in 1985 and was never marketed in the United States.

Other SSRIs developed during this period that have become household words include paroxetine (patented 1975 by Ferrosan to SmithKlineBeecham to GlaxoKline), citalopram (patented 1979 by Lindberg, licensed to Forest Labs), fluoxetine (patented 1982 by Lilly), and sertraline (patented 1985 by Pfizer).

Scientists at Lilly Research Laboratories synthesized more than 50 phenoxypropylamines derived from the antihistamine diphenhydramine (Benadryl) before discovering fluoxetine (21,22) (Fig. 18.2). The first of these compounds was nisoxetine, a potent SNRI (see Fig. 18.8) that was clinically developed but never marketed. Other derivatives that have since been marketed by Lilly include atomoxetine (an SNRI) and duloxetine (an NSRI).

Fluoxetine (Prozac) was heralded as the prototype for the next generation of SSRI antidepressants, possessing fewer adverse effects and with a greater margin of safety when overdoses are consumed compared with the TCAs and also lacking the food-interaction toxicity of MAOIs. Fluoxetine was marketed in 1987, and within a few years, it boasted worldwide sales of nearly $1.2 billion a year. During the past 20 years, nontricyclic selective NE or 5-HT reuptake inhibitors, reuptake inhibitors of both NE and 5-HT, and reversible selective MAOIs have been approved for use in depression. These newer additions allow exploration of the roles of NE versus 5-HT using treatments that are devoid of confounding receptor activities. Conscious targeting of more than one neurotransmitter activity (e.g., of serotonergic and noradrenergic mechanisms or of NE and DA), while retaining specificity, is the target for the development of the next generation of antidepressants.

The majority of antidepressants in current use selectively inhibit the reuptake of 5-HT and/or NE. Based on the previously neglected role proposed for DA in depression, it has been hypothesized that a "broad-spectrum" antidepressant will produce a more rapid onset and/or higher efficacy than agents inhibiting the reuptake of 5-HT and/or NE (23). Broad-spectrum antidepressants are compounds that inhibit the reuptake of NE, 5-HT, and DA, the three biogenic amines most closely linked to depression. The pharmacologic profile of one such compound, DOV 21947, an azabicyclo[3.1.0]hexane, has recently been described and is in phase III clinical trials (23,24). It is a potent inhibitor of NE, 5-HT, and DA reuptake by their corresponding membrane transporter proteins. The plasma concentrations of DOV 21947, following both single and multiple doses, appear to be sufficient to inhibit NE, 5-HT, and DA reuptake.

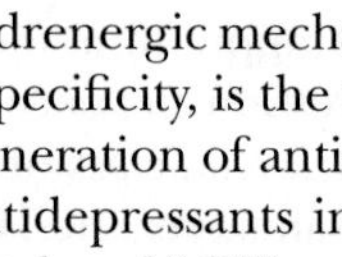

DOV 21947

S-(+)-Mecamylamine is a potent noncompetitive antagonist of nAChRs. Racemic mecamylamine was originally developed as a ganglionic-blocking agent for the treatment of moderately severe to severe essential hypertension (Chapter 24). However, it soon became apparent that mecamylamine was capable of crossing the blood–brain barrier and distributing itself into brain tissues, thus exerting CNS effects such as preventing nicotine-induced seizures in several animal species at doses lower than those necessary to reduce blood pressure or elicit other peripheral signs of postganglionic blocking activity. In contrast to its competitive blockade of preganglionic nAChRs in autonomic ganglia, mecamylamine is a noncompetitive inhibitor of neuronal nAChRs and binds to the $\alpha_4\beta_2$ nAChR subunit in the open channel of the receptor. Mecamylamine is in phase III clinical trials as an augmentative antidepressant strategy for patients with MDD who are refractory to SSRI treatment. If clinical trials are successful and the U.S. Food and Drug Administration (FDA) approves mecamylamine as an antidepressant, this new drug paves the way for further investigations using nAChRs as targets for the action of safer antidepressants and novel antiaddictive nicotine compounds.

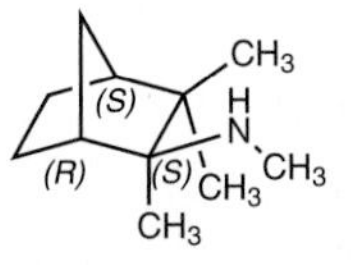

S(+)-Mecamylamine

The antiobesity agent, racemic (*R,S*)-sibutramine is a 5-HT and NE reuptake inhibitor and has an antidepressant profile similar to that of a "triple-acting" antidepressant in animals (25). It has two active metabolites, desmethylsibutramine and didesmethylsibutramine (the terms "desmethyl" and "demethyl" are used interchangeably). The half maximal inhibitory concentrations (IC_{50}) for the *R*-enantiomers of these metabolites were more potent as in vitro inhibitors of DA and NE reuptake than 5-HT (25). Both *R*-enantiomers had significantly greater anorectic effects than those of their respective *S*-enantiomers as well as that of (*R,S*)-sibutramine. The results suggest that these enantioselective metabolites of sibutramine could be safe and effective treatments for binge-eating disorder in obese patients.

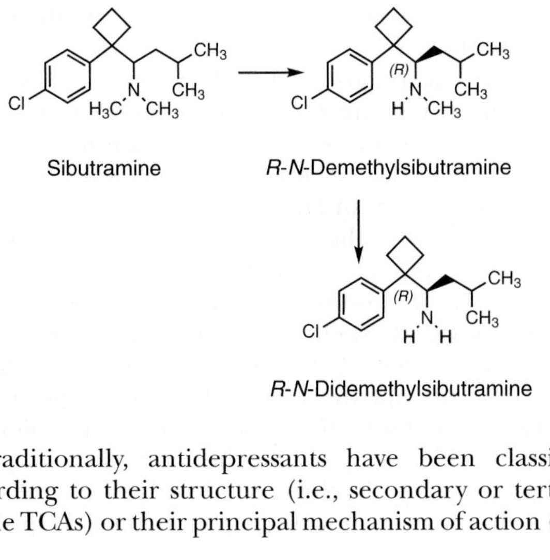

Sibutramine

R-*N*-Demethylsibutramine

R-*N*-Didemethylsibutramine

Traditionally, antidepressants have been classified according to their structure (i.e., secondary or tertiary amine TCAs) or their principal mechanism of action (i.e., MAOIs and SSRIs). With the appearance of increasing numbers of second- and third-generation antidepressants, however, a better way of classifying and describing the antidepressants was necessary. For the purposes of this chapter, the antidepressants are organized into eight classes plus mood stabilizers (Table 18.1) and discussed according to their distinct and different mechanisms of action (Fig. 18.3). Considerable overlap exists in their mechanism of actions and uses, but these different classes of antidepressants work by distinct mechanisms, have different side effect profiles, and may be favored for different types of depressive illnesses.

A key step that determines the intensity and duration of monoamine signaling at synapses is the reuptake of the released neurotransmitter into nerve terminals through high-affinity plasma membrane transporters (26). Reuptake is the process of rapidly removing the monoamine neurotransmitters from the synaptic cleft and allowing most of the released neurotransmitter to be recycled for further use. The advantage of reuptake is that it is faster than passive diffusion through the membrane. Any monoamine neurotransmitter remaining in the synaptic cleft is then absorbed and metabolized into inactive metabolites. The monoamine reuptake transporter protein binds the released neurotransmitter in the extracellular fluid and transports the monoamine across the presynaptic plasma membrane back into the intracellular fluid of the presynaptic neuron (Fig. 18.4). Monoamine transporters (Fig. 18.5; see the sidebar for more detail) are embedded in the plasma membrane of the nerve terminals (perisynaptically) of dopaminergic, noradrenergic, and serotonergic neurons rather than intrasynaptically (along the portion of the nerve terminal forming the synapse). They are members of a larger sodium-dependent transporter family and represent a major mechanism terminating the action of released monoamine neurotransmitters in the synaptic cleft. These transporters are important targets for many antidepressive drugs and substances of abuse (e.g., cocaine). Transporter proteins are specific to their respective neurotransmitter: serotonin reuptake transporter (SERT), norepinephrine reuptake transporter (NET), and dopamine reuptake transporter (DAT). None of the reuptake antidepressants exhibit significant affinity for DAT, which may be related to their ineffectiveness in types of depression that are resistant to the SNRIs, SSRIs, and NSRIs. The TCAs and nontricyclic NSRIs block both NET and SERT, the SSRIs selectively block SERT, and SNRIs selectively block NET. The antidepressant reuptake inhibitors also may contribute to relief of depression by decreasing the expression of their respective transporter proteins.

Figure 18.6 graphically illustrates the selectivity of the reuptake inhibitors for their respective transporters. The selectivity ratio for inhibiting SERT (ratio >1) is obtained by dividing the affinity of the inhibitor (K_i) for inhibiting SERT with its affinity (K_i) for inhibiting NET, whereas the selectivity ratio for inhibiting NET (ratio <1) is obtained by dividing its affinity (K_i) for inhibiting NET with the affinity (K_i) for inhibiting SERT. For example,

TABLE 18.1 Antidepressant Classes with Examples of Generic and Trade Names

Drug Classes	Abbreviation	Drug Examples	Trade Names
Selective Norepinephrine Reuptake Inhibitor	SNRIs	Amoxapine Atomoxetine Desipramine Maprotiline Nortriptyline Roboxetine	Asendin Strattera Norpramin Aventyl, Pamelor Vestra
Selective Serotonin Reuptake Inhibitor	SSRIs	Citalopram Escitalopram Fluoxetine Fluvoxamine Paroxetine Sertraline	Celexa Lexapro Prozac Luvox Paxil Zoloft
Norepinephrine and Serotonin Reuptake Inhibitor	NSRIs	Amitriptyline Clomipramine Desvenlaxine Doxepine Duloxetine Imipramine Milnacipran Trimipramine Venlafaxine	Elavil Anafranol Pristiq Sinequan Cymbalta Tofranil Ixel (in EU) Surmontil Effexor
Dopamine and Norepinephrine Reuptake Inhibitor	DNRIs	Bupropion	Wellbutrin, Zyban
Serotonin Receptor Modulators	SRMs	Aripipazole	Abilify
Serotonin-2 Antagonists/ Serotonin Reuptake Inhibitor	SARI	Trazodone Vilazodone	Desyrel, Oleptro Viibryd
α2 –Noradrenergic Antagonist/ Selective Serotonin Antagonist	NaSSA	Mirtazapine	Remeron
Monoamine Oxidase Inhibitors	MAOIs	Moclobemide Phenelzine Tranylcypramine	 Nardil Parnate
Mood Stabilizers		Lithium Valproic acid Carbamazepine	Eskalith, Lithobid Depakote, Depakene, Depacon Tegretol

a value of approximately 1 for amitriptyline means that amitriptyline will inhibit both NET and SERT at the same concentration (i.e., no selectivity with regard to their mechanism of antidepressant activity). The value of –30 for desipramine means that desipramine is 30 times more potent at inhibiting the NET than the SERT, although the SSRIs with selectivity ratio values of greater than 100 are more than 100 times more potent at inhibiting the SERT than the NET. Furthermore, because the selectivity ratio for most SSRIs is more than 100, a plasma concentration of any SSRI that will produce inhibition of the SERT will produce no physiologically meaningful inhibition of NET (27–29). The converse will be true regarding selectivity for the NET. Clinically, such selectivity ratios of greater than 100 translate into being able to produce all the physiologic effects mediated by inhibiting one transporter without causing any effects that will be produced by inhibiting the other uptake transporter. When the selectivity ratio is less than 30, such as with fluoxetine, the difference is small enough that inhibition of both reuptake transporters may occur under therapeutic doses and, thus, can contribute to the broad antidepressant activity of the drug.

Most scientists agree that MAOIs, SSRIs, SNRIs, and NSRIs improve depression by boosting the levels of NE and/or 5-HT in the brain, but what is not established is how increased concentrations of NE and 5-HT and their synergism translate into reducing depression. One problem with the original monoamine model was that whereas plasma concentrations of the antidepressant and binding to the monoamine transporter occur almost immediately, chronic administration of antidepressants is needed before clinical efficacy is attained (18). The therapeutic effect of an antidepressant is almost always observed after a period of 3 to 6 weeks of treatment. This suggests that certain adaptive changes are occurring with chronic administration of these drugs that may be important for their antidepressant

TRANSPORTER PROTEINS

The monoamine transporter protein (molecular weights, 60 to 80 kd) is a string of amino acids that weaves in and out of the presynaptic membrane 12 times (Fig. 18.4)—that is, 12 transmembrane domains (TMs) with a large extracellular loop between TM3 and TM4. Both the N- and C-termini of the transporters are located within the cytoplasm. There are six potential sites of phosphorylation by protein kinase A and protein kinase C, which regulate the transporters. The large extracellular loop and the cytoplasmic parts of the N- and C-termini do not appear to be the target sites for the transporter inhibitors (i.e., antidepressants). Rather, the areas important for selective monoamine affinity appear to be localized within TM1 to TM3 and TM8 to TM12 that project into the synapse, and these areas of the transporters have a common binding site for the monoamine and many of its inhibitors (Fig. 18.4). To transport protonated 5-HT (5-HT^+), SERT cotransports one sodium ion (Na^+) and one chloride ion (Cl^-) while countertransporting a potassium ion (K^+) (Fig. 18.5). The SERT then flips inside the cell, releasing the 5-HT^+ and the Na^+ and Cl^- into the cytoplasm of the neuron. On releasing the 5-HT^+ and the Na^+ and Cl^-, SERT flips back out, with the unoccupied binding site exposed to the synaptic cleft, ready to receive and transport another 5-HT^+ molecule. To transport protonated NE (NE^+), NET also cotransports Na^+ and Cl^- with intracellular K^+ stimulation and no K^+ efflux. The initial complex of the monoamine, Na^+, and Cl^- with the transporter protein creates a conformational change in the transporter protein. The driving force (electrical potential) for the energetically unfavorable transport of the monoamine is the Na^+ concentration gradient. The Na^+, K^+ transporter (Na^+, K^+-ATPase) maintains the extracellular Na^+ concentration as well as the intracellular K^+ concentration. The Na^+, K^+-ATPase transports three Na^+ ions for each two K^+ ions pumped into the cell. Unlike channels that stay open or closed, transporters undergo conformational changes (changes in their three-dimensional shape) and move one monoamine molecule in each cycle.

action (see previous Receptor Sensitivity Hypothesis section). This concept has been the motivating force for much of the development of alternative nonmonoamine theories. Over the years, mechanisms such as downregulation of β-adrenergic receptors, desensitization of presynaptic α_2-adrenoceptors, increased postsynaptic 5-HT receptor sensitivity, downregulation of 5-HT_2 receptors, and desensitization of presynaptic 5-HT_{1A} receptor have been cited either as the final common pathway or as one of many possible final common pathways.

It should be remembered that the neurotransmitter and downregulation hypotheses are incomplete explanations for how antidepressants work. Antidepressants most likely set off an intricate chain of reactions that occur between the time the patient first takes them and the following few weeks, when they finally produce their effect. What the neurotransmitter and downregulation hypotheses do provide are useful—if simplistic—models for comprehending at least some of the basic biochemical processes triggered by antidepressants.

ANTIDEPRESSANTS IN PSYCHOTHERAPY

The introduction of the second-generation classes of antidepressants in the 1980s and 1990s (SSRIs, SNRIs, NSRIs, and serotonin receptor modulators [serotonin antagonist/reuptake inhibitors {SARIs} and noradrenergic and specific serotonergic antidepressants {NaSSAs}]) (Table 18.1) has been regarded as the major pharmacologic advance in the treatment of depression since the appearance of the TCAs and MAOIs. The SSRIs, SNRIs, and NSRIs have proven to be effective for a broad range of depressive illnesses, dysthymia, several anxiety disorders, and bulimia. The SSRIs are the most widely prescribed antidepressant drugs and rank in the top 50 drugs in terms of total United States sales for 2004. In addition to being the usual first-line treatments for major depression, the SSRIs also are first-line treatments for panic disorder, obsessive-compulsive disorder, social phobia, posttraumatic stress disorder, and bulimia. They also may be the best medications for treatment of dysthymia and generalized anxiety disorder.

Differences in general tolerability of the different classes of antidepressants and in their side effect profiles are well known and generally accepted. Compared with the TCAs, the SSRIs cause significantly more nausea, diarrhea, agitation, sexual dysfunction, anorexia, insomnia, nervousness, and anxiety, whereas the TCAs cause more cardiotoxicity, dry mouth, constipation, dizziness, sweating, and blurred vision (18). Although the SSRIs, SNRIs, and NSRIs possess improved safety margins and lesser cardiovascular adverse effects than TCAs and utility for treating other nondepressive disorders, they offer no real gain in efficacy compared with the first-generation TCAs. Despite pharmacologic differences in their mechanisms of actions, the general view has been that all antidepressants are of equal efficacy. Only within the last 10 years has this general assumption come under serious challenge from comparisons of antidepressants with dual mechanisms of action that can be acting in a complementary and perhaps synergistic manner to improve depression versus those with a single mechanism of action (11). Often, a variety of antidepressants will be prescribed and the dosage adjusted before the most effective antidepressant or combination of antidepressants is found. Although some improvements may be seen during the first few weeks, the antidepressants must be taken regularly for 3 to 4 weeks (and, in some cases, for as many as 8 weeks) before the full therapeutic effect occurs. Patient compliance can become an issue, because patients often are tempted to stop medication too soon as a result of feeling better and, thus, thinking they no longer need the medication. They also may have problems with the adverse effects, or they may think

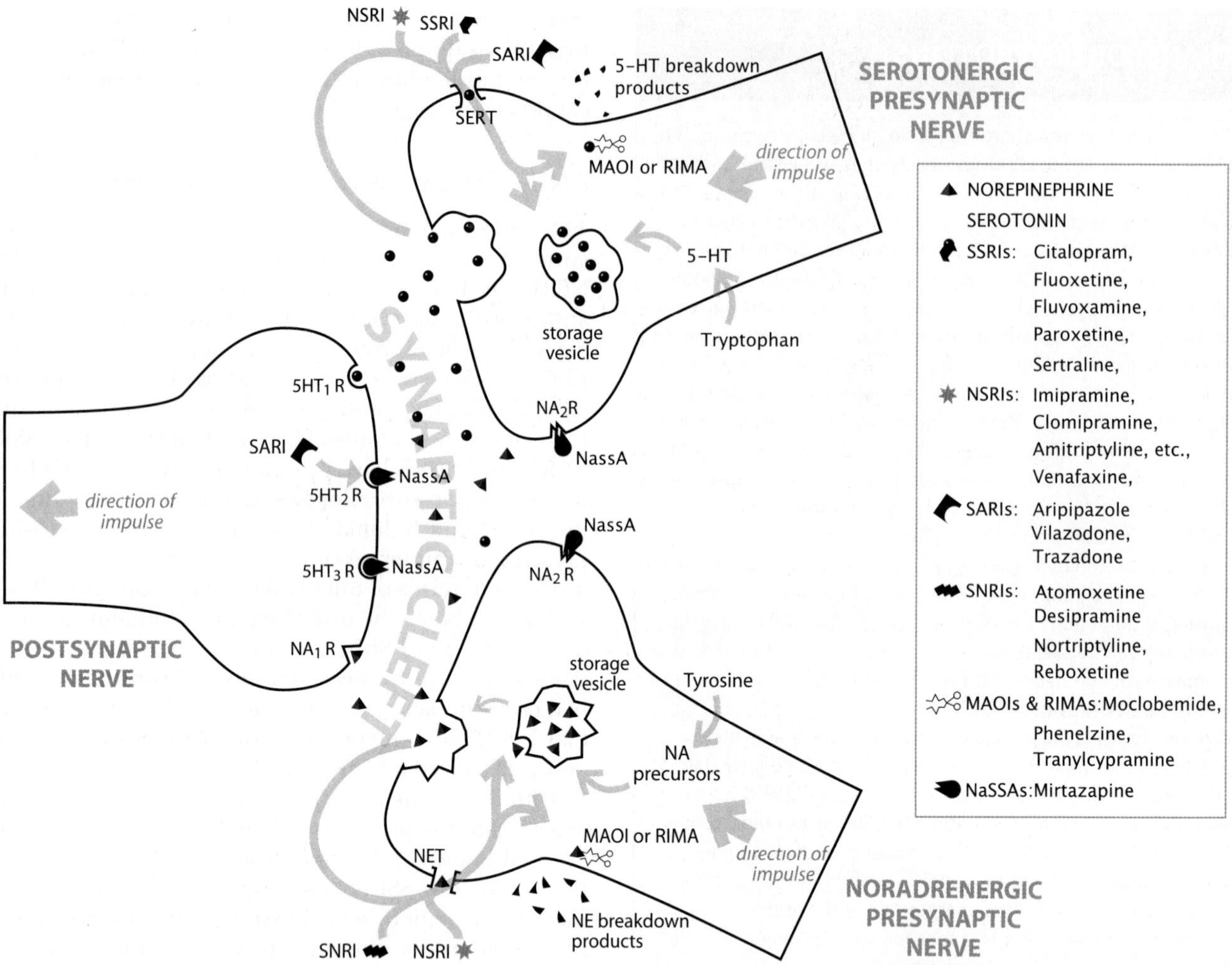

FIGURE 18.3 Sites of action of the antidepressants.

the medication is not helping at all. It is important for the patient to keep taking the antidepressant until it has a chance to work, although side effects often appear before antidepressant activity does. Once the individual is feeling better, it is important to continue the medication for at least 4 to 9 months (or longer) to prevent a recurrence of the depression. Antidepressants alter the brain chemistry; therefore, they must be stopped gradually to give the brain time to adjust. For some individuals with bipolar disorder or chronic major depression, antidepressant therapy may need to be maintained indefinitely (30). All patients who are prescribed antidepressants should be informed that although the drugs are not associated with tolerance and craving, discontinuation/withdrawal symptoms may occur on stopping, on missing doses, or occasionally, on reducing the dose of the drug. These symptoms usually are mild and self-limiting, but occasionally, they can be severe, particularly if the drug is stopped abruptly. Symptoms of antidepressant withdrawal include nausea, vomiting, anorexia, headache, restlessness, agitation, "chills," insomnia, and, sometimes, hypomania, panic-anxiety, and extreme motor restlessness, especially if an antidepressant (particularly an MAOI) is stopped suddenly after regular administration for 8 weeks or more.

Clinical trials have concluded that 2 or 3 of every 100 children and teenagers treated with antidepressants might be at higher risk of suicidal behavior. Data regarding suicidal behavior vary among the antidepressants, which leads to the conclusion that no antidepressant is free from risk at this time. Most of the suicides have occurred with the SSRIs, especially paroxetine (Paxil) and fluoxetine (Prozac); only fluoxetine has been proven to be effective and is approved for treating pediatric depression. Approximately 7% of antidepressant prescriptions are written for children. Thus, in 2007, the FDA approved that "black box labeling" be included on antidepressant product packaging, alerting physicians to avoid prescribing antidepressants to children because of possible risks of suicidal behavior and to watch for signs of worsening depression or suicidal thoughts in children who are taking any antidepressant.

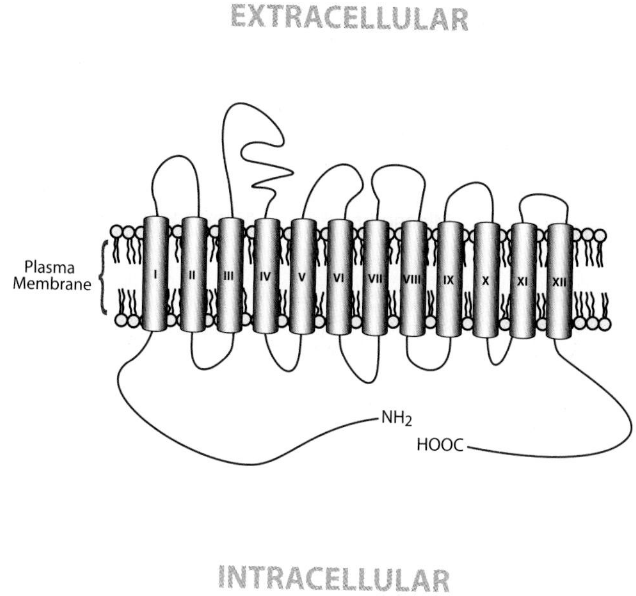

FIGURE 18.4 Monoamine reuptake transporter.

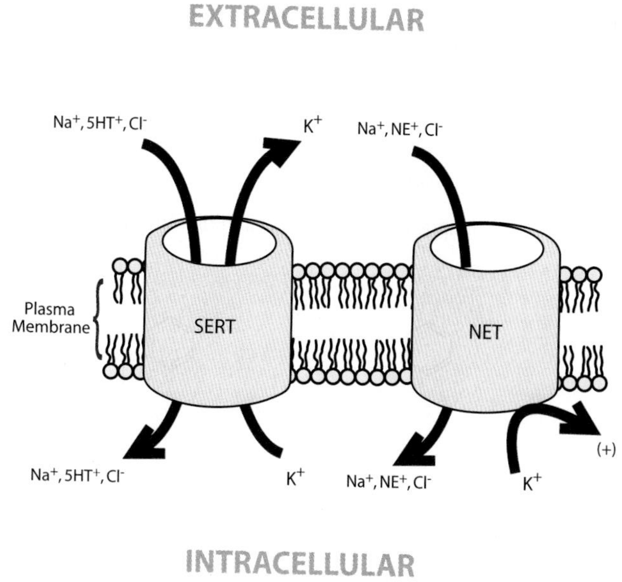

FIGURE 18.5 Model of the NET and SERT and the ion-coupled NE and 5-HT reuptake. Reuptake of 5-HT is dependent on the cotransport of Na^+ and Cl^- and countertransport of K^+. Reuptake of NE is dependent on the cotransport of Na^+ and Cl^- with intracellular K^+ stimulation but without K^+ efflux.

EFFECT OF PHYSIOCHEMICAL PROPERTIES AND STEREOCHEMISTRY ON ANTIDEPRESSANT EFFICACY

Small substituent changes in molecular structure can affect the pharmacokinetic and pharmacodynamic (clinical) properties of antidepressant drug molecules, resulting in profound differences between their transporter selectivity and their antidepressant effect—for example, a difference of a 2-chloro group between the structurally related antidepressants imipramine and clomipramine or the *o*- versus *p*-substituents between fluoxetine (SSRI) and atomoxetine (SNRI) (Fig. 18.7). Furthermore, a seemingly simple isosteric replacement of a sulfur atom in the central ring of chlorpromazine with an ethylene group to give a seven-membered azepine ring (clomipramine) or the replacement of the methylpiperidylidene at the 5-position for the antihistamine/5-HT antagonist cyproheptadine with a dimethylaminopropylidene for the antidepressant reuptake inhibitor amitriptyline has profound effects on the physicochemical properties, pharmacokinetics, mechanisms of action, and therapeutic activities (Fig. 18.7). On the other hand, the physicochemical differences can translate into differences in in vitro and in vivo pharmacologic and clinical properties, as exemplified between mianserin and mirtazapine (Fig. 18.7) (31). The isosteric replacement of a benzene ring (mianserin) with a pyridine (mirtazapine) resulted in significant changes in their dipole moments, lipophilicity (logP), pK_a values, and electronegativity, resulting in different mechanisms of action and regioselectivity in formation of hydroxylated metabolites.

Many antidepressants are stereoisomers and contain either a chiral center or a center of unsaturation by which chiral metabolites could result (32,33). Often, such drugs are marketed as a mixture of the resultant enantiomers (racemates) or of geometric isomers. These enantiomers or geometric isomers may differ markedly from each other with regard to their

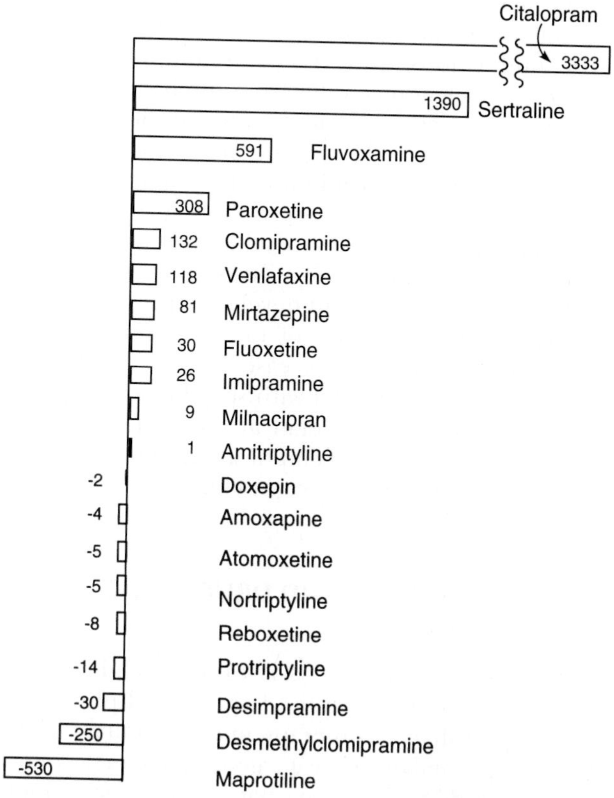

FIGURE 18.6 In vitro selectivity ratios for reuptake inhibitors.

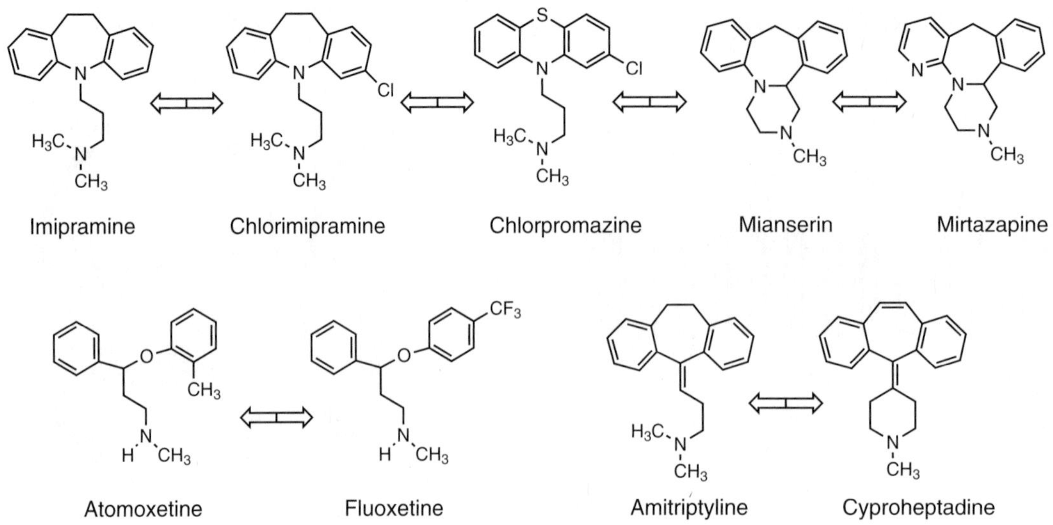

FIGURE 18.7 Structural relationship between selected molecular structures.

pharmacodynamic and/or pharmacokinetic properties. Increased knowledge about the molecular structure of specific drugs targets and an awareness of several possible advantages to using single enantiomers rather than racemic mixtures of drugs have led to an increased emphasis on understanding the role of chirality in drug development of antidepressant drugs. Several notable examples of antidepressants (the SSRIs) currently are available in which the individual enantiomers or geometric isomers differ considerably with regard to factors such as binding to SERTs and NETs, interactions with receptors and metabolizing enzymes, and clearance rates from the body. Examples of the effects of chiral centers or geometric centers on such properties include racemic mixtures (e.g., fluoxetine, citalopram, bupropion, and trimipramine), single enantiomers [e.g., (+)-sertraline, (−)-paroxetine, (−)-escitalopram, and (−)-atomoxetine]; or geometric isomers (e.g., *Z*-zimelidine, *Z*-doxepin, *E*-dosulepin, and *E*-fluvoxamine). Recent developments in analytical and preparative resolution of racemic and geometric drug mixtures as well as increased interest in developing new drugs that interact with specific targets, which have been described in detail at the molecular level, have resulted in increased emphasis on stereochemistry in antidepressant drug development.

DRUG METABOLISM AND DRUG–DRUG INTERACTIONS

Antidepressant treatment carries increased risks of adverse drug events because of age-related physiologic changes, polypharmacotherapy, and individual variability in drug metabolism (e.g., genetic factors, concurrent disease, diet, and eating habits). Pharmacokinetic drug–drug interactions occur when one medication (the precipitant drug) significantly affects the plasma concentration, half-life, or both of another medication (the object drug) by altering its absorption, distribution, metabolism, or elimination. For object drugs with narrow therapeutic indices, even small elevations in plasma drug concentration can cause potentially serious adverse reactions. Pharmacodynamic drug–drug interactions occur when the precipitant drug affects the ability of the object drug to bind with its therapeutic target (e.g., transporter protein) or receptor. Some compounds compete directly for binding to a receptor; others indirectly affect the ability of an object drug to interact with its site of action. Many medications can bind to multiple receptor types (e.g., first-generation TCAs), causing diverse adverse reactions. Thus, before adding a new drug to an existing antidepressant regimen, it is wise to determine whether any medications can be eliminated. Reduction of total drug burden, adjustment of dose levels, and careful selection of an appropriate agent are important steps toward avoiding adverse drug interactions. In addition, the documented and potential drug interactions of the various classes of antidepressants—and of the specific drugs within each class—should be considered. Each patient should be treated individually and monitored carefully during the initiation and maintenance of antidepressant therapy.

The infamous drug–drug interactions between mibefradil (Propulsid) and terfenadine (Seldane) and other drugs metabolized by cytochrome P450 (CYP) 3A4 resulted in these drugs being withdrawn from the market, which placed a spotlight on hepatic drug metabolism as a significant participant in drug–drug interactions. Nearly all the antidepressants are metabolized by at least one CYP isoform, and these drugs and their metabolites may be substrates or inhibitors for the CYPs (Table 18.2).

TABLE 18.2 Cytochrome P450 (CYP) Metabolism[a]

Antidepressant	Major CYP	Minor CYP	Metabolism Pathway	CYP Inhibitor
Amitriptyline	2D6	3A4, 2C19, 2C9, 1A2, and 2B6	2D6, 3A4, 2C19, and 1A2 *N*-demethylation 2D6 and 2B6 *E*-10-hydroxylation	2D6, 2C19, 1A2, and 2C9[b]
Clomipramine	2D6	3A4, 2C19, 1A2, and 2C9	2D6, 3A4, 2C19, 2C9, and 1A2 *N*-demethylation 2D6 2- and 8-hydroxylation	2D6
Desipramine	2D6	1A2 and 2C19	1A2 and 2C19 *N*-demethylation 2D6 and 2C19 2-hydroxylation	2D6 and 2C19[b]
E-Doxepin	2D6 and 2C9	3A4, 1A2, and 2C19	2D6 and 2C9 hydroxylation 3A4 and 1A2 *N*-demethylation	
Z-Doxepin	2C19	2C9, 3A4, and 1A2	2C19 and 2C9 *N*-demethylation 3A4 and 1A2 *N*-demethylation	
Imipramine	2D6	3A4, 2C19, 1A2, 2B6, and 2C9	1A2 and 2C19 *N*-demethylation 2D6, 1A2, 3A4, and 2C19 2- and 10-hydroxylation	1A2, 2D6, and 2C19
Maprotiline	2D6	1A2	2D6 and 1A2 *N*-demethylation	
Nortriptyline	2D6	3A4, 2C19, and 1A2	2D6, 3A4, 2C19, and 1A2 *N*-demethylation 2D6 *E*-10-hydroxylation	2D6 and 2C19[b]
Trimipramine	2D6	2C9 and 2C19	2-hydroxyl, 10-hydroxyl, and *N*-demethylation	2D6
(±)-Citalopram	2D6	1A2 and 2C19	2D6, 2C19, and 3A4 *N*-demethylation 2D6 *N*-oxidation	1A2[b] and 2D6[b]
Escitalopram	2D6	1A2 and 2C19	2D6, 2C19, and 3A4 *N*-demethylation 2D6 *N*-oxidation	
(±)-Fluoxetine	2D6	3A4, 2C9, 2C19, and 1A2	2D6 and 2C19 *N*-dealkylation 1A2 and 2C9 *O*-dealkylation	2D6 (*S*-fluoxetine) 1A2,[b] 2C19,[b] 3A4,[b] 2C9,[b] and 2D6[b]
Sertraline	3A4	2D6 and 2C19	3A4, 2C19, 2D6, and 2C9 *N*-demethylation	2C19,[b] 3A4,[b] and 2D6[b]
Fluvoxamine	1A2	3A4, 2C19, and 2D6	2D6 and 1A2 *O*-dealkylation	2C19, 1A2,[b] and 3A4[b]
Paroxetine	2D6	3A4, 1A2, and 2C9	2D6 cleavage methylene dioxy	2D6,[c] 2C19,[b] and 3A4[b]
Venlafaxine	2D6	3A4, 2C19, and 2C9	2D6, 2C19, and 2C9 *O*-demethylation 2C19, 2C9, and 3A4 *N*-demethylation	2D6[b]
Reboxetine	3A4		*O*-deethylation, aromatic ring hydroxylation	2D6 and 3A4
Atomoxetine	2D6	3A4, 2C19, and 1A2	2D6, 1A2, 2B6 and 2C19 4-hydroxylation 2C19, 3A4 and 2B6 *N*-demethylation	
Duloxetine	2D6		4- and 6-hydroxylation	2D6
Mirtazapine	2D6	3A4 and 1A2	2D6 and 1A2 8-hydroxylation 3A4 *N*-demethylation 3A4 and 1A2 *N*-oxidation	3A4[b] and 2D6[b]
Bupropion	2B6	2E1, 3A4, and 2D6	Hydroxylation t-butyl group	2D6[b]
Trazodone	3A4	2D6	*N*-dealkylation to chlorophenylpiperazine Aromatic ring hydroxylation	
Tranylcypromine		3A4, 2A6, 2D6, 2C19, and 2C9	Aromatic ring hydroxylation	2A6[c]
Moclobemide	2C19	2D6 and 1A2	Aromatic ring hydroxylation Morpholine ring oxidation	2D6[b]

[a]Rendic S. Human P450 metabolism database. Available at: http://www.gentest.com/human_p450_database. Accessed July 11, 2003.
[b]Weak CYP inhibitor.
[c]Mechanism-based inhibition.

When an antidepressant is metabolized by more than one CYP isoform in parallel, the antidepressant is unlikely to be affected by drug interactions or genetic polymorphisms and to cause clinically significant drug interactions via CYP isoform inhibition (34). However, if the drug is metabolized (depending on enzyme kinetics) primarily by CYP3A4 or the polymorphic CYP2C18 or CYP2D6 isoforms, the potential for drug–drug interactions increases. Therefore, knowledge regarding the metabolic pathways of antidepressants and knowledge about substrates and inhibitors of the CYP isoforms can assist in the selection of a proper drug and its dose, thus minimizing the risks of drug–drug interactions (35).

P-Glycoprotein Transporters

P-glycoprotein (P-gp) is a member of the adenosine triphosphate (ATP)-binding cassette superfamily of membrane transport proteins responsible for the efflux of many drugs (also see Chapter 5). It represents a major component of the blood–brain barrier and the intestinal barrier and contributes to renal and biliary elimination of drugs. At the blood–brain barrier, P-gp is localized in the apical membrane of brain capillary endothelial cells and transports substrates into the blood. Therefore, P-gp limits the penetration into and retention of numerous compounds, including the antidepressants, within the brain and thus modulates their effectiveness and CNS toxicity. Inhibition of P-gp could significantly increase drug concentrations in the CNS. Additionally, P-gp is highly expressed in the apical membrane of epithelial cells in the small and large intestine, where it transports drugs out of the cells into the intestinal lumen, thus limiting the bioavailability of compounds such as paclitaxel and HIV protease inhibitors.

The role of P-gp in affecting the pharmacokinetic parameters of antidepressants and contributing to numerous pharmacokinetic drug–drug interactions with coadministered drugs has not been thoroughly elucidated. Antidepressants, particularly TCAs, have a significant potential for inducing adverse drug reactions and, therefore, are subject to numerous drug–drug interactions. The role of P-gp in causing clinically relevant drug interactions is becoming more and more obvious (36). Concentrations of paroxetine and venlafaxine increased two to three times in the brains of mice without P-gp (i.e., knockout mice) after single-dose administration and after treatment for 11 days (34), suggesting that these antidepressants are P-gp substrates and that their pharmacokinetics might be influenced by coadministered P-gp inhibitors. In contrast, fluoxetine exhibited no P-gp substrate characteristics (34), indicating that not all antidepressants share these properties. For citalopram, the results are contradictory.

The potency of sertraline and its *N*-demethylated metabolite, desmethylsertraline, and paroxetine for inhibiting P-gp was comparable with that of quinidine (36). Fluoxetine, norfluoxetine, fluvoxamine, reboxetine, and *O*-demethylparoxetine showed intermediate inhibition, and citalopram, desmethylcitalopram, venlafaxine, and *N*-desmethylvenlafaxine showed only weak inhibition. No inhibition was found for *O*-desmethylvenlafaxine.

Inhibition of P-gp by drugs may play an important role in drug safety by increasing plasma and brain concentrations of coadministered drugs and, thus, causing adverse drug reactions. No evidence for a potent drug–drug interaction was found with fluoxetine, although sertraline and paroxetine exhibited the greatest potential for affecting the pharmacokinetics of coadministered drugs at the level of P-gp (36,37). At usual therapeutic doses of paroxetine and sertraline, however, the IC_{50} for the inhibition of P-gp is approximately 250 times higher than the plasma concentration for paroxetine and approximately 500 times higher than that for sertraline (37), suggesting that even if the accumulation of sertraline within the cell (e.g., in the biliary or renal system) is taken into account, the P-gp inhibition observed in vitro might not be clinically relevant. This is substantiated by the fact that sertraline, fluvoxamine, and citalopram did not have a clinically relevant influence on the pharmacokinetic parameters of digoxin, a P-gp prototype substrate. However, in addition to being an inhibitor of CYP2D6, paroxetine is a substrate for this same isoform, the activity of which is regulated by a genetic polymorphism. In individuals who lack this active enzyme (i.e., poor metabolizers), plasma paroxetine concentrations are up to 25 times higher than those in individuals who are extensive metabolizers. Therefore, one cannot exclude that in patients who are poor metabolizers, administration of high doses of paroxetine may translate into clinically relevant changes in the pharmacokinetics of concomitantly administered P-gp substrates.

It remains to be studied whether the inhibition of P-gp by the newer antidepressants might lead to drug–drug interactions in patients. Such interactions might, for instance, be relevant when drugs with low oral bioavailability because of substantial transport back into the gut lumen are to be coadministered, as has been shown for loperamide when given in combination with quinidine (38).

SPECIFIC DRUGS

Selective Norepinephrine Reuptake Inhibitors (SNRIs)

Despite the current popularity of the SSRIs for the treatment of depression, the noradrenergic neurons should not be overlooked, because they also influence the depressed mood (39). The noradrenergic system appears to be associated with increased drive, whereas the serotonergic system relates more to changes in mood (Fig. 18.1). Thus, the different symptoms of depression may benefit from drugs acting mainly on one or other of the neurotransmitter systems (18). The SNRIs (Fig. 18.8) seem to be at least as effective as the SSRIs in the treatment of depressive illness (39) by acting specifically at noradrenergic sites. Thus, the SSRIs and SNRIs influence

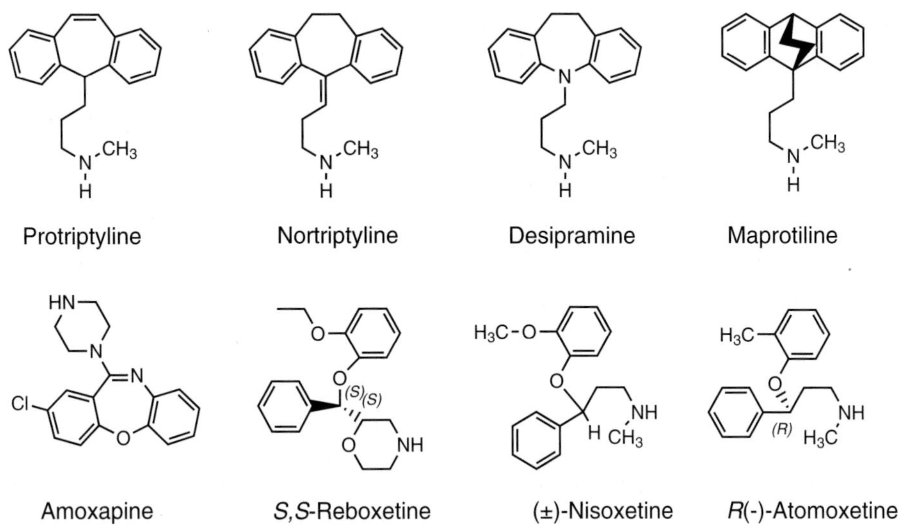

FIGURE 18.8 Selective norepinephrine reuptake inhibitors (SNRIs).

depression by parallel, independent pathways. The SNRIs have a role in the treatment of depression, either alone or as adjunct therapy. The SNRI antidepressants are well tolerated but possess different adverse event profiles.

The selectivity ratios (Fig. 18.6) show that the SNRIs, as a group, are potent selective inhibitors of the NET and that the secondary amine TCAs are substantially more potent with regard to their inhibition of NE reuptake compared with the SSRIs. Their in vitro affinity for inhibiting the NET essentially mirrors more or less their clinical efficacy as SNRIs (11): desipramine > protriptyline > amitriptyline = nortriptyline > reboxetine > maprotiline > amoxapine > imipramine > paroxetine. The level of affinity of the SNRIs for NET is not predictive for antidepressant activity.

Tricyclic Secondary Amine Antidepressants

Structure–Activity Relationship of the TCAs The tricyclic ring structure can be found in a variety of different drugs and, for the most part, represents a method for medicinal chemists to restrict the conformational mobility of two phenyl rings attached to a common carbon or hetero atom. The tricyclic ring structure is formed by joining the two phenyl rings into 6-6-6 or 6-7-6 ring systems, in which the central ring is either a six-membered or seven-membered carbocyclic or heterocyclic ring, respectively. Small molecular changes, such as ring flexibility, substituents, or heteroatoms in the tricyclic ring structure, can bring about significant changes in physicochemical, electronegativity (dipole moments), and pharmacodynamic properties (e.g., anticholinergics [antimuscarinic], cholinesterase inhibitors, antihistamine, antipsychotics, and antidepressants). This suggests that the tricyclic structure is not associated with affinity for any particular receptor but, rather, contributes to a range of multiple CNS pharmacodynamic (adverse) effects because of increased lipophilicity. The most common tricyclic ring found in drugs is the near-planar phenothiazine ring common to most of the antipsychotic drugs (Fig. 18.9). The TCAs are classified as such because they contain a 6-7-6 ring arrangement in which the central seven-membered ring is either carbocyclic or heterocyclic, saturated or unsaturated, which is fused to two phenyl rings (Fig. 18.8; also, see Fig. 18.17 for NSRIs). The side chain may be attached to any one of the atoms in the central seven-membered ring, but it must be three carbon atoms, either saturated (propyl) or unsaturated (propylidine), and have a terminal amine group (secondary or tertiary). The TCAs differ structurally from the antipsychotic phenothiazines in that the two phenyl (aromatic) rings are connected by a two-carbon link to form a central seven-membered ring instead of a sulfur bridge.

The TCAs are subdivided into a dihydrodibenzazepine ring (also known as iminodibenzyl, from which the name imipramine is derived); a dibenzocycloheptene ring, whereby the ring nitrogen of imipramine is replaced by an exocyclic olefinic group (e.g., amitriptyline); a dibenzoxepin ring as a bioisosteric modification of imipramine (e.g., doxepin); and a dibenzocycloheptriene ring, which replaces the dihydroethylene group of imipramine

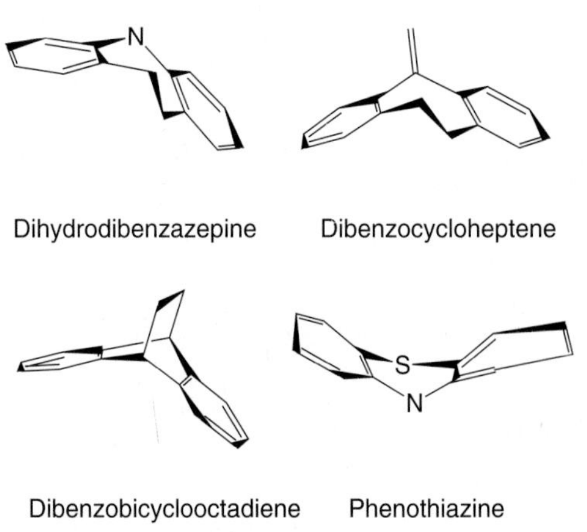

FIGURE 18.9 Three-dimensional models of the tricyclic and tetracyclic ring systems.

with an olefinic ethylene group (e.g., protriptyline) or a tetracyclic (bicyclic ring; e.g., maprotiline) derivative. The tricyclic ring system has little significance regarding selectivity for inhibiting the NET or SERT, but it appears to be important for DAT inhibition.

The secondary and tertiary amine TCAs differ markedly with regard to their selectivity ratios (Fig. 18.6) and their pharmacodynamic and/or pharmacokinetic properties (Tables 18.3, 18.8 and 18.9). Substituting a halogen (i.e., chlorine, clomipramine) or cyano group into the 3-position of the dihydrodibenzazepine ring enhances preferential affinity for SERT. 3-Cyanoimipramine was investigated as a potent SSRI but was never marketed as an antidepressant agent. It is used as a research probe for studying SERTs. Branching the propyl side chain with a 2-methyl group (as in trimipramine) significantly reduces the affinity (~100 times) of imipramine for both the SERT and NET. The *Z* (*cis*) geometry for the propylidine group in chiral TCAs appears to be important for transporter selectivity and affinity (e.g., doxepin).

Studies correlating the binding of the TCAs with the SSRIs found that the TCAs and SSRIs bind to different sites on the transporter and that the TCAs may act as a modulator of monoamine reuptake by producing conformational changes in the transporter, affecting affinity of the monoamine neurotransmitter (40).

Although similar in a two-dimensional plane to the antipsychotic (neuroleptic) phenothiazines, the ethylene bridge linking the two phenyl rings of the TCAs causes the two phenyl rings to be twisted out of the plane, leading to less rigid and more conformationally mobile molecular structures than the phenothiazines as shown in Fig 18.9. The conformational mobility for the TCAs, including ring inversion of the tricyclic ring system, flexing of the CH_2-X bridge (X = CH_2, O, N, or S) in the central seven-membered ring, and flexibility of the alkyl side chain, can result in substantial changes in the overall shape of the molecules. This, in turn, can affect transporter affinity and selectivity, diverse neuroreceptor affinity, and the drug's physicochemical properties. The rate of ring flexibility seems to be correlated with their differences in clinical potency. A dibenzazepine ring system exhibits a greater degree of conformational ring flexing, whereas the dibenzocycloheptene ring system and inserting heteroatoms into the benzylic position reduces the rate of ring flexing in TCAs and their potency (41). Thus, the differences in the pharmacologic activity between these TCAs allow selective binding to their respective transporter proteins. The angle between the two aromatic rings ranges from 106 to 110 degrees for the TCAs, and the large lipophilic ring enhances the affinity of TCA to block the CNS muscarinic, H_1-, and α_1-adrenergic receptors and to block sodium channels, contributing to its multiple pharmacodynamic effects.

TABLE 18.3 Pharmacokinetics of the Selective Norepinephrine Reuptake Inhibitors (SNRIs)

Parameters	Desipramine	Nortriptyline	Amoxapine	Protriptyline	Maprotiline	Reboxetine	Atomoxetine
Oral bioavailability (%)	60–70	32–79	ND	77–93	66–75	95	>70%
Lipophilicity ($logD_{7.4}$)	1.03	1.66	2.99	—	2.00	—	1.20
Protein binding (%)	91	92	92	92	88	>97	>97
Volume of distribution (L/kg)	17–42	14–22	ND	22	15–28	12–28	93–328 (250)
Elimination half-life (h)	30 (12–30)	30 (18–44)	8 (8–30)	67–89	43 (27–58)	12	4 (3–6) (EM)[a] 17–21 (PM)
Major active metabolites	None	10-*E*-hydroxy	8-OH (30 h) 7-OH (6.5 h)	None	(60–90 h)	None	4-Hydroxy
Peak plasma concentration (h)	4–6	7–9	90 min	24–30	8–24	12	1–2
Excretion (%)	Urine	Urine 40	Urine 60 (6 d)	Urine 50 (16 d)	Urine 65 (21 d)	Urine ~90%	Urine
	Feces	Feces minor	Feces 7–18	Feces minor	Feces 30	Feces minor	Feces
Plasma half-life (h)	14–62	18–93	8	54–198	21–52	2–4	4.3
Time to steady-state concentration	ND	ND	ND		7 d	ND	ND

ND, not determined.
[a]EM = extensive metabolizer; PM = poor metabolizer.

Pharmacokinetics Common to Secondary Amine TCAs The secondary amine TCAs are rapidly and well absorbed following oral administration. Although the pharmacokinetics are approximately similar within the tertiary and secondary amine groups, the pharmacokinetics are different between the two groups (Table 18.3; also see Table 18.9 for NSRIs). The secondary amine TCAs have relatively high bioavailability. Their primary routes of hepatic metabolism are *N*-demethylation to inactive primary amine metabolites and aromatic ring hydroxylation (Table 18.2). Despite the fact that serum plasma levels are reached within 1 to 2 days, their onset of antidepressant action typically is at least 2 to 3 weeks or longer. Their volume of distribution is very high, suggesting distribution into the CNS and protein binding. Elimination is primarily as metabolites and their conjugates via renal elimination. Renal and liver function can affect the elimination and metabolism of the parent secondary amine TCA and its metabolites, leading to increased potential for adverse effects, especially in patients (i.e., the elderly) with renal disease.

Mechanisms of Action Common to Secondary Amine TCAs The exact mechanism of action for the secondary TCAs is unclear, but the secondary amine TCAs exhibit substantially more affinity than the SSRIs and the tertiary TCAs for inhibiting the NE transporter. None of the secondary TCAs has significant affinity for the DA transporter. Blocking the reuptake of NE increases its concentration in the synaptic cleft and its ability to interact with synaptic NE receptors. When drugs are selective for a transporter, differences in potency become clinically irrelevant, because the plasma concentration can be dose adjusted to achieve inhibition of the desired transporter without affecting the other transporters. During chronic therapy with the TCAs, adaptive changes at the noradrenergic receptor occur (i.e., downregulation) as a result of neurotransmitter hypersensitivity from low concentrations of NE at the postsynaptic receptor. These changes involve the α_1-adrenergic receptor.

Therapeutic Uses Common to All TCAs The efficacy of the secondary and tertiary amine TCAs in the clinical treatment of depressive illness is recommended for various conditions, including major depressive episodes, dysthymia, panic disorder, social phobia, bulimia, narcolepsy, attention-deficit disorder with or without hyperactivity, migraine headache and various other chronic pain syndromes, enuresis in children, and obsessive-compulsive disorder (clomipramine). The TCAs possibly are useful as well for a broader range of depressive conditions described as dysthymia or depressive neurosis and even for prolonged or pathologic mourning, agoraphobia without panic attacks, and some of the symptoms (e.g., nightmares) in posttraumatic stress disorder.

Adverse Effects Common to All TCAs The family of TCAs has many undesirable side effects and behaves like "five drugs wrapped into one." They not only block the reuptake of NE and 5-HT but also block muscarinic receptors (anticholinergic), α_1-adrenergic receptors, H_1-receptors (antihistamine), and sodium channels. The common side effects and appropriate responses are given in Table 18.4.

Drug–Drug Interactions Common to the Secondary Amine TCAs The secondary amine TCAs were once first-line therapy for depression because of their efficacy in a broad range of depressive disorders. Today, however, these agents generally are reserved for second-line treatment because of their narrow therapeutic-to-toxicity ratios and troublesome adverse effect profiles. Even the better-tolerated nortriptyline is fatal in overdose and may have significant adverse effects at therapeutic dose levels. Most TCAs are metabolized by multiple CYP enzymes and, thus, are likely to be object drugs for many common medications. Because these TCAs have narrow therapeutic indices, any interference with their metabolism can lead to serious adverse reactions resulting from increased plasma concentrations (e.g., arrhythmias, seizures, and confusion). Such reactions are both more common and more likely to be life threatening in elderly patients because of age-related pharmacokinetic alterations. Therefore, although specific secondary amine TCAs are useful for some conditions (e.g., major depression), administration with other drugs should be done cautiously.

Concurrent administration of these TCAs and MAOIs is contraindicated, and at least 2 weeks should elapse between discontinuance of TCA therapy and initiation of MAOI therapy, and vice versa, to allow washout. Coadministration of SNRIs, TCAs, and MAOIs is potentially hazardous and may result in severe adverse effects associated with hypertension.

TABLE 18.4 Common Side Effects with Secondary Amine Tricyclic Antidepressants and Recommendations

Side Effects	Treatment Recommendations
Dry mouth	Drink sips of water; chew sugarless gum; clean teeth daily
Constipation	Diet rich in bran cereals, prunes, fruit, and vegetables
Bladder complaints (weak urine stream, emptying difficulty, painful urination)	Consult physician
Sexual problems	Consult physician
Blurred vision	Should pass with time
Dizziness	Rise slowly from the bed or chair
Daytime drowsiness	Do not drive; take medication at bedtime; commonly will pass with time

Because protein binding of secondary amine TCAs is high, displacement interactions with other highly protein-bound drugs with narrow therapeutic indices, although not yet fully evaluated, may be important. Concurrent use of the secondary amine TCAs with anticholinergic or sympathomimetic drugs requires close supervision and careful adjustment of the dosage because of potential additive anticholinergic effects (i.e., spastic colon) and increased blood pressure and heart rate. An additional disadvantage of these TCAs is their toxicity from overdosage, especially among those being treated for depression who may have suicidal thoughts.

In addition, secondary amine TCAs are inhibitors of sodium channels and, thus, can slow ventricular conduction at therapeutic doses. If the patient overdoses or drug interactions result in increased plasma concentration of the TCA, severe conduction block contributing to cardiotoxicity may result in ventricular arrhythmias. Also, changes in CNS conduction can result in seizures. Patients who are sensitive to one TCA may be sensitive to other TCAs.

The effect of smoking on the activity of CYP1A2 does not seem to have an effect on the plasma concentrations of the secondary TCAs because CYP1A is not involved with the *N*-dealkylation to their primary amine metabolites.

For common patient information and recommendations, see Table 18.5.

Unique Properties for the Specific Secondary Amine TCAs

Desipramine Desipramine is a dihydrodibenzazepine secondary amine TCA that also is the active metabolite of imipramine (Fig. 18.8). Desipramine appears to have a bioavailability comparable to the other secondary TCAs (Table 18.3). Desipramine is distributed into milk in concentrations similar to those present at steady-state in maternal plasma. This drug is metabolized primarily by CYP2D6 to its 2-hydroxy metabolite and by CYP1A2 and CYP2C19 to its *N*-demethylated (primary amine) metabolite (Table 18.2).

Desipramine exhibits a greater potency and selectivity for the NET than do the other secondary TCAs (Fig. 18.6). Its antidepressant effect results from increases in the level of NE in CNS synapses, and long-term administration causes a downregulation of α_1-adrenoceptors and desensitization of presynaptic α_2-receptors, equilibrating the noradrenergic system and, thus, correcting the dysregulated output of depressed patients. The SSRIs do not produce this effect. Desipramine also downregulates NET, but not SERT. Substantial loss of NET–binding sites takes 15 days to occur and is accompanied by a marked reduction of NET function in vivo. Desipramine has weak effects on 5-HT reuptake.

Nortriptyline Nortriptyline is a secondary amine dibenzocycloheptene TCA (Fig. 18.8) as well as the major metabolite of amitriptyline. Similar to desipramine, nortriptyline appears in mother's milk and is metabolized by CYP2D6 to the primary amine and by ring hydroxylation to its *E*-10-hydroxy metabolite (Table 18.2). Approximately one-third of a dose of nortriptyline is excreted in urine as metabolites within 24 hours, and small amounts are excreted in feces via biliary elimination.

Amoxapine Amoxapine is a dibenzoxazepine TCA (Fig 18.8) with antidepressant and antipsychotic effects that has shown therapeutic effectiveness in patients with delusional depression. Additionally, it is the *N*-desmethyl metabolite of the antipsychotic loxapine. Amoxapine differs structurally from the other secondary TCAs in that it has both a nitrogen and an oxygen atom in its seven-membered central ring and a piperazinyl ring rather than a propylamino side chain attached to the central ring.

Amoxapine is a less potent inhibitor of neuronal NE reuptake compared with the other secondary TCAs, with a mechanism of action similar to that of desipramine.

TABLE 18.5 Patient Information and Recommendations for Secondary Amines Tricyclic Antidepressants (TCAs)

Patient Information	Recommendations
Potential drug–drug and drug–health interactions	Share medical conditions, other medicines (including over-the-counter and herbal medicines), allergies to TCAs, fertility status, or breast-feeding with pharmacist
Seizures, breathing difficulties, fever and sweating, loss of bladder control, muscle stiffness, unusual weakness or tiredness	Discontinue therapy and consult physician (TCAs may increase risk of seizures)
Course of therapy	Complete full course of therapy
Discontinuance of therapy	Consult physician; abrupt discontinuance not recommended, because it may cause nausea, headache, and malaise
Alcohol use	Avoid alcohol
Central nervous system depressants	May exacerbate TCAs
Drowsiness, dizziness, blurred vision	Avoid driving or performing tasks requiring alertness and coordination
Sun/sunlamp exposure	Avoid prolonged exposure because of photosensitivity

Amoxapine shares the toxic potentials of the TCAs, and the usual precautions of TCA administration should be observed. Amoxapine resembles the atypical antipsychotic drugs in its intermediate affinity as an antagonist of DA-2 and of 5-HT_2 receptors.

Amoxapine is rapidly and almost completely absorbed from the gastrointestinal (GI) tract. Its pharmacokinetics are shown in Table 18.3. Amoxapine and its 8-hydroxyamoxapine metabolite have been detected in human milk at concentrations below steady-state therapeutic concentrations. Amoxapine has the shortest elimination time (~8 hours) of the secondary TCAs. It is metabolized in the liver principally to 8-hydroxyamoxapine and to 7-hydroxyamoxapine. Both of these metabolites are pharmacologically active and have half-lives of 30 and 6.5 hours, respectively. The hydroxylation of amoxapine is inhibited by ketoconazole, suggesting the involvement of CYP3A4.

Protriptyline Protriptyline is a dibenzocycloheptriene TCA that differs from the other tricyclics by having an unsaturated ethylene bridge joining the two aromatic rings and a secondary aminopropyl side chain (Fig. 18.8). Protriptyline is completely absorbed from the GI tract and slowly eliminated. Its pharmacokinetic data are shown in Table 18.3. Metabolism data are limited for protriptyline, but it is most likely metabolized via the same pathways as the other TCAs (Table 18.2). Very little drug is excreted in the feces via the bile.

Protriptyline exhibits high selectivity for the NET, but with less potency than desipramine. Its mechanism of action is similar to that of desipramine. Minimal effect on 5-HT reuptake has been observed.

Maprotiline Maprotiline is a secondary amine dibenzobicyclooctadiene (a tetracyclic antidepressant) that differs structurally from the TCAs by having an ethylene bridge in its central ring, resulting in a rigid bicyclomolecular skeleton (Fig. 18.8).

Maprotiline exhibits the highest affinity and selectivity for the NET (Fig. 18.6). Its antidepressant mechanism of action is similar to that of desipramine, with an onset of action of up to 2 to 3 weeks.

Maprotiline is slowly but completely absorbed from the GI tract, and like the other TCAs, it is metabolized by the polymorphic CYP2D6 and CYP2C19 isoforms in the liver, primarily to pharmacologically active *N*-desmethylmaprotiline and to maprotiline-*N*-oxide. Its pharmacokinetics are shown in Table 18.3. Maprotiline is distributed into breast milk at concentrations similar to those found at steady-state in maternal blood. The elimination half-life of maprotiline averages 43 hours (60 to 90 hours for its *N*-desmethyl metabolite).

Maprotiline shares the toxic potentials of the TCAs, and the usual precautions of TCA administration should be observed. Although most of the TCAs have been reported to induce seizures, it is generally recognized that maprotiline may be associated with a higher incidence of dose-dependent seizures compared with the other secondary TCAs. Maprotiline has been reported to produce sedation in depressed patients and to reduce aggressive behavior in animals. Maprotiline also shares the anticholinergic and cardiovascular effects of the secondary TCAs and may cause electrocardiographic changes, tachycardia, and postural hypotension.

NONTRICYCLIC SECONDARY AMINE ANTIDEPRESSANTS

Reboxetine Reboxetine is a nontricyclic SNRI in which the propylamine side chain of the TCAs is constrained into a morpholine ring (Fig. 18.8). It is a potent and selective ligand for the NET, with a mechanism of action similar to that of desipramine and with low affinity for β-adrenergic and muscarinic receptors. Reboxetine is used for the treatment of major depressive disorders. It is a chiral compound that is marketed as a racemic mixture of *R,R*- and *S,S*-reboxetine. The antidepressant activity for reboxetine appears to reside with the *S,S*-(+)-enantiomer, which has approximately twofold the inhibition potency of the *R,R*-enantiomer (42). It is well tolerated, with different adverse event profiles, and it seems to be at least as effective as the SSRIs in the treatment of depressive illness. Currently, it is available only in Europe and is under FDA review. It preferentially inhibits the reuptake of NE (5-HT:NE ratio = 8). Reboxetine is not metabolized by the polymorphic isoforms CYP2D6 or CYP2C19 and may offer a valuable alternative to the secondary amine TCAs in the treatment of major depression. Reboxetine is likely to become a promising alternative for patients who have failed treatment with or do not tolerate serotonergic antidepressants. Reboxetine has been shown to be effective and well tolerated in the treatment of panic disorder.

Reboxetine's oral bioavailability is greater than 90% for both *R,R*-(−)-reboxetine and *S,S*-(+)-reboxetine, indicating that stereoisomerism has no significant effect on absorption and first-pass metabolism. The pharmacokinetics of reboxetine are linear after multiple oral doses of 12 mg/d (Table 18.3). Food affects the rate but not the extent of absorption. In human liver microsomes, each reboxetine enantiomer was metabolized to one primary metabolite, *O*-desethylreboxetine, and three minor metabolites, two arising via oxidation of the ethoxy aromatic ring and a third yet-unidentified metabolite (43). The metabolism of both reboxetine enantiomers in humans is mediated principally via CYP3A4, and they are competitive inhibitors of CYP2D6 and CYP3A4. Less than 10% of the unmetabolized drug is cleared renally, with the other 90% being excreted hepatically.

After a single, 4-mg dose, the plasma concentration in the elderly (mean age, 81 years) was twice that of younger subjects, although in both groups, the plasma concentration was similar after 2 hours. The area under the curve (AUC) was nearly four times greater in the elderly than in the younger subjects, and the elimination half-life was twice as long (24 ± 6 vs. 12 ± 3 hours). Renal clearance also was reduced. The increased plasma concentrations of reboxetine observed in elderly subjects supports a reduction of the starting dose to 4 mg/d (in two divided doses) for elderly patients (44). Because of reduced metabolic clearance, reboxetine plasma concentrations also are increased in patients with hepatic or renal dysfunction. In these populations, reboxetine should be used with caution, and a dosage reduction is indicated. No ethnic differences have been observed with *R,R*-(−)- or *S,S*-(+)-reboxetine.

Drug Interactions. Reboxetine seems to be an antidepressant that has negligible interference with the pharmacokinetics of other drugs; thus, fewer drug–drug interactions are expected. It also may be possible to use reboxetine in combination with MAOIs, because it has no inhibitory effect on this enzyme, which would avoid tyramine-induced hypertensive reactions.

Adverse Effects. Reboxetine is relatively well tolerated, with insomnia, sweating, constipation, and dry mouth being commonly reported adverse events. Hypotension and urinary hesitancy occur at lower rates than with the TCAs. When compared with the SSRIs, reboxetine is associated with lower rates of nausea, somnolence, and diarrhea.

Structure–Activity Relationships for the Phenoxyphenylpropyl Amines

(±)-Nisoxetine Nisoxetine (Fig. 18.8) was the initial phenoxyphenylpropylamine synthesized in the Lilly research laboratories during the early 1970s from the rearrangement of an oxygen atom in diphenyhydramine, a diphenylmethoxyethylamine, to a phenoxyphenylpropylamine (Fig. 18.2). Nisoxetine was discovered to be a potent and very selective SNRI, with little affinity for other receptors. It underwent clinical studies as an alternative to Lilly's best-selling antidepressant, nortriptyline, but without the adverse effects associated with the tricyclic secondary amines. It was never marketed, however, because of a greater interest in developing its 4-trifluoromethyl analog, fluoxetine, an SSRI.

The type and position of the ring substitution plays a critical role in the mechanism of action for these phenoxyphenylpropylamines (see Table 18.6 for structure–activity relationships of the phenoxypropylamines). The unsubstituted molecule is a weak SSRI. However, 2-substitutions into the phenoxy ring (except for the 2-trifluoromethyl) yields compounds with high potency and selectivity for blocking NE reuptake (an SNRI), whereas the 4-substitution results in compounds having potent SSRI activity, with the 4-trifluormethyl group (fluoxetine) being the most potent and selective for SERT (28,29). The substantial changes in transporter selectivity for NET and SERT and the differences in affinity are more likely attributed to the bulky 2-(ortho)-substituted groups, which restrict the flexibility of the aromatic rings, thereby enhancing alignment of the hydrogen-bond acceptor group (the methoxy) with a donor group on the binding site on the NET for NE that is not available for the 5-HT binding site. The *R*-isomer of nisoxetine has 20 times greater affinity than its *S*-isomer for NET. The NET K_i for nisoxetine is 0.8 nM and is 40 times more selective for NET than for SERT. Its tertiary amine is approximately 100 times less effective at inhibiting NET. Increasing the size of the methylamino with ethyl or larger alkyl eliminates all activity. The 2- and 4-analogs exhibited weak effects on neuronal uptake of DA and lack affinity for other neuroreceptors at therapeutic concentrations. Substituting the 2-methoxy with the isosteric 2-methylthio (thionisoxetine) produced a more potent SNRI (K_i = 0.2 nM for the *R*-enantiomer) and 600 times more selective for NET than for SERT. Thionisoxetine is approximately 10 times more potent than nisoxetine at inhibiting NET, and unlike nisoxetine, it reduces food consumption in rodents and has been studied for the treatment of obesity and eating disorders. Substitution of the phenoxy group with a naphthyloxy group and the phenyl ring with the isosteric thienyl (thiophene) group results in a drug with dual inhibition of NE and 5-HT reuptake (i.e., duloxetine) (see Fig. 18.20 and the discussion of reuptake inhibitors of both NE and 5-HT for a description of duloxetine).

R-(−)-Atomoxetine *R*-(−)-Atomoxetine, 2-methylphenoxyphenylpropylamine, was marketed in 2003 as a "nonstimulant" treatment for attention-deficit hyperactivity disorder (ADHD) in both adults and children and for treatment of adult depression. The 2-methyl substitution (c.f., nisoxetine; Fig. 18.8) confers selectivity for inhibiting NE reuptake (Table 18.6) (21,22,45). The *R*-enantiomer is 10 times more potent than the *S*-enantiomer as a NET reuptake inhibitor. Atomoxetine has a low propensity for anticholinergic and adverse cardiovascular effects.

Pharmacokinetics. Atomoxetine is well absorbed from the GI tract and cleared primarily by metabolism, with the majority of the dose being excreted into the urine. Atomoxetine is metabolized primarily by CYP2D6 to its major active metabolite, 4-hydroxyatomoxetine, which is eliminated as its glucuronide (Fig. 18.10). Peak plasma concentrations of atomoxetine occur 1 to 2 hours after oral administration. Significant differences are seen in the elimination half-life between normal metabolizers, extensive metabolizers, and poor metabolizers (Table 18.3). Atomoxetine exhibited an elimination half-life of 3 to 6 hours for normal and extensive metabolizers and 17 to 21 hours for poor metabolizers (46). CYP2C19 is the other enzyme primarily responsible for the formation of its minor metabolite *N*-desmethylatomoxetine (46).

Adverse Effects. At therapeutic doses, no serious drug-related adverse effects have been encountered. Adverse

TABLE 18.6 Structure–Activity Relationships for Phenoxyphenylpropylamines

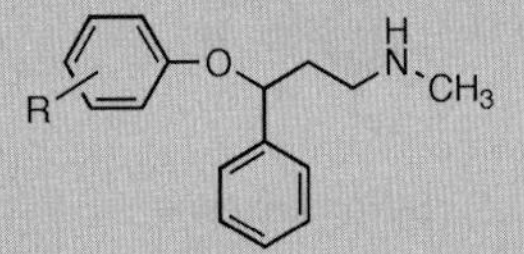

R (drug)	Inhibition of Reuptake (K_i nM) (20)	
	5-HT	NE
H	102	200
2-OCH_3 (nisoxetine)	1,371	2.4
2-SCH_3 (thionisoxetine)	130	0.2
2-CH_3 (atomoxetine)	390	3.4
2-F	898	5.3
2-I	25	0.4
2-CF_3	1,489	4,467
3-CF_3	16	1,328
4-CF_3 (fluoxetine)	17	2,703
4-CF_3 (norfluoxetine, NH_2)	17	2,176
4-CH_3	95	570
4-OCH_3	71	1,207
4-Cl	142	568
4-F	638	1,276

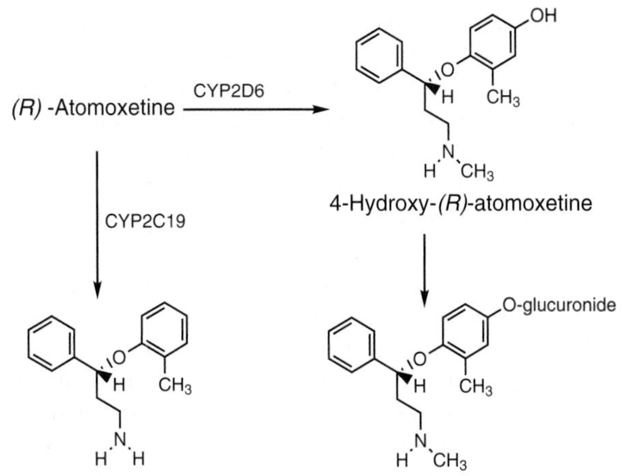

FIGURE 18.10 Metabolism of *R*-atomoxetine.

effects have included modest increases in diastolic blood pressure and heart rate, anorexia, weight loss, somnolence, dizziness, GI effects (nausea), dry mouth, and skin rash.

Therapeutic Uses. Atomoxetine is used as a safe and well-tolerated "nonstimulant" treatment of ADHD in both adults and children and of depression. Among children and adolescents age 8 to 18 years, atomoxetine was superior to placebo in reducing symptoms of ADHD and in improving social and family functioning symptoms. Oral atomoxetine is promoted as an alternative to conventional ADHD therapy with methylphenidate, dextroamphetamine, and pemoline. It also can be a replacement for bupropion or for TCAs. Onset of action is approximately 7 days.

Selective 5-HT Reuptake Inhibitors (SSRIs)

Serotonin Hypothesis of Depression

5-HT is a major player in depressive illness, and serotonergic pathways are closely related to mood disorders, especially depression (Fig. 18.1) (11,47). Thus, drugs affecting the 5-HT levels in the neural synapse and serotonergic pathways may lead to effective therapy of depression.

5-HT is synthesized from tryptophan, packaged into vesicles, and released into the synaptic cleft following an action potential (see Chapter 11). Once in the synaptic cleft, 5-HT interacts with both the pre- and postsynaptic serotonergic receptors. Evidence implicating multiple abnormalities in serotonergic pathways as a cause of depression includes:

1. Low urinary concentrations of 5-HT's major metabolite, 5-hydroxyindoleacetic acid.
2. A low density of brain and platelet SERT in depressed individuals.
3. A high density of brain and platelet 5-HT binding sites.
4. A low synaptic concentration of tryptophan, which is used in 5-HT synthesis.

Of these, the low level of SERTs in depressed patients has received the most attention in the development and synthesis of the SSRIs. The precise antidepressant mechanism of action for the SSRIs eludes neuroscientists, but the SSRIs have been shown to alleviate depression and are the most commonly used drugs in the therapy for depression. Claims of decreased adverse effects (adverse drug reactions) and less toxicity in overdose than both the MAOIs and the TCAs, together with increased safety, have led to their extensive use, and several are ranked in the top 50 prescription drugs dispensed in the United States during the year 2009.

The SSRIs are proven treatments for depression, obsessive-compulsive disorder, and panic disorder and are helpful in a variety of other conditions as well. The most substantial benefit to the SSRIs compared with the TCAs is their reduced adverse effect profile and the fact that they are better tolerated. Although the SSRIs have become the most commonly prescribed drugs for depression, there are clinical situations in which TCAs may be more appropriate (e.g., melancholic depression). Meaningful differences between the individual SSRIs are largely related to their pharmacokinetics, metabolism to active metabolites, inhibition of CYP isoforms, effect of drug–drug interactions, and the half-life of the individual SSRI.

The SSRIs are expensive, and it has been common to have noncompliant patients (especially elderly) relapse because they cannot afford their medications. Persuading the patient to take his or her medication as prescribed is extremely important for potentially suicidal patients with depression. Because of this, it is exceedingly important that patients receive the lowest effective (and, thereby, the most cost-effective) dose of any drug they are prescribed. Also, the SSRIs have a history of increased risk of suicide for reasons that are not clearly understood.

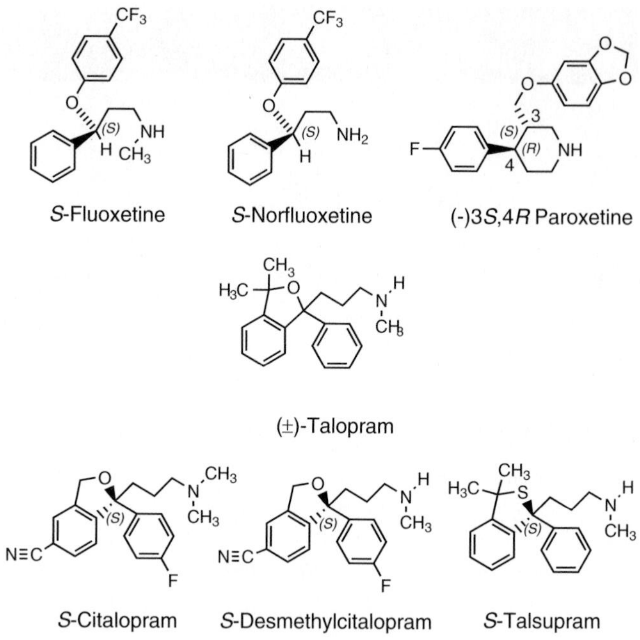

FIGURE 18.11 Phenoxyphenylalkylamine SSRIs.

The Discovery of SSRIs

Although the TCAs, as a group, are effective antidepressants, their adverse event profile and high potential for toxicity have limited their use. The early antidepressants indicated that 5-HT might play a significant role in depression. Therefore, medicinal chemists set out in search of the ideal SSRI with the goal for developing drugs with:

- High affinity and selectivity for the SERT.
- Ability to slow or inhibit the transporter when bound to it.
- Low affinity for the multiple neuroreceptors known to be responsible for many of the adverse effects of the TCAs (e.g., acetylcholine, histamine, and adrenergic receptors).
- No inhibition of the fast sodium channels that cause the cardiotoxicity problems associated with TCAs.

Initial success occurred with the synthesis of zimelidine, in which the central ring of amitriptyline was opened to form a diphenylpropylidine analog. *Z*-zimelidine displayed selective inhibition of 5-HT reuptake, with minimal inhibition of NE reuptake. Most importantly, zimelidine was without the adverse event profile exhibited by the TCAs. Thus, zimelidine became the template for the second-generation SSRIs as shown in Figure 18.11.

Mechanisms of Action Common to the SSRIs

The SSRIs preferentially act to inhibit SERT with minimal or no affinity for NET and DAT (11). These drugs have a high and selective affinity for SERT (Fig. 18.6) and, therefore, block 5-HT from binding to SERT and being absorbed into presynaptic cells. The excess 5-HT in the synaptic cleft means overactivation of the postsynaptic receptors. Over an extended period of time, this causes downregulation of pre- and postsynaptic receptors, a reduction in the amount of 5-HT produced in the CNS, and a reduction in the number of SERTs expressed. Long-term administration of SSRIs causes downregulation of the SERT, but not the NET. Substantial loss of SERT binding sites takes 15 days to occur and is accompanied by a marked reduction of SERT function in vivo. These compensatory responses at receptors and transporters are thought to produce the antidepressant effects of SSRIs. This onset delay may, in part, explain the delayed onset of action of SSRIs in the treatment of depression (48). Similar to the binding of 5-HT, SSRIs likely bind to SERT at the same site as 5-HT does, although it has not been determined conclusively. Although not as selective as the SSRIs, drugs of abuse, such as cocaine, fenfluramine, and 3,4-methylenedioxymethamphetamine ("Ecstasy"), are inhibitors of SERT.

The affinity data for the SSRIs show that the SSRIs, as a group, are very potent and selective inhibitors for SERT compared with their affinity for NET and DAT (Fig. 18.6) and are more potent inhibitors of 5-HT reuptake than are the tertiary amine TCAs, with the exception of clomipramine. None of the SSRIs has substantial effect on NET or DAT. Of the SSRIs, sertraline exhibits the most potent inhibition of DAT, although it is still 100 times less potent in terms of inhibiting DAT versus SERT. Therefore, the plasma concentration of sertraline would have to be increased by as much as 100 times to inhibit DAT. When drugs are this selective for reuptake transporters, differences in potency become clinically irrelevant because the plasma concentration can be dose-adjusted to achieve inhibition of the desired transporter without affecting the other transporters. Clomipramine displays less affinity for SERT than citalopram, fluvoxamine, paroxetine, or sertraline does and is more potent than fluoxetine. In terms of the ability to inhibit the NET, the SSRIs are two to three times less potent than the SNRI TCA, desipramine.

Their in vitro potency for selectively inhibiting the SERT more or less mirrors their clinical efficacy as SSRIs (11): paroxetine > sertraline > clomipramine > fluoxetine > citalopram > fluvoxamine > imipramine > amitriptyline > reboxetine > venlafaxine = milnacipran > desipramine. Clinically, however, all the SSRIs are equally effective over time, suggesting that these variations in potency do not affect efficacy or adverse effects. The SSRIs have less affinity for α_1, α_2, H_1, and muscarinic receptors, which may explain the adverse effect profile differences between TCAs and SSRIs.

The results in Table 18.7 show the therapeutic doses that produce approximately 70% to 80% inhibition of the SERT (48). The inhibition of SERT is relevant to the antidepressant efficacy of the SSRIs and suggests that approximately 70% to 80% inhibition of this SERT usually is necessary to produce an antidepressant effect. Higher doses of these drugs do not produce a greater antidepressant response on average (i.e., a flat dose–response curve for antidepressant efficacy) but do increase the incidence and severity of adverse effects mediated by excessive 5-HT reuptake inhibition. Obviously, the results shown in Table 18.7 pertain to the average patient. A patient who has a rapid clearance of the SSRI may need a higher-than-average dose to achieve an effective concentration, whereas a patient who has a slow clearance may do better in terms of the ratio of efficacy to adverse effects on a minimum dose.

The β-adrenergic blocker pindolol blocks the presynaptic 5-HT_{1A} receptors, thereby increasing 5-HT neuronal transmission. The 5-HT_{1A} receptors do not require prolonged exposure (several weeks) to excessive amounts of 5-HT to promote downregulation. This results in augmentation and acceleration of the antidepressant effect of the SSRIs when combined with a 5-HT_{1A} inhibitor. Bordet et al. (49) demonstrated the accelerated antidepressant response of pindolol with paroxetine.

TABLE 18.7 Relationship Between Dose, Plasma Level, Potency, and Serotonin Uptake

SSRI	Dose (mg/d)	Plasma Level	In Vitro Potency (IC_{50})	Inhibition of SERT
Citalopram	40	85 ng/mL (260 nM)	1.8	60%
Fluoxetine	20	200 ng/mL (300 nM/L)[a]	3.8	70%
Fluvoxamine	150	100 ng/mL (300 nM/L)	3.8	70%
Paroxetine	20	40 ng/mL (130 nM/L)	0.29	80%
Sertraline	50	25 ng/mL (65 nM/L)	0.19	80%

[a]Plasma level for fluoxetine represents the total of fluoxetine plus norfluoxetine given comparable effects on SERT; parent SSRI alone shown for all others. Also, plasma levels are a total of both enantiomers for citalopram and fluoxetine. Values for the parent drug and for the respective major metabolite are in parentheses.

Pharmacokinetics Common to the SSRIs

The SSRIs share a number of pharmacokinetic characteristics (48,50) (Table 18.8). They are well absorbed orally, although the presence of food in the stomach may alter the absorption of some SSRIs. Food, however, does not affect the AUC and does not appear to affect clinical efficacy. The SSRIs are highly lipophilic and are highly plasma protein bound.

Current SSRIs tend to be characterized by high volumes of distribution, which results in relatively long plasma concentration (typically 4 to 8 hours). The SSRIs display a range of elimination half-life values for the parent drugs, from half-life values of approximately 20 hours for paroxetine and fluvoxamine to 2 days for fluoxetine. Only sertraline and citalopram exhibit linear pharmacokinetics, whereas fluvoxamine, fluoxetine, and paroxetine exhibit nonlinear pharmacokinetics (i.e., changes in plasma concentration are not proportional to dose) as a result of their longer plasma half-lives within the usual therapeutic ranges (Table 18.8). Sertraline stands out as having the best effects on depression among all antidepressants. Fluoxetine and fluvoxamine are least likely to penetrate into breast milk. Thus, the SSRI antidepressants best suited for pharmacokinetic optimization of therapy are the following: sertraline, fluvoxamine, and citalopram. All the SSRIs are extensively metabolized by CYP isoforms to pharmacologically active *N*-demethylated metabolites, which are then excreted in urine and feces. Except for sertraline, the drugs fluoxetine, paroxetine, and fluvoxamine are metabolized by polymorphic CYP isoforms, a matter of concern for poor and extensive metabolizers who may need dose adjustments. Citalopram is metabolized almost equally by CYP2C19, CYP2D6, and CYP3A4 (Table 18.7). Peak plasma levels usually are reached in approximately 6 to 8 hours, and steady-state plasma levels are reached in approximately 7 to 10 days, except for fluoxetine (~4 weeks). The half-lives are variable depending on the specific SSRI and the presence and plasma concentration of an active metabolite, but the half-lives tend to be prolonged. No evidence indicates that serum drug monitoring of SSRIs is a useful strategy to predict response. The SSRIs in general exhibit a flat, dose-independent antidepressant response curve (i.e., the antidepressant activity does not improve with increasing dose, only side effects increase) (50).

Some of the key differences among the SSRIs are the result of differences in their pharmacokinetic properties and metabolism to active metabolites (Table 18.8). Fluoxetine is unique because of its long half-life and

TABLE 18.8 Pharmacokinetics of the Selective Serotonin Reuptake Inhibitors (SSRIs)

Parameters	(±)-Fluoxetine	(−)-Sertraline	(−)-Paroxetine	*E*-Fluvoxamine	(±)-Citalopram [(+)-Escitalopram]
Oral bioavailability (%)	70	20–36	50	>50	80 (51–93)
Lipophilicity (logD$_{7.4}$)	2.38	3.03	1.49	1.21	1.52
Protein binding (%)	95	96–98	95	77	~56 (70–80)
Volume of distribution (L/kg)	12–18	17 (9–25)	25 (12–28)	15–31	12–16
Elimination half-life (h)	50	24 (19–37)	22	15–20	36 (27–32); elderly ~48
Cytochrome P450 major isoform	2D6	3A4	2D6	2D6	2C19, 2D6, and 3A4
Major active metabolites	*O*-Desmethyl-fluoxetine (240 h)	*N*-Desmethyl (62–104 h)	None	None	*N*-Desmethylcitalopram (30 h)
	Norfluoxetine (96–364 h)				
Peak plasma concentration (h)	6–8	4–8	2–8	3–8	4 (1–6)
Excretion (%)	Urine 25–50	Urine 51–60	Renal ~50	Urine ~ 40 (24 h)	Feces 80–90
	Feces minor	Feces 24–32	Feces minor	Feces minor	Urine <5
Plasma half-life (h)	1–4 d (norfluoxetine 7–15 d)	22–35	24	7–63	36 (23–75)
Time to steady-state concentration	~4 wk	7–10 d; elderly 2–3 wk	7–14 d	10 d	7 d

the long half-life of its active metabolite norfluoxetine (48,50). Although sertraline also has an active metabolite, it is 10 times less potent than sertraline and probably is not clinically relevant (51). Fluvoxamine and paroxetine have no active metabolites. Because of the differences in half-lives and activities of metabolites, a much longer washout period is necessary when switching from fluoxetine (a long-acting SSRI) to another SSRI or MAOI. These differences can cause considerable therapeutic delays in the treatment of refractory patients.

Adverse Effects Common to the SSRIs

The SSRIs are reported to have fewer side effects than the TCAs, which have strong anticholinergic and cardiotoxic properties (50). Among the SSRIs, there are few differences in adverse effects. The adverse effects observed for the SSRIs include nausea, diarrhea, anxiety, agitation, insomnia, and sexual dysfunction. Fewer patients have discontinued SSRIs than TCAs (amitriptyline and imipramine and not nortriptyline, desipramine, doxepin, and clomipramine).

Sexual dysfunction is reported in both men and women, such as of decreased libido, anorgasmia, ejaculatory incompetence, ejaculatory retardation, or inability to obtain or maintain an erection. The basic pharmacologic similarities among the SSRIs suggest that the effects on sexual function should be similar for each drug and that no one SSRI was more likely to cause the reported sexual adverse effects than another. Moreover, evidence suggests that SSRI-induced sexual dysfunction may be dose related and may be treated by simply lowering its dose. In patients who cannot have their SSRI dosage reduced, another option is simply to wait and reassess sexual function after several months. If the above measures are ineffective in managing SSRI-induced sexual dysfunction, the next step is to consider an alternative antidepressant without serotonergic activity (e.g., bupropion). Orgasm difficulties and impotence occurred more frequently with paroxetine as compared with sertraline and fluoxetine. The addition of amantadine, cyproheptadine, yohimbine, or sildenafil has been reported to be effective in some patients with SSRI-induced sexual dysfunction.

Drug Interactions Common to the SSRIs

The most serious drug–drug interaction for the SSRIs is their potential to produce the "serotonin syndrome" (i.e., hyperserotonergic effect), which typically develops within hours or days following the addition of another serotonergic agent to a drug regimen that already includes serotonergic-enhancing drugs. Symptoms of the 5-HT syndrome include agitation, diaphoresis, diarrhea, fever, hyperreflexia, incoordination, confusion, myoclonus, shivering, or tremor.

The 5-HT syndrome interaction between MAOIs and SSRIs is the most important drug interaction for the SSRIs, necessitating a washout ranging from 2 to 5 weeks depending on the plasma half-life of the SSRI. These differences in washout times for the SSRIs when switching to an MAOI are key differences between SSRIs and should be remembered if an MAOI is planned as a possible subsequent treatment in the event of SSRI failure. The differences among SSRIs are not important when a patient is switched from an MAOI to an SSRI. However, in this case, a 10- to 14-day washout for the MAOI is necessary, regardless of which SSRI is used, to allow regeneration of monoamine oxidase. The drug interaction between TCAs and SSRIs is of particular importance because of the potential for the development of toxic TCA concentrations, 5-HT syndrome, and subsequent adverse effects (48,50).

Coadministration of the antihistamine cyproheptadine or other 5-HT antagonists with SSRIs might be expected to result in a pharmacodynamic interaction (i.e., reduced effectiveness for the SSRI). Cyproheptadine acts to block postsynaptic 5-HT. Lack of antidepressant efficacy has been reported when cyproheptadine was given concurrently with fluoxetine and paroxetine.

Clinically, the potency of the SSRIs to inhibit CYP2D6 decreases from paroxetine to fluoxetine to norfluoxetine and then to fluvoxamine, with sertraline and citalopram being metabolized by CYP3A4 and CYP2C19, respectively, explaining the extent of differences in pharmacokinetic interactions between the SSRIs and other CYP2D6 substrates. Fluvoxamine is associated with drug interactions from its inhibition of CYP1A2, CYP2C9, CYP2C19, and CYP3A4 (see Table 4.10 for inhibition drug interactions). Because all the SSRIs are extensively metabolized in the liver, it is possible that other drugs that inhibit or induce hepatic CYP microsomal enzyme systems may alter SSRI plasma concentrations (AUCs) (Table 18.7). The SSRIs may inhibit or interfere with the metabolism of other frequently prescribed drugs that are CYP hepatically metabolized, increasing the potential for drug–drug interactions (Table 18.2; see also Tables 4.5 and 4.6). Although similar drug interactions are possible with other SSRIs, there is considerable variability among the drugs in the extent to which they inhibit CYP2D6. Fluoxetine and paroxetine appear to be more potent in this regard than sertraline. The extent to which this potential interaction may become clinically important depends on the extent of inhibition of CYP2D6 by the SSRI and the therapeutic index of the concurrently administered drug. The drugs for which this potential interaction is of greatest concern are those that are metabolized principally by CYP2D6 and have a narrow therapeutic index. Caution should be exercised whenever concurrent therapy with fluoxetine and other drugs metabolized by CYP2D6 is considered. The clinical significance of these possible interactions with the CYP isoforms is questionable, however, because there is no known correlation between plasma concentration and therapeutic response for any of the SSRIs (50). If an interaction is suspected, the patient's SSRI dosage can be easily adjusted.

The SSRIs are highly protein bound and may affect the pharmacodynamic effect of other protein-bound drugs with narrow therapeutic indices (e.g., warfarin). The changes appear to be clinically significant, however, only for fluoxetine, fluvoxamine, and paroxetine (50). Close monitoring of prothrombin time and international normalized ratio is necessary if these drugs are used together.

The SSRIs have a high toxic to therapeutic ratio and, therefore, are safer than the TCAs or MAOIs in acute overdose. SSRI overdoses can result in drowsiness, tremor, nausea and vomiting, seizures, electrocardiographic changes, and coma. Fatalities are uncommon with pure SSRI overdoses.

Therapeutic Uses Common to the SSRIs

The primary uses for the SSRIs include MMD and bipolar depression (fluoxetine, paroxetine, sertraline, and citalopram), "atypical" depression (i.e., depressed patients with unusual symptoms such as hypersomnia, weight gain, and interpersonal rejection sensitivity; fluoxetine, paroxetine, sertraline, and citalopram), anxiety disorders, panic disorder (sertraline and paroxetine), dysthymia, premenstrual syndrome, postpartum depression, dysphoria, bulimia nervosa (fluoxetine), obesity, borderline personality disorder, obsessive-compulsive disorder (fluvoxamine, fluoxetine, paroxetine, and sertraline), alcoholism, rheumatic pain, and migraine headache. Among the SSRIs, there are more similarities than differences; however, the differences between the SSRIs could be clinically significant.

The SSRIs, such as paroxetine and fluoxetine, need stronger pediatric use warnings because of the possible risks of suicidal thoughts and behavior in some children and teenagers. Such risks may be unrelated to any specific SSRI. Recent clinical trials have concluded that 2 or 3 of every 100 young people treated with antidepressants might be at higher risk of suicidal behavior. Only fluoxetine has been proven to be effective and is approved for the treatment of pediatric depression.

Phenoxyphenylalkylamines

(±)-Fluoxetine

Structure–Activity Relationship Fluoxetine is a 3-phenoxy-3-phenylpropylamine that exhibits selectivity and high affinity for human SERT and low affinity for NET (Fig. 18.11). It is marketed as a racemic mixture of *R*- and

S-fluoxetine. Its selectivity for SERT inhibition depends on the position of the substituent in the phenoxy ring (Table 18.6). Mono-substitution in the 4-(para) position of the phenoxy group (with an electron-withdrawing group, e.g., trifluoromethyl group, as in fluoxetine) results in selective inhibition of 5-HT reuptake. Disubstitution (2,4- or 3,4-substitution) results in loss of SERT selectivity. Constraining fluoxetine into semirigid analogs, such as MDL28618A or a phenylpiperidine (i.e., femoxetine), maintains selectivity for SERT, but both have approximately 10% of the affinity of fluoxetine for SERT (52) (Fig. 18.12). The *trans*-(1*S*,2*S*)-MDL28618A stereoisomer is approximately 10 times more potent than the *cis*-(−)-enantiomer (52,53). The *trans*-(3*R*,4*S*)-(+)-enantiomer of femoxetine has approximately 10% the affinity of fluoxetine for SERT (54). *N*-Demethylation of femoxetine to its secondary amine enhances affinity for SERT by 10 times (comparable to fluoxetine). Femoxetine is an analog not only of fluoxetine and paroxetine but also of the (3*R*,4*S*)-diastereomer of a paroxetine analog.

Mechanism of Action Fluoxetine is a potent and selective inhibitor of 5-HT reuptake, but not of NE or DA uptake in the CNS. Its mechanism of action is common to the SSRIs. Fluoxetine does not interact directly with postsynaptic 5-HT receptors and has weak affinity for the other neuroreceptors. Both enantiomers of fluoxetine display similar affinities for human SERT. The NE:5-HT selectivity ratio, however, indicates that the *S*-enantiomer is approximately 100 times more selective for SERT inhibition than the *R*-enantiomer. The *R*-(+)-stereoisomer is approximately eight times more potent an inhibitor of SERT and has a longer duration of action than the *S*-(−)-isomer. However, the *S*-(−)-norfluoxetine metabolite is seven times more potent as an inhibitor of the 5-HT transporter than the *R*-(+)-metabolite, with a selectivity ratio approximately equivalent to that of *S*-fluoxetine (54,55).

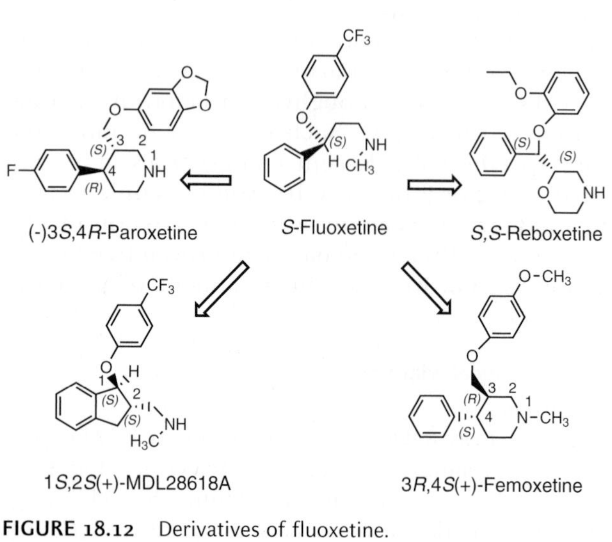

FIGURE 18.12 Derivatives of fluoxetine.

Pharmacokinetics The pharmacokinetics of fluoxetine fit the general characteristics of the SSRIs (Table 18.8). Of particular importance is its long half-life contributing to its nonlinear pharmacokinetics. In vitro studies show that fluoxetine and norfluoxetine are potent inhibitors of CYP2D6 and CYP3A4 and less potent inhibitors of CYP2C9, CYP2C19, and CYP1A2. Fluoxetine is metabolized primarily by CYP2D6 *N*-demethylation to its active metabolite norfluoxetine and, to a lesser extent, *O*-dealkylation to form the inactive metabolite *p*-trifluoromethylphenol. Following oral administration, fluoxetine and its metabolites are excreted principally in urine, with approximately 73% as unidentified metabolites, 10% as norfluoxetine, 10% as norfluoxetine glucuronide, 5% as fluoxetine *N*-glucuronide, and 2% as unmetabolized drug.

Both *R*- and *S*-norfluoxetine were less potent than the corresponding enantiomers of fluoxetine as inhibitors of NE uptake. Inhibition of 5-HT uptake in cerebral cortex persisted for more than 24 hours after administration of *S*-norfluoxetine similarly to fluoxetine. Thus, *S*-norfluoxetine is the active *N*-demethylated metabolite responsible for the persistently potent and selective inhibition of 5-HT uptake in vivo (54).

The pharmacokinetics of fluoxetine in healthy geriatric individuals do not differ substantially from those in younger adults. Because of its relatively long half-life and nonlinear pharmacokinetics, the possibility of altered pharmacokinetics in geriatric individuals could exist, particularly in those with systemic disease and/or in those receiving multiple medications concurrently. The elimination half-lives of fluoxetine and norfluoxetine do not appear to be altered substantially in patients with renal or hepatic impairment.

Drug Interactions Fluoxetine and its norfluoxetine metabolite, like many other drugs metabolized by CYP2D6, inhibit the activity of CYP2D6 and, potentially, may increase plasma concentrations of concurrently administered drugs that also are metabolized by this enzyme. Fluoxetine may make normal CYP2D6 metabolizers resemble poor metabolizers. Fluoxetine can inhibit its own CYP2D6 metabolism, resulting in higher-than-expected plasma concentrations during upward dose adjustments. Therefore, switching from fluoxetine to another SSRI or other serotonergic antidepressant requires a washout period of at least 5 weeks or a lower-than-recommended initial dose with monitoring for adverse events.

Fluoxetine is highly protein bound and may affect the free plasma concentration and, thus, the pharmacologic effect of other highly protein-bound drugs (e.g., warfarin sodium).

PAROXETINE

Structure–Activity Relationship Paroxetine is a costrained analog of fluoxetine in which the linear phenylpropy-lamine group has been folded into a piperidine ring (Fig. 18.11). Paroxetine contains two chiral centers, with the possibility of four stereoisomers. One of these stereoisomers, the (3*S*,4*R*)-(−)-enantiomer, is marketed as paroxetine. Paroxetine is a potent and selective inhibitor of SERT and displays high affinity for human SERT and little affinity for NET and DAT (Fig. 18.6). Converting the secondary amine of the piperidine ring into a tertiary amine with a methyl group reduces affinity for SERT by 100 times (Fig. 18.13). Substituting the 4-fluoro with either a hydrogen or methyl reduces affinity for human SERT by approximately 10 times; replacing the 3,4-methylenedioxy group with a 4-methoxy group in the phenoxy ring also reduces affinity by a factor of 10. Stereochemical factors affect affinity of the paroxetine molecule for SERT. Therefore, substitution into the 2-(ortho) position of either aromatic ring decreases affinity for rat SERT by as much as 10 to 100 times, with the greatest loss occurring with substitution in the phenoxy ring. In vitro binding studies suggest that paroxetine is a more selective and potent inhibitor of 5-HT reuptake than fluoxetine. The drug essentially has no effect on NE or DA reuptake and does not show affinity for other neuroreceptors. Its onset of action is 1 to 4 weeks.

Pharmacokinetics Paroxetine appears to be slowly but well absorbed from the GI tract after oral administration, with an oral bioavailability of approximately 50%, suggesting first-pass metabolism (Table 18.8), and reaching peak plasma concentrations in 2 to 8 hours. Food does not substantially affect the absorption of paroxetine. Paroxetine is distributed into breast milk. Approximately 80% of an oral dose of paroxetine is oxidized by CYP2D6 to a catechol intermediate, which is then either O-methylated or O-glucuronidated. These conjugates are then eliminated in the urine.

Paroxetine exhibits a preincubation-dependent increase in inhibitory potency of CYP2D6 consistent with a mechanism-based inhibition of CYP2D6 (55). The

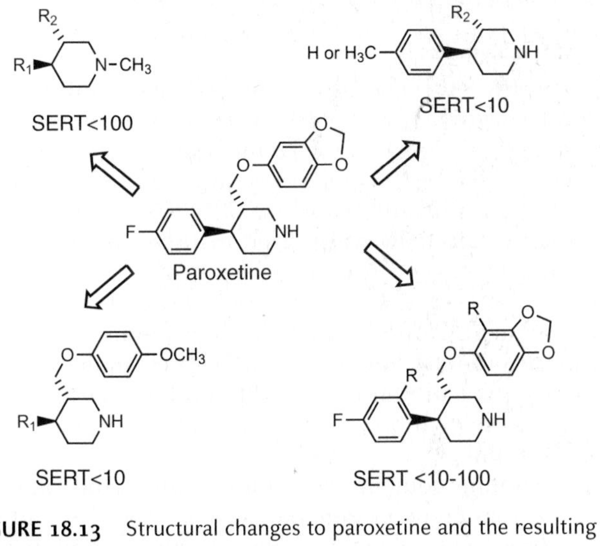

FIGURE 18.13 Structural changes to paroxetine and the resulting decrease in SERT affinity.

inactivation of CYP2D6 occurs via the formation of an o-quinonoid reactive metabolite.

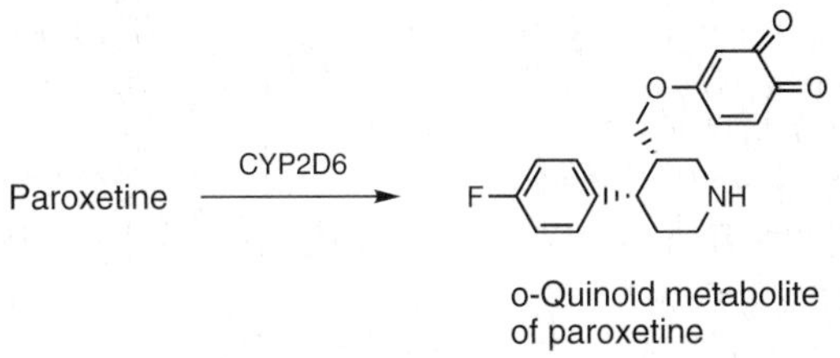

The methylenedioxy has been associated with mechanism-based inactivation of other CYP isoforms (56,57). In contrast, fluoxetine, a potent inhibitor of CYP2D6 activity, did not exhibit a mechanism-based inhibition of CYP2D6. As a result of mechanism-based inhibition, saturation of CYP2D6 at clinical doses appears to account for its nonlinear pharmacokinetics observed with increasing dose and duration of paroxetine treatment, which results in increased plasma concentrations of paroxetine at low doses. The elderly may be more susceptible to changes in doses and, therefore, should be started off at lower doses. After oral administration, paroxetine and its metabolites are excreted in both urine and feces.

Oral administration of a single dose resulted in unmetabolized paroxetine accounting for 2% and metabolites accounting for 62% of the excretion products. The effect of age on the elimination of paroxetine suggests that hepatic clearance of paroxetine can be reduced, leading to an increase in elimination half-life (e.g., to ~36 hours) and increased plasma concentrations. The metabolites of paroxetine have been shown to possess no more than 2% of the potency of the parent compound as inhibitors of 5-HT reuptake; therefore, they are essentially inactive.

Because paroxetine is a potent mechanism-based inhibitor of CYP2D6, this type of inhibition yields nonlinear and long-term effects on drug pharmacokinetics, because the inactivated or complexed CYP2D6 must be replaced by newly synthesized CYP2D6 protein. Thus, coadministration of paroxetine with CYP2D6-metabolized medications should be closely monitored or, in certain cases, avoided, as should upward dose adjustment of paroxetine itself.

(±)-CITALOPRAM In trying to create a new antidepressant to inhibit NE reuptake, Lundbeck chemists accidentally synthesized two new compounds (talopram and tasulopram) having the phenylspiro-isobenzofuran nucleus (Fig. 18.11). These compounds were potent SNRIs, but considering that a number of suicide attempts were reported during clinical studies with these compounds, Lundbeck discontinued the studies. Undeterred, the chemists subsequently modified talopram by addition of a 5-cyano to the phthalan ring and a 4-fluoro to the benzene ring in formation of citalopram (Fig. 18.11). Therapeutic activity for

(±)-citalopram resides in the *S*-(+)-isomer. Isosteric substitution of the isobenzofuran ring in citalopram with an isobenzothiophene yields talsupram, which changes selectivity from an inhibitor of SERT to a potent inhibitor of NET (Fig. 18.11). Citalopram was marketed in the United States in 1996 as the most selective SSRI and, therefore, as the least likely to cause the adverse effects observed with most of the other antidepressants (Fig. 18.6).

Mechanism of Action Citalopram, primarily through its *S*-enantiomer, blocks 5-HT reuptake, leading to potentiation of serotonergic activity in the CNS. Citalopram exhibits the greatest in vitro selectivity for 5-HT reuptake inhibition compared with the other SSRIs (Fig. 18.6). The drug essentially has no effect on NE or DA reuptake, nor does it show affinity for other neuroreceptors.

Pharmacokinetics The pharmacokinetics of citalopram are shown in Table 18.8. Unlike several of the other SSRIs, citalopram does not undergo first-pass metabolism; it has an oral bioavailability of approximately 80%. The drug is metabolized via hepatic *N*-demethylation to its major metabolite, *N*-desmethylcitalopram, almost equally by CYP2C19, CYP2D6, and CYP3A4 (Table 18.7). The major metabolite exhibits approximately 50% of the potency of citalopram as an inhibitor of 5-HT reuptake. Because the metabolite concentration in the plasma is lower than that of citalopram, it should not add significantly to citalopram's antidepressant effects. Citalopram exhibits dose-proportional linear pharmacokinetics in a dosage range of 10 to 60 mg/d; plasma levels increase proportionately with each increasing dose. Approximately 10% to 12% of an oral dose was recovered in the urine as unmetabolized drug. The clearance of orally administered citalopram was reduced by 37% and 17% in patients with hepatic and renal function impairment, respectively.

Citalopram and its desmethyl metabolite are weak inhibitors of the CYP isoforms, suggesting a low potential for drug interactions. Although no relevant in vivo interactions between citalopram and CYP2D6-metabolized medications have been reported, caution is advised when coadministering citalopram with potential object drugs, especially those having narrow therapeutic indices, in elderly patients. Because citalopram is metabolized in parallel by CYP2C19, CYP2D6, and CYP3A4, it would have little inhibitory effect on the metabolism of other drugs metabolized by these isoenzymes. Citalopram is less highly protein bound than the other SSRIs, reducing the potential for drug interactions with protein-bound drugs having narrow therapeutic indices.

ESCITALOPRAM Escitalopram is the *S*-enantiomer of citalopram that binds with high affinity and selectivity to the human SERT equivalent to (±)-citalopram. It has been reported that nearly all the activity resides in the *S*-enantiomer and that *R*-citalopram actually counteracts the action of the *S*-enantiomer (58,59). Studies show that escitalopram exhibits twice the activity of citalopram and is at least 27 times more potent than the *R*-enantiomer. The *R*-enantiomer inhibits the *S*-enantiomer at SERT (58,59). Escitalopram's mechanism of action is common to the SSRIs.

The pharmacokinetics for escitalopram do not exhibit stereoisomer selectivity and, therefore, are similar to those for citalopram (Table 18.7). Likewise, it exhibits linear pharmacokinetics so that plasma levels increase proportionately and predictably with increased doses, and its half-life of 27 to 32 hours is consistent with once-daily dosing. It also has been found that *R*-citalopram is cleared more slowly than the *S*-enantiomer. Therefore, when the drug is used as a racemic mixture (citalopram), the inactive isomer predominates at steady-state. This is an added incentive for use of the enantiomerically pure escitalopram. Escitalopram has negligible effects on CYP isoforms, suggesting a low potential for drug–drug interactions. Escitalopram is indicated for patients with major depressive disorder, generalized anxiety disorder, panic disorder, and social anxiety disorder.

Escitalopram is metabolized to *S*-desmethylcitalopram by CYP2C19 (37%), CYP2D6 (28%), and CYP3A4 (35%) and to *S*-didesmethylcitalopram (only by CYP2D6) in human liver microsomes and in expressed cytochromes. Escitalopram and its desmethyl metabolite are negligible inhibitors of CYP1A2, CYP2C9, CYP2C19, CYP2E1, and CYP3A and are weakly inhibited by CYP2D6. *R*-Citalopram and its metabolites have properties very similar to those of the corresponding *S*-enantiomers. Because escitalopram is biotransformed by three CYP isoforms in parallel, escitalopram is unlikely to be affected by drug interactions or genetic polymorphisms and is unlikely to cause clinically important drug interactions via CYP inhibition.

Phenylalkylamine

SERTRALINE Although sertraline appears to differ structurally from the other SSRIs, it is a phenylaminotetralin, in which the diphenylbutylamine nucleus is constrained into a rigid bicyclic ring system (Fig. 18.14). In the early work with the discovery of SSRIs at Pfizer, tametraline was initially synthesized in 1978. Animal studies showed it to be a stimulant and to block NE and DA uptake, a use that Pfizer was not interested in pursuing. Subsequently, one or two chlorine atoms were introduced into tametraline to produce new molecules that were potent inhibitors of 5-HT reuptake in the brain. One of the dichloro compounds was to become known as sertraline.

Sertraline contains two chiral centers and only the *S*,*S*-(+)-diastereomer is marketed. The *R*,*R*-, *R*,*S*-, and *S*,*R*-diastereomers are significantly weaker as inhibitors of 5-HT reuptake. Sertraline was marketed in the United

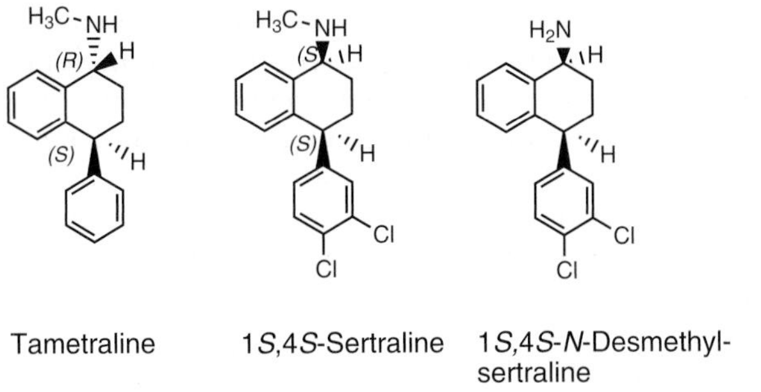

FIGURE 18.14 Phenylalkylamine SSRIs.

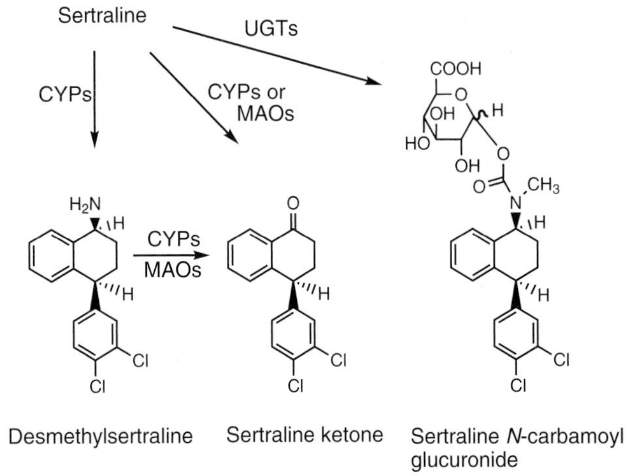

FIGURE 18.15 Metabolic products formed from sertraline metabolism.

States in 1992, emphasizing its pharmacokinetic differences from the other SSRIs.

Mechanism of Action Sertraline is a potent and selective inhibitor of the neuronal reuptake SERT. In vitro binding studies suggest that sertraline has a substantially higher selectivity for inhibiting 5-HT reuptake than other SSRIs or TCAs, including clomipramine (Fig. 18.6). It has only weak effects on neuronal uptake of NE and DA. Its mechanism of action is common to the SSRIs. Sertraline is very selective, lacking affinity for other neuroreceptors at therapeutic concentrations.

Pharmacokinetics Sertraline appears to be slowly but well absorbed from the GI tract after oral administration. The oral bioavailability of sertraline in humans ranges from 20% to 36% (Table 18.8), suggesting extensive first-pass metabolism to its *N*-desmethylated metabolite. Food enhances its oral absorption, decreasing the time to achieve peak plasma concentrations from approximately 8 to 6 hours. After multiple doses, steady-state plasma sertraline concentrations are proportional and linearly related to dose (half-life: single dose, 24 hours; multiple dose, 24 hours). *N*-Desmethylsertraline, sertraline's principal metabolite, exhibits dose-dependent pharmacokinetics. Sertraline and *N*-desmethylsertraline are distributed into breast milk. Although in elderly patients the elimination half-life is increased to approximately 36 hours, this effect does not appear to be clinically important and does not warrant dosing alterations. Sertraline is primarily metabolized to *N*-desmethylsertraline through the action of CYP2B6, CYP2C9, CYP2C19, CYP2D6, and CYP3A4 (Fig. 18.15). Of these, CYP2B6 appears to be the major isoform involved (60). *N*-Desmethylsertraline is approximately 5 to 10 times less potent as an inhibitor of 5-HT reuptake than sertraline. The formation of sertraline ketone can occur either through the action of CYP or MAO, but studies have not been reported to indicate the role of either or both. The formation of sertraline *N*-carbamoyl glucuronide is a unique product that was shown to form in vitro through the action primarily of UGT2B7. The involvement of multiple enzymes in the metabolism of sertraline suggests that no single drug could significantly alter sertraline pharmacokinetics and reduce any drug–drug interactions. Sertraline and *N*-desmethylsertraline undergo further metabolism via oxidative deamination and ring hydroxylation and glucuronide conjugation. *N*-Desmethylsertraline has an elimination half-life approximately 2.5 times that of sertraline. Following oral administration, sertraline and its conjugated metabolites are excreted in both urine and feces, and unmetabolized sertraline accounts for less than 5% of oral dose. Plasma clearance of sertraline was approximately 40% lower in geriatric patients. The elimination half-life of sertraline in patients with hepatic disease was prolonged to a mean of 52 hours, compared with 22 hours in individuals without hepatic disease.

Drug Interactions Sertraline is not a potent inhibitor of CYP3A4, and because CYP2D6 metabolism is a minor pathway for sertraline, drug–drug interactions with these isoforms are unlikely to be of clinical importance. Sertraline is metabolized by more than one CYP isoform in parallel; therefore, genetic polymorphisms are unlikely to cause clinically significant drug interactions via CYP isoform inhibition. Caution is advised, however, when coadministering sertraline with potential object drugs, especially those with narrow therapeutic indices in elderly patients. For example, sertraline has been shown to reduce the clearance of desipramine and imipramine as a result of CYP2D6 inhibition.

Because sertraline is highly protein bound, patients receiving it concurrently with any highly protein-bound drug should be observed for potential adverse effects associated with combined therapy.

Additional SSRIs

FLUVOXAMINE Fluvoxamine is a nontricyclic SERT inhibitor that is structurally unique among the SSRIs by being the (*E*)-isomer of a 2-aminoethyl oxime ether of

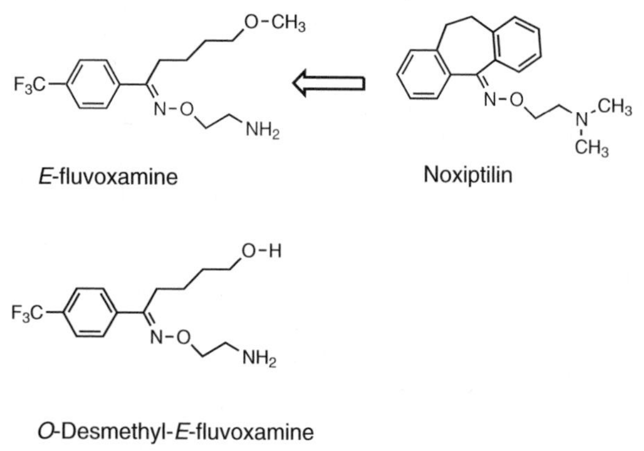

FIGURE 18.16 Miscellaneous SSRIs.

an aralkylketone (Fig. 18.16).The C=N double bond is isosteric with the propylidene group in amitriptyline and, thus, imparts geometric *E* or *Z* stereoisomerism to fluvoxamine. The oxime ether is found in a previously marketed analog of amitriptyline called noxiptilin (1966 by Bayer AG [Germany]). Thus, fluvoxamine may be considered to be an open-chain analog of the tricyclic noxipitilin. The 4-trifluoromethyl group or other electronegative group is essential for SERT affinity and selectivity. The C=N double bond also enhances the susceptibility of fluvoxamine to photoisomerization by ultraviolet (UV)-B light (290 to 320 nm). When fluvoxamine solutions were exposed to UV-B light, photoisomerization to the pharmacologically inactive *Z*-isomer occurred. Thus, fluvoxamine solutions should be protected from sunlight to prevent loss of antidepressant efficacy. No studies have been reported regarding its solid-state stability to UV-B light.

Mechanism of Action Fluvoxamine is a highly selective inhibitor of 5-HT reuptake at the presynaptic membrane. Potency data from in vitro affinity studies suggest that fluvoxamine is less potent than the other SSRIs (e.g., paroxetine, sertraline, and citalopram). Its mechanism of action is similar to that of the other SSRIs. Fluvoxamine appears to have little or no effect on the reuptake of NE or DA. In vitro studies have demonstrated that fluvoxamine possesses virtually no affinity for other neuroreceptors. Its onset of action is similar to the other SSRIs (2 to 4 weeks).

Pharmacokinetics Fluvoxamine is well absorbed, with a bioavailability of approximately 50%, probably because of first-pass metabolism (Table 18.8). At steady-state doses, fluvoxamine demonstrates nonlinear pharmacokinetics over a dosage range of 100 to 300 mg/d, which results in higher plasma concentrations at higher doses than would be predicted by lower dose kinetics (single dose, 15 hours; multiple dosing, 22 hours). Food does not significantly affect oral bioavailability. The mean apparent volume of distribution for fluvoxamine reflects its lipophilic nature, extensive tissue distribution, and protein binding. Fluvoxamine is distributed into breast milk. Fluvoxamine is preferentially metabolized by CYP2D6 in the liver by *O*-demethylation to its alcohol metabolite, which subsequently is oxidized to a carboxylic acid. Oxidative deamination and nine other metabolites have been identified, none of which shows significant pharmacologic activity.

Adverse Effects The adverse effects for fluvoxamine include symptoms of drowsiness, nausea or vomiting, abdominal pain, tremors, sinus bradycardia, and mild anticholinergic symptoms. Toxic doses could produce seizures and severe bradycardia.

Drug Interactions In vitro studies have shown fluvoxamine to be a potent inhibitor of CYP1A2, to inhibit CYP3A4 and CYP2C19, and to weakly inhibit CYP2D6. The bioavailability of fluvoxamine is significantly decreased in smokers compared with nonsmokers, possibly because of induction of CYP1A metabolism of fluvoxamine. Therefore, interactions with drugs that inhibit CYP1A2 also should be considered (e.g., theophylline and caffeine).

Therapeutic Uses Fluvoxamine is approved for use in obsessive-compulsive disorders.

Norepinephrine and Serotonin Reuptake Inhibitors (NSRIs)

The NSRI antidepressant drugs in this class block both the NET and SERT (i.e., they combine the mechanisms of action for both the SSRIs and SNRIs), exhibiting dual affinity for NET and SERT (low NE:5-HT potency ratio). These dual inhibitors, as a group, do not show a significant separation in selectivity for the NET and SERT reuptake transporter. Historically, the tertiary amine TCAs displayed dual inhibition of 5-HT and NE presynaptic reuptake, but they also bind to other types of neuroreceptors, which is responsible for their narrow therapeutic window and adverse effects. Clinical studies suggest that dual-acting inhibitors of 5-HT and NE reuptake may be more beneficial than selective inhibitors in managing depression. This has given impetus to the search for nontricyclic NSRIs and has led to a second group of NSRIs, such as venlafaxine and duloxetine.

Tricyclic Tertiary Amine Antidepressants

The TCAs in this class belong to the tertiary amine TCAs (Fig. 18.17). The relatively low bioavailability for the tertiary amine TCAs suggests first-pass metabolism (*N*-demethylation) to their secondary amine active metabolites (nor or desmethyl metabolites) and aromatic ring hydroxylation (Table 18.2). Despite the fact that steady-state serum plasma levels are reached within 1 to 2 days, their onset of antidepressant action typically is at least 2 to 3 weeks or longer. Their volume of distribution

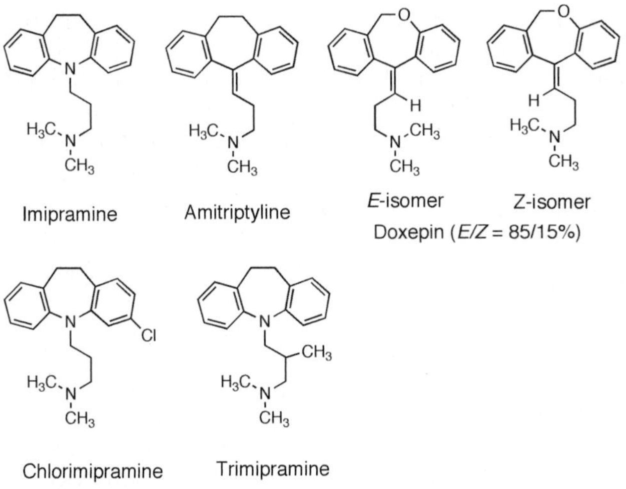

FIGURE 18.17 Tricyclic norepinephrine and serotonin reuptake inhibitors.

is very high, suggesting distribution into the CNS and protein binding. Excretion is primarily as metabolites via renal elimination. Renal and liver function can affect the elimination and metabolism of the parent TCA and its metabolites, leading to increased potential for adverse effects, especially in patients (i.e., elderly) with renal disease.

Meaningful differences between the tertiary TCAs are largely related to their pharmacokinetics, metabolism to active metabolites, inhibition of CYP isoforms, potential for drug–drug interactions, and half-life of the tertiary TCA.

Mechanisms of Action Common to the Tertiary Amine TCAs The exact mechanism of action for the tertiary TCAs is unclear, but it is known that the parent tertiary amine TCA exhibits dual inhibition of the NET and SERT. The result is an increase in both NE and 5-HT concentrations in the synaptic cleft. The in vivo antidepressant activity for these TCAs is more complex, however, because of the formation of secondary amine TCA metabolites, which in many cases annuls the 5-HT affinity of the parent TCA, leading to NET selectivity. The plasma concentrations for the secondary amine metabolites usually are higher than those of their parent tertiary amine TCA because of rapid *N*-demethylation metabolism. Note that none of the tertiary amine TCAs have any significant affinity for the DAT. During chronic therapy with the tertiary amine TCAs, downregulation of the noradrenergic and serotonergic receptors occurs, which is a result of neurotransmitter hypersensitivity caused by the continued high concentrations of NE and 5-HT at the postsynaptic receptor. The tertiary TCAs are less potent inhibitors than the SSRIs for SERT.

Therapeutic Uses Common to Tricyclic Tertiary Antidepressants For the most part, the therapeutic uses for the tertiary amine TCAs are very similar as a group, but these TCAs may be used in different cases of depression because of their variability in their dual mechanism of action as SNRIs and SSRIs. Their efficacy in treating depression suggests that mixed inhibition of NET and SERT influences depression by parallel and independent pathways. The tertiary TCAs may offer an option in the treatment of major depression for patients who have failed treatment with or who do not tolerate SNRIs or SSRIs.

Adverse Effects Common to Tertiary TCAs Because of their potent and multiple pharmacodynamic effects at histamine H_1, muscarinic, and α_1-adrenergic receptors, the tertiary TCAs exhibit greater anticholinergic, antihistaminic, and α_1-antiadrenergic adverse effects than the secondary TCAs do. Increased cardiotoxicity or frequency of seizures is higher for the tertiary TCAs than for the secondary TCAs, because they are potent inhibitors of sodium channels, leading to changes in nerve conduction. Cardiotoxicity can occur at plasma concentrations approximately 5 to 10 times higher than therapeutic blood levels. These concentrations can occur in individuals who take an overdose of the TCA or who are slow metabolizers and develop higher plasma concentrations on what usually are therapeutic doses.

Drug–Drug Interactions Common to Tertiary TCAs For the most part, drug–drug interactions for the tertiary amine TCAs are very similar to those for the secondary amine TCAs. These reactions, however, may be more pronounced.

The concurrent use of tertiary amine TCAs with SSRIs and other serotonergic drugs may result in 5-HT syndrome (see the discussion of drug interactions of SSRIs). Coadministration of a tertiary amine TCA with an MAOI is potentially hazardous and may result in severe adverse effects associated with 5-HT syndrome.

Because protein binding of the tertiary amine TCAs is high, displacement interactions with other highly protein-bound drugs and drugs with narrow therapeutic indices, although not fully evaluated, may be important. Concurrent use of tertiary amine TCAs with anticholinergic drugs requires close supervision and careful adjustment of the dosage because of potential additive anticholinergic effects (i.e., spastic colon). An additional disadvantage of TCAs is their toxicity from overdosage, especially in those who are being treated for depression who are having suicidal thoughts.

The plasma concentrations of tertiary amine TCAs usually are lower and plasma concentrations of their secondary amine metabolites usually are higher as a result of CYP1A induction.

Patient Information Common to the Tertiary Amine TCAs Common patient information and recommendations are similar to those given to patients who are prescribed secondary TCAs (Table 18.5).

Unique Properties of Specific Tertiary Amine TCAs

Amitriptyline Amitriptyline is a tertiary amine dibenzocycloheptadiene TCA with a propylidene side chain extending from the central carbocyclic ring (Fig. 18.17). The diarylpropylideneamine moiety for amitriptyline makes it sensitive to photo-oxidation; therefore, its hydrochloride solutions should be protected from light to avoid ketone formation and precipitation.

Pharmacokinetics. Amitriptyline is rapidly absorbed from the GI tract and from parenteral sites. Its pharmacokinetics are shown in Table 18.9. Amitriptyline and its active metabolite, nortriptyline, are distributed into breast milk. Amitriptyline is primarily (65%) metabolized by *N*-demethylation by CYP2D6 to nortriptyline and hydroxylation to its *E*-10-hydroxy metabolite. Nortriptyline is pharmacologically active as a secondary amine TCA. Amitriptyline shows approximately equal affinity for SERT and NET.

Imipramine Imipramine is a 10,11-dihydrodibenzazepine tertiary amine TCA (Fig. 18.17) that is marketed as hydrochloride and pamoate salts, both of which are administered orally. Although the hydrochloride salt may be administered in divided daily doses, imipramine's long duration of action suggests that the entire oral daily dose may be administered at one time. On the other hand, imipramine pamoate usually is administered as a single daily oral dose. Imipramine preferentially inhibits 5-HT reuptake over NE; however, the formation of its *N*-desmethyl metabolite removes whatever 5-HT activity imipramine had, with the net result of enhanced noradrenergic activity from inhibition of NE reuptake at the presynaptic neuronal membrane. Imipramine shares the pharmacologic and adverse effect profiles of the other tertiary TCAs.

The pharmacokinetics for imipramine are shown in Table 18.9. Imipramine is completely absorbed from the GI tract. Imipramine is primarily metabolized by CYP2D6 to its 2- and 10-hydroxylated metabolites and *N*-demethylated via CYP2C19 and CYP1A2 to desipramine, its *N*-monodemethylated metabolite, an SNRI.

Therapeutic Uses. Besides being used in the clinical treatment of depression, imipramine also has been used for the treatment of functional enuresis in children who are at least 6 years of age (25 mg daily administered 1 hour before bedtime, not to exceed 2.5 mg/kg daily).

Doxepin Doxepin is a tertiary amine dibenzoxepine derivative with an oxygen replacing one of the ethylene carbons in the bridge. The oxygen introduces

TABLE 18.9 Pharmacokinetics of the Tricyclic Norepinephrine and Serotonin Reuptake Inhibitors (NSRIs)

Parameters	Amitriptyline	Clomipramine	Doxepin	Imipramine	Trimipramine
Oral bioavailability (%)	31–61	~50	13–45	29–77	44
Lipophilicity ($\log D_{7.4}$)	2.53	2.52	2.49	2.28	2.35
Protein binding (%)	95	96–98	ND	89–95	95
Volume of distribution (L/kg)	12–18	17 (9–25)	12–28	23 (15–31)	~31
Elimination half-life (h)	10–26	32 (19–37)	11–16	11–25	9–11
Cytochrome P450 major isoform	2D6	2D6	2D6 and 2C19	2D6 and 2C19	2D6 and 2C19
Major active metabolites	Nortriptyline	Desclomipramine (54–77 h)	Nordoxepin (~30 h)	Desipramine	Desmethyltrimipramine (30 h)
Peak plasma concentration (h)	2–12	2–6 (4.7)	<2	1–2	<2
Excretion (%)	Urine 25–50	Urine 51–60 (14 d)	Renal ~50	Urine ~40 (24 h)	Feces 80–90
	Feces minor	Feces 24–32	Feces minor	Feces minor	Urine <5
Plasma half-life (h)	21 (10–46)	34 (22–84)	8–24	18 (9–24)	9
Time to steady-state concentration	—	1–2 wk	ND	ND	ND

ND, not determined.

asymmetry into the tricyclic ring system, resulting in the formation of two geometric isomers: *E* (*trans*) and *Z* (*cis*) (Fig. 18.17). No commercial attempt was made to separate the isomers; thus, doxepin is administered as an 85:15 mixture of *E*- and *Z*-stereoisomers, with the *Z*-isomer being the more active stereoisomer for inhibiting the reuptake of 5-HT (61). The *E*-isomer, on the other hand, inhibits the reuptake of NE. Unless otherwise specified, the reported in vitro and in vivo studies with doxepin were done with the 85:15 geometric mixture.

Mechanism of Action. Because doxepin is administered as an 85:15 mixture of geometric isomers, its mechanism of action and antidepressant properties reflect this ratio. Therefore, doxepin's selectivity for inhibiting presynaptic NE reuptake is most likely caused by the 85% presence of the *E*-isomer in the geometric mixture. Its antidepressant activity is similar to amitriptyline. Data suggest NE reuptake inhibitory potency comparable to imipramine and clomipramine; the fact that doxepin is an 85:15 mixture of *E*- and *Z*-geometric isomers clouds its true efficacy for SERT or NET. The formation of *N*-desmethyldoxepin results in inhibition of NE reuptake with enhanced noradrenergic activity. As a result of these mixed effects SERT and NET, doxepin shares the pharmacologic and adverse effect profiles of the other TCAs.

The pharmacokinetics for oral doxepin are described in Table 18.9. After oral dosing, no significant difference was found between the bioavailability of the *E*- and *Z*-isomers. The plasma concentrations of the doxepin isomers remained roughly those of the administered drug, whereas the ratio for the metabolites, *E*-*N*-desmethyldoxepin and *Z*-*N*-desmethyldoxepin, were approximately 1:1 (61,62). This similarity in ratios of metabolites is attributed to *E*-doxepin being primarily metabolized in parallel by CYP2D6 and CYP2C19, whereas *Z*-doxepin is primarily metabolized only by CYP2C19 and not at all by CYP2D6 (Table 18.2) (61). Its *Z*-*N*-demethylated metabolite is pharmacologically more active than its *E*-metabolite as an inhibitor of 5-HT and NE reuptake (61). Both isomers of doxepin showed large volumes of distribution and relatively short half-lives in plasma, suggestive of extensive distribution and/or tissue binding. Renal clearances did not differ for the isomers.

Clomipramine Clomipramine is considered to be the most powerful antidepressant ever made. This dihydrodibenzazepine TCA, with actions on both SERT and NET, was the last of the major TCAs to come to market. Initially, the FDA regarded it as another "me-too" drug, and accordingly, they did not license it. Subsequently, however, it was licensed for the treatment of obsessive-compulsive disorders. Clomipramine differs from imipramine only by the addition of a 3-chloro group (Fig. 18.17).

Mechanism of Action. Clomipramine is different from the other TCAs, exhibiting preferential selectivity for inhibiting the reuptake of 5-HT at the presynaptic neuronal membrane. Its antidepressant mechanism of action as an inhibitor of the SERT is reduced in vivo, however, because of the formation of its active metabolite, *N*-desmethylclomipramine, which inhibits the reuptake of NE. As a result of its common structure with the other TCAs, clomipramine shares the pharmacologic and adverse effect profiles of the other TCAs.

The efficacy of clomipramine relative to the other TCAs in the treatment of obsessive-compulsive disorder may be related to its potency in blocking 5-HT reuptake at the presynaptic neuronal membrane, suggesting a dysregulation of 5-HT for the pathogenesis of obsessive-compulsive disorder. Clomipramine appears to decrease the turnover of 5-HT in the CNS, probably because of a decrease in the release and/or synthesis of 5-HT.

Although in vitro studies suggest that clomipramine is approximately four times more potent than fluoxetine as a 5-HT reuptake inhibitor, in vivo studies suggest the opposite. This difference has been attributed to the relatively long elimination half-lives for fluoxetine and its principal serotonergic metabolite norfluoxetine. In addition, metabolism of clomipramine to its *N*-desmethyl secondary amine metabolite decreases the potency and selectivity of 5-HT reuptake inhibition of clomipramine, but not fluoxetine.

Pharmacokinetics. Clomipramine appears to be well absorbed from the GI tract following oral administration, with an oral bioavailability of approximately 50%, suggesting some first-pass metabolism (Table 18.9). Food does not appear to substantially affect its bioavailability. Clomipramine and its active metabolite, *N*-desmethylclomipramine, exhibit nonlinear pharmacokinetics at 25 to 150 mg daily. At dosages exceeding 150 mg daily, their elimination half-lives may be considerably prolonged, allowing plasma concentrations of both to accumulate, which may increase the incidence of plasma concentration–dependent adverse effects, particularly seizures. Because of the relatively long elimination half-lives of clomipramine and *N*-desmethylclomipramine, their steady-state plasma concentrations generally are achieved within approximately 1 to 2 weeks. Plasma concentrations of *N*-desmethylclomipramine generally are greater than those for clomipramine at steady-state conditions. Clomipramine crosses the placenta and is distributed into breast milk.

Clomipramine is primarily metabolized by CYP2D6 *N*-dealkylation to its pharmacologically active metabolite, the 2- and 8-hydroxylated metabolites and their glucuronides, and clomipramine *N*-oxide (Fig. 18.18). *N*-Dealkylation also involves CYP3A4, CYP2C19, CYP2C9, and CYP1A2. Like all the other secondary amine TCAs, *N*-desmethylclomipramine is significantly more potent

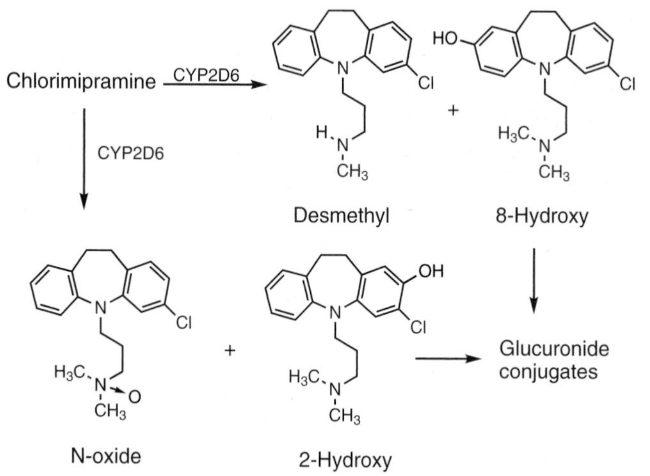

FIGURE 18.18 Metabolism of chlorimipramine.

as an inhibitor of NE reuptake than clomipramine. Although *N*-desmethylclomipramine is pharmacologically active, its efficacy in obsessive-compulsive disorder is not known. 8-Hydroxyclomipramine and 8-hydroxydesmethylclomipramine also are pharmacologically active, but their clinical importance remains unknown. The hydroxylation and *N*-demethylation of clomipramine highlight CYP2D6 polymorphism in healthy adults who were phenotyped as either extensive metabolizers or poor metabolizers of clomipramine. Interindividual variation in plasma concentrations may be caused by genetic differences in the metabolism of the drug. In addition, the CYP1A2 ring hydroxylates clomipramine. Less than 1% of an oral dose of clomipramine was excreted unmetabolized into the urine, with 8-hydroxyclomipramine glucuronide as the principal metabolite found in the urine. The effects of renal clearance suggest that clomipramine and desmethylclomipramine should be decreased in patients with renal impairment.

Pharmacogenetic differences in the metabolism of clomipramine after a single oral dose are apparent as increased plasma clomipramine concentrations in Indian and Pakistani patients compared with Caucasians. In Japanese patients, substantial interindividual variation in demethylation and hydroxylation of clomipramine was observed, although the prevalence of poor demethylators and poor hydroxylators of clomipramine has been estimated to be less than 1%.

If inhibition of SERT is critical to the desired clinical effect for clomipramine, then a patient may fail to respond because of higher levels of *N*-desmethylclomipramine as opposed to the parent drug. However, in a patient who has responded well and has stabilized to a dose of clomipramine, the drug might lose efficacy if exposed to an environmental agent that is capable of inducing CYP1A or CYP3A4.

Adverse Effects. Male patients taking clomipramine should be informed of sexual dysfunction as a side effect associated with antidepressants having significant serotonergic activity. Sexual dysfunction in men appears as ejaculatory incompetence, ejaculatory retardation, decreased libido, or inability to obtain or maintain an erection. Sexual dysfunction is dose related and may be treated simply by lowering the drug dose.

Trimipramine Trimipramine also is a dihydrodibenzazepine TCA that differs structurally from imipramine in that the 5-propyl side chain is branched by a methyl group creating a chiral center (Fig. 18.17). Trimipramine is marketed as a racemic mixture. No data are available regarding the activity of the enantiomers. Apparently, branching the propyl side chain reduces affinity by 100 times for both SERT and NET, but the selectivity ratio favors the SERT. Although trimipramine has the weakest binding affinity for the monoamine transporters, it shares the pharmacologic and toxicity actions of the other TCAs and is used primarily in the treatment of depression.

The pharmacokinetics for trimipramine are shown in Table 18.9. Trimipramine is rapidly absorbed. Trimipramine demonstrates stereoselectivity in its metabolism to its three major metabolites. (−)-Trimipramine is primarily metabolized via CY2D6 hydroxylation to 2-hydroxytrimipramine, whereas (+)-trimipramine is preferentially metabolized by CYP2C19 *N*-demethylation to desmethyltrimipramine. Desmethyltrimipramine is further hydroxylated to 2-hydroxydesmethyltrimipramine. (−)-Trimipramine is metabolized by CYP3A4/5 to an unknown metabolite (63,64). Most of the oral dose is excreted in urine in 72 hours, primarily as *N*-demethylated or hydroxylated and conjugated metabolites. The pharmacokinetics of trimipramine in geriatric individuals (≥65 years of age) do not differ substantially from those in younger adults.

Trimipramine is one of the antidepressants with the most pronounced differences in pharmacokinetics caused by the CYP2D6 genetic polymorphism (63,64). Its bioavailability and systemic clearance depend significantly on the CYP2D6 isoform with a linear dose relationship. Its mean bioavailability was 44% in individuals without CYP2D6 (poor metabolizers) but 16% and 12% in those individuals with two and three active genes of CYP2D6 (fast and ultrafast metabolizers), respectively. Consequently, the mean total clearances of the oral dose were 27, 151, and 253 L/h in poor, extensive, and ultrarapid metabolizers, respectively. The 44% bioavailability combined with low systemic clearance of trimipramine in poor metabolizers of CYP2D6 substrates results in a very high exposure to trimipramine with the risk of adverse drug reactions. However, the presystemic elimination may result in subtherapeutic drug concentrations in carriers of CYP2D6 gene duplications with a high risk of poor therapeutic response (63,64).

OTHER TRICYCLIC NSRIs Figure 18.19 shows two tricyclic 5-HT/NE reuptake inhibitors. One is an analog of imipramine, and the second is an isostere of doxepin.

Dosulepin Dosulepin (formerly dothiepin) is the thio isostere of doxepin and is marketed in Europe as its single *E*-geometric isomer (Fig. 18.19), in contrast to the active *Z*-geometric isomer for doxepin. Its antidepressant activity is mediated by inhibition of both the NET and SERT, with preferential affinity for SERT (65). It exhibits greater overall in vitro affinity for NET and SERT than its oxygen isostere doxepin, consistent with its greater potency. Its overall therapeutic efficacy is similar to that of amitriptyline.

Although dosulepin is readily absorbed from the GI tract, it is extensively first-pass metabolized by *S*-oxidation in the liver to its primary active metabolite, dosulepin *S*-oxide, and by *N*-demethylation to its minor metabolite, desmethyldosulepin (northiaden) (65). Dosulepin is excreted in the urine, mainly in the form of its metabolites; small amounts of the drug also are excreted in the feces and distributed into breast milk.

The incidence of anticholinergic side effects is less among patients treated with dosulepin than with amitriptyline and without cardiotoxicity at therapeutic doses. The sedative/anxiolytic activity of dosulepin is similar to that of amitriptyline. Dosulepin is an effective treatment for patients with depressive symptoms of varying severity and coexisting anxiety (65).

Lofepramine Lofepramine differs from imipramine by the attachment of a *p*-chlorophenacyl moiety to the *N*-aminopropyl side chain (Fig. 18.19). This change confers enhanced lipophilicity and the potential of more rapid distribution into the CNS with greater in vitro affinity and selectivity for NET. Its mechanism of antidepressant action is attributed to its rapid metabolism to the secondary amine metabolite, desipramine, which selectively inhibits the neuronal uptake of NE (66).

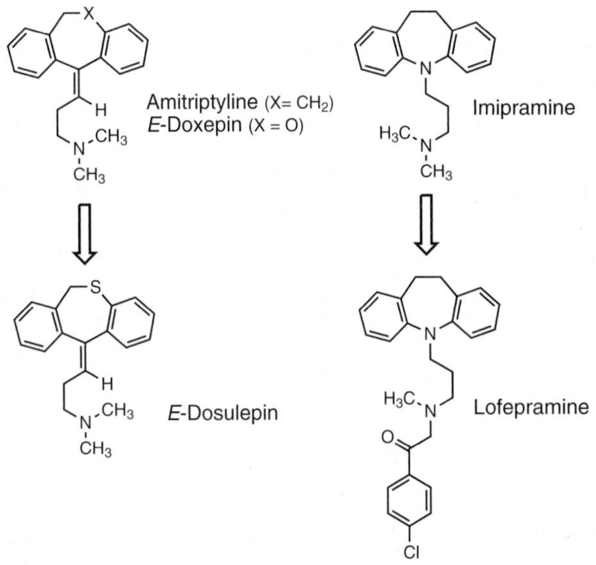

FIGURE 18.19 Future tricyclic NSRIs.

Lofepramine has an oral bioavailability of less than 10% as a result of the extensive first-pass metabolism. Most of a dose of lofepramine is excreted via the urine as metabolites, with a mean elimination half-life of approximately 2 hours. The adverse effects of lofepramine are similar to the secondary TCAs. Lofepramine displays reversible hepatotoxicity (jaundice and hepatitis), usually within 8 weeks of initiation of therapy.

Oral lofepramine is effective in the treatment of various types of depression and is similar in efficacy to imipramine and amitriptyline while inducing fewer adverse effects. This suggests its potential use in patients who are unable to tolerate other antidepressants.

NONTRICYCLIC NOREPINEPHRINE AND SEROTONIN REUPTAKE INHIBITORS Clinical studies suggest that compounds that increase the synaptic availability of both NE and 5-HT have greater efficacy than single-acting drugs in the treatment of major depression. Thus began the efforts to design a drug that combined the properties of SSRIs and SNRIs that only blocked SERTs and NETs and without the unwanted adverse effects of TCAs (67). Currently, the nontricyclic dual inhibitors of 5-HT and NE uptake are venlafaxine, milnacipran, and duloxetine (Fig. 18.20). A structurally related nontricyclic SNRI is atomoxetine. Based on preclinical studies, venlafaxine, milnacipran, and duloxetine inhibit the reuptake of 5-HT and NE both in vitro and in vivo in the following order of decreasing potency: duloxetine > milnacipran > venlafaxine. All the dual reuptake inhibitors exhibit low affinity at neuronal receptors of the other neurotransmitters, suggesting a low side effect potential. Venlafaxine, milnacipran, and duloxetine have repeatedly been shown to be as efficacious as TCA drugs in treating major depressive disorders. These nontricyclic antidepressants have been reported to produce a faster and greater antidepressant response than an SSRI alone, suggesting that these two mechanisms of action can be

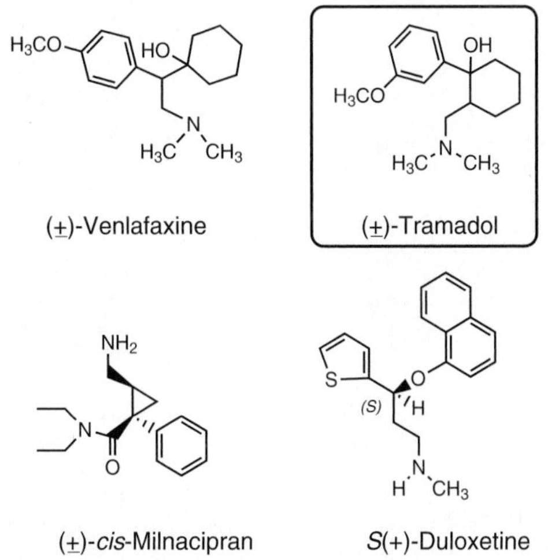

FIGURE 18.20 Nontricyclic NSRIs and related drug tramadol.

synergistic in terms of mediating antidepressant efficacy. Meaningful differences between the nontricyclic NSRIs are largely related to their pharmacokinetics, metabolism to active metabolites, inhibition of CYP isoforms, effect of drug–drug interactions, and the half-life of the nontricyclic NSRI.

Venlafaxine Venlafaxine is a methoxyphenylethylamine antidepressant that resembles an open TCA with one of the aromatic rings replaced by a cyclohexanol ring and a dimethylaminomethyl group rather than a dimethylaminopropyl chain (Fig. 18.20). It is structurally similar to the atypical opioid, tramadol (Ultram).

Venlafaxine and its active metabolite, *O*-desmethylvenlafaxine (ODV), have dual mechanisms of action, with preferential affinity for 5-HT reuptake and weak inhibition of NE and DA reuptake. Venlafaxine is approximately 30 times more potent as an inhibitor of SERT than of NET (68). Because of the 30-fold difference in transporter affinities, increasing the dose of venlafaxine from 75 to 375 mg/d can sequentially inhibit SERT and NET. Thus, venlafaxine displays an ascending dose-dependent antidepressant response in contrast to the flat dose–antidepressant response curve observed with the SSRIs. This sequential action for venlafaxine also is consistent with its dose-dependent adverse effect profile. Its mechanism of action is similar to imipramine.

Venlafaxine is rapidly and well absorbed (90%), but with a bioavailability of 15%, which has been attributed to first-pass metabolism (Table 18.10). Food delays its absorption but does not impair the extent of absorption. Venlafaxine is distributed into breast milk. Venlafaxine is primarily metabolized in the liver by CYP2D6 to its primary metabolite, ODV, which is approximately equivalent in pharmacologic activity and potency to venlafaxine. In vitro studies indicate that CYP3A4 also is involved in the metabolism of venlafaxine to its minor and less active metabolite, *N*-desmethylvenlafaxine (Fig. 18.21). Protein binding for venlafaxine and ODV is low and is not a problem for drug interactions. In patients with hepatic impairment, elimination half-lives were increased by approximately 30% for venlafaxine and approximately 60% for ODV (Table 18.10). In patients with renal function impairment, elimination half-lives were increased by approximately 40% to 50% for venlafaxine and for ODV. At steady-state doses, venlafaxine and ODV exhibit dose-proportional linear pharmacokinetics over the dose range of 75 to 450 mg/d. Steady-state concentrations of venlafaxine and ODV are attained within 3 days with regular oral dosing. Venlafaxine and its metabolites are excreted primarily in the urine (87%).

The potential for cardiotoxicity with venlafaxine during normal use and for various toxicities in overdose situations is a key concern. Venlafaxine displays minimal

TABLE 18.10 Pharmacokinetics of Nontricyclic Norepinephrine and Serotonin Reuptake Inhibitors (NSRIs)

Parameters	Venlafaxine	Desvenlafaxine (ODV)	Milnacipran	Duloxetine
Oral Bioavailability (%)	~15	80	90	>70
Lipophilicity ($logD_{7.4}$)	0.70	0.74	−0.53	3,09
Protein binding (%)	25–30	30	15–30	>90
Volume of distribution (L/kg)	8 (5–19)	3.4	17 (9–25)	1,940
Elimination half-life (hours)	4 (2–7)	11	~8	11–16
Cytochrome P450 major isoform	2D6	3A4	None	2D6/1A2
Major active metabolites	ODV	None	None	4-hydroxy
Peak plasma concentration (h)	2	7.5	32-48	6–10
Excretion (%)	Urine 87	Urine 45	Urine 90	Urine >70
	Feces 2		Feces, minor	Feces 15
Plasma half-life (h)	2		NA	
Time to steady-state concentration	3 d	3 d	32–48 h	3–7d

NA, not available.

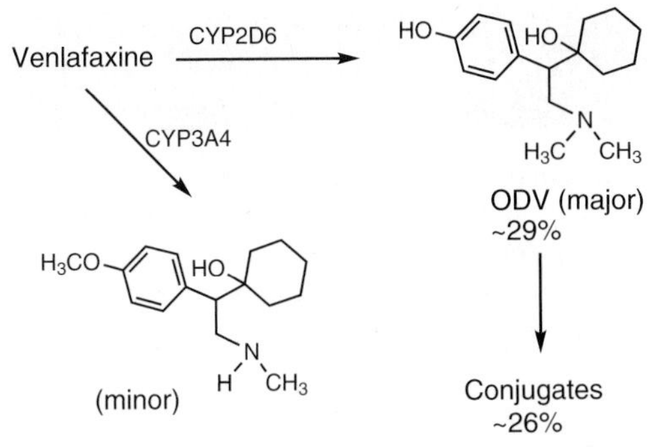

FIGURE 18.21 Metabolism of venlafaxine.

in vitro affinity for the other neural neurotransmitter receptors and, thus, a low probability for adverse effects. To minimize GI upset (e.g., nausea), venlafaxine can be taken with food without affecting its GI absorption. Venlafaxine should be administered as a single daily dose with food at approximately the same time each day. The extended-release capsules should be swallowed whole with fluid and should not be divided, crushed, chewed, or placed in water.

Whenever venlafaxine is being discontinued after more than 1 week of therapy, it generally is recommended that the patient be closely monitored and the dosage of the drug be tapered gradually to reduce the risk of withdrawal symptoms.

Although venlafaxine is a weak inhibitor of CYP2D6, variability has been observed in the pharmacokinetic parameters of venlafaxine in patients with hepatic or renal function impairment. As a precaution, elderly patients taking venlafaxine concurrently with a drug that has a narrow therapeutic index and also is metabolized by CYP2D6 should be carefully monitored. Concurrent use of CYP3A4 inhibitors with venlafaxine has been shown to interfere with its metabolism and clearance. Similar to the other antidepressants that block 5-HT reuptake, venlafaxine may interact pharmacodynamically to cause toxic levels of 5-HT to accumulate, leading to the 5-HT syndrome.

Desvenlafaxine Desvenlafaxine (ODV), as previously described, is the main active metabolite of venlafaxine, which is metabolized by CYP3A4 (*N*-demethylation) and *O*-glucuronidation.(Fig. 18.21). Similar to venlafaxine, desvenlafaxine is an antidepressant of the SNRI reuptake inhibitor class and has been approved for use in the United States and Canada as an antidepressant, but not approved for use in the European market. Non–FDA-approved (off-label) use is as a non–hormonal-based vasomotor (hot flash) treatment for menopause. The European Union has not approved desvenlafaxine for any indication because, in relation to its parent, venlafaxine, desvenlafaxine seemed to be less effective with no advantages in terms of safety and tolerability. Since venlafaxine is already approved for the treatment of MDD and is almost entirely transformed into desvenlafaxine, it would be expected that efficacy and safety of desvenlafaxine in the treatment of MDD would be very similar to those of venlafaxine. Desvenlafaxine is approximately 10-fold more potent at inhibiting 5-HT reuptake than NE reuptake. When most normal metabolizers take venlafaxine, approximately 70% of the parent drug is metabolized into desvenlafaxine, so the effects are very similar. Desvenlafaxine is structurally related to the atypical opioid tramadol (Ultram). The most common side effect of desvenlafaxine is nausea (30% to 50% vs. 9% to 11% for placebo), which is the most common reason for discontinuation. Other adverse reactions are dizziness, insomnia, sweating, constipation, somnolence, decreased appetite, priapism, night terrors, anxiety, and delayed ejaculation, which are consistent with the adverse reactions of other SNRIs. Suicidal risk was significant in some patients in each study.

Milnacipran (±)-Milnacipran is the cis-aminomethyl derivative of phenylcyclopropanecarboxamide (Fig. 18.20) that acts by inhibiting both NE and 5-HT reuptake. It is structurally different from the other NSRIs and currently is only available in Europe as a racemic mixture, with both enantiomers exhibiting antidepressant activity. Substituting the aminomethyl group of milnacipran with an aminopropyl gives a milnacipran homolog that exhibits antidepressant activity as a potent NMDA receptor antagonist. A glutamate hypothesis is being investigated as an alternative mechanism of depression (see the subsection on NMDA antagonists).

Milnacipran selectively inhibits the reuptake of 5-HT (selectivity ratio = 9) at the presynaptic membrane site, thus increasing the concentration of 5-HT in the synaptic cleft (69). Although milnacipran is not a TCA, its mechanism of action is similar to that of imipramine and its binding and reuptake inhibition profile more closely resembles that of the TCAs. Milnacipran has weak affinity for adrenergic, muscarinic, and H_1 receptors and, therefore, is expected to be devoid of the prominent side effects observed for the TCAs. In clinical studies, milnacipran showed antidepressant efficacy similar to that of TCAs and SSRIs.

In humans, milnacipran distinguishes itself from many other antidepressants by its simple pharmacokinetics. It is rapidly absorbed, with a high oral bioavailability, and it exhibits linear pharmacokinetics over a dose range of 25 to 200 mg/d (Table 18.10) (70). It circulates in the blood and distributes in the body principally as unmetabolized drug. Steady-state plasma levels are reached within 32 to 48 hours after twice-daily oral administration, and its metabolism does not involve the CYP enzyme system. Approximately 50% of the dose is excreted in urine as unmetabolized drug, and another 14% is excreted as its *N*-glucuronide conjugate. The remaining eliminated drug is composed of conjugated phase 1 inactive metabolites. Because the unmetabolized drug is the only compound responsible for the activity of milnacipran, no dosage adjustment is needed in patients presenting with liver impairment.

Milnacipran has proven to be a very safe drug, with an adverse event profile clearly superior to that of TCAs and, to a certain extent, that of SSRIs. Only approximately 10% of patients experience side effects, and only dysuria occurred more frequently (2%) with milnacipran than with TCAs or SSRIs. Therefore, milnacipran seems to be an antidepressant with a very favorable benefit–risk ratio, although with a slower onset of action than the TCAs.

Duloxetine Duloxetine (Fig. 18.20) has been approved for the treatment of depression and diabetic peripheral neuropathic pain. It is another analog in the line of fluoxetine-based products from Lilly, in which the phenyl and phenoxy groups of fluoxetine have been respectively replaced with the benzene isostere, thiophene, and a naphthyloxy group (previously described in the section on fluoxetine). Duloxetine exhibits dual inhibition with high affinity for the SERTs and NETs, with a fivefold preferential inhibition of the SERT (68). Duloxetine appears to be a more potent in vitro blocker of SERTs and NETs than venlafaxine. In humans, duloxetine has a low affinity for the other neuroreceptors, suggesting low incidence of unwanted adverse effects.

Duloxetine appears to be fairly well absorbed after oral doses, with peak plasma levels in 6 to 10 hours and linear pharmacokinetics (Table 18.10) (71). The drug is extensively metabolized in the liver to active metabolites, with 72% of an oral dose primarily excreted in the urine as conjugated metabolites and up to 15% appearing in the feces. Its elimination half-life, time to steady-state blood levels, and mean volume of distribution are shown in Table 18.10.

N-Demethylation to an active metabolite (CYP2D6) and hydroxylation of the naphthyl ring (CYP1A2) at the 4-, 5-, or 6-position are the main metabolic pathways for duloxetine. Its *O*-metabolites are primarily excreted into the urine as glucuronide, sulfate, and *O*-methylated conjugation products (Fig. 18.22). The major metabolites found in plasma also were found in the urine (71). A minor metabolite is oxidation of the thiophene ring to a reactive intermediate which reportedly leads to a jaundice-like condition. Preclinical data for 4-hydroxyduloxetine suggest it has a similar pharmacologic profile as duloxetine, with selective inhibition of SERT but less activity at NET.

Adverse effects have included insomnia, somnolence, headache, nausea, diarrhea, and dry mouth. Mild

VILOXAZINE

Viloxazine, which was originally developed for the treatment of depression and nocturnal enuresis, was withdrawn from consideration for business reasons. It deserves some discussion because of its early relationship with the development of the NE and 5-HT reuptake inhibitors.

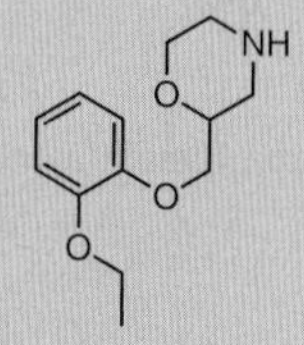

Viloxazine

Research scientists at ICI in England (now AstraZeneca) recognized that some β-blockers exhibited CNS 5-HT antagonist activity at high doses. To improve the CNS distribution for the β-blockers, the medicinal chemists at ICI constrained the ethanolamine side chain of the β-blockers into a morpholine ring, resulting in the synthesis of viloxazine.

Viloxazine selectively inhibits the presynaptic reuptake of NE reuptake (approximately half as potent as imipramine) and is a weak inhibitor of mouse brain 5-HT reuptake. No appreciable in vivo inhibition of MAO activity was observed. It differed from the TCAs in not exhibiting the TCA adverse effect profile. Viloxazine produces antidepressant activities both similar to and different from the tricyclics desimipramine, imipramine, and amitriptyline. These actions seem to be of relevance with respect to the antidepressant action of this drug.

Presently, viloxazine is classified as an orphan drug, under the trade name of Catatrol, for the treatment of narcolepsy and cataplexy.

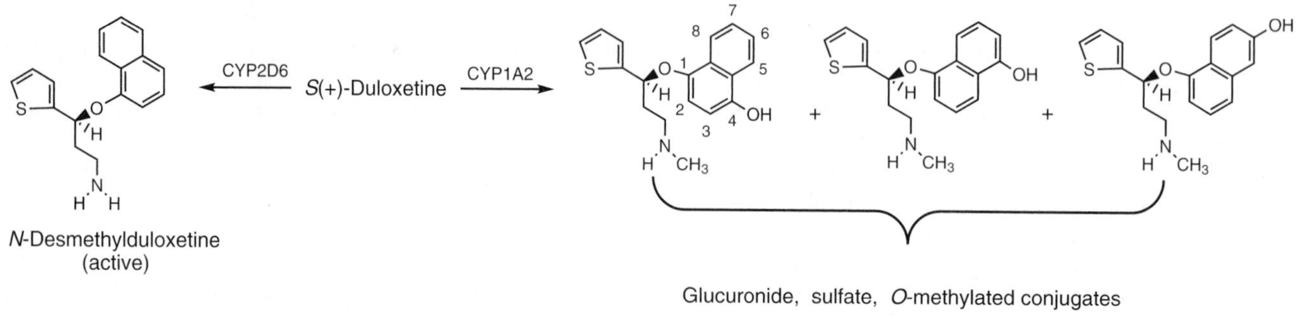

FIGURE 18.22 Metabolism of duloxetine.

OTHER USES FOR ANTIDEPRESSANT DRUGS

In addition to the wide use of antidepressants to treat depression, chronic neuropathic pain disorders, including fibromyalgia and diabetic and other peripheral neuropathic syndromes, have responded at least partly to treatment with tertiary TCAs and the NSRIs duloxetine, milnacipran, and venlafaxine. The NSRIs seem to be superior to the SSRIs (72).

withdrawal symptoms on abrupt discontinuation have been described in studies with healthy subjects.

Duloxetine is a moderately potent CYP2D6 inhibitor (intermediate between paroxetine and sertraline). Thus, duloxetine should be used with caution when CYP2D6 substrates and inhibitors are coadministered.

DA and Norepinephrine Reuptake Inhibitors

Bupropion Bupropion (amfebutamone) is a phenylisopropylaminoketone that is structurally related to the phenylisopropylamine CNS stimulant, methamphetamine; the phenylisopropylaminoketone, cathinone (a constituent in khat); and the anorexiant, diethylpropion (Fig. 18.23). Although structurally similar to the CNS stimulants, bupropion exhibits distinctive different pharmacologic and therapeutic effects mostly because of its metabolites. The absence of the tricyclic ring system in bupropion results in a better adverse effect profile than with the TCAs. The tertiary butyl group in bupropion prevents its *N*-dealkylation to metabolites that could possess sympathomimetic and/or anorexigenic properties.

Wellbutrin and Zyban (an aid in smoking cessation treatment) are trade name products for bupropion. Therefore, the potential exists for an overdose toxicity in a patient receiving multiple brand name and generic prescriptions containing bupropion for the treatment of depression, smoking cessation, and other off-label uses.

Mechanism of Action The mechanism of antidepressant action for bupropion is more complex because of its metabolism to its three principal metabolites (Fig. 18.23), which contribute to its antidepressant mechanism of action because their accumulated plasma concentrations are higher than those of bupropion, with a longer duration of action (see the discussion of pharmacokinetics below). Bupropion appears to be a selective inhibitor of DA reuptake at the DA presynaptic neuronal membrane and an SNRI (Table 18.2), and also induces the release of DA and NE. An additional mechanism of action for bupropion is as a noncompetitive antagonist of several nAChRs. Thus, the dual antidepressant and antinicotinic activity of bupropion is mediated by its stimulatory action on the DA and NE systems and inhibition of the neuronal nAChRs. The neuronal nAChRs are ligand-gated ion channels of the CNS that regulate synaptic activity from both pre- and postsynaptic sites. In addition, bupropion blocks noncompetitively the activation of $\alpha_3\beta_2$, $\alpha_4\beta_2$, and α_7 neuronal nAChRs and is approximately 50 and 12 times more effective blocking $\alpha_3\beta_2$ and $\alpha_4\beta_2$ (the brain nicotine binding site) than α_7 receptors. Bupropion at high concentration failed to displace nicotine from the $\alpha_4\beta_2$ receptors. Bupropion inhibition of $\alpha_3\beta_2$ and $\alpha_4\beta_2$ ion channel receptors on neuronal nAChRs involves initial binding to the ion channels in the resting state, decreasing the probability of the ion channels opening and further interaction with a binding domain in the ion channel shared with the tricyclic antidepressants. Bupropion does not exhibit clinically significant anticholinergic, antihistaminic, or α_1-adrenergic blocking activity or MAO inhibition.

Bupropion is also effective in nicotine dependence by blocking nicotine's pharmacologic effects,

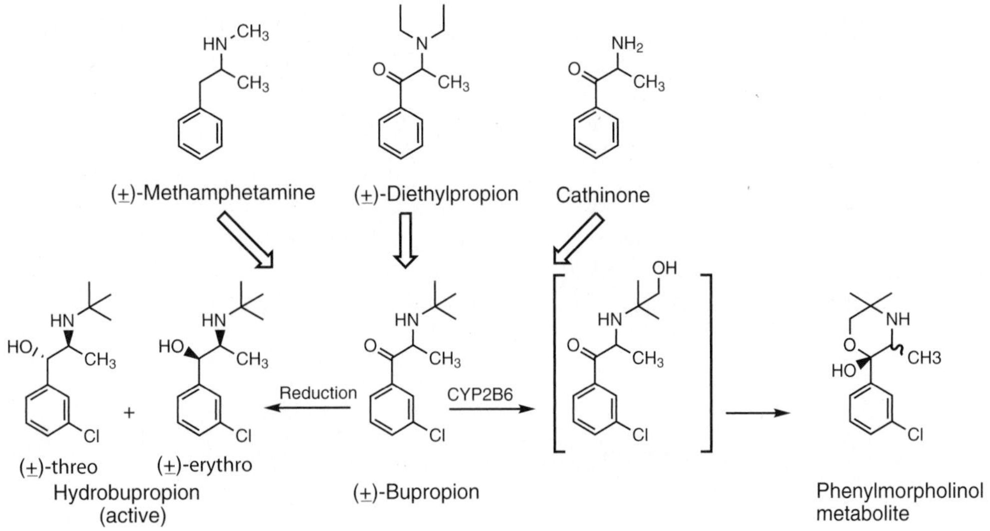

FIGURE 18.23 Bupropion, related derivatives, and metabolites.

suggesting that bupropion possesses some selectivity for neuronal nAChRs underlying these various nicotinic effects (73) and craving associated with smoking cessation, which suggests that the principal mode of action by bupropion as an aid in smoking cessation is on the withdrawal symptoms following smoking cessation. The efficacy of bupropion in smoking cessation does not appear to depend on the presence of depression. The current presumed mechanism of action of bupropion involves modulation of dopaminergic and noradrenergic systems that have been implicated by increasing extracellular CNS DA concentrations, most likely as a result of its inhibition of DAT and NET (Table 18.2). As nicotine CNS concentrations drop with smoking cessation, the firing rates of noradrenergic neurons increase, which may be the basis for the withdrawal symptoms. Thus, during withdrawal, bupropion and its active metabolite, hydroxybupropion, reduce the firing rates of these noradrenergic neurons in a dose-dependent manner, attenuating the symptoms of smoking cessation. Furthermore, its ability to block the nicotinic receptors also may prevent relapse by attenuating the reinforcing properties of nicotine but probably cannot acutely reduce smoking.

Bupropion is extensively metabolized in humans, with its three major hydroxylated metabolites reaching plasma levels higher than those of bupropion itself. These hydroxylated metabolites share many of the pharmacologic properties of bupropion, so they can play a greater role in attenuating the withdrawal and relapse by which bupropion exerts its activity in smoking cessation (73).

Pharmacokinetics Bupropion is absorbed from the GI tract, with a low oral bioavailability as a result of first-pass metabolism. The pharmacokinetic properties of bupropion are shown in Table 18.11. Food does not seem to substantially affect its peak plasma concentration or AUC. After oral administration, peak plasma concentrations usually are achieved within 2 hours for bupropion and 3 hours for sustained-released bupropion products, followed by a biphasic decline for bupropion. Plasma concentrations are dose proportional (linear pharmacokinetics) after single doses of 100 to 250 mg/d. The fraction of a dose excreted unmetabolized was less than 1%.

Bupropion hydroxylation of the tert-butyl group to hydroxypropion intermediate, which cyclizes to a phenylmorpholinol metabolite, is mediated exclusively by CYP2B6 (74,75). Other metabolites include reduction of the aminoketone to amino-alcohol isomers, *threo*-hydrobupropion, and *erythro*-hydrobupropion (Fig. 18.23). Further oxidation of the bupropion side chain results in the formation of *m*-chlorobenzoic acid, which is eliminated in the urine as its glycine conjugate. Hydroxybupropion is approximately 50% as potent as bupropion, whereas *threo*-hydrobupropion and *erythro*-hydrobupropion have 20% of the potency of bupropion. Peak plasma concentrations for hydroxybupropion are approximately 20 times the peak level of the parent drug at steady-state, with an elimination half-life of approximately 20 hours. Thus, CYP2B6-catalyzed bupropion hydroxylation is a clinically important bioactivation and elimination pathway. The times to peak concentrations for the *erythro*-hydrobupropion

TABLE 18.11 Pharmacokinetics of Dopamine and Norepinephrine Inhibitors

Parameters	Bupropion	Trazodone	Mirtazapine
Oral bioavailability (%)	5–20	65 (60–70)	~50
Lipophilicity ($logD_{7.4}$)	2.59	1.56	2.90
Protein binding (%)	80	90–95	85
Volume of distribution (L/kg)	19–21	0.84 (0.5–1.2)	107
Elimination half-life (h)	21 (14–16) ~20 (*S*,*S*)-hydroxy	7 (4–9)	16–40
Cytochrome P450 major isoform	2B6	3A4	3A4, 2D6
Major active metabolites	(*S*,*S*)-hydroxy	*m*-chlorophenylpiperazine	None
Peak plasma concentration (h)	2–3 8 (*S*,*S*)-hydroxy	1–2	2
Excretion (%)	Urine 87 Feces 10	Urine 70–75 Feces 25–30	Urine 75 Feces 15
Plasma half-life (h)	3–4 20 (*S*,*S*)-hydroxy	6 (4–8)	2
Time to steady-state concentration (d)	5 8 (S,S)-hydroxy	3–7	5

and *threo*-hydrobupropion metabolites are similar to that of the hydroxybupropion metabolite. The plasma levels of the *erythro*-hydrobupropion correlate with several side effects, such as insomnia and dry mouth. The elimination half-lives of *erythro*-hydrobupropion and *threo*-hydrobupropion, however, are longer (~33 and 37 hours, respectively), and the steady-state AUCs are 1.5 and 7.0 times that of bupropion, respectively. The hepatic clearance in patients with liver disease was increased from 19 to 29 hours. The median observed time to maximum plasma concentration was 19 hours for hydroxybupropion and 31 hours for *threo/erythro*-hydrobupropion. The mean half-lives for hydroxybupropion and *threo/erythro*-hydrobupropion were increased by 5 and 2 times, respectively, in patients with severe hepatic cirrhosis compared with healthy volunteers. Bupropion and its metabolites are distributed into breast milk.

In geriatric patients, the apparent half-life of hydroxybupropion averaged approximately 34 hours. Reduction in renal or hepatic function may affect elimination of the major metabolites, because these compounds are moderately polar and are likely to be metabolized further or conjugated in the liver before urinary excretion.

The pharmacokinetic parameters for bupropion and hydroxybupropion did not differ between smokers and nonsmokers, but adolescent girls exhibited increased AUCs and volume of distribution (normalized to body weight) and longer elimination half-life than did boys for bupropion and its major metabolite, hydroxybupropion. No differences in clearance between men and women, however, were observed.

Drug Interactions Inhibition studies with the SSRIs and bupropion suggest that bupropion is a potent CYP2D6 inhibitor (75). Bupropion hydroxylation was strongly inhibited by, in the following order: paroxetine > fluvoxamine > sertraline > desmethylsertraline > norfluoxetine > nefazodone > fluoxetine; it was only weakly inhibited by venlafaxine, ODV, citalopram, and desmethylcitalopram. The inhibition of bupropion hydroxylation in vitro by SSRIs suggests the potential for clinical drug interactions. Therefore, coadministration of drugs that inhibit CYP2D6 warrants careful monitoring. Because of its selective inhibition of DA reuptake, pharmacodynamic interactions with DA agonists (e.g., levodopa) and antagonists should be anticipated. Coadministration of bupropion with drugs that lower the seizure threshold should be avoided because of the risk of serious seizures. Drugs that affect metabolism by CYP2B6 (e.g., methadone, nicotine, and cyclophosphamide) also have the potential to interact with bupropion.

Therapeutic Uses Besides being used to treat depression, bupropion is a nonnicotine aid in the cessation of smoking. The efficacy of bupropion in smoking cessation is comparable to that of nicotine replacement therapy and should be considered as a second-line treatment in smoking cessation (72,73). It possesses a broad spectrum of infrequent adverse effects, however, with potential drug metabolism interactions with TCAs, β-adrenergic blocking drugs, and class Ic antiarrhythmics.

Serotonin Receptor Modulators

Serotonin Antagonist/Reuptake Inhibitors

General Mechanism of Action Serotonin receptor modulators are a class of antidepressants, the function of which is to modulate the concentration of 5-HT in the brain. A neuromodulator functions as a "volume control in the brain and nervous system," regulating the other neurotransmitters through its receptors in the brain in response to external stimuli. As previously described, the serotonergic system modulates a large number of physiologic events, such as temperature regulation, sleep, learning and memory, behavior, sexual function, hormonal secretions, and immune activity, and is implicated in stress, anxiety, aggressiveness, and depression disorders. Of the various types of 5-HT receptors (see Chapter 11) mediating serotonergic activity, the 5-HT_{1B} receptors play an important role in modulating the serotonergic system. The 5-HT_{1B} receptors are autoreceptors localized on serotonergic neuron terminals, where they inhibit the release of 5-HT and its biosynthesis; they also are heteroreceptors located on nonserotonergic terminals, where they inhibit the release of other neurotransmitters, such as ACh, GABA, and NE. Excessive amounts of 5-HT in the

MISCELLANEOUS NOREPINEPHRINE AND DA REUPTAKE INHIBITORS

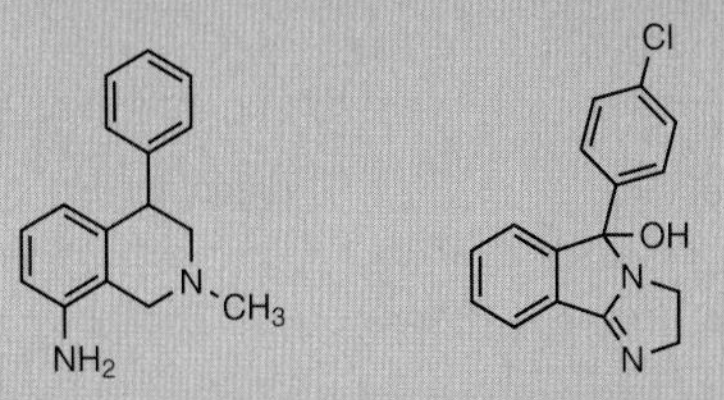

Nomifensine Mazindol

Nomifensine is a substituted phenylpiperidine (an aminophenyltetrahydroisoquinoline) structurally related to sertraline that was marketed as a stimulatory antidepressant in the mid-1970s but later withdrawn because of a high incidence of hemolytic anemia. Nomifensine inhibits the NET and DAT. It displays high affinity for NET (human pK_i = 7.8), moderate affinity for DAT (pK_i = 6.6), and a low affinity for SERT (5-HT:NE ratio = 65).

Mazindol (Sanorex) is a phenyl-substituted imidazobenzoisoindole that inhibits both NET and DAT. It exhibits high affinity for the NET (rat pK_i = 9.3), good affinity for DAT (rat pK_i = 7.8), and a 5-HT:NE ratio of 224. DA reuptake inhibitors suppress appetite; thus, mazindol is approved to be marketed as an appetite suppressant.

brain may cause relaxation, sedation, and a decrease in sexual drive; inadequate amounts of 5-HT can lead to psychiatric disorders. Therefore, the 5-HT receptor modulator antidepressants exert their antidepressant effects by mechanisms that enhance noradrenergic or serotonergic transmission by acting as mixed 5-HT_2 antagonists/5-HT reuptake inhibitors (SARI; trazodone) and α_2-adrenergic antagonists/5-HT_2 and 5-HT_3 antagonists (NaSSA; mirtazapine). Chronic antidepressant treatment with SARIs and NaSSAs modulate 5-HT receptor expression and, in turn, 5-HT function.

Arylpiperazines

Trazodone. Trazodone is a phenylpiperazine–triazolopyridine antidepressant (calculated logP = 2.8) that is structurally unrelated to most of the other antidepressant classes (Fig. 18.24). It acts as a dual 5-HT agonist and 5-HT reuptake inhibitor.

Mechanism of Action. Although the exact mechanism of action is unknown, trazodone acts as an antagonist at 5-HT_{2A} receptors and is a weak inhibitor of 5-HT reuptake at the presynaptic neuronal membrane, potentiating the synaptic effects of 5-HT. Its mechanism of action is complicated by the presence of its metabolite, *m*-chlorophenylpiperazine (Fig. 18.25), which is a 5-HT_{2C} agonist.

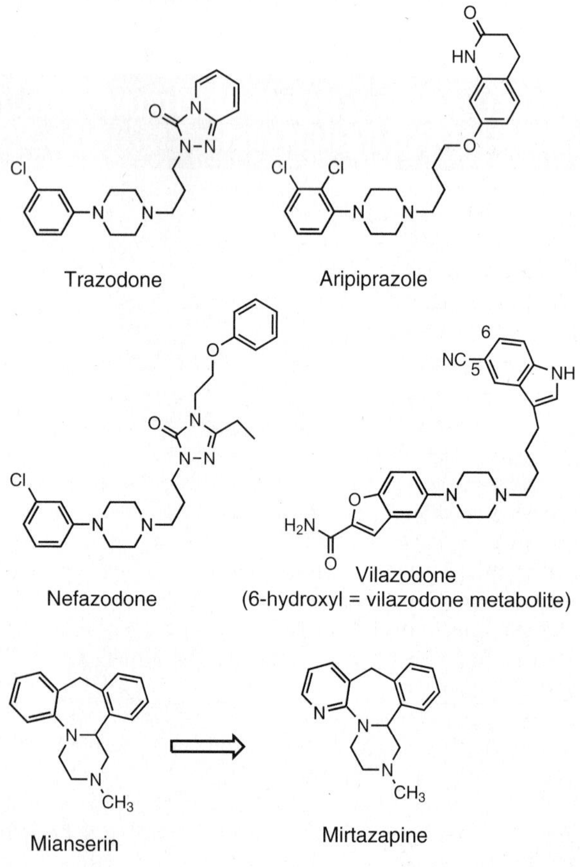

FIGURE 18.24 Serotonin receptor modulators.

At therapeutic dosages, trazodone does not appear to affect the reuptake of DA or NE within the CNS. It has little anticholinergic activity and is relatively devoid of toxic cardiovascular effects. The increase in serotonergic activity with long-term administration of trazodone decreases the number of postsynaptic serotonergic (i.e., 5-HT_2) and β-adrenergic binding sites in the brains of animals, decreasing the sensitivity of adenylate (or adenylyl) cyclase to stimulation by β-adrenergic agonists. It has been suggested that postsynaptic serotonergic receptor modification is mainly responsible for the antidepressant action observed during long-term administration of trazodone. Trazodone does not inhibit MAO and, unlike amphetamine-like drugs, does not stimulate the CNS.

Trazodone is rapidly and almost completely absorbed from the GI tract following oral administration, with an oral bioavailability of approximately 65% (Table 18.11). Peak plasma concentrations of trazodone occur approximately 1 hour after oral administration when taken on an empty stomach or 2 hours when taken with food. At steady-state, its plasma concentrations exhibit wide interpatient variation.

Trazodone is extensively metabolized in the liver by *N*-dealkylation to its primary circulating active metabolite, *m*-chlorophenylpiperazine (*m*-CPP), which subsequently undergoes aromatic hydroxylation to *p*-hydroxy-*m*-CPP (Fig. 18.25) (76). In vitro studies indicate that CYP3A4 is the major isoform involved in the production of *m*-CPP from trazodone (and CYP2D6 to a lesser extent). 4′-Hydroxy-*m*-CPP and oxotriazolopyridinepropionic acid (the major metabolite excreted in urine) are conjugated with glucuronic acid. Less than 1% of a dose is excreted unmetabolized. *m*-CPP is 4′-hydroxylated by CYP2D6. *m*-CPP is of significant interest because of its 5-HT_{2C} agonist and 5-HT_{2A} antagonist activities that may contribute to trazodone antidepressant action.

Trazodone therapy has been associated with several cases of idiosyncratic hepatotoxicity (see Chapter 4). Although the mechanism of hepatotoxicity remains unknown, the generation of an iminoquinone, an epoxide reactive metabolite, or both may play a role in the initiation of trazodone-mediated hepatotoxicity (Fig. 18.25) (76). Studies have shown that the bioactivation of trazodone involves, first, aromatic hydroxylation of the 3-chlorophenyl ring, followed by its oxidation to a reactive iminoquinone intermediate, which then reacts with glutathione. Alternately, the aromatic hydroxylated derivative is oxidized in the triazolopyridinone ring to an electrophilic epoxide followed by hydrolytic ring opening to the stable diol metabolite or nucleophilic conjugates through attachment by various nucleophiles (:Nu). The pathway involving trazodone bioactivation to the iminoquinone also has been observed with many para-hydroxyanilines (e.g., acetaminophen) (see Chapter 4), including the structurally related antidepressant nefazodone. The reactive intermediates consume the available glutathione, allowing the reactive intermediate to react with hepatic tissue, leading to liver damage.

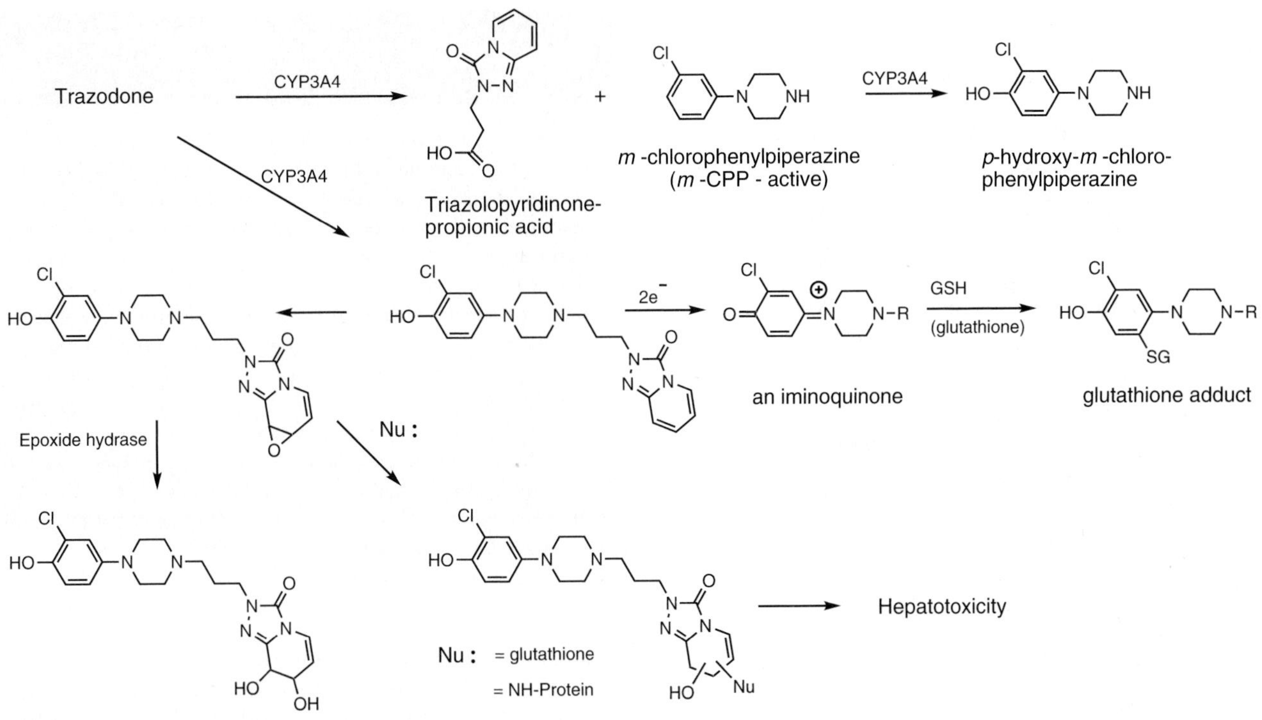

FIGURE 18.25 Metabolism of trazodone.

Unlike the TCAs, trazodone does not block the fast sodium channels and, thus, does not have significant arrhythmic activity. Compared with the SSRIs, it has a lesser tendency to cause drug-induced male sexual dysfunction as a side effect. Although trazodone displays α_1-adrenergic blocking activity, hypotension is relatively uncommon. Signs of overdose toxicity include nausea, vomiting, and decreased level of consciousness. Trazodone produces a significant amount of sedation in normal and mentally depressed patients (principally from its central α_1-adrenergic blocking activity and antihistaminic action).

Drug Interactions. Trazodone possesses serotonergic activity; therefore, the possibility of developing 5-HT syndrome should be considered in patients who are receiving trazodone and other SSRIs or serotonergic drugs concurrently. When trazodone is used concurrently with drugs metabolized by CYP3A4, caution should be used to avoid excessive sedation. Trazodone can cause hypotension, including orthostatic hypotension and syncope; concomitant administration of antihypertensive therapy may require a reduction in dosage of the antihypertensive agent.

The possibility of drug–drug interactions with trazodone and other substrates, inducers, and/or inhibitors of CYP3A4 exists (76).

Therapeutic Uses. Trazodone is used primarily in the treatment of insomnia, mental depression, or depression/anxiety disorders. The drug also has shown some efficacy in the treatment of benzodiazepine or alcohol dependence, diabetic neuropathy, and panic disorders.

Aripiprazole. Aripiprazole (Fig. 18.24) is an atypical antipsychotic but also an arylpiperazine antidepressant used for acute manic and mixed episodes associated with bipolar disorder in both pediatric patients age 10 to 17 years and adults and as an adjunct for major depression. In addition, it is often used as maintenance therapy in bipolar disorders in conjunction with a mood stabilizer such as lithium or valproate. Perhaps due to its dopaminergic mechanism of action, there is some evidence to suggest that aripiprazole blocks cocaine-seeking behavior in animal models without significantly affecting other rewarding behaviors (such as food self-administration).

Aripiprazole's mechanism of action is different from those of the other antidepressants but similar to trazodone as a partial agonist at the 5-HT_{1A} receptor and antagonist at the 5-HT_{2A} receptor. It is an antagonist at the 5-HT_7 receptor and acts as a partial agonist at the 5-HT_{2C} receptor, both with high affinity.

Aripiprazole undergoes extensive metabolism by CYP3A4 and CYP2D6 to produce its active circulating metabolites dehydroaripiprazole and 2,3-dichlorophenylpiperazine (DCPP), similar to *m*-CPP for trazodone and nefazodone (Fig. 18.26). It is unknown whether DCPP contributes to aripiprazole's antidepressant action, but the possibility cannot be excluded. Aripiprazole displays linear kinetics and has an elimination half-life of approximately 75 hours. Steady-state plasma concentrations are achieved in about 14 days. Peak concentration is achieved 3 to 5 hours after oral dosing. Bioavailability of the oral tablets is about 90%,

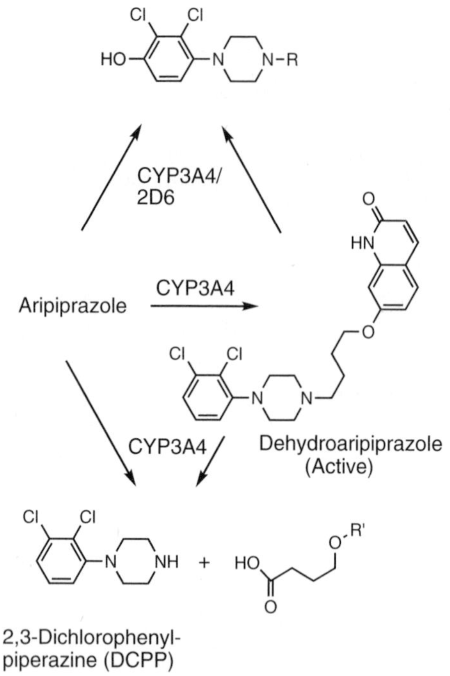

FIGURE 18.26 Major metabolites of aripiprazole.

NEFAZODONE

Nefazodone is a phenylpiperazine antidepressant structurally related to trazodone, but it differs pharmacologically from trazodone, the SSRIs, the MAOIs, and the TCAs (Fig. 18.24). When compared with trazodone, nefazodone displays approximately twice the affinity potency for SERT. Nefazodone therapy, however, was associated with life-threatening cases of idiosyncratic hepatotoxicity, and as a result, nefazodone was withdrawn from both the North American and European markets in 2003. The mechanism of hepatotoxicity remains unknown, but nefazodone, being structurally similar to trazodone (Fig. 18.24), is metabolized to *p*-hydroxynefazodone, *m*-CPP, and phenoxyethyltriazoledione. In turn, *p*-hydroxynefazodone is thought to be oxidized to an iminoquinone and/or an epoxide reactive metabolite, which may play a role in the initiation of nefazodone-mediated hepatotoxicity (78).

with approximately 40% of the aripiprazole plasma concentration being present as the dehydroaripiprazole, which are both excreted via feces and urine. The long half-life for aripiprazole is responsible for many of its adverse side effects. Recent studies suggest that the long half-life, which results in lower doses, may actually prevent formation of clinically significant hepatotoxic metabolites such as those that are responsible for the toxicity of nefazodone (77). Aripiprazole and its active metabolite dehydroaripiprazole have been identified as substrates for the efflux transporter P-gp in the brain, which contributes to wanted or unwanted clinical effects in patients treated with aripiprazole.

Vilazodone. Vilazodone is a phenylpiperazine–2-benzofurancarboxamide antidepressant that is structurally related to trazodone and aripiprazole with a calculated logP at pH 7.4 is 4.44 (Fig. 18.24). It acts as a dual 5-HT receptor partial agonist and 5-HT reuptake inhibitor (79).

Mechanism of Action. The mechanism of the antidepressant effect of vilazodone is not fully understood but could be related to its enhancement of CNS serotonergic activity through selective inhibition of 5-HT reuptake. In addition, vilazodone is also a partial agonist at 5-HT_{1A} receptors. Vilazodone binds with high affinity to the 5-HT reuptake site ($K_i = 0.1$ nM), but not to the NE ($K_i = 56$ nM) or DA ($K_i = 37$ nM) reuptake sites. Vilazodone is a potent and selective inhibitor of 5-HT reuptake ($IC_{50} = 1.6$ nM). As a 5-HT_{1A} receptor partial agonist, it binds selectively with high affinity to 5-HT_{1A} receptors ($IC_{50} = 2.1$ nM). Vilazodone does not prolong the QTc interval, as occurs with the TCAs, and is below the threshold for clinical concern. Clinical trials of vilazodone showed significant antidepressant efficacy with an onset of effect in 1 week, unlike other antidepressants. The 1-week onset of its antidepressant action has been linked to its partial agonist at the 5-HT_{1A} receptor.

Pharmacokinetics. The antidepressant activity for vilazodone activity is due primarily to the parent drug. Vilazodone exhibits dose-proportional linear pharmacokinetics, and steady-state is achieved in about 3 days. Elimination of vilazodone is primarily by hepatic metabolism, with a terminal half-life of approximately 25 hours. Peak plasma concentrations occur 4 to 5 hours after oral administration. The absolute bioavailability of vilazodone is 72% with food. The peak concentration of vilazodone with food (high-fat or light meal) increases oral bioavailability approximately 147% to 160%, and AUC is increased by approximately 64% to 85%. Vilazodone is widely distributed and approximately 96% to 99% protein bound. Vilazodone is extensively metabolized by CYP3A4 to 6-hydroxyvilazodone (inactive metabolite) with minor contributions from CYP2C19 and CYP2D6. In vitro studies have shown that CYP1A2, CYP2A6, CYP2C9, and CYP2E1 have minimal contribution to the metabolism of vilazodone. Non-CYP pathways include carboxylesterase. Unlike trazodone, no phenylpiperazine metabolite was observed. Only 1% of the oral dose is recovered in the urine and 2% is recovered in the feces as unchanged vilazodone. In vitro studies indicate that vilazodone is unlikely to inhibit or induce the metabolism of other CYP substrates (except for CYP2C8) and did not alter the pharmacokinetics CYP2C19, CYP2D6, and CYP3A4 substrates. Renal impairment or mild or moderate hepatic impairment did not affect the clearance of vilazodone; thus no dose adjustment is required. Coadministration of vilazodone with ethanol or with a proton pump inhibitor (e.g., pantoprazole) did not affect the rate or extent of vilazodone absorption. Vilazodone is excreted into the milk of lactating rats, and the effect on lactation and nursing in humans is unknown. Breast-feeding in women treated with vilazodone should be considered only if the potential benefit outweighs the potential risk to the child. A pharmacokinetic study in elderly (>65 years old) versus young (24 to 55 years old) subjects demonstrated that the pharmacokinetics were generally similar between the two age groups. No dose adjustment is recommended on the basis of age. Greater sensitivity of some older individuals to vilazodone cannot be ruled out. After adjustment for body weight, the systemic exposures between males and females are similar.

Adverse Effects. The most commonly observed adverse reactions in vilazodone-treated MDD patients with an incidence greater than 5% were diarrhea, nausea, vomiting, and insomnia. Sexual dysfunction was minimal with vilazodone. As with all antidepressants, use vilazodone cautiously in patients with a history or family history of bipolar disorder, mania, or hypomania. Vilazodone has safety risks associated with the induction of suicidal thoughts in young adults, adolescents, and children (a black box warning).

Drug Interactions. The risk of using vilazodone in combination with other CNS-active drugs has not been evaluated. Because of potential interactions with MAOIs, vilazodone should not be prescribed concomitantly with an MAOI or within 14 days of discontinuing or starting an MAOI. Based on the drug's mechanism of action and the potential for 5-HT toxicity (serotonin syndrome), caution is advised when coadministered with other drugs that may affect the serotonergic neurotransmitter systems (e.g., MAOIs, SSRIs, SNRIs, triptans, buspirone, tramadol, tryptophan products). Because 5-HT release by platelets plays an important role in hemostasis, concurrent use of a nonsteroidal anti-inflammatory drug or aspirin with vilazodone may potentiate the risk of abnormal bleeding. Altered anticoagulant effects, including increased bleeding, have been reported when SSRIs and SNRIs are coadministered with warfarin. Thus, patients receiving warfarin therapy should be carefully monitored when vilazodone is initiated or discontinued. Concomitant use of vilazodone and strong or moderate inhibitors of CYP3A4 (e.g., ketoconazole) can increase vilazodone plasma concentrations by approximately 50%, requiring a dosage adjustment. No dose adjustment is recommended when coadministered with mild inhibitors of CYP3A4 (e.g., cimetidine). Concomitant use of vilazodone with inducers of CYP3A4 has the potential to reduce vilazodone plasma levels. Concomitant administration of vilazodone with inhibitors of CYP2C19 and CYP2D6 is not expected to alter plasma concentrations of vilazodone. These isoforms are minor elimination pathways in the metabolism of vilazodone. Coadministration of vilazodone with substrates for CYP1A2, CYP2C9, CYP3A4, or CYP2D6 is unlikely to result in clinically significant changes in the concentrations of the CYP substrates. Vilazodone coadministration with mephenytoin resulted in a small (11%) increase in mephenytoin biotransformation, suggestive of a minor induction of CYP2C19. In vitro studies have shown that vilazodone is a moderate inhibitor of CYP2C19 and CYP2D6. In vitro studies also suggest that vilazodone may inhibit the biotransformation of substrates of CYP2C8; thus coadministration of vilazodone with a CYP2C8 substrate may lead to an increase in the plasma concentration of the CYP2C8 substrate. Chronic administration of vilazodone is unlikely to induce the metabolism of drugs metabolized by CYP1A1, CYP1A2, CYP2A6, CYP2B6, CYP2C9, CYP2C19, CYP2D6, CYP2E1, and CYP3A4/5. Because vilazodone is highly bound to plasma protein, administration to a patient taking another drug that is highly protein bound may cause increased free concentrations of the other drug.

Noradrenergic and Specific Serotonergic Antidepressants (NaSSAs)

Mirtazapine Mirtazapine is a pyrazinopyridobenazepine antidepressant that is an isostere of the antidepressant mianserin (Fig. 18.24). A seemingly simple isosteric replacement of an aromatic methine group (CH) in mianserin with a nitrogen to give a pyridine ring (mirtazapine) has significant effects on the physicochemical properties, pharmacokinetics, mechanisms of action, and antidepressant activities (Table 18.12) (31). Noteworty differences between receptor affinity and transporter affinity, pharmacokinetics, regioselectivity in the formation of metabolites, and toxicity are observed for mianserin and mirtazapine and their antidepressant mechanisms of action. The pyridine ring increases the polarity of the molecule and decreases the measured partition coefficient and the basicity. Mianserin is a potent inhibitor of NET, whereas mirtazapine has negligible effects on the inhibition of NET (pK_i = 7.1 vs. 5.8, respectively).

Mianserin is currently marketed in Europe as an antidepressant. Mianserin has not been approved for use in the United States because of its serious adverse effects

TABLE 18.12 Physicochemical Properties of Mirtazapine and Mianserin

Properties	Mirtazapine	Mianserin
pK_a	7.1	7.4
Lipophilicity ($logD_{7.4}$)	2.72	3.17
Polarity	2.63 debye	0.82 debye
NET affinity (pK_i)	5.8	7.1
5-HT release	Yes	No

of agranulocytosis and leukopenia. Mirtazapine has not exhibited this adverse effect

Mechanism of Action. Animal studies indicate that the efficacy of mirtazapine as an atypical antidepressant results from enhancing central noradrenergic and serotonergic activity, possibly through blocking central presynaptic α_2-adrenergic receptors. Blocking these receptors inhibits the negative feedback loop, which increases the release of NE into the synapse. Mirtazapine also is a potent antagonist at 5-HT_2 and 5-HT_3 receptors, and it shows no significant affinity for 5-HT_{1A} or 5-HT_{1B} receptors. Additionally, it displays some anticholinergic properties and produces sedative effects (because of potent histamine H_1 receptor antagonism) and orthostatic hypotension (because of moderate antagonism at peripheral α_1-adrenergic receptors). Its antidepressant effect is comparable to the TCAs and may be better than some SSRIs, especially in patients with depression of the melancholic type, but at higher doses, it may cause drowsiness and weight gain. The drug generally is well tolerated, producing no more adverse events (including anticholinergic events) than the SSRIs and fewer adverse events than the TCAs.

The pharmacokinetics for mirtazapine are shown in Table 18.11. Mirtazapine absorption is rapid and complete, with a bioavailability of approximately 50% as a result of first-pass metabolism. The rate and extent of mirtazapine absorption are minimally affected by food. Dose and plasma levels are linearly related over a dose range of 15 to 80 mg. The elimination half-life of the (−)-enantiomer is approximately twice that of the (+)-enantiomer. In woman of all ages, the elimination half-life is significantly longer than in men (mean half-life, 37 vs. 26 hours).

After oral administration, mirtazapine undergoes first-pass metabolism by *N*-demethylation and ring hydroxylation to its 8-hydroxy metabolite, followed by *O*-glucuronide conjugation (Fig. 18.27) (80). In vitro studies indicate that CYP2D6 and CYP1A2 are involved in the formation of the 8-hydroxy metabolite and that CYP3A4 is responsible for the formation of the *N*-desmethyl and *N*-oxide metabolites. The 8-hydroxy and *N*-desmethyl metabolites possess weak pharmacologic activity, but their plasma levels are very low and, thus, are unlikely to contribute to the antidepressant action of mirtazapine. Clearance for mirtazapine may decrease in patients with hepatic or renal impairment, increasing its plasma concentrations. Therefore, it should be used with caution in these patients. In vitro studies have shown mirtazapine to be a weak inhibitor of CYP1A2, CYP2D6, and CYP3A4.

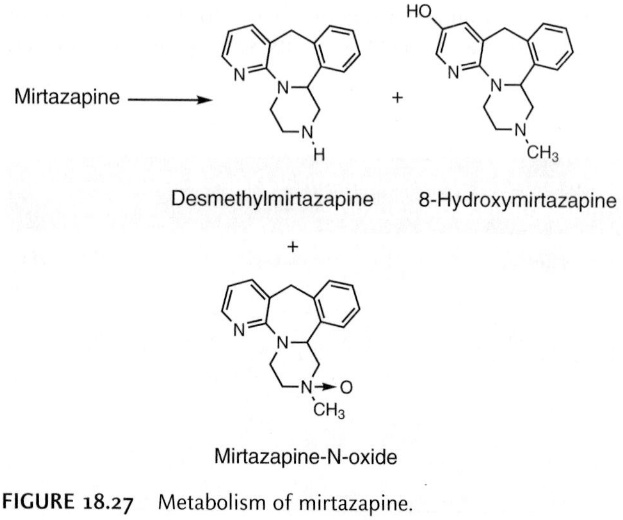

FIGURE 18.27 Metabolism of mirtazapine.

Monoamine Oxidase Inhibitors

The discovery of MAOIs resulted from a search for derivatives of isoniazid (isonicotinic acid hydrazide) (Fig.18.28) with antitubercular activity. During clinical trials with this hydrazine derivative, a rather consistent beneficial effect of mood elevation was noted in depressed patients with tuberculosis. Although no longer used clinically, iproniazid (Fig. 18.28), the first derivative to be synthesized, was found to be hepatotoxic at dosage levels required for antitubercular and antidepressant activity. The antidepressant activity of iproniazid, however, prompted a search for other MAOIs, which resulted in the synthesis of hydrazine and nonhydrazine MAOIs that were relatively less toxic than iproniazid.

The MAOIs can be classified as hydrazines (e.g., phenelzine) and nonhydrazines (e.g., tranylcypromine), which can block the oxidative deamination of naturally occurring monoamines. MAOIs can also be classified according to their ability to selectively inhibit MAO-A or MAO-B (nonselective inhibitors). The currently available MAOI antidepressants (phenelzine and tranylcypromine; Fig. 18.28) are considered to be irreversible inhibitors of both MAO-A and MAO-B. The mechanism of antidepressant action of the MAOIs suggests that an increase in free 5-HT and NE and/or alterations in other amine concentrations within the CNS are mainly responsible for their antidepressant effect.

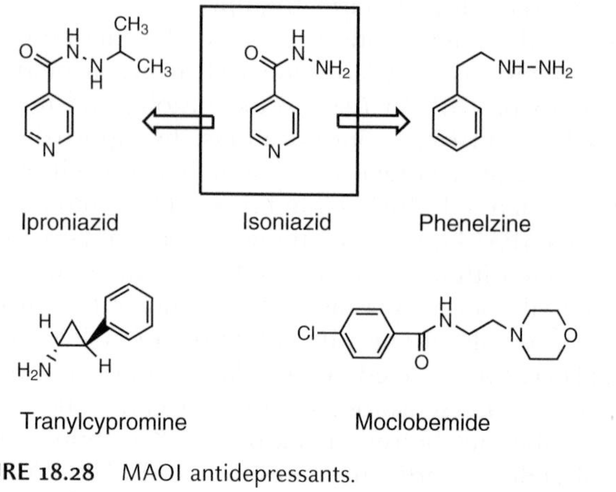

FIGURE 18.28 MAOI antidepressants.

Mechanisms of Action Common to MAOIs

An enzyme found mainly in nerve tissue and in the liver and lungs, MAO catalyzes the oxidative deamination of various amines, including epinephrine, NE, DA, and 5-HT. At least two isoforms of MAO exist, MAO-A and MAO-B, with differences in substrate preference, inhibitor specificity, and tissue distribution. The MAO-A substrates include 5-HT, and the MAO-B substrates include phenylethylamine. Tyramine, epinephrine, NE, and DA are substrates for both MAO-A and MAO-B. The cloning of MAO-A and MAO-B has demonstrated unequivocally that these enzymes consist of different amino acid sequences and also has provided insight regarding their structure, regulation, and function (51). Both MAO-A and MAO-B knockout mice exhibit distinct differences in neurotransmitter metabolism and behavior (51). The MAO-A knockout mice have elevated brain levels of 5-HT, NE, and DA, and they manifest aggressive behavior similar to human males with a deletion of MAO-A. In contrast, MAO-B knockout mice do not exhibit aggression, and only levels of phenylethylamine are increased. Both MAO-A and MAO-B knockout mice show increased reactivity to stress. These knockout mice are valuable models for investigating the role of monoamines in psychoses and in neurodegenerative and stress-related disorders.

The pharmacologic effects of MAOIs are cumulative. A latent period of a few days to several months may occur before the onset of the antidepressant action, and effects may persist for up to 3 weeks following discontinuance of therapy.

Adverse Effects Common to MAOIs

Common side effects for the nonselective MAOIs include difficulty getting to sleep and broken sleep, daytime insomnia, agitation, dizziness on standing that results in fainting (orthostatic hypotension), dry mouth, tremor (slight shake of muscles of arms and hands), syncope, palpitations, tachycardia, dizziness, headache, confusion, weakness, overstimulation including increased anxiety, constipation, GI disturbances, edema, dry mouth, weight gain, and sexual disturbances.

Drug Interactions Common to MAOIs

The most significant drug interaction limiting the efficacy of the nonselective MAOIs is with certain foods that have the potential to cause hypertensive crisis because of the release and potentiation of catecholamines. The severity and consequences of such interactions vary among individuals from only minor increases in blood pressure to substantial and rapid increases in blood pressure within 20 minutes. These patients may experience symptoms associated with brain hemorrhage or cardiac failure.

Hypertensive crises with MAOIs have occurred in some patients following ingestion of foods containing large amounts of tyramine or tryptophan. In general, patients taking MAOIs should avoid protein foods that have undergone protein breakdown by aging, fermentation, pickling, smoking, or bacterial contamination. Some of the common foods to avoid are shown in Table 18.13.

TABLE 18.13 Foods to Be Avoided Due to Potential Monoamine Oxidase Inhibitor–Food Interactions

Cheeses	**Meats**
Cheddar	Chicken livers
Camembert	Genoa salami
Stilton	Hard salami
Processed cheese	Pepperoni
Sour cream	Lebanon bologna
Spirits	**Fruit**
Chianti	Figs (overripe/canned)
Champagne	Raisins
Alcohol-free/reduced wines	Overripe bananas
Fish	**Dairy product**
Pickled herring	Yogurt
Anchovies	
Caviar	
Miscellaneous	**Vegetable products**
Shrimp paste	Yeast extract
Chocolate	Pods-broad beans
Meat tenderizers (papaya)	Bean curd
	Soy sauce
	Avocado

Patients should be warned against eating foods with a high tyramine content because hypertensive crisis may result. Excessive amounts of caffeine also reportedly may precipitate hypertensive crisis.

The MAOIs interfere with the hepatic metabolism of many prescription and nonprescription (over-the-counter) drugs and may potentiate the actions of their pharmacologic effects (i.e., cold decongestants, sympathomimetic amines, general anesthetics, barbiturates, and morphine).

Therapeutic Uses Common to MAOIs

The MAOIs are indicated in patients with atypical (exogenous) depression and in some patients who are unresponsive to other antidepressive therapy. They rarely are a drug of first choice. Unlabeled uses have included bulimia (having characteristics of atypical depression), treatment of cocaine addiction (phenelzine), night terrors, posttraumatic stress disorder, some migraines resistant to other therapies, seasonal affective disorder (30 mg/d), and some panic disorders. A list of information that should be transmitted to the patient concerning use of MAOIs is shown in Table 18.14.

Nonselective MAOI Antidepressants

PHENELZINE Phenelzine is a hydrazine MAOI (Fig. 18.28). Its mechanism of action is the prolonged, irreversible inhibition of MAO-A and MAO-B. Phenelzine has been used with some success in the management of bulimia nervosa. The MAOIs, however, are potentially dangerous in patients with binge eating and purging behaviors, and the American Psychiatric Association states that MAOIs should be used with caution in the management of bulimia nervosa.

Limited information is available regarding MAOI pharmacokinetics of phenelzine (Table 18.15). Phenelzine

TABLE 18.14 Common Information for Patients Taking Monoamine Oxidase Inhibitors (MAOIs)

Patient Information	Recommendation
Discontinuance of therapy or dose adjustment	Consult physician
Adding medication (prescription/over-the-counter)	Consult physician
Tyramine-containing foods and over-the-counter products	Avoid
Drowsiness, blurred vision	Avoid driving or performing tasks requiring alertness or coordination
Dizziness, weakness, fainting	Arise from sitting position slowly
Alcohol use	Avoid alcohol
Onset of action	Effects may be delayed for a few weeks
Severe headache, palpitation, tachycardia, sense of constriction in throat or chest, sweating, stiff neck, nausea or vomiting	Consult physician
New physician or dentist	Inform practitioner of MAOI use

seems to be well absorbed following oral administration; however, maximal inhibition of MAO occurs within 5 to 10 days. Acetylation of phenelzine to its inactive acetylated metabolite appears to be a minor metabolic pathway (79). Phenelzine is a substrate as well as an inhibitor of MAO, and major identified metabolites of phenelzine include phenylacetic acid and *p*-hydroxyphenylacetic acid. Phenelzine also elevates brain GABA levels, probably via its β-phenylethylamine metabolite. The clinical effects of phenelzine may continue for up to 2 weeks after discontinuation of therapy. Phenelzine is excreted in the urine mostly as its *N*-acetyl metabolite. Interindividual variability in plasma concentrations have been observed among patients who are either slow or fast acetylators. Slow acetylators of hydrazine MAOIs may yield exaggerated adverse effects after standard dosing. If adverse neurologic reactions occur during phenelzine therapy, phenelzine-induced pyridoxine deficiency should be considered. Pyridoxine supplementation can correct the deficiency while allowing continuance of phenelzine therapy.

TABLE 18.15 Pharmacokinetics of the Monoamine Oxidase Inhibitors (MAOIs)

Parameters	Phenelzine (Nardil)	Tranylcypromine (Parnate)	Moclobemide
Oral bioavailability (%)	NA	~50	50–90
Lipophilicity ($logD_{7.4}$)	1.10	0.54	1.47
Protein binding (%)	NA	NA	50
Volume of distribution (L/kg)	NA	1.1–5.7	1.2
Elimination half-life (h)	NA	2.5 (1.5–3.2)	1.5
Peak plasma concentration (h)	2–3	1.5 (0.7–3.5)	0.82
Excretion route	Urine	Urine Feces	Renal Feces

NA, not available.

Tranylcypromine Tranylcypromine is a nonhydrazine, irreversible MAO inhibitor antidepressant agent that was designed as the cyclopropyl analog of amphetamine (Fig. 18.28). Instead of exhibiting amphetamine-like stimulation, its mechanism of action is nonselective, irreversible inhibition of MAO. Its onset of antidepressant action is more rapid than for phenelzine. Tranylcypromine is well absorbed following oral administration (Table 18.15). Metabolism occurs via aromatic ring hydroxylation and *N*-acetylation (81). It is a competitive inhibitor of CYP2C19 and CYP2D6 and a noncompetitive inhibitor of CYP2C9. Most metabolism studies suggest that tranylcypromine is not metabolized to amphetamine, contrary to debate. Maximal MAO inhibition, however, occurs within 5 to 10 days. The GI absorption of the tranylcypromine shows interindividual variation and may be biphasic in some individuals, achieving an initial peak within approximately 1 hour and a secondary peak within 2 to 3 hours. It has been suggested that this apparent biphasic absorption in some individuals may represent different absorption rates. Following discontinuance of tranylcypromine, the drug is excreted within 24 hours. On withdrawal of tranylcypromine, MAO activity is recovered in 3 to 5 days (possibly in up to 10 days). However, concentrations of urinary tryptamine, an indicator of MAO-A inhibition, return to normal within 72 to 120 hours.

Reversible MAO-A Inhibitor Antidepressants

The major goal for developing new reversible inhibitors of MAO-A (RIMAs) is to avoid the severe, life-threatening hypertensive reactions that can occur with irreversible inhibitors. Irreversible inhibition of intestinal and hepatic MAO-A can lead to inhibition of tyramine degradation, thus allowing excessive amounts of naturally occurring tyramine to be absorbed from the food. Because these reversible compounds form unstable complexes with the MAO-A subtype, they can be easily displaced from MAO-A by tyramine. Thus, it becomes possible for ingested tyramine to be metabolized, diminishing the need for the dietary restrictions that plague the use of older irreversible nonselective MAOIs. This new class of selective and reversible inhibitors of MAO-A includes moclobemide (Fig. 18.28).

Moclobemide Moclobemide is a benzamide derivative containing a morpholine ring with a pK_a of 6.2 and a partition coefficient of 40 in an octanol/pH 7.4 buffer solution. Moclobemide is not currently available commercially in the United States but is available in the United Kingdom and Australia.

Mechanism of Action Moclobemide is an RIMA that preferentially inhibits MAO-A (~80%) and, to a lesser extent, MAO-B (20% to 30% inhibition), thereby increasing the concentration of 5-HT, NE, and other catecholamines in the synaptic cleft and in storage sites. During chronic therapy with the MAOIs, adaptive changes at the noradrenergic and serotonergic receptors occur ("downregulation") as a result of neurotransmitter hypersensitivity because of prolonged concentrations of NE and 5-HT at the postsynaptic receptor (see the discussion of the receptor sensitivity hypothesis for details). This mechanism is likely the basis for its antidepressant activity. Inhibition of MAO-A by moclobemide is short acting (maximum, 24 hours) and reversible. This is in contrast to phenelzine, which is long acting and irreversible in its binding to both MAO-A and MAO-B.

The pharmacokinetics (Table 18.15) for moclobemide are linear only up to 200 mg; at higher doses, nonlinear pharmacokinetics are observed (82). Although well absorbed from the GI tract, the presence of food reduces the rate but not the extent of absorption of moclobemide. Small quantities of moclobemide are distributed into human breast milk. Moclobemide undergoes a complex metabolism, initially involving morpholine carbon and nitrogen oxidation, deamination, and aromatic hydroxylation. The *N*-oxide and ring-opened metabolites retain some in vitro MAO-A inhibition. Moclobemide is a weak inhibitor of CYP2D6 in vitro. It is extensively metabolized in the liver by oxidation and is eliminated primarily into the urine as conjugates. Less than 1% of an administered dose of moclobemide is eliminated unmetabolized.

Because moclobemide is partially metabolized by the polymorphic isozymes CYP2C19 and CYP2D6, plasma concentrations of moclobemide may be affected in patients who are poor metabolizers. In patients who are slow metabolizers, the AUC for moclobemide is 1.5 times greater than the AUC in patients who are extensive metabolizers and receiving the same dose. This increase is within the normal range of variation (up to twofold) typically seen in patients.

Drug interactions for the RIMAs include interaction with SSRI antidepressants, which can cause the 5-HT syndrome (see the discussion of SSRIs). The effect of stimulant drugs, such as methylphenidate and dextroamphetamine (used to treat ADHD), may be increased. Some over-the-counter cold and hay fever decongestants (i.e., sympathomimetic amines) can have increased stimulant effects. Selegiline, a selective MAO-B used for Parkinson disease, should not be used concurrently with the RIMAs. Unlike the irreversible MAOIs, no significant interactions with foods occur because the selective inhibition of MAO-A does not stop the metabolism of tyramine. The RIMAs must not be taken concurrently with a nonreversible MAOI.

Mood Stabilizers

Manic depression, or bipolar affective disorder, is a prevalent mental disorder with a global impact. Mood stabilizers have acute and long-term effects and, at a minimum, are prophylactic for manic or depressive disorders. Lithium is the classic mood stabilizer and exhibits significant effects on mania and depression but may be augmented or substituted by some antiepileptic drugs. The biochemical basis for mood stabilizer therapies and the molecular origins of bipolar disorder are unknown. Lithium ion directly inhibits two signal transduction pathways. It suppresses inositol trisphosphate signaling through depletion of intracellular inositol and inhibits glycogen synthase kinase-3 (GSK-3), a multifunctional protein kinase. A number of GSK-3 substrates are involved in neuronal function and organization and, therefore, present plausible targets for manic depression. Despite these intriguing observations, it remains unclear how changes in inositol trisphosphate signaling underlie the origins of bipolar disorder (83).

Inositol (myo-inositol), a naturally occurring isomer of glucose, is a key intermediate of the phosphatidylinositol signaling pathway, a second messenger system used by noradrenergic, serotonergic, and cholinergic receptors. The suggestion that lithium might treat mania via its reduction of inositol levels led to experiments showing that oral doses of inositol reverse the behavioral effects of lithium in animals and the side effects of lithium in humans. Cerebrospinal fluid levels of inositol are low in depressed individuals (84). The effectiveness of inositol in treating manic depression was shown in a double-blind trial, which showed that large doses of inositol (12 g) increased inositol concentrations in human cerebrospinal fluid by 70% and led to improvement in depressed patients compared to placebo (84). Valproic acid and carbamazepine are antiepileptic drugs with mood-stabilizing properties that also inhibit inositol trisphosphate signaling through the inositol-depletion mechanism.

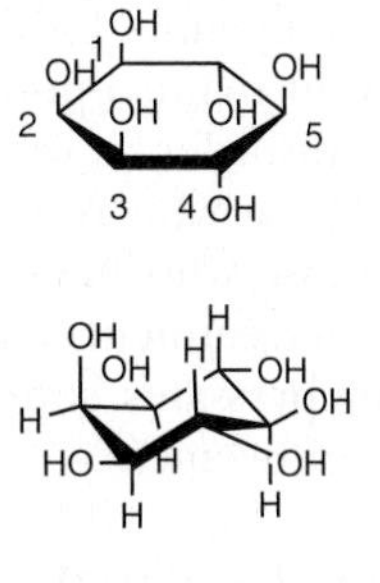

myo - inositol

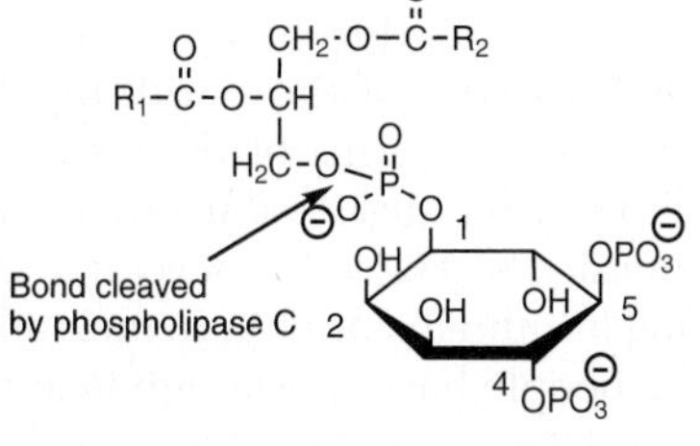

Phosphatidylinositol-4,5-triphosphate

Inositol significantly reduced the number of panic attacks per week in patients as compared to fluvoxamine and without the nausea and tiredness that are common with fluvoxamine. Inositol has few known side effects, thus making it attractive for administration to patients with manic depression who are ambivalent about taking other antidepressant drugs (83).

Lithium

Lithium (from the Greek word *lithos*, meaning "stone") is a monovalent cation that competes with sodium, potassium, calcium, and magnesium ions at intracellular binding sites; at sugar phosphatases; at protein surfaces; at carrier binding sites; and at transport sites. Lithium readily passes through sodium channels, and high concentrations can block potassium channels. In the 1870s, claims for the healthful effects of lithium fueled the markets for products such as Lithia Beer and Lithia Springs Mineral Water (in 1887, analysis of Lithia Springs Mineral Water proved the water to be rich not only in lithium but also in potassium, calcium, magnesium, fluoride, and other essential trace minerals). In 1890, the Lithia Springs Sanitarium (Georgia) was established using natural lithium water to treat alcoholism, opium addiction, and compulsive behavior, even though manic depression had not been identified as a form of mental illness until the early 1900s.

Lithium's mood-stabilizing properties were revitalized in the 1940s when an Australian physician, John Cade, hypothesized that a toxin in the blood was responsible for bipolar illness. Believing that uric acid would protect individuals from this toxin, he began studying the effects of a mixture of uric acid and lithium in rats. Lithium carbonate was used to dissolve the uric acid. He observed a calming effect of this combination on the rats and subsequently determined that the lithium, rather than the uric acid, was responsible for this calming effect. He then speculated that lithium might be useful in humans as a mood attenuator, subsequently administered lithium to a sample of patients with bipolar disorder, and discovered that lithium not only decreased the symptoms of mania but also prevented the recurrence of both depression and mania when taken regularly by these patients. After a decade of clinical trials, the FDA approved lithium for treatment of mania in 1970.

Lithium carbonate (Eskalith) is the most commonly used salt of lithium to treat manic depression. Lithium carbonate dosage forms are labeled in mg and mEq/dosage unit, and lithium citrate (Lithobid) is labeled as mg equivalent to lithium carbonate and mEq/dosage unit. Lithium is effectively used to control and prevent manic episodes in 70% to 80% of those with bipolar disorder as well as to treat other forms of depression. Those who respond to lithium for depression often are those who have not responded to TCAs after several weeks of treatment. When giving lithium in addition to their antidepressants, some of these people have shown significant improvement.

Mechanism of Action Lithium therapy for disorders is believed to be effective because of its ability to reduce signal transduction through the phosphatidylinositol signaling pathway (Fig. 18.29) (84,85). In this pathway, the second messengers diacylglycerol (DAG) and inositol 1,4,5-trisphosphate are produced from the enzymatic hydrolysis of phosphatidylinositol-4,5-bisphosphate (a membrane phospholipid) by the receptor-mediated activation of the membrane-bound, phosphatidylinositol-specific phospholipase C. The second messenger activity for inositol 1,4,5-trisphosphate is terminated by its hydrolysis in three steps by inositol monophosphatases to inactive inositol, thus completing the signaling pathway. To recharge the signaling pathway, inositol must be recycled back to phosphatidylinositol bisphosphate by inositol phospholipid–synthesizing enzymes in the CNS, because inositol is unable to cross the blood–brain barrier into the CNS in sufficient concentrations to maintain the signaling pathway. By uncompetitive inhibition of inositol phosphatases in the signaling pathway, the therapeutic plasma concentrations of lithium ion deplete the pool of inositol available for the resynthesis of phosphatidylinositol-4,5-bisphosphate, ultimately decreasing its cellular levels and, thereby, reducing the enzymatic formation of the second messengers. Thus, lithium ion restores the balance among aberrant signaling pathways in critical regions of the brain.

The effects of lithium ion on disorders are surprisingly specific because of the inability of inositol to cross the blood–brain barrier and replenish depleted inositol levels. Lithium ion exerts its greatest influence on this signaling pathway when the lithium ion concentration is at saturation conditions.

The clinical efficacy of lithium in the prophylaxis of recurrent affective episodes in bipolar disorder is characterized by a lag in onset and remains for weeks to months after discontinuation. Thus, the long-term therapeutic effect of lithium likely requires reprogramming of gene expression. Protein kinase C and GSK-3 signal transduction pathways are perturbed by chronic lithium at therapeutically relevant concentrations and have been implicated in modulating synaptic function in nerve terminals (85).

Pharmacokinetics The absorption of lithium is rapid and complete within 6 to 8 hours. The absorption rate of slow-release capsules is slower, and the total amount of lithium absorbed is lower than with other dosage forms. Lithium is not protein bound. The elimination half-life for elderly patients (39 hours) is longer than that for adult patients (24 hours), which in turn is longer than that for adolescent patients (18 hours). The time to peak serum concentration for lithium carbonate is dependent on the dosage form (tablets, 1 to 3 hours; extended tab, 4 hours; slow release, 3 hours). Steady-state serum concentrations are reached in 4 days, with the desirable dose targeted to give a maintenance lithium ion plasma concentration range of 0.6 to 1.2 mEq/L, with a level of 0.5 mEq/L for elderly patients. The risk of bipolar recurrence was approximately threefold greater for patients with lithium dosages that gave plasma concentrations of 0.4 to 0.6 mEq/L. Adverse reactions are frequent at therapeutic doses, and adherence is a big problem. Toxic reactions are rare at serum lithium ion levels of less than 1.5 mEq/L. Mild to moderate toxic reactions may occur at levels from 1.5 to 2.5 mEq/L, and severe reactions may be seen at levels from 2.0 to 2.5 mEq/L, depending on individual response. The onset of therapeutic action for clinical improvement is 1 to 3 weeks. Renal elimination of lithium ion is 95%, with 80% actively reabsorbed in the proximal tubule. The rate of lithium ion urinary excretion decreases with age. Fecal elimination is less than 1%.

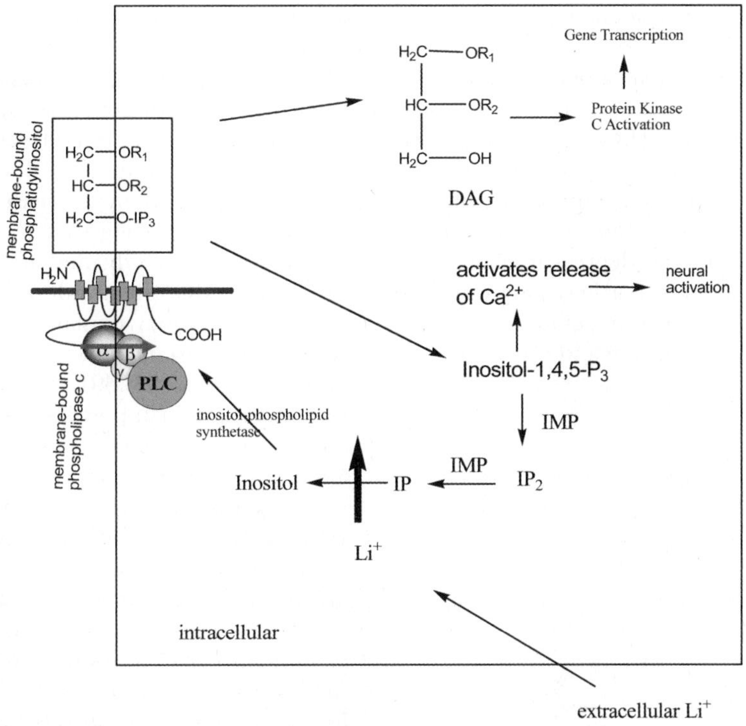

FIGURE 18.29 Intracellular phosphatidylinositol signaling pathway and site of action for lithium. Phospholipase C (PLC) is a membrane-bound enzyme. DAG, diacylglyceride; IMP, inositol monophosphatase; IP, inositol monophosphate.

Drug Interactions Lithium pharmacokinetics may be influenced by a number of factors, including age. Elderly patients require lower doses of lithium to achieve serum concentrations similar to those observed in younger adults as a result of reduced volume of distribution and reduced renal clearance. Lithium ion clearance decreases as the glomerular filtration rate decreases with increasing age. Reduced lithium ion clearance is expected in patients with hypertension, congestive heart failure, or renal dysfunction. Larger lithium ion maintenance doses are required in obese compared with nonobese patients. The most clinically significant pharmacokinetic drug interactions associated with lithium involve drugs that are commonly used in the elderly and that can increase serum lithium ion concentrations. People who are taking lithium should consult their physician before taking the following drugs: acetazolamide, antihypertensives, angiotensin-converting enzyme inhibitors, nonsteroidal anti-inflammatory drugs, calcium channel blockers, carbamazepine, thiazide diuretics, hydroxyzine, muscle relaxants, neuroleptics, table salt, baking powder, tetracycline, TCAs, MAOIs, and caffeine. The tolerability of lithium is lower in elderly patients. Lithium toxicity can occur in the elderly at concentrations considered to be "therapeutic" in the general adult populations. Serum concentrations of lithium ion need to be markedly reduced in the elderly population—and particularly so in the very old and frail.

Adverse Effects Common side effects of lithium include nausea, loss of appetite, and mild diarrhea, which usually taper off within the first few weeks. Dizziness and hand tremors also have been reported. Increased production of urine and excessive thirst are two common side effects that usually are not serious problems, but patients with kidney disease should not be given lithium. Taking the day's dosage of lithium at bedtime also seems to help with the problem of increased urination. Other side effects of lithium include weight gain, hypothyroidism, increased white blood cell count, skin rashes, and birth defects.

While on lithium, a patient's blood level must be closely monitored. If the blood level of lithium ion is too low, the patient's symptoms will not be relieved. If the blood level of lithium ion is too high, there is a danger of a toxic reaction.

Therapeutic Uses For many years, lithium has been the treatment of choice for bipolar disorder, because it can be effective in smoothing out the mood swings common to this condition. Its use must be carefully monitored, however, because the range between an effective and a toxic dose is small.

Nonmonoaminergic Antidepressants

N-Methyl-D-Aspartate Antagonists

Despite intensive research, the problems of treating antidepressant-resistant patients and that existing treatments for MDD usually take weeks to months to achieve response and remission of depression have not yet been solved. The past decade has seen a steady accumulation of evidence supporting a role for the excitatory amino acid neurotransmitter glutamate and its mGluR1 and mGluR5 receptors in depression and antidepressant activity (86,87). Glutamate plays an essential role as a neurotransmitter in many physiologic functions, and an increase in glutamate release can result in activation of NMDA receptors, an underlying cause for depression and anxiety. The NMDA receptor is a ligand-gated ion channel that mediates excitatory synaptic transmission in the CNS (Chapter 12). This channel opening and receptor activation are triggered by synaptically released glutamate and require the binding of glycine, which is a coagonist. Studies with NMDA receptor antagonists of mGluR1 and mGluR5 receptors, as well as positive modulators of AMPA receptors, have antidepressant-like activity in a variety of preclinical models. Furthermore, evidence implicates disturbances in glutamate metabolism, NMDA, and mGluR1/5 receptors in depression and suicidality.

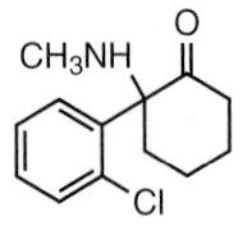

Ketamine

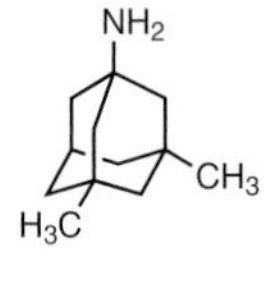

Memantine

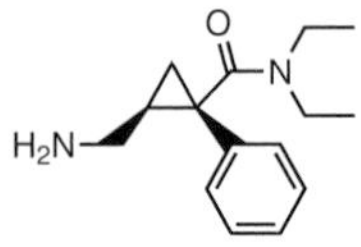

cis-Milnacipran

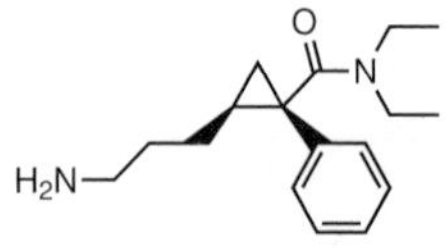

cis -1-Phenyl-2-[1-aminopropyl]-*N,N*-diethylcyclopropanecarboxamide

Several preclinical studies in the 1990s revealed an important role for NMDA receptor antagonists in the mechanism of action of antidepressants and have generated considerable interest in the NMDA receptor as a target for new antidepressant therapies (85–88). Recent human studies have shown that the NMDA receptor antagonist ketamine leads to rapid and relatively sustained antidepressant effects in patients with treatment-resistant major depression (88,89). These findings have given rise to the hypothesis that the NMDA antagonist ketamine (an anesthetic) (Chapter 16) might have potential as an antidepressant, which has been validated in drug-free patients with MDD. A significant reduction in depression was observed 3 hours after a single infusion of ketamine, and this effect was sustained for at least 72 hours (88). This rapid antidepressant effect of ketamine has been replicated using larger sample sizes and treatment-resistant patients with depression. This rapid effect has a high therapeutic value in depressed patients who are suicidal, who might benefit from such a rapid and marked effect because their acute mortality risk is not considerably diminished with conventional antidepressants due to their long delay in onset of action (usually 2 to 3 weeks). Suicidal thoughts were reduced 24 hours after a single ketamine infusion. Ketamine therapy could be extended to other disorders in which NMDA receptors are implicated in bipolar disorders and addiction. The use of ketamine for the treatment of bipolar disorder is currently in phase III clinical trials.

cis-1-Phenyl-2-[1-aminopropyl]-*N,N*-diethylcarboxamide, an NMDA receptor antagonist and homolog of milnacipran, produces sustained relief from depressive symptoms. Several studies have shown that chronic antidepressant treatment can modulate NMDA receptor expression and function. Preclinical studies with this and other NMDA receptor antagonists have demonstrated their potential antidepressant properties.

Thus, the therapeutic effects of monoaminergic antidepressants, ketamine, and other NMDA antagonists may be mediated by increased AMPA-to-NMDA glutamate receptor throughput in critical neuronal circuits, and ketamine directly mediates this throughput. Because the monoaminergic antidepressants work indirectly and gradually, this may explain, in part, the lag of onset of several weeks to months that is observed with traditional antidepressants (88,89). These studies suggest that an intimate relationship exists between regulation of monoaminergic and excitatory amino acid neurotransmission and antidepressant effects.

The combination of traditional antidepressant drugs (e.g., imipramine) and uncompetitive NMDA receptor antagonists (e.g., memantine) may produce enhanced antidepressive effects as a result of synergism. This observation may be of particular importance for the treatment of antidepressant-resistant patients. Most interesting was the observation that fluoxetine, which was inactive in the forced swimming test in rats when given alone, showed a positive effect when combined with memantine (2.5 and 5 mg/kg).

Melatonergic Receptor Agonist/Serotonin Antagonist

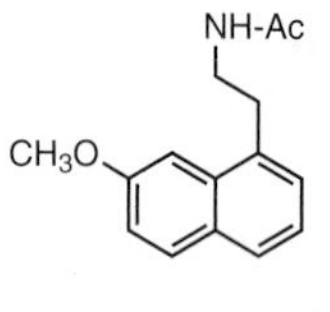

Agomelatine

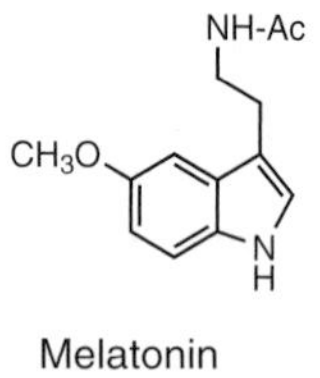

Melatonin

The discovery and development of melatonin receptor agonists as antidepressants was motivated by the need for more potent drugs with better pharmacokinetics, a shorter onset of antidepressant action, and lesser adverse effects than the traditional monoamine reuptake inhibitors. Melatonin receptor agonists are analogs of melatonin. The chemical structure of agomelatine is very similar to that of melatonin, except that the indole ring of melatonin has been replaced with the bioisosteric naphthalene ring. Agomelatine, a dual-acting melatonin agonist/5-HT_{2C} receptor antagonist, is the first antidepressant with a non–monoamine reuptake mechanism of action (14). In 2009, agomelatine was approved in Europe for the treatment of MDD in adults and is currently under review by FDA for approval in 2011.

Melatonin is the primary neurohormone secreted by the pineal gland in the brain that regulates the body's circadian (light/dark) rhythm. The two-step synthesis of melatonin from 5-HT is regulated by the light/dark cycle. Circadian rhythm is the body's internal 24-hour "clock" that plays a critical role in when we fall asleep and when we wake up. When it is dark, your body produces more melatonin; when it is light, the production of melatonin drops. Being exposed to bright lights in the evening or too little light during the day can disrupt the body's normal melatonin cycles. A core symptom of depression and a common problem in people with depression is a disruption in the normal melatonin sleep/wake rhythm.

Mechanism of Action Agomelatine is unique among FDA-approved melatonergic receptor agonists (e.g., ramelteon) because it exhibits affinity for both human melatonin receptor (MT) subtypes (MT_1 and MT_2) and has $5\text{-}HT_{2C}$ receptor antagonist properties (90). The antidepressant efficacy of agomelatine involves either complementary or synergistic actions on the MT and $5\text{-}HT_{2C}$ receptors. Binding studies indicate that it has no effect on monoamine reuptake and no affinity for α-adrenergic, β-adrenergic, histaminergic, cholinergic, dopaminergic, or benzodiazepine receptors. The MT_1 and MT_2 receptors are G protein–coupled, seven-membrane receptors responsible for the effects of melatonin on human circadian rhythms and on reproduction, which is also affected by the 24-hour sleep/wake cycle. These receptors are located in specific areas of the brain and in some peripheral organs. The MT_1 receptor is located in the hypothalamus, which is involved in circadian rhythm, and in the pituitary gland, which may be involved with melatonin's effect on reproduction. It can also be found in other areas of the brain. The MT_2 receptor is found mainly in the retina but can also be found in the lung, cardiovascular tissue, immune cells, duodenum, and adipocytes. When agomelatine binds to and activates both the MT_1 and MT_2 receptors, it triggers numerous physiologic processes, including the release of melatonin from the pineal gland, induction of sleep, and resynchronization of the altered sleep/wake circadian rhythm of depressed patients by delaying the sleep phase rhythm. It retains its antidepressant efficacy without the typical side effects of the other antidepressants such as sexual dysfunction and drug discontinuation symptoms commonly seen with the SSRIs and SNRIs (14). Hyperactivity of the $5\text{-}HT_{2C}$ receptors may contribute to the symptoms of MDD and may also be responsible for many of the negative side effects of SSRI and SNRI medications. Antagonism of $5\text{-}HT_{2C}$ receptors by agomelatine results in an increase in the release of DA and NE in the frontal cortex, the site most associated with depression in the brain, which may contribute to its overall antidepressant efficacy. Agomelatine does not affect the extracellular levels of 5-HT. The drug possesses a pharmacologic profile entirely distinct from SNRIs and SSRIs, making it a significant advance in the treatment of depression.

Pharmacokinetics Agomelatine is rapidly absorbed after oral administration, with an oral bioavailability of less than 5% at its therapeutic oral dose as a result of first-pass hepatic metabolism (90). Its bioavailability is increased in women who use oral contraceptives but is reduced by smoking, which induces CYP1A2. The peak plasma concentration is reached within 1 to 2 hours. In the therapeutic dose range, agomelatine exhibits linear pharmacokinetics, and at higher oral doses, a saturation of the first-pass effect occurs. Food intake does not modify its bioavailability or the absorption rate but is increased with high-fat food. Its steady-state volume of distribution is about 35 L, plasma protein binding is 95%, and its pharmacokinetics are not modified with age or in patients with renal impairment, but the free fraction is doubled in patients with hepatic impairment. Following oral administration, agomelatine is rapidly metabolized mainly via hepatic CYP1A2 with a minor contribution from CYP2C9 and CYP2C19. The major metabolites are hydroxylated and *O*-demethylated agomelatine, which are inactive and rapidly glucuronide conjugated and eliminated in the urine. Elimination is rapid, with a mean plasma half-life of 2 to 3 hours. Excretion is mainly (80%) urinary in the form of metabolites, whereas unchanged parent drug recovery in urine is negligible. The pharmacokinetics of agomelatine are not modified after repeated administration.

Therapeutic Uses A reduction in sleep disruption, a core symptom of depression and a common problem in people with depression, without any daytime sedation is one of the clinical benefits of agomelatine treatment. Agomelatine is indicated for the treatment of MDD episodes in adults and is not recommended for use in children and adolescents younger than 18 years of age due to a lack of data on safety and efficacy. Because only limited clinical data are available on the use of agomelatine in patients ≥65 years old who have MDD episodes, caution should be exercised when prescribing it to these patients. From the first week of treatment, its onset of antidepressant efficacy, as measured by onset of sleep and the quality of sleep, was significantly improved without daytime drowsiness as assessed by patients. Agomelatine at 25 to 50 mg has been shown to be effective in more severely depressed patients whatever the intensity of depressive symptoms. It has comparable antidepressant activity to venlafaxine (75 to 150 mg/d) and was more effective than 50 to 100 mg/d of sertraline. Agomelatine was superior to placebo for relapse prevention at 10 months, and treatment adherence rates were higher than with venlafaxine and sertraline over 6 months. The commonly reported adverse effects in the clinical trials of agomelatine are headache, nausea, and diarrhea. It is found to increase the level of liver enzymes, and thus, monitoring of enzyme level is warranted before starting therapy and every 6 weeks thereafter. It is also contraindicated in patients with hepatic impairment

Neuropeptides

The pharmacologic treatment of depressive illness has been dominated by drugs that directly target monoamine neurotransmitter systems. Monoamine transport inhibitors are first-line treatments for depression. Current antidepressants exhibit a delayed onset of therapeutic action, and a significant number of patients are nonresponsive to this treatment regimen (54). Moreover, many patients discontinue treatment because of adverse side effects, including nausea, sexual dysfunction, anorexia, mouth dryness, and cardiotoxicity. A complementary strategy is to identify other treatments that target other neurotransmitter and neuromodulators in the brain. Neuropeptides have been shown to be attractive targets for depression (91,92). Neuropeptides are short-chain amino acid neurotransmitters and neuromodulators often localized in brain regions that mediate emotional behaviors and the response to stress (91,92). The neuropeptides that have been identified in stress include the tachykinins (substance P and neurokinin A), corticotropin-releasing factor, vasopressin, galanin, brain-derived neurotrophic factor (BDNF), and melanocyte-inhibiting factor. Thus, drugs that are antagonists at these neuropeptide receptors might exhibit a lower incidence of adverse effects, because such antagonists would not be expected to bind to the NE and 5-HT neurotransmitter receptors. The expression of BDNF in individuals with MDD is decreased, suggesting that BDNF plays a role in the pathophysiology of depression as a regulator of neuronal signaling pathways. Antidepressant drugs increase the BDNF brain levels and, therefore, enhance the mechanism of action of the antidepressant drugs. Drugs that boost the levels of BDNF may lead to the development of novel therapeutic agents for the treatment of MDD and bipolar disorders.

Corticotropin-Releasing Factor Increasing evidence suggests that the neuroendocrine changes seen in patients suffering from affective disorders may be causally related to the course of depression. The most robustly confirmed neuroendocrine finding among patients with affective disorders is hyperactivity of the hypothalamic-pituitary-adrenocortical (HPA) system, resulting from hyperactive hypothalamic CRF neurons. Moreover, one of the most replicated findings in biologic psychiatry is that large numbers of unmedicated depressed patients exhibit HPA hyperactivity. The available evidence suggests that nAChRs play important roles in mediating stress-related and possibly depression-inducing neuroendocrine effects of ACh. ACh (hypercholinergic activity), in response to stress, can stimulate the HPA through activation of nAChRs. Abnormal HPA activity has been implicated in conditions related to stress, including HPA overactivation in depression, eating and substance abuse disorders, irritable bowel syndrome, inflammation, and cardiovascular dysfunction. Preclinical and clinical evidence suggests that both genetic and environmental factors contribute to the development of these HPA system abnormalities. CRF is a 41–amino acid neuropeptide that initiates and regulates the HPA axis response to stress, and it has been intensively studied in the pathophysiology and treatment of depression (93). In humans, the CRF system consists of CRF and two G protein–coupled CRF receptors (CRF_1 and CRF_2). The CRF_1 receptors play an important role in mediating the HPA response to stress. Additionally, CRF is capable of reproducing the hormonal changes that are characteristically seen in depressed patients. Postmortem and endocrine studies suggest that both hypothalamic and extrahypothalamic concentrations of CRF are elevated in proportion to antidepressant treatment. High CRF concentrations tend to reestablish the HPA imbalance. The careful manipulation of CRF concentrations with high-affinity CRF_1 antagonists, such as R121919, may hold therapeutic promise for sufferers of depression. Thus, antidepressants may reduce symptoms of depression, in part, through blockade of AChRs involved with stress-induced activation of the HPA (8).

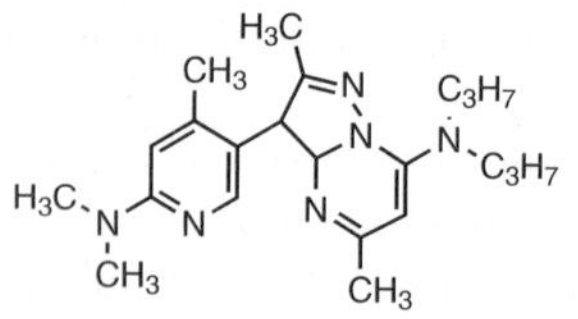

R121919

Substance P Substance P is an 11–amino acid neuropeptide belonging to the tachykinin family, mediating its biologic actions through activation of G protein–coupled tachykinin (neurokinin-1 [NK_1]) receptors. Its proposed physiologic roles include inflammation, pain, GI and respiratory function, stress responses, and emesis. Substance P is uniquely associated with the monoamine neurotransmitters 5-HT and NE. The 5-HT neurons coexpress substance P, and the firing of NE neurons is modulated by substance P. Preclinical studies have supported a role of the substance P–NK_1 receptor system in stress-related disorders, which has guided the antidepressant development of centrally active NK_1 receptor antagonists, such as aprepitant (94). Aprepitant (Emend) has been approved for the prevention of nausea and vomiting due to cancer chemotherapy. The NK_1 antagonists are generally well tolerated and exhibit less nausea and sexual dysfunction than some currently used antidepressants.

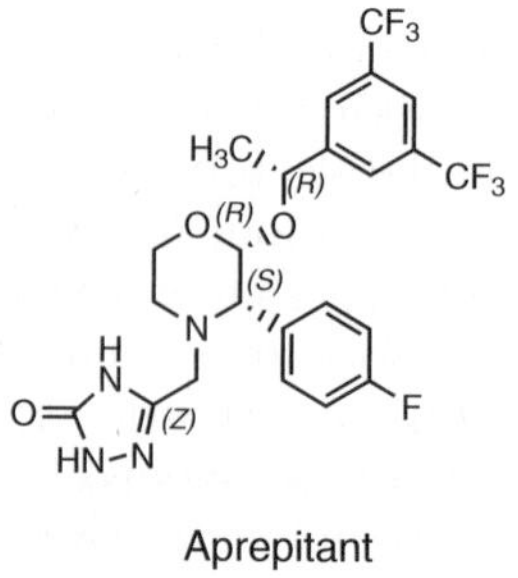

Aprepitant

Vasopressin The nonapeptide vasopressin is well known for its role on fluid metabolism (see Chapter 6), but it also is a key regulator of the HPA axis. Stress stimulates the release of vasopressin in the pituitary gland, where it strongly potentiates the effects of CRF on adrenocorticotropic hormone release. These findings suggest that HPA axis dysregulation in depression might be associated with the development of centrally acting vasopressin receptor antagonists for the treatment of depression.

Galanin Since its discovery in 1983, the neuropeptide galanin has been found to be involved in a wide range of functions, including pain sensation, sexual activity, feeding, and learning and memory (95). Galanin is widely distributed in the central and peripheral nervous systems and in the endocrine system, and it acts as an inhibitory neuromodulator of NE and 5-HT in the brain. The

29– to 30–amino acid sequence of galanin is conserved (almost 90% among species), indicating the importance of the molecule among species. Galanin is colocalized with ACh, 5-HT, and NE in neurons or in brain regions implicated in cognitive and affective behavior, suggesting a possible role in the regulation of 5-HT and NA neurotransmission in depressive states and during the course of antidepressant therapy. Three galanin receptor subtypes have been cloned and studied, but little is known about their specific contributions to behavioral processes. In the CNS, galanin inhibits ACh release, suggesting a possible role for galanin in cholinergic dysfunction; inhibits neurotransmitter release and neuronal firing rate; and inhibits signal transduction by inhibition of phosphatidylinositol hydrolysis, leading to symptoms of depression. Thus, blocking the inhibitory effects of galanin on monoamine neurotransmitters with galanin receptor antagonists would be predicted to mimic or augment the action of the other monoamine classes of antidepressants.

Melanocyte-Inhibiting Factor

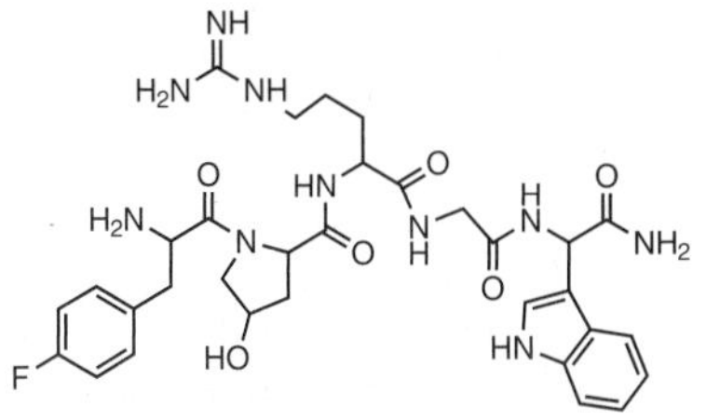

Nemifitide

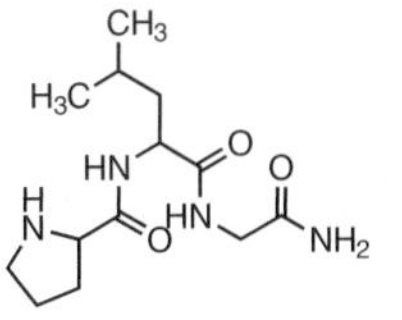

MIF-1

Nemifitide is a peptide analog of melanocyte-stimulating hormone release–inhibiting factor currently in clinical development for the potential treatment of moderate to severely depressed patients (96). It is rapidly absorbed, with a peak plasma concentration of 10 minutes and an elimination half-life of 15 to 30 minutes in most subjects. The pharmacokinetic results indicate that the dose is proportional in the dose range investigated. No evidence indicated systemic accumulation of drug following five daily doses. No serious adverse events or clinically significant systemic adverse events occurred at any of the doses investigated in the more than 100 subjects dosed in these studies. Drug-related adverse events were limited to local and transient skin reactions (pain and/or erythema) at the injection site, especially at the high doses administered. Melanocyte-stimulating hormone release–inhibiting factor-1 (MIF-1) has been shown to have antidepressant activity when administered subcutaneously (10 mg for 5 consecutive days) in a double-blind study of 20 depressed patients who all met the DSM-IIIR criteria for major depression. After the 5-day treatment with MIF-1, these patients all exhibited substantial improvement in their symptoms of depression (97). Moreover, the potential clinical efficacy of combining MIF-1 (0.01 mg/kg intraperitoneal [IP]) with small doses of the TCAs amitriptyline (5 mg/kg IP) or desipramine (1.25 mg/kg IP) may be of benefit in the therapy of depressed patients.

Herbal Therapy

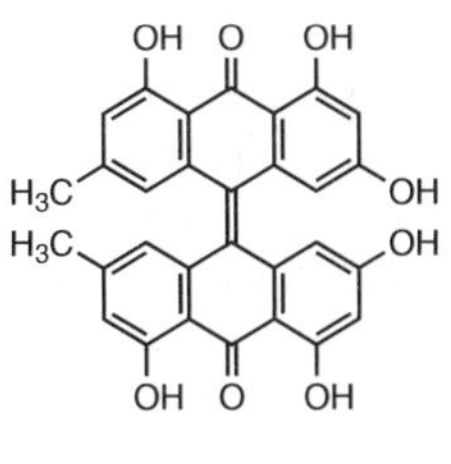

Hypericin

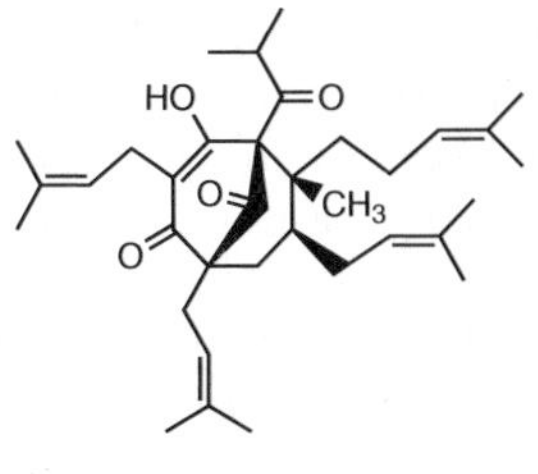

Hyperforin

During the past few years, much interest has been generated regarding the use of herbs in the treatment of both depression and anxiety (98). Recent studies, however, have revealed potentially fatal interactions between herbal remedies and traditional drugs.

St. John's wort (*Hypericum perforatum*), an herb used extensively in the treatment of mild to moderate depression in Europe, has aroused interest in the United States. A bushy, low-growing plant covered with yellow flowers in summer, St. John's wort has been used for centuries in many folk and herbal remedies. In Germany, *Hypericum* is used in the treatment of depression more than any other antidepressant. The scientific studies that have been conducted regarding its use have been short term, however, and have used several different doses. St. John's wort works like the SSRIs, in that it not only increases the availability of 5-HT in synaptic clefts by blocking its reuptake but also increases the availability of NE, which increases energy and alertness, and DA, which increases the feeling of well-being.

Ingestion of St John's wort increases the expression (i.e., upregulation) of intestinal P-gp and CYP3A4 in the liver and intestine, which impairs the absorption and stimulates the metabolism of other CYP3A4 substrates (e.g., the protease inhibitors indinavir and nevirapine, oral contraceptives, and TCAs [e.g., amitriptyline]), resulting in their subtherapeutic plasma levels. Hyperforin, the principal component in St. John's wort (2% to 4% in the fresh herb), contributes to the induction of CYP3A4. Furthermore, it not only inhibits the neuronal reuptake of 5-HT, NE, and DA, like many other antidepressants, but also inhibits GABA and L-glutamate uptake. This broad-spectrum effect is obtained by an elevation of the intracellular sodium ion concentration, probably resulting from activation of sodium conductive pathways not yet finally identified but most likely to be ionic channels. This makes hyperforin the first member of a new class of compounds with a preclinical antidepressant profile because of a completely novel mechanism of action (98,99). Hypericin, the other component in St. John's wort, also may exhibit inhibitor action on key neuroreceptors and may be responsible for the phototoxicity/photosensitivity of St. John's wort.

The National Institutes of Health conducted a double-blind, 3-year study of patients with major depression of moderate severity using St. John's wort and sertraline. This study did not support the use of St. John's wort in the treatment of major depression, but a possible role for St. John's wort in the treatment of milder forms of depression was suggested. Health care providers should alert their patients about potential drug interactions with St. John's wort. Some other frequently used herbal supplements that have not been evaluated in large-scale clinical trials are ephedra, gingko biloba, echinacea, and ginseng. Any herbal supplement should be taken only after consultation with the physician or other health care provider.

ELECTROCONVULSIVE THERAPY

Electroconvulsive therapy (ECT) has been in use since the late 1930s to treat a variety of severe mental illnesses, most notably major depression. Use of ECT is beneficial particularly for individuals whose depression is severe or life threatening or who cannot take antidepressant medication. Often, ECT is effective in cases where antidepressant drugs do not provide sufficient relief of symptoms.

ECT remains the "gold standard" for the treatment of major depression and a variety of other psychiatric and neurologic disorders (100). Because of the effectiveness and resurgence of ECT, more patients are considered to be good candidates for this treatment option. Overall, these patients are medication refractory and elderly and, thus, are more sensitive to polypharmacy. Additionally, these patients tend to have more coexisting medical problems.

In recent years, ECT has been much improved. A muscle relaxant is given before treatment, which is done under brief anesthesia. Electrodes are placed at precise locations on the head to deliver electrical impulses. The stimulation causes a brief (~30 seconds) seizure within the brain. The person receiving ECT does not consciously experience the electrical stimulus. For full therapeutic benefit, at least several sessions of ECT, typically given at the rate of three per week, are required. Electroconvulsive therapy appears to increase the sensitivity of postsynaptic 5-HT receptors and upregulation of 5-HT_{1A} postsynaptic receptors.

Side effects may result from the anesthesia, the ECT treatment, or both. Common side effects include temporary short-term memory loss, nausea, muscle aches, and headache. Some people may have longer-lasting problems with memory after ECT. Sometimes, a person's blood pressure or heart rhythm changes. If these changes occur, they are carefully watched during the ECT treatments and are immediately treated.

SCENARIO: OUTCOME AND ANALYSIS

Outcome

Nancy Ordonez, PharmD

There are several issues that need to be addressed during GP's current visit. GP's depressive symptoms have not improved even though the dose of venlafaxine has been increased to a total of 300 mg/d. In addition, GP's uncontrolled hypertension needs to be addressed as well as his worsening peripheral neuropathy. Venlafaxine can cause hypertension, especially in higher doses, and with GP's uncontrolled hypertension, venlafaxine may not be the best therapeutic option for his depression. Amitriptyline is indicated for peripheral neuropathy; however, it can cause sedation and has cardiovascular side effects. GP's venlafaxine will be gradually tapered and discontinued, and amitriptyline will be discontinued. Duloxetine was started at 20 mg twice daily and will be increased gradually. Duloxetine is indicated for depression and diabetic neuropathy. Blood pressures, blood glucose, as well as his signs of improvement of his depressive symptoms and peripheral neuropathy will be monitored. GP scheduled a follow-up visit in 3 weeks.

Chemical Analysis

Victoria F. Roche and S. William Zito

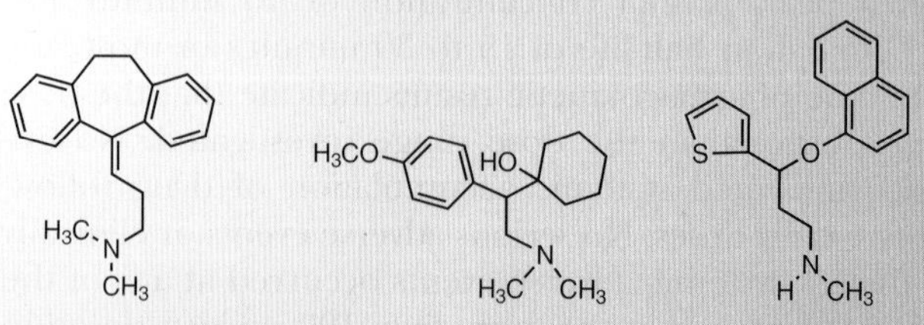

Amitriptyline Venlafaxine Duloxetine

Amitriptyline is a tertiary tricyclic antidepressant that acts in parent drug form to inhibit the reuptake of central serotonin. The increased serotonin in central synapses can lead to sedation, which explains GP's morning drowsiness. The strong structural overlap with antimuscarinic and antihistaminic agents also adds to the sedative potential of this agent, and it explains some of its

SCENARIO: OUTCOME AND ANALYSIS *(Continued)*

peripheral adverse effects including dry mouth, blurred vision, urinary retention, tachycardia, and orthostatic hypotension.

Venlafaxine and duloxetine both inhibit the reuptake of central norepinephrine as well as serotonin, with duloxetine being the more potent. Venlafaxine's tertiary amine structure may help explain its preference for blocking serotonin reuptake; however, selectivity will be lost at the high doses GP was taking. As norepinephrine concentrations in the CNS and periphery rise, so can blood pressure. Dependence can develop when venlafaxine is used chronically, which necessitates a step-down discontinuation regimen to avoid withdrawal symptoms. Venlafaxine is O-dealkylated by CYP2D6 to an equally active phenolic metabolite, desvenlafaxine. In addition to serving as a 2D6 substrate, venlafaxine inhibits this isoform. Both of these metabolic realities could lead to drug-drug interactions with other 2D6 substrates, such as metoprolol, which is the most highly dependent of all β-blockers on 2D6-mediated metabolism.

The secondary amine duloxetine is the more potent inhibitor of serotonin and norepinephrine reuptake and might be able to manage GP's depressive symptoms in lower doses. In therapeutic doses, it preferentially inhibits the serotonin reuptake transporter and, therefore, would be less likely to raise blood pressure than high doses of venlafaxine. Like venlafaxine, duloxetine has shown efficacy in the treatment of diabetic neuropathic pain. However, also like venlafaxine, it is both a substrate (N-dealkylation) and an inhibitor of CYP2D6, and a more pronounced antihypertensive effect may be noted from GP's maintenance dose of metoprolol.

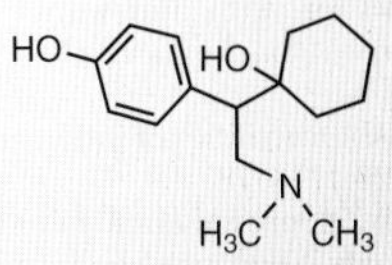

Desvenlafaxine (active metabolite)

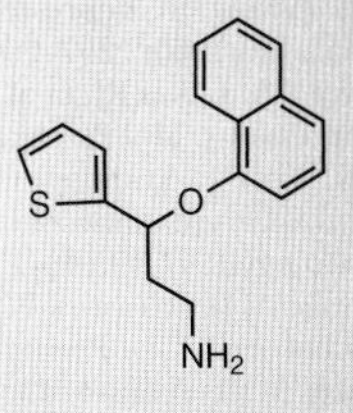

Desduloxetine (active metabolite)

As noted above, GP's blood pressure should be closely monitored and any needed adjustment in antihypertensive therapy made as he is stabilized on this new antidepressant medication.

CASE STUDY

Victoria Roche and S. William Zito

MF is a 32-year-old computer programmer who has struggled with depression for years. As an adolescent, he experienced suicidal ideation and once made an unsuccessful attempt to end his life. MF married 8 months ago and he and his wife, a marketing executive for a national chain of high-end wine and cheese shops, have moved to Bordeaux, France, for a 3-year opportunity related to her work. His wife is very loving and supportive, and he felt better than he had in years during their courtship and after the wedding. But now, with the move complete, those old feelings of despair and panic are starting to close in again. Never highly compliant with taking his medication, his wife urged him to resume his therapy, but he confides that his most currently prescribed antidepressant, amitriptyline, "just makes him feel bad all over." His current prescriptions also include low-dose amlodipine for modestly elevated blood pressure, another medication with which he is noncompliant.

With his wife at his side, MF has consulted with a psychiatrist in their new community about the return of his symptoms. This psychiatrist ordered a pharmacogenetic workup and it was found that MF is of the poor 2D6 metabolizer and slow acetylator phenotype. If you were lucky enough to be working as a pysch pharmacist in beautiful French "wine country," which of the three drugs drawn below would you recommend?

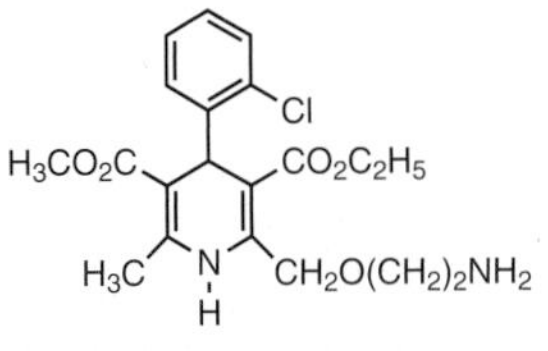

Amlodipine

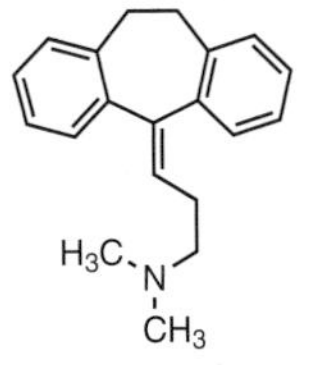

Amitriptyline

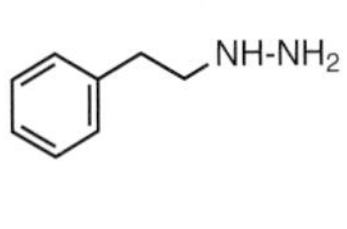

1

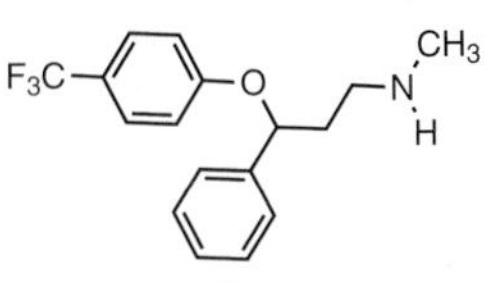

2

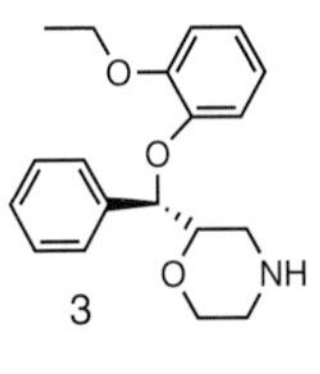

3

1. Conduct a thorough and mechanistic SAR analysis of the three therapeutic options in the case.
2. Apply the chemical understanding gained from the SAR analysis to this patient's specific needs to make a therapeutic recommendation.

References

1. National Institutes of Health. Depression. National Institutes of Health Publication 00-3561, 2000.
2. National Institutes of Health. Real men; real depression. National Institutes of Health Publication 03-4972, 2003.
3. Diagnostic and Statistical Manual of Mental Disorders, 4th Ed., Text Revision (DSM-IV-TR). Washington, DC: American Psychiatric Association, 2002.
4. Manji HK, Lenox RH. Signaling: cellular insights into the pathophysiology of bipolar disorder. Biol Psychiatry 2000;48:518–530.
5. Duman RS, Heninger GR, Nestler EJ. A molecular and cellular theory of depression. Arch Gen Psychiatry 1997;54:597–606.
6. Janowsky DS, Davis JM. Adrenergic-cholinergic balance in affective disorders. Psychopharmacol Bull 1978;14:58–60.
7. Schildkraut JJ, Klerman GL, Hammond R, et al. Excretion of 3-methoxymandelic acid (VMA) in depressed patients treated with antidepressant drugs. J Psychiatr Res 1965;2:257–266.
8. Shytle RD, Silver AA, Lukas RJ, et al. Nicotinic acetylcholine receptors as targets for antidepressants. Mol Psychiatry 2002;7:525–535.
9. van Praag HK, Korf J. Endogenous depression with and without disturbance of 5-hydroxytryptamine metabolism: a biochemical classification? Psychopharmacology 1971;19:148–152.
10. Coppen A, Prange AJ Jr, Whybrow PC, et al. Abnormalities of indoleamines in affective disorders. Arch Gen Psychiat 1972;26:474–478.
11. Lenox RH, Frazer A. Mechanism of action of antidepressants and mood stabilizers. In: Davis KL, Charney D, Coyle JT, et al., eds. Neuropsychopharmacology: The Fifth Generation of Progress. Baltimore, MD: Lippincott Williams & Wilkins, 2002;1139–1164.
12. Brown AS, Gershon S. DA and depression. J Neural Transm 1993;91:75–109.
13. Shopsin B, Gershon S, Goldstein M, et al. Use of synthesis inhibitors in defining a role for biogenic amines during imipramine treatment in depressed patients. Psychopharmacol Commun 1975;1:239–249.
14. de Bodinat C, Guardiola-Lemaitre B, Mocaër E, et al. Agomelatine, the first melatonergic antidepressant: discovery, characterization and development. Nat Rev Drug Discov 2010;9:628–642.
15. Mitchell AJ. The role of corticotropin-releasing factor in depressive illness: a critical review. Neurosci Biobehav Rev 1998;22:635–651.
16. Kuhn R. Uber Die Behandlung Depressives Zustande Mit Einem Iminobenzylderivat (G 22,355). Schweiz Med Wschr 1957;87:1135–1140.
17. Loomer HP, Saunders JC, Kline NS. A clinical and pharmacodynamic evaluation of iproniazid as a psychic energizer. Psychiatr Res Rep Am Psychiatr Assoc 1957;8:129–141.
18. Baldessarini RJ. Drug therapy of depression and anxiety disorders. In: Brunton LL, Lazo JS, Parker KL, eds. Goodman & Gilman's the Pharmacological Basis of Therapeutics, 11th Ed. New York: McGraw-Hill, 2006:429–460.
19. Hogberg T, Ulff B, Renyi AL, et al. Synthesis of pyridylallylamines related to zimelidine and their inhibition of neuronal monoamine uptake. J Med Chem 1981;24:1499–1507.
20. Ogren SO, Ross SB, Hall H, et al. The pharmacology of zimelidine: a 5-HT selective reuptake inhibitor. Acta Psychiatr Scand Suppl 1981;290:127–151.
21. Wong DT, Bymaster FP, Horng JS, et al. A new selective inhibitor for uptake of serotonin into synaptosomes of rat brain: 3-(p-trifluoromethylphenoxy). N-methyl-3-phenylpropylamine. J Pharmacol Exp Ther 1975;193:804–811.
22. Wong DT, Bymaster FP, Engleman EA. Prozac (fluoxetine, Lilly 110140), the first selective serotonin uptake inhibitor and an antidepressant drug: twenty years since its first publication. Life Sci 1995;57:411–441.
23. Skolnick P, Popik P, Janowsky A, et al. "Broad spectrum" antidepressants: is more better for the treatment of depression? Life Sci 2003;73:3175–3179.
24. Skolnick P, Popik P, Janowsky A, et al. Antidepressant-like actions of DOV 21,947: a "triple" reuptake inhibitor. Eur J Pharmacol 2003;461:99–104.
25. Glick SD, Haskew RE, Maisonneuve IM, et al. Enantioselective behavioral effects of sibutramine metabolites. Eur J Pharmacol 2000;397:93–102.
26. Torres GE, Gainetdinov RR, Caron MG. Plasma membrane monoamine transporters: structure, regulation and function. Nat Rev Neurosci 2003;4:13–25.
27. Owens MJ, Morgan WN, Plott SJ, et al. Neurotransmitter receptor and transporter binding profile of antidepressants and their metabolites. J Pharmacol Exp Ther 1997;283:1305–1322.
28. Hyttel J. Pharmacological characterization of selective serotonin reuptake inhibitors (SSRIs). Int Clin Psychopharmacol 1994;9(Suppl 1):19–26.
29. Sanchez C, Hyttel J. Comparison of the effects of antidepressants and their metabolites on reuptake of biogenic amines and on receptor binding. Cell Mol Neurobiol 1999;19:467–489.
30. Brunello N, Mendlewicz J, Kasper S, et al. The role of noradrenaline and selective noradrenaline reuptake inhibition in depression. Eur Neuropsychopharmacol 2002;12:461–475.
31. Kelder J, Funke C, De Boer T, et al. A comparison of the physicochemical and biological properties of mirtazapine and mianserin. J Pharm Pharmacol 1997;49:403–411.
32. Baker GB, Prior TI. Stereochemistry and drug efficacy and development: relevance of chirality to antidepressant and antipsychotic drugs. Ann Med 2002;34:537–543.
33. Lane RM, Baker GB. Chirality and drugs used in psychiatry: nice to know or need to know? Cell Mol Neurobiol 1999;19:355–372.
34. Venkatakrishnan K, Von Moltke LL, Greenblatt DJ. Human drug metabolism and the cytochromes P450: application and relevance of in vitro models. J Clin Pharmacol 2001;41:1149–1179.
35. Preskorn SH. Clinically relevant pharmacology of selective serotonin reuptake inhibitors. An overview with emphasis on pharmacokinetics and effects on oxidative drug metabolism. Clin Pharmacokinet 1997;32(Suppl 1):1–19.
36. Weiss J, Dormann SM, Martin-Facklam M, et al. Inhibition of P-glycoprotein by newer antidepressants. J Pharmacol Exp Ther 2003;305:197–204.
37. Ekins S, Kim RB, Leake BF, et al. Three-dimensional quantitative structure–activity relationships of inhibitors of P-glycoprotein. Mol Pharmacol 2002;61:964–973.
38. Sadeque AJ, Wandel C, He H, et al. Increased drug delivery to the brain by P-glycoprotein inhibition. Clin Pharmacol Ther 2000;68:231–237.
39. Eriksson E. Antidepressant drugs: does it matter if they inhibit the reuptake of noradrenaline or serotonin? Acta Psychiatr Scand Suppl 2000;402:12–17.
40. Norregaard L, Gether U. The monoamine neurotransmitter transporters: structure, conformational changes and molecular gating. Curr Opin Drug Discov Dev 2001;4:591–601.
41. Casarotto MG, Craik DJ. Ring flexibility within tricyclic antidepressant drugs. J Pharm Sci 2001;90:713–719.
42. Fleishaker JC. Clinical pharmacokinetics of reboxetine, a selective norepinephrine reuptake inhibitor for the treatment of patients with depression. Clin Pharmacokinet 2000;39:413–427.
43. Wienkers LC, Allievi C, Hauer MJ, et al. Cytochrome P-450–mediated metabolism of the individual enantiomers of the antidepressant agent reboxetine in human liver microsomes. Drug Metab Dispos 1999;27:1334–1340.
44. Bergmann JF, Laneury JP, Duchene P, et al. Pharmacokinetics of reboxetine in healthy, elderly volunteers. Eur J Drug Metab Pharmacokinet 2000;25:195–198.
45. Zerbe RL, Rowe H, Enas GG, et al. Clinical pharmacology of tomoxetine, a potential antidepressant. J Pharmacol Exp Ther 1985;232:139–143.
46. Sauer JM, Ponsler GD, Mattiuz EL, et al. Disposition and metabolic fate of atomoxetine hydrochloride: the role of CYP2D6 in human disposition and metabolism. Drug Metab Dispos 2003;31:98–107.
47. Cowen PJ. Serotonin hypothesis. In: Feighner JP, Boyer WR, eds. Selective Serotonin Reuptake Inhibitors, 2nd Ed. Chichester, United Kingdom: John Wiley & Sons, 1996:63–86.
48. Preskorn SH. Clinical pharmacology of SSRIs. Available at: http://www.preskorn.com. Accessed August 3, 2004.
49. Bordet R, Thomas P, Dupuis B. Effect of pindolol on onset of action of paroxetine in the treatment of major depression: intermediate analysis of a double-blind, placebo-controlled trial. Reseau de Recherche et d'Experimentation Psychopharmacologique. Am J Psychiatr 1998;155:1346–1351.
50. Brosen K, Rasmussen BB. Selective serotonin reuptake inhibitors: pharmacokinetics and drug interactions. In: Feighner JP, Boyer WR, eds. Selective Serotonin Reuptake Inhibitors, 2nd Ed. Chichester, United Kingdom: John Wiley & Sons, 1996:87–108.
51. Shih JC, Chen K, Ridd MJ. MAO: from genes to behavior. Annu Rev Neurosci 1999;22:197–217.
52. Olivier B, Soudjin W, van Wijngaarden I. Serotonin, DA and norepinephrine transporters in the CNS and their inhibitors. In: Jucker E, ed. Progress in Drug Research, Vol 54. Basel, Switzerland: Birkhäuser-Verlag, 2000:59–120.
53. Wong DT, Threlkeld PG, Robertson DW. Affinities of fluoxetine, its enantiomers and other inhibitors of serotonin uptake for subtypes of serotonin receptors. Neuropsychopharmacology 1991;5:43–47.
54. Wong DT, Bymaster FP, Reid LR, et al. Norfluoxetine enantiomers as inhibitors of serotonin uptake in rat brain. Neuropsychopharmacology 1993;8:337–344.
55. Bertelsen KM, Venkatakrishnan K, Von Moltke LL, et al. Apparent mechanism-based inhibition of human CYP2D6 in vitro by paroxetine: comparison with fluoxetine and quinidine. Drug Metab Dispos 2003;31:289–293.
56. Nakajima M, Suzuki M, Yamaji R, et al. Isoform selective inhibition and inactivation of human cytochrome P450s by methylenedioxyphenyl compounds. Xenobiotica 1999;29:1191–1202.
57. Bolton JL, Acay NM, Vukomanovic V. Evidence that 4-allyl-o-quinones spontaneously rearrange to their more electrophilic quinone methides: potential bioactivation mechanism for the hepatocarcinogen safrole. Chem Res Toxicol 1994;7:443–450.
58. Sanchez C, Bogeso KP, Ebert B, et al. Escitalopram versus citalopram: the surprising role of the R-enantiomer. Psychopharmacology 2004;174:163–176.
59. Owens MJ, Knight DL, Nemeroff CB. Second-generation SSRIs: human monoamine transporter binding profile of escitalopram and R-fluoxetine. Biol Psychiatry 2001;50:345–350.
60. Obach RS, Cox LM, Tremaine LM. Sertraline is metabolized by multiple cytochrome P450 enzymes, monoamine oxidases and glucuronyl transferase in human; an in vitro study. Drug Met Dispos 2005;33:262–270.
61. Haritos VS, Ghabrial H, Ahokas JT, et al. Role of cytochrome P450 2D6 (CYP2D6) in the stereospecific metabolism of *E*- and *Z*-doxepin. Pharmacogenetics 2000;10:591–603.
62. Yan JH, Hubbard JW, McKay G, et al. Absolute bioavailability and stereoselective pharmacokinetics of doxepin. Xenobiotica 2002;32:615–623.
63. Eap CB, Bender S, Gastpar M, et al. Steady-state plasma levels of the enantiomers of trimipramine and of its metabolites in CYP2D6-, CYP2C19- and CYP3A4/5-phenotyped patients. Ther Drug Monit 2000;22:209–214.

64. Kirchheiner J, Muller G, Meineke I, et al. Effects of polymorphisms in CYP2D6, CYP2C9 and CYP2C19 on trimipramine pharmacokinetics. J Clin Psychopharmacol 2003;23:459–466.
65. Lancaster SG, Gonzalez JP. Dothiepin: a review of its pharmacodynamic and pharmacokinetic properties and therapeutic efficacy in depressive illness. Drugs 1989;38:123–147.
66. Lancaster SG, Gonzalez JP. Lofepramine: a review of its pharmacodynamic and pharmacokinetic properties and therapeutic efficacy in depressive illness. Drugs 1989;37:123–140.
67. Wong DT, Bymaster FP. Dual serotonin and noradrenaline uptake inhibitor class of antidepressants potential for greater efficacy or just hype? Prog Drug Res 2002;58:169–222.
68. Bymaster FP, Dreshfield-Ahmad LJ, Threlkeld PG, et al. Comparative affinity of duloxetine and venlafaxine for serotonin and norepinephrine transporters in vitro and in vivo, human serotonin receptor subtypes and other neuronal receptors. Neuropsychopharmacology 2001;25:871–880.
69. Vaishnavi SN, Nemeroff CB, Plott SJ, et al. Milnacipran: a comparative analysis of human monoamine uptake and transporter binding affinity. Biol Psychiatry 2004;55:320–322.
70. Puozzo C, Panconi E, Deprez D. Pharmacology and pharmacokinetics of milnacipran. Int Clin Psychopharmacol 2002;17(Suppl 1):S25–S35.
71. Lantz RJ, Gillespie TA, Rash TJ, et al. Metabolism, excretion and pharmacokinetics of duloxetine in healthy human subjects. Drug Metab Dispos 2003;31:1142–1150.
72. Jensen TS, Madsen CS, Finnerup NB. Pharmacology and treatment of neuropathic pains. Curr Opin Neurol 2009;22:467–474.
73. Warner C, Shoaib M. How does bupropion work as a smoking cessation aid? Addict Biol 2005;10:219–231.
74. Coles R, Kharasch ED. Stereoselective metabolism of bupropion by cytochrome P4502B6 (CYP2B6) and human liver microsomes. Pharm Res 2008;25:1405–1411.
75. Hesse LM, Venkatakrishnan K, Court MH, et al. CYP2B6 mediates the in vitro hydroxylation of bupropion: potential drug interactions with other antidepressants. Drug Metab Dispos 2000;28:1176–1183.
76. Rotzinger S, Fang J, Baker GB. Trazodone is metabolized to m-chlorophenylpiperazine by CYP3A4 from human sources. Drug Metab Dispos 1998;26:572–575.
77. Bauman JN, Frederick KS, Sawant A, et al. Comparison of the bioactivation potential of the antidepressant and hepatotoxin nefazodone with aripiprazole, a structural analog and marketed drug. Drug Metab Dispos 2008;36:1016–1029.
78. Rotzinger S, Baker GB. Human CYP3A4 and the metabolism of nefazodone and hydroxynefazodone by human liver microsomes and heterologously expressed enzymes. Eur Neuropsychopharmacol 2002;12:91–100.
79. ViiBryd prescribing information. http://www.frx.com/pi/Viibryd_pi.pdf. Accessed January 30, 2011.
80. Stormer E, von Moltke LL, Shader RI, et al. Metabolism of the antidepressant mirtazapine in vitro: contribution of cytochromes P-450 1A2, 2D6 and 3A4. Drug Metab Dispos 2000;28:1168–1175.
81. Baker GB, Urichuk LJ, McKenna KF, et al. Metabolism of monoamine oxidase inhibitors. Cell Mol Neurobiol 1999;19:411–426.
82. Bonnet U. Moclobemide: evolution, pharmacodynamic and pharmacokinetic properties. CNS Drug Rev 2002;8:283–308.
83. Harwood AJ. Neurodevelopment and mood stabilizers. Curr Mol Med 2003;3:472–482.
84. Berridge MJ. The Albert Lasker Medical Awards. Inositol trisphosphate, calcium, lithium and cell signaling. JAMA 1989;262:1834–1841.
85. Lenox RH, Wang L. Molecular basis of lithium action: integration of lithium-responsive signaling and gene expression networks. Mol Psychiatry 2003;8:135–144.
86. Skolnick P, Popik P, Trullas R. Glutamate-based antidepressants: 20 years on. Trends Pharmacol Sci 2009;30:563–569.
87. Machado-Vieira R, Salvadore G, Diazgranados N, et al. Ketamine and the next generation of antidepressants with a rapid onset of action 2009. Pharmacol Ther 2009;123:143–150.
88. aan het Rot M, Collins KA, Murrough JW, et al. Safety and efficacy of repeated-dose intravenous ketamine for treatment-resistant depression. Biol Psychiatry 2010;67:139–145.
89. Ono S, Ogawa K, Yamashita K, et al. Conformational analysis of the NMDA receptor antagonist (1S,2R)-1-phenyl-2-[S-1-aminopropyl]-N,N-diethylcyclopropanecarboxamide (PPDC) designed by a novel conformational restriction method based on the structural feature of cyclopropane ring. Chem Pharm Bull (Tokyo) 2002;50:966–968.
90. Valdoxan. http://www.valdoxan.com/index.php/summary-of-product-characteristics/#E52. Accessed November 14, 2010.
91. Holmes A, Heilig M, Rupniak NM, et al. Neuropeptide systems as novel therapeutic targets for depression and anxiety disorders. Trends Pharmacol Sci 2003;24:580–588.
92. Hokfelt T, Bartfai T, Bloom F. Neuropeptides: opportunities for drug discovery. Lancet Neurol 2003;2:463–472.
93. De Souza EB, Grigoriadis DE. Corticotropin-releasing factor: physiology, pharmacology and role in central nervous system disorders. In: Davis KL, Charney D, Coyle JT, et al., eds. Neuropsychopharmacology: The Fifth Generation of Progress. Baltimore, MD: Lippincott Williams & Wilkins, 2002:91–109.
94. Kramer MS, Cutler N, Feighner J, et al. Distinct mechanism for antidepressant activity by blockade of central substance P receptors. Science 1998;281:1640–1645.
95. Vrontakis ME. Galanin: a biologically active peptide. Curr Drug Targets CNS Neurol Disord 2002;1:531–541.
96. Feighner JP, Nicolau G, Abajian H, et al. Clinical pharmacokinetic studies with INN 00835 (nemifitide), a novel pentapeptide antidepressant. Biopharm Drug Dispos 2002;23:33–39.
97. Ehrensing RH, Kastin AJ, Wurzlow GF, et al. Improvement in major depression after low subcutaneous doses of MIF-1. J Affect Disord 1994;31:227–233.
98. Ioannides C. Pharmacokinetic interactions between herbal remedies and medicinal drugs. Xenobiotica 2002;32:451–478.
99. Muller WE, Singer A, Wonnemann M. Hyperforin—antidepressant activity by a novel mechanism of action. Pharmacopsychiatry 2001;34(Suppl 1):S98–S102.
100. Christopher EJ. Electroconvulsive therapy in the medically ill. Curr Psychiatry Rep 2003;5:225–230.

Chapter 19

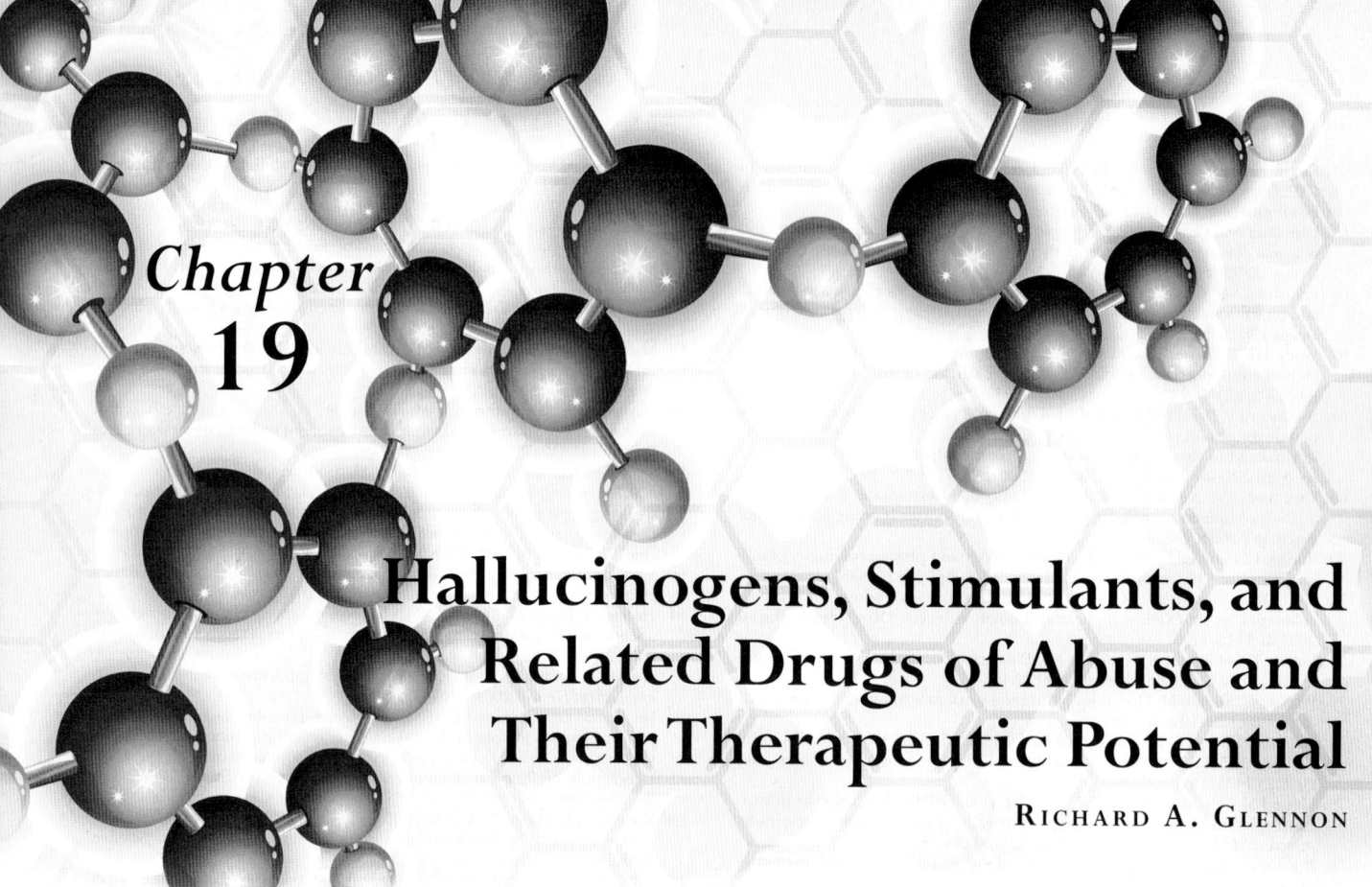

Hallucinogens, Stimulants, and Related Drugs of Abuse and Their Therapeutic Potential

RICHARD A. GLENNON

Abbreviations

A, adenosine
ADHD, attention-deficient hyperactivity disorder
2-AG, 2-arachidonylglycerol
cAMP, cyclic adenosine monophosphate
CB, cannabinoid
CBD, cannabidiol
DA, dopamine
DARPP-32, dopamine- and cAMP-regulated phosphoprotein, 32 kd
DET, *N,N*-diethyltryptamine
DMA, dimethoxyphenyl-2-aminopropane
DMH, 1,1-dimethylheptyl
DMT, *N,N*-dimethyltryptamine
DOB, 1-(4-bromo-2,5-dimethoxyphenyl)-2-aminopropane
DOI, 1-(2,5-dimethoxy-4-methylphenyl)-2-aminopropane
DOM, 1-(2,5-dimethoxy-4-methylphenyl)-2-aminopropane
DPT, *N,N*-di-*n*-propyltryptamine
d-TMP, d-*threo*-methylphenidate
ED_{50}, median effective dose
α-EtT, α-ethyltryptamine
FAAH, fatty acid amide hydrolase
GABA, γ-aminobutyric acid
GPCR, G protein–coupled receptor
5-HT, serotonin
IP_3, inositol triphosphate
LSD, lysergic acid diethylamide
MAGL, monoacylglycerol lipase
MAO, monoamine oxidase
MDA, 1-(3,4-methylenedioxyphenyl)-2-aminopropane
MDMA, *N*-methyl-1-(3,4-methylenedioxyphenyl)-2-aminopropane
MET, MethylEthylTryptamine or more correctly *N*-ethyl-*N*-methyltryptamine
α-MeT, α-methyltryptamine
NANM, *N*-allylnormetazocine
NE, norepinephrine
NMDA, *N*-methyl-D-aspartate
5-OMe α-Met, 5-methoxy-α-methyltryptamine
PCA, para-chloroamphetamine
PCP, phencyclidine
PDE, phosphodiesterase
PKA, phosphokinase A
PLC, phospholipase C
PMA, para-methoxyamphetamine
PMMA, *N*-methyl-1-(4-methoxyphenyl)-2-aminopropane
PP-1, protein phosphatase-1
PP-2A, protein phosphatase-2A
pTAP, 1-(para-tolyl)-2-aminopropane
REM, rapid eye movement
SAR, structure–activity relationship
Ser^{137}, $serine^{137}$
SSRI, selective serotonin reuptake inhibitor
Δ^9-THC, Δ^9-tetrahydrocannabinol
Thr^{34}, $threonine^{34}$
TMA, trimethoxyphenyl-2-aminopropane

SCENARIO

Mark D. Watanabe, PharmD, PhD, BCPP

JN, a 23-year-old male athlete from the United States, was offered some tablets of "flatliners" while at a dance club during a vacation in London. Having never tried them before, JN had heard that it was somehow related to "Ecstasy" and was willing to accept the offer. Shortly after ingestion, he felt his energy level increasing, his heart beating faster and stronger, and some of his anxiety about being in a foreign country going away. Eventually, he danced for several hours without stopping.

(The reader is directed to the clinical solution and chemical analysis of this case at the end of the chapter).

PSYCHOTOMIMETIC/HALLUCINOGENIC AGENTS

Why study psychotomimetic/hallucinogenic agents? It has been argued that investigations of such agents might shed light on mental illnesses and their potential treatment. Although studies with such agents have certainly contributed to our understanding of mental disorders, it is now recognized that there are many kinds of mental illnesses and that the actions—and putative mechanisms of action—of psychotomimetic/hallucinogenic agents are only tangentially related to their etiology or treatment. It has also been argued that investigations of psychotomimetic/hallucinogenic agents might contribute to a greater general understanding of basic neurochemical mechanisms and neurotransmitter function. This research approach has been much more rewarding. Studies with such agents have contributed *significantly* to what is currently known about G protein–coupled receptors (GCPRs) (e.g., cannabinoid receptors and serotonin [5-HT] receptors) and ion channel receptors (e.g., phencyclidine [PCP] receptors and excitatory amino acid receptors). Subsequent work with these receptors has identified new receptor subtypes that are being targeted for the development of novel therapeutic agents. Indeed, the past 10 to 20 years have witnessed an explosion of interest in the investigation of psychoactive substances because of their relevance to neurochemical mechanisms. Another important reason to study psychotomimetic agents is because they represent a large group of abused substances, and pharmacists are members of a health care team responsible for the dissemination of drug abuse prevention and treatment information. In addition, the past one to two decades have seen the popularization of controlled substance analogs (i.e., *designer drugs*), and the future will likely witness the introduction of yet more. So, yet another reason to study these agents is to prepare for the future: An understanding of presently available agents and their structure–activity relationships (SARs) will be instructive because many designer drugs emanate from the clandestine application of these same SAR principles at the street level. Also, some agents currently in clinical use possess abuse liability that is underrecognized. An understanding of how these drugs work can lead to new treatment modalities. Finally, investigations of these agents presage the development of novel therapies for the treatment of various neuropsychiatric, neurologic, and other disorders (see later discussion).

DEFINITIONS AND CLASSIFICATION

"Psychotomimetics" and "hallucinogens" are commonly used terms, and they are frequently used interchangeably. However, little agreement exists regarding what constitutes such agents or exactly what they do. Because the actions of these agents are largely subjective, the best information should come from those who experience these agents; yet, by experiencing their effect, one might not be in the best position to accurately describe the effects they produce (1b). In contrast, an "outside" observer can never fully and accurately describe the effects of these agents. This has led to problems of definition. The most widely accepted definition of a psychotomimetic substance is that provided by Hollister (2): Psychotomimetic/hallucinogenic agents are those that upon administration of a single effective dose consistently produce changes in thought, mood, and perception with little memory impairment; produce little stupor, narcosis, or excessive stimulation; produce minimal autonomic side effects; and are nonaddicting.

Although certain opioid analgesics occasionally produce psychotomimetic effects, they are effectively eliminated from this category of agents because they do not meet the necessary criteria (e.g., they can be addicting). Likewise, chronic administration of high doses of stimulants, such as amphetamine and cocaine, sometimes produce hallucinogenic episodes (i.e., amphetamine psychosis and cocaine psychosis). These agents are not considered to be hallucinogens, however, because multiple doses typically are required to produce this effect. The Hollister criteria served a very useful function in narrowing the list of agents that

CLINICAL SIGNIFICANCE

The manipulation of structure-activity relationships to alter pharmacological activity for recreational benefit lies at the heart of the "designer drug" concept. The clinical impact is clearly evident in the class of drugs discussed in this chapter, i.e., hallucinogens and stimulants. Many of the illicit street drugs intended to produce euphoria and enhanced awareness were developed based on an understanding of how specific modifications in chemical structure can lead to desired changes in bioavailability and pharmacodynamics. Unfortunately, although these approaches provide greater insight regarding the scientific basis of drug action, they are not without risk.

In a recent editiorial (1a), David Nichols, whose laboratory studied the MDMA ("ecstasy") analogue 4-methylthioamphetamine (4-MTA) in the 1990s, lamented the eventual consequences of his published research that resulted in motivating street chemists to synthesize 4-MTA for use as a club drug. Given the putative mechanism of action of 4-MTA, its inappropriate use has led to some potentially predictable fatalities due to elevated serotonin levels. Dr. Nichols' concerns highlight a central challenge of medicinal chemistry in drug development: for every alteration in molecular structure intended for improved therapeutic efficacy and safety, there is often a parallel possibility of increasing abuse and toxicity.

Mark D. Watanabe, PharmD, PhD, BCPP
Assistant Clinical Specialist
Department of Pharmacy Practice
Northeastern University
Boston, MA

belong to this category of drugs, and Hollister was able to identify several classes of psychotomimetic agents: lysergic acid derivatives (e.g., lysergic acid diethylamide [LSD]), phenylethylamines (e.g., mescaline), indolealkylamines (e.g., *N,N*-dimethyltryptamine), other indolic derivatives (e.g., ibogaine and the harmala derivatives), piperidyl benzilate esters (e.g., JB-329), phenylcyclohexyl compounds (e.g., PCP), and miscellaneous agents (e.g., kawain, dimethylacetamide, and cannabinoids) (2).

Over time, it was demonstrated that *psychotomimetic agents* represent a *behaviorally heterogeneous* class of psychoactive agents. For example, human subjects can readily differentiate between the actions produced by certain agents in this category, and cross-tolerance develops among some of these agents but not between others. Likewise, it is possible to differentiate between the actions of certain of these agents in humans and using various animal procedures. Subcategorization was necessary. Today, it is well recognized that some psychotomimetics/hallucinogens act primarily via a serotonergic mechanism, that cannabinoids produce many of their behavioral effects via cannabinoid receptors, and that PCP-like agents produce their effects via PCP receptors. This is not to imply that there now exists a full understanding of how these agents work, but it does support the concept that these agents do not belong to a homogeneous mechanistic class.

Human Versus Animal Studies: Applicability of Animal Models

Human subjects should be best suited to provide the most reliable assessment of the actions and potency of psychotomimetic agents, and considerable human data are available for some agents. However, much less information is available for most. Often, what human information is available comes from studies that were not well controlled, that included limited subject populations, or that investigated only a few drug doses. Some of what is known even comes from anecdotal reports. Very few clinical studies with psychotomimetic agents were sanctioned following the early 1960s. Although some human evaluations are once again being allowed, for a period of approximately 30 years, information concerning psychotomimetic substances relied—and continues to rely—heavily on the use of animal studies. This raises several questions: Do animal models exist that can accurately reflect human hallucinogenic activity? Indeed, do animals hallucinate? Many attempts have been made to develop animal models of psychotomimetic/hallucinogenic activity, but to date, no single animal model can account for the actions of these agents as a class (3).

Drug Discrimination Paradigm

One animal technique that has seen widespread application for the investigation of psychoactive agents is the drug discrimination paradigm (4). It must be emphasized at the outset that this method does not represent a model of psychotomimetic activity. Indeed, the technique has general applicability and has been employed to study a wide variety of centrally acting agents, including stimulants, antidepressants, barbiturates, anxiolytics, opiates, and many other drug classes. The technique may be viewed as a "*drug detection*" procedure. Specifically, animals (typically rats, pigeons, or monkeys) are trained to recognize or *discriminate* the stimulus effects of a training drug from vehicle; humans have also been used as subjects in some drug discrimination studies. Many centrally acting agents produce an interoceptive cue, or stimulus, that subjects recognize. When animals are used, they are taught to make a particular response (e.g., to respond on one lever of a two-lever operant apparatus or Skinner box) when administered a training drug and to make a different response (e.g., to respond on the second of the two levers) when administered saline vehicle. After a period of time, the animals learn the stimulus cue and associate it with one of the two levers; that is, the animals make >80% of their responses on the training-drug lever (i.e., >80% drug-appropriate responding) when administered the training dose of the training drug, and <20% of their responses on the same lever, when administered vehicle. Doses of training drug less than those of the training dose result in a decreased percentage of drug-appropriate responding. The effect is dose related, and a dose–response curve can be constructed. A median effective dose (ED_{50} value) can be calculated as a measure of potency.

Once trained, these animals can be used in what is referred to as tests of substitution or stimulus transfer (i.e., tests of stimulus generalization). In such tests, other agents (i.e., challenge drugs) are administered to the animals to determine if they produce stimulus effects similar to those of the training drug. Stimulus generalization is said to have occurred when animals make >80% of their responses on the training drug–appropriate lever following administration of some dose of challenge drug. Stimulus generalization or substitution implies that the *challenge drug* and the *training drug* are producing similar stimulus effects in the animals. It should be noted that no claim has ever been made that the agents—the training drug and a challenge drug—are producing identical effects; rather, there is an implication that the agents are capable of producing a common stimulus effect or a behavioral cue common to the two agents (e.g., a drug that produces effects A and B may be recognized by animals trained to a drug that produces effects B and C; although this is an uncommon occurrence, it should be recognized that it is possible). Thus, not only is it possible to determine if two agents are producing similar stimulus effects, it is also possible to compare their relative potencies by calculating an ED_{50} value for the challenge drug. Hence, results are qualitative and quantitative.

Other studies that can be conducted are tests of stimulus antagonism. That is, a specific training drug can be administered together with another agent; if the combination results in <20% training drug–appropriate responding, stimulus antagonism is said to have occurred. Although this technique can be used in the development of novel antagonists for a series of agents for which an antagonist is unknown, it is more common to use receptor-selective antagonists to investigate mechanisms of action. Drug discrimination, then, is a very powerful tool for investigating the actions and mechanisms of action of many different kinds of centrally acting agents. Specific examples of stimulus generalization and stimulus antagonists will be described later.

The drug discrimination procedure has seen broad application in the investigation of centrally acting agents, and a wide variety of different training drugs has been used. When a psychotomimetic/hallucinogenic agent is used as the training drug, it should be possible to identify other agents that produce similar stimulus effects (5). In this manner, it has been demonstrated that the psychotomimetics represent a behaviorally heterogeneous group of agents, much in the same way that humans have been able to differentiate the effects of these agents. Animals trained to discriminate LSD, for example, do not recognize PCP, and animals trained to discriminate PCP do not recognize LSD. Neither LSD- nor PCP-trained animals recognize tetrahydrocannabinol (Δ^9-THC). However, LSD-trained animals recognize mescaline, 1-(2,5-dimethoxy-4-methylphenyl)-2-aminopropane (DOM), and certain other hallucinogens. Using this technique, then, it has been possible to identify what are termed "*classical hallucinogens*" (6). The classical hallucinogens are LSD-like agents that share common discriminative stimulus properties and that might act via a common mechanism of action. The remaining psychotomimetic agents will be referred to here as nonclassical agents; these groups of agents act by different mechanisms and produce distinct effects common to members within each group.

PSYCHOACTIVE DRUGS OF ABUSE: NONCLASSICAL AGENTS

The term "*nonclassical agents*" is used here to differentiate these psychoactive agents from the *classical hallucinogens* that will be discussed later in this chapter. Several categories of agents are described here, but there is no implication that these classes of agents produce similar effects or act via similar mechanisms.

Cannabinoids

The marijuana or cannabis plant represents one of the oldest and most widely used psychoactive substances in the world and has been cultivated since approximately 6000 BC. Botanically, there are three major species of the plant—*Cannabis sativa*, *Cannabis indica*, and *Cannabis ruderalis*. Reference is made to three preparations, listed here in order of increasing potency: *Bhang* typically refers to the leaves and stems of the plant, *ganja* is prepared from the flowering tops of the plant, and *hashish* is the pure resin. Although marijuana is orally active, inhalation by smoking is more frequently used as a route of administration. One of the major active constituents of the plant is Δ^9-THC (often referred to simply as THC). Δ^9-THC is rapidly and efficiently absorbed by inhalation; it is absorbed into body tissue and is slowly released back into circulation. Deuterium-labeled Δ^9-THC has been detected in human plasma up to nearly 2 weeks postadministration. A major metabolite of Δ^9-THC is 11-hydroxy-Δ^9-THC. Evidence suggests that tolerance develops to Δ^9-THC and that it does not usually lead to physical dependence. Marijuana can produce impairment of performance, memory, and learning; controversy exists over whether it produces an amotivational syndrome.

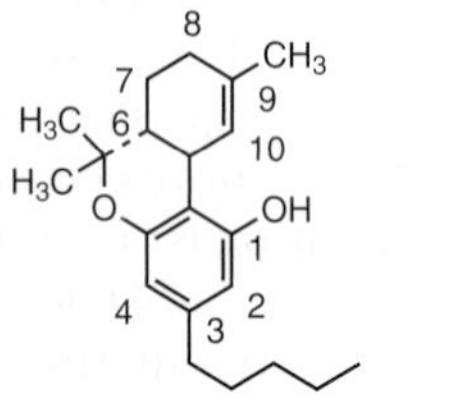

Δ^9-Tetrahydrocannabinol (Δ^9-THC)

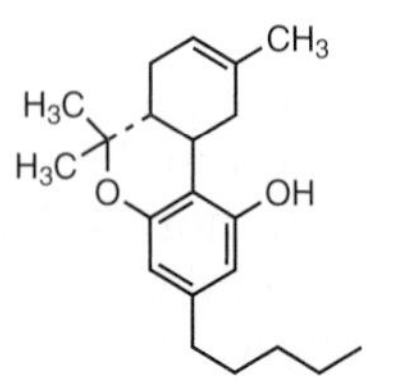

Δ^8-Tetrahydrocannabinol

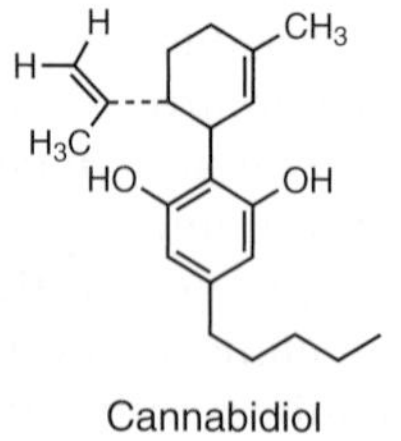

Cannabidiol

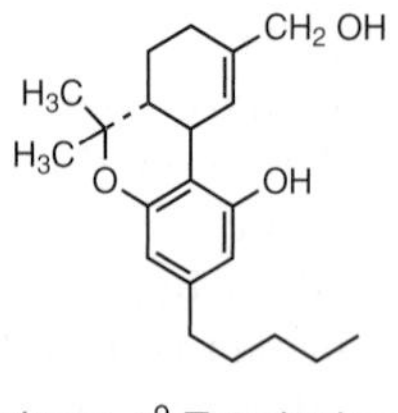

11–Hydroxy–Δ^9-Tetrahydrocannabinol (11-OH-Δ^9-THC)

Over the years, many cannabinoids and related structures (i.e., synthetic cannabinoids), such as CP-55,940 and nabilone (a mixture of *trans* isomers: *RR* and *SS*), were prepared and evaluated (7–9). Noncannabinoids, such as WIN-55,212-2 and JWH-018, can also produce THC-like actions. An herbal product commonly known as Spice or K2 has been shown to contain various synthetic cannabinoids including JWH-018.

The pyrazole analog rimonabant (SR141716A) was found to be one of the first cannabinoid antagonists, and extensive studies were conducted to help unravel the actions of cannabinoids such as Δ^9-THC (7,8). Rimonabant effectively attenuated the effects of Δ^9-THC and WIN-55,212-2 (7) as well as the discriminative stimulus effects of Δ^9-THC. Thus, in addition to cannabinoids and cannabinoid-related structures such as CP-55,940 and nabilone, there are other structural classes of cannabinoid ligands, including indolic derivatives such as WIN-55,212–2 and JWH-018, pyrazoles such as rimonabant, and fatty acid derivatives such as anandamide and 2-arachidonylglycerol (2-AG).

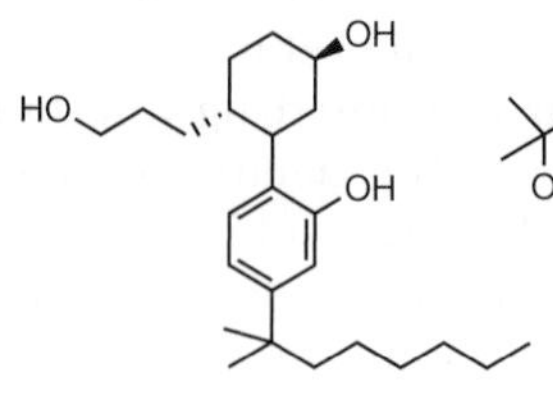

CP-55,940

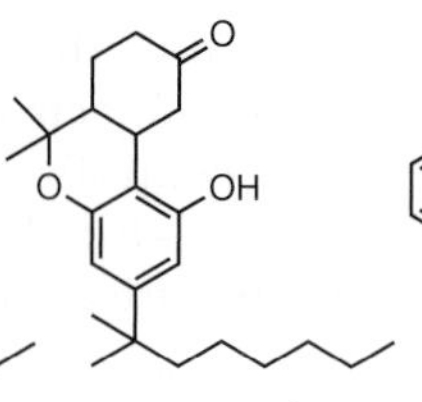

Nabilone (*trans* mixture)

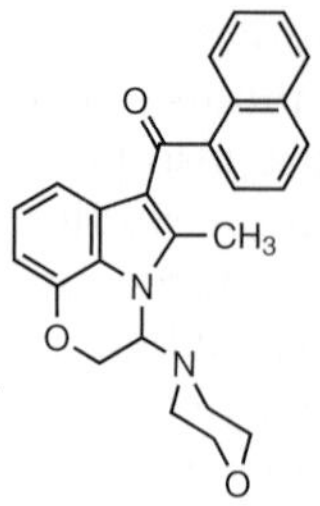

WIN-55,212-2

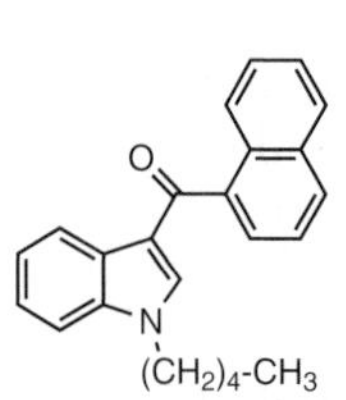

JWH-018

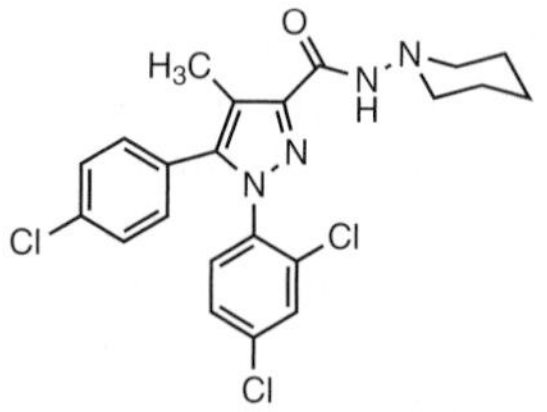

Rimonabant

Mechanism of Action

For many years, it was thought that Δ^9-THC acts in a nonspecific manner; however, in the early 1990s, two populations of cannabinoid (CB) receptors were identified: CB-1 and CB-2 receptors (8,9). Human forms of these receptors have been cloned, and both types are G protein–coupled, seven-helix transmembrane-spanning receptors. These receptors are differentially expressed: CB-1 receptors, which likely mediate the psychoactive effects of THC-related agents, are found primarily in the brain, whereas CB-2 receptors, which possibly are involved in immunomodulatory (and other) actions, are found almost exclusively in the periphery. The identification of such receptors suggested the possible existence of an endogenous ligand, and several now have been identified. The best investigated of these is the eicosanoid derivative arachidonylethanolamide or anandamide. Anandamide binds at CB-1 receptors with an affinity similar to that of Δ^9-THC (10). Related structures have also been identified including docosatetraenylethanolamide and homo-γ-linolenylethanolamide (10). Pharmacologically, anandamide seems to be a THC-like agent. Although the actions of anandamide may not be identical to those of Δ^9-THC, particularly regarding in vivo studies, differences may be related to the metabolic instability of anandamide. For example, in drug discrimination studies, a Δ^9-THC stimulus failed to consistently or reliably generalize to anandamide; however, the more metabolically stable methanandamide, a chain-methylated analog of anandamide, produced THC-like effects. Furthermore, methanandamide has been used as a training drug, and the methanandamide stimulus generalizes to Δ^9-THC (11). Another type of endocannabinoid is 2-AG (12). Despite their structural similarity, anandamide-type endocannabinoids are metabolized primarily by fatty acid amide hydrolase (FAAH), whereas

2-AG is metabolized mainly by monoacylglycerol lipase (MAGL) (8,9). It is now recognized that cannabinoids and synthetic cannabinoids influence the *endocannabinoid system.* The endocannabinoid system is composed of endogenous cannabinoids (i.e., endocannabinoids), enzymes that synthesize and degrade them, and cannabinoid receptors (12).

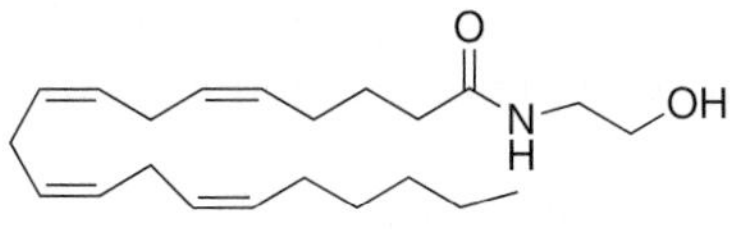

Anandamide

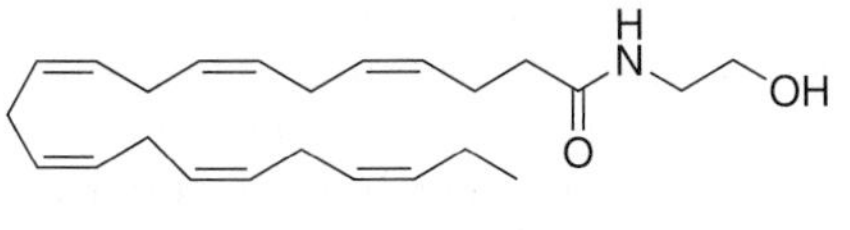

Docosatetraenoylethanolamide

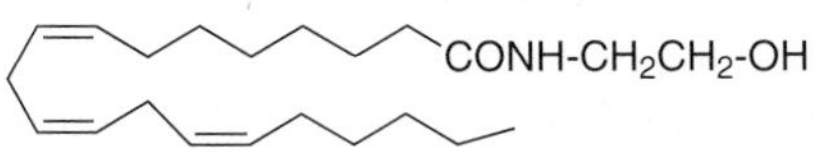

Homo-γ-linolenylethanolamide

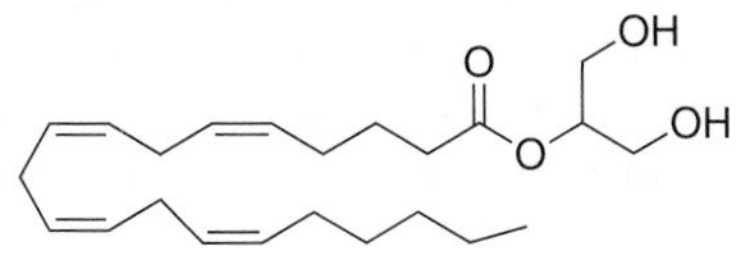

2-Arachidonylglycerol

Structure–Activity Relationships

Structure–activity relationships (SARs) both for THC-like actions and for CB receptor binding have been formulated (7,9). Structure–activity studies can be discussed on the basis of several different types of behavioral assays in rodents, and it has been shown for 60 cannabinoids that behavioral potencies are highly correlated with receptor binding affinities (13). THC-like discriminative effects probably offer a more specific method of detecting and measuring cannabimimetic effects and are particularly useful for formulating SARs (4). Using this approach, it has been demonstrated that SARs for THC-like stimulus effects are not necessarily identical to those for the analgesic, antiemetic, or anticonvulsant actions of cannabinoids. An early study showed that animals trained to discriminate intraperitoneal dosing of Δ^9-THC recognized hashish smoke and that animals trained to discriminate hashish smoke recognized Δ^9-THC, supporting the concept that Δ^9-THC likely accounts for the stimulus actions of hashish. A number of cannabinoids now have been evaluated. Cannabidiol (CBD), for example, does not produce THC-like stimulus effects. Relative to Δ^9-THC (ED_{50} = 0.43 mg/kg intraperitoneal), some 11-hydroxy metabolites are quite potent, such as 11-OH Δ^9-THC (ED_{50} = 0.10 mg/kg) and 11-OH Δ^8-THC (ED_{50} = 0.38 mg/kg). One of the more potent cannabinoids is Δ^8-THC-DMH (ED_{50} = 0.05 mg/kg), in which the 4-pentyl moiety of THC has been replaced with a 1,1-dimethylheptyl (DMH) group; its 11-hydroxyl analog, 11-OH Δ^8-THC-DMH (ED_{50} = 0.002 mg/kg), is even more potent (4). One of the most extensively studied cannabinoid ligands is WIN-55,212-2. Molecular modeling and site-directed mutagenesis studies suggest that cannabinoids, CP-55,940, and anandamide bind in a similar fashion but in a manner that differs from the binding of WIN-55,212-2.

Therapeutic Potential

The discovery of CB-1 and CB-2 receptors, CB receptor antagonists, agents showing selectivity between the two CB receptor populations, endocannabinoids, and novel chemical tools with which to investigate these receptors (7,9,14) has generated renewed interest in the cannabinoids. Already approved for use are dronabinol (Marinol) and nabilone (Cesamet). Dronabinol is the synthetic *trans*-(−)-isomer of Δ^9-THC, whereas nabilone is a synthetic chromenone derivative (a mixture of *RR* and *SS* isomers). Both are approved for treatment of chemotherapy-induced nausea and vomiting, as well as for the anorexia and weight loss seen in patients with AIDS. Sativex, whose major active ingredients are natural Δ^9-THC and CBD, is approved for use in several countries (not in the United States) for the treatment of neuropathic pain and spasticity associated with multiple sclerosis.

The CB-1 selective antagonist rimonabant was in clinical trials for the treatment of obesity, but its U.S. New Drug Application was withdrawn due to increased risk of suicidal ideation. Related analogs are still under investigation. CB-2 antagonists are being explored for their use in chronic pain, and several classes of FAAH inhibitors are being examined for their analgesic and anxiolytic actions (12). Various other compounds that influence the endocannabinoid system are being investigated for the treatment of glaucoma, Tourette syndrome, Parkinson disease, epilepsy, drug abuse, immune disorders, and several types of neuropsychiatric disorders (12,15).

PCP-Related Agents

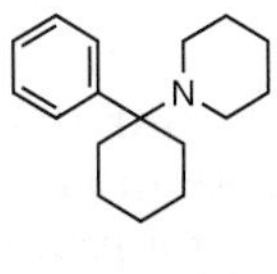

Phencyclidine (PCP)

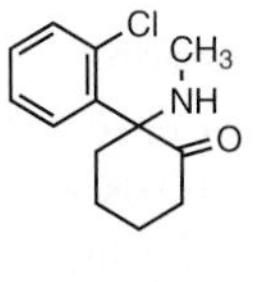

Ketamine

PCP [1-(1-phenylcyclohexyl)piperidine] was introduced as a dissociative anesthetic during the late 1950s. Shortly after its introduction, clinical studies were terminated because of the occurrence of schizophrenic-like psychotomimetic effects (i.e., PCP can be considered a true *psychotomimetic* agent), particularly during emergence from anesthesia. This might have been the end of the story except that additional attempts were made to exploit the anesthetic effects of PCP, leading to the development of novel agents such as ketamine; it was theorized that PCP-like states might provide a good model for investigating schizophrenia, leading to studies of PCP's mechanism of action; and PCP (e.g., "Angel Dust"), administered by inhalation, injection, ingestion, or smoking (as with PCP-laced parsley, tobacco, or marijuana), and ketamine (e.g., "Special K") emerged as drugs of abuse, leading to investigations of their abuse liability. Shortly thereafter, it was discovered that PCP behaves as an *N*-methyl-D-aspartate (NMDA) antagonist. Because NMDA receptors had been implicated in seizures and trauma, PCP and related arylcycloalkylamines were explored as potential antiepileptics and neuroprotective agents. Furthermore, because PCP is relatively easy to manufacture, it has become popular on the clandestine market, particularly being used among children and young adolescents (16,17).

Actions

In humans, PCP can produce disorientation, confusion, incoordination, delirium, impaired memory, and euphoria (17,18); higher doses produce additional adverse effects including death. PCP has a history of producing aggression and violent behavior. Because PCP often is consumed together with other substances, it sometimes has been difficult to establish exactly which effects are produced by PCP and which might be related to possible drug interactions. PCP has seen extensive investigation in animals, and it appears to produce effects similar to those of amphetamine-like stimulants and central depressants. PCP is self-administered by animals, and tolerance develops to its behavioral effects upon repeated exposure to the drug (18). PCP has both direct and indirect effects on dopaminergic systems; this might account, at least in part, for some of the amphetamine-like effects of PCP and might contribute to the production of its schizophrenic-like actions. The PCP model of schizophrenia was particularly attractive because PCP seemed to produce both the positive and negative symptoms associated with this disorder. PCP has also been widely investigated as a training drug in animals using drug discrimination studies (4).

Mechanism of Action

N-Allylnormetazocine (NANM; SKF-10047) produces some effects reminiscent of those produced by PCP. At one time, NANM was considered a prototypic σ opiate receptor ligand. It is now recognized that the σ receptors are *not* a class of opioid receptors and that the low-affinity NANM is only one of very few opiates that bind at these receptors. Subsequent structure–activity studies showed that NANM simply possesses certain minimal pharmacophoric features that are required for σ receptor binding (19). Nevertheless, the behavioral similarities between NANM and PCP led to early investigations regarding the binding of PCP at σ receptors, and because of its affinity (albeit low) for these receptors, the σ receptors were renamed NANM-PCP receptors or σ/PCP receptors. This confusion continued for several years until it was demonstrated that agents with much higher affinity and selectivity than PCP for σ receptors failed to produce PCP-like actions in animals (18). Later, it was shown that PCP antagonizes the effects of the excitatory amino acid NMDA. [^{3}H]PCP has been used to label putative PCP binding sites, and PCP binding and NMDA binding display similar regional distribution in brain. It is established that PCP is a noncompetitive NMDA receptor antagonist.

The NMDA receptor (Fig. 19.1) is a ligand-gated ion channel receptor that regulates the flow of cations (Na^+, Ca^{2+}) into certain neurons. The receptor complex possesses multiple binding sites, similar to the benzodiazepine/γ-aminobutyric acid (GABA) receptor complex that allows the binding of glutamate, glycine, polyamines, and other ligands that can modulate the actions of NMDA. Like the NMDA antagonist dizocilpine (MK-801), PCP binds at a site (i.e., the PCP site) that is believed to be located within the ion channel. Drug discrimination studies have shown that PCP-trained animals recognize NMDA antagonists that bind at PCP receptors; for example, MK-801 is nearly 10-fold more potent than PCP. Furthermore, animals trained to discriminate MK-801 recognize PCP and other PCP-related agents. Consistent with early findings that PCP produces a psychotic state in humans, PCP has been shown to produce a pattern of metabolic, neurochemical, and behavioral changes in animals that reproduce almost exactly those seen in patients with schizophrenia. Consequently, this provides new insight regarding the mechanisms underlying such disorders and offers an animal model for the evaluation of novel antipsychotic agents (20).

Structure–Activity Relationships

SARs for PCP-like actions have not been particularly well defined, and what little is known stems primarily from drug discrimination studies. The PCP stimulus does not generalize to opioids, sympathomimetic stimulants, anticholinergic agents, or classical hallucinogens and only partially generalizes to depressants, such as barbiturates. In general, the stimulus properties of PCP are not shared by members

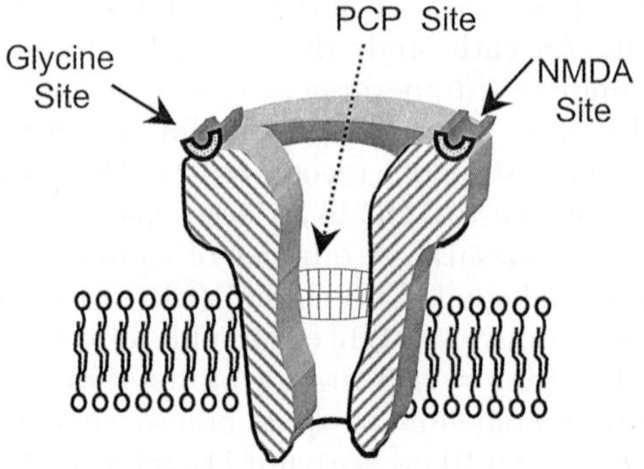

FIGURE 19.1 NMDA ion channel receptor showing binding sites for glycine, NMDA, and PCP.

of other drug classes (21). The PCP stimulus generalizes to ketamine and other structurally related derivatives of PCP, such as TCP, an analog of PCP in which the phenyl ring has been replaced by the isosteric 2-thienyl group.

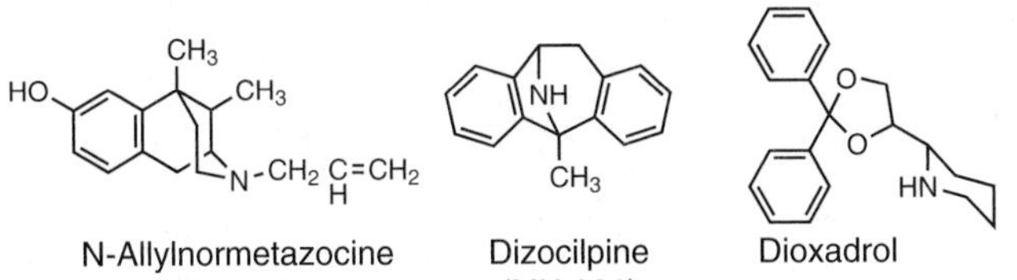

PCP does not possess a chiral center. Several 1,3-dioxolanes possessing an asymmetric center produce PCP-like effects and have proven to be useful for investigating PCP-like actions. Dioxadrol, or 2-(2,2-diphenyl-1,3-dioxolan-4-yl)piperidine, and etoxadrol (i.e., dioxadrol in which one of the phenyl groups has been replaced by an ethyl group) are examples of such dioxolanes. The (+)-isomer of dioxadrol, dexoxodrol, but not the (−)-isomer levoxadrol, binds at PCP receptors and is recognized by PCP-trained animals (21).

PSYCHOACTIVE DRUGS OF ABUSE: CLASSICAL HALLUCINOGENS

Classical hallucinogens are agents that meet the Hollister definition (2) and that, in addition, bind at 5-HT_2 receptors and are recognized by DOM-trained animals in tests of stimulus generalization (5). The classical hallucinogens all possess the general structure Ar-C-C-N, where Ar is a substituted phenyl, 3-indolyl, or substituted 3-indolyl moiety; C-C is an ethyl or branched ethyl chain; and N is a primary, secondary, or tertiary amine. This will be further discussed. (See Chapter 10 for additional information on 5-HT receptors.)

Classification

There are two major structural categories of classical or arylalkylamine hallucinogens: the *indolealkylamines* and the *phenylalkylamines.* The indolealkylamines are further divided into the simple *N*-substituted tryptamines, the α-alkyltryptamines, the ergolines (or lysergamides), and, tentatively, the β-carbolines. The phenylalkylamines consist of phenylethylamines and phenylisopropylamines. In humans, examples from the different categories seem to produce similar effects. It should be noted, however, that relatively few agents have been examined in comprehensive and carefully controlled clinical situations. Furthermore, no claim is made that these agents produce identical effects in humans. Each category—and, indeed, even certain examples from within a given category—may produce effects that make them somewhat different from the others. As if to underscore the behavioral similarity among these agents, however, examples from each of the above categories produce common DOM-like stimulus effects in animals (Table 19.1).

TABLE 19.1 Results of Stimulus Generalization Studies with Examples from the Various Categories of Classical Hallucinogens Using Animals Trained to Discriminate DOM from Vehicle

Category	Example	ED_{50} Value for DOM-Stimulus Generalization (mg/kg)[a]
N-Alkyltryptamines	DMT	5.8
α-Alkyltryptamines	α-MeT	3.1
Lysergamides	(+)LSD	0.05
β-Carbolines	Harmaline	6.2
Phenylethylamines	Mescaline	14.6
Phenylisopropylamines	DOB	0.2

[a]Data from Glennon and Young (4) and Glennon (5).
DMT, *N,N*-dimethyltryptamine; DOB, 2-(4-bromo-2,5-dimethoxyphenyl)-1-aminopropane; LSD, lysergic acid diethylamide; α-MeT, α-methyltryptamine.

Indolealkylamines

N-Alkyltryptamines

One of the best-investigated hallucinogens is *N,N*-dimethyltryptamine (DMT) (Table 19.2), which is the prototype of this subclass of agents. Although readily synthesized in the laboratory, DMT is also a naturally occurring substance. Its actions are characterized by a rapid onset (typically <5 minutes) and short duration of action (~30 minutes). Like some other members of this family, DMT is not active via oral administration; it is generally administered by inhalation or by smoking. Although less common, DMT can also be injected. Some indolealkylamines are sensitive to the acidic conditions of the stomach. The corresponding secondary amine, *N*-monomethyltryptamine, and primary amine, tryptamine, are inactive as psychoactive substances, both because they are not sufficiently lipophilic to readily penetrate the blood–brain barrier and because what little does get into the brain is rapidly metabolized by monoamine oxidase (MAO). Other tertiary amine derivatives, such as the *N*-ethyl-*N*-methyltryptamine, *N,N*-diethyltryptamine (DET), *N,N*-di-*n*-propyltryptamine (DPT), and some secondary amines, are also hallucinogenic in humans. If the *N*-alkyl or *N,N*-dialkyl substituents are bulky and lipophilic enough, these tryptamines can be orally active (Table 19.2).

The effect of substitution in the pyrrole portion of DMT has not been extensively investigated in humans. In contrast, substitution in the benzenoid ring can enhance or diminish potency depending on the specific nature and location of the substituents. Table 19.2 shows some of the more frequently encountered derivatives of DMT, their common names, and their approximate human potency. 5-HT is not hallucinogenic and does not readily penetrate the blood–brain barrier

TABLE 19.2 Psychoactive Indolealkylamine and Related Agents

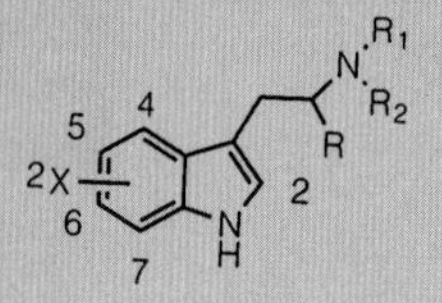

Agent	Common Name	R_1/R_2	R	X	Approximate Hallucinogenic Dose (mg)*	DOM Stimulus Generalization Poten cy(mg/kg)**
Tryptamine		H/H	H	H	Likely inactive	Inactive
N-Methyltryptamine	NMT	CH_3/H	H	H	Likely inactive	Inactive
(±)α-Methyltryptamine	α–MeT	H/H	CH_3	H	5–20 (smoked) 15–30 (po)	3.13
N,N-Dimethyltryptamine	DMT	CH_3/CH_3	H	H	60–100 (smoked) 4–30(iv)	5.80
N,N-Diethyltryptamine	DET	C_2H_5/C_2H_5	H	H	50–100 (po)	2.45
N-Ethyl-N-methyltryptamine	MET	C_2H_5/CH_3	H	H	Unknown	—
N,N-Di-n-propyltryptamine	DPT	$n\text{-}C_3H_7/n\text{-}C_3H_7$	H	H	100–250 (po)	2.20
N,N-Di-isopropyltryptamine	DIPT	$i\text{-}C_3H_7/i\text{-}C_3H_7$	H	H	25–100 (po)	2.60
(±)α-Ethyltryptamine	α-EtT	H/H	C_2H_5	H	100–150 (po)	6.62
4-Hydroxy DMT	Psilocin	CH_3/CH_3	H	4-OH	10–20 (po)	—
4-Methoxy DMT	4-OMe DMT	CH_3/CH_3	H	$4\text{-}OCH_3$	Unknown	3.53
5-Hydroxytryptamine	5-HT	H/H	H	5-OH	Inactive	Inactive
5-OH DMT	Bufotenine	CH_3/CH_3	H	5-OH	Likely inactive	Inactive
5-Methoxy DMT	5-OMe DMT	CH_3/CH_3	H	$5\text{-}OCH_3$	6–20 (smoked) 2–3 (iv)	1.22
(±)5-Methoxy-α-MeT	5-OMe α-MeT	H/H	CH_3	$5\text{-}OCH_3$	2.5–4.5 (po)	0.50
6-Methoxy DMT	6-OMe DMT	CH_3/CH_3	H	$6\text{-}OCH_3$	Likely inactive	Inactive
7-Methoxy DMT	7-OMe DMT	CH_3/CH_3	H	$7\text{-}OCH_3$	Likely inactive	Inactive

*Data primarily from reference 22. Key: po = oral, iv = intravenous.
**Drugs were administered via the ip route reference 5.

when administered systemically. *N,N*-Dimethylserotonin [bufotenine (5-OH DMT)] has been reported to be a weak hallucinogen, but the results of human studies are controversial. It, too, likely does not readily penetrate the blood–brain barrier and produces considerable peripheral effects (e.g., facial flushing and cardiovascular actions) that prevent evaluation of an extended dose range. *O*-Methylation of bufotenine results in 5-OMe DMT, one of the more potent *N*-alkyltryptamines. A naturally occurring substance, 5-OMe DMT is a constituent of a number of plants used in various concoctions prepared by South American Indians for ceremonial and visionary purposes. Bufotenine and 5-OMe DMT are also found in the skin of certain frogs and may have given rise to the phenomenon of "toad licking." Psilocin is 4-hydroxy DMT. Like bufotenine, with a polar hydroxyl group, psilocin might not have been expected to enter the brain, yet it is hallucinogenic. Although this phenomenon has never been adequately explained, it has been speculated that the 4-hydroxyl group forms a hydrogen bond with the terminal amine and that this reduces polarity just enough that psilocin penetrates the blood–brain barrier. Psilocin and its phosphate ester, psilocybin, are widely found in certain species of mushrooms and have given rise to the terms "shrooms" and "shrooming." There are no reports that 6-methoxy DMT or 7-methoxy DMT are hallucinogenic. It is quite difficult to make strict potency comparisons within this series because of the different routes of administration that have been used (Table 19.2).

In tests of stimulus generalization, the DOM stimulus has been shown to generalize to DMT, DET, DPT,

4-OMe DMT, 5-OMe DMT, and a number of other DMT analogs, but not to 5-OH DMT, 6-OMe DMT, or 7-OMe DMT.

The metabolism of these agents has not been well investigated. The indolealkylamine 5-HT is a substrate for oxidative deamination by MAO. What evidence exists suggests that other indolealkylamines are also substrates for this enzyme system.

α-Alkyltryptamines

Tryptamine is not psychoactive. Introduction of an α-methyl group seemingly enhances lipophilicity and sufficiently protects against metabolism such that α-methyltryptamine (α-MeT) (Table 19.2) is approximately twice as potent as DMT. As a general rule of thumb, α-MeTs, where such agents have been investigated, typically are twice as potent as their corresponding DMT counterpart. Otherwise, their SAR is essentially the same as that of the DMT analogs. For example, 5-methoxy-α-methyltryptamine (5-OMe α-MeT) is approximately twice as potent as 5-OMe DMT. Introduction of the α-methyl group results in the creation of an asymmetric center, and the *S*-(+)-isomers of α-MeTs are more potent than their *R*-(−)-enantiomers. Homologation of the α-methyl group to an α-ethyl group affords α-ethyltryptamines. α-Ethyltryptamine (α-EtT) has been reported to be hallucinogenic, with effects somewhat distinguishable by human subjects from those of LSD and mescaline (23). Interestingly, α-EtT was clinically available during the early 1960s as an antidepressant because of its actions as an MAO inhibitor; however, it was removed from the market about a year after its introduction. It may be the MAO inhibitory effect that allowed the actions of α-EtT to be distinguished from those of LSD and mescaline (see also the later section on designer drugs). During the mid-1990s, α-EtT made an appearance on the clandestine market as a designer drug (i.e., "ET"). (±)-α-Methyltryptamine, (±)-5-methoxy-α-methyltryptamine and both of its optical isomers, and (±)-α-ethyltryptamine are recognized by DOM-trained animals in tests of stimulus generalization (4).

Ergolines or Lysergamides

(+)-LSD (i.e., LSD) is perhaps the best known—and, certainly, one of the most potent—of the classical hallucinogens. Although LSD itself is not naturally occurring, many related ergolines are found in nature. In terms of potency, LSD is at least 3,000-fold more potent than mescaline, with doses of 100 μg showing activity. Certain structurally modified analogs of LSD retain hallucinogenic activity; although many derivatives are possible, relatively few have been investigated in humans. Structural changes often can reduce the activity of a pharmacologically active substance. Here is an instance in which a structural change resulting in even a 1,000-fold decrease in potency can afford a very active agent. Some work has been reported on the SAR of LSD (24,25).

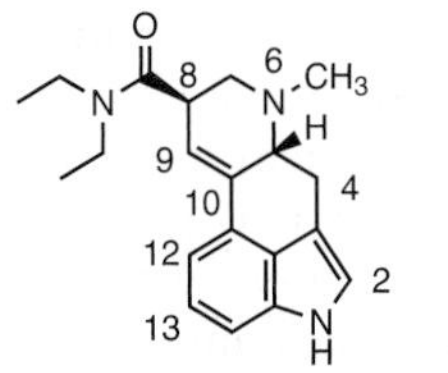

(+)Lysergic acid diethylamide
(LSD)

In humans, LSD has been thoroughly investigated (24); no other hallucinogen has been as extensively studied as this agent. Its actions in humans can be divided into three major categories: perceptual (altered shapes and colors and heightened sense of hearing), psychic (alterations in mood, depersonalization, visual hallucinations, and an altered sense of time), and somatic (nausea, blurred vision, and dizziness). In terms of principal effects, there seems to be little difference between LSD, psilocybin, and mescaline.

Although LSD has been sold on the clandestine market in tablet form, it is not uncommon to find this material available on "blotter paper" because of its high potency. A sheet of porous paper is impregnated with a solution of LSD, and the sheet can later be cut to afford the appropriate dose.

β-Carbolines

The β-carbolines represent a very interesting class of agents generally referred to as the harmala alkaloids. Several are naturally occurring. In South America, β-carbolines are constituents of certain vines and lianas (e.g., *Banisteriopsis caapi*), and in the Old World, β-carbolines are constituents of Syrian Rue (*Pegnum harmala*).

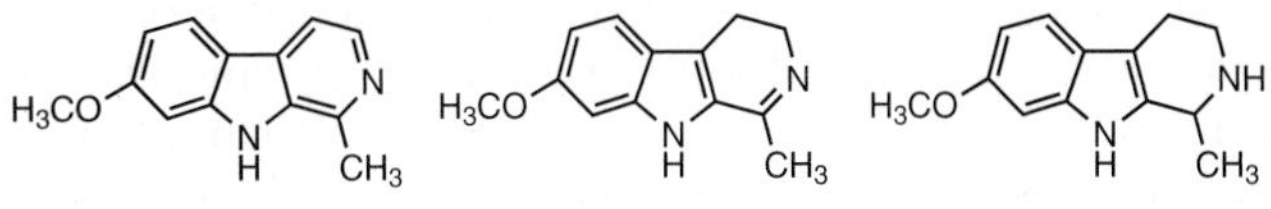

Harmine Harmaline Tetrahydroharmine

South American Indians prepare a variety of concoctions and snuffs, the most notable of which is ayahuasca, that are used for their hallucinogenic and visionary healing properties. In fact, the first written account of the use of these substances was made by a member of the Columbus expedition in 1493. There is little question that the concoctions are psychoactive; however, these plant preparations usually consist of admixtures in which certain tryptamines, such as DMT or 5-OMe DMT, sometimes have been identified. Some β-carbolines possess activity as MAO inhibitors; thus, the MAO inhibitory effect of the β-carbolines might be simply potentiating the effect of any other tryptaminergic hallucinogens present in the admixture by interfering with their metabolism. Studies with individual β-carbolines, especially under carefully controlled clinical settings, have been very limited. The three most commonly occurring β-carbolines are harmine, harmaline, and tetrahydroharmine, and evidence suggests that harmine and harmaline are hallucinogenic in humans (with potencies not greater than that of DMT) (26,27). Harmaline has seen some limited experimental application as an adjunct to psychotherapy (28). Like other classical hallucinogens, certain β-carbolines bind at 5-HT_{2A} receptors, and in animal studies, DOM stimulus generalization occurs to harmaline (28). Using harmaline-trained animals, harmaline stimulus generalization occurs to DOM. To date, however, few β-carbolines have been investigated, so they are only tentatively categorized as classical hallucinogens.

Although the scientific community has been aware of the psychoactive effects of the β-carbolines or β-carboline–containing natural substances for more than 100 years, only in the past decade or so have these agents become popular "on the street." The use of β-carboline–containing plants has moved out of the jungle and has given rise to a variety of religious movements in some South American cities. Recent books and movies are also helping to popularize the use of these preparations, and they are now being encountered in North America. In fact, as of 2006, the use of "ayahuasca tea" by certain religious groups has been permitted in the United States under the Religious Freedom Restoration Act.

Phenylalkylamines

Phenylalkylamines, phenylethylamines and phenylisopropylamines, represent the largest group of classical hallucinogens (29,30). The phenylethylamines are the α-desmethyl counterparts of the phenylisopropylamines; as with the indolealkylamines, the presence of the α-methyl group increases the agent's lipophilicity and reduces its susceptibility to metabolism by MAO. As a consequence, the phenylethylamines typically produce effects that are qualitatively similar to those of their corresponding phenylisopropylamines but typically less potent. Phenylethylamine counterparts of weak phenylisopropylamines might be inactive. Literally hundreds of analogs have been examined in human and animal studies (29).

Phenylethylamines Phenylethylamines are usually less potent analogs of the phenylisopropylamines. Some hallucinogenic phenylisopropylamines are claimed to possess some stimulant character that may be minimized or altogether absent in the corresponding phenylethylamines. The phenylisopropylamines also possess a chiral center that is absent in the phenylethylamines. Otherwise, the SARs of the two groups of agents are relatively similar; consequently, the phenylethylamines will not be discussed in detail here. The most common—and, indeed, one of the oldest known—phenylethylamine hallucinogen is mescaline. A constituent of peyote (and other) cactus, mescaline is a relatively weak hallucinogenic agent (total human dose ~350 mg). Like many of the hallucinogens, mescaline is listed as a Schedule I substance; however, the use of peyote in certain Native American Indian religious practices is sanctioned.

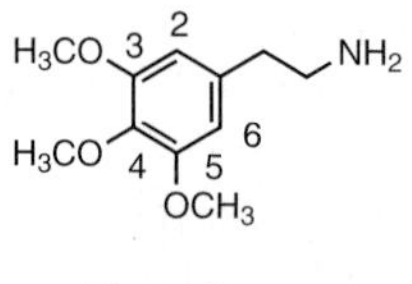

Mescaline

Phenylisopropylamines Structural modification of mescaline and related substances by introduction of an α-methyl group and by deletion or rearrangement of the position of its methoxy groups results in a series of agents known as the phenylisopropylamines. As might have been expected, introduction of an α-methyl group, to afford 3,4,5-trimethoxyphenyl-2-aminopropane (TMA) or α-methylmescaline, doubles the potency of mescaline. Although different nomenclatures exist for the dimethoxy- and trimethoxyphenylisopropylamines, the one used herein is a commonly used nomenclature: The position of methoxy groups is given by indicating its position, and the number of methoxy groups is indicated by a prefix. For example, α-methylmescaline is 3,4,5-TMA, indicating that it is a trimethoxy analog and that the methoxy groups are situated at the 3-, 4-, and 5-positions. Dimethoxy analogs are referred to as DMAs (dimethoxyphenyl-2-aminopropanes).

There are three possible monomethoxyphenylisopropylamines: the ortho-methoxy analog OMA, the meta-methoxy analog MMA, and the para-methoxy analog PMA (Table 19.3). Although PMA is specifically listed as a Schedule I substance, none of these three analogs is hallucinogenic. PMA possesses weak central stimulant actions and is an abused substance; several deaths have been attributed to PMA overdose within the past few years.

There are six isomeric DMA analogs. These have not been thoroughly investigated in humans, and few produce DOM-like stimulus effects in animals (Table 19.3). None is more potent than DOM. The most potent agent and one that has been evaluated in humans is 1-(2,5-dimethoxyphenyl)-2-aminopropane (2,5-DMA). There are also six different TMA analogs (Table 19.3). Here, most show some activity, but the 2,4,5-timethoxy analog 2,4,5-TMA (sometimes referred to simply as TMA) is the most potent of the series. Most of the trimethoxy analogs are recognized by DOM-trained animals, but none is more potent than DOM itself (5). The presence of the 2,5-methoxy substitution pattern in 2,5-DMA and 2,4,5-TMA might be noted.

The DMAs and TMAs are methoxy-substituted derivatives of the parent phenylisopropylamine known as amphetamine (Fig. 19.2). Amphetamine undergoes several different routes of metabolism; one of these is para-hydroxylation (a route that seems more important in rodents than in humans). Initially, it was thought that the greater potency of 2,4,5-TMA over that of 2,5-DMA might be related to the 4-position of the former being blocked to metabolism by para-hydroxylation. Keeping the 2,5-dimethoxy substitution intact, different 4-position

TABLE 19.3 Psychoactive Phenylisopropylamines and Related Agents

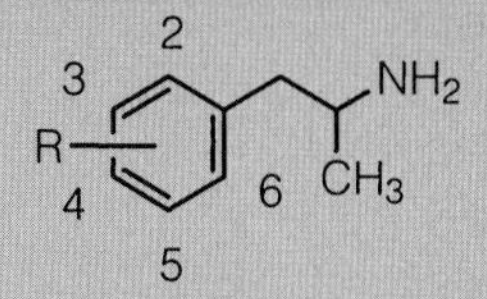

Agent	R_2	R_3	R_4	R_5	R_6	Human Hallucinogenic Dose (mg)*	DOM-stimulus Gen. Potency (umol/kg)†
Amphetamine	H	H	H	H	H	NH	NSG
OMA	OCH_3	H	H	H	H	NH	NSG
MMA	H	OCH_3	H	H	H	NH	NSG
PMA	H	H	OCH_3	H	H	NH	NSG
2,3-DMA	OCH_3	OCH_3	H	H	H	(?)	NSG
2,4-DMA	OCH_3	H	OCH_3	H	H	>60(?)	21.0
2,5-DMA	OCH_3	H	H	OCH_3	H	120 (80–160)	23.8
2,5-DMA, R(–)	OCH_3	H	H	OCH_3	H	(?)	14.0
2,6-DMA	OCH_3	H	H	H	OCH_3	(?)	NSG
3,4-DMA	H	OCH_3	OCH_3	H	H	>500 (?)	NSG
3,5-DMA	H	OCH_3	H	OCH_3	H	(?)	NSG
2,3,4-TMA	OCH_3	OCH_3	OCH_3	H	H	>100 (?)	29.8
2,3,5-TMA	OCH_3	OCH_3	H	OCH_3	H	>80 (?)	63.0
2,3,6-TMA	OCH_3	OCH_3	H	H	OCH_3	>30 (?)	—
2,4,5-TMA	OCH_3	H	OCH_3	OCH_3	H	30 (20–40)	13.7
2,4,6-TMA	OCH_3	H	OCH_3	H	OCH_3	38 (25–50)	13.9
3,4,5-TMA	H	OCH_3	OCH_3	OCH_3	H	175 (100–250)	24.2
MEM	OCH_3	H	OC_2H_5	OCH_3	H	35 (20–50)	22.9
DOM	OCH_3	H	CH_3	OCH_3	H	7 (3–10)	1.8
DOM, R(–)	OCH_3	H	CH_3	OCH_3	H	(?)	0.9
DOM, S(+)	OCH_3	H	CH_3	OCH_3	H	(?)	6.9
DOET	OCH_3	H	C_2H_5	OCH_3	H	4 (2.5–5)	0.9
DOPR	OCH_3	H	*n*-C_3H_7	OCH_3	H	4 (3–4.5)	0.6
DOIP	OCH_3	H	*i*-C_3H_7	OCH_3	H	(?)	2.9
DOBU	OCH_3	H	*n*-C_4H_9	OCH_3	H	(?)	3.2
DOAM	OCH_3	H	*n*-C_5H_{11}	OCH_3	H	(?)	NSG
DOT	OCH_3	H	SCH_3	OCH_3	H	8 (5–10)	—
DON	OCH_3	H	NO_2	OCH_3	H	4 (3–4.5)	2.7
DOF	OCH_3	H	F	OCH_3	H	(?)	5.8
DOC	OCH_3	H	Cl	OCH_3	H	2.5 (1.5–3)	1.2
DOB	OCH_3	H	Br	OCH_3	H	2 (1–3)	0.6
DOB, R(–)	OCH_3	H	Br	OCH_3	H	1.0–1.5 (?)	0.3
DOI	OCH_3	H	I	OCH_3	H	2.5 (1.5–3)	1.2
DOOC	OCH_3	H	COOH	OCH_3	H	(?)	NSG
DOOH	OCH_3	H	OH	OCH_3	H	(?)	NSG

*Data are primarily from reference 29. Where a dose range was reported in the literature, the arithmetic mean is also provided here for comparison (original range is fiven in parenthesis). The values should not be taken as a measure of precision. Doses are approximate and no implication is made that the different agents produce an identical effect. Key: NH = not hallucinogen, (?) = material has not been well studied or that its actions or potency are unknown.

†Drug discrimination data represent ED_{50} values and are from references 5,30. NSG = so stimulus generalization.

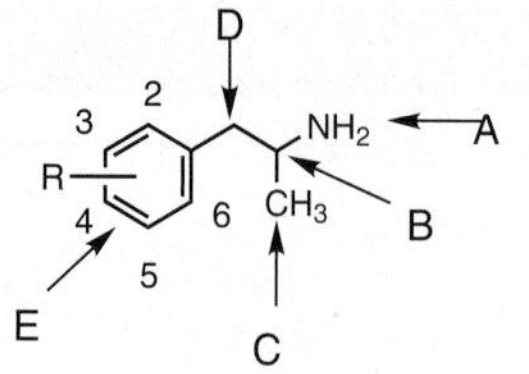

Position	Amphetamine-like action	DOM-like actions
A: Terminal amine	N-Methyl > NH_2 > NHR > NR_2	NH_2 > NHR > NR_2
B: Chiral center	S(+) > (±) > R(-)	R(-) > (±) > S(+)
C: α-Methyl group	Homologation decreases potency Replacement by H decreases potency	Homologation decreases potency Replacement by H decreases potency
D: β-Position	β-OH: reduces potency β =O: retains activity and potency	β-OH: not well investigated β =O: not well investigated
E: Aromatic substitution	Unsubstituted aromatic ring preferred	2,5-Dimethyl-substitution preferred 4-Substitution further modulates activity

FIGURE 19.2 Comparative structure–activity relationships for the amphetamine-like stimulant actions and the DOM-like action of the phenylisopropylamines (4,30).

substituents were examined. This led to a series of agents, such as DOM and 1-(4-bromo-2,5-dimethoxyphenyl)-2-aminopropane (DOB) (Table 19.3). These 4-substituted 2,5-dimethoxy analogs represent some of the most potent members of the series.

DOM represents the prototype member of this family of agents. Increasing the length of the 4-methyl group to an ethyl or *n*-propyl group (i.e., DOET and DOPR, respectively) results in enhanced potency on a molar basis. Further extension of the alkyl chain results in a decrease in potency or loss of action. Substitution at the 4-position by electron-withdrawing groups, particularly those with hydrophobic character, also results in active agents, such as DOB (Table 19.3), which is quite a potent agent and has been misrepresented on the clandestine market as LSD both in tablet and "blotter" form.

When optical isomers have been examined, activity resides primarily with the *R*-(−)-isomer; the *S*-(+)-isomers typically are less active, are inactive, or have received little study. For example, although not well investigated, it appears that *R*-(−)-DOM and *R*-(−)-DOB show activity at total human doses of less than 4 mg and less than 1 mg, respectively. *N*-Monomethylation reduces potency or abolishes activity; for example, the *N*-monomethyl analogs of DOM and DOB are approximately 10% as potent as their primary amine counterparts. The SARs for the DOM-like actions of phenylisopropylamines are summarized in Table 19.3 and Figure 19.2.

Table 19.3 also provides a comparison of the approximate human doses of various phenylisopropylamines when administered via the oral route. These agents represent a mere sampling of the agents that have been examined; it can be imagined, using only those functional groups shown in the table, how many different analogs are possible on the basis of structural rearrangement. There is no reason to suspect that each of these agents produces identical effects. In fact, the actions of some of these agents have been reported to be quite unique, ranging from hallucinations and closed-eye imagery to intellectual and sensory enhancement to erotic arousal (29).

Classical Hallucinogens: Mechanism of Action

Given that the arylalkylamines may not be producing identical effects, a common mechanism of action may not be expected. LSD was one of the first hallucinogens to be investigated mechanistically; another agent to see extensive investigation is mescaline. Interestingly, from a potency perspective, these two agents seem to represent opposite extremes. LSD has been proposed to produce its effects via numerous mechanisms, including those involving serotonergic, dopaminergic, histaminergic, adrenergic, and other receptors. LSD binds with high affinity at many different receptor populations and acts as an agonist at some, an antagonist at others, and a partial agonist at yet others. For many years, it was supposed that mescaline might be acting via a dopaminergic or adrenergic mechanism because of its structural similarity to dopamine (DA) and norepinephrine (NE). As early as the late 1950s, it was speculated, because of its structural similarity to 5-HT, that LSD might be working through a serotonergic mechanism. Significant experimental evidence supported this claim. Controversy existed, however, regarding whether LSD was a serotonergic agonist or antagonist. Furthermore, later studies revealed the existence of at least 14 populations of 5-HT receptors (see Chapter 10). With the subsequent availability of $5\text{-}HT_2$ selective antagonists, it was demonstrated that several of these antagonists (e.g., ketanserin and pirenperone) were particularly effective in blocking the stimulus effects of DOM and of DOM stimulus generalization to other hallucinogens, such as LSD, in tests of stimulus antagonism. It was later shown that the classical hallucinogens bind at 5-HT_2 receptors and that their receptor affinities were significantly correlated with both their DOM stimulus generalization potencies and their human hallucinogenic potencies (30). The classical hallucinogens are now thought to produce their effect by acting as agonists at 5-HT_2 receptors in the brain (i.e., the 5-HT_2 hypothesis of hallucinogen action). Radiolabeled analogs of DOB and DOI (e.g., $[^3H]$DOB and $[^{125}I]$DOI, respectively) are now available for the investigation of 5-HT_2 pharmacology.

More recently, it has been demonstrated that 5-HT_2 receptors actually represent a family of 5-HT receptors that consist of 5-HT_{2A}, 5-HT_{2B}, and 5-HT_{2C} receptor subpopulations. Fewer than three dozen arylalkylamines have been compared, but it appears that they show little selectivity for one subpopulation versus another. Various pharmacologic studies with selective antagonists or using antagonist correlation analysis, however, suggest that it may be the 5-HT_{2A} subtype that has a predominant role in the behavioral actions of these agents (30,31). Although the 5-HT_{2A} receptors might be responsible for those actions that the classical hallucinogens have in common, other neurochemical mechanisms may account for their differences. For example, LSD is a very promiscuous agent that binds with high affinity at many receptor populations for which most other classical hallucinogens show little to no affinity. Many of the indolealkylamines bind with high affinity at multiple populations of 5-HT receptors, and some display comparable or higher affinity at these receptors (e.g., 5-HT_{1A}, $h5\text{-HT}_{1D}$, and 5-HT_6) than they do at 5-HT_{2A} receptors. The phenylalkylamines are quite selective for 5-HT_2 receptors but, as mentioned earlier, display little selectivity for the three 5-HT_2 subpopulations. Some β-carbolines, although they bind at 5-HT_2 receptors, also possess activity as MAO inhibitors. Thus, these differences might account for their somewhat different actions. The one feature that all the classical hallucinogens have in common (i.e., the *common component hypothesis*) is that they bind at 5-HT_{2A} receptors (5).

CENTRAL STIMULANTS

Introduction, Classification, and Definitions

The ubiquitous term "stimulant" typically conjures up agents such as the tropane analog cocaine or the phenylisopropylamine stimulant amphetamine. However, stimulants can be divided into several categories. Terms such as "psychostimulant," "psychomotor stimulant," "behavioral stimulant," or, simply, "stimulant" typically refer to agents that produce a central stimulatory effect where actions are manifested mostly in motor activity, whereas the term "analeptic" refers to agents that have a stimulant effect primarily on autonomic centers such as those involved in the regulation of respiration and circulation. Nicotine and related nicotinic agents also possess stimulant properties but are best discussed with other cholinergic agents. Analeptics include agents such as nikethamide, strychnine, and pentylenetetrazol. The boundary between analeptics and psychomotor stimulants is not sharply defined. Caffeine, for example, has been classified as an analeptic but is also considered a psychomotor stimulant. Caffeine is probably the best known of a series of xanthines; in fact, caffeine, which is found in coffee, tea, chocolate, guarana, mate, and other naturally occurring substances, is probably the most widely used psychoactive substance in the world. Although analeptics have never represented significant abuse problems, evidence exists for caffeine abuse (32).

Xanthines and Caffeine-Related Stimulants

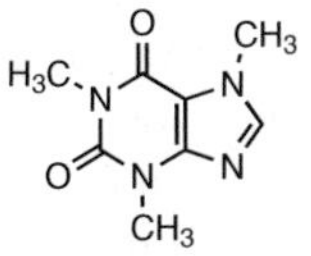

Caffeine

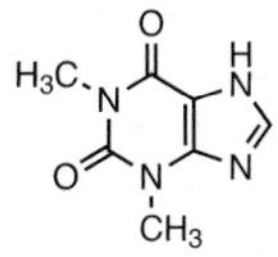

Theophylline

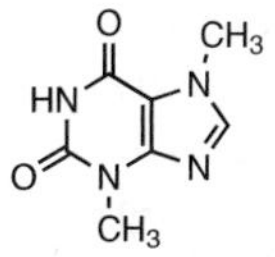

Theobromine

Caffeine (or 1,3,7-trimethylxanthine) is a naturally occurring methylated xanthine, as are its close relatives theophylline (1,3-dimethylxanthine) and theobromine (3,7-dimethylxanthine). A major metabolite of caffeine is paraxanthine, or 1,7-dimethylxanthine. All four compounds produce relatively similar, although not necessarily identical, effects (e.g., motor stimulation, relaxation of smooth muscle, stimulation of cardiac muscle). The different actions of the xanthines are thought to be mediated by (at least) one mechanism or, more commonly (depending on dose), a combination of mechanisms, at which some xanthines are more effective than others. In general, these xanthines act as nonselective competitive inhibitors at adenosine receptors (33) and of the enzyme(s) cyclic nucleotide phosphodiesterase (PDE; of which there are 14 human subtypes and >50 isoforms) (34); they can mobilize intracellular stores of calcium (e.g., from the endoplasmic reticulum) and bind with rather modest affinity at benzodiazepine binding sites on $GABA_A$ receptors (33). Other mechanisms might be involved. For example, the mechanism of action of the xanthines in the treatment of airway diseases probably involves their ability to cause bronchodilation via inhibition of PDE in the lung, whereas the immunomodulatory and anti-inflammatory actions of theophylline seem to result from induction of histone deacetylase (35,36).

The psychostimulant effects of caffeine-related xanthines are probably a direct consequence of their actions at adenosine receptors and, to a substantially lesser extent, on their ability to inhibit cyclic nucleotide PDE. Indeed, the stimulant properties of a series of xanthines have been correlated with their blockade of adenosine receptors (33). Adenosine receptors are now recognized to consist of a family of four subtypes (i.e., A_1–A_3): A_1 adenosine receptors, which are negatively coupled to adenylate cyclase; A_{2A} (with high affinity for agonists) and A_{2B} (with low affinity for agonists) receptors, which are positively coupled to adenylate cyclase; and A_3 receptors, which are coupled to phospholipase C (PLC) and also negatively coupled to adenylate cyclase; stimulation of PLC generates inositol triphosphate (IP_3), which, in turn, increases calcium levels (33). Adenosine binds with low affinity both at A_{2B} and A_3 receptors; in contrast, adenosine binds with higher affinity at A_1 and A_{2A} receptors, supporting a role for the latter in the stimulant actions of caffeine and related xanthines (33). The inhibitory control of neurotransmission exerted by A_1 receptor activation might account for the effects of caffeine on arousal and vigilance by its acting as a competitive antagonist (37). However, caffeine is believed to stimulate motor activity by countering the indirect tonic control exerted by activation of A_{2A} receptors on dopaminergic (primarily D_2) and glutamatergic transmission (37,38).

There are some similarities in the psychomotor stimulant actions of caffeine, amphetamine, and cocaine, and these involve both DA-dependent and DA-independent mechanisms; indeed, all ultimately seem to share a somewhat common component of action involving the modulation of DA- and cyclic adenosine monophosphate (cAMP)–regulated phosphoprotein (DARPP-32), a protein regulator of intracellular signaling (see Fig. 19.8). Direct activation of D_1 receptors by DA or DA agonists or indirect activation of these receptors by amphetamine and cocaine (e.g., by presynaptic release of DA or blockade of DA reuptake; see later sections) increases phosphorylation of DARPP-32 by protein kinase A (PKA) at a particular threonine moiety (i.e., Thr^{34}) to inhibit protein phosphatase-1 (PP-1); this results in enhanced signaling and increased psychomotor stimulation. Activation of these receptors also decreases phosphorylation of DARPP-32 at Thr^{75} by activation of a specific protein phosphatase (PP-2A); phosphorylation of Thr^{75} has an inhibitory effect on Thr^{34} phosphorylation (see Fig. 19.8). Stimulation of A_{2A} receptors has a similar effect, but activation of these receptors results in decreased motor activity in rodents; this is believed to be related to the tonic inhibitory control of dopaminergic and glutamatergic systems by A_{2A} receptors (38). Caffeine, being a competitive A_{2A} receptor antagonist, reduces its (i.e., adenosine's A_{2A} receptor–mediated) tonic activation of the cAMP/PKA pathway and produces a dose-dependent increase in phosphorylation of DARPP-32 at Thr^{75} (37). Caffeine also increases phosphorylation of Thr^{75} by inhibition of PP-2A, which, by having an inhibitory effect on phosphorylation of Thr^{34}, further amplifies its effect (37). The eventual outcome of blocking activation of A_{2A} adenosine receptors is disinhibition of its inhibitory control on dopaminergic and/or glutamatergic activity. Ultimately, then, amphetamine and cocaine indirectly regulate downstream effector mechanisms by having a particular effect on DARPP-32 via DA receptors, whereas caffeine regulates downstream effector mechanisms by having an effect on DARPP-32 via adenosine A_{2A} receptors. Both result in psychomotor stimulation. It might be noted that the psychomotor stimulant actions of caffeine are biphasic: Low doses produce A_{2A} receptor–mediated stimulation, whereas higher doses produce depression of activity. It has been speculated that higher caffeine doses result in blockade of A_1 adenosine receptors to produce this depressant effect (37).

Phenylisopropylamine Stimulants: Amphetamine-Related Agents

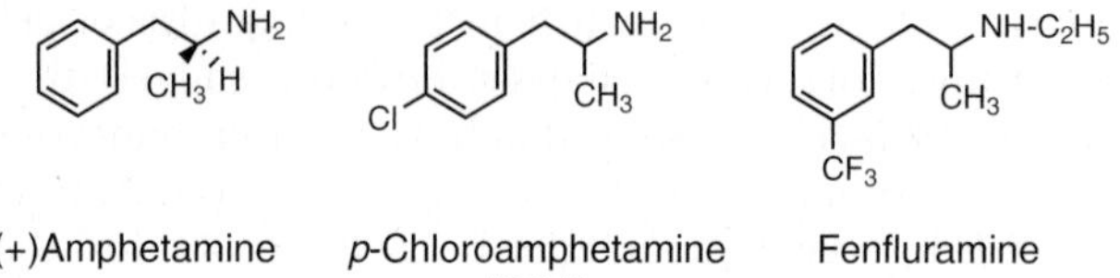

S(+)Amphetamine   *p*-Chloroamphetamine (PCA)   Fenfluramine

The simplest unsubstituted phenylisopropylamine, 1-phenyl-2-aminopropane, or amphetamine, serves as a common structural template for hallucinogens and psychostimulants. Amphetamine produces central stimulant, anorectic, and sympathomimetic actions, and it is the prototype member of this class (39). It is common to refer to amphetaminergic structures and amphetaminergic activity, but amphetamine may be more of an exception than a rule. Most substituted derivatives of amphetamine (i.e., phenylisopropylamine) lack central stimulant activity; in fact, pharmacologically, there are a greater number of "non–amphetamine-like" than "amphetamine-like" derivatives of amphetamine (e.g., see phenylisopropylamine hallucinogens). Relatively few derivatives of amphetamine retain the actions of amphetamine; still fewer retain the potency of amphetamine. This section will focus almost exclusively on the psychostimulant actions of amphetamine, and it should be recognized that these SARs are not necessarily identical to those for its anorectic or sympathomimetic actions.

Structure–Activity Relationships for Amphetamine-like Stimulant Action

In general, the SARs for amphetamine-like psychostimulant actions of the phenylisopropylamines are quite distinct from those for the DOM-like (or hallucinogenic) actions of the phenylisopropylamines, even though both share a common structural skeleton. The SARs for the two actions are summarized in Figure 19.2. The stimulus effects of amphetamine analogs have been reviewed elsewhere (4, 40).

Aryl-Substituted Derivatives In general, incorporation of substituents into the aromatic ring of amphetamine reduces or abolishes amphetamine-like psychostimulant activity. The sympathomimetic agent 4-hydroxyamphetamine lacks central stimulant action and is unlikely to penetrate the blood–brain barrier because of the presence of the polar aromatic hydroxyl group. Masking of the hydroxyl group in the form of its methyl ether affords the Schedule I substance *p*-methoxyamphetamine (PMA; also known as 4-methoxyamphetamine). PMA is a weak central stimulant with approximately 10% the potency of amphetamine. 4-Methylamphetamine (1-(*p*-tolyl)-2-aminopropane [pTAP]) has also been found on the clandestine market and is, at best, a weak central stimulant. Incorporation of electron-withdrawing substituents results in agents that generally lack central stimulant properties. For example, *p*-chloroamphetamine (PCA) is a 5-HT–releasing agent that saw evaluation as a potential antidepressant. Another related analog is the 5-HT–releasing agent fenfluramine, which was used for some time as an appetite suppressant. Both of these latter agents are still widely used as pharmacologic tools in basic neuroscience research.

Amine Substitution In general, the primary amines are more potent than the secondary amines, and the secondary amines are more potent than the tertiary amines, as central stimulants. With regard to secondary amines, as the length of the amine substituent increases, activity decreases; the *N*-monoethyl and *N*-mono-*n*-propyl amines retain stimulant character but are somewhat less potent than amphetamine itself. Larger *N*-substituents typically result in agents with little to no psychostimulant character. The one exception is the *N*-monomethyl derivative methamphetamine. Methamphetamine (e.g., "crystal," "ice," or "meth") is at least as potent as amphetamine as a central stimulant; in most studies, it may be two- to threefold more potent than amphetamine. Methamphetamine is the most widely abused synthetic substance in the world. *N*-Hydroxylation of amphetamine has little effect on stimulant action. *N*,*N*-Dimethylamphetamine has been seized from clandestine laboratories, but it has never been certain whether this agent was being prepared for its possible stimulant actions or was an undesired byproduct of methamphetamine synthesis.

α-Substituents Amphetamine possesses an α-methyl group. As already mentioned at the beginning of this chapter, α-demethylation (to afford phenylethylamine or 2-phenyl-1-aminoethane in the case of amphetamine) results in agents with decreased lipophilicity and increased susceptibility to metabolism. Phenylethylamine lacks central stimulant activity. Homologation of the α-methyl group to, for example, an α-ethyl or α-*n*-propyl group results in a decrease or loss of central stimulant activity. The presence of the α-methyl group in amphetamine creates a chiral center; hence, amphetamine exists as a pair of optical isomers. With respect to central stimulant actions, the *S*-(+)-isomer (i.e., dextroamphetamine) is several-fold more potent than its *R*-(−)-enantiomer (i.e., levoamphetamine); this is not necessarily the case with other actions produced by amphetamine, particularly those produced in the periphery, such as its cardiovascular actions.

β-Substituents The β-position has not been particularly well investigated. Perhaps the best-studied derivatives are ephedrine and norephedrine—and even these agents have not been especially well investigated. Ephedrine and norephedrine are phenylpropanolamines that may be viewed as the β-hydroxy analogs of methamphetamine and amphetamine, respectively. Actually, β-hydroxylation of amphetamine or methamphetamine results in the creation of a new chiral center; hence, a total of four optical isomers are possible in each case. These eight structures are shown in Figure 19.3. Relatively little comparative information is available regarding the central stimulant actions of these phenylpropanolamine isomers.

During the 1970s, there was a problem with what were termed "look-alike drugs." Look-alikes available on the clandestine market were made to resemble amphetamine and methamphetamine, both in action and physical appearance, to circumvent the control of amphetamine. The major constituents of these agents were various combinations of ephedrine, norephedrine, and caffeine. Although the look-alikes are no longer the problem they once were, the 1990s witnessed the introduction of "herbal dietary supplements." These supplements were—and still are—available in some health food and herbal shops, and even more so on the Internet; several dozen such preparations have appeared on the market. The major ingredients of many of these preparations are various combinations of ephedrine and caffeine (or of ephedrine-containing

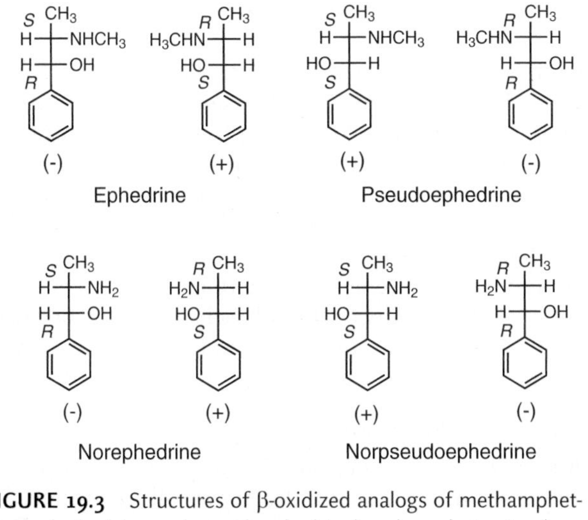

FIGURE 19.3 Structures of β-oxidized analogs of methamphetamine (ephedrine and pseudoephedrine) and amphetamine (norephedrine and norpseudoephedrine). Note that norpseudoephedrine is also known as cathine.

natural products [e.g., ma huang or ephedra] or caffeine-containing natural products [e.g., guarana or kola nut]). Interestingly, although ephedrine and caffeine possess stimulant character of their own, evidence suggests that these agents may potentiate one another's actions (41).

Although β-hydroxylation of amphetamine results in decreased central stimulant actions, this may be the result of the decreased ability of norephedrine to penetrate the blood–brain barrier, or it may be a clue that the presence of a β-oxygen substituent is inherently detrimental to activity. Support for the former is derived from the shrub *Catha edulis*. Commonly known as khat or kat, *C. edulis* is a plant indigenous to certain regions of the Middle East and eastern portions of Africa. The fresh shrub is sold openly in local markets and is used for its central stimulant character, much in the same way as the West uses coffee. Khat is used to prepare an infusion, or the fresh leaves are simply chewed. For more than 50 years, it was thought that the active constituent was the phenylpropanolamine cathine or (+)-norpseudoephedrine (Fig. 19.3). In the late 1970s, however, a more potent compound was isolated from fresh leaves and shown to be what is now called cathinone. Cathinone, which is simply β-ketoamphetamine or an oxidized analog of norephedrine, is at least as potent as amphetamine as a central stimulant.

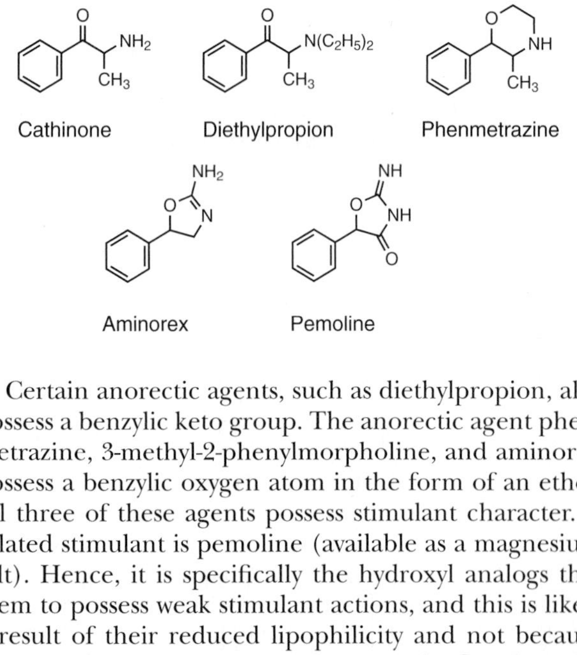

Certain anorectic agents, such as diethylpropion, also possess a benzylic keto group. The anorectic agent phenmetrazine, 3-methyl-2-phenylmorpholine, and aminorex possess a benzylic oxygen atom in the form of an ether. All three of these agents possess stimulant character. A related stimulant is pemoline (available as a magnesium salt). Hence, it is specifically the hydroxyl analogs that seem to possess weak stimulant actions, and this is likely a result of their reduced lipophilicity and not because they simply possess an oxygen atom at the β or benzylic position.

Metabolism of Amphetamine

In humans, (+)-amphetamine has a half-life of approximately 7 hours. Some of the metabolic products of amphetamine metabolism are shown in Figure 19.4. Although a significant portion of amphetamine is excreted unchanged, it also undergoes both phase 1 (functionalization to more polar derivatives) and phase 2 (conjugation) metabolism (42). The phase 1 metabolism of amphetamine analogs is catalyzed by two enzyme systems: cytochrome P450 and flavin monooxygenase. The latter system oxidizes secondary and tertiary amine analogs of amphetamine. Amphetamine undergoes hydroxylation on the α-carbon, the β-carbon, the terminal amine, and the aromatic ring. These metabolites are subsequently oxidized, where possible, or conjugated.

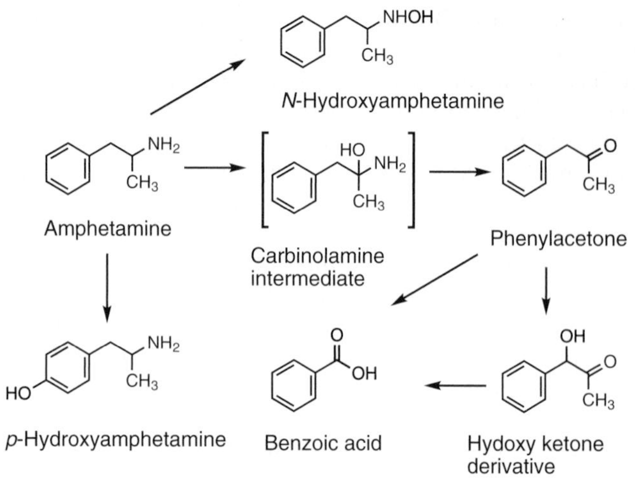

FIGURE 19.4 Some products of amphetamine metabolism.

Amphetamine is oxidized to phenylacetone (P2P) via a presumed carbinolamine intermediate. The phenylacetone is further oxidized directly to benzoic acid or, first, to a hydroxy keto analog that is subsequently converted to benzoic acid. Amphetamine can also undergo aromatic hydroxylation to *p*-hydroxyamphetamine. Initial work with rats indicated that *p*-hydroxylation is a major route of metabolism; however, subsequent studies showed that benzoic acid is the major metabolite in humans. Subsequent oxidation at the benzylic position by DA β-hydroxylase affords *p*-hydroxynorephedrine. Alternatively, direct oxidation of amphetamine by DA β-hydroxylase can afford norephedrine. Amphetamine and related derivatives also undergo *N*-hydroxylation, and the *N*-hydroxy derivatives can be further oxidized to nitroso, nitro, and oximino compounds. Some evidence suggests that the oximino derivative is hydrolyzed to phenylacetone. Additional metabolites are possible as well. In phase 2 reactions, ring-hydroxylated metabolites are conjugated to their corresponding glucuronides. Sulfation of the enol form of phenylacetone has been reported. Approximately 23% of methamphetamine is excreted unchanged, 18% is excreted as *p*-hydroxymethamphetamine, and 14% is excreted as the demethylated product (42).

Mechanism of Action of Amphetamine

Amphetamine is an indirect-acting dopaminergic and noradrenergic agonist; that is, amphetamine causes an

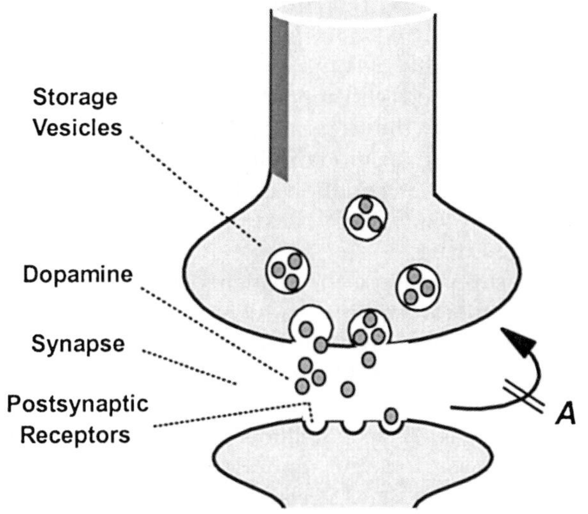

FIGURE 19.5 Schematic of a dopaminergic nerve terminal. Amphetamine increases synaptic concentration of DA primarily by causing its release from presynaptic terminals, whereas cocaine increases synaptic concentration by preventing its reuptake (*A*).

increase in the synaptic concentrations of the neurotransmitters DA and NE. Amphetamine enhances the release of DA and, to a lesser extent, prevents the reuptake of DA into presynaptic terminals (Fig. 19.5). The stimulant actions of amphetamine can be attenuated by the administration of DA antagonists, such as the antipsychotic phenothiazine chlorpromazine and the butyrophenone haloperidol. Chronic administration of high doses of amphetamine may result in "amphetamine psychosis," which exhibits symptoms similar to those of acute paranoid psychosis. This is consistent with a role for DA in the central actions of amphetamine and, further, with the DA antagonist mechanisms proposed for most antipsychotic agents (see also Chapter 14). Similar psychotic episodes have been associated with khat ("khat psychosis" or "cathinone psychosis") and cocaine ("cocaine psychosis").

Clinical Applications

Although phenylisopropylamines generally are known for their abuse liability, several have gained clinical acceptance. Indeed, certain agents display reduced stimulant character and/or are infrequently abused. Ephedrine (and, later, phenylpropanolamine) and amphetamine were two of the first agents used to treat obesity. Caffeine has also been used to treat obesity and, when given in combination with ephedrine (or amphetamine), the combination has a supra-additive effect (43,44). Alternatives to synthetic products include herbal preparations that contain ephedrine (e.g., ma huang) or caffeine (e.g., as in guarana). Recent studies indicate that ephedrine–caffeine combinations are associated with an increased risk of psychiatric, autonomic, cardiovascular, and other side effects (44). The central stimulant actions of phenylisopropylamines led to their structural modification and subsequent introduction of anorectic agents, such as diethylpropion, phenmetrazine, and phentermine. Despite a lack of widespread abuse, many of these agents retain central stimulant properties. (±)-Fenfluramine was developed in the 1960s and marketed as Pondimin. Although structurally related to amphetamine, fenfluramine is devoid of central stimulant character. Unlike amphetamine-related agents that act primarily via noradrenergic and dopaminergic mechanisms, fenfluramine is a 5-HT–releasing agent. The more potent isomer in reducing food intake, (+)-fenfluramine (i.e., dexfenfluramine), was introduced clinically during the 1980s. Fenfluramine was also available in combination with phentermine (i.e., phen-fen). Unfortunately, some patients treated with this combination displayed symptoms of valvular heart disease, resulting in the voluntary withdrawal from the market in 1997 of fenfluramine-containing anorectic agents. (±)-Fenfluramine is metabolized to its primary amine norfenfluramine, and evidence suggests that valvulopathy is the result of the agonist action of norfenfluramine on cardiac 5-HT_{2B} receptors (45,46). Today, it is not unusual for new drug candidates to be examined for 5-HT_{2B} agonist action during the early stages of their development in order to eliminate this side effect.

Other serotonergic agents have been evaluated for their antiobesity actions including selective serotonin reuptake inhibitors (SSRIs; e.g., fluoxetine; see Chapter 18) (43).

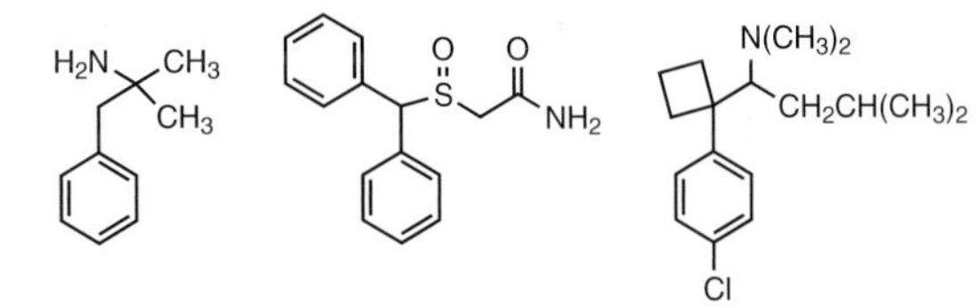

Phentermine — Modafinil (Provigil) — Sibutramine (Merida)

Sibutramine (Meridia), an agent with an amphetamine-like structural skeleton initially developed as an antidepressant, is an inhibitor of 5-HT and NE reuptake. Animal studies indicated that sibutramine reduces food intake by decreasing meal duration rather than feeding frequency, suggesting an effect on intrinsic satiation mechanisms (43). Sibutramine stimulates thermogenesis and effectively reduces amounts of visceral fat accumulation (47). Side effects of sibutramine include increased heart rate and increased blood pressure that have been attributed to its adrenergic action; in fact, because of its cardiovascular side effects, sibutramine was voluntarily withdrawn from the clinical market in 2010. These and other approaches and strategies to the treatment of obesity have been extensively reviewed (43,47).

Causes of excessive daytime sleepiness are numerous and include intrinsic sleep disorders, such as obstructive sleep apnea/hypopnea syndrome and narcolepsy;

circadian rhythm sleep disorders, such as jet lag; and sleep disorders associated with neuropsychiatric conditions, such as anxiety and depression (48–50). In many instances, excessive daytime sleepiness is commonly treated by addressing the underlying cause; however, the specific etiology of narcolepsy is unknown. Narcolepsy can also be characterized by brief periods of muscle paralysis (cataplexy). Hence, a need exists for agents that can effectively treat narcolepsy and cataplexy. Because of the increased behavioral activation (i.e., arousal, alertness, and motor activity) caused by psychostimulants, their use has been the mainstay for the treatment of narcolepsy. Agents such as methylphenidate (see later discussion) and amphetamine frequently are used, and methamphetamine and caffeine are used less commonly. Pemoline (Cyclert) has also seen some application but has been reported to produce liver toxicity (48–50) and was removed from the US market in 2005. Adderall, a combination of amphetamine salts [equal amounts of (+)-amphetamine saccharate, (+)-amphetamine sulfate, (±)-amphetamine aspartate, and (±)-amphetamine sulfate], was introduced in 1996; although used primarily for the treatment of attention-deficit hyperactivity disorder (ADHD), it is also used in the treatment of narcolepsy. Recently introduced for the treatment of ADHD is lisdexamfetamine (Vyvanse).

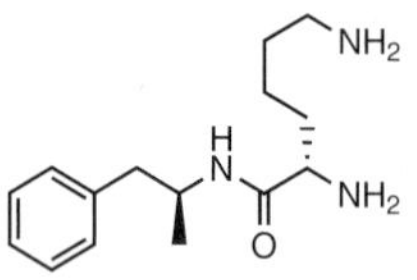

Lisdexamfetamine

Lisdexamfetamine is (+)-amphetamine acylated with an *N*-(L)-lysinyl function; in vivo, lisdexamfetamine is a prodrug that is slowly hydrolyzed to (+)-amphetamine. Newer agents for the treatment of narcolepsy include sodium oxybate ($HO\text{-}CH_2CH_2CH_2COO^- Na^+$; presumed to act through a GABAminergic mechanism) and modafinil. Modafinil (Provigil) is a new agent that seems to promote wakefulness without producing the arousing effects associated with many other stimulants; it has also been approved for the treatment of obstructive sleep apnea/hypopnea syndrome (51). The exact mechanism of action of modafinil is unknown but has been shown by various investigators to involve DA, NE, histamine, 5-HT, and/or GABA receptors; modafinil also binds at hypocretin (orexin receptors) (52,53). Modafinil showed reduced stimulant character relative to methylphenidate (see later discussion), and its potential for abuse in patients with narcolepsy has been demonstrated to be quite low (48). Nevertheless, modafinil binds at the DA transporter and is only about eightfold less potent than cocaine as an inhibitor of DA reuptake (54). Furthermore, its more potent *R*-isomer (armodafinil, Nuvigil), but not its *S*-isomer, is a potent D_2 receptor partial agonist (55). These dopaminergic actions might account for some of the stimulant actions associated with modafinil. Hepatic metabolism responsible for the clearance of modafinil includes amide hydrolysis to modafinilic acid, its primary inactive metabolite. *S*-Oxidation and aromatic ring hydroxylation occur via CYP2C9. Less than 10% is excreted as unchanged drug.

Motor suppression seen in patients with cataplexy is similar to the motor suppression seen in healthy individuals during rapid eye movement (REM) sleep. Consequently, agents previously found to decrease REM sleep have been evaluated for the treatment of cataplexy (50,52). Agents that suppress REM sleep include those that increase noradrenergic, serotonergic, and dopaminergic signaling. Tricyclic antidepressants, certain SSRIs, dual NE–serotonin reuptake inhibitors (e.g., venlafaxine), and MAO inhibitors have found application in the treatment of cataplexy, as has sodium oxybate (52,53). Psychostimulants also might be of some anticataplexic benefit, but modafinil generally produces little improvement (52).

Cocaine-Related Agents

There are eight possible stereoisomeric forms of methyl 3-(benzoyloxy)-8-methylazabicyclo[3.2.1]octan-2-carboxylate, of which one is simply referred to as "cocaine." Chemically, cocaine is 2*R*-carbomethoxy-3*S*-benzyloxy-1*R*-tropane. Cocaine is naturally occurring in a variety of plants, particularly the *Erythroxylon coca* species, which is indigenous to some countries in South America. In addition to its stimulant actions, cocaine possesses vasoconstrictor actions and is a local anesthetic; it has served as a template for the development of other therapeutically useful agents, including local anesthetics and $5\text{-}HT_3$ receptor antagonists.

Cocaine has a very interesting history. The coca plant has been used by South American Indians for religious and mystical purposes and as a stimulant, both to increase endurance and to alleviate hunger, for millennia. The plant was introduced into Europe during the 1800s, and at the end of the 19th century, cocaine use was quite popular and very socially acceptable. Various cocaine-containing preparations were available, and it was also used to "fortify" wines (e.g., *Vin Coca*). For a period of approximately 20 years, until just after the turn of the last century, it was a constituent of the soft drink Coca-Cola. Additionally, cocaine was used for therapeutic reasons but was later supplanted by amphetamine.

Cocaine is active via nearly every possible route of administration; however, insufflation of "snow" or "coke" represents one of the most popular routes. Administered in this manner, peak effects and plasma levels are achieved within 30 minutes (56). Smoking the freebase form of cocaine ("*crack*") results in an even more rapid effect. The freebase form, rather than the hydrochloride salt, is used for smoking, because the temperatures required for vaporization of the salt results in considerable decomposition (56). Intravenously administered cocaine can achieve peak blood levels within a few minutes. Cocaine is metabolized to benzoylecgonine, the methyl ester of ecgonine, and to a lesser extent, to ecgonine, norcocaine, and hydroxylated derivatives.

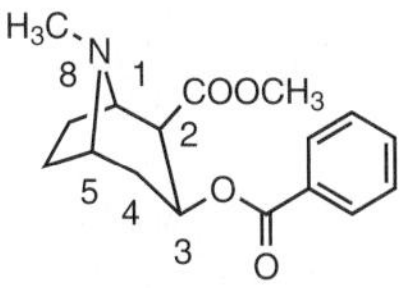

Cocaine

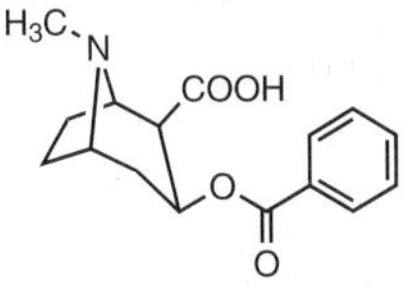

Benzoylecgonine

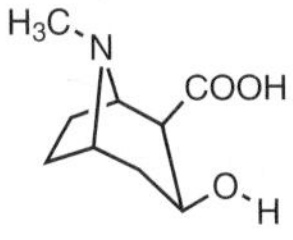

Ecgonine

Mechanism of Action of Cocaine

Cocaine has been shown to block the reuptake of NE, 5-HT, and DA; however, the reinforcing and stimulant nature of cocaine seems to be related primarily to blockade of DA reuptake, leading to the "dopamine hypothesis" of cocaine action (57). [^{3}H]Cocaine was used in an attempt to identify a "cocaine receptor," and this target was later shown to be similar to the DA transporter. Currently, it is thought that cocaine produces it reinforcing effects by interfering with DA reuptake (Fig. 19.5) by blocking the DA transporter (58). Although the human DA transporter has been cloned, it is unknown whether the DA and cocaine binding domains are identical or how much they overlap (57). There are also indications that NE might have a larger role in the actions of cocaine and other psychostimulants than previously appreciated.

Cocaine-Like Structure–Activity Relationships and Cocaine-Like Agents

Because cocaine binds at the DA transporter, this provides a convenient method for the investigation and formulation of SAR; these have been reviewed elsewhere (56,57). Important features for the binding of cocaine analogs include configuration, substituent at C_2, stereochemistry at C_2, substituent at N_8, and substituents at C_3. With respect to cocaine analogs, inversion of configuration can decrease activity. The C_2-position is quite important: Epimerization from β to α reduces activity by 30- to 200-fold, and hydrolysis of the ester to the acid (i.e., benzoylecgonine) reduces activity by more than 1,500-fold. Although an ester function seems to be important, the methyl group can be replaced by other substituents (e.g., phenyl or benzyl) with relatively little effect. A basic nitrogen atom appears to be optimal. Replacement of the N_8-methyl group by other substituents, such as a small alkyl or benzyl group, has only a small negative influence on activity, whereas quaternization or acylation (of norcocaine) reduces activity by 33- and 111-fold, respectively (57).

Other DA transport blockers are known, and their SARs have been investigated (58). One of the oldest and most widely investigated analogs is WIN-35,428, and [^{3}H] WIN-35,428 is commercially available as a radioligand. Others include methylphenidate (see next paragraph), benztropine, GBR 12909, and mazindol (58,59). These latter compounds produce varying degrees of cocaine-like actions and, thus, are being examined as structural leads for the development of therapies for the treatment of cocaine abuse (58). Because there are currently nearly 2 million cocaine users in the United States, various novel pharmacotherapies are being pursued, including GABAminergic agents, dopaminergic agents, adrenoceptor antagonists, vasodilators, and cocaine vaccines (60).

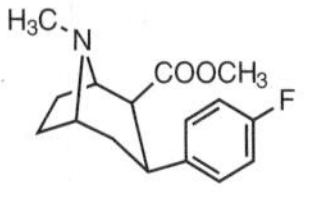

WIN 35,428

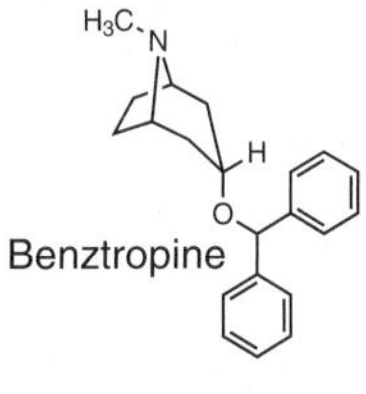

Benztropine

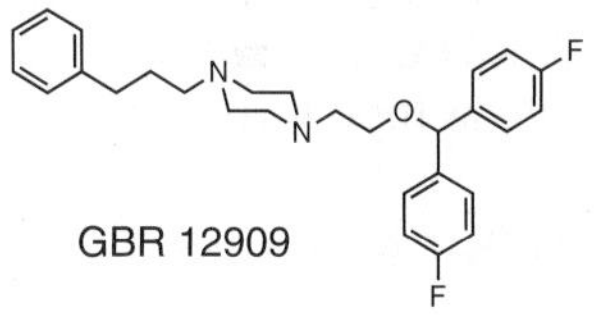

GBR 12909

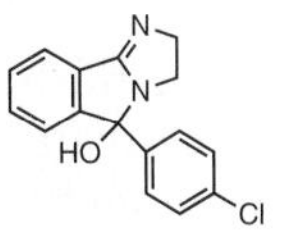

Mazindol

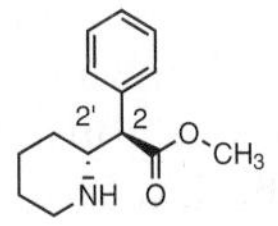

Methylphenidate

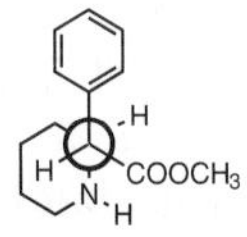

Anti conformation of d-TMP

Methylphenidate (Ritalin) is used for the treatment of ADHD and, to a lesser extent, for the treatment of narcolepsy. Methylphenidate possesses two chiral centers (i.e., one at the 2-position and one at the 2′-position) and, as such, exists as four possible isomers: a *threo* pair and an *erythro* pair (61). The SARs of methylphenidate isomers and analogs have been extensively investigated (62). X-ray crystallographic, conformational, computational, and other studies indicate the following stereochemistry for methylphenidate: (+)-*threo* = 2*R*,2′*R*, (−)-*threo* = 2*S*,2′*S*, (+)-*erythro* = 2*R*,2′*S*, and (−)-*erythro* = 2*S*,2′*R* (59–61). The structure of the (+)-*threo* isomer (i.e., d-*threo*-methylphenidate [d-TMP or (+)-TMP]) is shown; the *anti* conformation of d-TMP is particularly favored by a hydrogen bond between the piperidine nitrogen atom NH and the carbonyl oxygen atom of the ester group (61,63).

The psychostimulant action of methylphenidate (i.e., the actions desired for its use in ADHD) is associated exclusively with the *threo* isomeric pair; the *erythro* isomeric pair is essentially inactive in this regard (62). Ritalin, for example, is (±)-*threo*-methylphenidate. Following oral administration of (±)-*threo*-methylphenidate [(±)-TMP], it undergoes enantiomeric hepatic metabolism such that (-)-TMP is metabolized faster (to the corresponding ritalinic acid) than is the (+)-TMP (62,64). This is not necessarily the case following other routes of administration (e.g., transdermal) where first-pass hepatic metabolism is circumvented (64).

Studies have shown that (+)-TMP is the eutomeric form of the drug and that it is about 10 times more potent than (−)-TMP (62). Recently, (+)-TMP was introduced as dexmethylphenidate (Focalin; a Schedule II substance).

Methylphenidate (and its various isomers) has been around for more than 50 years, and its mechanism of action has been extensively investigated. (Note: Some studies were influenced by evaluation of various mixtures of its diastereomers or of enantiomeric pairs.) Methylphenidate blocks the reuptake of NE and DA. Although its actions are attributed mainly to its ability to block DA reuptake, it [i.e., (±)-TMP and d-TMP] is actually more potent as an inhibitor of NE than DA reuptake. However, there is evidence for a ceiling effect on NE, but not DA, shifting the actions to a more dopaminergic profile at higher drug doses (62).

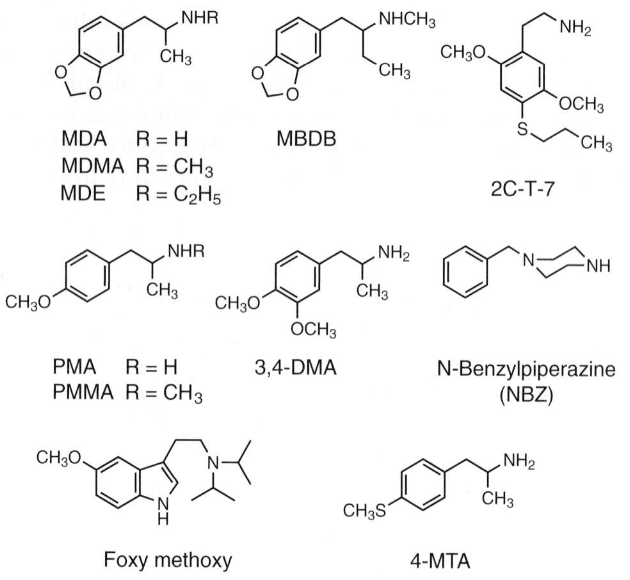

FIGURE 19.6 Examples of designer drugs.

DESIGNER DRUGS

Designer drugs, or controlled substance analogs, are the end result of the application of known SARs at the clandestine level. That is, knowledge of the established SARs of a particular class of abused substances can be applied at the clandestine level for the development of novel agents of abuse. What is particularly frightening about this concept is that the novel agents are not necessarily—or even commonly—examined for action or toxicity before they are put on the illicit market. The term "designer drug" was first introduced in reference to novel opiate-related analogs that appeared on the clandestine market approximately three decades ago; today, the term is applied more generically to any class of abusable substance. Furthermore, the term is now commonly applied to nearly any substance, novel or not to the scientific literature, that is new to the street scene. Designer drugs have appeared that are structurally related to the hallucinogens and stimulants discussed earlier; the present discussion will focus on some of these agents.

Specific Examples

Because some designer drugs result from the clandestine application of known hallucinogen or psychostimulant SARs, it should be possible to legitimately forecast the actions and, perhaps, even the approximate potencies of novel street drugs on the basis of available SAR data. In fact, this sometimes is the case. For example, "Nexus" made an appearance on the East Coast of the United States in the early 1990s. Nexus is α-desmethyl DOB, or 2-(4-bromo-2,5-dimethoxyphenyl)-1-aminoethane. Knowing that DOB is a potent phenylisopropylamine hallucinogen and that α-demethylation typically reduces the potency of phenylisopropylamines, it might have been suspected that Nexus would be a DOB-like hallucinogen with reduced potency. This has been supported by the results of drug discrimination studies in animals. Furthermore, this material, also known as 2C-B, has been shown to be active in humans at 12 to 24 mg relative to approximately 2 mg for DOB (29). In the last year or two, a number of related agents have been found on the clandestine market and, like 2C-B, are phenylethylamine analogs of their phenylisopropylamine counterparts; for example, 2C-C, 2C-I, 2C-N, 2C-E, and 2C-P are the phenylethylamine analogs of DOC, DOI, DON, DOET, and DOPR, respectively (Table 19.3 and Fig. 19.6). Another agent attracting recent attention is 2C-T-7 (e.g., "Blue Mystic" or "Tripstasy") (65), which has been recently controlled as a Schedule I substance. Recently controlled indolealkylamine analogs include α-MeT (AMT), α-EtT ("ET"), and 5-methoxy-*N,N*-diisopropyltryptamine ("Foxy Methoxy") (Fig. 19.6); these agents had been previously shown to produce DOM-like stimulus effects in animals (66).

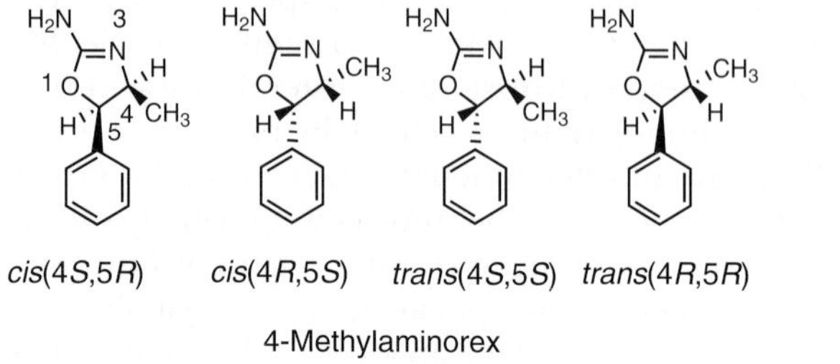

Stimulant designer drugs have also appeared. For example, CAT, or methcathinone, has been found on the illicit American market. Interestingly, it seems that methcathinone was a popular drug of abuse in the former Soviet Union (where it was known under a variety of names including ephedrone), but reports of this agent were never published in either the scientific or lay literature of that time. Methcathinone is the *N*-monomethyl analog of cathinone. Indeed, structurally, methcathinone is to cathinone what methamphetamine is to amphetamine. Methcathinone, which might be viewed as an oxidation product of ephedrine (hence the name ephedrone), is a potent central stimulant that is at least as potent as methamphetamine. Recently, a number of new cathinone analogs have appeared; the best known of these is 'bath salts'. Three common constituents of 'bath salts', mephedrone, methyenedioxypyrovalerone, and mephylone (or MDMC), were scheduled in 2011. Another example of a stimulant designer drug is 4-methylaminorex (U4Euh), which has been misrepresented on the illicit market as cocaine or methamphetamine. 4-Methylaminorex, an alkylated version of the anorectic/stimulant aminorex, contains two chiral centers and, hence, exists as four optical isomers. Typically, it is a mixture of the two *cis* isomers that has been confiscated by law enforcement officials, and *cis* 4-methylaminorex is now classified as a Schedule I substance. Interestingly, all four isomers behave as amphetamine-like agents, with the *trans*-(4S,5S) isomer being the most active, having a potency slightly greater than that of (+)-amphetamine itself (4). Yet other examples include piperazines. Several piperazine analogs have been reported to produce amphetamine-like effects in humans, and one in particular, *N*-benzylpiperazine (known either alone or in combination with other piperazines as "Rapture"), has been recently classified as a Schedule I substance (Fig. 19.6).

Not all designer drugs result in actions that are entirely predictable. One of the most popular of such agents is *N*-methyl-1-(3,4-methylenedioxyphenyl)-2-aminopropane (MDMA; e.g., "Ecstasy," "XTC," or "Adam") (Fig. 19.6). MDMA is the *N*-monomethyl analog of 1-(3,4-methylenedioxyphenyl)-2-aminopropane (MDA). MDA was popular during the 1960s, where it was known on the street as the "Love Drug." It was reported to produce effects in humans akin to a combination of cocaine and LSD. It has since been shown that MDA produces both amphetamine-like (i.e., central nervous system stimulant) and DOM-like (i.e., hallucinogen-lke) stimulus effects in animals and, furthermore, that animals trained to discriminate MDA recognize central stimulants, such as amphetamine and cocaine, as well as classical hallucinogens, such as LSD, mescaline, and DOM. Interestingly, the stimulant actions of MDA appear to be associated with the *S*-(+)-isomer, whereas the DOM-like actions are associated with the *R*-(−)-isomer. Knowing that *N*-monomethylation of phenylisopropylamine stimulants enhances their potency, whereas the corresponding change is detrimental to DOM-like actions, it would have been predicted that MDMA would probably behave as an amphetamine-like stimulant. Consistent with this prediction, amphetamine-trained (but not DOM-trained) animals recognized MDMA in tests of stimulus generalization. Furthermore, animals trained to discriminate MDMA recognized amphetamine but not DOM. However, MDMA was claimed to produce *empathogenic* effects in humans (i.e., increased empathy and sociability and enhanced feelings of well-being) and was used for several years as an adjunct to psychotherapy before emergency scheduling under the Controlled Substances Act as a Schedule I substance. It was argued that MDMA produces a unique, nonamphetamine-like effect (67). Although both optical isomers are active, the *S*-(+)-isomer is the more active of the two. A closely related agent is its *N*-ethyl homolog MDE ("Eve"). The general consensus today is that MDMA is probably an empathogen with amphetamine-like stimulant side effects. Homologation of the α-methyl group of phenylisopropylamine stimulants and hallucinogens typically diminishes their potency or abolishes their activity; however, the α-ethyl analog of MDMA [*N*-methyl-1-(3,4-methylenedioxyphenyl)-2-aminobutane] retains MDMA-like actions (68) (Fig. 19.6). Another agent, sold as a substitute for MDMA, is 4-MTA (e.g., "Flatliners" or "Golden Eagles") (Fig. 19.6); this agent produces MDMA-like stimulus effects in animals but did not produce either DOM-like or cocaine-like effects (65).

A closely related agent is *N*-methyl-1-(4-methoxyphenyl)-2-aminopropane (PMMA). PMMA is a hybrid structure of two phenylisopropylamine stimulants: PMA and methamphetamine (Fig. 19.6). Interestingly, PMMA lacks significant central stimulant actions, and unlike PMA and methamphetamine, PMMA is not recognized by (+)-amphetamine–trained animals. Because PMMA is structurally related to metabolites of MDMA, it was examined in MDMA-trained animals and found to be several times more potent than MDMA. Animals have been trained to discriminate PMMA from vehicle, and PMMA stimulus generalization occurred to (±)-MDMA and *S*-(+)-MDMA, but not to DOM, (+)-amphetamine, *R*-(−)-MDMA, or *R*-(−)-PMMA. Another psychoactive agent that has not been well investigated is 3,4-DMA (Table 19.3). 3,4-DMA may be viewed as an *O*-methyl ring-opened analog of MDA (Fig. 19.6). Although 3,4-DMA was not recognized by either DOM- or (+)-amphetamine–trained animals, it was recognized by MDA- and PMMA-trained animals. These results, coupled with the earlier discussion of MDMA, suggest that phenylisopropylamines might not best be described as merely central stimulants or hallucinogens; a third action needs to be accounted for. Although MDMA is widely abused, a contributing factor may be related to its amphetaminergic actions.

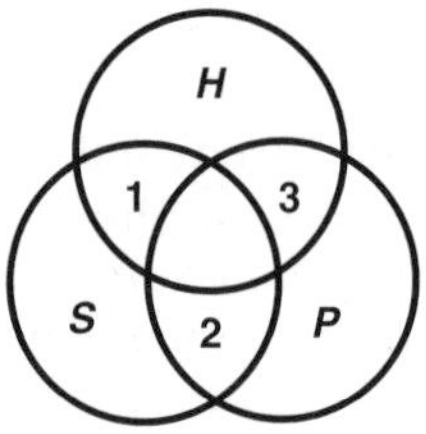

FIGURE 19.7 The behavioral effects of arylalkylamines may be described as falling into one or more of three different stimulus categories: classical hallucinogen (*H*), central stimulant (*S*), or PMMA-like (*P*). See text for further discussion.

It is not yet known if agents that fall into this third pharmacologic category possess abuse potential; consequently, they have been referred to simply as "other" agents. It has been proposed that the behavioral actions of the phenylisopropylamines can be described by the Venn diagram shown as Figure 19.7. As depicted in that figure, the three types of actions are classical hallucinogen (*H*), stimulant (*S*), and PMMA-like (*P*) (69). Because MDMA possesses both PMMA-like and (+)-amphetamine–like activity, it is perhaps best represented by Intersect 2. As mentioned earlier, *R*-(−)-MDA is hallucinogenic, and *S*-(+)-MDA is a stimulant. Both isomers possess PMMA-like activity. Thus, *R*-(−)-MDA is best represented by Intersect 3, whereas *S*-(+)-MDA is best represented by Intersect 2. The common intersect (shaded area) describes the actions of (±)-MDA. Using this classification system, it should be possible to classify the various phenylisopropylamines as falling into one or more categories. Furthermore, there is no reason to suspect that this classification system will be limited to the phenylisopropylamines; that is, there is evidence that the indolealkylamines might be classified in a similar manner. For example, *S*-(+)-α-EtT produces both DOM- and PMMA-like effects, but not (+)-amphetamine–like effects, whereas *R*-(−)-α-EtT produces (+)-amphetamine– and PMMA-like effects, but not DOM-like effects (70). The classification scheme suggests that there will be at least three different SARs and three different mechanisms of action. Certain agents, because they fall into more than one category, may represent mechanistic and structure–activity composites. The same may be said of arylalkylamine designer drugs; indeed, it may be the particular "mix" of actions that makes certain designer drugs so attractive as drugs of abuse.

Perhaps the most worrisome aspects about designer drugs are that almost none have been investigated under controlled clinical settings, that relatively little is known about their toxicity or long-term effects, and that medical professionals generally are unfamiliar with them (or with the treatment of their overdose) in emergency room settings. The situation is further exacerbated by the broad availability of Web sites describing such agents to potential users (71).

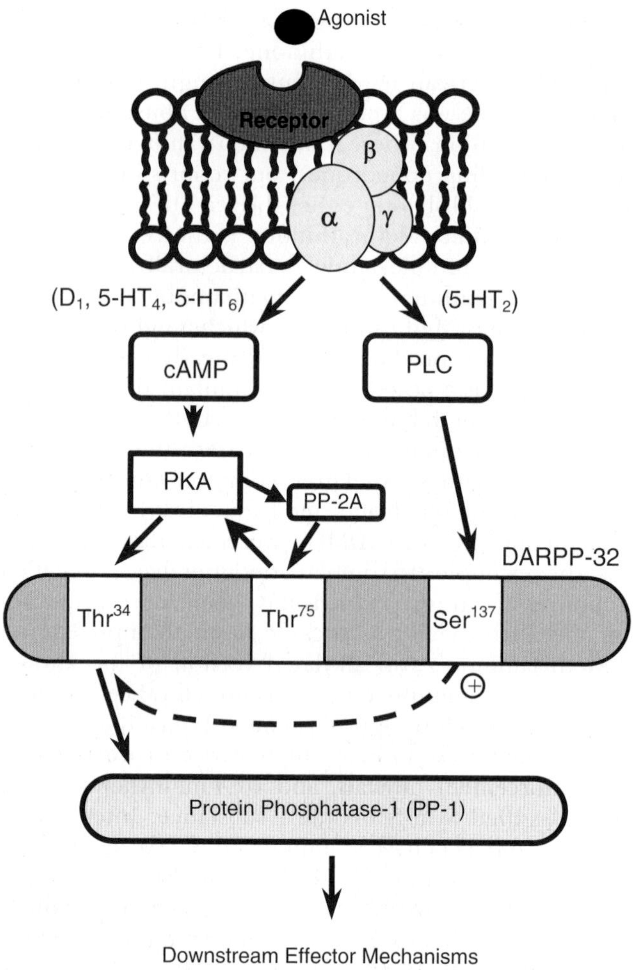

FIGURE 19.8 A simplistic schematic showing the proposed involvement of DARPP-32 in neurotransmission. Agonists (e.g., dopamine and serotonin) can interact with certain postsynaptic G protein–coupled receptors to activate second messenger systems. Agonist action at D_1 receptors increases cAMP levels and causes PKA to phosphorylate DARPP-32 at Thr^{34}; activation of D_1 receptors also decreases the phosphorylation state of DARPP-32 at Thr^{75} by what appears to involve PKA-dependent activation of a protein phosphatase (PP-2A). Likewise, the action of 5-HT at 5-HT_4 and 5-HT_6 receptors increases phosphorylation of Thr^{34} and decreases phosphorylation of Thr^{75}. Interaction of 5-HT at 5-HT_2 receptors activates PLC and promotes phosphorylation of DARPP-32 at Ser^{137}. Phosphorylation at Thr^{34} inhibits protein phosphatase-1 (PP-1). Inhibition of PP-1 enhances signaling. Phosphorylation of Thr^{75} has an inhibitory effect on Thr^{34} phosphorylation (conversely, decreased Thr^{75} phosphorylation disinhibits PKA to increase Thr^{34} phosphorylation), whereas phosphorylation of Ser^{137} prevents dephosphorylation of Thr^{34}. Other receptors can impinge on this mechanism (72–77).

NEURONAL PLASTICITY AND DRUGS OF ABUSE

Release of neurotransmitter from presynaptic terminals results in the activation of postsynaptic neurotransmitter receptors that are coupled to complex effector mechanisms. Through modulation of postsynaptic pathways, the state of the neuron can be altered such that neurons become more or less responsive to the neurotransmitter (72). This process is referred to as functional plasticity. One of the most exciting recent findings with implications for the treatment of drug abuse (as well as other neuropsychiatric disorders) involves the regulation of DARPP-32, an integrator of intracellular signaling (Fig. 19.8). Interaction of DA at D_1-like receptors (D_1/D_5) activates adenylate cyclase, which increases cAMP levels; this, in turn, regulates phosphorylation of DARPP-32 by PKA. Interaction of DA at D_2-like receptors ($D_2/D_3/D_4$, which are negatively coupled to cAMP) has an effect that is essentially opposite that of activation of D_1 receptors. Phosphorylation of a specific amino acid residue (i.e., threonine^{34} [Thr^{34}]), induced by D_1 agonists, converts DARPP-32 to an inhibitor of PP-1; thus, when phosphorylated at Thr^{34}, DARPP-32 behaves as an amplifier of PKA-mediated signaling through its ability to inhibit PP-1. The actions of DARPP-32 can also be modulated by phosphorylation (or dephosphorylation) of Thr^{75} (Fig. 19.8). Activation of D_1 receptors decreases the phosphorylation state of DARPP-32 at Thr^{75} by a process that involves PKA-dependent activation of protein phosphatase-2A (PP-2A); this disinhibits phosphorylation of Thr^{34} by PKA (i.e., results in enhanced phosphorylation of Thr^{34}). The result is potentiation of dopaminergic signaling. Together, PKA and PP-1 regulate the phosphorylation state of downstream neuronal effector proteins. Additionally, DARPP-32 can be phosphorylated at serine^{137} (Ser^{137}), and this phosphorylation decreases the rate of dephosphorylation of Thr^{34}.

5-HT causes an increase in phosphorylation of Thr^{34} (via activation of 5-HT_4 and 5-HT_6 receptors, which are positively coupled to cAMP) and Ser^{137} (via activation of 5-HT_2 receptors, which are coupled to phospholipase C) and a decrease in the phosphorylation of Thr^{75} (via activation of 5-HT_4 and 5-HT_6 receptors). Hence, 5-HT inhibits PP-1 through what might be considered a synergistic mechanism (73). Other receptors that might modulate DARPP-32 include glutamate, GABA, adenosine, nitrous oxide, and opioid receptors. Hence, it has been speculated that various drugs of abuse, including amphetamine, methamphetamine, cocaine, opioids (e.g., morphine), nicotine, and ethanol involve a DARPP-32 mechanism; caffeine was discussed earlier. Furthermore, agents such as antidepressants, antipsychotics, and antiparkinsonian drugs have been shown to influence phosphorylation of DARPP-32. Classical hallucinogens, as described earlier, are thought to act by activation of 5-HT_{2A} receptors. It has been shown that LSD increases phosphorylation of Ser^{137} (74). In theory, DARPP-32 should be modulated by various designer drugs that act via a dopaminergic or serotonergic mechanism. Only selected aspects of intracellular integration have been mentioned here, and others already have been implicated. The state of the art has been recently described (38,73–77). Nevertheless, the actions of many drugs of abuse might involve such postsynaptic events and certainly require further attention.

ACKNOWLEDGEMENT

Work from the author's laboratory was supported by PHS grant DA 01642.

SCENARIO: OUTCOME AND ANALYSIS

Outcome

Mark D. Watanabe, PharmD, PhD, BCPP

When JN took a break from the dance floor, he found that he was sweating profusely, short of breath, and quite dizzy. Given that he was in generally excellent physical shape from athletic training, he became alarmed about his weakened and disoriented state. Later, JN confided to a friend that although "flatliners" gave him a boost of energy, he was disappointed that he did not experience a more pleasant "buzz" as he had expected.

Chemical Analysis

S. William Zito and Victoria Roche

The designer drug offered to JN was referred to as "flatliners." It is structurally related to the arylisopropylamine classic hallucinogens. It is 4-MTA (4-methylthioamphetamine). JN was told it would act like Ecstacy. Ecstacy is *N*-Methyl-3,4-methylenedioxyamphetamine (MDMA). MDMA is the *N*-monomethyl analogue of MDA, or 1-(3,4-methylenedioxyphenyl)-2-aminopropane (also known as 3,4-methylenedioxyamphetamine).

MDA produces both amphetamine-like (i.e., CNS stimulant) and DOM-like (i.e., hallucinogen-like) stimulus effects in animals. Interestingly, the stimulant actions of MDA appear to be associated with the S-(+)-isomer, whereas the DOM-like actions are associated with the R-(−)-isomer. SAR studies have shown that *N*-monomethylation of phenylisopropylamine stimulants enhances their CNS-stimulant potency and decreases or eliminates their DOM-like actions, it is therefore predicted that MDMA probably behaves as an amphetamine-like stimulant. In addition, MDMA seems to have unique non–amphetamine-like effects referred to as *empathogenic* (i.e., increased empathy and sociability and enhanced feelings of well being) and was used for several years as an adjunct to psychotherapy. The general consensus today is that MDMA is probably an empathogen with amphetamine-like stimulant side effects. In this case, JN experienced the amphetamine-like effects of Ecstacy (increased energy, increased stamina, tachycardia, decreased anxiety) from 4-MTA; however, he was disappointed with the lack of hallucinogenic effects (the "buzz"). This is not surprising because 4-MTA has been shown to produce MDMA-like stimulus effects in animals but did not produce either DOM-like or cocaine-like effects.

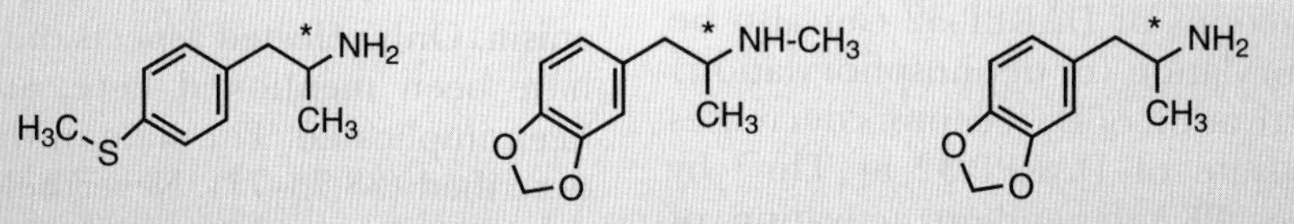

4-MTA MDMA MDA

CASE STUDY

S. William Zito and Victoria Roche

You are one of the lucky few students to draw the police forensic laboratory as one of your elective rotations. On your second day there, your preceptor asks you to evaluate a recent case involving JB, a young man who was arrested and charged with possession of a drug of abuse. Upon arrest, JB was red eyed, very thirsty, hungry, and bothered by bright light. Despite of the fix he was in, JB was laid back, laughing inappropriately and chuckling to himself. The forensic laboratory analyzed the confiscated substance and it was shown to contain the following three main compounds. Which one of them is responsible for JB's symptoms?

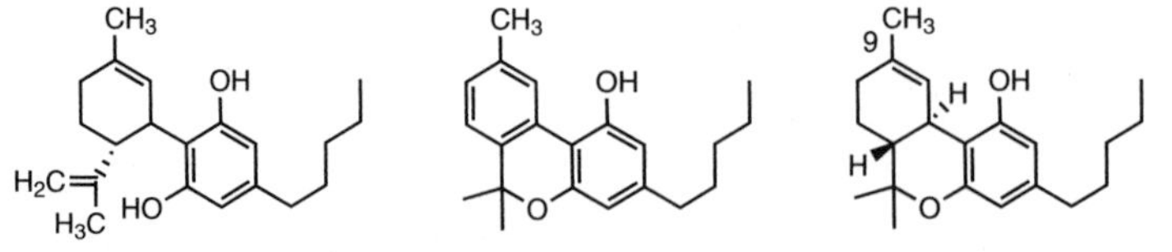

1 2 3

1. Conduct a thorough and mechanistic SAR analysis of the three therapeutic options in the case.
2. Apply the chemical understanding gained from the SAR analysis to this patient's specific needs to make a therapeutic recommendation.

References

1a. Nichols D. Legal highs: the dark side of medicinal chemistry. Nature 2011;469:7.
1b. Brimblecombe RW, Pinder RM. Hallucinogenic Agents. Bristol, UK: Wright-Scientechnica, 1975.
2. Hollister LE. Chemical Psychoses. Springfield, IL: Charles C. Thomas, 1968.
3. Glennon RA. Animal models for assessing hallucinogenic agents. In: Boulton AA, Baker GB, Wu PH, eds. Animal Models of Drug Addiction. Totowa, NJ: Humana Press, 1992:345–381.
4. Glennon RA, Young R, eds, Drug Discrimination: Applications to Medicinal Chemistry and Drug Studies, Hoboken, NJ; John Wiley and Sons, 2011.
5. Glennon RA. Discriminative stimulus properties of hallucinogens and related designer drugs. In: Glennon RA, Jarbe TUC, Frankenheim J, eds.

Drug Discrimination: Applications to Drug Abuse Research. Rockville, MD: National Institute on Drug Abuse, 1991:25–44.
6. Lin JC, Glennon RA, eds. Hallucinogens: An Update. Rockville, MD: National Institute on Drug Abuse, 1994.
7. Padgett LW. Recent developments in cannabinoid ligands. Life Sci 2005;77:1767–1798.
8. Pertwee RG. Cannabinoid pharmacology: the first 66 years. Br J Pharmacol 2006;147:S163–S171.
9. Reggio PH, ed. The Cannabinoid Receptors. Berlin: Springer, 2009.
10. Hanus L, Gopher A, Almog S, et al. Two new unsaturated fatty acid ethanolamides in brain that bind to the cannabinoid receptor. J Med Chem 1993;36:3032–3034.
11. Jarbe TUC, Lamb RL, Makriyannis A, et al. (R)-methanandamide as a discriminative stimulus in rats: tests with anandamide and Δ^9-THC. Behav Pharmacol 1998;9:S47.
12. Mackie K. Cannabinoid receptors as therapeutic targets. Ann Rev Pharmacol Toxicol 2006;46:101–123.
13. Martin BR. Marijuana. In: Bloom FE, Kupfer DJ, eds. Psychopharmacology: The Fourth Generation of Progress. New York: Raven Press, 1995:1757–1765.
14. Huffman JW. CB_2 receptor ligands. Mini Rev Med Chem 2005;5:641–649.
15. Corey S. Recent development in the therapeutic potential of cannabinoids. P R Health Sci J 2005;24:19–26.
16. Prem S. Overview of phencyclidine (PCP) intoxication in children and adolescents. UpToDate, http://www.uptodate.com/patients/content/topic.do?topicKey=~G5GcywxXRlFVI, 2010.
17. Bey T, Patel A. Phencyclidine intoxication and adverse effects: a clinical and pharmacological review of an illicit drug. West J Emerg Med 2007;8:9–14.
18. Balster RL, Willetts J. Phencyclidine: a drug of abuse and a tool for neuroscience research. In: Schuster CR, Kuhar MJ, eds. Pharmacological Aspects of Drug Dependence. Handbook of Experimental Pharmacology Series, Vol 118. Berlin: Springer, 1996:233–262.
19. Glennon RA. Pharmacophore identification for sigma-1(σ_1) receptor binding-application of the "deconstruction-reconstruction-elaboration" approach. Mini Rev Med Chem 2005;5:927–940.
20. Morris BJ, Cochran SM, Pratt JA. PCP: from pharmacology to modeling schizophrenia. Curr Opin Pharmacol 2005;5:101–106.
21. Balster RL. Discriminative stimulus properties of phencyclidine and other NMDA antagonists. In: Glennon RA, Jarbe TUC, Frankenheim J, eds. Drug Discrimination: Applications to Drug Abuse Research. Rockville, MD: National Institute on Drug Abuse, 1991:163–180.
22. Shulgin AT, Shulgin A. Tihkal. Berkeley, CA: Transform Press, 1997.
23. Murphree HB, Dippy RH, Jenney EH, et al. Effects in normal man of α-methyltryptamine and α-ethyltryptamine. Clin Pharmacol Ther 1961;2:722–726.
24. Siva Sankar DV, ed. LSD: a total study. Westbury, NY: PJD Publications, 1975.
25. Pfaff RC, Huang X, Marona-Lewicka D, et al. Lysergamides revisited. In: Lin JC, Glennon RA, eds. Hallucinogens: an update. Rockville, MD: National Institute on Drug Abuse, 1994:52–73.
26. Naranjo C. Psychotropic properties of harmala alkaloids. In: Efron DK, Holmstedt B, Kline NS, eds. Ethnopharmacologic search for psychoactive drugs. Washington, DC: U.S. Government Printing Office, 1967:385–391.
27. Naranjo C. The Healing Journey. New York: Pantheon Books, 1973.
28. Grella B, Dukat M, Young R, et al. Investigation of hallucinogenic and related β-carbolines. Drug Alcohol Depend 1998;50:99–107.
29. Shulgin AT, Shulgin A. Pihkal. Berkeley, CA: Transform Press, 1991.
30. Glennon RA. Classical hallucinogens. In: Schuster CR, Kuhar MJ, eds. Pharmacological Aspects of Drug Dependence. Handbook of Experimental Pharmacology Series, Vol 118. Berlin: Springer, 1996:343–371.
31. Nelson DL, Lucaites VL, Wainscot DB, et al. Comparisons of hallucinogenic phenylisopropylamine binding affinities at cloned human 5-HT_{2A}, 5-HT_{2B}, and 5-HT_{2C} receptors. Naunyn-Schmeideberg's Arch Pharmacol 1998;359:1–6.
32. Griffiths RR, Mumford GK. Caffeine reinforcement, discrimination, tolerance, and physical dependence in laboratory animals and humans. In: Schuster CR, Kuhar MJ, eds. Pharmacological Aspects of Drug Dependence. Handbook of Experimental Pharmacology Series, Vol 118. Berlin: Springer, 1996:315–341.
33. Daly JW. Caffeine analogs: biomedical impact. Cell Mol Life Sci 2007;64:2153–2169.
34. Essayan DM. Cyclic nucleotide phosphodiesterases. J Allergy Clin Immunol 2007;109:671–680.
35. Ito K, Lim S, Caramori G, et al. A molecular mechanism of action of theophylline: Induction of histone deacetylase activity to decrease inflammatory gene expression. Proc Natl Acad Sci U S A 2002;99:8921–8926.
36. Barnes PJ. Theophylline. New perspectives for an old drug. Am J Respir Crit Care Med 2003;167:813–818.
37. Fisone G, Borgkvist A, Usiello A. Caffeine as a psychomotor stimulant: mechanism of action. Cell Mol Life Sci 2004;61:857–872.
38. Sahin B, Galdi S, Hendrick T, et al. Evaluation of neuronal phosphoproteins as effectors of caffeine and mediators of striatal adenosine A_{2A} receptor signaling. Brain Res 2007;1129:1–14.
39. Cho AK, Segal DS, eds. Amphetamine and Its Analogues. San Diego: Academic Press, 1994:43–77.
40. Young R, Glennon RA. Discriminative stimulus properties of amphetamine and structurally related phenalkylamines. Med Res Rev 1986;6:99–130.
41. Young R, Gabryszuk M, Glennon RA. (−)-Ephedrine and caffeine mutually potentiate one another's amphetamine-like stimulus effects. Pharmacol Biochem Behav 1998;61:169–173.
42. Cho AK, Kumagai Y. Metabolism of amphetamine and other arylisopropylamines. In: Cho AK, Segal DS, eds. Amphetamine and Its Analogues. San Diego: Academic Press, 1994:43–77.
43. Finer N. Pharmacotherapy of obesity. Best Pract Res Clin Endocrinol Metab 2002;16:717–742.
44. Linne Y, Rossner S. Pharmacotherapy of obesity. Clin Dermatol 2004;22:319–324.
45. Rothman RB, Baumann MH, Savage JE, et al. Evidence for possible involvement of 5-HT_{2B} receptors in the cardiac valvulopathy associated with fenfluramine and other serotonergic medications. Circulation 2000;102:2836–2841.
46. Setola V, Dukat M, Glennon RA, et al. Molecular determinants for the interaction of the valvulopathic anorexigen norfenfluramine with the 5-HT_{2B} receptor. Mol Pharmacol 2005;68:20–33.
47. van Gaal L, Mertens I, Ballaux D, et al. Modern, new pharmacotherapy for obesity. Best Pract Res Clin Endocrinol Metab 2004;18:1049–1072.
48. Banerjee D, Vitiello MV, Grunstein RR. Pharmacotherapy for excessive daytime sleepiness. Sleep Med Rev 2004;8:339–354.
49. Boutrel B, Koob GF. What keeps us awake: the neuropharmacology of stimulants and wakefulness-promoting medications. Sleep 2004;27:1181–1194.
50. Black J, Guilleminault C. Medications for the treatment of narcolepsy. Expert Opin Emerg Drugs 2001;6:239–247.
51. Schwartz JR. Modafinil: new indications for wake promotion. Expert Opin Pharmacother 2005;6:115–129.
52. Houghton WC, Scammell TE, Thorpy M. Pharmacotherapy for cataplexy. Sleep Med Rev 2004;8:355–366.
53. Mignot E. An update on the pharmacotherapy of excessive daytime sleepiness and cataplexy. Sleep Med Rev 2004;8:333–338.
54. Zolkowska D, Jain R, Rothman RB, et al. Evidence for the involvement of dopamine transporters in the behavioral stimulant effects of modafinil. J Pharm Exp Ther 2009;329:738–746.
55. Seeman P, Guan H-C, Hirbec H. Dopamine D_2 receptors stimulated by phencyclidines, lysergic acid diethylamide, salvinorin A, and modafinil. Synapse 2009;63:698–704.
56. Fischman MW, Johanson CE. Cocaine. In: Schuster CR, Kuhar MJ, eds. Pharmacological Aspects of Drug Dependence. Handbook of Experimental Pharmacology Series, Vol 118. Berlin: Springer, 1996:159–195.
57. Carroll FI, Lewin AH, Boja JW, et al. Cocaine receptor: biochemical characterization and structure–activity relationships of cocaine analogues at the dopamine transporter. J Med Chem 1992;35:969–981.
58. Newman AH. Novel dopamine transporter ligands: the state of the art. Med Chem Res 1998;8:1–11.
59. Deutsch HM, Shi Q, Gruszecka-Kowalik E, et al. Synthesis and pharmacology of potential cocaine antagonists. 2. Structure–activity relationship studies of aromatic ring-substituted methylphenidate analogues. J Med Chem 1996;39:1201–1209.
60. Sofuoglu M, Kosten TR. Novel approaches to the treatment of cocaine abuse. CNS Drugs 2005;19:13–25.
61. Singh S. Chemistry, design, and structure-activity relationships of cocaine antagonists. Chem Rev 2000;100:925–1024.
62. Heal DJ, Pierce DM. Methylphenidate and it isomers. CNS Drugs 2006;20:713–738.
63. Froimowitz M, Patrick KS, Cody V. Conformational analysis of methylphenidate and its structural relationship to other dopamine reuptake blockers such as CFT. Pharmaceut Res 1995;12:1430–1434.
64. Srinivas NR, Hubbard JW, Korchinski ED, et al. Enantioselective pharmacokinetics of dl-threo-methylphenidate. Pharmaceut Res 1993;10:14–21.
65. Khorana N, Pullagurla M, Dukat M, et al. Stimulus effects of three sulfur-containing psychoactive agents. Pharmacol Biochem Behav 2004;78:821–826.
66. Glennon RA, Young R, Jacyno JM, et al. DOM-stimulus generalization to LSD and other hallucinogenic indolealkylamines. Eur J Pharmacol 1983;86:453–459.
67. Nichols DE, Oberlender R. Structure–activity relationships of MDMA-like substances. In: Ashgar K, De Souza E, eds. Pharmacology and Toxicology of Amphetamine and Related Designer Drugs. Washington, DC: U.S. Government Printing Office, 1989:1–29.
68. Oberlender R, Nichols DE. (+)-*N*-methyl-1-(1,3-benzodioxol-5-yl)-2-butanamine as a discriminative stimulus in studies of 3,4-methylenedioxyamphetamine-like behavioral activity. J Pharmacol Exp Ther 1990;255:1098–1106.
69. Glennon RA, Young R, Dukat M, et al. Initial characterization of PMMA as a discriminative stimulus. Pharmacol Biochem Behav 1997;57:151–158.
70. Glennon RA. Arylalkylamine drugs of abuse: an overview of drug discrimination studies. Pharmacol Biochem Behav 1999;64:251–256.
71. Wax PM. Just a click away: recreational drug web sites on the internet. Pediatrics 2002;109:96–100.
72. Benavides DR, Bibb JA. Role of Cdk5 in drug abuse and plasticity. Ann N Y Acad Sci 2004;1025:335–344.
73. Svenningsson P, Tzavara ET, Liu F, et al. DARPP-32 mediates serotonergic neurotransmission in the forebrain. Proc Natl Acad Sci U S A 2002;99:3188–3193.
74. Svenningsson P, Tzavara ET, Carruthers R, et al. Diverse psychotomimetics act through a common signaling pathway. Science 2003;302:1412–1415.
75. Svenningsson P, Nishi A, Fisone G, et al. DARPP-32: an integrator of neurotransmission. Ann Rev Pharmacol Toxicol 2004;44:269–296.
76. Nairn AC, Svenningsson P, Nishi A, et al. The role of DARPP-32 in the actions of drugs of abuse. Neuropharmacology 2004;47(Suppl 1):14–23.
77. Gould TD, Manji HK. DARPP-32: a molecular switch at the nexus of reward pathway plasticity. Proc Natl Acad Sci U S A 2005;102:253–254.

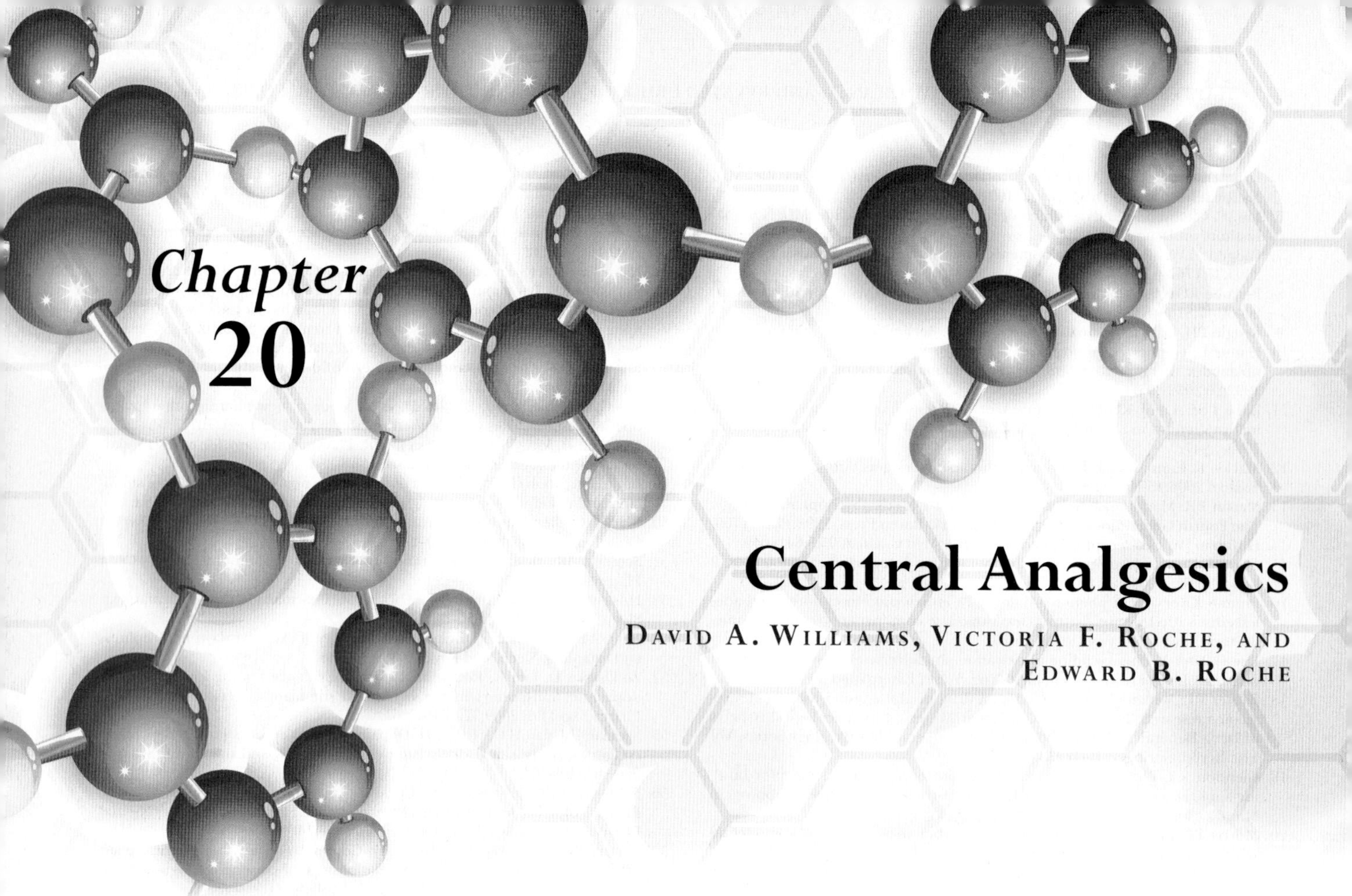

Chapter 20

Central Analgesics

David A. Williams, Victoria F. Roche, and Edward B. Roche

Drugs Covered in This Chapter

Nociceptive Analgesics

Multicyclic full μ agonists
- Codeine
- Hydrocodone
- Hydromorphone
- Levorphanol
- Morphine
- Oxycodone
- Oxymorphone

Multicyclic partial μ agonists
- Buprenorphine

Multicyclic κ agonists/μ antagonists
- Butorphanol
- Nalbuphine
- Pentazocine

Multicyclic opioid antagonists
- Methylnaltrexone bromide
- Nalmefene
- Naloxone
- Naltrexone

Flexible full μ agonists
- Alfentanil
- Fentanyl
- Meperidine
- Methadone
- Remifentanil
- Sufentanil

Dual-action analgesics
- Tapentadol
- Tramadol

Antidiarrheals
- Difenoxin
- Diphenoxylate
- Loperamide

Neuropathic Analgesics

First-line agents
- Desipramine
- Duloxetine
- Gabapentin
- Lidocaine
- Nortriptyline
- Pregabalin
- Venlafaxine

Second-line agents
- Methadone
- Morphine
- Oxycodone
- Tramadol

Third-line agents
- Bupropion
- Carbamazepine
- Oxcarbazepine
- Paroxetine

Future medications
- Cannabidiol
- Capsaicin
- Lacosamide
- Δ^9-Tetrahydrocannabinol

Medical food
- Metanx

Abbreviations

cAMP, cyclic adenosine monophosphate
CNS, central nervous system
DADLE, [D-Ala², D-Leu⁵] enkephalin
DPDPE, [D-Pen², D-Pen⁵] enkephalin
DSLET, [D-Ser², Leu⁵] enkephalin-Thr
FDA, U.S. Food and Drug Administration
GABA, γ-aminobutyric acid
GI, gastrointestinal
5-HT, serotonin
IUPHAR, International Union of Pharmacology

Abbreviations (Continued)

IV, intravenous
MAOI, monoamine oxidase inhibitor
NE, norepinephrine
NMDA, *N*-methyl-D-aspartate
N/OFQ, nociceptin/orphanin FQ
P-gp, P-glycoprotein
ppN/OFQ, preproN/OFQ
SAR, structure–activity relationship
SSRI, selective serotonin reuptake inhibitor
TCA, tricyclic antidepressant
TRPV1, transient receptor potential vanilloid 1

SCENARIO

Jill T. Johnson, PharmD, BCPS

JB is a 25-year-old African-American man with sickle cell disease who was admitted to the hospital for a vaso-occlusive crisis. He says his pain started in his low back and now includes his chest and abdomen. The pain is severe and gnawing, and the patient scored the pain as 10 out of 10. At home, he does not take opioids routinely but does take folic acid and hydroxyurea. He says he is allergic to morphine and codeine and has a history of rash when he takes either. He says intravenous pain medications work the best when he is in a crisis, and he prefers meperidine to hydromorphone.

(The reader is directed to the clinical solution and chemical analysis of this case at the end of the chapter.)

INTRODUCTION

This chapter begins by describing types of pain and the mechanisms by which noxious stimuli result in the perception of pain. The pharmacologic treatment of pain should target the specific mechanism of pain rather than suppressing the symptoms of pain. Nociceptive (acute), chronic, and neuropathic pain are caused by different neurophysiologic processes and therefore respond to different pharmacologic treatment modalities. Neuropathic pain can be one of the most debilitating forms of chronic pain. Therefore, accurate diagnosis and treatment of pain should be sought early, and appropriate treatment should be rendered to increase the likelihood of a good outcome (relief of pain), without restricting a person's quality of life and general well-being.

A number of classes of drugs are used to relieve nociceptive pain. The opioid analgesics, also inappropriately known as narcotics, are the first-line treatment for acute or nociceptive pain; thus, the use of the term antinociceptive to describe the opioids. Agents that decrease acute and some types of chronic pain are referred to as analgesics, or analgetics. Although analgetic is grammatically correct, common use has made analgesic preferable to analgetic for the description of the pain-killing drugs. On the other hand, neuropathic or chronic pain relieving agents include antidepressants, antiseizure agents, and local anesthetics. Narcotic analgesic literally means that the agents cause sleep or loss of consciousness (narcosis) in conjunction with their analgesic effect, something the opioids do not do. The term "narcotic" has become associated with the addictive properties of opioids and other central nervous system (CNS) depressants. Because the great therapeutic value of the opioids lies in their ability to induce analgesia without causing narcosis, and because not all opioids are addicting, the term "narcotic analgesic" is misleading and will not be used further in this chapter. The nonsteroidal anti-inflammatory agents have primarily a peripheral site of action as inhibitors of cyclooxygenase, are useful for mild to moderate pain, and often have an anti-inflammatory effect associated with their pain-killing action (Chapter 31). Local anesthetics inhibit pain transmission by inhibition of voltage-regulated sodium channels (Chapter 16). These agents are often highly toxic when used in concentrations sufficient to relieve chronic or acute pain in ambulatory patients. Dissociative anesthetics (ketamine) and other compounds that act as inhibitors of *N*-methyl-D-aspartate–activated glutamate receptors in the brain are effective antinociceptive agents when used alone or in combination with opioids (Chapter 16). Most CNS depressants (e.g., ethanol, barbiturates, and antipsychotics) will cause a decrease in pain perception. Current research into the antinociceptive effects of centrally acting α-adrenergic-, cannabinoid-, and nicotinic-receptor agonists may yield clinically useful analgesics working by nonopioid mechanisms.

The chapter concludes by describing the mechanism by which nerve damage results in neuropathic pain and the mechanisms of action of the major classes of drugs used for clinical neuropathic pain relief. Neuropathic pain can be very difficult to treat, with only 40% to 60% of patients achieving partial relief. Many of the pharmacologic treatments for chronic neuropathic pain decrease the sensitivity of nociceptors or desensitize C-fibers such that they transmit fewer signals. Agents for the treatment of neuropathic pain include the tricyclic and dual-acting reuptake inhibitor antidepressants (Chapter 18); these agents are useful either alone or in combination with opioids in treating certain cases of neuropathic pain, especially the anticonvulsants pregabalin (Lyrica) and gabapentin (Neurontin), which inhibit voltage-regulated Ca^{2+} ion channels (Chapter 17), and topical lidocaine (Chapter 16). Opioid analgesics, including the dual-action agent tramadol, are recognized as useful agents but are not recommended as first-line treatments. Tricyclic antidepressants and anticonvulsants have long been the mainstay of treatment of neuropathic pain.

Research in one or more of the above areas may lead to new drugs, but at present, severe acute and some types of chronic pain are generally treated most effectively with opioid agonists, and neuropathic pain is most effectively treated with antidepressants and antiseizure agents. The cannabinoid receptors and the endogenous cannabinoids have become the focus of chronic pain regulation.

OVERVIEW OF PAIN

Pain is defined as an unpleasant sensory and emotional experience associated with actual or potential tissue damage, or described in terms of such damage (1,2). Pain is part of the body's defense system producing a reflexive retraction from the painful stimulus and to protect the affected body part while it heals. Most pain resolves promptly once the painful stimulus is removed and the body has healed, but sometimes pain persists despite removal of the stimulus and apparent healing of the body (1). Pain sometimes arises in the absence of any detectable stimulus, damage, or disease. The experience of physical pain is familiar to everyone; however, the intensity, character, and tolerability of each person's pain are subjective. Differences in pain perception and tolerance thresholds are associated with, among other factors, ethnicity, genetics, and sex. For example, women have lower pain perception and tolerance thresholds than men, and this sex difference appears to apply to all ages, including newborn infants. Pain is essential for protection of our bodies from injury and recognition of the presence of injury (3). Pain is the most common reason for visiting the emergency department in more than 50% of cases and for 30% of family practice visits. According to the National Center for Health Statistics, 46 million Americans undergo inpatient surgical procedures each year and experience acute surgical pain; pain severity was reported as moderate to severe by 45% of patients in the emergency departments (4). Examples of clinical pain include pain following surgery and pain associated with injury. Pain management becomes more important as people approach death (5). Pain can significantly interfere with a person's quality of life and general well-being. Observation becomes critical when self-reporting of pain, and specific behaviors or types of pain (e.g., dull, throbbing, stabbing), location and intensity of pain, how and when it occurs, and the effects of pain are needed in order to recommend appropriate interventions (5). Because everyone feels pain differently, standardized pain scales are used in the clinic and in clinical trials to provide clues as to the intensity of a patient's pain. To help compensate for this problem, one common type of pain scale shows a series of numbered cartoon faces moving from 0 (smiling and pain-free) to 10 (weeping in agony). The person in pain is asked which face matches up with the intensity of the pain the patient is experiencing. These scales can be used to assess the progression of pain and/or the effectiveness of pain therapy (3).

An aging adult may not respond to pain in the way that a younger person would. Their ability to recognize pain may be blunted by illness or the use of multiple prescription drugs (3,5). Depression may also keep the older adult from reporting they are in pain. The older adult may refrain from reporting pain and also stop doing activities because they hurt too much. Decline in self-care activities (dressing, grooming, walking, etc.) may also be indicators that the older adult is experiencing pain.

Acute Pain

Acute pain is defined as the normal, predicted physiologic response to an adverse chemical, thermal, or mechanical stimulus associated with surgery, trauma, or acute illness (1). Acute pain results from activation of the pain receptors (nociceptors) at the site of tissue damage. This type of pain generally accompanies surgery, traumatic injury, tissue damage, and inflammatory processes. Acute pain provides a warning signal that something is wrong and in need of further examination. Acute pain is typically self-limiting and resolves over days to weeks, but it can persist for months or longer as healing occurs (3). Acute pain can activate the sympathetic branch of the autonomic nervous system to produce such responses as hypertension, tachycardia, sweating, shallow respiration, restlessness, facial grimacing, pallor, and pupil dilation, as well as unnecessary physical and emotional distress (2).

Pain can be divided into nociceptive and neuropathic pain (2). Nociceptive pain and neuropathic pain are caused by different neurophysiologic processes and therefore respond to different treatment modalities. Nociceptive pain is mediated by stimulation of nociceptors, which are located in skin, bone, connective tissue, muscle, and viscera and respond only to noxious stimuli approaching or exceeding harmful intensity (2). Nociceptors serve a biologically useful role at localizing noxious chemical (alcohol in an open wound), thermal (heat or cold), and mechanical (crushing, tearing, etc.) stimuli. Nociceptive pain can be divided into visceral, deep somatic, or superficial somatic pain (1–3). Visceral pain stems from nociceptors in the viscera (organs), tends to be vague in distribution, and is usually described as deep, aching, squeezing, and spasmodic. Examples of nociceptive pain include postoperative pain, pain associated with trauma, and the chronic pain of arthritis. Nociceptive pain usually responds to opioids and nonsteroidal anti-inflammatory drugs. Deep somatic pain originates from stimulation of nociceptors in ligaments, tendons, bones, blood vessels, fasciae, and muscles and is a constant pain described as sharp, aching, throbbing, or gnawing (6). Examples include sprains and broken bones.

Superficial pain is initiated by activation of nociceptors in the skin or superficial tissues and is sharp, well-defined, and clearly localized (also described as sharp, aching, throbbing, or gnawing). Examples of injuries that produce superficial somatic pain include minor wounds and minor (first-degree) burns (6). On the other hand, neuropathic pain (chronic pain) involves the abnormal processing of stimuli from nerve damage in the peripheral or central nervous system; it is believed to serve no useful purpose.

The nociceptive pain mechanism is highly complex (2). Initially, tissue damage releases chemical mediators, such as prostaglandins, bradykinin, serotonin, substance P, and histamine, which subsequently stimulate nociceptors, generating an action potential (an electrical impulse) (Fig. 20.1). The action potential travels from the site of peripheral injury along afferent neurons or fibers, designated C-fibers and A-delta (Aδ)-fibers, to receptors at the dorsal horn of the spinal cord, from where the action potential ascends the spinothalamic tract to the brainstem and onto the thalamus and the midbrain. Aδ-fibers are thinly myelinated and transmit the action potentials more rapidly (~20 m/s) than unmyelinated C-fibers (~2 m/s), but more slowly than more thickly myelinated A-fibers. Aδ-axons are associated with acute pain and therefore constitute the reflex process that results in "pulling away" from noxious stimuli (e.g., yanking hand away from hot stove). These fibers are associated with thermal and mechanical sensations. By contrast, the slowly conducting, unmyelinated C-fibers are responsible for the slow, dull, longer-lasting, second pain (2). The lack of myelination is the cause for the slow conduction of C-fibers. Because of their higher rate of conduction, Aδ-neurons are responsible for the sensation of the sharp first pain and respond to a low stimulus threshold. On the other hand, C-fibers respond to stronger stimulus intensity and cannot be normally activated, but become responsive during inflammation or intense mechanical, chemical, or thermal stimuli. Finally, from the thalamus, the nociceptive message is transmitted to the somatosensory cortex, parietal lobe, frontal lobe, and limbic system, where the stimulus is processed, causing perception of pain (2).

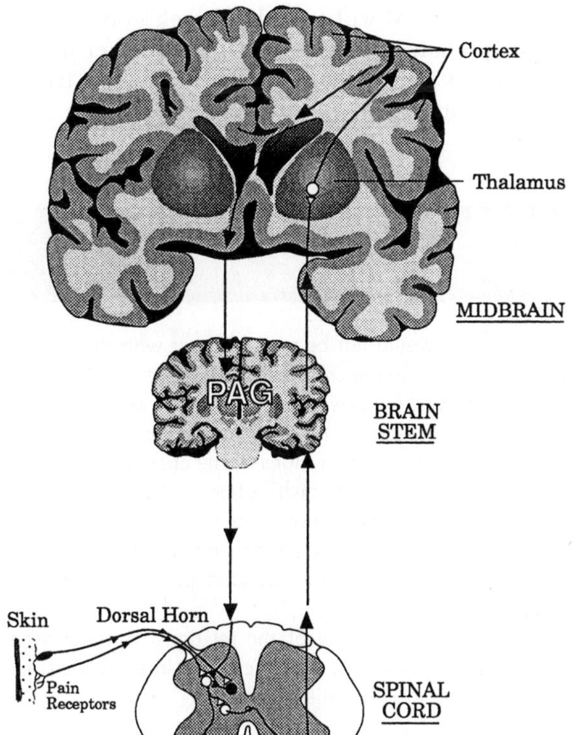

FIGURE 20.1 Location of endogenous opioid nerve tracts in the central nervous system. Endorphins and opioid receptors in the dorsal horn of the spinal cord, thalamus, and periaqueductal gray (PAG) areas are associated with the transmission of pain signals.

Chronic Pain

While acute pain is usually a transitory response to a noxious stimulus to nociceptors lasting only until the noxious stimulus is removed or the underlying damage or pathology has healed, chronic pain is different (7). Tens of millions suffer from chronic pain that is unrelenting, not self-limiting, and can persist from months to years and even decades after the initial injury heals. The pain can be refractory, mild, or excruciating, episodic or continuous, or inconvenient or incapacitating; is not a symptom that exists alone; and usually extends beyond the expected period of healing (3,6,7). Pain signals keep firing in the nervous system for weeks, months, or even years. Some painful conditions, such as rheumatoid arthritis, osteoporosis, endometriosis, scleroderma, peripheral neuropathy, cancer, and idiopathic pain, may persist for years. Chronic pain serves no protective biologic function (7). Rather than being the symptom of a disease process, chronic pain is itself a disease process. Other problems associated with chronic pain, if not properly treated, include fatigue, sleeplessness, withdrawal from activity, increased need to rest, weakened immune system, and changes in mood including hopelessness, fear, depression, irritability, anxiety, and stress, and disability (8). Chronic, nonmalignant pain is predominately neuropathic and involves damage either to the peripheral or central nervous systems (7). The most common sources of chronic pain result from headaches, joint pain, pain from injury, and backaches (9). Other sources of chronic pain include tendinitis, sinus pain, carpal tunnel syndrome, and pain affecting specific parts of the body, such as the shoulders, pelvis, and neck. Generalized muscle or nerve pain can also develop into a chronic condition. The symptoms of chronic pain include mild to severe pain that does not go away and pain that can be described as shooting, burning, aching, feeling of discomfort, soreness, tightness, or stiffness (9).

Chronic pain may originate with an initial trauma or injury such as a sprained back, serious infection, or head injury, or there may be an ongoing cause of pain, such as arthritis or cancer, but some people suffer chronic pain in the absence of any past injury or evidence of body damage (7). Common chronic pain complaints in older adults include headache, low back pain, cancer pain, arthritis pain, neurogenic pain (pain resulting from damage to the peripheral nerves or to the CNS itself), and psychogenic pain (pain not due to past disease or injury or any visible sign of damage inside or outside the nervous system) (10). A person may have two or more coexisting chronic pain conditions, such as chronic fatigue syndrome, endometriosis, fibromyalgia, inflammatory bowel disease, interstitial cystitis, or temporomandibular joint dysfunction. It is not known whether these disorders share a common cause. Medications and acupuncture are some treatments for chronic pain, which could include placebos, as well as using psychotherapy, relaxation, and behavioral modification.

Neuropathic pain is defined as pain arising as a direct consequence of a lesion or disease affecting the somatosensory system resulting in long-lasting pain (8) (to be discussed later in this chapter). Neuropathic pain is not one single disease but consists of a series of different diseases and conditions, such as nerve compression as a consequence of neoplasms, neuropathies due to metabolic disorders such as diabetes, and diseases of the CNS such as stroke and multiple sclerosis, that produce a common syndrome characterized by pain (10). An essential element in neuropathic pain is the combination of peripheral sensory loss and hypersensitivity in the painful area as consequence of an injury to the nervous system. As a result of damage to either C-fibers or Aδ-fibers, these fibers, in response to the injury, become abnormally sensitive due to a combination of degeneration and regeneration cellular changes with hypersensitization/hyperexcitability as the main factor causing the pain (8). Peripheral neuropathic pain is often described as a burning, tingling sensation, stabbing, or "pins and needles" (10). Phantom pain is a type of neuropathic pain from a part of the body that has been lost or from which the brain no longer receives signals (e.g., phantom limb pain is a common experience of amputees). Insensitivity to pain may also result from abnormalities in the nervous system as a result of damage to the nerves, such as spinal cord injury, or diabetes mellitus (diabetic neuropathy). These individuals are at risk of tissue damage due to undiscovered injury. People with diabetes-related nerve damage, for instance, sustain poorly healing foot ulcers as a result of decreased sensation (9).

OPIUM AND OPIOID ANALGESICS

History

The juice (*opium* in Greek) or latex from the unripe seed pods of the poppy *Papaver somniferum* is among the oldest recorded medications used by humans. The writings of Theophrastus around 200 BC describe the use of opium in medicine; however, evidence suggests that opium was used in the Sumerian culture as early as 3500 BC. The initial use of opium was as a tonic, or it was smoked. The pharmacist Surtürner first isolated an alkaloid from opium in 1803. He named the alkaloid morphine, after Morpheus, the Greek god of dreams. Codeine, thebaine, and papaverine are other medically important alkaloids that were later isolated from the latex of opium poppies.

CLINICAL SIGNIFICANCE

Central analgesics work to blunt painful stimuli operating through physiologically distinct nociceptive or neuropathic pathways. The most well-recognized centrally acting pain relievers are the opioid analgesics, which exert their agonist and/or antagonist action at defined receptors in the brain and spinal cord. Opioid agonists and partial agonist-antagonists generally act on μ and κ receptors to effect analgesia, and their structure–activity relationship (SAR) in the treatment of nociceptive pain is well defined. All of these receptors have subtypes that provide varying degrees of analgesia, euphoria or dysphoria, CNS depression, and perhaps the potential for tolerance. By modifying their structures, opioid agonist and antagonist properties can be changed to develop agents that require more or less hepatic metabolism, and thus, the duration of action, bioavailability, and risk of serious drug–drug interactions can be impacted. A simple change in nitrogen substituent can convert a potent μ agonist into a κ agonist/μ antagonist, an analgesic that would not be cross-tolerant with the original drug. Other changes in the chemical structures can yield agents with the same receptor selectivity profile but a much higher affinity, which corresponds to more potency on a milligram-to-milligram basis. Other alterations of the chemical structures can lead to improved central distribution profiles and/or positive changes related to respiratory depression liability, emesis, tolerance, and allergenicity. By altering the affinities for some receptors more than others, the addictive properties may also be manipulated.

Through an understanding of the relationship of chemical structures to biologic activity, the clinician can improve the selection of drug to the specific patient.

Jill T. Johnson, PharmD, BCPS
Associate Professor
Department of Pharmacy Practice
College of Pharmacy
University of Arkansas for Medical Sciences

Morphine was among the first compounds to undergo structure modification. Ethylmorphine (the 3-*O*-ethyl ether of morphine) was introduced as a medicine in 1898. Diacetylmorphine (heroin), which may be considered to be the first synthetic prodrug, was synthesized in 1874 and marketed as a nonaddicting analgesic, antidiarrheal, and antitussive agent in 1898.

OPIATE/OPIOID

The use of the terms "opiate" and "opioid" requires clarification. Until the 1980s, the term "opiate" was used extensively to describe any natural or synthetic agent that was derived from morphine. One could say an opiate was any compound that was structurally related to morphine. In the mid-1970s, the discovery of peptides in the brain with pharmacologic actions similar to morphine prompted a change in nomenclature. These peptides were not easily related to morphine structurally, yet their actions were like those produced by morphine. At this time, the term "opioid," meaning opium- or morphine-like in terms of pharmacologic action, was introduced. The broad group of opium alkaloids, synthetic derivatives related to the opium alkaloids, and the many naturally occurring and synthetic peptides with morphine-like pharmacologic effects are called opioids. In addition to having pharmacologic effects similar to morphine, a compound must be antagonized by an opioid antagonist, such as naloxone, to be classed as an opioid. The neuronal-located proteins to which opioid agents bind and initiate biologic responses are called opioid receptors.

Endogenous Opioid Peptides and Their Physiologic Functions

Scientists had postulated for some time that based on the rigid structural and stereochemical structure–activity requirements essential for the analgesic actions of morphine and related opioids, they produce their effects by binding with specific receptors to cause their actions. It was also reasoned that morphine and the synthetic opioid derivatives are not the natural ligands for the opioid receptors and that some analgesic substance must exist within the brain. Techniques to prove these two points were not developed until the mid-1970s. Hughes et al. (11) used the electrically stimulated contractions of guinea pig ileum and the mouse vas deferens, which are very sensitive to inhibition by opioids, as bioassays to follow the purification of compounds with morphine-like activity from mammalian brain tissue. These researchers were able to isolate and determine the structures of two pentapeptides, Tyr-Gly-Gly-Phe-Met (Met-enkephalin) and Tyr-Gly-Gly-Phe-Leu (Leu-enkephalin), that caused the opioid activity (Fig. 20.2). The compounds were named enkephalins after the Greek word *Kaphale,* which translates as "from the head."

At about the same time as Hughes and coworkers were making their discoveries, three other laboratories, using

Met-enkephalin	= Tyr-Gly-Gly-Phe-Met
Leu-Enkephalin	= Tyr-Gly-Gly-Phe-Leu
β-Endorphin	= Tyr-Gly-Gly-Phe-Met-Thr-Ser-Glu-Lys-Ser^{10}-Gln-Thr-Pro-Leu-Val-Thr-Leu-Phe-Lys- Asn^{20}-Ala-Ile-Ile-Lys-Asn-Ala-Tyr-Lys-Lys-Gly-GluOH^{31}
Dynorphin(dyn$^{1-17}$)	= Tyr-Gly-Gly-Phe-Leu-Arg-Arg-Ile-Arg-Pro-Lys-Leu-Lys-Trp-Asp-Asn-Gln
Dynorphin(dyn$^{1-8}$)	= Tyr-Gly-Gly-Phe-Leu-Arg-Arg-Ile
Dynorphin(dyn$^{1-13}$)	= Tyr-Gly-Gly-Phe-Leu-Arg-Arg-Ile-Arg-Pro-Lys-Leu-Lys
α-Neoenodorphin	= Tyr-Gly-Gly-Phe-Leu-Arg-Lys-Tyr-Pro-Lys
β-Neoendorphin	= Tyr-Gly-Gly-Phe-Leu-Arg-Lys-Tyr-Pro
Nociceptin	= Phe-Gly-Gly-Phe-Thr-Gly-Ala-Arg-Lys-Ser-Ala-Arg-Lys-Leu-Ala-Asn-Gln

FIGURE 20.2 Precursor proteins to the endogenous opioid peptides.

a different assay technique, were able to identify endogenous opioids and opioid receptors in the brain (12–14). These scientists used radiolabeled opioid compounds (radioligands), with high specific activity, to bind to opioid receptors in brain homogenates (15). They demonstrated saturable binding (i.e., the tissue contains a finite number of binding sites that can all be occupied) of the radioligands and that the receptor-bound radioligands could be displaced stereoselectively by nonradiolabeled opioids. Discovery of the enkephalins was soon followed by the identification of other endogenous opioid peptides, including β-endorphin (16), the dynorphins (17), and the endomorphins (18).

The opioid peptides isolated from mammalian tissue are known collectively as endorphins, a word that is derived from a combination of endogenous and morphine. The opioid alkaloids and all of the synthetic opioid derivatives are exogenous opioids.

Opioid Peptides

The endogenous opioid peptides are synthesized as part of the structures of large precursor proteins (19). There is a different precursor protein for each of the major types of opioid peptides (Fig. 20.2). Pro-opiomelanocortin is the precursor for β-endorphin. Proenkephalin A is the precursor for Met- and Leu-enkephalin. Proenkephalin B (prodynorphin) is the precursor for dynorphin and α-neoendorphin. The pronociceptin protein has been identified and contains only one copy of the active peptide, whereas the precursor protein for the endomorphins remains to be identified. All of the pro-opioid proteins are synthesized in the cell nucleus and transported to the terminals of the nerve cells from which they are released. The active peptides are hydrolyzed from the large proteins by proteases that recognize double basic amino acid sequences positioned just before and after the opioid peptide sequences.

Peptides with opioid activity have been isolated from sources other than mammalian brain. They include heptapeptide β-casomorphin (Tyr-Pro-Phe-Pro-Gly-Pro-Ile), which is found in cow's milk and is a μ-opioid agonist (20), and dermorphin (Tyr-D-Ala-Phe-Gly-Tyr-Pro-Ser-NH_2), which is a μ-selective peptide isolated from the skin of South American frogs and is approximately 100-fold more potent than morphine in in vitro tests (21).

The endogenous opioids exert their analgesic action at spinal and supraspinal sites (Fig. 20.1). They also produce analgesia by a peripheral mechanism of action associated with the inflammatory process. In the CNS, the opioids exert an inhibitory neurotransmitter or neuromodulator action on afferent pain-signaling neurons in the dorsal horn of the spinal cord and on interconnecting neuronal pathways for pain signals within the brain. In the brain, the arcuate nucleus, periaqueductal gray, and thalamic areas are especially rich in opioid receptors and are sites at which opioids exert an analgesic action. In the spinal cord, concentrations of endogenous opioids are high in laminae 1, laminae 2, and trigeminal nucleus areas. All of the endogenous opioid peptides and the three major classes of opioid receptors appear to be at least partially involved in the modulation of pain. The actions of opioids at the synaptic level are described in Figure 20.3.

Analgesia that results from acupuncture or is self-induced by a placebo or biofeedback mechanisms is caused by release of endogenous endorphins. Analgesia produced by these procedures can be prevented by the previous dosage of a patient with an opioid antagonist. Electrical stimulation from electrodes properly placed in the brain causes endorphin release and analgesia. This procedure is used for the "self-stimulated" release of endorphins in patients with chronic pain who do not respond to any other medical treatment. As with exogenously administered opioid drugs, tolerance develops to all procedures that work by release of endogenous opioids.

Structure–Activity Relationships of Opioid Peptides

Thousands of derivatives related to the endogenous opioid peptides have been prepared since the discovery of the enkephalins in 1975 (22) (Fig. 20.2). A thorough discussion of the SAR of these peptides would be a major task; however, some major trends have emerged and can easily be discussed. Some selected general SAR points for peptide opioids are as follows:

1. All of the endogenous opioid peptides, except for the endomorphins, have Leu- or Met-enkephalin as their first five amino acid residues.
2. The Tyr^1 at the first amino acid residue position of all the endogenous opioid peptides is essential for activity. Removal of the phenolic hydroxyl group or the basic nitrogen (amino terminus group) will abolish activity. The Tyr^1 free amino group may be alkylated (methyl or allyl groups to give agonists and antagonists), but it must retain its basic character. The structural resemblance between morphine and the Tyr^1 group of opioid peptides is especially obvious.
3. In addition to the phenol and amine groups of Tyr^1, the next most important moiety in the enkephalin structure is the phenyl group of Phe^4. Removal of this group or changing its distance from Tyr^1 results in full or substantial loss in activity.

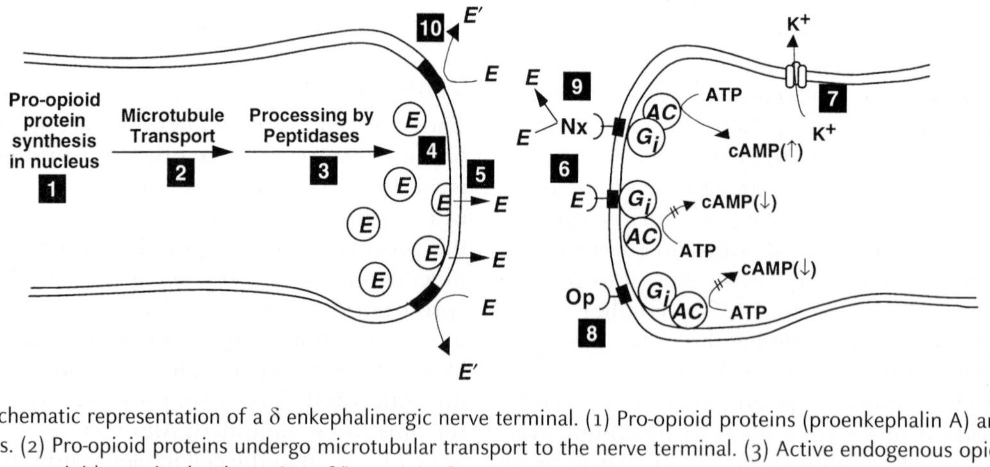

FIGURE 20.3 Schematic representation of a δ enkephalinergic nerve terminal. (1) Pro-opioid proteins (proenkephalin A) are synthesized in the cell nucleus. (2) Pro-opioid proteins undergo microtubular transport to the nerve terminal. (3) Active endogenous opioids (E) are cleaved from the pro-opioid proteins by the action of "processing" proteases. (4) The active peptides (E) are taken up and stored in presynaptic vesicles. (5) The peptides are released when the presynaptic neuron fires. (6) The endogenous opioid peptides bind to postsynaptic receptors and activate second messenger systems. (7) For all opioid receptors, the second messenger effect is primarily mediated by a G-inhibitory ($G_{i/o}$) protein complex, which promotes the inactivation of adenylate cyclase (AC), a decrease in intracellular cyclic adenosine-3′,5′-monophosphate (cAMP), and finally, an efflux of potassium ions (K^+) from the cell. The net effect is the hyperpolarization of the postsynaptic neuron and inhibition of cell firing. (8) Exogenous opioids (Op), such as morphine, combine with opioid receptors and mimic the actions of E. (9) Opioid antagonists, such as naloxone (Nx), combine with opioid receptors and competitively inhibit the actions of E or Op. (10) The action of E is terminated by a membrane-bound endopeptidase [EC3.4.24.11] (enkephalinase), which hydrolyzes the Gly3-Phe4 peptide bond of enkephalin. Other endopeptidases may be employed in the metabolism of different endogenous opioid peptides.

4. The enkephalins have several low-energy conformations, and different conformations likely are bound at different opioid receptor types and subtypes.
5. The replacement of the natural L-amino acids with unnatural D-amino acids can make the peptides resistant to the actions of several peptidases that generally rapidly degrade the natural endorphins. The use of a D-Ala in place of Gly^2 has been especially useful for protecting the peptides from the action of nonselective aminopeptidases. The placement of bulky groups into the structure (e.g., the addition of *N*-Me to Phe^4) will also slow the action of peptidases. When evaluating new peptides for opioid activity, it often is difficult to tell if changes are caused by metabolic stability or receptor affinity.
6. Conversion of the terminal carboxyl group into an alcohol or an amide will protect the compound from carboxy peptidases.
7. Any introduction of unnatural D- or L-amino acids or bulky groups into the enkephalin structure will affect its conformational stability. The resultant peptides will have an increase or decrease in affinity for each of the opioid receptor types. The right combination of increases and/or decreases in receptor affinity will result in selectivity for a receptor type.
8. Structural changes that highly restrict the conformational mobility of the peptides (e.g., substitution of proline for Gly^2 or cyclization of the peptide) have been especially useful for the discovery of receptor-selective opioid peptides.

For examples of the above SARs, see the structures of the peptides given in Figures 20.4 to 20.6.

Enkephalin Peptides The effect of lengthening the amino acid chain of the enkephalin peptides deserves special consideration. As previously noted, the endogenous opioids found in mammals most often have Leu- or Met-enkephalin at their amino terminus end. Lengthening the carboxyl terminus can give the peptide greater affinity or selectivity for an opioid receptor type. This effect can be illustrated by the dynorphins, for which incorporation of the basic amino acids (especially Arg^7) into the C-terminus chain results in a marked increase in affinity for κ receptors. The message-address analogy has been used to describe this effect. The first four amino acids (Tyr-Gly-Gly-Phe) are essential for peptide ligands to bind to and to activate all opioid receptor types. The N-terminus amino acids can then be referred to as carrying the "message" to the receptors. Adding additional amino acids to the C-terminus can "address" the message to a specific receptor type. The additional peptide chain may be affecting the address (selectivity) by providing new and favorable binding interactions to one of the

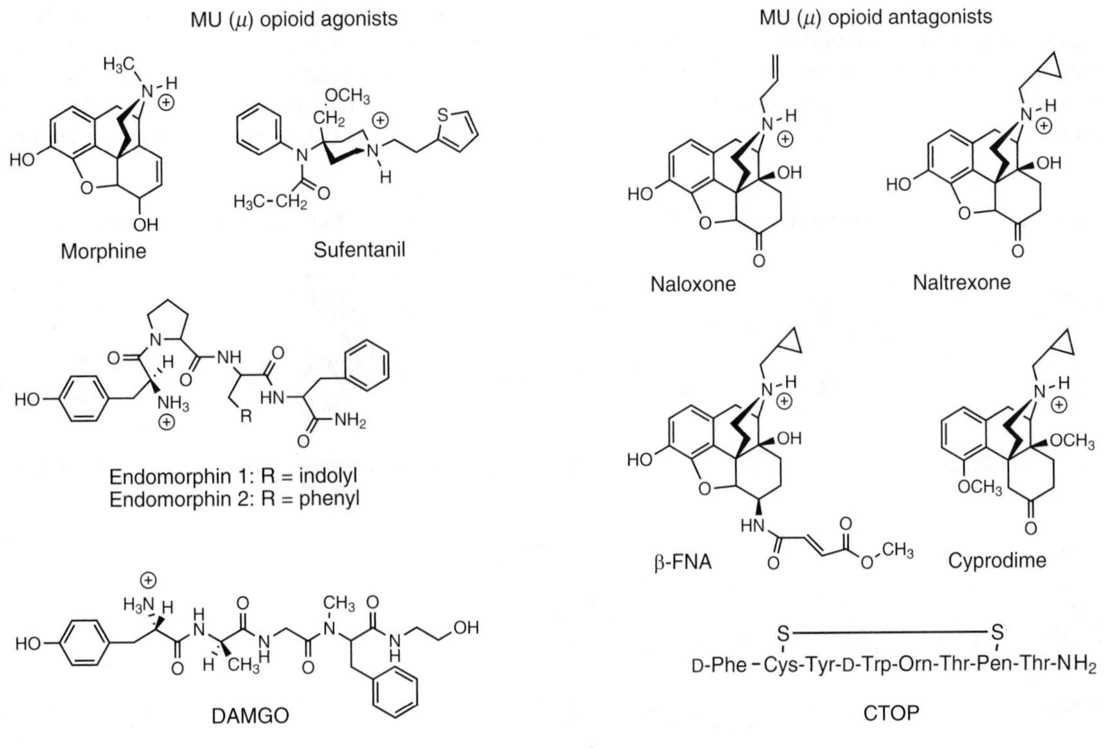

FIGURE 20.4 Structures of compounds selective for μ (OP_3) opioid receptors.

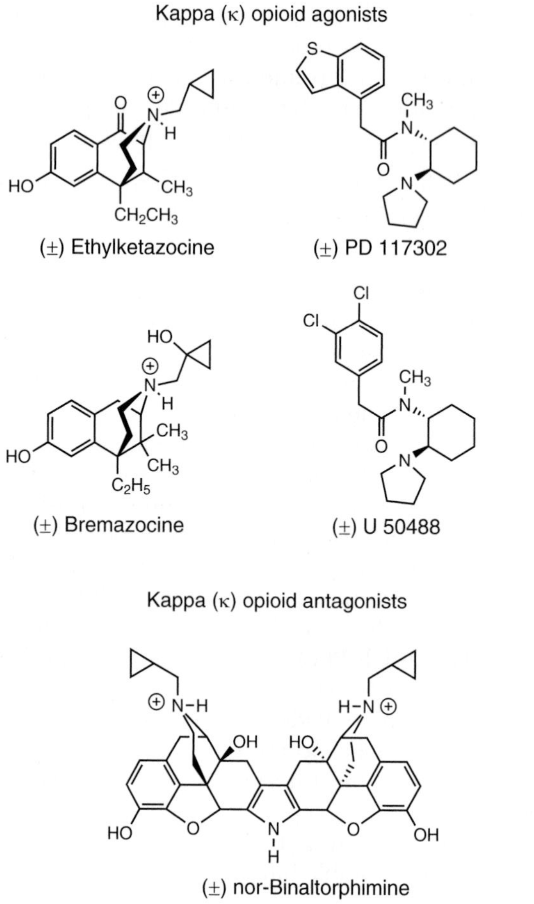

FIGURE 20.5 Structures of compounds selective for κ (OP_2) opioid receptors. (−)-Stereoisomers are the most active compounds.

receptor types. Alternatively, the additional peptide could be inducing a conformational change in the message portion of the peptide that favors interaction with one of the receptor types.

Opioid Receptors

Identification and Activation of Opioid Receptors

Identification of multiple opioid receptors has depended on the discovery of selective agonists and antagonists, the identification of sensitive assay techniques (23), and ultimately, the cloning of the receptor proteins (24). The techniques that have been especially useful are the radioligand binding assays on brain tissues and the electrically stimulated peripheral muscle preparations. Rodent brain tissue contains all three opioid receptor types, and special evaluation procedures (computer-assisted line fitting) or selective blocking (with reversible or irreversible binding agents) of some of the receptor types must be used to sort out the receptor selectivity of test compounds. The myenteric plexus–containing longitudinal strips of guinea pig ileum contain μ- and κ-opioid receptors. The contraction of these muscle strips is initiated by electrical stimulation and is inhibited by opioids. The vas deferens from mouse contains μ, δ, and κ receptors and reacts similarly to the guinea pig ileum to electrical stimulation and to opioids. Homogenous populations of opioid receptors are found in rat (μ), hamster (δ), and rabbit (κ) vas deferentia.

The signal transduction mechanism for μ, δ, and κ receptors is through $G_{i/o}$ proteins. Activation of opioid receptors is linked through the G protein to an inhibition of adenylate cyclase activity. The resultant decrease in cyclic adenosine monophosphate (cAMP) production, efflux of potassium ions, and closure of voltage-gated Ca^{2+} channels causes hyperpolarization of the nerve cell (25) and a strong inhibition of nerve firing.

It is now clear from work carried out in many laboratories over the last three decades that there are three major types of opioid receptors: μ, κ, and δ (26). All three of the receptor types have been well characterized and cloned (24). A nomenclature adopted by the International Union of Pharmacology (IUPHAR) in 1996 classifies the three opioid receptors by the order in which they were

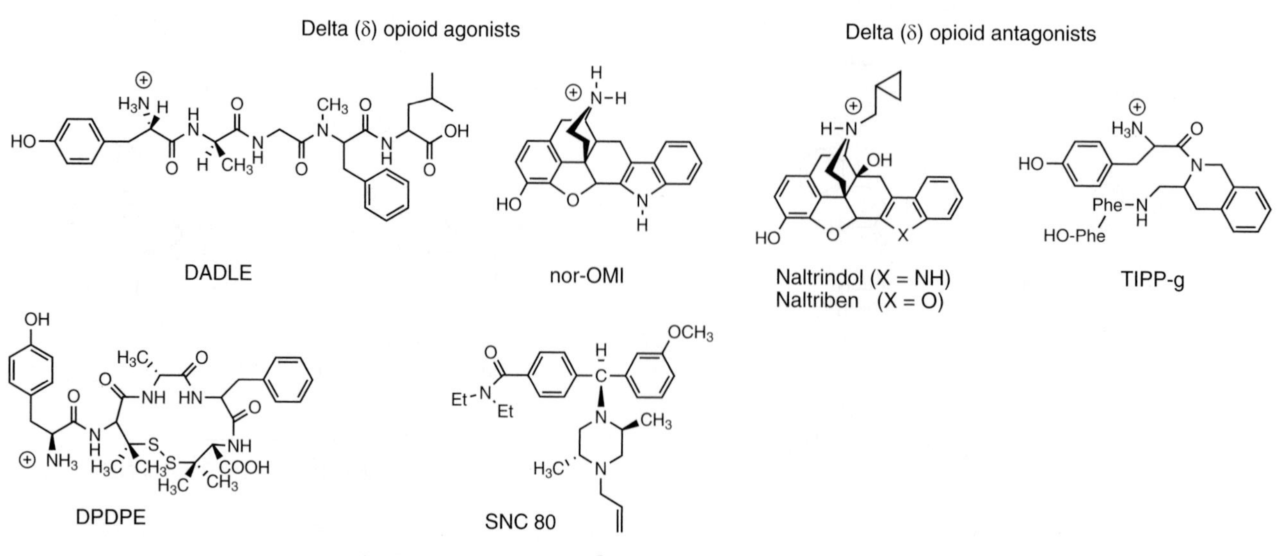

FIGURE 20.6 Structures of compounds selective for δ (OP_1) opioid receptors.

cloned (27). By this classification, δ-opioid receptors are OP_1 receptors, κ-opioid receptors are OP_2 receptors, and μ-opioid receptors are OP_3 receptors. The IUPHAR approved a new nomenclature in 2000, naming the receptors as MOP-μ, DOP-δ, and KOP-κ. In current literature, however, the opioid receptors often are referred to as DOR (δ), KOR (κ), and MOR (μ). There is evidence for subtypes of each of these receptors; however, the failure of researchers to find genomal evidence for additional receptors indicates that the receptor subtypes are posttranslational modifications (splice variants) of known receptor types (28). Receptor subtypes may also be known receptor types that are coupled to different signal transduction systems. A fourth opioid receptor family (NOP, nociception receptor; formerly opioid orphan receptor) was identified from cDNA encoding, which has a high degree of homology to the classical opioid receptors, and named after its endogenous ligand, nociceptin/orphanin FQ (N/OFQ) peptide receptor (29,30). Table 20.1 lists the opioid receptor types, their known physiologic functions, and selective agonists and antagonists for each of the receptors. All three of the major opioid receptor types are located in human brain or spinal cord tissues, and each has a role in the mediation of pain. At this time, only μ and κ agonists are in clinical use as opioid analgesic drugs.

TABLE 20.1 Opioid Receptors

Receptor Subtype	δ (delta, DOP, OP_1)	Κ (kappa, KOP, OP_2)	μ (mu, MOP, OP_3)	NOP (N/OFQ peptide, OP_4, ORL_1)
Transduction Mechanism	Inhibition of adenylate cyclase, activation of inwardly rectifying K+ channels, inhibition of Ca^{+2} channels, phospholipase C stimulation			
G protein	$G_{i/o}$	$G_{i/o}$	$G_{i/o}$	$G_{i/o}$
Localization	Olfactory bulb Nucleus accumbens Caudate putamen neocortex	Cerebral cortex Nucleus accumbens hypothalamus	CNS (neocortex, thalamus, nucleus accumbens, hippocampus, amygdala Vas deferens Myenteric gut neurons	Cortex, olfactory nucleus, hypothalamus, hippocampus, substantia nigra, locus coerulus, spinal cord, amygdala,
Endogenous Ligand	Enkephalins β-endorphin	Dynorphins β-endorphin	Endomorphin 1 Endomorphin 2 β-endorphin)	N/OFQ peptide
Likely physiological roles	Analgesia GI motility Olfaction Immune stimulation Respiratory depression (rate) Cognitive function Motor integration	Regulation of nociception Analgesia Sedation Miosis Diuresis Dysphoria Neuroendocrine secretions	Analgesia (morphine-like) Euphoria Increased gastrointestinal transit time thermo regulation Immune suppression Respiratory depression (volume) Emetic effects Tolerance Physical dependence	Motor and balance control Reinforcement and reward Nociception Stress response Sexual behavior Aggression Autonomic control of physiological processes
Key selective agonists	DADLE (D-Ala²-D-Leu⁵-enkephalin) DSLET (Tyr-D-Ser-Gly-Phe-Leu-Thr) DPDPE (D-Pen²-D-Pen⁵- DADLE ($δ_2$) D-Ala2-deltorphin II ($δ_2$)	Ethylketocyclazocine (EKC) Bremazocine Mr2034 dyn (1–17) Trifluadom U-50,488 ($κ_1$) Spiradoline (U-62,066)($κ_1$) U-69,593 ($κ_1$) PD 117302 ($κ_1$) dyn 1–17 ($κ_1$) NalBzOH ($κ_1$)	Morphine Sufentanil DAMGO (Tyr-D-Ala-MePhe-NH-$(CH_2)_2$ OH PLO17 (Tyr-Pro-MePhe-D-Pro-NH_2 BIT (affinity label) Meptazinol ($μ_1$ high affinity) Etonitazene	N/OFQ peptide Nociceptin (1–13)-NH_2
Key Selective Antagonists	ICI 174864 FIT (affinity label) SUPERFIT (affinitylabel) Naltrindole (NTI) BNTX Naltriben (NTB) Naltrindol isothiocyanate (NTII)	TENA nor-BNI UPHIT	Naloxone Naltrexone CTOP Cyprodime β-FNA (affinity label) Naloxonazine	(N-phe¹)-Nociceptin (1–13)-NH_2 J-113397 UFP-101

Mu (μ)-Opioid Receptors

Endomorphin-1 (Tyr[1]-Pro-Trp-Phe[4]-NH_2) and endomorphin-2 (Tyr[1]-Pro-Phe-Phe[4]-NH_2) are endogenous opioid peptides with a high degree of selectivity for μ (MOP) receptors (18). A number of therapeutically useful compounds have been found that are selective for μ-opioid receptors (Fig. 20.4). All of the opioid alkaloids and most of their synthetic derivatives are μ-selective agonists. Morphine, normorphine, and dihydromorphinone have 10- to 20-fold μ-receptor selectivity and were particularly important in early studies to differentiate the opioid receptors. Sufentanil and the peptides DAMGO (31) and dermorphin (32), all with 100-fold selectivity for μ over other opioid receptors, are frequently used in laboratory studies to demonstrate μ-receptor selectivity in cross-tolerance, receptor binding, and isolated smooth muscle assays. Studies with μ-receptor knockout mice have confirmed that all the major pharmacologic actions observed on injection of morphine (e.g., analgesia, respiratory depression, tolerance, withdrawal symptoms, decreased gastric motility, and emesis) occur by interactions with μ receptors (33).

Naloxone and naltrexone are antagonists that have weak (5- to 10-fold) selectivity for μ receptors. Cyprodime is a selective nonpeptide μ antagonist (~30-fold selective for μ over κ and 100-fold selective for μ over δ) available for laboratory use (34). CTOP, a cyclic peptide analog of somatostatin, is a selective μ antagonist (35). There is evidence that μ_1 receptors are high-affinity binding sites that mediate pain neurotransmission, whereas μ_2 receptors control respiratory depression. Naloxonazine is a selective inhibitor of μ_1-opioid receptors (36).

Kappa (κ)-Opioid Receptors

Ethylketazocine and bremazocine are 6,7-benzomorphan derivatives with κ-opioid receptor selectivity (Fig. 20.5). These two compounds were used in early studies to investigate κ (KOP) receptors. They are not highly selective, however, and their use in research has diminished. A number of arylacetamide derivatives, having a high selectivity for κ over μ or δ receptors, have been discovered. The first of these compounds, (±)-U50488, has a 50-fold selectivity for κ over μ receptors and has been extremely important in the characterization of κ-opioid activity (37). Other important agents in this class are (±) PD-117302 (38) and (–) CI-977 (39). Each of these agents has 1,000-fold selectivity for κ over μ or δ receptors. Evidence suggests that the arylacetamides bind to a subtype of κ receptors. In animals, including humans, κ agonists produce analgesia. Other prominent effects are diuresis, sedation, and dysphoria. Compared to μ agonists, κ agonists lack respiratory depressant, constipating, and strong addictive (euphoria and physical dependence) properties. It was hoped that κ agonists would become useful strong analgesics that lacked addictive properties; however, clinical trials with several highly selective and potent κ agonists were aborted because of the occurrence of unacceptable sedative and dysphoric side effects. κ-Selective opioids with only a peripheral action have been shown to be effective in relieving inflammation and the pain associated with it (40). Scientific evidence suggests there are κ_1, κ_2, and κ_3 subtypes of κ receptors; however, the physiologic effects initiated by the κ receptor subtypes are not well defined (41).

The peptides related to dynorphin are the natural agonists for κ receptors. Their selectivity for κ over μ receptors is not very high. Synthetic peptide analogs have been reported that are more potent and more selective than dynorphin for κ receptors (42,43).

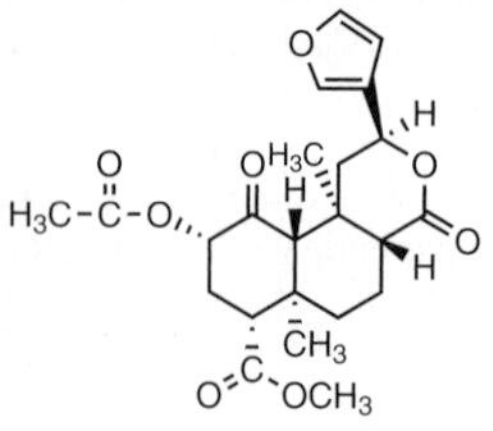

Salvinorin

The diterpene salvinorin A from *Salvia divinorum* has been reported to be a potent high-affinity and selective κ agonist (44,45). *Salvia divinorum* is a hallucinogenic plant in the mint family that has been used in traditional spiritual practices for its psychoactive properties by the Mazatecs of Oaxaca, Mexico, and its extracts have been used in the United States as legal hallucinogens. Salvinorin A thus represents the first known naturally occurring nonnitrogenous full κ agonist similar in efficacy to dynorphin, the naturally occurring peptide ligand for κ receptors. Results from structure–function studies suggested that the substituent at the 2-position of salvinorin A was critical for κ-opioid receptor binding and activation (45).

The major antagonist with good selectivity for κ receptors is norbinaltorphimine (46). This compound has approximately 100-fold selectivity for κ over δ receptors and an even greater selectivity for κ over μ receptors when tested during competitive binding studies in monkey brain homogenate. No medical use for a κ antagonist has been found.

Delta (δ)-Opioid Receptors

Enkephalins, the natural ligands at δ (DOP) receptors, are only slightly selective for δ over μ receptors. Changes in the amino acid composition of the enkephalins can give compounds with high potency and selectivity for δ receptors. The peptides most often used as selective δ receptor ligands (Fig. 20.6) are [D-Ala[2], D-Leu[5]] enkephalin (DADLE) (47), [D-Ser[2], Leu[5]] enkephalin-Thr (DSLET) (48), and the cyclic peptide [D-Pen[2],

D-Pen[5]] enkephalin (DPDPE) (49). These and other δ-receptor selective peptides have been useful for in vitro studies, but their metabolic instability and poor distribution properties (i.e., penetration of the blood–brain barrier is limited by their hydrophilicity) have limited their usefulness for in vivo studies. Nonpeptide agonists that are selective for δ receptors have been reported. Derivatives of morphindoles were the first nonpeptide molecules to show δ selectivity in in vitro assays (50). SNC-80 is a newer and more selective δ-opioid receptor agonist (51). This compound produces analgesia after oral dose in several rodent models, and side effects appear minimal. Clinical trials with SCN-80 and other nonpeptide δ receptor agonists were attempted and aborted, primarily because of the convulsant action of δ receptor agonists. Radioligand binding studies in rodent brain tissue and in electrically stimulated vas deferentia have provided evidence of δ_1 and δ_2 receptors (52). The functional significance of this differentiation has not been determined.

Naltrindol and naltriben are highly selective nonpeptide antagonist for δ receptors (53,54). Naltrindol penetrates the CNS and displays antagonist activity that is selective for δ receptors in in vitro and in vivo systems. Peptidyl antagonists TIPP and TIPP-ψ are selective for δ receptors (55,56); however, their usefulness for in vivo studies and as clinical agents is limited by their poor pharmacokinetic properties. The δ-opioid receptor antagonists have shown clinical potential as immunosuppressants and in treatment of cocaine abuse.

NOP Receptor

A fourth opioid receptor named after its endogenous ligand, N/OFQ peptide (NOP; OP_4) has been identified and cloned based on homology with the cDNA sequence of the known (μ, δ, and κ) opioid receptors (29,30). Despite the homology in cDNA sequence with known opioid receptors, NOP did not bind the classical opioid peptide or nonpeptide agonists or antagonists with high affinity. Thus, the receptor was initially called the orphan opioid receptor or opioid-like receptor (OPLR-1). In subsequent studies, two research groups found a heptadecapeptide (Phe-Gly-Gly-Thr-Gly-Ala-Arg-Lys-Ser-Ala-Lys-Ala-Asn-Gln) to be the endogenous peptide for this receptor and named it nociceptin because it caused hyperalgesia (nociception) after intracerebral ventricular injection in mice (57). Another research group (58) named the heptapeptide orphanin FQ, after its affinity for the "orphan opioid receptor," after the first and last amino acids in the peptide's sequence (i.e., F = Phe and Q = Gln). Thus, the OPRL-1 receptor was renamed the NOP or N/OFQ peptide receptor, and the current name for the endogenous ligand is N/OFQ peptide. Human N/OFQ peptide is derived from a precursor protein, prepro N/ OFQ (ppN/OFQ), which consists of 176 amino acids, and resembles dynorphin-A in structure, with the most notable difference being the replacement of the N-terminus Tyr[1] for dynorphin A with Phe[1] (58). Conflicting results have been published regarding the ability of N/OFQ peptide to produce hyperalgesia versus analgesia in rodent pain assay models. One study has established this compound to be a potent initiator of pain signals in the periphery, where it acts by releasing substance P from nerve terminals (59). N/OFQ peptide is thought to be an endogenous antagonist of dopamine transport that may act either directly on dopamine or by inhibiting γ-aminobutyric acid (GABA) to affect dopamine levels (60). Within the CNS, the actions of N/OFQ can be either similar or opposite to those of opioids depending on the location. It controls a wide range of biologic functions ranging from nociception to food intake, from memory processes to cardiovascular and renal functions, from spontaneous locomotor activity to gastrointestinal (GI) motility, and from anxiety to the control of neurotransmitter release at peripheral and central sites (57). Several commonly used opioid drugs, including etorphine and buprenorphine, have been demonstrated to bind to nociceptin receptors, but this binding is relatively insignificant compared to their binding at other opioid receptors. More recently, a range of selective ligands for NOP have been developed that show little or no affinity to other opioid receptors, which allows NOP-mediated responses to be studied in isolation (9). Injection of an N/OFQ peptide antagonist into the brains of laboratory animals results in an analgesic effect, raising hope for the use of these agents in the management of pain (57). The NOP receptors are widely distributed in the brain, and it is not surprising that many central actions of N/OFQ peptide have been suggested from animal studies, including supraspinal hyperalgesia, spinal analgesia, hyperphagia, depression, and inhibitions of anxiety, epilepsy, cough, motor activity, and learning and memory, as well as the regulation of cardiovascular, urogenital, GI, and immune systems. Many efforts have been endeavored in the development of agonists or antagonists of this novel member of the opioid receptor family. Table 20.1 summarizes the NOP receptor agonists and antagonists developed thus far.

Receptor Affinity Labeling Agents

A number of opioid receptor–selective affinity labeling agents (i.e., compounds that form an irreversible covalent bond with the receptor protein) have been developed (Fig. 20.7). These compounds have been important in the characterization and isolation of the opioid receptor types. Each of the affinity-labeling agents contains a pharmacophore that allows initial reversible binding to the receptor. Once reversibly bound to the receptor, an affinity labeling agent must have an electrophilic group positioned so that

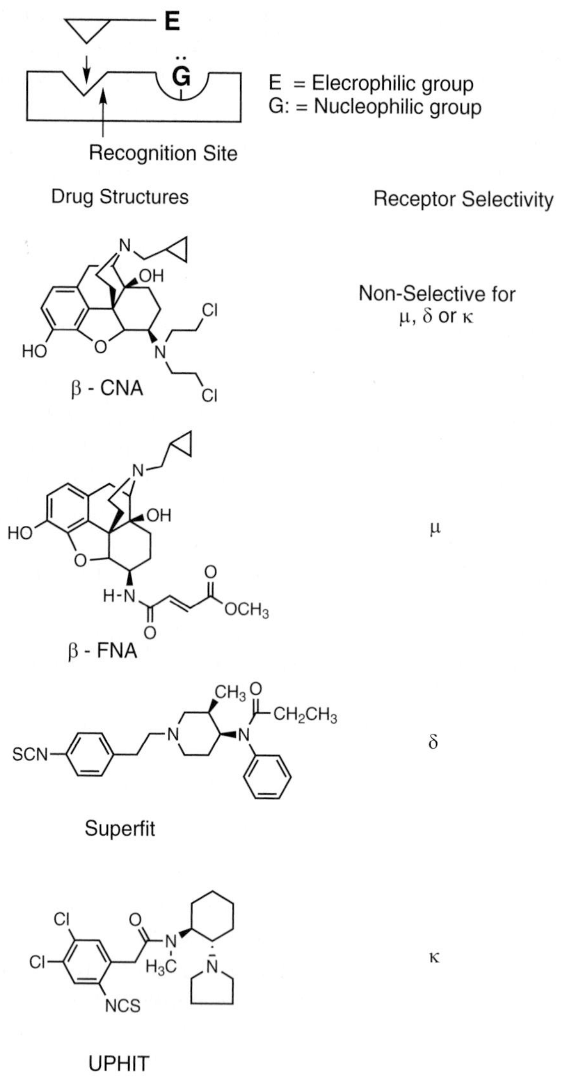

FIGURE 20.7 A representation of the concept of affinity labeling of receptors and affinity labeling agents for opioid receptors.

it can react with a nucleophilic group on the receptor protein. The receptor selectivity of these agents is dependent on 1) the receptor type selectivity of the pharmacophore, 2) the location of the electrophile within the pharmacophore structure so that when bound to the receptor it is positioned near a nucleophile, and 3) the relative reactivities of the electrophilic and nucleophilic groups.

An example of an important affinity labeling agent is β-CNA, which because of its highly reactive 2-chloroethylamine electrophilic group irreversibility binds to all three opioid receptor types (61). The structurally related compound β-FNA has a less reactive fumaramide electrophilic group and reacts irreversibly with only μ receptors (59). Derivatives of the fentanyl series, FIT and SUPERFIT, bind μ and δ receptors, but only the δ receptor is bound irreversibly (62,63). Apparently, when these agents are bound to μ receptors, the electrophilic isothiocyanate group is not oriented in proper juxtaposition to a receptor nucleophile for covalent bond formation to occur. Incorporation of the electrophilic isothiocyanate into the structure of the highly κ receptor–selective arylacetamides has provided affinity labeling agents (UPHIT and DIPPA) for κ receptors (64,65).

OPIOID THERAPEUTIC CHALLENGES

Tolerance, Dependence, and Withdrawal

Patients who take opioids on a chronic basis will experience tolerance to many of their pharmacologic actions, including analgesia, and a dependence on their presence in the CNS.

Tolerance is the situation where an increasingly larger dose of drug is required to produce the same degree of biologic response that had previously been obtained with a lower dose. In other words, the body has adapted to the presence of drug and needs a bigger dose to be able to experience its effect. Tolerance to μ-opioid agonists is related to the attenuating impact of these agents on intracellular cAMP. As cAMP levels decrease in response to μ-receptor occupation, analgesia is realized. However, over the course of several weeks or longer, upregulation of adenylate cyclase enzymes occurs in an attempt to overcome μ agonist–induced inhibition. It then takes a larger dose of agonist to inhibit both the original population of adenylate cyclase enzymes and those generated in response to the original dose (66). In addition to analgesia, tolerance occurs to μ-opioid–induced euphoria and respiratory depression, but not to the constipating or papillary (miosis) effects of these drugs.

Dependence is the need for a drug to maintain "normal" physiologic and psychological functioning. If a μ-opioid agonist used on a chronic basis is suddenly withdrawn, the inhibition of adenylate cyclase abruptly stops, and the "super-sized" enzyme population begins to produce cAMP. The elevated cAMP concentrations are believed responsible for the physiologic symptoms of opioid withdrawal, which include tremor, alternating chills and sweating, increased heart rate and blood pressure, and abdominal cramping. Withdrawal symptoms last until enzymatic homeostasis is regained, which can take days (67). Psychologically, withdrawal leads to often uncontrollable drug craving and drug-seeking behavior. Drug craving, a learned response, may last a lifetime, and it is the main reason why addicts in recovery relapse.

Cross Tolerance

There are times when practitioners intentionally put patients tolerant to and dependent on opioids into a

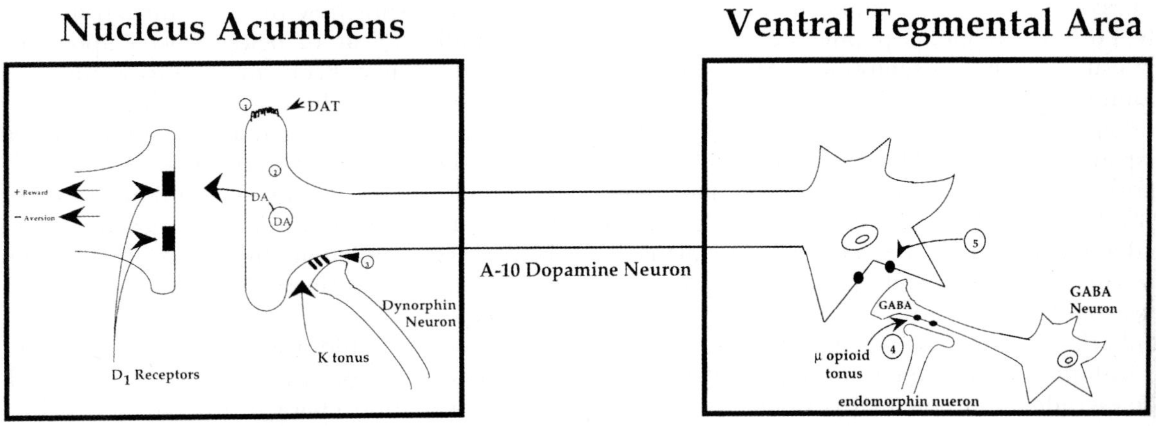

FIGURE 20.8 The neurochemical basis of drug abuse and addiction. The diagram is a representation of the brain's self-reward system. According to this theory, any agent that promotes stimulation of type 1 dopamine (D_1) receptors in the nucleus accumbens (NCA) potentiates self-reward and has the potential to be abused. Major drugs of abuse exert their actions at various sites within the self-reward system to increase dopamine (DA) in the NCA and stimulate D_1 receptors. Site 1: Cocaine blocks DA reuptake by the DA transporter (DAT) and greatly enhances DA action at D_1. Site 2: Amphetamine, methamphetamine, and related drugs cause DA release with the resultant stimulation of D_1. Site 3: Opioid κ agonists exert an inhibitory effect on DA neuronal firing, resulting in a decrease in DA release and aversion in animals. Site 4: Opioid μ agonists, such as morphine and heroin, exert an inhibitory action on γ-aminobutyric acid (GABA) interneurons in the DAT, thus removing the GABAergic inhibition on DA neuronal firing. Site 5: GABA agonists, such as gabapentin, enhance DA neuronal firing and DA release, and these agents may be useful in treating or preventing drug abuse and addiction. Other abused agents, such as nicotine and cannabis, also cause an increase in DA release in the NAC, but their exact neuronal connections to the self-reward system are not yet understood.

state of withdrawal, but these are few and far between. Unless you are attempting to rescue a patient from a life-threatening overdose or preparing to help an addicted patient on the road to recovery, withdrawal is an experience patients expect to avoid. Therefore, when abruptly switching a patient from one opioid agonist to another, practitioners must ensure that the two drugs are cross tolerant. Cross tolerance refers to the ability of one opioid agonist to substitute for another and produce the same biologic action without precipitating withdrawal symptoms. Cross-tolerant opioids exert their agonist effects through the same receptor subtype. In other words, one full μ agonist will be cross tolerant with another, but an analgesic that acts at the κ receptor will not be cross tolerant with another that works through the μ receptor. Similarly, a partial μ agonist would not be cross tolerant with a full μ agonist. Fortunately, opioid SARs will be explicit about receptor selectivity and intrinsic activity, so the chemically savvy practitioner will always be able to predict cross tolerance (or lack thereof) from a quick review of opioid structure.

Euphoria and Dysphoria

The ability of μ opioids to induce a profound euphoria is well known (68). Euphoria is a result of G_i-coupled μ-receptor stimulation in the thalamic, periaqueductal gray, and arcuate nucleus areas of the brain. The opioid-induced decrease in cAMP inhibits the release of the inhibitory neurotransmitter GABA from the ventral tegmental area, which is upstream of the nucleus accumbens. The nucleus accumbens is the brain's self-reward or pleasure center and is activated by dopamine. GABA normally inhibits dopamine release from this cerebral "candy land," so the decrease in GABA levels induced by μ-receptor stimulation enhances dopamine release from these terminals. The subsequent elevation in dopamine receptor stimulation in the nucleus accumbens is perceived as a feeling of intense well-being or euphoria.

In contrast, κ agonists have the potential to induce dysphoria, a feeling of intense discomfort. Kappa agonists act directly on receptors in the nucleus accumbens. Stimulation of these receptors results in a direct inhibitory effect on presynaptic dopaminergic neurons, resulting in a decrease in dopamine and an attenuation of pleasure-related responses that translates as dysphoria (69).

Addiction

Because of the euphoric effects that μ-opioid agonists produce, these agents have the potential for abuse. The destructive impact that drug abuse can have on individuals and society as a whole is undeniable, and the use of opioids, both prescribed and otherwise acquired, is on the rise. For example, despite representing only 4.6% of the global population, U.S. citizens are responsible for the consumption of 80% of opioids used around the world, including 99% of all available hydrocodone and two-thirds of all illicit drugs. In the decade spanning 1997 to 2007, the rise in the legal sale of euphoric opioids ranged from 222% for morphine to 1,293% for methadone, the latter of which is used in opioid addiction recovery as well as in the management of pain (70). Fortunately, patients using opioids for the treatment of pain are much less likely to experience euphoria or become addicted to these drugs than patients who do not need them for pain control (71). Nevertheless, addiction potential is viewed as a major use-limiting side effect by some health care providers, and patients, particularly those from underrepresented minority populations, can be undermedicated because of it (67,72–75). Fortunately, health care professionals are now recognizing the high importance of adequate pain control to quality of life and are taking steps to use opioids in more scientifically sound ways in patients who need them. The important role of the pharmacist in clinically competent pain management cannot be overestimated.

The above notwithstanding, opioid addiction is a serious social and health-related issue that merits additional discussion here. Addiction has been defined as "a primary, chronic neurobiologic disease with genetic, psychosocial and environmental factors influencing its development and manifestations," and it involves a complex set of physiologic and psychological responses to a drug's chemical message (76). The risk of addiction in chronic pain patients on opioids has been estimated at 3.3%, with genetic predisposition possibly accounting for 40% to 60% of that risk (77). Those interested in learning more about addiction as a disease state should consider viewing the program "Pleasure Unwoven," which was recently produced by the Institute for Addiction Study (78).

Although tolerance and dependence are components of addiction, these two phenomena by themselves are not sufficient to define it. As alluded to earlier, true addiction has a strong psychosocial and genetic component, leading to drug craving and drug-seeking behavior in the absence of pain. Individuals must engage in destructive behavior patterns before they can be classified as addicted. Such destructive behaviors can include intentional overuse or compulsive use of opioids in the face of negative mental and/or social consequences, forging prescriptions, social isolation, and abuse of other psychoactive drugs. The "4Cs" of true addiction have been coined, and they include **C**ompulsive use, inability to **C**ontrol the quantity taken, drug **C**raving, and **C**ontinued use despite negative consequences (77).

Patients taking opioids for chronic pain will be tolerant to and dependent on them, but practitioners should take care how they use the words "addiction" and "addict." Fear of being looked upon or labeled as an addict may keep some patients who need pain relief from taking the drugs that could best provide it (67,74). Clinicians should also take care to distinguish true addiction from pseudoaddiction, where patients with undertreated pain seek additional doses or "clock watch" until the time for their next dose of opioid. Unlike true addiction, the drug-seeking behavior of pseudoaddicted patients disappears when their pain is relieved (67,74).

Clinicians should also recognize that opioids used on a chronic basis can sometimes prompt hyperalgesia, a situation characterized by new pain, exacerbation of existing pain, or experiencing pain from nonpainful events (e.g., a light touch) (67,79,80). Hyperalgesia has been noted in patients with cancer, chronic nonmalignant pain, and neuropathic pain. Patients with hyperalgesia experience pain relief when their dose of opioid is decreased, rather than increased. When decreasing the dose of opioid in a hyperalgesic patient, care must be taken to avoid precipitating withdrawal. Clinicians should consider rotating to a different opioid that is cross tolerant with the original drug to re-establish optimum pain control (81). *N*-methyl-D-aspartate (NMDA) receptor antagonists may also have a therapeutic role to play, as the hyperalgesic response is believed to be mediated, at least in part, by the NMDA neurotransmitter system (82).

Frequent office visits or telephone calls to the pharmacy or requests for interim prescriptions of pain medication could signal hyperalgesia, worsening of (or new) pathology leading to untreated pain, a disorganized lifestyle leading to missed doses, or physical/psychological dependence (79). Each of these possibilities would demand a different response from the health care professional, illustrating the importance of patient-specific assessment whenever a change in the degree of pain control is reported. Establishing specific goals for chronic opioid therapy, monitoring patients closely and continuously, and maintaining a positive and open patient–practitioner relationship throughout are all of paramount importance to achieving optimum patient care outcomes.

Several avenues of recovery are available for patients with a true opioid addiction (83). Opioid-related therapeutic approaches can include blunting the pleasure response to μ agonists with opioid antagonist therapy (introduced after an opioid-free period of at least 7 days), initiating therapy with a partial μ agonist (buprenorphine) at the first sign of intentional withdrawal, or switching the patient from a highly euphoric μ agonist like heroin to a safer but still cross-tolerant μ agonist (methadone) and stair-stepping down to full recovery over the course of months or years. These therapeutic uses for analgesic opioids will be mentioned within the monographs of the drugs employed in addiction recovery. Common to all approaches is the need to work closely with the recovering patient so that he or she is ready from a physiologic, emotional, economic, and social support standpoint for a successful transition to each step in the recovery process.

Constipation

The GI tract has a high concentration of μ- and κ-opioid receptors. Stimulating intestinal μ receptors inhibits the release of acetylcholine from the myenteric plexus and halts propulsive peristalsis, resulting in constipation that can range from annoying to disabling. Because there is no tolerance to the effect of opioid agonists in the GI, the risk of GI complications with long-term opioid use is significant. Clinicians should recommend that all patients on chronic opioid therapy also use stool softeners and stimulant laxatives, such as Senna, bisacodyl, Milk of Magnesia or, when appropriate, magnesium citrate, to avoid fecal impaction (67).

PHYSICOCHEMICAL AND METABOLIC PROPERTIES OF OPIOIDS

Lipophilicity, pK_a, and Pharmacokinetics

The centrally mediated therapeutic actions of opioid analgesics and antagonists demand transport across the blood–brain barrier to reach receptors in the brain and spinal cord. In addition to having all critical receptor binding functional groups in the proper orientation, the most potent opioids will also be highly lipophilic structures (Table 20.2). The SAR discussion below will highlight the impact on potency of eliminating polar functional groups not needed at the receptor and/or adding carbon-rich functional groups to both promote central distribution and augment hydrophobic interactions at the receptor surface. The pharmacokinetic data for the opioids are listed in Table 20.2.

All opioids require a cationic amine for anchoring to the conserved Asp residue of the G protein–coupled opioid receptors. Most commonly, the pK_a of this amine is between 8 and 10. Multicyclic opioids (morphines, morphinans, benazazocines, and oripavines) will either have or must generate a phenolic hydroxyl moiety, making them ultimately amphoteric structures. With a pK_a of approximately 11, this phenolic group is predominantly un-ionized at physiologic pH and participates as a hydrogen donor in an essential bond with a hydrogen-accepting His residue on μ- and κ- opioid receptors (84).

Stereochemistry

Morphine, the prototypical opioid agonist, has five asymmetric centers. Naturally occurring levorotatory (–) morphine has the 5*R*,6*S*,9*R*,13*S*,14*R* absolute configuration, which is the most active isomeric form at μ-opioid receptors.

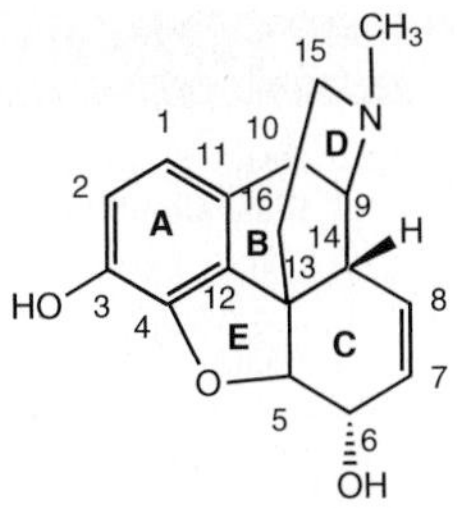

Morphine with 4-phenylpiperidine pharmacophore highlighted

Ring C of pentacyclic (morphines) and tetracyclic (morphinans) opioids is forced into a pseudoboat conformation due to the presence of the 7,8-double bond and the restraining furan (E) ring. Activity will increase if this structural element is eliminated to allow the C ring to assume the more stable chair conformation. The B/C ring fusion in naturally occurring levorotatory morphine is *cis*, placing rings B and C at right angles to one another. This gives morphine a decidedly nonplanar T-shaped conformation. The 14*R* (B/C *cis*) configuration is indicated in two-dimensional drawings by a $C_{14}\beta$ substituent (in front of the plane of the paper). An α substituent at C_{14} (indicated by a dotted line) would denote 14*S* stereochemistry and the more planar B/C *trans* ring fusion. Because the absolute configuration at C_{14} influences molecular conformation and degree of fit at the receptor surface, it is not surprising that the degree of fit also impacts analgesic activity. In pentacyclic opioids, the B/C *cis* fused system is 10-fold more potent than the B/C *trans* system. In contrast, the B/C *cis* isomer of tetracyclic morphinans is twofold less active than the B/C *trans*. In all multicyclic opioids, only the B/C *cis* form is marketed.

The aromatic A ring can be viewed as a substituent on the 4-position of the piperidine (D) ring. The 4-phenylpiperidine structure is considered the pharmacophore for opioid analgesic action. In multicyclic opioids, the A ring is held rigidly in an axial orientation relative to the D ring, which forces a van der Waals interaction with the μ-opioid receptor Trp^{293} residue that is expecting to see the Tyr^{1} residue of the enkephalins (84). For that reason, the aromatic A ring of analgesically active multicyclic opioids requires a phenolic hydroxyl group. If the orientation of the A ring can become equatorial to ring D (which occurs in flexible meperidine and anilidopiperidine-based opioids), then the phenyl ring will bind to the μ receptor Trp^{283} residue that normally binds with the enkephalin Phe^{4} residue (84). In that case, a phenolic OH is a binding liability.

Opioid receptors are highly stereoselective for the levorotatory isomers of morphine-like ligands. The dextrorotatory (+) isomers do not bind well to these receptors; however, both (+) and (–) isomers of many

TABLE 20.2 Pharmacokinetics of the Opioid Analgesics[a,b]

Opioid	Log $D_{pH7.4}$[c]	Oral Bioavailability (%)	Protein Binding (%)	V_d (L/kg)	$T_{1/2}$ (h)	Duration (h) of Analgesia	Excretion (%)	T_{max} (h) for Analgesia	Onset (min)of Analgesia
Codeine	0.82	Well	0	~3	2–3	4–6	90 Renal	2–4	30–60
Hydrocodone	1.36	-	-	-	4–5	4	70 Renal <24 h	2	60
Hydromorphone	1.56	24	10–30	~3	11	4	-	1–2	30
Levorphanol	1.76	Rapid	40–50	10	11	4	-	-	10–60
Morphine	0.48	20–40	20–40	~4	2–5	4–5 sc	10 Fecal 90 Renal	-	10–30 sc
Oxycodone	0.38	60–90	45	~3	3–4	3–6	80 renal 20 unc	1–2	60
Oxymorphone	0.32	10	~10	3	7–9	4–6 iv	90 Renal	-	10 iv
Buprenorphine	2.08	15 TD 90 im	96	430 iv	2–6	4–6 im 7 d TD	30 Renal 7-Fecal	60 min TD	20 TD
Butorphanol	2.61	20 oral 70 nasal	80	10–13	5–6 nasal	5–6 oral 3–4 iv	80 renal 15 fecal	4–5 iv	15 nasal 60 iv
Nalbuphine	0.28	-	-	~4	3–5	3–6	10 renal 80 fecal	-	2–3 iv
Pentazocine	3.22	~20	370–415	-	2–3	2–3	70 unc	1–3 oral	15–30 2–3 iv
Naloxone	1.46	Rapidly inactivated orally	10	2–4	<2	45 min iv	50 renal <6h	-	2–3 iv
Naltrexone	1.51	5–40	20	1350 IV	4	24 iv 3 days oral	60–80 renal 10 fecal	-	-
Alfentanil	2.11	NA	92	~1	~2	10 min	80 renal	15 min im	2–3 iv
Fentanyl	2.94	50–65 buccal 92 TD	85	4–6	3–12 iv 20–27 TD	72 TD ~1 iv	75 renal 10 fecal 10 unc	8 min iv 30–50 min	12–24 TD < 1 iv
Meperidine	1.17	~50	60–85	3–5	3–4	2–4 sc,iv	10 unc 60 renal	30–60 min	10 sc
Methadone	3.23	85	70–90	3–4 iv	23 iv 12–24	2–10	21 unc	-	120 oral 30 iv
Remifentanil	1.70	NA	70	30–60 IV	3–10 m	3–10 min	90 renal	-	1–3 iv
Sufentanil	3.54	NA	90	2–3	2–3	30 min	80 renal 20 unc	-	1–3 iv
Tapentadol	1.38	32	20	540	4	4–6	70 renal	1–2	-
Tramadol	0.62	75	20	~3	5–7	4–6	30 renal 60 fecal	2–3	60

Abbreviations key: V_d, volume of distribution; $T_{1/2}$ elimination half-life; T_{max}, time to maximum analgesic effect; TD, transdermal; unc, unchanged; iv, intravenous; im, intramuscular; sc, subcutaneous; min, minutes

[a]Data for oral administration unless otherwise noted

[b]Data from Thomson Reuters Micromedex 2.0, accessed June 10, 2011

[c]Log $D_{pH 7.4}$ calculated using ACD/LogP v.12 Advanced Chemistry Development, Toronto Canada

μ agonists are potent antitussives. For example, almost everyone has purchased dextromethorphan (e.g., Robitussin DM) to control cough because it is available over the counter. Despite the fact that its μ-opioid receptor binding is exceptionally low, its ready availability has made it a focus of abuse, with approximately 10% of U.S. teenagers admitting to using it in large quantities in an attempt to attain euphoria (85,86). The drug antagonizes NMDA and σ-1 receptors, and some studies have documented a neuroprotective role for this compound related to its ability to combat glutamate-induced neurotoxicity (87–89). The levorotatory enantiomer of this over-the-counter product is called levomethorphan, and it is a potent, full μ-receptor agonist. It is not marketed, although levorphanol (Levo-Dromeran), its chemical cousin, is. Levorphanol is a potent prescription μ agonist analgesic with all of the anticipated risks and adverse effects common to this class of therapeutic agents.

Common Metabolic Reactions

The common metabolic pathways of the opioids are predictable from their structure. Many μ agonists have an *N*-methyl group that is readily *N*-dealkylated by CYP3A4 (90). From a therapeutic standpoint, nor-metabolites have limited clinical relevance due to a decrease in distribution-enhancing lipophilicity and the loss of an agonist-promoting hydrophobic interaction with the receptor.

In contrast, CYP2D6-mediated *O*-dealkylation of the 3-methoxy group of codeine analogs is required to generate the phenolic OH group essential for μ-receptor binding. Patients deficient in this activating enzyme show little or no response to codeine-based analgesics (90,91). While no clinically marketed opioid analgesic has a C_3-ester, the need for metabolic liberation of the phenol would still hold true. For example, the 3-acetate ester of heroin is readily hydrolyzed in the CNS to generate the analgesically active monoacetylmorphine (Fig. 20.9). The 6-acetate ester is slower to cleave because its carbonyl carbon is less electrophilic due to a lack of resonance delocalization of electron density, but it will eventually succumb to hydrolysis to produce morphine.

Opioids are also subject to phase 2 metabolism prior to excretion. Phenols conjugate with either glucuronic acid or sulfate, and both conjugates are found in the urine of patients taking multicyclic opioids. These conjugates, like most, are inactive, and phase 2 conjugation in the GI tract impacts the oral bioavailability of many phenolic opioids (Table 20.2). Those administered by mouth must be given in doses higher than one would administer parenterally, and/or they are formulated to promote rapid absorption and limit exposure to intestinal transferase enzymes. Alcohols like those found at C_6 of morphine and codeine can also conjugate with

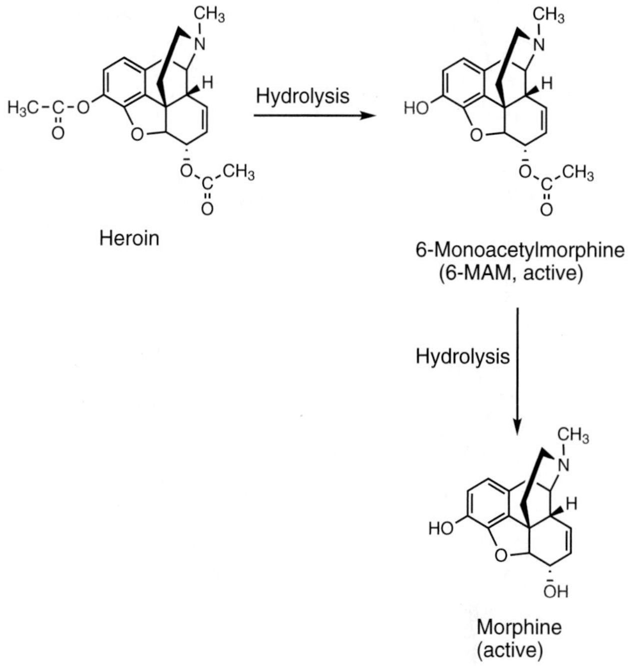

FIGURE 20.9 Heroin metabolism.

glucuronic acid. In a significant deviation from the norm, morphine's C_6-glucuronide actually has a higher affinity for the μ receptors than the free alcohol and is believed to be responsible for a significant amount of morphine's and codeine's analgesic action (90,92). Glucuronidation at both C_3 and C_6 is catalyzed by UGT2B7 (90).

The metabolic pathway of codeine is illuminating in that it contains essentially all of the aforementioned biotransformations and includes reactions that are activating, inactivating, attenuating, and augmenting with regard to analgesic action (Fig. 20.10).

STRUCTURE-ACTIVITY RELATIONSHIPS OF OPIOID AGONISTS AND ANTAGONISTS

In the following paragraphs, SARs that can be broadly applied to various chemical classes of opioid agonists and antagonists are presented. Several opioid molecules are "one of a kind," and their unique SAR will be presented within the individual drug monograph.

Multicyclic Opioids

Multicyclic opioids include those with pentacyclic (morphine), tetracyclic (morphinan), tricyclic (benzazocine), or bicyclic (oripavine) fused ring systems (Figs. 20.11 to 20.13). Although not every structural prototype will contain all of the functional groups identified

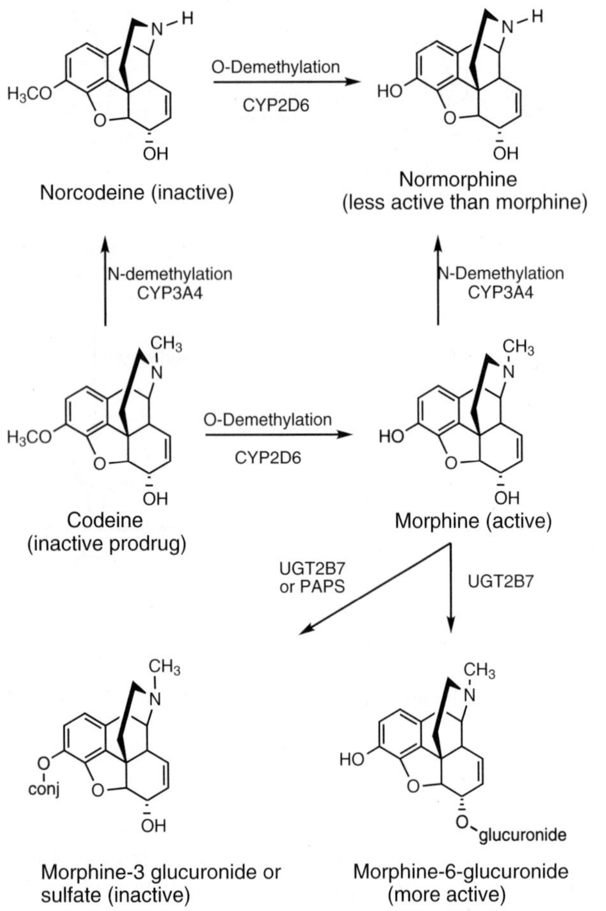

FIGURE 20.10 Codeine metabolism.

below, the following is a general discussion of key SARs that commonly apply to the multicyclic opioid analgesics and antagonists.

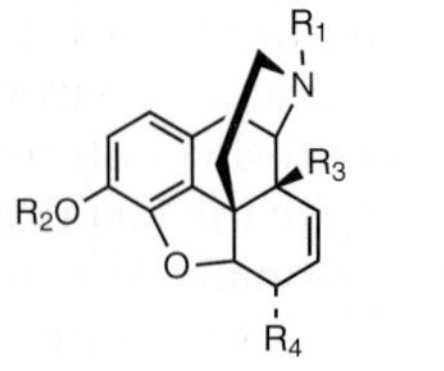

Multicyclic opioid pharmacophore

R_1

An amino nitrogen is an essential feature of all opioids because, in cationic conjugate acid form, it permits receptor anchoring through an essential electrostatic bond with the Asp residue conserved in all G protein–coupled receptors (84). With the exception of dezocine, an opioid agonist no longer available in the United States, only tertiary amines provide clinically significant opioid agonist or antagonist activity in the CNS.

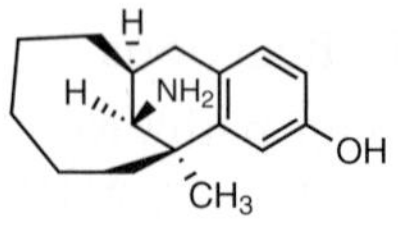

Dezocine

The nitrogen substituent found on tertiary μ selective multicyclic opioid agonists is most commonly CH_3. This group interacts hydrophobically with μ-receptor residues. An aralkyl substituent (e.g., phenethyl) would significantly enhance μ-receptor affinity and CNS distribution, but no such substituent is currently found on any multicyclic opioid.

Extending the length of the nitrogen substituent to three carbons or its equivalent and incorporating an area

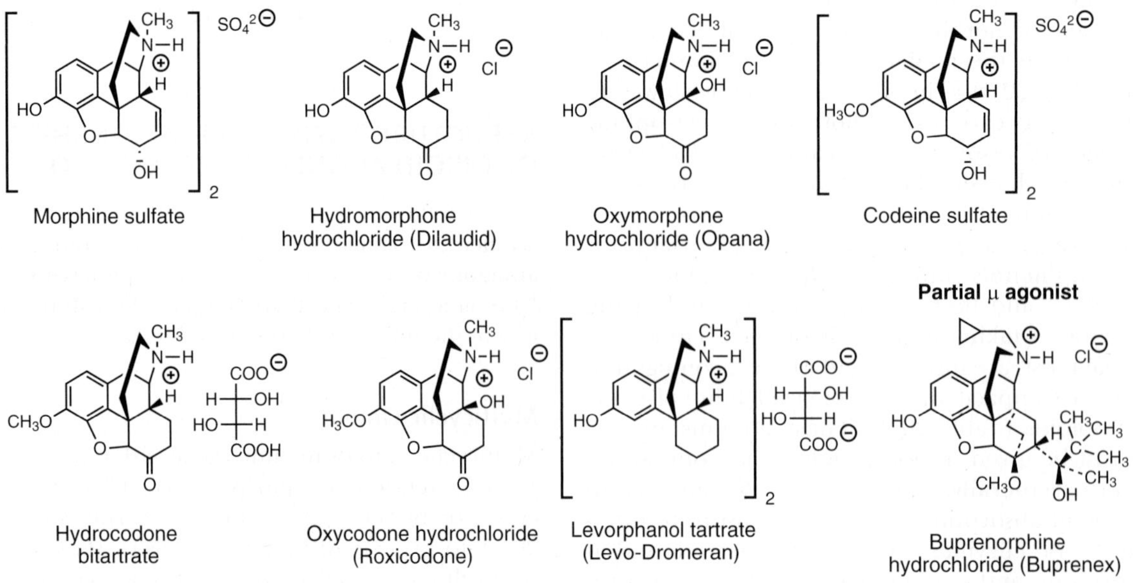

FIGURE 20.11 Multicyclic μ agonists.

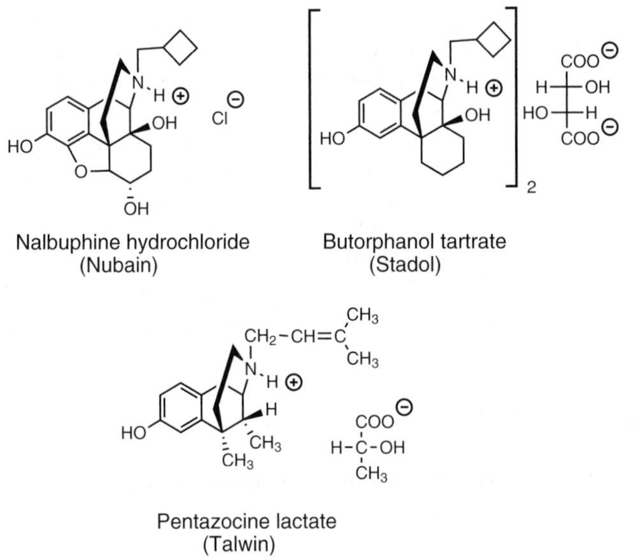

FIGURE 20.12 Multicyclic κ agonists/μ antagonists.

of high electron density two atoms away from the nitrogen shifts the μ-receptor activity profile from agonist to antagonist. The antagonist site on the μ receptor is a generally hydrophobic narrow pocket formed between the side chains of Asp, Met, Tyr, Ile, and Gly residues (84). If the moiety providing the high electron density is a double bond (R_1 = allyl) or a highly strained cyclopropane ring (R_1 = cyclopropylmethyl), μ antagonist activity is predominant. If found on a pentacyclic opioid framework containing a 14β-OH group and a 7,8-dihydro-6-one (or equivalent) C ring, allyl and cyclopropylmethyl substituents provide a pure opioid antagonist. Pure antagonists have their highest affinity for the μ receptor but, in higher doses, will block all other opioid receptor subtypes too. They provide no analgesic action at any receptor at any

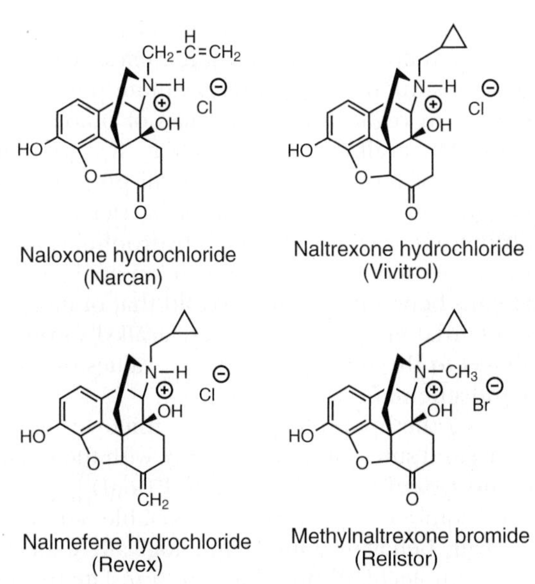

FIGURE 20.13 Multicyclic opioid antagonists.

dose. In other multicyclic systems, these two nitrogen substituents can provide κ agonism, but only in doses much higher than those needed to elicit μ antagonism. Strong dysphoria at these higher doses precludes their use as analgesics, and no such drugs are marketed.

If ring strain is eased as in cyclobutylmethyl, or if the allyl moiety is converted to dimethylallyl, significant μ antagonism remains but κ agonism (analgesia) becomes the therapeutically predominant action. While often potent, the level of μ antagonism exhibited by *N*-cyclobutylmethyl opioids will always be lower than that of their allyl or cyclopropylmethyl counterparts because of a less-than-optimal fit in (and affinity for) the narrow antagonist receptor cleft. However, because clinically significant μ antagonism will always accompany κ agonism, analgesics with cyclobutylmethyl or dimethylallyl nitrogen substituents will precipitate withdrawal in patients dependent on *N*-methyl– or *N*-aralkyl–substituted analgesics. In other words, these two chemically distinct classes of pain-relieving opioids are not cross tolerant.

R_2

A phenolic hydroxyl group or a methoxy ether will be found at C_3 of all marketed multicyclic opioids. As previously mentioned, the phenol is required for binding at μ and κ receptors, so the methoxy ethers (codeine analogs) are prodrugs. CYP2D6 *O*-dealkylation of these methoxy groups is activating, but it is a somewhat sluggish reaction. Only about 10% of a dose of codeine will be activated to morphine before activity-attenuating CYP3A4-mediated *N*-dealkylation occurs. Poor CYP2D6 metabolizers will not realize the full impact of codeine-based analgesics and require alternative analgesic therapy. Within the United States, the incidence of CYP2D6 deficiency has been estimated at 7.7% for Caucasians and between 1.9% and 7.3% for African Americans (93). These numbers are in line with estimates for these ethnic groups within the general population (94,95). Although the CYP2D6*3 and *4 alleles common in Caucasian poor metabolizers are present in only 1% or less of persons of Asian ancestry, the CYP2D6*10 allele associated with reduced CYP2D6 catalytic capability (intermediate metabolizer phenotype) is found in up to 50% of Asians (93–95).

The importance of CYP2D6 phenotype in the pharmacokinetics of 3-methoxy–substituted analgesics is powerfully illustrated by the tragic loss of life that occurred when a new mother, an ultrafast CYP2D6 metabolizer taking codeine for postpartum pain, nursed her newborn son who had the normal CYP2D6 metabolizer phenotype. Both mother and son were homozygous for the UGT2B7*2 (fast-metabolizing) allele of the C_6-glucuronidating transferase enzyme, meaning that both could rapidly convert morphine to the highly active and persistent 6-glucuronide metabolite. Over the course of 2 weeks, the infant was exposed to an excessive amount of morphine and its C_6-glucuronide metabolite, and he died of respiratory depression (96). One could envision the same tragic outcome if a CYP2D6 intermediate-metabolizer mother given high doses of codeine in an attempt to relieve pain breastfed a normal (extensive metabolizer) or ultrarapid CYP2D6-metabolizing infant.

When present, the phenolic OH group will be vulnerable to inactivating prehepatic GI and first-pass (liver) phase 2 metabolism. Premature conjugation with glucuronic acid or with 3′-phosphoadenylyl sulfate significantly compromises the oral bioavailability of many phenolic opioids. Phenols also undergo in vitro oxidation to therapeutically inactive quinones. Phenolic drugs, including active opioids, should always be protected from light, base, and oxygen in the air or, over time, they will decompose.

R_3

Multicyclic opioids currently on the market have either a 14β-H or OH moiety, which provides a B/C *cis* or equivalent configuration. The polar 14β-OH slows penetration of the blood–brain barrier, but the negative impact this would have on analgesic potency is more than overridden by a significant increase in receptor affinity. At μ, the 14β-OH H-bonds very effectively with a Tyr residue, whereas at κ receptors, the bonding residue is Glu (84). Overall, a two- to threefold increase in opioid activity is achieved through the addition of a 14β-OH. Interestingly, there is a decrease in antitussive (cough suppression) action (97), and 14β-OH opioids are not used for this therapeutic purpose.

R_4

The impact of the C_6 substituent of multicyclic opioids on pharmacologic action is tied to the presence or absence of the 7,8-double bond. The 6α-OH found in naturally occurring morphine and codeine is believed to engage in a hydrogen bond with a μ-receptor Asn residue (84), but the bond formed is not strong. Despite the loss of this drug–receptor interaction, removal of the alcoholic OH group results in an approximate 10-fold increase in activity due to a significant increase in molecular lipophilicity ($logD_{pH\ 7.4}$) (98). If the 6α-OH is oxidized to provide an α,β-unsaturated ketone, the H-bonding role of the 6-substituent converts from H-donor to H-acceptor. In the rigid pseudoboat C ring that is ensured by the 7,8-olefin, a marked decrease in receptor affinity occurs, and activity decreases threefold. However, if the 7,8-double bond is reduced, the C ring becomes significantly more flexible and can properly position the H-accepting C_6 ketone for high-affinity receptor binding. A sixfold gain in analgesic potency is achieved by changing C ring structure from the natural 7,8-dehydro-6α-ol to 7,8-dihydro-6-one.

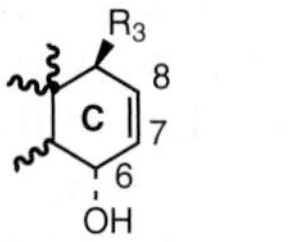

7,8-Dehydro-6α-ol

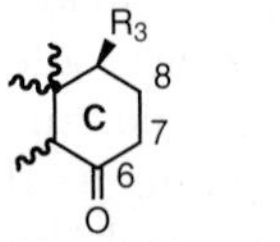

7,8-dihydro-6-one

The 6α-OH group of morphine and codeine (and the 6-glucuronide metabolite) is associated with mast cell degranulation and histamine release, which can lead to an allergic response involving hypotension, intense pruritus, and rash (99). The mechanism involves activation of protein kinase A and inositol triphosphate kinase, which not only releases histamine but also stimulates the production of proinflammatory chemokines in mast cells (100). This adverse effect is particularly intense with codeine, and as a result, parenteral administration of this analgesic is generally not recommended. The delayed allergic reaction is not reversed by opioid antagonists, indicating that it is not mediated through the μ receptor. Pruritus and hypotension are not generally observed with 6-keto or 6-desoxy opioids, and the risk of nausea may also be lowered.

Flexible Opioids: Anilidopiperidines

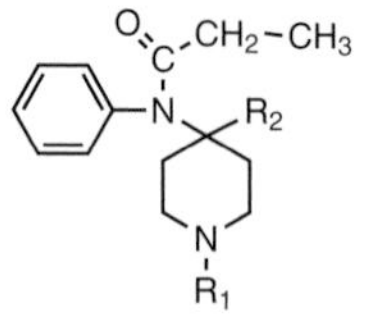

Anilidopiperidine pharmacophore

The anilidopiperidine (also called anilinopiperidine) analgesics, commonly known as the fentanyls, are the only class of flexible opioids with more than two members (Fig. 20.14). As the aromatic phenyl ring of the fentanyls is believed to interact with the μ receptor Trp^{283} residue that normally binds Phe^4 of enkephalin, no phenolic OH group is incorporated into their structures (84). These are highly lipophilic molecules that distribute rapidly across the blood–brain barrier, resulting in a fast and potent, albeit short-lived, analgesic response (101).

R_1

The SAR of the nitrogen substituent of all flexible opioids essentially parallels that of the multicyclics. *N*-Methyl or *N*-aralkyl substituents will always promote potent, selective μ agonism regardless of the class of opioids under discussion. The aralkyl substituents (e.g., R_1 = phenethyl, thienylethyl) of fentanyl and sufentanil promote a very fast penetration of the blood–brain barrier and a very high affinity at μ receptors through hydrophobic and van der Waals interactions. This results in an analgesic activity that runs between 80- and 800-fold that of morphine. The substantial lipophilicity of these aralkyl substituents contributes to the very high $logD_{pH\ 7.4}$ values of fentanyl (2.94) and sufentanil (3.54) (102).

Replacing the lipophilic phenyl or thienyl ring found in fentanyl and sufentanil, respectively, with the polar tetrazolinone system found in alfentanil ($logD_{pH\ 7.4}$ = 2.11) produces some complex but predictable changes in in vivo drug behavior. One might logically expect the decrease in molecular lipophilicity to translate to a more sluggish journey across the blood–brain barrier. However,

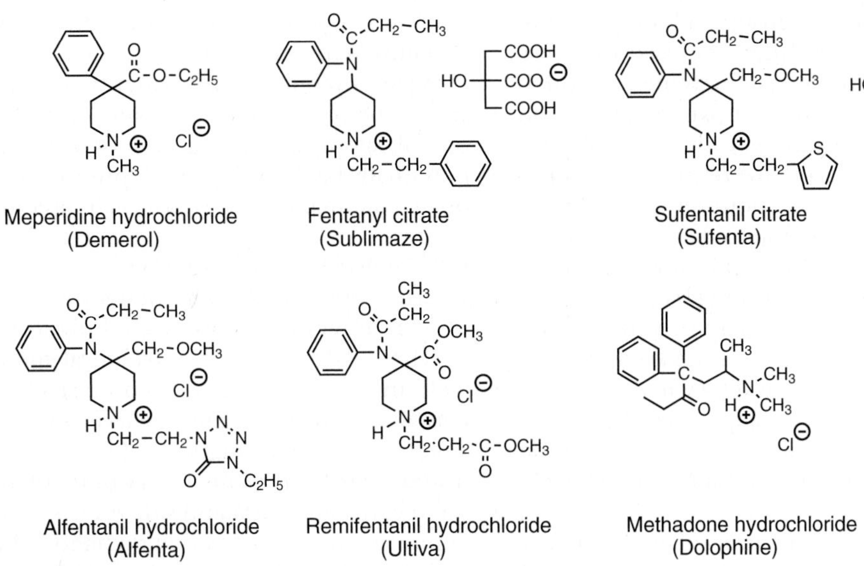

FIGURE 20.14 Flexible μ agonists.

this strongly electron-withdrawing ring system decreases the pK_a of the piperidino nitrogen atom to 6.5 compared to 8.4 for fentanyl's basic nitrogen atom, which significantly decreases the ratio of ionized to un-ionized conjugate forms in the bloodstream (103). Contrary to what would be expected from a simple comparison of $\log D_{pH\ 7.4}$ values, the lower pK_a allows for a faster penetration of the blood–brain barrier. However, this depressed ionized–to–un-ionized ratio is maintained at the receptor surface, which means less cationic drug is available for ion–ion anchoring with the μ receptor Asp. Therefore, despite a positive CNS distribution profile, the potency of alfentanil decreases to 25-fold that of morphine because of a lower μ-receptor affinity.

Mu antagonists are not found within the flexible opioid classes. The cyclopropylmethyl and allyl nitrogen substituents that provided such potent μ antagonism in the multicyclics simply attenuate agonist action in these less rigid structures, and they will not be encountered.

R_2

The methoxymethyl moiety at C_4 of the piperidine ring of sufentanil and alfentanil is lipophilic and promotes distribution to central sites of action. More importantly, its steric influence promotes high-affinity binding at the μ-receptor surface.

SPECIFIC DRUGS

Multicyclic Full μ Agonists (Fig. 20.11)

Morphine Sulfate

Morphine is the prototypical opioid agonist, and all synthetic multicyclic analgesics are based on the morphine nucleus to some degree. The presence of the *N*-CH_3 substituent, phenolic hydroxyl, and B/C *cis* configuration assure potent and selective μ agonism. Morphine has very poor oral bioavailability because of extensive prehepatic (GI) and first-pass (liver) metabolism to the inactive 3-glucuronide and 3-sulfate conjugates (Table 20.2). The C_3 glucuronide undergoes extensive enterohepatic cycling, so if oral administration is required, large initial doses must be given followed by lower maintenance doses. Morphine's $\log D_{pH\ 7.4}$ is low (0.48) (102), and opioids of higher lipophilicity exhibit better oral bioavailability as well as a faster onset of analgesic action (Table 20.2) (67). Polar and metabolically vulnerable morphine is about sixfold more active by the intramuscular route than the oral route.

Morphine is metabolized by CYP3A4-mediated *N*-dealkylation to normorphine (90) which, at 1/20 the activity of the parent, is theoretically active but not clinically relevant. Prior to excretion, glucuronic acid conjugation may occur at the C_6-OH group. As previously noted, this glucuronide retains activity at the receptor and is under investigation as a therapeutic agent for the relief of postoperative pain (104). A potency ratio between morphine-6-glucuronide and the parent morphine in humans has been estimated at up to 50:1 (105). That ratio can rise to 100:1 when the drug is administered directly into the brain of animals (106). Although this polar metabolite should be readily excreted, it can actually accumulate in patients with renal failure or poor renal function (e.g., elderly), increasing the risk of inadvertent overdose (90,107).

Morphine is one of the safest opioids to use to treat the pain of myocardial infarction, unstable angina, and other ischemic disorders because of its positive hemodynamic effects (108,109). Its negative chronotropic effect and venous and arterial vasodilation result in a decrease in myocardial oxygen demand. Morphine decreases blood pressure secondary to histamine release, an activity linked to the 6α-OH group and/or the active 6α-glucuronide metabolite, and must be used with caution in patients with hypovolemia. Extreme caution is advised with the use of all opioids in patients with head trauma because opioids can increase intracranial pressure, which in turn can exacerbate respiratory depression. Inhibition of cough reflex, however, is a valuable action in this situation because it helps keep intracranial pressure within defined limits. Because morphine lacks the 14β-OH group that attenuates cough suppression, it is an opioid of choice in the treatment of patients with head injury (110). A relatively recent study cautions that inflammation associated with head injury may downregulate efflux proteins such as P-glycoprotein (P-gp) and multidrug-resistant protein, resulting in an accumulation of morphine and the active 6-glucuronide, respectively, in cerebral tissue (110).

Morphine is available in a wide variety of dosage forms, including solution for injection, oral solution, tablets, controlled- and extended-release tablets, and extended-release capsules (the latter marketed as Avinza and Kadian). Extended-release formulations of any opioid should only be administered to opioid-tolerant patients. They must be swallowed whole and not chewed, crushed, or dissolved in liquid. If patients have difficulty swallowing, the pellets in some extended-release capsules may be sprinkled on food (e.g., applesauce) and swallowed without chewing. To take an extended-release opioid in any way other than prescribed risks releasing and absorbing a very large dose of active drug, which can result in death from respiratory depression. The consumption of alcohol while on opioid agonists is never advised, but it could prove fatal when taking extended-release capsules, because alcohol can promote rapid capsule dissolution in the GI tract.

Morphine sulfate in combination with the opioid antagonist naltrexone hydrochloride is on the market as Embeda. This trade name refers to the fact that a core of naltrexone is embedded in a pellet of extended-release morphine. A variety of strengths is available, but the milligram-to-milligram ratio of agonist-to-antagonist is consistently held at 25:1. As with Avinza and Kadian, this combination product is for use only when continuous long-term analgesia requiring "around the clock" opioid agonist therapy is warranted. Patients taking this and all extended-release products must not be opioid-naïve, or potentially fatal respiratory depression could result.

Combination products such as Embeda have also an abuse-deterrent purpose. If the capsules or their contents were crushed and the active constituents extracted for intravenous (IV) injection (e.g., in an attempt to get high), the naltrexone hydrochloride would be extracted along with the morphine salt. If injected, the antagonist would antagonize opioid receptors, thereby blocking any euphoric responses an abuser might be seeking. Fortunately, morphine-induced hemodynamic responses would also be blocked, at least to some extent. If a patient tolerant to opioids injected this illicit formulation, a naltrexone-induced withdrawal syndrome would most certainly be precipitated.

Again, opioid-tolerant patients are the only ones who should be prescribed this or any other extended-release opioid agonist. The risk of serious toxicity, specifically potentially fatal respiratory depression, prohibits the use of all extended-release products in opioid-naïve patients.

Hydromorphone Hydrochloride

Hydromorphone, known chemically as 7,8-dihydromorphone, differs from morphine only in the area of ring C. The 7,8-dihydro-6-one structural motif adds flexibility to the system and permits a more efficacious H-bond between the 6-ketone and the μ receptor. The increase in analgesic action arising from this single structural modification has been estimated at 6- to 10-fold. As μ receptor–elicited analgesia and side effects such as respiratory depression and constipation go hand-in-hand, the risk of toxicity with hydromorphone as compared to morphine also increases. Hydromorphone is available as a solution for injection, rectal suppositories, tablets, liquid for oral administration, and extended-release tablets. As with Avinza and Kadian, a black box warning has been issued for the extended-release formulation (Exalgo), because the potential for abuse and the risk of fatal respiratory depression are high. Like all extended-release opioids, Exalgo use is reserved for patients tolerant to and dependent on μ agonists who require high-potency pain management on a chronic basis.

Oxymorphone Hydrochloride

The addition of a hydroxyl group at 14β increases analgesic action approximately two- to threefold over hydromorphone secondary to an increase in μ-receptor affinity. This makes oxymorphone at least 12-fold more potent than morphine. It is available as a solution for injection, tablets, and extended-release tablets. All precautions previously outlined for extended-release morphine and hydromorphone apply to Opana ER, the extended-release formulation of oxymorphone.

Codeine Sulfate, Hydrocodone Bitartrate, and Oxycodone Hydrochloride

Codeine, hydrocodone, and oxycodone are the 3-methoxy analogs of morphine, hydromorphone, and oxymorphone, respectively, and they have the same potency relationship to one another as their parent structures demonstrated. All are prodrugs that must undergo CYP2D6-mediated activation to the phenolic structure required for binding to μ receptors. Codeine and oxycodone are available as single-drug products. Although the potency of each is about 10- to 12-fold lower than their phenolic counterpart, oral bioavailability is greatly enhanced (Table 20.2). Both are available in tablet form and as a solution for injection. As previously mentioned, the risk of a severe allergic reaction to parenterally administered codeine phosphate is high due to the presence of the 6α-OH group.

Oxycodone was one of the first μ agonist analgesics to be made available in controlled-release tablet form (Oxycontin), and there was much focus in the literature and lay press on the misuse of this drug by abusers when it was first released (111). Some abusers seek (and get) a very strong euphoric rush by dissolving a crushed Oxycontin tablet in alcohol. As can be imagined, this practice increases the likelihood of true addiction and/or death. It cannot be emphasized strongly enough that patients on opioids should avoid the consumption of alcohol due to the risk of additive CNS depressant actions, including coma and potentially fatal respiratory depression.

Hydrocodone is available only in analgesic combination with acetaminophen or aspirin and in some cough suppressant preparations (note the lack of the 14β-OH, which permits its use as a cough suppressant). With a potency approximately half that of morphine, its combination with a nonsteroidal anti-inflammatory drug or *p*-aminophenol–based analgesic attacks pain on two mechanistic fronts, presumably allowing for a lower dose of each potentially toxic drug to be used.

Codeine use for longer than 6 months has recently been associated with an increased risk of serious or fatal cardiovascular events, and an increased risk of all-cause mortality has been noted when used for more than 30 days (112). Oxycodone, but not hydrocodone, is also associated with these serious adverse effects. The risk-to-benefit ratio of long-term use of codeine, oxycodone, and other potentially cardiotoxic opioids must always be carefully evaluated, particularly in the elderly and other vulnerable patient populations.

Levorphanol Tartrate

Levorphanol is the only μ agonist in the tetracyclic (morphinan) class of multicyclic opioids. Unlike the pentacyclic morphines, the B/C *cis* (14*R*) configuration is twofold less active than the B/C *trans* (14*S*) isomer (113,114), but the B/C *cis* structure is the only isomeric form commercially available. The analgesic potency of levorphanol is approximately four- to eightfold that of morphine due to enhanced molecular flexibility from the loss of both the restraining E ring and the 7,8-double bond, which leads to increased μ-receptor affinity despite the lack of a 14β-OH. In addition, the loss of the E ring and 6-oxygen functions increases $\log D_{pH\ 7.4}$ (1.76) (102), which permits more facile transit across the blood–brain barrier. It is available as tablets and as a solution for injection.

Levorphanol's 6- to 8-hour duration of action is about twice that of morphine, which enhances utility in chronic pain. It has an 11- to 16-hour terminal half-life, however, and this allows the drug to accumulate over time. Patients should be monitored for unwanted or excessive sedation that might signal a build-up of drug in the blood and brain.

Multicyclic Partial μ Agonists

Buprenorphine Hydrochloride

This structurally unique opioid has an interesting and unique SAR (115–117). Despite the presence of the *N*-cyclopropylmethyl group, which normally promotes therapeutically useful μ antagonist action, buprenorphine is a very potent, but partial, μ agonist with an analgesic potency between 25- and 40-fold that of morphine (113,118). A 0.3- to 0.4-mg dose of this oripavine-based analgesic is equipotent with 10 mg of morphine. This superior potency is attributed to high lipophilicity and a higher-than-normal affinity for μ receptors because of the additional hydrophobic and hydrogen bonding capabilities of the C_7 side chain. Typical of its partial agonist action, a bell-shaped dose–response curve has been described for many of the actions of this bicyclic opioid (115,119–121). Although not used clinically for this purpose, buprenorphine also antagonizes κ receptors (121).

The μ-receptor binding of buprenorphine is strong enough to be classified as pseudoirreversible (121,122), which provides an exceptionally long half-life of 37 hours and permits once-daily dosing. In addition, the slow dissociation from μ receptors minimizes withdrawal symptoms even if the drug is abruptly discontinued (123). Any discomfort a patient experiences after abrupt withdrawal of buprenorphine normally occurs 5 days to 2 weeks after the last dose was taken. The down side of pseudoirreversible binding is that it is difficult to reverse receptor-mediated side effects (124). The most problematic adverse reaction associated with this drug is respiratory depression. This unwanted effect is less severe than can be observed with full μ agonists, and fortunately, it is rarely life-threatening, but it can be clinically significant. If respiratory depression occurs in a patient taking buprenorphine, it can take up to 10-fold the normal dose of naloxone to compete for the μ receptors and reverse it. The respiratory depression induced by buprenorphine can outlast naloxone's duration of action, making the impact of a single high dose of antagonist inconsistent (121). A regimen of 2 to 3 mg of naloxone followed by a 4-mg/h continuous infusion has been shown to restore normal breathing in respiratory-depressed patients within an hour, and kinetic models to explain this clinical observation have been published (121).

Because buprenorphine has only partial μ agonist action, it will precipitate withdrawal in patients dependent on full μ agonists (85,125), but it also suppresses the symptoms of full-blown withdrawal. In other words, if μ receptors are occupied by a full agonist, they will not tolerate a stepping down of receptor stimulation, but if they are already in "crisis mode," some μ agonism is viewed as better than none.

Buprenorphine undergoes significant first-pass metabolism. The CYP3A4-generated *N*-dealkylated metabolite norbuprenorphine retains some analgesic activity (40-fold less than the parent drug), but the C_3 glucuronide is predictably inactive (126,127). This drug is given IV or sublingually to avoid inactivating conjugation in the GI and on first pass. The dose of buprenorphine may need to be adjusted if coadministered with CYP3A4 substrates or inhibitors or benzodiazepines, or if alcohol use is known or suspected.

A transdermal patch formulation of buprenorphine, marketed as Butrans, has recently been made available in 5-, 10-, and 20-mcg/h strengths. The previously described precaution on using extended-release opioids only in opioid-tolerant patients also applies to transdermal buprenorphine. In addition, patients must be advised to avoid allowing the applied patch to become hot, as the release of drug from the patch matrix is temperature dependent. Although buprenorphine can be hepatotoxic in high doses secondary to inhibition of mitochondrial respiration and subsequent adenosine triphosphate depletion, the nor metabolite is apparently nontoxic (128).

In addition to its use as an analgesic, buprenorphine is also employed in opioid addiction recovery. As previously noted, opioid addiction affects millions of people in the United States and has a huge financial impact on health care economics. In 2003, over 8% of U.S. emergency room visits were related to heroin use. It has been estimated that 6% to 15% of people in the United States abuse drugs (85), and the National Institute on Drug Abuse has estimated that illicit drug abuse (including opioid abuse) consumes over half a trillion dollars each year (129). The number of individuals over 50 years of age seeking treatment for drug and alcohol addiction has been increasing at a rate disproportionate to the general population, and in 2008, almost a quarter million "baby boomers" (or older) sought professional help for substance abuse (130). In 2008, heroin was second only to alcohol as the most abused substance in this older population.

In 2-mg doses, buprenorphine blocks the euphoric effects of heroin and has been shown to be as active as 30 mg of methadone in addiction treatment programs. Doses between 2 and 32 mg daily are common, with an average daily dose of 16 mg. Treatment programs generally range from 6 months to over 2 years (83). Recovering addicts receiving their first dose of buprenorphine must be opioid-free for 7 to 10 days to avoid precipitation of a withdrawal episode. Alternatively, under the direct supervision of a physician, the patient can be allowed to enter the preliminary phase of opioid withdrawal and then be administered the first dose of buprenorphine, which will suppress the withdrawal symptoms (83). If a recovering addict relapses (common in the first years of abstinence) and increases the buprenorphine dose in an attempt to get euphoria, they will hit the partial agonist activity plateau, and their attempt to abuse will be thwarted (83). When the time comes, the patient can be withdrawn from buprenorphine with few, if any, withdrawal symptoms due to its slow dissociation from the receptors and slow disappearance from the body. The patient's receptors essentially wean themselves off of the drug.

Two sublingual formulations of buprenorphine are available for use in addiction recovery. Subutex contains only buprenorphine and is available in 2- and 8-mg strengths. Onset of action generally occurs within 30 to 60 minutes and peaks between 90 and 100 minutes. The same dose options are available for Suboxone, but these products contain 0.25 mg naloxone per mg of buprenorphine to block euphoria if the sublingual tablets are crushed, extracted, and injected IV by would-be abusers (83). Naloxone has limited activity by the sublingual (and oral) route.

The direct drug cost of Suboxone has been estimated at $250 per prescription, or about 10-fold that of methadone (85). However, the overall cost (which includes elements of adherence, regimen [every 2 to 3 days], and adverse events/toxicity), as well as the cost to patients, may actually be lower. The value of receiving therapy in one's own physician's office or pharmacy (greater accessibility, lower "stigma") cannot be overestimated. The addition of these products to the U.S. marketplace is significant in that it allows recovering addicts to receive care from the hands of their own physicians and pharmacists (131). Physicians who engage in office-based treatment of addiction must have completed a minimum of 8 hours of specialized training. They are issued special Drug Enforcement Administration numbers indicating authorization to prescribe buprenorphine. Physicians may dispense a small supply of Subutex to patients in the office, while pharmacies primarily stock Suboxone for long-term therapy. The need for appropriate sensitivity to patient privacy when counseling should be obvious (132).

Predictably, replacing the *N*-cyclopropylmethyl substituent of buprenorphine with a methyl group provides a full μ agonist. The *N*-methylated analog that has also replaced the *t*-butyl group within the C_7 side chain with *N*-propyl and oxidized the 6,14-endoethano bridge to endoetheno is known as etorphine. Etorphine has an analgesic potency estimated at up to 200-fold that of morphine in humans for reasons related to superior receptor affinity and central distribution properties. Although never marketed for human use in the United States, etorphine has been widely used in veterinary medicine and as an immobilizer to permit the safe capture and/or handling of zoo animals and large game. Marketed alone or in combination with the sedative antiemetic acetylpromazine, etorphine has enjoyed the descriptive trade names of Captivon and Immobilon, respectively. Buprenorphine can also be converted into a potent and pure opioid antagonist (diprenorphine) simply by replacing the *t*-butyl moiety on the C_7 side chain with methyl.

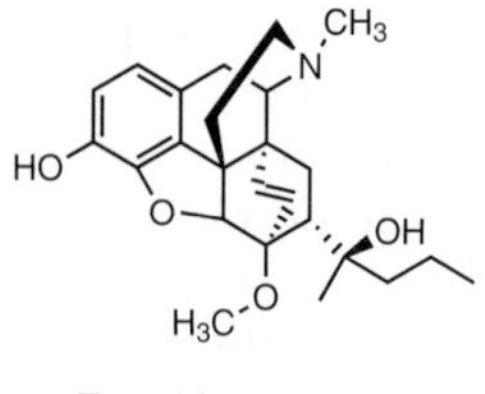

Etorphine

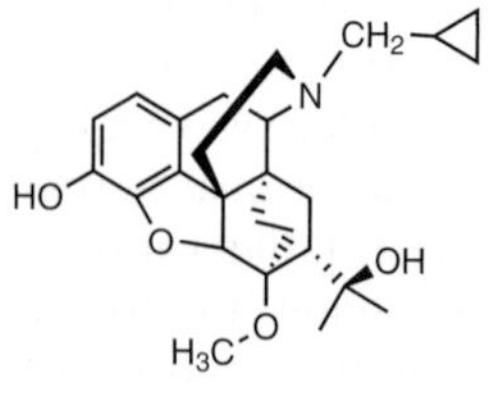

Diprenorphine

Multicyclic κ Agonists/μ Antagonists

Nalbuphine Hydrochloride

This pentacyclic *N*-cyclobutylmethyl opioid provides clinically useful analgesia elicited exclusively via the κ receptor. Potency is augmented by the lack of the 7,8-double bond and the presence of the 14β-OH group, and overall, it is between

0.5- and 1-fold as active as morphine in the relief of pain. It is administered only by injection. The μ antagonist component of its activity is approximately one-fourth that of the prototypical μ opioid antagonist naloxone. The κ agonist/μ antagonist activity profile assures a lack of cross tolerance with full or partial μ agonist analgesics, and patients stabilized on μ agonists cannot be switched to nalbuphine (or any other κ agonist) without precipitating withdrawal.

Kappa agonists produce less respiratory depression, constipation, euphoria, and potential for addiction than μ agonists (133). Sedation and diuresis are nalbuphine's major side effects. Like morphine, this analgesic decreases oxygen demand in the myocardium after infarct. Kappa receptor–related dysphoria is not as common with nalbuphine as with the other two marketed κ agonists, butorphanol and pentazocine.

Women often respond better to κ opioids than men (134), and these compounds are often used in obstetrics. Gender differences in response may be due to differences in types of pain, pain perception, threshold, and/or pathways, steroid influence on drugs or pain relief, and/or opioid receptor density. Some men have shown a pronounced antianalgesic response to low-dose (5 mg) nalbuphine (134).

Butorphanol Tartrate

Butorphanol is another *N*-cyclobutylmethyl κ agonist analgesic with μ antagonist actions. The lack of the furan oxygen and 6α-OH group provides a 5- to 10-fold higher analgesic potency compared to nalbuphine. This drug has enjoyed significant use in obstetrics and, while respiratory depression is possible, it is not usually a clinically significant problem. The ceiling effect for butorphanol-induced respiratory depression is lower than that observed with μ agonists, so the risk of fatality is slight, even when the drug is given in higher doses (135).

As with all κ agonists, receptor-mediated dysphoria and diuresis are possible with butorphanol, especially when higher doses are used (136,137). Although significant pulmonary hypertension and an increase in myocardial workload have been claimed (69), some indicate the hemodynamic impact of butorphanol is similar to morphine (138).

No oral dosage forms of butorphanol are available due to significant first-pass metabolism to an inactive *trans*-3′-hydroxy metabolite (139). However, a nasal spray is available for use when administration by injection is not warranted. The availability of this dosage form has increased the use of this analgesic in the outpatient setting.

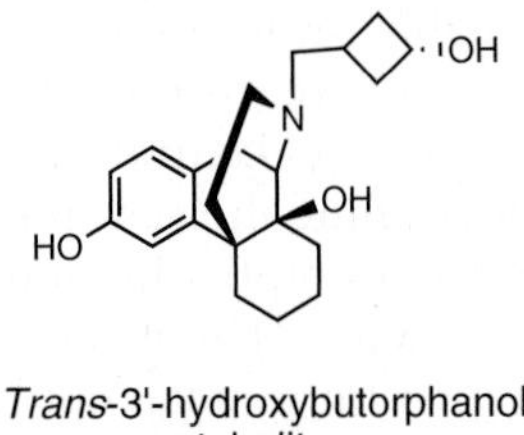

Trans-3'-hydroxybutorphanol metabolite

Pentazocine Lactate

The tricyclic (benzazocine) κ agonist pentazocine is missing carbons 6 and 7 of the C ring of multicyclic opioids, which compromises its ability to interact hydrophobically with opioid receptors. Although marketed as a racemic mixture, the analgesic action is found only in the levorotatory isomer, which is approximately half as active as morphine. Pentazocine is more likely than the other commercially available κ agonists to induce use-limiting dysphoria, especially at high doses (140). It also increases mean arterial and pulmonary arterial pressure and myocardial oxygen demand (138,141). This κ agonist should be avoided in myocardial infarction and congestive heart failure patients.

Pentazocine lactate is available as a solution for injection for the treatment of moderate to severe pain. Pentazocine hydrochloride is administered orally in combination with acetaminophen, but bioavailability is only 20% to 50% due to significant prehepatic and first-pass metabolism. Major inactivating reactions include phase 2 conjugation to the C_3-glucuronide and sulfate conjugates and hydroxylation of one of the terminal CH_3 groups of the dimethylallyl nitrogen substituent. The primary alcohol generated via hydroxylation can undergo further oxidation by alcohol and aldehyde dehydrogenase enzymes to provide a carboxylic acid metabolite.

An oral pentazocine hydrochloride/naloxone hydrochloride combination product designed to frustrate potential abusers is also commercially available. Marketed as Talwin NX, the philosophy behind its design is similar to buprenorphine/naloxone (Suboxone) and morphine/naltrexone (Embeda) combination products. If Talwin NX tablets are crushed in an attempt to extract pentazocine for IV injection, the antagonist would be extracted simultaneously. The injected naloxone would occupy the opioid receptors and block pentazocine-induced euphoria. If the drug is taken orally (as intended), the orally inactive naloxone antagonist will be destroyed on first pass so that the full analgesic effect of pentazocine can be realized.

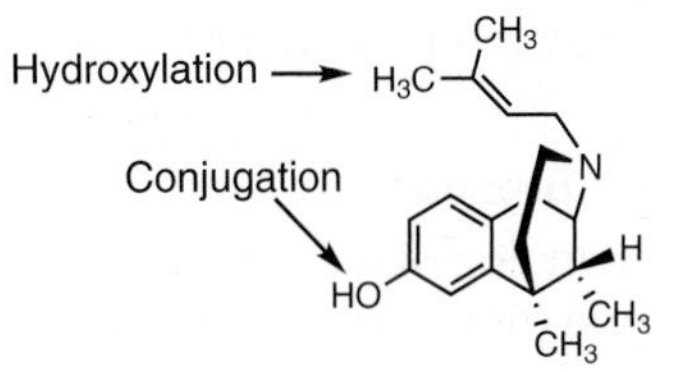

Sites of pentazocine metabolism

Multicyclic Opioid Antagonists

Naloxone Hydrochloride, Naltrexone Hydrochloride, and Nalmefene Hydrochloride (Fig. 20.13)

Three pure opioid antagonists are marketed to reverse the central actions of opioid agonists. They all have a classic antagonist-directing nitrogen substituent on a pentacyclic scaffold and contain the requisite 14β-OH and the

7,8-dihydro-6-one or 6-ene C ring. With a four-carbon *N*-cyclopropylmethyl substituent, naltrexone ($logD_{pH\ 7.4}$ = 1.51) is twice as potent as the allyl-substituted naloxone ($logD_{pH\ 7.4}$ = 1.46), presumably due to enhanced distribution to central sites of action. With the replacement of the polar C_6-keto of naltrexone with a lipophilic methylene moiety, nalmefene shows the anticipated rise in logP (2.66) and should distribute to the CNS at least as well as, if not better than, naltrexone.

Any of these opioid antagonists can be used IV to rescue patients from life-threatening opioid overdose. If administrated in this situation, they will precipitate withdrawal symptoms but can save a life. Naloxone is orally inactive due to rapid inactivating allylic oxidation and phase 2 conjugation in the GI tract and liver, and it is only used as an emergency opioid agonist antidote. In contrast, naltrexone and nalmefene have sufficient bioavailability for oral administration, although only naltrexone is available in an oral (tablet) dosage form. This enhances its utility in opioid addiction and alcoholism recovery.

In combination with a sustained-release formulation of the atypical antidepressant bupropion, sustained-release naltrexone is finding use in the treatment of obesity in adult populations (142), and low-dose (4.5 mg/d) naltrexone has also shown efficacy in healing bowel ulcerations and enhancing immunity in active Crohn's disease (143). Other off-label uses for naltrexone hydrochloride include facilitating smoking cessation, posttraumatic stress disorder, pathologic gambling, bulimia, and cholestasis and uremia-induced pruritus.

Although currently only indicated to reverse the life-threatening events associated with opioid agonist overdose, the high oral bioavailability of nalmefene could make it potentially useful in recovery therapy for opioid and alcohol addiction. Clinical trials have shown that oral nalmefene was effective in preventing relapse in recovering alcoholics (144), and it blocked the μ agonist effects of fentanyl (145). Nalmefene has an extremely long half-life compared to naloxone (11 vs. 1 to 2 hours) because it dissociates very slowly from the μ receptor. For this reason, it also produces prolonged withdrawal symptoms when administered to opioid-dependent patients.

Methylnaltrexone Bromide

This quaternary analog of naltrexone is incapable of penetrating the blood–brain barrier, but it is highly effective in reversing the unwanted actions of opioid agonists in areas outside of the CNS, most importantly constipation (146,147). Dosed by patient weight and administered subcutaneously on an every-other-day basis, it restores bowel function in patients on chronic opioid analgesic therapy. Because it cannot distribute to the CNS, the risk of displacing opioids from central receptors, which would abolish analgesia and precipitate withdrawal, is essentially nonexistent. If needed, the dosing frequency can be increased to a maximum of once daily. Because methylnaltrexone restores intestinal peristalsis, patients with bowel obstructions should not receive this drug until the blockage has been fully resolved.

Flexible μ Agonists (Fig. 20.14)

Meperidine Hydrochloride

Meperidine can be viewed as the "stripped down" opioid agonist pharmacophore, 4-phenylpiperidine. In protonated form, meperidine's amino nitrogen will anchor the drug to the anionic μ receptor Asp residue, and the *N*-CH_3 will bind by hydrophobic forces to the μ receptor agonist site, albeit via a different binding mode (and potentially different hydrophobic residues) than the multicyclic opioids.

Because it is not immobilized in a fused polycyclic "body cast," meperidine is structurally flexible and can adjust its conformation to fit the μ receptor in a way that is different from the multicyclics. Specifically, the phenyl ring at the piperidine C_4 can assume the more energetically stable equatorial conformation and bind to the μ receptor Trp^{283} residue that normally binds Phe^4 of the enkephalin pentapeptides, rather than to the Trp^{293} that normally binds the enkephalin Tyr^1 residue. Therefore, a phenolic hydroxyl group in flexible opioids is neither required nor desired. Another major structural difference between meperidine and multicyclic opioids is that this flexible μ agonist is achiral.

The analgesic activity of meperidine is about one-tenth that of morphine. As a full μ agonist, it shows all typical μ agonist effects except inhibition of GI motility and cough (148). Meperidine has poor oral bioavailability and a variable absorption after intramuscular injection. With an elimination half-life of 3 to 4 hours, it is considered short-acting. It has found use in obstetrics because of its rapid onset and short duration. The view that meperidine has a low fetal respiratory depression liability has been challenged (149).

Once hailed as "the most widely used opioid analgesic in the United States" (150), meperidine has fallen out of favor, and many are advocating its restricted use (149,151). Meperidine undergoes CYP3A4-mediated *N*-dealkylation to a nor metabolite that has about half the analgesic potency of meperidine. An oral dose of meperidine generates more nor metabolite than an equivalent IV dose. The nor metabolite has an extended half-life of 14 to 21 hours in patients with normal renal function and up to 35 hours in patients with renal disease. The extended half-life is clinically important because normeperidine can induce neurologic side effects that are not consistently or reliably reversed by naloxone. The most serious of these adverse reactions is grand mal seizures secondary to an increase in central serotonin (5-HT) levels. Therefore, meperidine therapy must not be initiated and/or it should be promptly discontinued in patients exhibiting CNS excitation. The risk of seizure is considered high if the ratio of nor metabolite to parent drug is greater than 1:1. Unfortunately, the dose of meperidine that can induce seizures in some patients overlaps with the dose commonly used in asymptomatic patients (260 to 540 mg/day), making it hard to predict when toxicity will manifest (151).

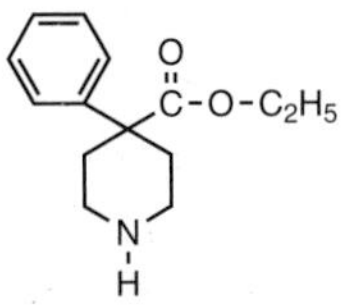

Normeperidine

The risk of serotonin syndrome–induced seizure, coma, and apnea (along with other potentially dangerous outcomes such as hypotension, cyanosis, and respiratory depression) is increased if meperidine is coadministered with monoamine oxidase inhibitors (MAOIs) (152). As might be expected, the risk of serious or fatal meperidine toxicity is significant if used in high doses, coadministered with cimetidine (which reduces meperidine clearance), or given to renally impaired patients (153,154). Urinary excretion of meperidine and normeperidine is pH dependent (154).

Like morphine and codeine, meperidine stimulates the release of histamine (155), although the mechanism does not appear to involve mast cell degranulation as is observed with the multicyclic analgesics (100). Meperidine can cause a precipitous drop in blood pressure, particularly in postsurgical patients or in those whose blood pressure is already compromised by disease or other hypotensive drugs.

The risk of potentially serious side effects and/or drug–drug interactions is prompting many hospitals to discourage and/or restrict meperidine use, especially in patient-controlled analgesia systems or when prolonged use is anticipated. Meperidine is still prescribed to treat postoperative or therapeutic hypothermia-related shivering (156), and it can be administered in low doses for short-term pain management. Treatment should be restricted to patients with normal renal function who have responded adversely to less toxic opioids, and the daily dose should be no greater than 600 mg. For more significant or prolonged pain, hydromorphone, morphine, or fentanyl is often recommended in place of meperidine.

Fentanyl Citrate

Fentanyl is a member of the anilidopiperidine class of opioid agonists and, as an *N*-phenethyl–substituted opioid structure, is a very sedative and euphoria-inducing analgesic with a potency approximately 50- to 100-fold that of morphine (157). The high activity of anilidopiperidines is due, in part, to their very high lipophilicity, which allows them to quickly penetrate the blood–brain barrier and concentrate in the CNS. Because they can leave the brain quickly too, their duration of analgesic action is short (30 to 60 minutes for fentanyl). They are most commonly administered IV as adjuncts to anesthesia.

Transmucosal, transdermal, and nasal spray formulations of fentanyl are available to treat chronic pain, including the pain of cancer (158,159). The metered-dose nasal spray provides rapid delivery of dry fentanyl citrate powder that is readily absorbed in the highly vascularized nasal passages. The bioavailability of fentanyl by this route is 71%. The onset of analgesia is approximately 5 minutes, making it useful for as-needed use in breakthrough pain, and the duration of action is approximately 1 hour (159). The transdermal patch formulation (Duragesic) releases fentanyl free base at a rate that maintains therapeutic blood levels for 72 hours, providing a convenient and reliable mechanism for chronic pain patients to achieve analgesia at home (158).

The transmucosal formulations are used to treat breakthrough pain in opioid-tolerant cancer patients and in pediatric burn patients undergoing painful cleansings and dressing changes. Fentanyl citrate is incorporated into the buccal film (Onsolis) and lozenge on a stick (buccal lollipop, Actiq) dosage forms, which are placed or held between the cheek and gum. Approximately 25% of the dose will be absorbed into the bloodstream from the buccal cavity at the normal salivary pH of about 6.4 (158). The remaining drug, when swallowed, will be inactivated in the GI tract.

The effervescent buccal tablet formulation of fentanyl base (Fentora) contains an alkalizing agent to raise the pH of the saliva and promote a faster and more complete absorption of the drug (~50% of the dose) (158). If there is a need to switch a patient from the lollipop or film to the effervescent tablet, the dose should be cut by 25% to 50% to avoid life-threatening toxicity (159). A sublingual tablet formulation of fentanyl base (Abstral) is also available which, when placed under the deepest sublingual area, disintegrates to release particles that cling to the mucosal surface, facilitating absorption (158). All transdermal and transmucosal dosage forms of fentanyl carry a black box warning related to unintentional overdose, toxicity, and intentional abuse.

Fentanyl is extensively biotransformed via CYP3A4-mediated *N*-dealkylation to an inactive metabolite and cannot be given orally (159). Because fentanyl is inactivated by this isoform, practitioners must be alert to the risk for potency-enhancing (CYP3A4 inhibitors or competitors) or attenuating (CYP3A4 inducers) interactions. Anilidopiperidines do not release histamine like meperidine and 6α-hydroxylated multicyclics do, and there is no risk of histamine-mediated allergic responses when fentanyl is administered IV (155). The fentanyl adverse reaction of greatest concern is respiratory depression. This potentially fatal reaction is persistent and can outlast the action of antagonists used to reverse it (114,160). Between April 2005 and March 2007, the Centers for Disease Control and Prevention estimated that more than 1,000 people died from the inappropriate use of fentanyl (161).

Patients experiencing fentanyl-induced respiratory depression should be closely monitored until a sustained, normal pattern of breathing returns. The risk is significantly lower with sufentanil and alfentanil, as respiratory depression generally occurs only at doses higher than those needed to relieve pain or support anesthesia.

Sufentanil Citrate

Sufentanil has replaced fentanyl's phenethyl nitrogen substituent with 2-thienylethyl, another aralkyl moiety that has a comparable affinity for μ receptors. The 4-methoxymethyl substituent augments the lipophilicity provided by the thienyl ring, and together they enhance potency approximately 5- to 10-fold over fentanyl (e.g., 600- to 800-fold compared with morphine) (157). Despite the positive impact on central distribution of this enhanced lipophilicity, the stereochemistry and steric influence of the 4-substituent appear to be more important to sufentanil's potency than its other chemical properties (157). Sufentanil redistributes from brain to periphery within 17 minutes (much faster than fentanyl), resulting in shorter postanesthesia recovery times. A transdermal patch designed to release sufentanil over a week's time is in clinical trials and may soon be available for the treatment of chronic pain.

Alfentanil Hydrochloride

The potency-attenuating impact of alfentanil's tetrazolinone ring system has been described previously. While still 25-fold as active as morphine as an analgesic, at 0.25-fold fentanyl, it is the least potent of the currently marketed anilidopiperidine opioids (157). However, because the ratio of un-ionized to ionized conjugates in the bloodstream is significantly higher compared to fentanyl and sufentanil, alfentanil distributes and redistributes across the blood–brain barrier more rapidly than either of its predecessors (162). Its onset of action is approximately fourfold faster than fentanyl, and its use is reserved for very short surgical procedures requiring anesthesia.

Remifentanil Hydrochloride

Remifentanil has a unique and interesting chemistry (107,163,164). Instead of the traditional μ agonist–promoting *N*-methyl or aralkyl substituent, remifentanil's nitrogen substituent contains an electron-withdrawing ester that functions in a manner similar to alfentanil's tetrazolinone ring in promoting the lipophilic un-ionized conjugate at pH 7.4. This drug distributes rapidly across the blood–brain barrier, where it induces a highly sedative analgesia of very short duration. Unlike the hindered ester at C_4, the ester incorporated within the nitrogen substituent is very vulnerable to hydrolysis by serum esterases to the inactive carboxylic acid. This rapid inactivation in the bloodstream eliminates any concern of drug accumulation in patients with suboptimal liver or kidney function. Remifentanil is used by the IV route to induce and/or maintain anesthesia. Its biologic half-life is a mere 3 to 10 minutes, which permits a rapid 3- to 5-minute onset of recovery from anesthesia.

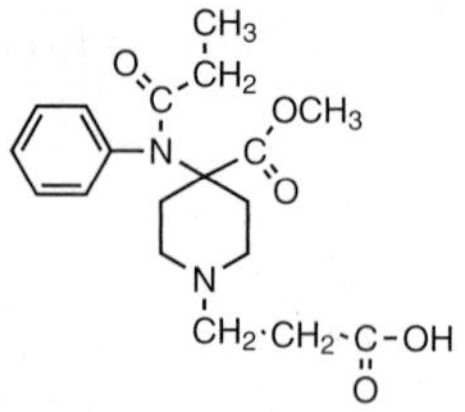

Remifentanil carboxylic acid
(Inactive metabolite)

Methadone Hydrochloride

Methadone is one of only three marketed opioid analgesics that do not contain a piperidine ring. However, its highly flexible structure could approximate the 4-phenylpiperidine pharmacophore in vivo through the formation of an intramolecular ion-dipole bond. The *N*-methyl substituent accurately predicts its μ agonist activity profile, and the activity-attenuating impact of ketone reduction supports a receptor binding role for the C_3 carbonyl oxygen.

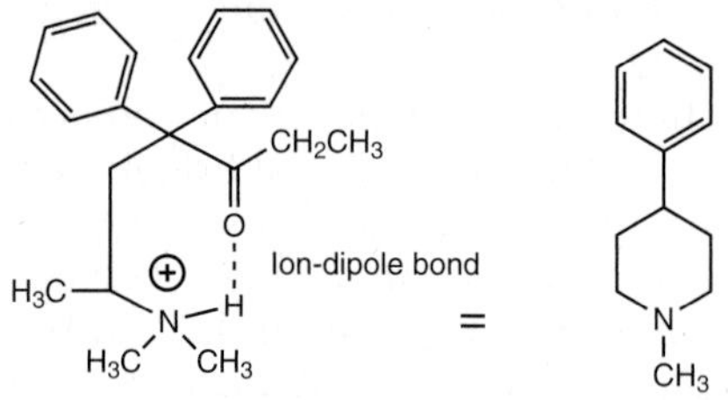

Methadone approximating the 4-phenylpiperidine pharmacophore

Methadone's lone chiral center, C_6, equates to the C_9 of morphine. While marketed as the racemic mixture, the *R*(−) isomer is responsible for methadone's analgesic action. The *S*(+) enantiomer antagonizes the NMDA receptor (165), which, although beneficial in neuropathic and opioid-resistant pain, may also be responsible for methadone's potentially serious cardiovascular toxicities such as a prolonged QT interval and torsades de pointes (83). The analgesic activity of methadone is shorter than its 15- to 60-hour terminal half-life would suggest, and it can induce respiratory depression that outlasts the analgesic phase. Methadone's naturally long half-life can be significantly increased in basified urine. Deaths from cardiac arrhythmia and respiratory depression have been noted, particularly as the drug is being introduced and/or the dose titrated. Dosing more frequently than once per day can allow drug accumulation, which sets the stage for serious and/or potentially fatal toxicity.

Methadone's prolonged duration is due to the generation of several active *N*-dealkylated and C_3-reduced (methadol) metabolites, some of which have long half-lives (Fig. 20.15). CYP2C19 catalyzes the stereoselective dealkylation of the active *R*(−) isomer of methadone and methadol, whereas CYP2B6 preferentially catalyzes

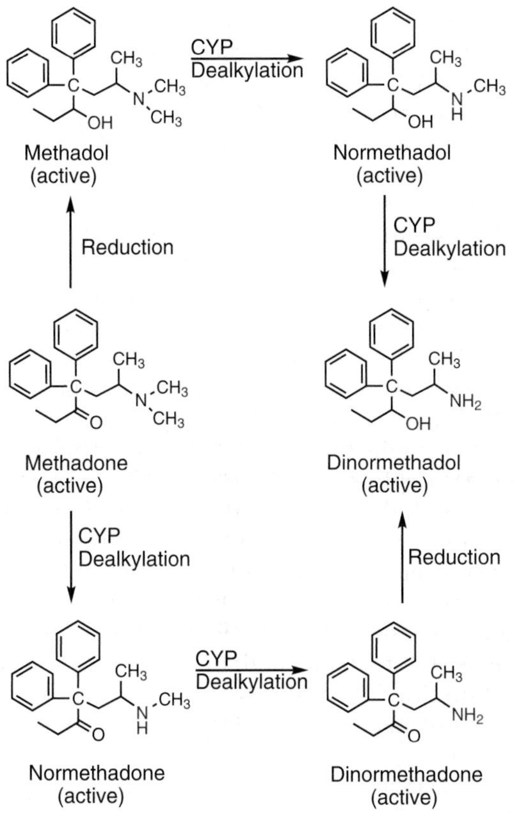

FIGURE 20.15 Methadone metabolism.

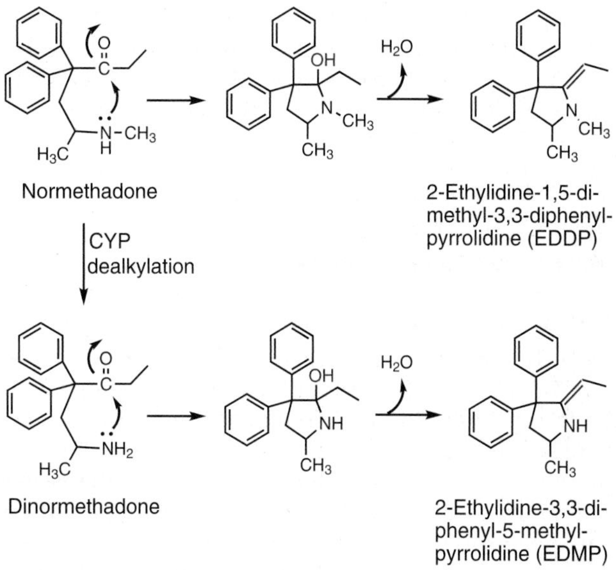

FIGURE 20.16 Formation of EDDP and EDMP.

the dealkylation of the inactive *S*(+) isomers. CYP3A4 (and other isoforms) dealkylate both enantiomers with equal ease (166). While many believe that CYP3A4 is the major isoform involved in methadone dealkylation (83), others suggest that these other isoforms could be important players in the methadone biotransformation process (167). Because of the risk of serious/fatal cardiac and respiratory toxicity, pharmacists should be vigilant with regard to monitoring for metabolism-related interactions with CYP competitors, inhibitors, and inducers.

The *N*-dealkylated metabolites of methadone (but not methadol) can cyclize to form inactive pyrrolidine-based structures that are found in the urine of patients on methadone (Fig. 20.16) (168,169). These compounds are commonly known as EDDP and EDMP, which are acronyms for their chemical names. Methadone is incapable of generating a cyclic pyrrolidine metabolite because the *N,N*-dimethyl substitution pattern of the parent drug provides steric hindrance to nucleophilic attack by the un-ionized amine at the electrophilic carbonyl carbon. EDDP, and to a lesser extent, EDMP have recently been shown to be mechanism-based inhibitors of CYP2C19 (167). EDDP has an elimination half-life of 40 to 48 hours.

Methadone can be used orally (tablets, oral solution) or by injection to treat pain. Methadone is most commonly given by the oral route, but patients who cannot swallow oral dosage forms can "swish and spit" solutions of methadone that have been treated with an alkalinizing agent to raise the pH of the saliva from 6.4 to 8.5. Holding the solution in the mouth for 2.5 minutes at a salivary pH of 8.5 results in the buccal absorption of 85% of the dose (99). First-pass metabolism would, of course, be avoided if methadone is given by the buccal route.

While certainly an effective analgesic, methadone has found its greatest use in addiction recovery ("methadone maintenance" or "methadone medication maintenance") programs (170). Its high oral bioavailability, long duration of action, daily dosing regimen, slow tolerance development, and relative lack of physical dependence are definitely advantages in its use as a heroin (or other potent μ agonist) substitute (Table 20.2). Unlike buprenorphine, methadone used in addiction recovery is administered in strictly regulated, federal- and state-licensed methadone clinics. Patients are titrated upward from an initial 20- to 30-mg daily dose to a maintenance daily dose that is most commonly between 80 and 120 mg (83). Therapy commonly continues over 1 to 2 (or more) years. Compliance can be tracked by quantifying urinary levels of EDDP and calculating the EDDP:urine creatinine ratio. This analytical technique provides results related to the consumed quantity of methadone that are independent of patient hydration status and resistant to attempts to adulterate the sample with agents like soap, bleach, or methadone itself (171). When the time is right to discontinue methadone, any withdrawal symptoms experienced will generally be mild due to the prolonged duration of action of the drug and active metabolites. However, the patient will still be both tolerant to and dependent on methadone, which, unlike buprenorphine, is not a pseudoirreversible μ agonist. Therefore, the protocol for medically supervised drug discontinuation involves a "stair-step" dose-attenuation process, with reductions of less than 10% of the maintenance dose taking place no sooner than every 10 to 14 days.

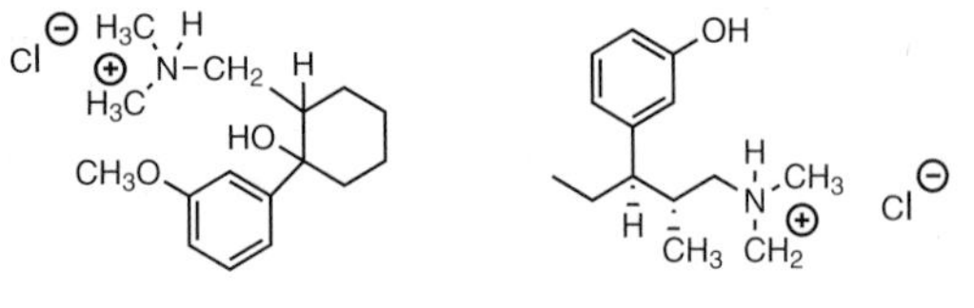

Tramadol hydrochloride (Ultram) Tapentadol hydrochloride (Nucynta)

FIGURE 20.17 Dual-action opioids.

Dual-Action Opioids (Fig. 20.17)

Two novel, orally active analgesics on the U.S. market work by dual mechanisms of action: μ-receptor stimulation and inhibition of norepinephrine (NE) or 5-HT reuptake in the CNS (172). Inhibiting central monoamine reuptake in descending nociceptive pathways has been shown to alleviate chronic pain. NE reuptake inhibition appears to provide the stronger analgesic response. The rationale for the development of these dual-action analgesics is to lower dependence on μ-receptor stimulation for full analgesic efficacy, thus decreasing the risk of uncomfortable or dangerous μ agonist side effects. While the risk of respiratory depression, constipation, sedation, tolerance, dependence, and addiction liability are markedly low, all precautions associated with the use of μ-opioid analgesics are advised with the use of these dual-action pain-relieving agents.

Tramadol Hydrochloride

Tramadol has two asymmetric centers and is marketed as the racemic mixture of *cis* isomers. Each enantiomer, plus the *O*-dealkylated phenolic dextrorotatory metabolite, has a role to play in the activity profile of this unique analgesic. Specifically, the 1*S*,2*S*-(−) isomer inhibits NE reuptake, the 1*R*,2*R*-(+) isomer inhibits 5-HT reuptake, and the dextrorotatory isomer of the *O*-dealkylated metabolite stimulates μ-opioid receptors to produce analgesia sixfold greater than the parent drug (172–175). The μ agonist potency of *O*-dealkylated tramadol has been estimated at 10% of morphine after parenteral administration (173).

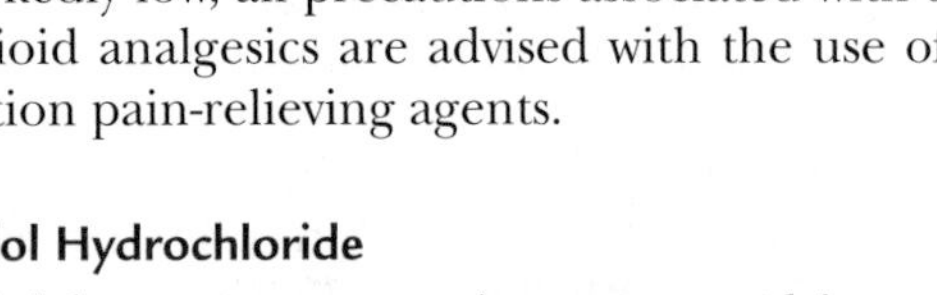

(1*R*,2*R*)-(+)-Tramadol (1*S*,2*S*)-(-)-Tramadol

The mechanism of tramadol's analgesic action is complex and time-dependent (173,174). Over time, as the parent isomers are *O*-dealkylated to phenolic metabolites, the μ-receptor agonist component of activity increases while the monoamine reuptake inhibition mechanism decreases. As in codeine analogs, CYP2D6 catalyzes the *O*-dealkylation reaction, and patients deficient in this isoform will not experience the μ agonist component of tramadol's action. Inactivating glucuronide or sulfate conjugation of the phenol will occur prior to urinary excretion. CYP3A4 and CYP2B6 catalyze inactivating *N*-dealkylation to secondary and primary amine metabolites (176).

Since the dextrorotatory (1*R*,2*R*) isomer of tramadol inhibits 5-HT reuptake, it has the potential to induce or exacerbate serotonin syndrome, a potentially life-threatening condition (172,177,178). The symptoms of serotonin syndrome can include agitation, coma, dangerous alterations in heart rate and blood pressure, hyperreflexia and loss of coordination, and GI distress. Tramadol also carries a risk of seizure, especially in patients taking drugs that increase central levels of monoamines (e.g., selective serotonin reuptake inhibitors [SSRIs], MAOIs, tricyclic antidepressants [TCAs]) or whose seizure risk threshold is otherwise reduced (179,180). Seizures have been documented in doses as low as 200 mg (which is close to the maintenance dose of 50 to 100 mg) and generally occur within 6 hours of drug ingestion (179). Withdrawal symptoms have been noted upon abrupt discontinuation of tramadol and, in addition to anticipated opioid withdrawal symptoms, can include paranoia, panic, sensory perception distortions, and hallucinations (172).

Tramadol is available in noninterchangeable immediate-release (every 4 to 6 hours) and extended-release (once daily) formulations. It is completely absorbed after oral administration and has a bioavailability of 75% (Table 20.2) (173). Drugs that increase central levels of 5-HT have been linked to suicide, and the tramadol manufacturer recently alerted the FDA and health care providers to the more stringent warnings related to suicide risk incorporated within the prescribing information for this dual-action analgesic (181,182).

Tapentadol Hydrochloride

Tapentadol was developed to couple time-independent μ-receptor agonism and selective NE reuptake inhibition and, in so doing, produce an analgesic with a consistently reliable therapeutic profile (183). Like tramadol, tapentadol has two chiral carbon atoms, but it is marketed as the pure 1*R*,2*R*-(−) isomer (174). A phenolic drug, it is selective for the μ-opioid receptor, and its overall analgesic potency is estimated at one-half to one-third that of morphine despite having a 50-fold lower affinity for μ receptors. The potency discrepancy is explained by the synergistic mechanism of analgesic action (184). Tolerance to tapentadol develops slowly (174), and there is less physical dependence when compared to morphine and other μ agonists. When chronic therapy is to be concluded, tapering doses can minimize the risk of withdrawal symptoms (172,175).

Despite the apparent vulnerability of the *N*,*N*-dimethylamino substituent to CYP-mediated metabolism, only about 10% to 13% of a dose undergoes dealkylation via CYP2C9 and CYP2C19. Tapentadol is preferentially metabolized by glucuronic acid (55%) or sulfate (15%)

conjugation of the phenolic OH group. All tapentadol metabolites are inactive (175,183).

Like all μ agonists, tapentadol can induce respiratory depression, and the drug should be used with caution or avoided altogether in elderly or debilitated patients or in patients with respiratory disease (e.g., chronic obstructive pulmonary disease, asthma, sleep apnea). Inhibition of GI motility, while less frequent than is observed with oxycodone, is still common, and the drug should not be used in patients with compromised intestinal function (e.g., paralytic ileus). Nausea and vomiting can occur, but some claim the risk is less than with oxycodone (172,183).

Tapentadol should not be used in patients taking MAOI antidepressants, because the synergistic increase in circulating NE levels could precipitate a hypertensive crisis. There should be a minimum 14-day MAOI "wash-out period" before initiating tapentadol therapy (183).

While the risk of serotonin syndrome should be less than that observed with tramadol, NE reuptake inhibitors can also induce this potentially fatal reaction, especially if other drugs that increase central levels of 5-HT are being coadministered (183). Likewise, although this drug has not been shown to increase seizure risk, it was not evaluated in patients with seizure disorder. Practitioners should be mindful of the possibility for these serious adverse reactions and employ all appropriate precautions when using this drug.

Opioid-Based Antidiarrheals (Fig. 20.18)

Constipation is undoubtedly one of the most discomforting and, at times, serious complications of opioid analgesic use. However, medicinal chemists, following the old adage "When life hands you lemons, make lemonade," have modified the structure of the flexible μ agonist meperidine to limit blood–brain barrier penetration without compromising GI mobility inhibition (185). Three peripherally selective μ agonists, diphenoxylate, difenoxin, and loperamide, have enjoyed significant therapeutic use as antidiarrheals for years.

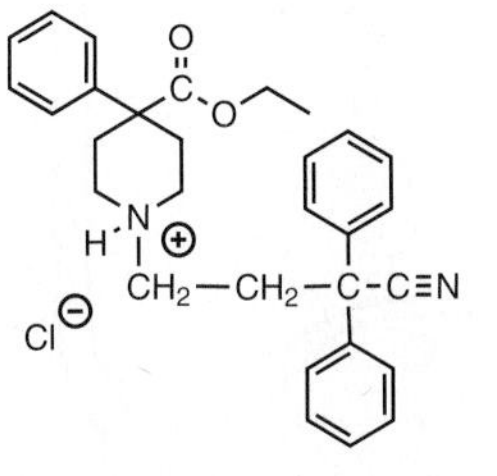

Diphenoxylate hydrochloride (Lomotil)

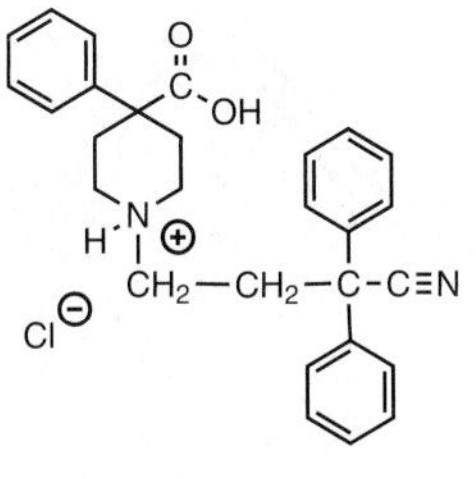

Difenoxin hydrochloride (Motofen)

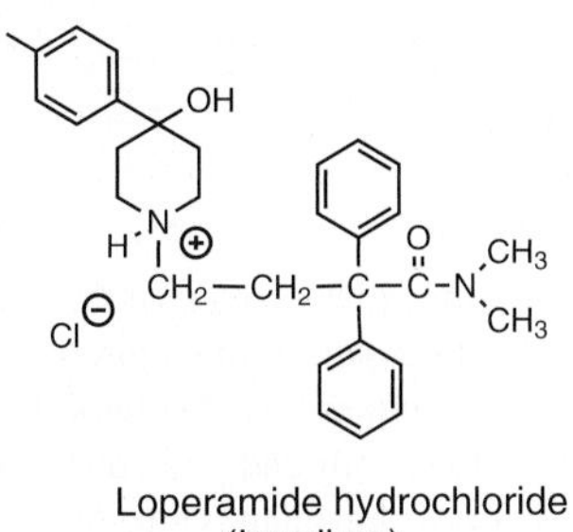

Loperamide hydrochloride (Imodium)

FIGURE 20.18 Opioid-based antidiarrheals.

Diphenoxylate Hydrochloride and Difenoxin Hydrochloride

Of the three opioid-based antidiarrheals, diphenoxylate bears the closest resemblance to the parent meperidine structure. The only chemical difference between the two compounds is the nature of the nitrogen substituent; meperidine has the prototypical μ agonist–directing methyl group, while diphenoxylate has a more complex 3,3,-diphenyl-3-cyanopropyl functional group. The ethylcarboxylate ester is readily cleaved by plasma esterases, yielding a carboxylic acid metabolite that is approximately fivefold as active as diphenoxylate as an antidiarrheal. The zwitterionic metabolite, which has been marketed as difenoxin, does not readily distribute into the CNS in therapeutic doses. In higher doses, the chemical reluctance to cross the blood–brain barrier is overcome, and central μ receptors can be stimulated.

For reasons both therapeutic (anticholinergic) and abuse related, diphenoxylate and difenoxin are only available in combination with atropine sulfate. If a potential abuser attempts to extract the antidiarrheal agent with the intent to inject and abuse, the atropine will be extracted and injected too, leading to nausea, weakness, sedation, and annoying peripheral effects such as dry mouth, blurred vision, and urinary retention. The diphenoxylate combination product is a Schedule V drug, indicating that there is a slight potential for abuse and/or addiction, whereas the difenoxin combination product is classified as Schedule IV (a medically useful drug with a low potential for abuse and/or addiction). If used alone, these antidiarrheals would be classified as Schedule II agents, indicating that they have a significant potential for abuse and/or addiction without the atropine "safety net."

Loperamide Hydrochloride

Loperamide is a nonhydrolyzable amide analog of meperidine. Meperidine's ethylcarboxylate ester has been replaced by a tertiary hydroxyl group, and the phenyl ring has been chlorinated at the *p* position. The nitrogen substituent is reminiscent of that incorporated into diphenoxylate and difenoxin, although a dimethylamide moiety has replaced the nitrile. While the highly lipophilic drug ($logD_{pH\ 7.4}$ = 5.47) acts as a full μ-receptor agonist, it lacks central μ agonist action because the efflux protein P-gp actively and extensively prevents drug uptake into the brain (186,187). This essentially abolishes its abuse potential and allows it to be available to patients without a prescription (188). Diphenoxylate, discussed earlier, is not a substrate for the P-gp efflux protein (189). In addition to and/or in concert with its μ agonist action, loperamide's GI motility inhibition has been linked to the μ agonist–mediated release of 5-HT (190) and calcium channel antagonism (191,192).

N-Demethylation of loperamide's tertiary amide group is catalyzed by CYP3A4 and CYP2C8 (193). Significant first-pass metabolism reduces oral bioavailability to approximately 40%. The desmethyl metabolite does not bind to μ receptors and is inactive as an antidiarrheal (194). Because loperamide also inhibits CYP3A4, there is risk of drug–drug interactions between this agent and other CYP3A4 substrates, although few have been reported in the literature. Loperamide has been compared favorably to diphenoxylate with regard to potency, duration and specificity of action, and safety margin (185).

NEUROPATHIC PAIN

Neuropathic pain generally arises from nerve damage due to physical injury or disease. A recent definition of neuropathic pain is "pain arising as a direct consequence of a lesion or disease affecting the somatosensory system" (8). It is estimated that 90% of neuropathic pain arises from peripheral injuries or diseases (e.g., postdiabetic neuralgia, postherpetic neuralgia, posttraumatic neuralgia, postpolio neuralgia, fibromyalgia, iatrogenic injuries). The remaining 10% is of central origin (e.g., stroke, Parkinson disease, multiple sclerosis, phantom limb pain) (195). This section will focus on peripheral neuropathic pain.

Nociceptive Versus Neuropathic Pain

Nociceptive pain is pain produced through disease or injury of nonneural tissues. Treatment of this kind of pain involves common analgesics (e.g., nonsteroidal anti-inflammatory drugs, opiates), and the pain subsides as the injury heals. As defined earlier, neuropathic pain emanates from lesions of the nervous system. There may be no observable injury, and the pain often increases in severity over time. However, regardless of the source of the lesion, the pain must involve the nociceptive pathways. The inverse of this is not true in that all lesions of the nociceptive pathways do not necessarily induce pain. Pain due to neuropathic processes generally has one or more of the following features: 1) widespread pain that is not explainable by nonneural injuries, 2) evidence of sensory deficit (e.g., numbness), 3) burning pain, 4) pain to light stroking of the skin, and 5) attacks of pain without seeming provocation (196).

Another descriptor of neuropathic pain is *allodynia* ("other power")—pain produced by a stimulus that does not normally produce pain.

Mechanisms of Neuropathic Pain

The mechanisms resulting in the characteristic persistence of neuropathic pain following nerve injury involve both functional and structural alterations in the nervous system. Figure 20.19 illustrates the involvement of both the primary afferent neurons and the CNS (2). Physiologic and transcriptional changes in the peripheral primary afferent sensory neurons that take place after the injury contribute to neuropathic pain. The alterations in

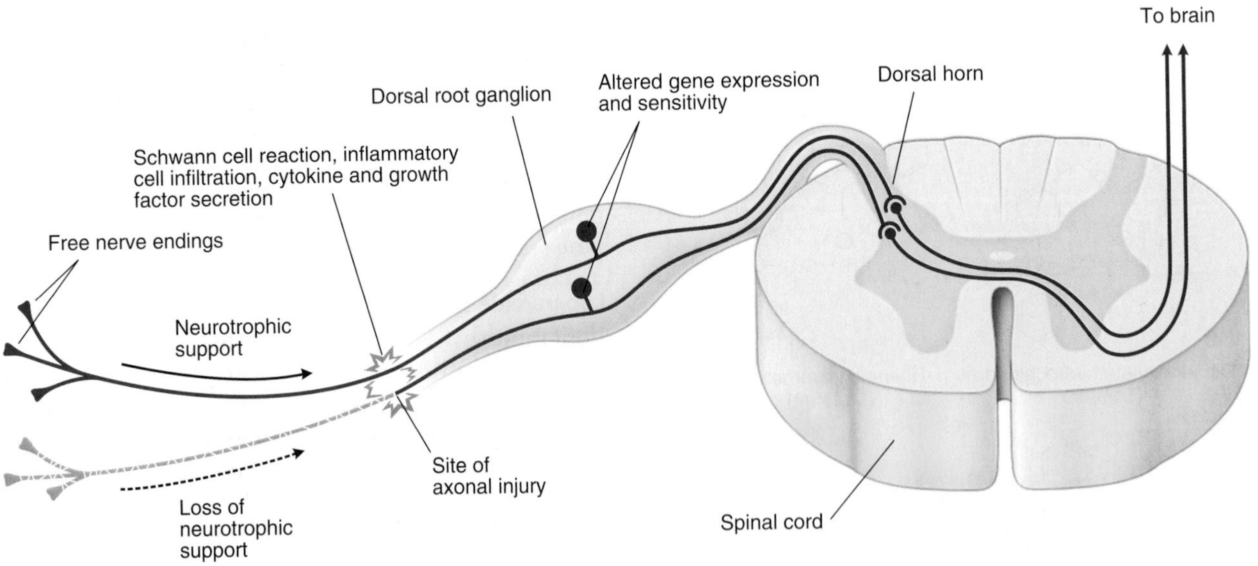

FIGURE 20.19 Schematization of neuropathic pain. Nerve injury results in a combination of negative signals and positive signals that alter the physiology of the nociceptive system. The loss of neurotrophic support alters gene expression in the injured nerve fiber, whereas the release of inflammatory cytokines alters gene expression in both the injured and adjacent uninjured nerve fibers. These changes in gene expression can lead to altered sensitivity and activity of nociceptive fibers and, thus, to the continued perception of injury that is characteristic of neuropathic pain. (Griffin RS, Woolf CJ. Pharmacology of analgesia. In: Golan DE, Tashjian AH Jr, Armstrong EJ, et al., eds. Principles of Pharmacology: The Pathophysiologic Basis of Drug Therapy, 2nd Ed. Philadelphia, PA: Lippincott Williams & Wilkins, 2008:272, with permission.)

neuronal function are induced by the release of inflammatory cytokines by macrophages. Alterations in the expression pattern of voltage-gated sodium channels are also seen in the injured sensory neurons. Specifically, $Na_v1.8$ and $Na_v1.9$ are downregulated, whereas $Na_v1.3$ is upregulated. The $Na_v1.3$ channels are normally not detectable in the primary sensory neurons, and their accelerated recovery from inactivation is thought to contribute to neuropathic pain. The efficacy of sodium channel blockers (e.g., local anesthetics and carbamazepine) in the treatment of trigeminal neuralgia is attributed to their role in the mechanism of neuropathic pain (2).

Structural changes caused by nerve injury also contribute to neuropathic pain. After peripheral nerve injury, there is an excitotoxic loss (via excessive stimulation by neurotransmitters) of inhibitory neurons in the dorsal horn. The resulting disinhibition contributes to the heightened pain sensitivity. In many respects, it is the loss of neuronal structures and supports that gives rise to the multiple targets and approaches to drug therapy (197). Although actual mechanisms in many cases are unknown, the preferred first-line medications either 1) support the inhibited nociceptive pathways modulated by NE and 5-HT (TCAs and dual-acting 5-HT–NE reuptake inhibitors), or 2) block the release of transmitters from the afferent peripheral neurons by binding to the α_2-δ subunit of the voltage-gated calcium channels or the voltage-gated sodium channels ($Na_v1.3$) (197,198).

Treatment of Neuropathic Pain

The Neuropathic Pain Special Interest Group of the International Association for the Study of Pain has developed evidence-based guidelines for the treatment of neuropathic pain (199). These guidelines consider clinical efficacy, adverse effects, effects on the health-related quality of life, convenience of dosing, and cost.

First-Line Medications

Antidepressants (Also see Chapter 18) Numerous studies have shown the efficacy and beneficial effects of TCAs in the treatment of neuropathic pain from many causes, leading to off-label use in these conditions. Antidepressants most often used in neuropathic pain treatment include the TCAs and dual-acting 5-HT–NE reuptake inhibitors (198,200). The tertiary TCAs (amitriptyline, imipramine) are characterized by their ability to inhibit the reuptake of both 5-HT and NE from presynaptic terminals as a result of *N*-monodealkylation to secondary TCAs (Chapter 18), and the secondary TCAs/5-HT–NE reuptake inhibitors (desipramine, nortriptyline) selectively inhibit the reuptake of NE. The TCAs relieve pain independent of their antidepressant effect. Of the TCAs, the tertiary TCAs have been shown to be more effective for painful diabetic neuropathy, nerve injury pain, fibromyalgia, and spinal cord injury pain due to their dual action. Although the presence of depression is not necessary for their use or efficacy as neuropathic analgesics, these agents are frequently used in comorbid patients suffering with neuropathic pain. The anticholinergic side effects associated with these TCA structures lead to a preference for the secondary amine derivatives (e.g., desipramine or nortriptyline). The cardiac toxicity associated with these compounds also limits their use. Studies have shown the SSRIs to have a weak analgesic effect.

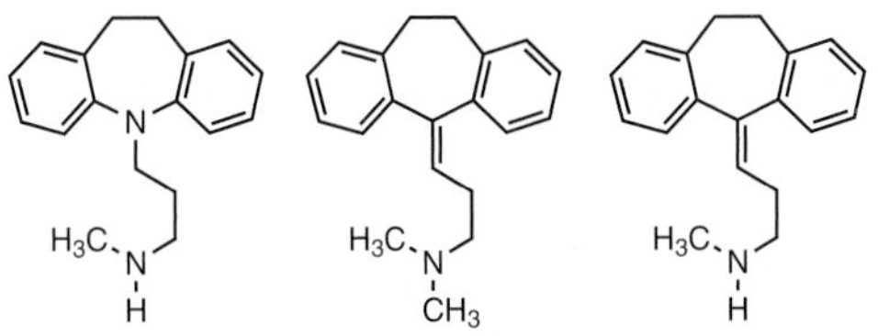

Desimipramine Amitriptyline Nortriptyline

Duloxetine (Cymbalta) and venlafaxine (Effexor) are potent reuptake inhibitors of both 5-HT and NE and are effective not only for the treatment of major depressive disorder, but also as neuropathic analgesics for diabetic neuropathic pain and fibromyalgia, without the adverse effects of the TCAs. Duloxetine is generally well tolerated, and is approved by the FDA specifically for the treatment of diabetic peripheral neuropathic pain. The drug has been shown to be superior to placebo at doses of 60 and 120 mg/d in treating diabetic peripheral neuropathic pain (201). Its analgesic effect for reducing 24-hour average pain is seen early, typically within the first week, as contrasted with its antidepressant effect. Its efficacy is comparable to that of the tertiary TCAs commonly used for the treatment of diabetic peripheral neuropathic pain. The standard approach to treatment of diabetic peripheral neuropathy has been to use a TCA as a first-line trial of treatment. Duloxetine was more effective than pregabalin in producing at least a 50% reduction in pain, whereas treatment with pregabalin resulted in a greater proportion of patients with a 30% to 50% reduction in pain. Patients taking duloxetine would be less likely to have a partial pain response and require additional therapy with other costly medications. Therefore, duloxetine is an acceptable initial or alternative treatment for patients with diabetic neuropathic pain (201).

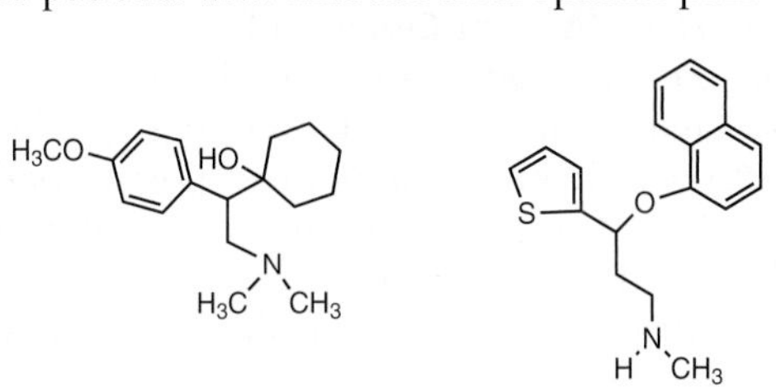

Venlafaxine Duloxetine

Calcium Channel α_2-δ Ligands (Also see Chapter 21)
Pregabalin (Lyrica) Pregabalin binds to the α_2-δ subunit of the voltage-gated calcium channels in the CNS and inhibits release of several neurotransmitters. It has a use in epilepsy as an adjunct in the control of partial seizures. However, its primary use is in the treatment of neuropathic pain in fibromyalgia, diabetic

neuropathies, and postherpetic neuropathy. Pregabalin is well absorbed orally and follows linear pharmacokinetics. Its metabolism in humans is negligible, leading to 90% being recovered in urine as unchanged pregabalin. The *N*-methylated derivative is the major metabolite, and accounts for only 0.9% of the dose. The lack of interaction with metabolizing enzymes and the absence of protein binding leads to essentially no drug interactions. However, synergism with other CNS depressants may be seen.

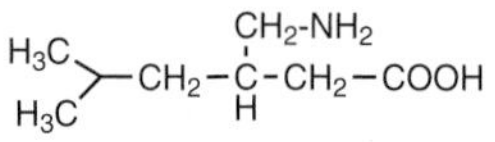

Pregabalin

Gabapentin (Neurontin) Gabapentin is listed in many reviews as a calcium channel α_2-δ subunit ligand. However, studies of binding to most major neurotransmitter receptor sites and voltage-gated ion channels have shown negative results (202). In addition, it does not affect $GABA_A$ or $GABA_B$ binding and is not converted to GABA or a GABA agonist or antagonist. Gabapentin's primary use is as an adjunct in the management of partial seizures in children and adults. Its use in neuropathic pain is off-label for diabetic neuropathic pain, fibromyalgia, and other chronic pain conditions. Gabapentin's bioavailability is not proportional to the dose, and it is not appreciably metabolized in humans.

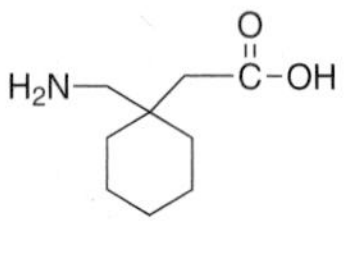

Gabapentin

Local Anesthetics (Also see Chapter 16).

Lidocaine Patch (Lidoderm) The lidocaine patch is a transdermal dosage form containing 5% lidocaine and is effective in the treatment of postherpetic neuropathic pain. It is also useful in the treatment of allodynia from different types of neuropathic pain. It is a more chemically and biochemically stable amide type of local anesthetic, and like all other local anesthetics, acts as a blocker of voltage-gated sodium channels, shutting down the ion fluxes necessary for the propagation of neuronal signals. As might be expected, it is more useful in localized, as opposed to central, neuropathic pain. It is not known whether lidocaine is metabolized in the skin. Hepatic metabolism produces two dealkylated metabolites, monoethylglycinexylidide and glycinexylidide, that are active but less potent than lidocaine.

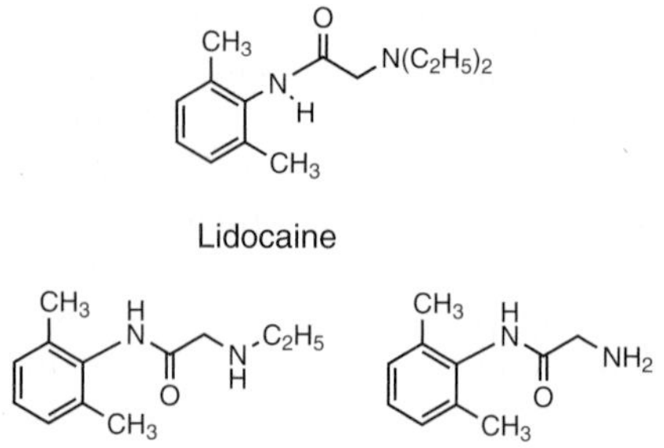

Lidocaine

MEGX GX

Second-Line Medications

This group of medications specifically involves the dual-action analgesic tramadol and μ-opioid analgesics and is recommended for use in patients who have not responded to first-line medications. They may be recommended as first-line medications in cases of acute neuropathic pain, neuropathic pain due to cancer, and central neuropathic pain.

Tramadol (Fig. 20.17) As discussed earlier in this chapter, tramadol is a dual-action analgesic that acts through inhibition of neurotransmitter (5-HT and NE) reuptake and μ-receptor agonism. It has shown efficacy in some neuropathic pain conditions (199). To some extent, its adverse effects match other opioids, but its effect on the reuptake of 5-HT can interact with other selective 5-HT–NE reuptake inhibitors used in neuropathic pain treatment, leading to potential toxicity.

Morphine, Oxycodone, and Methadone (Figs. 20.11 and 20.14) A number of clinical trials have compared the μ agonists morphine, oxycodone, and methadone with the first-line agents tricyclic antidepressants gabapentin and pregabalin and found them to be as effective (199,203). However, concerns about their long-term use and potential for abuse have placed them in the second-line category.

Third-Line Medications

This group of compounds should be reserved for patients who do not respond well to first- and second-line medications. The criteria for placement in this category is that they have shown activity in only one randomized clinical trial or have presented inconsistent results in multiple trials (199).

Bupropion (Wellbutrin, Zyban) (Also see Chapter 18)

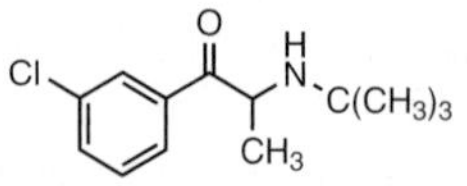

Bupropion

Bupropion is an antidepressant with weak reuptake inhibition of NE and dopamine. It showed neuropathic pain efficacy in two clinical trials of the extended-release dosage form. More studies need to be done to further prove efficacy (204,205).

Paroxetine (Paxil) (Also see Chapter 18)

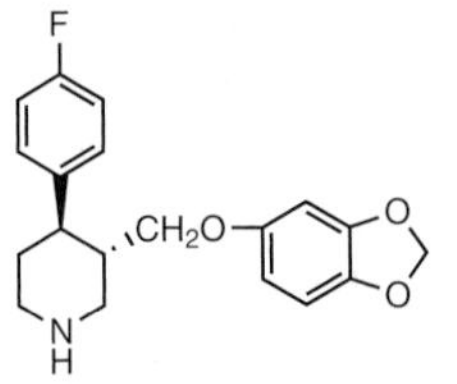

Paroxetine

Paroxetine is an SSRI antidepressant that may have analgesic properties. In a small number of clinical trials against diabetic neuropathic pain, it has shown efficacy greater than some first-line medications. However, more studies need to be done before it can be considered to be a first-line medication.

Carbamazepine (Tegretol) and Oxcarbazepine (Trileptal) (Also see Chapter 17)

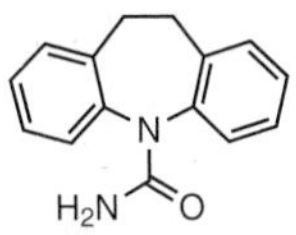

Carbamazepine

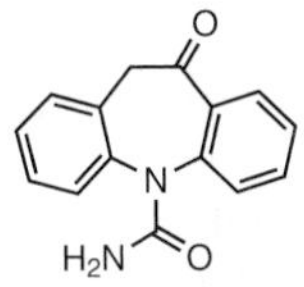

Oxcarbazepine

Carbamazepine and oxcarbazepine are both anticonvulsants. Oxcarbazepine is a derivative of carbamazepine with reduced toxicity. Carbamazepine has been studied in the treatment of postherpetic neuralgia, and oxcarbazepine has been studied in diabetic neuropathic pain. Inconsistent results in both cases lead to the need for further clinical study before any therapeutic recommendation on their use in neuropathic pain can be made.

Future Medications in the Treatment of Neuropathic Pain

Lacosamide (Vimpat) (Also see Chapter 17)

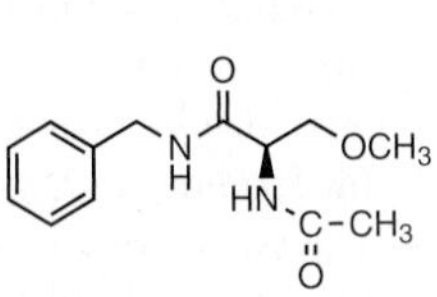

Lacosamide

Lacosamide is a new anticonvulsant that acts as a slow inactivator of sodium channels. Chemically, it is *N*^{2}-acetyl-*N*-benzyl-D-homoserinamide. Lacosamide has been studied in diabetic neuropathic pain and has presented evidence of efficacy. However, some later trials were inconclusive. Additional studies may provide the level of positive results needed for it to enter the mainstream of neuropathic pain treatments (198).

Capsaicin Patch (8%) (Qutenza)

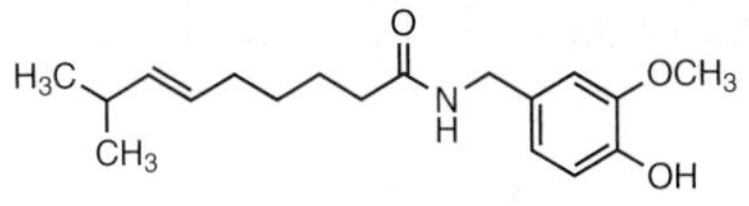

Capsaicin

Capsaicin is a natural compound isolated from Solanaceae family (chili peppers). The compound used in the patch is a synthetic equivalent of the natural substance. Capsaicin is an agonist for the transient receptor potential vanilloid 1 receptor (TRPV1), which is an ion channel-receptor complex expressed on nociceptive nerve fibers in the skin. Topical administration of capsaicin causes an initial enhanced stimulation of the TRPV1-expressing cutaneous nociceptors that may be associated with painful sensations. This is followed by pain relief thought to be mediated by a reduction in TRPV1-expressing nociceptive nerve endings. The efficacy of this patch in the treatment of postherpetic pain was shown in two multicenter studies. The activity in HIV neuropathic pain was inconsistent. The long-term effects of this treatment are not yet known (198).

Cannabinoids

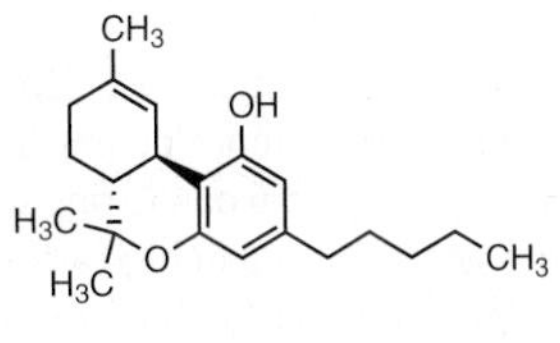

Δ^9-THC

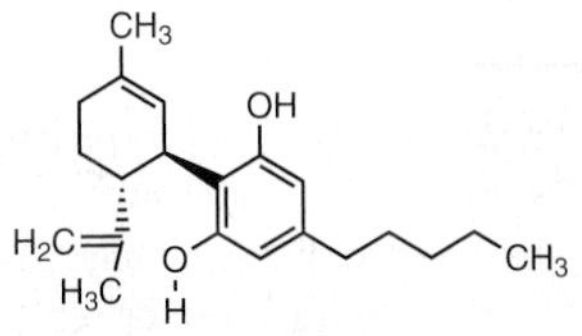

Cannabidiol

The development of analogs of Δ^9-tetrahydrocannabinol (Δ^9-THC) and cannabidiol, the two major components from *Cannabis sativa*, has brought forth some interesting agonists of the cannabinoid type 1 (CB_1) and type 2 (CB_2) receptors (206). The CB_1 receptor has been shown to play a role in peripheral pain. Although many studies have established an analgesic activity of cannabinoids on neuropathic pain, there have not been enough controlled trials comparing them with other medications known to be effective.

Medical Food for Diabetic Neuropathy

Metanx Metanx is a medical food under FDA Title 21. It is comprised of 6(*S*)-5-methyl-tetrahydrofolate calcium (3 mg), pyridoxal-5′-phosphate (35 mg), and methylcobalamin (methyl-B_{12}) (2 mg). All three of these ingredients are provided in their biologically active form and are indicated for the distinct nutritional requirements of patients with endothelial dysfunction with loss of protective sensation and neuropathic pain associated with diabetic peripheral neuropathy (207). Metanx relieves the numbness, tingling, and burning pain associated with diabetic neuropathic pain.

SCENARIO: OUTCOME AND ANALYSIS

Outcome

Jill T. Johnson, PharmD, BCPS

The pharmacist recommended IV hydration and IV hydromorphone 0.6 mg every 3 hours on a schedule with IV hydromorphone 0.2 mg every 3 hours as needed for breakthrough pain. The pharmacist avoided recommending meperidine due to the toxic metabolite, normeperidine, which has a longer duration but does not offer analgesia but instead puts the patient at risk for CNS stimulation including seizures. Although the pain medication was not enough at first, the dose was titrated upward to 1.2 mg every 3 hours. By the third day, the hydromorphone was changed to oral 2 mg every 4 hours. The patient was discharged with his pain almost completely resolved on day 5. The patient scored his pain severity as 2 out of 10. He was given a prescription for oxycodone 5 mg/acetaminophen 500 mg, one tablet every 6 hours as needed for pain. He was given 5 days of medication. He was also counseled to continue taking folic acid and hydroxyurea.

Chemical Analysis

Victoria Roche and S. William Zito

Morphine and codeine are naturally occurring opium alkaloids. The 6α-OH group found on each is associated with histamine release, and allergic responses to these analgesics can include rash, pruritus, and lowered blood pressure. Codeine is more problematic in this regard than morphine, especially if given parenterally. Opioids with a 6-keto group, such as oxymorphone and oxycodone, do not induce allergic reactions of this type.

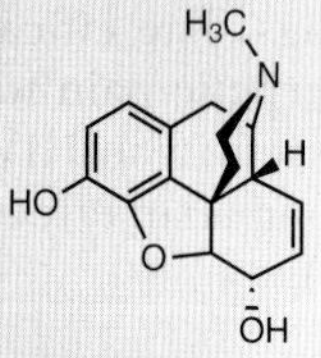

Morphine

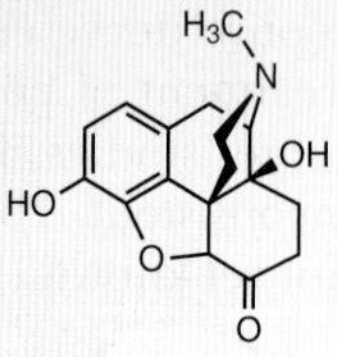

Oxymorphone

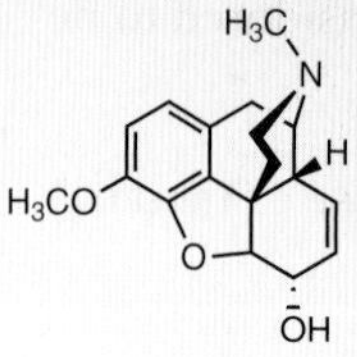

Codeine

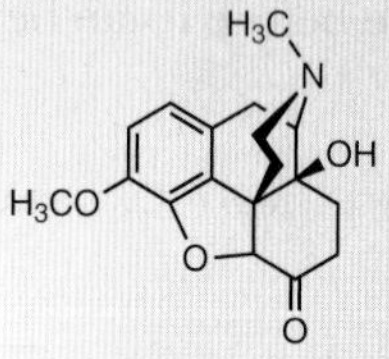

Oxycodone

The N-CH_3 substituent on all four structures documents that they selectively exert their analgesic effect at the μ receptor. Oxymorphone is approximately 10 to 12 times more potent than morphine as an analgesic due to the 7,8-dihydro-6-one C ring and the 14β-hydroxy substituent, both of which engage in high-affinity H-bonds with μ-receptor residues. Oxycodone is a prodrug of oxymorphone and requires CYP2D6-mediated activation to the essential C_3 phenol. Unless JB is a poor CYP2D6 metabolizer, he should get the analgesic relief he requires from this agent, as it is approximately as potent as morphine. The oral bioavailability of oxycodone is significantly higher than oxymorphone because the methoxy ether blocks glucuronide conjugation in the gut and liver. This inactivating phase 2 reaction is the major reason why most phenolic opioids are given parenterally, sublingually, or via nasal spray.

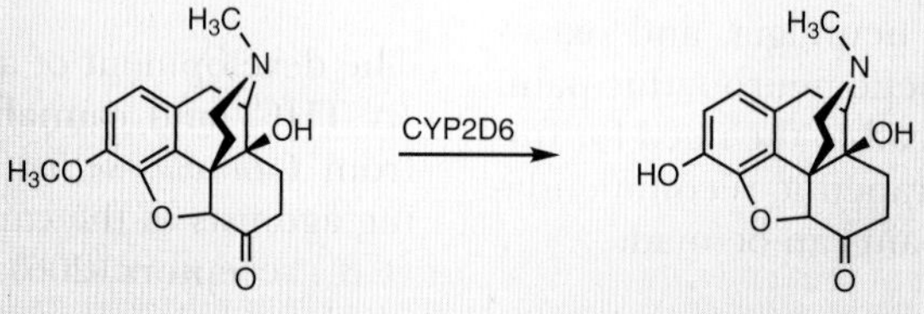

Oxycodone Oxymorphone

Avoiding meperidine was a wise decision. This flexible μ-opioid has an analgesic potency about one-tenth that of morphine. It is *N*-dealkylated by CYP3A4 to a toxic metabolite (normeperidine) that has only about half the analgesic action of the parent structure and can induce grand mal seizures. The actions of normeperidine are long lasting and not reversed by naloxone, the "gold standard" opioid antagonist. The risk of seizure is high if the ratio of normeperidine to meperidine exceeds 1.0, and it should not be used in renally impaired patients. The dose of meperidine that commonly induces seizures overlaps with that which elicits analgesia, making it very difficult to predict who will fall prey to this serious adverse reaction. In addition, like morphine and codeine, meperidine stimulates the release of histamine, and dangerous hypotensive episodes have occurred following its administration. The use of meperidine is generally restricted to patients with normal renal function whose pain cannot be controlled with less toxic agents or in the management of anesthesia-related shivering.

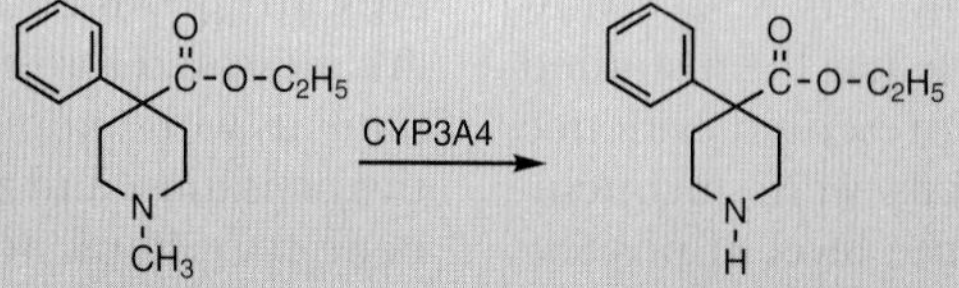

Meperidine Normeperidine

CASE STUDY

Victoria Roche and S. William Zito

EJ is a 27-year-old woman who currently works as clerk in a local discount megastore. Although she's managing fairly well now, her life has not been an easy one. She has suffered from depression serious enough to warrant drug therapy from the time she turned 16. Initially placed on an SSRI, she was switched to desipramine, a norepinephrine selective reuptake inhibitor, after the suicidal ideation she experienced while taking the SSRI prompted an unsuccessful attempt to end her life. During her young adulthood, EJ's depression was complicated by bulimia, and she has experienced myocardial damage from her years of binging and purging. She had an emergency appendectomy at age 22, and she remembers suffering a bad reaction to the codeine she was given during the later part of her recovery, which included an intensely itchy rash, low blood pressure, and visual hallucinations of dozens of multicolored parrots flying around her hospital room. She also remembers that the codeine seemed to do nothing for her pain.

EJ is now facing yet another health challenge. After months of painful and hemorrhagic periods, she was diagnosed with a benign ovarian cyst and has been scheduled for surgery to remove it. If all goes as planned, she will stay in the hospital for 1 day before being discharged. As the pharmacist consulting with the surgical team, you are presented with EJ's medical history and asked to make a recommendation on postsurgical analgesia. You initiate a risk:benefit ratio of the following three options.

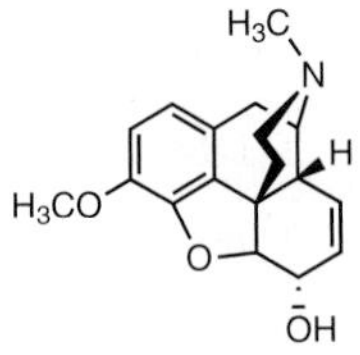

Codeine

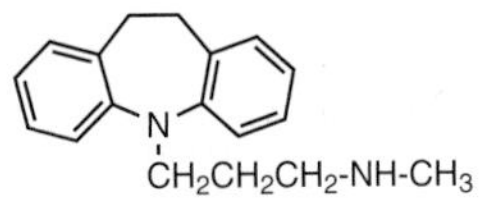

Desipramine

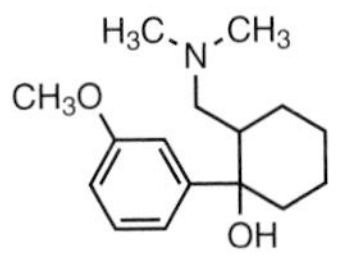

1

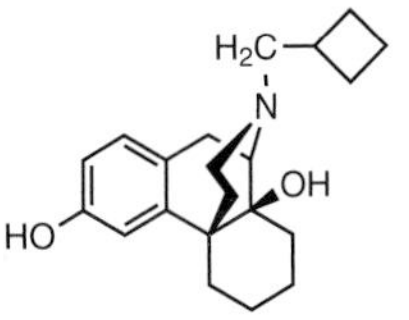

2

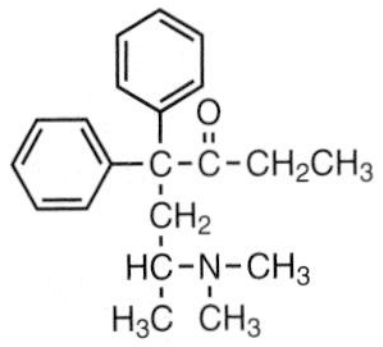

3

1. Conduct a thorough and mechanistic SAR analysis of the three therapeutic options in the case.
2. Apply the chemical understanding gained from the SAR analysis to this patient's specific needs to make a therapeutic recommendation.

References

1. Merskey H, Bogduk N, eds. Part III: Pain terms, a current list with definitions and notes on usage. In: Classification of Chronic Pain, 2nd Ed. Seattle, WA: International Association for the Study of Pain Press, 2004:209–214.
2. Griffen RS, Woolf CJ. Pharmacology of analgesia. In: Golan DE, Tashjian AH, Armstrong EJ, et al., eds. Principles of Pharmacology: The Physiologic Basis of Drug Therapy, 2nd Ed. Philadelphia: Lippincott Williams & Wilkins, 2008:263–273.
3. American Pain Foundation. Pain Resource Guide: Getting the Help You Need. Published 2007; revised 2009. Available at: http://www.painfoundation.org/learn/publications/files/PainResourceGuide2009.pdf. Accessed February 22, 2010.
4. National Center for Health Statistics. Health, United States, 2006 with Chartbook on Trends in the Health of Americans. Hyattsville, MD: National Center for Health Statistics, 2006. Available at: http://www.cdc.gov/nchs/data/hus/ hus06.pdf. Accessed March 6, 2010.
5. American Pain Foundation. Treatment Options: A Guide for People Living with Pain. Available at: http://www.painfoundation.org/learn/publications/files/TreatmentOptions2006.pdf. Accessed February 22, 2010.
6. Thienhaus O, Cole BE. Classification of pain. In: Weiner R, ed. Pain Management: A Practical Guide for Clinicians. Boca Raton, FL: CRC Press, 2002:28.
7. WebMD. Chronic pain: overview. Available at: http://www.webmd.com/pain-management/tc/chronic-pain-topic-overview. Accessed May 20, 2011.
8. Treede RD, Jensen TS, Campbell JN, et al. Neuropathic pain: redefinition and a grading system for clinical and research purposes. Neurology 2008;70:1630–1635.
9. Richeimer S, Macres SM. Understanding neuropathic pain. Available at: http://www.spineuniverse.com/conditions/understanding-neuropathic-pain. Accessed May 20, 2011.
10. WebMD. Chronic pain management. Available at: http://www.webmd.com/pain-management/guide/understanding-pain-management-chronic-pain. Accessed May 20, 2011.
11. Hughes J, Smith TW, Kosterlitz HW, et al. Identification of two related pentapeptides from the brain with potent opiate agonist activity. Nature 1975;258:577–579.
12. Terenius L. Stereospecific interaction between narcotic analgesics and synaptic plasma membrane fraction of rat cerebral cortex. Acta Pharmacol Toxicol 1973;32:317–320.
13. Pert CB, Snyder SH. Opiate receptor: demonstration in nervous tissue. Science 1973;70:2243–2247.
14. Waldhoer M, Bartlett SE, Whistler JL. Opioid receptors. Annu Rev Biochem 2004;73:953–990.
15. Eguchi M. Recent advances in selective opioid receptor agonists and antagonists. Med Res Rev 2004;24:182–212.
16. Li CH, Lemaire S, Yamashiro D, et al. The synthesis and opiate activity of β-endorphin. Biochem Biophys Res Commun 1976;71:19–25.
17. Goldstein A, Tachibana S, Lowney LI, et al. Procaine pituitary dynorphin: complete amino acid sequence of the biologically active heptadecapeptide. Proc Natl Acad Sci U S A 1979;76:6666–6670.

18. Zadina JE, Hackler L, Ge LJ, et al. A potent and selective endogenous agonist for the μ-opiate receptor. Nature 1997;386:499–502.
19. Akil H, Watson SJ, Young E, et al. Endogenous opioids: biology and function. Annu Rev Neurosci 1984;7:233–255.
20. Brantl V, Teshemacher H. A material with opioid activity in bovine milk and milk products. Naunyn Schmiedebergs Arch Pharmacol 1979;306:301–304.
21. Montecucchi PC, de Castiglioni R, Piani S, et al. Amino acid composition and sequence of dermorphin, a novel opiate-like peptide from the skin of *Phyllomedusa sauvagei*. Int J Pept Protein Res 1981;17:275–283.
22. Janecka A, Fichua J, Janecki T. Opioid receptors and their ligands. Curr Top Med Chem 2004;4:1–17.
23. Leslie FM. Methods used for the study of opioid receptors. Pharmacol Rev 1987;39:197–249.
24. Satoh M, Minami M. Molecular pharmacology of the opioid receptors. Pharmacol Ther 1995;68:343–364.
25. Connor M, Christie MD. Opioid receptor signaling mechanisms. Clin Exp Pharmacol Physiol 1999;26:493–499.
26. Lord JAH, Waterfield AA, Hughes J, et al. Endogenous opioid peptides: multiple agonists and receptors. Nature 1977;267:495–499.
27. Dhawan BN, Cesselin R, Raghbir R, et al. International Union of Pharmacology. XII. Classification of opioid receptors. Pharmacol Rev 1996;48:567–592.
28. Pan L, Xu J, Yu R, et al. Identification and characterization of six new alternatively spliced variants of the human mu opioid receptor gene, *Oprm*. Neuroscience 2005;133;209–220.
29. Henderson G, McKnight AT. The orphan opioid receptor and its endogenous ligand—nociceptin/orphanin FQ. Trends Pharmacol Sci 1997;18:293–300.
30. Meunier JC, Mollereau C, Toll L, et al. Isolation and structure of the endogenous agonist of opioid receptor-like ORL1 receptor. Nature 1995;377:532–535.
31. Handa BK, Land AC, Lord JA, et al. Analogues of β-LPH61–64 possessing selective agonist activity at μ-opiate receptors. Eur J Pharmacol 1981;70:531–540.
32. Negri L, Erspamer GF, Severini C, et al. Dermorphin-related peptides from the skin of *Phyllomedusa bicolor* and their amidated analogues activate two μ opioid receptor subtypes that modulate antinociception and catalepsy in the rat. Proc Natl Acad Sci U S A 1992;89:7203–7207.
33. Kieffer BL. Opioids: first lessons from knockout mice. Trends Pharmacol Sci 1999;20:19–25.
34. Schmidhammer H, Burkhard WP, Eggstein-Aeppi L, et al. Synthesis and biological evaluation of 14–alkoxymorphinans. 2. (–)-*N*-(cyclopropylmethyl)-4,14-dimethoxymorphinan-6-one, a selective μ opioid receptor antagonist. J Med Chem 1989;32:418–421.
35. Pelton JT, Kazmierski W, Gulya K, et al. Design and synthesis of conformationally constrained somatostatin analogues with high potency and specificity for μ opioid receptors. J Med Chem 1986;29:2370–2375.
36. Paul D, Pasternak GW. Differential blockade by naloxonazine of two mu opiate actions: analgesia and inhibition of gastrointestinal transit. Eur J Pharmacol 1988;149:403–404.
37. Szmuszkovicz J, Von Voigtlander PF. Benzeneacetamide amines: structurally novel non-μ opioids. J Med Chem 1982;25:1125–1126.
38. Clark CR, Halfpenny PR, Hill RG, et al. Highly selective κ opioid analgesics. Synthesis and structure–activity relationships of novel *N*-[(2-aminocyclohexyl)aryl]acetamide and *N*-[(2-aminocyclohexyl)aryloxy] acetamide derivatives. J Med Chem 1988;31:831–836.
39. Hunter JC, Leighton GE, Meecham KG, et al. CI-977, a novel and selective agonist for the κ-opioid receptor. Br J Pharmacol 1990;101:183–189.
40. Barber A, Bartoszyk GD, Bender HM, et al. A pharmacological profile of the novel, peripherally-selective κ-opioid receptor agonist, EMD 61753. Br J Pharmacol 1994;113:843–851.
41. Rothman RB, Bykov V, de Costa BR, et al. Evidence for four opioid κ binding sites in guinea pig brain. Prog Clin Biol Res 1990;328:9–12.
42. Choi H, Murray TF, DeLander GE, et al. N-terminal alkylated derivatives of [D-Pro10]dynorphin A-(1–11) are highly selective for κ-opioid receptors. J Med Chem 1992;35:4638–4639.
43. Lung FDT, Meyer JP, Li G, et al. Highly κ receptor–selective dynorphin A analogues with modifications in position 3 of dynorphin A(1–11)-NH_2. J Med Chem 1995;38:585–586.
44. Roth BL, Baner K, Westkaemper R, et al. Salvinorin A: a potent naturally occurring nonnitrogenous kappa opioid selective agonist. Proc Natl Acad Sci U S A 2002;99:11934–11939.
45. Chavkin C, Sud S, Jin W, et al. Salvinorin A, an active component of the hallucinogenic sage salvia divinorum is a highly efficacious kappa-opioid receptor agonist: structural and functional considerations. J Pharmacol Exp Ther 2004;308:1197–1203.
46. Portoghese PS, Lipkowski AW, Takemori AE. Bimorphinans as highly selective, potent κ opioid receptor antagonists. J Med Chem 1987;30:238–239.
47. James IF, Goldstein A. Site-directed alkylation of multiple opioid receptors. I. Binding selectivity. Mol Pharmacol 1984;25:337–342.
48. Gacel G, Fournie-Zaluski M-C, Roques BP. D-Tyr–Ser-Gly–Phe–Leu–Thr, a highly preferential ligand for δ-opiate receptors. FEBS Lett 1980;118:245–247.
49. Mosberg HI, Hurst R, Hruby VJ, et al. Bis-penicillamine enkephalins possess highly improved specificity toward δ opioid receptors. Proc Natl Acad Sci U S A 1983;80:5871–5874.
50. Portoghese PS, Larson DL, Sultana M, et al. Opioid agonist and antagonist activities of morphindoles related to naltrindole. J Med Chem 1992;35: 4325–4329.
51. Bilsky EJ, Calderon SN, Wang T, et al. SNC 80, a selective, nonpeptidic, and systemically active opioid δ agonist. J Pharmacol Exp Ther 1995;273:359–366.
52. Jiang Q, Takemori AE, Sultana M, et al. Differential antagonism of opioid δ antinociception by [D-Ala^2,Leu^5,Cys^6]-enkephalin and naltrindole 5′-isothiocyanate: evidence for δ receptor subtypes. J Pharmacol Exp Ther 1991;257:1069–1075.
53. Portoghese PS, Sultana M, Takemori AE. Naltrindole, a highly selective and potent nonpeptide δ opioid receptor antagonist. Eur J Pharmacol 1988;146:185–186.
54. Takemori AE, Sultana M, Nagase H, et al. Agonist and antagonist activities of ligands derived from naltrexone and oxymorphone. Life Sci 1992;149:1–5.
55. Schiller PW, Nguyen TM, Weltrowska G, et al. Differential stereochemical requirements of μ vs. δ opioid receptors for ligand binding and signal transduction: development of a class of potent and highly δ-selective peptide antagonists. Proc Natl Acad Sci U S A 1992;89:11871–11875.
56. Schiller PW, Weltrowska G, Nguyen TM, et al. TIPP[ψ]: a highly potent and stable pseudopeptide δ opioid receptor antagonist with extraordinary delta selectivity. J Med Chem 1993;36:3182–3187.
57. Zeilhofer HU, Calo G. Nociceptin/orphanin FQ and its receptor—potential targets for pain therapy. J Pharmacol Exp Ther 2003;306:423–429.
58. Chiou LC, Liao YY, Fan PC, et.al. Nociceptin/orphanin FQ peptide receptors: pharmacology and clinical implications. Curr Drug Targets 2007;8:117–135.
59. Portoghese PS, Larson DL, Sayre LM, et al. A novel opioid receptor site directed alkylating agent with irreversible narcotic antagonistic and reversible agonistic activities. J Med Chem 1980;23:233–234.
60. Calo G, Guerrini R, Rizzi A, et al. Pharmacology of nociceptin and its receptor: a novel therapeutic target. Br J Pharmacol 2000;129:1261–1283.
61. Portoghese PS, Larson DL, Jiang JB, et al. Synthesis and pharmacologic characterization of an alkylating analogue (chlornaltrexamine) of naltrexone with ultralong-lasting narcotic antagonist properties. J Med Chem 1979;22:168–173.
62. Burke TR Jr, Bajwa BS, Jacobson AE, et al. Probes for narcotic receptor mediated phenomena. 7. Synthesis and pharmacological properties of irreversible ligands specific for μ or δ opiate receptors. J Med Chem 1984;27:1570–1574.
63. Burke TR Jr, Jacobson AE, Rice KC, et al. Probes for narcotic receptor mediated phenomena. 12. *cis*-(+)-3-Methylfentanyl isothiocyanate, a potent site-directed acylating agent for δ opioid receptors. Synthesis, absolute configuration, and receptor enantioselectivity. J Med Chem 1986;29:1087–1093.
64. de Costa BR, Band L, Rothman RB, et al. Synthesis of an affinity ligand ('UPHIT') for in vivo acylation of the κ-opioid receptor. FEBS Lett 1989;249:178–182.
65. Chang AC, Takemori AE, Ojala WH, et al. κ Opioid receptor selective affinity labels: electrophilic benzeneacetamides as κ-selective opioid antagonists. J Med Chem 1994;37:4490–4498.
66. Sharma SK, Klee WA, Nirenberg M. Dual regulation of adenylate cyclase accounts for narcotic dependence and tolderance. Proc Natl Acad Sci U S A 1975;72:3092–3096.
67. Fakata KL, Lipman AG. Opioid pharmacotherapy for the management of moderate to severe pain: balancing clinical and risk management considerations. Accreditation Council for Pharmacy Education. Powerx-Pak CE, 2005. Available at: http://www.powerpak.com/index.asp?show=lesson&page=courses/10158/lesson.htm&lsn_id=10158.
68. Nesler EJ, Aghajanian GK. Molecular and cellular basis of addiction. Science 1997;278:58–63.
69. Fries DS. Opioid analgesics. In: Lemke TL, Williams DA, eds. Foye's Principles of Medicinal Chemistry, 6th Ed. Philadelphia: Lippincott Williams & Wilkins, 2008:659–660.
70. Manchikanti L, Fellows B, Ailinani H, et al. Therapeutic use, abuse and nonmedical use of opioids: a ten year perspective. Pain Physician 2010;13:401–435.
71. Zacny JP, Galinkin J. Psychotropic drugs used in anesthesia practice: abuse liability and epidemiology of abuse. Anaesthesiology 1999;90:269–288.
72. American Pharmacists Association. Overcoming Race-Based Disparities in Pain Management. Washington, DC: American Pharmacists Association, 2008:1–6.
73. Panda M, Staton LJ, Chen I, et al. The influence of discordance in pain assessment on the functional status of patients with chronic nonmalignant pain. Am J Med Sci 2006;332:18–23.

74. Brushwood DB, Finley R, Giglio JG, et al. Pharmacists' Responsibilities in Managing Opioids: A Resource. Washington, DC: American Pharmaceutical Association Special Report, Advisory Board, 2002:1–19.
75. Forman WB. Opioid analgesic drugs in the elderly. Clin Geriatr Med 1996;12:489–500.
76. American Pain Society. Definitions related to the use of opioids for the treatment of pain. Advocacy & Policy 2001. Available at: http://www.ampainsoc.org/advocacy/opioids2.htm. Accessed May 25, 2011.
77. Jan SA. Introduction: landscape of opioid dependence. J Manag Care Pharm 2010;16:S4–S8.
78. McCauley K. Pleasure unwoven: a personal journey about addiction. Institute for Addiction Study, Salt Lake City, UT, 2009. Available at: http://web.me.com/kevintmccauley/Pleasure_Unwoven/Home.html. Accessed May 25, 2011.
79. Ballantyne JC. Opioids for chronic nonterminal pain. South Med J 2006;99:1245–1255.
80. Axelrod DJ, Reville B. Using methadone to treat opioid-induced hyperalgesia and refractory pain. J Opioid Manag 2007;3:113–114.
81. Crespi-Lofton J. Identifying and managing opioid-induced hyperalgesia. Pharmacy Today 2008:35.
82. DuPen A, Shen D, Ersek M. Mechanisms of opioid-induced tolerance and hyperalgesia. Pain Manag Nurs 2007;8:113–121.
83. Nicholls L, Bragaw L, Ruetsch C. Opioid dependence: treatment and guidelines. J Manag Care Pharm 2010;16:S14–S21.
84. Pogozheva IR, Lomize A, Mosberg HI. Opioid receptor three-dimensional structures from distance geometry calculations with hydrogen bonding constraints. Biophys J 1998;75:612–632.
85. Ruetsch C. Empirical view of opioid dependence. J Manag Care Pharm 2010;16:S9–S13.
86. Schwartz RH. Adolescent use of dextromethorphan. Clin Pediatr 2005;44:565–568.
87. Kamal IR, Wendling WW, Chen D, et al. *N*-Methyl-(D)-aspartate (NMDA) antagonists–S(+)-ketamine, dextrorphan and dextromethorphan–act as calcium antagonists on bovine cerebral arteries. J Neurosurg Anesthesiol 2008;20:241–248.
88. Sellner J, Ringer R, Baumann P, et al. Effect of NMDA-receptor antagonist dextromethorphan in rat pneumococcal meningitis. Curr Drug Metab 2008;9:83–88.
89. Hollander D, Pradas J, Kaplan R, et al. High dose dextromethorphan in amyotrophic lateral sclerosis: phase 1 safety and pharmacokinetic studies. Ann Neurol 1994;36:920–924.
90. Coller JK, Christrup LL, Somogyi AA. Role of active metabolites in the use of opioids. Eur J Clin Pharmacol 2009;65:121–139.
91. Lotsch J, Skarke C, Liefhold J, et al. Genetic predictors of the clinical response to opioid analgesics: clinical utility and future perspectives. Clin Pharmacokinet 2004;43:983–1013.
92. Carrupt P-A, Testa B, Bechalany A, et al. Morphine 6-glucuronide and morphine-glucuronide as molecular chameleons with unexpected lipophilicity. J Med Chem 1991;34:1272–1275.
93. Bernard S, Neville KA, Nguyen AT, et al. Interethnic differences in genetic polymorphisms of CYP2D6 in the U.S. population: clinical implications. Oncologist 2006;11:126–135.
94. Zhou S-F. Polymorphism of human cytochrome P450 2D6 and its clinical significance. Part 1. 2009;48:689–723.
95. Matsui A, Azuma J, Witcher JW, et al. Pharmacokinetics, safety and tolerability of atomoxetine and effect of CYP2D6*10/*10 genotype in healthy Japanese men. J Clin Pharmacol 2011;online May 4:1–16. Available at: http://jcp.sagepub.com/content/early/2011/05/04/0091270011398657.full.pdf. Accessed May 25, 2011.
96. Madadi P, Koren G, Cairnes J, et al. Safety of codeine during breastfeeding. Can Fam Phys 2007;53:33–35.
97. Fries DS. Opioid analgesics. In: Lemke TL, Williams DA, eds. Foye's Principles of Medicinal Chemistry, 6th Ed. Philadelphia: Lippincott Williams & Wilkins, 2008:670.
98. Hassan HE, Mercer SL, Cunningham CW, et al. Evaluation of the P-glycoprotein (Abcb1) affinity status of a series of morphine analogs: comparative study with meperidine analogs to identify opioids with minimal P-glycoprotein interactions. Int J Pharmaceut 2009;375:48–54.
99. Latta K. "The Breakfast Club" gives a physician a pain management menu for his patient. Am Pharm 2006;May:23–25.
100. Sheen CH, Schleimer RP, Kulka M. Codeine induces mast cell chemokine and cytokine production: involvement of G-protein activation. Allergy 2007;62:532–538.
101. Taylor DR. The pharmacology of fentanyl and its impact on the management of pain. Medscape Neurol Neurosurg 2005;7:2.
102. National Library of Medicine. ChemIDplus Advanced. Available at: http://chem.sis.nlm.nih.gov/chemidplus/chemidheavy.jsp. Accessed May 26, 2011.
103. Williams DA. pKa values for some drugs and miscellaneous organic acids and bases. In: Lemke TL, Williams DA, eds. Foye's Principles of Medicinal Chemistry, 6th Ed. Philadelphia: Lippincott Williams & Wilkins, 2008:1343–1353.
104. Joshi GP. Morphine 6-glucuronide, an active morphine metabolite for the potential treatment of post-operative pain. Curr Opin Invest Drug 2008;9:786–799.
105. Abbott FV, Palmour RM. Morphine-6-gluruonide: analgesic effects and receptor binding profile in rats. Life Sci 1988;43:1685–1695.
106. Milo S, Ansonoff M, King M, et al. Codeine and 6-acetylcodeine analgesia in mice. Cell Molec Neurobiol 2006;26:1011–1019.
107. Wilhelm W, Kreuer S. The place for short-acting opioids: special emphasis on remifentanil. Crit Care 2008;12(Suppl 3):1–9.
108. Overbaugh KJ. Acute coronary syndrome. Am J Nursing 2009;109:42–52.
109. Kou V, Nassisi D. Unstable angina and non-ST segment myocardial infarction: an evidence-based approach to management. Mt Sinai J Med 2006;73:449–468.
110. Roberts DJ, Goralski KB, Renton KW, et al. Effect of acute inflammatory brain injury on the accumulation of morphine and morphine 3- and 6-glucuronide in the human brain. Crit Care Med 2009;37:2767–2774.
111. Prince V. OxyContin: myth and reality. Am Pharm 2003;October:81–86.
112. Soloman DH, Rassen JA, Glynn RJ, et al. The comparative safety of opioids of nnonmalignant pain in older adults. Arch Intern Med 2010;170:1979–1986.
113. Gates M, Webb WG. The synthesis and resolution of 3-hydroxy-*N*-methylisomorphinan. J Am Chem Soc 1958;80:1186–1194.
114. Kugita H, Takeda M, Inove E. Synthesis of B/C-*trans*-fused morphine structures III. Synthesis of B/C *trans* morphine. Tetrahedron 1969;25:1851–1862.
115. Jasinski DR, Pevnick JS, Griffith JD. Human pharmacology and abuse potential of the analgesic bupenorphine. Arch Gen Psychiatry 1978;35:501–516.
116. Heel RC, Brogden RN, Speight TM, et al. Buprenorphine: a review of its pharmacological properties and therapeutic efficacy. Drugs 1979;17:81–110.
117. Budd K, Raffa RB, eds. Buprenorphine: The Unique Opioid Analgesic. New York: Thieme Medical Publishers, 2005.
118. Mok MS, Lippman M, Steen SN. Multidose/observational, comparative clinical analgetic evaluation of buprenorphine. J Clin Pharmacol 1981;21:323–329.
119. Hoskins PJ, Hanks GW. Opioid agonist-antagonist drugs in acute and chronic pain states. 1991;41:326–344.
120. Cowan A, Friderichs E, Strassburger W, et al. Basic pharmacology of buprenorphine. In: Budd K, Raffa RB, eds. Buprenorphine: The Unique Opioid Analgesic. New York: Thieme Medical Publishers, 2007:3–21.
121. Dahan A, Aarts L, Smith TW. Incidence, reversal and prevention of opioid-induced respiratory depression. Anesthesiology 2010;112:226–238.
122. Thomas JM, Hoffman BB. Buprenorphine prevents and reverses the expression of chronic etorphine-induced sensitization of adenylyl cyclase in SK-N-SH human neuroblastoma cells. J Pharmacol Exp Ther 1993;264:368–374.
123. Fudala PJ, Jaffe JH, Dax EM, et al. Use of buprenorphine in the treatment of opioid addiction II. Physiologic and behavior effects of daily and alternate day administration and abrupt withdrawal. Clin Pharmacol Ther 1990;47:525–534.
124. Gal TJ. Naloxone reversal of buprenorphine-induced respiratory depression. Clin Pharmacol Ther 1989;45:66–71.
125. Donaher PA, Welsch C. Managing opioid addiction with buprenorphine. Am Fam Physician 2006;73:1573–1578.
126. Kobayashi K, Yamamoto T, Chiba K, et al. Human buprenorphine *N*-dealkylation is catalyzed by cytochrome P450 3A4. Drug Metab Dispos 1998;26:818–821.
127. Moore RA, Hand CW, McQuay HJ. Opiate metabolism and excretion. Bailliere's Clin Anaesthesiol 1987;1:829–858.
128. Berson A, Fau D, Fornacciari R, et al. Mechanisms for experimental buprenorphine hepatotoxicity: major role of mitochondria dysfunction versus metabolic activation. J Hepatol 2001;34:261–269.
129. Costello J. Buprenorphine-naloxone protocol eases opioid addiction. Pharm Pract News 2008;35:38.
130. Substance Abuse and Mental Health Services Administration. New release. Available at: http://www.samhsa.gov/newsroom/advisories/1009083541.aspx. Accessed May 27, 2011.
131. Fiellin DA, O'Connor PG. Office-based treatment of opioid-dependent patients. N Engl J Med 2002;347:817–823.
132. Crismon ML. Opioid dependency shifting to office-based care. Available at: http://www.pharmacist.com/AM/Template.cfm?Section=Pharmacy_Today2&Template=/CM/HTMLDisplay.cfm&ContentID=9311. Accessed May 27, 2011.
133. Kivell B, Prisinzano TE. Kappa opioids and the modulation of pain. Psychopharmacology 2010;210:109–119.
134. Gear RW, Miaskowski C, Gordon NC, et al. Significantly greater analgesia in females compared to males after kappa-opioids. Nature Med 1996;2:1248–1250.
135. Talbert RL, Peters JI, Sorrells SC, et al. Respiratory effects of high-dose butorphanol. Acute Care 1988;12(Suppl 1):47–56.
136. Roscow CE. Butorphanol in perspective. Acute Care 1988;12 (Suppl 1):21–27.

137. Walsh SL, Chausmer AE, Strain EC, et al. Evaluation of mu and kappa actions of butorphanol in humans through differential naltrexone blockade. Psychopharmacology 2008;196:143–155.
138. Mitaka C, Sakanichi N, Tsunoda Y, et al. Comparison of hemodynamic effects of morphine, butorphanol, buprenorphine and pentazocine on ICU patients. Bull Tokyo Med Dent Univ 1985;32:31–39.
139. Gaver RC, Vasiljev M, Wong H, et al. Disposition of parenteral butorphanol in man. Drug Metab Dispos 1980;8:230–235.
140. Walker DJ, Zacny JP, Galva KE, et al. Subjective, psychomotor, and physiological effects of cumulative doses of mixed-action opioids in healthy volunteers. Psychopharmacology 2001;155:362–371.
141. Lee G, DeMaria AN, Amsterdam EA, et al. Comparative effects of morphine, meperidine and pentazocine on cardiocirculatory dynamics in patients with acute myocardial infarction. Am J Med 1976;60:949–955.
142. Katsiki N, Hatzitolios AI, Mikhalidis DP. Naltrexone sustained-release (SR) + bupropion SR combination therapy for the treatment of obesity: "A new kid on the block"? Ann Med 2011;43:249–258.
143. Smith JP, Bingaman SI, Ruggiero F, et al. Therapy with the opioid antagonist naltrexone promotes mucosal healing in active Crohn's disease: a randomized placebo-controlled trial. Dig Dis Sci 2011;56:2088–2097.
144. Mason BJ, Ritivo EC, Morgan RO, et al. A double-blind, placebo-controlled pilot study to evaluate the efficacy and safety of oral nalmefene HCl for alcohol dependence. Alcohol Clin Exp Res 1994;18:1162–1167.
145. Gal TJ, DiFazio CA, Dixon R. Prolonged blockade of opioid effect with oral nalmefene. Clin Pharmacol Ther 1986;40:537–542.
146. Licup N, Baumrucker SJ. Methylnaltrexone: treatment for opioid-induced constipation. Am J Hosp Palliat Care 2011;28:59–61.
147. Leppert W. The role of opioid receptor antagonists in the treatment of opioid-induced constipation: a review. Adv Ther 2010;27:714–730.
148. Fries DS. Opioid analgesics. In: Lemke TL, Williams DA, eds. Foye's Principles of Medicinal Chemistry, 6th Ed. Philadelphia: Lippincott Williams & Wilkins, 2008:670.
149. Latta KS, Ginsberg B, Barkin RL. Meperidine: a critical review. Am J Ther 2002;9:53–68.
150. Eisendrath SJ, GoldmanB, Douglas J, et al. Meperidine-induced delirium. Am J Psychiatry 1987;144:1062–1065.
151. Stevenson JG, Mitchell JF. Reducing the use of meperidine in hospital practice. Pharm Pract News 2007;April:1–7.
152. Gillman PK. Monoamine oxidase inhibitors, opioid analgesics and serotonin toxicity. Br J Anaesth 2005;4:434–441.
153. Guay DR, Meatherall RC, Chalmers JL, et al. Cimetidine alters pethidine disposition in man. Br J Clin Pharmacol 1984;18:907–914.
154. Szeto HH, Inturrisi CE, Houde R, et al. Accumulation of normeperidine, an active metabolite of meperidine, in patients with renal failure or cancer. Ann Intern Med 1977;86:738–741.
155. Flacke JW, Flacke WE, Bloor BC, et al. Histamine release by four narcotics: a double-blind study in humans. Anesth Analg 1987;66:723–730.
156. Weant KA, Martin JE, Humphries RL, et al. Pharmacologic options for reducing the shivering response to therapeutic hypothermia. Pharmacotherapy 2010;38:830–841.
157. Vucovic S, Prostran M, Ivanovi M, et al. Fentanyl analogs: structure-activity relationship study. Curr Med Chem 2009;16:2468–2474.
158. Blasco A, Berzosa M, Iranzo V, et al. Update in cancer pain. Cancer Chemother Rev 2009;4:95–109.
159. Prommer E. The role of fentanyl in cancer-related pain. J Palliat Med 2009;12:947–954.
160. Adams AP, Pybus DA. Delayed respiratory depression after fentanyl use during anaesthesia. Br Med J 1798;1:278–279.
161. Dunham W. CDC reports 1,000 fentanyl overdoses in 2 years. Available at: http://www.caring4cancer.com/go/cancer/news?NewsItemId=20080724elin023.xml. Accessed May 28, 2011.
162. Clotz MA, Nahata MC. Clinical uses of fentanyl, sufentanil and alfentanil. Clin Pharm 1991;10:581–593.
163. Burkle H, Sunbar S, Van Aken H. Remifentanil: a novel, short-acting μ opioid. Anesth Analg 1996;83:646–651.
164. Stroumpos C, Manolaraki M, Paspatis GA. Remifentanil, a different opioid: potential clinical applications and safety aspects. Expert Opin Drug Saf 2010;9:355–364.
165. Inturrisi CE. Pharmacology of methadone and its isomers. Minerva Anesthesiol 2005;71:435–437.
166. Gerber JG, Rhodes RJ, Gal J. Stereoselective metabolism of methadone *N*-demethylation by cytochrome P4502B6 and 2C19. Chirality 2004;16:36–44.
167. Wenjie JL, Bies R, Kamden LK, et al. Methadone: a substrate and mechanism-based inhibitor of CYP2C19 (Aromatase). Drug Metab Dispos 2010;38:1308–1313.
168. Sullivan HR, Due SL. Urinary metabolites of dl-methadone in maintenance subjects. J Med Chem 1973;16:909–913.
169. Pohland A, Boaz HE, Sullivan HR. Synthesis and identification of metabolites resulting from the biotransformation of DL-methadone in man and in the rat. J Med Chem 1971;14:194–197.
170. King VL, Burke C, Stoller KB, et al. Implementing methadone medical maintenance in community-based clinics: disseminating evidence-based treatment. J Subst Abuse Treat 2008;35:312–321.
171. Larson MEM, Richards TM. Quantification of a methadone metabolite (EDDP) in urine: assessment of compliance. Clin Med Res 2009;7:134–141.
172. Nossaman VE, Ramadhyani U, Kadowitz PJ, et al. Advances in perioperative pain management: use of medications with dual action mechanisms, tramadol and tapentadol. Anesthesiol Clin 2010;28:647–666.
173. Grond S, Sablotzki A. Clinical pharmacology of tramadol. J Pharmacol Exp Ther 2004;43:879–923.
174. Tzschentke TM, Christoph T, Kogel B, et al. (−)-(1R,2R)-3-(3-Dimethylaminoe-1-ethyl-2-methyl-propyl)-phenol hydrochloride (Tapentadol HCl): a novel μ-opioid receptor agonist/norepinephrine reuptake inhibitor with broad-spectrum analgesic properties. J Pharmacol Exp Ther 2007;323:265–276.
175. Guay DR. Is tapentadol an advance over tramadol? Consult Pharm 2009;24:833–840.
176. Lotsch J. Opioid metabolites. J Pain Symptom Manag 2005;29(Suppl 5):S10–S24.
177. Takeshita J, Litzinger MH. Serotonin syndrome associated with tramadol. Prim Care Companion J Clin Psychiatry 2009;11:273.
178. Tashakori A, Afshari R. Tramadol overdose as a cause of serotonin syndrome: a case series. Clin Toxicol (Phila) 2010;48:337–341.
179. Marquardt KA, Alsop JA, Albertson TE. Tramadol exposures reported to a state-wide poison control system. Ann Pharmacother 2005;39:1039–1044.
180. Ripple MG, Pestaner JP, Levine BS, et al. Lethal combination of tramadol and multiple drugs affecting serotonin. Am J Forensic Med Pathol 2000;21:370–374.
181. Fass J. Comment: effect of scheduling tramadol as a controlled substance on poison center exposures to tramadol. Ann Phamacother 2010;44:1509.
182. U.S. Food and Drug Administration. Ultram (tramadol hydrochloride), Ultracet (tramadol hydrochloride/acetaminophen): label change. Available at: http://www.fda.gov/Safety/MedWatch/SafetyInformation/SafetyAlertsforHumanMedicalProducts/ucm213264.htm. Accessed May 29, 2011.
183. Conner CS, Metzger SE. New product bulletin: Nucynta (tapentadol HCl). Pharmacy Today 2009;September:3–16.
184. Schroder W, Tzschentke TM, Terlinden R, et al. Synergistic interaction between the two mechanisms of action of tapentadol in analgesia. J Pharmacol Exp Ther 2011;337:312–320.
185. Niemegeers CJ, McGuire JL, Heykants JJ, et al. Dissociation between opiate-like and antidiarrheal activities of antidiarrheal drugs. J Pharmacol Exp Ther 1979;210:327–333.
186. Sadeque AJ, Wandel C, He H, et al. Increased drug delivery to the brain by P-glycoprotein inhibition. Clin Pharmacol Ther 2000;68:231–237.
187. Schinkel AH, Wagenaar E, Mol CA, et al. P-glycoprotein in the blood-brain barrier of mice influences the brain penetration and pharmacological activity of many drugs. J Clin Invest 1996;97:2517–2524.
188. Baker DE. Loperamide: a pharmacological review. Rev Gastroenterol Disord 2007;7(Suppl 3):S11–S18.
189. Crowe A, Wong P. Potential roles of P-gp and calcium channels in loperamide and diphenoxylate transport. Toxicol Appl Pharmacol 2003;193:127–137.
190. De Luca A, Coupar IM. Difenoxin and loperamide: studies on possible mechanisms of intestinal antisecretory action. Naunyn-Schmiedeberg's Arch Pharmacol 1993;347:231–237.
191. Reynolds IJ, Gould RJ, Snyder SH. Loperamide: blockade of calcium channels as a mechanism for antidiarrheal effects. J Pharmacol Exp Ther 1984;231:628–632.
192. Church J, Fletcher EJ, Abdel-Hamid K, et al. Loperamide blocks high-voltage-activated calcium channels and *N*-methyl-D-aspartate-evoked responses in rat and mouse cultured hippocampal pyramidal neurons. Am Soc Pharmacol Exp Ther 1994;45:747–757.
193. Kim K-A, Chung J, Jung D-H, et al. Identification of cytochrome P450 isoforms involved in the metabolism of loperamide in human liver microsomes. Eur J Clin Pharmacol 2004;60:575–581.
194. He H, Sadeque A, Erve JCL, et al. Quantitation of loperamide and *N*-desmethyl-loperamide in human plasma using electrospray ionization with selected reaction ion monitoring liquid chromatograph-mass spectrometry. J Chromatog B 2000;744:323–331.
195. Dray A. Neuropathic pain: emerging treatments. Br J Anaesth 2008;101:48–58.
196. Campbell JN, Meyer RA. Mechanisms of neuropathic pain. Neuron 2006;52:77–92.
197. Finnerup NB, Sindrup SH, Jensen TS. Chronic neuropathic pain: mechanisms, drug targets and measurement. Fund Clin Pharmacol 2007;21:129–136.
198. Dworkin RH, O'Connor AB, Audette J, et al. Recommendations for the pharmacological management of neuropathic pain: an overview and literature update. Mayo Clin Proc 2010;85(Suppl):S3–S14.
199. Dworkin RH, O'Connor AB, Backonja M, et al. Pharmacologic management of neuropathic pain: evidence-based recommendations. Pain 2007;132:237–251.

200. Jensen TS, Madsen CS, Finnerup NB. Pharmacology and treatment of neuropathic pains. Curr Opin Neurol 2009;22:467–474.
201. Zilliox L, Russell JW. Maintaining efficacy in the treatment of diabetic peripheral neuropathic pain: role of duloxetine. Diabetes Metab Syndr Obes 2010;3:7–17.
202. Neurontin [package insert]. New York: Pfizer, April 2009.
203. Finnerup NB, Otto M, McQuay HJ, et al. Algorithm for neuropathic pain treatment: an evidence based proposal. Pain 2005;118:289–305.
204. Shah TH, Moradimehr A. Bupropion for the treatment of neuropathic pain. Am J Hosp Palliat Care 2010;27:333–336.
205. Semenchuk MR, Sherman S, Davis B. Double-blind, randomized trial of bupropion SR for the treatment of neuropathic pain. Neurology 2001;57:1583-1588.
206. Fontelles MIM, Garcia CG. Role of cannabinoids in the management of neuropathic pain. CNS Drugs 2008;22:645–653.
207. Metanx [package insert]. Covington, LA: Pamlab, February 2010.

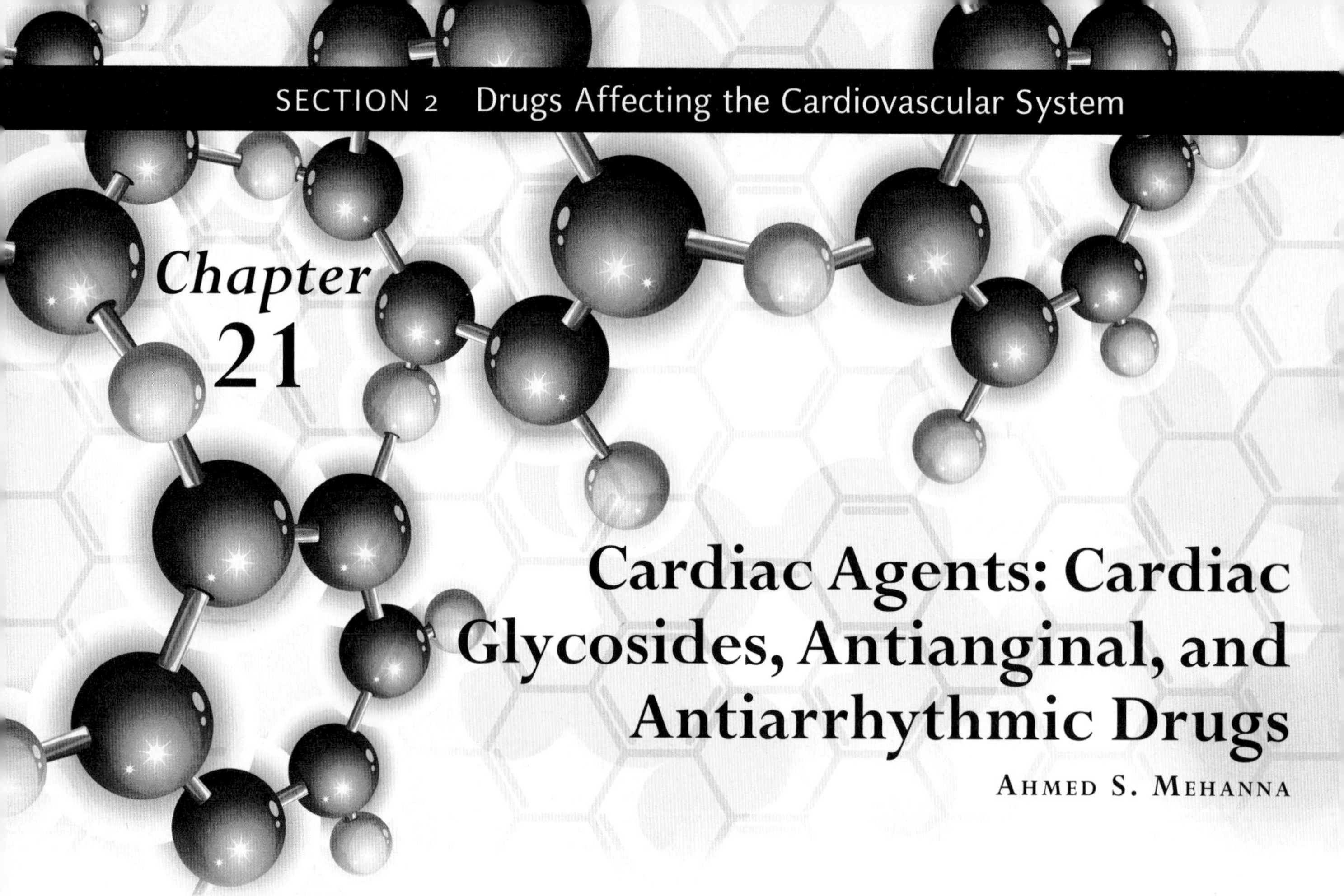

Chapter 21

Cardiac Agents: Cardiac Glycosides, Antianginal, and Antiarrhythmic Drugs

AHMED S. MEHANNA

*Drugs Covered in This Chapter**

CARDIAC GLYCOSIDES POSITIVE INOTROPIC DRUGS
- *Deslanatoside C (BP)*
- Digitalis products
- Digitoxin (BP)
- Digoxin
- Lanatoside C (BP)
- *Metildigoxin*
- *Ouabain (BP) (G-strophanthin)*

NONGLYCOSIDIC POSITIVE INOTROPIC DRUGS
- Dobutamine
- *Enoximone*
- Inamrinone
- Milrinone
- *Olprinone*
- *Pimobendan*
- *Vesnarinone*

ANTIANGINAL NITRATES AND NITRITES
- Amyl nitrite (isoamyl nitrite)
- Erythrityl tetranitrate
- Isosorbide dinitrate
- Nesiritide citrate
- *Nicorandil*
- Nitroglycerin
- Pentaerythritol tetranitrate

NITRIC OXIDE DONOR
- *Molsidomine*

CALCIUM CHANNEL BLOCKERS
- Amlodipine
- Bepridil
- Diltiazem
- Felodipine
- Nicardipine
- Nifedipine
- Nitrendipine
- Ranolazine
- Verapamil

ANTIARRHYTHMIC AGENTS
- Class IA
  - Disopyramide
  - Procainamide
  - Quinidine
- Class IB
  - Lidocaine
  - Mexiletine
  - Phenytoin
  - Tocainide
- Class IC
  - Encainide
  - Flecainide
  - Moricizine
  - Propafenone
- Class II
  - Propranolol
- Class III
  - Amiodarone
  - Bretylium
  - Dofetilide
  - Dronedarone
  - Ibutilide
  - Sotalol
- Class IV
  - Bepridil
  - Diltiazem
  - Verapamil

Abbreviations

ATP, adenosine triphosphate
ATPase, adenosine triphosphatase
AUC, area under the curve
AV, atrioventricular
cAMP, cyclic adenosine monophosphate
cGMP, cyclic guanosine monophosphate
CHF, congestive heart failure
COMT, catechol-*O*-methyltransferase
CYP, cytochrome P450
FDA, U.S. Food and Drug Administration
I_{Na}, sodium current
NO, nitric oxide

*Drugs listed include those available in the United States and outside the United States; drugs with the BP (British Pharmacopeia) designation are available only in Canada and countries other than the United States. Drugs in italics are not approved by the FDA.

Abbreviations (Continued)

PDE3, phosphodiesterase 3
PDE5, phosphodiesterase 5
P-gp, P-glycoprotein
SA, sinoatrial
SAR, structure–activity relationship

Scenario

Judy Cheng, PharmD

JS is a 58 year-old white man with a medical history of hypertension. He presented to the clinic today complaining of palpitation and dizziness for the past week. Electrocardiogram shows an irregular rhythm (i.e., atrial fibrillation) of 110 beats per minute. JS' blood pressure is 160/95 mmHg. He is diagnosed with new onset atrial fibrillation. His current medications include lisinopril 5 mg daily, but JS has a significant history of medication nonadherence.

(The reader is directed to the clinical solution and chemical analysis of this case at the end of the chapter).

INTRODUCTION

Heart diseases are grouped into three major disorders: cardiac failure or contractile dysfunction (congestive heart failure), ischemic heart disease (with angina as its primary symptom), and cardiac arrhythmia.

DRUGS FOR THE TREATMENT OF HEART FAILURE

Congestive Heart Failure

Cardiac failure can be described as the inability of the heart to pump blood effectively at a rate that meets the needs of metabolizing tissues. This is the direct result of reduced contractility of the cardiac muscles, especially those of the ventricles, which causes a decrease in cardiac output, increasing the blood volume of the heart (hence the term "congested"). As a result, systemic blood pressure and renal blood flow are both reduced, which often leads to the development of edema in the lower extremities and the lung (pulmonary edema) as well as renal failure. A group of drugs known as the cardiac glycosides were found to reverse most of these symptoms and complications.

Drugs for the Treatment of Congestive Heart Failure

Cardiac Glycosides: Positive Ionotropic Drugs Cardiac glycosides are an important class of naturally occurring drugs, the actions of which include both beneficial and toxic effects on the heart. Their desirable cardiotonic action is of particular benefit in the treatment of congestive heart failure (CHF) and associated edema, and their preparations have been used as medicinal agents, as well as poisons, since 1500 BC. This dual application serves to highlight the toxic potential for this class of life-saving drugs. Despite the extended use and obvious therapeutic benefits of the cardiac glycosides, it was not until the famous monograph by William Withering in 1785, "*An Account of the Foxglove and Some of Its Medical Uses*," that cardiac glycoside therapy started to become more standardized and rational (1–3). The therapeutic use of purified cardiac glycoside preparations has occurred only over the last century. Cardiac glycosides represent one of the most important drug classes available to the physician for the treatment of CHF.

Chemistry of the Cardiac Glycosides Cardiac glycosides and other similar glycosides are composed of two portions: the sugar moiety and the nonsugar (aglycone) moiety.

Aglycones. The aglycone portion of the cardiac glycosides is a steroid nucleus with a unique set of fused rings, which makes these agents easily distinguished from other steroids. Rings A-B and C-D are cis fused, whereas rings B-C have a trans configuration. Such ring fusion gives the aglycone nucleus of cardiac glycosides the characteristic "U-shape," as shown in Figure 21.1. The steroid nucleus also carries, in most cases, two angular methyl groups at C-10 and C-13. Hydroxyl groups are located at C-3, the site of the sugar attachment, and at C-14. The C-14 hydroxyl is normally unsubstituted. However, additional hydroxyl groups can be found at C-12 and C-16; the presence or absence of hydroxyl groups distinguishes the important differences in the genins: digitoxigenin, digoxigenin, and gitoxigenin (Fig. 21.2). These additional hydroxyl groups have significant impact on the partitioning and pharmacokinetics for each glycoside, to be discussed later. The lactone ring at C-17 is another major structural

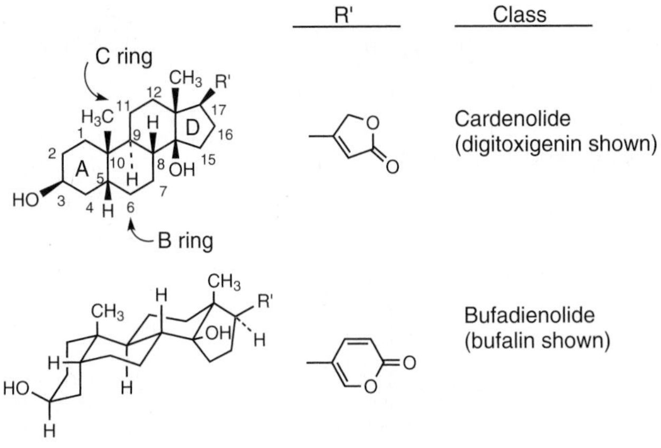

FIGURE 21.1 Cardenolide and bufadienolide aglycones.

CLINICAL SIGNIFICANCE

Digoxin, nitrates, and many antiarrhythmics are among the oldest cardiovascular agents around and still play an important role in managing different cardiovascular diseases. Cardiac glycosides such as digoxin have been used for decades for the management of heart failure as well as slowing down ventricular rate in patients with atrial fibrillation. Digoxin remains the only oral positive inotropic agent to date. Despite that, many questions still remain regarding the precise mechanism of action (beyond its positive inotropic effect), exactly what the most optimal therapeutic range should be, as well as what patient population will benefit the most from digoxin in terms of mortality and morbidity.

The role of nitrates in the management of angina is well established. However, the development of nitrate tolerance sometimes limits its long-term clinical benefits. Newer antianginals being developed have tried to overcome this issue by working as a direct nitric oxide donor (e.g., mosidomine). Others were developed to work through a completely different mechanism (e.g., ranolazine, a sodium channel blocker). Unlike other antianginals, ranolazine does not affect blood pressure and heart rate. It can benefit patients whose blood pressure and heart rate may be too low or slow to tolerate other antianginals.

In recent years, many antiarrhythmic agents have given way to implantable defibrillation and surgical ablation for potentially life-threatening arrhythmias. However, they are still commonly used as adjunct therapy. Antiarrhythmic agents, although effective in controlling arrhythmia, also possess serious and potential lethal adverse events, and some have numerous significant clinical drug interactions. Newer antiarrhythmic agents continued to be developed in an attempt to minimize the risk of these severe toxicities. For example, the development of dronedareone, by eliminating the iodine moiety from amiodarone, significantly reduces clinical incidence of development of thyroid disorders. Understanding the medicinal chemistry of these agents will allow pharmacists to understand how the structures of these agents contribute to their efficacy and toxicity and to make the most optimal choices for individual patient scenarios.

Judy Cheng, PharmD
Professor, Pharmacy Practice
School of Pharmacy-Boston
Massachusetts College of Pharmacy and Health Sciences

feature of the cardiac aglycones. The size and degree of unsaturation of the lactone ring vary with the source of the glycoside. In most cases, the cardiac glycosides of plant origin, also called cardenolides, possess a five-membered, α,β-unsaturated lactone ring, whereas those derived from animal origin, the bufadienolides, possess a six-membered lactone ring with two conjugated double bonds (usually referred to as α-pyrone).

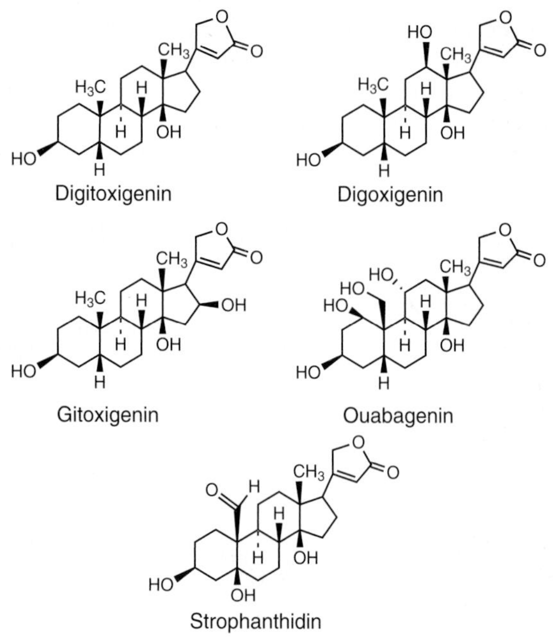

FIGURE 21.2 Major cardenolide aglycones.

Sugars. The hydroxyl group at C-3 of the aglycone portion is conjugated to a monosaccharide or a polysaccharide with β-1,4-glucosidic linkages. The number and identity of sugars vary from one glycoside to another, as detailed subsequently. The most commonly found sugars in the cardiac glycosides are D-glucose, D-digitoxose, L-rhamnose, and D-cymarose (Fig. 21.3). These sugars exist predominately in the cardiac glycosides in the β-conformation. In some cases, the sugars exist in the acetylated form. The presence of an *O*-acetyl group on a sugar greatly affects the lipophilic character and pharmacokinetics of the entire glycoside, as subsequently discussed.

Sources and Common Names of Cardiac Glycosides. The cardiac glycosides occur mainly in plants and, in rare cases,

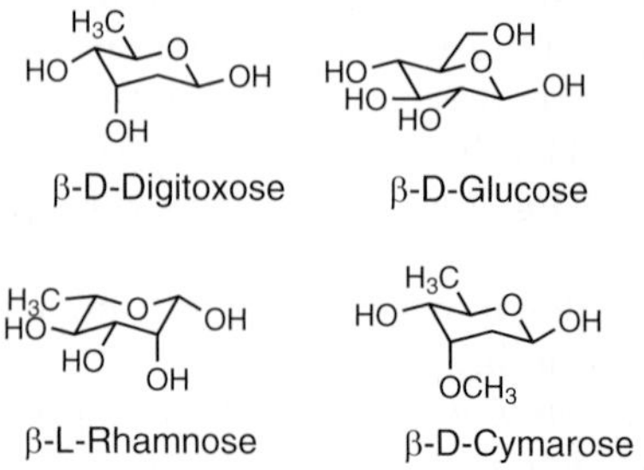

FIGURE 21.3 Selected sugars found in naturally occurring cardiac glycosides.

in animals, such as poisonous toads. *Digitalis purpurea* (foxglove plant), *Digitalis lanata, Strophanthus gratus*, and *Strophanthus kombe* are the major plant sources of the cardiac glycosides. Based on the nature and number of sugar molecules and the number of hydroxyl groups on the aglycone moiety, each combination of sugars and aglycones assumes different generic names. The site of the glycosides concentration in the plant, the types of glycosides, and the names of the structural components of these glycosides are summarized in Table 21.1.

Digitalis Lanata. Lanatoside A is composed of the aglycone digitoxigenin (genin indicates no sugar) connected to three digitoxose sugar molecules, the third of which carries a 3-acetyl group, and a terminal glucose molecule. In other words, the structure sequence is glucose$_4$-3-acetyldigitoxose$_3$-digitoxose$_2$-digitoxose$_1$-digitoxigenin.

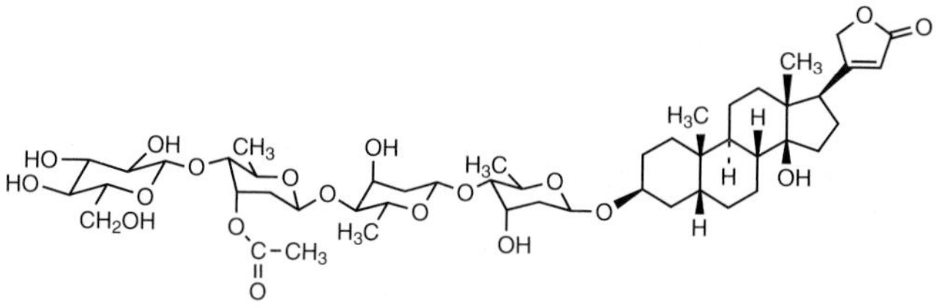

Lanatoside A

Lanatoside B has the identical sugar portion to lanatoside A, except that the aglycone has an extra hydroxyl group at C-16 and is given the name gitoxigenin. The structural sequence is glucose$_4$-3-acetyldigitoxose$_3$-digitoxose$_2$-digitoxose$_1$-gitoxigenin.

Lanatoside C has also the same sugars found in both lanatosides A and B; however, the aglycone has the steroid backbone of lanatoside A plus an additional hydroxyl group at C-12. This cardenolide is named digoxigenin. The structural sequence is glucose$_4$-3-acetyldigitoxose$_3$-digitoxose$_2$-digitoxose$_1$-digoxigenin.

Partial hydrolysis of the glucose molecule and the acetate group from lanatoside A and C produces, respectively, two new and most important cardiac glycosides, digitoxin and digoxin, with the following sequences: digitoxin, (digitoxose)$_3$-digitoxigenin; and digoxin, (digitoxose)$_3$-digoxigenin.

Digitalis Purpurea.

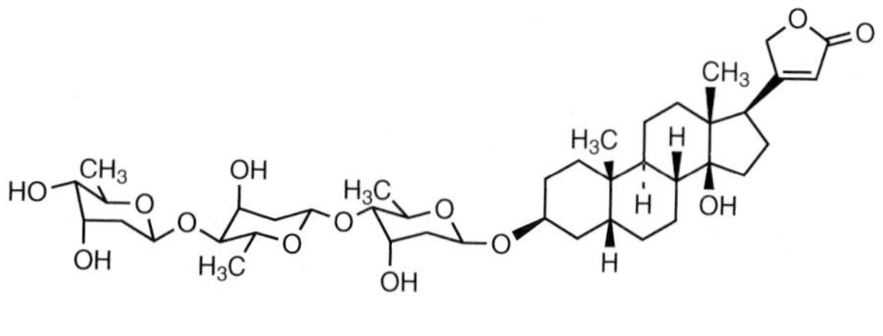

Digitoxin

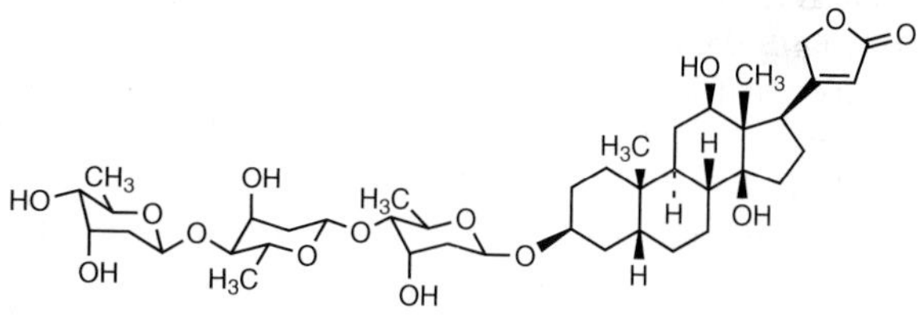

Digoxin

Purpurea glycosides A and B have structures identical to those of lanatosides A and B, but with no acetyl group on the third digitoxose. Therefore, the purpurea glycosides A and B are sometimes called desacetyl digilanides A and B. Their sequences are as follows: purpurea glycoside A, glucose-(digitoxose)$_3$-digitoxigenin; and purpurea glycoside B, glucose-(digitoxose)$_3$-gitoxigenin. There is no purpurea glycoside C.

TABLE 21.1 Selected Natural Cardiac Glycosides and Their Sources

Source	Glycoside	Aglycone	Sugar[a]
Digitalis lanata (leaf)	Lanatoside A (digilanide A)	Digitoxigenin	Glucose-3-acetyldigitoxose-digitoxose-digitoxose
	Lanatoside B (digilanide B)	Gitoxigenin	
	Lanatoside C (digilanide C)	Digoxigenin	
Digitalis purpurea (leaf)	Purpurea glycoside A (desacetyl digilanide A)	Digitoxigenin	Glucose-digitoxose-digitoxose-digitoxose
	Purpurea glycoside B (desacetyl digilanide B)	Gitoxigenin	
Strophanthus gratus (seed)	G-Strophanthin	Oubagenin	Rhamnose
Strophanthus kombe (seed)	k-Strophanthoside	Strophanthidin	Glucose-glucose-cymarose

[a]Conjugated with the C-3 hydroxyl of the aglycone via the sugar to the far right. All sugars are conjugated via β-1,4–glucosidic bond.

Strophanthus Gratus and Strophanthus Kombe.

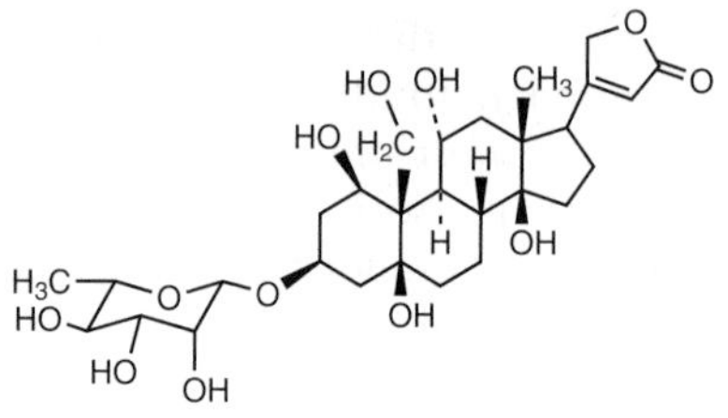

Ouabain

The glycosides extracted from the plants *Strophanthus gratus* and *Strophanthus kombe* are called G-strophanthin (or ouabain) and k-strophanthoside, respectively. The corresponding aglycone for ouabain is ouabagenin, and for k-strophanthoside, strophanthidin. Ouabagenin has a polyhydroxylated steroidal nucleus, and strophanthidin has an additional hydroxyl group at C-5 with an angular aldehyde group at C-10, replacing the traditional methyl group at that position (Fig. 21.2). Ouabagenin is conjugated only to a single molecule of L-rhamnose, whereas strophanthidin is conjugated to a molecule of cymarose, which is further linked to two molecules of glucose.

The medicinally used preparations are mainly obtained from *Digitalis purpurea* and *Digitalis lanata* plants. These glycosides are referred to as digitalis glycosides, cardiac glycosides, or simply, cardenolides. *Strophanthus* glycosides (e.g., ouabain) are no longer used therapeutically but were previously administered only intravenously because of poor oral absorption. Cardiac glycosides from animal sources (generally referred to as bufadienolides) are rare and of far less medicinal importance because of their high toxicity. Pharmaceutical preparations of whole plants and partially hydrolyzed glycosides of *Digitalis lanata* and *Digitalis purpurea* have been used clinically. Advancements in isolation and purification techniques, however, have made it possible to obtain highly purified digoxin preparations.

Pharmacology Cardiac glycosides affect the heart in a dual fashion, both directly (on the cardiac muscle and the specialized conduction system of sinoatrial [SA] node, atrioventricular [AV] node, and His-Purkinje system) and indirectly (on the cardiovascular system mediated by the autonomic nervous reflexes). The combined direct and indirect effects of the cardiac glycosides lead to changes in the electrophysiologic properties of the heart, including alteration of the contractility; heart rate; excitability; conductivity; refractory period; and automaticity of the atrium, ventricle, Purkinje fibers, AV node, and SA node. The heart response to the cardiac glycosides is a dose-dependent process and varies considerably between the normal heart and the heart with CHF. The cardio-effects observed after the administration of low doses of the cardiac glycosides (therapeutic doses) differ considerably from those observed at high doses (cardiotoxic doses). The pharmacologic effects discussed subsequently relate mainly to therapeutic doses administered to patients with CHF. The effects of cardiac glycosides on the properties of the heart muscle and different sites of the conduction system are summarized in Table 21.2. The increased force and rate of myocardial contraction (positive inotropic effect) and the prolongation of the refractory period of the AV node are the effects most relevant to the CHF problem. Both of these effects result from the direct action of the cardiac glycosides on the heart. The indirect effects are manifested as increased vagal nerve activity, which probably results from the glycoside-induced sensitization of the baroreceptors of the carotid sinus to changes in the arterial pressure; in other words, any given increase in the arterial blood pressure results in an increase in the vagal activity (parasympathetic) coupled with a greater decrease in the sympathetic activity. The vagal effect with uncompensated sympathetic response results in decreased heart rate and decreased peripheral vascular resistance (afterload). Therefore, cardiac glycosides reverse most of the symptoms associated with CHF as a result of increased sympathetic system activity, including increased heart rate, vascular resistance, and afterload. The administration of cardiac glycosides to a patient with CHF increases cardiac muscle contraction, reduces heart rate, and decreases both edema and the heart size.

Biochemical Mechanism of Action The mechanism whereby cardiac glycosides cause a positive inotropic effect and electrophysiologic changes is still not completely known despite years of active investigation. Several mechanisms have been proposed, but the most widely accepted mechanism involves the ability of cardiac glycosides to inhibit the membrane-bound Na^+/K^+–adenosine triphosphatase (Na^+/K^+-ATPase) pump responsible for sodium/potassium exchange. To better understand the correlation between the pump and the mechanism of action of cardiac glycosides on the heart muscle contraction, one has to consider the sequence of

TABLE 21.2 Effects of Cardiac Glycosides on the Heart

	Atrium	Purkinje Ventricle	AV Fiber	SA Node	Node
Contractility	↑	↑	—	—	—
Excitability	o	Variable	↑	—	—
Conductivity	↑	↑	↓	↓	—
Refractory period	↓	↓	↑	↑	—
Automaticity	—	—	↑	—	↓

AV, atrioventricular; SA, sinoatrial; ↑ increased action; ↓ decreased action; o, no action; —, no data available.

events associated with cardiac action potential that leads ultimately to muscular contraction. The process of membrane depolarization/repolarization is controlled mainly by the movement of the three ions, Na^+, K^+, Ca^{2+}, in and out of the cell.

At the resting state (no contraction), the concentration of sodium is high outside the cell. On membrane depolarization, Na^+ fluxes in, leading to an immediate elevation of the action potential. Elevated intracellular sodium triggers the influx of Ca^{2+}, which occurs slowly and is represented by the plateau region of the cardiac action potential. The influx of calcium results in the efflux of potassium out of the myocardium. The Na^+/K^+ exchange occurs at a later stage of the action potential to restore the membrane potential to its normal level (for further detail, see the discussion of antiarrhythmic agents and their classification at the end of this chapter). The Na^+/K^+ exchange requires energy and is catalyzed by the enzyme Na^+/K^+-ATPase. Cardiac glycosides are proposed to inhibit this enzyme, with a net result of reduced sodium exchange with potassium (i.e., increased intracellular sodium), which in turn results in increased intracellular calcium. Elevated intracellular calcium concentration triggers a series of intracellular biochemical events that ultimately result in an increase in the force of the myocardial contraction, or a positive inotropic effect. (The events that lead to muscle contraction are covered in further detail in the discussion of the mechanism of action of the calcium channel blockers later in this chapter.)

This mechanism of the cardiac glycosides via inhibiting the Na^+/K^+-ATPase pump is in agreement with the fact that the action of the cardiac glycosides is enhanced by low extracellular potassium and inhibited by high extracellular potassium. The cardiac glycosides–induced changes in the electrophysiology of the heart can also be explained based on the inhibition of Na^+/K^+-ATPase. It has been suggested that the intracellular loss of potassium because of inhibition of the pump causes a decrease in the cellular transmembrane potential approaching zero. This decrease in the membrane potential is sufficient to explain the increased excitability and other electrophysiologic effects observed after cardiac glycosides administration.

Structural Requirements for Intrinsic Activity Many hypotheses have been put forth to explain the cardiac glycoside structure–activity relationships (SARs). Some of the difficulty in arriving at a universally acceptable SAR model has been attributed to the early method of testing cardiac glycoside preparations and the lack of well-characterized cardiac glycoside "receptors." Until the early 1970s, nearly all the cardiac glycosides were evaluated based on their cardiac toxicity rather than on more therapeutically relevant criteria. This was partly because of the belief that cardiac toxicity was, in fact, an extension of the desired cardiotonic action. Thus, comparisons of cardiac glycoside preparations were based on the amount of drug required to cause cardiac arrest in test animals, usually anesthetized cats. More recently, most SAR studies have relied, at least initially, on results obtained with isolated cardiac tissue or whole-heart preparations. In these models, inotropic activity and contractility can be directly assessed. In addition, the recognition of cardiac Na^+/K^+-ATPase as the probable receptor for the cardiac glycosides has made the inhibition of this enzyme system an important criterion for the cardiac glycosides activity.

Much of the interest in the effects of structural modification on cardiotonic activity results from the desire to develop agents with less potential for toxicity. Early studies based primarily on cardiac toxicity testing data suggested the importance of the steroid "backbone" shape, the 14-β-hydroxyl and the 17-unsaturated lactone for activity. Other studies have been directed toward characterizing the interaction of the cardiac glycosides with Na^+/K^+-ATPase, the putative cardiac glycoside receptor. Using ATPase as a model for enzyme inhibition as the biologic end point, a number of hypotheses for cardiac glycoside receptor–binding interactions have been presented. Many of these hypotheses suggested that the 17-lactone has an important role in receptor binding. Using semisynthetic analogs, unsaturation in the lactone ring was discovered to be important, and the saturated lactone analog showed diminished activity (4,5). Further investigations of semisynthetic compounds in which the lactone was replaced with open-chain structures of varying electronic and steric resemblance to the lactone ring showed that the α,β-unsaturated lactone ring at C-17 was not an absolute requirement and that several α,β-unsaturated open-chain groups could be replaced with little or no loss in activity (4,5). For example, analogs possessing an α,β-unsaturated nitrile at the 17-β position had high activity. In light of this, most current theories point toward a key interaction of the carbonyl oxygen (or nitrile nitrogen) with the cardiac glycoside binding site on Na^+/K^+-ATPase (6,7).

Some controversy, however, exists regarding this point. The importance of the remainder of the cardiac glycoside molecule cannot be ignored. Despite the apparently dominant role of the 17-lactone, the steroid (A-B-C-D) ring system provides the lead structure for cardiac glycoside activity. Lactones, when not attached to the steroid ring system, show no Na^+/K^+-ATPase inhibitory activity. Some important steroid structural features have become apparent. The C-D *cis* ring juncture appears to be critical for activity in compounds possessing the unsaturated butyrolactone in the normal 17-β position. This requirement can be a reflection of changes in the spatial orientation of the 17-substituent (7). Moreover, the 14-β-OH is understood to be dispensable, and the contribution to activity previously attributed to this group is thought to be related to the need to retain the sp^3 and *cis* character of the C-D ring juncture. The earlier interpretation arose because the 14-deoxy analogs often had unsaturation in the D ring in place of the 14-β-OH. This double bond markedly influenced the position of the C-17 substituent, thereby complicating the importance of the 14-β-OH group on cardiotonic activity. Finally, the A-B *cis* ring juncture also appears not to be mandatory for cardiac glycoside activity. This feature, however, is characteristic of all clinically useful cardiac glycosides and conversion to an A-B *trans* ring system as a rule leads to a marked drop in activity unless compensating structural modifications are made elsewhere in the molecule.

Pharmaceutical Preparations The cardiac glycoside preparations that have been used therapeutically range from powdered digitalis leaf to purified individual glycosides, including gitalin, lanatoside C, its partially hydrolyzed product deslanatoside C (desacetyl lanatoside C), digoxin, and ouabain (Table 21.3). Digoxin is the only cardiac glycoside commercially available for therapeutic use in the United States. To arrive at an effective plasma concentration, a large initial dose of digoxin (i.e., digitalizing or loading dose) is often given. The purpose of this large initial dose is to achieve a therapeutic blood and tissue level in the shortest possible time. Depending on the condition of the patient and the desired therapeutic goal, the loading dose can be much less than, or almost equal to, the dose that is likely to cause toxicity. Once the desired effect is obtained, the amount of drug eliminated from the body per day is replaced with a maintenance dose.

Absorption, Metabolism, and Excretion The therapeutic effects of all cardiac glycosides on the heart muscle are qualitatively similar; however, the glycosides differ largely in their pharmacokinetic properties, which are greatly influenced by the lipophilic character of each glycoside. In general, cardiac glycosides with more lipophilic character are absorbed faster and exhibit a longer duration of action as a result of a slower urinary rate of excretion. The lipophilicity of a cardiac glycoside is measured by its partitioning between chloroform and water mixed with methanol: The higher the concentration of the cardiac glycoside in the chloroform phase, the higher its partition coefficient, and the more lipophilic it is. The partition coefficients for five cardiac glycosides are listed in Table 21.4. It is evident from a comparison of the coefficients that their lipophilicity is markedly influenced by the number of sugar molecules and the number of hydroxyl groups on the aglycone part of a given glycoside. Lanatoside C, with a partition coefficient of 16.2, is far less lipophilic than that of acetyldigoxin (partition coefficient, 98), which structurally differs only in lacking the terminal glucose molecule. Likewise, a comparison of digitoxin and digoxin structures reveals that they differ only by an extra hydroxyl in digoxin at C-12. This seemingly minor difference in their partition coefficients from 96.5 to 81.5 for digitoxin and digoxin, respectively, results in significant differences in their pharmacokinetic behavior (Table 21.5). Table 21.4 also illustrates that the presence of the 3-*O*-acetyl group on acetyldigoxin enhances its lipophilic character more than that of the desacetyl analog, digoxin (partition coefficients of 98 and 81.5, respectively). The glycoside G-strophanthin (ouabain) possesses a very low lipophilic character because of the presence of five free hydroxyl groups on the steroid nucleus of the aglycone ouabagenin.

Digoxin is the most frequently used cardiac glycoside. The absorption of digoxin from the gastrointestinal tract is a passive process that depends on the lipid solubility, dissolution, and membrane permeability of the drug. The oral bioavailability of digoxin following oral administration exhibits interindividual variability, ranging from 70% to 85% of an administered dose. This interindividual variability has been attributed to intestinal P-glycoprotein (P-gp) efflux and P-gp–dependent renal elimination. Although digoxin is not extensively metabolized, it is transported from intestinal enterocytes along its epithelium into the intestinal lumen (effluxed) by P-gp, which

TABLE 21.3 Cardiac Glycosides and Their Dosage Forms

Name[a]	Dosage Forms
Digoxin USP and BP	Tablets, elixir, pediatric
Digitalis powder (leaf) BP	Tablets, capsules
Digitoxin BP	Tablets, injection
Lanatoside C BP	Tablets
Ouabain BP	Injection (G-strophanthin)
Deslanatoside C BP	Injection (deacetyllanatoside C)

[a]Those cardiac glycosides with only the BP (British Pharmacopeia) designation are available only in Canada and other countries except the United States.

TABLE 21.4 Effect of Glycoside Structure on Partition Coefficient

Glycoside	Partition Coefficient ($CHCl_3$/16% aq.MeOH)
Lanatoside C (glucose-3-acetyldigitoxose–digitoxose$_2$–digoxigenin)	16.2
Digoxin (digitoxose$_3$-digoxigenin)	81.5
Digitoxin (digitoxose$_3$-digitoxigenin)	96.5
Acetyldigoxin (3-acetyldigitoxose-digitoxose$_2$-digoxigenin)	98.0
G-Strophanthin (rhamnose-ouabagenin)	Very low

TABLE 21.5 Comparison of the Pharmacokinetic Properties for Digoxin and Digitoxin

	Digoxin	Digitoxin
Gastrointestinal absorption	70%–85%	95%–100%
Average half-life	1–2 days	5–7 days
Protein binding	25%–30%	90%–95%
Enterohepatic cycling	5%	25%
Excretion	Kidneys; largely unchanged	Liver metabolism
Therapeutic plasma level	0.5–2.5 ng/mL	20–35 ng/mL
Digitalizing dose (mg)	Oral: 0.75–1.5 IV: 0.5–1.0	Oral: 0.8–1.2 IV: 0.8–1.2
Maintenance dose (oral mg)	0.125–0.5	0.05–0.2

IV, intravenous.

is also expressed in the kidney and liver. Alterations in P-gp transport can be the basis for several digoxin–drug interactions. For this reason, it is important to establish carefully the effective dose of digoxin for each patient to avoid digitalis toxicity.

Once the cardiac glycosides are absorbed, they bind to plasma proteins; digoxin has only 30% binding. The half-life of digoxin in patients with normal renal function is 1.5 to 2.0 days. Biliary excretion of digoxin is minimal. Digoxin is eliminated primarily unchanged by renal tubule excretion.

Contributing to the discontinuance of digitoxin as a therapeutic agent was a half-life range between 5 and 7 days because of its enterohepatic circulation. Approximately 25% of an absorbed dose of digitoxin is excreted in the bile unchanged, to be reabsorbed via enterohepatic circulation. Digitoxin, however, is extensively metabolized by the liver to a variety of metabolites, including (digitoxose)$_2$-digitoxigenin, (digitoxose)$_1$-digitoxigenin, and (digitoxose)$_1$-digitoxigenin. Trace amounts of digoxin have been discovered in the urine. The pharmacokinetic data for digoxin and digitoxin are summarized in Table 21.5.

Drug Interactions Digoxin–drug interactions are common causes of digitalis toxicity. Recently, the clinical significance of the P-gp–dependent renal tubular secretion of digoxin associated with the well-documented digoxin–quinidine interaction has been reported (8). The discovery that digoxin is actively secreted into the urine by the renal tubular cell via the P-gp efflux pump has led to the conclusion that the digoxin–quinidine interaction can be attributed to inhibition of renal tubular secretion of digoxin by quinidine (a P-gp substrate). Quinidine competitively binds to P-gp in the renal tubule, reducing the renal secretion of digoxin by as much as 60% and raising digoxin's plasma concentration to toxic levels. Other drugs that are substrates for renal P-gp are also likely to be associated with digoxin–drug interactions. Another documented digoxin–drug interaction associated with increased digoxin blood levels and toxicity is with verapamil. Unlike quinidine, verapamil inhibits intestinal P-gp efflux of digoxin, thereby blocking the intestinal secretion of digoxin into the lumen of the intestine and raising digoxin blood levels to toxic levels. On the other hand, the rifampin–digoxin interaction involves the rifampin induction of intestinal P-gp expression, thereby increasing the P-gp–mediated secretion of digoxin. This results in the lowering of digoxin blood levels to subtherapeutic concentrations. The P-gp transporters and their substrates, inhibitors, or inducers (see Table 4.16 for list) appear to play an important role in controlling the digoxin area under the curve (AUC) values through the renal tubular and intestinal secretion of digoxin and, subsequently, in digoxin–drug interactions and digitalis toxicity. Concurrent use of the cardiac glycosides with antiarrhythmics, sympathomimetics, β-adrenergic blockers, and calcium channel blockers, which are substrates for P-gp, can alter the control of arrhythmias.

The absorption of digoxin after oral administration can also be significantly altered by other drugs concurrently present in the gastrointestinal tract. For example, laxatives can interfere with the absorption of digoxin because of increased intestinal motility. The presence of the drug cholestyramine, an agent used to treat hyperlipoproteinemia, decreases the absorption of digoxin by binding to and retaining digoxin in the gastrointestinal tract. Antacids, especially magnesium trisilicate, and antidiarrheal adsorbent suspensions can also inhibit the absorption of the digoxin. Potassium-depleting diuretics, such as thiazides, can increase the possibility of digitalis toxicity because of the additive hypokalemia. Several other drugs that are known to bind to plasma proteins, such as thyroid hormones, have the potential to displace digoxin from its plasma-binding sites, thereby increasing its free drug concentration to a toxic level.

Therapeutic Uses Although the primary clinical use for digoxin is in the treatment of CHF, this agent is also used in cases of atrial flutter or fibrillation and paroxysmal atrial tachycardia.

Toxicity All cardiac glycosides preparations have the potential to cause toxicity. Because the minimal toxic dose of the glycosides is only two- to threefold the therapeutic dose, intoxication is quite common. In mild to moderate toxicity, the common symptoms are anorexia, nausea and vomiting, muscular weakness, bradycardia, and ventricular premature contractions. The nausea is a result of excitation of the chemoreceptor trigger zone in the medulla. In severe toxicity, the common symptoms are blurred vision, disorientation, diarrhea, ventricular tachycardia, and AV block, which can progress into ventricular fibrillation. It is usually accepted that the toxicity of the cardiac glycosides results from inhibition of the Na^+/K^+-ATPase pump, which results in increased intracellular levels of Ca^{2+}. Hypokalemia (decreased potassium), which can be induced by coadministration of thiazide diuretics, of glucocorticoids, or by other means, can be an important factor in initiating a toxic response. It has been shown that low levels of extracellular K^+ partially inhibit the Na^+/K^+-ATPase pump. In a patient stabilized on a cardiac glycoside, the Na^+/K^+-ATPase pump is already partially inhibited, and the hypokalemia only further inhibits the pump, causing an intracellular buildup of sodium, which leads to an increase in intracellular calcium levels. The high levels of calcium are responsible for the observed cardiac arrhythmias characteristic of the cardiac glycosides toxicity.

A common procedure used in treating cardiac glycoside toxicity is to administer potassium salts to increase extracellular potassium level, which stimulates the Na^+/K^+-ATPase pump, resulting in decreased intracellular sodium levels and, thus, decreased intracellular calcium. In treating any cardiac glycoside–induced toxicity, it is important to discontinue administration of the drug in addition to administering a potassium salt, such as potassium chloride. Other drugs that can be useful in treating the tachyarrhythmias present during toxicity are lidocaine, phenytoin, and propranolol. Specific antibodies directed toward digoxin (Dig-Bind) have been used experimentally and proven to be very effective.

Metildigoxin

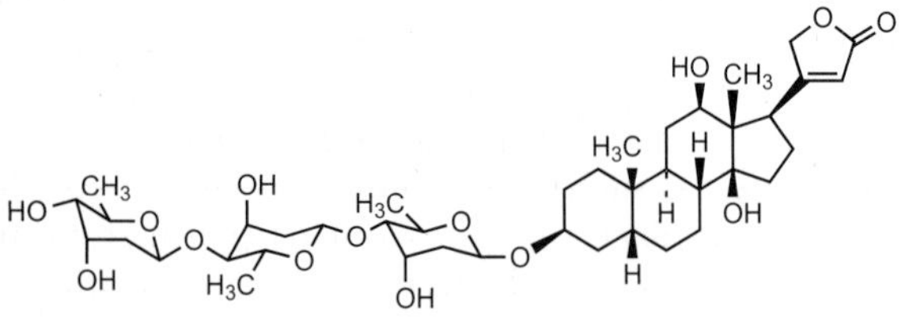

Digoxin

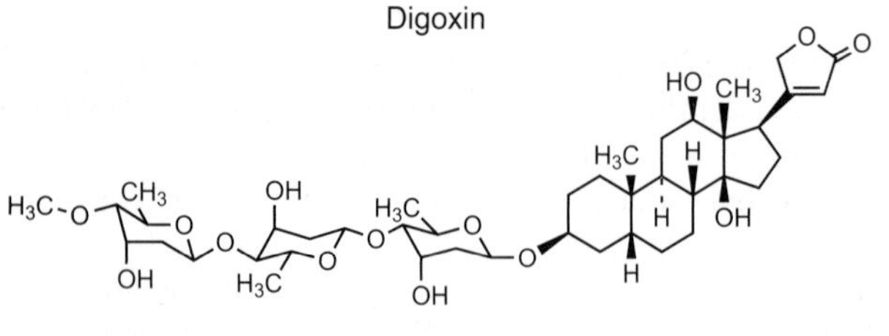

Metildigoxin

The drug is a semisynthetic derivative of digoxin, but with a methoxy group attached at position 4 of the terminal digitoxose molecule. The drug is marketed only in Europe and has not been approved by the U.S. Food and Drug Administration (FDA). The major advantage of metildigoxin over digoxin is its rapid and complete absorption after oral administration. After oral administration, some demethylation to digoxin occurs, but 60% of the administered dose (oral or injection) is excreted in urine unchanged.

Nonglycosidic Positive Inotropic Agents Nonglycosidic positive inotropic drugs can be divided into two main classes: those that act via stimulating the synthesis of cyclic adenosine monophosphate (cAMP), such as adrenergic and dopaminergic agonists; and those that inhibit the hydrolysis of cAMP, such as phosphodiesterase 3 (PDE3) inhibitors.

Phosphodiesterase 3 Inhibitors The mechanism of cardiac contraction involves a G protein signal transduction pathway, which regulates intracellular calcium concentrations. Activation of the G_s protein involves the formation of intracellular cAMP, which thereby increases intracellular calcium, stimulating cardiac muscle contraction. Relaxation occurs when the released cAMP is hydrolyzed by cytosolic cAMP-dependent PDE3, one of the phosphodiesterase isoforms. Therefore, inhibition of PDE3 increases intracellular cAMP, promoting cardiac muscle contraction but vasodilation of vascular smooth muscle.

The overall cardiostimulatory and vasodilatory actions of PDE3 inhibitors make them suitable for the treatment of heart failure, because vascular smooth muscle relaxation reduces ventricular wall stress and the oxygen demands placed on the failing heart. The cardiostimulatory effects of the PDE3 inhibitors increase inotropy, which further enhances stroke volume and ejection fraction. Clinical trials have shown that long-term therapy with PDE3 inhibitors increases mortality in heart failure patients. Therefore, these PDE3 inhibitors are not used for the long-term, chronic therapy of CHF. They are very useful, however, in treating acute, decompensated heart failure or temporary bouts of decompensated chronic failure. They are not used as a monotherapy. Instead, they are used in conjunction with other treatment modalities, such as diuretics, angiotensin-converting enzyme inhibitors, β-blockers, or cardiac glycosides. The PDE3 inhibitors contract cardiac muscle and are used for treating heart failure, whereas the phosphodiesterase 5 (PDE5) inhibitors are vasodilators and are also used for treating male erectile dysfunction (Chapter 40). Note that the generic names for PDE3 inhibitors end in "one," and those for the PDE5 inhibitors end in "fil."

Side Effects and Contraindications. The most common and severe side effects of PDE3 inhibitors are ventricular arrhythmias, some of which can be life threatening. Other side effects included headaches and hypotension, which are not uncommon for drugs that increase cAMP in cardiac and vascular tissues, with other examples being β-agonists.

Milrinone (Primacor) and Inamrinone (Inocor). Although the digitalis glycosides can be the principal therapeutic agents for the treatment of CHF, they are not the only positive inotropic agents available. Among the "nonglycoside" inotropic agents are the bipyridines, inamrinone and milrinone, which are selective PDE3 inhibitors (Fig. 21.4). Inamrinone and milrinone are positive inotropes and vasodilators indicated for the short-term intravenous management of CHF in patients who have not responded adequately to digitalis, diuretics, and/or vasodilators (9,10). Milrinone is the drug of choice from among the currently available PDE3 inhibitors because of its greater selectivity for PDE3, shorter half-life (30 to 60 minutes), and fewer side effects. Inamrinone is associated with thrombocytopenia in 10% of patients. Inamrinone was introduced in 1978, and it produces both positive inotropic and concentration-dependent vasodilatory effects. Despite similar positive inotropic action to the cardiac glycosides, the inotropic action involves inhibition of PDE3. Inamrinone was approved for the short-term intravenous administration in patients with severe heart failure refractory to other measures. Although inamrinone is orally active, several adverse side effects have dampened enthusiasm for long-term oral inamrinone therapy. These effects include gastrointestinal disturbances, thrombocytopenia, and impairment of the liver function. For intravenous infusion, inamrinone lactate and milrinone lactate injection solutions can be diluted in sodium chloride injection. Inamrinone lactate for injection is preserved with sodium metabisulfite and needs protection from light. It should not be diluted with solutions containing dextrose because a chemical reaction occurs in 24 hours. For milrinone, an immediate chemical interaction with furosemide with the formation of a precipitate is observed when furosemide is injected into an infusion of milrinone. Patients sensitive to bisulfites can also be sensitive to inamrinone lactate injection, which contains sodium metabisulfite.

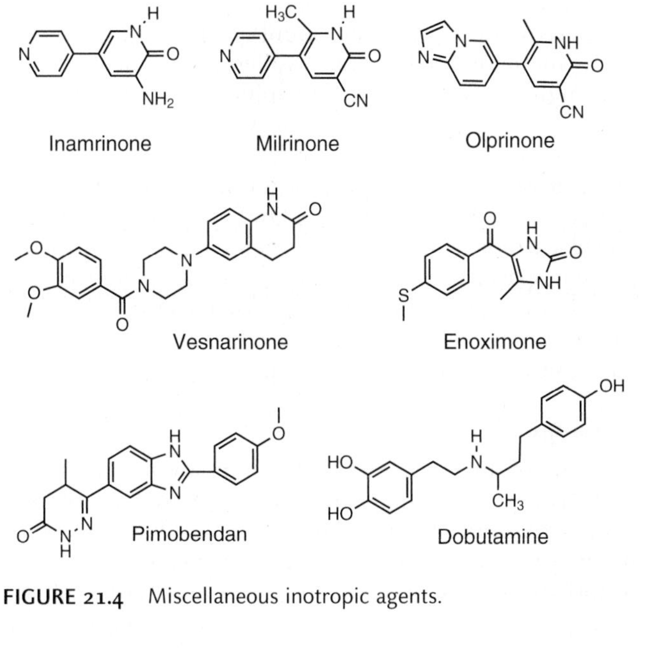

FIGURE 21.4 Miscellaneous inotropic agents.

The pharmacokinetics for inamrinone shows a half-life in healthy volunteers of approximately 3 to 4 hours, whereas in patients with CHF, the plasma half-life increases approximately 50% (5 to 8 hours). For infants younger than 4 weeks, the half-life life is 12.7 to 22.2 hours, and for infants older than 4 weeks, the half-life is 3.8 to 6.8 hours. Time to peak effect is less than 10 minutes, with its duration of action ranging from 30 minutes to 2 hours depending on the dosage. Approximately 63% of inamrinone is eliminated via the urine as unchanged drug, and 18% is eliminated in the feces. Elderly patients are more likely to have age-related impairment of renal function, which can require adjustment of dosage in patients receiving inamrinone.

The limited success of inamrinone led to the development of structurally related newer agents, such as milrinone, with a mechanism of action similar to inamrinone. Milrinone, however, is 10-fold more potent than inamrinone. Furthermore, preliminary reports show milrinone to be better tolerated, with no apparent thrombocytopenia or gastrointestinal disturbances. Milrinone is excreted largely unchanged in the urine, and accordingly, patients with impaired renal function require reduced dosages.

The pharmacokinetics for milrinone following intravenous injections to patients with CHF showed an elimination half-life of 2 to 3 hours. Its primary route of excretion is via the urine as unchanged milrinone (83%) and its *O*-glucuronide metabolite (12%). In patients with renal function impairment, elimination of unchanged milrinone is reduced, suggesting that a dosage adjustment can be necessary.

Phosphodiesterase 3 Inhibitors not Approved by FDA

Enoximone. Enoximone is a selective PDE3 inhibitor with vasodilating and positive inotropic activity that does not cause changes in myocardial oxygen consumption. It is used in patients with CHF. US clinical trials were halted because of significant adverse effects on the nervous system. The drug is approved for use in the United Kingdom, with an oral bioavailability of 50% and 85% protein binding. The drug is not recommended for long-term use and is given only by injection for short-term use.

Olprinone. Olprinone has positive inotropic and vasodilator effects, which improve myocardial mechanical efficiency. Additionally, the drug augments cerebral blood flow by a direct vasodilatory effect on cerebral arteries, especially in patients with impaired cerebral circulation. Olprinone improves inadequate redistribution of brain perfusion and may prevent cerebral metabolic abnormalities in heart failure. The drug is given intravenously during acute heart failure. The drug is currently marketed in Japan.

Vesnarinone. This drug is a mixed PDE3 inhibitor and ion channel modifier with modest, dose-dependent, positive inotropic activity but minimal negative chronotropic activity. Vesnarinone improves ventricular performance most in patients with the worst degree of heart failure. The drug was withdrawn from US phase III clinical trials but is marketed in Japan.

Pimobendan. Pimobendan is a selective inhibitor of PDE3, as well as a calcium sensitizer with positive inotropic and vasodilator effects. It is marketed in Japan for human use and also approved for the management of heart failure in dogs, most commonly caused endocardiosis or dilated cardiomyopathy. As a calcium sensitizer, it increases the binding efficiency of cardiac myofibrils to the calcium ions that are already present without increasing the consumption of oxygen and energy. These effects result in decreased pressure and decreased cardiac preload and afterload (decreases the failing heart's workload). Pimobendan is absorbed rapidly, with an oral bioavailability of 60% to 65%, and metabolized by the liver to an active metabolite. The plasma half-life is 0.5 hours, and the half-life of its metabolite is 2 hours. Elimination is by excretion in the bile and then feces. Pimobendan is 90% to 95% bound to plasma proteins in circulation, which has implications in patients who are on concurrent drug therapies that are also highly protein bound. The drug is used as an adjunct therapy with other agents, and as is the case with other phosphodiesterase inhibitors, prolonged use is reported to cause an increase in mortality rate.

β-Adrenergic Receptor Agonists Another promising area for the development of new positive inotropic agents is β-adrenergic receptor agonists (11) (see Chapter 10). The myocardium has mostly β_1-adrenergic receptors, and stimulation of these receptors by a variety of β-adrenergic agonists produces a potent positive inotropic response involving the G protein signal transduction process, increasing intracellular cAMP levels that lead to a cascade of events that ultimately produces an increase in intracellular Ca^{2+}, thereby increasing myocardial contractility (discussed in Chapters 7 and 10). Although many drugs possess β-adrenergic agonist activity, most have side effects that make them inappropriate for the treatment of CHF. For example, the well-known catecholamines, norepinephrine and epinephrine, are potent nonselective adrenergic receptor agonists. Because the actions of these agents are not limited to the myocardial β_1-receptors, however, they produce undesirable positive chronotropic effects, exacerbate arrhythmias, and result in vasoconstriction. These effects limit their utility in the treatment of CHF.

Dobutamine (Dobutrex). Among the most promising β_1-adrenergic agonists are those derived from dopamine, the endogenous precursor to norepinephrine. Dopamine is a potent stimulator of β_1-receptors, but with many of the undesirable side effects described in Chapter 10. The new analogs of dopamine that have been developed retain the potent inotropic effect but possess fewer effects on heart rate, vascular tone, and arrhythmias. Dobutamine is a prime representative of this group of agents. Dobutamine is a potent β_1-adrenergic agonist on the myocardium (as well as having α_1-agonist and -antagonist activities; see Chapter 10 for details concerning its mechanism of action) with beneficial effects, the composite of a variety of actions on the heart and the peripheral vasculature. Dobutamine is active only by the intravenous route because of its rapid first-pass metabolism via catechol-*O*-methyltransferase (COMT). Therefore, its use is limited to critical care situations. Nonetheless, its parenteral success has led to the search and development of orally active drugs. One of the major limitations associated with β_1-agonists is the phenomenon of myocardial β-receptor desensitization. This lowered responsiveness (desensitization) of the receptors appears to be due to a decrease in the number of β_1-receptors and partial uncoupling of the receptors from adenylate cyclase.

DRUGS FOR THE TREATMENT OF ANGINA

Angina Pectoris

Angina pectoris is the chronic disease affecting the coronary arteries, which supply oxygenated blood from the left ventricle to all heart tissues, including the ventricles themselves. When the lumen of the coronary artery becomes restricted, it becomes less efficient in supplying blood and oxygen to the heart, and the heart is said to be "ischemic" (oxygen deficient). Angina is the primary symptom of ischemic heart disease and is characterized by a sudden, severe pain originating in the chest, often radiating to the left shoulder and down the left arm. Angina is further subclassified into typical or variant angina based on the precipitating factors and the electrophysiologic changes observed during the attack. Typical angina is the result of an advanced state of atherosclerosis and is provoked by food, exercise, and emotional factors. It is characterized by low ST segment of the electrocardiogram. Variant or acute angina results from sudden spasm in the coronary artery unrelated to atherosclerotic narrowing of the coronary circulation and can occur at rest. It is characterized by an increase in the ST segment of the electrocardiogram.

Antianginal Drugs

Therapy of angina is directed mainly toward alleviating and preventing anginal attacks by altering the oxygen supply/oxygen demand ratio to the cardiac muscle or dilating the coronary vessels. Three classes of drugs are found to be very efficient in this regard, although via different mechanisms. These include organic nitrates, calcium channel blockers, and β-adrenergic blockers.

Organic Nitrates

Organic nitrates have dominated the treatment of acute angina over the last 100 years. Although the recent introduction of the calcium channel blockers and the β-blockers as antianginal agents has expanded the physician therapeutic arsenal, organic nitrates are still the class of choice in the treatment of acute anginal episodes.

Overview Organic nitrates are esters of simple organic alcohols or polyols with nitric acid. This class was developed after the antianginal effect of amyl nitrite (ester of isoamyl alcohol with nitrous acid) was first observed in 1857. Five members of this class are in clinical use today: amyl nitrite (amyl nitrite inhalant USP), nitroglycerin, isosorbide dinitrate, erythrityl tetranitrate, and pentaerythritol tetranitrate (Fig. 21.5). Two additional organic nitrates, tenitramine and propatylnitrate, are currently available in Europe (Fig. 21.5). This class is, as a rule, referred to as organic nitrates, because all of these agents, except amyl nitrite, are nitrate esters. It should be noted that the generic names do not always precisely describe the chemical nature of the drug but, rather, are used for simplicity. For example, the drug nitroglycerin is not really a nitro compound, because a nitro compound means a nitro group attached to a carbon atom (i.e., NO_2-C); the correct chemical name of nitroglycerin is glyceryltrinitrate. Another example is amyl nitrite, the structure of which indicates that it is an ester of isoamyl alcohol with nitrous acid; the correct chemical name of this drug is isoamyl nitrite.

The chemical nature of these molecules as esters constitutes some problems in formulating these agents for clinical use. The small lipophilic ester character makes them volatile. Volatility is an important concern in drug formulation because of the potential loss of the active principle from the dosage form. In addition, moisture should be avoided during storage to minimize the hydrolysis of the ester bond, which can lead to a decrease in the therapeutic effectiveness. Lastly, because these agents are nitrate esters, they possess explosive properties, especially in the pure concentrated form. Dilution in a variety of vehicles and excipients eliminates this potential hazard. The lipophilic nature of these esters, however, makes these agents very efficient in emergency treatment of anginal episodes as a result of their rapid absorption through biomembranes.

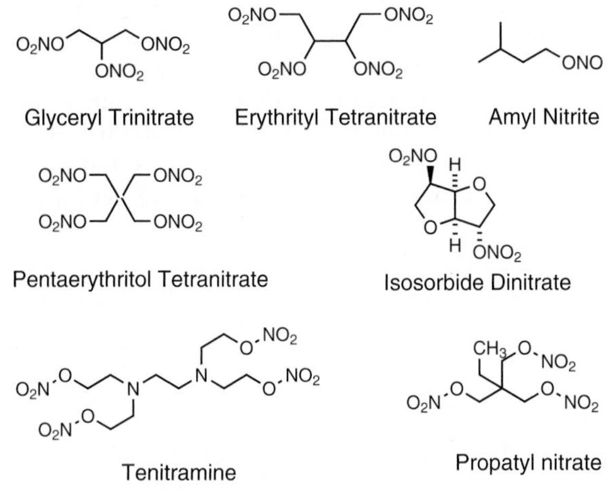

FIGURE 21.5 Organic nitrates and nitrites.

Pharmacologic Actions The oxygen requirements of the myocardial tissues are related to the workload (oxygen demand) of the heart, which is, in part, a function of the heart rate, the systolic pressure, and the peripheral resistance of the blood flow (oxygen supply). Myocardial ischemia occurs when the oxygen supply is insufficient to meet the myocardial oxygen demand. This can occur, as explained previously, because of atherosclerotic narrowing of the coronary circulation (typical) or vasospasm of the coronary artery (variant). The nitrates have been shown to be effective in treating angina resulting from either cause. The vasodilating effect of organic nitrates on the veins leads to pooling of the blood in the veins and decreased venous return to the heart (decreased preload), whereas vasodilation of the coronary arterioles decreases the resistance of the peripheral tissues (decreased afterload). The decrease in both preload and afterload results in a generalized decrease in the myocardial workload, which translates into a reduced oxygen demand by the myocardium. Organic nitrates restore the balance between oxygen supply by venous dilation and oxygen demand by decreasing the myocardial workload.

Biochemical Mechanism of Action The organic nitrates (Fig. 21.5) are pharmacologic sources of nitric oxide (NO) for the body. In the cardiovascular system, NO is naturally produced by vascular endothelial cells. This endothelial-derived NO has several important functions, including relaxation of vascular smooth muscle, inhibition of platelet aggregation (antithrombotic), and inhibition of leukocyte–endothelial interactions (anti-inflammatory). These actions involve NO-stimulated formation of cyclic guanosine monophosphate (cGMP) (see Chapter 24). Nitrodilators are drugs that mimic the actions of endogenous NO by releasing NO or forming NO within tissues. Free tissue sulfhydryl groups play a key role in the venodilation effect of nitroglycerin, which is supported by experimental evidence showing that prior administration of *N*-acetylcysteine, which should increase the availability of free sulfhydryl groups, resulted in an increase in the venodilating effect of organic nitrates. Similarly, pretreatment with reagents that react with free sulfhydryl groups, such as ethacrynic acid, blocked glyceryl trinitrate venodilation in vitro (12). A more complex mechanism for nitrate venodilation, however, was proposed by Ignarro et al. (14). They suggested that the nitrates act indirectly, by stimulating the enzyme guanylate (also known as guanylyl) cyclase and, thereby, producing elevated levels of cGMP, which in turn leads to venodilation. The initial stimulation of soluble guanylate cyclase is believed to be mediated by a nitrate-derived nitrosothiol metabolite produced intracellularly. In support of this mechanism is the observation that a variety of synthetic nitrosothiols were found to increase markedly soluble guanylate cyclase activity and to produce venodilation in vitro (15–19). Such a mechanism is consistent with the requirement for free sulfhydryl groups previously described. A unifying mechanism suggests that the organic nitrates, through the formation of NO via a nitrosothiol-intermediate, activate soluble guanylate cyclase, increasing intracellular cGMP concentrations, which in turn blocks the Ca^{2+}-catalyzed vascular contractions (Fig. 24.3) (20–23). Depletion of sulfhydryl groups during this metabolic process can be a major factor in the development of nitrate tolerance, along with compensatory physiologic mechanisms (13). Data also exist suggesting that organic nitrates increase intraplatelet cGMP concentrations, thereby inhibiting platelet aggregation. These pharmacologic actions of organic nitrates appear to preferentially occur within portions of blood vessels containing damaged endothelium, thus making them extremely useful in the pharmacotherapy of acute ischemic events.

Pharmaceutical Preparations and Dosage Forms Organic nitrates are administered by inhalation; by infusion; as sublingual, chewable, and sustained-release tablets; as capsules; as transdermal disks; and as ointments.

Absorption, Metabolism, and Therapeutic Effects Organic nitrates are used for both treatment and prevention of painful anginal attacks. The therapeutic approaches to achieve these two goals, however, are distinctly different. For the treatment of acute anginal attacks (i.e., attacks that have already begun), a rapid-acting preparation is required. In contrast, preventative therapy requires a long-acting preparation with more emphasis on duration and less emphasis on onset. The onset of organic nitrate action is influenced not only by the specific agent chosen but also by the route of administration. Sublingual administration is used predominantly for a rapid onset of action. The duration of nitrate action is strongly influenced by rate of metabolism. All of the organic nitrates are subject to rapid first-pass metabolism not only by the action of glutathione-nitrate reductase in the liver, but also in extrahepatic tissues, such as the blood vessel walls themselves (24,25). In addition, rapid uptake into the vessel walls plays a significant role in the rapid disappearance of organic nitrates from the bloodstream. Sublingual, transdermal, and buccal administration routes have been used in an attempt to avoid at least some of the hepatic metabolism.

Acute angina is most frequently treated with sublingual glyceryl trinitrate. This sublingual preparation is rapidly absorbed from the sublingual, lingual, and buccal mucosa and most commonly provides relief within 2 minutes. The duration of action is also short (~30 minutes). Other treatments include amyl nitrite by inhalation and sublingual isosorbide dinitrate. Amyl nitrite is by far the fastest-acting preparation, with an onset of action in approximately 15 to 30 seconds, but the duration of action is only approximately 1 minute. Isosorbide dinitrate is used as a long-acting agent and can be used to treat acute angina. Sublingually administered isosorbide dinitrate has a somewhat slower onset than glyceryl trinitrate (~3 minutes), but its action can last for 4 to 6 hours. Although the onset appears to be almost as rapid as that of glyceryl trinitrate, waiting an additional minute for relief can be deemed unacceptable by some patients.

To prevent recurring angina, long-acting organic nitrate preparations are used. Several agents fall into this category, such as orally administered isosorbide dinitrate, pentaerythritol tetranitrate, and erythrityl tetranitrate. In addition, a number of long-acting glyceryl trinitrate preparations are available. These include oral sustained-release forms, glyceryl trinitrate ointment, transdermal patches, and buccal tablets. Of these therapeutic options, isosorbide dinitrate and glyceryl trinitrate preparations are by far the most frequently used. At first, the whole concept of prophylactic nitrate use was met with skepticism by many physicians, both because early studies indicated that oral nitrates were almost completely broken down by first-pass metabolism (24,25) and because blood levels of the parent drug appeared to be virtually nil. These findings, in conjunction with several clinical studies showing equivocal efficacy, led Needleman et al. (25) to conclude, "There is no rational basis for the use of 'long-acting' nitrates (administered orally) in the prophylactic therapy of angina pectoris." More recent studies, however, suggest that oral prophylactic nitrates can be effective if appropriate doses are used (26). Moreover, some metabolites of long-acting nitrates are active as venodilators, albeit less potent than the parent drug. An example of this is isosorbide dinitrate, which is metabolized primarily in the liver by glutathione-nitrate reductase, which also participates in the metabolism of other organic nitrates, catalyzing the denitration of the parent drug to yield two metabolites, 2- and 5-isosorbide mononitrate (27). Of these, the 5-isomer is still a potent vasodilator, and its plasma half-life of approximately 4.5 hours is much longer than that of isosorbide dinitrate itself. The extended half-life, because of the metabolite's resistance to further metabolism, indicates that it can be contributing to the prolonged duration of action associated with use of isosorbide dinitrate (27).

Adverse Effects Most patients tolerate the nitrates fairly well. Headache and postural hypotension are the most common side effects of organic nitrates. Dizziness, nausea, vomiting, rapid pulse, and restlessness are among the additional side effects reported. These symptoms can be controlled by administering low doses initially and then gradually increasing the dose. Fortunately, tolerance to nitrate-induced headache develops after a few days of therapy. Because postural hypotension can occur in some individuals, advise the patient to sit down when taking a rapid-acting nitrate preparation for the first time. An effective dose of nitrate as a rule produces a fall in upright systolic pressure of 10 mm Hg and a reflex rise in heart rate of 10 beats per minute.

Another concern associated with prophylactic nitrate use is the development of tolerance (26,28). Tolerance, usually in the form of a shortened duration of action, is commonly observed with chronic nitrate use. The clinical importance of this tolerance is, however, a matter of controversy. Because tolerance to nitrates has not been reported to lead to a total loss of activity, some physicians feel that it is not clinically relevant. In addition, an adjustment in dosage can compensate for the reduced response (26). It has also been reported that intermittent use of long-acting and sustained-release preparations can limit the extent of tolerance development.

Drug Interactions The most significant interactions of organic nitrates are with those agents that cause hypotension, such as other vasodilators, alcohol, and tricyclic antidepressants, in which the potential for orthostatic hypotension can arise. On the other hand, concurrent administration with sympathomimetic amines, such as ephedrine and norepinephrine, can lead to a decrease in the antianginal efficacy of the organic nitrates.

Potassium Channel Opener

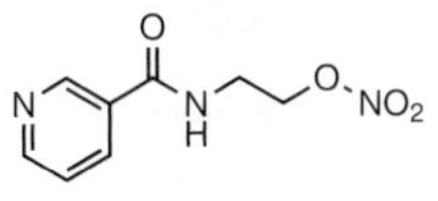

Nicorandil

Nicorandil is a nicotinamide-nitrate ester (Fig. 21.5) used for the treatment of angina pectoris and CHF in the United Kingdom and Europe, but is not approved by the FDA. It has a dual mechanism of action, and structurally, it is a hybrid between organic nitrates and potassium channel activators. Nicorandil, a nicotinamide derivative with a nitrate moiety, combines the smooth muscle–relaxing property of both nitrates and nicotinamide with its ability to increase potassium ion conductance. As a result, nicorandil has a direct (preload and afterload) vasodilating effect on normal and diseased coronary arteries and peripheral vessels. Although nicorandil contains a nitrate moiety, its pharmacologic properties differ from organic nitrates. The nicotinamide moiety is responsible for the effect on K^+-adenosine triphosphate (ATP) channels, which produces vascular smooth muscle relaxation by increasing potassium flux through ATP-sensitive sarcolemmal potassium channels. This leads to hyperpolarization of the cell membrane and subsequent decreases in levels of cytoplasmic calcium (calcium channel blockade) and dilation of arterial resistance vessels. Other agents in this class are minoxidil and diazoxide. The nitrate group explains its NO-like vasodilation on large coronary arteries, whereas its potassium channel–opening action is responsible for the dilatation of coronary resistance vessels, enabling it to decrease both preload and afterload and to increase coronary blood flow.

Nicorandil induces nitrate-like activation of soluble guanylate cyclase, increasing intracellular levels of cGMP with resultant dilation of venous capacitance vessels. Increases in cGMP are less than those observed with conventional nitrates, although the degree of vasodilation produced appears to be similar. Its oral bioavailability ranges from 75% to 80%. Food reduces the rate, but not the extent, of absorption. Nicorandil is extensively metabolized via denitration to inactive *N*-(2-hydroxyethyl)-nicotinamide, which undergoes further side-chain degradation to nicotinuric acid and, subsequently, nicotinamide and nicotinamide metabolites (e.g., nicotinic acid and *N*-methylnicotinamide). The nicotinamide derived from nicorandil merges into the endogenous pool of nicotinamide adenine dinucleoside coenzymes. Its elimination half-life is approximately 1 hour. Approximately 30% of nicorandil is excreted into the urine as metabolites, with less than 1% excreted unchanged.

Nitric Oxide Donor

Molsidomine (Corvaton) is an oral NO donor vasodilator known as a sydnone imine, a mesoionic compound that is soluble in both water and organic solvents.

Molsidomine is enzymatically metabolized by liver esterases to its active metabolite, linsodimine, which is spontaneously converted in the blood into its nitroso metabolite SIN-1A (Fig. 21.6). Molecular oxygen is required to release NO from SIN-1A. The beneficial effects of molsidomine in treatment of angina were recognized before the role of endogenous NO for causing vasodilation was identified. A possible explanation can revolve around activation of K^+ channels. Molsidomine has a slower onset and longer duration of action than conventional nitrates because of the relatively slow rate of conversion to linsodimine, which has a rapid onset and short duration of action. NO acts as a cellular messenger, leading to activation of soluble guanylate cyclase to

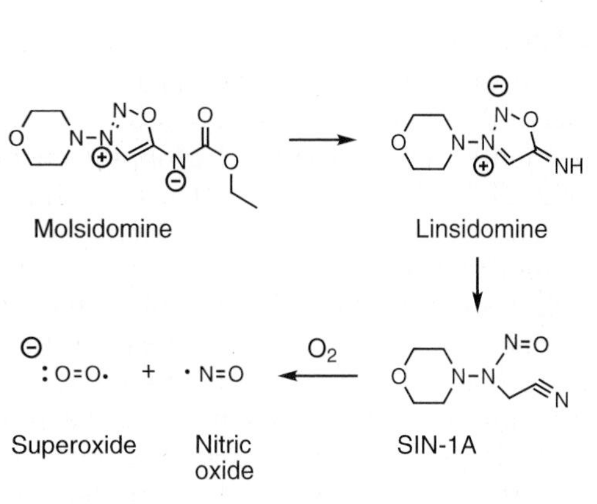

FIGURE 21.6 Molsidomine metabolism to nitric oxide.

release cGMP (see Chapter 24) and vasodilation. Because the metabolites of molsidomine generate NO without the need for enzymes or cofactors, other than the presence of oxygen, tolerance to prolonged exposure does not occur. This mechanism differs from organic nitrates in which cysteine or thiol donors are required for conversion into NO. It is believed that cysteine depletion is the major factor in the development of nitrate tolerance.

Molsidomine and lindosimine are therapeutic alternatives to traditional organic nitrates in treatment of stable angina, coronary vasospasm, and heart failure. Unlike organic nitrates, however, molsidomine and lindosimine have significant antiplatelet activity at therapeutic doses. The cogeneration of superoxide during the release of NO is a major concern limiting its therapeutic potential in the treatment of angina. Its short duration of action necessitates an increased dose frequency, which might be inconvenient in a clinical setting. The light sensitivity of molsidomine necessitates careful protection of infusion bags and tubing during administration.

The pharmacokinetics for molsidomine show 95% oral bioavailability, a plasma elimination half-life of approximately 5 hours (approximately 7 to 8 hours in the elderly), and volume of distribution of 98 L; 95% of the drug is renally eliminated. The pharmacokinetics and metabolism of molsidomine are impaired in the elderly, and thus, caution is warranted.

Calcium Channel Blockers

The second major therapeutic approach to the treatment of angina is the use of calcium channel blockers (29,30) (see also the corresponding subsection in Chapter 23). In the 1906s, it was recognized that inhibition of calcium ion (Ca^{2+}) influx into myocardial cells can be advantageous in preventing angina. Currently, the classes of calcium channel blockers approved for use in the prophylactic treatment of angina include the dihydropyridines nifedipine, nicardipine, and amlodipine; the benzothiazepine derivative diltiazem; the aralkyl amine derivative verapamil; the benzazepinone zatebradine, and the diaminopropanol ether bepridil (Fig. 21.7). These classes of drugs are reserved for treatment failures because serious arrhythmias can occur.

Zatebradine

The investigational drug zatebradine is structurally related to verapamil with a benzazepinone moiety replacing one of the dimethoxyphenyl groups seen in verapamil (Fig. 21.7). Despite its close structural similarity to verapamil, the drug has not been proven to have calcium channel–blocking activity or any effects on blood vessels. Zatebradine is reported to selectivity block the SA node and to reduce the hyperpolarization phase of the action potential with a net result of strong bradycardiac effects, hence its value in treating patients with stable angina. Zatebradine is available as oral tablets and as an oral solution. After oral administration, the drug has high oral absorption, undergoes hepatic first-pass metabolism, and

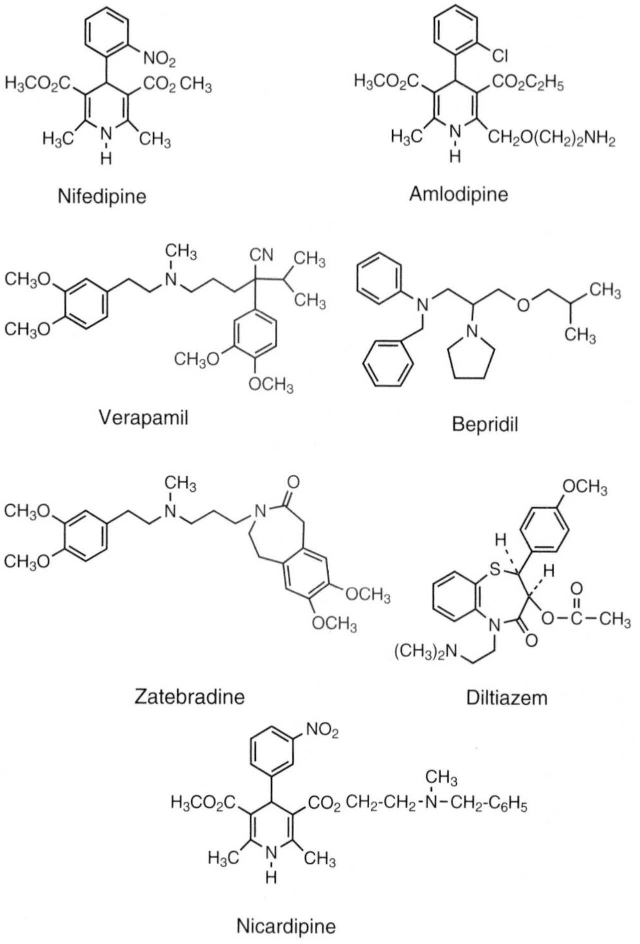

FIGURE 21.7 Calcium channel blockers.

is excreted in feces (40%). Several reports indicated that the drug causes severe visual adverse effects that may limit its clinical use for angina therapy.

Chemistry

The structural dissimilarity of these agents is apparent and serves to emphasize the fact that each is distinctly different from the others in its profile of effects. Although nifedipine and similar drugs belong to the dihydropyridine family, diltiazem belongs to the benzo[b-1,5]thiazepine family. Verapamil is structurally characterized by a central basic nitrogen to which alkyl and aralkyl groups are attached. It is noteworthy that diltiazem and verapamil are both chiral, possessing asymmetric centers. In each case, the dextro-rotatory [i.e., the (+)-enantiomer] is approximately one order of magnitude more potent as a calcium channel blocker than the levo-rotatory [i.e., (−)-enantiomer]. Zatebradine substitutes one of the dimethoxyphenyl moieties of verapamil with a benzazepinone group.

Pharmacologic Effects

Calcium ions are known to play a critical role in many physiologic functions. Physiologic calcium is found in a variety of locations, both intracellular and extracellular. Because calcium plays such a ubiquitous role in normal physiology, the overall therapeutic effect of the calcium channel blockers is often the composite of numerous pharmacologic actions in a variety of tissues. The most important of these tissues associated with angina are the myocardium and the arterial vascular bed. Because of the dependency of myocardial contraction on calcium, these drugs have a negative inotropic effect on the heart. Vascular smooth muscle depends also on calcium influx for contraction. Although the underlying mechanism is somewhat different, inhibition of calcium channel influx into the vascular smooth muscles by the calcium channel blockers leads to arteriolar vasodilation. The venous beds appear to be less affected by the calcium channel blockers. The negative inotropic effect and arterial vasodilation result in decreased heart workload and afterload, respectively. The preload is not affected because of a lesser sensitivity of the venous bed to the calcium channel blockers.

Mechanism of Action

The depolarization and contraction of the myocardial cells are mediated, in part, by calcium influx. As previously explained, the overall process consists of two distinct, inward ion currents: First, sodium ions flow rapidly into the cell through the "fast channels," and subsequently, calcium enters more slowly through the "slow channels." The calcium ions trigger contraction indirectly by binding and inhibiting troponin, a natural suppressor of the contractile process. Once the inhibitory effect of troponin is removed, actin and myosin can interact to produce the contractile response. The calcium channel blockers produce a negative inotropic effect by interrupting the contractile response. In vascular smooth muscles, calcium causes constriction by binding to a specific intracellular protein calmodulin to form a complex that initiates the process of vascular constriction. The calcium channel blockers inhibit vascular smooth muscle contraction by depriving the cell from the calcium ions.

The effects of the different classes of calcium channel blockers on the myocardium and the arteries vary from class to class. Although verapamil and diltiazem affect both the heart and the arteriolar bed, the dihydropyridines have much less effect on the cardiac tissues and higher specificity for the arteriolar vascular bed. Therefore, both verapamil and diltiazem are used clinically in the management of angina, hypertension, and cardiac arrhythmia, whereas the dihydropyridines are used more frequently as antianginal and antihypertensive agents. Because nicardipine has a less negative inotropic effect than nifedipine, it can be preferred over nifedipine for patients with angina pectoris or hypertension who have also CHF dysfunction.

The recognition of the pivotal role of calcium flux on biologic functions led to the reexamination of several therapeutic agents already in clinical use to see if their effects were also mediated through calcium-dependent mechanisms. Interestingly, many drugs were found to influence calcium movement and availability. In many cases, however, this effect was not found to contribute significantly to the desirable pharmacologic activity, with other mechanisms playing more dominant roles.

Pharmaceutical Preparations

Calcium channel blockers are administered as oral tablets and capsules as regular or sustained-release forms. Verapamil and diltiazem are also administered by injection.

Absorption, Metabolism, and Excretion

The calcium channel blockers are rapidly and completely absorbed after oral administration (see Table 25.11 for summary of their pharmacokinetic parameters). Prehepatic first-pass metabolism by CYP3A4 enzymes occurs with some orally administered calcium channel blockers, especially verapamil, with its low bioavailability of 20% to 35%. The bioavailability of diltiazem is 40% to 67%, of nicardipine 35%, of nifedipine 45% to 70%, and of amlodipine 64% to 90%.

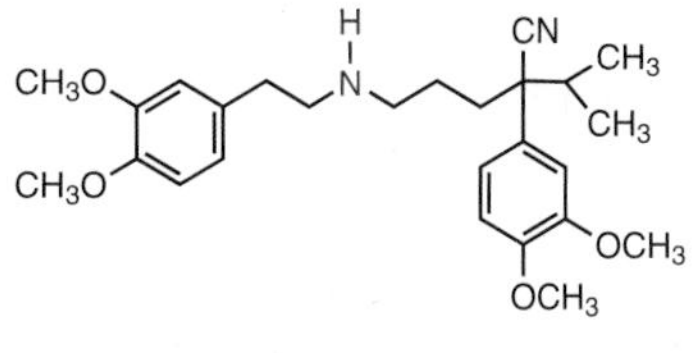

Norverapamil

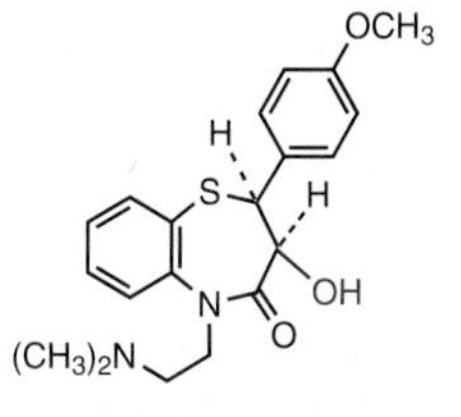

Desacetyldiltiazem

Verapamil is metabolized by CYP3A4 *N*-demethylation to its principal metabolite, norverapamil, which retains approximately 20% of the activity of verapamil, and by *O*-demethylation (CYP2D6) into inactive metabolites. Diltiazem is metabolized by enzyme hydrolysis to its primary metabolite, desacetyl derivative, which retains approximately 25% to 50% of the activity of diltiazem. The oral bioavailability of diltiazem and verapamil can be increased with chronic use and increasing dose (i.e., bioavailability is nonlinear). Diltiazem undergoes *N*-demethylation by CYP3A4 and *O*-demethylation by CYP2D6. The *N*-demethylated metabolism pathway results in mechanism-based inhibition of CYP3A4. The major metabolite, detected following oral and continuous intravenous administration but not following rapid intravenous administration, is desacetyl diltiazem, which has one-quarter to one-half the arteriolar vasodilation activity of the parent compound. Its elimination half-life ranges from 5 to 8 hours, depending on the dosage. Its onset of action following oral administration is 30 to 60 minutes; 2% to 4% is excreted unchanged. For extended-release capsules, the onset of action is 2 to 3 hours. CYP3A4 inhibition by diltiazem and a substrate for CYP2D6 provide a rational basis for pharmacokinetically significant interactions when they are coadministered with drugs that are cleared primarily by CYP3A4- or CYP2D6-mediated pathways. Considerable variability for verapamil can be observed in the elimination half-life of 1.5 to 7 hours. In addition, the plasma half-life cannot always accurately predict the duration of action because of the presence of active metabolites. Less than 5% of an orally administered dose of verapamil is excreted unchanged into the urine. Its protein binding is approximately 90%.

A well-documented drug interaction between digoxin and verapamil that increases the AUCs for digoxin has been attributed to verapamil blocking the intestinal P-gp efflux of digoxin (previously described in the section on digoxin–drug interactions). The fact that verapamil is a substrate for P-gp transport of drugs can be a potential source of other drug interactions. The oral coadministration of verapamil with CYP3A4 inhibitors (see Table 4.10 for a list of inhibitors) has resulted in at least a 100- to 200-fold increase in the blood AUCs for verapamil and, thereby, a toxic dose.

The dihydropyridines are metabolized largely to a variety of inactive metabolites. Their binding to plasma proteins is high, ranging from 70% to 98% depending on the individual agent: For verapamil, protein binding is 90%; for diltiazem, 70% to 80%; for nifedipine, 92% to 98%; for nicardipine, greater than 90%; and for amlodipine, greater than 90%. Less than 4% of the dihydropyridine dose is excreted unchanged into the urine. The duration of action of the calcium channel blockers ranges from 4 to 8 hours (verapamil, 4 hours; diltiazem, 6 to 8 hours; nifedipine, 4 to 8 hours; and nicardipine, 6 to 8 hours). Amlodipine has a 24-hour duration of action. Thus, it is the only calcium channel blocker that can be given once daily as a non–sustained-release product.

Adverse Effects

The most common side effects of the calcium channel blockers include dizziness, hypotension, headache, and peripheral and pulmonary edema. These symptoms are related mainly to the excessive vasodilation, especially with the dihydropyridines. Verapamil was reported to cause constipation to some patients.

Drug Interactions

Clinically significant drug interactions between calcium channel blockers and coadministration of CYP3A4 inhibitors, such as 6 to 8 oz. of grapefruit juice, HIV protease inhibitors, and erythromycin, have resulted in a 100- to 200-fold increase in the AUC for some calcium channel blockers (31). On the other hand, the coadministration of CYP3A4 inducers, such as rifampin or phenobarbital, result in an approximately 50% decrease in the AUC of calcium channel blockers. With other vasodilators, antihypertensive drugs, and alcohol, excessive hypotension can arise because of an additive effect. The high protein-binding nature of these drugs precipitates a potential for mutual plasma displacement with other drugs known to possess the same property, such as oral anticoagulants, digitalis glycosides, oral hypoglycemic agents, sulfa drugs, and salicylates. Dose adjustment can be necessary in some cases.

Therapeutic Uses

Calcium channel blockers are clinically used as antianginal, antiarrhythmic, and antihypertensive agents (see corresponding subsection in Chapter 25).

Late Sodium Current Inhibitor

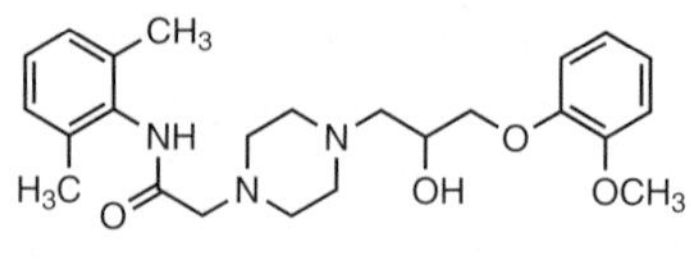

Ranolazine

Ranolazine (Ranexa) is used for chronic angina, and its mechanism of action is believed to alter the intracellular sodium level, which affects the sodium-dependent calcium channels during myocardial ischemia. Intracellular sodium and calcium overload play a key role in both electrical and contractility dysfunction of the heart in ischemia and heart failure. Inhibition of the late sodium current (I_{Na}) decreases intracellular sodium and calcium overload, thereby reducing their damaging effects on the heart. Ranolazine selectively inhibits late I_{Na} current and attenuates the abnormalities of ventricular repolarization and contractility associated with ischemia/reperfusion and heart failure. Thus, inhibition of late I_{Na} current may contribute to the cardioprotective effects of ranolazine. The drug indirectly prevents the calcium overload burden that causes cardiac ischemia without significantly changing blood pressure and heart rate. It is approved for the treatment of chronic angina in combination with calcium channels blockers, β-adrenoceptor antagonists, or nitrates in patients who have not achieved an adequate response with other antianginals. Its antianginal and anti-ischemic action is not dependent on heart rate or blood pressure reduction, and it does not increase myocardial workload.

The oral bioavailability of ranolazine from extended-release tablets is 76%, and plasma concentration is not affected by food. Metabolism is mainly by CYP3A4 and, to a lesser degree, by CYP2D6, with less than 5% being excreted unchanged in the urine and feces. After a single oral dose of ranolazine solution, approximately 75% of the dose is excreted in the urine and approximately 25% in feces. Its elimination half-life for extended-release tablets is 7 to 9 hours. Ranolazine is an inhibitor of P-gp transporter. Ranolazine plasma concentrations are increased by CYP3A4 inhibitors. The CYP2D6 inhibition has a negligible effect on ranolazine exposure.

β-Adrenergic Blocking Agents

The use of β-adrenergic blockers as antianginal agents is limited to the treatment of exertion-induced angina. Propranolol is the prototype drug in this class, but several newer agents have been approved for clinical use in the United States (see Chapter 10). Although these agents can be used alone, they are often used in combination therapy with nitrates, calcium channel blockers, or both. In several instances, combination therapy was found to provide more improvement than with either agent alone. This, however, is not always the case.

Miscellaneous Coronary Vasodilators

Another approach to the treatment of myocardial insufficiency is the use of the coronary vasodilators dipyridamole and papaverine. Dipyridamole, a PDE3 inhibitor (Fig. 21.8), causes a long-acting and selective coronary vasodilation by increasing coronary blood flow via selective dilation of the coronary arteries. The state of the coronary arteries can determine the effect of dipyridamole on coronary blood flow and metabolic responses. Blood flow increased by 80% in unobstructed coronary vessels, whereas in stenotic coronary arteries, flow increased by approximately 40%. In patients with single-vessel coronary artery disease, intravenous dipyridamole increases flow to the ischemic area, probably by increasing collateral blood flow. Dipyridamole increases intracellular concentrations of the coronary vasodilator adenosine and cAMP and inhibits adenosine metabolism and uptake by vascular endothelial cells. The increased concentration of adenosine in vascular smooth muscle stimulates adenylate cyclase activity, leading to increased cAMP synthesis and, consequently, to relaxation of vascular smooth muscle (vasodilation). The effect of dipyridamole might not result only from its effect on adenosine but also from its ability to increase prostacyclin (vasodilator and platelet inhibitor) production by increasing cAMP concentration. Dipyridamole also increases intracellular cAMP by inhibiting PDE3, decreasing cAMP breakdown. Adenosine is a natural vasodilatory substance released by the myocardium during hypoxic episodes. Some structural similarity of adenosine to dipyridamole is apparent and substantiates this mechanism. Dipyridamole is used prophylactically, but its efficacy in reducing the incidence and severity of anginal attacks is not universally accepted.

Papaverine (Fig. 21.8) is a benzoisoquinoline vasodilator (an alkaloid found in opium) that produces generalized, nonspecific arteriolar dilatation and smooth muscle relaxation. Its oral bioavailability ranges from 30% to 50%, suggesting first-pass 6-*O*-demethylation metabolism by CYP3A4. Increased levels of intracellular cAMP secondary to inhibition of phosphodiesterase can contribute to its vasodilatation and relaxation effects without involving nerve supply. Large doses of papaverine can cause hypotension and tachycardia. Other studies suggest that it also depresses cardiac conduction and prolongs the refractory period.

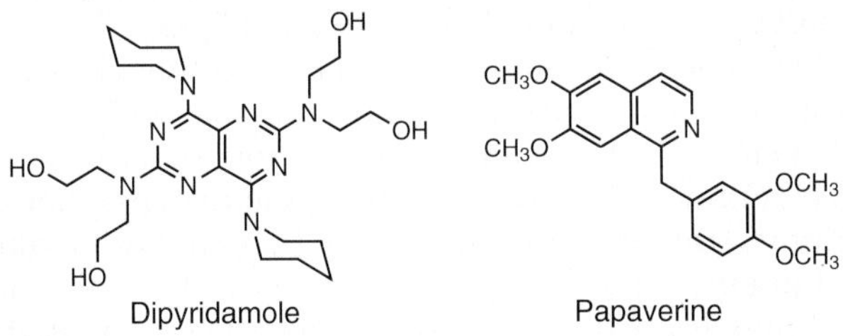

FIGURE 21.8 Miscellaneous coronary vasodilators.

The natriuretic polypeptide nesiritide (Natrecor) is manufactured in the United States using recombinant DNA technology for intravenous use to treat cases of angina and CHF. Nesiritide has the same amino acid sequence of the natural, 32-amino acid natriuretic peptide that normally is released during cardiac ischemia and acts as vasodilator. Nesiritide acts as a coronary vasodilator by binding to the soluble guanylate cyclase receptors in vascular smooth muscles, leading to increased intracellular concentrations of the vasodilator cGMP.

DRUGS FOR THE TREATMENT OF CARDIAC ARRHYTHMIA

Arrhythmia

Arrhythmia is an alteration in the normal sequence of electrical impulse rhythm that leads to contraction of the myocardium. It is manifested as an abnormality in the rate, in the site from which the impulses originate, or in the conduction through the myocardium. The rhythm of the heart normally is determined by a pacemaker site called the SA node, which consists of specialized cells that undergo spontaneous generation of action potentials at a rate of 100 to 110 action potentials ("beats") per minute. This intrinsic rhythm is strongly influenced by the vagus nerve, overcoming the sympathetic system at rest. This "vagal tone" brings the resting heart rate down to a normal sinus rhythm of 60 to 100 beats per minute. Sinus rates below this range are termed "sinus bradycardia," and sinus rates above this range are termed "sinus tachycardia." The sinus rhythm normally controls both atrial and ventricular rhythm. Action potentials generated by the SA node spread throughout the atria, depolarizing this tissue and causing atrial contraction. The impulse then travels into the ventricles via the AV node. Specialized conduction pathways within the ventricle rapidly conduct the wave of depolarization throughout the ventricles to elicit ventricular contraction. Therefore, normal cardiac rhythm is controlled by the pacemaker activity of the SA node. Abnormal or irregular cardiac rhythms (heartbeats) can occur when the SA node fails to function normally, when other pacemaker sites (e.g., ectopic pacemakers) trigger depolarization, or when a dysfunction occurs along the normal conduction pathways.

Causes of Arrhythmias

Many factors influence the normal rhythm of electrical activity in the heart. Arrhythmias can occur either because pacemaker cells fail to function properly or because of a blockage in transmission through the AV node. Underlying diseases, such as atherosclerosis, hyperthyroidism, or lung disease, can also be initiating factors. Some of the more common arrhythmias are those termed "ectopic," which occur when electrical signals spontaneously arise in regions other than the pacemaker and then compete with the normal impulses. Myocardial ischemia, excessive myocardial catecholamine release, stretching of the myocardium, and cardiac glycoside toxicity have all been shown to stimulate ectopic foci. A second mechanism for the generation of arrhythmias is from a phenomenon called reentry. This occurs when the electrical impulse does not die out after firing but, rather, continues to circulate and reexcite resting heart cells into depolarizing. The result of this reexcitation can be a single, premature beat or runs of ventricular tachycardia. Reentrant rhythms are common in the presence of coronary atherosclerosis.

Drugs for the Treatment of Arrhythmias and Their Classification

It is widely accepted that most currently available antiarrhythmic drugs can be classified into four categories, which are grouped on the basis of their effects on the cardiac action potential and, consequently, on the electrophysiologic properties of the heart. To understand the basis of classification and the pharmacology of these agents, an understanding of normal cardiac electrophysiology is necessary.

Normal Physiologic Action

Normal cardiac contractions largely are a function of the action of a single atrial pacemaker, a fast and usually uniform conduction in predictable pathways, and a normal duration of the action potential and refractory period. Figure 21.9 depicts a normal cardiac action potential from a Purkinje fiber. The resting cell has a membrane potential of approximately −90 mV, with the inside of the cell being electronegative relative to the outside of the cell. This is termed the "transmembrane resting potential." On excitation, the transmembrane potential reverses, and the inside of the membrane rapidly becomes positive with respect to the outside. On recovery from excitation, the resting potential is restored. These changes have been divided into five phases: Phase 0 represents depolarization and reversal of the transmembrane potential, phases 1 to 3 represent different stages of repolarization, and phase 4 represents the resting potential. During phase 0, which is also referred to as rapid depolarization, the permeability of the membrane for sodium ions increases, and sodium rapidly enters the cell, causing it to become depolarized. Phase 1 results from the ionic shift, which creates an electrochemical and concentration gradient that reduces the rate of sodium influx but favors the influx of chloride and efflux of potassium. Phase 2, the plateau phase, results from the slow inward movement of calcium, which is triggered by the rapid inward movement of sodium in phase 0. During this time, there is also an efflux of potassium that balances the influx of calcium, thus resulting in little or no change in membrane potential. Phase 3 is initiated by a slowing of the calcium influx coupled with a continued efflux of potassium. This continued efflux of potassium from the cell restores the membrane potential to normal resting potential levels. During phase 4, the Na^+, K^+-ATPase pump restores the ions to their proper local concentrations. The action potential is a coordinated sequence of ion movements in which sodium initially enters the cell, followed by a calcium influx, and finally, a potassium efflux returns the cell to its resting state. Several antiarrhythmic agents exert their effects by altering these ion fluxes.

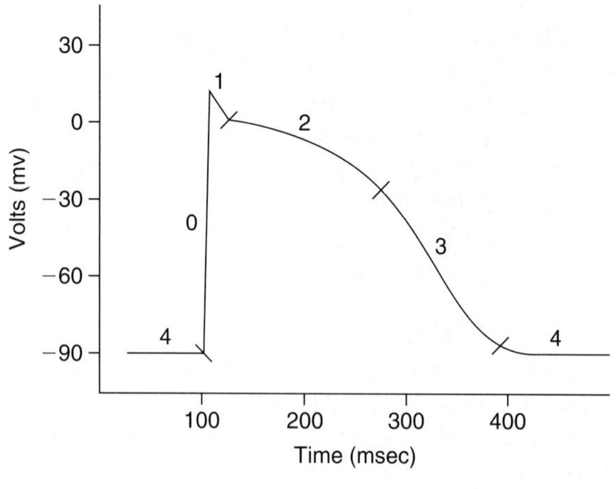

FIGURE 21.9 Cardiac action potential recorded from a Purkinje fiber.

Classification of Antiarrhythmic Drugs

Class I Sodium Channel Blockers

Class IA Antiarrhythmic Drugs This class of antiarrhythmic drugs includes local anesthetics acting on nerve and myocardial membranes to slow conduction by blocking fast Na^+ channels, inhibiting phase 0 of the action potential (Fig. 21.9). Myocardial membranes show the greatest sensitivity. Class IA drugs decrease the maximal rate of depolarization without changing the resting potential. They also increase the threshold of excitability, increase the effective refractory period, decrease conduction velocity, and decrease spontaneous diastolic depolarization in pacemaker cells. The decrease in diastolic depolarization tends to suppress ectopic foci activity. Prolongation of the refractory period tends to abolish reentry arrhythmias. Table 21.6 summarizes these effects. Quinidine is considered to be the prototype drug for class IA.

Quinidine. Quinidine (Fig. 21.10) is widely used for acute and chronic treatment of ventricular and supraventricular arrhythmias, especially supraventricular tachycardia. It is a member of a family of alkaloids found in Cinchona bark (*Cinchona officinalis* L.) and is the diastereomer of quinine. Despite their structural similarity, quinidine and quinine differ markedly in their effects on the cardiac muscles, with the effects of quinidine being much more pronounced. Structurally, quinidine is composed

TABLE 21.6 Summary of the Cardiac Physiologic Effects of the Antiarrhythmic Drugs

Classification	Mechanism of Action	Primary Sites of Action	Drug Examples
Class IA	Na^+ channel blockade		Quinidine
	Intermediate rate of dissociation from sodium channels		Procainamide
	Slows phase 0 depolarization	Atrial and ventricular tissue	Disopyramide
	Prolongs action potential duration		
	Slows conduction		
Class IB	Na^+ channel blockade		Lidocaine
	Rapid rate of dissociation from sodium channels		Mexiletine
	Shortens phase 3 repolarization	Ventricular tissue	Phenytoin
	Shortens action potential duration		Tocainide
Class 1C	Na^+ channel blockade	Ventricular tissue	Flecainide
	Slows rate of dissociation from sodium channels		Encainide
	Markedly slows phase 0 depolarization		Propafenone
	Slows conduction		Moricizine
Class II	Blocks sympathetic stimulation of β_1-adrenergic receptors	SA node	Propranolol
	Slows phase 4 depolarization	AV node	Sotalol
	Slows firing of SA node and conduction through AV node, prolonging repolarization		β_1-Blockers
Class III	K^+ channel blockade (block delayed rectifier current)	Atrial and ventricular tissue	Amiodarone
	Prolongs phase 3 repolarization		Dronedarone Sotalol
	Prolongs duration of action potential, which prolongs refractory period		Bretylium
Class IV	Ca^{+2} channel blockade	SA node	Verapamil
	Slows phase 4 depolarization	AV node	Diltiazem
	Slows firing of SA node and conduction through AV node, prolonging repolarization of AV node		

AV, atrioventricular; SA, sinoatrial.

of a quinoline ring and the bicyclic quinuclidine ring system, with a hydroxymethylene bridge connecting these two components. Examination of quinidine reveals two basic nitrogens, with the quinuclidine nitrogen (pK_a = 11) being the stronger of the two. Because of the basic character of quinidine, it is always used as water-soluble salt forms. These salts include quinidine sulfate, gluconate, and polygalacturonate. Good absorption (~95%) is observed with each of these forms after oral administration. In special situations, quinidine can be administered intravenously as the gluconate salt. The use of intravenous quinidine, however, is rare. The gluconate salt is particularly suited for parenteral use because of its high water solubility and lower irritant potential.

Quinidine's bioavailability appears to depend on a combination of metabolism and P-gp efflux. The bioavailabilities of quinidine sulfate and gluconate are 80% to 85% and 70% to 75%, respectively. Once absorbed, quinidine is subject to hepatic first-pass CYP3A4 metabolism and is approximately 85% plasma protein bound, with an elimination half-life of approximately 6 hours. Quinidine is metabolized mainly in the liver, and renal excretion of unchanged drug is also significant (~10% to 50%).

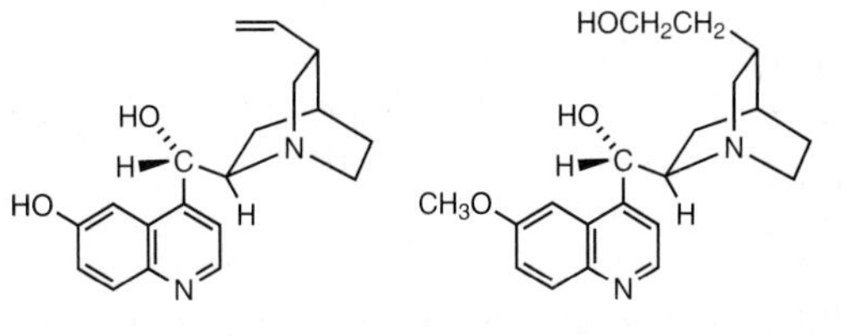

O-Demethylquinidine   Oxydihydroquinidine

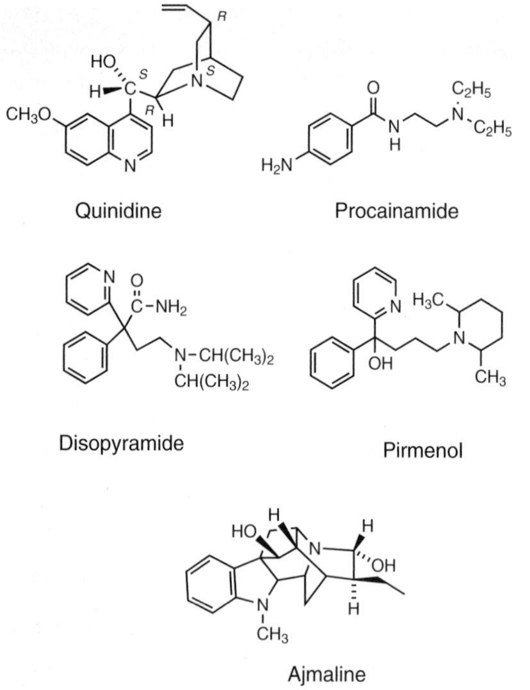

FIGURE 21.10 Class IA antiarrhythmics.

The metabolites are hydroxylated derivatives at either the quinoline ring through first-pass *O*-demethylation or at the quinuclidine ring through oxidation of the vinyl group. These metabolites possess only about one-third the activity of quinidine. Their contribution to the overall therapeutic effect of quinidine is unclear. The clinical significance of the well-documented digoxin–quinidine interaction was described previously in the section on digoxin–drug interactions. Apparently, quinidine (a P-gp substrate) inhibits the renal tubular secretion of digoxin via the P-gp efflux pump, resulting in increased plasma concentration for digoxin.

In addition, a common contaminant in quinidine preparations, dihydroquinidine, which is derived from reduction of the quinuclidine vinyl group at C-3 to an ethyl group, can also contribute to its activity (32). Although similar to quinidine in pharmacodynamic and pharmacokinetic behavior, this contaminant is both more potent as an antiarrhythmic and more toxic. Thus, levels of this contaminant can contribute to variability between commercial preparations. The most frequent adverse effects associated with quinidine therapy are gastrointestinal disturbances, such as nausea, diarrhea, and vomiting.

Procainamide. Procainamide (Fig. 21.10) is effective in the treatment of several types of cardiac arrhythmias. Its actions are similar to those of quinidine, yet procainamide can be effective in patients who are unresponsive to quinidine. The initial development of procainamide was stimulated by the observation that the local anesthetic procaine (the ester bio-isostere of procainamide), when administered intravenously, produced significant, although short-lived, antiarrhythmic effects. Unfortunately, considerable central nervous system toxicity, in addition to the short duration, limited the usefulness of this agent. Moreover, procaine is not active orally because of its short duration of action caused by both chemical and plasma esterase hydrolysis. A logical modification of this molecule was the isosteric replacement of the ester with an amide group. This produced orally active procainamide, which is more resistant to both enzymatic and chemical hydrolysis. Peak plasma levels of procainamide are observed within 45 to 90 minutes after oral administration, and approximately 70% to 80% of the dose is bioavailable. Approximately half of this dose is excreted unchanged, and the remaining half undergoes acetylation metabolism in the liver. Metabolites of procainamide include *p*-aminobenzoic acid and *N*-acetylprocainamide. Interestingly, the acetylated metabolite is also active as an antiarrhythmic. Its formation accounts for up to one-third of the administered dose and is catalyzed by the liver enzyme *N*-acetyltransferase. Because acetylation is strongly influenced by an individual's genetic background, marked variability in the amounts of this active metabolite can be observed from patient to patient. Renal excretion dominates, with approximately 90% of a dose excreted as unchanged drug and metabolites. The elimination half-life is approximately 3.5 hours. A substantial percentage (60% to 70%) of patients on procainamide show elevated levels of antinuclear antibodies after a few months. Of these patients, between 20% and 30% develop a drug-induced lupus syndrome if therapy is continued. These adverse effects, which are attributed to the aromatic amino group, are observed more frequently and more rapidly in "slow acetylators." As a rule, the symptoms associated with procainamide-induced lupus syndrome subside fairly rapidly after the drug is discontinued. These problems, however, have discouraged long-term procainamide therapy.

Disopyramide. Disopyramide phosphate (Norpace) is used orally for the treatment of certain ventricular and atrial arrhythmias. Despite its structural dissimilarity to procainamide (Fig. 21.10), its cardiac effects are very similar. Disopyramide is rapidly and completely absorbed from the gastrointestinal tract. Peak plasma level is, as a rule, reached within 1 to 3 hours, and a plasma half-life of 5 to 7 hours is common. Approximately half of an oral dose is excreted unchanged in the urine. The remaining drug undergoes hepatic CYP3A4 metabolism, principally to the corresponding *N*-dealkylated metabolite. This metabolite retains approximately half the antiarrhythmic activity of disopyramide and is also subject to renal excretion. Adverse effects of disopyramide frequently are observed. These effects are primarily anticholinergic in nature and include dry mouth, blurred vision, constipation, and urinary retention.

Ajmaline. Ajmaline (Fig. 21.10) inhibits sodium influx and prolongs phase 3. The drug is a natural product alkaloid obtained from the roots of *Rauwolfia serpentina* and is used in other parts of the world to treat ventricular tachyarrhythmia and supraventricular arrhythmias. Ajmaline is given orally, intramuscularly, and as intravenous infusion over a 5-minute period. Being a *Rauwolfia* alkaloid with similar effects on the neurotransmitters, the drug has also been used in the differential diagnosis of Wolff-Parkinson-White syndrome.

Pirmenol. Pirmenol (Fig. 21.10) is a class IA antiarrhythmic drug marketed in Japan, but not in the United States, for the control of the ventricular arrhythmias. The drug is structurally similar to disopyramide, except that the amide functionality has been replaced by a secondary alcohol and the basic nitrogen is incorporated in a piperidine heterocyclic ring.

Class IB Antiarrhythmic Drugs

Lidocaine. Lidocaine, similar to procaine, is an effective, clinically used local anesthetic (Fig. 21.11) (see Chapter 16). Its cardiac effects, however, are distinctly different from those of procainamide or quinidine. Lidocaine normally is reserved for the treatment of ventricular arrhythmias and, in fact, is typically the drug of choice for emergency treatment of ventricular arrhythmias. Its utility in these situations results from the rapid onset of antiarrhythmic effects on intravenous infusion. In addition, these effects cease soon after the infusion is terminated. Thus, lidocaine therapy can be rapidly modified in response to changes in the patient's status. Lidocaine is effective as an antiarrhythmic only when given parenterally, and the intravenous route is the most common. Antiarrhythmic activity is not observed after oral administration because of the rapid and efficient first-pass CYP3A4 and 2D6 metabolism by the liver. Parenterally administered lidocaine is approximately 60% to 70% plasma protein bound. Hepatic metabolism is rapid (plasma half-life, ~15 to 30 minutes) and primarily involves *N*-deethylation to yield monoethylglycinexylide, followed by amidase-catalyzed hydrolysis into *N*-ethylglycine and 2,6-dimethylaniline (2,6-xylidine) (Fig. 21.12).

Monoethylglycinexylide has good antiarrhythmic activity. It is not clinically useful, however, because it undergoes rapid enzymatic hydrolysis. The adverse effects of lidocaine include emetic and convulsant properties that predominantly involve the central nervous system and heart. The central nervous system effects can begin with dizziness and paresthesia and, in severe cases, ultimately lead to epileptic seizures.

Tocainide. Tocainide (Tonocard) (Fig. 21.11) is an α-methyl analog structurally related to monoethylglycinexylide, the active metabolite of lidocaine, which possesses very similar electrophysiologic effects to lidocaine. In contrast to lidocaine, tocainide is orally active, and its oral absorption is excellent. Like lidocaine, it is reserved for the treatment of ventricular arrhythmias. The α-methyl group is believed to slow the rate of metabolism and, thereby, to contribute to oral activity. The plasma half-life of tocainide is approximately 12 hours, and nearly 50% of the drug can be excreted unchanged in the urine. Adverse effects associated with tocainide are like those observed with lidocaine—specifically, gastrointestinal disturbances and central nervous system effects.

Mexiletine. Mexiletine (Mexitil) (Fig. 21.11) is similar to both lidocaine and tocainide in its effects and therapeutic application. It is used principally to treat and prevent ventricular arrhythmias. Like tocainide, mexiletine has very good oral activity and absorption properties. Clearance depends on CYP2D6 metabolism and renal excretion. A relatively long plasma half-life of approximately 12 to 16 hours is common. Adverse effects are similar to those experienced with tocainide and lidocaine.

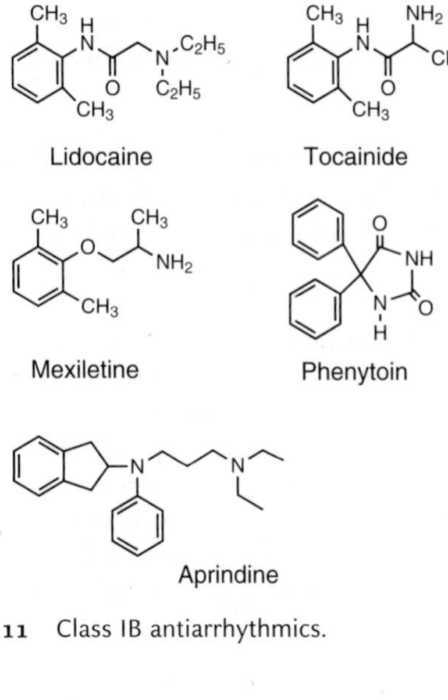

FIGURE 21.11 Class IB antiarrhythmics.

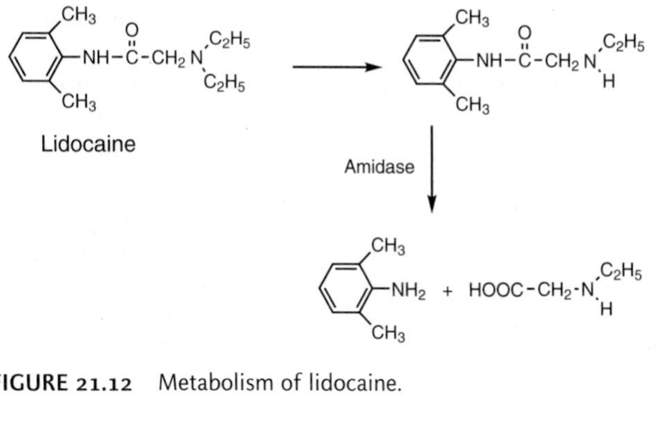

FIGURE 21.12 Metabolism of lidocaine.

Phenytoin. For 50 years, phenytoin (Fig. 21.11) has seen clinical use in the treatment of epileptic seizures (see Chapter 17). During this time, it was noticed that phenytoin also produced supposedly adverse cardiac effects. On closer examination, these adverse effects actually were found to be beneficial in the treatment of certain arrhythmias. Currently, phenytoin is used in the treatment of atrial and ventricular arrhythmias resulting from digitalis toxicity. It is not, however, officially approved for this use.

Phenytoin can be administered either orally or intravenously and is absorbed slowly after oral administration, with peak plasma levels achieved after 3 to 12 hours. It is extensively plasma protein bound (~90%), and the elimination half-life is between 15 and 30 hours. These large ranges reflect the considerable variability observed from patient to patient. Parenteral administration of phenytoin is limited to the intravenous route. Phenytoin for injection is dissolved in a highly alkaline vehicle (pH 12). This alkaline vehicle is required because phenytoin is weakly acidic and has very poor solubility in its un-ionized form. Reportedly, however, its phosphate ester fosphenytoin has water solubility advantages over phenytoin for injection. Intramuscular phenytoin is usually avoided, because it results in tissue necrosis at the site of injection and has erratic absorption as a result of of high alkalinity. In addition, intermittent intravenous infusion is required to reduce the incidence of severe phlebitis.

Phenytoin metabolism is relatively slow and predominantly involves aromatic hydroxylation by the CYP2C family of enzymes to *p*-hydroxylated inactive metabolites (see Chapter 17). Phenytoin also induces its own metabolism and is subject to large interindividual variability. The major metabolite, 5-*p*-hydroxyphenyl-5-phenylhydantoin, accounts for approximately 75% of a dose. This metabolite is excreted through the kidney as the β-glucuronide conjugate. Phenytoin clearance is strongly influenced by its metabolism; therefore, agents that affect phenytoin metabolism can cause intoxication. In addition, because phenytoin is highly plasma protein bound, agents that displace phenytoin can also cause toxicity.

Aprindine. Aprindine (Fig. 21.11) is classified as class IB antiarrhythmic agent due its inhibitory effects on the sodium current without affecting the duration of the action potential. The drug is available in Europe, but has not been approved by the FDA. Aprindine is administered both orally and intravenously to treat ventricular and supraventricular arrhythmias. The drug is well absorbed after oral administration with extensive binding (85% to 90%) to plasma proteins and is largely metabolized by hepatic CYP2D6 through aromatic hydroxylation. Adverse effects reported for the drug included hypersensitivity, inducing agranulocytosis and visual disturbances.

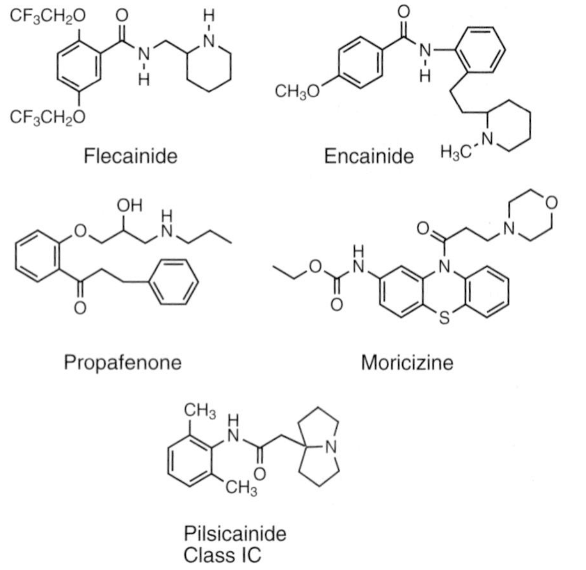

FIGURE 21.13 Class IC antiarrhythmics.

Class IC Antiarrhythmic Drugs

Flecainide. Flecainide (Tambocor) exhibits properties distinctly different from those of class IA or IB antiarrhythmic drugs. Flecainide is a fluorinated benzamide derivative (Fig. 21.13), available as the acetate salt. Flecainide has been approved by the FDA for the treatment of ventricular arrhythmias. Clinical studies suggest that this agent can be more effective than either quinidine or disopyramide in suppressing premature ventricular contractions. Oral flecainide is well absorbed, and the plasma half-life is approximately 14 hours. About half of an oral dose is CYP2D6 metabolized in the liver, and one-third is excreted unchanged in the urine. As with other antiarrhythmics, flecainide can produce adverse effects. The most severe is flecainide's occasional tendency to aggravate existing arrhythmias or to induce new ones. Although fewer than 10% of patients experience this effect, it can be life-threatening. Accordingly, it can be desirable to start therapy in the hospital. Other less serious side effects include blurred vision, headache, nausea, and abdominal pain.

Encainide. Encainide (Enkaid) (Fig. 21.13) represents another benzamide derivative, with similar pharmacologic properties to flecainide but with less negative inotropic effect.

Propafenone. Propafenone (Rythmol) (Fig. 21.13) is a class I, local anesthetic–type antiarrhythmic agent. Propafenone is structurally related to other class IC antiarrhythmic drugs and also to β-adrenergic receptor blockers. It is used primarily for ventricular and supraventricular arrhythmias. The drug is administered orally and intravenously; however, the parenteral dosage forms are not commercially available in the United States. After oral administration, the drug is rapidly and almost completely absorbed from the gastrointestinal tract. Propafenone metabolism involves hepatic CYP2D6 enzymes. Its rate of metabolism is genetically determined by an individual's ability to metabolize the so-called phenotype compounds (fast or slow metabolizers) (see Chapter 9).

Moricizine. Moricizine (Ethmozine) (Fig. 21.13) is a phenothiazine analog that processes the same electrophysiologic effects on the heart as those of class IC antiarrhythmics. Despite its short half-life after oral administration due to CYP1A2 metabolism, its antiarrhythmic effects can persist for many hours, suggesting that some of its metabolites can be active.

Pilsicainide. Pilsicainide (Fig 21.13) is an analog of lidocaine where the diethylamino group of lidocaine has been replaced with a pyrrollizidine bicyclic ring structure. Despite its structural similarity to lidocaine (Fig. 21.10), its electrophysiologic profile as a class IC antiarrhythmic is unlike that of lidocaine, which is a class IB antiarrhythmic drug. Apparently, class IC drugs prefer a bulky *N*-substituent. The drug is marketed in Japan and is not approved by the FDA. Pilsicainide is administered both orally and by injection to treat tachyarrhythmias and atrial fibrillation.

CLASS II ANTIARRHYTHMIC DRUGS Class II antiarrhythmic drugs (Fig. 21.14) are β-adrenergic receptor–blocking agents that block the role of the sympathetic nervous system in the genesis of certain cardiac arrhythmias. Their dominant electrophysiologic effect is to depress adrenergically enhanced calcium influx through β-receptor blockade. Drugs in this class decrease neurologically induced automaticity at normal therapeutic doses. At higher doses, these drugs can also exhibit anesthetic properties, which cause decreased excitability, decreased conduction velocity, and a prolonged effective refractory period. In normal therapeutic situations, the β-blocking effects are more important than any local anesthetic effects that these drugs can have. Propranolol is the prototype β-adrenergic blocker drug for class II (see Chapter 10).

Propranolol (+)-Propranolol, a nonselective β-adrenergic blocker, is the prototype for class II antiarrhythmics. Its pharmacology and pharmacokinetics are discussed in detail in Chapters 10 and 24. Its use as an antiarrhythmic is typically for the treatment of supraventricular arrhythmias, including atrial flutter, paroxysmal supraventricular tachycardia, and atrial fibrillation. Propranolol is also reported to be effective in the treatment of digitalis-induced ventricular arrhythmias. Moreover, beneficial results can be obtained when propranolol is used in combination with other agents. For example, in certain cases, quinidine and propranolol together have proved to be more successful in alleviating atrial fibrillation than either agent has alone. Few serious adverse effects are associated with propranolol therapy.

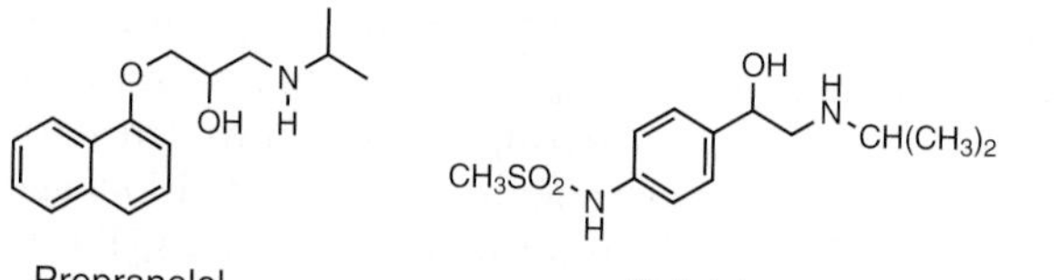

FIGURE 21.14 Class II inhibitors of depolarization.

Sotalol (±)-Sotalol (Betapace, Sotacor), a nonselective β-adrenergic blocker, is a methanesulfonanilide antiarrhythmic agent. As an antiarrhythmic, it is dually classified as class II and class III because of the similarity of its cardiac effects to both classes. Sotalol is used orally to suppress and prevent the recurrence of life-threatening ventricular arrhythmia.

CLASS III POTASSIUM CHANNEL BLOCKERS Class III drugs cause a homogeneous prolongation of the duration of the action potential. This results in a prolongation of the effective refractory period. It is believed that most of class III antiarrhythmic agents act through phase 3 of the action potential by blocking potassium channels. Figure 21.15 illustrates the chemical structures of members of class III. Bretylium is the prototype drug for this class.

Bretylium Tosylate Bretylium tosylate is a quaternary ammonium salt derivative (Fig. 21.15) originally developed for use as an antihypertensive. Its antiarrhythmic use is limited to emergency, life-threatening situations in which other agents, such as lidocaine and procainamide, have failed. Bretylium is used only in intensive care units and can be administered either intravenously or intramuscularly. The plasma elimination half-life is, as a rule, approximately 10 hours, and it is eliminated largely unchanged in the urine. The major adverse effect associated with bretylium tosylate is hypotension, including orthostatic hypotension, which can be very severe.

Amiodarone Initially developed as an antianginal (coronary vasodilator), amiodarone (Fig. 21.15) has antiarrhythmic effects that are somewhat similar to those of bretylium. It is approved by the FDA for the treatment of life-threatening ventricular arrhythmias that are refractory to other drugs. Its cardiac effects are not well characterized, but clinical studies indicate that it is primarily a class III agent but acts also as a class I, II, and IV antiarrhythmic. It has a unique mechanism of action that involves alteration of the lipid membrane in which ion channels and receptors are located. Its severe toxicity, however, makes it the drug of last choice. As with bretylium tosylate, use of this agent should be initiated in a hospital setting.

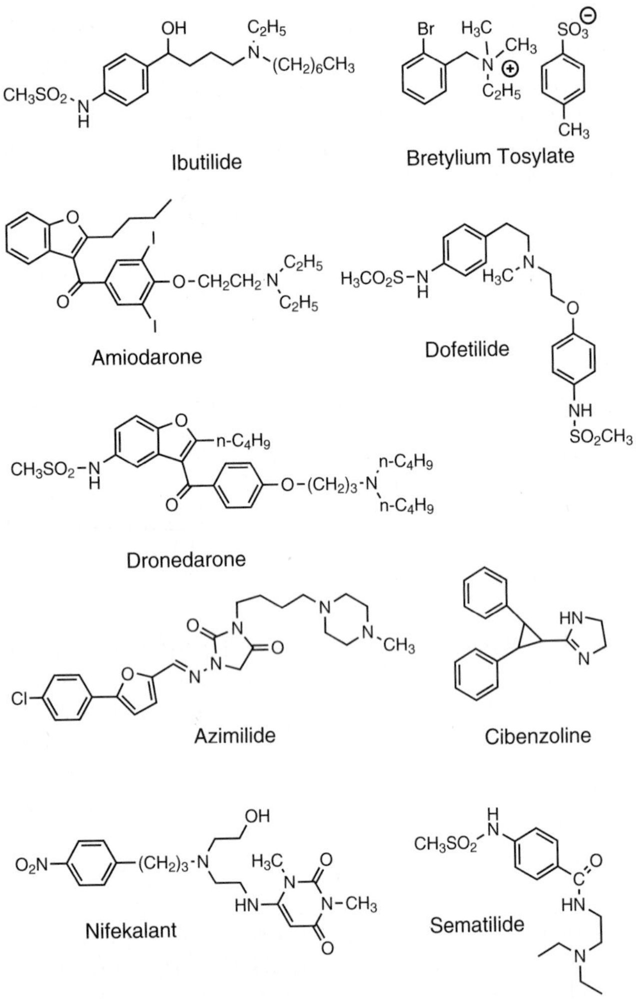

FIGURE 21.15 Class III antiarrhythmic agents.

Ibutilide Ibutilide (Corvert) is another methanesulfonanilide derivative (Fig. 21.15), but unlike sotalol, it lacks any β-adrenergic–blocking activity. Like sotalol, it exhibits electrophysiologic effects characteristic of class III. Ibutilide is used only by intravenous infusion as its fumarate salt.

Dofetilide Dofetilide (Tikosyn) is a bis-methanesulfonanilide derivative that is essentially the non–β-blocking moiety of the sotalol molecule (Fig. 21.15). It exhibits only class III electrophysiologic effects, but like ibutilide, it lacks any β-adrenergic–blocking activity. Dofetilide is used orally to suppress atrial fibrillation and flutter. It is more potent and selective than other class III methanesulfonanilides, including sotalol. Dofetilide is well absorbed from the gastrointestinal tract, with a bioavailability of 96% to 100%. The bioavailability of oral dofetilide is not affected by food or antacids. Protein binding is 60% to 70%. Dofetilide is metabolized by the hepatic CYP3A4 enzyme system via *N*-dealkylation and *N*-oxidation to inactive or minimally active metabolites. Of the approximately 80% of a dose excreted in urine, approximately 80% is excreted unchanged, with the other 20% excreted as metabolites.

Dronedarone (Multaq) Dronedarone was approved by the FDA in 2009 for the treatment of atrial fibrillation and atrial flutter. Dronedarone is the benzofuran noniodinated derivative of amiodarone, with two additional functional group differences including a methylsulfonamido group on the benzofuran ring and dibutyl substitution on the basic nitrogen. The iodine groups of amiodarone were removed to reduce toxic effects of amiodarone on the thyroid and other organs. The methylsulfonamido group was added to dronedarone to reduce lipophilicity and thus reduce neurotoxic effects. Dronedarone exhibits amiodarone-like class III antiarrhythmic activity in vitro and in clinical trials. Dronedarone is less lipophilic than amiodarone, has a much smaller volume of distribution, and has an elimination half-life of 24 hours, in contrast to amiodarone's half-life of several weeks. As a result of these pharmacokinetic characteristics, dronedarone dosing may be less complicated than amiodarone. The drug's bioavailability after oral administration is very poor (4%). Concurrent administration with high-fat meal improves the bioavailability to 15%. Accordingly, the drug is recommended to be taken with food. After oral absorption, the drug has 98% plasma protein binding and is metabolized by the liver by CYP3A4 *N*-debutylation into an active metabolite. Renal excretion is minimal (6%), and 84% of the administered dose is excreted in feces as either the parent drug or its metabolite.

Therapeutic Precaution. Because heart failure is a major serious adverse effect of dronedarone, the FDA approved the addition of a black box warning to the package insert, a summary of which is as follows:

> Warning: Heart failure: Multaq is contraindicated in patients with NYHA Class IV heart failure, or NYHA Class II–III heart failure with recent hospitalization or referral to a specialized heart failure clinic. In a placebo-controlled study in patients with severe heart failure requiring recent hospitalization or referral to a specialized heart failure clinic for worsening symptoms, patients given dronedarone had a greater than two-fold increase in mortality. Such patients should not be given dronedarone.

Azimilide Azimilide is a class III antiarrhythmic agent structurally unrelated to any of the other class III agents (Fig. 21.15). Azimilide is a potassium blocker similar to dofetilide or sotalol, but it blocks both I_{Kr} (rapid) and I_{Ks} (slow) inwardly rectifier potassium channels, which are responsible for repolarizing cardiac myocytes toward the end of the cardiac action potential. Blockages of both channels result in an increase of the QT interval and a prolongation of atrial and ventricular refractory periods. The drug does not perform as a β-blocker like sotalol. Azimilide has not been approved by the FDA and is only available in Europe. Following oral administration, the drug is completely absorbed, with no effect of food. Protein binding is 94%. The drug is metabolized in the liver to an active carboxylate metabolite, but its concentration in plasma is less than 5% of the parent compound. Thus, it is considered to be therapeutically inactive. Renal excretion is approximately 10%. Its elimination half-life is 3 to 4 days; thus, azimilide can be dosed once daily, limiting major fluctuations in blood levels.

Cibenzoline Cibenzoline (Fig. 21.15) is marketed in Japan and has not been approved by the FDA. The drug is structurally unrelated to any of the well-known nuclei of the other families of antiarrhythmic agents. Cibenzoline is a diphenyl-cyclopropyl-2-imidazoline derivative with electrophysiologic properties that make it difficult to categorize under a specific class. Although based on its electrophysiologic effects on the potassium current the drug is classified as class III antiarrhythmic agent, it is also reported to have characteristics that fit classes IA, IC, and IV. Cibenzoline is given orally and by injection for the management of ventricular and supraventricular arrhythmias. The drug is well absorbed after administration, with 90% bioavailability and moderate plasma protein binding (50% to 60%). The drug is excreted mostly unchanged in urine, which requires attention if given to patients with renal insufficiency. Cibenzoline is also associated with several adverse effects including gastrointestinal tract disturbances, neurologic side effects, and most notably, hypoglycemia.

Nifekalant Nifekalant (Fig. 21.15) is another class III antiarrhythmic agent developed and marketed in Japan that is not available in the United States. Nifekalant is used intravenously as a lifesaving drug for the treatment of life-threatening ventricular arrhythmias. The drug is a derivative of uracil (pyrimidindione), which is considered as a novel nucleus for class III antiarrhythmic agents. Very few clinical reports about the drug's adverse effects are available.

Sematilide Sematilide (Fig. 21.15) is an investigational class III antiarrhythmic drug that has not been approved by the FDA for clinical use. The drug is an analog of procainamide except that the aniline nitrogen has been substituted with a methylsulfone moiety. The methylsulfonamido procainamide derivative changed the molecule's selectivity from a sodium channel blocker (class IA antiarrhythmic) into a class III antiarrhythmic agent that selectively blocks the rapidly activating delayed rectifier K^+ current (I_{Kr}) in atrial myocytes, and evidence supports the usefulness of the drug as a class III antiarrhythmic agent. Further studies are needed to assess sematilide's place in antiarrhythmic therapy, including comparisons with prototypical class III agents (e.g., amiodarone, sotalol) and other pure class III agents (e.g., dofetilide).

Class IV Calcium Channel Blockers Class IV calcium channel antiarrhythmic drugs (Fig. 21.7) comprise a group of agents that selectively block the slow inward current carried by calcium (i.e., calcium channel blockers). The slow inward current in cardiac cells has been shown to be of importance for the normal action potential in SA node cells. It has also been suggested that this inward current is involved in the genesis of certain types of cardiac arrhythmias. Administration of a class IV drug causes a prolongation of the refractory period in the AV node and the atria, a decrease in AV conduction, and a decrease in spontaneous diastolic depolarization. These effects block conduction of premature impulses at the AV node and, thus, are very effective in treating supraventricular arrhythmias. Verapamil and diltiazem are prototype drugs for this class (Fig. 21.7), but dihydropyridine drugs are less effective in cardiac tissues. Refer to the section on calcium channel blockers under antianginal drugs for pharmacokinetic information.

SCENARIO: OUTCOME AND ANALYSIS

Outcome

Judy Cheng, PharmD

JS was initiated on diltiazem sustained release 240 mg daily for ventricular rate control and warfarin 5 mg daily to prevent a thromboembolic event that could be caused by atrial fibrillation. The sustained-release formulation was chosen to improve compliance. The lisinopril therapy was kept for now. Blood pressure will be monitored closely, and lisinopril may be discontinued if the patient's blood pressure becomes too low after the addition of diltiazem. JS will also go to a warfarin clinic to have his INR (International Normalized Ratio: prothrombin time) monitored.

Chemical Analysis

S. William Zito and Victoria Roche

Diltiazem is the only clinically useful benzo[*b*-1,5]thiazepine chemical class of calcium channel blockers. Diltiazem possesses asymmetric centers and the dextrorotatory (i.e., the (+)-enantiomer) is approximately one order of magnitude more potent as a calcium channel blocker than the levorotatory (i.e., (−)-enantiomer).

Diltiazem affects both the heart and the arteriolar bed by inhibiting the influx of extracellular calcium across both the myocardial and vascular smooth muscle cell membranes. This results in inhibition of the contractile processes and is used clinically in the management of angina, hypertension, and cardiac arrhythmias, often in combination with angiotensin-converting enzyme inhibitors such as lisinopril.

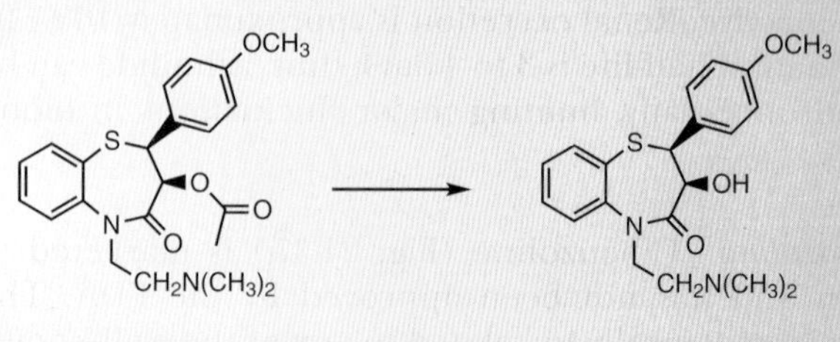

Diltiazem → Desacetyl diltiazem

Diltiazem is primarily metabolized by enzyme hydrolysis to its desacetyl derivative, which retains approximately 25% to 50% of the activity and adds to its duration of action. Diltiazem also undergoes *N*-demethylation by CYP3A4 and *O*-demethylation by CYP2D6. The *N*-demethylated metabolism pathway results in mechanism-based inhibition of CYP3A4. Because R-warfarin is metabolized by CYP 3A4 to yield 6-, 8-, and 10-hydroxylated metabolites, it is important that JR's INR be monitored.

CASE STUDY

S. William Zito and Victoria Roche

SB is a fairly active 45-year-old white man. He works for a shipping company and plays third base in the company softball league on weekends. SB was diagnosed with type 2 diabetes 5 years ago, which he successfully controls with diet and metformin (850 mg daily). Knowing that diabetics are prone to silent ischemic heart disease, his endocrinologist orders an exercise stress test as a routine screening measure. The test implies that SB has silent myocardial ischemia at a peak heart rate of 171 bpm and peak blood pressure of 195/85 mm Hg. These results suggest that SB may be at risk for sudden cardiac death, especially if he continues the high exertion associated with playing softball. The diagnosis was confirmed by the results of a Holter monitor that measured and recorded SB's electrocardiogram continuously for 48 hours and a thallium stress test. SB's physician suggests a reduction in physical activity and daily aspirin, and he wants to initiate combination drug therapy with a calcium channel blocker (nifedipine) and one of the three choices given below. Evaluate each choice in light of this case and make a recommendation.

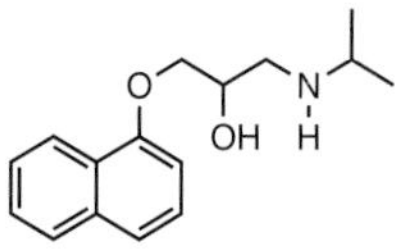

1

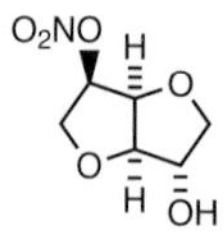

2

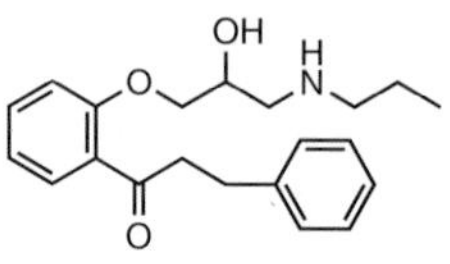

3

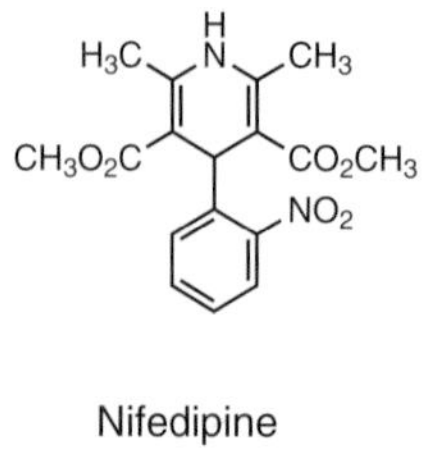

Nifedipine

1. Conduct a thorough and mechanistic SAR analysis of the three therapeutic options in the case.
2. Apply the chemical understanding gained from the SAR analysis to this patient's specific needs to make a therapeutic recommendation.

References

1. Smith TW, Antman EM, Friedman PL, et al. Digitalis glycosides: mechanisms and manifestations of toxicity. Part II. Prog Cardiovasc Dis 1984;26:495–540.
2. Smith TW, Antman EM, Friedman PL, et al. Digitalis glycosides: mechanisms and manifestations of toxicity. Part III. Prog Cardiovasc Dis 1984;27:21–56.
3. Rietbrock N, Woodcock BG. Two-hundred years of foxglove therapy: *Digitalis purpurea* 1785–1985. Trends Pharmacol Sci 1985;6:267–269.
4. Thomas R, Bontagy J, Gelbart A. Synthesis and biological activity of semisynthetic digitalis analogues. J Pharm Sci 1974;63:1649–1683.
5. Thomas R. Cardiac drugs. In: Wolff ME, ed. Burger's Medicinal Chemistry, 4th Ed., Part III. New York: John Wiley and Sons, 1981:47–102.
6. Repke K. New developments in cardiac glycoside structure–activity relationships. Trends Pharmacol Sci 1985;6:275–278.
7. Fullerton DS, Griffin JF, Rohrer DC, et al. Using computer graphics to study cardiac glycoside–receptor interactions. Trends Pharmacol Sci 1985;6:279–282.
8. Koren G, Woodland C, Ito S. Toxic digoxin–drug interactions: the major role of renal P-glycoprotein. Vet Human Toxicol 1998;40:45–46.
9. Colucci WS, Wright RF, Braunwald E. New positive inotropic agents in the treatment of congestive heart failure. 1. Mechanisms of action and recent clinical developments. N Engl J Med 1986;314:290–299.
10. Colucci WS, Wright RF, Braunwald E. New positive inotropic agents in the treatment of congestive heart failure. 2. Mechanisms of action and recent clinical developments. N Engl J Med 1986;314:349–358.
11. Westfall T, Westfall DP. Adrenergic agonists and antagonists. In: Brunton L, Lazo T, Barker K, eds. Goodman & Gilman's the Pharmacological Basis of Therapeutics, 11th Ed. New York: McGraw-Hill, 2006:237–296.
12. Needleman P, Jakschik B, Johnson EM Jr. Sulfhydryl requirement for relaxation of vascular smooth muscle. J Pharmacol Exp Ther 1973;187:324–331.
13. Needleman P, Johnson EM Jr. Mechanism of tolerance development to organic nitrates. J Pharmacol Exp Ther 1973;184:709–715.
14. Ignarro LJ, Lippton H, Edwards JC, et al. Mechanism of vascular smooth muscle relaxation by organic nitrates, nitrites, nitroprusside and nitric oxide: evidence for the involvement of S-nitrosothiols as active intermediates. J Pharmacol Exp Ther 1981;218:739–749.
15. Ignarro LJ, Barry BK, Gruetter DY, et al. Guanylate cyclase activation of nitroprusside and nitroguanidine is related to formation of S-nitrosothol intermediates. Biochem Biophys Res Commun 1980;94:93–100.
16. Ignarro LJ, Barry BK, Gruetter DY, et al. Selective alterations in responsiveness of guanylate cyclase to activation by nitroso compounds during enzyme purification. Biochim Biophys Acta 1981;673:394–407.
17. Ignarro LJ, Edwards JC, Gruetter DY, et al. Possible involvement of S-nitosothiols in the activation of guanylate cyclase by nitroso compounds. FEBS Lett 1980;110:275–278.
18. Ignarro LJ, Gruetter CA. Requirement of thiols for activation of coronary arterial guanylate cyclase by glyceryl trinitrate and sodium nitrite: possible involvement of S-nitrosothiols. Biochim Biophys Acta 1980;631:221–231.
19. Ignarro LJ, Kadowitz PJ, Baricos WH. Evidence that regulation of hepatic guanylate cyclase activity involves interactions between catalytic site -SH groups and both substrate and activator. Arch Biochem Biophys 1981;208:75–86.
20. Moncada S, Plamer RM, Higgs EA. Nitric oxide: physiology, pathophysiology, and pharmacology. Pharmacol Rev 1991;43:109–142.
21. Snyder SH, Bredt DS. Nitric oxide as a neuronal messenger. Trends Pharmacol Sci 1991;12:125–128.
22. McCall T, Vallance P. Nitric oxide takes centre-stage with newly defined roles. Trend Pharmacol Sci 1992;13:1–6.
23. Feldman PL, Criffen OW, Stuehr DJ. Surprising life of nitric oxide. Chem Eng News 1993;71:26–38.
24. Fung HL, Sutton SC, Kamiya A. Blood vessel uptake and metabolism of organic nitrates in the rat. J Pharmacol Exp Ther 1984;228:334–341.
25. Needleman P, Lang S, Johnson EM Jr. Organic nitrates: relationship between biotransformation and rational angina pectoris therapy. J Pharmacol Exp Ther 1972;181:489–497.
26. Abrams J. Pharmacology of nitroglycerin and long-acting nitrates. Am J Cardiol 1985;56:12A–18A.
27. Fung HL. Pharmacokinetics of nitroglycerin and long-acting nitrate esters. Am J Med 1983;72(Suppl):13–19.
28. Corwin S, Reiffel JA. Nitrate therapy for angina pectoris. Current concepts about mechanism of action and evaluation of currently available preparations. Arch Intern Med 1985;145:538–543.
29. Rahwan RG, Witiak DT, Muir WW. Newer antiarrhythmics. Annu Rep Med Chem 1981;16:257–268.
30. Yedinak KC. Use of calcium channel antagonists for cardiovascular disease. Am Pharm 1993;33:49–65.
31. Michalets EL. Update: clinically significant cytochrome P-450 drug interactions. Pharmacotherapy 1998;18:84–112.
32. Conn HL Jr, Luchi RJ. Some cellular and metabolic considerations relating to the action of quinidine as a prototype antiarrhythmic agent. Am J Med 1964;37:685–699.

Suggested Readings

Fozzard HA, Sheets MF. Cellular mechanism of action of cardiac glycosides. J Am Coll Cardiol 1985;5:10A–15A.

Hansten PD, ed. Drug Interactions: Clinical Significance of Drug–Drug Interactions, 5th Ed. Philadelphia: Lea and Febiger, 1985.

Kaplan HR. Advances in antiarrhythmic drug therapy: changing concepts. Federation Proc 1986;45:2184–2213.

Katz AM. Effects of digitalis on cell biochemistry: sodium pump inhibition. J Am Coll Cardiol 1985;5:16A–21A.

Kowey PR. Pharmacological effects of antiarrhythmic drugs. Arch Intern Med 1998;158:325–332.

Mangini RJ, ed. Drug Interaction Facts. St. Louis: J.B. Lippincott, 1983.

Michel T. Drugs used for the treatment of myocardial ischemia. In: Brunton L, Lazo T, Barker K, eds. Goodman and Gilman's the Pharmacological Basis of Therapeutics, 11th Ed. New York: McGraw-Hill, 2006:823–844.

Rocco T, Fong JG, Treatment of congestive heart failure. In: Brunton L, Lazo T, Barker K, eds. Goodman & Gilman's the Pharmacological Basis of Therapeutics, 11th Ed. New York: McGraw-Hill, 2006:869–898.

Thomas RE. Cardiac drugs. In: Wolff ME, ed. Burger's Medicinal Chemistry and Drug Discovery, 5th Ed., Part IIA, Vol 2. New York: John Wiley and Sons, 1996:153–261.

Chapter 22

Diuretics

PETER J. HARVISON AND GARY O. RANKIN

Drugs Covered in This Chapter*

OSMOTIC DIURETICS
- Glycerin
- Isosorbide
- Mannitol
- Sorbitol
- Urea

CARBONIC ANHYDRASE INHIBITORS
- Acetazolamide
- Brinzolamide/dorzolamide
- Methazolamide/ethoxzolamide/dichlorphenamide

THIAZIDE DIURETICS
- Bendroflumethiazide
- Benzthiazide
- Chlorothiazide
- Hydrochlorothiazide
- Hydroflumethiazide
- Methyclothiazide
- Polythiazide
- Trichlormethiazide

THIAZIDE-LIKE DIURETICS
- Chlorthalidone
- Indapamide
- Metolazone
- Quinethazone

LOOP DIURETICS
- *Azosemide/piretanide/tripamide*
- Bumetanide
- Ethacrynic acid
- Furosemide
- Torsemide

ALDOSTERONE ANTAGONISTS (MINERALOCORTICOID RECEPTOR ANTAGONISTS)
- *Canrenone*
- Eplerenone
- Spironolactone

POTASSIUM-SPARING DIURETICS
- Amiloride
- Triamterene

Abbreviations

AR, androgen receptor
ADH, antidiuretic hormone (vasopressin)
ENaC, epithelial sodium channel
GFR, glomerular filtration rate
GR, glucocorticoid receptor
MR, mineralocorticoid receptor
PR, progesterone receptor

*Drugs available outside the United States are shown in italics.

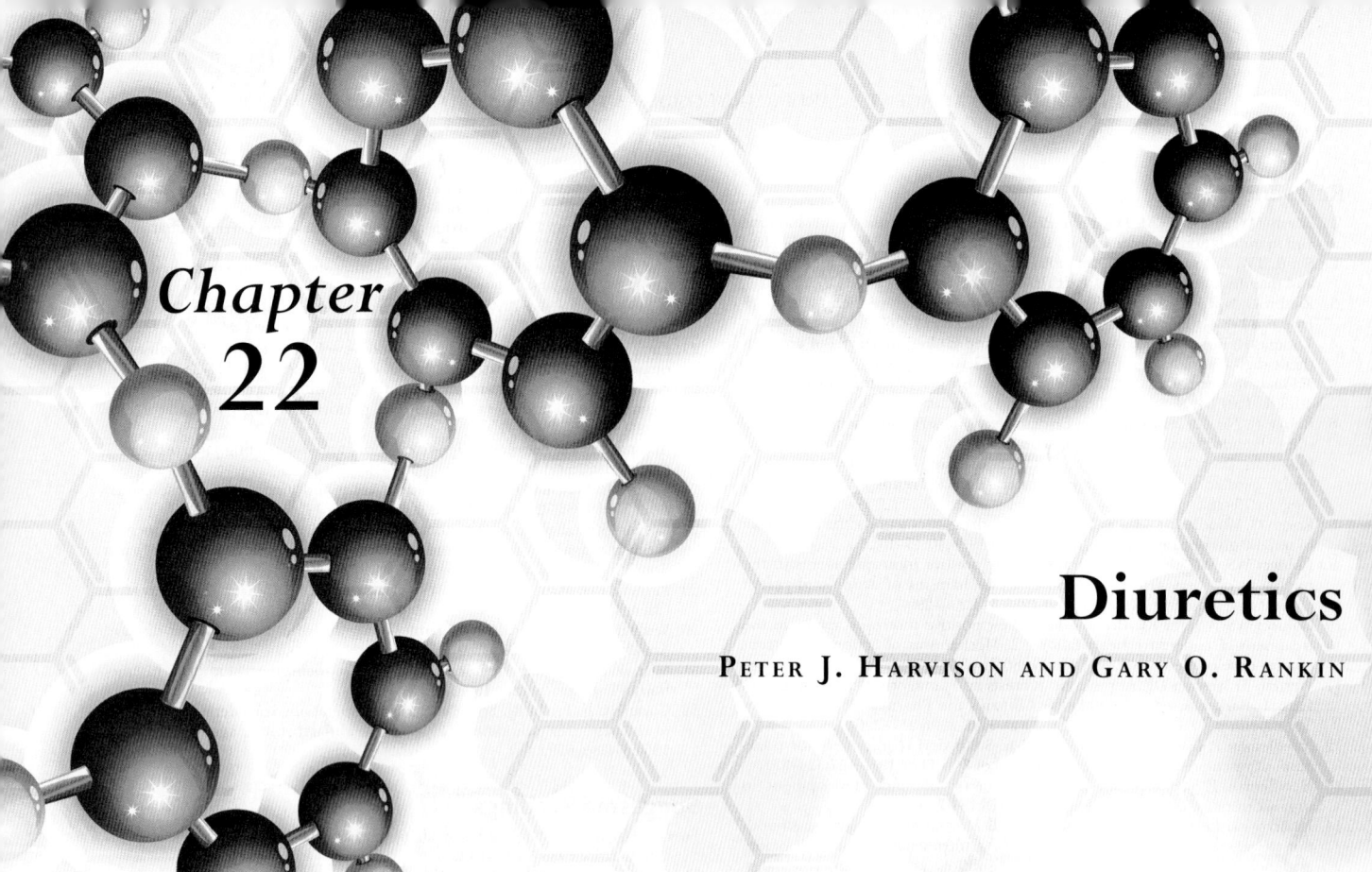

SCENARIO

Kim K. Birtcher, MS, PharmD, BCPS

TB, a 38-year-old white man, has been referred by his primary care physician (PCP) to the pharmacist-managed hypertension clinic. The patient states, "I was here for a physical. I haven't been to the doctor in awhile, and my wife encouraged me to come. I found out today that my blood pressure is a little high." The patient has no significant medical history or family history, and he is not taking any medications on a regular basis. His body mass index is 27, and his blood pressure is 162/92 mm Hg in the left arm and 164/88 mm Hg in the right arm. The baseline complete metabolic panel and fasting cholesterol panel from today are all within normal limits. The patient drinks wine occasionally with dinner, and he has never used tobacco. He works as an accountant. He is married and has two children living at home. The patient reports that he does not exercise on a regular basis, and he eats fast food for lunch during the week. The patient receives prescriptions and counseling for lisinopril 10 mg PO daily and HCTZ 12.5 mg PO daily. The patient is given information about the DASH diet and how to make healthier choices at the fast food restaurants. He is encouraged to do regular daily exercise, and he agrees to walk for at least 30 minutes each day during his lunch break. He is encouraged to lose weight. The patient agrees to buy a blood pressure cuff and to monitor his blood pressure at home. He agrees to fax his blood pressure logs to the office weekly so his medications could be titrated per protocol by the pharmacist.

(The reader is directed to the clinical solution and chemical analysis of this case at the end of the chapter).

INTRODUCTION

Diuretics are chemicals that increase the rate of urine formation (1). By increasing the urine flow rate, diuretic usage leads to increased excretion of electrolytes (especially sodium and chloride ions) and water from the body without affecting protein, vitamin, glucose, or amino acid reabsorption. These pharmacologic properties have led to the use of diuretics in the treatment of edematous conditions resulting from a variety of causes (e.g., congestive heart failure, nephrotic syndrome, and chronic liver disease) and in the management of hypertension. Diuretic drugs also are useful as the sole agent or as adjunct therapy in the treatment of a wide range of clinical conditions, including hypercalcemia, diabetes insipidus, acute mountain sickness, primary hyperaldosteronism, and glaucoma.

The primary target organ for diuretics is the kidney, where these drugs interfere with the reabsorption of sodium and other ions from the lumina of the nephrons, which are the functional units of the kidney. The amount of ions and accompanying water that are excreted as urine following administration of a diuretic, however, is determined by many factors, including the chemical structure of the diuretic, the site or sites of action of the agent, the salt intake of the patient, and the amount of extracellular fluid present. In addition to the direct effect of diuretics to impair solute and water reabsorption from the nephron, diuretics also can trigger compensatory physiologic events that have an impact on either the magnitude or the duration of the diuretic response. Thus, it is important to be aware of the normal mechanisms of urine formation and renal control mechanisms to understand clearly the ability of chemicals to induce diuresis.

NORMAL PHYSIOLOGY OF URINE FORMATION

Two important functions of the kidney are 1) to maintain a homeostatic balance of electrolytes and water and 2) to excrete water-soluble end products of metabolism. The kidney accomplishes these functions through the formation of urine by the nephrons (Fig. 22.1). Each kidney contains approximately 1 million nephrons and is capable of forming urine independently. The nephrons are composed of a specialized capillary bed called the glomerulus and a long tubule divided anatomically and functionally into the proximal tubule, loop of Henle, and distal tubule. Each component of the nephron contributes to the normal functions of the kidney in a unique manner; thus, all are targets for different classes of diuretic agents.

Urine formation begins with the filtration of blood at the glomerulus. Approximately 1,200 mL of blood per minute flows through both kidneys and reaches the nephron by way of afferent arterioles. Approximately 20% of the blood entering the glomerulus is filtered into Bowman's capsule to form the glomerular filtrate. The glomerular filtrate is composed of blood components with a molecular weight less than that of albumin (~69,000 daltons) and not bound to plasma proteins. The glomerular filtration rate (GFR) averages 125 mL/min in humans but can vary widely even in normal functional states.

The glomerular filtrate leaves the Bowman's capsule and enters the proximal convoluted tubule (S1, S2 segments; Fig. 22.1), where the majority (50% to 60%) of filtered sodium is reabsorbed osmotically. Sodium reabsorption is coupled electrogenetically with the reabsorption of glucose, phosphate, and amino acids and nonelectrogenetically with bicarbonate reabsorption. Glucose and amino acids are completely reabsorbed

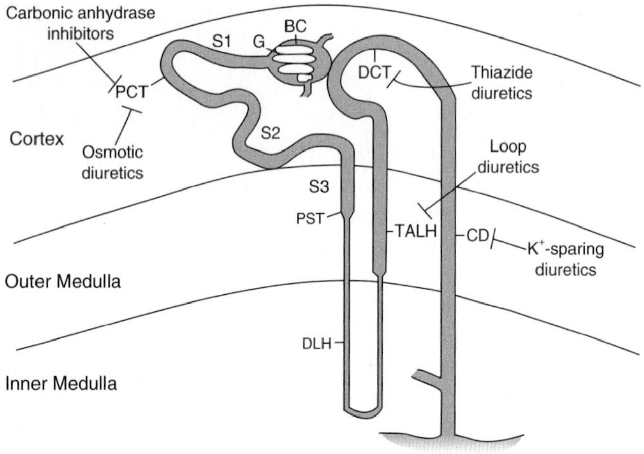

FIGURE 22.1 The nephron. BC, Bowman's capsule; CD, collecting duct; DCT, distal convoluted tubule; DLH, descending limb of the Loop of Henle; G, glomerulus; PCT, proximal convoluted tubule; PST, proximal straight tubule; TALH, thick ascending limb of the loop of Henle.

in this portion of the nephron, whereas phosphate reabsorption is between 80% and 90% complete. The early proximal convoluted tubule also is the primary site of bicarbonate reabsorption (80% to 90%), a process that is mainly sodium dependent and coupled to hydrogen ion secretion. The reabsorption of sodium and bicarbonate is facilitated by the enzyme carbonic anhydrase, which is present in proximal tubular cells and catalyzes the formation of carbonic acid from water and carbon dioxide. The carbonic acid provides the hydrogen ion, which drives the reabsorption of sodium bicarbonate. Chloride ions are reabsorbed passively in the proximal tubule, where they follow actively transported sodium ions into tubular cells.

The reabsorption of electrolytes and water also occurs isosmotically in the proximal straight tubule or pars recta (S3 segment; Fig. 22.1). By the end of the straight segment, between 65% and 70% of water and sodium, chloride, and calcium ions; 80% to 90% of bicarbonate and phosphate; and essentially 100% of glucose, amino acids, vitamins, and protein have been reabsorbed from the glomerular filtrate. The proximal tubule also is the site for active secretion of weakly acidic and weakly basic organic compounds. Thus, many of the diuretics can enter luminal fluid not only by filtration at the glomerulus but also by active secretion.

The descending limb of the loop of Henle is impermeable to ions, but water can freely move from the luminal fluid into the surrounding medullary interstitium, where the higher osmolality draws water into the interstitial space and concentrates luminal fluid. Luminal fluid continues to concentrate as it descends to the deepest portion of the loop of Henle, where the fluid becomes the most concentrated. The hypertonic luminal fluid next enters the water-impermeable, thick ascending limb of the loop of Henle. In this segment of the nephron, approximately 20% to 25% of the filtered sodium and chloride ions are reabsorbed via a cotransport system ($Na^+/K^+/2Cl^-$) on the luminal membrane. Reabsorption of sodium and chloride in the medullary portion of the thick ascending limb is important for maintaining the medullary interstitial concentration gradient. Reabsorption of sodium chloride in the cortical component of the thick ascending limb of the loop of Henle and the early distal

CLINICAL SIGNIFICANCE

It is important for the clinician to understand the medicinal chemistry of diuretics to appropriately use them in individual patients. This diverse group of medications is classified in many ways: mechanism of action, site of action, chemical class, and effect on urine contents. Knowledge of structure–activity relationships helps to predict indications, possible off-label uses, the magnitude of diuresis, potency, and the side effect profile.

Consequently, diuretics have a variety of uses. Thiazide diuretics may be used alone or in combination with other pharmacotherapy for the treatment of hypertension. Loop diuretics can provide immediate diuresis and are used for heart failure and in lieu of thiazides in patients with compromised renal function. In addition to more traditional uses, certain potassium-sparing diuretics provide added benefit to other pharmacotherapy in patients with primary hyperaldosteronism, heart failure, or who have had an acute myocardial infarction. Carbonic anhydrase inhibitors have limited use for diuresis; however, they may be used to reduce intraocular pressure and treat acute mountain sickness.

A thorough understanding of the medicinal chemistry, mechanisms of action, and pharmacokinetics helps the clinician appropriately use available diuretics. As new medications are developed, the clinician will rely on these basic concepts to continue tailoring therapy to the individual patient with the goals to maximize outcomes, improve quality of life, and minimize adverse events.

Kim K. Birtcher, MS, PharmD, BCPS
Clinical Associate Professor
Department of Clinical Sciences and Administration
University of Houston College of Pharmacy

convoluted tubule contributes to urinary dilution, and as a result, these two nephron sections sometimes are called the cortical diluting segment of the nephron.

Luminal fluid leaving the early distal tubule next passes through the late distal tubule and cortical collecting tubule (collecting duct), where sodium is reabsorbed in exchange for hydrogen and potassium ions. This process is partially controlled by mineralocorticoids (e.g., aldosterone) and accounts for the reabsorption of between 2% and 3% of filtered sodium ions. Although the reabsorption of sodium ions from these segments of the nephron is not large, this sodium/potassium/hydrogen ion exchange system determines the final acidity and potassium content of urine. Several factors, however, can influence the activity of this exchange system, including the amount of sodium ions delivered to these segments, the status of the acid-base balance in the body, and the levels of circulating aldosterone.

The urine formed during this process represents only approximately 1% to 2% of the original glomerular filtrate, with more than 98% of electrolytes and water filtered at the glomerulus being reabsorbed during passage through the nephron. Thus, a change in urine output of only 1% to 2% could double urine volume. Urine leaves the kidney through the ureters and travels to the bladder, where it is stored until urination removes it from the body.

NORMAL REGULATION OF URINE FORMATION

The body contains several control mechanisms that regulate the volume and contents of urine. These systems are activated by changes in solute or water content of the body, by changes in systemic or renal blood pressure, and by a variety of other stimuli. Activation of one or more of these systems by diuretic drugs can modify the effectiveness of these drugs to produce their therapeutic response and may require additional therapeutic measures to ensure a maximal response.

The kidney has the ability to respond to changes in the GFR through the action of specialized distal tubular epithelial cells called the macula densa. These cells are in close contact with the glomerular apparatus of the same nephron and detect changes in the rate of urine flow and luminal sodium chloride concentration. An increase in the urine flow rate at this site (as can occur with the use of some diuretics) activates the macula densa cells to communicate with the granular cells and vascular segments of the juxtaglomerular apparatus. Stimulation of the juxtaglomerular apparatus causes renin to be released, which leads to the formation of angiotensin II and subsequent renal vasoconstriction. Renal vasoconstriction leads to a decrease in GFR and, possibly, a decrease in the effectiveness of the diuretic. Renin release also can be stimulated by factors other than diuretics, including decreased renal perfusion pressure, increased sympathetic tone, and decreased blood volume.

Another important regulatory mechanism for urine formation is antidiuretic hormone (ADH), also known as vasopressin, which is released from the posterior pituitary in response to reduced blood pressure and elevated plasma osmolality. In the kidney, ADH acts on the collecting tubule to increase water permeability and reabsorption. As a result, the urine becomes more concentrated, and water is conserved in the presence of ADH.

DISEASE STATES

The diuretic drugs are used primarily to treat two medically important conditions, edema and hypertension (2–5). Both conditions are common, although some patients exhibit refractory disease states that require additional modification of the drug regimen to include alternative diuretics or addition of nondiuretic drugs. Edema (excessive extracellular fluid) normally results from disease to the heart, kidney, or liver. Decreased cardiac function (e.g., congestive heart disease) can result in decreased perfusion of all organs (e.g., kidney) and limbs and an accumulation of edema fluid in the extremities, particularly around the ankles and in the hands. Left-sided heart failure can lead to the development of acute pulmonary edema, which is a medical emergency. Right-sided heart failure shifts extracellular fluid volume from the arterial circulation to the venous circulation, which leads to general edema formation.

Kidney dysfunction can lead to edema formation as a result of decreased formation of urine and the subsequent imbalance of water and electrolyte (e.g., sodium ion) homeostasis. Retention of salt and water results in an expansion of the extracellular fluid volume and edema formation. Thus, when salt intake exceeds salt excretion, edema can form. Edema formation also is associated with deceased protein levels in blood, as seen in nephrotic syndrome and liver disease. Cirrhosis of the liver leads to increased lymph in the space of Disse. Eventually, the increased lymph volume results in movement of fluid into the peritoneal cavity and ascites develops.

Hypertension develops from many causes and will be discussed in more detail elsewhere (see Chapter 24). In general, hypertension occurs when blood pressure is sustained at greater than 140/90 mm Hg. At this blood pressure level, patients are at increased risk for developing cardiovascular disease. One key element in controlling blood pressure is sodium ion, and early antihypertensive effects of diuretics are related to increased salt and water excretion. Additionally, however, diuretics have long-term effects resulting in decreased vascular resistance that contribute to blood pressure control. Although effects on vascular calcium-activated potassium channels have been proposed as contributing to the chronic antihypertensive effects of thiazide diuretics, the exact mechanisms of long-term effects remain to be determined.

Diuretics also are useful in treating a number of other conditions including increased cranial (trauma or surgery) or intraocular (glaucoma) pressure (i.e., osmotic diuretics), diabetes insipidus (i.e., thiazides), hypercalcemia (i.e., loop diuretics), acute mountain sickness (i.e., carbonic anhydrase inhibitors), primary hyperaldosteronism (i.e., aldosterone antagonists), and osteoporosis (i.e., thiazides).

GENERAL THERAPEUTIC APPROACHES

Diuretic drugs may be administered acutely or chronically to treat edematous states. When immediate action to reduce edema (e.g., acute pulmonary edema) is needed, intravenous administration of a loop diuretic often is the approach of choice. Thiazide or loop diuretics normally are administered orally to treat nonemergency edematous states. The magnitude of the diuretic response is directly proportional to the amount of edema fluid that is present. As the volume of edema decreases, so does the magnitude of the diuretic response with each dose. If concern exists about diuretic-induced hypokalemia developing, then a potassium supplement or potassium-sparing diuretic may be added to the drug regimen. The development of hypokalemia is particularly important for patients with congestive heart failure who also are taking cardiac glycosides, such as digitalis. Digitalis has a narrow therapeutic index, and developing hypokalemia can potentiate digitalis-induced cardiac effects with potentially fatal results.

Diuretic drugs (thiazide and loop diuretics) are administered orally to help control blood pressure in the treatment of hypertension. Diuretics often are the first drugs used to treat hypertension, and they also may be added to other drug therapies used to control blood pressure with beneficial effects.

Diuretics have also been used illicitly by some athletes for "sport doping" (6). This is a consequence of the drugs' ability to quickly produce weight loss (via increased excretion of water) and masking of urine contents (via dilution of other drugs or metabolites that might be present in the urine). Furosemide, triamterene, and hydrochlorothiazide are the most commonly used diuretics for sport doping since they are eliminated rapidly and are therefore more difficult to detect in urine samples taken at later time points after use. Another consideration is that some diuretics can degrade in urine samples; for example, thiazides may hydrolyze to aminobenzenedisulfonamide derivatives (7). Use of diuretics by athletes without a documented therapeutic need has been banned since 1988, and routine monitoring for these drugs and their degradation products is commonplace. A list of banned drugs, including diuretics, is maintained and updated by the International Olympic Committee and the World Anti-Doping Agency.

DIURETIC DRUG CLASSES

History

Compounds that increase the urine flow rate have been known for centuries. One of the earliest substances known to induce diuresis is water, an inhibitor of ADH release. Calomel (mercurous chloride) was used as early as the 16th century as a diuretic, but because of poor absorption from the gastrointestinal tract and toxicity, calomel was replaced clinically by the organomercurials (e.g., chlormerodrin). The organomercurials represented the first group of highly efficacious diuretics available for clinical use. The need to administer these drugs parenterally, the possibility of tolerance, and their potential toxicity, however, soon led to the search for newer, less toxic diuretics. Today, the organomercurials are no longer used as diuretics, but their discovery began the search for many of the diuretics used today. Other compounds previously used as diuretics include the acid-forming salts (ammonium chloride) and methylxanthines (theophylline).

Structure Classification

The diuretics currently in use today (Table 22.1) are classified by their chemical class (thiazides), mechanism of action (carbonic anhydrase inhibitors and osmotics), site of action (loop diuretics), or effects on urine contents (potassium-sparing diuretics). These drugs vary widely in their efficacy (i.e., their ability to increase the rate of urine formation) and their site of action within the nephron. Efficacy often is measured as the ability of the diuretic to increase the excretion of sodium ions filtered at the glomerulus (i.e., the filtered load of sodium) and should not be confused with potency, which is the amount of the diuretic required to produce a specific diuretic response.

Efficacy is determined, in part, by the site of action of the diuretic. Drugs (e.g., carbonic anhydrase inhibitors) that act primarily on the proximal convoluted tubule to induce diuresis are weak diuretics because of the ability of the nephron to reabsorb a significant portion of the luminal contents in latter portions of the nephron. Likewise, drugs (potassium-sparing diuretics) that act at the more distal segments of the nephron are weak diuretics, because most of the glomerular filtrate has already been reabsorbed in the proximal tubule and ascending limb of the loop of Henle before reaching the distal tubule. Thus, the most efficacious diuretics discovered so far, the high-ceiling or loop diuretics, interfere with sodium chloride reabsorption at the ascending limb of the loop of Henle, which is situated after the proximal tubule but before the distal portions of the nephron and collecting tubule (Fig. 22.1).

Osmotic Diuretics

Mechanism of Action

Osmotic diuretics are low molecular weight compounds that are freely filtered through the Bowman's capsule into the renal tubules, are nonreabsorbable solutes, and are not extensively metabolized except for glycerin and urea (see Table 22.2 for their pharmacokinetic properties). Once in the renal tubule, osmotic diuretics have a limited reabsorption because of their high

TABLE 22.1 Diuretics: Sites and Mechanisms of Action

Class of Diuretic	Site of Action	Mechanism of Action
Osmotics	Proximal tubule	Osmotic effects decrease sodium and water reabsorption
	Loop of Henle	Increases medullary blood flow to decrease medullary hypertonicity and reduce sodium and water reabsorption
	Collecting tubule	Sodium and water reabsorption decreases because of reduced medullary hypertonicity and elevated urinary flow rate
Carbonic anhydrase inhibitors	Proximal convoluted tubule	Inhibition of renal carbonic anhydrase decreases sodium bicarbonate reabsorption
Thiazides and thiazide-like	Cortical portion of the thick ascending limb of loop of Henle and distal tubule	Inhibition of Na^+/Cl^- symporter
Loop or high-ceiling	Thick ascending limb of the loop of Henle	Inhibition of the luminal $Na^+/K^+/2Cl^-$ transport system
Potassium-sparing	Distal tubule and collecting duct	Inhibition of sodium and water reabsorption by competitive inhibition of aldosterone (spironolactone) and blockade of sodium channel at the luminal membrane (triamterene and amiloride)

water solubility. When administered as a hypertonic (hyperosmolar) solution, these agents increase intraluminal osmotic pressure, causing water to pass from the body into the tubule. Since the osmotic agent and associated water are not reabsorbed from the nephron, a diuretic effect is observed. Osmotic diuretics increase the volume of urine and the excretion of water and almost all of the electrolytes.

Polyols, such as mannitol, sorbitol, and isosorbide, provide this effect. Sugars, such as glucose and sucrose, also can have a diuretic effect by this mechanism. Although not a polyol, urea has a similar osmotic effect and has been used in the past as an osmotic diuretic.

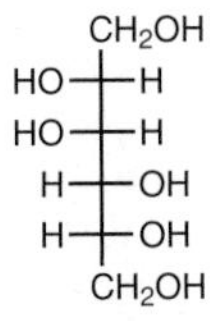
Mannitol

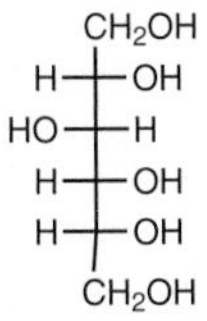
Sorbitol

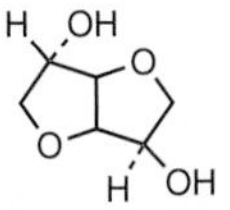
Isosorbide

Therapeutic Applications

Osmotic diuretics are not frequently used in medicine today except in the prophylaxis of acute renal failure, in which these drugs inhibit water reabsorption and maintain urine flow. They also may be helpful in maintaining urine flow in cases where urinary output is diminished because of severe bleeding or traumatic surgical experiences. The osmotic diuretics also have been used to acutely reduce increased intracranial or intraocular pressure. They are not considered to be primary diuretic agents in treating ordinary edemas, because osmotic diuretics can expand extracellular fluid volume.

Adverse Effects

Osmotic diuretics induce few adverse effects, but expansion of the extracellular fluid volume can occur, as noted earlier. Alteration of blood sodium levels can be seen, and these drugs should not be used in anuric or unresponsive patients. If cranial bleeding is present, mannitol or urea should not be used.

Specific Drugs

Mannitol Mannitol is the agent most commonly used as an osmotic diuretic. Sorbitol also can be used for similar reasons. These compounds can be prepared by the electrolytic reduction of glucose or sucrose.

Mannitol is administered intravenously in solutions of 5% to 50% at a rate of administration that is adjusted to maintain the urinary output at 30 to 50 mL/hour. Mannitol is filtered at the glomerulus and is poorly reabsorbed by the kidney tubule (8). The osmotic effect of mannitol in the tubule inhibits the reabsorption of water, and the rate of urine flow can be maintained. It also is used to reduce intracranial pressure by reducing cerebral intravascular volume.

Isosorbide Isosorbide is basically a bicyclic form of sorbitol that is used orally to cause a reduction in intraocular

TABLE 22.2 Pharmacokinetic Properties of the Nonthiazide Diuretics

Drug	Trade Name	Relative Potency	Oral Absorption (%)	Peak Plasma	Half-Life	Duration of Effect	Elimination
Osmotic diuretics							
Glycerin			>80	1–1.5 h	0.5–0.75 h	4–6 h	Urine, as metabolites
Isosorbide			>80	1–1.5 h	5–9.5 h	5–6 h	Urine, as parent drug
Mannitol			<20	1–3 h IV	0.5-1.5 h	6–8 h	Urine, as parent drug
Urea			<10	1–2 h IV	NA	5-6 h	Urine and bacterial urease in gut
Loop diuretics: high-ceiling diuretics							
Furosemide	Lasix	1	11–90[a]	4–5 h	0.5–4 h (>3 h)[b]	6–8 h	Urine/feces, as parent drug (60%–70%) and metabolites
Bumetanide	Bumex	40	80–100	<2 h	1–1.5 h (>3 h)[b]	5–6 h	Urine (major), as parent drug (~50%) and ~5 metabolites
Ethacrynic acid	Edecrin	0.7	>90	2 h	0.5–1 h	6–8 h	Urine/feces, as parent drug (30%–60%) and mercapturic acid
Torsemide	Demadex	3	80–100	1–2 h	0.8–4 h	6–8 h	Urine/feces (2:8), as parent drug
Carbonic anhydrase inhibitors							
Acetazolamide	Diamox		>90	1–3 h	6–9 h	8–12 h	Urine (major), as parent drug (70%–100%)
Methazolamide	Neptazane		>90	NA	~14 h	10–18 h	Urine, as parent drug (~25%) and metabolites
Ethoxzolamide	Cardrase		65	2.5–5.5 h			
Brinzolamide	Azopt		Topical use only (eye)	NA	~111 days[c]	8-12 h	Urine, as parent drug (major)
Dorzolamide	Truspot		Topical use only (eye)	NA	4 months[c]	8-12 h	Urine, as parent drug (major)
Potassium-sparing diuretics (inhibitors of renal epithelial Na^+ channels)							
Amiloride	Midamor	1	~50[a]	3–4 h	6–9 h normal (21 h)[b]	24 h	Urine/feces (5:4), as parent drug
Triamterene	Dyrenium	0.1	>70	2–4 h	2–3 h	>24 h	Urine, as parent drug and metabolites
Mineralocorticoid receptor antagonists							
Spironolactone	Aldactone	20–40	>90[d]	1–2 h	1–3 h (parent drug)	2–3 d	Urine/feces, as active metabolite(s)
Canrenone (7α-thiospironolactone)			NA	NA	3–4 h	13–24 h	Urine
Eplerenone	Inspra	1	70	1.5 h	4–6 h	NA	Urine/feces (2:1), as metabolites (>95%)

[a]Food affects bioavailability.
[b]In patients with renal insufficiency.
[c]Strongly bound to red blood cells.
[d]Formulation affects bioavailability.
IV, intravenous; NA, data not available.
Data from AHFS Drug Information (2010), American Society of Health-System Pharmacists; Lexicomp Online (2011), Lexicomp, Inc.; Facts and Comparisons (2010), Wolters Kluwer Health.

pressure in glaucoma cases. Although a diuretic effect is noted, its ophthalmologic properties are its primary value.

Carbonic Anhydrase Inhibitors

Mechanism of Action

In 1937, it was proposed that the normal acidification of urine was caused by secretion of hydrogen ions by the tubular cells of the kidney. These ions were provided by the action of the enzyme carbonic anhydrase, which catalyzes the formation of carbonic acid (H_2CO_3) from carbon dioxide and water.

$$CO_2 + H_2O \longrightarrow H_2CO_3 \longrightarrow H^{\oplus} + HCO_3^{\ominus}$$

It also was observed that sulfanilamide rendered the urine of dogs alkaline because of the inhibition of carbonic anhydrase. This inhibition of carbonic anhydrase resulted in a lesser exchange of hydrogen ions for sodium ions in the kidney tubule. Sodium ions, along with bicarbonate ions, and associated water molecules were then excreted, and a diuretic effect was noted. The large doses required and the side effects of sulfanilamide prompted a search for more effective carbonic anhydrase inhibitors as diuretic drugs.

It was soon learned that the sulfonamide portion of an active diuretic molecule could not be monosubstituted or disubstituted (9,10). It was reasoned that a more acidic sulfonamide would bind more tightly to the carbonic anhydrase enzyme. Synthesis of more highly acidic sulfonamides produced compounds with activities greater than 2,500-fold that of sulfanilamide. Acetazolamide was introduced in 1953 as an orally effective diuretic drug. Before that time, the organic mercurials, which commonly required intramuscular injection, were the principal diuretics available.

Carbonic anhydrase inhibitors induce diuresis by inhibiting the formation of carbonic acid within proximal (proximal convoluted tubule; S2) and distal tubular cells to limit the number of hydrogen ions available to promote sodium reabsorption. For a diuretic response to be observed, more than 99% of the carbonic anhydrase must be inhibited. Although carbonic anhydrase activity in the proximal tubule regulates the reabsorption of approximately 20% to 25% of the filtered load of sodium, the carbonic anhydrase inhibitors are not highly efficacious diuretics. An increased excretion of only 2% to 5% of the filtered load of sodium is seen with carbonic anhydrase inhibitors because of increased reabsorption of sodium ions by the ascending limb of the loop of Henle and more distal nephron segments.

Therapeutic Applications

With prolonged use of the carbonic anhydrase inhibitor diuretics, the urine becomes more alkaline, and the blood becomes more acidic. When acidosis occurs, the carbonic anhydrase inhibitors lose their effectiveness as diuretics. They remain ineffective until normal acid-base balance in the body has been regained. For this reason, this class of compounds is limited in its diuretic use. Today, they are most commonly used in the treatment of glaucoma, in which they inhibit carbonic anhydrase in the eye, reduce the rate of aqueous humor formation, and consequently, reduce intraocular pressure (11). These compounds also have found some limited use in the treatment of absence seizures, to alkalinize the urine, to treat familial periodic paralysis, to reduce metabolic alkalosis, and prophylactically, to reduce acute mountain sickness.

Adverse Effects

The carbonic anhydrase inhibitors generally do not produce serious side effects. However, monitoring for electrolyte disturbances may be necessary. Gastrointestinal (e.g., nausea, vomiting), nervous system (e.g., sedation, headache), and renal effects (kidney stones) have been reported. Although they contain sulfonamide groups, hypersensitivity reactions with other sulfonamide-containing drugs are not common. As noted earlier, these drugs can produce metabolic acidosis.

Specific Drugs

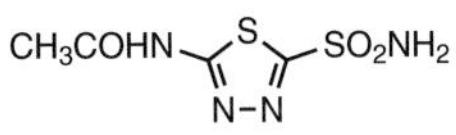

Acetazolamide

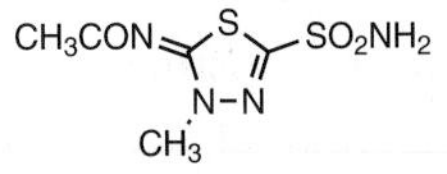

Methazolamide

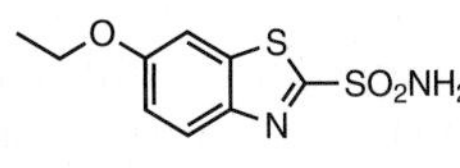

Ethoxzolamide

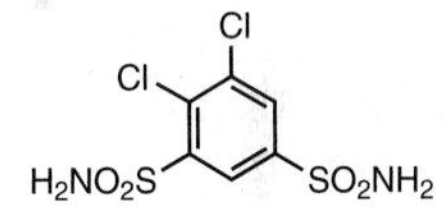

Dichlorphenamide

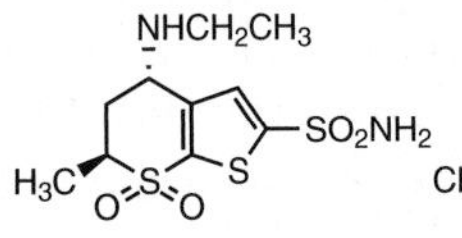

Dorzolamide

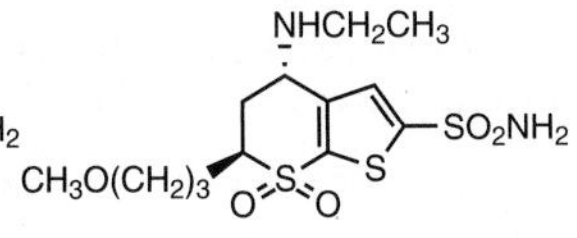

Brinzolamide

ACETAZOLAMIDE Acetazolamide, a thiadiazole derivative, was the first of the carbonic anhydrase inhibitors to be introduced as an orally effective diuretic, with a therapeutic effect that lasts approximately 8 to 12 hours (Table 22.2). As mentioned earlier, its diuretic action is limited because of the systemic acidosis it produces. The dose is 250 mg to 1 g per day.

METHAZOLAMIDE, ETHOXZOLAMIDE, AND DICHLORPHENAMIDE Methazolamide is a close structural analog of acetazolamide in which one of the active hydrogens in the thiadiazole ring has been replaced by a methyl group. This decreases polarity of the compound and permits a greater penetration into the ocular fluid, where it acts as a carbonic anhydrase inhibitor, reducing intraocular pressure. Its dose for glaucoma is 50 to 100 mg two to three times a day. Ethoxzolamide has a sulfonamide group attached to a fused 1,3-benzothiazole ring. Typical doses are 62.5 to 125 mg up to four times a day. Dichlorphenamide is a disulfonamide derivative that shares the same pharmacologic properties and clinical uses as the previously discussed compounds. The dose of dichlorphenamide is 25 to 100 mg one to three times a day. Distribution of these three drugs into the ocular compartment is not selective, and they can also inhibit multiple carbonic anhydrase isozymes in other tissues (11). Both of these properties can contribute to their side effects.

Brinzolamide and Dorzolamide Brinzolamide and dorzolamide contain ionizable amino groups and are the result of efforts to develop water-soluble carbonic anhydrase inhibitors that retain sufficient lipophilicity to penetrate the cornea (11). They are only indicated for topical eye administration in glaucoma patients. However, both drugs can be absorbed from ocular fluids into the blood. This results in prolonged half-lives (e.g., 111 days for brinzolamide in whole blood) because the drugs bind to carbonic anhydrase, especially in red blood cells.

Benzothiadiazine or Thiazide Diuretics

Mechanism of Action

Further study of the benzene disulfonamide derivatives was undertaken to find more efficacious carbonic anhydrase inhibitors. These studies provided some compounds with a high degree of diuretic activity. Chloro and amino substitution gave compounds with increased activity, but these compounds were weak carbonic anhydrase inhibitors. When the amino group was acylated, an unexpected ring closure took place. These compounds possessed a diuretic activity independent of the carbonic anhydrase inhibitory activity, and a new series of diuretics called the benzothiadiazines was discovered (9,10,12).

These diuretics are actively secreted in the proximal tubule and are carried to the loop of Henle and to the distal tubule. The major site of action of these compounds is in the distal convoluted tubule, where these drugs compete for the chloride binding site of the Na^+/Cl^- symporter and inhibit the reabsorption of sodium and chloride ions. For this reason, they are referred to as saluretics. They also inhibit the reabsorption of potassium and bicarbonate ions, but to a lesser degree.

Structure–Activity Relationship

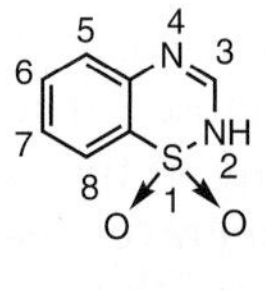

The thiazide diuretics are weakly acidic (see Appendix A for their pK_a values), with a benzothiadiazine 1,1-dioxide nucleus. The structure for the thiazide diuretics, relative activities, and pharmacokinetic properties for the thiazides are shown in Table 22.3. Chlorothiazide is the simplest member of this series, having a pK_a of 6.7 and 9.5. The hydrogen atom at the 2-N is the most acidic because of the electron-withdrawing effects of the neighboring sulfone group. The sulfonamide group that is substituted at C-7 provides an additional point of acidity in the molecule but is less acidic than the 2-N proton. These acidic protons make possible the formation of a water-soluble sodium salt that can be used for intravenous administration of the diuretics.

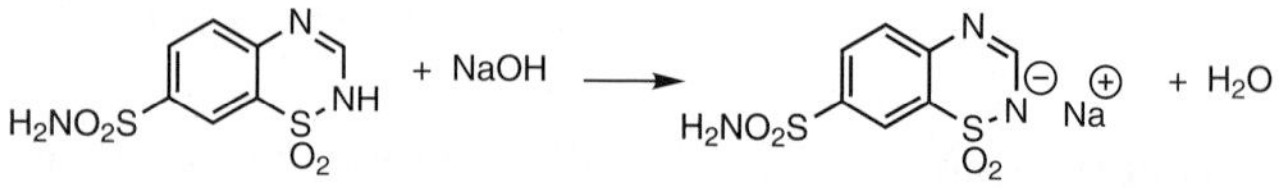

An electron-withdrawing group is necessary at position 6 for diuretic activity. Little diuretic activity is seen with a hydrogen atom at position 6, whereas compounds with a chloro or trifluoromethyl substitution are highly active (9,10,12). The trifluoromethyl-substituted diuretics are more lipid-soluble and have a longer duration of action than their chloro-substituted analogs. When electron-releasing groups, such as methyl or methoxyl, are placed at position 6, the diuretic activity is markedly reduced.

Replacement or removal of the sulfonamide group at position 7 yields compounds with little or no diuretic activity. Saturation of the double bond to give a 3,4-dihydro derivative produces a diuretic that is 10-fold more active than the unsaturated derivative. Substitution with a lipophilic group at position 3 gives a marked increase in the diuretic potency. Haloalkyl, aralkyl, or thioether substitution increases the lipid solubility of the molecule and yields compounds with a longer duration of action. Alkyl substitution on the 2-N position also decreases the polarity and increases the duration of diuretic action (Table 22.3). Although these compounds do have carbonic anhydrase activity, there is no correlation of this activity with their saluretic activity (excretion of sodium and chloride ions).

Therapeutic Applications

The thiazide diuretics are administered once a day or in divided daily doses. Some have a duration of action that permits administration of a dose every other day. Several of these compounds are rapidly absorbed orally and can show their diuretic effect in an hour (Table 22.3). These compounds are not extensively metabolized and are primarily excreted unchanged in the urine. Thiazide diuretics are used to treat edemas caused by cardiac decompensation as well as in hepatic or renal disease. They also commonly are used in the treatment of hypertension. Their effect may be attributed to a reduction in blood volume and a direct relaxation of vascular smooth muscle.

TABLE 22.3 Pharmacologic and Pharmacokinetic Properties for the Thiazide Diuretics

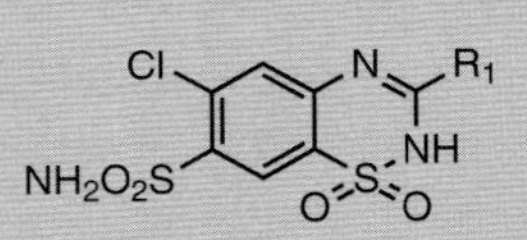

Structure I

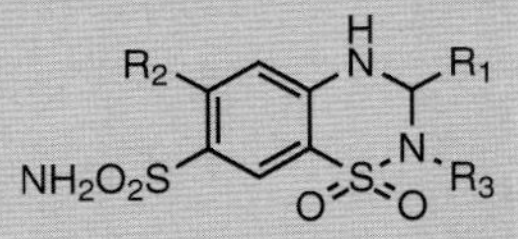

Structure II

Generic Name	Trade Name	Structure	Relative Potency[a]	Carbonic Anhydrase Inhibition[b]	Bioavailability	Peak Plasma (hours)	Half-life (hours)	Duration of Effect (hours)	Elimination
Chlorothiazide	Diuril	Structure I: R_1 = H	0.8	2×10^{-6}	<25%	4	0.75–2	12–16	U
Benzthiazide	Exna	Structure I: R_1 = 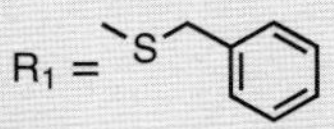	1.3	$\sim 10^{-7}$	NA	4	3–3.9	12–16	NA
Hydrochlorothiazide	HydroDiuril Esidrix	Structure II: R_1 = H, R_2 = Cl, R_3 = H	1.4	2×10^{-5}	>80%	4–6	6–15	12–16	U
Trichlormethiazide	Diurese Metahydrin Naqua	Structure II: R_1 = $CHCl_2$, R_2 = Cl; R_3 = H	1.7	6×10^{-5}	Var	6	2–7	24	U
Methyclothiazide	Enduron Aquatensen	Structure II: R_1 = CH_2Cl R_2 = Cl; R_3 = CH_3	1.8		Var	6	NA	>24	U
Polythiazide	Renese	Structure II: R_1 = $-CH_2-S-CH_2-CF_3$, R_2 = Cl, R_3 = CH_3	2.0	5×10^{-7}	Var	6	NA	24–48	U + 30% M
Hydroflumethiazide	Saluron Diucardin	Structure II: R_1 = H, R_2 = CF_3, R_3 = H	1.3	2×10^{-4}	Inc	3–4	17	18–24	U + M
Bendroflumethiazide	Naturetin	Structure II: R_1 = benzyl, R_2 = CF_3, R_3 = H	1.8	3×10^{-4}	>90%	4	8.5	6–12	U

[a]The numerical values refer to potency ratios (in humans) with the natriuretic response to that of a standard dose of meralluride, which is given a value of one;

[b]50% inhibition of carbonic anhydrase in vitro.

NA, data not available; Var, variable absorption; Inc, incomplete absorption.

Data from AHFS Drug Information (2010), American Society of Health-System Pharmacists; Lexicomp Online (2011), Lexicomp, Inc.; Facts and Comparisons (2010), Wolters Kluwer Health.

U, urine unchanged; M, metabolized.

Adverse Effects

Thiazide diuretics may induce a number of adverse effects, including hypersensitivity reactions, gastric irritation, nausea, and electrolyte imbalances, such as hyponatremia, hypokalemia, hypomagnesemia, hypochloremic alkalosis, hypercalcemia, and hyperuricemia. Individuals who exhibit hypersensitivity reactions to one thiazide are likely to have a hypersensitivity reaction to other thiazides and sulfamoyl-containing diuretics (e.g., thiazide-like and some high-ceiling diuretics). Potassium and magnesium supplements may be administered to treat hypokalemia or hypomagnesemia, but their use is not always indicated. These supplements usually are administered as potassium chloride, potassium gluconate, potassium citrate, magnesium oxide, or magnesium lactate. The salts are administered as solutions, tablets, or timed-release tablets. Generally, approximately 20 mEq of potassium is given daily. In cases of hypokalemia, 40 to 100 mEq/day may be administered. Potassium-sparing diuretics (e.g., triamterene or amiloride) also may be used to prevent hypokalemia. Combination preparations of hydrochlorothiazide or a potassium-sparing diuretic are available (e.g., Diazide and Moduretic).

Long-term use of thiazide diuretics also may result in decreased glucose tolerance and increased blood lipid (low-density lipoprotein cholesterol, total cholesterol, and total triglyceride) content.

Thiazide-like Diuretics

Mechanism of Action

This is a structurally diverse group of sulfonamide derivatives that do not contain benzothiadiazine rings (Table 22.4). Nevertheless, they have the same mechanism of action and similar therapeutic activities and adverse effects as the thiazide diuretics.

Specific Drugs

QUINAZOLINONE DERIVATIVES: METOLAZONE AND QUINETHAZONE

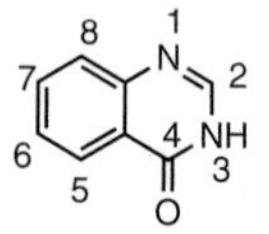

quinazolin-4-one

Overview The quinazolin-4-one molecule has been structurally modified in a manner similar to the modification of the thiazide diuretics. Metolazone and quinethazone (pK_a = 9.7) are examples of this class (Table 22.4). The structural difference between the quinazolinone diuretics is the replacement of the 4-sulfone group (—SO_2—) with a 4-keto group (—CO—). Because of their similar structures, it is not surprising that the quinazolinones have a diuretic effect similar to that of the thiazides.

TABLE 22.4 Pharmacokinetic Properties for the Thiazide-Like Diuretics

Generic name	Trade name	Structure	Bioavailability	Peak Plasma	Half-life (hours)	Duration (hours)	Route of Elimination
Metolazone	Zaroxylon	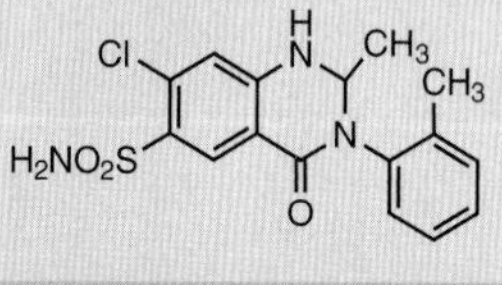	<65%	8–12 h	14	12–24	Urine/feces (8:2), as parent drug (>70%)
Quinethazone	Hydromox	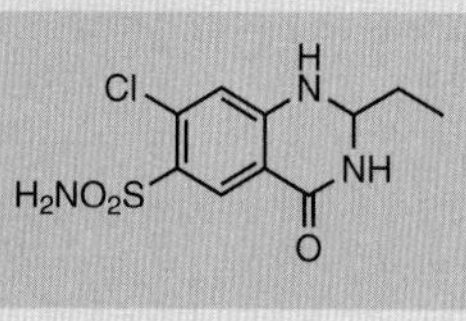	NA	6 h	6–15	18–24	Urine as parent drug
Chlorthalidone	Hygroton Thalitone#	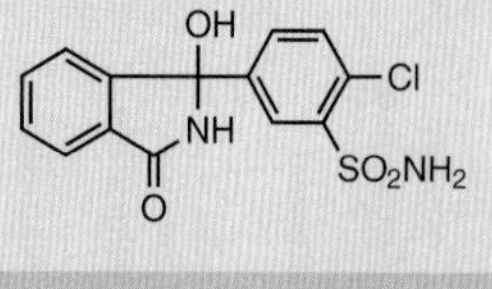	Inc/var. >90%	4 h 2 h	35–50*	48–72	Urine, as parent drug (50–65%)
Indapamide	Lozol	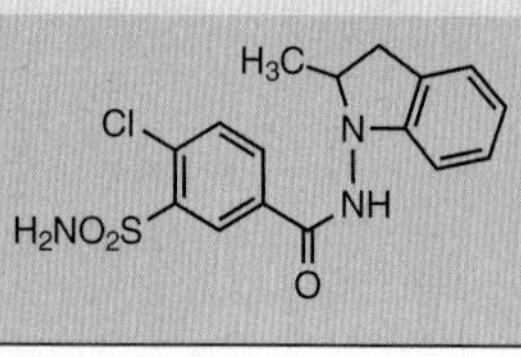	>90%	2–3 h	14–18	8 wks	Urine/feces (6:2), as parent drug (<10%) and metabolities

Data from AHFS Drug Information (2010). American Society of Health-System Pharmacists; Lexicomp Online (2011), Lexicomp, Inc.; Facts and Comparisons (2010), Wolters Kluwer Health.

*Strongly bound to red blood cells. #= not interchangable with similar drug. NA = data not available. var. = variable absorption. inc.= incomplete absorption.

Therapeutic Applications The pharmacokinetic properties for the quinazolinone diuretics are listed in Table 22.4. They have a long duration of action, usually as a result of protein binding. Although chlorothiazide has a duration of action of 6 to 12 hours, quinethazone has a duration of 18 to 24 hours, and metolazone has a duration of 12 to 24 hours. Metolazone has a bioavailability of 65% (Zaroxolyn) and a prolonged onset to reach peak plasma concentrations of action ranging from 8 to 12 hours. Another formulation of metolazone (Mykrox) was more rapidly absorbed and had improved bioavailability (>90%) compared to Zaroxolyn, but it has been discontinued in the United States and other countries. Approximately 50% to 70% of metolazone is bound to carbonic anhydrase in the erythrocytes. Metolazone also has an increased potency, and the mode of action for both compounds is similar to that of the thiazide derivatives. In contrast to thiazide diuretics, metolazone may be effective as a diuretic when the GFR falls below 40 mL/min. The dose of quinethazone is 50 to 100 mg daily and that of metolazone is 2.5 to 20 mg given as a single oral dose. Side effects are similar to adverse effects induced by the thiazide diuretics.

PHTHALIMIDINE DERIVATIVES: CHLORTHALIDONE

Overview Chlorthalidone (pK_a = 9.4) is an example of a diuretic in this class of compounds that bears a structural analogy to the quinazolinones (Table 22.4). This compound may be named as a 1-oxo-isoindoline or a phthalimidine. Although the molecule exists primarily in the phthalimidine form, the ring may be opened to form a benzophenone derivative. The benzophenone form illustrates the relationship to the quinazolinone series of diuretics.

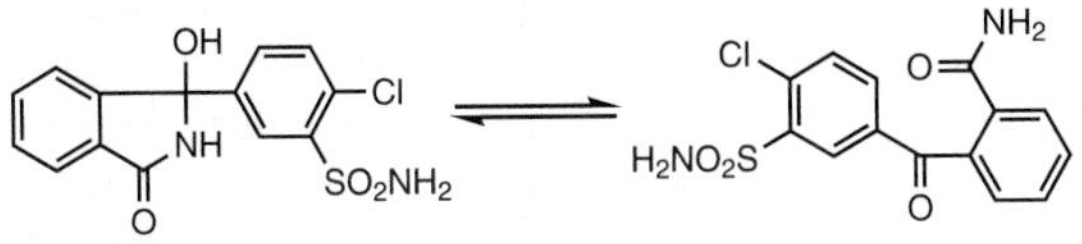

Therapeutic Application Chlorthalidone has a long duration of action (48 to 72 hours) (see Table 22.4 for its other pharmacokinetic properties). Although quinethazone and metolazone are administered daily, chlorthalidone may be administered in doses of 25 to 100 mg three times a week. When chlorthalidone is formulated with the excipient povidone, the product, Thalitone, has greater bioavailability (>90%) and reaches peak plasma concentrations in a shorter time compared with its other products. Similar to the quinazolinones, it also is extensively bound to carbonic anhydrase in the erythrocytes. Chlorthalidone-induced effects on urine content and side effects are similar to those induced by thiazide diuretics.

INDOLINES: INDAPAMIDE

Overview The prototypic indoline diuretic is indapamide, which was reported as a diuretic in 1984. Indapamide contains a polar chlorobenzamide moiety and a nonpolar lipophilic methylindoline group. In contrast to the thiazides, indapamide does not contain a thiazide ring, and only one sulfonamide group is present within the molecular structure (pK_a = 8.8). It is rapidly and completely absorbed from the gastrointestinal tract and reaches its peak plasma level in 2 to 3 hours, with a duration of action of up to 8 weeks. This prolonged duration of action is associated with its extensive binding to carbonic anhydrase in the erythrocytes. It exhibits biphasic kinetics, with a half-life of 14 to 18 hours and an elimination half-life of 24 hours. Indapamide is extensively metabolized (60% to 70%), with several of the metabolites being shown in Figure 22.2 (13,14). In vitro studies support aromatic hydroxylation as a metabolic route. Less than 10% of the drug is excreted unchanged, whereas the remaining 20% to 30% is eliminated via extrahepatic cycling.

Therapeutic Applications Uses of indapamide include the treatment of essential hypertension and edema resulting from congestive heart failure. Like metolazone, indapamide is an effective diuretic drug when GFR falls below 40 mL/min. The duration of action is approximately 24 hours, with the normal oral adult dosage starting at 2.5 mg given each morning. The dose may be increased to 5.0 mg/day, but doses beyond this level do not appear to provide additional results. Effects on urine content and side effects are similar to effects induced by thiazide diuretics.

High-Ceiling or Loop Diuretics

Mechanism of Action

This class of drugs is characterized more by its pharmacologic similarities than by its chemical similarities. Examples include furosemide, bumetanide, torsemide, and ethacrynic acid. These drugs produce a peak diuresis much greater than that observed with the other commonly used diuretics, hence the name high-ceiling diuretics. Their main

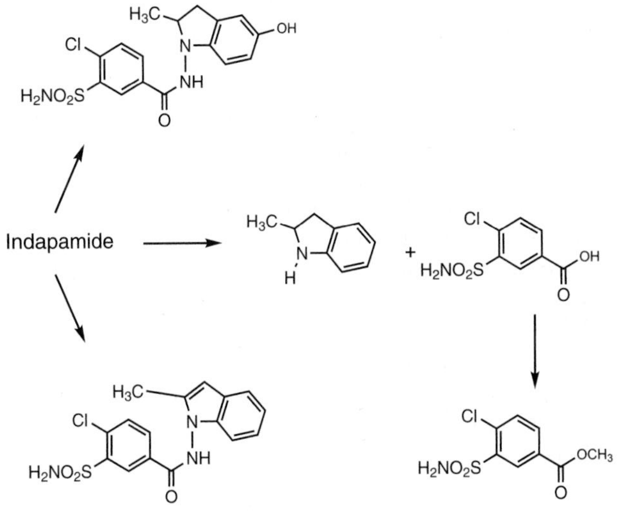

FIGURE 22.2 Metabolism of indapamide.

site of action is believed to be on the thick ascending limb of the loop of Henle, where they inhibit the luminal Na^+/K^+/$2Cl^-$ symporter. These diuretics are commonly referred to as loop diuretics. Additional effects on the proximal and distal tubules also are possible. High-ceiling diuretics are characterized by a quick onset and short duration of activity (15). Their diuretic effect appears in approximately 30 minutes and lasts for approximately 6 hours. The pharmacokinetic properties for the loop diuretics are listed in Table 22.2.

Specific Drugs

Furosemide

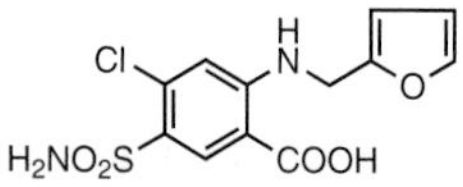

Furosemide

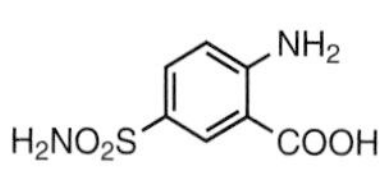

5-Sulfamoyl-anthranilic acid

Structure–Activity Relationships Furosemide is an example of a high-ceiling diuretic and may be regarded as a derivative of anthranilic acid or *o*-aminobenzoic acid. Research on 5-sulfamoylanthranilic acids at the Hoechst Laboratories in Germany showed them to be effective diuretics (10,12). The most active of a series of variously substituted derivatives was furosemide.

The chlorine and sulfonamide substitutions are features also seen in previously discussed diuretics. Because the molecule possesses a free carboxyl group, furosemide is a stronger acid than the thiazide diuretics ($pK_a = 3.9$). This drug is excreted primarily unchanged (16). A small amount of metabolism, however, can take place on the furan ring, which is substituted on the aromatic amino group (see Table 22.2 for its other pharmacokinetic properties).

Therapeutic Applications Furosemide has a saluretic effect 8- to 10-fold that of the thiazide diuretics; however, it has a shorter duration of action (~6 to 8 hours). Furosemide causes a marked excretion of sodium, chloride, potassium, calcium, magnesium, and bicarbonate ions, with as much as 25% of the filtered load of sodium excreted in response to initial treatment. It is effective for the treatment of edemas connected with cardiac, hepatic, and renal sites. Because it lowers the blood pressure similar to the thiazide derivatives, one of its uses is in the treatment of hypertension.

Furosemide is orally effective but may be used parenterally when a more prompt diuretic effect is desired, such as in the treatment of acute pulmonary edema. The dosage of furosemide, 20 to 80 mg/day, may be given in divided doses because of the short duration of action of the drug and carefully increased up to a maximum of 600 mg/day.

Adverse Effects Clinical toxicity of furosemide and other loop diuretics primarily involves abnormalities of fluid and electrolyte balance. As with the thiazide diuretics, hypokalemia is an important adverse effect that can be prevented or treated with potassium supplements or coadministration of potassium-sparing diuretics. Increased calcium ion excretion can be a problem for postmenopausal osteopenic women, and furosemide generally should not be used in these individuals. Hyperuricemia, glucose intolerance, increased serum lipid levels, ototoxicity, and gastrointestinal side effects might be observed as well. Hypersensitivity reactions also are possible with furosemide (a sulfonamide-based drug), and cross-reactivity with other sulfonamide-containing drugs is possible.

Bumetanide

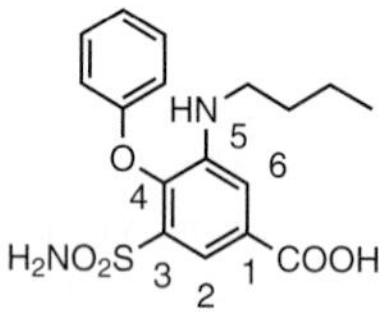

Bumetanide

Structure–Activity Relationships For bumetanide, a phenoxy group has replaced the customary chloro or trifluoromethyl substitutions seen in other diuretic molecules (17). The phenoxy group is an electron-withdrawing group similar to the chloro or trifluoromethyl substitutions. The amine group customarily seen at position 6 has been moved to position 5. These minor variations from furosemide produced a compound with a mode of action similar to that of furosemide, but with a marked increase in diuretic potency. The short duration of activity is similar, but the compound is approximately 50-fold more potent. Replacement of the phenoxy group at position 4 with a C_6H_5NH- or C_6H_5S- group also gives compounds with a favorable activity. However, when the butyl group on the C-5 amine is replaced with a furanylmethyl group, such as in furosemide, the results are not favorable.

Therapeutic Applications This compound also functions as a high-ceiling diuretic in the ascending limb of the loop of Henle. It's duration of action is approximately 4 hours. The uses of this compound are similar to those described for furosemide. The dose of bumetanide is 0.5 to 2 mg/day given as a single dose. Adverse effects are similar to those induced by furosemide.

Torsemide

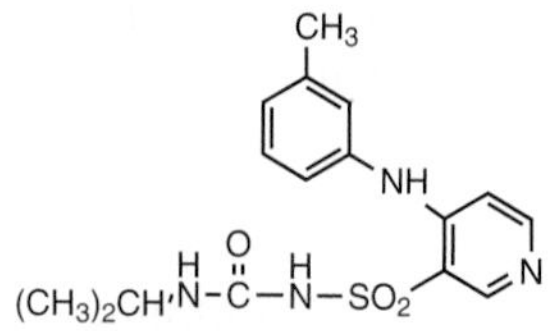

Torsemide

Overview Further modification of furosemide-like structures has led to the development of torsemide. Instead of the sulfonamide group found in furosemide and bumetanide, torsemide contains a sulfonylurea moiety.

Therapeutic Applications Similar to other high-ceiling diuretics, torsemide inhibits the luminal $Na^+/K^+/2Cl^-$ symporter in the ascending limb of the loop of Henle to promote the excretion of sodium, potassium, chloride, calcium, and magnesium ions and water. An additional effect on the peritubular side at chloride channels may enhance the luminal effects of torsemide. In contrast to furosemide and bumetanide, however, torsemide does not act at the proximal tubule and, therefore, does not increase phosphate or bicarbonate excretion. The oral bioavailability of torsemide is very good (~80%), and absorption is not affected by the presence of food in the gastrointestinal tract (18). Peak diuresis is observed 1 to 2 hours following oral or intravenous administration, with a duration of action of approximately 6 hours (Table 22.2). Torsemide is indicated for the treatment of edema resulting from congestive heart failure and for the treatment of hypertension. In patients with cirrhosis and ascites, torsemide should be used with caution. Adverse effects are similar to those induced by furosemide.

Ethacrynic Acid

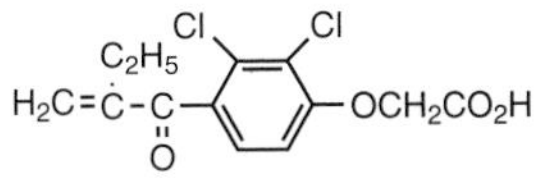

Ethacrynic acid

Mechanism of Action Another major class of high-ceiling diuretics is the phenoxyacetic acid derivatives, of which ethacrynic acid is the prototypical agent. These compounds were developed at about the same time as furosemide but were designed to act mechanistically similar to the organomercurials (i.e., via inhibition of sulfhydryl-containing enzymes involved in solute reabsorption). The mechanism of action of ethacrynic acid appears to be more complex than the simple Michael addition of the α,β-unsubstituted ketone of the drug to enzyme sulfhydryl groups. When the double bond of ethacrynic acid is reduced, the resulted compound is still active, although the diuretic activity is diminished. The sulfhydryl groups of the enzyme would not be expected to add to the drug molecule in the absence of the α,β-unsaturated ketone. Ethacrynic acid is the only loop diuretic that is not a sulfonamide derivative and may be useful in patients who are allergic to sulfonamides. The pharmacokinetic properties for ethacrynic acid are listed in Table 22.2.

Similar to the other high-ceiling diuretics, ethacrynic acid inhibits the $Na^+/K^+/2Cl^-$ symporter in the ascending limb of the loop of Henle to promote a marked diuresis. Sodium, chloride, potassium, and calcium excretion are increased following oral or intravenous administration of ethacrynic acid.

Structure–Activity Relationships Optimal diuretic activity was obtained when an oxyacetic acid group was positioned para to an α,β-unsaturated carbonyl (or other sulfhydryl-reactive group) and chloro or methyl groups were placed at the 2- or 3-position of the phenyl ring (19). In addition, hydrogen atoms on the terminal alkene carbon also provided maximum reactivity. Thus, a molecule with a weakly acidic group to direct the drug to the kidney and an alkylating moiety to react with sulfhydryl groups and lipophilic groups seemed to provide the best combination for a diuretic in this class. These features led to the development of ethacrynic acid as the prototypic agent in this class.

Therapeutic Applications Oral administration of this drug results in diuresis within 1 hour and a duration of action of 6 to 8 hours. Toxicity induced by ethacrynic acid is similar to that induced by furosemide and bumetanide. Ethacrynic acid is not widely used, however, because it induces a greater incidence of ototoxicity and more serious gastrointestinal effects than furosemide or bumetanide.

Azosemide, Piretanide, and Tripamide

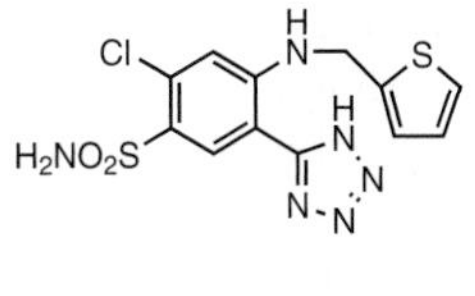

Azosemide

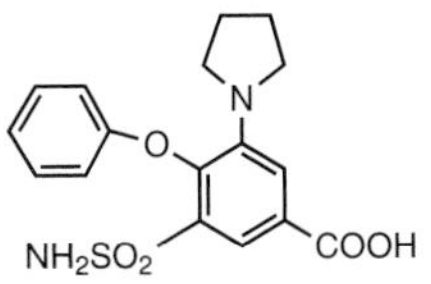

Piretanide

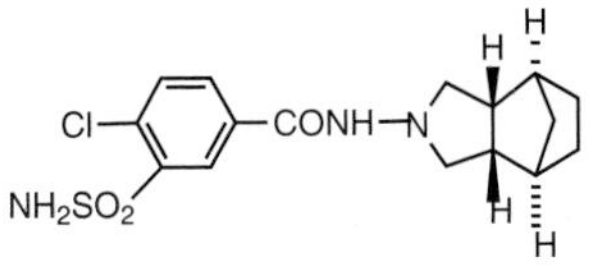

Tripamide

Three additional high-ceiling diuretics are azosemide, piretanide, and tripamide. Azosemide exerts a comparable diuretic effect to furosemide with oral dosing but is 5.5 to 8 times more potent following intravenous administration (20). Its low oral bioavailability (~10% to 15%) could be a consequence of high first-pass metabolism in the liver. Like bumetanide, piretanide is a sulfamoylbenzoic acid derivative. Piretanide exhibits diuretic potency greater than furosemide but lower than bumetanide (21). Acute side effects (pronounced diuresis, nausea, and thirst) with a conventional oral formulation appear to be more common than with furosemide and bumetanide. A sustained-release formulation of piretanide is better tolerated in patients. Similar to furosemide and azosemide, tripamide has a chloro group ortho to the sulfonamide functionality. At lower doses, tripamide exerts an antihypertensive effect without diuresis, whereas it exhibits both activities at higher doses, suggesting that it may affect other sites in the nephron (22). Azosemide, piretanide, and tripamide are not available in the United States but are used in other countries.

Mineralocorticoid Receptor Antagonists

Mechanism of Action

The adrenal cortex secretes a potent mineralocorticoid called aldosterone, which promotes salt and water retention and potassium and hydrogen ion excretion. Aldosterone exerts its biologic effects through binding to the mineralocorticoid receptor (MR), a nuclear transcription factor (23).

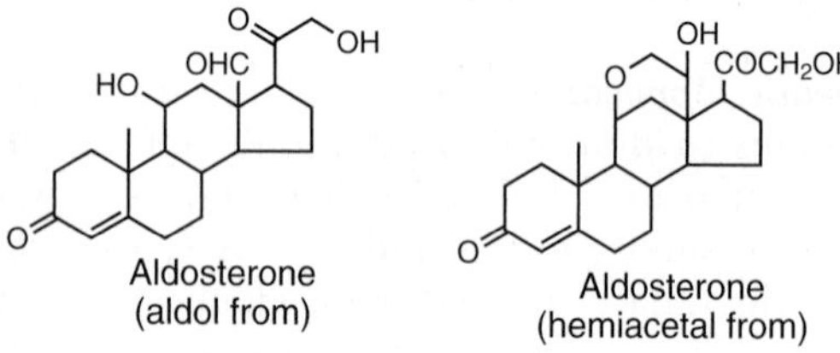

Other mineralocorticoids have an effect on the electrolytic balance of the body, but aldosterone is the most potent. Its ability to cause increased reabsorption of sodium and chloride ion and increased potassium ion excretion is approximately 3,000-fold that of hydrocortisone. A substance that antagonizes the effects of aldosterone could conceivably be a good diuretic drug. Spironolactone and eplerenone are examples of such antagonists. These drugs are also classified as potassium-sparing diuretics.

Specific Drugs

SPIRONOLACTONE

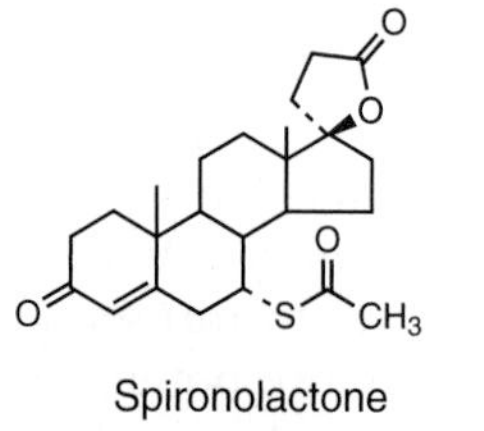

Overview Spironolactone competitively inhibits aldosterone binding to the MR, thereby interfering with reabsorption of sodium and chloride ions and the associated water. MR antagonist activity is dependent on the presence of a γ-lactone ring on C-17 and a substituent on C-7 in spironolactone and structurally related compounds (24,25). Interaction of C-7–unsubstituted agonists, such as aldosterone, with a methionine residue in the MR ligand binding domain is important for receptor activation and subsequent transcription. However, this interaction is sterically hindered by C-7 substituents on aldosterone antagonists, thereby leaving MR in an inactive conformation (24,25). The most important renal site of these receptors, and hence the primary site of action of spironolactone, is in the late distal convoluted tubule and collecting system (collecting duct).

Pharmacokinetics On oral administration, approximately 90% of the dose of spironolactone is absorbed and is significantly metabolized during its first passage through the liver to its major active metabolite, canrenone (see Table 22.2 for their pharmacokinetic properties), which is interconvertible with its canrenoate anion (Fig. 22.3) (26,27). Canrenone is an antagonist to aldosterone and exists in equilibrium with its ring-opened form, canrenoate.

The canrenoate anion is not therapeutically active but acts as an aldosterone antagonist because of its conversion back to canrenone, which exists in the lactone form. Canrenone has been suggested to be the active form of spironolactone as an aldosterone antagonist. The formation of canrenone, however, cannot fully account for the total activity of spironolactone (26,27). Both canrenone and potassium canrenoate are used as diuretics in other countries, but they are not available in the United States.

Therapeutic Applications Spironolactone is useful in treating edema resulting from primary hyperaldosteronism and refractory edema associated with secondary hyperaldosteronism. Spironolactone is considered to be the drug of choice for treating edema resulting from cirrhosis of the liver. The dose of spironolactone is 100 mg/day given in single or divided doses. Another use of spironolactone is coadministration with a potassium-depleting diuretic (e.g., a thiazide or loop diuretic) to prevent or treat diuretic-induced hypokalemia. However, it should not be combined with potassium-sparing diuretics (e.g., triamterene or amiloride). Spironolactone can be administered in a fixed-dose combination with

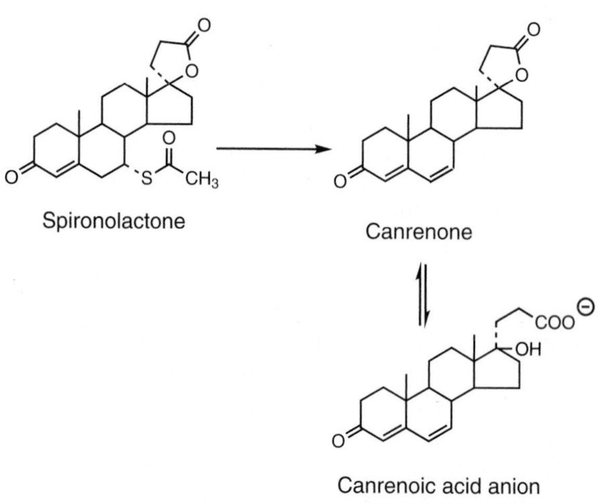

FIGURE 22.3 Metabolic conversion of spironolactone to canrenone.

hydrochlorothiazide for this purpose, but optimal individualization of the dose of each drug is recommended.

Adverse Effects The primary concern with the use of spironolactone is the development of hyperkalemia, which can be fatal. Spironolactone may cause hypersensitivity reactions, gastrointestinal disturbances and peptic ulcer. Sexual side effects (i.e., gynecomastia, decreased libido, and impotence) can also occur and are due to nonselective binding of spironolactone to the androgen receptor (AR), glucocorticoid receptor (GR), or progesterone receptor (PR). It also has been implicated in tumor production during chronic toxicity studies in rats, but human risk has not been documented.

EPLERENONE

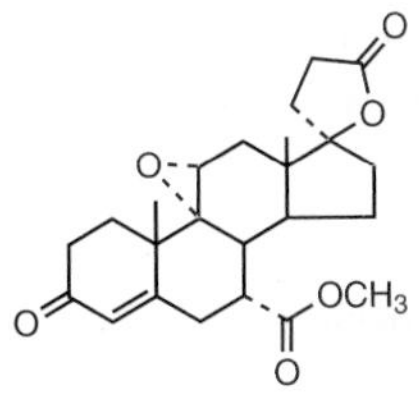

Overview Eplerenone is a newer drug that came out of efforts to develop spironolactone analogs with reduced adverse effects (28). In addition to the lactone ring and C-7 substituent (in this case, an acetyl group), which are important for MR antagonism, eplerenone has a 9α,11α-epoxy group as part of its structure. Like spironolactone, it binds to the MR and is an aldosterone antagonist. However, it has a 20- to 40-fold lower affinity for the MR than spironolactone (28). This reduced binding is believed to be due to the epoxy group (29,30). Nevertheless, eplerenone is an effective diuretic and has certain therapeutic advantages over spironolactone.

Pharmacokinetics Eplerenone has good (~70%) oral bioavailability and, unlike spironolactone, only undergoes limited first-pass metabolism (Table 22.2). Absorption is not affected by the presence of food in the gastrointestinal tract. In plasma, it is about 50% bound to plasma α_1-acid glycoprotein. Eplerenone has a half-life of approximately 5 hours and undergoes extensive metabolism by hepatic CYP3A4 to inactive metabolites (Fig. 22.4) (31). Combination with potent inhibitors of CYP3A4 (i.e., ketoconazole or erythromycin) can alter eplerenone pharmacokinetics (32). Elimination occurs in the urine and feces.

Therapeutic Applications Similar to spironolactone, eplerenone is used alone or with other diuretics for the treatment of hypertension or left ventricular systolic dysfunction and congestive heart failure after myocardial infarction. Single daily oral doses are 25 to 50 mg.

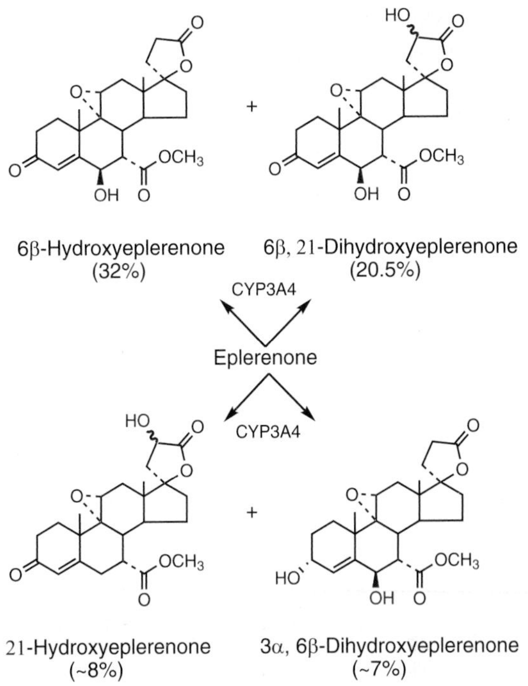

FIGURE 22.4 Major metabolic products formed from eplerenone.

Adverse Effects Hyperkalemia is a serious and potentially fatal side effect. In contrast to spironolactone, eplerenone has limited or no inhibitory effects on AR, GR, and PR and is, therefore, a more selective aldosterone antagonist (28). As a consequence, it has fewer sexual side effects.

Potassium-Sparing Diuretics

Mechanism of Action

Two drugs in this class of diuretics are triamterene and amiloride (Table 22.2). Individually, amiloride and triamterene exert a mild diuretic effect and are usually used in combination with thiazides or loop diuretics. In vitro experiments have shown that they exert a diuretic effect by blocking an epithelial sodium channel (ENaC) in principal cells of the late distal convoluted tubule and collecting duct (33,34). Both drugs are weak organic bases and inhibit ENaC in a voltage- and pH-dependent manner. Inhibition occurs because amiloride and triamterene bind to negatively charged regions of the sodium channel in the ENaC. The greater potency (approximately 100-fold in vitro) of amiloride is probably due to the fact that it is a stronger base ($pK_a = 8.7$) and is therefore more extensively protonated at physiologic pH than triamterene ($pK_a = 6.2$). Sodium channel inhibitors block the reabsorption of sodium ion and inhibit the secretion of potassium ion. The net result is increased sodium and chloride ion excretion in the urine and almost no potassium excretion. As a consequence, amiloride and triamterene can be used to offset the effect of other diuretics that result in loss of potassium.

Specific Drugs

Pteridines: Triamterene Pteridines have a marked potential for influencing biologic processes. Early screening of pteridine derivatives revealed that 2,4-diamino-6,7-dimethylpteridine was a fairly potent diuretic.

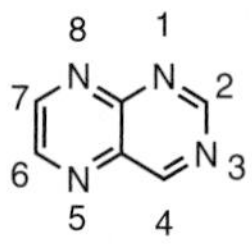

Pteridine

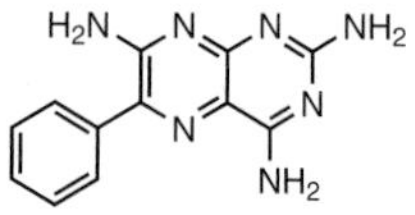

Triamterene

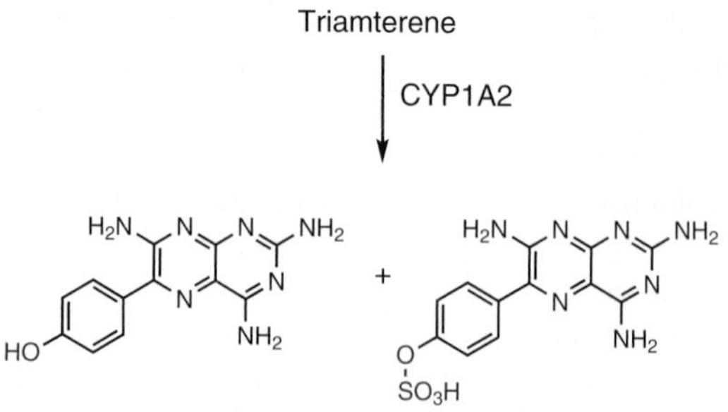

FIGURE 22.5 Metabolism of triamterene.

Overview Further structural modification of the pteridine nucleus led to the development of triamterene. Alterations of the triamterene structure are not usually beneficial in terms of diuretic activity. Activity is retained if an amine group is replaced with a lower alkylamine group. Introduction of a para-methyl group on the phenyl ring decreases the activity by approximately half.

Therapeutic Applications Triamterene is more than 70% absorbed on oral administration (see Table 22.2 for its other pharmacokinetic properties). The diuretic effect occurs rapidly (~30 minutes) and reaches a peak plasma concentration in 2 to 4 hours, with a duration of action of more than 24 hours. Triamterene is extensively metabolized to 4′-hydroxytriamterene and its sulfate conjugate, both of which (major metabolite) are still active as diuretics (Fig. 22.5) (35). Both the drug and its metabolites are excreted in the urine. Triamterene is useful in combination with a thiazide or loop diuretic in the treatment of edema or hypertension. Liddle syndrome, which is due to an inherited mutation in ENaC leading to increased activity of the receptor, also may be treated with a sodium channel–blocking drug, such as triamterene or amiloride. Triamterene is administered initially in doses of 100 mg twice a day. A maintenance dose for each patient should be individually determined. This dose may vary from 100 mg a day to as low as 100 mg every other day.

Adverse Effects The most serious side effect associated with the use of triamterene is hyperkalemia. For this reason, potassium supplements are contraindicated, and serum potassium levels should be checked regularly. Triamterene also is used in combination with hydrochlorothiazide. Here, the hypokalemic effect of the hydrochlorothiazide counters the hyperkalemic effect of the triamterene. Other side effects that are seen with the use of triamterene are nausea, vomiting, and headache.

Aminopyrazines: Amiloride

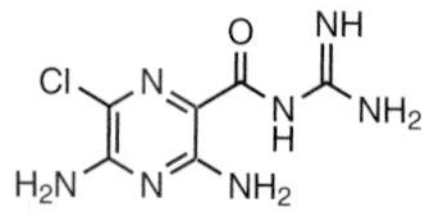

Amiloride is an aminopyrazine structurally related to triamterene as an open-chain analog. It has no effect on the action of aldosterone. Oral amiloride is approximately 50% absorbed (see Table 22.2 for its other pharmacokinetic properties), with a duration of action of 10 to 12 hours, which is slightly longer than that for triamterene. Although triamterene is extensively metabolized, approximately 50% of amiloride is excreted unchanged. Renal impairment can increase its elimination half-life. Like triamterene, amiloride combined with a thiazide or loop diuretic is used to treat edema or hypertension. Aerosolized amiloride has shown some benefit in improving mucociliary clearance in patients with cystic fibrosis. As with triamterene, the most serious side effect associated with amiloride is hyperkalemia, and it also has the other side effects associated with triamterene. The dose of amiloride is 5 to 10 mg/day. Amiloride also is combined with hydrochlorothiazide in a fixed-dose combination.

SCENARIO: OUTCOME AND ANALYSIS

Outcome

Kim K. Birtcher, MS, PharmD, BCPS

TB returns to the clinic after 12 weeks. He is taking lisinopril 20 mg daily and HCTZ 25 mg daily in the morning. His blood pressure is at goal (<130/80 mm Hg), and he has lost 10 lb. He reports eating a heart-healthy diet, and he walks at least 45 minutes/day. His K+ level is 4.8 mEq/L, his blood urea nitrogen level is 12 mg/dL, and his serum creatinine level is 1.0 ml/min. Because he has been stabilized on an appropriate dose of blood pressure medications, he is given a prescription for the combination product, lisinopril/HCTZ 20/25.

Chemical Analysis

Kim K. Birtcher, S. William Zito, and Victoria Roche

Thiazide diuretics are commonly used as initial or add-on therapy to treat hypertension. The thiazide diuretics decrease blood pressure by several mechanisms. They inhibit the Na+/Cl− symporter in the distal convoluted tubule and inhibit the reabsorption of sodium and chloride ions. They also promote water excretion, which decreases plasma volume and the workload of the heart. With chronic therapy, thiazides decrease peripheral vascular resistance. High amounts of sodium in the diet can counter the blood pressure–lowering effects of thiazides. To a lesser extent, thiazide diuretics also inhibit the reabsorption of potassium and bicarbonate ions. The clinician should periodically monitor K+ levels and clinical and laboratory parameters for dehydration.

Chemically, thiazides are1,2,4-benzothiadiazine-1,1-dioxide derivatives. Changes to their basic structure determines their potency and duration of action. For optimal activity, the sulfonamide group at position 7 is necessary (unsubstituted preferred), and there should be an electron withdrawing group at position 6. Saturation of the 3,4 double bond increases the diuretic activity (~10-fold) and alkyl substitutions at positions 2 and/or 3 increases activity as well as the duration of action.

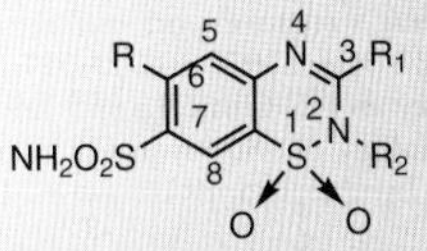

1,2,4-Benzothiadiazine-1,1-dioxide
(thiazide diuretic pharmacophore)

In the clinical scenario, the pharmacist chose to use a combination of an ACE inhibitor (see Chapter 23) and a thiazide diuretic to treat the patient's blood pressure. By doing this, the patient's blood pressure is lowered by different mechanisms of action. In addition, the K^+ lowering property of the hydrochlorothiazide may be countered with the K^+ raising property of the lisinopril.

CASE STUDY

S. William Zito and Victoria Roche

SY is a 63-year-old man who presents to the emergency room complaining of breathlessness for the past 3 days. His medical history shows that he had a myocardial infarction (MI) 3 years ago, which was followed by successful bypass surgery. SY has been asymptomatic since surgery with no complaints of chest pain. SY runs a small neighborhood grocery store and over the last 3 months has experienced shortness of breath while unloading groceries and climbing stairs. Two weeks ago he was unable to complete his daily 1-mile walk at the high school track, and 4 days ago he woke at 2 AM short of breath and had to sleep in his recliner the rest of the night. Yesterday, he became breathless walking from one room to another. He presents today with extreme shortness of breath and swelling in his feet and ankles, and he denies chest pain. A diagnosis of congestive heart failure (CHF) is made based on SY's symptoms, history of MI, and chest X-ray revealing cardiomegaly. The physician wants to initiate treatment with a diuretic to reduce edema before beginning treatment with digoxin for CHF. Evaluate the following three choices for appropriate use in this case.

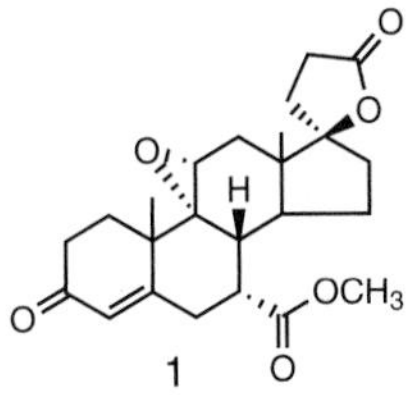

1

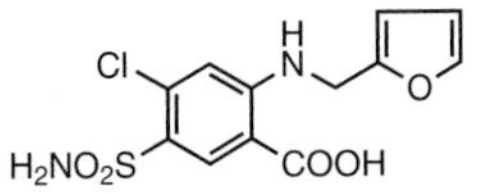

2

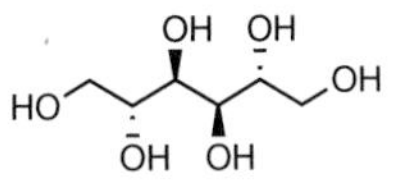

3

1. Conduct a thorough and mechanistic SAR analysis of the three therapeutic options in the case.
2. Apply the chemical understanding gained from the SAR analysis to this patient's specific needs to make a therapeutic recommendation.

References

1. Reilly RF, Jackson EK. Regulation of renal function and vascular volume. In: Brunton LL, Chabner BA, Knollmann BC, eds. Goodman and Gilman's the Pharmacological Basis of Therapeutics, 12th Ed. New York: McGraw-Hill, 2011:671–719.
2. Padilla MCA, Armas-Hernandez MJ, Hernandez RH, et al. Update of diuretics in the treatment of hypertension. Am J Ther 2007;14:154–160.
3. Supuran CT. Diuretics: from classical carbonic anhydrase inhibitors to novel applications of the sulfonamides. Curr Pharm Des 2008;14:641–648.
4. Ernst ME, Moser M. Use of diuretics in patients with hypertension. N Engl J Med 2009;361:2153–2164.
5. Ernst ME, Gordon JA. Diuretic therapy: key aspects in hypertension and renal disease. J Nephrol 2010;23:487–493.
6. Cadwallader AB, de la Torre X, Tieri A, et al. The abuse of diuretics as performance-enhancing drugs and masking agents in sport doping: pharmacology, toxicology and analysis. Br J Pharmacol 2010;161:1–16.
7. Deventer K, Baele G, Van Eenoo P, et al. Stability of selected chlorinated thiazide diuretics. J Pharm Biomed Anal 2009;49:519–524.
8. Nissenson AR, Weston RE, Kleeman CR. Mannitol. West J Med 1979;131:277–284.
9. Sprague JM. The chemistry of diuretics. Ann NY Acad Sci 1958;71:328–342.
10. Maren TH. Relations between structure and biological activity of sulfonamides. Annu Rev Pharmacol Toxicol 1976;16:309–327.
11. Mincione F, Menabuoni, Supuran CT. Clinical applications of carbonic anhydrase inhibitors in ophthalmology. In: Supuran CT, Scozzafava A, Conway J, eds. Carbonic Anhydrase: Its Inhibitors and Activators. Boca Raton, FL: CRC Press, 2004:243–254.
12. Fitzgerald D. Trails of discovery. A cornerstone of cardiovascular therapy: the thiazide diuretics. Dialogues Cardiovasc Med 2005;10:175–182.
13. Campbell DB, Taylor AR, Hopkins YW, et al. Pharmacokinetics and metabolism of indapamide: a review. Curr Med Res Opin 1977;5(Suppl 1):13–24.
14. Sun H, Moore C, Dansette PM, et al. Dehydrogenation of the indoline-containing drug 4-chloro-N-(2-methyl-1-indolinyl)-3-sulfamoylbenzamide (indapamide) by CYP3A4: correlation with in silico predictions. Drug Metab Dispos 2009;37:672–684.
15. Wargo KA, Banta WM. A comprehensive review of the loop diuretics: should furosemide be first line? Ann Pharmacother 2009;43:1836–1847.
16. Beermann B, Dalen E, Lindstrom B, et al. On the fate of furosemide in man. Eur J Clin Pharmacol 1975;9:57–61.
17. Feit PW. Bumetanide: the way to its chemical structure. J Clin Pharmacol 1981;21:531–536.
18. Blose JS, Adams KF Jr, Patterson JH. Torsemide: a pyridine-sulfonylurea loop diuretic. Ann Pharmacother 1995;29:396–402.
19. Koechel DA. Ethacrynic acid and related diuretics: relationship of structure to beneficial and detrimental actions. Annu Rev Pharmacol Toxicol 1981;21:265–293.
20. Suh OK, Kim SH, Lee MG. Pharmacokinetics and pharmacodynamics of azosemide. Biopharm Drug Dispos 2003;24:275–297.
21. Clissold SP, Brogden RN. Piretanide: a preliminary review of its pharmacodynamic and pharmacokinetic properties, and therapeutic efficacy. Drugs 1985;29:489–530.
22. Brater DC, Anderson S. Sites of action of tripamide. Clin Pharmacol Ther 1983;34:79–85.
23. Fogerson FM, Brennan FE, Fuller PJ. Mineralocorticoid receptor binding, structure and function. Mol Cell Endocrinol 2004;217:203–212.
24. Fagart J, Seguin C, Pinon GM, et al. The Met852 residue is a key organizer of the ligand-binding cavity of the human mineralocorticoid receptor. Mol Pharmacol 2005;67:1714–1722.
25. Huyet J, Pinon GM, Fay MR, et al. Structural basis of spironolactone recognition by the mineralocorticoid receptor. Mol Pharmacol 2007;72:563–571.
26. Ramsay L, Shelton J, Harrison I, et al. Spironolactone and potassium canrenoate in normal man. Clin Pharmacol Ther 1976;20:167–177.
27. Overdiek HWPM, Merkus FWHM. The metabolism and biopharmaceutics of spironolactone in man. Drug Metab Drug Interact 1987;5:273–302.
28. Garthwaite SM, McMahon EG. The evolution of aldosterone antagonists. Mol Cell Endocrinol 2004;217:27–31.
29. de Gasparo M, Joss, U, Ramjoue HP, et al. Three new epoxy-spironolactone derivatives: characterization in vivo and in vitro. J Pharmacol Exp Ther 1987;240:650–656.
30. Rogerson, FM, Yao Y, Smith BJ, et al. Differences in the determinants of eplerenone, spironolactone and aldosterone binding to the mineralocorticoid receptor. Clin Exp Pharmacol Physiol 2004;31:704–709.
31. Cook CS, Berry LM, Bible RH, et al. Pharmacokinetics and metabolism of [14C]eplerenone after oral administration to humans. Drug Metab Dispos 2003;31:1448–1455.
32. Craft J. Eplerenone (Inspra), a new aldosterone antagonist for the treatment of systemic hypertension and heart failure. Proc (Bayl Univ Med Cent) 2004;17:217–220.
33. Canessa CM, Schild L, Buell G, et al. Amiloride-sensitive epithelial Na+ channel is made of three homologous subunits. Nature 1994;367:463–467.
34. Busch AE, Suessbrich H, Kunzelmann K, et al. Blockade of epithelial Na+ channels by triamterenes: underlying mechanisms and molecular basis. Pflugers Arch Eur J Physiol 1996;432:760–766.
35. Fuhr U, Kober S, Zaigler M, et al. Rate-limiting biotransformation of triamterene is mediated by CYP1A2. Int J Clin Pharmacol Ther 2005;43:327–334.

Suggested Readings

Acara MA. Renal pharmacology—diuretics. In: Smith CM, Reynard AM, eds. Textbook of Pharmacology. Philadelphia: WB Saunders, 1992:554–588.

Brenner BM, Rector FC Jr, eds. The Kidney, 4th Ed. Philadelphia: WB Saunders, 1991.

Breyer J, Jacobson HR. Molecular mechanisms of diuretic agents. Annu Rev Med 1990;41:265–275.

Eaton DC, Pooler JP, eds. Vander's Renal Physiology, 6th Ed. New York: Lange Medical Books/McGraw Hill, 2004.

Friedman PA, Berndt, WO. Diuretic drugs. In: Craig CR, Stizel RE, eds. Modern Pharmacology with Clinical Applications, 6th Ed. Philadelphia: Lippincott Williams & Wilkins, 2004; pp 239–255.

Ives HE. Diuretic agents. In: Katzung BG, Masters SB, Trevor AJ, eds. Basic and Clinical Pharmacology, 11th Ed. New York: McGraw-Hill, 2009:251–267.

Kalantarinia K, Okusa MD. Diuretic drugs. In: Wecker L, Crespo LM, Dunaway G, et al., eds. Brody's Human Pharmacology; Molecular to Clinical, 5th Ed. Philadelphia: Elsevier Mosby, 2010:226–241.

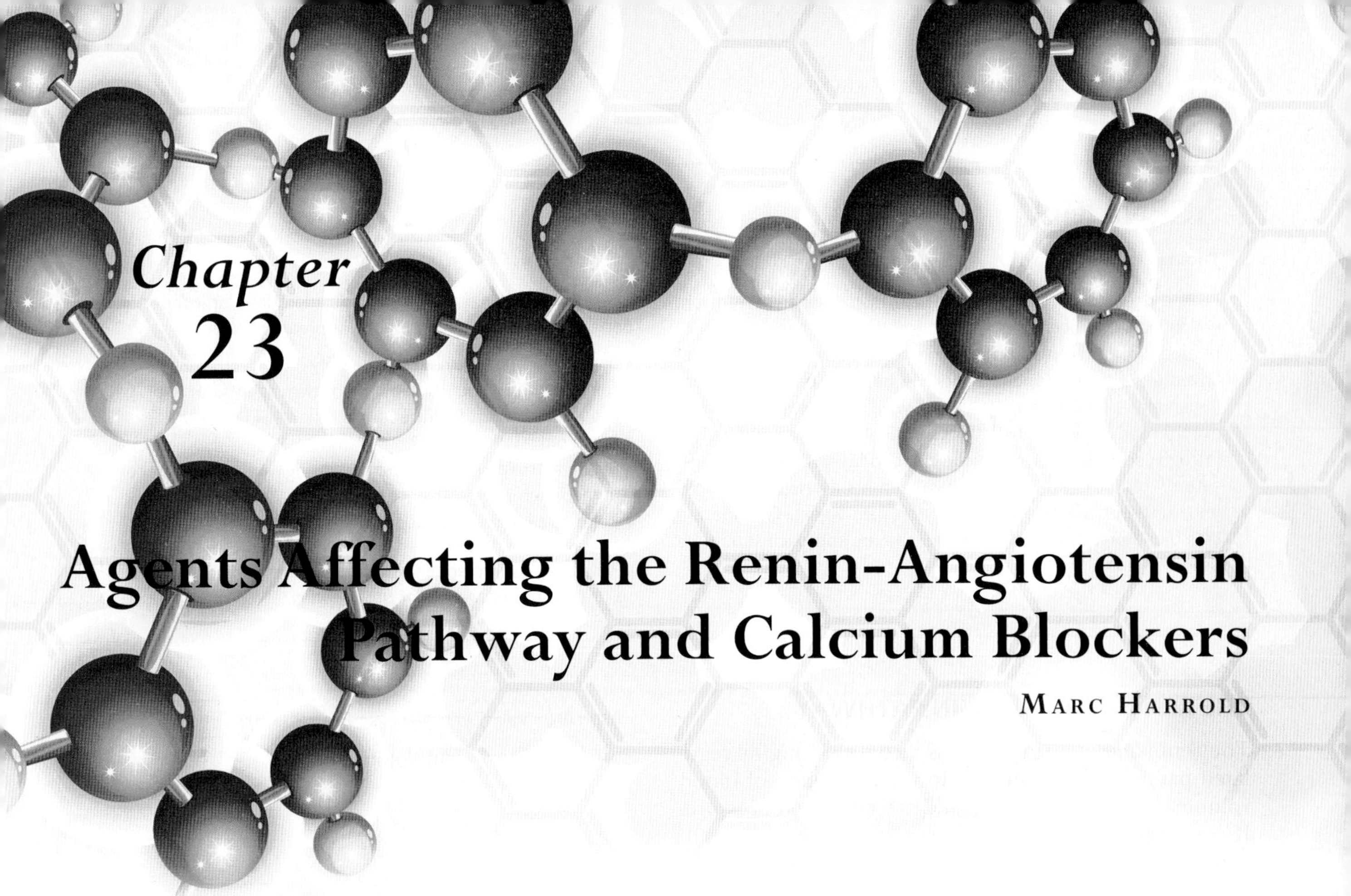

Chapter 23

Agents Affecting the Renin-Angiotensin Pathway and Calcium Blockers

Marc Harrold

*Drugs Covered in This Chapter**

Angiotensin-converting enzyme inhibitors
- Captopril
- Enalapril
- Fosinopril
- Lisinopril
- Moexipril
- Perindopril
- Quinapril
- Ramipril
- *Spirapril*
- Trandolapril

Angiotensin II receptor blockers
- Azilsartan
- Candesartan
- Eprosartan
- Irbesartan
- Losartan
- Olmesartan
- Telmisartan
- Valsartan

Calcium channel blockers
- Amlodipine
- *Bepridil*
- Clevidipine
- Diltiazem
- Felodipine
- Nicardipine
- Nifedipine
- Nimodipine
- Nisoldipine
- Verapamil
- Ziconotide

Renin inhibitor
- Aliskiren

Abbreviations

ACE, angiotensin-converting enzyme
ARB, angiotensin receptor blocker
AT_1, angiotensin II subtype 1 receptor
AT_2, angiotensin II subtype 2 receptor
AV, atrioventricular
BPF, bradykinin-potentiating factor
CNS, central nervous system
1,4-DHPs, 1,4-dihydropyridines
HVA, high-voltage activated
IC_{50}, half maximal inhibitory concentration
IV, intravenous
LVA, low-voltage activated
MI, myocardial infarction
PSVT, paroxysmal supraventricular tachycardia
SAR, structure–activity relationship

*Drugs listed include those available inside and outside of the United States; drugs available outside of the United States are shown in italics.

SCENARIO

Thomas L. Rihn, PharmD

LB is a 63-year-old man with a 4-year history of hypertension, which has not been well controlled. He has been primarily treated with attempts at lifestyle modification but has not followed up with his appointments. He has also been an insulin-dependent diabetic for 17 years (with proteinuria) and has experienced a few anginal attacks, which have been relieved by nitroglycerin. He presents at the clinic today with a blood pressure of 162/101 mm Hg (this has been his average, measured on three separate occasions over the past week). Considering LB's blood pressure level, what therapeutic approach should be used?

The following questions or considerations are important in deciding on an initial therapeutic approach:

- Begin treatment with a thiazide only?
- Consider initiating therapy with two agents, one of which should be a thiazide diuretic, the other ACEI?
- Begin only with an ARB?
- Begin a triple drug regimen to bring patient under control immediately?
- Refer to a hypertension specialist?

(The reader is directed to the clinical solution and chemical analysis of this case at the end of the chapter).

THE RENIN-ANGIOTENSIN PATHWAY

The renin-angiotensin system is a complex, highly regulated pathway that is integral in the regulation of blood volume, electrolyte balance, and arterial blood pressure. It consists of two main enzymes, renin and angiotensin-converting enzyme (ACE), the primary purpose of which is to release angiotensin II from its endogenous precursor, angiotensinogen (Fig. 23.1). Angiotensin II is a potent vasoconstrictor that affects peripheral resistance, renal function, and cardiovascular structure (1).

History and Overview of Pathway

Historically, the renin-angiotensin system dates back to 1898, when Tiegerstedt and Bergman demonstrated the existence of a pressor substance in crude kidney extracts. A little more than 40 years later, two independent research groups discovered that this pressor substance, which had previously been named renin, actually was an enzyme and that the true pressor substance was a peptide formed by the catalytic action of renin. This peptide pressor substance initially was assigned two different names, angiotonin and hypertensin; however, these names eventually were combined to produce the current designation, angiotensin. In the 1950s, it was discovered that angiotensin exists as both an inactive decapeptide, angiotensin I, and an active octapeptide, angiotensin II, and that the conversion of angiotensin I to angiotensin II is catalyzed by an enzyme distinct from renin (2).

Angiotensinogen is an α_2-globulin with a molecular weight of 58,000 to 61,000 daltons. It contains 452 amino acids, is abundant in the plasma, and is continually synthesized and secreted by the liver. A number of hormones, including glucocorticoids, thyroid hormone, and angiotensin II, stimulate its synthesis. The most important portion of this compound is the N-terminus, specifically the Leu^{10}-Val^{11} bond. This bond is cleaved by renin and

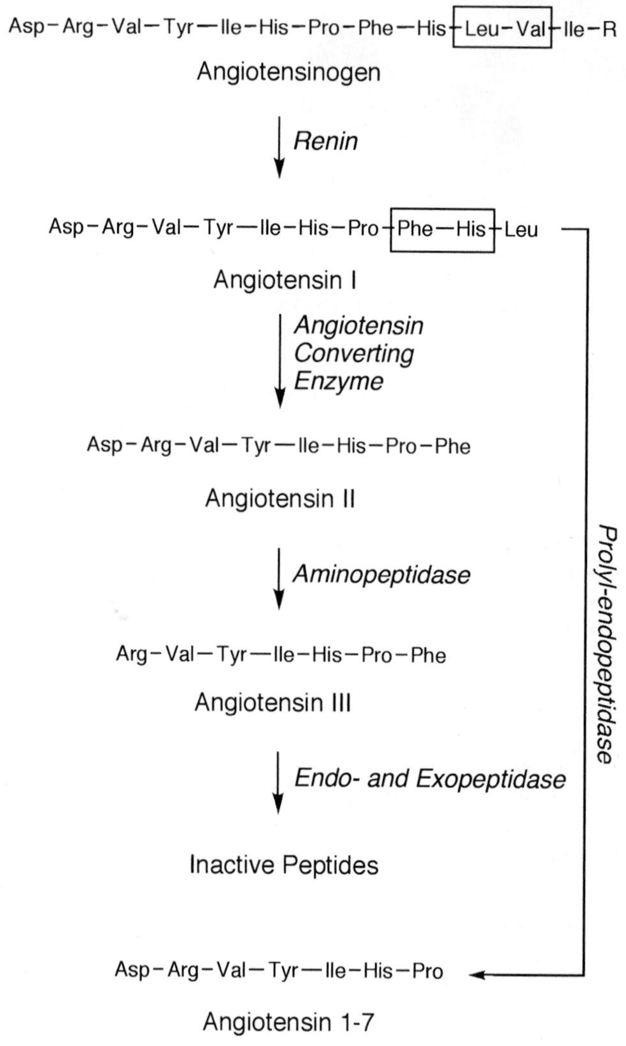

FIGURE 23.1 Schematic representation of the renin-angiotensin pathway. The labile peptide bonds of angiotensinogen and angiotensin I are highlighted.

CLINICAL SIGNIFICANCE

The treatment of hypertension and congestive heart failure (CHF) has improved significantly with the introduction of angiotensin-converting enzyme (ACE) inhibitors, angiotensin receptor blockers (ARBs), and calcium channel blockers. The SARs and structural modifications of these agents have produced major therapeutic advances. These drugs have become cornerstones of therapy today. For example, more than 30 years ago, captopril was the first ACE inhibitor to be developed. Subsequent molecular modifications led to the development of newer agents, such as lisinopril. Although lisinopril exerts comparable ACE inhibition, it possesses a superior pharmacokinetic profile. Instead of having to administer captopril three times daily, lisinopril can be administered once daily.

Medication compliance is notoriously poor in cardiovascular patients. Administering an ACE inhibitor such as lisinopril once daily results in greatly enhanced medication compliance. Clinical trials have clearly demonstrated that the therapeutic outcomes of patients with hypertension and CHF have improved immensely as a result. Similar molecular enhancements have been made with the ARBs and calcium channel blockers. Their therapeutic use today is also evidence-based.

The application of basic science in modifying the chemical structure of these agents has ultimately resulted in patients living longer and suffering fewer cardiovascular events, such as myocardial infarction or worsening CHF. Importantly, their day-to-day quality of life has improved as well.

Thomas L. Rihn, Pharm. D
Division Head and Associate Professor of Clinical Practice
Duquesne University
Mylan School of Pharmacy
Pittsburgh, Pennsylvania

produces the decapeptide angiotensin I. The Phe^8-His^9 peptide bond of angiotensin I is then cleaved by ACE to produce the octapeptide angiotensin II. Aminopeptidase can further convert angiotensin II to the active heptapeptide angiotensin III by removing the N-terminal arginine residue. Further actions of carboxypeptidases, aminopeptidases, and endopeptidases result in the formation of inactive peptide fragments. An additional compound can be formed by the action of a prolyl-endopeptidase on angiotensin I. Cleavage of the Pro^7-Phe^8 bond of angiotensin I produces a heptapeptide known as angiotensin 1-7. The actions of all of these compounds are discussed below.

Actions and Properties of Renin-Angiotensin Pathway Components

Renin is an aspartyl protease that determines the rate of angiotensin II production. It is a much more specific enzyme than ACE. Its primary function is to cleave the leucine-valine bond at residues 10 and 11 of angiotensinogen. The stimulation of renin release is controlled very closely by hemodynamic, neurogenic, and humoral signals (Fig. 23.2). Hemodynamic signals involve the renal juxtaglomerular cells. These cells are sensitive to the hemodynamic stretch of the afferent glomerular arteriole. An increase in the stretch implies a raised blood pressure and results in a reduced release of renin, whereas a decrease in the stretch increases renin secretion. Additionally, these cells also are sensitive to NaCl flux across the adjacent macula densa. Increases in NaCl flux across the macula densa inhibit renin release, but decreases in the flux stimulate release. Furthermore, neurogenic enhancement of renin release occurs via activation of β_1 receptors. Finally, a variety of hormonal signals influence the release of renin. Somatostatin, atrial natriuretic factor, and angiotensin II inhibit renin release, whereas vasoactive intestinal peptide, parathyroid hormone, and glucagon stimulate renin release (3).

In contrast, ACE, also known as kininase II, is a zinc protease that is under minimal physiologic control. It is not a rate-limiting step in the generation of angiotensin II and is a relatively nonspecific dipeptidyl carboxypeptidase that requires only a tripeptide sequence as a substrate. The only structural feature required by ACE is that the penultimate amino acid in the peptide substrate cannot be proline. For this reason, angiotensin II, which

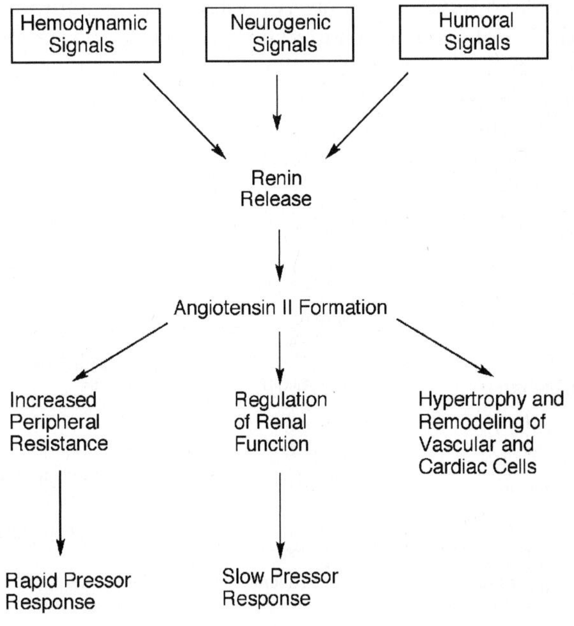

FIGURE 23.2 Summary of the factors involved in renin release and the effects mediated by angiotensin II.

contains a proline in the penultimate position, is not further metabolized by ACE. The lack of specificity and control exhibited by ACE results in its involvement in the bradykinin pathway (Fig. 23.3). Bradykinin is a nonapeptide that acts locally to produce pain, cause vasodilation, increase vascular permeability, stimulate prostaglandin synthesis, and cause bronchoconstriction. Similar to angiotensin II, bradykinin is produced by proteolytic cleavage of a precursor peptide. Cleavage of kininogens by the protease kallikrein produces a decapeptide known as either kallidin or lysyl-bradykinin. Subsequent cleavage of the N-terminal lysine by aminopeptidase produces bradykinin. The degradation of bradykinin to inactive peptides occurs through the actions of ACE. Thus, ACE not only produces a potent vasoconstrictor but also inactivates a potent vasodilator (1,3,4).

Angiotensin II is the dominant peptide produced by the renin-angiotensin pathway (Fig. 23.2). It is a potent vasoconstrictor that increases total peripheral resistance through a variety of mechanisms: direct vasoconstriction, enhancement of both catecholamine release and neurotransmission within the peripheral nervous system, and increased sympathetic discharge. The result of all these actions is a rapid pressor response. Additionally, angiotensin II causes a slow pressor response, resulting in long-term stabilization of arterial blood pressure. This long-term effect is accomplished by the regulation of renal function. Angiotensin II directly increases sodium reabsorption in the proximal tubule. It also alters renal hemodynamics and causes the release of aldosterone from the adrenal cortex. Finally, angiotensin II causes the hypertrophy and remodeling of both vascular and cardiac cells through a variety of hemodynamic and nonhemodynamic effects (1).

The secondary peptides, angiotensin III and angiotensin 1-7, can contribute to the overall effects of the renin-angiotensin pathway. Angiotensin III is equipotent with angiotensin II in stimulating aldosterone secretion; however, it is only 10% to 25% as potent in increasing blood pressure. In contrast, angiotensin 1-7 does not cause either aldosterone secretion or vasoconstriction, but it does have potent effects that are distinct from those of angiotensin II. Similar to angiotensin II, angiotensin 1-7 causes neuronal excitation and vasopressin release.

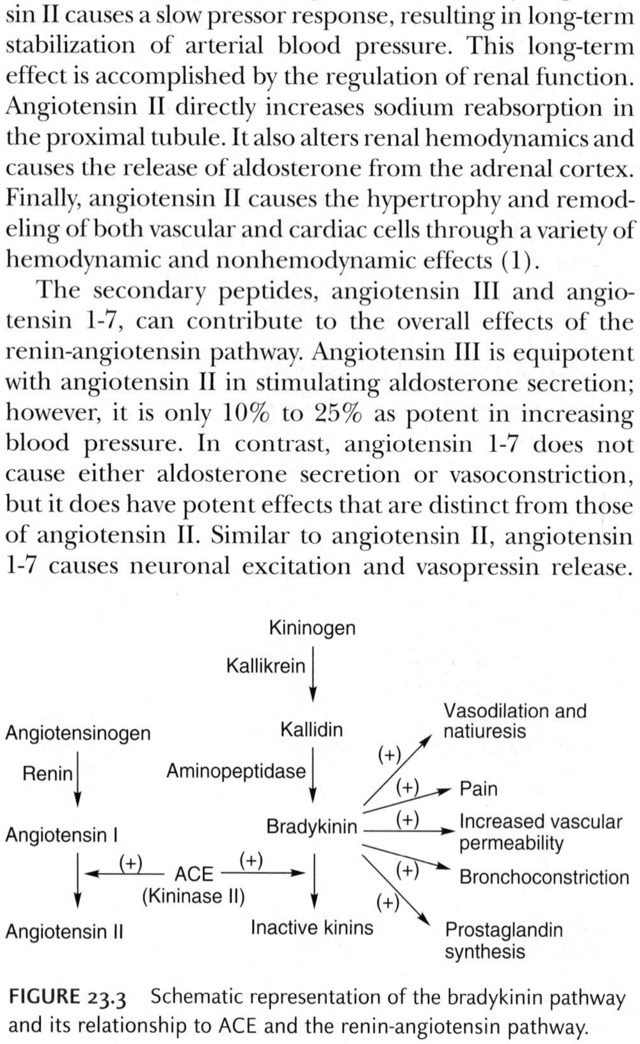

FIGURE 23.3 Schematic representation of the bradykinin pathway and its relationship to ACE and the renin-angiotensin pathway.

Additionally, it enhances the production of prostaglandins via a receptor-mediated process that does not involve an increase in intracellular calcium levels. It has been proposed to be important in the modulation of cell-to-cell interactions in cardiovascular and neural tissues (5).

ROLE OF THE RENIN-ANGIOTENSIN PATHWAY IN CARDIOVASCULAR DISORDERS

Because the renin-angiotensin pathway is central to the maintenance of blood volume, arterial blood pressure, and electrolyte balance, abnormalities in this pathway (e.g., excessive release of renin and overproduction of angiotensin II) can contribute to a variety of cardiovascular disorders. Specifically, overactivity of this pathway can result in hypertension or heart failure via the mechanisms previously described. Abnormally high levels of angiotensin II can contribute to hypertension through both rapid and slow pressor responses. In addition, high levels of angiotensin II can cause cellular hypertrophy and increase both afterload and wall tension. All of these events can cause or exacerbate heart failure.

High blood pressure is a relatively common disorder, affecting more than 50 million Americans. It is more prevalent in males than in females and in blacks than in Caucasians. Onset usually begins during the third, fourth, and fifth decades of life, and the incidence of the disorder increases with age. Hypertension is classified as either primary or secondary. Primary hypertension, also known as essential hypertension, is the most prevalent form of the disorder and is defined as high blood pressure of an unknown etiology. Most cases of primary hypertension are thought to result from a variety of underlying pathophysiologic mechanisms and not from a single, specific cause. Additionally, genetic factors appear to be important in the development of primary hypertension. Secondary hypertension is associated with a specific disorder (e.g., chronic renal disease, pheochromocytoma, and Cushing syndrome), is present in approximately 5% of individuals with high blood pressure, and, in some instances, is potentially curable. Secondary hypertension is much more common in children than in adults (6).

Heart failure (previously designated as congestive heart failure) affects approximately 5 million Americans and is the most common hospital discharge diagnosis in patients older than 65 years. The overall 5-year survival rate is approximately 50% for all patients, with women having an overall lower mortality rate than men. The disease results from conditions in which the heart is unable to supply blood at a rate sufficient to meet the demands of the body. Similar to hypertension, this pathophysiologic state can occur via a variety of mechanisms. Any pathophysiologic event that causes either systolic or diastolic dysfunction will result in heart failure. Systolic dysfunction, or decreased contractility, can be caused by dilated cardiomyopathies, ventricular hypertrophy, or a reduction in muscle mass. Diastolic dysfunction, or restriction in ventricular filling, can be caused by increased ventricular stiffness, mitral or tricuspid valve stenosis, or pericardial disease. Both ventricular hypertrophy and myocardial ischemia can contribute to increased ventricular stiffness. Angiotensin II causes and/or exacerbates heart failure by increasing systemic vascular resistance, promoting sodium retention, stimulating aldosterone release, and stimulating ventricular hypertrophy and remodeling (7).

OVERVIEW OF DRUG THERAPY AFFECTING THE RENIN-ANGIOTENSIN PATHWAY

Because angiotensin II produces the majority of the effects attributed to the renin-angiotensin pathway, compounds that can block either the synthesis of angiotensin II or the binding of angiotensin II to its receptor should attenuate the actions of this pathway. Indeed, enzyme inhibitors of both renin and ACE, as well as receptor antagonists of angiotensin II, have all been shown to produce beneficial effects in decreasing the actions of angiotensin II. Inhibitors of ACE were the first class of compounds to be marketed. This occurred in 1981 with the approval by the U.S. Food and Drug Administration of captopril. Fourteen years later, losartan was approved as the first angiotensin II receptor blocker (previous referred to as an angiotensin II receptor antagonist), and in 2007, aliskiren was approved as the first orally active renin inhibitor. The development, structure–activity relationships (SARs), physicochemical properties, interactions, and indications of these classes of drugs are discussed later in this chapter.

ANGIOTENSIN-CONVERTING ENZYME INHIBITORS

Currently, there are 11 ACE inhibitors approved for therapeutic use in the United States. These compounds can be subclassified into three groups based on their chemical composition: sulfhydryl-containing inhibitors (exemplified by captopril), dicarboxylate-containing inhibitors (exemplified by enalapril), and phosphonate-containing inhibitors (exemplified by fosinopril). Captopril and fosinopril are the lone representatives of their respective chemical subclassifications, whereas the majority of the inhibitors contain the dicarboxylate functionality. All of these compounds effectively block the conversion of angiotensin I to angiotensin II and have similar therapeutic and physiologic effects. The compounds differ primarily in their potency and pharmacokinetic profiles (1). Additionally, the sulfhydryl group in captopril is responsible for certain effects not seen with the other agents. Detailed descriptions of the rationale for the development of captopril, enalapril, and fosinopril are provided in the following sections.

Sulfhydryl-Containing Inhibitors: Development of Captopril

In 1965, Ferreira et al. (8) reported that the venom of the South American pit viper (*Bothrops jararaca*) contained factors that potentiated the action of bradykinin. These factors, originally designated as bradykinin-potentiating factors (BPFs), were isolated and found to be a family of peptides containing 5- to 13-amino acid residues. Their actions in potentiating bradykinin were subsequently linked to their ability to inhibit the enzymatic degradation of bradykinin. Soon thereafter, Bakhle et al. (9) reported that these same peptides also inhibited the enzymatic conversion of angiotensin I to angiotensin II. This latter enzyme, ACE, is now known to be identical with the former bradykininase enzyme (kininase II). Even at the time of these initial discoveries, however, BPFs were seen as lead compounds for the development of new antihypertensive agents, because they possessed dual activities—inhibition of the degradation of bradykinin, a potent vasodilator, and inhibition of the biosynthesis of angiotensin II, a potent vasoconstrictor (10).

A nonapeptide, SQ 20,881 (teprotide), isolated from the original BPFs, had the greatest in vivo potency in inhibiting ACE and was shown to consistently lower blood pressure in patients with essential hypertension. It also exerted beneficial effects in patients with heart failure; however, because of its peptide nature and lack of oral activity, teprotide had limited activity in the therapeutic treatment of these diseases (10,11).

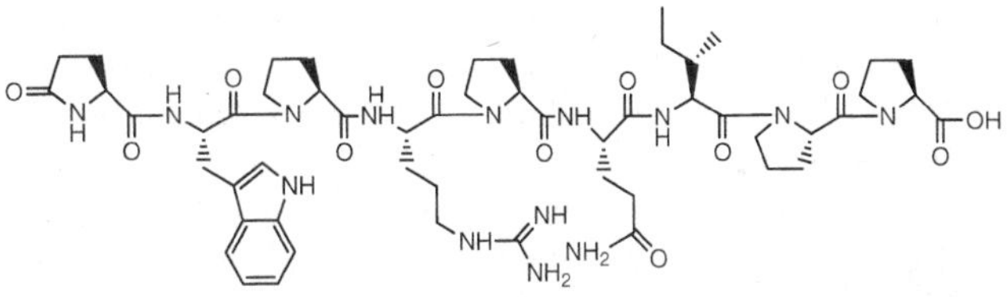

SQ 20,881

Cushman, Ondetti, and coworkers (12–14) used SQ 20,881 and other peptide analogs to provide an enhanced understanding of the enzymatic properties of ACE. Using knowledge of substrate-binding specificities and the fact that ACE has properties similar to those of pancreatic carboxypeptidases, these researchers developed a hypothetical model of the enzyme active site. Carboxypeptidase A, like ACE, is a zinc-containing exopeptidase. The binding of a substrate to carboxypeptidase A involves three major interactions (Fig. 23.4A). First, the negatively charged carboxylate terminus of the amino acid substrate binds to the positively charged Arg-145 on the enzyme. Second, a hydrophobic pocket in the enzyme provides specificity for a C-terminal aromatic or nonpolar residue. Third, the zinc atom is located close to the labile peptide bond and serves to stabilize the negatively charged tetrahedral intermediate, which results when a molecule of water attacks the carbonyl bond between the C-terminal and penultimate amino acid residues (15). Similarly, the binding of substrates to ACE was proposed to involve three or four major interactions (Fig. 23.4B). First, the negatively charged carboxylate terminus of angiotensin I and other substrates was assumed

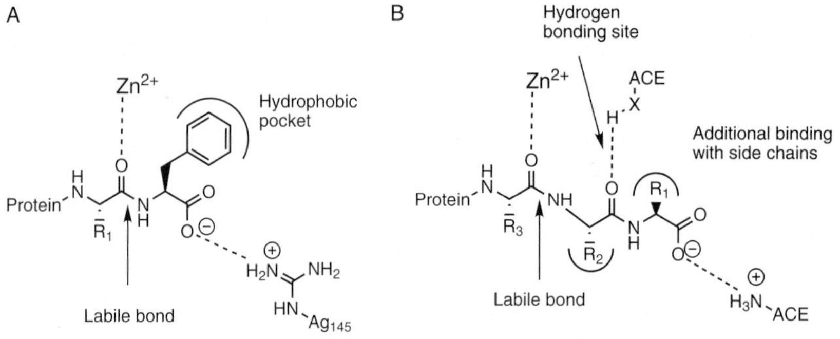

FIGURE 23.4 A model of substrate binding to carboxypeptidase A (A) and ACE (B). ACE substrate binding sites are highlighted in red.

to occur via an ionic bond with a positively charged amine on ACE. Second, the role of the zinc atom in the mechanism of ACE hydrolysis was assumed to be similar to that of carboxypeptidase A. Because ACE cleaves dipeptides instead of single amino acids, the position of the zinc atom was assumed to be located two amino acids away from the cationic center for it to be adjacent to the labile peptide bond. Third, the side chains R_1 and R_2 could contribute to the overall binding affinity; however, ACE, unlike carboxypeptidase A, does not show specificity for C-terminal hydrophobic amino acids and was not expected to have a hydrophobic binding pocket. Finally, the terminal peptide bond is nonlabile and was assumed to provide hydrogen bonding between the substrate and ACE.

The development of captopril and other orally active ACE inhibitors began with the observation that D-2-benzylsuccinic acid was an extremely potent inhibitor of carboxypeptidase A (12–14). The binding of this compound to carboxypeptidase A (Fig. 23.5A) is very similar to that seen for substrates with the exception that the zinc ion binds to a carboxylate group instead of the labile peptide bond. Byers and Wolfenden (16) proposed that this compound is a by-product analog that contains structural features of both products of peptide hydrolysis. Most of the structural features of the compound are identical to the terminal amino acid of the substrate (Fig. 23.4A), whereas the additional carboxylate group is able to mimic the carboxylate group that would be produced during peptide hydrolysis (16). Applying this concept to the hypothetical model of ACE described earlier resulted in the synthesis and evaluation of a series of succinic acid derivatives (Fig. 23.5B). Because proline was present as the C-terminal amino acid in SQ 20,881 as well as in other potent, inhibitory snake venom peptides, it was included in the structure of newly designed inhibitors. The first inhibitor to be synthesized and tested was succinyl-L-proline (Fig. 23.6). This compound proved to be somewhat disappointing. Although it provided reasonable specificity for ACE, it was only approximately 1/500 as potent as SQ 20,881.

Substitution of other amino acids in place of proline produced compounds that were even less potent; hence, all subsequent SAR studies were conducted using analogs of L-proline (Fig. 23.6). The addition of a methyl group to the 2-position of succinyl-L-proline to mimic the amino acid side chain, R_2, of the substrate enhanced activity, but only marginally. D-2-Methylsuccinyl-L-proline had effects similar to SQ 20,881 but was still only 1/300 as potent. The D-isomer, rather than the L-isomer normally seen for amino acids, was necessary because of the isosteric replacement of an NH_2 with a CH_2 present in succinyl-L-proline. A comparison of the R_2 group of the substrate (Fig. 23.4B) with the methyl group of D-2-methylsuccinyl-L-proline

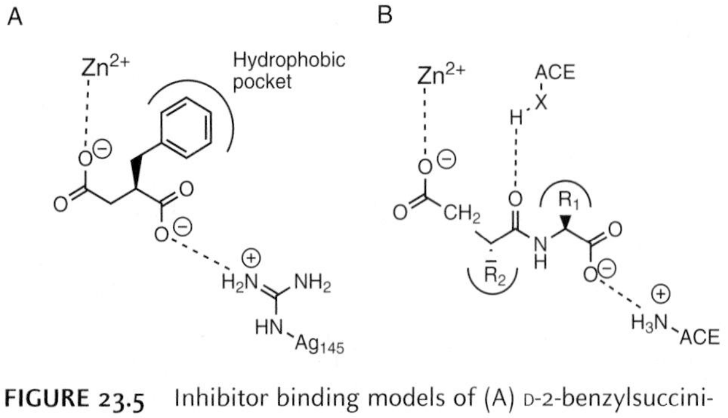

FIGURE 23.5 Inhibitor binding models of (A) D-2-benzylsuccinicacid to carboxypeptidase A and (B) succinic acid derivatives to ACE.

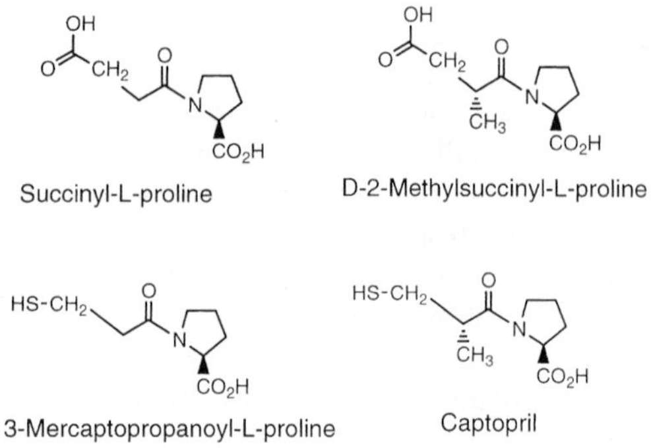

FIGURE 23.6 Compounds prepared in the development of captopril.

illustrates that this methyl group occupies the same binding site as the side chain of an L-amino group.

One of the most important alterations to succinyl-L-proline was the replacement of the succinyl carboxylate with other groups having enhanced affinity for the zinc atom bound to ACE. Replacement of this carboxylate with a sulfhydryl group produced 3-mercaptopropanoyl-L-proline. This compound has a half maximal inhibitory concentration (IC_{50}) value of 200 nmol/L and is greater than 1,000-fold more potent than succinyl-L-proline (Fig. 23.6). Additionally, it is 10- to 20-fold more potent than SQ 20,881 in inhibiting contractile and vasopressor responses to angiotensin I. Addition of a 2-D-methyl group further enhanced activity. The resulting compound, captopril (Fig. 23.6), is a competitive inhibitor of ACE with a K_i value of 1.7 nmol/L and was the first ACE inhibitor to be marketed.

The sulfhydryl group of captopril proved to be responsible not only for the excellent inhibitory activity of the compound but also for the two most common side effects, skin rashes and taste disturbances (e.g., metallic taste and loss of taste). These side effects usually subsided on dosage reduction or discontinuation of captopril. They were attributed to the presence of the sulfhydryl group, because similar effects had been observed with penicillamine, a sulfhydryl-containing agent used to treat Wilson disease and rheumatoid arthritis (17,18).

Dicarboxylate-Containing Inhibitors

Development of Enalapril

Researchers at Merck (19) sought to develop compounds that lacked the sulfhydryl group of captopril yet maintained some ability to chelate zinc. Compounds having the general structure shown below were designed to meet this objective.

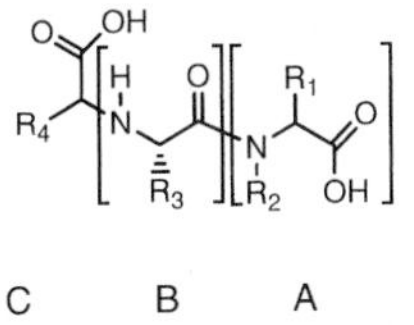

These compounds are tripeptide substrate analogs in which the C-terminal (A) and penultimate (B) amino acids are retained but the third amino acid is isosterically replaced by a substituted N-carboxymethyl group (C). Similar to the results seen in the development of captopril, C-terminal proline analogs provided optimum activity. The use of a methyl group at R_3 (i.e., B = Ala) and a phenylethyl group at R_4 resulted in enalaprilat (Fig. 23.7). In comparing the activity of captopril and enalaprilat, it was found that enalaprilat, with a K_i of 0.2 nmol/L, was approximately 10-fold more potent than captopril. Studies investigating the binding of enalaprilat revealed that its ability to chelate the enzyme-bound zinc atom was significantly less than that of captopril. The enhanced binding was proposed to be caused by the ability to mimic the transition state of angiotensin I hydrolysis. As shown in Figure 23.7, enalaprilat possess a tetrahedral carbon in place of the labile peptide bond. The secondary amine, the carboxylic acid, and phenylethyl groups all contribute to the overall binding of the compound to ACE. The secondary amine is located at the same position as the labile amide nitrogen, the ionized carboxylic acid can form an ionic bond with the zinc atom, and the phenylethyl group mimics the hydrophobic side chain of the Phe amino acid, which is present in angiotensin I.

Despite excellent intravenous (IV) activity, enalaprilat has very poor oral bioavailability. Esterification of enalaprilat produced enalapril (Fig. 23.8), a compound with superior oral bioavailability. The combination of structural features in enalaprilat, especially the two carboxylate groups and the secondary amine, is responsible for its overall low lipophilicity and poor oral bioavailability. Zwitterion formation also has been suggested to contribute to the low oral activity (20), and a comparison of the pK_a values for the secondary amine of enalaprilat and enalapril supports this explanation. Ionization of the adjacent carboxylate in enalaprilat greatly enhances the basicity of the secondary amine such that the pK_a of the amine in this compound is 8.02, whereas in enalapril, it is only 5.49. Thus, in the small intestine, the amine in enalaprilat will be primarily ionized and form a zwitterion with the adjacent carboxylate, but the amine in enalapril will be primarily un-ionized (21).

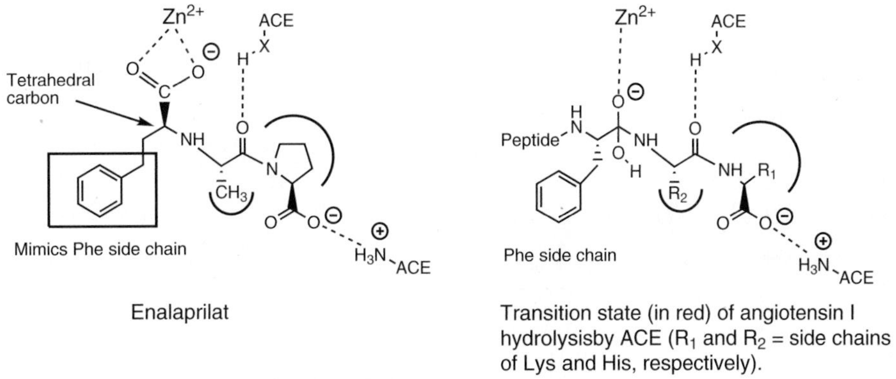

FIGURE 23.7 A comparison of enalaprilat and the transition state of angiotensin I hydrolysis by ACE.

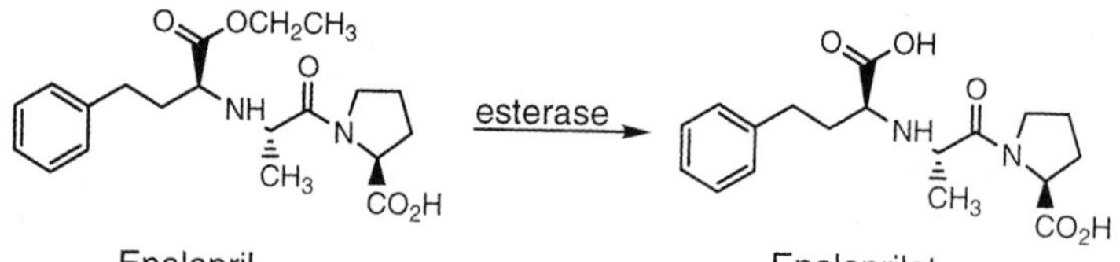

Enalapril Enalaprilat

FIGURE 23.8 Bioactivation of enalapril.

IV administration of either enalapril or enalaprilat produced similar effects on angiotensin II production despite the fact that enalapril showed a 1,000-fold decrease in in vitro activity. Subsequent studies showed that enalapril undergoes bioactivation and, thus, is a prodrug of enalaprilat. Because human plasma was reported to lack enalapril esterolytic activity, bioactivation by hepatic esterases (Fig. 23.8) has been suggested as the most probable mechanism for enalaprilat formation (22,23).

Additional Dicarboxylate Inhibitors

Eight other dicarboxylate inhibitors (Table 23.1) have been approved for various therapeutic indications; however, spirapril has never been marketed. Lisinopril is chemically unique in two respects. First, it contains the basic amino acid lysine (R_1 = $CH_2CH_2CH_2CH_2NH_2$) instead of the standard nonpolar alanine (R = CH_3) residue. Second, it does not require bioactivation, because neither of the carboxylic acid groups are esterified (i.e., R_2 = H). Lisinopril was developed at the same time as

TABLE 23.1 Additional Dicarboxylate-Containing Angiotensin-Converting Enzyme Inhibitors

General structure:

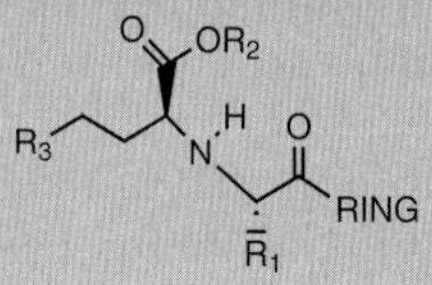

Benazepril

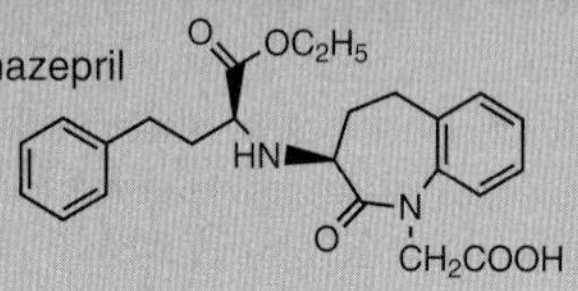

Compounds	Ring	R_1	R_2	R_3
Lisinopril	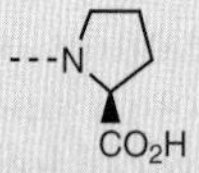	$(CH_2)_4NH_2$	H	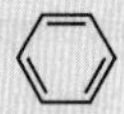
Moexipril	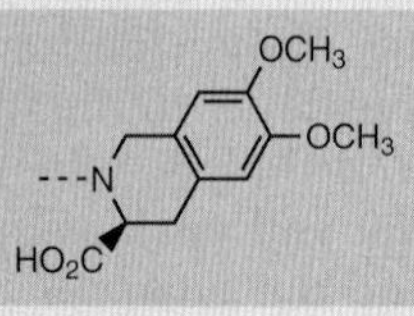	CH_3	CH_2CH_3	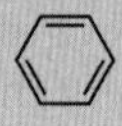
Perindopril	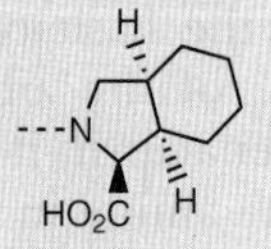	CH_3	CH_2CH_3	CH_3
Quinapril	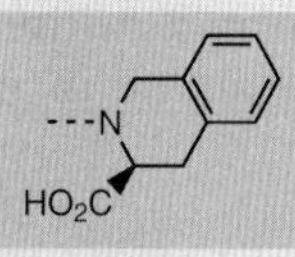	CH_3	CH_2CH_3	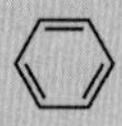
Ramipril	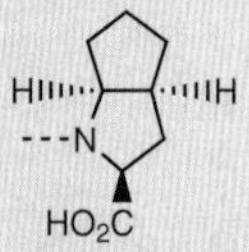	CH_3	CH_2CH_3	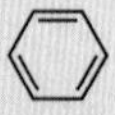
Spirapril	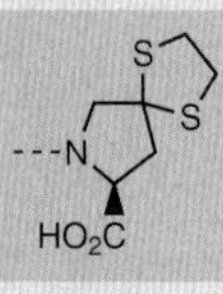	CH_3	CH_2CH_3	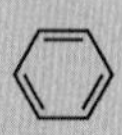
Trandolapril	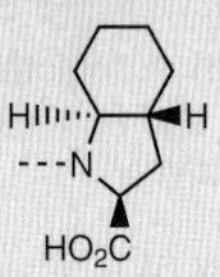	CH_3	CH_2CH_3	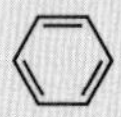

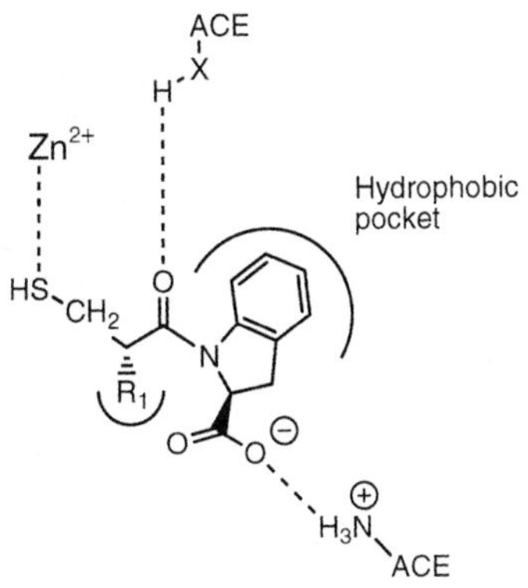

FIGURE 23.9 A modified model of ACE inhibitor binding.

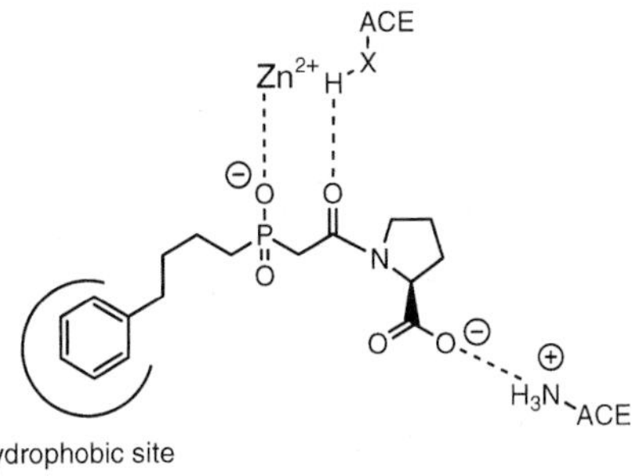

FIGURE 23.10 The binding of phosphinate analogs to ACE.

enalapril. Despite the addition of another ionizable group, the oral absorption of lisinopril was found to be superior to that of enalaprilat but less than that of enalapril. In vitro studies of enalaprilat and lisinopril showed lisinopril to be slightly more potent than enalaprilat (22,23). Currently, lisinopril and captopril are the only two ACE inhibitors that are not prodrugs.

The major structural difference among the remaining ACE inhibitors is in the ring of the C-terminal amino acid. Lisinopril, like enalapril and captopril, contains the pyrrolidine ring of proline, whereas all the other compounds contain larger bicyclic or spiro ring systems. Studies of indoline analogs of captopril indicated that a hydrophobic pocket similar to that seen in carboxypeptidase A also was present in ACE. This led to a modification (Fig. 23.9) of Ondetti and Cushman's original model and the development of inhibitors that contained larger hydrophobic ring systems (24). Although this modified model was proposed for captopril analogs, it is readily adaptable to include enalaprilat analogs. In general, the varied ring systems seen in benazepril, moexipril, perindopril, quinapril, ramipril, spirapril, and trandolapril provide enhanced binding and potency. They also lead to differences in absorption, plasma protein binding, elimination, onset of action, duration of action, and dosing among the drugs. These differences are discussed in more detail in a later section in this chapter, "Pharmacokinetic Properties."

Phosphonate-Containing Inhibitors: The Development of Fosinopril

The search for ACE inhibitors that lacked the sulfhydryl group also lead to the investigation of phosphorous-containing compounds (25). The phosphinic acid shown in Figure 23.10 is capable of binding to ACE in a manner similar to enalapril. The interaction of the zinc atom with the phosphinic acid is similar to that seen with sulfhydryl and carboxylate groups. Additionally, this compound is capable of forming the ionic, hydrogen, and hydrophobic bonds similar to those seen with enalapril and other dicarboxylate analogs. A feature unique to this compound is the ability of the phosphinic acid to more truly mimic the ionized, tetrahedral intermediate of peptide hydrolysis. Unlike enalapril and other dicarboxylate analogs, however, the spacing of this tetrahedral species is shorter, being only two atoms removed from the proline nitrogen. Additionally, the spacing between the proline nitrogen and the hydrophobic phenyl ring is one atom longer than that seen in the dicarboxylates.

Structural modification to investigate more hydrophobic, C-terminal ring systems, similar to that described earlier for the dicarboxylate compounds, led to a 4-cyclohexylproline analog of the original phosphinic acid. This compound, fosinoprilat (Fig. 23.11), was more potent than captopril but less potent than enalaprilat. The previously mentioned differences in the spacing of the phosphinic acid and phenyl groups may be responsible for this latter difference in potency. Similar to the dicarboxylates, fosinoprilat was too hydrophilic and exhibited poor oral activity. The prodrug fosinopril contains an (acyloxy)alkyl group that allows better lipid solubility and improved bioavailability (25). Bioactivation via esterase activity in the intestinal wall and liver produces fosinopril (Fig. 23.11).

Mechanism of Action

The ACE inhibitors attenuate the effects of the renin-angiotensin system by inhibiting the conversion of angiotensin I to angiotensin II (Fig. 23.1). They also inhibit the conversion of [des-Asp[1]]angiotensin I to angiotensin III; however, this action has only a minor role in the overall cardiovascular effects of these drugs. They are selective in that they do not directly interfere with any other components of the renin-angiotensin system; however, they do cause other effects that are unrelated to the decrease in angiotensin II concentration. Inhibitors of ACE increase bradykinin levels that, in turn, stimulate prostaglandin biosynthesis (Fig. 23.3). Both of these compounds have been proposed to contribute to the overall action of ACE inhibitors. Additionally, decreased angiotensin II levels increase the release of renin and the production of angiotensin I. Because ACE is inhibited, angiotensin I is shunted toward the production of angiotensin 1-7 and other peptides. The contribution of these peptides to the overall effect of ACE inhibitors is unknown (1).

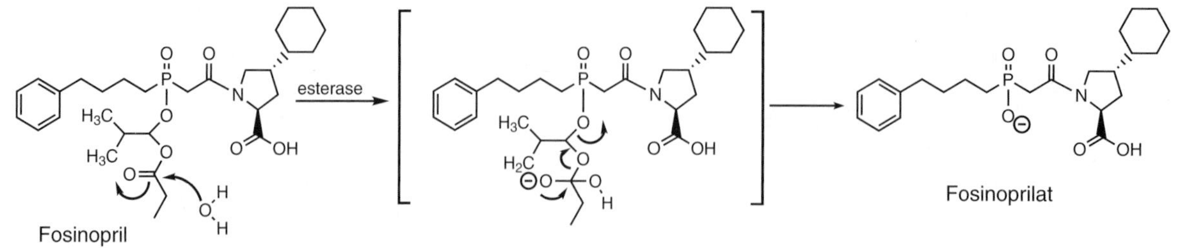

FIGURE 23.11 Bioactivation of fosinopril.

Structure–Activity Relationships

The structural characteristics for ACE inhibitory activity are given in Table 23.2. ACE is a stereoselective drug target. Because currently approved ACE inhibitors act as either di- or tripeptide substrate analogs, they must contain a stereochemistry that is consistent with the L-amino acids present in the natural substrates. This was established very early in the development of ACE inhibitors when compounds with carboxyl-terminal D-amino acids were discovered to be very poor inhibitors (26). Later work by Patchett et al. (19) reinforced this idea. They reported a 100- to 1,000-fold loss in inhibitor activity whenever the configuration of either the carboxylate or the R_1 substituent (Table 23.1) was altered. The *S,S,S*-configuration seen in enalapril and other dicarboxylate inhibitors meets the previously stated criteria and provides for optimum enzyme inhibition.

Physicochemical Properties

Captopril and fosinopril are acidic drugs, but all other ACE inhibitors are amphoteric. The carboxylic acid attached to the N-ring is a common structural feature in all ACE inhibitors. It has a pK_a in the range of 2.5 to 3.5 and will be primarily ionized at physiologic pH. As discussed earlier with enalapril, the pK_a and ionization of the secondary amine in the dicarboxylate series depend on whether the adjacent functional group is in the prodrug or active form. In the prodrug form, the amine is adjacent to an ester, is less basic, and is primarily un-ionized at physiologic pH. Following bioactivation, the amine is adjacent to an ionized carboxylic acid that enhances both the basicity and ionization of the amine. Similarly, the basic nitrogen enhances the acidity of the adjacent carboxylic acid such that it usually has a lower pK_a than the carboxylic acid attached to the N-ring. As an example, the pK_a values of enalapril are 3.39 and 2.30. These values correspond to the carboxylic acid on the N-ring and the carboxylic acid adjacent to the amine, respectively. The analogous values for these functional groups in lisinopril are 3.3 and 1.7 (21).

The calculated logP values (21) along with other pharmacokinetic parameters for the ACE inhibitors are shown

TABLE 23.2 Structure–Activity Relationship of ACE Inhibitors

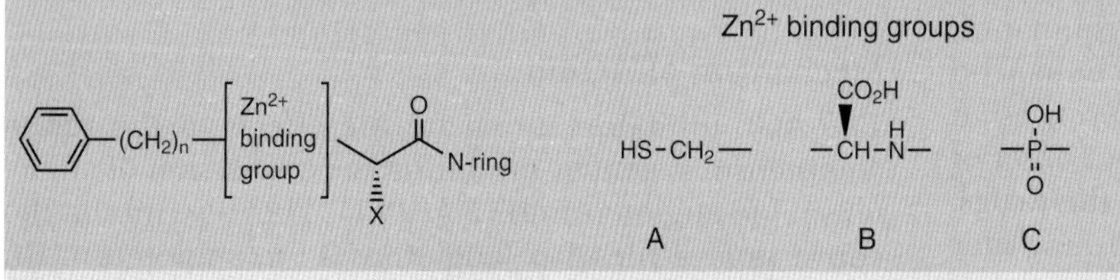

a. The N-ring must contain a carboxylic acid to mimic the C-terminal carboxylate of ACE substrates.
b. Large hydrophobic heterocyclic rings (i.e., the N-ring) increase potency and alter pharmacokinetic parameters.
c. The zinc binding groups can be either sulfhydryl (A), a carboxylic acid (B), or a phosphinic acid (C).
d. The sulfhydryl group shows superior binding to zinc (the side chain mimicking the Phe in carboxylate and phosphinic acid compounds partially compensates for the lack of a sulfhydryl group).
e. Sulfhydryl-containing compounds produce high incidence of skin rash and taste disturbances.
f. Sulfhydryl-containing compounds can form dimers and disulfides, which may shorten duration of action.
g. Compounds that bind to zinc through either a carboxylate or phosphinate mimic the peptide hydrolysis transition state and enhance binding.
h. Esterification of the carboxylate or phosphinate produces an orally bioavailable prodrug.
i. X is usually methyl to mimic the side chain of alanine. Within the dicarboxylate series, when X equals n-butylamine (lysine side chain), this produces a compound that does not require prodrug for oral activity.
j. Optimum activity occurs when stereochemistry of inhibitor is consistent with L-amino acid stereochemistry present in normal substrates.

in Table 23.3. With three notable exceptions, captopril, enalaprilat, and lisinopril, all of the compounds possess good lipid solubility. Compounds that contain hydrophobic bicyclic ring systems are more lipid soluble than those that contain proline. A comparison of the logP values of benazepril, fosinopril, moexipril, perindopril, quinapril, ramipril, spirapril, and trandolapril to those for captopril and enalapril illustrates this fact. As previously discussed, enalaprilat is much more hydrophilic than its ester prodrug and is currently the only ACE inhibitor marked for IV administration. In terms of solubility, lisinopril probably is the most interesting compound in that it is the most hydrophilic inhibitor, yet unlike enalaprilat, it is orally active. One possible explanation for this phenomenon is that in the duodenum, lisinopril will exist as a di-zwitterion in which the ionized groups can internally bind to one another. In this manner, lisinopril may be able to pass through the lipid bilayer with an overall net neutral charge.

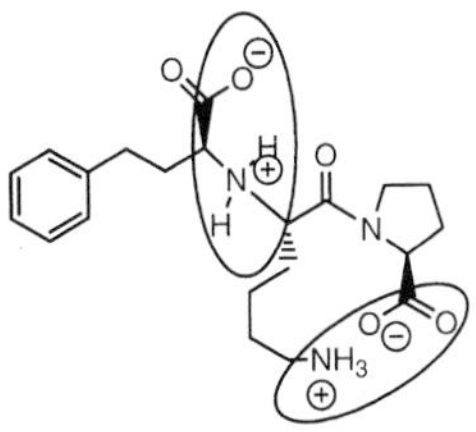

Metabolism

Lisinopril and enalaprilat are excreted unchanged, whereas all other ACE inhibitors undergo some degree of metabolic transformation (1,27–29). As previously discussed and illustrated (Figs. 23.8 and 23.11), all dicarboxylate and phosphonate prodrugs must undergo bioactivation via hepatic esterases. Additionally, based on their structural features, specific compounds can undergo metabolic inactivation via various pathways (Fig. 23.12). Because of its sulfhydryl group, captopril is subject to oxidative dimerization or conjugation. Approximately 40% to 50% of a dose of captopril is excreted unchanged, whereas the remainder is excreted as either a disulfide dimer or a captopril-cysteine disulfide. Glucuronide conjugation has been reported for benazepril, fosinopril, quinapril, and ramipril. This conjugation can occur either with the parent prodrug or with the activated drug. Benazepril, with the *N*-substituted glycine, is especially susceptible to this reaction because of a difference in steric hindrance. For all ACE inhibitors, except benazepril, the carbon atom directly adjacent to the carboxylic acid is part of a ring system and provides some steric hindrance to conjugation. The unsubstituted methylene group (i.e., $-CH_2-$) of benazepril provides less steric hindrance and, thus, facilitates conjugation. Moexipril, perindopril, and ramipril can undergo cyclization to produce diketopiperazines. This

TABLE 23.3 Pharmacokinetic Parameters of ACE Inhibitors

Drug	Calculated LogP	Oral Bioavailability (%)	Effect of Food on Absorption	Active Metabolite	Protein Binding (%)	Onset of Action (hours)	Duration of Action (hours)	Major Route(s) of Elimination
Benazepril	5.50	37	Slows absorption	Benazeprilat	>95	1	24	Renal (primary) Biliary (secondary)
Captopril	0.27	60–75	Reduced	NA	25–30	0.25–0.50	6–12	Renal
Enalapril	2.43	60	None	Enalaprilat	50–60	1	24	Renal/fecal
Enalaprilat	1.54	NA	NA	NA	—	0.25	6	Renal
Fosinopril	6.09	36	Slows absorption	Fosinoprilat	95	1	24	Renal (50%) Hepatic (50%)
Lisinopril	1.19	25–30	None	NA	25	1	24	Renal
Moexipril	4.06	13	Reduced	Moexiprilat	50	1	24	Fecal (primary) Renal (secondary)
Perindopril	3.36	65–95	Reduced	Perindoprilat	60–80	1	24	Renal
Quinapril	4.32	60	Reduced	Quinaprilat	97	1	24	Renal
Ramipril	3.41	50–60	Slows absorption	Ramiprilat	73	1–2	24	Renal (60%) Fecal (40%)
Spirapril	3.16	50	—	Spiraprilat	—	1	24	Renal (50%) Hepatic (50%)
Trandolapril	3.97	70	Slows absorption	Trandolaprilat	80	0.5–1.0	24	Fecal (primary) Renal (secondary)

NA, not applicable; —, data not available.

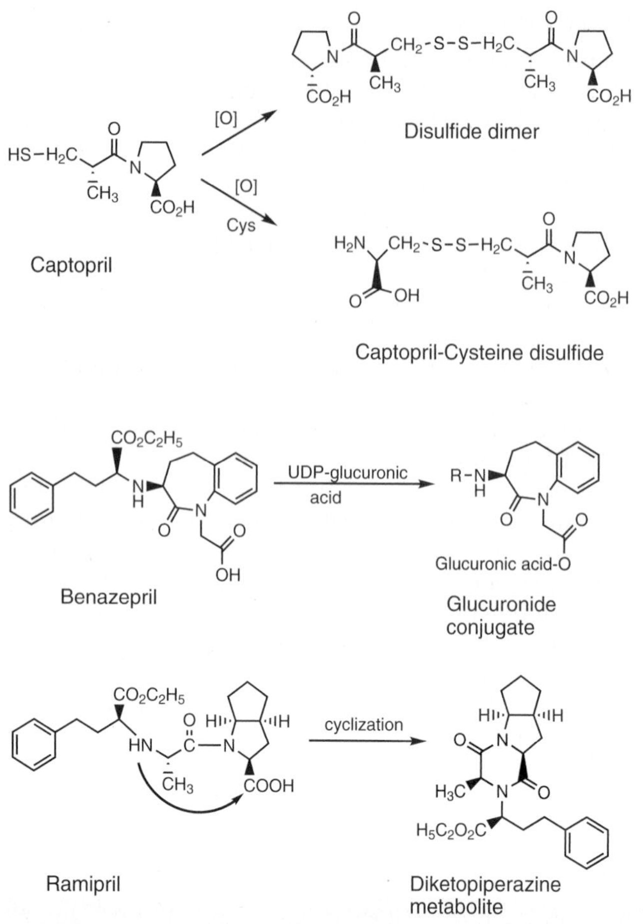

FIGURE 23.12 Metabolic routes of ACE inhibitors.

cyclization can occur with either the parent or active forms of the drugs.

A comparative study of the metabolism and biliary excretion of lisinopril, enalapril, perindopril, and ramipril revealed that whereas neither lisinopril nor enalapril underwent any appreciable metabolism beyond bioactivation of enalapril to enalaprilat, both perindopril and ramipril were extensively metabolized beyond the initial bioactivation. It was proposed that these differences in hepatic metabolism could be explained, in part, by the larger, more hydrophobic rings present on perindopril and ramipril (30).

Pharmacokinetic Parameters

The pharmacokinetic parameters and dosing information for ACE inhibitors are summarized in Tables 23.3 and 23.4, respectively (1,27–29). The oral bioavailability of this class of drugs ranges from 13% to 95%. Differences in both lipid solubility and first-pass metabolism are most likely responsible for this wide variation. Both parameters should be considered when comparing any two or more compounds. With the exceptions of enalapril and lisinopril, the concurrent administration of food adversely affects the oral absorption of ACE inhibitors. Product literature specifically instructs that captopril should be taken 1 hour before meals and that moexipril should be taken in the fasting state. Although not specifically stated, similar instructions also should benefit patients taking an ACE inhibitor whose absorption is affected by food.

The extent of protein binding also exhibits wide variability among the different compounds. The data suggest that this variation has some correlation with the calculated logP values for the compounds (Table 23.3). Three of the more lipophilic compounds—fosinopril, quinapril, and benazepril—exhibit protein binding of greater than 90%, whereas three of the least lipophilic compounds—lisinopril, enalapril, and captopril—exhibit much lower protein binding. The lack of a protein binding value for spirapril prevents a more definitive statement on this correlation.

Renal elimination is the primary route of elimination for most ACE inhibitors. With the exceptions of fosinopril and spirapril, altered renal function significantly diminishes the plasma clearance of ACE inhibitors, including those that are eliminated primarily by the feces. Therefore, the dosage of most ACE inhibitors should be reduced in patients with renal impairment (1). Studies of fosinopril in patients with heart failure demonstrated that it is eliminated by both renal and hepatic pathways and does not require a dosage reduction in patients with renal dysfunction (31). Spirapril also exhibits similar properties; however, it is not currently available for use. It should be noted that the literature data for routes of elimination are not always consistent. The designation of renal elimination is quite clear, but it is difficult to correlate what some sources call renal/hepatic elimination with what others call renal/fecal elimination. Additionally, it is uncertain whether the designation of fecal elimination also includes unabsorbed drug. As a result, there is some variability for major routes of elimination listed in Table 23.3.

With one exception, all ACE inhibitors have a similar onset of action, duration of action, and dosing interval. Captopril has a more rapid onset of action; however, it also has a shorter duration and requires a more frequent dosing interval than any of the other compounds. When oral dosing is inappropriate, enalaprilat can be used IV. The normal dose administered to hypertensive patients is 0.625 to 1.25 mg every 6 hours. The dose usually is administered over 5 minutes and may be titrated up to 5 mg IV every 6 hours.

Therapeutic Applications

The ACE inhibitors have been approved for the treatment of hypertension, heart failure, left ventricular dysfunction (either after myocardial infarction [MI] or

CHEMICAL/PHARMACOLOGIC CLASSES USED TO TREAT HYPERTENSION

Diuretics (see Chapter 22), ACE inhibitors, angiotensin II blockers, renin inhibitors, calcium channel blockers (present chapter), central α_2-agonists, peripheral α_1-antagonists, β-blockers, ganglionic blockers, and vasodilators (see Chapter 24).

TABLE 23.4 Dosing Information for Orally Available ACE Inhibitors

Generic Name	Trade Name(s)	Approved Indications	Dosing Range (Treatment of Hypertension)	Maximum Daily Dose	Dose Reduction with Renal Dysfunction	Available Tablet Strengths (mg)
Benazepril	Lotensin	Hypertension	40 mg once daily or b.i.d.	80 mg	Yes	5, 10, 20, 40
Captopril	Capoten	Hypertension, heart failure, left ventricular dysfunction (post-MI), diabetic nephropathy	25–150 mg b.i.d. or t.i.d.	450 mg	Yes	12.5, 25, 50, 100
Enalapril	Vasotec	Hypertension, heart failure, left ventricular dysfunction (asymptomatic)	2.5–40 mg once daily or b.i.d.	40 mg	Yes	2.5, 5, 10, 20
Fosinopril	Monopril	Hypertension, heart failure	10–40 mg once daily	80 mg	No	10, 20, 40
Lisinopril	Prinivil, Zestril	Hypertension, heart failure, improve survival post-MI	10–40 mg once daily	80 mg	Yes	2.5, 5, 10, 20, 30, 40
Moexipril	Univasc	Hypertension	7.5–30 mg once daily or b.i.d.	30 mg	Yes	7.5, 15
Perindopril	Aceon	Hypertension, stable CAD	4–8 mg once daily or b.i.d.	16 mg	Yes	2, 4, 8
Quinapril	Accupril	Hypertension, heart failure	10–80 mg once daily or b.i.d.	80 mg	Yes	5, 10, 20, 40
Ramipril	Altace	Hypertension, heart failure (post-MI), reduce risk of MI, stroke, and death from cardiovascular causes	2.5–20 mg once daily or b.i.d.	20 mg	Yes	1.25, 2.5, 5, 10
Trandolapril	Mavik	Hypertension, heart failure (post-MI), left ventricular dysfunction (post-MI)	1–4 mg once daily	8 mg	Yes	1, 2, 4

b.i.d., twice a day; CAD, coronary artery disease; MI, myocardial infarction; t.i.d., three times a day.

asymptomatic), improved survival after MI, stable coronary heart disease, diabetic nephropathy, and reduction of the risk of MI, stroke, and death from cardiovascular causes. Although all ACE inhibitors possess the same physiologic actions and, thus, should produce similar therapeutic effects, the approved indications differ among the currently available agents (Table 23.4). Inhibitors of ACE have been designated as first-line agents for the treatment of hypertension (32) and are effective for a variety of cardiovascular disorders. They can be used either individually or with other classes of compounds. They are especially useful in treating patients with hypertension who also suffer from heart failure, left ventricular dysfunction, or diabetes. Arterial and venous dilation seen with ACE inhibitors not only lowers blood pressure but also has favorable effects on both preload and afterload in patients with heart failure. Additionally, the ability of ACE inhibitors to cause regression of left ventricular hypertrophy has been demonstrated to reduce the incidence of further heart disease in patients with hypertension. The use of ACE inhibitors in patients with MI is similarly based on the ability of ACE inhibitors to decrease mortality by preventing postinfarction left ventricular hypertrophy and heart failure. Current recommendations to give ACE inhibitors to all patients with impaired left ventricular systolic impairment regardless of the presence of observable symptoms also are based on the ability of these inhibitors to block the vascular and cardiac hypertrophy and remodeling caused by angiotensin II. Inhibitors of ACE also have been reported to slow the progression of diabetic nephropathy and, thus, are preferred agents in the treatment of hypertension in patients with diabetes. It also has been suggested that ACE inhibitors be used in

COMBINATION PRODUCTS THAT INCLUDE AN ACE INHIBITOR

ACE Inhibitor/Diuretic: benazepril/hydrochlorothiazide, captopril/hydrochlorothiazide, enalapril/hydrochlorothiazide, fosinopril/hydrochlorothiazide, lisinopril/hydrochlorothiazide, moexipril/hydrochlorothiazide, and quinapril/hydrochlorothiazide

ACE Inhibitor/Calcium Channel Blocker: benazepril/amlodipine, enalapril/diltiazem, enalapril/felodipine, trandolapril/verapamil

UNLABELED USES

Hypertensive crises, renovascular hypertension, neonatal and childhood hypertension, stroke prevention, migraine prophylaxis, nondiabetic nephropathy, chronic kidney disease, scleroderma renal crisis, Raynaud phenomenon, and Bartter syndrome (27,28).

ADVERSE EFFECTS OF ACE INHIBITORS

Hypotension, hyperkalemia, cough, rash, taste disturbances, headache, dizziness, fatigue, nausea, vomiting, diarrhea, acute renal failure, neutropenia, proteinuria, and angioedema

patients with diabetic nephropathy regardless of the presence or absence or hypertension (1,6,7,28).

Adverse Effects and Drug Interactions

The most prevalent or significant side effects of ACE inhibitors are listed below, whereas drug interactions for ACE inhibitors are listed in Table 23.5 (1,27,28). Some adverse effects can be attributed to specific functional groups within individual agents, whereas others can be directly related to the mechanism of action of this class of compounds. The higher incidence of maculopapular rashes and taste disturbances observed among those using captopril have been linked to the presence of the sulfhydryl group in this compound. All ACE inhibitors can cause hypotension, hyperkalemia, and a dry cough. Hypotension results from an extension of the desired physiologic effect, whereas hyperkalemia results from a decrease in aldosterone secretion secondary to a decrease in angiotensin II production. Cough is by far the most prevalent and bothersome side effect seen with the use of ACE inhibitors. It is seen in 5% to 20% of patients, usually

PEPTIDE MIMETICS: DESIGN OF AGONISTS/ANTAGONISTS

Peptide mimetics have been defined as molecules that mimic the action of peptides, have no peptide bonds (i.e., no amide bonds between amino acids), and have a molecular weight of less than 700 daltons. In comparison with peptide drugs, peptide mimetics have numerous pharmaceutical advantages. Foremost among these are increased bioavailability and duration of action. The majority of known peptide mimetics have been discovered by random screening techniques; however, this process is costly, labor intensive, and unpredictable.

A more logical and rational approach is de novo peptide mimetic design (33), and an example of this approach is illustrated in Figure 23.13. In this example, the overall process is divided into three steps (A–C). Initially, the amino acids that comprise the pharmacophore of the peptide must be identified. Thus, a knowledge of the SARs for the peptide under consideration is essential. In Figure 23.13A, the side chains present on amino acid residues 1, 3, and 5 of a hypothetical heptapeptide are assumed to comprise the pharmacophore, and the remainder of the peptide is assumed to provide the proper structural support for these key groups. In the second step of this de novo design process, the proper spatial arrangement of the pharmacophoric groups must be elucidated. Nuclear magnetic resonance spectroscopy, x-ray diffraction studies, and molecular modeling programs that allow energy-minimization procedures and molecular dynamics simulation can be used to construct a model of the biologically active conformation. Returning to the example, the side chains representing the pharmacophore are assumed to be located on the inside of the peptide, whereas the remaining residues are assumed to be located on the outside of the peptide (Fig. 23.13B). In the final step of the process, the pharmacophoric groups must be mounted on a nonpeptide template in such a manner that they retain the proper spatial arrangement found in the original peptide. This is shown in Figure 23.13C, where side chains 1, 3, and 5 of the original peptide are connected to a rigid template (represented by the polygon). A variety of aromatic ring systems (e.g., benzene, biphenyl, phenanthrene, and benzodiazepine) can be used to provide the rigid template, and appropriately placed alkyl groups can be used to enhance spacing and increase flexibility. Additionally, isosteres of the original pharmacophoric groups may be used to circumvent specific synthetic problems (34).

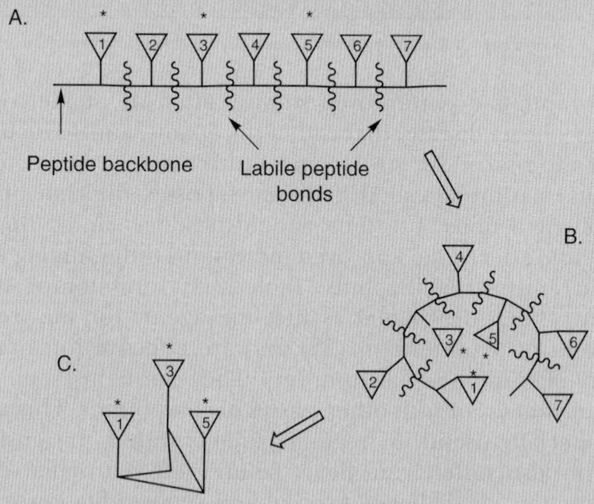

FIGURE 23.13 A general process for the rational design of peptide mimetics: (A) identification of crucial pharmacophoric groups, (B) determination of the spatial arrangement of these groups, and (C) use of a template to mount the key functional groups in their proper conformation. Groups highlighted with an asterisk comprise the pharmacophore of the heptapeptide. (From Harrold MW. Preparing students for future therapies: the development of novel agents to control the renin-angiotensin system. Am J Pharm Educ 1997;61:173–178, with permission.)

TABLE 23.5 Drug Interactions for ACE Inhibitors

Drug	ACE Inhibitor	Result of Interaction
Allopurinol	Captopril	Increased risk of hypersensitivity
Antacids	All	Decreased bioavailability of ACE inhibitor (more likely with captopril and fosinopril)
Capsaicin	All	Exacerbation of cough
Digoxin	All	Either increased or decreased plasma digoxin levels
Diuretics	All	Potential excessive reduction in blood pressure; the effects of loop diuretics may be reduced
Iron salts	Captopril	Reduction of captopril levels unless administration is separated by at least 2 hours
K^+ preparations or K^+-sparing diuretics	All	Elevated serum potassium levels
Lithium	All	Increased serum lithium levels
NSAIDs	All	Decreased hypotensive effects
Phenothiazides	All	Increased pharmacologic effects of ACE inhibitor
Probenecid	Captopril	Decreased clearance and increased blood levels of captopril
Rifampin	Enalapril	Decreased pharmacologic effects of enalapril
Tetracycline	Quinapril	Decreased absorption of tetracycline (may result from high magnesium content of quinapril tablets)

NSAIDs, nonsteroidal anti-inflammatory drugs.

is not dose related, and apparently results from the lack of selectivity of this class of drugs. As previously discussed, ACE inhibitors also prevent the breakdown of bradykinin (Fig. 23.3), and because bradykinin stimulates prostaglandin synthesis, prostaglandin levels also increase. The increased levels of both bradykinin and prostaglandin have been proposed to be responsible for the cough (35).

The use of ACE inhibitors during pregnancy is contraindicated. This class of compounds is not teratogenic during the first trimester, but administration during the second and third trimester is associated with an increased incidence of fetal morbidity and mortality. Inhibitors of ACE can be used in women of childbearing age; however, they should be discontinued as soon as pregnancy is confirmed.

ANGIOTENSIN II RECEPTOR BLOCKERS

From an historical perspective, the angiotensin II receptor was the initial target for developing compounds that could inhibit the renin-angiotensin pathway. Efforts to develop angiotensin II receptor antagonists began in the early 1970s and focused on peptide-based analogs of the natural agonist. The prototypical compound that resulted from these studies was saralasin, an octapeptide in which the Asp[1] and Phe[8] residues of angiotensin II were replaced with Sar (sarcosine, *N*-methylglycine) and Ile, respectively. Saralasin as well as other peptide analogs demonstrated the ability to reduce blood pressure; however, these compounds lacked oral bioavailability and expressed unwanted partial agonist activity. More recent efforts have used peptide mimetics to circumvent these inherent problems with peptide-based antagonists. The culmination of these efforts was the 1995 approval of losartan, a nonpeptide angiotensin II receptor blocker (ARB) (1,36).

Development of Losartan

The development of losartan can be traced back to two 1982 patent publications (37), which described the antihypertensive effects of a series of imidazole-5-acetic acid analogs. These compounds are exemplified by S-8308 (Fig. 23.14) and were later found to block the angiotensin II receptor specifically. Although these compounds were relatively weak antagonists, they did not possess the unwanted agonist activity previously seen in peptide analogs. A computerized molecular modeling overlap of angiotensin II with the structure of S-8308 revealed three common structural features: The ionized carboxylate of S-8308 correlated with the C-terminal carboxylate of angiotensin II, the imidazole ring of S-8308 correlated with the imidazole side chain of the His[6] residue, and the n-butyl group of S-8308 correlated with the hydrocarbon side chain of the Ile[5] residue (Fig. 23.14). The benzyl group of S-8308 was proposed to lie in the direction of the N-terminus of angiotensin II; however, it was not believed to have any significant receptor interactions.

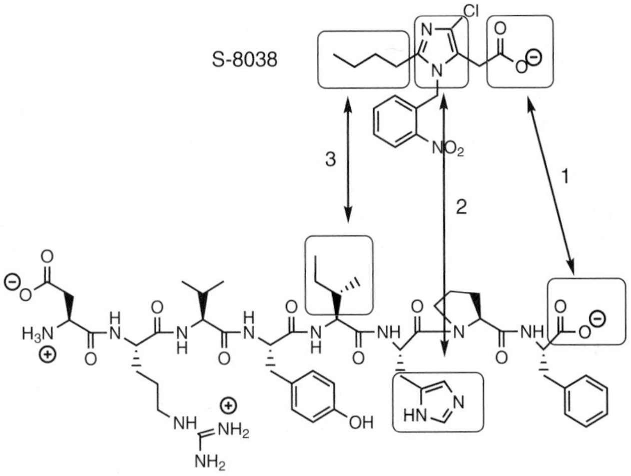

FIGURE 23.14 Structural comparison of S-8308, an imidazole-5-acetic acid analog, with angiotensin II. (Adapted from Timmermans PB, Wong PC, Chiu AT, et al. Angiotensin II receptors and angiotensin II receptor antagonists. Pharmacol Rev 1993;45:205–213, with permission.)

From S-8308, a number of molecular modifications were carried out in an attempt to improve receptor binding and lipid solubility, with the latter being important to assure adequate oral absorption. These changes resulted in the preparation of losartan, a compound with high receptor affinity (IC_{50} = 0.019 μmol/L) and oral activity (Fig. 23.15).

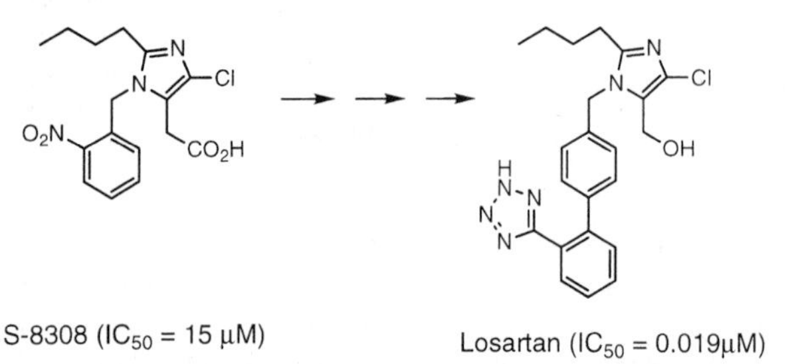

FIGURE 23.15 The development of losartan from S-8308.

Additional Angiotensin II Receptor Blockers

Valsartan, irbesartan, telmisartan, candesartan, olmesartan, and azilsartan are biphenyl analogs of losartan (Fig. 23.16). These compounds possess structural features that are similar to those seen in losartan. Valsartan, named for the valine portion of the compound, is the first nonimidazole-containing ARB and is slightly more potent (IC_{50} = 0.0089 μmol/L) than losartan. The amide carbonyl of valsartan is isosteric with the imidazole nitrogen of losartan and can serve as a hydrogen bond acceptor similar to the imidazole nitrogen. Irbesartan is a spiro-compound that lacks the primary alcohol of losartan but that has a 10-fold greater binding affinity (IC_{50} = 0.0013 μmol/L) for the angiotensin II receptor. Hydrogen bonding, or ion–dipole binding, of the carbonyl group can mimic the interaction of the primary alcohol of losartan, whereas the spirocyclopentane can provide enhanced hydrophobic binding. Azilsartan medoxomil, candesartan cilexetil, and telmisartan contain benzimidazole rings that provide some enhanced hydrophobic binding, similar to that seen with the spirocyclopentane ring of irbesartan. Azilsartan medoxomil, candesartan cilexetil, and olmesartan medoxomil are prodrugs that are rapidly and completely hydrolyzed during absorption from the gastrointestinal tract to their active carboxylic acid metabolites, azilsartan, candesartan, and olmesartan, respectively. These carboxylic acids lie in exactly the same locations as the hydroxyl group of losartan, the carboxylic acid of valsartan, and the ketone of irbesartan and can participate in both ionic and dipole interactions.

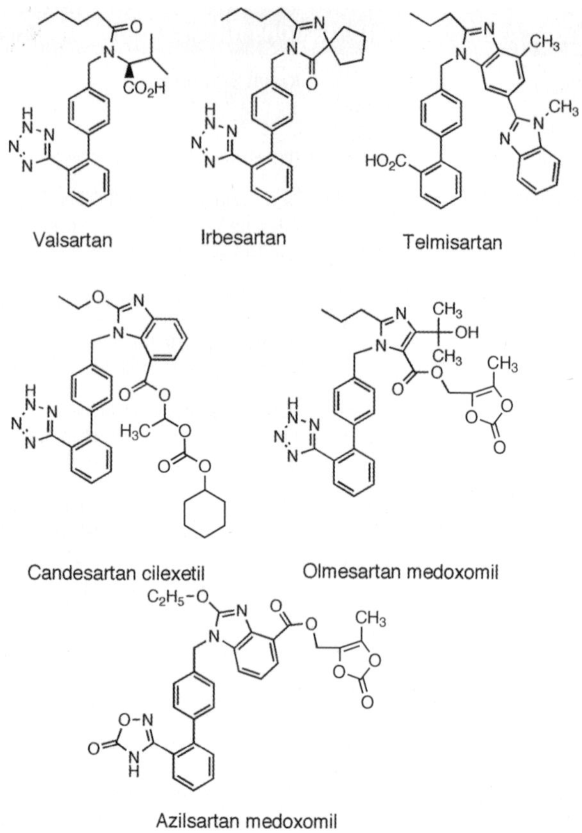

FIGURE 23.16. Structures of losartan analogs. The highlighted portions of candesartan cilexetil and olmesartan medoxomil are hydrolyzed via esterases to produce their respective active, carboxylate metabolites.

Eprosartan was developed using a different hypothesis than that for losartan (Fig. 23.17). Similar to the rationale for losartan, the carboxylic acid of S-8308 was thought to mimic the Phe[8] (i.e., C-terminal) carboxylate of angiotensin II. The benzyl group of S-8308 was proposed to be an important structural feature that mimicked the aromatic side chain of Tyr[4] present in the agonist. Thus, the major structural change was not an extension of the *N*-benzyl group but, rather, an enhancement of the compound's ability to mimic the C-terminal end of angiotensin II. This was accomplished by substituting the 5-acetic acid group with an α-thienylacrylic acid. In addition, a para-carboxylate (a functional group investigated during the development of losartan) also was added. The thienyl ring isosterically mimics the Phe[8] phenyl ring of angiotensin II and, along with the para-carboxylate, is responsible for the excellent potency (IC_{50} = 0.0015 μmol/L) of this compound (36).

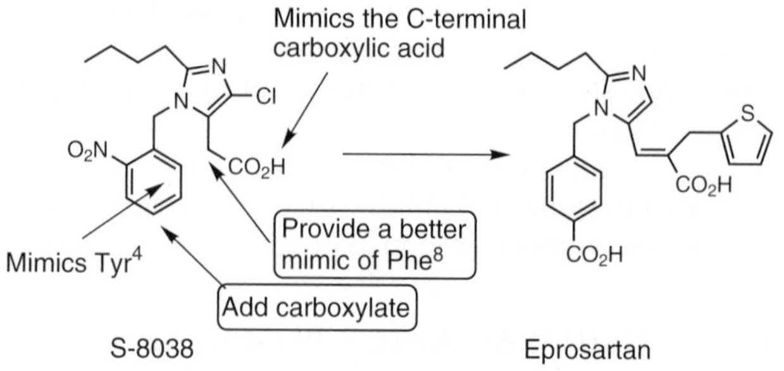

FIGURE 23.17 The development of eprosartan from S-8308. The Phe_8 residue of angiotensin II contains the C-terminal carboxylic acid.

Mechanism of Action

The angiotensin II receptor exists in at least two subtypes: type 1 (AT_1) and type 2 (AT_2). The AT_1 receptors are located in brain, neuronal, vascular, renal, hepatic, adrenal, and myocardial tissues and mediate the cardiovascular, renal, and central nervous system (CNS) effects of angiotensin II. All currently available ARBs are 10,000-fold more selective for the AT_1 receptor subtype and act as competitive antagonists at this site. In terms of relative affinity for the AT_1 receptor, azilsartan, candesartan, and olmesartan have the greatest affinity; irbesartan and eprosartan have a somewhat lower affinity; and telmisartan, valsartan, and losartan have the lowest affinity. All ARBs prevent and reverse all of the known effects of angiotensin II, including rapid and slow pressor responses, stimulatory effects on the peripheral sympathetic nervous system, CNS effects, release of catecholamines, secretion of aldosterone, direct and indirect renal effects, and all growth-promoting effects. The function of the AT_2 receptors is not as well characterized; however, they have been proposed to mediate a variety of growth, development, and differentiation processes. Some concern has arisen that unopposed stimulation of the AT_2 receptor in conjunction with AT_1 receptor antagonism may cause long-term adverse effects. As a result, compounds that exhibit balanced antagonism at both receptor subtypes are currently being sought (1,38).

Structure–Activity Relationships

All commercially available ARBs are analogs of the following general structure:

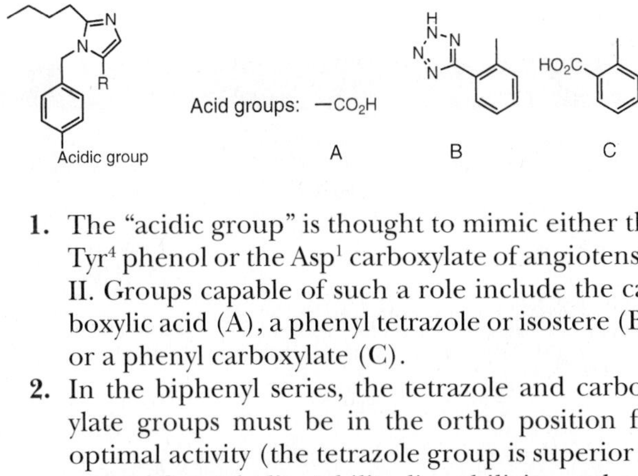

1. The "acidic group" is thought to mimic either the Tyr[4] phenol or the Asp[1] carboxylate of angiotensin II. Groups capable of such a role include the carboxylic acid (A), a phenyl tetrazole or isostere (B), or a phenyl carboxylate (C).
2. In the biphenyl series, the tetrazole and carboxylate groups must be in the ortho position for optimal activity (the tetrazole group is superior in terms of metabolic stability, lipophilicity, and oral bioavailability).
3. The n-butyl group of the model compound provides hydrophobic binding and, most likely, mimics the side chain of Ile[5] of angiotensin II. As seen with azilsartan, candesartan, telmisartan, and olmesartan, this n-butyl group can be replaced with either an ethyl ether or an n-propyl group.
4. The imidazole ring or an isosteric equivalent is required to mimic the His[6] side chain of angiotensin II.
5. Substitution can vary at the "R" position. A variety of R groups, including a carboxylic acid, a hydroxymethyl group, a ketone, or a benzimidazole ring, are present in currently available ARBs and are thought to interact with the AT_1 receptor through either ionic, ion–dipole, or dipole–dipole bonds.

Physicochemical Properties

All ARBs are acidic drugs. The tetrazole ring found in losartan, valsartan, irbesartan, candesartan, and olmesartan has a pK_a of approximately 6 and will be at least 90% ionized at physiologic pH. The carboxylic acids found on valsartan, candesartan, olmesartan, telmisartan, and eprosartan have pK_a values in the range of 3 to 4 and also will be primarily ionized. Currently, available agents have adequate, but not excellent, lipid solubility. As previously mentioned, the tetrazole group is more lipophilic than a carboxylic acid. Additionally, the four nitrogen atoms present in the tetrazole ring can create a greater charge distribution than that available for a carboxylic acid. These properties have been proposed to be responsible for the enhanced binding and bioavailability of the tetrazole-containing compounds (39). Similar to ACE inhibitors, the stereochemistry of valsartan is consistent with the L-amino acids in the natural agonist.

Metabolism

Approximately 14% of a dose of losartan is oxidized by the isozymes CYP2C9 and CYP3A4 to produce EXP-3174, a noncompetitive AT_1 receptor antagonist that is 10- to 40-fold more potent than losartan (Fig. 23.18). The overall cardiovascular effects seen with losartan result from the combined actions of the parent drug and the active metabolite; thus, losartan should not be considered to be a prodrug (1). As previously mentioned, azilsartan medoxomil, candesartan cilexetil, and olmesartan medoxomil are rapidly and completely hydrolyzed to azilsartan, candesartan, and olmesartan, respectively, in the intestinal wall.

None of the other compounds are converted to active metabolites. All of these compounds are primarily (80%) excreted unchanged. Approximately 20% of valsartan is metabolized to inactive compounds via mechanisms that do not appear to involve the CYP450 system. The primary circulating metabolites for irbesartan, telmisartan

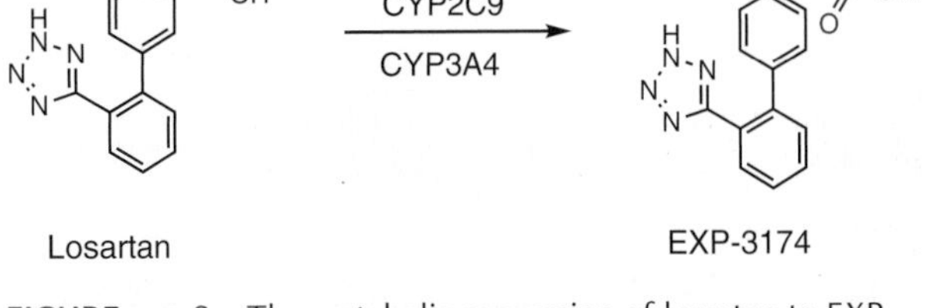

FIGURE 23.18 The metabolic conversion of losartan to EXP-3174 by cytochrome P450 isozymes.

and eprosartan, are inactive glucuronide conjugates. A small amount of irbesartan is oxidized by CYP2CP; however, irbesartan does not substantially induce or inhibit the CYP450 enzymes normally involved in drug metabolism (1,27–29,64). Azilsartan is primarily metabolized by CYP2C9 to an inactive O-dealkyated metabolite.

Pharmacokinetic Parameters

The pharmacokinetic parameters and dosing information for angiotensin receptor antagonists are summarized in Tables 23.6 and 23.7, respectively (27–29,64). With the exception of azilsartan medoxomil (60%), irbesartan (60% to 80%) and, possibly, telmisartan (42% to 58%), all of the compounds have low, but adequate, oral bioavailability (15% to 33%). Given the fact that most of the compounds are excreted unchanged, the most probable reasons for the low bioavailability are poor lipid solubility and incomplete absorption. The effect of food on the absorption of losartan, eprosartan, valsartan, and eprosartan is to reduce absorption; however, this effect has been deemed to be clinically insignificant; thus, the compounds can be taken either with or without food. All of the compounds have similar onsets, are highly protein bound, have elimination half-lives that allow once- or twice-daily dosing, and with the exception of olmesartan, are primarily eliminated via the fecal route. Candesartan and telmisartan appear to require a slightly longer time to reach peak plasma concentrations. As with ACE inhibitors, literature designation of fecal elimination is unclear regarding whether it includes unabsorbed drug.

Azilsartan medoxomil, candesartan cilexetil, losartan, and olmesartan medoxomil differ from the other compounds in several respects. They are the only compounds with active metabolites, and they have the highest renal elimination of all of the agents. Product labeling indicates that renal impairment does not require a dosage reduction for losartan, but area under the curve values are increased by 50% in patients with a creatinine clearance of less than 30 mL/min and are doubled in hemodialysis patients. These increases are not seen for the other agents. Losartan and telmisartan are the only two agents that require initial dose reductions in patients with hepatic impairment. Because of significantly increased plasma concentration, patients with impaired hepatic function or biliary obstructive disorders should avoid the use of telmisartan.

Therapeutic Applications

All ARBs are currently approved for the treatment of hypertension and, along with ACE inhibitors, diuretics, β-blockers, and calcium channel blockers, have been designated as first-line agents either alone or in combination with other antihypertensive agents (32). A number of other indications have also been approved. Irbesartan and losartan have been approved for the treatment of nephropathy in type 2 diabetes. Losartan has been approved for stroke prevention in hypertensive patients with left ventricular hypertrophy. Candesartan and valsartan have been approved for the treatment of heart failure. Telmisartan has been approved to reduce the risk of MI and stroke, while valsartan has been approved to reduce cardiovascular mortality in clinically stable patients with left ventricular failure or left ventricular dysfunction following MI. Based on their ability to attenuate the renin-angiotensin system, one should expect a gradual increase in the number of uses and approved indications for this class of agents.

TABLE 23.6 Pharmacokinetic Parameters of Angiotensin II Receptor Blockers

Drug	Oral Bioavailability (%)	Active Metabolite	Protein Binding (%)	Time to Peak Plasma Concentration (hours)	Elimination Half-Life (hours)	Major Route(s) of Elimination
Azilsartan Medoxomil	60	Azilsartan	99	1.5–3.0	11	Fecal (55%) Renal (42%)
Candesartan Cilexetil	15	Candesartan	99	3–4	9	Fecal (67%) Renal (33%)
Eprosartan	15	None	98	1–2	5–9	Fecal (90%) Renal (10%)
Irbesartan	60–80	None	90	1.5–2.0	11–15	Fecal (80%) Renal (20%)
Losartan	33	EXP-3174	98.7 (losartan) 99.8 (EXP-3174)	1 (losartan) 3–4 (EXP-3174)	1.5–2.0 (losartan) 6–9 (EXP-3174)	Fecal (60%) Renal (35%)
Olmesartan Medoxomil	26	Olmesartan	99	1.5–3.0	10–15	Fecal (35%–50%) Renal (50%–65%)
Telmisartan	42–58	None	100	5	24	Fecal (97%)
Valsartan	25	None	95	2–4	6	Fecal (83%) Renal (13%)

TABLE 23.7 Dose Information for Angiotensin II Receptor Blockers

Generic Name	Trade Name(s)	Approved Indications	Dosing Range (Treatment of Hypertension)	Maximum Daily Dose	Initial Dose Reduction with Hepatic Dysfunction	Dose Reduction with Renal Dysfunction	Available Tablet Strengths (mg)
Azilsartan Medoxomil	Edarbi	Hypertension	40–80 mg once daily	80 mg	No	No	40, 80
Candesartan Cilexetil	Atacand	Hypertension, heart failure	8–32 mg once daily	32 mg	No	Only with severe impairment	4, 8, 16, 32
Eprosartan	Teveten	Hypertension	400–800 mg once daily or b.i.d.	900 mg	No	Decrease maximum daily dose to 600 mg	400, 600
Irbesartan	Avapro	Hypertension, nephropathy in type 2 diabetics	150–300 mg once daily	300 mg	No	No	75, 150, 300
Losartan	Cozaar	Hypertension, nephropathy in type 2 diabetics, hypertension, stroke prevention in hypertensive patients with left ventricular hypertrophy	25–100 mg once daily or b.i.d.	100 mg	Yes (reduce to 25 mg once daily)	Adults, no Children, yes	25, 50, 100
Olmesartan Medoxomil	Benicar	Hypertension	20–40 mg once daily	40 mg	No	No	5, 20, 40
Telmisartan	Micardis	Hypertension, cardiovascular risk reduction of MI and stroke	40–80 mg once daily	80 mg	Yes (reduce to 20 mg once daily)	No	20, 40, 80
Valsartan	Diovan	Hypertension, heart failure, post-MI in patients with left ventricular failure or dysfunction	80–320 once daily	320 mg	No	No	40, 80, 160, 320

b.i.d., twice a day; MI, myocardial infarction.

Adverse Effects

The most prevalent side effects of ARBs are listed below (1,27–29). Overall, this class of agents is well tolerated, with CNS effects being the most commonly reported complaint. Similar to ACE inhibitors, some of the adverse effects are directly related to attenuation of the renin-angiotensin pathway. Notably absent are the dry cough and angioedema seen with ACE inhibitors. Because ARBs are specific in their actions, this class of drugs does not affect the levels of bradykinin or prostaglandins and, thus, does not cause these bothersome side effects. Like ACE inhibitors, the use of ARBs during pregnancy is contraindicated, especially during the second and third trimesters. The use of ARBs should be discontinued as soon as pregnancy is confirmed unless the benefits outweigh the potential risks.

COMBINATION PRODUCTS THAT INCLUDE AN ARB

ARB/Diuretic: candesartan/hydrochlorothiazide, eprosartan/hydrochlorothiazide, irbesartan/hydrochlorothiazide, losartan/hydrochlorothiazide, olmesartan/hydrochlorothiazide, telmisartan/hydrochlorothiazide, valsartan/hydrochlorothiazide

ARB/Calcium Channel Blocker: olmesartan/amlodipine, telmisartan/amlodipine, valsartan/amlodipine

ARB/Diuretic/Calcium Channel Blocker: olmesartan/hydrochlorothiazide/amlodipine, valsartan/hydrochlorothiazide/amlodipine

ARB/Renin Inhibitor: valsartan/aliskiren

Drug Interactions

Coadministration of ARBs with potassium salts, potassium-sparing diuretics, or drospirenone may cause

ADVERSE EFFECTS OF ANGIOTENSIN II RECEPTOR ANTAGONISTS

Headache, dizziness, fatigue, hypotension, hyperkalemia, dyspepsia, diarrhea, abdominal pain, upper respiratory tract infection, myalgia, back pain, pharyngitis, and rhinitis

hyperkalemia. Nonsteroidal anti-inflammatory drugs may alter the response to ARBs and other antihypertensive agents (including ACE inhibitors and calcium channel blockers) because of inhibition of vasodilatory prostaglandins. Studies have shown that indomethacin, naproxen, and piroxicam have a greater propensity for causing this interaction. Telmisartan has been reported to increase digoxin levels and to slightly decrease warfarin levels; however, the reduced warfarin levels were not sufficient to alter the international normalized ratio. Rifampin, because of its ability to induce CYP3A4, can decrease the plasma levels of losartan and its active metabolite, EXP-3174. The clinical significance of drug interactions between ARBs and compounds that can inhibit either CYP3A4 or CYP2C9 has yet to be established.

ALISKIREN, AN ORALLY ACTIVE RENIN INHIBITOR

Historical Overview

In 1957, Skeggs et al. (40) reported the activities of a purified amino acid sequence that could function as a renin substrate and proposed that the inhibition of renin would be beneficial in the treatment of hypertension. As previously mentioned in this chapter, renin is a very specific enzyme that recognizes the Pro^{7}-Phe^{8}-His^{9}- Leu^{10}-Val^{11}-Ile^{12}-His^{13}-Asn^{14} octapeptide sequence of angiotensinogen. Initial attempts to design renin inhibitors focused upon peptide analogs designed to mimic portions or all of this sequence. Many of these analogs, exemplified by compound A in Figure 23.19, showed effective inhibition of renin; however, susceptibility to proteolytic cleavage, poor or absent oral bioavailability, and short durations of action limited the therapeutic utility of these peptidic agents. Sequential structural modifications produced peptide-based compounds with the ability to mimic the transition state of angiotensinogen cleavage. Compounds such as zankiren (Fig. 23.19) possessed improved potency, favorable lipid solubility, and better oral bioavailability as compared to their predecessors. Unfortunately, the cost of synthetic preparation coupled with the success of newly approved ARBs temporarily curtailed commercial interest in this area. Success was finally obtained when the peptide backbone was abandoned and replaced with a nonpeptidic template. This template was used in the development of aliskiren (Fig 23.19), the first nonpeptide, low molecular weight, orally active, transition-state renin inhibitor (41–43).

Mechanism of Action

Aliskiren directly inhibits renin, thereby preventing the formation of angiotensin I and angiotensin II. As previously mentioned, this is the rate-limiting step in this pathway and is highly regulated by hemodynamic, neurogenic, and humoral signals. Studies have shown that there are two potential advantages of inhibiting this enzyme as compared to inhibiting ACE or using an ARB (41,44). Inhibition of the renin-angiotensin pathway through any of these mechanisms has been shown to cause a compensatory increase in renin concentrations; however, unlike ACE inhibitors and ARBs, the ability of renin inhibitors to directly bind to the enzyme blocks the increases in plasma renin activity seen with ACE inhibitors and ARBs. Additionally, alternate pathways, such as the chymostatin-sensitive pathway present in the heart, can convert angiotensin I to angiotensin II. While this alternate pathway could affect the efficacy of ACE inhibitors, it would not alter the effects of direct renin inhibition.

Physicochemical Properties

Aliskiren is a basic compound and is marketed as a hemifumarate salt. The calculated logP value for the unionized form of aliskiren is 4.32 (21); however, its salt form is highly water soluble. Aliskiren contains four chiral centers and is marketed as the pure 2S, 4S, 5S, 7S enantiomer (29).

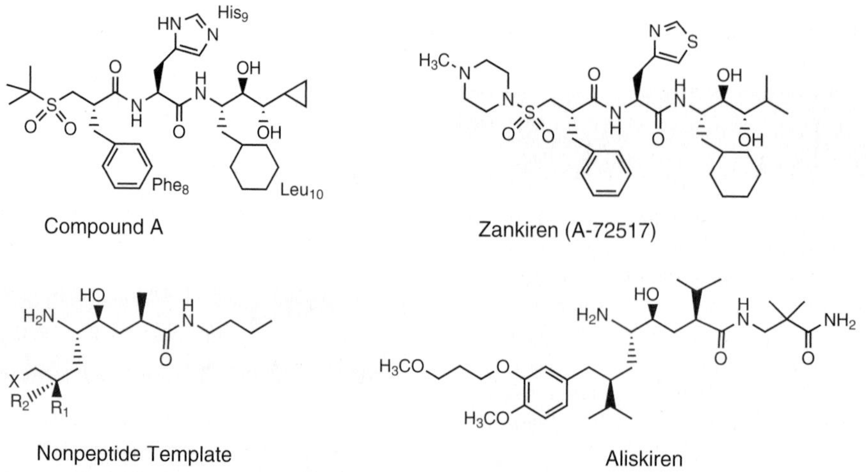

FIGURE 23.19 Aliskiren and predecessor compounds.

Metabolism

Approximately 90% of aliskiren is eliminated unchanged in the feces. Due to its poor bioavailability, the extent of systemic metabolism is unclear; however, clearance through the hepatobiliary tract appears to be the primary route of elimination. While metabolism is a minor pathway, the two major metabolites of aliskiren are an *O*-demethylated alcohol derivative and a carboxylic acid derivative. The primary metabolizing enzyme is CYP3A4. Aliskiren has not been shown to either inhibit or induce any of the CYP450 isoenzymes (27–29).

Pharmacokinetic Parameters

Aliskiren is a poorly absorbed and has a bioavailability of approximately 2.5%. Following oral administration, peak plasma concentrations are reached within 1 to 3 hours, and steady-state blood concentration is reached within 7 to 8 days.

The normal, initial dose of aliskiren is 150 mg once daily. This may be increased to 300 mg once daily in patients whose blood pressure is not adequately controlled. The antihypertensive effects are usually attained within 2 weeks. High-fat meals have been shown to significantly decrease absorption, and patients are encouraged to establish a fixed/routine time to take aliskiren. No adjustment in dose is required for elderly patients or those with renal impairment or hepatic insufficiency. Caution, however, should be used in dosing patients with severe renal impairment (27,28,44).

Therapeutic Applications

Aliskiren is approved for the treatment of hypertension, either as monotherapy or in combination with other antihypertensive agents. Aliskiren is available alone or in combination with hydrochlorothiazide (a diuretic), amlodipine (a calcium channel blocker), or valsartan (an ARB) (27).

Adverse Effects

Similar to ARBs, aliskiren does not affect the levels of bradykinin and prostaglandins and does not cause the dry cough or angioedema seen with ACE inhibitors. Pregnancy warnings are identical to those mentioned for ACE inhibitors and ARBs. Additionally and similar to ACE inhibitors and ARBs, aliskiren can cause hyperkalemia due to its ability to indirectly decrease aldosterone release. The most common adverse effects are mild and include diarrhea, abdominal pain, dyspepsia, gastroesophageal reflux, and rash (28,44).

Drug Interactions

Coadministration of aliskiren with irbesartan has been shown to decrease both the plasma levels and the efficacy of aliskiren. If these are used in combination, an adjustment of aliskiren may be required. Potent P-glycoprotein inhibitors, such as atorvastatin, cyclosporine, and ketoconazole, may increase the plasma levels of aliskiren. Coadministration of aliskiren and cyclosporine is not recommended. Aliskiren has been shown to decrease the area under the curve and maximum plasma concentration of furosemide (28,44).

ROLE OF CALCIUM AND CALCIUM CHANNELS IN VASCULAR SMOOTH MUSCLE CONTRACTION

Calcium is a key component of the excitation-contraction coupling process that occurs within the cardiovascular system. It acts as a cellular messenger to link internal or external excitation with cellular response. Increased cytosolic concentrations of Ca^{2+} result in the binding of Ca^{2+} to a regulatory protein, either troponin C in cardiac and skeletal muscle or calmodulin in vascular smooth muscle. This initial binding of Ca^{2+} uncovers myosin binding sites on the actin molecule, and subsequent interactions between actin and myosin result in muscle contraction. All of these events are reversed once the cytosolic concentration of Ca^{2+} decreases. In this situation, Ca^{2+} binding to troponin C or calmodulin is diminished or removed, myosin binding sites are concealed, actin and myosin can no longer interact, and muscle contraction ceases (45,46).

Mechanisms of Calcium Movement and Storage

The regulation of cytosolic calcium levels occurs via specific influx, efflux, and sequestering mechanisms (Fig. 23.20). The influx of calcium can occur through receptor-operated channels (site 1), the Na^+/Ca^{2+} exchange process (site 2), "leak" pathways (site 3), and potential-dependent channels (site 4). Influx via either receptor-operated or voltage-dependent channels has

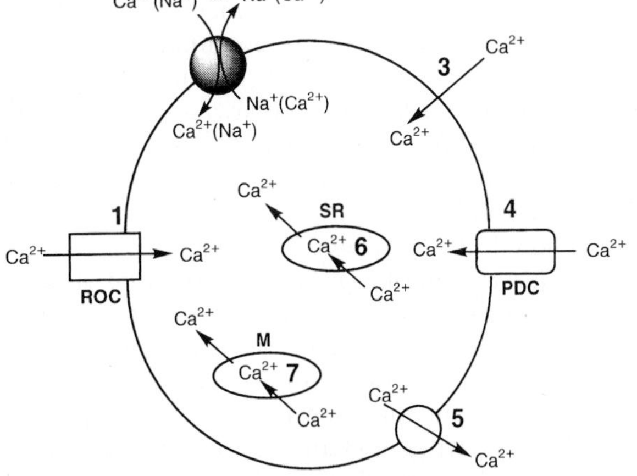

FIGURE 23.20 Cellular mechanisms for the influx, efflux, and sequestering of Ca^{2+}. M, mitochondria; PDC, potential-dependent Ca^{2+} channels; ROC, receptor-operated Ca^{2+} channels; SR, sarcoplasmic reticulum.

been proposed to be the major entry pathway for Ca^{2+}. Receptor-operated channels have been defined as those associated with cellular membrane receptors and activated by specific agonist–receptor interactions. In contrast, potential-dependent channels, also known as voltage-dependent or voltage-gated calcium channels, have been defined as those activated by membrane depolarization. The Na^+/Ca^{2+} exchange process can promote either influx or efflux, because the direction of Ca^{2+} movement depends on the relative intracellular and extracellular ratios of Na^+ and Ca^{2+}. The "leak" pathways, which include unstimulated Ca^{2+} entry as well as entry during the fast inward Na^+ phase of an action potential, play only a minor role in calcium influx.

Efflux can occur through either an adenosine triphosphate–driven membrane pump (site 5) or via the Na^+/Ca^{2+} exchange process previously mentioned (site 2). In addition to these influx and efflux mechanisms, the sarcoplasmic reticulum (site 6) and the mitochondria (site 7) function as internal storage/release sites. These storage sites work in concert with the influx and efflux processes to assure that cytosolic calcium levels are appropriate for cellular needs. Although influx and release processes are essential for excitation–contraction coupling, efflux and sequestering processes are equally important for terminating the contractile process and for protecting the cell from the deleterious effects of Ca^{2+} overload (47,48).

Potential-Dependent Calcium Channels

The pharmacologic class of agents known as calcium channel blockers produces their effects through interaction with potential-dependent channels. To date, six functional subclasses, or types, of potential-dependent Ca^{2+} channels have been identified: T, L, N, P, Q, and R. These types differ in location and function and can be divided into two major groups: low-voltage activated (LVA) channels and high-voltage activated (HVA) channels. Of the six types, only the T (transient, tiny) channel can be rapidly activated and inactivated with small changes in the cell membrane potential. It is thus designated as an LVA channel. All of the other types of channels require a larger depolarization and are thus designated as HVA channels. The L (long-lasting, large) channel is the site of action for currently available calcium channel blockers and, therefore, has been extensively studied. It is located in skeletal, cardiac, and smooth muscle and, thus, is highly involved in organ and vessel contraction within the cardiovascular system. The N channel is found in neuronal tissue and exhibits kinetics and inhibitory sensitivity distinct from both L and T channels. The functions, sensitivities, and properties of the other three types of channels are not as well known. The P channel has been named for its presence in the Purkinje cells, whereas the Q and R channels have been characterized by their abilities to bind to certain polypeptide toxins (49–51).

The L channel is a pentameric complex consisting of α_1, α_2, β, γ, and δ polypeptides (Fig. 23.21). The α_1 subunit is a transmembrane-spanning protein that consists of four domains and that functions as the pore-forming subunit. The α_1 subunit also contains binding sites for all the currently available calcium channel blockers. The other four subunits surround the α_1 portion of the channel and contribute to the overall hydrophobicity of the pentamer. This hydrophobicity is important in that it allows the channel to be embedded in the cell membrane. Additionally, the α_2, δ, and β subunits modulate the α_1 subunit. Other types of potential-dependent channels are similar to the L channel. They all have a central α_1 subunit; however, molecular cloning studies have revealed that there are at least six α_1 genes: α_{1S}, α_{1A}, α_{1B}, α_{1C}, α_{1D}, and α_{1E}. Three of these genes, α_{1S}, α_{1C}, and α_{1D}, have been associated with L channels. The L channels found in skeletal muscle result from the α_{1S} gene; those in the heart, aorta, lung, and fibroblast result from the α_{1C} gene; and those in endocrine tissue result from the α_{1D} gene. Both α_{1C} and α_{1D} are used for L channels in the brain. Thus, there are some differences among the L channels located in different organs and tissues. Additionally, differences in α_1 genes and differences among the other subunits are responsible for the variations seen among the other five types of potential-dependent channels. As an example, the N channel lacks the γ subunit and contains an α_1 subunit derived from the α_{1B} gene (49,51).

CARDIOVASCULAR DISORDERS ASSOCIATED WITH POTENTIAL-DEPENDENT CALCIUM CHANNELS

As described earlier, the movement of calcium underlies the basic excitation–contraction coupling process. Thus, vascular tone and contraction primarily are determined by the availability of calcium from extracellular or intracellular sources. Potential-dependent Ca^{2+} channels are important in regulating the influx of Ca^{2+}; therefore, inhibition of Ca^{2+} flow through these channels results in both vasodilation and decreased cellular response to contractile stimuli. Arterial smooth muscle is more sensitive to this action than venous smooth muscle. Additionally, coronary and cerebral arterial vessels are more sensitive than other arterial beds (48,51). As a result of these actions, calcium channel blockers are useful in the treatment of hypertension and ischemic heart disease. A brief overview of hypertension is provided in the renin-angiotensin section of this chapter.

The term "ischemic heart disease," or coronary heart disease, encompasses a variety of syndromes. These include angina pectoris, silent myocardial ischemia, acute coronary insufficiency, and MI. The overall incidence of coronary heart disease is higher in men than in women

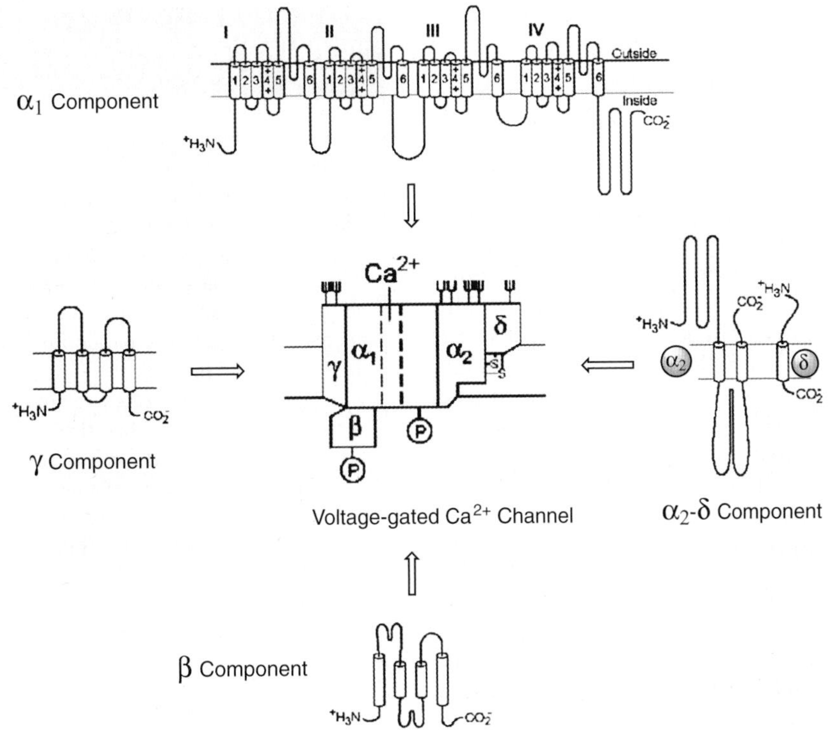

FIGURE 23.21 Representation of the structure of the voltage-gated Ca^{2+} channel (L channel) composed of several subunits—α_1, α_2–δ, β, γ—organized as depicted in the central area.

and increases with age. MI is the primary initial event in men, whereas angina is the most common initial presentation in women. Approximately 1.25 million individuals suffer new or recurrent episodes annually. Statistics published in 2006 from the American Heart Association estimate the prevalence of angina at approximately 10.2 million individuals (52).

Angina pectoris is a clinical manifestation that results from coronary atherosclerotic heart disease. It is characterized by a severe constricting pain in the chest that often radiates to the left shoulder, the left arm, or the back. Clinically, angina pectoris can be classified as either exertional, variant, or unstable. Exertional angina, otherwise known as stable angina or exercise-induced angina, is the most common form and results from an imbalance between myocardial oxygen supply and demand. Variant angina, otherwise known as Prinzmetal angina, results from the vasospasm of large, surface coronary vessels or branches. Unstable angina is the most difficult to treat and may occur as a result of advanced atherosclerosis and coronary vasospasm (53).

Excitation–contraction coupling in the heart is different from that in vascular smooth muscle in that a portion of the inward current is carried by Na^+ through the fast channel. In the sinoatrial and atrioventricular (AV) nodes, however, depolarization depends primarily on the movement of Ca^{2+} through the slow channel. Attenuation of this Ca^{2+} movement produces a negative inotropic effect and decreased conduction through the AV node. This latter effect is especially useful in treating paroxysmal supraventricular tachycardia (PSVT), an arrhythmia primarily caused by AV nodal reentry and AV reentry (51).

CALCIUM CHANNEL BLOCKERS

Historical Overview

Identification of compounds that could block the inward movement of Ca^{2+} through slow cardiac channels occurred in the early 1960s. Verapamil and other phenylalkylamines were shown to possess negative inotropic and chronotropic effects that were distinct from other coronary vasodilators. Further investigations revealed that these agents mimicked the cardiac effects of Ca^{2+} withdrawal: They reduced contractile force without affecting the action potential. The effects of these compounds could be reversed by the addition of Ca^{2+}, thus suggesting that the negative inotropic effect was linked to an inhibition of excitation–contraction coupling. Subsequently, derivatives of verapamil, as well as other chemical classes of compounds, were shown to competitively block Ca^{2+} movement through the slow channel and, thus, alter the cardiac action potential. Therefore, calcium channel blockers also are known as slow channel blockers, calcium entry blockers, and calcium antagonists (47,51).

Chemical Classifications

Overview

Currently, 10 calcium channel blockers are available for therapeutic use. These compounds have diverse chemical structures and can be grouped into one of four chemical classifications (Fig. 23.22), each of which produces a distinct pharmacologic profile: 1,4-dihydropyridines (1,4-DHPs; e.g., nifedipine), phenylalkylamines (e.g., verapamil), benzothiazepines (e.g., diltiazem), and diaminopropanol ethers (e.g., bepridil). The majority of calcium channel blockers are 1,4-DHPs, and a detailed description of the SAR for this chemical class is provided below. In contrast, verapamil, diltiazem, and bepridil are the lone representatives of their respective chemical classes and, thus, are discussed as individual agents. Verapamil and diltiazem are discussed along with the 1,4-DHPs. Bepridil is a nonselective agent that is no longer available in the United States.

1,4-Dihydropyridines

History and Development The chemistry of dihydropyridines can be traced back to an 1882 paper in which Hantzsch described their utility as intermediates in the synthesis of substituted pyridines. Fifty years later, interest in this chemical class of compounds increased when it was discovered that a 1,4-DHP ring was responsible for the "hydrogen-transfer" properties of the coenzyme NADH. Numerous biochemical studies followed this discovery; however, it was not until the early 1970s that the pharmacologic properties of 1,4-DHPs were fully investigated. Loev and coworkers at Smith, Klein & French laboratories investigated the activities of "Hantzsch-type" compounds. As shown in Figure 23.23, the Hantzsch reaction produced a symmetrical compound in which both the esters (i.e., CO_2R_2) and the C_2 and C_6 substituents (i.e., CH_3) are identical with each other. Structural requirements necessary for activity were identified by sequentially modifying the C_4 substituent (i.e., the R_1 group), the C_3- and C_5-esters (i.e., the R_2 groups), the C_2- and C_6-alkyl groups, and the N_1-H substituent (54–57).

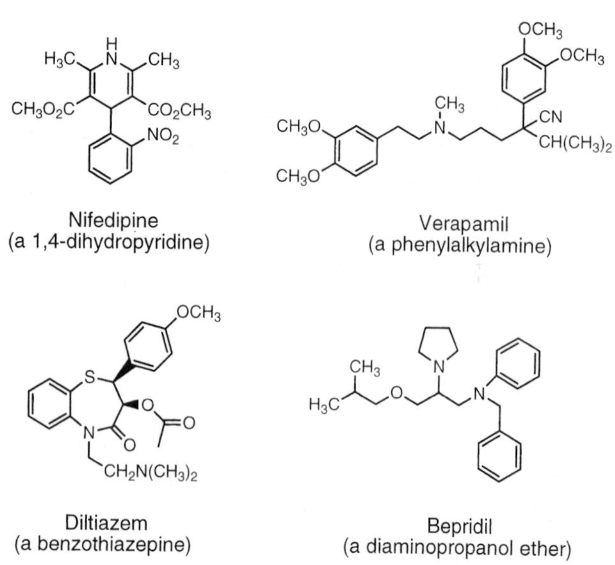

FIGURE 23.22 Chemical classes of calcium channel blockers.

> **BEPRIDIL**
>
> Bepridil is unique among all the calcium channel blockers in that its actions are not based solely on its ability to block potential-dependent L-type (i.e., slow) Ca^{2+} channels (27,51). Unlike other calcium channel blockers, bepridil also blocks fast Na^+ channels as well as receptor-operated calcium channels. These additional actions are responsible for bepridil's ability to inhibit cardiac conduction, to slow AV nodal conduction, to increase the refractory period, to slow the heart rate, and to prolong the QT interval.
>
> Bepridil was indicated for the oral treatment of chronic stable angina pectoris; however, its manufacturer voluntarily removed it from the US market, primarily because of its ability to cause torsades de pointes. It also should be noted that bepridil was never highly prescribed, most likely because of the significant number of cardiovascular warnings and contraindications associated with its use.

Structure–Activity Relationships The SARs for 1,4-DHP derivatives (see *General Structure* in Table 23.8) indicate that the following structural features are important for activity:

1. A substituted phenyl ring at the C_4 position optimizes activity (heteroaromatic rings, such as pyridine, produce similar therapeutic effects but are not used because of observed animal toxicity), and C_4 substitution with a small nonplanar alkyl or cycloalkyl group decreases activity.
2. Phenyl ring substitution (X) is important for size and position rather than for electronic nature. Compounds with ortho or meta substitutions possess optimal activity, whereas those that are unsubstituted or that contain a para substitution show a significant decrease in activity. Despite the fact that all commercially available 1,4-DHPs have electron-withdrawing ortho and/or meta substituents, this

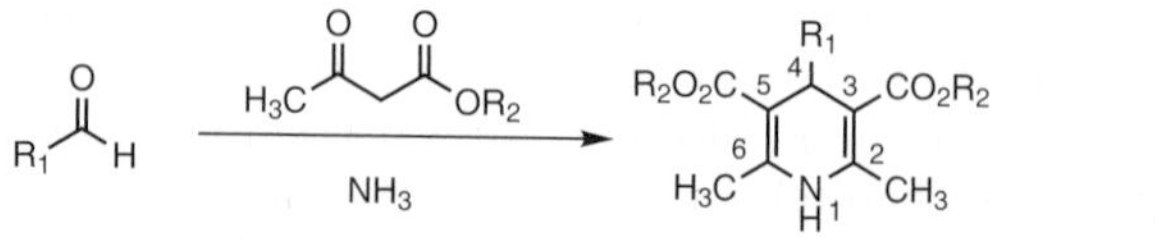

FIGURE 23.23 Synthesis of 1,4-DHPs using the Hantzsch reaction.

TABLE 23.8 Structure of the Dihydropyridine Ca^{2+} Channel Blockers

General structure:

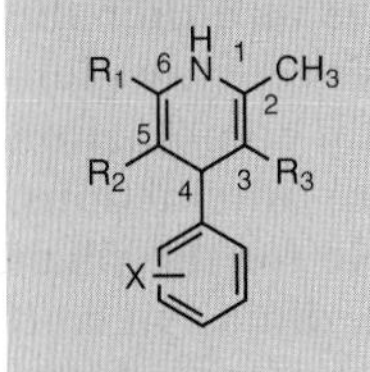

Isradipine:

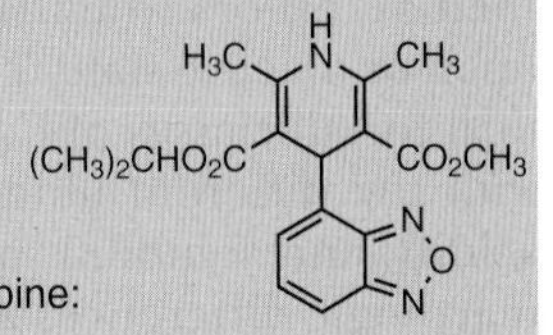

Compounds	R_1	R_2	R_3	X
Amlodipine	$CH_2O(CH_2)_2NH_2$	$CO_2CH_2CH_3$	CO_2CH_3	2-Cl
Clevidipine	CH_3	$CO_2CH_2O\text{-}C(=O)\text{-}nC_3H_7$	CO_2CH_3	2,3-Cl_2
Felodipine	CH_3	$CO_2CH_2CH_3$	CO_2CH_3	2,3-Cl_2
Nicardipine	CH_3	$CO_2(CH_2)_2\text{-}N(CH_3)\text{-}H_2C\text{-}C_6H_5$	CO_2CH_3	3-NO_2
Nifedipine	CH_3	CO_2CH_3	CO_2CH_3	2-NO_2
Nimodipine	CH_3	$CO_2CH_2CH_2OCH_3$	$CO_2CH(CH_3)CH_3$	3-NO_2
Nisoldipine	CH_3	$CO_2CH_2CH(CH_3)_2$	CO_2CH_3	2-NO_2

is not an absolute requirement. Compounds with electron-donating groups at these same positions also have demonstrated good activity. The importance of the ortho and meta substituents is to provide sufficient bulk to "lock" the conformation of the 1,4-DHP such that the C_4 aromatic ring is perpendicular to the 1,4-DHP ring (Fig. 23.24). This perpendicular conformation has been proposed to be essential for the activity of the 1,4-DHPs.

3. The 1,4-DHP ring is essential for activity. Substitution at the N_1 position or the use of oxidized (piperidine) or reduced (pyridine) ring systems greatly decreases or abolishes activity.
4. Ester groups at the C_3 and C_5 positions optimize activity. Other electron-withdrawing groups show decreased antagonist activity and may even show agonist activity. For example, the replacement of the C_3 ester of isradipine with a NO_2 group produces a calcium channel activator, or agonist (Fig. 23.25). Thus, the term "calcium channel modulators" is a more appropriate classification for the 1,4-DHPs.
5. When the esters at C_3 and C_5 are nonidentical, the C_4 carbon becomes chiral, and stereoselectivity between the enantiomers is observed. Additionally, evidence suggests that the C_3 and C_5 positions of the dihydropyridine ring are not equivalent positions. Crystal structures of nifedipine, a symmetrical 1,4-DHP, have shown that the C_3 carbonyl is synplanar to the C_2-C_3 bond but that the C_5 carbonyl is antiperiplanar to the C_5-C_6 bond (Fig. 23.26). Asymmetrical compounds have shown enhanced selectivity for specific blood vessels and are being preferentially developed. Nifedipine, the first 1,4-DHP to be marketed, is the only symmetrical compound in this chemical class.
6. With the exception of amlodipine, all 1,4-DHPs have C_2 and C_6 methyl groups. The enhanced

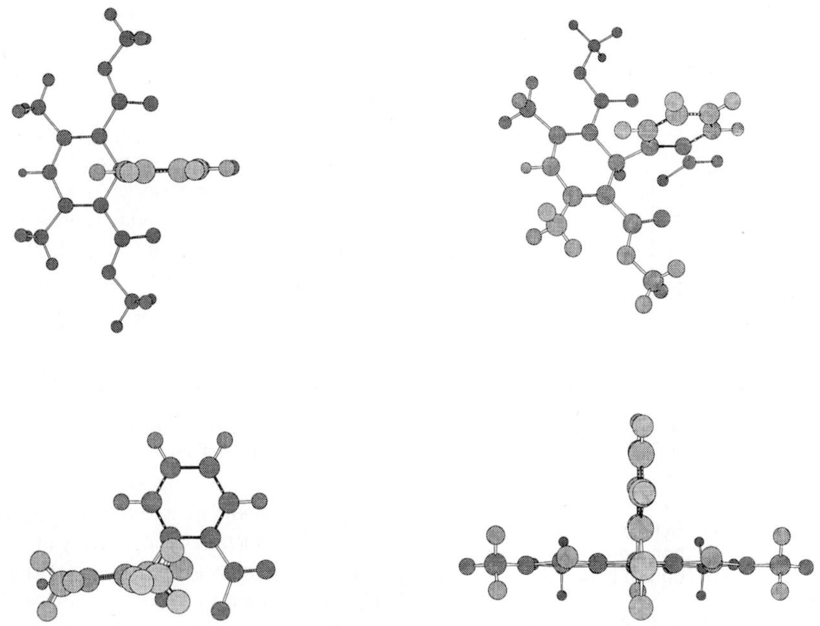

FIGURE 23.24 Molecular models of nifedipine. The ortho-nitro group of nifedipine provides steric bulk and ensures that the required perpendicular nature of the phenyl and dihydropyridine rings is maintained.

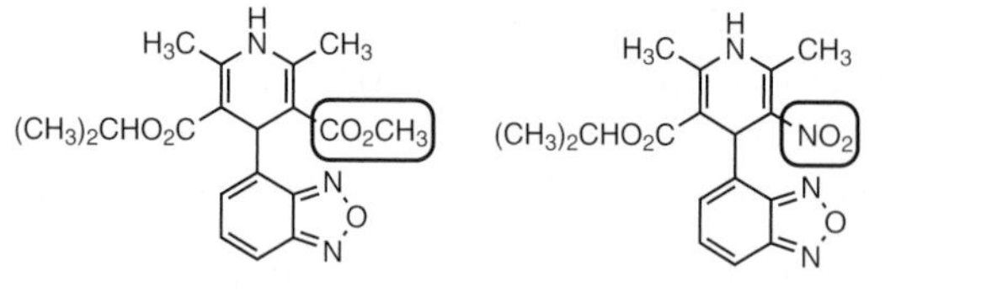

Isradipine (Calcium channel blocker) PN 202.791 (Calcium channel activator)

FIGURE 23.25 Structures of isradipine and its analogous 3-nitro derivative.

potency of amlodipine (vs. nifedipine) suggests that the 1,4-DHP receptor can tolerate larger substituents at this position and that enhanced activity can be obtained by altering these groups.

Mechanism of Action

Despite the name, calcium channel blockers do not simply "plug the hole" and physically block the Ca^{2+} channel. Instead, they exert their effects by binding to specific receptor sites located within the central α_1 subunit of L-type, potential-dependent channels. Three distinct, but allosterically interacting, receptors have been identified for verapamil, diltiazem, and the 1,4-DHPs. As shown in Table 23.9, the binding of verapamil to its receptor inhibits the binding of both diltiazem and the 1,4-DHPs to their respective receptors. Likewise, the binding of either diltiazem or the 1,4-DHPs inhibits the binding of verapamil. In contrast, diltiazem and the 1,4-DHPs mutually enhance the binding of each other (54).

Potential-dependent channels can exist in one of three conformations: a resting state, which can be stimulated by membrane depolarization; an open state, which allows the Ca^{2+} to enter; and an inactive state, which is refractory to further depolarization. Calcium channel blockers have been shown to be more effective when membrane depolarization is either longer, more intense, or more frequent. This use dependency suggests that these compounds preferentially interact with their receptors when the Ca^{2+} channel is in either the open or inactive state. This state dependence is not identical for all classes of Ca^{2+} blockers and, in combination with the different binding sites, allosteric interactions, acidity, and solubility, may be responsible for the pharmacologic differences among verapamil, diltiazem, and the 1,4-DHPs. A summary of these differences is listed in Table 23.10. The 1,4-DHPs are primarily vasodilators,

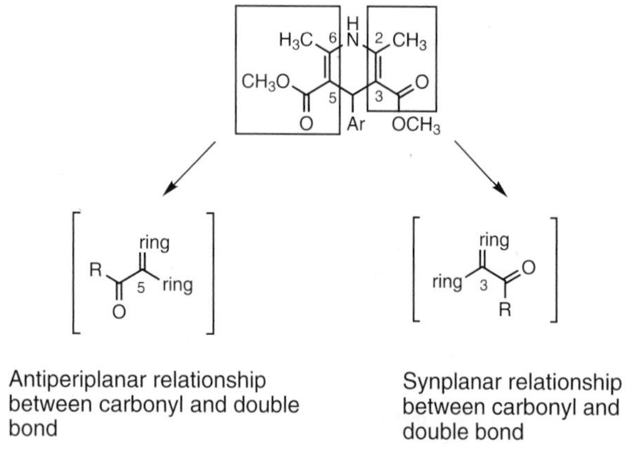

FIGURE 23.26 Conformation of the C_3 and C_5 esters of nifedipine (Ar = 2-nitrophenyl). The C_3 carbonyl is synplanar to the C_2-C_3 bond, and the C_5 carbonyl antiperiplanar to the C_5-C_6 bond.

ZICONOTIDE: AN N-TYPE CALCIUM CHANNEL BLOCKER

Ziconotide (Prialt) is a synthetic analog of a naturally occurring conopeptide found in the piscivorous marine snail (*Conus magus*). It is structurally, mechanistically, and therapeutically different from the other calcium channel blockers discussed in this chapter. Structurally, it is a polybasic peptide containing 25 amino acids and three disulfide bridges.

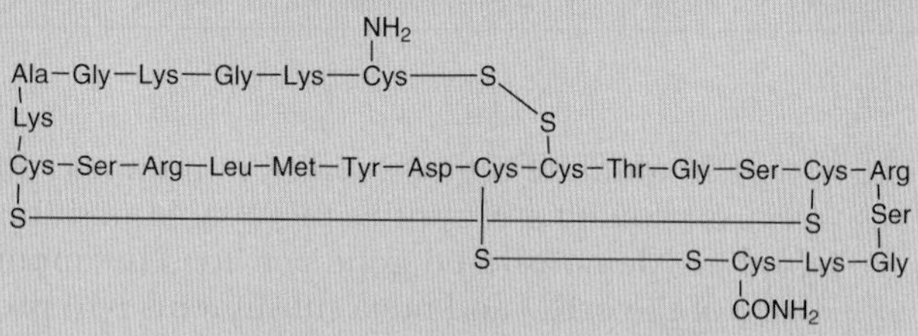

It selectively binds to N-type potential-dependent calcium channels located on the primary nociceptive (A-d and C) afferent nerves in the superficial layers (Rexed laminae I and II) of the dorsal horn in the spinal cord. Analgesic effects result from a blockade of neurotransmitter release and a disruption of normal nociceptive signal transmission. Ziconotide is indicated for the management of severe chronic pain in patients who are intolerant of or refractory to other systemic analgesics, adjunct therapies, or intrathecal morphine. Because of its peptide structure, ziconotide is not effective orally. It is administered by continuous intrathecal infusion. The initial recommended dose is 2.4 μg/day (0.1 μg/hour) and can be titrated up to a maximum daily dose of 19.2 mg (0.8 μg/hour). Ziconotide has a half-life of approximately 4.5 hours. It is metabolized by endopeptidases and exopeptidases in numerous organs and tissues. Common adverse effects of ziconotide include dizziness, nausea, confusion, headache, somnolence, nystagmus, asthenia, and pain. The most serious adverse effects appear to be the development of severe psychiatric symptoms and neurologic impairment. As a result, ziconotide should not be used in patients with a preexisting history of psychosis. Frequent monitoring for evidence of cognitive impairment, hallucinations, or changes in mood or consciousness is essential. These effects are potentially additive with those of other CNS-depressant drugs (27,28,58).

TABLE 23.9 Actions of Calcium Channel Blockers and Interactions among Their Receptor Sites

Calcium Channel Blocker	Effect on Ca^{2+} Channel	Allosteric Effect on the Binding of:		
		Verapamil	Diltiazem	1,4-Dihydropyridines
Verapamil	Antagonist; blocks channel	NA	Inhibits	Inhibits
Diltiazem	Antagonist; blocks channel	Inhibits	NA	Enhances
1,4-Dihydropyridines	Antagonist/agonist; can either block or open channel	Inhibits	Enhances	NA

NA, not applicable.

whereas verapamil and diltiazem have both vasodilator and cardiodepressant actions. The increased heart rate seen with the 1,4-DHPs results from a reflex mechanism that tries to overcome the vasodilation and subsequent drop in blood pressure caused by these drugs. In contrast, the compensatory mechanism does not occur to the same extent with either verapamil or diltiazem. This difference is the result of the ability of verapamil and diltiazem to block AV nodal conductance and the increased ability of 1,4-DHPs to activate the baroreceptor reflex. Ultimately, these pharmacologic differences are reflected in the clinical use of these agents (48,53,54).

Physicochemical Properties

A comparison of the acid-base properties of verapamil, diltiazem, and the 1,4-DHPs reveals that whereas all of the compounds are basic, the 1,4-DHPs are considerably less basic than verapamil and diltiazem. Verapamil and diltiazem both contain tertiary amines with pK_a values of 8.9 and 7.7, respectively (21). In contrast, the nitrogen of the 1,4-DHPs is part of a conjugated carbamate. Its electrons are involved in resonance delocalization and are much less available for protonation. Thus, at physiologic pH, verapamil and diltiazem are primarily ionized, whereas 1,4-DHPs are primarily un-ionized. There are two exceptions to this. Amlodipine and nicardipine contain basic amine groups as part of the side chains connected to the 1,4-DHP ring. Although the 1,4-DHP ring of these compounds is un-ionized, the side-chain amines will be primarily ionized at physiologic pH. Because ionic attraction often is the initial interaction between a drug and its receptor, the differences in basicity between the 1,4-DHP ring and the tertiary amines of verapamil and diltiazem are consistent with the previously noted fact that the binding site for the 1,4-DHPs is distinct from those for verapamil and diltiazem.

TABLE 23.10 Similarities and Differences among 1,4-Dihydropyridines (DHPs), Verapamil, and Diltiazem

Cardiovascular Effect	1,4-DHPs	Verapamil and Diltiazem
Peripheral vasodilation	Increase	Increase
Blood pressure	Decrease	Decrease
Heart rate	Increase	Decrease or no effect
Atrioventricular node conduction	No effect	Decrease
Contractility	No effect or moderate increase	Decrease

The calculated logP values for the calcium channel blockers are listed in Table 23.11 (21,59). As evidenced by the data, all of these compounds possess good lipid solubility and, hence, excellent oral absorption (not shown in Table 23.11). Within the 1,4-DHP class, enhanced lipid solubility occurs in compounds that contain either larger ester groups or disubstituted phenyl rings. A comparison of the logP values of nifedipine and nisoldipine illustrates this fact. It should be noted that the calculated logP values listed in Table 23.11 are for the un-ionized compounds. These values significantly decrease for the ionized forms of amlodipine, nicardipine, verapamil, and diltiazem such that the latter three agents possess sufficient water solubility to be used both orally and parenterally.

All calcium channel blockers, with the exception of nifedipine, contain at least one chiral center; however, they are all marketed as their racemic mixtures. As previously noted, 1,4-DHPs with asymmetrically substituted esters exhibit stereoselectivity between the enantiomers. Additionally, the *S*-(−)-enantiomers of verapamil and other phenylalkylamines are more potent than the *R*-(+)-enantiomers. Very few SAR studies are available for diltiazem; however, the *cis* arrangement of the acetyl ester and the substituted phenyl ring is required for activity (54).

Metabolism

With the exception of clevidipine, all calcium channel blockers undergo extensive first-pass metabolism in the

TABLE 23.11 Pharmacokinetic Parameters of Calcium Channel Blockers

Drug	Calculated LogP	Oral Bioavailability (%)	Effect of Food on Absorption	Active Metabolite	Protein Binding (%)	T_{max} (hours)	Elimination Half-Life (hours)	Major Route(s) of Elimination
1,4-Dihydropyridines								
Amlodipine	2.76	64–90	None	None	93–97	6–12	35–50	Renal (60%) Fecal (20%–25%)
Clevidipine	2,96	NA	NA	None	>99	2–4 (min)	0.15	Renal (63%–74%) Fecal (7%–22%)
Felodipine	4.69	10–25	Increase	None	>99	2.5–5.0	11–16	Renal (70%) Fecal (10%)
Isradipine	3.19	15–24	Reduced rate, same extent	None	95	7–18 (CR)	8	Renal (60%–65%) Fecal (25%–30%)
Nicardipine	4.27	35	Reduced	None	>95	0.5–2.0 (IR) 1–4 (SR)	2–4	Renal (60%) Fecal (35%)
Nifedipine	2.40	45–70 86 (SR)	None	None	92–98	0.5 (IR) 6 (SR)	2–5 (IR) 7 (SR)	Renal (60%–80%) Biliary/fecal (15%)
Nimodipine	3.14	13	Reduced	None	>95	1	8–9	Renal
Nisoldipine	3.86	5	High-fat meal increases immediate release but lowers overall amount	Hydroxylated analog	>99	6–12	7–12	Renal (70%–75%) Fecal (6%–12%)
Phenalkylamines								
Verapamil	3.53	20–35	Reduced (SR form only)	Norverapamil	90	1–2 (IR) 7–11 (SR) 0.1–0.2 (IV)	3–7 (IR) 12 (SR)	Renal (70%) Fecal (16%)
Benzothiazepines								
Diltiazem	3.55	40–60	None	Deacetyl-diltiazem	70–80	2–4 (IR) 6–14 (SR)	3.0–4.5 (IR) 4.0–9.5 (SR) 3.4 (IV)	Renal (35%) Fecal (60%–65%)

CR, controlled-release product; IR, immediate-release product; IV, intravenous administration; NA, not applicable; SR, sustained-release product; T_{max}, time to maximum blood concentration.

liver and are substrates for the CYP3A4 isozyme (27,29). Additionally, several of these compounds can inhibit CYP3A4. Clevidipine was designed to have an ultra-short duration of action. Upon IV infusion, clevidipine exerts its antihypertensive actions within 2 to 4 minutes. Rapid ester hydrolysis (Fig. 23.27) inactivates the compound

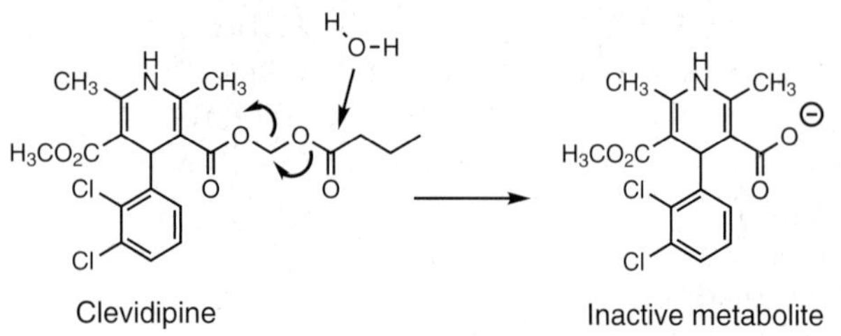

FIGURE 23.27 In vivo metabolitic hydrolysis of clevidipine to an inactive metabolite.

and allows it to be used in patients with either renal or hepatic dysfunction without any dosage adjustments (27). All other 1,4-DHPs are oxidatively metabolized to a variety of inactive compounds. In many cases, the dihydropyridine ring is initially oxidized to an inactive pyridine analog (Fig. 23.28). These initial metabolites are then further transformed by hydrolysis, conjugation, and additional oxidation pathways. Nisoldipine also is subject to these processes; however, hydroxylation of its isobutyl ester produces a metabolite that retains 10% of the activity of the parent compound. In addition to the drug–drug interactions listed below (see Table 23.13), an interesting drug–food interaction occurs with the 1,4-DHPs and grapefruit juice (60). Coadministration of 1,4-DHPs with grapefruit juice produces an increase systemic concentration of the 1,4-DHPs. The mechanism of this interaction appears to result from inhibition of intestinal CYP450 by flavonoids and furanocoumarins

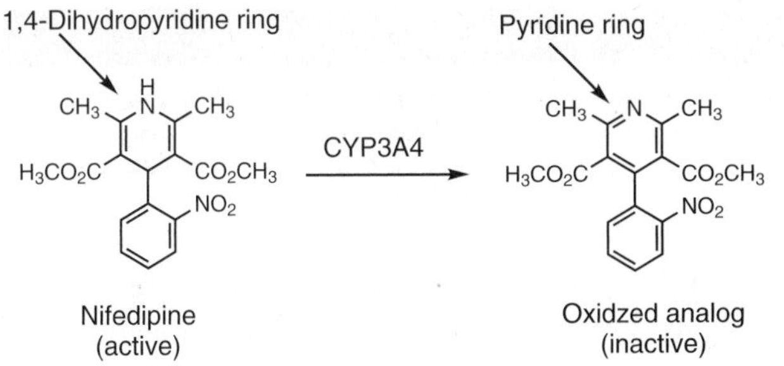

FIGURE 23.28 Oxidation of the 1,4-dihydropyridine ring of nifedipine.

specifically found in grapefruit juice. It has been proposed that limiting daily intake to either an 8-oz. glass of grapefruit juice or half of a fresh grapefruit would likely avoid significant drug interactions with most CYP3A4-metabolized drugs (61).

Verapamil is primarily metabolized to the *N*-demethylated compound, norverapamil, which retains approximately 20% of the pharmacologic activity of verapamil and can reach or exceed the steady-state plasma levels of verapamil. Interestingly, the more active *S*-(−)-isomer undergoes more extensive first-pass hepatic metabolism than does the less active *R*-(+)-isomer. This is important to note, because when given IV, verapamil prolongs the PR interval of the electrocardiogram to a greater extent than when it is given orally (62). This is because the preferential metabolism of the more active enantiomer does not occur with parenteral administration. Diltiazem is primarily hydrolyzed to deacetyldiltiazem. This metabolite retains 25% to 50% of the coronary vasodilatory effects of diltiazem and is present in the plasma at levels of 10% to 45% of the parent compound.

Pharmacokinetic Parameters

The pharmacokinetic parameters and oral dosing information for calcium channel blockers are summarized in Tables 23.11 and 23.12, respectively (27–29). Some doses (specifically, those for diltiazem and verapamil) may vary for either specific indications (i.e., hypertension vs. angina) or different brand names, and the reader should consult the product literature for additional information. The primary differences among the compounds are onset of action, half-life, and oral bioavailability. All calcium channel blockers have excellent oral absorption; however, because they also are subject to rapid first-pass metabolism in the liver, the actual oral bioavailability of these compounds varies considerably depending on the extent of metabolism. All compounds are highly plasma protein bound and primarily eliminated as inactive metabolites in the urine. Because of extensive hepatic transformation, calcium channel blockers should be used cautiously in patients with hepatic disease. Recommendations for these patients include dosage reductions, careful titrations, and close therapeutic monitoring. Diltiazem and verapamil also require dosage adjustments in patients with renal dysfunction, because renal impairment can significantly increase the concentrations of the active metabolites of these compounds. Dosage adjustments usually are not required for the other eight compounds, because seven of them produce inactive metabolites and nisoldipine produces active metabolites with significantly lower activity.

Felodipine and nisoldipine are only available as sustained-release (or extended-release) formulations, and amlodipine and nimodipine are only available as immediate-release formulations. Nifedipine, isradipine, nicardipine, verapamil, and diltiazem are available as both immediate-release and sustained-release formulations. The latter three compounds also are available as parenteral preparations, as is clevidipine. Unlike regular tablets and capsules, sustained-release (or extended-release) formulations cannot be chewed or crushed, because this may lead to an immediate, rather than a sustained, release of the compound. This effect not only will decrease the duration of the dose but also could produce an overdose and subsequent toxicities in the patient. Parenteral preparations of nicardipine and verapamil are incompatible with IV solutions containing sodium bicarbonate. In each case, sodium bicarbonate increases the pH of the solution, resulting in the precipitation of the calcium channel blocker. Although this interaction is not listed for diltiazem, it is reasonable to assume that a similar interaction may occur. Additionally, nicardipine is incompatible with lactated Ringer's solution, and verapamil will precipitate in solutions having a pH greater than or equal to 6 (27,28).

Therapeutic Applications

As illustrated in Table 23.12, calcium channel blockers have been approved for the treatment of hypertension, angina pectoris, subarachnoid hemorrhage, and specific types of arrhythmias (27,28). All calcium channel blockers cause vasodilation and decrease peripheral resistance. With the exceptions of nimodipine, all are approved to treat hypertension. Recent studies have indicated that immediate-release formulations of short-acting calcium channel blockers, especially nifedipine, can cause an abrupt vasodilation that can result in MI. As a result, only the sustained-release formulations of nifedipine and diltiazem should be used in the treatment of essential hypertension (63). Five of the 10 agents are approved for the treatment of angina pectoris. Verapamil is the most versatile agent in that it is indicated for all three types of angina: vasospastic, chronic stable, and unstable. Amlodipine, nifedipine, and diltiazem are indicated for both vasospastic and

CHEMICAL/PHARMACOLOGIC CLASSES USED TO TREAT ANGINA PECTORIS

Organic nitrates, β-blockers (see Chapter 21), and calcium channel blockers

TABLE 23.12 Oral Dosing Information for Calcium Channel Blockers

Generic Name	Brand Name(s)	Approved Indications	Normal Dosing Range	Maximum Daily Dose	Precautions with Hepatic Dysfunction	Available Tablet or Capsule Strengths (mg)
1,4-Dihydropyridines						
Amlodipine	Norvasc	Angina (V, CS), hypertension	5–10 mg once daily	10 mg	Reduce dosage	2.5, 5, 10
Clevidipine	Cleviprex	Hypertension	4–6 mg/hr IV	32 mg/hr IV	None	25 mg/50 mL emulsified suspension
Felodipine	Plendil	Hypertension	2.5–10.0 mg once daily	10 mg	Reduce dosage	ER: 2.5, 5, 10
Isradipine	DynaCirc CR	Hypertension	5–20 mg once daily	20 mg	Titrate dosage	2.5, 5 (CR: 5, 10)
Nicardipine	Cardene, Cardene IV	Angina (CS), hypertension	20–40 mg t.i.d. (SR: 30–60 mg b.i.d.) (IV: 5–15 mg/hour)	120 mg	Titrate dosage	20, 30 (ER: 30, 45, 60) (IV: 2.5 mg/mL)
Nifedipine	Procardia, Adalat	Angina (V, CS), hypertension	10–20 mg t.i.d. (SR: 30–60 mg once a day)	180 mg (SR: 90 mg)	Reduce dosage	10, 20 (ER: 30, 60, 90)
Nimodipine	Nimotop	Subarachnoid hemorrhage	60 mg every 4 hours for 21 days	360 mg	Reduce dosage	30
Nisoldipine	Sular	Hypertension	17–34 mg once daily	34 mg	Closely monitor blood pressure	ER: 8.5, 17, 20, 25.5, 30, 34, 40
Phenylalkylamines						
Verapamil	Calan, Covera, Isoptin, Verelan	Angina (V, CS, U), hypertension, atrial fibrillation/flutter, PSVT	80–120 mg t.i.d. or q.i.d. (SR: 240–480 mg once daily or b.i.d.)	480 mg (540 mg for Covera HS only)	Reduce dosage	40, 80, 120 (SR: 100, 120, 180, 200, 240, 300, 360) (IV: 2.5 mg/mL)
Benzothiazepines						
Diltiazem	Cardizem, Cartia Dilacor, Taztia, Tiazac	Angina (V, CS), hypertension, atrial fibrillation/flutter, PSVT	30–120 mg t.i.d. or q.i.d. (SR: 120–480 mg once daily)	480 mg (SR: 540 mg)	Reduce dosage	30, 60, 90, 120 (SR: 60, 90, 120,180, 240, 300, 360, 420) (IV: 5 mg/mL)

b.i.d., twice a day; CR, controlled release; CS, chronic stable angina; ER, extended release; IV, intravenous; PSVT, paroxysmal supraventricular tachycardia; q.i.d., four times a day; SR, sustained release; t.i.d., three times a day; U, unstable angina; V, vasospastic angina.

chronic stable angina, whereas nicardipine is indicated only for chronic stable angina. Nimodipine is unique in that it has a greater effect on cerebral arteries than on other arteries. As a result, nimodipine is indicated for the improvement of neurologic deficits because of spasm following subarachnoid hemorrhage from ruptured congenital intracranial aneurysms in patients otherwise in good neurologic condition after the episode. Verapamil and diltiazem are pharmacologically different from the 1,4-DHPs in that they block sinus and AV nodal conduction. As a result, IV formulations of verapamil and diltiazem are indicated for the treatment of atrial fibrillation, atrial flutter, and PSVT. Verapamil also can be used orally, either alone (for prophylaxis of repetitive PSVT) or in combination with digoxin (for atrial flutter or atrial fibrillation).

Adverse Effects and Drug Interactions

The most prevalent or significant side effects of calcium channel blockers are listed below (27,28,48,51,53). Drug interactions for calcium channel blockers are listed in Table 23.13. In most instances, these side effects do not cause long-term complications, and they often resolve with time or dosage adjustments. Many of these effects are simply extensions of the pharmacologic effects of

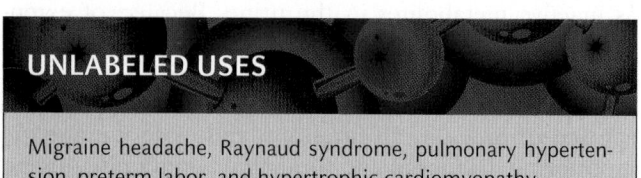

UNLABELED USES

Migraine headache, Raynaud syndrome, pulmonary hypertension, preterm labor, and hypertrophic cardiomyopathy

this class of compounds. Excessive vasodilation results in edema, flushing, hypotension, nasal congestion, headache, and dizziness. Additionally, the palpitations, chest pain, and tachycardia seen with 1,4-DHPs are a result of sympathetic responses to the vasodilatory effects of this chemical class. The use of a β-blocker in combination with a 1,4-DHP can minimize these compensatory effects and can be very useful in treating hypertension. Verapamil and diltiazem can cause bradycardia and AV block because of their ability to depress AV nodal conduction. Because of risks associated with additive cardiodepressive effects, they should not be used in combination with β-blockers. Clevidipine is formulated as an oil-in-water emulsion that contains soybean oil, glycerin, and purified egg yolk phospholipids. As a result, this compound is contraindicated in patients with egg hypersensitivity or soya lecithin hypersensitivity. Additionally, the emulsion used in this formulation can aggravate preexisting disorders of lipid metabolism.

ADVERSE EFFECTS OF CALCIUM CHANNEL BLOCKERS

Edema, flushing, hypotension, nasal congestion, palpitations, chest pain, tachycardia, headache, fatigue, dizziness, rash, nausea, abdominal pain, constipation, diarrhea, vomiting, shortness of breath, weakness, bradycardia, and AV block

TABLE 23.13 Drug Interactions for Calcium Channel Blockers

Drug	Calcium Blocker(s)	Result of Interaction
α_1-Blockers (prazosin, terazosin)	Verapamil	Increased prazosin and terazosin levels
Amiodarone	Diltiazem, verapamil	Increased bradycardia and cardiotoxicity; decreased cardiac output
Aspirin	Verapamil	Increased incidence of bruising
Azole antifungals	Felodipine, isradipine, nifedipine, nisoldipine	Increased serum concentrations of the calcium channel blockers
Barbiturates	Felodipine, nifedipine, verapamil	Decreased pharmacologic effects of the calcium channel blockers
β-Blockers	All	Coadministration may cause additive or synergistic effects; increased cardiodepressant effects (more extensive with verapamil and diltiazem); inhibition of β-blocker metabolism by diltiazem, isradipine, nicardipine, nifedipine, and verapamil
Buspirone	Diltiazem, verapamil	Increase buspirone levels
Carbamazepine, oxcarbazepine	Felodipine, diltiazem, verapamil	Carbamazepine and oxcarbazepine decrease felodipine levels; verapamil and diltiazem increase carbamazepine levels
Cimetidine	All	Increased 1,4-DHP levels
Cyclosporine	Felodipine, nicardipine, nifedipine, diltiazem, verapamil	Increased cyclosporine levels when used with all of these except for nifedipine; cyclosporine increases felodipine and nifedipine levels
CYP3A4 Inhibitors	All	Potentially can increase the plasma levels of calcium channel blockers
Digoxin	Nifedipine, diltiazem, verapamil	Increased digoxin levels
Disopyramide, flecainide	Verapamil	Additive cardiodepressant effects
Dofetilide	Verapamil	Increased dofetilide levels
Doxorubicin	Verapamil	Increased doxorubicin levels
Erythromycin, clarithromycin	All	Increased 1,4-DHP levels and increased toxicity
Fentanyl	All	Severe hypotension and/or bradycardia
General anesthetics	All	Potentiation of the cardiac effects and vascular dilation associated with anesthetics
HMG-CoA reductase inhibitors	Diltiazem, verapamil	Increase levels of HMG-CoA reductase inhibitor
Imipramine	Diltiazem, verapamil	Increased imipramine levels
Lithium	Diltiazem, verapamil	Decreased lithium levels with verapamil; neurotoxicity with diltiazem

TABLE 23.13 Drug Interactions for Calcium Channel Blockers *(Continued)*

Drug	Calcium Blocker(s)	Result of Interaction
Lovastatin	Isradipine	Decreased effects of lovastatin
Melatonin	All	Decreased therapeutic effects of calcium channel blockers
Methylprednisolone	Diltiazem, verapamil	Increased methylprednisolone levels
Midazolam, triazolam	Diltiazem, verapamil	Increased effects of these benzodiazepines
Moricizine	Diltiazem	Increased moricizine levels; decreased diltiazem levels
Phenobarbital	All	Decreased bioavailability of calcium channel blocker
Phenytoin	All	Decreased effectiveness of calcium channel blocker due to induction of metabolism
Quinidine	Diltiazem, nifedipine, nisoldipine, verapamil	Variable responses: quinidine decreases AUC of nisoldipine, but increases actions of nifedipine; diltiazem and verapamil increase the effects of quinidine; nifedipine decreases quinidine levels and actions
Rifampin	Diltiazem, isradipine, nicardipine, nifedipine, verapamil	Decreased levels of calcium channel blocker
Sirolimus, tacrolimus	Diltiazem, nifedipine, verapamil	Increased sirolimus and tacrolimus levels
St. John's wort	Nifedipine	Decreased nifedipine levels (St. John's wort most likely increases the metabolism of all calcium channel blockers)
Theophylline	Diltiazem, verapamil	Increased theophylline levels and toxicity
Valproic acid	Nimodipine	Increased nimodipine levels
Vecuronium	Verapamil	Increased vecuronium levels
Vincristine	Nifedipine	Increased vincristine levels

AUC, area under the curve; HMG-CoA, 3-hydroxy-3-methyl-glutaryl–coenzyme A.

SCENARIO: OUTCOME AND ANALYSIS

Outcome

Thomas L. Rihn, PharmD

According to the National Institutes of Health Joint National Committee VII Practice Guidelines for High Blood Pressure, LB has stage 2 hypertension (systolic blood pressure >160 mm Hg and diastolic blood pressure >100 mm Hg). A thiazide diuretic is indicated for LB; however, the vast majority of patients with this level of high blood pressure will require a two-drug regimen. Considering LB's longstanding diabetes and proteinuria, an ACE inhibitor should be administered in addition to the diuretic. Lisinopril would be a drug of choice because of its pharmacokinetic profile (once daily therapy) and relatively low cost to the patient. It will allow for better blood pressure control and will likely favorably lower the level of proteinuria and perhaps slow the progression of diabetic nephropathy. Although an ARB could be given, the preferred approach generally would be to add an ACE inhibitor before an ARB. If the patient is intolerant to the ACEI (e.g., cough), an ARB could be substituted. It is not necessary to begin with a three-drug regimen. This would be reserved for patients for sustained severe elevations in blood pressure or in whom end organ damage has occurred. Finally, there would be no need to refer LB to a hypertension specialist at this point in time. Only if he developed refractory hypertension would he be preferred to a specialist.

Chemical Analysis

S. William Zito and Victoria Roche

A two-drug regime is recommended for this patient. A thiazide diuretic (see Chapter 22) and an ACE inhibitor. The added ACE inhibitor will contribute to lowering LB's blood pressure as well as aid in controlling his diabetic nephropathy. The natural substrate for ACE is the decapeptide, angiotensin I (Asp-Arg-Val-Tyr-Ile-His-Pro-Phe-His-Leu). The catalytic site of ACE contains an arginine (Arg) residue that binds the carboxyl group of the terminal Leu, and a Zn^{2+} that coordinates with a carbonyl (Phe) to orient angiotensin I so that it can be hydrolyzed to angiotensin

II by attack of the carboxylate anion from Glu. Therefore an ACE inhibitor must have affinity for the ACE active site, have an anionic group to bind to the cationic Arg residue, be capable of binding to the Zn^{2+} and stable to the hydrolytic attack of the Glu carboxylate anion. These structural features are incorporated into a general pharmacophore which represents a di- or tripeptide and contains a stereochemical center with an L-amino acid representation.

Lisinopril contains those structural features that make it an ACE inhibitor. The carboxyl group on the proline can bind to the Arg, a second carboxyl group that can bind to the Zn^{2+}, and a chiral center that can represent an L-amino acid configuration. In addition, lisinopril contains an phenylethyl group and an amino butyl moiety that enhance pharmacokinetics making it have good oral absorption due to the possible formation of zwitterions, no metabolic transformation, and quick onset and long duration of action resulting in once-a-day dosing.

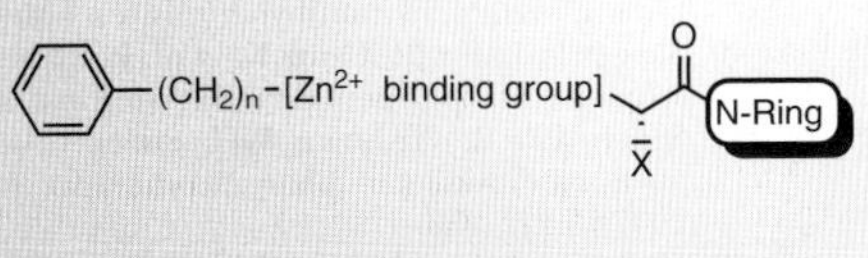

ACEI pharmacophore

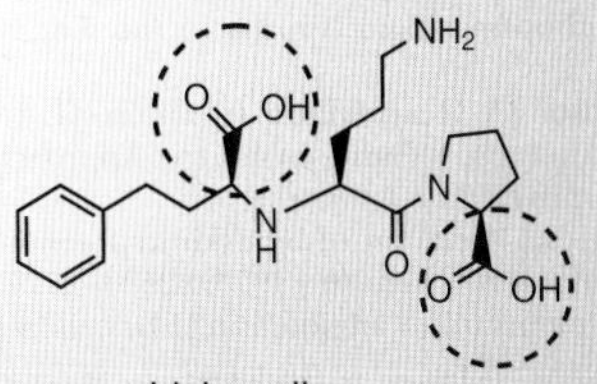

Lisinopril

CASE STUDY

S. William Zito and Victoria Roche

JB is a 46-year-old white man who presents to his local physician for a routine check-up. He is a professional opera singer. He has no complaints except for mild shortness of breath when singing tenor arias on stage. He also says that he experiences shortness of breath when walking long distances or up a flight of stairs. JB's medical history reveals that he has had type 2 diabetes for the past 6 years, which has been successfully treated with glipizide 10 mg po bid. His current blood pressure is 146/101 mm Hg, which is consistent with blood pressure measured during a previous visit. JB has a family history of hypertension and dyslipidemia. His laboratory tests reveal proteinuria and elevated cholesterol. His physician has diagnosed JB's hypertension as stage 2 according to JNC VII guideline and needs to prescribe a two-drug therapeutic regimen. The drug of choice for hypertension is a thiazide diuretic, and JB's physician prescribes hydrochlorthiazide 25 mg daily but is undecided as to which one of the following three antihypertensives to use as the second drug that would best fit JB's needs.

1. Conduct a thorough and mechanistic SAR analysis of the three therapeutic options in the case.
2. Apply the chemical understanding gained from the SAR analysis to this patient's specific needs to make a therapeutic recommendation.

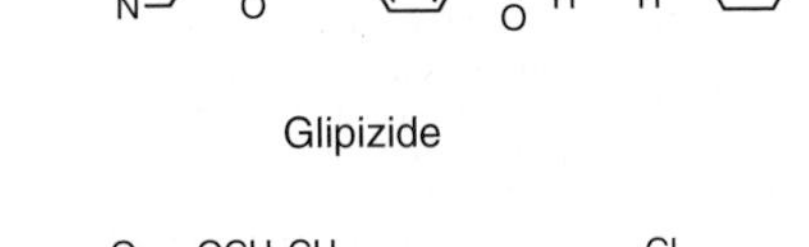

Glipizide

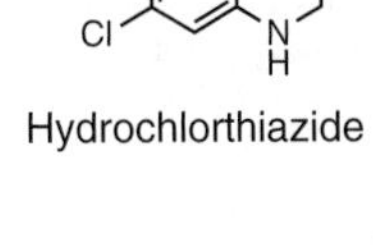

Hydrochlorthiazide

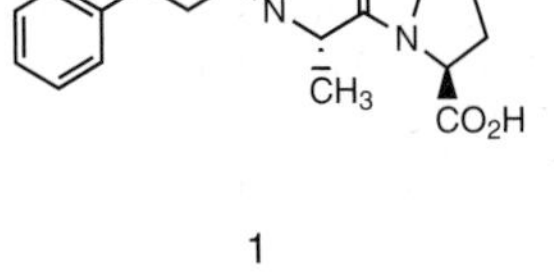

1

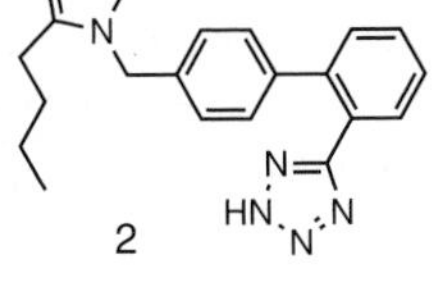

2

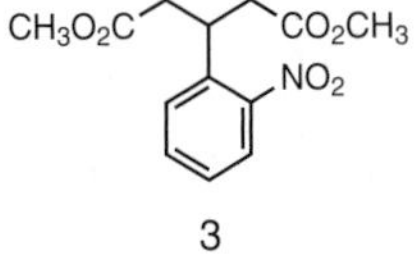

3

References

1. Jackson EK. Renin and angiotensin. In: Brunton L, Lazo J, Parker K, et al., eds. Goodman & Gilman's the Pharmacological Basis of Therapeutics, 11th Ed. New York: McGraw-Hill, 2006:789–821.
2. Skeggs L. Historical overview of the renin-angiotensin system. In: Doyle AE, Bearn AG, eds. Hypertension and the Angiotensin System: Therapeutic Approaches. New York: Raven Press, 1984:31–45.
3. Vallotton MB. The renin-angiotensin system. Trends Pharmacol Sci 1987;8:69–74.
4. Skidgel RA, Erdos EG. Histamine, bradykinin, and their antagonists. Brunton L, Lazo J, Parker K, et al., eds. Goodman & Gilman's the Pharmacological Basis of Therapeutics, 11th Ed. New York: McGraw-Hill, 2006:629–651.
5. Ferrario CM, Brosnihan KB, Diz DI, et al. Angiotensin-(1-7): a new hormone of the angiotensin system. Hypertension 1991;18(5 Suppl):126–133.
6. Saseen JJ, Carter BL. Hypertension. In: Dipiro JT, Talbert RL, Yee GC, et al., eds. Pharmacotherapy: A Pathophysiologic Approach, 6th Ed. New York: McGraw-Hill, 2005:185–217.
7. Parker RB, Patterson JH, Johnson JA. Heart failure. In: Dipiro JT, Talbert RL, Yee GC, et al., eds. Pharmacotherapy: A Pathophysiologic Approach, 6th Ed. New York: McGraw-Hill, 2005:219–260.
8. Ferreira SH, Bartelt DC, Lewis LJ. Isolation of bradykinin-potentiating peptides from *Bothrops jararaca* venom. Biochemistry 1970;9:2583–2593.
9. Bakhle YS. Conversion of angiotensin I to angiotensin II by cell-free extracts of dog lung. Nature 1968;220:919–921.
10. Garrison JC, Peach MJ. Renin and angiotensin. In: Gilman AG, Rall TW, Nies AS, et al., eds. The Pharmacological Basis of Therapeutics, 8th Ed. New York: Pergamon Press, 1990:749–763.
11. Silverman RB. The Organic Chemistry of Drug Design and Drug Action. San Diego: Academic Press, 1992:162–170.
12. Ondetti MA, Rubin B, Cushman DW. Design of specific inhibitors of angiotensin-converting enzyme: new class of orally active antihypertensive agents. Science 1977;196:441–444.
13. Cushman DW, Cheung HS, Sabo EF, et al. Design of potent competitive inhibitors of angiotensin-converting enzyme. Carboxyalkanoyl and mercaptoalkanoyl amino acids. Biochemistry 1977;16:5484–5491.
14. Ondetti MA, Cushman DW. Enzymes of the renin-angiotensin system and their inhibitors. Annu Rev Biochem 1982;51:283–308.
15. Stryer L. Biochemistry, 4th Ed. New York: Freeman and Company, 1995: 218–222.
16. Byers LD, Wolfenden R. Binding of the by-product analogue benzylsuccinic acid by carboxypeptidase A. Biochemistry 1973;12:2070–2078.
17. Klaassen CD. Heavy metals and heavy-metal antagonists. Brunton L, Lazo J, Parker K, et al., eds. Goodman & Gilman's the Pharmacological Basis of Therapeutics, 11th Ed. New York: McGraw-Hill, 2006:1753–1775.
18. Atkinson AB, Robertson JIS. Captopril in the treatment of clinical hypertension and cardiac failure. Lancet 1979;ii:836–839.
19. Patchett AA, Harris E, Tristram EW, et al. A new class of angiotensin-converting enzyme inhibitors. Nature 1980;288:280–283.
20. Gringauz A. Introduction to Medicinal Chemistry. New York: Wiley, 1997:450–461.
21. SciFindeer. Calculated using Advanced Chemistry Development (ACD/Lab) Software V8.14 for Solaris (1994–2005 ACD/Lab) (V8.19 used for Perindolpril).
22. Gross DM, Sweet, CS, Ulm EH, et al. Effect of N-[(S)-1-carboxy-3-phenylpropyl]-L-Ala-L-Pro and its ethyl ester (MK-421) on angiotensin converting enzyme in vitro and angiotensin I pressor responses in vivo. J Pharmacol Exp Ther 1981;216:552–557.
23. Ulm EH, Hichens M, Gomez HJ, et al. Enalapril maleate and a lysine analogue (MK-521): disposition in man. Br J Clin Pharmacol 1982;14:357–362.
24. Kim DH, Guinosso CJ, Buzby GC Jr, et al. (Mercaptopropanoyl)indoline-2–carboxylic acids and related compounds as potent angiotensin-converting enzyme inhibitors and antihypertensive agents. J Med Chem 1983;26:394–403.
25. Krapcho J, Turk C, Cushman DW, et al. Angiotensin-converting enzyme inhibitors. Mercaptan, carboxyalkyl dipeptide, and phosphinic acid inhibitors incorporating 4-substituted prolines. J Med Chem 1988;31:1148–1160.
26. Oparil S, Koerner T, Tregear GW, et al. Substrate requirements for angiotensin I conversion in vivo and in vitro. Circ Res 1973;32:415–423.
27. Clinical Pharmacology Online. Gold Standard Elsevier, 2010. Available at: http://clinicalpharmacology.com. Accessed October 6, 2010.
28. Facts & Comparisons eAnswers. St. Louis, MO: Wolters Kluwer Health. Available at: http://www.factsandcomparisons.com. Accessed October 6, 2010.
29. Micromedex Healthcare Series. Thomson Reuters (Healthcare) Inc. Available at: http://www.thomsonhc.com. Accessed October 6, 2010.
30. Drummer OH, Nicolaci J, Iakovidis D. Biliary excretion and conjugation of diacid angiotensin-converting enzyme inhibitors. J Pharmacol Exp Ther 1990;252:1202–1206.
31. Kostis JB, Garland WT, Delaney C, et al. Fosinopril: pharmacokinetic and pharmacodynamics in congestive heart failure. Clin Pharmacol Ther 1995;58:660–665.
32. Chobanian AV, Bakris GI, Black HR, et al., and the National High Blood Pressure Education Program Coordinating Committee. The Seventh Report of the Joint National Committee on Prevention, Detection, Evaluation, and Treatment of High Blood Pressure. JAMA 2003;289:2560–2572.
33. Moore GJ. Designing peptide mimetics. Trends Pharmacol Sci 1994;15:124–129.
34. Harrold MW. Preparing students for future therapies: the development of novel agents to control the renin-angiotensin system. Am J Pharm Educ 1997;61:173–178.
35. Lacourciere Y, Brunner H, Irwin R, et al. Effects of modulators of the renin-angiotensin-aldosterone system on cough. Losartan Cough Study Group. J Hypertens 1994;12:1387–1393.
36. Timmermans PB, Wong PC, Chiu AT, et al. Angiotensin II receptors and angiotensin II receptor antagonists. Pharmacol Rev 1993;45:205–213.
37. Furakawa Y, Kishimoto S, Nishikawa K. Hypotensive imidazole derivatives and hypotensive imidazole-5-acetic acid derivatives. U.S. Patents 4,340,598 and 4,355,040. Osaka, Japan, 1982.
38. Bauer JH, Reams GP. The angiotensin II type 1 receptor antagonists: a new class of antihypertensive drugs. Arch Intern Med 1995;155:1361–1368.
39. Carini DJ, Duncia JV, Aldrich PE, et al. Nonpeptide angiotensin II receptor antagonists: the discovery of a series of N-(biphenylylmethyl)imidazoles as potent, orally active antihypertensives. J Med Chem 1991;35:2525–2547.
40. Skeggs L, Kahn JR, Lentz K, et al. Preparation, purification and amino acid sequence of a polypeptide renin substrate. J Exp Med 1957;106:439–453.
41. Sepehrdad R, Frishman WH, Steier C, et al. Direct inhibition of renin as a cardiovascular pharmacotherapy: focus on aliskiren. Cardiol Rev 2007;15:242–256.
42. Maibaum J, Stutz S, Goschke R, et al. Structural modification of the P2' position of 2,7-dialkyl-substituted 5(S)-amino-4(S)-hydroxy-8-phenyl-octanecarboxamides: the discovery of aliskiren, a potent nonpeptide human renin inhibitor active after once daily dosing in marmosets. J Med Chem 2007;50:4832–4844.
43. Fisher NDL, Hollenberg NK. Renin inhibition: what are the therapeutic opportunities? J Am Soc Nephrol 2005;16:592–599.
44. Aliskiren (Tekturna) for hypertension. Med Lett Drugs Ther 2007;49:29–31.
45. Cutler SJ. Cardiovascular agents. In: Block JH, Beale, JM, eds. Wilson and Gisvold's Textbook of Organic Medicinal and Pharmaceutical Chemistry, 12th Ed. Philadelphia: Lippincott Williams & Wilkins, 2011:617–665.
46. Silverthorn DU. Human Physiology: An Integrated Approach. Upper Saddle River, NJ: Prentice Hall, 1998:325–361.
47. Janis RA, Triggle DJ. New developments in Ca^{2+} channel antagonists. J Med Chem 1983;26:775–785.
48. Swamy VC, Triggle DJ. Calcium channel blockers. In: Craig CR, Stitzel RE, eds. Modern Pharmacology with Clinical Applications, 5th Ed. Boston: Little, Brown, 1997:229–234.
49. Varadi G, Mori Y, Mikala G, et al. Molecular determinants of Ca^{2+} channel function and drug action. Trends Pharmacol Sci 1995;16:43–49.
50. Gilmore J, Dell C, Bowman D, et al. Neuronal calcium channels. Annu Rep Med Chem 1995;30:51–60.
51. Michel T. Treatment of myocardial ischemia. In: Brunton L, Lazo J, Parker K, et al., eds. Goodman and Gilman's the Pharmacological Basis of Therapeutics, 11th Ed. New York: McGraw-Hill, 2006:823–844.
52. American Heart Association. Heart attack and angina statistics. Available at: http://www.americanheart.org/presenter.jhtml?identifier=4591. Accessed October 29, 2010.
53. Vaghy PL. Calcium antagonists. In: Brody TM, Larner J, Minneman KP, et al., eds. Human Pharmacology: Molecular to Clinical, 2nd Ed. St. Louis: Mosby, 1994:203–213.
54. Triggle DJ. Drugs acting on ion channels and membranes. In: Hansch C, Sammes PG, Taylor JB, eds. Comprehensive Medicinal Chemistry, Vol 3. Oxford, UK: Pergamon Press, 1990:1047–1099.
55. Loev B, Ehrreich SJ, Tedeschi RE. Dihydropyridines with potent hypotensive activity prepared by the Hantzsch reaction. J Pharm Pharmacol 1972;24: 917–918.
56. Loev B, Goodman MM, Snader KM, et al. "Hantzsch-type" dihydropyridine hypotensive agents. J Med Chem 1974;17:956–965.
57. Triggle AM, Shefter E, Triggle DJ. Crystal structures of calcium channel antagonists: 2,6-dimethyl-3,5-dicarbomethoxy-4-[2-nitro, 3-cyano-, 4-(dimethylamino)-, and 2,3,4,5,6-pentafluorophenyl]-1,4-dihydropyridine. J Med Chem 1980;23:1442–1445.
58. Product information for Prialt. Available at: http://www.prialt.com. Accessed November 1, 2005.
59. Calculated using ChemBioDraw Ultra Software V12.0 (1986–2009), Cambridge Soft, http://www.cambridgesoft.com.
60. Bailey DG, Arnold JMO, Spence JD. Grapefruit juice and drugs: how significant is the interaction? Clin Pharmacokinet 1994;26:91–98.
61. Drug interactions with grapefruit juice. Med Lett Drugs Ther 2004;46:2–4.
62. Roden DM. Antiarrhythmic drugs. In: Brunton L, Lazo J, Parker K, et al., eds. Goodman & Gilman's the Pharmacological Basis of Therapeutics, 11th Ed. New York: McGraw-Hill, 2006:899–932.
63. Safety of calcium-channel blockers. Med Lett Drugs Ther 1997;39:13–14.
64. Product information for Edarbi. Available at http://www.edarbi.com. Accessed November 16, 2011.

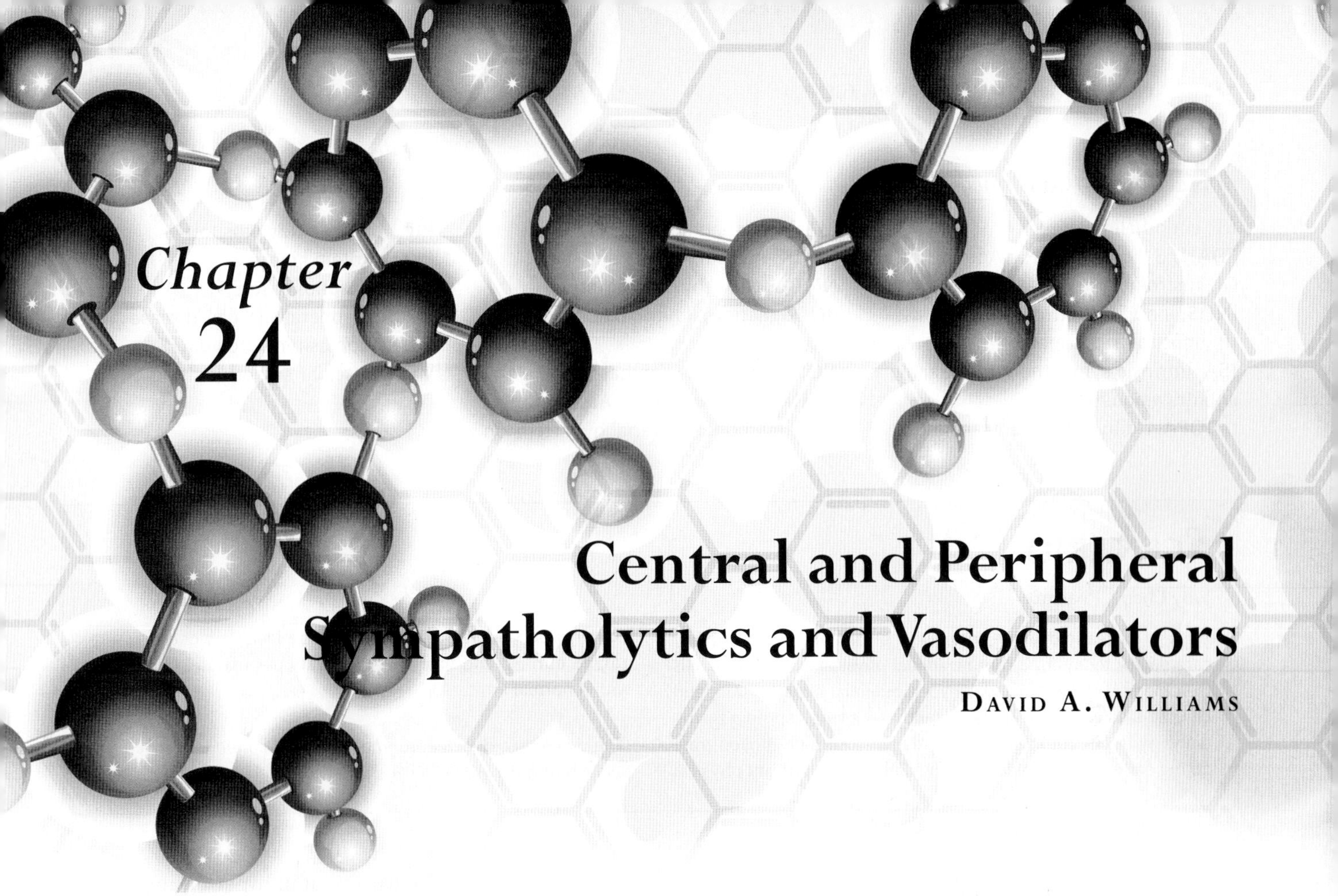

Chapter 24

Central and Peripheral Sympatholytics and Vasodilators

DAVID A. WILLIAMS

*Drugs Covered in This Chapter**

β-NONSELECTIVE BLOCKERS
- Bucindolol
- Carteolol
- Levobunolol
- Nadolol
- Penbutolol
- Pindolol
- Propranolol
- Timolol

β_1-SELECTIVE BLOCKERS
- Acebutolol
- Atenolol
- Betaxolol
- Bisoprolol
- Esmolol
- Metoprolol
- Nebivolol

α_1-BLOCKERS
- Prazosin
- Doxazosin
- Terazosin

MIXED α/β-BLOCKERS
- Carvedilol
- Labetalol

CENTRALLY ACTING SYMPATHOLYTICS
- Methyldopa
- Clonidine
- *Moxonidine*
- *Rilmenidine*
- Guanabenz
- Guanfacine
- Metyrosine

ADRENERGIC NEURON BLOCKING AGENTS
- Reserpine
- Guanethidine
- Guanadrel

VASODILATORS
- Hydralazine
- Minoxidil
- Diazoxide

PHOSPHODIESTERASE INHIBITORS
- Inamrinone
- Milrinone
- Sildenafil

NITRODILATOR
- Sodium nitroprusside

GANGLIONIC BLOCKERS
- Mecamylamine
- Trimethaphan

ENDOTHELIAL ANTAGONISTS
- Bosentan
- Ambrisentan
- *Sitaxsentan*

PROSTANOIDS
- Epoprostenol
- Treprostinil
- *Beraprost*
- *Iloprost*

Abbreviations

ACE, angiotensin-converting enzyme
ACEI, angiotensin-converting enzyme inhibitor
ADHD, attention-deficit hyperactivity disorder
ARB, angiotensin receptor blocker
AT-II, angiotensin II
ATP, adenosine triphosphate
BB, β-blocker
CaM, calmodulin
cAMP, cyclic adenosine monophosphate
cGMP, cyclic guanosine monophosphate
CCB, calcium channel blocker
CNS, central nervous system
COMT, catechol-*O*-methyltransferase
COX-2, cyclooxygenase-2
CSF, cerebrospinal fluid
DAG, diacylglycerol
eNOS, endothelial nitric oxide synthase

*Drugs listed include those available inside and outside of the United States; drugs available outside of the United States are shown in italics.

Abbreviations (Continued)

ET, endothelin
FDA, U.S. Food and Drug Administration
GI, gastrointestinal
iNOS, inducible nitric oxide synthase
IP_3, inositol triphosphate
ISA, intrinsic sympathomimetic activity
IV, intravenous
L-DOPA, L-dihydroxyphenylalanine
MAO, monoamine oxidase
MLCK, myosin light-chain kinase
NMDA, *N*-methyl-D-aspartate
nNOS, neuronal nitric oxide synthase
NO, nitric oxide
NOS, nitric oxide synthase
NYHA, New York Heart Association
PAH, pulmonary arterial hypertension
PIP_2, phosphatidylinositol
PKC, protein kinase C
PLC, phospholipase C
PVD, peripheral vascular disease
SR, sarcoplasmic reticulum
VSM, vascular smooth muscle

SCENARIO

Judy Cheng, PharmD

AJ is a 62-year-old white male who presented to his primary care doctor today for a routine annual physical examination. His past medical history includes hyperlipidemia, hypertension, and chronic stable angina. He is currently receiving aspirin 325 mg daily, hydrochlorothiazide 25 mg daily, isosorbide mononitrate 30 mg daily, and simvastatin 40 mg daily. His significant physical examination findings at the clinic today include blood pressure 165/98 mm Hg and heart rate 80 beats per minute. Others are within normal limit.

(The reader is directed to the clinical solution and chemical analysis of this case at the end of the chapter).

CARDIOVASCULAR HYPERTENSION

Hypertension is the most common cardiovascular disease and is the major risk factor for coronary artery disease, heart failure, stroke, and renal failure. Approximately 50 million Americans have a systolic or diastolic blood pressure ≥ 140/90 mm Hg. The onset of hypertension is defined as having a blood pressure of 140/90 mm Hg or greater and most commonly appears during the fourth, fifth, and sixth decades of life (1).

The importance of controlling blood pressure is well documented (1), although the rates of awareness, treatment, and control of hypertension have not risen as expected in the National Health and Nutrition Examination Survey (2). This survey showed that 68% of Americans are aware that they have high blood pressure but that only 53% are receiving treatment and only 27% have their blood pressure under control. Since 1976, there has been a significant improvement in the rates of awareness, treatment, and control of hypertension; however, since 1990, whatever progress had been achieved has now reached a plateau (2). Although the age-adjusted death rates from stroke and coronary heart disease during this period have fallen by 59% and 53%, respectively, these rates of decline also appear to have reached a plateau (2). These troubling trends should awaken clinicians to be more aggressive in the treatment of patients with hypertension.

When the decision to initiate hypertensive therapy is made, physicians often are presented with the dilemma of which of more than 80 antihypertensive products, representing more than 8 different drug classes, to use for their patients (Table 24.1) (1,3). Those factors that can affect the outcomes from the treatment of hypertension, including potential adverse effects, clinically significant drug–drug interactions (especially when so many different drug classes are involved), patient compliance, affordability, risk/benefit ratios, and dosing frequency, must be considered (3). Having considered these factors, the health care provider (clinician or pharmacist) arrives at an appropriate choice of antihypertensive drug (3). Once the patient is stabilized with an antihypertensive medication, some of these issues need to be reevaluated. Patients should be continually asked about side effects, because many of the antihypertensive drugs possess side effects that the patient cannot tolerate (1). This problem and the cost of drug therapy can affect compliance to drug therapy especially for the elderly and those on fixed incomes (4).

Drug therapy in the management of hypertension must be individualized and adjusted based on coexisting risk factors, including the degree of blood pressure elevation, severity of the disease (e.g., presence of target organ damage), presence of underlying cardiovascular or other risk factors, response to therapy (single or multiple drugs), and tolerance to drug-induced adverse effects (1,3). Antihypertensive therapy is generally reserved for patients who fail to respond to nondrug therapies along with lifestyle modifications, such as diet including sodium restriction and adequate potassium intake, regular aerobic physical activity, moderation of alcohol consumption, and weight reduction (3).

It is not surprising that compliance with antihypertensive therapy can be as low as 40% when one considers that the patient, if he or she has other chronic diseases, can be taking as many as 10 different drugs and up to 40 tablets

CLINICAL SIGNIFICANCE

Cardiovascular diseases continue to be the number one cause of death in many industrialized nations, as a result of risk factors such as hypertension, coronary artery diseases, and heart failure. Sympatholytic agents play an important role in managing these diseases, not only by reducing blood pressure, angina, and other clinical symptoms, but also by reducing mortality. β-Blockers are now considered part of the standard of care in patients with coronary artery disease and heart failure and one of the drugs of first choice in hypertension management.

However, not all sympatholytic agents have the same pharmacologic and chemical properties or equal amounts of clinical evidence to support their use in every clinical indication. For instance, carvedilol, metoprolol, and bisoprolol have the most clinical evidence related to improving heart failure mortality, and nonselective β-blockers are probably more detrimental than others in patients with reactive airway disease, peripheral arterial diseases, and cocaine overdose, due to their β_2-antagonistic effect (which can be predicted by their chemical structure). Newer generation β-blockers such as nebivolol, which is the only β-blocker that structurally differs fundamentally from that derived from propranolol, also possess additional effects in relaxing smooth muscle by the nitric oxide pathway and may be less harmful in these situations.

The sympathetic nervous system of our body plays important roles in many disease processes. New medications continue to be discovered that augment our sympathetic nervous system activities. Newer agents are designed with a hope to reduce the side effect profiles of older agents and to enhance their therapeutic effects. Understanding the medicinal chemistry of these agents will allow us to select the specific agent that is most optimal for a particular patient situation.

Judy Cheng, PharmD
Professor, Pharmacy Practice
School of Pharmacy-Boston
Massachusetts College of Pharmacy and Health Sciences

or capsules per day (4). To achieve better compliance requires educating the patient and simplifying the drug regimen by reducing the number of drugs being taken.

Hypertension in pregnancy presents a formidable therapeutic challenge and requires comprehensive management with close monitoring for both maternal and fetal welfare (5). Mechanisms involved with pregnancy-related hypertension include a hyperadrenergic state, plasma volume reduction, reduction in uteroplacental perfusion, hormonal control of vascular reactivity, and prostacyclin deficiency and can result from or activate the mechanisms that elevate blood pressure. Effective blood pressure control for pregnancy-related hypertension can often be achieved with methyldopa (recommended), β-blockers (BBs), or mixed α/β-blockers (dual combination of α- and β-blocker activity). The vasodilating agent hydralazine is used to treat hypertensive emergencies associated with eclampsia (1,6). The presence or development of proteinuria (preeclampsia) in a hypertensive pregnant woman implies a major increase in risk to the fetus and warrants immediate admission to a hospital for specialist management (5).

Patients with diabetes mellitus have a much higher rate of hypertension than would be expected in the general population. Regardless of the antihypertensive agent used, a reduction in blood pressure helps to prevent or reduce diabetic microvascular and macrovascular complications, such as blindness and kidney failure. Angiotensin-converting enzyme (ACE) inhibitors

TABLE 24.1 Classification of Antihypertensive Activity According to Mechanism of Action

	Drug Class	Drug Subclass
I	Diuretics (Chapter 22)	
II	Sympatholytic drugs	1. Centrally acting drugs (methyldopa, clonidine, guanabenz, guanfacine) (Chapter 24) 2. Ganglionic blocker drugs (Chapter 24) 3. Adrenergic neuron blocking drugs (Chapter 24) 4. β-Adrenergic blocking drugs (Chapters 10 and 24) 5. α-Adrenergic blocking drugs (Chapters 10 and 24) 6. Mixed α/β-adrenergic blocking drugs (Chapters 10 and 24)
III	Vasodilator (Chapter 24)	Arterial (hydralazine, minoxidil, diazoxide) Arterial and venous (sodium nitroprusside)
IV	Calcium channel blockers (Chapter 23)	
V	Angiotensin-converting enzyme inhibitors (Chapter 23)	
VI	Angiotensin receptor antagonists (Chapter 23)	

(ACEIs) and angiotensin receptor blockers (ARBs) are considered first-line therapy in patients with diabetes and hypertension because of their well-established renal protective effects. Most diabetic patients with hypertension require combination therapy with low-dose diuretics and BBs to achieve optimal blood pressure goals.

Combination Antihypertensive Therapy

It is well-documented that monotherapy adequately controls hypertension only in approximately 50% of patients (7,8). Therefore, a large percentage of patients will require at least a combination of two drugs to control their blood pressure and symptoms of hypertension. By combining different antihypertensive drug classes in low doses, their different mechanisms of action result in synergistic blood pressure lowering as well as in minimizing the adverse effects and improving compliance issues (1,8). For example, the addition of a low-dose thiazide diuretic dramatically increases the response rates to methyldopa, ACEIs, and BBs without producing the undesirable side effects. In the latest guidelines for treatment of hypertension, the Joint National Committee for Prevention, Detection, Evaluation and Treatment of High Blood Pressure (JNC-7), clinicians are encouraged to begin initially as stage 1 with thiazide-type diuretics and can also consider adding ACEIs, ARBs, BBs, or calcium channel blockers (CCBs) or combinations of these drugs in hypertensive patients without compelling risk factors (Table 24.2). These drug classes have been shown to decrease morbidity and mortality in long-term clinical trials (2). In patients with compelling risk factors such as heart disease, clinical manifestations of cardiovascular diseases or diabetes, other antihypertensive classes are considered as well as including the stage 1 agents (Table 24.2). In these patients with compelling risk factors for cardiovascular disease, treatment should be more aggressive, with the goal of reducing blood pressure to less than 130/80 mm Hg (Table 24.3). These recommendations reflect the current awareness of the importance of addressing other cardiovascular conditions aside from just lowering the blood pressure.

Arterial pressure is the product of cardiac output and peripheral vascular resistance and, therefore, can be lowered by decreasing or inhibiting either or both of these physiologic responses with the drug classes represented in Table 24.1 and summarized in Figure 24.1. This chapter will discuss those antihypertensives that are classified as either sympatholytics (i.e., having a central or peripheral mechanism of action) or vasodilators. These classes of drugs are less commonly used today because of the higher incidence of side effects associated with inhibition of the sympathetic nervous system (sympathoinhibition) or vasodilation. In many instances, they have been replaced because of availability of newer and more effective antihypertensive drugs with fewer side effects, such as ACEIs and ARBs.

Overview of Vascular Tone (1)

Before beginning the discussion of the sympatholytics and vasodilators, it is important to review the nature of vascular tone. The term "vascular tone" refers to the degree of constriction experienced by a blood vessel relative to its maximally dilated state. All resistance (arteries) and capacitance (venous) vessels under basal conditions exhibit some degree of smooth muscle contraction, which determines the diameter and, hence, the tone of the vessel.

Basal vascular tone varies among organs. Those organs having a large vasodilatory capacity (e.g., myocardium, skeletal muscle, skin, and splanchnic circulation) have high vascular tone, whereas organs having relatively low vasodilatory capacity (e.g., cerebral and renal circulations) have low vascular tone. Vascular tone is determined by many different competing vasoconstrictor and vasodilator influences acting on the blood vessel. Influences such as sympathetic nerves and circulating angiotensin II regulate arterial blood pressure by increasing vascular tone (i.e., vasoconstriction). On the other hand, mechanisms for local blood flow regulation within an organ include

TABLE 24.2 Initial Drug Choices (JNC-7)

Without Compelling Risk Factors		With Compelling Risk Factors
Blood pressure goal in age ≥50 years, <140/90 mm Hg		Blood pressure goal, <130/80 mm Hg
Stage 1 Hypertension	**Stage 2 Hypertension**	**Compelling risk factors include:**
SBP 140–159 or DBP 90–99 mm Hg	SBP ≥160 or DBP ≥100 mm Hg	Heart failure After myocardial infarction High coronary disease risk Diabetes Chronic kidney disease Recurrent stroke prevention
Thiazide-type diuretics + may consider adding ACEIs, ARBs, BBs, CCBs, or combinations	Two drug combinations + may consider adding thiazide-type diuretics, ACEIs, ARBs, BBs, CCBs	Drugs for compelling indications: Stage 1 drugs and other antihypertensive drugs
Not at Blood Pressure Goal		
Optimize stage 2 drug treatment, or add additional classes of antihypertensive drugs until blood pressure goal is achieved		

TABLE 24.3 Risk Factors for Cardiovascular Disease

Correctable	Noncorrectable
Cigarette smoking	Age >60 years
Hypertension	Sex (men and postmenopausal women)
Elevated cholesterol	Family history of cardiovascular disease or stroke (women <65 years, men <55 years)
Reduced HDL cholesterol	
Diabetes mellitus	
Obesity	Target oral damage

HDL, high-density lipoprotein.

endothelial factors (e.g., nitric oxide [NO] and endothelin [ET]) or local hormones/chemical substances (e.g., prostanoids, thromboxanes, histamine, and bradykinin) that can either increase or decrease tone. The mechanisms by which the above influences either constrict or relax blood vessels involve a variety of signal transduction mechanisms that, ultimately, influence the interaction between actin and myosin in the smooth muscle.

Overview of the Regulation of Vascular Smooth Muscle Contraction and Relaxation (1)

The contractile characteristics and the mechanisms that cause contraction of vascular smooth muscle (VSM) are very different from those of cardiac muscle. The VSM undergoes slow, sustained, tonic contractions, whereas cardiac muscle contractions are rapid and of relatively short duration (a few hundred milliseconds). Whereas VSM contains actin and myosin, it does not have the regulatory protein troponin, as is found in the heart. Furthermore, the arrangement of actin and myosin in VSM is not organized into distinct bands, as it is in cardiac muscle. This is not to imply that the contractile proteins of VSM are disorganized and not well developed. Actually, they are highly organized and well suited for their role in maintaining tonic contractions and reducing lumen diameter.

Contraction of the VSM can be initiated by mechanical, electrical, and chemical stimuli. Passive stretching of VSM can cause contraction that originates from the smooth muscle itself and, therefore, is termed a "myogenic response." Electrical depolarization of the VSM cell membrane also elicits its contraction, most likely by opening voltage-dependent calcium channels (L-type calcium channels) and causing an influx (increase) in the intracellular concentration of calcium ion. Finally, a number of chemical stimuli, such as norepinephrine, angiotensin II, vasopressin, endothelin-1, and thromboxane A_2, can cause contraction. Each of these substances bind to specific receptors on the VSM cell (or to receptors on the endothelium adjacent to the VSM), which then leads to VSM contraction. The mechanism of contraction involves different signal transduction pathways, all of which converge to increase intracellular Ca^{+2}.

The mechanism by which an increase in intracellular Ca^{+2} stimulates VSM contraction is illustrated in the left panel of Figure 24.1. An increase in free intracellular Ca^{+2} results from either increased flux of Ca^{+2} into the VSM cell through calcium channels or by release of Ca^{+2} from intracellular stores of the sarcoplasmic reticulum (SR). The

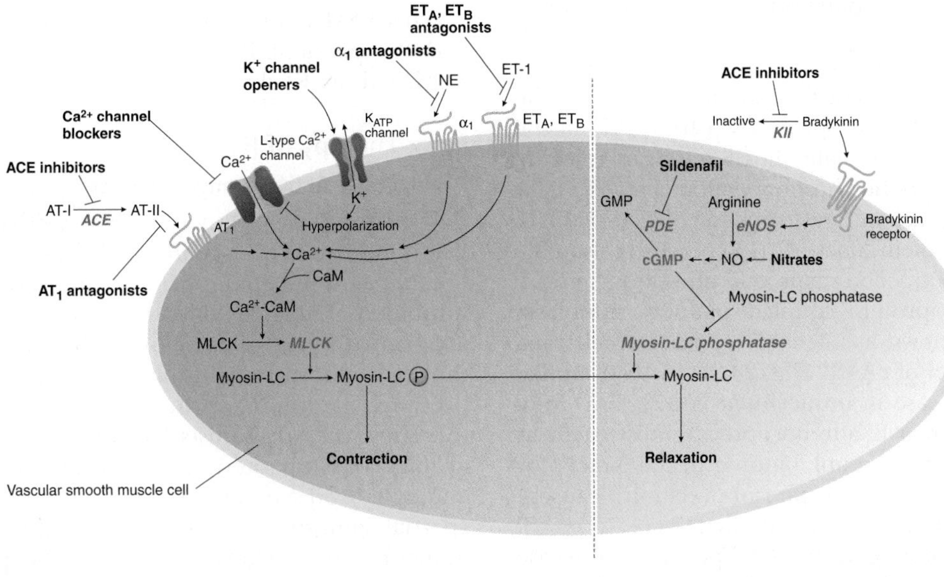

FIGURE 24.1 Calcium second messenger mechanism of vascular smooth muscle contraction and relaxation and sites of action of the peripheral and centrally acting sympatholytics and vasodilators. ACE, angiotensin-converting enzyme; AT, angiotensin; CaM, calmodulin; ET-1, endothelin peptide; ET_A and ET_B, endothelin receptors; eNOS, endothelial nitric oxide synthase; KII, kininase II or ACE; MLCK, myosin light chain kinase; PDE, phosphodiesterase. (From Yeh DC, Michel T. Pharmacology of vascular tone. In: Golan DE, Tashjian A, Armstrong E, et al., eds. Principles of Pharmacology: The Pathophysiologic Basis of Drug Therapy, 2nd Ed. Baltimore, MD: Wolters Kluwer/Lippincott Williams & Wilkins, 2008:367–385, with permission.)

SR is an internal membrane system within the VSM that functions as the major regulator of Ca^{+2} for managing VSM contractility and relaxation. The SR releases Ca^{+2} during contraction, and the released free intracellular Ca^{+2} binds to a special calcium binding protein called calmodulin (CaM), which in turn activates myosin light-chain kinase (MLCK), an enzyme that phosphorylates the myosin light chains by means of adenosine triphosphate (ATP). Phosphorylation of the myosin light chain leads to actin–myosin cross-bridge formation between the myosin heads and the actin filaments and, hence, VSM contraction. Dephosphorylation of the phosphorylated myosin light chain by myosin light-chain phosphorylase yields myosin light chain, which results in relaxation of the VSM. The concentration of intracellular Ca^{+2} depends on the balance between the Ca^{+2} that enters the VSM cells, the Ca^{+2} released by the SR, and the removal of Ca^{+2} either transported by an ATP-dependent calcium pump back into SR where the Ca^{+2} is resequestered or removed from the VSM cell to the external environment by an ATP-dependent calcium pump or by the sodium–calcium exchanger.

The activation of the calcium second messenger system by hormones, neurotransmitters, local mediators, and sensory stimuli is very important in regulating VSM contraction. Several signal transduction mechanisms modulate intracellular calcium concentration and, therefore, the state of vascular tone. These calcium second messenger systems are the phosphatidylinositol (PIP_2)/ G_q protein–coupled pathway, the cyclic adenosine monophosphate (cAMP)/G_s protein–coupled pathway, and the NO/cyclic guanosine monophosphate (cGMP) pathway.

The PIP_2 pathway in VSM is similar to that found in the heart (Fig. 24.2). The VSM membrane is lined with specific receptors for norepinephrine (α_1-adrenoceptors), angiotensin II (AT-II), or endothelin-1 (ET-1, which binds one of two receptors ET_A or ET_B), that stimulate G_q protein, activating phospholipase C (PLC) and resulting in the formation of inositol triphosphate (IP_3) from PIP_2 in the membrane. Then, IP_3 stimulates the SR to release calcium, which in turn activates the phosphorylation of myosin light chain, causing contraction. The formation of diacylglycerol (DAG) activates protein kinase C (PKC), which also contributes to VSM contraction via protein phosphorylation.

The cAMP/G_s protein–coupled pathway stimulates adenylate (also known as adenylyl) cyclase, which catalyzes the formation of cAMP (Fig. 24.2). In VSM, unlike the heart, an increase in intracellular cAMP concentrations stimulated by a β_2-adrenoceptor agonist, such as epinephrine or isoproterenol, binding to the β-receptor inhibits myosin light-chain phosphorylation, causing VSM relaxation. Therefore, drugs that increase cAMP (e.g., β_2-adrenoceptor agonists, PDE3 phosphodiesterase inhibitors) cause vasodilation. On the other hand, stimulation of G_i protein inhibits adenylyl cyclase.

A third mechanism that is also very important in regulating VSM tone is the NO/cGMP pathway (Fig. 24.1, right panel). The formation of NO in the endothelium activates guanylate (also known as guanylyl) cyclase, which causes increased formation of cGMP and vasodilation. The precise mechanisms by which cGMP relaxes VSM is unclear; however, cGMP can activate a cGMP-dependent PKC, inhibit calcium entry into the VSM, activate K^+ channels, and decrease IP_3.

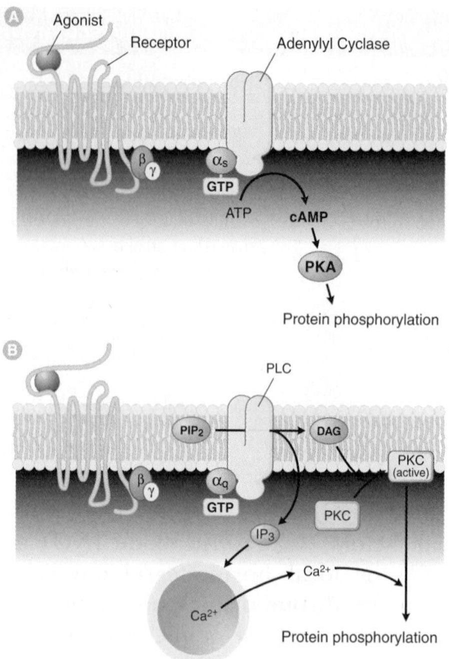

FIGURE 24.2 The mechanism of activation of the cyclic adenosine monophosphate (cAMP)/G_s protein–coupled pathway and the phospholipase C/phosphatidylinositol (PIP_2) pathway in vascular smooth muscle. PKA, protein kinase A; DAG, diacylglycerol; IP_3, inositol triphosphate. (From Yeh DC, Michel T. Pharmacology of vascular tone. In: Golan DE, Tashjian A, Armstrong E, et al., eds. Principles of Pharmacology: The Pathophysiologic Basis of Drug Therapy. Baltimore, MD: Wolters Kluwer/Lippincott Williams & Wilkins, 2008:367–385, with permission.)

Drug Therapy of Hypertension

Peripherally Acting Sympatholytics

β-Adrenergic Receptor Blockers BBs are drugs that bind to β-adrenoceptors and, thereby, block the binding of norepinephrine and epinephrine to these receptors, causing inhibition of normal sympathetic effects. Therefore, BBs are sympatholytic drugs. Some BBs, when they bind to the β-adrenoceptor, partially activate the receptor while preventing norepinephrine from binding to the receptor. These partial agonists therefore provide some "background" of sympathetic activity while preventing normal and enhanced sympathetic activity. These particular BBs (partial agonists) are said to possess intrinsic sympathomimetic activity (ISA). Some BBs also possess what is referred to as membrane-stabilizing activity. This effect is similar to the membrane-stabilizing activity of sodium channel blockers that represent class I antiarrhythmics.

The first generation of BBs were nonselective, meaning that they blocked both β_1- and β_2-adrenoceptors (Fig. 24.3). Second-generation BBs are more cardioselective, because they are relatively selective for

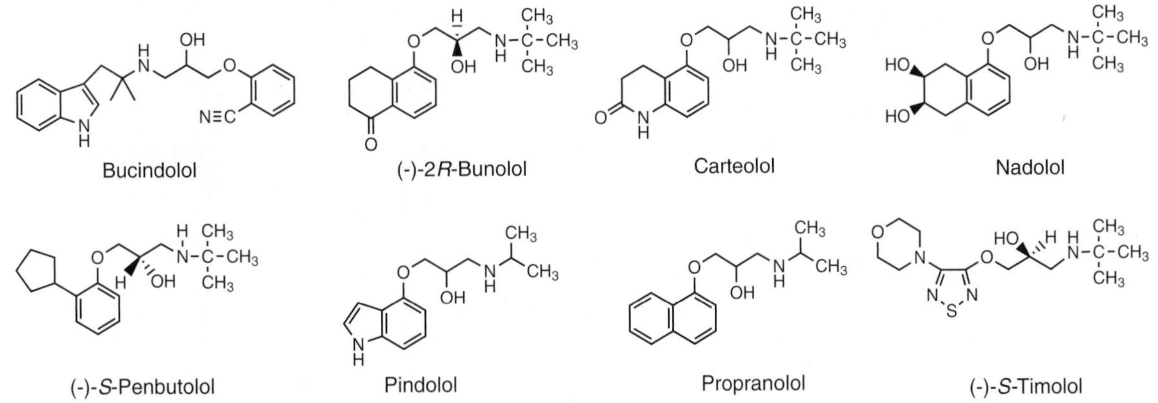

FIGURE 24.3 Nonselective β-adrenergic blockers.

β_1-adrenoceptors (Fig. 24.4). Note that this relative selectivity can be lost at higher drug doses. Finally, the third-generation BBs are drugs that also possess vasodilator actions through blockade of vascular α-adrenoceptors (mixed α_1/β_1-adrenergic blockers) (see Fig. 24.6). Their structure–activity relationship, pharmacokinetics, and metabolism are discussed in Chapter 10 and are also presented in Table 24.4. In addition to uncomplicated hypertension, they can also be used as monotherapy in the treatment of angina, arrhythmias, mitral valve prolapse, myocardial infarction, migraine headaches, performance anxiety, excessive sympathetic tone, or "thyroid storm" in hyperthyroidism (6).

Mechanism of Action The VSMs are lined with β_2-adrenoceptors that normally are activated by norepinephrine released from sympathetic adrenergic nerves or by circulating epinephrine. These receptors, like those in the heart, are coupled to a G_s protein, which stimulates the formation of cAMP. Although increased cAMP enhances cardiac contraction, with VSM an increase in cAMP leads to smooth muscle relaxation (Fig. 24.2). Therefore, increases in intracellular cAMP caused by β_2-agonists inhibit MLCK, thereby producing less contractile force (i.e., promoting relaxation). Inhibition of cardiac β_1- and β_2-adrenoceptors reduces the contractility of the myocardium (negative inotropic), decreasing heart rate (negative chronotropic), blocking sympathetic outflow from the central nervous system (CNS), and suppressing renin release (9). The antianginal and antiarrhythmic effects of the BBs are discussed in Chapter 21.

Therapeutic Applications (1,6,10) BBs decrease arterial blood pressure by reducing cardiac output. Many forms of hypertension are associated with an increase in blood volume and cardiac output. Therefore, reducing cardiac output by β-blockade can be an effective treatment for hypertension, especially when used in conjunction with a diuretic. Hypertension in some patients is caused by emotional stress, which causes enhanced sympathetic activity. BBs are very effective in these patients and are especially useful in treating hypertension caused by a pheochromocytoma, which results in elevated circulating catecholamines. BBs have an additional benefit as a treatment for hypertension in that they inhibit the release of renin by the kidneys (the release of which is partly regulated by a β_1-adrenoceptors in the kidney). Decreasing circulating plasma renin leads to a decrease

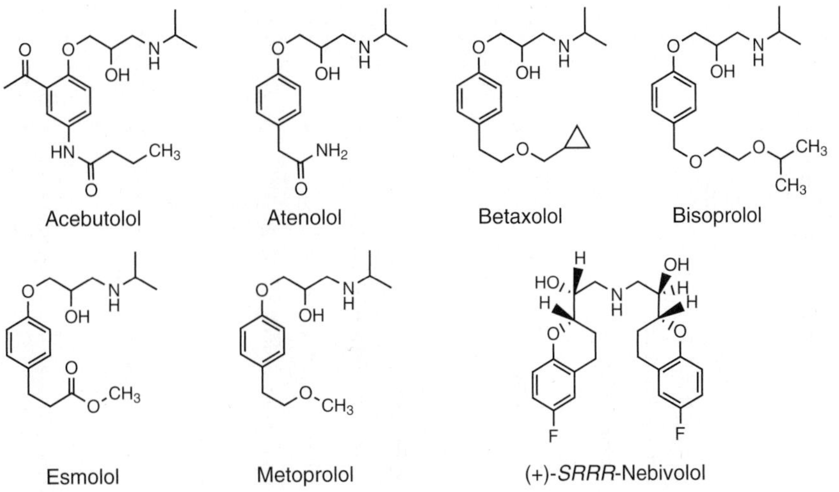

FIGURE 24.4 β_1-Selective adrenergic blockers.

TABLE 24.4 Pharmacologic/Pharmacokinetic Properties of Antihypertensive β-Adrenergic Blocking Agents

Drug	Adrenergic Receptor Blocking Activity	Membrane-Stabilizing Activity	Intrinsic Sympathomimetic activity	Lipophilicity[e] ($logD_{pH 7.4}$)	Extent of Absorption (%)	Absolute Oral Bioavailability (%)	Half-Life (h)	Protein Binding (%)	Metabolism/Excretion
Acebutolol (Sectral)	β_1[a]	+	+	−0.09	90	20–60	3–4	26	Hepatic; renal excretion 30%–40%, nonrenal excretion 50%–60% (bile)
Atenolol (Tenormin)	β_1[α]	0	0	−2.01	50	50–60	6–9	5–16	~50% excreted unchanged in feces
Betaxolol (Kerlone)	β_1[α]	0	0	2.4	~100	89	14–22	50	Hepatic; >80% recovered in urine, 15% unchanged
Bisoprolol (Zebeta)	β_1[α]	0	0	2.2	≥0	80	9–12	30	~50% excreted unchanged in urine, remainder as inactive metabolites; <2% excreted in feces
Esmolol (Brevibloc)	β_1[α]	0	0	1.7	NA	NA	0.15	55	Rapid metabolism by esterases in cytosol of red blood cells
Metoprolol (Lopressor)	β_1[α]	0[b]	0	−0.24	95	40–50	3–7	12	Hepatic; renal excretion, <5% unchanged
Metoprolol, LA			—	—	77	—			
Nebivolol (Bystolic)	β_1[α]	0	0	2.34	NA	12-fast metabolizers 96-poor metabolizers	12–19	98	Hepatic; glucuronidation, *N*-dealkylation and oxidation by CYP2D6 Renal: 38%–67%; <1% renal unchanged; fecal 13%–44%
Carteolol (Cartrol, Occupress)	β_1 β_2	0	+ +	−1.56	80	85	6	23–30	50%–70% excreted unchanged in urine
Levobunolol (Betagan)	β_1 β_2	0	0	0.19	NA	NA	NA	NA	Ophthalmic
Nadolol (Corgard)	β_1 β_2	0	0	−1.43	30	30–50	20–24	30	Urine, unchanged
Penbutolol (Levatol)	β_1 β_2	0	+	2.06	~100	>90	5	80–98	Hepatic (conjugation, oxidation); renal excretion of metabolites (17% as conjugate)
Pindolol (Visken)	β_1 β_2	+	+ + +	−0.36	95	>90	3–4[c]	40	Urinary excretion of metabolites (60%–65%) and unchanged drug (35%–40%)
Propranolol (Inderal)	β_1 β_2	+ +	0	1.41	90	30	3–5	90	Hepatic; <1% excreted unchanged in urine
Propranolol, LA						9–18	8–11		
Timolol (Blocadren, Timoptic)	β_1 β_2	0	0	0.03	90	75	4	10	Hepatic; urinary excretion of metabolites and unchanged drug
Labetalol[d] (Normodyne)	β_1 β_2 α_1	0	0	1.08	100	30–40	5.5–8.0	50	55%–60% excreted in urine as conjugates or unchanged drug
Carvedilol (Coreg)	β_1 β_2 α_1	0	0	3.53	>90	25–35	7–10	98	

[a]Inhibits β_2-receptors (bronchial and vascular) at higher doses.
[b]Detectable only at doses much greater than required for β-blockade.
[c]In elderly hypertensive patients with normal renal function; half-life variable, 7–15 h.
[d]Not labetalol monograph.
[e]Measured logD at pH 7.4 from Avdeef A. Absorption and Drug Development. Hoboken, NJ: Wiley-Interscience, 2003:59–66.
Adapted from Drug Facts and Comparison 2000; with permission.
NA, not applicable (available as intravenous only); 0, none; +, low; + +, moderate; + + +, high.

in angiotensin II and aldosterone, which enhances renal loss of sodium and water and further diminishes arterial pressure. Acute treatment with a BB is not very effective in reducing arterial pressure because of a compensatory increase in systemic vascular resistance. This can occur because of baroreceptor reflexes working in conjunction with the removal of β_2 vasodilatory influences that normally offset, to a small degree, α-adrenergic–mediated vascular tone. Chronic treatment with BB lowers arterial pressure more than acute treatment, possibly because of reduced renin release and effects of β-blockade on central and peripheral nervous systems.

Several of the nonselective BBs are also used to reduce intraocular pressure in the treatment of glaucoma. These include carteolol (Occupress), levobunolol (Betagan), and timolol (Timoptic).

The selection of oral BBs as monotherapy for stage 1 or 2 hypertension without compelling risk factors (Table 24.2) is based on several factors, including their cardioselectivity and preexisting conditions, ISA, lipophilicity, metabolism, and adverse effects (exception is esmolol) (Table 24.4). Esmolol is a very short-acting cardioselective β_1-blocker administered by infusion because of its rapid hydrolysis by plasma esterases to a rapidly excreted zwitterionic metabolite (plasma half-life, 9 minutes). After the discontinuation of esmolol infusion, blood pressure returns to preexisting conditions in approximately 30 minutes. The elderly hypertensive patient (age, ≥65 years) cannot tolerate or respond to these drugs because of their mechanism of lowering cardiac output and increasing systemic vascular resistance (11).

Adverse Effects Common adverse effects for the BBs include decreased exercise tolerance, cold extremities, depression, sleep disturbance, and impotence, although these side effects can be less severe with the β_1-selective blockers, such as metoprolol, atenolol, or bisoprolol (12). The use of lipid-soluble BBs, such as propranolol (Table 24.4), has been associated with more CNS side effects, such as dizziness, confusion, or depression (1,6). These side effects can be avoided, however, with the use of hydrophilic drugs, such as nadolol or atenolol. The use of β_1-selective drugs also helps to minimize adverse effects associated with β_2-blockade, including suppression of insulin release and increasing the chances for bronchospasms (asthma) (1,6). It is important to emphasize that none of the BBs, including the cardioselective ones, are cardiospecific. At high doses, these cardioselective BBs can still adversely affect asthma, peripheral vascular disease, and diabetes (1,6). Nonselective BB are contraindicated in patients with bronchospastic disease (asthma), and β_1-selective blockers should be used with caution in these patients. BBs with ISA, such as acebutolol, pindolol, carteolol, or penbutolol (Table 24.4), partially stimulate the β-receptor while also blocking it (13). The proposed advantages of BBs with ISA over those without ISA include less cardiodepression and resting bradycardia as well as neutral effects on lipid and glucose metabolism. Neither cardioselectivity nor ISA, however, influences the efficacy of BBs in lowering blood pressure (6).

Unlike the conventional cardioselective β_1-receptor blocker, nebivolol also exhibits NO-potentiating vasodilatory effect for the treatment of hypertension. Chemically, it is a mixture of stereoisomers (+)-nebivolol [(+)-*SRRR* nebivolol] and (−)-nebivolol [(−)-*RSSS* nebivolol] that differs chemically and pharmacologically from other BBs. The selective β_1-blocking effect is determined almost exclusively by the (+)-stereoisomer. The combination of (+)-nebivolol and (−)-nebivolol acts synergistically to produce a cardiovascular profile that differs noticeably from that of conventional BBs with respect to enhanced blood pressure reduction at lower doses. The drug is highly cardioselective at low doses, but at higher doses, it loses its cardioselectivity and blocks both β_1- and β_2-receptors. The (−)-stereoisomer has minimal effect on systolic and diastolic blood pressure. Nebivolol is unique among the conventional BBs by stimulating endothelial NO synthesis, thereby producing a sustained vasodilation in VSM, which results in decreased peripheral resistance and blood pressure. The (−)-stereoisomer indirectly increases NO availability by the inhibition of endothelial NO synthase, thereby reducing NO inactivation. Neither nebivolol nor its stereoisomers show any intrinsic sympathomimetic activity, without the undesirable BB effects, such as a decrease in cardiac output. Nebivolol is also not cardioselective when taken by patients who are poor CYP2D6 metabolizers of nebivolol (and other drugs). As many as 1 in 10 whites and even more blacks are poor CYP2D6 metabolizers and therefore would not be likely to benefit from nebivolol's cardioselectivity.

α_1-ADRENERGIC BLOCKERS The structures for the available α_1-receptor blockers are shown in Figure 24.5. These include prazosin ($logD_{7.4}$ = 1.70), doxazosin ($logD_{7.4}$ = 1.97), terazosin ($logD_{7.4}$ = 2.13), and alfuzosin ($logD_{7.4}$ = 0.87). The structure–activity relationships of these drugs were previously discussed in Chapter 10, along with their pharmacokinetics and metabolism.

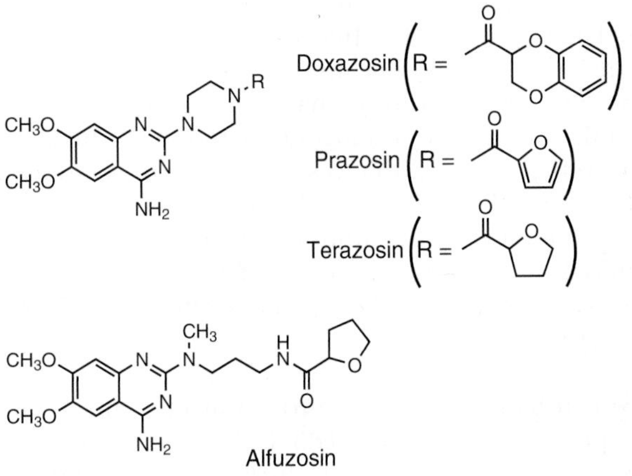

FIGURE 24.5 α_1-Selective adrenergic blockers.

Mechanism of Action These drugs block the effect of sympathetic nerves on blood vessels by selectively binding to α_1-adrenoceptors located on the VSM (Fig. 24.1), which then stimulate the G_q protein, activating smooth muscle contraction through the IP_3 signal transduction pathway. Most of these drugs act as competitive antagonists by competing with the binding of norepinephrine to α_1-adrenergic receptors on VSM. Some α-blockers are noncompetitive (e.g., phenoxybenzamine) (see Chapter 10), which greatly prolongs their action. Prejunctional α_2-adrenoceptors located on the sympathetic nerve terminals serve as a negative feedback mechanism for norepinephrine release.

α-Blockers dilate both arteries and veins, because both vessel types are innervated by sympathetic adrenergic nerves. The vasodilator effect is more pronounced, however, in the arterial resistance vessels. Because most blood vessels have some degree of sympathetic tone under basal conditions, these drugs are effective dilators. They are even more effective under conditions of elevated sympathetic activity (e.g., during stress) or during pathologic increases in circulating catecholamines caused by an adrenal gland tumor (pheochromocytoma) (9). α_2-Adrenoceptors are also abundant in the smooth muscle of the bladder neck and prostate and, when inhibited, cause relaxation of the bladder muscle, increasing urinary flow rates and the relief.

Therapeutic Applications (6,14) α_1-Blockers are effective agents for the initial management of hypertension and are especially advantageous for older men who also suffer from symptomatic benign prostatic hyperplasia. They have been shown to be as effective as other major classes of antihypertensives in lowering blood pressure in equivalent doses. α_1-Blockers possess a characteristic "first-dose" effect, which means that orthostatic hypotension frequently occurs with the first few doses of the drug. This side effect can be minimized by slowly increasing the dose and by administering the first few doses at bedtime.

Side Effects and Contraindications The most common side effects are related directly to α_1-adrenoceptor blockade. These side effects include dizziness, orthostatic hypotension (because of loss of reflex vasoconstriction on standing), nasal congestion (because of dilation of nasal mucosal arterioles), headache, and reflex tachycardia (especially with nonselective α-blockers). Fluid retention is also a problem that can be rectified by use of a diuretic in conjunction with the α_1-blocker. α-Blockers have not been shown to be beneficial in heart failure or angina and should not be used in these conditions.

MIXED α/β-BLOCKERS The two available mixed α/β-receptor blockers are carvedilol (15) and labetalol (16) (Fig. 24.6), and their structure–activity relationships were previously discussed in Chapter 10 along with their pharmacokinetics and metabolism (Table 24.4). The α-methyl substituent attached to the *N*-arylalkyl group appears to be responsible for the α-adrenergic blocking effect. Carvedilol is administered as its racemate; its *S*-(−)-enantiomer is both an α- and nonselective β-blocker, whereas its *R*-(+)-enantiomer is an α_1-blocker. Labetalol possesses two chiral centers and, therefore, is administered as a mixture of four stereoisomers, of which $R(CH_3)$,*R*(OH) is the active β-blocker diastereomer with minimal α_1-blocking activity and the $S(CH_3)$,*R*(OH) diastereomer is predominantly an α_1-blocker. The *R,R* diastereomer is also known as dilevalol, which was not approved by the FDA because of hepatotoxicity. The $S(CH_3)$,*S*(OH) and $R(CH_3)$,*S*(OH) diastereomers are both inactive. The comparative potency for labetalol reflects the fact that 25% of the diastereomeric mixture is the active *R,R*-diastereomer.

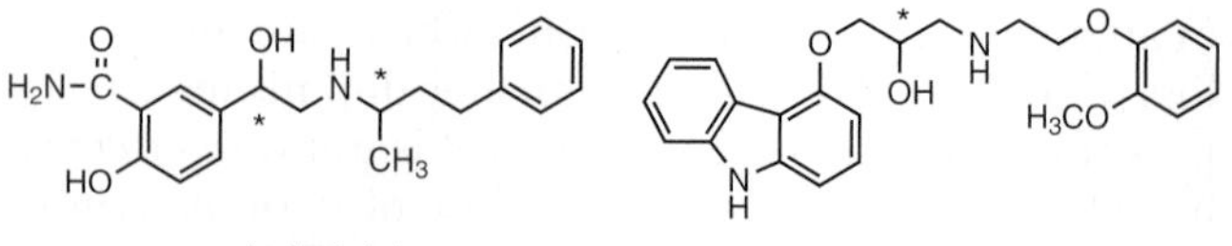

FIGURE 24.6 Mixed α/β-selective adrenergic blockers.

Mechanism of Action The mixed α/β-receptor blocking properties in the same molecule confer some advantages in the lowering of blood pressure. Vasodilation via α_1-blockade lowers peripheral vascular resistance to maintain cardiac output, thus preventing bradycardia more effectively when compared to BBs (17). β-Blockade helps to avoid the reflex tachycardia sometimes observed with the other vasodilators listed later in this chapter.

Therapeutic Applications Monotherapy with these mixed-acting antihypertensive drugs reduces blood pressure as effectively as other major antihypertensives and their combinations (15–17). Selection of mixed α/β-blockers is recommended for management of hypertension when the stage 2 family of drugs cannot be used alone or when a compelling indication (Table 24.2) is present that requires the use of a specific drug. Both drugs effectively lower blood pressure in essential and renal hypertension. Carvedilol is also effective in ischemic heart disease.

Adverse Effects Any adverse effects are usually related to β_1- or α_1-blockade. The β effects are usually less bothersome, because the α_1-blockade reduces the effects of β-blockade.

Centrally Acting Sympatholytics

The sympathetic adrenergic nervous system plays a major role in the regulation of arterial pressure. Activation of these nerves to the heart increases the heart rate (positive chronotropy), contractility (positive inotropy), and velocity of electrical impulse conduction (positive chronotropy). Within the medulla are located preganglionic sympathetic excitatory neurons, which travel from the spinal cord to the ganglia. They have significant basal activity, which generates a level of sympathetic tone to the heart and vasculature even under basal conditions. The sympathetic neurons within the medulla receive input from other neurons within the medulla, and together, these neuronal systems regulate sympathetic (and parasympathetic) outflow to the heart and vasculature. Sympatholytic drugs can block this sympathetic adrenergic system on three different levels. First, peripheral sympatholytic drugs, such as α-adrenoceptor and β-adrenoceptor antagonists, block the influence of norepinephrine at the effector organ (heart or blood vessel). Second, there are ganglionic blockers that block impulse transmission at the sympathetic ganglia. Third, centrally acting sympatholytic drugs block sympathetic activity within the brain. Centrally acting sympatholytics block sympathetic activity by binding to and activating α_2-adrenoceptors, which reduces sympathetic outflow to the heart, thereby decreasing cardiac output by decreasing heart rate and contractility. Reduced sympathetic output to the vasculature decreases sympathetic vascular tone, which causes vasodilation and reduced systemic vascular resistance, which in turn decreases arterial pressure.

Specific Drugs

Methyldopa and Methyldopate Ester Hydrochloride

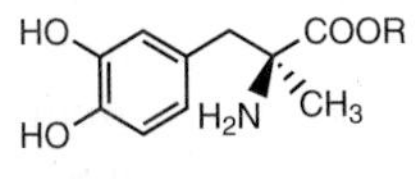

L-Methyldopa R = H
Methyldopate ethyl ester hydrochloride R = C_2H_5

Physicochemical Properties Methyldopa is structurally and chemically related to L-dihydroxyphenylalanine (L-DOPA) and the catecholamines. To increase its water solubility for parenteral administration, the zwitterion methyldopa is esterified and converted to its hydrochloride salt, methyldopate ethyl ester hydrochloride (referred to as methyldopate). Methyldopate ester hydrochloride is used to prepare parenteral solutions of methyldopa, having a pH in the range of 3.5 to 6.0. Methyldopa is unstable in the presence of oxidizing agents (i.e., air), alkaline pH, and light. Being related to the catecholamines, which are subject to air oxidation, metabisulfite/sulfite can be added to dosage formulations to prevent oxidation. Some patients, especially those with asthma, can exhibit sulfite-related hypersensitivity reactions. Methyldopate hydrochloride injection has been reported to be physically incompatible with drugs that are poorly soluble in an acidic medium (e.g., sodium salts of barbiturates and sulfonamides) and with drugs that are acid labile. Incompatibility depends on several factors (e.g., concentrations of the drugs, specific diluents used, resulting pH, and temperature).

Mechanism of Action As discussed in Chapter 10, the central mechanism for the antihypertensive activity of the prodrug methyldopa is not caused by its inhibition of norepinephrine biosynthesis but, rather, by its metabolism in the CNS to α-methylnorepinephrine, an α_2-adrenergic agonist (Fig. 24.7) (9). Other more powerful inhibitors of aromatic L-amino acid decarboxylase (e.g., carbidopa) have proven to be clinically useful, but not as antihypertensives. Rather, these agents are used to inhibit the metabolism of exogenous L-DOPA administered in the treatment of Parkinson disease (see Chapter 13).

The mechanism of the central hypotensive action for methyldopa is attributed to its transport into the CNS via an aromatic amino acid transport mechanism, where it is decarboxylated and hydroxylated into α-methylnorepinephrine (Fig. 24.7) (9). This active metabolite of methyldopa decreases total peripheral resistance, with little change in cardiac output and heart rate, through its stimulation of central inhibitory α_2-adrenoceptors. A reduction of plasma renin activity can also contribute to the hypotensive action of methyldopa. Postural hypotension and sodium and water retention are also effects related to a reduction in blood pressure. If a diuretic is not administered concurrently with methyldopa, tolerance to the antihypertensive effect of the methyldopa during prolonged therapy can result.

Pharmacokinetics (18) The oral bioavailability of methyldopa ranges from 20% to 50% and varies among individuals. Optimum blood pressure response occurs in 12 to 24 hours in most patients. After withdrawal of the drug, blood pressure returns to pretreatment levels within 24 to 48 hours. Methyldopa and its metabolites are weakly bound to plasma proteins. Although 95% of a dose of methyldopa is eliminated in hypertensive patients with normal

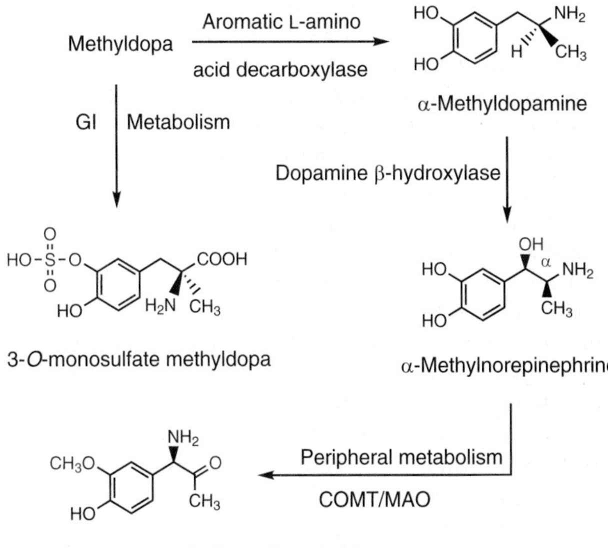

FIGURE 24.7 Metabolism of methyldopa.

renal function, with a plasma half-life of approximately 2 hours, in patients with impaired renal function, the half-life is doubled to approximately 3 to 4 hours, with about 50% of it excreted. Orally administered methyldopa undergoes presystemic first-pass metabolism in the gastrointestinal (GI) tract to its 3-*O*-monosulfate metabolite (Fig. 24.7). Sulfate conjugation occurs to a greater extent when the drug is given orally than when it is given intravenously (IV). Its rate of sulfate conjugation is decreased in patients with renal insufficiency. Methyldopa is excreted in urine as its mono-*O*-sulfate conjugate. Any peripherally decarboxylated α-methylnorepinephrine is metabolized by catechol-*O*-methyltransferase (COMT) and monoamine oxidase (MAO) (Fig. 24.7).

Methyldopate is slowly hydrolyzed in the body to form methyldopa. The hypotensive effect of IV methyldopate begins in 4 to 6 hours and lasts 10 to 16 hours.

Therapeutic Applications (1,6) Methyldopa is used in the management of moderate to severe hypertension and is reserved for patients who fail to achieve blood pressure goals with stage 2 drugs. Methyldopa is also coadministered with diuretics and other classes of antihypertensive drugs, permitting a reduction in the dosage of each drug and minimizing adverse effects while maintaining blood pressure control. Methyldopa has been used in the management of hypertension during pregnancy without apparent substantial adverse effects on the fetus and also for the management of pregnancy-induced hypertension (i.e., preeclampsia) (5).

Intravenous methyldopate can be used for the management of hypertension when parenteral hypotensive therapy is necessary. Because of its slow onset of action, however, other agents, such as sodium nitroprusside, are preferred when a parenteral hypotensive agent is employed for hypertensive emergencies.

Adverse Effects (6) The most common adverse effect for methyldopa is drowsiness, which occurs within the first 48 to 72 hours of therapy and can disappear with continued administration of the drug. Sedation commonly recurs when its dosage is increased. A decrease in mental acuity, including impaired ability to concentrate, lapses of memory, and difficulty in performing simple calculations, can occur and usually necessitates withdrawal of the drug. Patients should be warned that methyldopa can impair their ability to perform activities requiring mental alertness or physical coordination (e.g., operating machinery or driving a motor vehicle). Nightmares, mental depression, orthostatic hypotension, and symptoms of cerebrovascular insufficiency can occur during methyldopa therapy and are indications for dosage reduction. Orthostatic hypotension can be less pronounced with methyldopa than with guanethidine but can be more severe than with reserpine, clonidine, hydralazine, propranolol, or thiazide diuretics. Nasal congestion commonly occurs in patients receiving methyldopa. Positive direct antiglobulin (Coombs') test results have been reported in approximately 10% to 20% of patients receiving methyldopa, usually after 6 to 12 months of therapy. This phenomenon is dose related. Methyldopa should be used with caution in patients with a history of previous liver disease or dysfunction, and it should be stopped if unexplained drug-induced fever and jaundice occur. These effects commonly occur within 3 weeks after initiation of treatment.

Dosage forms of methyldopa and methyldopate can contain sulfites, which can cause allergic-type reactions, including anaphylaxis and life-threatening or less severe asthmatic episodes. These allergic reactions are observed more frequently in asthmatic than in nonasthmatic individuals. Methyldopa is contraindicated in patients receiving MAO inhibitors.

α_2-Adrenergic Agonists The mechanism of action, therapeutic applications, and adverse effects common to the α_2-adrenergic agonists clonidine, guanabenz, and guanfacine (Fig. 24.8) will be discussed together, but any significant differences between these specific agents will be included in the discussions of the individual drugs.

Agmatine (Fig 24.8), an aminoguanidine, is an endogenous neurotransmitter found in the brain with high affinity for the G protein–coupled imidazoline receptors, I_1 and I_2, α_2, and glutaminergic *N*-methyl-D-aspartate (NMDA) receptor channels, where it binds as an antagonist. It is biosynthesized by the decarboxylation of the amino acid, arginine, metabolized by agmatase to the polyamine, putrescine, which binds to NMDA receptor channels (Fig. 24.9). As a neurotransmitter, agmatine is stored in vesicles in neurons and released upon neuronal depolarization. It also irreversibly inhibits neuronal nitric oxide synthase. Agmatine is released from storage vesicles in response to stress (e.g., hypoxic-ischemia) and/or inflammation. The sympathoinhibition of agmatine involves α_2-adrenoceptors and imidazoline I_1 receptors. Despite binding like clonidine to α_2-adrenergic receptors and imidazoline I_1 and I_2 receptors, agmatine does not replicate the central

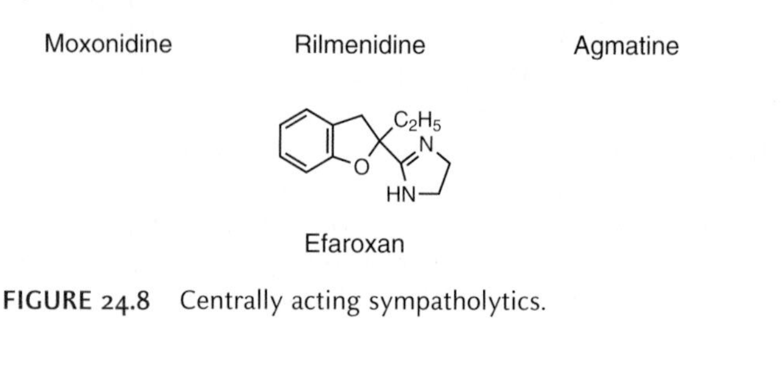

FIGURE 24.8 Centrally acting sympatholytics.

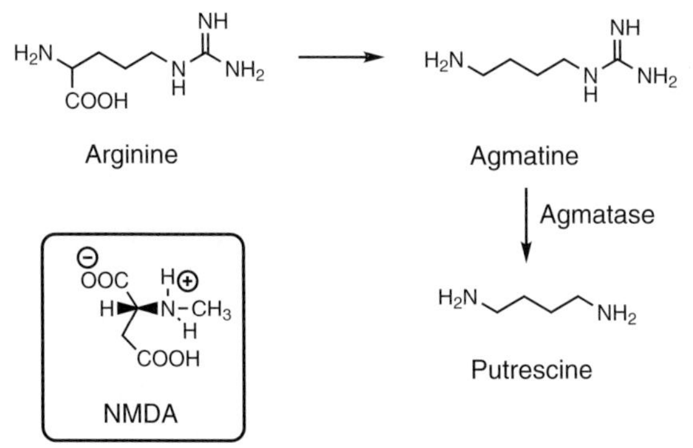

FIGURE 24.9 Biosynthesis and metabolism of agmatine.

or peripheral actions of clonidine. Agmatine appears to be a CNS endogenous neurotransmitter or neuromodulator (not reabsorbed by the presynaptic neuron or metabolized into inactive products) in stress-related disorders, such as depression, anxiety, and posttraumatic stress disorder. Although the physiologic role of agmatine in normal brain function is still unknown, it also blocks the development of morphine tolerance and exhibits antidepressant-like effects in depression models. Agmatine, administered intracerebroventricular or intraperitoneal in animal models, has not been shown to lower arterial pressure, thus ruling out the possibility of α_2-adrenergic receptor activation in this action of agmatine.

Mechanism of Action The overall mechanism of action for the centrally active sympatholytics, clonidine, guanabenz, and guanfacine, appears to be stimulation of α_2-adrenoceptors and specific binding to nonadrenergic imidazoline I_1 receptors in the CNS (mainly in the medulla oblongata), causing inhibition of sympathetic output (sympathoinhibition) (19,20). This effect results in reduced peripheral and renovascular resistance and leads to a decrease in systolic and diastolic blood pressure. Through the use of imidazoline and α_2-adrenergic antagonists, specific I_1 receptors have recently been characterized in CNS control of blood pressure (21). The I_1 receptors are pharmacologically distinct from α_2-receptors, because they are not activated by catecholamines but characterized by their high affinity for 2-iminoimidazolines (or 2-aminoimidazolines) and low affinity for guanidines (21). Thus, the central hypotensive action for clonidine, other 2-aminoimidazolines, and structurally related compounds needs both the I_1 and α_2-adrenoceptors to produce their central sympatholytic response (20). As a result of this discovery, a new generation of centrally acting antihypertensive agents selective for the I_1 receptor has been developed and includes moxonidine (a pyrimidinyl aminoimidazoline) and rilmenidine (an alkylaminooxazoline) (Fig. 24.8). Rilmenidine and moxonidine are both highly selective for the I_1 receptor while having low affinity for α_2-adrenoceptors, and both control blood pressure effectively without the adverse effects associated with binding to α_2-receptors (e.g., sedation, bradycardia, and mental depression) (20). Clonidine appears to be more selective for α_2-adrenoceptors than for I_1 receptors. Another antihypertensive is efaroxan, which exhibits good affinity for I_1 receptor but is an antagonist at α_2-receptors.

Pharmacokinetics The effective oral dose range for rilmenidine is 1 to 3 mg, with a dose-dependent duration of action of 10 to 20 hours. Moxonidine is administered once a day at a dose range of 0.2 to 0.4 mg. The oral bioavailability of moxonidine in humans is greater than 90%, with approximately 40% to 50% of the oral dose excreted unmetabolized in the urine (22,23). The principal route of metabolism for moxonidine is oxidation of the 2-methyl group in the pyrimidine ring to 2-hydroxymethyl and 2-carboxylic acid derivative as well as the formation of corresponding glucuronides. After an oral dose of moxonidine, peak hypotensive effects occur within 2 hours, with an elimination half-life of greater than 8 hours (23,24). Rilmenidine is readily absorbed from the GI tract, with an oral bioavailability greater than 95%. It is poorly metabolized and is excreted unchanged in the urine, with an elimination half-life of 8 hours (25,26).

After IV or oral administration of these drugs in normotensive patients, an initial hypertensive response to the drug occurs that is caused by activation of the peripheral α_2-adrenoceptors and the resulting vasoconstriction. This response is not observed, however, in patients with hypertension.

Therapeutic Applications (1,6) The selection of these drugs for monotherapy or in the combination therapy is based on several factors, including their similar mechanism of action, preexisting or compelling conditions, pharmacokinetics, distribution, and metabolism. The α_2-adrenergic antagonists show a similarity in adverse effects.

Clonidine, guanabenz, and guanfacine are used in the management of mild to moderate hypertension or when stage 2 drugs have been ineffective in achieving blood pressure goals (1,6). They have been used as monotherapy or to achieve lower dosages in combination with other classes of antihypertensive agents. The centrally acting sympatholytics are generally reserved for patients who fail to respond to therapy with a stage 1 drug (e.g., diuretics, β-adrenergic blocking agents, ACEIs, or ARBs). Clonidine, guanabenz, and guanfacine can be used in combination with diuretics and other stage 1 hypotensive agents, permitting a reduction in the dosage of each drug, which minimizes adverse effects while maintaining blood pressure control. Geriatric patients, however, cannot tolerate the adverse cognitive effects of these sympatholytics. All three drugs reduce blood pressure to essentially the same extent in both supine and standing patients; thus, orthostatic effects are mild and infrequently encountered. Exercise does not appear to affect the blood pressure response to guanabenz and guanfacine in patients with hypertension. Plasma renin activity can be unchanged or reduced during long-term therapy with these drugs.

Adverse Effects (6) Overall, the frequency of adverse effects produced by clonidine, guanabenz, and guanfacine are similar and appear to be dose related. Drowsiness, tiredness, dizziness, weakness, bradycardia, headache, and dry mouth are common adverse effects for patients receiving clonidine, guanabenz, and guanfacine. The sedative effect for these centrally acting sympatholytics can result from their central α_2-agonist activity. The dry mouth induced by these drugs can result from a combination of central and peripheral α_2-adrenoceptor mechanisms, and the decreased salivation can involve inhibition of cholinergic transmission via stimulation of peripheral α_2-adrenoceptors. Orthostatic hypotension does not appear to be a significant problem with these drugs, because there appears to be little difference between supine and standing systolic and diastolic blood pressures in most patients. Other adverse effects include increased urinary frequency (nocturia), urinary retention, sexual dysfunction (e.g., decreased libido, erectile dysfunction, and impotence), nasal congestion, tinnitus, blurred vision, and dry eyes. These symptoms most often occur within the first few weeks of therapy and tend to diminish with continued therapy, or they can be relieved by a reduction in dosage. Although adverse effects of the drug are generally not severe, discontinuance of therapy has been necessary in some patients because of intolerable sedation or dry mouth. Sodium and fluid retention can be avoided or relieved by administration of a diuretic.

Drug Interactions (6) The hypotensive actions for clonidine, guanabenz, and guanfacine can be additive with, or can potentiate the action of, other CNS depressants, such as opiates or other analgesics, barbiturates or other sedatives, anesthetics, or alcohol. Coadministration of opiate analgesics with clonidine can also potentiate the hypotensive effects of clonidine. Tricyclic antidepressants (i.e., imipramine and desipramine) have reportedly inhibited the hypotensive effect of clonidine, guanabenz, and guanfacine, and the increase in blood pressure usually occurs during the second week of tricyclic antidepressant therapy. Dosage should be increased to adequately control hypertension if necessary. Sudden withdrawal of clonidine, guanabenz, and guanfacine can result in an excess of circulating catecholamines; therefore, caution should be exercised in concomitant use of drugs that affect the metabolism or tissue uptake of these amines (MAO inhibitors or tricyclic antidepressants, respectively). Because clonidine, guanabenz, and guanfacine can produce bradycardia, the possibility of additive effects should be considered if these drugs are given concomitantly with other drugs, such as hypotensive drugs or cardiac glycosides.

Specific Drugs

Clonidine. Clonidine is an aryl-2-aminoimidazoline that is more selective for α_2-adrenoceptors than for I_1 receptors (Fig. 24.8) in producing its hypotensive effect. It is available as oral tablets, injection, or a transdermal system.

Mechanism of Action. In addition to its central stimulation of I_1 receptors and α_2-adrenoceptors (20,21), clonidine (as well as other α_2-adrenergic agonists), when administered epidurally, produces analgesia by stimulation of spinal α_2-adrenoceptors, inhibiting sympathetically mediated pain pathways that are activated by nociceptive stimuli, thus preventing transmission of pain signals to the brain (9) (also see Chapter 20). The administration of clonidine, while blocking opiate withdrawal, causes sympathetic inhibition and reduction in arterial pressure. The actions of clonidine on morphine pain response and withdrawal are most likely mediated by its ability to block NMDA receptor channels. Analgesia resulting from clonidine therapy is not antagonized by opiate antagonists. Activation of α_2-adrenoceptors also apparently stimulates acetylcholine release and inhibits the release of substance P, an inflammatory neuropeptide.

Pharmacokinetics. Clonidine has an oral bioavailability of more than 90%, with a $\log D_{7.4}$ of 1.82. It is well absorbed when applied topically to the eye and is well absorbed percutaneously following topical application of a transdermal system to the arm or chest (27–29). Following application of a clonidine transdermal patch, therapeutic plasma concentrations are attained within 2 to 3 days. Studies have indicated that release of clonidine from the patch averages from 50% to 70% after 7 days of wear. Plasma clonidine concentrations attained with the transdermal systems are generally similar to twice-daily oral dosing regimens of the drug. Percutaneous absorption of the drug from the upper arm or chest is similar, but less drug is absorbed from the thigh (29). Replacement of the transdermal system at a different site at weekly intervals continuously maintains therapeutic plasma clonidine concentrations. After discontinuance of transdermal therapy, therapeutic plasma drug concentrations persist for approximately 8 hours and then decline slowly over several days; over this time period, blood pressure returns gradually to pretreatment levels.

Blood pressure begins to decrease within 30 to 60 minutes after an oral dose of clonidine, with the maximum decrease in approximately 2 to 4 hours (6). The hypotensive effect lasts up to 8 hours. Following epidural administration of a single bolus dose of clonidine, it is rapidly absorbed into the systemic circulation and into cerebrospinal fluid (CSF), with maximal analgesia within 30 to 60 minutes. Although the CSF is not the presumed site of action of clonidine-mediated analgesia, the drug appears to diffuse rapidly from the CSF to the dorsal horn of the spinal cord. After oral administration, clonidine appears to be well distributed throughout the body, with the lowest concentration in the brain. Clonidine is approximately 20% to 40% bound to plasma proteins, and it crosses the placenta. The plasma half-life of clonidine is 6 to 20 hours in patients with normal renal

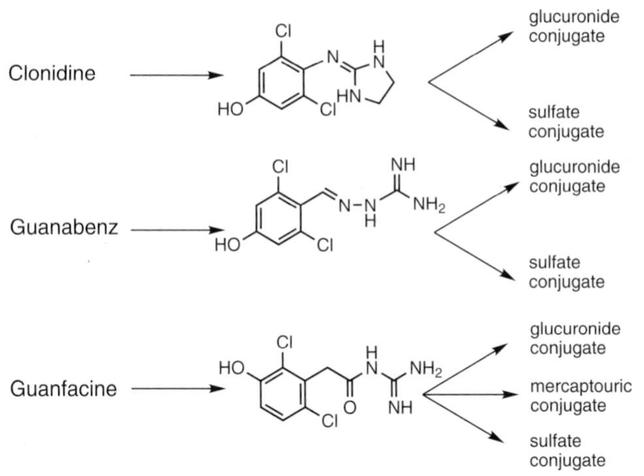

FIGURE 24.10 Metabolites formed from clonidine, guanabenz, and guanfacine.

function and 18 to 41 hours in patients with impaired renal function. Clonidine is metabolized in the liver to its inactive major metabolite 4-hydroxyclonidine and its glucuronide and sulfate conjugates (10% to 20%) (Fig. 24.10). In humans, 40% to 60% of an oral or IV dose of clonidine is excreted in urine as unchanged drug within 24 hours. Approximately 85% of a single dose is excreted within 72 hours, with 20% of the dose excreted in feces, probably via enterohepatic circulation.

Therapeutic Applications (6). Clonidine is administered twice a day for the management of mild to moderate hypertension in those patients not achieving the blood pressure goal with stage 2 drugs (6). Transdermal clonidine has also been successfully substituted for oral clonidine in some patients with mild to moderate hypertension whose compliance with a daily dosing regimen can be a problem (28).

When administered by epidural infusion, clonidine is used as adjunct therapy in combination with opiates for the management of severe cancer pain not relieved by opiate analgesics alone. Other nonhypertensive uses for clonidine include the prophylaxis of migraine headaches, the treatment of severe dysmenorrhea, menopausal flushing, rapid detoxification in the management of opiate withdrawal in opiate-dependent individuals, in conjunction with benzodiazepines for the management of alcohol withdrawal, and for the treatment of tremors associated with the adverse effects of methylphenidate in patients with attention-deficit hyperactivity disorder (ADHD). Clonidine has been used to reduce intraocular pressure in the treatment of open-angle and secondary glaucoma.

Clonidine, a nonstimulant drug, is also used in reducing the symptoms of ADHD and bipolar disorders, whose mechanism of action is thought to regulate norepinephrine release from the locus ceruleus, part of the brain stem involved with physiologic responses to stress and panic. Clonidine can also reduce symptoms of aggression as with patients with bipolar disorders and reduce the insomnia associated with CNS stimulants such as methylphenidate. Once stabilized, children on larger doses can be switched to the transdermal clonidine patch.

Adverse Effects (6). Adverse effects occurring with transdermal clonidine generally appear to be similar to those occurring with oral therapy (28,29). They have been mild and have tended to diminish with continued treatment. Hypotension has occurred in patients receiving clonidine by epidural infusion as adjunct therapy with epidural morphine for the treatment of cancer pain. With the transdermal system, localized skin reactions, such as erythema and pruritus, have occurred in some patients. The use of clonidine and methylphenidate in combination for managing ADHD can adversely affect cardiac conduction and increase risk for arrhythmias. ADHD patients need to be closely monitored and screened for a patient or family history of rhythm disturbances, and periodic monitoring of blood pressure, heart rate, and rhythm is recommended.

Within 2 to 3 hours following the abrupt withdrawal of oral clonidine therapy, a rapid increase in systolic and diastolic blood pressures occurs, and blood pressures can exceed pretreatment levels. Associated with the clonidine withdrawal syndrome, the symptoms observed include nervousness, agitation, restlessness, anxiety, insomnia, headache, sweating, palpitations, increased heart rate, tremor, and increased salivation. The exact mechanism of the withdrawal syndrome following discontinuance of α_2-adrenergic agonists has not been determined but can involve increased concentrations of circulating catecholamines, increased sensitivity of adrenoceptors, enhanced renin-angiotensin system activity, decreased vagal function, failure of autoregulation of cerebral blood flow, and failure of central α_2-adrenoceptor mechanisms to regulate sympathetic outflow from the CNS (6). The clonidine withdrawal syndrome is more pronounced after abrupt cessation of long-term therapy and with administration of high oral dosages (>1.2 mg daily). Withdrawal symptoms have been reported following discontinuance of transdermal therapy or when absorption of the drug is impaired because of dermatologic changes (e.g., contact dermatitis) under the transdermal system. Epidural clonidine can prolong the duration of the pharmacologic effects, including both sensory and motor blockade, of epidural local anesthetics.

Guanabenz Acetate. Guanabenz, a centrally active hypotensive agent, is pharmacologically related to clonidine but differs structurally from clonidine by the presence of an aminoguanidine side chain rather than an aminoimidazoline ring (Fig. 24.8). Guanabenz (pK_a = 8.1; log$D_{7.4}$ = 2.42) is largely (~80%) in the nonionized, lipid-soluble base form. Guanabenz can be given as a single daily dose administered at bedtime to minimize adverse effects.

Pharmacokinetics (30). The oral bioavailability of guanabenz is 70% to 80%. After an oral dose, the hypotensive effect of guanabenz begins within 1 hour, peaks within

2 to 7 h, and is diminished within 6 to 8 hours. It has an elimination half-life averaging 4 to 14 hours. The blood pressure response can persist for at least 12 hours. After IV dosing, guanabenz is distributed into the CNS, with brain concentrations 3 to 70 times higher than concurrent plasma concentrations. Guanabenz is approximately 90% bound to plasma proteins. In patients with hepatic or renal impairment, its elimination half-life can be prolonged.

Guanabenz is metabolized principally by hydroxylation to its inactive metabolite, 4-hydroxyguanabenz, which is eliminated in the urine as its glucuronide (major) and sulfate conjugates (Fig. 24.10). Guanabenz and its inactive metabolites are excreted principally in urine, with approximately 70% to 80% of its oral dose excreted in urine within 24 hours and approximately 10% to 30% excreted in feces via enterohepatic cycling. Approximately 40% of an oral dose of guanabenz is excreted in urine as 4-hydroxyguanabenz and its glucuronide, and less than 5% is excreted unchanged. The remainder is excreted as unidentified metabolites and their conjugates.

Therapeutic Applications (6,30). The therapeutic applications for guanabenz are similar to those of clonidine and other α_2-adrenergic agonists. One advantage for guanabenz is its once-a-day dosing schedule. Guanabenz has been used in diabetic patients with hypertension without adverse effect on the control of or therapy for diabetes, and it has been effective in hypertensive patients with chronic obstructive pulmonary disease, including asthma, chronic bronchitis, or emphysema. Guanabenz has been used alone or in combination with naltrexone in the management of opiate withdrawal in patients physically dependent on opiates and undergoing detoxification. Guanabenz has also been used as an analgesic in a limited number of patients with chronic pain.

Adverse Effects (6,30). Overall, the frequency of adverse effects produced by guanabenz is similar to that produced by clonidine and the other α_2-adrenergic agonists, but the incidence is lower. As with the other centrally active sympatholytics (e.g., clonidine), abrupt withdrawal of guanabenz can result in rebound hypertension, but the withdrawal syndrome symptoms appear to be less severe.

Guanfacine Hydrochloride. Guanfacine, a phenylacetyl guanidine derivative ($pK_a = 7.1$; $logD_{7.4} = 1.52$) (Fig. 24.8), is a centrally acting sympatholytic that is more selective for α_2-adrenoceptors than is clonidine. Its mechanism of action is similar to clonidine and is an effective alternative to that of the other centrally acting antihypertensive drugs. Although guanfacine is 5- to 20-fold less potent than clonidine on a weight basis, comparable blood pressure–lowering effects have been achieved when the two drugs were given in equipotent dosages. Its relatively long elimination half-life permits a once-a-day dosing schedule. Guanfacine activates peripheral α_2-adrenoceptors because a transient increase in blood pressure is observed in normotensive, but not in hypertensive, patients.

Pharmacokinetics (31–33). The pharmacokinetic properties for guanfacine differ from those of clonidine, guanabenz, and α-methyldopa. At pH 7.4, guanfacine is predominately (67%) in the nonionized, lipid-soluble base form, which accounts for its high oral bioavailability (>80%). Following an oral dose, peak plasma concentrations occur in 1 to 4 hours, with a relatively long elimination half-life of 14 to 23 hours. The maximum blood pressure response occurs in 8 to 12 hours after oral administration and is maintained up to 36 hours after its discontinuation. After IV dosing, guanfacine achieves the highest concentrations in liver and kidney, with low concentrations in the brain. Guanfacine is 64% bound to plasma proteins. In patients with hepatic or renal impairment, its elimination half-life can be prolonged.

Guanfacine is metabolized principally by hepatic hydroxylation to its inactive metabolite, 3-hydroxyguanfacine (20%), which is eliminated in the urine as its glucuronide (30%), sulfate (8%), or mercapturic acid conjugate (10%), and 24% to 37% is excreted as unchanged guanfacine (Fig. 24.10). Its nearly complete bioavailability suggests no evidence of any first-pass effect. Guanfacine and its inactive metabolites are excreted principally in urine, with approximately 80% of its oral dose excreted in urine within 48 hours.

Therapeutic Applications (6,32). The therapeutic applications for guanfacine are similar to those of the other centrally acting α_2-adrenergic agonists and methyldopa. It has been effective as monotherapy in the treatment of patients with mild to moderate hypertension. One advantage for guanfacine is its once-a-day dosing schedule. The use of diuretics to prevent accumulation of fluid can allow a reduction in the dosage for guanfacine. Somnolence and sedation were commonly reported adverse events in clinical trials. The most common adverse events associated with guanfacine treatment include somnolence/sedation, abdominal pain, dizziness, hypotension/decreased blood pressure, dry mouth, and constipation.

Guanfacine extended-release tablets (Intuniv) have been FDA approved for the non-stimulant treatment of ADHD in children and adolescents age 6 to 17 years. Although the mechanism of action for treatment of ADHD is unknown, guanfacine is thought to directly bind to postsynaptic α_2-adrenoceptors in the prefrontal cortex of the brain, an area of the brain that has been linked to ADHD. Stimulation of these adrenoceptors is theorized to strengthen working memory, reduce susceptibility to distraction, improve attention regulation, improve behavioral inhibition, and enhance impulse control. Guanfacine treatment can cause decreases in blood pressure and heart rate, which can lead to syncope. This drug should be used with caution in ADHD patients with a history of hypotension, heart block, bradycardia, cardiovascular disease, syncope, orthostatic hypotension, or dehydration and should be used with caution in patients being treated concomitantly with antihypertensive agents or other drugs that reduce blood pressure or heart rate or increase the risk of syncope. Guanfacine extended-release tablets should not be crushed, chewed, or broken before they are swallowed and not substituted for immediate-release tablets. ADHD patients should be reevaluated periodically for the long-term usefulness of this drug. When ADHD therapy with guanfacine is discontinued, the dose should be tapered over a period of 7 days.

Adverse Effects (6,32). Overall, although the frequency of troublesome adverse effects produced by guanfacine is similar to that produced by clonidine and the other centrally acting sympatholytics, their incidence and severity are lower with guanfacine. Unlike clonidine, abrupt discontinuation of guanfacine rarely results in rebound hypertension. When a withdrawal syndrome has occurred, its onset was slower and its symptoms less severe than the syndrome observed with clonidine.

Metyrosine.

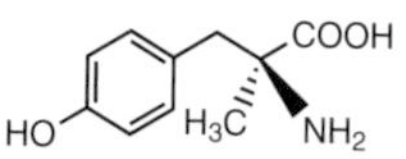

Metyrosine

Hypothetically, inhibitors of any of the three enzymes involved in the conversion of L-tyrosine to norepinephrine (see Fig. 10.1) could be used as drugs to moderate adrenergic transmission. Inhibitors of the rate-limiting enzyme tyrosine hydroxylase would be the most logical choice. One inhibitor of tyrosine hydroxylase, metyrosine or α-methyl-L-tyrosine, a competitive inhibitor of tyrosine hydroxylase, is in limited clinical use to help control hypertensive episodes caused by excess catecholamine biosynthesis. The drug can also control other symptoms of catecholamine overproduction in patients with the rare adrenal tumor pheochromocytoma. Although metyrosine is useful in treating hypertension associated with pheochromocytoma, it is not useful for treating essential hypertension. The drug metyrosine is the *S*-enantiomer of α-methyltyrosine. The *R*-enantiomer does not bind to the active site of tyrosine hydroxylase and, thus, has no useful pharmacologic activity.

Adrenergic Neuron Blocking Agents

Reserpine, bretylium, guanethidine and guanadrel are four drugs with similar mechanisms of action involving norepinephrine storage granules. These drugs are transported into the adrenergic neurons by uptake-1, where they bind to the storage vesicles and prevent release of neurotransmitter in response to a neuronal impulse. Reserpine, guanethidine, and guanadrel are orally active antihypertensives that actually replace norepinephrine in the storage vesicles, resulting in a slow release in the amount of norepinephrine that is present. At usual doses, guanethidine and guanadrel act as "false neurotransmitters" in that they are released into the synapse but do not effectively stimulate the receptors. At higher acute doses, their principal mechanism is a poorly understood inhibition of neurotransmitter release. Bretylium is a quaternary ammonium salt and must be given IV, because it has poor oral absorption. Initially, it can cause a release of norepinephrine and a transient rise in blood pressure, but its clinical utility is limited to cardiac arrhythmias and so will not be discussed in this chapter (see Chapter 21).

Reserpine

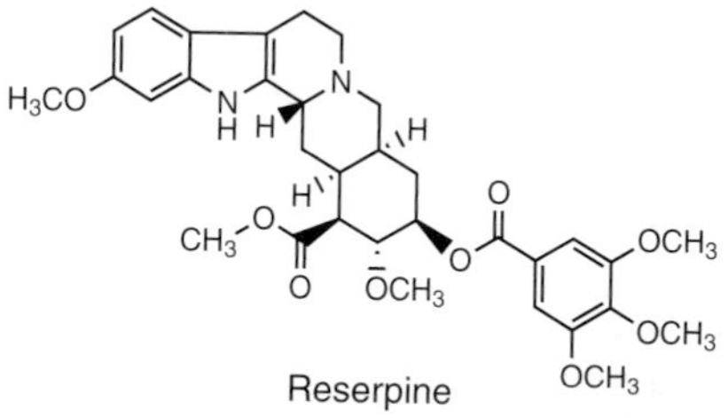

Reserpine

An old and historically important drug that affects the storage and release of norepinephrine is reserpine. Reserpine (p*Ka* = 6.6; $\log D_{7.4}$ = 3.14) is one of several indole alkaloids isolated from the roots of *Rauwolfia serpentina*; these roots were used in India for centuries both as a remedy for snake bites and as a sedative. The antihypertensive effects of the root extracts were first reported in India in 1918 and in the West in 1949. Shortly thereafter, reserpine was isolated and identified as the principal active agent. Reserpine was the first effective antihypertensive drug introduced into Western medicine, but it has largely been replaced in clinical use by agents with fewer side effects.

Mechanism of Action (9) Reserpine acts to replace and deplete the adrenergic neurons of their stores of norepinephrine by inhibiting the active transport Mg-ATPase responsible for sequestering norepinephrine and dopamine within the storage vesicles. The norepinephrine and dopamine that are not sequestered in vesicles are destroyed by MAO. As a result, the storage vesicles contain little neurotransmitter, adrenergic transmission is dramatically inhibited, and sympathetic tone is decreased, leading to vasodilation. Reserpine has the same effect on epinephrine storage in the adrenal medulla. Reserpine readily enters the CNS, where it also depletes the stores of norepinephrine and serotonin. The CNS neurotransmitter depletion led to the use of reserpine in treating certain mental illnesses.

Pharmacokinetics (6,9) Limited information is available regarding the pharmacokinetics of reserpine. Peak blood concentrations for reserpine occur within 2 hours following oral administration, and the full effects for reserpine are usually delayed for at least 2 to 3 weeks. Both CNS and cardiovascular effects can persist for several days to several weeks after chronic oral therapy is discontinued.

Reserpine appears to be widely distributed in body tissues, especially adipose tissue; crosses the blood–brain barrier and the placenta; and is distributed into milk. The elimination of reserpine appears to be biphasic, with a plasma half-life averaging 4.5 hours during the first phase and approximately 11.3 days during the second phase. Reserpine is metabolized to unidentified inactive compounds. Unchanged reserpine and its metabolites are excreted slowly in urine and feces, with an average of 60% reserpine recovered in feces within 96 hours after oral administration of 0.25 mg of radiolabeled reserpine.

Therapeutic Application (6) Reserpine has been used in the management of mild to moderate hypertension, but because of very significant CNS adverse effects and its cumulative action in the adrenergic neurons, reserpine is rarely used. Reserpine and related *Rauwolfia* alkaloids have been used in the symptomatic treatment of agitated psychotic states, such as schizophrenic disorders, although other antipsychotic agents have generally replaced reserpine and the alkaloids.

Adverse Effects (6) The common adverse CNS effects for reserpine include drowsiness, fatigue, and lethargy. Mental depression is one of the most serious potential adverse effects for reserpine, which can be severe enough to require hospitalization or result in suicide attempts. Reserpine-induced depression can persist for several months after the drug is discontinued.

GUANETHIDINE MONOSULFATE

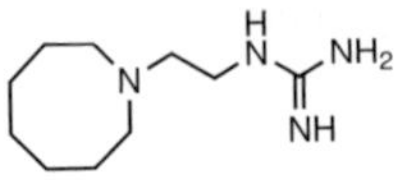

Guanethidine

Guanethidine contains two basic nitrogen atoms with pK_a values of 9.0 and 12.0 and, therefore, can form guanethidine monosulfate ($C_{10}H_{22}N_4 \cdot H_2SO_4$) or guanethidine sulfate [$(C_{10}H_{22}N_4)_2 \cdot H_2SO_4$] salts. Caution should be exercised when interchanging between these sulfate forms, because the potency of guanethidine can be expressed in terms of guanethidine sulfate or guanethidine monosulfate, a significant difference in molecular weight.

Mechanism of Action Guanethidine is an adrenergic neuronal blocking agent that produces a selective block of peripheral sympathetic pathways by replacing and depleting norepinephrine stores from adrenergic nerve endings, but not from the adrenal medulla (6,9). It prevents the release of norepinephrine from adrenergic nerve endings in response to sympathetic nerve stimulation. The chronic administration of guanethidine results in an increased sensitivity of these effector cells to catecholamines. Following the oral administration of usual doses of guanethidine, depletion of the catecholamine stores from adrenergic nerve endings occurs at a very slow rate, producing a more gradual and prolonged fall in systolic blood pressure than in diastolic pressure. Associated with the decrease in blood pressure is an increase in sodium and water retention and expansion of plasma volume (edema). If a diuretic is not administered concurrently with guanethidine, tolerance to the antihypertensive effect of the guanethidine during prolonged therapy can result.

Pharmacokinetics (6) Guanethidine is incompletely absorbed ($\log D_{7.4}$ = –0.24) from the GI tract and is metabolized in the liver to several metabolites, including guanethidine *N*-oxide from flavin mononucleotide. These metabolites of guanethidine are excreted in the urine and have less than 10% of its hypotensive activity. The amount of drug that reaches the systemic circulation after oral administration is highly variable from patient to patient and can range from 3% to 50% of a dose. Guanethidine accumulates in the neurons with an elimination half-life of 5 days.

Therapeutic Applications (6) Guanethidine is used in the management of moderate to severe hypertension and in the management of renal hypertension. Guanethidine is for patients with compelling indications or who fail to respond adequately to an antihypertensive regimen that includes stage 2 drugs. Its coadministration with other hypotensive agents permits a reduction in the dosage of each drug and a minimization of adverse effects while maintaining blood pressure control. It has been administered as ophthalmic drops in the treatment of chronic open-angle glaucoma and for endocrine ophthalmopathy, ophthalmoplegia, lid lag, and lid retraction.

Adverse Effects (6) Adverse effects of guanethidine frequently are dose related, including dizziness, weakness, lassitude, and syncope resulting from postural or postexercise hypotension. A hot environment (i.e., a hot bath) can aggravate postural hypotension. Patients should be warned about possible orthostatic hypotension and about the effect of rapid postural changes on blood pressure (e.g., arising in the morning) that can cause fainting, especially during the initial period of dosage adjustment. Sodium retention (edema) is usually controlled by the coadministration of a diuretic.

Drug Interactions (6) Diuretics and other hypotensive drugs can potentiate the hypotensive effects of guanethidine. Reportedly, MAO inhibitors antagonize the hypotensive effect of guanethidine. Oral sympathomimetics, nasal decongestants, and other vasopressor agents should be used cautiously in patients receiving guanethidine, because guanethidine can potentiate their pressor effects. The mydriatic response to ophthalmic administration of phenylephrine is markedly increased in patients receiving guanethidine either ophthalmically or orally. Tricyclic antidepressants and some phenothiazines block the uptake of guanethidine into adrenergic neurons and, thus, prevent the hypotensive activity of guanethidine. Orthostatic hypotension can be increased by concomitant administration of alcohol with guanethidine, and patients receiving guanethidine should be cautioned to limit alcohol intake.

GUANADREL SULFATE

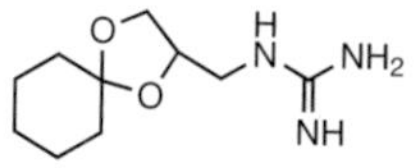

Guanadrel

Guanadrel sulfate is an adrenergic neuronal blocking agent that is structurally and pharmacologically related to guanethidine: Both are guanidine derivatives. Guanadrel ($logD_{7.4}$ = −4.80) differs structurally from guanethidine by the presence of a dioxaspirodecyl ring system linked to guanidine by a methyl group rather than a hexahydroazocinyl ring linked by an ethyl group.

Mechanism of Action Guanadrel, like guanethidine, produces a selective block of efferent, peripheral sympathetic pathways by replacing and depleting norepinephrine stores from adrenergic nerve endings, thus preventing the release of norepinephrine from adrenergic nerve endings in response to sympathetic nerve stimulation (9,34). Unlike guanethidine, it does not release norepinephrine from the adrenal medulla and reportedly depletes norepinephrine stores in the GI tract to a lesser extent than guanethidine does. Guanadrel decreases systolic blood pressure more than diastolic blood pressure.

Pharmacokinetics (34) Guanadrel, unlike guanethidine, is rapidly and almost completely absorbed following oral administration. Following oral administration, its peak plasma concentrations are usually achieved in approximately 2 hours, and its hypotensive effect usually has an onset of 0.5 to 2.0 hours, with peak activity at 4 to 6 hours and a duration of action of 4 to 14 hours. Approximately 20% of guanadrel is bound to plasma proteins, and little, if any, of the drug crosses the blood–brain barrier or distributes into the eye. Guanadrel has a plasma half-life of approximately 2 hours and an elimination half-life of approximately 10 to 12 hours in patients with normal renal function. Approximately 40% to 50% of guanadrel is metabolized in the liver to 2,3-dihydroxypropylguanidine and several unidentified metabolites, which are excreted principally in the urine (Fig. 24.11). Unlike guanethidine, approximately 85% of an oral dose of the drug is excreted in the urine within 24 hours, with 40% to 50% of the dose excreted in the urine unchanged. In patients with impaired renal function, the half-life of guanadrel is prolonged, and apparent total-body clearance and renal clearances are decreased.

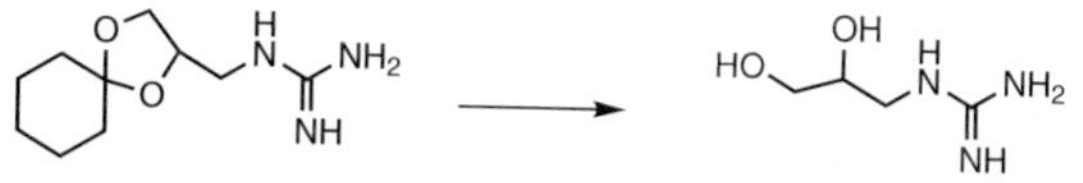

Guanadrel

FIGURE 24.11 Metabolism of guanadrel.

Therapeutic Application (6,34) Guanadrel is used in the management of hypertension, and its efficacy is similar to that of guanethidine. Guanadrel is reserved for patients with compelling indications who fail to respond to therapy with stage 2 drugs or for cases requiring more prompt or aggressive therapy. Postural and postexercise hypotension is common in patients receiving guanadrel, and it is also likely that heat-induced vasodilation will augment its hypotensive effect. There is a possibility that geriatric patients cannot tolerate the postural hypotensive effects of guanadrel. Being a peripheral adrenergic neuron blocking drug, guanadrel shares the toxic potentials of guanethidine, and the usual precautions of this drug should be observed.

Adverse Effects (6) Overall, the frequency of adverse effects produced by guanadrel is similar or less than those produced by guanethidine and by methyldopa. In patients with impaired renal function, the elimination half-life of unmetabolized guanadrel is prolonged and its clearance decreased, thus increasing the incidence of adverse effects if the usual dosage is maintained in these patients.

Drug Interactions Being a peripheral adrenergic neuron blocking drug, guanadrel shares the same potential for drug interactions as guanethidine, and the usual precautions of this drug should be observed.

Vasodilators

Vasodilator drugs relax the smooth muscle in blood vessels, which causes the vessels to dilate. Dilation of arterial vessels leads to a reduction in systemic vascular resistance, which leads to a fall in arterial blood pressure. Dilation of venous vessels decreases venous blood pressure.

Arterial dilator drugs are used to treat systemic and pulmonary hypertension, heart failure, and angina. They reduce arterial pressure by decreasing systemic vascular resistance, thereby reducing the afterload on the left ventricle and enhancing stroke volume and cardiac output. They also decrease the oxygen demand of the heart and, thereby, improve the oxygen supply/demand ratio. The primary functions of venous dilators in treating cardiovascular hypertension include reduction in venous pressure, thus reducing preload on the heart and decreasing cardiac output and capillary fluid filtration and edema formation (a decrease in capillary hydrostatic pressure). Therefore, venous dilators sometimes are used in the treatment of heart failure along with other drugs, because they help to reduce pulmonary and/or systemic edema that results from heart failure.

There are three potential drawbacks in the use of vasodilators: First, vasodilators can lead to a baroreceptor-mediated reflex stimulation of the heart (increased heart rate and inotropy) from systemic vasodilation and arterial pressure reduction. Second, they can impair the normal baroreceptor-mediated reflex vasoconstriction when a person stands up, which can lead to orthostatic hypotension and syncope on standing. Third, they can lead to renal retention of sodium and water, increasing blood volume and cardiac output.

Vasodilator drugs are classified either based on their site of action (arterial vs. venous) or, more commonly, by their primary mechanism of action.

Direct-Acting Vasodilators

Hydralazine Hydrochloride

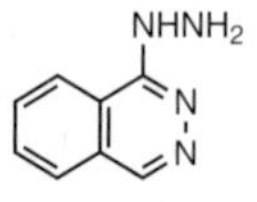

Hydralazine

Mechanism of Action. The only drug in this group, hydralazine, does not fit neatly into the other mechanistic classes, in part because its mechanism of action is not entirely clear. It seems to have multiple, direct effects on the VSM. Hydralazine, a phthalazine-substituted hydrazine antihypertensive drug with a pK_a of 7.3 and log$D_{7.4}$ of 0.52, is highly specific for arterial vessels, producing its vasodilation by a couple of different mechanisms. First, it causes smooth muscle hyperpolarization, quite likely through the opening of K^+ channels. Activation therefore increases the efflux of potassium ions from the cells, causing hyperpolarization of VSM cells and, thus, prolonging the opening of the potassium channel and sustaining a greater vasodilation on arterioles than on veins (9). It can also inhibit the second messenger, IP_3-induced release of calcium from the smooth muscle SR (the PIP_2 signal transduction pathway) (Fig. 24.2). Finally, hydralazine stimulates the formation of NO by the vascular endothelium, leading to cGMP-mediated vasodilation (Fig. 24.1). The arterial vasodilator action of hydralazine reduces systemic vascular resistance and arterial pressure. Diastolic blood pressure is usually decreased more than systolic pressure is. The hydralazine-induced decrease in blood pressure and peripheral resistance causes a reflex response, which is accompanied by increased heart rate, cardiac output, and stroke volume and an increase in plasma renin activity. It has no direct effect on the heart (6). This reflex response could offset the hypotensive effect of arteriolar dilation, limiting its antihypertensive effectiveness. Hydralazine also causes sodium and water retention and expansion of plasma volume, which could develop tolerance to its antihypertensive effect during prolonged therapy. Thus, coadministration of a diuretic improves the therapeutic outcome.

Pharmacokinetics (6,9). Hydralazine is well absorbed from the GI tract and is metabolized in the GI mucosa (prehepatic systemic metabolism) and in the liver by acetylation, hydroxylation, and conjugation with glucuronic acid (Fig. 24.12; see Table 4.17). Little of the hydralazine dose is excreted unchanged while most of the dose appears as metabolites in the urine which are without significant therapeutic activity. A small amount of hydralazine is reportedly converted to a hydrazone, most likely with vitamin B_6 (pyridoxine), which can be responsible for some its neurotoxic effects. Following the oral administration of hydralazine, its antihypertensive effect begins in 20 to 30 minutes and lasts 2 to 4 hours. The plasma half-life of hydralazine is generally 2 to 4 hours but, in some patients, can be up to 8 hours (i.e., slow acetylators). In slow acetylator patients or those with impaired renal function, the plasma concentrations for hydralazine are increased and, possibly, prolonged. Approximately 85% of hydralazine in the blood is bound to plasma proteins following administration of usual doses.

First-pass acetylation in the GI mucosa and liver is related to genetic acetylator phenotype (8). Acetylation phenotype is an important determinant of the plasma concentrations of hydralazine when the same dose of hydralazine is administered orally. Slow acetylators have an autosomal recessive trait that results in a relative deficiency of the hepatic enzyme *N*-acetyl transferase, thus prolonging the elimination half-life of hydralazine (see Chapter 4). This population of hypertensive patients will require an adjustment in dose to reduce the increased overactive response. Approximately 50% of African Americans and whites and the majority of American Indians, Eskimos, and Orientals are rapid acetylators of hydralazine. This population of patients will have subtherapeutic plasma concentrations of hydralazine because of its rapid metabolism to inactive metabolites and shorter elimination times. Patients with hydralazine-induced systemic lupus erythematosus frequently are slow acetylators.

Therapeutic Applications (6). Hydralazine is used in the management of moderate to severe hypertension. Hydralazine is reserved for patients with compelling indications and who fail to respond adequately to a stage 2 antihypertensive regimen. This drug is recommended for use in conjunction with cardiac glycosides and other

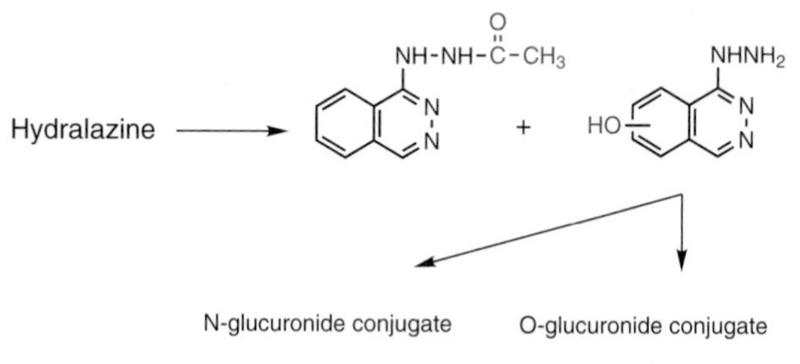

FIGURE 24.12 Metabolism of hydralazine.

vasodilators for the short-term treatment of severe congestive heart failure. Patients who engage in potentially hazardous activities, such as operating machinery or driving motor vehicles, should be warned about possible faintness, dizziness, or weakness. Hydralazine should be used with caution in patients with cerebrovascular accidents or with severe renal damage.

Parenteral hydralazine can be used for the management of severe hypertension when the drug cannot be given orally or when blood pressure must be lowered immediately. Other agents (e.g., sodium nitroprusside) are preferred for the management of severe hypertension or hypersensitive emergencies when a parenteral hypotensive agent is employed.

Drug Interactions. The coadministration of diuretics and other hypotensive drugs can have a synergistic effect, resulting in a marked decrease in blood pressure.

Potassium Channel Openers

Specific Drugs

Minoxidil Although several potassium channel openers have been used in research for many years, only one, minoxidil, is approved for use in humans for treating hypertension. Minoxidil is the *N*-oxide of a piperidinopyrimidine hypotensive agent, has a pK_a 4.6 and $logD_{7.4}$ of 0.62, and is not an active hypotensive drug until it is metabolized by hepatic thermolabile phenol sulfotransferase (SULT1A1) to minoxidil *N-O*-sulfate (9).

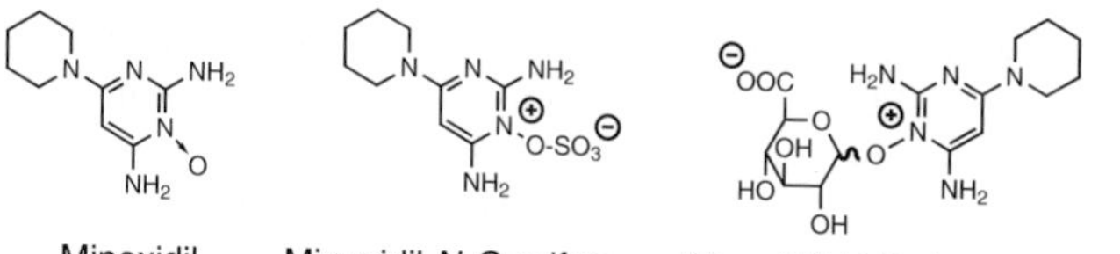

Minoxidil Minoxidil *N-O*-sulfate Minoxidil *N-O*-glucuronide

Mechanism of Action. Potassium channel openers are drugs that activate (i.e., open) ATP-sensitive K^+ channels in the VSM (Fig. 24.1) (35). By opening these potassium channels, there is increased efflux of potassium ions from the cells, causing hyperpolarization of VSM, which closes the voltage-gated calcium channels and, thereby, decreases intracellular calcium. With less calcium available to combine with calmodulin, there is less activation of MLCK and phosphorylation of myosin light chains. This leads to relaxation and vasodilation. Because small arteries and arterioles normally have a high degree of smooth muscle tone, these drugs are particularly effective in dilating these resistance vessels, decreasing systemic vascular resistance, and lowering arterial pressure. The fall in arterial pressure leads to reflex cardiac stimulation (baroreceptor-mediated tachycardia).

Minoxidil, as its active metabolite minoxidil *O*-sulfate, prolongs the opening of the potassium channel, sustaining greater vasodilation on arterioles than on veins. The drug decreases blood pressure in both the supine and standing positions, and there is no orthostatic hypotension. Associated with the decrease in peripheral resistance and blood pressure is a reflex response that is accompanied by increased heart rate, cardiac output, and stroke volume, which can be attenuated by the coadministration of a BB (6). Along with this decrease in peripheral resistance is increased plasma renin activity and sodium and water retention, which can result in expansion of fluid volume, edema, and congestive heart failure. The sodium- and water-retaining effects of minoxidil can be reversed by coadministration of a diuretic. When minoxidil is used in conjunction with a β-adrenergic blocker, pulmonary artery pressure remains essentially unchanged.

Pharmacokinetics (36). Minoxidil is absorbed from the GI tract and is metabolized to its active sulfate metabolite. Plasma concentrations for minoxidil sulfate peak within 1 hour and then decline rapidly. Following an oral dose of minoxidil, its hypotensive effect begins in 30 minutes, is maximal in 2 to 8 hours, and persists for approximately 2 to 5 days. The delayed onset of the hypotensive effect for minoxidil is attributed to its metabolism to its active metabolite. The drug is not bound to plasma proteins. The major metabolite for minoxidil is its N-O-glucuronide, which unlike the sulfate metabolite, is inactive as a hypotensive agent. Approximately 10% to 20% of an oral dose of minoxidil is metabolized to its active metabolite, minoxidil O-sulfate, and approximately 20% of minoxidil is excreted unchanged.

Therapeutic Applications.

Hypertension (6,36). Being effective arterial dilators, potassium-channel openers are used in the treatment of hypertension. These drugs are not first-line therapy for hypertension because of their side effects; therefore, they are relegated to treating refractory, severe hypertension. They are generally used in conjunction with a BB and a diuretic to attenuate the reflex tachycardia and retention of sodium and fluid, respectively.

Minoxidil is used in the management of severe hypertension. It is reserved for resistant cases of hypertension that have not been managed with maximal therapeutic dosages of a diuretic and two other hypotensive drugs or for patients who have failed to respond adequately with hydralazine. To minimize sodium retention and increased plasma volume, minoxidil must be used in conjunction with a diuretic. A BB must be given before beginning minoxidil therapy and should be continued during minoxidil therapy to minimize minoxidil-induced tachycardia and increased myocardial workload.

Androgenetic Alopecia (6,37). Minoxidil is used topically to stimulate regrowth of hair in patients with androgenic alopecia (male pattern alopecia, hereditary alopecia, or common male baldness) or alopecia areata. Commercially available topical minoxidil preparations should be used rather than the extemporaneous topical formulations from tablets to reduce the potential of minoxidil being absorbed systemically.

Drug Interactions. When minoxidil is administered with diuretics or other hypotensive drugs, the hypotensive effect of minoxidil increases, and concurrent use can cause profound orthostatic hypotensive effects.

Diazoxide

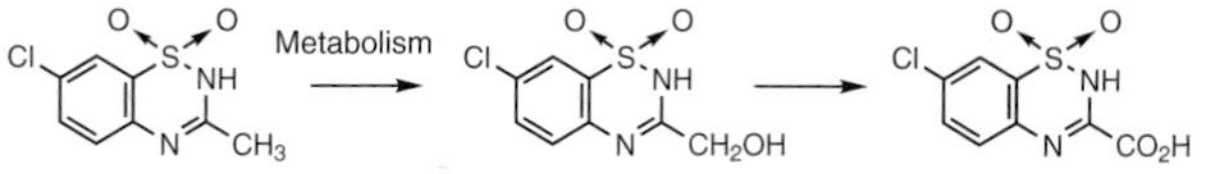

Diazoxide

Diazoxide is a nondiuretic hypotensive and hyperglycemic agent that is structurally related to the thiazide diuretics. Being a sulfonamide with a pK_a of 8.5 and $logD_{7.4}$ of 1.28, it can be solubilized in alkaline solutions (pH of injection is 11.6). Solutions or oral suspension of diazoxide are unstable to light and will darken when exposed to light. Such dosage forms should be protected from light, heat, and freezing. Darkened solutions can be subpotent and should not be used.

Mechanism of Action. Diazoxide reduces peripheral vascular resistance and blood pressure by a direct vasodilating effect on the VSM with a mechanism similar to that described for minoxidil by activating (opening) the ATP-modulated potassium channel (36). Thus, diazoxide prolongs the opening of the potassium channel, sustaining greater vasodilation on arterioles than on veins (9). The greatest hypotensive effect is observed in patients with malignant hypertension. Although oral or slow IV administration of diazoxide can produce a sustained fall in blood pressure, rapid IV administration is required for maximum hypotensive effects, especially in patients with malignant hypertension (6). Diazoxide-induced decreases in blood pressure and peripheral vascular resistance are accompanied by a reflex response, resulting in an increased heart rate, cardiac output, and left ventricular ejection rate. In contrast to the thiazide diuretics, diazoxide causes sodium and water retention and decreased urinary output, which can result in expansion of plasma and extracellular fluid volume, edema, and congestive heart failure, especially during prolonged administration.

Diazoxide increases blood glucose concentration (diazoxide-induced hyperglycemia) by several different mechanisms: by inhibiting pancreatic insulin secretion, by stimulating release of catecholamines, or by increasing hepatic release of glucose (6,9). The precise mechanism of inhibition of insulin release has not been elucidated but, possibly, can result from an effect of diazoxide on cell-membrane potassium channels and calcium flux.

Pharmacokinetics (6). After rapid IV administration, diazoxide produces a prompt reduction in blood pressure, with maximum hypotensive effects occurring within 5 minutes. The duration of its hypotensive effect varies from 3 to 12 hours, but ranges from 30 minutes to 72 hours have been observed. The elimination half-life of diazoxide following a single oral or IV dose has been reported to range from 21 to 45 hours in adults with normal renal function. In patients with renal impairment, the half-life is prolonged. Approximately 90% of the diazoxide in the blood is bound to plasma proteins. Approximately 20% to 50% of diazoxide is eliminated unchanged in the urine, along with its major metabolites, resulting from the oxidation of the 3-methyl group to its 3-hydroxymethyl- and 3-carboxyl-metabolites.

Therapeutic Applications.

Severe Hypertension (6). Intravenous diazoxide has been used in hypertensive crises for emergency lowering of blood pressure when a prompt and urgent decrease in diastolic pressure is required in adults with severe nonmalignant and malignant hypertension and in children with acute severe hypertension. However, other IV hypotensive agents are preferred for the management of hypertensive crises. Diazoxide is intended for short-term use in hospitalized patients only. Although diazoxide has also been administered orally for the management of hypertension, its hyperglycemic and sodium-retaining effects make it unsuitable for chronic therapy.

Hypoglycemia (6). Diazoxide is administered orally in the management of hypoglycemia caused by hyperinsulinism associated with inoperable islet cell adenoma or carcinoma or extrapancreatic malignancy in adults.

Phosphodiesterase Inhibitors

MECHANISM OF ACTION OF cAMP-DEPENDENT PHOSPHODIESTERASE INHIBITORS (PDE3) PDE3 is one of the isoforms of phosphodiesterase found in the heart and VSM. The mechanism by which cAMP and cGMP relaxes VSM has been described previously in the section on VSM contraction and relaxation (Figs. 24.1 and 24.2). The cAMP released is broken down by a cAMP-dependent phosphodiesterase (PDE3). Therefore, inhibition of PDE3 increases intracellular cAMP, which further inhibits MLCK, thereby producing less contractile force (i.e., promoting relaxation). The overall cardiac and vascular effects of cAMP-dependent phosphodiesterase inhibitors cause cardiac stimulation, increasing cardiac output and reducing systemic vascular resistance, thereby lowering arterial pressure. Because cardiac output increases and systemic vascular resistance decreases, the change in arterial pressure depends on the relative effects of the phosphodiesterase inhibitor on the heart versus the VSM. At normal therapeutic doses, PDE3 inhibitors, such as milrinone, have a greater effect on VSM than cardiac muscle so that arterial pressure is lowered in the presence of augmented cardiac output. Because of the dual cardiac and vascular effects of these compounds, they sometimes are referred to as inodilators.

MECHANISM OF ACTION OF cGMP-DEPENDENT PHOSPHODIESTERASE INHIBITORS (PDE5) A second isoenzyme form of phosphodiesterase found in VSM is PDE5, a cGMP-dependent phosphodiesterase, which is also found in the corpus cavernosum of the penis (erectile dysfunction). This enzyme is responsible for breaking down cGMP that forms in response to increased NO (Fig. 24.1). Increased cGMP leads to smooth muscle relaxation primarily by reducing calcium entry into the cell. Inhibitors of cGMP-dependent phosphodiesterase increase intracellular cGMP, thereby enhancing VSM relaxation and vasodilation.

Therapeutic Indications The cardiostimulatory and vasodilatory actions of PDE3 inhibitors make them suitable for the treatment of heart failure, because VSM relaxation reduces ventricular wall stress and the oxygen demands placed on the failing heart. The cardiostimulatory effects of the PDE3 increase inotropy, which further enhances stroke volume and ejection fraction. A baroreceptor reflex, which occurs in response to hypotension, can contribute to the tachycardia. Clinical trials have shown that long-term therapy with PDE3 inhibitors increases mortality in patients with heart failure; therefore, these drugs are not used for long-term, chronic therapy. They are very useful, however, in treating acute, decompensated heart failure or temporary bouts of decompensated chronic failure. They are not used as a monotherapy. Instead, they are used in conjunction with other treatment modalities, such as diuretics, ACEIs, BBs, or digitalis. The somewhat selective vasodilatory actions of PDE5 inhibitors have made these compounds very useful in the treatment of male erectile dysfunction and as a combination therapy for pulmonary hypertension. The PDE3 inhibitors are used for treating heart failure, whereas the PDE5 inhibitors are used for treating male erectile dysfunction. Note that the generic names for PDE3 inhibitors end in "one" and those for the PDE5 inhibitors end in "fil."

Specific Drugs

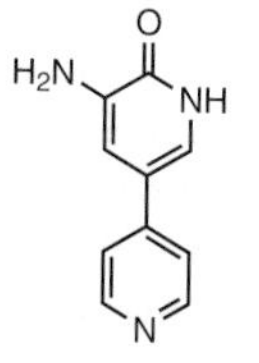

Inamrinone

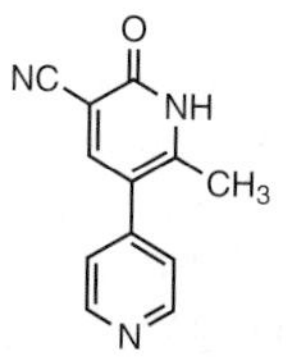

Milrinone

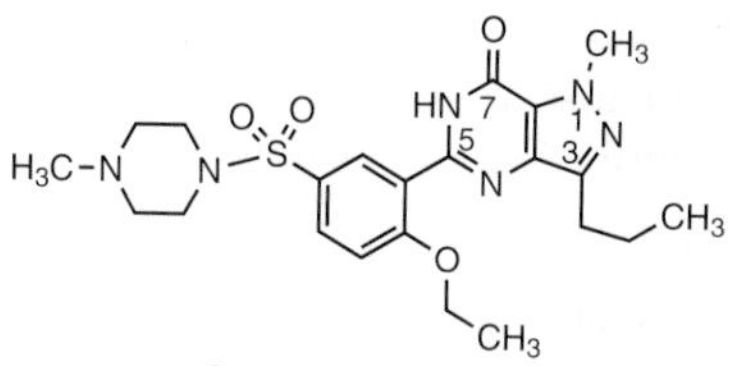

Sildenafil

Milrinone (Primacor as Lactate Salt) and Inamrinone (Inocor as Lactate Salt) Inamrinone and milrinone ($logD_{7.4}$ = −1.89) are positive inotropes and vasodilators indicated for the short-term IV management of congestive heart failure in patients who have not responded adequately to digitalis, diuretics, and/or vasodilators.

For IV infusion, inamrinone lactate and milrinone lactate injection solutions can be diluted in sodium chloride solution for injection. Inamrinone lactate for injection is preserved with sodium metabisulfite and needs protection from light. It should not be diluted with solutions containing dextrose, because a chemical interaction occurs over 24 hours. For milrinone, an immediate chemical interaction with furosemide with the formation of a precipitate is observed when furosemide is injected into an infusion of milrinone. Patients who are sensitive to bisulfites can also be sensitive to inamrinone lactate injection, which contains sodium metabisulfite.

The pharmacokinetics for inamrinone shows protein binding from 10% to 49%. Its half-life in healthy volunteers is approximately 3.6 hours, whereas in patients with congestive heart failure, the plasma half-life increases to approximately 5.0 to 8.3 hours. For infants younger than 4 weeks, the half-life is 12.7 to 22.2 hours, and for infants older than 4 weeks, the half-life is 3.8 to 6.8 hours. Time to peak effect is less than 10 minutes. Its duration of action is dose related, ranging from 30 minutes at low dose to 2 hours at the higher dosages. Approximately 63% of the administered dose is eliminated via the urine as unchanged drug, and 18% is eliminated in the feces. Elderly patients are more likely to have age-related renal function impairment, which can require adjustment of dosage in patients receiving inamrinone.

The pharmacokinetics for milrinone following IV injections to patients with congestive heart failure showed a volume of distribution of 0.38 to 0.45 L/kg, a mean terminal elimination half-life of 2.3 hours, and a clearance of 0.13 L/kg/hour. These pharmacokinetic parameters were not dose dependent, and the area under the plasma concentration versus time curve following injections was significantly dose dependent. Milrinone is approximately 70% bound to human plasma protein. The primary route of excretion for orally administered milrinone is via the urine, with unchanged milrinone (83%) and its *O*-glucuronide metabolite (12%) being present. Elimination in normal subjects via the urine is rapid, with approximately 60% recovered within the first 2 hours following dosing and approximately 90% within the first 8 hours following dosing. In patients with renal function impairment, elimination of unchanged milrinone is reduced, suggesting that a dosage adjustment can be necessary.

The selective PDE5 inhibitor most commonly used is sildenafil (Viagra as citrate) ($logD_{7.4}$ = 1.85). Studies in vitro have shown that sildenafil is selective for PDE5. Its effect is more potent on PDE5 than on other known phosphodiesterases (10 times for PDE6, >80 times for PDE1, and >700 times for PDE2, PDE3, PDE4, PDE7, PDE8, PDE9, PDE10, and PDE11). The approximately 4,000 times selectivity for PDE5 versus PDE3 is important because PDE3 is involved in control of cardiac contractility. Sildenafil is only approximately 10 times as potent for PDE5 compared to PDE6, an enzyme found in the retina that is involved in the phototransduction pathway of the retina. This lower selectivity is thought to be the basis for abnormalities related to color vision observed with higher doses or plasma levels. (For a complete discussion of the pharmacokinetics including drug metabolism, see Chapter 40.)

Side Effects and Contraindications The most common and severe side effect for PDE3 inhibitors is ventricular arrhythmias, some of which can be life-threatening. Other side effects include headaches and hypotension, which are not uncommon for drugs that increase cAMP in cardiac and vascular tissues (e.g., β-agonists).

In addition to human corpus cavernosum smooth muscle, PDE5 is also found in lower concentrations in other tissues, including platelets, vascular and visceral smooth muscle, and skeletal muscle. The inhibition of PDE5 in these tissues by sildenafil can be the basis for the enhanced platelet antiaggregatory activity of NO observed in vitro, an inhibition of platelet thrombus formation in vivo, and peripheral arterial-venous dilatation in vivo. The most common side effects for PDE5 inhibitors include headache and cutaneous flushing, both of which are related to vascular dilation caused by increased vascular cGMP. Clinical evidence suggests that nitrodilators can interact adversely with PDE5 inhibitors. The reason for this adverse reaction is that nitrodilators stimulate cGMP production, whereas PDE5 inhibitors inhibit cGMP degradation. When combined, these two drug classes greatly potentiate cGMP levels, which can lead to hypotension and impaired coronary perfusion.

Nitrodilators

Mechanism of Action NO, a molecule produced by many cells in the body, has several important actions. NO is a highly reactive gas that participates in many chemical reactions. It is one of the nitrogen oxides ("NOx") in automobile exhaust and plays a major role in the formation of photochemical smog, but NO has also many physiologic functions. It is synthesized within cells by an enzyme NO synthase (NOS). There are three isoenzymes, neuronal NOS (nNOS or NOS-1), inducible NOS (iNOS or NOS-2) found in macrophages, and endothelial NOS (eNOS or NOS-3) found in the endothelial cells that line the lumen of blood vessels. Whereas the levels of nNOS and eNOS are relatively steady, expression of iNOS genes awaits an appropriate stimulus. All types of NOS produce NO from arginine with the aid of molecular oxygen and NADPH. Because NO diffuses freely across cell membranes, there are many other molecules with which it can interact, and NO is quickly consumed close to where it is synthesized. Thus, NO affects only cells adjacent to its point of synthesis. NO relaxes the smooth muscle in the walls of the arterioles. At each systole, the endothelial cells that line the blood vessels release a puff of NO, which diffuses into the underlying smooth muscle cells, causing them to relax and, thus, to permit the surge of blood to pass through easily. The signaling functions of NO begin with its binding to protein receptors on or in the cell, triggering the formation of cGMP from soluble guanylyl cyclase (Fig. 24.1). Mice in which the genes for the NOS found in endothelial cells (eNOS) have been "knocked out" suffer from hypertension. Nitroglycerin, which is often prescribed to reduce the pain of angina, does so by generating NO, which relaxes venous walls and arterioles, improving the oxygen supply/demand ratio (see Chapter 21). NO also inhibits the aggregation of platelets and, thus, keeps inappropriate clotting from interfering with blood flow. Other actions on smooth muscle include penile erection and peristalsis aided by the relaxing effect of NO on the smooth muscle in intestinal walls. NO also inhibits the contractility of the smooth muscle wall of the uterus, but at birth, the production of NO decreases, allowing contractions to occur. Nitroglycerin has helped some women who were at risk of giving birth prematurely to carry their baby to full term. The NO from iNOS inhibits inflammation in blood vessels by blocking the release of mediators of inflammation from the endothelial cells, macrophages, and T lymphocytes. The NO from iNOS has been shown to *S*-nitrosylate cyclooxygenase-2 (COX-2), increasing its activity, and drugs that prevent this interaction could work synergistically with the nonsteroidal anti-inflammatory drugs inhibiting COX-2. NO affects hormonal secretion from several endocrine glands. Hemoglobin transports NO at the same time that it carries oxygen, and when it unloads oxygen in the tissues, it also unloads NO. Fireflies use NO to turn on their flashers.

Since the dawn of recorded human history, nitrates have been used to preserve meat from bacterial spoilage. Harmless bacteria in our throat convert nitrates in our food into nitrites. When the nitrites reach the stomach, the acidic gastric juice (pH ~1.4) generates NO from these nitrites, killing almost all the bacteria that have been swallowed in our food.

In the cardiovascular system, NO is produced primarily by vascular endothelial cells. This endothelial-derived NO has several important functions, including relaxing VSM (vasodilation), inhibiting platelet aggregation (antithrombotic), and inhibiting leukocyte–endothelial interactions (anti-inflammatory). These actions involve NO-stimulated formation of cGMP (Fig. 24.1). Nitrodilators are drugs that mimic the actions of endogenous NO by releasing NO or forming NO within tissues. These drugs act directly on the VSM to cause relaxation and, therefore, serve as endothelial-independent vasodilators.

Sodium Nitroprusside (Sodium Nitroferricyanide; Nitropress; Nipride)

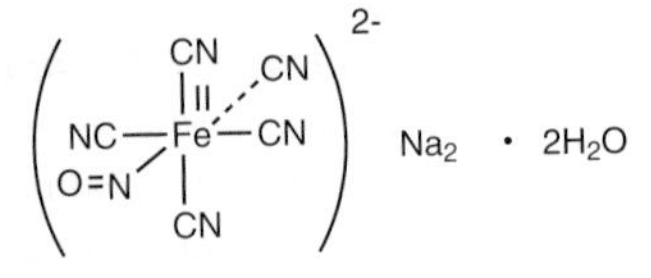

Sodium nitroprusside

There are two basic types of nitrodilators: those that release NO spontaneously (e.g., sodium nitroprusside) and those that require an enzyme activation to form NO (organic nitrates). Sodium nitroprusside is a direct-acting vasodilator on VSM, producing its vasodilation by the release of NO. Since 1929, it has been known as a rapidly acting hypotensive agent when administered as an infusion. It is chemically and structurally unrelated to other available hypotensive agents. As a reminder in preparing extemporaneous infusions, the potency of sodium nitroprusside is expressed in terms of the dihydrated drug. When reconstituted with 5% dextrose injection, sodium nitroprusside solutions are reddish-brown in color, with a pH of 3.5 to 6.0. Its crystals and solutions are sensitive and unstable to light and should be protected from extremes of light and heat. The exposure of sodium nitroprusside solutions to light causes deterioration, which can be evidenced by a change from a reddish-brown to a green to a blue color, indicating a rearrangement of the nitroso to the inactive isonitro form. Sodium nitroprusside solutions in glass bottles undergo approximately 20% degradation within 4 hours when exposed to fluorescent light and even more rapid degradation in plastic bags. Sodium nitroprusside solutions should be protected from light by wrapping the container with aluminum foil or other opaque material. When adequately protected from light, reconstituted solutions are stable for 24 hours. Trace metals, such as iron and copper, can catalyze the degradation of nitroprusside solutions, releasing cyanide. Any change in color for the nitroprusside solutions is an indication of degradation, and the solution should be discarded. No other drug or preservative should be added to stabilize sodium nitroprusside infusions.

Mechanism of Action Sodium nitroprusside is not an active hypotensive drug until metabolized to its active metabolite, NO, the mechanism of action of which has been previously described (Fig. 24.1). Studies with sodium nitroprusside suggest that it releases NO by its interaction with glutathione or with sulfhydryl groups in the erythrocytes and tissues to form a *S*-nitrosothiol intermediate, which spontaneously produces NO, which in turn freely diffuses into the VSM, thereby increasing intracellular cGMP concentration (6,9). NO also activates K^+ channels, which leads to hyperpolarization and relaxation.

The hypotensive effect of sodium nitroprusside is augmented by concomitant use of other hypotensive agents and is not blocked by adrenergic blocking agents. It has no direct effect on the myocardium, but it can exert a direct coronary vasodilator effect on VSM. When sodium nitroprusside is administered to hypertensive patients, a slight increase in heart rate commonly occurs, and cardiac output is usually decreased slightly. Moderate doses of sodium nitroprusside in patients with hypertension produce renal vasodilation without an appreciable increase in renal blood flow or decrease in glomerular filtration (6).

Intravenous infusion of sodium nitroprusside produces an almost immediate reduction in blood pressure. Blood pressure begins to rise immediately when the infusion is slowed or stopped and returns to pretreatment levels within 1 to 10 minutes.

Pharmacokinetics Sodium nitroprusside undergoes a redox reaction that releases cyanide (6,9). The cyanide that is produced is rapidly converted into thiocyanate in the liver by the enzyme thiosulfate sulfotransferase (rhodanase) and is excreted in the urine (6,9). The rate-limiting step in the conversion of cyanide to thiocyanate is the availability of sulfur donors, especially thiosulfate. Toxic symptoms of thiocyanate begin to appear at plasma thiocyanate concentrations of 50 to 100 mg/mL. The elimination half-life of thiocyanate is 2.7 to 7.0 days when renal function is normal but longer in patients with impaired renal function.

Therapeutic Applications (6) Intravenous sodium nitroprusside is used as an infusion for hypertensive crises and emergencies. The drug is consistently effective in the management of hypertensive emergencies, irrespective of etiology, and can be useful even when other drugs have failed. It can be used in the management of acute congestive heart failure.

Adverse Effects (6) The most clinically important adverse effects of sodium nitroprusside are profound hypotension and the accumulation of cyanide and thiocyanate. Thiocyanate can accumulate in the blood of patients receiving sodium nitroprusside therapy, especially in those with impaired renal function. Thiocyanate is mildly neurotoxic at serum concentrations of 60 μg/mL and can be life-threatening at concentrations of 200 μg/mL. Other adverse effects of thiocyanate include inhibition of both the uptake and binding of iodine, producing symptoms of hypothyroidism.

Sodium nitroprusside can bind to vitamin B_{12}, interfering with its distribution and metabolism, and it should be used with caution in patients having low plasma vitamin B_{12} concentrations. Excess cyanide can also bind to hemoglobin, producing methemoglobinemia.

Ganglionic Blockers

Mechanism of Action Ganglionic blockers block impulse transmission at the sympathetic ganglia. Neurotransmission within the sympathetic and parasympathetic ganglia involves the release of acetylcholine from preganglionic efferent nerves, which binds to nicotinic receptors on the postganglionic efferent nerves. Ganglionic blockers inhibit autonomic activity by interfering with neurotransmission within autonomic ganglia. This reduces sympathetic outflow to the heart, thereby decreasing cardiac output by decreasing heart rate and contractility. Reduced sympathetic output to the vasculature decreases sympathetic vascular tone, which causes vasodilation and reduced systemic vascular resistance, which decreases arterial pressure. Parasympathetic outflow is also reduced by ganglionic blockers.

THERAPEUTIC INDICATIONS Ganglionic blockers are not commonly used in the treatment of chronic hypertension or in patients with compelling indications largely because of their side effects and because numerous more effective and safer antihypertensive drugs can be used. They are, however, occasionally used for hypertensive emergencies. The ganglionic blockers available for clinical use include trimethaphan camsylate, and mecamylamine, which are competitive antagonists at $\alpha_4\beta_2$-nicotinic acetylcholine receptor.

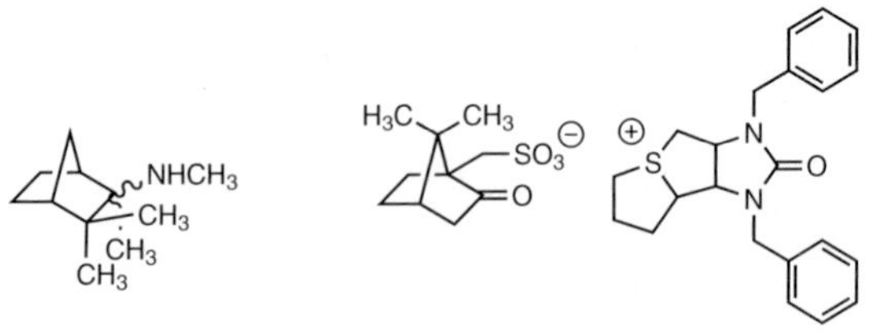

± Mecamylamine Trimethaphan camsylate

Trimethaphan is a tertiary sulfonium ion and cannot cross lipid cell membranes, whereas mecamylamine is a secondary amine with pKa of 11.2 and $\log D_{7.4}$ of −1.1. Therefore, trimethaphan is a short-acting peripheral direct vasodilator that must be given as an IV infusion, whereas mecamylamine can be given orally. *S*-(+)-Mecamylamine is the active enantiomer for the $\alpha_4\beta_2$-nicotinic acetylcholine receptor. Mecamylamine rapidly disappears from the blood with a plasma half-life of 1 hour and crosses the blood–brain barrier into the CNS. Trimethaphan is rapidly excreted in unchanged form by the kidney. Mecamylamine is excreted by the kidney much more slowly. Trimethaphan is the drug of choice for managing acute aortic dissection and for hypertensive emergencies. Both drugs are of limited use, because of the availability of more specific acting vasodilators. Mecamylamine has been used for labeling CNS nicotinic receptors and crosses into the CNS, where it can block neuronal $\alpha_4\beta_2$-nicotinic acetylcholine receptors. Mecamylamine has been studied for use with nicotine for smoking cessation and as an antidepressant.

SIDE EFFECTS AND CONTRAINDICATIONS Side effects of trimethaphan include prolonged neuromuscular blockade and potentiation of neuromuscular blocking agents. It can produce excessive hypotension and impotence (because of its sympatholytic effect) as well as constipation, urinary retention, and dry mouth (because of its parasympatholytic effect).

PULMONARY ARTERIAL HYPERTENSION

Pulmonary hypertension, which was once a rare life-threatening disease, reportedly affects about 160,000 people today. Pulmonary arterial hypertension (PAH) is defined as a group of diseases characterized by a progressive increase of pulmonary vascular resistance, leading to right ventricular failure. It includes a variety of pulmonary hypertensive diseases with different etiologies but similar clinical presentation (36). Primary pulmonary hypertension can occur without any apparent cause (idiopathic), or it can be inherited. PAH is a disease of the small pulmonary arteries, characterized by progressive narrowing of the pulmonary vascular bed. Vasoconstriction and scarring (or fibrosis) cause the pulmonary wall to become stiffer and thicker, contributing to an increased pulmonary vascular resistance. This extra stress causes the heart to enlarge and become less flexible. Less blood flows from the heart, through the lungs and into the body, resulting in additional symptoms. One direct effect of these abnormally elevated pressures is blood leakage from the pulmonary vessels. A blood-producing cough often is an indicator of leakage from the pulmonary vessels. The pulmonary arterial walls produce a substance called endothelin, which causes these blood vessels to constrict. The reasons for this overproduction are unknown. In some cases, the cause is genetically programmed or the person is predisposed genetically to primary pulmonary hypertension after being exposed to a certain drug (e.g., the diet drugs Fen-Phen [fenfluramine/phentermine], Redux [dexfenfluramine], or Pondimin [fenfluramine]).

Often, primary pulmonary hypertension is not diagnosed in a timely manner, because its early symptoms can be confused with those of many other conditions (Table 24.5). To establish a diagnosis of pulmonary hypertension, a series of tests are performed that show how well a person's heart and lungs are working. These tests can include assessment of daily living tasks, such as a 6-minute walk test, a computed tomography scan to rule out a pulmonary embolism or lung disease, a pulmonary function test to rule out obstructive lung disease, a formal sleep study to rule out sleep apnea, and laboratory tests to rule out hepatitis, collagen disease, HIV, or other conditions.

Rationale for Pharmacologic Treatment

If PAH has an identifiable cause, then measures can be taken to correct the underlying problem. If the diagnosis is primary PAH, then pharmacologic intervention is required to reduce the pressure. This is done using vasodilator drugs to decrease pulmonary vascular resistance and, thereby, to lower the pressure. Adjunct therapy can include diuretics to reduce blood volume, which will reduce central venous pressure and right

TABLE 24.5 Symptoms of Primary Pulmonary Hypertension

Breathlessness or shortness of breath
Feeling tired all the time
Dizziness, especially when climbing stairs or standing up
Fainting (often the symptom that brings people to their doctors)
Swollen ankles and legs
Chest pain, especially during physical activity

ventricular stroke volume, as well as to reduce some of the signs and symptoms of edema and shortness of breath associated with PAH. Anticoagulants are administered to prevent the formation of pulmonary thrombi. Patients with cardiovascular hypertension are generally treated with antihypertensive drugs that reduce blood volume (which reduces central venous pressure and cardiac output), reduce systemic vascular resistance, or reduce cardiac output by depressing heart rate and stroke volume.

Drugs Used to Treat Pulmonary Hypertension

Classes of drugs used in the treatment of PAH include thiazide diuretics, loop diuretics, vasodilators, calcium channel blockers, prostaglandins, endothelin receptor antagonists, NO, and PDE5 inhibitors (38,39). During the last decade, substantial improvements in the therapeutic options for PAH have emerged that target the mechanisms involved in the pathogenesis of this devastating disease. Intravenous epoprostenol was the first drug to improve symptoms and survival of patients with PAH. Novel prostanoids, including subcutaneous treprostinil and inhaled iloprost, have beneficial effects in many patients, although their long-term efficacy is less well known. Among the newer treatments for PAH, endothelin receptor antagonists and PDE5 inhibitors have reshaped clinical practice for PAH. The endothelin receptor antagonist bosentan is recommended as first-line treatment for patients with PAH and New York Heart Association (NYHA) functional class III heart failure (i.e., patients with marked limitation of activity; they are comfortable only at rest). Other endothelin receptor antagonists include sitaxsentan sodium and ambrisentan. The combination of the PDE5 inhibitor sildenafil and iloprost, a prostacyclin analog, is being studied in patients with pulmonary hypertension. Targeting a single pathway cannot be expected to be uniformly successful, because PAH is a complex disorder. Thus, combining drugs with different modes of action is expected to improve symptoms, hemodynamics, and survival in PAH patients, although combination therapy has yet to undergo the scrutiny of large randomized clinical trials.

Specific Drugs

Phosphodiesterase Inhibitors

SILDENAFIL (REVATIO) Sildenafil has been approved for treatment of PAH through its inhibition of cGMP and smooth muscle relaxation of the pulmonary vasculature.

Endothelin Receptor Antagonists

MECHANISM OF ACTION ET-1 is a 21–amino acid peptide that is produced by the vascular endothelium. It is a very potent vasoconstrictor that binds to VSM endothelin receptors ET_A and ET_B (Fig. 24.13) (40). The ET-1 receptors are linked to the G_q protein and IP_3 signal transduction pathway (Fig. 24.1). Therefore, ET-1 causes SR release of calcium, increasing the VSM contractility. Vascular endothelial cells secrete the majority of ET-1, which binds to two receptor subtypes: ET_A and ET_B. In vascular tissue, ET_A is located predominantly on smooth muscle cells, whereas ET_B is found on both endothelial and smooth muscle cells. Activation of ET_A by ET-1 leads to potent vasoconstriction resulting from an increase in cytosolic calcium levels via influx of extracellular calcium and release from

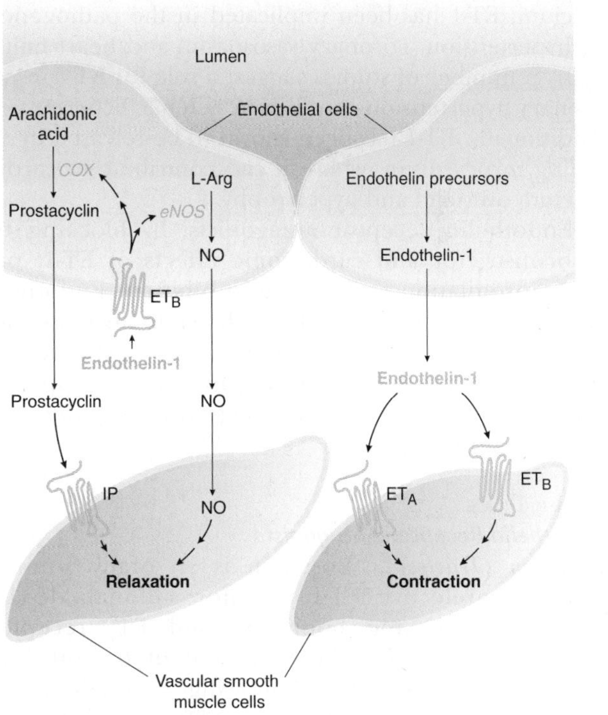

FIGURE 24.13 The effects of endothelin-1, prostacyclin, and nitric oxide on the contraction and relaxation (vasodilation) of vascular smooth muscle cells. ET, endothelin receptor; IP, isoprostenoid receptor; L-Arg, L-arginine; NO, nitric oxide. (From Yeh DC, Michel T. Pharmacology of vascular tone. In: Golan DE, Tashjian AH, Armstrong E, et al., eds. Principles of Pharmacology: The Pathophysiologic Basis of Drug Therapy. Baltimore: Lippincott Williams & Wilkins, 2008, with permission)

intracellular SR stores (Fig. 24.1). The actions of ET_B are more complicated. Like ET_A, ET-1 activation of ET_B on VSM cells leads to vasoconstriction. Furthermore, some studies suggest that in the pulmonary hypertensive state, blockade of both ET_A and ET_B is necessary to achieve maximal vasodilation. Activation of ET_B by ET-1 stimulates COX, which catalyzes the formation of prostacyclin from arachidonic acid. Prostacyclin then binds to and activates the isoprostanoid receptor on VSM. ET-1 also activates ET_B, which stimulates eNOS (eNOS) to produce NO from L-arginine. Both prostacyclin and NO are potent vasodilators of VSM (relaxation). Additionally, ET-1 binds to the ET_B receptors on the endothelium of pulmonary smooth muscle to stimulate the formation of NO, which produces vasodilation in the absence of smooth muscle ET_A and ET_B receptor activation. This receptor distribution helps to explain the phenomenon that ET-1 administration causes transient vasodilation (initial endothelial ET_B activation) and hypotension, followed by prolonged vasoconstriction (smooth muscle ET_A and ET_B activation) and hypertension.

Therapeutic Indications Because of its powerful vasoconstrictor properties and its effects on intracellular calcium, ET-1 has been implicated in the pathogenesis of hypertension, coronary vasospasm, and heart failure (40). A number of studies suggest a role for ET-1 in pulmonary hypertension as well as in systemic hypertension. Additionally, ET-1 has been shown to be released by the failing myocardium, where it can contribute to cardiac calcium overload and hypertrophy.

Endothelin receptor antagonists, by blocking the vasoconstrictor and cardiotonic effects of ET-1, produce vasodilation and cardiac inhibition. Endothelin receptor antagonists have been shown to decrease mortality and to improve hemodynamics in experimental models of heart failure. At present, the only approved indication for endothelin antagonists is pulmonary hypertension.

Specific Drugs

Endothelin Receptor Antagonists

Bosentan (Tracleer). Bosentan is an orally administered, nonselective ET-1 receptor sulfonamide-class antagonist blocking both ET_A and ET_B receptors and is approved for the treatment of patients with PAH (Fig. 24.14) (41). Following oral administration, bosentan attains peak plasma concentrations in approximately 3 hours, with an absolute bioavailability of approximately 50%. Food has no clinically relevant effect on its absorption recommended doses. Bosentan is approximately 98% bound to albumin, with a volume of distribution of 30 L. Its terminal half-life after oral administration is 5.4 hours and is unchanged at steady-state. Steady-state concentrations are achieved within 3 to 5 days after multiple-dose administration. Bosentan is mainly eliminated from the body by hepatic metabolism and subsequent biliary excretion of the metabolites. Three metabolites have been identified, formed by CYP2C9 and CYP3A4 (Fig. 24.15). The pharmacokinetics of bosentan are dose proportional up to 500 mg/d (multiple doses). The pharmacokinetics of bosentan in pediatric patients with PAH are comparable to those in healthy subjects, whereas adult patients with PAH show a two-fold increase in clearance. Severe renal impairment and mild hepatic impairment do not have a clinically relevant influence on its pharmacokinetics. Bosentan should generally be avoided in patients with moderate or severe hepatic impairment and/or elevated liver

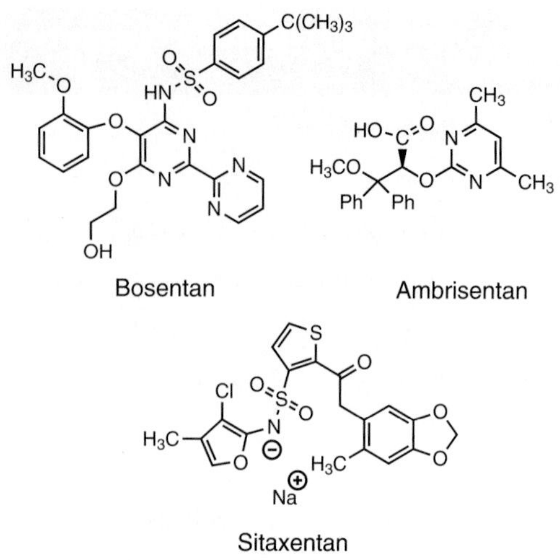

FIGURE 24.14 Endothelin receptor antagonists.

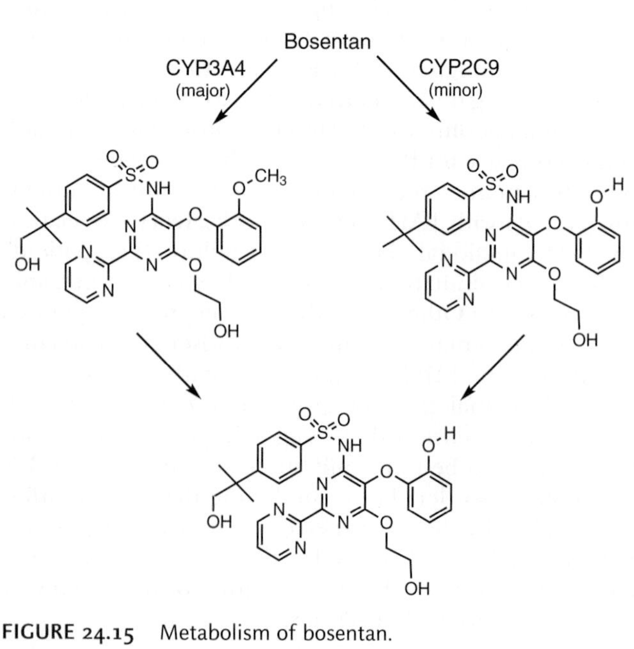

FIGURE 24.15 Metabolism of bosentan.

aminotransferases. Inhibitors of CYP3A4 increase the plasma concentration of bosentan and cause an increase in the clearance of drugs metabolized by CYP3A4 and CYP2C9. The drug induces CYP2C9 expression. The possibility of reduced efficacy of CYP2C9 and CYP3A4 substrates coadministered with bosentan is increased. No clinically relevant interaction was detected for P-glycoprotein. Bosentan can increase plasma levels of ET-1. Adverse effects include hypotension, headache, flushing, increased liver aminotransferases, leg edema, and anemia. Bosentan is teratogenic in animal models and therefore can cause birth defects and is contraindicated in pregnancy. Bosentan can also cause liver injury. Patients with hypersensitivity to sulfonamides should be excluded.

When prescribing any endothelin receptor antagonist, it is important to be aware of potential interactions with concomitant medications. Patients with PAH frequently require anticoagulant therapy, and bosentan affects warfarin metabolism. Because bosentan induces CYP2C9, the principal hepatic enzyme involved in the metabolism of warfarin, bosentan reduces prothrombin clotting time (as measured by international normalized ratio) in patients receiving warfarin. Increases in warfarin dose may be necessary to maintain a desirable clotting time. Thus, monitoring of coagulation status is warranted when bosentan is prescribed.

Ambrisentan (Letairis). Ambrisentan has been FDA approved for the treatment of PAH (Fig. 24.14). The drug is a selective antagonist of the ET_A receptor with a 77-fold selectivity for the ET_A receptor as compared to the ET_B receptor (42,43). The drug is significantly more selective for the ET_A receptor than bosentan (20:1). Ambrisentan exhibits two major adverse warnings. First, it is classified as a category X drug that must not be used in pregnant women because of its known teratogenicity in animal models, and pregnancy must be excluded before the start of treatment and prevented thereafter by the use of a reliable contraceptive method. Second, ambrisentan shows hepatotoxicity, and liver function tests for alanine aminotransferase and aspartate aminotransferase levels should be monitored before and during therapy.

Ambrisentan is administered orally and shows an 80% oral bioavailability. The drug is highly bound to plasma protein (99%). The drug is a substrate for P-glycoprotein and primarily undergoes glucuronidation of the carboxyl group catalyzed by UGT1A9, UGT2B7, and UGT1A3 to form an acyl glucuronide. Ambrisentan does not appear to undergo significant metabolism via CYP3A4/5 and CYP2C9 isoforms and is therefore unlikely to affect the pharmacokinetics of P450 metabolism of the drug. The FDA new drug application identifies two additional metabolites, which include oxidation of the 4-methyl group to the 4-hydroxymethyl group and the formation of a diglucuronide metabolite of the 4-hydroxymethyl and carboxyl groups. Biliary excretion is the primary route of elimination for ambrisentan (~36%) and metabolites (~30%), with another 20% of the metabolites appearing in the urine. Elimination half-life is 15 hours, thus allowing for dose accumulation.

Sitaxsentan Sodium (Thelin). Sitaxsentan is an orphan drug approved for marketing in the European Union (August 2006), Canada, and Australia (March 2007) and undergoing phase III clinical trials in the United States for the treatment of PAH. If FDA approved, sitaxsentan will join bosentan and ambrisentan, which are presently available in the United States for treatment of PAH (Fig. 24.14).

Sitaxsentan is a potent sulfonamide-class inhibitor of the ET_A receptor, exhibiting 6,500-fold selectivity for the ET_A receptor as compared to the ET_B receptor, blocking the action of endothelin (44,45). This selective antagonist of the ET_A receptor increases vascular blood flow and reverses vasoconstriction in human clinical studies. Clinical trials have shown that the efficacy of sitaxsentan is much the same as bosentan, a nonselective ET antagonist, but with reduced liver toxicity, although it carries a black box warning in the Canadian drug-approved labeling. Alanine aminotransferase and aspartate aminotransferase levels should be monitored using liver function tests before and during therapy

When administered orally, sitaxsentan was rapidly and extensively absorbed, with an oral bioavailability of approximately 55%. The drug can be taken with or without food. Sitaxsentan has a volume of distribution of greater than 60 L and a half-life of 6 to 7 hours and is greater than 98% protein bound. Sitaxsentan or its metabolites did not effectively cross the blood–brain barrier, but it was found in rat breast milk. In vitro tests have shown that sitaxsentan is primarily metabolized by CYP2C9 and, to a lesser extent, CYP3A4/5. It is a strong inhibitor of CYP2C9 and a lesser inhibitor of CYP2C19 and CYP3A4/5. The two main circulating metabolites were identified as 1,2-diketositaxsentan and 1-keto-2-hydroxy-sitaxsentan, which account for approximately 3% and 9% of the parent drug, respectively (Fig. 24.16) (45). These two metabolites were 20 to 30 times less active than sitaxsentan on ET_A receptors and inactive on ET_B receptors. The main routes of excretion were renal (49% to 62%) and fecal (34% to 48%). Renal clearance was decreased in PAH patients compared to healthy individuals.

The coadministration of sitaxsentan did not alter the pharmacokinetic disposition of cyclosporin, which is extensively metabolized by CYP3A4/5 (45). Although this coadministration resulted in a sixfold increase in the plasma concentrations of sitaxsentan, the mechanism for

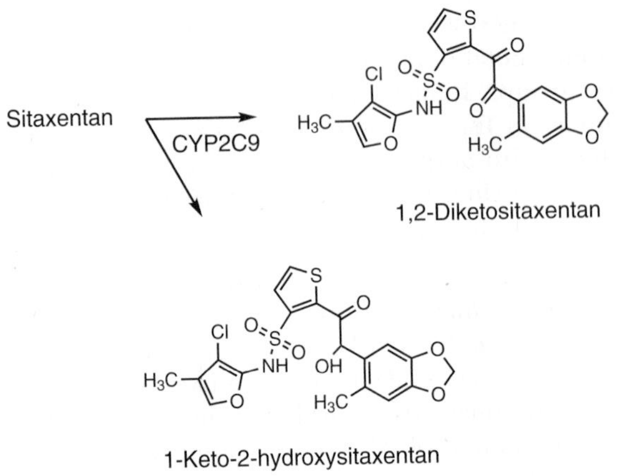

FIGURE 24.16 Metabolism of sitaxsentan.

this interaction is not known but may be due to cyclosporin inhibition of CYP3A4/5. Because of this increase in sitaxsentan exposure, its use in patients receiving cyclosporin is contraindicated.

When prescribing any endothelin receptor antagonist, patients with PAH frequently require anticoagulant therapy, and sitaxsentan affects warfarin metabolism or similar anticoagulants. Sitaxsentan is a potent inhibitor of CYP2C9 and therefore increases the area under the curve and maximum plasma concentration of drugs metabolized by CYP2C9 (45). When sitaxsentan is coadministered with warfarin, the area under the curve of warfarin was increased by approximately 96%, and clearance was decreased by approximately 63%. An enhanced effect on prothrombin clotting times was observed, consistent with the increase in plasma levels of warfarin. Therefore, because sitaxsentan inhibits the metabolism of warfarin, a warfarin dose adjustment is needed when coadministered with sitaxsentan. The dose of warfarin should be decreased by 80% when starting sitaxsentan, and then increased in increments of no greater than 0.5 mg/d while titrating to the desired clotting time. Thus, monitoring of coagulation status is warranted when sitaxsentan is prescribed.

Like other endothelin receptor antagonists, sitaxsentan is also teratogenic, and pregnancy must be excluded before the start of treatment and prevented thereafter by using a reliable contraceptive method. The drug has been associated with a reversible, dose-related increase in the liver enzymes aspartate aminotransferase and alanine aminotransferase, accompanied in some cases by elevated bilirubin (hepatotoxicity). Therefore, testing of liver aminotransferases prior to starting treatment and monthly thereafter is recommended. Patients with hypersensitivity to sulfonamides should be excluded.

The most commonly reported adverse events were headache, peripheral edema, nasal congestion, and nausea.

Prostanoids (46).

Epoprostenol (Flolan). Prostacyclin and its analogs (prostanoids) (Fig. 24.17) are potent vasodilators and possess antithrombotic and antiproliferative properties. Prostacyclin is derived from the endothelium of VSM, and its synthesis is reduced in patients with PAH. Its physiologic antagonist, thromboxane A_2, is increased, however, causing vasoconstriction. Prostacyclin produces its vasodilation via activation of the PIP_2 signal transduction pathway, increasing concentrations of cAMP (Fig. 24.2). Epoprostenol is the sodium salt of prostacyclin and is administered as an implanted continuous IV infusion because of its very short duration of action (2 to 3 minutes). It must be reconstituted with a special glycine buffer diluent, giving a reconstituted solution with pH 10 to 11 that is stable for 15 minutes at 4°C and for less than 10 minutes at 37°C. Its injection solution is unstable at a lower pH because of acid-catalyzed hydrolysis of the vinyl-ether structure to 6-oxo-$PGF_{1\alpha}$ (Fig. 24.17). It is short acting because of rapid metabolism at the 15-hydroxy group to the inactive 15-oxo metabolite.

Treprostinil (Remodulin). Treprostinil (Fig. 24.17) is a synthetic, stable form of prostacyclin for the treatment of advanced pulmonary hypertension with NYHA class III or IV symptoms, as well as for late-stage peripheral vascular disease (PVD). Its sodium salt injectable form is administered either as a continuous subcutaneous infusion directly into the skin or, if the subcutaneous infusion is not tolerated, as a continuous IV infusion without an implanted catheter. Treprostinil is rapidly absorbed from the subcutaneous site of infusion, with an almost 100% bioavailability and a mean half-life of 85 minutes (34 minutes for the IV infusion). The IV solution must be diluted with normal saline or sterile water before starting the infusion. Unlike epoprostenol, treprostinil is stable at room temperature for up to 5 years, with vasodilation action lasting from 4 to 6 hours, compared with the short, 2- to 3-minute action for epoprostenol. Because of its long life in the body, it can be administered under the skin with a microinfusion subcutaneous infusion pump rather than into the bloodstream and, thus, without hospitalization, as contrasted with the central IV infusion of epoprostenol.

Side effects include jaw pain, headaches, nausea, diarrhea, flushing, and localized pain at the delivery site under the skin. This pain has been reported as slight to severe irritation. Patients using the drug seem to experience improvement in their condition, including decreased fatigue, decreased shortness of breath, and decreased pulmonary artery pressures, as well as overall improvement in quality of life.

Beraprost. Beraprost is an oral formulation of a prostacyclin analog for the treatment of early-stage pulmonary hypertension as well as early-stage PVD (Fig. 24.17).

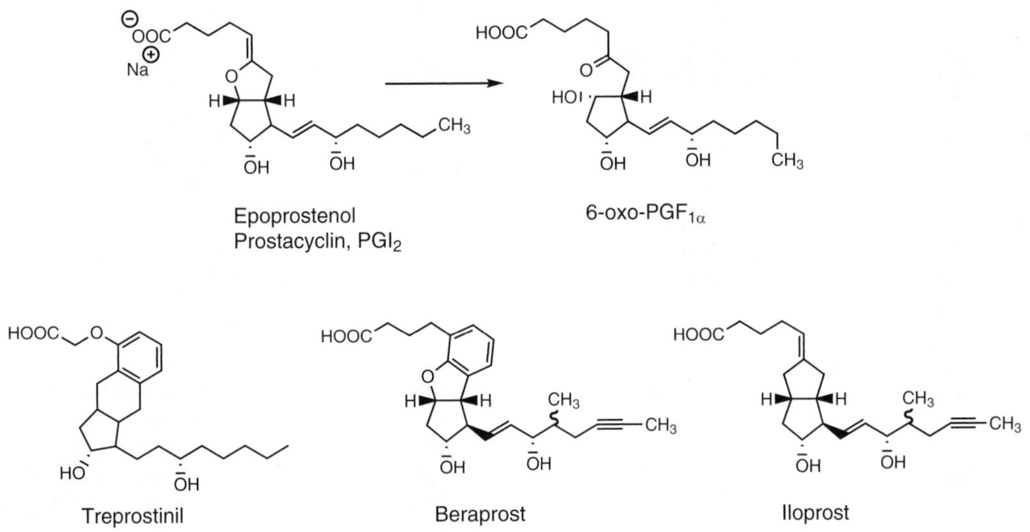

FIGURE 24.17 Prostacyclin analogs.

Beraprost is a chemically stable, oral form of prostacyclin that is readily absorbed from GI tract. Like natural prostacyclin, beraprost dilates blood vessels, prevents platelet aggregation, and prevents proliferation of smooth muscle cells surrounding blood vessels. It can be an important treatment for early-stage PVD and early-stage pulmonary hypertension. Intermittent oral doses of beraprost, however, do not seem to provide the consistent blood levels necessary to treat the advanced stages of pulmonary hypertension. Beraprost has proven to be safe and effective for the treatment of PVD in the clinical studies conducted and has been approved for the treatment of PVD in Japan since 1994. It will soon be available for use in patients with pulmonary hypertension in the United States. Adverse effects include headache, flushing, jaw pain, and diarrhea.

Iloprost (Ventavis). Iloprost is administered as an inhalation solution of a prostacyclin analog for the treatment of NYHA class III and class IV PAH (Fig. 24.17). The drug can also be administered as an IV infusion. It is stable at room temperature and to light, with a body half-life of 30 minutes. Iloprost has approximately 10 times greater potency than prostacyclin as a vasodilator of the pulmonary blood vessels; this greater potency of inhaled iloprost results from coating of the drug on the alveoli of the lungs. It relieves pulmonary vascular resistance. Patients inhale six to eight puffs every 2 to 3 hours. Each puff lasts approximately 15 minutes. This therapy is used mainly in Europe and is not available in United States. Studies have reported minor side effects, such as coughing, headaches, and jaw pain.

SCENARIO: OUTCOME AND ANALYSIS

Outcome

Judy Cheng, PharmD

An additional antihypertensive agent is necessary to better control blood pressure. Because AJ has also history of chronic stable angina, adding a β-blocker will not only help control the patient's blood pressure (his goal needs to be at least <140/90 mm Hg) and his heart rate (his goal needs to be 50 to 60 beats per minute to minimize risk of chest pain), but it is also a good antianginal agent for AJ. It is recommended that metoprolol succinate 25 mg once daily be added to the patient's regimen.

Chemical Analysis

Victoria Roche and S. William Zito

Metoprolol succinate is a β_1-selective adrenergic antagonist commonly used to decrease heart rate and force of myocardial contraction. The aryloxypropanolamine pharmacophore contains all of the functional groups required by adrenoceptors of their endogenous neurotransmitter norepinephrine, but separates the critical binding moieties (aromatic ring, carbinol OH, cationic amino nitrogen) by distances that are longer than what is observed in the agonist. The flexibility of the side chain permits access to key adrenoceptor binding residues but disallows receptor stimulation. Strong competitive antagonism is the pharmacologic result.

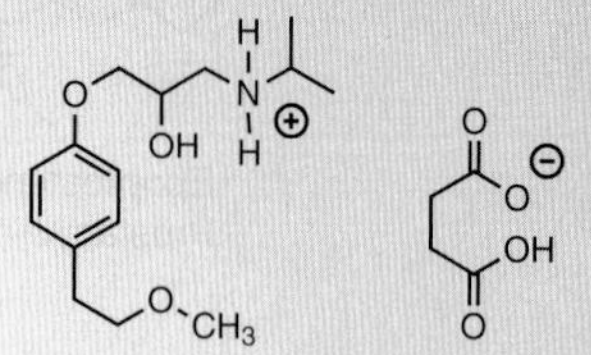

Metoprolol succinate

Metoprolol targets β-adrenoceptors rather than α-receptors because the *N*-isopropyl moiety binds with high affinity to the hydrophobic binding site at β sites but encounters affinity-destroying steric hindrance at α sites. The selectivity is further defined by the *p*-substituent on the aromatic ring, which directs the molecule to β_1-receptors in the heart over β_2-receptors in the lung. The lack of problematic bronchoconstriction in therapeutic doses enhances the safety of this agent, particularly in patients with compromised lung function.

Metoprolol and other β_1-selective agents can attenuate the symptoms of angina because, with the decrease in cardiac workload, the coronary vessels have more time to fill with blood during diastole, leading to improved coronary artery perfusion. Of importance to AJ is that β_1-selective blockers do not negatively impact serum lipid levels to the extent that nonselective β-blockers do. They are commonly coadministered with diuretics like hydrochlorothiazide in the treatment of hypertension.

CASE STUDY

Victoria Roche and S. William Zito

HP is a 72-year-old retiree who lives with his wife in a beachside community in south Florida. HP was born and raised in Iowa, and he was a very successful pig farmer for all of his adult life. As a result of his exposure to organic dusts and gases associated with his agricultural occupation, he has compromised lung function that manifests as chronic bronchitis and emphysema. Like many men his age, he suffers from benign prostatic hypertrophy, which he manages through the use of the nutraceutical saw palmetto. HP and his wife love hitting the open road on day trips to see the south Florida sights. They still enjoy a healthy sexual relationship, although he depends on the PDE5 inhibitor sildenafil (Viagra) to overcome age-related erectile dysfunction.

Always borderline hypertensive, HP had been able to keep his blood pressure in check with a proper diet and the active lifestyle that was a natural part of his farm-related occupation. However, now that he's taking life easy (and eating out more often), his pressure is elevated to the point where pharmacotherapy is appropriate. When advising HP's physician about a good starting therapy, you make note that, in addition to Viagra, his patient profile includes Symbicort, a combination product containing budesonide (an inhaled corticosteroid), and formoterol fumerate (a long-acting β_2-adrenoceptor agonist). Which of the three blood pressure–lowering agents below would you recommend for this "young-at-heart" retiree?

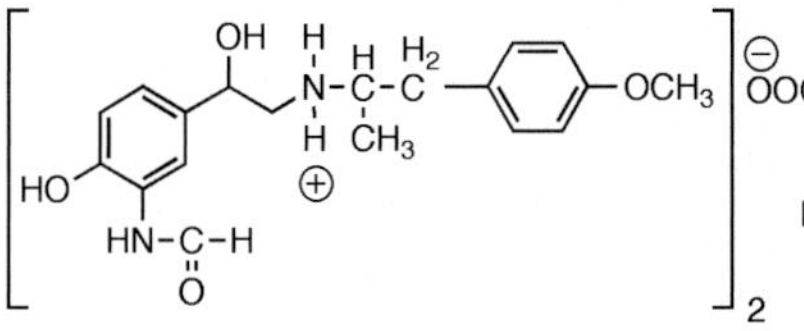

Formoterol fumarate

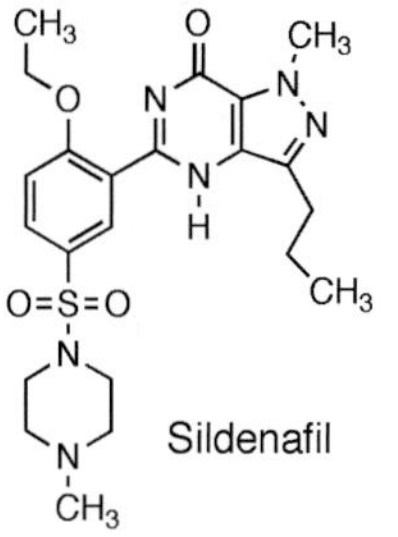

Sildenafil

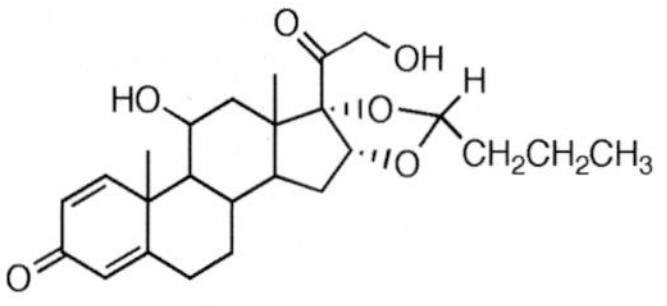

Budesonide

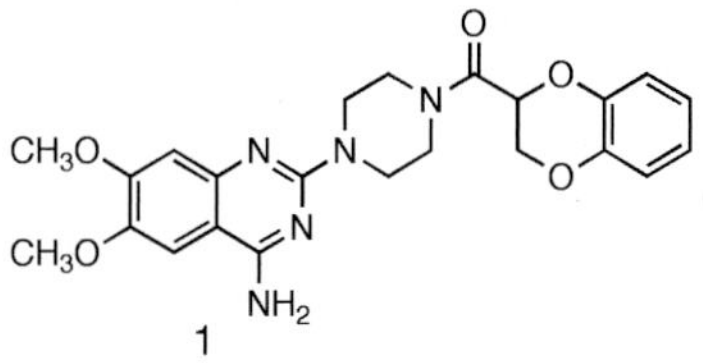

1

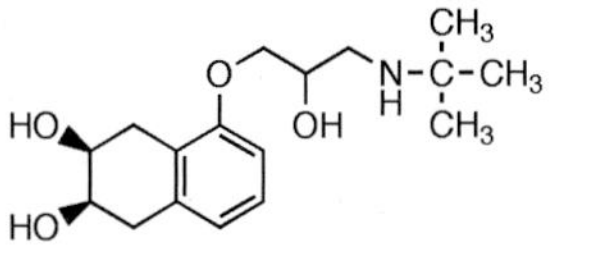

2

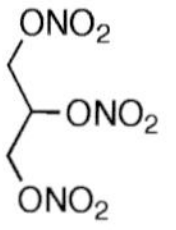

3

1. Conduct a thorough and mechanistic SAR analysis of the three therapeutic options in the case.
2. Apply the chemical understanding gained from the SAR analysis to this patient's specific needs to make a therapeutic recommendation.

References

1. Yeh D, Michel T. Pharmacology of vascular tone. In: Goan DE, Tashjian A, Armstrong E, et al., eds. Principles of Pharmacology: The Pathophysiologic Basis of Drug Therapy. Baltimore, MD: Lippincott Williams & Wilkins, 2004:317–330.
2. Weibert RT. Hypertension. In: Herfindal ET, Gourley DR, eds. Textbook of Therapeutics: Drug and Disease Management, 7th Ed. Baltimore, MD: Lippincott Williams & Wilkins, 2000:795–824.
3. The Sixth Report of the Joint National Committee on Prevention, Detection, Evaluation and Treatment of High Blood Pressure (JNC VI). Arch Intern Med 1997;157:2413–2446.
4. Brown MJ, Haydock S. Pathoetiology, epidemiology and diagnosis of hypertension. Drugs 2000;59(Suppl 2):1–12.
5. Sibai B. Treatment of hypertension in pregnant women. N Engl J Med 1996;335:257–265.
6. McEvoy GK, ed. AHFS 2000 Drug Information. Bethesda, MD: American Society of Health-System Pharmacists, 2000:1658–1726.
7. Kaplan NM. Combination therapy for systemic hypertension. Am J Cardiol 1995;76:595–597.
8. Abernethy DR. Pharmacological properties of combination therapies for hypertension. Am J Hypertens 1997;10:13S–16S.
9. Hoffman B. Therapy of hypertension. In: Brunton LL, Lazo JS, Parker KL, eds. Goodman and Gilman's The Pharmacologic Basis of Therapeutics, 11th Ed. New York: McGraw-Hill, 2006:845–869.
10. Robertson JIS. State-of-the-art review: β-blockade and the treatment of hypertension. Drugs 1983;25(Suppl 2):5–11.
11. Freis ED, Papademetriou V. Current drug treatment and treatment patterns with antihypertensive drugs. Drugs 1996;52:1–16.
12. Husserl FE, Messerli FH. Adverse effects of antihypertensive drugs. Drugs 1981;22:188–210.
13. Goldberg M, Fenster PE. Clinical significance of intrinsic sympathomimetic activity of beta blockers. Drug Therapy 1991:35–43.
14. Cauffield JS, Gums JG, Curry RW. Alpha blockers: a reassessment of their role in therapy. Am Fam Physician 1996;54:263–270.
15. Dunn CJ, Lea AP, Wagstaff AJ. Carvedilol. A reappraisal of its pharmacologica properties and therapeutic use in cardiovascular disorders. Drugs 1997;54:161–185.
16. Goa KL, Benfield P, Sorkin EM. Labetalol: a reappraisal of its pharmacology, pharmacokinetics and therapeutic use in hypertension and ischemic heart disease. Drugs 1989;37:583–627.
17. Van Zwieten PA. An overview of the pharmacodynamic properties and therapeutic potential of combined α- and β-adrenoreceptor antagonists. Drugs 1993;45:509–517.
18. Skerjanec A, Campbell NRC, Robertson S, et al. Pharmacokinetics and presystemic gut metabolism of methyldopa in healthy human subjects. J Clin Pharmacol 1995;35:275–280.
19. Bousquet P, Feldman J. Drugs acting on imidazoline receptors. A review of their pharmacology, their use in blood pressure control and their potential interest in cardioprotection. Drugs 1999;58:799–812.
20. Piletz JE, Regunathan S, Ernsberger P. Agmatine and imidazolines: their novel receptors and enzymes. Ann N Y Acad Sci 2003;1009–1043.
21. Dardonville C, Rozas I. Imidazoline binding sites and their ligands: an overview of the different chemical structures. Med Res Rev 2004;24:639–661
22. Ziegler D, Haxhiu MA, Kaan EC, et al. Pharmacology of moxonidine, an I_1-imidazoline receptor agonist. J Cardiovascular Pharmacol 1996;27(Suppl 3):S26–S37.
23. Theodor R, Weimann HJ, Weber W, et al. Absolute bioavailability of moxonidine. Eur J Drug Metab Pharmacokinet 1991;16:153–159.
24. Chrisp P, Faulds D. Moxonidine: a review of its pharmacology and therapeutic use in essential hypertension. Drugs 1992;44:993–1012.
25. Genissel P, Bromet N, Fourtillan JB, et al. Pharmacokinetics of rilmenidine in healthy subjects. Am J Cardiol 1988;61:47D–53D.
26. Genissel P, Bromet N. Pharmacokinetics of rilmenidine. Am J Med 1989;87:8S–23S.
27. Langley MS, Heel RC. Transdermal clonidine. A preliminary review of its pharmacodynamic properties and therapeutic efficacy. Drugs 1988;35:123–142.
28. Fujimura A, Ebihara A, Ohashi K-I, et al. Comparison of the pharmacokinetics, pharmacodynamics and safety of oral (Catapres) and transdermal (M-5041T) clonidine in healthy subjects. J Clin Pharmacol 1994;34:260–265.
29. Ebihara A, Fujimura A, Ohashi K-I, et al. Influence of application site of a new transdermal clonidine, M-5041T, on its pharmacokinetics and pharmacodynamics in healthy subjects. J Clin Pharmacol 1993;33:1188–1191.
30. Holmes B, Brogden RN, Heel RC, et al. Guanabenz. A review of its pharmacodynamic properties and therapeutic efficacy in hypertension. Drugs 1983;26:212–225.
31. Sorkin EM, Heel RC. Guanfacine: a review of its pharmacodynamic and pharmacokinetic properties and therapeutic efficacy in the treatment of hypertension. Drugs 1986;31:301–336.
32. Cornish LA. Guanfacine hydrochloride. A centrally acting antihypertensive agent. Clin Pharm 1988;7:187–197.
33. Carchman SH, Crowe JT Jr, Wright GJ. The bioavailability and pharmacokinetics of guanfacine after oral and intravenous administration to healthy volunteers. J Clin Pharmacol 1987;27:762–767.
34. Finnerty FA Jr, Brogden RN. Guanadrel. A review of its pharmacodynamic and pharmacokinetic properties and therapeutic use in hypertension. Drugs 1985;30:22–31.
35. Duty S, Weston AH. Potassium channel openers. Pharmacological effects and future uses. Drugs 1990;40:785–791.
36. Campese VM. Minoxidil: a review of its pharmacological properties and therapeutic use. Drugs 1981;22:257–278.
37. Clissold SP, Heel RC. Topical minoxidil: a preliminary review of its pharmacodynamic properties and therapeutic efficacy in alopecia areata and alopecia androgenetica. Drugs 1987;33:107–122.

38. Golpon HA, Welte T, Hoeper MM. Pulmonary arterial hypertension: pathobiology, diagnosis and treatment. Minerva Med 2005;96:303–314.
39. Hoeper MM. Drug treatment of pulmonary arterial hypertension: current and future agents. Drugs 2005;65:1337–1354.
40. Kawanabe Y, Nauli SM. Endothelin. Cell Mol Life Sci 2011;68:195–203.
41. Dhillon S, Keating GM. Bosentan: a review of its use in the management of mildly symptomatic pulmonary arterial hypertension. Am J Cardiovasc Drugs 2009;9:331–350.
42. Newman JH, Kar S, Kirkpatrick P. Ambrisentan. Nat Rev Drug Discov 2007;6:697–698.
43. Vatter H, Seifert V. Ambrisentan, a non-peptide endothelin receptor antagonist. Cardiovasc Drug Rev 2006;24:63–76.
44. Wittbrodt ET, Abubakar A. Sitaxsentan for treatment of pulmonary hypertension. Ann Pharmacother 2007;41:100–105.
45. Pfizer. Prescription products. http://www.pfizer.ca/en/our_products/products/monograph/170. Accessed: November 29, 2010.
46. Olschewski H, Rose F, Schermuly R, et al. Prostacyclin and its analogues in the treatment of pulmonary hypertension. Pharmacol Ther 2004;102:139–153.

Chapter 25

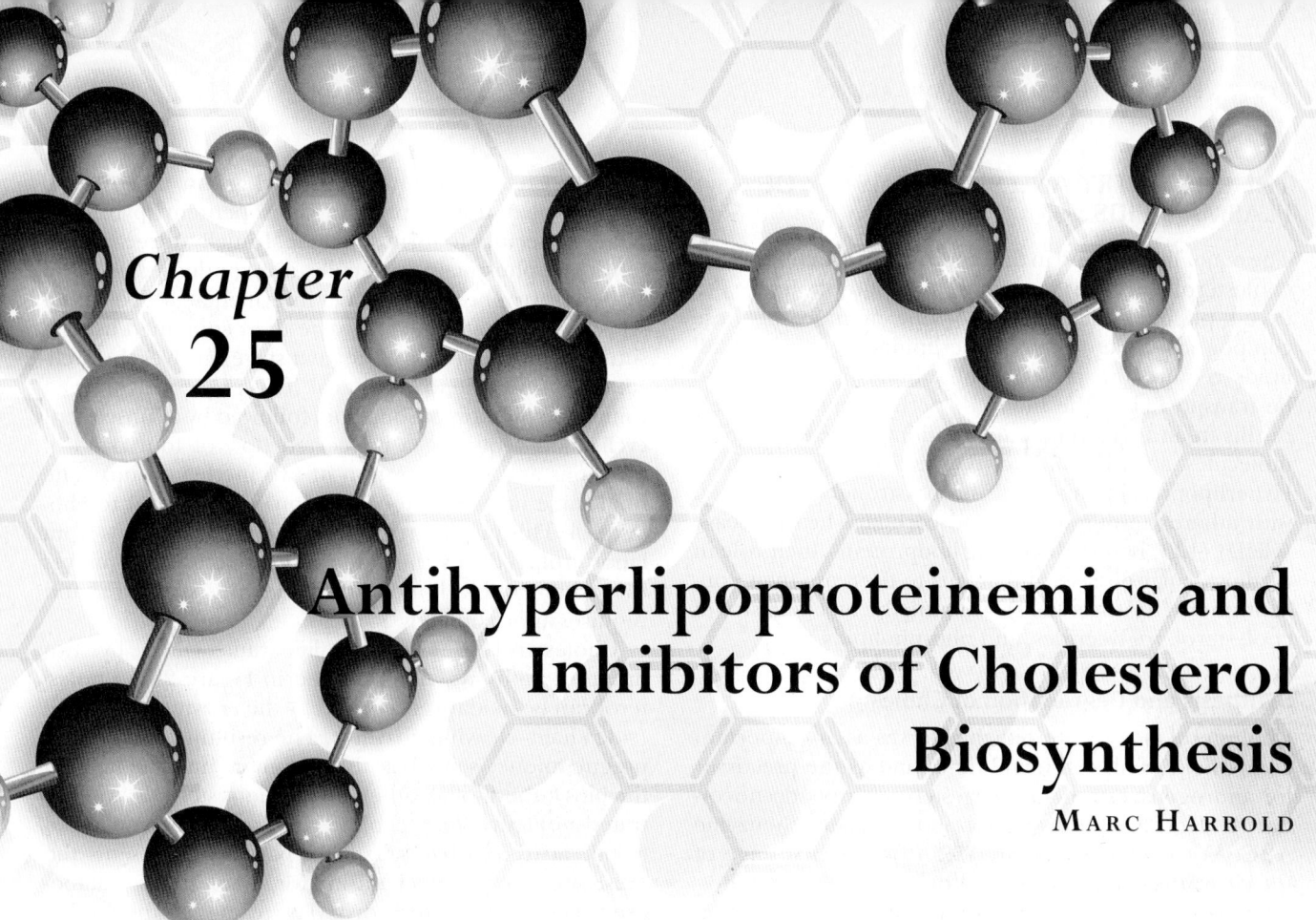

Antihyperlipoproteinemics and Inhibitors of Cholesterol Biosynthesis

MARC HARROLD

*Drugs Covered in This Chapter**

- Atorvastatin
- *Bezafibrate*
- Cholestyramine
- *Ciprofibrate*
- *Clofibric acid*
- Colesevelam
- Colestipol
- Ezetimibe
- Fenofibric acid
- Fluvastatin
- Gemfibrozil
- Lovastatin
- Mevastatin
- Nicotinic acid/niacin
- Pitavastatin
- Pravastatin
- Rosuvastatin
- Simvastatin

Abbreviations

ACAT, acyl CoA–cholesterol acyltransferase
ALT, alanine transaminase
apo, apolipoprotein
AST, aspartate transaminase
CETP, cholesterol ester transfer protein
CHD, coronary heart disease
CoA, coenzyme A
FDA, U.S. Food and Drug Administration
HDL, high-density lipoprotein
HMG, 3-hydroxy-3-methylglutaryl
HMGRIs, HMG-CoA reductase inhibitors
IDL, intermediate-density lipoprotein
LDL, low-density lipoprotein
NAD⁺, nicotinamide adenine dinucleotide
NADP⁺, nicotinamide adenine dinucleotide phosphate
PPAR, peroxisome proliferator-activated receptor
SAR, structure–activity relationship
RCT, reverse cholesterol transport
VLDL, very-low-density lipoprotein

SCENARIO

Thomas L. Rihn, PharmD

TN is a 66-year-old man with a 2-year history of angina and an 8-year history of non–insulin-dependent diabetes mellitus. He also has fairly severe peripheral vascular disease. TN returned to his primary care physician for follow-up after experiencing several recent bouts of chest pain upon exertion. Blood work during that visit revealed the following lipid profile:

- Total Chol. 272 mg/dL
- LDL-C 197 mg/dL
- HDL-C 46 mg/dL
- Normal triglycerides

TN has insurance for prescription coverage.

(The reader is directed to the clinical solution and chemical analysis of this case at the end of the chapter).

*Drugs listed include those available inside and outside of the United States; drugs available outside of the United States are shown in italics.

THE CHEMISTRY AND BIOCHEMISTRY OF PLASMA LIPIDS

The major lipids found in the bloodstream are cholesterol, cholesterol esters, triglycerides, and phospholipids. An excess plasma concentration of one or more of these compounds is known as hyperlipidemia. Because all lipids require the presence of soluble lipoproteins to be transported in the blood, hyperlipidemia ultimately results in an increased concentration of these transport molecules, a condition known as hyperlipoproteinemia. Hyperlipoproteinemia has been strongly associated with atherosclerotic lesions and coronary heart disease (CHD) (1,2). Before discussing lipoproteins, their role in cardiovascular disease, and agents to decrease their concentrations, it is essential to examine the biochemistry of cholesterol, triglycerides, and phospholipids.

Synthesis and Degradation of Cholesterol

Cholesterol is a C_{27} steroid that serves as an important component of all cell membranes and as the precursor for androgens, estrogens, progesterone, and adrenocorticoids (Fig. 25.1). It is synthesized from acetyl coenzyme A (CoA), as shown in Figure 25.2 (3). The first stage of the biosynthesis is the formation of isopentenyl pyrophosphate from three acetyl CoA molecules. The conversion of 3-hydroxy-3-methylglutaryl (HMG)–CoA to mevalonic acid is especially important, because it is a primary control site for cholesterol biosynthesis. This reaction is catalyzed by HMG-CoA reductase and reduces the thioester of HMG-CoA to a primary hydroxyl group. The second stage involves the coupling of six isopentenyl pyrophosphate molecules to form squalene. Initially, three isopentenyl pyrophosphate molecules are condensed to form farnesyl pyrophosphate, a C_{15} intermediate. Two farnesyl pyrophosphate molecules are then combined using a similar type of reaction. The next stage involves the cyclization of squalene to lanosterol. This process involves an initial epoxidation of squalene, followed by a subsequent cyclization requiring a concerted flow of four pairs of electrons and the migration of two methyl groups. The final stage involves the conversion of lanosterol to cholesterol. This process removes three methyl groups from lanosterol, reduces the side-chain double bond, moves the other double bond within the ring structure, and requires approximately 20 steps.

Cholesterol is enzymatically transformed by two different pathways. As illustrated in Figure 25.1, cholesterol can be oxidatively cleaved by the enzyme desmolase (side chain–cleaving enzyme). The resulting compound, pregnenolone, serves as the common intermediate in the biosynthesis of all other endogenous steroids. As illustrated in Figure 25.3, cholesterol also can be converted to bile acids and bile salts. This pathway represents the most important mechanism for cholesterol catabolism. The enzyme 7α-hydroxylase catalyzes the initial, rate-limiting step in this metabolic pathway and, thus, is the key control enzyme for this pathway. Cholic acid and its derivatives are primarily (99%) conjugated with either glycine (75%) or taurine (24%). Bile salts, such as

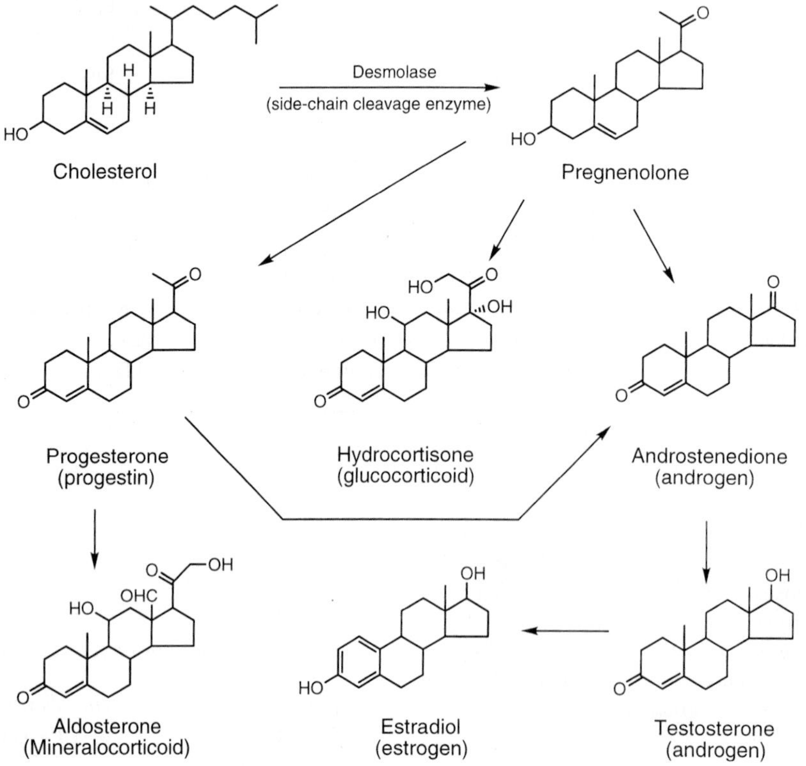

FIGURE 25.1 Cholesterol's role as a key intermediate in the biosynthesis of endogenous steroids.

SQUALENE SYNTHASE: A POTENTIAL DRUG TARGET

Inhibitors of squalene synthase, the enzyme responsible for catalyzing the two-step conversion of two molecules of farnesyl pyrophosphate to squalene, are currently being investigated as antihyperlipidemic agents. Squalene synthase catalyzes the first committed step in sterol biosynthesis and offers some potential advantages over HMG-CoA reductase as a drug target. The latter group of compounds inhibits cholesterol synthesis at an early stage of the pathway and, thus, lacks specificity. Mevalonic acid, the immediate product of HMG-CoA reductase, is a common intermediate in the biosynthesis of other isoprenoids, such as ubiquinone (an electron carrier in oxidative phosphorylation), dolichol (a compound involved in oligosaccharide synthesis), and farnesylated proteins (the farnesyl portion targets the protein to cell membrane as opposed to the cytosol). Inhibitors of squalene synthase target an enzyme involved in a later stage of cholesterol biosynthesis and could potentially accomplish the same desired outcomes as currently available agents without interfering with the biosynthesis of other essential, nonsteroidal compounds. One class of compounds currently under investigation is the squalestatins. These compounds were originally isolated as fermentation products produced by a species of *Phoma*. Squalestatin 1 is a potent inhibitor of squalene synthetase and has been shown to produce a marked decrease in serum cholesterol. Additional analogs and other structural classes continue to be investigated and, ultimately, may produce alternatives to currently available therapy (4,5).

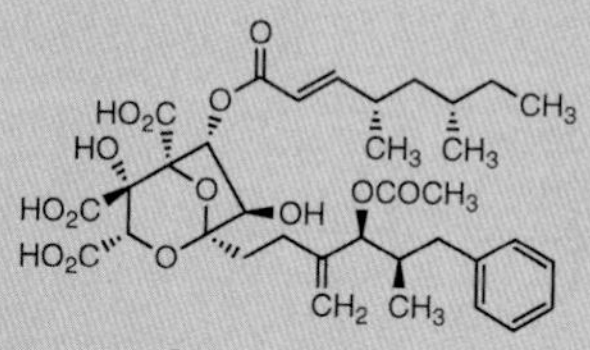

Squalestatin 1

glycocholate, are surface-active agents that act as anionic detergents.

The bile salts are synthesized in the liver, stored in the gallbladder, and released into the small intestine, where they emulsify dietary lipids and fat-soluble vitamins. This solubilization promotes the absorption of these dietary compounds through the intestinal mucosa. Bile salts are predominantly reabsorbed through the enterohepatic circulation and returned to the liver, where they exert a negative feedback control on 7α-hydroxylase and, thus, regulate any subsequent conversion of cholesterol (3,6).

The terms "bile acid" and "bile salt" refer to the un-ionized and ionized forms, respectively, of these compounds. For illustrative purposes only, Figure 25.3 shows cholic acid as a un-ionized bile acid and glycocholate as an ionized bile salt (as the sodium salt). At physiologic and intestinal pH values, both compounds would exist almost exclusively in their ionized forms.

Overview of Triglycerides and Phospholipids

Triglycerides (or, more appropriately, triacylglycerols) are highly concentrated stores of metabolic energy. They are formed from glycerol 3-phosphate and acylated CoA (Fig. 25.4) and accumulate primarily in the cytosol of adipose cells. When required for energy production, triglycerides are hydrolyzed by lipase enzymes to liberate free fatty acids that are then subjected to β-oxidation, the citric acid cycle, and oxidative phosphorylation.

Phospholipids, or phosphoglycerides, are amphipathic compounds that are used to make cell membranes, generate second messengers, and store fatty acids for use in the generation of prostaglandins. They can be synthesized from phosphatidate, an intermediate in triglyceride synthesis. Two common phospholipids, phosphatidyl choline and phosphatidyl inositol, are shown below (3).

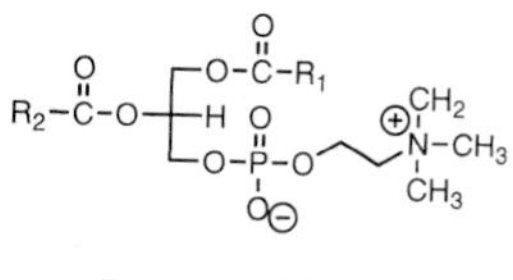

Phosphatidyl choline

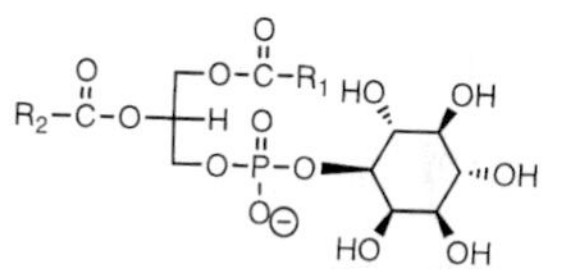

Phosphatidyl inositol

Lipoproteins and Transport of Cholesterol and Triglycerides

Cholesterol, triglycerides, and phospholipids are freely soluble in organic solvents, such as isopropanol, chloroform, and diethyl ether, but are relatively insoluble in aqueous, physiologic fluids. To be transported within the blood, these lipids are solubilized through association with macromolecular aggregates known as lipoproteins. Each lipoprotein is associated with additional proteins, known as apolipoproteins, on their outer surface. These apolipoproteins provide structural support and stability, bind to cellular receptors, and act as cofactors for enzymes involved in lipoprotein metabolism. The compositions and primary functions of the six major lipoproteins are listed in Table 25.1 (6,7).

Lipoprotein nomenclature is based on mode of separation. When preparative ultracentrifugation is used, lipoproteins are separated according to their density and identified as very-low-density lipoproteins (VLDLs), intermediate-density lipoproteins (IDLs), low-density lipoproteins (LDLs), and high-density lipoproteins (HDLs). When electrophoresis is used in the separation, lipoproteins are designated as pre-β, β, and α. The IDLs are mainly found in the pre-β fraction as a second electrophoretic band and are currently believed to be an intermediate lipoprotein in the catabolism of VLDL to LDL. Chylomicron remnants and IDLs may show similar electrophoretic and ultracentrifugation separation characteristics. In general, VLDL, LDL, and HDL correspond to pre-β, β, and α lipoprotein, respectively.

The interrelationship among the lipoproteins is shown in Figure 25.5 (7,8). As illustrated, the pathway can be divided into both exogenous (dietary intake) and endogenous (synthetic) components. The exogenous

CLINICAL SIGNIFICANCE

The development and availability of cholesterol and triglyceride-lowering agents has evolved significantly over the past 10 to 15 years. The structure–activity relationships and structural modifications of bile acid sequestrants, fibrates, nicotinic acid, and, in particular, 3-hydroxy-3-methylglutaryl–coenzyme A reductase inhibitors form the basis for this evolution and the therapeutic advances that have resulted.

The most widely used cholesterol-lowering agents in cardiovascular medicine today are the "statins" (vastatins). Lovastatin was the first statin to be used clinically on a large scale. Structural modifications of the early statin molecules have produced superior agents in terms of their pharmacokinetic profile, potency, drug interactions, and, perhaps, selective adverse effects. This has resulted in the widespread clinical use of superior agents, such as atorvastatin. In randomized clinical trials, such agents have been demonstrated to exert a potent effect in lowering low-density lipoprotein cholesterol as well as an important anti-inflammatory action.

The net effect of applying basic science in modifying the chemical structure of cholesterol-lowering drugs is that negative patient outcomes such as death, myocardial infarction, and other cardiovascular events have been greatly reduced. This is clearly a situation in which the application of basic and clinical science has produced a profound effect on tens of millions of patients.

Thomas L. Rihn, PharmD
Senior Vice President and Chief Clinical Officer
University Pharmacotherapy Associates and Associate Professor of Clinical Pharmacy
Duquesne University
School of Pharmacy
Pittsburgh, Pennsylvania

pathway begins after the ingestion of a fat-containing meal or snack. Dietary lipids are absorbed in the form of cholesterol and fatty acids. The fatty acids are then reesterified within the intestinal mucosal cells and, along with the cholesterol, are incorporated into chylomicrons, the largest lipoprotein. During circulation, chylomicrons are degraded into remnants by the action of lipoprotein lipase, a plasma membrane enzyme located on capillary endothelial cells in adipose and muscle tissue. The interaction of chylomicrons with lipoprotein lipase requires apolipoprotein (apo) C-II, and the absence of either the enzyme or the apolipoprotein can lead to hypertriglyceridemia and pancreatitis. The liberated free acids are then available for either storage or energy

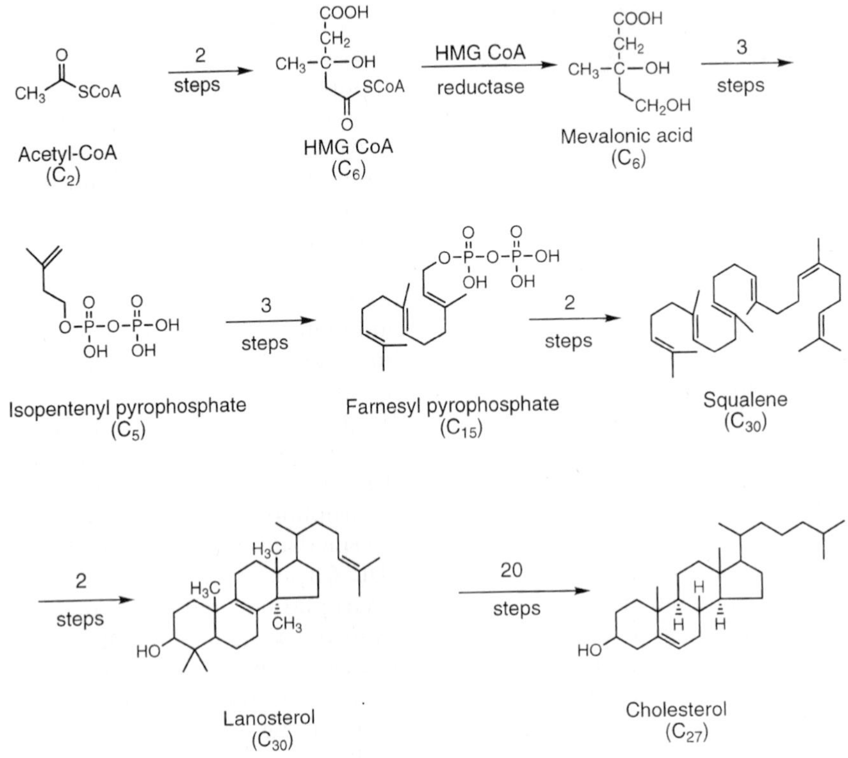

FIGURE 25.2 The biosynthesis of cholesterol.

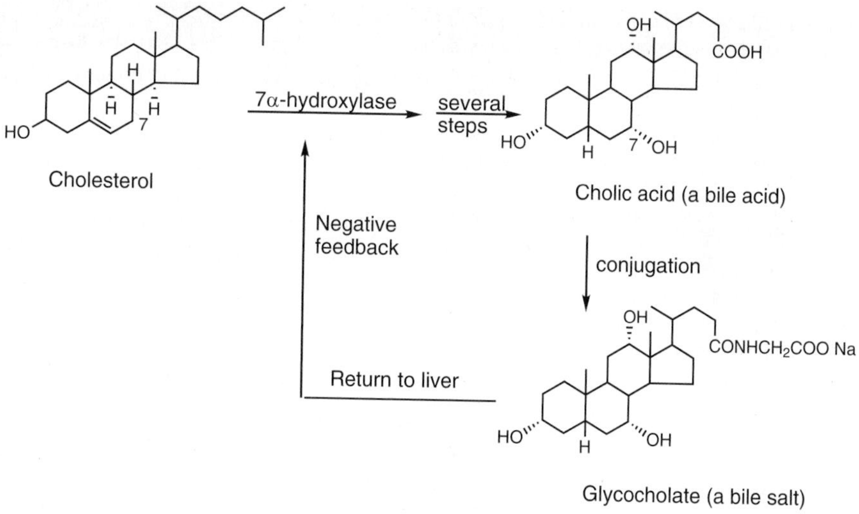

FIGURE 25.3 The conversion of cholesterol to bile acids and bile salts.

generation by these tissues. The remnants are predominantly cleared from the plasma by liver parenchymal cells via recognition of the apoE portion of the carrier.

The endogenous pathway begins in the liver with the formation of VLDL. Similar to chylomicrons, triglycerides are present in a higher concentration than either cholesterol or cholesterol esters; however, the concentration difference between these lipids is much less than that seen in chylomicrons. The metabolism of VLDL also is similar to chylomicrons in that lipoprotein lipase reduces the triglyceride content of VLDL and increases the availability of free fatty acids to the muscle and adipose tissue. The resulting lipoprotein, IDL, either can be further metabolized to LDL or can be transported to the liver for receptor-mediated endocytosis. This latter effect involves an interaction of the LDL receptor with the apolipoproteins, apoB-100 and apoE, on IDL. The amount of IDL delivered to the liver is approximately the same as that converted to LDL. The half-life of IDL is relatively short as compared to that of LDL and, thus, accounts for only a small portion of total plasma cholesterol. In contrast, LDL accounts for approximately two-thirds of total plasma cholesterol and serves as the primary source of cholesterol for both hepatic and extrahepatic cells. As with IDL, the uptake of LDL by these cells is mediated by a receptor interaction with the apoB-100 on LDL. The number of LDL receptors on the cell surface mediates regulation of cellular LDL uptake. Cells requiring increased amounts of cholesterol will increase the biosynthesis of LDL receptors. Conversely, it has been demonstrated that increased hepatic concentrations of cholesterol will inhibit both HMG-CoA reductase as well as the production of LDL receptors. As previously discussed, hepatic cholesterol can be converted to bile acids and bile salts and reenter the endogenous pathway through the bile and enterohepatic circulation.

Synthesized in the liver and intestine, HDL initially exists as a dense, phospholipid disk composed primarily of apoA-I. The primary function of HDL is to act as a scavenger to remove cholesterol from extrahepatic cells and to facilitate its transport back to the liver. Nascent HDL accepts free, unesterified cholesterol. A plasma enzyme, lecithin-cholesterol acyltransferase, then esterifies the cholesterol. This process allows the resulting cholesterol esters to move from the surface to the core and results in the production of spherical HDL_3 particles. As cholesterol content is added, HDL_3 is converted to HDL_2, which is larger and less dense than HDL_3. The ultimate return of cholesterol from HDL_2 to the liver is known as

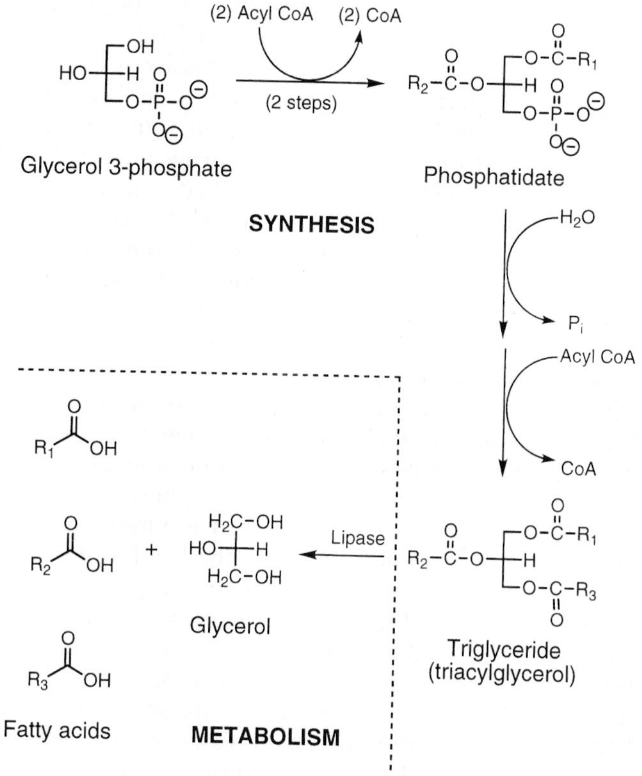

FIGURE 25.4 The biosynthesis and metabolism of triglycerides.

TABLE 25.1 Classification and Characteristics of Major Plasma Lipoproteins

Classification	Composition	Major Apolipoproteins	Primary Function(s)
Chylomicrons	Triglycerides 80%–95%, free cholesterol 1%–3%, cholesterol esters 2%–4%, phospholipids 3%–9%, apoproteins 1%–2%	apoA-I, apoA-IV, apoB-48, apoC-I, apoC-II, apoC-III	Transport dietary triglycerides to adipose tissue and muscle for hydrolysis by lipoprotein lipase
Chylomicron remnants	Primarily composed of dietary cholesterol esters	apoB-48, apoE	Transport dietary cholesterol to liver for receptor-mediated endocytosis
VLDL	Triglycerides 50%–65%, free cholesterol 4%–8%, cholesterol esters 16%–22%, phospholipids 15%–20%, apoproteins 6%–10%	apoB-100, apoE, apoC-I, apoC-II, apoC-III	Transport endogenous triglycerides to adipose tissue and muscle for hydrolysis by lipoprotein lipase
IDL	Intermediate between VLDL and LDL	apoB-100, apoE, apoC-II, apoC-III	Transport endogenous cholesterol for either conversion to LDL or receptor-mediated endocytosis by the liver
LDL	Triglycerides 4%–8%, free cholesterol 6%–8%, cholesterol esters 45%–50%, phospholipids 18%–24%, apoproteins 18%–22%	apoB-100	Transport endogenous cholesterol for receptor-mediated endocytosis by either the liver or extrahepatic tissues
HDL	Triglycerides 2%–7%, free cholesterol 3%–5%, cholesterol esters 15%–20%, phospholipids 26%–32%, apoproteins 45%–55%	apoA-I, apoA-II, apoE, apoC-I, apoC-II, apoC-III	Removal of cholesterol from extrahepatic tissues via transfer of cholesterol esters to IDL and LDL

apo, apolipoprotein; HDL, high-density lipoprotein; IDL, intermediate-density lipoprotein; LDL, low-density lipoprotein; VLDL, very-low-density lipoprotein.

reverse cholesterol transport and is accomplished via an intermediate transfer of cholesterol esters from HDL_2 to either VLDL or IDL. This process regenerates spherical HDL_3 molecules that can recirculate and acquire excess cholesterol from other tissues. In this manner, HDL serves to prevent the accumulation of cholesterol in arterial cell walls and other tissue and may serve as the basis for its cardioprotective properties (6,7).

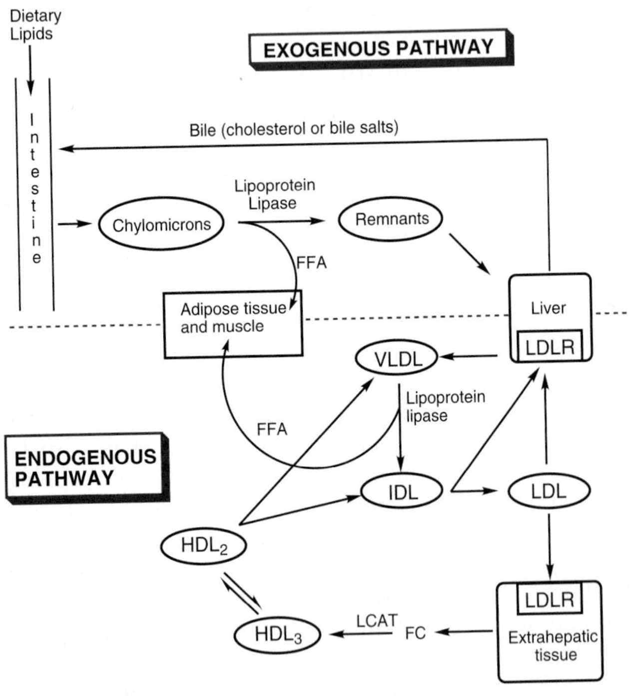

FIGURE 25.5 Endogenous and exogenous pathways for lipid transport and metabolism. FC, free unesterified cholesterol; FFA, free fatty acids; LCAT, lecithin-cholesterol acyltransferase; LDLR, low-density lipoprotein receptor.

Classification of Hyperlipoproteinemias

Hyperlipoproteinemia can be divided into primary and secondary disorders. Primary disorders are the result of genetic deficiencies or mutations, whereas secondary disorders are the result of other conditions or diseases. Secondary hyperlipoproteinemia has been associated with diabetes mellitus, hypothyroidism, renal disease, liver disease, alcoholism, and certain drugs (1,6,7).

In 1967, Fredrickson et al. (8) classified primary hyperlipoproteinemias into six phenotypes (I, IIa, IIb, III, IV, and V) based on which lipoproteins and lipids were elevated. Current literature and practice, however, appear to favor the more descriptive classifications and subclassifications listed in Table 25.2. Primary disorders are currently classified as those that primarily cause hypercholesterolemia, those that primarily cause hypertriglyceridemia, and those that cause a mixed elevation of both cholesterol and triglycerides. Subclassifications are based on the specific biochemical defect responsible for the disorder. Classifications developed by Fredrickson have been included in Table 25.2 under the heading *Previous Classification* for comparative and reference purposes.

As shown in Table 25.2, some disorders are well characterized, whereas others are not (1,6,7). Familial hypercholesterolemia is caused by a deficiency of LDL receptors. This results in a decreased uptake of IDL and LDL by hepatic and extrahepatic tissues and an elevation in plasma LDL levels. The homozygous form of this disorder is rare but results in extremely high LDL levels

TABLE 25.2 Characteristics of the Major Primary Hyperlipoproteinemias

Current Classification	Biochemical Defect	Elevated Lipoproteins	Previous Classification
Hypercholesterolemias			
Familial hypercholesterolemia	Deficiency of LDL receptors	LDL	IIa
Familial defective apoB-100	Mutant apoB-100	LDL	IIa
Polygenic hypercholesterolemia	Unknown	LDL	IIa
Hypertriglyceridemias			
Familial hypertriglyceridemia	Unknown	VLDL	IV
Familial lipoprotein lipase deficiency	Deficiency of lipoprotein lipase	Chylomicrons, VLDL	I (chylomicron elevation only), V
Familial apoC-II deficiency	Deficiency of apoC-II	Chylomicrons, VLDL	I (chylomicron elevation only), V
Mixed hypercholesterolemia and hypertriglyceridemia			
Familial combined hyperlipidemia	Unknown	VLDL, LDL	IIb
Dysbetalipoproteinemia	Presence of $apoE_2$ isoforms	VLDL, IDL	III

apo, apolipoprotein; IDL, intermediate-density lipoprotein; LDL, low-density lipoprotein; VLDL, very-low-density lipoprotein.

and early morbidity and mortality because of the total lack of LDL receptors. A related disorder, familial defective apoB-100, also results in elevated LDL levels but is caused by a genetic mutation rather than a deficiency. Alteration of apoB-100 decreases the affinity of LDL for the LDL receptor and thus hinders normal uptake and metabolism. Elevations in chylomicron levels can result from a deficiency of either lipoprotein lipase or apoC-II. These deficiencies cause decreased or impaired triglyceride hydrolysis and result in a massive accumulation of chylomicrons in the plasma. Dysbetalipoproteinemia results from the presence of an altered form of apoE and is the only mixed hyperlipoproteinemia with a known cause. Proper catabolism of chylomicron and VLDL remnants requires apoE. The presence of a binding-defective form of apoE, known as $apoE_2$, results in elevated levels of VLDL and IDL triglyceride and cholesterol levels.

DISEASES AND DISORDERS CAUSED BY HYPERLIPIDEMIAS

CHD, which includes acute myocardial infarction, ischemic heart disease, and angina pectoris, is the leading cause of mortality in the United States. In 2006, CHD was responsible for 425,00 deaths. In addition, mortality from CHD often occurs rapidly, either in an emergency room or before hospitalization. The highest mortality is seen in patients older than 65 years; however, the vast majority of deaths in patients younger than 65 years occur during an initial attack. Risk factors associated with CHD include hypertension, cigarette smoking, elevated plasma cholesterol levels, physical inactivity, diabetes, and obesity (9).

Atherosclerosis, which is named from the Greek terms for "gruel" (*athere*) and "hardening" (*sclerosis*), is the underlying cause of CHD. It is a gradual process in which an initial accumulation of lipids in the arterial intima leads to thickening of the arterial wall, plaque formation, thrombosis, and occlusion (10–12). The involvement of LDL cholesterol in this process is shown in Figure 25.6. Within the extracellular space of the intima, LDL is more susceptible to oxidative metabolism, because it is no longer protected by plasma antioxidants. This metabolism alters the properties of LDL such that it is readily scavenged by macrophages. Unlike normal LDL, the uptake of oxidized LDL is not regulated; thus, macrophage cells can readily become engorged with oxidized LDL. Subsequent metabolism produces free cholesterol, which either can be released into the plasma or reesterified by the enzyme acyl CoA–cholesterol acyltransferase (ACAT). Cholesterol released into plasma can be scavenged by HDL_3 and returned to the liver, thus preventing any accumulation or damage. In this manner, HDL acts as a cardioprotective agent, because high concentrations of reesterified cholesterol can morphologically change macrophages into foam cells. Accumulation of lipid-engorged foam cells in the arterial intima results in the formation of fatty streaks, the initial lesion of atherosclerosis. Later, the deposition of lipoproteins, cholesterol, and phospholipids causes the formation of softer, larger plaques. Associated with this lipid deposition is the proliferation of arterial smooth muscle cells into the intima and the laying down of collagen, elastin, and glycosaminoglycans, leading to fibrous plaques. Ultimately, the surface of the plaque deteriorates, and an atheromatous ulcer is formed with a fibrous matrix, accumulation of necrotic tissue, and appearance of cholesterol and cholesterol ester crystals. A complicated lesion also shows calcification and hemorrhage with the formation of organized mural thrombi. Thrombosis results from changes in the arterial walls and in the blood-clotting mechanism.

Obviously, individuals with higher cholesterol and LDL levels are more susceptible to these detrimental effects than those with normal cholesterol and LDL levels. Total plasma cholesterol levels less than 200 mg/dL are considered desirable. Levels above 240 mg/dL are considered high, and levels between 200 and 239 mg/dL are considered borderline. For LDL, plasma levels of less than 100 mg/dL are considered optimal, plasma levels equal to or greater than 160 are considered high, plasma levels between 130 and 159 mg/dL are considered

POTENTIAL DRUG TARGETS: ACAT AND CEPT

Inhibitors of ACAT are currently being investigated as cholesterol-lowering or antiatherosclerotic agents. In addition to its role in foam cell formation, ACAT also is required for esterification of cholesterol in intestinal mucosal cells and for synthesis of cholesterol esters in hepatic VLDL formation. Thus, ACAT inhibitors have the potential of providing three beneficial effects in patients with hypercholesterolemia: decreased cholesterol absorption, decreased hepatic VLDL synthesis, and decreased foam cell formation. Initial successes at inhibiting ACAT were dampened by the discovery of accompanying adrenal toxicity. Subsequent structural modifications have led to the development of potent, orally active ACAT inhibitors that lack this toxicity. Two promising compounds are shown below. These and other analogs and efforts have given new hope that inhibitors of this enzyme may provide an alternative treatment of atherosclerotic disorders (11,13,14).

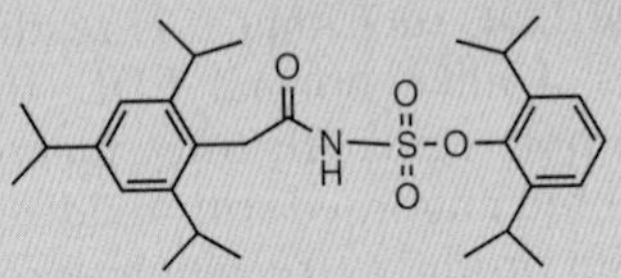

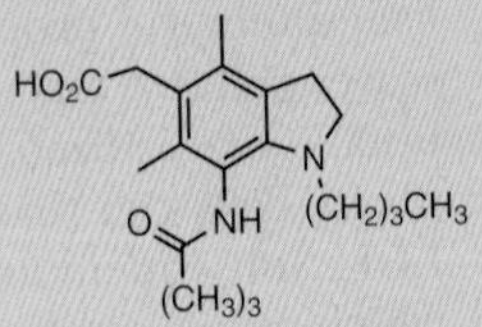

Cholesterol ester transfer protein (CETP) interacts with HDL, LDL, and VLDL to mediate the transfer of cholesterol esters from HDL (primarily HDL_2) to LDL and VLDL while balancing this exchange in a 1:1 fashion with a transfer of triglycerides from LDL and VLDL to HDL. The end result of this process is a higher concentration of LDL cholesterol and a lower concentration of HDL cholesterol. It has been postulated that CETP inhibitors would produce a therapeutic benefit due to their ability to prevent these transfers and favorably increase HDL cholesterol and lower LDL cholesterol. The initial development of potent CETP inhibitors proved to be challenging due to the nonenzymatic nature of a transport protein, the lack of a transition state and/or tightly bound intermediates, and the lack of potent natural and synthetic inhibitors. A number of chemical classes of compounds have been investigated, including thiol-based irreversible inhibitors and tetrahydroquinoline-based reversible inhibitors. Drug development at Pfizer produced torcetrapib, a potent oral CETP inhibitor that was evaluated in a phase III clinical outcomes trial. Unfortunately, torcetrapib caused increased blood pressure as well as increased circulating aldosterone levels and altered serum electrolyte levels. Further studies verified that these effects were not related to the inhibition of CETP and thus would not necessarily be seen with other agents. Another structurally related compound, anacetrapib (Merck), is currently in phase III clinical trials and has been shown to reduce LDL by up to 40% and increase HDL by up to 138% with a more acceptable side effect profile than originally seen with torcetrapib. Since CETP is also involved in reverse cholesterol transport (RCT), the process by which HDL promotes the efflux of cholesterol from macrophages, there has been some debate as to whether inhibition of CETP would cause the production of cholesterol-laden HDL molecules that would be less efficient in the RCT atheroprotective process. Clinical trials involving both torcetrapib and anacetrapib have shown that isolated HDL particles from patients involved in these studies are still capable of promoting this efflux. Additional studies are needed prior to the approval of anacetrapib or another CETP inhibitor (15,16).

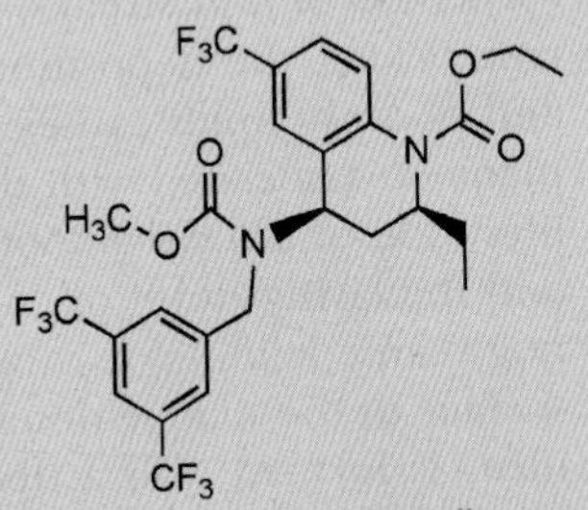

Torcetrapib

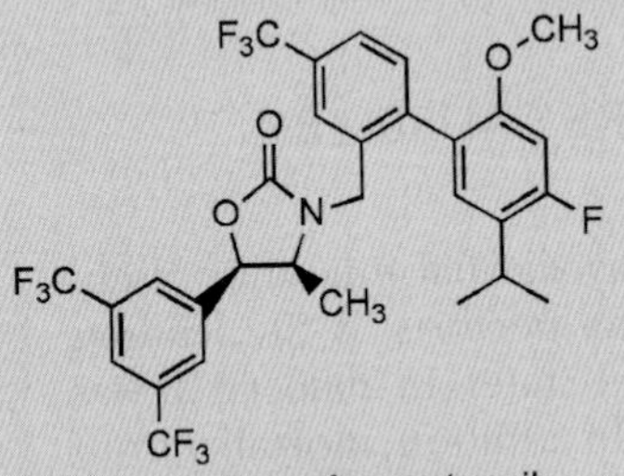

Anacetrapib

borderline, and plasma levels between 100 and 129 mg/dL are considered above optimal. Current guidelines (8,13) also recommend an LDL level below 70 mg/dL as a goal for very high-risk patients (i.e., those with multiple risk factors and known cardiovascular disease).

Elevated plasma triglyceride levels can contribute to atherosclerosis and CHD in mixed hyperlipoproteinemias, whereas pure hypertriglyceridemias are primarily associated with pancreatitis and show little to no relationship to CHD (6,7).

OVERVIEW OF DRUG THERAPY AFFECTING LIPOPROTEIN METABOLISM

Bile acid sequestrants, HMG-CoA reductase inhibitors (HMGRIs), ezetimibe, fibrates, and niacin are all used in the treatment of hyperlipoproteinemia. In general, successful use of these compounds depends on proper identification and classification of the hyperlipoproteinemia affecting the patient. With the possible exceptions of niacin, atorvastatin, and rosuvastatin, currently

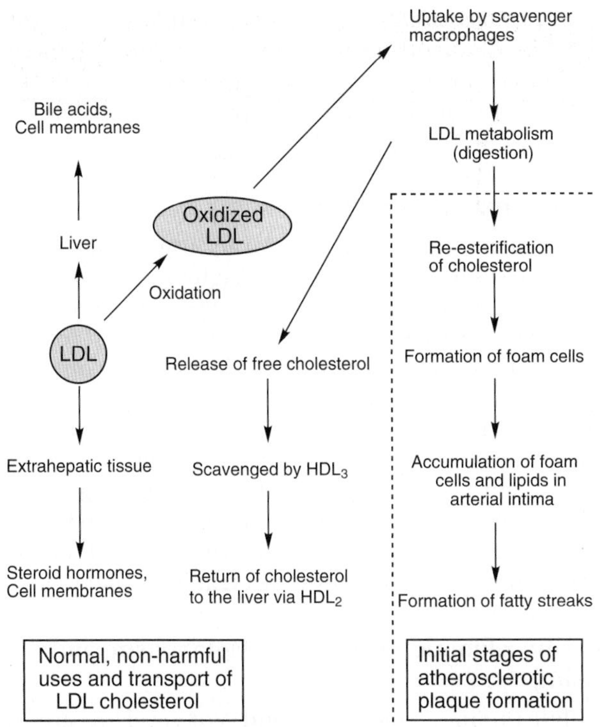

FIGURE 25.6 The role of LDL cholesterol in the development of atherosclerotic plaques. The mechanism by which HDL provides a cardioprotective action also is shown.

available compounds do not have equal efficacy in reducing both hypercholesterolemia and hypertriglyceridemia and, thus, are used primarily for their ability to decrease either cholesterol or triglyceride levels. Bile acid sequestrants, inhibitors of HMG-CoA reductase, and ezetimibe are effective in decreasing plasma cholesterol and LDL levels. The fibrates also have some actions on plasma cholesterol; however, their main effect is to stimulate lipoprotein lipase and to increase the clearance of triglycerides. Niacin, through its ability to decrease VLDL formation, has been shown to decrease the plasma levels of both triglycerides and cholesterol. All of these compounds are discussed in the following sections. References for these sections have been limited to current reviews and texts, selected papers, and product literature, both traditional and electronic. Readers requiring additional references for any of these compounds should consult either the previous edition of this text or the references contained within the cited reviews and texts.

BILE ACID SEQUESTRANTS

Historical Overview

Cholestyramine was originally developed in the 1960s to treat pruritus secondary to elevated plasma concentrations of bile acids in patients with cholestasis. Its ability to bind (i.e., to hold or to sequester) bile acids and to increase their fecal elimination was subsequently shown to produce beneficial effects in lowering serum cholesterol levels. In 1973, cholestyramine was approved for the treatment of hypercholesterolemia in patients who do not respond to dietary modifications. Colestipol and colesevelam, which retain the key structural features required to bind bile acids, were approved in 1977 and 2000, respectively (6,17).

Cholestyramine, colestipol, and colesevelam are chemically classified as anion-exchange resins. This term arises from their ability to selectively bind and exchange negatively charged atoms or molecules with one another. The selectivity comes from the fact that these positively charged resins do not bind equally to all anions. For example, the chloride ion of cholestyramine can be displaced by, or exchanged with, other anions (e.g., bile acids) that have a greater affinity for the positively charged functional groups on the resin.

Mechanism of Action

Cholestyramine, colestipol, and colesevelam lower plasma LDL levels by indirectly increasing the rate at which LDL is cleared from the bloodstream. Under normal circumstances, approximately 97% of bile acids are reabsorbed into the enterohepatic circulation. As previously discussed, these compounds are returned to the liver where they regulate their own production. Bile acid sequestrants are not orally absorbed but, rather, act locally within the gastrointestinal tract to interrupt this process. They bind the two major bile acids, glycocholic acid and taurocholic acid, and greatly increase their fecal excretion. As a result, decreased concentrations of these compounds are returned to the liver. This removes the feedback inhibition of 7α-hydroxylase and increases the hepatic conversion of cholesterol to bile acids (Fig. 25.3). The decrease in hepatic cholesterol concentrations leads to several compensatory effects: increased expression of LDL receptors, increased hepatic uptake of plasma LDL, induction of HMG-CoA reductase, and increased biosynthesis of cholesterol. The latter two effects are insufficient to counteract the increases in cholesterol clearance and catabolism; however, concurrent use of an HMGRI can provide an additive effect in lowering LDL cholesterol. Bile acid sequestrants do not alter the removal of plasma LDL by nonreceptor-mediated mechanisms and, thus, are ineffective in treating homozygous familial hypercholesterolemia (6,17–19).

The decreased return of bile acids to the liver also will produce an increase in triglyceride synthesis and a transient rise in VLDL levels. Subsequent compensatory mechanisms will increase VLDL removal, most likely through the increased LDL receptors, and return VLDL levels to predrug levels. For those patients with preexisting hypertriglyceridemia, the compensatory mechanisms are inadequate, and a persistent rise in VLDL levels occurs (6).

Structure–Activity Relationships

Cholestyramine (Fig. 25.7) is a copolymer consisting primarily of polystyrene, with a small amount of divinylbenzene as the cross-linking agent. In addition, it contains approximately 4 mEq of fixed quaternary ammonium groups per gram of dry resin. These positively charged groups function as binding sites for anions. Virtually all of these sites are accessible to bile acids. Increasing the amount of divinylbenzene from 2% to 4% to 8% increases the cross-linkage and reduces the porosity of the resin. This prevents binding of bile acids to interior sites and decreases the efficacy of the compound.

Colestipol (Fig. 25.7) is a copolymer of tetraethylenepentamine and epichlorhydrin and is commercially marked as its hydrochloride salt. The key functional groups on colestipol are the basic secondary and tertiary amines. Although the total nitrogen content of colestipol is greater than that of cholestyramine, the functional anion-exchange capacity of the resin depends on intestinal pH and may be less than cholestyramine. Comparative in vitro studies indicate that cholestyramine has a higher adsorption capacity than colestipol for bile salts (20). Quaternization of colestipol with methyl iodide increases the capacity in vitro for glycocholate (21).

Colesevelam is a more diverse polymer; however, its initial formation is similar to colestipol. In the case of colesevelam, poly(allyamine) is initially cross-linked with epichlorhydrin and then alkylated with 1-bromodecane and (6-bromohexyl)-trimethylammonium bromide. The resulting polymer contains four basic and/or quaternary functional groups, as shown in Figure 25.7. Fragment A is a primary amine, fragment B contains a secondary amine and a quaternary ammonium group, fragment C contains a pair of secondary amines, and fragment D is a decylated amine. The overall polymer is a hydrophilic gel and is insoluble in water (6).

Physicochemical Properties

All bile acid sequestrants are large, hygroscopic, water-insoluble resins. The molecular weight of cholestyramine is reported to be greater than 1,000,000 daltons; however, no specific molecular weight has been assigned to either colestipol or colesevelam. Cholestyramine contains a large number of quaternary ammonium groups and has multiple permanent positive charges. Colestipol contains a large number of secondary and tertiary amines, whereas colesevelam contains quaternary ammonium groups as well as primary and secondary amines. Normal pK_a values for the amines range from 9.0 to 10.5; thus, all of these groups should be primarily ionized at intestinal pH.

Pharmacokinetic Parameters, Metabolism, and Dosing

Cholestyramine, colestipol, and colesevelam are not orally absorbed and are not metabolized by gastrointestinal enzymes. They are excreted in the feces as an insoluble complex with bile acids. Their onset of action occurs

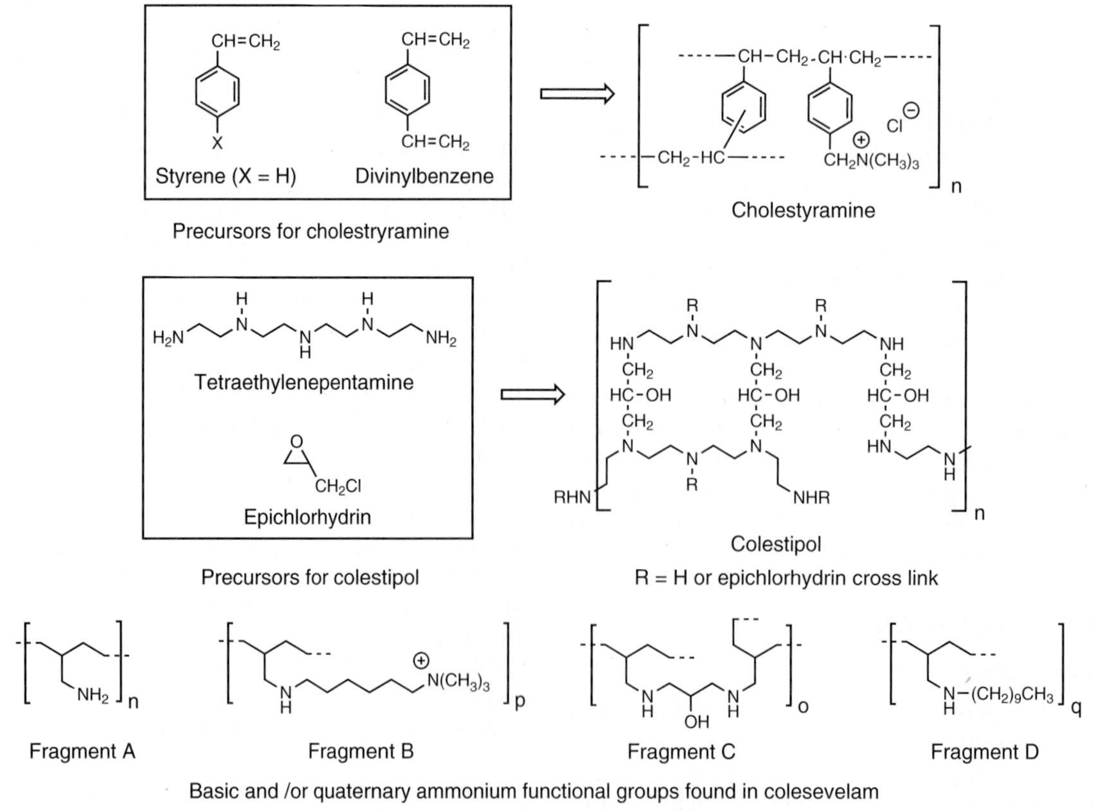

FIGURE 25.7 Structures of cholestyramine, colestipol, and precursors for these polymeric resins. Also included are the basic and quaternary functional groups found on colesevelam. Note that cholestyramine will contain a fraction of unsubstituted aromatic rings (i.e., those that are neither cross-linked nor contain a quaternary ammonium group).

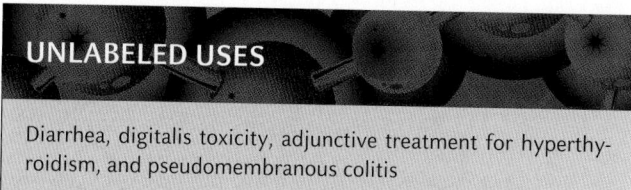

UNLABELED USES

Diarrhea, digitalis toxicity, adjunctive treatment for hyperthyroidism, and pseudomembranous colitis

within 24 to 48 hours; however, it may take up to 1 month to achieve peak response (6,17,22).

Cholestyramine is available as a powder that is mixed with water, juice, or other noncarbonated beverages to create a slurry to drink. Patients should experiment with various liquids to find the most palatable combination; however, patient acceptance and compliance with this dosage formulation can limit its use. Each packet or scoop of cholestyramine is equivalent to 4 g of cholestyramine. The recommended daily dose for the treatment of hypercholesterolemia is 8 to 16 g (two to four packets or scoops) per day divided into two doses and taken with meals. The maximum daily dose for hypercholesterolemia is 24 g. Colestipol is available as either granules or 1-g tablets. The granules should be taken in a manner similar to that described for the cholestyramine powder. The starting dose for the granules is 5 g once or twice daily. This dose can be increased in 5-g increments every 1 to 2 months until therapeutic goals or a maximum of 30 g/d has been reached. The starting dose for the tablets is 2 g once or twice daily. This dose can then be increased in 2-g segments up to a maximum daily dose of 16 g. Patients must be advised that colestipol tablets should not to be chewed, crushed, or cut and should be taken with plenty of water (17,23). Colesevelam is available as a 625-mg tablet and a 3.75-g powder for suspension. Both formulations should be taken with a meal. The starting dose is three tablets (1.875 g) twice a day, six tablets (3.75 g) once a day, or one 3.75-g powder packet once a day. The dose may be increased to a maximum of seven tablets per day (4.375 g).

Therapeutic Applications

Bile acid sequestrants are indicated for the treatment of hypercholesterolemia in patients who do not adequately respond to dietary modifications. They may be used either alone or in combination with HMGRIs or niacin. These combinations often can achieve a 50% reduction in plasma LDL levels. Cholestyramine is also approved for the relief of pruritus associated with partial biliary obstruction, whereas colestipol and colesevelam are approved for use as adjunct agents to improve glycemic control in patients with type 2 diabetes mellitus. Bile acid sequestrants should not be used to treat hypertriglyceridemias or mixed hyperlipoproteinemias in which hypertriglyceridemia is the primary concern. These compounds also are contraindicated in patients with cholelithiasis or complete biliary obstruction because of the impaired secretion of bile acids caused by these conditions. Finally, cholestyramine and colestipol are contraindicated in patients with primary biliary cirrhosis, because this can further raise serum cholesterol (6,17,23).

Adverse Effects

Because bile acid sequestrants are not orally absorbed, they produce minimal systemic side effects and, thus, are one of the safest drugs to use for hypercholesterolemia. Constipation is by far the most frequent patient complaint. Increasing dietary fiber or using bulk-producing laxatives, such as psyllium, often can minimize this adverse effect. Other gastrointestinal symptoms, such as bloating and abdominal discomfort, usually disappear with continued use; however, the possibility of fecal impaction requires that extreme caution be used in patients with preexisting constipation. All three of these compounds release chloride ions as part of their exchange mechanism and can cause hyperchloremic acidosis. This is not a common occurrence, but it may limit the use of bile acid sequestrants in patients with renal disease. Hypoprothrombinemia and bleeding are caused by the ability of bile acid sequestrants to bind with and impair the absorption of dietary vitamin K. These effects also are rare, but they may limit the use of these agents in patients with preexisting clotting disorder and in those being concurrently treated with anticoagulants (2,6,17,23).

Drug Interactions

Because of their mechanism of action, bile acid sequestrants can potentially bind with and decrease the oral absorption of almost any other drug. Because these anion-exchange resins contain numerous positive charges, they are much more likely to bind to acidic compounds than to basic compounds or nonelectrolytes. This is not an absolute, however, because cholestyramine and colestipol have been reported to decrease the oral absorption of propranolol (a base) and the lipid-soluble vitamins A, D, E, and K (nonelectrolytes). As a result, the current recommendation is that all other oral medication should be administered at least 1 hour before or 4 hours after cholestyramine and colestipol. Interestingly, this drug interaction has been used in a beneficial manner to treat digitalis overdose and toxicity.

Colesevelam seems to be less likely to interfere with the absorption of concurrently administered drugs. No significant decreases in absorption were seen when colesevelam was coadministered with digoxin, lovastatin, warfarin, metoprolol, quinidine, or valproic acid. Because of potential interactions, especially for drugs with a low therapeutic index, the administration of drugs that have not been directly studied in combination with colesevelam should be spaced accordingly, as described earlier for cholestyramine and colestipol (6,17).

HMGCoA REDUCTASE INHIBITORS

Currently, seven HMGRIs are approved for therapeutic use in the United States. Chemically, they can be divided

ADVERSE EFFECTS OF BILE ACID SEQUESTRANTS

Bloating, abdominal discomfort, constipation, bowel obstruction, steatorrhea, anorexia, cholelithiasis, pancreatitis, hyperchloremic acidosis, hypoprothrombinemia, and bleeding

into two groups, natural products and synthetic agents. All of these compounds effectively block the conversion of HMG-CoA to mevalonic acid and have similar effects on plasma cholesterol levels. The compounds differ somewhat in their indications, potencies, and pharmacokinetic profiles. They often are referred to as statins or vastatins. Because of the potential confusion of the terms "statin" and "statine" (i.e., a stable dipeptide mimic [see Chapter 23]), it is suggested here that classifying an HMGRI as a vastatin is preferable to classifying it as a statin.

Historical Overview and Development

The development and use of HMGRIs began in 1976 with the discovery of mevastatin. Originally named compactin, this fungal metabolite was isolated from two different species of *Penicillium* and demonstrated potent, competitive inhibition of HMG-CoA reductase. Its affinity for the enzyme was shown to be 10,000-fold greater than that of the substrate HMG-CoA (24). Several years later, a structurally similar compound was isolated from *Monascus ruber* and *Aspergillus terreus*. This compound was originally known as mevinolin, was later renamed lovastatin, and was more than twofold more potent than mevastatin (Fig. 25.8). Structurally, it differed from mevastatin only by the presence of a methyl group at the 6′ position of the bicyclic ring. As illustrated in Figure 25.8, mevastatin and lovastatin can bind very tightly with HMG-CoA reductase, because their hydrolyzed lactones mimic the tetrahedral intermediate produced by the reductase enzyme (6). Studies published in 1985 confirmed this theory and also established that the bicyclic portions of these compounds bind to the CoA site of the enzyme (25). Clinical trials of mevastatin were halted after reports of altered intestinal morphology in dogs (26); however, lovastatin received approval by the U.S. Food and Drug Administration (FDA) in 1987, representing the first HMGRI to be available in the United States for therapeutic use.

Structure–Activity Relationship

Mevastatin and lovastatin served as lead compounds in the development of additional HMGRIs. Initial research published by Merck Pharmaceuticals examined alterations of the lactone and bicyclic rings as well as the ethylene bridge between them. The results demonstrated that the activity of HMGRIs is sensitive to the stereochemistry of the lactone ring, the ability of the lactone ring to be hydrolyzed, and the length of bridge connecting the two ring systems. Additionally, it was found that the bicyclic

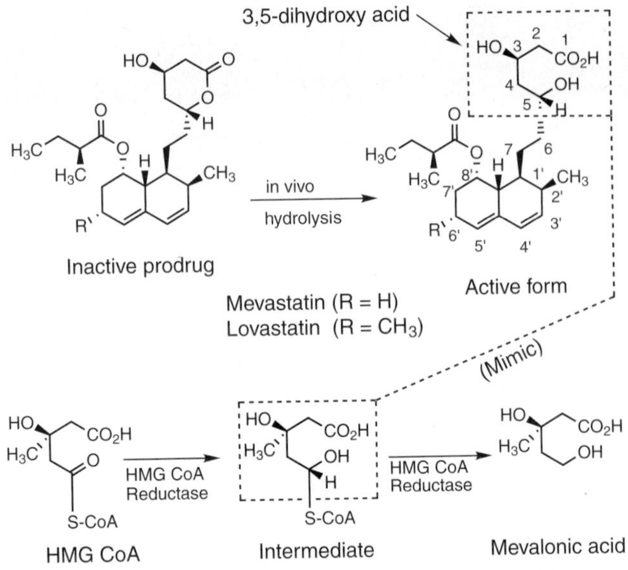

FIGURE 25.8 Mechanism of action of mevastatin and lovastatin. Hydrolysis of these prodrugs produces a 3,5-dihydroxy acid that mimics the tetrahedral intermediate produced by HMG-CoA reductase.

ring could be replaced with other lipophilic rings and that the size and shape of these other ring systems were important to the overall activity of the compounds (27).

Minor modifications of the bicyclic ring and side-chain ester of lovastatin produced simvastatin and pravastatin (Fig. 25.9). Pravastatin, a ring-opened dihydroxy acid with a 6′α-hydroxyl group, is much more hydrophilic than either lovastatin or simvastatin. Proposed advantages of this enhanced hydrophilicity are minimal penetration into the lipophilic membranes of peripheral cells, better selectivity for hepatic tissues, and a reduction in the incidence of side effects seen with lovastatin and simvastatin (28,29).

The replacement of the bicyclic ring with various substituted, aromatic ring systems led to the development of atorvastatin, fluvastatin, pitavastatin, and rosuvastatin (Fig. 25.9). The initial rationale centered on a desire to simplify the structures of mevastatin and lovastatin. The 2,4-dichlorophenyl analog (compound A) was one of the first compounds to demonstrate that this type of substitution was possible; however, compound A was considerably less potent than mevastatin. Subsequent research investigated a variety of aromatic substitutions and heterocyclic ring systems to optimize HMGRI activity. The substituted pyrrole (compound B) retained 30% of the activity of mevastatin (30) and was a key intermediate in the development of atorvastatin. The 4-fluorophenyl and isopropyl (or cyclopropane) substitutions found in compound B also are seen in the indole, quinoline, and pyrimidine ring systems of fluvastatin, pitavastatin, and rosuvastatin, respectively, and most likely represent the optimum substitutions at their respective positions. The design of all four of these compounds included the ring-opened dihydroxy acid functionality first seen in pravastatin.

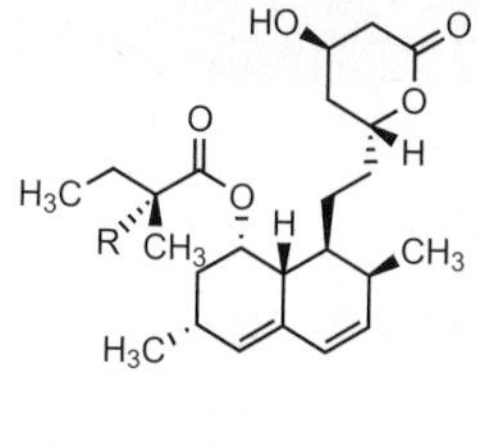

Lovastatin (R = H)
Simvastatin (R = CH_3)

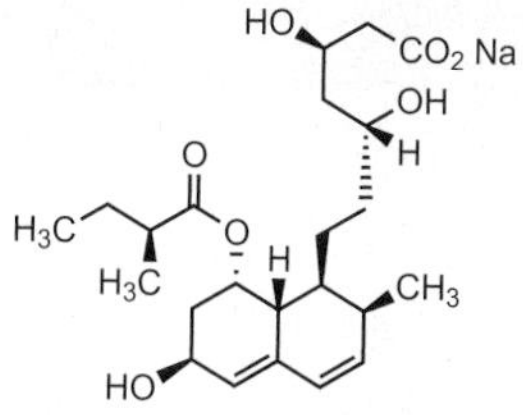

Pravastatin

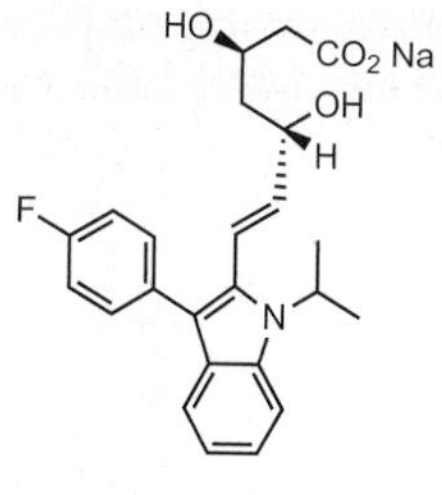

Fluvastatin

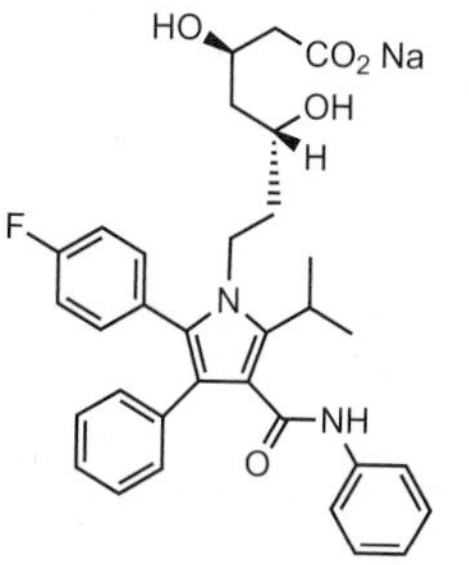

Atorvastatin

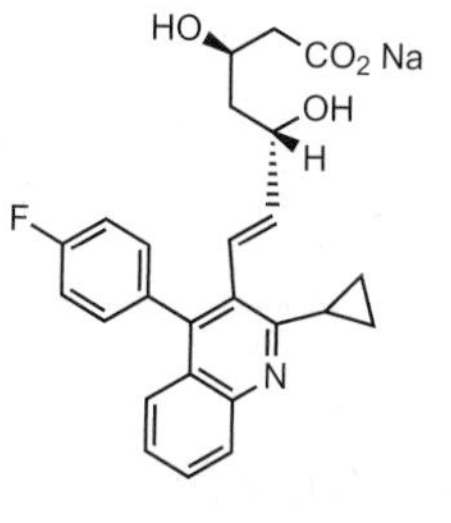

Pitavastatin

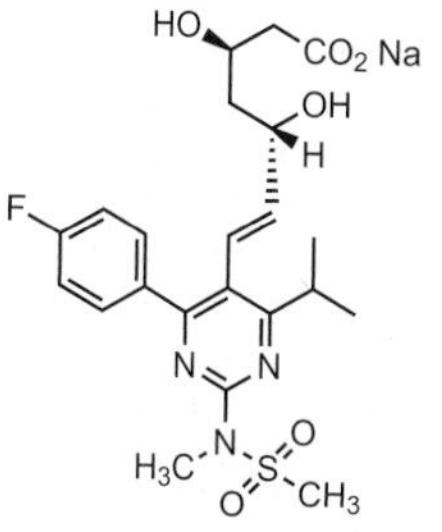

Rosuvastatin

FIGURE 25.9 Commercially available HMG-CoA reductase inhibitors.

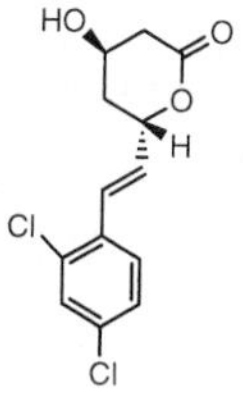

Compound A

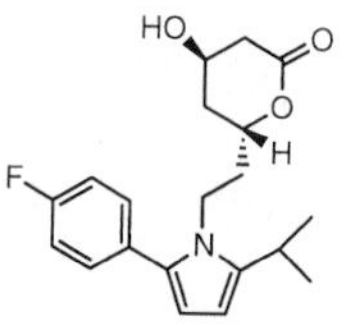

Compound B

All HMGRIs can be chemically classified as 7-substituted-3,5-dihydroxyheptanoic acids, the general structure of which is shown in Table 25.3. Additionally, these compounds can be subclassified based on their lower ring. Compounds structurally related to the natural products mevastatin and lovastatin have structural features common to ring A, whereas those that are completely synthetic have structural features common to ring B (27,29–37).

Mechanism of Action

Inhibitors of HMG-CoA reductase lower plasma cholesterol levels by three related mechanisms: inhibition of cholesterol biosynthesis, enhancement of receptor-mediated LDL uptake, and reduction of VLDL precursors (17,23). As previously discussed, HMG-CoA reductase is the rate-limiting step in cholesterol biosynthesis. Inhibition of this enzyme causes an initial decrease in hepatic cholesterol. Compensatory mechanisms result in an enhanced expression of both HMG-CoA reductase and LDL receptors. The net result of all these effects is a slight to modest decrease in cholesterol synthesis, a significant increase in receptor-mediated LDL uptake, and an overall lowering of plasma LDL levels. Evidence to support the theory that enhanced LDL receptor expression is the primary mechanism for lowering LDL levels comes from the fact that most statins do not lower LDL levels in patients who are unable to produce LDL receptors (i.e., homozygous familial hypercholesterolemia). The increased number of LDL receptors also may increase the direct removal of VLDL and IDL. Because these lipoproteins are precursors to LDL, this action may contribute to the overall lowering of plasma LDL cholesterol. Finally, all HMGRIs can produce a modest (8% to 12%) increase in HDL (17).

Atorvastatin, rosuvastatin, and simvastatin appear to have some effects beyond those seen with the other HMGRIs. These compounds have been shown to decrease plasma LDL levels in patients with homozygous familial hypercholesterolemia, an effect that is proposed to result from their ability to produce a more significant decrease in the hepatic production of LDL cholesterol. Additionally, atorvastatin and rosuvastatin can produce a significant lowering in plasma triglycerides. In the case of atorvastatin, this effect has been attributed to its ability to produce an enhanced removal of triglyceride-rich VLDL (17,38,39).

Physicochemical Properties

In their active forms, all HMGRIs contain a carboxylic acid. This functional group is required for inhibitory activity, has a pK_a in the range of 2.5 to 3.5, and will be primarily ionized at physiologic pH. Lovastatin and simvastatin are neutral, lactone prodrugs and should be classified as nonelectrolytes. Pravastatin, fluvastatin, and atorvastatin can be classified as acidic drugs. The nitrogen atoms in the indole and pyrrole rings of fluvastatin and atorvastatin, respectively, are aromatic nitrogens that are not ionizable. This is because the lone pair electrons of these atoms are

TABLE 25.3 Structure–Activity Relationship of HMG-CoA Reductase Inhibitors

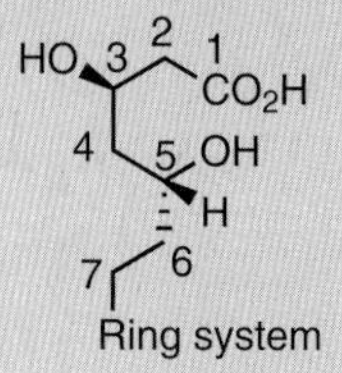

7-substituted-3,5-dihydroxyheptanoic acid

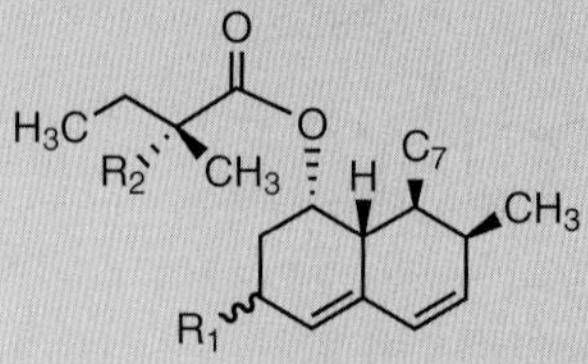

Ring A

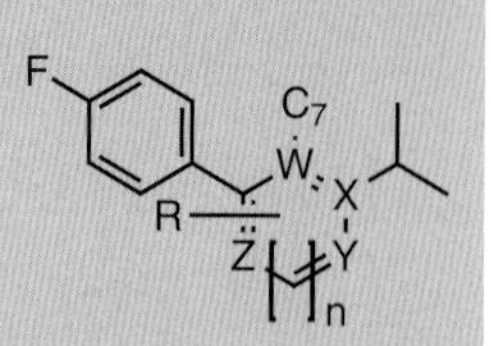

Ring B

Common for all HGMIs	1. The 3,5-dihydroxycarboxylate is essential for inhibitory activity. Compounds containing a lactone are prodrugs requiring in vivo hydrolysis. 2. The absolute stereochemistry of the 3- and 5-hydroxyl groups must be the same as that found in mevastatin and lovastatin. 3. Altering the two-carbon distance between C5 and the ring system diminishes or fails to improve activity. 4. A double bond between C6 and C7 can either increase or decrease activity. The ethyl group provides optimal activity for compounds containing ring A and some heterocyclic rings (e.g., pyrrole ring of atorvastatin). The ethenyl group is optimal for compounds with other ring systems, including the indole, quinoline, and pyrimidine rings seen in fluvastatin, pitavastatin, and rosuvastatin, respectively.
Ring A subclass	1. The decalin ring is essential for anchoring the compound to the enzyme active site. Replacement with a cyclohexane ring resulted in a 10,000-fold decrease in activity. 2. Stereochemistry of the ester side chain is not important for activity; however, conversion of this ester to an ether results in a decrease in activity. 3. Methyl substitution at the R_2 position increases activity (i.e., simvastatin is more potent than lovastatin). 4. β-Hydroxyl group substitution at the R_1 position enhances hydrophilicity and may provide some cellular specificity.
Ring B subclass	1. Substituents W, X, Y, and Z can be either carbon or nitrogen; n is equal to either zero or one (i.e., five- or six-member heterocyclic). 2. The para-fluorophenyl cannot be coplanar with the central aromatic ring. (Structural restraints to cause coplanarity have resulted in a loss of activity). 3. R substitution with aryl groups, hydrocarbon chains, amides, or sulfonamides enhances lipophilicity and inhibitory activity.

involved in maintaining the aromaticity of their respective rings and are not available to bind protons. Pitavastatin and rosuvastatin are amphoteric compounds; however, their quinoline and pyrimidine rings are weakly basic and will primarily be un-ionized at physiologic pH.

The calculated logP values for the HMGRIs are shown in Table 25.4. Although some variation exists among the values for lovastatin, pravastatin, and simvastatin, the general trends are the same regardless of what program was used to calculate the values. Atorvastatin, fluvastatin, pitavastatin, and the prodrugs lovastatin and simvastatin have a much higher lipid solubility than either pravastatin and rosuvastatin. Hydrolysis of the lactone ring for the two prodrugs produces a 3,5-dihydroxycarboxylate with significantly improves water solubility.

The HMG-CoA reductase enzyme is stereoselective. The 3*R*,5*R* stereochemistry seen in the active forms of mevastatin and lovastatin (Fig. 25.8) is required for inhibitory activity and is present in all other HMGRIs. Stereochemistry of the substituents on the bicyclic rings of lovastatin, simvastatin, and pravastatin is less crucial to activity, as indicated in the summary of the structure–activity relationships (SARs).

Metabolism

As previously mentioned, lovastatin and simvastatin are inactive prodrugs that must undergo in vivo hydrolysis to produce their effects (Fig. 25.8). The active forms of these two compounds as well as most HMGRIs undergo extensive first-pass metabolism (15,20,36,37). The CYP3A4 isozyme is responsible for the oxidative metabolism of atorvastatin, lovastatin, and simvastatin. In the case of atorvastatin, the *ortho-* and *para*-hydroxylated metabolites are equiactive with the parent compound and contribute significantly to the overall activity of the drug (Table 25.4). Rosuvastatin is metabolized to a limited extent by CYP2C9 to form an *N*-desmethyl metabolite that can contribute to activity, but is sevenfold less potent. In contrast, the activity of lovastatin and simvastatin resides primarily in the initial hydrolysis product (i.e., further oxidation decreases activity). Fluvastatin is metabolized by the CYP2C9 and CYP3A4 isozymes to active hydroxylated metabolites; however, these metabolites do not circulate systemically and do not contribute to the overall activity. Pravastatin also undergoes oxidative metabolism, but the resulting compounds retain only minimal activity and are not significant. Neither pitavastatin, pravastatin, nor rosuvastatin is metabolized by CYP3A4; therefore, these drugs are potentially advantageous for patients who must take concurrent medication that alters the activity of this isozyme. Pitavastatin is primarily metabolized by CYP2CP and undergoes lactonization to an inactive compound.

Pharmacokinetic Parameters

The pharmacokinetic parameters and dosing information for HMGRIs are summarized in Tables 25.4 and 25.5, respectively (2,6,17,21,22,38,40,41). With a few exceptions, all of these compounds have similar onsets of action, durations of action, dosing intervals, and plasma protein binding. Despite the ability to attain a peak plasma concentration in 1 to 4 hours, HMGRIs require approximately 2 weeks to demonstrate an initial lowering of plasma cholesterol. Peak reductions of plasma cholesterol occur after 4 to 6 weeks of therapy for most compounds. Studies with atorvastatin, however, indicate that it may only need 2 weeks to produce its peak reduction. Atorvastatin and rosuvastatin also are unique in that they have much longer durations of action than the other compounds. With the exception of pravastatin, which is one of the more hydrophilic compounds in this class, most HMGRIs bind extensively to plasma proteins.

Because of first-pass metabolism, the oral bioavailability of this class of drugs generally is low and does not reflect the actual absorption of the individual drugs. For example, 60% to 80% of a dose of simvastatin is orally absorbed, but only 5% is actually available to produce an effect. The same is true with fluvastatin, pravastatin, and lovastatin, which have oral absorptions of 90%, 34%, and 35%, respectively, but much lower bioavailabilities. Pitavastatin has the highest oral bioavailability in this class of compounds (Table 25.4). With the exception of lovastatin, the concurrent administration of food does not affect the overall therapeutic effects of HMGRIs. Lovastatin should always be administered with food to maximize oral bioavailability. Failure to do this results in a 33% decrease in plasma concentrations. In general, HMGRIs should be administered in the evening or at bedtime to counteract the peak cholesterol synthesis, which occurs in the early morning hours. Exceptions to this are atorvastatin and rosuvastatin, which because of their long half-lives are equally effective regardless of when they are administered.

The primary route of elimination of these compounds is through the feces. Because of extensive hepatic transformation and the ability to elevate hepatic enzymes, HMGRIs are contraindicated in patients with active hepatic disease or unexplained persistent elevations in serum aminotransferase concentrations. Dosage reductions in patients with renal dysfunction depend on the individual agent. Atorvastatin, which has minimal renal excretion, requires no dosage reduction and may be the best agent for patients with renal disorders. Fluvastatin, rosuvastatin, and simvastatin require dosage reductions only in cases of severe renal impairment and are better choices than lovastatin, pitavastatin, and pravastatin, which require dosage reductions in mild or moderate impairment.

Therapeutic Applications

All HMGRIs are approved for the treatment of primary hypercholesterolemia and familial combined hyperlipidemia, or mixed dyslipidemia (Fredrickson type IIa and IIb) (Table 25.2) in patients who have not responded to diet, exercise, and other nonpharmacologic methods (Table 25.6) (17,23). They may be used either alone or in combination with bile acid sequestrants, ezetimibe, or niacin. As previously mentioned, they should be administered at least 1 hour before or 4 to 6 hours after bile acid sequestrants when this combination is desired. Atorvastatin, fluvastatin, lovastatin, pravastatin, and simvastatin have been specifically indicated to reduce the mortality of CHD and stroke. By

TABLE 25.4 Pharmacokinetic Parameters of HMG-CoA Reductase Inhibitors

Drug	Calculated LogP[a]	Oral Bioavailability (%)	Active Metabolite(s)	Protein Binding (%)	Time to Peak Concentration (h)	Elimination Half-Life (h)	Major Route(s) of Elimination
Atorvastatin	4.13	12–14	*ortho*- and *para*-hydroxylated	98	1–2	14–19	Biliary/fecal (>90%) Renal (<2%)
Fluvastatin	3.62	20–30	None	98	0.5–1.0	1	Biliary/fecal (95%) Renal (5%)
Lovastatin	4.07 (4.04)[b]	5	3,5-Dihydroxy acid	>95	2	3–4	Fecal (83%) Renal (10%)
Pravastatin	1.44 (0.5)[b]	17	None	43–55	1.0–1.5	2–3	Fecal (70%) Renal (20%)
Pitavastatin	3.45	51	None	>99	1	12	Fecal (79%) Renal (15%)
Rosuvastatin	0.42	20	*N*-Desmethyl	88	3–5	19–20	Fecal (90%) Renal (10%)
Simvastatin	4.42 (4.2)[b]	5	3,5-Dihydroxy acid	95	4	3	Fecal (60%) Renal (13%)

[a]A commercial program was used for calculated values (47).
[b]Calculated using the CLOG program (40).

TABLE 25.5 Dosing Information for HMG-CoA Reductase Inhibitors

Generic Name	Brand Name(s)	Dosing Range	Maximum Daily Dose	Dose Reduction with Renal Dysfunction	Tablet Strengths (mg)
Atorvastatin	Lipitor	10–80 mg once daily	80 mg	No	10, 20, 40,80
Fluvastatin	Lescol Lescol XR	20–80 mg once daily or b.i.d.	80 mg	Caution in severe impairment	20, 40, 80 (XR)
Lovastatin	Mevacor Altoprev (XR)	10–80 mg once daily or b.i.d.	80 mg (60 mg if XR) (20 mg with fibrate)	Yes	10, 20, 40, 20 (XR), 40 (XR), 60 (XR)
Pitavastatin	Livalo	1-4 mg once daily	40 mg	Yes	1, 2, 4
Pravastatin	Pravachol	10–80 mg once daily	80 mg	Yes	10, 20, 40, 80
Rosuvastatin	Crestor	5–40 mg once daily	40 mg (10 mg with fibrate)	Only with severe impairment	5, 10, 20, 40
Simvastatin	Zocor	5–40 mg once daily	80 mg (10 mg with fibrate)	Only with severe impairment	5, 10, 20, 40, 80

b.i.d., twice a day; XR, extended release.

reducing plasma LDL levels, these compounds slow the progression of atherosclerosis and reduce the risk of myocardial infarction and other ramifications of vascular occlusion. Atorvastatin, rosuvastatin, and simvastatin have been shown to be effective in homozygous familial hyperlipidemia and are indicated for this use. Additionally, atorvastatin, pravastatin, rosuvastatin, and simvastatin are indicated for primary dysbetalipoproteinemia (Fredrickson type III) (Table 25.2). Finally, with the exception of lovastatin, all HMGRIs are indicated for the treatment of hypertriglyceridemia.

Inhibitors of HMG-CoA reductase are contraindicated in pregnancy. Fetal development requires cholesterol as a precursor for the synthesis of steroids and cell membranes; thus, inhibition of its synthesis may cause fetal harm. Additionally, HMGRIs are excreted in breast milk and should not be used by nursing mothers.

Adverse Effects

The most prevalent or significant side effects of HMGRIs are listed below (6,17,23). In general, this class of drugs is well tolerated. Gastrointestinal disturbances are the most common complaint; however, these and other adverse reactions tend to be mild and transient. Elevations in hepatic transaminase levels can occur with all HMGRIs. These increases usually occur shortly after the initiation of therapy and resolve after the discontinuation of medication. In a small percentage of patients, these levels can increase to more than threefold the upper limit of normal. Therefore, liver function tests should be done at the initiation of therapy, at 6 and 12 weeks after the initiation of therapy, and at periodic intervals (e.g., every 6 months) thereafter. Similar testing should be done with dosage increases. Approximately 5% to 10% of patients will experience mild increases in creatine phosphokinase levels; however, less than 1% will develop symptoms of myalgia and myopathy (e.g., fever, muscle aches or cramps, and unusual tiredness or weakness). Tests for creatine phosphokinase levels should be performed in patients reporting muscle complaints. Rhabdomyolysis (i.e., massive muscle necrosis with secondary acute renal failure) has occurred, but this is rare. The risk of this very serious adverse effect increases when an HMGRI is taken with certain other medications, such as cyclosporine, erythromycin, niacin, or fibrates (Table 25.7). Specific dosage reductions have been suggested for the combination use of fibrates with lovastatin, rosuvastatin, or simvastatin (17).

EZETIMIBE, A CHOLESTEROL ABSORPTION INHIBITOR

Historical Overview

The discovery of ezetimibe and its mechanism of action began with a desire to develop novel ACAT inhibitors, a potential target for hypercholesterolemia described earlier in this chapter (43). Compound C was one of the initial azetidinones tested for the ability to inhibit ACAT and to

COMBINATION PRODUCTS THAT INCLUDE AN HMGRI

HMGRI and antithrombotic
- Pravastatin/aspirin (Pravigard Pac)

HMGRI and calcium channel blocker
- Atorvastatin/amlodipine (Caduet)

HMGRI and additional antihypercholesterolemic agent
- Lovastatin/niacin (Advicor)
- Simvastatin/niacin (Simcor)
- Simvastatin/ezetimibe (Vytorin)

TABLE 25.6 Approved Therapeutics Conditions for HMG-CoA Reductase Inhibitors

Therapeutics Condition	Atorvastatin	Fluvastatin	Lovastatin	Pitavastatin	Pravastatin	Rosuvastatin	Simvastatin
Primary hypercholesterolemia	√	√	√	√	√	√	√
Primary dysbetalipoproteinemia	√				√	√	√
Mixed dyslipidemia	√	√	√	√	√	√	√
Hypertriglyceridemia	√	√		√	√	√	√
Homozygous familial hyperlipidemia	√					√	√
Primary prevention of cardiovascular events	√		√		√	√	√
Secondary prevention of cardiovascular events	√	√	√		√		√

lower plasma cholesterol. Interestingly, this compound's ability to decrease plasma cholesterol exceeded its ability to inhibit ACAT. Further SAR studies resulted in the development of compound D and confirmed that the cholesterol-lowering activity of this class of compounds was independent of its ability to inhibit ACAT. Using compound D as a lead, as well as in vivo data suggesting that metabolic transformations produced the active compound ultimately responsible for the cholesterol-lowering effect, structural modifications were made that, eventually, led to the development of ezetimibe. The most important changes involved the introduction of hydroxyl groups to help localize the compound in the intestine and the introduction of *p*-fluoro groups to block undesirable metabolism.

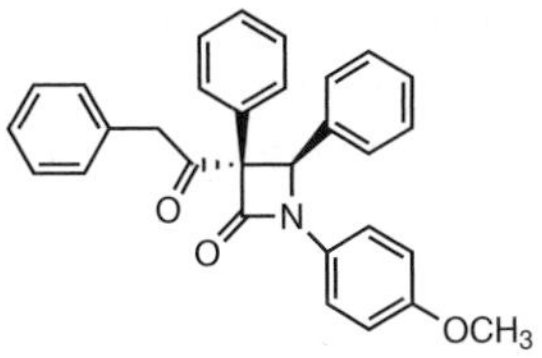

Compound C

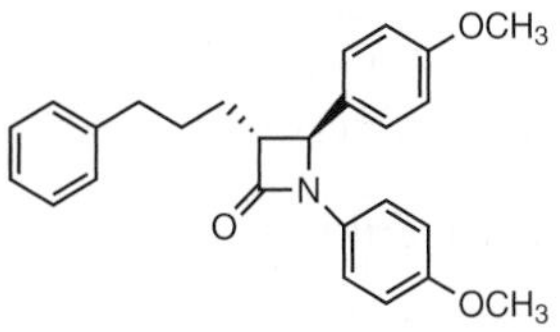

Compound D

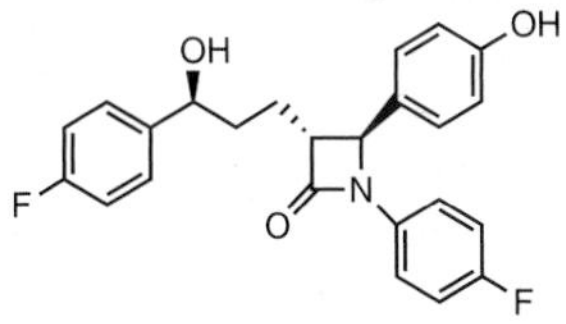

Ezetimibe

POTENTIAL NON–LIPID-LOWERING USES OF HMGRIS

Cellular metabolites derived from mevalonic acid are required for cell proliferation. Cholesterol is an essential component of cell membranes, farnesyl pyrophosphate is required to covalently bind to intracellular proteins and modify their function, ubiquinone is required for mitochondrial electron transport, and dolichol phosphates are required for glycoprotein synthesis.

Farnesyl pyrophosphate (Fig. 25.2) is an intermediate in the biosynthesis of cholesterol, ubiquinone, and dolichol phosphates. Based on their site of action, HMGRIs will decrease the availability of all four of these compounds and, thus, decrease cell proliferation. Potential applications of this antiproliferative effect include the prevention of restenosis following angioplasty, prevention of glomerular injury in renal disease, treatment of malignant disease, and prevention of organ transplantation rejection (42).

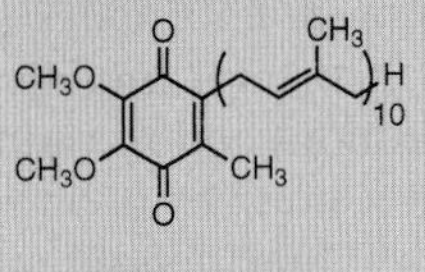

Ubiquinone

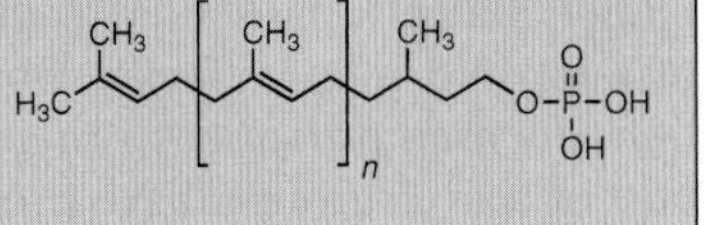

Dolichol phosphate (n = 15-19)

Mechanism of Action

Ezetimibe lowers plasma cholesterol levels by inhibiting the absorption of cholesterol at the brush border of the small intestine (17,23). Specifically, ezetimibe has been proposed to bind to a specific transport protein located in the wall of the small intestine, resulting in a reduction of cholesterol transport and absorption (44). Ezetimibe appears to be selective in its actions in that it does not interfere with the absorption of triglycerides, lipid-soluble vitamins, or other nutrients. The decreased absorption

ADVERSE EFFECTS OF HMGRIS

Constipation, flatulence, dyspepsia, abdominal pain, diarrhea, nausea, vomiting, headache, rhinitis, sinusitis, elevated hepatic enzymes, arthralgia, myalgia, myopathy, muscle cramps, rhabdomyolysis, and chest pain

of cholesterol eventually leads to enhanced receptor-mediated LDL uptake similar to that seen with bile acid sequestrants and HMGRIs. When used as monotherapy, the decreased absorption of cholesterol causes a compensatory increase in cholesterol biosynthesis. This is similar to that described for bile acid sequestrants and is insufficient to override the overall LDL-lowering effects of ezetimibe.

Physicochemical Properties

Ezetimibe is a crystalline powder that is practically insoluble in water but is freely soluble in ethanol and other organic solvents. Its calculated logP value is 3.50 (40). The phenol present in ezetimibe allows this compound to be classified as an acidic compound; however, the phenol has a pK_a of 9.72 and is predominantly un-ionized at physiologic pH.

Metabolism

After oral administration, ezetimibe is rapidly and extensively metabolized in the intestinal wall and the liver to its active metabolite, a corresponding phenol glucuronide (Fig. 25.10). This glucuronide is reexcreted in the bile back to its active site. A small amount (<5%) of ezetimibe undergoes oxidation to covert the benzylic hydroxyl group to a ketone; however, ezetimibe does not appear to exert any significant effect on the activity of CYP450 enzymes (17,22,44).

Pharmacokinetic Parameters

Ezetimibe is administered orally; however, its absolute bioavailability cannot be determined because of its aqueous insolubility and the lack of an injectable formulation. Based on area under the curve values, the oral absorption ranges from 35% to 60%. Mean peak concentrations of the active glucuronidated metabolite are reached within 1 to 2 hours. Both ezetimibe and its glucuronide conjugate are extensively bound (>90%) to plasma proteins. The relative plasma concentrations of ezetimibe and its glucuronide conjugate range from 10% to 20% and from 80% to 90%, respectively. Both compounds have a long half-life of approximately 22 hours. The coadministration of food with ezetimibe has no effect on the extent of absorption.

The normal dose of ezetimibe is 10 mg once daily. Dosage reduction for patients with renal impairment, intermittent hemodialysis, or mild hepatic impairment is not necessary. Because of insufficient data, the use of ezetimibe is not recommended in patients with moderate to severe hepatic impairment (17,22,23).

Therapeutic Applications

Ezetimibe is indicated as monotherapy or in combination with an HMGRI for the reduction of elevated total cholesterol, LDL cholesterol, and apoB in patients with primary (heterozygous familial and nonfamilial) hypercholesterolemia, homozygous familial sitosterolemia, or homozygous familial hypercholesterolemia. When used as monotherapy, ezetimibe reduces LDL cholesterol by approximately 18%. When used in combination therapy with an HMGRI, LDL levels are reduced by 25% to 65% depending on the dose of the HMGRI inhibitor. Ezetimibe is also indicated for combination use with fenofibrate to treat hypercholesterolemia in patients with mixed hyperlipoproteinemia. All indications are for patients who have not responded to diet, exercise, and other nonpharmacologic methods.

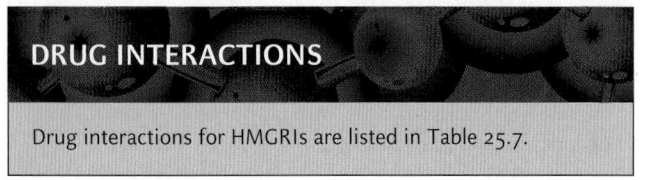

DRUG INTERACTIONS

Drug interactions for HMGRIs are listed in Table 25.7.

ADVERSE EFFECTS OF EZETIMIBE

Abdominal pain, diarrhea, arthralgia, back pain, cough, pharyngitis, sinusitis, fatigue, and viral infection

Adverse Effects

Ezetimibe generally is well tolerated. The most common adverse effects are listed above. Whenever ezetimibe is used in combination with an HMGRI, the incidence of myopathy or rhabdomyolysis does not increase above that seen with HMGRI monotherapy (17,23). Drug interactions for ezetimibe are listed in Table 25.8.

FIBRATES

Historical Overview and Development

The use of this class of drugs to treat hyperlipoproteinemias can be traced back to 1962 and thus predates the use of bile acid sequestrants and HMGRIs. A random screening test on a series of aryloxyisobutyric acids demonstrated that these compounds could lower both plasma cholesterol and total lipid levels (45). The compound that produced the best balance between activity and toxicity was ethyl *p*-chlorophenoxyisobutyrate (Fig. 25.11). Later renamed clofibrate, this compound was subsequently shown to be a prodrug for *p*-chlorophenoxyisobutyric acid (clofibric acid). It was approved for therapeutic use in 1967, and for a time, it was a very popular and widely prescribed drug. Results from a 1978 World Health Organization trial changed the acceptance of clofibrate and dramatically decreased its use. These trials indicated that despite a 9% lowering of cholesterol, patients taking clofibrate showed no reduction of cardiovascular events and actually had an increase in overall mortality (6). Although clofibrate is no longer available in the United States, it has served as the prototype for the design of safer and more effective fibrates. Structural modifications, focused primarily on ring substitutions and the addition of spacer groups, have produced a number of active compounds (Fig. 25.11). Gemfibrozil and fenofibrate became available for therapy in 1981 and 1998, respectively. Fenofibrate was actually approved in 1993; however,

TABLE 25.7 Drug Interactions for HMG-CoA Reductase Inhibitors (HMGRIs)

Drug	HMGRIs	Result of Interaction
Amiodarone	Lovastatin, simvastatin	Increased risk of myopathy
Antacids	Atorvastatin, rosuvastatin	Decreased levels of atorvastatin, rosuvastatin; no change in plasma LDL reduction; administer rosuvastatin at least 2 h after antacid
Azole antifungal agents	All	Increased risk of severe myopathy or rhabdomyolysis; increased plasma levels of atorvastatin, lovastatin, and simvastatin because of inhibition of CYP3A4; additive decreases in concentrations or activity of endogenous steroid hormones
Bile acid sequestrants	All	Decreased bioavailability of HMGRI if administration is not adequately spaced
Cimetidine	Fluvastatin	Increase in plasma fluvastatin levels
Cyclosporine	All	Increased risk of severe myopathy or rhabdomyolysis
Danazol	Lovastatin	Increased risk of severe myopathy or rhabdomyolysis
Digoxin	Atorvastatin, fluvastatin, simvastatin	Slight elevation in plasma concentrations of digoxin
Diltiazem	Atorvastatin, lovastatin, simvastatin	Increased risk of severe myopathy
Erythromycin, clarithromycin	All	Increased risk of severe myopathy or rhabdomyolysis; increased plasma levels of atorvastatin, lovastatin, and simvastatin because of inhibition of CYP3A4
Ethanol	Fluvastatin, lovastatin	Increased risk of hepatotoxicity
Fibrates	All	Increased risk of severe myopathy or rhabdomyolysis
Grapefruit juice (>1 quart/d)	Atorvastatin, lovastatin, simvastatin	Elevated plasma levels of the HMGRIs and increased risk of myopathy
HIV protease inhibitors	Atorvastatin, lovastatin, pitavastatin, simvastatin	Elevated plasma levels of the HMGRIs and increased risk of myopathy
Isradipine	Lovastatin	Increased clearance of lovastatin and its metabolites
Itraconazole	Pitavastatin	Decreased plasma levels of pitavastatin
Niacin	All	Increased risk of severe myopathy or rhabdomyolysis
Omeprazole	Fluvastatin	Increase in plasma fluvastatin levels
Oral contraceptives	Atorvastatin, rosuvastatin	Increased plasma concentrations of norethindrone and ethinyl estradiol
Phenytoin	Fluvastatin	Increased plasma concentrations of both compounds because of CYP2C9 interaction
Ranitidine	Fluvastatin	Increase in plasma fluvastatin levels
Rifampin	Fluvastatin, pitavastatin	Increased plasma clearance of fluvastatin
Ritonavir, saquinavir	Pravastatin	Decreased plasma levels of pravastatin
Spironolactone	All	Additive decreases in concentrations or activity of endogenous steroid hormones
St. John's wort	Lovastatin, simvastatin	Decreased HMGRI plasma levels
Warfarin	Fluvastatin, lovastatin, rosuvastatin, simvastatin	Anticoagulant effect of warfarin may be increased

its marketing was voluntarily delayed until a more bioavailable, micronized formulation of the drug was available (46). Both of these compounds are safer and more effective than clofibrate in lowering plasma triglyceride levels and increasing plasma HDL levels. Additional compounds, such as ciprofibrate and bezafibrate, are not currently available in the United States but have been used in other countries.

Mechanism of Action

Overall, fibrates decrease plasma triglyceride levels much more dramatically than they decrease plasma cholesterol levels. They significantly decrease VLDL levels, cause a moderate increase in HDL levels, and have variable effects on LDL concentrations. As an example of this latter point, gemfibrozil will raise LDL levels in patients with hypertriglyceridemia but lower LDL levels in patients with normal triglyceride levels. The exact mechanisms for these actions have not been fully elucidated; however, studies have shown that this class of compounds can produce a variety of beneficial effects on lipoprotein metabolism. Many of these effects have been proposed to be mediated through the activation of peroxisome proliferator-activated receptors (PPARs) and an alteration of gene expression. Specifically, fibrates bind to PPARα (6,17,29,46).

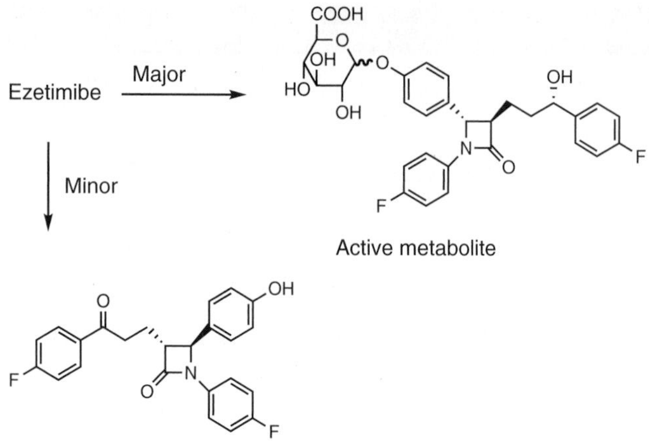

FIGURE 25.10 Metabolism of ezetimibe to its active and inactive metabolites.

TABLE 25.8 Drug Interactions for Ezetimibe

Drug	Result of Interaction
Antacid	Aluminum and magnesium-containing antacids decrease the maximum plasma concentration of ezetimibe
Bile acid sequestrants	Decreased bioavailability of ezetimibe if administration is not adequately spaced
Cyclosporine	Increased ezetimibe concentration
Fibrates	Increased ezetimibe concentration and possible increased risk of cholelithiasis. With the exception of fenofibrate, concomitant use is not recommended.

Decreases in plasma VLDL primarily result from the ability of these compounds to stimulate the activity of lipoprotein lipase, the enzyme responsible for removing triglycerides from plasma VLDL (Fig. 25.5). Additionally, fibrates can lower VLDL levels through PPARα-mediated stimulation of fatty acid oxidation, inhibition of triglyceride synthesis, and reduced expression of apoC-III. This latter effect enhances the action of lipoprotein lipase because apoC-III normally serves as an inhibitor of this enzyme. Favorable effects on HDL levels appear to be related to increased transcription of apoA-I and apoA-II as well as a decreased activity of cholesteryl ester transfer protein.

All fibrates accelerate the turnover and removal of cholesterol from the liver. This increases the biliary secretion of cholesterol, enhances its fecal excretion, and may cause cholelithiasis (i.e., gallstone formation).

Structure–Activity Relationships

Fibrates can be chemically classified as analogs of phenoxyisobutyric acid. Literature references to the SARs for this class of drugs are sparse; however, all compounds are analogs of the following general structure.

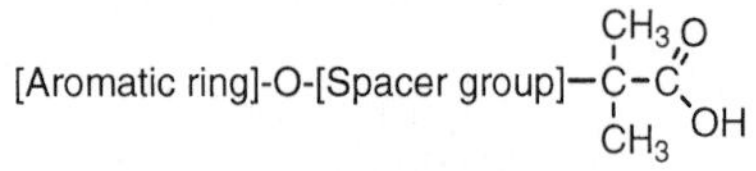

The isobutyric acid group is essential for activity. Fenofibrate, which contains an ester, is a prodrug and requires in vivo hydrolysis. Substitution at the para position of the aromatic ring with a chloro group or a chlorine-containing cyclopropyl ring produces compounds with significantly longer half-lives. Although most compounds contain a phenoxyisobutyric acid, the addition of an *n*-propyl spacer, as seen in gemfibrozil, results in an active drug.

Physicochemical Properties

Similar to HMGRIs, the active forms of all fibrates contain a carboxylic acid. The pK_a of this functional group on clofibric acid is reported to be 3.5 (47), and thus, it will be primarily ionized at physiologic pH. Although not reported, the pK_a and ionization values of gemfibrozil and fenofibric acid can reasonably be assumed to be similar. Both clofibrate and fenofibrate are neutral, ester prodrugs and should be classified as nonelectrolytes. Gemfibrozil can be classified as an acidic drug. The calculated logP values for fenofibrate and gemfibrozil are shown in Table 25.9 (47). Both compounds are highly lipid soluble despite the fact that gemfibrozil contains a water-soluble carboxylic acid. This can be partially explained by examining the π values for the substituents on fenofibrate and gemfibrozil (48). The 2,5-dimethyl ring in gemfibrozil is predicted to be much more hydrophobic than the 4-chloro ring of fenofibrate. Additionally, the propyl bridge seen in gemfibrozil, but not in fenofibrate, significantly adds to its hydrophobicity. The isopropyl ester as well as the additional aromatic ring account for the enhanced lipid solubility of fenofibrate. All currently available fibrates are achiral molecules and not subject to stereochemical concerns.

Metabolism

The prodrug fenofibrate undergoes rapid hydrolysis to produce fenofibric acid. This active metabolite can then be further metabolized by oxidative or conjugative pathways. Gemfibrozil is slightly different in that it does not require initial bioactivation; however, similar to fenofibric acid, it can be oxidized or conjugated. Oxidation of the aromatic methyl groups produces inactive hydroxymethyl and carboxylic acid analogs. As a drug class, fibrates and their oxidized analogs are primarily excreted as glucuronide conjugates in the urine. Oxidization requires the CYP3A4 isozyme; however, because of the ability of these compounds to be conjugated and eliminated either with or without oxidation, drug interactions with other compounds affecting the CYP3A4 system are less important here than with other drug classes.

Pharmacokinetic Parameters

The pharmacokinetic parameters and dosing information for the fibrates are summarized in Tables 25.9 and 25.10, respectively (6,17,22,23,47). The prodrug, fenofibrate,

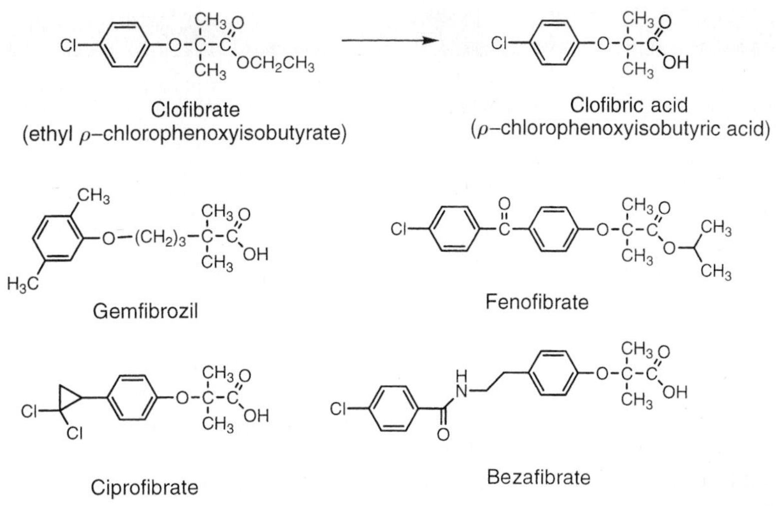

FIGURE 25.11 Bioactivation of clofibrate and chemical structures of other fibrates.

requires a longer time to reach peak concentrations compared with gemfibrozil. Because of differences in aromatic substitution, fenofibrate also has a much longer half-life than gemfibrozil. As previously mentioned, the 2,5-dimethyl substitution in gemfibrozil is much more susceptible to oxidative metabolism than the para-chloro group present in fenofibrate. Similar to HMGRIs, changes in lipid levels are not seen immediately, and up to 2 months may be required to reach maximal clinical effects and to determine the overall clinical efficacy.

Fibrates have excellent bioavailability and are extensively bound to plasma proteins. Because food can significantly enhance their oral absorption, these compounds should be taken either with or just before meals. Fenofibrate was available in Europe and elsewhere as standard tablet and capsule formulations for many years before its approval and marketing in the United States, where it was introduced only after the development of a micronized formulation that allowed better oral absorption, a lower daily dose, and once-daily administration. A variety of formulations and doses of fenofibrate have been developed. Specific dosing ranges, maximum daily doses, and available strengths are noted in Table 25.10.

Renal elimination is the primary route through which these compounds are excreted from the body. Patients with mild renal dysfunction often can be managed with minor dosage adjustments, whereas those with severe impairment or renal failure may have to discontinue its use.

Therapeutic Applications

Fibrates are approved to treat hypertriglyceridemia and familial combined hyperlipidemia (Fredrickson types IIa, IIb, IV, and V) (Table 25.2) in patients who are at risk of pancreatitis and have not responded to dietary adjustments or in patients who are at risk of CHD and have not responded to weight loss, dietary adjustments, and other pharmacologic treatment. They can be used either alone or in combination with niacin, bile acid sequestrants, or HMGRIs. If used with bile acid sequestrants, fibrates must be taken either 1 hour before or 4 to 6 hours after the sequestrant. As discussed previously and reemphasized below, caution should be used if fibrates are combined with HMGRIs. Fibrates are not effective in the treatment of hypertriglyceridemia associated solely to elevated chylomicron levels (Fredrickson type I).

Adverse Effects

The most prevalent or significant side effects caused by the fibrates are listed below (6,17,23). Despite the potential to cause serious side effects, fibrates usually are well tolerated. Gastrointestinal complaints are the most common but do not usually cause discontinuation of therapy. In general, gemfibrozil and fenofibrate appear to be less problematic than the original compound, clofibrate. In fact, many of the concerns regarding fibrate therapy are based on the effects of clofibrate and the results of a 1978 clinical trial in which patients taking clofibrate had a significantly higher morbidity and mortality from causes other than CHD. These causes included malignancy, gallbladder disease, pancreatitis, and postcholecystectomy complications. Studies with gemfibrozil and fenofibrate have not shown similar increases; however, because all fibrates have similar pharmacologic actions, cautions and contraindications generally are applied to the entire drug class. As an example, even though gemfibrozil and fenofibrate have not demonstrated a significant increase in gallbladder disease, as seen with clofibrate, all three of these compounds are contraindicated in patients with preexisting gallbladder disease or cholelithiasis. Similar to HMGRIs, fibrates can cause myopathy, myositis, and rhabdomyolysis. Although rare, the risk of these serious effects increases when these two classes of agents are used together. Fibrates also cause increases in plasma aspartate transaminase (AST), alanine transaminase (ALT), and creatine phosphokinase levels.

Drug interactions for fibrates are listed in Table 25.11.

TABLE 25.9 Pharmacokinetic Parameters of Fibrates

Drug	Calculated LogP	Oral Bioavailability (%)	Active Metabolite	Protein Binding (%)	Time to Peak Concentration (h)	Elimination Half-Life (h)	Major Route(s) of Elimination
Fenofibrate	5.24	60–90	Fenofibric acid	99	4–8	20–22	Renal (60%–90%) Fecal (5%–25%)
Gemfibrozil	3.9	>90	None	99	1–2	1.5	Renal (70%) Fecal (6%)

NICOTINIC ACID

Historical Overview

The history of nicotinic acid (niacin) began in 1867, when it was first synthesized by oxidation of nicotine. The name niacin was derived later from the words *ni*cotinic *ac*id and vitam*in* in an effort to avoid confusing nicotinic acid and nicotinamide with nicotine. Although the terms "niacin" and "nicotinic acid" are today used interchangeably, only the more chemically descriptive term, "nicotinic acid," will be used in the following discussions.

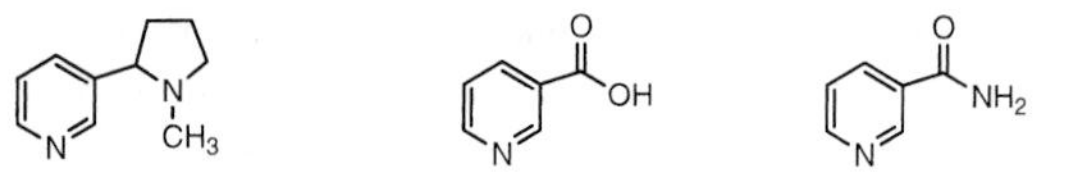

Nicotine Nicotinic acid Nicotinamide

Discovery of the biochemical and pharmacologic actions of nicotinic acid began in the early 1900s, when brewer's yeast was demonstrated to prevent pellagra in humans. The subsequent isolation of nicotinic acid from brewer's yeast established its role as an essential dietary requirement. In the 1930s, its amide metabolite, nicotinamide, was isolated from liver extracts and found to be a required structural feature of nicotinamide adenine dinucleotide phosphate ($NADP^+$), a cofactor involved in electron transport and intermediary metabolism (49). In 1955, Altschul et al. (50) observed that high doses of nicotinic acid lowered cholesterol levels in humans, an activity unrelated to its properties as a vitamin. Subsequent studies have shown that nicotinic acid also lowers serum triglyceride levels and is effective against a variety of hyperlipoproteinemias. None of these antihyperlipidemic effects are seen with nicotinamide.

Mechanism of Action

Nicotinic acid exerts a variety of effects on lipoprotein metabolism (6,18,51). One of its most important actions is the inhibition of lipolysis in adipose tissue. This initial inhibition, like those of previously discussed antihyperlipidemic agents, produces a sequence of events that ultimately result in the lowering of plasma triglycerides and cholesterol. Impaired lipolysis decreases the mobilization of free fatty acids, thus reducing their plasma levels and their delivery to the liver. In turn, this decreases hepatic triglyceride synthesis and results in a decreased production of VLDL. Enhanced clearance of VLDL through stimulation of lipoprotein lipase also has been proposed to contribute to the reduction of plasma VLDL levels. Because LDL is derived from VLDL (Fig. 25.5), the decreased production of VLDL ultimately leads to a decrease in LDL levels. The sequential nature of this process has been clinically demonstrated. The reduction in triglyceride levels occurs within several hours after initiation of nicotinic acid therapy, whereas the reduction in cholesterol does not occur until after several days of therapy. Nicotinic acid also increases HDL levels because of a reduction in the clearance of apoA-I, an essential component of HDL. Unlike bile acid sequestrants and HMGRIs, nicotinic acid does not have any effects on cholesterol catabolism or biosynthesis.

TABLE 25.10 Dosage Information for Fibrates

Generic Name	Brand Name	Dosing Range	Maximum Daily Dose	Dose Reduction with Renal Dysfunction	Tablet/Capsule Strengths (mg)
Fenofibrate	TriCor	48–145 mg once daily	145 mg	Only with severe impairment	48, 145
	Lofibra	54–160 mg once daily	160 mg		54, 160
	Lipofen	50–150 mg once daily	150 mg		50, 150
	Triglide	50–160 mg once daily	160 mg		50, 160
	Antara (micronized)	43–130 mg once daily	130 mg		67, 134, 200
	Lofibra (micronized)	67–200 mg once daily	200 mg		43, 130
Gemfibrozil	Lopid	600 mg b.i.d.	1200 mg	Yes	600

b.i.d., twice a day.

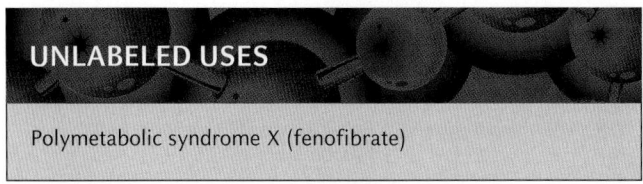

UNLABELED USES

Polymetabolic syndrome X (fenofibrate)

Physicochemical Properties

Nicotinic acid (niacin) is a stable, nonhygroscopic, white, crystalline powder. Its carboxylic acid has a pK_a of 4.76 and, thus, is predominantly ionized at physiologic pH. The pyridine nitrogen is a very weak base ($pK_a = 2.0$) and, therefore, primarily exists in the un-ionized form. Nicotinic acid is freely soluble in alkaline solutions and has a measured logP of –0.20 at pH 6.0 (47).

Metabolism

Nicotinic acid is a B-complex vitamin that is converted to nicotinamide, nicotinamide adenine dinucleotide (NAD^+), and $NADP^+$. The latter two compounds are coenzymes and are required for oxidation/reduction reactions in a variety of biochemical pathways. Additionally, nicotinic acid is metabolized to a number of inactive compounds, including nicotinuric acid and *N*-methylated derivatives. Normal biochemical regulation and feedback prevent large doses of nicotinic acid from producing excess quantities of NAD^+ and $NADP^+$. Thus, small doses of nicotinic acid, such as those used for dietary supplementation, will be primarily excreted as metabolites, whereas large doses, such as those used for the treatment of hyperlipoproteinemia, will be primarily excreted unchanged by the kidney (17).

Pharmacokinetic Parameters

Nicotinic acid is readily absorbed. Peripheral vasodilation is seen within 20 minutes, and peak plasma concentrations occur within 45 minutes. The half-life of the compound is approximately 1 hour, thus necessitating frequent dosing or an extended-release formulation. Extended-release tablets produce peripheral vasodilation within 1 hour, reach peak plasma concentrations within 4 to 5 hours, and have a duration of 8 to 10 hours.

ADVERSE EFFECTS

Abdominal pain, dyspepsia, nausea, vomiting, diarrhea, constipation, cholestasis, jaundice, cholelithiasis, pancreatitis, headache, dizziness, drowsiness, blurred vision, mental depression, impotence, decreased libido, myopathy, myositis, rhabdomyolysis, anemia, leukopenia, eosinophilia, pruritus, and rash

Dosing of nicotinic acid should be titrated to minimize adverse effects. An initial dose of 50 to 100 mg three times a day often is used with immediate-release tablets. The dose then is gradually increased by 50 to 100 mg every 3 to 14 days, up to a maximum of 6 g/day, as tolerated. Therapeutic monitoring to assess efficacy and prevent toxicity is essential until a stable and effective dose is reached. Similar dosing escalations are available for extended-release products, with doses normally starting at 500 mg once daily at bedtime. (6,17,23).

Therapeutic Applications

Nicotinic acid is approved for the treatment of hypercholesterolemia, hypertriglyceridemia, and familial combined hyperlipidemia (Fredrickson types IIa, IIb, IV, and V) (Table 25.2) in patients who have not responded to diet, exercise, and other nonpharmacologic methods. It also is approved for nutritional supplementation, for the prevention of pellagra, and as adjunct therapy for peripheral vascular disease and circulatory disorders. It is contraindicated in patients with hepatic disease and peptic ulcer disease. Additionally, because of its ability to elevate glucose and uric acid levels, especially when taken in large doses, nicotinic acid should be used with caution in patients who have or are predisposed to diabetes mellitus and gout (17,22,23).

TABLE 25.11 Drug Interactions for Fibrates

Drug	Fibrate	Result of Interaction
Antidiabetic agents	All	Increased hypoglycemic effect through increased sensitivity and decreased glucagon secretion
Bexarotene	Gemfibrozil	Increased bexarotene plasma concentrations
Bile acid sequestrants	All	Decreased bioavailability of fibrate if administration is not adequately spaced
Cyclosporine	Fenofibrate	Increased potential for nephrotoxicity
Ezetimibe	All	Increased ezetimibe concentration and possible increased risk of cholelithiasis; concomitant use is not recommended
HMG-CoA reductase inhibitors	All	Increased risk of severe myopathy or rhabdomyolysis
Oral anticoagulants	All	Increased hypoprothrombinemic effect
Repaglinide	Gemfibrozil	Increased repaglinide plasma concentrations
Ursodiol	All	Increased hepatic cholesterol secretion, which may increase the possibility of gallstone formation and counteract the effectiveness of ursodiol

ADVERSE EFFECTS OF NIACIN

Flushing, pruritus, headache, nausea, vomiting, diarrhea, flatulence, hepatic dysfunction, jaundice, hyperglycemia, hyperuricemia, blurred vision, and tachycardia

Adverse Effects

The most common (and, often, dose-limiting) side effects of nicotinic acid treatment are cutaneous vasodilation (flushing and pruritus) and gastrointestinal intolerance, which may occur in 20% to 50% of treated patients. Flushing and pruritus are prostaglandin-mediated effects and may be prevented by taking aspirin or indomethacin before nicotinic acid. Gastrointestinal side effects, such as flatulence, nausea, vomiting, and diarrhea, can be minimized if nicotinic acid is taken either with or immediately after meals. As previously mentioned, all of these effects can be minimized by slowly titrating the dose of nicotinic acid. Hepatic dysfunction is one of the more serious complications of high-dose nicotinic acid. Plasma AST, ALT, lactate dehydrogenase, and alkaline phosphatase levels often are elevated but usually return to normal when therapy is either adjusted or discontinued (6,17,23).

Drug interactions for nicotinic acid are listed in Table 25.12.

TABLE 25.12 Drug Interactions for Nicotinic Acid

Drug	Result of Interaction
Adrenergic blocking agents	Enhanced vasodilation and postural hypotension
Bile acid sequestrants	Decreased bioavailability of nicotinic acid if administration is not adequately spaced
Ethanol	Potential enhanced hepatotoxicity and excessive peripheral or cutaneous vasodilation
HMG-CoA reductase inhibitors	Increased risk of myopathy and rhabdomyolysis
Vasodilating agents (calcium channel blockers, epoprostenol, nitrates)	Enhanced cutaneous vasodilation

SCENARIO: OUTCOME AND ANALYSIS

Outcome

Thomas L. Rihn, PharmD

The therapeutic goal in this case is to achieve low-density lipoprotein cholesterol (LDL-C) level of at least <100 mg/dL. The most recent guidelines for a patient like TN—one with extensive vascular disease and diabetes—would suggest lowering the LDL-C even further to <70 mg/dL. Given TN's current lipid profile, a potent statin such as atorvastatin would be the preferred choice. TN does have a prescription plan to cover the cost of the medication. Beginning the patient on atorvastatin 10–20 mg daily and titrating the dose over time to achieve the therapeutic goal would be the treatment of choice. This is a case where the application of medicinal chemistry in the development of newer, more potent statins and their clinical use in a patient would result in a much more rapid and predictable control of the lipid abnormality. The net result is a better patient health outcome and avoidance of adverse cardiovascular events.

Chemical Analysis

Victoria F. Roche and S. William Zito

Atorvastatin is a good antihyperlipidemic candidate for this patient. Its unesterified carboxylic acid moiety confirms its ability to immediately initiate binding at the target enzyme, HMG CoA reductase (HMGR), through an ion-ion bond with an anchoring Lys residue. The C_3 and C_5 hydroxyls, *p*-fluorine and isopropyl moieties make important contributions to high affinity binding, and these groups are common to many (and, in the case of the hydroxyl groups, all) statin structures. A particularly strong hydrogen bond is formed between the carbonyl oxygen of atorvastatin's unique amide moiety and an HMGR Ser residue. Collectively, these high-affinity interactions make atorvastatin one of the most potent of the marketed statins. Once it is bound to HMGR, atorvastatin inhibits the biosynthesis of cholesterol and stimulates the receptor-mediated uptake of LDL, which results in a lowering of serum LDL levels. The different statins have a variable impact on high-density lipoprotein cholesterol elevation, but all are able to lower triglyceride levels to some extent. The ability of statins to inhibit C-reactive protein, a major biomarker of inflammation, only adds to their value in the treatment of inflammation-based diseases, including coronary artery disease.

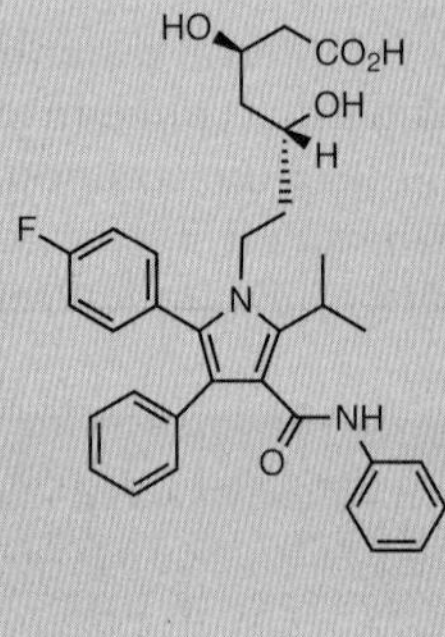

Atorvastatin

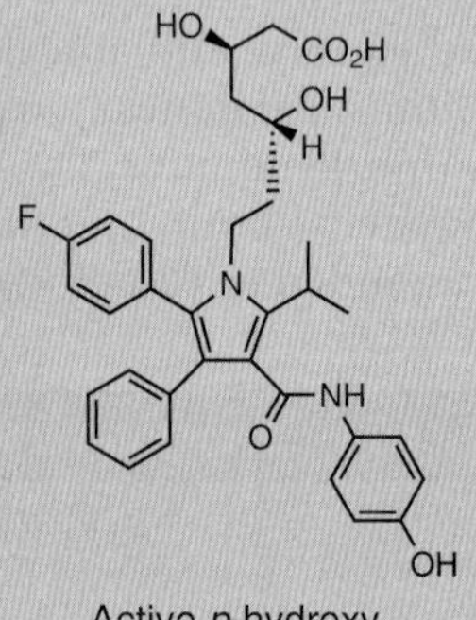

Active *p*-hydroxy metabolite

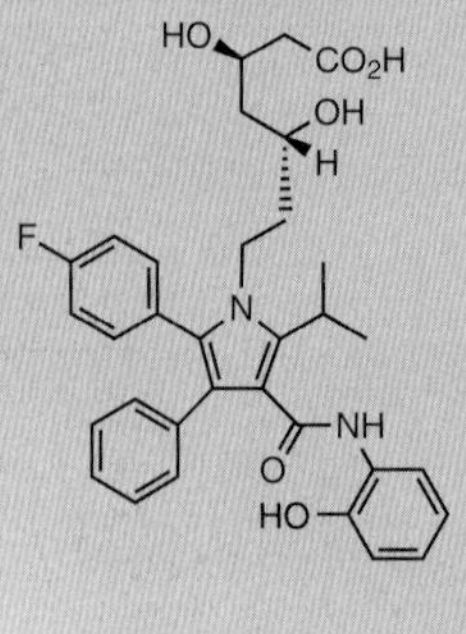

Active *o*-hydroxy metabolite

SCENARIO: OUTCOME AND ANALYSIS (*Continued*)

In addition to high affinity HMGR binding and LDL-lowering potency, atorvastatin has a long duration of action due to CYP3A4-mediated hydroxylation to two equally active metabolites. The 14-hour half-life permits convenient once-daily dosing without regard to time of day.

If TN is taking other medications that compete for or inhibit the 3A4 isoform, he may be at increased risk for statin-induced myopathy. Depending on the level of risk and/or TN's susceptibility to muscle toxicity, a highly potent, long-acting statin alternative that is not metabolized by CYP3A4 (e.g., rosuvastatin) could be considered. Rosuvastatin is vulnerable to CYP2C9-mediated N-demethylation, but only about 10% of a dose undergoes this sluggish reaction. Through hydrogen bonding with the aforementioned Ser and an Arg HMGR residue, the sulfonamide oxygen atoms of rosuvastatin make this drug the most potent of all currently marketed statin antihyperlipidemic agents.

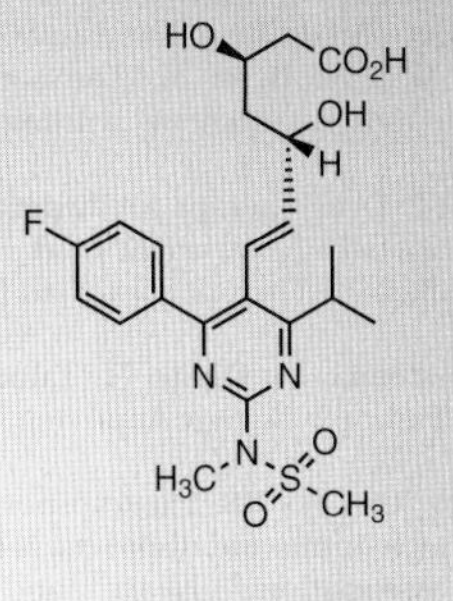

Rosuvastatin

CASE STUDY

Victoria Roche and S. William Zito

JC is a 60-year-old waitress at "The Southern Comfort," a restaurant famous for its fried chicken and homemade biscuits (always served with lots of butter and honey). JC lives alone and, after a hard day on her feet, just wants to "take a load off." She has a difficult time resisting this comfort food and, with the blessing of the restaurant manager, often takes her dinner home in a box to eat in front of the TV. JC has been blessed throughout her life with general good health, although lately she's been experiencing significant gastrointestinal upset that she's self-treating with over-the-counter omeprazole (a proton pump inhibitor). She's also taking low-dose, extended-release diltiazem for mildly elevated blood pressure and pravastatin for hypercholesterolemia.

During her most recent checkup, JC's physician noted a rise in her LDL and total serum cholesterol levels. Her serum HDLs are low to normal and her serum triglycerides levels are in the acceptable range. A decision is made to alter her therapy. You remind the physician of the other drugs JC is taking and that diltiazem is an inhibitor of CYP3A4. The physician asks for your opinion about which of the therapeutic choices drawn below would be the best way to go. She wants to either replace pravastatin with compound 1 or add compound 2 or 3 to her pravastatin regimen.

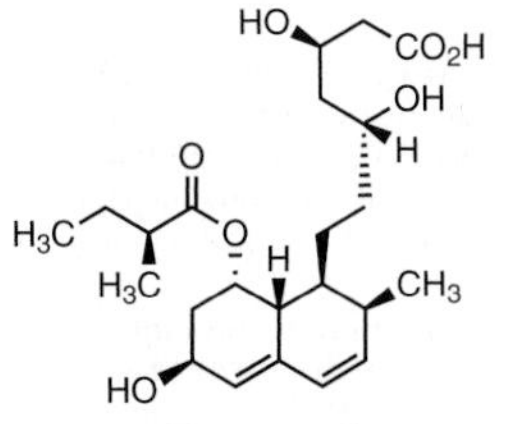

Pravastatin

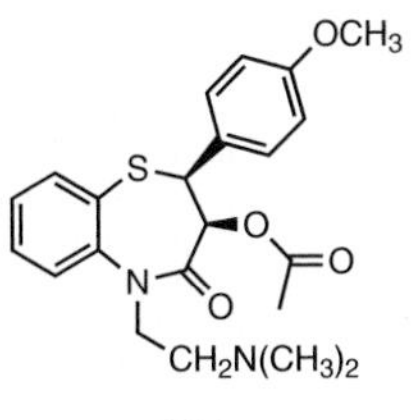

Diltiazem

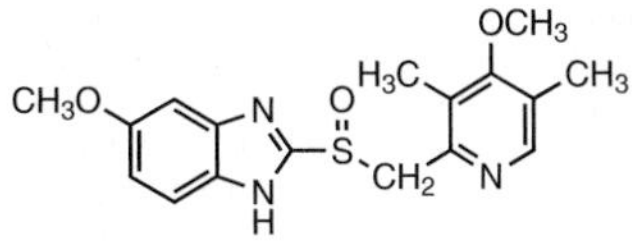

Omeprazole

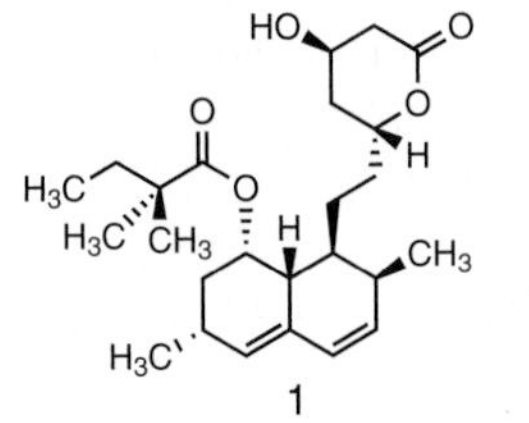

1

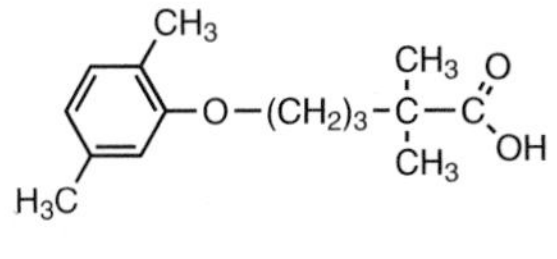

2

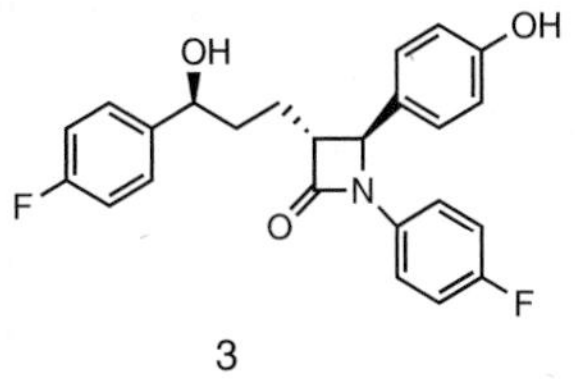

3

1. Conduct a thorough and mechanistic SAR analysis of the three therapeutic options in the case.
2. Apply the chemical understanding gained from the SAR analysis to this patient's specific needs to make a therapeutic recommendation.

References

1. Ginsberg HN, Goldberg IJ. Disorders of lipoprotein metabolism. In: Fauci AS, Braunwald E, Isselbacher KJ, et al., eds. Harrison's Principles of Internal Medicine, 14th Ed. New York: McGraw-Hill, 1998:2138–2149.
2. Drugs for lipids. Treat Guidel Med Lett 2008;6:9–16.
3. Berg JM, Tymoczko JL, Stryer L. Biochemistry, 5th Ed. New York: Freeman and Company, 2002:715–743.
4. Kourounakis AP, Charitos C, Rekka EA, et al. Lipid-lowering (hetero)aromatic tetrahydro-1,4-oxazine derivatives with antioxidant and squalene synthase inhibitory activity. J Med Chem 2008;51:5861–5865.
5. Chan C, Andreotti D, Cox B, et al. The squalestatins: decarboxy and 4-deoxy analogues as potent squalene synthase inhibitors. J Med Chem 1996;39:207–216.
6. Mahley RW, Bersot TP. Drug therapy for hypercholesterolemia and dyslipidemia. In: Brunton L, Lazo J, Parker K, et al., eds. Goodman & Gilman's the Pharmacological Basis of Therapeutics, 11th Ed. New York: McGraw-Hill, 2006:933–966.
7. Talbert RL. Hyperlipidemia. In: Dipiro JT, Talbert RL, Yee GC, et al., eds. Pharmacotherapy: A Pathophysiologic Approach, 6th Ed. New York: McGraw-Hill, 2005:429–452.
8. Fredrickson DS, Levy RI, Lees RS. Fat transport in lipoproteins—an integrated approach to mechanisms and disorders. N Engl J Med 1967;276:34–42.
9. American Heart Association. Heart and stroke statistics—2010 update. Available at: http://www.americanheart.org/downloadable/heart/1265665152970DS-3241%20HeartStrokeUpdate_2010.pdf. Accessed September 7, 2010.
10. Libby P. Atherosclerosis. In: Fauci AS, Braunwald E, Isselbacher KJ, et al., eds. Harrison's Principles of Internal Medicine, 14th Ed. New York: McGraw Hill, 1998:1345–1352.
11. Sliskovic DR, White AD. Therapeutic potential of ACAT inhibitors as lipid lowering and antiatherosclerotic agents. Trends Pharmacol Sci 1991;12:194–199.
12. Grundy SM, Cleeman JI, Bairey CN, et al. Implications of recent clinical trials for the National Cholesterol Education Program Adult Panel III guidelines. Circulation 2004;110:227–239.
13. Roth B. ACAT inhibitors: evolution from cholesterol-absorption inhibitors to antiatherosclerotic agents. Drug Discov Today 1998;3:19–25.
14. Takahashi K, Kasai M, Ohta M, et al. Novel indoline-based acyl-CoA:cholesterol acyltransferase inhibitor with antiperoxidative activity: improvement of physicochemical properties and biological activities by introduction of carboxylic acid. J Med Chem 2008;51:4823–4833.
15. Sikorski JA. Oral cholesteryl ester transfer protein (CETP) inhibitors: a potential new approach for treating coronary artery disease. J Med Chem 2006;49:1–22.
16. Cannon CP, Shah S, Dansky HM, et al. Safety of anacetrapib in patients with or at high risk for coronary heart disease. N Engl J Med 2010;363:2406–2415.
17. Clinical Pharmacology Online. Gold Standard Elsevier, 2010. Available at: http://clinicalpharmacology.com. Accessed September 10, 2010.
18. Cendella RJ. Cholesterol and hypocholesterolemic drugs. In: Craig CR, Stitzel RE, eds. Modern Pharmacology with Clinical Applications, 5th Ed. Boston: Little, Brown and Co., 1997:279–289.
19. Brown MS, Goldstein JL. A receptor-mediated pathway for cholesterol homeostasis. Science 1986;232:34–47.
20. Zhu XX, Brown GR, St-Pierre LE. Polymeric sorbents for bile acids. I: comparison between cholestyramine and colestipol. J Pharm Sci 1992;81:65–69.
21. Clas SD. Quaternized colestipol, an improved bile salt adsorbent: in vitro studies. J Pharm Sci 1991;80:128–131.
22. Micromedex Healthcare Series. Thomson Reuters (Healthcare) Inc. Available at: Avhttp://www.thomsonhc.com. Accessed September 10, 2010.
23. Facts & Comparisons eAnswers. St. Louis, MO: Wolters Kluwer Health. Available at: http://www.factsandcomparisons.com. Accessed September 10, 2010.
24. Heathcock CH, Hadley CR, Rosen T, et al. Total synthesis and biological evaluation of structural analogues of compactin and dihydromevinolin. J Med Chem 1987;30:1858–1873.
25. Adams JL, Metcalf BW. Therapeutic consequences of the inhibition of sterol metabolism. In: Hansch C, Sammes PG, Taylor JB, eds. Comprehensive Medicinal Chemistry, Vol 2. Oxford, UK: Permagon Press, 1990:333–363.
26. Cutler SJ, Cocolas GH. Cardiovascular agents. In: Block JH, Beale, JM, eds. Wilson and Gisvold's Textbook of Organic Medicinal and Pharmaceutical Chemistry, 11th Ed. Philadelphia, PA: Lippincott Williams & Wilkins, 2004:657–663.
27. Stokker GE, Hoffman WF, Alberts AW, et al. 3-Hydroxy-3-methylglutaryl–coenzyme A reductase inhibitors. 1. Structural modification of 5-substituted 3,5-dihydroxypentanoic acids and their lactone derivatives. J Med Chem 1985;28:347–358.
28. Sliskovic DR, Blankley CJ, Krause BR, et al. Inhibitors of cholesterol biosynthesis. 6. *trans*-5-[2-(-*N*-heteroaryl-3,5-disubstituted-pyrazol-4-yl) ethyl/ethenyl]tetrahydro-4-hydroxy-2*H*-pyran-2-ones. J Med Chem 1992;35:2095–2103.
29. Bone EA, Davidson AH, Lewis CN, et al. Synthesis and biological evaluation of dihydroeptastatin, a novel inhibitor of 3-hydroxy-3-methylglutaryl–coenzyme A reductase. J Med Chem 1992;35:3388–3393.
30. Roth BD, Ortwine DF, Hoefle ML, et al. Inhibitors of cholesterol biosynthesis. 1. *trans*-6-(2-pyrrol-1-ylethyl)-4-hydroxypyran-2-ones, a novel series of HMG-CoA reductase inhibitors. 1. Effects of structural modifications at the 2-and 5-positions of the pyrrole nucleus. J Med Chem 1990;33:21–31.
31. Hoffman WF, Alberts AW, Cragoe EJ Jr, et al. 3-Hydroxy-3-methylglutaryl–coenzyme A reductase inhibitors. 2. Structural modification of 7-(substituted aryl)-3,5-dihydroxy-6-heptenoic acids and their lactone derivatives. J Med Chem 1986;29:159–169.
32. Stokker GE, Alberts AW, Anderson PS, et al. 3-Hydroxy-3-methylglutaryl-coenzyme A reductase inhibitors. 3. 7-(3,5-Disubstituted [1,1′-biphenyl]-2-yl)-3,5-dihydroxy-6-heptenoic acids and their lactone derivatives. J Med Chem 1986;29:170–181.
33. Heathcock CH, Davis BR, Hadley CR. Synthesis and biological evaluation of a monocyclic, fully functional analogue of compactin. J Med Chem 1989;32:197–202.
34. Lee TJ, Holtz WJ, Smith RL, et al. 3-Hydroxy-3-methylglutaryl–coenzyme A reductase inhibitors. 8. Side chain ether analogues of lovastatin. J Med Chem 1991;34:2474–2477.
35. Hoffman WF, Alberts AW, Anderson PS, et al. 3-Hydroxy-3-methylglutaryl-coenzyme A reductase inhibitors. 4. Side chain ester derivatives of mevinolin. J Med Chem 1986;29:849–852.
36. Stokker GE, Alberts AW, Gilfillan JL, et al. 3-Hydroxy-3-methylglutaryl–coenzyme A reductase inhibitors. 5. 6-(Fluoren-9-yl)- and 6-(fluoren-9-ylidenyl)-3,5-dihydroxyhexanoic acids and their lactone derivatives. J Med Chem 1986;29:852–855.
37. Procopiou PA, Draper CD, Hutson JL, et al. Inhibitors of cholesterol biosynthesis. 2. 3,5-Dihydroxy-7-(*N*-pyrrolyl)-6-heptenoates, a novel series of HMG-CoA reductase inhibitors. J Med Chem 1993;36:3658–3662.
38. Atorvastatin—a new lipid-lowering drug. Med Lett Drugs Ther 1997;39:29–31.
39. Rosuvastatin—a new lipid-lowering drug. Med Lett Drugs Ther 2003;45:81–83.
40. Craig PN. Drug compendium. In: Hansch C, Sammes PG, Taylor JB, eds. Comprehensive Medicinal Chemistry, Vol 6. Oxford, UK: Permagon Press, 1990:237–991.
41. Zocor (simvastatin) product literature. Merck, 1999.
42. Wheeler DC. Are there potential nonlipid-lowering uses of statins? Drugs 1998;56:517–522.
43. Clader JW. The discovery of ezetimibe: a view from outside the receptor. J Med Chem 2004;47:1–9.
44. Kosoglou T, Statkevich P, Johnson-Levonas AO, et al. Ezetimibe: a review of its metabolism, pharmacokinetics, and drug interactions. Clin Pharmacokinet 2005;44:467–494.
45. Thorp JM, Waring WS. Modification and distribution of lipids by ethyl chlorophenoxyisobutyrate. Nature 1962;194:948–949.
46. Hussar DA. New drugs of 1998. J Am Pharm Assoc 1999;39:170–172.
47. Values calculated by author using ACD/ChemSketch, Version 12.01, 2010. Obtained from Advanced Chemistry Development, Inc. Available at: http://www.acdlabs.com.
48. Hansch C, Leo A. Substituent constants for correlation analysis in chemistry and biology. New York: Wiley, 1979:49–54.
49. Garrett RH, Grisham CM. Biochemistry. Fort Worth, TX: Saunders College Publishing, 1995:468–473.
50. Altschul R, Hoffer A, Stephen JD. Influence of nicotinic acid on serum cholesterol in man. Arch Biochem 1955;54:558–559.
51. Drood JM, Zimetbaum PJ, Frishman WH. Nicotinic acid for the treatment of hyperlipoproteinemia. J Clin Pharmacol 1991;31:641–650.

Chapter 26

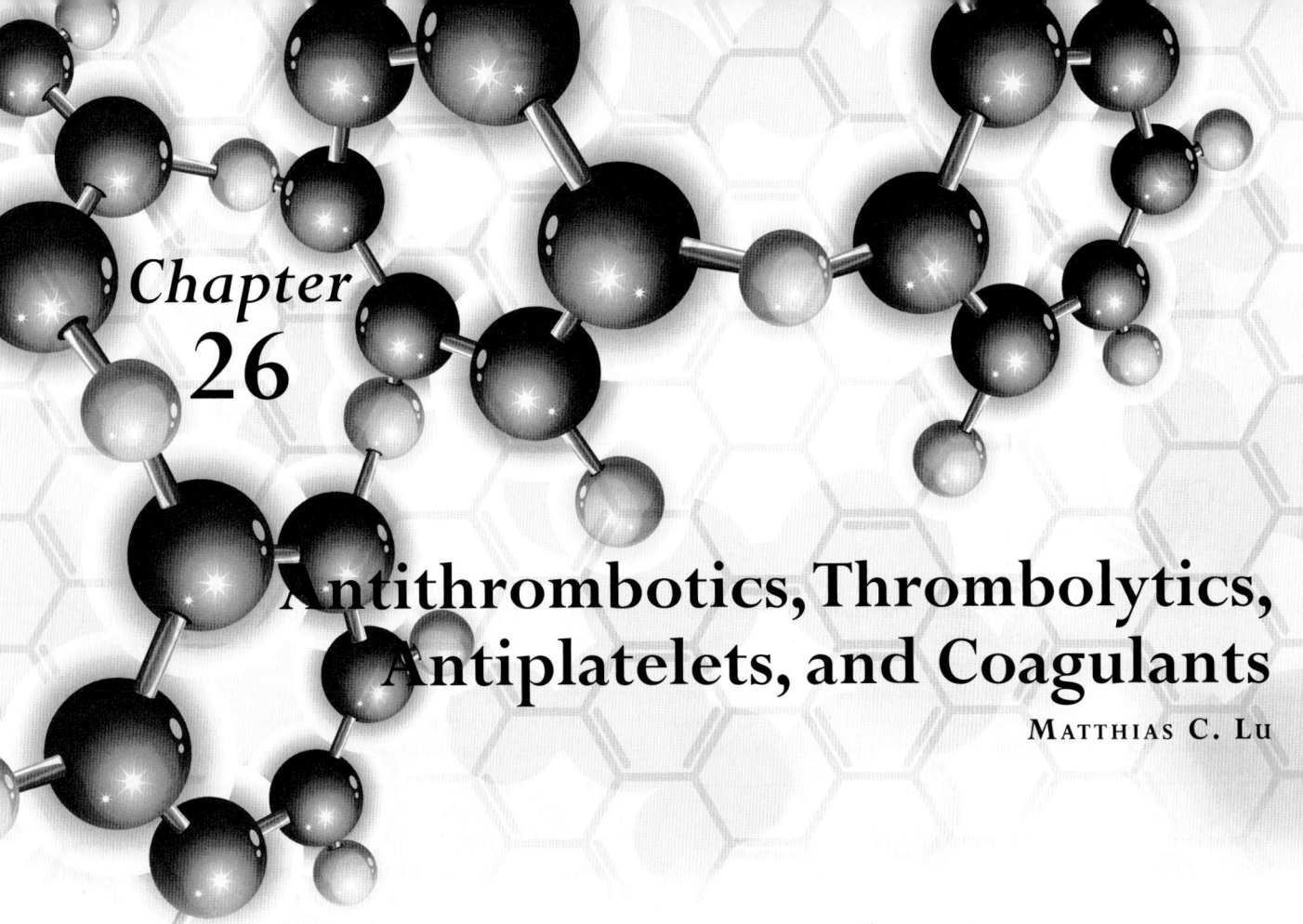

Antithrombotics, Thrombolytics, Antiplatelets, and Coagulants

Matthias C. Lu

Drugs Covered in This Chapter*

Warfarin

Heparins

- High molecular weight heparin
- Low molecular weight heparin
  - Ardeparin
  - Dalteparin
  - Enoxaparin
  - Tinzaparin
- Fondaparinux

Direct thrombin inhibitors

- Argatroban
- Bivalirudin
- Desirudin
- Lepirudin
- Dabigatran etexilate
- Rivaroxaban

Antiplatelet drugs

- Abciximab
- Aspirin
- Cilostazol
- Clopidogrel
- Dipyridamole
- Eptifibatide
- *Indobufen*
- Prasugrel
- Ticagrelor
- Ticlopidine
- Tirofiban
- *Triflusal*

Thrombolytic drugs

- Alteplase
- Prourokinase
- Reteplase
- Streptokinase
- Tenecteplase
- Urokinase

Coagulants

- Protamine
- Vitamin K

Thrombopoietin receptor agonists

- Eltrombopag
- Romiplositim

Antifibrinolytic agents

- Aprotinin

Abbreviations

ADP, adenosine diphosphate
aPTT, activated partial thromboplastin time
ATP, adenosine triphosphate
a-Xa U, antifactor Xa units
cAMP, cyclic adenosine monophosphate
COX, cyclooxygenase
CYP, cytochrome P450
DTI, direct thrombin inhibitor
DVT, deep vein thrombosis
FDA, U.S. Food and Drug Administration
FXa, activated factor X
GP, glycoprotein
HIT, heparin-induced thrombocytopenia
5-HT, serotonin
HTB, 2-hydroxy-4-trifluoromethylbenzoic acid
IC_{50}, half maximal inhibitory concentration
INR, international normalized ratio
ITP, idiopathic thrombocytopenia purpura
KH_2, vitamin K hydroquinone
LMWH, low molecular weight heparin
NSAID, nonsteroidal anti-inflammatory drug
PAI-1, plasminogen activator inhibitor-1

*Drugs listed include those available inside and outside of the United States; drugs available outside of the United States are shown in italics.

Abbreviations (Continued)

PAR-1, protease-activated receptor-1
PDE, phosphodiesterase
PE, pulmonary embolism
PF4, platelet factor 4
PGI_2, prostacyclin
PT, prothrombin time
TF, tissue factor
TFPI, tissue factor pathway inhibitor
tPA, tissue-type plasminogen activator
TXA_2, thromboxane A_2
USP, U.S. Pharmacopeia
V_d, volume of distribution
VKORC1, vitamin K 2,3-epoxide reductase complex 1
VTE, venous thromboembolism
vWF, von Willebrand factor

SCENARIO

Kim K. Birtcher, PharmD

JF, a 46-year-old white man, came to the emergency department by ambulance complaining of crushing chest pain, which radiated down his left arm and started 1 hour ago while he was watching television. The patient's wife called 911, and the paramedics gave him an aspirin, sublingual nitroglycerin, and oxygen en route to the hospital. Clinical and laboratory parameters showed that the patient had a non–ST-segment elevation myocardial infarction.

The patient was started on a heparin infusion and intravenous eptifibatide and was sent for cardiac catheterization. The patient received a loading dose of clopidogrel, and a drug-eluting stent was placed in the patient's left anterior descending artery.

(The reader is directed to the clinical solution and chemical analysis of this case at the end of the chapter).

Venous thromboembolism (VTE) is a complicating condition responsible for high morbidity and mortality worldwide (1). This disease is commonly linked to advanced age but has both hereditary and acquired risk factors, such as surgery, any form of trauma, and childbirth, associated with it. It encompasses an avoidable condition of deep vein thrombosis (DVT) that may result in pulmonary embolism (PE). It is estimated that 2 million people in the United States develop DVT each year with approximately one-third of these patients progressing to PE, leading to 200,000 deaths annually. Preventative therapy consists of the use of two different classes of antithrombotic agents, namely anticoagulants and antiplatelet drugs (2,3).

Heparin was discovered serendipitously in 1916 by a young coal miner turned medical student, Jay McLean, while working in the research laboratory of Professor W.H. Howell (4). Its beneficial effects were not realized until the early 1970s, when Kakkar et al. (5) established in a prospective, double-blind trial that low doses of heparin can prevent DVT after major surgery. In 1933, Dr. K.P. Link discovered that hydroxycoumarins are contained in sweet clover after finding cattle hemorrhaging to death (4). This discovery led to the development of orally active anticoagulants for prophylaxis in VTE and other thrombotic disorders. Optimal therapy with warfarin and other coumarin derivatives is not easy, however, because of their narrow therapeutic indexes. The need to carefully assess the benefit and risks for anticoagulation with frequent drug monitoring and dose adjustment also is troublesome (1,6). Thus, further development of novel antithrombotic agents with greater specificity on the coagulation cascade, with more predictable pharmacodynamic and pharmacokinetic profiles, and with fewer or no laboratory monitoring requirements is still needed for optimal treatment of thrombotic disorders (7–10).

Thrombolytics, on the other hand, are drugs needed to dissolve the newly formed thrombi in conditions such as DVT, acute PE, or myocardial infarction. Because of their lack of specificity, however, these agents actually may cause internal bleeding and, thus, are contraindicated with the use of many other therapeutic agents.

A variety of pathologic and toxicologic conditions can result in excessive bleeding from inadequate coagulation. Depending on the etiology and severity of the hemorrhagic episode, select coagulants that induce blood coagulation are therapeutically used to prevent excessive bleeding in these conditions.

DISEASE STATES REQUIRING ANTITHROMBOTIC THERAPY

A number of serious medical conditions are thrombotic in nature. In fact, in Western society, thrombotic conditions are the major cause of morbidity and mortality, and it is speculated that these disorders will be the leading cause of death worldwide within 20 years (2,8). As would be expected from the gravity of thrombotic disorders, many of the conditions involve the major vasculature, heart, brain, and lungs.

In the heart, a thrombotic condition may be involved in the disease state of acute myocardial infarction, valvular heart disease, unstable angina, and atrial fibrillation as well as surgical procedures, such as percutaneous transluminal coronary angioplasty and prosthetic heart valve replacement. Thrombotic conditions involving the vasculature include VTE, primary and secondary prevention of arterial thromboembolism, and peripheral vascular disease. The most significant such condition involving the lungs is PE and, in the brain, cerebrovascular accidents. Anticoagulation therapy is indicated for all of these conditions.

CLINICAL SIGNIFICANCE

The treatment, management, and prevention of thrombogenesis are complex. Clinicians must understand the steps of the clotting cascade, the basics of clot formation and lysis, and the differences between the individual medications that affect these processes. The clinician's knowledge of the mechanisms of action and pharmacokinetics of the anticoagulants will facilitate safe and effective treatment for individual patients. For example, it takes several days for warfarin to deplete the vitamin K–dependent clotting factors, so warfarin should be given in combination with unfractionated heparin or low molecular weight heparin when initiating treatment of VTE. Using low molecular weight heparin for this indication may allow the patient to receive outpatient therapy, whereas the use of unfractionated heparin requires continuous intravenous infusion in the hospital. In addition, the onset, duration of action, and predictability of anticoagulant effects of the low molecular weight heparins make them safer alternatives to warfarin during the perioperative period. The combined actions of aspirin; a thienopyridine; heparin, low molecular weight heparin, fondaparinux, or bivalirudin; a glycoprotein II_b/III_a inhibitor; and/or a fibrinolytic agent are necessary to manage thrombosis formation during an acute myocardial infarction.

Knowledge of structure–activity relationships helps predict site of action, duration of activity, potency, and side effect profile. As new medications are developed, the clinician will rely on this knowledge to tailor therapy to the individual patient. For example, the low molecular weight heparins' short pentasaccharide-containing heparin chains bind to antithrombin, so they have a greater relative affinity against factor Xa than the large pentasaccharide-containing heparin chains, which bind to both antithrombin and thrombin. Unfractionated heparin and bivalirudin are both antithrombotic agents, so they should not be used at the same time. Fondaparinux, a synthetic pentasaccharide, is not long enough to bind with thrombin, so it must be combined with heparin to prevent thrombus formation during percutaneous coronary intervention procedures. Dabigatran, a direct thrombin inhibitor, may be a safer and more convenient alternative to warfarin for some patients, because it does not require the same frequent laboratory monitoring as warfarin.

Kim K. Birtcher, MS, PharmD, BCPS
Clinical Associate Professor
Department of Clinical Sciences and Administration
University of Houston College of Pharmacy

Venous Thromboembolism and Pulmonary Embolism

VTE occurs when red bloods cells, fibrin, and, to a lesser extent, platelets and leukocytes coagulate to form a thrombus within an intact cardiovascular system (11). A patient undergoing orthopedic surgery incurs the greatest risk for VTE (3,12). PE occurs when a segment of a thrombus within the deep venous system detaches itself from the blood vessel, travels to the lungs, and lodges within the pulmonary arteries. Both of these conditions, if not properly detected and treated, can have serious consequences, such as sudden death or recurrent VTE and postthrombotic syndrome characterized by persistent pain, swelling, and skin discoloration or necrosis and ulceration of the affected limb (7,8).

Atrial Fibrillation

Atrial fibrillation is the most common cardiac arrhythmia, being found in more than 2 million Americans. It is characterized as a storm of electrical energy that travels in spinning wavelets throughout the atria, causing the upper chambers to quiver or fibrillate. It also is one of the leading risk factors for ischemic stroke for those individuals older than 50 years (13–15). Atrial fibrillation is more prevalent in men than in women, and the median age of patients with atrial fibrillation is approximately 72 years. Anticoagulation with warfarin and lifestyle modification are the most effective treatment modalities for patients with atrial fibrillation.

Pathophysiology of Thrombogenesis

Arterial thrombosis usually is initiated by the exposure of the thrombogenic material as a result of spontaneous or mechanical rupture of an atherosclerotic plaque (16,17). Arterial thrombi usually form in medium-sized vessels as a result of surface lesions on endothelial cells roughened by atherosclerosis. In most cases, circulating platelets adhere to the areas of abnormal vascular endothelium. More platelets then aggregate with those stuck to the vascular wall, forming a clot known as an occlusive thrombus (16). The formation of the occlusive thrombus at the site of the lesion is the major cause of complications of stroke and myocardial infarction. Venous thrombosis results from either an excessive activation of the coagulation cascade (hypercoagulability) or from some disease process or venous pooling (stasis) of the blood. Venous thrombus is initiated in the same fashion as the arterial thrombus formation, except that the bulk of the clot is formed of long fibrin tails that enmesh red blood cells. Venous thrombosis also can occur from vascular trauma caused by damage to the vessel wall, especially after major orthopedic surgery (11). Hypercoagulability, venous stasis, and vascular injury are known as Virchow's triad. As a general rule, arterial thrombi cause serious conditions through localized occlusive ischemia, whereas venous thrombi fragments give rise to pleural embolic complications.

Biochemical Mechanism of Blood Coagulation: The Coagulation Cascade

The formation of a blood clot is the result of an intricate and elegant cascade of biochemical events (Fig. 26.1).

The coagulation in arteries or veins is triggered by tissue factor (TF), a small molecular weight glycoprotein that initiates the TF pathway (previous known as the extrinsic clotting cascade) (1,17). The TF glycoprotein is expressed on the surface of macrophages, and TF is a major initiating factor of arterial thrombogenesis. TF binds and activates factor VII to form TF/VIIa complex, which in turn activates factor IX and factor X from either the intrinsic or extrinsic pathways shown in Figure 26.1.

Initiation of the contact activation pathway (also known as the intrinsic pathway) involves the sequential activation of factors XII, XI, and IX. (The activated form of a coagulation factor is indicated by a lowercase "a.") In the presence of calcium, factor IXa binds to an activated factor VIII on the surface of activated platelets to form an intrinsic Xase complex, which initiates the activation of factor X to Xa. In addition, initiation of the tissue factor pathway involves activation of factor VII by TF to form TF/VIIa, which, like factor IXa, also catalyzes the conversion of factor X to Xa. The underlying purpose of the contact activation pathway is maintenance of homeostasis, whereas the tissue factor pathway is activated by trauma. The TF and contact activation pathways come together with the conversion of

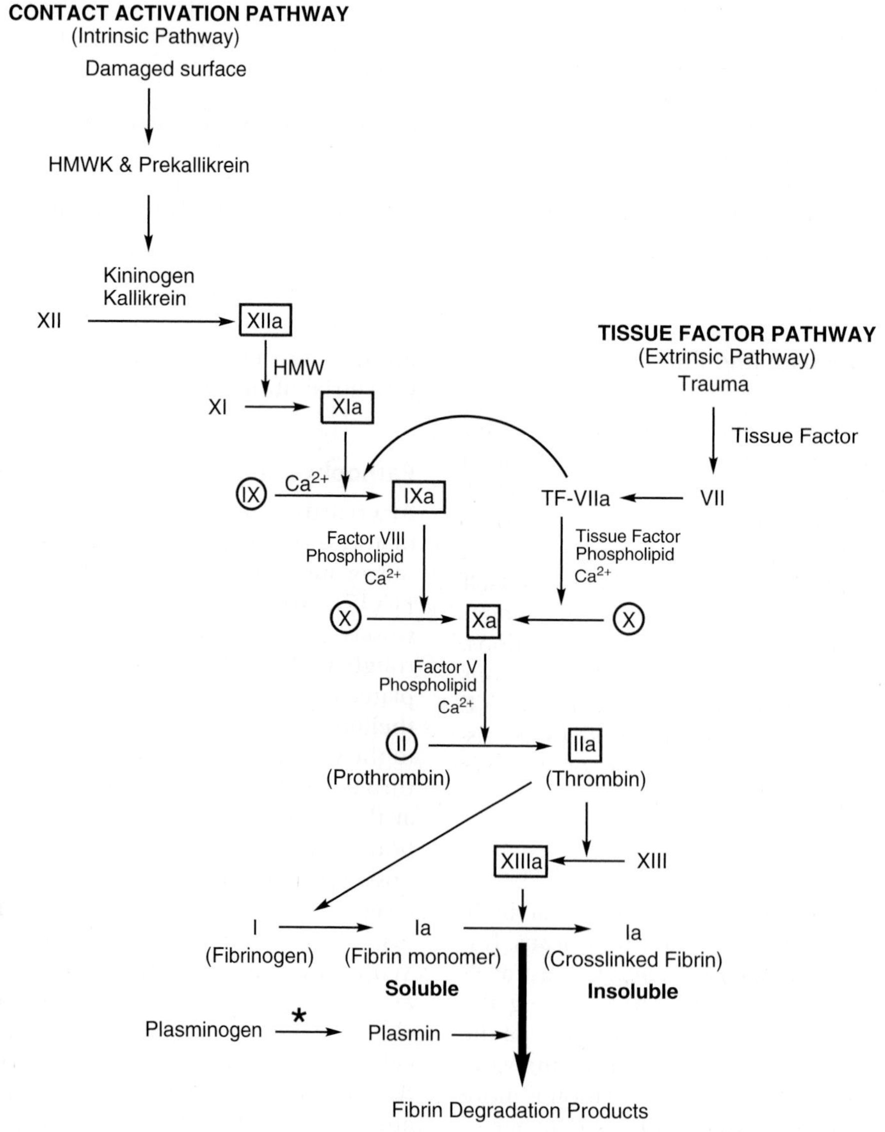

FIGURE 26.1 The coagulation cascade. *Circled factors* are those inhibited by warfarin-like drugs; *boxed factors* are those affected by heparin. The *star* indicates the site of action of thrombolytic drugs, such as streptokinase and urokinase.

factor X to its activated form, factor Xa. The coagulation cascade is unique in that the product of a given reaction (i.e., activated form of a specific factor) catalyzes the activation of the next factor in the cascade. The final steps in the coagulation cascade involve the conversion of prothrombin (factor II) to thrombin (factor IIa) by prothrombinase complex, consisting of factor Xa and activated factor V (Fig. 26.2). In turn, thrombin catalyzes the conversion of fibrinogen to soluble fibrin, which then becomes insoluble fibrin through the action of factor XIIIa. In its activated state, factor XIIIa actually is a transamidase enzyme. This enzyme catalyzes the formation of isopeptide bonds between lysine and glutamine side chains of distinct fibrin molecules, resulting in cross-linked (insoluble) fibrin aggregates (Fig. 26.3) (18).

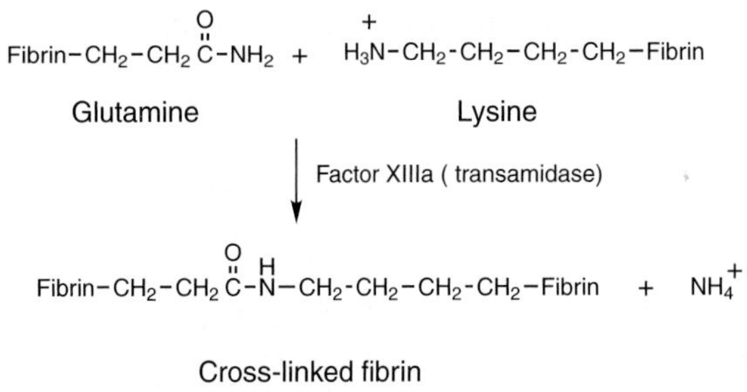

FIGURE 26.3 Cross-linking of soluble fibrin monomers (factor Ia) through the activity of factor XIIIa, a transamidase enzyme.

Strategies for Regulating Coagulation

Coagulation can be regulated at several levels (1,17). These include TF pathway inhibitor (TFPI), antithrombin, and the protein C pathways. Because the designs of many new anticoagulant drugs are aimed at enhancing endogenous anticoagulant or fibrinolytic mechanisms, a brief review of these pathways is warranted here.

TFPI is now recognized as a major physiologic inhibitor of TF-initiated coagulation (19). Its main role is to modulate factor VIIa/TF catalytic activity by a two-step process. First, TFPI binds and inactivates factor Xa by forming a TFPI/factor Xa complex. Then, the inactivated factor Xa/TFPI complex binds factor VIIa within the TF/VIIa complex to modulate its catalytic activity. Additionally, TFPI potentiates the effect of heparins (i.e., TFPI is released from the vascular endothelium after injection of either unfractionated heparin or low molecular weight heparins [LMWHs]), which may then provide high concentrations of TFPI at sites of tissue damage and ongoing thrombosis (20). The propagation of coagulation occurs when TFPI concentrations are low (17).

Antithrombin is a potent inhibitor of thrombin and factors IXa and Xa. It also has inhibitory actions on other activated clotting factors, including the TF/VIIa complex. In the absence of heparin, however, the action of antithrombin is slow. The action of antithrombin is enhanced more than 2,000-fold in the presence of heparin (1). It should be pointed out that even though heparin is not normally found in the blood, the vascular endothelium is rich in heparin sulfate, which contains the antithrombin-binding pentasaccharide sequence of the heparin. Drugs such as fondaparinux and idraparinux block the propagation of coagulation by inactivating factor Xa and, thereby, inhibiting the thrombin formation (1,17). Direct thrombin inhibitors, such as hirudin and argatroban, work by inhibiting both the clot-bound and free thrombin and, thus, preventing fibrin formation, the final step in the coagulation cascade (1,17).

In the protein C pathway, thrombin also is inhibited by binding to thrombomodulin, a thrombin receptor found in the endothelium. On binding to thrombomodulin, thrombin changes conformation, converting it from a procoagulant into a potent activator of protein C, a vitamin K–dependent protein, which degrades and inactivates factors Va and VIIa, thereby attenuating thrombogenesis (21,22).

GENERAL APPROACHES TO ANTICOAGULANT THERAPY

Overview

Because current clinically available antithrombotic drugs target only a few specific areas within the coagulation cascade, the selection of an appropriate anticoagulant for a given patient should be based on the patient's medical and drug history, age and location of the clot, underlying diagnosis of the disease state, and ultimate goal of the therapeutic intervention. If dissolving of an existing clot is needed, activation of plasminogen with the thrombolytic agents, which degrades insoluble fibrin, is the

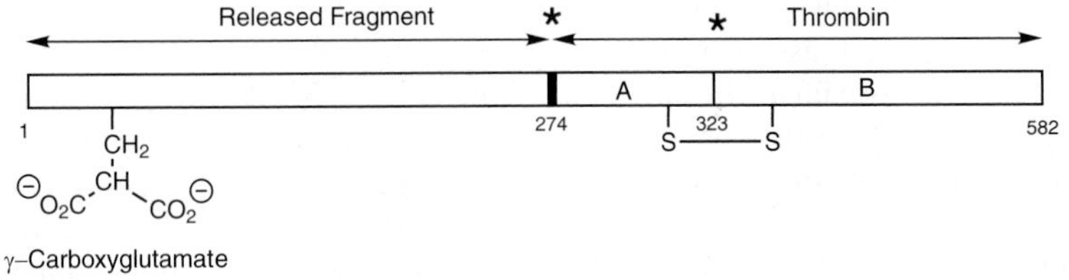

FIGURE 26.2 Structure of prothrombin. Thrombin is liberated through the cleavage of the Arg 274–Thr 275 and Arg 323–Ile 324 peptide bonds (indicated by the *red stars*). The γ-carboxyglutamate residues are in the released N-terminal portion of prothrombin and are not part of thrombin. The A and B chains of thrombin are joined by a disulfide bond.

typical approach. If the therapeutic goal is prevention of thrombus formation or extension, however, inhibition of factor activation higher in the cascade with heparin and other oral anticoagulants is the most appropriate.

An ideal anticoagulant should have reproducible pharmacodynamic and pharmacokinetic properties such that no coagulation monitoring is necessary (9). It also should have a wide therapeutic window, a rapid onset and offset of action, and minimal adverse effects, particularly with minimal interactions with food and other drugs (9).

Laboratory Assessment and Monitoring

Anticoagulant drug dosing represents a fine balance between reducing the morbidity and mortality associated with the thrombotic condition and minimizing the risk of serious hemorrhage from excessive therapeutic anticoagulation. Because of the potentially life-threatening consequences of either inadequate or excessive anticoagulation, patients receiving antithrombotic medications, such as warfarin and unfractionated heparin, often are closely monitored with specific clinical laboratory assays. A baseline assessment of the patient's coagulation features is performed before the initiation of anticoagulant therapy. This allows detection of congenital coagulation factor deficiencies, thrombocytopenia, hepatorenal insufficiency, and vascular abnormalities, which could prove to be catastrophic if anticoagulant therapy was instituted empirically.

For monitoring oral anticoagulant therapy (i.e., vitamin K antagonists), the prothrombin time (PT) is measured (23–25). This test is used to assess the activity of the vitamin K–dependent clotting factors (II, VII, IX, and X). The PT is particularly sensitive to factor VII, which is not of great clinical significance by itself but serves as a rough estimate for the ability of the liver to synthesize proteins or the extent of vitamin K depletion from warfarin therapy. The PT assay measures the time that it takes for a clot to form in citrated plasma after the addition of tissue thromboplastin and calcium. In normal (i.e., warfarin-free) plasma, this clot formation takes 10 to 13 seconds (23–25). Because of variances in commercially available thromboplastins, most clinical laboratories now report PT results in terms of international normalized ratios (INRs). Patients on warfarin therapy are optimally maintained with an INR of 2.0 to 3.0. In cases of patients who have had mechanical prosthetic heart valves placed, an INR of 2.5 to 3.5 often is recommended. At the initiation of warfarin therapy, daily PTs are performed. As the drug dosage is adjusted appropriately based on these results, the length of time between PT assessments can be extended to weekly. Finally, after warfarin therapy has been optimized and the patient's PT results have stabilized within an acceptable range, monthly or bimonthly PT checks are reasonable.

Heparin directly deactivates clotting factors II and X. Therapy with this drug is monitored based on the activated partial thromboplastin time (aPTT) assay (23–25). This assay monitors factors II and X as well as several others. Deficiencies of clotting factors that affect the aPTT result can be of little clinical significance (e.g., prekallikrein and factor XII), of potential clinical significance (e.g., factor XI), or of great clinical significance (e.g., factors VIII and IX and the hemophilic factors). In the aPTT assay, a surface activator, such as elegiac acid, kaolin, or silica, is used to activate the intrinsic pathway. When this activator comes in contact with citrated plasma in the presence of calcium and phospholipid, clot formation begins. As with the PT, the time taken for this clot to form is measured. In normal (nonheparinized) plasma, the average aPTT result is 25 to 45 seconds. A therapeutic aPTT in a patient receiving heparin typically is 70 to 140 seconds. In vivo, the platelet membrane rather than the phospholipid is the source of several clotting factors and the site of many of the coagulation reactions in the intrinsic pathway. The phospholipid used in the aPTT assay does not completely substitute for the in vivo actions of the platelets. Although this phospholipid does potentiate the intrinsic pathway, it does so without activating factor VII. This "partial activation" of the intrinsic pathway is the genesis of the name of the assay (aPTT).

Several other laboratory assays are used to assess function at various points within the clotting cascade. Quantitative levels of fibrinogen and fibrin degradation products are used to assess the extent of the effects of conditions such as acute inflammation, disseminated intravascular coagulation, and severe liver disease. The specific clotting factors in which a given patient may be deficient also can be determined using various mixing studies (23–25). These assessments are far more specialized and performed much less frequently than the PT and aPTT.

ORAL ANTICOAGULANTS

There are two different chemical classes of orally active anticoagulants, namely coumarin derivatives and 1,3-indandiones. It has been known since 1921 that cattle eating spoiled sweet clover hay often would die from uncontrollable bleeding after suffering a very minor injury. This discovery and other subsequent findings eventually led to the isolation of bishydroxycoumarin (i.e., dicoumarol) in 1934 by Link and Campbell and its use in humans in 1954 as the first orally active anticoagulant drug (26).

Coumarin Derivatives

Warfarin and other vitamin K antagonists have been the mainstay of oral anticoagulant therapy for more than 50 years (1). Although their effectiveness in the prophylaxis of thrombotic disorders has been established through many well-designed clinical trials, their use in clinical practice is challenging because of their narrow therapeutic index, potential for drug–drug/drug–food interactions, and patient variability including genetic polymorphisms (CYP2C9, VKORC1) that require close assessment and drug monitoring (24,25,27).

Mechanism of Action

Vitamin K antagonists, such as warfarin, produce their effect on blood coagulation by interfering with the cyclic interconversion of vitamin K and vitamin K 2,3-epoxide (Fig. 26.4) (28). Vitamin K is an essential cofactor necessary for the posttranslational carboxylation of the glutamic acid residues on the N-terminal portions of the specific clotting factors (II, VII, IX, and X) and anticoagulant proteins, such as protein C (21). This γ-glutamyl carboxylation results in a new amino acid, γ-carboxyglutamate, which through chelation of calcium ions causes the proteins to undergo a conformational change. This change in tertiary structure allows the four vitamin K–dependent clotting factors to become activated and bind to the negatively charged phospholipid membranes during clotting cascade activation.

The specific enzyme that carboxylates vitamin K–dependent coagulation factors requires a reduced form of vitamin K (vitamin K hydroquinone [KH_2]), molecular oxygen, and carbon dioxide as cofactors. In the process of this reaction, KH_2 is oxidized to vitamin K 2,3-epoxide. The return of the epoxide to the active KH_2 form is the result of a two-step reduction. First, the epoxide is reduced to vitamin K quinone, the rate-limiting step, by vitamin K 2,3-epoxide reductase complex 1 (VKORC1), in the presence of NADH (29). This quinone intermediate is then further reduced back to KH_2 by vitamin K quinone reductase. The warfarin-like anticoagulants (i.e., vitamin K antagonists) exert their anticoagulant activity through the inhibition of VKORC1 and, possibly, through inhibition of vitamin K quinone reductase, which in turn inhibits activation of the four affected coagulation factors. Unlike heparin, and as a direct result of their mechanism of action, the vitamin K antagonists only inhibit blood coagulation in vivo.

Structure–Activity Relationship of Coumarin Derivatives

All of the coumarin derivatives (Fig. 26.5) are water-insoluble lactones. Structure–activity relationship requirements typically are based on substitution of the lactone ring, specifically in positions 3 and 4. Although coumarin is a neutral compound, the clinically available derivatives are weakly acidic because of the presence of a 4-hydroxy substitution. The acidity of the proton on the 4-hydroxy group allows formation of water-soluble sodium salts for commercial preparations. Furthermore, warfarin (and, possibly, acenocoumarol) also can exist in

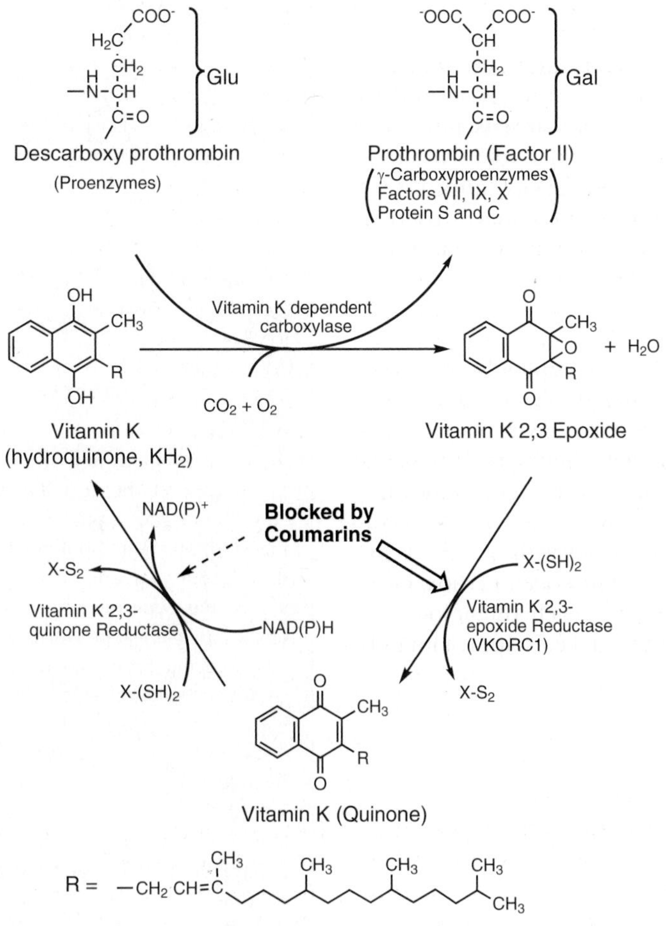

FIGURE 26.4 Redox cycling of vitamin K in the activation of blood clotting, which involves conversion of glutamate residues to γ-carboxyglutamates.

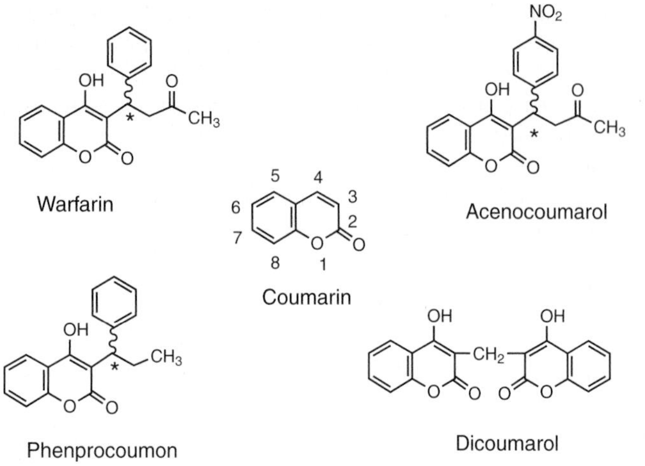

FIGURE 26.5 Chemical structures of coumarin and coumarin-derived drugs.

solution as two diastereomeric cyclic hemiketal conformers in addition to its open-chain conformer (Fig. 26.6). Because it has been suggested that vitamin K forms an active hemiketal in vivo, the cyclic hemiacetals of the vitamin K antagonists, such as warfarin, also may be the active conformers in vivo (30).

Pharmacokinetics

The substituents at position 3 greatly affect the pharmacokinetic and toxicologic properties of warfarin and its derivatives (Table 26.1) (31). Dicoumarol is not completely absorbed in the gastrointestinal tract, often is associated with gastrointestinal discomfort, and is very rarely used clinically. Today, the only coumarin used in the United States is warfarin, but phenprocoumon and acenocoumarol are used in Europe.

Warfarin

Warfarin sodium is rapidly and completely absorbed (~100% bioavailability) following oral, intramuscular, intravenous, or rectal administration. Peak plasma concentrations occur at approximately 3 hours. Its anticoagulant effect is not immediately present, however, following initiation of therapy. Instead, a delay in onset of anticoagulation occurs while the clotting factors with normal activity are cleared and those that have not been carboxylated because of the actions of warfarin reach physiologically significant levels. On average, this delay is approximately 5 hours for factor V turnover and 2 to 3 days for factor II (thrombin). Consequently, because of the rapid decline in protein C levels, the anticoagulated state frequently is preceded by a period of hypercoagulability (32).

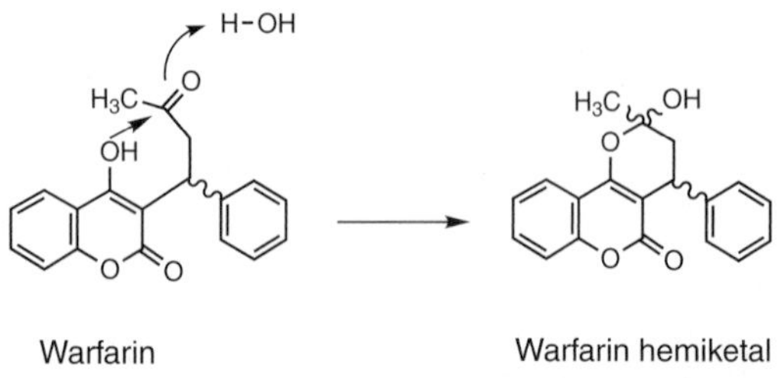

FIGURE 26.6 Formation of a cyclic hemiketal of warfarin.

Warfarin also is highly protein bound (95% to 99%) and, as a result, has numerous interactions with other drugs. The free drug (i.e., that not bound to plasma proteins) is the active constituent. Therefore, any other substance that displaces bound drug from protein binding sites increases the levels of free drug and, as a result, can cause warfarin toxicity, which usually is manifested by hemorrhage. The volume of distribution is quite small (0.1 to 0.2 L/kg), and the plasma half-life is quite long, both of which presumably result from the high degree of plasma protein binding (24,33).

"SUPERWARFARIN" RODENTICIDES

Brodifacoum is a member of the second-generation anticoagulant rodenticides known as "superwarfarins" (34). This compound and others like it (e.g., bromadiolone and difenacoum) were developed to combat rodent resistance to warfarin (34).

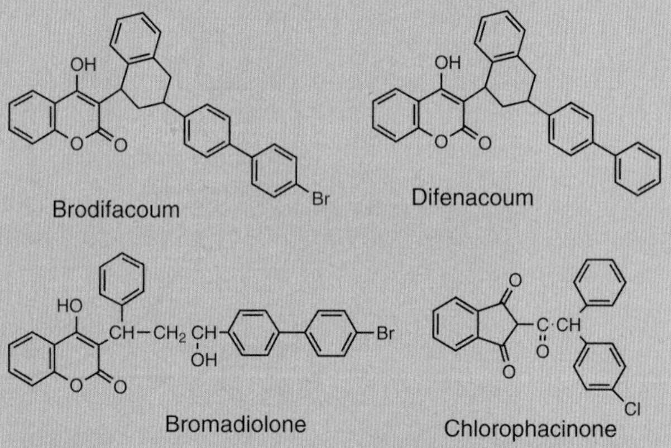

Human ingestion of brodifacoum typically is accidental in children but usually is intentional in adults (i.e., to commit suicide) (35). In cases when large quantities are ingested, severe and potentially fatal hemorrhaging can result. Brodifacoum is readily available over the counter in hardware stores and supermarkets, and it is marketed under numerous trade names in North America, Europe, Australia, and New Zealand. Brodifacoum, like warfarin, is thought to exhibit its anticoagulant effects through inhibition of vitamin K epoxide reductase. Despite the similarity in mechanism of action between brodifacoum and warfarin, brodifacoum is at least fivefold more potent as an anticoagulant rodenticide (34,36). The half-life of brodifacoum in humans is approximately 24.2 days, which is roughly ninefold longer than that of warfarin (34,37). Brodifacoum also has a volume of distribution roughly six times that of warfarin (37). For these reasons, vitamin K therapy may be needed for weeks to months after ingestion of a superwarfarin rodenticide (38).

TABLE 26.1 Pharmacokinetic Properties of the Coumarins and Anisindione

Drug	Trade Name	Onset (hours)	Duration (days)	Half-Life (days)	Time to Peak Plasma Concentration (hours)
Warfarin	Coumadin	1.5–3.0	2–5	0.62–2.5	4
Dicoumarol		1–5	2–10	1–4	1–9
Phenprocoumon	Marcumar[a]		7–14	5–6	
Acenocoumarol	Sinthrom[a]		2	0.3–1.0	1–3
Anisindione	Miradon	~6	1–3	3–5	2–3

[a]Not available in the United States but available in Europe.

The clinically used preparation of warfarin is racemic, but the (*S*)- and (*R*)-enantiomers are not equipotent. In fact, (*S*)-warfarin is at least fourfold more potent as an anticoagulant than (*R*)-warfarin. The difference in the activities and metabolism of the enantiomers is the key to understanding several stereoselective drug interactions. Similar stereochemical properties are noted for the other asymmetric coumarins (Fig. 26.5). In the case of acenocoumarol, the (*R*)-isomer is responsible for the majority of its activity.

Hepatic CYP2C9 isozyme is responsible for metabolizing (*S*)-warfarin and other coumarin derivatives to give 6- and 7-hydroxywarfarins as the major inactive metabolites, whereas hepatic CYP3A4, CYP1A2, and CYP2C19 isozymes inactivate (*R*)-warfarin, the less active enantiomer, to give 4′-, 6-, and 8-hydroxywarfarins, respectively (39). Warfarin also undergoes, to a lesser extent, reductive metabolism of the ketone on the C-3 side chain to a pair of pharmacologically active, diastereomeric 2′-hydroxywarfarins (Fig. 26.7). Almost no unchanged drug is excreted in the urine. As expected, those individuals with compromised hepatic function are at greater risk for warfarin toxicity secondary to diminished clearance. Furthermore, individuals with VKORC1 and CYP2C9 variants may require a much lower warfarin maintenance dose to avoid serious bleeding complications (40). Many of the drug–drug interactions are associated with enhanced or inhibited metabolism of warfarin via CYP2C9 induction or inhibition. Many additional drugs and conditions have profound effects on warfarin therapy. A partial list of these factors is shown in Table 26.2 (31).

Indandiones

Indane-1,3-dione derivatives (Fig. 26.8), such as phenindione and anisindione, are orally active anticoagulants having a similar mechanism of action to the coumarins but are rarely used clinically today because of their significant renal and hepatic toxicities. Furthermore, because of the structural similarity, patients who are allergic to warfarin will experience cross-sensitivity with anisindione and other indandione anticoagulants (41). Although anisindione reportedly has fewer significant side effects, most clinicians still prefer warfarin for oral anticoagulation. The pharmacokinetic properties also are similar to those of the coumarins (Table 26.1). Most of the newer indandione drugs, such as chlorophacinone, are marketed as potent rodenticides.

HEPARIN-BASED ANTICOAGULANTS

Chemistry

The heparin anticoagulants are represented by a variety of structures, including the natural heparan sulfate that lines the vascular endothelium, unfractionated heparin, LWMHs, and most recently, the synthetic pentasaccharide

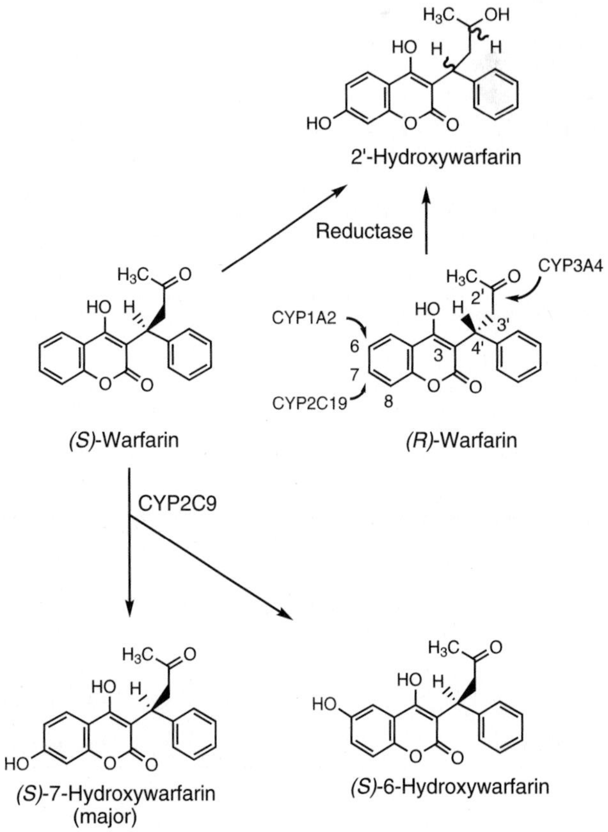

FIGURE 26.7 Metabolism of warfarin.

TABLE 26.2 Factors Affecting Warfarin Therapy

Potentiate Anticoagulation		**Antagonize Anticoagulation**
Drugs:		**Drugs:**
Acetaminophen	Miconazole	Alcohol (chronic abuse)
Alcohol/ethanol (acute intoxication)	Nalidixic acid	Aminoglycosides
Allopurinol	Naproxen	Antacid
Amiodarone	Omeprazole	Antihistamines
Anabolic and androgenic steroids	Oral hypoglycemics	Barbiturates
Aspirin	Pentoxifylline	Carbamazepine
Bromelains	Phenylbutazone	Chlordiazepoxide
Cephalosporins	Phenytoin	Cholestyramine
Chenodiol	Piroxicam	Colestipol
Chloral hydrate	Propafenone	Corticosteroids
Cimetidine	Propranolol	Dextrothyroxine
Clofibrate	Quinidine, quinine	Griseofulvin
Chlorpropamide	Sulfamethoxazole–trimethoprim	Haloperidol
Cotrimoxazole	Sulfinpyrazone	Meprobamate
Dextran	Sulfonylureas	Nafcillin
Diazoxide	Sulindac	Oral contraceptives
Diflunisal	Tamoxifen	Penicillins (large doses)
Disulfiram	Thyroxine	Phenytoin
Erythromycin	Ticlopidine	Primidone
Ethacrynic acid	Tolmetin	Rifampin
Fenoprofen	Tricyclic antidepressants	Sucralfate
Fluconazole		Trazodone
Glucagon	**Other Factors:**	Vitamin K (large doses)
Heparin	Fever	
Ibuprofen	Stress	**Other Factors:**
Indomethacin	Congestive heart failure	High–vitamin K diet: spinach, cheddar cheese, cabbage
Inhalation anesthetics	Radioactive compounds	Edema
Isoniazid	Diarrhea	Hypothyroidism
Ketoconazole	Cancer	Nephrotic syndrome
Lovastatin	X-rays	
Mefenamic acid	Hyperthyroidism	
Metronidazole	Hepatic dysfunction	

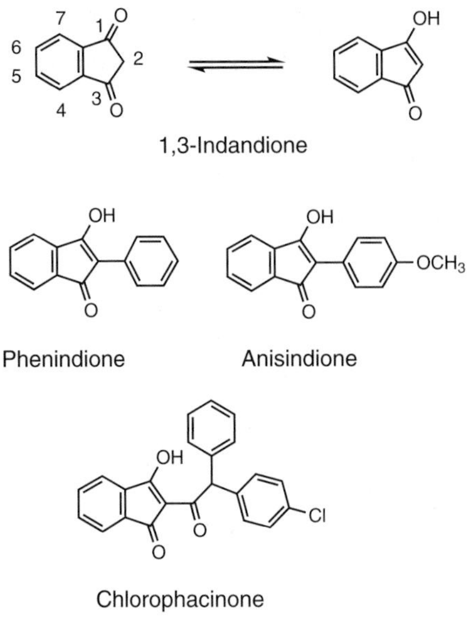

FIGURE 26.8 Chemical structures of 1,3-indandione and 1,3-indandione–derived drugs.

fondaparinux. Heparin is composed of a heterogeneous mixture of straight-chain, sulfated, and negatively charged mucopolysaccharides of a molecular weight range of 5 to 30 kd, isolated from bovine lung or porcine intestinal mucosa. Heparin, also known as heparinic acid, is an acidic molecule similar to chondroitin and hyaluronic acid. The polysaccharide polymer chains are composed of two alternating sugar units, *N*-acetyl-D-glucosamine and uronic acid (either D-glucuronic or L-iduronic), linked by α, 1 → 4 bonds (Fig. 26.9) (42).

These chains are called glycosaminoglycans and typically are composed of 200 to 300 monosaccharide units. In mast cells, approximately 10 to 15 of these chains are bound to a core protein to yield a proteoglycan (i.e., a protein/sugar conglomerate molecule) with a molecular weight of 750 to 1,000 kd. Before the molecule is capable of binding to antithrombin, the proteoglycan must undergo a series of structural modifications (42). These modifications include *O*-sulfation and *N*-sulfation of the D-glucosamine residues at carbons 6 and 2, respectively; *O*-sulfation of the D-glucuronic acid at carbon 2; epimerization of the D-glucuronic acid at carbon 5 to form L-iduronic acid; *O*-sulfation at carbon 2 of the L-iduronic acid; and *N*-deacetylation of the glucosamine and *O*-sulfation of the glucosamine at position 3. None of these reactions goes to completion, so the resulting polysaccharide chains are structurally quite diverse (43,44). The heparin proteoglycan then undergoes degradation by an endo-β-glucuronidase in mast cell granules to release the active 5- to 30-kd polysaccharide chains.

Under physiologic pH conditions, heparin exists primarily as polysulfate anions and, therefore, usually is administered as a salt. In clinical use, standard heparin most often is the sodium salt, but calcium heparin also is effective. Lithium heparin is used in blood sample collection tubes to prevent clotting of the blood samples in vitro but not in vivo. The use of heparin salts also is important to maintain aqueous solubility, which is necessary for injection. Heparin can be administered intravenously or subcutaneously but not orally, because the polysaccharide chains are broken down by gastric acid. Intramuscular injection of heparin is associated with a high risk of hematoma formation and is not recommended.

Mechanism of Action

Heparin (unfractionated heparin) was the first parenteral anticoagulant to show efficacy in the treatment of VTE and has been in use since 1937. Heparin acts at multiple sites in the coagulation cascade (42). Anticoagulation occurs when heparin binds, via a distinct pentasaccharide sequence in its molecule, to the circulating antithrombin III (a serine protease inhibitor) and potentates the antithrombin III–mediated inhibition of thrombin (factor IIa) and factor Xa, two of the key proteases in the blood coagulation cascade (Fig. 26.10) (45,46). The binding between heparin and antithrombin III consists of ionic bonding between sulfate and carboxylate anions in the pentasaccharide chain of heparin and arginine and lysine cations in the antithrombin III (46,47). Antithrombin III works by forming a stable 1:1 complex with both thrombin and factor Xa. Although the rates of these reactions (with IIa and Xa) are slow in the absence of heparin, binding is accelerated more than 2,000-fold when heparin is added (1,46). The reason for this enhancement is that when heparin binds to the antithrombin III, it induces a conformational change, resulting in increased accessibility of its active site and more rapid interaction with its protease substrates (i.e., thrombin and factor Xa). It should be noted that the ability of heparin to expose the active sites of antithrombin III is related to the large molecular size of heparin. With smaller molecules, such as LMWH and fondaparinux, the binding of antithrombin to

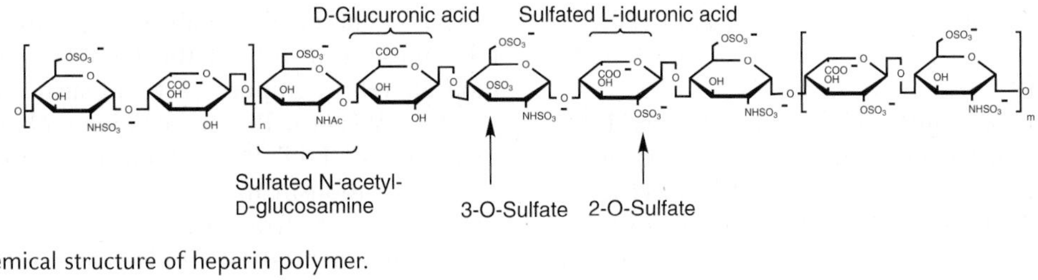

FIGURE 26.9 Chemical structure of heparin polymer.

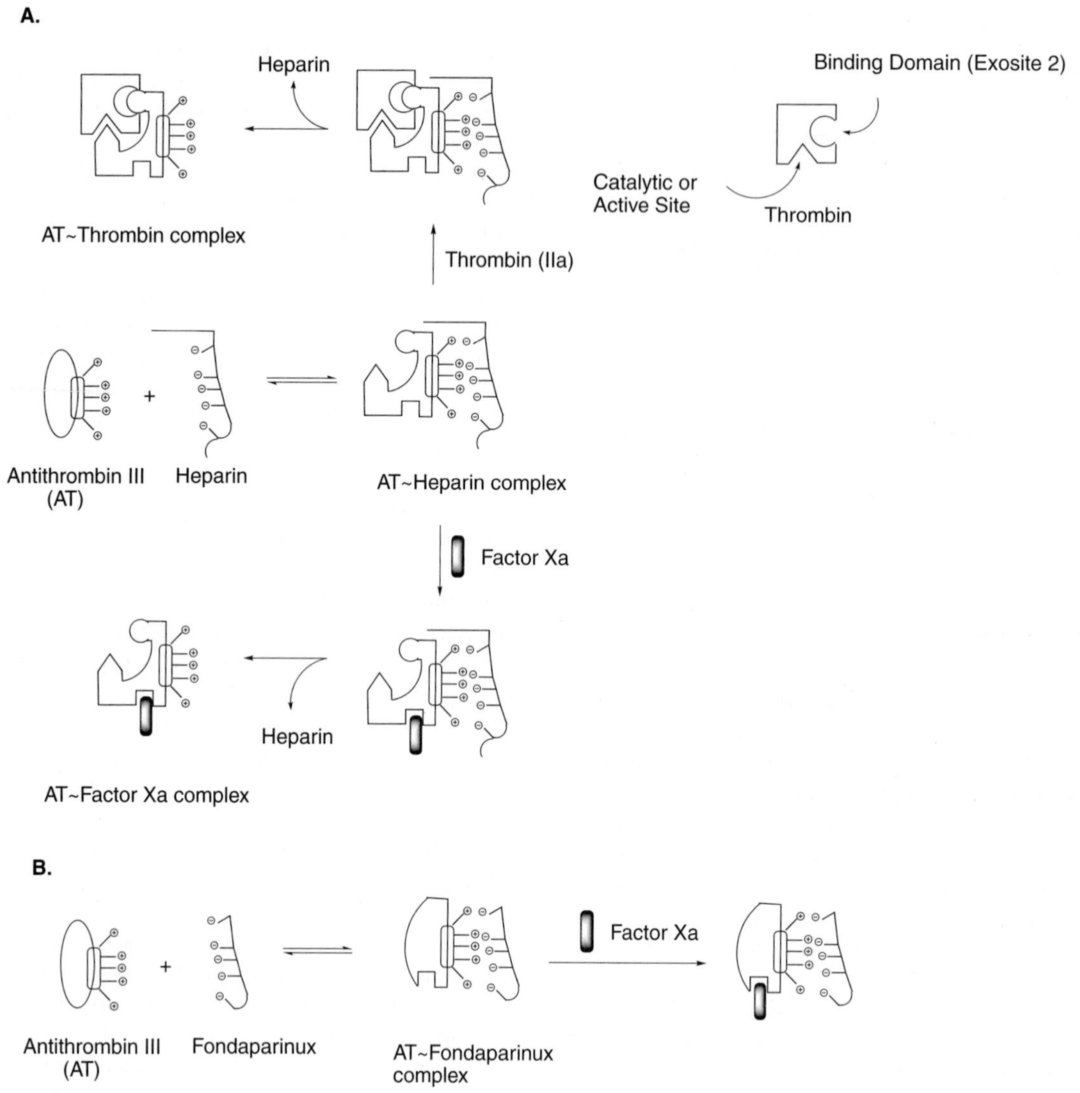

FIGURE 26.10 Schematic representation of catalytic role of the heparin drugs in promoting **(A)** antithrombin-factor Xa and antithrombin–thrombin complexes and **(B)** antithrombin–fondaparinux complex.

thrombin is diminished, and the drugs become more selective (see discussions of LMWH and fondaparinux). Interestingly, the role of heparin in this process is only catalytic in nature (i.e., it is not consumed, inactivated, or degraded by the reaction). In fact, once the complex of antithrombin and protease is formed, the heparin is released, with no loss of activity, to catalyze formation of more antithrombin/protease complexes (Fig. 26.10) (45). Additional effects of heparin on the coagulation of blood are a result of heparin's effects on plasminogen activator inhibitor, protein C inhibitor, and TFPI (20,21).

Pharmacokinetics

The pharmacokinetic profiles of heparin and LMWHs are quite different. Whereas heparin is only 30% absorbed following subcutaneous injection, 90% of LMWH is systemically absorbed (40,48). The binding affinity of heparin to various protein receptors, such as those on plasma proteins, endothelial cells, platelets, platelet factor 4 (PF4), and macrophages, is very high and is related to the high negative-charged density of heparin (44). This high nonspecific binding decreases bioavailability and patient variability. Additionally, heparin's nonspecific binding to PF4 may account for heparin's narrow therapeutic window and heparin-induced thrombocytopenia (HIT), a major limitation of heparin (46,49). These same affinities are quite low, however, in the case of LMWHs. These parameters explain several of the benefits of the LMWHs. The favorable absorption kinetics and low protein binding affinity of the LMWHs result in a greater bioavailability compared with heparin. The lowered affinity of LMWHs for PF4 seems to correlate with a reduced incidence of HIT (44). Heparin is subject to fast zero-order metabolism in the liver, followed by slower first-order clearance from the kidneys (50,51). The LMWHs are renally cleared and follow first-order kinetics. This makes the clearance of LMWHs more predictable as well as resulting in a prolonged half-life. Finally, the incidence of heparin-mediated osteoporosis is significantly diminished with use of LMWHs as opposed to heparin.

Metabolism

Independent of molecular weight, the metabolic fate of the heparins is essentially the same. The distribution of the compounds is limited primarily to the circulation, but heparins also are taken up by the reticuloendothelial system (33). Once this uptake occurs, rapid depolymerization of the polysaccharide chains ensues, resulting in products that are inactive as anticoagulants. Desulfation also occurs in mononuclear phagocytes, which also produces inactive metabolites. These metabolites, as well as some of the parent compound, are then excreted in the urine (33). Because of the depolymerization of heparin in the liver and ultimate renal elimination of both metabolites and parent drug, half-life is prolonged in patients with hepatic or renal dysfunction. Another heparin-like medication is danaparoid sodium (52). The drug is composed of 84% heparan sulfate, 12% dermatan sulfate, and 4% chondroitin sulfate. The average molecular weight is 5.5 kd, and like the LMWHs, danaparoid is dosed in terms of antifactor Xa activity (with target anti-Xa levels of 0.5 to 0.7 U/mL). Danaparoid is completely bioavailable intravenously or subcutaneously and attains maximal antifactor Xa activity 2 to 12 hours after administration, without bleeding or thromboembolic events during treatment in patients with suspected HIT (52). The elimination half-life is approximately 24 hours, and clearance is through the kidneys. Coagulation assays (e.g., PT and aPTT) are not routinely monitored in patients who are receiving danaparoid therapy.

Specific Heparin Drugs

High Molecular Weight Heparin (Unfractionated Heparin)

Standard heparin is unfractionated and contains mucopolysaccharides ranging in molecular weight from 5 to 30 kd (mean, ~15 kd) and is referred to as high molecular weight heparin (Table 26.3). This group of compounds has a very high affinity for antithrombin III and causes significant in vivo anticoagulant effects. Because heparin is a heterogeneous mixture of polysaccharides with different affinities for the target receptor, dosing based on milligrams of drug is inappropriate (i.e., there frequently is a limited correlation between the concentration of heparin given and the anticoagulant effect produced). Therefore, heparin is dosed in terms of standardized activity units that must be established by bioassay. One U.S. Pharmacopeia (USP) unit for heparin is the quantity of heparin required to prevent 1.0 mL of citrated sheep blood from clotting for 1 hour after the addition of 0.2 mL of 1% calcium chloride (23). Commercially available heparin sodium USP must contain at least 120 USP units per milligram. Heparin therapy typically is monitored by the aPTT. A therapeutic aPTT is represented by a clotting time in the assay that is 1.5- to 2.5-fold the normal mean aPTT (23). Monitoring therapy with laboratory testing is critical.

Low Molecular Weight Heparins

In the past two decades, an increased interest has surfaced in a group of compounds known as LMWHs (50). The LMWHs typically are in the 4- to 6-kd molecular weight range and are isolated as fractions from heparin using gel filtration chromatography or differential precipitation with ethanol (46). The LMWHs have more favorable pharmacokinetic and pharmacodynamic profiles relative to standard heparins (Table 26.3) (53,54). The mechanism of action of LMWHs is similar to conventional heparin, but the binding of LMWHs is more selective (i.e., LMWHs have more targeted activity against activated factor Xa and less against activated factor IIa [thrombin]) (Fig. 26.10). The reason for this difference is that even though LMWHs still possess the exact same specific pentasaccharide sequence as that of heparin needed for binding and potentiating the antithrombin

TABLE 26.3 Properties of Heparin Derivatives

Drug	Trade Name	Dosing	Molecular Weight (daltons)	Binding Ratio
Unfractionated heparin				
Heparin	Calciparine, Calcilean	bid, tid	5–30	1:1
Low molecular weight heparins				
Ardeparin	Normiflo	bid	5.6–6.4	2
Dalteparin	Fragmin	qd	3–8	2.2:1
Enoxaparin	Lovenox	qd, bid	3.5–5.5	2.7-3.9:1
Tinzaparin	Innohep	qd	5.5–7.5	2.8:1
Pentasaccharide				
Fondaparinux	Arixtra	qd	1.728	Xa only

bid, twice a day; qd, every day; tid, three times a day.

III–mediated inhibition of activated factor Xa, most of the LMWH/antithrombin III complex is of insufficient length to bind and inhibit factor Xa and thrombin at the same time (53). Thus, although all LMWHs inactivate factor Xa, only 25% to 50% of these molecules also inactivate thrombin (50). This factor selectivity typically is defined as a higher factor Xa:thrombin (anti-Xa:anti-IIa) activity ratio. In fact, although standard (unfractionated) heparin has an anti-Xa:anti-IIa ratio of 1:1, the same ratio in the LMWHs varies from 2:1 to 4:1 (Table 26.3) (50).

Four LWMHs are commercially available in the United States. The LWMHs are shown in Table 26.3. These drugs differ slightly in their medical indications for use as well as in their molecular weight ranges. All four compounds are indicated for perioperative thromboembolism prevention for specific abdominal and orthopedic surgeries. Enoxaparin and dalteparin are approved for use, in combination with aspirin, for the prophylaxis of ischemic complications of unstable angina and non–Q-wave myocardial infarction (55). Enoxaparin also is used in therapy for DVT with or without concomitant PE (55,56). Because of the increased homogeneity of enoxaparin compared to heparin, dosing of this drug is based on drug weight rather than on USP unitage. A typical dosing scheme for enoxaparin is the administration of 1 mg/kg once or twice daily. In the cases of dalteparin and ardeparin, dosage is based on antifactor Xa units (a-Xa U). Dalteparin is given as a once-daily subcutaneous injection at a dose of 2,500 to 5,000 a-Xa U. Typical dosing for tinzaparin is 175 a-Xa U/kg once daily, but the U.S. Food and Drug Administration (FDA) has issued a warning for using this product in elderly patients with impaired renal function. The LMWHs have a limited anticoagulant effect on in vitro clotting assays, such as the aPTT. In contrast to heparin, coagulation parameters, such as aPTT, usually are not monitored in patients receiving LMWHs; in addition, monitoring these assays is not really necessary because the LMWHs have a highly predictable dose–response relationship (50,53).

Newer Heparin Developments

Many recent studies involving heparin have been directed toward either increasing oral bioavailability or decreasing unwanted side effects (43,57). The poor bioavailability of heparin results from its high molecular weight and high anionic charge density. These properties, combined with the instability of the polysaccharides to gastric acid, make penetration of biologic membranes, such as the gut wall, extremely difficult for heparin. Various approaches to increase heparin absorption following oral administration have been investigated (58). Combinations of heparin with assorted calcium-binding substances and non–α-amino acids (*N*-acylated aminoalkanoic acids) for simultaneous oral administration also have been studied (58). Attempts to use structural modifications to heparin to attenuate undesirable side effects also have been investigated (57,59). HIT is caused by the interaction of heparin with PF4. The PF4 binding domain appears to be distinct from the thrombin binding domain. Therefore, it should be possible to use shorter oligosaccharides that bind specifically to the thrombin inhibitory sites without binding to PF4 (57). These observations were used to develop and synthetically produce a series of oligosaccharides with good thrombin binding profiles that have limited interaction with PF4. This preliminary work is quite promising, but these compounds are not yet clinically available.

Fondaparinux

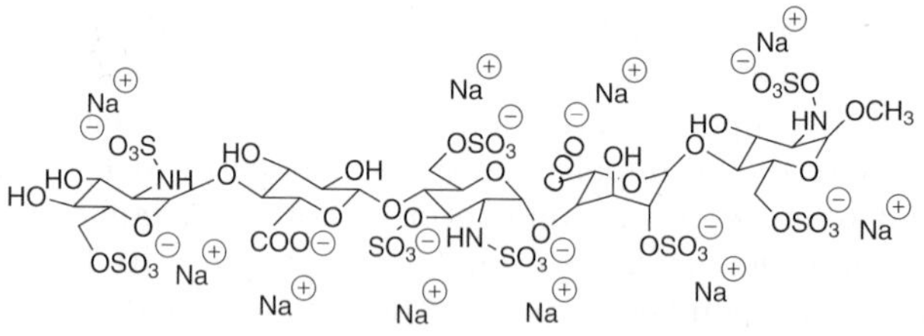

Fondaparinux is a prototype of a novel class of anticoagulants with significant advantages compared to their structurally related heparin (60). Based on the active site of the heparins, fondaparinux is a synthetic, highly sulfonated pentasaccharide. The immediate advantage of fondaparinux is that as a synthetic drug, its composition will not change, which results in improved pharmacokinetics and a more selective anticoagulant action.

Mechanism of Action The development of fondaparinux, a synthetically derived pentasaccharide that binds specifically to and activates antithrombin III, is a further refinement on the mechanism of action of heparin (61). Fondaparinux and a related analog, idraparinux, are specific, indirect inhibitors of activated factor Xa via their activation of antithrombin (Fig. 26.10). Fondaparinux has strategically located sulfonates that bind to antithrombin. Fondaparinux is structurally related to the antithrombotic binding site of heparin (62,63). Unlike heparin or LMWHs, however, these inhibitors have no effect on thrombin, because they lack the longer saccharide chains required for binding to thrombin. The highly sulfated heparins exhibit nonselective binding to a number of additional proteins, resulting in decreased bioavailability and significant variation in activity.

Therapeutic Application Fondaparinux is the first selective factor Xa inhibitor that is approved for the prophylaxis of DVT, which may occur in patients undergoing hip fracture surgery or hip or knee replacement surgery (64). The most common side effect is major and minor bleeding, and the patient must be carefully monitored because its anticoagulant effect cannot be neutralized by protamine sulfate (8). The drug is not to be used when spinal anesthesia or spinal puncture is employed because of the potential for developing a blood clot in the spine.

IDRABIOTAPARINUX

Idrabiotaparinux is a biotinylated and polymethylated derivative of fondaparinux that is long-acting yet its anticoagulant effect is easily reversible with intravenous administration of avidin, a tetrameric protein derived from egg whites (7,67,68). Avidin binds with high affinity to the biotin moiety of idrabiotaparinux to form a 1:1 stoichiometric complex that is rapidly cleared via the kidneys (68). Like fondaparinux, this drug is an indirect inhibitor of factor Xa, which binds to antithrombin with very high affinity for antithrombin (K_d <1 nmol/L) (67). The drug can be given subcutaneously on a once-weekly regimen. Idrabiotaparinux, like fondaparinux, is 100% bioavailable and does not bind to other plasma proteins.

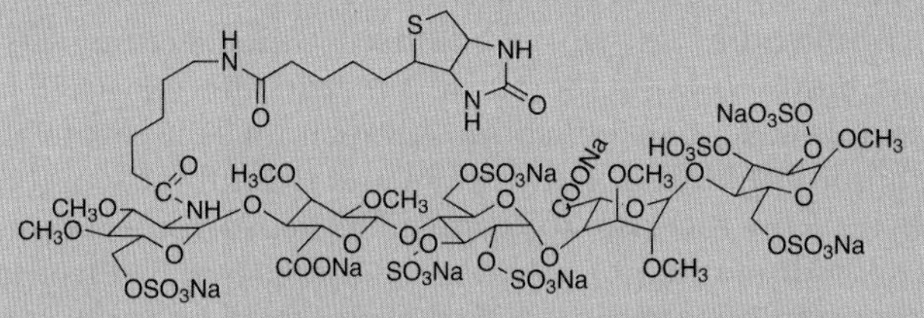

Idrabiotaparinux

Fondaparinux has not been reported to cause thrombocytopenia, a condition seen with heparin (61,64–66). It is 100% bioavailable, with little or no protein binding.

Pharmacokinetics Fondaparinux is administered via subcutaneous injection with a single daily dose and shows complete absorption. The drug is highly bound to antithrombin III (~94%), with no significant binding to other plasma proteins. Because of the predictable anticoagulant effect, the drug does not require routine coagulation monitoring (66). The drug is not metabolized and is excreted in the urine unchanged within 72 hours in patients with normal renal function. Fondaparinux has an elimination half-life of 17 hours. Presently, no clinically significant drug interactions have been reported.

DIRECT THROMBIN INHIBITORS

In the last 10 years, with a better understanding of the molecular mechanisms of blood coagulation, the availability of molecular modeling and recombinant technologies, and the structure-based drug design strategies, many new anticoagulants that target almost every step in the coagulation pathway have been developed (17,69). Among these, five direct thrombin inhibitors (DTIs; hirudin, lepirudin, desirudin, bivalirudin, and argatroban) have been approved for clinical use in recent years (Table 26.4). Many other anticoagulants that act on the endogenous anticoagulation mechanisms, such as activated protein C pathway, TFPI, and additional orally active DTIs, currently are undergoing clinical trials (15,69,70).

Discovery and Design of Direct Thrombin Inhibitors

Hirudin, the lead compound for the design of DTIs, is a small protein (65 amino acids) that was originally isolated from the salivary glands of the medicinal leech, *Hirudo medicinalis* (71). This protein has potent and specific inhibitory effects on thrombin through the formation of a 1:1 complex with the clotting factor. The anticoagulant activity of hirudin seems to be contained within its highly anionic C-terminus. Several clinical studies have compared hirudin and a small peptidomimetic analog, hirulog, with heparin in the treatment of several thrombotic disorders. In many cases, hirudin seems to be more efficacious and the responses to it more predictable. Furthermore, some of the studies also indicate a lower incidence of bleeding complications with hirudin compared with heparin. Hirudin is now produced by recombinant technology, and many hirulogs continue to be screened (72,73). Significant progress in the design and development of direct thrombin inhibition has been achieved. The recent emergence of orally active DTIs may simplify the prevention and treatment of various thrombotic disorders (74–76).

Mechanism of Action

The DTIs bind and inactivate both free thrombin and thrombin bound to fibrin. Unlike heparin, DTIs, such as lepirudin, bivalirudin, and argatroban, bind directly

TABLE 26.4 Direct Thrombin Inhibitors (DTIs)

Drugs	Trade Name	Route of Administration	Site of Binding	Reversibility	Half-Life (minutes)	Route of Excretion	Protein Binding
Hirudin		IV	CS, Exosite I	Irreversible			
Leprirudin	Refludan	IV	CS, Exosite I	Irreversible	80		
Desirudin	Revasc	SC	CS, Exosite I	Irreversible	120–180	Kidney	0
Bivalirudin	Angiomax	IV	CS, Exosite I	Reversible	25	Kidney	0
Argatroban	Novastan	IV	CS	Reversible	39–51	Hepatobiliary	54%

CS, catalytic site; IV, intravenous; PO, oral; SC, subcutaneous.

and reversibly to the active site of thrombin. Unlike the heparins, these inhibitors do not require an activated antithrombin III as a cofactor for their anticoagulant activity. Furthermore, contrary to the heparins, these agents inhibit only the activity of thrombin, whereas heparin indirectly inhibits factors IIa (thrombin), IXa, Xa, XIa, and XIIa (77). There are three different domains where DTIs bind to and block the action of thrombin: the active site (or catalytic site, CS) as well as two additional exosites. Exosite-1 acts as a dock for substrates such as fibrin and, thereby, orients the appropriate peptide bonds in the active site for its biotransformation. Exosite-2 is the heparin binding domain. Bivalent DTIs, such as lepirudin and bivalirudin, block thrombin at the active site and exosite-1, whereas argatroban is a univalent DTI and, thus, binds only to the active site of the thrombin.

Specific Drugs

Recombinant Hirudin Derivatives: Lepirudin (Refludan) and Desirudin (Revasc)

Lepirudin and desirudin have been approved for the treatment of HIT and of HIT with thrombotic syndrome (78). Both lepirudin and desirudin are recombinant hirudin derivatives that consists of a 65–amino acid protein (79,80). Lepirudin is related to the recombinant product desirudin differing in the two N-terminal amino acids. The N-terminal amino acids in lepirudin are leucine-1 and threonine-2, whereas in desirudin, the N-terminal amino acids are valine-1 and valine-2. Additionally, desirudin lacks a sulfated tyrosine at amino acid 63. The antithrombin activity of the two drugs is slightly different.

Lepirudin and desirudin are both bivalent DTIs that bind to both the active site and the exosite-1 of thrombin. The result of this binding is that they create a nearly irreversible inhibition of thrombin. Lepirudin and desirudin inhibit both free thrombin and thrombin bound to fibrin (81).

Lepirudin is administered via intravenous bolus injection, followed by continuous infusion, whereas desirudin is administered subcutaneously twice daily (Table 26.4) (80,82). The drugs are cleared via the kidneys. Lepirudin is nearly totally degraded before excretion (~90%), whereas desirudin is excreted 50% unchanged. Lepirudin has immunogenic properties, and a significant number of patients develop antihirudin antibodies. In addition, hemorrhages may occur in patients treated with lepirudin. The drug half-life is approximately 1.3 hours (83).

Bivalirudin (Angiomax, Angiox)

Bivalirudin, a 20–amino acid peptide, has been approved for use in patients with unstable angina undergoing percutaneous coronary intervention (Fig. 26.11) (84).

Bivalirudin is a rapid-onset, short-acting DTI that binds to both the active site and the exosite-1 of thrombin. Unlike lepirudin, bivalirudin is a reversible inhibitor of both free thrombin and thrombin bound to fibrin. This reversibility is possible because the bound bivalirudin undergoes cleavage at the second N-terminal proline to release the portion of the drug bound to the active site. The carboxyl-terminal portion of bivalirudin dissociates from thrombin to regenerate thrombin (Fig. 26.11) (83). Bivalirudin does not bind to plasma protein.

Bivalirudin is administered via intravenous bolus injection, followed by continuous infusion (Table 26.4). The drug exhibits a rapid onset and a short duration of action. Bivalirudin is eliminated by renal excretion. It has been suggested that dosage adjustments be made in patients with severe renal impairment and in patients undergoing dialysis. Approximately 30% is eliminated unchanged along with proteolytic cleavage products. Because of the reversible nature of bivalirudin, the drug exhibits less risk of bleeding than other antithrombotics,

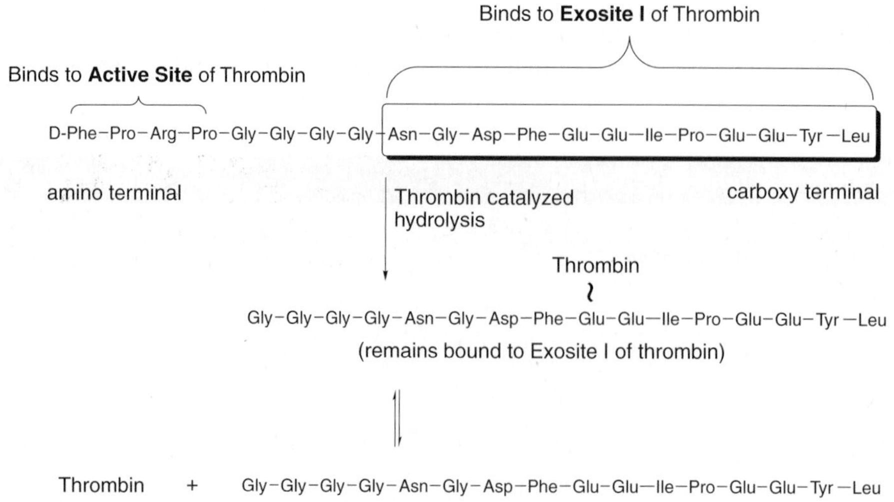

FIGURE 26.11 Chemical structure of bivalirudin, binding sites to thrombin, and release from thrombin.

and there have been no reported cases of antibody formation to bivalirudin (85).

Argatroban

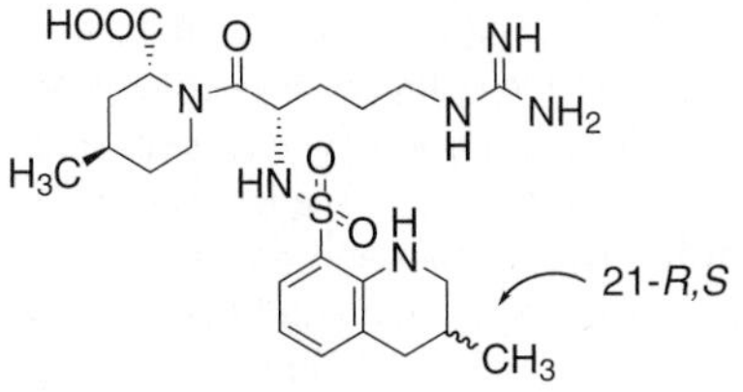

Argatroban

Argatroban has been approved for the prophylaxis and treatment of thrombosis in patients with HIT (86). Argatroban is a peptidomimetic that binds selectively to the catalytic site of thrombin as a univalent competitive DTI (Fig. 26.12). Argatroban is available as a mixture of 21-(*R*) and 21-(*S*) diastereomers (64:36), with the (*S*)-isomer approximately twice as potent as the (*R*)-isomer (87). The drug is a reversible inhibitor of both free thrombin and clot-bound thrombin.

Pharmacokinetics (Table 26.4) Argatroban is administered subcutaneously because of the low lipophilicity of the drug. The drug is bound to plasma protein and is metabolized via CYP3A4/5 to the aromatized metabolite and the two hydroxylated metabolites (Fig. 26.13). The M-1 metabolite retains 20% to 30% of the antithrombotic activity. Coadministration of argatroban with inhibitors of CYP3A4 does not appear to produce clinically significant effects. Argatroban is eliminated via biliary secretion into the feces (88).

Dabigatran Etexilate (Pradaxa)

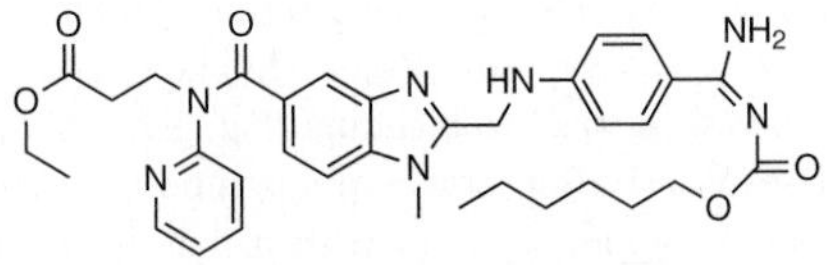

Dabigatran etexilate

Dabigatran etexilate, an orally active DTI, has recently been approved for the prevention of stroke and blood clots in individuals with atrial fibrillation. Dabigatran etexilate is a nonpeptidomimetic prodrug that gives

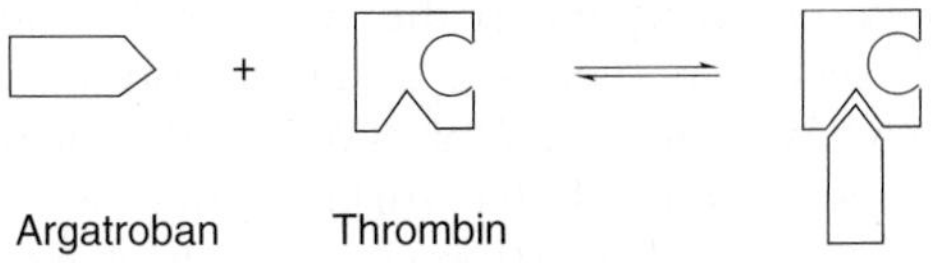

FIGURE 26.12 Schematic representation of mechanism of action of argatroban.

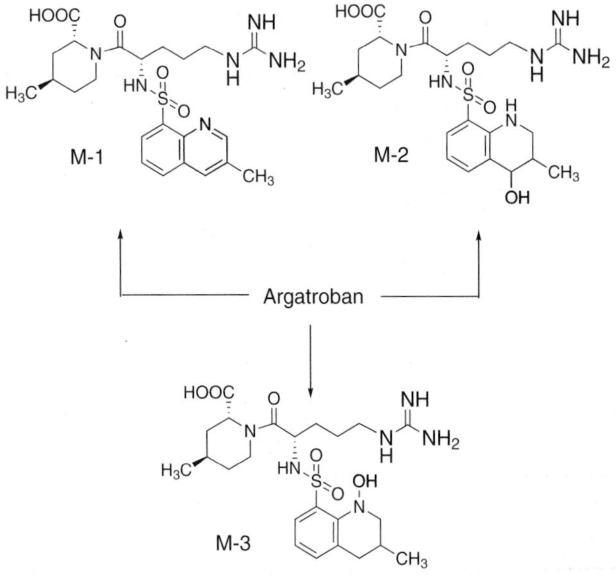

FIGURE 26.13 Metabolism of argatroban.

rise to dabigatran (Fig. 26.14), a reversible, basic benzamidine-based direct thrombin inhibitor that binds and inactivates both free and fibrin-bound thrombins (89,90). The drug is available in the European Union and Canada, where it is approved for treatment of VTE in patients undergoing hip or knee replacement surgery, and it is being studied for treatment of DVT and PE.

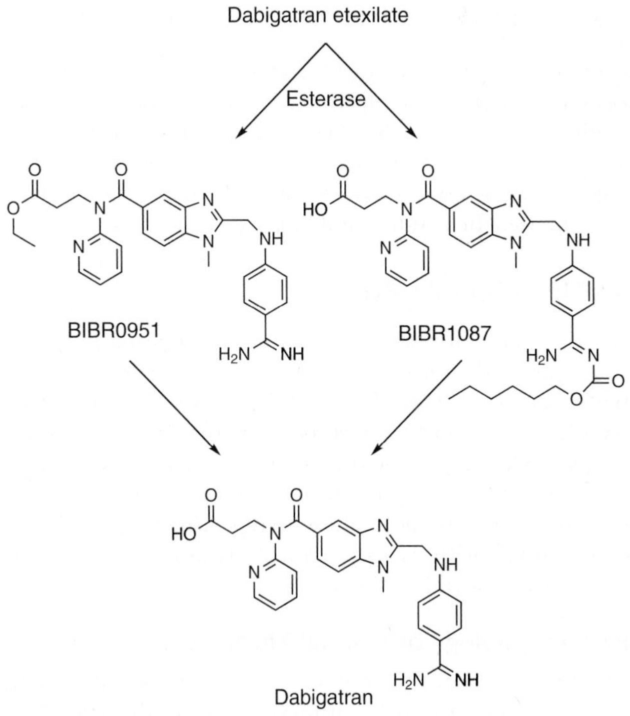

FIGURE 26.14 Metabolic activation of dabigatran etexilate to dabigatran.

PHARMACOKINETICS Dabigatran etexilate has a rapid onset of action, reaching maximum plasma concentrations within 0.5 to 2 hours after oral administration, and is quickly converted to dabigatran by plasma esterases (89,91). Very little dabigatran etexilate or the intermediate metabolites (BIBR0951-1087) are detectable in plasma. Dabigatran itself is quite hydrophilic due to the strongly basic amidine group and, at physiologic pH, exists as a charged species. As a result, dabigatran is not absorbed orally. The less basic etexilate is readily absorbed from the stomach and small intestine, but requires an acid environment. To promote an acidic microenvironment, the dabigatran etexilate is coated on tartaric acid pellets within the drug capsule, which creates an acidic environment thus promoting absorption and reducing variability due to different gastric pH in the individual. Dabigatran etexilate has a low bioavailability (~6.5%), which is offset by the administration of a large dose (75 to 150 mg twice a day). Up to 80% of dabigatran is eliminated unchanged in the kidneys with the remainder excreted via the biliary system as its acylglucuronides (91). Dabigatran etexilate was reported to have no clinically relevant interactions with drugs metabolized by cytochrome P450 (CYP) isozymes; thus, it can be given in fixed doses without coagulation monitoring (89). However, because dabigatran etexilate is excreted predominantly in the kidneys, it is not recommended for patients with severe renal dysfunction (70). Dosage is based on creatinine clearance: For patients with creatinine clearance greater than 30 mL/minute, the recommend dose is 150 mg twice a day, whereas for patients with a creatinine clearance of 15 to 30 mL/min, the recommended dose is 75 mg twice a day. Due to dabigatran's rapid onset and rapid offset, the drug does not require coagulation monitoring, which represents a major advantage over other anticoagulant therapy. However, the drug is reported to produce a significant increase in risk of major gastrointestinal bleeding, and the patient should be made aware of this side effect. It is reported that there is a significant reduction in life-threatening and total bleeding. Other side effects reported include dyspepsia, stomach pain, nausea, heartburn, and bloating.

ORALLY ACTIVE DIRECT THROMBIN INHIBITORS IN THE PIPELINE

Several additional orally active small-molecule inhibitors that specifically target thrombin or activated factor X (FXa) are in various stages of their clinical development for VTE, atrial fibrillation, and other thrombotic diseases (1,2,8,15,70,89). Two of these agents that are in the late stages of their clinical development are rivaroxaban and apixaban. The former was approved in the European Union and Canada in 2008 for prevention and treatment of VTE in patients undergoing elective hip or knee surgery.

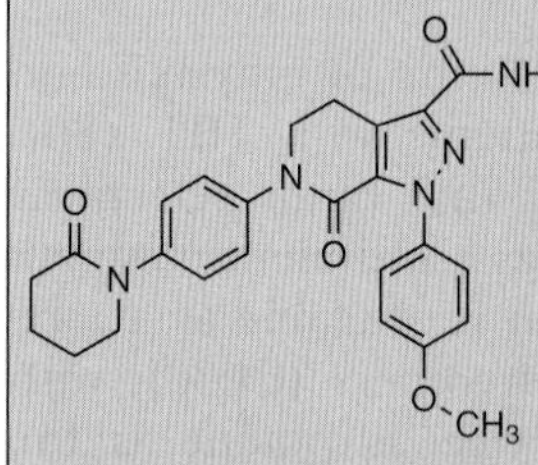

Apixaban

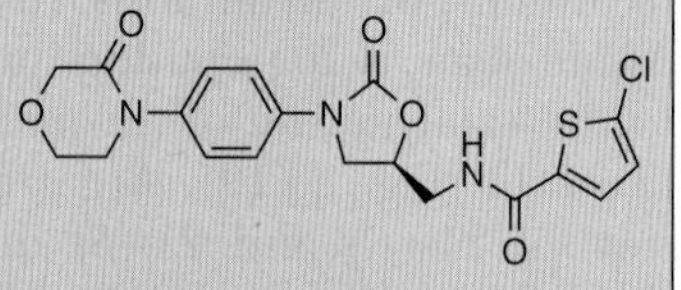

Rivaroxaban (Xarelto)

Orally active direct thrombin inhibitors

Rivaroxaban was the first orally active, direct coagulation FXa inhibitor with the most published clinical trials data showing similar efficacy and safety to enoxaparin in preventing VTE in major orthopedic surgery (92,93). It has received approvals for the prevention of VTE associated with major surgery in several countries and has been recently approved for use in the United States (94). Rivaroxaban is a highly selective and reversible inhibitor of direct FXa (K_i = 0.4 nmol/L) that binds to the active site of both free and prothrombinase-bound FXa. It is rapidly absorbed, reaching maximum plasma concentrations 3 hours after oral administration, and has a half-life ranging from 5 to 9 hours in young adults and 11 to 13 hours in the elderly.

Apixaban is the second selective and potent oral direct FXa inhibitor (K_i = 0.8 nmol/L) that exhibits a superior risk-to-benefit ratio with respect to bleeding than enoxaparin (93,95). It is well absorbed after oral administration, reaching peak plasma levels in about 3 hours with a half-life of 12 hours. Metabolic profile studies have revealed that apixaban is the major drug-related component in plasma, urine, and feces in humans, with the *O*-demethylapixaban sulfate as a stable, water-soluble inactive metabolite (96).

ANTIPLATELET DRUGS

Another site for regulating blood coagulation and subsequent thrombus formation is at the level of the platelets (97). Antiplatelet drugs work by inhibiting platelet activation via a number of different mechanisms (97,98). The major role of antiplatelet drugs is in the prevention of ischemic complications in patients with coronary diseases (99,100). These drugs also are effective in combination with moderate-intensity anticoagulants for patients with atrial fibrillation.

Pathophysiology of Arterial Thrombosis

The pivotal role of platelets in thrombus formation and potential sites for drug interventions is illustrated in Figure 26.15 (98,100). Normal endothelial cells in the vascular wall synthesize and release prostacyclin (PGI_2), which stimulates the conversion of adenosine triphosphate (ATP) to cyclic adenosine monophosphate (cAMP), thus preventing platelet aggregation and degranulation. In the case of an injury to the vascular wall, glycoprotein (GP) receptors (i.e., GPI_a and GPI_b) bind substances such as von Willebrand factor (vWF) and collagen from the exposed subendothelial surface, thereby activating the platelets. The $GPII_b/III_a$ receptors (also known as the fibrinogen receptor or integrin αIIbβ3 receptor) then mediate the final step of platelet aggregation by binding

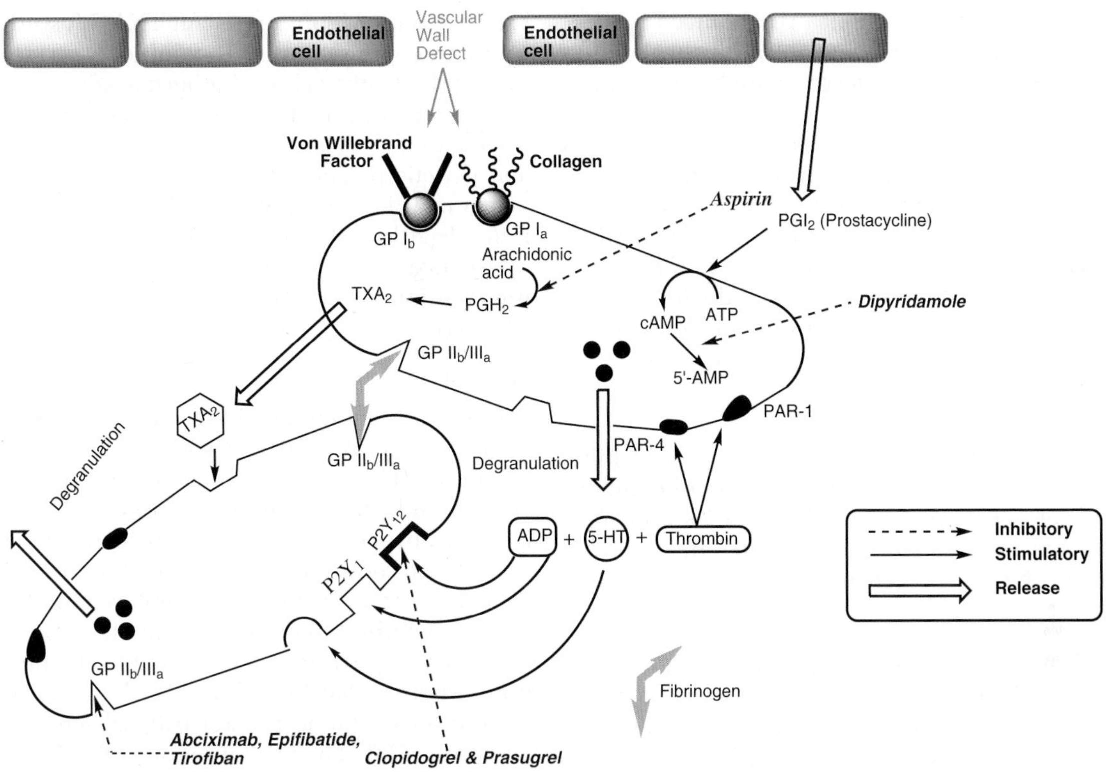

FIGURE 26.15 Scheme describing platelet activation as it relates to blood clot formation. The thrombus is formed at the site of a damaged wall in the vasculature. Normal endothelial cells in the vascular wall provide prostacyclin, which stimulates the conversion of adenosine triphosphate (ATP) to cyclic adenosine monophosphate (cAMP), preventing platelet aggregation. In injury, glycoprotein (GP) receptors bind substances such as von Willebrand factor and collagen, activating the platelet. The $GPII_b/III_a$ receptors cross-link platelets via fibrinogen binding. As the platelet degranulates, additional aggregating substances, including thromboxane A_2 (TXA_2), serotonin (5-HT), and adenosine diphosphate (ADP), are released. ADP, by binding to $P2Y_1$ and $P2Y_{12}$, promotes and sustains platelet aggregation, respectively. Also shown (in *italics*) are drugs and sites of inhibition of platelet aggregation.

to fibrinogen or vWF, thus cross-linking platelets to form aggregates (Fig. 26.15).

The adherent platelets degranulate and release additional aggregating substances, such as thromboxane A_2 (TXA_2), serotonin (5-HT), thrombin, and adenosine diphosphate (ADP). These substances serve as secondary chemical messengers to recruit more platelets to the site of vascular injury and, thereby, amplify platelet aggregation (98,100). For example, thrombin production releases ADP, which is a potent inducer of platelet aggregation and stimulates prostaglandin synthesis from arachidonic acid in the platelet. The prostaglandins synthesized, PGI_2 and TXA_2, have opposite effects on thrombogenesis. PGI_2 is synthesized in the walls of the vasculature and inhibits thrombus formation. Conversely, TXA_2, which is synthesized in the platelets, induces vasoconstriction and thrombogenesis. Serotonin, which also is released from the platelets, has similar and additive effects to those of TXA_2.

This rapid platelet aggregation and thrombus formation at the site of vascular injury is the main mechanism of hemostasis (stoppage of bleeding, a normal process of wound healing). When platelets are activated on the ruptured atherosclerotic plaques or in regions of restricted blood flow, however, it can lead to thromboembolic complications that contribute to common diseases, such as myocardial infarction or ischemic stroke.

Mechanism of Action of Antiplatelet Drugs

Most of the current available antiplatelet drugs, such as aspirin, dipyridamole, and ticlopidine, exert their actions by affecting only the secondary platelet aggregation pathways (97,101). For example, aspirin inhibits the biosynthesis of TXA_2 in the platelets by irreversibly and permanently inactivating cyclooxygenase (COX)-1 through covalent acetylation of a serine residue in close proximity to the active site of the enzyme. A cumulative inactivation effect occurs on platelets with long-term aspirin therapy in doses as low as 30 mg/d (99), because platelets do not synthesize new COX (i.e., platelets are unable to synthesize, via de novo pathway, COX-1, because they are anucleated cells). Therefore, the effects of aspirin last for the lifetime of the platelet (7 to 10 days). Dipyridamole interrupts platelet function through its effect of increasing cellular concentration of cAMP by inhibiting phosphodiesterase, an enzyme needed for degradation of cAMP. Dipyridamole also may stimulate PGI_2 release and inhibits TXA_2 formation. Ticlopidine, clopidogrel, and prasugrel selectively inhibit ADP-induced platelet aggregation with no direct action on prostaglandin production. New and more selective antiplatelet drugs, such as thrombin receptor (or protease-activated receptor-1 [PAR-1]) antagonists, integrin αIIbβ3 receptor antagonists ($GPII_a/III_b$ blockers), thromboxane synthase inhibitor, and TXA_2 receptor antagonists, are currently being developed (7,101). Recent trials with the PAR-1 antagonists have indicated that these agents may provide a better overall platelet inhibition without the liability of increased bleeding when used with aspirin or clopidogrel therapy (100).

COX-1 Inhibitors

Because TXA_2 is a potent vasoconstrictor as well as a labile platelet aggregation inducer, inhibition of production of TXA_2 effectively blocks platelet aggregation. Aspirin and related analogs (Fig. 26.16) exhibit their effectiveness through such a blocking mechanism.

Aspirin

Aspirin is a well-established antiplatelet drug in the treatment of atherothrombotic vascular disease (7,97–99). As stated earlier, aspirin works by its ability to acetylate and irreversibly deactivate platelet COX (COX-1), and its antithrombotic effect remains for the life span of the platelet (7 to 10 days) (Fig. 26.17). Aspirin also has been shown to have other antithrombotic effects that are unrelated to its action on COX-1 (97). These effects include the dose-dependent inhibition of platelet function, the enhancement of fibrinolysis, and the suppression of blood coagulation.

Aspirin is rapidly absorbed in the stomach and quickly degraded by plasma cholinesterases (half-life, 15 to 20 minutes). A once-daily dose of 50 to 100 mg of aspirin, which is much lower than dosages needed for its anti-inflammatory/analgesic actions, is sufficient to completely inactivate platelet COX-1 irreversibly (97,99). Higher doses of aspirin only contribute to its side effects, especially internal bleeding and upper gastrointestinal irritations.

In recent years, the term "aspirin resistance" has been used to denote those situations in which the use of aspirin is unable to protect a patient from thrombotic complications, to cause a prolongation of the bleeding time, or to produce an anticipated effect on one or more in vitro tests of platelet function (97,99,102). One possible explanation for aspirin-resistant TXA_2 biosynthesis is the transient expression of COX-2 in newly formed platelets (103). Many other clinical, pharmacodynamic, biologic, and genetic factors, however, such as tobacco use, drug interaction, alternate pathways for platelet activation, and genetic polymorphism or mutations of the COX-1 gene, may be involved (104). Currently, many questions regarding the biochemical mechanism, diagnosis, prevalence, clinical relevance, and optimal therapeutic intervention for aspirin resistance remain unanswered (97,104).

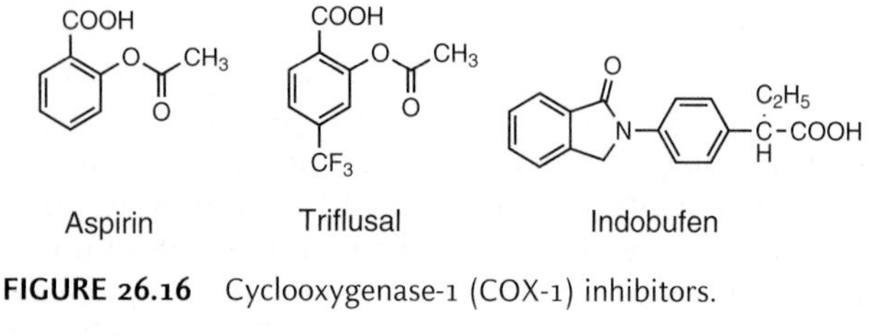

FIGURE 26.16 Cyclooxygenase-1 (COX-1) inhibitors.

Triflusal

Triflusal (2-acetoxy-4-trifluoromethyl benzoic acid) is an antiplatelet drug that despite its structural similarity to aspirin (Fig. 26.16) exhibits quite different pharmacologic and pharmacokinetic properties (105). Unlike aspirin, 2-hydroxy-4-trifluoromethylbenzoic acid (HTB), the deacetylated metabolite of triflusal, retains significant antiplatelet activity. Triflusal is rapidly absorbed and metabolized. The area under the concentration–time curve for triflusal is 20.26 mg/L/h after a 900-mg dose, whereas that for HTB is 42.27 mg/L/h. Much of the pharmacokinetic data for triflusal activity are associated with HTB. The inhibition of COX, as measured by reduced production of thromboxane B_2, is 25% after 2 hours and 85% after 7 days with triflusal, whereas the effect of aspirin on thromboxane B_2 is more than 90% reduction after 2 hours and is maintained at this level after 7 days (106). It would appear that the presence of a 4-trifluoromethyl group also greatly enhances triflusal's ability to inhibit the activation of nuclear factor-κB, which in turn regulates the expression of the mRNA of vascular cell adhesion molecule-1 (107) needed for platelet aggregation. In addition, triflusal increases nitric oxide synthesis in neutrophils, which results in an increased vasodilatory potential (108). Finally, an additional site of action for triflusal/HTB is the inhibition of cAMP phosphodiesterase, leading to increased levels of cAMP. Elevated cAMP levels decrease platelet aggregation through decreased mobilization of calcium. Aspirin and salicylic acid do not significantly increase cAMP levels.

Although recent trials comparing triflusal and aspirin for the prevention of vascular events in patients following a stroke revealed no significant differences between these two antiplatelet drugs, triflusal's use was associated with a significantly lower rate of hemorrhagic complications (105).

Indobufen

Many nonsteroidal anti-inflammatory drugs (NSAIDs) also inhibit TXA_2-dependent platelet function through a competitive, reversible inhibition of COX-1. At a conventional analgesic dosage, these drugs only inhibit COX-1 activity by 70% to 90%, which is inadequate for controlling platelet aggregation. Thus, unlike aspirin, most of

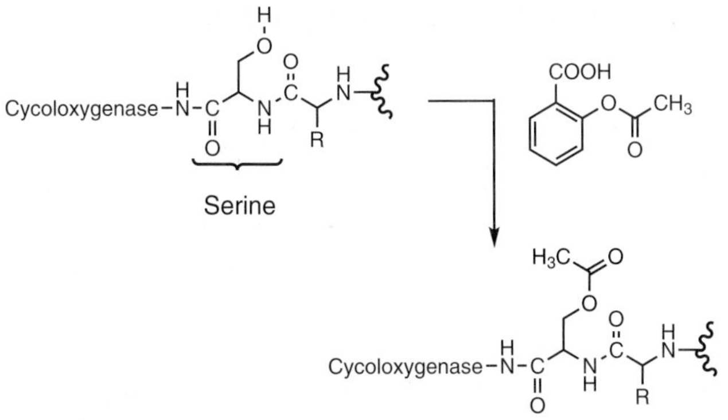

FIGURE 26.17 Irreversible acetylation of serine 530 in cyclooxygenase-1 by aspirin.

the clinically available NSAIDs are not used clinically for their antithrombotic properties.

In contrast, indobufen (Fig. 26.16), a reversible but very potent inhibitor of platelet COX-1 activity, was shown to have comparable clinical efficacy to that of aspirin in prevention of DVT after myocardial infarction and in blocking exercise-induced increase in platelet aggregation (109). In the secondary prevention of thromboembolic events, 100 or 200 mg of indobufen twice daily is as effective as warfarin or aspirin in patients with or without atrial fibrillation (110). Currently, indobufen is only available for routine clinical use in Europe.

Phosphodiesterase Inhibitors

Phosphodiesterase-3 (PDE3) is an enzyme responsible for degradation of cAMP to adenosine monophosphate in platelets and blood vessels. Selective cAMP PDE3 inhibitors, such as dipyridamole and cilostazol (Fig. 26.17), inhibit the degradation of cAMP, thereby increasing cellular concentration of cAMP and leading to inhibition of platelet aggregation and vasodilation (111).

Dipyridamole (Aggrenox)

Dipyridamole is a pyrimidopyrimidine derivative with vasodilatory and antiplatelet properties (Fig. 26.18). Dipyridamole exerts its antiplatelet function by increasing cellular concentrations of cAMP via its inhibition of the degradating enzyme, cyclic nucleotide PDE3. It also blocks adenosine uptake, which acts at A_2 adenosine receptors to stimulate platelet adenyl cyclase. Less common uses for this drug include inhibition of embolization from prosthetic heart valves when used in combination with warfarin (the only currently recommended use) and reduction of thrombosis in patients with thrombotic disease when used in combination with aspirin. Alone, dipyridamole has little, if any, benefit in the treatment of thrombotic conditions (97,112).

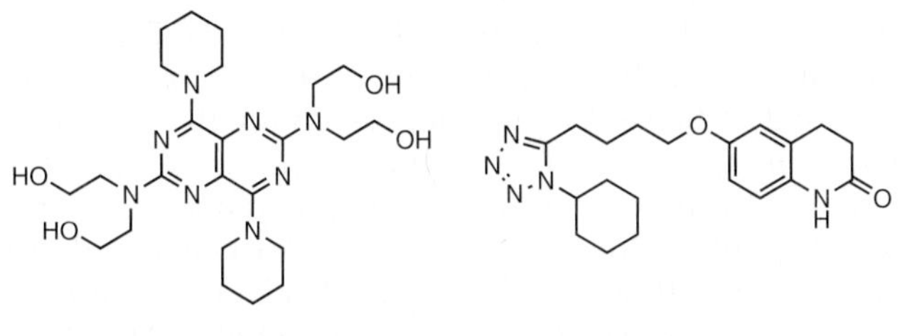

Dipyridamole Cilostazol

FIGURE 26.18 Chemical structures of phosphodiesterase inhibitors.

Cilostazol (Pletal)

Cilostazol, a quinolinone derivative, is a potent orally active antiplatelet drug approved for the treatment of intermittent claudication (a peripheral artery disease resulting from blockage of blood vessels in the limbs). Cilostazol exhibits greater selectivity than dipyridamole as an inhibitor of PDE3A (Fig. 26.19) (112). The drug does not affect the other PDEs (PDEs 1, 2, or 4). Cilostazol reversibly inhibit platelet aggregation induced by a number of stimuli, such as thrombin, ADP, collagen, or stress from exercise (113,114). Additionally, cilostazol inhibits adenosine uptake, leading to increased activity of adenosine at A_1 and A_2 receptors. Adenosine's action on A_2 receptors in platelets increases cAMP levels, which, as previously indicated, leads to decreased platelet aggregation (115).

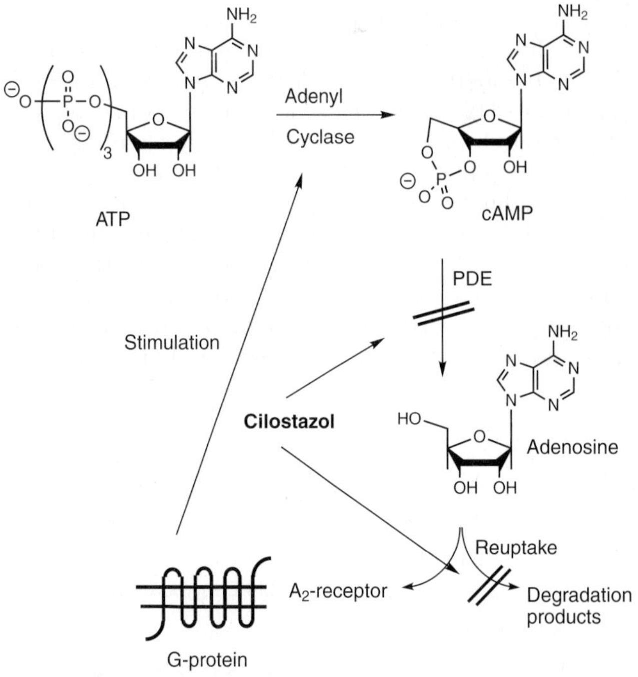

FIGURE 26.19 Sites of action of cilostazol, blocking phosphodiesterase 3A (PDE) and adenosine uptake, leading to increased levels of cyclic adenosine monophosphate (cAMP) directly by inhibition of cAMP breakdown and indirectly through adenosine binding to adenosine 2 receptors (A_2-receptor), which, through G protein coupling, stimulate adenyl cyclase.

Cilostazol is rapidly absorbed after oral administration, particularly with a high-fat meal, which greatly increases its bioavailability to approximately 90%. It is extensively metabolized in the liver by various cytochromes. The most important cytochromes appear to be CYP3A4 and, to lesser extent, CYP2C19, with an elimination half-life of approximately 11 to 13 hours. Among the various metabolites produced (11 metabolites are known), the two major metabolites are 3,4-dehydrocilostazol and 4′-trans-hydroxycliostazol (Fig. 26.20). These two metabolites are pharmacologically active. Studies indicate that the concomitant administration of cilostazol with CYP3A inhibitors can greatly increase cilostazol blood concentrations, and a dose reduction may be required (116). Similar results are seen when CYP2C19 is inhibited, leading to decreased formation of 4-trans-hydroxycliostazol and significant increases in cilostazol and 3,4-dehydrocilostazol (117).

Platelet P2Y Purinergic Receptor

The crucial role that ADP plays in platelet activation and aggregation has been extensively investigated (98,118). The molecular targets of ADP in the platelet are G protein–coupled P2Y purinergic receptors. There are three nucleotide receptors: $P2X_1$, a cation channel receptor activated by ATP, and purinergic receptors $P2Y_1$ and $P2Y_{12}$, both of which are activated by ADP. Initial binding of ADP to the $P2Y_1$ purinergic receptor (373–amino acid protein) induces platelet shape changes, causes intracellular calcium mobilization, and initiates aggregation. Subsequent binding of ADP to the $P2Y_{12}$ purinergic receptors (342 amino acids) leads to sustained platelet aggregation by inhibiting adenylate cyclase and, thereby, decreasing cellular cAMP levels (119). The $P2Y_{12}$ receptor is coupled to the $G\alpha_{i2}$ G protein. The antithrombotic drugs ticlopidine and clopidogrel are irreversible antagonists of this $P2Y_{12}$ purinergic receptor (118,120). The clinical relevance of this $P2Y_{12}$ receptor as a new target for antiplatelet drug development of novel reversible antagonists has been extensively reviewed (120–122).

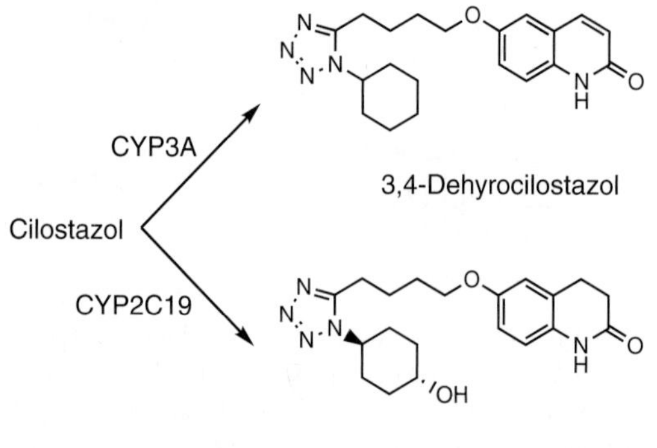

FIGURE 26.20 Metabolism of cilostazol.

Ticlopidine (Ticlid) and Clopidogrel (Plavix)

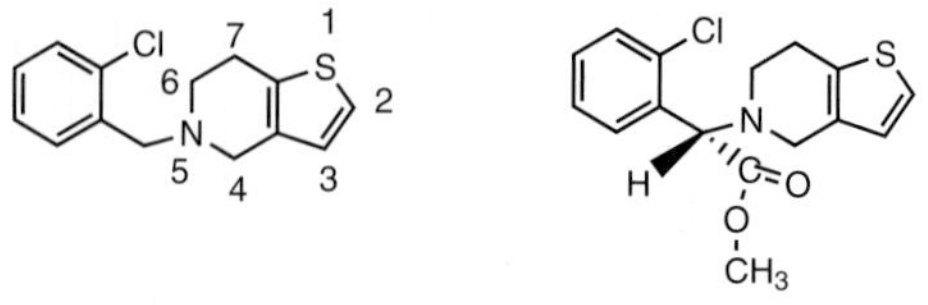

Ticlopidine and clopidogrel are thienopyridines, which through inhibition of platelet aggregation prolong bleeding time and delay clot retraction (97,122). The thienopyridines are prescribed for reduction of myocardial infarction and stroke, for treatment of peripheral arterial disease, and in combination with aspirin for acute coronary syndromes. This latter utility appears to result from the fact that both aspirin and the thienopyridines block major amplification pathways, leading to platelet aggregation and, thus, producing enhanced effectiveness. Ticlopidine has major safety concerns in that in a small population (1% to 2%), neutropenia occurs that is potentially fatal, may cause thrombotic thrombocytopenic purpura, and is largely replaced with clopidogrel. These same side effects are rare with clopidogrel. Additional side effects include diarrhea, nausea, vomiting, and skin rash (123).

The thienopyridine class exhibits selective inhibition of ADP-induced platelet aggregation. The actions of ticlopidine and clopidogrel appear to be irreversible in that there is still antiplatelet activity for 7 to 10 days after discontinuation of the medications (124). Support of the theory of irreversible inhibition of $P2Y_{12}$ is provided by the observation that ticlopidine is not effective in blocking platelet aggregation in vitro when compared to the effect of the drug on the platelets of people taking ticlopidine. The thienopyridines function as prodrugs requiring cytochrome P450 activation. The thienopyridines are rapidly absorbed and extensively metabolized in the liver. The most significant metabolites of clopidogrel are shown in Figure 26.21. An inactive carboxylic acid represents the major circulating metabolite, while activation occurs through oxidation by CYP3A4 (with possible involvement of other cytochrome isoforms) giving rise to the 2-oxo derivative, which in turn is hydrolyzed to the thiol. The thiol binds irreversibly to $P2Y_{12}$ by forming a disulfide bridge to a cysteine in $P2Y_{12}$ (125–127). Specially, clopidogrel is thought to bind to Cys17 or Cys270 and, thus, block the binding of the agonist. In the case of ticlopidine, oxidative activation occurs, but additional metabolites have been identified, dihydrothienopyridinium (M5) and thienodihydropyridinium metabolites (M6). These short-lived metabolites may be responsible for the toxic adverse reactions (128).

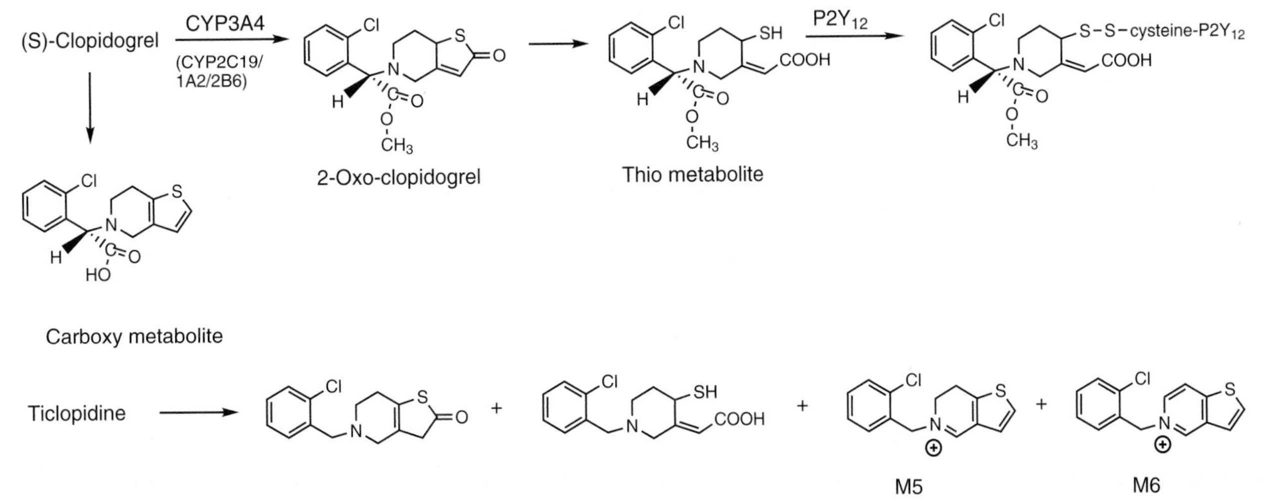

FIGURE 26.21 Metabolism of clopidogrel and ticlopidine. Irreversible reaction of clopidogrel with $P2Y_{12}$ is shown in *red*.

Prasugrel (Effient)

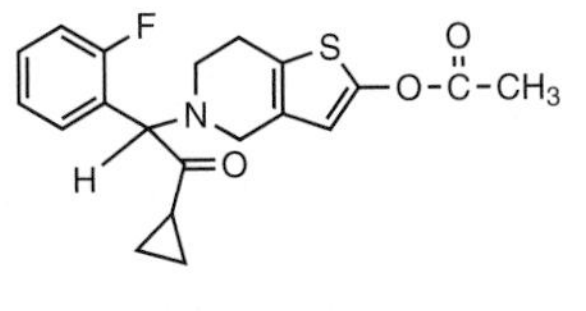

Prasugrel

Prasugrel has recently been approved for treatment of acute coronary syndrome when managed with percutaneous coronary intervention (129–131). The drug has also been shown to reduce the rate of thrombotic cardiovascular events in unstable angina and some forms of myocardial infarction. Prasugrel joins clopidogrel and ticlopidine in the prevention of platelet aggregation.

As with ticlopidine and clopidogrel, prasugrel is a prodrug that, upon activation, serves as an irreversible inhibitor of $P2Y_{12}$ receptors. Unlike the previous agents, prasugrel's activation involves hydrolysis to the thiolactone, which is then hydrolyzed to the thiol intermediate, which is the active metabolite and reacts irreversibly with $P2Y_{12}$ (Fig. 26.22) (122,132–134).

Several reports in the literature suggest a role for various cytochromes in this activation (CYP3A4 and CYP2B6), as is the case with clopidogrel and ticlopidine, but this does not appear to be true with prasugrel. R-138727, the active metabolite of prasugrel, is metabolically inactivated via *S*-methylation. Additional minor metabolites have been isolated, and they may be formed through CYP-catalyzed reactions.

Prasugrel is rapidly absorbed following oral administration, reaching peak plasma concentration of R-138727 within 30 minutes. High-fat diets may slow the time to reach maximum plasma concentration, and it is recommended that the drug be taken on an empty stomach. R-138727 is highly bound to serum albumin (~98%) and is excreted as the inactive metabolite via both the urine (68%) and fecal route (27%).

Prasugrel is commonly used in combination with aspirin and is reported to be more effective than clopidogrel in treatment of unstable angina or myocardial infarction. Prasugrel does have a higher rate of major bleeding and life-threatening bleeding than does clopidogrel (135).

REVERSIBLE P2Y PURINERGIC RECEPTOR INHIBITORS

Even though prasugrel has a faster onset and reduced interpatient variability than clopidogrel, newer agents are still needed because prasugrel works via an irreversible inhibition of $P2Y_{12}$ purinergic receptors and it appears to have a higher rate of bleeding incidences than clopidogrel. Ticagrelor and cangrelor are two reversible inhibitors of the $P2Y_{12}$ purinergic receptors in their advanced stages of development (122,136,137). Ticagrelor is the first oral reversible $P2Y_{12}$ antagonist that has improved pharmacokinetic and pharmacodynamic profiles than currently available drugs for treating acute coronary syndromes (138,139). Cangrelor, on the other hand, is being developed as a short-term, intravenous $P2Y_{12}$ antagonist with a very fast onset and offset, which may provide advantages over current drugs (99,136,140). Recently ticagrelor has been approved by the USFDA for prevention of thrombotic events in patients with acute cornary syndromes.

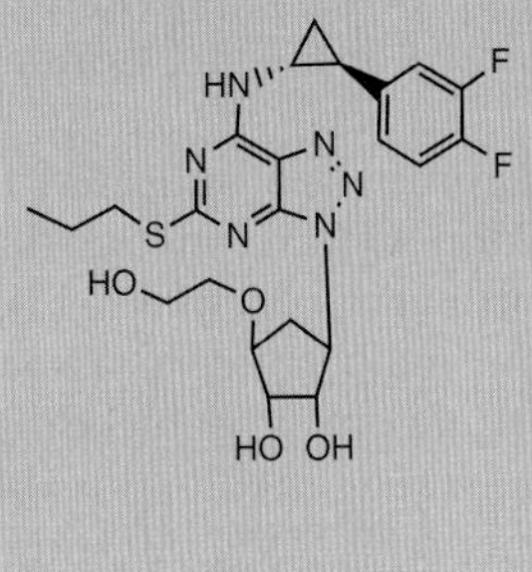

Ticagrelor (Brilinta)

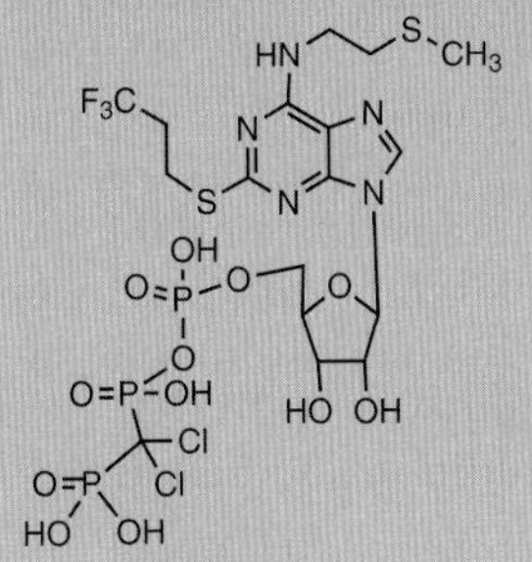

Cangrelor

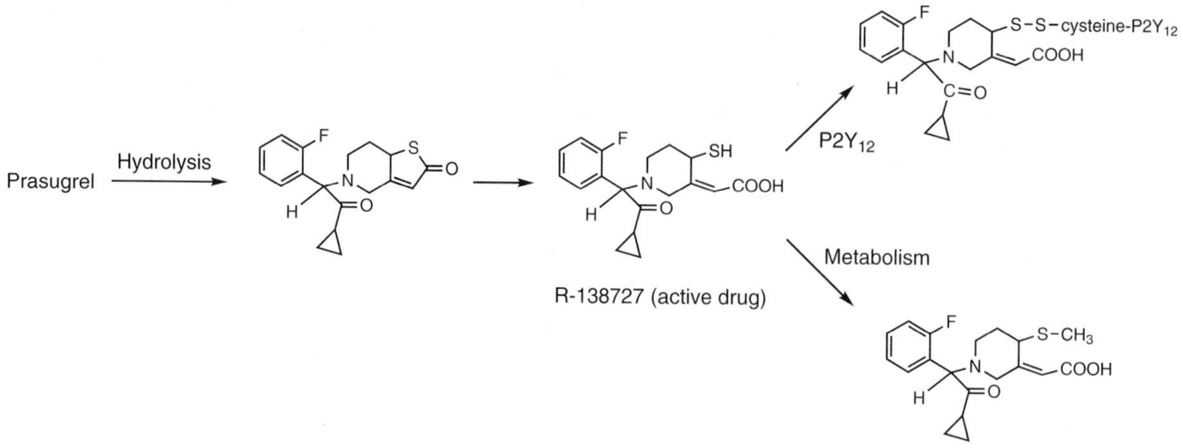

FIGURE 26.22 Activation of prasugrel to R-128727 followed by irreversible binding to P2Y_{12} or metabolic methylation to inactive metabolite.

Glycoprotein II_b/III_a Receptor Antagonists

One of the newest groups of antithrombotic agents is the platelet receptor $GPII_b/III_a$ antagonists (97,145,146). This novel class of compounds has been shown to provide more comprehensive inhibition of platelet aggregation than the usual combination of aspirin and heparin (140). The final common pathway in platelet aggregation is the expression of functional $GPII_b/III_a$ (integrin αIIbβ3) receptors. These protein receptors are expressed regardless of the origin of the stimulus initiating the clotting cascade. The normal substrate for the $GPII_b/III_a$ receptor is fibrinogen. One fibrinogen molecule acts to cross-link two platelets via binding to the $GPII_b/III_a$ receptors on the platelet surfaces (Fig. 26.15). If the platelet surface receptors are occupied by another substrate that prevents fibrinogen binding and cross-linking, platelet aggregation will not occur. To this end, a number of novel compounds representing diverse structural groups have been prepared as $GPII_b/III_a$ receptor antagonists (Fig. 26.23) (147,148). Included in this list of antagonists are monoclonal antibodies against the natural $GPII_b/III_a$ receptor, naturally occurring peptides isolated from snake venom that contain the Arg-Gly-Asp (RGD) sequence, synthetic peptides containing either the RGD or Lys-Gly-Asp (KGD) sequences, and peptidomimetic and nonpeptide RGD mimetics that compete with fibrinogen and other ligands for occupancy of the receptor (97). The natural binding ligands, such as vWF and fibronectin, contain the natural RGD sequence.

The $GPII_b/III_a$ receptor antagonists are indicated in therapy for unstable angina, non–Q-wave myocardial infarction, and percutaneous coronary procedures. Like other antithrombotic agents, the main concern associated with $GPII_b/III_a$ receptor antagonists is bleeding. Additionally, these drugs have been suggested to possibly increase the risk of thrombocytopenia (97,149). Although a number of orally active $GPII_b/III_a$ receptor antagonists have been prepared and evaluated, their clinical efficacy in acute treatment of patients with unstable angina and in those undergoing angioplasty has not been fully established (147).

Abciximab (ReoPro)

The initial antibodies against the $GPII_b/III_a$ receptor were murine in origin. Because of concerns about the antigenicity of a pure murine antibody, a chimeric human–mouse 7E3 Fab was developed (150,151). This chimera, marketed as abciximab, is the clinically available form of the antibody that is widely studied in patients undergoing percutaneous coronary intervention (151). For an adult patient, the usual dosing scheme is 0.25 mg/kg as an intravenous bolus given 10 to 60 min before percutaneous coronary intervention, followed by the continuous infusion of 0.125 μg/kg/minute for 12 hours to a maximum of 10 μg/kg. Elimination of abciximab is biphasic. The initial phase has a half-life of 10 minutes, whereas the half-life of the second phase is approximately 30 minutes and results from platelet binding. Platelet function returns to normal within 48 hours after infusion, even though abciximab is bound to circulating platelets for approximately 2 weeks (Table 26.5) (152,153).

Eptifibatide (Integrilin)

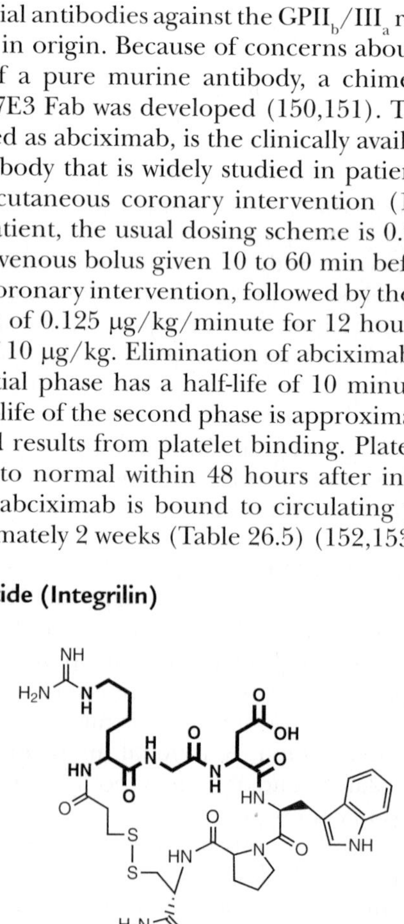

Eptifibatide (red indicates KGD portion of drug)

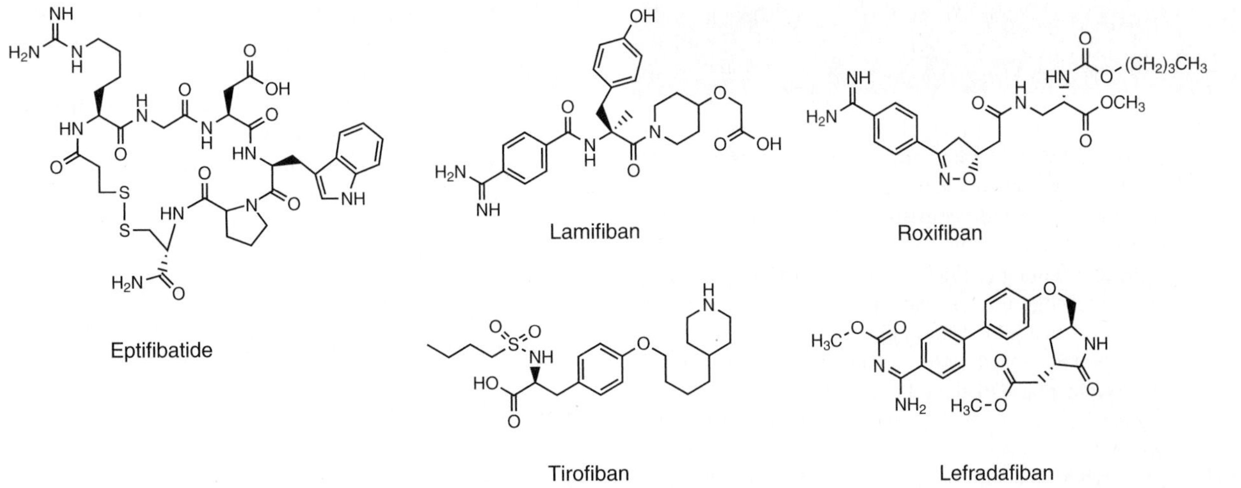

FIGURE 26.23 Structures of selected glycoprotein (GP) II_b/III_a receptor agonists.

Eptifibatide is a cyclic heptapeptide composed of six amino acids and one mercaptopropionyl residue. The cyclization is completed via a disulfide linkage between the cysteine and the mercaptopropionyl moieties. The lysine-glycine-aspartate component of eptifibatide is highly specific for the $GPII_b/III_a$ receptor, with low binding affinity, as indicated by the rapid dissociation constant (Table 26.5). Because of this, eptifibatide is a reversible, parenterally administered antagonist of platelet aggregation.

The drug is eliminated primarily via renal mechanisms as eptifibatide and deaminated eptifibatide. The clinical importance of eptifibatide and its benefits in comparison with other therapeutic agents used in the treatment of acute coronary syndromes and percutaneous coronary intervention have recently been reviewed by Curran and Keating (154).

Tirofiban (Aggrastat)

Tirofiban is a member of a new class of antithrombotic agents known as the "fibans" (Fig. 26.23). These compounds have a structural similarity to disintegrin, which was originally isolated from snake venoms. The location of the $-COO^-$ and NH_3^+ in the fibans is identical to the distance between the same functional groups of the RGD loop of disintegrin, and as a result, the fibans are able to effectively block the binding of fibrinogen to the $GPII_b/III_a$ receptor in a reversible manor. Tirofiban, like eptifibatide, has a rapid dissociation constant (Table 26.5). Tirofiban is a peptidomimetic (nonpeptide) that is parenterally administered and exhibits a reduced risk of bleeding because of its shorter biologic half-life than abciximab (155). Additionally, it is less costly than other $GPII_b/III_a$ receptor antagonists. The clinical use of tirofiban in ST elevation for myocardial infarction is effective and has an acceptable safety profile (155,156). The remaining fibans shown in Figure 26.23 are in various stages of development. Lamifiban is administered parenterally, whereas roxifiban and lefradafiban are used orally.

New Developments in Antiplatelet Drugs

Several newer approaches to antiplatelet drug development have been recently discovered (157). These include inhibitions of the vWF/GPI_b interaction, the platelet/collagen interaction, and the thrombin-induced platelet activation. Other approaches to platelet inhibition include the use of serotonin antagonists (because serotonin induces platelet aggregation), nitric oxide–donating antiplatelet agents, phosphodiesterase inhibitors, and inducers of adenyl cyclase.

TABLE 26.5 Pharmacokinetic Properties of the Glycoprotein IIb/IIIa Receptor Antagonists

Drug	Trade Name	Molecular Weight (daltons)	Dissociation Constant (nmol/L)	Plasma Half-Life (h)	Protein Binding (%)
Abciximab	ReoPro	47,615	5	72	
Eptifibatide	Integrelin	800	120	4	25
Tirofiban	Aggrastat	495	15	3–4	65

PAR-1 ANTAGONISTS

Despite the effectiveness of aspirin, clopidogrel, and other newer $P2Y_{12}$ antagonists for the treatment and prevention of atherothrombotic events in patients with acute coronary syndrome, myocardial infarction, and other existing peripheral arterial diseases, the risk of bleeding events, potential drug resistance, and other factors contributing to the interpatient variability remain a therapeutic challenge in these patients (99). Two novel oral antiplatelet agents that inhibit thrombin-mediated platelet activation via G protein–linked PAR-1 antagonists have recently advanced to pivotal phase III clinical trials (100,101,141).

Vorapaxar is a potent, highly selective, himbacined-based PAR-1 antagonist that has greater than 90% oral bioavailability and is well tolerated in patients undergoing nonurgent percutaneous coronary intervention (141,142). It binds competitively with high affinity (K_i = ~8 nmol/L) yet in a slowly reversible manner to PAR-1 (142). Vorapaxar is primarily metabolized and eliminated via biliary and gastrointestinal routes by CYP3A4 isozymes at a very slow rate (141). Preliminary clinical trial data further indicate that vorapaxar, unlike prasugrel, improves ischemic outcomes without significantly increasing the bleeding liability (99–101).

Another PAR-1 antagonist that has demonstrated similar antiplatelet effects without increasing bleeding times is E-5555 (143). Interestingly, E-5555 also inhibits thrombin-induced release of interleukin-6 (half maximal inhibitory concentration [IC_{50}] = 0.19 nmol/L) and P-selectin expression (IC_{50} = 16 nmol/L) in human coronary artery smooth muscles, thereby preventing vascular spasm in an animal model studies (144).

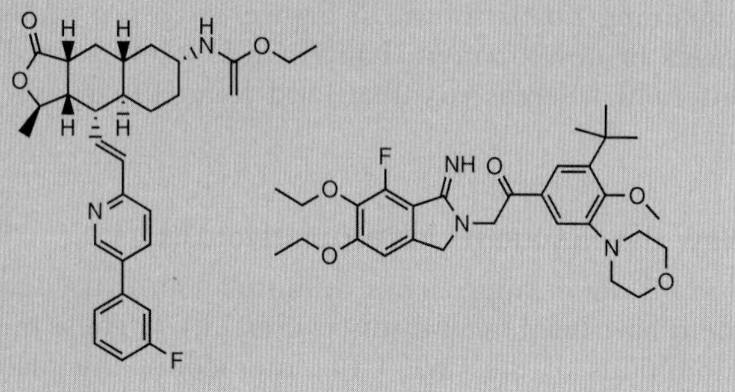

Vorapaxar E-5555

Specific inhibitors of thromboxane synthase have been tested for their ability to block this enzyme without inhibiting the entire arachidonic acid cascade (99,158). This allows an accumulation of prostaglandin G_2 and prostaglandin H_2, which can then be channeled into an increased production of PGI_2, which also has antithrombotic activity.

THROMBOLYTIC DRUGS

Early application of reperfusion therapy with thrombolytic agents has significantly improved the outcomes of acute myocardial infarction and other conditions, such as PE, DVT, arterial thrombosis, acute thrombosis of retinal vessel, extensive coronary emboli, and peripheral vascular thromboembolism (159).

Although, the beneficial effect of the thrombolytic drugs, such as streptokinase and urokinase, for dissolving newly formed thrombus in patients with acute myocardial infarction were first reported in 1958, their full acceptance into clinical practice was not realized until the early 1980s as a result of several prospective, randomized, controlled trials. Today, with the approval of many second- and third-generation thrombolytic drugs, thrombolytic therapy has become a standard treatment for patients presenting with acute myocardial infarction or stroke (159,160).

Mechanism of Action

Normally, newly formed blood clots (fibrin) are dissolved by the actions of the fibrinolytic system, the purpose of which is the removal of unwanted clots without damaging the integrity of the vascular system. This system works via a relatively nonspecific protease enzyme called plasmin, the function of which is to digest fibrin (the very last step of the coagulation cascade) (Fig. 26.1). The lack of substrate specificity of plasmin is illustrated by the fact that it degrades fibrin clots as well as some plasma proteins and coagulation factors.

The fibrinolytically active plasmin is produced from the circulating inactive "proenzyme" plasminogen following the cleavage of a single peptide bond by a group of trypsin-like serine proteases known as the plasminogen activators. The principal activator, tissue-type plasminogen activator (tPA), is released from the vascular endothelium. Thrombolytic drugs, such as streptokinase and urokinase, act like a plasminogen activator that converts this proenzyme to the active plasmin. Endogenously, plasmin activity is regulated by two specific inactivators known as tPA inhibitors 1 and 2.

SNAKE VENOM–INDUCED COAGULOPATHY

The venom of snakes of the Crotalinae family, which includes rattlesnakes, produces a state of impaired coagulation. This can lead to both local and systemic hemorrhagic events. Venom consists of many components, including phospholipases and hemolysins, which cause cell lysis by disrupting platelet and red blood cell membranes. The venoms also contain procoagulant components that induce the formation of intravascular clots as well as hemorrhagins that destroy vascular integrity. Typically, both PT and aPTT are elevated with total fibrin levels being lowered and fibrin degradation products being increased. All of the findings are consistent with a consumptive coagulopathy. Because of the multiple mechanisms affecting coagulation, coagulopathies caused by snake venom are best managed using antivenin.

First-Generation Thrombolytic Agents

Streptokinase (Streptase)

Streptokinase, an exocellular protein produced by several strains of β-hemolytic streptococci, is a drug of choice for thrombolytic therapy based on its cost-effectiveness consideration, and it is the only thrombolytic drug approved by the FDA for peripheral vascular disease (161). The drug is approved for treatment of myocardial infarction but rarely is used for this condition today, having been replaced with the fibrin-specific agents discussed below (162).

Mechanism of Action Streptokinase is a protein purified from culture broths of group C β-hemolytic streptococci bacteria. Streptokinase contains a single polypeptide chain of 414–amino acid residues with a molecular weight of 47 kd (161). Streptokinase by itself has no intrinsic enzymatic activity. To be active, it must bind with plasminogen to form an activator complex (1:1 complex). This complex then acts to convert uncomplexed plasminogen to the active fibrinolytic enzyme, plasmin. The streptokinase/plasminogen complex not only degrades fibrin clots but also catalyzes the breakdown of fibrinogen and factors V and VII (159,161). As a result, streptokinase is considered to be a fibrin-nonspecific drug.

Pharmacokinetics Unfortunately, the half-life of the activator complex is less than 30 minutes, which frequently is too short to completely lyse a thrombus. Anistreplase (APSAC; Eminase) is a 1:1 streptokinase/lysine-plasminogen complex that has been acylated with an anisoyl group at the active-site serine within the lysine-plasminogen. Anistreplase is inactive as such, but following complexation with fibrin, the anisoyl group is slowly cleaved, exposing the active site and, thus, leading to degradation of fibrin. The prodrug nature of anistreplase exhibits an improved pharmacokinetic profile, with anistreplase acting as a semiselective lysis agent at the clot site. The inactivity of the circulating anistreplase also allows this drug to be given as a very rapid intravenous infusion (typically, 30 U over 3 to 5 minutes). Tissue reperfusion following anistreplase therapy compares favorably to streptokinase because of the extended half-life (90 minutes).

Side Effects Because it is a foreign protein, streptokinase is associated with significant hypersensitivity reactions. Most people have, at some point in their lives, had a streptococcal infection and, therefore, have developed circulating antistreptococcal antibodies. These antibodies frequently are active against streptokinase as well. The response of the streptokinase to these antibodies can vary widely, from inactivation of the fibrinolytic properties of the protein to rash, fever, and rarely, anaphylaxis. Significant allergic reactions to streptokinase occur in approximately 3% of patients.

Urokinase (Abbokinase)

Urokinase is an enzyme with the ability to directly degrade fibrin and fibrinogen. It is now isolated from cultures of human fetal kidney cells and is composed of two polypeptide chains with molecular weights of 32 and 54 kd. This method of isolation is much more efficient than the original isolation of urokinase from human urine (163). Because of its source, the human body does not see urokinase as a foreign protein. Therefore, it lacks the antigenicity associated with streptokinase and frequently is used for patients with a known hypersensitivity to streptokinase (164). Plasmin cannot be used directly because of the presence of naturally occurring plasmin antagonists in plasma. No such inhibitors of urokinase exist in the plasma, however, allowing this enzyme to have clinical utility. Even so, urokinase is much more expensive (threefold the price of streptokinase) and has an even shorter half-life (15 minutes). Urokinase also has other fibrin-nonspecific actions similar to streptokinase.

Currently, urokinase is only approved for treatment of PE.

Second-Generation Thrombolytic Agents

Alteplase (Activase)

Alteplase (tPA) is a serine protease with a low affinity for free plasminogen but a very high affinity for the plasminogen bound to fibrin in a thrombus (fibrin-specific agent) (Fig. 26.24). Both streptokinase and urokinase lack this specificity (i.e., are nonspecific) and act on free plasminogen, inducing a generalized thrombolytic state. Alteplase also has a greater specificity for older clots compared with newer clots relative to streptokinase and urokinase. Alteplase was originally isolated from cultures of human melanoma cells but is now produced commercially using recombinant DNA technology. Alteplase is unmodified human tPA, whereas reteplase (see below) is human tPA that has had several specific amino acid sequences removed (165). At low doses, alteplase is quite selective for degrading fibrin without concomitant lysis of other proteins, such as fibrinogen. At the higher doses currently used therapeutically, however, alteplase activates free plasminogen to some extent and, therefore, can cause hemorrhage. Many of the therapeutic indications for the other thrombolytic agents also are indications for alteplase (i.e., myocardial infarction, massive PE, and acute ischemic stroke). The half-life of alteplase is very short (~5 minutes), necessitating its administration as a 15-mg intravenous bolus, followed by a 85-mg intravenous infusion over 90 minutes, or as 60 mg infused over the first hour, with the remaining 40 mg given at a rate of 20 mg/h.

Prourokinase (scuPA, r-ProUK)

Prourokinase is a single-chain, urokinase-like plasminogen activator of 411 amino acids that displays clot-lysis activity yet does not interfere with hemostasis (166). It is nonimmunogenic and has a more favorable dose-related safety and efficacy profile than both urokinase and streptokinase. Thus, it is a potentially useful thrombolytic drug in the treatment of peripheral vascular occlusion (167).

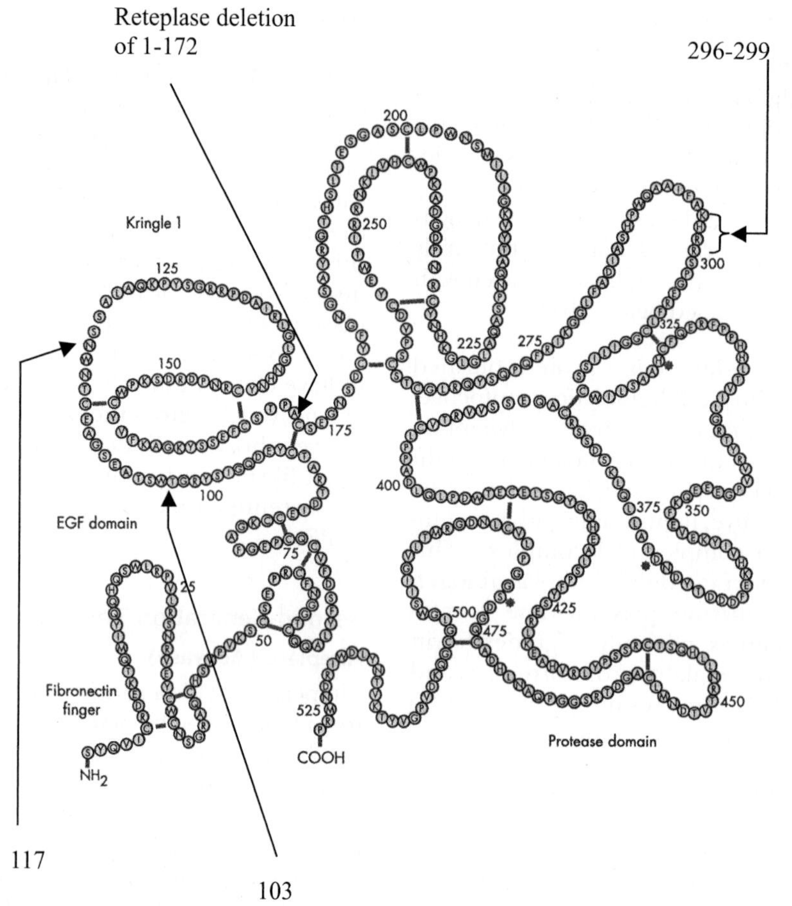

FIGURE 26.24 Schematic diagram of alteplase, reteplase (removal of amino acids 1 to 172), and tenecteplase in which threonine (T) at position 103 is replaced with asparagines, asparagine (N) at position 117 is replaced with glutamine, and lysine (K)-histidine-arginine-asparagine at positions 296 to 299 are replaced with four alanines. (Adapted with permission from Nordt TK, Bode C. Thrombolysis: newer thrombolytic agents and their role in clinical medicine. Heart 2003;89:1358–1362.)

Third-Generation Thrombolytic Agents

Many third-generation thrombolytic agents currently are under clinical trials. These agents are derived from structural modifications of the basic plasminogen activators (tPA or other tPA of animal origins) using technologies such as mutations, conjugation with monoclonal antibodies, or hybridization with another thrombolytic agent. Some of these agents are amediplase (hybrid of tPA and prourokinase), lanoteplase (mutant tPA), and staphylokinase (from bacterial tPA) (160).

Reteplase (Retavase)

Reteplase is a recombinant deletion mutant of tPA lacking the finger, epidermal growth factor, kringle 1 domain, and carbohydrate side chain (Fig. 26.24) (168). As a highly fibrin-specific thrombolytic agent, reteplase is missing the first 172 amino acids that are present in alteplase and has 355 amino acids with a molecular weight of 39 kd. Because of the removal of the finger kringle 1 domain, reteplase binding to fibrin is reduced from that of alteplase, and reteplase has reduced fibrin selectivity. In addition, the structural modification reduces hepatic elimination, leading to a longer half-life (reteplase, 14 to 18 minutes; alteplase, 3 to 4 minutes).

Administered as a double bolus of 10 U every 30 minutes, reteplase is approved for use in acute myocardial infarction.

Tenecteplase (TNKase)

Tenecteplase is composed of 527 amino acids with 17 disulfide bridges. It differs structurally from alteplase by three point mutations (Fig. 26.24). The mutations were bioengineered to occur at amino acid 103, where threonine (T) is replaced by asparagine; at amino acid 117, where asparagine (N) is replaced by glutamine; and at amino acids 296 to 299, where lysine (K)-histidine-arginine-arginine are replaced with four alanines. Thus, the name TNK is derived from the mutations. The replacement of these amino acids along with their attached carbohydrate side chains results in a prolonged half-life (~17 minutes) and allows a single bolus application (168). These point-mutation changes also change the binding of tenecteplase to plasminogen activator inhibitor-1 (PAI-1) by 80-fold, thus improving activity. A physiologic enzyme, PAI-1 inhibits fibrinolysis. Finally, tenecteplase shows a 15-fold higher fibrin specificity. The drug is still eliminated via hepatic mechanisms.

TOXICITY OF ANTITHROMBOTICS AND THROMBOLYTICS

Antithrombotic Toxicity

Recall that warfarin exhibits its anticoagulation effects by preventing γ-carboxylation of specific glutamate residues necessary for vitamin K–dependent coagulation (Fig. 26.4). However, γ-carboxyglutamate proteins are not unique to coagulation factors. These types of proteins are synthesized in bone as well. As would be expected, warfarin also interferes with the carboxylation of these proteins, resulting in an inhibition of the effects of vitamin K on osteoblast development. It has been suggested that this is the mechanism responsible for bone abnormalities in neonates born to mothers who were treated with warfarin while pregnant (169). No evidence suggests that bone metabolism or development is affected by warfarin when the drug is administered to children or adults. Because of the mechanism of action of the warfarin-like drugs, the management of their toxicity is based largely on vitamin K therapy (see "Coagulants," later in this chapter).

Unlike warfarin, heparin is safe for anticoagulant therapy during pregnancy (169). Although warfarin is known to cause serious fetal malformations when used in pregnancy, heparin does not cross the placental barrier and has shown no tendency to induce fetal damage. Furthermore, heparin does not increase fetal mortality or prematurity. To minimize the risk of postpartum hemorrhage, it is recommended that heparin therapy be withdrawn 24 hours before delivery.

Despite its safety in pregnancy, several potential problems are associated with heparin therapy. Because heparins (high molecular weight heparins and LMWHs) are isolated from animal sources, the chance of antigenic hypersensitivity exists but is rarely observed. Heparin competitively binds many other plasma proteins (i.e., vitronectin and PF4) in addition to the antithrombin, resulting in inactivation of the heparin as an anticoagulant (44). This may be the reason for heparin resistance and for a serious condition known as HIT. Typically, this condition occurs 7 to 14 days after initiation of heparin therapy, but it may occur earlier in some patients who have had previous exposures to heparin. In these cases, heparin-induced platelet aggregation occurs and may result in the production of antiplatelet antibodies. Development of this condition necessitates termination of heparin therapy and institution of antiplatelet drugs or oral anticoagulants. On withdrawal of heparin, the thrombocytopenia usually is reversible. Mild increases in liver function tests frequently are associated with heparin therapy. Long-term use of full therapeutic doses of heparin (>20,000 U/d for 3 to 6 months) has been associated with osteoporosis, and spontaneous vertebral fractures have been infrequently reported (44).

Hemorrhagic complications of heparin therapy are managed, in part, with the specific antagonist protamine sulfate (44). This agent is discussed in greater detail in the "Coagulants" section of this chapter.

The structural and mechanistic diversity of the antiplatelet drugs disallows a cohesive description of their toxicities. Hemorrhage is certainly a concern, but other, more drug-specific toxicities may be of greater immediate concern. It is suggested that toxicity information for antiplatelet medications be obtained from appropriate references for the specific agent in question and from the most recent reviews of antiplatelet agents (97,99).

Thrombolytic Toxicities

As discussed earlier, plasmin, because of its lack of specificity, not only digests fibrin but also degrades many other plasma proteins, including several coagulation factors and the anticoagulating factor, activated protein C. Thus, as expected, most thrombolytic drugs not only attack pathologic clots but also exert their actions on any other site of compromised vascular integrity. The dissolution of necessary clots results in the principal side effect of thrombolytic therapy, hemorrhage. Its action on the activated protein C also may be responsible for their neurovascular toxicities (170).

Multiple studies have examined the incidence of life-threatening hemorrhage (i.e., intracranial hemorrhage) with the various thrombolytic medications. These studies indicate that the rate of significant hemorrhagic complication is essentially the same (0.1% to 0.7%) regardless of the specific therapeutic agent used. Supportive care is indicated in cases of thrombolytic toxicity. No specific antagonist exists to manage thrombolytic medication-induced hemorrhage, but antifibrinolytic drugs, such as aminocaproic acid and tranexamic acid, often are used. These compounds are described in detail in the following "Coagulants" section of this chapter.

COAGULANTS

A variety of pathologic and toxicologic conditions can result in excessive bleeding from inadequate coagulation. Depending on the etiology and severity of the hemorrhagic episode, several possible blood coagulation inducers can be therapeutically employed.

Vitamin K

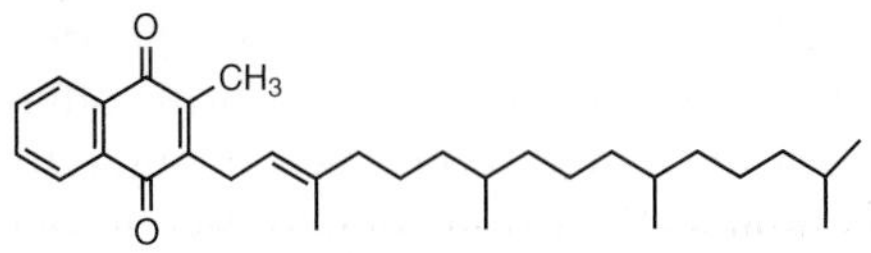

Vitamin K_1

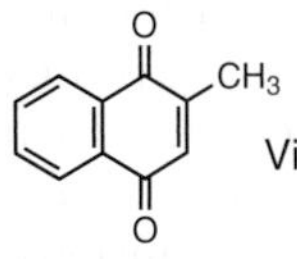

Vitamin K_3

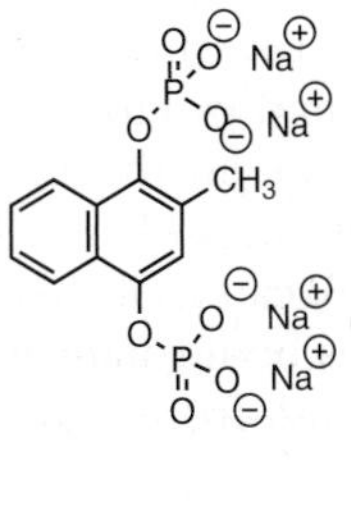

Vitamin K_4

Because the orally active anticoagulants, such as warfarin and the indandiones, act through interruption of the normal actions of vitamin K, it stands to reason that vitamin K should be effective in the treatment of bleeding induced by these agents (157). Vitamin K_1 (phytonadione, Mephyton) is the form of vitamin K most often used therapeutically. Vitamin K_1 is safe for use in infants, pregnant women, and patients with glucose-6-phosphate deficiency. Furthermore, phytonadione, being more lipid soluble, has a faster onset than other vitamin K preparations and requires smaller doses than vitamin K_3 (menadione) or vitamin K_4 (menadiol sodium diphosphate). Both vitamins K_3 and K_4 may produce hyperbilirubinemia and kernicterus in neonates as well as hemolysis in neonates and glucose-6-phosphate–deficient patients. In fact, the only advantage of vitamins K_3 and K_4 over vitamin K_1 is that whereas absorption of vitamin K_1 requires the presence of bile, absorption of vitamins K_3 and K_4 does not, because they are absorbed via a passive process directly from the intestine (157). This may be a slight advantage for patients with cholestasis or severe pancreatic dysfunction. Only vitamin K_1, however, is appropriate therapy for bleeding associated with warfarin and superwarfarin anticoagulation. Vitamin K_2 is not used therapeutically.

Vitamin K_1 is effective at inducing coagulation when administered orally, subcutaneously, intramuscularly, or intravenously. Although the oral route is preferred, it is not always practical in a patient who is critically hemorrhaging. The other routes of administration, though used clinically, all have significant potential drawbacks. Larger doses (e.g., volume >5 mL) are not appropriate for subcutaneous administration, and intramuscular injection generally is avoided in patients who are at risk for significant hematoma formation (e.g., hemophiliacs). Intravenous dosing of vitamin K has been associated with severe anaphylactoid reactions (including death) presumably secondary to colloidal formulation.

The half-life of vitamin K_1 is quite short—only 1.7 hours via the intravenous route and 3 to 5 hours via the oral route. When given orally, vitamin K_1 is absorbed directly from the proximal small intestine in an energy-dependent and saturable process that requires the presence of bile salts. These kinetic features argue for administration in divided doses rather than larger, single daily doses. The typical starting point for adults with drug-induced hypoprothrombinemia is 2.5 to 10 mg of vitamin K_1 orally, repeating in 12 to 48 hours if needed. In cases of ingestion of long-acting superwarfarin rodenticides (e.g., brodifacoum), therapy may be 125 mg/d for weeks or months. Practically speaking, because vitamin K_1 is dispensed as 5-mg tablets, superwarfarin-poisoned patients may require 10 to 30 tablets every 6 hours.

Because of the short half-life of vitamin K_1, dosing must be repeated two to four times per day for the duration of treatment. Furthermore, regardless of the route of administration, coagulant effects are not evident for up to 24 hours. Because of this delay in onset, severe acute hemorrhage is better managed initially with intravenous infusion of fresh-frozen plasma, followed by vitamin K therapy.

Protamine

Mechanism of Action

Protamine sulfate has been approved in the United States as a specific antagonist to heparin since 1968 (169). Protamines are an arginine-rich, highly basic group of simple proteins derived from salmon sperm. The highly acidic heparin polysaccharides exhibit their anticoagulant activity through binding to antithrombin III. Because of the basicity of protamine, heparin has an increased affinity for protamine relative to antithrombin III. In fact, its binding affinity for protamine is so much greater than that of antithrombin III that protamine actually will induce dissociation of the heparin/antithrombin III complex. If protamine is administered in the absence of heparin, it can have marked effects on coagulation. Protamine is not completely selective for heparin and, in vivo, also interacts with fibrinogen, platelets, and other plasma proteins causing anticoagulation. For this reason, the minimal amount of protamine necessary to antagonize heparin-associated bleeding should be used (usually 1 mg of protamine intravenously for every 100 U of heparin remaining in the patient).

Side Effects

Anaphylaxis also has been associated with the use of protamine. Although development of protamine anaphylaxis is not limited to diabetics, those patients with diabetes who have used protamine-containing insulin (NPH or protamine zinc) do have a slightly increased risk of anaphylaxis. Some less common reactions to protamine include pulmonary vasoconstriction, hypotension, and thrombus formation.

Thrombopoietin Receptor Agonists

Chronic idiopathic thrombocytopenia purpura (ITP), unlike HIT, is an autoimmune disorder characterized by persistent thrombocytopenia that involves antibody-mediated platelet destruction and decreased platelet production leading to life-threatening bleeding (171,172). The disease is characterized by platelet counts of less than 30,000 platelets/μL (normal platelet count, ~150,000 to 450,000 platelets/μL). Successful treatment is indicated by platelet counts of 200,000 platelets/μL. The diagnosis and management of this autoimmune disorder is a challenge to clinicians because the pathophysiology of ITP is not completely understood (171,173). Recent evidence supports the coexistence of antibody-induced megakaryocyte abnormalities that impair proliferation and differentiation of megakaryocytes, decreased proplatelet formation, and subsequent platelet release in ITP patients (173).

Romiplostim and eltrombopag are two thrombopoietin receptor agonists that have recently been approved for the short-term treatment of thrombocytopenia in patients with chronic ITP (174,175). These drugs work by binding to the transmembrane domain of the human thrombopoietin receptor (c-Mpl) on the platelet surface as well as megakaryocytes and megakaryocyte precursor cells, thereby activating a number of signaling pathways, including tyrosine phosphorylation of c-Mpl, Janus kinase 2, and signal transduction and activation of transcription, which results in an increase in the synthesis of new platelets (174,176).

Romiplostim (Nplate)

Romiplostim is an Fc-peptide fusion protein analog of thrombopoietin with a molecular weight of 59 kd that is administered subcutaneously in a dose range of 3 to 15 μg/kg/wk, based on the patient's platelet count (174,177). It was approved in 2003 by the FDA as an orphan drug and subsequently in 2008 for long-term treatment of adult chronic ITP, especially in relapsed postsplenectomy patients (177). Romiplostim is generally well tolerated with many major adverse events that could be attributed to the drug (178). The serum half-life of romiplostim ranges from 1 to 34 days (median, 3.5 days) following subcutaneous injection.

Eltrombopag (Promacta)

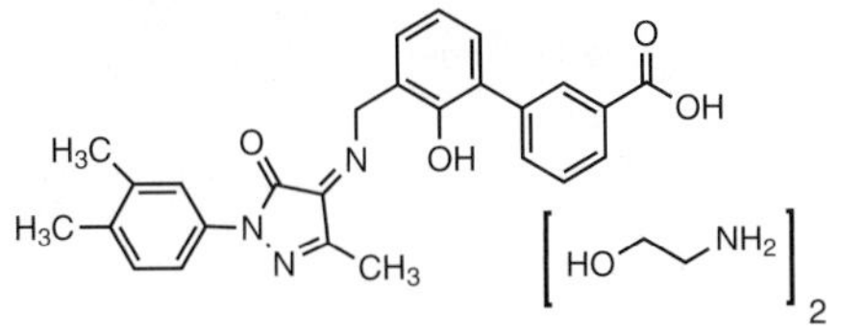

Eltrombopag

Eltrombopag has been approved for the treatment of thrombocytopenia in patients with chronic immune ITP. It is the first orally active low molecular weight agent approved in 2008 (175,179).

Eltrombopag is rapidly absorbed, reaching maximum plasma concentrations in 3 to 6 hours, and is highly bound to plasma protein (~99%). Coadministration of eltrombopag with heavy metals found in antacids results in reduced (~70%) systemic exposure, whereas the fat content of food does not affect eltrombopag absorption. The drug should be administered on an empty stomach. Eltrombopag is metabolized in the liver, although only minor CYP-catalyzed oxidation is reported, and some glucuronidation also occurs. The half-life of eltrombopag is approximately 26 to 35 hours, with elimination occurring through the feces (~59%) and urine (~31%). Systemic exposure to eltrombopag is reported to be increased in individuals of East Asian decent, and the initial dose should be decreased in these patients.

Eltrombopag is reported to cause hepatotoxicity, and patients must have liver function tests done every 2 weeks during initial drug therapy and monthly after establishment of a maintenance dose. The drug is only available in pharmacies that are part of the PROMACTA CARES program, and patients must be registered with this program.

Antifibrinolytic Agents

Mechanism of Action

Control of a variety of fibrinolytic states can be achieved using a number of synthetic antifibrinolytic agents, such as tranexamic acid (Cyklokapron) and ε-aminocaproic acid (Amicar), that completely inhibit plasminogen activation. Plasmin binds to fibrin through a lysine binding site to activate the final stages of fibrinolysis (Fig. 26.1). Aminocaproic acid, a lysine analog, and tranexamic acid are antifibrinolytic agents with high affinity for the five lysine binding sites of plasminogen, thus effectively competing and preventing the binding of plasmin to fibrin.

$H_2N-CH_2-CH_2-CH_2-CH_2-CH_2-COOH$

Aminocaproic acid

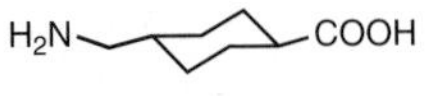

Tranexamic acid

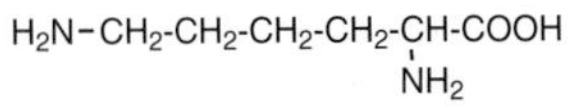

Lysine

Pharmacokinetics

Both ε-aminocaproic acid and tranexamic acid are readily absorbed when administered orally. They also can be given intravenously, although significant hypotension can result if the infusion is given too quickly. Elimination of the drugs is primarily renal, with little metabolism taking place. The half-lives of ε-aminocaproic acid and tranexamic acid are each approximately 2 hours.

Therapeutic Use

These drugs find clinical utility in settings such as prevention of rebleeding in intracranial hemorrhages, as adjunctive therapy in hemophilia, and of course, in treatment of bleeding associated with fibrinolytic therapy. In most bleeding conditions, however, ε-aminocaproic acid therapy has not been shown to be of definitive benefit. In recent trials, tranexamic acid was found to reduce red cell transfusion better than ε-aminocaproic acid or placebo in patients undergoing liver transplantation (180).

Side Effects

The major risk associated with ε-aminocaproic or tranexamic acid therapy is intravascular thrombosis as a direct result of the inhibition of plasminogen activator. Thrombi that form during therapy are not easily lysed and, therefore, can have additional ischemic consequences. Additional possible complications include hypotension, abdominal discomfort, and rarely, myopathy and muscle necrosis.

Aprotinin (Traysylol)

Operative procedures, such as heart valve replacement, frequently have effects on platelet function and endogenous coagulation factors (181). These effects may result in significant peri- or postoperative bleeding. Aprotinin is a serine protease inhibitor that blocks kallikrein and plasmin and provides some protection to platelets from mechanical injury. The inhibition of fibrinolysis results in profound antihemorrhagic effects (181). Side effects of aprotinin therapy usually are minor, but anaphylaxis has possibly been implicated in a small population (<0.5%). For this reason, it is suggested that a small test dose be given before initiation of the therapeutic infusion.

Plasma Fractions

Spontaneous bleeding can result from dysfunction or deficiencies of specific coagulation factors. A list of coagulation factors and deficiency states is given in Table 26.6.

TABLE 26.6 Clotting Factors

Factor	Common Name	Deficiency State	Source	Half-Life of Infused Factor (days)	Target for Action of
I	Fibrinogen	Afibrinogenemia, defibrination syndrome	Liver	4	
II	Prothrombin	Prothrombin deficiency	Liver (requires vitamin K)	3	Heparin (IIa), warfarin (synthesis)
III	Tissue thromboplastin, thrombokinase, tissue factor		Liver (may require vitamin K)		
IV	Calcium (Ca^{2+})				
V	Proaccelerin, labile factor	Factor V deficiency	Liver	1	
VI	Deleted factor				
VII	Proconvertin, stable factor	Factor VII deficiency	Liver (requires vitamin K)	0.25	Heparin (VIIa); warfarin (synthesis)
VIII	Antihemophilic A factor (AHF), antihemophilic globulin (AHG)	Hemophilia A (classic) von Willebrand disease	Liver	0.5 Unknown	
IX	Antihemophilic B factor, plasma thromboplastin component (PTC), Christmas factor	Hemophilia B (Christmas disease)	Liver (requires vitamin K)	1	Heparin (IXa); warfarin (synthesis)
X	Stuart or Stuart-Prower factor	Stuart-Prower defect	Liver (requires vitamin K)	1.5	Heparin (IXa); warfarin (synthesis)
XI	Plasma thromboplastin antecedent (PTA)	PTA deficiency	Unknown	3	
XII	Hageman factor, contact factor	Hageman defect	Unknown	Unknown	
XIII	Fibrin-stabilizing factor, fibrinase	Fibrin-stabilizing factor deficiency	Unknown	6	
	Fletcher factor, prekallikrein factor		Liver		
	Fitzgerald factor, high molecular weight kininogen		Liver		
Antithrombin III Proteins C & S Plasminogen		Antithrombin III deficiency		3	Warfarin (synthesis) Thrombolytic enzymes, aminocaproic acid

Spontaneous bleeding usually occurs when the activity of coagulation factors falls below 5% of normal. Typically, these deficiencies are the result of a chronic disease state, such as von Willebrand disease or hemophilia. Management of an acute hemorrhagic event in a coagulation factor–deficient patient includes administration of the appropriate factors in concentrated form. The most common inherited clotting factor deficiencies involve factor VIII (classic hemophilia A) and factor IX (hemophilia B, or Christmas disease).

Two forms of factor VIII concentrate are clinically available, cryoprecipitate and lyophilized factor VIII concentrate. Cryoprecipitate is a factor VIII–rich plasma protein fraction prepared from whole blood that also contains approximately 300 mg of fibrinogen per unit. Immediately before infusion, the required number of cryoprecipitate units are thawed in a sterile saline/citrate solution and pooled. The lyophilized factor VIII concentrates are prepared from large plasma pools and also are rich in fibrinogen. Lyophilized factor VIII concentrates are not useful in therapy for von Willebrand disease, because during the extraction and lyophilization process, the polymeric structure of factor VIII in the von Willebrand protein that supports platelet adhesion is destroyed, rendering the preparation inactive. Because of the pooling of blood from multiple donors in the preparation of lyophilized factor VIII concentrates, it generally is held that cryoprecipitate, which is isolated from a single donor, is safer.

The major concern associated with the use of concentrated clotting factors is the risk of viral transmission (primarily HIV and hepatitis B). This fear has somewhat attenuated the use of concentrated plasma fractions, even in diseases such as hemophilia. Ultrapure factor VIII concentrates produced using recombinant DNA technology have been approved for use. Frequently, however, the expense of these recombinant agents is the reason why the more traditional plasma isolates are used—despite the possibility of viral transmission.

Lyophilized preparations of prothrombin, factor IX, and factor X also are available. The manufacturing process involves plasma extraction with solvents and detergents that renders the preparations virally inactive but still able to activate clotting factors. To prevent excessive thrombus formation in these situations, heparin often is added to the therapeutic regimen.

At times, a hemorrhagic event is possible, but the patient does not require immediate coagulation therapy. For example, if a patient with mild hemophilia A needs to have a dental extraction performed, the potential for hemorrhage exists. In these cases, it is possible to increase the activity of the endogenous factor VIII through pretreatment with desmopressin acetate. This preoperative measure may alleviate the need for clotting factor replacement.

SCENARIO: OUTCOME AND ANALYSIS

Outcome

Kim K. Birtcher, MS, PharmD, BCPS

During the hospitalization, the patient received aspirin, clopidogrel, and other evidence-based therapies. He was enrolled in a cardiac rehabilitation program and received instructions for lifestyle modifications to decrease his risk of future cardiovascular events. He was discharged to his home after 3 days. His discharge medications included aspirin, clopidogrel, an angiotensin-converting enzyme inhibitor, a β-blocker, a statin, and fish oil. The pharmacist provided discharge counseling and emphasized the importance of continuous adherence to the dual antiplatelet therapy with aspirin and clopidogrel therapy for at least a year after drug-eluting stent placement to prevent stenosis.

Chemical Analysis

Kim E. Birtcher, Victoria Roche and S. William Zito

Myocardial infarction is commonly caused by the rupture of an unstable atherosclerotic plaque and the subsequent formation of a platelet-mediated thrombus. Shortly after plaque rupture, platelets adhere to collagen fibrils through the GPIa/IIa receptors. Tissue factor and collagen are exposed, which induces adhesion and activation of platelets and the release of ADP and TXA2. The GPIIb/IIIa receptors change, allowing fibrin bridges to form between the platelets. The extrinsic coagulation pathway is also activated. Thrombin is produced and converts fibrinogen to fibrin. The fibrin stabilizes the thrombus and catches red blood cells.

The use of antiplatelet agents and anticoagulants for the treatment of myocardial infarction in the clinical scenario matches the complexity of clot formation. Aspirin's acetoxy moiety (unique among NSAIDs) irreversibly deactivates platelet COX-1 through acetylation of a COX-1 Ser residue, thus rapidly inhibiting the synthesis of TXA_2 and attenuating platelet aggregation. Clopidogrel, a thienopyridine, is a prodrug that requires activation by cytochrome 2C19 to exert its antiplatelet effect. The active metabolite, the thiol product of the hydrolysis of the CYP2C19-generated thioester, selectively and irreversibly inhibits the binding of ADP to its platelet P2Y12 receptor, which impairs the ADP-mediated activation of the $GPII_b/III_a$ complex and ultimately inhibits platelet aggregation.

Unfractionated heparin binds to antithrombin and inhibits the activity of clotting factors Xa and IIa (thrombin). The lysine-glycine-aspartate component of eptifibatide is highly specific for the $GPII_b/III_a$ receptor. Eptifibatide is a reversible inhibitor of the receptor, since it has a low binding affinity for the receptor. The combined actions of these medications provide comprehensive management of the thrombus formed during myocardial infarction.

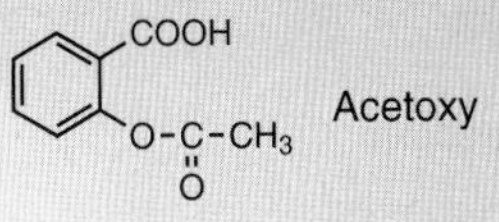

Aspirin

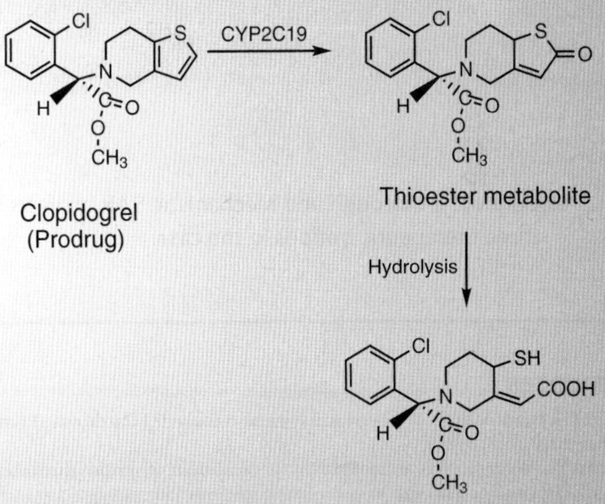

Clopidogrel (Prodrug)

Thioester metabolite

Thiol metabolite

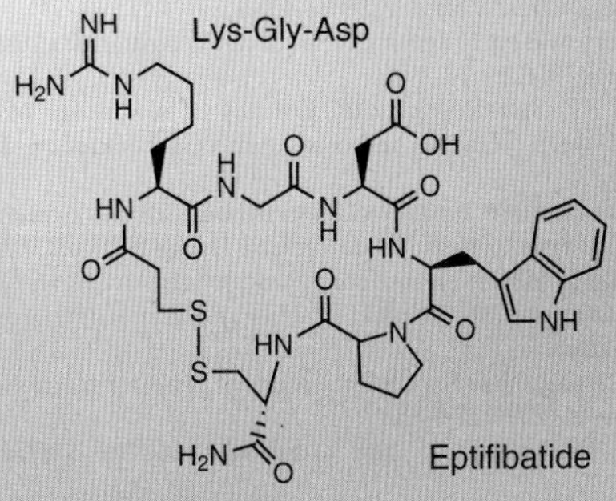

Eptifibatide

CASE STUDY

Matthis C. Lu

DY is a 78-year-old Asian woman who was admitted to the hospital because she needs to have hip-replacement surgery because she fell in her house recently. Her significant medical history includes chronic renal failure (creatine clearance, 14 mL/min), osteoarthritis, hypertension, and congestive heart failure. Her current medication list includes furosemide 20 mg po daily, spironolactone 12.5 mg po daily, imidapril 2.5 mg po bid, and celecoxib 200 mg po bid. Unfractionated heparin therapy at a subcutaneous dosage of 5,000 units tid was initiated after surgery for deep vein thrombosis prophylaxis. Five days after surgery, DY complained of pain and swelling in her left leg. A compression ultrasound reading demonstrated superficial femoral and popliteal vein thrombosis. A laboratory evaluation for heparin-induced thrombocytopenia (serotonin release assay) was ordered and yielded a positive result. Her physician wants to change her unfractionated heparin to a different anticoagulant and asks your opinion of the choices 1–3.

(continued)

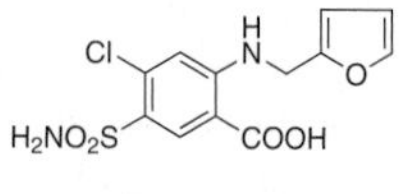

Furosemide

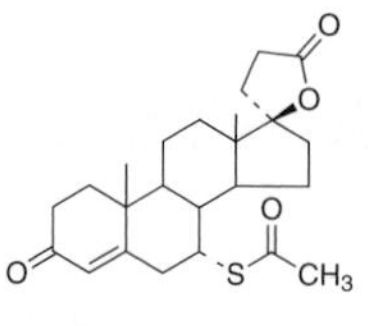

Spironolactone

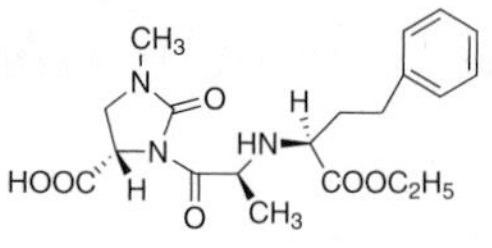

Imidapril

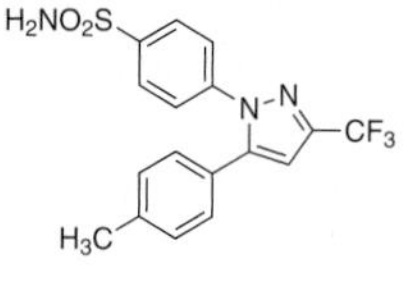

Celecoxib

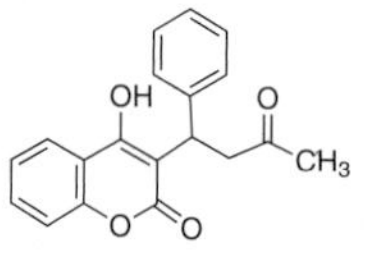

1

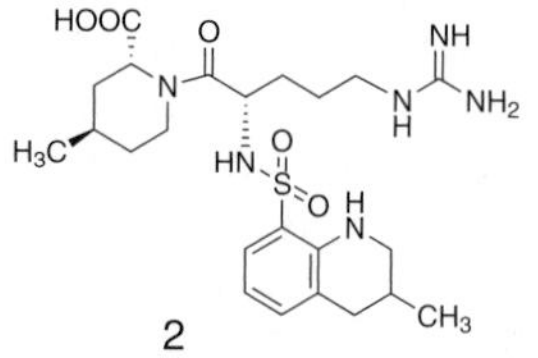

2

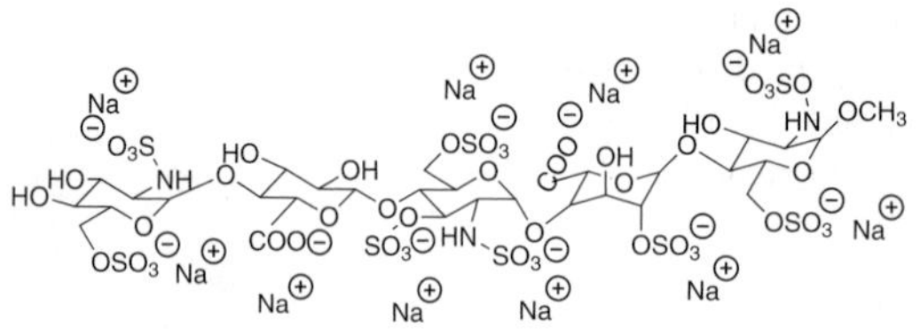

3

1. Conduct a thorough and mechanistic SAR analysis of the three therapeutic options in the case.
2. Apply the chemical understanding gained from the SAR analysis to this patient's specific needs to make a therapeutic recommendation.

References

1. Ruff CT, Braunwald E. Will warfarin ever be replaced? J Cardiovasc Pharmacol Ther 2010;15:210–219.
2. Gross PL, Weitz JI. New anticoagulant for treatment of venous thromboembolism. Arterioscler Thromb Vasc Biol 2008;28:380–386.
3. Geerts WH, Bergqvist D, Pineo GF, et al. Prevention of venous thromboembolism: American College of Chest Physicians evidence-based clinical practice guidelines (8th edition). Chest 2008;133:381S–453S.
4. Wright IS. The discovery and early development of anticoagulants: a historical perspective. Circulation 1959;19:73–134.
5. Kakkar VV, Corrigan TP, Spindler J, et al. Efficacy of low doses of heparin in prevention of deep vein thrombosis after major surgery. Lancet 1972;300:101–106.
6. Blanchard E, Ansell J. Extended anticoagulation therapy for the primary and secondary prevention of venous thromboembolism. Drugs 2005;65:303–311.
7. Weitz JI, Hirsh J, Samama MM. New anticoagulant drugs: American College of Chest Physicians evidence-based clinical practice guidelines (8th edition). Chest 2008;133:234S–256S.
8. Weitz JI. Emerging anticoagulants for the treatment of venous thromboembolism. Thromb Haemost 2006;96:274–284.
9. Bates SM, Weitz JI. The status of new anticoagulants. Br J Haematol 2006;134:3–19.
10. Garcia D. Novel anticoagulants and the future of anticoagulation. Thromb Res 2009;4:550–555.
11. Kyrle PA, Eichinger S. Deep vein thrombosis. Lancet 2005;365:1163–1174.
12. Geerts WH, Pineo GF, Heit JA, et al. Prevention of venous thromboembolism: the Seventh ACCP Conference on Antithrombotic and Thrombolytic Therapy. Chest 2004;126:338S–400S.
13. Lane DA, Lip GYH. Atrial fibrillation and mortality: the impact of antithrombotic therapy. Eur Heart J 2010;31:2075–2076.
14. Nutescu EA, Helgason CM. Concomitant drug, dietary, and lifestyle issues in patients with atrial fibrillation receiving anticoagulation therapy for stroke prophylaxis. Curr Treat Options Cardiovasc Med 2005;7:241–250.
15. Turpie AGG. New oral anticoagulants in atrial fibrillation. Eur Heart J 2007;29:155–165.
16. Khrenov AV, Anayeva NM, Griffin JH, et al. Coagulation pathways in atherothrombosis. Trends Cardiovasc Med 2002;12:317–324.
17. Weitz JI, Hirsh J, Samama MM. New anticoagulant drugs: the Seventh ACCP Conference on Antithrombotic and Thrombolytic Therapy. Chest 2004;126:265–286.
18. Stryer L. Biochemistry, 3rd Ed. New York: W.H. Freeman and Company, 1988.
19. Broze GJ Jr. Tissue factor pathway inhibitor. Thromb Haemost 1995;74:90–93.
20. Sandset PM, Bendz B, Hansen JB. Physiological function of tissue factor pathway inhibitor and interaction with heparins. Haemostasis 2000;30:48–56.
21. Esmon CT. The protein C pathway. Chest 2003;124:26S–32S.
22. Mosnier LO, Zlokovic BV, Griffin JH. The cytoprotective protein C pathway. Blood 2007;109:3161–3172.
23. Brookoff D. Hematologic evaluation. In: Flomenbaum N, Goldfrank L, Jacobson S, eds. Emergency Diagnostic Testing, 2nd Ed. St. Louis, MO: Mosby, 1995.
24. Ansell J, Hirsh J, Poller L, et al. The pharmacology and management of the vitamin K antagonists: the Seventh ACCP Conference on Antithrombotic and Thrombolytic Therapy. Chest 2004;126:204S–233S.
25. Jones M, McEwan P, Morgan CL, et al. Evaluation of the pattern of treatment, level of anticoagulation control, and outcome of treatment with warfarin in patients with non-valvar atrial fibrillation: a record linkage study in a large British population. Heart 2005;91:472–477.
26. O'Reilly RA. Vitamin K and the oral anticoagulant drugs. Annu Rev Med 1976;27:245–261.
27. Le Cam-Duchez V, Frétigny M, Cailleux N, et al. Algorithms using clinical and genetic data (CYP2C9, VKORC1) are relevant to predict warfarin dose in patients with different INR targets. Thromb Res 2010;126:e235–e237.
28. Hirsh J, Dalen JE, Anderson DR, et al. Oral anticoagulants: mechanism of action, clinical effectiveness, and optimal therapeutic range. Chest 2001;119:8S–21S.
29. Wajih N, Sane DC, Hutson SM, et al. Engineering of a recombinant vitamin K-dependent gamma-carboxylation system with enhanced gamma-carboxyglutamic forming capacity: evidence for a functional CXXC redox center in the system. J Biol Chem 2005;280:10540–10547.
30. Valente EJ, Lingafelter EC, Porter WR, et al. Structure of warfarin in solution. J Med Chem 1977;20:1489–1493.
31. USPDI Drug Information for the Health Care Professional, 16th Ed. Rockville, MD: United States Pharmacopeial Convention, Inc., 1996:236–246.
32. Ansell J, Hirsh J, Dalen J, et al. Managing oral anticoagulant therapy. Chest 2001;119:22S–38S.
33. Baselt RC, ed. Disposition of Toxic Drugs and Chemicals in Man, 5th Ed. Foster City, CA: Chemical Toxicology Institute, 2000.
34. Hollinger BR, Pastoor TP. Case management and plasma half-life in a case of brodifacoum poisoning. Arch Intern Med 1993;153:1925–1928.
35. Palmer RB, Alakija P, Cde Baca JE, et al. Fatal brodifacoum rodenticide poisoning: autopsy and toxicologic findings. J Forensic Sci 1999;44:851–855.
36. Redfern R, Gill JE, Hadler MR. Laboratory evaluation of WBA8119 (brodifacoum) as a rodenticide for use against warfarin-resistant and non-resistant rats and mice. J Hygiene 1976;77:419–426.
37. Bachmann KA, Sullivan TJ. Dispositional and pharmacodynamic characteristics of brodifacoum in warfarin-sensitive rats. Pharmacology 1983;27:281–288.
38. Laposata M, Van Cott EM, Lev MH. Case 1-2007: a 40-year old women with epistaxis, hematemesis and altered mental status. N Engl J Med 2007;356:174–182
39. Rettie AE, Tai G. The pharmacogenomics of warfarin: closing in on personalized medicine. Mol Interv 2006;6:223–227.
40. Pasmant E, de Beauvoir C, Plessier A, et al. VKROC1 and CYP2C9 genetic polymorphisms in hepatic or portal vein thrombosis. Thromb Res 2010;126:e134–e136.
41. Spyropoulos AC, Hayth KA, Jenkins P. Anticoagulation with anisindione in a patient with a warfarin-induced skin eruptions. Pharmacotherapy 2003;23:533–536.
42. Linhardt RJ. Heparin: structure and activity. J Med Chem 2003;46:2551–2554.

43. Codée JDC, Overkleeft HS, Van der Marel GA, et al. The synthesis of well-defined heparin and heparin sulfate fragments. Drug Discov Today 2004;1:317–326.
44. Hirsh J, Raschke R. Heparin and low-molecular weight heparin: the Seventh ACCP Conference on Antithrombotic and Thrombolytic Therapy. Chest 2004;126:188S–203S.
45. De Kort M, Buijsman RC, Van Boeckel CAA. Synthetic heparin derivatives as new anticoagulant drugs. Drug Discov Today 2005;10:769–779.
46. Desai UR. New antithrombin-based anticoagulants. Med Res Rev 2004;24:151–181.
47. Jin L, Abrahams JP, Skinner R, et al. The anticoagulant activity of antithrombin by heparin. Proc Natl Acad Sci U S A 1997;94:14683–14688.
48. Weitz JI. Low-molecular-weight heparins. N Engl J Med 1997;337:688–698.
49. Reilly RF. The pathophysiology of immune-mediated heparin-induced thrombocytopenia. Semin Dial 2003;16:54–60.
50. Hovanessian HC. New generation anticoagulants: the low-molecular-weight heparins. Ann Emerg Med 1999;34:768–779.
51. Rosenberg RD. Biochemistry and pharmacology of low-molecular-weight heparin. Semin Hematol 1997;4(Suppl 4):2–8.
52. de Pont AJM, Hofstra JH, Pik DR, et al. Pharmacokinetics and pharmacodynamics of danaparoid during continuous venovenous hemofiltration: a pilot study. Crit Care 2007;11:R102.
53. Kakkar AK. Low- and ultralow-molecular-weight heparins. Best Pract Res Clin Hematol 2004;17:77–87.
54. Louzada ML, Majeed H, Wells PS. Efficacy of low-molecular-weight-heparin versus vitamin K antagonists for long term treatment of cancer-associated venous thromboembolism in adults: a systematic review of randomized controlled trials. Thromb Res 2009;123:837–844.
55. Siddiqui MAA, Wagstaff AJ. Enoxaparin—a review of its use as thromboprophylaxis in acutely ill, nonsurgical patients. Drugs 2005;65:1025–1036.
56. Sinnaeve P, Van de Werf F. Enoxaparin and fibrinolysis: ExTRACTing prognosis from bleeding complications. Eur Heart J 2010;31:2077–2079.
57. Petitou M, Herault J, Bernat A, et al. Synthesis of thrombin-inhibiting heparin mimetics without side effects. Nature 1999;398:417–422.
58. Leone-Bay A, Paton DR, Freeman J, et al. Synthesis and evaluation of compounds that facilitate the gastrointestinal absorption of heparin. J Med Chem 1998;41:1163–1171.
59. Eom JS, Koh KS, Al-Hilal TA, et al. Antithrombotic efficacy of an oral low molecular weight heparin conjugated with deosycholic asset on microsurgical anastomosis in rats. Thromb Res 2010;126:e220–e224.
60. Nutescu EA. Evolving concepts in the treatment of venous thromboembolism: the role of factor Xa inhibitors. Pharmacotherapy 2004;24:82S–87S.
61. Bauer KA. Fondaparinux: a new synthetic and selective inhibitor of factor Xa. Best Pract Res Clin Hematol 2004;17:89–104.
62. Koopman MMW, Buller HR. Short- and long-acting synthetic pentasaccharides. J Intern Med 2003;254:335–342.
63. Petitou M, Duchaussoy P, Jaurand G, et al. Synthesis and pharmacological properties of a close analogue of an antithrombotic pentasaccharide (SR 90107A/ORG 31540). J Med Chem 1997;40:1600–1607.
64. Cheng JWM. Fondaparinux: a new antithrombotic agent. Clin Ther 2002;24:1757–1769.
65. Dager WE, Andersen J, Nutescu EA. Special considerations with fondaparinux therapy: heparin-induced thrombocytopenia and wound healing. Pharmacotherapy 2004;7:88S–94S.
66. Hawkins D. Limitation of traditional anticoagulants. Pharmacotherapy 2004;7:62S–65S.
67. Savi P, Herault JP, Duchaussoy P, et al. Reversible biotinylated oligosaccharides: a new approach for a better management of anticoagulant therapy. J Thromb Haemot 2008;6:1697–1706.
68. Paty I, Trellu M, Destors JM, et al. Reversibility of the anti-Fxa activity of idrabiotaparinux (biotinylated idraparinux) by intravenous avidin infusion. J Thromb Haemost 2010;8:722–729.
69. Hirsh J, O'Donnell M, Eikelboom JW. Beyond unfractionated heparin and warfarin: current and future advances. Circulation 2007;116:552–560.
70. Garcia D, Libby E, Crowther MA. The new oral anticoagulants. Blood 2010;115:15–20.
71. Johnson PH. Hirudin: clinical potential of a thrombin inhibitor. Annu Rev Med 1994;45:165–177.
72. Krstenansky JL, Owen TJ, Yates MT, et al. Design, synthesis, and antithrombin activity for conformationally restricted analogues of peptide anticoagulants based on the C-terminal region of the leech peptide, hirudin. Biochim Biophys Acta 1988;957:53–59.
73. Maraganore JM, Bourdon P, Jablonski J, et al. Design and characterization of hirulogs: a novel class of bivalent peptide inhibitors of thrombin. Biochemistry 1990;29:7095–7101.
74. Nutescu EA, Shapiro, NL. New anticoagulant agents: direct thrombin inhibitors. Clin Geriatr Med 2006;22:33–56.
75. Agnelli G. Clinical potential of oral direct thrombin inhibitors in the prevention and treatment of venous thromboembolism. Drugs 2004;64:47S–52S.
76. Haas S. Oral direct thrombin inhibition: an effective and novel approach for venous thromboembolism. Drugs 2004;64:7S–16S.
77. Nisio MD, Middeldorp S, Buller HR. Direct thrombin inhibitors. N Engl J Med 2005;353:1028–1040.
78. Eikelboom JW, French J. Management of patients with acute coronary syndromes. What is the clinical role of direct thrombin inhibitors? Drugs 2002;62:1839–1852.
79. Greinacher A, Lubenow N. Recombinant hirudin in clinical practice. Focus on lepirudin. Circulation 2001;103:1479–1484.
80. Matheson AJ, Goa KL. Desirudin: a review of its uses in the management of thrombotic disorders. Drugs 2000;60:679–700.
81. Hirsh J. Current anticoagulant therapy—unmet clinical needs. Thromb Res 2003;109:S1–S8.
82. Levy JH. Novel intravenous antithrombins. Am Heart J 2001;141:1043–1047.
83. Warkentin TE. Bivalent direct thrombin inhibitors: hirudin and bivalirudin. Best Pract Res Clin Hematol 2004;17:105–125.
84. Caron MF, McKendall GR. Bivalirudin in percutaneous coronary intervention. Am J Health Syst Pharm 2003;60:1841–1849.
85. Curran MP. Bivalirudin: in patients with ST-segment elevation myocardial infarction. Drugs 2010;70:909–918.
86. Saugel B, Phillip V, Moessmer G, et al. Argatroban therapy for heparin-induced thrombocytopenia in ICU patients with multiple organ dysfunction syndrome: a retrospective study. Crit Care 2010;14:R90.
87. Nagashima H. Studies on the different modes of action of the anticoagulant protease inhibitors DX-9065a and argatroban. J Biol Chem 2002;277: 50439–50449.
88. Hauptmann J. Pharmacokinetics of an emerging new class of anticoagulant/antithrombotics drugs. Eur J Clin Pharmacol 2002;57:751–758.
89. Eriksson BI, Quinlan DJ, Weitz JI. Comparative pharmacodynamics and pharmacokinetics of oral direct thrombin and factor Xa inhibitors in development. Clin Pharmacokinet 2009;48:1–22.
90. Baetz BE, Spinler SA. Dabigatran etexilate: an oral direct thrombin inhibitor for prophylaxis and treatment of thromboembolic diseases. Pharmacotherapy 2008;28:1354–1373.
91. Blech S, Ebner T, Ludwig-Schwellinger E, et al. The metabolism and disposition of the oral direct thrombin inhibitor, dabigatran, in humans. Drug Metab Dispos 2008;36:386–399.
92. Imberti D, Dall'Asta C, Pierfranceschi MG. Oral factor Xa inhibitors for thromboprophylaxis in major orthopedic surgery: a review. Intern Emerg Med 2009;4:471–477.
93. Turpie AGG. Oral, direct factor Xa inhibitors in development for the prevention and treatment of thromboembolic diseases. Arterioscler Thromb Vasc Biol 2007;27:1238–1247.
94. Morell J, Sullivan B, Khalabuda M, et al. Role of orally available antagonists of factor Xa in the treatment and prevention of thromboembolic disease: focus on rivaroxaban. J Clin Pharmacol 2010;50:986–1000.
95. Lassen MR, Raskob GE, Gallus A, et al; the ADVANCE-2 investigators. Apixaban versus enoxaparin for thromboprophylaxis after knee replacement (ADVANCE-2): a randomised double-blind trial. Lancet 2010;375:807–815.
96. Raghavan N, Frost CE, Yu Z, et al. Apixaban metabolism and pharmacokinetics after oral administration to humans. Drug Metab Dispos 2009;37:74–81.
97. Patrono C, Baigent C, Hirsh J, et al. Antiplatelet drugs: American College of Chest Physicians evidence-based clinical practice guidelines (8th edition). Chest 2008;133:199S–233S.
98. Davi G, Patrono C. Platelet activation and atherothrombosis. N Engl J Med 2007;357:2482–2494.
99. Coccheri S. Antiplatelet drugs: do we need new options? Drugs 2010;70:887–908.
100. Leonardi S, Tricoci P, Becker RC. Thrombin receptor antagonists for the treatment of atherothrombosis: therapeutic potential of vorapaxar and E-5555. Drugs 2010;70:1771–1783.
101. Angiolillo DJ, Capodanno D, Goto S. Platelet thrombin receptor antagonist and atherothrombosis. Eur Heart J 2010;31:17–28.
102. Sztriha LK, Sas K, Vecsei L. Aspirin resistance in stroke: 2004. J Neurol Sci 2005;229–230:163–169.
103. Rocca B, Secchiero P, Ciabattoni G, et al. Cyclooxygenase-2 expression is induced during human megakaryopoiesis and characterizes newly formed platelets. Proc Natl Acad Sci U S A 2002;99:7634–7639.
104. Mason PJ, Jacobs AK, Freedman JE. Aspirin resistance and atherothrombotic disease. J Am Coll Cardiol 2005;46:986–993.
105. Matías-Guiu J, Ferro JM, Alvarez-Sabin J, et al. Comparison of triflusal and aspirin for prevention of vascular events in patients after cerebral infarction. Stroke 2003;34:1–8.
106. McNeely W, Goa KL. Triflusal. Drugs 1998;55:823–833.
107. Bayón Y, Alonso A, Crespo MS. 4-Trifluoromethyl derivatives of salicylate, triflusal and its main metabolite 2-hydroxy-4-trifluoromethylbenzoic acid, are potent inhibitor of nuclear factor κB activation. Br J Pharmacol 1999;126:1359–1466.
108. Sanzhez de Miguel L, Jimenez A, Monton M, et al. A 4-trifluoromethyl derivative of salicylate, triflusal, stimulates nitric oxide production by human neutrophils: role in platelet function. Eur J Clin Invest 2000;30:811–817.
109. Eligini S, Violi F, Banfi C, et al. Indobufen inhibits tissue factor in human monocytes through a thromboxane-mediated mechanism. Cardiovas Res 2006;69:218–226.
110. Bhana N, McClellan KJ. Indobufen: an updated review of its use in the management of atherothrombosis. Drugs Aging 2001;18:369–388.
111. Lee S-W, Park S-W, Hong M-K, et al. Triple versus dual antiplatelet therapy after coronary stenting. J Am Coll Cardiol 2005;46:1833–1837.
112. Diener H-C, Bogousslavsky J, Brass LM, et al. Aspirin and clopidogrel compared with clopidogrel alone after recent ischemic stroke or transient ischemic attack in high-risk patients (MATCH): randomized, double-blind, placebo-controlled trial. Lancet 2004;364:331–337.
113. Lee SW, Park SW, Hong MK, et al. Comparison of cilostazol versus ticlopidine therapy after successful coronary stenting. Am J Cardiol 2005;95:859–862.

114. Ahn JC, Song WH, Kwon JA, et al. Effects of cilostazol on platelet activation in coronary stenting patients who already treated with aspirin and clopidogrel. Korean J Intern Med 2004;19:230–236.
115. Schror K. The pharmacology of cilostazol. Diabetes Obes Metab 2002;4(Suppl 2):S14–S19.
116. Suri A, Forbes WP, Bramer SL. Effects of CYP3A inhibition on the metabolism of cilostazol. Clin Pharmacokinet 1999;37(Suppl 2):61–68.
117. Suri A, Bramer SL. Effect of omeprazole on the metabolism of cilostazol. Clin Pharmacokinet 1999;37(Suppl 2):53–59.
118. Gachet C. The platelet P2 receptor as molecular targets for old and new antiplatelet drugs. Pharmacol Ther 2005;108:180–192.
119. Nguyen TA, Diodati JG, Pharand C. Resistance to clopidogrel: a review of the evidence. J Am Coll Cardiol 2005;45:1157–1164.
120. Van Giezen JJJ. Opitmizing platelet inhibition. Eur Heart J 2008;10:D23–D29.
121. Gachet C. P2 receptors, platelet function and pharmacological implications. Thromb Haemost 2008;99:466–472.
122. Wallentin L. $P2Y_{12}$ inhibitors: differences in properties and mechanisms of action and potential consequences for clinical use. Eur Heart J 2009;30:1964–1977.
123. Dorsam RT, Murugappan S, Ding Z, et al. Clopidogrel: interactions with the P2Y12 receptor and clinical relevance. Hematology 2003;8:359–365.
124. Cattaneo M. Advances in antiplatelet therapy: overview of new P2Y12 receptor antagonists in development. Eur Heart J 2008;10:133–137.
125. Savi P, Zachayus JL, Delesque-Touchard N, et al. The active metabolite of clopidogrel disrupts P2Y12 receptor oligomers and partitions them out of lipid rafts. Proc Natl Acad Sci USA 2006;103:11069–11074.
126. Savi P, Pereillo JM, Uzabiaga MF, et al. Identification and biological activity of the active metabolites of clopidogrel. Thromb Haemost 2000;84:891–896.
127. Ding Z, Kim S, Dorsam RT, et al. Inactivation of the human P2Y12 receptor by thiol reagents requires interaction with both extracellular cysteine residues, Cys17 and Cys270. Blood 2003;101:3908–3914.
128. Dalvie DK, O'Connell TN. Characterization of novel dihydrothienopyridinium and thienopyridinium metabolites of ticlopidine in vitro: role of peroxidases, cytochromes P450, and monoamine oxidases. Drug Metab Dispos 2004;32:49–57.
129. Wiviott SD, Antman EM, Winters KJ, et al. Randomized comparison of prasugrel (CS-747, LY640315), a novel thienopyridine P2Y12 antagonist, with clopidogrel in percutaneous coronary intervention: results of the joint utilization of medications to block platelets optimally (JUMBO)-TIMI 26 trial. Circulation 2005;111:3366–3373.
130. Duggan ST, Keating GM. Prasugrel: a review of its use in patients with acute coronary syndromes undergoing percutaneous coronary intervention. Drug 2009;69:1707–1726.
131. Jakubowski JA, Winters KJ, Naganuma H, et al. Prasugrel: a novel thienopyridine antiplatelet agent. A review of preclinical and clinical studies and the mechanistic basis for its distinct antiplatelet profiles. Cardiovasc Drug Rev 2007;4:357–374.
132. Farid NA, Smith RL, Gillespie TA, et al. The disposition of prasugrel, a novel thienopyridine, in humans. Drug Metab Dispos 2007;35:1096–1104.
133. Nishiya Y, Hagihara K, Ito T, et al. Mechanism-based inhibition of human cytochrome P-450 2B6 by ticlopidine, clopidogrel, and thiolactone metabolite of prasugrel. Drug Metab Dispos 2009;37:589–593.
134. Farid NA, Kurihara A, Wrighton SA. Metabolism and disposition of the thienopyridine antiplatelet drugs ticlopidine, clopidogrel, and prasugrel in humans. J Clin Pharmacol 2010;50:126–142.
135. Veverka A, Hammer JM. Prasugrel: a new thienopyridine inhibitor. J Pharm Pract 2009;22:158–165.
136. Oliphant CS, Doby JB, Das K, et al. Emerging $P2Y_{12}$ receptor antagonists: role in coronary artery disease. Curr Vasc Pharmacol 2010;8:93–101.
137. Moser M, Bode C. Antiplatelet therapy for atherothrombotic disease: how can we improve the outcomes? J Thromb Thrombolysis 2010;30:240–249.
138. Anderson SD. Efficacy and safety of ticagrelor: a reversible $P2Y_{12}$ receptor antagonist. Ann Pharmacother 2010;44:524–537.
139. Wallentin L, Becker R, Budaj A, et al. Ticagrelor versus clopidogrel in patients with acute coronary syndromes. N Engl J Med 2009;361:1045–1057.
140. Dovlatova NL, Jakubowski JA, Sugidachi A, et al. The reversible P2Y12 antagonist cangrelor influences the ability of the active metabolites of clopidogrel and prasugrel to produce irreversible inhibition of platelet function. J Thromb Haemost 2008;6:1153–1159.
141. Becker RC, Moliterno DJ, Jennings LK, et al. Safety and tolerability of SCH 530348 in patients undergoing non-urgent percutaneous coronary intervention: a randomised, double-blind, placebo-controlled phase II study. Lancet 2009;373:919–928.
142. Chackalamannil S, Wang Y, Greenlee WJ, et al. Discovery of a novel, orally active himbacine-based thrombin receptor antagonist (SCH 530348) with potent antiplatelet activity. J Med Chem 2008;51:3061–3064.
143. Chackalamannil S. Thrombin receptor (protease activated receptor-1) antagonists as potent antithrombotic agents with strong antiplatelet effects. J Med Chem 2006;49:5389–5403.
144. Kai Y, Hirano K, Maeda Y, et al. Prevention of the hypercontractile response to thrombin by proteinase-activated receptor-1 antagonist in subarachnoid hemorrhage. Stroke 2007;38:3259–3265.
145. Proimos G. Platelet aggregation inhibition with glycoprotein IIb-IIIa inhibitors. J Thromb Thrombolysis 2001;11:99–110.
146. Berger PB. The glycoprotein IIb/IIIa inhibitor wars. J Am Coll Cardiovasc 2010;56:476–478.
147. Mousa SA. Antiplatelet therapies: from aspirin to GPIIb/IIIa-receptor antagonists and beyond. Drug Discov Today 1999;4:552–561.
148. Hashemzadeh M, Furukawa M, Goldberry S, et al. Chemical structures and mode of action of intravenous glycoprotein IIb/IIIa receptor blockers: a review. Exp Clin Cardiol 2008;13:192–197.
149. Moliterno DJ, Ziada KM. The safety and efficacy of glycoprotein IIb/IIIa inhibitors for primary angioplasty: more option to choose and more time to decide. J Am Coll Cardiol 2008:51:536–537.
150. Reverter JC, Beguin S, Kessels H, et al. Inhibition of platelet-mediated, tissue factor–induced thrombin generation by the mouse/human chimeric 7E3 antibody: potential implications for the effect of c7E3 Fab treatment on acute thrombosis and "clinical restenosis." J Clin Invest 1996;98:863–874.
151. Vergara-Jimenez J. Safety and efficacy of abciximab as an adjunct to percutaneous coronary intervention. Vascular Health Risk Manage 2010;6:39–45.
152. Genetta TB, Mauro VF. ABCIXIMAB: a new antiaggregant used in angioplasty. Ann Pharmacother 1996;30:251–257.
153. Tam SH, Sassoli PM, Jordan RE, et al. Abciximab (ReoPro, chimeric 7E3 Fab) demonstrates equivalent affinity and functional blockade of glycoprotein IIb/IIIa and $\alpha v \beta 3$ integrins. Circulation 1998;98:1085–1091.
154. Curran MP, Keating GM. Eptifibatide. Drugs 2005;65:2009–2035.
155. Van't Hof AW, Valgimigli M. Defining the role of platelet glycoprotein receptor inhibitors in STEMI: focus on tirofiban. Drugs 2009;69:85–100.
156. Juwana YB, Suryapranata H, Ottervanger JP, et al. Tirofiban for myocardial infarction. Expert Opin Pharmacother 2010;11:861–866.
157. Gresele P, Agnelli G. Novel approaches to the treatment of thrombosis. Trends Pharmacol Sci 2002;23:25–32.
158. De la Cruz JP, Villalobos MA, Escalante R, et al. Effects of the selective inhibition of platelet thromboxane synthase on the platelet-subendothelium interaction. Br J Pharmacol 2002;137:1082–1088.
159. Khan IA, Gowda RM. Clinical perspective and therapeutics of thrombolysis. Int J Cardiol 2003;91:115–127.
160. Baruah DB, Dash RN, Chaudhari MR, et al. Plasminogen activators: a comparison. Vascular Pharmacol 2006;44:1–9.
161. Banerjee A, Chisti Y, Banerjee UC. Streptokinase—a clinically useful thrombolytic agent. Biotechnol Adv 2004;22:287–307.
162. Perler B. Thrombolytic therapies: the current state of affairs. J Endovasc Ther 2005;12:224–232.
163. Hansen AP, Petros AM, Meadows RP, et al. Solution structure of the amino terminal fragment of urokinase-type plasminogen activator. Biochemistry 1994;33:4847–4864.
164. Belkin M, Belkin B, Buckman CA, et al. Intra-arterial fibrinolytic therapy, efficacy of streptokinase vs urokinase. Arch Surg 1986;121:769–773.
165. Antman EM, Braunwald E. Coronary thrombosis. In: Braunwald E, Zipes DP, Libby P, eds. Baunwald's Textbook of Cardiovascular Medicine, 6th Ed. Philadelphia: WB Saunders, 2001:1145–1218.
166. Orsini G, Brandazza A, Sarmientos P, et al. Efficient renaturation and fibrinolytic properties of prourokinase and a deletion mutant expressed in *Escherichia coli* as inclusion bodies. Eur J Biochem 1991;195:691–697.
167. Ouriel K, Kandarpa K, Schuerr DM, et al. Prourokinase versus urokinase for recanalization of peripheral occlusions, safety and efficacy: the purpose trial. J Vasc Interv Radiol 1999;10:1083–1091.
168. Nordt TK, Bode C. Thrombolysis: newer thrombolytic agents and their role in clinical medicine. Heart 2003;89:1358–1362.
169. Bates SM, Greer IA, Hirsh J, et al. Use of antithrombotic agents during pregnancy: the Seventh ACCP Conference on Antithrombotic and Thrombolytic Therapy. Chest 2004;126:627S–644S.
170. Liu D, Cheng T, Guo H, et al. Tissue plasminogen activator neurovascular toxicity is controlled by activated protein C. Nat Med 2004;10:1379–1383.
171. Rank A, Weigert O, Ostermann H. Management of chronic immune thrombocytopenic purpura: targeting insufficient megakaryopoiesis as a novel therapeutic principle. Biologics 2010;4:139–145.
172. Schwartz RS. Immune thrombocytopenic purpura: from agony to agonist. N Engl J Med 2007;357:2299–2301.
173. Pruemer J. Epidemiology, pathophysiology, and initial management of chronic immune thrombocytopenic purpura. Am J Health Syst Pharm 2009;66:S4–S10.
174. Frampton JE, Lyseng-Williamson KA. Romiplostim. Drugs 2009;69:307–317.
175. Garnock-Jones KP, Keam SJ. Eltrombopag. Drugs 2009;69:567–576.
176. Burzynski J. New options after first-line therapy for chronic immune thrombocytopenic purpura. Am J Health Syst Pharm 2009;66:S11–S23.
177. Bussel JB, Kuter DJ, George JN, et al. AMG 531, a thrombopoiesis-stimulating protein, for chronic ITP. N Engl J Med 2006;355:1672–1681.
178. Kuter DJ, Bussel JB, Lyons RM, et al. Efficacy of romiplostim in patients with chronic immune thrombocytopenic purpura: a double-blind randomized controlled trial. Lancet 2008;371:395–403.
179. Rice L. Treatment of immune thrombocytopenic purpura: focus on eltrombopag. Biologics 2009;3:151–157.
180. Dalmau A, Sabate A, Acosta F, et al. Tranexamic acid reduces red cell transfusion better than epsilon-aminocaproic acid or placebo in liver transplantation. Anesth Analg 2000;91:29–34.
181. Greilich PE, Okada K, Latham P, et al. Aprotinin but not ε-aminocaproic acid decreases interleukin-10 after cardiac surgery with extracorporeal circulation: randomized, double-blind, placebo-controlled study in patients receiving aprotinin and ε-aminocaproic acid. Circulation 2001;104 (Suppl I):265–269

Chapter 27

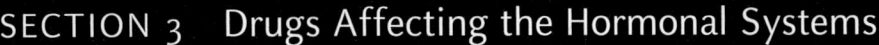

Insulin and Drugs Used to Treat Diabetes

S. William Zito

Drugs Covered in This Chapter*

ACARBOSE

AMYLIN

EXENATIDE

INSULIN
- Aspart
- Detemir
- Glulisine
- Glargine
- Lispro

LIRAGLUTIDE

LINAGLIPTIN

METFORMIN

MIGLITOL

NATEGLINIDE

PIOGLITAZONE

PRAMLINTIDE

REPAGLINIDE

ROSIGLITAZONE

SAXAGLIPTIN

SITAGLIPTIN

SULFONYLUREAS
- Acetohexamide
- Chlorpropamide
- Glimepiride
- Glipizide
- Glyburide
- Tolazamide
- Tolbutamide

TROGLITAZONE

Vildagliptin

VOGLIBOSE

Abbreviations

ADA, American Diabetes Association
ADP, adenosine diphosphate
AGE, advanced glycation end-product
Arg, arginine
Asp, aspartate
ATP, adenosine triphosphate
DAG, diacylglycerol
DPP-IV, dipeptidyl peptidase-IV
FDA, U.S. Food and Drug Administration
FFA, free fatty acid
FPG, fasting plasma glucose
GAPDH, glyceraldehyde-3-phosphate dehydrogenase
GIP, glucose-dependent insulinotropic polypeptide
GLP-1, glucagon-like peptide-1
Glu, glutamate
GLUT, facilitative glucose transporter
Gly, glycine
HbA$_{1c}$, hemoglobin A$_{1c}$
HLA, human leukocyte antigen
IRS, insulin receptor substrate
Lys, lysine
NPH, neutral protamine Hagedorn
OGTT, oral glucose tolerance test
PARP, poly(ADP-ribose) polymerase
PKC, phosphokinase C
PPAR, peroxisome proliferator–activated receptor
PTP, protein tyrosine phosphatase
Ser, serine
SGLT, sodium-glucose co-transporters
SUR, sulfonylurea receptor
Thr, threonine
TNF-α, tumor necrosis factor-α
TZD, thiazolidinedione
UPD, uridine diphosphate

*Drugs listed include those available inside and outside of the United States; drugs available outside of the United States are shown in italics.

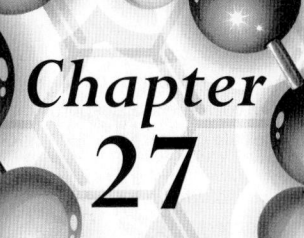

SCENARIO

JL is a 57-year-old Hispanic man who was initially prescribed metformin 500 mg PO BID, but his doctor increased it to 1000 mg PO BID 4 months ago. He is also taking glipizide 10 mg BID. His body mass index is 35 and hemoglobin A1c value is 7.7%. He is very reluctant to use insulin because he thinks it is too complicated, he fears hypoglycemia, and has heard that insulin use is associated with weight gain. He monitors his blood glucose one to two times daily, including after meals. His fasting blood glucose levels are approximately 140 mg/dL; most postprandial values are greater than 200 mg/dL.

(The reader is directed to the clinical solution and chemical analysis of this case at the end of the chapter).

INTRODUCTION

The history of diabetes dates back to antiquity and is probably a disease that has always afflicted humankind. The recorded history of medicine begins with the Egyptian and Greek civilizations. The discovery of the Ebers Papyrus, written in 1550 BC, contains descriptions of a number of diseases including an account resembling the signs and symptoms of diabetes (1). Aretaeus of Cappadocia (81–138 AD) used the term "diabetes" in connection with this disease, which means "to run through" or "siphon," and Galen (131–201 AD) described the disease as "diarrhea urinosa" (diarrhea of urine) and "dipsakos" (the disease of thirst). In the 5th and 6th centuries, a number of cultures (Indian, Chinese, and Japanese) described the sweetness of the urine of diabetics, but it was not until the 16th century that the term "mellitus" (Latin for "honey" or "sweet") was applied to distinguish it from a similar polyuric disease, diabetes insipidus, where the urine was tasteless (insipid) (2). Sugar was positively identified in the urine of diabetics by Dobson in 1776, the cause of which was attributed by him and others as being associated with defects in the blood, kidney, and liver. Two seminal discoveries guided the understanding of the etiology of diabetes. The first was the identification of a polysaccharide in the liver termed "glycogen" by Claude Bernard in1875. The second was the discovery, in 1889 by Oskar Minkowski, that when the pancreas was removed from a dog, the animal developed all the signs and symptoms of diabetes mellitus (2,3). In 1869, Paul Langerhans noticed small clusters of ductless cells on the pancreas but gave no function to them, and in 1902, the work of Eugene Opie clearly linked these ductless cells, which by now were called the isles of Langerhans, to diabetes mellitus. Although a hypothetical secretion of the islet cells was postulated and called insulin (from insula, which means island), it took the work of Frederick Banting, Charles Best, and John Macloud to isolate insulin and use it as a diabetes medication. In 1923, Banting and Macloud shared the Nobel Prize in medicine, and Banting subsequently shared his prize with Best (2–4). Since the discovery of insulin, a number of types have been developed to improve its pharmacokinetics. The amino acid sequence of insulin was identified by Sanger and Tuppy in 1951 (5,6), and the total synthesis of active insulin was accomplished in 1963 by Katsoyannis et al. (7). The late 1970s saw recombinant DNA technology applied to the synthesis of human insulin in *Escherichia coli* (8), and the use of small, nonprotein molecules for the treatment of diabetes was developed from the discovery by Janbon et al. in 1942 that the sulfonamide 2-(*p*-aminobenzenesulfonamide)-5-isopropylthiadiazole induced hypoglycemia (9).

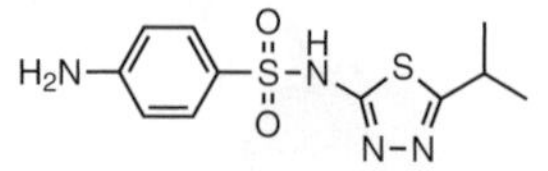

IPTD

DIABETES MELLITUS

Diabetes mellitus is a metabolic disorder characterized by hyperglycemia and associated with impaired fat, carbohydrate, and protein metabolism. The disease is the result of defects in insulin secretion and/or insulin action, which progressively leads to chronic microvascular, macrovascular, and neuropathic complications (10). There are two major types of diabetes, type 1 and type 2. In addition diabetes mellitus is associated with certain other hyperglycemic conditions, including gestational diabetes, maturity-onset diabetes of youth, diabetes secondary to other disease states, and drug- or chemical-induced diabetes (11).

Type 1 was formerly called insulin-dependent diabetes mellitus or juvenile-onset diabetes. It accounts for 5% to 10% of patients with diabetes and is largely recognized as an autoimmune disease whereby the β-cells are destroyed by the body's own antibodies. Because the pancreas can no longer produce insulin, type 1 diabetics have an absolute requirement for exogenous insulin. The symptoms of type 1 diabetes often come on suddenly, can be severe, and include polydipsia (thirst), polyuria (frequent urination), polyphagia (hunger), weight loss, fatigue, and diabetic ketoacidosis (12).

Type 2 diabetes (formerly called non–insulin-dependent diabetes mellitus or adult-onset diabetes) accounts for 90% to 95% of adult cases of diabetes. Type 2 diabetes slowly progresses from a state where the patient develops insulin resistance to a state where the pancreas loses its ability to produce enough insulin to compensate for the insulin resistance of peripheral tissues. Insulin resistance is the state where tissues do not utilize insulin properly. Insulin resistance is associated with a number of physiologic risk factors (hyperinsulinemia, hypertension, dyslipidemia, hypercoagulation, proinflammatory state, and abdominal obesity) most commonly referred to as "the metabolic syndrome." Nondiabetic patients with metabolic syndrome (Table 27.1) are at high risk for the development of type 2 diabetes, which then gives these patients a two to four times greater risk of developing coronary heart disease and stroke (13). In addition, type 2 diabetes is usually associated with race, lack of physical activity, and a family history of the disease (14,15). Unlike some traits, diabetes does not seem to be inherited in a simple pattern. Yet clearly, some people inherit a greater predisposition for diabetes than others.

Gestational diabetes is usually diagnosed during pregnancy. It occurs more often in women who are obese, have a family history of diabetes, and are members of a high-risk ethnic group (African American, Hispanic/Latino, Asian/Pacific Islander, and American Indian). Gestational diabetes requires treatment to control the hyperglycemia and to avoid complications to the infant. Most women return to normal postpartum; however, there is increased risk of developing diabetes in the next 10 years (16).

Maturity-onset diabetes of youth is characterized by faulty secretion of insulin, is rare (<5% of type 2 diabetes), and is associated with a number of genetic defects of β-cell function. These defects are inherited and occur at six chromatin loci identified on chromosomes 20q, 7p, 12q, 13q, 17q, and 2q (11). This form of diabetes is the result of impaired secretion of insulin, and there is no evidence that insulin action on tissue targets is decreased.

TABLE 27.1 International Diabetes Federation Worldwide Definition of Metabolic Syndrome (13)

Central obesity	Waist circumference* (race and gender specific) U.S. male: 40 inches U.S. female: 35 inches *If body mass index (BMI) is >30 kg/m^2, then central obesity is assumed. Plus any *two* of the following:
Triglycerides	≥150 mg/dL or if under treatment for this dyslipidemia
HDL cholesterol	Males : <40 mg/dL Females: <50 mg/dL or if under treatment for this dyslipidemia
Blood pressure	≥130/85 mm Hg of if under treatment for hypertension
Fasting plasma glucose	≥100 mg/dL or previously diagnosed with type 2 diabetes

HDL, high-density lipoprotein.

Diagnosis of Diabetes

The American Diabetes Association (ADA) has established four criteria for the diagnosis of diabetes: 1) a fasting plasma glucose (FPG) ≥126 mg/dL; 2) a 2-hour oral glucose tolerance test (OGTT) of ≥200 mg/dL; 3) in patients with overt symptoms of hyperglycemia (polyphagia, polyuria, polydipsia, weight loss), a random plasma glucose of ≥200 mg/dL; or 4) hemoglobin A_{1c} (HbA_{1c}) of ≥6.5%. In addition, the ADA has recognized a prediabetic state for patients who are

CLINICAL SIGNIFICANCE

Diabetes is a condition wherein the body no longer produces insulin (β-cell dysfunction) or uses insulin efficiently (insulin resistance). Insulin is a hormone that is needed to convert carbohydrates and other food into energy needed for life. The cause of diabetes remains unknown, although genetics and environmental factors, such as obesity and a sedentary lifestyle, seem to play important roles.

Many oral diabetes medications are available with different mechanisms of action. Combination therapy, using medications from different classes to address the deficiencies seen in diabetes, is standard in diabetes care.

Differences in the structures and structure-activity relationships account for the differences in the secretegogues, such as the sulfonylureas and the meglitinides. Both of these classes increase pancreatic insulin secretion, but their structures allow for different binding capacities and adverse effect profiles. Metformin blocks hepatic output of glucose and is a modification of phenformin, which causes a significant amount of lactic acidosis. Thiazolidinediones enhance insulin sensitivity. The initial concern about the hepatoxicity of thiazolidinediones has been relaxed, with few cases being reported with available agents, especially after troglitazone was removed from the market. Differences in the structure-activity of the two remaining agents, pioglitazone and rosiglitazone, may account for the reported difference is adverse events, such as myocardial infarction and impact in lipids.

With the introduction of the incretin mimetics, the first new class of diabetes agents in nearly 20 years is now available. Incretins improve glucose control but also have the potential to improve insulin resistance and to restore β-cell function. Many drugs affecting the incretin system are in development and are all modifications or mimetics of endogenous incretins.

With every new medication being developed and new structure modifications being pursued, there will be more options in our arsenal to treat a disease that is very prevalent and complex.

Nathan A. Painter, PharmD
Assistant Clinical Professor of Pharmacy Practice
Skaggs School of Pharmacy and Pharmaceutical Science
La Jolla, CA

at risk of developing diabetes. The criteria include an FPG of 100 to 125 mg/dL, referred to as impaired fasting glucose, and/or a 2-hour OGTT of 140 to 199 mg/dL (impaired glucose tolerance), and/or an HbA_{1c} of 5.7% to 6.4%. The HbA_{1c} is perhaps the most accurate indicator of glucose because it reflects plasma glucose levels over the previous 2 to 3 months and is now accepted as the ideal standard for assessing glycemic control (17,18).

Epidemiology

Diabetes is a global health problem. More than 220 million people worldwide have diabetes. In 2004, an estimated 3.4 million people died from consequences of high blood sugar, and most of the deaths occurred in low- to middle-income countries. The World Health Organization projects that diabetes deaths will double between 2005 and 2030. The most recent data from the ADA report that 23.5 million children and adults have diabetes (19). The total prevalence includes 5.7 million people who are undiagnosed and does not include the 57 million people who are defined as prediabetics. The ADA also predicts that 1.6 million new cases of diabetes will be diagnosed each year. Relatively few diabetics (~0.2%) are under the age of 20, and approximately 1 in 500 of them has type 1 diabetes. Of the diabetics over the age of 20 (23.5 million), more than half are 60 years or older. There is an almost equal distribution between adult men and women with diabetes (12 million vs. 11.5 million, respectively).

There are race and ethnic differences in the prevalence of diabetes in adults. Figure 27.1 shows that non-Hispanic blacks have the highest prevalence (11.8%), followed closely by Hispanics, which include Cubans, Mexican Americans, and Puerto Ricans (10.4%). The prevalence of diabetes in Asian Americans is 7.5%, whereas non-Hispanic whites have a prevalence of 6.6%.

Diabetes was the seventh leading cause of death in the United States in 2006. Diabetes is not likely to be reported as the cause of death because the cause of death might be listed as being due to one of the many complications associated with diabetes, such as heart disease, hypertension, kidney disease, and nervous system disease. It is most likely that the risk of death for people with diabetes is twice that of people without diabetes (16).

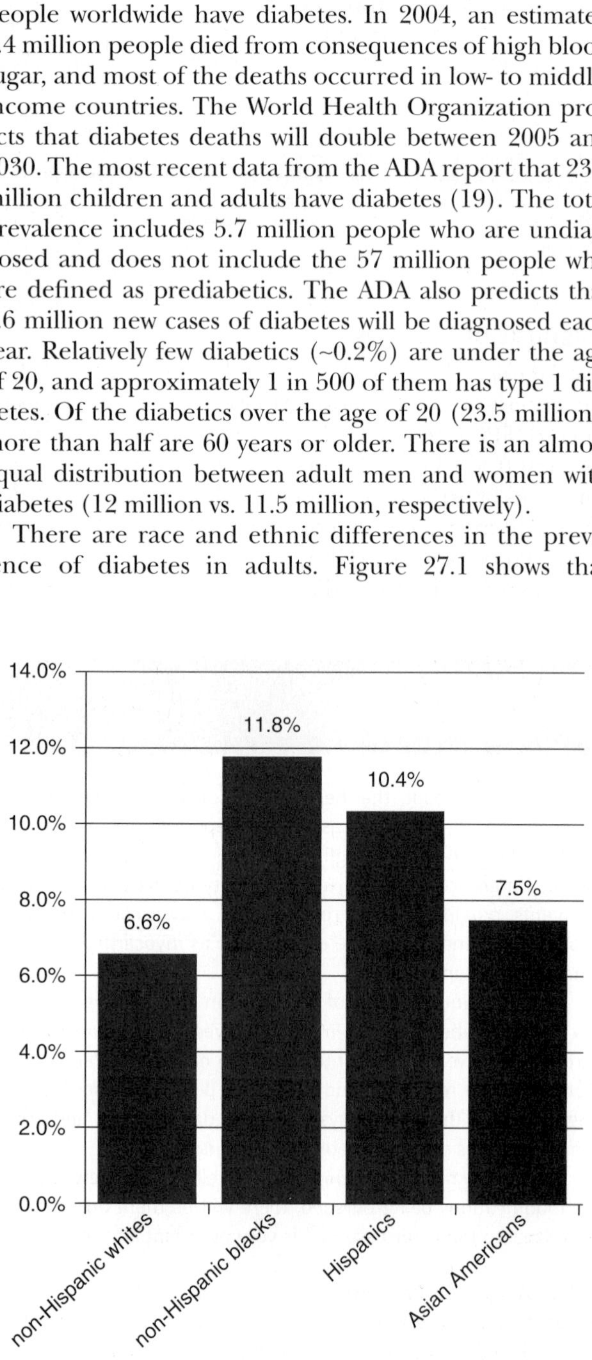

FIGURE 27.1 Prevalence of diabetes in adults by race/ethnicity—United States 2007.

Biochemistry of Diabetes

Regulation of Glucose Homeostasis

Glucose is the primary source of cellular energy, and therefore, plasma glucose concentration is tightly controlled, normally between 65 and 104 mg/dL. Glucose homeostasis is maintained by a number of hormones, the most important being insulin and glucagon. Insulin is secreted by β-cells when blood glucose concentration rises. Insulin reduces blood glucose levels either by inhibition of hepatic glucose production (glycogenolysis and gluconeogenesis) or by increasing glucose uptake into liver, muscle, and fat tissue. Glucagon is secreted by pancreatic α-cells in response to low concentrations of glucose. It acts principally at the liver and antagonizes the effects of insulin by increasing glycogenolysis and gluconeogenesis. In addition to glucagon, cortisol (hydrocortisone) and catecholamines also raise plasma glucose levels.

Other hormones also function in maintaining normal plasma glucose levels. These include amylin (a 37–amino acid peptide), glucagon-like peptide-1 (GLP-1) (a 30–amino acid peptide), and glucose-dependent insulinotropic polypeptide (GIP) (a 42–amino acid peptide). Amylin is actually co-secreted with insulin from β-cells and functions in decreasing gastric emptying, which enhances glucose absorption following a meal. GLP-1 and GIP are incretins, or gut-derived peptides, which have a multitude of effects, the primary of which is to promote the synthesis and secretion of insulin from β-cells (20).

It is surprising that such an essential nutrient as glucose is not freely absorbed from the intestines or by cells that require it for energy. Instead, glucose must be transported across membranes by glucose transporters. The glucose transporters are a family of membrane-bound glycoproteins divided into two main types: sodium-glucose co-transporters (SGLT) and facilitative glucose transporters (GLUT). The SGLT1 type is expressed in the absorptive epithelial cells of the intestines and transports glucose against its concentration gradient. SGLT1 is composed of 664 amino acids arranged into 14-transmembrane helices, and both the N- and C-terminals face the extracellular fluid. The SGLT2 type is expressed in the brush border membrane of the kidney and is the major transporter involved in the reabsorption of glucose from the glomerular filtrate. There are as many as six SGLTs found in a variety of tissues including liver, brain, lung, and heart (21).

In contrast to the SGLTs, the GLUT family of transporters is sodium independent and composed of 12 membrane-spanning α-helices connected through hydrophilic loops with their N- and C-terminals on the cytoplasmic side of the cell membrane. Helices 7, 8, and 11 are believed to form an aqueous pore providing a channel for substrate passage. Mammalian cells have 12 transporters (GLUT1 to GLUT12). GLUT1, GLUT3, and GLUT4 have D-glucose specificity, whereas GLUT2 and GLUT5 have specificity for D-fructose. The GLUT4 transporter is by far the most abundant type, is expressed in adipose and muscle (heart, smooth, and skeletal), and is responsible for insulin-stimulated transport of glucose (22). GLUT4 has been the only insulin-responsive GLUT transporter characterized to date (Fig. 27.2).

When insulin binds to its receptor on sensitive cells, it sets off a complicated cascade of events involving both the phosphatidylinositol-3-kinase and protein kinase Akt or protein kinase B pathways that result in the release of GLUT4 from storage vesicles and its translocation to the cell membrane (Fig. 27.3). The insulin receptor is a transmembrane glycoprotein composed of two α-subunits and two β-subunits linked by disulfide bonds (23). The α-subunits contain the insulin binding site and are located extracellularly. The β-subunits contain tyrosine kinase activity, which is activated by insulin binding–induced autophosphorylation. When insulin binds to the receptor's two α-subunits, it enables a conformational change that allows for adenosine triphosphate (ATP) binding to the β-subunit's intracellular domain. ATP binding activates receptor autophosphorylation, which, in turn, enables the receptor's tyrosine kinase to phosphorylate insulin receptor substrates (IRS). The IRS family of

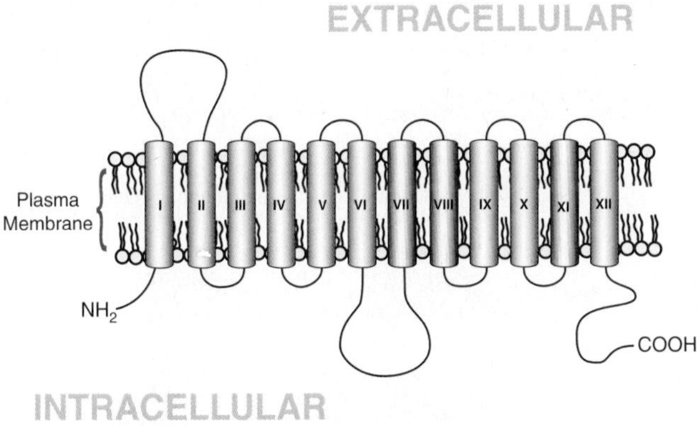

FIGURE 27.2 Schematic representation of the GLUT receptor, showing the membrane-spanning α-helices (1–12). Helices 7, 8, and 11 (*red*) are believed to form the hydrophilic channel, and the extracellular loop between helices 1 and 2 is the location of glycosylation.

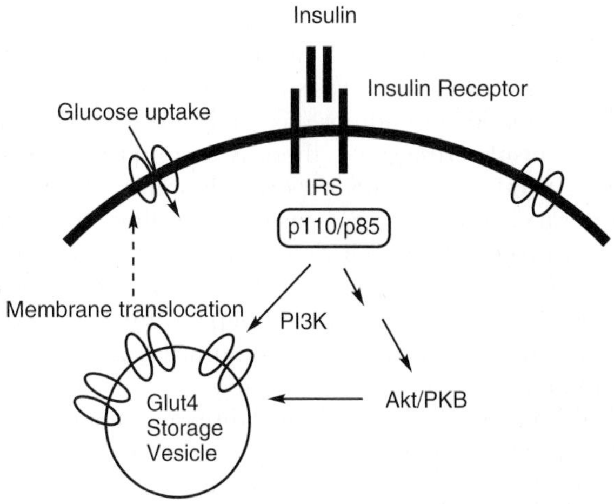

FIGURE 27.3 Overview of insulin signaling pathway leading to translocation of the GLUT4 transporter from storage vesicles. Akt, protein kinase Akt; IRS, insulin receptor substrates; p110, catalytic subunit of PI3K; p85, regulatory subunit of PI3K; PI3K, phosphatidylinositol-3-kinase; PKB, protein kinase B.

proteins consists of four closely related members (IRS-1 to IRS-4) and the related homolog Gab-1. These IRS proteins act as intracellular messengers that begin the cascade of events that result in the translocation of GLUT4 to the cell surface as well as other processes necessary for cell survival (24).

Pathogenesis of Diabetes

Type 1 Diabetes

It is well established that type 1 diabetes results from immunologic destruction of the insulin-producing β-cells of the pancreas. However, abnormal response to external factors can have also a role in disease pathogenesis including damage caused by viruses (e.g., mumps, coxsackie B4, enteroviruses), cytotoxins, and antibodies released from lymphocytes and environmental chemical exposure. It is now understood that type 1 diabetes results from the interplay between genetic susceptibility and certain external triggers such as viruses, environmental toxins (nitrosamines), or foods (e.g., cow's milk proteins, cereals, gluten). Genetic susceptibility to type 1 diabetes is linked to two genes found on chromosome 6. These genes code for the production of human leukocyte antigens (HLAs) DR3 and DR4. Most but not all of patients with type 1 diabetes have both of these antigens. Interestingly, patients who carry HLA-DQA1*0102 or HLA-DQB1*0602 antigens are actually resistant to type 1 diabetes. Type 1 diabetes is characterized by a long preclinical period marked by the presence of immune markers such as circulating antibodies, islet cell antibodies, and insulin autoantibodies. It is not known as to just when the interplay between genetic susceptibility and environmental factors combine to develop the full blown disease with the result in an absolute insulin deficiency (25,26).

Type 2 Diabetes

The pathogenesis of type 2 diabetes is complex but typically begins with insulin resistance at target organs such as liver, muscle, and adipose tissue. In order to compensate for insulin resistance, there is an initial increase in insulin production. This hyperinsulinemic state is only temporary, and over time, insulin secretion diminishes due to progressive β-cell deterioration. The combined effect of insulin resistance and β-cell dysfunction results in a diminished capacity to limit hepatic glucose production and the ability to uptake and utilize glucose in muscle and adipose tissue.

Insulin resistance is a complex disease that typifies the metabolic syndrome and is likely caused by a number of defects along the insulin signaling cascade (27). Other factors include increased concentrations of free fatty acids (FFAs), tumor necrosis factor-α (TNF-α), and the hormone resistin (27). The increase in plasma FFAs produces insulin resistance by inhibiting glucose uptake and its glycolysis in skeletal muscle and also increases hepatic gluconeogenesis. Both TNF-α and resistin are produced by adipose tissue in greater amounts in obese diabetic individuals. TNF-α impairs insulin action, whereas resistin is known to antagonize the effects of insulin.

Increased hepatic glucose production in type 2 diabetes is attributed to both hepatic insulin resistance and increased glucagon levels (28). β-Cells compensate for this insulin resistance by secreting more insulin. The hyperinsulinemic state is only temporary, because β-cells cannot maintain insulin levels required to maintain normal plasma glucose levels. Impaired insulin secretion and increased glucagon contribute to continued hepatic glucose output, resulting in elevated fasting glucose levels. When insulin resistance can no longer be overcome, transition to type 2 diabetes occurs.

Hyperglycemia can be caused by a number of other mechanisms. Some patients have abnormal hormone levels including elevated glucagon, somatostatin, growth hormone, cortisol, and epinephrine. Of special importance for the treatment of diabetes is the effect of certain drugs on plasma glucose levels. Table 27.2 lists drugs that both increase and decrease plasma glucose levels.

Diabetic Complications

All types of diabetics constantly battle to control their chronic hyperglycemia. If high levels of plasma glucose are uncontrolled or poorly controlled, it will result in the development of both acute and chronic pathologies. The short-term effects are usually those symptoms usually associated with type 1 diabetics, such as polydipsia, polyuria, polyphagia, blurred vision, urinary tract infections, weight loss, and fatigue. Although these acute effects are relatively minor, they can lead to two rather serious complications: diabetic ketoacidosis and a hyperosmolar hyperglycemic state.

Diabetic ketoacidosis can be life threatening. Insulin blocks the action of lipases that hydrolyze stored fats to free fatty acids. The diabetic with diminished or no insulin, therefore, has increased free fatty acids, which are oxidized to acetone, acetoacetic acid, and β-hydroxybutyric acid, presumably to make up for lack of glucose for oxidative energy (glycolysis). These keto acids can be metabolized, but in prolonged periods of insulin deficiency, the body cannot keep up with their production,

TABLE 27.2 Drugs that Alter Plasma Glucose Levels

Drugs that Increase Plasma Glucose	Drugs that Decrease Plasma Glucose
Acetazolamide	Alcohol (ethanol)
Birth control pills	Anabolic steroids
Atypical antipsychotics: clozapine; olanzapine, risperidone	ACE inhibitors
β-Adrenergic blockers	Chloramphenicol
Caffeine	Clofibrate
Calcium Channel blockers	Coumadin when coadministered with oral hypoglycemic agents
Clonidine	Gatifloxin
Diuretics: thiazides > loop > K-sparing	MAO inhibitors
Glucocorticoids	Saquinavir
Niacin	
Phenytoin	
Rifampin	
Thyroid hormones	

ACE, angiotensin-converting enzyme; MAO, monoamine oxidase.

and ketoacidosis occurs. Decreased insulin levels also allow for unchecked glucagon activity to increase plasma glucose by gluconeogenesis and glycogenolysis. The lowering of plasma pH by keto acids and hyperglycemia lead to symptoms of ketoacidosis, including vomiting, dehydration, hyperventilation, confusion, and possibly coma and death.

When plasma glucose levels become higher than 600 mg/dL, increased amounts of glucose are excreted in the urine, leading to development of hyperglycemic state characterized by dehydration, hyperosmolarity, and electrolyte imbalance. Symptoms of hyperglycemic state include tachycardia, dry skin, and orthostatic hypotension, which if not treated can lead to death in as many as 30% of those afflicted (20).

The long-term effects of diabetes are serious and often not detected until they become overt. Both microvascular and macrovascular effects occur. The microvascular pathologies involve the retina, renal glomerulus, and peripheral nerves, and as a consequence, diabetes is a leading cause of blindness, end-stage renal disease, and painful neuropathies. The macrovascular effects involve arteries that supply the heart, brain, and lower extremities. Therefore diabetics have a much higher risk of cardiovascular disease, including atherosclerosis, myocardial infarct, stoke, and limb amputation (17).

The essential question now is how does diabetes result in so many diverse microvascular and macrovascular pathologies? The answer centers around four main molecular mechanisms, all related to the diabetic hyperglycemic state and all seemingly related to the overproduction of superoxide by the mitochondrial electron-transport chain. The four biochemical mechanisms are increased polyol pathway flux; increased advanced glycation end-product (AGE) formation; activation of protein kinase C (PKC) isoforms; and increased hexosamine pathway flux (29,30).

The polyol pathway (Fig. 27.4) involves the reduction of aldehydes generated by reactive oxygen species to inactive alcohols, and glucose is reduced to sorbitol by the enzyme aldose reductase. Aldose reductase is a cytosolic oxidoreductase that uses NADPH. The sorbitol produced is oxidized by sorbitol dehydrogenase to fructose using NAD^+ as cofactor. When glucose levels are high, the activation of the polyol pathway can deplete reduced glutathione, leading to cellular oxidative stress. The effect of polyol pathway flux is implicated in the formation of cataracts in the eye as well as development of peripheral neuropathies (31).

Increased levels of AGEs have been found in both retinal blood vessels and renal glomeruli. They arise from intracellular hyperglycemia by the auto-oxidation of glucose to glyoxal and the subsequent formation of 3-deoxyglucosone and dephosphorylation of glyceraldehydes 3-phosphate and dihydroxyacetone phosphate to methylglyoxal (Fig. 27.5). These products are often referred to as dicarbonyls, and they react with protein amino groups of lysine (Lys), arginine (Arg), and the thiol group of cysteine to form AGEs. AGEs damage vascular cells and also alter several cellular functions, including changes in gene expression in endothelial cells and macrophages (32).

Activation of the family of PKC enzymes is brought about by the secondary messenger, diacylglycerol (DAG). In hyperglycemic cells, DAG is increased by de novo synthesis from reduction of dihydroxyacetone phosphate to glycerol-3-phosphate followed by stepwise acylation. PKCs can also be activated indirectly through ligation of AGE receptors and increased activity of the polyol pathway (30). PKC, when increased in cells, is involved in a significant number of biochemical pathways, leading to blood flow abnormalities, vascular permeability and angiogenesis, capillary and vascular occlusion, proinflammatory gene expression, and reactive oxygen species elevation (Table 27.3). Elevated levels of PKCs, primarily the α- and β-isoforms, have been found in the retina and renal glomeruli of diabetic animals as well as in cultured vascular cells (33).

When intracellular glucose levels are in excess, glucose gets shunted into the hexosamine pathway.

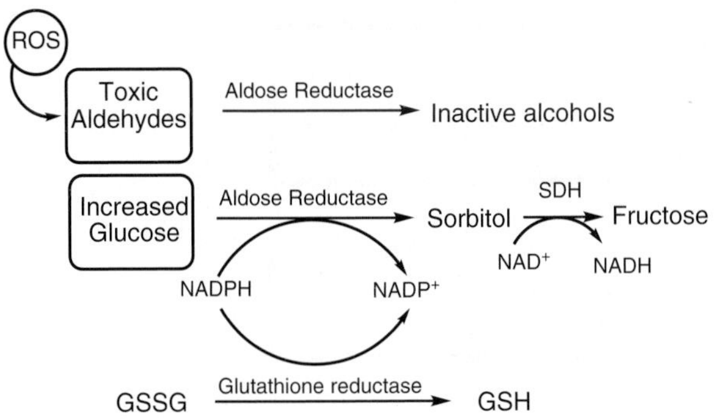

FIGURE 27.4 The polyol pathway showing the role of aldose reductase in reducing toxic aldehydes and glucose to sorbitol. GSH, reduced glutathione; ROS, reactive oxygen species; SHD, sorbitol dehydrogenase.

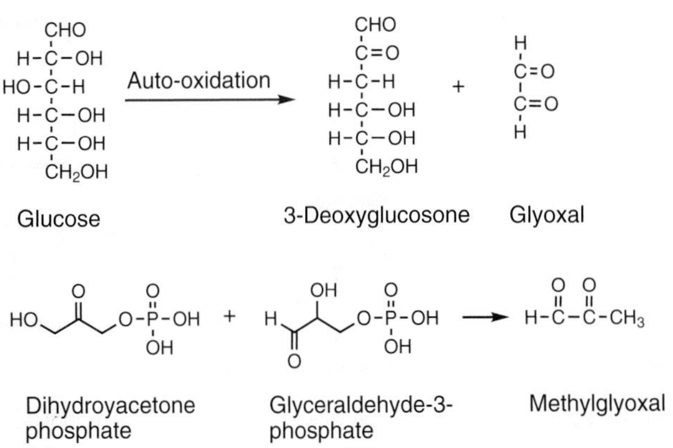

FIGURE 27.5 Formation of advanced glycation end-product precursors: glyoxal, 3-deoxyglucosone, and methylglyoxal.

TABLE 27.3 Pathologic Consequences of Protein Kinase C Activation

Factor Effected	Pathology
↓ Enthodelial nitric oxide synthase (eNOS)	Blood flow abnormalities
↑ Endothelin-1 (ET-1)	Blood flow abnormalities
↑ Vascular endothelial growth factor (VEGF)	Vascular permeability and angiogenesis
↑ Collagen	Capillary occlusion
↑ Fibronectin	Capillary occlusion
↑ Plasminogen activator inhibitor-1 (PAI-1)	↓ Fibrinolysis and vascular occlusion
↑ Nuclear factor κ light-chain enhancer of activated B cells (NF-κB)	Proinflammatory gene expression
↑ NAD(P)H oxidases	Increased reactive oxygen species and multiple effects

In this pathway, fructose-6-phosphate is converted to glucosamine-6-phosphate and then to uridine diphosphate (UDP)–*N*-acetylglucosamine by the rate-limiting enzyme glutamine:fructose-6-phosphate amidotransferase (Fig. 27.6). UDP-*N*-acetylglucosamine is coupled to intracellular protein serine (Ser) and threonine (Thr) residues by *O*-linked *N*-acetylglucosamine transferase. Because both phosphorylation and *O*-linked *N*-acetylglucosamine transferase acylation compete for the same substrates, the two processes can compete for sites. The increased linkage of *N*-acetylglucosamine to Ser and Thr residues on transcription factors leads to alteration in both gene expression and protein function, which together contribute to the pathologies of diabetic complications.

Each of the four different pathogenic mechanisms is activated by a single hyperglycemic event, that is, overproduction of superoxide by the mitochondrial electron transport chain (30). It is now believed that the overproduction of superoxide activates the four pathogenic pathways (Fig. 27.6). Excess superoxide inhibits the glycolytic enzyme glyceraldehyde-3-phosphate dehydrogenase (GAPDH) through its effect on poly(adenosine diphosphate [ADP]-ribose) polymerase (PARP). This inhibition causes intermediate metabolites of the glycolysis to accumulate. Thus, the inhibition of the conversion of glyceraldehyde-3-phosphate to 1,3-diphosphoglycerate results in increased amounts of dihydroxyacetone phosphate, which in turn increases DAG, the intracellular activator of PKC. In addition, the increase in DAG also results in the formation of methylglyoxal, the main precursor to AGEs. Earlier in the glycolytic chain, increased levels of fructose-6-phosphate are shunted into the hexosamine pathway, producing UDP-*N*-acetylglucosamine, which in turn forms *O*-linked glycoproteins that affect transcription. Finally, increased amounts of glucose are diverted through the polyol pathway, which consumes NADPH and depletes glutathione. It was originally thought that superoxide itself directly inhibited GAPDH; however, further investigations revealed that GAPDH is actually

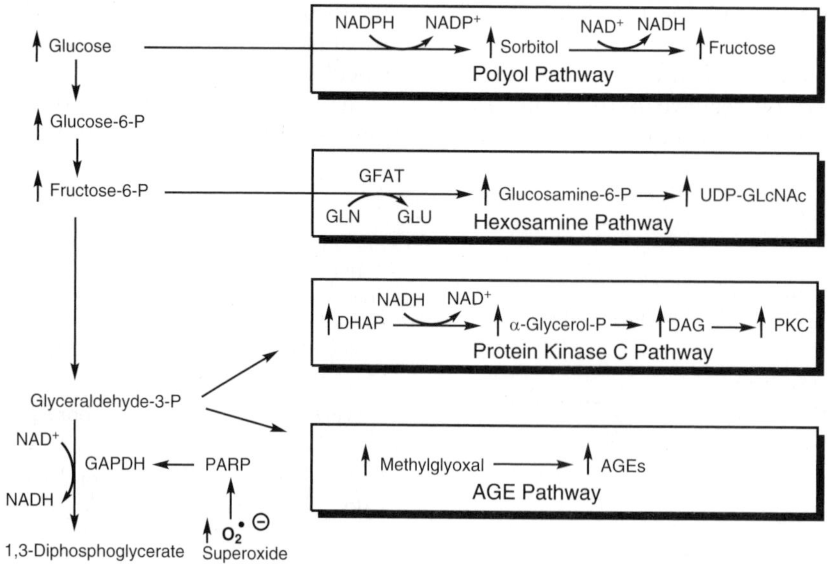

FIGURE 27.6 The role of hyperglycemia-induced mitochondrial excess superoxide in activation of the four pathways involved in diabetic microvascular and macrovascular damage. AGEs, advanced glycation end-products; DAG, diacylglycerol; DHAP, dihydroxyacetone phosphate; GAPDH, glyceraldehyde-3-phosphate dehydrogenase; GFAT, glutamine:fructose-6-phosphate amidotransferase; Gln, glutamine; GLcNAc, *N*-acetylglucosamine; PARP, poly(ADP-ribose)polymerase; PKC, protein kinase C.

inhibited by PARP. PARP is a DNA repair enzyme found in the nucleus. PARP is activated in response to DNA strand breaks caused by superoxide radicals. Once activated, PARP splits NAD^+ into nicotinic acid and ADP-ribose. PARP then makes polymers of ADP-ribose, which accumulate on GAPDH, inhibiting its activity (29,34).

Therapeutic Approaches to the Treatment of Diabetes

Diabetes is a complex chronic disease with no cure. Therefore, therapy is directed at controlling hyperglycemia and reducing the symptoms and morbidities associated with microvascular and macrovascular complications. Early diagnosis and aggressive maintenance of euglycemia (normal blood glucose levels) will go a long way to moderate the microvascular pathologies (35); however, reduction of the risk for macrovascular pathologies requires management of cardiovascular risk factors, such as smoking cessation, treatment for dyslipidemia, control of hypertension, and antiplatelet therapy. The ADA recommends that appropriate medical care for the diabetic requires setting goals for glycemia, as well as for therapeutic lifestyle changes (diet and exercise) along with control of blood pressure, plasma lipids, and the use of appropriate medications (36).

Glycemic control involves two primary techniques, patient self-monitoring and measurement of HbA_{1c}. HbA_{1c} is perhaps the most accurate indicator of glucose because it reflects plasma glucose levels over the previous 2 to 3 months and is now accepted as the gold standard for assessing glycemic control. HbA_{1c} is formed by the glycosylation of hemoglobin's amino terminal valine residue and has a half-life equivalent to that of an erythrocyte. The United Kingdom Prospective Diabetes Study and the Diabetes Control and Complications Trial/Epidemiology of Diabetes Interventions and Complications Study have established that if a patient's HbA_{1c} is maintained below 7%, the development and progression of neuropathy, nephropathy, retinopathy, and cardiovascular disease in type 1 or 2 patients can be significantly decreased (37–39).

Pharmacologic treatment for type 1 diabetics requires intensive insulin therapy. The large number of short- and long-acting insulin analogs allows for the use of multiple doses of basal and prandial (at meals) doses of insulin. Therefore, patients can match their dose of prandial insulin to carbohydrate intake, premeal plasma glucose, and anticipated activity. The most common side effect of the use of insulin is severe hypoglycemia; however, the development of quick-acting and long-acting insulin analogs has moderated this side effect while still maintaining equal HbA_{1c} lowering (36).

Medical treatment of the type 2 diabetic requires management of hyperglycemia as measured by the patient's HbA_{1c} below 7%. Along with lifestyle interventions, the array of different classes of hypoglycemic drugs offers the physician many different treatment options. Obesity and sedentary lifestyle are the major risk factors for diabetes; therefore, weight loss, dietary changes, and increased activity levels should be the initial approach to treating the type 2 diabetic. In fact, morbidly obese patients who have undergone weight-loss surgery and who have maintained at least a 40-pound weight loss have shown elimination of the disease (40). When diet and exercise are insufficient to maintain the patient's HbA_{1c} below 7%, it then becomes necessary to initiate blood glucose–lowering medications. In addition to insulin, there are several classes of oral hypoglycemic agents available. They include the insulin secretagogues (sulfonylureas, meglitinides), biguanides (metformin), insulin sensitizers (glitazones or thiazolidinediones), α-glucosidase inhibitors, GLP-1 analogs, dipeptidyl peptidase-IV (DPP-IV) inhibitors, amylin antagonists, and a number of new drugs in development.

Currently, ADA recommends beginning medication therapy with metformin along with lifestyle interventions (Fig. 27.7). If this therapy fails to maintain or sustain glucose levels, then another medication should be added, usually a sulfonylurea or insulin. Insulin (intermediate or long acting) is indicated for patients who have trouble decreasing their HbA_{1c} level below 8.5%. If lifestyle, metformin, and sulfonylurea or insulin do not result in achievement of target glycemia, the next step is to intensify the insulin therapy. This usually consists of additional injections of a short- or rapid-acting insulin analog given before meals. At this stage, insulin secretagogues (sulfonylureas or meglitinides) should be terminated because they are not considered to be synergistic. Under certain conditions (e.g., patients who have hazardous jobs, allergic to sulfonylureas, promotion of weight loss), the addition of pioglitazone or exenatide to metformin can be considered. The addition of a third medication to metformin/pioglitazone or metformin/exenatide can be considered if target HbA_{1c} is not reached. The use of amylin agonists, α-glucosidase inhibitors, meglitinides, and DPP-IV inhibitors is usually reserved for patients who cannot tolerate the first-line drugs, because these drugs do not have equivalent glucose-lowering ability and are relatively expensive and there are limited clinical data demonstrating effectiveness (41).

Therapeutic Classes of Drugs Used to Treat Diabetes

Insulin

Insulin was isolated in crystalline form by Abel in 1926, only 5 years after it was isolated from the canine pancreas by Banting, Best, Collip, and Macleod. Banting and Macleod received the 1923 Nobel Prize for their work, and Banting announced that he would share his prize with Best; Macleod did the same with Collip. In 1958, Sanger received the Nobel Prize for the determination of the amino acid sequence of insulin, and Hodgkin received the Nobel Prize in 1964 for determining its three-dimensional structure. The development of an immunoassay for insulin by Berson and Yallow in 1960 earned Yallow the Nobel Prize in 1977, after Berson had passed away.

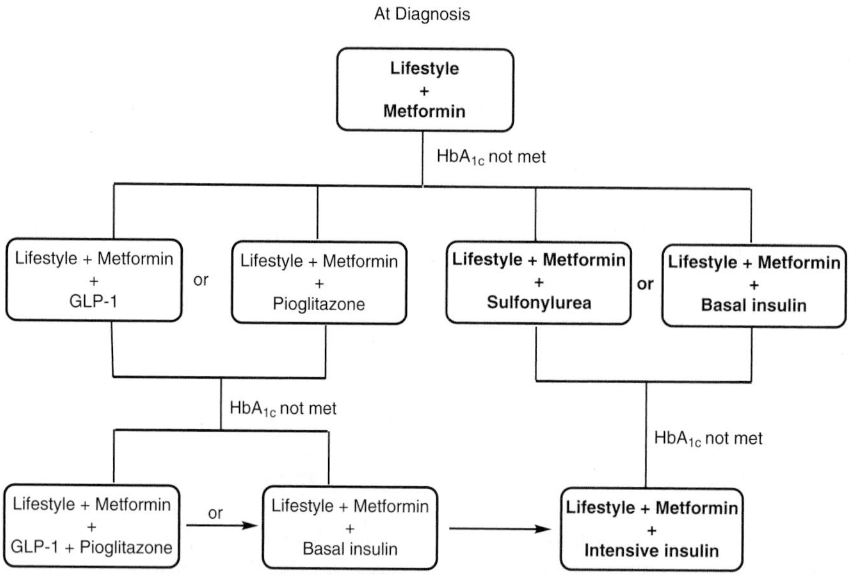

FIGURE 27.7 Decision tree for the management of type 2 diabetes. Lifestyle interventions are reinforced at every step, and HbA_{1c} is recommended to be less than 7%. The path in *red* represents first-line treatment protocols recommended by the consensus of the American Diabetes Association and the European Associations for the Study of Diabetes (41).

Clearly, the awarding of so many Nobel Prizes points to the importance of insulin-related research throughout the 20th century (42).

The insulin molecule is composed of two polypeptide chains (A and B) linked together by two disulfide bonds. There is an additional disulfide bond in chain A. Chain A contains 21 amino acid residues, and chain B has 30 amino acids, giving a molecular weight of 5,734 Daltons. Insulin is biosynthesized in the β-cells of the pancreas from preproinsulin, a 110–amino acid chain with a molecular weight of 12,000 Daltons. Preproinsulin is cleaved in the endoplasmic reticulum, losing a 24–amino acid unit from the N-terminus. The product is called proinsulin (molecular weight = 9,000 Daltons), which folds to allow the disulfide bonds to form and undergoes further proteolytic modification in the Golgi apparatus, losing four basic amino acids (Arg^{B31}, Arg^{B32}, Lys^{A64}, and Arg^{A65}) and releasing connector C-chain by the action of prohormone convertases PC1 and PC2 (Fig. 27.8) (43,44).

The biologically active form of insulin is the monomer. However, in solution, insulin can exist as a dimer and as a hexamer (six monomeric units attached together). The hexamer is formed by its coordination with two zinc ions, the storage form of insulin in the granules of the β-cells. When released from the granules, the hexamer gets diluted in the plasma (nanomolar) and dissociates into monomers. Secretion of insulin is primarily regulated by glucose, but many other nutrients and hormones also have a role. Amino acids, fatty acids, and ketone bodies promote the secretion of insulin. On the other hand, stimulation of the α_2-adrenergic receptors on the β-cells inhibits secretion, whereas β_2-adrenergic receptor stimulation and vagal nerve stimulation enhance the release of insulin. It follows that any physiologic condition that activates the sympathetic system causes a decrease in the secretion of insulin via stimulation of the α_2-adrenergic receptors. Such conditions include exercise, hypothermia, surgery, hypoxia, and of course, hypoglycemia. In addition, α_2-adrenergic receptor antagonists will be expected to increase basal insulin levels and β_2-adrenergic receptor blockers to decrease basal insulin levels (45).

Glucose enters the β-cell facilitated by GLUT2 transport, is phosphorylated to glucose-6-phosphate by a specific isoform of glucokinase, and enters glycolysis ultimately generating ATP. The increase in ATP changes the ratio of ATP to ADP and prevents an ATP-sensitive K^+ channel from functioning, which in turn leads to depolarization of the β-cells. This prompts activation of a voltage-gated calcium channel, and calcium flows into the β-cells. The elevated intracellular calcium concentration causes activation of phospholipases A_2 and C and increased levels of inositol triphosphate, an intracellular second messenger. Inositol triphosphate facilitates additional release of calcium into the cytosol, and concentrations of calcium are now sufficiently high to promote insulin secretion from the β-cells. The ATP-sensitive K^+ channel is an octameric hetero-complex consisting of four pore-forming inwardly rectifying K^+ channel subunits (Kir6.2) and four regulatory sulfonylurea receptor subunits (SUR1). ATP binding to Kir6.2 closes the channel. Binding of sulfonylureas and the meglitinides to SUR1 also closes the channel, whereas binding of ADP to SUR1 opens the channel (46). Therefore sulfonylurea binding to SUR1 causes the same effect as an increase in the ATP/ADP ratio, which is to close the channel leading to the depolarization of the β-cell membrane and the ultimate secretion of insulin (Fig. 27.9).

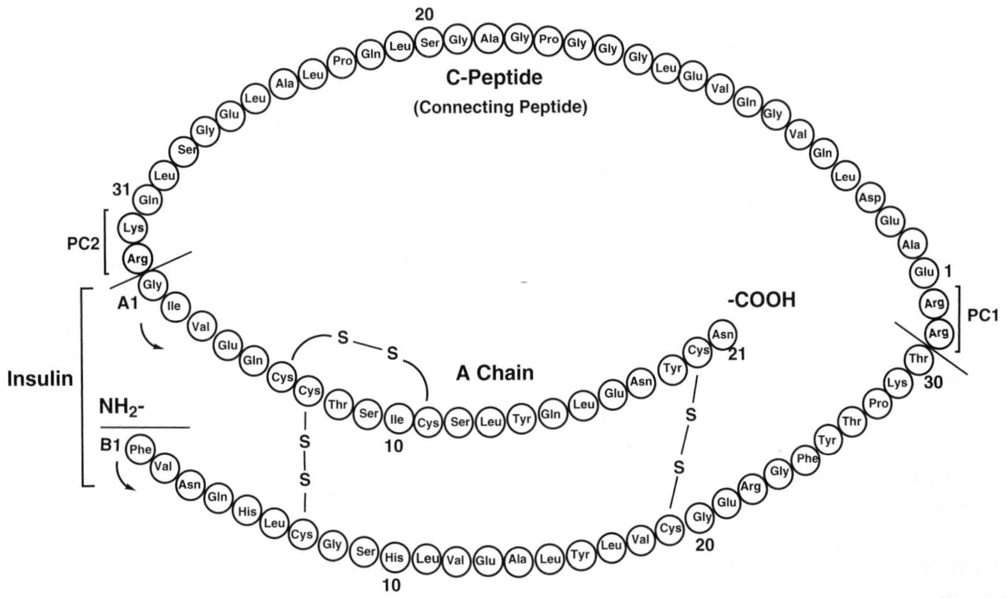

FIGURE 27.8 Schematic structure of proinsulin. Prohormone convertases (PC1 and 2) cleave dipetptides (*red*) to form insulin.

Fifty percent of the insulin secreted from the pancreas is degraded in the liver and never reaches the general circulation. Hepatic degradation of insulin is the result of the action of a thiol metalloproteinase, which can also be involved in the degradation of glucagon. Insulin is internalized into the hepatocyte by receptor-mediated endocytosis and stored along with its receptor in small vesicles termed endosomes. Insulin is filtered by the renal glomeruli to be reabsorbed by the renal tubules, which also degrade it. Insulin is also degraded at the cell surface of insulin-sensitive tissues (45).

The primary target cells for insulin are liver, muscle, and adipocytes. Insulin interacts with amino acid residues of the α-subunit of its receptor via key amino acid residues on both the A and B chains. Table 27.4 shows that the N-terminus and C-terminus of the A and B chains are involved in receptor binding (45). Insulin binding to its receptor activates a series of intracellular events that lead to translocation of the GLUT4 transporter to the cell surface. The details of this process have previously been described (Fig. 27.3).

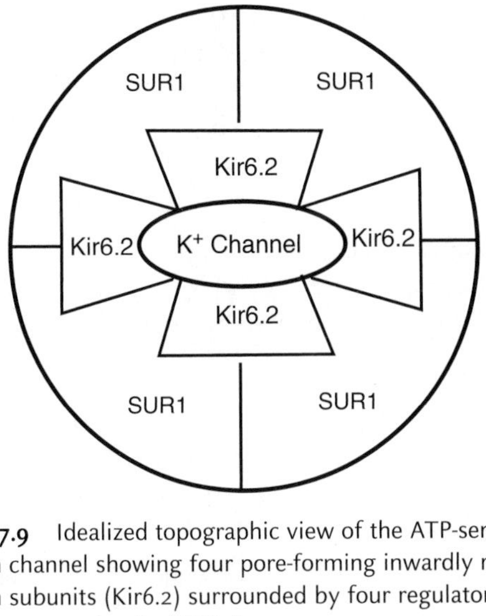

FIGURE 27.9 Idealized topographic view of the ATP-sensitive potassium channel showing four pore-forming inwardly rectifying potassium subunits (Kir6.2) surrounded by four regulatory sulfonylurea receptor subunits (SUR1).

Sources and Stability of Insulin Historically, patients only had the option of administering either bovine-based or porcine-based insulin, which were alternatives to human insulin because their amino acid sequence homology between species was superb. However, animal sources have become less relevant and have fallen into disuse. Today, the following sources of insulin are available: biosynthetic human, semisynthetic human, and analogs of human insulin. Human insulin is the least antigenic of the available insulins and tends to be more soluble than animal insulin. Human insulin and insulin analogs are formed by recombinant DNA techniques carried out by inserting the human or a modified human gene for proinsulin into *Escherichia coli* or yeast. These genetically altered organisms are fermented and produce proinsulin, which is harvested and enzymatically altered to produce insulin. Human insulin is also produced semisynthetically

TABLE 27.4 Amino Acid Interactions with Insulin Receptor

Chain	N-Terminus	C-Terminus
A	Gly A1, Glu A4, Gln A5	Tyr A19, Asn A21
B	Val B12	Tyr B16, Gly B23, Phe B24, Phe B25, Tyr B26

by the enzymatic transpeptidation of pork insulin at position 30 of the B chain with the substitution of the amino acid threonine for alanine (20).

Only the insulin monomer is able to interact with insulin receptors, and native insulin exists as a monomer at low, physiologic concentrations (<0.1 μmol/L). Insulin dimerizes at the higher concentrations (0.6 mmol/L) found in pharmaceutical preparations. At neutral pH in the presence of zinc ions, hexamers will form, the storage form of insulin in β-cells. At concentrations greater than 0.2 mmol/L, hexamers form even in the absence of zinc ions. Changes in the concentration of insulin can profoundly change absorption after subcutaneous administration. The monomer form of insulin is the only absorbable form, so when insulin is administered subcutaneously at concentrations when dimers and hexamers exist, it is absorbed significantly more slowly (43).

The importance of zinc ions for stabilizing insulin preparations has been known since the first reported crystallization of insulin in the presence of zinc ions in 1934. Presently, all pharmaceutical preparations are either solutions of zinc insulin or suspensions of insoluble forms of zinc insulin. A longer-acting and more stable form of insulin is protamine zinc insulin, which is prepared by precipitating insulin in the presence of zinc ions and protamine, a basic protein. This precipitate is known to contain two zinc ions per insulin hexamer. A somewhat shorter-acting and more useful preparation is neutral protamine Hagedorn (NPH) insulin, which includes *m*-cresol as a preservative. Six *m*-cresol molecules occupy cavities in the hexamer involving the B1-B8 helix formed as a result of the presence of the *m*-cresol. Later, it was reported that when small additional amounts of zinc ions were added to hexameric two-zinc insulin in neutral acetate buffer, insulin could be made to crystallize in several forms with varying rates of dissolution in water. Thus, the slowly soluble lente insulin is a two-zinc insulin, and the crystalline, more slowly soluble ultralente insulin is a four-zinc form.

Fibrils (partially unfolded insulin) are a viscous or insoluble insulin precipitate. Shielding of hydrophobic domains is the principal driving force for the aggregation. Further studies revealed that when the exposed hydrophobic domain (A2, A3, B11, and B15) interacts with the normally buried aliphatic residues (A13, B6, B14, and B18) in the hexameric structure, fibrils form. Insulin fibrils do not resuspend on shaking; thus, they are pharmaceutically inactive. Insulin fibril formation is particularly important with the advent of infusion pumps to deliver insulin. In these devices, insulin is exposed to elevated temperatures, the presence of hydrophobic surfaces, and shear forces—all factors that increase insulin's tendency to aggregate. These problems can be overcome if the insulin is prepared with phosphate buffer or other additives. Another physical stability problem associated with insulin is adsorption to tubing and other surfaces. This normally occurs if the insulin concentration is less than 5 IU/mL (0.03 mmol/L), and it can be prevented by adding albumin to the dosage form if a dilute insulin solution must be used (43).

There also are chemical instability issues associated with insulin. For many years, the only rapid-acting form of insulin was a solution of zinc insulin, with pH 2 to 3. If this insulin is stored at 4°C, deamidation of the AsnA21 occurs at a rate of 1% to 2% per month. The C-terminal Asn, under acidic conditions, undergoes cyclization to the anhydride, which in turn reacts with water, leading to deamidation to aspartate. The anhydride also can react with the *N*-terminal phenylalanine of another chain to yield a cross-linked molecule. If insulin is stored at 25°C, the inactive deamidated derivative constitutes 90% of the total insulin protein after 6 months (Fig. 27.10).

If a solution of insulin is stored at neutral pH, a different reaction can occur. Deamidation occurs on the AsnB3, and the products, the aspartate (Asp) and isoaspartate-containing insulins, are equiactive with native insulin (Fig. 27.10). More problematic transformations are possible, including chain cleavage between ThrA8 and SerA9 and covalent cross-linking, either with a second insulin chain or with protamine, if added to the solution. These processes are relatively slow compared to the deamidations, but they have the potential of leading to products that can cause allergic reactions (43).

Types of Insulin The insulin analogs available for treatment of diabetes are classified according to their rate of onset and duration of action. Structure–activity relationship

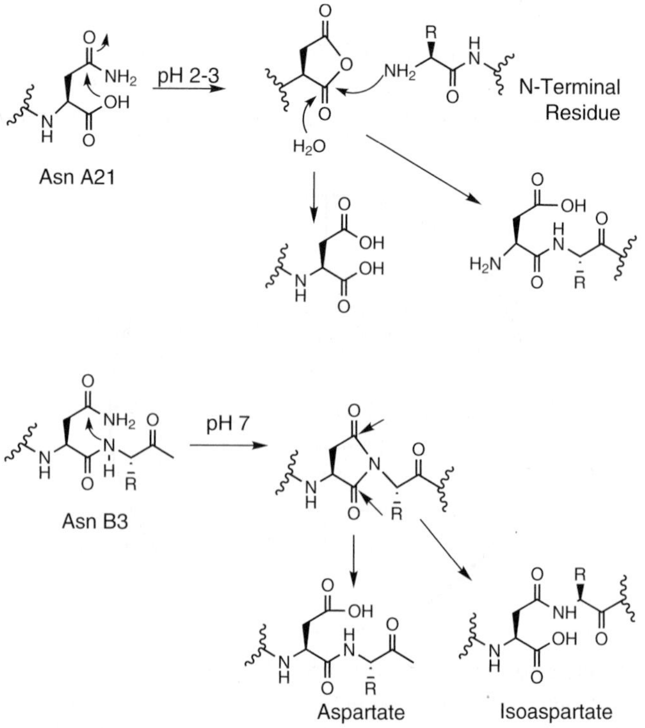

FIGURE 27.10 Chemical degradation of insulin.

studies revealed that variations or removal of amino acid residues from the C-terminus of the B chain could influence the rate of dimer formation while not drastically changing the biologic activity. Inhibiting dimer formation can allow for rapid-acting insulin. Thus, the various insulin analogs that have been developed have substitutions in or additions to the C-terminus of the B chain starting at residue B28. The resulting analogs have either a faster onset or a longer duration of action relative to native insulin. These analogs are all produced by recombinant DNA technology using a modified DNA template. The available insulin preparations are summarized in Table 27.5.

Rapid-acting insulin analogs include insulin lispro, insulin aspart, and insulin glulisine. All have changes made to the amino acid residues in the C-terminus of the B chain (Table 27.6). In insulin lispro, the LysB29 is switched with ProB28, whereas in insulin aspart, the ProB28 has been substituted with an Asp. Glulisine's ValB3 is substituted with a Lys, and LysB29 is changed to a glutamate (Glu). These modifications, as already stated, result in insulin analogs that do not form dimers in solution and that dissociate immediately into monomers, producing a very quick onset of action. Pharmacodynamically, lispro, aspart, and glulisine bind as well to insulin receptors as human insulin and have a low mitogenic potency. Mitogenic activity is the ability of insulin to induce cell division and is believed to be associated with insulin's binding to insulin-like growth factor receptors I and II (47). Lispro, aspart, and glulisine have an onset of action within 15 minutes, peak activity at 30 to 90 minutes, and duration of action of 3 to 4 hours (Table 27.5).

Regular human insulin is the prototype of short-acting insulin. Its onset of action is 30 to 60 minutes, its peak effect 2 to 3 hours after injection, and its duration of action ranges from 4 to 6 hours. Its slow onset requires it to be administered 30 to 60 minutes before meals, which is not convenient, but its slow onset also occurs via intravenous administration, making regular insulin a good choice for intravenous treatment of diabetics.

Intermediate-acting insulin is prepared by adding stoichiometric (equal) amounts of the positively charged polypeptide protamine to regular insulin, forming a poorly soluble insulin–protamine complex. The complex is known as NPH insulin. NPH insulin has an onset of action of 2 to 4 hours, a peak effect of 4 to 12 hours, and a duration of action of 18 to 26 hours after injection. However, most patients receive little effect after 13 to 15 hours (48). Another way to prepare intermediate-acting insulin is to combine regular insulin and zinc in an acetate buffer to form a crystalline complex that dissolves slowly in subcutaneous fluids. This product is termed insulin lente and has a similar onset, peak effect, and duration of action as NPH insulin.

The first long-acting insulin analog to be introduced to the market was insulin glargine. This analog results from the replacement of AsnA21 by glycine (Gly) and the addition of two Arg amino acids to the C-terminus of the B chain (Table 27.6). The resulting analog has an isoelectric point close to 7, but is formulated at an acidic pH 4, where it is completely water soluble. After subcutaneous injection of the acidic solution into tissue at physiologic pH (approximately 7.4), the increase in pH to 7.4 causes the analog to precipitate from solution, forming microcrystals of insulin hexamers, which then slowly dissociate into insulin monomers. The slow dissolution of the hexamer to monomeric insulin from the site of injection results in an onset of 1 to 4 hours, a peak between 5 and 24 hours, and a duration of 20 to 24 hours, which represents a fairly constant release of insulin glargine over 24 hours, giving an almost peakless profile. It has been demonstrated to be comparable or slightly better than NPH insulin at maintaining or reducing HbA_{1c} levels without nocturnal hypoglycemia (43). Insulin ultralente is a long-acting insulin that is a four-zinc acetate crystalline product that has an even slower dissolution rate than the two-zinc acetate insulin lente. Insulin detemir is the newest long-acting analog. This analog results from *N*-acylation of the LysB29 with the 14-carbon myristic acid (Table 27.6). The fatty acid side chain complexes

TABLE 27.5 Classification, Appearance, and Pharmacokinetics of Insulin Preparations

Type	Appearance	Onset (hours)	Peak (hours)	Duration (hours)
Rapid-acting				
Lispro	Clear	<0.25	0.5–1.5	3–4
Aspart	Clear	<0.25	0.5–1.5	3–4
Glulisine	Clear	<0.25	0.5–1.5	3–4
Short-acting				
Human insulin	Clear	0.5–1	2–3	4–6
Intermediate-acting				
Lente	Cloudy	2–4	6–12	18–26
NPH	Cloudy	2–4	4–12	18–26
Long-acting				
Ultralente	Cloudy	4–8	10–30	>36
Glargine	Clear	1–4	5–24	20–24
Detemir	Cloudy	1–4	5–24	20–24

TABLE 27.6 Insulin Analogs

Generic Name	Trade Name	Change in A Chain	Change in B Chain
Lispro	Humalog	None	B28 Pro → Lys B29 Lys → Pro
Aspart	NovoLog	None	B28 Pro → Asp
Glulisine	Apidra	None	B3 Val → Lys B29 Lys → Glu
Glargine	Lantus	A21 Asn → Gly	Add: B31 Arg and B32 Arg
Detemir	Levemir	None	Remove: B30 Thr Add: C14 fatty acid to B29 Lys

with plasma albumin to produce a depot and longer duration of action. It has approximately the same duration of action as insulin glargine, when administered in appropriate doses.

A new long-acting insulin analog currently in phase III clinical trials is insulin degludec. Insulin degludec is an ultra long–acting insulin that can be administered daily or three times a week and is comparable to glargine and detemir in onset and duration of action. Insulin degludec results from the removal of GluB30 and *N*-acylation of LysB29 with L-γ-Glu amidated with hexadecandioic acid. The long duration of action of insulin degludec is believed to be due to the combination of the formation of soluble multihexamer assemblies upon subcutaneous administration, which slowly release monomers, and hexadecandioic acid side chain binding to plasma albumin to produce a depot (49).

An important difference between glargine, ultralente, and detemir is that glargine is a clear solution, whereas the others are cloudy. This can be a problem for patients who rely on the physical appearance of their insulin to distinguish NPH, lente, and ultralente from regular, lispro, aspart, glulisine, or glargine, which are all clear (Table 27.5).

Different types of insulin can be premixed in the same syringe and are usually prescribed for patients needing a simple insulin treatment plan. NPH insulin can be premixed with either aspart or lispro rapid-acting insulins. Mixtures of NPH and lispro can be 50:50 or 75:25, whereas NPH and aspart are available in a 70:30 ratio. A 70:30 NPH/regular insulin premix is also available. The benefit of using premixed insulin is that rapid-acting and long-acting insulin can be administered at the same time and can be given twice a day, usually at breakfast and supper. The drawback of using such a regimen is that to be effective, the amount of carbohydrate to be eaten at each meal is preset. Therefore this works best for patients who can follow strict adherence to a consistent schedule of meals and activity and are able to follow a prescribed diet (49).

Oral Hypoglycemic Agents

The hallmark characteristic of type 2 diabetes is diminished insulin secretion due to impaired β-cell function and/or insulin resistance of peripheral tissues such as liver, adipose, and skeletal muscle, which causes hyperglycemia. The current approach to treatment of type 2 diabetes is to institute lifestyle changes and to initiate therapy with suitable pharmacologic agents (Fig 27.7). The current line of treatment includes: 1) insulin secretagogues, 2) insulin sensitizers, 3) DPP-IV inhibitors, 4) biguanides, 5) α-glucosidase inhibitors, and 6) hormone-related drugs and drugs in development.

Insulin Secretagogues The insulin secretagogues include the sulfonylureas and meglitinides, and both increase insulin release from the pancreas by a common mechanism. Sulfonylureas and meglitinides stimulate insulin secretion by binding to the sulfonylurea receptor (SUR) of the ATP-sensitive K^+ channel on the pancreatic β-cells.

Sulfonylureas The discovery of the ability of the sulfonylureas to lower plasma glucose resulted from research done in 1942 that noted the hypoglycemic effect of sulfonamides used to treat typhoid fever (50). Subsequent investigations revealed that modifying the sulfonamide antibacterial agents with a urea moiety resulted in sulfonylureas with significant hypoglycemic effects, and consequently, the first-generation oral hypoglycemic drugs were born, which include tolbutamide, chlorpropamide, tolazamide, and acetohexamide (Fig. 27.11).

The first-generation sulfonylureas differ structurally in that they have a small lipophilic substituent on the para position of the phenyl ring (R_1 of the pharmacophore) and an alkyl or cyclic lipophilic substituent on the non–sulfonyl-attached urea nitrogen (R_2 of the pharmacophore) as shown in Figure 27.11. However, these structural modifications do little to increase their binding efficiency to the ATP-sensitive K^+ channel, thus requiring relatively high doses to achieve effectiveness and therefore increasing the potential for adverse events. In addition, the plasma half-life of these first-generation sulfonylureas is fairly long (5 to 36 hours), which also increases their potential for adverse effects.

The second-generation sulfonylureas (Fig. 27.11) developed out of research efforts intended to design hypoglycemic agents with increased potency and that possessed a more rapid onset, shorter plasma half-lives, and longer durations of action. Thus, glyburide, glipizide, and glimepiride are 50 to 100 times more active, with plasma half-lives of 1 to 4 hours and durations of action up to 24 hours. This enhancement of activity is the result of the strong binding affinity to the ATP-sensitive K^+ channel associated with the larger *p*-(β-arylcarboxyamidoethyl) group, which replaces the small lipophilic *p*-substituents found in the first-generation agents (Fig. 27.11).

As mentioned previously, the mechanism of action of all the sulfonylureas is to stimulate the release of insulin from β-cells of the pancreas. These cells metabolize

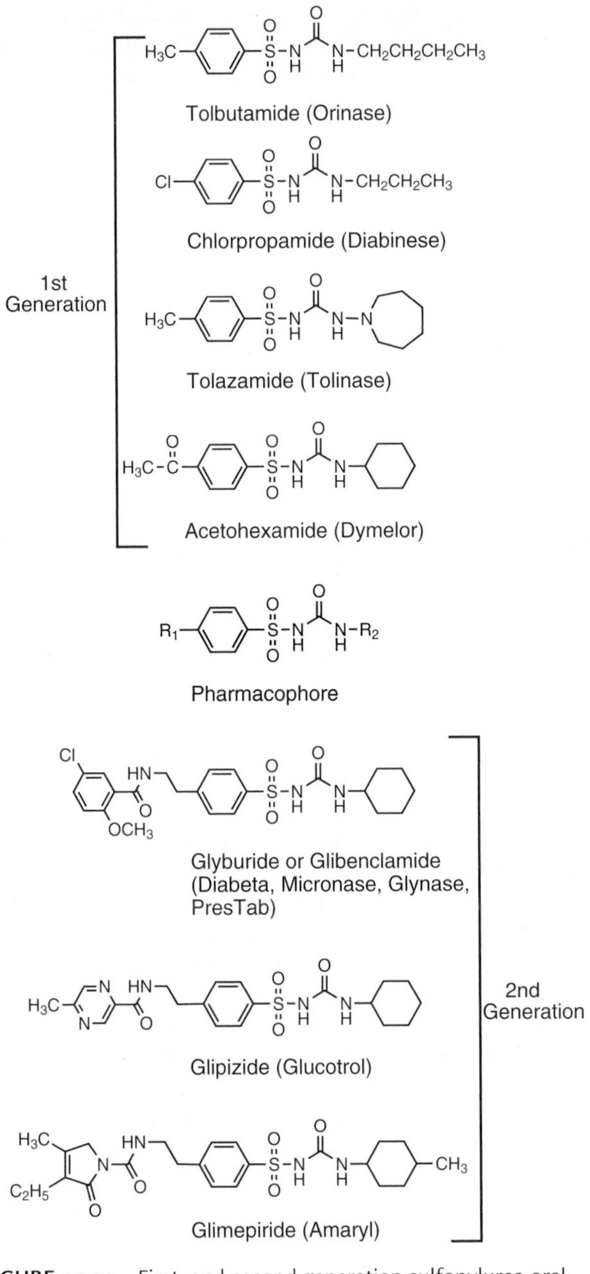

FIGURE 27.11 First- and second-generation sulfonylurea oral hypoglycemics.

glucose in the mitochondria to produce ATP, which increases the intracellular ratio of ATP/ADP, resulting in the closure of the ATP-sensitive K^+ channel on the plasma membrane. Closure of this channel triggers the opening of voltage-sensitive Ca^{2+} channels, leading to rapid influx of Ca^{2+}. Increased intracellular Ca^{2+} causes an alteration in the cytoskeleton and stimulates translocation of insulin-containing granules to the plasma membrane and the exocytotic release of insulin (51).

The ATP-sensitive K^+ channel is an octameric heterocomplex consisting of two units of the binding site for both sulfonylureas and ATP designated as the sulfonylurea receptor type 1 (SUR1) and an inwardly rectifying K^+ channel (Kir6.2) (46). Sulfonylurea binding to the SUR1 causes the same effect as an increase in the ATP/ADP ratio, which is to close the channel leading to the secretion of insulin. The ATP-sensitive K^+ channels are not only found in the plasma membrane of β-cells of the pancreas but also in the vasculature (SUR2B) and the cardiac myocytes (SUR2A). The binding of sulfonylureas to vascular and cardiac SURs, like the binding to the β-cell receptors, has a number of physiologic consequences. In cardiac myocytes, binding to the SUR2B prevents the opening of these channels, which prevents the reduction of Ca^{2+} influx and results in myocardial cell death. In vascular cells, blocking the SUR2B by sulfonylureas increases muscular tone, resulting in decreased flow. Both of these effects are detrimental to the heart during an ischemic attack (52). Furthermore, inhibition of SUR2A in the heart prevents ischemic preconditioning. Ischemic preconditioning results in reducing the size of an infarct and is a protection resulting from repeated ischemic episodes (53).

Meyer et al. (54) have studied the structure–activity relationships of the sulfonylureas for interaction with SUR subtypes. They concluded that the anionic groups (p*Ka* ~5) on these compounds were key to their interaction with the three subtypes of SUR1, SUR2A, and SUR2B. Their selectivity for the SUR1 subtype is due to the lipophilic substituents (cyclohexyl, azepinyl, butyl, propyl) on the non–sulfonyl-attached urea nitrogen. Most interestingly, they found that the *p*-(β-arylcarboxyamidoethyl) groups on the second-generation sulfonylureas, which greatly enhanced binding affinity (54,55), contributed little to their selectivity for the SUR1 subunit.

Sulfonylurea Pharmacokinetics and Metabolism Sulfonylureas are highly protein bound, primarily to albumin, which leads to a large volume of distribution (~0.2 L/kg) (Table 27.7). Food can delay the absorption of these drugs but does not typically affect bioavailability. Metabolism takes place in the liver, and the metabolites are renal excreted.

Chlorpropamide has a considerably longer half-life than the other sulfonylureas and, as a result, has a greater tendency for adverse effects. One explanation for the long half-life is that its metabolism (ω and ω-1 hydroxylation of the propyl group) is slow. A significant amount of the drug (~20%) is excreted unchanged.

In contrast, tolbutamide and tolazamide undergo a more rapid benzylic oxidation, leading to an inactive benzoic acid derivative (Fig. 27.12). An alternative hydroxylation of the aliphatic ring of tolazamide to an active metabolite results in a prolonged duration of action relative to tolbutamide.

The major metabolite of acetohexamide is reduction of the keto group, forming an alcohol. The hydroxy metabolite exhibits 2.5-fold the hypoglycemic activity of the parent molecule. An additional reported metabolite results from hydroxylation of the cyclohexyl group at the 4′-position, leading to inactivity.

TABLE 27.7 Pharmacokinetic Properties of the Sulfonylureas

Drug (sulfonylureas)	Equivalent Dose (mg)	Serum Protein Binding (%)	Half-Life (hours)	Duration (hours)	Renal Excretion (%)
Tolbutamide	1,000	95–97	4.5–6.5	6–12	100
Chlorpropamide	250	88–96	36	Up to 60	80–90
Tolazamide	250	94	7	12–14	85
Acetohexamide	500	65–88	6–8	12–18	60
Glyburide	5	99	1.5–3.0	Up to 24	50
Glipizide	5	92–97	4	Up to 24	68
Glimepiride	2	99	2–3	Up to 24	40

Glipizide and glyburide are extensively metabolized (Fig. 27.13) to less active or inactive metabolites. Glipizide metabolites are excreted primarily in the urine, whereas glyburide metabolites are excreted equally in the urine and bile.

Glimepiride is metabolized in the liver, primarily by CYP2C9, to the active metabolite M-1 (Fig. 27.14), which is then further metabolized to the inactive metabolite M-2.

Meglitinides Meglitinide is the prototype structure that defines this class of insulin secretagogues. It is the benzoic acid derivative of the non-sulfonylurea moiety of glibenclamide [i.e., the *p*-(β-arylcarboxyamidoethyl)] group (Fig. 27.15). These agents exert their effects by inducing closure of the ATP-sensitive K^+ channel found on the plasma membrane of the pancreatic β-cells (56).

Repaglinide is an analog of meglitinide containing additional substituents (*m*-ethoxy, isobutyl and piperidine ring) added to the basic benzoic acid structure. Repaglinide stimulates insulin secretion by binding to three different receptors on the β-cells; one of them is the SUR1, whereas the other two receptors have been identified via Western blots but have yet to be completely characterized (57). Repaglinide is not tissue specific and binds well to SUR1, SUR2A, and SUR2B found on cardiac and smooth muscle cells, therefore conferring extrapancreatic effects in addition to the stimulation of insulin in much the same way as glimepiride (58).

Repaglinide has a rapid onset and short duration of action compared to other hypoglycemic drugs. It is not associated with the prolonged hyperinsulinemia seen with the sulfonylureas, and possibly for this reason, it produces fewer side effects, including weight gain and potentially dangerous hypoglycemia. Repaglinide is at least 5-fold more potent than glyburide on intravenous administration and nearly 10-fold more active on oral administration.

Nateglinide is a phenylalanine analog of meglitinide where the phenyl carboxyl group is transposed to the α-carbon of the ethyl side chain, creating the amino acid functionality. Nateglinide binds selectively to the SUR1 on the β-cells and has a much lower affinity for cardiac and skeletal muscle tissue (59). Nateglinide is a rapidly absorbed insulin secretagogue that has a mechanism of action similar to that of repaglinide, with effects appearing within 20 minutes following oral dosing. Bioavailability is

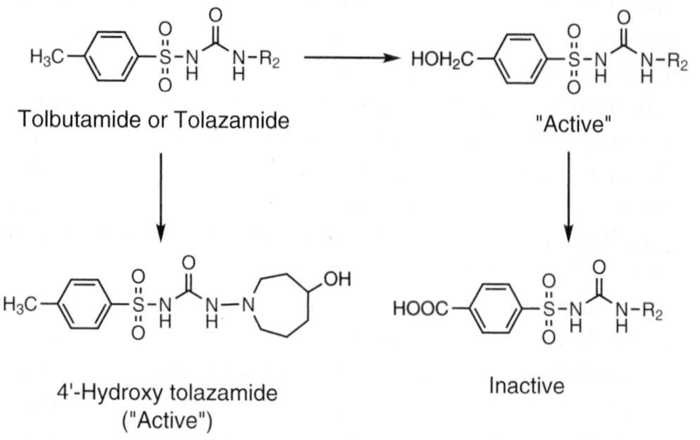

FIGURE 27.12 Metabolism of tolbutamide and tolazamide.

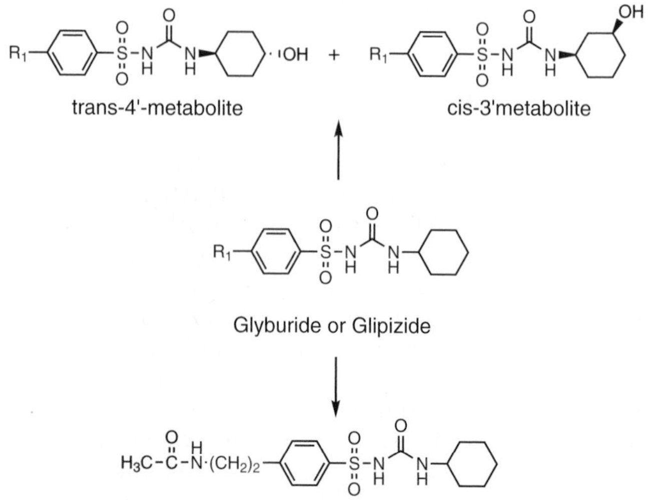

FIGURE 27.13 Metabolism of glyburide and glipizide.

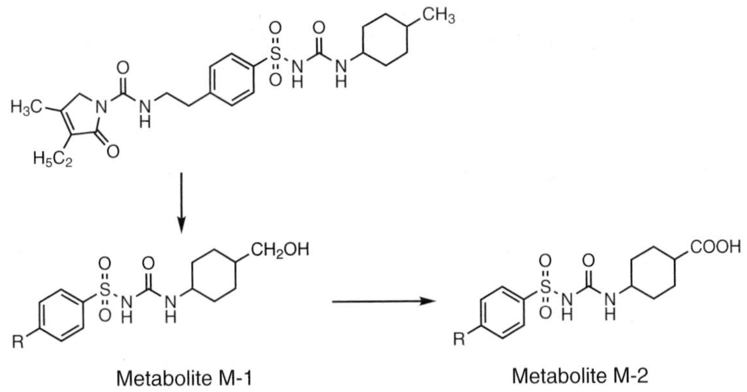

FIGURE 27.14 Metabolism of glimepiride.

73%, and it is 98% protein bound, primarily to albumin. Nateglinide is tissue selective, with low affinity for cardiac and skeletal muscle. It is metabolized in the liver, with 16% excreted in the urine unchanged. The major metabolites are hydroxyl derivatives (CYP2C9, 70%; CYP3A4, 30%) that are further conjugated to glucuronide derivatives (Fig. 27.16). The drug has an elimination half-life of 1.5 hours.

Molecular modeling studies have shown that there is a similar conformation between the sulfonylurea hypoglycemics, glibenclamide and glimepiride, and the meglitinides, which might be important in the interaction of these drugs with the SUR1 on the β-cells. Specifically, these agents display a common U-shape formed by the hydrophobic interaction between the saturated hydrocarbon cyclic moieties, such as cyclohexyl, that are located at the extremity of these molecules and a peptide bond at the bottom of the U. Moreover, the inactive analogs of the meglitinides, including the inactive enantiomer of repaglinide, are unable to adopt this U-shape and thus cannot bind effectively to the SUR1 (60).

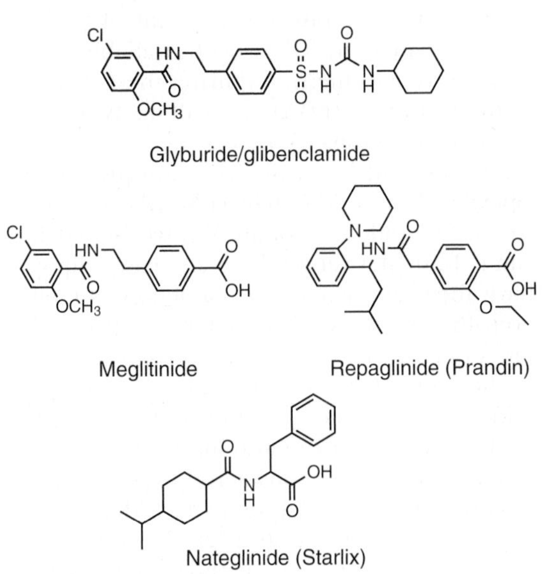

FIGURE 27.15 The meglitinide hypoglycemic agents.

Biguanides Oral hypoglycemic agents from the biguanide chemical class primarily act by reducing hepatic glucose production and by enhancing insulin sensitivity. Although the mechanism of action is not completely understood, biguanides reduce hepatic glucose output by decreasing gluconeogenesis and stimulating glycolysis (61,62). They also increase insulin signaling, which means an increase in insulin receptor activity, as well as metabolic responsiveness by both, the liver and skeletal muscle (61). Unlike the insulin secretagogues, insulin secretion is not directly affected by the biguanides, so they do not cause hypoglycemia. Importantly, biguanides do not induce weight gain, which is very useful for insulin-resistant obese patients (63). They are also considered to have antihypertriglyceridemic effects and to possess vasoprotective properties, which are important actions in treating cardiovascular complications (64). In addition, the biguanides block the breakdown of fatty acids through the activation of AMP-dependent protein kinase.

The use of biguanides can be traced back to medieval times. The plant *Galega officinalis* was not only traditionally used for promoting perspiration during plague epidemics and as a galactagogue (a substance that stimulates lactation) in animals like cows, but it was also prescribed for the relief of intense urination associated with diabetes. *G. officinalis* has several common names, including Goat's rue, French lilac, and Italian fitch. This plant contains active compounds, such as galegine (isoamylene guanidine), that have been shown to have blood glucose–lowering effects (65). The hypoglycemic properties of the plant ultimately led to the synthesis of the biguanide compounds. The biguanides are chemically represented by the linkage of two guanidine groups with different side chains. Despite the toxicity associated with guanidine, the biguanides were shown to exert beneficial effects and quickly became available therapeutic agents for diabetes in the 1950s.

The biguanides (Fig. 27.17) include metformin, phenformin, and buformin. Approved in 1995, metformin is currently the only available biguanide in the United States and is considered to be the first-line treatment for

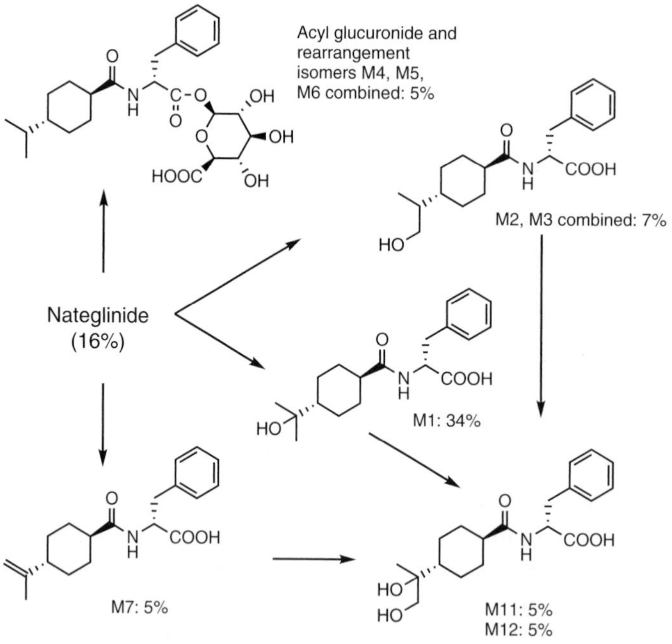

FIGURE 27.16 Urinary metabolites of nateglinide.

type 2 diabetes. It is widely used as monotherapy or in combination with oral agents from the class of sulfonylureas or thiazolidinediones (66).

Metformin makes peripheral muscle tissues more sensitive to insulin for glucose uptake, resulting in the lowering of blood glucose levels. In addition to improving insulin sensitivity in the muscle and liver, it decreases hepatic glucose production by gluconeogenesis, as well as increases oxidative metabolism and even glucose utilization by the intestine through nonoxidative metabolism (64). Metformin can also contribute to the translocation of glucose transporters to the cell surface (65). Although the mechanism of action is not clear, studies provide support showing AMP-dependent protein kinase to be its primary target. Metformin is also useful in treating other types of conditions, such as the insulin resistance experienced by women with polycystic ovary syndrome (67). Side effects include diarrhea, which can be minimized with food intake, mild gastrointestinal distress, and lactic acidosis (68). Metformin is quickly absorbed from the small intestine. Bioavailability is from 50% to 60%, and the drug is not protein bound. Peak plasma concentrations occur at approximately 2 hours. The drug is widely distributed in the body and accumulates in the wall of the small intestine. This depot of drug serves to maintain plasma concentrations. Metformin is excreted in the urine, via tubular excretion, as unmetabolized drug with a half-life of approximately 2 to 5 hours; therefore, renal impairment and hepatic disease are contraindications for the drug. One key drug–drug interaction of note is the competitive inhibition of renal excretion of metformin by cimetidine, which can lead to increased metformin blood levels (43).

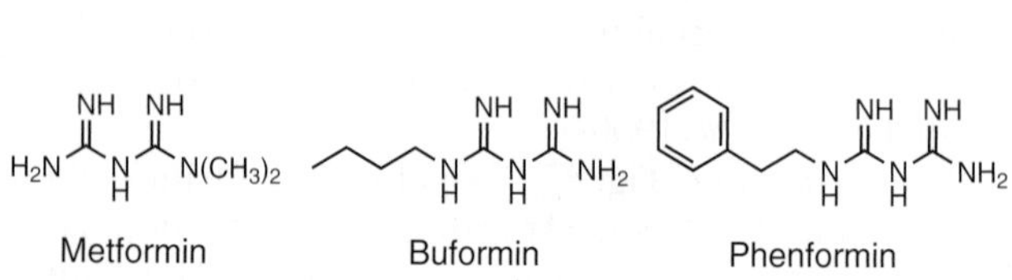

FIGURE 27.17 Chemical structures of the biguanides.

The other two antidiabetic drugs from the biguanide class are phenformin and buformin (Fig. 27.17). Although relatively popular in the 1960s, they were withdrawn from the market in the early 1970s due to toxic lactic acidosis effects and an increased incidence of cardiac mortality. Despite the removal of phenformin from the U.S. market, it has been available illegally as a metformin replacement, requiring the U.S. Food and Drug Administration (FDA) to recall many phenformin-containing medications (69).

Phenformin and buformin are derivatives of metformin. Specifically the addition of a phenyl ring yields phenformin, and the addition of an *N*-butyl side chain yields buformin. Both derivatives have increased lipophilicity and have the same mechanism of action as metformin. However, they both have the major drawback of a high frequency of lactic acidosis in diabetic patients. Lactic acidosis is the result of the accumulation of lactic acid associated with the decreased gluconeogenesis caused by the biguanides. Metformin can also induce such a complication; however, the risk is considered to be minimal when administered at a proper dose. In fact, diabetic subjects taking phenformin are at 10 to 20 times higher risk of developing lactic acidosis than those taking metformin (70). Nevertheless, metformin is not recommended for type 2 diabetic patients who are inclined toward metabolic ketoacidosis due to certain conditions including hepatic disease, heart failure, respiratory disease, hypoxemia, severe infection, alcohol abuse, or renal disease (61).

Insulin Sensitizers (Peroxisome Proliferator–Activated Receptor [PPAR] Agonists) Activators of PPARγ in the treatment of insulin resistance and type 2 diabetes mellitus are a much sought after target, because PPARs are central regulators of lipid, carbohydrate, and inflammatory pathways and help maintain homeostasis (71). They belong to the nuclear hormone receptor superfamily of ligand-activated transcription factors and are closely related to steroid, retinoid, and thyroid hormone receptors. This receptor family is comprised of three members: PPARα, δ, and γ. PPARδ is ubiquitously present in tissues of adult mammals, whereas the α subtype is abundantly present in tissues catalyzing lipid oxidation, which include the liver, kidney, and heart (72). PPARγ is primarily expressed in adipose tissue, where it helps control its differentiation.

The thiazolidinediones (TZDs) are classic examples of PPARγ agonists and are commonly referred to as the "glitazones." These agents were developed when clofibric acid analogs were being screened for antihyperglycemic and lipid-lowering activity. Although initially the mechanism of action of the TZDs was unclear, it was soon discovered that they enhanced adipocyte differentiation by activation of the nuclear hormone receptor superfamily, PPAR (73). A ligand, which can be endogenous, upon binding to PPAR, induces a conformational change in the receptor, thus stabilizing the interaction with the retinoid X receptor and, in turn, resulting in the stimulation of transcription of target genes (74). The endogenous ligands for PPARγ have not been identified; however, studies suggest that certain arachidonic acid metabolites and long-chain unsaturated fatty acids such as linoleic acid are the intrinsic agonists (Fig. 27.18) (75).

PPARγ agonists, such as the glitazones, act by increasing the sensitivity of cells to insulin. The glitazones also decrease both systemic fatty acid production and fatty acid uptake, which contribute to increased sensitization of cells to insulin. Patients with type 2 diabetes are known to have high triglyceride and low high-density lipoprotein levels. The glitazones increase the lipolysis of triglycerides in very low–density lipoproteins and, as a result, increase high-density lipoprotein levels. However, during the lipolysis of very low–density lipoproteins, the production of low-density lipoproteins could be a major drawback to the use of these drugs (76,77).

PPARγ activation improves glucose uptake by skeletal muscle and, at the same time, reduces glucose production by slowing down gluconeogenesis. Hence, these drugs improve metabolism of glucose in not only diabetic patients, but also in obese individuals who have impaired glucose tolerance (71). As mentioned earlier, the first PPARγ agonists to be introduced were the glitazones. The pharmacophore responsible for activity is the thiazolidinedione moiety outlined in red in

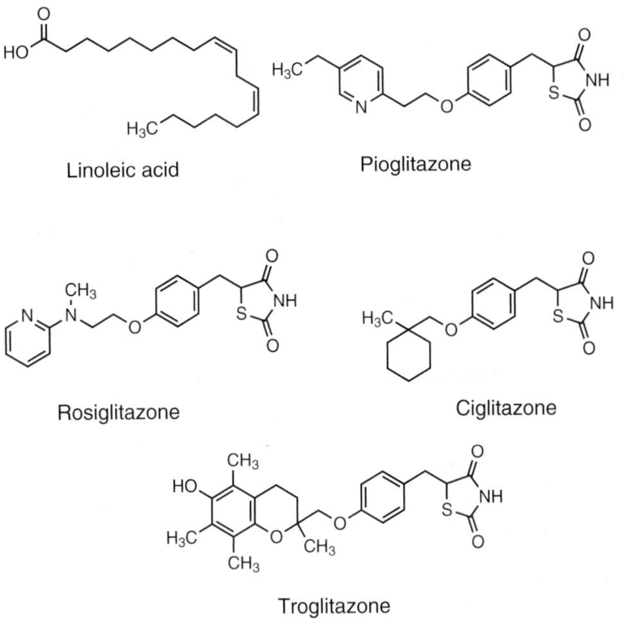

FIGURE 27.18 Linoleic acid and thiaxolidinedione (TDZ) PPARγ agonists (glitazones).

Figure 27.18. A phenyl ring attached to the central nucleus via a methylene group is essential for activity, and in many instances, a saturated linker is found to be more potent than the unsaturated counterpart. The first generation of TZDs includes pioglitazone, rosiglitazone, and ciglitazone. The rationale used for the development of these agents was the fact that the structure of troglitazone (the first drug in this class to be marketed) includes the structure of α-tocopherol, an antioxidant, which retards the oxidation of low-density lipoproteins (78). However, due to severe drug-induced hepatotoxicity and cardiovascular effects, troglitazone and rosiglitazone have been withdrawn, leaving pioglitazone as the only clinically used drug in the TZD family (79). The metabolism of pioglitazone has been studied in rats and dogs and has led to the discovery of up to eight metabolic products. These products result from oxidation at either carbon adjacent to the pyridine ring and are found as various conjugates in the urine and bile (Fig. 27.19). Metabolites M-1, M-2, and M-3 appear to contribute to the biologic activity of pioglitazone (43).

Recently, dual PPARα/γ agonists have become much sought after targets, and many research groups are actively involved in synthesizing such bioactive compounds as novel antidiabetic agents. Combined activation of PPARα and PPARγ is believed to induce complementary and synergistic action on lipid metabolism, insulin sensitivity, and inflammation control, possibly circumventing or reducing the side effects of PPARγ. Cotreatment was shown to improve overall metabolic parameters including free fatty acids, glycemia, and insulin resistance. In addition, edema associated with rosiglitazone treatment was reduced, and a lowering of

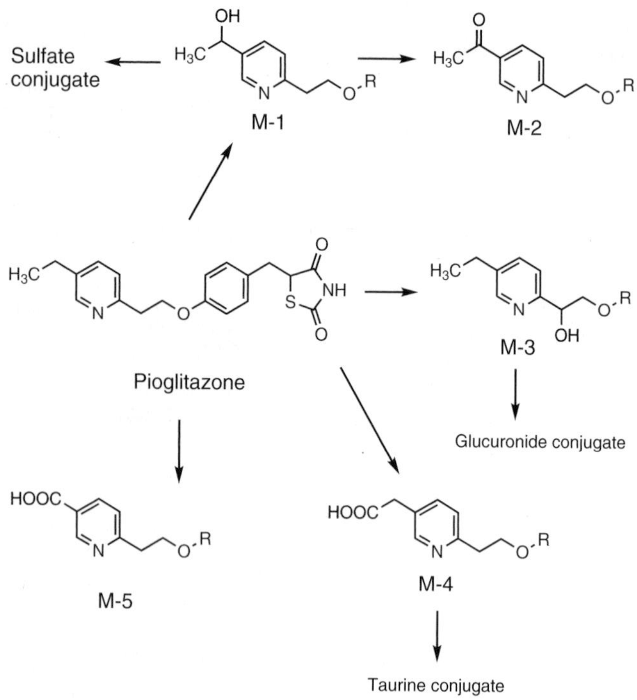

FIGURE 27.19 Metabolic pathway of pioglitazone.

HbA_{1c} levels was more effective than with rosiglitazone used alone. Ragaglitizar and muraglitazar (Fig. 27.20) are examples of dual PPARα/γ agonists; however, the latter was withdrawn from clinical trials due to cardiovascular toxicity (80,81). Several 2,4-thiazolidinedione derivatives of 1,3-benzoxazinone were synthesized and evaluated in the ob/ob mouse model. DRF-2519, the most active analog, is being further developed, due to its equivalence in activity to the existing TZDs and significant improvement in lipid parameters in fat-fed rats, in which it tested better than the fibric acid antihyperlipidemics (82).

α-Glucosidase Inhibitors α-Amylase (EC 3.2.1.1) and α-glucosidase (EC 3.2.1.20) are key enzymes responsible for the metabolism of carbohydrates. The salivary and pancreatic α-amylases are responsible for the breakdown of complex polysaccharides into oligo- and disaccharides, preparing them for intestinal absorption. α-Glucosidase, which consists of maltase, sucrase, isomaltase and glucoamylase, is a membrane-bound enzyme present in the brush border of the small intestine in relatively high concentrations in the proximal part of the jejunum. This enzyme catalyzes the conversion of the disaccharides sucrose and maltose into glucose. The resulting monosaccharides are then absorbed by the enterocytes of the jejunum and enter systemic circulation, as well as various biochemical pathways for the production of energy (83). Thus, inhibiting α-glucosidase will delay the process of carbohydrate absorption in the gut by moving these undigested disaccharides into the distal sections of the small intestine and colon. The result is the prevention of glucose production, thereby reducing postprandial hyperglycemia. All known α-glucosidase inhibitors are excreted unchanged in the feces, obviating metabolic drug interactions (84).

The α-glucosidase inhibitors were first introduced in 1996 with the drug acarbose (Fig. 27.21) (85). Acarbose is an oligosaccharide obtained from *Actinomyces utahensis* and is the drug of choice in this category. It is a competitive inhibitor with a high affinity for sucrase and a lesser affinity for glucoamylase and pancreatic α-amylase in humans (86). When used in monotherapy, there is no risk of hypoglycemia and weight gain, as seen with the first- and second-generation sulfonylureas. However, gastrointestinal irritation, bloating, and flatulence caused by fermentation of undigested sugars in the large bowel by intestinal microflora are some drawbacks common to all α-glucosidase inhibitors (83). These side effects can be minimized to a certain extent by gradual dose titration

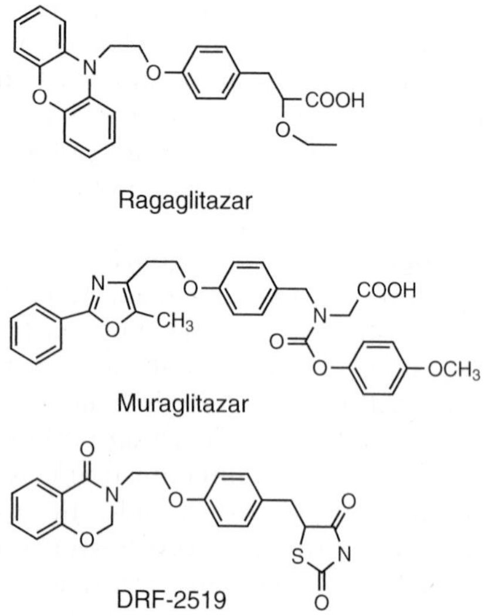

FIGURE 27.20 Examples of dual PPARα/γ agonists.

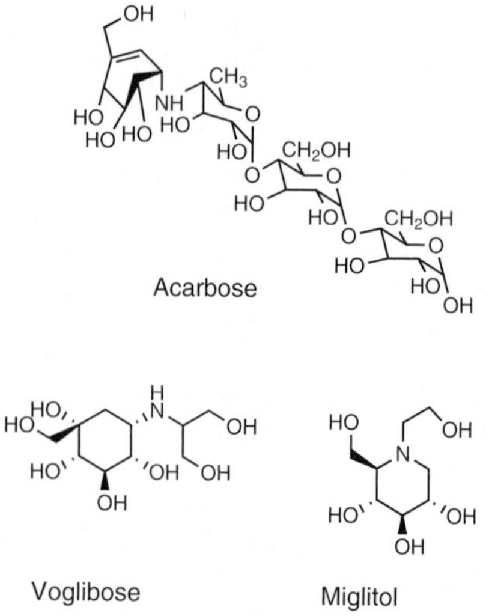

FIGURE 27.21 Clinically useful α-glucosidase inhibitors.

and the right combination therapy with other orally active hypoglycemic drugs.

Voglibose and miglitol are other α-glucosidase inhibitors in clinical use in the management of diabetes. α-Glucosidase inhibitors reduce postprandial hyperglycemia to a lesser extent as compared to other oral antidiabetic agents, and clinical trials with acarbose have shown that the reduction in HbA_{1c} levels is 0.5% to 1% when compared to placebo (85). Therefore, these agents are seldom used as monotherapy and frequently find use in combination therapy especially with sulfonylureas (86). Apart from their use in diabetes, their use can be extended to the treatment of glycosphingolipid lysosomal storage disease, HIV infections, and certain tumors (87,88).

A number of iminosugars isolated from plants were found to have potent α-glucosidase inhibitory activity. The presence of polyhydroxy groups on these compounds is critical for α-glucosidase inhibition activity, because most mimic the natural substrates maltose and sucrose (87). A polyhydroxy piperidine compound, nojirimycin (Fig. 27.22), isolated from *Bacillus* species, was the first compound representative of this family. Research modifying the structure of iminosugars yielded the most potent compound 1-deoxynojirimycin, which is now clinically used in the treatment of Gaucher syndrome (87).

Naturally occurring compounds from different chemical classes have been identified to have α-glucosidase inhibitory activity. Genistein (Fig. 27.22) is a potent isoflavone isolated from soy fermentation broths of *Streptomyces* species and has been demonstrated to be a reversible, noncompetitive α-glucosidase inhibitor (89).

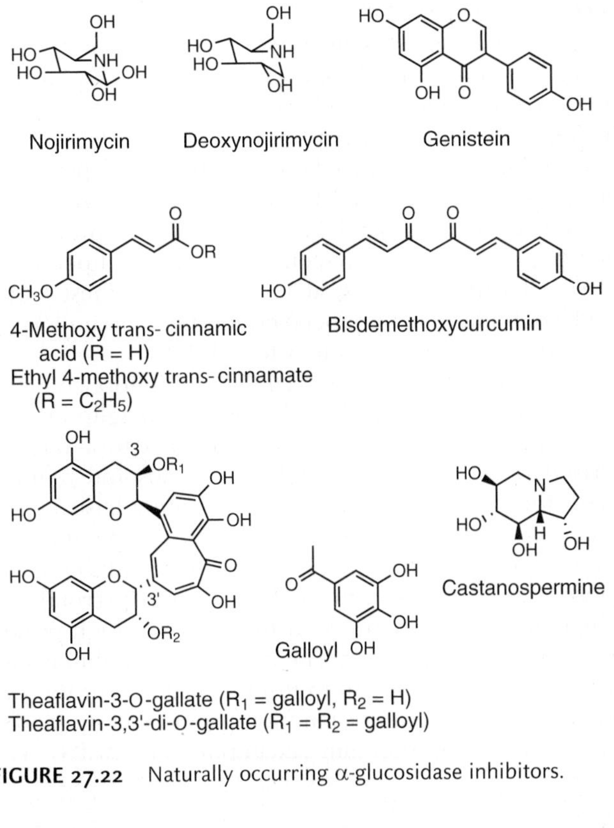

FIGURE 27.22 Naturally occurring α-glucosidase inhibitors.

Some cinnamic acid analogs of particular interest have been isolated from the rhizomes of *Kaempferia galangal*. A 4-methoxy-transcinnamic acid and its corresponding ethyl ester are inhibitors of maltase (K_i = 0.05 mmol/L) (Fig. 27.22). Both of these methoxy derivatives of cinnamic acid showed improved enzyme inhibitory activity, but replacing the electron-rich hydroxy groups on the molecule or introduction of an electron-withdrawing nitro group renders them inactive (90). Closely related to the cinnamic acids is the noncompetitive inhibitor bisdemethoxycurcumin (Fig. 27.22), isolated from rhizomes of *Curcuma longa*, which was found to be twice as active as the clinically used pseudotetrasaccharide acarbose (91).

Green tea, which is an excellent source of polyphenols such as flavonoids, catechins, and theaflavins, has been studied extensively in the control of blood glucose by inhibition of the carbohydrate-metabolizing enzymes. Among the theaflavin derivatives, 3-*O*-gallate and its 3,3′ di-*O*-gallate analog are potent inhibitors of rat and porcine intestinal maltase (92) (Fig. 27.22).

The alkaloid castanospermine (Fig. 27.22), an indolizine that closely resembles 1-deoxynojirimycin, was isolated from the seeds of *Castanospermum australe*. This has been one of the few isolated compounds that, in addition to its α- and β-glucosidase–inhibiting properties, inhibits β-glucocerebrosidase and viral replication of HIV (87).

Although there are few α-glucosidase inhibitors that have been approved by the FDA, current literature shows an increasing awareness in the field of these carbohydrate-metabolizing enzyme inhibitors, which can lead to novel α-glucosidase inhibitors in the near future.

GLP-1 Agonists and DPP-IV Inhibitors GLP-1 is a 36–amino acid peptide secreted by L-cells of the gut in response to a meal. It exerts control over glucose levels by promoting insulin secretion in a glucose-dependent manner (93). The role of GLP-1 was first proposed based on the observation that the amount of insulin secreted following an oral glucose dose exceeded that of an equivalent glucose dose administered intravenously in both diabetic and nondiabetic individuals (94). This observation was termed the incretin effect and is the result of two gut hormones, GLP-1 and GIP (95). GLP-1 secretion from L-cells is similar to that of glucose-induced insulin secretion from pancreatic β-cells. Metabolism of glucose in the intestinal L-cells leads to closure of ATP-linked potassium (K^+) channels, resulting in depolarization of the membrane and entry of Ca^{2+}, which leads to the secretion of GLP-1 (96). GLP-1 is rapidly metabolized, with a half-life of 1 to 2 minutes, by an aminopeptidase enzyme, DPP-IV, yielding an inactive peptide that is two amino acids shorter (97,98). It follows, therefore, that GLP-1 agonists or DDP-IV inhibitors would be effective agents to control blood glucose levels in diabetic patients.

GLP-1 Analogs GLP-1 is deactivated by DPP-IV, which removes a dipeptide from the N-terminus. One of the principal reasons why GLP-1 is so susceptible to DPP-IV is because it contains an alanine in the penultimate N-terminal position. Substitution in this position should result in analogs with increased stability. Indeed, substitution of the Ala with Thr (half-life = 197 minutes), Gly (half-life = 159 minutes), Ser (half-life = 174 minutes), or α-aminoisobutyric acid each gives analogs that are more stable in vitro than GLP-1 (half-life = 28 minutes) under the same conditions (99). In fact, the α-aminoisobutyric acid analog exhibited no degradation even after 6 hours. While such analogs are found to be more stable to DPP-IV in vitro, the in vivo half-life is increased only from 1 to 2 to 3 to 4 minutes, and this is attributed to rapid elimination by the kidneys. Interestingly, these analogs still retained binding affinity to the GLP-1 receptor, with the α-aminoisobutyric analog almost twice as potent as GLP-1. More useful in vivo analogs, therefore, require both DPP-IV resistance and decreased renal elimination.

This was achieved with the introduction of the GLP-1 analog exenatide as a parenteral therapy into the market in April 2005. Exenatide is a 39–amino acid peptide analog of GLP-1, isolated from the saliva of the Gila monster (*Heloderma suspectum*), that is resistant to the action of DPP-IV and is a GLP-1 receptor agonist. It has a glycine instead of alanine in the penultimate N-terminal position, is 53% homologous to human GLP-1, and has an in vivo half-life of approximately 3 hours.

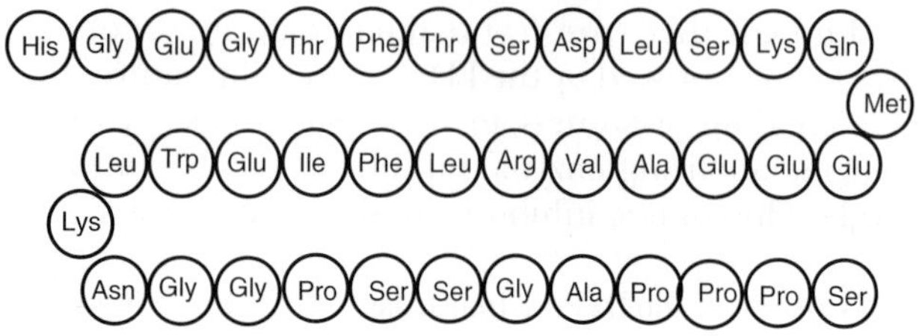

Exenatide (Byetta)

Exenatide has been shown to reduce HbA_{1c} levels in sulfonylurea-treated patients with type 2 diabetes and is associated with weight loss (100). This weight loss is probably due to a decrease in appetite. In *db/db* mice, it increased β-cell mass and delayed the onset of diabetes, so it can even have a prophylactic use (101).

Several other DPP-IV–resistant GLP-1 analogs are currently undergoing human clinical trials. The most promising was liraglutide (102). Liraglutide, which represents amino acid residues 7 to 37 of GLP-1, was developed from a series of acylated GLP-1(7-37) derivatives. Several positions of GLP-1 were substituted with different acyl moieties ranging in length from 12 to 18 carbons. However, the C16 derivative, α-L-glutamoyl-(*N*-α-hexadecanoyl)-$Lys^{26}Arg^{34}$-GLP-1 (liraglutide) was found to have the best combination of albumin binding to retard renal elimination and resistance to DPP-IV degradation due to the replacement of Lys34 with Arg (103,104). This analog of GLP-1(7-37) has multiple actions in addition to reduction of hyperglycemia, including, suppression of inappropriate glucagon secretion, slowing of gastric emptying, and enhancement of β-cell function and mass (105). Liraglutide was approved for marketing under the name Victoza by the FDA in 2010; however, due to a possible link to the production of thyroid C-cell tumors, the product label has a Black Box Warning with the recommendation that it be used only in patients for whom the potential benefits outweigh the potential risk (106).

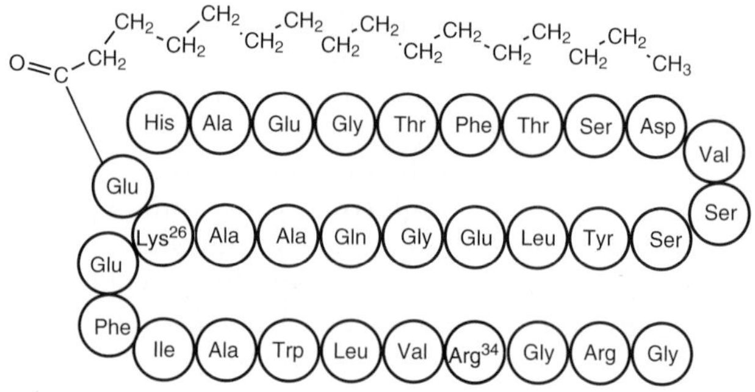

Liraglutide (Victoza)

The major problem with GLP-1 analogs is their need for subcutaneous administration, which can limit patient compliance. Also, GLP-1 analogs, as with any peptide drug, have the potential to be immunogenic. Therefore, this stimulated the search for small-molecule inhibitors of DPP-IV.

DPP-IV Inhibitors DPP-IV (EC 3.4.14.5) is a serine protease that exists as both a membrane-bound and a plasma-soluble form. It is a proline-specific aminopeptidase responsible for the degradation of a number of biologically important peptides other than GLP-1 and GIP. DPP-IV belongs to a family of dipeptidyl peptidase enzymes, including DPP-VI to DPP-IX, DPP-X, fibroblast protein-a, acylaminoacyl carboxypeptidase, prolyl carboxypeptidase, and quiescent cell proline dipeptidase (107). Because the clinical importance of these other prolyl peptidases has not been established, it is important that inhibitors have specificity for DPP-IV.

There are currently four DPP-IV inhibitors commercially available: sitagliptin, vildagliptin, linagliptin, and saxagliptin. The development of many structural variants has led to the knowledge that there is an absolute requirement for all DPP-IV inhibitors to contain a basic amino function in the position equivalent to the penultimate amino acid (alanine) in GLP-1. Most active inhibitors are therefore peptide derivatives of α-aminoacylpyrrolidines, which also takes advantage of the enzyme's high preference for proline binding. The most active inhibitors also have an electrophilic group in the 2-position of the pyrrolidine ring. The most common group is cyano and is present in vildagliptin and saxagliptin (Fig. 27.23). The

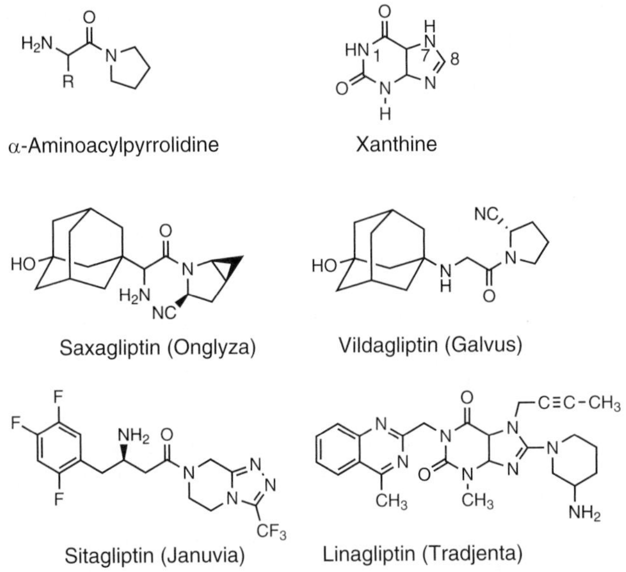

FIGURE 27.23 α-Aminoacylpyrrolidine/thiazolidine pharmacophore and currently available DPP-IV inhibitors.

cyano group forms a covalent imidate adduct with the active site Ser[630] to irreversibly inactivate it. Sitagliptin has a piperazine ring fused to a pyrazole in place of the pyrrole ring but still contains the α-amino acyl moiety and the amide bond. Recently, linagliptin, a novel xanthine-derived, potent, and selective DPP-IV inhibitor, has been developed (Fig. 27.23). It contains an N-1 quinazoline, a C-8 aminopiperidine, and an N-7 butynyl substiutent, all of which play an important role in binding to the enzyme active site. The primary amine of the C-8 aminopiperidine occupies the recognition site for the amino terminus of peptide substrates for DPP-IV and hydrogen bonds to Glu[205], Glu[206], and Tyr[662]. The butynyl substituent occupies a hydrophobic pocket, and the xanthine scaffold is positioned above Tyr[547] and held in place via π-stacking aromatic interactions with the phenol of the Tyr[547]. The C-6 xanthine carbonyl hydrogen bonds with the backbone NH of Tyr[631], and the quinazoline moiety at N-1 interacts by π-stacking with the aromatic ring of Trp[629] on a hydrophobic surface area of the protein (108,109).

Sitagliptin was approved by the FDA in 2006 for monotherapy or in combination with metformin, TZDs, or sulfonylureas for treatment of type 2 diabetes. Sitagliptin has a good oral bioavailability of 87% with no effect from food. It is protein bound only to about 37%, and 80% is excreted unchanged in the urine. It is important to have high specificity for DPP-IV, as inhibition of DPP-8 and DPP-9 has been shown to cause severe toxicity in animal studies. The selectivity of sitagliptin for DPP-IV compared to DPP-VIII and DPP-IX is greater than 2,600-fold. Sitagliptin has no effect on glucose levels in healthy patients; however, it reduces HbA_{1c} about 0.6%R to 0.9% in type 2 diabetics. Sitagliptin has a number of side effects including upper respiratory tract infection, nasopharyngitis, and headache. Patients experience nausea when sitagliptin is taken with metformin, leg swelling when taken with TZDs, and hypoglycemia when administered with a sulfonylurea. There have also been reports of anaphylaxis, angioedema, and rashes, although a causal link has not been established (110).

Vildagliptin was approved in 2008 by the European Medicines Agency for use in the European Union, but the manufacturer has withdrawn its intent to submit it for FDA approval because the FDA demanded additional clinical data assuring that skin lesions and kidney impairment seen in animal studies were not seen in humans. In phase III clinical trials, vildagliptin showed good oral bioavailability of 85% and low protein binding (9.3%), and was 21% excreted unchanged in the urine. It has a high specificity for DPP-IV compared to DPP-VIII and DPP-IX of 32- to 250-fold. In clinical trials, no patients discontinued medication due to adverse effects, which are similar to sitagliptin (i.e., upper respiratory tract infections, diarrhea, nausea, and hypoglycemia) (110).

The FDA approved saxagliptin in 2009. It is 10 times more potent an inhibitor of DPP-IV than either vildagliptin or sitagliptin. It shows a higher specificity for DPP-IV compared to DPP-VIII and DPP-IX (400- and 75-fold, respectively). Trials using doses of 2.5 to 10 mg have shown reductions of HbA_{1c} of 0.5% to 0.8%, with no significant weight gain. Saxagliptin was well tolerated, with side effects equivalent to placebo and a very low incidence of hypoglycemia (110).

Linagliptin was approved by the FDA in 2011 as an oral treatment for type 2 diabetes either as a stand-alone medication or in combination with other therapies. Linagliptin should not be prescribed for patients with type 1 diabetes or those who have diabetic ketoacidosis. Its most common adverse effects are upper respiratory tract infection, stuffy or runny nose, sore throat, muscle pain, and headache. Linagliptin has high selectivity for DPP-IV versus the related enzymes DPP-VIII and DPP-IX and inhibits plasma DPP-IV activity by more than 80% over 24 hours. Linagliptin binds extensively to plasma proteins and is not significantly metabolized, with approximately 85% excreted unchanged via the feces (111).

Amylin Agonists Amylin is a hormone that consists of a single chain of 37 amino acids and is released from pancreatic β-cells, co-secreted with insulin, and primarily involved in controlling postprandial glucose levels. Amylin, like insulin, shows similar fasting and postprandial patterns in healthy individuals by a variety of mechanisms, including delayed gastric emptying and suppression of glucagon secretion (not normalized by insulin alone), which leads to a suppression of endogenous glucose output from the liver (112). Amylin also regulates food intake by modulating the appetite center of the brain. The observation that amylin was deficient in both type 1 and type 2 diabetics stimulated research and development of amylin analogs that would be able to control postprandial glucose levels by 1) modulation of gastric emptying, 2) prevention of postprandial rise in glucagon, and 3) inhibition of caloric intake and potential weight gain. Amylin itself is unsuitable as a drug because it aggregates and is insoluble in solution, which encouraged development of chemical analogs (113).

Pramlintide is a chemical analog of amylin given enhanced water solubility and reduced aggregation liability by replacing the Ala^{25}, Ser^{28}, and Ser^{29} of the amylin peptide chain with prolines (114). The subcutaneous administration of 15 mcg of the drug shows optimum peak effect within 20 minutes, thus permitting the drug to be used before meals. Pramlintide has a duration of action of 150 minutes, no significant accumulation liability with repetitive administration, and a renal clearance rate of 1 to 2 L/min. The drug is primarily metabolized in the kidneys, with an elimination half-life of 30 to 50 minutes. Pramlintide is used together with insulin for those who are unable to achieve their target postprandial blood sugar levels on insulin alone (115,116). Pramlintide delays gastric emptying, suppresses glucagon release, and has a central nervous system anorectic effect via unknown mechanisms. The nucleus accumbens and dorsal vagal complex of the brain have been shown to contain the amylin receptor, which can be involved in the central effects of this hormone. Because of the wide differences between the pH of pramlintide and insulin products (4.0 vs. 7.8, respectively), concurrent mixing within the same syringe is not recommended. To avoid severe hypoglycemia with initial drug titration, only short or rapid insulin dosage forms should be used together with pramlintide. In this case, the dose of insulin should be reduced by 50% (117).

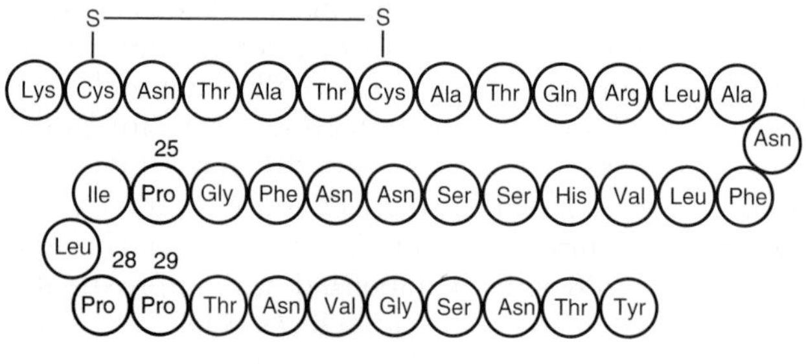

Pramlintide (Symlin)

Drugs in Development

Considering the medical and economic importance of type 2 diabetes and the need for improvement over existing treatments, new agents for existing targets and the development of new therapeutic targets are being actively pursued in the laboratory and the clinic. Many promising targets are only in the early stages of preclinical development (e.g., small-molecule insulin mimetics or glucagon antagonists, glucokinase activators, and β-cell potassium channel openers). The following are selected new classes of therapeutics, some of which are in clinical trials or earlier in research.

Glucagon Antagonists Glucagon is an important counter-regulator protein to the actions of insulin in glucose regulation. The disruption of the glucagon–insulin bimodal relationship is believed to contribute to diabetes mellitus. Glucagon is synthesized in the α-cells of the pancreatic islet cells and consists of a single 29–amino acid chain (118). The hormone is produced by proteolytic cleavage of a 69–amino acid peptide called glicentin. Glicentin, glucagon, GLP-1, and GLP-2 are all members of the enteroglucagon peptide family (119). Glucagon binds to receptors in the liver, leading to a G_s protein–coupled elevation in adenylyl cyclase activity, resulting in an increase in blood glucose as a result of a breakdown of stored glycogen, increased ketogenesis, and gluconeogenesis. Skeletal muscle glycogen does not appear to be affected by glucagon, probably as a result of the lack of specific receptors at this tissue site. Glucagon can also cause pancreatic β-cell insulin release, catecholamine release from adrenal tumors, and calcium release from medullary tumors (120).

Because diabetic hypoglycemic glucose control is antagonized by glucagon and the diabetic patient exhibits high basal glucagon levels, research has been directed toward the development of glucagon antagonists. Recent research has identified several nonpeptide antagonists (121–128). These antagonists cover a variety of chemical classes (Fig. 27.24). These include, but are not limited to, bi-phenyl and 4-phenyl pyridine derivatives, tri-aryl imidazoles and pyrroles, isoxadiazole thiophenes, alkylidene hydrazides, tri-substituted ureas and their methylene analogs, and a 2-thio benzimidazole derivative. Currently the glucagon antagonists NNC92-1687 and Bay27-9955 are in clinical trials. Bay27-9955 appears to be the most promising agent, with a glucagon-binding half maximal inhibitory concentration of approximately 110 nmol/L and a glucagon-stimulated cyclic adenosine monophosphate accumulation in cells reported as approximately 46 nmol/L (129).

Protein Tyrosine Phosphatase 1B Inhibitors Protein tyrosine phosphatase (PTB1B) and its potential role in the treatment of type 2 diabetes was first discovered in mice lacking the *PTB1B* gene in 1999. Studies using the PTB1B knockout mice demonstrated enhanced sensitivity to insulin due to the prolonged phosphorylation of the insulin receptor. In addition, a lack of PTB1B activity is associated with an increased ability to clear glucose in both glucose and insulin tolerance tests, as well as to cause a decrease in plasma insulin levels. In addition, mice lacking the *PTB1B* gene were resistant to weight gain when placed on a high-fat diet, in which no increase in total plasma triglycerides and cholesterol levels were detected (130,131). Since then, PTB1B has become an attractive, novel drug target in the development of potent and selective inhibitors for the treatment of both type 2 diabetes and obesity (132).

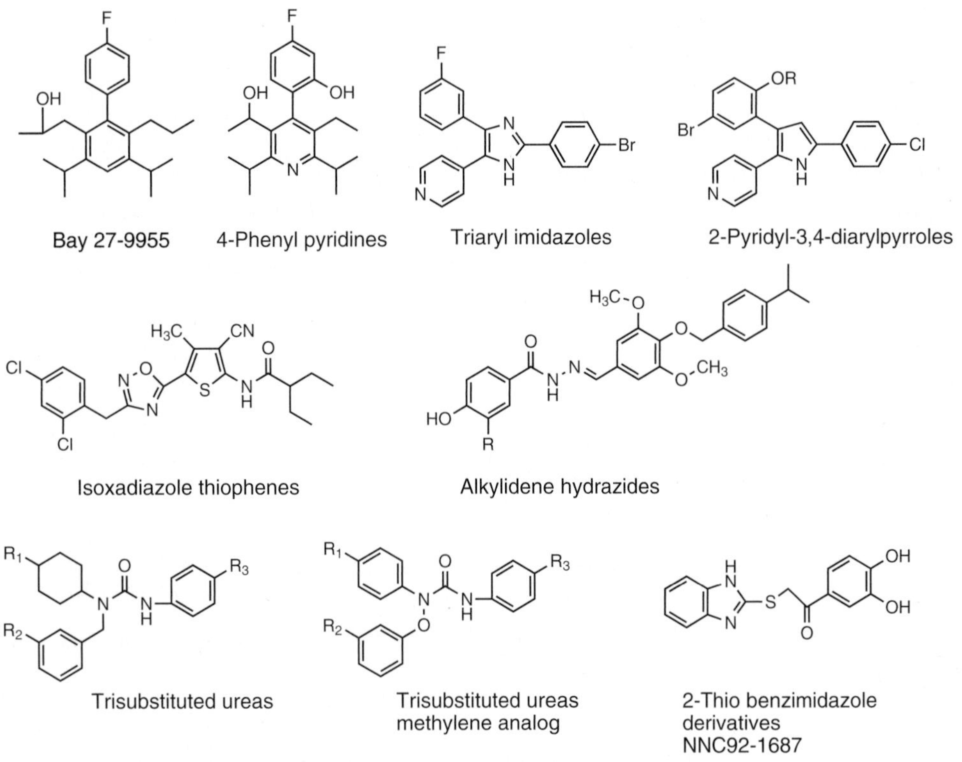

FIGURE 27.24 Structures of representative glucagon antagonists.

The PTPs belong to a superfamily of enzymes that catalyze protein tyrosine dephosphorylation. The importance of this class of enzymes is as modulators in various signal transduction pathways (133). Sequence analysis of the human genome indicates the existence of 107 PTP genes as compared to 90 human protein tyrosine kinase genes (134). The PTP superfamily of enzymes consists of three major subfamilies, which are divided according to their substrate specificity: classical phosphotyrosine-specific PTPs, dual specific PTPs, and low molecular weight PTPs. Currently, there are 38 PTPs belonging to the classical subfamily, and as the name suggests, they target proteins containing phosphotyrosine. The dual specific PTPs recognize proteins that contain phosphothreonine, phosphoserine, and phosphotyrosine residues (134,135).

PTB1B belongs to the subclass of classical phosphotyrosine-specific PTPs. PTB1B was first isolated from human placental tissue and is found on the cytoplasmic face of the endoplasmic reticulum. It is universally expressed and is found in insulin-targeted tissues including the liver, muscle, and fat (136,137). PTB1B plays an important role in the regulation of signal transduction networks. These signaling pathways are regulated by protein tyrosine kinases that catalyze the tyrosine phosphorylation cascade, a major posttranslational modification used by cells. To counterbalance the kinases, the PTPs are responsible for dephosphorylation processes, which control the rate and duration of a particular response. Therefore, both the protein tyrosine kinases and PTPs are equally important in signaling pathways, and an imbalance or defective operation of these networks can cause abnormal tyrosine phosphorylation, the consequence of which is often seen by the development of human diseases (133–135).

Type 2 diabetics have an inability to propagate the insulin signaling pathway, resulting in insulin resistance (130,138). One possible explanation for insulin resistance would be abnormalities of the insulin signaling events downstream from the receptor (138). In the complex insulin signaling pathway, PTB1B participates by dephosphorylating the tyrosine residues on the activated β subunit of the insulin receptor, as well as dephosphorylating the IRSs (130,132). Therefore, PTB1B acts as a negative regulator in the insulin signal transduction pathway (139). In fact, an overexpression of PTB1B has been shown to cause a decrease in the insulin-stimulated pathway, and thus contributes to diabetes and obesity. Therefore, inhibition of PTB1B activity would prove to be advantageous in augmenting insulin-initiated signaling events. Therefore, there is interest in development of PTB1B inhibitors as a potential treatment for type 2 diabetes.

Numerous PTB1B inhibitors have been synthesized with the hope of developing treatments for type 2 diabetes and obesity. Figure 27.25 shows the variety of chemical structures of some PTB1B inhibitors in development (132). Designing effective PTB1B inhibitors poses multiple challenges to drug development. The first and major challenge is that in order to design selective active site–directed compounds, they must mimic the negatively

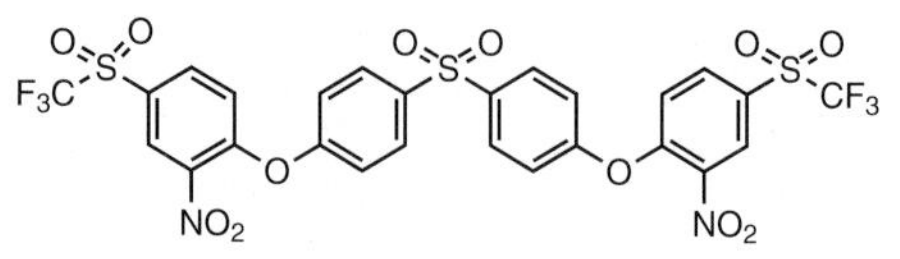

Trifluoromethyl sulfonyl derivatives (IC_{50}=400nM)

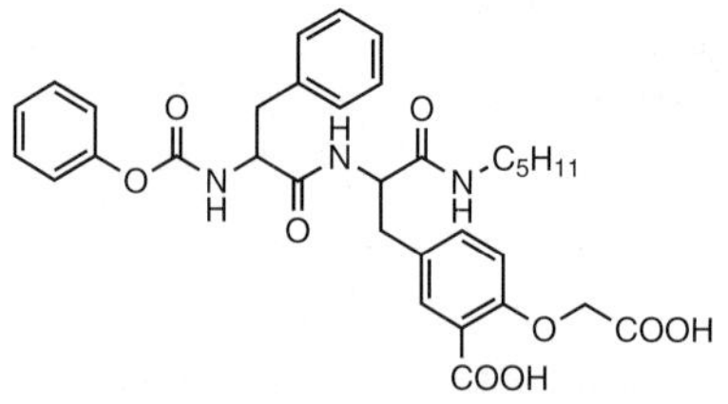

3'-Carboxy-4'-(O-carboxymethyl)tyrosine derivative (Ki = 870nM)

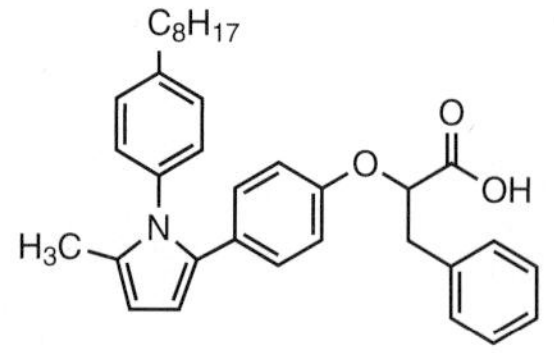

Pyrrole phenoxy proprionic acid derivative (CI_{50}=90nM)

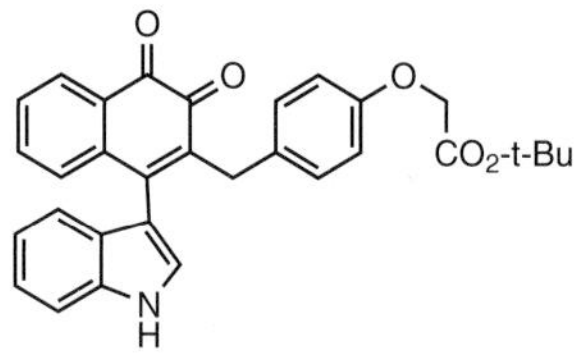

1,2-Naphthoquinone derivative (IC_{50}=650nM)

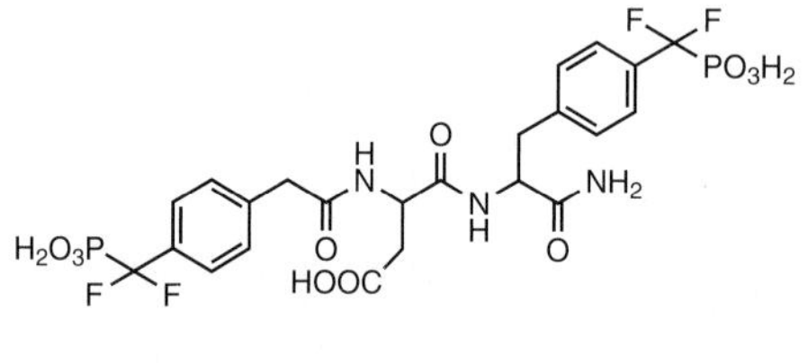

4'-Phosphonyldifluoromethyl-phenylalanine derivative (Ki=2.4nM)

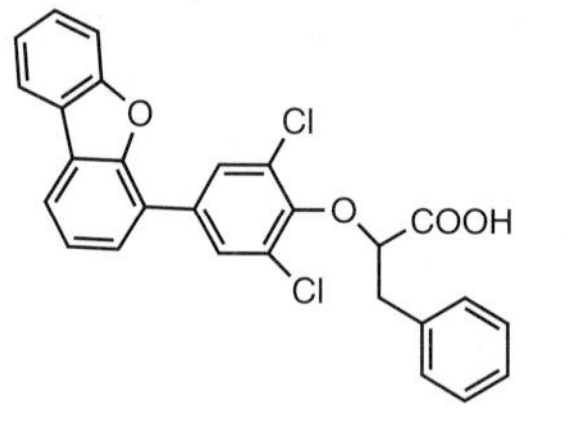

4-Dichlorophenyloxy-dibenzofuran derivative (IC_{50}=14uM)

FIGURE 27.25 Structures of PTB1B inhibitors in development. (Adapted from Rotella DP. Novel "second-generation" approaches for the control of type 2 diabetes. J Med Chem 2004;47:4111–4112.)

charged phosphotyrosine residues. Highly charged molecules rarely make good drug candidates primarily because they demonstrate poor pharmacokinetics, being poorly absorbed and distributed in the body. Fortunately, research has discovered that the active site of PTB1B contains subpockets (allosteric sites) that can be targeted for inhibitor development. This has led to the concept known as bidentate ligand binding, which aims to design inhibitors that bind to both the active site and a unique adjacent peripheral site (133). The bioavailability issue has been addressed by charge reduction, increasing the molecule's hydrophobicity, or targeting the subpocket sites only (133).

The development of PTB1B inhibitors continues to be an active area of research, and although as far as we know, there are no compounds in clinical trials, it is most likely that effective PTB1B-selective inhibitors with improved pharmacokinetics will be developed in the near future.

SCENARIO: OUTCOME AND ANALYSIS

Outcome

Nathan A. Painter, PharmD

JL has both fasting and postprandial hyperglycemia; however, the postprandial values are primarily responsible for increasing the hemoglobin A1c values. Even though insulin is a good choice for JL, his concerns of hypoglycemia and weight gain are real. Of the other options available, the drug exenatide is most likely to reduce postprandial glucose values. Because exenatide stimulates insulin secretion in a glucose-dependent manner, there is no risk of hypoglycemia when this medication is used alone. When used in combination with a sulfonylurea, however, the risk of hypoglycemia is increased, so the dosage of sulfonylurea may be reduced. Exenatide also promotes weight loss.

Increasing glipizide to 20 mg twice daily offers no benefit; sulfonylureas reach maximal therapeutic benefit at approximately half the maximum recommended dosage. Increasing metformin to 2550 mg daily offers little added benefit for similar reasons. Adding a thiazolidinedione may lower her hemoglobin A1C value an additional percentage point but may be associated with weight gain, congestive heart failure, and myocardial infarction (rosiglitazone).

Chemical Analysis

S. William Zito and Victoria Roche

Exenatide is the recommended choice in this case to help bring JL's fasting and postprandial hyperglycemia down to normal levels. Exenatide is a glucagon-like peptide 1 (GLP-1) receptor agonist. GLP-1 is a 36 amino acid peptide secreted by L-cells of the gut in response to a meal. It exerts control over glucose levels by promoting insulin secretion in a glucose-dependent manner. Exenatide is a 39-amino acid peptide analog of GLP-1 and is isolated from the saliva of the gila monster (Heloderma suspectum). It is resistant

SCENARIO: OUTCOME AND ANALYSIS (Continued)

to the proteolytic action of DPP-IV, which removes a dipeptide from the N-terminus because it has a glycine instead of alanine in the penultimate N-terminal position and is 53% homologous to human GLP-1. It has an in vivo half-life of approximately 3 hours.

Exenatide has been shown to reduce HbA1c levels in sulfonylurea treated patients with type 2 diabetes and is associated with weight loss. This weight loss is probably due to a decrease in appetite. In db/db mice it increased β-cell mass and delayed the onset of diabetes, so it may even have a prophylactic use. Exenatide is available as a sterile 250 mcg/ml solution for subcutaneous injection using a pen-injector. Dosing should be initiated at 5 mcg twice daily any time within 60 minutes before the morning and evening meals.

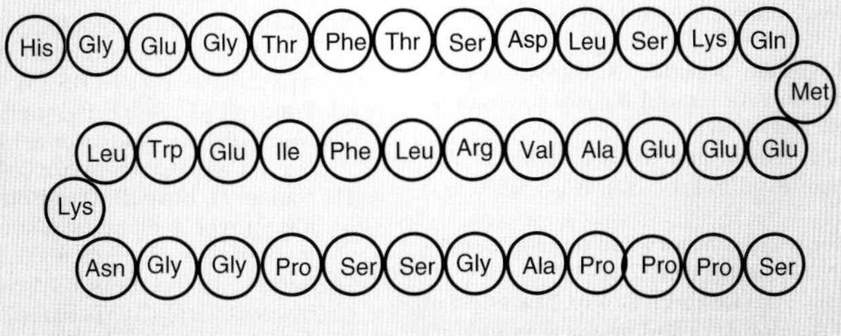

Exenatide (Byetta)

CASE STUDY

S. William Zito and Victoria Roche

MJ is a 45-year-old Native American male ironworker. Ironworkers are construction workers who build steel structural skeletons for skyscrapers and bridges. MJ is proud of his heritage as one of a long line of Mohawk ironworkers who have been building bridges and buildings all across the United States since the late 1800s. MJ has been a type 2 diabetic since he was 30 years old and has mild hypertension and hyperlipidemia, both of which are under control with enalapril and lovastatin, respectively. He visits his physician complaining that he has been unable to control his blood glucose levels even though he carefully watches what he eats and is conscientious about taking his glyburide every day (10 mg twice a day). His last glucose test revealed a level of 195 mg/dL 2 hours after breakfast. In addition, he is very concerned that he has become thirsty, tired, and always wanting to urinate, all of which makes it dangerous for him to "walk the steel." After eliminating any secondary causes of poor glycemic control (e.g., infection, other medications), and because MJ is currently taking the maximum dose of glyburide, his physician concludes he has most likely developed a "tolerance" to this drug. He would like to add another oral hypoglycemic drug to his therapy. What is your advice as to the following three choices?

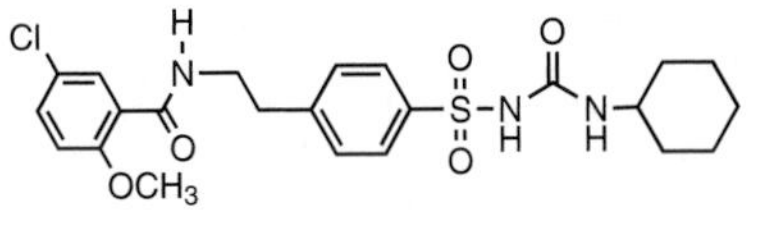

Glyburide

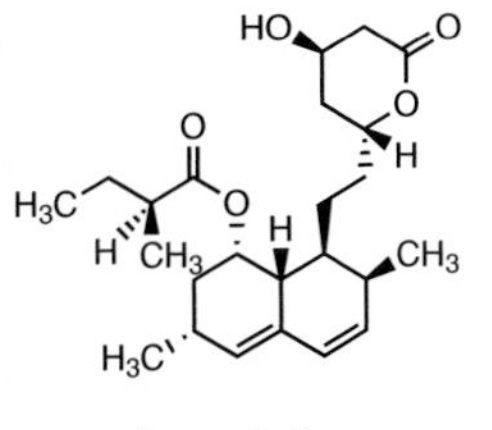

Lovastatin

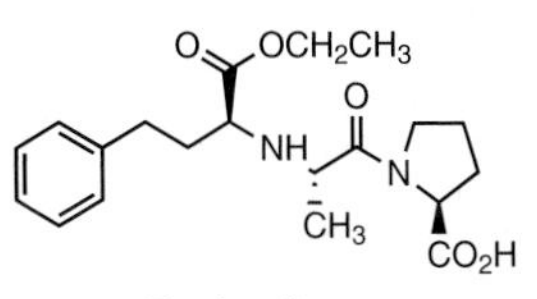

Enalapril

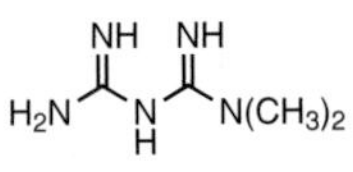

1

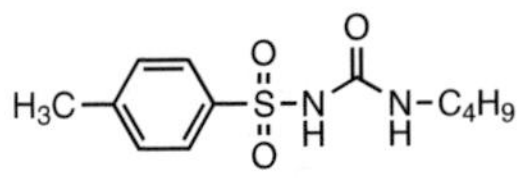

2

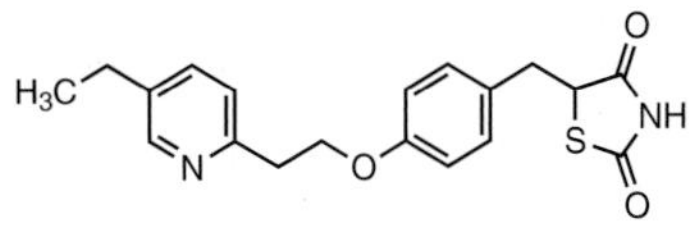

3

1. Conduct a thorough and mechanistic SAR analysis of the three therapeutic options in the case.
2. Apply the chemical understanding gained from the SAR analysis to this patient's specific needs to make a therapeutic recommendation.

References

1. Carpenter S, Rigaud M, Barile M, et al. An Interlinear Transliteration and English Translation of Portions of the Ebers Papyrus. Possibly Having to Do with Diabetes. Annandale-on Hudson, NY: Bard College, 1998.
2. Ali H, Anwar M, Ahmad T, et al. Diabetes mellitus from antiquity to present scenario and contribution of greco-arab physicians. J Int Soc Hist Islamic Med 2006;5:46–50.
3. Farmer L. Notes on the history of diabetes mellitus. Bull N Y Acad Med 1952;28:408–416.
4. Thayer A. Insulin. Chem Eng News 2005;83:74–75.
5. Sanger F, Tuppy H. The amino-acid sequence in the phenylalanyl chain of insulin. 1. The identification of lower peptides from partial hydrolysates. Biochem J 1951;49:463–481.
6. Sanger F, Tuppy H. The amino-acid sequence in the phenylalanyl chain of insulin. 2. The investigation of peptides from enzymic hydrolysates. Biochem J 1951;49:481–490.
7. Katsoyannis P, Tometsko A, Kukua K. Insulin peptides IX: the synthesis of the A-chain of insulin and its combination with natural B-chain to generate insulin activity. J Am Chem Soc 1963;85:2863–2865.
8. Goeddel DV, Kleid DG, Bolivar F, et al. Expression in Escherichia coli of chemically synthesized genes for human insulin. Proc Natl Acad Sci U S A 1979;76:106–110.
9. Loubatieres A. The hypoglycemic sulfonamides: history and development of the problem from 1942 to 1955. Ann N Y Acad Sci 1957;71:4–11.
10. The Diabetes Control and Complications Trial Research Group. The effect of intensive treatment of diabetes on the development and progression of long-term complications in insulin-dependent diabetes mellitus. N Engl J Med 1993;329:977–986.
11. Triplitt C, Reasoner CA, Isley WL. Diabetes mellitus. In: DiPiro J, Talbert RL, Yee GC, et al., eds. Pharmacotherapy. A Pathopysiologic Approach. New York: McGraw-Hill, 2008.
12. Oki J, Isley WL. Diabetes mellitus. In: DiPiro J, Talbert RL, Yee GC, et al., eds. Pharmacotherapy. A Pathopysiologic Approach. New York: McGraw-Hill, 2002:1335–1357.
13. Alberti KGMM, Zimmet P, Shaw J. Metabolic syndrome—a new world-wide definition. A Consensus Statement from the International Diabetes Federation. Diabetic Med 2006;23:469–480.
14. Kahn S, Hull RL, Utzschneider KM. Mechnisms linking obesity to insulin resistance and type 2 diabetes. Nature 2006;444:840–846.
15. Andrikopoulos S. Obesity and type 2 diabetes: slow down! Can metabolic deceleration protect the islet beta cell from excess nutrient-induced damage? Mol Cell Endocrinol 2010;316:140–146.
16. Centers for Disease Control and Prevention. National diabetes fact sheet: general information and national estimates on diabetes in the United States, 2007. Available from: http://www.cdc.gov/diabetes/pubs/factsheet07.htm.
17. American Diabetes Association. Diagnosis and classification of diabetes mellitus. Diabetes Care 2010;33(Suppl 1):S62–S69.
18. Nyenwe E, Jerkins TW, Umpierrez GE, et al. Management of type 2 diabetes: evolving strategies for the treatment of patients with type 2 diabetes. Metabolism 2011;60:1–23.
19. American Diabetes Association. Diabetes statistics. Available from: http://www.diabetes.org/diabetes-basics/diabetes-statistics.
20. Setter SW, Cambell RK. Diabetes. In: Helms R, Quan DJ, Herfindal ET, et al., eds. Textbook of Therapeutics. Drug and Disease Management. Baltimore: Lippincott Williams & Wilkins, 2006:1042–1075.
21. Wright E, Turk E. The sodium/glucose cotransport family SLC5. Plugers Arch-Eur J Physiol 2004;447:510–518.
22. Mueckler M. Facilitative glucose transporters. Eur J Biochem 1994;219:713–725.
23. Kido Y, Nakae J, Accili D. The insulin receptor and its cellular targets. J Clin Endocrinol Metab 2001;86:972–979.
24. Stumvoll M, Goldstein BJ, van Haeften TW. Type 2 diabetes: principles of pathogenesis and therapy. Lancet 2005;365:1333–1346.
25. Atkinson MA, Eisenbarth GS. Type 1 diabetes: new perspectives on disease pathogenesis and treatment. Lancet 2001;358:221–229.
26. Daneman D. Type 1 diabetes. Lancet 2006;367:847–858.
27. Moneva MH, Dagogo-Jack S. Multiple drug targets in the management of type 2 diabetes. Curr Drug Targets 2002;3:203–221.
28. Triplitt C, Wright A, Chiquette E. Incretin mimetics and dipeptidyl peptidase-IV inhibitors: potential new therapies for type 2 diabetes mellitus. Pharmacotherapy 2006;26:360–374.
29. Brownlee M. The pathological implications of protein glycation. Clin Invest Med 1995;18:275–281.
30. Brownlee M. Biochemistry and molecular cell biology of diabetic complications. Nature 2001;414:813–820.
31. Lee AYW, Chung SSM. Contributions of polyol pathway to oxidative stress in diabetic cataract. FASEB J 1999;13:23–30.
32. Degenhardt T, Thorpe SR, Baynes JW. Chemical modifications of proteins by methylglyoxal. Cell Mol Biol 1998;44:1139–1145.
33. Xia P, Inoguchi T, Kern TS, et al. Characterization of the mechanism for the chronic activation of diacylglycerol-protein kinase C pathway in diabetes and hypergalactosemia. Diabetes 1994;43:1122–1129.
34. Brownlee M. The pathobiology of diabetic complications. A unifying mechanism. Diabetes 2005;54:1615–1625.
35. Bergenstal RM, Bailey CJ, Kendall DM. Type 2 diabetes: assessing the relative risks and benefits of glucose-lowering medications. Am J Med 2010;123:374.e9–374.e18.
36. American Diabetes Assocaition. Standards of medical care in diabetes—2011. Diabetes Care 2011;34(Suppl 1):S11–S61.
37. The Diabetes Control and Complications Trial Research Group. The effect of intensive treatment of diabetes on the development and progression of long-term complications in insulin-dependent diabetes mellitus. N Engl J Med 1993;329:977–986.
38. Diabetes Control and Complications Trial/Epidemiology of Diabetes Interventions and Complications Study Research Group. Intensive diabetes treatment and cardiovascular disease in patients with type 1 diabetes. N Engl J Med 2005;353:2643–2653.
39. UKPDS. Intensive blood-glucose control with sulphonylureas or insulin compared with conventional treatment and risk of complications in patients with type 2 diabetes (UKPDS 33). Lancet 1998;352:837–853.
40. Pontiroli AE, Folli F, Paganelli M, et al. Laparoscopic gastric banding prevents type 2 diabetes and arterial hypertension and induces their remission in morbid obesity. Diabetes Care 2005;28:2703–2709.
41. Nathan D, Buse JB, Davidson MB, et al. Medical management of hyperglycemia in type 2 diabetes: a consensus algorithm for the initiation and adjustment of therapy. Diabetes Care 2009;32:193–203.
42. Kahn C, Roth J. Berson, Yallow and the JCI: the agony and the ecstasy. J Clin Invest 2004;114:1051–1054.
43. Zavod R, Krstenansky JL, Currie BL. Insulin and drugs used for the treatment of diabetes. In: Lemke T, Williams DA, Roche VF, et al., eds. Foye's Principles of Medicinal Chemistry. Philadelphia: Lippincott Williams & Wilkins, 2008.
44. Powers A, D Alessio D. Endocrine pancreas and pharmacotherapy of diabetes mellitus and hypoglycemia. In: Brunton L, Chabner, BA, Knollman BC, eds. Goodman and Gilman's The Pharmacological Basis of Therapeutics. New York: McGraw-Hill, 2011.
45. Davis S. Insulin, oral hypoglycemic agents and the pharmacology of the endocrine pancreas. In: Brunton L, Lazo JS, Parker KL, eds. Goodman and Gilman's The Pharmacological Basis of Therapeutics. New York: McGraw-Hill. 2006.
46. Aguilar-Bryan L, Clement JP, Gonzalez G, et al. Toward understanding the assembly and structure of KATP channels. Physiol Rev 1998;78:227–245.
47. De Vroede MA, Rechler MM, Nissley SP, et al. Mitogenic activity and receptor reactivity of hybrid molecules containing portions of the insulin-like growth factor I (IGF-I), IGF-II, and insulin molecules. Diabetes 1986;35:355–361.
48. Herbst KL, Hirsch IB. Insulin strategies for primary care providers. Clin Diabetes 2002;20:11–17.
49. University of California, San Francisco. Diabetes education online. Available from: http://www.deo.ucsf.edu/type2/diabetes-treatment/.
50. Mulder H, Schopman W Sr, van der Lely AJ. Extrapancreatic insulin effect of glibenclamide. Eur J Clin Pharmacol 1991;40:379–381.
51. Meglasson MD, Matschinsky FM. Pancreatic islet glucose metabolism and regulation of insulin secretion. Diabetes Metab Rev 1986;2:163–214.
52. Thisted H, Johnsen SP, Rungby J. Sulfonylureas and the risk of myocardial infarction. Metabolism 2006;55(Suppl 1):S16–S19.
53. Downey JM. An explanation for the reported observation that ATP dependent potassium channel openers mimic preconditioning. Cardiovasc Res 1993;27:1565.
54. Meyer M, Chudziak F, Schwanstecher C, et al. Structural requirements of sulphonylureas and analogues for interaction with sulphonylurea receptor subtypes. Br J Pharmacol 1999;128:27–34.
55. Inagaki N, Gonoi T, Clement JP, et al. A family of sulfonylurea receptors determines the pharmacological properties of ATP-sensitive K+ channels. Neuron 1996;16:1011–1017.
56. Malaisse WJ. Stimulation of insulin release by non-sulfonylurea hypoglycemic agents: the meglitinide family. Horm Metab Res 1995;27:263–266.
57. Bakkali Nadi A, Zhang TM, Malaisse WJ. Effects of the methyl esters of pyruvate, succinate and glutamate on the secretory response to meglitinide analogues in rat pancreatic islets. Pharmacol Res 1996;33:191–194.
58. Proks P, Reimann F, Green N, et al. Sulfonylurea stimulation of insulin secretion. Diabetes 2002;51(Suppl 3):S368–S376.
59. Akiyoshi M, Kakei M, Nakazaki M, et al. A new hypoglycemic agent, A-4166, inhibits ATP-sensitive potassium channels in rat pancreatic beta-cells. Am J Physiol 1995;268:E185–E193.
60. Lins L, Brasseur R, Malaisse WJ. Conformational analysis of non-sulfonylurea hypoglycemic agents of the meglitinide family. Biochem Pharmacol 1995;50:1879–1884.
61. Golan DE, Tashjian J, Armstrong E, et al. Principles of Pharmacology: The Pathophysiologic Basis of Drug Therapy. New York: Lippincott Williams and Wilkins, 2007:540–541.
62. Plutzky J, Viberti G, Haffner S. Atherosclerosis in type 2 diabetes mellitus and insulin resistance: mechanistic links and therapeutic targets. J Diabetes Compl 2002;16:401–415.
63. Augusti KT, Sunil NP, Andrews A, et al. A comparative study on the effects of diet and exercise, metformin and metformin + pioglitazone treatment on NIDDM patients. Indian J Clin Biochem 2007;22:65–69.

64. Bailey CJ. Biguanides and NIDDM. Diabetes Care 1992;15:755–772.
65. Witters LA. The blooming of the French lilac. J Clin Invest 2001;108:1105–1107.
66. Coustan DR. Pharmacological management of gestational diabetes: an overview. Diabetes Care 2007;30(Suppl 2):S206–S208.
67. Nestler JE. Metformin for the treatment of the polycystic ovary syndrome. N Engl J Med 2008;358:47–54.
68. Bolen S, Feldman L, Vassy J, et al. Systematic review: comparative effectiveness and safety of oral medications for type 2 diabetes mellitus. Ann Intern Med 2007;147:386–399.
69. Fimognari FL, Pastorelli R, Incalzi RA. Phenformin-induced lactic acidosis in an older diabetic patient: a recurrent drama (phenformin and lactic acidosis). Diabetes Care 2006;29:950–951.
70. Hulisz DT, Bonfiglio MF, Murray RD. Metformin-associated lactic acidosis. J Am Board Fam Pract 1998;11:233–236.
71. Bragt MC, Popeijus HE. Peroxisome proliferator-activated receptors and the metabolic syndrome. Physiol Behav 2008;94:187–197.
72. Murphy GJ, Holder JC. PPAR-gamma agonists: therapeutic role in diabetes, inflammation and cancer. Trends Pharmacol Sci 2000;21:469–474.
73. Reginato M, Lazar M. Mechanisms by which thiazolidinediones enhance insulin action. Trends Endocrinol Metab 1999;10:9–13.
74. Schoonjans K, Auwerx J. Thiazolidinediones: an update. Lancet 2000;355:1008–1010.
75. Nolte RT, Wisely G, Westin S, et al. Ligand binding and co-activator assembly of the peroxisome proliferator-activated receptor-gamma. Nature 1998;395:137–143.
76. Schwartz S, Raskin P, Fonesca V, et al. Effect of troglitazone in insulin-treated patients with type II diabetes mellitus. Troglitazone and Exogenous Insulin Study Group. N Engl J Med 1998;338:861–866.
77. Suter SL, Nolan J, Wallace P, et al. Metabolic effects of new oral hypoglycemic agent CS-045 in NIDDM subjects. Diabetes Care 1992;15:193–203.
78. Parker JC. Troglitazone: the discovery and development of a novel therapy for the treatment of type 2 diabetes mellitus. Adv Drug Deliv Rev 2002;54:1173–1197.
79. Chan J, Ilag L,Tan M. Effects of thiazolidinediones on the triad of type 2 diabetes mellitus, insulin resistance and cardiovascular disease. Diabetes Res Clin Pract 2007;78S:S3–S13.
80. Gross B, Staels B. PPAR agonists: multimodal drugs for the treatment of type-2 diabetes. Best Pract Res Clin Endocrinol Metab 2007;21:687–710.
81. Nissen SE, Wolski K, Topol EJ. Effect of muraglitazar on death and major adverse cardiovascular events in patients with type 2 diabetes mellitus. JAMA 2005;294:2581–2586.
82. Madhavan GR, Chakrabarti R, Reddy K, et al. Dual PPAR-alpha and -gamma activators derived from novel benzoxazinone containing thiazolidinediones having antidiabetic and hypolipidemic potential. Bioorg Med Chem 2006;14:584–591.
83. Cheng A, Josse R. Intestinal absorption inhibitors for type 2 diabetes mellitus: prevention and treatment. Drug Discov Today 2004;1:201–206.
84. Bell DS. Type 2 diabetes mellitus: what is the optimal treatment regimen? Am J Med 2004;116:23S–29S.
85. Inzucchi SE. Oral antihyperglycemic therapy for type 2 diabetes: scientific review. JAMA 2002;287:360–372.
86. Emilien G, Maloteaux JM, Ponchon M. Pharmacological management of diabetes: recent progress and future perspective in daily drug treatment. Pharmacol Ther 1999;81:37–51.
87. Borges de Melo E. Alpha and beta glucosidase inhibitors: chemical structure and biological activity. Tetrahedron 2006;62:10277–10302.
88. Platt FM, Butters TD. Substrate deprivation: a new therapeutic approach for the glycosphingolipid lysosomal storage diseases. Expert Rev Mol Med 2000;2:1–17.
89. Lee DS, Lee SH. Genistein, a soy isoflavone, is a potent alpha-glucosidase inhibitor. FEBS Lett 2001;501:84–86.
90. Adisakwattana S, Sookkongwaree K, Roengsumran S, et al. Structure-activity relationships of trans-cinnamic acid derivatives on alpha-glucosidase inhibition. Bioorg Med Chem Lett 2004;14:2893–2896.
91. Du ZY, Liu RR, Shao WY, et al. Alpha-glucosidase inhibition of natural curcuminoids and curcumin analogs. Eur J Med Chem 2006;41:213–218.
92. Matsui T, Tanaka T, Tamura S, et al. Alpha-glucosidase inhibitory profile of catechins and theaflavins. J Agric Food Chem 2007;55:99–105.
93. Holst JJ, Orskov C, Nielson OV, et al. Truncated glucagon-like peptide I, an insulin-releasing hormone from the distal gut. FEBS Lett 1987;211:169–174.
94. Perley MJ, Kipnis DM. Plasma insulin responses to oral and intravenous glucose: studies in normal and diabetic sujbjects. J Clin Invest 1967;46:1954–1962.
95. Dupre J, Ross S, Watson D, et al. Stimulation of insulin secretion by gastric inhibitory polypeptide in man. J Clin Endocrinol Metab 1973;37:826–828.
96. Reimann F, Gribble FM. Glucose-sensing in glucagon-like peptide-1-secreting cells. Diabetes 2002;51:2757–2763.
97. Deacon CF, Johnsen AH, Holst JJ. Degradation of glucagon-like peptide-1 by human plasma in vitro yields an N-terminally truncated peptide that is a major endogenous metabolite in vivo. J Clin Endocrinol Metab 1995;80:952–957.
98. Mentlein R, Gallwitz B, Schmidt WE. Dipeptidyl-peptidase IV hydrolyses gastric inhibitory polypeptide, glucagon-like peptide-1(7-36)amide, peptide histidine methionine and is responsible for their degradation in human serum. Eur J Biochem 1993;214:829–835.
99. Deacon CF, Knudsen L, Madsen K, et al. Dipeptidyl peptidase IV resistant analogues of glucagon-like peptide-1 which have extended metabolic stability and improved biological activity. Diabetologia 1998;41:271–278.
100. Buse JB, Henry R, Han J, et al. Effects of exenatide (exendin-4) on glycemic control over 30 weeks in sulfonylurea-treated patients with type 2 diabetes. Diabetes Care 2004;27:2628–2635.
101. Wang Q, Brubaker PL. Glucagon-like peptide-1 treatment delays the onset of diabetes in 8 week-old db/db mice. Diabetologia 2002;45:1263–1273.
102. Arulmozhi DK, Portha B. GLP-1 based therapy for type 2 diabetes. Eur J Pharm Sci 2006;28:96–108.
103. Elbrond B, Jacobsen G, Larsen S, et al. Pharmacokinetics, pharmacodynamics, safety, and tolerability of a single-dose of NN2211, a long-acting glucagon-like peptide 1 derivative, in healthy male subjects. Diabetes Care 2002;25:1398–1404.
104. Knudsen LB. Glucagon-like peptide-1: the basis of a new class of treatment for type 2 diabetes. J Med Chem 2004;47:4128–4134.
105. Sturis J, Gotfredsen C, Romer J, et al. GLP-1 derivative liraglutide in rats with beta-cell deficiencies: influence of metabolic state on beta-cell mass dynamics. Br J Pharmacol 2003;140:123–132.
106. U.S. Food and Drug Administration. Postmarket drug safety information. Available from: http://www.fda.gov/Drugs/DrugSafety/PostmarketDrugSafetyInformationforPatientsandProviders/ucm198543.htm.
107. Rosenblum JS, Kozarich JW. Prolyl peptidases: a serine protease subfamily with high potential for drug discovery. Curr Opin Chem Biol 2003;7:496–504.
108. Thoma R, Loffler B, Stihle M, et al. Structural basis of proline-specific exopeptidase activity as observed in human dipeptidyl peptidase-IV. Structure 2003;11:947–959.
109. Eckhardt M, Langkopf E, Mark M, et al. 8-(3-(R)-Aminopiperidin-1-yl)-7-but-2-ynyl-3-methyl-1-(4-methyl-quinazolin-2-ylmethyl)-3,7-dihydropurine-2,6-dione (BI 1356), a highly potent, selective, long-acting, and orally bioavailable DPP-4 inhibitor for the treatment of type 2 diabetes. J Med Chem 2007;50:6450–6453.
110. Tahrani A, Piya M, Kennedy A, et al. Glycaemic control in type 2 diabetes: targets and new therapies. Pharmacol Ther 2010;125:328–361.
111. Blech S, Ludwig-Schwellinger E, Gräfe-Mody EU, et al. The metabolism and disposition of the oral dipeptidyl peptidase-4 inhibitor, linagliptin, in humans. Drug Metab Dispos 2010;38:667–678.
112. Ryan GJ, Jobe LJ, Martin R. Pramlintide in the treatment of type 1 and type 2 diabetes mellitus. Clin Ther 2005;27:1500–1512.
113. Kruger DF, Gloster MA. Pramlintide for the treatment of insulin-requiring diabetes mellitus: rationale and review of clinical data. Drugs 2004;64:1419–1432.
114. Heptulla RA, Rodriguez LM, Bomgaars L, et al. The role of amylin and glucagon in the dampening of glycemic excursions in children with type 1 diabetes. Diabetes 2005;54:1100–1107.
115. Owen SK. Amylin replacement therapy in patients with insulin-requiring type 2 diabetes. Diabetes Educ 2006;32(Suppl 3):105S–110S.
116. Pullman J, Darsow T, Frias JP. Pramlintide in the management of insulin-using patients with type 2 and type 1 diabetes. Vasc Health Risk Manag 2006;2:203–212.
117. Singh-Franco D, Robles G, Gazze D. Pramlintide acetate injection for the treatment of type 1 and type 2 diabetes mellitus. Clin Ther 2007;29:535–562.
118. Burcelin R, Katz EB, Charron MJ. Molecular and cellular aspects of the glucagon receptor: role in diabetes and metabolism. Diabetes Metab 1996;22:373–396.
119. Cascieri MA, Fong TM, Strader CD. Molecular characterization of a common binding site for small molecules within the transmembrane domain of G-protein coupled receptors. J Pharmacol Toxicol Methods 1995;33:179–185.
120. Christophe J. Glucagon receptors: from genetic structure and expression to effector coupling and biological responses. Biochim Biophys Acta 1995;1241:45–57.
121. Chang LL, Sidler K, Cascieri M, et al. Substituted imidazoles as glucagon receptor antagonists. Bioorg Med Chem Lett 2001;11:2549–2553.
122. de Laszlo SE, Hacker C, Li B, et al. Potent, orally absorbed glucagon receptor antagonists. Bioorg Med Chem Lett 1999;9:641–646.
123. Duffy JL, Kirk BA, Konteatis Z, et al. Discovery and investigation of a novel class of thiophene-derived antagonists of the human glucagon receptor. Bioorg Med Chem Lett 2005;15:1401–1405.
124. Kurukulasuriya R, Sorensen B, Link J, et al. Biaryl amide glucagon receptor antagonists. Bioorg Med Chem Lett 2004;14:2047–2050.
125. Ladouceur GH, Cook J, Hertzog D, et al. Integration of optimized substituent patterns to produce highly potent 4-aryl-pyridine glucagon receptor antagonists. Bioorg Med Chem Lett 2002;12:3421–3424.
126. Liang R, Abrardo L, Brady E, et al. Design and synthesis of conformationally constrained tri-substituted ureas as potent antagonists of the human glucagon receptor. Bioorg Med Chem Lett 2007;17:587–592.
127. Ling A, Hong Y, Gonzalez J, et al. Identification of alkylidene hydrazides as glucagon receptor antagonists. J Med Chem 2001;44:3141–3149.
128. Ling A, Plewe M, Gonzalez J, et al. Human glucagon receptor antagonists based on alkylidene hydrazides. Bioorg Med Chem Lett 2002;12:663–666.
129. Petersen KF, Sullivan JT. Effects of a novel glucagon receptor antagonist (Bay 27-9955) on glucagon-stimulated glucose production in humans. Diabetologia 2001;44:2018–2024.

130. Montalibet J, Kennedy BP. Therapeutic strategies for targeting PTB1B in diabetes. Drug Discov Today 2005;2:129–135.
131. Rotella DP. Novel "second-generation" approaches for the control of type 2 diabetes. J Med Chem 2004;47:4111–4112.
132. Hooft van Huijduijnen R, Bombrun A, Swinnen D. Selecting protein tyrosine phosphatasesas drug targets. Drug Discov Today 2002;7:1013–1019.
133. Zhang S, Zhang Z-Y. PTB1B as a drug target: recent developments in PTB1B inhibitor discovery. Drug Discov Today 2007;12:373–381.
134. Koren S, Fantus IG. Inhibition of the protein tyrosine phosphatase PTB1B: potential therapy for obesity, insulin resistance and type-2 diabetes mellitus. Best Pract Res Clin Endocrinol Metab 2007;21:621–640.
135. Zhang Z-Y. Protein tyrosine phosphatases: prospects for therapeutics. Curr Opin Chem Biol 2001;5:416–423.
136. Tonks NK, Diltz CD, Fischer EH. Purification of the major protein-tyrosine-phosphatases of human placenta. J Biol Chem 1988;263:6722–6730.
137. Forsell PKAL, Boie Y, Montalibet J, et al. Genomic characterization of the human and mouse protein tyrosine phosphatase-1B genes. Gene 2000;260:145–153.
138. Saltiel AR, Kahn CR. Insulin signalling and the regulation of glucose and lipid metabolism. Nature 2001;414:799–806.
139. Patankar SJ, Jurs PC. Classification of inhibitors of protein tyrosine phosphatase 1B using molecular structure based descriptors. J Chem Info Comput Sci 2003;43:885–899.

Chapter 28

Adrenocorticoids

DUANE D. MILLER, ROBERT W. BRUEGGEMEIER, AND JAMES T. DALTON

Drugs Covered in This Chapter

GLUCOCORTICOSTEROIDS
- Betamethasone
- Dexamethasone
- Fludrocortisone
- Hydrocortisone and derivatives
- Methylprednisolone
- Prednisone and prednisolone
- Triamcinolone

GLUCOCORTICOSTEROIDS USED TOPICALLY OR FOR INHALATION
- Beclomethasone dipropionate
- Budesonide
- Ciclesonide
- Clobetasol propionate
- Flunisolide
- Fluocinolone acetonide
- Fluocinonide
- Fluorometholone
- Flurandrenolide
- Fluticasone propionate
- Halcinonide
- Halobetasol propionate
- Mometasone furoate
- Triamcinolone acetonide

MINERALOCORTICOSTEROIDS
- Aldosterone
- 11-Desoxycorticosterone

ADRENOCORTICOID ANTAGONISTS
- Spironolactone
- Eplerenone
- Aminoglutethimide
- Metyrapone
- Trilostane

Abbreviations

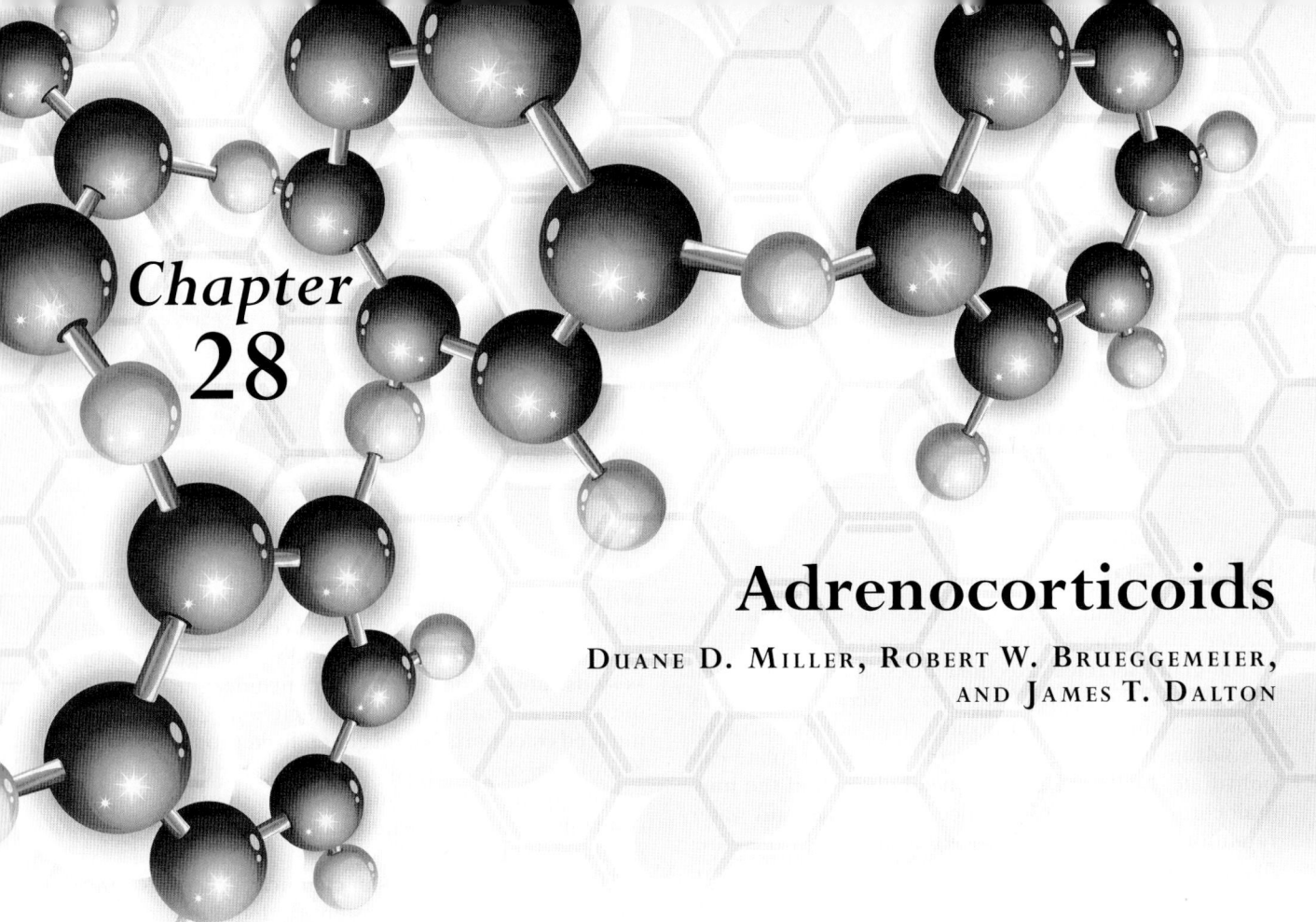

ACTH, adrenocorticotropic hormone
BDP, betamethasone dipropionate
17-BMP, beclomethasone 17α-monopropionate
21-BMP, beclomethasone 21-monopropionate
cAMP, cyclic adenosine monophosphate
CRF, corticotropin-releasing factor
COPD, chronic obstructive pulmonary disease
des-CIC, desisobutyrylciclesonide
DPI, dry powder inhaler
GI, gastrointestinal
GR, glucocorticoid receptor
HPA, hypothalamic-pituitary-adrenal
HRE, hormone-responsive elements
11β-HSD1, type 1 11β-hydroxysteroid dehydrogenase
11β-HSD2, type 2 11β-hydroxysteroid dehydrogenase
3β-HSD, 5-ene-3β-hydroxysteroid dehydrogenase
IL, interleukin
IM, intramuscular
IV, intravenous

SCENARIO

Jeffrey T. Sherer, PharmD, MPH, BCPS, CGP

LT is a 74-year-old woman with chronic obstructive pulmonary disease due to a 55 pack-year history of cigarette smoking. As an outpatient, she is maintained on a regimen including inhaled tiotropium and inhaled salmeterol. Over the past several days, she has experienced an increase in shortness of breath and a change in the color and quantity of her sputum. A chest radiograph shows hyperinflated lungs but no evidence of pneumonia. She is admitted to the hospital with a diagnosis of acute exacerbation of chronic obstructive pulmonary disease.

(The reader is directed to the clinical solution and chemical analysis of this case at the end of the chapter).

INTRODUCTION

The adrenal glands are flattened, cap-like structures located above the kidneys. The inner core (medulla) of the gland secretes catecholamines, whereas the shell (cortex) of the gland synthesizes steroid hormones known as the adrenocorticoids. The adrenocorticoid steroids include the glucocorticoids, which regulate carbohydrate, lipid, and protein metabolism, and the mineralocorticoids, which influence salt balance and water retention. A third class of steroids produced by the adrenal glands is called the adrenal androgens, which have weak androgenic activity in men and women and can serve as precursors to the sex hormones, estrogens and androgens.

The adrenocorticoids and sex hormones have much in common. All are steroids; consequently, the rules that define their structures, chemistry, and nomenclature are the same. The rings of these biochemically dynamic and physiologically active compounds have a similar stereochemical relationship. Changes in the geometry of the ring junctures usually result in inactive compounds regardless of the biologic category of the steroid. Similar chemical groups are used to render some of these agents water soluble or active when taken orally or to modify their absorption.

In addition, the adrenocorticoids and the sex hormones, which include the estrogens, progestins, and androgens, are mainly biosynthesized from cholesterol, which in turn is synthesized from acetyl–coenzyme A. Cholesterol and steroid hormone catabolism takes place primarily in the liver. Although the products found in the urine and feces depend on the hormone undergoing catabolism, many of the metabolic reactions are similar for these compounds. For example, reduction of double bonds at positions 4 and 5 or 5 and 6, epimerization of 3α-hydroxyl groups, reduction of 3-keto groups to the 3α-hydroxyl function, and oxidative removal of side chains are transformations common to these agents.

The adrenocorticoids have many clinical uses. Glucocorticoids and mineralocorticoids may be used for the treatment of adrenal insufficiency (hypoadrenalism), which results from failure of the adrenal glands to synthesize adequate amounts of the hormones. Major pharmacologic uses of glucocorticoids include the treatment of rheumatoid diseases, symptomatic relief from asthma and allergic conditions, topical application for various dermatologic disorders, and cancer therapy. Toxicities arise when corticosteroids are used for longer than brief periods, and toxic effects can include glucocorticoid-induced adrenocortical insufficiency, glucocorticoid-induced osteoporosis, and generalized protein depletion. Knowledge of the numerous steroid products, structure–activity relationships, and available dosage forms will result in significant benefits for patients with minimal troublesome toxicities.

Despite the similarities in chemical structures and stereochemistry, each class of steroids demonstrates unique and distinctively different biologic activities. Minor structural modifications to the steroid nucleus, such as changes in or insertion of functional groups at different positions, cause marked changes in physiologic activity. The first part of this chapter focuses on the similarities among the steroids and reviews steroid nomenclature, stereochemistry, and general mechanism of action. The second portion of the chapter focuses on the adrenocorticoids and discusses the biosynthesis, metabolism, medicinal chemistry, pharmacology, and pharmacokinetics of endogenous steroid hormones, synthetic agonists, and synthetic antagonists.

STEROID NOMENCLATURE AND STRUCTURE

Steroids consist of four fused rings (A, B, C, and D) (Fig. 28.1). Chemically, these hydrocarbons are cyclopentanoperhydrophenanthrenes; they contain a five-membered cyclopentane (D) ring plus the three rings of phenanthrene. A perhydrophenanthrene (rings A, B, and C) is the completely saturated derivative of phenanthrene. The polycyclic hydrocarbon known as 5α-cholestane will be used to illustrate the numbering system for a steroid (Fig. 28.1). The term "cholestane" refers to a steroid with 27 carbons that includes a side chain of eight carbons at position 17. Numbering begins in ring A at C1 and proceeds around rings A and B to C10, then into ring C beginning with C11, and snakes around rings C and D to C17. The angular methyl groups are numbered 18 (attached to C13) and 19 (attached to C10). The 17 side chain begins with C20, and the numbering

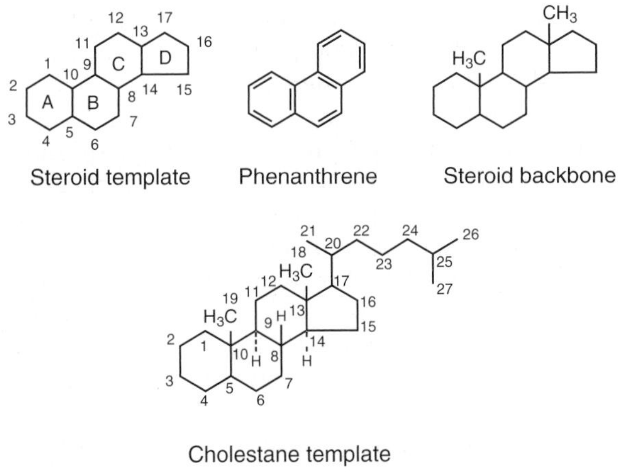

FIGURE 28.1 Basic steroid structure and numbering system.

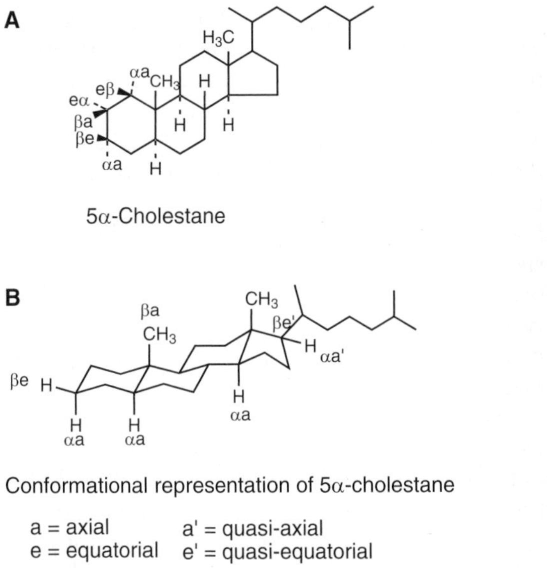

FIGURE 28.2 Planar and conformational structures of 5α-cholestane.

finishes in sequential order. Using the rigid planar representation for drawing the steroid structure (Fig. 28.2A), the basic steroid structure becomes a plane with two surfaces: The top or β surface is pointing out toward the reader, and the bottom or α surface is pointing away from the reader. Hydrogens or functional groups on the β side of the molecule are denoted by solid lines; those on the α side are designated by dotted lines. The 5α notation is used to denote the configuration of the hydrogen atom at C5, which is opposite from the C19 angular methyl group, making the A/B ring juncture *trans.* The C19 angular methyl group is assigned the β side of the molecule. Similarly, the configuration of the 8β and 9α hydrogens, and the 14α hydrogen and C18 angular methyl group, denote *trans* fusion for rings B/C and C/D. The side chains at position 17 are always β unless indicated by dotted lines or in the nomenclature of the steroid (e.g., 17β or 17α).

Just as cyclohexane can be drawn in a chair conformation, the three-dimensional representation for 5α-cholestane is shown by the following conformational formula (Fig. 28.2B). Although cyclohexane may undergo a flip in conformation, steroids are rigid structures, because they generally have at least one *trans* fused ring system and these rings must be diequatorial to each other.

If one is aware that the angular methyl groups at positions 18 and 19 are β and have an axial orientation (i.e., perpendicular to the plane of the rings), the conformational orientation of the remaining bonds of a steroid can be easily assigned. For example, in 5α-cholestane, the C19 methyl group attached at position 10 is always β-axial (βa); the two bonds at position 3 must be β-equatorial (βe) and α-axial (αa), as indicated. The orientation of the remaining bonds on a steroid may be determined if one recalls that groups on a cyclohexane ring that are positioned on adjacent carbon atoms (vicinal, —C_1H—C_2H—) of the ring (i.e., 1,2 to each other) are *trans* if their relationship is 1,2-diaxial or 1,2-diequatorial and are *cis* if their relationship is 1,2-equatorial-axial.

CLINICAL SIGNIFICANCE

Few groups of drugs can rival the adrenocorticoids, which are used for the widest variety of conditions. From asthma to rheumatologic diseases to dermatologic disorders, the adrenocorticoids are commonly prescribed for their beneficial action. Unfortunately, they also exhibit significant toxicity. Only by understanding their complicated mechanisms of action can pharmacists help maximize the therapeutic benefits while minimizing the numerous adverse effects of these agents.

Pharmacists must be familiar with the numerous steroid products and dosage forms that are available as well as with the structure–activity relationships that determine their effects at different receptors. By understanding these factors, the likelihood that patients will derive significant benefits without untoward toxicities is significantly increased.

Jeffrey T. Sherer, PharmD, MPH
Clinical Associate Professor
University of Houston College of Pharmacy
Houston, Texas

Steroid chemists often refer to the series of carbon–carbon bonds shown with heavy lines as the backbone of the steroid (Fig. 28.1). The *cis* or *trans* relationship of the four rings may be expressed in terms of the backbone. The compound 5α-cholestane (Fig. 28.2) is said to have a *trans-anti-trans-anti-trans* backbone. In this structure, all the fused rings have *trans* (diequatorial) stereochemistry; in other words, the A/B fused ring, the B/C fused ring, and the C/D fused ring are *trans*. The term *anti* is used in backbone notation to define the orientation of rings that are connected to each other and have a *trans*-type relationship. For example, the bond equatorial to ring B, at position 9, which forms part of ring C, is *anti* to the bond equatorial to ring B, at position 10, which forms part of ring A. 5β-Cholestane (Fig. 28.3) has a *cis-anti-trans-anti-trans* backbone in which the A/B rings are fused *cis*. The term *syn* is used in a similar fashion as *anti* to define a *cis*-type relationship. No natural steroids exist with a *syn*-type geometry, although such compounds can be chemically synthesized. Thus, the conventional drawing of the steroid nucleus is the natural configuration and does not show the hydrogens at 8β, 9α, or 14β positions. If the carbon at position 5 is saturated, the hydrogen is always drawn as either 5α or 5β. Also, the conventional drawing of a steroid molecule has the C18 and C19 methyl groups shown only as solid lines (no CH_3 drawn).

The stereochemistry of the rings markedly affects the biologic activity of a given class of steroids. Nearly all biologically active steroids have the cholestane-type backbone. In most of the important steroids discussed in this chapter, a double bond is present between positions 4 and 5 or 5 and 6; consequently, there is no *cis* or *trans* relationship between rings A and B. The symbol Δ is often used to designate a carbon–carbon double bond (C=C) in a steroid. If the C=C is between positions 4 and 5, the compound is referred to as a Δ^4-steroid. If the C=C is between positions 5 and 10, the compound is designated a $\Delta^{5(10)}$-steroid.

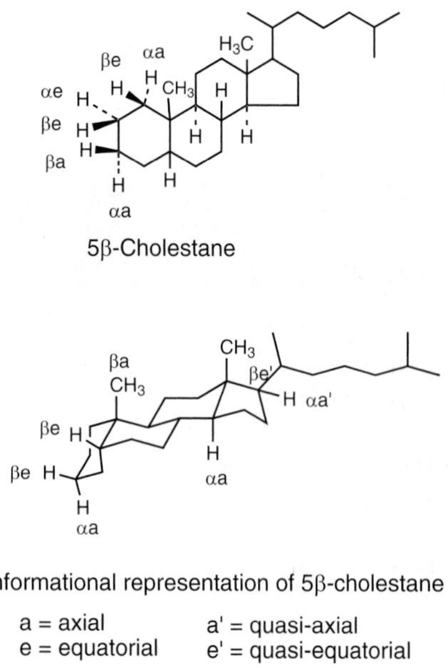

FIGURE 28.3 Planar and conformational structures of 5β-cholestane.

Cholesterol (cholest-5-en-3α-ol) is a Δ^5-steroid or, more specifically, a Δ^5-sterol, because it is an unsaturated alcohol. Biologically active compounds include members of the 5α-pregnane, 5α-androstane, and 5α-estrane steroid classes (Fig. 28.4). Pregnanes are steroids with 21 carbon atoms, androstanes 19 carbon atoms, and estranes 18 carbon atoms, with the C19 angular methyl group at C10 replaced by hydrogen. Numbering is the same as in 5α-cholestane.

The adrenocorticoids (adrenal cortex hormones) are pregnanes and are exemplified by cortisone, which is a 17α,21-dihydroxypregn-4-ene-3,11,20-trione. The acetate ester is named 17α,21-dihydroxypregn-4-ene-3,11,20-trione 21-acetate (cortisone acetate) (Fig. 28.4). Progesterone (pregn-4-ene-3,20-dione), a female sex hormone synthesized by the corpus luteum, is also a pregnane analog. The male sex hormones (androgens) are based on the structure of 5α-androstane. Testosterone, an important and naturally occurring androgen, is named 17β-hydroxyandrost-4-en-3-one. Dehydroepiandrosterone is the major adrenal androgen and is named 3β-hydroxyandrost-5-en-17-one (Fig. 28.4). The estrogens, which are female sex hormones synthesized by the graafian follicle of the ovaries, are estrane analogs containing an aromatic A ring. Although the A ring does not contain isolated C=C groups, these analogs are named as if the bonds were in the positions shown in 17β-estradiol. Hence, 17β-estradiol, a typical member of this class of drugs, is named estra-1,3,5,(10)-triene-3,17β-diol. Other examples of steroid nomenclature are found throughout this chapter.

Aliphatic side chains at position 17 are always assumed to be β when cholestane or pregnane nomenclature is employed. Hence, the notation 17β need not be used when naming these compounds. If a pregnane has a 17α chain, however, this should be indicated in the nomenclature. Finally, the final "e" in the name for the parent steroid hydrocarbon is always dropped when it precedes a vowel, regardless of whether a number appears between the two parts of the word (e.g., note the nomenclature for cholesterol and testosterone versus that for cortisone). For a more extensive discussion of steroid nomenclature, consult the literature (1).

MECHANISM OF STEROID HORMONE ACTION

In addition to their structural similarities, adrenocorticoids, estrogens, progestins, and androgens share a common mode of action. They are present in the body only in extremely low concentrations (e.g., 0.1 to 1.0 nmol/L), where they exert potent physiologic effects on sensitive tissues, and they bind with high affinity to intracellular receptors. Extensive research activities directed at elucidation of the general mechanism of

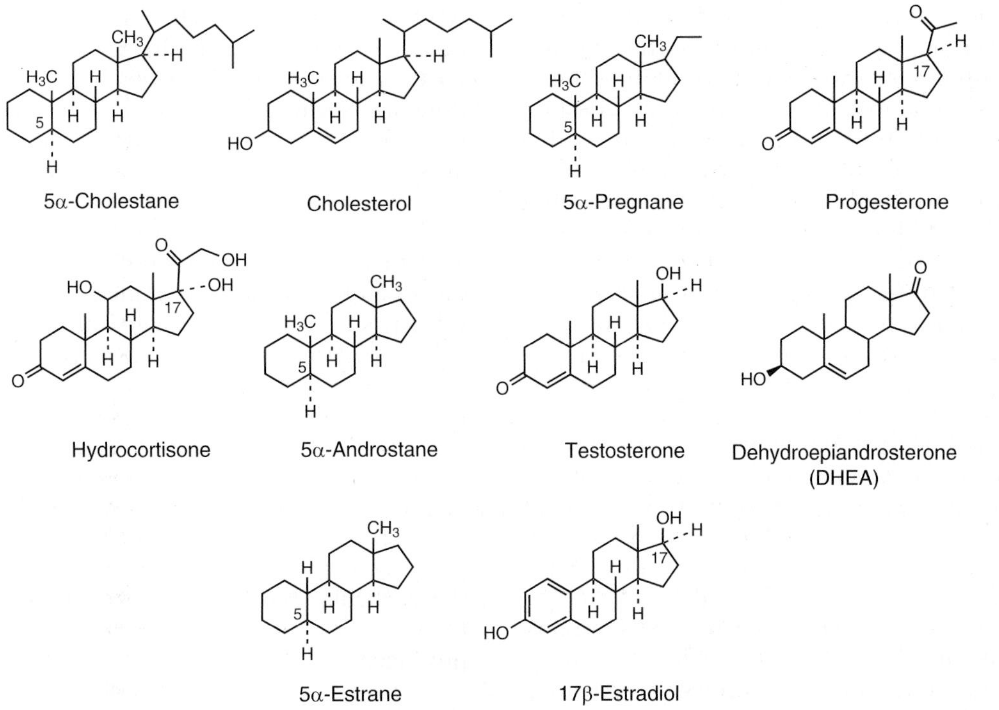

FIGURE 28.4 Steroid classes and corresponding natural hormones.

steroid hormone action have been performed for several decades, and many reviews have appeared (2–7).

Steroid hormones act on target cells to regulate gene expression and protein biosynthesis via the formation of steroid–receptor complexes and subsequent transactivation of gene expression, as outlined in Figure 28.5. The lipophilic steroid hormones are carried in the bloodstream, with the majority of the hormones reversibly bound to serum carrier proteins. The free steroids can diffuse through the cell membrane and enter cells. Those cells sensitive to the particular steroid hormone (referred to as target cells) contain steroid receptors capable of high-affinity binding with the steroid. These receptors are soluble intracellular proteins that can both bind steroid ligands with high affinity and act as transcriptional factors via interaction with specific DNA sites. Early studies

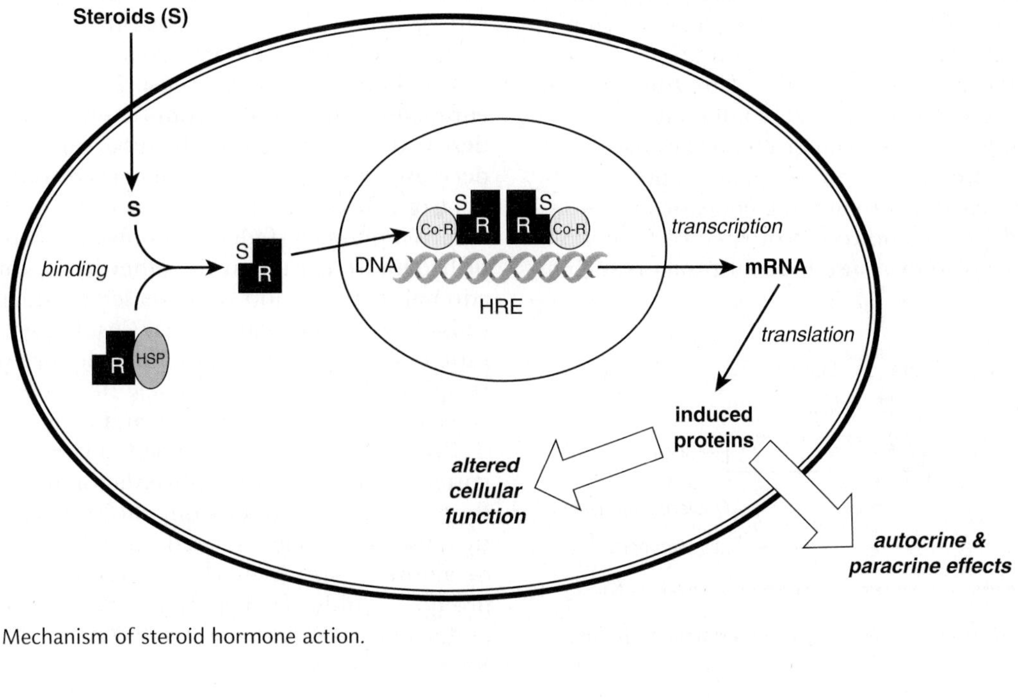

FIGURE 28.5 Mechanism of steroid hormone action.

suggested that the unoccupied steroid receptors were located solely in the cytosol of target cells. Investigations on estrogen, progestin, and androgen action, however, indicate that active, unoccupied receptors are also present in the nucleus of the cell (2,7). Before the binding of the steroid, the steroid receptor is complexed with heat shock proteins. In the current model, the steroid enters the cell and binds to the steroid receptor in the cytoplasm or nucleus. This binding initiates a conformational change and dissociation of the heat shock protein, allowing steroid receptor dimerization and translocation to the nucleus. The receptor dimer interacts with particular regions of the cellular DNA, referred to as hormone-responsive elements (HRE), and with various coactivators and nuclear transcriptional factors. Binding of the nuclear steroid–receptor complex to DNA initiates transcription of the DNA sequence to produce mRNA. Finally, the elevated levels of mRNA lead to an increase in protein synthesis in the endoplasmic reticulum. These proteins include enzymes, receptors, and secreted factors that subsequently result in the steroid hormonal response regulating cell function, growth, and differentiation and playing central roles in normal physiologic processes as well as in many important diseases.

The primary amino acid sequences of the various steroid hormone receptors have been deduced from cloned cDNA (3,5). The steroid receptor proteins are part of a larger family of nuclear receptor proteins that also include receptors for vitamin D, thyroid hormones, and retinoids. The overall structures of the receptors have strong similarities (Fig. 28.6). A high degree of homology (sequence similarities) in the steroid receptors is found in the DNA binding region that interacts with the HRE. The DNA binding region has critically placed cysteine amino acids that chelate zinc ions, forming finger-like projections, called zinc fingers, that bind to the DNA. Structure–function studies of cloned receptor proteins also identify regions of the molecules that are important for interactions with nuclear transcriptional factors, coactivator or corepressor proteins, activation of gene transcription, and protein-to-protein interactions.

More recently, steroid–receptor complexes have demonstrated negative regulation of gene expression by interacting at negative response elements or by transrepression via direct or indirect protein–protein interactions with other known transcriptional proteins such as AP-1 and NFκB (8,9). This can be critical for cross-talk between signaling pathways within the cell and may have an important role in feedback systems. Additional evidence suggests that steroid receptors can activate transcription in the absence of hormone, an effect that appears to depend on the phosphorylation of the receptor via cross-talk with membrane-bound adrenergic and/or growth factor receptors (10). The interactions necessary for formation of the steroid–receptor complexes and subsequent activation or repression of gene transcription are complicated, involve multistage processes, and leave many unanswered questions. Lastly, nongenomic mechanisms involving cytosolic and/or membrane-bound steroid receptors have been identified to explain rapid onset actions of steroid hormones (8).

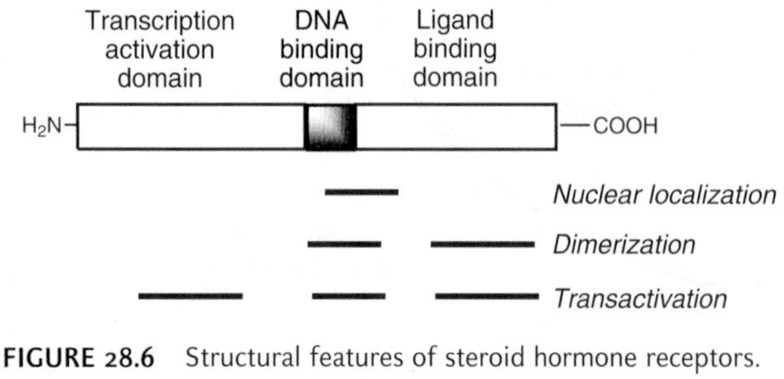

FIGURE 28.6 Structural features of steroid hormone receptors.

The basic mechanism of steroid hormone action on target cells is similar for the various classes of agents. Differences in the actions of adrenocorticoids, estrogens, progestins, and androgens arise from the specificity of the particular receptor proteins, the particular genetic processes initiated, and the specific cellular proteins produced.

HISTORY AND DISEASE STATES

The importance of the adrenal glands was recognized long ago. Addison disease, Cushing disease, and Conn syndrome are pathologic conditions related to the adrenal cortex and the hormones produced by the gland.

Addison disease was named after Thomas Addison. In 1855, Addison described a syndrome in which the physiologic significance of the adrenal cortex was emphasized (11). This disease is characterized by extreme weakness, anorexia, anemia, nausea and vomiting, low blood pressure, hyperpigmentation of the skin, and mental depression resulting from decreased secretion of steroid hormones by the adrenal cortex. Addison disease is a rare affliction that affects roughly 1 in 100,000 people and is seen equally in both sexes and in all age groups.

Conditions of this type, usually referred to as hypoadrenalism, can result from several causes, including destruction of the cortex by tuberculosis or atrophy or decreased secretion of adrenocorticotropin (adrenocorticotropic hormone [ACTH]) because of diseases of the anterior pituitary (adenohypophysis). Cushing disease, or hyperadrenalism, on the other hand, can result from adrenal cortex tumors or increased production of ACTH caused by pituitary carcinoma. Cushing syndrome is also rare, occurring in only 2 to 5 people for every 1 million people each year. Approximately 10% of newly diagnosed cases are observed in children and teenagers.

Conn syndrome is caused by an inability of the adrenal cortex to carry out 17α-hydroxylation during the biosynthesis of the hormones from cholesterol. Consequently, the disease is characterized by a high secretory level of aldosterone, which lacks a 17α-hydroxyl functional group. In addition, hypernatremia, polyuria, alkalosis, and hypertension are observed (12).

The importance of the adrenocorticoids is most dramatically observed in adrenalectomized animals. There is an increase of urea in the blood, muscle weakness (asthenia), decreased liver glycogen, decreased resistance to insulin, lowered resistance to trauma (e.g., cold and mechanical or chemical shock), and electrolyte disturbances. Potassium ions are retained, and excretion of Na^+, Cl^-, and water is increased. Adrenalectomy in small animals causes death in a few days.

After Addison's observations in 1855, physiologists, pharmacologists, and chemists from many countries contributed to our understanding of adrenocorticoids. It was not until 1927, however, that Rogoff and Stewart found that extracts of adrenal glands, administered by intravenous (IV) injection, kept adrenalectomized dogs alive.

Since that discovery, similar experiments have been repeated many times. Originally, the biologic activity of the extract was thought to result from a single compound. Later, 47 compounds were isolated from such extracts, and some were highly active. Among the biologically active corticoids isolated, hydrocortisone (as called cortisol), corticosterone, aldosterone, cortisone, 11-desoxycorticosterone (17α-hydroxyprogesterone), 11-dehydrocorticosterone (11-desoxycortisol), and 17α-hydroxy-11-desoxycorticosterone were found to be most potent (13). The biosynthesis of these steroids is described below.

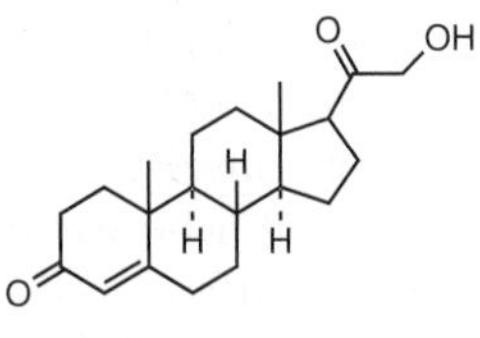

11-Desoxycorticosterone

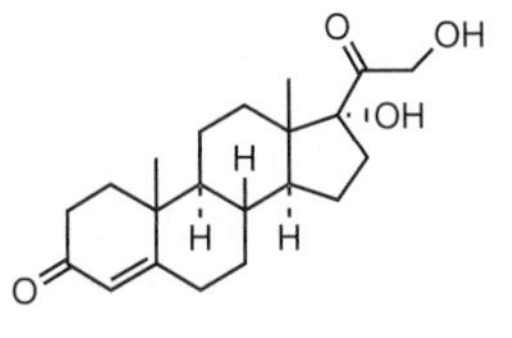

17α-Hydroxy-11-desoxy-corticosterone

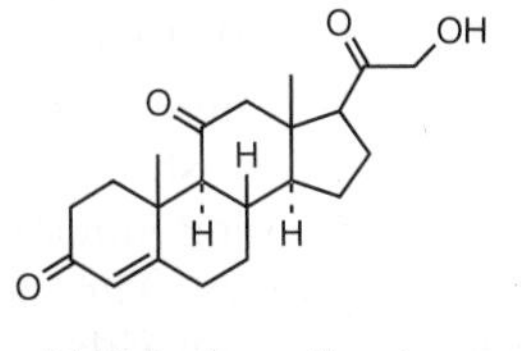

11-Dehydrocorticosterone

BIOSYNTHESIS

Pregnenolone Formation

In the adrenal glands, cholesterol is converted by enzymatic cleavage of its side chain to pregnenolone, which serves as the biosynthetic precursor of the adrenocorticoids (Fig. 28.7). This biotransformation is performed by a mitochondrial cytochrome P450 enzyme complex. This enzyme complex found in the mitochondrial membrane consists of three proteins: CYP11A1 (also known as $P450_{SCC}$), adrenodoxin, and adrenodoxin reductase (14). Defects in CYP11A1 lead to a lack of glucocorticoids, feminization, and hypertension. Three oxidation steps are involved in the conversion, and three moles of NADPH and molecular oxygen are consumed for each

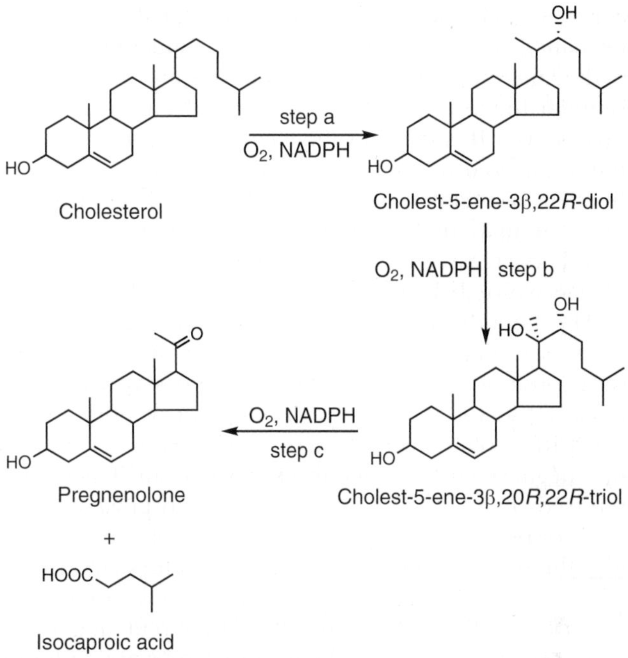

FIGURE 28.7 Biosynthesis of pregnenolone from cholesterol.

mole of cholesterol converted to pregnenolone. The first oxidation results in the formation of cholest-5-ene-3β,22R-diol (step a), followed by the second oxidation yielding cholest-5-ene-3β,20R,22R-triol (step b). The third oxidation step catalyzes the cleavage of the C20-C22 bond to release pregnenolone and isocaproic acid (step c).

Pregnenolone serves as the common precursor in the formation of the adrenocorticoids and other steroid hormones. This C21 steroid is converted via enzymatic oxidations and isomerization of the double bond to a number of physiologically active C21 steroids, including the female sex hormone progesterone and the adrenocorticoids hydrocortisone, corticosterone, and aldosterone. Oxidative cleavage of the two-carbon side chain of pregnenolone and subsequent enzymatic oxidations and isomerization lead to C19 steroids, including the androgens testosterone and dihydrotestosterone. The final group of steroids, the C18 female sex hormones, are derived from oxidative aromatization of the A ring of androgens to produce estrogens. More detailed information regarding these biosynthetic pathways is provided in this and the following chapters under the particular class of steroid hormones.

Pregnenolone to Glucocorticoids and Mineralocorticoids

The biosynthesis of the glucocorticoids and mineralocorticoids is regulated by independent mechanisms. The glucocorticoids, such as hydrocortisone (also known as cortisol), are biosynthesized and released under the influence of peptide hormones secreted by the hypothalamus and anterior pituitary (adenohypophysis) to activate the adrenal cortex (the hypothalamic-pituitary-adrenal [HPA] axis). Removal of the pituitary results in atrophy of the adrenal cortex and a marked decrease in the rate of glucocorticoid formation and secretion. On the other hand, the secretion of the mineralocorticoids, corticosterone and aldosterone, is under the influence of the octapeptide, angiotensin II. Angiotensin II is the active metabolite resulting from the renin-catalyzed proteolytic hydrolysis of plasma angiotensinogen to angiotensin I in the blood. In hypophysectomized animals, the rate of secretion of aldosterone is only slightly decreased or remains unchanged. Consequently, the electrolyte balance remains nearly normal.

The peptide hormone in the anterior pituitary that influences glucocorticoid biosynthesis is ACTH, whereas the peptide hormone in the hypothalamus is corticotropin-releasing factor (CRF). The production of both ACTH and CRF is regulated by the central nervous system and by a negative corticoid feedback mechanism. The CRF is released by the hypothalamus and is transported to the anterior pituitary, where it stimulates the release of ACTH into the bloodstream. Then, ACTH is transported to the adrenal glands, where it stimulates the biosynthesis and secretion of the glucocorticoids. The circulating levels of glucocorticoids act on the hypothalamus and anterior pituitary to regulate the release of both CRF and ACTH. As the levels of glucocorticoids rise, smaller amounts of CRF and ACTH are secreted, and a negative feedback is observed (HPA suppression). Stimuli, such as pain, noise, and emotional reactions, increase the secretion of CRF, ACTH, and consequently, the glucocorticoids. Once the stimulus is alleviated or removed, the negative feedback mechanism inhibits further production and helps to return the body to a normal hormonal balance (15,16).

ACTH acts at the adrenal gland by binding to a receptor protein on the surface of the adrenal cortex cell to stimulate the biosynthesis and secretion of glucocorticoids. The only steroid stored in the adrenal gland is cholesterol, found in the form of cholesterol esters stored in lipid droplets. ACTH stimulates the conversion of cholesterol esters to glucocorticoids by initiating a series of biochemical events through its surface receptor. The ACTH receptor protein is coupled to a G protein and to adenylate cyclase. Binding of ACTH to its receptor leads to activation of adenylate cyclase via the G protein. The result is an increase in intracellular cyclic adenosine monophosphate (cAMP) levels. One of the processes influenced by elevated cAMP levels is the activation of cholesterol esterase, which cleaves cholesterol esters and liberates free cholesterol. Another process is the rapid induction of steroidogenic acute regulatory protein, referred to as StAR, which transfers cholesterol into the mitochondrial membrane.

Free cholesterol is then converted within mitochondria to pregnenolone via the side-chain cleavage reaction described earlier (Fig. 28.7). Pregnenolone is converted to adrenocorticoids by a series of enzymatic oxidations and isomerization of the double bond (Fig. 28.8). The next several enzymatic steps in the biosynthesis of glucocorticoids occur in the endoplasmic reticulum of the adrenal cortex cell. Hydroxylation of pregnenolone at position 17 by the enzyme 17α-hydroxylase (CYP17) produces 17α-hydroxypregnenolone (step b). The 17α-hydroxyl group is important for adrenocorticoid hormone action. In one step, 17α-hydroxypregnenolone is oxidized to a 3-keto intermediate and isomerized to 17α-hydroxyprogesterone by the action of a single enzyme, 5-ene-3β-hydroxysteroid dehydrogenase (3β-HSD) (step c). Another hydroxylation occurs by the action of 21-hydroxylase (CYP21) to give rise to 11-deoxycortisol, which contains the physiologically important ketol (—$COCH_2OH$) side chain at the 17β position (step d). A lack of CYP21 prevents hydrocortisone biosynthesis, diverting excess 17α-hydroxypregnenolone and 17α-hydroxyprogesterone into overproduction of C19 androgens. The final step in the biosynthesis of hydrocortisone is catalyzed by the enzyme 11β-hydroxylase, a mitochondrial cytochrome P450 enzyme complex (CYP11B2). This last enzymatic step (step e) results in the formation of hydrocortisone (cortisol), the most potent endogenous glucocorticoid secreted by the adrenal cortex. Approximately 15 to 20 mg of hydrocortisone are biosynthesized daily. Several reviews (14,15,17–19) provide more detailed discussions about the enzymology and regulation of adrenal steroidogenesis.

The pathway for the formation of the potent mineralocorticoid molecule, aldosterone, is similar to that for hydrocortisone and uses several of the same enzymes (Fig. 28.8). The preferred pathway involves the conversion of pregnenolone to progesterone by 3β-HSD (step c). Hydroxylation at position 21 of progesterone by 21-hydroxylase results in 21-hydroxyprogesterone (11-deoxycorticosterone) (step d). Again, these first conversions occur in the endoplasmic reticulum of the cell, whereas the next enzymatic steps occur in the mitochondria. 11β-Hydroxylase (CYP11B2) catalyzes the conversion of 21-hydroxyprogesterone to corticosterone (step e), which exhibits mineralocorticoid activity. The final two oxidations involve hydroxylations at the C18 methyl group and are catalyzed by 18-hydroxylase (step f). These reactions produce first 18-hydroxycorticosterone (not shown) and then aldosterone, the most powerful endogenous mineralocorticoid secretion of the adrenal cortex. The aldehyde at C18 of aldosterone exists in equilibrium with its hemiacetal form.

METABOLISM

Hydrocortisone (hormonally active) and cortisone (the inactive metabolite of hydrocortisone) are biochemically interconvertible by the enzyme 11β-hydroxysteroid dehydrogenase (Fig. 28.9). Two isozymes of 11β-hydroxysteroid dehydrogenase are present, type 1 11β-hydroxysteroid dehydrogenase (11β-HSD1), referred to as the "liver" isozyme, and type 2 11β-hydroxysteroid dehydrogenase (11β-HSD2), referred to as the "kidney" isozyme (20–22). The 11β-HSD1 isozyme is a bidirectional enzyme, which readily interconverts hydrocortisone and cortisone, and is found in many tissues in the body. This isozyme has an important role in the regulation of hepatic gluconeogenesis in the liver and in fat production in adipose tissues. By contrast, the 11β-HSD2 isozyme is only unidirectional,

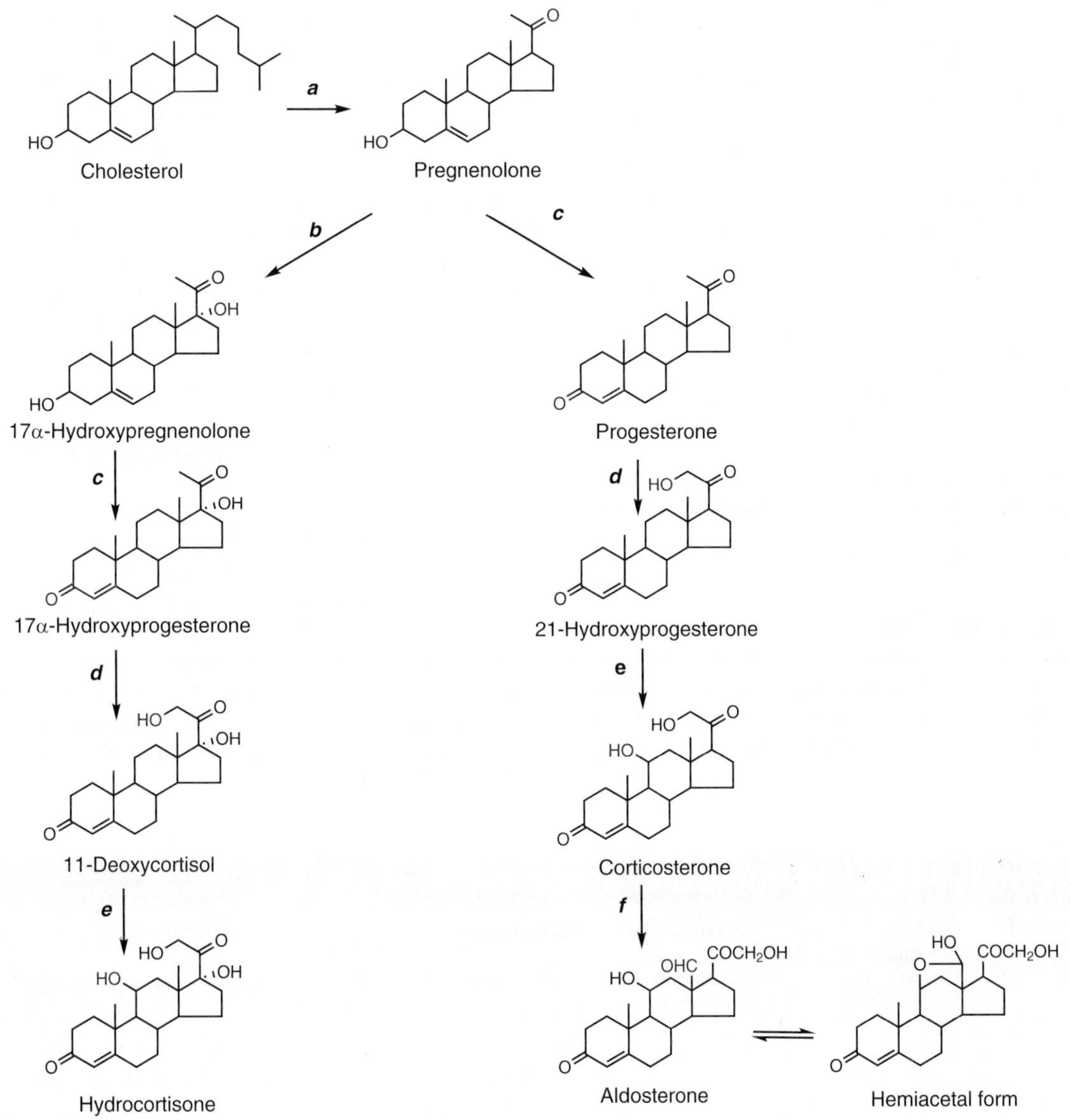

FIGURE 28.8 Biosynthesis of the adrenocorticoids from cholesterol.

catalyzing the 11β-dehydrogenation of hydrocortisone to give cortisone. The 11β-HSD2 is present in placenta and in kidney, specifically the distal convoluted tubules and cortical collecting ducts in the kidney. The 11β-HSD2 isozyme has an important role in the rapid metabolism of hydrocortisone, thus preventing hydrocortisone from binding to the mineralocorticoid receptors present in the same kidney tissues. A deficiency of 11β-HSD2 is associated with the inherited genetic disease, apparent mineralocorticoid excess, which is characterized by hypertension, excessive salt retention, and hypokalemia caused by the elevated hydrocortisone levels in the kidney.

Hydrocortisone is metabolized by the liver following administration by any route, with a half-life of approximately 1.0 to 1.5 hours (23). Hydrocortisone is mainly excreted in the urine as inactive *O*-glucuronide conjugates and minor *O*-sulfate conjugates of urocortisol, 5β-dihydrocortisol, and urocortisone (Fig. 28.9). The tetrahydro metabolite urocortisol is the major metabolite formed and has the 5β-pregnane geometry and 3α-hydroxyl function. The 5β configuration is similar to the ring geometry for the nonhormonal bile acids. Several compounds of this type have been isolated (24,25). All of the biologically active adrenocorticoids contain a ketone at the 3-position and a double bond in the 4,5-position. The formation of inactive 5β-metabolites from hydrocortisone is characterized by reduction of the 4,5-double bond to a 5β geometry for rings A and B (a *cis* configuration) by 5β-reductase or reduction of the 3-ketone by 3α-hydroxysteroid dehydrogenase (3α-hydroxyl configuration) or 3β-hydroxysteroid dehydrogenase (3β-hydroxyl configuration). These reactions represent the major pathways of metabolism for the glucocorticoids and their endogenous counterparts for terminating glucocorticoid activity. Urocortisol and urocortisone are named after cortisol (hydrocortisone) and cortisone. Reversible oxidation of the 11β-hydroxyl

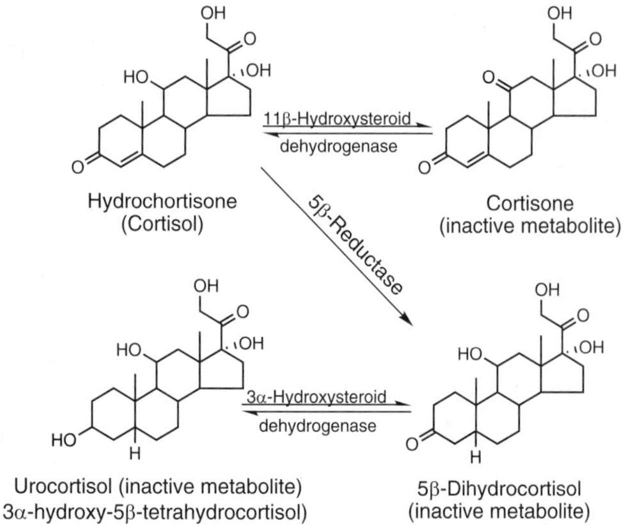

FIGURE 28.9 Major routes of metabolism for hydrocortisone.

group of many glucocorticoids (e.g., hydrocortisone, prednisolone, and methylprednisolone, but not dexamethasone and other 9α-fluorinated glucocorticoids) by 11β-hydroxysteroid dehydrogenase inactivates these drugs and limits their mineralocorticoid activity in the kidneys. Other routes of metabolism include 6β-hydroxylation (CYP3A4) and reduction of the 20-ketone (e.g., prednisolone) to form 20-hydroxyl analogs as well as oxidation of the 17-ketol side chain to 17β-carboxylic acids and loss of the 17-ketol side chain, resulting in 11β-hydroxy-17-keto-C19 steroids with the geometry of either 5α-androstane or 5β-androstane (15,17–19). In addition, some ring A aromatic adrenocorticoid metabolites that resemble the estrogens have been isolated (26). Biliary and fecal excretion contributes little to the elimination of the adrenocorticoids. The rate of formation of 6β-hydroxyhydrocortisone is a biomarker for determining the level of HPA suppression and adrenal insufficiency.

DEVELOPMENT OF ADRENOCORTICOID DRUGS

Systemic Corticosteroids

The route of administration depends on the disease being treated and the physicochemical, pharmacologic, and pharmacokinetic properties of the drug (Table 28.1). The clinically available adrenocorticoids may be administered by IV injection, oral tablets or solutions, topical formulations, intra-articular administration, and oral or nasal inhalation (Table 28.2). Only a handful of corticosteroids

TABLE 28.1 Pharmacological and Pharmacokinetic Properties for Some Adrenocorticoids

Adrenocorticoid	Oral Glucocorticoid Dose[a] (mg)	Potency Relative to Hydrocortisone		Protein Binding (%)[d]	Half-life (hours)		Duration of Action (days)
		Glucocorticoid Activity[b]	Mineralocorticoid Activity[c]		Plasma	Biologic (tissue)	
Short-acting							
Hydrocortisone	20	1	2+	>90	1.5–2.0	8–12	1.0–1.5
Cortisone	25	0.8	2+	>90	0.5	8–12	1.0–1.5
Intermediate-acting							
Prednisone	5	3.5	1+	>90	3.4–3.8	18–36	1.0–1.5
Prednisolone	5	4	1+	>90	2.1–3.5	18–36	1.0–1.5
Methylprednisolone	5	5	0[e]	>90	>3.5	18–36	1.0–1.5
Triamcinolone	5	5	0[e]		2–5	18–36	1.0–1.5
Long-acting							
Dexamethasone	0.75	20–30	0[e]	>90	3.0–4.5	36–54	2.8–3
Betamethasone	0.6	20–30	0[e]	>90	3–5	36–54	2.8–3
Fludrocortisone	Not employed	10	10	<90	3.5	18–36	1–2
Fluprednisolone	1.6	10	0[e]				
Aldosterone	Not employed	0.2	800				
11-Desoxycorticosterone	Not employed	0	40				
Corticosterone	IM	0.5	5				

[a]Based on the oral dose of an anti-inflammatory agent in rheumatoid arthritis.
[b]Anti-inflammatory, immunosuppressant, and metabolic effects.
[c]Sodium and water retention and potassium depletion effects.
[d]Hydrocortisone binds to transcortin (corticosteroid binding globulin [CBG]) and to albumin. Prednisone also binds to CBG, but betamethasone, dexamethasone and tramincinolone do not.
[e]Although these glucocorticoids are considered not to have significant mineralocorticoid activity, hypokalemia and/or sodium and fluid retention may occur depending on the dosage, duration of use, and patient predisposition.

TABLE 28.2 Adrenocorticoids, Their Trade Names, and Their Routes of Administration

Adrenocorticoid	Trade Name	PO	IV	IM	Inhaled/Intranasal	Topical
Alclometasone dipropionate	Alclovate					•
Amcinonide	Cyclocort					•
Beclomethasone dipropionate	Beclovent, Vanceril, Beconase				•	
Beclomethasone dipropionate monohydrate	Beconase AQ, Vancenase AQ				•	
Betamethasone	Celestone, Diprolene, Luxiq	•				
Betamethasone dipropionate	Diprosone, Maxivate					•
Betamethasone sodium phosphate	Celestone Phosphate			•		
Betamethasone valerate	BetaVal, Valisone,					•
Budesonide	Pulmicort, Rhinocort				•	
Ciclesonide	Alvesco, Omnaris				•	
Clobetasol propionate	Clobex, Cormax, Olux, Temovate					•
Clocortolone pivalate	Cloderm					•
Cortisone acetate		•		•		
Desonide	Desonate					•
Dexamethasone	Decadron	•				•[a]
Dexamethasone acetate	Decadron-LA, Dalalone, Dexasone			•		
Dexamethasone sodium phosphate	Decadron Phosphate		•	•	•	
Desoximetasone	Topicort					•
Diflorasone diacetate	ApexiCon					•
Fludrocortisone acetate		•				
Flumethasone pivalate						•
Flunisolide	Aerobid				•	
Fluocinolone acetonide	Retisert, Drema-Smoothe					•
Fluocinonide	Capex					•
Fluorometholone	FML					•[a]
Fluorometholone acetate	Flarex					•[a]
Flurandrenolide	Cordran					•
Fluticasone propionate	Cutivate, Flovent, Flonase				•	•
Halcinonide	Halog					•
Halobetasol propionate	Ultravate					•
Hydrocortisone		•				•[b]
Hydrocortisone acetate				•		•[c]
Hydrocortisone buteprate						•
Hydrocortisone butyrate						•
Hydrocortisone cypionate		•				
Hydrocortisone sodium phosphate			•	•		

(Continued)

TABLE 28.2 Adrenocorticoids, Their Trade Names, and Their Routes of Administration (*Continued*)

Adrenocorticoid	Trade Name	PO	IV	IM	Inhaled/Intranasal	Topical
Hydrocortisone sodium succinate			•	•		
Hydrocortisone valerate						•
Methylprednisolone	Medrol	•				
Methylprednisolone acetate	Depo-Medrol			•		•
Methylprednisolone sodium succinate	Solu-Medrol		•	•		
Mometasone furoate	Elocon					•
Mometasone furoate monohydrate	Nasonex				•	
Prednicarbate	Dermatop					•
Prednisolone	Deltacortef	•				
Prednisolone acetate	Predcor, Predalone	•		•		
Prednisolone acetate	Pred-Mild, Pred-Forte					•[a]
Prednisolone sodium phosphate	Pediapred, Orapred,	•		•		•[a]
Prednisolone tebutate				•		
Prednisone		•				•
Triamcinolone acetonide	Aristocort, Kenacort	•				
Triamcinolone acetonide	Kenalog, Triderm, Delta-Tritex, Flutex					•
Triamcinolone acetonide	Azmacort, Nasacort, Nasacort AQ				•	
Triamcinolone diacetate	Aristocort Forte, Triam Forte			•		
Triamcinolone hexacetonide	Aristospan			•		

[a]Ophthalmic formulations.
[b]Also in otic, ophthalmic, and rectal formulations (Cortenema).
[c]Also in intrarectal foam (Cortifoam).
IM, intramuscular; IV, intravenous; PO, oral.

are used clinically by the oral route, including hydrocortisone, prednisone, prednisolone, methylprednisolone and dexamethasone (Fig. 28.10). These corticosteroids are often described as short-acting, intermediate-acting, or long-acting according to their biologic half-life and duration of action (Table 28.1). They are well-absorbed, undergo little first-pass metabolism in the liver, and demonstrate oral bioavailabilities of 70% to 80%, except for triamcinolone (Table 28.3). The larger volume of distribution for methylprednisolone compared to prednisolone is thought to result from a combination of increased lipophilicity, decrease in metabolism, and better tissue penetration. Glucocorticoids vary in the extent to which they are bound to the plasma proteins, albumin, and corticosteroid-binding globulin (transcortin) (Table 28.3) (27).

Hydrocortisone is extensively bound to the plasma proteins, primarily to transcortin (corticosteroid-binding globulin), with only 5% to 10% of plasma hydrocortisone unbound. Prednisolone and methylprednisolone, but not the 9α-fluoro analogs betamethasone, dexamethasone, or triamcinolone, have a high affinity for transcortin and, thus, compete with hydrocortisone for this binding protein. The 9α-halo analogs bind primarily to albumin. Only the unbound fraction of hydrocortisone and the synthetic corticosteroids are biologically active. As a rule, the amount of transcortin in the plasma determines the distribution of glucocorticoids between free and bound forms, and free glucocorticoid concentrations determine the drug's half-life. Glucocorticoids cross the placenta and can be distributed into milk.

The degree of systemic side effects is dose-dependent, related to the half-life of the drug, frequency of administration, time of day when administered, and route of administration. In other words, the higher the plasma corticosteroid concentration and longer the half-life, the greater will be the systemic side effects.

Regardless of the route of administration, all the synthetic adrenocorticoids are excreted from the body in a manner similar to the endogenous adrenocorticoids

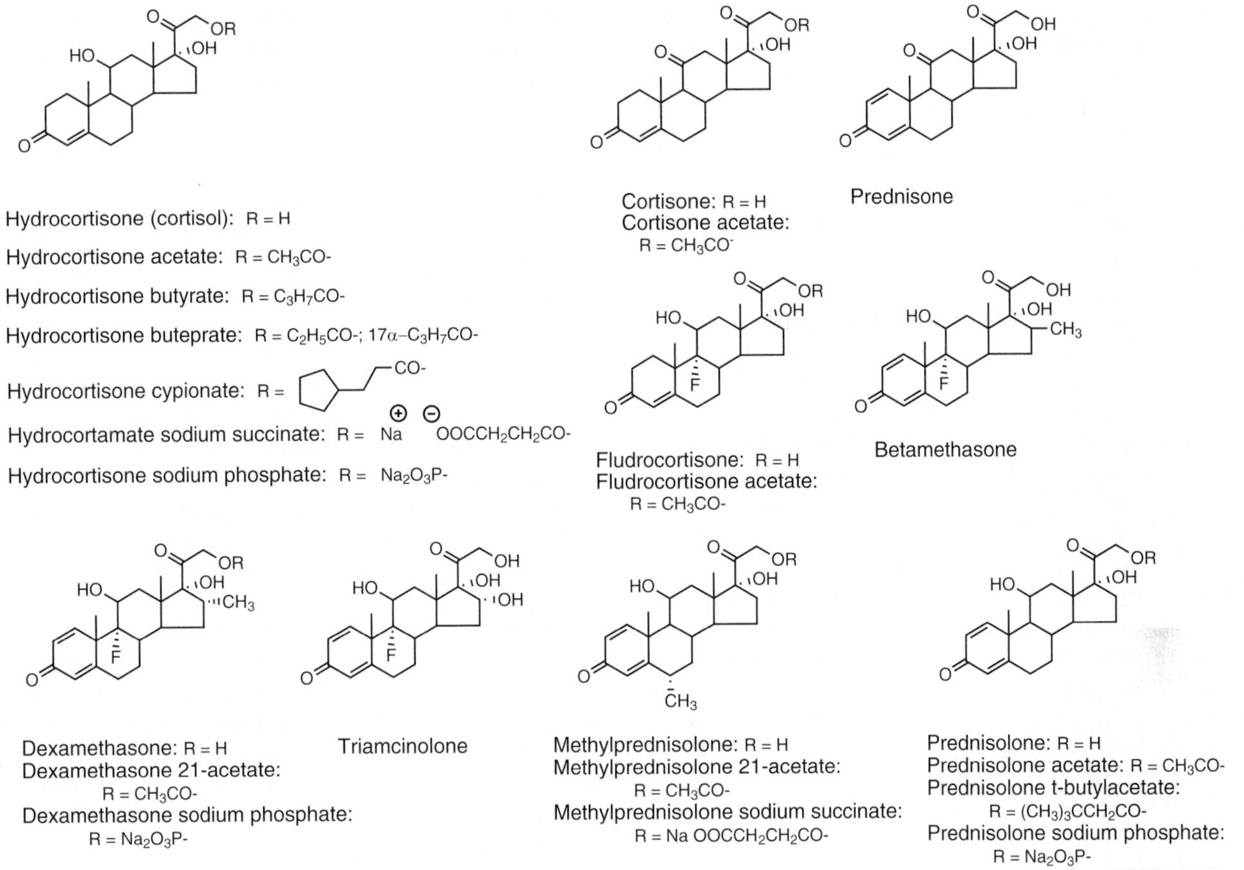

FIGURE 28.10 Systemic corticosteroids.

(i.e., they are metabolized in the liver and excreted into the urine primarily as glucuronide conjugates but also as sulfate conjugates) (28). In fact, hepatic oxidative metabolism rapidly converts many of the systemic and topical corticosteroids to inactive metabolites and, thus, serves to protect patients from the HPA-suppressive effects of these drugs on endogenous steroid production. The corticosteroids are metabolized in many tissues, including the liver, muscles, and red blood cells (15,18,29); however, the liver metabolizes them most rapidly. The fact that many of the endogenous corticosteroids are rapidly metabolized by the liver precludes their administration by the oral route. Catabolic products can be isolated from the urine and bile and can be formed in tissue preparations in vitro (30,31).

Specific Drugs

11-Desoxycorticosterone was the first naturally occurring corticoid to be synthesized. It was prepared, before its isolation from the adrenal cortex, by Steiger and Reichstein (32).

TABLE 28.3 Pharmacokinetics of Commonly Used Oral Adrenocorticoids

Adrenocorticoid	Bioavailability (%)	Half-Life (hours)	Protein Binding (%)	Volume Distribution (L/kg)	LogP (experimental)	Clearance (mL/min/70 g)
Dexamethasone	78	3.0	90–95	0.2	1.83	260
Hydrocortisone	96	1.7	90	0.5	1.61	400
Methylprednisolone	90	2.3	90–95	1.5	1.76	430
Prednisone	80	3.6	~90	1.0	1.46	250
Prednisolone	82	2.8	90–95	0.7–1.5	1.62	60
Triamcinolone	23	2.96	~90	1.3	1.16	61

As a result of his synthesis of 11-desoxycorticosterone and other early work with corticoids, Reichstein later shared the Nobel Prize with Kendall, another chemist who was instrumental in carrying out early steroid syntheses, and with Hench, a rheumatologist who in 1929 discovered that cortisone is effective in the treatment of rheumatoid arthritis. Kendall's basic research ultimately led to the synthesis of cortisone from naturally occurring bile acids (33).

Cortisone, Hydrocortisone, and Their Derivatives After the synthesis of 11-desoxycorticosterone in 1937, all the corticoids were synthesized and their structures confirmed. The first synthesis of cortisone from methyl 3α-hydroxy-11-ketobisnorcholanate was reported by Sarett (34) in 1946. Earlier work of Kendall and coworkers involving its preparation from the methyl ester of desoxycholic acid was used in his research (35). Later, several chemists, including Sarett (36), Kendall, and Tishler, found ways to improve the yields and to decrease the labor involved in the multistep conversion of bile acids to cortisone acetate. In 1949, Merck sold limited quantities of this glucocorticoid to physicians at $200 per gram for treating rheumatoid arthritis. Subsequent improvements in the methods of synthesis reduced the price to $10 per gram by 1951. In 1955, Upjohn used an efficient process involving the synthesis of cortisone acetate from progesterone, with the latter steroid being prepared from diosgenin (a steroid sapogenin isolated from the tubers of the *Dioscorea* wild yam). This further reduced the price to $3.50 per gram. In 2005, the cost was $8 per gram. Other pharmaceutical companies also began to sell cortisone synthesized from bile acids by a well-developed but lengthy procedure (33).

Cortisone is administered orally or by intramuscular (IM) injection as its 21-acetate (cortisone acetate). Cortisone acetate or hydrocortisone (acetate) are usually the corticosteroid of choice for replacement therapy in patients with adrenocortical insufficiency, because these drugs have both glucocorticoid and mineralocorticoid properties. Following oral administration, cortisone acetate and hydrocortisone acetate are completely and rapidly deacetylated by first-pass esterase metabolism (37). Much of the oral cortisone, however, is inactivated by oxidative metabolism (Fig. 28.9) before it can be converted to hydrocortisone in the liver. The pharmacokinetics for hydrocortisone acetate are indistinguishable from those of orally administered hydrocortisone. Oral hydrocortisone is completely absorbed, with a bioavailability of greater than 95% and a half-life of 1 to 2 hours (23). The metabolism of hydrocortisone (Fig. 28.9) has been previously described. Cortisone acetate is slowly absorbed from IM injection sites over a period of 24 to 48 hours and is reserved for patients who are unable to take the drug orally. The acetate ester derivative demonstrates increased stability and has a longer duration of action when administered by IM injection. Thus, smaller doses can be used. Similarly, hydrocortisone may be dispensed as its 21-acetate (hydrocortisone acetate), which is superior to cortisone acetate when injected intra-articularly. Systemic absorption of hydrocortisone acetate from intra-articular injection sites is usually complete within 24 to 48 hours. When administered intrarectally, hydrocortisone is poorly absorbed (38,39).

Other ester derivatives that are available include hydrocortisone cypionate [21-(3-cyclopentylpropionate) ester], hydrocortisone butyrate (17α-butyrate ester), hydrocortisone buteprate (17α-butyrate, 21-propionate esters), hydrocortisone valerate (17α-valerate ester), hydrocortisone sodium succinate (21-sodium succinate ester), and hydrocortisone sodium phosphate (the 21-sodium phosphate ester) (Fig. 28.10). The water-insoluble hydrocortisone cypionate is used orally in doses expressed in terms of hydrocortisone for slower absorption from the gastrointestinal (GI) tract. The extremely water-soluble 21-sodium succinate and 21-sodium phosphate esters are used for IV or IM injection in the management of emergency conditions that can be treated with anti-inflammatory steroids. The phosphate ester is completely and rapidly metabolized by phosphatases, with a half-life of less than 5 minutes (38). Peak hydrocortisone levels are reached in approximately 10 minutes. The sodium succinate ester is slowly and incompletely hydrolyzed, and peak hydrocortisone levels are attained in 30 to 45 minutes (38). Hydrocortisone butyrate, hydrocortisone buteprate, and hydrocortisone valerate are used topically.

After the introduction of cortisone (1948) and, later, hydrocortisone (1951) for the treatment of rheumatoid arthritis, many investigators began to search for superior agents having fewer side effects. When these drugs are used in doses necessary to suppress symptoms of rheumatoid arthritis, they also affect other metabolic processes. Side effects, such as excessive sodium retention and potassium excretion, negative nitrogen balance, increased gastric acidity, edema, and psychosis, are exaggerated manifestations of the normal metabolic functions of the hormones.

It was hoped that a compound with high glucocorticoid and low mineralocorticoid activity could be synthesized. Because it was recognized early from structure–activity relationships that a carbonyl group at C3, a double bond between carbons 4 and 5, an oxygen (C=O or β-OH) at carbon 11, and a β-ketol side chain at position 17 are necessary for superior glucocorticoid activity, investigators began to synthesize analogs containing these functions. Additional groups were inserted into other positions of the basic steroid structure, with the expectation that these new substituents might modify the glucocorticoid and mineralocorticoid activities of the parent drugs.

However, the first potent analogs discovered, did not result from a concentrated effort to find a better drug but, rather, from basic chemical research concerned with the preparation of hydrocortisone from 11-epicortisol (11α-hydrocortisone).

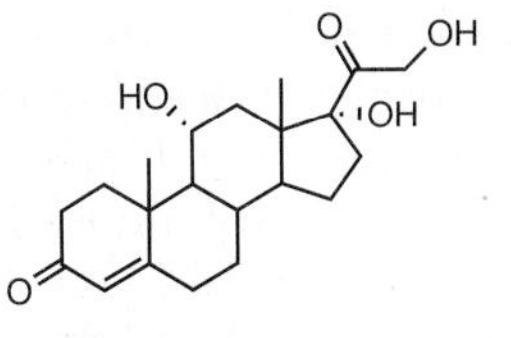

11-Epicortisol

Fludrocortisone A 9α-bromo analog was prepared that had one-third the glucocorticoid activity of cortisone acetate (40). Other halogens were introduced into the 9α-position, and it was soon observed that glucocorticoid activity is inversely proportional to the size of the halogen at carbon 9. The 9α-fluoro analog (fludrocortisone) is approximately 11-fold as potent as cortisone acetate (Fig. 28.10). Fludrocortisone is orally administered as its 21-acetate derivative. When tested clinically in patients with rheumatoid arthritis, it was found to be effective at approximately one-tenth the dose of cortisone acetate. Although glucocorticoid activity is increased 11-fold by insertion of the 9α-fluoro substituent, mineralocorticoid activity is increased 300- to 800-fold (27). Because of its intense sodium-retaining activity, fludrocortisone is contraindicated in all conditions except those that require a high degree of mineralocorticoid activity, because it leads to edema. Fludrocortisone acetate is used orally for mineralocorticoid replacement therapy in patients with adrenocortical insufficiency, such as Addison disease. This drug, introduced in 1954, helped to provide the impetus for the synthesis and biologic evaluation of newer halogenated analogs.

Prednisone, Prednisolone, and Its Derivatives One year after the introduction of fludrocortisone, the Δ-corticoids were brought forth into clinical medicine. Investigators at Schering observed that the 1-dehydro derivatives of cortisone and hydrocortisone—namely, prednisone and prednisolone—are more potent antirheumatic and antiallergenic agents than the parent compounds and produced fewer undesirable side effects at lower dosages. These compounds are known as Δ^1-corticoids, because they contain an additional double bond between positions 1 and 2 (Fig. 28.10).

The Δ^1-corticoids, which can be prepared by microbial dehydrogenation of cortisone or hydrocortisone with *Corynebacterium simplex* (41) and by several synthetic methods (33), represent the first chemical innovation leading to the creation of a modified compound that could be prescribed for rheumatoid arthritis. One high-yield route involves oxidation of 5α- or 5β-pregnane precursors that have appropriate oxygen substitutions with selenium dioxide (42).

Both prednisone and prednisolone were found to have adrenocortical activity (measured by eosinopenic response, liver glycogen decomposition, and thymus involution in adrenalectomized mice). In these tests, prednisone and prednisolone were found to be three- or fourfold more potent than cortisone and hydrocortisone. Antiphlogistic (anti-inflammatory) strengths in human subjects were similarly augmented, but their electrolyte activities were not proportionately increased.

The increased potency reflects the effect in the change in geometry of ring A caused by the introduction of C1=C2 function on glucocorticoid receptor (GR) affinity and altered pharmacokinetics (primarily metabolism). Although the remaining portions of the steroid are essentially unchanged (except for less easily visualized molecular perturbations), the conformation of ring A changes from a chair, as in 5α-pregnan-3-one, to a half-chair (pregn-4-en-3-one) and to a flattened boat (pregna-1,4-dien-3-one) on introduction of unsaturation (Fig. 28.11). The order of GR affinity is dexamethasone (10×) > triamcinolone (5×) > methylprednisolone (4×) > prednisolone (2×) > hydrocortisone (1×) (43).

When orally administered, prednisone and prednisolone are almost completely absorbed, with a bioavailability of greater than 80% (Table 28.3) (44,45). As with the relationship between cortisone and hydrocortisone, prednisone and prednisolone are interconvertible by 11β-hydroxysteroid dehydrogenase in the liver. For practical purposes, prednisone and prednisolone are equally potent and can be used interchangeably. When prednisone or prednisolone is used in the treatment of rheumatoid arthritis, smaller doses are required than with hydrocortisone. The usual dose is 5 mg two to four times a day. Prednisolone is metabolized into a number of hydrophilic and less active metabolites, as shown in Figure 28.12, except there is no reduction of ring A as with hydrocortisone. The major metabolites (6β- and 16β-hydroxy) are primarily excreted as glucuronide conjugates in the urine. Prednisolone acetate is available in suspension and ointment forms for use externally. As with hydrocortisone, several other 21-esters of prednisolone are available. Prednisolone tert-butylacetate (3,3-dimethylbutyrate) is used in suspension form and by injection for the same reasons the 21-ester derivatives of hydrocortisone are employed. The butylacetate ester, which is suitable only for use by injection, has a long duration of action because of low water solubility and a slow rate of hydrolysis. The drug is administered in doses of 4 to 20 mg.

Prednisolone sodium phosphate is the water-soluble sodium salt of the 21-phosphate ester, with a half-life of less than 5 minutes because of rapid hydrolysis by

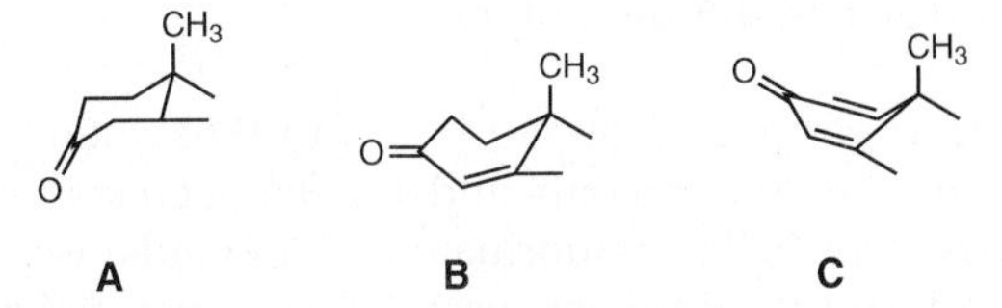

FIGURE 28.11 Ring A conformations for 5α-pregnan-3-one (A), for pregn-4-en-3-one (B), and for pregna-1,4-dion-3-one (C).

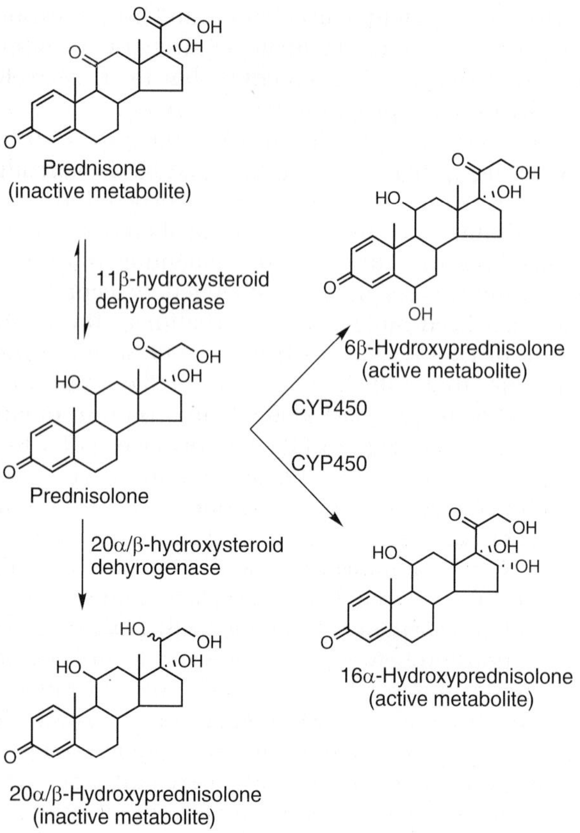

FIGURE 28.12 Major routes of metabolism for prednisolone.

phosphatases (44,46). Peak plasma levels for prednisolone are attained in approximately 10 minutes following its administration by injection (usual dose of 20 mg IV or IM). Topically, one or two drops of a 0.5% solution may be used four to six times daily for its anti-inflammatory action in the eye.

When doses of equivalent antirheumatic potency are given to patients not treated with steroids, the Δ^1-corticoids promote the same pattern of initial improvement as hydrocortisone. Statistical results of the improvement status during the first few months of therapy have been similar with prednisolone, prednisone, and hydrocortisone. The results of longer-term therapy have been significantly better with the modified compounds. Studies indicate that the Δ^1-corticoids can be used continuously in patients with rheumatoid arthritis without undue GI hazard. Although the Δ^1-corticoids are considered not to have significant mineralocorticoid activity, hypokalemia and sodium and fluid retention can occur, depending on the dosage and duration of use.

Methylprednisolone Between 1953 and 1962, many derivatives of the Δ^1-corticoids and the halogen-containing analogs (especially 9α-fluorinated compounds) were synthesized, and some became useful clinical agents. Studies with methylcorticoids revealed 2α-methyl derivatives to be inactive, whereas the 2α-methyl-9α-fluoro analogs had potent mineralocorticoid activity. Methylprednisolone (6α-methyl derivative of prednisolone) was synthesized in 1956 and introduced into clinical medicine (Fig. 28.10). Methylprednisolone is extensively metabolized, with approximately 10% recovered unchanged in urine (47). The metabolic pathways include reduction of the C20 ketone, oxidation of 17β-ketol group to C21-COOH and C20-COOH, and 6β-hydroxylation (CYP3A4). These compounds potentiated glucocorticoid activity with negligible salt retention for short-term therapy (Table 28.2) (48).

In human subjects, the metabolic effects did not differ appreciably from those of prednisolone. Its activities with respect to nitrogen excretion, ACTH suppression, and reduction of circulating eosinophils were similar to those of prednisolone. The sodium retention and potassium loss were slightly less than with prednisolone (49).

Methylprednisolone is administered IV as its water-soluble sodium salt of the 21-succinate ester. The succinate ester is slowly and incompletely hydrolyzed. Peak plasma levels for methylprednisolone are attained in approximately 30 to 60 minutes following its IV administration, and approximately 15% of its IV dose is recovered unchanged in urine (45,46). CYP3A4 inhibitors such as the antifungals, ketoconazole, and itraconazole can potentiate the effects of prednisolone.

Triamcinolone The original interest in 16α-hydroxycorticosteroids stemmed from their isolation from the urine of a boy with an adrenal tumor. The desire of chemists to synthesize these corticoids, and the hope that such analogs might have potent biologic activity furthered their development (50–52). Therefore, inserting a 16α-hydroxy group into 9α-fluoroprednisolone resulted in triamcinolone with glucocorticoid activity equivalent to prednisolone but with decreased mineralocorticoid activity. In fact, 16α-hydroxy analogs of natural corticoids retain glucocorticoid activity and have a considerably reduced mineralocorticoid activity. Thus, a natural extension of corticoid research involved examination of compounds containing a 9α-fluoro group, a double bond between positions 1 and 2, and a 16-hydroxy group. Triamcinolone introduced in 1958 combines the structural features of a Δ^1-corticoid and a 9α-fluoro corticoid plus a 16α-hydroxy group (Fig. 28.10). As mentioned previously, the 9α-fluoro group increases the anti-inflammatory potency, but also markedly increases the mineralocorticoid potency. This is undesirable if the drug is to be used internally for the treatment of rheumatoid arthritis. However, by inserting a 16α-hydroxy group into the molecule, one decreases the mineralocorticoid activity.

The lower-than-expected oral anti-inflammatory potency for triamcinolone (Table 28.1) has been attributed to its low oral bioavailability (Table 28.3), in part because of increased hydrophilicity from the 16α-hydroxy group and first-pass metabolism, primarily to its 6β-hydroxy metabolite. These glucocorticoids actually can cause sodium excretion rather than sodium retention. Triamcinolone diacetate (17,21-diacetate) and its hexacetonide [16α, 17α-methylenedioxy-21-(3,3-dimethylbutyrate)] esters are administered IM or intra-articularly for a prolonged release of triamcinolone. Triamcinolone diacetate has a duration of action depending on its route of administration from 1 to 8 weeks, and triamcinolone hexacetonide has a duration of action of 3 to 4 weeks (53,54).

On a weight-for-weight basis, the antirheumatic potency of triamcinolone is greater than that of prednisolone (~20%) and approximately the same as that of methylprednisolone. Initial improvement following administration of triamcinolone is similar to that noted with other compounds. Reports in the literature, however, indicate that the percentage of patients maintained satisfactorily for long periods has been distinctly smaller than that with prednisolone.

Although triamcinolone has an apparently decreased tendency to cause salt and water retention and edema and can induce sodium and water diuresis, it causes other unwanted side effects, including anorexia, weight loss, muscle weakness, leg cramps, nausea, dizziness, and a general toxic feeling (55). IM triamcinolone is reportedly effective and safe in the treatment of dermatoses, and in combination with folic acid antagonists, it is effective in the treatment of psoriasis (56,57).

Dexamethasone Research with 16-methyl substituted corticoids was initiated in part because investigators hoped to stabilize the 17 β-ketol side chain to metabolism in vivo and improve bioavailability (Fig. 28.10). These studies led to the clinical development of dexamethasone, which combines the structural features of a Δ^1-corticoid and a 9α-fluoro corticoid plus a 16α-methyl group (Fig. 28.10). A 16α-methyl group decreases the reactivity of the 20-keto group to carbonyl reagents and increases the stability of the drug in human plasma in vitro (58,59). Unlike 16α-hydroxylation, a methyl group increases the anti-inflammatory activity by increasing lipophilicity and, consequently, receptor affinity. Like the 16α-hydroxyl group, the methyl group reduces markedly the salt-retaining properties of the corticosteroids (Table 28.2) (60–62). The activity of dexamethasone, as measured by glycogen deposition, is 20-fold greater than that of hydrocortisone. It has fivefold the anti-inflammatory activity of prednisolone. Clinical data indicate that this compound has sevenfold the antirheumatic potency of prednisolone. It is roughly 30-fold more potent than hydrocortisone. Its pharmacokinetics are presented in Table 28.3. Routes of metabolism for dexamethasone are similar to those for prednisolone, with its primary 6β-hydroxy metabolite being recovered in urine (63). Dexamethasone sodium phosphate is the water-soluble sodium salt of the 21-phosphate ester, with an IV half-life of less than 10 minutes because of rapid hydrolysis by plasma phosphatases (64). Peak plasma levels for dexamethasone usually are attained in approximately 10 to 20 minutes following its IV administered dose. A similar reaction occurs when the phosphate ester is applied topically or by inhalation.

In practical management, 0.75 mg of dexamethasone promotes a therapeutic response equivalent to that from 4 mg of triamcinolone or methylprednisolone, 5 mg of prednisolone, and 20 mg of hydrocortisone. Clinical investigations with small groups of patients indicate that this compound could control patients who did not respond well to prednisolone. Over long periods, the improved status of some patients deteriorated.

In summarizing the biologic properties of this drug, it seems clear that with doses of corresponding antirheumatic strength, this steroid has approximately the same tendency as prednisolone to produce facial mooning, acne, and nervous excitation. Peripheral edema is uncommon (7%) and mild. The more common and most objectionable side effects are excessive appetite and weight gain, abdominal bloating, and distention. The frequency and severity of these symptoms vary with the dose (1 mg maximum for females, and 1.5 mg maximum for males). The longer biologic half-life for dexamethasone significantly increases the potential for glucocorticoid-induced adrenal insufficiency (see *Adverse Effects*).

The striking increase in potency does not confer a general therapeutic index on dexamethasone that is higher than that of prednisolone. Again, this drug probably is best employed as a special-purpose corticoid. It can be useful when other steroids are no longer effective or when increased appetite and weight gain are desirable (64–69). Its efficacy may be increased when it is used in combination with cyproheptadine as an antiallergenic, antipyretic, and anti-inflammatory agent (60).

Betamethasone Shortly after the introduction of dexamethasone, betamethasone, which differs from dexamethasone only in configuration of the 16-methyl group (Fig. 28.10), was made available for the treatment of rheumatic diseases and dermatologic disorders. This analog, which contains a 16β-methyl group, has received sufficient clinical trial examination to indicate that it is as effective as dexamethasone or, perhaps, even slightly more active. Although this drug has been reported to be less toxic than other steroids, some clinical investigators suggest that it is best used for short-term therapy. Toxic side effects, such as increased appetite, weight gain, and facial mooning, occur with prolonged use. A 0.5-mg tablet of betamethasone is equivalent to a 5.0-mg tablet of prednisolone, which is on par with dexamethasone (70).

Selective Glucocorticoid Receptor Modulators

The long-term use of glucocorticoids is associated with severe adverse effects (see *Adverse Effects*), including osteoporosis, hyperglycemia, muscle wasting, hypertension, and impaired wound healing. Improved glucocorticoids that demonstrate potent anti-inflammatory activity without these serious side effects would provide a significant therapeutic advance and are the focus of intense research efforts by the pharmaceutical industry.

The molecular mechanism of the GR makes it a particularly suitable target for this effort. The majority of unwanted side effects of the glucocorticoids arise from the interaction of the GR with DNA (i.e., GR-mediated transcription), whereas the anti-inflammatory effects are mediated via protein–protein interactions between the GR and proinflammatory transcription factors (i.e., AP-1 and NFκB) that result in repression of the inflammatory response. A variety of selective GR modulators with the ability to repress inflammation but with lesser ability to elicit GR-mediated transcription have been reported (71–75). Early investigations indicate that a variety of different nonsteroidal pharmacophores (e.g., spirocyclic dihydropyridines, triphenylmethanes, pyrazoles, and benzoindazoles) bind with high affinity and selectivity to the GR. Importantly, some of these analogs demonstrate preferential ability to repress proinflammatory genes and a lesser ability to induce GR-mediated transcription. Although these nonsteroidal ligands have yet to be evaluated in clinical studies, these drugs may someday prove to be the first members of an improved class of anti-inflammatory drugs.

Topical Glucocorticoids

Topically applied glucocorticoids are also capable of being systemically absorbed, although to a much smaller extent. The extent of absorption of topical adrenocorticoids is determined by several factors, including the type of cream or ointment, the condition of the skin to which it is being applied, and the use of occlusive dressings. Previous studies with halobetasol propionate showed that approximately 6% of the drug was systemically absorbed after topical application. Although this is a small fraction of the dose, the very high potency of halobetasol propionate contributed to its ability to cause mild adrenal suppression in some patients. The relative potency of the topical glucocorticoids is commonly determined using topical vasoconstriction assays and is dependent on the intrinsic activity of the drug, its concentration in the formulation, and the vehicle in which it is applied (Table 28.4).

Once absorbed through the skin, topical corticosteroids are handled through metabolic pathways similar to the systemically administered corticosteroids. They are metabolized, primarily in the liver, and are then excreted into the urine or in the bile (76). The fact that circulating levels of the topical glucocorticoids are often well below the level of detection does not reduce the risk for potential adverse effects from systemic exposure of topical corticosteroids. The structures for the glucocorticoids applied topically are shown in Figure 28.13 and their relative potencies in Table 28.4. Topical dermatologic products with a low potency ranking have a modest anti-inflammatory effect and are safest for chronic application. Those products with a medium potency ranking are used in moderate inflammatory dermatoses of limited duration. High potency preparations are used in more severe inflammatory dermatoses, but only for a short duration of treatment. Very high potency products are used primarily as an alternative to systemic corticosteroid therapy when local areas are involved and for only a short duration of therapy and on small surface areas.

TABLE 28.4 Potency Ranking for Topical Corticosteroids

Potency Ranking	Topical Corticosteroids
I. Very high potency	Augmented betamethasone dipropionate Clobetasol propionate Diflorasone diacetate Halobetasol propionate
II. High potency	Amcinonide Augmented betamethasone dipropionate Betamethasone dipropionate Betamethasone valerate Desoximetasone Diflorasone diacetate Fluocinolone acetonide Fluocinonide Halcinonide Triamcinolone acetonide
III. Medium potency	Betamethasone benzoate Betamethasone dipropionate Betamethasone valerate Clocortolone pivalate Desoximetasone Fluocinolone acetonide Flurandrenolide Fluticasone propionate Hydrocortisone butyrate Hydrocortisone valerate Mometasone furoate Triamcinolone acetonide
IV. Low potency	Alclometasone dipropionate Desonide Dexamethasone Dexamethasone sodium phosphate Fluocinolone acetonide Hydrocortisone Hydrocortisone acetate Prednicarbate

The relative potency is based on the drug concentration, type of vehicle used, and the vasoconstrictor assay as a measure of topical anti-inflammatory activity.

Triamcinolone to be used topically is usually dispensed as its more potent and lipophilic acetonide, a 16α,17α-methylenedioxy cyclic ketal or isopropylidene derivative (Fig. 28.14) (see *Inhaled and Intranasal Glucocorticoids*). It is effective in the treatment of psoriasis and other corticoid-sensitive dermatologic conditions. Topically, triamcinolone acetonide is a more potent derivative of triamcinolone and is approximately eightfold more active than prednisolone. The side effects of the drug, however, have occurred with sufficient frequency to discourage its routine use for rheumatoid patients requiring steroid therapy. The drug can be employed advantageously as a special-purpose steroid for instances in which salt and water retention (from other corticoids, hypertension, or

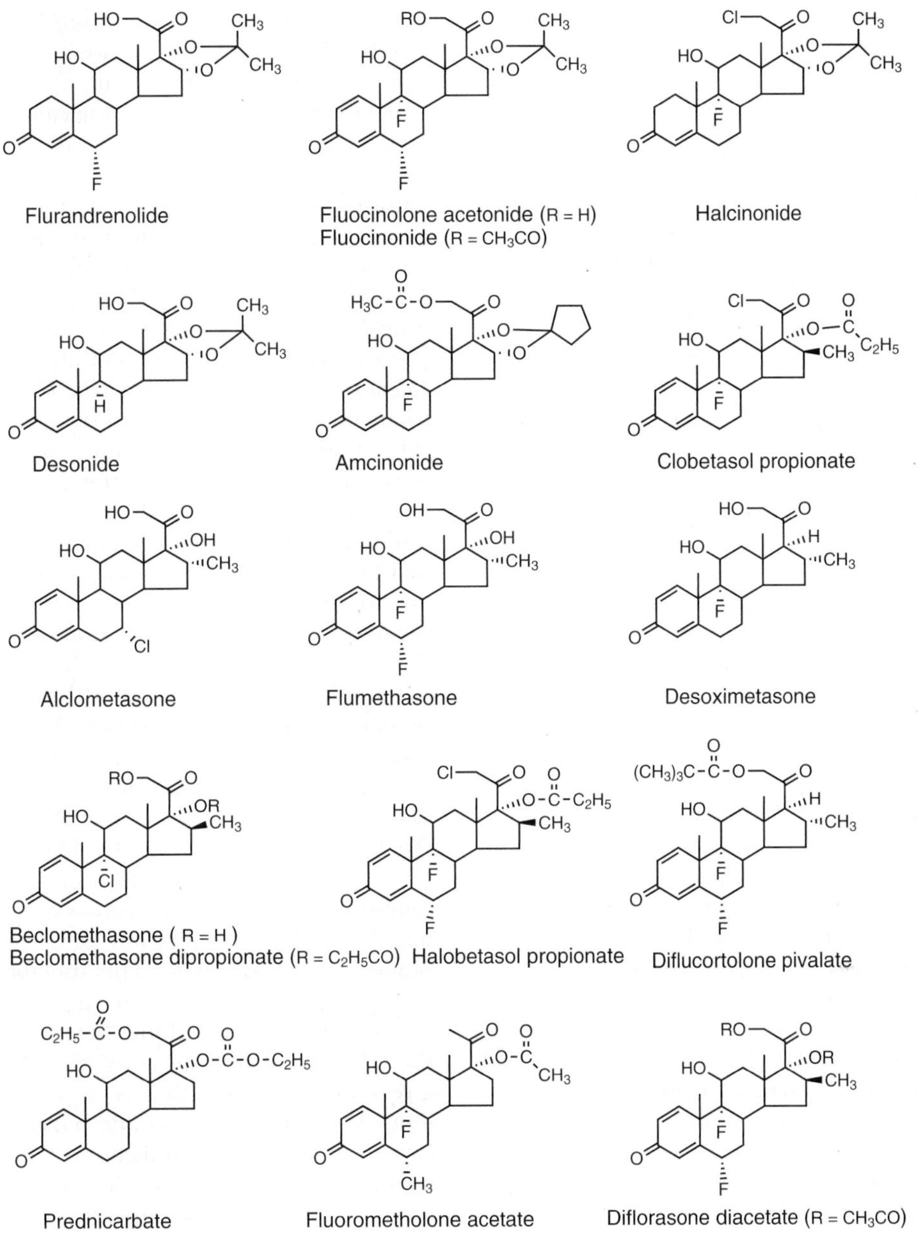

FIGURE 28.13 Topical corticosteroids.

cardiac compensation) or excessive appetite and weight gain are problems in management.

Newer synthetic glucocorticoids have incorporated chlorine atoms onto the steroid molecule as fluorine substitutes. Beclomethasone, a 9α-chloro analog of betamethasone, is a potent glucocorticoid with approximately half the potency of its fluoro analog. It is used topically as its dipropionate derivative in inhalation aerosol therapy for asthma and rhinitis (see *Inhaled and Intranasal Glucocorticoids*) but not for treatment of steroid-responsive dermatoses (77). The topical anti-inflammatory potency for beclomethasone dipropionate (BDP) is approximately 5,000-fold greater than hydrocortisone, 500-fold greater than betamethasone or dexamethasone, and approximately 5-fold greater than fluocinolone acetonide or triamcinolone acetonide, as measured by vasoconstrictor assay. Another potent topical glucocorticoid that contains a 7α-chloro group is alclometasone (78).

Additional mono- and difluorinated analogs for topical application include fluorometholone (a 6α-methyl-9α-fluoro; ophthalmic use), flurandrenolide (a 6α-fluoro-16α,17α-acetonide), fluocinolone acetonide (a 6α, 9α-difluoro-16α,17α-acetonide), and fluocinonide (a 21-acetate ester of fluocinolone acetonide) (Fig. 28.13). These compounds are classified as high- to medium-potency anti-inflammatory agents depending on the concentration and vehicle used (Table 28.4). The acetonide (ketal) derivatives at the 16,17-position enhance lipophilicity to provide potent topical anti-inflammatory agents (Table 28.4).

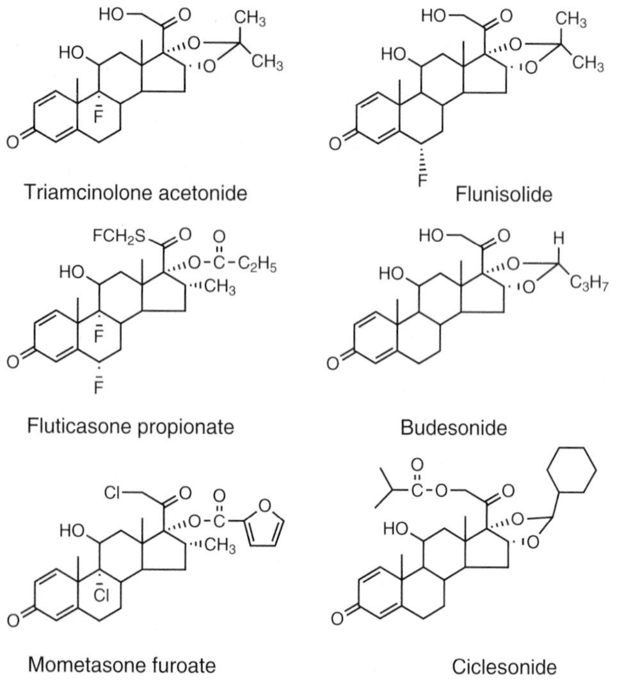

FIGURE 28.14 Inhaled and intranasal corticosteroids.

Psoriasis is one of the few inflammatory dermatoses that has not responded to routine topical steroid therapy, but these more potent steroids appear to work if a special occlusive dressing is used. In this technique, a thin layer of cream or ointment containing flurandrenolide is applied to the individual patch of psoriasis. The area is then covered with plastic food wrap or a similar pliable plastic film.

Clinical investigations show (0.05%) flurandrenolide to be more effective than 1% hydrocortisone acetate and to have approximately the same activity as 0.1% triamcinolone acetonide. Some investigators believe that its greater activity results from an increased biologic half-life. In other words, these analogs are not metabolized as readily. Fluocinolone acetonide has about the same anti-inflammatory activity as fluorometholone.

Clobetasol propionate, halcinonide, halobetasol propionate, and mometasone furoate are examples of 21-chlorocorticoids, in which the 21-chloro group replaces the 21-hydroxyl group (79–82) (Figs. 28.13 and 28.14). Clobetasol propionate, the 21-chloro analog of betamethasone 17-propionate, is approximately eightfold more active as topical anti-inflammatory agent than betamethasone 17α-valerate, the standard of comparison for topical vasoconstrictor/anti-inflammatory activity. Mometasone furoate, a 9α,21-dichloro derivative (see *Inhaled and Intranasal Glucocorticoids*), is also approximately eightfold more active than betamethasone 17α-valerate as a topical anti-inflammatory agent. Thus, substitution of a chlorine (or a fluorine) atom for the 21-hydroxyl group on the glucocorticoids greatly enhances topical anti-inflammatory activity (80). Clobetasol propionate and halobetasol propionate are classified as very high–potency topical corticosteroid preparations (Table 28.4). The HPA suppression has occurred following the topical application of 2 g of the 0.05% clobetasol propionate ointment or cream (1 mg of clobetasol propionate total) daily. Because of its high potency and potential for causing adverse systemic effects during topical therapy, the usual dosage for very high–potency topical steroids should not be exceeded. Fluticasone propionate is similar to the 21-chloro steroids, except that it has a 17α-fluoromethylcarbothioate group instead of the 17-ketol group derivative (see *Inhaled and Intranasal Glucocorticoids*) (Fig. 28.14). Although mometasone furoate and fluticasone propionate are very lipophilic and have the highest binding affinity for the GR (see *Inhaled and Intranasal Glucocorticoids*) when compared to triamcinolone acetonide and dexamethasone, their topical potency is listed as medium, in part because of their insolubility and poor dissolution into inflamed tissue.

Several nonfluorinated analogs of triamcinolone acetonide with the potency-enhancing cyclic ketal moiety are marketed, suggesting that halogens are not always necessary for topical activity. These nonfluorinated cyclic ketals include desonide and amcinonide (Table 28.13) and the cyclic acetal ciclesonide (Fig. 28.14). Amcinonide's potency is greatly enhanced by the more lipophilic cyclopentanone ketal and 21-acetate. A recent addition to the nonhalogenated prednisolone derivatives is prednicarbate, a 17,21-diester (17α-ethylcarbonate-21-propionate) derivative of prednisolone (Fig. 28.13), which is used for the local treatment of corticoid-sensitive skin diseases (83). Any prednicarbate that is absorbed systemically is readily metabolized by hydrolysis of the 21-ester to its primary and pharmacologically active metabolite, prednisolone-17-ethylcarbonate. This metabolite has a half-life of approximately 1 to 2 hours and is further metabolized by the liver to prednisolone. In vitro binding studies with the GR suggest that the ethyl carbonate metabolite has a receptor binding affinity comparable to that of dexamethasone. The low systemic bioavailability for prednicarbate after dermal application has been attributed to its metabolism to less active prednisolone, which can be a factor for the low systemic side effects of prednicarbate.

Inhaled and Intranasal Glucocorticoids

It is generally accepted that the anti-inflammatory effect of glucocorticosteroids cannot be separated from their adverse effects at the receptor level. Therefore, pulmonary and nasal pharmacokinetics become important determinants for the potential of an inhaled or nasally applied corticosteroid to cause systemic effects, because the lung and nasal tissue provide an enormous surface area from which drug absorption can occur into the systemic circulation (84,85). The main areas of concern with regard to drug-induced systemic effects include HPA axis suppression, change in bone mineral density and growth retardation in children, cataracts, and glaucoma. The degree of systemic side effects is dose-dependent, related to the half-life of the drug, the frequency of administration, the time of day when administered, and the route of administration; in other words, the higher the plasma corticosteroid concentration and longer the half-life, the greater will be the systemic side effects (86).

Thus, the search is to develop inhaled/intranasal corticosteroids with the following desirable pharmacokinetic qualities: They would exhibit fast systemic clearance following GI absorption (high degree of first-pass intestinal/hepatic metabolism), short half-life, lack of active metabolites, and high affinity for the corticosteroid receptor. These qualities determine the proportion of the drug that reaches the target cells as well as the fraction of the dose that reaches the systemic circulation to produce side effects.

Modification of the pharmacokinetics through structural alterations has provided several new steroids with a better GR affinity and therapeutic index and a lower bioavailability than the older drugs (Fig. 28.14). The new inhaled/intranasal glucocorticosteroids like mometasone furoate, budesonide, and fluticasone propionate are more lipophilic than those used in oral and systemic therapy and have greater affinity for the GR than does dexamethasone as a consequence of their greater lipophilicity (43). Several of the topical corticosteroids, such as mometasone furoate, BDP, triamcinolone acetonide, and flunisolide, were reintroduced as inhalation and intranasal dosage forms for treatment of respiratory diseases (e.g., asthma or rhinitis). Inhaled budesonide and flunisolide are readily absorbed from the airway mucosa into the blood and are rapidly biotransformed in the liver into inactive metabolites. Mometasone furoate and fluticasone propionate are very potent anti-inflammatory steroids with an oral bioavailability of less than 1%. Obviously, the risk of systemic side effects for these newer corticosteroids is greatly reduced when compared with the older glucocorticosteroids (e.g., dexamethasone). Beclomethasone dipropionate was discovered to be a prodrug, and this discovery led to the reexamination of other 17α-monoesters as the active form of the corticosteroid esters. The absorption of budesonide, fluticasone propionate, and BDP into the airway tissue was 25- to 130-fold greater than that for dexamethasone and hydrocortisone (86). The GR affinity and the pharmacokinetic properties for the inhaled and intranasal corticosteroids are listed in Table 28.5.

It is generally recognized that when administered by oral inhalation, 10% to 30% of a dose of the corticosteroid is deposited in the respiratory tract depending on type of inhaler (metered dose inhaler or dry powder inhaler [DPI]) and spacer used (87,88). The remainder of the dose is deposited primarily in the mouth and throat to be swallowed into the GI tract, where the drug can be absorbed, metabolized, and eliminated unchanged in the feces. Thus, systemic bioavailability of the inhaled/intranasal steroids is determined by the fraction of the dose absorbed from the lungs/nasal mucosa and the GI tract into systemic circulation and the degree of first-pass metabolism. Although these corticosteroids are very lipid soluble, they display variable degrees of absorption from respiratory and GI tissues, in part because of dissolution problems. When systemically absorbed, they are capable of suppressing the HPA and adrenal function with high and chronic dosing regimens (88,89). Although as much as 40% of the dose for the high-potency adrenocorticoids flunisolide, mometasone furoate, fluticasone propionate, or ciclesonide is absorbed into airway and nasal tissues during oral inhalation, the remainder of the drug is swallowed to undergo extensive first-pass metabolism in the liver to essentially inactive metabolites, with no apparent suppression effects on adrenal function with long-term therapy.

Lipophilicity can positively or negatively alter the pharmacokinetic and pharmacodynamic actions of the inhaled/intranasal steroids (90). The lipophilic substituents attached to the corticosteroid nucleus can improve receptor affinity (Table 28.5), or they can affect pharmacokinetic properties, such as absorption, protein and tissue binding, distribution, and excretion. The inhaled/intranasal corticosteroids are inhaled as microcrystals and need sufficient water solubility to be dissolved in the nasal or lung epithelial tissue for local anti-inflammatory activity to occur. Lipophilicity, however, can delay their rate of dissolution into these tissues, which can be advantageous, by prolonging their retention within these tissues, affecting their onset and duration of action, or a disadvantage, by facilitating their transport away from these tissues via mucociliary clearance before full dissolution can occur. The systemic steroids prednisolone and hydrocortisone are less effective as inhaled/intranasal steroids because of their higher water solubility and lower lipophilicity. For inhaled/intranasal steroids, there is a sharp drop in water solubility when the lipophilicity is $\log P \geq 4$ ($P = 10{,}000$), which is the case for BDP, ciclesonide, fluticasone propionate, and mometasone furoate. High lipophilicity correlates well with low oral bioavailability and high protein binding (Table 28.5).

The use of dexamethasone sodium phosphate inhalation aerosol is not recommended because of the potential for extensive systemic absorption and the long metabolic half-life for dexamethasone after absorption, resulting in an increased risk of adverse effects with usual inhalation doses (27). Following the oral inhalation of dexamethasone sodium phosphate, a cumulative dose of 1,200 mcg/day will result in the systemic absorption of 400 to 600 mcg of dexamethasone, which is sufficient to cause HPA suppression. Dexamethasone sodium phosphate nasal aerosol delivers 100 mcg per metered spray. The total daily adult nasal dose is 1,200 mcg.

Specific Drugs

Triamcinolone Acetonide Triamcinolone acetonide is frequently used by inhalation for the treatment of lung diseases (e.g., asthma). After inhalation, triamcinolone acetonide can become systemically available when the inhaled formulation is swallowed and absorbed unchanged from the GI tract, causing undesirable systemic effects (91–93). Triamcinolone acetonide that is swallowed is metabolized to 6β-hydroxytriamcinolone acetonide, 21-carboxytriamcinolone acetonide, and 21-carboxy-6β-hydroxytriamcinolone acetonide, all of which are more hydrophilic than their parent drug. Only approximately 1% of the dose was recovered from the urine as triamcinolone acetonide (94). Triamcinolone is not a major metabolite of triamcinolone acetonide in humans, suggesting that acetonide is resistant to hydrolytic cleavage. Triamcinolone acetonide is approximately eightfold more potent than prednisolone.

TABLE 28.5 Pharmacokinetics of Inhaled and Intranasal Corticosteroids

Parameters	Beclomethasone Dipropionate	Budesonide	Flunisolide[a]	Triamcinolone Acetonide	Fluticasone Propionate	Mometasone Furoate[a]
Receptor binding affinity[b]	0.4 13.5[c]	9.4 22R, 11.2 22S, 4.2	1.8	3.6	18	25–27
Relative lipophilicity[d]	79,432 25,120 BMP	3,980	2,512	2,515	31,622	50,120[e]
Pulmonary bioavailability	~20%[f]	~39%	40%	25%[g]	~30% (aerosol)	<1% (aerosol)
Nasal bioavailability	~20%[f]	<20%	50%	25%[g]	13–16% (powder)	Not detectable (powder)
Oral bioavailability (systemic)	15–20%	~10%, oral	6–10%	23%	<2%	<1%
Protein binding	87% (transcortin & albumin)	85–90% (albumin)	Moderate (transcortin & albumin)	68%[g] (albumin)	91% (albumin)	90%
Half-life	30 min IV 10 min inhaled 6.5 hr BMP IV 2–7 hr BMP inhaled	2–3 hr IV	1–2 hr IV	1–2 hr IV 1–7 hr nasal 3.1 hr solution	~7.8 hr IV ~14 hr inhaled	4–6 h IV Aerosol (not detectable) Inhaled (not detectable)
Metabolism	Lung and liver esterase, liver (CYP3A4) first pass	Liver (CYP3A) first pass	Liver first pass	Liver first pass	Liver (CYP3A4) first pass	Liver
Onset of action	3–7 d	2–3 d	3–7 d	4–7 d	2–3d	7 hr
Excretion	Feces, urine 12–15%	~60% urine ~30% feces	~50% renal ~40% feces	~40% urine ~60% feces	80–90% feces <5% urine	50–90% feces 6–10% urine

BMP, beclomethasone IV, intravenous.
Data from McEvoy GK ed. AHFS 2001 Drug Information. Bethesda, MD: American Society of Health-System Pharmacists, 2001.
[a]Nasarel and Nasalide are not bioequivalent. Total absorption of Nasarel was 25% less, and the peak plasma concentration was 30% lower, than that of Nasalide. The clinical significance of this is likely to be small, however, because clinical efficacy is dependent on local effects on the nasal mucosa.
[b]Binding affinity to human glucocorticoid receptors in vitro relative to dexamethasone. Data from Kelly HW. Establishing a therapeutic index for the inhaled corticosteroids. Part 1: Pharmacokinetic pharmacodynamic comparison of the inhaled corticosteroids. J Allergy Clin Immunol 1998;102:S36–S51.
[c]Beclomethasone dipropionate is converted in the liver to the more active beclomethasone monopropionate.
[d]Measured from reverse-phase high-performance liquid chromatographic technique. Log k′ data from Brattsand R. Eur Respir Rev 1997;7:356–361 were converted to antilogs. k′ values: water = 1, hydrocortisone = 794, prednisolone = 316, dexamethasone = 400.
[e]Calculated log P for mometasone furoate = 4.7.
[f]Estimated for inhaled beclomethasone aerosol.
[g]Data from oral inhalation administration.

Triamcinolone acetonide inhalation aerosol for pulmonary delivery is a microcrystalline suspension in a chlorofluorocarbon propellant that delivers 200 mcg per metered spray, which is equivalent to 100 mcg delivered at the mouthpiece. The total daily adult nasal dose for triamcinolone acetonide is 1.6 mg. Triamcinolone acetonide nasal aerosol is a microcrystalline suspension in a chlorofluorocarbon propellant that delivers 55 mcg per metered spray. The total daily dose for triamcinolone acetonide is 440 mcg.

Beclomethasone 17,21-dipropionate Beclomethasone dipropionate is used primarily as an inhalation aerosol therapy for asthma and rhinitis (77). A breakthrough in the discovery of new inhalation corticosteroids with reduced risks from systemic absorption was that the 17α-monopropionate ester of beclomethasone (17-BMP) was more active than BDP and beclomethasone 21-monopropionate (21-BMP) esters (95). Thus, BDP is a prodrug that is rapidly metabolized by esterases in the lung and other tissues to its more active metabolite, 17-BMP, which has 30-fold greater affinity for the GR than BDP and approximately 14-fold greater affinity than dexamethasone (Table 28.5) (43).

Whether orally administered or swallowed from inhalation, BDP undergoes rapid first-pass metabolism of the unhindered 21-ester via enzymatic hydrolysis in the liver or GI tract primarily to 17-BMP but more slowly to 21-BMP and to beclomethasone and other unidentified metabolites and polar conjugates (96,97). The terminal half-life for 17-BMP is 6.5 hours. The portion of the inhaled dose of BDP that enters the lung is rapidly metabolized to 17-BMP in the respiratory tract before reaching systemic circulation, where it can be further metabolized by the liver. Following oral administration, BDP and its metabolites are excreted mainly in feces via biliary elimination, and 12% to 15% of a 4-mg dose of BDP is excreted in urine as free and conjugated metabolites. The usual therapeutic dose (<1,200 mcg/day) for BDP oral inhalation does not produce systemic glucocorticoid effects, probably because the drug is rapidly metabolized to less active metabolites. At doses greater than 1,200 mcg/day, HPA suppression has been observed (27).

The BDP monohydrate nasal suspension is available as an aqueous microcrystalline suspension of BDP, which delivers 42 mcg per metered spray. The BDP nasal aerosol or inhalation aerosol consists of microcrystalline suspension of BDP in chlorofluorocarbon propellant, both of which deliver 42, 50, or 84 mcg per metered spray. The total daily adult dose for BDP is 600 mcg from the nasal spray or nasal inhaler and 336 to 1,000 mcg for the aerosol inhaler. Doses exceeding 2,000 mcg/day need to be monitored for HPA suppression.

Flunisolide When administered intranasally or by inhalation, flunisolide (Fig. 28.14) is rapidly absorbed from nasal or lung tissue (Table 28.5) (94). This corticosteroid is efficiently metabolized by the liver to inactive metabolites with no apparent effects on adrenal function with long-term therapy. Flunisolide that is swallowed undergoes extensive first-pass metabolism in the liver, and that which is absorbed directly from the nasopharyngeal mucosa or lung bypasses this initial metabolism (98). It is not known if the drug undergoes metabolism in the GI tract. Flunisolide is rapidly hydroxylated by CYP3A4 at the 6β position, followed by elimination of the 6α-fluoro group to its more polar 6β-hydroxy metabolite, which attains plasma concentrations that usually are greater than those for flunisolide (94,98).

Following IV administration of flunisolide, the 6β-hydroxy metabolite has 1/100 the potency of flunisolide and a plasma half-life of 3.9 to 4.6 hours. Flunisolide and its 6β-hydroxy metabolite are conjugated in the liver to inactive glucuronides and sulfates. After intranasal administrations of 100 mcg, the plasma levels for flunisolide were undetectable within 4 hours. The duration of its systemic effects is short because of its short half-life.

Flunisolide nasal solution is available in an aqueous solubilized form, which delivers 25 mcg per spray. The total daily adult dose for flunisolide from the nasal spray is 200 to 400 mcg. Flunisolide inhalation aerosol for pulmonary delivery is a microcrystalline suspension in a chlorofluorocarbon propellant that delivers 250 mcg per metered spray. The total daily adult inhalation dose for flunisolide is 1,000 mcg. Doses exceeding 2,000 mcg/day need to be monitored for HPA suppression.

Budesonide Budesonide is a highly potent, nonhalogenated glucocorticoid intended for the local treatment of lung disease and rhinitis. It was designed to have a high ratio between local and systemic effects. Budesonide is composed of a 1:1 mixture of epimers of the 16,17-butylacetal, creating a chiral center (Fig. 28.14) (99). The 22*R*-epimer binds to the GR with higher affinity than does the 22*S*-epimer (Table 28.5) (43). The butyl acetal chain provided the highest potency for the homologous acetal chains. Its rate of topical uptake into epithelial tissue is more than 100-fold faster than that for hydrocortisone and dexamethasone. Approximately 85% of the orally inhaled dose of budesonide undergoes extensive first-pass hepatic metabolism by CYP3A4 to its primary metabolites, 6β-hydroxybudesonide and 16α-hydroxyprednisolone, which have approximately 1/100 the potency of budesonide (100,101). This is an important inactivation step in limiting budesonide's systemic effect on adrenal suppression. Budesonide was metabolized three- to sixfold more rapidly than triamcinolone acetonide. The pharmacokinetics of budesonide after inhalation, oral, and IV administration displayed a mean plasma half-life of 2.8 hours and a systemic bioavailability of approximately 10% after oral administration (Table 28.5) (101). Pulmonary bioavailability is less than 40% after inhalation (70% to 75% after correction for the amounts of budesonide deposited in the inhalation device and oral cavity). No oxidative metabolism was observed in the lung. When given by inhalation, 32% of the dose is excreted in the urine as metabolites, 15% is excreted in the feces, and 41% remains in the mouthpiece of the inhaler. Following intranasal administration, very little of intranasal budesonide is absorbed from the nasal mucosa. Much of the intranasal dose (~60%) was swallowed, however, and remained in the GI tract to be excreted unchanged in the feces, whereas that fraction of the intranasal dose that was absorbed was extensively metabolized.

Inhaled budesonide, despite its lower lipophilicity, exhibits greater retention within the airways than other inhaled corticosteroids do (100,101). This unusual behavior for inhaled budesonide has been attributed to the subsequent formation of intracellular fatty acid esters of the 21-hydroxy group of budesonide in the airway and lung tissue (102,103). Following inhalation, approximately 70% to 80% of budesonide was reversibly esterified by free fatty acids in the airway tissue. These inactive esters behave like an intracellular depot drug by slowly regenerating free budesonide. Thus, this reversible esterification prolongs the local anti-inflammatory action of budesonide in the airways and may contribute to the high efficacy and safety of budesonide in the treatment of mild asthma when inhaled once daily.

The systemic availability of budesonide in children was estimated to be 6.1% of the nominal dose, and the terminal half-life was 2.3 hours (104,105). Approximately 6% of the nominal dose reached the systemic circulation of young children after inhalation of nebulized budesonide. This is approximately half the systemic availability found in healthy adults using the same nebulizer.

Budesonide nasal aerosol is supplied as a micronized suspension using a chlorofluorocarbon propellant, which delivers 32 mcg from the nasal adapter supplied per metered spray. The total daily adult dose for budesonide is 256 mcg. Budesonide powder for pulmonary inhalation uses micronized dry powder in a turboinhaler (DPI) that delivers 200 mcg per metered sprayed. The total daily adult dose for budesonide from the DPI is 200 to 800 mcg. Full benefit is attained in approximately 1 to 2 weeks.

Ciclesonide The newest third-generation nonhalogenated prednisolone analog approved in 2006 is ciclesonide (Fig 28.13). Ciclesonide is the 21-isobutyrate ester, and the 16α,17α-acetal of cyclohexanecarboxaldehyde of prednisolone creates an epimeric center. The *R*-epimer binds to the GR with high affinity (Table 28.5). The 21-isobutyrate ester and 16α,17α-acetal of cyclohexanecarboxaldehyde greatly enhance its lipid solubility. Ciclesonide is a prodrug that is converted locally in airways by carboxylesterases to produce the active metabolite, desisobutyrylciclesonide (des-CIC). Des-CIC has a 100-fold greater relative GR binding affinity than ciclesonide itself (relative glucocorticoid receptor binding affinities are 1,200 and 12, respectively; dexamethasone is 100). If any ciclesonide or des-CIC enters the circulation, it is highly protein bound (99%) and undergoes extensive first-pass hepatic metabolism by CYP3A4 to 6β-hydroxy metabolites, resulting in very low systemic exposure. Clinical studies demonstrate that ciclesonide is used in inhalation aerosol therapy for asthma and rhinitis (see *Inhaled and Intranasal Glucocorticoids*).

Ciclesonide is supplied as an aqueous inhalation solution pump that dispenses 50 mcg per 70 μL spray for seasonal allergies or delivered in solution form via a hydrofluoroalkane metered-dose inhaler with a once-daily dosing schedule, which facilitates asthmatic patient compliance. The total daily dose is 200 mcg for seasonal allergies and 80 to 160 mcg for asthma. Following inhalation administration, ciclesonide and des-CIC are not detected in the plasma. Ciclesonide has a half-life of less than 1 hour, and des-CIC has a half-life of 6 to 7 hours and an oral bioavailability of less than 1% due to extensive plasma protein binding (Table 28.5). Ciclesonide produces potent anti-inflammatory effects with an onset of action of approximately 2 to 4 weeks. It is extensively metabolized, with less than 20% of the administered dose recovered in the urine as des-CIC. The majority of the oral inhalation for ciclesonide is deposited in the airway passages and swallowed without absorption in the GI tract until eliminated in the feces (~60% of the administered dose is recovered in the feces). The portion of the inhalation dose that is absorbed is extensively metabolized. These results indicate that inhaled ciclesonide has negligible systemic bioavailability and is extensively metabolized, with reduced risk for causing systemic adrenal suppression effects.

Mometasone Furoate The development of mometasone furoate resulted from reexamination of the effect of 17α-ester functionalities on topical anti-inflammatory potency relative to the potent 17-benzoate ester of betamethasone. The structure–activity relationship study involved substitution of the 17-benzoate ester with heteroaromatic furoic, thienoic, and pyrrolic esters (81,106). Of the numerous 17α-heteroaryl esters studied, the 2-furoate ester displayed the greatest increase in potency. Therefore, combining the 17α-(2-furoate) ester with the potency-enhancing effect of the 21-chloro group, the resultant glucocorticoid (mometasone furoate) (Fig. 28.14) was 5- to 10-fold more potent than the betamethasone benzoate ester, with a more rapid onset of action. Mometasone furoate was originally marketed as a topically applied corticosteroid, but because of its low systemic bioavailability, it was found to be more useful in the treatment of allergic disorders and lung diseases (107). It has the greatest binding affinity for the GR (Table 28.5), followed by fluticasone propionate, budesonide, triamcinolone acetonide, and dexamethasone (43). Mometasone furoate has strong local anti-inflammatory activity equivalent to that of fluticasone propionate. It has a quick onset of action relative to the other inhaled/intranasal steroids with the least systemic availability and, consequently, the fewest systemic side effects.

After IV suspension or inhalation administration, mometasone furoate was detected in the plasma for up to 8 hours, with a half-life of 4 to 6 hours (Table 28.5) and an oral bioavailability of less than 1%. It is extensively metabolized with less than 10% of the administered dose recovered in the urine unchanged (108). Among the polar metabolites (~80%) and their conjugates (42%) that were recovered were 6β-hydroxymometasone furoate and its 21-hydroxy metabolite. In contrast, following intranasal administration, its plasma concentrations were below the limit of quantification, and the systemic bioavailability by this route was estimated to be less than 1%. The majority of the intranasal dose for mometasone furoate is deposited in the nasal mucosa and swallowed without absorption in the GI tract until eliminated in the feces (~50% to 90% of the intranasal dose is recovered in the feces). That portion of the intranasal dose that was absorbed was extensively metabolized. These results indicate that inhaled mometasone furoate has negligible systemic bioavailability and is extensively metabolized, with reduced risk for causing systemic adrenal suppression effects.

Mometasone furoate nasal suspension is supplied as an aqueous suspension with an atomizing pump that dispenses 50 mcg per metered spray. The total daily dose for mometasone furoate is 200 mcg.

ANDROSTANE 17β-CARBOXYLATES AND 17β-CARBOTHIOATES

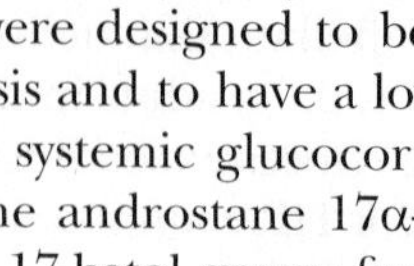

Androstane-17β-carboxylates (R = OCH_2F)
Androstane-17β-carbothioates (R = SCH_2F)
(X = acetate or propionate)

The androstane 17β-hydroxyl-17β-carboxylates and 17β-carbothioates were designed to be metabolically susceptible to hydrolysis and to have a low systemic bioavailability to minimize systemic glucocorticoid-induced adrenal suppression. The androstane 17α-hydroxyl-17β-carboxylates lacked the 17-ketol group found in most of the systemic corticosteroids. When these 17β-carboxylates were esterified to their 17α/β-diesters, however, they proved to be extremely potent anti-inflammatory corticosteroids, whereas the parent carboxylic acids were inactive (109). Thus, enzymatic hydrolysis of the 17-carboxylate ester function by intestinal or liver esterases would lead to formation of inactive metabolites. The greatest anti-inflammatory activity was observed with 17α-acetoxy and 17α-propionoxy groups and simple alkyl carboxylate esters, although the fluoromethyl esters showed the highest activity. Superseding the androstane 17β-carboxylates were the corresponding 17β-carbothioates (thioesters) derived from flumethasone. The 17β-fluoromethylcarbothioate when combined with the 17α-propionoxy group yielded fluticasone (Fig. 28.14) (110). The androstane 17β-carbothioates proved not only to be very potent anti-inflammatory agents but also to exhibit weak HPA suppression in the rat. Both the androstane 17β-carboxylates and the androstane 17β-carbothioates are very lipophilic and exhibit minimal oral bioavailability and very low systemic activity after inhalation because of intestinal and hepatic enzymatic hydrolysis to inactive metabolites, which have 1/2,000 the activity of the parent molecule (111).

Fluticasone Propionate Fluticasone propionate, a trifluorinated glucocorticoid based on the androstane 17β-carbothioate nucleus (Fig. 28.14), was designed to be metabolically susceptible to hydrolysis and to have a low systemic bioavailability to minimize the systemic effects on plasma hydrocortisone levels. Its susceptibility to metabolic hydrolysis is doubly enhanced by the combination of a thioester and the high electronegativity of the fluorine group. Fluticasone propionate is approximately as lipophilic as BDP, eightfold more lipophilic than budesonide, and fourfold more lipophilic than triamcinolone acetonide (Table 28.5). It also displays high in vitro selectivity for the GR and a relative receptor affinity 1.5-fold that of 17-BMP and ciclesonide, about equal to mometasone furoate, 2-fold that of budesonide, 18-fold that of dexamethasone, 10-fold that of flunisolide, and 5-fold that of triamcinolone acetonide (43). The rate of association for fluticasone dipropionate with the receptor is faster, and the rate of dissociation is slower, than the other corticosteroids. The half-life of the fluticasone propionate active steroid–receptor complex is greater than 10 hours, compared with approximately 5 hours for budesonide, 7.5 hours for 17-BMP, and 4 hours for triamcinolone acetonide (43).

After topical application to the nasal mucosa or after inhalation, fluticasone propionate produces potent anti-inflammatory effects, with an onset of action of approximately 2 to 3 days. The topical anti-inflammatory potency for fluticasone propionate is approximately equal to that for mometasone furoate, 13-fold greater than that for triamcinolone acetonide, 9-fold greater than that for fluocinolone acetonide, 3-fold greater than that for betamethasone 17-valerate, and 2-fold greater than that for BDP (111). Because of its low systemic bioavailability when administered intranasally or by inhalation and nondetectability in plasma, most pharmacokinetic data for fluticasone propionate are based on IV or oral administration (Table 28.5). Its rate of topical uptake into epithelial tissue is more than 100-fold faster than that for hydrocortisone and dexamethasone but is similar to BDP and budesonide.

As a consequence of its high lipophilicity (Table 28.5), fluticasone propionate is very insoluble and, therefore, is poorly absorbed from the respiratory (10% to 13%) and GI tracts following nasal inhalation of the drug (112–114). The majority of the intranasal dose for fluticasone propionate is deposited in the nasal mucosa and swallowed into the GI tract until eliminated in the feces (~80% to 90% of the intranasal dose is recovered metabolized and unchanged in the feces). After administration of an IV suspension, fluticasone propionate displayed a systemic bioavailability of less than 2% and underwent extensive hydrolysis and CYP3A4 first-pass metabolism in the liver, with an elimination half-life of approximately 3 hours. Its primary hydrolysis product is 17β-carboxylate metabolite, which has 1/2,000 the affinity for the GR and can be recovered from the urine along with other unidentified hydroxy metabolites and their conjugates. Following oral administration of 1 to 40 mg, fluticasone propionate is poorly absorbed from the GI tract because of hydrolysis and its insolubility, with an oral bioavailability of less than 1%. Less than 5% of the oral dose is excreted unchanged in the urine. Fluticasone propionate was not detected in plasma for up to 6 hours after IV or oral administration (113). Approximately 80% to 90% of the oral dose is excreted unchanged in the feces, of which approximately 3% to 40% is the hydrolyzed 17β-carboxylate metabolite. Pulmonary bioavailability ranges between 16% and 30% depending on the inhalation device used, with an elimination half-life of approximately 14 hours, increasing its potential for drug accumulation with repeated dosing (114). The long elimination half-life for fluticasone propionate results, in part, from its very high lipophilicity and very poor water solubility and, consequently, slow dissolution into lung tissue. Some suppression of overnight hydrocortisone levels has been reported with inhaled fluticasone propionate at higher dosages (indicative of HPA axis suppression) (115).

Fluticasone propionate nasal suspension and inhalation aerosol are both available as micronized suspensions in a chlorofluorocarbon propellant that delivers 50 mcg per metered spray. The total daily adult dose for fluticasone propionate is 200 mcg for the nasal suspension and 880 mcg for the inhalation aerosol.

SUMMARY OF STRUCTURE–ACTIVITY RELATIONSHIPS

The structure in Figure 28.15 depicts the ring conformation and the absolute configuration of hydrocortisone and prednisolone. The all-*trans* (B/C and C/D) backbone that is necessary for activity is very evident.

As previously pointed out, the adrenocorticoids are classified as either glucocorticoids, which affect intermediary metabolism and are associated with inhibition of the inflammatory process, or mineralocorticoids. In fact, most

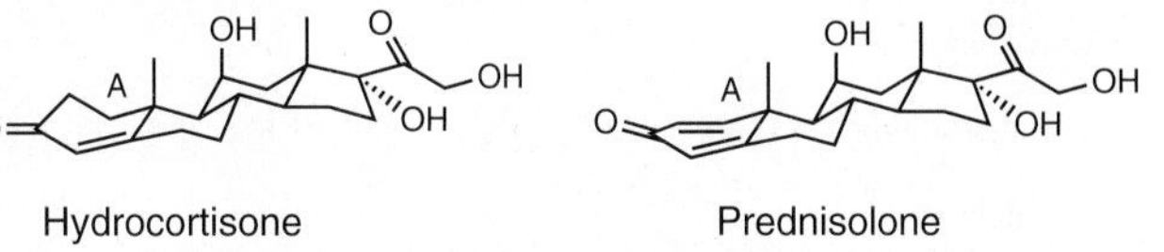

FIGURE 28.15 Conformations of hydrocortisone and prednisolone.

naturally occurring and semisynthetic analogs exhibit both of these actions. The 17β-ketol (—$COCH_2OH$) side chain and the Δ^4-3-ketone functions are found in clinically used adrenocorticoids, and these groups contribute to the potency of the drugs. Modifications of these groups result in derivatives that retain biologic activity. For example, replacement of the 21-OH group with fluorine increases glucocorticoid and sodium-retaining activities, whereas substitution with chlorine or bromine abolishes activity. Some compounds that do not contain the Δ^4-3-ketone system have appreciable activity. It has been suggested that this group makes only a minor contribution to the specificity of action by these drugs or to the steroid–receptor association constant (116).

Based on structure–activity studies, the C and D rings, involving positions 11, 12, 13, 16, 17, 18, 20, and 21, are more important for receptor binding than the A and B rings. As a rule, insertion of bulky substituents on the β-side of the molecule abolishes glycogenic activity, whereas insertion on the α-side does not. It has been suggested that association of these steroids with receptors involves β-surfaces of rings C and D and the 17β-ketol side chain (116). It is possible, however, that association with the α-surface of rings A, C, and D, as well as with the ketol side chain, is essential for sodium-retaining activity. Many functional groups, such as 17α-OH, 17α-CH_3, 16α-CH_3, 16β-CH_3, 16α-CH_3O, and 16α-OH substituents, abolish or reverse this activity in 11-desoxycorticosterone and 11-oxygenated steroids. Discussions of exceptions of these generalities are found in the literature (116).

Although some steroids cause sodium retention, many have glucocorticoid and either sodium-retaining or sodium-excreting action. Difficulties in correlating the structures of adrenocorticoids with biologic action are compounded because of differences in assay methods, species variation, and mode of drug administration. For example, whereas liver glycogen and anti-inflammatory assays in the rat correlate well, some drugs show high anti-inflammatory action in the rat but little or no antirheumatic activity in humans. The 9α-F analog, fludrocortisone acetate, is more active than the 9α-Cl analog in terms of sodium retention in the dog; the reverse is true in the rat. Although 16α-methylation and 16β-methylation enhance glucocorticoid activity, anti-inflammatory action is increased disproportionately to glycogenic action in both series.

In humans, eosinopenic and hyperglycemic potencies are essentially the same. There is a close correlation in efficacy ratios derived from these tests and antirheumatic potency (Table 28.6). Because the eosinopenic–hyperglycemic activity and antirheumatic potency show excellent agreement, it has been suggested that these assays afford advantages in the preliminary estimation of anti-inflammatory potency (27).

Structure–activity studies of glucocorticoids have been carried out mainly in animals and are not necessarily applicable to clinical efficacy in man. Relative activity and

TABLE 28.6 Biologic Potencies of Modified Adrenocorticoids in the Rat and Humans

Adrenocorticoid	Thymus Involution	Potency Relative to Hydrocortisone (Cortisol)			
		Rats		Humans	
		Liver Glycogen Deposition	Eosinopenic Potency	Hyperglycemic Potency	Antirheumatic Potency
Corticosterone	—	0.8	0.06	0.06	<0.1
Prednisone	—	3	—	4	4
Prednisolone	2	3.9	4	4	4
Methylprednisolone	10	11	5	5	5
Triamcinolone	4	47	5	5	5
Paramethasone	—	150	12	12	11
Dexamethasone	56	265	28	28	29
Fludrocortisone acetate	6	9	8	8	10
Fluprednisolone	6	81	9	9	10
Triamcinolone acetonide	33	242	3	3	3
Flurandrenolone	4	—	1	—	2
Fluorometholone	25	115	10	10	—
Fluocinolone	19	112	5	6	9

Data from Ringer I. Steroidal activity in experimental animals and man. In: Dorfman RI, ed. Methods of Hormone Research, Vol 3, Part A. New York: Academic Press, 1964.

dose correlations for the clinically useful drugs are found in Table 28.1.

Several other compounds have been studied in animals and used to derive structure–activity relationships. For example, insertion of a double bond between positions 1 and 2 in hydrocortisone increases glucocorticoid activity. The Δ^1-corticoids have a much longer half-life in the blood than hydrocortisone. Ring A is much more slowly metabolized, but it is oxidatively metabolized at other positions, especially the 6β position and the 17β-ketol (Fig. 28.12). If, however, a double bond is inserted between positions 9 and 11 (no oxygen function at 11), a decrease in glucocorticoid activity is observed. Except for cortisone, which results in an analog with decreased glucocorticoid activity when a double bond is inserted between position 6 and 7, such modification of other glucocorticoids generally produces no change in activity (16).

Insertion of α-CH_3 groups at positions 2 (in 11β-OH analogs), 6, and 16 increases glucocorticoid activity in animals. Again, insertion of a 2α-CH_3 group into the glucocorticoid almost completely prevents reduction of the Δ^4-3-ketone system in vivo and in vitro. Substitutions at positions 4α, 7α, 9α, 11α, and 21 decrease activity.

Although some analogs, such as 16α,17α-isopropylidinedioxy-6α-methylpregna-1,4-diene-3,20-dione and the 1,2-dihydro derivative, are 11-desoxysteroids and biologically active, the 11β-OH group of hydrocortisone does seem to be involved in the drug–receptor interaction (116). Cortisone, which contains an 11-keto function, is reduced in vivo to hydrocortisone. The drug 2α-methylhydrocortisone exhibits high glucocorticoid activity, probably because of steric hindrance to reduction (i.e., C=O → C-β-OH) by the methyl group, thus rendering the analog inactive (40,117,118). Insertion of α-OH groups into most other positions (1, 6, 7, 9, 14, and 16) or reduction of the 20-ketone, however, decreases glucocorticoid activity, in part because of increased hydrophilicity.

The 9α-F group increases glucocorticoid activity and nearly prevents metabolic oxidation of the 11β-OH group to a ketone. Redox metabolism of Δ^4-steroids is mainly restricted to the Δ^4-3-ketone, 6 and 16 positions, and 17β-ketol side chains, whereas for Δ^4-steroids, it is only the 6 and 16 positions and 17β-ketol side chains. The 9α-F group increases activity by an inductive effect, which increases the acidic dissociation constant of the 11β-OH group and, thereby, increases the ability of the drug to hydrogen bond to GRs.

A 6α-F group also increases glucocorticoid activity, but it has less effect than the 9α-F function on sodium retention. Insertion of 2α-, 11α- (no OH group at 11), or 21-F groups decreases glucocorticoid activity. Of particular interest is a 12α-F group. When this function is inserted into corticosterone, which has no 17α-OH group, it potentiates activity to the same extent as a 9α-F group. Insertion of a 12α-F group into a 16α,17α-dihydroxy steroid, however, renders the compound inactive. A 9α-F group potentiates activity in such analogs.

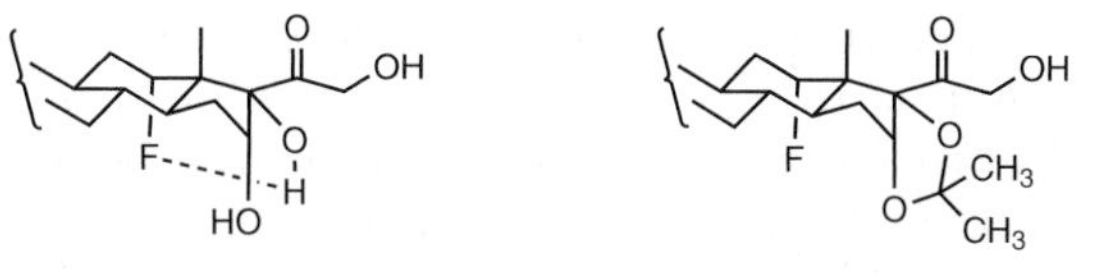

16α, 17α-Dihydroxy steroid   16α, 17α-Isopropylidenedioxy steroid

FIGURE 28.16 Hydrogen bonding between 17α-hydroxyl and 12α-fluoro groups.

It has been proposed that hydrogen bonding between the 12α-F and 17α-OH groups renders the analog inactive (Fig. 28.16). Conversion to the 16α,17α-isopropylidinedioxy (acetonide) derivative, which cannot hydrogen bond, restores biologic activity (119).

The mineralocorticoid activity of adrenocorticoids is another action of major significance. Many toxic side effects, making it necessary to withdraw steroid therapy in rheumatoid patients, are a result of this action. Highly active, naturally occurring mineralocorticoids have no OH function in positions 11 and 17. In fact, OH groups in any position reduce the sodium-retaining activity of the adrenocorticoid.

9α-F, 9α-Cl, and 9α-Br substitution usually causes increased retention of urinary sodium with an order of activity in which F > Cl > Br, but species differences do exist. For these reasons, such compounds are not used internally in the treatment of diseases such as rheumatoid arthritis. Insertion of a 16α-OH group into the molecule affects the sodium retention activity so markedly that it not only negates the effect of the 9α-F atom but also causes sodium excretion.

A double bond between positions 1 and 2 (Δ^1-corticoids) also reduces the sodium retention activity of the parent drug. However, this functional group contributes to the parent drug approximately one-fifth the sodium-excreting tendency of a 16α-OH group (120).

The 12α-F, 2α-CH_3, and 9α-Cl substitutions contribute equally to sodium retention. A 21-OH group, found in all these drugs, contributes to this action to the same degree. Because 21-OH groups also contribute to glucocorticoid activity, it is easy to understand why it is difficult to develop compounds with only one major action.

A 2α-CH_3 group is approximately threefold, and a 21-F substituent twofold, as effective as unsaturation between positions 1 and 2 in reducing sodium retention. Other substituents reported to inhibit sodium retention include 16α-CH_3, 16β-CH_3, 16α-CH_3O, and 6α-Cl functions. A 17α-OH group, which is present in naturally occurring and semisynthetic analogs, reduces sodium retention to about the same extent as does unsaturation between positions 1 and 2.

Conversion of the 17α-hydroxy to either a 17α-ester or an ether, as with 16α,17α-isopropylidinedioxy (acetonide), greatly enhances the anti-inflammatory potency and GR affinity (Table 28.5). As evidenced with BDP, however, esterifying the 21-hydroxy group reduces activity and receptor affinity. On the other hand, 21-halogens or 21-halomethylene groups greatly increase topical anti-inflammatory activity with no change or a decrease in mineralocorticoid activity. Perhaps a hydrogen bonding group at position 21 enhances or retains mineralocorticoid receptor affinity.

ADRENOCORTICOID ANTAGONISTS

Antagonists of adrenocorticoids include agents that compete for binding to steroid receptors (antiglucocorticoids or antimineralocorticoids) and inhibitors of adrenosteroid biosynthesis. The action of adrenal steroids can be blocked by antagonists that compete with the endogenous steroids for binding sites on their respective cytosolic receptor proteins. The antagonist–receptor complexes are unable to stimulate the production of new mRNA and protein in the target tissues and, thus, are unable to elicit the biologic responses of the hormone agonist. Spironolactone, eplerenone (Fig. 28.17), and related analogs bind to the mineralocorticoid receptor in the kidney and result in the diuretic response of increased Na^+ excretion and K^+ retention. The 3-keto-4-ene A ring is essential for this antagonistic activity, and the opening of the lactone ring dramatically reduces activity. The 7α-substituent increases both intrinsic activity and oral activity (121,122). Progesterone has also shown antimineralocorticoid activity at 10^{-4} molar concentrations.

Receptor antagonists of glucocorticoids have been described that are derivatives of 19-nortestosterone (123). Mifepristone, also referred to as RU-486 (Fig. 28.17), was originally developed as an antiprogestin and also exhibits very effective antagonism of glucocorticoids.

Several inhibitors of adrenocorticoid biosynthesis have been described, with the majority of nonsteroidal agents inhibiting one or more of the cytochrome P450 enzyme complexes involved in adrenosteroid biosynthesis (Fig. 28.18). Metyrapone reduces hydrocortisone biosynthesis by primarily inhibiting mitochondrial

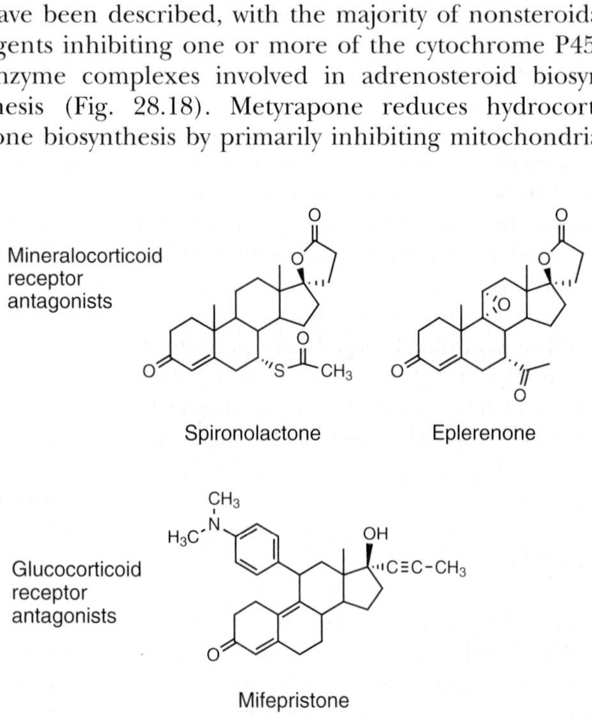

FIGURE 28.17 Adrenocorticoids receptor antagonists.

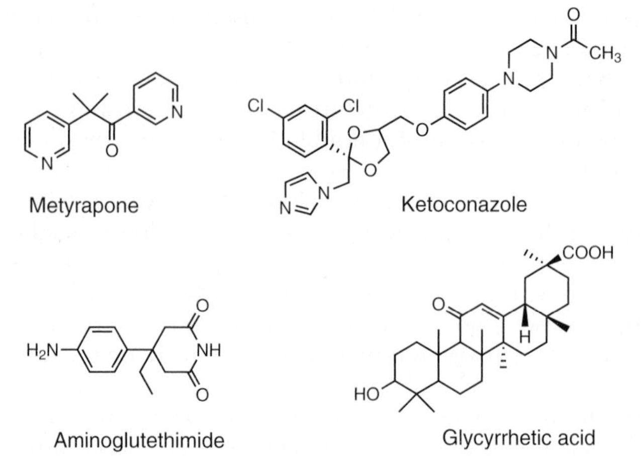

FIGURE 28.18 Inhibitors of adrenocorticoid biosynthesis.

11β-hydroxylase (124,125). It also inhibits, to a lesser degree, 18-hydroxylase and side-chain cleavage. This agent is used to test pituitary–adrenal function and the ability of the pituitary to secrete ACTH (125). Aminoglutethimide inhibits side-chain cleavage (125) and has been used as a medical adrenalectomy. Several azole antifungal drugs inhibit adrenocorticoid biosynthesis. Ketoconazole is one example of a potent inhibitor of fungal sterol biosynthesis at low concentrations; however, at higher doses, ketoconazole inhibits CYP3A4 in adrenosteroid biosynthesis (126). Trilostane is a steroidal inhibitor of 3β-hydroxysteroid dehydrogenase (127) and has been used in the treatment of Cushing syndrome.

Inhibition of the two 11β-hydroxysteroid dehydrogenase isozymes has been described. Excessive ingestion of licorice, an extract of the roots of *Glycyrrhiza glabra*, produces undesirable mineralocorticoid-like intoxication (hypertension, excessive salt retention, and hypokalemia). The active components of licorice, glycyrrhetic acid (Fig. 28.17), and carbenoxolone inhibit both 11β-HSD isozymes (128), with the undesirable side effects resulting from inhibition of 11β-HSD2 in the kidney. Bile acids, such as chenodeoxycholic acid and lithocholic acid, have recently shown selective inhibition of 11β-HSD1 (129,130), and nonsteroidal arylsulfoamidothiazoles also recently have been reported as 11β-HSD1 inhibitors (131). Such enzyme inhibitors may be useful in the treatment of metabolic syndromes to reduce elevated glucose concentrations and as possible antidiabetic agents.

MECHANISMS OF ADRENOCORTICOID ACTION

Molecular Interaction

Glucocorticoid action is mediated through the GR, which is found primarily in the cytosol of the cell when not bound to glucocorticoids. The GR is stabilized in the cytosol by complexation with phosphorylated proteins, including a 90-kilodalton protein referred to as a heat shock protein 90 (132). The steroid molecule binds to the GR, resulting in a conformational change of the receptor to dissociate the other proteins and initiate translocation of the steroid–receptor complex into the nucleus. The steroid–nuclear GR complex interacts with particular HRE regions of the cellular DNA, referred to as glucocorticoid-responsive elements, and initiates transcription of the DNA sequence to produce mRNA. Finally, the elevated levels of mRNA lead to increased protein synthesis in the endoplasmic reticulum. These proteins then mediate glucocorticoid effects on carbohydrate, lipid, and protein metabolism. An alternative isoform of the GR has been identified. This isoform of the receptor does not bind known glucocorticoids, and its function remains to be determined (133,134). Some of the specific proteins induced by glucocorticoids have been identified and are discussed later. Mineralocorticoid effects are observed in several tissues, and specific mineralocorticoid receptors have been characterized that mediate mineralocorticoid functions (135). Steroid–receptor complexes have also demonstrated negative regulation of gene expression by interacting at negative response elements or by transrepression via direct or indirect protein–protein interactions with other known transcriptional proteins such as AP-1 and NFκB (8,9). Lastly, nongenomic mechanisms involving cytosolic and/or membrane-bound steroid receptors have been identified to explain rapid onset actions of steroid hormones (8).

Physiologic Effects

Glucocorticoids

Corticosteroids influence all tissues of the body and produce numerous and varying effects in cells (16). These steroids regulate carbohydrate, lipid, and protein biosynthesis and metabolism (glucocorticoid effects), and they influence water and electrolyte balance (mineralocorticoid effects). Hydrocortisone is the most potent glucocorticoid secreted by the adrenal gland, and aldosterone is the most potent endogenous mineralocorticoid. Both naturally occurring glucocorticoids and related, semisynthetic analogs can be evaluated in terms of their ability to sustain life, to stimulate an increase in blood glucose concentrations and a deposition of liver glycogen, to decrease circulating eosinophils (136), and to cause thymus involution in adrenalectomized animals (137,138). In addition, corticosteroids can affect immune system functions, inflammatory responses, and cell growth.

The primary physiologic function of glucocorticoids is to maintain blood glucose levels and, thus, ensure glucose-dependent processes critical to life, particularly brain functions. Hydrocortisone and related steroids accomplish this by stimulating the formation of glucose, by diminishing glucose use by peripheral tissues, and by promoting glycogen synthesis in the liver to increase carbohydrate stores for later release of glucose. For glucose formation, glucocorticoids mobilize amino acids and promote amino acid metabolism and gluconeogenesis. These steroids, acting via the GR mechanism, induce the production of a variety of enzymes important for glucose formation. The synthesis of tyrosine aminotransferase increases within 30 minutes of glucocorticoid exposure (139–141). This enzyme promotes the transfer of amino groups from tyrosine to α-ketoglutarate to form glutamate and hydroxyphenylpyruvate. Another amino acid–metabolizing enzyme induced rapidly by glucocorticoids is tryptophan oxidase (142). This enzyme oxidizes tryptophan to formylkynurenine, which is subsequently converted to alanine. Alanine transaminase is also induced by glucocorticoids (143). Alanine and, to a lesser extent, glutamate are important for gluconeogenesis in the liver (144).

Several other enzymes important in gluconeogenesis and glycogen formation are elevated for several hours following glucocorticoid administration; these include glycogen synthetase, pyruvate kinase, phosphoenolpyruvate carboxykinase, and glucose-6-phosphate kinase (16,145,146). The delayed increases in these enzymes suggest that their biosyntheses are not regulated directly by glucocorticoids. In peripheral tissues, glucocorticoid-induced inhibition of phosphofructokinase is observed (146). This enzyme catalyzes the formation of D-fructose-1,6-diphosphate from D-fructose-6-phosphate during glycolysis. Inhibition of this enzyme decreases glucose utilization by peripheral tissues and results in maintaining blood glucose levels. Reviews of the multiple effects of glucocorticoids on carbohydrate metabolism have been published (16,146).

Additional effects of glucocorticoids in the body are preventing or minimizing inflammatory reactions and suppressing immune responses. These steroids interfere with both early events in inflammation (e.g., release of mediators, edema, and cellular infiltration) and later stages (e.g., capillary infiltration and collagen formation). Only a few of the mechanisms involved in glucocorticoid suppression of inflammation are known. Hydrocortisone will induce the production of lipocortin and related proteins by increasing gene expression through the GR mechanism (147,148). Lipocortin inhibits the activity of phospholipase A_2, which liberates arachidonic acid and leads to the biosynthesis of eicosanoids (e.g., prostaglandins and leukotrienes) (149). Lipocortin also mediates the decreased production and release of platelet-activating factor (150), and glucocorticoids can suppress the expression of interleukin (IL)-1, tumor necrosis factor, and inducible nitric oxide synthase (151–153). These eicosanoids and peptide factors are important as mediators in the inflammatory response. Some of these factors also have important roles in cellular infiltration and capillary permeability in the inflamed region. Suppression of the immune responses is mediated by inhibition of the synthesis and release of important mediators as well. In macrophages, glucocorticoids inhibit IL-1 synthesis and, thus, interfere with proliferation of B lymphocytes, which are important for antibody production (154). Additionally, IL-1 is important for activation of resting T lymphocytes, which are important for cell-mediated immunity. The activated T cells produce IL-2, the biosynthesis of which is also reduced by glucocorticoids (154).

Mineralocorticoids

The primary physiologic function of mineralocorticoids is to maintain electrolyte balances in the body by enhancing Na^+ reabsorption and increasing K^+ and H^+ secretion in the kidney. Similar effects on cation transport are observed in a variety of secretory tissues, including the salivary glands, sweat glands, and mucosal tissues of the GI tract and the bladder. Aldosterone is the most potent endogenous mineralocorticoid. Deoxycorticosterone is approximately 20-fold less potent than aldosterone. Hydrocortisone exhibits weak mineralocorticoid activity in vivo because of rapid metabolism of hydrocortisone by 11β-hydroxysteroid dehydrogenase. The mechanism of action of aldosterone involves binding of the steroid to the mineralocorticoid receptor and initiation of gene transcription, mRNA biosynthesis, and protein production. A protein referred to as aldosterone-induced protein is produced through this mechanism and is thought to aid in Na^+ retention. One possible mode of action of aldosterone-induced protein is to act as a permease to increase the permeability of the cell membrane to Na^+ (155). This results in an accelerated rate of Na^+ influx and elevated activity of Na^+, K^+-ATPase to pump Na^+ into extracellular space (156).

PHARMACOLOGIC EFFECTS AND CLINICAL APPLICATIONS

In addition to their natural hormonal actions, the adrenocorticoids have many clinical uses. Glucocorticoids and mineralocorticoids can be used for the treatment of adrenal insufficiency (hypoadrenalism), which results from failure of the adrenal glands to synthesize adequate amounts of the hormones. Adrenocorticoids are also used to maintain patients who have had partial or complete removal of their adrenal glands or adenohypophysis (adrenalectomy and hypophysectomy, respectively). Glucocorticoids can cross the placenta and can be distributed into milk.

Two major uses of glucocorticoids are in the treatment of rheumatoid diseases and allergic manifestations. Their use in the treatment of severe asthma is well documented, as is the utility of glucocorticoids in sepsis and acute respiratory distress syndrome (157,158). They are effective in the treatment of rheumatoid arthritis, acute rheumatic fever, bursitis, spontaneous hypoglycemia in children, gout, rheumatoid carditis, sprue, allergy (including contact dermatitis), and other conditions. The treatment of chronic rheumatic diseases and allergic conditions with glucocorticoids is symptomatic and continuous. Symptoms return after withdrawal of the drug.

In addition, these drugs are moderately effective in the treatment of ulcerative colitis, dermatomyositis, periarteritis nodosa, idiopathic pulmonary fibrosis, idiopathic thrombocytopenic purpura, regional ileitis, acquired hemolytic anemia, nephrosis, cirrhotic ascites, neurodermatitis, and temporal arteritis. The newer analogs with medium to high potency rankings (Table 28.4), such as diflorasone diacetate, desoximetasone, flurandrenolide, and fluocinonide (Fig. 28.12), are effective topically in the treatment of psoriasis. Glucocorticoids can be combined with antibiotics to treat pneumonia, peritonitis, typhoid fever, and meningococcemia.

When dosages with equivalent antirheumatic potency are given to patients not treated with steroids, the Δ^1-corticoids (prednisone and prednisolone) promote the same pattern of initial improvement as hydrocortisone. Statistical results of improvement during the first few months of therapy have been similar with prednisone, prednisolone, and hydrocortisone. The results of longer-term therapy have been significantly better with the modified compounds.

Satisfactory rheumatic control, lost after prolonged hydrocortisone therapy, may be regained in an appreciable number of patients by changing to prednisone, prednisolone, or other modified drugs. Of patients whose conditions deteriorate below adequate levels during hydrocortisone administration, nearly half reach their previous level of improvement after Δ^1-corticoids (in doses slightly larger in terms of antirheumatic strength) are used. With further prolongation of steroid therapy, improvement again wanes in some patients, but in other patients, such management is successful for longer than 2 years. In some instances, the improvement is attributed to increased effectiveness of the drug because of correction of salt and water retention; in other instances, there is no adequate explanation.

When these drugs are administered in doses that have similar antirheumatic strengths, the general incidence of adverse reactions with prednisone and prednisolone is about the same as that with hydrocortisone. The compounds differ, however, in their tendencies to induce individual side effects. The incidence and degree of salt and water retention and blood pressure elevation are less with the Δ^1-corticoids. Conversely, these analogs are more likely to promote digestive complaints, peptic ulcer, vasomotor symptoms, and cutaneous ecchymosis.

Although these analogs have unwanted side effects, most clinical investigators prefer the Δ^1-corticoids to hydrocortisone for rheumatoid patients who require steroid therapy. The reasons are that these drugs have less tendency to cause salt and water retention and potassium loss and that they restore improvement in a significant percentage of patients whose therapeutic control has been lost during hydrocortisone therapy.

It seems desirable to administer prednisone and prednisolone in conjunction with nonabsorbable antacids. This affords improvement of long-term therapy. It appears that the therapeutic indices of these two analogs, especially when used in conjunction with nonabsorbable antacids, are higher than those for the naturally occurring glucocorticoids.

Most important, glucocorticoids should not be withdrawn abruptly in cases of acute infections or severe stress, such as surgery or trauma. Myasthenia gravis, peptic ulcer, diabetes mellitus, hyperthyroidism, hypertension, psychological disturbances, pregnancy (first trimester), and infections may be aggravated by glucocorticoid administration. Hormone therapy is contraindicated in these conditions and should be used only with the utmost precaution.

Semisynthetic analogs exhibiting high mineralocorticoid activity are not employed in the treatment of rheumatic disorders because of toxic side effects resulting from a disturbance of electrolyte and water balance. Some newer synthetic steroids (Table 28.2) are relatively free of sodium-retaining activity. They can show other toxic manifestations, however, and eventually need to be withdrawn.

Glucocorticoids sometimes are used in the treatment of scleroderma, discoid lupus, acute nephritis, osteoarthritis, acute hepatitis, hepatic coma, Hodgkin disease, multiple myeloma, lymphoid tumors, acute leukemia, metastatic carcinoma of the breast, and chronic lymphatic leukemia. Glucocorticoids may be more or less effective in these diseases depending on the clinical condition.

Some modified compounds have been recommended for use when other analogs are no longer effective or when it is desirable to promote increased appetite and weight gain. Triamcinolone can be used advantageously when salt and water retention (from other glucocorticoids, hypertension, or cardiac compensation) or excessive appetite and weight gain are problems in management.

One factor must not be overlooked when applying potent anti-inflammatory agents with high mineralocorticoid activity to the skin. Consideration must be given to percutaneous absorption. Sodium retention and edema occur in patients with dermatitis who apply as much as 75 mg of fludrocortisone acetate (i.e., 30 mL of a 0.25% lotion) to the skin in 24 hours. The relative rate of percutaneous absorption, administered as a cream in rats, was triamcinolone acetate ≥ hydrocortisone > dexamethasone, but dexamethasone was deposited in skin longer than the other two drugs. Hydrocortisone disappeared most rapidly (159).

Topical Applications

Topical dermatologic products with a low potency ranking have a modest anti-inflammatory effect and are safest for chronic application (Table 28.4). These products are also the safest products for use on the face with occlusion and in infants and young children. Those products with a medium potency ranking are used in moderate inflammatory dermatoses, such as chronic hand eczema and atopic eczema, and may be used on the face and intertriginous areas (areas where skin comes into contact with itself, such as the armpits, in the groin, and beneath the breasts, which are more prone to infections and rashes because they are hot and often sweaty) for a limited duration. High-potency preparations are used in more severe inflammatory dermatoses, such as severe eczema and psoriasis. They can be used for a limited duration and for longer periods in areas with thickened skin because of chronic conditions. High-potency preparations may also be used on the face and intertriginous areas, but only for a short treatment duration. Very high–potency products are used primarily as an alternative to systemic corticosteroid therapy when local areas are involved. Examples of conditions for which very high–potency products frequently are used include thick, chronic lesions caused by psoriasis, lichen simplex chronicus, and discoid lupus erythematosus. They may be used for only a short duration of therapy and on small surface areas. Occlusive dressings should not be used with these products. It has been suggested that patients using a lotion or ointment containing these drugs be instructed to apply them sparingly and to spread them lightly over the affected areas. The extent and frequency of applications should be carefully considered. A lotion vehicle is more effective when treating a dermatitis, but a greater degree of percutaneous absorption occurs than when ointments are used.

Intranasal and Inhaled Applications

The pulmonary and nasal bioavailabilities are important determinants for the potential of an inhaled or nasally applied corticosteroid to cause systemic effects, because the lung and nasal tissue provide an enormous surface area from which drug absorption can occur into the systemic circulation. The main areas of concern with regard to systemic effects include HPA axis suppression, change in bone mineral density and growth retardation in children, cataracts, and glaucoma. The degree of systemic side effects is dose-dependent, related to the half-life of the drug, frequency administration, time of day when administered, and route of administration; in other words, the higher the plasma corticosteroid concentration and longer the half-life, the greater will be the systemic side effects (Table 28.5) (27). The amount of an inhaled or nasal corticosteroid reaching the systemic circulation is the sum of the drug concentration available following absorption from the lungs/nasal mucosa, from the GI tract, and the extent of plasma protein binding. The fraction deposited in the mouth will be swallowed, and the systemic availability will be determined by its absorption from the GI tract and the degree of first-pass metabolism and protein binding.

Delivery devices can produce clinically significant differences in activity by altering the dose deposited in the lung (10% to 25%) and, for orally absorbed drugs, the amount deposited in the oropharynx and swallowed (75% to 90%). Clinical studies have shown the following relative potency differences: ciclesonide > mometasone furoate > fluticasone propionate > budesonide = BDP > triamcinolone acetonide = flunisolide. Potency differences can be overcome by giving larger doses of the less potent drug, which increases risks from systemic effects. Adrenal suppression may be associated with high doses of inhaled corticosteroids (>1.5 mg/day, or >0.75 mg/day for fluticasone propionate), although there is a considerable degree of interindividual susceptibility.

All currently used inhaled corticosteroids are rapidly cleared from the body but show varying levels of oral bioavailability, with fluticasone propionate having the lowest (Table 28.5). Following inhalation, there is also considerable variability in the rate of absorption from the lung, and pulmonary residence times are greatest for fluticasone propionate and triamcinolone acetonide and shortest for budesonide and flunisolide. Adrenal suppression has not been observed when intranasal fluticasone propionate was administered in dosages of 200 to 4,000 mcg daily for up to 12 months.

Adverse Effects

Although short-term administration of corticosteroids is unlikely to produce harmful effects, these drugs, when used for longer than brief periods, can produce a variety of devastating effects, including glucocorticoid-induced adrenocortical insufficiency, glucocorticoid-induced osteoporosis, and generalized protein depletion (16,27). The duration of anti-inflammatory activity of glucocorticoids approximately equals the duration of HPA axis suppression. The durations of HPA axis suppression after a single oral dose of glucocorticoids in one study are shown in Table 28.7. When given for prolonged periods, glucocorticoids suppress the HPA axis, thereby decreasing secretion of endogenous corticosteroids and adrenal atrophy. Glucocorticoids inhibit ACTH production by the adenohypophysis, and in turn, this reduces endogenous glucocorticoid production. With time, atrophy of the adrenal glands takes place. The degree and duration of adrenocortical insufficiency produced by the synthetic glucocorticoids is highly variable among patients and depends on the dose, frequency, and time of administration, and duration of glucocorticoid therapy. This effect can be minimized by use of alternate-day therapy.

Patients who develop drug-induced adrenocortical insufficiency may require higher corticosteroid dosage when they are subjected to stress (e.g., infection, surgery, or trauma). In addition, acute adrenal insufficiency (even death) can occur if the drugs are withdrawn abruptly or if patients are transferred from systemic glucocorticoid therapy to oral inhalation therapy. Therefore, the drugs should be withdrawn very gradually following long-term therapy with pharmacologic dosages. Adrenal suppression can persist up to 12 months in patients who receive large dosages for prolonged periods. Until recovery occurs, patients may show signs and symptoms of adrenal insufficiency when they are subjected to stress, and replacement therapy may be required. Because mineralocorticoid secretion can be impaired, sodium chloride or a mineralocorticoid also should be administered.

TABLE 28.7 Effect of an Oral Single Dose on the Duration of HPA Suppression

Adrenocorticoid	Duration of Suppression (days)
Hydrocortisone (250 mg)	1.25–1.5
Cortisone (250 mg)	1.25–1.5
Methylprednisolone (40 mg)	1.25–1.5
Prednisone (50 mg)	1.25–1.5
Prednisolone (50 mg)	1.25–1.5
Triamcinolone (40 mg)	2.25
Dexamethasone (5 mg)	2.75
Betamethasone (6 mg)	3.25

Although side effects and toxicities vary with the drug and, sometimes, with the patient, facial mooning, flushing, sweating, acne, thinning of the scalp hair, abdominal distention, and weight gain are observed with most glucocorticoids. Protein depletion (with osteoporosis and spontaneous fractures), myopathy (with weakness of muscles of the thighs, pelvis, and lower back), and aseptic necrosis of the hip and humerus are other side effects. These drugs can cause psychological disturbances, headache, vertigo, and peptic ulcer, and they can suppress growth in children.

Patients with well-controlled diabetes must be closely monitored and their insulin dosage increased if glycosuria or hyperglycemia ensues either during or following glucocorticoid administration. Patients should also be watched for signs of adrenocorticoid insufficiency after discontinuation of glucocorticoid therapy. Individuals with a history of tuberculosis should receive prophylactic doses of antituberculosis drugs.

Osteoporosis is one of the most serious adverse effects of long-term glucocorticoid therapy. Moderate- to high-dose glucocorticoid therapy is associated with loss of bone and an increased risk of fracture that is most rapid during the initial 6 months of therapy. These adverse effects of glucocorticoids appear to be both dose- and duration-dependent, with oral prednisone dosages of 7.5 mg or more daily for 6 months or longer often resulting in clinically important bone loss and increased fracture risk. Bone loss has even been associated with oral inhalation of glucocorticoids and is of great concern in children. Most patients receiving long-term glucocorticoid therapy will develop some degree of bone loss, and more than 25% will develop osteoporotic fractures. Vertebral fractures have been reported in 11% of patients with asthma who are receiving systemic glucocorticoids for at least 1 year, and glucocorticoid-treated patients with rheumatoid arthritis are at increased risk of fractures of the hip, rib, spine, leg, ankle, and foot. Muscle wasting or weakness and atrophy of the protein matrix of the bone resulting in osteoporosis are manifestations of protein catabolism, which can occur during prolonged therapy with glucocorticoids. These adverse effects can be especially serious in debilitated patients, in geriatric populations, and in postmenopausal women who are especially prone to osteoporosis.

To minimize the risk of glucocorticoid-induced bone loss (osteoporosis) and in those with low mineral bone density, the smallest possible effective dosage and duration should be used. Topical and inhaled preparations should be used whenever possible. The immunosuppressive effects of glucocorticoids increase the susceptibility to and mask the symptoms of infections and can result in activation of latent infection or exacerbation of intercurrent infections. The most common adverse effect of oral inhalation therapy with glucocorticoids is fungal infections of the mouth, pharynx, and occasionally, the larynx. The mineralocorticoid effects are less frequent with synthetic glucocorticoids (except fludrocortisone) than with hydrocortisone but may occur, especially when synthetic glucocorticoids are given in high dosage for prolonged periods.

SCENARIO: OUTCOME AND ANALYSIS

Outcome

Jeffrey T. Sherer, PharmD, MPH, BCPS, CGP

LT is started on intravenous antibiotics and albuterol plus ipratropium administered through a nebulizer. She is also started on intravenous methylprednisolone 25 mg every 12 hours. After 2 days, her symptoms improve dramatically, and she is eating and drinking well. The pharmacist recommends changing her intravenous antibiotic to an oral equivalent and that her intravenous methylprednisolone be switched to oral prednisone 40 mg daily. Her symptoms continue to improve, and she is discharged 2 days later with a short course of oral prednisone plus her usual inhaled medications.

Chemical Analysis

Victoria Roche and S. William Zito

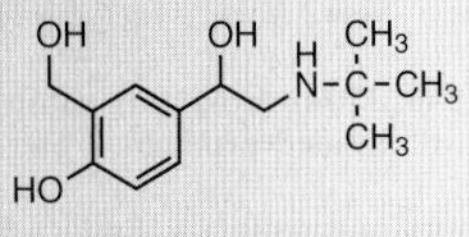

Albuterol

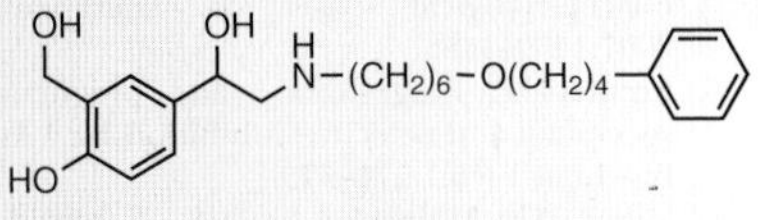

Salmeterol

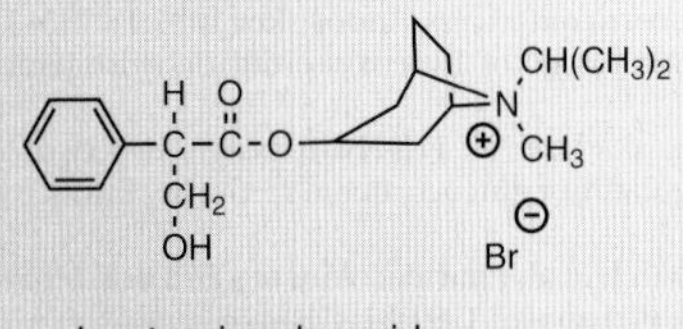

Ipratropium bromide

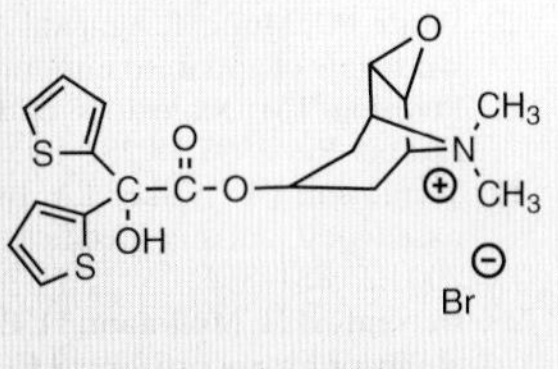

Tiotropium bromide

Salmeterol and albuterol are both β_2-selective adrenergic agonists that, in therapeutic doses, dilate bronchi without unwanted stimulation of the heart (a β_1-receptor–mediated response). Both structures are phenethylamines with a β_2-directing salicyl alcohol aromatic ring and a bulky β_2-directing substituent on the tertiary amino nitrogen. Both contain the carbinol OH group essential to high affinity β-adrenoceptor binding. β_2-Adrenoceptor agonists are beneficial in the treatment of chronic obstructive pulmonary disease (COPD) due to their ability to relax bronchial smooth muscle and decrease airway resistance.

Tiotropium and ipratropium are quaternary amine-containing antimuscarinic agents based on the structure of naturally occurring Belladonna alkaloids. They are useful in the treatment of COPD due to their antisecretory actions and ability to inhibit acetylcholine-mediated bronchoconstriction. Tiotropium's slower dissociation from muscarinic receptors leads to a longer duration of action compared to ipratropium, but it has also a slower onset of action.

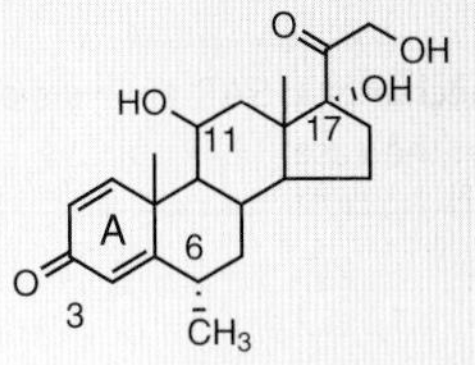

Methylprednisolone

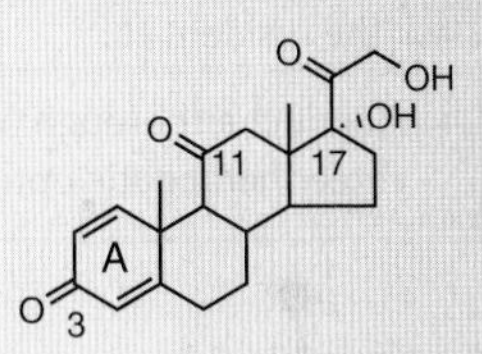

Prednisone

Methylprednisolone and prednisone are gluco-selective adrenocorticoids that act to decrease airway inflammation in patients with asthma and COPD. The 17β-ketol, 17α-OH, and Δ^4-3-one A ring are essential to corticoid action of all kinds. Both methylprednisolone and prednisone have the Δ^1-double bond that flattens ring A and provides higher affinity for gluco receptors compared to mineralo receptors. The addition of this conjugated double bond also makes the A ring more resistant to inactivating reduction. Methylprednisolone contains a 6α-CH_3 group, which essentially abolishes mineralo side effects (e.g., fluid retention, electrolyte imbalance) in therapeutic doses and provides some steric hindrance to the reduction of the already-resistant A ring. The hydroxyl moiety at 11β (found on methylprednisolone) forms an important affinity-enhancing H-bond with the glucocorticoid receptor, but the 11-keto (found on prednisone) is rapidly converted to the 11β-OH via the hepatic enzyme 11β-hydroxysteroid dehydrogenase. The equilibrium established between these two forms ensures an equivalent potency of compounds otherwise identical in structure. Although methylprednisolone is available in an oral dosage form, the switch to prednisone (a glucocorticoid with a slightly decreased potency) is a chemically viable alternative for maintenance therapy.

CASE STUDY

Victoria Roche and S. William Zito

You are next door neighbors with LK, a friendly guy who owns a relatively new but increasingly successful lawn service business in your community. LK recently landed a contract with an exclusive real estate company to landscape some model homes in a wooded area being developed on the south side of town. Against his better judgment, LK hired DK, his 22-year-old nephew, for the summer and put him to work on the job. After clearing a large section of one wooded lot of weeds and vines as LK had directed him to do, DK started a controlled burn of the organic debris while his uncle was off inspecting another part of the development property. Fortunately, his uncle returned in time to halt the burning shortly after it began. Unfortunately there was poison ivy in the cleared vegetation and DK was directly exposed to the urushiol from the plant itself and, briefly, to the smoke from the burning leaves. He is experiencing a significant reaction to the allergen and is thoroughly miserable. Because of the potential for urushiol-induced lung irritation, his uncle knew to seek medical attention, and they are now in the emergency room of the hospital where you practice. While the attending is examining DK, you talk with LK about an anticipated therapeutic plan that will include an oral corticosteroid to provide much-needed anti-inflammatory/antiallergic relief.

Back in the pharmacy, you challenge your ambulatory care resident to employ his understanding of corticosteroid SAR by selecting the most likely drug candidate from three potential adrenocorticoid structures you draw on the whiteboard.

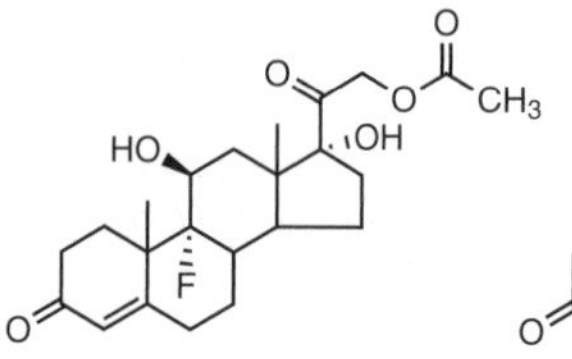

1

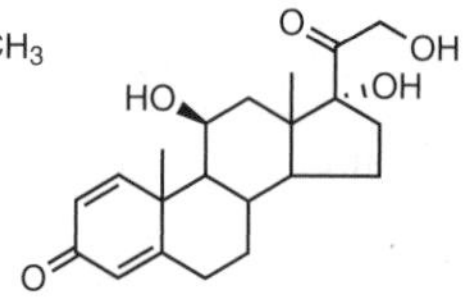

2

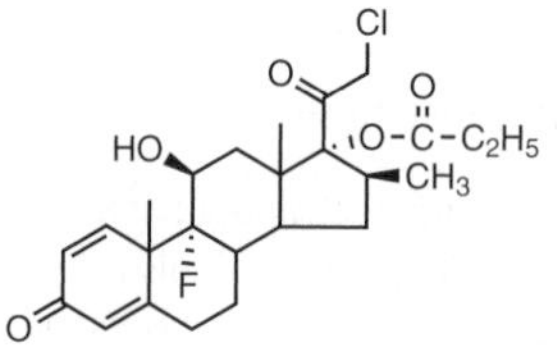

3

You ask the resident to:

1. Conduct a thorough and mechanistic SAR analysis of the three therapeutic options in the case.
2. Apply the chemical understanding gained from the SAR analysis to this patient's specific needs to make a therapeutic recommendation.

References

1. IUPAC-IUB Joint Commission on Biochemical Nomenclature (JCBN). The nomenclature of steroids. Recommendations 1989. Eur J Biochem 1989;186:429–458. [Published erratum appears in Eur J Biochem 1993;213:2.]
2. Gustafsson JA, Carlstedt-Duke J, Poellinger L, et al. Biochemistry, molecular biology, and physiology of the glucocorticoid receptor. Endocr Rev 1987;8:185–234.
3. Evans RM. The steroid and thyroid hormone receptor superfamily. Science 1988;240:889–895.
4. Ringold G, University of California Los Angeles. Steroid Hormone Action: Proceedings of a UCLA Symposium, Held in Park City, Utah, January 17–23, 1987. New York: Liss, 1988.
5. Beato M. Gene regulation by steroid hormones. Cell 1989;56:335–344.
6. O'Malley B. The steroid receptor superfamily: more excitement predicted for the future. Mol Endocrinol 1990;4:363–369.
7. Carson-Jurica MA, Schrader WT, O'Malley BW. Steroid receptor family: structure and functions. Endocr Rev 1990;11:201–220.
8. Stahn C, Lowenberg M, Hommes DW, et al. Molecular mechanisms of glucocorticoid action and selective glucocorticoid receptor agonists. Mol Cell Endocrinol 2007;275:71–78.
9. van der Laan S, Meijer OC. Pharmacology of glucocorticoids: beyond receptors. Eur J Pharmacol 2008;585:438–491.
10. Eickelberg O, Roth M, Lorx R, et al. Ligand-independent activation of the glucocorticoid receptor by β_2-adrenergic receptor agonists in primary human lung fibroblasts and vascular smooth muscle cells. J Biol Chem 1999;274:1005–1010.
11. Addison T. On the Constitutional and Local Effects of Disease of the Suprarenal Capsules by Thomas Addison. Special Ed. Birmingham, AL: Classics of Medicine Library, 1980.
12. Murison PJ. Hyperfunctioning adrenocortical diseases. Med Clin North Am 1967;51:883–901.
13. Shoppee CW. Chemistry of the Steroids, 2nd Ed. London: Butterworths, 1964.
14. Simpson ER. Cholesterol side-chain cleavage, cytochrome P450, and the control of steroidogenesis. Mol Cell Endocrinol 1979;13:213–227.
15. Simpson ER, Waterman MR. Regulation of the synthesis of steroidogenic enzymes in adrenal cortical cells by ACTH. Annu Rev Physiol 1988;50:427–440.
16. Schimmer BP, Parker KL. Adrenocorticotropic hormones. In: Hardman JG, Limbird LE, Molinoff PB, et al., eds. Goodman & Gilman's The Pharmacological Basis of Therapeutics. New York: McGraw-Hill, 2001:1459–1485.
17. Kremers P. Progesterone and pregnenolone 17α-hydroxylase: substrate specificity and selective inhibition by 17α-hydroxylated products. J Steroid Biochem 1976;7:571–575.
18. Miller WL. Molecular biology of steroid hormone synthesis. Endocr Rev 1988;9:295–318.
19. Miller WL, Auchus RJ. Molecular biology, biochemistry, and physiology of human steroidogenesis and its disorders. Endocr Rev 2011;32:81–151.
20. White PC, Mune T, Agarwal AK. 11β-Hydroxysteroid dehydrogenase and the syndrome of apparent mineralocorticoid excess. Endocr Rev 1997;18:135–156.
21. Penning TM. Molecular endocrinology of hydroxysteroid dehydrogenases. Endocr Rev 1997;18:281–305.
22. Tomlinson JW, Walker EA, Bujalska IJ, et al. 11β-Hydroxysteroid dehydrogenase type 1: a tissue-specific regulator of glucocorticoid response. Endocr Rev 2004;25:831–866.
23. Derendorf H, Mollmann H, Barth J, et al. Pharmacokinetics and oral bioavailability of hydrocortisone. J Clin Pharmacol 1991;31:473–476.
24. Romanoff LP, Morris CW, Welch PW, et al. The metabolism of cortisol-4-C14 in young and elderly men. I. Welch secretion rate of cortisol and daily excretion of tetrahydrocortisol, allotetrahydrocortisol, tetrahydrocortisone, and cortolone (20α and 20β). J Clin Endocrinol Metab 1961;21:1413–1425.
25. Fukushima DK, Leeds NS, Bradlow HL, et al. The characterization of four new metabolites of adrenocortical hormones. J Biol Chem 1955;212:449–460.
26. Chang E, Dao TL. Adrenal estrogens. II. Further characterizations of isolated urinary 11β-hydroxyesterone and 11β-hydroxyestradiol. Biochim Biophys Acta 1962;57:609–612.
27. AHFS Drug Information 2006. Bethesda, MD: American Society of Health-System Pharmacists, 2006.
28. Gray CH, Green MA, Holness NJ, et al. Urinary metabolic products of prednisone and prednisolone. J Endocrinol 1956;14:146–154.
29. Robbins ED, Burton SD, Byers SO, et al. Hydrocortisone metabolism in the perfused isolated rat liver. J Clin Endocrinol Metab 1957;17:111–115.
30. Stevens W, Berliner DL, Dougherty TF. Conjugation of steroid by liver, kidney, and intestine of mice. Endocrinology 1961;68:875–877.

31. Glick JH. The isolation of two corticosteroids from cattle bile. Endocrinology 1957;60:368–375.
32. Steiger M, Reichstein T. Desoxy-cortico-steron (21-Oxy-progesteron) aus Δ^5-3-Oxy-ätio-cholensäure. Helv Chim Acta 1937;20:1164–1179.
33. Fieser LF, Fieser M. Steroids. New York: Reinhold, 1959.
34. Sarett LH. Partial synthesis of pregnene-4-triol-17(b),20(b),21-dione-3,11 and pregnene-4-diol-17(b),21-trione-3,11,20 monoacetate. J Biol Chem 1946;162:601–631.
35. McKenzie BF, Marttox VR, Engel LL, et al. Steroids derived from bile acids. VI. An improved synthesis of methyl 3,9-epoxy- Δ^{11}-cholenate from desoxycholic acid. J Biol Chem 1948;173:271–281.
36. Sarett LH. Preparation of pregnane-17α,21-diol-3,11,20-trione acetate. J Am Chem Soc 1949;71:2443–2444.
37. Heazelwood VJ, Galligan JP, Cannell GR, et al. Plasma cortisol delivery from oral cortisol and cortisone acetate: relative bioavailability. Br J Clin Pharmacol 1984;17:55–59.
38. Lima JJ, Jusko WJ. Bioavailability of hydrocortisone retention enemas in relation to absorption kinetics. Clin Pharmacol Ther 1980;28:262–269.
39. Mollmann H, Barth J, Mollmann C, et al. Pharmacokinetics and rectal bioavailability of hydrocortisone acetate. J Pharm Sci 1991;80:835–836.
40. Bush IE, Mahesh VB. Metabolism of 11-oxygenated steroids. 2. 2-Methyl steroids. Biochem J 1959;71:718–742.
41. Nobile A, Charney W, Perlman PL, et al. Microbiological transformation of steroids. I. Δ-1,4-diene-3-ketosteroids. J Am Chem Soc 1955;77:4184.
42. Meystre C, Frey H, Voser W, et al. Gewinnung von 1,4-bisdehydro-3-oxosteroiden. Über Steroide, 139. Mitteilung. Helv Chim Acta 1956;39:734–742.
43. Smith CL, Kreutner W. In vitro glucocorticoid receptor binding and transcriptional activation by topically active glucocorticoids. Arzneimittelforschung 1998;48:956–960.
44. Barth J, Damoiseaux M, Mollmann H, et al. Pharmacokinetics and pharmacodynamics of prednisolone after intravenous and oral administration. Int J Clin Pharmacol Ther Toxicol 1992;30:317–324.
45. Rohatagi S, Barth J, Mollmann H, et al. Pharmacokinetics of methylprednisolone and prednisolone after single and multiple oral administration. J Clin Pharmacol 1997;37:916–925.
46. Mollmann H, Rohdewald P, Barth J, et al. Pharmacokinetics and dose linearity testing of methylprednisolone phosphate. Biopharm Drug Dispos 1989;10:453–464.
47. Vree TB, Verwey-van Wissen CP, Lagerwerf AJ, et al. Isolation and identification of the C6-hydroxy and C20-hydroxy metabolites and glucuronide conjugate of methylprednisolone by preparative high-performance liquid chromatography from urine of patients receiving high-dose pulse therapy. J Chromatogr B Biomed Sci Appl 1999;726:157–168.
48. Spero GB, Thompsin JL, Lincoln FH, et al. Adrenal hormones related compounds. V. Fluorinated 6-methyl steroids. J Am Chem Soc 1957;79:1515–1516.
49. Boland EW. Clinical comparison of the newer anti-inflammatory corticosteroids. Ann Rheumatic Dis 1962;21:176–187.
50. Hirschmann H, Hirschmann FB, Farrel GL. Partial synthesis of 16α,21-diacetoxyprogesterone. J Am Chem Soc 1953;75:4862–4863.
51. Allen WS, Bernstein S. Steroidal cyclic ketals. XII. The preparation of Δ^{16}-steroids. J Am Chem Soc 1955;77:1028–1032.
52. Allen WS, Bernstein S. Steroidal cyclic ketals. XX. 16-hydroxylated steroids. III. The preparation of 16α-hydroxyhydrocortisone and related compounds. J Am Chem Soc 1956;78:1909–1913.
53. Hochhaus G, Portner M, Barth J, et al. Oral bioavailability of triamcinolone tablets and a triamcinolone diacetate suspension. Pharm Res 1990;7:558–560.
54. Portner M, Mollmann H, Barth J, et al. [Pharmacokinetics of triamcinolone following oral administration]. Arzneimittelforschung 1988;38:1838–1840.
55. Boland EW. The treatment of rheumatoid arthritis with adrenocorticosteroids and their synthetic analogs: an appraisal of certain developments of the past decade. Ann N Y Acad Sci 1959;82:887–901.
56. Weiner AL. Intramuscular triamcinolone diacetate therapy of dermatoses: preliminary report. Antibiot Chemother 1962;12:360–366.
57. Dobes WL. The use of folic acid antagonists and steroids in treatment of psoriasis. South Med J 1963;56:187–192.
58. Arth GE, Johnson DBR, Fried J, et al. 16-Methylated steroids. I. 16α-Methylated analogs of Johnson cortisone, a new group of anti-inflammatory steroids. J Am Chem Soc 1958;80:3160–3161.
59. Oliveto EP, Rausser R, Nussbaum AL, et al. 16-Alkylated corticoids. I. 16α-Methylprednisone and 16β-methylprednisone. J Am Chem Soc 1958;80:4431.
60. Sperber PA. Cyproheptadine-dexamethasone combination in the treatment. Curr Ther Res 1962;4:70–73.
61. Silber RH. The biology of anti-inflammatory steroids. Ann N Y Acad Sci 1959;82:821–833.
62. Tolksdorf S. Laboratory evaluation of anti-inflammatory steroids. Ann N Y Acad Sci 1959;82:829–835.
63. Rohdewald P, Mollmann H, Barth J, et al. Pharmacokinetics of dexamethasone and its phosphate ester. Biopharm Drug Dispos 1987;8:205–212.
64. Nierman MM. Management of steroid-responsive dermatologic disorders with betamethasone. Clin Med 1962;69:1311–1320.
65. Cohen A, Coldman J. Use of a new corticosteroid in rheumatoid arthritis. Penn Med J 1962;65:347–350.
66. Cohen AI. Treatment of allergy with oral betamethasone in 141 patients. Antibiot Chemother 1962;12:91–96.
67. Glyn JH, Fox DB. Preliminary clinical assessment of β-methasone. BMJ 1961;1:876–877.
68. Glyn JH, Fox DB. Betamethasone. BMJ 1961;2:650–651.
69. Wilkinson DS. Betamethasone. BMJ 1961;1:1319–1320.
70. Irwin GW, Priebe FH, Ridolfo AS. Metabolic effects of paramethasone acetate. Metabolism 1961;10:852–858.
71. Buijsman RC, Hermkens PH, van Rijn RD, et al. Nonsteroidal steroid receptor modulators. Curr Med Chem 2005;12:1017–1075.
72. Einstein M, Greenlee M, Rouen G, et al. Selective glucocorticoid receptor nonsteroidal ligands completely antagonize the dexamethasone mediated induction of enzymes involved in gluconeogenesis and glutamine metabolism. J Steroid Biochem Mol Biol 2004;92:345–356.
73. Miner JN, Hong MH, Negro-Vilar A. New and improved glucocorticoid receptor ligands. Expert Opin Investig Drugs 2005;14:1527–1545.
74. Cole TJ, Mollard R. Selective glucocorticoid receptor ligands. Med Chem 2007;3;494–506.
75. De Bosscher K. Selective glucocorticoid receptor modulators. J Steroid Biochem Mol Biol 2010;120:96–104.
76. Andersson P, Lihne M, Thalen A, et al. Effect of structural alterations on the biotransformation rate of glucocorticosteroids in rat and human liver. Xenobiotica 1987;17:35–44.
77. Brogden RN, Heel RC, Speight TM, et al. Beclomethasone dipropionate. A reappraisal of its pharmacodynamic properties and therapeutic efficacy after a decade of use in asthma and rhinitis. Drugs 1984;28:99–126.
78. Green MJ, Berkenkopf J, Fernandez X, et al. Synthesis and structure–activity relationships in a novel series of topically active corticosteroids. J Steroid Biochem 1979;11:61–66.
79. Asche H, Botta L, Rettig H, et al. Influence of formulation factors on the availability of drugs from topical preparations. Pharm Acta Helv 1985;60:232–237.
80. Bodor N, Harget AJ, Phillips EW. Structure–activity relationships in the anti-inflammatory steroids: a pattern-recognition approach. J Med Chem 1983;26:318–333.
81. Popper TL, Gentles MJ, Kung TT, et al. Structure–activity relationships of a series of novel topical corticosteroids. J Steroid Biochem 1987;27:837–843.
82. Shapiro EL, Gentles MJ, Tiberi RL, et al. 17-Heteroaroyl esters of corticosteroids. 2. 11β-Hydroxy series. J Med Chem 1987;30:1581–1588.
83. Barth J, Lehr KH, Derendorf H, et al. Studies on the pharmacokinetics and metabolism of prednicarbate after cutaneous and oral administration. Skin Pharmacol 1993;6:179–186.
84. Kelly HW. Comparison of inhaled corticosteroids. Ann Pharmacother 1998;32:220–232.
85. Derendorf H. Pharmacokinetic and pharmacodynamic properties of inhaled corticosteroids in relation to efficacy and safety. Respir Med 1997;91(Suppl A):22–33.
86. Derendorf H, Hochhaus G, Meibohm B, et al. Pharmacokinetics and pharmacodynamics of inhaled corticosteroids. J Allergy Clin Immunol 1998;101:S440–S446.
87. Wales D, Makker H, Kane J, et al. Systemic bioavailability and potency of high-dose inhaled corticosteroids: a comparison of four inhaler devices and three drugs in healthy adult volunteers. Chest 1999;115:1278–1284.
88. Shaw RJ. Inhaled corticosteroids for adult asthma: impact of formulation and delivery device on relative pharmacokinetics, efficacy, and safety. Respir Med 1999;93:149–160.
89. Lipworth BJ. Systemic adverse effects of inhaled corticosteroid therapy: a systematic review and meta-analysis. Arch Intern Med 1999;159:941–955.
90. Greiff L, Andersson M, Svensson C, et al. Effects of orally inhaled budesonide in seasonal allergic rhinitis. Eur Respir J 1998;11:1268–1273.
91. Rohatagi S, Hochhaus G, Mollmann H, et al. Pharmacokinetic and pharmacodynamic evaluation of triamcinolone acetonide after intravenous, oral, and inhaled administration. J Clin Pharmacol 1995;35:1187–1193.
92. Argenti D, Shah B, Heald D. A pharmacokinetic study to evaluate the absolute bioavailability of triamcinolone acetonide following inhalation administration. J Clin Pharmacol 1999;39:695–702.
93. Derendorf H, Hochhaus G, Rohatagi S, et al. Pharmacokinetics of triamcinolone acetonide after intravenous, oral, and inhaled administration. J Clin Pharmacol 1995;35:302–305.
94. Mollmann H, Derendorf H, Barth J, et al. Pharmacokinetic/pharmacodynamic evaluation of systemic effects of flunisolide after inhalation. J Clin Pharmacol 1997;37:893–903.
95. Seale JP, Harrison LI. Effect of changing the fine particle mass of inhaled beclomethasone dipropionate on intrapulmonary deposition and pharmacokinetics. Respir Med 1998;92(Suppl A):9–15.
96. Lipworth BJ, Jackson CM. Pharmacokinetics of chlorofluorocarbon and hydrofluoroalkane metered-dose inhaler formulations of beclomethasone dipropionate. Br J Clin Pharmacol 1999;48:866–868.
97. Harrison LI, Soria I, Cline AC, et al. Pharmacokinetic differences between chlorofluorocarbon and chlorofluorocarbon-free metered dose inhalers of beclomethasone dipropionate in adult asthmatics. J Pharm Pharmacol 1999;51:1235–1240.
98. Dickens GR, Wermeling DP, Matheny CJ, et al. Pharmacokinetics of flunisolide administered via metered dose inhaler with and without a spacer

device and following oral administration. Ann Allergy Asthma Immunol 2000;84:528–532.
99. Thalen BA, Axelsson BI, Andersson PH, et al. 6α-Fluoro- and 6α, 9α-difluoro-11β, 21-dihydroxy-16α, 17α-propylmethylenedioxypregn-4-ene-3,20-dione: synthesis and evaluation of activity and kinetics of their C-22 epimers. Steroids 1998;63:37–43.
100. Ryrfeldt A, Andersson P, Edsbacker S, et al. Pharmacokinetics and metabolism of budesonide, a selective glucocorticoid. Eur J Respir Dis Suppl 1982;122:86–95.
101. Szefler SJ. Pharmacodynamics and pharmacokinetics of budesonide: a new nebulized corticosteroid. J Allergy Clin Immunol 1999;104:175–183.
102. Miller-Larsson A, Mattsson H, Hjertberg E, et al. Reversible fatty acid conjugation of budesonide. Novel mechanism for prolonged retention of topically applied steroid in airway tissue. Drug Metab Dispos 1998;26:623–630.
103. Miller-Larsson A, Jansson P, Runstrom A, et al. Prolonged airway activity and improved selectivity of budesonide possibly due to esterification. Am J Respir Crit Care Med 2000;162:1455–1461.
104. Pedersen S, Steffensen G, Ekman I, et al. Pharmacokinetics of budesonide in children with asthma. Eur J Clin Pharmacol 1987;31:579–582.
105. Agertoft L, Andersen A, Weibull E, et al. Systemic availability and pharmacokinetics of nebulized budesonide in preschool children. Arch Dis Child 1999;80:241–247.
106. Shapiro EL, Gentles MJ, Tiberi RL, et al. Synthesis and structure–activity studies of corticosteroid 17-heterocyclic aromatic esters. 1. 9α,11β-Dichloro series. J Med Chem 1987;30:1068–1073.
107. Onrust SV, Lamb HM. Mometasone furoate. A review of its intranasal use in allergic rhinitis. Drugs 1998;56:725–745.
108. Affrime MB, Cuss F, Padhi D, et al. Bioavailability and metabolism of mometasone furoate following administration by metered-dose and dry-powder inhalers in healthy human volunteers. J Clin Pharmacol 2000;40:1227–1236.
109. Phillipps GH, Bailey EJ, Bain BM, et al. Synthesis and structure–activity relationships in a series of antiinflammatory corticosteroid analogs, halomethyl androstane-17β-carbothioates and -17β-carboselenoates. J Med Chem 1994;37:3717–3729.
110. Harding SM. The human pharmacology of fluticasone propionate. Respir Med 1990;84(Suppl A):25–29.
111. Johnson M. Development of fluticasone propionate and comparison with other inhaled corticosteroids. J Allergy Clin Immunol 1998;101:S434–S439.
112. Mollmann H, Wagner M, Meibohm B, et al. Pharmacokinetic and pharmacodynamic evaluation of fluticasone propionate after inhaled administration. Eur J Clin Pharmacol 1998;53:459–467.
113. Mackie AE, Ventresca GP, Fuller RW, et al. Pharmacokinetics of intravenous fluticasone propionate in healthy subjects. Br J Clin Pharmacol 1996;41:539–542.
114. Thorsson L, Dahlstrom K, Edsbacker S, et al. Pharmacokinetics and systemic effects of inhaled fluticasone propionate in healthy subjects. Br J Clin Pharmacol 1997;43:155–161.
115. Rohatagi S, Bye A, Falcoz C, et al. Dynamic modeling of cortisol reduction after inhaled administration of fluticasone propionate. J Clin Pharmacol 1996;36:938–941.
116. Bush IE. Chemical and biological factors in the activity of adrenocortical steroids. Pharmacol Rev 1962;14:317–336.
117. Glenn EM, Stafford RO, Lyster SC, et al. Relation between biological activity of hydrocortisone analogs and their rates of inactivation by rat liver enzyme systems. Endocrinology 1957;61:128–142.
118. Dulin WE, Bowman BJ, Stafford RO. Effects of 2-methylation on glucocorticoid activity of various C-21 steroids. Proc Soc Exp Biol Med 1957;94:303–305.
119. Fried J, Borman A. Synthetic derivatives of cortical hormones. Vitam Horm 1958;16:303–374.
120. Funder JW, Feldman D, Highland E, et al. Molecular modifications of antialdosterone compounds: effects on affinity of spirolactones for renal aldosterone receptors. Biochem Pharmacol 1974;23:1493–1501.
121. Peterfalvi M, Torelli V, Fournex R, et al. Importance of the lactonic ring in the activity of steroidal antialdosterones. Biochem Pharmacol 1980;29:353–357.
122. Duval D, Durant S, Homo-Delarche F. Effect of antiglucocorticoids on dexamethasone-induced inhibition of uridine incorporation and cell lysis in isolated mouse thymocytes. J Steroid Biochem 1984;20:283–287.
123. Agarwal MK, Hainque B, Moustaid N, et al. Glucocorticoid antagonists. FEBS Lett 1987;217:221–226.
124. Napoli JL, Counsell RE. New inhibitors of steroid 11β-hydroxylase. Structure–activity relationship studies of metyrapone-like compounds. J Med Chem 1977;20:762–766.
125. Shaw MA, Nicholls PJ, Smith HJ. Aminoglutethimide and ketoconazole: historical perspectives and future prospects. J Steroid Biochem 1988;31:137–146.
126. Sonino N. The use of ketoconazole as an inhibitor of steroid production. N Engl J Med 1987;317:812–818.
127. Potts GO, Creange JE, Hardomg HR, et al. Trilostane, an orally active inhibitor of steroid biosynthesis. Steroids 1978;32:257–267.
128. Monder C, Stewart PM, Lakshmi V, et al. Licorice inhibits corticosteroid 11β-dehydrogenase of rat kidney and liver: in vivo and in vitro studies. Endocrinology 1989;125:1046–1053.
129. Diederich S, Grossmann C, Hanke B, et al. In the search for specific inhibitors of human 11β-hydroxysteroid-dehydrogenases (11β-HSDs): chenodeoxycholic acid selectively inhibits 11β-HSD-I. Eur J Endocrinol 2000;142:200–207.
130. Buhler H, Perschel FH, Fitzner R, et al. Endogenous inhibitors of 11β-OHSD: existence and possible significance. Steroids 1994;59:131–135.
131. Barf T, Vallgarda J, Emond R, et al. Arylsulfonamidothiazoles as a new class of potential antidiabetic drugs. Discovery of potent and selective inhibitors of the 11β-hydroxysteroid dehydrogenase type 1. J Med Chem 2002;45:3813–3815.
132. Pratt WB. Transformation of glucocorticoid and progesterone receptors to the DNA-binding state. J Cell Biochem 1987;35:51–68.
133. de Castro M, Elliot S, Kino T, et al. The nonligand binding β-isoform of the human glucocorticoid receptor (hGRβ): tissue levels, mechanism of action, and potential physiologic role. Mol Med 1996;2:597–607.
134. Bamberger CM, Bamberger AM, de Castro M, et al. Glucocorticoid receptor β, a potential endogenous inhibitor of glucocorticoid action in humans. J Clin Invest 1995;95:2435–2441.
135. Marver D. Aldosterone action in target epithelia. Vitam Horm 1980;38:55–117.
136. Speirs RS, Meyer RK. A method of assaying adrenal cortical hormones based on a decrease in the circulating eosinophil cells of adrenalectomized mice. Endocrinology 1951;48:316–326.
137. Ringer I, Brownfield R. The thymolytic activities of 16α, 17α ketals of triamcinolone. Endocrinology 1960;66:900–902.
138. Dorfman RI, Dorfman AS. The relative thymolytic activities of corticoids using the ovariectomized-adrenalectomized mouse. Endocrinology 1961;69:283–291.
139. Sereni F, Kenny FT, Kretchmer N. Factors influencing the development of tyrosine-α-ketoglutarate transaminase activity in rat liver. J Biol Chem 1959;234:609–612.
140. Kupfer D. Alteration in the magnitude of induction of tyrosine transaminase by glycocorticoids. The effects of phenobarbital, o,p'-DDD and β-diethylaminoethyl diphenylpropylacetate (SKF 525A). Arch Biochem Biophys 1968;127:200–206.
141. Lee K, Kenney FT. Induction of alanine transaminase by adrenal steroids in cultured hepatoma cells. Biochem Biophys Res Commun 1970;40:469–476.
142. Feigelson P, Beato M, Colman P, et al. Studies on the hepatic glucocorticoid receptor and on the hormonal modulation of specific mRNA levels during enzyme induction. Recent Prog Horm Res 1975;31:213–242.
143. Kenney F, Lee KL, Reel JR, et al. Regulation of tyrosine α-ketoglutarate transaminase in rat liver. IX. Studies of the mechanisms of hormonal inductions in cultured hepatoma cells. J Biol Chem 1970;245:5806–5812.
144. Felig P, Pozefsky T, Marliss E, et al. Alanine: key role in gluconeogenesis. Science 1970;167:1003–1004.
145. Landau BR. Adrenal steroids and carbohydrate metabolism. Vitam Horm 1965;23:1–59.
146. McMahon M, Gerich J, Rizza R. Effects of glucocorticoids on carbohydrate metabolism. Diabetes Metab Rev 1988;4:17–30.
147. Goulding NJ, Godolphin JL, Sharland PR, et al. Anti-inflammatory lipocortin 1 production by peripheral blood leucocytes in response to hydrocortisone. Lancet 1990;335:1416–1418.
148. Peers SH, Smillie F, Elderfield AJ, et al. Glucocorticoid and nonglucocorticoid induction of lipocortins (annexins) 1 and 2 in rat peritoneal leucocytes in vivo. Br J Pharmacol 1993;108:66–72.
149. Solito E, Parente L. Modulation of phospholipase A_2 activity in human fibroblasts. Br J Pharmacol 1989;96:656–660.
150. Parente L, Flower RJ. Hydrocortisone and 'macrocortin' inhibit the zymosan-induced release of lyso-PAF from rat peritoneal leucocytes. Life Sci 1985;36:1225–1231.
151. Beutler B, Cerami A. Cachectin: more than a tumor necrosis factor. N Engl J Med 1987;316:379–385.
152. Radomski MW, Palmer RM, Moncada S. Glucocorticoids inhibit the expression of an inducible, but not the constitutive, nitric oxide synthase in vascular endothelial cells. Proc Natl Acad Sci U S A 1990;87:10043–10047.
153. Lew W, Oppenheim JJ, Matsushima K. Analysis of the suppression of IL-1α and IL-1β production in human peripheral blood mononuclear adherent cells by a glucocorticoid hormone. J Immunol 1988;140:1895–1902.
154. Goodwin JS, Atluru D, Sierakowski S, et al. Mechanism of action of glucocorticosteroids. Inhibition of T cell proliferation and interleukin 2 production by hydrocortisone is reversed by leukotriene B_4. J Clin Invest 1986;77:1244–1250.
155. Sharp GW, Leaf A. Studies on the mode of action of aldosterone. Recent Prog Horm Res 1966;22:431–471.
156. Koeppen BM, Biagi BA, Giebisch GH. Intracellular microelectrode characterization of the rabbit cortical collecting duct. Am J Physiol 1983;244:35–47.
157. Meduri GU, Kanangat S. Glucocorticoid treatment of sepsis and acute respiratory distress syndrome: time for a critical reappraisal [editorial; comment]. Crit Care Med 1998;26:630–633.
158. Meduri GU, Headley AS, Golden E, et al. Effect of prolonged methylprednisolone therapy in unresolving acute respiratory distress syndrome: a randomized controlled trial [see comments]. JAMA 1998;280:159–165.
159. Suzuki M. [Percutaneous absorption and systemic distribution of corticosteroids.] Nippon Hifuka Gakkai Zasshi 1982;92:757–776.

Chapter 29

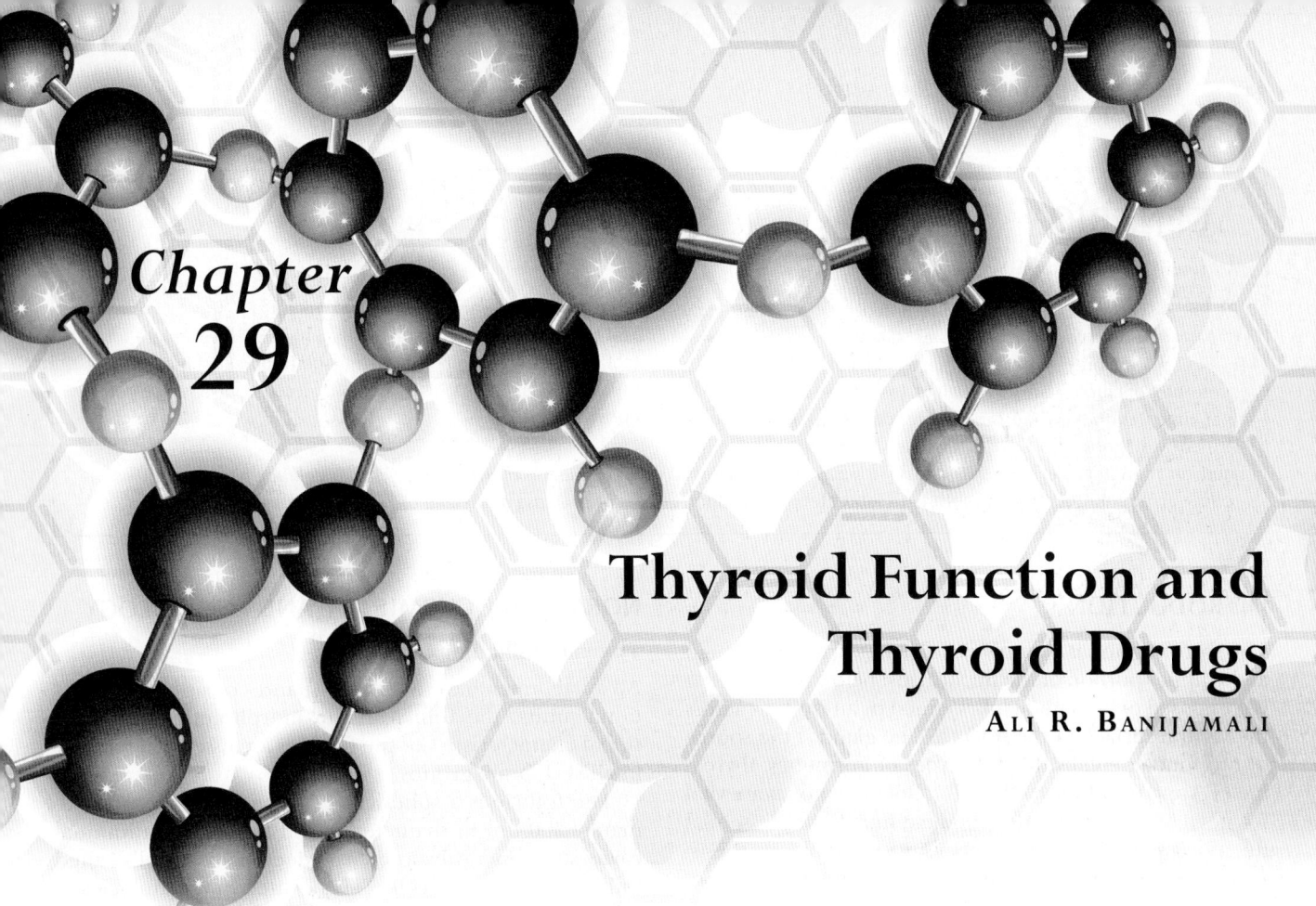

Thyroid Function and Thyroid Drugs

ALI R. BANIJAMALI

Drugs Covered in This Chapter

DRUGS FOR TREATMENT OF HYPOTHYROIDISM
- Levothyroxine
- Liothyronine
- Liotrix
- Thyroid gland products

DRUGS FOR TREATMENT OF HYPERTHYROIDISM
- Iodide
- Perchlorate
- Radioiodine
- 1-Methyl-2-mercaptoimidazole
- Propylthiouracil

Abbreviations

BMR, basal metabolic rate
cAMP, cyclic adenosine monophosphate
DIT, diiodo-L-tyrosine
dT_4, dextrothyroxine
FAD, flavin adenine dinucleotide
GRTH, generalized resistance to thyroid hormone
HSA, human serum albumin
99mTcO_4–, radioactive pertechnetate
MIT, monoiodo-L-tyrosine
MMI, 1-methyl-2-mercaptoimidazole
NADPH, reduced form of nicotinamide adenine dinucleotide phosphate
NIS, sodium/iodide symporter
PTU, propylthiouracil
rT_3, 3,3′,5′-triiodo-L-thyronine (reverse T_3)
SAR, structure–activity relationship
T_2, 3,3′-diiodo-L-thyronine
T_3, Levo or L-triiodothyronine, Liothyronine
T_4, Levo or L-thyroxine
TBG, thyroxine-binding globulin
Tg, thyroglobulin
TPO, thyroperoxidase
TRH, thyroid-releasing hormone
TSH, thyrotropin (thyroid-stimulating hormone)
TTR, transthyretin
USP, U.S. Pharmacopeia

SCENARIO

Autumn Stewart, PharmD

PA, a 43-year-old white man, presented to the emergency department with complaints of fever, sleeplessness, and a "racing heart." PA presented to his physician 1 month prior with symptoms including anxiety, weight loss, and tachycardia. At that time, laboratory and radioactive iodine uptake tests confirmed a diagnosis of Graves' disease. The patient was initiated on methimazole 5 mg TID and instructed to schedule a follow-up appointment in 1 month with laboratory tests. Upon admission in the emergency department, PA's heart rate was 160 beats per minute and irregular; his TSH levels were undetectable and thyroid-stimulating antibodies remained significantly elevated. PA's white blood cell counts were within normal limits.

(The reader is directed to the clinical solution and chemical analysis of this case at the end of the chapter).

INTRODUCTION

The thyroid gland is a highly vascular, flat structure located at the upper portion of the trachea, just below the larynx. It is composed of two lateral lobes joined by an isthmus across the ventral surface of the trachea. The gland is the source of two fundamentally different types of hormones, thyroxine (T_4) and triiodothyronine (T_3). Both hormones are vital for normal growth and development and control essential functions, such as energy metabolism and protein synthesis.

The word thyroid, meaning shield-shaped, was introduced by Wharton in his description of the gland (1). Like many before him, he attributed a solely cosmetic function to it because of the more frequent presence of enlarged glands in women, giving the throat region a more beautiful roundness. Later, however, it was observed that some characteristic symptoms for diseases always were accompanied by an obvious change in the size of the thyroid. This change was correctly interpreted as evidence that this structure plays a major role in normal body function.

An important step in the understanding of thyroid function was taken by Baumann (2), who discovered that the thyroid gland was the only organ in mammals that had the capability to incorporate iodine into organic substances. That discovery was important in research concerning the phylogeny of the thyroid.

Major clues to the physiologic roles of thyroid hormones were provided when normal and abnormal thyroid functions were related to oxygen uptake (3) and when thyroid hormones were found to induce metamorphosis in tadpoles (4). The first discovery led to investigations regarding the role of thyroid hormone in metabolism and calorigenesis, and the second inspired research concerning specific receptors as points of initiation of thyroid hormone expression. A patient lacking thyroid hormones may be treated with synthetic hormones or natural preparations. Better agents to treat hyperthyroidism are still being sought. Presently available drugs, other compounds affecting thyroid function, and current approaches in the search for new drugs are presented in this chapter within the context of thyroid biochemistry and physiology.

NORMAL BIOCHEMISTRY AND PHYSIOLOGY

Thyroid Follicular Cells

All vertebrates have a thyroid gland consisting of functional units, the follicles. The morphologic and functional characteristics of the follicles are essentially similar in all vertebrate groups.

The follicle is a spherical, cyst-like structure approximately 300 μm in diameter, and it consists of a luminal cavity surrounded by a one-cell-deep layer of cells called follicular or acinar cells. The center of the follicles is filled with a gelatinous colloid, the main component of which is a glycoprotein called thyroglobulin. The follicular cells contain an extensive network of rough endoplasmic reticulum, a well-developed Golgi apparatus, and lysosomes of various sizes (5). Thyroglobulin is synthesized in the rough endoplasmic reticulum of the follicular cells and transported by way of the Golgi complex to the apical membrane and then secreted into the follicle lumen.

The follicular cell contains two major assembly lines operating in opposite directions (6). One line moves in an apical direction (towards the lumen of the cell) and produces thyroglobulin that is delivered to the follicle lumen; the other line begins at the apical cell surface (cell surface facing the lumen of the cell) with endocytosis of thyroglobulin and ends by delivering hormones at the basolateral cell membrane. Therefore, the follicular cell seems to fulfill the functions of secretory and absorptive cells simultaneously. In addition to the functions associated with these two lines, the follicle has the specific ability to metabolize iodine, comprising the accumulation of iodide, iodination of tryosyl residues in thyroglobulin, and coupling of the iodinated tyrosyls to form thyroid hormones.

Parafollicular cells, also called light cells or C cells, are located individually or in clusters between follicular cells but do not border on the colloid. These cells produce thyrocalcitonin, a peptide hormone involved in calcium homeostasis (see also Chapter 30). The extrafollicular space of the gland is occupied by blood vessels, capillaries, lymphatic vessels, and connective tissue.

CLINICAL SIGNIFICANCE

Differences in the activity profiles of available treatments for thyroid disorders make patient-specific drug selection extremely important. The development of synthetic thyroid hormones has significantly improved treatment of hypothyroidism by decreasing the variations in levothyroxine and liothyronine blood levels that often resulted from inconsistent bovine and porcine sources. Once-daily or once-weekly dosing, which has been associated with improved patient compliance, is another clinically significant benefit of synthetic T_4, resulting from its extended half-life. Knowledge of levothyroxine's pharmacokinetic profile has also prompted patient counseling efforts promoting premeal administration because of marked reduction in absorption when combined with meals. The understanding of structure–activity relationships also enabled the development of synthetic T3 (liothyronine), the metabolically more active form of thyroid hormone with a much shorter duration of action. This is especially useful for patients with thyroid carcinoma who are to undergo radioiodine imaging and possible treatment. Because of a half-life of only 24 hours, liothyronine substitution enables more timely radioiodine imaging and treatment; as a result, patients experience less symptomatic hypothyroidism.

The study of medicinal chemistry has improved the treatment of thyroid disorders by reducing variability in plasma concentrations of T_3 and T_4 and by increasing the reliability of available monitoring methods. Accurate monitoring and therapy adjustments have resulted in fewer complications and increased quality of life among the millions of patients with thyroid disorders.

Autumn Stewart, PharmD
Assistant Professor of Pharmacy Practice
Duquesne University
School of Pharmacy
Pittsburgh, Pennsylvania

Hormones of the Thyroid Gland

Thyroid hormones are essential for normal development, differentiation, growth, and metabolism of every cell in the body. Thyroid hormones are iodinated amino acids derived from L-tyrosine. They are synthesized in the thyroid gland and stored as amino acid residues of thyroglobulin. The first known biologically active iodine-containing compound of the thyroid gland was isolated from thyroid extracts and named L-thyroxine (T_4). Later, its structure was established as the 3,5,3′,5′-tetraiodo-L-thyronine (T_4) (Fig. 29.1), and its synthesis was accomplished. Twenty-five years later, with the availability of chromatographic techniques and radioactive iodine, researchers discovered another major thyroid hormone, 3,5,3′-triiodo-L-thyronine (T_3) (Fig. 29.1), which is derived mainly from T_4 deiodination by deiodinase enzymes outside the thyroid. The body is therefore able to use a dose of T_4 to produce its own T_3.

T_4 and T_3 play numerous and meaningful roles in regulating metabolism, growth, and development and in maintaining homeostasis. Their reactions and products influence carbohydrate metabolism, protein synthesis and breakdown, and cardiovascular, renal, and brain function. It is usually believed that these actions result from effects of thyroid hormones on protein synthesis.

The thyroid gland also contains two quantitatively important iodinated amino acids, diiodo-L-tyrosine (DIT) and monoiodo-L-tyrosine (MIT). In addition, there are small amounts of other iodothyronines, such as 3,3′-diiodo-L-thyronine (T_2) and 3,3′,5′-triiodo-L-thyronine (reverse T_3 [rT_3]). None of the latter compounds possesses any significant hormonal activity. Chemically, MIT is 3-iodo-L-tyrosine, and DIT is 3,5-diiodo-L-tyrosine. The coupling of the two outer rings of DIT or of one outer ring of DIT with that of MIT (each with the net loss of alanine) leads to the formation of the two major thyroid hormones, T_4 and T_3, respectively.

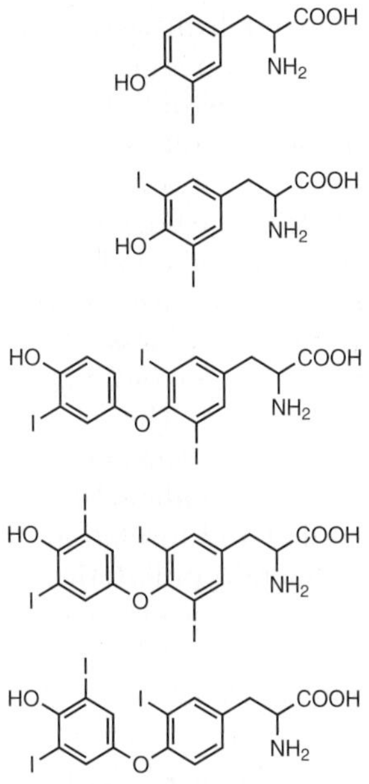

MIT

DIT

T3

T4

r-T3

FIGURE 29.1 Structure of the iodinated compounds of the thyroid gland.

Thyroglobulin (Tg) is of special importance, because it serves as the matrix for the synthesis of T_4 and T_3 and as the storage form of the hormones and iodide. Tg, a large glycoprotein with a molecular weight of 660,000 daltons, accounts for about one-third of the weight of the thyroid gland. Tg carries an average of 6 tyrosyl residues as MIT, 5 residues as DIT, 0.3 residues as T_3, and 1 residue as T_4. From these values, it can be estimated that a 20-g thyroid stores roughly 10 μmole (7.8 mg) of T_4 and 3 μmole (2.0 mg) of T_3 and that the normal human thyroid gland contains enough potential T_4 to maintain a euthyroid state for 2 months without new synthesis. The structures of the iodinated compounds of the thyroid gland are shown in Figure 29.1.

Biosynthesis of Thyroid Hormones

The thyroid contains two hormones, L-thyroxine (T_4) and L-triiodothyronine (T_3). Iodine is an indispensable component of the thyroid hormones, comprising 65% of the weight of T_4 and 58% of the weight of T_3. The thyroid hormones are the only iodine-containing compounds with established physiologic significance in vertebrates. Ingested iodine is absorbed through the small intestine and transported in the plasma to the thyroid, where it is concentrated, oxidized, and then incorporated into Tg to form MIT and DIT and later T_4 and T_3. After a variable period of storage in thyroid follicles, Tg is subjected to proteolysis, and the released hormones are secreted into the circulation, where specific binding proteins carry them to target tissues.

The synthesis of the thyroid hormones, T_3 and T_4, is regulated by thyrotropin (also known as thyroid-stimulating hormone [TSH]), which stimulates the synthesis of Tg, thyroperoxidase (TPO), and hydrogen peroxide. The formation of the thyroid hormones depends on an exogenous supply of iodide. The thyroid gland is unique in that it is the only tissue of the body able to accumulate iodine in large quantities and incorporate it into hormones. Approximately 25% of the body's supply of iodide is located in the thyroid gland. The iodine atoms play a unique role in the conformational preferences for T_3 and T_4 because of their large steric bulkiness. The metabolism of iodine is so closely related to thyroid function that the two must be considered together. The formation of thyroid hormones involves the following complex sequence of events: 1) active uptake of iodide by the follicular cells, 2) oxidation of iodide and formation of iodotyrosyl residues of Tg, 3) formation of iodothyronines from iodotyrosines, 4) proteolysis of Tg and release of T_4 and T_3 into blood, and 5) conversion of T_4 to T_3. These processes are summarized in Figure 29.2 (7).

Active Uptake of Iodide by Follicular Cells

The first step in the synthesis of the thyroid hormones is the uptake of iodide from the blood by the thyroid gland. An adequate intake of iodide is essential for the synthesis of sufficient thyroid hormone. Ingested iodine is absorbed through the small intestine and transported in the plasma to the thyroid, where it is concentrated, oxidized, and then incorporated into Tg. Blood iodine is present in a steady state in which dietary iodide, iodide "leaked" from the thyroid gland, and reclaimed hormonal iodide provide the iodide input. Thyroid gland iodide uptake, renal elimination, and a small biliary excretion provide iodide loss. The thyroid gland regulates both the fraction of circulating iodide that it takes up and the amount of iodide that it leaks back into the circulation. A simplified scheme of iodide metabolism is shown in Figure 29.3.

The mechanism enabling the thyroid gland to concentrate blood iodide against a gradient into the follicular cell is the iodide pump (NIS, sodium/iodide symporter), which is regulated by TSH. Decreased stores of thyroid iodine enhance iodide uptake; conversely, dietary iodide can reverse this process. The iodide pump maintains a ratio of thyroid iodide to serum iodide (T:S ratio) of about 20:1 under basal conditions but of more than 100:1 in hyperactive gland. Iodide uptake may be blocked by several inorganic ions, such as thiocyanate (SCN^-) and perchlorate. Because iodide uptake involves concurrent uptake of potassium, it can also be blocked by cardiac glycosides that inhibit potassium accumulation.

Oxidation of Iodide and Formation of Iodotyrosines

To serve as an iodinating agent, iodide must be oxidized to a higher oxidation state, a step that is hydrogen peroxide dependent and is catalyzed by TPO, a membrane-bound heme-enzyme that utilizes hydrogen peroxide as the oxidant. In addition to catalyzing the oxidation of iodide, TPO is essential for the incorporation of iodide into tyrosine residues in Tg (aromatic iodination) and coupling of the iodotyrosyl residues from DIT to form T_4 and T_3. The activity of TPO is increased by TSH from increased synthesis of TPO.

The second step in the synthesis of the thyroid hormones is a concerted reaction at the apical membrane in which the iodide in the follicle lumen is oxidized by TPO in the presence of hydrogen peroxide to an active iodine species that, in turn, iodinates selected tyrosyl residues of Tg. Consistent with the conditions necessary for aromatic halogenation, the iodination of the tyrosyl residues requires the iodinating species to be in a higher oxidation state compared with the iodide anion. The iodinating species is thought to be hypoiodate (OI^-) (7). The two-electron oxidation of iodide to its hypoiodate reactive species is accomplished by TPO. Although the diiodotyrosyl residues constitute the major products, some MIT peptides are also produced. TSH stimulates the generation of hydrogen peroxide and, thus, the process of iodination.

Hydrogen peroxide is an essential and limiting factor in the oxidation of iodide, aromatic iodination of tyrosyl residues, and the coupling reaction. The hydrogen peroxide–generating system is localized at the apical membrane, and its generation involves the oxidation of

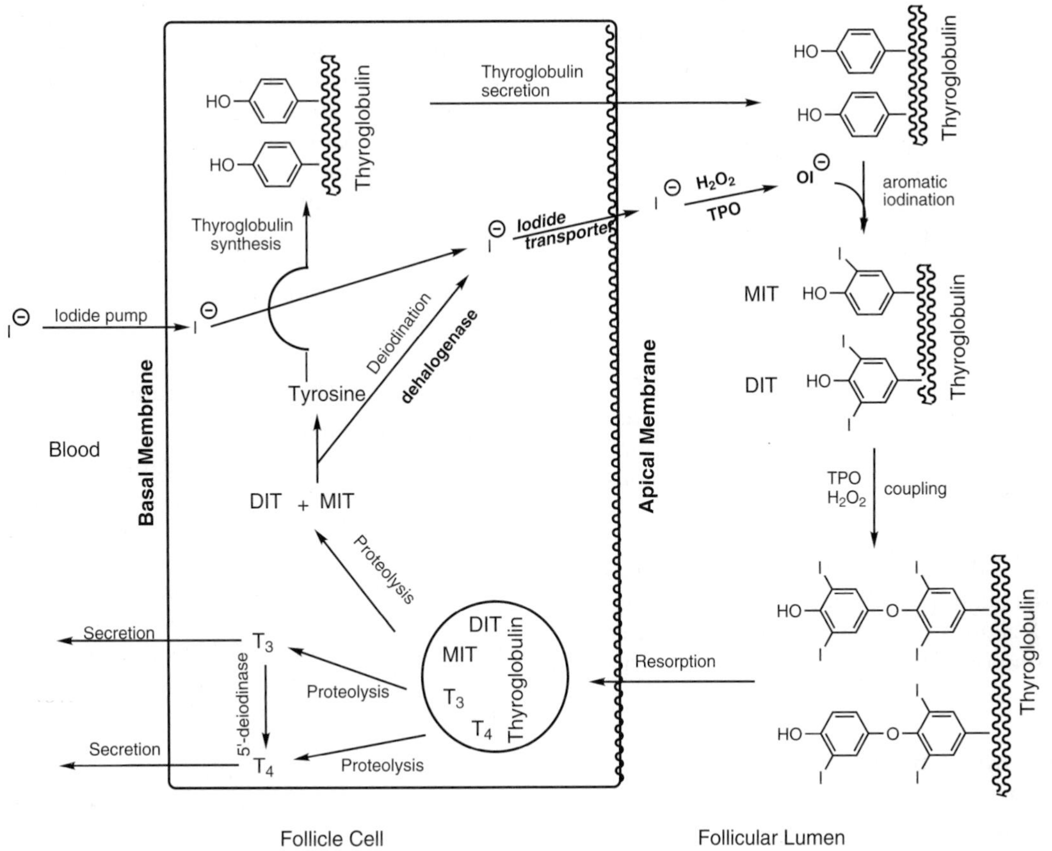

FIGURE 29.2 Summary of the major pathways for the biosynthesis and secretion of the thyroid hormones. When thyrotropin (TSH) binds to the TSH receptor at the basal membrane of the follicular cell, the biosynthesis of thyroglobulin (TG) is stimulated, as is that of thyroperoxidase (TPO) and the production of hydrogen peroxide. Noniodinated TG is synthesized by the rough endoplasmic reticulum of the follicular cell and secreted through the apical membrane of the follicular cell into the follicular lumen. Iodide enters the follicular cell by the iodide pump (NIS, sodium/iodide symporter) and is then transported into the follicular lumen. In the lumen, the iodide is oxidized by TPO-O (a π-cation radical intermediate formed from TPO and hydrogen peroxide) at the apical membrane to form hypoiodate anion (OI^-), followed by aromatic iodination of selected tyrosyl residues on TG to form diiodotyrosyl (DIT) and monoiodotyrosyl (MIT) residues. The tyrosyl ring of DIT couples with adjacent DIT and MIT residues with an ether linkage to form the outer ring of thyroxine (T_4) and of triiodothyronine (T_3), both of which remain attached to TG. Although shown as a sequential reaction, the iodination and coupling reactions occur simultaneously via TPO and hydrogen peroxide. Hydrogen peroxide is generated by a NADPH/FAD thyroid oxidase (THOX) at the apical membrane. Low plasma levels for T_4 cause the iodinated TG to be resorbed into the follicular cell, where complete proteolysis occurs by lysosomal protease to T_4, T_3, DIT, MIT, and noniodinated amino acids. Both T_4 and T_3 are secreted by the cell into the blood; T_4 is deiodinated to active T_3. Both DIT and MIT are recycled by a dehalogenase (or deiodinase) to free tyrosine and iodide, both of which are recycled back into iodinated thyroglobulin.

the reduced form of nicotinamide adenine dinucleotide phosphate (NADPH) by an NADPH/flavin adenine dinucleotide (FAD) oxidase called thyroid oxidase. The reaction product of TPO with hydrogen peroxide is described as TPO-P, a π-cation radical, which generates hypoiodate. The generation of hydrogen peroxide is concentration controlled by iodide, which permits efficient hormone synthesis when iodide is scarce while avoiding excessive hormone synthesis when iodide is abundant. Deficient generation of hydrogen peroxide has been proposed as one explanation for goiter and decreased aromatic iodination in euthyroid patients. The in vitro addition of a hydrogen peroxide–generating system to thyroid homogenates or slices from these patients restored normal organification.

In the thyroid follicular cell, intracellular iodide taken up from blood is bound in organic form in a few minutes, so less than 1% of the total iodine of the gland is found as iodide. Therefore, inhibition of the iodide transport system requires blockade of organic binding. This can be achieved by the use of antithyroid drugs, of which n-propyl-6-thiouracil and 1-methyl-2-mercaptoimidazole (MMI) are the most potent.

Coupling of Iodotyrosine Residues

Coupling is also catalyzed by TPO at the apical membrane, and although shown in Figure 29.2 as sequential steps, they occur simultaneously. This coupling reaction takes place at Tg and involves the coupling of the two outer rings from DIT residues to become T_4, whereas the

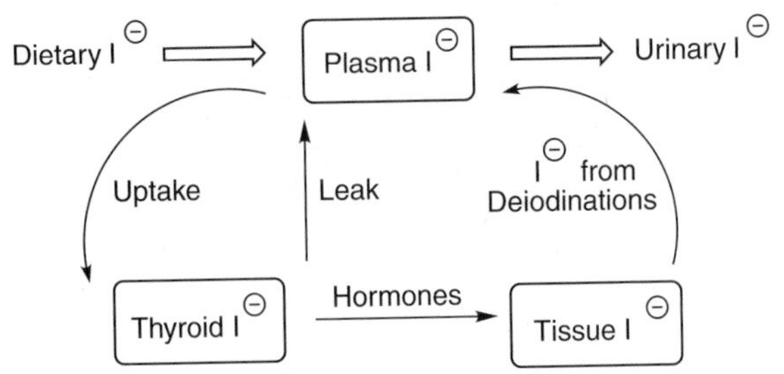

FIGURE 29.3 Simplified scheme of iodide metabolism.

coupling of the outer ring from MIT with DIT results in the formation of T_3. During the coupling reaction as shown in Figure 29.2, a tyrosyl residue donates its iodinated phenyl group as a DIT radical to become the outer ring of the iodothyronine amino acid at an acceptor site, leaving dehydroalanine at the donor site. The location of the iodotyrosyl residues within Tg creates an optimal spatial alignment, facilitating the coupling reaction. These reactions are catalyzed by TPO and can be blocked by compounds such as thiourea, thiouracils, and sulfonamides.

Proteolysis of Thyroglobulin and Release of Iodothyronines

In response to demand for thyroid hormones, the release of thyroid hormones from Tg begins with the resorption of Tg via endocytosis into the follicular epithelial cells and its subsequent complete proteolysis by the lysosomal digestive enzymes of the follicular cells. Tg proteolysis yields MIT, DIT, T_3, and T_4. Although MIT and DIT are formed, they do not leave the thyroid but, instead, are selectively deiodinated to tyrosine and recycled into new Tg. The iodide is recycled into hypoiodate for subsequent iodination, conserving the essential nutrients for the thyroid gland. Both T_3 and T_4 are secreted by the cell into the circulation. A defect in the recyclization of MIT and DIT can lead to hypothyroidism and goiter by increasing their elimination in the urine.

Conversion of Thyroxine to Triiodothyronine

Although T_4 is by far the major thyroid hormone secreted by the thyroid (~8 to 10 times the rate of T_3), it is usually considered to be a prohormone. Because T_4 has a longer half-life, much higher levels of T_4 than of T_3 are in the circulation. The enzymatic conversion of T_4 to T_3 is an obligate step in the physiologic action of thyroid hormones in most extrathyroidal tissues. In the peripheral tissues, approximately 33% of the T_4 secreted undergoes 5′-deiodination to give T_3, and another 40% undergoes deiodination of the inner ring to yield the inactive material rT_3 (8). The 5′-deiodination of T_4 is a reductive process catalyzed by a group of enzymes named iodothyronine 5′deiodinases, referred to as 5′-deiodinases and symbolized by 5′-D, which are found in a variety of cells. Approximately 80% of the T_3 is derived from circulating T_4.

Three types of 5′-deiodinases are currently known, and these are distinguished from each other primarily based on their location, substrate preference, and susceptibility to inhibitors. Type I 5′-deiodinase is found in liver and kidney and catalyzes both inner ring and outer ring deiodination (i.e., T_4 to T_3 and rT_3 to 3,3′-T_2). Type II 5′-deiodinase catalyzes mainly outer ring deiodination (i.e., T_4 to T_3, and T_3 to 3,3′-T_2) and is found in brain and the pituitary. Type III 5′-deiodinase is the principal source of rT_3 and is present in brain, skin, and placenta (9).

Transport of Thyroid Hormones

Transport in the Blood

More than 99% of the circulating thyroid hormone is bound to plasma proteins but can be liberated rapidly for entry into cells. The thyroid hormone-binding proteins are comprised of thyroxine-binding globulin (TBG), transthyretin (TTR or thyroxine-binding prealbumin), human serum albumin (HSA), and lipoproteins. Their functions are most probably to ensure a constant supply of thyroid hormones to the cells and tissues by preventing urinary loss, protect the organism against abrupt changes in thyroid hormone production and degradation, protect against iodine deficiency, and target the amount of thyroid hormone delivery by ensuring a site-specific, enzymatic alteration of TBG.

Thyroxine-Binding Globulin

TBG carries the major part of both circulating T_4 and T_3 (as well as rT_3), and therefore, quantitative or qualitative changes in TBG concentration have a high impact on total serum T_4 and T_3. The protein is encoded by a single gene on the X chromosome and is produced and cleared by the liver. It has a single iodothyronine-binding site with higher affinity for T_4 compared to T_3. When TBG is fully saturated, it carries approximately 20 μg T_4/L. The TBG concentration in serum is between 11 and 21 mg/L (180 to 350 nM), present from the 12th week of fetal life and 1.5 times higher in newborns and children until 2 to 3 years of age. Estrogen has a marked effect on TBG by prolonging the biologic half-life from the normal 5 days, thus resulting in increased plasma concentrations of TBG and total thyroid hormones, whereas testosterone has the opposite effect (10). In children and adolescents, this may have an implication in diseases with a severe sex hormone overproduction related to age, as well as oral contraceptive use and pregnancy in adolescent girls.

Transthyretin

TTR (previously called thyroxine-binding prealbumin) binds only about 15% to 20% of the circulating thyroid hormones and has a lower affinity for the hormones, thus dissociating from them more rapidly, and is responsible for much of the immediate delivery of T_4 and T_3. TTR is the major thyroid hormone-binding protein in cerebrospinal fluid. It is synthesized in the liver and the choroid plexus and secreted into the blood and cerebrospinal fluid, respectively. Only 0.5% of the circulating TTR is occupied by T_4, and it has a rapid turnover of 2 days in plasma. Acquired abnormalities in TTR include major illness, nephrotic syndrome, liver disease, cystic fibrosis, protein fasting, and hyperthyroidism. However, changes in TTR concentrations have little effect on the serum concentrations of thyroid hormones (10).

Albumin

HSA binds about 5% of the circulating T_4 and T_3. Its affinity for the hormones is even lower, and because HSA associates with a wide variety of substances, including a number of different hormones and drugs, the association between thyroid hormones and HSA can hardly be regarded as specific. Even marked fluctuations in serum HSA concentrations have no effect on thyroid hormone levels.

Lipoproteins

Lipoproteins transport a minor fraction of circulating T_4 and to some extent T_3. The binding site for thyroid hormones on apolipoprotein A1 is distinct from that which binds to cellular protein receptors.

Consequences of Abnormal Binding Protein Concentrations

Abnormalities of the thyroid hormone-binding proteins do not cause alterations in the metabolic state of the individual and do not result in thyroid disease. Thus, abnormal concentrations of these binding proteins, due to changed synthesis, degradation, or stability, result in maintaining normal free thyroid hormone concentrations.

Metabolism and Excretion

As discussed earlier, T_4 is considered to be a prohormone, and its peripheral metabolism occurs in two ways: outer ring deiodination by the enzyme 5′-D, which yields T_3, and inner ring deiodination by the enzyme 5-D, which yields rT_3, for which there is no known biologic function (Fig. 29.4). In humans, deiodination is the most important metabolic pathway of the hormone, not only because of its dual role in the activation and inactivation of T_4 but also in quantitative terms.

A second pathway of thyroid hormone metabolism involves the conjugation of the phenolic hydroxyl group of the outer phenolic ring with sulfonate or glucuronic acid. These conjugation reactions occur primarily in the liver and to a lesser degree in the kidney and result in biotransformation of T_4 and T_3. The iodothyronine glucuronides are rapidly excreted in bile, but after hydrolysis in intestine by bacterial β-glucuronidases, at least part of the liberated iodothyronine is reabsorbed, constituting an enterohepatic cycle. In contrast, little iodothyronine sulfate appears as a rule in the bile or in the serum because the sulfate esters are rapidly deiodinated

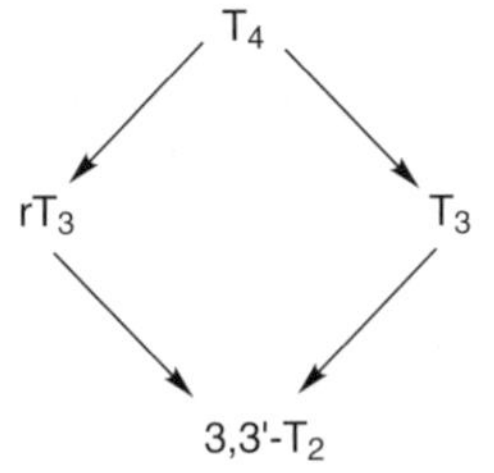

FIGURE 29.4 Deiodination of thyroxine (T_4).

in the liver. Sulfonate conjugation is the primary step in irreversible deactivation of thyroid hormones. Thyroid hormones can also undergo deamination and decarboxylase reactions in the liver, resulting in the formation of so-called acetic acid analogs. These reactions occur at the alanine side chain of the inner tyrosyl ring. Although these analogs are thought to be metabolically active, little is known about the quantities produced or their contribution to hormone activity in humans. The reactions through which thyroid hormone is metabolized are summarized in Figure 29.5.

Physiologic Actions of Thyroid Hormones—Oxygen Consumption and Calorigenesis

The two most important actions of thyroid hormone are those related to oxygen consumption and those related to protein synthesis. A respiratory component of the action of thyroid hormones was first observed almost a century ago. Respiratory exchange was depressed in patients diagnosed as hypothyroid and increased in patients diagnosed as hyperthyroid (3). The increase in respiration that follows the administration of thyroid hormone reflects an increase in metabolic rate, and thyroid function has, indeed, long been assessed by measuring the basal or resting metabolic rate (BMR), a test in which the oxygen consumed, as measured in an individual at rest, is used to calculate total-body energy production. The BMR of a hyperthyroid individual is above the normal range, or positive, and that of a hypothyroid individual is below the normal range, or negative.

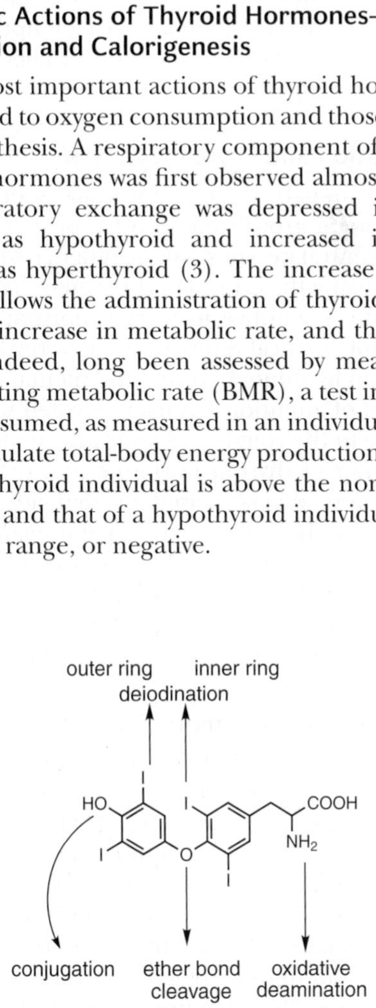

FIGURE 29.5 Metabolic pathways for thyroxine.

Because most of the energy produced by cellular respiration eventually appears as heat, an increase in cellular respiration necessarily leads to an increase in heat production (i.e., to a thermogenic or calorigenic effect). Thus, to the degree that thyroid hormones control BMR, they also control thermogenesis (11).

Clinically, the inability to adjust to environmental temperature is symptomatic of departure from the euthyroid status. Patients with myxedema frequently have subnormal body temperature, have cold and dry skin, and tolerate cold poorly; the thyrotoxic patient, who compensates for excess heat production by sweating (warm, moist hands), does not easily tolerate a warm environment.

Thyroid hormones regulate the turnover of carbohydrates, lipids, and proteins. They promote glucose absorption, hepatic and renal gluconeogenesis, hepatic glycogenolysis, and glucose utilization in muscle and adipose tissue (12). Thyroid hormones are anabolic when present at normal concentrations; they then stimulate the expression of many key enzymes of metabolism. Thyroid hormones at the levels present in hyperthyroidism are catabolic; they lead to the mobilization of tissue protein and, especially, of muscle tissue protein for gluconeogenetic processes (13). Thus, the depletion of liver glycogen, the increased breakdown of lipids, and the negative nitrogen balance observed in hyperthyroidism represent toxic effects.

Differentiation and Protein Synthesis

In young mammals, thyroid hormone is necessary not only for general growth but also for proper differentiation of the central nervous system. A deficiency of thyroid hormone during the critical period when the developing human brain is sensitive to thyroid hormone results in an irreversible clinical entity termed cretinism, which is characterized by stunted growth and mental retardation. A great deal of attention has been devoted to the events taking place in the roughly 48-hour interval between the administration of thyroid hormone and the manifestation of certain effects caused by that administration. After Tata (14) had observed that the anabolic effects observed in rats given T_4 could be blocked by inhibitors of protein synthesis, further investigations led Tata and Widnell (15) to the conclusion that thyroid hormones were activating protein synthesis at the ribosomal level.

Control of Thyroid Hormone Biosynthesis

The primary role of thyroid is to produce thyroid hormones. The primary regulator of thyroid function and growth is the pituitary hormone TSH, a glycoprotein with a molecular weight of approximately 28,000 daltons. The most important controller of TSH secretion is thyroid-releasing hormone (TRH). TRH is secreted by hypothalamic neurons into hypothalamic-hypophyseal portal blood and finds its receptors in the anterior pituitary, stimulating the secretion of TSH. TRH is three amino acids long (a tripeptide). Its basic sequence is *pyro*-glutamyl-histidine-proline amide. Secretion of TRH and, hence, TSH, is inhibited by high blood levels of thyroid hormones in a classical negative feedback loop.

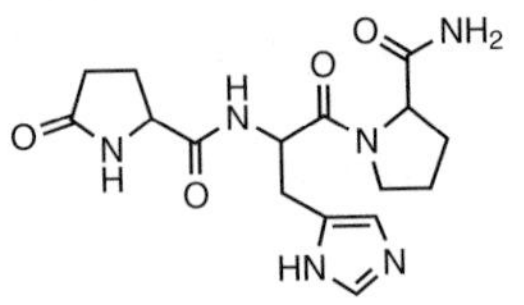

TRH

The amount of thyroid hormone circulating in body fluids and present in tissues remains fairly constant. Accounting for this constancy are the relatively long biologic half-life of the thyroid hormones, the regulation of gland activity by the pituitary-hypothalamic system, and the availability of iodide. Thyroid hormone research points toward T_3 as the thyroid hormone; therefore, factors affecting peripheral T_3 formation by the 5′-D enzymes are highly relevant.

T_4 is greater than 99.9% bound to plasma proteins. Thus, T_4 has a biologic half-life of 1 week, as compared to 1 day for the less firmly bound T_3.

The biosynthesis and secretion of TSH is regulated by TRH and, thus, the quantity of thyroid hormone in circulation through feedback control. The ability of thyroid hormones to prevent the release of TSH is referred to as feedback regulation. The amount of iodide available to the gland for hormone synthesis is also an important regulator of thyroid function. The efficiency of the thyroid pump mechanism and the rate of Tg and TPO synthesis are all TSH dependent. In cases of iodide deficiency, the production of thyroid hormone is lowered, and TSH rises through the pituitary feedback mechanism previously described. The effect of the increased TSH is to produce more thyroid hormone by increasing efficiency of the iodide pump and increasing Tg and TPO synthesis. Thus, in iodide deficiency, there is an increased uptake of iodide (16) and larger MIT-to-DIT ratios, which lead to larger T_3-to-T_4 ratios. T_3 is the more rapidly acting hormone, mitigating the effect of iodide deficiency. When iodide deficiency is severe, a persistent rise in TSH is observed. This then results in thyroid gland growth.

In the presence of an excess of circulating iodide, the absolute amount of iodide taken up by the thyroid gland remains approximately constant, which is compensated by a decrease in the fraction of the total iodide taken up and an increase in the amount of iodide leaked from the thyroid gland. In addition, there may be a decrease in the formation of iodinated Tg residues and in the release of hormones from the gland. The decrease in the formation of iodinated Tg residues that occurs at excessive physiologic doses of iodide has been called the Wolff-Chaikoff block (17). This block may be caused by an interaction of iodide with NADPH (18), which depletes follicular NADPH and, in turn, depletes the hydrogen

position. The suggested maintenance dosages are 50 to 800 mg daily for PTU and 5 to 30 mg daily for MMI.

Pharmacokinetics PTU is rapidly absorbed from the gastrointestinal tract, reaching peak serum levels after 1 hour. The bioavailability of 50% to 80% may be due to incomplete absorption or a large first-pass effect in the liver. The volume of distribution approximates total-body water with accumulation in the thyroid gland. Most of an ingested dose of PTU is excreted by the kidney as the inactive glucuronide within 24 hours. In contrast, MMI is completely absorbed but at variable rates. It is readily accumulated by the thyroid gland and has a volume of distribution similar to that of PTU. Excretion is slower than with PTU; 65% to 70% of a dose is recovered in the urine in 48 hours. The short plasma half-life of these agents (1.5 hours for PTU and 6 hours for MMI) has little influence on the duration of the antithyroid action or the dosing interval because both agents are accumulated by the thyroid gland. For PTU, giving the drug every 6 to 8 hours is reasonable since a single 100-mg dose can inhibit iodine organification by 60% for 7 hours. Since a single 30-mg dose of MMI exerts an antithyroid effect for longer than 24 hours, a single daily dose is effective in the management of mild to moderate hyperthyroidism. The two drugs differ in their binding to serum proteins. MMI is essentially free in serum, whereas 80% to 90% of PTU is bound to albumin.

Efforts to improve the taste and decrease the rate of release of MMI led to the development of 1-carbethoxy-3-methylthioimidazole (carbimazole). Carbimazole, the prodrug derivative of MMI, gives rise to MMI in vivo and is used in the same dosage.

The side effects of thioamides include diarrhea, vomiting, jaundice, skin rashes, and at times, sudden onset of agranulocytosis. There does not appear to be a great difference in toxicity among the compounds currently in use.

Antithyroid drugs are associated with a variety of minor side effects, as well as potentially life-threatening or even lethal complications. Side effects of MMI are dose related, whereas those of PTU are less clearly related to dose. This may favor use of low-dose MMI rather than PTU in the average patient with hyperthyroidism. Adverse reactions to the thioamides occur in 3% to 12% of treated patients. Most reactions occur early, especially nausea and gastrointestinal distress. An altered sense of taste or smell may occur with MMI. The most common adverse effect is a maculopapular pruritic rash (4% to 6%), at times accompanied by systemic signs such as fever.

Both PTU and MMI are concentrated several-fold by the thyroid gland and inhibit the iodination and coupling reactions of TPO (7). Taurog (40) described the thioureylenes as potent inhibitors of Tg iodination. He suggested that a thioureylene, such as PTU (PTU-SH), would irreversibly inhibit TPO-catalyzed iodination of Tg when the thioureylene-to-iodide ratio was high and reversibly when the PTU-SH-to-iodide ratio was low. In the course of the iodination reaction, the thioureylene PTU-SH would be oxidized (41), possibly to a disulfide dimer, such as PTU-SS-PTU. Iodination of tyrosyl residues resumes once oxidation of the drug to disulfide products occurs by either hypoiodate (OI^-) or an enzyme-hypoiodate complex (EOI^-). Under these conditions, the thioureylenes act as competitive inhibitors by competing with tyrosyls for hypoiodate. Conversely, at high drug concentrations, the thioureylenes are only partially oxidized, and the partially oxidized intermediate can presumably inactivate TPO by covalent binding of an oxidized form of the drug to the prosthetic heme group of TPO to prevent formation of the hydrogen peroxide–TPO complex. As a result, iodination is irreversibly blocked. Data obtained from rats fed an iodide-deficient diet are consistent with this in vitro model in that intrathyroidal metabolism is radiolabeled PTU and MMI is decreased.

Thioureylene drugs also effectively inhibit the coupling of the DIT/MIT residues on Tg to yield T_4 and T_3. This effect has been related to an alteration of the conformation of Tg brought on by the binding of the thioureylene to Tg (i.e., by the formation of a compound such as TPO-S-S-PTU) (42).

After the observation that PTU inhibited the peripheral deiodination of T_4 (37,43), attempts to relate deiodinase inhibitory activity to structural parameters were undertaken (43). These studies emphasized the need for tautomerization to a thiol form and for the presence of a polar hydrogen on the nitrogen adjacent to the sulfur-bearing carbon. A study of the relation of chemical structure to 5′-D-I inhibitory activity related to similar studies of structural requirements for TPO inhibition could prove fruitful in the design of improved antithyroid drugs.

Toxicity Agranulocytosis is the most feared side effect of antithyroid drug therapy. Agranulocytosis (an absolute granulocyte count of <500/mm^3) occurred in 0.37% of patients receiving PTU and in 0.35% receiving MMI. Agranulocytosis must be distinguished from the transient, mild granulocytopenia (a granulocyte count of <1,500/mm^3) that occasionally occurs in patients with Graves disease, in some patients of African descent, and occasionally in patients treated with antithyroid drugs. A baseline differential white blood cell count should be obtained before initiation of therapy.

Most cases of agranulocytosis occur within the first 90 days of treatment, but this complication can occur even a year or more after starting therapy. It is important to note that agranulocytosis can develop after a prior uneventful course of drug therapy, a finding that is important since renewed exposure to the drug frequently occurs when patients have a relapse and undergo a second course of antithyroid therapy. Agranulocytosis is thought to be autoimmune mediated, and antigranulocyte antibodies are shown by immunofluorescence and cytotoxicity assays. Agranulocytosis induced by PTU is evidence of a drug-dependent antibody reacting with granulocytes, monocytes, and hematopoietic progenitor cells. All patients should be instructed to discontinue the antithyroid drug and contact a physician immediately if fever or sore throat develops. Hepatotoxicity is another major side effect of antithyroid drugs. Estimates regarding the frequency of this condition are imprecise, but it probably ranges from 0.1% to 0.2%. The recognition of PTU-related hepatotoxicity may be difficult, since in up to 30% of patients with normal baseline aminotransferase levels who are treated with PTU, transient acute increases in those levels develop, ranging from 1.1 to 6 times the upper limit of normal levels, that resolve while therapy is continued. In addition, asymptomatic elevations in serum aminotransferase levels occur frequently in untreated patients with hyperthyroidism and are not predictive of further increases after the institution of PTU therapy.

Propylthiouracil-Induced Hepatotoxicity

Vasculitis is the third major toxic reaction seen with antithyroid drug treatment, more commonly found in connection with PTU than with MMI. Serologic evidence consistent with lupus erythematosus develops in some patients, fulfilling the criteria for drug-induced lupus. Antineutrophil cytoplasmic antibody–positive vasculitis has also been reported, especially in Asian patients treated with PTU. Most patients have perinuclear antineutrophil cytoplasmic antibodies, with a majority of them having anti-myeloperoxidase antineutrophil cytoplasmic antibodies. It has been hypothesized that antithyroid drugs, especially PTU, can react with myeloperoxidase to form reactive intermediates that promote autoimmune inflammation.

Thyrotoxicosis

Hyperthyroidism is the term for overactive tissue within the thyroid gland causing an overproduction of thyroid hormones. Hyperthyroidism is thus a cause of thyrotoxicosis (44), the clinical condition of increased thyroid hormones in the blood. It is important to note that hyperthyroidism and thyrotoxicosis are not synonymous. For instance, thyrotoxicosis could instead be caused by ingestion of exogenous thyroid hormone or inflammation of the thyroid gland, causing it to release its stores of thyroid hormones. Because symptoms of thyrotoxicosis resemble those of adrenergic overstimulation, attempts to decrease such symptoms by adrenergic blockade have been undertaken. Reserpine and guanethidine, both of which are depleters of catecholamines, and propranolol, a β-blocking agent, have been used effectively to decrease the tachycardia, tremor, and anxiety of thyrotoxicosis. Because of its less serious side effects, propranolol has become the drug of choice in this adjunctive therapy. Reports of decreased T_3 plasma levels during propranolol treatment suggest that blocking of the peripheral deiodination of T_4 may contribute to the beneficial effects of propranolol. The use of propranolol as a preventive drug in acute thyrotoxicosis has been found to be beneficial by some investigators, but not by others. Hyperthyroidism has become a common and well-recognized disorder of middle-aged to older cats, and treatment with these antithyroid drugs has been equally effective in the long-term control of the feline hyperthyroidism.

Goitrogens and Drugs Affecting Thyroid Function

The presence of environmental goitrogens was suggested by the resistance of endemic goiters to iodine prophylaxis and iodide treatment in Italy and Colombia. In the past, endemic outbreaks of hypothyroidism have pointed toward calcium as a source of waterborne goitrogenicity, and it is presently believed that calcium is a weak goitrogen able to cause latent hypothyroidism to come to the surface.

Lithium salts have been used as safe adjuncts in the initial treatment of thyrotoxicosis (45). Lithium is concentrated by the thyroid gland (46), with a thyroid-to-serum ratio of more than 2:1, suggesting active transport. Lithium ion inhibits adenylate cyclase, which forms cAMP. Formed in response to TSH, cAMP is a stimulator of the processes involved in thyroid hormone release from the gland. Inhibition of hormone secretion by lithium has proved to be a useful adjunct in treatment of hyperthyroidism (47).

In view of the role of cysteine residues in the conformation of Tg, the mode of action of TPO, and the deiodination of T_4, the effect of sulfur-containing compounds on thyroid hormone formation is hardly surprising. Most naturally occurring sulfur compounds are derived from glucosinolates (formerly referred to as thioglucosides) (48), which are present in foods such as cabbage, turnip, mustard seed, salad greens, and radishes (most of these are from the genus *Brassica* or *Cruciferae*) as well as in the milk of cows grazing in areas containing *Brassica* weeds. Chemically, glucosinolates can give rise to many components, primarily to isothiocyanate (SCN^-) and lesser extent to thiocyanate (CNS^-), isothiocyanate (SCN^-), nitriles (RCN), and thiooxazolidones. Thiocyanate is a large anion that competes with iodide for uptake by the thyroid gland; its goitrogenic effect can be reversed by iodide intake. Goitrin, 5-*R*-vinyloxazolidine-2-thione, is a potent thyroid peroxidase inhibitor (49) that is claimed to be more effective than PTU in humans (50) and is held to be the cause of a mild goiter endemia in Finland. In rats, goitrin is actively taken up by the thyroid gland and appears to inhibit the coupling of Tg diiodotyrosyl residues (51). Many workers, however, believe that the goitrogenic effects of *Brassica* result from the additive effects of all goitrogenic components present.

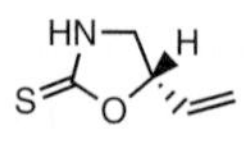

Goitrin

Other compounds affecting thyroid function include sulfonamides, anticoagulants, and oxygenated and iodinated aromatic compounds. The hypoglycemic agent carbutamide and the diuretic acetazolamide (Diamox) are examples of sulfonamides. Of the anticoagulants, heparin appears to interfere with the binding of T_4 to plasma transport proteins (52), but warfarin (Coumadin) and dicoumarol are competitive inhibitors of the substrate T_4 or rT_3 in the 5′-D reaction, with a dissociation constant in the micromolar range (53). Other oxygenated compounds affecting the 5′-D include resorcinol, long known to be a goitrogen, and phloretin, a dihydrochalocone with a half maximal inhibitory concentration of 4 mol/L.

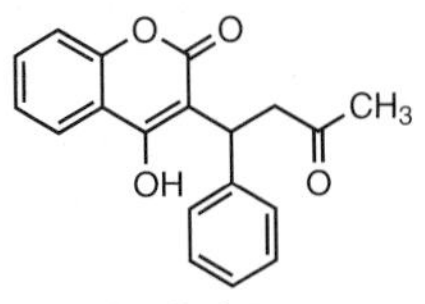

Warfarin

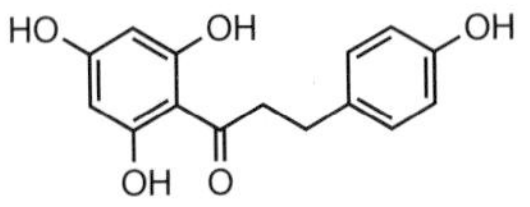

Phloretin

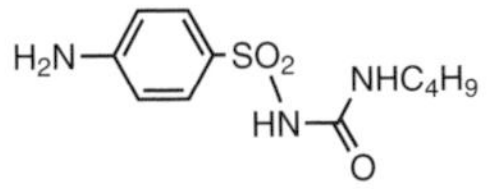

Carbutamide

The ability of oxidation products of 3,4-dihydroxy-cinnamic acid to prevent the binding of TSH to human thyroid membranes (54) suggests that other oxygenated phenols may interfere with thyroid hormone function in more than one way. Examples of iodinated drugs affecting thyroid function are the antiarrhythmic agent amiodarone and the radiocontrasting agent iopanoic acid. All of these compounds interfere with the peripheral deiodination of T_4 and are being tested as adjuncts in the treatment of hyperthyroidism.

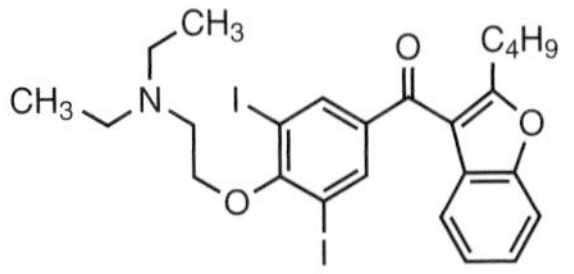

Amiodarone

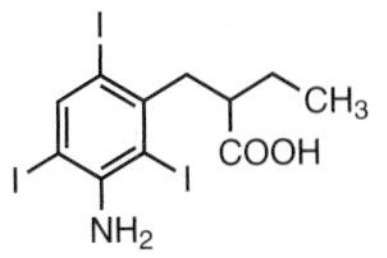

Iopanoic acid

The binding of thyroid hormones to plasma carrier proteins is affected by endogenous agents or by drugs that can change the concentration of these proteins or compete with thyroid hormones for binding sites. Examples of the first group are testosterone and related anabolic agents, which are able to decrease the concentration of T_4 binding globulin, and estrogens and related contraceptive agents, which are able to increase the concentration of T_4 binding globulin. Salicylates, diphenylhydantoin, and heparin are members of the large group competing with thyroid hormones for binding sites. Alterations in the binding of T_3 and T_4 are of no large physiologic consequence, because the steady-state concentrations of free hormone are rapidly restored by homeostatic mechanisms. Knowledge regarding the presence of agents affecting thyroid hormone binding, however, is important for the interpretation of diagnostic tests assessing the presence of free or total hormone in plasma.

STRUCTURE–ACTIVITY RELATIONSHIPS OF THYROID ANALOGS

The synthesis and biologic evaluation of a wide variety of T_4 and T_3 analogs allowed a significant correlation of structural features with their relative importance in the production of hormonal responses. The key findings are summarized in Table 29.2. In general, only compounds with the appropriately substituted phenyl-X-phenyl nucleus (as depicted in the structure at the top of Table 29.2) have shown significant thyroid hormonal activities. Both single ring compounds such as DIT and a variety of its aliphatic and alicyclic ether derivatives showed no T_4-like activity in the rat antigoiter test (55), the method most often used in determining thyromimetic activity in vivo (56). The SARs are discussed in terms of single structural variations of T_4 in the 1) alanine side chain, 2) 3- and 5-positions of the inner ring, 3) bridging atom, 4) 3′- and 5′-positions of the outer ring, and 5) 4′-phenolic hydroxyl group.

Aliphatic Side Chain

The naturally occurring hormones are biosynthesized from L-tyrosine and possess the L-alanine side chain. The L-isomers of T_4 and T_3 (compounds 1 and 3 in Table 29.2) are more active than the D-isomers (compounds 2 and 4 in Table 29.2). The carboxylate ion and the number of atoms connecting it to the ring are more important for activity than is the intact zwitterionic alanine side chain. In the carboxylate series, the activity is maximum with the two-carbon acetic acid side chain (compounds 7 and 8) but decreases with either the shorter formic acid (compounds 5 and 6) or the longer propionic and butyric acid analogs (compounds 9 to 12). The ethylamine side chain analogs of T_4 and T_3 (compounds 13 and 14) are less active than the corresponding carboxylic acid analogs. In addition, isomers of T_3 in which the alanine side chain is transposed with the 3-iodine or occupies the 2-position were inactive in the rat antigoiter test (57), indicating a critical location for the side chain in the 1-position of the inner ring.

Alanine-Bearing Ring

The phenyl ring bearing the alanine side chain, called the inner ring or α-ring, is substituted with iodine in the 3- and 5-positions in T_4 and T_3. As shown in Table 29.2, removal of both iodine atoms from the inner ring to form 3′,5′-T_2 (compound 15) or 3′-T_1 (compound 16) produces analogs devoid of T_4-like activity, primarily because of the loss of the perpendicular orientation of diphenyl ether conformation. Retention of activity observed on replacement of the 3- and 5-iodine atoms with bromine (compounds 17 and 18) implies that iodine does not play a unique role in thyroid hormone activity. Moreover, a broad range of hormone activity found with halogen-free analogs (compounds 19 and 20) indicates that a halogen atom is not essential for activity. In contrast to T_3, 3′-isopropyl-3,6- dimethyl-L-thyronine (compound 20) has the capacity to cross the placental membrane and exerts thyromimetic effects in the fetus after administration to the mother. This could prove to be useful in treating fetal thyroid hormone deficiencies or in stimulating lung development (by stimulating lung to synthesize special phospholipids [surfactant], which ensure sufficient functioning of the infant's lungs at birth)

TABLE 29.2 Structure–Activity Relationships of Thyromimetics

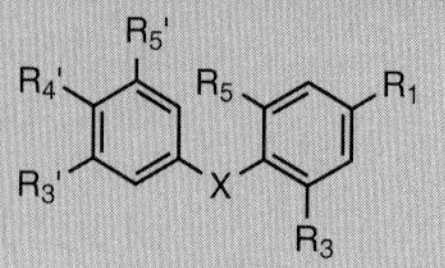

Compound	R_1	R_3	R_5	X	$R_{3'}$	$R_{5'}$	$R_{4'}$	Antigoiter Activity[a]
1. L-T_4	L-Ala	I	I	O	I	I	OH	100
2. D-T_4	D-Ala	I	I	O	I	I	OH	17
3. L-T_3	L-Ala	I	I	O	I	H	OH	550
4. D-T_3	D-Ala	I	I	O	I	H	OH	41
5.	COOH	I	I	O	I	I	OH	0.1
6.	COOH	I	I	O	I	H	OH	0.4
7.	CH_2COOH	I	I	O	I	I	OH	50
8.	CH_2COOH	I	I	O	I	H	OH	36
9.	$(CH_2)_2COOH$	I	I	O	I	I	OH	15
10.	$(CH_2)_2COOH$	I	I	O	I	H	OH	20
11.	$(CH_2)_3COOH$	I	I	O	I	I	OH	4
12.	$(CH_2)_3COOH$	I	I	O	I	H	OH	5
13.	$(CH_2)_2NH_2$	I	I	O	I	I	OH	0.6
14.	$(CH_2)_2NH_2$	I	I	O	I	H	OH	6
15.	L-Ala	H	H	O	I	I	OH	<0.01
16.	L-Ala	H	H	O	I	H	OH	<0.01
17.	DL-Ala	Br	Br	O	I	H	OH	93
18.	L-Ala	Br	Br	O	iPr	H	OH	166
19.	L-Ala	Me	Me	O	Me	H	OH	3
20.	L-Ala	Me	Me	O	iPr	H	OH	20
21.	DL-Ala	iPr	iPr	O	I	H	OH	0
22.	DL-Ala	sBu	sBU	O	I	H	OH	0
23.	DL-Ala	I	I	—	I	I	OH	0
24.	DL-Ala	I	I	S	I	H	OH	132
25.	DL-Ala	I	I	CH_2	I	H	OH	300
26.	L-Ala	I	I	O	H	H	OH	5
27.	L-Ala	I	I	O	OH	H	OH	1.5
28.	L-Ala	I	I	O	NO_2	H	OH	<1
29.	DL-Ala	I	I	O	F	H	OH	6
30.	L-Ala	I	I	O	Cl	H	OH	27
31.	DL-Ala	I	I	O	Br	H	OH	132
32.	L-Ala	I	I	O	Me	H	Oh	80
33.	L-Ala	I	I	O	Et	H	OH	517
30.	L-Ala	I	I	O	iPr	H	OH	786
35.	L-Ala	I	I	O	nPr	H	OH	200
36.	DL-Ala	I	I	O	Phe	H	OH	11
37.	DL-Ala	I	I	O	F	F	OH	2.3
38.	L-Ala	I	I	O	Cl	Cl	OH	21
39.	L-Ala	I	I	O	I	H	NH_2	<1.5
40.	DL-Ala	I	I	O	I	H	H	>150
41.	DL-Ala	I	I	O	CH_3	H	CH_3	0
42.	L-Ala	I	I	O	I	H	CH_3O	225

[a]See Ekins (68) and Ahmad et al. (69). In vivo activity in rats relative to L-T_4 = 100% or DL-T_4 = 100% for goiter prevention.

immediately before premature birth (58). Substitution in the 3- and 5-positions by alkyl groups significantly larger and less symmetric than methyl groups, such as isopropyl and secondary butyl moieties, produces inactive analogs (compounds 21 and 22). These results show that 3,5-disubstitution by symmetric, lipophilic groups not exceeding the size of iodine is required for activity.

Bridging Atom

Several analogs have been synthesized in which the ether oxygen bridge has been removed or replaced by other atoms. The biphenyl analog of T_4 (compound 23 in Table 29.2), formed by removal of the oxygen bridge, is inactive in the rat antigoiter test. The linear biphenyl structure is a drastic change from the normal diphenyl ether conformation found in the naturally occurring hormones. Replacement of the bridging oxygen atom by sulfur (compound 24) or by a methylene group (compound 25) produces highly active analogs. This provides evidence against the Niemann quinoid theory, which postulates that the ability of a compound to form a quinoid structure in the phenolic ring is essential for thyromimetic activity, and emphasizes the importance of the three-dimensional structure and receptor fit of the hormones. Attempts to prepare amino- and carbonyl-bridged analogs of T_3 and T_4 have been unsuccessful (59,60).

Phenolic Ring

The phenolic ring, also called the outer or β-ring, of the thyronine nucleus is required for hormonal activity. Variations in 3′- or 3′,5′-substituents on the phenolic ring have dramatic effects on biologic activity and affinity for the nuclear receptor. The unsubstituted parent structure of this series T_2 (compound 26 in Table 29.2) possesses low activity. Substitution at the 3′-position by polar hydroxyl or nitro groups (compounds 27 and 28) causes a decrease in activity as a consequence of both lowered lipophilicity and intramolecular hydrogen bonding with the 4′-hydroxyl (61). Conversely, substitution by nonpolar halogen or alkyl groups results in an increase in activity in direct relation to the bulk and lipophilicity of the substituent—for example, F < Cl < Br < I (compounds 29 to 31) and CH_3 < CH_2CH_3 < $CH(CH_3)_2$ (compounds 32 to 34). Although 3′-isopropylthyronine (compound 34) is the most potent analog known, being approximately 1.4 times as active as T_3, *n*-propylthyronine (compound 35) is only about one-fourth as active as isopropyl, apparently because of its less compact structure. As the series is further ascended, activity decreases with a further reduction for the more bulky 3′-phenyl substituent (compound 36). Substitution in both 3′- and 5′-positions by the same halogen produces less active hormones (compounds 37 and 38) than the corresponding 3′-monosubstituted analogs (compounds 29 and 30). The decrease in activity has been explained as resulting from the increase in phenolic hydroxyl ionization and the resulting increase in binding to TBG (the primary carrier of thyroid hormones in human plasma) (62). In general, a second substituent adjacent to the phenolic hydroxyl (5′-position) reduces activity in direct proportion to its size.

Phenolic Hydroxyl Group

A weakly ionized phenolic hydroxyl group at the 4′-position is essential for optimum hormonal activity. Replacement of the 4′-hydroxyl with an amino group (compound 39 in Table 29.2) results in a substantial decrease in activity, presumably as a result of the weak hydrogen bonding ability of the latter group. The retention of activity observed with the 4′-unsubstituted compound (compound 40) provides direct evidence for metabolic 4′-hydroxylation as an activating step. Introduction of a 4′-substituent that cannot mimic the functional role of a phenolic group, such as a methyl group (compound 41), and that is not metabolically converted into a functional residue results in complete loss of hormonal activity. The thyromimetic activity of the 4′-methyl ether (compound 42) was ascribed to the ready metabolic cleavage to form an active 4′-hydroxyl analog. The pK_a of 4′-phenolic hydroxyl group is 6.7 for T_4 (90% ionized at pH 7.4) and 8.5 for T_3 (~10% ionized). The greater acidity for T_4 is reflective of its stronger affinity for plasma proteins and, consequently, of its longer plasma half-life.

Conformational Properties of Thyroid Hormones and Analogs

The importance of the diphenyl ether conformation for biologic activity was first proposed by Zenker and Jorgensen (63,64). Through molecular models, they showed that a perpendicular orientation of the planes of the aromatic

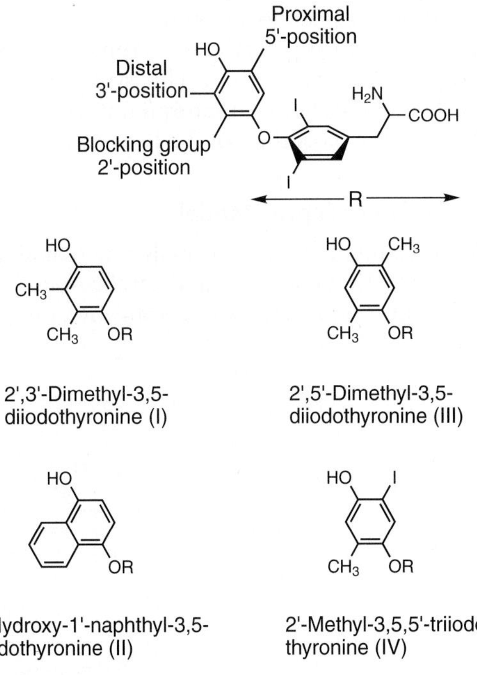

FIGURE 29.6 Structures of representative distal and proximal compounds.

rings of 3,5-diiodothyronines would be favored to minimize interactions between the bulky 3,5-iodines and the 2′,6′-hydrogens. In this orientation, the 3′- and 5′-positions of the ring are not conformationally equivalent, and the 3′-iodine of T_3 could be oriented either distal (away from) or 5′ proximal (closer) to the side chain–bearing ring (Fig. 29.6). Because the activity of compounds such as 3′,5′-dimethyl-3,5-diiodothyronine had demonstrated that alkyl groups could replace the 3′- and 5′-iodine substituents, model compounds bearing alkyl groups in the 3′-position and alkyl or iodine substituents in the 5′-position (in addition to the blocking 2′-methyl group) were synthesized for biologic evaluation (64).

Biologic evaluation of 2′,3′- and 2′,5′-substituted diiodothyronines (65) revealed that 3′-substitution was favorable for thyromimetic activity but that 5′-substitution was not. The structures of representative distal analogs, 2′,3′-dimethyl-3,5-DL-diiodothyronine (compound I) and O-(4′-hydroxy-1′-naphthyl)-3,5-DL-diiodotyrosine (compound II), and of the proximal analogs, 2′,5′-dimethyl-3,5-DL-diiodothyronine (compound III) and 2′-methyl-3, 5,5′-DL-triiodothyronine (compound IV), are given in Figure 29.6. The effectiveness of these compounds in rat antigoiter assay (66) is presented in Table 29.3. These results clearly indicate that in 2′-blocked analogs, a distal 3′-substitution is favorable for thyromimetic activity, but a proximal 5′-substitution is not.

In addition to being perpendicular to the inner ring, the outer phenolic ring can adopt conformations relative to the alanine side chain, which would be *cis* or *trans*. In other words, the cisoid and transoid conformations result from the methine group in the alanine side chain being either *cis* or *trans* to the phenolic ring (Fig. 29.7). Although the bioactive conformation of the alanine side chain in thyroid hormone analogs has not yet been defined, these conformations appear to be similar in energy, because both are found in thyroactive structures as determined by x-ray crystallography (67). The synthesis of conformationally fixed cyclic or unsaturated analogs may allow evaluation of the bioactivity of the two conformers.

TABLE 29.3 Effectiveness of Distal and Proximal Compounds Antigoiter Assay

Compound[a]	Dose (mg/kg/day)	% T_4 activity
I	0.025	50
II	0.013	>100
III	2.3	<1
IV	0.5	2

[a]See text for specific descriptions of compounds I to IV.

Transthyretin Receptor Model

An additional tool in structural analysis and analog design has been TTR. TTR is a serum and cerebrospinal fluid carrier of T_4 and retinol. This is how transthyretin gained its name—**trans**ports **thy**roxine and **retin**ol. TTR was originally called *prealbumin* because it ran faster than albumins on electrophoresis gels. TTR, a plasma protein, binds as much as 27% of plasma T_3 (68). The amino acid sequence of the TTR-T_3 binding site is known, and the protein has therefore served as a model, although admittedly an approximate model, for the T_3 receptor. The TTR model portrays the T_3 molecule as placed in an envelope near the axis of symmetry of the TTR dimer. In this envelope, hydrophobic residues, such as those of leucine, lysine, and alanine, are near pockets accommodating the 3,5,3′- and 5′-positions of T_3, whereas the hydrophilic groups of serine and threonine (hydrogen bonded to water), are between the 3′-substituent and the 4′-phenolic group. Taking this model into account, Ahmad et al. (69) suggested that 3′-acetyl-3,5-diiodothyronine might be a good analog or a good inhibitor of T_3, because the carbonyl group of the 3′ acetyl substituent would form a strong hydrogen bond with the 4′ phenolic hydrogen, thereby preventing its bonding with the hydrated residue of the putative receptor.

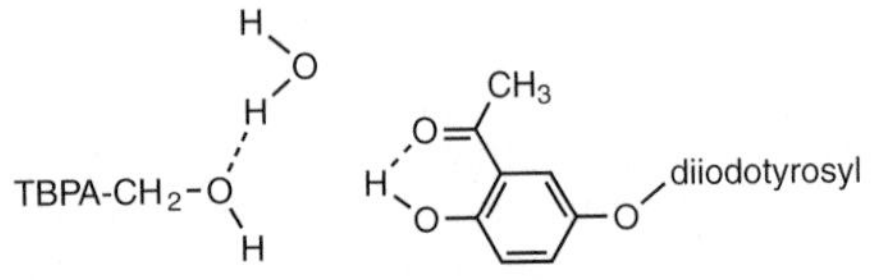

This compound, prepared by Benson et al. (70), was found to be indistinguishable from T_3 in oxygen uptake and glycerophosphate activity tests and to be half as active as T_3 in displacing labeled T_3 from rat liver nuclei in specific in vivo conditions.

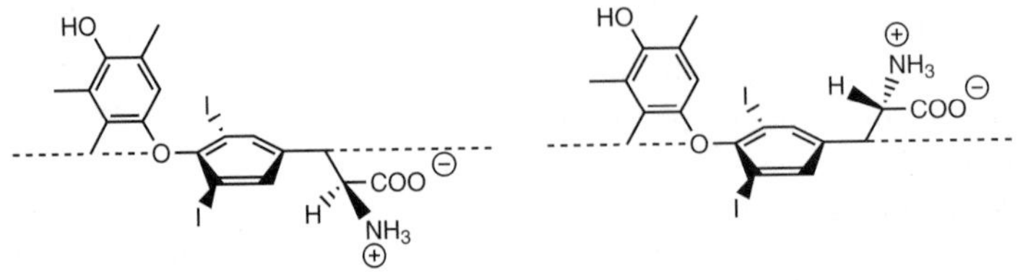

FIGURE 29.7 Side-chain conformations of thyroid hormones: transoid (left) and cisoid (right).

SCENARIO: OUTCOME AND ANALYSIS

Outcome

Autumn Stewart, PharmD

Agranulocytosis ruled out; PA was diagnosed with "thyroid storm" and was stabilized. Upon review of medications at discharge, the clinical pharmacist recommended discontinuation of methimazole and initiation of propylthiouracil 200 mg every 8 hours as an alternative. PA was discharged on propylthiouracil and propranolol 80 mg BID and referred for treatment with radioactive iodine (^{131}I).

Chemical Analysis

S. William Zito and Victoria Roche

PA's "thyroid storm" was stabilized in the emergency department, and at discharge he was changed from methimazole to propylthiouracil and placed on propranolol 80 mg BID to control arrhythmia. The change to propylthiouracil was made because of its ability to inhibit the enzyme 5′-iodothyronine deiodinase (i.e., inhibits the peripheral deiodination of T_4 to T_3). Propylthiouracil also inhibits the intrathyroidal formation of thyroid hormones. Taken together, this makes propylthiouracil the drug of choice for the emergency treatment of thyroid storm. Single doses of propylthiouracil in excess of 300 mg are capable of almost total blockage of peripheral T_3 production.

Methimazole and propylthiouracil are classed as thionamides or thioureylenes, which are five- or six-membered heterocyclic derivatives of thiourea. This chemical class contains the major drugs for treatment of thyrotoxicosis and hyperthyroidism. Their mechanism of action is to inhibit thyroperoxidase, which is responsible for the iodination of tyrosine residues of thyroglobulin and the coupling of iodotyrosine residues to form iodothyronines. These drugs have no effect on the iodide pump or on thyroid hormone release. The uptake of these drugs into the thyroid gland is stimulated by thyroid-stimulating hormone and inhibited by iodide.

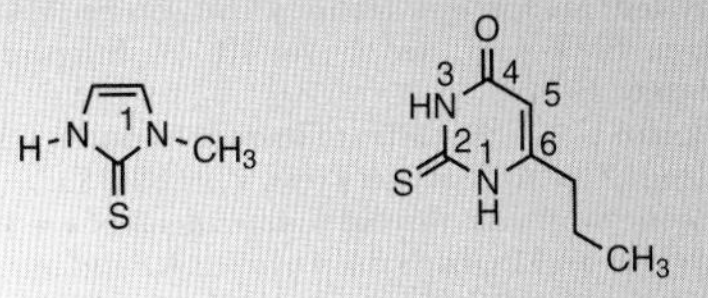

Methimazole Propylthiouracil

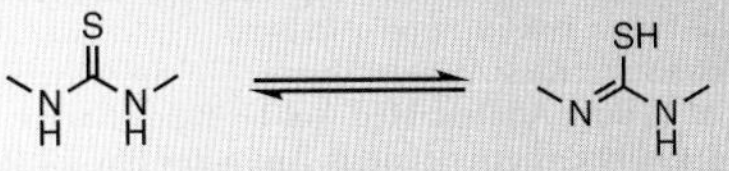

Thioureylene tautomers

The essential chemical grouping in the thioureylenes is N-CS-N- which can tautomerize to either the thioketo or thioenol forms. Structure–activity relationships of the thioureas indicate that they are inhibitors of outer ring deiodinase. The C_2 thioketo/thioenol group and an unsubstituted N_1 position are essential for activity. The enolic hydroxyl group at C_4 in propylthiouracil and the presence of alkyl group at C_5 and C_6 enhance the inhibitory potency. Methimazole has more thyroperoxidase inhibitory activity and is longer-acting than propylthiouracil but, in contrast to propylthiouracil, is not able to inhibit the peripheral deiodination of T_4, presumably because of the presence of the methyl group at N_1 position. The suggested maintenance dosages are 50 to 800 mg daily for propylthiouracil and 5 to 30 mg daily for methimazole.

CASE STUDY

S. William Zito and Victoria Roche

ST is brought to the emergency room of the local hospital. He is approximately 35 years old and homeless; he was found in an alley and was unresponsive to verbal questioning. Upon arrival at the emergency room ST was sweating, thrashing, screaming, and displayed combative behavior. His temperature was 102°F, his blood pressure was 144/68, and he had a pulse of 158 beats per minute. He was restrained until his behavior was controlled with intramuscular haloperidol. An electrocardiogram revealed sinus tachycardia and he was treated with propranolol. Based on clinical laboratory values indicating elevated free T_4 and T_3 (5.42 and 458 ng/dL, respectively) and decreased thyroid-stimulating hormone (<0.01 UIU/mL), and after eliminating other possible diagnoses (severe anxiety disorder, neuroleptic malignant syndrome, drug toxicity and meningitis), his condition was diagnosed as thyroid storm. In addition, ST had also elevated thyroid-stimulating immunoglobulin (281 ng/dL), indicating that there was new hormone synthesis, likely from Graves' disease. Evaluate the following three drugs for treatment of ST's thyroid storm.

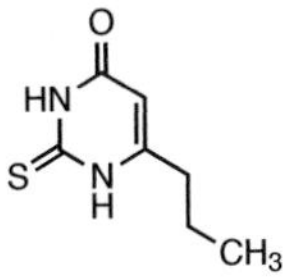

1

NaI

2

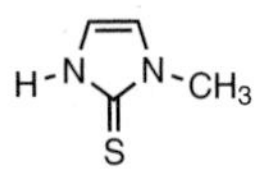

3

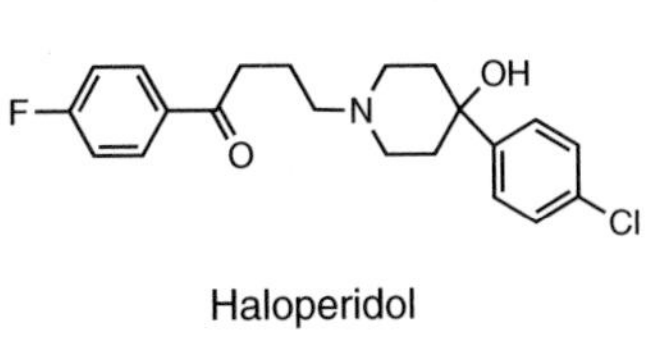

Haloperidol

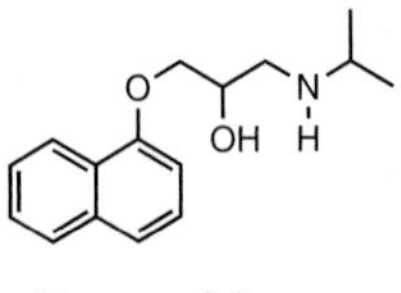

Propranolol

1. Conduct a thorough and mechanistic SAR analysis of the three therapeutic options in the case.
2. Apply the chemical understanding gained from the SAR analysis to this patient's specific needs to make a therapeutic recommendation.

References

1. Harington CR. Biochemical basis of thyroid function. Lancet 1935;I:1199–1204, 1261–1266.
2. Baumann E. Uber das normale vorkommen von jod in tierkorper. Zeitschr Physiol Chem 1896;21:319.
3. Magnus-Levy A. Uber den respiratorischen gewechsel unter dem einfluss der thyroidea sowie unter verschiedenen pathologischen zustanden. Berl Klin Wchnschr 1895;32:650.
4. Gudernatsch JF. Feeding experiments on tadpoles. Arch Entwicklungsmechanik der Organismen 1912;35:457.
5. Nadler NJ. Thyroid anatomical features. In: Greer MA, Solomon DH, eds. Handbook of Physiology, Sec 7, Vol III. Washington, DC: American Physiological Society, 1974.
6. Ekholm R, Bjorkman U. Biochemistry of thyroid hormones. In: Martini L, ed. The Thyroid Gland. New York: Raven Press, 1990:83–125.
7. Taurog A. Hormone synthesis: thyroid iodine metabolism. In: Braverman L, Utiger R, eds. Werner and Ingbar's the Thyroid: A Fundamental and Clinical Text, 8th Ed. Philadelphia, PA: Lippincott Williams & Wilkins, 2000:61–85.
8. Chopra IJ, Solomon DH, Chopra U, et al. Pathways of metabolism of thyroid hormones. Recent Prog Horm Res 1978;34:521–567.
9. Visser TJ, Docter R, Krenning EP, et al. Regulation of thyroid hormone bioactivity. Endocrinol Invest 1986;9(Suppl 4):17–26.
10. Krassas GE, Rivkees SA, Kiess W, eds. Diseases of the Thyroid in Childhood and Adolescence. Pediatr Adolesc Med. Vol 11. Basel: Karger, 2007:80–103.
11. Himms-Hagen J. Cellular thermogenesis. Annu Rev Physiol 1976;38:315–351.
12. Muller MJ, Seitz HJ. Thyroid hormone action on intermediary metabolism. Part I: respiration, thermogenesis, and carbohydrate metabolism. Klin Wochenschr 1984;62:11–18.
13. Muller MJ, Seitz HJ. Thyroid hormone action on intermediary metabolism. Part III. Protein metabolism in hyper- and hypothyroidism. Klin Wochenschr 1984;62:97–102.
14. Tata JR. Inhibition of the biological action of thyroid hormones by actinomycin D and puromycin. Nature 1963;197:1167–1168.
15. Tata JR, Widnell CC. Ribonucleic acid synthesis during the early action of thyroid hormones. Biochem J 1966;98:604–620.
16. Greenspan FS, Forsham PH. Basic and Clinical Endocrinology. Los Altos, CA: Lange Medical, 1983:141.
17. Wolff J, Chaikoff IL. Plasma inorganic iodide as homeostatic regulator of thyroid function. J Biol Chem 1948;174:555–564.
18. Virion A, Michot JL, Deme D, et al. NADPH oxidation catalyzed by the peroxidase/H_2O_2 system. Iodide-mediated oxidation of NADPH to iodinated NADP. Eur J Biochem 1985;148:239–248.
19. Leonard JL, Kaplan MM, Visser TJ, et al. Cerebral cortex responds rapidly to thyroid hormones. Science 1981;214:571–573.
20. McConnon J, Row VV, Volpe R. The influence of liver damage in man on the distribution and disposal rates of thyroxine and triiodothyronine. J Clin Endocrinol Metab 1972;34:144–153.
21. Lim VS, Fang VS, Katz AI, et al. Thyroid dysfunction in chronic renal failure. A study of the pituitary-thyroid axis and peripheral turnover kinetics of thyroxine and triiodothyronine. J Clin Invest 1977;60:522–530.
22. Carter JN, Eastmen CJ, Corcoran JM, et al. Inhibition of conversion of thyroxine to triiodothyronine in patients with severe chronic illness. Clin Endocrinol 1976;5:587–594.
23. Spaulding SW, Chopra IJ, Sherwin RS, et al. Effect of caloric restriction and dietary composition of serum T_3 and reverse T_3 in man. J Clin Endocrinol Metab 1976;42:197–200.
24. Chacon MA, Tildon JT. Mode of death and post-mortem time effects on 3,3′,5-triiodothyronine levels—relevance to elevated post-mortem T_3 levels in SIDS. Fed Proc 1984;43:866–868.
25. Heyma P, Larkins RG, Campbell DG. Inhibition by propranolol of 3,5,3′-triiodothyronine formation from thyroxine in isolated rat renal tubules: an effect independent of β-adrenergic blockade. Endocrinology 1980;106:1437–1441.
26. Silva JE, Larsen PR. Adrenergic activation of triiodothyronime production in brown adipose tissue. Nuture 1983;305:712–713.
27. Zenker N, Chacon MA, Tildon JT. Mode of death effect on rat liver iodothyronine 5′-deiodinase activity: role of adenosine 3′,5′-monophosphate. Life Sci 1984;35:2213–2217.
28. Nakazawa D. The Autoimmune Epidemic. New York: Simon & Schuster, 2008:32–35.
29. Weiss B, Landrian PJ. The developing brain and the environment: an introduction. Environ Health Prospect 2000;108(Suppl 3):373–374.
30. Hauser P, Zametkin AJ, Martinez P, et al. Attention-deficit hyperactivity disorder in people with generalized resistance to thyroid hormone. N Engl J Med 1993;328:997–1001.
31. Mitchell RS, Kumar V, Abbas AK, et al. Robbins Basic Pathology, 8th Ed. Philadelphia: Saunders, 2007.
32. Jackson IM, Cobb WE. Why does anyone still use desiccated thyroid USP? Am J Med 1978;64:284–288.
33. Pittman JA Jr. In: Selenkow HA, Hoffman F, eds. Diagnosis and Treatment of Common Thyroid Disease. Amsterdam: Excerpta Medica, 1971:72–73.
34. Agency for Toxic Substances and Disease Registry, U.S. Department of Health and Human Services. Draft Toxicological Profile for Perchlorates. Washington, DC: U.S. Department of Health and Human Services, September 2005.
35. Lamas L, Ingbar SH. In: Robbins J, Braverman LE, eds. Thyroid Research. Amsterdam: Excerpta Medica, 1976:213.
36. Pittman JA Jr. Diagnosis and Treatment of Thyroid Disease. Philadelphia, PA: FA Davis, 1963:48.
37. Morreale de Escobar G, Escobar del Rey R. Extrathyroid effects of some antithyroid drugs and their metabolic consequences. Rec Prog Horm Res 1967;23:87–137.
38. Cooper DS, Saxe VC, Meskell M, et al. Acute effects of PTU (PTU) on thyroidal iodide organification and peripheral iodothyronine deiodination: correlation with serum PTU levels measured by radioimmunoassay. J Clin Endocrinol Metab 1982;54:101–107.
39. Visser TJ, van Overmeeren E, Fekkes D, et al. Inhibition of iodothyronine 5′-deiodinase by thioureylenes: structure–activity relationship. FEBS Lett 1979;103:314–318.
40. Taurog A. The mechanism of action of the thioureylene antithyroid drugs. Endocrinology 1976;98:1031–1046.
41. Nakashima T, Taurog A, Riesco G. Mechanism of action of thioureylene antithyroid drugs: factors affecting intrathyroidal metabolism of PTU and MMI in rats. Endocrinology 1978;103:2187–2197.
42. Papapetrou PD, Mothon S, Alexander WD. Binding of the 35-S of 35-S-propylthiouracil by follicular thyroglobulin in vivo and in vitro. Acta Endocrinol 1975;79:248–258.
43. Chopra IJ, Chua Teco GN, Eisenberg JB, et al. Structure–activity relationships of inhibition of hepatic monodeiodination of thyroxine to 3,5,3′-triiodothyronine by thiouracil and related compounds. Endocrinology 1982;110:163–168.
44. Kittisupamongkol W. Hyperthyroidism or thyrotoxicosis? Cleve Clin J Med 2009;76:152.
45. Turner JG, Brownlie BE, Sadler WA, et al. An evaluation of lithium as an adjunct to carbimazole treatment in acute thyrotoxicosis. Acta Endocrinol 1976;83:86–92.
46. Berens SC, Wolff J, Murphy DL. Lithium concentration by the thyroid. Endocrinology 1970;87:1085–1087.
47. Temple R, Berman M, Robbins J, et al. The use of lithium in the treatment of thyrotoxicosis. J Clin Invest 1972;51:2746–2756.
48. Tookey HL, Van Ettén CH, Daxenbichler ME. Glucosinolates. In: Liener IE, ed. Toxic Constituents of Plant Foodstuffs. New York: Academic Press, 1980:103–142.
49. Langer P, Michajlovskij N. Effect of naturally occurring goitrogens on thyroid peroxidase and influence of some compounds on iodide formation during the estimation. Endocrinol Exp 1972;6:97–103.
50. Greer MA. Natural occurrence of goitrogenic agents. Rec Prog Hormone Res 1962;18:187–219.
51. Elfving S. Studies on the naturally occurring goitrogen 5-vinyl-2-thiooxazolidone. Metabolism and antithyroid effect in the rat. Ann Clin Res 1980;12(Suppl 28):7–47.
52. Tabachnick M, Hao YL, Korcek L. Effect of oleate, diphenylhydantoin, and heparin on the binding of ^{125}I-thyroxine to purified thyroxine-binding globulin. J Clin Endocrinol Metab 1973;36:392–394.
53. Goswami A, Leonard JL, Rosenberg IN. Inhibition by coumadin anticoagulants of enzymatic outer ring monodeiodination of iodothyronine. Biochem Biophys Res Commun 1982;104:1231–1238.
54. Auf'mkolk M, Amir SM, Kubota K, et al. The active principles of plant extracts with antithyrotropic activity: oxidation products of derivatives of 3,4-dihydroxycinnamic acid. Endocrinology 1985;116:1677–1686.
55. Jorgensen EC, Lehman PA. Thyroxine analogues. IV. Synthesis of aliphatic and alicyclic ethers of 3,5-diiodo-DL-tyrosine. J Org Chem 1961;26:894.
56. Mussett MV, Pitt-Rivers R. The physiologic activity of thyroxine and triiodothyronine analogs. Metab Clin Exper 1957;6:18–25.
57. Jorgensen EC, Reid JAW. Thyroxine analogues. XI. Structural isomers of 3,5,3′-triiodo-DL-thyronine. J Med Chem 1964;7:701–705.
58. Gluckman PD, Ballard PL, Kaplan SL, et al. Prolactin in umbilical cord blood and the respiratory distress syndrome. J Pediatr 1978;93:1011–1014.
59. Tripp SL, Block FB, Barile G. Synthesis of methylene- and carbonyl-bridged analogues of iodothyronine and iodothyroacetic acids. J Med Chem 1973;66:60–64.
60. Mukherjee R, Block P Jr. Thyroxine analogues: synthesis and nuclear magnetic resonance spectral studies of diphenylamines. J Chem Soc (C) 1971;9:1596–1600.
61. Leeson PD, Ellis D, Emmett JC, et al. Thyroid hormone analogues. Synthesis of 3′-substituted 3,5-diiodo-L-thyronines and quantitative structure–activity studies of in vitro and in vivo thyromimetic activities in rat liver and heart. J Med Chem 1988;31:37–54.
62. Jorgensen EC. Thyroid hormones and analogs II. Structure–activity relationships. In: Li CH, ed. Hormonal Proteins and Peptides, Vol 6. New York: Academic Press, 1978:107–204.
63. Jorgensen EC. Thyroid hormones. In: Wolff ME, ed. Burger's Medicinal Chemistry, Part 3, 4th Ed. New York: Wiley, 1981:103–148.

64. Zenker N, Jorgensen EC. Thyroxine analogues. I. Synthesis of 3,5-diiodi-4-(2′-alkylphenoxy)-DL-phenylalanine. J Am Chem Soc 1959;81:4643–4647.
65. Jorgensen EC, Zenker N, Greenberg C, et al. Thyroxine analogues. III. Antigoitrogenic and calorigenic activity of some alkyl substituted analogues of thyroxine. J Biol Chem 1960;235:1732–1737.
66. Jorgensen EC, Lehman PA, Greenberg C, et al. Thyroxine analogues. VII. Antigoitrogenic, calorigenic, and hypocholesteremic activities of same aliphatic, alicyclic, and aromatic ethers of 3,5-diiodotyrosine in the rat. J Biol Chem 1962;237:3832–3838.
67. Cody V. Thyroid hormones: crystal structure, molecular conformation, binding, and structure-function relationships. Rec Prog Horm Res 1978;34:437–475.
68. Ekins R. Methods for the measurement of free thyroid hormones. In: Ekins R, Faglia G, Pennisi F, et al., eds. International Symposium on Free Thyroid Hormones. Amsterdam: Excerpta Medica, 1979:7–29.
69. Ahmad P, Fyfe CA, Mellors A. Parachors in drug design. Biochem Pharmacol 1975;24:1103–1110.
70. Benson MG, Ellis D, Emmett JC, et al. 3′-Acetyl-3,5-diiodo-L-thyronine: a novel highly active thyromimetic with low receptor affinity. Biochem Pharmacol 1984;33:3143–3149.

Suggested Readings

Gilbert ES, Tarone R, Bouville A, et al. Thyroid cancer rates and I-131 doses from Nevada atmospheric nuclear bomb tests. J Natl Cancer Inst 1998;90:1654–1660.
Ladenson PW, Braverman LE, Mazzaferri EL, et al. Comparison of administration of recombinant human thyrotropin with withdrawal of thyroid hormone for radioactive iodine scanning in patients with thyroid carcinoma. N Engl J Med 1997;337:888–896.
McCowen KC, Garber JR, Spark R. Elevated serum thyrotropin in thyroxine-treated patients with hypothyroidism given sertraline. N Engl J Med 1997;337:1010–1011.

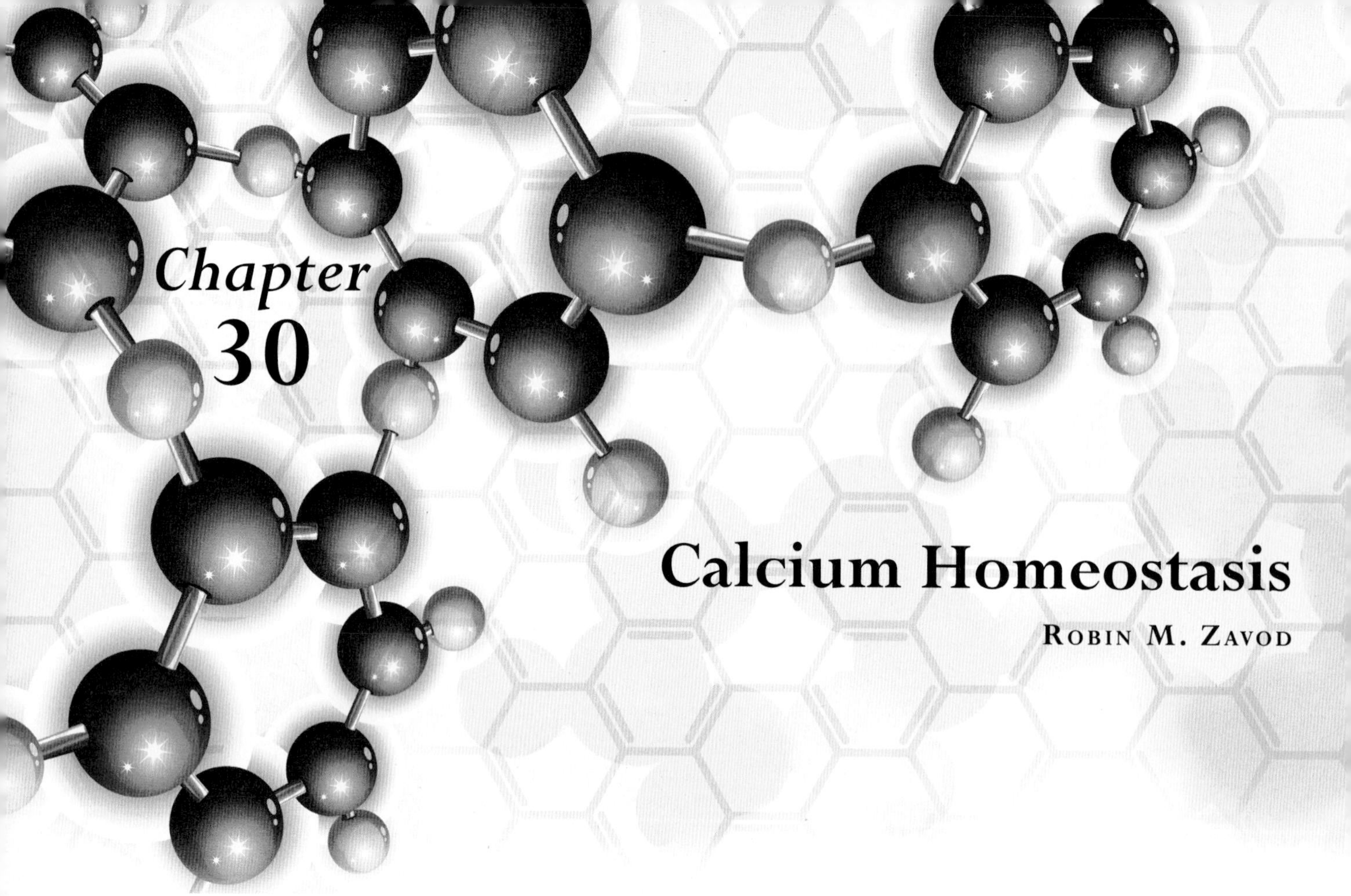

Chapter 30

Calcium Homeostasis

Robin M. Zavod

Drugs Covered in This Chapter[*]

Selective estrogen receptor modulators
- Bazedoxifene acetate
- *Lasofoxifene*
- Raloxifene hydrochloride
- Toremifene citrate

Bisphosphonates
- Alendronate sodium
- *Clodronate tetrasodium*
- *Etidronate disodium*
- Ibandronate sodium
- Pamidronate disodium
- Risedronate sodium
- Tiludronate disodium
- Zoledronic acid

Calcitonin

Cinacalcet hydrochloride

Teriparatide

Monoclonal antibody
- Denosumab

Inorganic salts
- Calcium salts
- Gallium nitrate
- Sodium fluoride
- *Strontium ranelate*

Abbreviations

AF-2, activation factor-2
ATP, adenosine triphosphate
BMD, bone mineral density
CaSR, calcium-sensing receptor
DIOP, drug-induced osteoporosis
DNA, deoxyribonucleic acid
ER, estrogen receptor
ERE, estrogen responding element
ERT, estrogen replacement therapy
FDA, U.S. Food and Drug Administration
HMG-CoA, hydroxymethylglutaryl–coenzyme A
IM, intramuscular
IV, intravenous
NaF, sodium fluoride
NHANES III, National Health and Nutrition Examination Survey III
$1,25(OH)_2D_3$, 1,25-dihydroxycholecalciferol
$25(OH)D_3$, 25-hydroxycholecalciferol
PPARγ2, peroxisome proliferator-activated receptor γ2
PTH, parathyroid hormone
RANKL, receptor activator of nuclear factor-κB ligand
RRE, raloxifene responding element
SAR, structure–activity relationship
SC, subcutaneous
SERM, selective estrogen receptor modulator
UGT, uridine diphosphate glucuronosyltransferase

[*]Drugs listed include those available inside and outside of the United States; drugs available outside of the United States are shown in italics.

SCENARIO

Kathryn Neill, PharmD

PJ is a 70-year-old woman with hypertension, gastroesophageal reflux, and osteoporosis. She was prescribed alendronate and calcium 6 months ago, but the resulting improvement in bone density is less than expected. The pharmacist interviews PJ. Her current medications are alendronate 10 mg daily, calcium carbonate 500 mg three times daily with meals, omeprazole 20 mg daily, and ramipril 5 mg daily.

PJ takes alendronate each morning with only a glass of water. After 30 minutes she takes ramipril, omeprazole, and calcium with coffee. Additional calcium doses are taken with lunch and supper. PJ has lost weight the last few months due to an unsettled stomach.

(The reader is directed to the clinical solution and chemical analysis of this case at the end of the chapter).

INTRODUCTION

Three primary hormones—calcitonin, parathyroid hormone, and vitamin D—control the homeostatic regulation of calcium and its principle counterion, inorganic phosphate. Homeostatic control of these ions is essential not only for the moderation of longitudinal bone growth and bone remodeling but also for blood coagulation, neuromuscular excitability, plasma membrane structure and function, muscle contraction, glycogen and adenosine triphosphate (ATP) metabolism, neurotransmitter/hormone secretion, and enzyme catalysis (1). In an average 70-kg adult, approximately 1 kg of calcium is found, 99% of which is located in the bone. The principle calcium salt contained in the hydroxyapatite crystalline lattice of teeth and bones is $Ca_{10}(PO_4)_6(OH)_2$. Similarly, approximately 500 to 600 g of phosphate are present, 85% of which is found in the bone. The normal plasma concentration of calcium is approximately 4.5 to 5.7 mEq/L, 50% of which is protein bound. The remainder of the calcium is either complexed to corresponding counterions (46%) or exists in its ionized form (4%). It is only the ionized form of calcium that is tightly hormonally regulated (varies less than 5% to 10%) (1,2). Because serum calcium concentrations fluctuate, so do the plasma levels of the hormones associated with calcium homeostasis. Serum phosphorous levels vary with age, diet, and hormonal status. The most common form of phosphate in the blood (pH 7.4) is HPO_4^{2-}.

The bone is composed of two distinct tissue structures: cortical (compact) bone and trabecular (cancellous) bone (3). Eighty percent of the skeleton is composed of cortical bone (e.g., long bones such as the humerus, radius, and ulna) (4,5), which is a relatively dense tissue (80% to 90% calcified) (4) that provides structure and support (3). Bone marrow cavities, flat bones, and the ends of long bones are all composed of trabecular bone, which is considerably more porous (5% to 20% calcified) (4,5). To maintain healthy, well-mineralized bone, a continuous process of bone resorption (loss of ionic calcium from bone) and bone formation occurs along the bone surface. Cortical bone is remodeled at the rate of 3% per year, whereas 25% of trabecular bone, which has a considerably higher surface area, is remodeled annually (3). In terms of calcium turnover in bone, approximately 500 mg are removed and replaced on a daily basis.

Both inorganic and organic components are present in the bone. The highly crystalline inorganic component is hydroxyapatite, and the collagen matrix comprises the major portion (90%) of the organic component. The collagen matrix serves as the foundation for hydroxyapatite mineralization. Osteocalcin and osteonectin are minor organic constituents that promote binding of hydroxyapatite and calcium to the collagen matrix and regulate the rate of bone mineralization, respectively (5).

In general, peak bone mass occurs between 30 and 40 years of age (3,6) and is dependent on genetic factors as well as proper intake of calcium, maintenance of quality nutrition, and participation in weight-bearing exercise (6). Thereafter, peak bone mass progressively declines at the rate of 0.3% to 0.5% of cortical bone per year (3). After menopause, bone loss is accelerated (2% per year in the spine) (6) for a period of 5 to 10 years because of the loss of estrogen. This can result in up to a 30% decrease in bone mineral density.

HORMONAL REGULATION OF SERUM CALCIUM LEVELS

Arnaud has developed a "butterfly model" that provides a diagrammatic view of the complex interrelationships among the three hormones (parathyroid, calcitonin, and vitamin D) that control calcium homeostasis (serum concentrations of ionic calcium) and their target organs (bone, kidney, and intestine) (Fig. 30.1) (7). The right side (B loops) of the butterfly model describes the processes that increase the serum calcium concentration in response to hypocalcemia; the left side (A loops) depicts the events that occur in response to hypercalcemia.

CLINICAL SIGNIFICANCE

As our knowledge about the development and risk factors associated with disruptions in calcium homeostasis has increased, so too have the modalities available to prevent and/or treat these disease processes. In general, disorders of calcium homeostasis involve the development of bone disease and/or alterations in serum calcium concentration. In the most basic sense, the development of bone disease is simply an inequity between bone breakdown and bone formation, which also may result in an altered serum calcium concentration. In addition to bone disease, disruptions in normal serum calcium concentrations may be related to an imbalance in calcium intake and renal calcium elimination. These disturbances can result from various factors, including increased activity of cells that cause bone breakdown, decreased activity of cells that form new bone, decreased absorption of calcium, or irregularities in levels of hormones that affect calcium absorption and influence cells involved in bone maintenance. An increased understanding of these physiologic pathways has led to the development of multiple classes of agents targeting the different mechanisms for evolution of these disease processes, including selective estrogen receptor modulators, bisphosphonates, and various calcium salts.

Application of the principles of medicinal chemistry has resulted in the formulation of agents with additional routes of administration, increased potency, and decreased frequency of dosing. These advances have increased the utility of these agents and improved the quality of life for countless individuals affected by calcium homeostasis disorders. Understanding the development of individual disease processes involved in disorders of calcium homeostasis (e.g., osteoporosis, osteopetrosis, hyperparathyroidism, and Paget's disease) and the pharmacodynamic effects of individual compounds used to treat these disorders is paramount for the practitioner making therapeutic decisions. Incorporation of these factors into the therapeutic plan is necessary to target the valued pharmacodynamic effects of these agents while minimizing unwanted or harmful effects. For example, the selection of raloxifene to treat osteoporosis in a patient with severe gastroesophageal reflux disease, as opposed to an oral bisphosphonate, which could increase the likelihood of developing erosive esophagitis. Finally, it is also important for the clinician to recognize the capacity of certain entities used to treat calcium disorders to be allergenic or more prone to produce adverse effects so that selection of the best agent for an individual patient is facilitated.

Kathryn Neill, PharmD
Hospital Experiential Director
Assistant Professor
Critical Care Specialist
Department of Pharmacy Practice
College of Pharmacy
University of Arkansas for Medical Sciences
Little Rock, Arkansas

Calcitonin

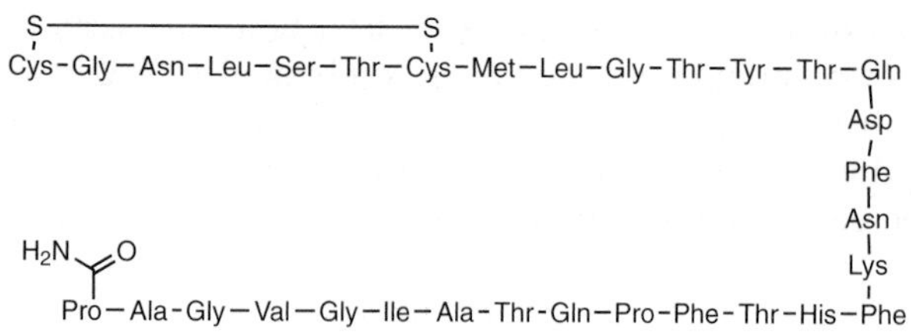

Human calcitonin

Human calcitonin is a 32–amino acid peptide (molecular weight, 3,527 daltons) biosynthesized in the parafollicular "C" cells found within the thyroid gland. This hormone contains a critical disulfide bridge between residues 1 and 7, with the entire amino acid sequence required for biologic activity. The carboxy-terminal residue is a proline amide. "Procalcitonin," a precursor peptide, has been identified and proposed to facilitate intracellular transport and secretion. Calcitonin is secreted in response to elevated serum calcium concentrations (>9 mg/100 mL) and serves to oppose the hormonal effects of parathyroid hormone. In response to a hypercalcemic state (Fig. 30.1, B loops), increased calcitonin secretion drives serum calcium concentrations down via stimulation of urinary excretion of both calcium and phosphate (loop 3B), prevention of calcium resorption from the bone via inhibition of osteoclast activity (loop 1B), and inhibition of intestinal absorption of calcium (loop 2B). When serum calcium concentrations are low (hypocalcemia), the release of calcitonin is slowed, thereby activating loops 1A, 2A, and 3A.

Parathyroid Hormone

Parathyroid hormone (PTH) is biosynthesized as a 115–amino acid preprohormone in the rough endoplasmic reticulum of the parathyroid gland and is cleaved to the prohormone (90 amino acids) in the cisternal space of the reticulum (Fig. 30.2). The active hormone is finally produced (84 amino acids; molecular weight, 9,500 daltons) in the Golgi complex and is stored in secretory granules in the parathyroid gland. This gland is exquisitely sensitive to serum calcium concentrations and is able to monitor these levels via calcium-sensing receptors

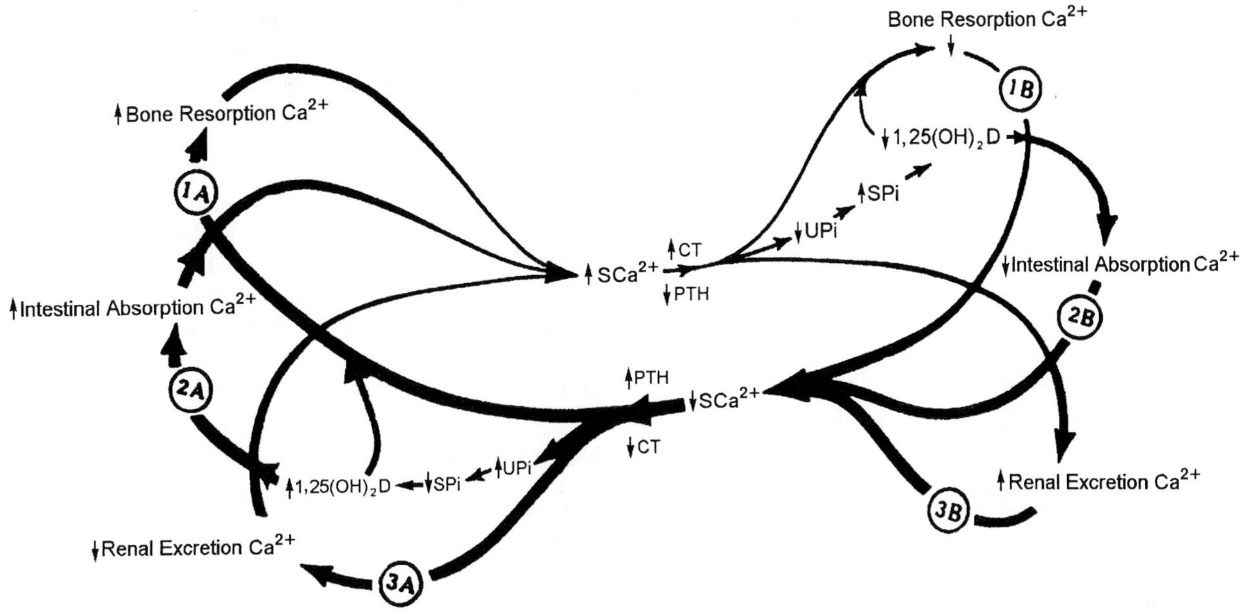

FIGURE 30.1 The Arnaud's butterfly model for regulating calcium homeostasis consists of three overlapping loops that interlock and relate to one another through the serum concentrations of ionic calcium (SCa), parathyroid hormone (PTH), and calcitonin (CT). The right side (B loops, where B refers to the effects of CT) of the model describes the physiologic processes that increase the serum calcium concentration in response to hypocalcemia; the left side (A loops, where A refers to the effects of PTH) of the model depicts the events that decrease the serum calcium concentration in response to hypercalcemia. Loop 1 bone resorption; loop 2 intestinal absorption; loop 3 renal excretion; SPi, serum inorganic phosphate; UPi, urinary inorganic phosphate. (Adapted from Arnaud CD. Calcium homeostasis: regulatory elements and their integration. Fed Proc 1978;37:2557–2560, with permission).

(CaSR). These cell surface receptors help cells to react to micromolar changes in the concentration of ionized calcium in the serum (8). Binding of calcium to these receptors facilitates activation of phospholipase C and, ultimately, inhibition of PTH secretion. The relatively short-acting PTH is secreted from the parathyroid gland chief cells in response to a hypocalcemic state and serves to oppose the hormonal effects of calcitonin (1). Unlike calcitonin, the biologic activity of PTH resides solely in residues 1 to 34 in the amino terminus.

PTH decreases renal excretion of calcium (Fig. 30.1, loop 3A), indirectly stimulates intestinal absorption of calcium (Fig. 30.1, loop 2A), and in combination with active vitamin D, promotes bone resorption (Fig. 30.1, loop 1A). PTH stimulates bone resorption by several mechanisms: 1) transformation of osteoprogenitor cells into osteoclasts is stimulated in the presence of PTH, 2) PTH promotes the deep osteocytes to mobilize calcium from perilacunar bone, and 3) surface osteocytes are stimulated by PTH to increase the flow of calcium out of the bone. In addition, the secretion of PTH stimulates the biosynthesis, activation, and release of the third hormone associated with calcium homeostasis, vitamin D. When serum calcium concentrations are high, the release of PTH is inhibited.

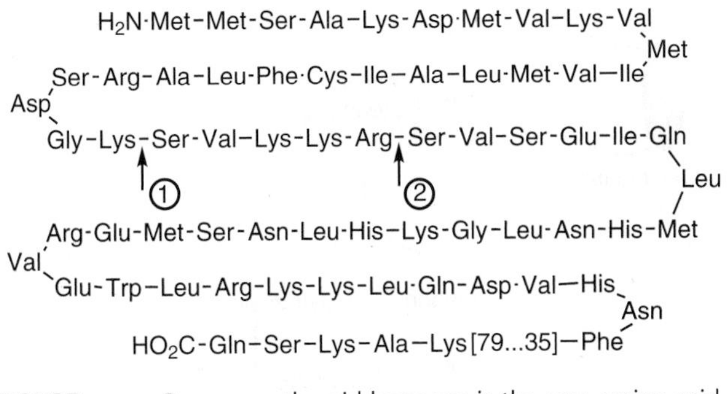

FIGURE 30.2 Preproparathyroid hormone is the 115–amino acid protein indicated above. Cleavage at site 1 gives rise to proparathyroid hormone (89 amino acids), whereas cleavage at site 2 gives rise to parathyroid hormone (PTH, 84 amino acids). The protein shown in *red* is teriparatide (34 amino acids).

Vitamin D

Derived from cholesterol, vitamin D is biosynthesized from its prohormone cholecalciferol (D_3), the product of solar ultraviolet irradiation of 7-dehydrocholesterol in the skin (2). In 1966, it was first recognized that vitamin D must undergo activation via two oxidative metabolic steps (Fig. 30.3). The first oxidation to 25-hydroxycholecalciferol [25(OH)D_3: calcifediol; Calderol] occurs in the endoplasmic reticulum of the liver and is catalyzed by vitamin D 25-hydroxylase. This activation step is not regulated by plasma calcium concentrations. The major circulating form (10 to 80 μg/mL) is 25(OH)D_3, which also is the primary storage form of vitamin D (2). In response to a hypocalcemic state and the secretion of PTH, a second oxidation step is activated in the mitochondria of the

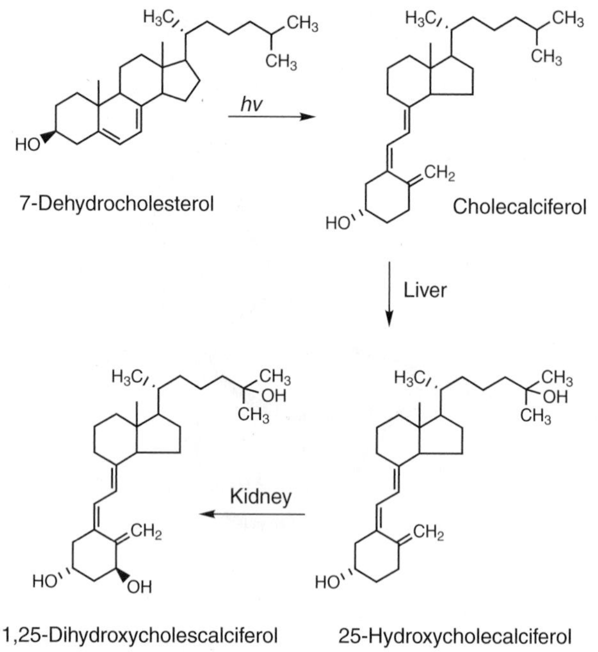

FIGURE 30.3 Bioactivation of vitamin D.

kidney, catalyzed by vitamin D 1α-hydroxylase (2,9). The product of this reaction, 1,25-dihydroxycholecalciferol [1,25$(OH)_2D_3$: 1,25-calcitriol; Rocaltrol, Calcijex] is the active form of vitamin D. Its concentration in the blood is 1/500 that of its monohydroxylated precursor. The biosynthesis of vitamin D is tightly regulated based on the serum concentrations of calcium, phosphate, PTH, and active vitamin D (2).

Sterol-specific cytoplasmic receptor proteins (vitamin D receptor) mediate the biologic action of vitamin D (9). The active hormone is transported from the cytoplasm to the nucleus via the vitamin D receptor, and as a result of the interaction of the hormone with target genes, a variety of proteins are produced that stimulate the transport of calcium in each of the target tissues. Active vitamin D works in concert with PTH to enhance active intestinal absorption of calcium, to stimulate bone resorption, and to prohibit renal excretion of calcium (2,9). If serum calcium or 1,25-calcitriol concentrations are elevated, then vitamin D 24-hydroxylase (in renal mitochondria) is activated to oxidize 25$(OH)D_3$ to inactive 24,25-dihydroxy-cholecalciferol and to further oxidize active vitamin D to the inactive 1,24,25-trihydroxylated derivative. Both the 1,24,25-trihydroxylated and the 24,25-dihydroxylated products have been found to suppress PTH secretion as well. Several factors have been identified in the regulation of the biosynthesis of vitamin D, including low phosphate concentrations (stimulatory) as well as pregnancy and lactation (stimulatory).

NORMAL PHYSIOLOGY

During growth periods in childhood and early adulthood, bone formation characteristically exceeds bone loss. In young adulthood, bone formation and bone resorption are nearly equal. After the age of 40 years, however, bone resorption is slightly greater than bone formation, and this results in a gradual decline in skeletal mass. Osteoblasts, osteoclasts, and osteocytes are the three types of cells that make up the bone remodeling unit or bone metabolizing unit and, therefore, are largely responsible for the bone remodeling process (3,4).

The bone remodeling process is comprised of two opposing activities, bone resorption and bone formation. Bone resorption is launched when osteocytes and those cells that line the bone surface release cytokines and growth factors (Fig. 30.4). These endogenous substances signal osteoblasts to release receptor activator of nuclear factor-κB ligand (RANK-ligand or RANKL), a cytokine (10). This ligand interacts with and activates its receptor (RANK) found on 1) the surface of osteoclast precursor cells, which stimulates osteoclast differentiation, and 2) the surface of mature osteoclasts, which promotes activation (10). RANKL also decreases osteoclast apoptosis.

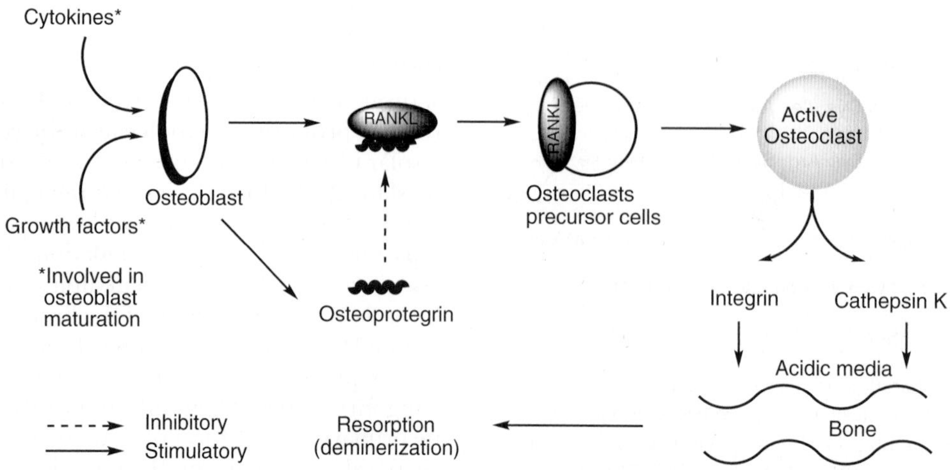

FIGURE 30.4 Bone resorption involving receptor activator of nuclear factor-κB ligand (RANKL).

Osteoclasts are the large multinucleated cells of hemopoietic origin that are responsible for carrying out the bone resorption or destroying process (6). Cytokines (including RANKL), PTH, and the active form of vitamin D are responsible for activation of these cells. Bone-lining flat cells, derived from "retired" osteoclasts and osteoblasts, are located on the bone surface (3). The function of these flat cells is thought to serve to identify areas of the bone that have become weakened or misshapen and to send a signal to the bone remodeling unit to prepare the bone. Lining cells then digest the outer layer of the bone matrix in preparation for bone remodeling. As part of the bone resorption process, the osteoclast membrane comes into contact with the bone surface and, in the presence of integrin, forms an impermeable "sealing zone" of approximately 500 to 1,000 μm in size (2,6). The ruffled border of the osteoclast membrane secretes hydrogen ions, H^+ ATPase, and the cysteine protease cathepsin K (11). As a result, this microenvironment becomes acidified, and ultimately, bone demineralization occurs (6). Several types of lysosomal enzymes have been proposed to digest the collagen matrix, thereby pitting the bone surface to a depth of 50 μm (3–6).

Osteoblasts, which are of mesenchymal origin and are formed in the bone marrow, stimulate bone formation (6). In the maturation process, osteoblasts undergo multiple cell divisions and, in so doing, express the gene products that are needed to form the bone matrix or osteoid, as well as those products responsible for mineralization of that tissue (3,6). It is in the rough endoplasmic reticulum that the biosynthesis of the bone matrix protein occurs (4). Multiple endogenous substances are involved in osteoblast maturation, including many cytokines (interleukins and granulocyte-macrophage colony-stimulating factor), as well as hormones and growth factors.

Not only are osteoblasts involved in bone formation, but they also have a role in limiting bone resorption. Produced by osteoblasts, osteoprotegerin binds to RANKL and therefore prevents its interaction with its RANK receptors on the osteoclast (11). As a result, osteoclast differentiation and bone resorption are inhibited.

Quantification of bone mineral density (BMD) can be measured by noninvasive radiographic tests, such as single-photon or dual-photon absorptiometry (spine, hip, and total body), dual-energy x-ray absorptiometry (spine, hip, and total body), peripheral dual-energy x-ray absorptiometry (wrist, heel, and finger), single energy x-ray absorptiometry (wrist or heel), quantitative computed tomography (spine), peripheral quantitative computed tomography (wrist), and quantitative ultrasound (heel, shin bone, and knee cap) (3,12–14). Dual-energy x-ray absorptiometry is considered to be the gold standard for measuring bone density and has an accuracy that exceeds 95% (4). These techniques measure the attenuation of x-rays or gamma rays as they cross the spine, hip, or radius before they reach the detector (6). Other methods under development that measure BMD include ultrasound, traditional x-rays, and blood/urine tests (6). Traditional x-rays can identify the site of fracture, but they cannot measure BMD (3). Blood/urine tests can identify if the patient is suffering from a medical condition that is contributing to the loss of BMD and can identify important biochemical markers that can assess the rate of bone resorption and bone turnover. The measurement of serum calcium, phosphorous, and vitamin D levels also may provide insight regarding the cause of decreased BMD (3). Often, patients suffer from multiple vertebral compression fractures without seeking treatment other than an over-the-counter analgesic, and the diagnosis of osteoporosis occurs only after the patient has already lost significant (as much as 30%) bone mass.

DISEASE STATES ASSOCIATED WITH ABNORMAL CALCIUM HOMEOSTASIS

Osteoporosis

Osteoporosis is a skeletal disease that is characterized by loss of bone mass as well as microarchitectural deterioration of the bone tissue. This disease is associated with increased bone fragility and susceptibility to fracture. It is a condition that is characterized not by inadequate bone formation but, rather, by a deficiency in the production of well-mineralized bone mass. Whereas no medical cause typically is evident in primary osteoporosis (3), secondary osteoporosis classically stems from medical illness or medication use. There are two types of primary adult osteoporosis, type I, or postmenopausal, and type II, or senile (Table 30.1) (15,16). In type I osteoporosis, there is an accelerated rate of bone loss via enhanced resorption at the onset of menopause. In this form of the disease, the loss of trabecular bone is threefold greater than the loss of cortical bone. This disproportionate loss of bone mass is the primary cause of the vertebral crush fractures and the wrist and ankle fractures experienced by postmenopausal women. In type II osteoporosis, which is associated with aging, the degree of bone loss is similar in both trabecular and cortical bone and is caused by decreased bone formation by the osteoblasts (5).

Drug- or disease-induced, or type III, osteoporosis (Table 30.2) accounts for up to 30% of the cases of vertebral fractures reported annually. It can be caused by a variety of factors, including long-term suppression of osteoblast function, an inhibition of calcium absorption from the gut, altered vitamin D metabolism, or excessive loss of calcium in the urine (17). Disease states or pharmacologic therapies that result in estrogen deficiency, hyperparathyroidism, hyperthyroidism, or hypogonadism have been correlated with the development of osteoporosis (6,13,17,18). Drug-induced osteoporosis (DIOP) is associated with the use of glucocorticoids, thyroid hormone replacement, lithium,

TABLE 30.1 Classification of Osteoporosis (15)

Etiology	Type I (postmenopausal) Increased Osteoclast Activity and Bone Resorption	Type II (senile) Decreases Osteoblast Activity and Bone Formation; Decreased GI Ca Absorption	Type II(secondary) Drug Therapies; Disease States
Typical age at diagnosis (years)	50–75	>70	Any age
Gender ratio (women:men)	6:1	2:1	1:1
Typical fracture site	Vertebrae, distal radius	Femur, neck, hip	Vertebrae, hip, extremities
Bone morphology	Decreased trabecular bone	Decreased trabecular and normal cortical bone	Decreases cortical bone
Rate of bone loss (per year)	2%–3%	0.3%–0.5%	Variable

antiepileptic agents, selective serotonin reuptake inhibitors, proton pump inhibitors, thiazolidinediones, methotrexate, cyclosporine, aromatase inhibitors, gonadotropin-releasing hormone agonists, and immunosuppressive therapy (6,17–21). See Table 30.3 for a list of the drug-specific mechanisms associated with DIOP (17).

After estrogen deficiency related to menopause, long-term therapy with glucocorticoids represents the most prevalent cause of DIOP. As much as 3% to 27% of total bone loss can occur within the first 6 to 12 months of glucocorticoid therapy (17). From a mechanistic perspective, glucocorticoids cause an initial increase in bone resorption as a result of their ability to increase RANKL and macrophage colony-stimulating factor. This results in an increase in osteoclastogenesis and a decrease in osteoclast apoptosis. With the ability of the glucocorticoids to cause an increase in peroxisome proliferator-activated receptor γ2 (PPARγ2) signaling and a decrease in Wnt signaling protein, a decrease in osteoblast formation and function and an increase in osteoblast apoptosis result, and there is a decrease in bone formation (22).

Vitamin D deficiency, as the cause of pseudohyperparathyroidism, is a common cause of osteoporosis in elder persons who are institutionalized and lack adequate sunlight exposure (2). Many of the older antiepileptic agents induce cytochrome P450 24A1 (CYP24A1) enzymes, which catalyze the conversion of vitamin D to inactive metabolites (17).

According to the National Health and Nutrition Examination Survey III (NHANES III) the National Osteoporosis Foundation estimates that more than 10 million Americans have osteoporosis and an additional 33.6 million have low BMD of the hip (23). It is projected that by 2020, these numbers will increase to 14 and 47 million, respectively (24). With these increases, it is anticipated that the number of hip fractures will double or triple by 2040. Approximately 40% of United States white women and 13% of United States white men will experience at least one fracture related to low BMD in their lifetime. The chance of a 50-year-old woman experiencing a hip, vertebral, or forearm fracture is 17%, 15%, and 16%, respectively. It is predicted that by age 80, 27% of women will be osteopenic and 70% will be osteoporotic. It has been estimated that approximately 20% of hip fracture patients will require long-term nursing home care. A surprising 60% of hip fracture patients do not regain full function, and within 3 to 4 months of hip fracture, as many as 25% die as a result of secondary complications (e.g., pneumonia or infection). Mortality also is increased 17% after both femoral and vertebral fractures. Whereas postmenopausal African Americans have the lowest rate of osteoporosis (4%), Native Americans have the highest (12%) with Hispanic and Asian postmenopausal women falling in between (10% for both) (25). Additional risk factors associated with osteoporosis are presented in Table 30.4. Given these statistics, osteoporosis should be considered a significant health problem that only stands to worsen unless appropriate interventions are pursued.

TABLE 30.2 Causes of Secondary (Type III) Osteoporosis

Gastrointestinal diseases	Anorexia nervosa, chronic liver disease, malabsorption syndromes (e.g., celiac disease, Crohn disease, gastric bypass, short bowel disease)
Nutritional excesses or deficiencies	Alcoholism, calcium, vitamin D, protein deficiency, excess vitamin A, total parenteral nutrition.
Endocrine-based diseases	Acromegaly, diabetes mellitus (types 1 and 2), disease-related elevated hormone levels (hypercortisolism, hyperthyroidism, hyperparathyroidism), disease-related suppressed hormone levels
Other disease states	Chronic obstructive pulmonary disease, hemophilia, myeloma, and some other cancers
Drugs	Corticosteroids, aromatase inhibitors, thiazolidinediones, antiepileptic agents

TABLE 30.3 Mechanisms Related to Drug-Induced Osteoporosis

Drug Therapy	Proposed Mechanism Leading to Altered Bone Mineral Density (BMD)	Citations in Reference 17
Aromatase inhibitors	Inhibit conversion of androgens to estrogen	62
Gonadotropin-releasing hormone agonists	Antiandrogenic effect on pituitary gland suppressing testosterone (results in hypogonadism)	70
Thyroid hormone replacement therapy	Increase in osteoclast activation and RANKL	81
Antipsychotic agents	Stimulation of prolactin secretion lowers estrogen and testosterone levels (results in hypogonadism)	99, 100
Lithium	Hyperparathyroidism	104–106
Thiazolidinediones	Decreases osteoblast differentiation and function via PPARγ activation	117–119
Loop diuretics	Enhances renal calcium excretion	15

Osteopetrosis

Osteopetrosis, also known as marble bone disease, describes a group of heritable disorders that are centered on a defect in osteoclast-mediated bone resorption. There are four autosomal recessive forms and one autosomal dominant form of osteopetrosis (Table 30.5) (26). It generally is characterized by abnormally dense, brittle bone and increased skeletal mass. Unlike osteoporosis, this disorder results from decreased osteoclast activity, which has an effect on both the shape and structure of the bone. In very extreme cases, the medullary cavity, which houses bone marrow, fills with new bone, and production of hematopoietic cells is hampered. Like osteoporosis, this disease can be detected radiographically and appears as though there is a "bone within a bone." There is limited evidence that bisphosphonates can induce osteopetrosis via their inhibition of osteoclast activity (27).

Hypocalcemia

Hypocalcemia can be caused by PTH deficiency, vitamin D deficiency, various pharmacologic agents, and miscellaneous disorders (Table 30.6) (28). A state of hypocalcemia will inhibit calcitonin release. This results in an elevation of PTH biosynthesis and release and indirectly causes an increase in the production of vitamin D. The left wing of Arnaud's butterfly model (Fig. 30.1) is then activated to increase serum calcium concentrations. In the absence of calcitonin, osteoclast activity is unregulated; therefore, bone resorption is accelerated. In acute cases of hypocalcemia, specifically in the case of hypocalcemic tetany, PTH is administered to correct the hormonal imbalance.

TABLE 30.4 Lifestyle and Genetic Risk Factors for Osteoporosis

Lifestyle Factors	Genetic Factors
Smoking	Female
Sedentary lifestyle	Family history
Calcium intake	Small frame
Milk intolerance	Early menopause
Excessive caffeine	
Excessive alcohol	
Nulliparity	

Hypercalcemia

A state of hypercalcemia (Table 30.7) will promote calcitonin biosynthesis and release. As a result, PTH biosynthesis and its secretion are inhibited, as is the production of vitamin D. The right wings of Arnaud's butterfly model (Fig. 30.1, B loops) are then activated to decrease serum calcium concentrations. In the presence of calcitonin, osteoclast activity is inhibited, so bone resorption is slowed. In acute cases of hypercalcemia, calcitonin is administered to reestablish calcium homeostasis. Hypercalcemia also can be treated with sulfate salts, ethylenediaminetetraacetic acid (EDTA), furosemide, ethacrynic acid, glucocorticoids, and plicamycin.

Hypoparathyroidism

Hypoparathyroidism is caused by decreased serum PTH concentrations. It is characterized by hypocalcemia, hyperphosphatemia, and reduced levels of circulating vitamin D. The right wing of Arnaud's butterfly model predominates (Fig. 30.1), and serum calcium concentrations precipitously decrease. Administration of intravenous (IV) calcium gluconate and PTH serves to acutely correct plasma calcium levels. Chronic oral administration of active vitamin D as well as calcium supplements has been effective in maintaining appropriate serum calcium concentrations.

Pseudohypoparathyroidism

In this disease state, levels of PTH are normal or even elevated; however, serum calcium concentrations are low. End-organ insensitivity to PTH has been proposed to be the cause of the hypocalcemic state. Treatment of this

TABLE 30.5 Human Osteopetrosis Genotypes

Gene Involved	Function of Gene	Clinical Symptoms	Patients Affected (%)
Autosomal recessive disorders			
CAII	Carbonic acid and proton production	Less severe: may improve with age, short stature, no hematologic failure	<5
TCIRG1	Proton pump	Severe: apparent in infancy, visual impairment, hypocalcemia, death by 10 years of age	~60
CLCN7	Chloride channel	Severe: apparent in infancy, similar to *TCIRG1* symptoms	~15
		Intermediate: apparent in infancy but less aggressive, osteomyelitis, fractures	
Gl/gl	Unknown	Extremely severe: death within months	<5
Autosomal dominant disorder			
CLCN7	Chloride channel	Frequent fractures, osteomyelitis, some more severe (like recessive disorders)	

condition with calcium and vitamin D has proven to be successful.

Hyperparathyroidism

Increased levels of PTH lead to moderately to severely elevated serum calcium concentrations and, as a result, a significant loss of calcium from the bone (2). Deposits of calcium salts in soft tissue, as well as formation of renal calculi, also can result from this hormonal imbalance. Treatment of this condition with salmon calcitonin, loop diuretics, or other classical treatments for hypercalcemia has been favorable. The IV vitamin D analog paricalcitol, which is used for both prevention and treatment of hyperparathyroidism secondary to chronic renal failure, has been shown to reduce PTH levels by an average of 30% after 6 weeks of treatment. Whereas paricalcitol is a fully active form of vitamin D, doxercalciferol requires activation by the liver.

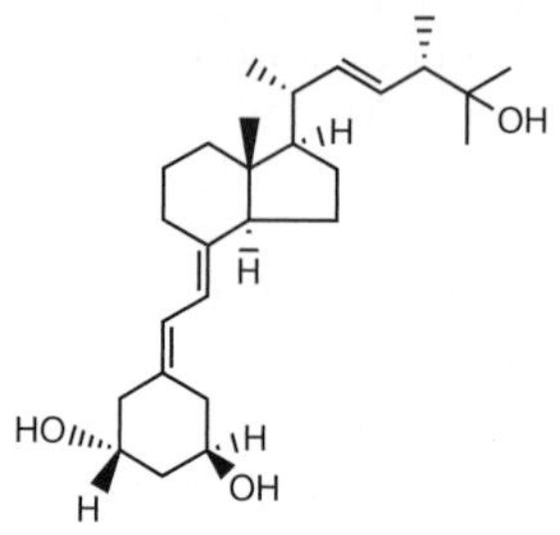

Paricalcitol (Zemplar)

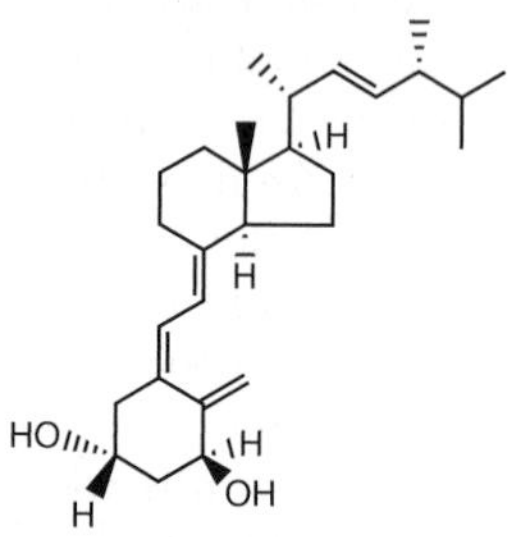

Doxercalciferol (Hectorol)

This analog also is indicated for the treatment of secondary hyperparathyroidism. Doxercalciferol capsules should be administered three times weekly at the time of dialysis along with close monitoring of calcium and phosphate levels. Treatment of secondary hyperparathyroidism with vitamin D therapy is problematic, however, because it often leads to hypercalcemia,

TABLE 30.6 Causes of Hypocalcemia

PTH Deficiency	Vitamin D Deficiency	Drugs	Miscellaneous
Hypoparathyroidism	Nutritional deficiency	Chemotherapeutic agents	Osteoblastic metastases
Pseudohypoparathyroidism	Gastrointestinal malabsorption	Diuretics Furosemide	Phosphate infusion
Hypomagnesemia	Renal Failure Tubule disorders Nephrotic syndrome Hepatobiliary disease (decreases synthesis) Pancreatic disease (malabsorption) Anticonvulsant therapy (malabsorption, abnormal metabolism)	Inhibitors of bone resorption	Rapid infusion of citrate buffered plasma or blood or large amounts of albumin

TABLE 30.7 Calcium Homeostasis-Related Disorders

Type of Disorder	Treatment	Examples
Disorders leading to hypercalcemia	Fluids, low-calcium diet, sulfate, loop diuretics, glucocorticoids, calcitonin, EDTA	Hyperparathyroidism Hypervitaminosis D Sarcoidosis Neoplasia Hyperthyroidism Immobilization Paget disease of the bone
Disorders of bone remodeling	Bisphosphonates, calcitonin, estrogen, calcium, fluoride, PTH + vitamin D	Osteoporosis

EDTA, ethylenediaminetetraacetic acid.

hyperphosphatemia, or both because of increased intestinal absorption of both calcium and phosphorous (29). In patients with chronic renal failure, CaSR agonists are able to limit progression of hyperparathyroidism and growth of the parathyroid gland.

Rickets and Osteomalacia

During the Industrial Revolution, there was widespread incidence of rickets in both children and adults, because inadequate exposure to sunlight prevented the biosynthesis of the precursor to active vitamin D in the skin. Both rickets and osteomalacia are metabolic bone diseases that are characterized by poor bone mineralization. Without adequate plasma levels of vitamin D and calcium, deposition of the calcium salts in the bone markedly decreases. Vitamin D supplementation (to improve intestinal absorption of calcium and mineralization of the bone) as well as oral calcium supplementation are required to treat these diseases once established. The incidence of rickets in the United States dropped dramatically through vitamin D–supplemented food programs. The increased use of milk substitutes (e.g., soy) and reduced exposure to sunlight has recently led to a rise in rickets. Rickets is still considered to be a worldwide health problem.

In addition to the classical environmental or nutritional cause of these diseases, both osteomalacia and rickets can have a pharmacologic origin as a result of chronic treatment with anticonvulsants (phenobarbital and phenytoin) or glucocorticoids. These agents interfere with intestinal absorption of calcium and, thereby, cause pseudohyperparathyroidism. As a result, an increase in bone turnover and a decrease in the formation of appropriately mineralized bone are observed. In these patients, treatment with vitamin D improves calcium absorption, ultimately enhancing mineralization of the bone.

Paget Disease of the Bone

Paget disease of the bone (Table 30.7) is characterized by excessive bone resorption, followed by replacement of the normally mineralized bone with soft, poorly mineralized tissue (30). It has been determined that the osteoclasts have an abnormal structure, are hyperactive, and are present at elevated levels. Patients afflicted with this painful condition often suffer from multiple compression fractures. Administration of calcitonin and oral calcium and phosphate supplements had been the treatment of choice until the bisphosphonate risedronate sodium was approved by the U.S. Food and Drug Administration (FDA). Daily administration of risedronate sodium (see later discussion of bisphosphonates) results in a decreased rate of bone turnover and a decrease in the levels of serum alkaline phosphatase and urinary hydroxyproline, two biochemical markers of bone turnover (4,30). A significant advantage to treatment with the bisphosphonates is long-term suppression of the disease. Calcium supplementation, which often is necessary in these patients, must be dosed separately from risedronate sodium, because calcium- and aluminum- or magnesium-containing antacids interfere with absorption of the bisphosphonates.

DRUG THERAPIES USED TO TREAT OSTEOPOROSIS

Agents used in the treatment and prevention of osteoporosis are categorized as antiresorptive agents or bone-forming agents depending on the primary mechanism of action (31). For most of the effective therapies, bone mass is observed to increase for the first few years of treatment. Eventually, however, all the pits or lacunae will be filled in with new bone, and no additional increase in bone mass will occur. Antiresorptive agents have been shown to increase bone mass by as much as 8% to 9% at the lumbar spine and 3% to 6% in the femoral neck. Once a diagnosis of osteoporosis and the likely cause has been established, it is important to consider both patient fracture history and general medical history when selecting the appropriate treatment for a given patient (Table 30.8) (32).

Antiresorptive Agents

Estrogen Analogs—Estrogen Replacement Therapy

Mechanism of Action The precise mechanism by which estrogen prevents bone resorption has not been elucidated;

TABLE 30.8 Osteoporosis Treatment Selection Criteria (32)

Patient Data	Alendronate	Risedronate	Raloxifene	Calcitonin	Teriparatide
PM women: (+) osteoporosis/(+) fracture	X	X	X	X	X
PM women: (+) osteoporosis/(–) fracture	X				
Men: (+) osteoporosis	X				X
Corticosteroid-induced osteoporosis	X		X		
(+) Esophageal or upper GI disorder	(–)	(–)	X	X	
(+) Vasomotor symptoms	X	X	(–)	X	
(+) Venous thromboembolic event	X	X	(–)	X	
(+) Vertebral compression fracture pain				X	

X, recommended; (–), not recommended; GI, gastrointestinal; PM, postmenopausal.

however, it has been proposed to be associated with inhibition of osteoclast activity. Limited evidence supports the presence of estrogen-specific receptors (present on osteoclasts) having a biochemical role in the regulation of bone remodeling (15). Estrogen improves calcium absorption, promotes calcitonin biosynthesis, and increases the vitamin D receptors on osteoclasts. Although the primary mechanism of action remains unclear and its use is controversial at best, estrogen replacement therapy (i.e., 17β-estradiol, estrone sodium sulfate, or 17-ethinyl estradiol) has value in the treatment and prevention of osteoporosis (31,33–35).

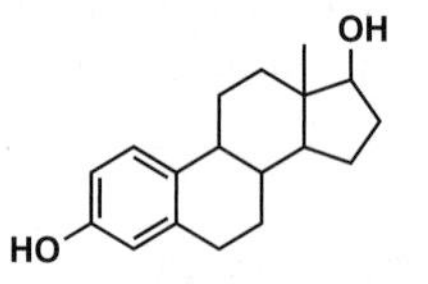

17β-estradiol

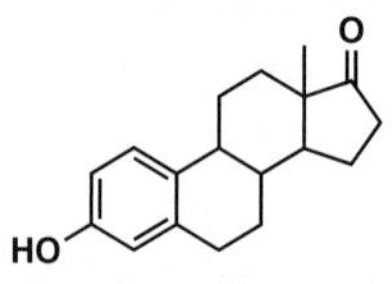

Estrone

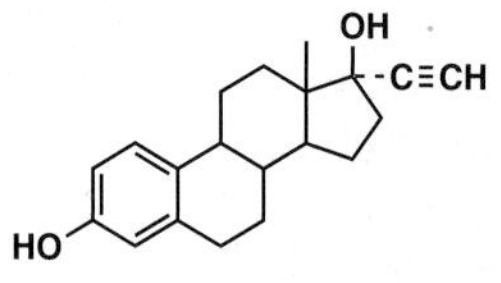

17-Ethinyl estradiol

In light of the findings of the Women's Health Initiative study, the FDA recommends the use of short-term hormone replacement therapy (estrogen and progestin) in the prevention of osteoporosis only in select cases. The pharmacokinetics of the estrogens are covered in detail in Chapter 41 (33,34).

Therapeutic Effects Fractures of the spine, wrist, and hips decrease by 50% to 70%, and spinal bone density increases by 5%, in those women treated with estrogen within 3 years of the onset of menopause and for 5 to 10 years thereafter (5,13,36,37). The minimum dose required and that which is considered to be standard therapy is 0.625 mg/d of conjugated estrogens (Premarin); however, a 0.3 mg/d dose of esterified estrogen (e.g., Menest) has been shown to be adequate for the prevention of osteoporosis (5). Estrogen replacement therapy (ERT) is available in several types of formulations, including transdermal patches (e.g., 17β-estradiol: Climera, Estraderm, Menostar, or Vivelle).

Initiated at the onset of menopause, this therapy also has favorable effects on serum cholesterol levels (reduces low-density lipoprotein and elevates high-density lipoprotein levels). Women taking ERT have found relief from hot flashes, vaginal dryness, and urinary stress incontinence (31). It is recommended that the estrogen be combined with a progestin for those women with an intact uterus so as to decrease the risk of endometrial cancer (15).

Selective Estrogen Receptor Modulators

Raloxifene (Evista) Tamoxifen citrate, classified chemically as a triarylethylene, was developed as an antiestrogenic agent and as a selective estrogen receptor modulator (SERM). It is indicated as adjuvant therapy in the treatment of axillary node–negative or –positive breast cancer following partial or full mastectomy. Raloxifene hydrochloride, a benzothiophene derivative, also may be considered a semirigid analog of tamoxifen (Fig. 30.5) (36).

The two drugs are similar in that they both possess agonist activity in certain tissues (e.g., bone and cardiovascular) and antagonist activity in others (e.g., breast and uterus) (see Chapter 41) (6,31). Raloxifene hydrochloride, the first SERM approved for the prevention of osteoporosis in postmenopausal women, acts as an estrogen agonist on receptors in osteoblasts and osteoclasts but as an antagonist at breast and uterine estrogen receptors. This selective action means that this agent does not increase the risk of endometrial or breast cancer, as is the case with long-term tamoxifen therapy. Because this

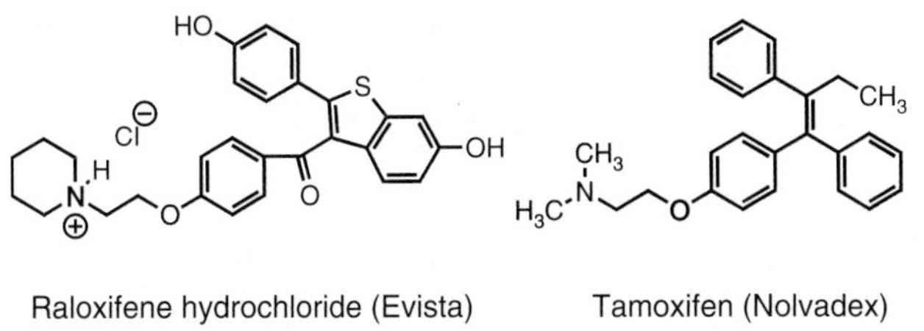

FIGURE 30.5 Structures of raloxifene and tamoxifen highlighting the structural similarity between the two drugs.

agent does not have a stimulatory effect at its receptors on most tissues, it does not prevent the hot flashes and other symptoms of menopause as estrogen does (5).

Therapeutic Action Clinical trials have shown that raloxifene hydrochloride, in combination with oral calcium supplementation, decreases the risk of vertebral fracture and promotes bone formation, albeit to a lesser extent than with estrogen. Raloxifene hydrochloride has been shown to have a beneficial effect on lipid profiles (13). Raloxifene hydrochloride should not be administered in combination with cholestyramine (decreased absorption), warfarin (prothrombin times and international normalized ratios must be monitored more closely), and those drugs that are highly protein bound, such as clofibrate, diazepam, ibuprofen, indomethacin, and naproxen.

Structure–activity Relationship From a structural perspective, the only pure antiestrogens are 7α-substituted estrogens (31). In the triarylethylene class of agents (e.g., tamoxifen), the A ring phenol is critical for interaction with the portion of the estrogen receptor (ER) protein referred to as the activation factor-2 (AF-2) region, because it mimics the essential 3-phenol group found in estrogen (31). This interaction initiates a change in protein conformation to the form of the receptor able to interact with a specific deoxyribonucleic acid (DNA) sequence known as the estrogen responding element (ERE). As a result, activation of a specific group of genes occurs, and protein biosynthesis ensues. The orientation of the three aryl rings in a propeller type of arrangement also is important for tight receptor binding and biologic activity (31). In raloxifene hydrochloride, the substituted benzothiophene ring mimics the estrogen A ring; however because of the presence of a semirigid, amine-containing side chain, raloxifene is unable to interact with AF-2 (38,39). As a result, interaction with ERE is prevented and antiestrogenic action is observed in reproductive tissues. The raloxifene hydrochloride–ER complex, in concert with specific adapter proteins, is also able to interact with and activate a raloxifene responding element (RRE). Activation of this DNA sequence facilitates activation of another group of genes responsible for the production of proteins that allows for agonist action in nonreproductive tissues (38,39).

Pharmacokinetics Raloxifene hydrochloride is rapidly absorbed following oral administration, with an estimated 60% absorption, but it has a very low bioavailability (2%), associated with extensive phase II metabolism. The metabolites are excreted via the bile, with potential enterohepatic recycling that could account for the interaction with cholestyramine. Supportive of the enterohepatic recycling is the half-life of 28 hours. Metabolism of raloxifene hydrochloride occurs to a great extent in the intestine and consists of glucuronide conjugation catalyzed by uridine diphosphate glucuronosyltransferase (UGT) (40–42). The UGT1A family is responsible for intestinal human metabolism, as shown in Figure 30.6. Efflux by intestinal cells of the resulting glucuronide occurs via P-glycoprotein and multidrug resistance–related protein. The combination of rapid metabolism and efflux can account for the low bioavailability.

Lasofoxifene (Fablyn) Lasofoxifene is a very potent second-generation SERM in clinical trials in the United States and approved in the European Union for the treatment and prevention of osteoporosis in postmenopausal women (Fig. 30.7). At low doses, this agent has been shown to prevent bone loss and decrease serum cholesterol (dose range, 0.01 to 20.0 mg/day). In early clinical trials, lasofoxifene improved BMD in the lumbar spine by 3% (after 12 months of therapy), which is twice the improvement observed with similar treatment using raloxifene. Improvement in hip BMD was similar for both agents. Interestingly, a more pronounced reduction in low-density lipoprotein cholesterol was observed with lasofoxifene treatment than with raloxifene treatment. Despite the fact that phase III clinical trial data indicate that there is an increase in deaths from stroke and cancer, lasofoxifene was approved by the European Commission in March 2009 for the treatment of osteoporosis fractures in postmenopausal women.

Ospemifene Ospemifene is a SERM in clinical trials for the treatment of postmenopausal osteoporosis and

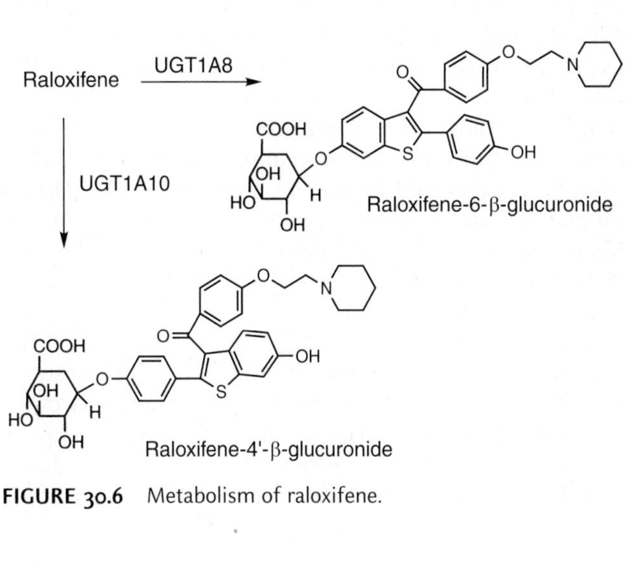

FIGURE 30.6 Metabolism of raloxifene.

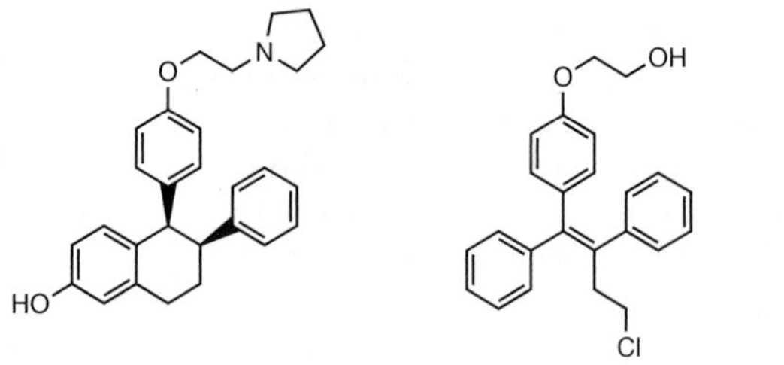

Lasofoxifene Ospemifene

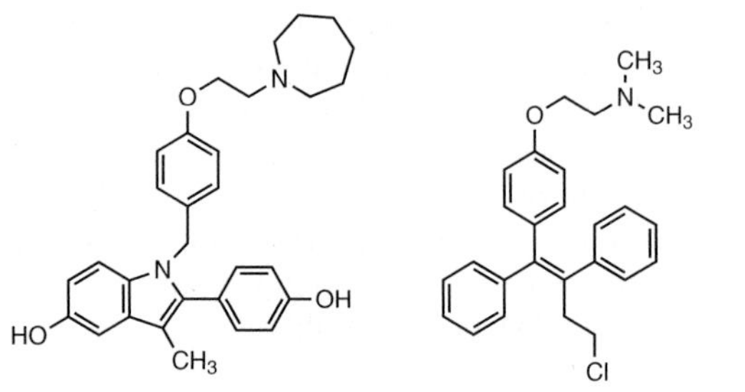

Bazedoxifene Toremifene

FIGURE 30.7 Investigational second-generation selective estrogen receptor modulators.

postmenopausal vaginal atrophy (Fig. 30.7). It is a known metabolite of toremifene, a triphenylethylene derivative used to treat breast cancer. Ospemifene has been shown to have beneficial effects on the bone without significant estrogen-related side effects. The beneficial effect observed on bone stems from this agent's ability to increase osteoblast proliferation and, as a result, to enhance bone mineralization as well as bone formation. Unlike tamoxifen, ospemifene does not induce osteocyte apoptosis (43). Presently the New Drug Application submitted to the FDA under the trade name of Ophena lists treatment of postmenopausal vaginal atrophy as the only indication.

Bazedoxifene (Viviant) Bazedoxifene is an indole-based SERM that is under investigation for the treatment and prevention of postmenopausal osteoporosis (Fig. 30.7). It also is being evaluated in combination with Premarin (conjugated estrogens). Bazedoxifene acetate displaces 17β-estradiol from ERs and has excellent binding affinity for the receptor itself. Unlike raloxifene hydrochloride, this agent does not cause hot flashes at the doses required to have a beneficial effect on bone. In addition, it does not cause uterine or mammary gland stimulation (44). Wyeth received approvable letters from the FDA for the use of bazedoxifene acetate in the prevention and treatment of postmenopausal osteoporosis in 2007 and 2008, respectively.

Toremifene Toremifene citrate (Fig. 30.7), a SERM approved for the treatment of breast cancer (Fareston), is under investigation in patients undergoing androgen-deprivation therapy in the treatment of advanced prostate cancer. Preliminary results from phase III clinical trials indicate a 50% reduction in the rate of osteoporotic fractures, as well as an increase in BMD in the lumbar spine, hip, and femur. Presently, the drug has not been approved for treatment of osteoporosis.

Bisphosphonates

Mechanism of Action The bisphosphonates are synthetic in origin and are designed to mimic pyrophosphate, where the oxygen in P-O-P is replaced with a carbon atom to create a nonhydrolyzable backbone (Fig. 30.8) (36,37). Because pyrophosphate is a normal constituent of bone, these analogs selectively bind to the hydroxyapatite portion of the bone and can bind to and stabilize calcium phosphate effectively (37,45). The bisphosphonates (Fig. 30.9) effectively inhibit osteoclast proliferation, decrease osteoclast activity, reduce osteoclast life span, and as a result, decrease the number of sites along the bone surface where bone resorption occurs (37). This is largely accomplished via inhibition of the mevalonate pathway within osteoclasts, as well as via inhibition of ATP-dependent enzymes. By these three mechanisms, the bisphosphonates are able to limit bone turnover and allow the osteoblasts to form well-mineralized bone without opposition (3). The precise mechanisms of action of these antiresorptive agents have not been elucidated; it is equally uncertain whether all the bisphosphonates act by a similar mechanism (37). To date, cell surface receptors have not been identified, nor has a second messenger system been detected. There is evidence that bisphosphonates inhibit the mevalonate pathway (specifically farnesyl diphosphate synthase) within osteoclasts, as well as inhibit ATP-dependent enzymes (impairing cellular energetics), both of which are associated with inhibition of osteoclast activity.

Structure–Activity Relationships From a structural perspective, the bisphosphonates have been proposed to have specific molecular interactions with their biologic target for drug action, even though precise structure–activity relationships (SARs) have not been elucidated. In fact, the exact molecular target is still under investigation. The central carbon of the geminal phosphonate has been substituted with a variety of functional groups to yield a large family of compounds with differing physicochemical and biologic properties (37). The SAR studies (Fig. 30.8) have concluded that a hydroxyl substituent (R_1) maximizes the affinity of the agent for the hydroxyapatite as

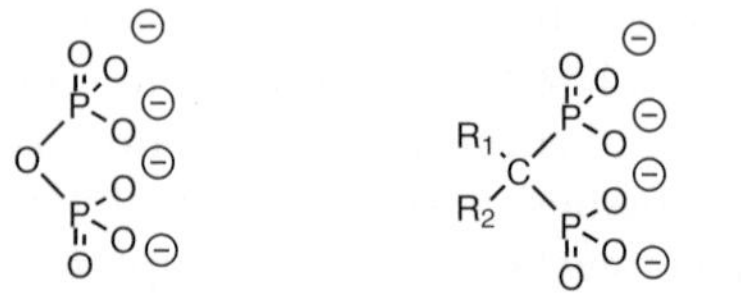

Pyrophosphate

Bisphosphonate
R_1 = hydroxy
R_2 = varies

FIGURE 30.8 Bisphosphonate structure–activity relationships.

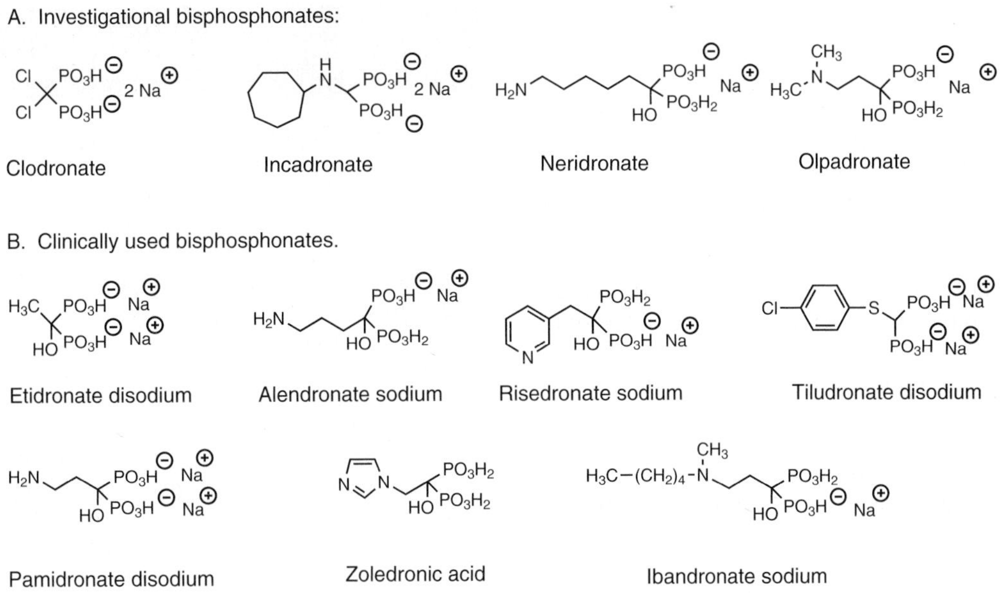

FIGURE 30.9 Bisphosphonates, both investigational and clinically used.

well as improves the antiresorptive character of the agent (31,46). The character of the R_2 substituent varies widely and clearly has a significant influence on the potency of this class of compounds (Fig. 30.9). The R_2 amino–substituted bisphosphonates (pamidronate disodium, alendronate sodium, and neridronate) are more potent than etidronate disodium and clodronate disodium (not available in the United States). The R_2 3-carbon amino linear chain for alendronate sodium is more potent than the R_2 2-carbon derivative pamidronate disodium and the R_2 6-carbon analog neridronate (31). Alkylation of the amine functional group improves potency as is demonstrated by compounds with *N* substituted amino alkyls at R_2 (e.g., olpadronate and ibandronate sodium) and those that contain rings at R_2 (e.g., risedronate sodium, incadronate, tiludronate disodium, and zoledronic acid). The third-generation analogs contain a basic heterocyclic side chain at R_2 tethered to the central carbon by a variety of linkages (potency: NH > CH_2 > S > O) (31,46). Because structural variation of R_2 has a significant effect on potency, it can be surmised that R_2 interacts at an "active site" and participates in a specific molecular interaction. The bisphosphonate itself as well as the hydroxyl group at R_1 also should be included as critical SAR features (31).

Pharmacokinetics To date, four generations of bisphosphonates have been developed for the treatment of osteoporosis (Fig. 30.9). Absorption of these agents from the gut is quite poor (1% to 5%) because of their polar nature, and as a therapeutic class, they have limited cellular penetration (13). Up to 50% of the actual absorbed dose is taken up specifically by the bone within 4 to 6 hours, and the rest is exclusively excreted by the kidney (6,36). Uptake of these agents in the bone is concentrated in areas of the bone that are actively undergoing remodeling (45). Between the selective uptake and the rapid rate of clearance, the bisphosphonates enjoy a short circulating half-life and very limited drug exposure to nontarget tissues (37). Because the bisphosphonates are only released from the bone when the bone is resorbed, they have a tissue half-life of 1 to 10 years; however, these agents remain pharmacologically active only while they are exposed on bone resorption surfaces (45).

Specific Drugs

Etidronate Disodium (Didronel) and Tiludronate Disodium (Skelid) Agents in the first generation of bisphosphonates that were dosed continuously produced poorly mineralized bone, because there was no interval for appropriate bone mineralization to occur (3). Subsequent studies that used a cyclic dosing schedule (400 mg/d for 2 weeks, followed by 2.5 months of calcium supplementation only) showed improvement in bone mineralization (13,43). Both of these bisphosphonates have been approved for treatment of Paget disease of the bone but not for the treatment of osteoporosis (5). Tiludronate disodium is approximately 10-fold more potent than etidronate disodium and, when given orally for 6 months (200, 400, or 800 mg/d), increases BMD by 2% (Fig. 30.9) (6). No further bone loss was detected in patients 6 months after cessation of therapy.

Alendronate Sodium (Fosamax) The second-generation agent alendronate sodium was the first bisphosphonate agent approved by the FDA for the prevention and treatment of osteoporosis and Paget disease of the bone and is 1,000-fold more potent than etidronate disodium (Fig. 30.9) (45,47). Alendronate sodium is also indicated for the treatment of glucocorticoid-induced osteoporosis. This derivative, when dosed continuously (5 to 10 mg/d for osteoporosis and 40 mg/d for Paget disease of the bone) and given with oral calcium supplements (500 mg/d), produced well-mineralized bone and significantly improved BMD (7% in the spine and 4% in the hip) within 18 months (6). In addition, the vertebral fracture rate was shown to decrease by 47%. A side effect associated with alendronate sodium, chemical esophagitis, has been attributed to inadequate intake of water and lying down after taking the medication (2,3,13,36). Specific patient instructions were developed to limit the incidence of upper gastrointestinal problems and include: 1) taking the medication with 6 to 8 ounces of water on arising in the morning, 2) remaining in an upright position for at least 30 minutes after taking the medication, and 3) delaying drinking other liquids/eating for at least 30 minutes, if not 1 to 2 hours, to allow maximal absorption of the agent. To enhance absorption, calcium supplements and any aluminum- or magnesium-containing antacids should be dosed separately from agents in this class. These agents are not recommended in patients with renal impairment (serum creatinine, <2.5 mg/dL), a history of esophageal disease, gastritis, or peptic ulcer (5). In an attempt to address the inconvenience associated with tablet administration, a once-weekly, 70-mg buffered effervescent formulation of alendronate is under investigation.

Risedronate Sodium (Actonel) The third-generation agent risedronate sodium has been approved for the treatment of osteoporosis (both postmenopausal and in men), Paget disease of the bone, and glucocorticoid-induced osteoporosis (Fig. 30.9). Risedronate sodium is 1,000- to 5,000-fold more potent than etidronate disodium. At the end of an 18-month study, 53% of patients who took risedronate sodium for 2 months remained in remission, as compared to 14% of patients who took etidronate disodium, an earlier-generation bisphosphonate, for 6 months. Oral administration of this agent suffers from the same problems as that of other bisphosphonate agents. Risedronate sodium should not be given to patients with creatinine clearance of less than 30 mL/min. A once-weekly, delayed-release formulation (Atelvia) that can be taken immediately after breakfast with 4 ounces of water was approved by the FDA in October 2010. Other oral formulations of risedronate sodium include tablets to be consumed daily (5 mg), weekly (35 mg), and monthly (150 mg).

Ibandronate Sodium (Boniva) Ibandronate sodium is approved for the treatment and prevention of osteoporosis in postmenopausal women and has a mechanism of action that is identical to the other bisphosphonate agents (Fig. 30.9). Administered daily (2.5 mg), ibandronate sodium has been clinically shown to reduce the risk of vertebral fractures by 62% (48). If administered on an intermittent basis (20 mg), it reduces the risk of vertebral fractures by 50%. Ibandronate sodium (2.5 mg daily), along with 500 mg of supplemental calcium, has been clinically shown to increase BMD in the hip (1.8%), femoral neck (2.0%), and lumbar spine (3.1%). A 150-mg formulation has been approved by the FDA for once-monthly administration as well as a 3-mg IV formulation for quarterly administration.

ADDITIONAL DOSAGE FORMS

A unique formulation of alendronate sodium, FOSAMAX PLUS D, includes 70 mg of alendronate sodium and 2,800 IU or 5,600 IU of vitamin D_3 (i.e., a 7-day supply of both the bisphosphonate and vitamin D). This formulation should not be used in patients with severe kidney disease or low serum calcium levels and should not be the only therapy used to correct a vitamin D deficiency.

Risedronate sodium with calcium carbonate (Actonel with Calcium) represents an additional type of packaging for this class of agents. It addresses the Surgeon General's Report on Bone Health and Osteoporosis, which states that treatments for osteoporosis need to be made simpler and more structured. Sold in units that contain a 1-month supply, each week of therapy includes a total of seven tablets, including one 35-mg tablet of risedronate and six 500-mg tablets of calcium carbonate.

The oral bioavailability of this agent is extremely poor (0.6%) and is adversely affected by the presence of food, beverages other than water, and other medications, including calcium or vitamin D supplements and antacids. Because of the increased calcium content in mineral water, patients should not take this medication with this type of water. Drugs that inhibit gastric acid secretion (e.g., H_2 antagonists and proton pump inhibitors) actually promote ibandronate sodium absorption. Like the other agents in this therapeutic class, ibandronate sodium is not metabolized, and that which is not bound to the bone (40% to 50% of the absorbed dose) is eliminated renally unchanged. It does not inhibit the CYP450 isozymes. This agent does not require any dosage adjustment for patients with hepatic impairment or mild to moderate renal impairment (creatinine clearance, >30 mL/min). Ibandronate sodium should not be prescribed for patients with severe renal impairment (creatinine clearance, <30 mL/min).

Zoledronic Acid (Reclast) Zoledronic acid is approved for the treatment of glucocorticoid-induced osteoporosis and prevention and treatment of postmenopausal osteoporosis, male osteoporosis, and Paget disease of the bone (Fig. 30.9). For the treatment of osteoporosis, zoledronic acid is formulated as a 5-mg, once-yearly IV infusion. The frequency of IV infusion decreases to 5 mg every 2 years for the prevention of osteoporosis. In order to prevent hypocalcemia, concomitant calcium (1,500 mg) and vitamin D (800 to 1,000 IU) intake and/or supplementation is recommended in patients being treated for osteoporosis. On the day of treatment, patients should drink at least two glasses of water and eat normally.

Osteonecrosis of the jaw has been reported in patients receiving IV bisphosphonate therapy (49). The majority of the patients who developed osteonecrosis of the jaw were undergoing chemotherapy (typically for multiple myeloma, breast, prostate, or lung cancers), taking corticosteroids, and had undergone a dental procedure (e.g., tooth extraction). The FDA recommends that patients receive a thorough dental examination before initiation of IV bisphosphonate therapy and that they avoid invasive dental work during treatment.

In October 2010, the FDA approved safety labeling changes for the bisphosphonates in response to reports of an increase in risk of atypical femur fracture in patients undergoing long-term bisphosphonate therapy (50,51). In addition, an increase in the risk of developing esophageal cancer has surfaced in patients with approximately 5 years of oral bisphosphonate use. Because of these adverse effects, it is recommended that clinicians weigh the benefits against the potential risks.

The remaining bisphosphonates, pamidronate disodium and zoledronic acid, are approved for treatment of hypercalcemia of malignancy as well as other cancer conditions and will be discussed later in the chapter.

Calcitonin (Calcimar [IV, subcutaneous]; Miacalcin and Fortical [nasal spray])

Calcitonin (see earlier discussion in this chapter) has been approved for the treatment of postmenopausal osteoporosis, hypercalcemia of malignancy, and Paget disease of the bone. Several sources are available (e.g., eel, human, salmon, and porcine). The calcitonin isolated from salmon is the preferred source, because it has greater receptor affinity and a longer half-life than the human hormone (3,7). Calcitonin is commercially available as synthetic calcitonin-salmon, which contains the same linear sequence of 32 amino acids, as occurs in natural calcitonin-salmon. Calcitonin-salmon differs structurally from human calcitonin at 16 of 32 amino acids (see Fig. 30.10 for primary structure differences between human and salmon calcitonin). The pharmacologic activity of these calcitonins is the same, but calcitonin-salmon is approximately 50-fold more potent on a weight basis than human calcitonin with a longer duration of action. The duration of action for calcitonin salmon is 8 to 24 hours following intramuscular (IM) or subcutaneous (SC) administration and 0.5 to 12.0 hours following IV administration. The parenteral dose required for the treatment of osteoporosis is 100 IU/d (46). Initially only available by IM or SC injection, the peptide hormone calcitonin-salmon is available as a nasal spray (Miacalcin) and as a rectal suppository (6). A recombinant DNA form of calcitonin-salmon (Fortical) is available as a nasal spray. The bioavailability of calcitonin-salmon nasal spray shows great variability (range, 0.3% to 30.6% of an IM dose). It is absorbed rapidly from the nasal mucosa, with peak plasma concentrations appearing 30 to 40 minutes after nasal administration, compared with 16 to 25 minutes following parental dosing. Calcitonin-salmon is readily metabolized in the kidney, with an elimination half-life calculated at 43 minutes. As a result, the intranasal dose required is 200 IU/d (3). Once the Miacalcin nasal pump has been activated, the bottle may be kept at room temperature until the medication is finished (2 weeks).

Therapeutic Application Calcitonin therapy requires the concomitant oral administration of elemental calcium (500 mg/d, see Table 30.9). Clinical studies have shown that the combination of intranasal calcitonin-salmon (200 IU/d), oral calcium supplementation (>1,000 mg/d of elemental calcium), and vitamin D (400 IU/d) has decreased the rate of new fractures by more than 75% and has improved vertebral BMD by as much as 3% annually (3). Calcitonin prevents the abnormal bone turnover characteristic of Paget disease of the bone and has antiresorptive activity. In the presence of calcitonin, the osteoclast brush borders disappear, and the osteoclasts move away from the bone surface undergoing remodeling (52). Side effects are significantly more pronounced when calcitonin-salmon is administered by injection and can include nausea, vomiting, anorexia, and flushing. Because calcitonin-salmon is protein in nature, the possibility of a systemic allergic reaction should be considered, and appropriate measures for treatment of hypersensitivity reaction should be readily available. Although calcitonin-salmon does not cross the placenta, it may pass into breast milk. Calcitonin-salmon is a possible alternative to ERT; however, only limited evidence suggests that it has efficacy in women who already have fractures. Resistance to calcitonin-salmon can result from the development of neutralizing antibodies (53).

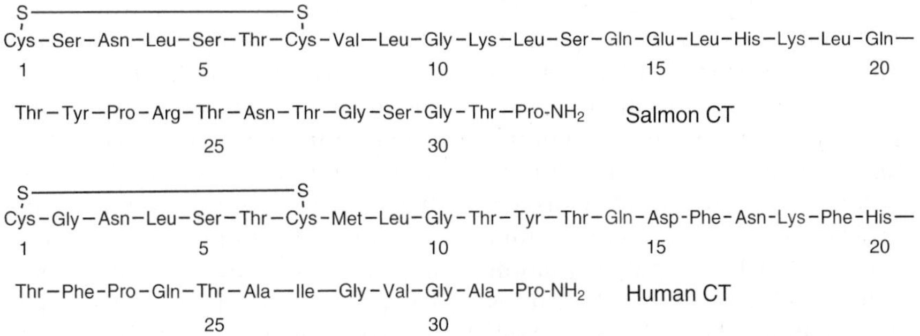

FIGURE 30.10 Primary structures of salmon and human calcitonin (CT). Similarities are highlighted in *red*.

In addition to its antiresorptive action via suppression of osteoclast activity, calcitonin-salmon exhibits a potent analgesic effect and has provided considerable relief to those patients suffering from the pain associated with Paget disease of the bone and osteoporosis. This analgesic effect is a result of calcitonin-stimulated endogenous opioid release. The potency of this analgesic effect has been demonstrated to be 30- to 50-fold that of morphine in selected patients. Calcitonin is preferred over estrogen and the bisphosphonates when treatment of both osteoporosis and related bone pain is warranted.

Bone-Forming Agents

Teriparatide (Forteo)

In 2002, the FDA approved teriparatide for the treatment of postmenopausal osteoporosis in patients who have a high risk of fracture, for the treatment of glucocorticoid-induced osteoporosis, and to increase bone mass in men with primary or hypogonadal osteoporosis who have a high risk of fracture (54). Teriparatide is recombinant human PTH 1-34 (Fig. 30.2), the biologically active portion of the endogenously produced preprohormone. Unlike the bisphosphonates, which are classified as bone restorative agents, teriparatide is the first approved bone-forming agent. Bone formation is possible because of the ability of this agent to increase the number of osteoblasts. Although teriparatide enhances the function of both osteoclasts and osteoblasts, the exposure incidence dictates its effect on the skeleton. If administered once daily or intermittently, teriparatide preferentially enhances osteoblastic function, and bone formation occurs. Continuous exposure to endogenous PTH may result in poor skeletal composition because of enhanced osteoclast-mediated bone resorption (52). After 18 months of treatment, lumbar BMD increased up to 12% in postmenopausal women. After 10 months of treatment, 53% of men had an increase of 5% or greater in spine BMD. The risk for developing new vertebral fractures was reduced by 65% after 21 months of treatment, and the number of nonvertebral fragility fractures was reduced by 53% (35). There is limited evidence that teriparatide can regrow jaw bone that has been damaged by osteonecrosis and periodontitis.

A black box warning from the FDA advises that treatment with teriparatide should be avoided in patients with an increased baseline risk for osteosarcoma and that treatment should not exceed 2 years in duration.

Administered as a once-daily, 20-μg SC injection in the thigh or abdominal wall, teriparatide is a clear, colorless liquid that is available as a 750 μg/3 mL, prefilled, disposable pen that requires refrigeration. Concurrent calcium (1,000 mg) and vitamin D (400 IU) supplementation is recommended. Treatment for longer than 2 years is not recommended. Teriparatide is rapidly absorbed, demonstrates 95% bioavailability, and is quickly eliminated via both hepatic and extrahepatic routes. The half-life is 1 hour when administered SC. Metabolic studies have not been performed on teriparatide; however, the entire PTH preprohormone has been shown to undergo enzyme-mediated transformations in the liver. Dizziness and leg cramps are the most commonly reported adverse side effects.

Temporary increases in serum calcium levels occur following administration of teriparatide. As a result, this agent is contraindicated in patients who are predisposed to hypercalcemia. Some evidence suggests that these elevations in serum calcium levels may cause a patient who is taking digitalis to experience digitalis toxicity (55). Teriparatide should not be prescribed to patients with Paget disease of the bone, children, young adults, women who are pregnant or nursing, and patients who have received skeletal radiation therapy (52). Because of an increased incidence of osteosarcoma (malignant bone tumors) observed in rats, teriparatide also carries a black box warning.

Inorganic Salts

Calcium Salts Appropriate intake of calcium during childhood, adolescence, and early adulthood increases peak BMD and may reduce the overall risk of developing osteoporosis. For those who are at low risk of developing osteoporosis and have adequate BMD, consumption of the recommended amounts of calcium (1,300 mg/d of elemental calcium for teenagers, 1,000 mg/d for premenopausal women and men, and 1,200 mg/d for postmenopausal women) typically is sufficient to prevent bone loss (56,57). This often can be accomplished by eating a well-balanced diet. For patients with established osteoporosis or areas of poorly mineralized bone, calcium supplementation alone is not sufficient to reverse the bone loss or to significantly improve mineralization of the bone (13).

It should be noted that a study conducted by Bolland et al. (58) reported that calcium supplementation in postmenopausal women may be correlated with significant increases in the rates of vascular events.

The actual amount of elemental calcium that is present in the available calcium salts varies considerably; however, no one particular salt has been identified as an exceptional source of elemental calcium (Table 30.9). Absorption of calcium from the gastrointestinal tract (25% to 40%) improves under acidic conditions; therefore, those medications that change the acidic environment of the stomach (e.g., H_2 antagonists and proton pump inhibitors) have an adverse effect on calcium absorption (3). Total daily doses of elemental calcium that exceed 500 mg should be spaced out over the day to improve absorption (5,56). The more water soluble and, therefore, more easily absorbed salts (e.g., citrate, lactate, and gluconate) are less dependent on the acidic environment for appropriate absorption and would be

TABLE 30.9 Percent of Elemental Calcium Content in Various Salts (3)

Salt	Calcium (%)	Elemental Calcium (mg/tablet)
Calcium carbonate	40	
Tums (500 mg chewable)		200 mg
Titilac (1 g/5 mL suspension)		400 mg/5 mL
Alka-Mints (850 mg chewable)		340 mg
Os-Cal 500 (1,250 mg tablet)		500 mg
Viactive (1,250 mg chewable)		500 mg
Tricalcium phosphate	39	
Calcium chloride	27	
Tribasic calcium phosphate	23	
Posture (1,565.2 mg tablets)		600 mg
Calcium citrate	21	
Citrical (950 mg tablets)		200 mg
Citrical Liquitab (2,376 mg effervescent tablets)		500 mg
Calcium lactate	13	
Generics (325 mg tablets)		42 mg
Generics (650 mg tablets)		84 mg
Calcium gluconate	9	
Neo-Calglucon (1.8 g/5 mL syrup)		115 mg/5 mL

appropriate alternatives for patients who produce low levels of acid. Calcium carbonate is a poorly soluble form of calcium, but it is inexpensive and only requires the patient to take a few tablets per day with acidic food or beverages like citrus juice (56).

Sodium Fluoride Sodium fluoride (NaF) promotes the proliferation and activity of osteoblasts and is classified as a nonhormonal bone-forming agent. Because treatment with NaF induces bone formation, it is essential that this therapy be coupled with oral calcium supplementation (1,000 mg/d). Additionally, NaF exhibits moderate antiresorptive activity, because it inhibits osteoclastic activity when it is absorbed into the bone matrix. In the treatment of osteoporosis, the therapeutic window for this agent is fairly narrow: Doses less than 45 mg/d are subtherapeutic, and doses in excess of 75 mg/d impair bone mineralization. In addition, the bone that is formed in the presence of NaF is neither as well mineralized nor as strong as normal bone tissue. In fact, some studies have demonstrated that patients taking sodium fluoride have increased bone fragility despite the increase in bone mass and, as a result, have an increased nonvertebral fracture rate as compared to the placebo group (5,31,46). As a result, its use in the treatment of osteoporosis has not been approved and is considered to be somewhat controversial. Several studies have examined the benefits of continuous versus cyclic dosing of NaF in the treatment of osteoporosis. Intermittent dosing (25 mg twice a day for 12 months, followed by 2 months of calcium supplementation alone) of a slow-release formulation of NaF with 400 mg of calcium citrate was shown to effectively improve bone mass (vertebra, 5% per year; femoral neck, 2% per year) and to decrease the number of vertebral fractures (59,60).

Monoclonal Antibody-Based Therapies

RANKL Inhibitor

Denosumab (Prolia) Denosumab (Prolia) has been approved by the FDA for the treatment of postmenopausal women with osteoporosis at high risk for fracture. Denosumab is a fully human monoclonal antibody to RANKL, where it functions as a RANKL inhibitor (Fig. 30.4). The RANKL receptor is expressed on the surface of osteoclasts and osteoclast precursors. When bound to its receptor, RANKL promotes the formation and activation of osteoclasts. To balance the effects of RANKL, osteoblasts produce osteoprotegerin, which binds to RANKL and prevents it from binding to and activating its receptor, modulating the production and activation of osteoclasts (61). When an individual develops osteoporosis, this balance is "disrupted," and RANKL overwhelms osteoprotegerin activity, causing significant bone loss. Denosumab was designed to mimic the biochemical effects of osteoprotegerin. Studies show that denosumab is more effective in improving BMD (4% to 7%) than weekly administration of alendronate (5%) (61). Denosumab is reported to reduce the risk of vertebral fraction (68%), hip fracture (40%), and nonvertebral facture (20%). This agent is administered subcutaneously once every 6 months and has been associated with adverse events including back pain (35%), serious infections, hypocalcemia, and osteonecrosis of the jaw.

Cathepsin K Inhibitor

Odanacatib Odanacatib selectively inhibits cathepsin K, a cytosolic cysteine protease. Produced by osteoclasts, this protease is responsible for degradation of the collagen matrix found in bone tissue.

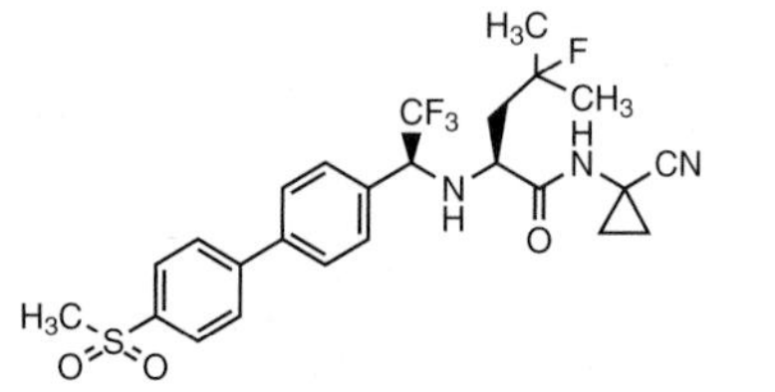

Odanacatib

Phase II clinical studies with odanacatib show that treatment for 2 years resulted in an increase in BMD at the lumbar spine and hip (62). Odanacatib is being evaluated in large-scale phase III clinical trials on vertebral, hip, and nonvertebral fractures.

Miscellaneous Therapies

Strontium ranelate (Protelos) is an orally active agent that can be classified as both an antiresorptive agent and a bone-forming agent (63,64).

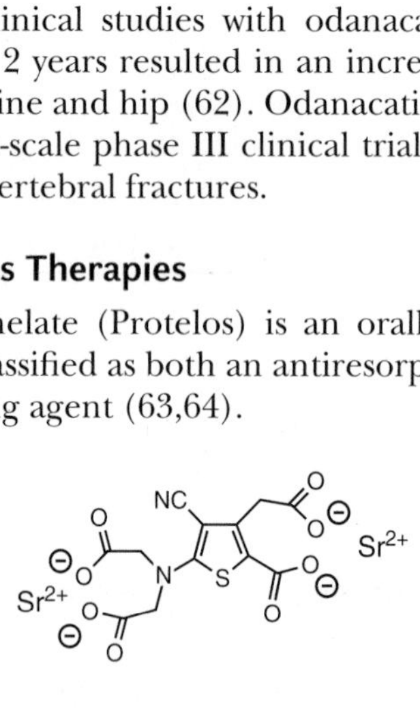

Strontium ranelate

It is able not only to stimulate replication of preosteoblastic cells to promote bone formation but also is able to decrease osteoclastic activity to prevent bone resorption. Biochemical markers for bone formation (e.g., bone-specific alkaline phosphatase), which normally decrease in the presence of antiresorptive therapy, are elevated in the presence of strontium ranelate (65). Strontium ranelate is active by virtue of the strontium cation and not the anion portion of the drug. Lumbar spine BMD increased 11.4% in patients treated with this new agent. Although approved as second-line therapy for the treatment of osteoporosis in a number of European nations, Protelos is not FDA approved (66).

The hydroxymethylglutaryl–coenzyme A (HMG-CoA) reductase inhibitors, otherwise known as the statins, have been found to increase bone formation via enhanced activity of the bone morphogenic protein 2 (*BMP-2*) gene. This gene increases osteoblast differentiation. In addition, by inhibiting HMG-CoA reductase, the statins not only prevent the biosynthesis of cholesterol but also prevent the formation of compounds associated with osteoclast activation (67). Unfortunately, clinical data from several large studies conflict, and further study is warranted before the statins can be considered as a viable treatment for osteoporosis (68).

There are a number of investigational agents in the pipeline that act through very novel mechanisms of action (Table 30.10). These include calcilytic inhibitors, inhibitors of protein tyrosine kinase C-src, and Dkk1 monoclonal antibodies (66,69).

DRUG THERAPIES USED TO TREAT HYPERPARATHYROIDISM

Increased levels of PTH lead to moderately to severely elevated serum calcium concentrations and alterations in phosphorous metabolism (2). To modulate the levels of PTH released from the parathyroid gland chief cells, regulation of CaSR sensitivity is required. An agonist at this receptor, a calcimimetic, serves to activate the receptor, whereas an antagonist at this receptor is classified as a calcilytic. There are two types of calcimimetic agents: those that activate the CaSR directly (type I), and those that require the presence of a cation, such as calcium or magnesium (type II), for activation (70). Type I calcimimetics are polycations (e.g., magnesium and neomycin). The first and second generations of type II calcimimetics are phenylalkylamine based. They have an indirect/allosteric action on CaSR mediated by a conformational alteration of these receptors.

Cinacalcet Hydrochloride (Sensipar)

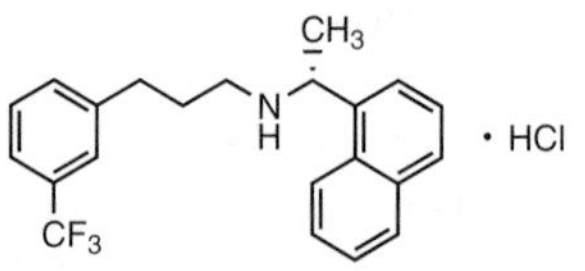

Cinacalcet hydrochloride (Sensipar)

TABLE 30.10 Classes of Experimental Agents for Treatment of Abnormal Calcium Homeostasis

Class	Action
Antiresorptive Agents	
Cathepsin K inhibitors	Prevent degradation of collagen matrix
C-src kinase inhibitors	Prevent formation of osteoclast sealing zone
Bone-Forming Agents	
Calcilytic agents	Inhibit calcium-sensing receptors to promote PTH release
Dkk1 monoclonal antibody	Inhibitor of negative regulators of Wnt signaling

Cinacalcet is the first type II calcimimetic agent approved that improves CaSR sensitivity to calcium (29,71). When calcium is bound to the CaSR, phospholipase C is activated, and the secretion of PTH is inhibited. In the presence of cinacalcet, not only is a decrease in PTH levels observed, but a decrease in serum calcium and phosphorous levels is also observed. This represents a significant therapeutic advantage over vitamin D–based treatments for secondary hyperparathyroidism (29). Cinacalcet hydrochloride is a second-generation calcimimetic approved for the treatment of secondary hyperparathyroidism in patients with chronic kidney disease on dialysis and for the treatment of hypercalcemia in patients with parathyroid cancer. It can be used alone, with vitamin D, and/or with a phosphate binder (72).

DRUG THERAPIES USED TO TREAT HYPERCALCEMIA OF MALIGNANCY

Zoledronic Acid (Zometa)

Zoledronic acid, a bisphosphonate, was approved by the FDA in 2001 for the treatment of hypercalcemia of malignancy, a metabolic complication that can be life-threatening (Fig. 30.9). Hypercalcemia of malignancy can occur in up to 50% of patients diagnosed with advanced breast cancer, multiple myeloma, and non–small-cell lung cancer. This condition arises when chemical moieties produced by the tumor cause overstimulation of osteoclasts. When there is an increase in bone degradation, there is a concomitant release of calcium into the plasma. When serum concentrations of calcium rapidly elevate, the kidneys are unable to handle the overload, and hypercalcemia results. This can lead to dehydration, nausea, vomiting, fatigue, and confusion. Zoledronic acid effectively decreases plasma calcium concentrations via inhibition of bone resorption (inhibition of osteoclastic activity and induction of osteoclast apoptosis). It also prevents the increase in osteoclastic activity caused by tumor-based stimulatory factors. In addition, zoledronic acid has been approved by the FDA for the treatment of multiple myeloma and bone metastases associated with solid tumor–based cancers (e.g., prostrate and lung) (73).

Cancer treatment–induced bone loss is a major adverse effect associated with endocrine-based cancer therapies. These therapies may depress ovarian function (e.g., goserelin acetate), decrease ER activation (e.g., ER antagonist), and/or inhibit estrogen biosynthesis (e.g., aromatase inhibition) all of which will lead to significant bone loss. Zoledronic acid has demonstrated efficacy in reducing or delaying these complications.

The maximum recommended dose for the treatment of hypercalcemia of malignancy is 4 mg every 3 to 4 weeks. A clinically significant deterioration in renal function occurs when single doses of this agent exceed 4 mg and the infusion duration is less than 15 minutes (74). It is recommended that patients be well hydrated before infusion. If serum calcium levels do not fall to normal levels, retreatment is appropriate, but retreatment is not recommended until 7 days have elapsed from the initial treatment. For the treatment of multiple myeloma and metastatic bone lesions, a 4-mg initial dose is recommended, followed by additional doses every 3 to 4 weeks for 9 to 15 months (prostate cancer, 15 months; breast cancer, 12 months; other solid tumors, 9 months).

Zoledronic acid is a white, crystalline powder that is available in vials for reconstitution for IV infusion over at least 15 minutes. It does not undergo metabolic transformation and does not inhibit CYP450 enzymes. Clearance of this agent is dependent on the patient's creatinine clearance, not on dose. Serum creatinine levels should be evaluated prior to every treatment. Zoledronic acid is contraindicated in patients with severe renal impairment.

Zoledronic acid should not be mixed with infusion solutions that contain calcium (e.g., lactated Ringer's) and should be administered via IV infusion in its own line. Because of the possibility of a serious deterioration in renal function, the manufacturer requires strict adherence to the infusion duration being no less than 15 minutes.

Pamidronate Disodium (Aredia)

Pamidronate disodium, a second-generation bisphosphonate, is 100-fold more potent than etidronate disodium for the treatment of hypercalcemia of malignancy (Fig. 30.9) (6). It has also been approved for the treatment of Paget disease of the bone and for osteolytic bone metastases of breast cancer and osteolytic lesions of multiple myeloma. When used to treat bone metastases, pamidronate disodium decreases osteoclast recruitment, decreases osteoclast activity, and increases osteoclast apoptosis (75). Administered by IV infusion, a single dose is typically sufficient for the treatment of hypercalcemia and Paget disease of the bone. In the treatment of osteolytic lesions of multiple myeloma, monthly administration is indicated. Pamidronate disodium is cleared renally and therefore is contraindicated in patients with deteriorated renal function.

Gallium Nitrate (Ganite)

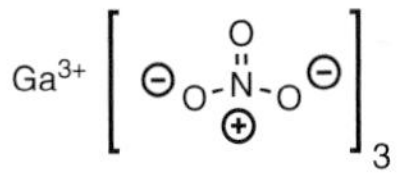

Gallium nitrate has been approved for the treatment of hypercalcemia of malignancy in patients who do not respond to hydration (46). Its effectiveness stems from its ability to inhibit bone resorption despite the presence of tumor-derived factors that promote calcium loss from the bone. Administered by infusion over 24 hours, the typical dose is 200 mg/m^2/day for 5 consecutive days. A lower dose is recommended if the symptoms of hypercalcemia are mild (100 mg/m^2/d for 5 days). Steady-state is achieved in 24 to 48 hours. Maintenance of patient hydration is essential during treatment. Gallium nitrate is not significantly metabolized and is largely excreted through the kidneys. It is contraindicated in patients with severe renal impairment. Renal function should be closely monitored in all patients receiving this agent.

DRUG THERAPY USED IN THE TREATMENT OF HYPOPARATHYROIDISM

Parathyroid Hormone [rDNA 1-84] (Preos)

In 2007, the FDA Office of Orphan Products Development granted orphan drug designation for Preos for the treatment of hypoparathyroidism (Fig. 30.2). Structurally identical to endogenous PTH, the recombinant human PTH is administered once daily as an SC injection. Although Preos shares a common mechanism of action with teriparatide, it has been suggested that the C-terminal region may possess valuable biologic activity mediated by a novel receptor that specifically interacts with this portion of the peptide hormone.

SCENARIO: OUTCOME AND ANALYSIS

Outcome

Kathryn Neill, PharmD

The pharmacist recommends changing the calcium carbonate to calcium citrate 200 mg with 200 IU of vitamin D (two tablets three times daily); limiting caffeine intake to no more than two servings daily; and separating the administration of ramipril from calcium by 2 hours.

Chemical Analysis

Victoria F. Roche and S. William Zito

The oral bioavailability of calcium ranges from approximately 5% to 45%. Absorption is dependent on salt form, dose, presence of gastric acid, and presence of activated vitamin D. Calcium absorption is increased when administered with meals as a result of increased secretion of gastric acid in response to a food bolus. The increased gastric acidity releases calcium from water insoluble salt forms (like calcium carbonate) and allows its absorption. For example, calcium carbonate absorption increases as much as 30% when taken with a meal. Absorption of calcium citrate is greater than other salt forms because it is freely water soluble and does not require the action of strong acid to break down the salt to release the calcium. Therefore, it is the most efficacious calcium supplement for patients with achlorhydria.

$CaCO_3$	$CaCl_2$
Calcium carbonate	Calcium citrate

As it dissolves in the gastric acid, calcium carbonate can create gas (CO_2) in the stomach, resulting in stomach upset. Because it is not a CO_2 generator, this adverse effect is not commonly experienced with calcium citrate. Absorption of calcium in the duodenum is dependent upon active vitamin D. Dietary vitamin D intake is rarely adequate to meet the recommended 800–1,000 units per day (some researchers now recommend 2000 units per day), and supplementation is usually necessary, especially for seniors who may have even higher daily requirements.

Calcium should be separated from doses of other medications by 2 hours to prevent chelation, which can result in decreased absorption and therapeutic effects. As a divalent cation, calcium will be chelated by electron-rich (nucleophilic) atoms like oxygen. Both ramipril and alendronate have many nucleophilic oxygen atoms that could sequester calcium ion, as shown below.

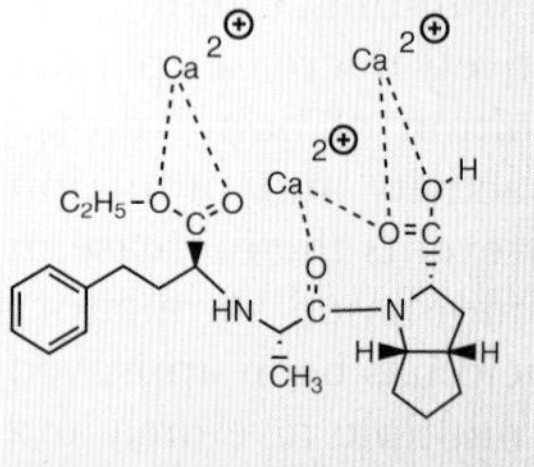

Calcium chelated by ramipril

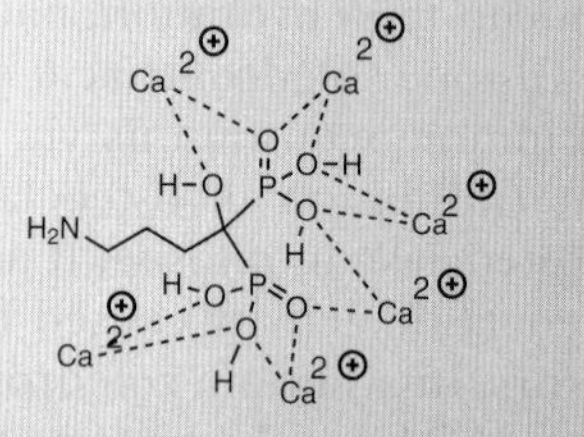

Calcium chelated by alendronate

It would be important to counsel PJ to take alendronate with a full glass of water and to remain in a sitting or standing position for at least 30 minutes because this bisphosphonate can induce a chemical esophagitis that could exacerbate the distress PJ is experiencing from other GERD-related pathologies.

CASE STUDY

Victoria Roche and S. William Zito

JA is a 73-year-old woman who had polio 58 years ago. Although she had maintained a very active lifestyle throughout her youth and most of her adulthood, postpolio syndrome (PPS) has significantly restricted her mobility and she now uses a wheelchair at home and a power chair to get around outside. JA's relative lack of activity during the past 5 years has caused a troublesome weight gain, and she now carries close to 185 pounds on a 5′5″ frame. The extreme fatigue that is a hallmark of PPS is complicated by osteoarthritis in the joints of her upper extremities that came from years of walking in full leg braces with the aid of canes. Some days the fatigue and the joint pain are so disabling that she just stays in bed and sleeps, saying it is the only place she is comfortable.

JA was recently diagnosed with Paget's disease of the bone, a disorder characterized by the deterioration and demineralization of bone. In addition to exacerbating osteoarthritis and leading to loss of hearing, Paget's disease predisposes patients to the development of osteosarcoma, a rare and therapeutically challenging bone cancer. It is important that JA be treated for this disease because, in addition to these serious complications and the compounding of her pain, she would be at high risk for compression fractures from the stress she must put on her arms when she transfers to and from her wheelchair and power chair.

JA's current medications include the proton pump inhibitor pantoprazole sodium (Protonix) for gastric hyperacidity and pregabalin (Lyrica) for neuropathic pain in her feet. She takes 1,000 mg of elemental calcium daily (2 Viactiv calcium chews) and 2,000 IU of vitamin D. She is depending on you, her ambulatory care pharmacist, to select the right therapy to keep her going in the face of this newest health challenge. You contemplate the structures of three potential drug candidates shown below.

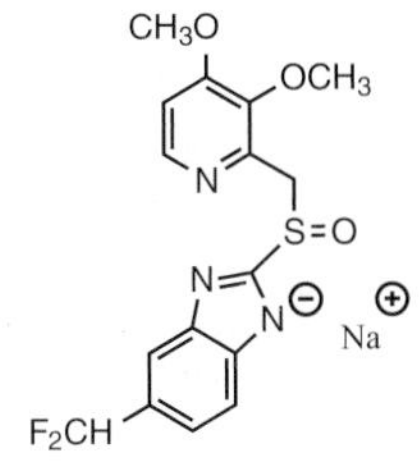

Pantoprazole sodium

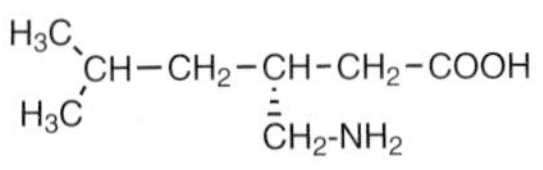

Pregabalin

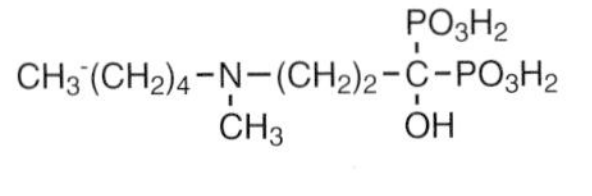

1

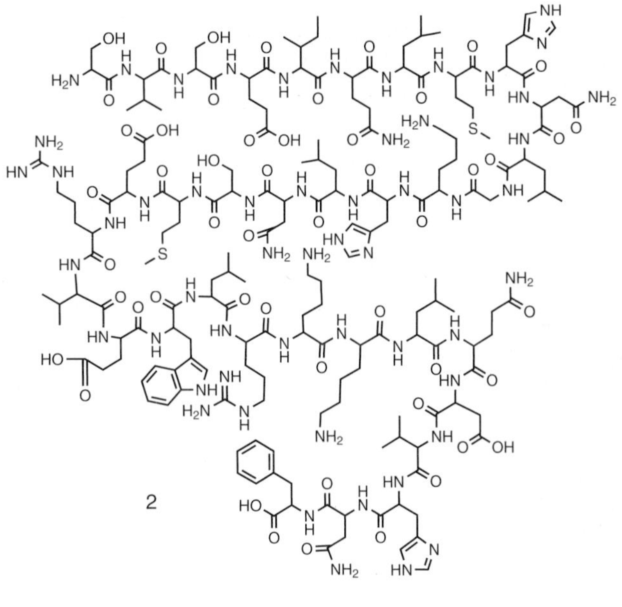

2

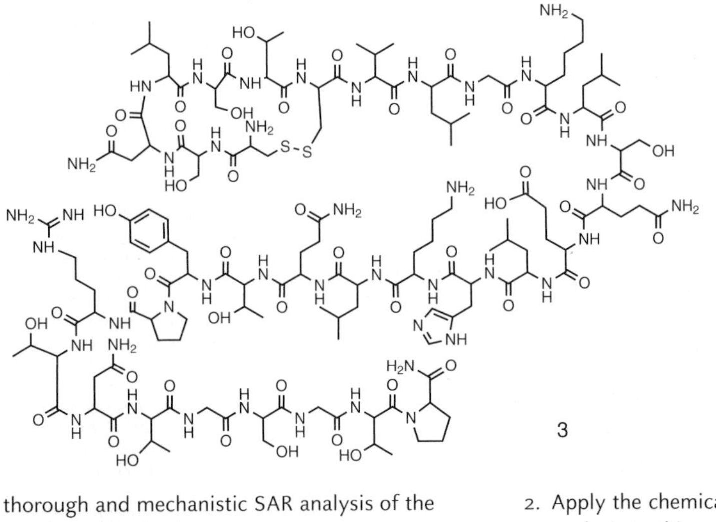

3

1. Conduct a thorough and mechanistic SAR analysis of the three therapeutic options in the case.
2. Apply the chemical understanding gained from the SAR analysis to this patient's specific needs to make a therapeutic recommendation.

References

1. Copp DH. Calcitonin: discovery, development, and clinical application. Clin Invest Med 1994;17:268–277.
2. Bouillon R, Carmeliet G, Boonen S. Aging and calcium metabolism. Bailliere's Clin Endocrinol Metab 1997;11:341–365.
3. Haines ST, Caceres B, Yancey L. Alternatives to estrogen replacement therapy for preventing osteoporosis. J Am Pharm Assoc 1996;36:707–715.
4. Christenson RH. Biochemical markers of bone metabolism: an overview. Clin Biochem 1997;30:573–593.
5. Miller DR, Hanel HJ. Prevention and treatment of osteoporosis. US Pharmacist 1999;24:81–90.
6. Rodan GA. Emerging therapies in osteoporosis. Ann Rpts Med Chem 1994;29:275–285.
7. Arnaud CD. Calcium homeostasis: regulatory elements and their integration. Fed Proc 1978;37:2557–2560.
8. Iqbal J, Zaidi M, Schneider AE. Cinacalcet hydrochloride. IDrugs 2003;6:587–592.
9. DeLuca HF, Zierold C. Mechanisms and functions of vitamin D. Nutr Rev 1998;56:S4–S10.
10. Raisz LG. Pathogenesis of osteoporosis: concepts, conflicts and prospects. J Clin Invest 2005;115:3318–3325.
11. U.S. Department of Health and Human Services. Chapter 2: the basics of bone in health and disease. In: Bone Health and Osteoporosis: A Report of the Surgeon General (2004). Available at: http://www.surgeongeneral.gov/library/bonehealth/. Accessed January 19, 2011.
12. Schaefer B, Cone S. Increasing awareness of osteoporosis: a community pharmacy's experience. US Pharmacist 1998;23:72–85.
13. Francis RM. Management of established osteoporosis. Br J Clin Pharmacol 1998;45:95–99.
14. Saljoughian M. Postmenopausal osteoporosis. US Pharmacy 2003;28:18–35.
15. Hansen LB, Follin Vondracek S. Prevention and treatment of nonpostmenopausal osteoporosis. Am J Health Syst Pharm 2004;61:2637–2656.
16. Watts NB, Bilezikian JP, Camacho PM, et al. American Association of Clinical Endocrinologists medical guidelines for clinical practice for the diagnosis and treatment of postmenopausal osteoporosis. Endocr Pract 2010;16(Suppl 3):1–37.
17. O'Connell MB, Borgelt LM, Bowles SK, et al. Drug-induced osteoporosis in the older adult. Aging Health 2010;6:501–518.
18. Reid DM, Harvie J. Secondary osteoporosis. Bailliere's Clin Endocrinol Metab 1997;11:83–99.
19. Diem SJ, Blackwell TL, Stone KL, et al. Use of antidepressants and rates of hip bone loss in older women. Arch Intern Med 2007;167:1240–1245.
20. Gray SL, LaCroix AZ, Larson J, et al. Proton pump inhibitor use, hip fracture and change in bone mineral density in postmenopausal women. Arch Intern Med 2010;179:765–771.
21. Riche DM, King ST. Bone loss and fracture risk associated with thiazolidinedione therapy. Pharmacotherapy 2010;30:716–727.
22. van Brussel MS, Bultink IE, Lems WF. Prevention of glucocorticoid-induced osteoporosis. Exp Opin Pharmacother 2009;10:997–1005.
23. National Osteoporosis Foundation. Clinicians guide to prevention and treatment of osteoporosis, revised January 2010. Available at: http://www.nof.org/sites/default/files/pdfs/NOF_ClinicianGuide2009_v7.pdf. Accessed January 10, 2011.
24. International Osteoporosis Foundation. Facts and statistics about osteoporosis and its impact. Available at: http://www.iofbonehealth.org/facts-and-statistics.html. Accessed January 10, 2011.
25. Barrett-Connor E, Siris ES, Wehren LE, et al. Osteoporosis and fracture risk in women of different ethnic groups. J Bone Miner Res 2005;20:185–194.
26. Tolar J, Teitelbaum SL, Orchard PJ. Osteopetrosis. N Engl J Med 2004;351:2839–2849.
27. Whyte MP, Wenkert D, Clements KL, et al. Bisphosphonate-induced osteoporosis. N Engl J Med 2003;349:457–463.
28. Suneja M. Hypocalcemia. Available at: http://www.emedicine.com/med/topic1118.htm. Updated September 3, 2010. Accessed January 21, 2011.
29. Block GA, Martin, KJ, De Francisco AL. Cinacalcet for secondary hyperparathyroidism in patients receiving hemodialysis. N Engl J Med 2004;350:1516–1525.
30. Reginster J-YL, LeCart M-P. Efficacy and safety of drugs for Paget's disease of bone. Bone 1995;17:485S–488S.
31. De Silva Jardine P, Thompson D. Antiosteoporosis agents. Ann Rpts Med Chem 1996;31:211–220.
32. Hisel TM, Phillips BB. Update on the treatment of osteoporosis. Formulary 2003;38:223–243.
33. Rossouw JE, et al. Risks and benefits of estrogen plus progestin in healthy postmenopausal women. Principal results from the Women's Health Initiative randomized controlled trial. JAMA 2002;288:321–333.
34. Women's Health Initiative Steering Committee. Effects of conjugated equine estrogen in postmenopausal women with hysterectomy. JAMA 2004;291: 1701–1712.
35. Greenblatt D. Treatment of postmenopausal osteoporosis. Pharmacotherapy 2005;25:574–584.
36. Francis RM. Bisphosphonates in the treatment of osteoporosis in 1997: a review. Curr Ther Res 1997;58:656–678.
37. Yates AJ, Rodan GA. Alendronate and osteoporosis. Drug Discov Today 1998;3:69–78.
38. Grese TA, Sluka JP, Bryant HU, et al. Benzopyran selective estrogen receptor modulators (SERMs): pharmacological effects and structural correlation with raloxifene. Bioorg Med Chem Lett 1996;6:903–908
39. Bryant HU, Glasebrook AL, Yang NN, et al. A pharmacologic review of raloxifene. J Bone Miner Metab 1996;14:1–9.
40. Kemp DC, Fan PW, Stevens JC. Characterization of raloxifene glucuronidation in vitro: contribution of intestinal metabolism to presystemic clearance. Drug Metab Dispos 2002;30:694–700.
41. Jeong EJ, Lin H, Hu M. Disposition mechanisms of raloxifene in the human intestinal Caco-2 model. J Pharmacol Exp Ther 2004;310:376–386.
42. Jeong EJ, Liu Y, Lin H, et al. Species- and disposition model-dependent metabolism of raloxifene in gut and liver: role of UGT1A10. Drug Metab Dispos 2005;33:785–794.
43. Gennari L. Ospemifene. Curr Opin Invest Drugs 2004;5:448–455.
44. Gruber C, Gruber D. Bazedoxifene. Curr Opin Invest Drugs 2004;5:1086–1093.
45. Diener KM. Bisphosphonates for controlling pain from metastatic bone disease. Am J Health Syst Pharm 1996;53:1917–1927.
46. Caggiano TJ, Zask A, Bex F. Recent advances in bone metabolism and osteoporosis research. Ann Rpts Med Chem 1991;26.
47. Ashworth L. Focus on alendronate. Formulary 1996;31:23–30.
48. Riley TN, DeRuitter J. New drug review. US Pharmacist 2003:95–104.
49. King AE, Umland EM. Osteonecrosis of the jaw in patients receiving intravenous or oral bisphosphonates. Pharmacotherapy 2008;28:667–677.
50. U.S.FoodandDrugAdministration.Bisphosphonates(osteoporosisdrugs):label change—atypical fractures update. Available at: http://www.fda.gov/Safety/MedWatch/SafetyInformation/SafetyAlertsforHumanMedicalProducts/ucm229244.htm. Accessed January 14, 2011.
51. Schmidt GA, Horner KE, McDanel DL, et al. Risks and benefits of long-term bisphosphonate therapy. Am J Health Syst Pharm 2010;67:e12–e19.
52. Reginster J. Calcitonin for prevention and treatment of osteoporosis. Am J Med 1993;95(Suppl 5A):44S–47S.
53. Gennari C, Agnusdei D, Camporeale A. Long-term treatment with calcitonin in osteoporosis. Horm Metab Res 1993;25:484–485.
54. Freeman TR. Teriparatide: a novel agent that builds new bone. J Am Pharm Assoc 2003;43:535–537.
55. LoBuono C. New osteoporosis drug is first to form bone. Drug Topics 2003:24.
56. American Pharmaceutical Association. Special Report. Therapeutic Options for Osteoporosis. Washington, DC: American Pharmaceutical Association, 1993.
57. Institute of Medicine, National Academy of Sciences. Dietary reference intakes for calcium and vitamin D. Available at: http://iom.edu/Reports/2010/Dietary-Reference-Intakes-for-Calcium-and-Vitamin-D/DRI-Values.aspx. Updated November 20, 2010.
58. Bolland MJ, Barber PA, Doughty RN, et al. Vascular events in healthy older women receiving calcium supplementation: randomized controlled trial. BMJ 2008;336:262–266.
59. American Pharmaceutical Association. New product bulletin. Miacalcin nasal spray. Washington, DC: American Pharmaceutical Association, 1996.
60. Pak CYC, Sakhaee K, Rubin C, et al. Update of fluoride in the treatment of osteoporosis. Endocrinologist 1998;8:15–20.
61. Bekker PJ, Holloway DL, Rasmussen AS, et al. A single-dose placebo-controlled study of AMG 162, a fully human monoclonal antibody to RANKL in postmenopausal women. J Bone Miner Res 2004;19:1059–1066.
62. Bone HG, McClung MR, Roux C, et al. Odanacatib, a cathepsin-K inhibitor for osteoporosis: a two year study in postmenopausal women with low bone density. J Bone Miner Res 2010;25:934–936.
63. Meunier PJ, Roux C, Seeman E, et al. The effects of strontium ranelate on the risk of vertebral fracture in women with postmenopausal osteoporosis. N Engl J Med 2004;350:459–468.
64. Reginster J-Y, Lecart M-P, Deroisy R, et al. Strontium ranelate—a new paradigm in the treatment of osteoporosis. Expert Opin Investig Drugs 2004;13:857–864.
65. Marie PJ. Strontium ranelate: a novel mode of action optimizing bone formation and resorption. Osteoporosis Int 2005;16(Suppl 1):S7–S10.
66. Gogakos AI, Cheung MS, Bassett JHD, et al. Bone signaling pathways and treatment of osteoporosis. Expert Rev Endocrinol Metab 2009;4:639–650.
67. Gonyeau M. Statins and osteoporosis: a clinical review. Pharmacotherapy 2005;25:229–243.
68. Richard AA, Harrison TM. Efficacy of HMG-CoA reductase inhibitors in treating osteoporosis. Am J Health Syst Pharm 2002;59:372–377.
69. Burkiewicz J, O'Connell MB. New approaches to the management of osteoporosis. American Pharmacists Association Highlights Newsletter 2010;13:S1–S12
70. Joy MS, Kshirsagar A, Franceschini N. Calcimimetics and the treatment of primary and secondary hyperparathyroidism. Ann Pharmacother 2004;38:171–180.
71. Franceschini N, Joy MS, Kshirsagar A. Cinacalcet HCl: a calcimimetic agent for the treatment of primary and secondary hypoparathyroidism. Expert Opin Investig Drugs 2003;12:1413–1421.
72. Hussar DA. New drugs of 2004. J Am Pharm Assoc 2005;45:185–218.
73. Michaelson MD, Smith MR. Bisphosphonates for treatment and prevention of bone metastases. J Clin Oncol 2005;23:8219–8224.
74. Zometa prescribing information. Available at: http://www.pharma.us.novartis.com/product/pi/pdf/Zometa.pdf. Updated October 2009. Accessed January 20, 2011.
75. Van Poznak CH. The use of bisphosphonates in patients with breast cancer. Cancer Control 2002;9:480–489.

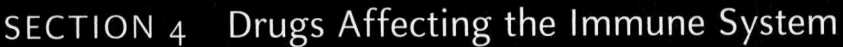

Chapter 31

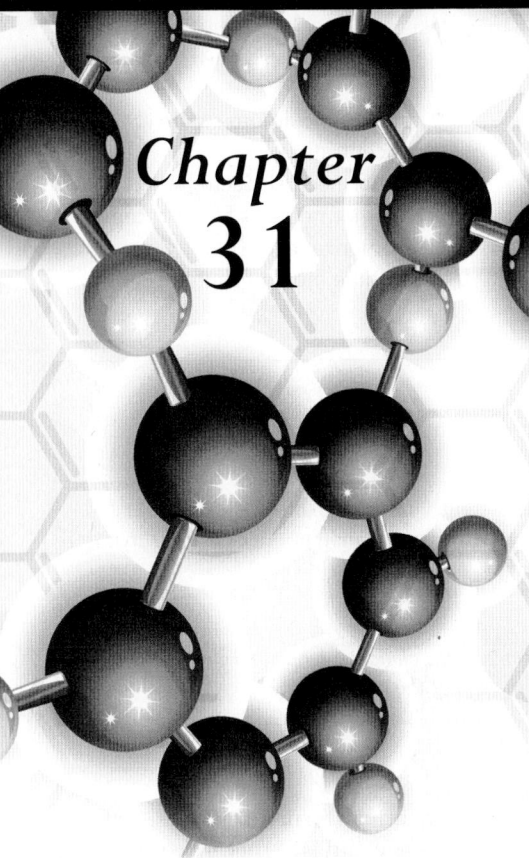

Nonsteroidal Anti-Inflammatory Drugs

RONALD BORNE, MARK LEVI, AND NORMAN WILSON

Drugs Covered in This Chapter

ANTIPYRETIC ANALGESICS
- Acetaminophen

ANTI-INFLAMMATORY ANALGESICS
- Aspirin and other salicylates
- Bromfenac
- Diclofenac
- Diflunisal
- Etodolac
- Fenoprofen
- Flurbiprofen
- Ibuprofen
- Indomethacin
- Ketoprofen
- Ketorolac
- Mefenamic acid
- Meclofenamic acid
- Meloxicam
- Nabumetone
- Naproxen
- Oxaprozin
- Piroxicam
- Sulindac
- Suprofen
- Tolmetin

COX-2 INHIBITORS
- Celecoxib

DISEASE-MODIFYING DRUGS FOR ARTHRITIS
- Abatacept
- Adalimumab
- Anakinra
- Certolizumab
- Etanercept
- Gold salts
- Golimumab
- Hydroxychloroquine
- Infliximab
- Leflunomide
- Methotrexate
- Rituximab
- Sulfasalazine
- Tocilizumab

DRUGS FOR THE TREATMENT OF GOUT
- Allopurinol
- Colchicine
- Febuxostat
- Pegloticase
- Probenecid
- Sulfinpyrazone

Abbreviations

APC, antigen-presenting cell
5-ASA, 5-aminosalicylic acid
AUC, area under the curve
C_{max}, maximum plasma concentration
C_{mim}, minimum plasma concentration
CNS, central nervous system
COX, cyclooxygenase
CTLA-4, cytotoxic T-lymphocyte antigen-4
CYP, cytochrome P450
DMARD, disease-modifying antirheumatic drug
ED_{50}, median effective dose
FAAH, fatty acid amide hydrolase
FDA, U.S. Food and Drug Administration
GI, gastrointestinal
GPCR, G protein–coupled receptor
HPETE, hydroperoxy-eicosatetraenoic acid
IC_{90}, 90% of maximal inhibitory concentration
ID_{50}, half maximal inhibitory concentration
Ig, immunoglobulin
IL, interleukin
IM, intramuscular
IV, intravenous
JAK, Janus activated kinase
LT, leukotriene
6MNA, 6-methoxynaphthalene-2-acetic acid

Abbreviations (Continued)

μM, micromoles/L
mPEG, monomethoxypoly(ethylene glycol)
NF-κB, nuclear factor-κB
NSAID, nonsteroidal anti-inflammatory drug
OTC, over the counter
PEG, polyethylene glycol
PG, prostaglandin
SRS-A, slow reacting substance of anaphylaxis
T_{max}, time to maximum serum concentration
TNF, tumor necrosis factor
TNFR, tumor necrosis factor receptor
TX, thromboxane
UMP, uridine monophosphate

SCENARIO

Jill T. Johnson, PharmD, BCPS

EB is a 53-year-old woman who has had rheumatoid arthritis for the past 20 years. She occasionally wakes with swollen joints but is relatively well controlled with methotrexate and hydroxychloroquine. She does not feel she is severe enough to require anti–tumor necrosis factor drugs at this point. On days she has painful joints, she takes a nonsteroidal drug. Recently she has become fearful of developing a stomach ulcer because she has to take nonsteroidal drugs quite often. She usually takes naproxen but wonders if there is another effective drug that is safer.

(The reader is directed to the clinical solution and chemical analysis of this case at the end of the chapter).

INTRODUCTION

The classification of drugs covered in this chapter as nonsteroidal anti-inflammatory drugs (NSAIDs) is somewhat misleading, because many of these entities possess antipyretic and analgesic properties in addition to anti-inflammatory properties, which are useful in the treatment of a number of rheumatic disorders. On the other hand, there are drugs that possess analgesic/antipyretic properties but are essentially devoid of anti-inflammatory activity. Additionally, drugs that possess uricosuric properties useful in the treatment of gout will be covered here. The prototype agent of the NSAIDs is acetylsalicylic acid, aspirin, which has therapeutically useful analgesic, antipyretic, and anti-inflammatory actions; other drugs to be covered can possess only one or two of these properties. The corticosteroids that are useful anti-inflammatory drugs are covered separately in Chapter 28.

NSAIDs continue to be one of the more widely used groups of therapeutic drugs. The medicinal drugs covered in this chapter represent a major market in both prescription and nonprescription drugs. Other than caffeine or ethyl alcohol, aspirin remains the most widely used of all drugs (1). As a class, NSAIDs represent one of the most widely used prescription and over-the-counter (OTC) drugs. Rheumatic diseases (Table 31.1) (2) are inflammatory disorders affecting more individuals than any chronic illness and are the most common form of disability in the United States. Based on data obtained from 2003-5 from the National Health Interview Survey, the Centers for Disease Control and Prevention (3,4) estimates that over 46 million adults have self-reported doctor-diagnosed arthritis, whereas 19 million have arthritis and arthritis-attributable limited activity. Women report significantly higher age-related prevalence than men in nearly all forms of arthritis. Arthritis prevalence increases with age and is higher in women than men in every age group. Arthritis affects all race and ethnic groups with whites being affected approximately nine times more than blacks and Hispanics. Approximately 300,000 children under the age of 18 have some form of arthritis or rheumatoid illness. Individuals who are overweight or obese report more physician-diagnosed arthritis than individuals possessing a lower body mass index. Almost two-thirds of adults with arthritis are overweight, whereas only 16% of those who are underweight or normal weight are affected by the disorder. Osteoarthritis is the most common form of arthritis in the United States, whereas rheumatoid arthritis affects approximately 1.3 million Americans. Because the number of Americans reporting a disability has increased approximately 8% in the past decade, the use of NSAIDs will increase as Americans experience a greater life expectancy. However, the development of new NSAIDs has slowed down because of recent controversies surrounding the safety of selective cyclooxygenase (COX)-2 inhibitors.

The diseases mentioned are considered to be host defense mechanisms. Inflammation is a normal and essential response to any noxious stimulus that threatens the host and can vary from a localized response to a generalized response (5). The resulting inflammation can be summarized as follows: 1) initial injury causing release of inflammatory mediators (e.g., histamine, serotonin, leukokinins, SRS-A, lysosomal enzymes, lymphokinins, and prostaglandins); 2) vasodilation; 3) increased vascular permeability and exudation; 4) leukocyte migration, chemotaxis, and phagocytosis; and 5) proliferation of connective tissue cells. The most common sources of chemical mediators include neutrophils, basophils, mast cells, platelets, macrophages, and lymphocytes. The etiology of inflammatory and arthritic diseases has received a great deal of recent attention but remains, for the most part, unresolved, hindering the development of new agents that are curative in nature. Currently available drugs relieve the symptoms of the disease but are not considered curative.

Anti-inflammatory drugs can act by interfering with any one of several mechanisms, including immunologic mechanisms such as antibody production or antigen–antibody complexation, activation of complement, cellular activities such as phagocytosis, interference with the formation and release of the chemical mediators of inflammation, or stabilization of lysosomal membranes. The complement system (6–9) is one component of the host defense system that aids in the elimination of various microorganisms and antigens from blood and tissues. Although complement normally has a functional role in the development of disease states, excessive complement activation, by promoting inflammation locally, is detrimental. Individuals with a deficiency of individual complement proteins, however, either acquired or hereditary, are more susceptible to infections caused by pyrogenic bacteria and diseases resulting from the generation of autoantibodies and immune complexes. Complement proteins are numbered C1 to C9, and their cleavage products are indicated by the suffixes a, b, and so on. The complement system consists of two activating pathways (an antibody-mediated classical pathway and a nonimmunologically activated alternate pathway), a single termination pathway, regulatory proteins, and complement receptors and involves approximately 30 membrane and plasma proteins (7). A major function of complement is to mark antigens and microorganisms with C3 fragments that direct them to cells containing C3 receptors, such as phagocytic cells (7). Complement has been implicated

TABLE 31.1 Classification of Rheumatic Diseases

Classification	Diseases
Acute and chronic polyarthritis and other synovial diseases	Rheumatoid arthritis
Infection-related rheumatic diseases	Septic arthritis Osteomyelitis Lyme disease Rheumatic fever
Spondyloarthropathies	Ankylosing spondylitis Reactive arthritis Psoriatic arthritis Enteropathic spondyloarthropathy (arthritis of inflammatory bowel disease)
Osteoarthritis and related degenerative diseases	
Crystal-induced arthropathies	Gout (monosodium urate) Calcium pyrophosphate dehydrate, apatite, and other calcium crystals deposited in the joint
Metabolic bone disease	Osteoporosis
Connective tissue disease	Systemic lupus erythematosus Scleroderma/polymyositis Mixed connective tissue disease
Musculoskeletal diseases (regional pain syndromes)	Neck, lower back, and lumbar spine stenosis, shoulder, elbow, wrist and hand, hip, and knee
Inflammatory muscle (nonarticular) diseases	Fibromyalgia Bursitis Tendinitis
Vasculitis	Polymyalgia rheumatica
Sjögren syndrome	
Neoplasms	
Drug-induced rheumatologic syndromes	Systemic lupus erythematosus Glucocorticoid-induced arthritis Scleroderma (acrosclerosis) Vasculitis Statin-induced myositis

From Klippel JH, Wayand CM, Wortmann R, et al., eds. Primer on the Rheumatic Diseases, 12th Ed. Atlanta, GA: Arthritis Foundation, 2001; with permission.

CLINICAL SIGNIFICANCE

The arachidonic acid pathway that leads to the production of inflammatory mediators provides several targets for intervention on inflammation. The most widely used nonsteroidal anti-inflammatory agents NSAIDs in practice today are drugs such as aspirin, naproxen, ibuprofen, and diclofenac, which inhibit the cyclo-oxygenase enzymes. Although specific NSAIDs have found their niches in particular disease states, the NSAIDs work by the same mechanism with few exceptions. Aspirin, a salicylate, is somewhat different from the other agents; its property of irreversibly inhibiting platelet homeostasis works to its advantage and broadens its use in coronary artery disease prophylaxis, for which it has been shown to reduce mortality, whereas the others have not. Other salicylate varieties lack the ability to irreversibly inhibit platelet function and are therefore not clinically useful in this way.

Variations of the molecular structures have provided improved side effect profiles of agents used. For example, although phenacetin and acetaminophen are not anti-inflammatory agents, they are included in this chapter because they are analgesics and antipyretics and illustrate the point that improvement in molecular structure from phenacetin to acetaminophen helped to reduce the hepatotoxicity and risk for drug-induced hemolytic anemia, with which phenacetin was associated when it was on the market in the past.

Changes to the currently available NSAIDs drugs are being made constantly, hence the abundance of "me-too" drugs. Gastrointestinal (GI) bleeding and complications are the most feared consequence of taking these drugs; therefore, emphasis on minimizing these risks has been one of the motivations to develop less offensive agents. Gastrointestinal side effects are believed to be related to indirect toxic effects (inhibiting COX enzymes) and direct toxic effects (local irritation to the GI mucosa). Molecular changes have been made to the various NSAIDs to produce more potent compounds, reduce the direct irritant effects, and to create prodrugs that lack the direct irritant effect altogether. Other changes have resulted in compounds with no more potency but with lower incidence of GI side effects, which still represents a therapeutic advantage.

As can be seen, a through understanding and appreciation of the chemical nature of the NSAIDs is directly linked to clinically significant endpoints and positive therapeutic outcomes.

Jill T. Johnson, Pharm.D., BCPS
Associate Professor
Department of Pharmacy Practice
College of Pharmacy
University of Arkansas for Medical Sciences
Little Rock, Arkansas

in numerous diseases, including allergic, hematologic, dermatologic, infectious, renal, hepatic inflammatory (rheumatoid arthritis and systemic lupus erythematosus), pulmonary, and others (e.g., multiple sclerosis and myasthenia gravis). Complement activation can induce the synthesis or release of inflammatory mediators, such as interleukin-1 (a potent proinflammatory cytokine) and prostaglandins (e.g., PGE_2). Leukotrienes (e.g., LTB_4) and thromboxanes are also released. Complement also aids the immigration of phagocytes associated with inflammation. Thus, inhibition of the complement system by controlling its activation or inhibiting those active fragments that are produced should be beneficial in reducing or eliminating tissue damage associated with inflammatory diseases.

ROLE OF CHEMICAL MEDIATORS IN INFLAMMATION

As indicated previously, a number of chemical mediators have been postulated to have important roles in the inflammatory process. Before 1971, the proposal by Shen (10,11) that the NSAIDs exert their effects by interacting with a hypothetical anti-inflammatory receptor was widely accepted. The topography of the proposed receptor was based on known structure–activity relationships primarily within the series of indole acetic acid derivatives, of which indomethacin was the prototype. Most NSAIDs, whether they be salicylates, arylalkanoic acids, oxicams, or anthranilic acid derivatives, possess the common structural features of an acidic center, an aromatic or heteroaromatic ring, and an additional center of lipophilicity in the form of either an alkyl chain or an additional aromatic ring. The proposed receptor to which indomethacin was postulated to bind consisted of a cationic site to which the carboxylate anion would bind, a flat area to which the indole ring would bind through van der Waals forces, and an out-of-the-plane trough to which the benzene ring of the *p*-chlorobenzoyl group would bind through hydrophobic or charge-transfer interactions. Additional binding sites for the methoxy and carbonyl groups were also suggested. In 1971, Vane (12) published a classic paper in which he reported that indomethacin, aspirin, and salicylate, in descending order of potency, inhibited the biosynthesis of prostaglandins from arachidonic acid using cell-free preparations of guinea pig lung, and he further suggested that the clinical actions of these drugs resulted from the inhibition of prostaglandins. Vane's theory has become the most widely accepted mechanism of action of NSAIDs. Gund and Shen (13) subsequently modified Vane's hypothesis and proposed that the earlier anti-inflammatory receptor model actually described the active site of the key enzyme in prostaglandin biosynthesis (i.e., prostaglandin cyclooxygenase). However, the complexity of the arachidonic acid pathway and the existence of several isoforms of the cyclooxygenase system have limited the relevance of this model.

Prostaglandins, Thromboxanes, Prostacyclin, and Leukotrienes

Prostaglandins

Prostaglandins are naturally occurring, 20-carbon, cyclopentano–fatty acid derivatives produced in mammalian tissue from polyunsaturated fatty acids. They belong to the class of eicosanoids, a member of the group of autocoids derived from membrane phospholipids. The eicosanoids are derived from unsaturated fatty acids and include the following groups of compounds: prostaglandins, thromboxanes, prostacyclin, and leukotrienes. They have been found in essentially every compartment of the body. In 1931, Kurzrok and Lieb (14) reported that human seminal fluid possessed potent contractile and relaxant effects on uterine smooth muscle. Shortly thereafter, Goldblatt (15) in England and von Euler (16) in Sweden independently reported vasodepressor and smooth muscle–contracting properties in seminal fluid (semen); von Euler identified the active constituent as a lipophilic acidic substance, which he termed "prostaglandin." These observations attracted little attention during World War II, but shortly thereafter, primarily through the efforts of Bergstrom and Samuelsson (17), it was realized that von Euler's prostaglandin was actually a mixture of a number of structurally related fatty acids. The first report of the structure of the prostaglandins in 1962 stimulated several studies relating to the chemical and biologic properties of these potent substances.

Prostaglandin Structure

The general structure of the prostaglandins is shown in Figure 31.1. All naturally occurring prostaglandins possess the following substitution pattern: a 15α-hydroxy group and a *trans* double bond at C-13. Unless a double bond occurs at the C-8, C-12 positions, the two side chains (the carboxyl-bearing chain termed the α-chain and the hydroxyl-bearing chain termed the β-chain) are of the *trans* stereochemistry depicted in Figure 31.1. The prostaglandins are classified by the capital letters A, B, C, D, E, F, G, H, and I (e.g., PGA, PGB, and so on) depending on the nature and stereochemistry of oxygen substituents at the 9- and 11-positions. For example, members of the PGE series possess a keto function at C-9 and an α-hydroxyl group at C-11, whereas members of the PGF series possess α-hydroxyl groups at both of these positions. Members of the PGG and PGH series are cycloendoperoxide intermediates in the biosynthesis of prostaglandins, as depicted in Figure 31.2. The number of double bonds in the side chains connected to the cyclopentane ring is designated by subscripts 1, 2, or 3, indicative of the nature of the fatty acid precursor. The subscript 2 indicates an additional *cis* double bond at the C-5, C-6 positions, and the subscript 3 indicates a third double bond of *cis* stereochemistry at the C-17, C-18 positions.

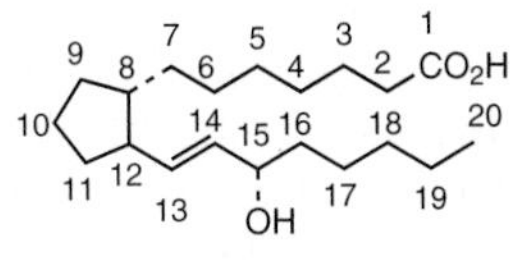

FIGURE 31.1 General structure of prostaglandins.

Prostaglandin Biosynthesis

Prostaglandins are derived biosynthetically from unsaturated fatty acid precursors (Fig. 31.2). The number of double bonds contained in the naturally occurring prostaglandins reflects the nature of the biosynthetic precursors. Those containing one double bond are derived from 8,11,14-eicosatrienoic acid, those with two double bonds from arachidonic acid (5,8,11,14-eicosatetraenoic acid), and those with three double bonds from 5,8,11,14,17-eicosapentenoic acid. The most common of these fatty acids in humans is arachidonic acid; hence, prostaglandins of the 2 series have an important biologic role. Arachidonic acid is derived from dietary linoleic acid or is ingested from the diet (18) and esterified to phospholipids (primarily phosphatidylethanolamine or phosphatidylcholine) in cell membranes. Various initiating factors interact with membrane receptors coupled to G proteins (guanine nucleotide–binding regulatory proteins) activating phospholipase A_2, which in turn hydrolyzes membrane phospholipids resulting in the release of arachidonic acid. Other phospholipases (e.g.,

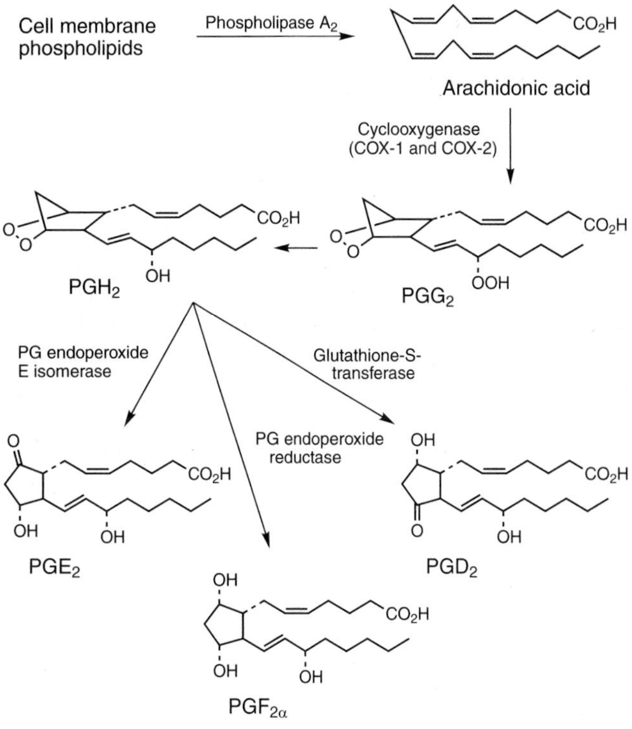

FIGURE 31.2 Biosynthesis of prostaglandins from arachidonic acid.

phospholipase C) are also involved. Phospholipase C differs from phospholipase A_2 by inducing the formation of 1,2-diglycerides from phospholipids with the subsequent release of arachidonic acid by the actions of mono- and diglyceride lipases on the diglyceride (16). A polypeptide produced by leukocytes, interleukin-1, which mediates inflammation, increases phospholipase activity and, thus, prostaglandin biosynthesis. The steroidal anti-inflammatory drugs (corticosteroids) appear to act, in part, by inhibiting these phospholipases, particularly phospholipase A_2. The liberated arachidonic acid can then be acted on by two major enzyme systems: by arachidonic acid cyclooxygenase (prostaglandin endoperoxide synthetase, COX) to produce prostaglandins, thromboxanes, and prostacyclin, or by lipoxygenases to produce leukotrienes.

Cyclooxygenases

Interaction of arachidonic acid with cyclooxygenase (COX) in the presence of oxygen and heme produces, first, the cyclic endoperoxide, PGG_2, and then, through its peroxidase activity, PGH_2, both of which are chemically unstable and decompose rapidly (half-life, 5 minutes). The PGE_2 is formed by the action of PGE isomerase and PGD_2 by the actions of isomerases or glutathione-*S*-transferase on PGH_2, whereas $PGF_{2\alpha}$ is formed from PGH_2 via an endoperoxide reductase system (Fig. 31.2). It is the COX step at which the NSAIDs inhibit prostaglandin biosynthesis to prevent inflammation. Because PGG_2 and PGH_2 themselves can possess the ability to mediate the pain responses and produce vasoconstriction and because PGG_2 can mediate the inflammatory response, COX inhibition would have a profound effect on the reduction of inflammation.

To date, three isoforms of COX have been identified: COX-1, COX-2, and COX-3. COX was first purified in 1976 (19). Among the more significant advances of the past decade was the isolation of a second isoform of the COX enzyme, COX-2, the expression of which is inducible by cytokines and growth factors (20–24). In 2002, a third distinct COX isoform, COX-3 was reported (25) in addition to two smaller COX-1–derived proteins (partial COX-1, or PCOX-1, proteins, termed PCOX-1α and PCOX-1β). The primary mechanism by which NSAIDS are held to produce their pharmacologic effects is attributed to inhibition of the COX-1 and COX-2 enzymes. Both isoforms carry out the same two reactions in the PG biosynthetic pathway: the double dioxygenation of arachidonic acid to PGG_2 at the cyclooxygenase active site and the subsequent reduction to PGH_2 at the peroxidase site (26).

It has been long known that acetaminophen possesses analgesic and antipyretic activity but little, if any, anti-inflammatory activity. Thus, the identification of COX-3 can be of importance, because COX-3 is selectively inhibited by analgesic/antipyretic drugs and is potently inhibited by some NSAIDs. Inhibition of COX-3 can represent a primary central mechanism by which acetaminophen decreases pain and fever (discussed later).

Both COX-1 and COX-2 are very similar in structure (27,28) and almost identical in length, varying from 599 (human) to 602 (mice) amino acids for COX-1 and from 603 (mice) to 604 (human) amino acids for COX-2. Both isoforms possess molecular masses of 70 to 74 kd and contain just over 600 amino acids, with an approximately 60% homology within the same species (29,30). Cyclooxygenase-2 contains an 18–amino acid insert near the C-terminal end of the enzyme that is not present in COX-1, but all other residues that have been previously identified as being essential to the catalytic activity of COX-1 are present in COX-2. Both isoforms have been cloned from various species, including human, and are heme-containing membrane proteins that exist as dimers (29). The three-dimensional radiographic crystal structure of COX-2 derived from human or murine sources can be superimposed on that of COX-1. Residues that form the substrate binding channel, the catalytic sites, and those residues immediately adjacent are essentially identical with the exception of two minor differences. The isoleucine at positions 434 and 523 in COX-1 is exchanged for valine in COX-2. The smaller size of Val^{523} in COX-2 allows inhibitor access to a side pocket off the main substrate channel, whereas the longer side chain of Ile in COX-1 sterically blocks inhibitor access. The available space in the binding pocket of COX-2 is 20% to 25% larger than the COX-1 binding site because of the replacement of the smaller Val^{523} in COX-2 for the larger Ile^{523} in COX-1. A major difference between COX-1 and COX-2 is that COX-2 lacks a sequence of 17 amino acids from the N-terminus but contains a sequence of 18 amino acids at the C-terminus. The sequence differences cause a disparity in the numbering systems of the two isoforms such that the serine residue acetylated by aspirin in COX-1 is numbered Ser^{530}, whereas in COX-2, the serine residue acetylated is Ser^{516}. Yet, the amino acid residues that are thought to be responsible for providing the catalytic role are the same, with both isoforms displaying similar ability to convert arachidonic acid to PGH_2. COX-1 appears to be more specific than COX-2 for fatty acid substrates, because COX-2 accepts a wider range of fatty acid substrates than COX-1. COX-1 primarily metabolizes arachidonic acid, and COX-2 metabolizes C-18 and C-20 fatty acid substrates. Selective inhibitors of COX-2 do not bind to Arg-120, which is used by the —COOH of arachidonic acid and the carboxylic acid selective or nonselective COX-1 inhibitors. The active site cavities of COX-1 and COX-2 are illustrated in Figure 31.3 (27).

From a therapeutic standpoint, the major difference between COX-1 and COX-2 lies in physiologic function rather than in structure. Little COX-2 is present in resting cells, but its expression can be induced by cytokines in vascular smooth muscle, fibroblasts, and epithelial cells, leading to the suggestion that COX-1 functions to produce prostaglandins that are involved in normal cellular activity (protection of gastric mucosa, maintenance of kidney function) and COX-2 to produce prostaglandins at inflammatory sites (31). Inducible COX-2 linked

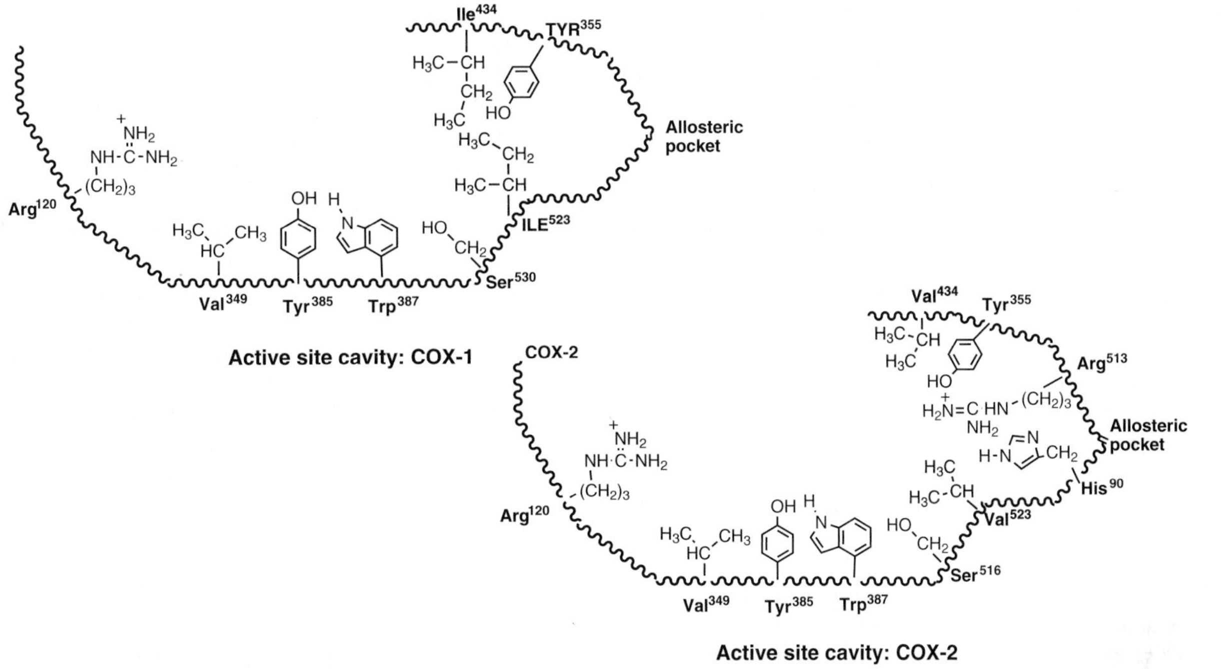

FIGURE 31.3 Representations of COX-1 and COX-2 active sites. (From Roche VF. A receptor-grounded approach to teaching nonsteroidal anti-inflammatory drug chemistry and structure-activity relationhips. Am J Pharm Educ 2009;78:143.)

to inflammatory cell types and tissues is believed to be the target enzyme in the treatment of inflammatory disorders by NSAIDs. Until recently, most NSAIDs inhibited both COX-1 and COX-2, but with varying degrees of selectivity. Selective COX-2 inhibitors can eliminate side effects associated with NSAIDs because of COX-1 inhibition, such as gastric and renal effects.

Prostaglandin Metabolism

Prostaglandins are rapidly metabolized and inactivated by various oxidative and reductive pathways. The initial step involves rapid oxidation of the 15α-OH to the corresponding ketone by the prostaglandin-specific enzyme, prostaglandin 15-OH dehydrogenase, which is followed by reduction of the C-13, C-14 double bond by prostaglandin Δ^{13}-reductase to the corresponding dihydro ketone, which for PGE_2 represents the major metabolite in plasma. Subsequently, enzymes normally involved in β- and ω-oxidation of fatty acids more slowly cleave the α-chain and oxidize the C-20 terminal methyl group to the carboxylic acid derivative, respectively. Hence, dicarboxylic acid derivatives containing only 16 carbon atoms are the major excreted metabolites of PGE_1 and PGE_2.

The effects of prostaglandins on the gastrointestinal (GI) tract deserve special mention. The PGEs and PGI_2 inhibit gastric secretion that can be induced by gastrin or histamine. Prostaglandins appear to have a major cytoprotective role in maintaining the integrity of gastric mucosa. PGE_1 exerts a protective effect on gastroduodenal mucosa by stimulating secretion of an alkaline mucus and bicarbonate ion and by maintaining or increasing mucosal blood flow. Thus, inhibition of prostaglandin formation in joints produces favorable results, as indicated by a reduction in fever, pain, and swelling. Inhibition of prostaglandin biosynthesis in the GI tract is unfavorable, however, because it can cause disruption of mucosal integrity, resulting in peptic ulcer disease that, as will be discussed later, is commonly associated with the use of NSAIDs and aspirin.

Prostaglandins as Drugs

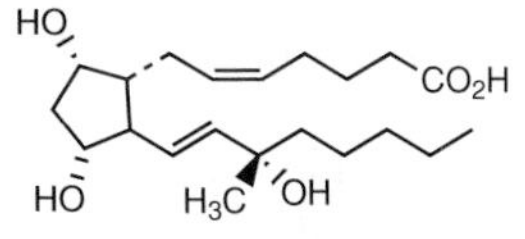

Carboprost tromethamine

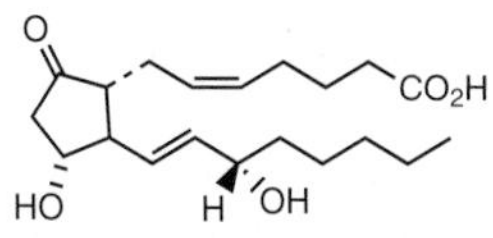

Dinoprostone (PGE_2)

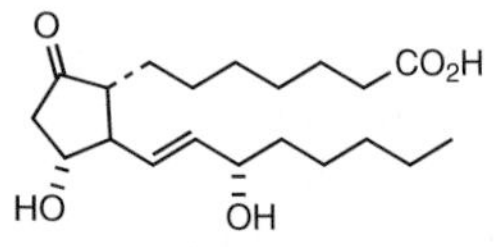

Alprostadil (PGE_1)

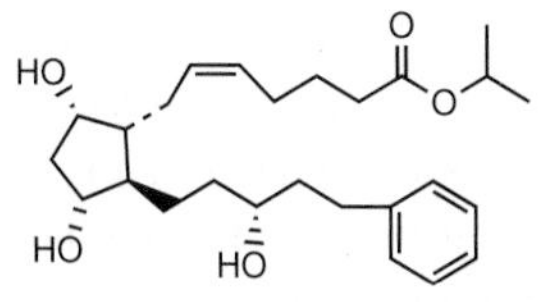

Latanoprost

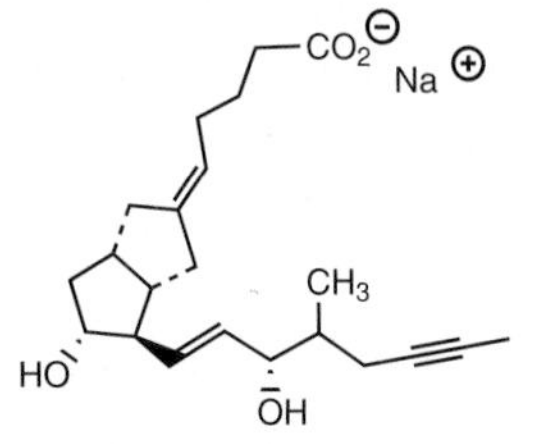

Iloprost

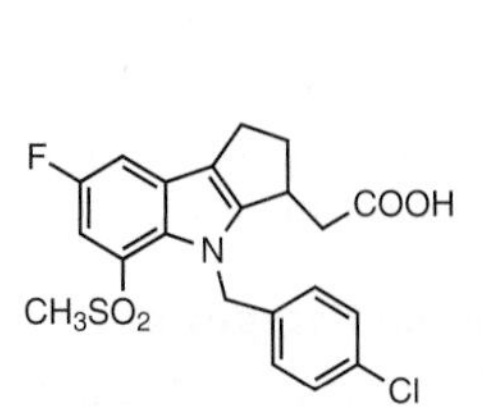

Laropiprant (approved in EU)

The promise of prostaglandins as therapeutically effective drugs has been limited because of the pharmacologic diversity displayed by prostaglandins and the metabolic instability observed with their administration. The pharmacologic actions of the various prostaglandins are quite diverse. When administered intravaginally, PGE_2 will stimulate the endometrium of the gravid uterus to contract in a manner similar to uterine contractions observed during labor. Thus, PGE_2 is therapeutically available as dinoprostone (Prostin E2) for use as an abortifacient at 12 to 20 weeks of gestation and for evacuation of uterine content in missed abortion or intrauterine fetal death up to 28 weeks of gestation. Additionally, PGE_2 is a potent stimulator of smooth muscle of the GI tract and can elevate body temperature in addition to possessing potent vasodilating properties in most vascular tissue while possessing constrictor effects at certain sites. The PGEs in general cause pain when administered via the intradermal route. Many of these properties are shared by $PGF_{2\alpha}$, which is also therapeutically available as an abortifacient at 16 to 20 weeks of gestation and is available as dinoprost tromethamine (Prostin F2α). The synthetic 15-methyl derivative of $PGF_{2\alpha}$, carboprost, is also available as the tromethamine salt (Prostin 15/M) as an abortifacient at 13 to 20 of weeks gestation. However, $PGF_{2\alpha}$ differs from PGE_2 in that it does not significantly alter blood pressure in humans. PGD_2 causes both vasodilation and vasoconstriction. The PGEs produce a relaxation of bronchial and tracheal smooth muscle, but the PGFs and PGD_2 cause contraction. PGE_1 is available as alprostadil (Prostin VR Pediatric) to maintain patency of the ductus arteriosus in neonates until surgery can be performed to correct congenital heart defects.

Prostaglandins have been shown to reduce intraocular pressure by increasing the outflow of aqueous humor, and structurally modified prostaglandin analogs have thus found a place in the treatment of glaucoma. The most widely used of these agents is latanoprost (Xalatan), but travaprost (Travatan), bimatoprost (Lumigan), and unoprostone (Rescula) are also available.

Iloprost (Ventavis), a synthetic analog of the metabolically unstable prostacyclin, is indicated for the treatment of pulmonary arterial hypertension, scleroderma, Raynaud phenomenon, and ischemia. It is marketed as the side chain 3*S*, 4-*RS*-isomer but the 4*S*-isomer is substantially more potent than the 4*R*-isomer.

Antagonists at prostaglandin receptors also hold therapeutic promise. Laropiprant, an antagonist at the PGD_2 receptor subtype 1 (DP1), is effective in suppressing niacin-induced vasodilation, an adverse effect of niacin that limits its use in dyslipidemia. A combination of nicotinic acid and laropiprant has been approved in Europe as a lipid-modifying therapy for patients with dyslipidemia and primary hypercholesterolemia.

Prostanoid Receptors

The existence of distinct prostaglandin receptors can explain the broad spectrum of action displayed by the prostaglandins (32,33). Prostaglandins exert their various effects by activating G protein–coupled receptors (GPCRs). Ten members of the prostanoid receptor family have been identified (DP_{1-2}, EP_{1-4}, FP, IP_{1-2}, and TP). The nomenclature of these receptors is based on the affinity displayed by natural prostaglandins, prostacyclin, or thromboxanes at each receptor type. Thus, EP receptors are those receptors for which the PGEs have high affinity, FP receptors are those for PGFs, DP receptors are those for PGDs, IP receptors are those for PGI_2, and TP receptors are those for thromboxane (TX) A_2. These receptors are coupled through G proteins to effector mechanisms that include stimulation of adenylate (or adenylyl) cyclase and, hence, increased cyclic adenosine monophosphate levels and phospholipase C, which results in increased levels of inositol-1,4,5-triphosphate. Three distinct receptors for leukotrienes have been identified as well.

Nonprostanoid Products of the Arachidonic Acid Pathway

In addition to forming the various prostaglandins, nonprostanoids can also be formed from PGH_2, as illustrated in Figure 31.4. Thromboxane synthetase acts on PGH_2 to produce TXA_2, whereas prostacyclin synthetase converts PGH_2 to prostacyclin (PGI_2), both of which possess short biologic half-lives. A potent vasoconstrictor and inducer of platelet aggregation, TXA_2 has a biologic half-life of approximately 30 seconds, being rapidly nonenzymatically converted to the more stable, but inactive, TXB_2. Prostacyclin, a potent hypotensive and inhibitor of platelet aggregation, has a half-life of approximately 3 minutes and is nonenzymatically converted to 6-keto-$PGF_{1\alpha}$. Platelets contain primarily thromboxane synthetase, whereas endothelial cells contain primarily prostacyclin synthetase. Considerable research efforts are being expended in the development of stable prostacyclin analogs and thromboxane antagonists as cardiovascular drugs. The pharmacologic effects of some prostaglandins, TXA_2, and prostacyclin are summarized in Table 31.2.

Leukotrienes Lipoxygenases are a group of enzymes that oxidize polyunsaturated fatty acids possessing two *cis* double bonds separated by a methylene group to produce lipid hydroperoxides (34). Arachidonic acid is thus metabolized to a number of hydroperoxy-eicosatetraenoic acid (HPETE) derivatives. Lipoxygenases differ in the position at which they peroxidize arachidonic acid and in their tissue specificity. For example, platelets possess only a 12-lipoxygenase, whereas leukocytes possess both a 12-lipoxygenase and a 5-lipoxygenase (35). The HPETE derivatives are not stable, being rapidly converted to a number of metabolites. Leukotrienes are products of the 5-lipoxygenase pathway and are divided into two major classes: hydroxylated eicosatetraenoic acids (LTs), represented by LTB_4, and peptidoleukotrienes (pLTs), such as LTC_4, LTD_4, and LTE_4. 5-Lipoxygenase will produce

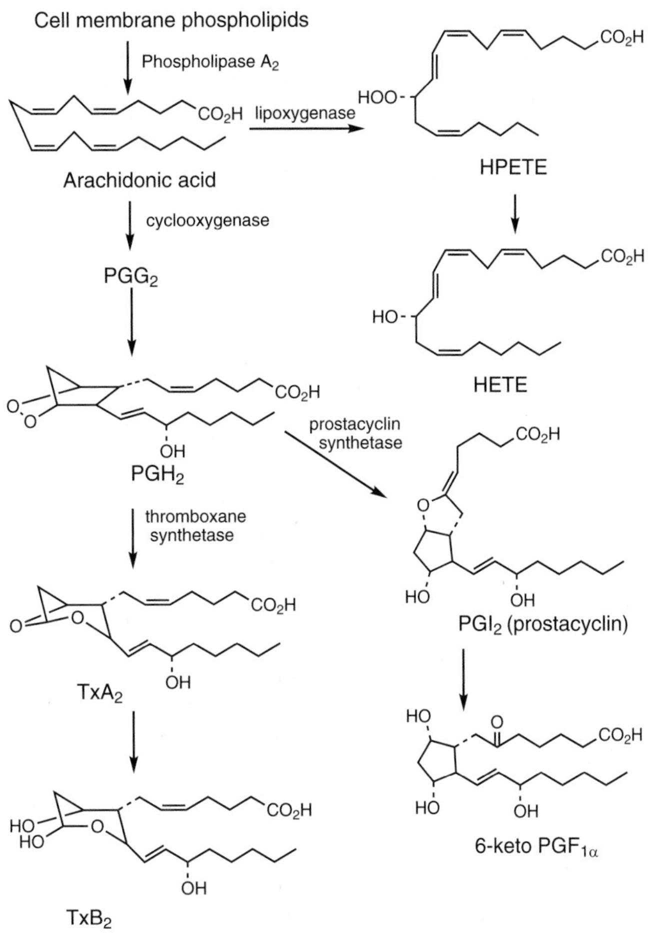

FIGURE 31.4 Biosynthesis of thromboxanes, prostacyclin, and leukotrienes.

leukotrienes from 5-HPETE, as shown in Figure 31.5. LTA synthetase converts 5-HPETE to an unstable epoxide called LTA_4 that can be converted by LTA hydrolase to the leukotriene LTB_4 or by glutathione-*S*-transferase to LTC_4. Other cysteinyl leukotrienes (e.g., LTD_4, LTE_4, and LTF_4) can then be formed from LTC_4 by the removal of glutamic acid and glycine and then reconjugation with glutamic acid, respectively. The cysteinyl leukotrienes produce airway edema, smooth muscle constriction, and altered cellular activity associated with the inflammatory process, all of which are associated with the pathophysiology of asthma (see also Chapter 39). Cysteinyl leukotrienes activate at least two receptors, designated as $CysLT_1$ and $CysLT_2$. A long-recognized mediator of inflammation, slow-reacting substance of anaphylaxis (SRS-A), is primarily a mixture of two leukotrienes, LTC_4 and LTD_4. The physiologic roles of the various leukotrienes are becoming better understood. LTB_4 is a potent chemotactic agent for polymorphonuclear leukocytes, causes the accumulation of leukocytes at inflammation sites, and leads to the development of symptoms characteristic of inflammatory disorders. Both LTC_4 and LTD_4 are potent hypotensives and bronchoconstrictors. Because of the role played by LTs and pLTs in inflammatory conditions and asthma, it is not surprising that intensive research is being conducted in this area. Zafirlukast (Acccolate), the first marketed cysteinyl leukotriene receptor antagonist (termed "lukasts"), was approved in 1996 for the prophylaxis and chronic treatment of asthma (Fig. 31.6). It is a selective and competitive receptor antagonist of the cysteinyl leukotrienes, LTD_4 and LTE_4. In humans, pretreatment with single oral doses of zafirlukast inhibited bronchoconstriction caused by sulfur dioxide and cold air and reduced the both early and late-phase

TABLE 31.2 Pharmacologic Properties of Prostaglandins, Thromboxane, and Prostacyclin

	PGE_2	$PGF_{2\alpha}$	PGI_2	TXA_2
Uterus	Oxytocic dilation	Oxytocic constriction		
Bronchi	Dilates	Constricts		Constricts
Platelets			Inhibits	Aggregation
Blood vessels	Dilation	Constriction	Dilation	Constriction

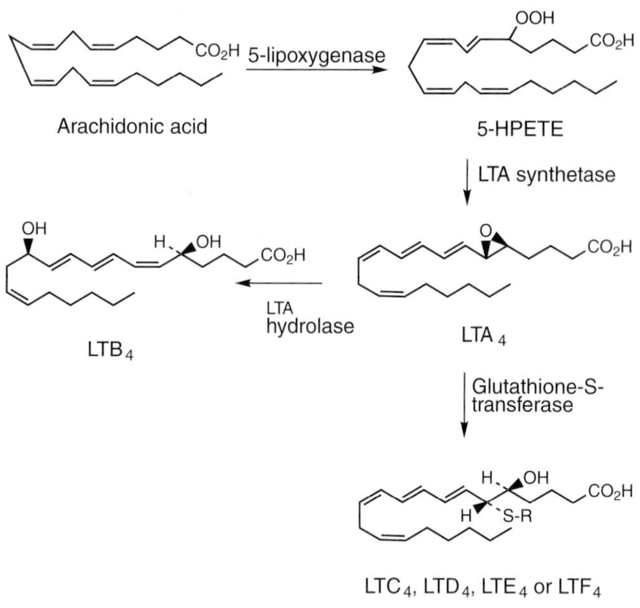

FIGURE 31.5 Biosynthesis of leukotrienes.

reaction in patients with asthma caused by inhalation of various antigens, such as grass, cat dander, and ragweed. Zafirlukast reduced the increase in bronchial hyperresponsiveness to inhaled histamine that followed inhaled allergen challenge. It is rapidly absorbed, but food reduces bioavailability to approximately 40%. Zafirlukast is extensively metabolized via hydroxylation reactions mediated primarily by CYP2C9, and to a minor extent CYP3A4, to essentially inactive metabolites. Excretion is 90% fecal and 10% via urine with an elimination half-life of approximately 10 hours. A second leukotriene antagonist, montelukast (Singulair) (Fig. 31.6), was approved shortly thereafter for prophylaxis and chronic treatment of asthma as an antagonist of LTD_4 at the $CysLT_1$ receptor. Its oral bioavailability ranges from 60% to 75% depending on the dosage form used. On oral administration, the time to peak concentration ranges from 2 to 4 hours. Food can reduce its bioavailability, prolonging

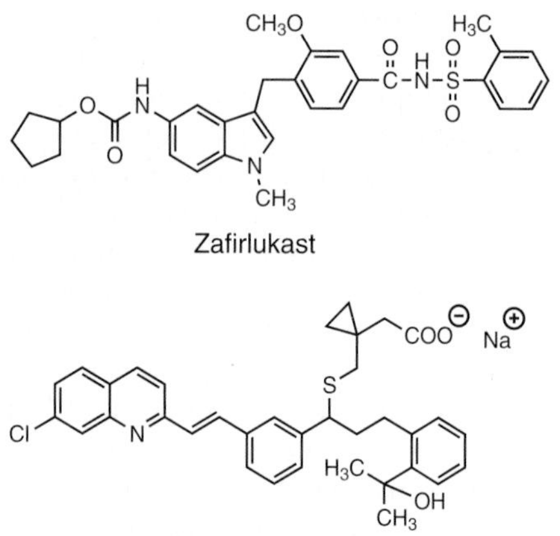

FIGURE 31.6 Leukotriene antagonists.

time to maximum plasma concentration. Protein binding is more than 99%. Like zafirlukast, montelukast is also extensively metabolized via hydroxylation reactions mediated by CYP2C9 and CYP3A4 to essentially inactive metabolites. Montelukast is excreted primarily in feces (86%), with an elimination half-life of 3 to 6 hours. The convenience of once-daily dosing provides montelukast an advantage over zafirlukast in the treatment of asthma.

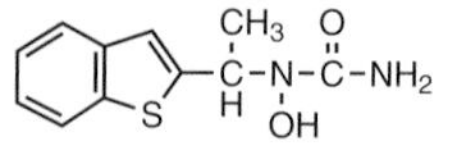

Zileuton

The first marketed inhibitor of leukotriene biosynthesis, zileuton (Zyflo), was approved shortly after zafirlukast for prophylaxis and chronic treatment of asthma. Zileuton is a specific inhibitor of 5-lipoxygenase and, thus inhibits the formation of LTB_4, LTC_4, LTD_4, and LTE_4. The *R*(+)- and *S*(−)-enantiomers equally inhibit 5-lipoxygenase so the drug is marketed as the racemic mixture. Zileuton is metabolized primarily to two diasteromeric glucuronide conjugates and the *N*-dehydroxylated metabolite. The use of zileuton is limited because of reports of liver toxicity, whereas the leukotriene receptor antagonists appear to produce little toxicity.

THERAPEUTIC APPROACH TO ARTHRITIC DISORDERS

The goal of drug treatment in early rheumatoid arthritis is to induce remission or at least eliminate evidence of disease activity. Rheumatoid arthritis was traditionally treated with a stepwise approach starting with NSAIDs and progressing through more potent drugs such as glucocorticoids, disease-modifying antirheumatic drugs (DMARDs), and biologic response modifiers. The DMARDs were avoided early in the disease because of their potentially serious side effects and were usually reserved for individuals who showed signs of joint damage. Over time, however, this strategy of avoiding DMARDs was recognized as being faulty, because people treated early with DMARDs have better long-term outcomes, with greater preservation of joint function and less work disability.

The current approach, therefore, is to treat rheumatoid arthritis aggressively with DMARDs and biologic response modifiers soon after diagnosis. Treating rheumatoid arthritis early with DMARDs, within 3 to 6 months after symptoms begin, controls inflammation better and is the best way to stop or slow progression of the disease and bring about remission and long-term prevention of joint disease. Methotrexate is the cornerstone of DMARD therapy. Long-term treatment with methotrexate and biologic response modifiers can offer the best control of rheumatoid arthritis for the majority of people, which can eliminate the need for other NSAID medications.

A large number of NSAIDs, inhibitors to varying degrees of COX-1 and COX-2, are therapeutically available for the treatment of pain and inflammation associated with arthritic disorders, differing in efficacy but, perhaps more importantly, differing also in overall toxicity. As a group, NSAIDs can cause GI toxicity, such as dyspepsia, abdominal pain, heartburn, gastric erosion leading to wall perforation, peptic ulcer formation, bleeding, diarrhea, renal disorders (e.g., acute renal failure, tubular necrosis, and analgesic nephropathy), and other effects (e.g., tinnitus and headache). Gastric damage produced by NSAIDs usually involves a dual insult mechanism (Fig. 31.7). Most NSAIDs are acidic substances that produce a primary insult because of direct acid damage, an indirect contact effect, and a back diffusion of hydrogen ions. The secondary insult results from inhibition of prostaglandin biosynthesis in the GI tract, where prostaglandins exert a cytoprotective effect. The dual insult leads to gastric damage. A report from the Arthritis, Rheumatism, and Aging Medical Information System Post-Marketing Surveillance Program, before the introduction of COX-2–selective drugs, ranked the overall toxicity of NSAIDs in the following decreasing order: indomethacin > tolmetin > meclofenamate > ketoprofen > fenoprofen > salsalate > aspirin.

THERAPEUTIC CLASSIFICATIONS

Antipyretic Analgesics

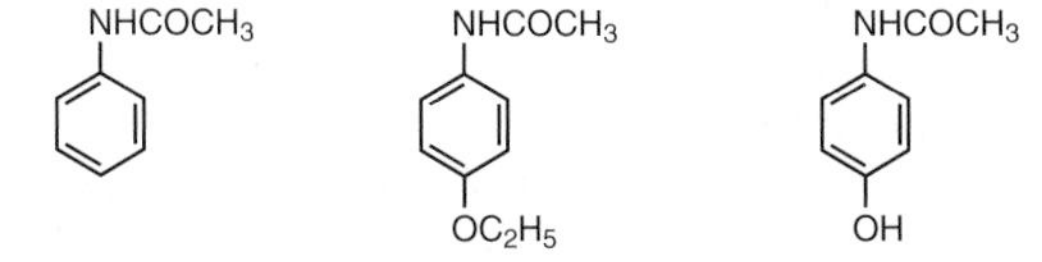

Acetanilide Phenacetin Acetaminophen

Mechanism of Action

Drugs included in this class possess analgesic and antipyretic actions but lack anti-inflammatory effects. Antipyretics interfere with those processes by which pyrogenic factors produce fever, but they do not appear to lower body temperature in afebrile subjects. It had been historically accepted that the antipyretics exert their actions within the central nervous system (CNS), primarily at the hypothalamic thermoregulatory center, but more recent evidence suggests that peripheral actions can also contribute. Endogenous leukocytic pyrogens can be released from cells that have been activated by various stimuli, and antipyretics can act by inhibiting the activation of these cells by an exogenous pyrogen or by inhibiting the release of endogenous leukocytic pyrogens from the cells once they have been activated by the exogenous pyrogen. Substantial evidence exists suggesting a central antipyretic mechanism, an antagonism that can result from either a direct competition of a pyrogen and the antipyretic agent at CNS receptors, or an inhibition of prostaglandins in the CNS (36). Despite the extensive use of acetaminophen, the mechanism of action has not been fully elucidated. Acetaminophen can inhibit pain impulses by exerting a depressant effect on peripheral receptors; an antagonistic effect on the actions of bradykinin can have a role. The antipyretic effects might not result from inhibition of release of endogenous pyrogen from leukocytes but, rather, from inhibiting the action of released endogenous pyrogen on hypothalamic thermoregulatory centers. The fact that acetaminophen is an effective antipyretic/analgesic but an ineffective anti-inflammatory agent can result from its greater inhibition of prostaglandin biosynthesis via inhibition of the COX-3 isoform in the CNS compared with that in the periphery.

Recent research in dogs has revealed a splice variant of COX-1 that was sensitive to inhibition by acetaminophen. This novel variant of the COX system was named COX-3, and it was hypothesized that inhibition of COX-3 could represent a primary CNS mechanism by which acetaminophen and phenacetin exerted their analgesic and antipyretic effects (25). The ability of selected analgesic/antipyretic drugs to inhibit COX-1, COX-2, and COX-3 is shown in Table 31.3 (25).

Further studies revealed that similar COX variants were present in rodents and humans, but these did not appear to be inhibited by acetaminophen (37,38). These

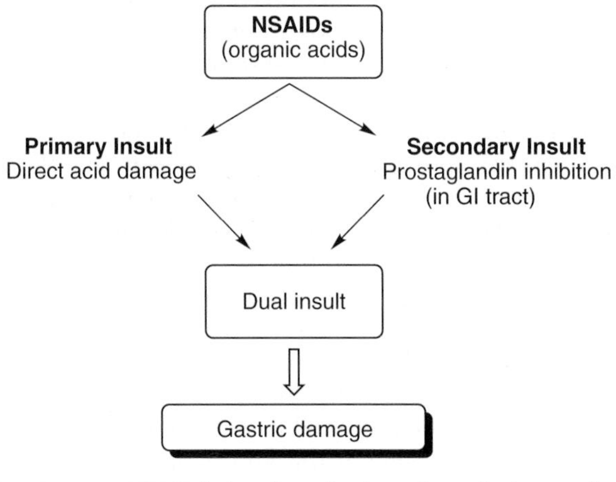

FIGURE 31.7 NSAID-induced production of gastric damage by a dual-insult mechanism.

TABLE 31.3 Binding Constants (IC50, μM) of Selected NSAIDs for the COX Enzymes

Drug	COX-1	COX-2	COX-3
Acetaminophen	>1,000	>1,000	460
Phenacetin	>1,000	>1,000	102
Aspirin	10	>1,000	3.1
Diclofenac	0.035	0.041	0.008
Ibuprofen	2.4	5.7	0.24
Indomethacin	0.010	0.66	0.016

COX variants are proposed to be COX-active, however, and to have a role in the biochemistry of these species (39,40). There is substantial nonhomology between the human, canine, and rodent COX-3 proteins.

Because PGE_2 is crucial to induction of fever, the antipyretic activity of this class is probably due to some degree of inhibition of COX enzymes. The same pertains to the analgesic effects of acetaminophen, where PGE_2 in particular synergizes greatly with other pain-producing mediators such as bradykinin and histamine. However, it appears that not all COX types are inhibited by this class of drugs, and the lack of anti-inflammatory activity suggests that acetaminophen is subtly different from the other NSAIDs. The apparently plausible hypothesis that there is a COX variant (COX-3) sensitive to acetaminophen has been challenged (41). Recent results have shown that acetaminophen increases the levels of endocannabinoids in traumatized tissues by inhibition of the endocannabinoid metabolizing enzyme(s) and that this could be an important mechanism for analgesia. Several, if not all, NSAIDs display the ability to inhibit fatty acid amide hydrolase (FAAH) and raise the levels of endocannabinoids. The body of evidence is such that it is now appropriate to raise the awareness of this mechanism of action (42). The novel proposal that endocannabinoids make a major contribution to the mechanism of action of acetaminophen is based on the observation that ibuprofen and several other NSAIDs inhibited FAAH (43). Further research has augmented this view and can explain the anomalous activity of acetaminophen, since agonists at cannabinoid receptors are known to have analgesic and hypothermic actions (44,45). Further support of the expanding role of endocannabinoids in acetaminophen activity is the observation (46) that the known FAAH inhibitor, AM404, can be formed from the deacylated metabolite of acetaminophen (Fig. 31.8). Interestingly, esters of acetaminophen were recently found to inhibit FAAH (47).

Additionally, it is known that opioids in combination with cannabinoids, for pain relief, display a large synergistic effect that also decreases the propensity for drug dependence of both drug classes (48). In light of the acetaminophen results, the use of cannabinoid agonists as analgesics should be reconsidered, especially in

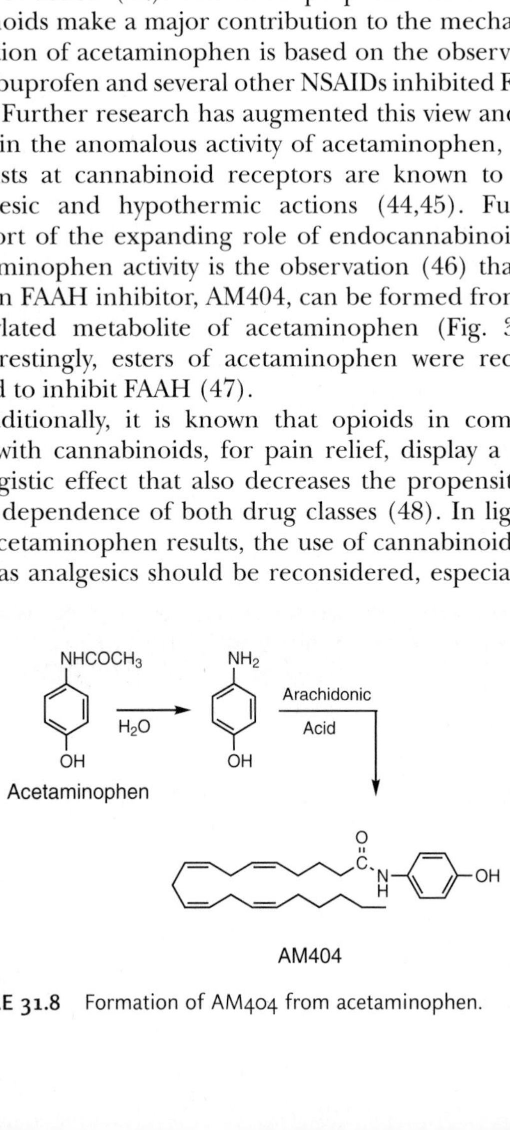

FIGURE 31.8 Formation of AM404 from acetaminophen.

combination with NSAIDs and in situations where opioids are inappropriate because of their more highly addictive character (49). A fuller discussion of the pharmacology of the endocannabinoid system in relation to NSAIDs and other biosystems is available (50).

It is now appreciated that many NSAIDs also reduce the immune response and that patients should not use these drugs after vaccination unless unbearable pain is experienced (51). The reduction in the immune response also fits well with the known agonist effects on the cannabinoid receptors, which modulate the immune system via both CB1 and CB2 receptors. There can be little doubt that the potential medical benefits of actions on this ubiquitous and abundant receptor system in mammals have been much attenuated by traditional abuse of phytocannabinoids. Ajulemic acid, a phytocannabinoid analog, has been studied as a cannabinoid agonist for the possible treatment of arthritis, multiple sclerosis, CNS injury, and analgesia in neuropathic pain (52,53).

Lipoxins, Resolvins, and Protectins

Lipoxins, naturally occurring eicosanoid mediators in mammals, derived from arachidonic acid by specific trihydroxylation, appear to be involved in inflammation resolution by action on specific GPCRs (54). The observation that resolution of inflammation is not a passive action but requires positive signaling by lipoxin-type mediators is an important potential breakthrough.

Similar substances to the lipoxins derived from timnodonic acid (eicosapentaenoic acid) or docosahexaenoic acid have been termed "resolvins" (RvE and RvD, respectively). Dihydroxylated lipids derived from these important polyunsaturated acids have been termed protectins and maserins and add to the spectrum of inflammation-resolving actions (55). These specialized proresolution lipid mediators, or similar substances with anti-inflammatory action, can be generated by COX enzymes that have been only partially inhibited by NSAIDs. Aspirin in particular has been identified as having the ability to increase lipoxin levels by irreversible inhibitory action on the COX system, thereby preventing the normal prostaglandin formation but still allowing oxidation reactions producing lipoxins or lipoxin-related substances (54). This activity can possibly be absent in acetaminophen, and this could explain its low anti-inflammatory effect. It is at present unclear if other NSAIDs have the effect of increasing lipoxins as a major component of their anti-inflammatory mechanism (56,57). However endocannabinoids also increase lipoxin levels, and therefore, typical NSAIDs can also do this via this mechanism.

Therefore, the mode of action of acetaminophen is still in question. Certainly, the analgesic and antipyretic properties parallel the decrease in PGE_2 levels in the CNS caused by acetaminophen. COX-1–deleted, but not the COX-2–deleted, mice showed a decrease in these actions (58). The authors suggest that in this species, it is COX-1, or a variant of it, that is affected by acetaminophen. Unlike other NSAIDs, such as ibuprofen or aspirin, acetaminophen does not have significant anti-inflammatory, antiplatelet, or gastric ulcerogenic activity. Other authors claim that the mechanism of action of acetaminophen is thought to involve inhibition of COX-2, and this fits with the therapeutic profile of the recently discovered, powerful, and selective COX-2 inhibitors (59). Acetaminophen is only effective, however, when COX-2 activity is at a low level. This view partially explains the lack of anti-inflammatory action, because COX-2 activity will be high in this situation (60).

Graham and Scott (60) have also put forward the interesting hypothesis that acetaminophen acts by depletion of the stores of glutathione, which is a known cofactor for PGE synthase. This would explain the decrease in PGE production and the concomitant analgesic effect. The depletion of glutathione is the main cause of acetaminophen toxicity. The highly reactive benzoquinoneimine, formed by CYP2E1 isoform, must be conjugated with glutathione before it can react with other crucial cell components. In overdose, failure of this molecular mechanism results in serious liver damage. The depletion of the body's supply of glutathione also should affect the biosynthesis of the inflammatory mediator leukotriene C4. Depletion of the body's supply of glutathione does not seem to be significant with therapeutic levels of acetaminophen.

A review article discussing the dichotomies of the acetaminophen mechanism and COX-3 is available (41).

Historical Background

Acetanilide was introduced into therapy in 1886 under the name antifebrin as an antipyretic/analgesic agent but was subsequently found to be too toxic (methemoglobinemia and jaundice), particularly at high doses, to be useful. Phenacetin was introduced the following year and remained in use until the 1960s because of reports of nephrotoxicity. Phenacetin is longer acting than acetaminophen despite the fact that it is metabolized to acetaminophen but is a weaker antipyretic. Shortly thereafter, acetaminophen (paracetamol) was introduced in 1893 but remained unpopular for more than 50 years, until it was observed that it is a metabolite of both acetanilide and phenacetin. It remains the only useful agent of this group and is widely used as a nonprescription antipyretic/analgesic under a variety of trade names (Tylenol, Patrol, and Tempera). The analgesic activity of acetaminophen is comparable to that of aspirin, but acetaminophen lacks useful anti-inflammatory activity. Its advantage over aspirin as an analgesic, however, is that individuals who are hypersensitive to salicylates usually respond well to acetaminophen.

Structure–Activity Relationships

The structure–activity relationships of *p*-aminophenol derivatives have been widely studied. Based on the comparative toxicity of acetanilide and acetaminophen, aminophenols are less toxic than the corresponding aniline derivatives, although *p*-aminophenol itself is too toxic for therapeutic purposes. Etherification of the phenolic function with methyl or propyl groups produces derivatives with greater side effects than with ethyl groups. Substituents on the nitrogen atom that reduce basicity reduce activity unless that substituent is metabolically labile (e.g., acetyl). Amides derived from aromatic acids (e.g., *N*-phenylbenzamide) are less active or inactive.

ACETAMINOPHEN USP Acetaminophen is weakly acidic (phenolic $pK_a = 9.51$) and synthesized by the acetylation of *p*-aminophenol. It is weakly bound to plasma proteins (18% to 25%). Acetaminophen is indicated for use as an antipyretic/analgesic, particularly in individuals displaying an allergy or sensitivity to aspirin. It does not possess anti-inflammatory activity, but it will produce analgesia in a wide variety of arthritic and musculoskeletal disorders. It is available in various formulations, including suppositories, tablets, capsules, granules, and solutions. The usual adult dose is 325 to 650 mg every 4 to 6 hours. Doses greater than 2.6 g/d are not recommended for long-term therapy because of potential hepatotoxicity issues. Acetaminophen, unlike aspirin, is stable in aqueous solution, making liquid formulations readily available, and particularly advantageous in pediatric cases. Because acetaminophen is water insoluble, liquid formulations are prepared with solvents such as propylene glycol to keep acetaminophen in solution; otherwise, the formulation would be a suspension.

Metabolism and Toxicity The metabolism of acetanilide, acetaminophen, and phenacetin is illustrated in Figure 31.9 (61). As indicated earlier, both acetanilide and phenacetin are metabolized to acetaminophen. Additionally, both undergo hydrolysis to yield aniline derivatives that produce directly, or through their conversion to hydroxylamine derivatives, significant methemoglobinemia and hemolytic anemia, which resulted in their removal from the US market. It has been known for more than 30 years that CYP450-mediated metabolism is responsible for the hepatotoxicity of acetaminophen (62) (see also Chapter 4). However, acetaminophen undergoes rapid first-pass metabolism in the GI tract primarily by conjugation reactions, with the *O*-sulfate being the primary metabolite in children and the *O*-glucuronide being the primary metabolite in adults. A minor, but significant, product of both acetaminophen and phenacetin is the *N*-hydroxyamide produced by CYP2E1 and CYP3A4. CYP2E1 is the rate-limiting enzyme that initiates the cascade of events leading to acetaminophen hepatotoxicity; in the absence of this cytochrome P450 (CYP) enzyme, toxicity will only be apparent at high concentrations. Both CYP2E1 and CYP3A4 are induced by the ingestion of alcohol (63), accounting for the increase in acetaminophen toxicity, especially among alcoholics, observed upon the concomitant consumption of alcoholic beverages with acetaminophen. The *N*-hydroxyamide is then converted to a reactive toxic metabolite, an acetimidoquinone—*N*-acetyl-*p*-benzoquinoneimine—that has been suggested (64)

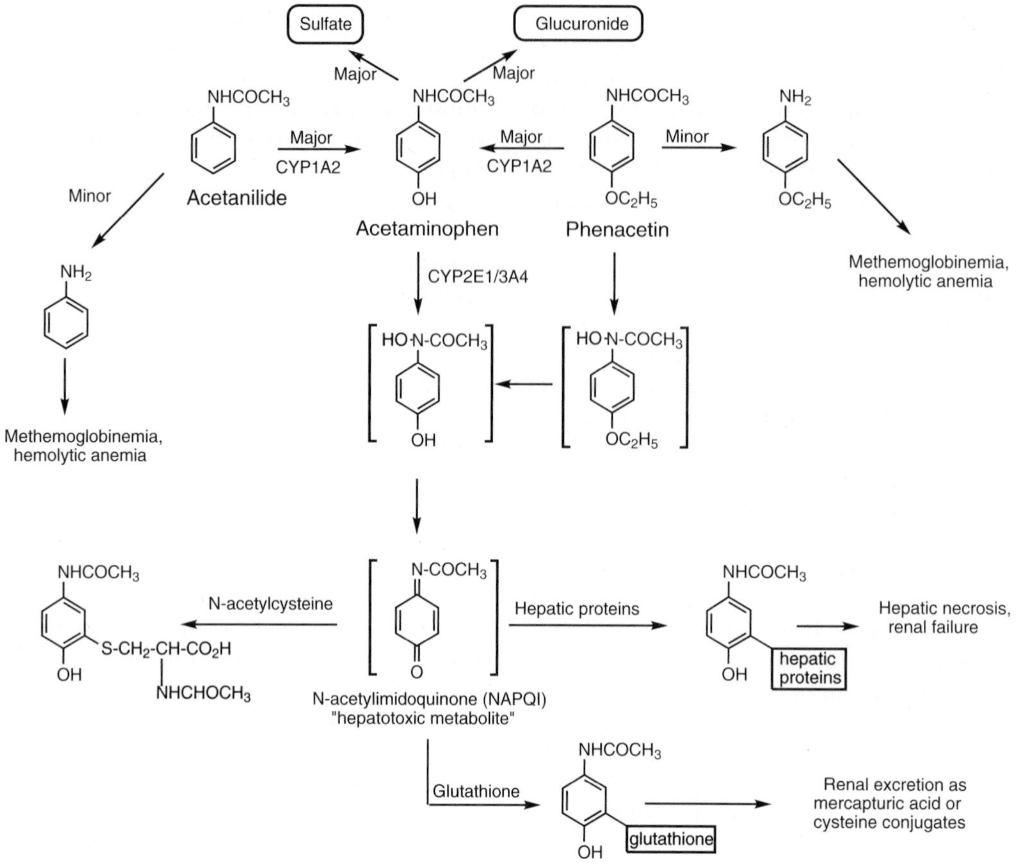

FIGURE 31.9 Metabolism of acetaminophen.

to produce the nephrotoxicity and hepatotoxicity associated with acetaminophen and phenacetin. Normally, this iminoquinone is detoxified by conjugation with hepatic glutathione. In cases of ingestion of large doses or overdoses of acetaminophen, however, hepatic stores of glutathione can be depleted by more than 70%, allowing the reactive quinone to interact with soft nucleophilic functional groups, primarily —SH groups, on hepatic proteins, resulting in the formation of covalent adducts that produce hepatic necrosis. Overdoses of acetaminophen can lead to fulminant acute liver failure, renal tubular necrosis, and hypoglycemic coma. Various sulfhydryl-containing compounds were found to be useful as antidotes to acetaminophen overdoses. The most useful of these antidotes is *N*-acetylcysteine (Mucomyst, Acetadote), which serves as a substitute for the depleted glutathione by enhancing hepatic glutathione stores and/or by enhancing disposition by nontoxic sulfate conjugation (65). *N*-Acetylcysteine can also inhibit the formation of the toxic iminoquinone metabolite (66). In cases of acetaminophen overdoses, *N*-acetylcysteine is administered as a 5% solution in water, soda, or juice or intravenously (IV) at 140 mg/kg followed by 17 maintenance doses of 70 mg/kg every 5 hours.

Drug Interactions Hepatic necrosis develops at much lower doses of acetaminophen in some heavy drinkers than would be expected (61), perhaps because of the induction of the CYP2E1 system, depletion of glutathione stores, or aberrations in the primary sulfate and glucuronide conjugation pathways. At 4 g/d, acetaminophen has been reported to potentiate the response to oral anticoagulants, increasing prothrombin time (international normalized ratio values) two to three times. Interactions with warfarin (Coumadin), dicumarol, anisindione, and diphenadione have been suggested. The mechanism of these interactions has not been fully elucidated but can be associated with competition for plasma protein binding sites, because acetaminophen is a weak acid and is weakly bound, but can also interfere with the enzymes involved in vitamin K–dependent coagulation factor synthesis. The absorption of acetaminophen is enhanced by polysorbate and sorbitol and is reduced by anticholinergics and narcotic analgesics. Chemical incompatibilities have also been reported based on hydrolysis by strong acids or bases or by phenolic oxidation in the presence of oxidizing agents. Acetaminophen forms "sticky" mixtures with diphenhydramine HCl and discolors under humid conditions in the presence of caffeine or codeine phosphate.

Anti-Inflammatory Drugs

SALICYLATES The use of salicylates dates back to the 19th century. Salicylic acid itself was first obtained in 1838 from salicin, a glycoside present in most willow and poplar bark. Interestingly, Hippocrates prescribed chewing willow bark for pain relief in the fifth century AD. In 1860, Kolbe synthesized salicylic acid from sodium phenoxide and carbon dioxide, a method that inexpensively produced large quantities. Derivatives of salicylic acid began to receive medical attention shortly thereafter. Sodium salicylate was employed as an antipyretic/antirheumatic agent in 1875, and the phenyl ester was used in 1886. Acetylsalicylic acid was prepared in 1853 but was not used medicinally until 1899. The term "aspirin" was given to acetylsalicylic acid by Dreser, the director of pharmacology at Frederich Bayer and Company in Germany, as a contraction of the letter "a" from acetyl and "spirin," an older name given to salicylic acid (spiric acid) that was derived from a natural source in spirea plants. Since then, numerous derivatives of salicylic acid have been synthesized and evaluated pharmacologically, yet only a relatively few derivatives have achieved therapeutic utility.

In addition to possessing antipyretic, analgesic, and anti-inflammatory properties, salicylates possess other actions that have been proven to be therapeutically beneficial. Because salicylates promote the excretion of uric acid, they are useful in the treatment of gouty arthritis. More recent attention has been given to the ability of salicylates to inhibit platelet aggregation, which can contribute to heart attacks and stroke. Aspirin appears to inhibit prostaglandin COX in platelet membranes, thus blocking formation of the potent platelet-aggregating factor TXA_2 in a manner that is irreversible. The Physicians Health Study concluded that in a group of 22,071 participants, there was a 44% reduction in the risk of myocardial infarction in the group taking a single 325-mg aspirin tablet taken every other day versus the placebo group (67). The role of aspirin in reducing cardiac mortality has been reviewed (68). Also, aspirin and other NSAIDs might be protective against colon cancer (69). Thus, the therapeutic utility of aspirin continues to increase. Unfortunately, a number of side effects are associated with the use of salicylates, most notably GI disturbances such as dyspepsia, gastroduodenal bleeding, gastric ulcerations, and gastritis.

Mechanism of Action A number of possible mechanisms of action have been proposed for salicylates over the years. Among those that have been suggested are inhibition of the biosynthesis of histamine, antagonism of the actions of various kinins, inhibition of mucopolysaccharide biosynthesis, inhibition of lysosomal enzyme release, and inhibition of leukocyte accumulation. The most widely accepted mechanism of action currently is the ability of these drugs to inhibit the biosynthesis of prostaglandins at the cyclooxygenase stage discussed earlier. Aspirin is the only NSAID that covalently modifies COX by acetylating Ser^{530} of COX-1 and Ser^{516} of COX-2. Aspirin, however, is 10 to 100 times more potent against COX-1 than against COX-2 (70). Aspirin's actions on COX-1 prevent both endoperoxide and 15-peroxidation of arachidonic acid, but its action on COX-2 does not prevent formation of 15-OOH arachidonic acid (29).

Structure–Activity Relationships Despite the vast effort that has been expended in the search to find a "better" aspirin—that is, one possessing fewer GI side effects but a greater potency and a longer duration of action yet is inexpensive and an antipyretic, analgesic, and anti-inflammatory agent that is overall superior to aspirin—none has yet to be discovered. The following structure–activity relationships have been established:

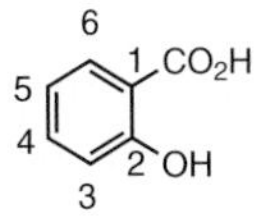

Salicylic acid

The active moiety appears to be the salicylate anion. The side effects of aspirin, particularly the GI effects, appear to be associated with the carboxylic acid function. Reducing the acidity of this group (e.g., converting to an amide, salicylamide) maintains the analgesic actions of salicylic acid derivatives but eliminates the anti-inflammatory properties. Substitution on either the carboxyl or phenolic hydroxyl groups can affect potency and toxicity. Benzoic acid itself has only weak anti-inflammatory activity. Placing the phenolic hydroxyl group meta or para to the carboxyl group abolishes this activity. Substitution of halogen atoms on the aromatic ring enhances potency and toxicity. Substitution of aromatic rings at the 5-position of salicylic acid increases anti-inflammatory activity (e.g., diflunisal).

Absorption and Metabolism Most salicylates are rapidly and effectively absorbed on oral administration, with the rate of absorption and bioavailability being dependent on a number of factors, including the dosage formulation, gastric pH, food contents in the stomach, gastric emptying time, the presence of buffering agents or antacids, and particle size. Because salicylates are weak carboxylic acids (acetylsalicylic acid $pK_a = 3.5$), absorption takes place primarily from the small intestine and, to a lesser extent, from the stomach by the process of passive diffusion of un-ionized molecules across the epithelial membranes of the GI tract. Thus, gastric pH is an important factor in the rate of absorption of salicylates. Any factor that increases gastric pH (e.g., buffering agents, proton pump inhibitors) will slow its rate of absorption, because more of the salicylate will be in the ionized form. The differences in the rates of absorption of aspirin, salicylate salts, and the numerous buffered preparations of salicylates are actually quite small, with absorption half-times in humans ranging from approximately 20 minutes for buffered preparations to 30 minutes for aspirin itself. The presence of food in the stomach also slows the rate of absorption. Formulation factors can contribute to the differences in absorption rates of the various brands of plain and buffered salicylate preparations. Tablet formulations consisting of small particles are absorbed faster than those of larger particle size. The bioavailability of salicylate from enteric-coated preparations can be inconsistent. Absorption of salicylate from rectal suppositories is slower and incomplete and is not recommended when high salicylate levels are required. Topical preparations of salicylic acid ester (e.g., methyl salicylate) are effective because the rate of salicylate absorption from the skin is rapid. However, 3% to 5% solutions of salicylic acid are also applied topically as a keratolytic agent.

Salicylates are highly bound to plasma protein albumin, with binding being concentration dependent. At low therapeutic concentrations of 100 μg/mL, approximately 90% of aspirin is plasma protein bound, whereas at higher concentrations of approximately 400 μg/mL, only 76% binding is observed. Plasma protein binding is a major factor in the drug interactions observed for salicylates.

The major metabolic routes of esters and salts of salicylic acid are illustrated in Figure 31.10. The initial route of metabolism of these derivatives is their conversion to salicylic acid, which can be excreted in the urine as the free acid (10%) or undergo conjugation with either glycine, to produce the major metabolite salicyluric acid (75%), or with glucuronic acid, to form the glucuronide ether and ester (15%). In addition, small amounts of metabolites resulting from microsomal aromatic hydroxylation are found. The major hydroxylation metabolite, gentisic acid, was once thought to be responsible for the anti-inflammatory actions of the salicylates, but its presence in trace quantities would rule out a major role for gentisic acid, or the other hydroxylation metabolites, in the pharmacologic action of salicylates. The metabolism of pharmacokinetic properties of salicylates has been extensively reviewed (71).

Side Effects The most commonly observed side effects associated with the use of salicylates relate to disturbances of the GI tract. Nausea, vomiting, epigastric discomfort, intensification of symptoms of peptic ulcer disease (e.g., dyspepsia and heartburn), gastric ulcerations, erosive gastritis, and GI hemorrhage occur in individuals on high doses of aspirin. The incidence of these side effects is rarer at low doses, but a single dose of aspirin can cause GI distress in 5% of individuals. Gastric bleeding induced by salicylates is usually painless but can lead to fecal blood loss and can cause a persistent iron deficiency anemia. At dosages that are useful in anti-inflammatory therapy, aspirin can lead to a loss of 3 to 8 mL/d of blood. The mechanism by which salicylates cause gastric mucosal cell damage can be caused by a number of factors, including gastric acidity, ability of salicylates to damage the normal mucosal barrier that protects against the back diffusion of hydrogen ions, ability of salicylates to inhibit the formation of prostaglandins (particularly those of the PGE series, which normally inhibit gastric acid secretion), and inhibition of platelet aggregation (leading to an increased tendency toward bleeding). Thus, salicylate use before surgery or tooth extraction is contraindicated.

Reye syndrome is an acute condition that can follow influenza and chickenpox infections in children from infancy to their late teens, with the majority of cases occurring between the ages of 4 and 12 years. It is characterized by symptoms including sudden vomiting, violent headaches, and unusual behavior in children who appear to be recovering from an often mild viral illness. Although a rare condition (60 to 120 cases per year, or an incidence of 0.15 per 100,000 population of those ≤18 years), it can be fatal, with a death rate of between 20% and 30%. Fortunately, the number of cases

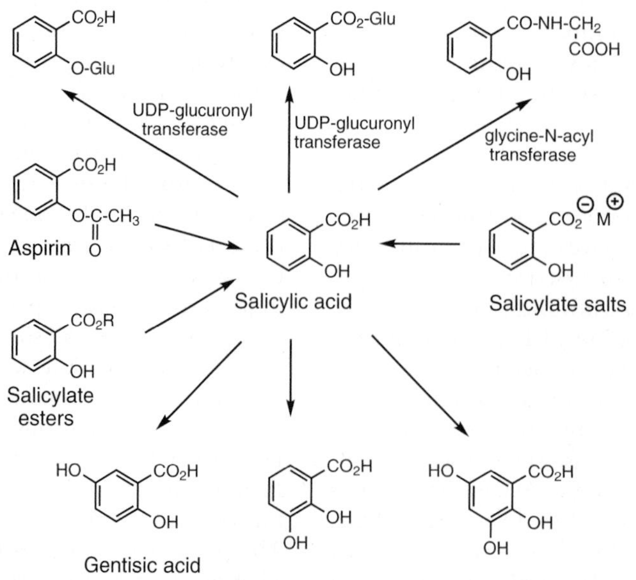

FIGURE 31.10 Metabolism of salicylic acid derivatives. Glu, glucuronide conjugate.

is declining, partly because of the observation that more than 90% of children with Reye syndrome were on salicylate therapy during a recent viral illness. Based on these observations, the FDA has proposed that aspirin and other salicylates be labeled with a warning against their use in children younger than 16 years with influenza, chickenpox, or other flu-like illness. Acetaminophen would appear to be the drug of choice in children with these conditions.

Salicylates account for approximately 25% of all accidental poisonings in the United States.

Drug Interactions Because of the widespread use of salicylates, it is not surprising that interactions with many other drugs used in therapeutic combinations have been observed. Several of these interactions are clinically significant. More data are available for aspirin than for any other specific salicylate product. As mentioned previously, acetylsalicylic acid is a weak acid that is highly bound to plasma proteins (50% to 80%), and it will compete for these plasma protein binding sites with other drugs that are highly bound to these sites. The interaction that results from the combination of salicylates with oral anticoagulants represents one of the most widely documented clinically significant drug interactions reported to date. The plasma concentration of free anticoagulant increases in the presence of salicylates, necessitating a possible decrease in the dosage of anticoagulant required to produce a beneficial therapeutic effect. The ability of salicylates to produce GI ulcerations and bleeding, coupled with the inhibition of the clotting mechanism, results in a clinically significant drug interaction. In addition, salicylates can inhibit the synthesis of prothrombin by antagonizing the actions of vitamin K. Additionally, NSAIDs can produce these interactions. The competition for plasma protein binding sites can also lead to an increase in free methotrexate levels (thus enhancing the toxicity of methotrexate), enhanced toxicity of long-acting sulfonamides, and a hypoglycemic effect (resulting from displacement of oral hypoglycemic drugs). In large doses, salicylates given concomitantly with uricosuric drugs, such as probenecid and sulfinpyrazone, can lead to a retention of uric acid and, thus, antagonize the uricosuric effect, despite the fact that salicylates when used alone increase urinary excretion of uric acid. The diuretic activity of aldosterone antagonists, such as spironolactone, can be antagonized by salicylates. Corticosteroids can decrease blood levels of salicylates because of their ability to increase the glomerular filtration rate. The incidence and severity of GI ulcerations can be increased if corticosteroids, salicylates, and NSAIDs are administered together. The GI bleeding induced by salicylates can be enhanced by the ingestion of ethanol. Numerous other interactions have been reported, but their clinical significance has not been fully established.

Salicylate hypersensitivity, particularly to aspirin, is relatively uncommon but must be recognized, because severe and potentially fatal reactions can occur. Signs of aspirin hypersensitivity appear soon after administration and include skin rashes, watery secretions, urticaria, vasomotor rhinitis, edema, bronchoconstriction, and anaphylaxis. Less than 1% of the US population can experience aspirin hypersensitivity; this group consists primarily of middle-aged individuals. Females are more likely to experience aspirin intolerance or hypersensitivity. Aspirin-sensitive patients with asthma are especially at high risk. Mild salicylism can occur after repeated administration of large doses. Symptoms include dizziness, tinnitus, nausea, vomiting, diarrhea, and mental confusion. Doses of 10 to 30 g have been known to cause death in adults, but some individuals have ingested up to 130 g without fatality. More than 10,000 cases of serious salicylate toxicity occur in the United States each year.

Available Preparations The structures of the marketed preparations of salicylic acid are presented in Figure 31.11.

Aspirin USP. Acetylsalicylic acid, or aspirin, is a white powder that is stable in a dry environment but that is hydrolyzed to salicylic acid and acetic acid under humid or moist conditions. Hydrolysis can also occur when aspirin is combined with alkaline salts or with salts containing water of hydration. Stable aqueous solutions of aspirin are thus unobtainable despite the addition of modifying drugs that tend to decrease hydrolysis. Aspirin is rapidly absorbed largely intact from the stomach and upper small intestine on oral administration but is rapidly hydrolyzed by plasma esterases. Peak plasma levels are usually achieved within 2 hours after administration. Increasing the pH of the stomach by the addition of buffering agents can affect absorption, because the degree of ionization will be increased.

Aspirin is indicated for the relief of minor aches and mild to moderate pain (325 to 650 mg every 4 hours), for arthritis and related arthritic conditions (3.2 to

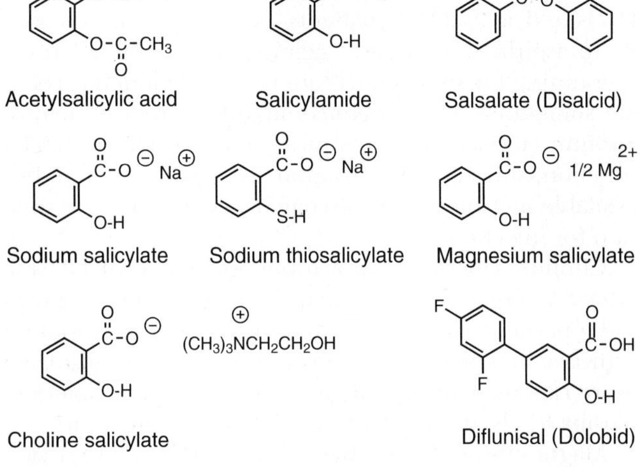

FIGURE 31.11 Structures of marketed derivatives of salicylic acid.

6.0 g/d), to reduce the risk of transient ischemic attacks (1.3 g/d), for myocardial infarction prophylaxis (300 to 325 mg/d), and as a platelet aggregation inhibitor (80 to 325 mg/d). It is available in a large number of dosage forms and strengths as tablets, suppositories, capsules, enteric-coated tablets, and buffered tablets.

Salicylamide. Salicylamide is less acidic (pK_a = 8.2) than other salicylic acid derivatives. Although poorly soluble in water, stable solutions can be formed at pH 9 through ionization of the phenolic group. It is absorbed from the GI tract on oral administration and is rapidly metabolized to inactive metabolites by intestinal mucosa, but not by hydrolysis. Activity appears to reside in the intact molecule. Salicylamide is approximately 40% to 55% plasma protein bound, and it competes with other salicylates and acetaminophen for glucuronide conjugation, decreasing the extent of conjugation of these other drugs. Excretion occurs rapidly, primarily in the urine. The major advantages of salicylamide are its general lack of gastric irritation relative to aspirin, and its use in individuals who are hypersensitive to aspirin. Salicylamide enters the CNS more rapidly than other salicylates and will cause sedation and drowsiness when administered in large doses. Whereas salicylamide is reported to be as effective as aspirin as an analgesic/antipyretic and is effective in relieving pain associated with arthritic conditions, it does not appear to possess useful anti-inflammatory activity (72). Thus, indications for the treatment of arthritic disease states are unwarranted, and its use is restricted to the relief of minor aches and pain at a dosage of 325 to 650 mg three or four times per day. Its effects in humans are not reliable, however, and its use is not widely recommended.

Salicylate Salts. Several salts of salicylic acid, sodium salicylate USP, choline salicylate USP, and magnesium salicylate USP, and one salt of thiosalicylic acid, sodium thiosalicylate USP, are available. These salts are used primarily to decrease GI disturbances or because they form stable aqueous solutions. Sodium salicylate is half as potent, on a weight basis, as aspirin as an analgesic/antipyretic, but it produces less GI irritation and equivalent blood levels and is useful in patients exhibiting hypersensitivity to aspirin. It generates salicylic acid in the GI tract, accounting for some GI irritation, and sodium bicarbonate sometimes is given concomitantly to reduce acidity. Sodium salicylate, unlike aspirin, does not affect platelet function, although prothrombin times are increased. It is available as tablets, enteric-coated tablets, and as a solution for injection.

Choline salicylate has a lower incidence of GI side effects compared with aspirin, and it has been shown to be particularly useful in treating juvenile rheumatoid arthritis, in which aspirin was ineffective. It is absorbed more rapidly than aspirin and produces higher salicylate plasma levels. It is available as a mint-flavored liquid.

Magnesium salicylate has a low incidence of GI side effects. Both sodium salicylate and magnesium salicylate should be used cautiously in individuals in whom excessive amounts of these electrolytes might be detrimental. The possibility of magnesium toxicity in individuals with renal insufficiency exists. It is available as tablets, but its safety in children under 12 years of age has not been fully determined.

Sodium thiosalicylate (Solate) is administered intramuscularly (IM) for the treatment of rheumatic fever, muscular pain, and acute gout.

Salsalate (Disalcid). Salsalate, or salicylsalicylic acid, (pK_a = 3.5 [COOH], 9.8 [AR-OH]) is a dimer of salicylic acid. It is insoluble in gastric juice but is soluble in the small intestine, where it is partially hydrolyzed to two molecules of salicylic acid and absorbed. On a molar basis, it produces 15% less salicylic acid than aspirin. It does not cause GI blood loss and can be given to aspirin-sensitive patients. Salsalate is available as capsules and tablets.

Diflunisal (Dolobid). Diflunisal (pK_a = 3.3) was introduced in the United States in 1982 and has gained considerable acceptance as an analgesic and as a treatment of rheumatoid arthritis and osteoarthritis. Diflunisal is metabolized primarily to ether and ester glucuronide conjugates. No metabolism involving changes in ring substituents has been reported. It is more potent than aspirin but produces fewer side effects and has a biologic half-life three to four times greater than that of aspirin. It is rapidly and completely absorbed on oral administration, with peak plasma levels being achieved within 2 to 3 hours of administration. It is highly bound (99%) to plasma proteins after absorption. Its elimination half-life is 8 to 12 hours, and it is excreted into urine primarily as glucuronide conjugates. The most frequently reported side effects include disturbances of the GI system (e.g., nausea, dyspepsia, and diarrhea), dermatologic reactions, and CNS effects (e.g., dizziness and headache).

Diflunisal is a moderately potent inhibitor of prostaglandin biosynthesis, but it differs from the manner in which aspirin inhibits the cyclooxygenase system in that the inhibition is competitive and reversible in nature. Diflunisal does not have an appreciable effect on platelet aggregation, however, and does not significantly produce gastric or intestinal bleeding.

ARYLALKANOIC ACIDS

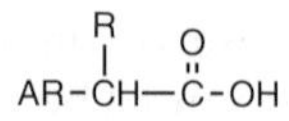

R = H, CH_3 or alkyl
AR = aryl or heteroaryl

The largest group of NSAIDs is represented by the class of arylalkanoic acids as typified by the general chemical structure, and several factors have caused this to be one of the most active areas of drug development in recent years. The impact that the introduction of phenylbutazone in the 1950s had on arthritis therapy was more than matched by the interest generated by the introduction of indomethacin in the mid-1960s. As a result of a study designed to investigate the anti-inflammatory activity of 350 indole acetic acid derivatives related structurally to serotonin and metabolites of serotonin, the Merck group led by Shen (73) reported the synthesis and antipyretic and anti-inflammatory activity of the most potent compound in the series, indomethacin. The observation that indomethacin possessed 1,085-fold the anti-inflammatory activity and 20-fold the antipyretic activity of phenylbutazone (and 10-fold the antipyretic activity of aminopyrine) generated considerable interest in the development of other aryl and heteroaryl acetic acid and propionic acid derivatives. The marketplace was ripe for new anti-inflammatory drugs, and most pharmaceutical companies joined in the search for new arylalkanoic acids. The introduction of ibuprofen in the 1970s by Upjohn was quickly followed by the appearance of fenoprofen calcium, naproxen, and tolmetin. Sulindac, an analog of indomethacin, was introduced in the late 1970s. The 1980s produced zomepirac, benoxaprofen, ketoprofen, flurbiprofen, suprofen, and diclofenac sodium. The 1990s produced ketorolac, etodolac, nabumetone, and most significantly, the development of selective COX-2 inhibitors, celecoxib, rofecoxib, and valdecoxib, which reached the market during the period from 1997 to 2000. This rapid development was accompanied by some setbacks, however. Zomepirac, introduced in 1980 as an analgesic, was withdrawn in 1983 because of severe anaphylactoid reactions, particularly in patients sensitive to aspirin.

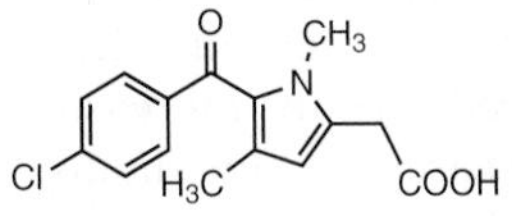

Zomepirac

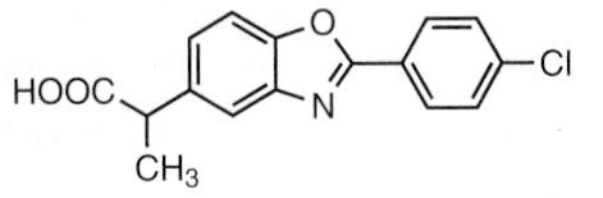

Benoxaprofen

Benoxaprofen was withdrawn within 6 months of its introduction in 1982 because of several deaths caused by cholestatic jaundice in Europe and the United States. In addition, benoxaprofen produced photosensitivity reactions in patients when they were exposed to sunlight and onycholysis (loosening of the fingernails) in some patients. Suprofen, introduced as an analgesic in 1985, was removed from the market 2 years later because of flank pain and transient renal failure. In 1989, however, it was reintroduced for ophthalmic use. Numerous other arylalkanoic acids currently are being evaluated in various stages of clinical trials.

As discussed earlier, most NSAIDs possess a number of biochemical and pharmacologic actions. As was the case for the salicylates, the arylalkanoic acids share, to various extents, the property of inhibition of prostaglandin biosynthesis by inhibiting COX-1 and COX-2 with varying degrees of selectivity (Table 31.3).

General Structure–Activity Relationships Drugs of this class share a number of common structural features. These general structure–activity relationships will be discussed here as they pertain to the proposed mechanism of action. Specific structure–activity relationships for each drug or drug class will be presented separately, where appropriate.

All nonselective COX inhibitors possess a center of acidity, which can be represented by a carboxylic acid function, an enolic function, a hydroxamic acid function, a sulfonamide, or a tetrazole ring. The relationship of this acid center to the carboxylic acid function of arachidonic acid is obvious. The activity of ester and amide derivatives of carboxylic acids is usually attributed to the metabolic hydrolysis products. One nonacidic drug, nabumetone, has been recently introduced in the United States, but as will be discussed later, its activity is attributed to its bioactivation to an active acid metabolite. The center of acidity is usually located one carbon atom adjacent to a flat surface represented by an aromatic or heteroaromatic ring. The distance between these centers is crucial, because increasing this distance to two or three carbons usually diminishes activity.

R-COOH	Carboxylic acid; pKa 4-6
R-CONHOH	Hydroxamic acids; pKa (NH) 8-9
R-SO_2NH_2	Sulfonamide; pKa (NH) 9-10
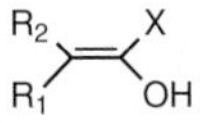	Enolic (phenol); pKa (OH) 8-10
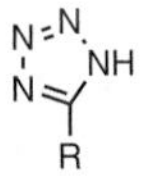	Tetrazoles; pKa (NH) 4-6

Derivatives of aryl or heteroaryl acetic or propionic acids are most common. This aromatic system appears to correlate with the double bonds at the 5- and 8-positions of arachidonic acid. Substitution of a methyl group on the carbon atom separating the acid center from the aromatic ring tends to increase anti-inflammatory activity. The resulting α-methyl acetic acid, or 2-substituted propionic acid, analogs have been given the class name "profens" by the U.S. Adopted Name Council. Groups larger than methyl decrease activity, but incorporation of this methyl group as part of an alicyclic ring system does not drastically affect activity. Introduction of a methyl group creates a center of chirality. Anti-inflammatory activity in those cases in which the enantiomers have been separated and evaluated, whether determined in vivo or in vitro by COX assays, is associated with the *S*-(+)-enantiomer. Interestingly, in those cases in which the propionic acid is administered as a racemic mixture, in vivo conversion of the *R*-enantiomer to the biologically active *S*-enantiomer is observed to varying degrees. A second area of lipophilicity that is noncoplanar with the aromatic or heteroaromatic ring usually enhances activity. This second lipophilic area can correspond to the area of the double bond in the 11-position of arachidonic acid. This lipophilic function can consist of an additional aromatic ring or alkyl groups either attached to or fused with the aromatic center.

General Metabolism Essentially all the arylalkanoic acid derivatives that are therapeutically available are extensively metabolized. Metabolism occurs primarily through hepatic microsomal enzyme systems and can lead to deactivation or bioactivation of the parent molecules. Metabolism of each drug will be treated separately.

Drug Interactions All the arylalkanoic acids are highly bound to plasma proteins and, thus, can displace other drugs from protein binding sites, resulting in an enhanced activity and toxicity of the displaced drugs. Interestingly, despite the high degree of plasma protein binding, indomethacin does not display this characteristic drug interaction. The most commonly observed interaction is that between the arylalkanoic acid and oral anticoagulants, particularly warfarin (Coumadin). Coadministration can prolong prothrombin time. Potential interactions with other acidic drugs, such as hydantoins, sulfonamides, and sulfonylureas, should be monitored. Concomitant administration of aspirin decreases plasma levels of arylalkanoic acids by as much as 20%. Probenecid, on the other hand, tends to increase these plasma levels. Interactions with drugs that can induce hepatic microsomal enzyme systems, such as phenobarbital, can enhance or diminish anti-inflammatory activity depending on whether the arylalkanoic acid is metabolically bioactivated or inactivated by this enzyme system. Certain diuretics, such as furosemide, inhibit the metabolism of prostaglandins by 15-hydroxy-prostaglandin dehydrogenase, and the resulting increase in PGE_2 levels induces plasma renin activity. Because the arylalkanoic acids block the biosynthesis of prostaglandins, the effects of furosemide can be antagonized, in part, offering a potentially significant drug interaction.

ARYL- AND HETEROARYLACETIC ACIDS The structures of the aryl- and heteroarylacetic acid derivatives and the aryl- and heteroarylpropionic acids ("profens") available are presented in Figure 31.12.

Indomethacin Aqueous solutions of indomethacin are not stable because of the ease of hydrolysis of the *p*-chlorobenzoyl group. The original synthesis of indomethacin by Shen et al. (73) involved the formation of 2-methyl-5-methoxyindole acetic acid and subsequent acylation after protection of the carboxyl group as the *t*-butyl ester. It was introduced in the United States in 1965. It is still one of the most potent NSAIDs in use. It is also a more potent antipyretic than either aspirin or acetaminophen, and it possesses approximately 10 times the analgesic potency of aspirin. The analgesic effect, however, is widely overshadowed by concern over the frequency of side effects.

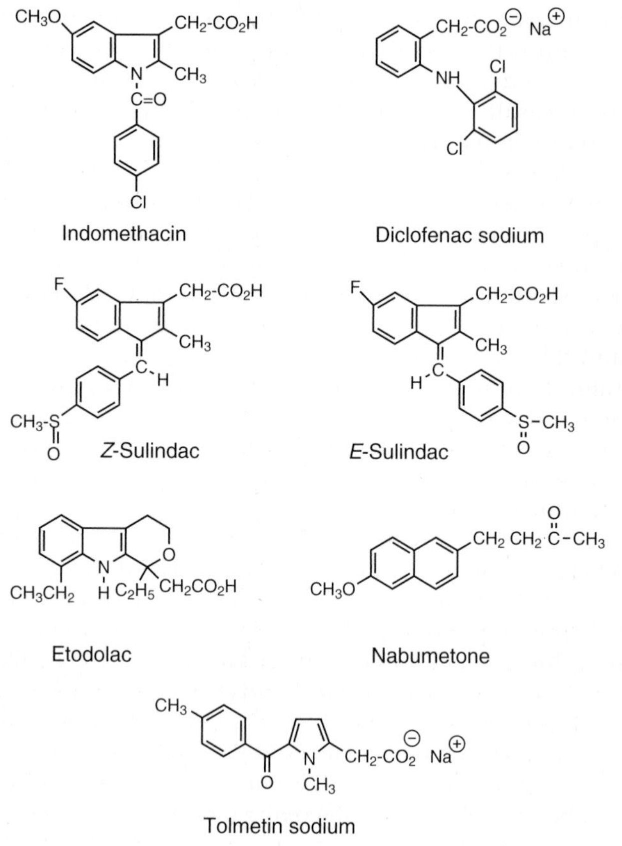

FIGURE 31.12 Structures of aryl- and heteroarylacetic acid derivatives.

Structure–Activity Relationships. Replacement of the carboxyl group with other acidic functionalities decreases activity. Anti-inflammatory activity usually increases as the acidity of the carboxyl group increases and decreases as the acidity is decreased. Amide analogs are inactive. Acylation of the indole nitrogen with aliphatic carboxylic acids or aralkylcarboxylic acids results in amide derivatives that are less active than those derived from benzoic acid. *N*-Benzoyl derivatives substituted in the para-position with fluoro, chloro, trifluoromethyl, or thiomethyl groups are the most active. The 5-position of the indole ring is most flexible with regard to the nature of substituents that enhance activity. Substituents such as methoxy, fluoro, dimethylamino, methyl, allyloxy, and acetyl are more active than the unsubstituted indole ring. The presence of an indole ring nitrogen is not essential for activity, because the corresponding 1-benzylidenylindene analogs (e.g., sulindac) are active. Alkyl groups, especially methyl, at the α-position are more active than aryl substituents. Substitution of a methyl group at the α-position of the acetic acid side chain (to give the corresponding propionic acid derivative) leads to equiactive analogs. The resulting chirality introduced in the molecules is important. Anti-inflammatory activity is displayed only by the *S*-(+)-enantiomer. The conformation of indomethacin appears to have a crucial role in its anti-inflammatory actions. The acetic acid side chain is flexible and can assume a large number of different conformations. The preferred and lower-energy conformation of the *N-p*-chlorobenzoyl group is one in which the chlorophenyl ring is oriented away from the 2-methyl group (or *cis* to the methoxyphenyl ring of the indole nucleus) and is noncoplanar with the indole ring because of steric hindrance produced by the 2-methyl group and the hydrogen atom at the 7-position. These conformations are represented as follows:

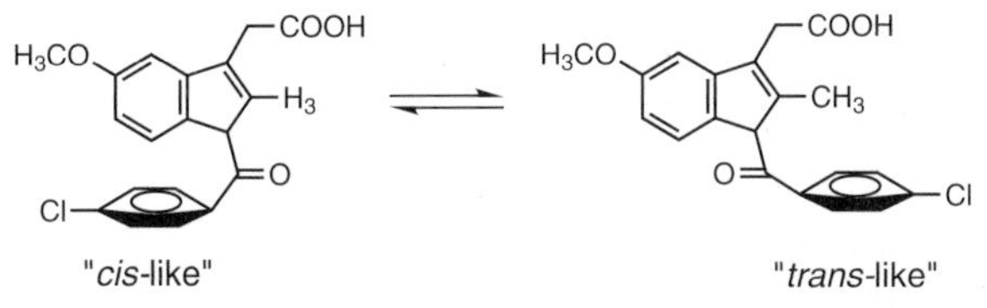

Indomethacin

Absorption and Metabolism. Absorption of indomethacin occurs rapidly on oral administration, and peak plasma levels are obtained within 2 to 3 hours. Being an acidic substance (pK_a = 4.5), it is highly bound to plasma proteins (97%). Indomethacin is converted to inactive metabolites; approximately 50% of a single dose is 5-*O*-demethylated by CYP2C9 and 10% is conjugated with glucuronic acid. Nonhepatic enzyme systems hydrolyze indomethacin to *N*-deacylated metabolites. The metabolism of indomethacin is illustrated in Figure 31.13. The ability of indomethacin to potently inhibit prostaglandin biosynthesis can account for its anti-inflammatory, antipyretic, and analgesic actions.

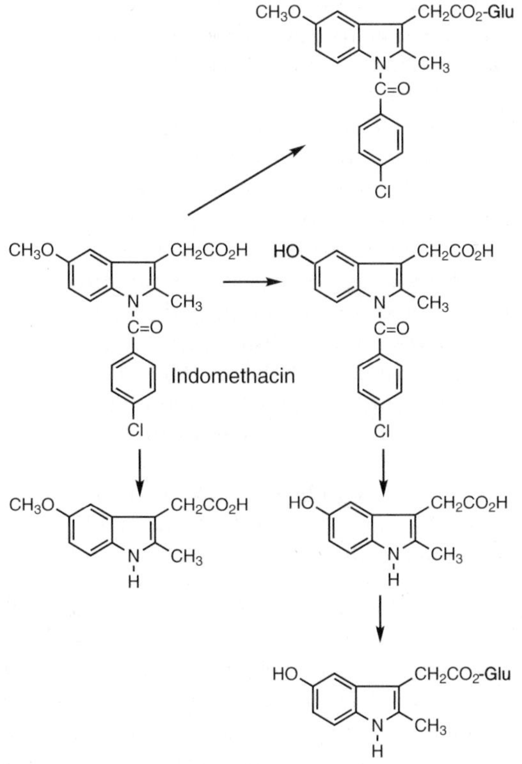

FIGURE 31.13 Metabolism of indomethacin.

Adverse Effects. Pronounced side effects are frequently observed at antirheumatic doses. A large number of individuals taking indomethacin, especially those over the age of 70, experience undesirable effects of the GI tract (e.g., nausea, dyspepsia, diarrhea, erosion/ulceration of the stomach walls), CNS (e.g., headache, dizziness, and vertigo), and ears (e.g., tinnitus). Thus, many patients must discontinue its use. As with other arylalkanoic acids, administration of indomethacin with food or milk decreases GI side effects.

Indomethacin is available for the short-term treatment of acute gouty arthritis, acute pain of ankylosing spondylitis, and osteoarthritis. An injectable form to be reconstituted is also available as the sodium trihydrate salt for IV use in premature infants with patent ductus arteriosus. Because of its ability to suppress uterine activity by inhibiting prostaglandin biosynthesis, indomethacin also has an unlabeled use to prevent premature labor.

Sulindac Sulindac was introduced in the United States in 1978 by Merck as a result of chemical studies designed to produce an analog without the side effects commonly associated with the use of indomethacin, particularly GI irritation. It achieved wide popularity and remains a widely used NSAID. Its synthesis was also reported by Shen et al. (74). Sulindac is a prodrug and is converted to a metabolite that appears to inhibit the COX system approximately eightfold as effectively as aspirin. In anti-inflammatory and antipyretic assays, it is only about half as potent as indomethacin but is equipotent in analgesic assays.

Structure–Activity Relationships. The use of classical bioisosteric changes in medicinal chemistry drug design was invoked in the design of sulindac. The isosteric replacement of the indole ring with the indene ring system resulted in a derivative with therapeutically useful anti-inflammatory activity and fewer CNS and GI side effects but with other undesirable effects, particularly poor water solubility and resultant crystalluria. The replacement of the *N-p*-chlorobenzoyl substituent with a benzylidiene function resulted in active derivatives. However, when the 5-methoxy group of the indene isostere was replaced with a fluorine atom, enhanced analgesic effects were observed. The decreased water solubility of the indene isostere was alleviated by replacing the chlorine atom of the phenyl substituent with a sulfinyl group. The importance of stereochemical features in the action of sulindac, introduced by the benzylidene double bond, is evidenced by the observation that the *Z*-isomer is a much more potent anti-inflammatory agent than the corresponding *E*-isomer (Fig. 31.12). This *cis*-relationship of the phenyl substituent to the aromatic ring bearing the fluoro substituent is similar to the proposed conformation of indomethacin, suggesting that both indomethacin and sulindac assume similar conformations at the active site of arachidonic acid COX. Although sulindac contains a chiral sulfoxide entity, it is marketed as the racemate because of its reduction to the active, achiral sulfide.

Absorption and Metabolism. Sulindac is well absorbed on oral administration (90%), reaches peak plasma levels within 2 to 4 hours, and being acidic (pK_a = 4.5), is highly bound to serum proteins (93%). The metabolism of sulindac has a major role in its actions, because all of the pharmacologic activity is associated with its major metabolite. Sulindac is, in fact, a prodrug, the sulfoxide function being reduced to the active sulfide metabolite. Sulindac is absorbed as the sulfoxide, which is not an inhibitor of prostaglandin biosynthesis in the GI tract. As discussed earlier, prostaglandins exert a protective effect in the GI tract, and inhibition of their synthesis here leads to many of the GI side effects noted for most NSAIDs. Once sulindac enters the circulatory system, it is reduced to the active sulfide, which is an inhibitor of prostaglandin biosynthesis in the joints. Thus, sulindac produces less GI side effects, such as bleeding, ulcerations, and so on, than indomethacin and many other NSAIDs. In addition, the active metabolite has a plasma half-life approximately twice that of the parent compound (~16 hours vs. 8 hours), which favorably affects the dosing schedule. In addition to the sulfide metabolite, sulindac is oxidized to the corresponding sulfone, which is inactive. A minor product results from hydroxylation of the benzylidene function and the methyl group at the 2-position. Glucuronides of several metabolites are also found. Sulindac and the sulfide and the sulfone metabolites are all highly protein bound. Despite the fact that the sulfide metabolite is a major activation product and is found in high concentration in human plasma, it is not found in human urine, perhaps because of its high degree of protein binding. The major excretion product is the sulfone metabolite and its glucuronide conjugate. The metabolism of sulindac is illustrated in Figure 31.14.

Whereas the toxicity of sulindac is lower than that observed for indomethacin and other NSAIDs, the spectrum of adverse reactions is very similar. The most frequent side effects reported are associated with irritation of the GI tract (e.g., nausea, dyspepsia, and diarrhea), although these effects are generally mild. Effects on the CNS (e.g., dizziness and headache) are less common. Dermatologic effects are less frequently encountered.

Sulindac is indicated for long-term use in the treatment of rheumatoid arthritis, osteoarthritis, ankylosing spondylitis, and acute gouty arthritis. The usual maximum dosage is 400 mg/d, with starting doses recommended at 150 mg twice a day. It is recommended that sulindac be administered with food.

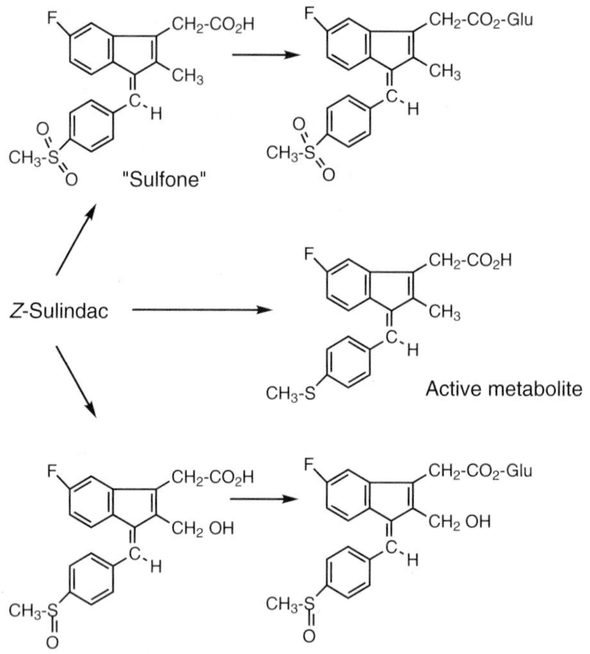

FIGURE 31.14 Metabolism of sulindac. Glu, glucuronide.

Tolmetin Sodium Tolmetin is synthesized straightforwardly from 1-methylpyrrole (75). It was introduced in the United States in 1976, and like other NSAIDs, inhibits prostaglandin biosynthesis. Tolmetin, however, also inhibits polymorph migration and decreases capillary permeability. Its anti-inflammatory activity, as measured in the carrageenan-induced rat paw edema and cotton pellet granuloma assays, is intermediate between those of phenylbutazone and indomethacin.

Structure–Activity Relationships. The relationship of tolmetin to indomethacin is clear, with each containing a noncoplanar *p*-chlorobenzoyl group and an acetic acid function. Tolmetin possesses a pyrrole ring instead of the indole ring in indomethacin. Replacement of the 5-*p*-toluoyl group with a *p*-chlorobenzoyl moiety produced little effect on activity, whereas introduction of a methyl group in the 4-position of the pyrrole ring produced interesting results. The 4-methyl-5-*p*-chlorobenzoyl analog is approximately four times as potent as tolmetin. Substitution of the *p*-methyl group of tolmetin with a *p*-chloro group blocked oxidative metabolism, increasing duration of action to approximately 24 hours. McNeil marketed this *p*-chloro compound in 1980 as zomepirac, an analgesic that was removed from the market in 1983 because of severe anaphylactic reactions, particularly in patients sensitive to aspirin. Unlike the previous structure–activity relationships discussed for arylalkanoic acids, the propionic acid analog is slightly less potent than tolmetin.

Absorption and Metabolism. Tolmetin sodium is rapidly and almost completely absorbed on oral administration, with peak plasma levels being attained within the first hour of administration. It has a relatively short plasma half-life of approximately 1 hour because of extensive first-pass metabolism, involving hydroxylation of the *p*-methyl group to the primary alcohol, which is

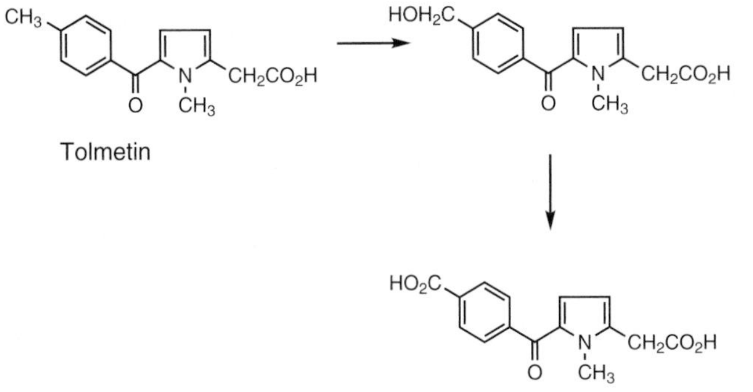

FIGURE 31.15 Metabolism of tolmetin.

subsequently oxidized to the dicarboxylic acid (Fig. 31.15). This metabolite is inactive in standard in vivo anti-inflammatory assays. The free acid (pK_a = 3.5) is highly bound to plasma proteins (99%), and excretion of tolmetin and its metabolites occurs primarily in the urine. Approximately 15% to 20% of an administered dose is excreted unchanged, and 10% is excreted as the glucuronide conjugate of the parent drug. Conjugates of the dicarboxylic acid metabolite account for the majority of the remaining administered drug.

The most frequently adverse reactions are those involving the GI tract (e.g., abdominal pain, discomfort, and nausea) but appear to be less than those observed with aspirin. The CNS effects (e.g., dizziness and drowsiness) are also observed. Few cases of overdosage have been reported, but in such cases, recommended treatment includes elimination of the drug from the GI tract by emesis or gastric lavage and elimination of the acidic drug from the circulatory system by enhancing alkalinization of the urine with sodium bicarbonate.

Tolmetin sodium is indicated for the treatment of rheumatoid arthritis, juvenile rheumatoid arthritis, and osteoarthritis.

Diclofenac Sodium Diclofenac is synthesized from *N*-phenyl-2,6-dichloroaniline (76). It is available in 120 different countries and, perhaps, is the most widely used NSAID in the world. It was introduced in the United States in 1989 but was first marketed in Japan in 1974. It ranks among the top prescription drugs in the United States. Diclofenac possesses structural characteristics of both arylalkanoic acid and the anthranilic acid classes of anti-inflammatory drugs, and it displays anti-inflammatory, analgesic, and antipyretic properties. In the carrageenan-induced rat paw edema assay, it is twice as potent as indomethacin and 450 times as potent as aspirin. As an analgesic, it is six times more potent than indomethacin and 40 times as potent as aspirin in the phenyl benzoquinone–induced writhing assay in mice. As an antipyretic, it is twice as potent as indomethacin and more than 350 times as potent as aspirin in the yeast-induced fever assay in rats. Diclofenac is unique among the NSAIDs in that it possesses three possible mechanisms of action: 1) inhibition of the arachidonic acid COX system (3 to 1,000 time more potent than other NSAIDs on a molar basis), resulting in a decreased production of prostaglandins and thromboxanes; 2) inhibition of the lipoxygenase pathway, resulting in decreased production of leukotrienes, particularly the proinflammatory LKB_4; and 3) inhibition of arachidonic acid release and stimulation of its reuptake, resulting in a reduction of arachidonic acid availability.

Structure–Activity Relationships. Structure–activity relationships in this series have not been extensively studied. It does appear that the function of the two *o*-chloro groups is to force the anilino-phenyl ring out of the plane of the phenylacetic acid portion, this twisting effect being important in the binding of NSAIDs to the active site of the COX, as previously discussed. A selective COX-2 inhibitor, lumiracoxib, which is closely related structurally to diclofenac, was briefly marketed in 2007 but quickly withdrawn from the market because of hepatotoxicity.

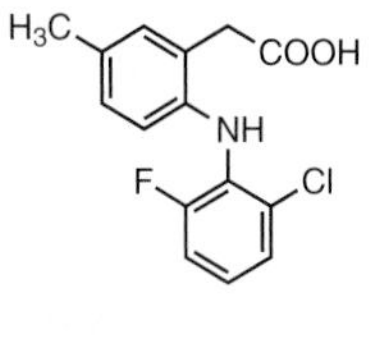

Lumiracoxib

Absorption and Metabolism. Diclofenac is rapidly and completely (~100%) absorbed on oral administration, with peak plasma levels being reached within 1.5 to 2.5 hours. The free acid (pK_a = 4.0) is highly bound to serum proteins (99.5%), primarily albumin. Only 50% to 60% of an oral dose is bioavailable because of extensive hepatic metabolism. Four major metabolites resulting from aromatic hydroxylation have been identified. The major metabolite via CYP3A4 is the 4′-hydroxy derivative and accounts for 20% to 30% of the dose excreted, whereas the 5-hydroxy, 3′-hydroxy, and 4′,5-dihydroxy metabolites via CYP2C9 account for 10% to 20% of the excreted dose. The remaining drug is excreted in the form of sulfate conjugates. Although the major metabolite is much less active than the parent compound, it can exhibit significant biologic activity, because it accounts for 30% to 40% of all of the metabolic products. The metabolism of diclofenac is illustrated in Figure 31.16. Also, diclofenac has been reported to produce reactive benzoquinone imine intermediates (77) similar to that reported in the metabolism of acetaminophen. These reactive intermediates are also normally inactivated via conjugation with glutathione.

Diclofenac sodium is indicated for the treatment of rheumatoid arthritis, osteoarthritis, and ankylosing spondylitis.

Etodolac Etodolac was promoted as the first of a new chemical class of anti-inflammatory drugs, the pyranocarboxylic acids. Although not strictly an arylacetic acid

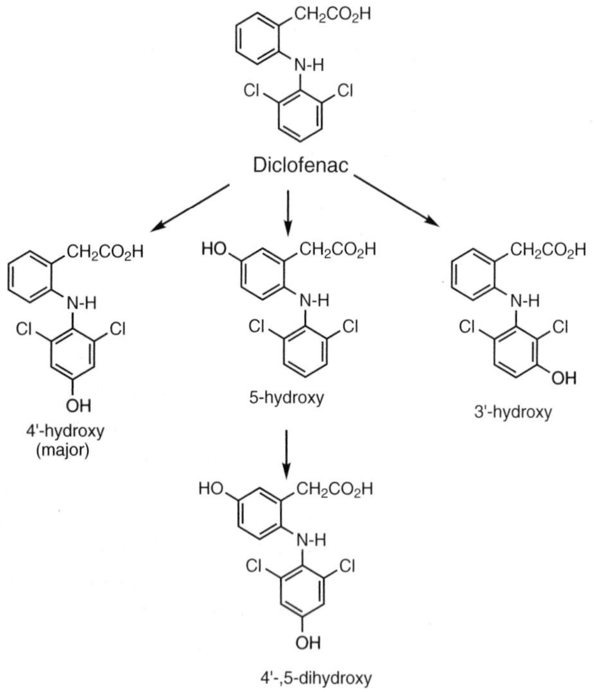

FIGURE 31.16 Metabolism of diclofenac.

derivative (because there is a two-carbon atom separation between the carboxylic acid function and the heteroaromatic ring) (Fig. 31.12), the drug still possesses structural characteristics similar to those of the heteroarylacetic acids and is classified here. It was introduced in the United States in 1991 for acute and long-term use in the management of osteoarthritis and as an analgesic and also possesses antipyretic activity. Etodolac is marketed as a racemic mixture, although only the *S*-(+)-enantiomer possesses anti-inflammatory activity in animal models. Etodolac also displays a high degree of enantioselectivity in its inhibitory effects on the arachidonic acid COX system. With regard to its anti-inflammatory actions, etodolac was approximately 50 times more active than aspirin, three times more potent than sulindac, and one-third as active as indomethacin. The ratio of the anti-inflammatory activity (inhibitory dose [ID_{50}]) to the median effective dose (ED_{50}) for gastric ulceration or erosion was more favorable for etodolac (ID_{50}/ED_{50} = 10) than for aspirin, naproxen, sulindac, or indomethacin (ID_{50}/ED_{50} = 4). At 2.5 to 3.5 times the effective anti-inflammatory dose, etodolac was reported to produce less GI bleeding than indomethacin, ibuprofen, or naproxen. The primary mechanism of action appears to be inhibition of the biosynthesis of prostaglandins at the cyclooxygenase step, with no inhibition of the lipoxygenase system. Interestingly, etodolac is highly selective for COX-2 yet possesses a high safety profile. Etodolac, however, possesses a more favorable ratio of inhibition of prostaglandin biosynthesis in human rheumatoid synoviocytes and chondrocytes than by cultured human gastric mucosal cells compared to ibuprofen, indomethacin, naproxen, diclofenac, and piroxicam. Thus, although etodolac is no more potent an NSAID than many others, the lower incidence of GI side effects represents a potential therapeutic advantage.

Structure–Activity Relationships. During a search for newer, more effective antiarthritic drugs in the 1970s, the Ayerst group led by Humber investigated a series of pyranocarboxylic acids of the general structure shown below (78,79). Structure–activity relationship studies indicated that alkyl groups at R_1 and an acetic acid function at R_2 enhanced anti-inflammatory activity.

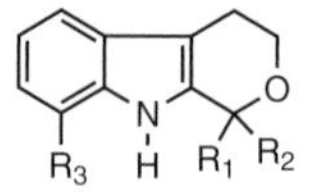

Lengthening the acid chain, or ester or amide derivatives, gave inactive compounds. The corresponding α-methylacetic acid derivatives were also inactive. Increasing the chain length of the R_1 substituent to ethyl or *n*-propyl gave derivatives that were 20 times more potent than methyl. A number of aromatic substituents in the aromatic ring were evaluated, and substituents at the 8-position were most beneficial. Among the most active were the 8-ethyl, 8-*n*-propyl, and 7-fluoro-8-methyl derivatives. Etodolac was found to possess the most favorable anti-inflammatory to gastric distress properties among these analogs.

Absorption and Metabolism. Etodolac is rapidly absorbed following oral administration, with maximum serum levels being achieved within 1 to 2 hours, and it is highly bound to plasma proteins (99%) with a pK_a of 4.7. The penetration of etodolac into synovial fluid is greater than or equal to that of tolmetin, piroxicam, or ibuprofen. Only diclofenac appears to provide greater penetration. Etodolac is metabolized to three inactive hydroxylated metabolites (Fig. 31.17) and to glucuronide conjugates, none of which possesses important pharmacologic activity. Metabolism appears to be the same in the elderly as in the general population, so no dosage adjustment appears necessary.

Etodolac is indicated for the management of the signs and symptoms of osteoarthritis and for the management of pain.

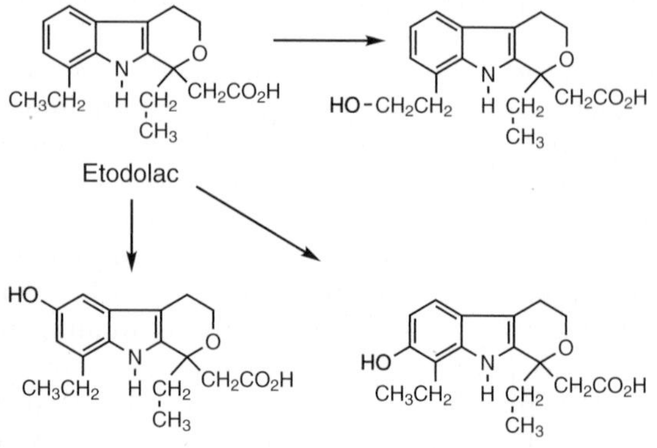

FIGURE 31.17 Metabolism of etodolac.

Nabumetone Nabumetone is unique among the NSAIDs in that it represents a new class of nonacidic prodrugs, being rapidly metabolized after absorption to form a major active metabolite, 6-methoxynaphthaleneacetic acid. It was introduced in the United States in 1992 and is synthesized from 2-acetyl-6-methoxynaphthalene (80). Nabumetone, being nonacidic, does not produce a significant primary insult and is an ineffectual inhibitor of prostaglandin COX in gastric mucosa, thus producing minimum secondary insult. The result is that gastric side effects of nabumetone appear to be minimized. Once the parent drug enters the circulatory system, however, it is metabolized to an active metabolite, 6-methoxynaphthalene-2-acetic acid (6MNA), which is an effective inhibitor of COX in joints. Nabumetone thus represents a classic example of the prodrug approach in drug design.

In the carrageenan-induced rat paw assay, nabumetone is approximately 13 times more potent than aspirin, one-third as active as indomethacin, and half as active as diclofenac. It is only half as active as aspirin as an analgesic, as measured by the phenylquinone-induced writhing assay in mice. Despite its lower potency, the advantages of nabumetone can reside in its favorable gastric irritancy profile. The ratio of gastric irritancy dose in rats to anti-inflammatory activity in rats (ED_{50}) for nabumetone is 21.25, whereas this ratio is 0.41 for aspirin, 0.55 for indomethacin, 0.72 for diclofenac, 3.00 for tolmetin, and 7.85 for zomepirac.

Structure–Activity Relationships. Introduction of methyl or ethyl groups on the butanone side chain greatly reduced anti-inflammatory activity. The ketone function can be converted to a dioxolane with retention of activity, whereas converting the ketone to an oxime reduced activity. Removal of the methoxy group at the 6-position reduced activity, but replacement of the methoxy with a methyl or chloro group gave active compounds. Replacement of the methoxy with hydroxyl, acetoxy, or *N*-methylcarbamoyl groups, or positional isomers of the methoxy group at the 2- or 4-positions, greatly reduced activity. The active metabolite, 6MNA, is closely related structurally to naproxen, differing only by the lack of an α-methyl group. The ketone precursor, 4-(6-methoxy-2-naphthyl)pentan-2-one, that would be expected to produce naproxen as a metabolite was inactive in chronic models of inflammation.

Absorption and Metabolism. Nabumetone is absorbed primarily from the duodenum. Milk and food increase the rate of absorption and the bioavailability of the active metabolite. Plasma concentrations of unchanged drug are too low to be detected in most subjects after oral administration, so most pharmacokinetic studies have involved the disposition of the active metabolite. Pharmacokinetic properties are altered in elderly patients, with higher plasma levels of the active metabolite being noted. Nabumetone undergoes rapid and extensive metabolism in the liver, with a mean absolute bioavailability of the active metabolite of 38%. The metabolism of nabumetone is illustrated in Figure 31.18. The major, most active metabolite is 6MNA, but the initial alcohol metabolite, a minor product, and its esters also possess significant anti-inflammatory properties.

Nabumetone is indicated for the acute and chronic treatment of the signs and symptoms of osteoarthritis and rheumatoid arthritis. The recommended starting dosage is 1,000 mg as a single dose with or without food. More symptomatic relief of severe or persistent symptoms can be obtained at doses of 1,500 or 2,000 mg/d.

Bromfenac Bromfenac was recently approved by the FDA for the treatment of postoperative inflammation and reduction of ocular pain in patients who have undergone cataract extraction. It will be available as a 0.09% ophthalmic solution for once-daily dosing. Bromfenac was originally approved by the FDA as a NSAID, but in 1998, 6 months after its approval, the FDA added a "black box" warning that the drug should not be taken for more than 10 days because of the risk of liver failure and hepatitis. Shortly thereafter, bromfenac was removed from the market because of reports of 4 deaths, 8 cases of liver transplantation, and 12 reports of liver damage associated with its use.

Aryl- and Heteroarylpropionic Acids Members of this class represent the most widely used NSAIDs because several members of the class are available OTC. The introduction of the α-methyl group in the carboxylic acid side chain results in a chiral carbon atom and thus the existence of enantiomers, with oxaprozin being the sole exception. As will be detailed for each drug, pharmacologic activity resides in the *S*-enantiomer, but most drugs of this class are marketed as racemates because of the rapid epimerization of the *R*-enantiomer to the active

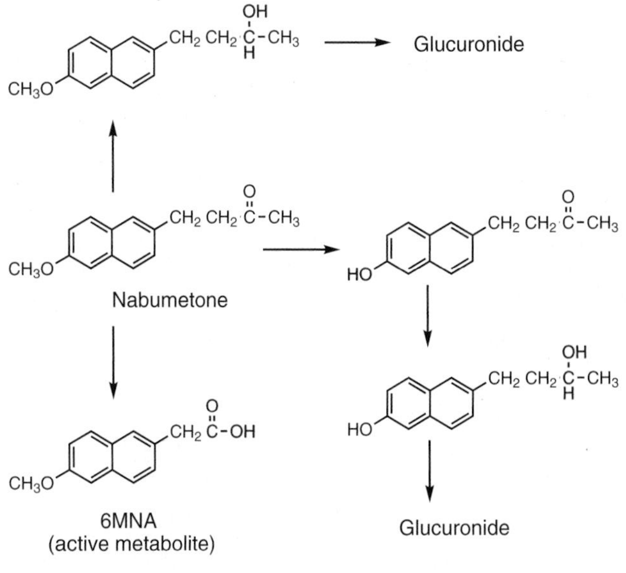

FIGURE 31.18 Metabolism of nabumetone.

S-enantiomer. Structures of aryl- and heteroarylpropionic acid derivatives are shown in Figure 31.19.

Ibuprofen The synthesis of ibuprofen was originally reported in 1964 from *p*-isobutylacetophenone (81), but the drug was not marketed in the United States until 1974, despite the fact that it had been available for several years in Europe. It was the first NSAID approved since indomethacin and was immediately accepted into therapy. Its success precipitated the introduction of many new drugs in the 1970s. This chemical class currently comprises the largest group of NSAIDs. Ibuprofen became the first prescription NSAID to become available as a nonprescription (OTC) analgesic in almost 30 years and is available under a number of brand names. It is marketed as the racemic mixture, although biologic activity resides almost exclusively in the *S*-(+)-isomer. Ibuprofen is more potent than aspirin but less potent than indomethacin in anti-inflammatory and prostaglandin biosynthesis inhibition assays, and it produces moderate degrees of gastric irritation.

Structure–Activity Relationships. The substitution of an α-methyl group on the alkanoic acid portion of acetic acid derivatives enhances anti-inflammatory actions and reduces many side effects. For example, the acetic acid analog of ibuprofen, ibufenac (*p*-isobutylphenylacetic acid), is less potent and more hepatotoxic than ibuprofen. The stereochemistry associated with the chiral center in the arylpropionic acids, but lacking in the acetic acid derivatives, has an important role in both the in vivo and in vitro activities of these drugs. As indicated earlier, although marketed as a racemic mixture, the (+)-enantiomer of ibuprofen possess greater activity in vitro than the (−)-isomer. The eudismic (*S*/*R*) ratio for the inhibition of bovine prostaglandin synthesis is approximately 160, but in vivo, the two enantiomers are equiactive (see next section on absorption and metabolism). The (+)-enantiomer of ibuprofen—and of most of the arylpropionic acids under investigation—has been shown to possess the *S*-absolute configuration.

Absorption and Metabolism. Ibuprofen is rapidly absorbed on oral administration, with peak plasma levels being usually attained within 2 hours and a duration of action of less than 6 hours. As with most of these acidic NSAIDs, ibuprofen (pK_a = 4.4) is extensively bound to plasma proteins (99%) and will interact with other acidic drugs that are protein bound. Metabolism occurs rapidly, and the drug is nearly completely excreted in the urine as unchanged drug and oxidative metabolites within 24 hours after administration (Fig. 31.20).

Metabolism by CYP2C9 (90%) and CYP2C19 (10%) involves primarily ω-, ω_1-, and ω_2-oxidation of the *p*-isobutyl side chain, followed by alcohol oxidation of the primary alcohol resulting from ω-oxidation to the corresponding carboxylic acid. All metabolites are inactive. When ibuprofen is administered as the individual enantiomers, the major metabolite isolated is the *S*-(+)-enantiomer whatever the configuration of the starting enantiomer. Interestingly, the *R*-(−)-enantiomer is inverted to the *S*-(+)-enantiomer in vivo via an acetyl–coenzyme A intermediate, accounting for the observation that the two enantiomers are bioequivalent in vivo. This is a metabolic phenomenon that has been also observed for other arylpropionic acids, such as ketoprofen, benoxaprofen, fenoprofen, and naproxen (82).

Ibuprofen is indicated for the relief of the signs and symptoms of rheumatoid arthritis and osteoarthritis, the

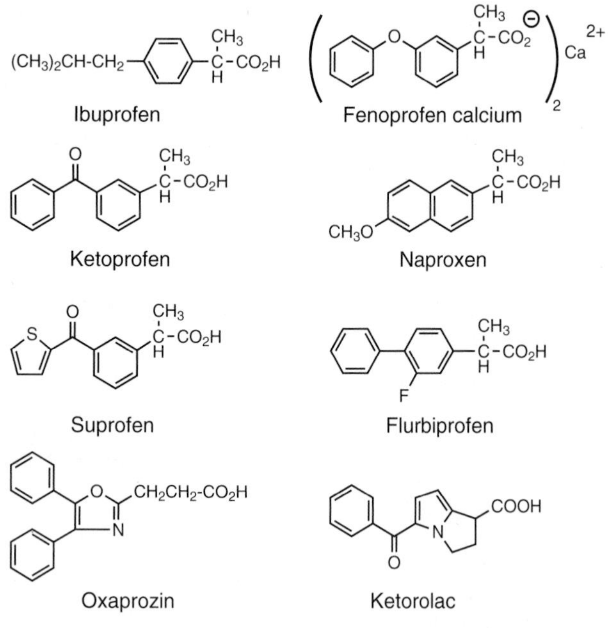

FIGURE 31.19 Structures of aryl- and heteroarylpropionic acid derivatives.

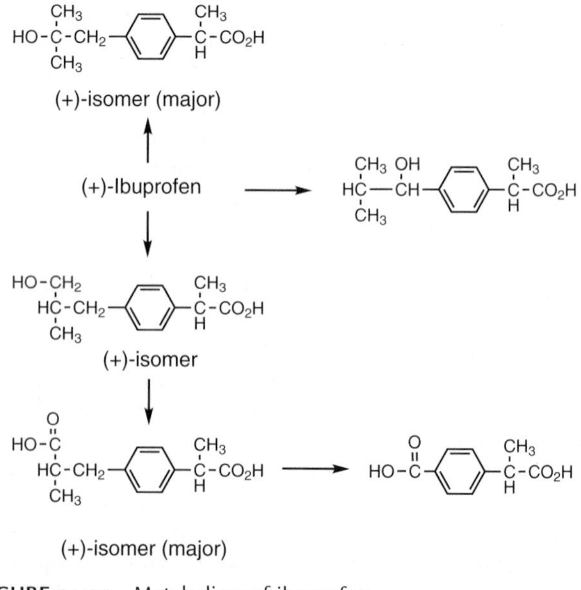

FIGURE 31.20 Metabolism of ibuprofen.

relief of mild to moderate pain, the reduction of fever, and the treatment of dysmenorrhea.

Fenoprofen Calcium The calcium and sodium salts of fenoprofen possess similar bioavailability, distribution, and elimination characteristics. It is the calcium salt that is marketed, however, because it has the advantage of being less hygroscopic. Its original synthesis was reported in 1970 (83), and it was marketed in the United States in 1976. Fenoprofen is less potent in anti-inflammatory assays than ibuprofen, indomethacin, ketoprofen, or naproxen. As an inhibitor of prostaglandin biosynthesis, it is much less potent than indomethacin, more potent than aspirin, and about equipotent with ibuprofen. Fenoprofen also possesses analgesic and antipyretic activity. It possesses other pharmacologic properties, such as inhibition of phagocytic and complement functions and stabilization of lysosomal membranes. Fenoprofen is marketed as a racemic mixture, because no differences have been observed in the in vivo anti-inflammatory or analgesic properties of the individual enantiomers. The ability of *R*-(−)-arylpropionic acids to undergo inversion to the *S*-(+)-enantiomers, however, can be involved. Like other NSAIDs, in vitro prostaglandin synthesis assays indicate that the *S*-(+)-enantiomer is more potent than the *R*-(−)-isomer.

Structure–Activity Relationships. Placing the phenoxy group in the ortho- or para-position of the arylpropionic acid ring markedly decreases activity. Replacement of the oxygen bridge between the two aromatic rings with a carbonyl group results in a marketed analog (ketoprofen).

Absorption and Metabolism. Fenoprofen is readily absorbed (85%) on oral administration and is highly bound (99%) to plasma proteins. Peak plasma levels are attained within 2 hours of administration. The free acid has a pK_a of 4.5, which is within the range of the other arylalkanoic acids. Fenoprofen is rather extensively metabolized, primarily through glucuronide conjugation with the parent drug and the CYP2C9 4′-hydroxy metabolite (84).

Fenoprofen calcium is indicated for treatment of rheumatoid arthritis and osteoarthritis and for the relief of mild to moderate pain.

Ketoprofen Ketoprofen was synthesized from 2-(*p*-aminophenyl)propionic acid via a thiaxanthone intermediate (85) and was introduced in 1986. Ketoprofen, unlike many NSAIDs, inhibits the synthesis of leukotrienes and leukocyte migration into inflamed joints in addition to inhibiting the biosynthesis of prostaglandins. It stabilizes the lysosomal membrane during inflammation, resulting in decreased tissue destruction. Antibradykinin activity has been also observed. Bradykinin is released during inflammation and can activate peripheral pain receptors. In addition to anti-inflammatory activity, ketoprofen also possesses antipyretic and analgesic properties. Although it is less potent than indomethacin as an anti-inflammatory agent and an analgesic, its ability to produce gastric lesions is about the same (86).

Absorption and Metabolism. Ketoprofen is rapidly and nearly completely absorbed on oral administration, reaching peak plasma levels within 0.5 to 2 hours. It is highly plasma protein bound (99%) despite a lower acidity (pK_a = 5.9) than some other NSAIDs. Wide variation in plasma half-lives has been reported. There are no known active metabolites of ketoprofen. It is metabolized by glucuronidation of the carboxylic acid, CYP3A4 and CYP2C9 hydroxylation of the benzoyl ring, and reduction of the keto function.

Ketoprofen is indicated for the long-term management of rheumatoid arthritis and osteoarthritis, for mild to moderate pain, and for primary dysmenorrhea.

Naproxen Naproxen is synthesized from 2-methoxynaphthalene and the (+)-isomer obtained by resolution with cinchonidine (87). It was introduced in the United States in 1976 and, as a generic drug, has consistently been among the more popular NSAIDs. It is marketed as the *S*-(+)-enantiomer, but interestingly, the sodium salt of the (−)-isomer is also on the market as Anaprox. As an inhibitor of prostaglandin biosynthesis, it is 12 times more potent than aspirin, 10 times more potent than phenylbutazone, 3 to 4 times more potent than ibuprofen, and 4 times more potent than fenoprofen, but it is approximately 300 times less potent than indomethacin. In vivo anti-inflammatory assays are consistent with this relative order of potency. In the carrageenan-induced rat paw edema assay, it is 11 times more potent than phenylbutazone and 55 times as potent as aspirin, but only 0.7 times as potent as indomethacin. In the phenylquinone writhing assay for analgesia, it is 9 times as potent as phenylbutazone and 7 times as potent as aspirin, but only 10% as potent as indomethacin. In the yeast-induced pyrexia assay for antipyretic activity, it is 7 times as potent as phenylbutazone, 22 times as potent as aspirin, and equipotent as indomethacin. The order of gastric ulcerogenic activity is sulindac < naproxen < aspirin, indomethacin, ketoprofen, and tolmetin.

Structure–Activity Relationships. In a series of substituted 2-naphthylacetic acids, substitution in the 6-position led to maximum anti-inflammatory activity. Small lipophilic groups, such as Cl, CH_3S, and CHF_2O, were active analogs, with CH_3O being the most potent. Larger groups were found to be less active. Derivatives of 2-naphthylpropionic acids are more potent than the corresponding acetic acid analogs. Replacing the carboxyl group with functional groups capable of being metabolized to the carboxyl function (e.g., —CO_2CH_3, —CHO, or —CH_2OH) led to a retention of activity. The *S*-(+)-isomer is the more potent enantiomer. Naproxen is the only arylalkanoic acid NSAID currently marketed as optically active isomers.

Absorption and Metabolism. Naproxen is almost completely absorbed following oral administration. Peak plasma levels are achieved within 2 to 4 hours following administration with a duration of action ~12 hours. Like most of the acidic NSAIDs (pK_a = 4.2), it is highly bound (99.6%) to plasma proteins. Approximately 70% of an administered dose is eliminated as either unchanged drug (60%) or as conjugates of unchanged drug (10%). The remainder is converted to the 6-*O*-desmethyl metabolite by both CYP3A4 and CYP1A2 and, further, to the glucuronide conjugate of the demethylated metabolite. The 6-*O*-desmethyl metabolite lacks anti-inflammatory activity. Like most of the arylalkanoic acids, the most common side effect associated with the use of naproxen is irritation to the GI tract. The most common other adverse reactions are associated with CNS disturbances (e.g., nausea and dizziness).

Naproxen is indicated for the treatment of rheumatoid arthritis, osteoarthritis, juvenile arthritis, ankylosing spondylitis, tendinitis, bursitis, acute gout, and primary dysmenorrhea and for the relief of mild to moderate pain.

Suprofen Suprofen is a white, microcrystalline powder that is slightly soluble in water.

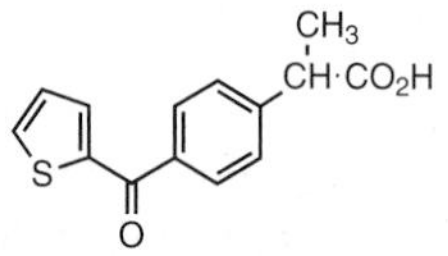

Suprofen

Suprofen is a thiophene isostere of ketoprofen. It was originally synthesized from thiophene in 1974 (88) and was introduced in the United States in 1985 for the treatment of dysmenorrhea and as an analgesic for mild to moderate pain. Reports of severe flank pain and transient renal failure appeared, however, with the syndrome being noted abruptly within several hours after one or two doses of the drug; therefore, suprofen was removed from the US market in 1987. Obviously, clinical trials are not always sufficient to determine a drug's safety, and postmarketing surveillance becomes most important. Suprofen was reintroduced in the United States in 1990 as a 1% ophthalmic solution for the prevention of surgically induced miosis during cataract extraction. Miosis complicates the removal of lens material and implantation of a posterior chamber intraocular lens that thus increases the risk of ocular trauma. The mechanism of action also involves inhibition of prostaglandin synthesis, because prostaglandins constrict the iris sphincter independent of a cholinergic mechanism. Additionally, prostaglandins also break down the blood–aqueous barrier, allowing the influx of plasma proteins into aqueous humor, resulting in an increase in intraocular pressure.

Flurbiprofen Flurbiprofen synthesis was originally reported in 1974 (89). During a study of the pharmacologic properties of a large number of substituted phenylalkanoic acids, including ibuprofen and ibufenac, the most potent were found to be substituted 2-(4-biphenyl)propionic acids. Further toxicologic and pharmacologic studies indicated that flurbiprofen possessed the most favorable therapeutic profile, so it was selected for further clinical development. It was not marketed until 1987, when it was introduced as the sodium salt as Ocufen, the first topical NSAID indicated for ophthalmic use in the United States. The indication for Ocufen is the same as that for Profenal—that is, to inhibit intraoperative miosis induced by prostaglandins in cataract surgery. Thus, flurbiprofen is an inhibitor of prostaglandin synthesis. Unlike other members of this class, there is no *R*- to *S*-epimerization observed in rats or humans, although epimerization has been observed in mice (90,91). The oral form was introduced in 1988 as Ansaid (another NSAID) and gained immediate acceptance. In acute inflammation assays in adrenalectomized rats, flurbiprofen was found to be 536-fold more potent than aspirin and 100-fold more potent than phenylbutazone. Orally, it was half as potent as methylprednisolone. As an antipyretic, it was 403 times as potent as aspirin in the yeast-induced fever assay in rats and was 26 times more potent than ibuprofen as an antinociceptive.

Absorption and Metabolism. Flurbiprofen is well absorbed after oral administration, with peak plasma levels being attained within 1.5 hours. Food alters the rate of absorption but not the extent of its bioavailability. It is extensively bound to plasma proteins (99%) and has a plasma half-life of 2 to 4 hours. Metabolism is extensive, with 60% to 70% of flurbiprofen and its metabolites being excreted as sulfate and glucuronide conjugates. Flurbiprofen shows some interesting metabolic patterns, with 40% to 47% as the 4′-hydroxy metabolite, 5% as the 3′,4′-dihydroxy metabolite, 20% to 30% as the 3′-hydroxy- 4′-methoxy metabolite, and the remaining 20% to 25% of the drug being excreted unchanged. None of these metabolites demonstrates significant anti-inflammatory activity. The metabolism of flurbiprofen is presented in Figure 31.21.

Flurbiprofen is indicated as an oral formulation for the acute or long-term treatment of rheumatoid arthritis and osteoarthritis and as an ophthalmic solution for the inhibition of intraoperative miosis. The *R*-enantiomer has been proposed to have potential use in the prophylaxis and treatment of colon cancer (92) and Alzheimer disease (93).

Ketorolac Tromethamine Ketorolac represents a cyclized, heteroarylpropionic acid derivative, with the α-methyl group being fused to the pyrrole ring. It was introduced in 1990 and is indicated as a peripheral analgesic for short-term use and for the relief of ocular itching caused by seasonal allergic conjunctivitis, although it exhibits anti-inflammatory and antipyretic activity as well. It was initially introduced only in an injectable form, but recently, an oral formulation has been made available. Its analgesic activity

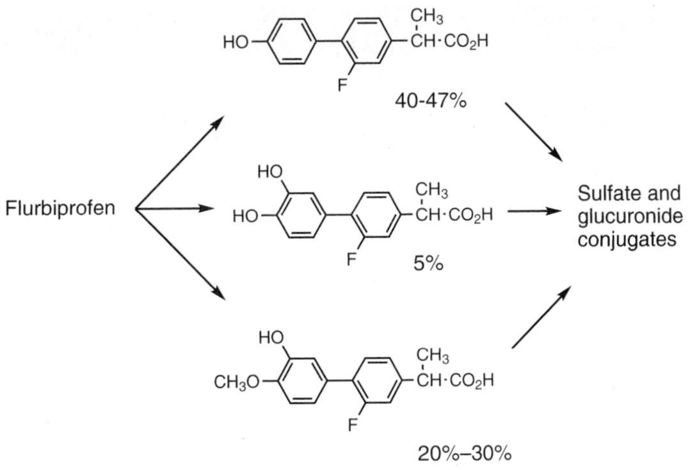

FIGURE 31.21 Metabolism of flurbiprofen.

resembles that of the centrally acting analgesics, with 15 to 30 mg of ketorolac producing analgesia equivalent to a 12-mg dose of morphine, and it has become a widely accepted alternative to narcotic analgesia. Ketorolac inhibits prostaglandin synthesis. Although the analgesic effect is achieved within 10 minutes of injection, peak analgesia lags behind peak plasma levels by 45 to 90 minutes. The free acid has a pK_a of 3.5, and it is not surprising that it is highly plasma protein bound (>99%). Ketorolac is metabolized by CYP2C9 to its *p*-hydroxy derivative and to conjugates that are excreted primarily in the urine.

Oxaprozin Oxaprozin was marketed in 1993 for acute and long-term use in the management of signs and symptoms of osteoarthritis and rheumatoid arthritis. Oxaprozin is synthesized by condensing benzoin with succinic anhydride and cyclizing the resulting benzoin hemisuccinate with ammonium acetate. Although not formally a propionic acid of the α-methylacetic acid type, it appears to be similar to the other propionic acid derivatives considered here. Oxaprozin is well absorbed (100%) after oral administration, but maximum plasma concentrations are not reached until 3 to 5 hours following ingestion. Oxaprozin is an anti-inflammatory agent possessing a rapid onset of action and a prolonged duration of action. In both the carrageenan-induced rat paw edema assay and analgesic tests, it was equipotent with aspirin. Oxaprozin has been associated with the appearance of rash and/or mild photosensitivity. Some patients experience an increased incidence of rash on sun-exposed skin during clinical testing. Oxaprozin, aspirin, ibuprofen, indomethacin, naproxen, and sulindac have comparable efficacy in the treatment of rheumatoid arthritis, whereas oxaprozin, aspirin, naproxen, and piroxicam have comparable efficacy in osteoarthritis. It is highly bound to plasma proteins (99%), is highly lipophilic, and undergoes little first-pass metabolism. Metabolism is via hepatic microsomal oxidation and glucuronidation. Two hydroxylated phenolic metabolites that are produced (<5%) have been shown to possess anti-inflammatory activity (94) but do not appear to contribute significantly to the overall pharmacologic activity of oxaprozin.

Oxaprozin possesses a relatively long elimination half-life of 59 hours (range, 26 to 92 hours), enabling once-daily dosing. Administration with food appears to delay absorption but not bioavailability.

Several properties of the NSAIDs are summarized in Table 31.4.

***N*-ARYLANTHRANILIC ACIDS (FENAMIC ACIDS)** The anthranilic acid class of NSAIDs is the result of the application of classical medicinal chemistry bioisosteric drug design concepts, because these derivatives are nitrogen isosteres of salicylic acid. Additionally, they could be considered structural analogs of the arylacetic acid derivative, diclofenac. In the early 1960s, the Parke-Davis research group reported the development of a series of *N*-substituted anthranilic acids that have since been given the chemical class name of fenamic acids. The fact that this class of compounds possesses little advantage over the salicylates with respect to their anti-inflammatory and analgesic properties has diminished interest in their large-scale development relative to the arylalkanoic acids. Mefenamic acid was introduced in the United States in 1967 as an analgesic, and this remains the primary indication despite the fact that it possesses modest anti-inflammatory activity. Flufenamic acid has been available in Europe as an antirheumatic agent, but there are no apparent plans to introduce this drug in the United States. With regard to anti-inflammatory activity, mefenamic acid is approximately 1.5 times as potent as phenylbutazone and half as potent as flufenamic acid. Meclofenamic acid was introduced in the United States as its sodium salt in 1980, primarily as an antirheumatic agent and analgesic. The structures of these fenamic acids are shown in Figure 31.22.

The fenamic acids share a number of pharmacologic properties with the other NSAIDs. Because these drugs are potent inhibitors of prostaglandin biosynthesis, it

TABLE 31.4 Some Properties of the NSAIDs

Drug	Year Introduced	Anti-Inflammatory Dose (mg)	Onset (Duration) of Action	Peak Plasma Levels (h)	Protein Binding (%)	Biotransformation	Elimination Half-Life (h)	pK_a
Aspirin	1899	3,200–6,000	ND	2	90	Plasma hydrolysis and hepatic	<30 minutes	3.5
Diclofenac (Voltaren)	1989	100–200	30 min (~8 h)	1.5–2.5	99	Hepatic; first-pass metabolism: 3A4	1–2	4.0
Diflunisal (Dolobid)	1982	500–1,000	1 h (8–12 h)	2–3	99	Hepatic	8–12	3.3
Etodolac (Lodine)	1991	800–1,200	30 min (4–6 h)	1–2	99	Hepatic: 2C9	6–7	4.7
Fenoprofen calcium (Nalfon)	1976	1,200–2,400	NR	2	99	Hepatic: 2C9	3	4.5
Flurbiprofen (Ansaid)	1988	200–300	NR	1.5	99	Hepatic: 2C9	6 (2–12)	4.2
Ibuprofen (Motrin, Advil)	1974	1,200–3,200	30 min (4–6 h)	2	99	Hepatic; first-pass metabolism: 2C9, 2C19	~2	4.4
Indomethacin (Indocin)	1965	75–150	2–4 h (2–3 d)	2–3	97	Hepatic: 2C9	5 (3–11)	4.5
Ketoprofen (Orudis)	1986	150–300	NR	0.5–2	99	Hepatic: 2C9, 3A4	~2	5.9
Meclofenamate sodium (Meclomen)	1980	200–400	1 h (4–6 h)	4.0	99	Hepatic: 2C9	2–3	NR
Mefenamic acid (Ponstel)	1967	1,000	NR	2–4	79	Hepatic: 2C9	2	4.2
Meloxicam (Mobic)	2000	7.5–15	NR	4–5	99	Hepatic 2C9	15–20	1.1, 4.2
Nabumetone[a] (Relafen)	1992	1,500–2,000	NR	2.5 (1–8) 6MNA	99[b]	Hepatic; first-pass metabolism to 6MNA	6MNA, 23	Neutral
Naproxen (Naprosyn, Anaprox)	1976	500–1,000	NR	2–4	99	Hepatic: 3A4, 1A2	13	4.2
Oxaprozin (Daypro)	1993	1,200	NR	3–5	99	Hepatic: 2C9	25	4.3
Piroxicam (Feldene)	1982	20	2–4 h (24 h)	2	99	Hepatic: 2C9	50	1.8, 5.1
Sulindac[a] (Clinoril)	1978	400	NR	2–4	93	Hepatic; sulfide metabolite active	50	4.5
Tolmetin (Tolectin)	1976	1,200	NR	<1	99	Hepatic	5	3.5

6MNA, 6-methoxynaphthalene-2-acetic acid; ND, not determined; NR, not reported.
[a]Prodrug.

is tempting to speculate that this represents their primary mechanism of action. Scherrer, like Shen, had proposed a hypothetical receptor for NSAIDs and later modified (95) the receptor to represent the active site of arachidonic acid COX. Structurally, the fenamic acids fit the proposed active site of arachidonic acid COX proposed by Shen (10), because they possess an acidic function connected to an aromatic ring along

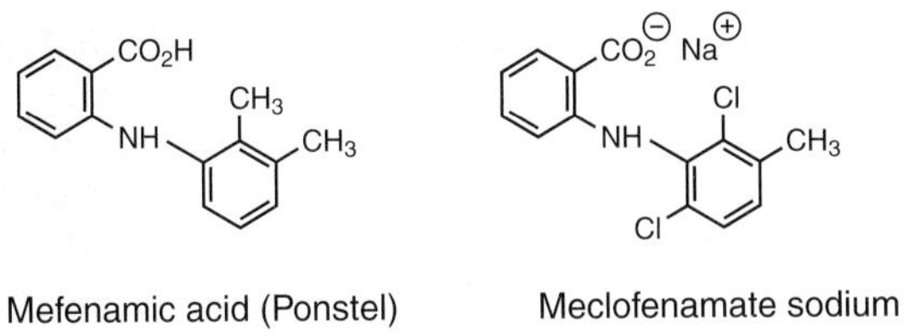

FIGURE 31.22 Structures of *N*-arylanthranilic acids (fenamic acids).

with an additional lipophilic binding site—in this case, the *N*-aryl substituent. The greater anti-inflammatory activity of meclofenamic acid compared to that of mefenamic acid correlates well with its ability to inhibit prostaglandin synthesis. Scherrer (96) compared the in vivo anti-inflammatory activities, clinical anti-inflammatory doses in humans, and in vitro inhibition of prostaglandin synthesis activities of mefenamic acid, meclofenamic acid, phenylbutazone, indomethacin, and aspirin and suggested an important role of prostaglandin synthesis inhibition in the production of therapeutic effects of the fenamic acids.

Side effects are those primarily associated with GI disturbances (e.g., dyspepsia, discomfort, and especially, diarrhea), some CNS effects (e.g., dizziness, headache, and drowsiness), skin rashes, and transient hepatic and renal abnormalities. Isolated cases of hemolytic anemia have been reported.

General Structure–Activity Relationships Substitution on the anthranilic acid ring reduces activity, whereas substitution of the *N*-aryl ring can lead to conflicting results. In the ultraviolet erythema assay for anti-inflammatory activity, the order of activity is usually 3′ > 2′ >> 4′ for monosubstitution, with the 3′-CF_3 derivative (flufenamic acid) being particularly potent.

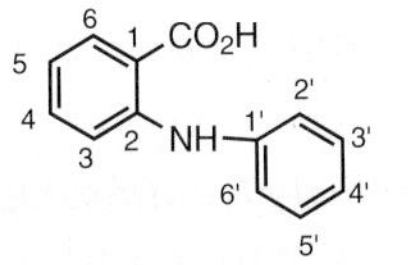

The opposite order of activity was observed, however, in the rat paw edema assay, with the 2′-Cl derivative being more potent than the 3′-Cl analog. In disubstituted derivatives, in which the nature of the two substituents is the same, 2′,3′-disubstitution appears to be the most effective. A plausible explanation can be found in an examination of the proposed topography of the active sites of arachidonic acid COX using either the Shen or Sherrer models. Proposed binding sites include a hydrophobic trough to which a lipophilic group, noncoplanar with the ring bearing the carboxylic acid function, binds. Substituents on the *N*-aryl ring that force this ring to be noncoplanar with the anthranilic acid ring should enhance binding at this site and, thus, activity. This can account for the enhanced anti-inflammatory activity of meclofenamic acid, which has two ortho-substituents forcing this ring out of the plane of the anthranilic acid ring, over flufenamic acid (no ortho-substituents) and mefenamic acid (one ortho-substituent). Meclofenamic acid possesses 25 times greater anti-inflammatory activity than mefenamic acid. The NH-moiety of anthranilic acid appears to be essential for activity, because replacement of the NH function with O, CH_2, S, SO_2, N-CH_3, or N-$COCH_3$ functionalities significantly reduces activity. Finally, the position, rather than the nature, of the acidic function is critical for activity. Anthranilic acid derivatives are active, whereas the *m*- and *p*-aminobenzoic acid analogs are not. Replacement of the carboxylic acid function with the isosteric tetrazole moiety has little effect on activity.

Drug Interactions The pK_a values of the *N*-arylanthranilic acids (4.0 to 4.2) resemble those of the arylalkanoic acids; thus, it is not surprising that they are strongly bound to plasma proteins and that interactions with other highly protein bound drugs are very probable. The most common interactions reported are those of mefenamic acid and meclofenamic acid with oral anticoagulants. Concurrent administration of aspirin results in a reduction of plasma levels of meclofenamic acid.

Specific Drugs

Mefenamic Acid. Mefenamic acid is synthesized from *o*-chlorobenzoic acid and 2,3-dimethylaniline under catalytic conditions (97). Mefenamic acid is the only fenamic acid derivative that produces analgesia centrally and peripherally. Mefenamic acid is indicated for the short-term relief of moderate pain and for primary dysmenorrhea.

Mefenamic acid is absorbed rapidly following oral administration, with peak plasma levels being attained within 2 to 4 hours. It is highly bound to plasma proteins (78.5%) and has a plasma half-life of 2 to 4 hours. Metabolism occurs through regioselective oxidation of the 3′-methyl group and glucuronidation of mefenamic acid and its metabolites. Urinary excretion accounts for approximately 50% to 55% of an administered dose, with unchanged drug accounting for 6%, the 3′-hydroxymethyl metabolite (primarily as the glucuronide) accounting for 25%, and the remaining 20% as the dicarboxylic acid (of which 30% is the glucuronide conjugate) (Fig. 31.23). These metabolites are essentially inactive.

Meclofenamate Sodium. Meclofenamate sodium is rapidly and almost completely absorbed following oral administration, reaching peak plasma levels within 2 hours. It is highly bound to plasma proteins (99%) and has a plasma half-life of 2 to 4 hours. Metabolism involves oxidation of the methyl group, aromatic hydroxylation, monodehalogenation, and conjugation. Urinary excretion accounts for approximately 75% of the administered dose. The major metabolite is the product of 3′-methyl oxidation

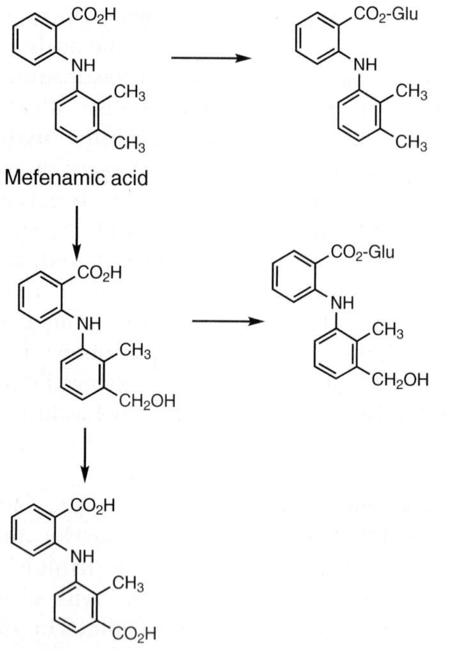

FIGURE 31.23 Metabolism of mefenamic acid.

and has been shown to possess anti-inflammatory activity (Fig. 31.24).

Meclofenamate sodium is indicated for the relief of mild to moderate pain, the acute and chronic treatment of rheumatoid arthritis and osteoarthritis, the treatment of primary dysmenorrhea, and the treatment of idiopathic, heavy menstrual blood loss.

Oxicams The enolic acid class of NSAIDs has been termed "oxicams" by the U.S. Adopted Name Council to describe the series of 4-hydroxy-1,2-benzothiazine carboxamides that possess anti-inflammatory and analgesic properties. These structurally distinct substances resulted from extensive studies by the Pfizer group in an effort to produce noncarboxylic acid, potent, and well-tolerated anti-inflammatory drugs. Several series were prepared, including 2-aryl-1,3-indanediones, 2-arylbenzothiophen-3-(2*H*)-one 1,1-dioxides, dioxoquinoline-4-carboxamides, and 3-oxa-2*H*-1,2-benzothiazine-4-carboxamide 1,1-dioxides, and evaluated. These results, combined with the previously known activity of 1,3-dicarbonyl derivatives, such as phenylbutazone, led to the development of the oxicams. The first member of this class, piroxicam, was introduced in the United States in 1982 as Feldene and gained immediate acceptance.

Piroxicam is potent in standard in vivo assays, being 200 times more potent than aspirin and at least 10 times as potent as any other standard agent in the ultraviolet erythema assay, as potent as indomethacin and more potent than phenylbutazone or naproxen in the carrageenan-induced rat paw edema assay, and equipotent with indomethacin and 15 times more potent than phenylbutazone in the rat adjuvant arthritis assay. It is less potent than indomethacin, equipotent with aspirin, and more potent than fenoprofen, ibuprofen, naproxen, and phenylbutazone as an analgesic in the phenylquinone writhing assay. Piroxicam inhibits the migration of polymorphonuclear cells into inflammatory sites and inhibits the release of lysosomal enzymes from these cells. It also inhibits collagen-induced platelet aggregation. It is an effective inhibitor of arachidonic acid COX, being almost equipotent with indomethacin and more potent than ibuprofen, tolmetin, naproxen, fenoprofen, phenylbutazone, and aspirin in the inhibition of prostaglandin biosynthesis by methylcholanthrene-transformed mouse fibroblasts (MC-5) assay. A template for designing anti-inflammatory compounds based on CPK space-filling models of the peroxy radical precursor of PGG and inhibitors of COX was proposed (98), and the ability of oxicams, particularly piroxicam, to inhibit this enzyme was subsequently rationalized on the ability of oxicams to assume a conformation resembling that of the peroxy radical precursor (99).

Approximately 20% of individuals on piroxicam report adverse reactions. Not unexpectedly, the greatest incidence of side effects results from GI disturbances. The reported incidence of peptic ulcers, however, is less than 1%.

As will be discussed later, a new oxicam derivative, meloxicam, has been approved as a selective COX-2 inhibitor for the treatment of osteoarthritis.

General Structure–Activity Relationships Within the series of 4-hydroxy-1,2-benzothiazine carboxamides represented by the general structure shown below, optimum activity was observed when R1 was a methyl substituent. The carboxamide substituent, R, is usually an aryl or heteroaryl substituent, because alkyl substituents are less active.

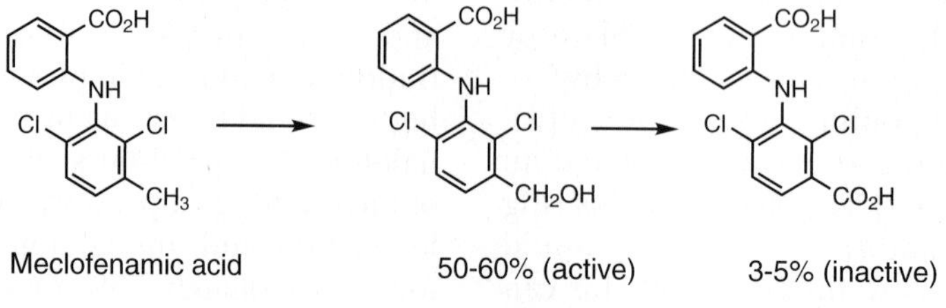

FIGURE 31.24 Metabolism of meclofenamic acid.

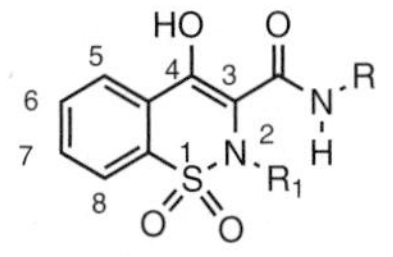

Oxicams are acidic compounds, with pK_a values in the range of 4 to 6. *N*-Heterocyclic carboxamides are more acidic than the corresponding *N*-aryl carboxamides, and this enhanced acidity was attributed (100) to stabilization of the enolate anion by the pyridine nitrogen atom, as illustrated in tautomer A and additional stabilization by tautomer B:

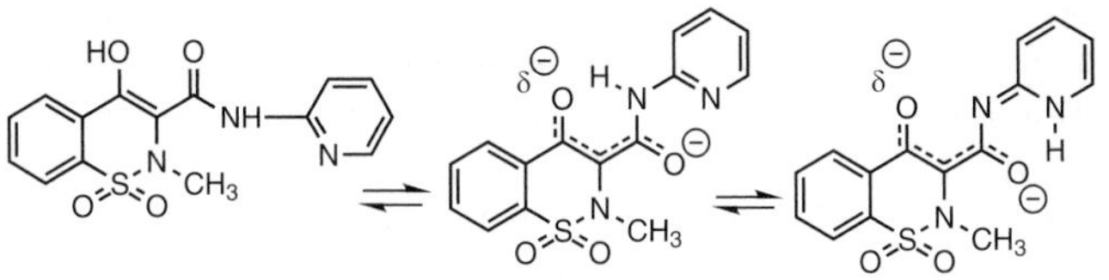

Piroxicam A B

This explains the observation that primary carboxamides are more potent than the corresponding secondary derivatives, because no N–H bond would be available to enhance the stabilization of the enolate anion. When the aryl group is *o*-substituted, variable results were obtained, whereas *m*-substituted derivatives are usually more potent than the corresponding *p*-isomers. In the aryl series, maximum activity is observed with an *m*-Cl substituent. No direct correlations were observed between acidity and activity, partition coefficient, and electronic or spatial properties in this series. Two major differences, however, are observed when R = heteroaryl rather than aryl: The pK_a values are usually two to four units lower, and anti-inflammatory activity is increased as much as sevenfold. The greatest activity is associated with the 2-pyridyl (as in piroxicam), 2-thiazolyl, or 3-(5-methyl) isoxazolyl ring systems, with the latter derivative (isoxicam) having been withdrawn from the European market in 1985 following several reports of severe skin reactions. In addition to possessing activity equal to or greater than indomethacin in the carrageenan-induced rat paw edema assay, the heteroaryl carboxamides also possess longer plasma half-lives, providing an improvement in dosing scheduling regimens.

Drug Interactions Few reports of therapeutically significant interactions of oxicams with other drugs have appeared. Concurrent administration of aspirin has been shown to reduce piroxicam plasma levels by approximately 20%, whereas the anticoagulant effect of acenocoumarin is potentiated, presumably as a result of plasma protein displacement.

Specific Drugs

Piroxicam. Piroxicam was synthesized by ring-expansion reactions of saccharin derivatives (101). Piroxicam is readily absorbed on oral administration, reaching peak plasma levels in approximately 2 hours. Peak plasma levels appear to be lower when given with food at low doses (30 mg), with no differences appearing with a 60-mg dose, but in general, food does not markedly affect bioavailability. Being acidic (pK_a = 6.3), it is highly bound to plasma proteins (99%). Piroxicam possesses an extended plasma half-life (38 hours), making single daily dosing possible. Piroxicam is indicated for long-term use in rheumatoid arthritis and osteoarthritis.

Metabolism Although the metabolism of piroxicam varies quantitatively from species to species, qualitative similarities are found in the metabolic pathways of humans, rats, dogs, and rhesus monkeys. It is extensively metabolized in humans, with less than 5% of an administered dose being excreted unchanged. The major metabolites in humans result from CYP2C9 hydroxylation of the pyridine ring and subsequent glucuronidation; other metabolites are of lesser importance (Fig. 31.25). Aromatic hydroxylation at several positions of the aromatic benzothiazine ring also occurs; two hydroxylated metabolites have been extracted from rat urine. Based on nuclear magnetic resonance deuterium-exchange studies, hydroxylation at the 8-position was ruled out, indicating that hydroxylation occurs at two of the remaining positions. Other novel metabolic reactions occur. Cyclodehydration gave a tetracyclic metabolite (the major metabolite in dogs), whereas ring contraction following amide hydrolysis and decarboxylation eventually yields saccharin. All the known metabolites of piroxicam lack anti-inflammatory activity. For example, the major human metabolite is 1,000-fold less effective as an inhibitor of prostaglandin biosynthesis than piroxicam itself. Related oxicams undergo different routes of metabolism. For example, sudoxicam (the *N*-2-thiazolyl analog) undergoes primarily hydroxylation of the thiazole ring, followed by ring

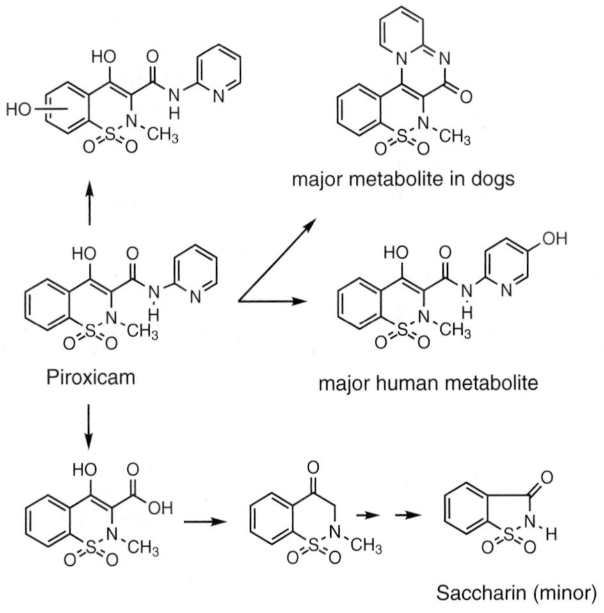

FIGURE 31.25 Metabolism of piroxicam.

opening, whereas isoxicam undergoes primarily cleavage reactions of the benzothiazine ring.

Meloxicam. In April 2000, the FDA approved meloxicam for the treatment of osteoarthritis in the United States. When meloxicam was initially introduced in the United Kingdom, it was promoted as a selective COX-2 inhibitor. Meloxicam, however, is less selective for COX-2 than is celecoxib. Meloxicam is readily absorbed when administered orally and is highly bound to plasma proteins. It is extensively metabolized in the liver, primarily by CYP2C9 and, to a lesser extent, by CYP3A4. The advantages of meloxicam over celecoxib in the treatment of osteoarthritis (or rheumatoid arthritis) are not readily apparent.

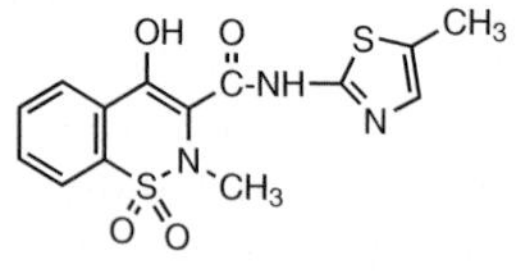

Meloxicam

Metabolism. Unlike the metabolism of piroxicam, the metabolism of meloxicam in humans is rather straightforward. Oxidation of the thiazole methyl group mediated by CYP2C9 (CYP3A4 is involved to a much lesser extent), followed by subsequent oxidation to the carboxylic acid, yields metabolites that have not been shown to possess anti-inflammatory activity. The metabolism of meloxicam is shown in Fig. 31.26.

Gastroenteropathy Induced by Nonselective COX NSAIDs

The effectiveness and popularity of the NSAIDs in the United States and Europe make this class one of the most commonly used classes of therapeutic entities. Unfortunately, until the introduction of the selective COX-2 inhibitors, almost all of the current drugs, which are essentially nonselective COX-1 and COX-2 inhibitors, share the undesirable property of producing damaging effects to gastric and intestinal mucosa, resulting in erosion, ulcers, and GI bleeding, and these represent the major adverse reactions to the use of NSAIDs. As many as 20,000 deaths and 100,000 hospitalizations per year have been associated with GI complications resulting from the use of NSAIDs. Approximately 30% to 40% of patients taking NSAIDs report some type of gastric injury, and approximately 10% discontinue therapy because of these effects. These acute and chronic injuries to gastric mucosa result in a variety of lesions referred to as NSAID gastropathy, which differs from peptic ulcer disease by localization of lesions more frequently in the stomach rather than in the duodenum. Additionally, NSAID-induced lesions occur more frequently in the elderly than typical peptic ulcers. Normally, the stomach protects itself from the harmful effects of hydrochloric acid and pepsin by a number of protective mechanisms referred to as the gastric mucosal barrier, which consists of epithelial cells, the mucous and bicarbonate layer, and mucosal blood flow. Gastric mucosa is actually a gel consisting of polymers of glycoprotein, which limit the diffusion of hydrogen ions. These polymers reduce the rate at which hydrogen ions (produced in the lumen) and bicarbonate ions (secreted by the mucosa) mix; thus, a pH gradient is created across the mucus layer. Normally, gastric mucosal cells are rapidly repaired when they are damaged by factors such as food, ethanol, or acute ingestion of NSAIDs. Among the cytoprotective mechanisms is the ability of prostaglandins of the PGE series, particularly PGE_1, to increase the secretion of bicarbonate ion and mucus and to maintain mucosal blood flow. The prostaglandins also decrease acid secretion, permitting the gastric mucosal barrier to remain intact. The use of PGE_1 to reduce NSAID-induced gastric damage is limited by the fact that it is ineffective orally and degrades rapidly on parenteral administration, primarily by oxidation of the 15-hydroxy group. To overcome these limitations, misoprostol was synthesized as a prostaglandin prodrug analog in which oral activity was achieved by administering the drug as the methyl ester, allowing the bioactive acid to be liberated after absorption. Oxidation of the 15-hydroxy group was overcome by moving the hydroxy group to the 16-position, thus "fooling" the enzyme prostaglandin 15-OH dehydrogenase. Oxidation was further limited by the introduction of a methyl group at the 16-position, producing a tertiary alcohol that is more difficult to oxidize than the secondary alcohol group of the prostaglandins. Misoprostol was introduced in 1989 as a mixture of stereoisomers at the 16-position as Cytotec for the prevention of NSAID-induced gastric ulcers (but not duodenalulcers) in patients at high risk of complications from a gastric ulcer, particularly the elderly and patients with concomitant debilitating disease and in individuals with a history of gastric ulcers.

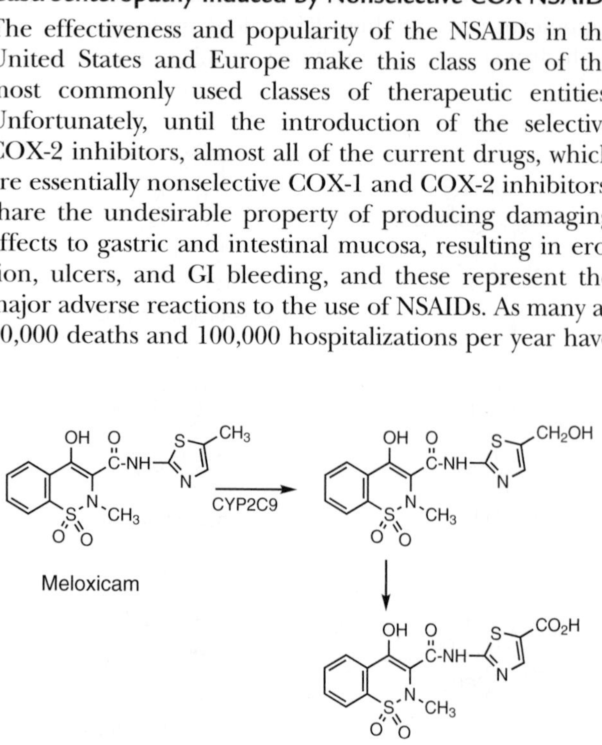

FIGURE 31.26 Metabolism of meloxicam.

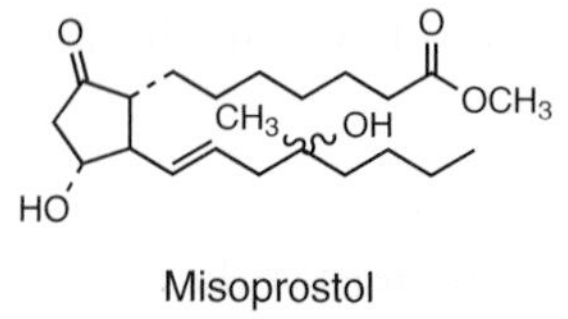

Misoprostol

As mentioned earlier, Figure 31.7 illustrates the ability of aspirin and NSAIDs to induce gastric damage by a dual-insult mechanism. Aspirin and the NSAIDs are acidic substances that can damage the GI tract, even in the absence of hydrochloric acid, by changing the permeability of cell membranes, allowing a back diffusion of hydrogen ions. These weak acids remain un-ionized in the stomach, but the resulting lipophilic nature of these substances allows accumulation or concentration in gastric mucosal cells. Once inside these cells, however, the higher pH of the intracellular environment causes the acids to dissociate and become "trapped" within the cells. The permeability of the mucosal cell membrane is thus altered, and the accumulation of hydrogen ions causes mucosal cell damage. This gastric damage is a result, therefore, of the primary insult of acidic substances. As detailed earlier in this chapter, the primary mechanism of action of the NSAIDs is to inhibit the biosynthesis of prostaglandins at the cyclooxygenase step. The resulting nonselective inhibition of prostaglandin biosynthesis in the GI tract prevents the prostaglandins from exerting their protective mechanism on gastric mucosa; thus, the NSAIDs induce gastric damage through this secondary insult mechanism.

Selective COX-2 Inhibitors As previously discussed, the most notable achievement in the development of NSAIDs has been in the area of selective COX-2 inhibitors ("coxibs"). Classic NSAIDs share similar side effect profiles, particularly on the GI tract, many of which have been attributed to the inhibition of COX, the rate-limiting step in prostaglandin biosynthesis. With the discovery of two isoforms of COX, COX-1 and COX-2, and the realization that COX-1 is beneficial in maintaining normal processes in the GI tract by producing cytoprotective prostaglandins, stimulating bicarbonate secretion and mucus, and producing an overall reduction in acid secretion, the search for drugs that selectively inhibit the COX-2 isoform has received much attention. The traditional NSAIDs inhibit COX-1, COX-2, and thromboxane synthetase to varying degrees of selectivity. Decreased gastric mucosal protection (resulting in an enhanced risk of ulceration) and stress-induced decreased renal perfusion result from nonselective inhibition of COX, whereas inhibition of thromboxane synthesis results in increased prostaglandin synthesis and a reduction in platelet aggregation and, thus, an increased bleeding tendency. Those NSAIDs with a greater selectivity for COX-1 as a rule cause greater GI bleeding and renal toxicity than those with greater selectivity for COX-2.

These early studies led to extensive efforts by many laboratories to develop selective inhibitors of the COX-2 isoform with the goal of developing an "ideal" NSAID—that is, one that selectively inhibits COX-2, thus reducing the inflammatory response, but does not interfere with the GI-protective functions of COX-1. Two early lead compounds were developed, NS-398 and DuP 697, which have served as the basis of the development of two widely explored chemical classes. NS-398 and nimesulide are the prototypes of compounds known as "sulides," whereas DuP 697 is the prototype of a class of COX-2 inhibitors termed "coxibs."

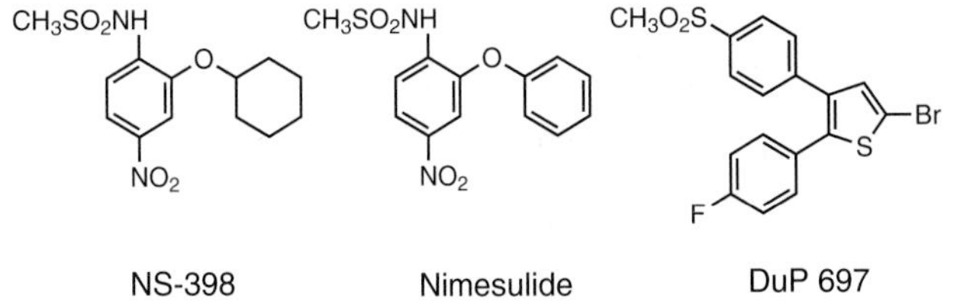

These efforts led to the introduction of several selective COX-2 inhibitors in the US market (celecoxib, rofecoxib, lumiracoxib, and valdecoxib), but safety risks and cardiovascular side effects led to the removal of all coxibs except celecoxib, and the development of other selective COX-2 inhibitors such as parecoxib and etoricoxib has been halted (Fig. 31.27). An excellent review of the various chemical classes of selective COX-2 inhibitors has been published (102). Selective COX-2 inhibitors were designed to take advantage of the much larger NSAID binding site on COX-2 compared to the NSAID binding site on COX-1, resulting from the substitution of the smaller amino acid valine in COX-2 for isoleucine at position 523 in COX-1 (see earlier discussion). In COX-1, the larger isoleucine residue near the active site restricts access by larger, relatively rigid side-chain substituents, such as sulfamoyl or sulfonyl side chains usually seen in the selective COX-2 inhibitors.

A comparison of the selectivity of several NSAIDs and selective COX-2 inhibitors has been presented (Fig. 31.28) (103). In this study, rofecoxib displayed greater than 50-fold selectivity for COX-2 versus COX-1,

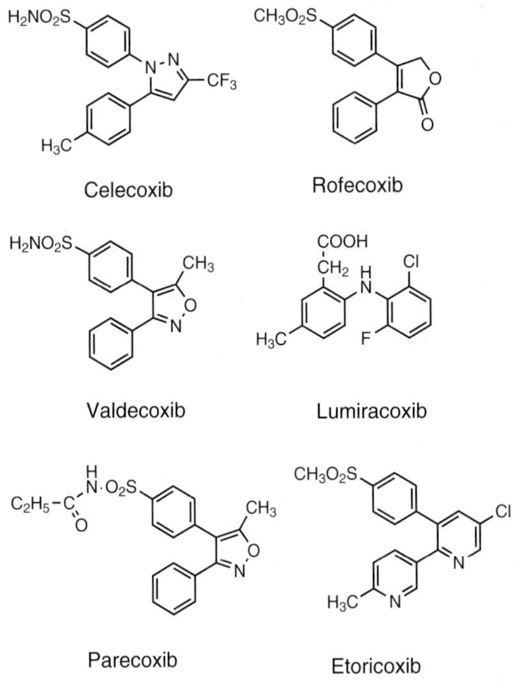

FIGURE 31.27 Structures of selective COX-2 inhibitors.

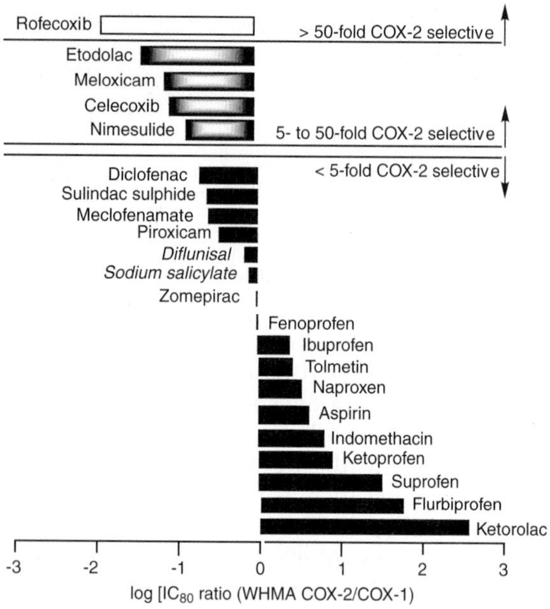

FIGURE 31.28 Selectivity of COX-2 inhibitors and NSAIDs given as log inhibitory concentration (IC_{80}) ratio. The "o" line indicates equipotency. (Adapted from Warner TD, Giuliano F, Vojnovic I, et al. Nonsteroid drug selectivities for cyclooxygenase-1 rather than cyclooxygenase-2 are associated with human gastrointestinal toxicity: a full in vitro analysis. Proc Natl Acad Sci U S A 1999;96:7563–7568, with permission.)

whereas celecoxib displayed 5- to 550-fold selectivity. In another study regarding the pharmacologic and biochemical profile of a new investigational selective COX-2 inhibitor, etoricoxib, the comparison of COX-1/COX-2 selectivity for several selective and nonselective inhibitors in human whole blood assays was reported (Table 31.5) (104).

Perhaps as interesting as the role that COX-2 selective inhibitors have in reducing the incidence of GI side effects among NSAIDs are the reports of other potential therapeutic uses for this new class of drugs, including potential use in the treatment of Alzheimer disease and carcinomas of various types. COX-2 appears to be induced in inflammatory plaques that are evident in the CNS in Alzheimer disease. Several reports have appeared indicating that patients taking NSAIDs have a lower incidence and a decreased rate of progression of Alzheimer disease. Epidemiologic studies suggest a significant reduction in the risk for colon cancer in patients regularly taking aspirin. Additionally, NSAIDs have been reported to reduce the growth rate of polyps in the colon in humans as well as the incidence of tumors of the colon in animals. The expression of COX-2 appears to be significantly upregulated in carcinoma of the colon. The effectiveness of NSAIDs in the prevention and treatment of other cancers, such as prostate cancer and mammary carcinoma, has been reported as well. This effectiveness is more noticeable among COX-2 selective drugs.

TABLE 31.5 A Comparison of IC50 (μmole) Binding Constants for Selective Versus Nonselective Cyclooxygenase (COX) Inhibitors

Drug	COX-1	COX-2	COX-1/COX-2 Ratio
Etoricoxib	116	1.1	106
Rofecoxib	18.8	0.53	35
Valdecoxib	26.1	0.87	30
Celecoxib	6.7	0.87	7.6
Nimesulide	4.1	0.56	7.3
Diclofenac	0.15	0.05	3.0
Etodolac	9.0	3.7	2.4
Meloxicam	1.4	0.70	2.0
Indomethacin	0.19	0.44	0.4
Ibuprofen	4.8	24.3	0.2
6MNA	28.9	154	0.2
Piroxicam	0.76	9.0	0.08

IC_{50}, half maximal inhibitory concentration; 6MNA, 6-methoxynaphthalene-2-acetic acid.

Despite the promise of therapeutic effectiveness of the selective COX-2 inhibitors, the potential for severe cardiovascular effects prompted a critical review of these drugs. This concern was initiated through the revelation of long-term clinical trials of rofecoxib that indicated an increased risk of heart attack. One study completed in 2000, named VIGOR (105), showed an increased risk of myocardial infarction. A later retrospective analysis (106) of 1.4 million patients showed that daily rofecoxib doses of greater than 25 mg increased the risk of heart problems by 3.6-fold as compared with older NSAIDs. The coxibs were found (107) to suppress the formation of PGI_2, which can result in elevated blood pressure and accelerated atherogenesis and predispose patients on coxib therapy to a heightened thrombotic response on the rupture of an atherosclerotic plaque (108). These effects can be related to the different consequences of inhibition of COX-1 and COX-2. Whereas COX-1 mediates the production of prostaglandins and the platelet aggregate stimulator TXA_2, COX-2 can mediate the production of the platelet aggregate inhibitor prostacyclin. In an excellent review of the adverse cardiovascular effects of selective COX-2 inhibitors, it was suggested that the apparent consequence of selective inhibition of COX-2 is a significant reduction in the production of prostacyclins, whereas the production of TXA_2 by COX-1 is unaffected (109). Of practical interest is a report that resveratrol, an *m*-hydroxyquinone present in red wine that has been suggested to be one agent responsible for the cardioprotective effects observed with the consumption of red wine (i.e., the "French Paradox"), inhibits COX-1 with no apparent effect on COX-2 (110, 111). Thus, the design of highly selective inhibitors of

COX-2 would not be as desirable therapeutically as drugs that preferentially inhibit COX-2 but also inhibit COX-1 to a lesser extent.

In one of the most publicized drug withdrawals, Merck voluntarily withdrew rofecoxib from the US market in September 2004, followed by Pfizer's withdrawal of valdecoxib in April 2005 and the removal of lumiracoxib by Novartis in 2007. These drugs were voluntarily withdrawn because of safety concerns from increased risk of serious cardiovascular thrombotic events, myocardial infarction, and stroke, which can be fatal. This risk can increase with duration of use. Thus, the future of selective COX-2 inhibitors in the treatment of inflammatory disorders remains clouded.

Specific Drugs

Celecoxib (Celebrex). Celecoxib is synthesized by condensing 4-methyl-acetophenone and ethyltrifluoroacetate with sodium methoxide and the resulting butanedione derivative cyclized with 4-hydrazinophenylsulfonamide (111). It was the first NSAID to be marketed as a selective COX-2 inhibitor. Celecoxib is well absorbed from the GI tract, with peak plasma concentrations normally being attained within 3 hours of administration. Peak plasma levels in geriatric patients can be increased, but dosage adjustments in elderly patients are usually not required unless the patient weighs less than 50 kg. Celecoxib is excreted in the urine and feces primarily as inactive metabolites, with less than 3% of an administered dose being excreted as unchanged drug. Metabolism occurs primarily in the liver by CYP2C9 and involves hydroxylation of the 4-methyl group to the primary alcohol, which is subsequently oxidized to its corresponding inactive carboxylic acid, the major metabolite (73% of the administered dose) (Fig. 31.29). The carboxylic acid is conjugated, to a slight extent, with glucuronic acid to form the corresponding glucuronide. None of the isolated metabolites have been shown to exhibit pharmacologic activity as inhibitors of either COX-1 or COX-2.

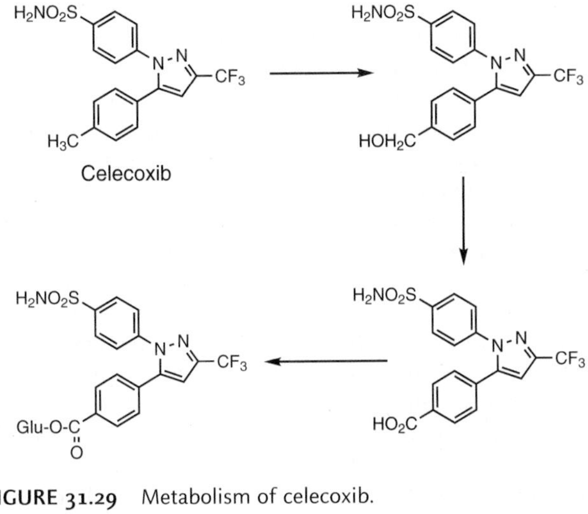

FIGURE 31.29 Metabolism of celecoxib.

> **ADVERSE EFFECTS**
>
> Celecoxib can cause an increased risk of serious cardiovascular thrombotic events, myocardial infarction, and stroke, which can be fatal. All NSAIDs can have a similar risk. This risk can increase with duration of use. Patients with cardiovascular disease or risk factors for cardiovascular disease can be at greater risk. The NSAIDs, including celecoxib, cause an increased risk of serious GI adverse events, including bleeding, ulceration, and perforation of the stomach or intestines, which can be fatal. These events can occur at any time during use and without warning symptoms. Elderly patients are at greater risk for serious GI events.

Celecoxib also inhibits CYP2D6; thus, the potential of celecoxib to alter the pharmacokinetic profiles of other drugs inhibited by this isoenzyme exists. Celecoxib, however, does not appear to inhibit other CYP isoforms, such as CYP2C19 or CYP3A4. Other drug interactions related to the metabolic profile of celecoxib have been noted, particularly with other drugs that inhibit CYP2C. For example, coadministration of celecoxib with fluconazole can significantly increase plasma concentration of celecoxib, because fluconazole inhibits CYP2C9.

Celecoxib is currently indicated for the relief of signs and symptoms of osteoarthritis and rheumatoid arthritis and to reduce the number of adenomatous colorectal polyps in familial adenomatous polyposis as an adjunct to usual care. Celecoxib is at least as effective as naproxen in the symptomatic management of osteoarthritis and at least as effective as naproxen and diclofenac in the symptomatic treatment of rheumatoid arthritis, and it is less likely to cause adverse GI effects. Celecoxib appears to be effective in the management of pain associated with both of these arthritic conditions, but effectiveness in acute or chronic pain has not been fully demonstrated. Unlike aspirin, celecoxib does not exhibit antiplatelet activity. Concomitant administration of aspirin and celecoxib can increase the incidence of GI side effects. Another notable potential drug interaction with celecoxib is its ability, like other NSAIDs, to reduce the blood pressure response to angiotensin-converting enzyme inhibitors. A more detailed discussion of the chemical, pharmacologic, pharmacokinetic, and clinical aspects of celecoxib is available (112).

DISEASE-MODIFYING ANTIRHEUMATIC DRUGS

The drugs previously discussed as NSAIDs, both the nonselective COX and selective COX-2 inhibitors, have proven to be beneficial as analgesics and for the symptomatic treatment of arthritic disorders. Despite their effectiveness and popularity, however, it should be remembered that none of these drugs are effective in preventing or inhibiting the underlying pathogenic, chronic inflammatory processes. Recent interest has been generated by drugs that are effective in the treatment of arthritic disorders yet fail to demonstrate significant activity in the standard screening assays for antiarthritic drugs. Disease-modifying antirheumatic drugs (DMARDs) differ from the previously discussed drugs in that they are drugs that retard or halt the underlying progression, limiting the amount of joint damage that occurs in rheumatoid arthritis while lacking the anti-inflammatory and analgesic effects observed with NSAIDs. Although both NSAIDs and DMARDs improve symptoms of active rheumatoid arthritis, only DMARDs have been shown to alter the disease course and to improve radiographic outcomes. The DMARDs have an effect on rheumatoid arthritis that is different and more delayed in onset than either NSAIDs or corticosteroids. Once persistent disease activity (chronic synovitis) is established, a DMARD should be considered. The development of erosions or joint space narrowing on radiographs of the involved joints is a clear indication for DMARD therapy; however, one should not wait for radiographic changes to occur. DMARDs are much slower acting, taking as long as 3 months for measurable clinical benefits to be observed. Although these drugs also possess potentially dangerous adverse side effects, which in many cases limit their long-term use, DMARDs are effective in reducing joint destruction and the progression of early rheumatoid arthritis.

A 2004 study reported that taking DMARDs at early stages in the development of rheumatoid arthritis is especially important to slow the disease and to save the joints and other tissues from permanent damage (113). Typically, DMARDs are used with an NSAID or a corticosteroid. The NSAID or corticosteroid handles the immediate symptoms and limits inflammation, and the DMARD goes to work on the disease itself.

The DMARDS can be divided into two general categories: synthetic DMARDS, which can be taken orally, and biologic DMARDS, which are given by IV infusion or subcutaneously, that target and inactivate cell proteins (cytokines) and T lymphocytes (T cells) from causing joint inflammation. The DMARD methotrexate, in combination with the biologic DMARDs, can offer the best control of rheumatoid arthritis for the majority of people, eliminating the need for NSAID medications.

Synthetic Disease-Modifying Antirheumatic Drugs

The synthetic DMARDs include gold salts, hydroxychloroquine, and sulfasalazine. Less common synthetic DMARDs are penicillamine and minocycline. Synthetic immunosuppressants used for the treatment of inflammatory diseases include the antimetabolites methotrexate, leflunomide, and azathioprine.

Gold Compounds

Historical Background At the end of the 19th century, the chemotherapeutic applications of heavy metal derivatives were receiving considerable interest. Among those metals gaining the greatest attention were gold compounds (or gold salts). The first of these, gold cyanide, was effective in vitro against *Mycobacterium tuberculosis*. This discovery prompted others to extend the use of gold compounds in other disease states that are thought to be tubercular in origin. Early clinical observations had suggested similarities in the symptoms of tuberculosis and rheumatoid arthritis, and some thought rheumatoid arthritis to be an atypical form of tuberculosis. In 1927, aurothioglucose was found to relieve joint pain when used to treat bacterial endocarditis. The area of chrysotherapy had begun. Subsequent investigations led to an extensive study of gold compounds in Great Britain by the Empire Rheumatism Council, which reported in 1961 that sodium aurothiomalate was effective in slowing the development of progressive joint diseases. Both aurothioglucose and sodium aurothiomalate are orally ineffective and are administered by IM injection. In 1985, the first orally effective gold compound for arthritis, auranofin, was introduced in the United States. Several other gold compounds have been evaluated clinically but do not appear to offer advantages in terms of efficacy or toxicity.

Mechanism of Action The biochemical and pharmacologic properties shared by gold compounds are quite diverse. The mechanism by which they produce their antirheumatic actions has not been totally determined. The earlier observations that gold compounds were effective in preventing arthritis induced by hemolytic streptococci and by pleuropneumonia-like organisms led to the postulation that they acted through an antimicrobial mechanism. The inability of gold compounds to consistently inhibit mycoplasmal growth in vitro while inhibiting the arthritic process independent of microbial origins, however, suggested that they did not directly produce their effects by this mechanism. The involvement of immunologic processes in the pathogenesis of arthritis suggested that a direct suppression of the immunologic response by gold compounds was involved. Available evidence, however, suggests that whereas enzymatic mediators released as a result of the immune response can be inhibited, no direct effect on either immediate or delayed cellular responses is evident to suggest any immunosuppressive mechanism. Suggestions have been made that protein denaturation and macroglobulin formation cause the proteins to become antigenic, thus initiating the immune response and producing biochemical changes in connective tissue, which ultimately leads to rheumatoid arthritis. The possibility that gold compounds inhibit the aggregation of macroglobulins and, in turn, inhibit the formation of immune complexes can account for their ability to slow connective tissue degradation. Interaction with collagen fibrils and, thus, reduction of collagen reactivity that alters the course of the arthritic process has been also postulated. Perhaps the most widely accepted mechanism of action is related to the ability of gold compounds to inhibit lysosomal enzymes, the release of which promotes the inflammatory response. The lysosomal enzymes glucuronidase, acid phosphatase, collagenase, and acid hydrolases are inhibited, presumably through a reversible interaction of gold with sulfhydryl groups on the enzymes. Gold thiomalate inhibits glucosamine-6-phosphate synthetase, a rate-limiting step in mucopolysaccharide biosynthesis and a property shared, to a lesser extent, by several NSAIDs. Gold sodium thiosulfate is a potent uncoupler of oxidative phosphorylation. Gold sodium thiomalate is also a fairly effective inhibitor of prostaglandin biosynthesis in vitro, but the relationship of this effect to the antiarthritic actions of gold compounds has not been clarified.

More recent studies suggest that auranofin suppressed the TLR4-mediated activation of the transcription factors by nuclear factor-κB (NF-κB) and IRF3, thus preventing the expression of cytokines and COX-2 (114). Previously it was shown that zinc is a necessary component of NF-κB for DNA binding and that gold ion can block this binding by oxidizing custeines associated with zinc (115). Auranofin has also been shown to decrease tumor necrosis factor (TNF)-α–induced NF-κB activation, suggesting that effective inhibitors of NF-κB can be useful immunosuppressive and anti-inflammatory agents (116).

Side Effects Toxic side effects have been associated with the use of gold compounds, with the incidence of reported adverse reactions in patients on chrysotherapy being as high as 55%. Serious toxicity occurs in 5% to 10% of reported cases. The most common adverse reactions include dermatitis (e.g., erythema, papular, vesicular, and exfoliative dermatitis), mouth lesions (e.g., stomatitis preceded by a metallic taste and gingivitis), pulmonary disorders (e.g., interstitial pneumonitis), nephritis (e.g., albuminuria and glomerulitis), and hematologic disorders (e.g., thrombocytopenic purpura, hypoplastic and/or aplastic anemia, and eosinophilia; blood dyscrasias are rare in incidence but can be severe). Less commonly reported reactions are GI disturbances (e.g., nausea, anorexia, and diarrhea), ocular toxicity (e.g., keratitis with inflammation and ulceration of the cornea and subepithelial deposition of gold in the cornea), and hepatitis. In those cases in which severe toxicity occurs, excretion of gold can be markedly enhanced by the administration of chelating agents, the two most common of which are dimercaprol (British Anti-Lewisite) and penicillamine. Corticoids also suppress the symptoms of gold toxicity and the concomitant administration of dimercaprol, and corticosteroids have been recommended in cases of severe gold intoxication.

General Structure–Activity Relationships Structure–activity relationships of gold compounds have not received a great amount of attention. Two important relationships, however, have been established: 1) Monovalent gold (aurous ion [Au^+]) is more effective than trivalent gold (auric ion [Au^{3+}]) or colloidal gold; and 2) only those compounds in which aurous ion is attached to a sulfur-containing ligand are active (Fig. 31.30). The nature of the ligands affects tissue distribution and excretion properties and are usually highly polar, water-soluble functions. Aurous ion has only a brief existence in solution and is rapidly converted to metallic gold or auric ion. Aqueous solutions decompose on standing at room temperature, posing a stability problem for the two injectable gold compounds therapeutically available (aurothioglucose and gold sodium thiomalate). Complexation of Au^+ with phosphine ligands stabilizes the reduced valence state and results in both nonionic complexes that are soluble in organic solvents and an enhancement of oral bioavailability. Other changes also occur. In the phosphine-Au-S compounds, gold has a coordination number of 2, and the molecules are nonconducting monomers in solution. The injectable gold compounds are monocoordinated. Whereas nongold phosphine compounds are ineffective in arthritic assays, the nature of the phosphine ligand in the gold coordination complexes appears to have a greater role in antiarthritic activity than the other groups bound to gold. Within a homologous series, the triethylphosphine gold derivatives provide greatest activity.

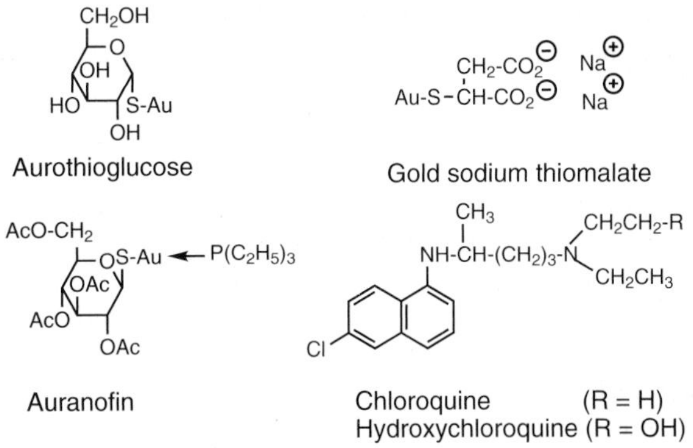

FIGURE 31.30 Structures of disease-modifying antirheumatic drugs (DMARDs).

The structures of the three therapeutically available gold compounds in the United States are shown in Figure 31.30.

Absorption and Metabolism Gold compounds are rapidly absorbed following IM injection, and the gold is widely distributed in body tissues, with the highest concentrations found in the reticuloendothelial system and in adrenal and renal cortices. Binding of gold from orally administered gold to red blood cells is higher than that of injectable gold. Gold accumulates in inflamed joints, where high levels persist for at least 20 days after injection. Although gold is excreted primarily in the urine, the bulk of injected gold is retained. Gold can be found in the urine months later.

Drug Interactions The only significant drug interactions reported are the concurrent administration of drugs that also produce blood dyscrasias (most notably phenylbutazone and the antimalarial and immunosuppressive drugs).

Specific Drugs

Gold Sodium Thiomalate Gold sodium thiomalate (actually a mixture of mono- and disodium salts of gold thiomalic acid) is very water soluble. It is available as a light-sensitive, aqueous solution of pH 5.8 to 6.5. The gold content is approximately 50%. It is administered IM, because it is not absorbed on oral administration and is highly bound (95%) to plasma proteins.

Gold sodium thiomalate is indicated in the treatment of active adult and juvenile rheumatoid arthritis as one part of a complete therapy program. It is recommended that injections be given to patients only when they are in a supine position. They must remain so for 10 minutes following injection.

Aurothioglucose Aurothioglucose is highly water soluble, and its aqueous solutions decompose on long standing. Therefore, it is available as a suspension in sesame oil. Gold content is approximately 50%. After IM injection, it is highly protein bound (95%), and peak plasma levels are achieved within 2 to 6 hours. After a single 50-mg dose, the biologic half-life ranges from 3 to 27 days, but following successive weekly doses, the half-life increases to 14 to 40 days after the third dose. The therapeutic effect does not correlate with serum plasma gold levels but appears to depend on total accumulated gold. Aurothioglucose is indicated for the adjunctive treatment of adult and juvenile rheumatoid arthritis.

Auranofin Auranofin contains approximately 29% gold. The carbohydrate portion assumes a chair conformation, with all substituents occupying the equatorial position. It is the first orally effective gold compound used to treat rheumatoid arthritis. On a milligram of gold per kilogram basis, it is reported to be as effective in the rat adjuvant arthritis assay as the parenterally effective drugs. Daily oral doses produce a rapid increase in kidney and blood gold levels for the first 3 days of treatment, with a more gradual increase on subsequent administration. Plasma gold levels are lower than those attained with parenteral gold compounds. The major route of excretion is via the urine. Auranofin can produce fewer adverse reactions than parenteral gold compounds, but its therapeutic efficacy can also be less.

Auranofin is indicated in adults with active rheumatoid arthritis who have not responded sufficiently to one or more NSAIDs.

Aminoquinolines

Background The 4-aminoquinoline class of antimalarial drugs has been known to possess pharmacologic actions that are beneficial in the treatment of rheumatoid arthritis. Two of these drugs, chloroquine and hydroxychloroquine (Fig. 31.30), have been used as antirheumatics since the early 1950s. The corneal and renal toxicity of chloroquine, however, has resulted in its discontinuance for this purpose, although it is still indicated as an antimalarial agent and an amebicide. Whereas hydroxychloroquine is less toxic, it is also less effective than chloroquine as an antirheumatic. The mechanism of action of these drugs as an antirheumatic remains unresolved. Interestingly, most of the data available relate to chloroquine rather than hydroxychloroquine but are assumed to be applicable to the latter. The spectrum of action of the 4-aminoquinolines differs from the NSAIDs in that chloroquine appears to be an antagonist of certain preformed prostaglandins. This effect, however, would indicate an acute, rather than a chronic, antirheumatic effect, whereas chloroquine has been shown to be similar to gold compounds in that it possesses a slow onset of action. Beneficial effects are noted only after 1 to 2 months of administration. Chloroquine inhibits chemotaxis of polymorphonuclear leukocytes in vitro but not in vivo. Its effects on collagen metabolism in connective tissue are also unclear. The most widely accepted mechanism of action of chloroquine and, presumably, of hydroxychloroquine is related to its ability to accumulate in lysosomes. Although evidence indicating stabilization of lysosomal membranes is not convincing, it can inhibit the activity of certain lysosomal enzymes, such as cartilage chondromucoprotease and cartilage cathepsin B. The possibility that chloroquine can prevent the release of TNFα from phagocytes has been proposed (117). There does not appear to be a correlation of the antirheumatic effects of the 4-aminoquinolines with their antimalarial activity.

Hydroxychloroquine Sulfate Hydroxychloroquine sulfate is highly water soluble and exists in two different forms of different melting points. It is readily absorbed on oral administration, reaching peak plasma levels within 1 to 3 hours. It concentrates in organs such as the liver, spleen, kidneys, heart, lung, and brain, thereby prolonging elimination. Hydroxychloroquine is metabolized by *N*-dealkylation of the tertiary amines, followed by oxidative deamination of the resulting primary amine to the carboxylic acid derivative. In addition to possessing corneal and renal toxicity, hydroxychloroquine can also cause CNS, neuromuscular, GI, and hematologic side effects. Hydroxychloroquine sulfate is indicated for the treatment of rheumatoid arthritis, lupus erythematosus, and malaria.

Immunosuppressants

The discovery of drugs that modify the immune response, whether as immunoregulatory, immunostimulatory, or immunosuppressive agents, has been the focus of much recent research activity. Several substances that suppress the immune system have been explored as antirheumatic drugs, because the etiology of rheumatoid arthritis can involve a destructive immune response. Thus, unlike drugs previously discussed,

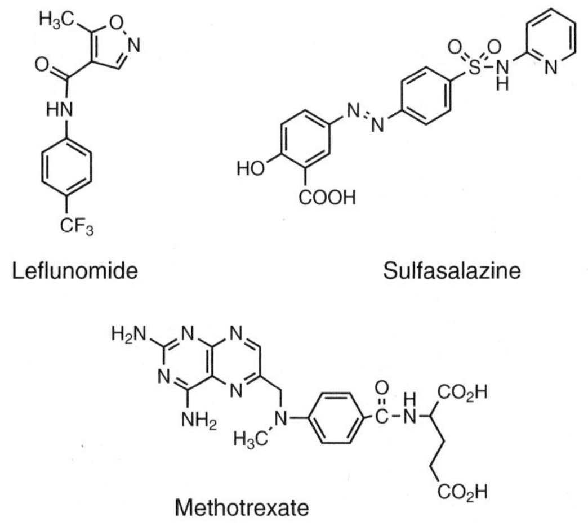

FIGURE 31.31 Structures of DMARD immunosuppressants.

immunosuppressive drugs can act at the steps involved in the pathogenesis of the inflammatory disorders. As a group, however, these drugs are cytotoxic, as evidenced by the initial development of these drugs as anticancer agents. Among the more widely employed immunosuppressants for rheumatoid arthritis are leflunomide, methotrexate, and sulfasalazine (Fig. 31.31). Others that have been explored include azathioprine and cyclophosphamide. All of these drugs are quite toxic and, are indicated for rheumatoid arthritis only in patients with severe, active disease who have not responded to full-dose NSAID therapy and at least one DMARD and a corticosteroid. Interestingly, although aspirin and NSAIDs are effective in only one-third of children with juvenile arthritis, methotrexate, when given only once a week at low doses (<20 mg) to minimize side effects, is effective. Cyclosporine (Sandimmune) has been investigated in rheumatoid arthritis and appears to offer short-term benefits, although its toxic effects also limit its long-term use. Cyclosporine appears to inhibit the proliferation of T-helper/inducer lymphocytes, blocking the signaling pathway involved in the etiology of rheumatoid arthritis.

A new class of oral small-molecule immunosuppressants with anti-inflammatory and antiallergic properties that can be administered orally are the Janus activated kinase (JAK) 3 inhibitors, which includes tofacitinib, a pyrrolo[2,3-d]pyrimidine analog. The Janus tyrosine kinases (JAK1, JAK2, JAK3, and Tyk2), named after the Roman god of gates and doors ("Janus"), regulate the signal transduction pathways of numerous cytokines including the interleukins, and therefore have a central role in immunosuppression and immunomodulation. Of the four JAK enzymes, JAK3 controls the signaling pathways of the multiple interleukin cytokines important for various B- and T-cell functions. JAK3 was identified as a target for immunosuppression because its expression is limited to lymphoid cells. Thus inhibition of JAK3 by tofacitinib in clinical trials has shown promising activity in the treatment of rheumatoid arthritis, inflammatory bowel disease, ankylosing spondylitis, psoriasis, and psoriatic arthritis and for the prevention of transplant rejection (118).

Specific Drugs

Leflunomide Leflunomide is a DMARD with anti-inflammatory and immunosuppressive activity used for the management of rheumatoid arthritis. It retards structural damage associated with arthritis in adults who have moderate to severe active rheumatoid arthritis. Leflunomide is also being investigated for use in patients with solid tumors and in organ transplant recipients.

Leflunomide is a prodrug that is rapidly and almost completely metabolized (half-life, <60 minutes) after oral administration to teriflunomide, the pharmacologically active α-cyanoenol metabolite (Fig. 31.32). The C_3-H of the isoxazole ring is essential for the ring opening to its active metabolite. The reaction is similar to the CYP1A2-catalyzed dehydration of aldoximes. The exact mechanism of action of leflunomide in the management of rheumatoid arthritis has not been fully elucidated but appears to principally involve inhibition of B-lymphocyte (B-cell) proliferation, reducing antibody formation. Activated lymphocytes must proliferate and synthesize large quantities of cytokines, requiring increased de novo synthesis of uridine monophosphate (UMP) and other pyrimidine nucleotides for its cell life cycle. Therefore, any substance that reduces the intracellular concentration of pyrimidine nucleotides will affect the growth of these activated cells.

Leflunomide itself lacks activity, but teriflunomide inhibits pyrimidine de novo synthesis at low therapeutic doses by inhibiting dihydroorotate dehydrogenase (the rate-determining enzyme for the synthesis of UMP), decreasing DNA and RNA synthesis, and arresting the cell proliferation cycle and production of antibodies. The reduction of dihydroorotate to orotate occurs concurrently with the reduction of its cofactor, ubiquinone (coenzyme Q) (Fig. 31.33).

The inhibition of dihydroorotate dehydrogenase by teriflunomide demonstrates noncompetitive and uncompetitive kinetics. Administration of leflunomide in patients with rheumatoid arthritis results in progressive removal of B cells and downregulation of the immune

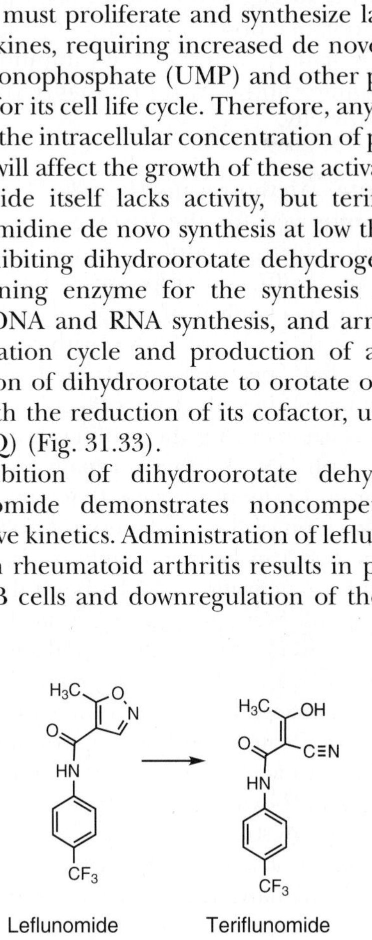

FIGURE 31.32 Metabolism of leflunomide.

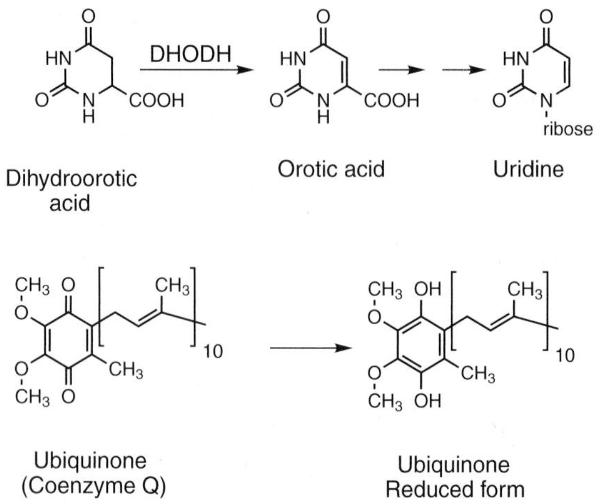

FIGURE 31.33 Dihydroorotate dehydrogenase (DHOH) pathway with cofactor, coenzyme Q.

process. Teriflunomide not only inhibits B-cell proliferation but also T-cell proliferation, blocking the synthesis of immunosuppressive cytokines. At high therapeutic doses, leflunomide inhibits protein tyrosine kinases.

Leflunomide is administered orally as a single daily dose without regard to meals. Therapy can be initiated with a loading dosage given for 3 days, followed by the usual maintenance dose. It undergoes primarily enterohepatic circulation, extending its duration of action. Cholestyramine can be used to enhance its elimination in cases of toxicity.

Methotrexate Methotrexate (Fig. 31.31) is an antifolate drug approved for the treatment of severe active rheumatoid arthritis in adults who are intolerant to or have had an insufficient response to first-line therapy. Although the mechanism of action of methotrexate in rheumatoid arthritis is not known with certainty, several mechanisms have been proposed. Methotrexate blocks pyrimidine biosynthesis by reversibly inhibiting dihydrofolate reductase, blocking the proliferation of B cells by interfering with DNA synthesis, repair, and replication. Other actions of methotrexate that can be involved include inhibition of the production of polyamines such as spermine that can be responsible for inducing tissue damage and the activation of NF-κB. Oral absorption is dose dependent, being well absorbed at doses of 7.5 to 25 mg once a week. At this dose, oral bioavailability is approximately 60%, and food can delay absorption and reduce peak concentration. The volume of distribution is 0.4 to 0.8 L/kg. Protein binding is approximately 50%. It is metabolized to active metabolites, methotrexate polyglutamates, and 7-hydroxymethotrexate. Some metabolism occurs by intestinal flora after oral administration. Methotrexate is actively transported into the urine (80% to 90% unchanged in the urine within 24 hours) via the folate transporter, an organic anion transporter (hOAT3). Its elimination half-life is 3 to 10 hours.

Life-threatening drug interactions are known to occur between methotrexate and NSAIDs, probenecid, and penicillin G. The NSAIDs (salicylate, ibuprofen, ketoprofen, piroxicam, and indomethacin), probenecid, and penicillin G dose dependently inhibited methotrexate elimination into urine by human organic anion transporters (hOAT1, hOAT3, and hOAT4) (Chapter 5). The inhibitory effects of these drugs on hOAT3 were comparable, with therapeutically relevant plasma concentrations of unbound drugs. Thus, patients with rheumatoid arthritis should not take NSAIDs while taking methotrexate.

Methotrexate therapy requires monitoring of liver enzymes and is contraindicated in those with hepatic disease and in women considering pregnancy.

Sulfasalazine (Azulfidine) Sulfasalazine is a prodrug that is not active in its ingested form; rather, it is hydrolyzed by colonic bacteria into 5-aminosalicylic acid (5-ASA; mesalamine) and sulfapyridine (Fig. 31.34). Some controversy exists regarding which of these two products is responsible for the activity of Azulfidine. 5-Aminosalicylic acid, like acetylsalicylic acid, is an inhibitor of prostaglandin biosynthesis and is known to have therapeutic benefit. However, it is not clear whether sulfapyridine adds any further benefit. It was shown to inhibit purine biosynthesis by inhibiting 5-aminoimidazole-4-carboxamisoribonucleotide transformylase and to enhance adenosine release, enhancing the ability of adenosine to decrease inflammation by binding to A_2 adenosine receptors on inflammatory cells (119). Sulfasalazine and/or its metabolites have been shown to inhibit the release of inflammatory cytokines and TNFα. In the colon, the products created by the breakdown of sulfasalazine work as anti-inflammatory agents for treating colon inflammation. The beneficial effect of sulfasalazine is believed to result from a local effect on the bowel, although there can also be a beneficial systemic immunosuppressant effect. Sulfasalazine was approved in 1950.

Following oral administration, sulfasalazine is poorly absorbed, with approximately 20% of the ingested sulfasalazine reaching the systemic circulation. The remainder of the ingested dose is metabolized by colonic bacteria into its components, sulfapyridine and mesalamine (5-ASA). Most of the sulfapyridine metabolized

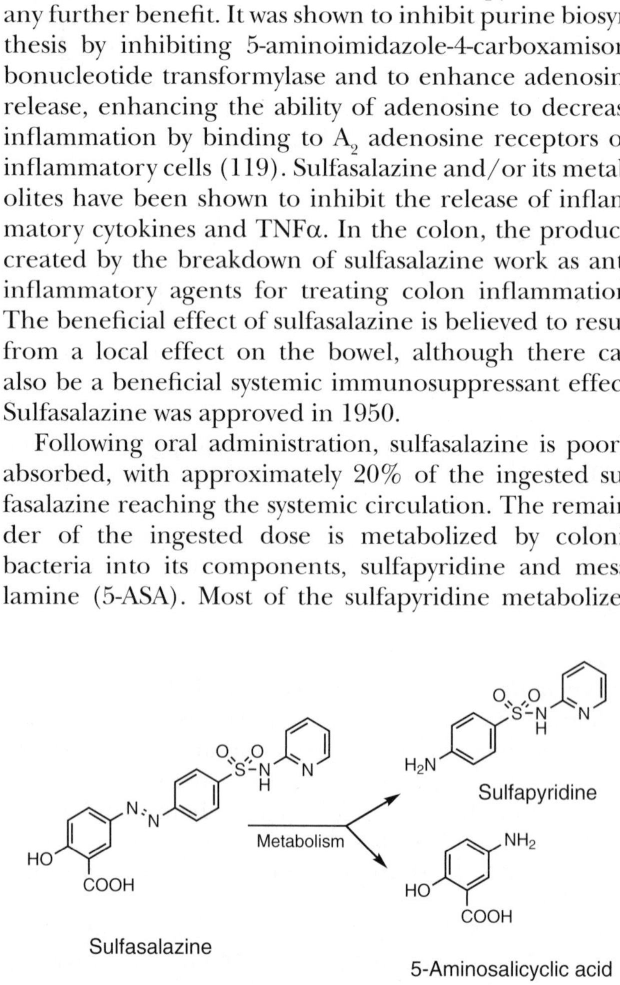

FIGURE 31.34 Metabolism of sulfasalazine.

from sulfasalazine (60% to 80%) is absorbed in the colon following oral administration, and approximately 25% of the 5-ASA metabolized from sulfasalazine is absorbed in the colon. The apparent volume of distribution of sulfasalazine in eight healthy volunteers was 64 L/kg, and that of sulfapyridine was 0.4 to 1.2 L/kg. Protein binding is approximately 99% for sulfasalazine, approximately 50% for sulfapyridine, and approximately 43% for 5-ASA. The absorbed sulfapyridine is acetylated and hydroxylated in the liver, followed by conjugation with glucuronic acid and, for 5-ASA, acetylation in the intestinal mucosal wall and the liver. The elimination half-life is 5 to 10 hours for sulfasalazine and 6 to 14 hours for sulfapyridine, depending on acetylator status of the patient, and 0.6 to 1.4 hours for 5-ASA. Time to peak serum concentration is 1.5 to 6 hours for oral sulfasalazine and 9 to 24 hours for oral sulfapyridine; for enteric-coated tablets, time to peak serum concentration is 3 to 12 hours for sulfasalazine and 12 to 24 hours for sulfapyridine. Approximately 5% of sulfapyridine and approximately 67% of mesalamine are eliminated in the feces, and 75% to 91% of sulfasalazine and sulfapyridine metabolites are excreted in urine within 3 days, depending on the dosage form used. 5-ASA is excreted in urine mostly in acetylated form.

Sulfasalazine is used for the treatment of mild to moderate ulcerative colitis; as adjunct therapy in the treatment of severe ulcerative colitis; for the treatment of Crohn disease; and for the treatment of rheumatoid arthritis or ankylosing spondylitis. Contraindications include hypersensitivity to sulfa drugs, salicylates, intestinal or urinary obstruction, and porphyria.

Tofacitinib Tofacitinib (Orencia) (formerly known as tasocitinib) is an orally active immunosuppressant implicated in the pathogenesis and used for treatment of rheumatoid arthritis, inflammatory bowel disease, ankylosing spondylitis, psoriasis, and psoriatic arthritis and for the prevention of transplant rejection. Tofacitinib specifically inhibits JAK3, blocking proinflammatory cytokine signaling, thus preventing the expression of both B and T cells. Tofacitinib is an investigational drug in FDA phase III trials, which suggest this new drug to be as effective as TNFα inhibitors. Dose-dependent decreases in white blood cell counts and increases in low-density lipoprotein cholesterol, high-density lipoprotein cholesterol, total cholesterol, and serum creatinine levels were observed in patients treated with tofacitinib. The most frequent treatment-related adverse events (<5%) were urinary tract infection, diarrhea, bronchitis, and headache. Some hepatic metabolism of tofacitinib conducted in human liver microsomes and hepatocytes was observed by CYP3A4/5 and CYP2C19. The low clearance of the drug in humans occurred via a combination of renal excretion of unchanged drug and low hepatic metabolic clearance. Volume of distribution in humans was 1.9 L/kg, with a terminal elimination half-life of 7 hours. Pharmacokinetics support daily or twice a day dosing (118).

Biologic Disease-Modifying Antirheumatic Drugs

Cytokine Inhibitors

Tumor Necrosis Factor Blockers T lymphocytes (T cells), a type of white blood cell, are important cells of the immune system. Patients with rheumatoid arthritis have increased numbers of T cells within the inflamed joints. These T cells are "activated"—that is, they multiply and release chemicals (cytokines) that promote the destruction of tissues surrounding the joints and cause the signs and symptoms of rheumatoid arthritis (120).

As discussed earlier in this chapter (see also Chapter 6 for a detailed discussion of cytokines), there is considerable expression of the cytokines, interleukin (IL)-1, IL-6, and TNFα by the rheumatoid synovium. TNFα is a proinflammatory cytokine (cell protein) that has a major role in the pathologic inflammatory process of rheumatoid arthritis. TNF is an important mediator of local inflammation, and the release of TNFα from T cells produces increased vascular permeability, release of nitric oxide with vasodilation, local activation of vascular endothelium, increased expression of adhesion molecules on endothelial blood vessels, and increased platelet activation and adhesion. As TNFα builds up in the joints, it leads to joint inflammation, which ultimately results in joint destruction. Because of its role in the progression of rheumatoid arthritis, methods for rendering TNFα inactive have become a key focus of therapies for rheumatoid arthritis (119). Patients with rheumatoid arthritis display elevated levels of the cytokines, TNFα, IL-1, and IL-6 in synovial fluid and tissue, and there appears to be a correlation between the amount of these products present and the severity of the disease. A significant advance in the treatment of arthritic diseases was the observation that therapy directed toward diminishing the effects of TNFα appeared to also improve the symptoms of ankylosing spondylitis and psoriatic arthritis.

Two different approaches have been developed to decrease TNF activity that has resulted in marketable drugs: administration of soluble TNF receptors (TNFRs; etanercept), and treatment with anti-TNFα antibodies (e.g., infliximab, adalimumab). These compounds are designed to target and neutralize the effects of TNF, helping to reduce pain, morning stiffness, and tender or swollen joints, usually within 1 or 2 weeks after treatment begins. Evidence suggests that TNF blockers can also halt the progression of the disease. These medications work synergistically with methotrexate and therefore are often taken with methotrexate. TNF blockers approved for treatment of rheumatoid arthritis are etanercept, infliximab, adalimumab, and rituximab. Potential side effects include injection site irritation (adalimumab and etanercept), worsening congestive heart failure (infliximab), blood disorders, lymphoma, demyelinating diseases, and increased risk of infection. These drugs should not be taken if an active infection is present. Effectiveness is lost if the drugs are discontinued.

Because TNF is also important for host defense against infections, the effects of long-term use on toxicity require further study. Substantial improvements in the course of the disease have been noted with both therapeutic approaches.

Structural illustrations of the anti-TNF agents etanercept, infliximab, adalimumab, and rituximab are provided in Figure 31.35. Two new anti-TNFα antibodies have been introduced recently (certolizumab and golimumab) for rheumatoid arthritis and other forms of inflammatory arthritis.

Etanercept (Enbrel) Etanercept is produced by recombinant DNA technology in a Chinese hamster ovary mammalian cell line and is the first biotechnology-derived drug to be introduced for the reduction of the signs and symptoms of moderately to severely active rheumatoid arthritis in patients who have not adequately responded to one or more of the synthetic DMARDs. It is a dimeric soluble form of the p75 TNFR capable of binding to two TNF molecules in the circulation. It consists of the extracellular ligand binding portion of the 75-kd human TNFR fused to the Fc portion of human immunoglobulin (Ig) G1. The Fc component of etanercept contains the C_H2 domain, the C_H3 domain, and the hinge region, but not the C_H1 domain of IgG1. It consists of 934 amino acids and has an apparent molecular weight of approximately 150 kd. Two TNFRs have been identified, a 75-kd protein and a 55-kd protein, that occur as monomeric molecules on cell surfaces and soluble forms in the blood. The biologic activity of TNF requires its binding to either of the two cell surface TNFRs. Etanercept can bind specifically to two molecules of TNFα in the circulation, preventing its interaction with cell surface TNFRs. Etanercept also binds TNFβ. It can be used as monotherapy or in combination with methotrexate. Some concern exists because of reports that etanercept can, in some cases, cause serious infections and could have contributed to the deaths of several patients using the drug. An excellent review of the properties and use of etanercept is available (121).

Etanercept is available as a powder for injection in single-use vials containing 25 mg of the drug. The reconstituted solution is administered twice a week at 25 mg or once a week at 50 mg as a clear and colorless subcutaneous injection.

Etanercept has been approved for reducing signs and symptoms, inhibiting the progression of structural damage, and improving physical function in patients with moderately to severely active rheumatoid arthritis; for reducing signs and symptoms in patients with active arthritis and patients with psoriatic arthritis; and for reducing signs and symptoms in patients with active ankylosing spondylitis.

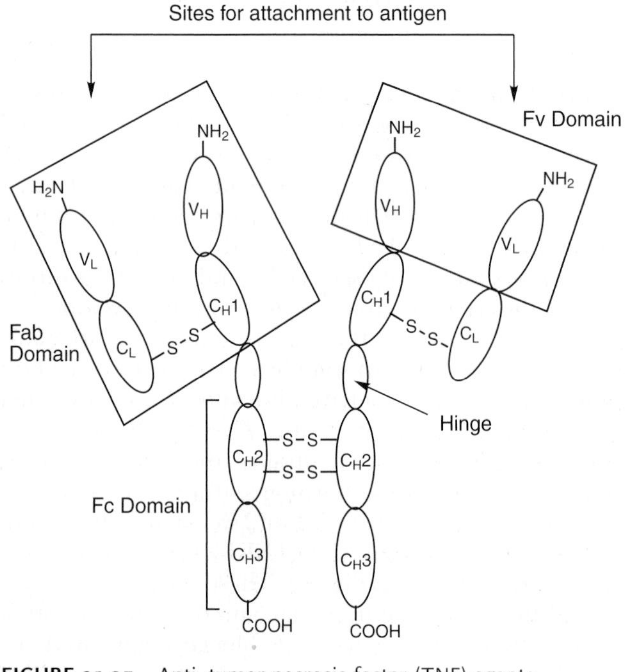

FIGURE 31.35 Anti–tumor necrosis factor (TNF) agents. Etanercept is the extracellular portion of the human TNF receptor fused to the Fc domain of human immunoglobulin (Ig) G1. Infliximab is a partially humanized monoclonal antibody against TNFα. The Fv domains are derived from mouse antihuman sequences, whereas the Fc domain is composed of human IgG1 sequences. Adalimumab is fully humanized antibody to human TNFα (Fv and Fc derived from human sequences). Rituximab is a partially humanized monoclonal antibody against CD40. The Fv domains are derived from mouse antihuman sequences, and the Fc domain is composed of human IgG1 sequences.

Infliximab (Remicade) Infliximab is a chimeric ("humanized") IgG1κ monoclonal antibody to human TNFα (see Chapter 6 for detailed discussions of monoclonal antibodies). By combining the Fv domain of the mouse antibody responsible for recognizing TNFα with parts of the human Fc domain of IgG1 (IgG1κ), the fused protein looks more like normal human IgG1 molecule ("humanized"), so there is a better chance the fused protein will not be destroyed by the patient's own immune system. Infliximab has an approximate molecular weight of 149,100 daltons and binds specifically, with high affinity, to both the transmembrane and soluble forms of TNFα in the blood, thus neutralizing its biologic activity. It does not bind to TNFβ (lymphotoxin A), a related cytokine that uses the same receptors as TNFα. Infliximab is produced by a recombinant cell line cultured by continuous perfusion and is purified by a series of steps that includes measures to inactivate and remove viruses. Cells expressing transmembrane TNFα bound by infliximab can be lysed. The TNFα antibodies decrease synovitis and joint erosions in a murine model of collagen-induced arthritis and, when administered after disease onset, allow eroded joints to heal.

After treatment with infliximab, patients with rheumatoid arthritis or Crohn disease exhibited reduced infiltration of inflammatory cells and TNFα production in inflamed tissues and decreased levels of serum IL-6 and C-reactive protein compared to baseline. In psoriatic arthritis, treatment with infliximab resulted in a reduction in the number of T cells and blood vessels in the synovium and psoriatic skin as well as a reduction of macrophages in the synovium. Single IV infusions showed a linear relationship between the dose administered and the maximum serum concentration. The volume of distribution at steady-state was independent of dose and indicated that infliximab was distributed primarily within the vascular compartment. The terminal half-life of infliximab is 8.0 to 9.5 days. No systemic accumulation of infliximab occurred on continued repeated treatment at 4- or 8-week intervals.

Infliximab is supplied as a sterile, white, lyophilized powder formulated for IV infusion. Following reconstitution with Sterile Water for Injection, the solution should be used immediately after reconstitution, because the vials do not contain antibacterial preservatives. The reconstituted solution should be colorless to light yellow and opalescent.

Infliximab is indicated for the treatment of rheumatoid arthritis in combination with methotrexate and for Crohn disease. Long-term use can be associated with the development of anti-infliximab antibodies, an effect that does not appear when it is used with methotrexate. Warnings associated with the use of infliximab include risks of autoimmunity, infections, and hypersensitivity reactions. An excellent review of the properties and use of infliximab has recently appeared (122). Infliximab is more specific than etanercept, because etanercept binds to both TNFα and TNFβ, whereas infliximab is an antibody that binds only to TNFα. Infliximab possesses a longer half-life giving a dosing schedule of approximately every 6 to 8 weeks.

Infliximab, in combination with methotrexate, is indicated for reducing signs and symptoms, inhibiting the progression of structural damage, and improving physical function in patients with moderately to severely active rheumatoid arthritis; for reducing signs and symptoms and maintaining clinical remission in patients with moderately to severely active Crohn disease who have had an inadequate response to conventional therapy; for reducing signs and symptoms in patients with active arthritis and in patients with psoriatic arthritis; for reducing signs and symptoms in patients with active ankylosing spondylitis; and for reducing the signs and symptoms of ulcerative colitis.

Adalimumab (Humira) Adalimumab is a recombinant human IgG1 monoclonal antibody targeted for human TNFα. Adalimumab is produced by recombinant DNA technology in a mammalian cell expression system using a protein-engineering strategy for creating a TNFα antibody with human-derived, heavy- and light-chain variable regions (Fab) and human IgG1κ constant regions. It consists of 1,330 amino acids and has a molecular weight of approximately 148 kd. Adalimumab, as an antibody, works by targeting and binding TNFα, thus neutralizing the effect of TNFα and, thereby, reducing the symptoms of rheumatoid arthritis and slowing the progression of structural joint damage caused by the disease. Adalimumab does not bind or inactivate TNFβ.

Adalimumab is supplied in single-use, prefilled, glass syringes as a sterile, preservative-free, colorless solution for subcutaneous administration. The pharmacokinetics of adalimumab were linear over the dose range of 0.5 to 10.0 mg/kg following a single IV dose. The mean elimination half-life was approximately 2 weeks.

Rituximab (Rituxan) Rituximab is a genetically engineered, fused mouse/human anti-CD40 monoclonal antibody that targets B lymphocytes by binding specifically to CD20 antigen, a protein found on the surface of B cells at certain stages in their life cycle. Rituximab is composed of two heavy chains of 451 amino acids and two light chains of 213 amino acids with an approximate molecular weight of 145 kd (Fig. 31.30). Its binding affinity for the CD20 antigen is approximately 8.0 nmol/L. The mouse light- and heavy-chain Fab domains of rituximab, which bind to the CD20 antigen on B cells, are linked to the human Fc domains of IgG1κ. Once the rituximab molecule attaches to the B cells, it initiates B-cell lysis, inducing rapid and profound depletion of peripheral B cells, with patients showing near complete B-cell depletion within 2 weeks after receiving the first dose of rituximab. Because rituximab does not target B cells at the earliest stages of their development, however, these B-cell depletions are usually temporary. In clinical trials, the majority of patients showed peripheral B-cell depletion for at least 6 months, followed by subsequent gradual recovery. A small proportion of patients (4%) had prolonged peripheral B-cell depletion lasting more than 3 years after a single course of treatment.

Rituximab is a sterile, clear, colorless, preservative-free, liquid concentrate formulated for IV administration. It has changed the treatment of rheumatoid arthritis by showing that targeted B-cell therapy in combination with methotrexate can reduce signs and symptoms of rheumatoid arthritis in adult patients with moderately to severely active rheumatoid arthritis who have had an inadequate response to one or more TNF antagonist therapies. Although B cells once were considered to be one of the main contributing factors in the pathogenesis of rheumatoid arthritis, recent evidence has shown that T cells, dendritic cells, and macrophages are also involved. Rituximab has rekindled interest in B cells, highlighting their important role in perpetuating the inflammatory process and showing how they can interact with other cell types and contribute to joint inflammation.

For rheumatoid arthritis, rituximab is given as two 1,000-mg IV infusions separated by 2 weeks. Glucocorticoids are also recommended to reduce the incidence and severity of infusion reactions. Rituximab is given in combination with methotrexate. Its administration has been associated with hypersensitivity reactions (non–IgE-mediated reactions), which can respond to adjustments in the infusion rate and in medical management. People who have not found relief using TNF blockers might consider using rituximab. Side effects include flu-like signs and symptoms such as fever, chills, and nausea. Some people experience an "infusion-reaction complex," such as difficulty breathing and heart problems, that can result in death.

Although originally approved for use in people with non-Hodgkin lymphoma, rituximab was approved for rheumatoid arthritis in 2006. A review of the clinical applications of rituximab is available (123).

Certolizumab Pegol (Cimzia) Certolizumab is a monoclonal antibody directed against TNFα (124). It selectively neutralizes TNFα with an IC_{90} of 4 ng/mL while not neutralizing lymphotoxin A (TNF). Certolizumab is composed of a humanized anti-TNFα antibody Fab′ fragment, which is linked to polyethylene glycol (PEG). The Fab′ fragment is composed of a light chain with 214 amino acid residues and a heavy chain with 229 amino acids. The antibody lacks an Fc portion and thus binds to only TNFα, without having to bind to the cell surface receptors for antibodies. The drug is produced in higher yields in *Escherichia coli* in only 2 to 3 days; thus, certolizumab offers a lower cost of production with a more reliable supply. The purpose of linking the antibody to PEG (pegolate) is to reduce the immunogenicity of the antibody; increase the circulating half-lives of antibodies, thereby increasing the dosing range to once every 4 weeks, rather than every 2 weeks with several of the other monoclonal antibodies; and enhance TNFα targeting.

Absorption and Metabolism. Subcutaneous and single IV dosing studies of certolizumab demonstrate predictable dose-related plasma concentrations with a linear relationship between the dose administered and maximum plasma concentration (C_{max}) and area under the curve (AUC) versus time. A mean C_{max} of 43 to 49 mcg/mL occurred at week 5 during the initial dosing period, which led to the development of the dosing regimen of 400 mg subcutaneously at weeks 0, 2, and 4 followed by 200 mg biweekly. Metabolism of the Fab′ fragment is unknown, whereas the PEG moiety is excreted in the urine.

Adverse Effects. The major adverse effects are mild and include upper respiratory infections, rash, and urinary tract infections.

Golimumab (Symponi) Golimumab is a human IgG1k monoclonal antibody specific for human TNFα. Its molecular mass is 150 to 151 kd (125). It is an alternative to etanercept, adalimumab, and infliximab for the treatment of rheumatoid arthritis. Golimumab binds to both the soluble and transmembrane bioactive forms of human TNFα, with affinities of 17 pmol by surface plasmon resonance and 1.4 pmol in solution (126).

Absorption, Metabolism, and Dose. Median time to reach maximum serum concentrations (T_{max}) is 2 to 6 days, whereas the median terminal half-life is 2 weeks. Metabolism is unknown. Dosing of 50 mg subcutaneously every 4 weeks leads to steady-state serum concentrations by week 12. The advantage golimumab possesses over other anti-TNFα agents is dosing (injected subcutaneously once a month, whereas adalimumab is injected subcutaneously every other week, etanercept is injected subcutaneously weekly, and infliximab is injected by IV infusion every 8 weeks).

Adverse Effects. The most frequent adverse reactions are upper respiratory tract infection, sore throat, and nasopharyngitis. However, serious infections can occur along with lymphomas and other malignancies. Labeling includes a black box warning that alerts patients to the risk of tuberculosis and invasive fungal infections.

Interleukin-1 Receptor Antagonist

Anakinra (Kineret) Anakinra is a recombinant, nonglycosylated form of the human IL-1 receptor antagonist (IL-1Rα) that neutralizes the inflammatory activity of IL-1 by competing with IL-1 for binding to its IL-1 type 1 receptor (IL-1R1). IL-1 is a cytokine for which production is induced in response to inflammatory stimuli and that mediates various physiologic responses, including inflammatory and immunologic responses that promote inflammation. When IL-1 binds to IL-1R1, a signal is produced that increases the formation of nitric oxide, PGE_2, and collagenase in synovial cells, resulting in cartilage degradation and stimulation of bone resorption. Thus, IL-1Rα has an important role for regulating synovial proinflammatory IL-1 activity by preventing IL-1 from binding to IL-1R1. Analysis of synovial fluid suggests that the rheumatoid synovium is characterized by an overexpression of IL-1. The resulting imbalance between IL-1 and IL-1Rα has been implicated in perpetuating the proinflammatory response and destructive tide of events in rheumatoid arthritis. If IL-1 is prevented from binding to IL-1R1, the inflammatory response decreases. The levels of the naturally occurring IL-lRα in synovium and synovial fluid from rheumatoid arthritis patients are insufficient to compete with the elevated amount of locally produced IL-1.

Therefore, anakinra neutralizes the proinflammatory activity of IL-1 by competitively inhibiting the binding of IL-1 to IL-1RI, similar to the endogenous antagonist, IL-1Rα. In vitro studies have shown that anakinra inhibits the induction of the inflammatory mediators, nitric oxide and PGE_2, and collagenase. Anakinra differs from native human IL-1Rα in that it has the addition of a single methionine residue at its amino terminus. Anakinra consists of 153 amino acids and has a molecular weight of 17.3 kd. It is produced by recombinant DNA technology using an *E. coli* bacterial expression system.

Anakinra is the first IL-1Rα to be approved for use in adults with moderate to severe active rheumatoid arthritis who have not responded adequately to conventional DMARD therapy. It can be used either alone or in combination with methotrexate. Anakinra is supplied in single-use, prefilled, glass syringes as sterile, clear, preservative-free solution that is administered daily as a self-administered subcutaneous injection under the skin. Some potential side effects include injection site reactions, decreased white blood cell counts, headache, and an increase in upper respiratory infections. There can be a slightly higher rate of respiratory infections in people who have asthma or chronic obstructive pulmonary disease. Persons with an active infection are advised not to use anakinra. Its elimination half-life after subcutaneous administration is 4 to 6 hours.

TOCILIZUMAB (ACTEMRA) Tocilizumab is a recently introduced recombinant humanized antihuman monoclonal antibody that binds to solubilized and membrane-bound IL-6 receptors and inhibits IL-6–mediated signaling (127). It is a member of the IgG1κ subclass with a typical H_2L_2 (two heavy and two light chains) polypeptide structure. Each light chain consists of 214 amino acids, whereas the heavy chain contains 448 residues. The four polypeptide chains are linked by disulfide bonds both intra- and intermolecularly. Tocilizumab is the first monoclonal antibody that targets IL-6 and offers an alternative to patients not adequately responding to TNFα blockers. It has a molecular weight of approximately 148 kd.

Absorption, Metabolism, and Dose With a dose of tocilizumab (4 mg/kg IV) given every 4 weeks, the predicted mean steady-state AUC, minimum plasma concentration (C_{min}), and C_{max} of tocilizumab were 13,000 mcg/hour/mL, 1.49 mcg/mL, and 88.3 mcg/mL, respectively. Steady-state was reached following the first administration for C_{max} and AUC, respectively, and after 16 weeks for C_{min}. At 8 mg/kg given every 4 weeks, the predicted mean steady-state AUC, C_{min}, and C_{max} of tocilizumab were 35,000 mcg/h/mL, 9.74 mcg/mL, and 183 mcg/mL, respectively. The half-life is concentration dependent and is 11 days for the 4 mg/kg dose and 13 days for the 8 mg/kg dose. Metabolism is unknown, and the total dose should not exceed 800 mg per infusion.

Adverse Effects The most frequent adverse effects are upper respiratory tract infection, headache, hypertension, increased alanine transaminase, and nasopharyngitis. All precautions for using an immunosuppressant should be taken.

COSTIMULATION MODULATORS Two signals are required to activate a T-cell response to an antigen, called costimulation. Regulation of costimulatory molecules can be a mechanism whereby the immune system limits the extent of an immune response. If an unactivated antigen-presenting cell (APC; a cell that "presents" an antigen complex that is recognized by the T-cell receptor) presents an antigen to a T cell in the absence of an appropriate costimulatory signal, the T cell does not respond and becomes unreactive and nonresponsive to any further antigenic stimuli (Fig. 31.36). The T-cell costimulatory activation pathway is initiated, however, when an activated APC presents both an antigen and a costimulatory ligand, such as B7 (CD86), that interacts with CD28 on the surface of the T cell to form B7-CD28 complex, initiating T-cell proliferation and differentiation in response to the antigenic stimulus. This stimulus releases cytokines that bind to the T cell, further enhancing its activation. A counterbalance to CD28 is cytotoxic T-lymphocyte antigen-4 (CTLA-4), both of which are expressed on the surface of T cells. The CTLA-4, which is homologous with CD28, becomes expressed on T-cell activation, where it then competes with CD28 for binding to B7 ligands on the surface of APCs. The B7 ligands bind with much greater affinity to CTLA-4 than to CD28, preventing delivery of the costimulatory signal. This built-in limit prevents T-cell activation from spiraling out of control. The CTLA-4 is not expressed constitutively, and its expression is upregulated on T-cell activation. Eventually, however, CD28 is downregulated.

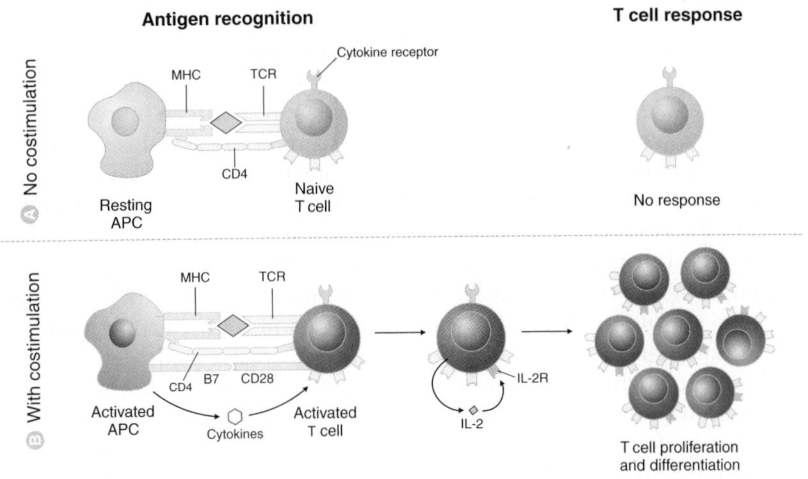

FIGURE 31.36 Costimulation in the T-cell activation pathway.

Because the formation of a B7-CD28 complex between the APC and the T cell results in T-cell proliferation and the release of inflammatory cytokines, whereas the B7–CTLA-4 interaction inhibits the T-cell responses, the design of a pharmacologic agent that prevents costimulation would preferentially inhibit only reactive T cells and be effective in treatment of rheumatoid arthritis—thus, the discovery of abatacept.

Abatacept (Orencia) Abatacept, the first in a new class of immunosuppressant agents, known as costimulation modulators, acts by downregulating T-cell activation for the treatment of rheumatoid arthritis (128). Abatacept is a novel chimeric CTLA-4–IgG1 fused protein created from the fusion of the extracellular domain of the mouse CTLA-4 with the modified heavy-chain constant region of human IgG1.

Abatacept, therefore, acts like an antibody that binds with great affinity to B7 ligands, preventing these ligands from interacting with CD28 on activated T cells. In patients with rheumatoid arthritis, blocking this response by abatacept prevents the generation of positive costimulation signals and stimulation of T-cell activation, suppressing the proliferation of reactive T-cells and the release of more cytokines that destroy tissue, causing the symptoms and signs of arthritis. The extracellular CTLA-4 portion of abatacept is responsible for the affinity of B7. Thus, abatacept slows the damage to bones and cartilage and relieves the symptoms and signs of arthritis.

People with moderate to severe active rheumatoid arthritis who have not been helped by TNF blockers might consider abatacept, which is administered IV monthly. Side effects can include headache, nausea, and mild infections, such as upper respiratory tract infections. Serious infections, such as pneumonia, can occur. There is some concern that blocking of the suppressive signal from B7 to CTLA-4 can have a negative effect on regulatory T cells and, thus, eventually, promote autoimmunity.

Herbs

At least a dozen different herbs are used to ease the symptoms of rheumatoid arthritis; most are considered to be anti-inflammatories. Herbs that have been tried include powdered ginger, borage seed oil, or devil's claw to reduce pain and swelling. Stinging nettles or turmeric can also lessen pain, stiffness, and inflammation. Because these herbs can interact with each other or with prescription comedications, lack of careful studies means that little is known about long-term effects and drug interactions.

Ayurvedic medicine also uses herbal compounds both internally and externally for symptom relief. Topical curcumin can relieve the inflammation of rheumatoid arthritis. When taken in capsule form, it can reduce morning stiffness and boost endurance. A combination of *Withania somnifera*, *Boswellia serrata*, and *Cucurma longa* also caused a significant drop in pain and disability for study participants with osteoarthritis.

Two herbs that have been used for centuries to treat headaches, fever, sore muscles, and rheumatism are white willow bark and meadowsweet, commonly described as "Nature's aspirin." White willow bark (*Salix alba*) contains salicin, a glycoside of salicylic acid. Once in the stomach, the salicin hydrolyzes into salicylic acid, which is the active principle for reducing pain and fever. White willow bark has been mentioned in ancient Egyptian, Assyrian, Greek, and Chinese manuscripts, and it was used to treat pain and fever by the ancient physicians Galen, Hippocrates, and Dioscorides. Native Americans used it for headaches, fever, sore muscles, rheumatism, and chills. In the mid-1700s, it was used to treat malaria. Salicin was isolated and identified in the early 1830s, but it was not conclusively shown to reduce the aches and soreness of rheumatism until 1874. White willow bark is recommended for headaches, backache, nerve pain, toothache, and injuries.

Meadowsweet (*Filipendula ulmaria*) is a common wild plant in Britain, Europe, and North America that also contains salicin, but it is not as potent as willow bark, which has a higher salicin content. Its primary medicinal actions are antirheumatic, anti-inflammatory, carminative, antacid, antiemetic, astringent, and diuretic. The flower buds of meadowsweet are the source for salicin and methyl salicylate. Ingestion of the flower buds in a tea results in the breakdown of salicin to salicylic acid. Nicholas Culpeper, a 17th-century English pharmacist, mentioned the use of meadowsweet flower buds to help break fevers and promote sweating during a cold or flu.

A review of the role of traditional Chinese medicine in treating rheumatoid arthritis is available (129).

DRUGS USED TO TREAT GOUT

Pathophysiology

Gout, an ancient and common form inflammatory arthritis, is characterized by elevated levels of uric acid (as urate ion) in the plasma and urine and can take two forms, acute and chronic. It is the most common inflammatory arthritis in men with the incidence occurring in black males at almost twice that of white males. Risk factors include obesity, hypertension, ingestion of alcohol, the use of diuretics, and diets rich in meats and seafood. Gout is associated with an increased risk of kidney stones (130).

Acute gouty arthritis results from the accumulation of needle-like crystals of monosodium urate monohydrate within the joints, synovial fluid, and periarticular tissue and usually appears without warning. Initiating factors can be minor trauma, fatigue, emotional stress, infection, overindulgence in alcohol or food, or drugs, such as penicillin or insulin. Chronic gout symptoms develop as permanent erosive joint deformity appears. The increase in extracellular urate can result from increased uric acid biosynthesis, decreased urinary excretion of uric acid, or perhaps, a combination of both. The formation of uric acid from adenine and guanine is illustrated in Figure 31.37. Uric acid is formed by the oxidation of xanthine by the

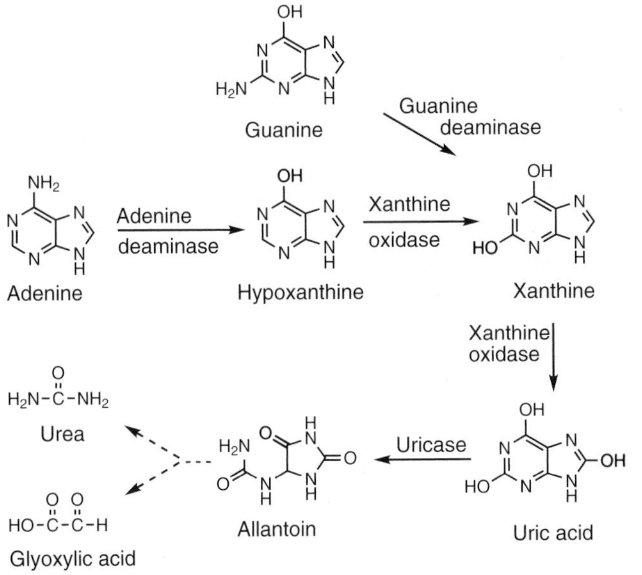

FIGURE 31.37 Formation of uric acid, urea, and glyoxylic acid from purines.

enzyme xanthine oxidase. Xanthine is a metabolic product of adenine (via hypoxanthine) and guanine formed by the enzymes adenine deaminase and guanine deaminase, respectively. Thus, uric acid is the excretory product of purine metabolism in humans as well as the scavenging of potential harmful oxygen free radicals in the body. In other mammals, uric acid is hydrolyzed to allantoin by the enzyme uricase, which is then subsequently hydrolyzed by allantoinase to allantoic acid. Hydrolysis of allantoic acid by allantoicase yields the final products, urea and glyoxylic acid.

Normal pool levels of uric acid are approximately 1,000 to 1,200 mg in males and half that in females. In patients suffering from gout, these levels can be as high as two or three times the normal levels. Uric acid is a weak acid with two pK_a values (5.7 and 10.3), with very low water solubility (~6 mg/100 mL). At physiologic pH, it exists primarily as the monosodium salt, which is approximately 50 times more soluble in aqueous media than the free acid. Blood levels of urate are maintained by a careful balance between its formation and excretion. The kidney has a dominant role in urate elimination, excreting about 70% of the daily urate production. The excretion of urate has been implicated in the development of hyperuricemia that leads to gout. In humans, the excretion of urate requires the urate anion transporter (URAT1) located in renal proximal tubule cells, which has a central role in urate homeostasis. The URAT1 is targeted by uricosuric and antiuricosuric agents that affect urate excretion.

When levels of uric acid in the body increase, either as a result of decreased excretion or increased formation, the solubility limits of sodium urate are exceeded, and precipitation of the salt from the resulting supersaturated solution causes deposits of urate crystals to form. It is the formation of these urate crystals in joints and connective tissue that initiate attacks of gouty arthritis.

The control of gout has been approached from the following therapeutic strategies: 1) control of acute attacks by drugs that reduce inflammation caused by the deposition of urate crystals (these drugs can possess only an anti-inflammatory component, such as colchicine, or both anti-inflammatory and analgesic actions, such as indomethacin, phenylbutazone, and naproxen), 2) increasing the rate of uric acid excretion (by definition, these drugs are termed "uricosuric drugs" and include probenecid and sulfinpyrazone), and 3) inhibiting the biosynthesis of uric acid by inhibiting the enzyme xanthine oxidase by drugs such as allopurinol.

The structures of the drugs used to treat gout are shown in Figure 31.38.

Treatment of Acute Gout

The management of gout has been approached with the following therapeutic strategies: 1) control of acute attacks with drugs that reduce inflammation caused by the deposition of urate crystals, and 2) control of chronic gout by increasing the rate of uric acid excretion ("uricosuric drugs") and inhibiting the biosynthesis of uric acid by inhibiting the enzyme xanthine oxidase. Treatment of acute gout includes NSAIDs, such as indomethacin, colchicines, and glucocorticoids. The choice of an NSAID is usually based on the side effect profile.

Colchicine

Colchicine is a pale-yellow powder that is obtained from various species of *Colchicum*, primarily *Colchicum autumnale* L. Its total chemical synthesis has been achieved, but the primary source of colchicine currently remains alcohol extraction

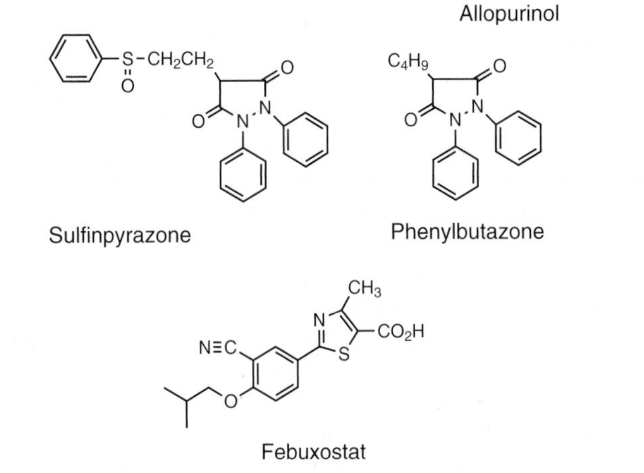

FIGURE 31.38 Structures of agents used to control gout.

of the alkaloid from the corm and seed of *C. autumnale* L. It darkens on exposure to light and possesses moderate water solubility. Colchicine has a pK_a of 12.4. Its use in the treatment of gout dates back to the sixth century AD. Unlike the drugs that will be discussed next, colchicine does not alter serum levels of uric acid. It does, however, appear to retard the inflammation process initiated by the deposition of urate crystals. Acting on polymorphonuclear leukocytes and diminishing phagocytosis, it inhibits the production of lactic acid, causing an increase in the pH of synovial tissue and, thus, a decrease in urate deposition, because uric acid is more soluble at the higher pH. Additionally, colchicine inhibits the release of lysosomal enzymes during phagocytosis that also contributes to the reduction of inflammation. Because colchicine does not lower serum urate levels, it has been found to be beneficial to combine colchicine with a uricosuric agent, particularly probenecid. It is a potent drug, being effective at doses of approximately 1 mg, but doses as small as 7 mg have caused fatalities.

The FDA approved the first single-ingredient oral colchicine formulation, Colcrys, for the treatment of acute gout flares in 2010. The drug is also approved for the treatment of familial Mediterranean fever.

Absorption and Metabolism Colchicine is absorbed on oral administration, with peak plasma levels being attained within 0.5 to 2 hours after dosing. Plasma protein binding is only 31%. It concentrates primarily in the intestinal tract, liver, kidney, and spleen and is excreted primarily in the feces, with only 20% of an oral dose being excreted in the urine. It is retained in the body for considerable periods of time, being detected in the urine and leukocytes for 9 to 10 days following a single dose. Metabolism occurs primarily in the liver, with the major metabolite being the amine resulting from amide hydrolysis.

Side Effects Colchicine can produce bone marrow depression, with long-term therapy resulting in thrombocytopenia or aplastic anemia. At maximum dose levels, GI disturbances (e.g., nausea, diarrhea, and abdominal pain) can occur. Acute toxicity is characterized by GI distress, including severe diarrhea resulting in excessive fluid loss, respiratory depression, and kidney damage. Treatment normally involves measures that prevent shock as well as morphine and atropine to diminish abdominal pain. A number of drug interactions have been reported. In general, the actions of colchicine are potentiated by alkalinizing substances and are inhibited by acidifying drugs, consistent with its mechanism of action of increasing the pH of synovial fluid. Responses to CNS depressants and to sympathomimetic drugs appear to be enhanced. Clinical tests can be affected; most notably, elevated alkaline phosphatase and serum glutamate oxaloacetate transaminase values and decreased thrombocyte values can be obtained. Because colchicine is a P-gp and CYP3A4 substrate, life-threatening and fatal drug interactions have been reported as a result of significant increases in colchicine plasma levels in patients treated with P-gp and strong CYP3A4 inhibitors.

Dosing Colchicine is indicated for the treatment of acute attacks of gout and is very effective. The usual dose is 1.0 to 1.2 mg, followed by 0.5 to 1.2 mg every 1 to 2 hours until either pain relief is observed or symptoms of GI distress are observed. When a rapid response is required, or if GI reactions warrant discontinuance of oral administration, IV administration (usually 2 mg initially) can be indicated. It is available as 0.5- or 0.6-mg tablets and as an injectable solution of 1 mg in 2-mL ampoules. It often is given in combination with probenecid, and combination products of the two are available in tablets containing 500 mg of probenecid and 0.5 mg of colchicine.

Treatment of Chronic Gout

Drugs That Increase Uric Acid Secretion

Probenecid Probenecid is insoluble in water and acidic solutions but is soluble in alkaline solutions buffered to pH 7.4. Probenecid initially was synthesized as a result of studies in the 1940s on sulfonamides that indicated the sulfonamides decreased the renal clearance of penicillin, extending the half-life of penicillin as supplies diminished. Probenecid thus was initially used—and is still indicated—for that purpose. Probenecid promotes the excretion of uric acid by inhibiting the urate anion exchange transporter (URAT1), decreasing the reabsorption of uric acid in the proximal tubules. The overall effect is to decrease plasma uric acid concentrations, thereby decreasing the rate and extent of urate crystal deposition in joints and synovial fluids. Within the series of *N*-dialkylsulfamyl benzoates from which probenecid is derived, renal clearance of these compounds is decreased as the length of the *N*-alkyl substituents is increased. Uricosuric activity increases with increasing size of the alkyl group in the series methyl, ethyl, and propyl.

Probenecid is essentially completely absorbed from the GI tract on oral administration, with peak plasma levels observed within 2 to 4 hours. Like most acidic compounds, probenecid (pK_a = 3.4) is extensively plasma protein bound (93% to 99%). The primary route of elimination of probenecid and its metabolites is the urine. It is extensively metabolized in humans, with only 5% to 10% being excreted as unchanged drug. The major metabolites detected result from glucuronide conjugation of the carboxylic acid, ω-oxidation of the *n*-propyl side chain and subsequent oxidation of the resulting alcohol to the carboxylic acid derivative, ω-oxidation of the *n*-propyl group, and *N*-dealkylation (Fig. 31.39). Those metabolites possessing a free carboxylic acid functional group usually possess some uricosuric activity. The glycine conjugates possess high affinity to the organic anion transport system thus preventing the reabsorption of uric acid. Probenecid appears to be well tolerated, with few adverse reactions. The major side effect is GI distress (e.g., nausea, vomiting, and anorexia), but these occur in only 2% of patients at low doses. Other effects include headache, dizziness, urinary frequency, hypersensitivity reactions, sore gums, and anemia. Overdosages do not appear to present major

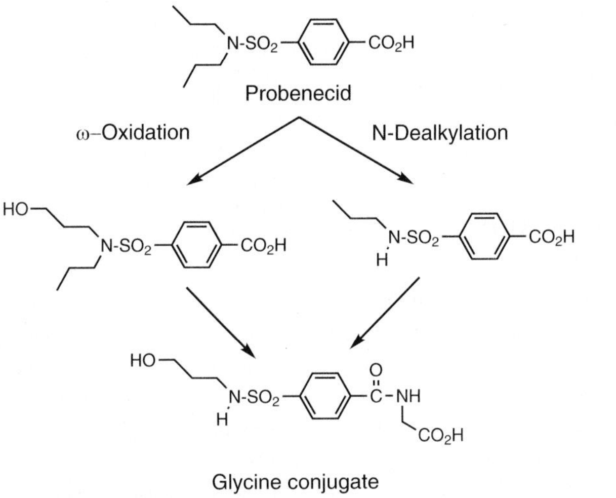

FIGURE 31.39 Metabolism of probenecid.

difficulties; a case of a 49-year-old man who recovered from the ingestion of 47 g in a suicide attempt has been reported. Should overdosage occur, treatment consists of emesis or gastric lavage, short-acting barbiturates (if CNS excitation occurs), and epinephrine (for anaphylactic reactions). A number of drug interactions have been reported. Despite the high degree of plasma protein binding, displacement interactions with other drugs bound to plasma proteins do not appear to occur to any significant extent. Salicylates counteract the uricosuric effects of probenecid. Because probenecid inhibits their renal excretion, increased plasma levels of the following drugs can be observed: aminosalicylic acid, methotrexate, sulfonamides, dapsone, sulfonylureas, naproxen, indomethacin, rifampin, and sulfinpyrazone. (The effects on penicillin plasma levels were discussed previously.)

Probenecid is indicated for the treatment of hyperuricemia associated with gout and gouty arthritis and for the elevation and prolongation of plasma levels of penicillins and cephalosporins. In gout, treatment should not begin until an acute attack has subsided. It is not recommended in individuals with known uric acid kidney stones or blood dyscrasias or for children younger than 2 years of age.

SULFINPYRAZONE Sulfinpyrazone is soluble in alkaline solutions. Its structure and synthesis are similar to that of phenylbutazone (131) (Fig. 31.38). It produces its uricosuric effect in a manner similar to that of probenecid. A dose of 35 mg produces a uricosuric effect equivalent to that produced by 100 mg of probenecid, whereas 400 mg/d of sulfinpyrazone produces an effect comparable to that obtained with doses of 1.5 to 2 g of probenecid. It also possesses, not surprisingly, some of the properties of phenylbutazone. It is an inhibitor of human platelet prostaglandin synthesis at the cyclooxygenase step, resulting in a decrease in platelet release and a reduction in platelet aggregation. This antiplatelet effect suggests a role for sulfinpyrazone in reducing the incidence of sudden death, which can occur in the first year following a myocardial infarction; however, it lacks the analgesic and anti-inflammatory effects of phenylbutazone.

Sulfinpyrazone is a strong acid (enolic OH pK_a = 2.8), a factor that is important in the production of the uricosuric effect, because within a series of pyrazolidinedione derivatives, the stronger the acid, the more potent the uricosuric effect. Polar substitution on the side chain also influences uricosuric activity, as discussed previously with regard to the pyrazolidinediones.

Oral administration results in rapid and essentially complete absorption, with peak plasma levels being attained within 1 to 2 hours of administration. It is highly bound (98% to 99%) to plasma proteins, and it is excreted in the urine primarily (50%) as unchanged drug.

The metabolites produced result from sulfoxide reduction, sulfur and aromatic oxidation, and C-glucuronidation of the heterocyclic ring in a manner similar to that for phenylbutazone (Fig. 31.40). The metabolite resulting from *p*-hydroxylation of the aromatic ring possesses uricosuric effects in humans. The sulfide metabolite, a major metabolic product, can contribute to the antiplatelet effects of sulfinpyrazone but

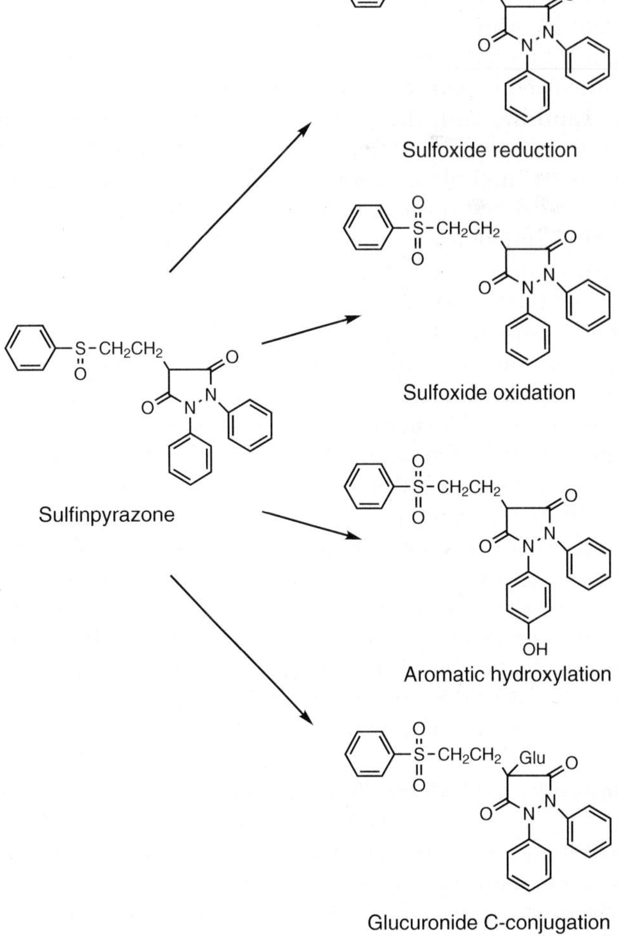

FIGURE 31.40 Metabolism of sulfinpyrazone.

not to the uricosuric effects. The most frequent adverse reactions are GI disturbances; however, the incidence is relatively low. It has been suggested that sulfinpyrazone is a much weaker inhibitor of prostaglandin synthesis in bovine stomach microsomes than either aspirin or indomethacin, a factor that can account for its gastric tolerance. Much rarer have been reports of blood dyscrasias and rash. Overdosage produces symptoms that are primarily GI in nature (e.g., nausea, diarrhea, and vomiting) but can also involve impaired respiration and convulsions. Treatment consists of emesis or gastric lavage and supportive care. Like probenecid, its uricosuric effects are antagonized by salicylates, and probenecid markedly inhibits the renal tubular secretion of sulfinpyrazone. It potentiates the actions of other drugs that are highly plasma protein bound, such as coumarin-type oral anticoagulants, antibacterial sulfonamides, and hypoglycemic sulfonylureas.

Sulfinpyrazone is indicated for the treatment of chronic and intermittent gouty arthritis.

Drugs That Decrease Uric Acid Formation

Allopurinol

Mechanism of Action The biosynthesis of uric acid from the immediate purine precursor xanthine that results from adenine, via the intermediate hypoxanthine, or from guanine is illustrated in Figure 31.37. The enzyme xanthine oxidase (a molybdenum hydroxylase enzyme) is involved in two steps, the conversion of hypoxanthine to xanthine and, the final step, the conversion of xanthine to uric acid. Allopurinol originally was designed as an antineoplastic antimetabolite to antagonize the actions of key purines inasmuch as it differs from normal purines only by the inversion of the nitrogen and carbon atoms at the 7- and 8-positions of the purine ring system but was found to have little or no effect on experimental tissues. It was subsequently found that allopurinol serves as a substrate for xanthine oxidase (15 to 20 times the affinity of xanthine) and reversibly inhibits that enzyme. Normally, uric acid is a major metabolic end product in humans. When allopurinol is administered, however, xanthine and hypoxanthine are elevated in the urine, and uric acid levels decrease. When the synthesis of uric acid is inhibited, plasma urate levels decrease, supersaturated solutions of urate are no longer present, and urate crystal deposits dissolve, eliminating the primary cause of gout. The increased plasma levels of hypoxanthine and xanthine pose no real problem, because they are more soluble than uric acid and are readily excreted.

Absorption and Metabolism Allopurinol was synthesized in 1956 as part of a study of purine antagonists (132). It is well absorbed on oral administration, with peak plasma concentrations appearing within 1 hour. Decreases of uric acid can be observed within 24 to 48 hours. Excretion of allopurinol and its metabolite occurs primarily in the urine,

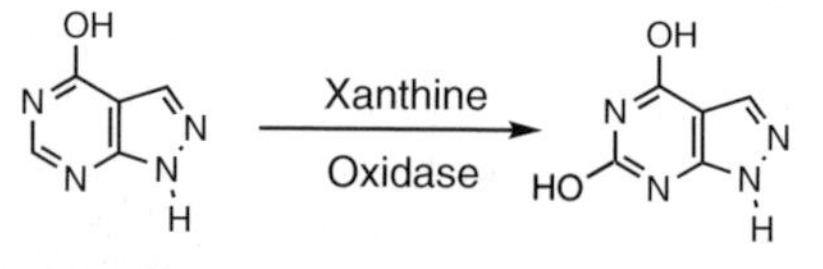

FIGURE 31.41 Metabolism of allopurinol.

with approximately 20% of a dose being excreted in the feces. Allopurinol is rapidly metabolized via oxidation and the formation of numerous ribonucleoside derivatives (Fig. 31.41). The major oxidation metabolite, alloxanthine or oxypurinol, has a much longer half-life (18 to 30 hours vs. 2 to 3 hours) than the parent drug and is an effective, although less potent, inhibitor of xanthine oxidase. The longer plasma half-life of alloxanthine results in an accumulation in the body during chronic administration, thus contributing significantly to the overall therapeutic effects of allopurinol. The major adverse effects are primarily dermatologic in nature (e.g., skin rash and exfoliative lesions). Other effects, such as GI distress (e.g., nausea, vomiting, and diarrhea), hematopoietic effects (e.g., aplastic anemia, bone marrow depression, and transient leukopenia), neurologic disorders (e.g., headache, neuritis, and dizziness), and ophthalmologic effects (e.g., cataracts) are less commonly encountered. Allopurinol can also initiate attacks of acute gouty arthritis during the early stages of therapy and can require the concomitant administration of colchicine. Drug interactions include those drugs that normally are also metabolized by xanthine oxidase. For example, the oxidation of 6-mercaptopurine, a useful antineoplastic agent, is inhibiting, permitting a reduction in the therapeutic dose. Allopurinol also has an inhibitory effect on liver microsomal enzymes, thus prolonging the half-lives of drugs, such as oral anticoagulants, that normally are metabolized and inactivated by these enzymes, although this effect is quite variable. The incidence of ampicillin-related skin rashes increases with the concurrent administration of allopurinol.

Allopurinol is indicated for the treatment of primary and secondary gout, for malignancies such as leukemia and lymphoma, and for the treatment of patients with recurrent calcium oxalate calculi.

Febuxostat

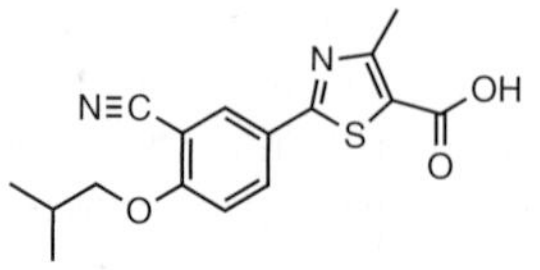

Febuxostat (Uloric)

Febuxostat, the first new drug to be approved for the treatment of gout in over 40 years, is the first nonpurine, selective xanthine oxidase inhibitor marketed in the

United States (Uloric; Adenuric in European Union). Unlike allopurinol, febuxostat noncompetitively blocks the channel leading to the active site of both the oxidized and reduced forms of xanthine oxidase, thereby inhibiting the synthesis of uric acid (133,134). It was synthesized in seven steps from 4-hydroxy-3-nitrobenzaldehyde (135). Structurally, febuxostat does not contain or mimic a purine or pyrimidine; thus, it does not inhibit enzymes involved in pyrimidine or purine metabolism, resulting in fewer adverse events relative to allopurinol.

Absorption and Metabolism Febuxostat is well absorbed on oral administration, with peak plasma concentrations appearing within 1 to 1.5 hours and a half-life of 5 to 8 hours. Febuxostat is extensively metabolized by conjugation by glucuronosyltransferase enzymes including UGT1A1, UGT1A3, UGT1A9, and UGT2B7, as well as by oxidation by CYP1A1, CYP1A2, CYP2C8, and CYP2C9 and non-CYP enzymes to produce metabolites resulting from ω-oxidation, ω-1 oxidation, *O*-dealkylation, and alcohol oxidation (136,137). Excretion of febuxostat, as various metabolites and their conjugates, occurs primarily in the urine (49%) and feces (45%). From an administered dose, only 3% and 12% are recovered as unchanged drug in urine and feces, respectively. The metabolism of febuxostat is shown in Figure 31.42.

Adverse Effects and Dosing The major adverse effects are primarily liver function abnormalities. Initial dosing with febuxostat can initiate gout flares and can require the concomitant administration of an NSAID or colchicine. Drug interactions include those drugs that normally are also metabolized by xanthine oxidase, such as azathioprine, mercaptopurine, and theophylline.

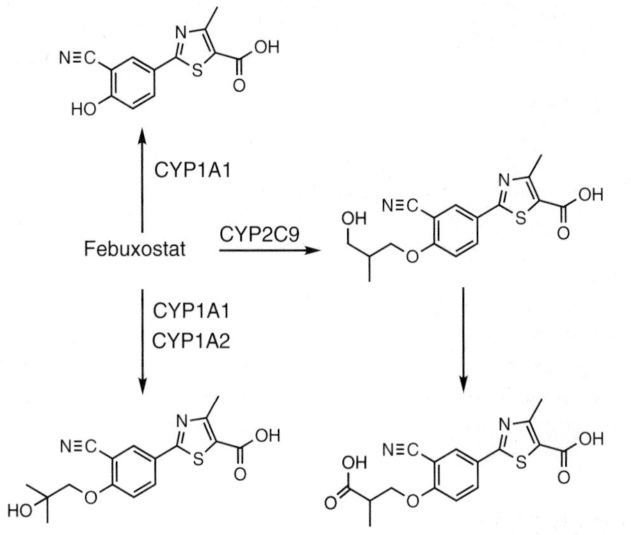

FIGURE 31.42 Metabolism of febuxostat.

Febuxostat is indicated for the chronic management of hyperuricemia in patients with gout and for patients who cannot tolerate allopurinol. Dosing is recommended at 40 or 80 mg once daily. A review of the clinical properties of febuxostat as a new treatment option has recently appeared (138,139).

Drugs Acting by Enhancing the Degradation of Uric Acid

Pegloticase Pegloticase was recently approved in the United States for the treatment of chronic gout in patients for whom traditional small-molecule therapy does not prove effective. Unlike allopurinol or febuxostat, pegloticase does not block the formation of uric acid but enhances the excretion of uric acid by converting it into a more excretable metabolite. The active agent is a recombinant porcine-like uricase (uric oxidase) that catalyzes the oxidation of uric acid to the inert allantoin. Allantoin is more soluble than uric acid and more readily excreted (Fig. 31.37). Pegloticase is a uric acid–specific enzyme that consists of recombinant modified mammalian urate oxidase (uricase) produced by a genetically modified strain of *E. coli* and polyethylene-glycolated (PEGylated). Uricase is covalently conjugated to monomethoxypoly(ethylene glycol) (mPEG) (10 kd molecular weight). The cDNA coding for uricase was derived from mammalian sequences. Each uricase subunit weighs approximately 34 kd (34,000 MW). The average molecular weight of pegloticase (tetrameric enzyme conjugated to mPEG) is approximately 540 kd.

Absorption As would be expected from the administration of an active enzyme, the duration of suppression of plasma uric acid was positively associated with the dose of pegloticase. As for clearance and volume of distribution, the significant covariates were antipegloticase antibodies and body surface area.

Dosing and Adverse Effects The recommended dose of pegloticase is 8 mg IV every 2 weeks. See prescribing information for specific instructions because the drug must not be diluted until it will be administered slowly, over more than 120 minutes. Prior to beginning the infusion, premedication of the patient with antihistamines and corticosteroids is recommended to prevent anaphylaxis and infusion reactions, which are thought to result from cytokine release. During the first 3 months of treatment, gout flares are likely to occur, and thus, NSAIDs and/or colchicine should be started at least 1 week prior to pegloticase therapy.

SCENARIO: OUTCOME AND ANALYSIS

Outcome

Jill T. Johnson, PharmD, BCPS

For pain relief, there are no significant short-term (<6 months) differences among oral NSAIDs. For serious harms such as cardiovascular events, celecoxib does not seem to be associated with higher risk compared with nonselective NSAIDs. All nonselective NSAIDs except naproxen are associated with similar increased risk for serious cardiovascular events. Naproxen has a lower cardiovascular risk than nonselective NSAIDs. Compared to nonselective NSAIDS, celecoxib is gastroprotective in the short term (6 months) but not in the long term (at 12 months) in causing clinically significant upper GI events. Nonselective NSAIDs are similar to each other regarding their increased risks of serious GI events, but the partially selective NSAID nabumetone is gastroprotective compared to nonselective NSAIDs.

EB could take nabumetone or celecoxib, which would afford her short-term decreased risk for a stomach ulcer caused by NSAID drug therapy. Because she has a chronic illness necessitating NSAID use, she will require long-term therapy. After 6 months of use, celecoxib failed to be superior to nonselective NSAIDs regarding clinically significant upper GI events; so, in the long term, celecoxib may not provide an advantage over her original therapy. The other alternative is to select an NSAID that relieves her pain and to give her a proton pump inhibitor or a prostaglanvdin analogue such as misoprostol to protect her stomach from ulcer formation.

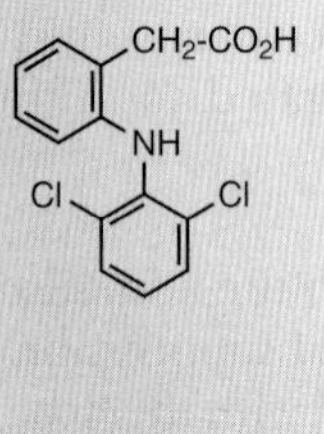

Diclofenac

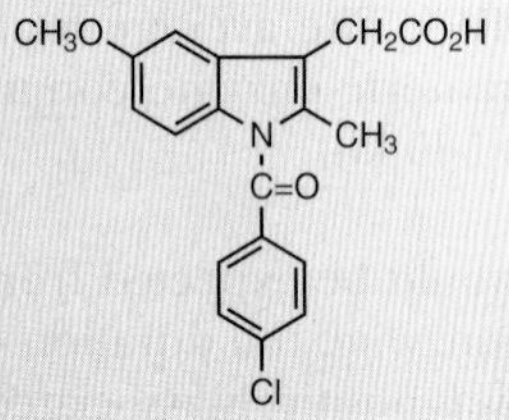

Indomethacin

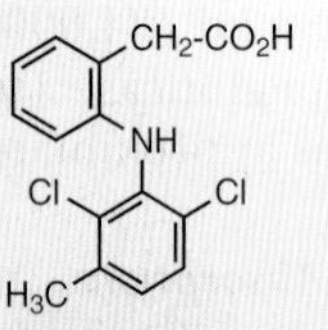

Meclofenamic acid

Chemical Analysis

Victoria Roche and S. William Zito

With the exception of aspirin and the COX-2 selective NSAIDs (the "coxibs"), NSAIDs have a similar pharmacophoric nucleus because they all bind to the same active site on the COX enzyme. To bind to this site, the NSAID must anchor to a cationic Arg residue (Arg^{120}) and, therefore, must contain an acidic functional group with a pKa low enough to generate a significant amount of anionic conjugate base at pH 6.8, the pH of inflamed tissue. Two conjugated aromatic rings capable of assuming a noncoplanar orientation are ideal for binding to aromatic and aliphatic residues in the active site cavity, although one aromatic system provides therapeutically useful anti-inflammatory activity.

Much of the remaining NSAID SAR relates to increasing potency by enhancing distribution through membranes to reach COX receptors (lipophilic groups) or promoting the ideal noncoplanar conformation between aromatic rings (appropriately placed large groups). For example, a chlorine atom placed at the o-position of one aromatic ring would increase potency significantly over a nonsubstituted analog because it would enhance potency via both mechanisms. This substitution pattern is observed in NSAIDs such as diclofenac and meclofenamate. Another chemical strategy for enhancing NSAID activity is to block degradative metabolism, e.g., through the addition of a *p*-substitutent (preferably a lipophilic one) to an aromatic ring. Indomethacin is a good example of this strategy.

COX-1 is found in the gut, and inhibition of this isoform is responsible for much of the GI distress induced by NSAIDs. When gastric COX-1 is inhibited, the synthesis of the cytoprotective PGE$_1$ ceases. Coxibs bind selectively to the allosteric site of the COX-2 isoform in inflamed tissue and kidney. The allosteric site of COX-1 is more sterically restricted than COX-2, which denies the coxib drugs access to the binding residues of this isoform. Because they have a lower affinity for gastric COX-1, coxibs claim to have a decreased risk of GI ulceration and hemorrhage, although this holds true mostly in the short term. Celecoxib was the original COX-2 selective NSAID and its anionic sulfonamide group helps it bind securely into the COX-2 allosteric site through an ion-ion interaction with an Arg residue. Many coxibs are diarylheteroaromatic compounds, and the two aromatic rings of these structures enhance affinity for COX-2 through van der Waals bonds with Tyr, His and other aromatic residues in or near the allosteric site. Note the two distinct binding sites on the COX-2 enzyme cartoon below; the active site (which would bind nonselective NSAIDs such as diclofenac, indomethacin, and meclofenamate) and the allosteric site (which binds the coxibs).

Though the degree of inherent COX-2 preference in nonselective (noncoxib) NSAIDs is hard to predict, the lower GI distress of nabumetone can be directly related to its prodrug status. To inhibit COX-1 in the gut, NSAIDs have to bind to the active site Arg^{120} residue, and this requires an anionic drug. Nabumetone has no acidic functional group and can only generate the active anionic form after it has been absorbed from the gut and metabolized via beta-oxidation in the liver. As a nonacidic prodrug, it does not inhibit gastric COX-1, nor can it physically irritate the gastric mucosa as all acidic NSAIDs are capable of doing.

SCENARIO: OUTCOME AND ANALYSIS *(Continued)*

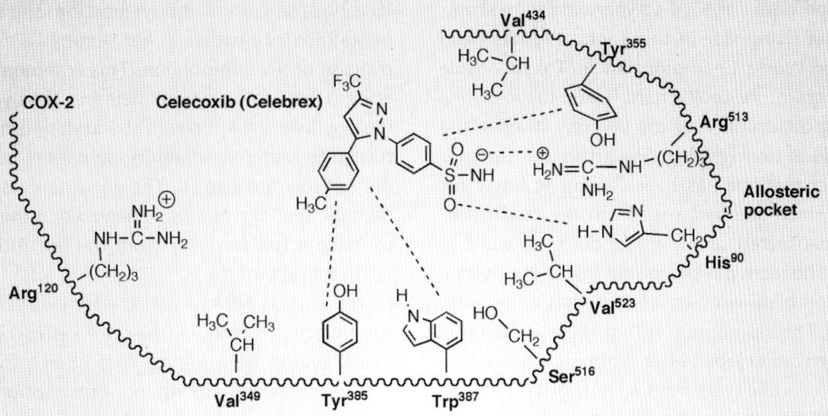

Active site cavity

Although it is not as potent as some other NSAIDs because it has only one aromatic moiety, it is often gentler on the stomach. This is an acceptable trade off in mild inflammatory disease.

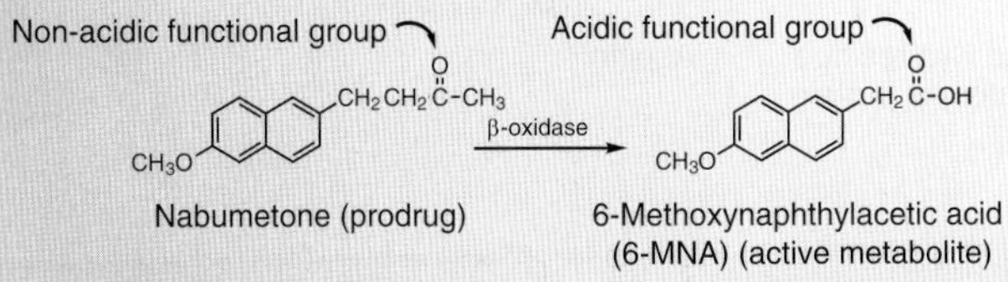

The original NSAID EB was taking (naproxen) is similar to nabumetone in that it has only one aromatic moiety (a methoxy-substituted naphthylene ring system), but it is significantly different in that it has the carboxylic acid functional group that would permit inhibition of gastric COX-1 and direct gastric mucosal irritation. The GI distress of naproxen would be anticipated to be greater than its chemical cousin nabumetone. It should be noted that the α-CH_3 group of naproxen is a potency-enhancing feature.

Misoprostol, a PGE_1 analog, protects the gastric mucosa from distress by serving as a replacement for the endogenous gastric PGE_1 inhibited by the use of nonselective NSAIDs. Proton pump inhibitors are cytoprotective in the stomach because they stop all gastric acid secretion by irreversibly inhibiting the adenosine triphosphatase that is responsible for the secretion of acid into the stomach lumen.

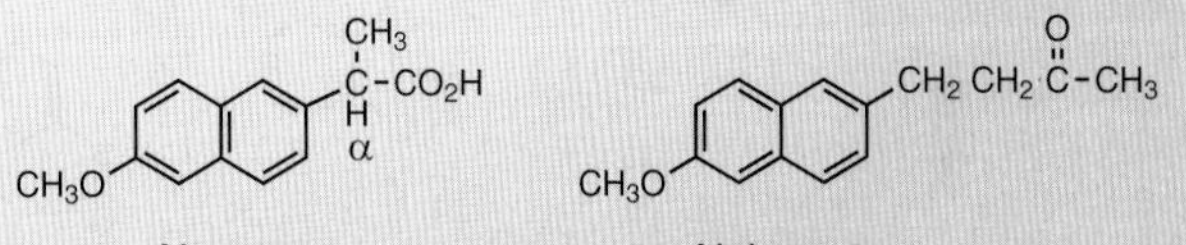

CASE STUDY

Victoria Roche and S. William Zito

This has not been a good week for IG, a 17-year-old figure skater from Minnesota. IG is a rising star in this sport, and has been competing in the 2011 World Championship in Tokyo. While practicing her long program, she took a hard fall on the ice while attempting to execute a quadruple axel and severely strained the adductor (groin) muscle of her right leg. She attributed the mishap, in part, to the fact that she has been feeling so lousy for the past week or so, which she had kept from her coach. Her joints ache, she feels nauseated, and she just does not want to eat much of anything. The team physician sent her to the nearby medical center for a complete workup, and she has been diagnosed with hepatitis A. The assumption is that she acquired this illness when she first arrived in Japan after grabbing a quick bite from a small family-run noodle restaurant a short distance from her downtown hotel.

IG is no stranger to liver dysfunction; she experienced significant heptatotoxicity earlier in her skating career through the chronic overuse of acetaminophen. This common pain reliever can generate a hepatotoxic quinoneimine (known as NAPQI) that can destroy liver cells through the arylation of cysteine residues. IG turned to acetaminophen for pain relief because her GI tract just did not tolerate aspirin. The good news is that her drug-induced heptatic damage has since healed and the physicians expect her to make a full recovery from the hepatitis infection within the next several months.

IG now needs NSAID therapy for her severely strained adductor muscle. Which of the three prescription NSAIDs drawn below would be a logical first choice for this young athlete? She is currently taking no prescription or over-the-counter drugs.

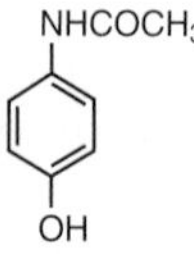

Acetaminophen

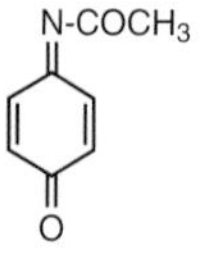

NAPQI

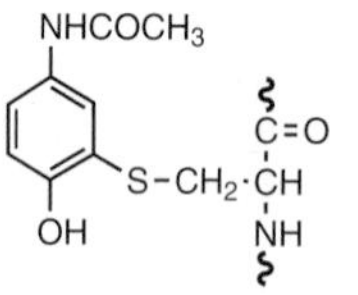

Arylated Cys residue of hepatocyte protein

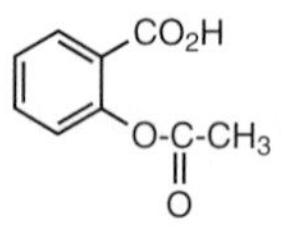

Aspirin

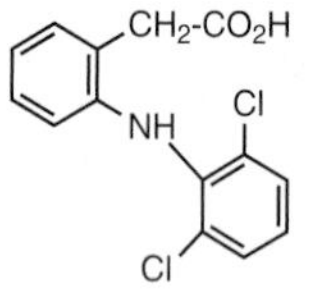

1

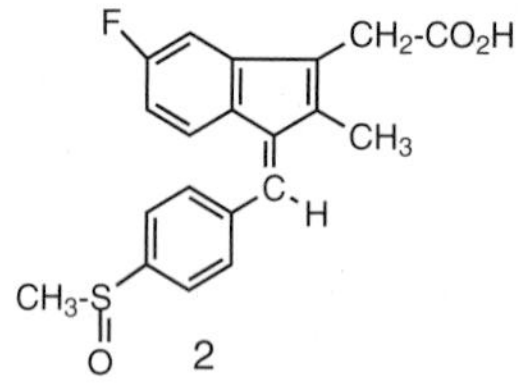

2

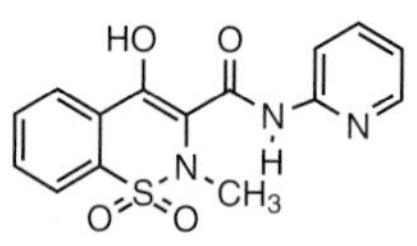

3

1. Conduct a thorough and mechanistic SAR analysis of the three therapeutic options in the case.
2. Apply the chemical understanding gained from the SAR analysis to this patient's specific needs to make a therapeutic recommendation.

References

1. Borne RF. Non-steroidal anti-inflammatory agents, antipyretics, and uricosuric agents. In: Verderame M, ed. Handbook of Cardiovascular and Anti-Inflammatory Agents. Boca Raton, FL: CRC Press, 1986:27–104.
2. Klippel JH, Stone JH, Crofford LJ, et al., eds. Primer on the Rheumatic Diseases, 13th Ed. New York: Springer-Verlag, 2008.
3. Hootman J, Bolen J, Helmick C, et al. Prevalence of doctor-diagnosed arthritis and arthritis-attributable activity limitation—United States, 2003–2005. Morbid Mortal Wkly Rep 2006;55:1089–1092.
4. Hootman JM, Helmick CG. Projections of U.S. prevalence of arthritis and associated activity limitations. Arthritis Rheum 2006;54:266–229.
5. Hamor GH. Non-steroidal anti-inflammatory drugs. In: Foye WO, ed. Principles of Medicinal Chemistry, 3rd Ed. Philadelphia, PA: Lea & Febiger, 1989:503–530.
6. Walport M. Complement. In: Roitt IM, Brostoff J, Male DK, eds. Immunology, 2nd Ed. St. Louis, MO: C.V. Mosby Co., 1989.
7. Kinoshita T. Biology of complement: the overture. Immunol Today 1991;12:291–295.
8. Frank MM, Fries LF. The role of complement in inflammation and phagocytosis. Immunol Today 1991;12:322–326.
9. Frank MM, Hester CG. Complement and arthritis: another step in understanding. Arthritis Res Ther 2008;10:104–110.
10. Shen TY. Proc. Int. Symp. Milan, 1964. In: Grattini S, Dukes MNG, eds. Excerpta Medica, Amsterdam, 1965;18.
11. Shen TY. Anti-inflammatory agents. Top Med Chem 1967;1:29–38.
12. Vane JR. Inhibition of prostaglandin synthesis as a mechanism of action for aspirin-like drugs. Nat New Biol 1971;231:232–235.
13. Gund P, Shen TY. A model for the prostaglandin synthetase cyclooxygenation site and its inhibition by antiinflammatory arylacetic acids. J Med Chem 1977;20:1146–1152.
14. Kurzrok R, Lieb C. Biochemical studies of human semen II the action of semen on the human uterus. Proc Soc Exptl Biol NY 1931;28:268.
15. Goldblatt MW. Properties of human seminal plasma. J Physiol (London) 1935;84:208–218.
16. von Euler US. The specific vasodilating and plain muscle-stimulating substances from accessory genital glands in man and certain animals (prostaglandin and vesiglandin). J Physiol (London) 1936;88:213–234.
17. Bergstrom S, Samuelsson B. The prostaglandins. Endeavour 1968;27:109–113.
18. Campbell WB. Lipid-derived autacoids: eicosanoids and platelet-activating factor. In: Gilman AG, Rall TW, Nies AS, et al., eds. Goodman and Gilman's the Pharmacological Basis of Therapeutics, 8th Ed. New York: Pergamon Press, 1990:600–601.
19. Miyamoto T, Ogino N, Yaamamoto S, et al. Purification of prostaglandin endoperoxide synthetase from bovine vesicular gland microsomes. J Biol Chem 1976;251:2629–2632.

20. Xie W, Chipman JG, Robertson DL, et al. Expression of a mitogen-responsive gene encoding prostaglandin synthase is regulated by mRNA splicing. Proc Natl Acad Sci U S A 1991;88:2692–2696.
21. Hla T, Nielson K. Human cyclooxygenase-2 cDNA. Proc Natl Acad Sci U S A 1992;89:7384–7388.
22. Jones DA, Carlton DP, McIntyre TM, et al. Molecular cloning of human prostaglandin endoperoxide synthase type II and demonstration of expression in response to cytokines. J Biol Chem 1993;268:9049–9054.
23. Kennedy B, Chan C-C, Culp S, et al. Cloning expression of rat prostaglandin endoperoxide synthase (cyclooxygenase)-2 cDNA. Biochem Biophys Res Commun 1993;197:494–500.
24. Kujubu DA, Fletcher BS, Varnum C, et al. TIS10, a phorbol ester tumor promoter-inducible mRNA from Swiss 3T3 cells, encodes a novel prostaglandin synthase/cyclooxygenase homologue. J Biol Chem 1991;266:12866–12872.
25. Chandrasekharan NV, Dai H, Roos K, et al. COX-3, a cyclooxygenase-1 variant inhibited by acetaminophen and other analgesic/antipyretic drugs: cloning, structure, and expression. Proc Natl Acad Sci U S A 2002;99:13926–13931.
26. Blobaum AL, Marnett LJ. Structural and functional basis of cyclooxygenase inhibition. J Med Chem 2007;50:1425–1440.
27. Roche VF. A receptor-grounded approach to teaching nonsteroidal anti-inflammatory drug chemistry and structure-activity relationships. Am J Pharm Educ 2009;73:143–149.
28. Flower RJ. The development of COX2 inhibitors. Nat Rev Drug Discov 2003;2:179–191.
29. Chang HW, Jahng Y. Selective cyclooxygenase-2 inhibitors as anti-inflammatory agents. Korean J Med Chem 1998;8:48–79.
30. Vane JR, Bakhle YS, Botting YM. Cyclooxygenases 1 and 2. Ann Rev Pharmacol Toxicol 1998;38:97–120.
31. Botting JH. Nonsteroidal anti-inflammatory agents. Drugs Today 1999;35:225–235.
32. Hata AN, Breyer RM. Pharmacology and signaling of prostaglandin receptors: multiple roles in inflammation and immune modulation. Pharmacol Ther 2004;103:147–166.
33. Tsuboi K, Sugimoto Y, Ichikawa A. Prostanoid receptor subtypes. Prostaglandins Other Lipid Mediat 2002;68–69:535–556.
34. Smyth EM, Burke A, Fitzgerald GA. Lipid-derived autocoids: eicosanoids and platelet-activating factor. In: Brunton LI, Lazo JS, Parker KI, eds. Goodman and Gilman's the Pharmacological Basis of Therapeutics, 11th Ed. New York: Pergamon Press, 2006:653–670.
35. Okazaki T, Sagawa N, Okita, JR, et al. Diacylglycerol metabolism and arachidonic acid release in human fetal membranes and decidua vera. J Biol Chem 1981;256:7316–7321.
36. Clark WG. Mechanisms of antipyretic action. Gen Pharmacol 1979;10:71–77.
37. Hersh EV, Lally ET, Moore PA. Update on cyclooxygenase inhibitors: has a third COX isoform entered the fray? Curr Med Res Opin 2005;21:1217–1226.
38. Qin N, Zhang SP, Reitz TL, et al. Cloning, expression, and functional characterization of human COX-1 splicing variants: evidence for intron-1 retention. J Pharmacol Exp Ther 2005;315:1298–1305.
39. Nurmi JT, Puolakkainen PA, Rautonen NE. Intro-1 retaining cyclooxygenase-1 splice variant is induced by osmotic stress in human intestinal epithelial cells. Prostaglandins Leukot Essent Fatty Acids 2005:73:343–350.
40. Snipes JA, Kis B, Shelness GS, et al. Cloning and characterization of cyclooxygenase-1b (putative cyclooxygenase-3) in rat. J Pharmacol Exp Ther 2005;313:668–676.
41. Kis B, Snipes JA, Busija DW. Acetaminophen and the cyclooxygenase-3 puzzle: sorting out facts, fictions, and uncertainties. J Pharmacol Exp Ther 2005;315:1–7.
42. Hamza M, Dione RA. Mechanisms of non-opioid analgesics beyond cyclooxygenase enzyme inhibition. Curr Mol Pharmacol 2005;2:1–14.
43. Fowler CJ, Stenström A, Tiger G. Ibuprofen inhibits the metabolism of the endogenous cannabimimetic anandamide. Pharmacol Toxicol 1997;80:103–107.
44. Holt S, Paylor B, Boldrup L, et al. Inhibition of fatty acid amide hydrolase, a key cannabinoid metabolizing enzyme, by analogues of ibuprofen and indomethacin. Eur J Pharmacol 2007;565:26–32.
45. Schlosberg JE, Kinsey SG, Lichtman AH. Targeting fatty acid amide hydrolase (FAAH) to treat pain and inflammation. AAPS J 2009;11:39–44.
46. Hogestatt ED, Jonsson BAG, Ermund A, et al. Conversion of acetaminophen to the bioactive N-acylphenolamine AM404 via fatty acid amide hydrolase-dependent arachidonic acid conjugation in the nervous system. J Biol Chem 2005;280:31405–31412.
47. Onnis V, Congiu C, Bjorklund E, et al. Synthesis and evaluation of paracetamol esters as novel fatty acid amide hydrolase inhibitors. J Med Chem 2010;53:2286–2298.
48. Smith PA, Selley DE, Sim-Selley LJ, et al. Low dose combination of morphine and D9-tetrahydrocaannabinol circumvents antinociceptive tolerance and apparent desensitization of receptors. Eur J Pharmacol 2007;571:129–137.
49. Ahn DK, Choi HS, Yeo SP, et al. Blockade of central cyclooxygenase (COX) pathways enhances the cannabinoid-induced antinociceptive effects on inflammatory temporomandibular joint (TMJ) nociception. Pain 2007;132:23–32.
50. Fowler CJ, Holt S, Nilsson, et al. The endocannabinoid signaling system: pharmacological and therapeutic aspects. Pharmacol Biochem Behav 2005;81:248–262.
51. Bancos S, Bernard MP, Topham DL, et al. Ibuprofen and other widely used non-steroidal antiinflammatory drugs inhibit antibody production in human cells. Cell Immunol 2009;258:18–28.
52. Vann RE, Cook CD, Martin BR, et al. Cannabimimetic properties of ajulemic acid. J Pharmacol Exp Ther 2007;320:678–686.
53. Klein TW, Newton CA. Therapeutic potential of cannabinoid-based drugs. Adv Exp Med Biol 2007;601:395–413.
54. Chiang N, Serhaan CN, Dahlen S-E, et al. The lipoxin receptor ALX: potent-ligand-specific and stereoselective actions in vivo. Pharmacol Rev 2006;58:463–487.
55. Bannenberg G, Serhan CN. Specialized pro-resolving lipid mediators in the inflammatory response: an update. Biochim Biophys Acta 2010;180:1260–1267.
56. Zurier RB, Sun Y-P, Kerri L, et al. Ajulemic acid, a synthetic cannabinoid, increases formation of the endogenous proresolving and anti-inflammatory eicosanoid, lipoxin A4. FASEB J 2009;23:1503–1509.
57. Burnstein SH, Zurier RB. Cannabinoids, endocannabinoids, and related analogs in inflammation. AAPS J 2009;11:109–118.
58. Botting R, Ayoub SS. COX-3 and the mechanism of action of paracetamol/acetaminophen. Prostaglandins Leukot Essent Fatty Acids 2005;72:85–87.
59. Kis B, Snipes JA, Simandle SA, et al. Acetaminophen-sensitive prostaglandin production in rat cerebral endothelial cells. Am J Physiol 2005;288:R897–R902.
60. Graham GC, Scott RF. Mechanism of action of paracetamol. Am J Ther 2005;12:46.
61. Kunkel DB. Emergency Medicine. Basel: Geigy Pharmaceuticals, July 15, 1985.
62. Mitchell JR, Jollow DJ, Potter WZ, et al. Acetaminophen-induced hepatic necrosis. I. Role of drug metabolism. J Pharmacol Exp Ther 1973;187:185–194.
63. Sinclair J, Jeffery E, Wrighton S, et al. Alcohol-mediated increase in acetaminophen hepatotoxicity. Biochem Pharmacol 1998;55:1557–1565.
64. Calder IC, Creek MJ, Williams PJ, et al. *N*-Hydroxylation of *p*-acetophenetidide as a factor in nephrotoxicity. J Med Chem 1973;16:499–502.
65. Buckpitt AR, Rollins DE, Mitchell JR. Varying effects of sulfhydryl nucleophiles on acetaminophen oxidation and sulfhydryl adduct formation. Biochem Pharmacol 1979;28:2941–2946.
66. Smilkstein MJ, Knapp GL, Kulig KW, et al. Efficacy of oral *N*-acetylcysteine in the treatment of acetaminophen overdose. Analysis of the national multicenter study (1976 to 1985). New Engl J Med 1988;319:1557–1562.
67. Hennekens CH, Buting JE. Final report on the aspirin component of the ongoing physicians' health study. New Engl J Med 1989;321:129–135.
68. Gossel TA. Aspirin's role in reducing cardiac mortality. U.S. Pharmacist 1988;13:34.
69. Thun MJ, Namboodiri MM, Heath CW. Unsuccessful emergency medical resuscitation: are continued efforts in the emergency department justified? New Engl J Med 1991;325:1393–1398.
70. Kalgutkar AS, Crews BC, Rowlinson SW, et al. Aspirin-like molecules that covalently inactivate cyclooxygenase-2. Science 1998;280:1268–1270.
71. Davison C. Salicylate metabolism in man. Ann N Y Acad Sci 1971;179:249–268.
72. Paulus HE, Whitehouse MW. Some relevant clinical conditions and the available therapy. In: Rubin AA, ed. Search for New Drugs, Vol. 6. New York: Marcel Dekker, 1972:11–40.
73. Shen TY, Ellis RL, Windholz TB, et al. Non-steroid anti-inflammatory agents. J Am Chem Soc 1963;85:488–489.
74. Shen TY, Witzel BE, Jones H, et al. U.S. Patent 3,654,349,971. Chem Abstr 1971;74:141379v.
75. Carson JR, McKinstry DN, Wong S. 5-Benzoyl-1-methylpyrrol-2-acetic acids as anti-inflammatory agents. J Med Chem 1971;14:646–647.
76. Sallman A, Pfister R. Ger. Patent 1,815,802. 1969. Chem Abstr 1970;72:12385d.
77. Poon GK, Chen Q, Teffera Y, et al. Bioactivation of diclofenac via benzoquinone imine intermediates: identification of urinary mercapturic acid derivatives in rats and humans. Drug Metab Disp 2001;29:1608–1613.
78. Demerson CA, Humber LG, Dobson TA, et al. Chemistry and anti-inflammatory activities of prodolic acid and related 1,3,4,9-tetrahydropyrano[3,4,-*b*] indole-1-alkanoic acids. J Med Chem 1975;18:189–191.
79. Demerson CA, Humber LG, Phillip AH, et al. Etodolic acid and related compounds. Chemistry and anti-inflammatory actions of some potent di- and tri-substituted 1,3,4,9-tetrahydropyrano [3,4-*b*]indole-1-acetic acids. J Med Chem 1976;19:391–395.
80. Goudie AC, Gaster LM, Lake AW, et al. 4-(6-Methoxy-2-naphthyl)butan-2-one and related analogues, a novel structural class of anti-inflammatory compounds. J Med Chem 1978;21:1260–1264.
81. Nicholson JS, Adams SS. Brit. Patent. 971,700. Chem Abstr 1964;61:14591d.
82. Hutt AJ, Caldwell J. The metabolic chiral inversion of 2-arylpropionic acids: a novel route with pharmacological consequences. J Pharm Pharmacol 1983;35:693–704.
83. Marshall WS. French Patent 2,015,728. 1970. Chem Abstr 1971;75:48707m.
84. Rubin A, Warrick P, Wolen RL, et al. Physiological disposition of fenoprofen in man. III. Metabolism and protein binding of fenoprofen. J Pharmacol Exp Ther 1972;183:449–457.

85. Farge D, Messer MN, Moutonnier C. U.S. Patent 3,641,127. 1972. Chem Abstr 1974;81:50040f.
86. Ueno K, Kubo S, Tagawa H, et al. 6,11-Dihydro-11-oxodibenz[b,e] oxepinacetic acids with potent antiinflammatory activity. J Med Chem 1976;19:941–946.
87. Harrison IT, Lewis B, Nelson P, et al. Nonsteroidal antiinflammatory agents. I. 6-Substituted 2-naphthylacetic acids. J Med Chem 1970;13:203–205.
88. Janssen PAJ, Van Deale GHP, Boey JM. Ger. Patent 2,353,375. 1974. Chem Abstr 1973;79:104952j.
89. Adams SS, Bernard J, Nicholson JS, et al. U.S. Patent 3,755,427. 1975. Chem Abstr 1974;81:49433e.
90. Menzel-Soglowek S, Geisslinger G, Beck WS, et al. Variability of inversion of (R)-flurbiprofen in different species. J Pharm Sci 1992;81:888–891.
91. Geisslinger G, Lotsch J, Menzel S, et al. Stereoselective disposition of flurbiprofen in healthy subjects following administration of single enantiomers. Br J Clin Pharmacol 1994;37:392–394.
92. Wechter WJ, Kantoci D, Murray ED Jr, et al. R-Flurbiprofen chemoprevention and treatment of intestinal adenomas in the APC(Min)/+ mouse model: implications for prophylaxis and treatment of colon cancer. Cancer Res 1997;57:4316–4324.
93. Morihara T, Chu T, Ubeda O, et al. Selective inhibition of Abeta42 production by NSAID *R*-enantiomers. J Neurochem 2002;83:1009–1012.
94. Davies NM. Clinical pharmacokinetics of oxaprozin. Clin Phrmacokinetics 1998;35:425–436.
95. Scherrer RA. Introduction to the chemistry of antiinflammatory and antiarthritic agents. In: Scherrer RA, Whitehouse MW, eds. Anti-Inflammatory Agents, Vol. 1. New York: Academic Press, 1974:35–55.
96. Scherrer RA. Aryl- and heteroarylcarboxylic acids. In: Scherrer RA, Whitehouse MW, eds. Anti-Inflammatory Agents, Vol. 1. New York: Academic Press, 1974:56–74.
97. Winder CV, Wax J, Scotti L, et al. Anti-inflammatory, antipyretic and antinociceptive properties of *N*-(2,3-xylyl) anthranilic acid (mefenamic acid). J Pharmacol Exp Ther 1962;138:405–413.
98. Appleton RA, Brown K. Conformational requirements at the prostaglandin cyclooxygenase receptor site: a template for designing non-steroidal antiinflammatory drugs. Prostaglandins 1979;18:29–34.
99. Carty TJ, Stevens JS, Lombardino JG, et al. Piroxicam, a structurally novel antiinflammatory compound. Mode of prostaglandin synthesis inhibition. Prostaglandins 1980;19:671–682.
100. Lombardino JG, Wiseman EH. Piroxicam and other antiinflammatory oxicams. Med Res Rev 1982;2:127–152.
101. Lombardino JG, Wiseman EH, Chiaini J. Potent anti-inflammatory *N*-heterocyclic 3-carboxamides of 4-hydroxy-2-methyl-2*H*-1,2-benzothiazine 1,1-dioxide. J Med Chem 1973;16:493–496.
102. Black WC. Selective cyclooxygenase-2 inhibitors. Ann Rep Med Chem 2004;39:125–138.
103. Warner TD, Giuliano F, Vojnovic I, et al. Nonsteroid drug selectivities for cyclo-oxygenase-1 rather than cyclo-oxygenase-2 are associated with human gastrointestinal toxicity: a full in vitro analysis. Proc Natl Acad Sci USA 1999;96:7563–7568.
104. Chan CC, Boyce S, Brideau C, et al. Rofecoxib [Vioxx, MK-0966; 4-(4'-methylsulfonylphenyl)-3-phenyl-2-(5*H*)-furanone]: a potent and orally active cyclooxygenase-2 inhibitor. Pharmacological and biochemical profiles. J Pharmacol Exp Ther 1999;290:551–560.
105. Bombardier C, Laine L, Reicin A, et al. Comparison of upper gastrointestinal toxicity of rofecoxib and naproxen in patients with rheumatoid arthritis. N Engl J Med 2000;343:1520–1528.
106. Aw T-J, Haas SJ, Liew D, et al. Meta-analysis of cyclooxygenase-2 inhibitors and their effects on blood pressure. Arch Intern Med 2005;165:1–7.
107. Fitzgerald GA. Coxibs and cardiovascular disease. N Engl J Med 2004;351:1709–1711.
108. Topol EJ. Failing the public health-rofecoxib, Merck, and the FDA. N Engl J Med 2004;351:1707–1709.
109. Dogne J-M, Supuran CT, Pratico D. Adverse cardiovascular effects of the coxibs. J Med Chem 2005;48:2251–2257.
110. Szewczuk LM, Penning TM. Mechanism-based inactivation of COX-1 by red wine m-hydroquinones. A structure-activity relationship study. J Nat Prod 2004;67:1777–1782.
111. Szewczuk LM, Forti L, Stivala LA, Penning TM. Resveratrol is a peroxidase-mediated inactivator of COX-1 but not COX-2 - A Mechanistic approach to the design of COX-1 selective agents. J. Biol. Chem 2004;279: 22727-22737.
112. Penning TD, Talley JJ, Bertenshaw SR, et al. Synthesis and biological evaluation of the 1,5-diarylpyrazole class of cyclooxygenase-2 inhibitors: identification of 4-[5-(4-methylphenyl)-3-(trifluoromethyl)-1*H*-pyrazol-1-yl]benzenesulfonamide (SC-58635, celecoxib). J Med Chem 1997;40:1347–1365.
113. McEvoy GK, ed. American Hospital Formulary Service Drug Information 2011. STAT!Ref Online Electronic Medical Library. Available at: http://www.statref.com/. Accessed January 14, 2011.
114. Korpela M, Laasonen L, Hannonen P, et al. Retardation of joint damage in patients with early rheumatoid arthritis by initial aggressive treatment with disease-modifying antirheumatic drugs: five year experience from the FIN-RACo study. Arthr Rheumat 2004;50:2072–2081.
115. Youn HS, Lee JY, Saitoh SI, et al. Auranofin, as an antirheumatic gold compound suppresses LPS-induced homodimerization of TLR4. Biochem Biophys Res Comun 2006;350:866–871.
116. Yang JP, Merin JP, Nakano T, et al. Inhibition of the DNA binding activity of NF-kappa B by gold compounds in vitro. FEBS Lett 1995;321:89–96.
117. Bratt J, Belcher J, Vercellotti GM, et al. Effects of antirheutmatic gold salts on NF-kB mobilization and tumor necrosis factor-alpha (TNF-a)-induced neutrophil-dependent cytotoxicity for human endothelial cells. Clin Exp Immunol 2000;120:79–84.
118. Weber SM., Levitz SM. Chloroquine interferes with lipopolysaccharide-induced TNF- gene expression by a nonlysosomotropic mechanism. J Immunol 2000;165:1534–1540.
119. Flanagan ME, Blumenkopf TA, Brissette WH et al. Discovery of CP-690,550: a potent and selective Janus kinase (JAK) inhibitor for the treatment of autoimmune diseases and organ transplant rejection. J Med Chem 2010;53:8468–8484.
120. Gadangi P, Longaker M, Naime D, et al. The anti-inflammatory mechanism of sulfasalazine is related to adenosine release. J Immunol 1996;156:1937–1941.
121. Gadangi P, Longaker M, Naime D, et al. The anti-inflammatory mechanism of sulfasalazine is related to adenosine release. J Immunol 1996;156:1937–1941.
122. Naguwa SM. Tumor necrosis factor inhibitor therapy for rheumatoid arthritis. NY Acad Sci 2005;1051:709–715.
123. Jarvis B, Faulds D. Etanercept: a review of its use in rheumatoid arthritis. Drugs 1999;57:945–966.
124. Markham A, Lamb HM. Infliximab: a review of its use in the management of rheumatoid arthritis. Drugs 2000;59:1341–1359.
125. King KM, Younes A. Rituximab; review and clinical applications focusing on non-Hodgkin's lymphoma. Expert Rev Anticancer Ther 2001;1:177–186.
126. Kaushik VV, Moots RJ. CDP-870 (certolizumab) in rheumatoid arthritis. Expert Opin Biol Ther 2005;5:601–606.
127. McCluggage LK, Scholtz JM. Golimumab: a tumor necrosis factor alpha inhibitor for the treatment of rheumatoid arthritis. Ann Pharmacother 2010;44:135–144.
128. Shealy D, Cai A, Nesspor T, et al. Characterization of golimumab (CNTO 148), a novel monoclonal antibody specific for human TNF-α. Ann Rheum Dis 2007;66(Suppl 2):151.
129. Oldfield V, Dhillon S, Plosker GL. Tocilizumab: a review of its use in the management of rheumatoid arthritis. Drugs 2009;69:609–632.
130. Kaine JL. Abatacept for the treatment of rheumatoid arthritis. Curr Ther Res 2007;68:379–399.
131. Zhang P, Li J, Han Y, et al. Traditional Chinese medicine in the treatment of rheumatoid arthritis. Rheumatol Int. 2010;30:713–718.
132. Centers for Disease Control and Prevention. Gout. Available at: http://www.cdc.gov/arthritis/basics/gout.htm.
133. Pfister R, Häflinger F. Über derivate und analoġe de phenylbutazoins IV analoġemit schwefelhaltiġen seitenkitten. Helv Chim Acta 1961;44: 232–237.
134. Robins RK. Potential purine antagonist. I. Synthesis of some 4,6-substituted pyrazolo[3,4-d] pyrimidines. J Am Chem Soc 1956;78:784–790.
135. Stamp LK, O'Donnell JL, Chapman PT. Emerging therapies in the long-term management of hyperuricaemia and gout. Intern Med J 2007;37:258–266.
136. Bruce SP. Febuxostat: a selective xanthine oxidase inhibitor for the treatment of hyperuricemia and gout. Ann Pharmacother 2006;40: 21187–21194.
137. Sorbera LA, Casta FR, Rabasseda X, et al. Synthesis of TMX-67. Drugs Fut 2001;26:32.
138. Grabowski BA, Khosravan R, Vernillet L, et al. Metabolism and excretion of [14C] febuxostat, a novel nonpurine selective inhibitor of xanthine oxidase, in healthy male subjects. J Clin Pharmacol 2011;51:189–201.
139. Mukoyoshi M, Nishimura S, Hoshide S, et al. In vitro drug-drug interaction studies with febuxostat, a novel non-purine selective inhibitor of xanthine oxidase: plasma protein binding, identification of metabolic enzymes and cytochrome P450 inhibition. Xenobiotica 2008;38:496–510.
140. Avena-Woods C, Hilas O. Febuxostat (Uloric), a new treatment option for gout. Pharm Therapeut 2010;35:82–85.

Chapter 32

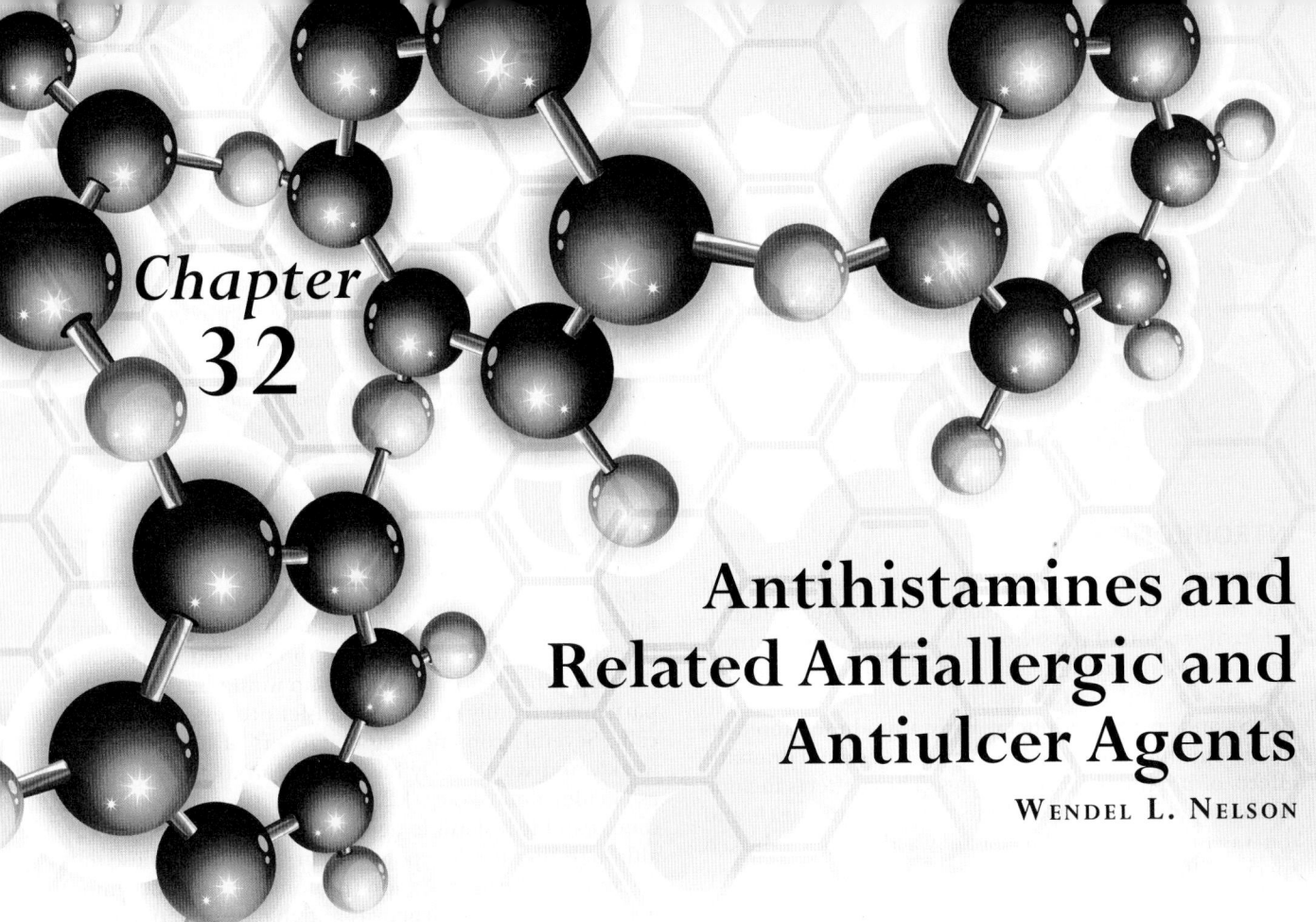

Antihistamines and Related Antiallergic and Antiulcer Agents

WENDEL L. NELSON

Drugs Covered in This Chapter[*]

ANTIHISTAMINES

- Acrivastine
- Azelastine
- Bepotastine
- *Bilastine*
- *Carebastine*
- Cetirizine
- Cromolyn
- Desloratadine
- *Ebastine*
- Emedastine
- Epinastine
- Fexofenadine
- Ketotifen
- Levocabastine
- Levocetirizine
- Lodoxamide
- Loratadine
- *Mizolastine*
- Nedocromil
- Olopatadine
- Pemirolast
- *Rupatadine*
- *Terfenadine*

ANTIULCER AGENTS

- Cimetidine
- Dexlansoprazole
- Esomeprazole
- Famotidine
- Lansoprazole
- Metoclopramide
- Misoprostol
- Nizatidine
- Omeprazole
- Pantoprazole
- Rabeprazole
- Ranitidine
- *Revaprazan*
- Sucralfate

Abbreviations

ADO, aldehyde oxidase
ATP, adenosine triphosphate
AUC, area under the curve
cAMP, cyclic adenosine monophosphate
CNS, central nervous system
FDA, U.S. Food and Drug Administration
GERD, gastroesophageal reflux disease
hERG, human ether-a-go-go
Ig, immunoglobulin
IL, interleukin
IP_3, inositol-1,4,5-triphosphate
LTC_4, leukotriene C_4
MAO, monoamine oxidase
NF-κB, nuclear factor-κB
NSAID, nonsteroidal anti-inflammatory drug
OTC, over the counter
PGD_2, prostaglandin D_2
PPI, proton pump inhibitor
T_H1, T-helper type 1
T_H2, T-helper type 2
TNF, tumor necrosis factor

[*]Drugs listed include those available inside and outside of the United States; drugs available outside of the United States are shown in italics.

SCENARIO

Anne Pace, PharmD

CP, a 70-year-old white man, walked into the pharmacy with a chief complaint of itchy eyes, running nose, and sneezing for the past 2 days. CP states that he experiences these symptoms usually in the spring. His past medical history includes benign prostatic hyperplasia. His current medication is tamsulosin 0.4 mg daily. CP does not have time to visit his physician and wants a recommendation from the pharmacist.

(The reader is directed to the clinical solution and chemical analysis of this case at the end of the chapter).

INTRODUCTION

Histamine (2-[imidazol-4-yl]ethylamine) was synthesized and its effects in model biologic systems were studied before it was found physiologically. Its synthesis occurs in many tissues, including mast cells, parietal cells of the gastric mucosa, and neurons of the central nervous system (CNS) and in the periphery. Early hypotheses about its physiologic function were based on the observed dramatic effects of histamine in guinea pigs. These effects include massive bronchial spasm and effects on smooth muscle and the vasculature resembling anaphylactic shock. Marked species differences in the observed effects occur however, and these dramatic effects are not observed in humans.

Histamine is located in many tissues, and upon release, its effects are principally local ones, as it functions as an autocoid or paracrine (1). Its physiologic function is complex and not completely understood. Histamine is one of the many mediators involved in allergic inflammatory responses, and it has an important role in the regulation of the secretion of gastric acid. These observations have led to development of many important drugs that antagonize its effects and are useful in treatment of allergic inflammatory disorders (H_1 antihistamines) and in the treatment of gastric hypersecretory disorders (H_2 antihistamines).

Besides its role in allergic inflammatory processes and gastric acid secretion, a physiologic role at axons in several regions of the CNS has established its role in the regulation of sleeping and waking, in energy and endocrine homeostasis, and in cognition and memory. Histamine modulates the release of neurotransmitters via H_3 auto- and heteroreceptors located at histaminergic and nonhistaminergic neurons centrally and peripherally. A novel H_4 receptor has also been described where histamine facilitates synthesis and release of other proinflammatory mediators and modulates chemotactic responses principally at mast cells and eosinophils.

CHEMISTRY

Histamine has pK_a values of 5.80 (imidazole) and 9.40 (aliphatic primary amine) (2). At physiologic pH, it exists as an equilibrium mixture of tautomeric cations, with the monocation making up more than 96% of the total and the dication about 3%, with only a very small amount of the nonprotonated species. At lower pHs (e.g., the pH of acidic lipids), a much larger proportion of the dication exists. The two protonated species (monocation and dication) are often considered the biologically active forms. Penetration of membranes by histamine would be expected to occur via the nonprotonated species, and the unprotonated imidazole group would be expected to participate readily in proton transfer processes physiologically. Several aromatic ring congeners of histamine with weakly and very weakly basic heteroaromatic rings, such as 4-chloroimidazole, 1,2,4-triazole, thiazole, and pyridine, exhibit histamine agonist activity (Table 32.1) (2), although they are less potent than histamine. These data suggest that the monocation (protonated aliphatic amine) is sufficient for agonist activity and that protonation of the heterocyclic ring is not an absolute requirement.

In aqueous solutions, the tautomeric equilibrium of the imidazole ring apparently favors the N^{τ}-H tautomer by about 4:1. The free base also prefers the N^{τ}-H tautomer. However, in the crystal of the monohydrochloride salt of histamine, where intermolecular crystal packing forces are important, the N^{π}-H tautomer is preferred. Changes in tautomeric composition of analogs occur with changes in the 4-substituent (e.g., Me vs. Cl), where the proportion of N^{τ}-H tautomer is decreased in the chlorine-substituted congener to 12% versus 70% for 4-methylhistamine, and decreased agonist potency is observed. An interpretation of these results is that tautomeric composition might be important in the agonist–receptor interaction (3).

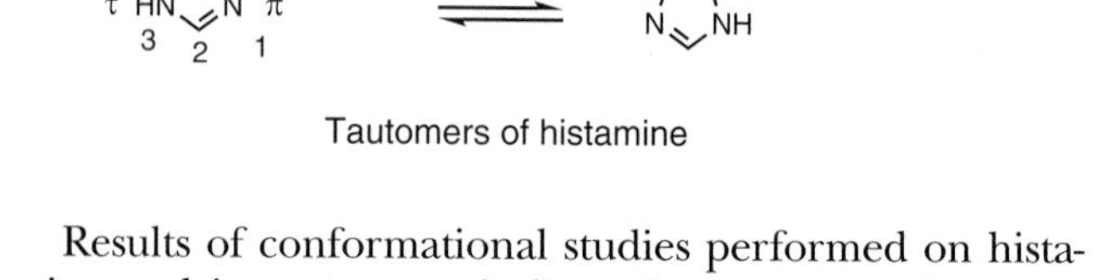

pKa of histamine

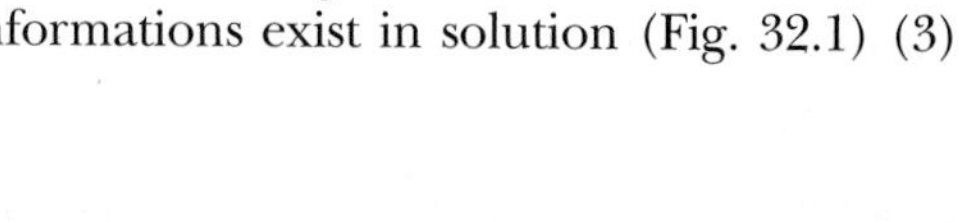

Tautomers of histamine

Results of conformational studies performed on histamine and its congeners indicate both trans and gauche conformations exist in solution (Fig. 32.1) (3). However,

TABLE 32.1 Histamine-Related Agonists

	Relative H1 activity vs. histamine	Relative H2 activity vs. histamine	Relative H3 activity vs. histamine
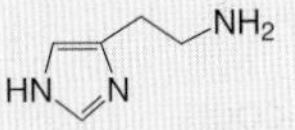	100	100	100
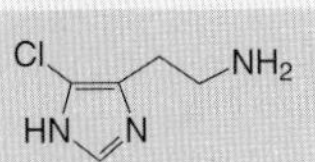	1.7	12	ND[b]
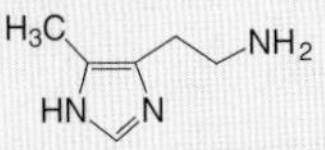	0.23	39	<0.008
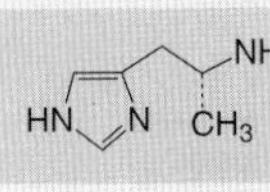	0.49	1.0	1550
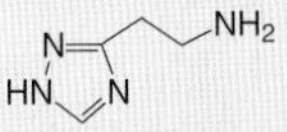	12.7	13.7	ND
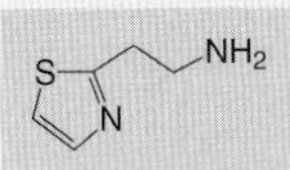	26	~0.3	<0.008
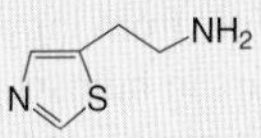	0.01	~0.1	ND
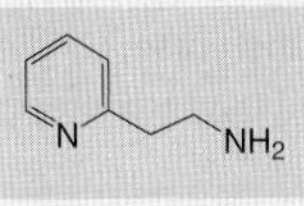	5.6	2.5	<0.06
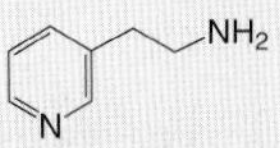	Inactive	Inactive	ND
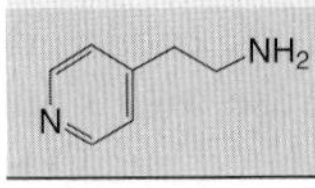	~0	~0.4	ND

ND = not determined.
[a]Activity expressed relative to histamine = 100, determined in vitro on guinea pig ileum (H_1), guinea pig atrium (H_2) and rat cerebral cortex (H_3)(3).

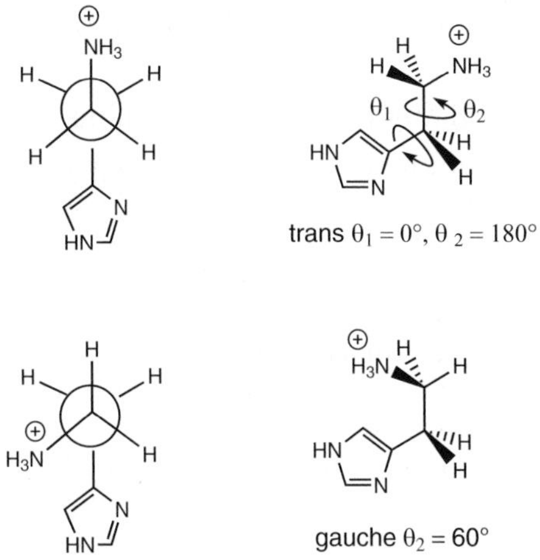

FIGURE 32.1 Conformers of histamine.

the trans conformation of 4-methylhistamine, which is a selective H_2 agonist, cannot readily adopt the fully extended trans conformation because of interaction of the 4-methyl group with the aliphatic two-carbon chain. Since α- and β-methylhistamine exist predominantly as gauche conformers and both are very weak H_1 and H_2 agonists, it has been suggested that trans conformation of histamine is preferred at both H_1 and H_2 receptors. A gauche conformation has been suggested for histamine at the H_3 receptor because α-methylhistamine and some other more conformationally restricted analogs are potent H_3 agonists.

Addition of other alkyl substituents onto the histamine molecule generally produces compounds with decreased potency at H_1 and H_2 receptors. 2-Methylhistamine is a selective H_1 agonist (vs. 4-methylhistamine, a selective H_2 agonist), but imidazole *N*-substitution (*N^1* or *N^3*) with methyl groups results in nearly inactive agents. Similarly, aliphatic amine nitrogen substitution results in decreasing activity (NH_2 > NHMe > NMe_2 > N^+Me_3 [quaternary ammonium salt]) at both H_1 and H_2 receptors (3,4).

CLINICAL SIGNIFICANCE

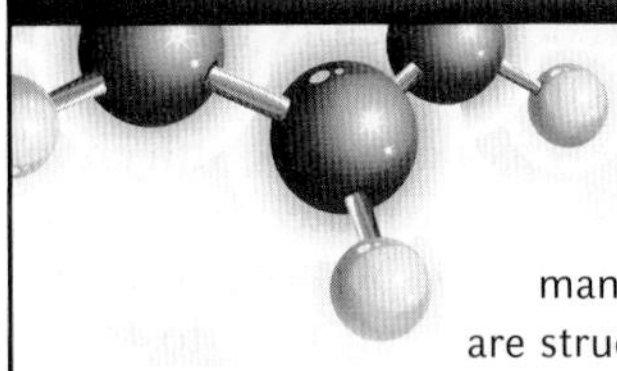

This chapter describes a wide array of medications that have a myriad of different uses. Although many of the compounds presented are structurally similar, their subtle differences in chemical structure produce vastly different pharmacologic effects, potency, and side effect profiles. As a result, the compounds presented are used to treat a variety of conditions, including allergies, motion sickness, and gastroesophageal reflux disease. Studying and understanding the different structures of these compounds allows the reader to distinguish the differences in their pharmacologic effects, potency, and side effects of each of the medications. Many of these drugs are available over the counter and present an opportunity for pharmacists to be an integral part of the patient's health care. Therefore, only when armed with patient-specific information and a thorough understanding of the drugs, including their chemical structure, can the pharmacist identify the proper medicine and make the best recommendation for their patients.

Anne Pace, PharmD
Assistant Professor
College of Pharmacy
University of Arkansas for Medical Sciences
Little Rock, AR

PHYSIOLOGIC CHARACTERISTICS OF HISTAMINE

Synthesis and Metabolism of Histamine

Histamine is synthesized in the Golgi apparatus of mast cells and basophils by enzymatic decarboxylation of histidine. This conversion is catalyzed by L-histidine decarboxylase, with pyridoxal phosphate serving as a cofactor for this process (5). The reaction mechanism for this decarboxylation probably involves the formation of an imine intermediate followed by the loss of carbon dioxide, a mechanism demonstrated to occur for decarboxylation of many α-amino acids (Fig. 32.2). Pyridoxal phosphate provides an important catalytic function, and in the final step, the product is released by hydrolysis of the enzyme-bound Schiff base of histamine. Mechanism-based inhibitors of this process, such as α-fluoromethylhistidine, decrease the rate of synthesis of histamine, and thus deplete cells of histamine. As such, α-fluoromethylhistidine is an important pharmacologic tool (4). This approach has not been successfully developed into agents for the treatment of allergic inflammatory disorders, peptic ulcer, or motion of sickness.

Once released, histamine is rapidly metabolized in vivo (based on products from radiolabeled histamine administered intradermally) to nearly inactive metabolites by two major pathways: *N*-methylation and oxidation (Fig. 32.3). Methylation (*S*-adenosylmethionine), which is catalyzed by the intracellular enzyme *N*-methyltransferase, yields an inactive metabolite. A portion of the *N*-methylated metabolite is oxidized sequentially via monoamine oxidase (MAO) and then via aldehyde oxidase (ADO) to the corresponding *N*-methylimidazole acetic acid. Histamine is also oxidized to imidazole acetic acid by diamine oxidase (histaminase). A small amount of this acid intermediate is converted to the corresponding ribotide, an unusual metabolite (6).

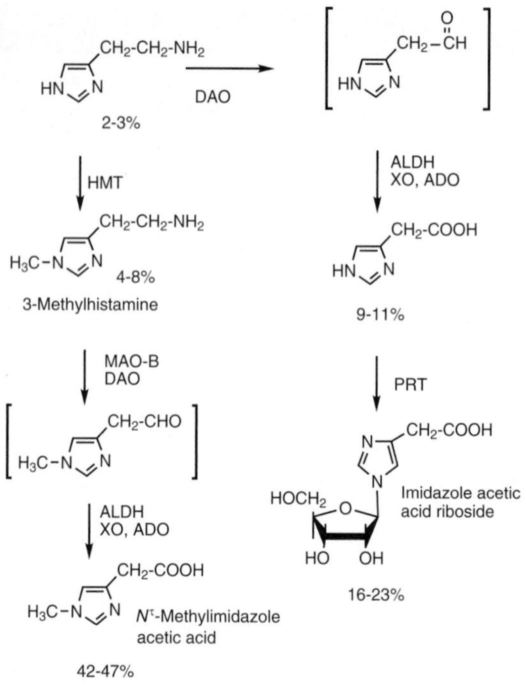

FIGURE 32.3 Major metabolic pathways of histamine, from intradermal histamine as measured in the urine in 12 hours in human men (6). ADO, aldehyde oxidase; ALDH, aldehyde dehydrogenase; DAO, diamine oxidase; HMT, histamine *N*-methyltransferase; MAO-B, monoamine oxidase type B; PRT, phosphoribosyl transferase; XO, xanthine oxidase.

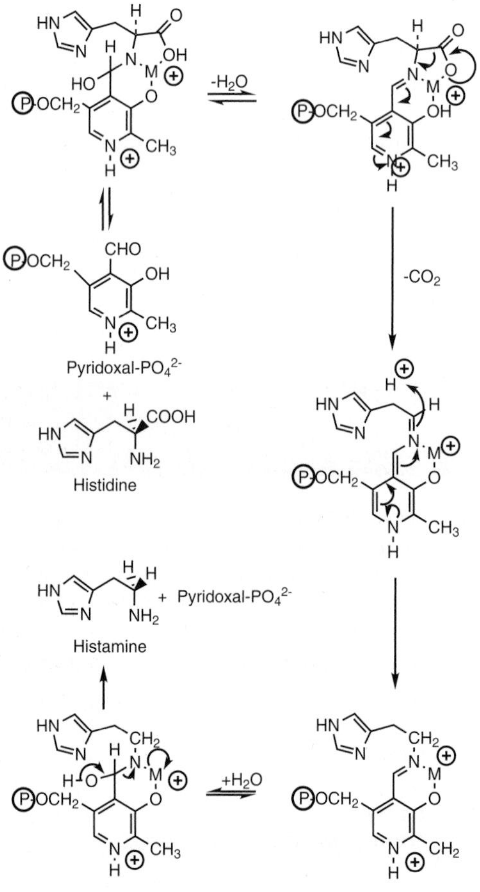

FIGURE 32.2 Formation of histamine by decarboxylation of histidine.

Storage and Release of Histamine

In mast cells, histamine is stored in secretory granules as a complex with acidic residues of the proteoglycan heparin, and in basophils in the blood as a complex with chondroitin sulfate (7,8). Mast cells are distributed in areas of skin and mucous membranes of the respiratory, gastrointestinal, and genitourinary tracts and adjacent to blood and lymph vessels. Although histamine is secreted at low levels from these mast cells and basophils, the primary mechanism of release is associated with cell activation by immunoglobulin (Ig) E–mediated hypersensitivity processes (Fig. 32.4). Immediate hypersensitivity is initiated when allergen molecules crosslink to Fab components of adjacent IgE antibody molecules bound to high-affinity FcεRI receptors on the surface of these cells ($Fc\varepsilon RI^+$ cells). Dimerization of occupied IgE-Fc receptors results in several membrane and cytosolic events. These include release

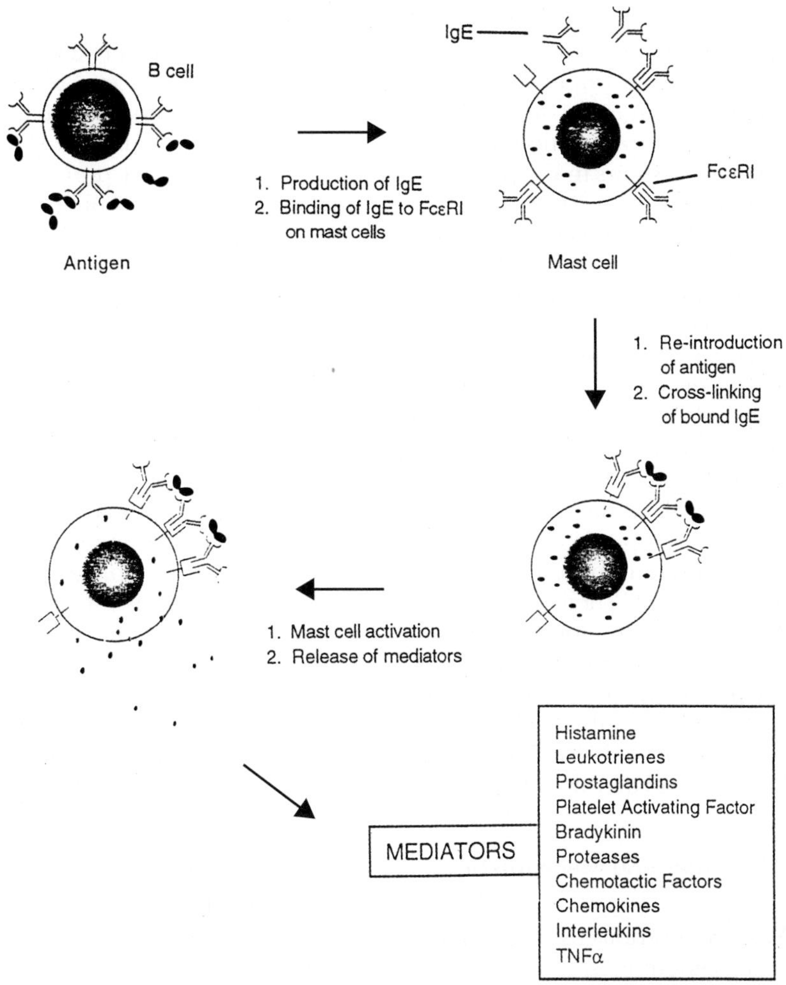

FIGURE 32.4 Sequence of events in immediate hypersensitivity. Initial contact with an antigen leads to specific IgE synthesis by B cells. Secreted IgE binds to mast cells or basophils through high-affinity Fcε receptors (FcεRI). On subsequent exposure to the antigen, an immediate hypersensitivity reaction is triggered by cross-linking the IgE molecules.

of preformed mediators from secretory granules by exocytosis, synthesis and release of chemotactic mediators and neutral proteases (e.g., tryptase), synthesis and release of lipid mediators (leukotrienes and prostaglandins), and stimulation of synthesis of cytokines and their subsequent release. Other cell activation stimuli for the release of histamine include concanavalin A, substance P, polyamines, opiates, and several lymphokines and cytokines. There are different subpopulations of cells that respond differently to these stimuli. With the exocytotic response, histamine rapidly dissociates from the partially solubilized granule matrix. In basophils, the release process may be slightly different, occurring without degranulation. Other cell types, including lymphocytes, platelets, neutrophils, monocytes, and some macrophages, secrete histamine-releasing factors. These cells also have distinct low-affinity receptors for IgE, which when occupied result in secretion of mediators that selectively recruit and activate secondary effector cells in the inflammatory process. More complete exposition of these processes is available (9,10).

Mast cells play an important role in the early response to allergens, and they provide mediators that lead to initial and late stages of the process and subsequently to chronic inflammatory reactions (11,12). Early stages appear to be related to degranulation and the release of many mediators, including histamine, prostaglandin D_2 (PGD_2), leukotriene C_4 (LTC_4), platelet activating factor, adenosine triphosphate (ATP), kinins, and some enzymes (e.g., tryptase and chymase). Thus, additional important mediators other than histamine have very significant roles. These mediators include platelet activation factor, substance P, neurokinin A, and others. Besides processes of vasodilation and edema, activation of secondary inflammatory cells, adherence of neutrophils, and migration of eosinophils and T cells to postcapillary venule endothelial cells occur. Specific cell adhesion molecules mediate this process. A further array of mediators and cellular responses follows. A series of interleukins are generated and secreted by subtypes of T cells. Stimulation of many nuclear factor-κB (NF-κB)–mediated gene transcription pathways occurs via H_1-receptor activation. Important cytokines are produced and liberated, including tumor necrosis factor (TNF)-α, interleukin (IL)-4, IL-5, IL-1, and IL-6, which are involved in chemokine secretion and regulation of cell maturation and proliferation processes, changes that occur in late-stage inflammatory processes. Thus, the inflammatory cascade is a complex and intricate one, and the effects of histamine are only a small part of the process. Inhibition of the production of many of the proinflammatory cytokines occurs in the presence of many of the H_1 antihistamines.

As a result of occupation of H_1 receptors by histamine, constriction of bronchial and gastrointestinal smooth muscle occurs. Spasm of the bronchi to inhaled histamine at one time was a test for airway reactivity. Intradermal injection of histamine produces vasodilation of arterioles, as the first step in the "triple response," mediated via H_1 and H_2 receptors. A flare response follows this stimulation, resulting in release of substance P and other neuropeptides. Edema from exudation of plasma fluids follows due to contraction of endothelial cells of the postcapillary venules. The wheal and flare responses are mostly H_1 receptor mediated.

Histamine affects the maturation of the immune system cells altering their activation, chemotactic, and effector functions via H_1-receptor activation. Histamine regulates functions of monocytes, dendritic cells, and antigen-specific T-helper type 1 (T_H1) and T-helper type 2 (T_H2) cells, as well as regulating antibody responses. These cells synthesize high amounts of histamine, where the synthesis of histamine is modulated by interleukins and other cytokines (13,14).

Histamine Receptors: Molecular and Mechanistic Aspects

Histamine receptors are found in various tissues. Among these are the H_1 receptors in smooth muscle of the bronchi, gut, and uterus. Contraction of the bronchi leads to restriction of air flow in the lungs. Histamine increases the permeability of capillary walls. Plasma constituents flow into extracellular spaces due to contraction of endothelial cells; this process leads to edema. At the level of the CNS, histamine secretion appears to be associated with wakefulness, as H_1-receptor antagonism centrally is associated with drowsiness. In the stomach, parietal cell stimulation increases production and secretion of acid, mediated through H_2 receptors. The H_2 receptors play a minor role in allergic inflammatory processes. The H_3 receptor is principally an autoreceptor in the CNS at histaminergic neurons, and it is a heteroreceptor on neurons that release other neurotransmitters, also in the brain. The H_4 receptor is expressed primarily on eosinophils and mast cells where it is associated with chemotactic responses.

All of the histamine receptors appear to have constitutive receptor G protein signaling activity independent of the presence of histamine (15). Most of the antihistamines studied are not antagonists, but are inverse agonists. They reduce constitutive G protein signaling activity. Occasionally, some antihistamines are neutral antagonists (i.e., they do not reduce the constitutive G protein–coupled activity of the receptor). A two-state model of inactive and active conformations of the receptor is consistent with this observation.

Histamine H_1 receptors are expressed widely. They are found on nerve cells, airway and vascular smooth muscle, hepatocytes, chondrocytes, endothelial cells, eosinophils, monocytes, macrophages, dendritic cells, and T and B lymphocytes. The human H_1-receptor gene encodes for a 487–amino acid protein with the signature structural features of G protein–coupled receptors (seven transmembrane domains, *N*-terminal glycosylation sites, phosphorylation sites for protein kinase A and C, and a large intracellular loop with several serine and threonine residues) (15,16). It is coupled (via $G_{q/11}$ proteins) to phosphatidylinositol turnover as the second messenger system. The H_1 receptor shows 40% homology with the muscarinic M_1 receptor and the M_2 receptor. An aspartic acid in the third transmembrane domain is highly conserved in several species, and it is suggested as a recognition site for the protonated aliphatic amine function of histamine, at both H_1 and H_2 receptors. Based on mutation studies and homologous positions to α-adrenergic receptors, suggestions for sites of binding of the imidazole portion of histamine to amino acids threonine and/or asparagine in the fifth transmembrane have been made.

Signal transduction processes begin with $G_{q/11}$-coupled hydrolysis of phosphatidylinositide to IP_3 (inositol-1,4,5-triphosphate) and 1,2-diacylglycerol, which occurs via activation of phospholipase C. Elevation of intracellular calcium ion from intracellular stores occurs. Voltage-gated calcium channels may be opened by activation of ion channels permeable to Na^+ and K^+ ions. Calcium channel antagonists block some effects of histamine on intestinal smooth muscle. In addition, the H_1 receptor can activate other signaling pathways, including phospholipase D and phospholipase A_2, and stimulate NF-κB–mediated gene transcription.

Histamine H_2 receptors are widely distributed like H_1 receptors. They are found at airway and vascular smooth muscle cells, hepatocytes, chondrocytes, epithelial cells, neutrophils, eosinophils, monocytes, dendritic cells, and T and B lymphocytes. T-cell responses in general are negatively regulated by activation of H_2 receptors.

The H_2 receptor is a 359–amino acid protein in humans. It has some features similar to the H_1 protein (e.g., *N*-terminal glycosylation sites and phosphorylation sites in the C-terminal). An aspartic acid residue in the third transmembrane loop appears to be critical to agonist and antagonist binding, and threonine/aspartate and tyrosine/aspartate couples in the fifth transmembrane domain appear to be important for interaction of the imidazole part of the histamine molecule. It is positively coupled via $G_{\alpha s}$ to activate adenylyl cyclase for synthesis of cyclic adenosine monophosphate (cAMP) as second messenger. In some systems, it is coupled through G_q proteins to stimulate phospholipase C. It appears in some cells that other processes, such as the breakdown of phosphoinositides, control of intracellular calcium ion levels, and phospholipase A_2 activity, can be regulated by other cAMP-independent pathways.

The highest density of H_3 receptors in nerve cells occurs in the brain, principally in the striatum, substantia nigra, and the cortex, and to a much lesser extent at peripheral nerve terminals. The H_3 receptors also occur in eosinophils, dendritic cells, and monocytes. Low expression of these receptors occurs in peripheral tissues. In the brain, the H_3 receptor is a presynaptic auto- and heteroreceptor where activation leads to a decrease in neurotransmitter release. The most widely studied H_3 receptor is 445 amino acids, but many splice variants have been observed (17). It is activated via $G_{\alpha i/o}$-coupled proteins (negatively to adenylyl cyclase) to the activation of protein kinase A to modulate gene transcription. H_3 receptors, via $G_{\alpha i/o}$ G proteins, may activate phospholipase A_2, mitogen-activated protein kinase, and phosphotidylinositol-3-kinase. The H_3 receptors have low sequence homology with H_1 and H_2 receptors (~20% each). Activation of histaminergic neurons centrally, which promotes arousal and attention and improves learning in animals, is a potential target for H_3-receptor antihistamines. Like the H_1 and H_2 antihistamines, the H_3 antihistamines function primarily as inverse agonists.

H_4 receptors are expressed by cells of the hematopoietic system, with expression occurring primarily on eosinophils, neutrophils, dendritic cells, and T cells. The H_4 receptors are also reported at mast cells. Low expression is reported in nerve cells, hepatocytes, and the periphery. Histamine stimulation results in a chemotactic response, cell migration. The presence of H_4 receptors on these cells suggests that this receptor plays a role in the inflammatory response. Evidence suggests that it may be regulation via inflammatory stimulation of TNF-α and cytokine IL-6. The H_4 receptor has a sequence of 390 amino acids; it is coupled via $G_{\alpha i/o}$ to inhibition of adenylyl cyclase. It has highest homology with the H_3 receptor (~35% to 40%), with greater homology (58%) of the transmembrane segments. Thus, antihistamines could be useful agents to antagonize the inflammatory response. Agents studied to date also appear to be inverse agonists.

INHIBITORS OF HISTAMINE RELEASE

Mechanism of Action

The bronchodilatory activity of khellin, a chromone obtained from a plant source (*Ammi visnaga*) used by ancient Egyptians for spasmolytic activity, stimulated the search for related compounds with similar pharmacologic properties (18). From a study of many bischromones, cromolyn sodium was developed and marketed (Fig. 32.5). Although it prevents bronchospasm, cromolyn sodium does not reverse antigen-induced bronchiolar constriction. Thus, it and other agents like it that followed prevent the release of histamine but do not block the effects of histamine at its receptors.

The mechanism by which cromolyn and nedocromil inhibit degranulation of mast cells has been investigated (19). Both agents stimulate phosphorylation of moesin, a 78-kd protein that is phosphorylated by isozymes of protein kinase C. It is suggested that phosphorylation at serine hydroxyl groups results in conformational changes that expose domains that promote association with actin and other proteins of the secretory granules. This association results in immobilization of the granules and inhibition of exocytosis. Cromolyn and nedocromil (vide infra) apparently inhibit function of cells other than mast cells; these effects may occur in later stages of inflammatory responses. Cromolyn does not have intrinsic antihistaminic or anti-inflammatory activity.

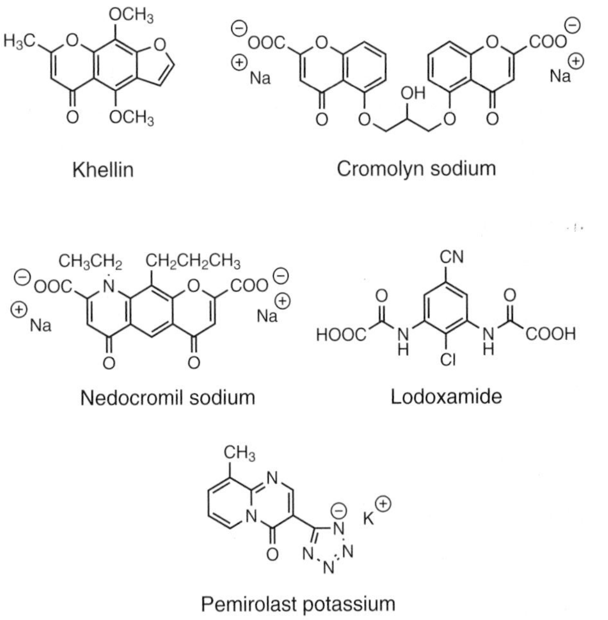

FIGURE 32.5 Mast cell degranulation inhibitors.

Therapeutic Applications of Specific Drugs

Cromolyn (Intal, Nasalcrom, Gastrocrom)

Cromolyn is usually used prophylactically for bronchial asthma (as an inhaled powder), for prevention of exercise-induced bronchospasm, and for seasonal and perennial allergic rhinitis (nasal solution). Topically, it is also used as eye drops for allergic conjunctivitis and keratitis. In the management of asthmatic conditions, it is administered using a power-operated nebulizer. The bioavailability is very low on oral administration because of poor absorption. By inhalation, the powder is irritating to some patients. After inhalation, much less than 10% of the dose reaches the systemic circulation. An oral dosage form is used for mastocytosis.

Nedocromil (Alocril)

Nedocromil is a chromone analog used as an ophthalmic solution for the treatment of seasonal and perennial allergic conjunctivitis. Aerosols have previously been used in the prophylaxis of asthma and in reversible obstructive airway disease.

Lodoxamide (Alomide)

Lodoxamide, which shows some structural similarities to cromolyn and nedocromil, is also a mast cell stabilizer that inhibits the immediate hypersensitivity reaction, preventing increases in vascular permeability associated with antigen-IgE–mediated responses. Its precise mechanism(s) of action is (are) not completely understood. It is used topically in the eye principally for conjunctivitis and keratitis associated with vernal allergens.

Pemirolast (Alamast)

Pemirolast, with an acidic tetrazole isosteric replacement for a carboxylic acid functionality, is used topically in the eye to prevent itching associated with allergic conjunctivitis. It is an inhibitor of release of histamine and other inflammatory mediators, including leukotrienes.

INHIBITORS OF RELEASED HISTAMINE

Historical Background

The first antihistamine was discovered by Forneau and Bovet, who observed that piperoxan protected guinea pigs against histamine-induced bronchospasm (20). The sensitivity of the guinea pig was initially thought to make it a good model for anaphylaxis. Piperoxan also has important effects related to antagonism of norepinephrine at α-adrenergic receptors.

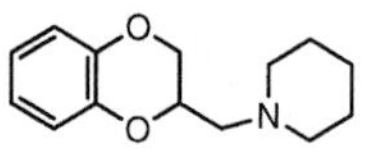

Piperoxan

Antihistamines, specifically H_1 antihistamines (14,21), are useful in the treatment of allergy and inflammatory disorders, where many effects are mediated via histamine. Compounds that had antagonistic effects in these assays did not antagonize the effects of histamine on the stomach (acid secretion) and heart (positive chronotropic and inotropic effects). These differences led to suggestion of the presence of H_1 and H_2 receptors and, ultimately, to the development of selective H_2 antihistamines to diminish the secretion of gastric acid. A third class of histamine receptors, H_3 receptors, appears primarily to be autoreceptors that control the synthesis and release of histamine presynaptically and heteroreceptors that control the release of other transmitters, primarily in the CNS. The most recently discovered histamine receptors, H_4 receptors, are expressed principally on eosinophils and mast cells where they may play a role in the inflammatory response, especially in late stages. Classical H_1 antihistamines do not bind to this histamine receptor, and H_4 receptors do not modulate degranulation of mast cells.

The first-generation H_1 antihistamines are useful and effective in the treatment of allergic responses (e.g., hay fever, rhinitis, urticaria, and food allergy). These agents also have effects at cholinergic, adrenergic, dopaminergic, and serotonergic receptors. Adverse central effects include sedation, drowsiness, decreased cognitive ability, and somnolence. Peripheral side effects associated with cholinergic blockade include blurred vision, dry mouth, urinary retention, and constipation. Other effects observed have included appetite stimulation, muscle spasm, anxiety, confusion, and occasionally irritability, tremor, and tachycardia. Of all the side effects, CNS depression is the most common, and it can be so pronounced that some of these agents with short durations of action are used as over-the-counter (OTC) sleep aids. The separation of CNS depressant and anticholinergic effects from peripheral antihistaminic effects in later agents led to the second-generation antihistamines (vide infra).

Structural classes of H_1 antihistamines can be represented by a general structure of two aromatic groups linked through a short chain to a tertiary aliphatic amine (Fig. 32.6). The aromatic groups (Ar_1, Ar_2) are usually phenyl or substituted phenyl, thienyl, or pyridyl. These aryl substituents are attached to the X group, which is a nitrogen atom in the ethylenediamines, a carbon attached to an ether oxygen atom in the ethanolamine ether series, or only a carbon atom in the alkyl amine series. The spacer is usually two or three carbons in length, and it may be in a ring, branched, and saturated or unsaturated. The R groups attached to the aliphatic amine are usually simple alkyl groups, usually methyl, or occasionally aralkyl groups. One of the early thiophene-containing analogs was carcinogenic in rats. After thiophene versus benzene replacement in other series of compounds demonstrated some toxic effects, thiophene has been relegated to one of the low-priority choices for isosteric replacement of a phenyl group.

Most H_1 antihistamines are inverse agonists rather than neutral antagonists. Like other histamine receptors, H_1 receptors have constitutive G protein–coupled activity in the absence of the agonist histamine that results in activation of second messenger signaling pathways (e.g., phospholipase C activity and NF-κB–mediated gene transcription) (22). A model of active and inactive conformations of histamine receptors has been advanced to accommodate these biochemical findings. Inverse agonists bind to the inactive conformation of the receptor shifting the equilibrium toward the inactive state. Neutral antagonists interact with both conformations of the receptor.

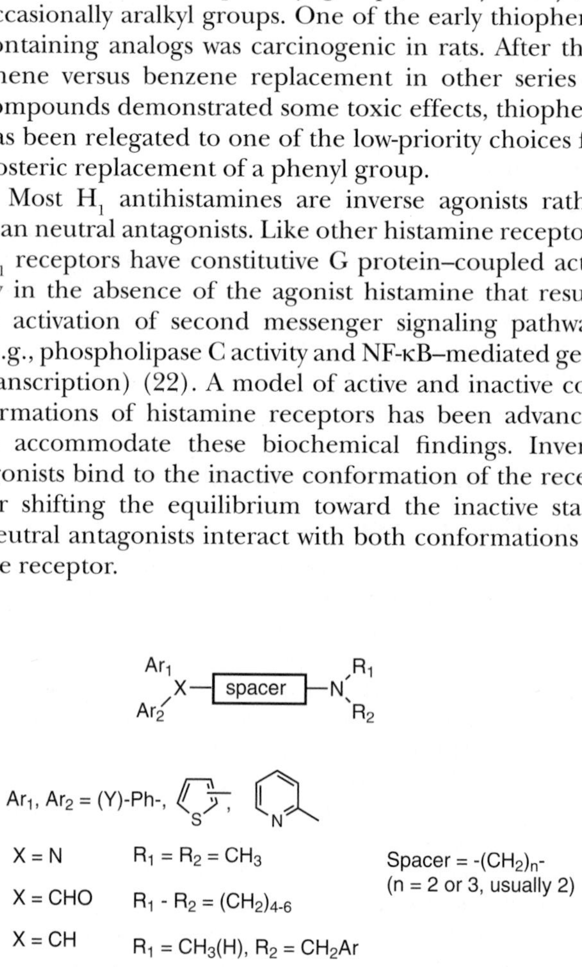

FIGURE 32.6 General structure of first-generation antihistamines.

First-Generation H_1 Antihistamines

Ethylenediamines

The earliest series of H_1 antihistamines is the ethylenediamines. Two two-carbon spacers may appear between the two nitrogen atoms in the piperazine series (vide infra). Examples of agents in the ethylenediamine class, of which phenbenzamine was the first of these agents, appear in Table 32.2. Compounds with several different but closely related aromatic rings are useful and include phenyl, 2-pyridyl, halogen- and methoxy-substituted phenyl, or pyrimidyl. Thiazole-, furanyl-, and thiophene-ring congeners have also been available in the past. The small alkyl substituents on basic nitrogen are usually methyl groups. A number of these agents are still used. With the exception of antazoline, all have the ethylenediamine spacer. In antazoline, the alkyl tertiary amine in phenbenzamine is replaced with an imidazoline group. CNS effects, usually sedation, are very common among agents in this class.

Information on pharmacokinetic and metabolic disposition is limited because this early group of compounds was not studied in great depth. Only later, with the development of second-generation H_1 antihistamines, and/or where issues of potential toxicity have arisen concerning some of the early compounds, have metabolic disposition and pharmacokinetic properties been examined more completely. Thus, the available information on the metabolism of these early antihistamines is sparse. From some of the ethylenediamines, expected products of *N*-demethylation and subsequent deamination have been reported. In addition, some produce quaternary *N*-glucuronides as urinary metabolites, a process that occurs to some extent in many relatively unhindered tertiary aliphatic amines among the antihistamines and also in other lipophilic aliphatic tertiary amine drug classes.

TABLE 32.2 Examples of Ethylenediamine Antihistamines

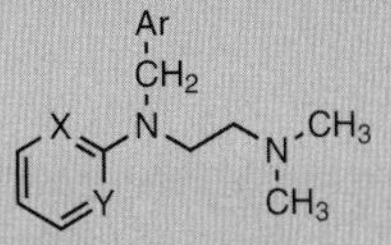

Drugs	X	Y	Ar
Phenbenzamine	CH	CH	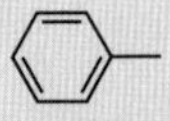
Tripelennamine	N	CH	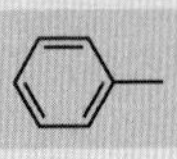
Methapyrilene	N	CH	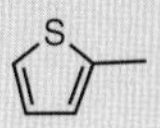
Thonzylamine	N	N	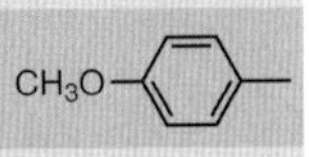 CH3O
Related compound:		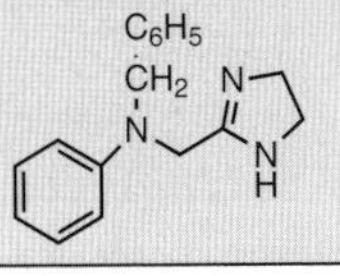 C6H5 CH2 N N N H	Antazoline

Ethanolamine Ethers

Structure–Activity Relationships The prototype of the aminoalkyl ethers is diphenhydramine, a benzhydryl ether still widely used for allergic conditions more than a half-century after its introduction. Structural analogs with various ring substituents (Me, OMe, Cl, Br) in one of the aromatic rings have also been developed, as have compounds with a 2-pyridyl group replacing one of the phenyl groups (Table 32.3).

Significant anticholinergic side effects are observed among members of the group (i.e., dry mouth, blurred vision, tachycardia, urinary retention, constipation). Sedative properties are also very common. Sedation, accompanied with a short half-life and a wide margin of safety, allows some of these compounds to be used as OTC sleep aids. The 8-chlorotheophyllinate salt of diphenhydramine is marketed as dimenhydrinate for use in the treatment of motion sickness. The compound with the *p*-Cl-Ph and 2-pyridyl aryl groups is carbinoxamine, a potent antihistamine. Substitution of a methyl group at the carbon α to the ether function affords the related compound doxylamine, in which the aryl groups are phenyl and 2-pyridyl. Clemastine, a homolog with an additional carbon atom between the oxygen and the basic nitrogen, which is incorporated into a ring, has less sedative properties, as does the drug setastine in which the alkyl amine substituent is incorporated into a seven-membered hexahydroazepine ring.

Antihistaminic Versus Anticholinergic Activity Besides the structural analogs in Table 32.3 that possess increased selectivity for histamine H_1 receptors over muscarinic receptors, introduction of alkyl substituents at C-2′ or C-4′ of one aromatic ring results in significant changes

TABLE 32.3 Ethanolamine Ether Antihistamines

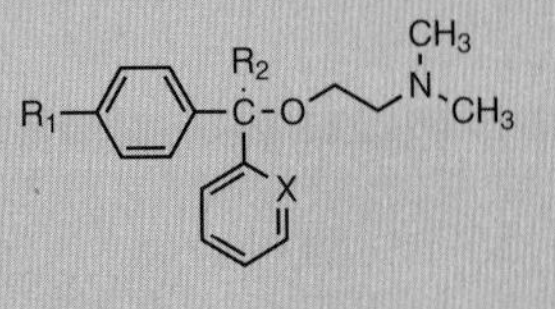

Drugs	Trade Name	R_1	R_2	X
Diphenhydramine Dimenhydrinate	Benadryl Dramamine	H	H	CH
Bromodiphenhydramine		Br	H	CH
Chlorodiphenhydramine		Cl	H	CH
Carbinoxamine		Cl	H	N
Doxylamine	Decapryn	H	CH_3	N
	Unisom			

Related compounds:

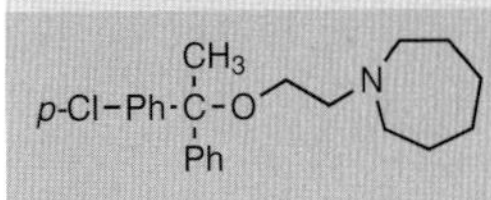

Setastine

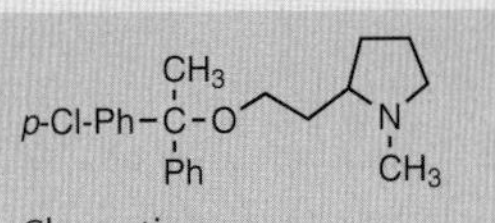

Clemastine

in selectivity in tissue-based assays for antihistaminic versus anticholinergic activity. With increasing alkyl group size (Me, Et, *i*Pr, *t*Bu) at C-2′, large decreases in antihistaminic activity and increases in anticholinergic activity are observed (23). With larger alkyl groups, the possible spatial orientations of the two aromatic rings with regard to each other are limited due to increasing rotameric restrictions. Introduction of these alkyl substituents at C-4′ decreases anticholinergic activity and yields small increases in antihistaminic activity. A chiral center is introduced with these changes, and differences in pharmacologic properties of the enantiomers of each compound are observed; two examples are shown in Table 32.4.

Stereochemical and Structural Effects This change in receptor selectivity (histaminergic vs. cholinergic) stimulated the synthesis of a large number of related homologs. However, diphenhydramine itself is also used in the treatment of parkinsonism because of its central anticholinergic properties. Other anticholinergic agents that are structurally related to the benzhydryl ether antihistamines are also used in the treatment of parkinsonism. Compounds with central anticholinergic and antihistaminic effects have been used as one approach to the treatment of Parkinson disease (see Chapter 13).

The observed differences in potency of enantiomers in tissue-based assays suggest significant stereoselective interactions of antagonists at the receptor level. Differences in affinity of 60- to 200-fold are noted between enantiomers in several analogs where the chiral center results because of differences in the two aromatic rings (e.g., Ph and 2-pyridyl, or Ph and *p*-Br-Ph) (24). Enantiomers with the *S*-absolute configuration are usually more potent. Clemastine, a more complex homolog, is marketed as the *R*,*R*-enantiomer, which is the more potent of the *R*,*R*- and *S*,*S*-enantiomeric pair, and more potent than either the *R*,*S*- and *S*,*R*-enantiomers of the other diastereomer (25). Consistent with results from related compounds, the chiral center at the benzhydryl carbon has a significant influence on potency, whereas the one in the pyrrolidine ring is of lesser importance (Table 32.5).

Very small changes in the arrangement of aromatic groups in the members of the ethanolamine ether series significantly alter the scope of their pharmacologic properties. Previous work has shown that the two aromatic rings in diphenhydramine can be located slightly differently with respect to each other as in phenyltoloxamine, a potent antihistamine. However, a retro arrangement of carbon and oxygen atoms, prepared in an attempt to investigate structural requirements for antihistamines, afforded significantly different pharmacologic properties and ultimately led to a series of very important selective serotonin reuptake inhibitors, like fluoxetine (Fig. 32.7). Unlike the bioisosteric oxygen to nitrogen atom replacement, conversion of the oxygen atom to a sulfur atom in the diphenhydramine series results in a compound with greatly decreased antihistaminic activity (26).

Metabolism Only limited information on the metabolic disposition of this group of compounds is available. As expected, sequential *N*-demethylations (formation of the corresponding secondary and the primary amines) followed by subsequent deamination (formation of the carboxylic acid metabolite) is a major pathway for diphenhydramine (Fig. 32.8) and some of its analogs. Although the early experiments are relatively incomplete, it appears that the *N*-demethylation products have shorter half-lives than the corresponding parent drugs, and they probably contribute very little to the observed antihistaminic

TABLE 32.4 Antihistamine and Anticholinergic Activity of Enantiomers of Ring-Substituted Ethanolamine Ethers

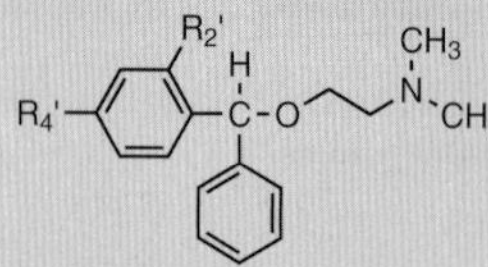

		Antihistaminic Activity		Anticholinergic Activity	
$R_{2'}$	$R_{4'}$	pD_2	Ratio of Potency of (+)- to (−)-Isomer	pD_2	Ratio of Potency of (+)- to (−)-Isomer
$(CH_3)_3C$	H	(+) 8.76[a] (−) 6.87	78	(+) 6.14 (−) 5.89	1.9
H	CH_3	(+) 6.36 (−) 6.00	2.3	(+) 6.03 (−) 8.12[a]	0.008[b]

[a]Most potent enantiomer in each assay.
[b](−)-Enantiomer is ~125 times as potent as the (+)-enantiomer.

TABLE 32.5 Antihistamine Activity of Stereoisomers of Clemastine

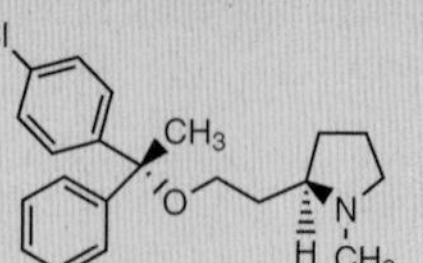

Drug	Diastereomers	pA_2	ED_{50}[a]
Clemastine	(*R*, *R*)	9.45	0.04 mg/kg
	(*S*, *S*)	7.99	5.0
	(*R*, *S*)	9.40	0.28
	(*S*, *R*)	8.57	11.0

[a]ED_{50} vs. lethal dose of histamine in guinea pigs (22).

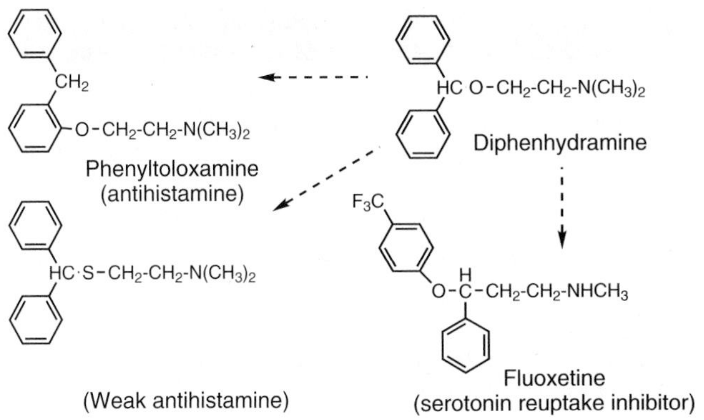

FIGURE 32.7 Structural similarities among diphenhydramine-related structures.

properties. Minor metabolites that are conjugates of the carboxylic acid or of ether cleavage products have been found in some animal species. Compounds with shorter half-lives, like diphenhydramine, when used as antihistamines, require repeated administration, but a very short half-life is an advantage when the same drugs are used as sleep aids (21,27).

Alkyl Amines

A third class of analogs includes those compounds in which a carbon atom replaces the heteroatom spacer in the general structure (Fig. 32.6). Examples are pheniramine, chlorpheniramine, brompheniramine, and the *E*-isomers of olefinic homologs (Fig. 32.9). The ring halogen-substituted compounds are widely used OTC antihistamines for mild seasonal allergies. These agents are characterized by a long duration of antihistaminic action and by a decreased incidence of central sedative side effects, when compared to the ethylenediamines and ethanolamine ether series. This structural change introduces a chiral carbon when the two aromatic rings are different (e.g., Ph and 2-pyridyl). These were the most extensively used antihistamines until the more selective second-generation antihistamines appeared.

Structural and Stereochemical Effects *E*- and *Z*-isomers of the alkenes in this series show very large differences in potency in tissue-based assays (e.g., *E*-pyrobutamine is more potent than its *Z*-isomer by 165-fold and *E*-triprolidine is more potent than its *Z*-isomer by about 1,000-fold) (Fig. 32.9) (3). Dimethindene has many of the structural features of both of these two agents in a more complex cyclized structure. The observed difference in potency between the *E*- and *Z*-isomers of triprolidine shows that the two aromatic rings probably have quite different binding environments at the receptor (28). Phenindamine, also a related cyclic analog, was also an effective antihistamine. These observations provide evidence suggesting that a 5 to 6 Å distance between the tertiary aliphatic amine and one of the aromatic rings is required at the site of receptor binding (Fig. 32.10) (29).

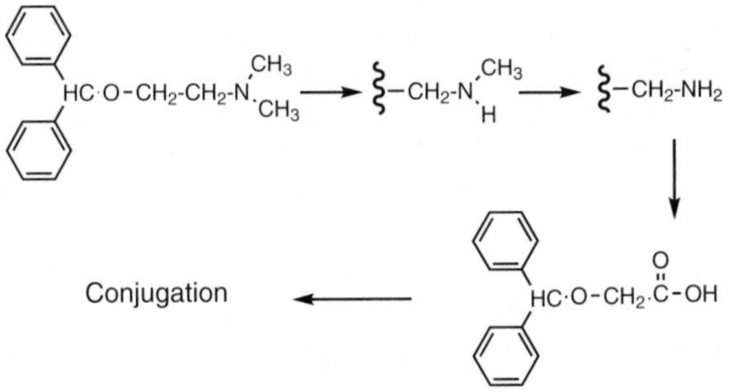

FIGURE 32.8 Metabolism of diphenhydramine.

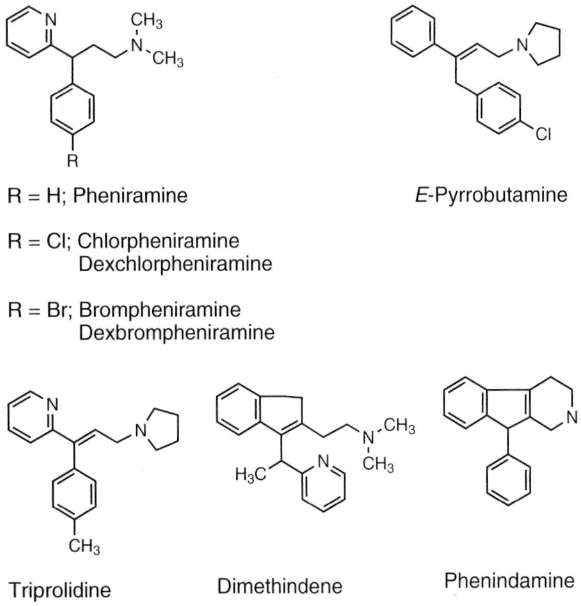

FIGURE 32.9 Examples of alkane and alkene antihistamines.

Differences in potency between the enantiomers of the conformationally mobile amino-alkanes have also been observed. The *S*-enantiomers have greater affinity for H_1 histamine receptors, occasionally by very large amounts [e.g., by 200 to 1,000 fold in radioligand displacement assays and in tissue-based assays for (+)-*S*- vs. (−)-*R*-chlorpheniramine], with the (+)-enantiomer being more potent (Ar = X-Ph, 2-pyridyl). Greater selectivity for H_1 receptors versus muscarinic and adrenergic receptors is also observed. For members of the series, the chiral center of the more potent enantiomer correlates

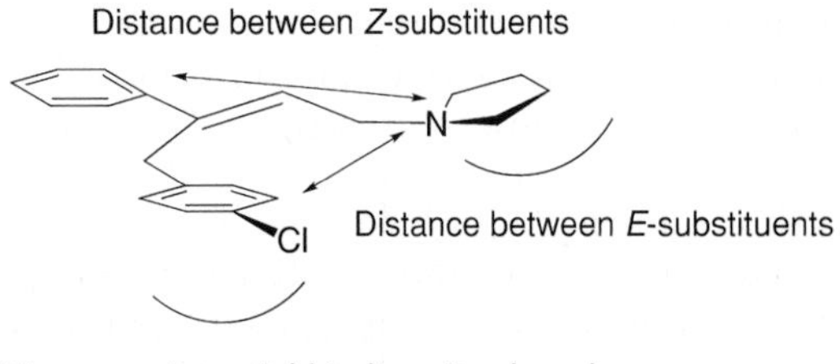

FIGURE 32.10 Potential binding sites based on *E*/*Z*-configurations.

stereochemically with the more active enantiomer of the oxygen congener carbinoxamine (Ar = Ph, Ar = *p*-Br-Ph) (Table 32.3) (3,30). Single enantiomers of these agents are available in the case of dexchlorpheniramine and dexbrompheniramine.

HALF-LIFE AND METABOLISM The alkyl amines have significantly less CNS depressant effects than benzhydryl ethers of ethanolamines. Additionally, these compounds have long half-lives and extended durations of action. These agents have decreased antiemetic effects and decreased anticholinergic properties compared to ethanolamine ethers. Many are available in OTC preparations for hay fever and other mild allergic conditions, sometimes in combination with decongestants. Most are suitable for once-a-day dosing because of their long half-lives, up to 24 hours, although they are routinely administered more frequently.

Information on the metabolic disposition of several of these agents has been reported. As expected, *N*-dealkylation is a major pathway with the corresponding secondary and primary amines being found in the plasma, as well as the parent drug. In cases where *O*-methyl aryl ethers are present, expected *O*-demethylation products have been reported.

TABLE 32.6 Examples of Piperazine Antihistamines

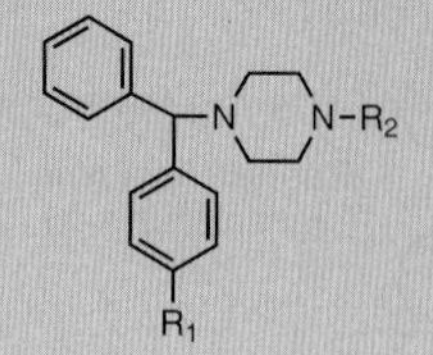

Drugs	Trade name	R_1	R_2
Cyclizine	Marezine, Bonine	H	CH_3
Chlorcyclizine	Mantadil	Cl	CH_3
Meclizine	Antivert	Cl	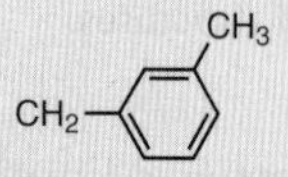
Buclizine	Bucladin-S	Cl	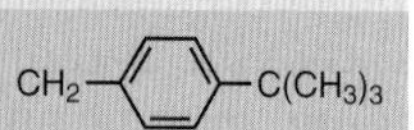
Oxatomide	Tinset	H	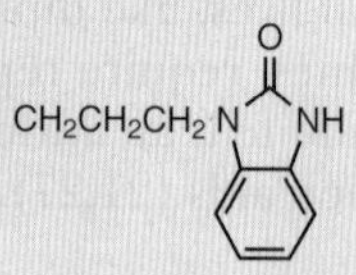
Hydroxyzine	Vistaril	Cl	$CH_2CH_2OCH_2CH_2OH$
Cetirizine	Zyrtec	Cl	$CH_2CH_2OCH_2COOH$

Piperazines

Members of the piperazine class of agents are structurally related to both the ethylenediamines and the benzhydryl ethers of ethanolamines. Their structures include the two-carbon separation between nitrogen atoms, which is incorporated into the piperazine ring (Table 32.6).

Diarylmethylene groups (benzhydryl substituents, like in diphenhydramine) are attached to one of the nitrogen atoms, and an alkyl or aralkyl substituent is attached to the other nitrogen. Early compounds, like cyclizine, chlorcyclizine, meclizine, buclizine, and hydroxyzine, have been widely used as antihistamines and as agents for treatment of motion sickness because they have useful central antiemetic effects.

These agents also have significant anticholinergic and antihistaminic properties. Anticholinergic side effects and drowsiness are common. The primary use of these compounds remains as treatment of motion sickness and vertigo and for suppression of nausea and vomiting. Although teratogenic effects of cyclizine and meclizine have been observed in rodents, large studies have not demonstrated adverse fetal effects in humans. However, these agents are used cautiously in pregnant women and children. Oxatomide is used in Europe principally in allergic rhinitis, urticaria, and in combination with albuterol in asthma. Drowsiness and sedation are noted. Hydroxyzine is used in treatment of pruritus, and at higher dosages, it is used in the management of anxiety and emotional stress. Its acid metabolite, cetirizine, which is formed from oxidation of the terminal primary alcohol to the corresponding carboxylic acid, is usually classified with the second-generation nonsedating antihistamines. The amphoteric nature of cetirizine, having both the tertiary aliphatic amine and carboxylic acid functional groups, appears to be associated with decreased, but not absent, sedative side effects.

Tricyclic H_1 Antihistamines

The two aromatic groups noted in several of the classes of antihistamines can be connected to each other through additional atoms such as the heteroatoms sulfur or oxygen or through a short one- or two-carbon chain. They have a general structure shown in Figure 32.11. The earliest potent tricyclic antihistamines (Table 32.7) were phenothiazines (Y = S, X = N). The phenothiazine antihistamines contain a two- or three-carbon branched alkyl chain between the nonbasic phenothiazine nitrogen and the aliphatic amine. They differ from the antipsychotic phenothiazine derivatives in which the side chain is usually three carbons long and unbranched, and usually without substituents in the aromatic ring. Most had pronounced sedative effects and long durations of action. Other uses included the treatment of nausea and vomiting associated with anesthesia, the treatment of motion sickness, and as antipruritic agents in the treatment of urticaria.

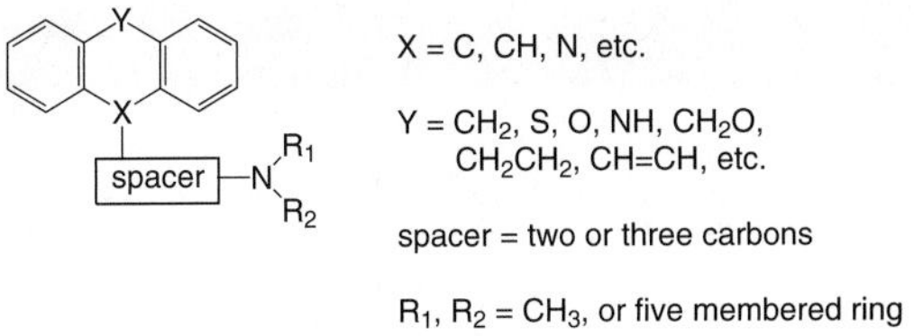

FIGURE 32.11 General structure of tricyclic antihistamines.

Conformational and Stereochemical Effects In the active agents, the steric restrictions and decreased degrees of conformational freedom resulting from the connection of the two aromatic rings together suggests that certain spatial relationships between these two rings are acceptable in the drug receptor interaction of H_1 antihistamines. These ring systems are not flat, but are somewhat puckered with the two aromatic rings not in the same plane. However, the conformations usually undergo rapid intraconversion. In some closely related systems, where this intraconversion is very slow, conformational enantiomers (atropisomers) have been obtained and studied, including cyproheptadine, doxepin, and hydroxylated metabolites of loratadine (31,32). The enantiomers of 3-methoxycyproheptadine have significantly different pharmacologic potency as antihistamine, antiserotonin, and anticholinergic agents (Fig. 32.12) (33). The (−)-isomer retained antihistaminic, antiserotonin, and appetite-stimulating effects similar to cyproheptadine, whereas the (+)-enantiomer had greater anticholinergic potency. Differences of 9- to 60-fold were observed in the reported assays.

Promethazine has many useful pharmacologic effects other than being an antihistamine. It has significant antiemetic and anticholinergic properties. It is has sedative-hypnotic properties and has been used to potentiate the effects of analgesic drugs.

TABLE 32.7 Examples of Tricyclic Antihistamines

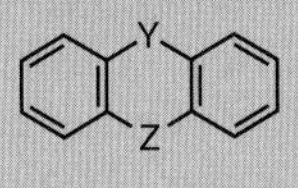

Drugs	Y	Z
Promethazine	S	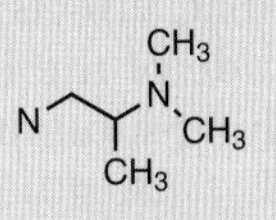
Pyrathiazine	S	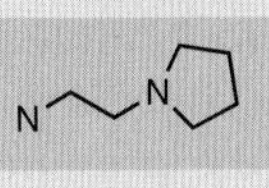
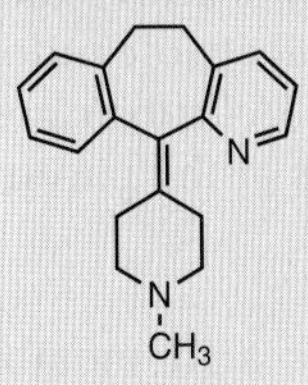 Cyproheptadine		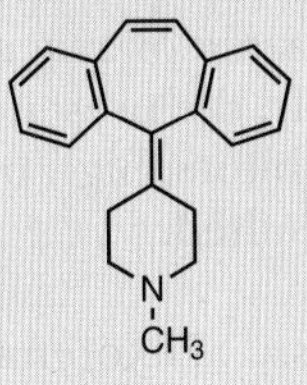 Azatadine

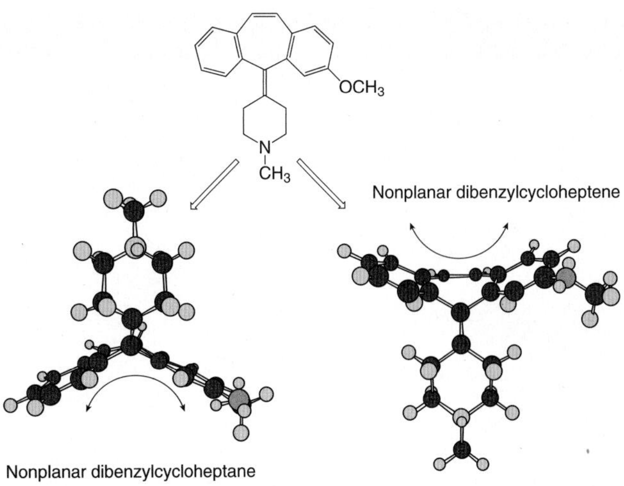

FIGURE 32.12 Enantiomers (atropisomers) of 3-methoxycyproheptadine.

Compounds in which the sulfur atom is replaced with another bridge (e.g., two methylene groups) are also available. Some have a pyridine ring replacing one of the benzenoid systems. Cyproheptadine, with a two-carbon spacer between the aromatic rings, also has anticholinergic, antiserotonergic, and appetite-stimulating properties, which are useful in treatment of anorexia nervosa and cachexia. The pyridine analog apparently lacks most of these qualities. Doxepin, an oxygen-containing congener of cyproheptadine, also has significant affinity for other receptors and has CNS-depressant qualities. It exists as a mixture of *Z*- and *E*-isomers (15:85) in its olefinic nonpiperidine side chain. In tissue-based assays, the *Z*-isomer is more potent than the *E*-isomer by more than threefold (31). Loratadine and desloratadine are widely used, nonsedating, second-generation antihistamines (vide infra).

Metabolism Information on the metabolic disposition and pharmacokinetic properties of agents in this group is limited, including incomplete identification of primary metabolic pathways, results of liver microsomal metabolic experiments, and only occasionally pharmacokinetic information. In humans, products from the phenothiazines include products of *N*-demethylation, aromatic hydroxylation, and occasionally sulfoxidation. From tricyclic analogs, metabolites resulting from *N*-demethylation, aromatic hydroxylation, and formation of *N*-quaternary glucuronides have been reported (34).

Second-Generation Nonsedating H_1 Antihistamines

Background

The second-generation antihistamines, marketed over the last 25 years, have improved H_1 selectivity, have little or no sedative qualities, and may have antiallergic effects apart from antihistaminic activity (35). They vary widely in structure (Table 32.8), but less so in pharmacologic

TABLE 32.8 Second-Generation Nonsedating Antihistamines

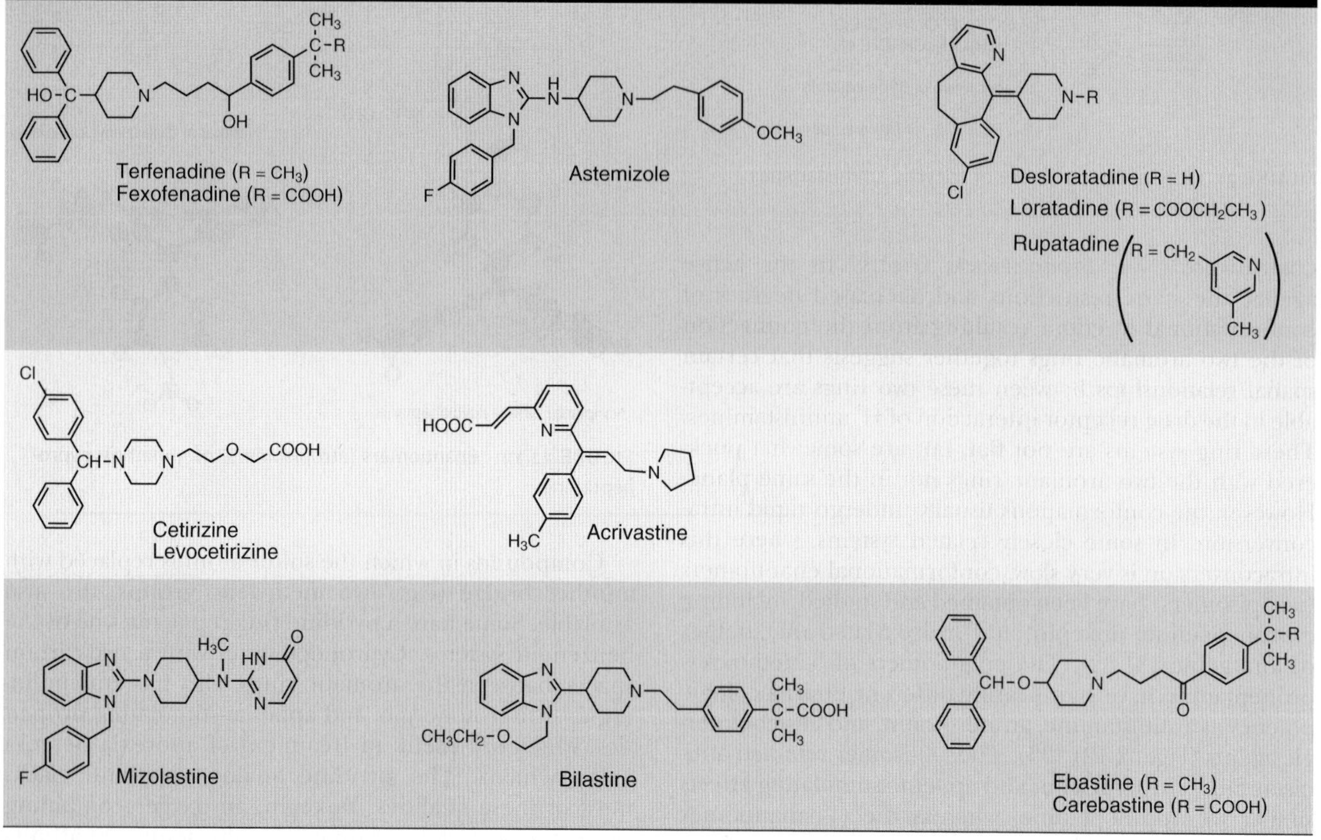

properties, having effects principally in the periphery. Structural resemblance to the first-generation H_1 antagonists is not always obvious as some of these agents were discovered while investigating new molecular structures for other pharmacologic targets. These agents possess selective peripheral H_1 antihistaminic effects, and they usually have less anticholinergic activity. Furthermore, they also have decreased affinity for adrenergic and/or serotonergic receptors and have limited CNS effects. The active agents apparently do not penetrate the blood–brain barrier significantly, perhaps because of their amphoteric nature (most are zwitterionic at physiologic pH) and partitioning characteristics and/or they are substrates for the drug efflux P-glycoprotein transporter or organic anion transporter proteins. Some of these agents have very slow rates of dissociation from H_1 receptors. Several have antiallergic properties that are separate from their antihistaminic properties, which are not thoroughly understood. In most cases, the parent drug or its important metabolites have half-lives sufficiently long to account for the extended duration of action (36). Most are administered once daily.

Specific Drugs

Terfenadine and Fexofenadine (Allegra)

Pharmacologic Effects This group of nonsedating antihistamines is usually thought to include fexofenadine and its parent terfenadine, astemizole, cetirizine, and loratadine and its metabolite desloratadine. Terfenadine was synthesized as an analog of azacyclanol in a search for antipsychotic agents. The initial reports of its antihistaminic properties included the observation of similar effects of its acid metabolite fexofenadine (37). Although terfenadine is no longer available, it was once a very widely used nonsedating antihistamine. Extensive clinical experience resulted in the reports of dangerous cardiac arrhythmias occurring occasionally when certain other drugs were taken concomitantly (38). These cardiac arrhythmias included prolongation of the QT interval and torsades de pointes, a life-threatening ventricular arrhythmia. These cardiac effects are now known to be associated with blockade of the hERG (human ether-a-go-go) gene product, the α-subunit of an inward rectifying cardiac K^+ channel (I_{Kr}) (39,40). These effects are associated only with the parent molecule. The side effects occur primarily at high concentrations of this lipophilic amine and usually in the presence of other CYP3A4 substrates like ketoconazole or macrolide antibiotics (triacetyloleandomycin). In the presence of competing CYP3A4 substrates and inhibitors, high plasma concentrations of the parent agent resulted.

Metabolism Fexofenadine, the carboxylic acid metabolite of terfenadine, is widely available (Fig. 32.13).

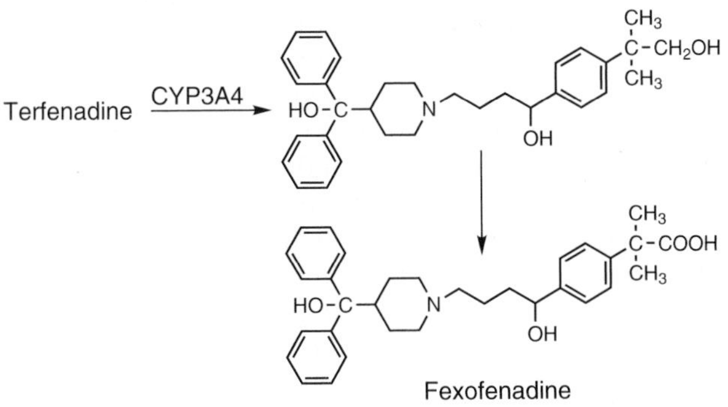

FIGURE 32.13 Metabolism of terfenadine leading to fexofenadine.

It accounted for the antihistaminic properties of terfenadine, which is very rapidly metabolized via CYP3A4-catalyzed processes. Although the enantiomers of terfenadine are reported to have approximately equal antihistaminic activity (41), no data on the activity of the enantiomers of fexofenadine were found. Members of the organic anion transporter protein family and the drug efflux transporter P-glycoprotein are involved in the disposition of fexofenadine. A higher plasma concentration of the *R*-enantiomer is reported, showing some stereoselectivity in this process (42,43). Fexofenadine does not have the antiarrhythmic side effects of terfenadine.

Terfenadine and other lipophilic amines (e.g., astemizole, another second-generation antihistamine that is not longer marketed, grepafloxacin, thioridazine, sertindole, and cisapride) are all lipophilic aliphatic amines containing one or more aromatic groups (40). Each has been associated with life-threatening cardiac arrhythmias associated with binding to the hERG K^+ ion channel. The disposition of each depends significantly on CYP3A4 for its oxidative metabolism so that in the presence of inhibitors or competitive substrates, significantly elevated plasma levels are observed. Screening of potential drug candidates for hERG K^+ ion channel affinity is done routinely to aid in attempts to develop safe new drugs. Similarly, proof of safety of agents that are primarily CYP3A4 substrates is required. Studies on the effect of ketoconazole on the plasma levels of the drug in vivo are routinely required by the U.S. Food and Drug Administration (FDA).

Astemizole

Astemizole (Table 32.8), like terfenadine, produced cardiac arrhythmias via interaction with the hERG K^+ ion channel. Study of its primary metabolites (products of *O*-demethylation and *N*-dealkylation) as possible agents to avoid these effects did not lead to marketing of any of them as drugs.

Loratadine (Claritin) and Desloratadine (Clarinex)

PHARMACOLOGIC EFFECTS Loratadine (Table 32.8) is related to the first-generation tricyclic antihistamines and to antidepressants. It is nonsedating, and neither it nor its major metabolite, desloratadine (descarboethoxyloratadine), is associated with the potentially cardiotoxic effects reported for terfenadine and astemizole. Upon chronic dosing, the area under the curve (AUC; plasma concentration vs. time curve) for the metabolite is greater than for the parent drug, and its half-life is longer. Desloratadine is a more potent H_1 antagonist and a more potent inhibitor of histamine release. This metabolite probably contributes significantly to the antihistaminic effects of administered loratadine. Desloratadine has a slow off-rate from the H_1 receptor in vitro, nearly 100 times slower than first-generation antihistamines (44). One of the hydroxylated metabolites, 3′-hydroxydesloratadine, may contribute to the pharmacologic properties of desloratadine (45).

METABOLISM The metabolic conversion of loratadine to descarboethoxyloratadine occurs via an oxidative process and not via direct hydrolysis (Fig. 32.14). CYP2D6 and CYP3A4 appear to be the CYP450 isozymes catalyzing this oxidative metabolic process (46). Apparently the metabolite does not reach the CNS in significant concentrations. Among the nonsedating second-generation antihistamines, this metabolite appears to be the only nonzwitterionic species. Although the failure of zwitterionic molecules to reach CNS sites in significant concentrations can be rationalized readily, a similar explanation is not apparent for loratadine or its metabolite. Competitive substrates for CYP3A4 do not produce a significant drug–drug interaction because the parent molecule lacks effects on hERG K^+ channel in cardiac tissue.

When desloratadine is administered, its terminal phase half-life is greater than 24 hours, with about half of the administered dose being excreted in the urine and a similar amount in the feces (47,48). The principal hydroxylated metabolite is 3′-hydroxydesloratadine, but a number of other aliphatic and aromatic hydroxylation products have been identified, many appearing as *O*-glucuronides in vivo (49,50).

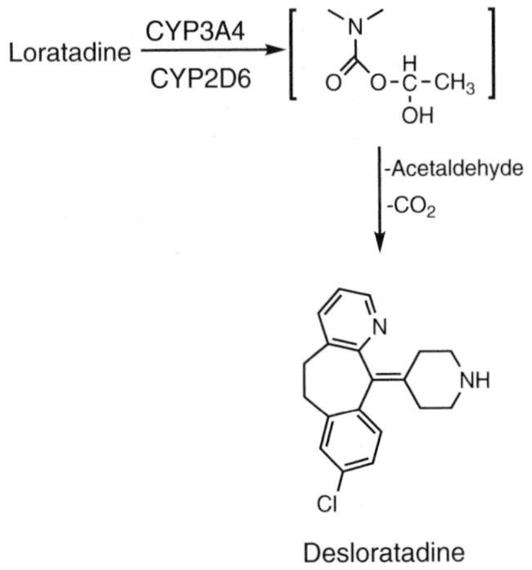

FIGURE 32.14 Metabolism of loratadine.

Rupatadine (Rupafin)

Rupatadine (Table 32.8) is a selective oral H_1-receptor antagonist available in Europe and in other countries that is also used in seasonal and perennial allergic rhinitis and in chronic idiopathic urticaria. It is dosed once daily. Like loratadine, it is metabolized to desloratadine and to 3′-hydroxydesloratadine. The parent molecule has a terminal phase half-life of 5 to 6 hours. A majority of the metabolites are excreted in the feces. Rupatadine is reported to be more effective than desloratadine in inhibiting release of TNF-α and IL-6 in mast cells and to be an antagonist to platelet-activating factor in vitro, an activity not observed with other second-generation H_1 antagonists. In reported clinical trials, this agent has actions similar to desloratadine, cetirizine, and ebastine (51).

Cetirizine (Zyrtec) and Levocetirizine (Xysal, Xusal)

Cetirizine, the acid metabolite from oxidation of the primary alcohol of the antihistamine hydroxyzine (Fig. 32.15; see also Table 32.6), is a widely used antihistamine (52). It has a long duration of action and is highly selective for H_1 receptors. No cardiotoxicity has been reported, but some drowsiness occurs. The *R*-enantiomer of cetirizine, levocetirizine, is now marketed. Levocetirizine has higher affinity than its *S*-enantiomer for the H_1 receptor (>30-fold) and is more slowly dissociated by more than 20-fold from the receptor (53). Thus the antihistaminic properties of cetirizine are probably accounted for by the *R*-enantiomer. Similar large differences in ratios of dissociation rates and K_i values for closely related enantiomers are also reported. It is excreted primarily unchanged. Only a small amount of levocetirizine is reported as metabolites, including expected products of glucuronidation and aromatic hydroxylation (54).

Acrivastine (Semprex)

Acrivastine (Table 32.8), an acidic congener of triprolidine in which a carboxylic acid–substituted chain has been attached, is also a second-generation nonsedating antihistamine. Penetration of the blood–brain barrier is limited, and it is less sedating than triprolidine. It is used principally in a combination with a decongestant.

Ebastine (Kestine) and Carebastine

Benzhydryl ethers of piperidinols are also useful antihistamines. Those with large *N*-substituents, like those in terfenadine and other nonsedating antihistamines, are most successful. Ebastine (Table 32.8), structurally similar to terfenadine, is a potent selective H_1 antihistamine as measured in radioligand displacement assays. In these assays, its acid metabolite has significantly higher affinity than the parent molecule. It is nonsedating and apparently free of anticholinergic effects (55). Like some other second-generation antihistamines, ebastine blocks release of PGD_2 and LTC_4/D_4 in cellular assays. Pharmacokinetic data indicate that its acid metabolite carebastine is responsible for its antihistaminic properties, because the parent drug has a very short half-life and the active metabolite a much longer one (Fig. 32.16). In an animal model of torsades de pointes, ebastine, at a high dose, produced significant cardiac conduction abnormalities (e.g., prolongation of the QT interval), whereas the metabolite did not. At lower doses, these effects occurred only in the presence of competitive CYP3A4 substrates. However, some in vitro data suggest that CYP450 isozymes other than CYP3A4 may be important in the initial hydroxylation. The pharmacologically active acid metabolite carebastine is metabolically analogous to fexofenadine (oxidation of a *t*-butyl group), the acid metabolite of terfenadine. Ebastine is marketed in several countries outside the United States.

Mizolastine (Mizollen)

Mizolastine (Table 32.8) is a second-generation nonsedating antihistamine that structurally resembles astemizole (56). Its half-life is long. It is primarily conjugated, and only small amounts of the compound are metabolized oxidatively. The AUC increases about twofold in the presence of ketoconazole, a CYP3A4 substrate and inhibitor. Only weak interaction with the hERG K^+ channel and with muscarinic receptors is reported. It is available in Europe.

Bilastine

Bilastine is structurally related to other second-generation H_1 antihistamines, being an amino acid with structural resemblance to parts of fexofenadine and astemizole (Table 32.8). It is being developed for the treatment of symptoms of seasonal and perennial allergic rhinitis and

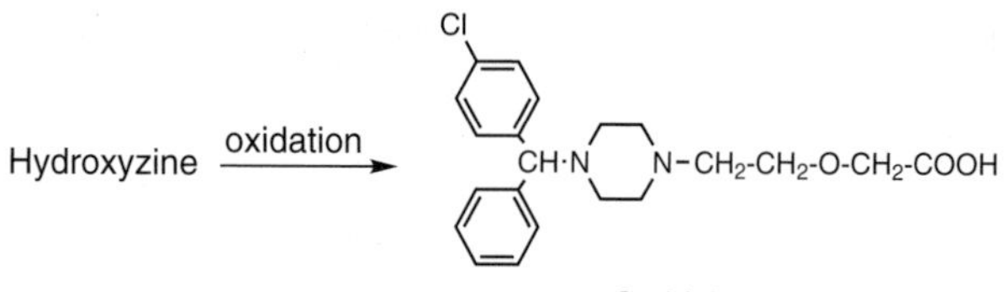

Cetirizine

FIGURE 32.15 Metabolism of hydroxyzine to cetirizine.

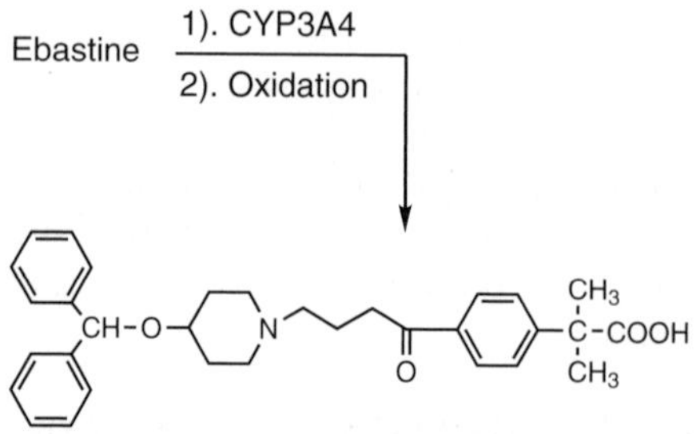

Carebastine

FIGURE 32.16 Metabolism of ebastine to carebastine.

chronic idiopathic urticaria. Comparison with cetirizine, fexofenadine, and desloratadine has shown similar effectiveness and safety characteristics. It has a long duration of action allowing once-daily dosing (57). Bilastine has recently received approval for use in Europe.

Topical H_1 Antihistamines

Therapeutic Applications

Topical application of H_1 antihistamines to the eye relieves itching, congestion of the conjunctiva, and erythema (19,58). The density of mast cells in the conjunctiva is high, and the histamine concentrations in tear film are significant in the ocular allergic response. From eye drops, only small amounts of the antihistamine (1% to 5%) penetrate the cornea. More of the compound is absorbed via the conjunctiva and nasal mucosa, and still more ends up swallowed from tear duct and nasal drainage. Until recently, topical ocular antihistamines were limited to two classical agents: antazoline (Table 32.2) from the ethylenediamine series and pheniramine (Fig. 32.9) from the alkylamine series. Both are used in combination with sympathomimetic vasoconstrictors.

A slow rate of receptor dissociation of H_1 antagonists is associated with long duration of action systemically, which occurs with the more recently available ocular antihistamines. Based on correlations of pK_a values and lipophilicity data, it appears that compounds with a logD (the sum of the partition coefficients of both the ionized and nonionized species) near 1.0 ± 0.5 at pH 7.4 are most efficacious and their water-soluble salts also show a low incidence of ocular irritation. Relationships between partitioning characteristics of these and other antihistamines indicate receptor affinity (moderate at least) and a particular range of lipophilicity is optimum for topical ocular antihistamines with minimum ocular irritation (59). Some of these compounds are currently available (Table 32.9) or are being evaluated as nasal sprays, and some are also occasionally used as systemic antihistamines.

TABLE 32.9 Topical Antihistamines

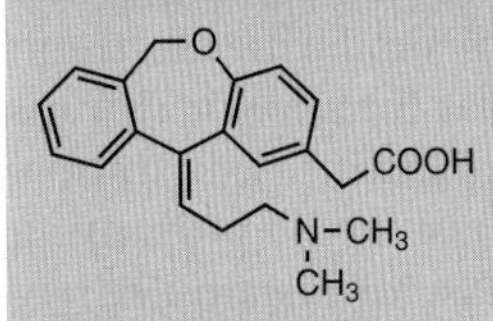
Olopatadine

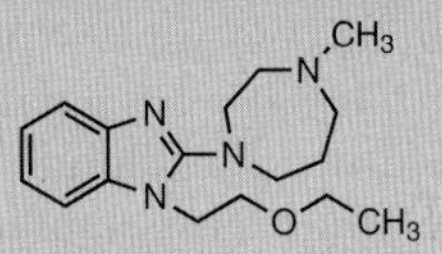
Emedastine

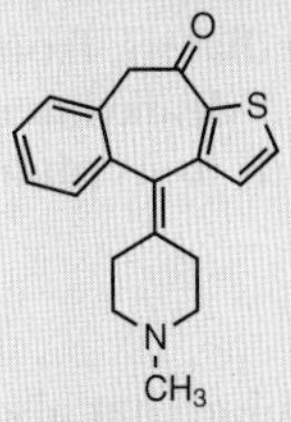
Ketotifen

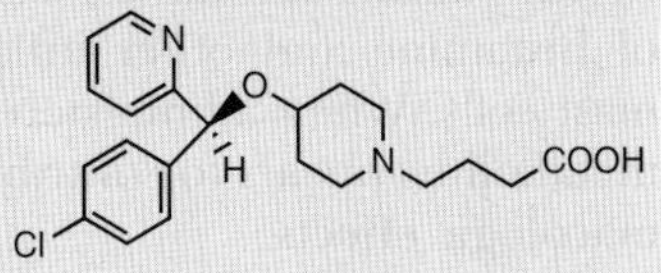
Bepotastine

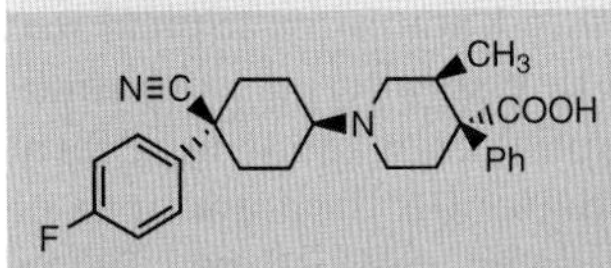
Levocabastine

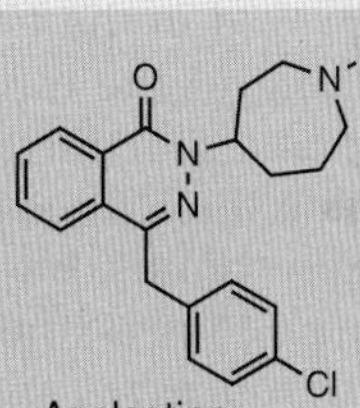
Azelastine

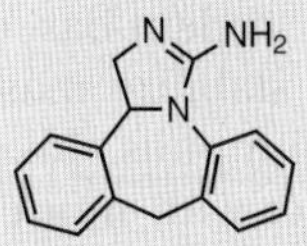
Epinastine

Olopatadine (Patanol)

Olopatadine (Table 32.9) is structurally related to the tricyclic antihistamines. It is available as an eye drop and more recently also as a nasal spray. It has a long duration of action when applied topically, and it appears to also inhibit the release of inflammatory mediators (e.g., histamine, tryptase, PGD_2) from mast cells. Its selectivity for H_1 receptors in tissue assays (over H_2 and H_3 receptors) is very high, and its selectivity for H_1-receptor blockade over α-adrenergic, dopaminergic, serotonergic, and muscarinic receptors is also very high. Olopatadine is reported to have a rapid onset of action and a long duration of action, consistent with high histamine receptor affinity and a slow rate of receptor dissociation. The presence of the carboxylic acid side chain is apparently responsible for the observed lack of muscarinic receptor affinity. This feature may also be responsible for limited penetration. Olopatadine is also a mast cell stabilizer. The mechanism for this activity has not been delineated, but it has been shown to stabilize model cell membranes by interaction with phospholipid monolayers.

Levocabastine (Livostin)

Levocabastine (Table 32.9) is a potent selective H_1-receptor antagonist used topically in eye drops for seasonal allergic conjunctivitis. A small amount of systemic absorption of the compound is reported. The agent also prevents release of transmitters from mast cells. A nasal spray used for allergic rhinitis is available outside the United States.

Emedastine (Emadine)

Emedastine (Table 32.9) is also a newer antihistamine used topically in the eye for conjunctivitis. It has very high H_1-receptor selectivity characteristics and is structurally related to the benzimidazoles such as astemizole. Inhibition of mast cell release of inflammatory mediators has been noted.

Azelastine (Astelin)

Azelastine, although not a close structural analog to the benzimidazoles, has some structural similarities to them (Table 32.9). It is used as a nasal spray for allergic rhinitis and as eye drops for allergic conjunctivitis. Like olopatadine, azelastine also stabilizes mast cells, preventing degranulation and subsequent release of histamine, leukotrienes, and PGD_2. It is available in Europe for systemic use for the treatment of asthma and seasonal allergies. Besides antihistaminic effects, it may also block release of histamine and other inflammatory mediators from mast cells. When administered orally, the *N*-dealkylated metabolite appears to contribute significantly to its pharmacologic effects.

Ketotifen (Zaditor)

Ketotifen is a potent selective H_1 antihistamine that also prevents release of transmitters from mast cells (Table 32.9). It is approved in the United States for topical use to prevent itching of the eye due to allergic conjunctivitis. It is used as a systemic antiallergy agent in several countries outside the United States for the treatment of seasonal allergic rhinitis, hay fever, and asthma. Being structurally analogous to the cyproheptadine-like antihistamines, differences in activity of the two enantiomers (atropisomers) have been noted, being about six- to sevenfold in ligand displacement and rodent-based assays (60). Ketotifen has been shown to stabilize mast cells and to inhibit degranulation of eosinophils. Like olopatadine, it has been shown to interact with model membranes, stabilizing them by interaction with phospholipids monolayers.

Epinastine (Elestat)

Epinastine (Table 32.9) is a potent, long-acting H_1 antihistamine and an inhibitor of release of histamine and other transmitters from mast cells. It has some affinity for H_2 receptors, as well. It is used as an eye drop for allergic conjunctivitis. It does not penetrate into the CNS and is classified as a nonsedating antihistamine.

Bepotastine (Bepreve)

Bepotastine is a potent selective H_1 antihistamine that decreases the production of proinflammatory cytokines from mast cells and prevents eosinophil migration (Table 32.9). In the United States, it is approved for topical use to prevent itching of the eye due to allergic conjunctivitis. It is approved in Japan as a systemic antihistamine used for allergic rhinitis, urticaria, and pruritus.

Antiulcer Agents

Background

The secretion of gastric acid occurs at the level of parietal cells of the oxyntic gland in the gastric mucosa (Fig. 32.17), producing 2 to 3 L of gastric juice daily (pH 1 in hydrochloric acid). Ultimately, this secretory process occurs via an H^+/K^+-ATPase that exchanges hydronium ion (H_3O^+) with uptake of a potassium ion. Several mediators regulate this secretion by way of receptor systems on the basolateral membrane. The H_2 histaminergic pathway is cAMP dependent. Gastrin and muscarinic receptors also regulate the secretion of gastric acid through calcium ion–dependent pathways. In parietal cells, E series prostaglandins work in opposition to the histaminergic pathway, inhibiting histamine-stimulated adenylyl cyclase activity. Other epithelial cells in the mucosal lining under the influence of prostaglandin-mediated pathways secrete bicarbonate and mucus, both of which are important in protecting the gastric lining from the effects of acid secretion. In many cases, hypersecretion of gastric acid appears to be associated with *Helicobacter pylori* infection, which may contribute to defects in mucosal protective defenses. There is evidence that some H_2 antihistamines, particularly cimetidine and ranitidine, have regulatory effects on T-cell lymphocyte proliferation by augmenting cytokine production and immunoglobulin production. These effects may not be associated with histamine receptors and may not be shared by nizatidine and famotidine.

Therapeutic Applications of H_2 Antihistamines

H_2 antihistamines are used in the treatment of duodenal ulcers, gastric ulcers, gastroesophageal reflux disease (GERD), pathologic hypersensitivity disorders, and upper gastrointestinal bleeding in critically ill patients and are sold OTC for acid indigestion (61). They are also included in multidrug treatment protocols for eradication of *H. pylori* in treatment of peptic ulcers and prior to surgery to prevent aspiration pneumonitis. Like H_1 antihistamines, H_2 antihistamines are inverse agonists that block the basal level of activity at this receptor. Combinations of H_1 and H_2 antihistamines are useful in idiopathic urticaria not responding to H_1 antihistamines alone and to treat itching and flushing of anaphylaxis, pruritus, and contact dermatitis.

Structural Requirements H_2 antihistamines specifically designed to decrease the secretion of gastric acid are based on an extensive investigative approach to drug design that began from the structures of partial agonist molecules very closely related to histamine (62). Ultimately, this work resulted in the development of cimetidine (Table 32.10), in which the imidazole ring like that of histamine is maintained. The imidazole ring is substituted with a C-4 methyl group, which in histamine agonists affords H_2 selectivity, a four-atom side chain that includes one sulfur atom (the sulfur atom increases potency compared to carbon and oxygen congeners), and a terminal polar nonbasic unit, in this case an N-cyanoguanidine substituent. Guanidines substituted with electron-withdrawing groups have significantly decreased basicity compared to guanidine, and they are neutral (nonprotonated) at physiologic pH. Thus, these are logical substituents to replace the terminal thiourea feature in unsuccessful earlier homologous candidates, metiamide and burimamide. The former agent was not marketed due to untoward effects, including agranulocytosis, and the latter agent lacked significant

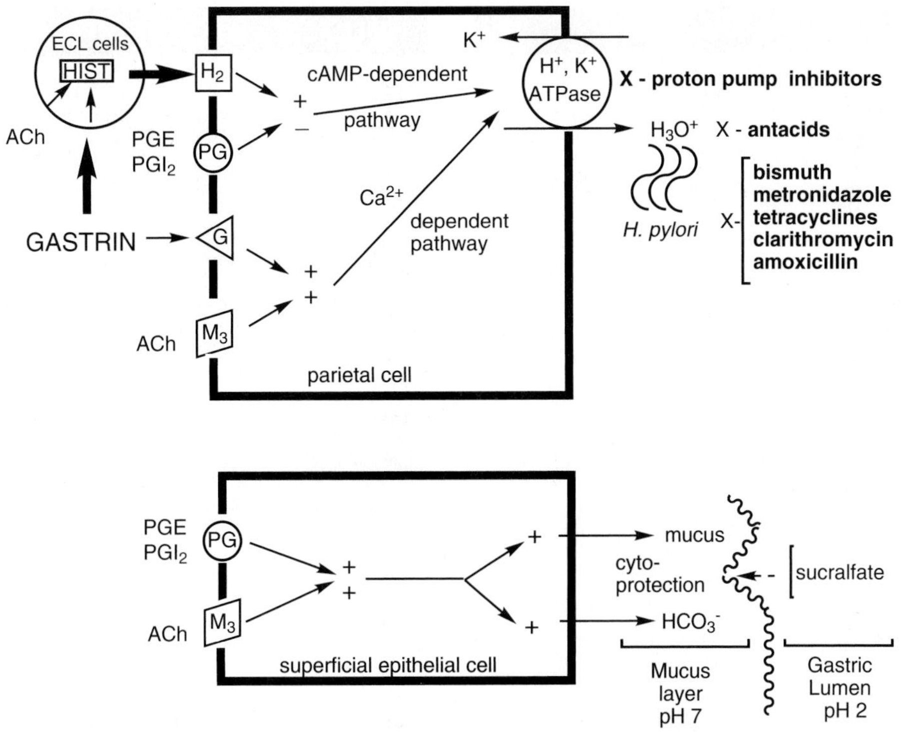

FIGURE 32.17 Secretion of gastric acid and peptic ulcer disease. Histamine is secreted from an endochromaffin-like (ECL) cell, which is innervated by muscarinic receptors (M) via the enteric nervous system and by gastrin receptors (G). Agonist occupation of histamine H_2 receptors in parietal cells leads to gastric acid secretion. Other input at parietal cells includes the prostaglandins (PGs), gastrin, and muscarinic receptors. (Adapted from Hoogerwerf WA, Pasricha PJ. Pharmacotherapy of gastric acidity, peptic ulcers, and gastroesophageal reflux disease. In: Hardman JG, Limbird LE, Mollinoff PB, et al., eds. Goodman and Gilman's the Pharmacological Basis of Therapeutics, 11th Ed. New York: McGraw-Hill, 2005:968, with permission.)

oral bioavailability. Subsequently, the nitromethylene unit was a replacement of the *N*-cyanoimino group in the substituted guanidine analogs, affording compounds of increased potency. Replacement for the imidazole ring with other heteroaromatic rings resulted in other useful analogs.

Metabolism Cimetidine, ranitidine, and famotidine are subject to first-pass metabolism, and each has oral bioavailability of about 50%. The oral bioavailability of nizatidine is about 90%. All have half-lives of 1.5 to 4 hours, with that of nizatidine being the shortest. Significant amounts of each of these H_2 antihistamines are excreted unchanged, with small amounts of urinary products of sulfoxidation being a common metabolic feature. As expected, hydroxylation of the imidazole C-4 methyl group of cimetidine occurs. Ranitidine is excreted largely unchanged, but minor metabolic pathways include *N*-demethylation and *N*- and *S*-oxidation. The metabolites are not thought to contribute to the therapeutic properties of the parent drugs, with the exception of nizatidine from which the *N*-desmethyl metabolite retains H_2 antihistamine activity (63).

Side Effects and Drug Interactions Cimetidine, the earliest of these agents, shows the greatest number of drug interactions (64). Among them are somnolence and confusion in elderly patients with decreased renal function. Gynecomastia, presumably related to increased prolactin secretion, has been reported. Cimetidine inhibits CYP450-dependent metabolic processes, affording increased concentration of several agents, the most important being those having narrow therapeutic concentration windows (e.g., phenytoin, theophylline, some benzodiazepines, warfarin, quinidine). Inhibition of several CYP450 oxidative processes is associated with the presence of the imidazole ring of cimetidine, which apparently replaces the histidine that serves as a ligand to the porphyrin iron in CYP450 enzymes. Other agents in this group contain heterocyclic rings other than imidazole and do not show this effect. Cimetidine is an inhibitor of renal tubular secretion of some drugs including procainamide. These tubular secretion effects are less prevalent or absent with other agents in this class. The other agents in the group are more potent than cimetidine, and significant differences are noted among them. Of these, ranitidine is the most widely used. The H_2 antihistamines have OTC status and are widely available for gastric hyperacidity.

Proton Pump Inhibitors

Proton pump inhibitors (PPIs) are widely used in the treatment of duodenal and gastric ulcers, erosive esophagitis, GERD, GERD-related laryngitis, and hypersecretory conditions (Zollinger-Ellison syndrome) (65,66). Some of the generic agents are available OTC for the treatment

TABLE 32.10 H_2-Receptor Antihistamines

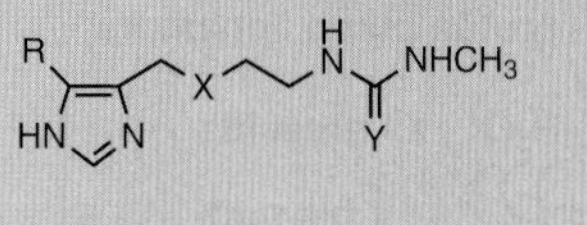

Drug	Trade name	R	X	Y
Burimamide		H	CH_2	S
Metiamide		CH_3	S	S
Cimetidine	Tagamet	CH_3	S	N–C≡N

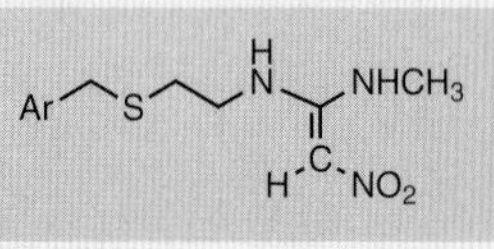

Drug	Trade name	Ar
Ranitidine	Zantac	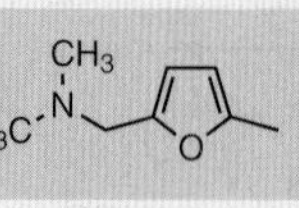
Nizatidine	Axid	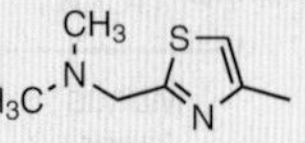

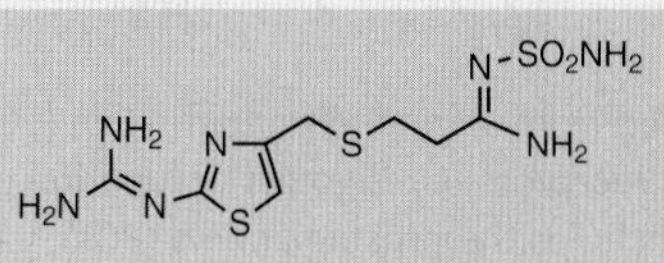

Famotidine (Pepcid)

TABLE 32.11 H^+/K^+-ATPase Proton Pump Inhibitors

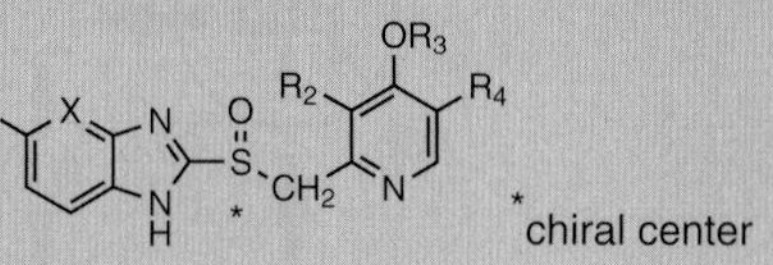

Drugs	Trade name	X	R_1	R_2	R_3	R_4
Omeprazole	Prilosec	CH	OCH_3	CH_3	CH_3	CH_3
Esomeprazole (*S*-enantiomer)	Nexium	CH	OCH_3	CH_3	CH_3	CH_3
Tenatoprazole		N	OCH_3	CH_3	CH_3	CH_3
Lansoprazole	Prevacid	CH	H	CH_3	CH_2CF_3	H
Dexlansoprazole (*R*-enantiomer)	Dexilant	CH	H	CH_3	CH_2CF_3	H
Rabeprazole	Aciphex	CH	H	CH_3	$(CH_2)_3OCH_3$	H
Pantoprazole	Protonix	CH	$OCHF_2$	OCH_3	CH_3	H

of acid reflux disorders. The final step in acid secretion in parietal cells of the gastric mucosa is a process mediated by H^+/K^+-ATPase, the gastric proton pump, an enzyme with significant homology to Na^+/K^+-ATPase. This H^+/K^+-ATPase has some similarities to the H^+/K^+-ATPase in osteoclasts, which is involved in bone resorption. Gastric acid secretion can be inhibited in many ways. These include by antagonists at muscarinic, gastrin, or histamine H_2 receptors; by agonists at inhibitory receptors for prostaglandins and somatostatin; by PPIs; or by carbonic anhydrase inhibitors.

Mechanism of Action Omeprazole and related analogs (Table 32.11), produce inhibition of stimulated gastric acid secretion irrespective of the receptor stimulation process. Nearly all of the compounds are close structural relatives, being weakly basic 2-pyridylmethylsulfinylbenzimidazoles. An analog, tenatoprazole, which is an imidazopyridine isostere, is in clinical trial.

Only a few successful changes of the heterocyclic rings are possible (67). These agents have irreversible effects on the secretion of gastric acid because the molecule rearranges in the strongly acidic environment of the parietal cell. Covalent binding of the rearranged inhibitor to the H^+/K^+-ATPase results in inactivation of the catalytic function of the proton pump. A number of cysteine sulfhydryl groups are potential sites. There is evidence that two molecules of the intermediate from omeprazole are bound to the active site, and one of these sites has been identified as cysteine-813 (and probably cysteine-892 and/or -822) of the cysteine-rich H^+/K^+-ATPase (68). These cysteines are in different environments (e.g., exposed to the lumen or in the membrane), and different PPIs bind differentially to them and other sulfhydryl groups. In the covalent binding, disulfide bonds with it are formed. Analogous, but slightly different results are reported for lansoprazole, pantoprazole, and rabeprazole (69). A chemical mechanism for the process is shown in Figure 32.18.

Because the initial rearrangement only occurs at a strongly acidic pH, acid-stable oral dosage forms are used that allow for dissolution, release, and absorption of drug in the duodenum (enteric-coated granules in capsules or enteric-coated tablets). More recently, granular preparations of lansoprazole (enteric-coated granules) and omeprazole (with sodium bicarbonate) have become available. Intravenous dosage forms of lansoprazole and pantoprazole are also available. The acid-catalyzed rearrangement of absorbed drug then occurs selectively in the acidic environment of the canaliculus as it is secreted into the gastric lumen from the parietal cells. Some differences may occur in the molecular sites of binding of the agents, and differences have been noted in recovery times, with rabeprazole having a shorter duration of action (70). Tenatoprazole has the longest plasma half-life and, in testing, appears to offer better control of nocturnal hyperacidity (71).

CYP450 Metabolism Metabolism of omeprazole and other PPIs occurs primarily in the liver (Fig. 32.19). The sulfone, sulfide, and hydroxylated and *O*-demethylated metabolites have been reported as products.

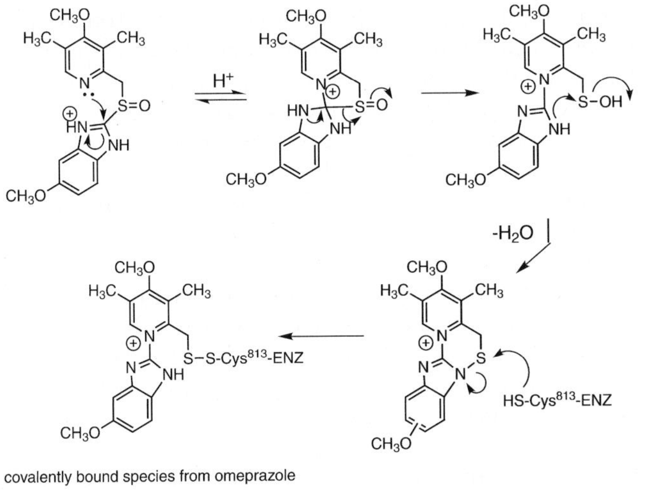

FIGURE 32.18 Acid-catalyzed activation of omeprazole to reactive sulfenamide. At the parietal cell, H^+/K^+-ATPase, a cysteine residue, reacts to form disulfide-attached enzyme inhibitor.

Omeprazole is a substrate primarily for CYP2C19 and may elevate concentrations of other substrates for this enzyme (diazepam) when given concurrently. CYP3A4 contributes to a lesser extent. Further oxidation of the sulfone affords additional metabolites, which are excreted in the feces. Lansoprazole is metabolized by analogous routes (72). Fewer drug interactions with lansoprazole have been reported, although it is also a substrate for CYP2C19.

These sulfoxides have a chiral sulfur atom, and recent work has been reported on the effects of stereochemistry on pharmacologic and dispositional characteristics. The oxidative metabolism of omeprazole is catalyzed principally by CYP2C19 (primarily 5′-hydroxylation and to a lesser extent benzimidazole *O*-demethylation) (73). In human liver microsomes, the *R*-(+)-enantiomer is cleared more rapidly, and it is almost exclusively metabolized by CYP2C19. The clearance of the *S*-(−)-enantiomer is dependent both on oxidation by CYP2C19 and to a lesser extent on CYP3A4-mediated metabolism, primarily sulfone formation. The marketed single enantiomer, esomeprazole, provides greater bioavailability in CYP2C19 extensive metabolizers and less interindividual variation between extensive and slow CYP2C19 metabolizer populations (~3% of Caucasians and up to 15% to 20% of Asians). Thus the impact of variant alleles of CYP2C19 is less on the *S*-(−)-enantiomer than on the parent racemate. Higher blood levels and greater AUCs are observed in extensive metabolizers, and increases in the duration of gastric pH >4.0 are observed, which are correlated with healing rates. Esomeprazole, the *S*-(−)-enantiomer of omeprazole, has been marketed.

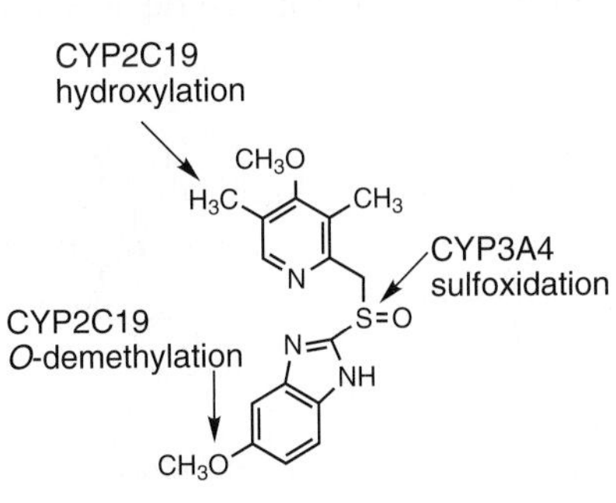

FIGURE 32.19 Oxidation sites and CYP450 isozymes in the metabolism of omeprazole.

Different PPIs depend differently on CYP2C19 for oxidative metabolism, and the enantiomers show variation in dependence on CYP2C19 and other pathways (principally CYP3A4). Pantoprazole and lansoprazole show greater metabolism via CYP2C19, with the enantiomers being affected differently, and rabeprazole is metabolized to a lesser extent by oxidative CYP450 enzymes. Lansoprazole, pantoprazole, and rabeprazole all lack the pyridyl 5-methyl group, a major site of CYP2C19 oxidation, but CYP2C19 oxidations occur at other sites in each of them.

Risk of adverse outcomes associated with concomitant use of clopidogrel with PPIs following acute coronary syndrome has been reported. Platelet antiaggregatory activity of clopidogrel is dependent on CYP2C19 oxidation to a reactive metabolite; thus PPIs are competitive substrates with clopidogrel via this pathway (see Chapter 26).

Single-Enantiomer Proton Pump Inhibitors

The development of single enantiomers has been of interest in this class of compounds for more than 15 years. The primary reasons for such development are to obtain more optimal treatment and specificity of effects, potentially resulting in exposure of nontarget tissues to lower drug concentrations. The development of improved stereoselective syntheses and assay techniques has facilitated these efforts. A quantitative difference in pharmacologic effects of the two enantiomers provides impetus to develop the enantiomer with higher affinity or potency, assuming it is has no increased adverse pharmacologic effects or toxicity and/or no undesirable pharmacokinetic properties (74). When only one enantiomer has desirable pharmacologic properties, the term "isomeric ballast" has been used to characterize the much less active or inactive enantiomer, because it contributes little to the observed effects. However, for the benzimidazole sulfoxide PPIs, the enantiomers are approximately equiactive in vitro. The chemical process to the reactive intermediate occurs with loss of the chiral center (Fig. 32.18).

For omeprazole, exposure of the target (H^+/K^+-ATPase at the parietal cell) as represented by the AUC was correlated to inhibition of gastric acid secretion, as expected in a normal log-linear dose–effect relationship curve (75). Differential metabolism of the enantiomers of omeprazole by the important isozymes CYP2C19 and CYP3A4 occurs. From racemic omeprazole, the AUCs of the *S*-enantiomer differed about threefold between extensive and slow metabolizer genotypes and about 7.5-fold for the *R*-enantiomer, thus arguing that esomeprazole would offer an advantage of less interindividual variability and improved therapeutic effect. Higher bioavailability of esomeprazole occurs in extensive metabolizers, and lower exposure occurs in poor metabolizers (76,77).

From lansoprazole, dexlansoprazole, the *R*-enantiomer, has been marketed. It has a higher plasma concentration (six- to ninefold) than the *S*-enantiomer when the racemate is administered to both extensive and poor metabolizer CYP2C19 genotypes, and the AUCs from the enantiomers differ about fivefold in both populations (*R*>*S*). Administering the *R*-enantiomer to both populations would not be expected to decrease the interindividual variability between these groups, but it does have the potential to decrease the exposure to off-target effects (potential toxicity). Other factors such as differences in protein binding between enantiomers and potential enantiomer–enantiomer interaction are not considered in this analysis. Additionally, the two enantiomers of lansoprazole are not interconverted in man via sulfoxide reduction to sulfide and subsequent reoxidization to the sulfoxide, another potential complicating feature. Changes are made in the available dexlansoprazole dosage form; it is a dual delayed-release formulation to provide two releases of the drug to extend the absorption phase.

Upon administration of racemic pantoprazole, no stereoselectivity is noted in extensive metabolizer phenotypes. About equal AUCs of the two enantiomers are observed. However in poor metabolizers, the AUC of the *S*-enantiomer is lower than that of the *R*-enantiomer (*S*/*R* ratio = 0.3 to 0.4). The CYP2C19 pathway appears to be primarily *O*-demethylation (pyridine 4-methyl ether) followed by sulfoxide formation. The *S*-enantiomer, which would be expected to generate less interindividual variability between slow and fast metabolizers, has been marketed in India (78).

Upon administration of racemic rabeprazole, small differences are noted in plasma concentration and AUCs of the enantiomers, with the *R*-enantiomer exceeding the *S*-enantiomer by about twofold in both slow and fast metabolizers. Rabeprazole is nonenzymatically reduced to the sulfide, and in microsomal experiments, stereoselective oxidation of *R*-rabeprazole by both CYP2C19 and CYP3A4 occurs, with the latter isozyme showing a greater intrinsic clearance of the racemic sulfide. CYP2C19 appears to catalyze *O*-demethylation of the side chain terminal ether. A single enantiomer of *R*-rabeprazole was launched in India (79).

Tenatoprazole, as previously noted, has a much longer half-life than the other PPIs, about 7 to 8 hours. Thus, it is expected to exhibit an extended duration of acid suppression with smaller differences between day and night time effectiveness. The *S*-enantiomer is currently in clinical trial (78,80).

Combination Therapy in *Helicobacter Pylori* Infections The majority of peptic ulcers are related to *H. pylori* infections and nonsteroidal anti-inflammatory drug (NSAID) therapy. *H. pylori* apparently penetrates the layer of gastric mucus by producing ammonia and carbon dioxide (urease catalyzed hydrolysis of urea) to withstand the acidic environment of the stomach. More than 90% of duodenal ulcer patients, excluding those with gastrinoma or taking NSAIDs, show the presence of *H. pylori*. Determination of *H. pylori* infection is routinely performed by measuring production of carbon dioxide (breath) or bicarbonate (blood) after oral administration of ^{13}C- or ^{14}C-labeled urea. Endoscopic examination and antigen-based serologic tests may be used as confirmation (81). Eradication of *H. pylori* markedly decreases the incidence of ulcer recurrence. Several regimens of antibiotic therapy, widely used with PPIs or less commonly with H_2 antagonists, are effective. Double and triple drug combinations (e.g., PPIs with amoxicillin and clarithromycin or metronidazole) are used.

Drug Safety In 2010, the FDA revised the prescription and OTC labels of the PPIs to include safety information about a possible increased risk of fractures of the hip, wrist, and spine with use of these medications. The agency reviewed several epidemiologic studies that reported these risks. The increased risk of fractures occurred primarily in patients 50 years of age and older. Use of OTC PPIs is indicated for short-term therapy, up to 14 days of continuous use.

Competitive K^+ Inhibitors

Newer agents that block gastric acid secretion at the H^+/K^+-ATPase by binding as competitive inhibitors at the K^+ binding site are under development (Fig. 32.20) (61,66). An initial compound SCH 28080 was hepatotoxic. Newer agents followed. Each of them binds ionically to the proton pump at or near the K^+ binding site. From this work, revaprazan has been marketed in Korea. It is used for the treatment of peptic and duodenal ulcers and gastritis (82,83).

Prokinetic Agents

Prokinetic drugs, such as metoclopramide, cisapride, and related compounds, increase esophageal sphincter pressure and enhance peristalsis and gastric emptying, thus counteracting factors that lead to esophagitis (Table 32.12) (84). These agents are 5-HT_4 agonists in the enteric nervous system leading to release of acetylcholine. Enterochromaffin cells of the gastrointestinal mucosa secrete large amounts of histamine after a meal, with the excess moving into the portal circulation and intestinal lumen. In addition, metoclopramide is a dopamine D_2

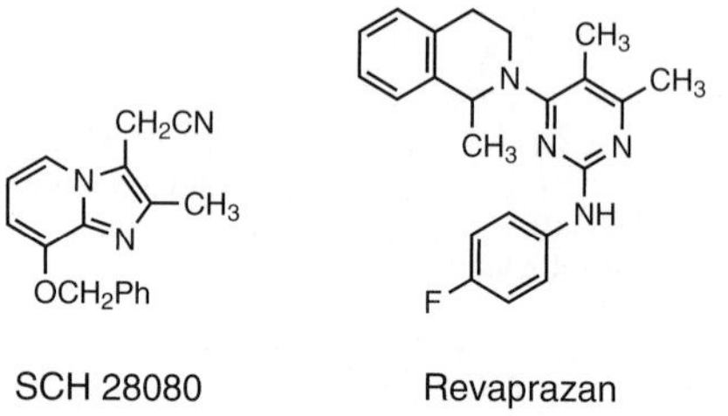

SCH 28080 Revaprazan

FIGURE 32.20 Examples of proton pump competitive K^+ inhibitors.

TABLE 32.12 Examples of Prokinetic Agents

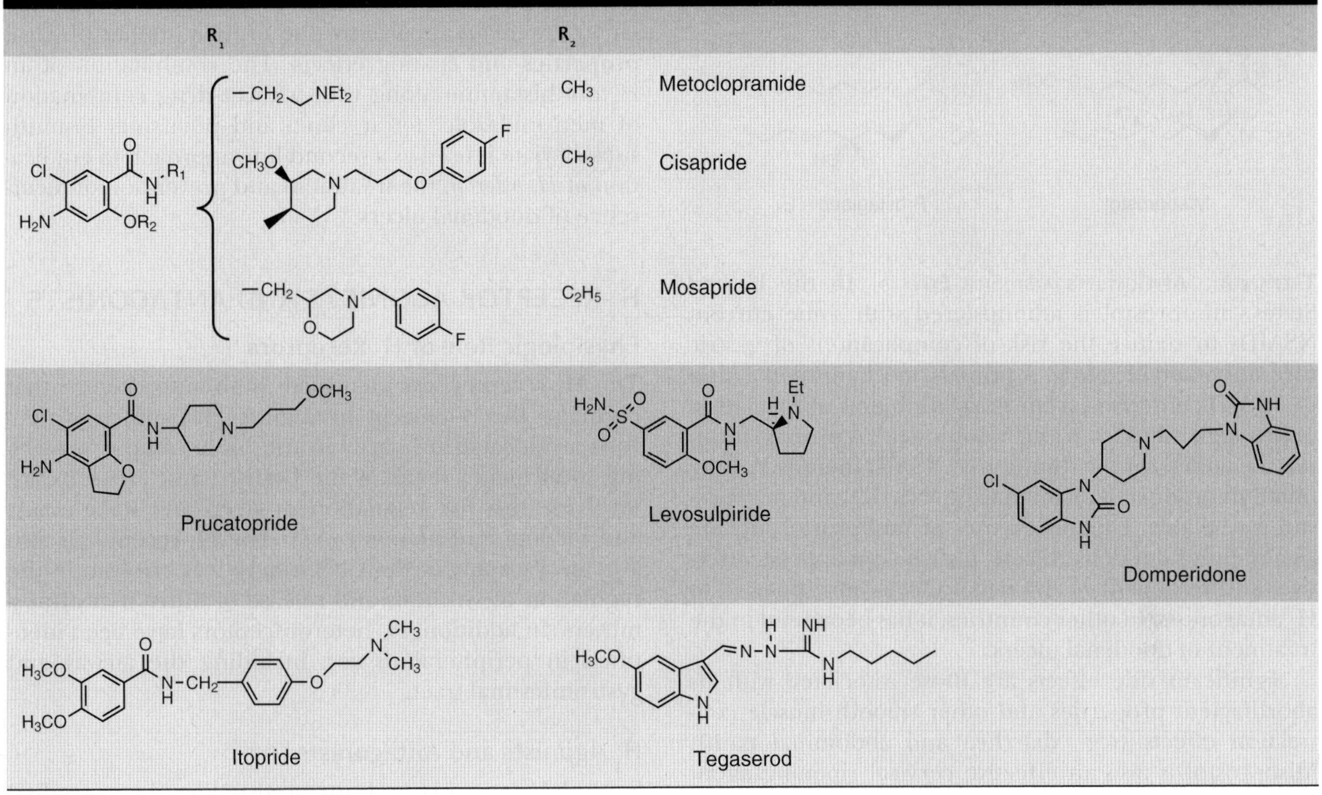

antagonist. Metoclopramide and some other prokinetic drugs also have 5-HT_3 antagonism effects. Metoclopramide is used in GERD, diabetic gastroparesis, and nausea and vomiting caused by emetogenic cancer chemotherapy.

Cisapride was removed from the US prescription market because of metabolism-based interactions. In the presence of competing CYP3A4 substrates, high concentrations of the parent molecule lead to life-threatening cardiac arrhythmias via interaction with the hERG K^+ channel, similar to H_1 antihistamines terfenadine and astemizole. It is available only through an investigational limited access program.

Structurally related agents, some of which are available outside the United States, are in clinical trial. Among them are prucalopride, a potent and selective 5-HT_4 receptor agonist used for chronic constipation (85); mosapride, which is used primarily for gastritis (86); and itopride, which is also being tried for gastritis (87). Tegaserod is also a selective 5-HT_4 partial agonist that is used in irritable bowel syndrome in women and has been used successfully in critically ill patients with gastroparesis.

Other agents (e.g., domperidone, a specific peripheral D_2-receptor antagonist) also have effects on the upper gastrointestinal tract similar to metoclopramide and are used for antiemetic effects and the treatment of gastroparesis and pediatric gastroesophageal reflux. Domperidone is available as an investigational drug for patients with severe gastrointestinal disorders who are refractory to other therapies.

Erythromycin, a macrolide antibiotic (Chapter 33), is also used as a prokinetic agent. It is a motilin receptor agonist. Motilin is a polypeptide hormone in endocrine cells of the distal stomach and the duodenum. It increases lower esophageal sphincter pressure and is responsible for the migrating motor complex (i.e., the process of irregular and subsequently regular contractions that clear the stomach of undigested food).

Prostaglandins

Prostaglandins have antisecretory effects on gastric acid (Fig. 32.17). Besides inhibiting adenylyl cyclase activity in parietal cells that results in secretion of gastric acid, prostaglandins stimulate secretion of mucus and bicarbonate in adjacent superficial cells. Cytoprotective effects of endogenous E series prostaglandins and of other more stable synthetic congeners are observed. The only available oral prostaglandin in the United States is misoprostol. The orally administered carboxylic acid ester is hydrolyzed to the pharmacologically active carboxylic acid. It is a synthetic analog of prostaglandin E_1, in which structural changes at C-13, C-14, C-15, and C-16 are made to prevent rapid metabolic conversion to inactive products. The presence of the tertiary alcohol one carbon removed to C-16 obviates the usual conversion of the allylic secondary alcohol ($\Delta^{13,14}$-15-alcohol) of prostaglandins to the corresponding saturated ketones. A mixture of diastereomers of misoprostol is used; most of the activity arises from the 11*R*,16*S*-isomer (88). Misoprostol reduces basal levels of gastric acid secretion, but it has considerable smooth muscle contraction effects.

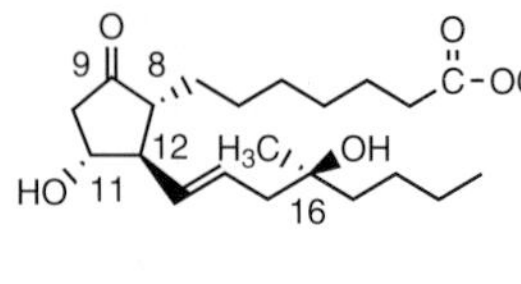

Misoprostol

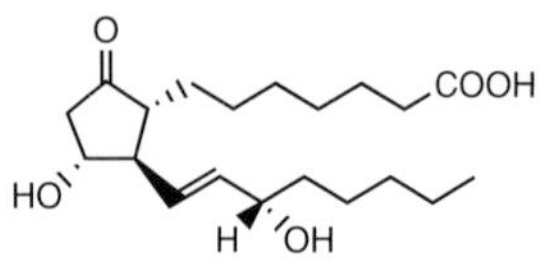

Prostaglandin E_1

Therapeutic Applications and Side Effects In the United States, misoprostol is administered with some current NSAIDs to reduce the risk of complications of gastric ulceration and bleeding. A primary mechanism of action of NSAIDs is derived from their inhibition of formation of prostaglandins from arachidonic acid. A prostaglandin may be added for the duration of NSAID therapy. A combination product of diclofenac (an NSAID) and misoprostol is available. Unlabelled uses of misoprostol include treatment of duodenal ulcers, for which it appears effective, and treatment of duodenal ulcers unresponsive to H_2 antagonists. In other countries, it has been used in the treatment of duodenal ulcers.

Significant side effects are those associated with its abortifacient properties and other smooth muscle contraction effects (e.g., diarrhea and abdominal pain). Misoprostol is also an effective cervical ripening agent (by vaginal application) for the induction of labor. Other unlabeled uses include the treatment of postpartum hemorrhage and, with mifepristone, pregnancy termination.

Sucralfate and Insoluble Bismuth Preparations

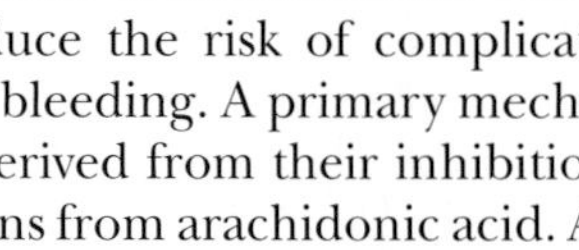

Sucralfate $R = SO_3[Al_2(OH)_5]$

Sucralfate is a complex of the sulfuric acid ester of sucrose and aluminum hydroxide. Secondary polymerization with aluminum hydroxide forms intermolecular bridges between molecules of sulfate esters with aluminum (89). Limited dissociation of the complex occurs in gastric acid, but these anionic sulfate esters form insoluble adherent complexes with the proteinaceous exudate at the abraded surface of a crater of the ulcerated area in the stomach. This physical complex protects the ulcer from the erosive action of pepsin and bile salts. Sucralfate also stimulates synthesis and release of prostaglandins, bicarbonate, and epidermal and fibroblast growth factors. Significant ulcer healing effects are noted in placebo-controlled trials. Only small amounts of sucralfate are absorbed systemically. In renal impairment, there is a risk of accumulation of absorbed aluminum from the drug. Sucralfate reduces absorption of other drugs including H_2 antihistamines, quinolone antibiotics, phenytoin, and perhaps warfarin (90).

Bismuth-containing preparations (those containing colloidal salts of bismuth subsalicylate) have effects similar to sucralfate apparently due to their similar physical properties and coating effects. The combination of an H_2 antihistamine along with a three-drug combination of metronidazole, tetracycline, and potassium bismuth subsalicylate is used as a second-line approach to eradication of *H. pylori* in the treatment and prevention of recurrence of duodenal ulcers.

H_3-RECEPTOR AGONISTS AND ANTAGONISTS

Physiologic Role of H_3 Receptors

The H_3 receptor was identified as an autoreceptor that regulates the release of histamine. Histaminergic neurons are located primarily in the hippocampus projecting to all major areas of the brain. These neurons are involved with the regulation of sleep and wakefulness and feeding and memory (17). The H_3 receptor is also a heteroreceptor in the CNS, where it is involved in the regulation of synthesis and release of other neurotransmitters. In addition, H_3 heteroreceptors have been identified in peripheral tissues, including the airway and gastrointestinal tract.

H_3 Agonists and Antagonists

Several H_3 agonists and antagonists have been studied (Table 32.13). *R*-α-Methylhistamine is a more potent agonist than is histamine. The addition of methyl groups to the side chain or to the aliphatic amine nitrogen of histamine usually results in potent H_3 agonists (e.g., α,α-dimethylhistamine, *R*-α,*S*-β-dimethylhistamine, and *N*-methyl- and *N*-ethylhistamine), unlike the deleterious effect of these changes on H_1 and H_2 agonist activity. Other selective agonists are the isothiourea imetit, immepip and its *N*-methyl analog methimepip, both substituted piperidines, immethridine, a pyridine congener of immepip, and SCH 50971. All retain the imidazole ring of histamine.

Early H_3 antagonists, like thioperamide and clobenpropit analogs of immepip and imetit, respectively, are primarily pharmacologic tools. Like the H_3 agonists, these agents retain the imidazole group but possess widely varying *N*-substituents. Some of the imidazole-containing agonist and antagonist analogs have affinity for other receptors (e.g., some α-adrenergic receptor subtypes), and they have the potential to interact with CYP450 enzymes as an iron-porphyrin ligand. Thus, non–imidazole-containing ligands have been sought.

Centrally acting H_3 antagonists are under study by several drug companies. Agents are sought for a variety of disorders. These include treatment of depression, mild cognitive impairment, Alzheimer disease, schizophrenia, narcolepsy, obesity, and attention-deficient hyperactivity disorder. Examples of lead compounds, some of which have entered clinical trial, are tiprolisant, JNJ 1018146, and GSK-189254 (91,92).

TABLE 32.13 Examples of H_3 Agonists and Antagonist

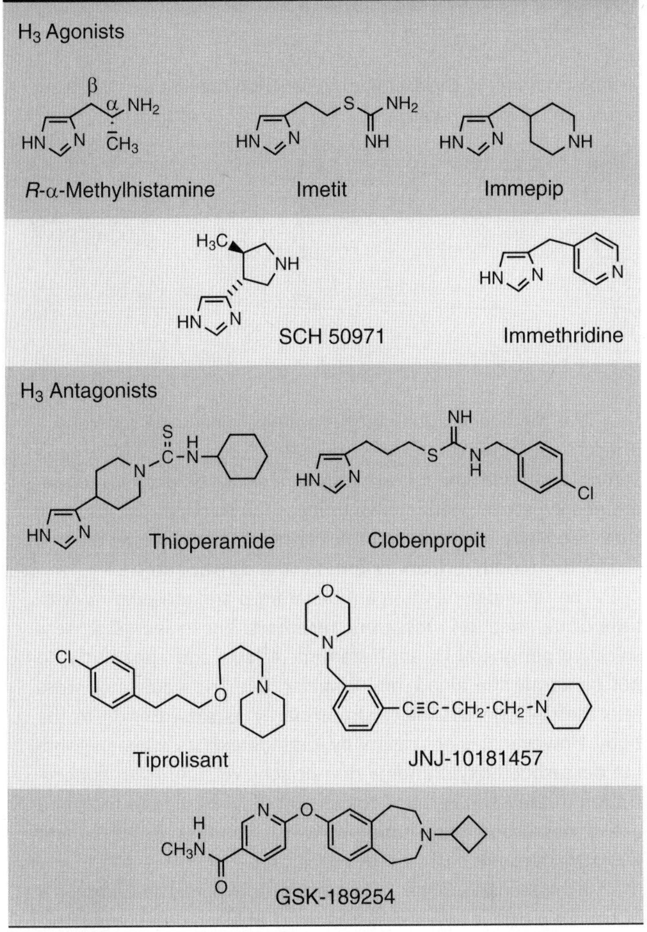

H_4-RECEPTOR AGONISTS AND ANTAGONISTS

Physiologic Role of H_4 Receptors

The H_4 receptor is expressed in mast cells, eosinophils, and other cells of hematopoietic lineage, including basophils and T cells. It is a relatively recent discovery; thus, much is not yet understood about its physiologic role. It is thought to play a role in inflammatory responses, especially in the mediation of chemotactic responses. Its sequence homology is greatest with H_3 receptor (35% to 40%) and is very low versus H_1 and H_2 receptors (93).

The localization of H_4 receptors largely in hematopoietic cells such as dendritic cells, mast cells, monocytes, eosinophils, basophils, and T cells, with a role in chemotaxis and mediator release, led to reevaluation of their role in physiologic effects in altered responses to inflammatory stimuli. As such, histamine has taken on a larger role in T-cell responses (94,95).

H_4 Agonists and Antagonists

Classical leukocyte chemoattractant effects that occur are blocked by thioperamide, an H_3/H_4 antihistamine. Other H_3 receptor ligands such as *R*-α-methylhistamine and imetit are also agonists at H_4 receptors, but they have lower affinity than at H_3 receptors (Table 32.13). Clobenpropit is a partial agonist at H_4 receptors, but it is an H_3 antihistamine (inverse agonist). Thioperamide is an inverse agonist at H_4 receptors and at H_3 receptors. 4-Methylhistamine (Fig. 32.21) has greater affinity (>100-fold) for H_4 receptors than other histamine receptor subtypes (96).

Selective H_4 antihistamines have been reported, beginning from JNJ 7777120 (Fig. 32.21). It blocks many mediated functions, including histamine-induced chemotaxis in mast cells and eosinophils (97). Conditions in which H_4 antagonists may be useful include several autoimmune inflammatory and allergic disorders, including rheumatoid arthritis, asthma, allergic rhinitis, pruritus, and inflammatory bowel disease. Nasal stuffiness and blockage in allergic rhinitis, conditions that are poorly treated with H_1 and H_2 antihistamines, can also possibly be treated using H_4 antihistamines. Analogs of JNJ 7777120 and congeners in related nitrogen-containing heterocyclic systems are being investigated (98,99).

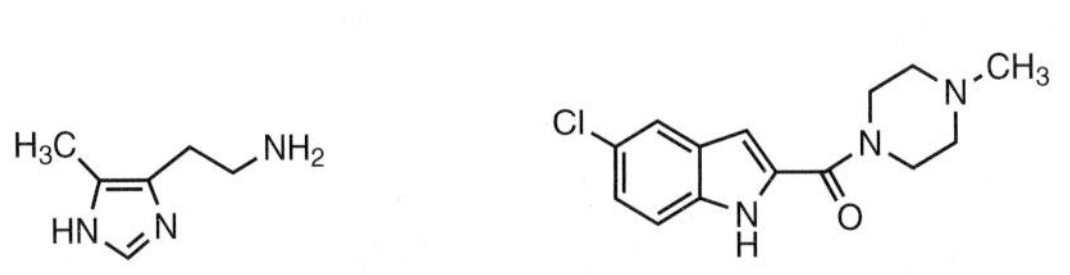

4-Methylhistamine JNJ 7777120

FIGURE 32.21 Other ligands at the H_4 receptor.

SCENARIO: OUTCOME AND ANALYSIS

Outcome

Anne Pace, PharmD

The pharmacist assesses the patient as having seasonal allergies and recommends one of the over-the-counter second-generation antihistamines, loratadine or cetirizine. The pharmacist does not recommend one of the first-generation antihistamines because of a drug–disease interaction. CP has benign prostatic hyperplasia, which causes urinary retention that will be worsened if CP uses a first-generation antihistamine.

Chemical Analysis

S. William Zito and Victoria Roche

H_1 antihistamines were thought of as reversible competitive inhibitors of the interaction of histamine with the H_1 receptors. However, it is now recognized that they are inverse agonists that bind to the inactive conformation of the H_1 receptor shifting the active-inactive equilibrium of the receptor toward the inactive state. All H_1-receptor antagonists have the following pharmacophore:

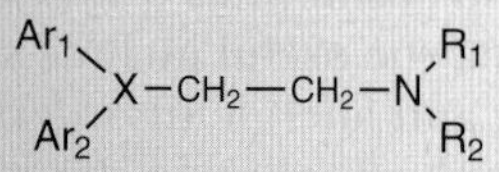

The X group defines the chemical classes:

Aminoalkyl ether	X = CH_2-O-
Ethylenediamines	X = -N-, phenothiazines, piperazines
Alkylamines	X = -C-(sp^3), -C= (sp^2)

Both aromatic rings are necessary for antagonistic activity at the H_1 receptor. Having only one aromatic ring makes these compounds more like histamine, and therefore, they might have agonist activity. Sometimes the two aromatic rings are bridged, as in loratadine, or the aminoethyl function may be part of a ring structure, as in cetirizine.

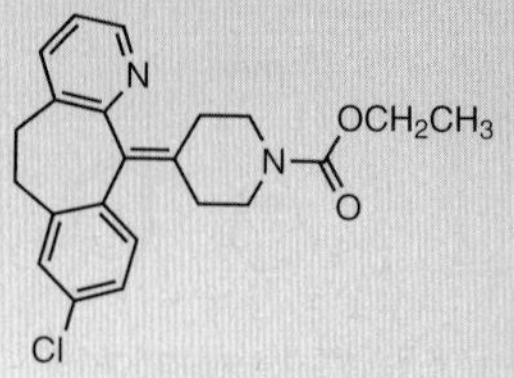

Loratadine

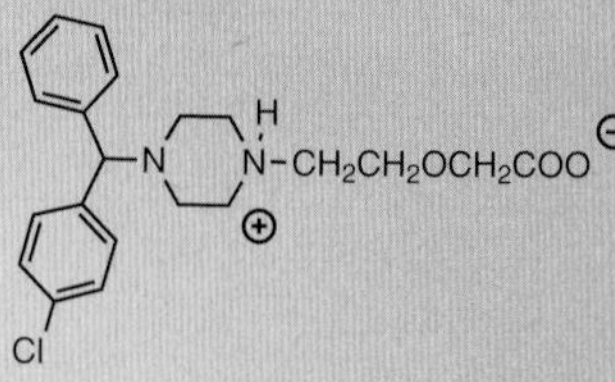

Cetirizine

The first-generation antihistamines have adverse central effects (sedation, drowsiness, decreased cognitive ability, and somnolence) with the following general order of sedative action: aminoalkyl ethers > ethylenediamines > alkylamines. In addition, they also have significant antimuscarinic action including blurred vision, dry mouth, urinary retention, and constipation.

The second-generation antihistamines are nonsedating with little or no effect on muscarinic receptors. These agents possess selective peripheral H_1 antihistaminic effects and apparently do not penetrate the blood–brain barrier. Cetirizine does not cross into the CNS because it exists primarily as a zwitterion in the body. However, it is not clear why loratadine or its active metabolite descarboethoxyloratidine do not achieve significant concentration in the CNS. Perhaps conversion of loratadine to the more active descarboethoxyloratidine, which requires CYP3A4 and CYP2D6, does not easily occur in the CNS.

In this scenario, CP has benign prostatic hyperplasia. Symptoms of benign prostatic hyperplasia are those of bladder outlet obstruction (i.e., weak stream, hesitancy, urinary frequency, urgency, nocturia, incomplete emptying, terminal dribbling, overflow or urge incontinence, and complete urinary retention). Therefore, the first-generation H_1 antihistamines, especially the aminoalkyl ethers, are contraindicated because of their antimuscarinic activity, which can slow urine flow and exacerbate urinary retention.

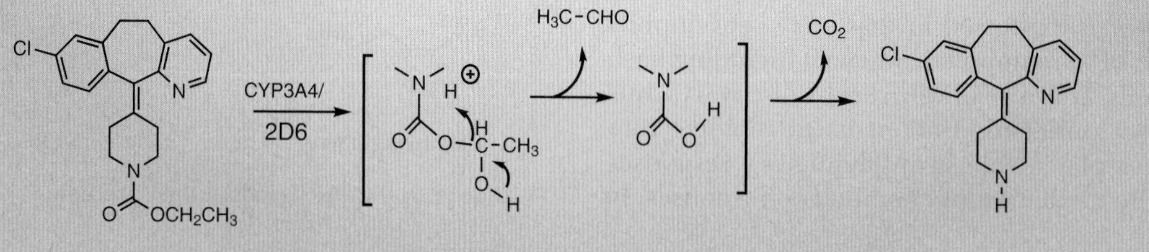

Loratadine

Descarboethoxyloratadine

CASE STUDY

S. William Zito and Victoria Roche

FT is a 45-year-old man who visits his ear, nose, and throat specialist complaining of severe allergic rhinitis and itching, burning, and tearing in both eyes that is affecting his vision. FT is a New York City taxi driver and is worried about his ability to drive safely. A review of FT's medical records reveals he has a family history of allergic diseases. He has glaucoma and often suffers from bouts of eczema. The glaucoma is treated with 0.25% timolol maleate (1 gtt bid), and eczema flares respond well to treatment with an over-the-counter topical steroid. FT states that these recent symptoms began shortly after he picked up a woman at the local airport who was relocating from the Midwest and transporting four cats to her new home in New York. His physician diagnoses FT with an exacerbation of atopic keratoconjunctivitis (AKC). He prescribes fluticasone (nasal spray) to treat the allergic rhinitis but is reluctant to prescribe steroid eye drops to treat the AKC because ocular steroids can promote further development of FT's glaucoma. Which of the following antihistamines would be the best choice in this case?

1. Conduct a thorough and mechanistic SAR analysis of the three therapeutic options in the case.
2. Apply the chemical understanding gained from the SAR analysis to this patient's specific needs to make a therapeutic recommendation.

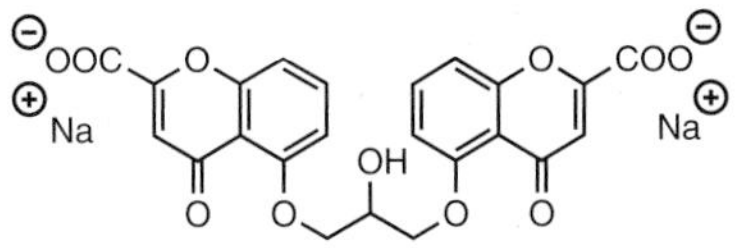

1

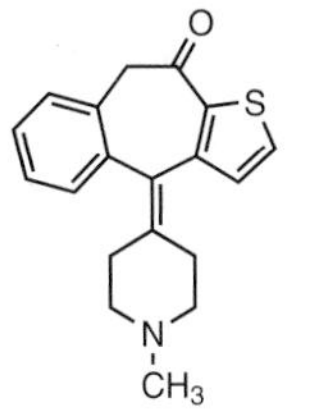

2

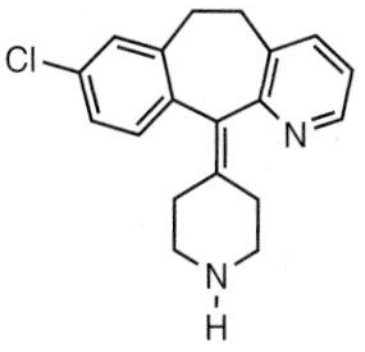

3

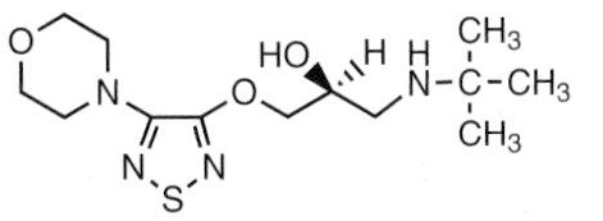

Timolol

References

1. Babe KSJ, Serafin WE. Histamine, bradykinin, and their antagonists. In: Hardman JG, Limbird LE, Mollinoff PB, et al., eds. Goodman and Gilman's the Pharmacological Basis of Therapeutics, 9th Ed. New York: McGraw-Hill, 1995:581–600.
2. Zhang M-Q, Leurs R, Timmerman H. Histamine H_1-receptor antagonists. In: Wolff ME, ed. Burger's Medicinal Chemistry and Drug Discovery, 5th Ed. New York: John Wiley & Sons, 1997:495–559.
3. Cooper DG, Young RC, Durant GJ, et al. Histamine receptors. In: Emmett JC, ed. Comprehensive Medicinal Chemistry: The Rational Design, Mechanistic Study, and Therapeutic Application of Chemical Compounds, Vol 3: Membranes and Receptors. Oxford, UK: Pergamon Press, 1990:343–421.
4. Watanabe T, Yamatodani A, Maeyama K, et al. Pharmacology of a-fluoromethylhistidine, a specific inhibitor of histidine decarboxylase. Trends Pharmacol Sci 1990;11:363–367.
5. Moya-Garcia AA, Pino-Angeles A, Gil-Redondo R, et al. Structural features of mammalian histidine decarboxylase reveal the basis for specific inhibition. Br J Pharmacol 2009;157:4–13.
6. Schayer RC, Cooper JAD. Metabolism of ^{14}C histamine in man. J Appl Physiol 1956;9:481–483.
7. Marone G, Genovese A, Granata F, et al. Pharmacological modulation of human mast cells and basophils. Clin Exp Allergy 2002;32:1682–1689.
8. Oliver JM, Kepley CL, Ortega E, et al. Immunologically mediated signaling in basophils and mast cells: finding therapeutic targets for allergic diseases in the human FceR1 signaling pathway. Immunopharmacology 2000;48:269–281.
9. Bischoff SC. Role of mast cells in allergic and non-allergic immune responses: comparison of human and murine data. Nat Rev Immunol 2007;7:93–104.
10. Kalesnikoff J, Galli SJ. New developments in mast cell biology. Nat Immunol 2008;9:1215–1223.
11. Church MK, Shute JK, Jensen HM. Mast cell-derived mediators. In: Adkinson NF, Yunginer JW, Busse WW, eds. Middleton's allergy: principles and practice, 6th Ed. Philadelphia: Mosby, 2003:189–212.
12. Goetzl EJ. Lipid mediators of hypersensitivity and inflammation. In: Adkinson NF, Yunginer JW, Busse WW, eds. Middleton's allergy: principles and practice, 6th Ed. Philadelphia: Mosby, 2003:213–230.
13. Jutel M, Akdis M, Akdis CA. Histamine, histamine receptors and their role in immune pathology. Clin Exp Allergy 2009;39:1786–1800.
14. Simons FER, Akdis CA. Histamine and H_1-antihistamines. In: Adkinson NF, Bochner BS, Busse WW, eds. Middleton's Allergy: Principles and Practice, 7th Ed. Philadelphia: Mosby, 2009:1517–1547.
15. Bakker RA, Timmerman H, Leurs R. Histamine receptors: specific ligands, receptor biochemistry, and signal transduction. In: Simons FER, ed. Histamine and H_1-Antihistamines in Allergic Disease, 2nd Ed. New York: Marcel Dekker, Inc., 2002:27–64.
16. Leurs R, Vollinga RC, Timmerman H. The medicinal chemistry and therapeutic potentials of ligands of the histamine H_3 receptor. Prog Drug Res 1995;45:107–165.
17. Leurs R, Bakker RA, Timmerman H, et al. The histamine H_3 receptor: from gene cloning to H_3 receptor drugs. Nat Rev Drug Discov 2005;4:107–120.
18. Edwards AM, Holgate ST. The chromones: cromolyn sodium and neodocromil sodium. In: Adkinson NF, Bochner BS, Busse WW, et al., eds. Middleton's Allergy: Principles and Practice, 7th Ed. Philadelphia: Mosby, 2009:1591–1601.
19. Cook EB, Stahl JL, Barney NP, et al. Mechanisms of antihistamines and mast cell stabilizers in ocular allergic inflammation. Med Chem Rev 2004;1:333–347.
20. Forneau E, Bovet D. Recherches sur l'action sypmathicolytique d'un nouveau derive du dioxane. Arch Int Pharmacodyn 1933;46:1781–191.
21. Simons FER. Advances in H_1-antihistamines. N Engl J Med 2004;351:2203–2217.
22. Leurs R, Church MK, Taglialatela M. H_1-Antihistamines: inverse agonism, anti-inflammatory actions and cardiac effects. Clin Exp Allergy 2002;32:489–498.
23. Ariens EJ. Stereoselectivity of bioactive agents: general aspects. In: Ariens EJ, Soudijn W, Timmermans PBM, eds. Stereochemistry and Biological Activity. Oxford, UK: Blackwell Scientific Publications, 1983:11–32.
24. Casy AF, Ganellin CR, Mercer AD, et al. Analogues of triprolidine: structural influences upon antihistamine activity. J Pharm Pharmacol 1992;44:791–795.
25. Ebnöther A, Weber HP. Synthesis and absolute configuration of clemastine and its isomers. Helv Chim Acta 1976;59:2462–2468.
26. Timmerman H, Rekker RF, Harms AF, et al. Effect of alkyl substitution in drugs. XXII. Antihistaminic and anticholinergic activity of a series of thio ether analogs of substituted diphenhydramines. Arzneim-Forsch 1970;20:1258–1259.
27. Simons FER. Antihistamines. In: Adkinson NF, Yunginer JW, Busse WW, eds. Middleton's Allergy: Principles and Practice, 6th Ed. Philadelphia: Mosby, 2003:834–869.
28. Towart R, Sautel M, Moret E, et al. Investigation of the antihistaminic action of dimethindene maleate (Fenistil) and its optical isomers. In: Timmerman H, van der Goot H, eds. Agents Actions Supplements, Vol. 33: New Perspectives in Histamine Research, 1991:403–408.
29. Hanna PE, Ahmed AE. Conformationally restricted analogs of histamine H_1 receptor antagonists: *trans-* and *cis-*1,5-diphenyl-3-dimethylaminopyrrolidine. J Med Chem 1973;16:963–968.
30. Shafi'ee A, Hite G. The absolute configurations of the pheniramines, methyl phenidates, and pipradrols. J Med Chem 1969;12:266–270.
31. Otsuki I, Ishiko J, Sakai M, et al. Pharmacological activities of doxepin hydrochloride in relation to its geometrical isomers. Oyo Yakuri 1972;6:973–984.
32. Piwinski JJ, Wong JK, Chan TM, et al. Hydroxylated metabolites of loratadine: an example of conformational diastereomers due to atropisomerism. J Org Chem 1990;55:3341–3350.

33. Remy DC, Rittle KE, Hunt CA, et al. (+)- and (−)-3-Methoxycyproheptadine. A comparative evaluation of the antiserotonin, antihistaminic, anticholinergic, and orexigenic properties with cyproheptadine. J Med Chem 1977;20:1681–1684.
34. Hawes EM. N+-Glucuronidation, a common pathway in human metabolism of drugs with a tertiary amine group. Drug Metab Dispos 1998;26:830–837.
35. Golightly LK, Greos LS. Second-generation antihistamines: actions and efficacy in the management of allergic disorders. Drugs 2005;65:341–384.
36. Molimard M, Diquet B, Strolin-Benedetti M. Comparison of pharmacokinetics and metabolism of desloratadine, fexofenadine, levocetirizine and mizolastine in humans. Fund Clin Pharmacol 2004;18:399–411.
37. Garteiz DA, Hook RH, Walker BJ, et al. Pharmacokinetics and biotransformation studies of terfenadine in man. Arzneim-Forsch 1982;32:1185–1190.
38. Soldovieri MV, Miceli F, Taglialatela M. Cardiotoxic effects of antihistamines: from basics to clinics (...and back). Chem Res Toxicol 2008;21:997–1004.
39. Aronov AM. Predictive in silico modeling for hERG channel blockers. Drug Discov Today 2005;10:149–155.
40. Pearlstein R, Vaz R, Rampe D. Understanding the structure-activity relationship of the human ether-a-go-go-related gene cardiac K^+ channel. A model for bad behavior. J Med Chem 2003;46:2017–2022.
41. Zhang MQ, Caldirola P, Timmerman H. Chiral manipulation of drug selectivity: studies on a series of terfenadine-derived dual antagonists of H_1-receptors and calcium channels. Agents Actions 1994;41(Spec. Conf. Issue):C140–C142.
42. Miura M, Uno T, Tateishi T, et al. Pharmacokinetics of fexofenadine enantiomers in healthy subjects. Chirality 2007;19:223–227.
43. Sakugawa T, Miura M, Hokama N, et al. Enantioselective disposition of fexofenadine with the P-glycoprotein inhibitor verapamil. Br J Clin Pharmacol 2009;67:535–540.
44. DuBuske LM. Pharmacology of desloratadine: special characteristics. Clin Drug Investigation 2002;22(Suppl 2):1–11.
45. Gupta S, Banfield C, Kantesaria B, et al. Pharmacokinetic and safety profile of desloratadine and fexofenadine when coadministered with azithromycin: a randomized, placebo-controlled, parallel-group study. Clin Ther 2001;23:451–466.
46. Yumibe N, Huie K, Chen KJ, et al. Identification of human liver cytochrome P450 enzymes that metabolize the nonsedating antihistamine loratadine. Formation of descarboethoxyloratadine by CYP3A4 and CYP2D6. Biochem Pharmacol 1996;51:165–172.
47. Dizdar EA, Sekerel BE, Tuncer A. Desloratadine: a review of pharmacology and clinical efficacy in allergic rhinitis and urticaria. Therapy 2008;5:817–828.
48. Murdoch D, Goa KL, Keam SJ. Desloratadine: an update of its efficacy in the management of allergic disorders. Drugs 2003;63:2051–2077.
49. Ramanathan R, Reyderman L, Kulmatycki K, et al. Disposition of loratadine in healthy volunteers. Xenobiotica 2007;37:753–769.
50. Ramanathan R, Reyderman L, Su AD, et al. Disposition of desloratadine in healthy volunteers. Xenobiotica 2007;37:770–787.
51. Keam SJ, Plosker GL. Rupatadine a review of its use in the management of allergic disorders. Drugs 2007;67:457–474.
52. Curran MP, Scott LJ, Perry CM. Cetirizine: a review of its use in allergic disorders. Drugs 2004;64:523–561.
53. Gillard M, Van Der Perren C, Moguilevsky N, et al. Binding characteristics of cetirizine and levocetirizine to human H_1 histamine receptors: contribution of Lys191 and Thr194. Mol Pharmacol 2002;61:391–399.
54. Benedetti MS, Plisnier M, Kaise J, et al. Absorption, distribution, metabolism and excretion of [^{14}C]levocetirizine, the R enantiomer of cetirizine, in healthy volunteers. Eur J Clin Pharmacol 2001;57:571–582.
55. van Cauwenberge P, De Belder T, Sys L. A review of the second-generation antihistamine ebastine for the treatment of allergic disorders. Expert Opin Pharmacother 2004;5:1807–1813.
56. Lebrun-Vignes B, Diquet B, Chosidow O. Clinical pharmacokinetics of mizolastine. Clin Pharmacokinet 2001;40:501–507.
57. Kuna P, Bachert C, Nowacki Z, et al. Efficacy and safety of bilastine 20 mg compared with cetirizine 10 mg and placebo for the symptomatic treatment of seasonal allergic rhinitis: a randomized, double-blind, parallel-group study. Clin Exp Allergy 2009;39:1338–1347.
58. Bielory L, Lien KW, Bigelsen S. Efficacy and tolerability of newer antihistamines in the treatment of allergic conjunctivitis. Drugs 2005;65:215–228.
59. Sharif NA, Hellberg MR, Yanni JM. Antihistamines, topical ocular. In: Wolff ME, ed. Burger's Medicinal Chemistry and Drug Discovery, 5th Ed. New York: John Wiley & Sons, Inc., 1997:255–279.
60. Polivka Z, Budesinsky M, Holubek J, et al. 4H-Benzo[4,5-cyclohepta[1,2-b] thiophenes and 9,10-dihydro derivatives. Sulfonium analogs of pizotifen and ketotifen. Chirality of ketotifen. Synthesis of the 2-bromo derivative of ketotifen. Collect Czech Chem Commun 1989;54:2443–2469.
61. Roberts S, McDonald IM. Inhibitors of gastric acid secretion. In: Abraham DJ, ed. Burger's Medicinal Chemistry and Drug Discovery, Vol. 4: Autocoids, Diagnostics, and Drugs from New Biology, 6th Ed. Hoboken, NJ: Wiley-Interscience, 2003:85–127.
62. Ganellin CR. Discovery of cimetidine. In: Roberts SM, Price BJ, eds. Medicinal Chemsitry: The Role of Organic Chemistry in Drug Research. London: Academic Press, 1985:93–118.
63. Price AH, Brogden RN. Nizatidine. A preliminary review of its pharmacodynamic and pharmacokinetic properties, and its therapeutic use in peptic ulcer disease. Drugs 1988;36:521–539.
64. Somogyi A, Muirhead M. Pharmacokinetic interactions of cimetidine. Clin Pharmacokinet 1987;12:321–366.
65. Robinson M. Proton pump inhibitors: update on their role in acid-related gastrointestinal diseases. Int J Clin Pract 2005;59:709–715.
66. Vakil N. Review article: new pharmacological agents for the treatment of gastroesophageal reflux disease. Aliment Pharmacol Ther 2004;19:1041–1049.
67. Lindberg P, Brandstrom A, Wallmark B, et al. Omeprazole: the first proton pump inhibitor. Med Res Rev 1990;10:1–54.
68. Shin JM, Cho YM, Sachs G. Chemistry of covalent inhibition of the gastric (H^+,K^+)-ATPase by proton pump inhibitors. J Am Chem Soc 2004;126:7800–7811.
69. Besancon M, Simon A, Sachs G, Shin JM. Sites of reaction of the gastric H,K-ATPase with extracytoplasmic thiol reagents. J Biol Chem 1997;272:22438–2246.
70. Horn J. Review article: relationship between the metabolism and efficacy of proton pump inhibitors—focus on rabeprazole. Aliment Pharmacol Ther 2004;20(Suppl 6):11–19.
71. Galmiche JP, des Varannes SB, Ducrotte P, et al. Tenatoprazole, a novel proton pump inhibitor with a prolonged plasma half-life: effects on intragastric pH and comparison with esomeprazole in healthy volunteers. Aliment Pharmacol Ther 2004;19:655–662.
72. Andersson T. Pharmacokinetics, metabolism and interactions of acid pump inhibitors. Focus on omeprazole, lansoprazole and pantoprazole. Clin Pharmacokinet 1996;31:9–28.
73. Andersson T. Single-isomer drugs: true therapeutic advances. Clin Pharmacokinet 2004;43:279–285.
74. Agranat I, Caner H, Caldwell J. Putting chirality to work: the strategy of chiral switches. Nat Rev Drug Discov 2002;1:753–768.
75. Lind T, Cederberg C, Ekenved G, et al. Effect of omeprazole, a gastric proton pump inhibitor, on pentagastrin stimulated acid secretion in man. Gut 1983;24:270–276.
76. Lind T, Rydberg L, Kyleback A, et al. Esomeprazole provides improved acid control vs. omeprazole in patients with symptoms of gastro-esophageal reflux disease. Aliment Pharmacol Ther 2000;14:861–867.
77. Andersson T, Weidolf L. Stereoselective disposition of proton pump inhibitors. Clin Drug Invest 2008;28:263–279.
78. Zhou Q, Yan X-F, Pan W-S, et al. Is the required therapeutic effect always achieved by racemic switch of proton-pump inhibitors? World J Gastroenterol 2008;14:2617–2619.
79. Jain SC. A postmarketing surveillance study of dexrabeprazole in the treatment of acid peptic disorders. J Indian Med Assn 2009;107:111–113.
80. Hunt RH, Armstrong D, Yaghoobi M, et al. The pharmacodynamics and pharmacokinetics of S-tenatoprazole-Na 30 mg, 60 mg and 90 mg vs. esomeprazole 40 mg in healthy male subjects. Aliment Pharmacol Ther 2010;31:648–657.
81. Chisholm MA. Pharmacotherapy of duodenal and gastric ulcerations. Am J Pharm Ed 1998;62:196–203.
82. Andersson K, Carlsson E. Potassium-competitive acid blockade: a new therapeutic strategy in acid-related diseases. Pharmacol Ther 2005;108:294–307.
83. Kim H-K, Park S-H, Cheung D-Y, et al. Clinical trial: inhibitory effect of revaprazan on gastric acid secretion in healthy male subjects. J Gastroenterol Hepatol 2010;25:1618–1625.
84. De Maeyer JH, Lefebvre RA, Schuurkes JAJ. 5-HT_4 receptor agonists: similar but not the same. Neurogastroenterol Motil 2008;20:99–112.
85. Frampton JE. Prucalopride. Drugs 2009;69:2463–2476.
86. Curran MP, Robinson DM. Mosapride in gastrointestinal disorders. Drugs 2008;68:981–991.
87. Holtmann G, Talley NJ, Liebregts T, et al. A placebo-controlled trial of itopride in functional dyspepsia. N Engl J Med 2006;354:832–840.
88. Won-Kim S, Kachur JF, Gaginella TS. Stereospecific actions of misoprostol on rat colonic electrolyte transport. Prostaglandins 1993;46:221–231.
89. Nagashima R, Yoshida N. Sucralfate, a basic aluminum salt of sucrose sulfate. I. Behaviors in gastroduodenal pH. Arzneim-Forsch 1979;29:1668–1676.
90. Marks IN. Sucralfate: worldwide experience in recurrence therapy. J Clin Gastroenterol 1987;9(Suppl 1):18–22.
91. Chazot PL. Therapeutic potential of histamine H_3 receptor antagonists in dementias. Drug News Perspect 2010;23:99–103.
92. Raddatz R, Tao M, Hudkins RL. Histamine H_3 antagonists for treatment of cognitive deficits in CNS diseases. Current Topics Med Chem 2010;10:153–169.
93. Jablonowski JA, Carruthers NI, Thurmond RL. The histamine H_4 receptor and potential therapeutic uses for H_4 ligands. Mini-Revs Med Chem 2004;4:993–1000.
94. Thurmond RL, Gelfand EW, Dunford PJ. The role of histamine H_1 and H_4 receptors in allergic inflammation: the search for new antihistamines. Nat Rev Drug Discov 2008;7:41–53.
95. Zampeli E, Tiligada E. The role of histamine H_4 receptor in immune and inflammatory disorders. Br J Pharmacol 2009;157:24–33.
96. Lim HD, van Rijn RM, Ling P, et al. Evaluation of histamine H_1-, H_2-, and H_3-receptor ligands at the human histamine H_4 receptor: identification of 4-methylhistamine as the first potent and selective H_4 receptor agonist. J Pharmacol Exp Ther 2005;314:1310–1321.
97. Thurmond RL, Desai PJ, Dunford PJ, et al. A potent and selective histamine H_4 receptor antagonist with anti-inflammatory properties. J Pharmacol Exp Ther 2004;309:404–413.
98. Engelhardt H, Smits RA, Leurs R, et al. A new generation of anti-histamines: histamine H_4 receptor antagonists on their way to the clinic. Curr Opin Drug Discov Dev 2009;12:628–643.
99. Smits RA, Leurs R, de Esch IJP. Major advances in the development of histamine H_4 receptor ligands. Drug Discov Today 2009;14:745–753.

Chapter 33

Antibiotics and Antimicrobial Agents

ELMER J. GENTRY

*Drugs Covered in This Chapter**

ANTIBACTERIALS

- Fosfomycin
- Methenamine
- Metroindazole
- Nitrofurantoin
- Quinolone class
  - Besifloxacin
  - Ciprofloxacin
  - Gatifloxacin
  - Gemifloxacin
  - Levofloxacin, ofloxacin
  - Moxifloxacin
  - Norfloxacin
- Sulfonamide class
  - Silver sulfadiazine
  - Sulfacetamide
  - Sulfamethoxazole
  - Sulfisoxazole
- Trimethoprim

ANTIBIOTICS

- Penicillin class
  - Amoxicillin
  - Ampicillin
  - *Bacampicillin*
  - Benzylpenicillin
  - *Carbenicillin and indanyl carbenicillin*
  - Dicloxacillin
  - *Methicillin*
  - *Mezlocillin*
  - Nafcillin
  - Oxacillin
  - Phenoxymethylpenicillin
  - Piperacillin
  - Ticarcillin
- β-Lactamase Inhibitors
  - Clavulanic acid
  - Sulbactam
  - Tazobactam
- Cephalosporin class
  - Cefaclor
  - Cefadroxil
  - Cefazolin
  - Cefdinir
  - Cefditoren pivoxil
  - Cefepime
  - Cefixime
  - Cefotaxime
  - Cefotetan
  - Cefoxitin
  - Cefpodoxime proxetil
  - Cefprozil
  - Ceftaroline
  - Ceftazidime
  - Ceftibuten
  - Ceftizoxime
  - Ceftriaxone
  - Cefuroxime
  - Cephalexin
- Carbapenems
  - Doripenem
  - Ertapenem
  - Imipenem/cilastatin
  - Meropenem
- Monobactams
  - Aztreonam
- Aminoglycosides
  - Amikacin
  - Gentamicin
  - Kanamycin
  - Neomycin
  - *Spectinomycin*
  - Streptomycin
  - Tobramycin
- Macrolides and ketolides
  - Azithromycin
  - Clarithromycin
  - *Erythromycin estolate*
  - Erythromycin ethylsuccinate
  - Erythromycin stearate
  - Telithromycin
- Lincosamides
  - Clindamycin
  - Lincomycin
- Tetracyclines and glycylcyclines
  - Demeclocycline
  - Doxycycline
  - Minocycline

*Drugs listed include those available inside and outside of the United States; drugs available outside of the United States are shown in italics.

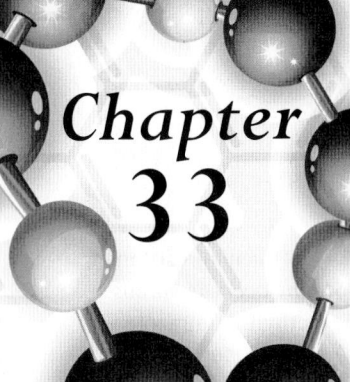

- Tetracycline
- Tigecycline
- Special Purpose Antibiotics
  - Bacitracin
  - Chloramphenicol
  - Daptomycin
  - Linezolid
  - Mupirocin
  - Polymyxin B
  - Quinupristin/dalfopristin
  - Retapamulin
  - Telavancin
  - Vancomycin

Abbreviations

AAC, aminoglycoside acetylase
ANT, aminoglycoside nucleotide transferase
6-APA, 6-aminopenicillanic acid
APH, aminoglycoside phosphorylase
ATP, adenosine triphosphate
CNS, central nervous system
GABA, γ-aminobutyric acid
GI, gastrointestinal
HABA, L-hydroxyaminobutyryl amide
MIC, minimum inhibitory concentration
MRSA, methicillin-resistant *Staphylococcus aureus*
MTT, methylthiotetrazole
PABA, *p*-aminobenzoic acid
PBP, penicillin-binding protein

SCENARIO

Elizabeth Coyle, PharmD

ER is a 24-year-old man who is in the intensive care unit after being in a motor vehicle accident 5 days ago. He sustained a laceration of his spleen, which was removed during surgery shortly after his arrival at the hospital. ER has been mechanically ventilated since surgery and has been stable for the last 96 hours; however, on rounds this morning the nurse states that ER spiked a fever (103°F) at 6 AM and his respiratory secretions have become more mucopurulent compared with yesterday. The team reviews the chest radiograph and appreciates new diffuse, bilateral infiltrates. Cultures are taken from his respiratory secretions, and ER is started empirically on cefepime 2 g every 8 hours and vancomycin 1 g every 12 hours. Two days later ER is not improving and the culture results come back as *Escherichia coli* that is sensitive only to carbapenems and aminoglycosides and has intermediate susceptibility to cefepime and pipericillin/tazobactam. The results also note that the *E. coli* is an extended spectrum beta-lacatmase (ESBL)–producing organism.

(The reader is directed to the clinical solution and chemical analysis of this case at the end of the chapter).

INTRODUCTION

Antibiotics are microbial metabolites or synthetic analogs inspired by them that, in small doses, inhibit the growth and survival of microorganisms without serious toxicity to the host. Selective toxicity is the key concept. Antibiotics are among the most frequently prescribed medications today, although microbial resistance due to evolutionary pressures and misuse threatens their continued efficacy. In many cases, the utility of natural antibiotics has been improved through medicinal chemical manipulation of the original structure, leading to broader antimicrobial spectrum, greater potency, lesser toxicity, more convenient administration, and additional pharmacokinetic advantages. Synthetic substances that are unrelated to natural products but still inhibit or kill microorganisms are referred to as antimicrobial agents.

All of the parts of our bodies that are in contact with the environment support microbial life. It is estimated that our body contains approximately 10 times more bacterial cells than human cells. These organisms are generally harmless to the host and actually provide a number of benefits. However, all of our internal fluids, organs, and body structures are sterile under normal circumstances, and the presence of bacteria, fungi, viruses, or other organisms in these places is diagnostic evidence of infection. When mild microbial disease occurs, an otherwise healthy patient will often recover without requiring treatment because their immune system is called upon to kill invasive microorganisms. When this is insufficient to protect us, appropriate therapeutic intervention is indicated.

HISTORY

Humankind has been subject to infection by microorganisms since before recorded history. One presumes that mankind has been searching for suitable therapy for nearly as long. This was a desperately difficult enterprise given the acute nature of most infections and the nearly total lack of understanding of their origins until the 19th century. Although one can find indications in ancient medical writings of folkloric use of plant and animal preparations, these factors were inefficiently applied, and they often failed. Until the discovery of bacteria by van Leeuwenhoek in 1676 and subsequent understanding of their role in infection about 150 years later, there was no hope for rational therapy.

In the 19th century, Robert Koch showed that specific microorganisms could always be isolated from the excreta and tissues of people with particular infectious diseases and that these same microorganisms were usually absent in healthy individuals. They could then be

CLINICAL SIGNIFICANCE

The treatment of bacterial infections is one of the few disease states that all clinicians are guaranteed to be challenged with at some time in their career. Because bacteria are constantly changing, the selection of appropriate antimicrobial therapy is crucial in providing efficacious treatment of infections. It is of the utmost importance that clinicians understand the medicinal chemistry of antimicrobial agents to choose the most effective therapy for their patients. Antimicrobial resistance trends are constantly changing and vary from institution to institution; therefore, a complete understanding of the structural relationship differences between antibiotics, even within the same class, is helpful when selecting the most appropriate therapy for an individual patient. In addition, side chains and subtle structural differences within antimicrobial classes can change the side effect profiles of these agents. The informed clinician can optimize treatment choices from patient to patient while avoiding severe adverse effects.

The development of newer and more effective antimicrobial agents is essential in the fight against infectious diseases. Understanding the medicinal chemistry of the older and newer antimicrobial agents helps the clinician to comprehend their differences in antimicrobial spectrum and side effect profile. Newer antibiotics are continuously being developed; however, many of them are from antimicrobial classes already established with small changes on the functional groups and/or side chains, leading to dramatic differences in their antimicrobial spectra. As stated previously, bacteria are constantly changing, as are antimicrobial susceptibility patterns. To optimize patient care, the clinician needs to stay informed of the effects of the medicinal chemistry differences as newer drugs come to market and antimicrobial resistance trends change.

Elizabeth Coyle, PharmD
Clinical Associate Professor
Department of Clinical Sciences & Administration
University of Houston College of Pharmacy

grown on culture media and be administered to healthy individuals so as to reproduce in healthy individuals all of the classic symptoms of the same disease. Finally, the identical microorganism could then be isolated from this deliberately infected person. Following these rules, at long last, a chain of evidence connecting cause and effect was forged between certain microorganisms and specific infectious diseases. This work laid the foundation for rational prevention and therapy of infectious diseases.

Louis Pasteur reported in 1877 that when what he termed "common bacteria" were introduced into a pure culture of anthrax bacilli, the bacilli died, and that an injection of deadly anthrax bacillus into a laboratory animal was harmless if "common bacteria" were injected along with it. This did not always work but led to the appreciation of antibiosis, wherein two or more microorganisms competed with one another for survival (1). However, it was more than a half century later that the underlying mechanisms began to be appreciated and applied to achieve successful therapy.

The modern anti-infective era opened with the discovery of the sulfonamides in France and Germany in 1936 as an offshoot of Paul Ehrlich's earlier achievements in treating infections with organometallics and his theories of vital staining (2). The well-known observation of a clear zone of inhibition (lysis) in a bacterial colony surrounding a colony of contaminating airborne *Penicillium* mold by Alexander Fleming in England in 1929 and the subsequent purification of penicillin from it in the late 1930s and early 1940s by Florey, Chain, Abraham, and Heatley, provided important additional impetus (3,4). With the first successful clinical trial of crude penicillin in 1941 and the requirements of war times, an explosion of successful activity ensued that continues into the 21st century. In rapid succession, deliberate searches of the metabolic products of a wide variety of soil microbes led to discovery of tyrothricin (1939), streptomycin (1943), chloramphenicol (1947), chlortetracycline (1948), neomycin (1949), and erythromycin (1952). These discoveries ushered in the age of the so-called miracle drugs. The discovery of antibiotics is widely considered to be one of the top five discoveries/inventions of the 20th century.

Microbes of soil origin remain to this day one of the more fruitful sources of antibiotics, although the specific means employed for their discovery are more sophisticated today than those employed 70 years ago. Initially, extracts of fermentations were screened simply for their ability to kill pathogenic microorganisms in vitro. Those that did were pushed along through ever more complex pharmacologic and toxicologic tests in attempts to discover clinically useful agents. Today, many thousands of such extracts of increasingly unusual microbes are tested each year, and the tests now include sophisticated assays for agents operating through particular biochemical mechanisms or possessing particular properties.

Combinatorial chemical synthesis coupled with high-throughput screening today make it possible to screen hundreds of thousands of compounds in a short time for antimicrobial activity. This is coupled with dramatic advances in all of the relevant sciences. One would logically suppose that this would lead to the emergence of a large number of new antimicrobial agents. That this is yet to happen is a measure of the complexity of the task. The impact of genomics and proteomics is predicted to have a larger effect on this effort. The genome of *Haemophilus influenzae* was determined in 1995, and currently more than 1,000 microbial genomes have been deciphered and are publicly available (5,6). Of the more than 1,700 genes of *H. influenzae*, it is thought that 642 are essential and thus are potential targets for antimicrobial drug development (7). These exciting new possibilities have yet to yield practical results due to the inherent complexity of the task.

This picture has an increasing dark side, however, because of the increasing impact of bacterial resistance. Intrinsic resistance to antimicrobial agents (resistance present before exposure to antibiotics) was recognized from the beginning. Some bacteria are immune to treatment from the outset because they do not take up the antibiotic or lack a susceptible target. Starting in the 1940s, however, and encountered with increasing frequency to this day, bacteria that were previously expected to respond were found to be resistant, many bacteria became resistant during the course of chemotherapy, and others were simultaneously resistant to several different antibiotics. The organisms were found to be capable of passing this trait on to other bacteria, even to those belonging to different genera. The spread of this phenomenon is aided by microorganisms' short generation time (sometimes measured in fractions of an hour) and genetic versatility, as well as by poor antibiotic prescribing and utilization practices. Some authorities predict an impending return to the defenseless days of the preantibiotic era. An understanding of these phenomena and the devising of appropriate practical response measures are important contemporary priorities.

GENERAL THERAPEUTIC APPROACH

Drug Nomenclature

The names given to antimicrobials and antibiotics are as varied as their inventor's taste, and yet some helpful unifying conventions are followed. For example, the penicillins are derived from fungi and have names ending in the suffix -cillin, as in the term ampicillin. The cephalosporins are likewise fungal products, although their names mostly begin with the prefix cef- (or sometimes, following the English practice, spelled ceph-). The synthetic fluoroquinolones mostly end in the suffix -floxacin. Although helpful in many respects, this nomenclature does result in many related substances possessing quite similar names. This can make remembering them quite difficult. Most of the remaining antibiotics are produced by fermentation of soil microorganisms belonging to various *Streptomyces* species. By convention, these have names ending in the suffix -mycin, as in streptomycin. Some prominent antibiotics are produced by fermentation of various soil microbes known as *Micromonospora* sp. These antibiotics have names ending in -micin (e.g., gentamicin).

In earlier times, the terms "broad spectrum" and "narrow spectrum" had specific clinical meaning. The widespread emergence of microbes resistant to single agents and multiple agents has made these terms less meaningful. It is, nonetheless, still valuable to remember that some antimicrobial families have the potential of inhibiting a wide range of bacterial genera belonging to both gram-positive and gram-negative cultures and so are called broad spectrum (such as the tetracyclines). Others inhibit only a few bacterial genera and are termed narrow spectrum (such as the glycopeptides, typified by vancomycin, which are used almost exclusively for a few gram-positive and anaerobic microorganisms).

The Importance of Identification of the Pathogen

Empiric-Based Therapy

Fundamental to appropriate antimicrobial therapy is an appreciation that individual species of bacteria are associated with particular infective diseases and that specific antibiotics are more likely to be useful than others for killing them. Sometimes this can be used as the basis for successful empiric therapy. For example, first-course community-acquired urinary tract infections in otherwise healthy individuals are commonly caused by gram-negative *Escherichia coli*. Even just knowing this much can give the physician several convenient choices for useful therapy. Likewise, skin infections, such as boils, are commonly the result of infection with gram-positive *Staphylococcus aureus*. In most other cases, the cause of the disease is less obvious and so likewise is the agent that might be useful against it. It is important to determine the specific disease one is dealing with in these cases and what susceptibility patterns are exhibited by the causative microorganism. Knowing these factors enables the clinician

GRAM STAIN

Hans C. J. Gram, a Danish microbiologist, developed the Gram staining method for staining bacteria so that they were more readily visible under the microscope. The term has proven to be particularly useful in describing antibiotics as well because antibiotics are conveniently classified by their activity against microorganisms depending on their reaction to this method. Gram-positive microorganisms are stained purple by contact with a methyl violet-iodine process. This is largely a consequence of their lack of an outer membrane and the nature of the thick cell wall surrounding them. Gram-negative microorganisms do not retain the methyl violet-iodine stain when washed with alcohol but rather are colored pink when subsequently treated with the red dye safranin. The lipopolysaccharides on their outer membrane apparently are responsible for the staining behavior of gram-negative cells.

Since the Gram stain is dependent on the outer layers of bacterial cells and this also strongly influences the ability of antimicrobial agents to reach their cellular targets, knowing the Gram staining behavior of infectious bacteria helps one decide which antimicrobial might be effective in therapy.

Not all bacteria can be stained by the Gram procedure. These often require special staining processes for visualization. Among the more prominent of these for our purposes are the mycobacteria (the causative agents of tuberculosis, for example). These very waxy cells are called acid-fast and are stained by carbol fuchsin instead.

to narrow the range of therapeutic choices. The only certainty, however, is that inability of a given antibiotic to kill or inhibit a given pathogen in vitro is a virtual guarantee that the drug will fail in vivo. Unfortunately, activity in vitro often also results in failure to cure in vivo, but in these cases, at least, there is a significant possibility of success. Before the emergence of widespread bacterial resistance, identification of the causative microorganism often was sufficient for selecting a useful antibiotic. Now this is only a useful first step, and much more detailed laboratory studies are needed in order to make a successful choice.

Experimentally Based Therapy

The modern clinical application of Koch's discoveries to the selection of an appropriate antibiotic involves sampling infectious material from a patient before instituting anti-infective chemotherapy, culturing the microorganism on suitable growth media, and identifying its genus and species. The bacterium in question is then grown in the presence of a variety of antibiotics to see which of them will inhibit its growth or survival and what concentrations will be needed to achieve this result. This is expressed in minimum inhibitory concentration (MIC) units. The term MIC refers to the concentration that will inhibit 99% or more of the microbe in question and represents the minimum quantity that must reach the site of the infection in order to be useful. These concepts are illustrated in Figure 33.1. To "cure" the infection, it is usually desirable to have several multiples of the MIC at the site of infection. This requires not only an understanding of the MIC, but also an understanding of pharmacokinetic and pharmacodynamic considerations as well as the results of accumulated clinical experience. The choice of anti-infective agent is made from among those that are active. One of the most convenient experimental procedures is that of Kirby and Bauer. With this technique, sterile filter paper disks impregnated with fixed doses of commercially available antibiotics are placed on the seeded Petri dish. The dish is then incubated for a period of time. If the antibiotic is active against the particular strain of bacterium isolated from the patient, a clear zone of inhibition will be seen around the disk. If a given antimicrobial agent is ineffective, the bacterium may even grow right up to the edge of the disk. The diameter of the inhibition zone is directly proportional to the degree of sensitivity of the bacterial strain and the concentration of the antibiotic in question. Currently, a given zone size in millimeters is dictated above which the bacterium is sensitive and below which it is resistant. When the zone size obtained is near this break point (the break point represents the maximum clinically achievable concentration of an anti-infective agent), the drug is regarded as intermediate in sensitivity, and clinical failure can occur. This powerful methodology gives the clinician a choice of possible antibiotics to use. This method is illustrated in Figure 33.2. The widespread occurrence of resistance of certain strains of bacteria to given antibiotics reinforces the need to perform susceptibility testing. Other laboratory methods can be employed for similar purposes. Of particular note is the Epsilometer test (E test), which uses the same idea but employs a gradient of drug concentrations on a filter paper strip. This high level of scientific medicine requires significant expertise and equipment and thus is practiced mainly in medical centers. In

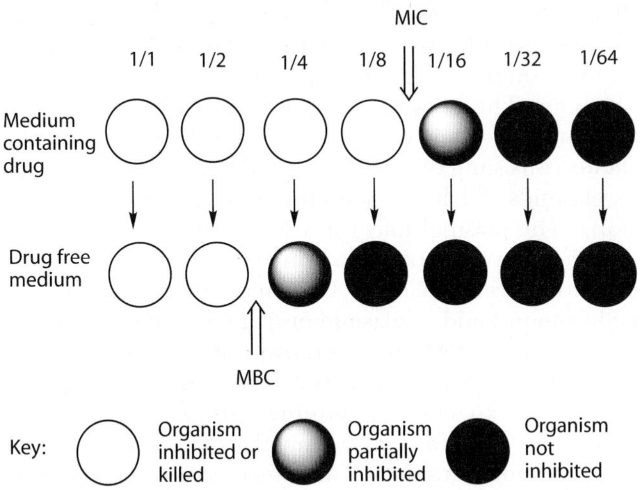

FIGURE 33.1 In the top tubes (viewed from the top), a serially decreasing amount of antimicrobial agent is added to a suitable growth medium inoculated with a microorganism. Following incubation, microbial growth is detected by turbidity. The last concentration that produces no visible growth is scored as the minimum inhibitory concentration (MIC) (1/8). Next, a loopful is taken from each tube and placed in fresh medium (bottom row). In tubes where the organisms were killed by the drug, there is no resumption of growth. Where the organisms were inhibited but not killed, removal of drug allows for resumption of growth. The last concentration that produces no visible growth under these conditions is scored as the minimum bactericidal concentration (MBC) (1/2).

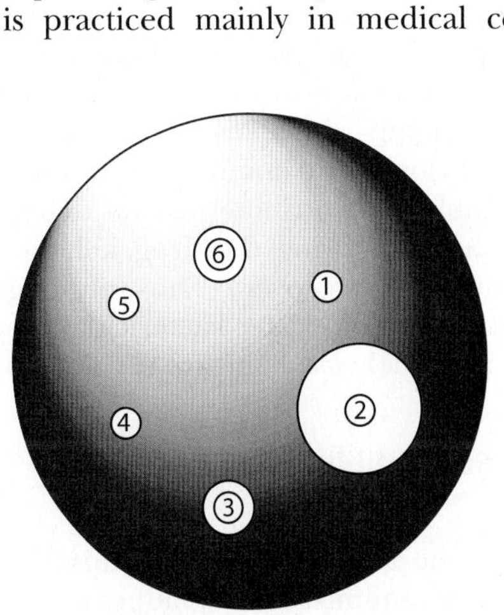

FIGURE 33.2 Looking down on a Petri dish containing solidified nutrient agar to which had been added a suspension of a bacterial species. Next, six filter paper disks containing six different antimicrobials were added, followed by overnight incubation. The antimicrobials in disks 1, 4, and 5 were inactive. Of the active agents in disks 2, 3, and 6, antibiotic 2 was much more active because the microorganism was not able to grow as near this impregnated disk.

outpatient practice, the choice of antimicrobial agents is more commonly made empirically.

Bactericidal Versus Bacteriostatic

Almost all antibiotics have the capacity to be bactericidal in vitro; that is, they will kill bacteria if the concentration or dose is sufficiently high. In the laboratory, it is almost always possible to use such doses. Subsequent inoculation of fresh, antibiotic-free media with a culture that has been so treated will not produce growth of the culture because the cells are dead. When such doses are achievable in live patients, such drugs are clinically bactericidal. At somewhat lower concentrations, bacterial multiplication is prevented even though the microorganism remains viable (bacteriostatic action).

The smallest concentration that will kill a bacterial colony is the minimum bactericidal concentration. The difference between a minimum bactericidal dose and a bacteriostatic dose is characteristic of given families of antibiotics. With gentamicin, for example, doubling or quadrupling the dose changes the effect on bacteria from bacteriostatic to bactericidal. Such doses are usually achievable in the clinic, so gentamicin is termed bactericidal. However, the difference between bactericidal and bacteriostatic doses with tetracycline is approximately 40-fold, and it is not possible to achieve such doses safely in patients, so tetracycline is referred to as bacteriostatic. If a bacteriostatic antibiotic is withdrawn prematurely from a patient, the microorganism can resume growth, and the infection can reestablish itself because the organism is still viable. When a patient is immunocompetent or the infection is not severe, a bacteriostatic concentration will break the fulminating stage of the infection (when bacterial cell numbers are increasing at a logarithmic rate). With *E. coli*, for example, the number of cells doubles approximately every 2 hours. A bacteriostatic agent will interrupt this rapid growth and give the immune system a chance to deal with the disease. Cure usually follows if the numbers of live bacteria are not excessive at this time. Obviously, in immunocompromised patients who are unable to contribute natural defenses to fight their own disease, having the drug kill the bacteria is more important for recovery. Thus, although it is preferred that an antibiotic be bactericidal, bacteriostatic antibiotics are widely used and are usually satisfactory.

Microbial Susceptibility

Resistance

Resistance is the failure of microorganisms to be killed or inhibited by antimicrobial treatment. Resistance can either be intrinsic (be present before exposure to drug) or acquired (develop subsequent to exposure to a drug). Resistance of bacteria to the toxic effects of antimicrobial agents and to antibiotics develops fairly easily both in the laboratory and in the clinic and is an ever-increasing public health hazard. Challenging a culture in the laboratory with sublethal quantities of an antibiotic kills the most intrinsically sensitive percentage of the strains in the colony. Those not killed or seriously inhibited continue to grow and have access to the remainder of the nutrients. A mutation to lower sensitivity also enables individual bacteria to survive against the selecting pressure of the antimicrobial agent. If the culture is treated several times in succession with sublethal doses in this manner, the concentration of antibiotic required to prevent growth becomes ever higher. When the origin of this form of resistance is explored, it is almost always found to be due to an alteration in the biochemistry of the colony so that the molecular target of the antibiotic has become less sensitive, or it can be due to decreased uptake of antibiotic into the cells. This is genomically preserved and passes to the next generation. The altered progeny may be weaker than the wild strain so that they die out if the antibiotic is not present to give them a competitive advantage. In some cases, additional compensatory mutations can occur that restore the vigor of the resistant organisms. Resistance of this type is usually expressed toward other antibiotics with the same mode of action and thus is a familial characteristic; most tetracyclines, for example, show extensive cross-resistance with other agents in the tetracycline family. This is very enlightening with respect to discovery of the molecular mode of action but is not very relevant to the clinical situation.

In the clinic, resistance more commonly takes place by resistance (R) factor mechanisms. In this case, enzymes are elaborated that attack the antibiotic and inactivate it. Mutations leading to resistance occur by many mechanisms. They can result from point mutations, insertions, deletions, inversions, duplications, and transpositions of segments of genes or by acquisition of foreign DNA from plasmids, bacteriophages, and transposable genetic elements. The genetic material coding for this form of resistance is often carried on extra chromosomal elements consisting of small circular DNA molecules known as plasmids. A bacterial cell may have many plasmids or none. The plasmid may carry DNA for several different enzymes capable of destroying structurally dissimilar antibiotics. Such plasmid DNA may migrate within the cell from plasmid to plasmid or from plasmid to chromosome by a process known as transposition. Such plasmids may migrate from cell to cell by conjugation (passage through a sexual pilus), transduction (carriage by a virus vector), or transformation (uptake of exogenous DNA from the environment). These mechanisms can convert an antibiotic-sensitive cell to an antibiotic-resistant cell. This can take place many times in a bacterium's already short generation time. The positive selecting pressure of inadequate levels of an antibiotic favors explosive spread of R-factor resistance. This provides a rationale for conservative but aggressive application of appropriate antimicrobial chemotherapy. Bacterial resistance is generally mediated through one of three mechanisms: failure of the drug to penetrate into or stay in the cell, destruction of the drug by defensive enzymes, or alterations in the cellular target of the drug. It is rarely an all-or-nothing effect. In many cases, a resistant microorganism can still be controlled by achievable, although higher, doses than are required to control sensitive populations.

Persistence

Sensitive bacteria may not all be killed. Survivors are thought to have been resting (not metabolizing) during the drug treatment time and are still viable. These bacteria are still sensitive to the drug even though they survived an otherwise toxic dose. Some bacteria also can aggregate in films. A poorly penetrating antibiotic may not reach the cells lying deep within such a film. Such cells, although intrinsically sensitive, may survive antibiotic treatment. Bacteria living in host cells, living in cysts, or existing as an abscess are also harder to reach by drugs and thus are more difficult to control.

Combination Therapy

It could be assumed that use of combinations of antibiotics would be superior to the use of individual antibiotics because this would broaden the antimicrobial spectrum and make less critical the accurate identification of the pathogen. It has been found, however, that many times such combinations are antagonistic. A useful generalization, but one that is not always correct, is that one can often successfully combine two bactericidal antibiotics, particularly if their molecular mode of action is different. A common example is the use of a β-lactam antibiotic and an aminoglycoside for empiric therapy of overwhelming sepsis of unknown etiology. Therapy must be instituted as soon as a specimen is obtained or the patient may die. This often does not allow the microbiologic laboratory sufficient time to identify the offending microorganism or to determine its antibiotic susceptibility. Both of the antibiotic families applied in this example are bactericidal in readily achievable parenteral doses. As will be detailed later in this chapter, the β-lactams inhibit bacterial cell wall formation, and the aminoglycosides interfere with protein biosynthesis and membrane function. Their modes of action are supplementary. Because of toxicity considerations and the potential for adverse effects, this empiric therapy is replaced by suitable specific monotherapy at the first opportunity after the sensitivity of the bacterium is experimentally established.

One may also often successfully combine two bacteriostatic antibiotics for special purposes, for example, a macrolide and a sulfonamide. This combination is occasionally used for the treatment of an upper respiratory tract infection caused by *Haemophilus influenzae* because the combination of a protein biosynthesis inhibitor and an inhibitor of DNA biosynthesis results in fewer relapses than the use of either agent alone. However, the use of a bacteriostatic agent, such as tetracycline, in combination with a bactericidal agent, such as a β-lactam, is usually discouraged. The β-lactam antibiotics are much more effective when used against growing cultures, and a bacteriostatic agent interferes with bacterial growth, often giving an indifferent or antagonistic response when such agents are combined. Additional possible disadvantages of combination chemotherapy are higher cost, greater likelihood of adverse effects, and difficulties in demonstrating synergism. The rising rate of clinical failure due to antibiotic resistance is overcoming these reservations, and combination therapy is becoming more common.

Serum Protein Binding

The influence of serum protein binding on antibiotic effectiveness is fairly straightforward. It is considered in most instances that the percentage of antibiotic that is protein bound is not available at that moment for the treatment of infections so must be subtracted from the total blood level in order to get the effective blood level. The tightness of the binding is also a consideration. Thus a heavily and firmly serum protein-bound antibiotic would not generally be a good choice for the treatment of septicemias or infections in deep tissue, even though the microorganism involved is susceptible in in vitro tests. If the antibiotic is rapidly released from the protein, however, this factor decreases in importance, and the binding becomes a depot source. Distinguishing between these two types of protein binding is accomplished by comparing the percentages of binding to the excretion half-life. A highly bound but readily released antibiotic will have a comparatively short half-life and work well for systemic infections. An antibiotic that is not significantly protein bound will normally be rapidly excreted and have a short half-life. Thus, some protein binding of poorly water-soluble agents is normally regarded as helpful.

Preferred Means of Dosing

Under ideal circumstances, it is desirable for an antibiotic to be available in both parenteral and oral forms. Whereas there is no question that the convenience of oral medication makes this ideal for outpatient and community use, very ill patients often require parenteral therapy. It would be consistent with today's practice of discharging patients sooner to send them home from the hospital with an efficacious oral version of the same antibiotic that led to the possibility of discharge in the first place. In this way, the patient would not have to come back to the hospital at intervals for drug administration and would not have to risk treatment failure by starting therapy with a new drug.

COST

Antibiotics are often expensive, but so is morbidity and mortality. For many patients, however, cost is a significant consideration. The pharmacist is in an ideal position to guide the physician and the patient on the question of possible alternative equivalent treatments that might be more affordable. The most frequent comparisons are based on the cost of the usual dose of a given agent for a single course of therapy (usually the wholesale cost to the pharmacist for 10 days' worth of drug).

Agricultural Use of Antibiotics

It is estimated that more than half of the antibiotics of commerce are used for agricultural purposes. Their use for treatment of infections of plants and animals is not to be discouraged so long as drug residues from the treatment do not contaminate foods. In contamination, problems such as penicillin allergy or subsequent infection higher up the food chain by drug-resistant microbes can occur. Animals demonstrably grow more rapidly to marketable size when antibiotics are added to their feed even though the animals have no apparent infection. This is believed to be due in large part to suppression of subclinical infections that would consequently divert protein biosynthesis from muscle and tissue growth into proteins needed to combat the infection. Under appropriate conditions, antibiotic feed supplementation is partly responsible for the comparative wholesomeness and cheapness of our food supplies. This practice has the potential, however, to contaminate the food we consume or to provide reservoirs of drug-resistant enteric microorganisms. Occasionally, infections are traced to this cause, and resistance genes can originate in this manner and pass from strain to strain and even to other species.

THERAPEUTIC CLASSES

Synthetic Antimicrobial Agents

Synthetic antimicrobial agents have not been modeled after any natural product, so they may not properly be called "antibiotics." Some synthetics are extremely effective for treatment of infections and are widely used. Very few antibiotics are known to work in precisely the same way as these agents in antibacterial action.

Sulfonamides

The antibacterial properties of the sulfonamides were discovered in the mid-1930s after an incorrect hypothesis, but after observing the results carefully and drawing correct conclusions. Prontosil rubrum, a red dye, was one of a series of dyes examined by Gerhard Domagk of Bayer of Germany in the belief that it might be taken up selectively by certain pathogenic bacteria and not by human cells, in a manner analogous to the way that the Gram stain works, and thus serve as a selective poison to kill these cells (2). The dye, indeed, proved active in vivo against streptococcal infections in mice. Curiously, it was not active in vitro. Trefouel and others soon showed that the urine of prontosil rubrum–treated animals was bioactive in vitro (8). Fractionation led to identification of the active substance as *p*-aminobenzenesulfonic acid amide (sulfanilamide), a colorless cleavage product formed by reductive liver metabolism of the administered dye. Today, we would call prontosil rubrum a prodrug.

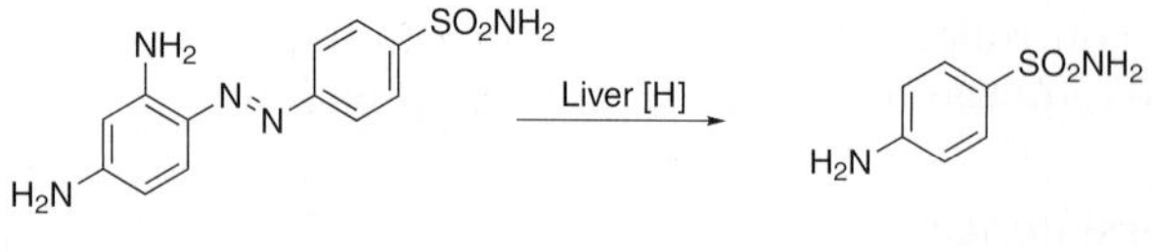

The discovery of sulfanilamide's in vivo antibacterial properties ushered in the modern anti-infective era, and Domagk was awarded a Nobel Prize for medicine in 1939.

Once mainstays of antimicrobial chemotherapy, the sulfonamides have decreased enormously in popularity and are now comparatively minor drugs. The relative inexpensiveness of the sulfonamides is one of their most attractive features and accounts for much of their persistence on the market.

Mechanism of Action The sulfonamides are bacteriostatic when administered to humans in achievable doses. They inhibit the enzyme dihydropteroate synthase, an important enzyme needed for the biosynthesis of folic acid derivatives and, ultimately, the thymidine required for DNA (9). They do this by competing at the active site with *p*-aminobenzoic acid (PABA), a normal structural component of folic acid derivatives. PABA is otherwise incorporated into the developing tetrahydrofolic acid molecule by enzyme-catalyzed condensation with 6-hydroxymethyl-7,8-dihydropterin-pyrophosphate to form 7,8-dihydropteroate and pyrophosphate. Thus, sulfonamides may also be classified as antimetabolites (Fig. 33.3). Indeed, the antimicrobial efficacy of sulfonamides can be reversed by adding significant quantities of PABA into the diet (in some multivitamin preparations and as metabolites of certain local anesthetics) or into the culture medium. Most susceptible bacteria are unable to take up preformed folic acid from their environment and convert it to a tetrahydrofolic acid but, instead, synthesize their own folates de novo. Folates are essential intermediates for the biosynthesis of thymidine without which bacteria cannot multiply. Thus, inhibition of the dihydropteroate synthase is bacteriostatic. Humans are unable to synthesize folates from component parts, lacking the necessary enzymes (including dihydropteroate synthase), and folic acid is supplied to humans in our diet. Sulfonamides consequently have no similarly lethal effect on human cell growth, and the basis for the selective toxicity of sulfonamides is clear.

In a few strains of bacteria, however, the picture is somewhat more complex. Here, sulfonamides are attached to the dihydropteroate diphosphate in place of the normal PABA. The resulting unnatural product, however, is not capable of undergoing the next necessary reaction, condensation with glutamic acid. This false metabolite is also an enzyme inhibitor, and the net result is inability of the bacteria to multiply when the folic acid in their cells is used up, and further nucleic acid biosynthesis becomes impossible. The net result is the same, but the molecular basis of the effect is somewhat different in these strains (Fig. 33.3).

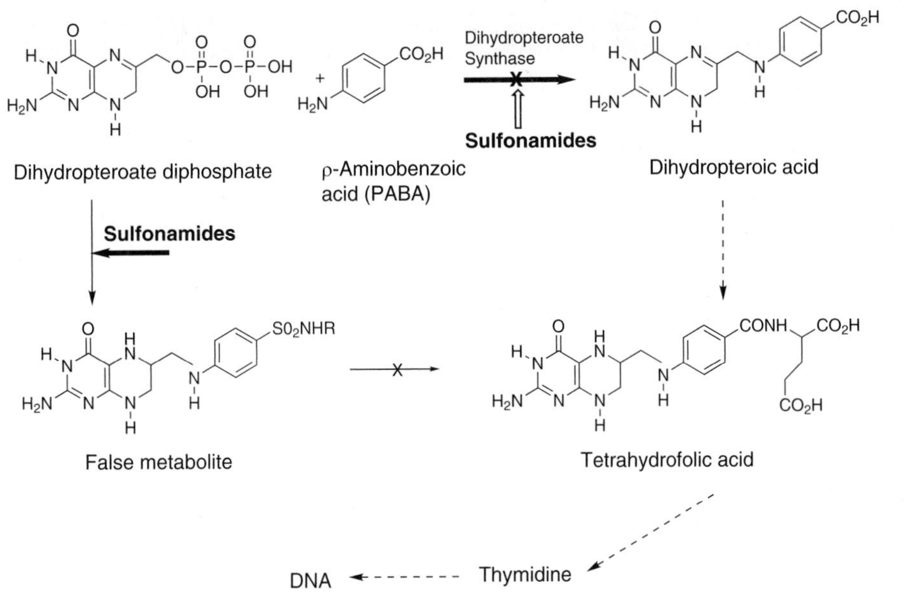

FIGURE 33.3 Microbial biosynthetic pathway leading to tetrahydrofolic acid synthesis and major site of action (⟹) of sulfonamides as well as the site of action seen in some bacteria (⟵), resulting in incorporation of sulfonamide as a false metabolite.

Bacteria that are able to take up preformed folic acid into their cells are intrinsically resistant to sulfonamides.

Structure–Activity Relationships The basis of the structural resemblance of sulfonamides to PABA is clear. The functional group that differs in the two molecules is the carboxyl of PABA and the sulfonamide moiety of sulfanilamide. The strongly electron-withdrawing character of the aromatic SO_2 group makes the nitrogen atom to which it is directly attached partially electropositive. This, in turn, increases the acidity of the hydrogen atoms attached to the nitrogen so that this functional group is slightly acidic (pK_a = 10.4). The pK_a of the carboxyl group of PABA is approximately 4.9. It was soon found that replacement of one of the NH_2 hydrogens by an electron-withdrawing heteroaromatic ring enhanced the acidity of the remaining hydrogen and dramatically enhanced potency. With suitable groups in place, the pK_a is reduced to the same range as that of PABA itself. Not only did this markedly increase the antibacterial potency of the product, but it also dramatically increased the water solubility under physiologic conditions. The pK_a of sulfisoxazole, one of the sulfonamides in present use, is approximately 5.0. The poor water solubility of the earliest sulfonamides led to occasional crystallization in the urine (crystalluria) and resulted in kidney damage because the molecules were un-ionized at urine pH values. It is still recommended to drink increased quantities of water to avoid crystalluria when taking certain sulfonamides, but this form of toxicity is now comparatively uncommon with the more important agents used today because they form sodium salts that are at least partly ionized and hence reasonably water soluble at urinary pH values. They are poorly tolerated on injection, however, because these salts are corrosive to tissues.

Structural variation among the clinically useful sulfonamides is restricted primarily to installation of various heterocyclic aromatic substituents on the sulfonamide nitrogen.

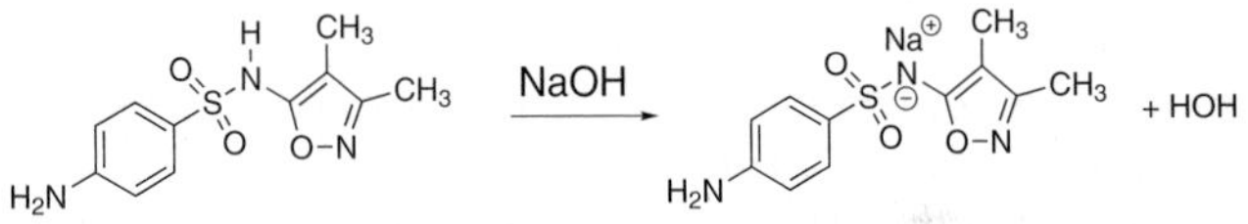

Sulfisoxazole. pKa = 5 Sodium Sulfisoxazole.

Pharmacokinetics

The orally administered sulfonamides are well absorbed from the gastrointestinal (GI) tract, distributed fairly widely, and excreted by the kidney. The drugs are bound to plasma protein (sulfisoxazole 30% to 70%, sulfamethoxazole 70%) and, as such, may displace other protein-bound drugs as well as bilirubin. The latter phenomenon disqualifies them for use in late-term pregnancy because they can cause neonatal jaundice. Sulfonamides are partly deactivated by acetylation at N-4 and glucuronidation of the anilino nitrogen in the liver (10).

Plasmid-mediated resistance development is common, particularly among gram-negative microorganisms and usually takes the form of decreased sensitivity of dihydropteroate synthase or increased production of PABA (11).

Therapeutic Applications

Of the thousands of sulfonamides that have been evaluated, only a few are still available and are often used in combination with other agents. The surviving sulfonamides (Table 33.1) include sulfisoxazole, which is used in combination with erythromycin. It has a comparatively

TABLE 33.1 Clinically Relevent Sulfonamides

Generic Name	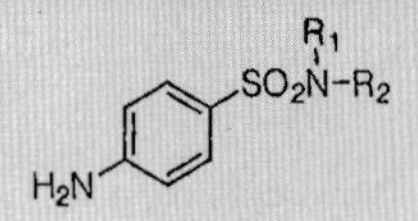 R₁	R₂	pKa
Sulfamethoxazole	H	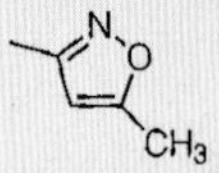	5.6
Silver Sulfadiazine	$Ag^{\oplus}$	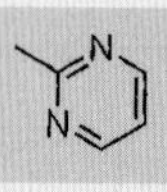	
Sulfisoxazole	H	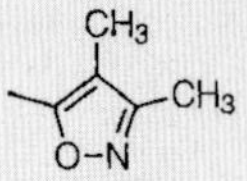	5.0
Sulfacetamide	H	$COCH_3$	5.4

broad antimicrobial spectrum in vitro, especially against gram-negative organisms, but clinical use is generally restricted due to the development of bacterial resistance. Susceptible organisms may include Enterobacteriaceae (*E. coli*, *Klebsiella*, and *Proteus*) and *Streptococcus pyogenes*, *Streptococcus pneumoniae*, and *Haemophilus* (12). Sulfamethoxazole in combination with trimethoprim is more commonly seen and is further described in the discussion of trimethoprim.

The remaining sulfonamides are not used systemically. Sulfadiazine in the form of its silver salt is used topically for treatment of burns and is effective against a range of bacteria and fungus, whereas sulfacetamide is used ophthalmically for treatment of eye infections caused by susceptible organisms. Sulfasalazine stands out from the typical sulfonamide because although it is administered orally, the drug is not absorbed in the gut, so the majority of the dose is delivered to the distal bowel. In addition, the drug is a prodrug that undergoes reductive metabolism by gut bacteria converting the drug into sulfapyridine and 5-aminosalicyclic acid, the active component (Fig. 33.4). The liberation of 5-aminosalicylic acid (mesalamine), an anti-inflammatory agent, is the purpose for administering this drug. This agent is used to treat ulcerative colitis and Crohn disease (13). Direct administration of salicylates is otherwise irritating to the gastric mucosa.

Adverse Effects

Allergic reactions are the most common and take the form of rash, photosensitivity, and drug fever. Less common problems are kidney and liver damage, hemolytic anemia, and other blood problems. The most serious adverse effect is the Stevens-Johnson syndrome characterized by sometimes fatal erythema multiforme and ulceration of mucous membranes of the eye, mouth, and urethra (10). Fortunately, these effects are comparatively rare.

Trimethoprim

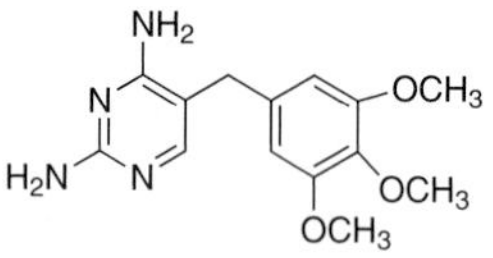

Trimethoprim (Proloprim, Trimpex)

Mechanism of Action A further step in the pathway leading from the pteroates to folic acid and on to DNA bases requires the enzyme dihydrofolate reductase. Exogenous folic acid must be reduced stepwise to dihydrofolic acid and then to tetrahydrofolic acid, an important cofactor essential for supplying a one-carbon unit in thymidine

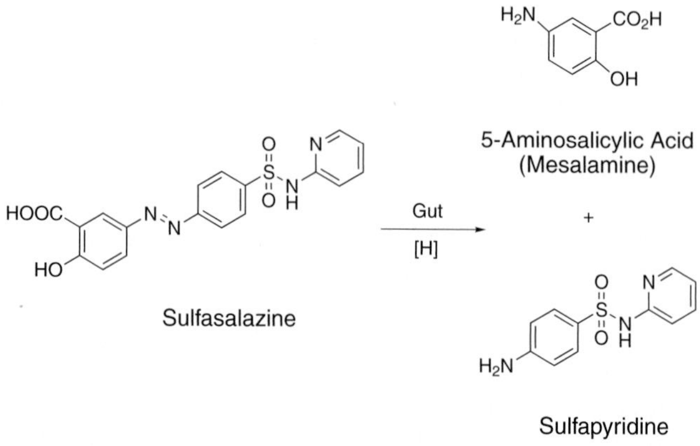

FIGURE 33.4 Activation of sulfasalazine to 5-aminosalicylic acid.

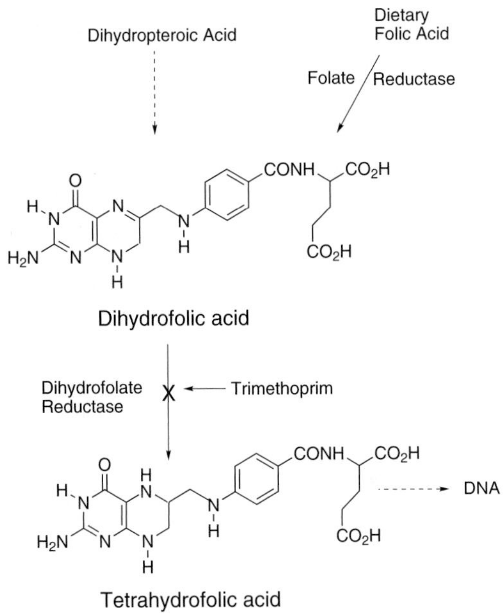

FIGURE 33.5 Site of action of trimethoprim.

biosynthesis and ultimately for DNA synthesis (Fig. 33.5). The same enzyme must also reduce endogenously produced dihydrofolate. Inhibition of this key enzyme had been widely studied in attempts to find anticancer agents by starving rapidly dividing cancer cells of needed DNA precursors. Antifolates such as methotrexate arose from such studies. Methotrexate, however, is much too toxic to be used as an antibiotic. Subsequently, however, trimethoprim was developed in 1969 by George Hitchings and Gertrude Elion (who shared a Nobel Prize for this and other contributions to chemotherapy in 1988). This inhibitor prevents tetrahydrofolic acid biosynthesis and results in bacteriostasis. Trimethoprim selectivity between bacterial and mammalian dihydrofolate reductases results from the subtle but significant architectural differences between these enzyme systems. Whereas the bacterial enzyme and the mammalian enzyme both efficiently catalyze the conversion of dihydrofolic acid to tetrahydrofolic acid, the bacterial enzyme is sensitive to inhibition by trimethoprim by up to 100,000 times lower concentrations than is vertebrate enzyme (14). This difference explains the useful selective toxicity of trimethoprim.

Therapeutic Application Trimethoprim can be used as a single agent clinically for the oral treatment of uncomplicated urinary tract infections caused by susceptible bacteria (predominantly community-acquired *E. coli* and other gram-negative rods) (15). It is, however, most commonly used in a 1:5 fixed concentration ratio with the sulfonamide sulfamethoxazole (Bactrim, Septra). This combination is not only synergistic in vitro but is less likely to induce bacterial resistance than either agent alone. It is rationalized that microorganisms not completely inhibited by sulfamethoxazole at the pteroate condensation step will not likely be able to push the lessened amount of substrates that leak through past a subsequent blockade of dihydrofolate reductase. Thus these agents block sequentially at two different steps in the same essential pathway, and this combination is extremely difficult for a naive microorganism to survive. It is also comparatively uncommon that a microorganism will successfully mutate to resistance at both enzymes during the course of therapy. However, if the organism is already resistant to either drug at the outset of therapy, much of the advantage of the combination is lost.

Pairing these two particular antibacterial agents was based on pharmacokinetic factors. For such a combination to be useful in vivo, the two agents must arrive at the necessary tissue compartment where the infection is at the correct time and in the right ratio. In this context, the optimum ratio of these two agents in vitro is 1:20. Administration of the 1:5 combination of the two drugs orally produces the desired 1:20 ratio in the body once steady-state is reached (10). The combination is used for oral treatment of urinary tract infections, shigellosis, otitis media, traveler's diarrhea, community-acquired methicillin-resistant *Staphylococcus aureus* (MRSA), acute exacerbations of chronic bronchitis, and pneumocystis pneumonia (10). The pneumonia-causing fungus *Pneumocystis jiroveci* (previously classified as *Pneumocystis carinii*) is an opportunistic pathogen for immunocompromised individuals.

The most frequent side effects of trimethoprim-sulfamethoxazole are rash, nausea, and vomiting. Blood dyscrasias are less common, as is pseudomembranous colitis (caused by non–antibiotic-sensitive opportunistic gut anaerobes, often *Clostridium difficile*) (10). Despite a significant effort, no structurally related analog has emerged to compete with trimethoprim.

Resistance Bacterial resistance to trimethoprim is increasingly common. In pneumococcal infections, it can result from a single amino acid mutation (Ile-100 to Leu) in the dihydrofolate reductase enzyme. Overexpression of dihydrofolate reductase by *Staphylococcus aureus* has also been reported in resistant strains (11).

Quinolones

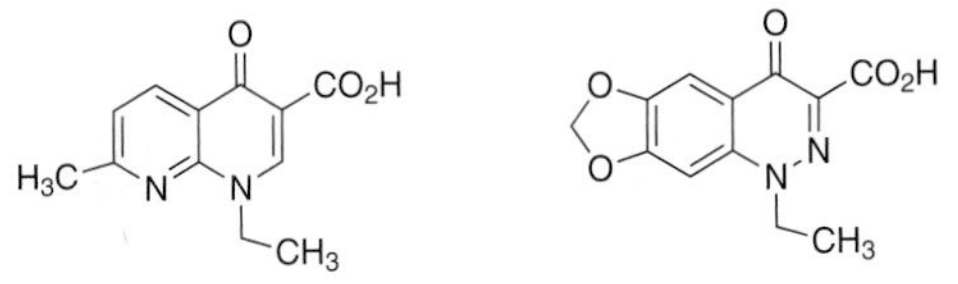

Nalidixic Acid

Cinoxacin

The quinolone antimicrobials comprise a group of synthetic substances possessing in common an *N*-1-alkylated 3-carboxypyrid-4-one ring fused to another aromatic ring, which itself carries other substituents. The first quinolone to be marketed was nalidixic acid, which has since been discontinued. Nalidixic acid was classified as a first-generation quinolone based on its spectrum of activity and pharmacokinetic properties. The spectrum of activity was limited to a small number of gram-negative organisms. Thus, the quinolones were of little clinical significance until the discovery that the addition of a fluoro group to the 6 position of the basic nucleus greatly increased the biologic activity (16). Agents that contain the 6-fluoro substitution are referred to as fluoroquinolones and represent an important therapeutic class of antimicrobials. Norfloxacin was approved for use in 1986 and represents the first of the second-generation quinolones; it is considered to be broad spectrum and equivalent in potency to many of the fermentation-derived antibiotics (16). Following its introduction, intense research ensued, and over a thousand analogs have now been made. Ciprofloxacin, gemifloxacin, norfloxacin, ofloxacin, levofloxacin, and moxifloxacin are currently marketed for systemic use in the United States. In addition, ciprofloxacin, levofloxacin, moxifloxacin, and ofloxacin along with besifloxacin and gatifloxacin are available for ophthalmic use (Fig. 33.6).

Mechanism of Action The quinolones are rapidly bactericidal, largely as a consequence of inhibition of DNA gyrase and topoisomerase IV, key bacterial enzymes that dictate the conformation of DNA (17). Using the energy generated by adenosine triphosphate (ATP) hydrolysis, DNA is progressively wound about itself in a positive supercoil. In the absence of ATP, the process is reversed, relaxing the molecule. It must also be partially unwound so that the cell has access to the genetic information it contains. This requires reversible conformational changes so that it can be stored properly, unwound, replicated, repaired, and transcribed on demand. DNA gyrase alters the conformation of DNA by catalyzing transient double-strand cuts, passing the uncut portion of the molecule through the gap, and resealing the molecule back together (Fig. 33.7) (17). In this way, DNA gyrase alters the degree of twisting of DNA by introducing negative DNA supercoils releasing tensional stress in the molecule. DNA topoisomerase IV, on the other hand, decatenates (unties) enchained daughter DNA molecules produced through replication of circular DNA (17). Inhibition of DNA gyrase and topoisomerase IV makes a cell's DNA inaccessible and leads to cell death, particularly if the cell must deal with other toxic effects at the same time. Different quinolones

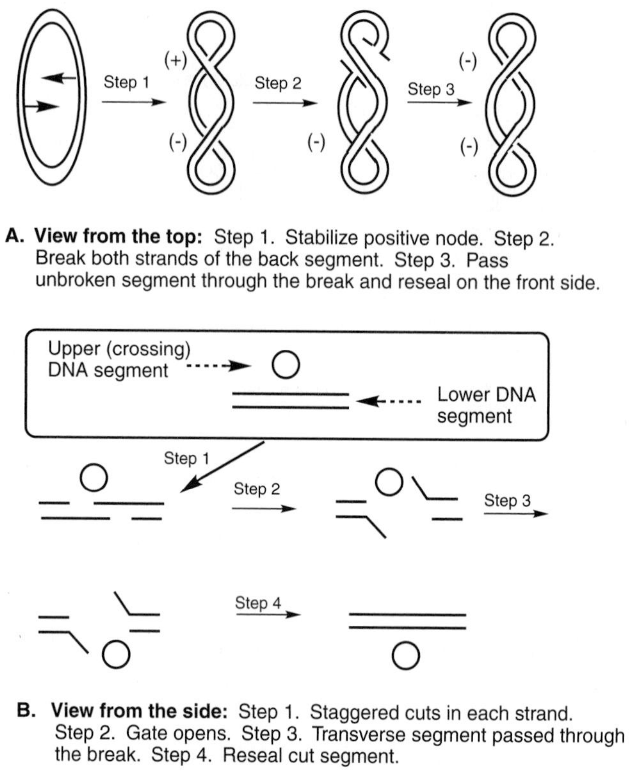

FIGURE 33.7 Schematic depicting supercoiling of circular DNA catalyzed by DNA gyrase.

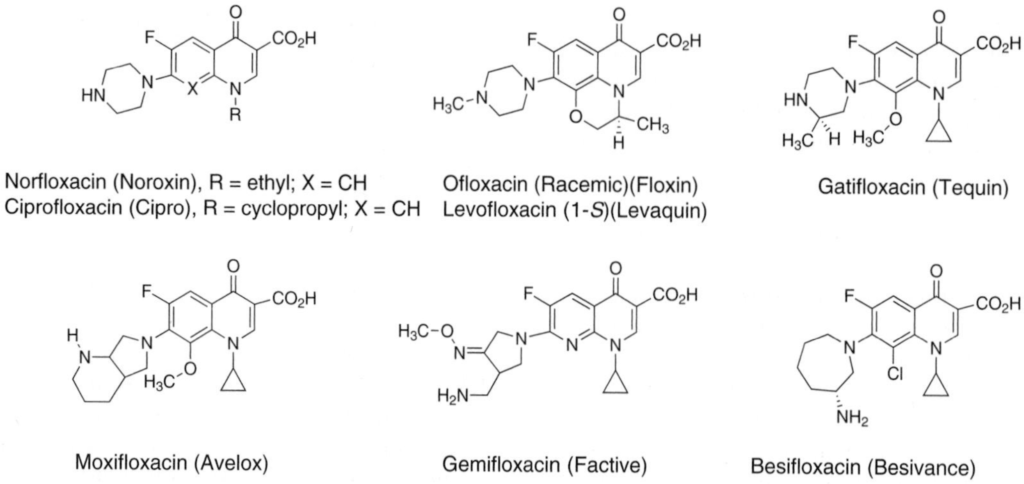

FIGURE 33.6 Second-, third-, and fourth-generation quinolones.

inhibit these essential enzymes to different extents, which explains some of the differences in the spectrum of activity of the fluoroquinolones. Topoisomerase IV seems more important to some gram-positive organisms, and DNA gyrase seems more important to some gram-negative organisms.

Humans shape their DNA with a topoisomerase II, an analogous enzyme to DNA gyrase that, however, does not bind quinolones at normally achievable doses, so the quinolones of commerce do not kill host cells.

Structure–Activity Relationship The structural features of the quinolones strongly influence the antimicrobial and pharmacokinetic properties of this class of drugs (18). The essential pharmacophore for activity is the carboxy-4-pyridone nucleus (Fig. 33.8). Apparently, the carboxylic acid and the ketone are involved in binding to the DNA/DNA-gyrase enzyme system. Reduction of the 2,3-double bond or the 4-keto group inactivates the molecule, and substitution at C-2 interferes with enzyme–substrate complexation. Fluoro substitution at the C-6 position greatly improves antimicrobial activity by increasing the lipophilicity of the molecule, which in turn improves the drug's penetration through the bacterial cell wall. C-6 fluoro also increases the DNA gyrase/topoisomerase IV inhibitory action. An additional fluoro group at C-8 further improves drug absorption and half-life, but also increases drug-induced photosensitivity. Substitution of a methoxy group at C-8 reduces the photosensitivity (moxifloxacin and gatifloxacin). Heterocyclic substitution at C-7 improves the spectrum of activity especially against gram-negative organisms. The piperazinyl (ciprofloxacin) and pyrrolidinyl (moxifloxacin) represent the most significant antimicrobial improvement. Unfortunately, the piperazinyl group at C-7 also increases binding to central nervous system (CNS) γ-aminobutyric acid (GABA) receptors, which accounts for CNS side effects. Alkyl substitution on the piperazine nitrogen (ofloxacin and levofloxacin) is reported to decrease binding to GABA. The cyclopropyl substitution at N-1 appears to broaden activity of the quinolones to include activity against atypical bacteria including *Mycoplasma, Chlamydia,* and *Legionella* species. Substitution of a 2,4-difluorophenyl at N-1 also improves antimicrobial potency, but agents with this substitution (trovafloxacin and temafloxacin) have been withdrawn from the market due to serious adverse effects.

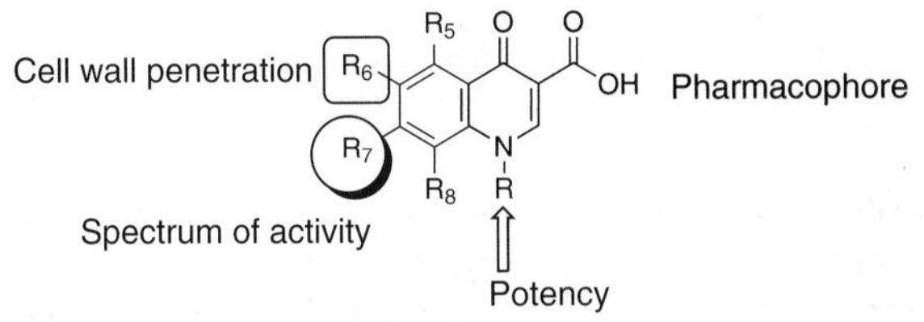

FIGURE 33.8 Major structure–activity relationship features of 4-quinolones.

The introduction of a third ring to the nucleus of the quinolones gives rise to ofloxacin. Additionally, ofloxacin has an asymmetric carbon at the C-3′ position. The *S*-(−)-isomer (levofloxacin) is twice as active as ofloxacin and 8 to 128 times more potent than the *R*-(+)-isomer resulting from increased binding to the DNA gyrase.

Finally, a chemical incompatibility common to all of the quinolones involves the ability of these drugs to chelate polyvalent metal ions (Ca^{2+}, Mg^{2+}, Zn^{2+}, Fe^{2+}, Al^{3+}), resulting in decreased solubility and reduced drug absorption. Chelation occurs between the metal and the 3-carboxylic acid and 4-keto groups. Agents containing polyvalent metals should be administered separately from the quinolones.

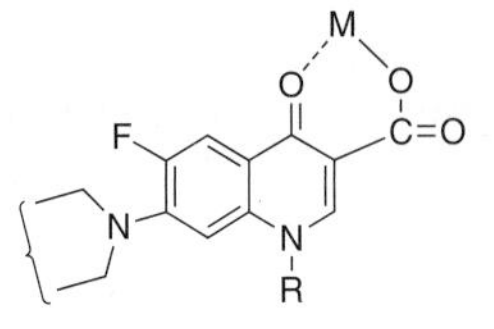

Pharmacokinetics The fluoroquinolones are well absorbed following oral administration, with excellent bioavailability. The maximum plasma concentration is usually reached within a few hours, and the drugs are moderately bound to plasma protein, leading to comparatively long half-lives (Table 33.2). Earlier quinolones were rapidly excreted into the urine, which limited their therapeutic application to urinary tract infections, whereas the newer drugs are distributed to alveolar macrophages, bronchial mucosa, epithelial lining fluid, and saliva, improving the use in various systemic infections.

Therapeutic Applications The quinolones therapeutically fall into one of four classifications (Table 33.3). The specific drugs within each classification include nalidixic acid and cinoxacin as first-generation agents with utility limited to uncomplicated urinary tract infections. The second-generation quinolones include norfloxacin and

TABLE 33.2 Pharmacokinetic Properties for Select Quinolones

Drug	Bioavailability (%)	Protein Binding (%)	Half-Life (hours)
Ciprofloxacin	70	30	3.5
Enoxacin	90	40	3–6
Gatifloxacin	96	20	8.0
Gemifloxacin	71	60–70	8.0
Levofloxacin	99	31	6.9
Moxifloxacin	86	47	12.1
Norfloxacin	30–40	10–15	3–4
Ofloxacin	98	32	9

TABLE 33.3 Therapeutic Classification of Quinolones

Generation	Characteristics
First generation	Poor serum and tissue concentration Not valuable for systemic infections Lack activity against *Pseudomonas aeruginosa*, gram-positive organisms, and anaerobes
Second generation	Adequate serum and tissue concentration Good for systemic infections Active against gram-negative organisms including *P. aeruginosa*; weak activity against *Streptococcus pneumoniae*; and no activity against anaerobes
Third generation	Once-daily dosing Active against *S. pneumoniae* and atypical bacteria; less active against *P. aeruginosa*
Fourth generation	Active against anaerobes and aerobic gram-positive and gram-negative organisms

ciprofloxacin. Norfloxacin is mainly used for urinary tract infections (*Enterobacter*, *Enterococcus*, or *Pseudomonas aeruginosa*), prostatitis, and gonorrhea, whereas ciprofloxacin is also used for upper respiratory tract infections, bone infections, septicemia, staphylococcal and pseudomonal endocarditis, meningitis, and anthrax infections (19,20). The third-generation quinolones include levofloxacin, gatifloxacin, and gemifloxacin. These agents find use in the treatment of bacterial exacerbation of chronic bronchitis and community-acquired pneumonia (21). Levofloxacin is also used to treat respiratory infections caused by *Legionella*, *Chlamydia*, and *Mycoplasma* as well as other nosocomial pneumonias. Additional indications for levofloxacin include skin and skin structure infections and acute sinusitis caused by *Streptococcus pneumoniae*, *Haemophilus influenzae*, and *Moraxella catarrhalis* (22). The fourth-generation quinolones include moxifloxacin and have a spectrum of activity that includes *Bacteroides fragilis* (23). Moxifloxacin and levofloxacin are also recommended as second-line agents for tuberculosis as an off-label use (22,23).

Resistance Resistance to the quinolones is becoming more frequent and is associated with spontaneous mutations in genes (*gyrA* and *gyrB*) that encode for the quinolone target protein, DNA gyrase, and genes (*parC* and *parE*) that encode for topoisomerase IV (17). A single mutation can lead to low-level resistance, whereas mutations in more than one gene lead to high-level resistance. This mechanism of resistance would be expected to produce differing levels of cross-resistance within the class of quinolones. In addition, there are suggestions that resistance may be associated with an increase in drug efflux or a decrease in outer membrane permeability affecting drug influx. Such a mechanism of resistance would be expected to be more common in gram-negative organisms with a more complex cell wall than in gram-positive organisms with their cell envelope.

Adverse Effects The quinolone class is associated with more side effects than the β-lactam and macrolide classes, but nonetheless see very widespread medicinal use. All of the fluoroquinolones have a black box warning for possible tendonitis and tendon rupture. They are also not for use in myasthenia gravis patients. Another side effect associated with quinolones is a proconvulsant action, especially when coadministered with nonsteroidal anti-inflammatory drugs. Other CNS problems include hallucinations, insomnia, and visual disturbances. Some patients also experience diarrhea, vomiting, abdominal pain, and anorexia. The quinolones are associated with erosion of the load-bearing joints of young animals. As a precaution, these drugs are not used casually in children less than 18 years of age or in sexually active females of childbearing age. They are also potentially damaging in the first trimester of pregnancy because of a risk of severe metabolic acidosis and of hemolytic anemia. Some of the quinolones may potentiate the action of theophylline and should be monitored closely. They also have been linked to QT prolongation and may increase the risk of torsades de pointes when used with other QT-prolonging agents such as some antiarrhythmic agents (20–24).

Severe Toxicities Certain members of the fluoroquinolone family were marketed for a while but were subsequently severely limited in use or withdrawn because of the unacceptable toxicities experienced by some patients. These agents, because of their breadth of spectrum and potency against resistant microorganisms, were introduced with great hope. Temafloxacin, for example, was removed from the market because of hemolysis, renal failure, and thrombocytopenia (the hemolytic uremic syndrome). These effects only became apparent when large numbers of patients received the drug. Severe liver toxicity led to the removal from the market of trovafloxacin. Grepafloxacin was introduced on the market in late 1997 as a broad-spectrum fluoroquinolone and withdrawn from the market in 1999 because of cardiovascular toxicity. Analogs with a C-8 chloro substituent, such as clinafloxacin and sitafloxacin, were also very potent but have been withdrawn due to excessive phototoxicity.

Miscellaneous Agents

Nitroheteroaromatic Compounds

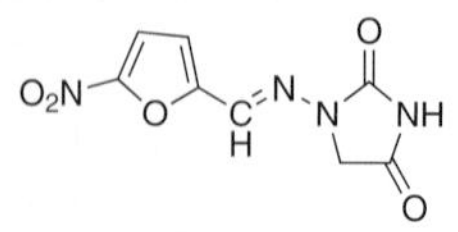

Nitrofurantoin
(Furadantin, Macrodantin)

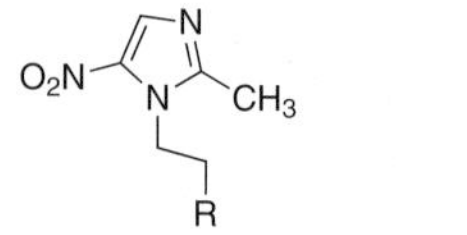

Metronidazole, R = OH (Flagyl)
Tinidazole R = $SO_2C_2H_5$(Fasigyn)

Nitrofurantoin, a widely used oral antibacterial nitrofuran, has been available since World War II. It is used for prophylaxis or treatment of acute urinary tract infections when kidney function is not impaired, and it inhibits kidney stone growth. Nausea and vomiting are common side effects. This is avoided in part by slowing the rate of absorption of the drug through use of wax-coated large particles (Macrodantin). Nitrofurantoin inhibits DNA and RNA functions through mechanisms that are not well understood, although bioreductive activation is suspected to be an important component of this. There is little acquired resistance to this agent. Severe side effects can be experienced when using this drug (acute pulmonary reactions, peripheral neuropathy, hemolytic anemia, liver toxicity, and fertility impairment) (25).

Metronidazole was initially introduced for the treatment of vaginal infections caused by amoeba. This nitroimidazole is also useful orally for the treatment of trichomoniasis, giardiasis, and *Gardnerella vaginalis* infections. It has found increasing use of late in the parenteral treatment of anaerobic infections and for treatment of pseudomembranous colitis due to *Clostridium difficile*. *C. difficile* is an opportunistic pathogen that occasionally flourishes as a consequence of broad-spectrum antibiotic therapy, and infections can be life-threatening. The drug is believed to be metabolically activated by reduction of its nitro group to produce metabolites that interfere with DNA and RNA function. Metronidazole is also a component of a multidrug cocktail used to treat *Helicobacter pylori* infections associated with gastric ulcers (26). Tinidazole, another nitroimidazole, has been introduced primarily as an antiprotozoal agent (27). Because of the similarities in structure and action, tinidazole is believed to have a similar spectrum to metronidazole. Both drugs can cause disulfiram-like adverse reactions when alcohol is consumed. Metronidazole use is associated with allergic rashes and CNS disturbances, including convulsions, in some patients. It is carcinogenic in rodents (26).

METHENAMINE

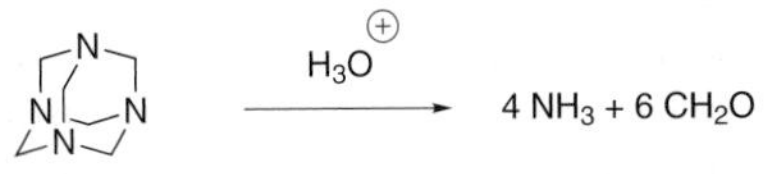

Methenamine
(Prosed, Urimax, Urised, Uroqid-Acid)

Methenamine is a drug that can be used for the disinfection of acidic urine. Structurally it is a low molecular weight polymer of ammonia and formaldehyde which reverts to its components under mildly acid conditions. Formaldehyde is the active antimicrobial component. Methenamine can be used for recurrent urinary tract infections. The drug is available in various dosage forms as well as various salts including the hippurate and mandelate.

FOSFOMYCIN

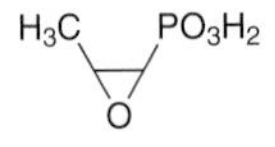

Phosphomycin (Monurol)

Fosfomycin (also known as phosphomycin) inhibits enolpyruvial transferase, an enzyme catalyzing an early step in bacterial cell wall biosynthesis. Inhibition results in reduced synthesis of peptidoglycan, an important component in the bacterial cell wall. Fosfomycin is bactericidal against *Escherichia coli* and *Enterobacter faecalis* infections. It is used for treatment of uncomplicated urinary tract infections by susceptible organisms.

Antibiotics: Inhibitors of Bacterial Cell Wall Biosynthesis

THE BACTERIAL CELL WALL Bacterial cells are enclosed within a complex and largely rigid cell wall. This differs dramatically from mammalian cells that are surrounded by a flexible membrane whose chemical composition is dramatically different. This provides a number of potentially attractive targets for selective chemotherapy of bacterial infections. For one thing, enzymes that have no direct counterpart in mammalian cells construct the bacterial cell wall. Three of the main functions of the bacterial cell wall are: 1) to provide a semipermeable barrier interfacing with the environment through which only desirable substances may pass; 2) to provide a sufficiently strong barrier so that the bacterial cell is protected from changes in the osmotic pressure of its environment; and 3) to prevent digestion by host enzymes. The initial units of the cell wall are constructed within the cell, but soon the growing and increasingly complex structure must be extruded; final assembly takes place outside of the inner membrane. This circumstance makes the enzymes involved in late steps more vulnerable to inhibition because they are at or near the cell surface. Whereas individual bacterial species differ in specific details, the following generalized picture of the process is sufficiently accurate to illustrate the process.

Gram-Positive Bacteria The cell wall of gram-positive bacteria, although complex enough, is simpler than that of gram-negative organisms. A schematic representation is shown in Figure 33.9. On the very outside of the cell is a set of characteristic carbohydrates and proteins that together make up the antigenic determinants that differ from species to species and that also cause adherence to particular target cells. There may also be a lipid-rich capsule surrounding the cell (not shown in the diagram). The next barrier that the wall presents is the peptidoglycan layer. This is a spongy, gel-forming layer consisting of a series of alternating sugars (*N*-acetylglucosamine and *N*-acetylmuramic acid) linked (1,4)-β in a long chain (Fig. 33.10). To the lactic acid carboxyl moieties of the *N*-acetylmuramic acid units is attached, through an amide linkage, a series of amino acids of which L-alanyl-D-glutamyl-L-lysyl-D-alanine is typical of *Staphylococcus aureus*. One notes the D-stereochemistry of the glutamate and the terminal alanine. This feature is presumably important in protecting the peptidoglycan from hydrolysis by host peptidases, particularly in the GI tract.

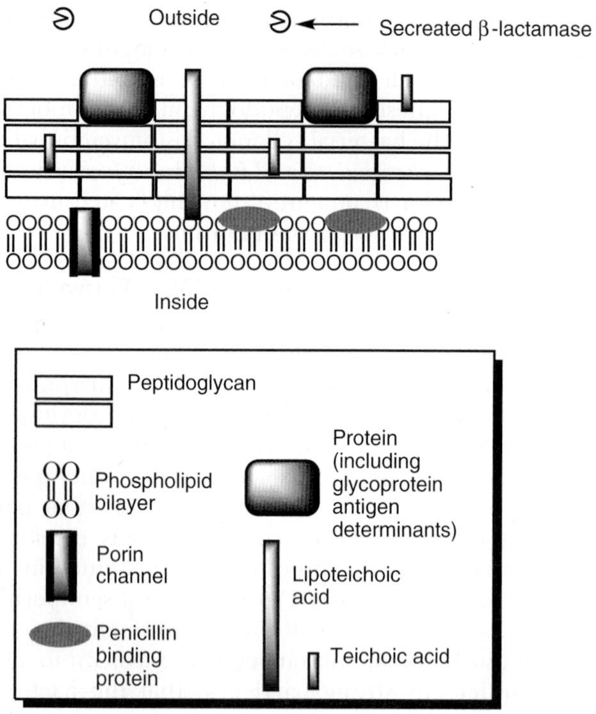

FIGURE 33.9 Schematic of some features of the gram-positive bacterial cell wall.

The early steps in the biosynthesis of the peptidoglycan unit result in formation of a complex polymeric sheet. This is then cross-linked to form a thickened wall. This bonds the terminal D-alanyl unit to the lysyl unit

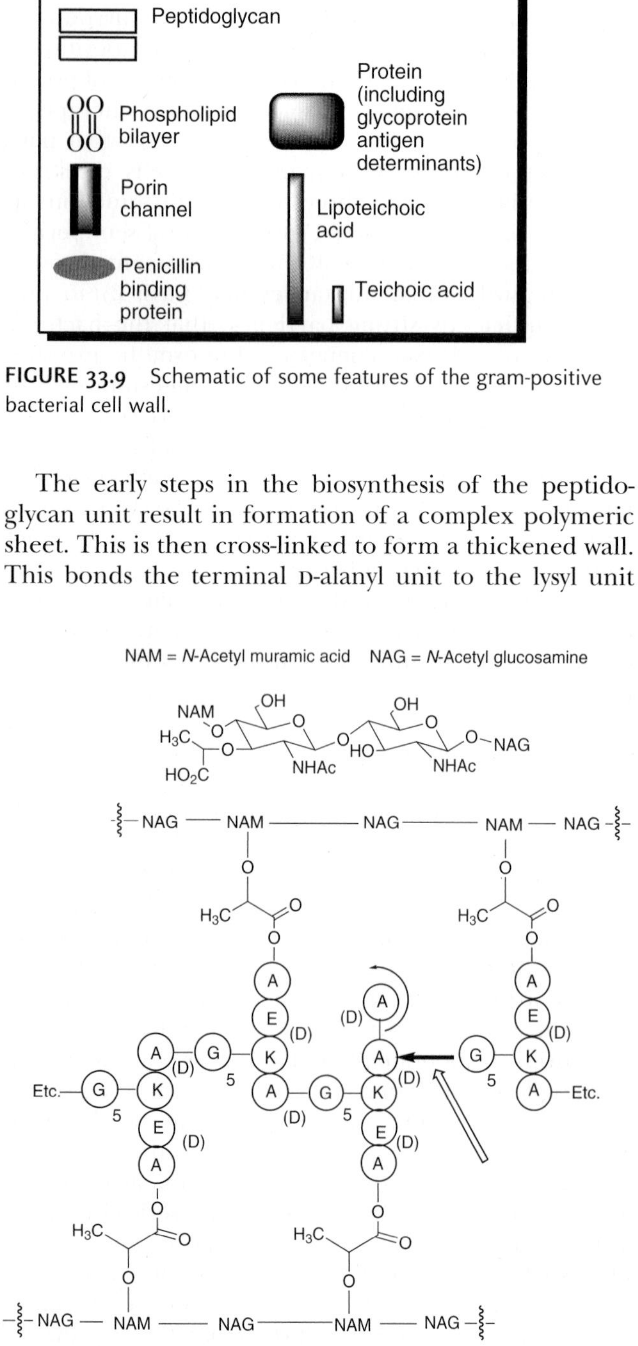

FIGURE 33.10 Schematic of cell wall cross-linking. Pentaglycyl group replaces terminal D-alanine.

of an adjacent tetrapeptide strand through a pentaglycyl unit. This last step is an enzyme-catalyzed transamidation by which the terminal amino moiety on the last glycine unit of the A strand displaces the terminal D-ala unit on the nearby B strand. The cell wall transamidase, one of the penicillin-binding proteins (PBPs), forms a transient covalent bond during the synthesis phase with a particular serine hydroxyl on the enzyme. Completion of the catalytic cycle involves displacement of the enzyme by a glycine residue, which regenerates the enzyme. This process gives the wall additional rigidity. This strong barrier protects against osmotic stress and accounts for the retention of characteristic morphologic shape of gram-positive bacteria (globes and rods, for example). This step is highly sensitive to inhibition of β-lactam antibiotics. It is also the target of the glycopeptide antibiotics (such as vancomycin), as will be discussed later.

The peptidoglycan layer is traversed by complex glycophospholipids called teichoic and teichuronic acids. These are largely responsible for the acid mantle of gram-positive bacteria. Beneath the peptidoglycan layer is the lipoidal cytoplasmic cell membrane in which a number of important protein molecules float in a lipid bilayer. Among these proteins are the β-lactam targets, the PBPs (28). These are enzymes that are important in cell wall formation and remodeling. In gram-positive bacteria, the outer layers are relatively ineffective in keeping antibiotics out. The inner membrane and its protein components provide the principal barrier to uptake of antibiotics. There are a number of different types of PBPs (PBP-1a, PBP-1b, PBP-2, PBP2a, PBP-3, etc), and their function is dependent on the species of bacteria and has been more fully reviewed elsewhere (29). The functions of all of the PBPs are not entirely understood, but they are important in construction and repair of the cell wall. β-Lactam antibiotics bind to these proteins and kill bacteria by preventing the biosynthesis of a functional cell wall. Various β-lactam antibiotics display different patterns of binding to the PBPs. These proteins must alternate in a controlled and systematic way between their active and inert states so that bacterial cells can grow and multiply in an orderly manner. Selective interference by β-lactam antibiotics with their functioning prevents normal growth and repair and creates serious problems for bacteria, particularly young cells needing to grow and mature cells needing to repair damage or to divide.

Gram-Negative Bacteria With the gram-negative bacteria, the cell wall is more complex and more lipoidal (Fig. 33.11). These cells usually contain an additional outer lipid membrane that differs considerably from the inner membrane. The outer layer contains complex lipopolysaccharides that encode antigenic responses, cause septic shock, provide the serotype, and influence morphology. This exterior layer also contains a number of enzymes and exclusionary proteins. Important among these are the porins. These are transmembranal supermolecules made up of two or three monomeric proteins.

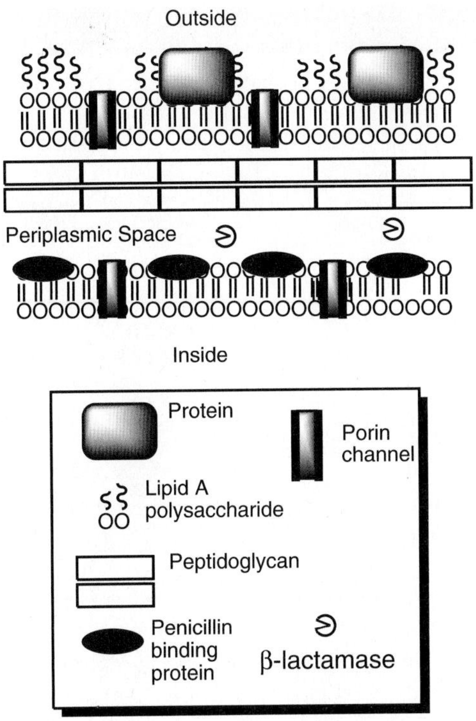

FIGURE 33.11 Schematic of some features of the gram-negative bacterial cell wall.

The center of this array is a transmembranal pore of various dimensions. Some allow many kinds of small molecules to pass, and others contain specific receptors that allow only certain molecules to come in. The size, shape, and lipophilicity of drugs are important considerations controlling porin passage. Antibiotics have greater difficulty in penetrating into gram-negative bacterial cells as a consequence. Next comes a periplasmic space containing a somewhat less impressive and thinner, as compared to gram-positive organisms, layer of peptidoglycan. Also present is a phospholipid-rich cytoplasmic membrane in which floats a series of characteristic proteins with various functions. The β-lactam targets (PBPs) are found here.

Other inner membrane proteins are involved in transport, energy, and biosynthesis. In many such cells, there are proteins that actively pump out antibiotics and other substances at the expense of energy and that may require the simultaneous entrance of oppositely charged materials to maintain an electrostatic balance.

β-Lactam Antibiotics

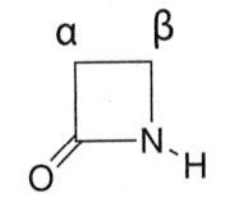

β -lactam
azetidinone

The name lactam is given to cyclic amides and is analogous to the name lactone given to cyclic esters. In an older nomenclature, the second carbon in an aliphatic carboxylic acid was designated alpha, the third beta, and so on. Thus a β-lactam is a cyclic amide with four atoms in its ring. The contemporary name for this ring system is azetidinone. This structural feature was very rare when it was found to be a feature of the structure of the penicillins, so the name β-lactam came to be a generic descriptor for the whole family. Ultimately, this ring proved to be the main component of the pharmacophore, so the term possesses medicinal as well as chemical significance. The penicillin subclass of β-lactam antibiotics is characterized by the presence of a substituted five-membered thiazolidine ring fused to the β-lactam ring. This fusion and the chirality of the β-lactam ring result in the molecule roughly possessing a "V" shape. This drastically interferes with the planarity of the lactam bond and inhibits resonance of the lactam nitrogen with its carbonyl group. Consequently the β-lactam ring is much more reactive and thus more sensitive to nucleophilic attack when compared with normal planar amides.

History The general story of the discovery of the penicillins was previously discussed. The earliest penicillins were produced by fungi from media constituents. The bicyclic heterocyclic nucleus of 6-aminopenicillanic acid is constructed by a process catalyzed by enzymes. The side chain was added essentially intact from media constituents. It was discovered that certain arylacetic acids, when added to the medium, were used to form the side chain amide moiety and that this was very important for stability and breadth of spectrum (30). It was later discovered that exclusion of such materials from the medium allowed the production of 6-aminopenicillanic acid without a side chain (31). Chemists could then add a wider variety of side chains without being limited by the specific requirements of the fungal enzymes. With this breakthrough, the penicillin field expanded to include orally active, broad-spectrum, and enzymatically stable penicillins. The cephalosporins were discovered as secondary metabolites of a different fungal species (32). Because it was stable to many activity-destroying β-lactamases, its core nucleus, 7-aminocephalosporanic acid was substituted with a wide variety of unnatural side chains, and three generations of clinically useful analogs have resulted. Later work produced the carbapenems, monobactams, and β-lactamase inhibitors (33–35). Many thousands of these compounds have been prepared by partial or total chemical synthesis, and a significant number of these remain on the market many years after their discovery.

Penicillins The medicinal classifications, chemical structures, and generic names of the penicillins currently available are provided in Table 33.4.

Preparation of Penicillins. The original fermentation-derived penicillins were produced by growth of the fungus *Penicillium chrysogenum* on complex solid media with

TABLE 33.4 Commercially Significant Penicillins and Related Molecules

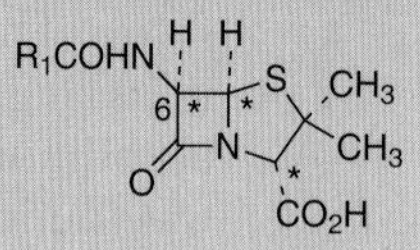

Generic Name	Trade Name	R_1
Fermentation-Derived Penicillins		
6-Aminopenicillanic acid		H
Benzylpenicillin (Penicillin G)	Generic	C_6H_5-CH_2
Phenoxymethylpenicillin (Penicillin V)	Generic	C_6H_5-OCH_2
Semi-Synthetic Penicillinase-Resistant Parenteral Penicillins		
Methicillin[a]		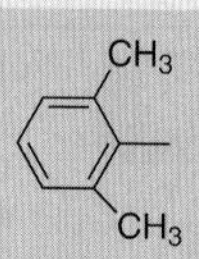
Nafcillin	Nallpen, Unipen	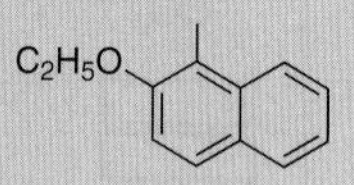
Semi-Synthetic Penicillinase-Resistant Oral Penicillins		
Oxacillin (X = Y = H) Dicloxacillin (X = Y = Cl)	Bactocill Generic	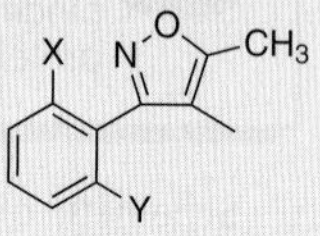
Semi-Synthetic Penicillinase-Sensitive, Broad Spectrum, Parenteral Penicillins		
Carbenicillin[a] (R_2 = H) Carbenicillin indanyl[a] (R_2 = 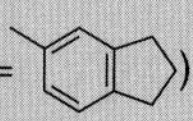)		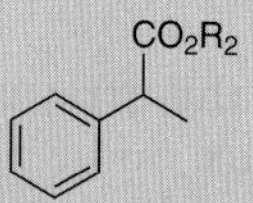
Ticarcillin (in combination with clavulanic acid)	Timentin	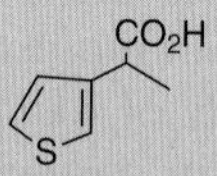
Mezlocillin[a]		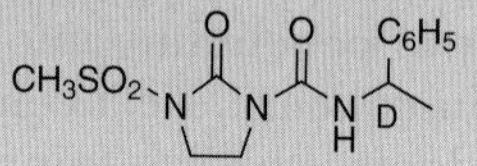
Piperacillin (in combination with tazobactam)	Zosyn	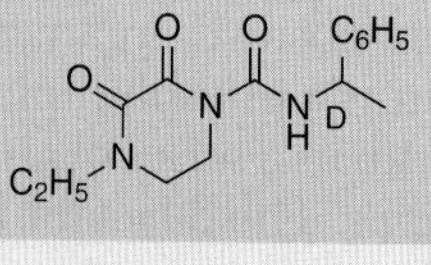
Semi-Synthetic Penicillinase-Sensitive, Broad-Spectrum, Oral Penicillins		
Ampicillin (X = H) Amoxicillin (X = OH)	Generic Amoxil, Trimox	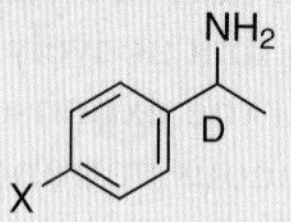

[a]Not currently available in U.S.

the result that they were mixtures differing from one another in the identity of the side chain moiety. When a sufficient supply of phenylacetic acid is present in liquid media, this is preferentially incorporated into the molecule to produce mainly benzylpenicillin (penicillin G in the old nomenclature). Use of phenoxyacetic acid instead leads to phenoxymethyl penicillin (penicillin V). More than two dozen different penicillins have been made in this way, but these two are the only ones that remain in clinical use. The complete exclusion of side chain precursor acids from the medium produces the fundamental penicillin nucleus, 6-aminopenicillanic acid (6-APA), but in poor yield. By itself, 6-APA has only very weak antibiotic activity, but when substituted on its primary amino group with a suitable acid to give amide side chains, its potency and antibacterial spectrum are profoundly enhanced. With this key precursor isolated, limitations caused by enzyme specificities in biosynthesis could be overcome by use of partial chemical synthesis.

The sodium and potassium salts of penicillins are crystalline, hydroscopic, and water soluble. They can be employed orally or parentally. When dry, they are stable for long periods, but they hydrolyze rapidly when in solution. Their best stability is noted at pH values between 5.5 and 8, especially at pH 6.0 to 7.2. The procaine and benzathine salts of benzylpenicillin, on the other hand, are water insoluble. Because they dissolve slowly, they are used for repository purposes following injection when long-term blood levels are required.

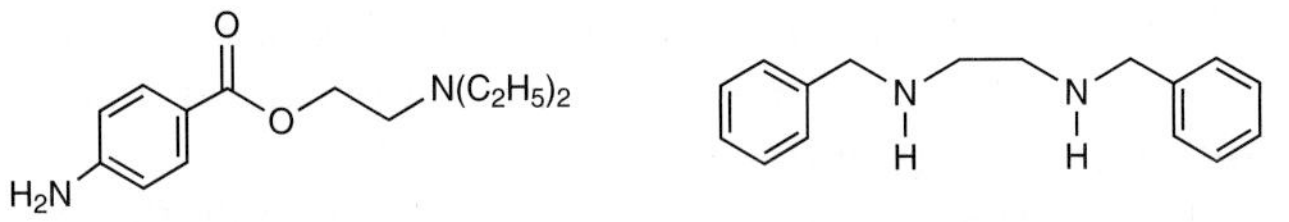

Procaine Benzathine

Nomenclature. The nomenclature of the penicillins, as with most antibiotics, is complex. The Chemical Abstracts system is definitive and unambiguous but too complex for ordinary use (Fig. 33.12). For example, the chemical name for benzylpenicillin sodium is monosodium (2*S*,5*R*,6*R*)-3,3-dimethyl-7-oxo)-6-(2-phenylacetamido)-4-thia-l-azabicyclo[3.2.0]heptane-2-carboxylate. A simpler system has stood the test of time and involves taking the repeating unit, carbonyl-6-APA, and adding to this the chemical trivial name for the added radical that completes the structure. The use of the names benzylpenicillin and phenoxymethylpenicillin makes practical sense. There are three asymmetric centers in the benzylpenicillin molecule as indicated by the asterisk in Table 33.4. This absolute stereochemistry must be preserved for useful antibiotic activity.

Clinically Relevant Chemical Instabilities. The most unstable bond in the penicillin molecule is the highly strained and reactive β-lactam amide bond. This bond cleaves moderately slowly in water unless heated, but breaks down much more rapidly in alkaline solutions to produce penicilloic acid, which readily decarboxylates to produce penilloic acid (Fig. 33.13). Penicilloic acid has a negligible tendency to reclose to the corresponding penicillin, so this reaction is essentially irreversible under physiologic conditions. Because the β-lactam ring is an essential portion of the pharmacophore, its hydrolysis deactivates the antibiotic. A fairly significant degree of hydrolysis also takes place in the liver. The bacterial enzyme, β-lactamase, catalyzes this reaction also and is a principal cause of bacterial resistance in the clinic. Alcohols and amines bring about the same cleavage reaction, but the products are the corresponding esters and amides. These products are inactive.

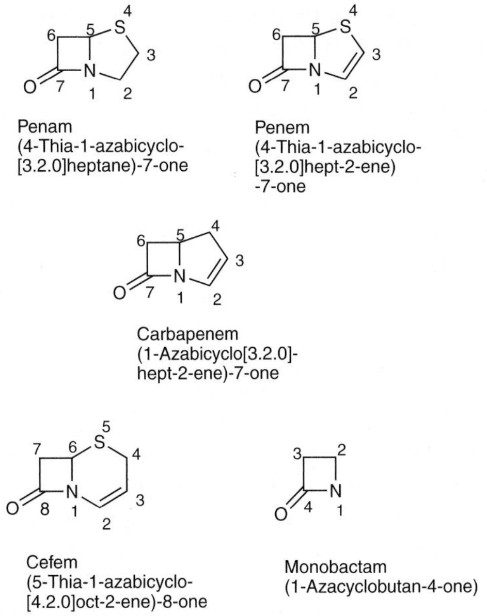

FIGURE 33.12 Ring and numbering systems of clinically available β-lactam antibiotic types.

A reaction with a specific primary amino group of aminoglycoside antibiotics is of clinical relevance as it inactivates penicillins and cephalosporins and will be discussed later in the chapter. When proteins serve as the nucleophiles in this reaction, the antigenic conjugates that cause many penicillin allergies are produced. Small molecules that are not inherently antigenic but react with proteins to produce antigens in this manner are called haptens. Commercially available penicillin salts may be contaminated with small amounts of these antigenic penicilloyl proteins derived from reaction

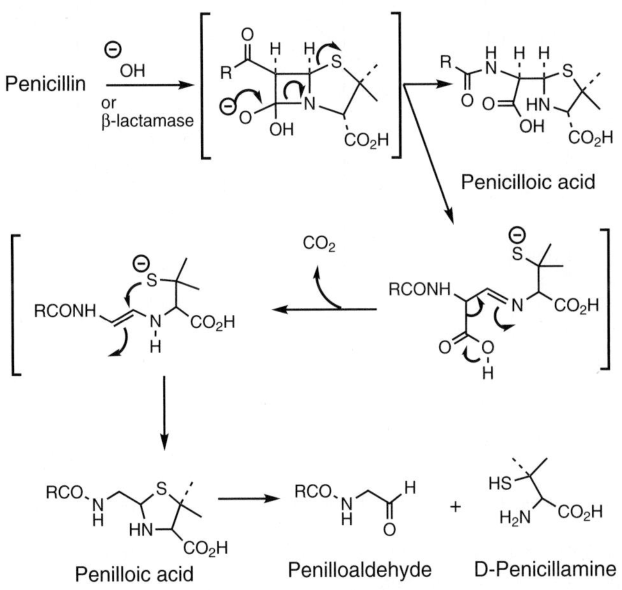

FIGURE 33.13 Instability of β-lactams to nucleophiles.

with proteins encountered in their fermentative production or by high molecular weight self-condensation–derived polymers resulting when penicillins are concentrated and react with themselves. Both of these classes of impurities are antigenic and may sensitize some patients.

In acidic solutions, the hydrolysis of penicillins is complex. Hydrolysis of the β-lactam bond can be shown through kinetic analysis to involve participation of the side chain amide oxygen because the rate of this reaction differs widely depending on the nature of the R group. The main end products of the acidic degradation are penicillamine, penilloic acid, and penilloaldehyde (Fig. 33.14). The intermediate penicillenic acid is highly unstable and undergoes subsequent hydrolysis to the corresponding penicilloic acid. An alternate pathway involves sulfur ejection to a product that in turn fragments to liberate penicilloic acid also. Penicilloic acid readily decarboxylates to penilloic acid. The latter hydrolyzes to produce penilloaldehyde and penicillamine (itself used clinically as a chelating agent). Several related fragmentations to a variety of other products take place. None of these products has antibacterial activity. At gastric pH (~2.0) and temperature of 37°C, benzyl penicillin has a half-life measured in minutes. The less water-soluble amine salts are more stable.

Structure–Activity Relationship. The chemical substituents attached to the penicillin nucleus can greatly influence the stability of the penicillins as well as the spectrum of activity. It is important to recognize whether the structural changes affect drug stability on the shelf or in the GI tract (in vivo), improve stability toward bacterial metabolism, or enlarge the spectrum of activity.

The substitution of a side-chain R group on the primary amine of 6-APA with an electron-withdrawing group decreases the electron density on the side-chain carbonyl and protects these penicillins in part from acid degradation. This property has clinical implications because these compounds survive passage through the stomach better and many can be given orally for systemic purposes. The survival of passage and degree of absorption under fasting conditions is shown in Table 33.5.

In addition, in vitro degradation reactions of penicillins can be retarded by keeping the pH of solutions between 6.0 and 6.8 and by refrigerating them. Metal ions such as mercury, zinc, and copper catalyze the degradation of penicillins so they should be kept from contact with penicillin solutions. The lids of containers used today are routinely made of inert plastics in part to minimize such problems.

The more lipophilic the side chain of a penicillin, the more serum protein bound is the antibiotic (Table 33.6). Although this has some advantages in terms of protection from degradation, it does reduce measurably the effective bactericidal concentration of the drug in whole blood. The degree of serum protein binding of the penicillins has comparatively little influence on their half-lives. The penicillins are actively excreted into the urine via an active transport system for weak acids, and the rate of release from their protein-bound form is sufficiently rapid that the controlling rate is the

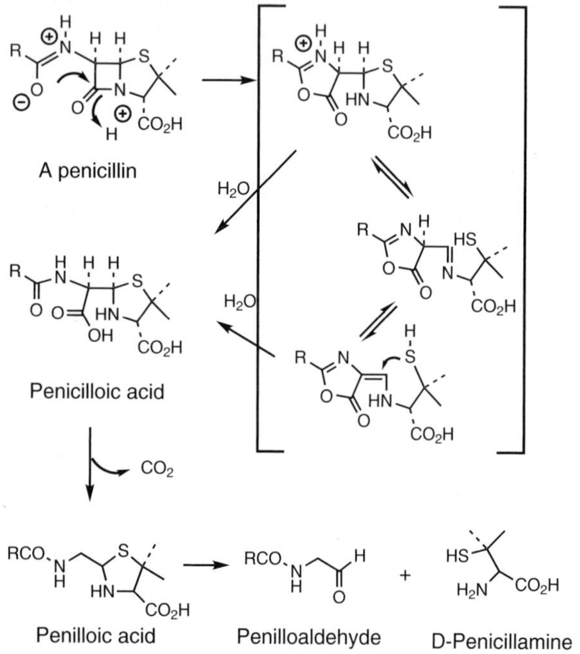

FIGURE 33.14 Instability of penicillins in acid. Hydrolysis involves the C-6 side chain.

TABLE 33.5 Improved Acid Stability and Absorption of Substituted Penicillins

Drug	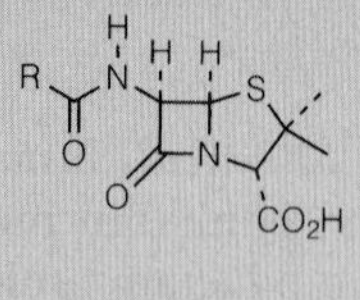 R	% Absorption intact drug
Benzylpenicillin	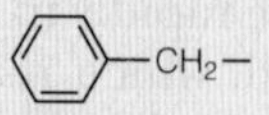	15–30
Pen V	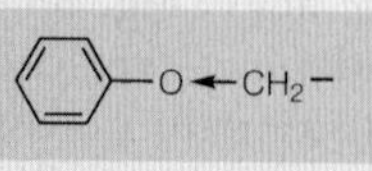	60–73
Ampicillin	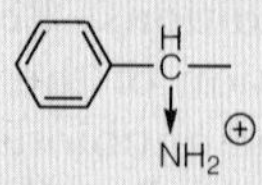	30–50
Amoxicillin	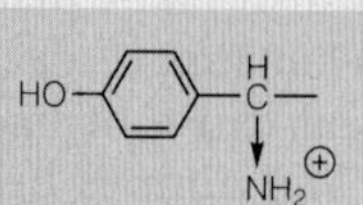	75–90

TABLE 33.6 Protein Binding of Penicillins

Penicillin	Protein Binding (%)
Benzyl penicillin	45–68
Phenoxymethyl penicillin	75–89
Methicillin	35–80
Ampicillin	25–30
Amoxicillin	25–30
Carbenicillin	~50
Oxacillin	>90
Cloxacillin	>90

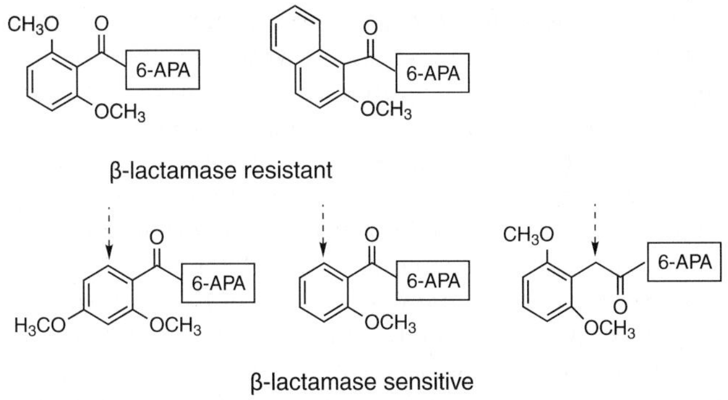

FIGURE 33.15 β-Lactamase resistant/sensitive structural features.

kidney secretion rate. The serum half-life of penicillin G is about 0.4 to 0.9 hours, and that of phenoxymethyl penicillin is about 0.5 hours. Both are excreted into the urine by tubular excretion. Probenecid, when present, competes effectively for excretion and thus prolongs the half-life.

Stability of the penicillins toward β-lactamase is influenced by the bulk in the acyl group attached to the primary amine. β-Lactamases are much less tolerant to the presence of steric hindrance near the side-chain amide bond than are the PBPs. The stability of methicillin to β-lactamases is an example of this. When the aromatic ring is attached directly to the side chain carbonyl and both ortho-positions are substituted by methoxy groups, β-lactamase stability results (Fig. 33.15). Movement of one of the methoxy groups to the para position or replacing one of them with a hydrogen results in an analog sensitive to β-lactamases. Putting in a methylene between the aromatic ring and 6-APA likewise produces a β-lactamase–sensitive agent (Fig. 33.15). These findings provide strong support for the hypothesis that its resistance to enzyme degradation is based on differential steric hindrance. Prime examples of this effect are seen in nafcillin, oxacillin, and dicloxacillin (Table 33.4).

Mechanism of Action. The molecular mode of action of the β-lactam antibiotics is a selective and irreversible inhibition of the enzymes processing the developing peptidoglycan layer (Fig. 33.16). Just before cross-linking

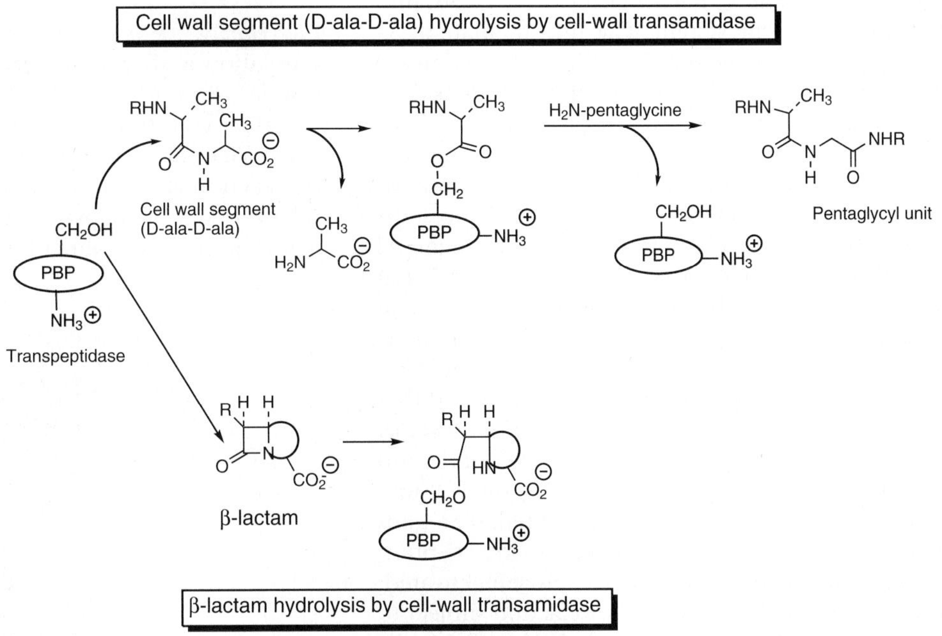

FIGURE 33.16 Cell wall cross-linking and mechanism of action of β-lactams.

occurs, the peptide pendant from the lactate carboxyl of a muramic acid unit terminates in a D-alanyl-D-alanine unit. The terminal D-alanine unit is exchanged for a glycine unit on an adjacent strand in a reaction catalyzed by a cell wall transamidase. This enzyme is one of the PBPs (carboxypeptidases, endopeptidases, and transpeptidases) that normally reside in the bacterial inner membrane and perform construction, repair, and housekeeping functions, maintaining cell wall integrity and playing a vital role in cell growth and division. They differ significantly from bacterium to bacterium, and this is used to rationalize different potency and morphologic outcomes following β-lactam attack on the different bacteria. The cell wall transamidase uses a serine hydroxyl group to attack the penultimate D-alanyl unit forming a covalent ester bond, and the terminal D-alanine, which is released by this action, diffuses away. The enzyme–peptidoglycan ester bond is attacked by the free amino end of a pentaglycyl unit of an adjacent strand, regenerating the transpeptidase's active site for further catalytic action and producing a new amide bond, which connects two adjacent strands together.

The three-dimensional geometry of the active site of the enzyme perfectly accommodates to the shape and separation of the amino acids of its substrate. Because the substrate has unnatural stereochemistry at the critical residues, this enzyme is not expected to attack host peptides or even other bacterial peptides composed of natural amino acids.

The penicillins and the other β-lactam antibiotics have a structure that closely resembles that of acylated D-alanyl-D-alanine. The enzyme mistakenly accepts the penicillin as though it were its normal substrate. The highly strained β-lactam ring is much more reactive than a normal amide moiety, particularly when fused into the appropriate bicyclic system. The intermediate acyl–enzyme complex, however, is rather different structurally from the normal intermediate in that the hydrolysis does not break penicillin into two pieces as it does with its normal substrate. In the penicillins, a heterocyclic residue is still covalently bonded and cannot diffuse away as the natural terminal D-alanine unit does. This presents a steric barrier to approach by the nearby pentaglycyl unit and thus keeps the enzyme's active site from being regenerated and the cell wall precursors from being cross-linked. The result is a defective cell wall and an inactivated enzyme. The relief of strain that is obtained on enzymatic β-lactam bond cleavage is so pronounced that there is virtually no tendency for the reaction to reverse. Water is also an insufficiently effective nucleophile and cannot hydrolyze the complex either. Thus, the cell wall transamidase is stoichiometrically inactivated. The gaps in the cell wall produced by this covalent interruption are not filled in because the enzyme is now inactivated. The resulting cell wall is structurally weak and subject to osmotic stress. Cell lysis can result, and the cell rapidly dies assisted by another class of bacterial enzymes, the autolysins (36).

Resistance. The first literature reports of a penicillinase were published in 1940 (37). This phenomenon was rare at the time and caused no particular alarm. Resistance to β-lactam antibiotics is unfortunately increasingly common and is rather alarming. It can be intrinsic and involve decreased cellular uptake of drug, or involve lower binding affinity to the PBPs. This is particularly the case with MRSA. MRSA produces a mutated PBP-2 (PBP-2a) that does not efficiently bind methicillin any longer. More common, however, is the elaboration of a β-lactamase. β-Lactamases are enzymes (usually serine proteases) elaborated by microorganisms that catalyze hydrolysis of the β-lactam bond and inactivate β-lactam antibiotics to penicilloic acids before they can reach the PBPs (Fig. 33.17). They somewhat resemble the cell wall transamidase, which is the usual target. Hydrolytic regeneration of the active site is dramatically more facile with β-lactamases than is the case with cell wall transamidase, so that the enzyme can turn over many times and a comparatively small amount of enzyme can destroy a large amount of drug. With gram-positive bacteria, such as staphylococci, the β-lactamases are usually shed continuously into the medium and meet the drug outside the cell wall. They are biosynthesized in significant quantities. With gram-negative bacteria, a more conservative course is followed. Here the β-lactamases are secreted into the periplasmic space between the inner and outer membrane so, while still distal to the PBPs, they do not readily escape into the medium and need not be resynthesized as often. Numerous β-lactamases with various antibiotic substrate specificities are now known. Various classification systems are used for β-lactamases and have been extensively reviewed (29). Elaboration of β-lactamases is often R-factor mediated and, in some cases, is even induced by the presence of β-lactam antibiotics.

Allergenicity. It is estimated that 2% to 8% of the U.S. population is allergic to β-lactam antibiotics. The actual number is very difficult to determine due to overreporting. Most commonly, the allergy is expressed as a mild drug rash or itching and is of delayed onset. Occasionally, the reaction is immediate and profound. It may include cardiovascular collapse and shock and can result in death. Sometimes penicillin allergy can be anticipated

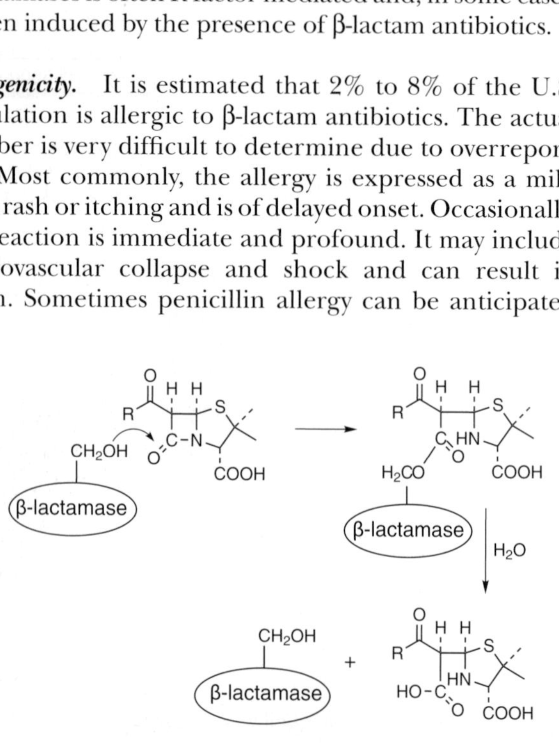

FIGURE 33.17 β-Lactamase–catalyzed hydrolysis of penicillins.

by taking a medication history, and often, patients likely to be allergic are those with a history of hypersensitivity to a wide variety of allergens (e.g., foods and pollens). A prior history of allergy to penicillins is a contraindicating factor to their use. Skin tests are available when there is doubt. When an allergic reaction develops, the drug must be discontinued and, because cross-sensitivity is relatively common, other β-lactam families should be used carefully. Considering all therapeutic categories, penicillins are probably the drugs most associated with allergy. Erythromycin and clindamycin are useful alternate choices for therapy in many cases of penicillin allergy.

In some cases, the patient may have become sensitized without knowing it due to prior passive exposure through contaminated foodstuffs or cross-contaminated medications. Penicillins are manufactured in facilities separate from those used to prepare other drugs in order to prevent cross contamination and possible sensitization. Animals treated with penicillins are required to be drug free for a significant time before products prepared from them can be consumed. Because the origin of the allergy is a haptenic reaction with host proteins and the responsible bond in the drug is the β-lactam moiety, this side effect is caused by the pharmacophore of the drug and is unlikely to be overcome by molecular manipulation.

Individual Penicillins. The penicillins are usually discussed under various groups based on spectrum of activity and sensitivity or resistance toward β-lactamase. One of the earliest and still most commonly used penicillins is benzylpenicillin.

Benzylpenicillin Group.

Benzylpenicillin (Penicillin G, Table 33.4) With the exception of *Neisseria gonorrhoeae* and *Haemophilus influenzae*, and a few bacteria encountered less frequently, the useful antimicrobial spectrum of benzylpenicillin is primarily against gram-positive cocci. Because of its cheapness, efficacy, and lack of toxicity (except for acutely allergic patients), benzylpenicillin remains a remarkably useful agent for treatment of diseases caused by susceptible microorganisms. As with most antibiotics, susceptibility tests must be performed because many formerly highly sensitive microorganisms are now comparatively resistant. Infections of the upper and lower respiratory tract and the genitourinary tract are the particular province of benzylpenicillin. Infections caused by group A β-hemolytic streptococci (pharyngitis, scarlet fever, cellulitis, pelvic infections, and septicemia) are commonly responsive. Group B hemolytic streptococci infections, especially of neonates (acute respiratory distress, pneumonia, meningitis, septic shock, and septicemia), also may respond. Pneumococcal pneumonia, *H. influenzae* pneumonia of children, *Streptococcus pneumoniae*– and *Streptococcus pyogenes*–caused otitis media and sinusitis, meningococcal meningitis and brain abscess, meningococcal and pneumococcal septicemia, streptococcal endocarditis (often by *Streptococcus viridans*), pelvic inflammatory disease (often by *Neisseria gonorrhoeae* and *S. pyogenes*), uncomplicated gonorrhea (*N. gonorrhoeae*), meningitis (*Neisseria meningitidis*), syphilis (*Treponema pallidum*), Lyme disease (*Borrelia burgdorferi*), gas gangrene (*Clostridium perfringens*), and tetanus (*Clostridium tetani*) are among the diseases that may respond to benzylpenicillin therapy, either alone or sometimes with other drugs used in combination. Nonpenicillinase-producing *Staphylococcus aureus* and *Staphylococcus epidermidis* are quite sensitive but are very rare today. Other, less common, bacterial diseases also respond, such as those caused by *Bacillus anthracis* (anthrax) and *Corynebacterium diphtheriae* (diphtheria).

Because of its low cost, mild infections with susceptible microorganisms can be treated with comparatively large oral doses, although the most effective route of administration is parenteral because five times the blood level can be regularly achieved in this manner. As previously discussed (see previous section *Clinically relevant chemical instabilities*), penicillin G is unstable under the acidic conditions of the stomach.

Very water-insoluble penicillin salts form with procaine and with *N,N'*-bibenzyl ethylenediamine. These find therapeutic application for intramuscular injections. This produces lower but prolonged levels of penicillin as the drug slowly diffuses from the injection site.

The need to improve defects in benzylpenicillin stimulated an intense research effort that persists to this day. Overcoming such negative features as comparative instability (particularly to acid), comparatively poor oral absorption, allergenicity, sensitivity to β-lactamases, and relatively narrow antimicrobial spectrum has been an objective of this work.

Phenoxymethyl Penicillin (Penicillin V, Table 33.4) Penicillin V is produced by fermentation where the medium is enriched in phenoxyacetic acid. It can also be prepared by semisynthesis. It is considerably more acid stable than benzylpenicillin as indicated by oral absorption (Table 33.5). This is rationalized as being due to the electronegative oxygen atom in the C-7 amide side chain inhibiting participation in β-lactam bond hydrolysis. In any case, penicillin V was the first of the so-called oral penicillins giving higher and more prolonged blood levels than penicillin G itself. Its antimicrobial and clinical spectrum is roughly the same as that of benzylpenicillin, although it is somewhat less potent and is not used for acutely serious infections. Penicillin V has approximately the same sensitivity to β-lactamases and allergenicity as penicillin G.

Penicillinase-Resistant Penicillins.

Methicillin (Table 33.4) Methicillin is now archaic but was the first of the penicillinase-resistant agents to reach the clinic (38). It is unstable to gastric acid, having a half-life of 5 minutes at pH 2, so it has to be administer via injection. As discussed previously, increased bulk resulting from the addition of the dimethoxybenzoyl group to 6-APA leads to methicillin being a β-lactamase–resistant drug. Methicillin has significantly narrower antimicrobial spectrum and less potency, so it was restricted to clinical use primarily for parenteral use in infections due to β-lactamase–producing *S. aureus* and a few other infections. An increasing number of infections are caused by MRSA. In these organisms, an altered PBP is formed that has a very low affinity for β-lactams, excluding ceftaroline. Furthermore, methicillin is an efficient inducer of penicillinases. Consequently this drug fell out of favor, and methicillin has now been replaced.

Nafcillin (Table 33.4) Nafcillin has a 2-ethoxynaphthyl side chain. This bulky group serves to inhibit destruction by β-lactamases analogous to methicillin. Although slightly more acid stable than methicillin, it is clinically virtually identical to it.

Oxacillin and Dicloxacillin Using a substituted isoxazolyl ring as a bioisosteric replacement for the benzene ring of penicillin G produces the isoxazolyl penicillins. Currently, oxacillin and dicloxacillin (Table 33.4) are available. Chemically, they differ from one another by chlorine substituents on the benzene ring. Like methicillin, these are generally less potent than benzylpenicillin against gram-positive microorganisms (generally staphylococci and streptococci) that do not produce a β-lactamase but retain their potency against those that do. An added bonus exists in that they are somewhat more acid stable; thus they may be taken orally, and they are more potent as well. Because they are highly serum protein bound (Table 33.6), they are not good choices for treatment of septicemia. Microorganisms resistant against methicillin are also resistant to the isoxazolyl group of penicillins. Like nafcillin, the isoxazolyl group of penicillins is primarily used against penicillinase-producing *Staphylococcus aureus* (39,40).

Penicillinase-Sensitive, Broad-Spectrum, Oral Penicillins.
Ampicillin The first member of this group, ampicillin, is a benzylpenicillin analog in which one of the hydrogen atoms of the side chain methylene has been replaced with a primary amino group to produce an *R*-phenylglycine moiety (Table 33.4). In addition to significant acid stability enhancing its successful oral use, the antimicrobial spectrum is shifted so that many common gram-negative pathogens are sensitive to ampicillin. This is believed to be due to greater penetration of ampicillin into gram-negative bacteria. The acid stability is generally believed to be caused by the electron-withdrawing character of the protonated primary amine group reducing participation in hydrolysis of the β-lactam bond as well as to the comparative difficulty of bringing another positively charged species (H_3O^+) into the vicinity of the protonated amino group. The oral activity is also enhanced, in part, to active uptake by the dipeptide transporters (41). It unfortunately lacks stability toward β-lactamases, and resistance is increasingly common. To assist with this, several β-lactamase inhibitors for coadministration (discussed below) have been developed that restore many penicillinase-producing strains to the clinical spectrum of the aminopenicillins.

Ampicillin is essentially equivalent to benzyl penicillin for pneumococcal, streptococcal, and meningococcal infections and many strains of gram-negative *Salmonella, Shigella, Proteus mirabilis,* and *Escherichia coli,* as well as many strains of *Haemophilus influenzae* and *Neisseria gonorrhoeae* respond well to oral treatment with ampicillin.

Bacampicillin

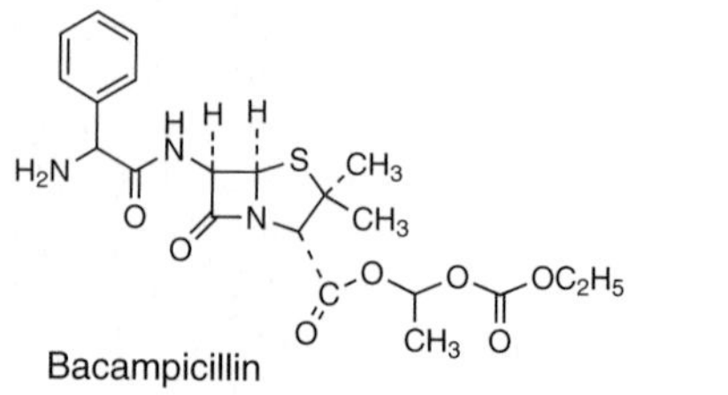

Bacampicillin

Although comparatively well absorbed, ampicillin's oral efficacy for systemic infections can be enhanced significantly through the preparation of prodrugs. In contrast to ampicillin itself, which is amphoteric, bacampicillin is a weak base and is very well absorbed in the duodenum. Enzymatic ester hydrolysis in the gut wall liberates carbon dioxide and ethanol followed by spontaneous loss of acetaldehyde and production of ampicillin. The acetaldehyde is metabolized oxidatively by alcohol dehydrogenase to produce acetic acid, which joins the normal metabolic pool. Amoxicillin, which has better oral availability than ampicillin has made the clinical use of bacampicillin unnecessary, and it is no longer available in the United States.

Amoxicillin (Table 33.4) Amoxicillin is a close analog of ampicillin in which a para-phenolic hydroxyl group has been introduced into the side-chain phenyl moiety. This adjusts the isoelectric point of the drug to a more acidic value and is believed to be partially responsible, along with the intestine dipeptide transporter, for the enhanced blood levels obtained with amoxicillin compared with ampicillin itself (Table 33.5). Better oral absorption leads to less disturbance of the normal GI flora and, therefore, less drug-induced diarrhea. The antimicrobial spectrum and clinical uses of amoxicillin are approximately the same as those of ampicillin.

The addition of clavulanic acid (below) to amoxicillin gives a combination (Augmentin) in which the clavulanic acid serves to protect amoxicillin to a considerable extent against β-lactamases. This expands the spectrum of activity to include organisms and strains that produce β-lactamases.

Clavulanic Acid

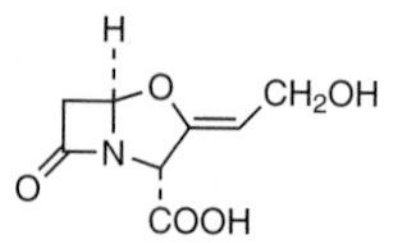

Clavulanic acid

Clavulanic acid is a mold product that has only weak intrinsic antibacterial activity but is an excellent irreversible

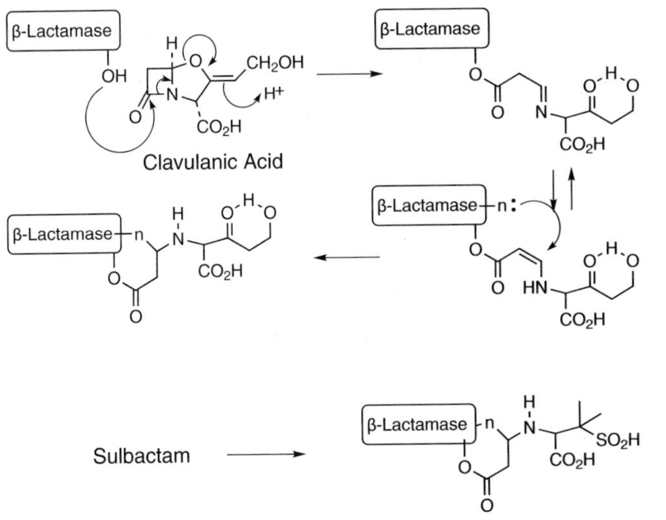

FIGURE 33.18 Speculative mechanism for irreversible inactivation of β-lactamase by clavulanic acid and sulbactam.

inhibitor of most β-lactamases. It is believed to acylate the active site serine by mimicking the normal substrate. While hydrolysis occurs with some β-lactamases, in many cases, subsequent reactions occur that inhibit the enzyme irreversibly. This leads to its classification as a mechanism-based inhibitor (or so-called suicide substrate). The precise chemistry is not well understood (Fig. 33.18), but when clavulanic acid is added to amoxicillin and ticarcillin preparations, the potency against β-lactamase–producing strains is markedly enhanced.

Sulbactam

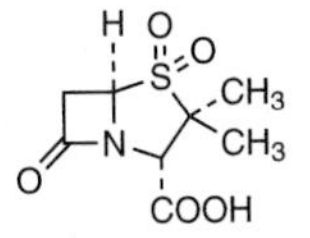

Sulbactam

Another β-lactamase inhibitor is sulbactam. Sulbactam is prepared by partial chemical synthesis from penicillins. The oxidation of the sulfur atom to a sulfone greatly enhances the potency of sulbactam. The combination of sulbactam and ampicillin (Unasyn) is also clinically popular. Not all β-lactamases are sensitive to the presence of clavulanic acid or sulbactam.

Penicillinase-Sensitive, Broad-Spectrum, Parenteral Penicillins. *Mezlocillin and Piperacillin* Mezlocillin and piperacillin are ampicillin derivatives in which the D-side chain amino group has been converted by chemical processes to a variety of substituted urea analogs (Table 33.4). These are known as acylureidopenicillins and preserve the useful anti–gram-positive activity of ampicillin but have higher anti–gram-negative potency. Some strains of *Pseudomonas aeruginosa* are sensitive to these agents. It is speculated that the added side-chain moiety mimics a longer segment of the peptidoglycan chain than ampicillin does. This cell wall fragment is usually a tetrapeptide, so there is expected to be room for an extension in this direction. This would give more possible points of attachment to the penicillin-binding proteins, and perhaps these features are responsible for their enhanced antibacterial properties. These agents are used parenterally with particular emphasis on gram-negative bacteria, especially *Klebsiella pneumoniae* and the anaerobe, *Bacteroides fragilis* (42). Resistance due to β-lactamases is a prominent feature of their use, so disk testing and incorporation of additional agents (such as an aminoglycoside) for the treatment of severe infections are advisable. Mezlocillin is not marketed in the United States.

Piperacillin and Tazobactam Combination (Zosyn)

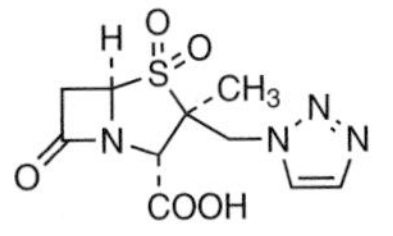

Tazobactam

Tazobactam is often coadministered with piperacillin because of tazobactam's ability to inhibit β-lactamases. Tazobactam, like other β-lactamase inhibitors, has little or no antibacterial activity. This effect is analogous to that of clavulanic acid and sulbactam discussed earlier. This combination is the broadest spectrum penicillin currently available (43).

Carbenicillin and Indanyl Carbenicillin Carbenicillin is a benzyl penicillin analog in which one of the methylene hydrogens of the side chain has been substituted with a carboxylic acid moiety (Table 33.4). The specific stereochemistry of this change is not very important as both diastereoisomers are configurationally unstable and mutarotate with time to produce the same mixture of epimers. The introduction of the side-chain carboxyl produces enhanced anti–gram-negative activity. In fact, carbenicillin is intrinsically one of the broadest-spectrum penicillins. Carbenicillin is an order of magnitude less potent than the acylureidopenicillins. The drug is susceptible to β-lactamases and is acid unstable and thus must be given by injection.

Because it is a malonic acid hemiamide with a carbonyl (amide) moiety beta to the carboxyl group, carbenicillin can decarboxylate readily to produce benzyl penicillin (Fig. 33.19). While still an antibiotic, this degradation product has no activity against the organisms for

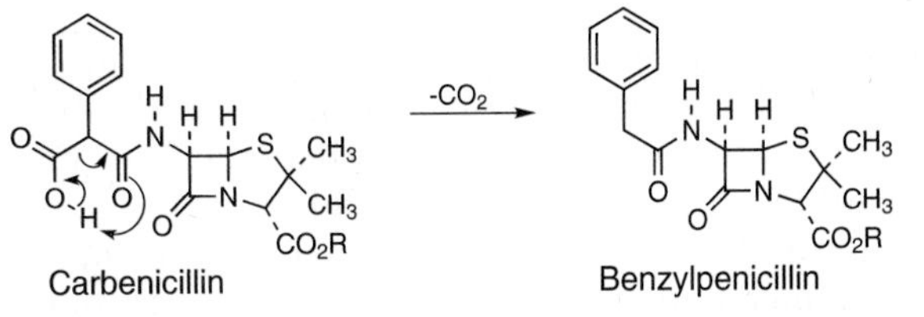

FIGURE 33.19 Decarboxylation of carbenicillin to benzylpenicillin.

which carbenicillin would be indicated. In addition, the large doses of carbenicillin sodium that have to be used (multigrams per day) result in ingestion of a significant amount of sodium ion, which could be a consideration for patients. Indanyl carbenicillin is an oral prodrug form. Due to these issues, neither form is currently available, and these drugs have been replaced by ticarcillin.

Ticarcillin Ticarcillin is a sulfur-based bioisostere of carbenicillin that cannot decarboxylate as the carboxyl group of carbenicillin does (Table 33.4). This agent is somewhat more potent against pseudomonads than is indanyl carbenicillin.

When potassium clavulanate is added to ticarcillin (Timentin), the combination has enhanced spectrum due to its enhanced stability to lactamases (44).

Summary. The penicillins ushered in the era of powerful antibiotics, and their use transformed the practice of antimicrobial chemotherapy. A significant percentage of the population that is alive today owes their longevity and relative freedom from morbidity to the use of these agents. The pace of discovery has fallen off dramatically, and no new penicillin has been introduced into the market for many years. Instead, although retaining their important place in contemporary medicine, research has turned elsewhere for novel agents.

Cephalosporins

History. In contrast to the discovery of the penicillins, in which the first agent had such outstanding biologic antibiotic properties that it entered clinical use with comparatively little modification, the cephalosporins are remarkable for the level of persistence required before their initial discovery yielded economic returns. Abraham and Newton described the structure of the first cephalosporin, cephalosporin C (32). The compound was interesting because, although it was not very potent, it had activity against some penicillin-resistant cultures due to its stability to β-lactamases. Cephalosporin C is not potent enough to be a useful antibiotic, but removal, through chemical means, of the natural side chain produced 7-aminocephalosporanic acid, which, analogous to 6-APA, could be fitted with unnatural side chains (Fig. 33.20). Many of the compounds produced in this way are remarkably useful antibiotics. They differ from one another in antimicrobial spectrum, β-lactamase stability, absorption from the GI tract, metabolism, stability, and side effects as detailed below.

Chemical Properties. The cephalosporins have their β-lactam ring annealed to a six-membered dihydrothiazine ring, in contrast to the penicillins where the β-lactam ring is fused to a five-membered thiazolidine ring. As a consequence of the bigger ring, the cephalosporins should be less strained and less reactive/potent. However, much of the reactivity loss is made up by possession of an olefinic linkage at C-2,3 and a methyleneacetoxy or other leaving group at C-3. When the β-lactam ring is opened by hydrolysis, the leaving group can be ejected, carrying away the developing negative charge. This greatly reduces the energy required for the process. Thus the facility with which the β-lactam bond of the cephalosporins is broken is modulated both by the nature of the C-7 substituent (analogous to the penicillins) as well as the nature of the C-3 substituent and its ability to serve as a leaving group. Considerable support for this hypothesis comes from the finding that isomerization of the olefinic linkage to C-3,4 leads to great losses in antibiotic activity. In practice, most cephalosporins are comparatively unstable in aqueous solutions, and the pharmacist is often directed to keep injectable preparations frozen before use. Being carboxylic acids, they form water-soluble sodium salts, whereas the free acids are comparatively water insoluble.

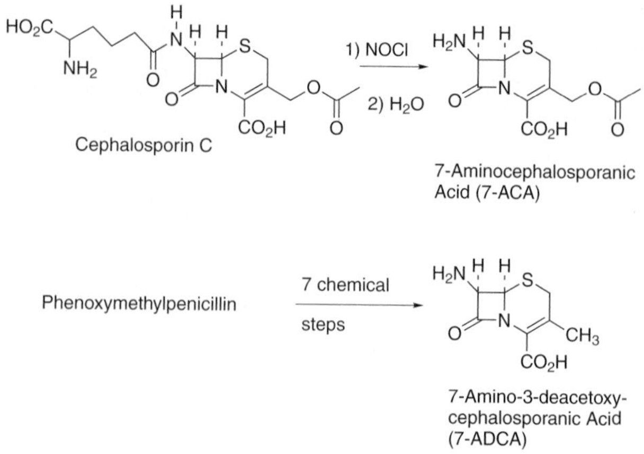

FIGURE 33.20 Chemical preparation of 7-aminocephalosporanic acid (7-ACA) and 7-amino-3-deacetoxycephalosporanic acid (7-ADCA).

Clinically Relevant Chemical Instabilities. The principal chemical instability of the cephalosporins is associated with β-lactam bond hydrolysis. The role of the C-7 and C-3 side chains in these reactions was discussed previously. Ejection of the C3 substituent following β-lactam–bond cleavage is usually drawn for convenience as though this is an unbroken (concerted) process, although ejection of the side chain may at certain times and with specific cephalosporins involve a discrete intermediate with the β-lactam bond broken, but the C-3 substituent not yet eliminated, while other cephalosporins have nonejectable C-3 substituents. The methylthiotetrazole (MTT) group, found in a number of cephalosporins, is capable of elimination. When this happens, this moiety is believed to be responsible in part for clotting difficulties and acute alcohol intolerance in certain patients. The role of the C-7 side chain in all of these processes is clearly important, but active participation of the amide moiety in a manner analogous to the penicillins is rarely specifically invoked. The same considerations that modulate the chemical stability of cephalosporins are also involved in dictating β-lactamase sensitivity, potency, and allergenicity.

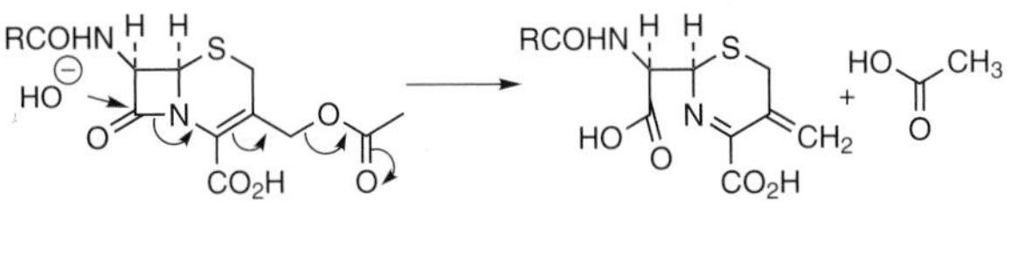

Metabolism. Those cephalosporins that have an acetyl group in the side chain are subject to enzymatic hydrolysis in the body. The result is molecules with a hydroxymethyl moiety at C-3. A hydroxy moiety is a poor leaving group, so this change is considerably deactivating with respect to breakage of the β-lactam bond. In addition, the particular geometry of this part of the molecule leads to facile lactonization with the carboxyl group attached to C-2 (Fig. 33.21). In principle, this should result in formation of a different but reasonable leaving group. The result is, instead, inactivation of the drugs involved. The PBPs have an absolute requirement for a free carboxyl group to mimic that of the terminal carboxyl of the D-alanyl-D-alanine moiety in their normal substrate. Lactonization masks this docking functional group, and as a result, blocks affinity of the inhibitor for the enzyme.

Structure–Activity Relationship.

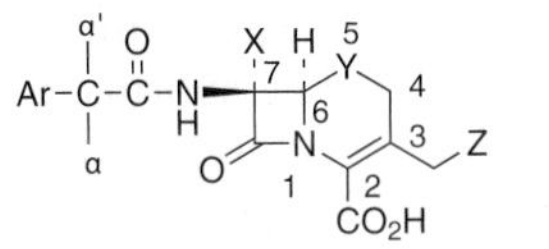

As with the penicillins, various molecular changes in the cephalosporin can improve in vitro stability, antibacterial activity, and stability toward β-lactamases (45). The addition of an amino and a hydrogen to the α and α′ positions, respectively, results in a basic compound that is protonated under the acidic conditions of the stomach.

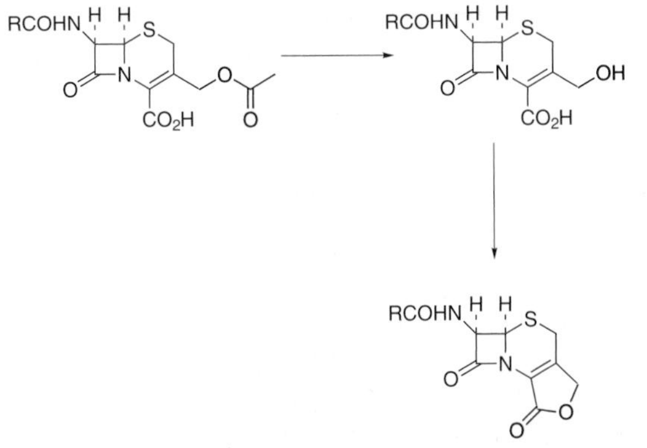

FIGURE 33.21 Metabolism of C-3-acetyl–substituted cephalosporins.

The ammonium ion improves the stability of the β-lactam of the cephalosporin, leading to orally active drugs.

The 7β amino group is essential for antimicrobial activity (X = H), whereas replacement of the hydrogen at C-7 (X = H) with an alkoxy (X = OR) results in improvement of the antibacterial activity of the cephalosporin. Within specific cephalosporin derivatives, the addition of a 7α methoxy also improves the drugs stability toward β-lactamase. The derivatives where Y = S exhibit greater antibacterial activity than if Y = O, but the reverse is true when stability toward β-lactamase is considered. The 6α hydrogen is essential for biologic activity. And finally, antibacterial activity is improved when *Z* is a five-membered heterocycle versus a six-membered heterocycle.

In a study examining stability of cephalosporins toward β-lactamase, it was noted that the following changes improved β-lactamase resistance: 1) the L-isomer of an α amino α′ hydrogen derivative of a cephalosporin was 30 to 40 times more stable than the D-isomer; 2) the addition of a methoxyoxime to the α and α′ positions increased stability nearly 100-fold; and 3) the *Z*-oxime was as much as 20,000-fold more stable than the *E*-oxime (Fig. 33.22) (45). These changes have been incorporated into a number of marketed and experimental cephalosporins (e.g., cefuroxime, ceftizoxime, ceftazidime, cefixime).

Mechanism of Action. The cephalosporins are believed to act in a manner analogous to that of the penicillins by binding to the penicillin-binding proteins followed by cell lysis (Fig. 33.16). Cephalosporins are bactericidal in clinical terms.

Resistance. Analogous to the penicillins, susceptible cephalosporins can be hydrolyzed by β-lactamases before they reach the penicillin-binding proteins. Certain β-lactamases are constitutive (chromosomally encoded) in certain strains of gram-negative bacteria (*Citrobacter, Enterobacter, Pseudomonas,* and *Serratia*) and are normally repressed. These are induced (or derepressed) by certain β-lactam antibiotics (e.g., imipenem, cefotetan, and cefoxitin). As with the penicillins, specific examples will be seen below wherein resistance to β-lactamase hydrolysis is conveyed by strategic steric bulk near the side-chain amide linkage. Penetration barriers to the cephalosporins are also known.

Allergenicity. Allergenicity is less commonly experienced and is less severe with cephalosporins than with penicillins. Cephalosporins are frequently administered to patients

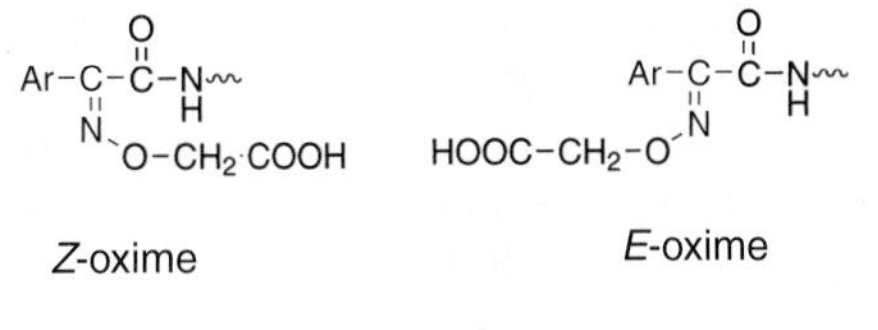

FIGURE 33.22 *Z*- and *E*-oxime configuation.

who have had a mild or delayed penicillin reaction; however, cross allergenicity is possible, and this should be done with caution for patients with a history of allergies. Patients who have had a rapid and severe reaction to penicillins should not be treated with cephalosporins.

Nomenclature and Classification. Most cephalosporins have generic names beginning with cef- or ceph-. This is convenient for classification but makes discriminating between individual members a true memory test. The cephalosporins are classified by a trivial nomenclature system loosely derived from the chronology of their introduction but more closely related to their antimicrobial spectrum. The first-generation cephalosporins are primarily active in vitro against gram-positive cocci (penicillinase-positive and -negative *Staphylococcus aureus* and *Staphylococcus epidermis*), group A β-hemolytic streptococci (*Streptococcus pyogenes*), group B streptococci (*Streptococcus agalactiae*), and *Streptococcus pneumoniae*. They are not effective against MRSA. They are not significantly active against gram-negative bacteria, although some strains of *Escherichia coli*, *Klebsiella pneumoniae*, *Proteus mirabilis*, and *Shigella* sp. may be sensitive (46). The second-generation cephalosporins generally retain the anti–gram-positive activity of the first-generation agents but include *Haemophilus influenzae* as well and add to this better anti–gram-negative activity, so that some strains of *Acinetobacter*, *Citrobacter*, *Enterobacter*, *E. coli*, *Klebsiella*, *Neisseria*, *Proteus*, *Providencia*, and *Serratia* are also sensitive (47). Cefotetan and cefoxitin also have antianaerobic activity as well (48). The third-generation cephalosporins are less active against staphylococci than the first-generation agents but are much more active against gram-negative bacteria than either the first- or the second-generation drugs (49). They are frequently particularly useful against nosocomial multidrug-resistant hospital-acquired strains. *Morganella* sp. and *Pseudomonas aeruginosa* can also be added to the list of species that are often sensitive. The fourth-generation cephalosporins have an antibacterial spectrum like the third-generation drugs but add some enterobacteria that are resistant to the third-generation cephalosporins. They are also more active against some gram-positive organisms (50).

Therapeutic Application. The incidence of cephalosporin resistance is such that it is usually preferable to do sensitivity testing before instituting therapy. Infections of the upper and lower respiratory tract, skin and related soft tissue, urinary tract, bones, and joints, as well as septicemias, endocarditis, intra-abdominal, and bile tract infections caused by susceptible gram-positive organisms are usually responsive to cephalosporins. When gram-positive bacteria are involved, a first-generation agent is preferable. When the pathogen is gram-negative and the infection is serious, parenteral use of a third-generation agent is recommended.

Adverse Effects. Aside from mild or severe allergic reaction, the most commonly experienced cephalosporin toxicities are mild and temporary nausea, vomiting, and diarrhea associated with disturbance of the normal flora. Rarely, a life-threatening pseudomembranous colitis diarrhea associated with the opportunistic and toxin-producing anaerobic pathogen, Clostridium difficile, can be experienced. Rare blood dyscrasias, which can even include aplastic anemia, can also be seen. Certain structural types (details below) are associated with prolonged bleeding times and a disulfiram-like acute alcohol intolerance.

First-generation Cephalosporins (Table 33.7).
Cefazolin. Cefazolin has the natural acetyl side chain at C-3 replaced by a thio-linked thiadiazole ring. Although this group is an activating leaving group, the moiety is not subject to the inactivating host hydrolysis reaction. At C-7, it possesses a tetrazoylmethylene unit. Its dosing should be reduced in the presence of renal impairment. It is comparatively unstable and should be protected from heat and light.

Cephalexin. Use of the ampicillin-type side chain conveys oral activity to cephalexin. Whereas it no longer has an activating side chain at C-3, and as a consequence is somewhat less potent, it does not undergo metabolic deactivation and thus maintains potency. It is rapidly and completely absorbed from the GI tract and has become quite popular. Somewhat puzzling is the fact that the use of the ampicillin side chain in the cephalosporins does not result in a comparable shift in antimicrobial spectrum. Cephalexin, like the other first-generation cephalosporins is active against many gram-positive aerobic cocci but is limited against gram-negative bacteria. It is a widely used drug, particularly against gram-negative bacteria causing urinary tract infections, gram-positive infections (*S. aureus*, *S. pneumoniae*, and *S. pyogenes*) of soft tissues, pharyngitis, and minor wounds (46).

Cefadroxil. Cefadroxil has an amoxicillin-like side chain at C-7 and is orally active. The prolonged biologic half-life of cefadroxil allows for once-a-day dosage.

Second-Generation Cephalosporins (Table 33.8). Some of the second-generation cephalosporins contain an *N*-methyl-5-thiotetrazole (commonly referred to by the acronym, MTT) at the C-3 position.

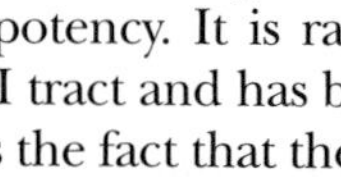

MTT

Loss of the MTT group is associated with prothrombin deficiency and bleeding problems, as well as with a disulfiram-like acute alcohol intolerance (51). However, this grouping enhances potency and prevents metabolism by deacetylation.

Cefuroxime. Cefuroxime has a *Z*-oriented methoxyimino moiety as part of its C-7 side chain (Fig. 33.22). This

TABLE 33.7 First Generation Cephalosporins

Generic Names	Trade Names	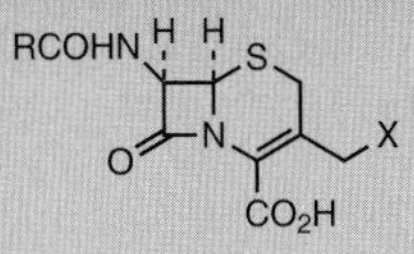 R	X	Salt
Parenteral agents:				
Cefazolin	Ancef, Kefzol, Zolicef	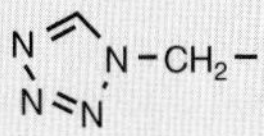	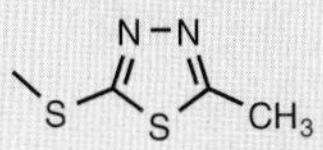	Na
Oral agents:				
Cephalexin	Keflex, Biocef Keftab	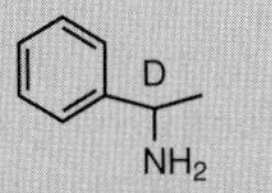	H	HCl
Cefadroxil	Duricef	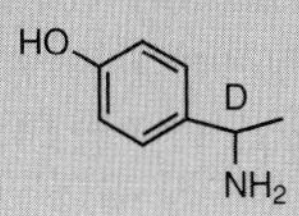	H	–

conveys considerable resistance to attack by many β-lactamases but not by all. This is believed to result from the steric demands of this group. Resistance by *Pseudomonas aeruginosa,* on the other hand, is attributed to lack of penetration of the drug rather than to enzymatic hydrolysis. The carbamoyl moiety at C-3 is intermediate in metabolic stability between the classic acetyl moieties and the thiotetrazoles.

In the form of its axetil ester (1-[acetyloxy]ethyl ester) prodrug, cefuroxime axetil, a more lipophilic drug is produced that results in satisfactory blood levels on oral administration. The ester bond is cleaved metabolically,

TABLE 33.8 Second Generation Cephalosporins

Generic Name	Trade Name	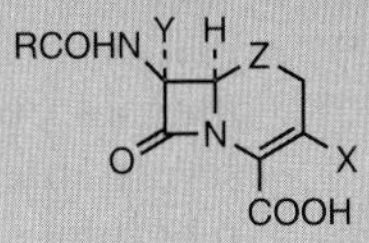 R	X	Y	Z	Salt
Parenteral agents						
Cefuroxime	Ceftin Kefurox Zinacef	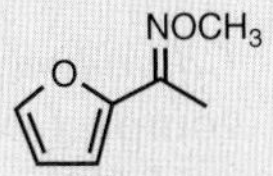	$-CH_2OCONH_2$	H	S	Na
Cefoxitin	Mefoxin	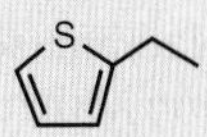	$-CH_2OCONH_2$	OCH_3	S	Na
Cefotetan	Cefotan	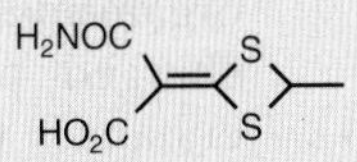	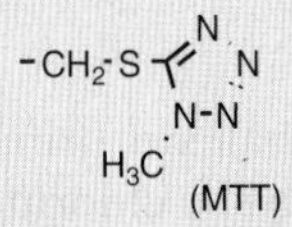 (MTT)	OCH_3	S	diNa
Oral agents						
Cefaclor	Ceclor	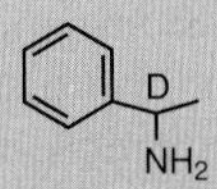	Cl	H	S	–
Cefprozil	Cefzil	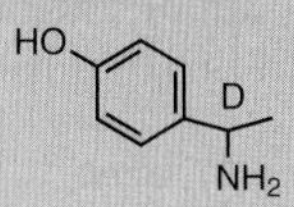	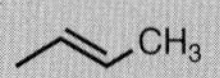	H	S	–

and the resulting intermediate form loses acetaldehyde spontaneously to produce cefuroxime itself. The axetil is officially labeled for treatment of Lyme disease (although doxycycline is often the first choice) (47).

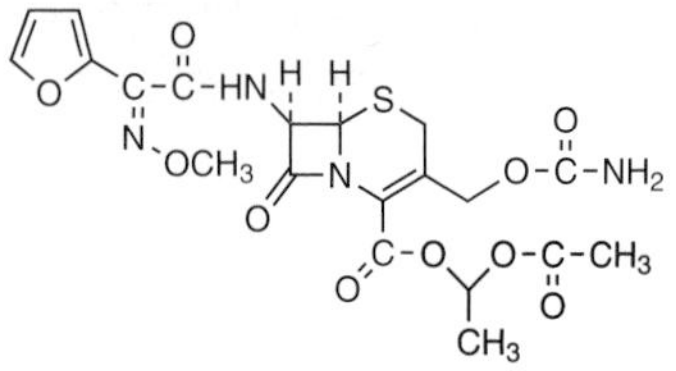

Cefuroxime axetil

Cefoxitin. The most novel chemical feature of cefoxitin is the possession of an α-oriented methoxyl group in place of the normal H-atom at C-7. This increased steric bulk conveys very significant stability against β-lactamases. The inspiration for these functional groups was provided by the discovery of the naturally occurring antibiotic cephamycin C derived from fermentation of *Streptomyces lactamdurans* (52). Cephamycin C itself has not seen clinical use but provided the structural clue that led to useful agents such as cefoxitin. Agents that contain this 7α methoxy group are commonly referred to as cephamycins.

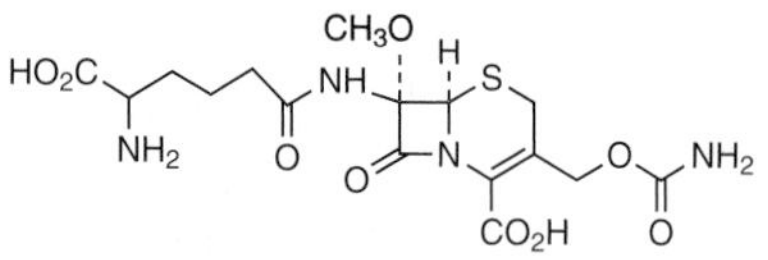

Cephamycin C

Cefoxitin has useful activity against gonorrhea and against some anaerobic infections (including *Bacteroides fragilis*) as compared with its second-generation relatives. On the negative side, cefoxitin has the capacity to induce certain broad-spectrum β-lactamases.

Cefotetan. Cefotetan is also a cephamycin but has a rather unusual sulfur-containing C-7 side-chain amide. Possession of two carboxyl groups leads to its marketing as a disodium salt. The C-3 MTT side chain suggests caution in monitoring bleeding as well as care in ingesting alcohol when using this agent. Like cefoxitin, cefotetan has better activity against anaerobes than the rest of this group. Like cefoxitin, it is stable to a wide range of β-lactamases but is also an inducer in some bacteria.

Cefaclor. Cefaclor differs from cephalexin primarily in the bioisosteric replacement of methyl by chlorine at C-3 and is quite acid stable, allowing for oral administration. It is also quite stable to metabolism. It is less active against gram-negative bacteria than the other second-generation cephalosporins but is more active against gram-negative bacteria than the first-generation drugs.

Cefprozil. Cefprozil has an amoxicillin-like side chain at C-7, but at C-3, there is now a l-propenyl group conjugated with the double bond in the six-membered ring. The double bond is present in its two geometric isomeric forms, both of which are antibacterially active. Fortunately, the predominant *trans* form (illustrated in Table 33.8) is much more active against gram-negative organisms. Cefprozil most closely resembles cefaclor in its properties but is a little more potent.

Third-Generation Cephalosporins (Table 33.9).

Cefotaxime. Cefotaxime, like cefuroxime, has a *Z*-methoxyimino moiety at C-7 that conveys significant β-lactamase resistance. The oxime moiety of cefotaxime is connected to an aminothiazole ring. Like other third-generation cephalosporins, it has excellent anti–gram-negative activity. It has a metabolically vulnerable acetoxy group attached to C-3 and loses about 90% of its activity when this is hydrolyzed. This metabolic feature also complicates the pharmacokinetic data because both structures are present and have different properties. Cefotaxime should be protected from heat and light and may color slightly without significant loss of potency. Like other third-generation cephalosporins, cefotaxime has less activity against staphylococci but has greater activity against gram-negative organisms (53).

Ceftizoxime. In ceftizoxime, the whole C-3 side chain has been omitted to prevent deactivation by hydrolysis. It rather resembles cefotaxime in its properties; however, not being subject to metabolism, its pharmacokinetic properties are much less complex.

Ceftriaxone. Ceftriaxone has the same C-7 side-chain moiety as cefotaxime and ceftizoxime, but the C-3 side chain consists of a metabolically stable and activating thiotriazinedione in place of the normal acetyl group. The C-3 side chain is sufficiently acidic that at normal pH, it forms an enolic sodium salt, and thus the commercial product is a disodium salt. It is useful for many severe infections and notably in the treatment of some meningitis infections caused by gram-negative bacteria. It is quite stable to many β-lactamases but is sensitive to some inducible chromosomal β-lactamases (49).

Ceftazidime. In ceftazidime, the oxime moiety is more complex, containing two methyl groups and a carboxylic acid. This assemblage conveys even more pronounced β-lactamase stability, greater anti–*Pseudomonas aeruginosa* activity, and increased activity against gram-positive organisms. The C-3 side chain has been replaced by a charged pyridinium moiety. The latter considerably enhances water solubility and also highly activates the β-lactam bond toward cleavage. It is not stable under some conditions, such as in the presence of aminoglycosides and vancomycin. It is also attacked readily in sodium bicarbonate solutions. Resistance is mediated by chromosomally mediated β-lactamases and also by lack of penetration into target bacteria. Otherwise, it has a very broad antibacterial spectrum (54).

Cefixime. In cefixime, in addition to the β-lactamase stabilizing *Z*-oximino acidic ether at C-7, the C-3 side chain

TABLE 33.9 Third Generation Cephalosporins

Generic Name	Trade Name	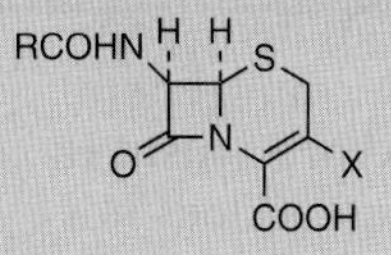 R	X	Salt
Parenteral agents				
Cefotaxime	Claforan	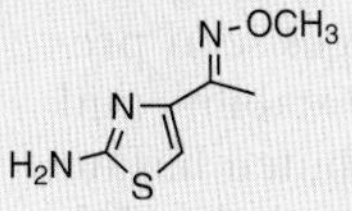	CH_2OAc	Na
Ceftizoxime	Cefizox	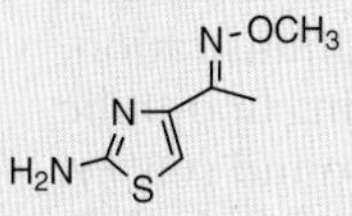	H	Na
Ceftriaxone	Rocephin	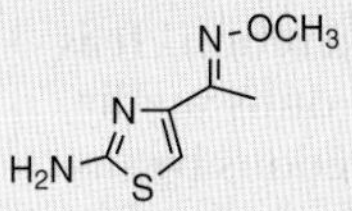	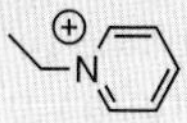	diNa
Ceftazidime	Fortaz Tazicef	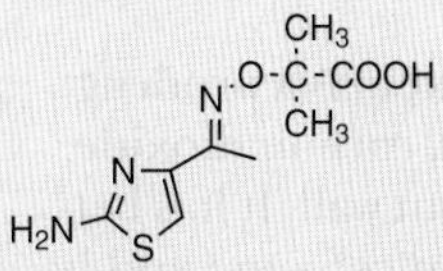	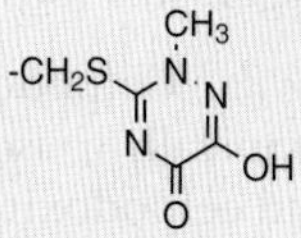	H or Na
Oral agents				
Cefixime	Suprax	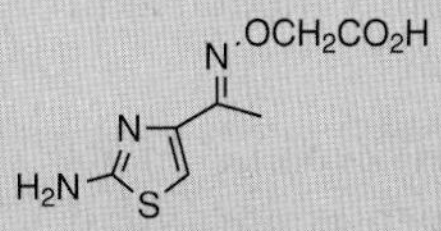	—CH=CH_2	–
Ceftibuten	Cedax	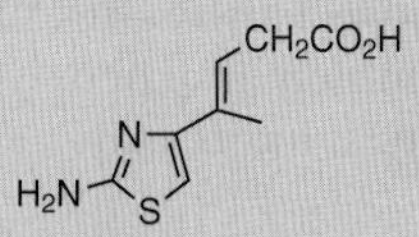	H	–
Cefpodoxime proxetil 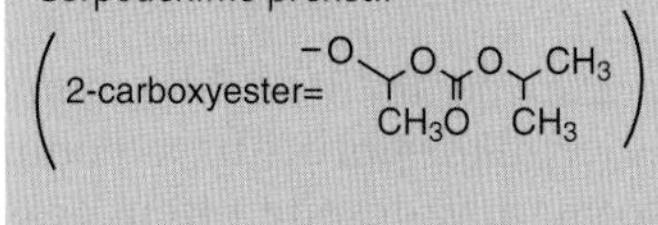	Vantin	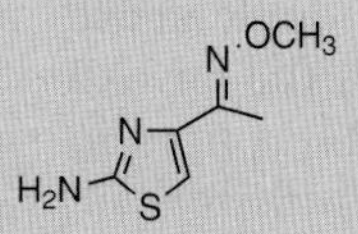	$-CH_2OCH_3$	–
Cefdinir	Omnicef	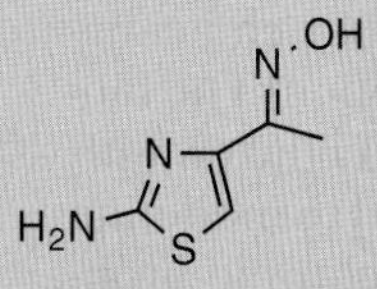	-CH=CH_2	–
Cefditoren pivoxil 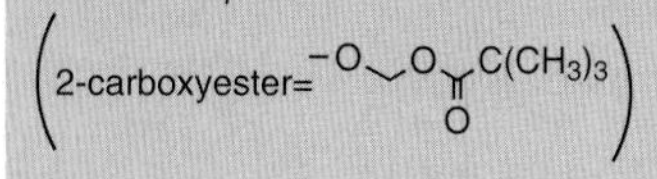	Spectracef	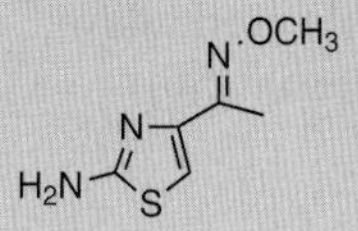	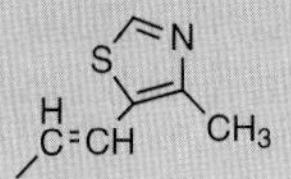	–

is a vinyl group analogous to the propenyl group of cefprozil. This is believed to contribute strongly to the oral activity of the drug. Cefixime has anti–gram-negative activity intermediate between that of the second-generation and third-generation agents described previously. It is poorly active against staphylococci because it does not bind satisfactorily to a specific PBP (PBP-2).

Ceftibuten. Ceftibuten has a *Z*-ethylidinecarboxyl group at C-7 instead of the *Z*-oximino ether linkages seen previously. This conveys enhanced β-lactamase stability and may contribute to oral activity as well. Ceftibuten has no C-3 side chain and thus is not measurably metabolized. It is highly (75% to 90%) absorbed on oral administration, but this is decreased significantly by food. Being lipophilic and acidic, it is significantly serum protein bound (65%). Some isomerization of the geometry of the olefinic linkage appears to take place in vivo before excretion. It is mainly used for respiratory tract infections, otitis media, and pharyngitis, as well as urinary tract infections by susceptible microorganisms (55).

Cefpodoxime Proxetil. Cefpodoxime proxetil is a prodrug. It is cleaved enzymically to isopropanol, carbon dioxide, acetaldehyde, and cefpodoxime in the gut wall. It has better anti–*Staphylococcus aureus* activity than cefixime and is used to treat pharyngitis, urinary tract infections, upper and lower respiratory tract infections, otitis media, skin and soft tissue infections, and gonorrhea.

Cefdinir. Cefdinir has an unsubstituted *Z*-oxime in its C-7 side chain, the consequence of which is attributed to its somewhat enhanced anti–gram-positive activity—its main distinguishing feature. It has a vinyl moiety attached to C-3 that is associated with its oral activity. It has reasonable resistance to β-lactamases.

Cefditoren Pivoxil. Cefditoren pivoxil is an orally active prodrug. Similar to cefpodoxime proxetil, the pivoxil ester is hydrolyzed following intestinal absorption to release the active drug, cefditoren, along with formaldehyde and pivalic acid. Cefditoren pivoxil should not be administered with drugs that reduce stomach acidity because this may result in decreased absorption. The bioavailability of cefditoren pivoxil is increased if taken with food. Cefditoren pivoxil is indicated for mild to moderate infections in adults and adolescents with chronic bronchitis, pharyngitis/tonsillitis, and uncomplicated skin infections associated with gram-negative bacteria (56).

Fourth-Generation Cephalosporins.
Cefepime.

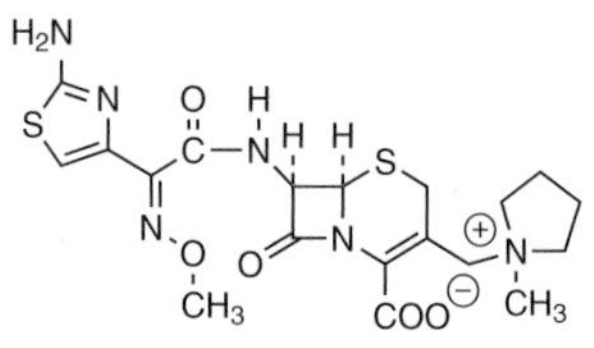

Cefepime (Maxipime)

Cefepime is a semisynthetic agent containing a *Z*-methoxyimine moiety and an aminothiazolyl group at C-7, broadening its spectrum, increasing its β-lactamase stability, and increasing its antistaphylococcal activity. The quaternary *N*-methylpyrrolidine group at C-3 seems to help penetration into gram-negative bacteria. The fourth-generation cephalosporins are characterized by enhanced antistaphylococcal activity and broader anti–gram-negative activity than the third-generation group. Cefepime is used intramuscularly and intravenously against urinary tract infections, skin and skin structure infections, pneumonia, and intra-abdominal infections (50).

Newer Cephalosporins.
Ceftaroline Fosamil.

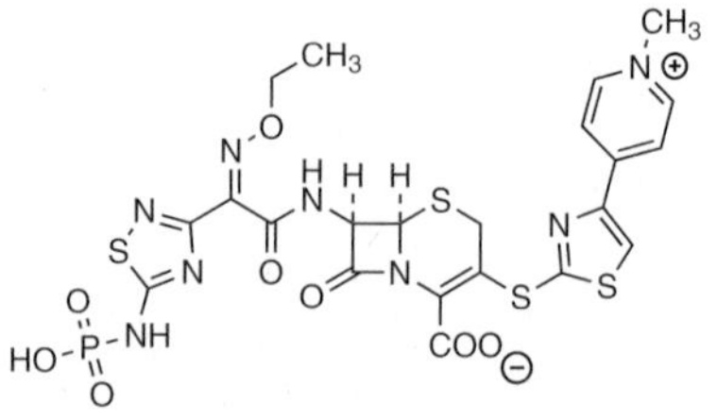

Ceftaroline fosamil (Teflaro)
(prodrug of ceftaroline)

Ceftaroline fosamil was approved in 2010. It is currently unique among the marketed β-lactams because of its affinity for "abnormal" PBPs, in addition to having affinity for normal PBPs. It is bactericidal against MRSA due to its affinity for PBP-2a and against *Streptococcus pneumoniae* due to its affinity for PBP-2x. It can be used to treat MRSA infections of skin and soft tissues. It is administered as a water-soluble prodrug that is readily hydrolyzed to the active ceftaroline (loss of the phosphate ester). The most common adverse effects are nausea, diarrhea, and rash (57).

Summary. With their broader spectrum including many very dangerous bacteria, the cephalosporins have come to dominate β-lactam chemotherapy, despite often lacking oral activity. Because the cephalosporin field is still being very actively pursued, the student can expect additional introduction of new agents in the future.

Carbapenems.

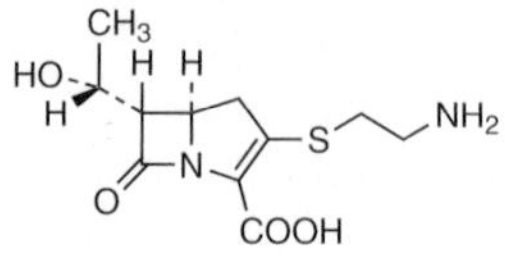

Thienamycin

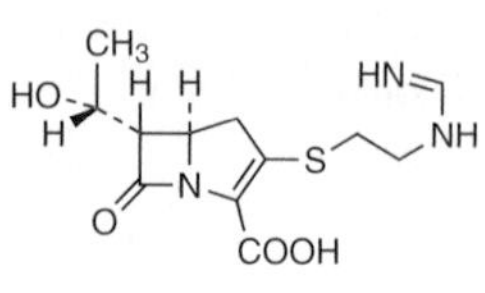

Imipenem

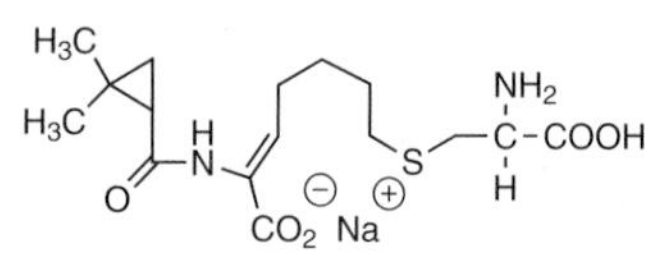

Cilastatin sodium

Thienamycin, the first of the carbapenems, was isolated from *Streptomyces cattleya* (58). Because of its extremely intense and broad-spectrum antimicrobial activity and its ability to inactivate β-lactamases, it combines in one molecule the functional features of the best of the β-lactam antibiotics as well as the β-lactamase inhibitors. It differs structurally in several important respects from the penicillins and cephalosporins. The sulfur atom is not part of the five-membered ring but rather has been replaced by a methylene moiety at that position. Carbon is roughly half the molecular size of sulfur. Consequently, the carbapenem ring system is highly strained and very susceptible to reactions cleaving the β-lactam bond. The sulfur atom is now attached to C-3 as part of a functionalized side chain. The endocyclic olefinic linkage also enhances the reactivity of the β-lactam ring. Both make thienamycin unstable, and this caused difficulties in the original isolation studies. The terminal amino group in the side chain attached to C-3 is nucleophilic and attacks the β-lactam bond of nearby molecules destroying activity (Fig. 33.23). Ultimately, this problem was overcome by changing the amino group to a less nucleophilic *N*-formiminoyl moiety by a semisynthetic process to produce imipenem. At C-6, there is a 2-hydroxyethyl group attached with α-stereochemistry. Thus the absolute stereochemistry of the molecule is 5*R*,6*S*,8*S*. With these striking differences from the penicillins and cephalosporins, it is not surprising that thienamycin analogs bind differently to the penicillin-binding proteins (especially strongly to PBP-2), but the result is very potent broad-spectrum activity (59). However, none of the current carbapenems have activity against MRSA.

Imipenem. Imipenem, as well as thienamycin, penetrates very well through porins and is very stable, even inhibitory, to many β-lactamases. Imipenem is not, however, orally active. Renal dehydropeptidase-l hydrolyzes imipenem through hydrolysis of the β-lactam and deactivates it. An inhibitor for this enzyme, cilastatin, is coadministered with imipenem to protect it (59). Inhibition of human dehydropeptidase does not seem to have deleterious consequences to the patient, making this combination highly efficacious.

The combination of imipenem and cilastatin (Primaxin) is about 25% serum protein bound. On injection, it penetrates well into most tissues, but not cerebrospinal fluid, and it is subsequently excreted in the urine. This very potent combination is especially useful for treatment of serious infections by aerobic gram-negative bacilli, anaerobes, and *Staphylococcus aureus.* It is used clinically for a number of significant infections. The more

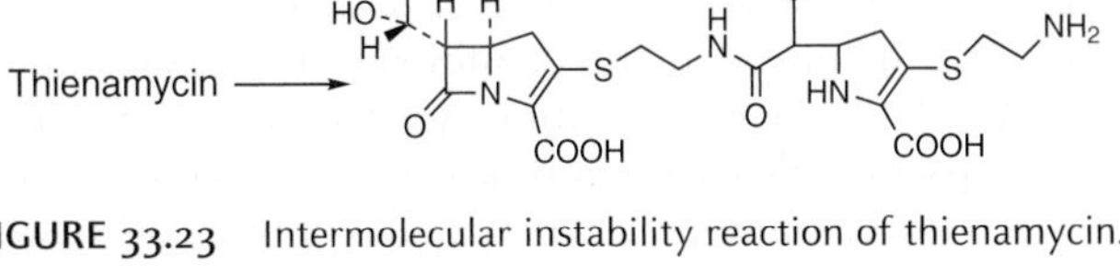

FIGURE 33.23 Intermolecular instability reaction of thienamycin.

common adverse effects are irritation at the infusion site, nausea, vomiting, diarrhea, and pruritus. Of greater concern is the ability of imipenem to induce seizures. The risk factors for seizure development include impaired renal function, preexisting CNS disease or infection, and use of large doses (60).

Meropenem.

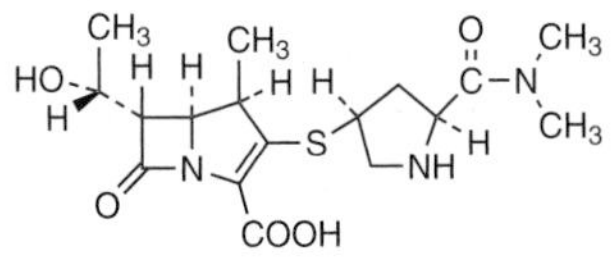

Meropenem (Merrem)

Meropenem is a synthetic carbapenem possessing a complex side chain at C-3. It also has a chiral methyl group at C-4. This methyl group conveys intrinsic resistance to hydrolysis by dehydropeptidase-1 (61). As a consequence, it can be administered as a single agent for the treatment of severe bacterial infections. While the common adverse effects are similar to imipenem/cilastatin, the risk of seizures is significantly less (62).

Doripenem.

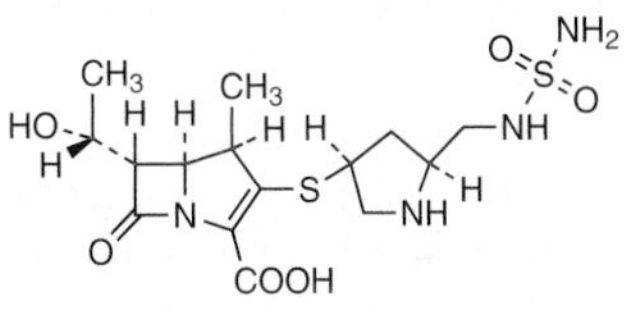

Doripenem (Doribax)

Doripenem is the newest of the approved carbapenems. It also contains the 4-β-methyl group, which confers stability toward dehydropeptidase-1, so it is given as a single agent. It is similar in spectrum to imipenem and meropenem but is considered more potent against *Pseudomonas* species (63).

Ertapenem.

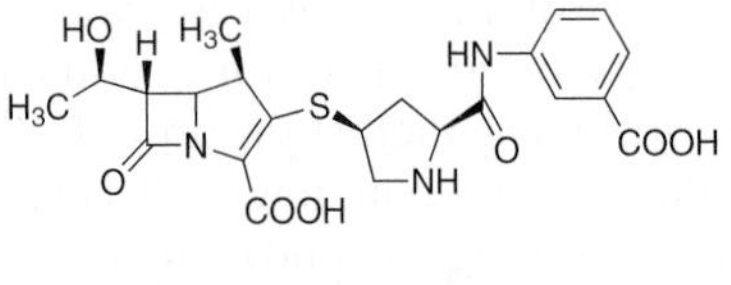

Ertapenem (Invanz)

Ertapenem is another synthetic carbapenem with a rather complex side chain at C-3. As with meropenem and doripenem, the 4-β-methyl group confers stability toward dehydropeptidase-1. It is not active against *Pseudomonas* or *Acinetobacter* and thus should not be substituted for other carbapenems for these organisms (63). This class of antimicrobial agents is under intensive investigation, and several analogs are currently in various phases of preclinical investigation, including tebipenem, an oral prodrug carbapenem (64).

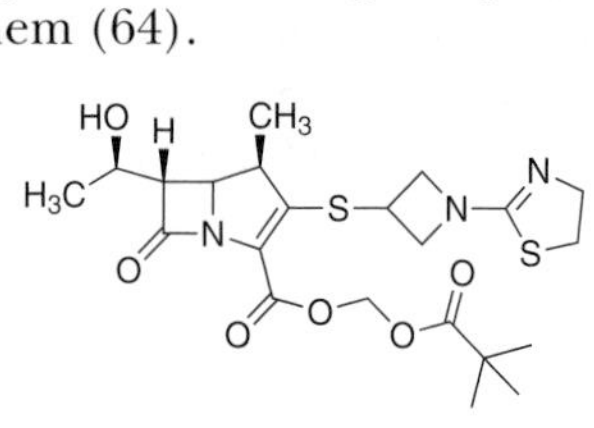

Tebipenem pivoxil

Monobactams.
Aztreonam.

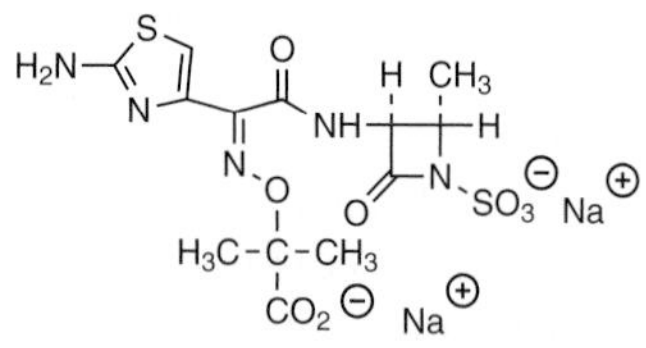

Aztreonam disodium (Azactam)

Fermentation of unusual microorganisms led to the discovery of a class of monocyclic β-lactam antibiotics, named monobactams (34,35). None of these natural molecules have proven to be important, but the group served as the inspiration for the synthesis of aztreonam. Aztreonam is a totally synthetic parenteral antibiotic whose antimicrobial spectrum is devoted almost exclusively to gram-negative microorganisms, and it is capable of inactivating some β-lactamases. Its molecular mode of action is closely similar to that of the penicillins, cephalosporins, and carbapenems, the action being characterized by strong affinity for PBP-3, producing filamentous cells as a consequence. Whereas the principal side chain closely resembles that of ceftazidime, the sulfamic acid moiety attached to the β-lactam ring was unprecedented. Remembering the comparatively large size of sulfur atoms, this assembly may sufficiently spatially resemble the corresponding C-2 carboxyl group of the precedent β-lactam antibiotics to confuse the PBPs. The strongly electron-withdrawing character of the sulfamic acid group probably also makes the β-lactam bond more vulnerable to hydrolysis. In any case, the monobactams demonstrate that a fused ring is not essential for antibiotic activity. The α-oriented methyl group at C-2 is associated with the stability of aztreonam toward β-lactamases.

The protein binding is moderate (~50%), and the drug is nearly unchanged by metabolism. Aztreonam is given by injection and is primarily excreted in the urine. The primary clinical use of aztreonam is against severe infections caused by gram-negative microorganisms, especially those acquired in the hospital. These are mainly urinary tract, upper respiratory tract, bone, cartilage, abdominal, obstetric, and gynecologic infections and septicemias. The drug is well tolerated, and adverse effects are infrequent (65). Interestingly, allergy would not be unexpected, but cross-allergenicity with penicillins and cephalosporins has not often been reported (65).

Antibiotics: Inhibitors of Protein Biosynthesis

Basis for Selectivity Once the bacterial cell wall is traversed, complex cellular machinery deeper within the cell becomes available to antibiotics. Some of the most successful antibiotic families exert their lethal effects on bacteria by inhibiting ribosomally mediated protein biosynthesis. At first glimpse, this may seem problematic because eukaryotic organisms also construct their essential proteins on ribosomal organelles and the sequence of biochemical steps is closely analogous to that in prokaryotic microorganisms. At a molecular level, however, the apparent anomaly resolves itself because the detailed architecture of prokaryotic ribosomes is rather different. In *Escherichia coli*, for example, the 70S ribosomal particle is composed not only of three RNA molecules, but also of 55 different structural and functional proteins arranged in a nonsymmetrical manner. The small (30S) subunit has a 16S rRNA molecule and about 20 different proteins. The large subunit has a 23S and a 5S rRNA and over 30 proteins. The x-ray crystal structure of the components of the bacterial ribosome has been determined (66,67). This was a landmark achievement given the size and complexity of this organelle. The picture is still not complete but allows one to unravel the molecular details not only of how proteins are biosynthesized but also where important antibiotics bind when they interrupt this process. The functioning parts of the ribosome organize and catalyze some portions of the biosynthetic cycle. The tRNA molecules bind roughly at the interface where the 50S and 30S subparticles come together. The codon–anticodon interaction with mRNA takes place in the 30S subunit, and the incoming amino acid and the growing peptide chain being made lies in the 50S subunit. Upsetting the view held for decades that the antibiotics bind to ribosomal proteins, it is now known that they bind to the rRNA instead. Aside from this important fact, most of the other key beliefs are still valid. Of key importance is the repeated movement of the tRNA bases, which mostly take place near interfaces between the individual rRNA molecules where this would be easiest. In agreement with this theory, it has been found that this region is comparatively disordered, which is consistent with that movement (Fig. 33.24).

At normal doses, antibiotics do not bind to or interfere with the function of eukaryotic 80S ribosomal particles. The basis for the selective toxicity of these antibiotics is apparent. Interference with bacterial protein biosynthesis prevents repair, cellular growth, and reproduction and can be clinically bacteriostatic or bactericidal.

Aminoglycosides and Aminocyclitols

Introduction. The aminoglycoside/aminocyclitol class of antibiotics contains a pharmacophoric 1,3-diaminoinositol moiety consisting either of streptamine, 2-deoxystreptamine, or spectinamine (Fig. 33.25). Several of the alcoholic functions of the 1,3-diaminoinositol are substituted through glycosidic bonds with characteristic amino sugars to form pseudo-oligosaccharides. The chemistry, spectrum, potency, toxicity, and pharmacokinetics of these agents are a function of the specific identity of the diaminoinositol

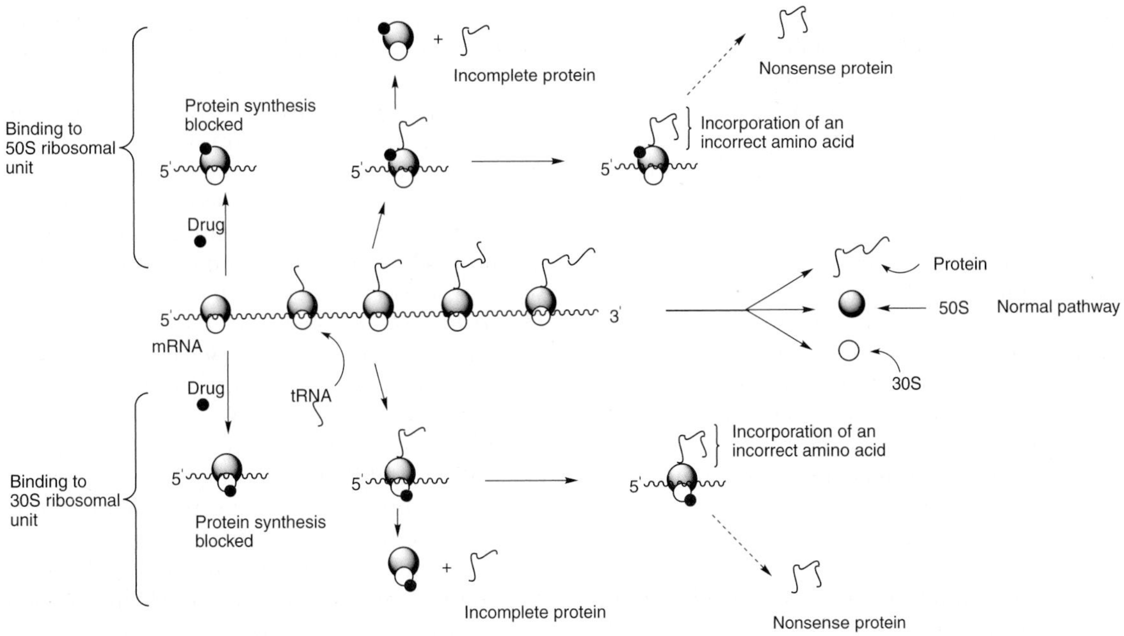

FIGURE 33.24 General mechanism of action of drugs that block protein synthesis by binding to ribosomal units.

unit and the arrangement and identity of the attachments. The various aminoglycoside antibiotics are freely water soluble at all achievable pHs, are basic and form acid salts, are not absorbed in significant amounts from the GI tract, and are excreted in active form in fairly high concentrations in the urine following injection. When the kidneys are not functioning efficiently, the dose must be reduced to prevent accumulation to toxic levels. When given orally, their action is confined to the GI tract. Aminoglycosides are used topically as solutions or ointments for ophthalmic infections. They can be given intramuscularly but are more commonly delivered by intravenous infusion. Tobramycin is available for inhalation to treat *Pseudomonas aeruginosa* infections in cystic fibrosis patients (68). This route of administration results in significantly reduced toxicity to the patient. These agents have intrinsically broad antimicrobial spectra, but their toxicity potential limits their clinical use to infections

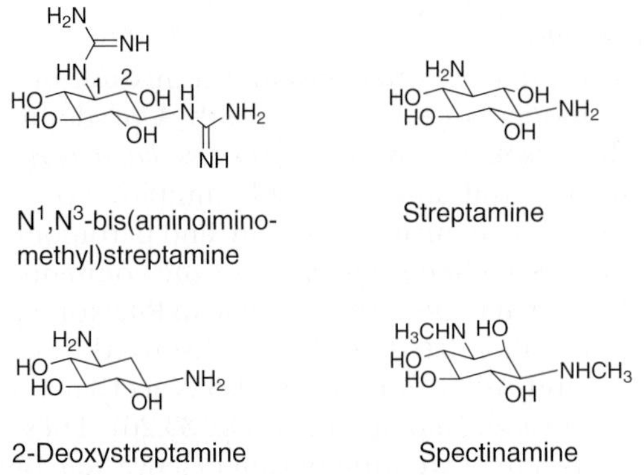

FIGURE 33.25 1,3-Diaminoinositol moieties present in aminoglycosides.

by gram-negative bacteria. The aminoglycoside antibiotics are widely distributed (mainly in extracellular fluids) and have low levels of protein binding.

Mechanism of Action. The aminoglycosides are bactericidal due to a combination of toxic effects. At less than toxic doses, they bind to the 16S ribosomal DNA portion of the 30S ribosomal subparticle, impairing the proofreading function of the ribosome. A conformational change occurs in the peptidyl A site of the ribosome upon aminoglycoside binding. This leads to mistranslation of RNA templates and the selection of wrong amino acids and formation of so-called nonsense proteins (Fig. 33.24). The most relevant of these unnatural proteins are involved in upsetting bacterial membrane function. Their presence destroys the semipermeability of the membrane, and this damage cannot be repaired without de novo programmed protein biosynthesis. Among the substances that are admitted by the damaged membrane are large additional quantities of aminoglycoside. At these increased concentrations, protein biosynthesis ceases altogether. These combined effects are devastating to the target bacterial cells. Given their highly polar properties, the student may wonder how these agents can enter bacterial cells at all. Aminoglycosides apparently bind initially to external lipopolysaccharides and diffuse into the cells in small amounts. The uptake process is inhibited by Ca^{2+} and Mg^{2+} ions. These ions are, then, partially incompatible therapeutically. Passage through the cytoplasmic membrane is dependent on electron transport and energy generation. At high concentrations, eukaryotic protein biosynthesis can also be inhibited by aminoglycoside/aminocyclitol antibiotics (69,70).

Bacterial Resistance. Bacterial resistance to aminoglycoside antibiotics in the clinic is most commonly due to bacterial elaboration of R-factor–mediated enzymes that *N*-acetylate (aminoglycoside acetylase [AAC]), *O*-phosphorylate (aminoglycoside phosphorylase [APH]), and *O*-adenylate (aminoglycoside nucleotide transferase [ANT]) specific functional groups, preventing subsequent ribosomal binding (Fig. 33.26).In some cases, chemical deletion of the functional groups transformed by these enzymes leaves a molecule that is still antibiotic but no longer a substrate; thus agents with intrinsically broader spectrum can be made semisynthetically in this way. In other cases, novel functional groups can be attached to remote functionality, which converts these antibiotics to poorer substrates for these R-factor–mediated enzymes, and this expands their spectra, as discussed later in this chapter. It is important to note that resistance mediated in this way is not necessarily class-wide, so susceptibility testing with multiple aminoglycosides should be used. Resistance can also involve point mutations of the ribosomal A site. These involve single nucleotide residues at specific positions (70). The substituent at position 6′ of the aminoglycoside, the number of protonated amino groups, and the linkage between the sugar rings and the central deoxystreptamine moiety are particularly important in the interactions with the rRNA.

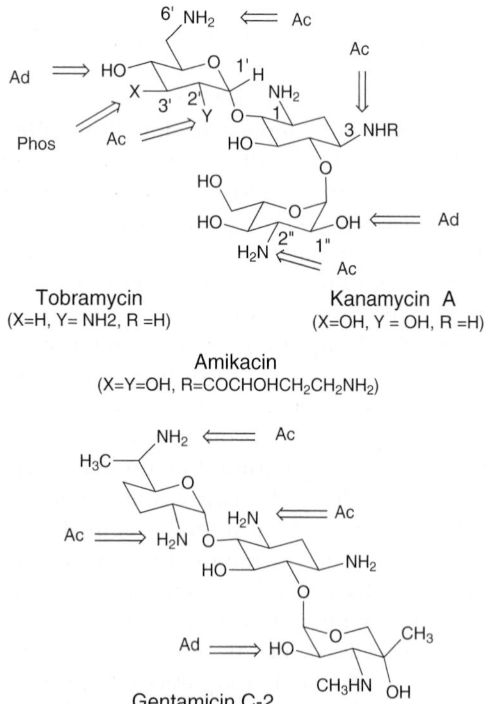

FIGURE 33.26 Commercially important 2-desylstreptamine–containing aminoglycosides. Some points of inactivating attack by specific R-factor–mediated enzymes are indicated by the following: Ac, acetylation; Ad, adenylation; Phos, phosphorylation. APH(3′)-1, for example, is an acronym for an enzyme that phosphorylates aminoglycosides at the 3′-OH position.

Resistance due to decreased aminoglycoside/aminocyclitol uptake into bacterial cells is also encountered.

Therapeutic Application. Intrinsically, aminoglycosides have broad antibiotic spectra against aerobic gram-positive and gram-negative bacteria but are reserved for use in serious infections caused by gram-negative organisms because of serious toxicities that are often delayed in onset. They are active against gram-negative aerobes such as *Acinetobacter* sp., *Citrobacter* sp., *Enterobacter* sp., *Escherichia coli*, *Klebsiella* sp., *Proteus vulgaris*, *Providencia* sp., *Pseudomonas aeruginosa*, *Salmonella* sp., *Serratia marcesans*, *Shigella* sp. and gram-positive aerobes such as *Staphylococcus epidermidis* (70).

Streptomycin and spectinomycin differ from the others in their useful antimicrobial spectra. Streptomycin is most commonly used for the treatment of tuberculosis and spectinomycin for treatment of gonorrhea, although it is no longer marketed in the United States. Some aminoglycoside antibiotics in present clinical use are illustrated in Figure 33.26, along with some of their sites of enzymatic inactivation.

Adverse Effects. The toxicities associated with the aminoglycosides involve toxicity to functions mediated by the eighth cranial nerve, such as hearing loss and vertigo. Their use can also lead to kidney tubular necrosis, producing decreases in glomerular function. These toxic effects are related to blood levels and are apparently mediated by the special affinity of these aminoglycosides to kidney cells and to the sensory cells of the inner ear (71). The effects may have a delayed onset, making them all the more dangerous because the patient can be injured significantly before symptoms appear. Less common is a curare-like neuromuscular blockade believed to be caused by competitive inhibition of calcium ion–dependent acetylcholine release at the neuromuscular junction. This effect can exaggerate the muscle weakness of myasthenia gravis and parkinsonian patients (72). In current practice, all of these toxic phenomena are well known; therefore, creatinine clearance should be determined and the dose adjusted downward accordingly so that these adverse effects are less common and less severe.

Specific Agents.

Kanamycin (Kantrex). Kanamycin is a mixture of at least three components (A, B, and C, with A predominating; Fig. 33.26), isolated from *Streptomyces kanamyceticus*. In addition to typical aminoglycoside antibiotic properties, it, along with gentamicin, neomycin, and paromomycin, is among the most chemically stable of the common antibiotics. Kanamycin is, however, unstable to R-factor enzymes, being *O*-phosphorylated on the C-3′ hydroxyl by enzymes APH(3′)-I and APH(3′)-II and is also *N*-acetylated on the C-6′ amino group, among others (Fig. 33.26). These transformation products are antibiotically inactive. Kanamycin is used parenterally against some gram-negative bacteria, but *Pseudomonas aeruginosa* and anaerobes are usually resistant

(73). Although it can also be used in combination with other agents against certain mycobacteria (*Mycobacterium kansasii, Mycobacterium marinum,* and *Mycobacterium intracellulare*), its popularity for this use is fading.

Amikacin (Amikin). Amikacin is made semisynthetically from kanamycin A (Fig. 33.26). Interestingly, the L-hydroxyaminobutyryl amide (HABA) moiety attached to N-3 inhibits adenylation and phosphorylation in the distant amino sugar ring (at C-2′ and C-3′) even though the HABA substituent is not where the enzymatic reaction takes place. This effect is attributed to decreased binding to the R-factor–mediated enzymes. With this change, potency and spectrum are strongly enhanced, and amikacin is used for the treatment of sensitive strains of *Mycobacterium tuberculosis, Yersinia tularensis,* and severe *Pseudomonas aeruginosa* infections resistant to other agents (74).

Tobramycin (Nebcin). Tobramycin is one component of a mixture produced by fermentation of *Streptomyces tenebrarius* (Fig. 33.26). Lacking the C-3′ hydroxyl group, it is not a substrate for APH(3′)-I and –II, and thus has an intrinsically broader spectrum than kanamycin. It is a substrate, however, for adenylation at C-2′ by ANT(2′) and acetylation at C-3 by AAC(3)-I and –II and at C-2′ by AAC(2′) (Fig. 33.26). It is used parenterally for difficult infections, especially those by gentamicin-resistant *Pseudomonas aeruginosa* (75).

Gentamicin (Garamycin). Gentamicin is a mixture of several antibiotic components produced by fermentation of *Micromonospora purpurea* and other related soil microorganisms (hence its name is spelled with an "i" instead of a "y"). Gentamicins C-l, C-2, and C-1a are most prominent (gentamicin C-2 is shown in Fig. 33.26). Gentamicin was one of the first antibiotics to have significant activity against *Pseudomonas aeruginosa* infections. This water-loving opportunistic pathogen is frequently encountered in burns, pneumonias, and urinary tract infections. It is highly virulent. As noted earlier, some of the functional groups that serve as targets for R-factor–mediated enzymes are missing in the structure of gentamicins, so their antibacterial spectrum is enhanced. They are, however, inactivated through C-2′ adenylation by enzyme ANT(2′) and acetylation at C-6′ by AAC(6′), at C-l by AAC(1)-I and -II, and at C-2′ by AAC(2′). Gentamicin is often combined with other anti-infective agents, and an interesting incompatibility has been uncovered. With certain β-lactam antibiotics, the two drugs react with each other so that *N*-acylation on C-l of gentamicin by the β-lactam antibiotic takes place, thus inactivating both antibiotics (Fig. 33.27). The two agents should not, therefore, be mixed in the same solution and should ideally be administered into different tissue compartments to prevent this. This incompatibility is likely to be associated with other aminoglycoside antibiotics as well. Gentamicin is used for urinary tract infections, burns, some pneumonias, and bone and joint infections caused by susceptible gram-negative bacteria (72).

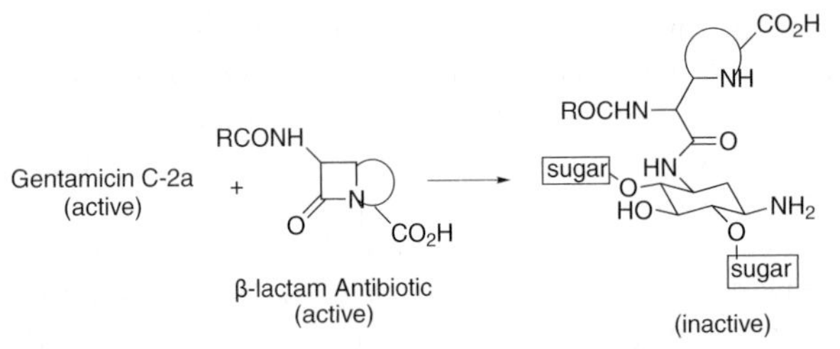

FIGURE 33.27 A chemical drug–drug incompatibility between gentamicin C-2a and β-lactams.

Spectinomycin (Trobicin).

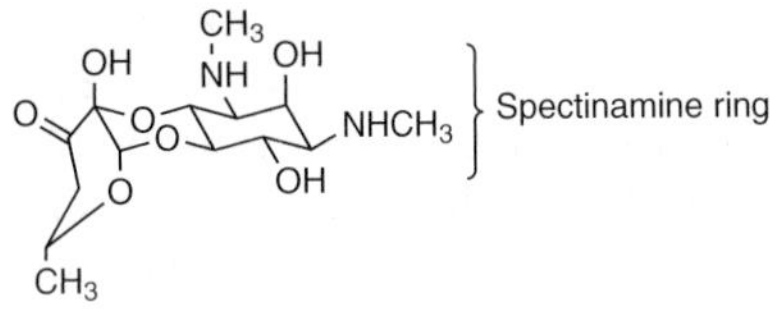

Spectinomycin

An unusual aminoglycoside antibiotic, spectinomycin is produced by fermentation of *Streptomyces spectabilis* and differs substantially in its clinical properties from the others. The diaminoinositol unit (spectinamine) contains two mono-*N*-methyl groups, and the hydroxyl between them has a stereochemistry opposite to that in streptomycin. The glycosidically attached sugar is also unusual in that it contains three consecutive carbonyl groups, either overt or masked, and is fused by two adjacent linkages to spectinamine to produce an unusual fused three-ring structure. Spectinomycin is bacteriostatic as normally employed. It is almost exclusively used in a single bolus injection intramuscularly against *Neisseria gonorrhea,* especially penicillinase-producing strains, in cases of urogenital or oral gonorrhea and does not apparently produce any serious oto- or nephrotoxicity when used in this way. It is particularly useful for the treatment of patients allergic to penicillin and patients not likely to comply well with a medication scheme. It would likely be more widely used except that syphilis and chlamydia do not respond to it. It causes significant mistranslation following ribosomal binding but does not cause much inhibition of overall programmed protein biosynthesis. As mentioned previously, spectinomycin is no longer marketed in the United States.

Streptomycin.

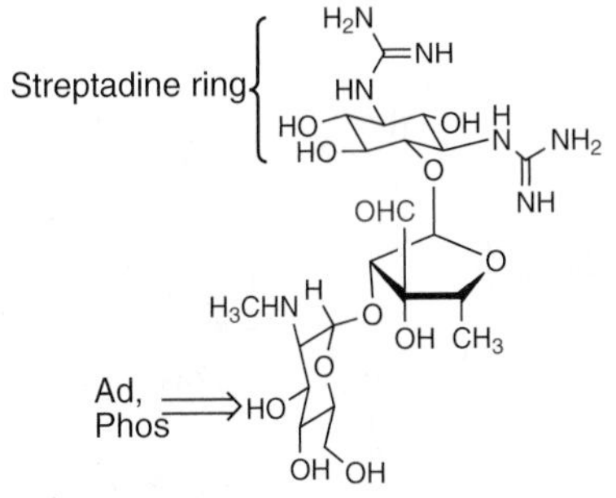

Streptomycin

Streptomycin is produced by fermentation of *Streptomyces griseus* and several related soil microorganisms. It was introduced in 1943 primarily for the treatment of tuberculosis (see Chapter 36). It was the first antibiotic effective for this devastating disease, and Selmon Waksman, the discoverer of streptomycin, received a Nobel Prize in 1952 (76). Streptomycin differs from the typical aminoglycosides with a modified pharmacophore in that the diaminoinositol unit is streptamine, and streptomycin has an axial hydroxyl group at C-2 and two highly basic guanido groups at C-l and C-3 in place of the primary amine moieties of 2-deoxystreptamine. It is possible that the unusual pharmacophore of streptomycin accounts in large measure for its unusual antibacterial spectrum. Another molecular feature, the α-hydroxyaldehyde moiety, is a center of instability such that streptomycin cannot be sterilized by autoclaving, so streptomycin sulfate solutions that need sterilization are made by ultrafiltration. Streptomycin is rarely used today as a single agent. Resistance to streptomycin takes the familiar course of *N*-acetylation, *O*-phosphorylation, and *O*-adenylation of specific functional groups.

Orally Used Aminoglycosides. Neomycin, as part of a combination of agents, finds some oral use for the suppression of gut flora in preparation for bowel surgery. Paromomycin (Humatin) is also used for the oral treatment of amoebic dysentery. Amoebas are persistent pathogens causing chronic diarrhea and are acquired most frequently by travelers who consume food supplies contaminated with human waste.

Neomycin.

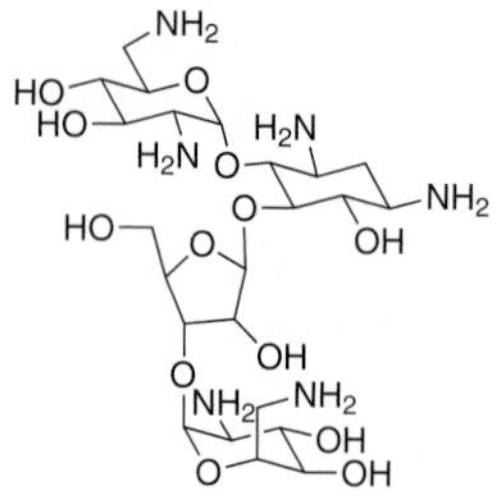

Neomycin B

Neomycin is a mixture of three compounds produced by fermentation of *Streptomyces fradiae*, with neomycin B predominating. Although it is not normally considered to have systemic absorption when administered orally, neomycin now has a black box warning related to systemic toxicities due to absorption in ulcerated or denuded areas of the GI tract (77). It is also found in nonprescription ointments and used topically for treatment of bacterial skin infections. When applied to intact skin, the drug is not absorbed, but if applied to large denuded areas, systemic absorption occurs with the potential to cause toxic side effects.

Macrolide Antibiotics The term macrolide is derived from the characteristic large lactone (cyclic ester) ring found in these antibiotics. The clinically important members of this antibiotic family (Fig. 33.28) have two or more characteristic sugars (usually cladinose and desosamine) attached to the 14-membered ring. One of these sugars usually carries a substituted amino group, so their overall chemical

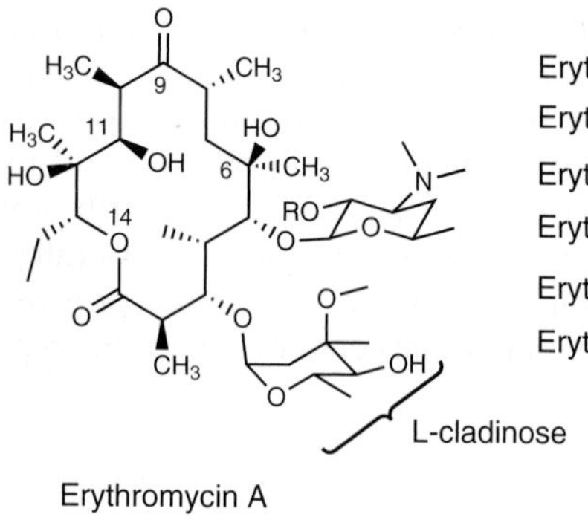

Erythromycin A

	R	Salt
Erythromycin base	H	—
Erythromycin hydrochloride	H	HCl
Erythromycin estolate	$COCH_2CH_3$	$CH_3(CH_2)_{11}OSO_3H$
Erythromycin ethylsuccinate	$CO(CH_2)CO_2C_2H_5$	—
Erythromycin lactobionate	H	Structure A
Erythromycin stearate	H	$CH_3(CH_2)_{16}CO_2H$

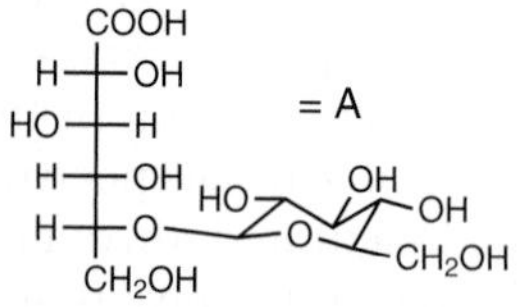

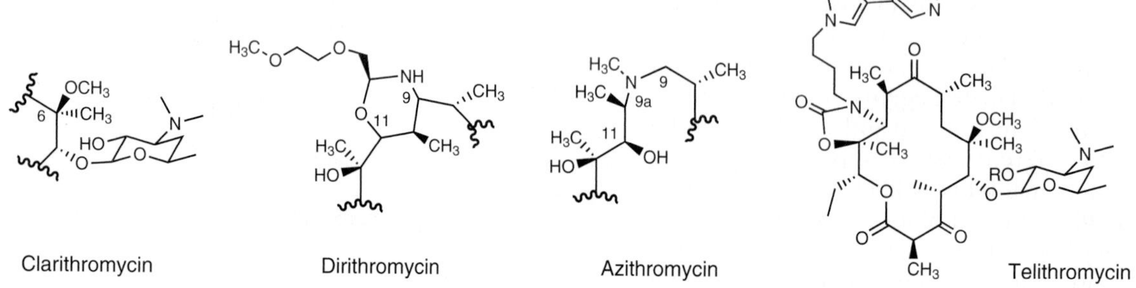

FIGURE 33.28 Clinically important macrolide antibiotic.

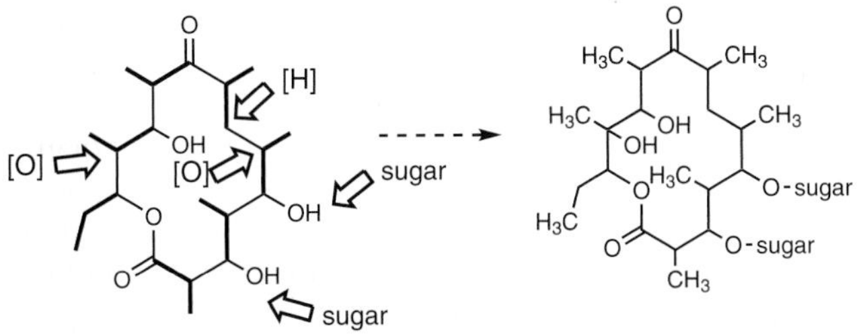

FIGURE 33.29 Biosynthetic pathway to erythromycins from propionic acid units. → refers to modifications to the basic ring skeleton.

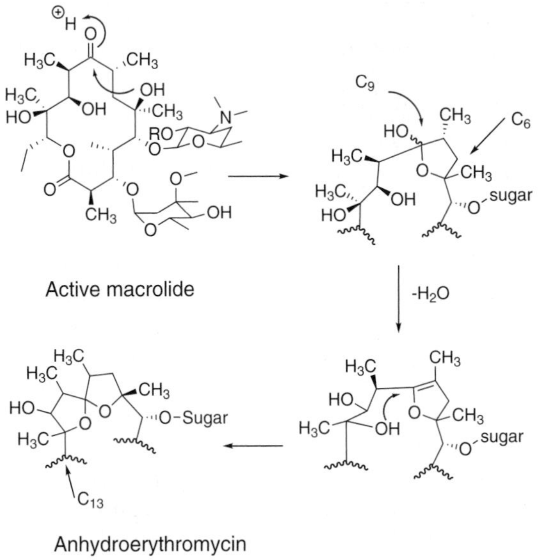

FIGURE 33.30 Acid-catalyzed intramolecular ketal formation with erythromycin.

character is weakly basic (pK_a ~8). They are not very water soluble as free bases, but salt formation with certain acids (glucoheptonic and lactobionic acids in Fig. 33.28) increases water solubility, whereas other salts decrease solubility (laurylsulfate and stearic). Macrolide antibiotics with 16-membered rings are popular outside the United States, but one example, tylosin, finds extensive agricultural use in the United States. The 14-membered ring macrolides are biosynthesized from propionic acid units so that every second carbon of erythromycin, for example, bears a methyl group and the rest of the carbons, with one exception, are oxygen bearing. Two carbons bear so-called "extra" oxygen atoms introduced later in the biosynthesis (not present in a propionic acid unit), and two hydroxyls are glycosylated (Fig. 33.29) (78).

Chemical Properties. The early macrolides of the erythromycin class are chemically unstable due to rapid acid-catalyzed internal cyclic ketal formation, leading to inactivity (Fig. 33.30). This reaction, which occurs in the GI tract, is clinically important. Most acid-susceptible macrolides are administered in coated tablets to minimize this. Analogs have been prepared semisynthetically that are structurally incapable of undergoing this reaction and have become very popular in the clinic (79).

Many macrolides have an unpleasant taste, which is partially overcome with water-insoluble dosage forms that also reduce acid instability and the gut cramps. Enteric coatings are also beneficial in reducing these adverse effects.

Mechanism of Action. The macrolides inhibit bacteria by interfering with programmed ribosomal protein biosynthesis by binding to the 23S rRNA in the polypeptide exit tunnel adjacent to the peptidyl transferase center in the 50S ribosomal subunit (Fig. 33.24). This prevents the growing peptide from becoming longer than a few residues, resulting in the dissociation of peptidyl tRNA molecules. Clindamycin, lincomycin, and chloramphenicol bind in the same vicinity, leading to extensive cross-resistance between them.

Resistance. Developed bacterial resistance is primarily caused by bacteria possessing R-factor enzymes that methylate a specific guanine residue on their own ribosomal RNA making them somewhat less efficient at protein biosynthesis but comparatively poor binders of macrolides (80). The erythromycin-producing soil organism uses the same ribosomal methylation technique to protect itself against the toxic effects of its own metabolite (80). This leads to the speculation that the origin of some antibiotic resistance genes may lie in the producing organism itself and that this genetic material is acquired by bacteria from this source. A second mechanism of resistance is associated with the mutation of adenine to guanine that occurs in domain V at A2058. This change results in a 10,000-fold reduction of binding capacity of erythromycin and clarithromycin to the 23S rRNA (80). Some bacterial strains, however, appear to be resistant to macrolides due to the operation of an active efflux process in which the drug is expelled from the cell at the cost of energy (80). Intrinsic resistance of gram-negative bacteria is primarily caused by lack of penetration as the isolated ribosomes from these organisms are often susceptible.

Drug Interactions. Drug–drug interactions with macrolides are comparatively common and usually involve inhibition of CYP3A4 of the cytochrome P450 oxidase family (81). There is also evidence suggesting that these interactions are intensified by the inhibition of P-glycoprotein (82). These interactions can have severely negative consequences for the patient. The result of this interaction is a longer half-life and enhanced potential toxicity by increasing the effective dose over time. The main product of liver metabolism of erythromycin is the *N*-demethylated analog.

Therapeutic Application. The macrolides are among the safest of the antibiotics in common use and are often used for the treatment of upper and lower respiratory tract and soft tissue infections primarily caused by gram-positive microorganisms like *Streptococcus pyogenes* and *Streptococcus pneumoniae,* Legionnaire disease, prophylaxis of bacterial endocarditis by *Streptococcus viridans,* upper respiratory tract and lower respiratory tract infections, otitis media caused by *Haemophilus influenzae* (with a sulfonamide added), mycoplasmal pneumonia, and *Mycobacterium avium* complex infections in AIDS patients (in combination with rifabutin). They are also used for certain sexually transmitted diseases, such as gonorrhea and pelvic inflammatory disease, caused by mixed infections involving cell wall–free organisms such as *Chlamydia trachomatis*. Clarithromycin is also used to treat gastric ulcers due to *Helicobacter pylori* infection as a component of multidrug cocktails. The macrolides have a comparatively narrow antimicrobial spectrum, reminiscent of the medium-spectrum penicillins, but the organisms involved include many of the more commonly encountered community-acquired microorganisms. The utility of the macrolides against upper respiratory tract infections is enhanced by their particular affinity for these tissues. Tissue levels in the upper respiratory tract are often several times those seen in the blood. They are considered bacteriostatic against most organisms in achievable concentrations.

Specific Agents.

Erythromycin Esters and Salts.

ESTOLATE One of the erythromycin prodrugs, erythromycin estolate, is a C-2′-propionyl ester, *N*-laurylsulfate salt (Fig. 33.28). Administration of erythromycin estolate produces higher blood levels following metabolic regeneration of erythromycin. In a small number of cases, a severe, dose-related, cholestatic jaundice occurs in which the bile becomes granular in the bile duct, impeding flow so that the bile salts back up into the circulation. This seems to be partly allergic and partly dose-related. If the drug causes hepatocyte damage, perhaps this releases antigenic proteins that promote further damage. When cholestatic jaundice occurs, the drug must be replaced by another, nonmacrolide antibiotic such as one of the penicillins, one of the cephalosporins, or clindamycin. This form is no longer available in the United States.

ETHYLSUCCINATE (ERYPED, EES) Erythromycin ethyl succinate is a mixed double-ester prodrug in which one carboxyl of succinic acid esterifies the C-2′ hydroxyl of erythromycin and the other ethanol (Fig. 33.28). This prodrug is frequently used in an oral suspension for pediatric use largely to mask the bitter taste of the drug. Film-coated tablets are also used to deal with this. Some cholestatic jaundice is associated with the use of erythromycin ethyl succinate (83).

STEARATE Erythromycin stearate is a very insoluble salt form of erythromycin. The water insolubility helps mask the taste of the drug and enhances its stability in the stomach.

LACTOBIONATE Erythromycin lactobionate is a salt with enhanced water solubility that is used for injections.

Clarithromycin (Biaxin). Clarithromycin differs from erythromycin in that the C-6 hydroxy group has been converted semisynthetically to a methyl ether (Fig. 33.28). The C-6 hydroxy group is involved in the process, initiated by protons, leading to internal cyclic ketal formation in erythromycin that results in drug inactivation (Fig. 33.30). This ketal, or one of the products of its subsequent degradation, is also associated with GI cramping. Conversion of the molecule to its more lipophilic methyl ether prevents internal ketal formation, which not only gives better blood levels through chemical stabilization, but also results in less gastric upset. An extensive saturable first-pass liver metabolism of clarithromycin leads to formation of its C-14 hydroxy analog, which has even greater antimicrobial potency, especially against *Haemophilus influenzae* (84). The enhanced lipophilicity of clarithromycin also allows for lower and less frequent dosage for mild infections.

Azithromycin (Zithromax, Zmax). Azithromycin, called an "azalide," has been formed by semisynthetic conversion of erythromycin to a ring-expanded analog in which an *N*-methyl group has been inserted between carbons 9 and 10 and the carbonyl moiety is thus absent (Fig. 33.28). Azithromycin has a 15-membered lactone ring. This new functionality does not form a cyclic internal ketal. Not only is azithromycin more stable to acid degradation than erythromycin, but it also has a considerably longer half-life, attributed to greater and longer tissue penetration, allowing once-a-day dosage (85). A popular treatment schedule with azithromycin is to take two tablets on the first day and one a day for the following 5 days and then to discontinue treatment. This is convenient for patients who comply poorly. The drug should be taken on an empty stomach. Azithromycin tends to be broader spectrum than either erythromycin or clarithromycin. Azithromycin has a significant postantibiotic effect against a number of pathogens (85). Azithromycin is now commonly the first choice for treatment of infections that require a macrolide.

Ketolides. Research activity in the macrolide antibiotic class has been intense recently in attempts to reduce side effects and to broaden their antimicrobial spectra. The ketolides are a group of agents that are characterized by oxidation of the 3 position from an alcohol to a ketone. They are active against a significant number of erythromycin-resistant microorganisms.

Telithromycin (Ketek). Telithromycin (Fig. 33.28) is orally effective in the treatment of community-acquired pneumonia, acute bacterial exacerbations of chronic bronchitis, and acute sinusitis. Its principle advantage is activity against macrolide-resistant infections mediated by the methylation mechanisms. Significant controversy about the safety of this agent arose after approval by the U.S. Food and Drug Administration and ultimately led to additional warning information about liver toxicity and a black box warning regarding use in myasthenia gravis patients (86). The toxicity reported for telithromycin appears to be associated with the pyridine portion of the molecule and the antagonist action of the drug on cholinergic receptors. Ketolides under investigation that do not contain a pyridine are devoid of the reported toxicities.

Lincosamides

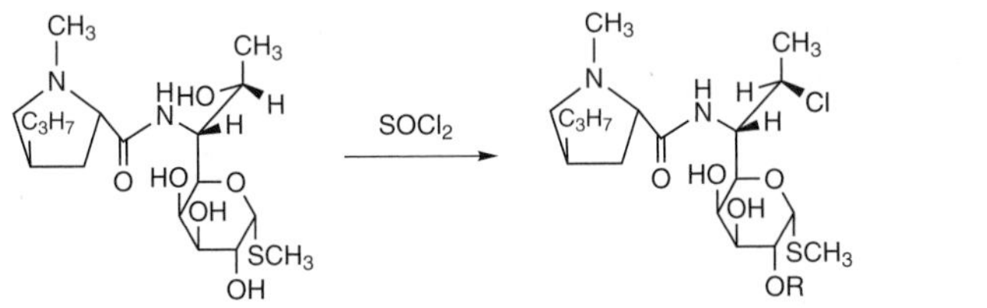

Lincomycin

Clindamycin, R = H (Cleocin)
Clindamycin phosphate, R = PO_3H

The lincosamides contain an unusual 8-carbon sugar, a thiomethyl amino-octoside (*O*-thio-lincosamide), linked by an amide bond to an *n*-propyl substituted *N*-methylpyrrolidylcarboxylic acid (*N*-methyl-*n*-propyl-*trans*-hygric acid). Lincosamides are weakly basic and form clinically useful hydrochloric acid salts. They are chemically distinct from the macrolide antibiotics but possess many pharmacologic similarities to them. The lincosamides bind to 50S ribosomal subparticles at a site partly overlapping with the macrolide site and are mutually cross-resistant with macrolides and work through essentially the same molecular mechanism of action (Fig 33.24). The lincosamides undergo extensive liver metabolism resulting primarily in *N*-demethylation. The *N*-desmethyl analog retains biologic activity.

Specific Agents.
Lincomycin (Lincocin). Lincomycin is a natural product isolated from fermentations of *Streptomyces lincolnensis.* It is active against gram-positive organisms including some anaerobes. It is indicated for treatment of serious infections caused by sensitive strains of streptococci, pneumococci, and staphylococci (87). It is generally reserved for penicillin-allergic patients due to the increased risk of pseudomembranous colitis (described below). It also serves as the starting material for the synthesis of clindamycin (by an S_N-2 reaction that inverts the *R* stereochemistry of the C-7 hydroxyl to a C-7 *S*-chloride).

Clindamycin (Cleocin). The substitution of the chloride for the hydroxy group consequently makes clindamycin more bioactive and lipophilic than lincomycin, and thus, it is better absorbed following oral administration. It is about 90% absorbed when taken orally. Clindamycin has a clinical spectrum rather like the macrolides, although it distributes better into bones. Clindamycin works well for gram-positive coccal infections, especially in patients allergic to β-lactams, and also has generally better activity against anaerobes. However, as with lincomycin, it is associated with GI complaints (nausea, vomiting, cramps, and drug-related diarrheas) (88). The most severe of these (black box warning) is pseudomembranous colitis caused *Clostridium difficile,* an opportunistic anaerobe. Its overgrowth results from suppression of the normal flora whose presence otherwise preserves a healthier ecologic balance. The popularity of clindamycin in the clinic has decreased even though pseudomembranous colitis is comparatively rare and is also associated with several other broad-spectrum antibiotics. A less common side effect is exudative erythema multiform (Stevens-Johnson syndrome). Clindamycin has excellent activity against *Propionibacterium acnes* when applied topically (88). A very water-insoluble palmitate hydrochloride prodrug of clindamycin is also available (lacks bitter taste).

Tetracyclines and Glycylcyclines The tetracycline family is widely but not intensively used in office practice. Of the agents in this family, minocycline and doxycycline are still frequently prescribed in the United States. This family of antibiotics is characterized by a highly functionalized, partially reduced naphthacene (four linearly fused six-membered rings) ring system from which both the family name and numbering system are derived.

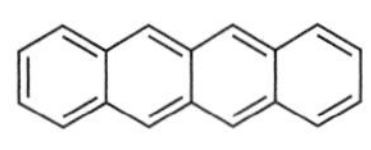

Naphthacene

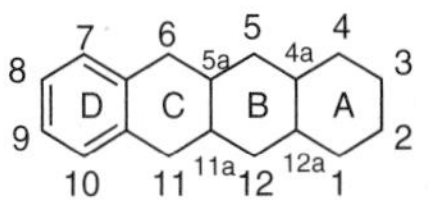

Tetracycline
(1,2,3,4,4a,5,5a,6,11,11a ,12,12a-dodecahydronaphthacene)

They possess a number of adverse effects, although most of them are annoying rather than dangerous. Because their antimicrobial spectrum is broad enough to include many of the pathogens encountered in a community setting, they were once very widely used. The advent of other choices and the high incidence of resistance that has developed have greatly decreased their medicinal prominence in recent years. Presently, they are recommended primarily for use against *Rickettsia, Chlamydia, Mycoplasma,* anthrax, plague, and *Helicobacter.*

Chemical Properties. The tetracyclines are amphoteric substances with three pK_a values revealed by titration (2.8 to 3.4, 7.2 to 7.8, and 9.1 to 9.7) and have an isoelectric point at about pH 5. The basic function is the C-4-α-dimethylamino moiety. Commercially available tetracyclines (Table 33.10) are generally administered as comparatively water-soluble hydrochloride salts. The conjugated phenolic enone system extending from C-10 to C-12 is associated with the pK_a at about 7.5, whereas the conjugated trione system extending from C-1 to C-3 in ring A is nearly as acidic as acetic acid (pK_a ~3) (89). These resonating systems can be drawn in a number of essentially equivalent ways with the double bonds in alternate positions. The formulae normally shown are those settled upon by popular convention.

Chelation. Chelation is an important feature of the chemical and clinical properties of the tetracyclines. The acidic functions of the tetracyclines are capable of forming salts through chelation with metal ions. The salts of polyvalent metal ions, such as Fe^{2+}, Ca^{2+}, Mg^{2+}, and Al^{3+}, are all quite insoluble at neutral pHs (Fig. 33.31). This

TABLE 33.10 Commercially Available Tetracyclines

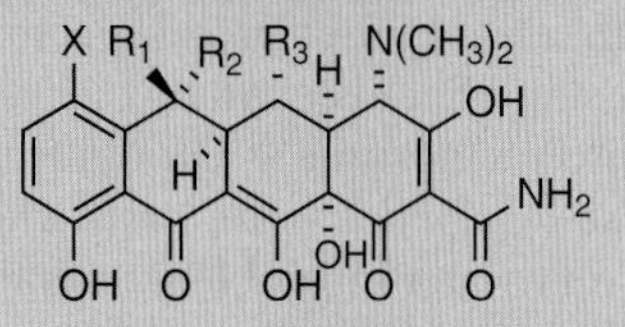

Generic Name	Trade Name	X	R_1	R_2	R_3
Tetracycline	Generic	H	OH	CH_3	H
Demeclocycline	Declomycin	Cl	OH	H	H
Minocycline	Minocin	$N(CH_3)_2$	H	H	H
Doxycycline	Vibramycin	H	H	CH_3	OH

insolubility is not only inconvenient for the preparation of solutions, but also interferes with blood levels on oral administration.

Consequently, the tetracyclines are incompatible with coadministered multivalent ion-rich antacids, and concomitant consumption of daily products rich in calcium ion is also contraindicated (89). When concomitant oral therapy with tetracyclines and incompatible metal ions must be done, the ions should be given 1 hour before or 2 hours after the tetracyclines. Further, the bones, of which the teeth are the most visible, are calcium-rich structures at nearly neutral pHs and so accumulate tetracyclines in proportion to the amount and duration of therapy when bones and teeth are being formed. Because the tetracyclines are yellow, this leads to a progressive and essentially permanent discoloration in which, in advanced cases, the teeth are even brown. The intensification of discoloration with time is thought to be a photochemical process. This is cosmetically unattractive but does not seem to be deleterious except in extreme cases where so much antibiotic is taken up that the structure of bone is mechanically weakened. To avoid this, tetracyclines are not normally given to children (89).

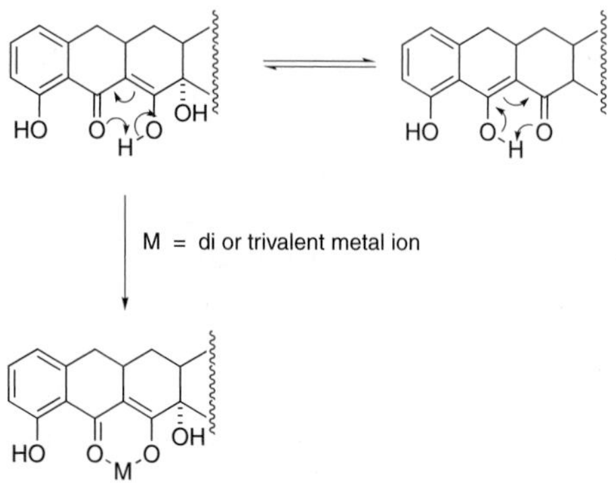

FIGURE 33.31 Metal chelation with the tetracyclines.

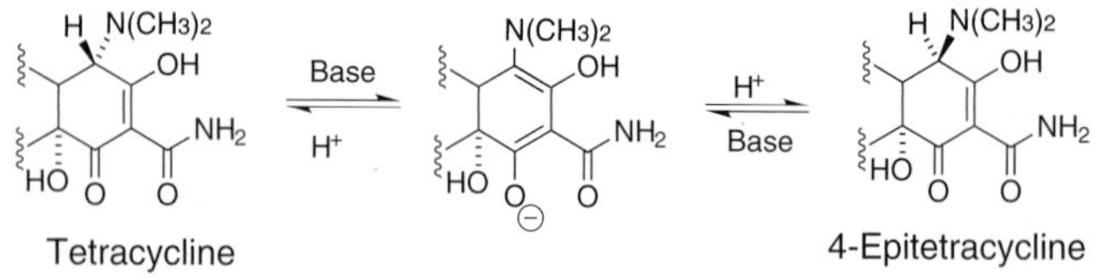

FIGURE 33.32 Epimerization of tetracyclines

Epimerization. The α-stereo orientation of the C-4 dimethylamino moiety of the tetracyclines is essential for their bioactivity. The presence of the tricarbonyl system of ring A allows enolization involving loss of the C-4 hydrogen (Fig. 33.32). Reprotonation can take place from either the top or bottom of the molecule. Reprotonation from the top of the enol regenerates tetracycline. Reprotonation from the bottom, however, produces inactive 4-epitetracycline. At equilibrium, the mixture consists of nearly equal amounts of the two diastereomers.

Dehydration. Most of the natural tetracyclines have a tertiary and benzylic hydroxyl group at C-6. This function has the ideal geometry for acid-catalyzed dehydration involving the C-5a α-oriented hydrogen (antiperiplanar *trans*). The resulting product is a naphthalene derivative, so there are energetic reasons for the reaction proceeding in that direction (Fig. 33.33). C-5a,6-Anhydrotetracycline is much deeper in color than tetracycline and is biologically inactive.

Not only can inactive 4-epitetracyclines dehydrate to produce 4-epianhydrotetracyclines, but also anhydrotetracycline can epimerize to produce the same product. This degradation product is toxic to the kidneys and produces a Fanconi-like syndrome that, in extreme cases, has been fatal (90). Tetracyclines that have no C-6-hydroxyl groups, such as minocycline and doxycycline, cannot undergo dehydration and thus are completely free of this toxicity.

Cleavage in Base. Another untoward degradation reaction involving a C-6-hydroxyl group is cleavage of the C-ring in alkaline solutions at or above pH 8.5 (Fig. 33.34).

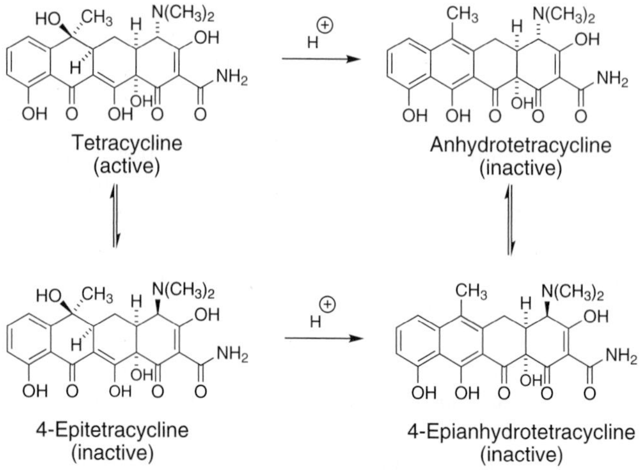

FIGURE 33.33 Acid-catalyzed instability of tetracyclines.

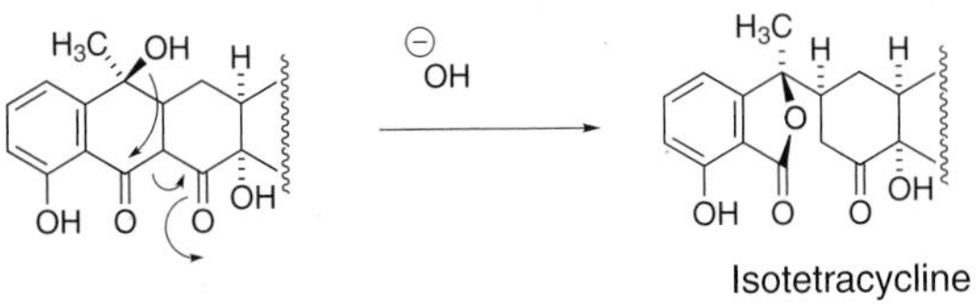

FIGURE 33.34 Base-catalyzed instability of tetracyclines.

The lactonic product, an isotetracycline, is inactive. The clinical impact of this degradation under normal conditions is uncertain.

Phototoxicity. Certain tetracyclines, most notably those with a C-7-chlorine, absorb light in the visible region, leading to free radical generation and potentially causing severe erythema to sensitive patients on exposure to strong sunlight. Patients should be advised to be cautious about such exposure for at least their first few doses to avoid potentially severe sunburn. This effect is comparatively rare with most currently popular tetracyclines (90).

Mechanism of Action. The tetracyclines of clinical importance interfere with protein biosynthesis at the ribosomal level, leading to bacteriostasis. Tetracyclines bind to rRNA in the 30S subparticle with the possible cooperation of a 50S site by a process that remains imprecisely understood despite intensive study (Fig. 33.24). There is more than one binding site, but only one is believed to be critical for its action. The points of contact with the rRNA are those associated with antibiosis, with the puzzling exception of the dimethylamino function (Fig. 33.35). This latter is known to be essential for activity but does not appear to bind in the x-ray structures that are available (91–93). Once the tetracycline binds, it inhibits subsequent binding of aminoacyltransfer-RNA to the ribosomes, resulting in termination of peptide chain growth. The more lipophilic tetracyclines, typified by minocycline, are also capable of disrupting cytoplasmic membrane function, causing leakage of nucleotides and other essential cellular components from the cell, and have bactericidal properties.

Resistance. Resistance to tetracyclines results in part from an unusual ribosomal protection process involving elaboration of bacterial proteins. These proteins associate with the ribosome, thus allowing protein biosynthesis to proceed even in the presence of bound tetracycline, although exactly how this works is not well understood. Another important resistance mechanism involves R-factor–mediated, energy-requiring, active efflux of tetracyclines from the bacterial cells (94). Some of the efflux proteins have activity that is limited to older tetracyclines, whereas others confer resistance to the entire family with the exception of glycylcyclines. Certain other microbes, such as *Mycoplasma* and *Neisseria*, seem to have modified membranes that either accumulate fewer tetracyclines or have porins through which tetracyclines have difficulty passing. Because resistance is now widespread,

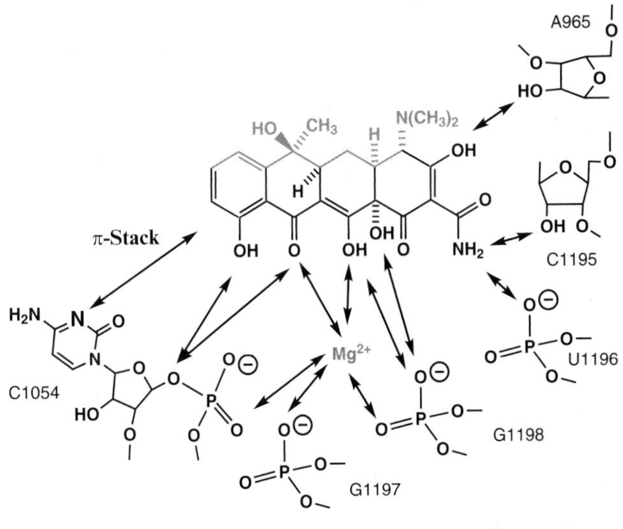

FIGURE 33.35 Schematic representation of the primary binding site for a tetracycline and the sugar phosphate groups of 16S rRNA, which also involves a magnesium ion and the critical functional groups on the "southern" and "eastern" face of the tetracycline. (Redrawn and modified from Brodersen DE, Clemons WM Jr, Carter AP, et al. The structural basis for the action of the antibiotics tetracycline, pactamycin, and hygromycin B on the 30S ribosomal subunit. Cell 2000;103:1143–1154).

these once extremely popular antibiotics are falling into comparative disuse.

Therapeutic Application. The tetracyclines possess very wide bacteriostatic antibacterial activity. Because of the resistance phenomenon and the comparative frequency of troublesome side effects, they are rarely the drugs of first choice. The differences between the antimicrobial spectra of various tetracyclines are not large, although greater resistance to older agents limits their use. They are used for low-dose oral and topical therapy for acne, first-course community-acquired urinary tract infections (largely due to *Escherichia coli*), brucellosis, borreliosis, sexually transmitted diseases (especially chlamydia), rickettsial infections, mycoplasmal pneumonia, prophylaxis of malaria, prevention of traveler's diarrhea, cholera, *Enterobacter* infections, as part of *Helicobacter* cocktails, Lyme disease, Rocky Mountain spotted fever, anthrax, and many other less common problems (90). The tetracyclines are also widely used for agricultural purposes.

Adverse Effects. In addition to the adverse effects mentioned earlier (tooth staining, phototoxicity, and potential kidney damage with outdated drug), the tetracyclines are associated with nausea, vomiting, diarrhea, and some CNS effects (dizziness and vertigo). Rapid administration or prolonged intravenous use can lead to thrombophlebitis, so tetracyclines are generally administered orally because they are well absorbed. They also distinguish imperfectly between the bacterial 70S ribosomes and the mammalian 80S ribosomes, so in high doses or special situations (i.e., intravenous use during pregnancy), these drugs also demonstrate a significant antianabolic effect. In cases of significant renal impairment, higher serum levels of tetracyclines can lead to azotemia. Additionally, inducers of CYP450 metabolism (i.e., rifampin, barbiturates, carbamazepine) increase metabolism of tetracyclines (especially doxycycline), so the dose of the tetracycline may require adjustment (90).

Specific Agents (Table 33.10).

Tetracycline (Sumycin). Tetracycline is produced by fermentation of *Streptomyces aureofaciens* and related species or by catalytic reduction of chlortetracycline. The blood levels achieved on oral administration are often irregular. Food and milk lower absorption by about 50% (89).

Demeclocycline (Declomycin). Demeclocycline lacks the C-6-methyl of tetracycline and is produced by a genetically altered strain of *S. aureofaciens.* Because it is a secondary alcohol, it is more chemically stable than tetracycline against dehydration. Food and milk co-consumption decrease absorption by half, although it is 60% to 80% absorbed by fasting adults. It is the tetracycline most highly associated with phototoxicity and also has been shown to produce dose-dependent, reversible diabetes insipidus with extended use. Demeclocycline is commonly used off label for treatment of inappropriate secretion of antidiuretic hormone.

Minocycline (Minocin and Others). An important antibiotic produced by semisynthesis from demeclocycline is minocycline. It is much more lipophilic than its precursors, gives excellent blood levels following oral administration (90% to 100% available), and can be given once a day. Its absorption is lowered by about 20% when taken with food or milk. It is less dependent on active uptake mechanisms and has a somewhat broader antimicrobial spectrum. It has vestibular toxicities (e.g., vertigo, ataxia, and nausea) not generally shared by other tetracyclines (95).

Doxycycline (Vibramycin and Others). It is produced by semisynthesis from other tetracycline molecules and is the most widely used of the tetracycline family. Doxycycline is well absorbed on oral administration (90% to 100% when fasting; reduced by 20% by co-consumption with food or milk), has a half-life permitting once-a-day dosing for mild infections, and is excreted partly in the feces and partly in the urine.

Tigecycline (Tygacil).

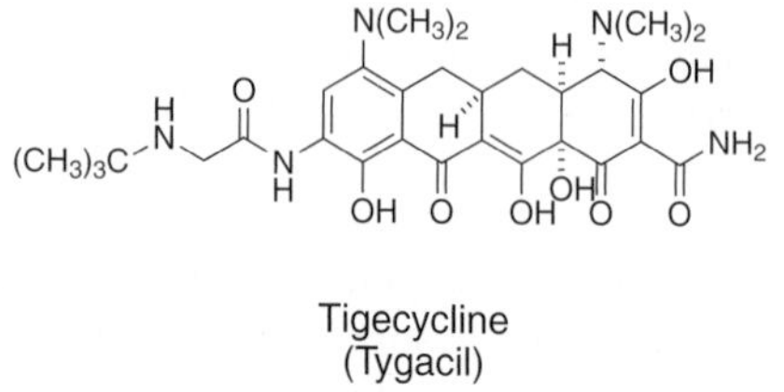

Tigecycline
(Tygacil)

The increased incidence of resistance to the tetracyclines led to a renewed research effort to find novel agents within this class. This effort led to the discovery of a new class of antibiotics, the glycylcyclines, that are closely structurally related to the tetracyclines but lack many of the clinical resistance issues (96,97). They are characterized by having an additional glyclamido substitution at the 9 position. Tigecycline is the first of these agents to be marketed. Although it has limited indications, treatment of complicated skin/skin structure and complicated intra-abdominal infections, this agent is a broad-spectrum antibiotic based on the in vitro data. It is administered intravenously and, like the tetracyclines, can cause injection site pain and thrombophlebitis. It has other adverse effects similar to the tetracyclines.

Special Purpose Antibiotics This group of antibiotics consists of a miscellaneous collection of structural types whose toxicities or narrow range of applicability give them a more specialized place in antimicrobial chemotherapy than those covered to this point. They are generally reserved for special purposes.

Chloramphenicol (Chloromycetin).

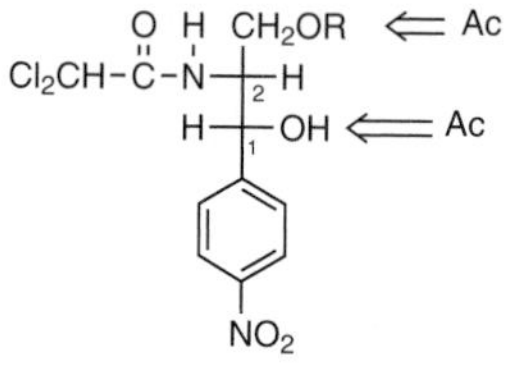

R = H	Chloramphenicol (Chloromycetin)
R = $COCH_2CH_2CO_2H$	Chloramphenicol hemisuccinate
R = $CO(CH_2)_{12}CH_3$	Chloramphenicol palmitate

Chloramphenicol was originally produced by fermentation of *Streptomyces venezuelae,* but its comparatively simple chemical structure soon resulted in several efficient total chemical syntheses. With two asymmetric centers, it is one of four diastereomers, only one of which (1*R*,2*R*) is significantly active. Because total synthesis produces a mixture of all four, the unwanted isomers must be removed before use. Chloramphenicol is a neutral substance only moderately soluble in water because both nitrogen atoms are nonbasic under physiologic conditions (one is an amide and the other a nitro moiety). It was the first broad-spectrum oral antibiotic used in the United States (1947) and was once very popular. Severe potential blood dyscrasia has greatly decreased its use in North America, although its cheapness and efficacy make it still very popular in much of the rest of the world where it can often be purchased over the counter without a prescription.

Mechanism of Action. Chloramphenicol is bacteriostatic by virtue of inhibition of protein biosynthesis in both bacterial and, to a lesser extent, in the host ribosomes. Chloramphenicol binds to the 50S subparticle in a region near where the macrolides and lincosamides bind (Fig. 33.24).

Resistance is mediated by several R-factor enzymes that catalyze acetylation of the secondary and, to some extent, the primary hydroxyl groups in the aliphatic side chain (98). These products no longer bind to the ribosomes and thus are inactivated. *Escherichia coli* is frequently resistant due to chloramphenicol's lack of intercellular accumulation.

Metabolism. When given orally, chloramphenicol is rapidly and completely absorbed but has a fairly short half-life. It is mainly excreted in the urine in the form of its metabolites, which are C-3 and C-1 glucuronides, and, to a lesser extent, its deamidation product and the product of dehalogenation and reduction. These metabolites are all inactive. The aromatic nitro group is also reduced metabolically, and this product can undergo amide hydrolysis. The reduction of the nitro group, however, does not take place efficiently in humans but primarily occurs in the gut by the action of the normal flora (99). Chloramphenicol potentiates the activity of some other drugs by inducing liver metabolism. Such agents include anticoagulant coumarins, sulfonamides, oral hypoglycemics, and phenytoin (99).

Prodrug Forms. Two prodrug forms of chloramphenicol are available (only the injectable form is available in the United States). The drug is intensively bitter. This can be masked for use as a pediatric oral suspension by use of the C-3 palmitate, which is cleaved in the duodenum to liberate the drug.

Chloramphenicol's poor water solubility is largely overcome by conversion to the C-3 hemisuccinoyl ester, which forms a water-soluble sodium salt. This is cleaved in the body by lung, liver, kidney, and blood esterases to produce active chloramphenicol. Because cleavage in muscles is slow, this prodrug is used intravenously rather than intramuscularly.

Therapeutic Applications. Despite potentially serious limitations, chloramphenicol is an effective drug when used carefully. Its special value is in typhoid fever, *Haemophilus* infections (especially epiglottitis and meningitis, when given along with ampicillin), and rickettsial infections, and in cases where susceptible organisms have proven resistant to other therapies. Safer antibiotics should be used whenever possible. It is about 60% serum protein bound and diffuses well into tissues, especially into inflamed cerebrospinal fluid, and is, therefore, of value for meningitis. It also penetrates well into lymph and mesenteric ganglions, rationalizing its particular value in typhoid fever.

Adverse Effects. Toxicities prevent chloramphenicol from being more widely used. Blood dyscrasias are seen in patients predisposed to them (99). The more serious form is a pancytopenia of the blood that is fatal in about 70% of cases and is believed to be caused by one of the reduction products of the aromatic nitro group. This side effect is known as aplastic anemia and has even occurred following use of the drug as an ophthalmic ointment. There seems to be a genetic predisposition toward this in a very small percentage of the population. Less severe, but much more common, is a reversible inhibition of hematopoiesis, seen in older patients or in those with renal insufficiency. If cell counts are taken, this can be controlled because it is dose-related and marrow function will recover if the drug is withdrawn.

The so-called "gray" or "gray baby" syndrome, a form of cardiovascular collapse, is encountered when chloramphenicol is given to young infants (especially premature infants) when liver glucuronidation is underdeveloped, and successive doses will lead to rapid accumulation of the drug due to impaired excretion. A dose-related profound anemia accompanied by an ashen gray pallor is seen, as are vomiting, loss of appetite, and cyanosis. Deaths have resulted, often involving cardiovascular collapse.

A variety of cyclic peptides are utilized for their antibiotic properties. The usual physiologically significant peptides are linear. Several bacterial species, however, produce antibiotic mixtures of cyclic peptides, some with uncommon amino acids and some with common amino acids but with the D absolute stereochemistry. These cyclic substances often have a pendant fatty acid chain as well. One of the consequences of this unusual architecture is that these glycopeptide agents are not readily metabolized. These drugs are usually water soluble and are highly lethal to susceptible bacteria because they attach themselves to the bacterial membranes and interfere with their semipermeability so that essential metabolites leak out and undesirable substances pass in. Unfortunately, they are also highly toxic in humans, so their use is reserved for serious situations where there are few alternatives or to topical uses. Bacteria are rarely able to develop significant resistance to this group of antibiotics. They are generally unstable, so solutions should be protected from heat, light, and extremes of pH.

Vancomycin (Vancocin, Generic).

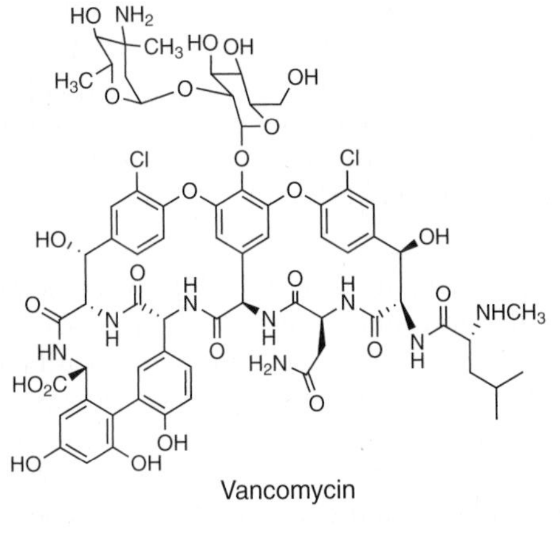

Vancomycin

Vancomycin is produced by fermentation of *Amycolatopsis orientalis* (formerly called *Nocardia orientalis*). It has been available for about 40 years, but its popularity has increased significantly with the emergence of MRSA in the early 1980s. Chemically, vancomycin has a glycosylated hexapeptide chain rich in unusual amino acids, many of which contain aromatic rings cross-linked by aryl ether bonds into a rigid molecular framework.

Mechanism of Action Vancomycin is a bacterial cell wall biosynthesis inhibitor. There is evidence that the active species is a homodimer of two vancomycin units. The binding site for its target is a peptide-lined cleft having high affinity for acetyl-D-alanyl-D-alanine and related peptides through five hydrogen bonds (100). It inhibits both transglycosylases (inhibiting the linking between muramic acid and acetyl glucosamine units) and transpeptidase (inhibiting peptide cross-linking) activities in cell wall biosynthesis (Fig. 33.10). Thus, vancomycin functions like a peptide receptor and interrupts bacterial cell wall biosynthesis at the same step as does the β-lactams but by a different mechanism. By covering the substrate for cell wall transamidase, it prevents cross-linking, resulting in osmotically defective cell walls.

Resistance Only recently, despite decades of intensive use, have some vancomycin-resistant bacteria emerged (vancomycin-resistant *Enterococcus* and vancomycin-resistant *Staphylococcus aureus*) (101). The mechanism of resistance appears to be alteration of the target D-alanyl-D-alanine units on the peptidoglycan cell wall precursors to D-alanyl-D-lactate. This results in lowered affinity for vancomycin. It is greatly feared that this form of resistance will become common in the bacteria for which vancomycin presently is used for successful chemotherapy.

Therapeutic Applications Although a number of adverse effects can result from intravenous infusion (see below), vancomycin has negligible oral activity. It can be used orally for action in the GI tract, especially in cases of *Clostridium difficile* overgrowth. The useful spectrum is restricted to gram-positive pathogens with particular utility against multiply resistant coagulase-negative staphylococci and MRSA, which causes septicemias, endocarditis, skin and soft tissue infections, and infections associated with venous catheters (102).

Adverse Effects Vancomycin is highly associated with adverse infusion-related events. These are especially prevalent with higher doses and a rapid infusion rate. Rapid infusion rate has been shown to cause anaphylactoid reactions, including hypotension, wheezing, dyspnea, urticaria, and pruritus. A significant drug rash (the so-called red man syndrome) can also occur. These events are much less frequent with a slower infusion rate.

In addition to the danger of infusion-related events, higher doses of vancomycin can cause nephrotoxicity and auditory nerve damage. The risk of these effects is increased with elevated, prolonged concentrations, so vancomycin use should be monitored, especially in patients with decreased renal function. The ototoxicity may be transient or permanent and more commonly occurs in patients on high doses, those who have underlying hearing loss, and those treated concomitantly with other ototoxic agents (i.e., aminoglycosides) (102).

Telavancin (Vibativ).

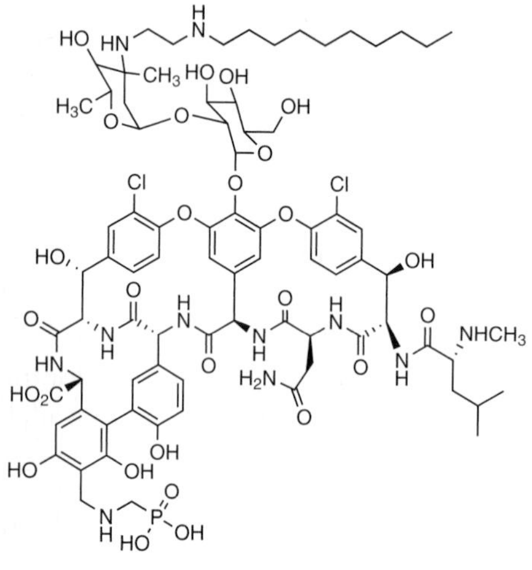

Televancin

Telavancin is a semisynthetic derivative of vancomycin that is more properly called a lipoglycopeptide. Although it does inhibit cell wall biosynthesis in the same manner as vancomycin, it appears to also disrupt cell membrane integrity as part of its mechanism. This is suspected to be why telavancin retains some activity against vancomycin-resistant strains (103). Telavancin is indicated for treatment of complicated skin and soft tissue infections by gram-positive organisms including MRSA. It should not be used in pregnancy, and like vancomycin, it requires dose adjustment with renal impairment. Telavancin also produces infusion-related toxicities, so slow infusion is recommended (104).

Daptomycin (Cubicin).

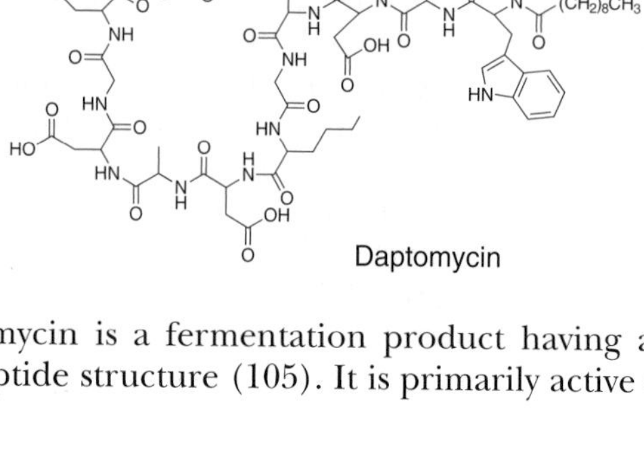

Daptomycin

Daptomycin is a fermentation product having a cyclic lipopeptide structure (105). It is primarily active against gram-positive infections, especially skin and skin structure infections. It is given intravenously but must be administered over a period of 30 minutes or more. It binds to cell membranes and causes depolarization, which interrupts protein, DNA, and RNA synthesis. Daptomycin is bactericidal. Although resistance can be achieved in vitro, resistance has been slow to emerge in the clinic. Patients should be monitored for muscle pain or weakness because some incidence of elevated serum creatinine phosphokinase is associated with its use. Daptomycin is eliminated primarily by the kidney, so dose adjustment may be necessary in cases of renal insufficiency (106).

Quinupristin/Dalfopristin (Synercid).

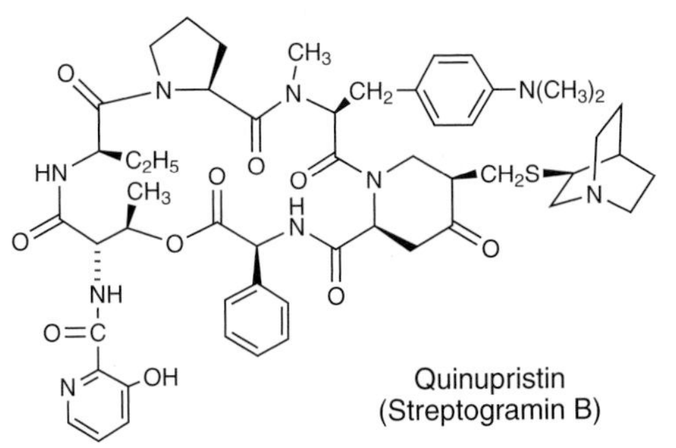

Quinupristin
(Streptogramin B)

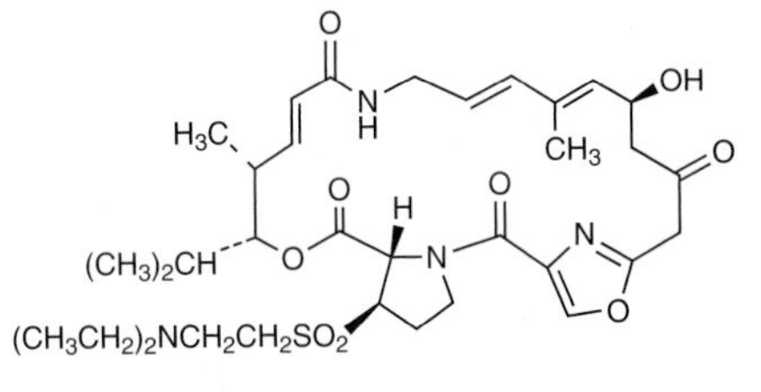

Dalfopristin
(Streptogramin A)

A combination of the streptogramins quinupristin and dalfopristin is approved for intravenous use in the treatment of infections caused by vancomycin-resistant *Enterococcus faecium* bacteremia as well as skin and skin structure infections caused by methicillin-sensitive *Staphylococcus aureus* and *Streptococcus pyogenes.* Certain strains of *E. faecium* are resistant to essentially all other antibiotics, including vancomycin. Dalfopristin binds to the 70S ribosomal subparticle at the A and P sites, thus interfering with substrate attachment. Quinupristin binds to the A and P sites, also causing a misalignment of the tRNA in the P site (107). Thus, they bind to nearly the same place in the ribosome (Fig. 33.24). The two drugs are bacteriostatic when administered individually but are found to act synergistically when combined (quinupristin:dalfopristin [30:70 w/w]) to produce a bactericidal effect. It appears that dalfopristin binding creates a high-affinity binding site for quinupristin, accounting for the synergy. The combination is found to inhibit protein synthesis by binding to the 70S ribosome that is thought to account for the mechanism of action. Synercid is a strong inhibitor of the CYP3A4 isozyme, and a number of drug interactions are to be expected. Although the combination does not appear to prolong the QT_c interval, it inhibits the metabolism of a number of agents that have been shown to have this effect, so concomitant administration should be avoided. Synercid also can produce a number of other adverse effects including infusion site reactions (pain, edema, and inflammation), arthralgia and myalgia, and hyperbilirubinemia (108).

Polymyxin B.

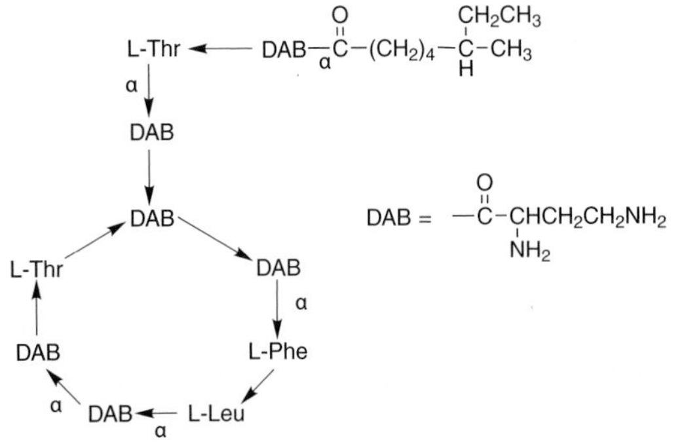

Polymyxin B is produced by fermentation of *Bacillus polymyxa.* It is separated from a mixture of related cyclic peptides and is primarily active against gram-negative microorganisms. It apparently binds to phosphate groups in bacterial cytoplasmic membranes and disrupts their integrity. It is used intramuscularly or intravenously as a sulfate salt to treat serious urinary tract infections, meningitis, and septicemia primarily caused by *Pseudomonas aeruginosa,* but some other gram-negative bacteria will also respond. It is also used orally to treat enteropathogenic *E. coli* and *Shigella* sp. diarrheas. Irrigation of the urinary bladder with solutions of polymyxin B sulfate is also employed by some to reduce the incidence of infections subsequent to installation of indwelling catheters. When given parenterally, the drug is neuro- and nephrotoxic and thus is used only after other drugs have failed.

Bacitracin.

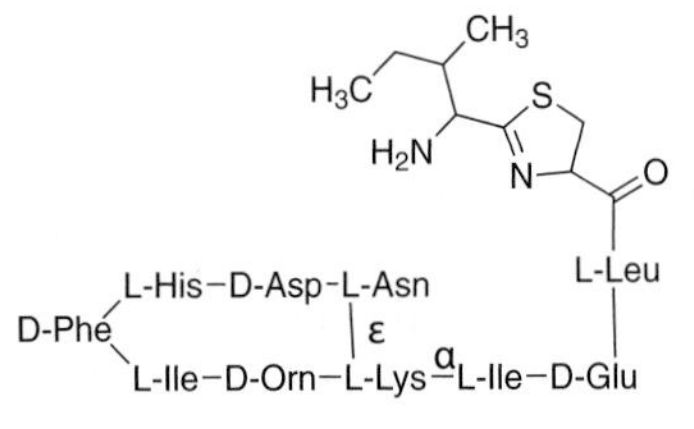

Bacitracin A

Bacitracin is a mixture of similar peptides produced by fermentation of the bacterium *Bacillus subtilis.* The A component predominates. Its mode of action is to inhibit both peptidoglycan biosynthesis at a late stage (probably at the dephosphorylation of the phospholipid carrier step) and disruptions of plasma membrane function. It is predominantly active against gram-positive microorganisms, and parenteral use is limited to intramuscular injection for infants with pneumonia and empyema caused by staphylococci resistant to other agents. It is rather neuro- and nephrotoxic and thus is used in this manner with caution. Bacitracin is also widely used topically to prevent infection in minor cuts, scrapes, and burns.

Linezolid (Zyvox).

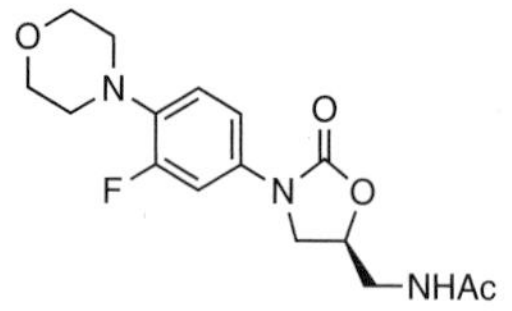

Linezolid

Linezolid is a bacteriostatic (bactericidal against some bacteria) antibacterial agent effective against primarily gram-positive bacteria. This drug is a member of the oxazolidinone class of agents and represents a new synthetic class of antibacterials. It is available in injectable, tablet, and oral suspension dosage forms; is effective against MRSA; and is used to treat nosocomial pneumonia, community-acquired pneumonia, complicated and uncomplicated skin and skin structure infections, and vancomycin-resistant *Enterococcus faecium* infections (109).

The mechanism of action of linezolid is associated with inhibition of protein synthesis, but at a stage different from that of other protein synthesis inhibitors. The oxazolidinones inhibit the initiation of protein synthesis by binding to the 50S subparticle, preventing the formation of a functional initiation complex including *N*-formylmethionyl-tRNA ($tRNA^{fMet}$), the 30S subunit, mRNA, and initiation factors. It is believed that the drug distorts the binding site for the initiator-tRNA, which overlaps both 30S and 50S ribosomal subunits (110). The result of this is that translation of the mRNA is prevented. The other prominent ribosomal protein biosynthesis inhibitors inhibit after a functional initiation complex forms. In those cases, mRNA translation begins, but elongation of the growing peptide chain is blocked.

Resistance to oxazolidinones is encountered in the clinic due to a mutation in the 23S rRNA associated with the 50S ribosomal subunit (111). This is believed to distort the linezolid binding site. Gram-negative microorganisms are intrinsically resistant to linezolid due to the presence of endogenous efflux pumps that keep them from accumulating in the cells.

Linezolid is well absorbed orally and is generally well to moderately well tolerated; however, some severe cases of reversible blood dyscrasias have been noted, resulting in a package insert warning that complete blood counts should be monitored weekly, especially in patients with poorly draining infections and who are receiving prolonged therapy with the drug (109). Linezolid is an inhibitor of monoamine oxidase, so patients should be cautious about eating tyramine-containing foods. Coadministration with adrenergic and serotonergic agents is also unadvisable. Significant oxidative metabolism occurs by oxidation of the morpholine ring, and the antimicrobially inactive metabolites are excreted primarily in the urine (109).

Mupirocin (Bactroban).

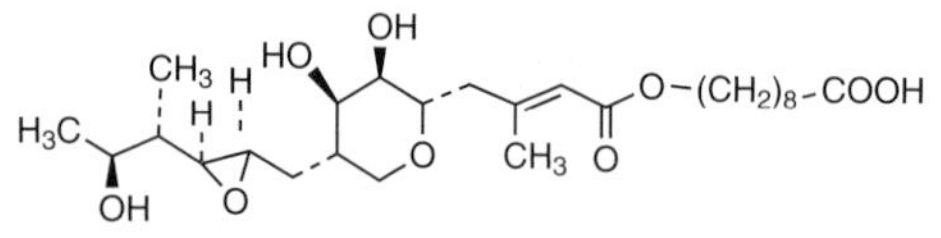

Mupirocin

Mupirocin is a member of a group of lipid acids produced by fermentation of *Pseudomonas fluorescens.* It can only be used topically because of hydrolysis in vivo that inactivates the drug. It is intrinsically broad spectrum, but its primary indication is topically against staphylococcal and streptococcal skin infections. Mupirocin binds to bacterial isoleucyl tRNA synthase, preventing incorporation of isoleucine into bacterial proteins. Resistance is due to alterations of the synthase target such that the enzyme still functions but does not bind mupirocin.

Retapamulin (Altabax).

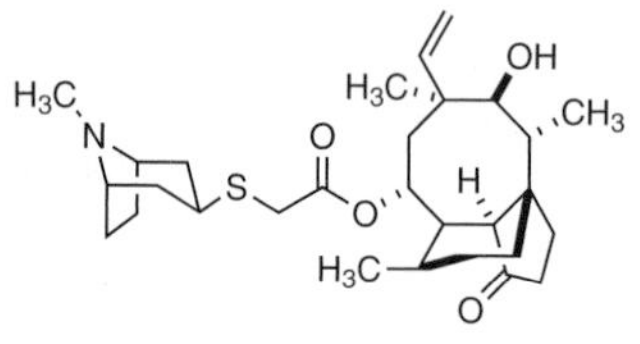

Retapamulin

Retapamulin is approved for use in adults and children over the age of 9 months for the treatment of impetigo caused by methicillin-susceptible *Staphylococcus aureus* and *Streptococcus pyogenes.* Impetigo is a highly contagious infection found most commonly in children involving the upper layers of the skin and spread through close contact. Retapamulin is a semisynthetic diterpene derivative of the naturally occurring pleuromutilins, a group of chemicals produced by the fungus *Pleurotus mutilus* (also referred to as *Clitopilus scyphoides*) (112).

Retapamulin is a bacteriostatic topically used drug that inhibits protein synthesis by binding to the 50S ribosomal subunit. It is a semisynthetic derivative of the natural product mutilin (alcohol at C-14) and pleuromutilin (C-14 hydroxyacetate). The drug is selective for inhibiting translational bacterial protein syntheses and is inactive in eukaryotic translation. Retapamulin is active at a site distinct from that occupied by macrolide antibiotics, both of which inhibit protein synthesis at the 50S ribosomal subunit. It inhibits ribosomal peptidyl transferase, thus preventing peptide bond formation. The C-14 sulfamylacetate moiety appears important for binding to the peptidyl transferase center in the 50S ribosomal subunit of the susceptible bacteria. By occupying this site, the pleuromutilins block peptide bond formation, thus inhibiting bacterial protein synthesis. The pleuromutilins interact with the 23S RNA domain V. There are indications because of the unique binding of retapamulin to the 50S ribosomal subunit that bacterial resistance will be low. Additionally, it has been reported that retapamulin inhibits the biosynthesis of the 50S ribosomal subunit itself in susceptible gram-positive bacteria, leading to the suggestion of a duel antibacterial action (113–115).

Retapamulin is well tolerated, with minimal adverse events. The most common adverse effects are pruritus, diarrhea, and nasopharyngitis. The drug does not appear to be absorbed to any great degree when applied topically, although it is a substrate for CYP3A4 (112).

SCENARIO: OUTCOME AND ANALYSIS

Outcome

Elizabeth Coyle, PharmD

Although the organism has intermediate susceptibility to cefepime, the treatment would likely fail because the ability of ESBL to hydrolyze the cephalosporin. Carbapenems are the drugs of choice for infections caused by ESBL-producing organisms because of their stability in the presences of ESBLs. The team changes ER's antibiotics to meropenem 1 g every 8 hours and discontinues the vancomycin.

Chemical Analysis

Victoria Roche and S. William Zito

The antibacterial agent decided upon in this scenario is a second generation carbapenem. Carbapenems are novel β-lactam antibiotics derived from thienamycin which was isolated from fermentations of *Streptomyces cattleya*. Aside from meropenem, there are other carbapenems, i.e., imipenem, biapenem (approved in Japan in 2001), ertapenem, and doripenem (approved in the United States in 2007). Carbapenems are similar to penicillins and cephalosporins in that they have a fused bicyclic ring system containing a β-lactam ring and an equivalent 3-carboxyl group. However, they differ in that the fused system contains a 5-membered ring that has a methylene group instead of the sulfur atom found in penicillins and cephalosporins. The sulfur atom is attached to C-3 as part of the side chain. In addition, the 5-membered ring contains a double bond. Both of these structural changes result in a strained carbapenem that can be hydrolysed easily at the β-lactam bond.

Early carbapenems suffered from both chemical and metabolic instability. The amino group in thienemycin can attack the β-lactam bond of another molecule through an intermolecular reaction deactivating activity. Imipenem and all the other carbapenems do not have this problem; however, imipenem was found to be hydrolyzed by renal dehydropeptidase-1, causing loss of antibacterial activity. Meropenem, on the other hand, is resistant to both chemical and biological deactivation. Its resistance to renal dehydropeptidase-1 is caused by the methyl group at C-4 of the bicyclic ring system. Meropenem is not active orally and must be administered parenterally. It is excreted primarily unchanged (70–80%) in the urine; the remainder is the inactive β-lactam hydrolysis product.

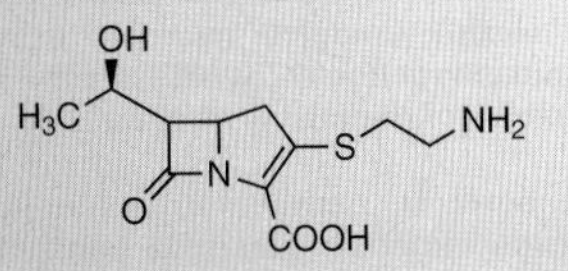

Thienamycin

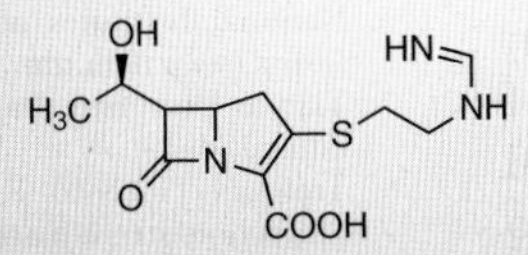

Imipenem

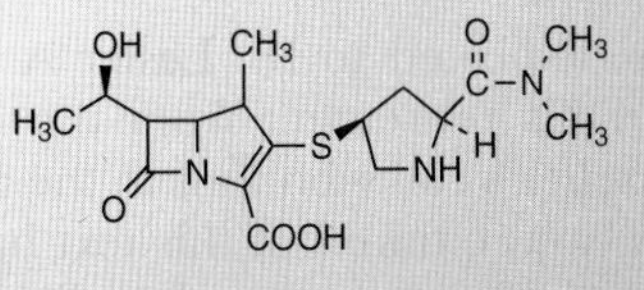

Meropenem (Merrem)

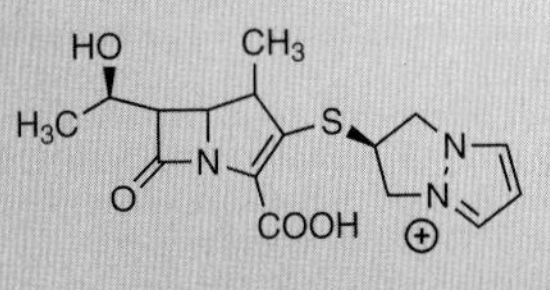

Biapenem

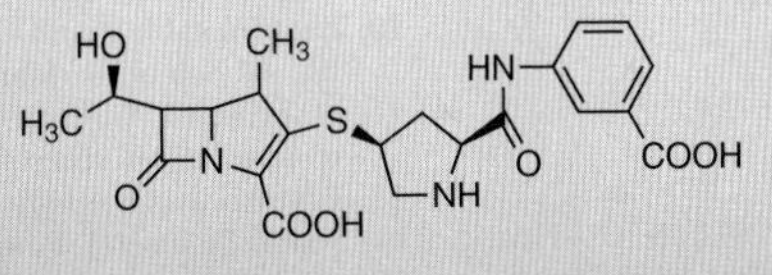

Ertapenem

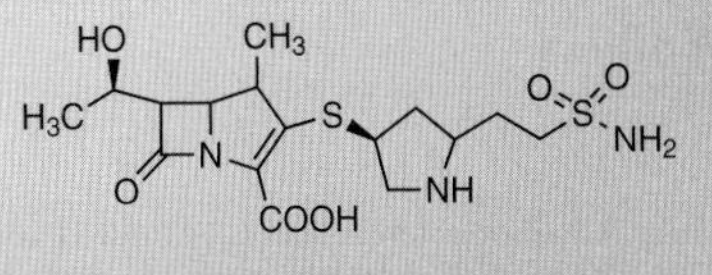

Doripenem

CASE STUDY

S. William Zito and Victoria Roche

YU, a 42-year-old man, presents to the clinic where you work. He states that he has a sore throat and lumps in his neck. He had some nausea and vomiting the previous evening. YU states that these symptoms have been going on for more than a week and he "just feels really bad." He denies any shortness of breath, difficulty breathing, chest pain, light headedness, dizziness, or loss of consciousness.

YU is 5′4″ and weighs 142 lb. His blood pressure is 135/92 mm Hg, his pulse is 121 beats per minute, and his temperature is 100.1°F. YU's sinuses are not tender and his nares are normal. His throat is very red. His neck is supple, with two tender lymph nodes on the right. During questioning, YU states that he has been taking felodipine (10mg/daily) for hypertension for the past 2 years and has no side effects. YU recalls that several years ago he developed a rash when he was treated with bactrim (sulfamethoxazole/trimethoprim) for a bladder infection and had to be switched to another antibiotic. The rapid strep test is positive, and therefore YU is assessed with a Strep throat. Given the following three therapeutic choices, which would you recommend?

1. Conduct a thorough and mechanistic SAR analysis of the three therapeutic options in the case.
2. Apply the chemical understanding gained from the SAR analysis to this patient's specific needs to make a therapeutic recommendation.

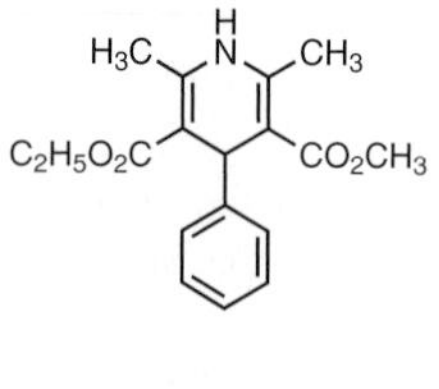

Felodipine

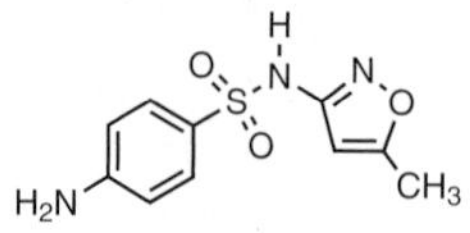

Sulfamethoxazole

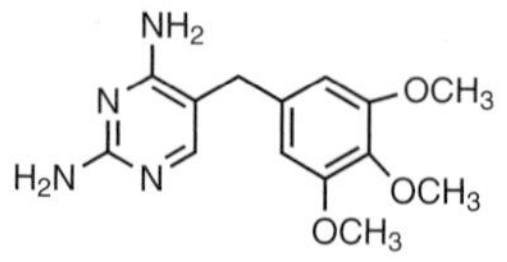

Trimethoprim

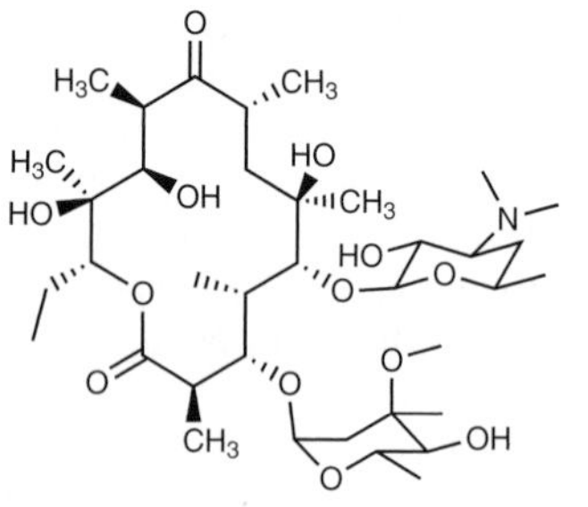

1

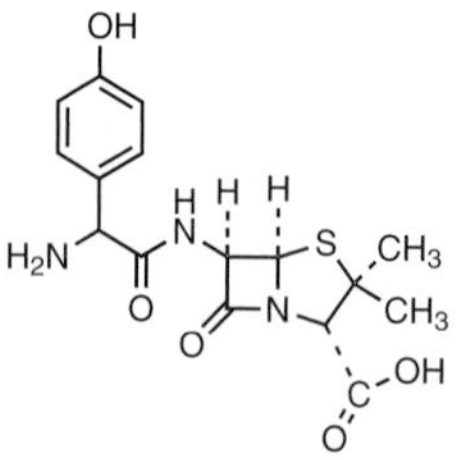

2

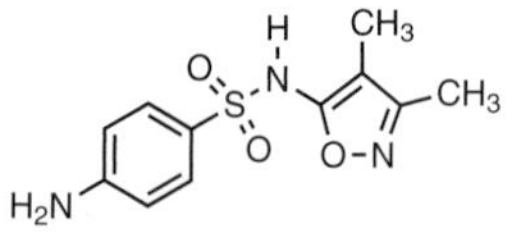

3

ACKNOWLEDGMENT

This chapter is dedicated to Dr. Lester A. Mitscher on the occasion of his retirement from the University of Kansas. Dr. Mitscher's contributions to the antimicrobial field and to previous editions of this text have served to educate thousands of pharmacy and medicinal chemistry students on the significance and intrigue of antibiotics. Thank you for your many years of commitment to the education of others.

References

1. Pasteur L, Joubert J. Charbon et septicemia. CR Acad Sci Paris 1877;85:101–115.
2. Domagk GJ. Ein Beitrag zur chemotherapie der bakteriellen infektionen. Dtsch Med Wochenschr 1935;61:250–253.
3. Fleming A. On the antibacterial action of cultures of a penicillum, with special reference to their use in the isolation of *B. influenza*. Br J Exp Pathol 1929;10:226–236.
4. Abraham EP, Chain E, Fletcher CM, et al. Further observations on penicillin. Eur J Clin Pharmacol 1941;42:3–9.
5. Fleischmann RD, Adams MD, White O, et al. Whole-genome random sequencing and assembly of *Haemophilus influenzae* Rd. Science 1995;269:496–512.
6. National Institutes of Health. Complete microbial genomes. Available at: http://www.ncbi.nlm.nih.gov/genomes/lproks.cgi?view=1.
7. Tianjin University. Database of essential genes. Available at: http://tubic.tju.edu.cn/deg/.
8. Tréfouël JT, Nitti F, Bovet D. Activité du *p*-aminophénylsulfamide sur l'infection streptococcique expérimentale de la souris et du lapin. CR Soc Biol 1935;120:756.
9. Seydel, JK. Sulfonamides, structure-activity relationship, and mode of action. Structural problems of the antibacterial action of 4-aminobenzoic acid (PABA) antagonists. J Pharm Sci 1968;57:1455–1478.
10. Bactrim tablets and double strength tablets [package insert]. Philadelphia, PA: AR Scientific, March 2005.
11. Huovinen P, Sundstrom L, Swedberg G, et al. Trimethoprim and sulfonamide resistance. Antimicrob Agents Chemother 1995;39:279–289.
12. Erythromycin ethylsuccinate and sulfisoxazole acetyl for oral suspension [package insert]. Pomona, NY: Duramed, March 2007.
13. Azulfidine [package insert]. Kalamazoo, MI: Pharmacia & Upjohn, August 2002.
14. Roberts VA, Dauber-Osguthorpe P, Osguthorpe DJ, et al. A comparison of the binding of the ligand trimethoprim to bacterial and vertebrate dihydrofolate reductases. Israel J Chem 1986;27:198–210.
15. Proloprim [package insert]. Bristol, TN: Monarch Pharmaceuticals, February 2003.

16. Appelbaum PC, Hunter PA. The fluoroquinolone antibacterials: past, present, and future. Int J Antimicrob Agents 2000;1:5–15.
17. Drlica K, Zhao X. DNA gyrase, topoisomerase IV and the 4-quinolones. Microbiol Mol Biol Rev 1997;61:377–392.
18. Domagala JM. Structure-activity and structure-side effect relationships for the quinolone antibacterials. J Antimicrob Chemother 1994;33:685–706.
19. Noroxin [package insert]. Whitehouse Station, NJ: Merck & Co, October 2008.
20. Cipro [package insert]. Kenilworth, NJ: Schering-Plough, October 2008.
21. Factive [package insert]. Waltham, MA: Oscient Pharmaceuticals, October 2008.
22. Levaquin [package insert]. Raritan, NJ: Ortho-McNeil-Janssen Pharmaceuticals, September 2008.
23. Avelox [package insert]. Kenilworth, NJ: Schering-Plough Corp., March 2010.
24. Kang J, Wang L, Chen X, et al. Interactions of a series of fluoroquinolone antibacterial drugs with the human cardiac K^+ channel HERG. Mol Pharmacol 2001;59:122–126.
25. Macrodantin (nitrofurantoin macrocrystals) [package insert]. Cincinnati, OH: Procter & Gamble Pharmaceuticals, June 2003.
26. Flagyl [package insert]. New York: Pfizer, July 2009.
27. Tindamax [package insert]. San Antonio, TX: Mission Pharmacal Company, May 2007.
28. Wise EM, Park JT. Penicillin: its basic site of action as an inhibitor of a peptide cross-linking reaction in cell wall mucopeptide synthesis. Proc Natl Acad Sci USA 1965;54:75–81.
29. Kong KF, Schneper L, Mathee K. Beta-lactam antibiotics: from antibiosis to resistance and bacteriology. APMIS 2010;118:1–36.
30. Behrens OK, Corse JW, Jones RG, et al. U.S. Patent 2479297, 1949.
31. Peter DF, Charles NJH, Newbolt RG. U.S. Patent 2941995, 1960.
32. Abraham EP, Newton GGF. The structure of cephalosporin-C. Biochem J 1961;79:377–393.
33. Nagarajan R, Boeck LD, Gorman M, et al. Beta-lactam antibiotics from *Streptomyces*. J Am Chem Soc 1971;93:2308–2310.
34. Imada A, Kitano K, Kintaka K, et al. Sulfazecin and isosulfazecin, novel beta-lactam antibiotics of bacterial origin. Nature 1981;289:590–591.
35. Sykes RB, Cimarusti CM, Bonner DP, et al. Monocyclic beta-lactam antibiotics produced by bacteria. Nature 1981;291:489–491.
36. Tomasz A, Waks S. Mechanism of action of penicillin: triggering of the pneumococcal autolytic enzyme by inhibitors of cell wall synthesis. Proc Natl Acad Sci U S A 1975;72:4162–4166.
37. Abraham EP, Chain E. An enzyme from bacteria able to destroy penicillin. Nature 1940;146:837–838.
38. Fairbrother RW, Taylor G. Sodium methicillin in routine therapy. Lancet 1961;1:473–476.
39. Nafcillin [package insert]. Princeton, NJ: Sandoz Pharmaceuticals, June 2008.
40. Oxacillin [package insert]. Princeton, NJ: Sandoz Pharmaceuticals, October 2009.
41. Ganapathy ME, Brandsch M, Prasad PD, et al. Differential recognition of β-lactam antibiotics by intestinal and real peptide transporters, PEPT 1 and PEPT 2. J Biol Chem 1995;270:25672–25677.
42. Piperacillin for injection [package insert]. Schaumberg, IL: American Pharmaceutical Partners, November 2003.
43. Zosyn [package insert]. Philadelphia, PA: Wyeth Pharmaceuticals, November 2007.
44. Timentin [package insert]. Research Triangle Park, NC: GlaxoSmithKline, January 2007.
45. Dunn GL. Ceftizoxime and other third generation cephalosporins: structure-activity relationships. J Antimicrob Chemother 1982;10(suppl C):1–10.
46. Keflex capsules [package insert]. Germantown, MD: Advancis, May 2006.
47. Ceftin [package insert]. Research Triangle Park, NC: GlaxoSmithKline, January 2010
48. Cuchural GJ, Tally FP, Jacobus NV, et al. Comparative activities of newer β-lactam agents against members of the *Bacteroides fragilis* group. Antimicrob Agents Chemother 1990;3:479–480.
49. Rocephin [package insert]. Nutley, NJ: Roche Pharmaceuticals, August 2008.
50. Maxipime [package insert]. Princeton, NJ: Bristol-Meyers Squibb Company, March 2009.
51. Lipsky JJ. Mechanism of the inhibition of γ-carboxylation of glutamic acid by *N*-methylthiotetrazole antibiotics. Proc Natl Acad Sci U S A 1984;81:2893–2897.
52. Wildman GT, Datta R. U.S. Patent 4137405, 1979.
53. Claforan [package insert]. Bridgewater, NJ: Aventis Pharmaceuticals, July 2004.
54. Fortaz [package insert]. Research Triangle Park, NC: GlaxoSmithKline, April 2007.
55. Cedax [package insert]. Gonzales, LA: Pernix Therapeutics, February 2011.
56. Spectracef [package insert]. Stamford, CT: Purdue Pharmaceutical Products, August 2003.
57. Teflaro [package insert]. St. Louis, MO: Forest Pharmaceuticals, November 2010.
58. Kahan JS, Kahan FM, Goegelman R, et al. Thienamycin, a new beta-lactam antibiotic I. Discovery, taxonomy, isolation, and physical properties. J Antibiot 1979;32:1–12.
59. Birnbaum J, Kahan FM, Kropp H, et al. Carbapenems, a new class of beta-lactam antibiotics. Discovery and development of ipenem/cilastatin. Am J Med 1985;78(6A):3–21.
60. Primaxin [package insert]. Whitehouse Station, NJ: Merck, April 2008.
61. Tsuji M, Ishii Y, Ohno A, et al. In vitro and in vivo antibacterial activities of S-4661, a new carbapenem. Antimicrob Agents Chemother 1998;42:94–99.
62. Norrby SR. Neurotoxicity of carbapenem antibiotics: consequences for their use in bacterial meningitis. J Antimicrob Chemother 2000;45:5–7.
63. Zhanel GC, Wiebe R, Dialy L, et al. Comparative review of the carbapenems. Drugs 2007;67:1027–1052.
64. Kobayashi R, Komoni M, Hasegawa K, et al. In vitro activity of tebipenem, a new oral carbapenem antibiotic, against penicillin-nonsusceptible *Streptococcus pneumoniae*. Antimicrob Agents Chemother 2005;49:889–994.
65. Azactam [package insert]. Princeton, NJ: Bristol-Myers Squibb Company, January 2007.
66. Schuwirth BS, Borovinskava MA, Hau CW, et al. Structures of the bacterial ribosome at 3.5A resolution. Science 2005;310:827–834.
67. Selmer M, Dunham CM, Murphy FV 4th, et al. Structure of the 70S ribosome complexed with mRNA and tRNA. Science 2006;313:1935–1942.
68. Tobi [package insert]. East Hanover, NJ: Novartis Pharmaceuticals Corporation, November 2009.
69. Jana S, Deb JK. Molecular understanding of aminoglycoside action and resistance. Appl Microbiol Biotechnol 2006;70:140–150.
70. Magnet S, Blanchard JS. Molecular insights into aminoglycoside action and resistance. Chem Rev 2005;105:477–497.
71. Kahlmeter G, Dahlager JI. Aminoglycoside toxicity: a review of clinical studies published between 1975 and 1982. J Antimicrob Chemother 1984;13 (Suppl A):9–22.
72. Gentamicin [package insert]. Lake Forest, IL: Hospira, August 2005.
73. Kantrex [package insert]. Princeton, NJ: Bristol-Myers Squibb, December 2002.
74. Amikacin [package insert]. Irvine, CA: Sicor Pharmaceuticals, June 2005.
75. Tobramycin injection [package insert]. Lake Forest, IL: Hospira, July 2004.
76. Schatz A, Bugie E, Waksman SA. Streptomycin, a substance exhibiting antibiotic activity against Gram-positive and Gram-negative bacteria. Proc Soc Exp Biol Med 1944;55:66–69.
77. Neomycin sulfate tablets [package insert]. Amityville, NY: Hi-Tech Pharmacal Company, October 2009.
78. Stauton J, Wilkinson B. Biosynthesis of erythromycin and rapamycin. Chem Rev 1997;97:2611–2629.
79. Fiese EF, Steffen SH. Comparison of the acid stability of azithromycin and erythromycin A. J Antimicrob Chemother 1990;25(Suppl A):39–47.
80. Roberts MC, Sutcliffe J, Courvalin P, et al. Nomenclature for macrolide and macrolide-lincosamide-streptogramin B resistance determinants. Antimicrob Agents Chemother 1999;43:2823–2830.
81. Westphal JF. Macrolide-induced clinically relevant drug interactions with cytochrome P-450A (CYP) 3A4: an update focused on clarithromycin, axithromycin, and dirythromycin. Br J Clin Pharmacol 2000;50:285–295.
82. Yasuda K, Lan L, Sanglard D, et al. Interaction of cytochrome P450 3A inhibitors with P-glycoprotein. J Pharmacol Exp Ther 2002;303:323–332.
83. Ery-Ped [package insert]. North Chicago, IL: Abbott Laboratories, September 2006.
84. Biaxin Filmtab, Biaxin XL Filmtab, Biaxin Granules [package insert]. North Chicago, IL: Abbott Laboratories, August 2007.
85. Zithromax [package insert]. New York: Pfizer Labs, January 2009.
86. Ketek [package insert]. Bridgewater, NJ: Sanofi-Aventis, February 2007.
87. Lincocin [package insert]. New York: Pfizer, February 2006.
88. Cleocin [package insert]. New York: Pharmacia & Upjohn, June 2007.
89. Chopra I, Roberts M. Tetracycline antibiotics: mode of action, applications, molecular biology, and epidemiology of bacterial resistance. Microbial Mol Biol Rev 2001;65:232–260.
90. Tetracycline hydrochloride capsules [package insert]. Corona, CA: Watson Pharma, September 2010.
91. Broderson DE, Clemons WM Jr, Carter AP, et al. The structural basis for the action of the antibiotics tetracycline, pactamycin, and hygromycin B on the 30S ribosomal subunit. Cell 2000;103:1143–1154.
92. Pioletti M, Schlunzen F, Harms J, et al. Crystal structures of complexes of the small ribosomal subunit with tetracycline, edeine, and IF3. EMBO J 2001;20:1829–1839.
93. Anokhina MM, Barta A, Nierhaus KH, et al. Mapping of the second tetracycline binding site on the ribosomal small subunit of *E. coli*. Nucl Acids Res 2004;92:2594–2597.
94. Speer BS, Shoemaker NB, Salyers AA. Bacterial resistance to tetracycline: mechanisms, transfer, and clinical significance. Clin Microbiol Rev 1992;5:387–399.
95. Minocin [package insert]. Cranford, NJ: Triax Pharmaceuticals, February 2007.
96. Goldstein FW, Kitzis MD, Acar JF. *N,N*-Dimethylglycyl-amido derivative of minocycline and 6-demethyl-6-desoxytetracycline, two new glycylcyclines highly effective against tetracycline-resistant Gram-positive cocci. Antimicrob Agents Chemother 1994;38:2218–2220.
97. Sum PE, Peterson P. Synthesis and structure-activity relationship of novel glycylcycline derivative leading to the discovery of GAR-936. Bioorg Med Chem Lett 1999;9:1459–1462.
98. Shaw WV, Packman LC, Burleigh BD, et al. Primary structure of a chloramphenicol acetyltransferase specified by R plasmids. Nature 1979;282: 870–872.
99. Chloramphenicol sodium succinate [package insert], Bristol, TN: Monarch Pharmaceuticals, April 2007.

100. Barna JCJ, Williams DH. The structure and mode of action of glycopeptide antibiotics of the vancomycin group. Annu Rev Microbiol 1984;38:339–357.
101. Arthur M, Courvalin P. Genetics and mechanisms of glycopeptide resistance in enterococci. Antimicrob Agents Chemother 1993;37:1563–1571.
102. Vancomycin hydrochloride [package insert]. Deerfield, IL: Baxter Healthcare Corp., February 2009.
103. Higgins DL, Chang R, Debabov DV, et al. Telavancin, a multifunctional lipoglycopeptide, disrupts both cell wall synthesis and membrane integrity in methicillin-resistant *Staphylococcus aureus*. Antimicrob Agents Chemother 2005;49:1127–1134.
104. Vibativ [package insert]. Deerfield, IL: Astellas Pharma; August 2009.
105. Tally FP, DeBruin MF. Development of daptomycin for Gram positive infections. J Antimicrob Chemother 2000;46:523–526.
106. Cubicin [package insert]. Lexington, MA: Cubist Pharmaceuticals, November 2010.
107. Vasquez D. The streptogramin family of antibiotics. In: Gottlieb D, Shaw PD, eds. Antibiotics. New York: Springer-Verlag, 1967:387–403.
108. Synercid [package insert]. Bristol, TN: Monarch Pharmaceuticals, November 2007.
109. Zyvox [package insert]. New York: Pharmacia and Upjohn, December 2009.
110. Colca JR, McDonald WG, Waldon DJ, et al. Cross-linking in the living cell locates the site of action of oxazolidinone antibiotics. J Biol Chem 2003;278:21972–21979.
111. Lincopan N, de Almeida LM, Elmor de Araújo MR, et al. Linezolid resistance in Staphylococcus epidermidis associated with a G2603T mutation in the 23S rRNA gene. Int J Antimicrob Agents 2009;34:281–282.
112. Altabax [package insert]. Research Triangle Park, NC: GlaxoSmithKline, June 2010.
113. Yan K, Madden L, Choudhry AE, et al. Biochemical characterization of the interactions of the novel pleuromutilin derivative retapamulin with bacterial ribosomes. Antimicrob Agents Chemother. 2006;50:3875–3881.
114. Davidovich C, Bashan A, Auerbach-Nevo T, et al. Induced-fit tightens pleuromutilins binding to ribosomes and remote interactions enable their selectivity. Proc Nat Acad Sci U S A 2007;104:4291–4296.
115. Champney WS, Rodgers WK. Retapamulin inhibition of translation and 50S ribosomal subunit formation in *Staphylococcus aureus* cells. Antimicrob Agents Chemother 2007;51:3385–3387.

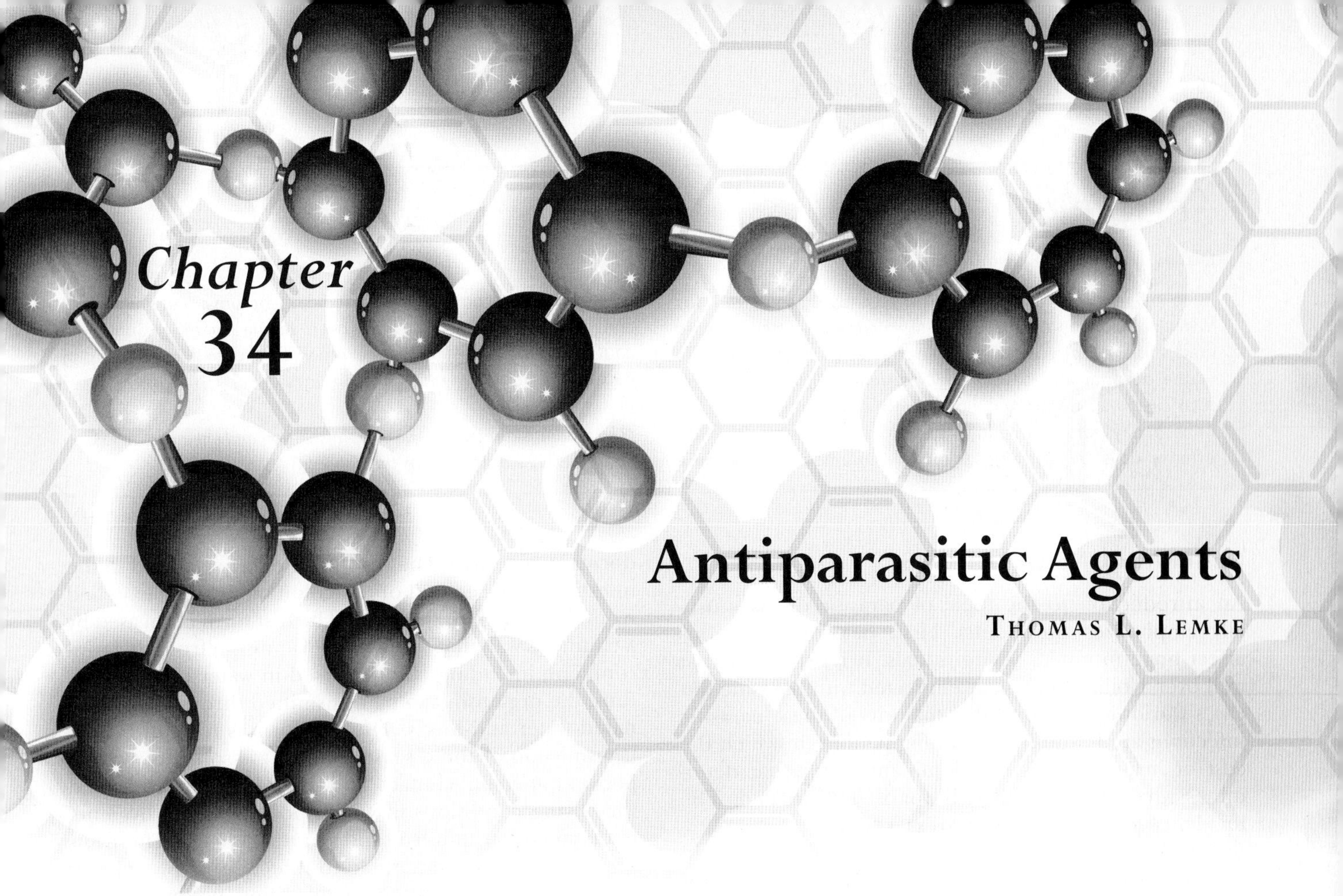

Chapter 34

Antiparasitic Agents

Thomas L. Lemke

Drugs Covered in This Chapter

Drug treatment of amebiasis, giardiasis, trichomoniasis

- Diloxanide furoate
- Metronidazole
- Nitazoxanide
- Tinidazole

Treatment of pneumocystis

- Atovaquone
- Pentamidine isethionate
- Sulfamethoxazole–trimethoprim
- Trimetrexate glucuronate

Treatment of trypanosomiasis

- *Benznidazole*
- Eflornithine
- Melarsoprol
- Nifurtimox
- Pentamidine isethionate
- Suramin sodium

Treatment of leishmaniasis

- *Sodium stibogluconate*
- Miltefosine

Antimalarials

- Artemisinins (arteether, artemether, artesunate, dihydroartemisinin)
- Atovaquone–proguanil
- Chloroquine
- Halofantrine
- Lumefantrine
- Mefloquine
- Pyrimethamine
- Quinine

Anthelmintics

- Albendazole
- Diethylcarbamazine
- Ivermectin
- Mebendazole
- Oxamniquine
- Praziquantel
- Pyrantel pamoate
- Thiabendazole

Scabicides and pediculocides

- Crotamiton
- Lindane
- Permethrin
- Pyrethrin
- Spinosad

Abbreviations

ACT, artemisinin-based combination therapy
ADH, alcohol dehydrogenase
ALDH, aldehyde dehydrogenase
CDC, Centers for Disease Control and Prevention
CDI, *Clostridium difficile* infection
CNS, central nervous system
DDT, dichlorodiphenyltrichloroethane
DEC, diethylcarbamazine
DFMO, difluoromethyl ornithine
DHFR, dihydrofolate reductase
FDA, U.S. Food and Drug Administration
GABA, γ-aminobutyric acid
GI, gastrointestinal
HM, 2-hydroxymethylmetronidazole
IV, intravenous
IVM, ivermectin
NTZ, nitazoxanide
ODC, ornithine decarboxylase
PCP, pneumocystis pneumonia
PABA, *p*-aminobenzoic acid
PZQ, praziquantel
RBC, red blood cell
ROS, reactive oxygen species
TIZ, tizoxanide
TMQ, trimetrexate
WHO, World Health Organization

SCENARIO

Elizabeth B. Hirsch, PharmD, BCPS

JB, a 67-year-old white man, was recently hospitalized for 5 weeks following complications after coronary artery bypass graft surgery. He received multiple courses of antibiotics while in the hospital and developed *Clostridium difficile* infection (CDI). He was discharged home with a prescription to continue 7 days of treatment with oral metronidazole for CDI. After 4 days of metronidazole, he presents to his primary care physician complaining of cold symptoms (cough and congestion) for which he had been taking over-the-counter cough medicine. Last night, he reported experiencing severe nausea and vomiting with some dizziness.

(The reader is directed to the clinical solution and chemical analysis of this case at the end of the chapter.)

GENERAL CONSIDERATIONS

An introduction to the topic of parasitic diseases usually emphasizes two points. First, parasitic infections affect huge numbers of individuals. It is estimated that well over 1 billion people are infected with parasitic diseases worldwide. Second, the majority of these parasitic infections are found in developing nations, in which the cost of health care is the dominant factor that determines whether the patient is (or is not) treated. The incidence of some parasitic diseases can exceed 80% of the population. The high cost of drug discovery and the low incidence of many of the parasitic infections in affluent Western countries have combined to reduce the incentive for both the study of the diseases and the development of effective therapy. This may be changing, however, because of global travel, improved communications, and growth of the developing countries, leading to an increased demand for more effective treatments.

The diseases associated with parasitic infections represent a large and diverse number of conditions, some common and some relatively unheard of by the general population. Included under the title of parasitic infections are the numerous types of protozoal infections: amebiasis, giardiasis, babesiosis, Chagas disease, leishmaniasis, malaria, sleeping sickness, toxoplasmosis, trichomoniasis, and pneumocystosis (also considered to be a fungal infection). Helminth infections (worms) are also considered to be parasitic infections and can be caused by any of three classes of helminths: nematodes, cestodes, and trematodes. Insect infections, such as scabies, lice (pediculosis), chiggers, and bedbugs (Cimicidae family), are also considered to be parasitic infections.

PROTOZOAL DISEASES

Amebiasis

Amebiasis is a disease of the large intestine caused by *Entamoeba histolytica.* The disease occurs mainly in the tropics, but it is also seen in temperate climates. Amebiasis can be carried without significant symptoms or can lead to severe, life-threatening dysentery. The organism exists in one of two forms, the motile trophozoite form or the dormant cyst form. The trophozoite form is found in the intestine or in the wall of the colon and can be expelled from the body with the feces. The cyst form is encased by a chitinous wall that protects the organism from the environment, including chlorine used in water purification; thus, the organism can be transmitted through contaminated water and foods. The cyst form is responsible for transmission of the disease. The cyst is spread by direct person-to-person contact and is commonly associated with living conditions in which poor personal hygiene, poor sanitation, poverty, and ignorance exist. The hosts can be rendered susceptible to infection by preexisting conditions, such as protein malnutrition, pregnancy, HIV infection, or high-carbohydrate intake. Under these conditions, the organism is capable of invading body tissue. The protozoal invasion is not well understood, but it does appear to involve the processes indicated in Table 34.1. Symptoms can range from intermittent diarrhea (foul-smelling loose/watery stools) to tenderness and enlargement of the liver (with the extraintestinal form) to acute amoebic dysentery. Many patients can experience no symptoms, and the organism remains in the bowels as a commensal organism.

Giardiasis

Giardiasis is a disease that shows considerable similarity to amebiasis. It is caused by *Giardia lamblia,* an organism that can be found in the duodenum and jejunum. The organism exists in a motile trophozoite form and an infectious cyst form. The cyst form can be deposited in water (lives up to 2 months), and the contaminated

TABLE 34.1 *Entamoeba histolytica* Invasion of Host

Intestinal form	a. Disintegration of cyst wall in small intestine b. Movement of trophozoites into the colon c. Adhesion of trophozoite to cells of the host, which involves a change in composition and production of mucus
Extraintestinal form	d. Penetration of intestinal lining and entrance into portal circulation e. Invasion of liver tissue

CLINICAL SIGNIFICANCE

Parasitic infections affect more than half the world's population and are responsible for significant health complications, particularly throughout the developing world. Efforts to control parasitic infections often use a broad approach that includes strategies for prevention, treatment, and control. Drug therapy for parasitic infections can be quite challenging to practitioners for multiple reasons. They are often more prevalent in specific high-risk groups, so practitioners may lack experience with these agents and may be unfamiliar with the toxicities and monitoring parameters associated with these drugs. Certain agents are available in only a limited number of countries, and opinions regarding safety and efficacy vary greatly among practitioners. Understanding the medicinal chemistry, pharmacokinetics, and pharmacodynamics of these agents is of utmost importance.

Despite efforts of vaccine development, drug therapy remains the most effective means to control parasitic infections. Limited introduction of new antiparasitic agents and drug shortages make the treatment of parasitic infestations challenging. Understanding which drugs work at different parts of the life cycle of the parasite must also be taken into consideration. Lastly, clinicians must stay up to date on the rapid evolution of drug resistance to ensure their patients receive the most efficacious treatment regimens.

Elizabeth B. Hirsch, PharmD, BCPS
Assistant Professor
Department of Pharmacy Practice
Northeastern University College of Pharmacy
Boston, Massachusetts

water can then be ingested by the human. The trophozoite, if expelled from the gastrointestinal (GI) tract, normally will not survive. *Giardia lamblia* is the single most common cause of waterborne diarrhea in the United States. Giardiasis is a common disease among campers who drink water from contaminated streams. It can also be spread between family members, children in day care centers, and dogs and their masters. The organism can attach to the mucosal wall via a ventral sucking disk, and similar to amebiasis, the patient can be asymptomatic or develop watery diarrhea, abdominal cramps, distention and flatulence, anorexia, nausea, and vomiting. Usually, the condition is self-limiting in 1 to 4 weeks.

Trichomoniasis

Trichomoniasis is a protozoal infection caused by *Trichomonas vaginalis,* which exists only in a trophozoite form. The organs most commonly involved in the infection include the vagina, urethra, and prostate; thus, the disease is considered to be a venereal infection. The condition is transmitted by sexual contact, and it is estimated that trichomoniasis affects 180 million individuals worldwide. Infections in the male can be asymptomatic, whereas in the female, the symptoms can consist of vaginitis, profuse and foul-smelling discharge, burning and soreness on urination, and vulvar itching. Diagnosis is based on microscopic identification of the organism in fluids from the vagina, prostate, or urethra.

ORGANISMS THAT COMMONLY CAUSE VAGINITIS

Vaginitis may also be caused by *Haemophilus vaginalis* (bacteria) or *Candida albicans* (fungus), which are treated differently from the protozoal infection.

Pneumocystis

The disease pneumocystis, commonly referred to as pneumocystis pneumonia (PCP), incorrectly derived its name from what was thought to be the causative organism, *Pneumocystis carinii* and the disease state of pneumonia. The organism *P. carinii* was originally isolated and reported to grow in both humans and rats. The organism itself was difficult to characterize since it had morphologic characteristics of a protozoan (i.e., lack of ergosterol in its cell membrane), but its rRNA and mitochondrial DNA pattern resembles that of fungi. It was only later recognized that the organism infecting humans and responsible for the disease PCP was actually *Pneumocystis jirovecii,* a yeast-like fungus that can only be cultured in humans. Acute pneumocystis rarely strikes healthy individuals, although the organism is harbored in most humans without any apparent adverse effect. *P. jirovecii* becomes active only in individuals who have a serious impairment of their immune systems. Thus, the organism is considered to be an opportunistic pathogen. More recently, this disease has appeared in patients with HIV/AIDS, 80% of whom ultimately contract *P. jirovecii* pneumonia, as one of the main causes of death. The disease also occurs in those receiving immunosuppressive drugs to prevent rejection following organ transplantation or for the treatment of malignant disease. Additionally, pneumocystis is seen in malnourished infants whose immunologic systems are impaired. The disease is thought to be transmitted via an airborne route. PCP is characterized by a severe pneumonia caused by rapid multiplication of the organisms, almost exclusively in lung tissue, with the organism lining the walls of the alveoli and gradually filling the alveolar spaces. Untreated, the acute form of the disease is generally fatal. Even patients who recover from pneumocystosis are at risk of recurrent episodes. Patients with AIDS experience a recurrence rate of approximately 50%.

Extrapulmonary pneumocystosis—that is, pneumocystosis outside of the lungs—is also known to exist and can be more common than presently recognized. This infection can be complicated by the presence of coinfectious organisms. Fortunately, drug therapy used for treatment of the pulmonary infection is beneficial for the extrapulmonary condition, although intravenous (IV) administration of the drugs can be necessary.

The common therapy for PCP uses antibacterial and antiprotozoal drugs.

Tritryps

Three protozoan pathogens that belong to the family Trypanosomatidae, the order Kinetoplastida, and the genus *Trypanosoma* are *Leishmania major*, which is responsible for leishmaniasis; *Trypanosoma brucei*, which is responsible for African trypanosomiasis (African sleeping sickness); and *Trypanosoma cruzi*, which is responsible for Chagas disease. Referred to as the "tritryps," these eukaryotic organisms share characteristic subcellular structures of a kinetoplast and glycosomes, are unicellular motile protozoa, are transmitted by various insect vectors, and infect mammalian hosts. The genomes of tritryps have recently been reported (1–3). Together, they infect hundreds of millions of people annually.

Trypanosomiasis (4)

There are two distinct forms of trypanosomiasis: Chagas disease and African sleeping sickness.

Chagas Disease Chagas disease, also known as American trypanosomiasis, is caused by the parasitic protozoa *T. cruzi* and is found only in the Americas, primarily in Brazil but also in the southern United States. The protozoa lives in mammals and is spread by the bloodsucking insect known as the reduviid bug, assassin bug, or kissing bug. The insect becomes infected by drawing blood from an infected mammal and releasing the protozoa with discharged feces. The pathogen then enters the new host through breaks in the skin. Inflammatory lesions are seen at the site of entry. The disease can also be spread through transfusion with contaminated blood. Signs of initial infection can include malaise, fever, anorexia, and skin edema at the site where the protozoa entered the host. The disease ultimately can invade the heart, where after decades of infection with chronic Chagas disease, the patient can experience an infection-associated heart attack. It is estimated that 5% of the Salvadorian and Nicaraguan immigrants to the United States can have chronic Chagas disease.

African Trypanosomiasis African trypanosomiasis, or sleeping sickness, is caused by several subspecies of *T. brucei* (*T. brucei rhodesiense* [east African sleeping sickness] and *T. brucei gambiense* [west African sleeping sickness]). In this case, the infected animal is bitten by the bloodsucking tsetse fly, which in turn transmits the protozoa via inoculation during a subsequent bite of a human. The protozoa, initially present in the gut of the vector, appear in the salivary gland for inoculation during the subsequent biting of a human. It is estimated that some 50 million people are at risk of African sleeping sickness, with 300,000 to 500,000 cases occurring in sub-Saharan Africa each year. The infection progresses through two stages. Stage I can present as fever and high temperatures lasting several days; hematologic and immunologic changes occur during this stage. Stage II occurs after the organism enters the central nervous system (CNS) and can involve symptoms suggesting the disease name—daytime somnolence, loss of spontaneity, halting speech, listless gaze, and extrapyramidal signs (e.g., tremors and choreiform movements). A breakdown of neurologic function leading to coma and death can occur. Death can occur within weeks if untreated (*T. brucei rhodesiense*) or only after several years (*T. brucei gambiense*).

It should be noted that the sole source of energy for the trypanosomal organism is glycolysis, which in turn can account for the hypoglycemia seen in the host. In addition, the migration of the organism into the CNS can be associated with the organism's search for a rich source of available glucose.

Leishmaniasis

Leishmaniasis is a disease caused by a number of protozoa in the genus *Leishmania*. The protozoa can be harbored in diseased rodents, canines, and various other mammals and transmitted from the infected mammal to man by bites from female sandflies of the genus *Phlebotomus* and then appear in one of four major clinical syndromes: visceral leishmaniasis, cutaneous leishmaniasis, mucocutaneous leishmaniasis, or diffuse cutaneous leishmaniasis. The sandfly, the vector involved in spreading the disease, breeds in warm, humid climates; thus, the disease is more common in the tropics. As many as 12 million individuals worldwide are infected by this organism.

The visceral leishmaniasis, also known as kala azar (black fever), is caused by *Leishmania donovani*. This form of the disease is systemic and is characterized in patients by fever, typically nocturnal, diarrhea, cough, and enlarged liver and spleen. The skin of the patient can become darkened. Without treatment, death can occur in 20 months and is commonly associated with diarrhea, superinfections, or GI hemorrhage. Visceral leishmaniasis is most commonly found in India and Sudan.

Both cutaneous and monocutaneous leishmaniasis are characterized by single or multiple localized lesions. These slow-healing and, possibly, painful ulcers can lead to secondary bacterial infections. The Old World cutaneous leishmaniasis is caused by *Leishmania topica*, which is found most commonly in children and young adults in regions bordering the Mediterranean, the Middle East, Southern Russia, and India. *Leishmania major* is endemic to desert areas in Africa, the Middle East, and Russia, whereas *Leishmania aethiopica* is found in the Kenyan highlands and Ethiopia. The New World disease caused by *Leishmania peruviana*, *Leishmania braziliensis*, and *Leishmania panamensis* is found in South and Central America, whereas *Leishmania mexicana* can be endemic to south-central Texas. The incubation period for cutaneous leishmaniasis ranges from a few weeks to several months. The slow-healing lesions can be seen on the skin in various regions of the body depending on the specific strain of organism. Usually, these conditions exhibit spontaneous healing, but this can also occur over an extended period of time (1 to 2 years).

Malaria

Malaria is transmitted by the infected female *Anopheles* mosquito. The specific protozoan organisms causing malaria are from the genus *Plasmodium*. Only 4 of approximately 100 species cause malaria in humans. The remaining species affect birds, monkeys, livestock, rodents, and reptiles. The four species that affect humans are *Plasmodium falciparum*, *Plasmodium vivax*, *Plasmodium malariae*, and *Plasmodium ovale*. Concurrent infections by more than one of these species are seen in endemically affected regions of the world. Such multiple infections further complicate patient management and the choice of treatment regimens.

It is estimated that 2 billion individuals are at risk of developing malaria and that the disease affects as many as 500 million humans globally and causes more than 2 million deaths annually. It is estimated that a third of these fatalities occur in children younger than 5 years. Although this disease is found primarily in the tropics and subtropics, it has been observed far beyond these boundaries. Malaria was virtually eradicated from the United States between 1947 and 1951 through the use of the insecticide DDT (dichlorodiphenyltrichloroethane), which destroyed the insect vector, and in 1955, the World Health Organization (WHO) lunched a program titled the Global Malaria Eradication Program. The program intended to eradicate the disease worldwide through the use of DDT and disease treatment with chloroquine, but due to the development of DDT-resistant *Anopheles* mosquitoes, drug-resistant plasmodium, and political resistance, WHO abandoned its program in 1972. Recently, there has been an increase in global interest in fighting the disease through the use of preventative measures and development of multidrug treatments, although at present, nearly nothing new has reached the market.

While malaria has essentially been eradicated in most temperate-zone countries, more than 1,000 cases of malaria were documented recently in U.S. citizens returning from travel abroad. Today, malaria is found in most countries of Africa, Central and South America, and Southeast Asia. It is reported to be on the increase in Afghanistan, Bangladesh, Brazil, Burma, Cambodia, Colombia, China, Iran, India, Indonesia, Mexico, the Philippines, Thailand, and Vietnam. Infection from plasmodia can cause anemia, pulmonary edema, renal failure, jaundice, shock, cerebral malaria, and if not treated in a timely manner, even death.

Types of Malaria

Malarial infections are known according to the species of the parasite involved.

Plasmodium Falciparum Infection with *Plasmodium falciparum* has an incubation period (time from mosquito bite to clinical symptoms) of 1 to 3 weeks (average, 12 days). The *P. falciparum* life cycle in humans begins with the bite of an infected female mosquito. The parasites in the sporozoite stage enter the circulatory system, through which they can reach the liver in approximately 1 hour. These organisms grow and multiply 30,000- to 40,000-fold by asexual division within liver cells in 5 to 7 days. Then, as merozoites, they leave the liver to reenter the blood stream and invade the erythrocytes, or red blood cells (RBCs), where they continue to grow and multiply further for 1 to 3 days. Specific receptors on the surface of the erythrocytes serve as binding sites for the merozoite. These infected RBCs rupture, releasing merozoites in intervals of approximately 48 hours. Chemicals released by the ruptured cell in turn cause activation and release of additional substances associated with the patient's symptoms. The clinical symptoms include chills, fever, sweating, headaches, fatigue, anorexia, nausea, vomiting, and diarrhea. Some of the released merozoites are sequestered in vital organs (brain and heart), where they continue to grow. Recurrence of the clinical symptoms on alternate days leads to the terminology of tertian malaria. The *P. falciparum* parasite can also cause RBCs to clump and adhere to the wall of blood vessels. Such a phenomenon has been known to cause partial obstruction and, sometimes, restriction of the blood flow to vital organs like the brain, liver, and kidneys. Reinfection of RBCs can occur, allowing further multiplication and remanifestation of the malaria symptoms. Some merozoites develop into male and female sexual forms, called gametocytes, which can then be acquired by the female mosquito after biting the infected human. Gametocytes mature in the mosquito's stomach to form zygotes. Growth of the zygotes leads to the formation of oocysts (spherical structures located on the outside wall of the stomach). Sporozoites develop from the oocysts, are released into the body cavity of the mosquito, and migrate to the salivary gland of the insect, from which they can be transmitted to another human following a mosquito bite. The life cycle of the malaria parasites is shown in the Figure 34.1. The genome of the *P. falciparum*, as well as that of the *Anopheles* mosquito, is now known and is expected to provide potential new avenues

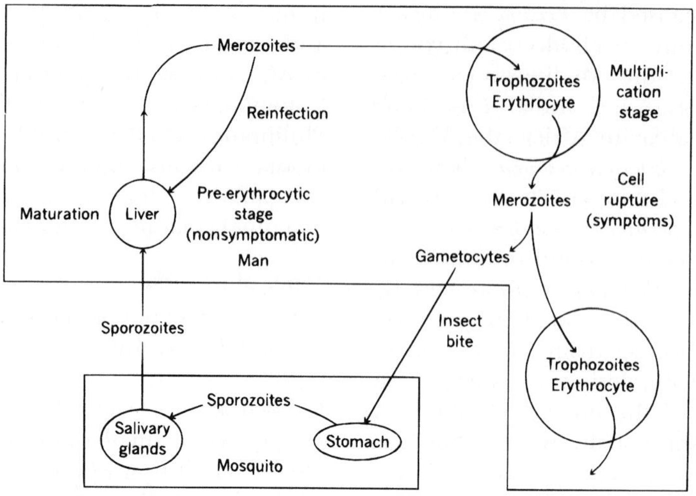

FIGURE 34.1 Life cycle of malarial protozoa.

for drug development. Genome information is also expected to give insight regarding the mechanisms of resistance and improve drug treatment.

Plasmodium Vivax *Plasmodium vivax* (benign tertian) is the most prevalent form of malaria. It has an incubation period of 1 to 4 weeks (average, 2 weeks). This form of malaria can cause spleen rupture and anemia. Relapses (renewed manifestations of erythrocytic infection) can occur. This results from the periodic release of dormant parasites (hypnozoites) from the liver cells. The erythrocytic forms are usually considered to be susceptible to treatment.

Plasmodium Malariae *Plasmodium malariae* is responsible for quartan malaria. It has an incubation period of 2 to 4 weeks (average, 3 weeks). The asexual cycle occurs every 72 hours. In addition to the usual symptoms, this form also causes nephritis. This is the mildest form of malaria and does not relapse. The RBC infection associated with *P. malariae* can last for many years. The *P. malariae* is quite unlikely to become resistant.

Plasmodium Ovale Infection with *Plasmodium ovale* has an incubation period of 9 to 18 days (average, 14 days). Relapses have been known to occur in individuals infected with this plasmodium. The relapse can be indicative of ovale tertian malaria and is associated with the ability of the organism to lie dormant (hypnozoites) in hepatic tissue for extended periods of time.

Types of Chemotherapy

Drug Classification Generally, the antimalarial drugs are classified by the life cycle stage (see Fig. 34.1) that the drugs are effective against. Listed in the following sections are the theoretical approaches of how drugs might be able to intervene in destroying the organism. Presently, the majority of drugs act on the intracellular erythrocytic form of the disease.

Tissue Schizonticides These drugs eradicate the exoerythrocytic liver-tissue stages of the parasite, which prevents the parasite's entry into the blood. Drugs of this type are useful for prophylaxis. Some tissue schizonticides can act on the long-lived tissue form (hypnozoites of *P. vivax* and *P. ovale*) and, thus, can prevent relapses.

Blood Schizonticides These drugs destroy the erythrocytic stages of parasites and can cure cases of falciparum malaria or suppress relapses. This is the easiest phase to treat, because drug delivery into the bloodstream can be accomplished rapidly.

Gametocytocides Agents of this type kill the sexual forms of the plasmodia (gametocytes), which are transmittable to the *Anopheles* mosquito, thereby preventing transmission of the disease.

Sporontocides (Sporozooiticides) These drugs act against sporozoites and are capable of killing these organisms as soon as they enter the bloodstream following a mosquito bite.

It should be noted that antimalarials can operate against more than one form of the organism and can be effective against one species of plasmodium but lack efficacy against others. In addition, antimalarial drugs can be classified according to their structural types.

Despite the history of malaria, the epidemiology and clinical features of the disease are not that well documented. In many parts of Africa, the diagnosis of the disease is not routinely done, and therefore, the success of prevention and treatment cannot be known. For more details on these difficulties, the reader is directed to the *Suggested Readings*, especially the article by Greenwood et al.

GENERAL APPROACHES TO PROTOZOAL THERAPY

Amebiasis and Giardiasis

The most appropriate approach for treatment of this type of protozoal infection is through prevention. Because the infection usually occurs by consumption of contaminated drinking water and food, avoidance is the key to prevention. Drinking bottled water, or boiling or disinfecting the water, will reduce the risk. Improvement in personal hygiene and general sanitation are also beneficial.

Trypanosomiasis, Leishmaniasis, and Malaria

For these diseases that are spread by insect vectors, the use of insecticides, protective clothing, and insect repellents can greatly reduce the incidence of the disease. Unfortunately, many of these protozoal infections can also infect other hosts beside humans; thus, even the most successful insect irradiation methods cannot destroy all the reservoirs of the protozoa. The use of insect repellents and protective clothing can be useful for visitors to regions with endemic infections, but these procedures can prove to be ineffective for those living in the area. For such individuals, early detection and drug therapy are the methods of treatment.

DRUG THERAPY FOR PROTOZOAL INFECTIONS

Treatment of Amebiasis, Giardiasis, and Trichomoniasis

Metronidazole (Flagyl, Metryl, Satric)

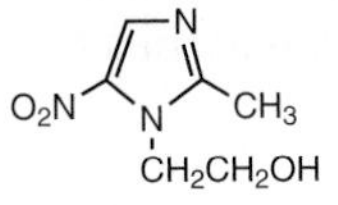

Metronidazole

Metronidazole was initially introduced for the treatment of vaginal infections caused by *Trichomonas vaginalis* but has since been shown to be effective for treatment of amebiasis, giardiasis, and anaerobic bacterial infections, including *Clostridium difficile*.

MECHANISM OF ACTION Despite the availability of metronidazole since the late 1950s, the mechanism of action of the drug is still unknown. It is generally agreed that metronidazole is a prodrug and that anaerobic organisms reduce the nitro group in metronidazole to a hydroxylamine, as shown in Figure 34.2, during which a reactive derivative or reactive species is produced that causes destructive effects on cell components (i.e., DNA, proteins, and membranes). Specifically, DoCampo (5) has

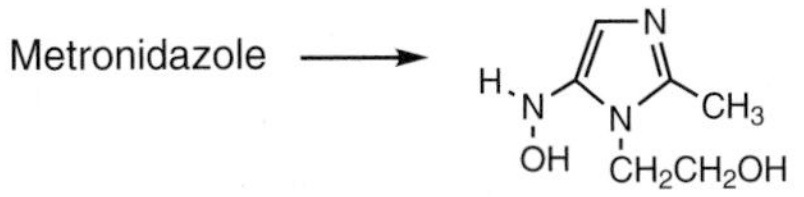

FIGURE 34.2 Metabolic activation of metronidazole.

reported that nitroaryl compounds (nitroimidazoles, metronidazole, nitrofurans, nifurtimox) are reduced to nitro radical anions, which in turn react with oxygen to regenerate the nitroaryl and the superoxide radical anion (Fig. 34.3). Further reduction of superoxide radical anion leads to hydrogen peroxide, and homolytic cleavage of the latter leads to hydroxyl radical formation. Superoxide radical anion, hydrogen peroxide, and hydroxyl radicals are referred to as reactive oxygen species (ROS) and are the reactive substances that are implicated in damage to critical cellular components of the parasite.

METABOLISM Liver metabolism of metronidazole leads to two major metabolites: hydroxylation of the 2-methyl group to 2-hydroxymethylmetronidazole (HM) and its oxidation to metronidazole acetic acid (6). Both compounds possess biologic activity. Additionally, HM is found in the urine as glucuronide and sulfate conjugates. In addition, a small amount of metronidazole is oxidized to acetamide, a known carcinogen in rats but not in humans, and to the oxalate derivative shown in Figure 34.4 (7).

PHARMACOKINETICS (6) Metronidazole is available in a variety of dosage forms, including IV, oral, rectal, and vaginal suppositories. The bioavailability of metronidazole is nearly 100% when administered orally but is significantly less when administered via the rectal route (67% to 82%) or the vaginal route (19% to 56%). The drug is not bound to plasma protein. Distribution of the drug is fairly uniform throughout the body, including mother's milk.

THERAPEUTIC APPLICATION Metronidazole is considered to be the drug of choice for treatment for the protozoal infections amebiasis (intestinal and extraintestinal), giardiasis, and trichomoniasis (8). It is the drug of choice for treatment of the gram-positive bacilli *Clostridium difficile* and, in combination, is an alternative therapy for *Helicobacter pylori* infections (9,10). The common side effects exhibited with metronidazole include abdominal distress, a metallic taste,

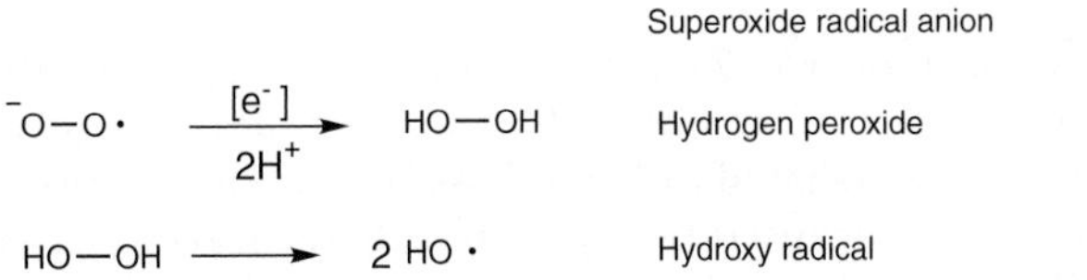

FIGURE 34.3 Formation of ROS from nitroaryl compounds.

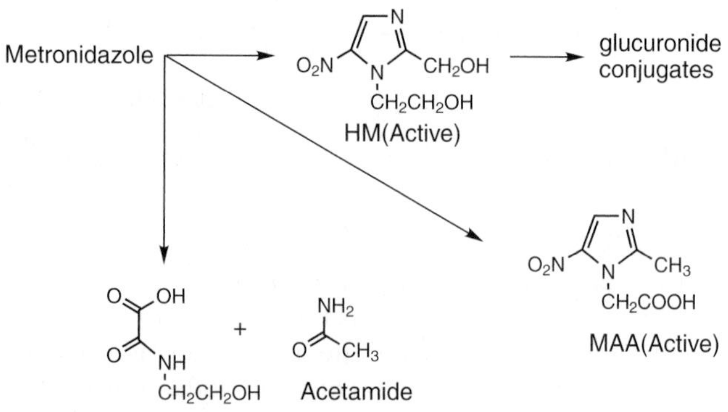

FIGURE 34.4 Metabolism of metronidazole.

and a disulfiram-like effect if taken with alcohol. The drug is reported to be carcinogenic in mice, possibly related to the metabolite acetamide, and as a result should not be used during the first trimester of pregnancy.

Tinidazole (Tindamax)

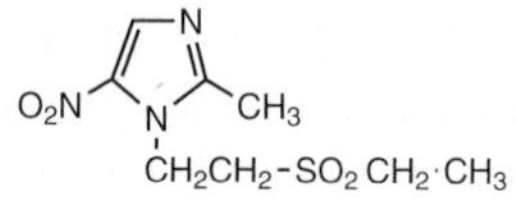

Tinidazole

Tinidazole has been approved by the U.S. Food and Drug Administration (FDA) for the treatment of amebiasis, giardiasis, and trichomoniasis. It appears also to be highly effective against *Helicobacter pylori* infections, although it is not approved for this use. The drug is rapidly and completely absorbed following oral administration and can be administered with food to reduce GI disturbance. Tinidazole has a mechanism of action that parallels that of metronidazole as well as a similar metabolic pathway leading to hydroxylation at the 2-methyl group catalyzed by CYP3A4. Basically, tinidazole appears to mimic the actions of metronidazole, although there are reports that it is effective against some protozoa that are resistant to metronidazole.

Nitazoxanide (Alinia)

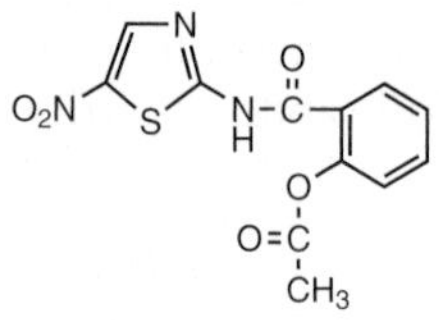

Nitazoxanide

Nitazoxanide (NTZ) has been approved as an orphan drug for the treatment of diarrhea in children (age 1 to 11 years) associated with giardiasis, but it is also approved for diarrhea caused by cryptosporidiosis in patients with AIDS. Cryptosporidiosis is a protozoal infection caused by *Cryptosporidium parvum*. The condition is uncommon in healthy individuals but can be life-threatening in immunosuppressed patients and those with HIV infections.

Mechanism of Action (10) NTZ is a prodrug that is metabolically converted into the deacetylated drug tizoxanide (TIZ) (Fig. 34.5). TIZ then undergoes a four-electron reduction of the 5-nitro group giving various short-lived intermediates, which can include the hydroxylamine derivative. These reduced products represent the active forms of NTZ. Whereas these intermediates would suggest that NTZ has the same mechanism of action as metronidazole, this does not appear to be the case. NTZ is thought to inhibit the enzyme pyruvate:ferredoxin oxidoreductase in *Trichomonas vaginalis*, *Entamoeba histolytica*, and *Clostridium perfringens*. The result of this inhibition is disruption of the bioenergetics of these organisms. Unlike metronidazole and tinidazole, which fragment DNA and are suspected mutagenic agents, NTZ and TIZ do not cause DNA fragmentation and are not considered to be mutagenic. This might be associated with the higher redox potential found for NTZ, a nitrothiazole, in comparison with very low redox potential found for the nitroimidazoles, such as metronidazole and tinidazole. Additional metabolites of TIZ include the glucuronide, which shows some biologic activity, and small amounts of an aromatic hydroxylation product (Fig. 34.5).

Pharmacokinetics NTZ is available as powder that is reconstituted and dispensed as an oral suspension. The drug is well absorbed from the GI tract and rapidly metabolized, with elimination products appearing in the urine and feces. The only identified products in the plasma are TIZ and its glucuronide (11). The product can be taken with food.

Therapeutic Application Although NTZ has only been approved for treatment of diarrhea in children caused by *Giardia lamblia* and diarrhea caused by *Cryptosporidium*

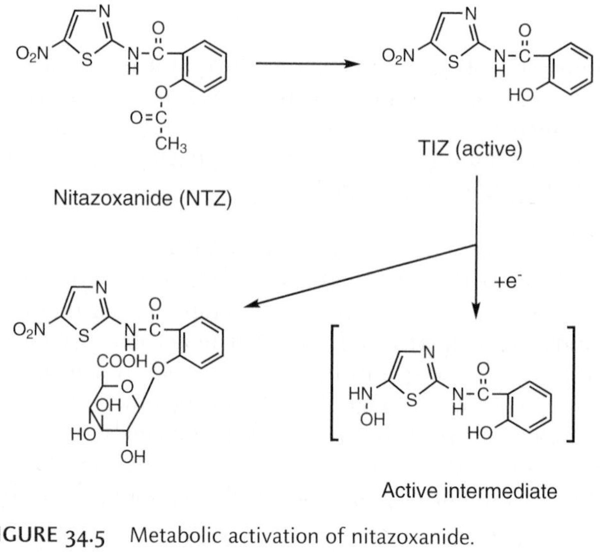

FIGURE 34.5 Metabolic activation of nitazoxanide.

parvum, the drug might soon be approved for adults suffering from diarrhea caused by *Giardia lamblia.* In addition, the drug has been shown to be effective against the protozoa *Entamoeba histolytica* and *Trichomonas vaginalis,* the bacteria *Helicobacter pylori* and *Clostridium perfringens,* and various helminths, including *Ascaris lumbricoides, Enterobius vermicularis, Ancylostoma doudenale,* and *Strongyloides stercoralis* (12).

Diloxanide Furoate

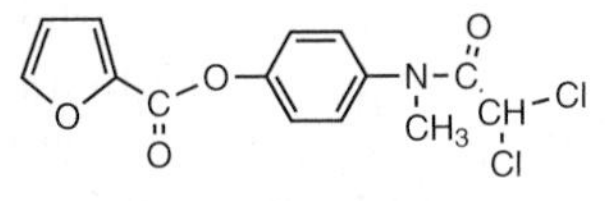

Diloxanide furoate

Diloxanide furoate (available from the Centers for Disease Control and Prevention [CDC]) is prescribed for the treatment of asymptomatic amebiasis but is ineffective as a single agent for the extraintestinal form of the disease. The drug is administered orally and is hydrolyzed in the gut to give diloxanide, which is considered to be the active drug. Diloxanide is the only form identified in the bloodstream. The drug is found in the urine as the glucuronide (Fig. 34.6).

Treatment of Pneumocystis (13,14)

Sulfamethoxazole–Trimethoprim; Cotrimoxazole (Bactrim, Septra, Cotrim)

The combination of sulfamethoxazole and trimethoprim has proven to be the most successful method for treatment and prophylaxis of pneumocystis in patients with AIDS. This combination was first reported as being effective against PCP in 1975, and by 1980, it had become the preferred method of treatment, with a response rate of 65% to 94%. The combination is effective against both pneumocystic pneumonia and the extrapulmonary disease. *P. jirovecii* appears to be especially susceptible to the sequential blocking action of cotrimoxazole, which inhibits both the incorporation of *p*-aminobenzoic acid (PABA) into folic acid as well as the reduction of dihydrofolic acid to tetrahydrofolic acid by dihydrofolate reductase (DHFR). (A detailed discussion of the mechanism of action and the structure–activity relationship of these drugs can be found in Chapter 33.) Depending on the severity of the infection, the combination is administered in doses of 20 mg/kg/d of trimethoprim and 100 mg/kg/d of sulfamethoxazole in four divided doses over a period of 14 to 21 days. The incidence of side effects of this combination is high and reflects generally the effects of the sulfa drug component. Side effects can be significant enough to terminate treatment.

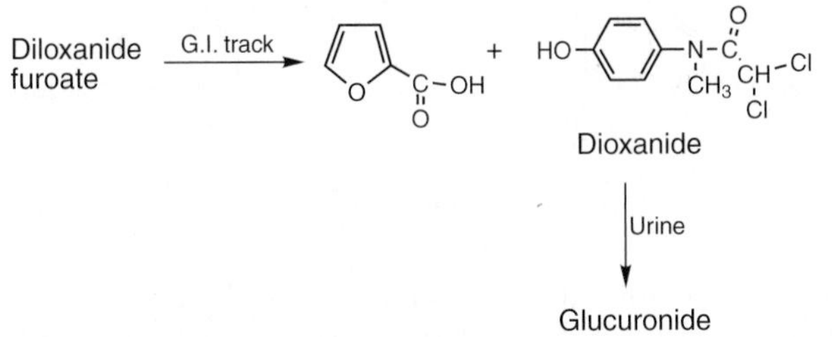

FIGURE 34.6 Metabolism of diloxanide furoate.

Pentamidine Isethionate (Pentam 300, Nebupent)

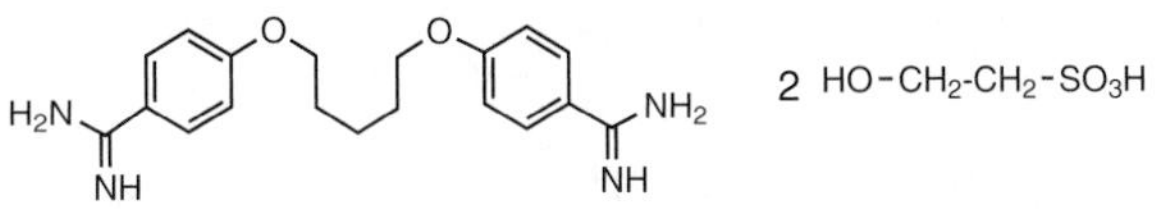

Pentamidine isethionate

Pentamidine is available as the water-soluble isethionate salt, which is used both IV and as an aerosol. The drug can be used via the intramuscular route, but significant complications have been reported, and therefore, this route of administration is not recommended. The drug has fungicidal and antiprotozoal activity but is used primarily for treatment of PCP.

Mechanism of Action The mechanism of action of pentamidine is not known with certainty, but strong evidence supports various mechanisms of action for pentamidine. Pentamidine selectively binds to the DNA in the *Trypanosoma* parasite (see below). Pentamidine has also been shown to inhibit topoisomerase in *P. jirovecii,* which leads to double-strand cleavage of DNA in *Trypanosoma* (12–14). It has been suggested that pentamidine's mechanism of action might be different in different organisms and, therefore, that the actions reported for *Trypanosoma* might not carry over to pneumocystis.

Pharmacokinetics Pentamidine must be administered IV and, after multiple injections daily or on alternate days, accumulates in body tissue. Plasma concentrations were measured up to 8 months following a single, 2-hour IV infusion. The accumulation aids in treatment as well as in prophylaxis. The drug shows poor penetration of the CNS.

Therapeutic Application Pentamidine is used as a second-line agent either by itself or in combination for the treatment and prophylaxis of PCP. For prophylaxis, the aerosol form of the drug is indicated and has minimum

ORPHAN DRUG PRODUCT

Dapsone plus trimethoprim also has been used for the treatment of pneumocystis, with effectiveness nearly equal to that of cotrimoxazole.

toxicity. The limitation of pentamidine—that is, the need for IV administration—can be associated with the potential for severe toxicity, which includes breathlessness, tachycardia, dizziness, headache, and vomiting. These symptoms can occur in as many as 50% of the patients. These effects are thought to be associated with a too rapid IV administration, resulting in the release of histamine.

Atovaquone (Mepron)

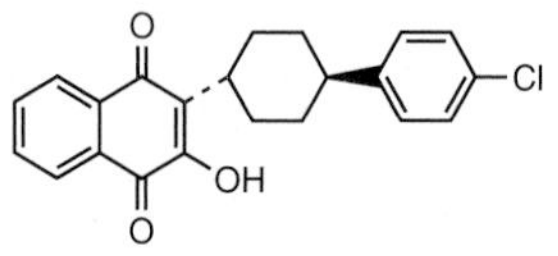

Atovaquone

Atovaquone, a chemical with structural similarity to the ubiquinone metabolites, was initially synthesized and investigated as an antimalarial, a use for which it has recently gained acceptance when used in combination therapy with other antimalarial agents. Today, its usefulness is primarily directed toward the treatment of PCP.

Mechanism of Action Atovaquone is thought to produce its antiparasitic action by virtue of its ability to inhibit the mitochondrial respiratory chain. More specifically, atovaquone is a ubiquinone reductase inhibitor, inhibiting at the cytochrome bc_1 complex (15). This action leads to a collapse of the mitochondrial membrane potential. The compound shows stereospecific inhibition, with the *trans* isomer being more active than the *cis* isomer.

Pharmacokinetics Atovaquone is poorly absorbed from the GI tract because of its poor water solubility and high fat solubility, but the absorption can be significantly increased if taken with a fat-rich meal. The drug is highly bound to plasma protein (94%) and does not enter the CNS in significant quantities. It is not significantly metabolized in humans and is exclusively eliminated in feces via the bile.

Therapeutic Applications With as many as 70% of patients with AIDS developing pneumocystis and, of these, nearly 60% of the patients on cotrimoxazole developing serious side effects to this combination, atovaquone is an important alternative drug (16). Atovaquone also has been reported to be effective for the treatment of toxoplasmosis caused by *Toxoplasma gondii,* although it has not been approved for this use.

Trimetrexate Glucuronate (Neutrexin)

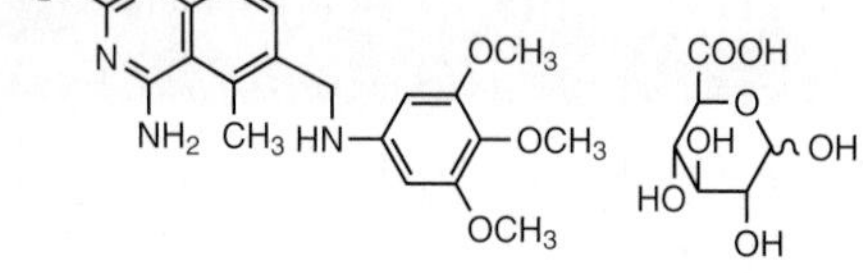

Trimetrexate glucuronate

Trimetrexate (TMQ) has been approved for the treatment of *P. jirovecii* in patients with AIDS and also exhibits antiprotozoal activity against *T. cruzi.* The drug is available as a single-ingredient medication, but it can be administered along with folinic acid in much the same way that methotrexate is administered with calcium leucovorin in cancer chemotherapy. TMQ is a derivative of methotrexate.

Mechanism of Action TMQ is considered to be a nonclassical folate antagonist, whereas methotrexate, the structurally similar analog of TMQ, is a classical folate antagonist. The difference between these two drugs is that methotrexate, with its polar glutamate side chain, is transported into the cell via a carrier-mediated transport system, whereas TMQ, without the glutamate moiety, is absorbed by the cell via a passive diffusion. Once in the cell, TMQ inhibits DHFR. TMQ binds to *P. jirovecii* DHFR 1,500 times more strongly than trimethoprim and somewhat more strongly than methotrexate. It has also been reported that TMQ readily enters the *P. jirovecii* cell because of the lipophilic nature of this drug (17). Methotrexate and leucovorin are not able to enter the cell, however, because the cell membrane of *P. jirovecii* does not possess the transporter protein (17).

Therapeutic Application TMQ, when combined with the cytoprotective agent leucovorin (folinic acid), is more effective and better tolerated than pentamidine in the treatment of PCP (18). Because the first- and second-line agents are successful in only 50% to 75% of these cases and because adverse reactions severely limit the use of some of the older agents, TMQ can offer some advantages in treatment. TMQ is administered by IV infusion over 60 to 90 minutes and should be combined with the cytoprotective drug leucovorin. The leucovorin protects against bone marrow suppression and against renal and hepatic dysfunction. Leucovorin administration should continue for 72 hours after the last dose of TMQ. Additionally, TMQ has been reported to be effective in the treatment of Chagas disease.

Treatment of Trypanosomiasis (19)

Suramin Sodium (Available from the CDC)

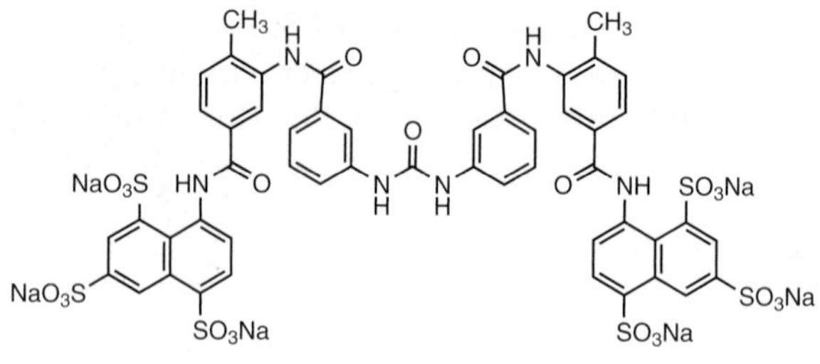

Suramin Sodium

Introduced into therapy for the treatment of early trypanosomiasis in the 1920s, suramin, a bis-hexasulfonatednaphthylurea, is still considered to be the drug of choice for treatment of non–CNS-associated African trypanosomiasis.

Mechanism of Action The mechanism of action of suramin is unproven, but the drug is known to have a high affinity for binding to a number of critical enzymes in the pathogen. Among the enzymes to which suramin has been shown to bind are several dehydrogenases and kinases. As a result of binding, suramin has been shown to be an inhibitor of DHFR, a crucial enzyme in folate metabolism, and thymidine kinase. In addition, suramin is an inhibitor of glycolytic enzymes in *Trypanosoma brucei,* with binding constants much lower than those seen in mammalian cells. Inhibition of glycolysis would be expected to block energy sources of the pathogen, leading to lysis. Whether one or more of these inhibitor actions represent the toxic action of suramin on the pathogen remains unproven.

Pharmacokinetics Suramin sodium is a water-soluble compound that is poorly absorbed via oral administration and must be administered IV in multiple injections. Because of its highly ionic nature, suramin will not cross the blood–brain barrier and, therefore, is ineffective for the treatment of trypanosomal infections that reach the CNS. In addition, suramin is tightly bound to serum albumin. Despite this binding, the drug is preferentially absorbed by trypanosomes through a receptor-mediated endocytosis of serum protein. Because the drug remains in the bloodstream for an extended period of time, suramin has value as a prophylactic drug.

Therapeutic Application Suramin sodium is effective against east African trypanosomiasis, but it has limited value against west African trypanosomiasis. As indicated, because the drug will not enter the CNS, the drug is only useful for the treatment of early stages of the disease. The drug exhibits a wide variety of side effects, which can be severe in debilitated individuals, and include nausea, vomiting, and fatigue.

Pentamidine, Isethionate (Pentam 300, Nebupent)

First introduced as a therapy for trypanosomiasis in 1937, pentamidine is now used in a variety of protozoal and fungal infections and finds use in the treatment of trypanosomiasis, leishmaniasis, and pneumocystis (PCP). The drug is primarily used for treatment of PCP. When used for trypanosomiasis, pentamidine is only effective against *Trypanosoma brucei rhodesiense* (east African sleeping sickness) and, even then, only during the early stage of the disease, because the drug does not readily cross the blood–brain barrier.

Mechanism of Action As indicated earlier, several biochemical actions have been reported for pentamidine. The drug has been shown to bind to DNA through hydrogen-bonding of the amidine proton with the adenine-thymine–rich regions of DNA. More specifically, pentamidine binds to the N-3 of adenine, spans four to five base pairs, and binds to a second adenine to form interstrand cross-bonding (20). In addition to and, possibly, separate from this action, pentamidine appears to be a potent inhibitor of type II topoisomerase of mitochondria DNA (kinetoplast DNA) of the *Trypanosoma* parasite (21). The mitochondrial DNA is a cyclic DNA. This inhibition leads to double-stand breaks in the DNA and linearization of the DNA. The relationship between binding to specific regions of the DNA and inhibition of topoisomerase is unclear.

In the case of *T. brucei,* resistant strains are common. It is thought that resistance develops through an inability of the drug to reach the mitochondrial DNA (22). Transport into the mitochondria is a carrier-mediated process, with the absence of carrier in the resistant strains.

Eflornithine (Ornidyl)

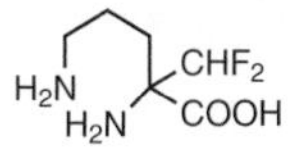

Eflornithine

Metcalf et al. (23) reported the synthesis of eflornithine (difluoromethyl ornithine [DFMO]) in 1978. Their interest arose from the desire to prepare ornithine decarboxylase (ODC) inhibitors as tools for studying the role of polyamines as regulators of growth processes. ODC catalyzes the conversion of ornithine to putrescine (1,4-diaminobutane), which in turn leads to the formation of the polyamines, spermine, and spermidine. It was not until 1980 that Bacchi et al. (24) demonstrated the potential of DFMO in the treatment of trypanosomiasis.

Mechanism of Action DFMO is a suicide inhibitor of ODC, a pyridoxal phosphate–dependent enzyme, as shown in Figure 34.7. Evidence suggests that cysteine-360 in ODC is the site of eflornithine alkylation (25). Alkylation of ODC blocks the synthesis of putrescine, the rate-determining step in the synthesis of polyamines. Mammalian ODC can also be inhibited, but because the turnover of ODC is so rapid in mammals, eflornithine does not produce serious side effects.

Pharmacokinetics Eflornithine can be administered either IV or orally. Administration IV requires large doses and frequent dosing, whereas poor oral absorption and rapid excretion because of the zwitterionic nature of the drug (an amino acid) has limited the oral route of administration. The drug does not bind to plasma protein and enters the CNS readily, most likely via an amino acid transport system. As a result, the drug can be used for both early and late stages of trypanosomiasis.

Therapeutic Application Eflornithine is indicated for the treatment of west African trypanosomiasis caused by *T. brucei gambiense* but has proven to be ineffective

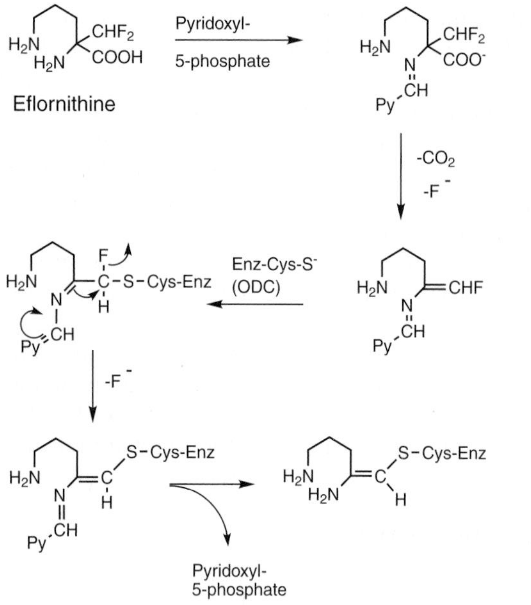

FIGURE 34.7 Inhibition of ornithine decarboxylase (Enz-Cys-SH) by eflornithine.

against east African trypanosomiasis. The cause of this ineffectiveness remains a mystery, although evidence suggests that in the resistant organism, endogenous ornithine plus increased activity of *S*-adenosylmethionine decarboxylase allows sufficient synthesis of spermidine and spermine to support cell division, thus bypassing the need for organism-synthesized ornithine (26). Side effects reported for eflornithine consist of anemia, diarrhea, and leukopenia.

Nifurtimox (Lampit)

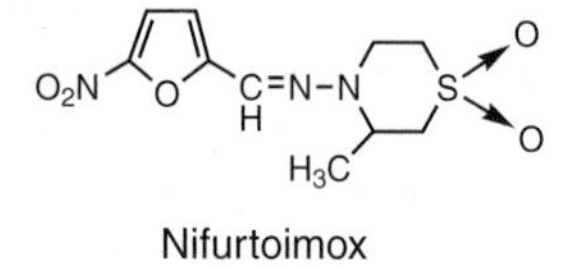

Nifurtoimox

Another of the nitroaryl compounds, nifurtimox has proven to be useful as a drug for the treatment of trypanosomiasis. It is one of two drugs approved for use in treatment of Chagas disease.

Mechanism of Action As discussed for metronidazole, nifurtimox is thought to undergo reduction followed by oxidation and, in the process, generate ROS, such as the superoxide radical anion, hydrogen peroxide, and hydroxyl radical (Fig. 34.3) (5). These species are potent oxidants, producing oxidative stress that can produce damage to DNA and lipids that can affect cellular membranes. In addition, Henderson et al. (27) have reported that nifurtimox inhibits trypanothione reductase, which results in the inhibition of trypanothione formation (93% inhibition). Trypanothione is a critical protective enzyme found uniquely in trypanosomal parasites.

Therapeutic Application Nifurtimox is the drug of choice for the treatment of acute Chagas disease. The drug is not effective for the chronic stages of the disease. In the acute stage, the drug has an 80% cure rate. Side effects of the drug include hypersensitivity reactions, GI complications (nausea and vomiting), myalgia, and weakness.

Benznidazole (Rochagan)

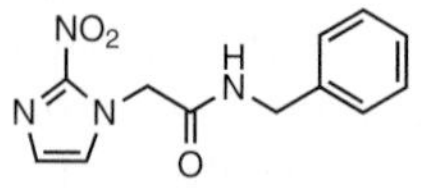

Benznidazole

Benznidazole is the second of the drugs approved for treatment of Chagas disease. Like nifurtimox, it is effective against the circulating form of *Trypanosoma cruzi* during the acute phase of the disease, but also like nifurtimox, it is ineffective during the chronic stage of the disease.

Mechanism of Action Studies suggest that benznidazole does not catalyze the formation of ROS and, therefore, has a mechanism of action different from that of nifurtimox. It has been proposed that benznidazole undergoes a one-electron transfer to the nitro group, which in turn dismutates to give back the nitroimidazole and a nitrosoimidazole (28). The latter product can then undergo an electrophilic addition to trypanothione, which leads to depletion of trypanothione, an essential enzyme system in *T. cruzi* (Fig. 34.8).

Benznidazole is not available in the United States but is available in South American countries. It is administered orally in a tablet form.

Melarsoprol (Available from the CDC)

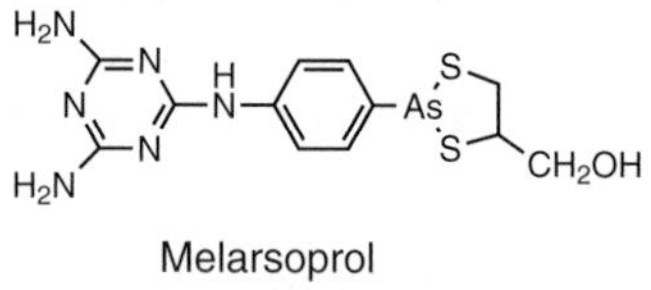

Melarsoprol

Knowingly or unknowingly, arsenic-containing drugs have been used for treatment of parasitic conditions for thousands of years. In the late 1800s and early 1900s, Paul Ehrlich introduced the use of trivalent arsenicals. Melarsoprol, an organoarsenical, came into use in the late 1940s, and it remains the first-choice drug in the treatment of trypanosomiasis. Until 1990, it also was the only treatment for late-stage sleeping sickness.

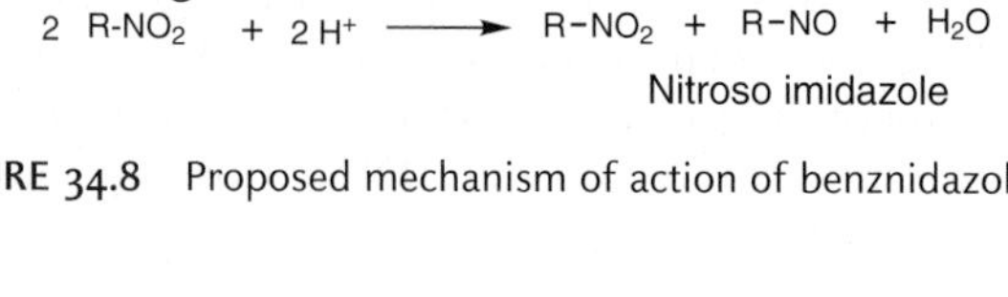

FIGURE 34.8 Proposed mechanism of action of benznidazole.

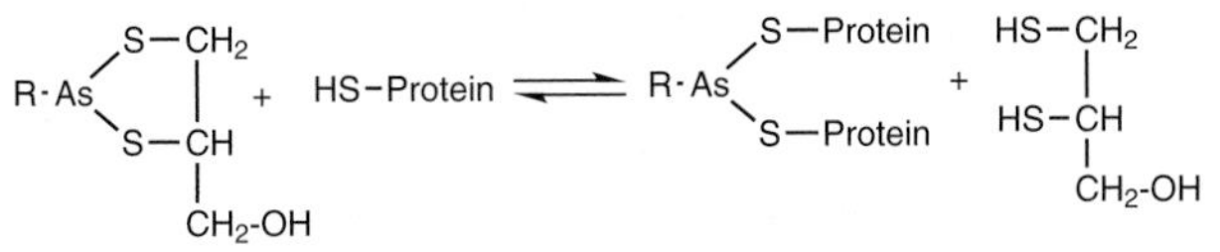

FIGURE 34.9 Mechanism of action of trivalent arsenic compounds with trypanosome organism.

MECHANISM OF ACTION It is known that trivalent arsenic reacts rapidly and reversibly with sulfhydryl-containing proteins, as shown in Figure 34.9. It is generally accepted that the enzyme with which melarsoprol reacts is an enzyme involved in glycolysis, and as a result, inhibition of pyruvate kinase occurs. It is argued, however, that the inhibition might not occur at pyruvate kinase but, rather, at a step before the pyruvate kinase. Blockage of glycolysis would be expected to lead to loss of motility and cell lysis. More recently, Fairlamb et al. (29) have proposed a mechanism of action that results in the inhibition of trypanothione reductase through the formation of a stable complex between melarsoprol and trypanothione. Melarsoprol reacts with the cysteine sulfhydryl of trypanothione to form the stable adduct shown in Figure 34.10. Supportive of this mechanism is the synergistic action of melarsoprol with eflornithine, two drugs that produce sequential blockage of the synthesis of trypanothione.

PHARMACOKINETICS Melarsoprol is administered IV in multiple doses and multiple sessions. Its major metabolite in humans is the lipophilic melarsen oxide, which can penetrate into the CNS. This metabolite apparently is responsible for the protein-binding characteristic for melarsoprol.

THERAPEUTIC APPLICATION Melarsoprol is the drug of choice for the treatment of late-stage meningoencephalitic trypanosomiasis caused by the west and east African strains of the disease. Because the drug has the potential for serious nervous system toxicities (e.g., convulsions, acute cerebral edema, and coma), the drug is usually administered in a hospital setting with supervision. An additional problem with melarsoprol is the development of resistance by the parasite.

Treatment of Leishmaniasis

Sodium Stibogluconate (Pentostam; Available from the CDC)

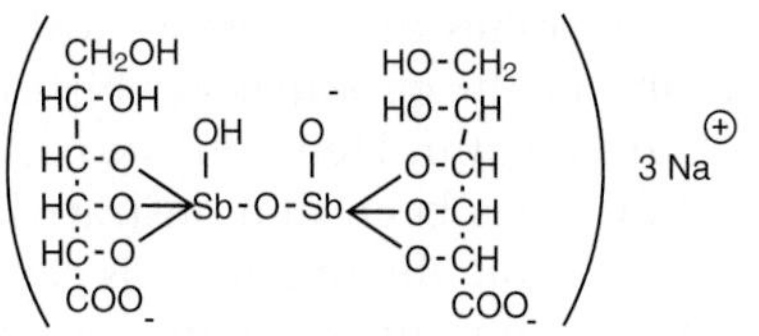

Sodium stibogluconate

Leishmaniasis was first described in the medical literature by Deishman and Donovan in 1903, and shortly after that, antimony-based drugs were introduced as therapeutic agents to treat this disease (30). Although the structure of sodium stibogluconate is commonly drawn as shown, the actual compound probably is much more complex. The drug is a water-soluble preparation that is administered intramuscularly or IV. Pentavalent antimony compounds are thought to inhibit bioenergetic processes in the pathogen, with catabolism of glucose and inhibition of glycolytic enzymes being the primary sites of action (glucose catabolism is 86% to 94% inhibited). This in turn results in inhibition of adenosine triphosphate/guanosine triphosphate formation. Sodium stibogluconate is the drug of choice for the treatment of most forms of leishmaniasis (or meglumine antimonate, another pentavalent antimony agent). The recommended dose is 20 mg antimony/kg/d, not to exceed 850 mg antimony/d. A number of other drugs have been reported to be effective in the treatment of leishmaniasis, and these include pentamidine, amphotericin B, paromomycin, alkylphosphocholine analogs, rifampicin, and ketoconazole (31,32).

Miltefosine (Impavido)

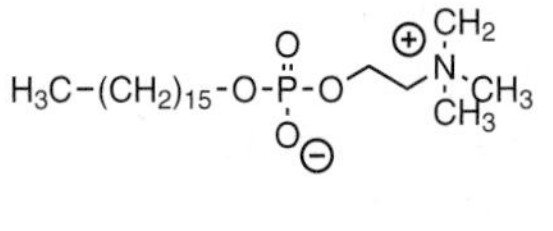

Miltefosine

Miltefosine is an orally active drug that is effective against visceral and cutaneous leishmaniasis. Although the drug has not been approved by the FDA, a compassionate use protocol is pending. This drug is especially important since the only other drug available is sodium stibogluconate, which is administered intramuscularly or IV, thus limiting its utility, and has a high potential for toxicity associated with the antimony component of the drug. Miltefosine has been reported to exhibit activity in vitro against a broad range of leishmanial strains. Although the mechanism of action of the drug remains unknown, it has been suggested that the drug acts directly on the promastigote and amastigote stages of the parasite and not through stimulation of the immune system (33). This distinction is important because patients who are immunocompromised may also suffer from leishmaniasis.

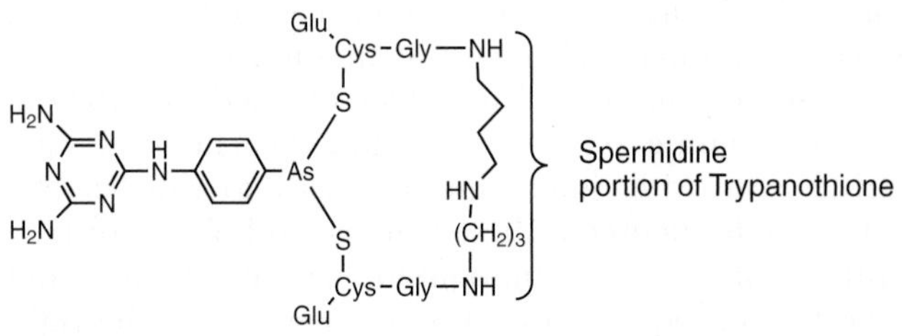

FIGURE 34.10 Structure of melarsoprol trypanothione complex.

The drug is well absorbed via the oral route and well distributed, with a half-life of 6 to 8 days.

Treatment of Malaria

Historical Background

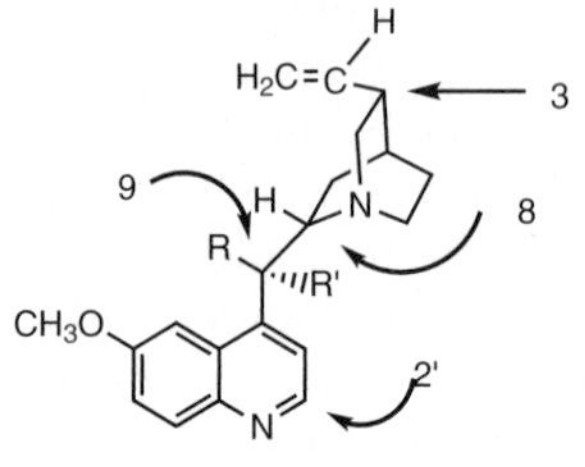

Quinine (R = OH, R' = H)
Quinidine (R = H, R' = OH)

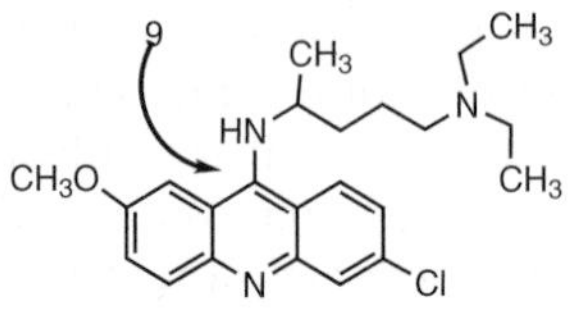

Quinacrine

Quinine was the first known antimalarial. It is a 4-quinolinemethanol derivative bearing a substituted quinuclidine ring. The use of quinine in Europe began in the 17th century, after the Incas of Peru informed the Spanish Jesuits about the antimalarial properties of the bark of an evergreen mountain tree they called quinquina (later called cinchona, after Dona Franciscoa Henriquez de Ribera [1576–1639], Countess of Chinchon and wife of the Peruvian Viceroy). The bark, when made into an aqueous solution, was capable of curing most forms of malaria. It was listed in the London Pharmacopeia of 1677. The alkaloid derived from the bark, quinine, was isolated in the mid-1820s. Quinine, a very bitter substance, has been used by millions of malaria sufferers. Recently, it has been employed successfully to treat chloroquine-resistant strains of *Plasmodium falciparum* and is considered to be the drug of choice for these resistant strains.

Quinidine, the C-9 stereoisomer of quinine, is also an effective antimalarial, but suffers from the fact that it is considerably more toxic than quinine. Its use is usually limited to treatment of severe malarial infections. Quinidine is also used as an antiarrhythmic agent.

A second class of chemicals that played a role in the development of synthetic antimalarials were the 9-aminoacridines. 9-Aminoacridine was known to exhibit antibacterial activity, whereas a derivative of 9-aminoacridine synthesized in 1934, quinacrine, was found to possess weak antimalarial activity.

With the beginning of World War II and concern about an interruption in the supply of cinchona bark from the East Indies, a massive effort was begun to search for synthetic alternatives to quinine and to develop more effective antimalarial agents than quinacrine. With a basic understanding of the structure–activity relationship of quinine (see *Quinine*) and the chemical similarities seen with quinacrine, it is easy to visualize the relationship between these agents and the synthetic antimalarials. The 4-aminoquinolines, chloroquine and hydroxychloroquine, are structurally similar to the right half of quinacrine (Fig. 34.11). The 8-aminoquinolines,

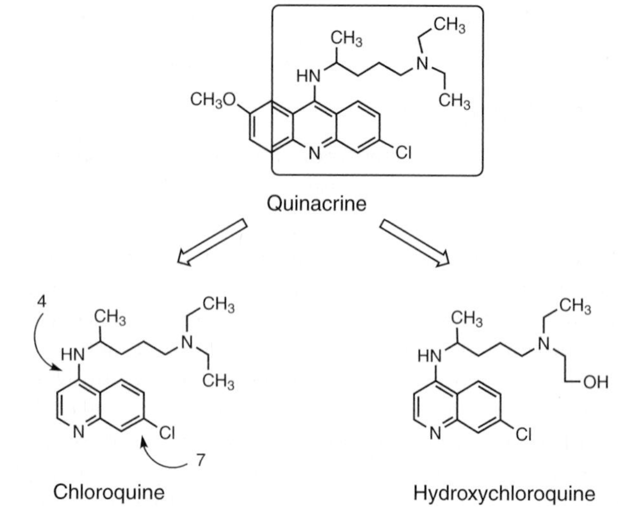

FIGURE 34.11 Structural similarity between quinacrine and the 4-aminoquinolines.

pamaquine and primaquine, retain the methoxyquinoline nucleus of quinine and quinacrine (Fig. 34.12). The quinoline-4-methanols, mefloquine and halofantrine, show similarity to the 4-quinolinemethanol portion of quinine (Fig. 34.12).

4-Substituted Quinolines

Six compounds can be considered within this class of drugs: quinine, chloroquine, and hydroxychloroquine, mefloquine, halofantrine, and lumefantrine (Figs. 34.11 and 34.12). These compounds not only share a structural similarity but are also thought to have similar mechanisms of action, are effective on the same stage of the parasite, and can share similar mechanisms of resistance.

Mechanism of Action The mechanism of action of chloroquine has been studied in depth, and the results of these studies have been assumed to be applicable to the other 4-substituted quinolines (34). Various mechanisms of actions have been offered to explain the action of this class of drugs, including the DNA intercalation mechanism, the weak base hypothesis, and the ferriprotoporphyrin hypothesis. The present understanding about the mechanism of action would appear to use various aspects of each of these previous mechanisms. It is known that hemoglobin is transported into the food vacuoles of the plasmodium (Figs. 34.13 and 34.14), where digestion of the hemoglobin supplies the organism with a source of amino acids. One of the products of this digestion is a free heme called hematin. Hematin is toxic to the plasmodium cell, but it has been demonstrated that within the plasmodium vacuole the organism is capable of converting the hematin to nontoxic hemozoin. While it was initially thought that hemozoin was a polymeric form of hematin, it is now thought that the detoxification occurs through biocrystallization (35,36). The dimeric hemozoin as a biocrystal is insoluble and chemically inert and

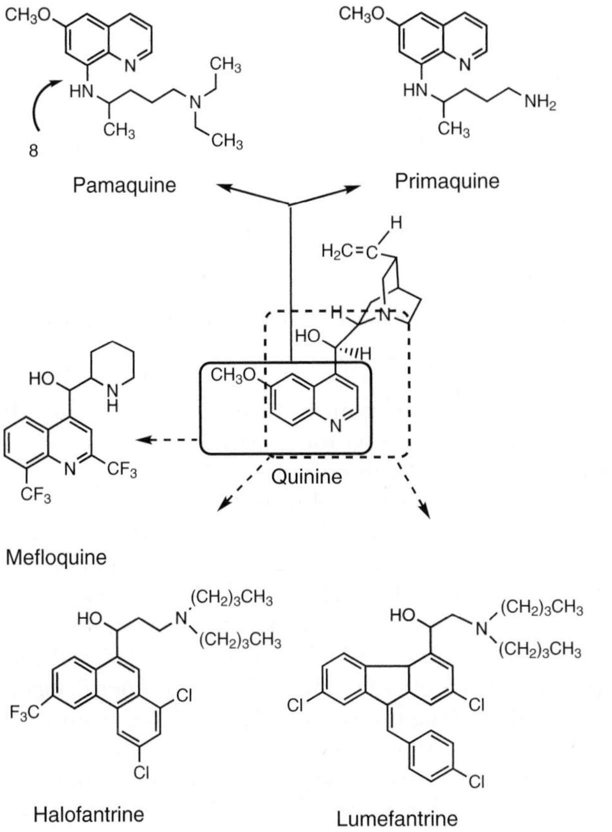

FIGURE 34.12 Structural similarity between quinine and the 8-aminoquinolines (- - -➤) and between quinine and the quinoline-4-methanols (- - -➤).

therefore has no biologic effect on the plasmodium. The quinolines bind to hematin through a drug–heme complex in which the aromatic quinoline ring π-bonds to the porphyrin nucleus (37). This drug–heme complex blocks further biocrystallization. The result of this complexation is that newly formed, free toxic hematin is now present, which leads to the death of the plasmodium. Additionally since heme is not a component of plasmodium, it appears unlikely that the organism will be capable of developing a resistance mechanism to this type of activity. The accumulation of the 4-substituted quinolines in the acidic food vacuoles (pH 4.8 to 5.2) is based on the fact that these drugs are weak bases, as indicated by their pK_a values. The extracellular fluid of the parasite is at pH 7.4, and as a result, the weak base will move toward the more acidic pH of the vacuoles, reaching concentrations hundreds of times those in the plasma. Additionally, the binding of the quinoline to the heme draws additional quantities into the vacuole.

Mechanism of Resistance A limiting factor for most of the antimalarial drugs is the development of resistant strains of plasmodium. It should be noted that resistance differs from region to region, and in some cases, a resistant strain can develop to a particular drug without that

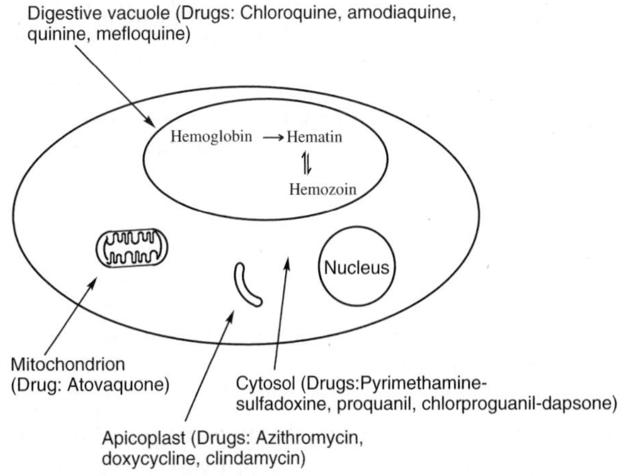

FIGURE 34.13 *Plasmodium* parasite cell as present within the erythrocyte and sites of drug action.

drug ever having been introduced to the region (possible cross-resistance). The development of resistance is thought to be a spontaneous gene mutation. Several mechanisms of resistance appear to be operating. One of these mechanisms is based on the *Plasmodium falciparum* chloroquine-resistance transporter (*pfcrt*) mechanism, which is sufficient and necessary to impart resistance (38). A gene encodes for a transmembrane transporter protein found in the membrane of the food vacuole. Multiple mutations within a specific region in this gene result in reduced accumulation of chloroquine, resulting from the increased efflux of the drug. Additional transporter proteins may also be involved in resistance.

Rapid metabolism of the antimalarials by resistant strains of plasmodium also might be considered to play a significant role in the development of resistance. It has been shown that cytochrome P450 activity parallels increased resistance to specific drugs.

Therapeutic Application The 4-substituted quinolines are referred to as rapidly acting blood schizonticides, with activity against plasmodium in the erythrocytic stage. Chloroquine is the drug of choice, but unfortunately, the incidence of chloroquine-resistant infections is extremely common today. The spread of chloroquine resistance has reached almost all malarious areas of the world. In addition, multidrug-resistant and cross-resistant strains of plasmodium are now common. The drug of choice for the treatment of malaria caused by *Plasmodium falciparum, Plasmodium ovale, Plasmodium vivax,* and *Plasmodium malariae* in regions infected by chloroquine-resistant *P. falciparum* is quinine, in combination with traditional antibiotics, mefloquine, or various other combinations as alternative treatment agents (Table 34.2). Of interest is the observation that after years of nonuse of chloroquine, a reemergence of chloroquine-sensitive parasites has been found.

The 4-substituted quinolines, depending on the specific drug in question, can also be used for prophylaxis

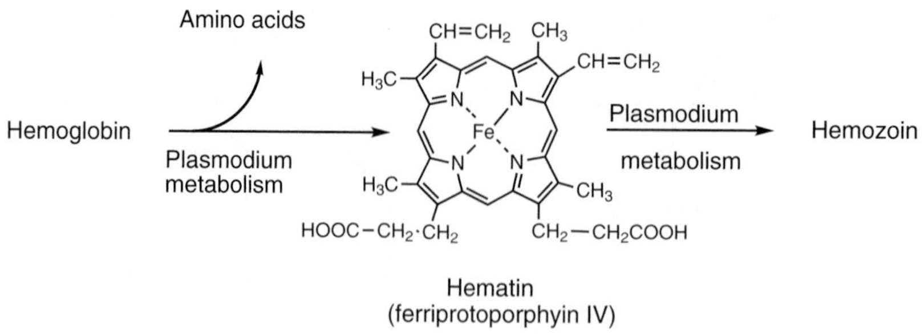

FIGURE 34.14 Proteolytic degradation of hemoglobin by the *Plasmodium* organism to the potentially toxic hematin and then to the nontoxic dimer hemozoin.

of malaria. Two types of prophylaxis are possible: causal prophylaxis and suppressive prophylaxis. The former prevents the establishment of hepatic forms of the parasite, whereas the latter eradicates the erythrocytic parasites but has no effect on the hepatic forms. Several of the 4-substituted quinolines are effective suppressive prophylactics.

Specific 4-substituted Quinolines

Quinine. Quinine is the most prevalent alkaloid present in the bark extracts (~5%) of cinchona. Four stereochemical centers exist in the molecule (at C-3, C-4, C-8, and C-9) (Fig. 34.12). Quinine (absolute configuration of 3R:4S:8S:9R), quinidine (absolute configuration of 3R:4S:8R:9S), and their optical isomers all have antimalarial activity, whereas their C-9 epimers (i.e., the epi-series having either 3R:4S:8R:9R or 3R:4S:8S:9S configurations) are inactive. Modification of the secondary alcohol at C-9, through oxidation, esterification, or similar processes, diminishes activity. The quinuclidine portion is not necessary for activity; however, an alkyl tertiary amine at C-9 is important.

Quinine is metabolized in the liver to the 2′-hydroxy derivative, followed by additional hydroxylation on the quinuclidine ring, with the 2,2′-dihydroxy derivative as the major metabolite. This metabolite has low antimalarial activity and is rapidly excreted. The metabolizing enzyme of quinine is CYP3A4. With the increased use of quinine and its use in combination with other drugs, the potential for drug interactions based on the many known substrates for CYP3A4 (see Chapter 4) is of concern (39).

A quinine overdose causes tinnitus and visual disturbances; these side effects disappear on discontinuation of the drug. Quinine can also cause premature contractions during the late stages of pregnancy. Although quinine is suitable for parenteral administration, this route is considered to be hazardous because of its ability to cause hemolysis. Quinidine, the (+)-isomer of quinine, has been

TABLE 34.2 Guidelines for Treatment of Malaria in the United States[a]

Clinical Diagnosis	Sensitivity	Drug Recommendation
Uncomplicated malaria	Chloroquine sensitive	Chloroquine phosphate
P. falciparum	Chloroquine resistant or unknown	A. Atovaquone–proguanil (Malarone) B. Artemether–lumefantrine (Coartem) C. Quinine sulfate + one of the following: Doxycycline Tetracycline Clindamycin D. Mefloquine
Uncomplicated malaria *P. malariae, P. knowlesi*	Chloroquine sensitive	A. Chloroquine B. Hydroxychloroquine
Uncomplicated malaria *P. vivax* or *P. ovale*	Chloroquine sensitive	Chloroquine phosphate + primaquine phosphate
Uncomplicated malaria *P. vivax*	Chloroquine resistant	A. Quinine sulfate + doxycycline or tetracycline B. Atovaquone–proguanil C. Mefloquine + primaquine phosphate
Severe malaria	Chloroquine sensitive/resistant	Quinidine gluconate (parenteral) + one of the following: Doxycycline Tetracycline Clindamycin

[a]Information taken from the CDC Guideline for Treatment of Malaria in the United States. For more details, including infectious region and dosing, go to http://www.cdc.gov/malaria/diagnosis_treatment/index.html.

shown to be more effective in combating the disease, but it has undesirable cardiac side effects. When used for severe malaria, the quinidine gluconate is administered IV.

Chloroquine (Aralen). Chloroquine is the most effective of the hundreds of 4-aminoquinolines synthesized and tested during World War II as potential antimalarials. Structure–activity relationships demonstrated that the chloro at the 8-position increased activity, whereas alkylation at C-3 and C-8 diminished activity. The replacement of one of its *N*-ethyl groups with a hydroxyethyl produced hydroxychloroquine, a compound with reduced toxicity that is rarely used today except in cases of rheumatoid arthritis.

Chloroquine is commonly administered as the racemic mixture, because little is gained by using the individual isomers. The drug is well absorbed from the GI tract and distributed to many tissues, where it is tightly bound and slowly eliminated. The drug is metabolized by *N*-dealkylation by CYP2D6 and CYP3A4 isoforms. It has been reported that the level of metabolism correlates closely with the degree of resistance. The suggestion has been made to coadminister chloroquine with CYP2D6 and CYP3A4 inhibitors to potentate activity and reduce resistance. Although this can be possible, it is not commonly practiced.

Chloroquine is an excellent suppressive agent for treating acute attacks of malaria caused by *Plasmodium vivax* and *Plasmodium ovale*. The drug is also effective for cure and as a suppressive prophylactic for the treatment of *Plasmodium malariae* and susceptible *Plasmodium falciparum*.

Chloroquine is generally a safe drug, with toxicity occurring at high doses of medication if the drug is administered too rapidly via parenteral routes. With oral administration, the side effects primarily are GI effects, mild headache, visual disturbances, and urticaria.

Mefloquine (Lariam) (40). Mefloquine, which was synthesized with the intent of blocking the site of metabolism in quinine with the chemically stable CF_3 group, exists as four optical isomers of nearly equal activity. The drug is active against chloroquine-resistant strains of plasmodium, yet cross-resistance is not uncommon. Metabolism is cited as the possible mechanism of resistance. Mefloquine is slowly metabolized through CYP3A4 oxidation to its major inactive metabolite, carboxymefloquine (Fig. 34.15). Most of the parent drug is excreted unchanged into the urine. Its coadministration with CYP3A4 inhibitors (e.g., ketoconazole) has increased the area under the curve for mefloquine by inhibiting its metabolism to carboxymefloquine.

Mefloquine is only available in an oral dosage form, which is well absorbed. The presence of food in the GI tract affects the pharmacokinetic properties of the drug, usually enhancing absorption. The lipophilic nature of the drug accounts for the extensive tissue binding and low clearance of total drug, although the drug does not accumulate after prolonged administration. The drug has a high affinity for erythrocyte membranes.

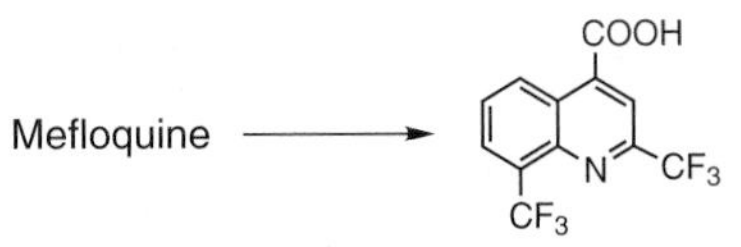

FIGURE 34.15 *Plasmodium falciparum* metabolism of mefloquine.

Mefloquine is an effective suppressive prophylactic agent against *Plasmodium falciparum* both in nonimmune populations (travelers coming into regions of malaria) and in resident populations. The drug has also high efficacy against falciparum malaria, with a low incidence of recrudescence. The drug is ineffective against sexual forms of the organism.

The incidence of side effects with mefloquine is considered to be high. The effects are classified as neuropsychiatric, GI, dermatologic, and cardiovascular. The neuropsychiatric effects can be serious (e.g., suicidal tendencies or seizures) or minor (e.g., dizziness, vertigo, ataxia, and headaches). GI side effects included nausea, vomiting, and diarrhea, whereas the dermatologic effects include rash, pruritus, and urticaria. Finally, cardiovascular side effects can include bradycardia, arrhythmias, and extrasystoles.

Halofantrine (Hafan). Halofantrine (40–42), a member of the 9-phenanthrenemethanol class (Fig. 34.12), originally came out of a synthesis program dating to World War II, but this particular agent was not fully developed until the 1960s. Halofantrine has one chiral center and has been separated into its enantiomers. There appears to be little difference between the enantiomers; thus, the drug is used as a racemic mixture.

Halofantrine is considered to be an alternative drug for treatment of both chloroquine-sensitive and chloroquine-resistant *Plasmodium falciparum* malaria, but its efficacy in mefloquine-resistant malaria can be questionable. It is generally believed that halofantrine acts through a mechanism similar to that of the 4-aminoquinolines. The drug is metabolized via *N*-dealkylation to desbutylhalofantrine by CYP3A4 (Fig. 34.16). The metabolite appears to be several-fold more active than the administered drug.

At present, halofantrine is only available in a tablet form, which has significant implications as it relates to its insolubility and drug absorption (bioavailability). Animal studies have shown that following oral administration, the drug is eliminated in feces, suggesting poor oral absorption. Its oral suspensions leads to as much as

ADDITIONAL THERAPEUTIC INDICATIONS FOR CHLOROQUINE

Chloroquine is also prescribed for treatment of rheumatoid arthritis, discoid lupus erythematosus, and photosensitivity diseases.

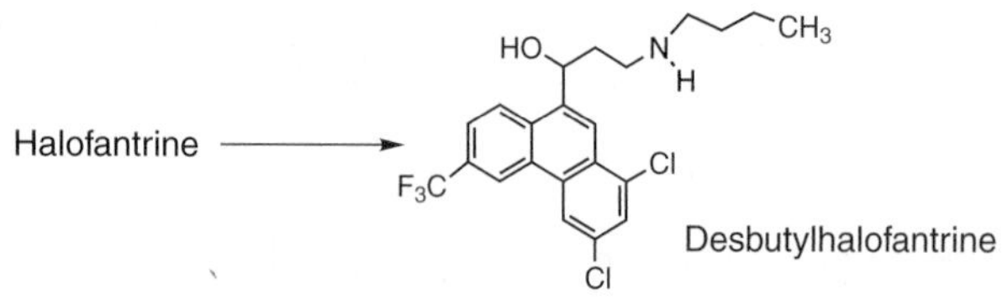

FIGURE 34.16 Metabolism of halofantrine.

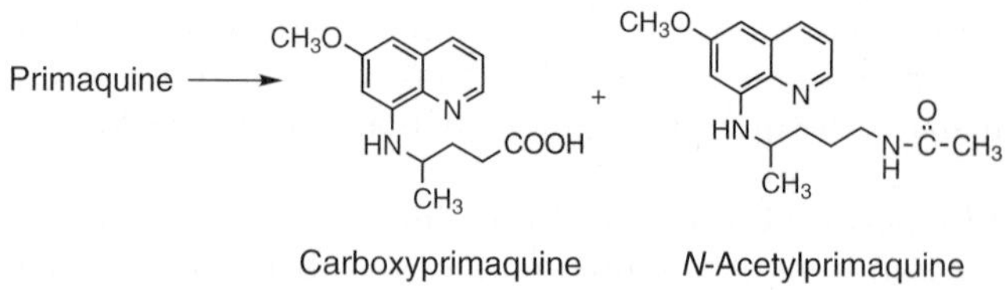

FIGURE 34.17 Metabolism of primaquine.

30% lower plasma levels of the drug in comparison with the tablet. A micronized form of the drug has shown improved bioavailability. Its administration with or without food in the stomach also leads to considerable variation in plasma levels. A high lipid content in a meal taken 2 hours before dosing leads to substantial increases in the rate and extent of absorption. Several cases of drug treatment failure appear to be related to poor absorption. Incomplete absorption and, as a result, low plasma levels can play a role in the development of organism resistance. The elimination half-lives of halofantrine and desbutylhalofantrine tend to be prolonged, which can be another factor in the development of resistance. Low levels of the drug can increase the likelihood of augmenting the emergence of halofantrine resistance.

Absorption problems with halofantrine cannot be solved by increasing the dosage of halofantrine because of significant toxicity problems. Toxicity, although minimal with short-term low doses, can be severe with high doses of halofantrine. GI side effects include nausea, vomiting, diarrhea, and abdominal pain. Cardiovascular toxicity includes orthostatic hypotension and dose-dependent lengthening of QTc intervals.

Lumefantrine. Lumefantrine, an effective erythrocytic schizonticide, is a derivative of halofantrine that has been reported to exhibit antimalarial activity when combined with artemether in the treatment of multidrug-resistant *Plasmodium falciparum* (Fig. 34.12). The drug is only used in combination with artemether (artemisinin-based combination therapies) in which a synergistic effect has been noted (see below). Lumefantrine has a relatively long half-life of 3 to 6 days, which makes it ideal for combining with the short half-life artemisinins. The drug is quite lipophilic, and a diet rich in fat increases the bioavailability of the drug. Unfortunately, many patients suffering from malaria do not tolerate food, and therefore, the bioavailability of lumefantrine is not very high. No evidence of cardiotoxicity has been reported with this combination, which can offer promise for successful treatment of resistant organisms.

8-Aminoquinolines.

Pamaquine/primaquine Pamaquine, an 8-aminoquinoline, was first introduced for treatment of malaria in 1926 and has since been replaced with primaquine (Fig. 34.12). Primaquine is active against latent tissue forms of *Plasmodium vivax* and *Plasmodium ovale,* and it is active against the hepatic stages of *Plasmodium falciparum.* The drug is not active against erythrocytic stages of the parasite but does possess gametocidal activity against all strains of plasmodium.

Mechanism of Action. The mechanism of action of the 8-aminoquinolines is unknown, but primaquine can generate ROS via an auto-oxidation of the 8-amino group. The formation of a radical anion at the 8-amino group has been proposed by Augusto et al. (43). As a result, cell-destructive oxidants, such as hydrogen peroxide, superoxide, and hydroxyl radical, can be formed, as shown in Figure 34.3, leading to oxidative damage to critical cellular components.

Metabolism. Primaquine is almost totally metabolized by CYP3A4 (99%), with the primary metabolite being carboxyprimaquine (Fig. 34.17) (44). Trace amounts of *N*-acetylprimaquine plus aromatic hydroxylation and conjugation metabolites also have been reported.

Therapeutic Application. Primaquine is classified as the drug of choice for the treatment of relapsing vivax and ovale forms of malaria and will produce a radical cure of the condition. It is recommended that the drug be combined with chloroquine to eradicate the erythrocytic stages of malaria. Primaquine is not given for long-term treatment because of potential toxicity and sensitization. The sensitivity appears most commonly in individuals who have glucose-6-phosphate dehydrogenase deficiency. In these cases, hemolytic anemia can develop.

TAFENOQUIN

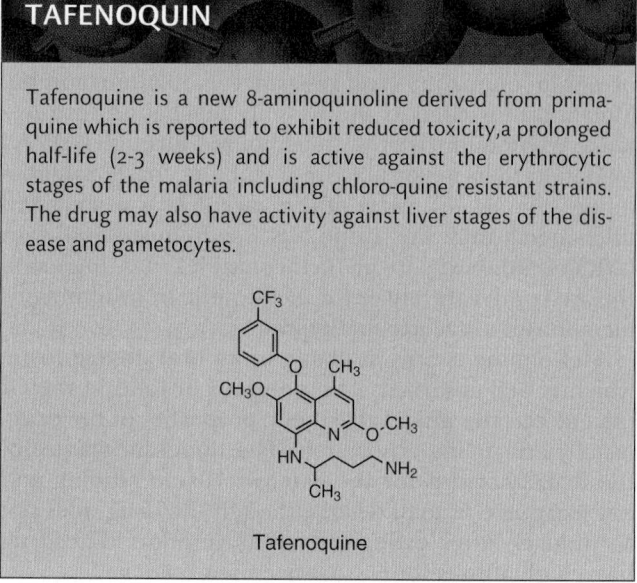

Tafenoquine is a new 8-aminoquinoline derived from primaquine which is reported to exhibit reduced toxicity,a prolonged half-life (2-3 weeks) and is active against the erythrocytic stages of the malaria including chloro-quine resistant strains. The drug may also have activity against liver stages of the disease and gametocytes.

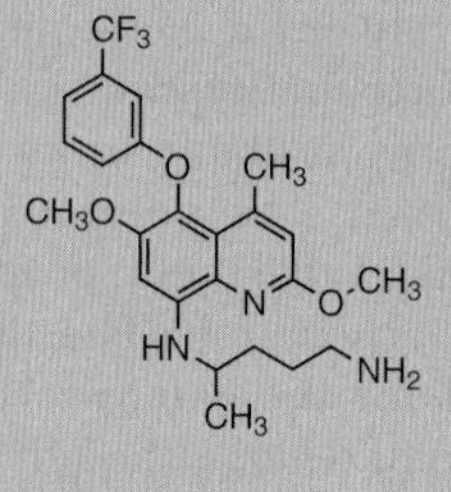

Tafenoquine

Pyrimethamine (Daraprim)

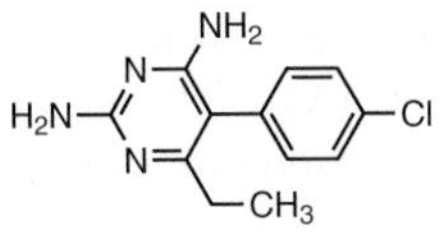

Pyrimethamine

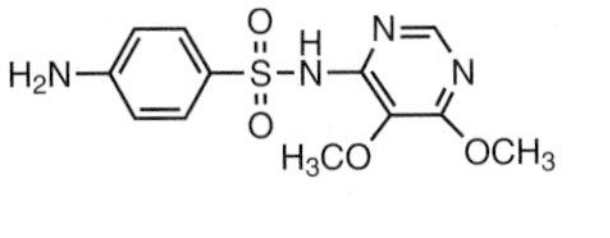

Sulfadoxine

Pyrimethamine is a potent inhibitor of DHFR (45). The drug has been shown to have a significantly higher affinity for binding to the DHFR of plasmodium than to the host enzyme (>1,000 times in *Plasmodium berghei*) and, as a result, has been used to selectively treat plasmodium infections. The combination of pyrimethamine with a long-acting sulfonamide, sulfadoxine, which blocks dihydrofolate synthesis by blocking incorporation of PABA into the dihydrofolate, is called Fansidar, which produces sequential blockage of tetrahydrofolate synthesis similar to that reported for treatment of bacterial infections (see Chapter 33). It should be noted that the site of action of this combination is in the cytosol of the plasmodium (Fig. 34.13). *Plasmodium* enzymes catalyzing folic acid synthesis differ from those enzymes found in other organisms. A single bifunctional protein present in *Plasmodium* sp. catalyzes the phosphorylation of 6-hydroxymethyl-7,8-hydropterin (a pyrophosphokinase) and the incorporation of PABA into dihydropteroic acid. A second bifunctional enzyme catalyzes the reduction of dihydropteroic acid and thymidylic acid synthesis. As a result, the drug combination (Fansidar) appears to have improved drug-mediated disruption of folic acid in *Plasmodium* sp. (34,46). This combination has been used with quinine for the treatment and prevention of chloroquine-resistant malaria (*Plasmodium falciparum, Plasmodium ovale, Plasmodium vivax,* and *Plasmodium malaria*). The combination therapy (Fansidar) has the added advantage of being inexpensive, which is essential for successful therapy in developing countries. When used on its own, pyrimethamine is a blood schizonticide without effects on the tissue stage of the disease.

The mechanism of resistance to the folate inhibitor combination has been shown to be associated with point mutations in both DHFR and the dihydropteroate synthase enzymes (35).

Atovaquone–proguanil

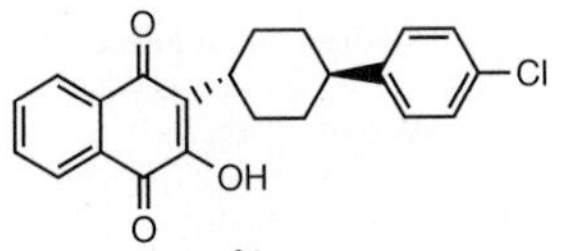

Atovaquone

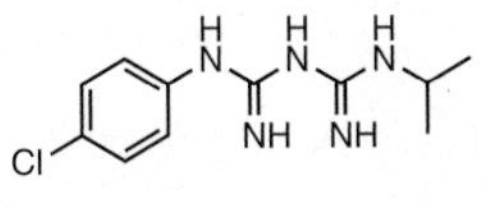

Proguanil

Atovaquone was originally developed as an antimalarial, but because of the high failure rate (~30%), it is not prescribed as a single chemical entity but, rather, is used to treat pneumocystis (see page XX). More recently, however, atovaquone has been combined with proguanil as an effective prophylactic and therapeutic antimalarial (38). The two drugs together (Malarone) exhibit synergy in which proguanil reduces the effective concentration of atovaquone needed to damage the mitochondrial membrane and atovaquone increases the effectiveness of proguanil but not its active metabolite (for the mechanism of action of atovaquone, see page XX). Proguanil was developed decades earlier as a folic acid antagonist and functions as a prodrug. The active form of proguanil is cycloguanil, which acts as a DHFR inhibitor (Fig. 34.18). Later, this discovery led to the development of pyrimethamine. The sites of action of this combination involve two different locations. Atovaquone is active within the mitochondrion of the plasmodium, while proguanil as an antifolate is active in the cytosol (Fig. 34.13).

Resistance to atovaquone used as a monotherapy might have been associated with the pharmacokinetics of the drug. Atovaquone is quite lipophilic and has slow uptake, resulting in the pathogen experiencing low concentrations of the drug over an extended period of time, both of which encourage the development of resistance. A single point mutation appears to be sufficient for resistance (47). To date, resistance to the combination has not been reported.

ARTEMISININS (48–51)

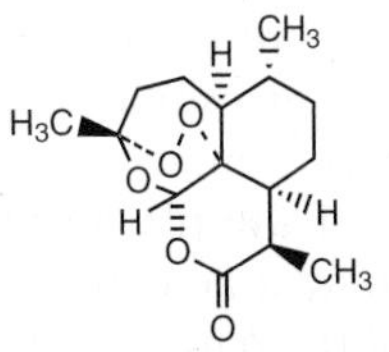

Artemisinin

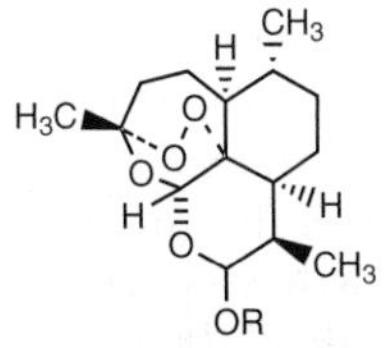

Artemether (R = CH_3)
Arteether/Artemotil (R = C_2H_5)
Dihydroartemisinin (R = H)

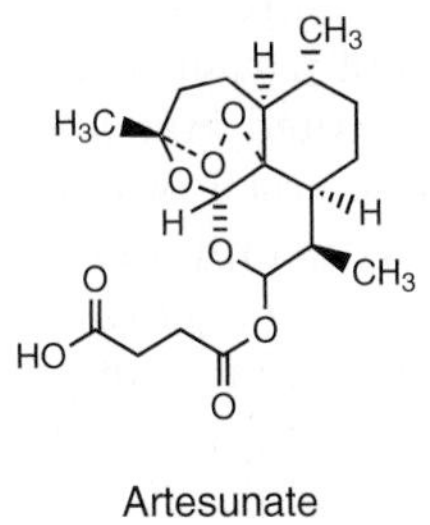

Artesunate

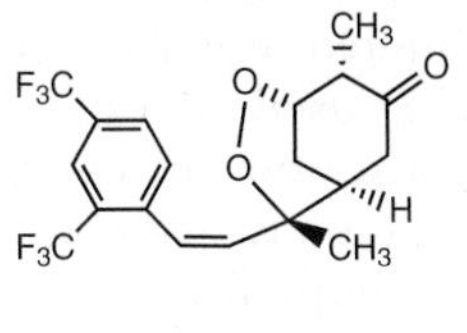

Arteflene

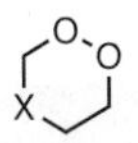

1,2,4-Trioxane (X = O) and 12-Dioxane (X = CH_2) rings

The most recent additions to the drug therapy for malaria are artemisinin and its derivatives. Isolated from *Artemisia annua* (qinghao, sweetworm wood), this material has been used by Chinese herbalists since 168 BC. Artemisinin and the synthetic and semisynthetic derivatives, artemether, arteether, arteflene, and artesunate, are active by virtue of the endoperoxide. The artemisinin derivatives are built on the 1,2,4-trioxanes or 1,2-dioxane ring systems.

Mechanism of Action Two mechanisms have been suggested to account for the antimalarial action of the

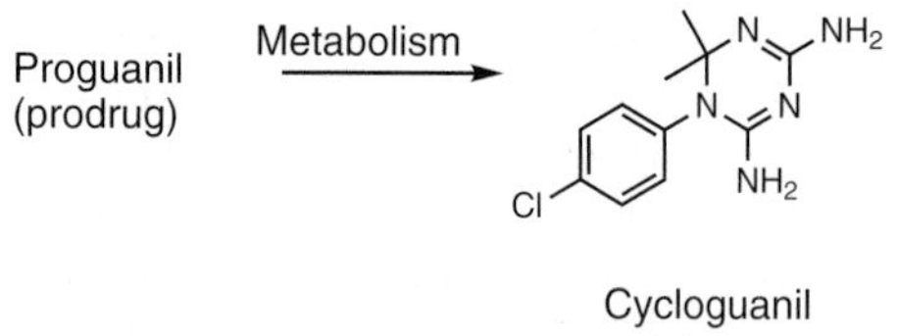

FIGURE 34.18 Activation of proguanil leading to cycloguanil.

artemisinins. In the first mechanism, the artemisinins appear to kill the parasite by a free radical mechanism—not by the generation of ROS but, rather, by virtue of a free radical associated with the endoperoxide, possibly involving a carbon radical. It is proposed that the heme in the form of hemozoin within the digestive vacuole is a source of Fe^{II}, which reacts with the peroxide to generate an oxy radical and Fe^{III}. A carbon radical is formed from the oxy radical, which is then lethal to the plasmodium within the erythrocyte. The second mechanism suggests endoperoxide activation via an iron-dependent mechanism, but the activated artemisinins target sarcoplasmic/endoplasmic reticulum Ca^{2+}-ATPase of the *Plasmodium falciparum* (PfATP6), altering calcium stores (52,53). The artemisinins actually can form covalent adducts to specific membrane-associated proteins after concentrating in infected erythrocytes.

Therapeutic Application The artemisinins are hydrophobic in nature with the exception of artesunate, which is available as a water-soluble hemisuccinate salt, and are partitioned into the membrane of the plasmodium. These compounds have gametocytocidal activity as well as activity against all asexual stages of the parasites. These agents are short acting, with relatively short half-lives. Little or no cross-resistance has been reported, with the drugs rapidly clearing the blood of parasites. The drugs have limited availability in the United States, but they are being used elsewhere as commercial or experimental agents, often in combination therapy (Table 34.3). Combination therapy has the goal of reducing resistance with the hope for synergism and, when combined with longer-acting drugs, an improved therapy.

Among the combinations reportedly used are artesunate–fosmidomycin, artemether–lumefantrine (Coartem), amodiaquine–artesunate, chloroquine–artemisinin, and artesunate–sulfadoxine–pyrimethamine (54). These combinations are referred to as artemisinin-based combination therapy (ACT). These ACTs have been reported to show cure rates of greater than 90%. The fixed-dose combination Coartem has been used in more than 10 million treatments, with significant increases being forecast.

The use of the artemisinins and artemisinin derivatives in other parasitic infections has received recent attention (53). Specifically, several derivatives of artemisinin exhibited activity as antileishmaniasis agents, in treatment of schistosomiasis, and in treatment of trypanosomiasis. Combinations of artesunate–sulfamethoxypyrazine–pyrimethamine and artemether–lumefantrine are effective against *Schistosoma mansoni*, and artemisinin was reported to show activity against *Trypanosoma brucei rhodesiense*, *Trypanosoma cruzi*, and *Leishmania donovani* in vitro.

Antibiotics

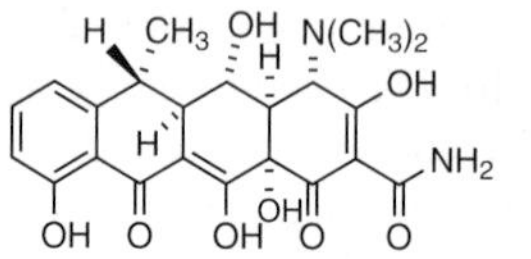

Doxycycline (Vibramycin)

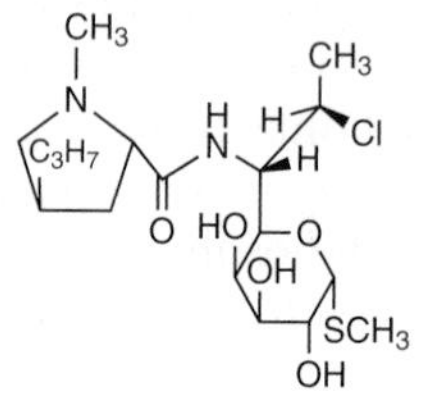

Clindamycin (Cleocin)

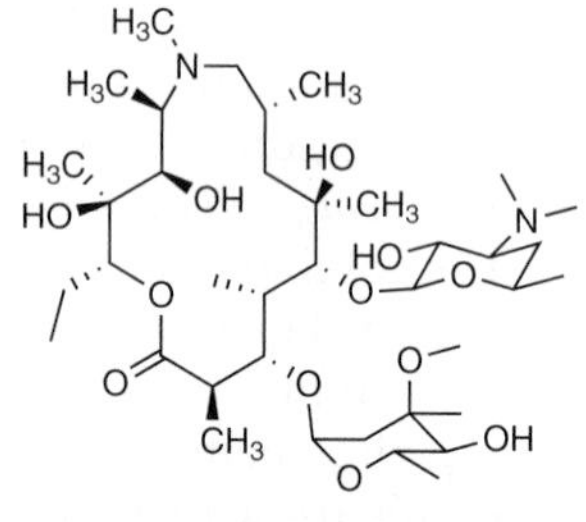

Azithromycin (Zithromax, Zmax)

TABLE 34.3 Examples of Commercially Available Artemisinins

Artemisinin	Trade Name	Dose/Route of Administration	Treatment Condition	Patients
Arteether or artemotil	Artecef	50 mg/IM 150 mg/IM	Severe *P. falciparum*	Children and adolescents
Artemether–lumefantrine	Coartem	20 mg artemether/120 mg lumefantrine PO	Acute uncomplicated *P. falciparum*	Weight >5 kg
Artesimate	IND in United States	IV used in combination	Severe *P. falciparum*	
Artemether	Gvither, Artenam	300 mg/100 mL PO and injectable 180 mg/60 mL PO	Multidrug-resistant *P. falciparum*	
Dihydroartemisinin	Alaxin	60 mg PO tablet 160 mg/80 mL PO suspension 20/40/80 mg suppository	*P. falciparum* *P. falciparum, vivax, malariae*	Adults and children

IM, intramuscular; IND, investigational new drug; IV, intravenous; PO, oral.

Various antibiotics have proven useful in the treatment of malaria. They can be used alone as prophylaxis or in combination with quinine or artesunate as treatment measures. The most commonly used antibiotics are doxycycline, clindamycin, and azithromycin (55).

Their mechanisms of action are the same as those seen when treating a bacterial infection and involve interference in protein synthesis. What is unique about the use of the antibiotics is the site of action. The antibiotics affect protein synthesis within the apicoplast (Fig. 34.13). The apicoplast is an organelle found in most Apicomplexa (a group of eukaryotic microorganisms which include plasmodium). The apicoplast is a nonphotosynthesizing plastid with undefined function, although it does contain tRNAs, rRNAs, RNA polymerases, and ribosomal protein and is essential to the parasite's survival. Interference with protein synthesis blocks replication of the apicoplast organelle and therefore prevents a second replication of the life cycle of the plasmodium and thus the prophylactic action. Limitations on the use of doxycycline include children and pregnant women, two major groups of malarial patients; thus, clindamycin and azithromycin are used as back-up drugs. Azithromycin has proven valuable in prophylaxis against *Plasmodium vivax.*

HELMINTH INFECTIONS

Helminthiasis, or worm infestation, is one of the most prevalent diseases—and one of the most serious public health problems—in the world. Many worms are parasitic in humans and cause serious complications. Hundreds of millions (if not billions) of human infections by helminths exist worldwide, and with increased world travel and immigration from developing countries, one might expect to see this pattern of infection continue. It is estimated that one-fourth of the world population may be infected. It is interesting to note that helminths differ from many other parasites in that these organisms multiply outside of the definitive host and have the unique ability to evade host immune defenses for reasons that are not fully understood. As a result, helminth infections tend to be chronic, possibly lasting for the entire lifetime of the host (for a discussion of the uniqueness of helminth infections, see Maizels et al. in *Suggested Readings*). Helminths that infect human hosts are divided into two categories, or phyla: Platyhelminthes (flatworms), and Aschelminthes or nematodes (roundworms). The flatworms include the classes Cestode (tapeworms) and Trematode (flukes or schistosomes). The nematode class includes helminths common to the United States: roundworm, hookworm, pinworm, and whipworm. These worms are cylindrical in shape, with significant variations in size, proportion, and structure.

Nematode Infections

Ancylostomiasis or Hookworm Infection

The two most widespread types of hookworm in humans are the American hookworm (*Necator americanus*) and the "Old World" hookworm (*Ancylostoma doudenale*). The life cycles of both are similar. The larvae are found in the soil and are transmitted either by penetrating the skin or being ingested orally. The circulatory system transports the larvae via the respiratory tree to the digestive tract, where they mature and live for 9 to 15 years if left untreated. These worms feed on intestinal tissue and blood. Infestations cause pulmonary lesions, skin reactions, intestinal ulceration, and anemia. The worms are most prevalent in regions of the world with temperatures of 23°C to 33°C, abundant rainfall, and well-drained, sandy soil.

Enterobiasis or Pinworm Infection (*Enterobius vermicularis*)

These worms are widespread in temperate zones and are a common infestation of households and institutions. The pinworm lives in the lumen of the GI tract, attaching itself by the mouth to the mucosa of the cecum. Mature worms reach 10 mm in size. The female migrates to the rectum, usually at night, to deposit her eggs. This event is noted by the symptom of perianal pruritus. The eggs infect fingers and contaminate nightclothes and bed linen, where they remain infective for up to 3 weeks. Eggs resist drying and can be inhaled with household dust to continue the life cycle. Detection of the worm in the perianal region can be accomplished by means of a cellophane tape swabbed in the perianal region in the evening. The worms can be visible with the naked eye. The eggs can be collected in a similar manner but can only be seen under a microscope.

Ascariasis or Roundworm Infections (*Ascaris lumbricoides*)

These roundworms are common in developing countries, with the adult roundworm reaching 25 to 30 cm in length and lodging in the small intestine. Some infections are without symptoms, but abdominal discomfort and pain are common with heavy infestation. Roundworm eggs are released into the soil, where they incubate and remain viable for up to 6 years. When the egg is ingested, the larvae are released in the small intestine, penetrate the intestinal walls, and are carried via the blood to the lungs. The pulmonary phase of the disease lasts approximately 10 days, with the larvae passing through the bronchioles, bronchi, and trachea before being swallowed and returning to the small intestine. Some patients have reported adult worms exiting the esophagus through the oral cavity, and it is not unusual for live ascaris to be expelled with a bowel movement. Poor or lacking sanitary facilities expose the population to infestation through contaminated foods and beverages.

Trichuriasis or Whipworm Infections (*Trichuris trichiura*)

Infections by this parasite are caused by swallowing eggs from contaminated foods and beverages. The eggs are passed with the feces from an infected individual. These eggs can live in the soil for many years. The ingested eggs hatch in the small intestine, and the larvae embed in the intestinal wall. The worms then migrate to the large intestine, where they mature. Adult worms, which reach approximately 5 cm in length, thread their bodies into the epithelium of the colon. They feed on tissue fluids and blood. Infections from this worm cause symptoms of irritation and inflammation of the colonic mucosa, abdominal pain, diarrhea, and distention. Infections can last 5 or more years if not treated. Whipworm infections are commonly seen in individuals returning from visits to the subtropics and are more common in rural areas of the southeastern United States.

Trichinosis or Trichina Infection (*Trichinella spiralis*)

Trichinella spiralis produces an infection that can be both intestinal and systemic. The worm is found in muscle meat, where the organism exists as an encysted larvae. Traditionally, the worm has been associated with domestic pork that feeds on untreated garbage. More recently, outbreaks have occurred in individuals eating infected game, such as wild boar, bear, or walrus. Trichinosis infections are more likely to occur after consumption of homemade pork or wild-game sausages. After ingestion, the larvae are released from the cyst form and then migrate into the intestinal mucosa. After maturation and reproduction, the newly released larvae penetrate the mucosal lining and are distributed throughout the body, where they enter skeletal muscle. During the adult intestinal stage, diarrhea, abdominal pain, and nausea are the most common symptom, whereas the muscular form of the disease has symptoms that can include muscle pain and tenderness, edema, conjunctivitis, and weakness.

Filariasis

The term "filariasis" denotes infections with any of the Filarioidea, although it is commonly used to refer to lymphatic-dwelling filariae, such as *Wuchereria bancrofti, Brugia malayi,* and *Brugia timori.* Other filarial infections include *Loa loa* and *Onchocerca volvulus.* The latter two are known as the eyeworm and the river blindness worm, respectively. Elephantiasis is the most common disease associated with filariasis. These parasites vary in length from 6 cm for brugia to 50 cm for onchocerca. The incubation periods also vary from 2 months for brugia to 12 months for bancroftian filaria. It is estimated that 400 million persons are infected with human filarial parasites. Depending on the specific organism, various intermediate hosts are involved in spreading the infection. Mosquitoes are involved with the spread of *Wuchereria bancrofti, Brugia malayi,* and *Brugia timori,* whereas the female blackfly spreads river blindness. The larvae released by the female filaria are referred to as microfilariae and commonly can be found in the lymphatics.

Cestode and Trematode Infections

Cysticercosis or Tapeworm Infection

Helminths of this class that are of concern as potential parasites in humans include:

- **Beef tapeworm (*Taenia saginata*).** This worm is found worldwide and infects people who eat undercooked beef. The worm reaches a length of more than 5 m, and it contains approximately 100 segments/m. Each of these segments contains its own reproductive organs.
- **Pork tapeworm (*Taenia solium*).** Pork tapeworms sometimes are called bladder worms and occasionally are found in uncooked pork. The worm attaches itself to the intestinal wall of the human host. The adult worm reaches 5 m in length and, if untreated, survives in the host for many years.
- **Dwarf tapeworm (*Hymenolepis nana*).** This infection is transmitted directly from one human to another without an intermediate host. *Hymenolepis nana* reaches only 3 to 4 cm in length. It is found in temperate zones, and children are most frequently infected.
- **Fish tapeworm (*Diphyllobothrium latum*).** The fish tapeworm reaches a length of 10 m and contains approximately 400 segments/m. These tapeworms attach themselves to the intestinal wall and rob the host of nutrients. They especially absorb vitamin B_{12} and folic acid. Depletion of these critical nutrients, especially vitamin B_{12}, can lead to pernicious anemia. Tapeworm eggs are passed in the patient's feces, and contamination of food and drink can result in transmission of the infection.

Schistosomiasis or Blood Flukes

Three primary trematode species cause schistosomiasis in humans: *Schistosoma hematobium, Schistosoma mansoni,* and *Schistosoma japonicum.* Infections result from the penetration of normal skin by living (free-swimming) cercariae (the name given to the infectious stage of the parasite) with the aid of secreted enzymes. The cercariae develop to preadult forms in the lungs and skin. Then, these parasites travel in pairs via the bloodstream and invade various tissues. The adult worm reaches approximately 2 cm in length. The female deposits her eggs near the capillary beds, where granulomas form. Some of the eggs will move into the lumen of the intestines, bladder, or ureters and are released into the environmental surrounding, where the parasite will seek out the intermediate snail vector. Asexual reproduction occurs in the snail. After a period of time, the cercariae are again released from the snail to continue the cycle. The patients might experience headache, fatigue, fever, and GI disturbances during the early stages of the disease. Hepatic fibrosis and ascites occur during later stages. Untreated patients can harbor as many as 100 pairs of worms. Untreated worms can live 5 to 10 years within the host. As many as 200 million persons worldwide are estimated to be infected with schistosomes. Depending on the species of schistosome, the disease is found in parts of South America, the Caribbean Islands, Africa, and the Middle East.

Drug Therapy for Helminth Infections (56)

Helminths represent a biologically diverse group of parasitic organisms differing in size, life cycle, site of infection (local and systemic), and susceptibility to chemotherapy. With such variation in infectious organisms, it is not surprising that the drugs used to control helminth infections also represent a varied group of chemical classes. As indicated in Table 34.4, the drugs can have fairly narrow spectra of activity (pyrantel pamoate) or a broad spectra of activity (benzimidazoles).

TABLE 34.4 Therapeutic Application of Anthelmintics for Specific Helminth Infections

	M	A	DEC	IVM	PZQ	PP
Nematode Infections:						
Necator americanus	√	√				
Ancylostoma doudenale	√	√				√
Enterobius vermicularis	√			√		√
Ascaris lumbricoides	√	√		√		√
Trichuris trichiura	√	√		√		
Trichinella spiralis	√	√				
Wuchereria bancrofti			√	√		
Brugia malayi			√	√		
Brugia timori.			√			
Loa Loa		√	√	√		
Onchocerca volvulus		√	√	√		
Cestode Infections:						
Taenia saginata	√	√				
Taenia solium	√	√			√√	
Hymenolepis nana	√					
Diphyllobothrium latum					√√	
Trematode Infections:						
Schistosoma hematobium						
Schistosoma mansoni					√√	
Schistosoma japonicum					√	

Benzimidazoles: A, albendazole; DEC, diethylcarbamazine; IVM, ivermectin; M, mebendazole; PP, pyrantel pamoate; PZQ, praziquantel.

Benzimidazoles

The benzimidazoles (Table 34.5) are a broad-spectrum group of drugs discovered in the 1960s with activity against GI helminths. Several thousand benzimidazoles have been synthesized and screened for anthelmintic activity, with albendazole, mebendazole, and thiabendazole representing the benzimidazoles marketed today. The development and chemistry of this class of agents have been reviewed by Townsend and Wise (57).

MECHANISM OF ACTION Two mechanisms have been proposed to account for the action of the benzimidazoles. Fumarate reductase is an important enzyme in helminths that appears to be involved in oxidation of NADH to NAD. The benzimidazoles are capable of inhibiting fumarate reductase (58). Inhibition of fumarate reductase ultimately uncouples oxidative phosphorylation, which is important in adenosine triphosphate production.

A second mechanism and, probably, the primary action of the benzimidazoles is associated with the ability of these drugs to bind to the protein tubulin and, thus, prevent tubulin polymerization to microtubules (59,60). Tubulin is a dimeric protein that is in dynamic equilibrium with the polymeric microtubules. Binding to the tubulin prevents the self-association of subunits and creates a "capping" of the microtubule at the associating end of the microtubule. The microtubulin continues to dissociate from the opposite end, with a net loss of microtubule length. What is interesting is the unique selectivity of the benzimidazoles. Benzimidazole can also bind to mammalian tubulin, but when used as anthelmintics, these drugs are destructive to the helminth, with minimal toxicity to the host. It has been suggested that the

TABLE 34.5 BENZIMIDAZOLE ANTHELMINITICS

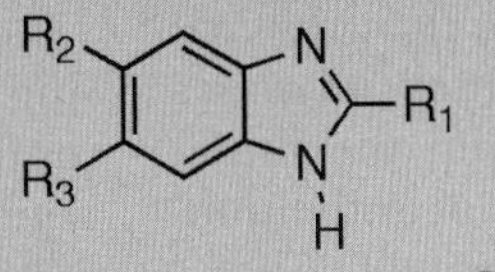

Drugs	Trade name	R1	R2	R3
Thiabendazole	Mintezol	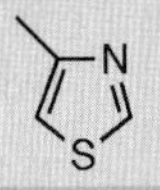	—H	H
Mebendazole	Vermox	—N(H)-C(=O)-OCH$_3$	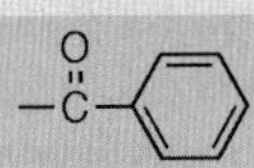	H
Albendazole	Zental	—N(H)-C(=O)-OCH$_3$	—SCH$_2$CH$_2$CH$_3$	H
Triclabendazole	Egaten[1] Fasinex*	—S-CH$_3$	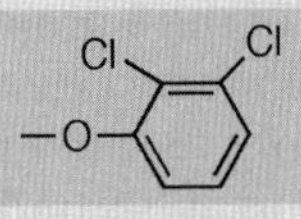	Cl
Fenbendazole	Several brand names*	—N(H)-C(=O)-OCH$_3$	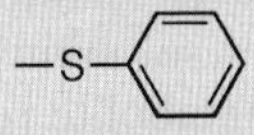	H
Flubendazole		—N(H)-C(=O)-OCH$_3$	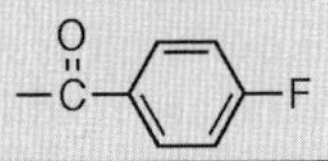	

[1]Egaten has recently been shown to be useful for treatment of fascioliasis by WHO. *Used in veterinary practice for protection and treatment of parasite and worm infections.

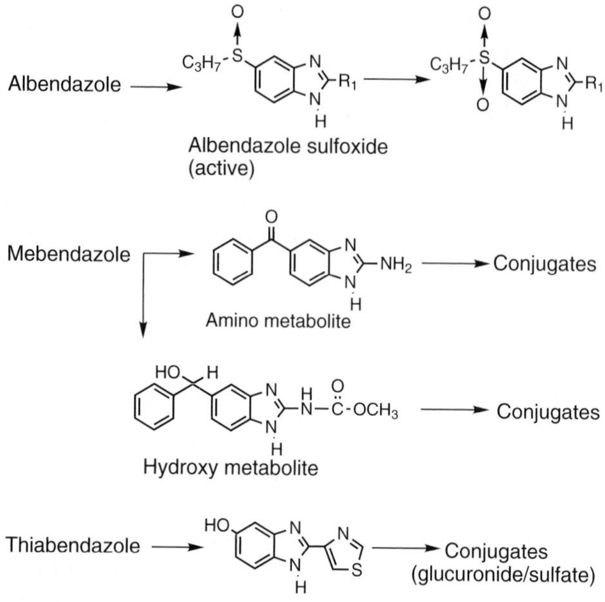

FIGURE 34.19 Metabolism of benzimidazoles.

selectivity is associated with differing pharmacokinetics between binding to the two different tubulin proteins.

Metabolism The benzimidazoles have limited water solubility and, as a result, are poorly absorbed from the GI tract (a fatty meal will increase absorption). Poor absorption can be beneficial, because the drugs are used primarily to treat intestinal helminths. To the extent that the drugs are absorbed, they undergo rapid metabolism in the liver and are excreted in the bile (Fig. 34.19) (61,62). In most cases, the parent compound is rapidly and nearly completely metabolized with oxidative and hydrolytic processes predominating. The phase 1 oxidative reaction commonly is a cytochrome P450–catalyzed reaction, which can then be followed by a phase 2 conjugation.

Albendazole is unique in two ways. First, the presence of a thioether substituent at the five position increases the likelihood of sulfur oxidation. Second, the initial metabolite, albendazole sulfoxide, is a potent anthelmintic. This initial oxidation is catalyzed principally (70%) by CYP3A4 and CYP1A2 and (30%) by flavin-containing monooxygenase, giving rise to a compound that is bound to plasma protein. This intermediate has an expanded utility in that it has been shown to be active against the hydatid cyst found in echinococciasis, a tapeworm disease (63). Further oxidation by cytochrome P450 leads to the inactive sulfone. Additional metabolites of the sulfone have been reported that include carbamate hydrolysis to the amine and oxidation of the 5-propyl side chain. These reactions occur only to a minor extent.

Metabolism of mebendazole occurs primarily by reduction of the 5-carbonyl to a secondary alcohol, which greatly increases the water solubility of this compound. An additional phase 1 metabolite resulting from carbamate hydrolysis has been reported as well. Both the secondary alcohol and the amine are readily conjugated (a phase II metabolism). Evidence would suggest that the anthelmintic activity of mebendazole resides in the parent drug and none of the metabolites.

Thiabendazole is metabolized through aromatic hydroxylation at the five position catalyzed by CYP1A2. The resulting phenol is conjugated to 5-hydroxythiabendazole glucuronide and 5-hydroxythiabendazole sulfate, respectively. The initial metabolite and minor amount of N_1-methylthiabendazole (from a methylation phase 2 reaction) have been reported to be teratogenic in mice and rats.

Therapeutic Application As indicated in Table 34.4, mebendazole and albendazole have a wide spectrum of activity against intestinal nematodes. The drugs are useful and effective against mixed infections. The adverse reactions are commonly GI in nature (nausea, vomiting, and diarrhea). Both drugs have been reported to be teratogenic in rats and, therefore, should not be used during the first trimester of pregnancy. A third drug of this class is thiabendazole, which remains of some value in treatment of strongyloidiasis, as an alternate drug, and cutaneous larva migrans (creeping eruption), for which it is the drug of choice. Thiabendazole is commonly used in veterinary medicine. The drug is less commonly used because of associated toxicity. Thiabendazole has been reported to cause Stevens-Johnson syndrome and has the potential for hepatotoxicity and crystalluria.

Diethylcarbamazine (Hetrazan)

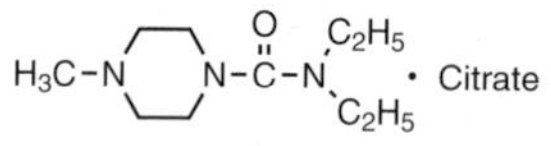

Diethylcarbamazine citrate

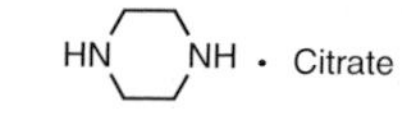

Piperazine citrate

Discovered in the 1940s, diethylcarbamazine (DEC) has proven to be especially effective as a filaricidal agent. The incidence of filariasis among American troops during World War II necessitated a search for drugs with an antifalarial spectrum of activity. The once-popular piperazine also was discovered during these initial screenings. Although chemically similar, the activity again helminths is quite different. Piperazine is active against nematodes, whereas DEC is active against falaria and microfalaria (64).

Mechanism of Action Although studied extensively, the mechanism of action of DEC remains unknown. DEC appears to be the active form of the drug, with a very rapid onset of action (within minutes), but of interest is the fact that the drug is inactive in vitro, suggesting that activation of a cellular component is essential to the filaricidal action. Three mechanisms have been suggested. The first is involvement of blood platelets triggered by the action of filarial excretory antigens. A complex reaction is thought to occur between the drug, the antigen, and platelets (65). Although these authors were unable to show a direct action of the drug on the microfalaria, a more recent study showed that DEC produced morphologic damage to the microfalaria. The damage consisted of the loss of the cellular sheath, exposing antigenic determinants to immune defense mechanisms. Severe damage then occurred to microfalaria organelles, leading to death (66). The second is inhibition of microtubule polymerization and disruption of preformed microtubules (67). The third is interference with arachidonic acid metabolism (68). DEC is known to have anti-inflammatory action, which appears to involve blockage at cyclooxygenase and leukotriene A_4 synthase (leukotriene synthesis). This action appears to alter vascular and cellular adhesiveness and cell activation. This latter action would suggest a possible relationship between the first and third mechanism.

METABOLISM The metabolism of DEC leads to the compounds shown in Figure 34.20 plus trace amounts of methylpiperazine and piperazine. Nearly all of the metabolites appear in the urine. As much as 10% to 20% of the drug is excreted unchanged. As indicated by the rapid action of the drug, it would appear that none of the metabolites are involved in the therapeutic action of DEC.

THERAPEUTIC APPLICATION DEC citrate is freely soluble in water, is rapidly absorbed, and is effective against microfilariae. The drug does not appear to be effective against the adult worm. In general, the drug has mild adverse effects, but under some conditions, it can produce severe adverse reactions, including anaphylactic reactions, intense pruritus, and ocular complications (69). The severe anaphylactic reaction is known as the Mazzotti reaction, and it appears to be an immune response related to the presence of dead microfilariae. This reaction is more common in individuals who have a high-load microfilarial infection, and it can preclude the use of DEC in some patient populations (56).

Ivermectin (Stromectol)

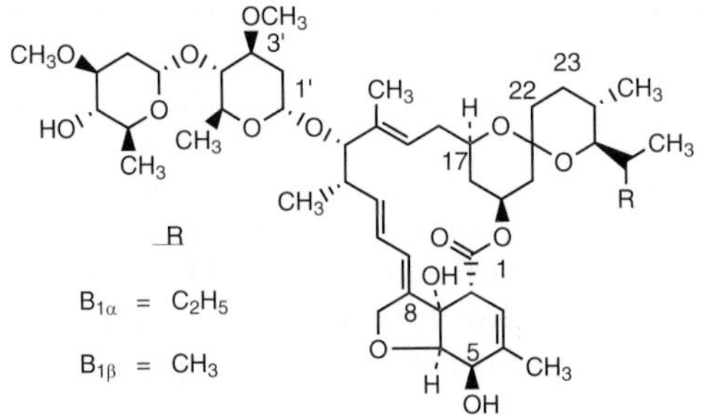

Ivermectin

Extracted from the soil actinomycete *Streptomyces avermitilis,* the natural avermectins are 16-membered macrocyclic lactones that are an 80:20 mixture of avermectin $B_{1\alpha}$ and $B_{1\beta}$, respectively, and are used under the generic name abamectin. As such the product is used for the control of various insects, mite pests, fire ants and as a veterinary antihelminthic. Reduction of the $C_{22\text{-}23}$ double bond gives

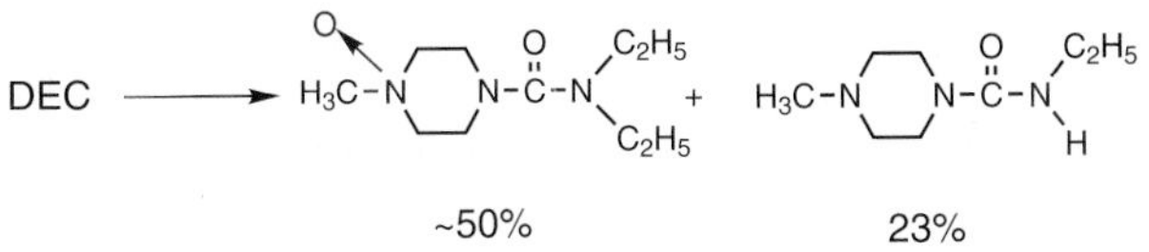

FIGURE 34.20 Metabolism of diethylcarbamazine (DEC).

rise to ivermectin (IVM), which is an 80:20 mixture of dihydroavermectin $B_{1\alpha}$ and $B_{1\beta}$, respectively. The natural avermectins have minimal biologic activity, but IVM has proven to be quite beneficial in the treatment of various nematode infections.

MECHANISM OF ACTION Two mechanisms of action are thought to be involved in the action of IVM (56,70). The first is an indirect action in which motility of microfalaria is reduced, which in turn allows cytotoxic cells of the host to adhere to the parasite, resulting in elimination from the host. This action can occur by virtue of the ability of IVM to act either as a γ-aminobutyric acid (GABA) agonist or as an inducer of chloride ion influx, leading to hyperpolarization and muscle paralysis. The chloride ion influx appears to be the more plausible mechanism (71). Recently, it has been shown that IVM binds irreversibly to the glutamate-gated chloride channel of the nematode *Haemonchus contortus,* whereas the channel is in an open conformation. The binding then remains locked in the open conformation, allowing ions to cross the membrane, leading to the paralytic action of IVM (72). The result of this action is a rapid decrease in microfilarial concentrations.

A second action of IVM leads to the degeneration of microfilariae in utero. This action would result in fewer microfilariae being released from the female worms, and it occurs over a longer period of time. The presence of degenerated microfilariae in utero prevents further fertilization and production of microfilariae.

METABOLISM IVM is rapidly absorbed, is bound to a great extent to plasma protein, and is excreted in the urine or feces either unchanged or as the 3′-*O*-demethyl-22,23-dihydroavermectin $B_{1\alpha}$ or as the dihydroavermectin $B_{1\alpha}$ monosaccharide. The absorption of IVM is significantly affected by the presence of alcohol. Administration of IVM as an alcoholic solution can result in as much as a 100% increase in absorption.

THERAPEUTIC APPLICATION Although IVM has activity against a variety of microfalaria, including *Wuchereria bancrofti, Brugia malayi, Loa loa,* and *Mansonella ozzardi,* as well as activity against *Strongyloides stercoralis,* the drug is used primarily in the treatment of onchocerciasis (African river blindness) caused by *Onchocerca volvulus.* It is estimated that 20 million people are affected by this condition and an additional 123 million are at risk of the infection. The drug is effective against both the eyeworm as well as skin infections of *O. volvulus*. IVM has the distinct advantage over DEC in that IVM can be used as a single dose (150 μg/kg) once a year (although there is support for dosing every 6 months), has far less likelihood of causing the potentially fatal anaphylactic reaction (Mazzotti reaction), and can be used for mass treatment programs.

Praziquantel (Biltricide)

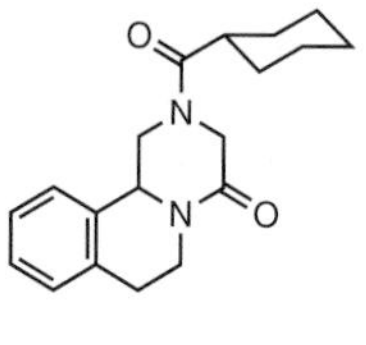

Praziquantel

Praziquantel (PZQ) is an isoquinoline derivative with most of the biologic activity found in the levo enantiomer. The compound has no activity against nematodes, but it is highly effective against cestodes and trematodes.

Mechanism of Action More than one mechanism of action can exist for PZQ, possibly depending on the type of parasite being treated. The mechanism of action appears to involve Ca^{2+} redistribution either directly or indirectly. In the case of helminths found in the lumen of the host (cestode infection), the drug leads to muscle contraction and paralysis, leading in turn to worm expulsion. Additionally, PZQ has been shown to inhibit phosphoinositide metabolism, which by an undetermined mechanism leads to the worm paralysis (73). With intravascular-dwelling schistosomes, PZQ leads to drug-induced damage of the tegument of the worm. As a result, antigens in the helminth are subject to attack by immune antibodies of the host (74,75). An antigen–antibody immunologic reaction leads to the death of the parasite. Finally, PZQ affects glycogen content and energy metabolism (76,77).

Metabolism PZQ is rapidly absorbed and undergoes hepatic first-pass metabolism. The metabolites are either less active or inactive and consist of hydroxylated compounds. In the serum, the major metabolite appears to be the monohydroxylated 4-hydroxycyclohexylcarboxylate, whereas in the urine, 50% to 60% of the initial PZQ exists as dihydroxylated products (Fig. 34.21) (78). These hydroxylation reactions are catalyzed by CYP2B6 and CYP3A4. The metabolites would be expected to exist in the conjugated form in the urine.

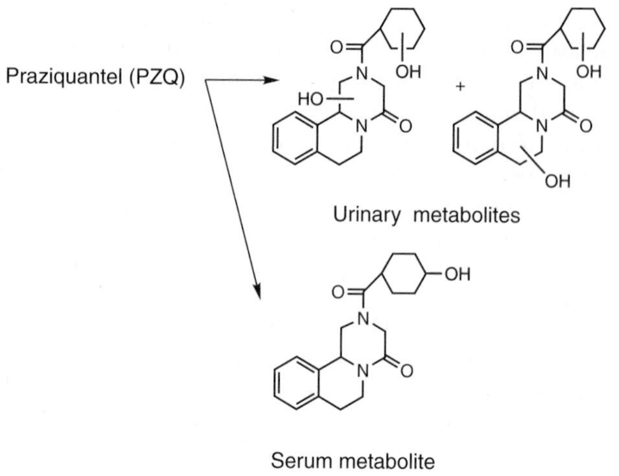

FIGURE 34.21 Metabolism of praziquantel (PZQ).

Therapeutic Application PZQ is the drug of choice for treatment of schistosomiasis and liver flukes (trematode and cestode infections). The drug is stage specific, with activity against the invasive stages, which includes the cercariae and young schistosomula and the mature worms, but not against the liver stages. Although an approved drug, PZQ is considered to be an investigational drug by the FDA in the treatment of schistosomiasis and liver flukes. The drug has a bitter taste and, therefore, should not be chewed. The side effects are usually not severe and consist of abdominal discomfort (pain and diarrhea). Mounting evidence suggests that resistance can become a significant problem.

Oxamniquine (Mansil, Vansil)

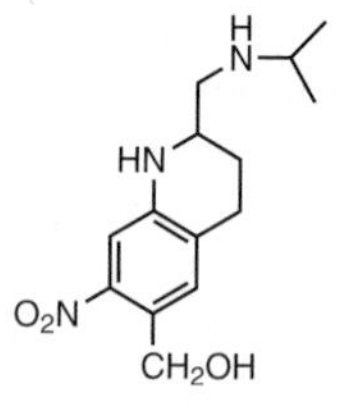

Oxamniquine

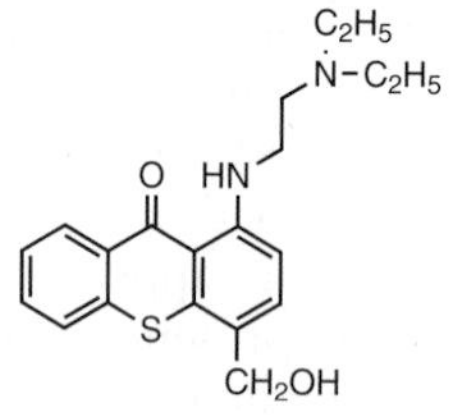

Hycanthone

Oxamniquine was originally investigated in the 1960s and was found to have limited antiprotozoal activity, with activity against *Schistosoma mansoni* but no activity against the other two schistosomal organisms. In addition, the drug is stage specific, with activity against cercariae and very young schistosomula and adult worms. For unknown reasons, the drug is more effective against adult male worms than against female worms. The drug has structural similarity to hycanthone, which is no longer used because of severe toxicity and teratogenic effects.

Mechanism of Action Oxamniquine is activated by the organism via esterification to a biologic ester that spontaneously dissociates to an electrophile, which alkylates the helminth DNA, leading to irreversible inhibition of nucleic acid metabolism (Fig. 34.22) (77). Resistant helminths do not esterify oxamniquine; therefore, activation does not occur. Other metabolic reactions consist of oxidative reactions, leading to inactivation (Fig. 34.22). The metabolites are excreted primarily in the urine.

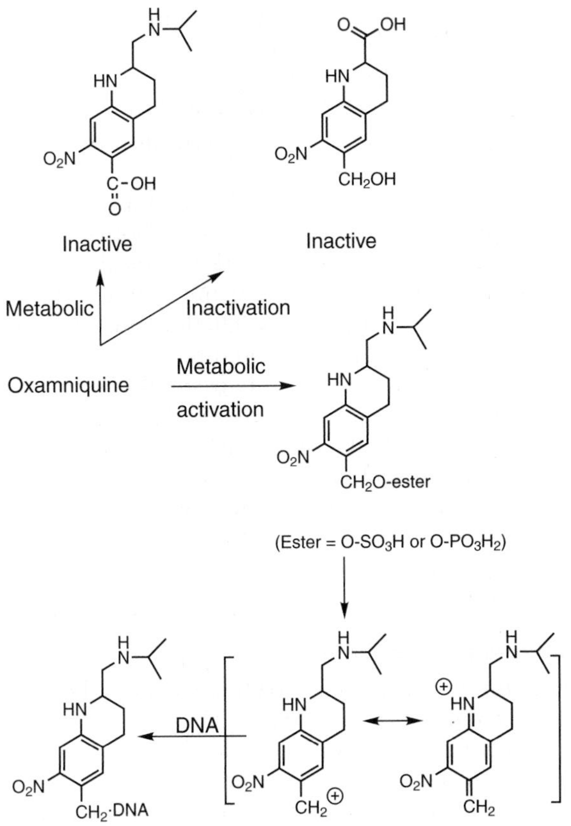

FIGURE 34.22 Metabolism of oxamniquine accounting for the mechanism of action and inactivation.

THERAPEUTIC APPLICATION Oxamniquine is readily absorbed following oral administration and has a relatively short half-life. The drug has been highly effective against *Schistosoma mansoni* native to Brazil, where it is marketed under the trade name Mansil. It is also beneficial against west African *S. mansoni* and is supplied under the trade name Vansil. Side effects are minimal, with transient dizziness being reported. The major drawback is its high cost. Encouraging outcomes have been reported with the combination of oxamniquine and PZQ.

Pyrantel Pamoate (Antiminth)

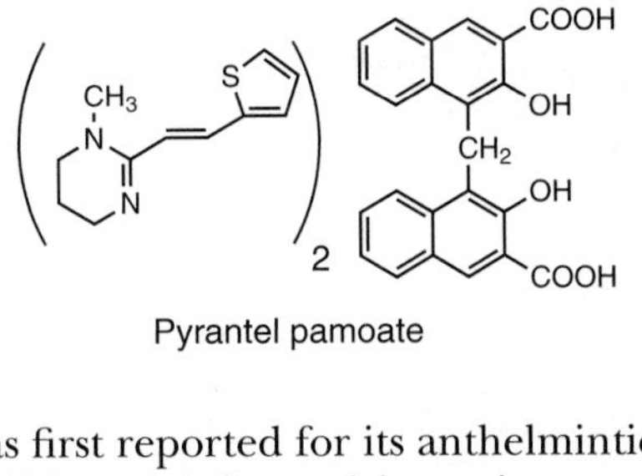

Pyrantel pamoate

Pyrantel was first reported for its anthelmintic activity in 1966 (79). Although it has activity against most intestinal roundworm infections, it has not been approved by the FDA for treatment of these infestations. It is considered to be the drug of choice in the treatment of pinworms. The drug is used as the pamoate salt, which is quite insoluble and, as a result, is not readily absorbed. This property improves the usefulness of the drug for treatment of intestinal helminths. In addition to its value in treating enterobiasis, the drug is effective for hookworm and roundworm (ascariasis) infections. Pyrantel acts as a depolarizing neuromuscular blocking agent that activates nicotinic receptors and inhibits cholinesterase, ultimately leading to worm paralysis.

ECTOPARASITIC INFECTIONS

Three parasitic organisms that cause common topical infections are *Sarcoptes scabiei,* which is responsible for scabies, *Pediculus humanus,* which is responsible for lice infections, and *Cimex lectularius,* which is the common bedbug, an insect living exclusively on the blood of warm-blooded animals. This latter organism has shown a recent reemergence, and although its bite normally is not responsible for a primary or secondary infection, the topical irritation and the social implications can be quite disturbing to the patient. The only treatment is the use of antipruritics and the hiring of a professional exterminator.

Scabies

Scabies, commonly referred to as the "seven-year itch," is a condition caused by *Sarcoptes scabiei,* or the itch mite. The condition is commonly spread by direct, person-to-person contact, although the organism is capable of living for 2 to 3 days in clothing, bedding, or house dust. Sharing of clothing is a common means whereby the condition spreads. The organism burrows into the epidermis, usually in the folds of the skin of the fingers, the elbows, female breast, penis, scrotum, and buttocks. The female parasite lays eggs in the skin, which then hatch and mature to adults. The itch mite can live for 30 to 60 days. The infections are most common in children, but they may also be found in adults in institutional settings. The primary symptom of severe itching can foster secondary infections at the site of scratching. Because of the potential for spread to other members of a family, it is common to treat all members of the family. This will prevent reinfection from a second family member after successful therapy of the first family member.

Lice

Pediculosis, or lice, is caused by any of the following parasites: *Pediculus humanus capitis,* the head louse; *Pediculus humanus corporis,* the body louse; or *Phthirus pubis,* the crab louse (found in the genital area). Lice are bloodsucking insects that live for 30 to 40 days on the body of the host. The organisms reproduce, and the female lays her eggs, the nits, which become attached to hair. The nits are white in color and hatch in 8 to 10 days. For the parasite to live, it must feed on blood, which it sucks through punctures in the skin. A hypersensitivity reaction occurs at these puncture sites, which then leads to pruritus, host scratching, and possible secondary infection. In addition to the scalp and skin, the eyebrows, eyelids, and beard can become sites of infection. The transfer of infection can occur through person-to-person contact and from infected clothing, on which the organism can survive for up to 1 week. The sharing of clothing is a common means for the spread of body lice. Head lice are quite common among children in grade school, whereas crab lice are common among individuals who are sexually active. Treatment of family members is recommended, and clothing and bed linens should be removed and washed in very hot water.

Drug Therapy for Scabies and Pediculosis

Lindane (Kwell)

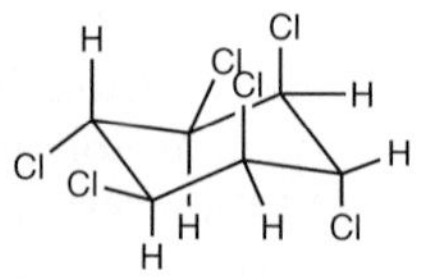

γ-Benzene hexachloride

Chlorination and reduction of benzene leads to a mixture of hexachlorocyclohexanes. The insecticidal activity resides primarily in the γ-isomer of hexachlorocyclohexane (γ-benzene hexachloride). The compound is thought to produce its insecticidal action by virtue of a CNS stimulatory action that occurs by blockage of GABA. The compound is readily absorbed through the chitinous exoskeleton of the parasite. Unfortunately, lindane is also readily absorbed through intact human skin, especially the scalp, and has the potential for systemic neurotoxicity in the host. Infants and children and, possibly, the elderly are most prone to the neurotoxic effects of the drug. Because the lindane is quite lipophilic and is applied to the scalp as a shampoo, it can be absorbed, where upon it can readily enter the CNS of the patient producing signs of neurotoxicity (convulsions, dizziness, clumsiness, and unsteadiness).

The drug is available in a lotion and a shampoo and is recommended for the treatment of both pediculosis and scabies. When using the lotion topically, it should be applied to dry skin, covering the entire surface and being left in place for 8 hours. The lindane then should be removed by washing thoroughly. If the shampoo is used for *Pediculosis capitis,* the hair should be cleaned of oil and dried before application of the lindane shampoo. The shampoo is then worked into the hair and scalp, being applied in such a way as to prevent other parts of the body from coming into contact with the drug. After approximately 4 minutes, the drug is removed by washing with water, and the hair is dried and then combed with a fine-toothed comb to remove nits.

Pyrethrum and Pyrethroids

The naturally occurring pyrethrums have been used as insecticides since the 1800s. These compounds are extracted from the flowering portion of the chrysanthemum plant. The flowers produced in Kenya have, on average, 1.3% pyrethrins. These pyrethrum extracts are a major agricultural product for that country.

Chemistry The chrysanthemum extract is a mixture of esters consisting of the acids chrysanthemic and pyrethric and the alcohols pyrethrolone and cinerolone (Fig. 34.23). The esters are prone to hydrolysis and oxidation and, as a result, should be stored in the cold and protected from light. Because of the high cost, limited availability, and rapid degradation, synthetic derivatives

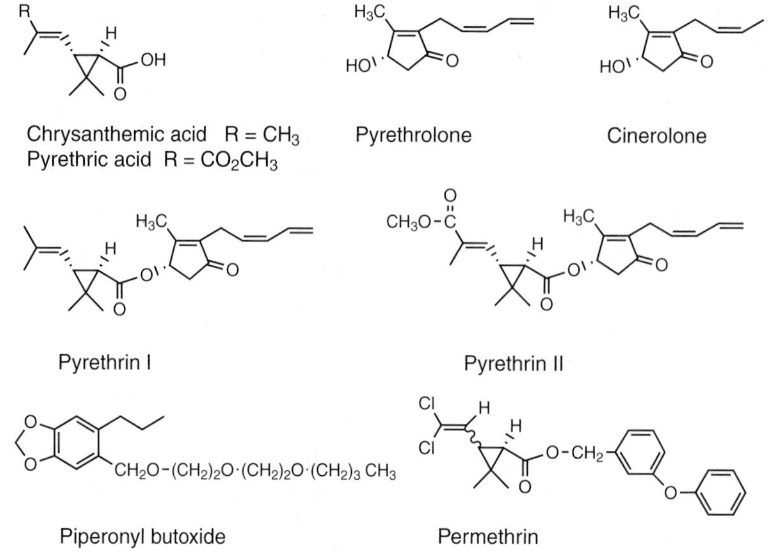

FIGURE 34.23 Structures of pyrethrum and pyrethroid.

have been investigated. The result has been the preparation of pyrethroids, the synthetic derivatives of pyrethrins. The compound used therapeutically is permethrin, which exists as a 60:40 mixture of *trans:cis* isomers.

Mechanism of Action (80–83) The pyrethrins and pyrethroids (permethrin) are nerve membrane sodium channel toxins that do not affect potassium channels. The compounds bind to specific sodium channel proteins and slow the rate of inactivation of the sodium current elicited by membrane depolarization and, as a result, prolong the open time of the sodium channel. At low concentrations, the pyrethroids produce repetitive action potentials and neuron firing; at high concentrations, the nerve membrane is depolarized completely and excitation blocked.

The receptor interaction of the pyrethrums with the sodium channel complex is stereospecific and dependent on the stereochemistry of the carboxylic acid. In the case of the pyrethroids, the most active isomers are the *1R*,3-*cis*- and *1R*,3-*trans*-cyclopropanecarboxylates. The *1S*-*cis*- and -*trans*-isomers are inactive and actually are antagonists to the action of the *1R*-isomers.

Metabolism A property that enhances the usefulness of the pyrethrums and pyrethroids is that these compounds are highly toxic to the ectoparasites but relatively nontoxic to mammals if absorbed. The apparent lack of toxicity is associated with the rapid metabolism of these drugs through hydrolysis and or oxidation (Fig. 34.24) (84,85). The nature of the metabolism (i.e., hydrolysis vs. oxidation) is dependent on the structure of the pyrethrins or pyrethroids. Oxidation of the *trans*-methyl of the isobutylene in the carboxyl moiety initially gives an alcohol, which then proceeds to the carboxylic acid, whereas epoxidation of the terminal alkene of the alcohol portion of pyrethrin I gives either the 1,2-diol or the 1,4-diol. No ester hydrolysis is reported. Permethrin is hydroxylated on the terminal aromatic ring at either the 4- or 2-position, is oxidized on the methyl group of the dimethylcyclopropane, and is hydrolyzed at the ester moiety. The rapid breakdown of these agents also accounts for their low persistence in the environment.

Therapeutic Application

Pyrethrins (A-200, RID) Because of the high cost and rapid degradation of the pyrethrins, they are usually combined with piperonyl butoxide, a synergist (Fig. 34.23). Piperonyl butoxide has no insecticidal activity in its own right but is thought to inhibit the cytochrome P450 enzyme of the insect, thus preventing an oxidative inactivation of the pyrethrins by the parasite. The combination is used in a 10:1 ratio of piperonyl butoxide to pyrethrins. The mixture is used for treatment of *Pediculus humanus capitis*, *Pediculus humanus corporis*, and *Phthirus*

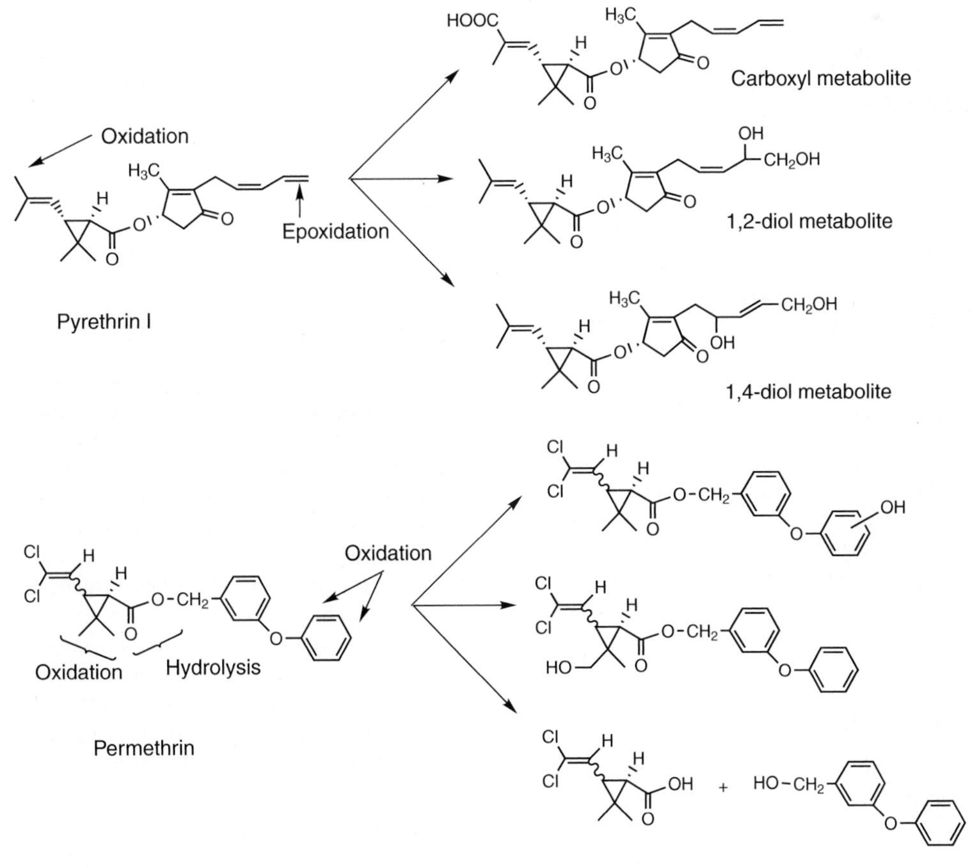

FIGURE 34.24 Metabolism of pyrethrin I and permethrin.

pubis. Various dosage forms are available, including a gel, shampoo, and topical solution.

Permethrin (Nix-1% lotion, Elimite-5% Cream) Permethrin, because of its increased stability and its availability synthetically, is not used with a synergist. The compound is used in a 1% lotion for the treatment of pediculosis capitis and in a 5% cream as a scabicide.

CROTAMITON Crotamiton is available as a 10% cream for the treatment of scabies, although it is less effective than pyrethrins or permethrin (86,87). Because crotamiton may need to be applied a second time for successful treatment of scabies but the pyrethrins or permethrin require a single application, poor patient compliance with crotamiton can reduce its effectiveness. The advantage of crotamiton over lindane comes from the fact that lindane has potential neurotoxicity if absorbed, especially in infants and children, whereas crotamiton has less systemic neurotoxicity. The most common side effect reported for crotamiton is skin irritation.

SPINOSAD (NATROBA)

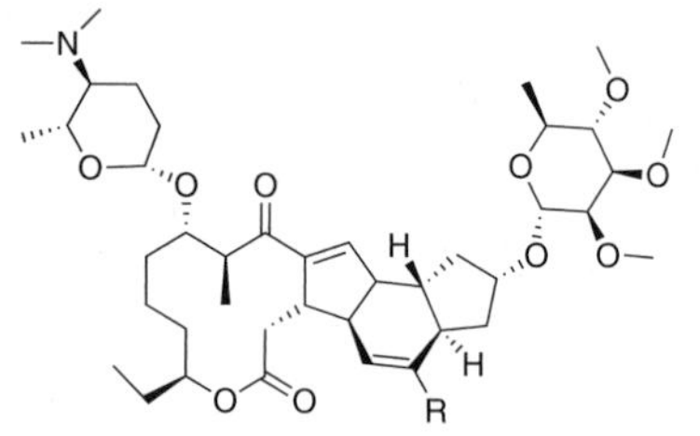

Spinosad (Natroba)

(Spinosyn A R = H, Spinosyn D, R = CH_3)

Spinosad is a newly FDA-approved treatment for head lice infestation (*Pediculus humanus capitis*). The product is available as a 0.9% topical suspension, which is applied to a dry scalp and hair for a period of 10 minutes and is then rinsed with water. Because spinosad has ovicidal activity, nit combing is not required. Studies suggest that spinosad, which requires a single treatment, is more effective (~80%) than permethrin (~45%), especially after a single treatment. Fewer topical adverse events were noted with spinosad versus permethrin, and presently resistance, a growing problem with the permethrin, has not been reported for spinosad (88).

Spinosad is a naturally occurring 12-member macrolide that consists of a mixture of spinosyn A and D produced by the bacterium *Saccharopolyspora spinosa*, a member of the actinomycete family. The product was a serendipitous discovery isolated from a soil sample found in an abandoned rum distillery on a Caribbean island by an employee of Eli Lilly. The mixture has a broad spectrum of activity and was approved for agricultural use by the Environmental Protection Agency in 1995 (89).

The mechanism of action has been investigated and found to lead to death of the insect via rapid excitation of the insect's nervous system. Spinosad is an insecticide by virtue of its ability to act as an agonist at the nicotinic acetylcholine receptors and, more specifically, at the Da6 subunit (90,91). Thus, spinosad has a novel mechanism of action compared to other insecticides. The results are that spinosad creates prolonged hyperexcitation of the CNS of the insects and eventually paralysis and death of the organism.

SCENARIO: OUTCOME AND ANALYSIS

Outcome

Elizabeth B. Hirsch, PharmD, BCPS

After reviewing JB's medication list, it was discovered that the over-the-counter nighttime cough syrup he started taking yesterday contained a small amount of alcohol (ethanol). It is believed the oral metronidazole in combination with the ethanol caused a disulfiram-like reaction, resulting in nausea, vomiting, and dizziness. The pharmacist advised JB to discontinue the offending cough syrup and recommended another safer non–ethanol-containing medication.

Chemical Analysis

Victoria Roche and S. William Zito

Ethanol is primarily metabolized by sequential hepatic oxidation, first to acetaldehyde by alcohol dehydrogenase (ADH) and then to acetic acid by aldehyde dehydrogenase (ALDH). Certain antibacterials, including metronidazole, have been implicated in the ability to act similarly to disulfiram, causing a disulfiram-like reaction. Disulfiram irreversibly inhibits the oxidation of acetaldehyde, causing a considerable increase in acetaldehyde concentrations following ethanol ingestion; this is known as the disulfiram–ethanol reaction. Disulfiram's ability to react with sulfhydryl groups on essential proteins (generating diethyldithiocarbamate in the process) is believed to be important to its activity. Signs and symptoms of a disulfiram–ethanol reaction are due to high acetaldehyde concentrations and include facial and body warmth and flushing, conjunctival injection, pruritus, urticaria, diaphoresis, lightheadedness, vertigo, headache, nausea, vomiting, and abdominal pain. Cardiac effects include dyspnea, palpitations, and chest pain.

(*Continued*)

SCENARIO: OUTCOME AND ANALYSIS *(Continued)*

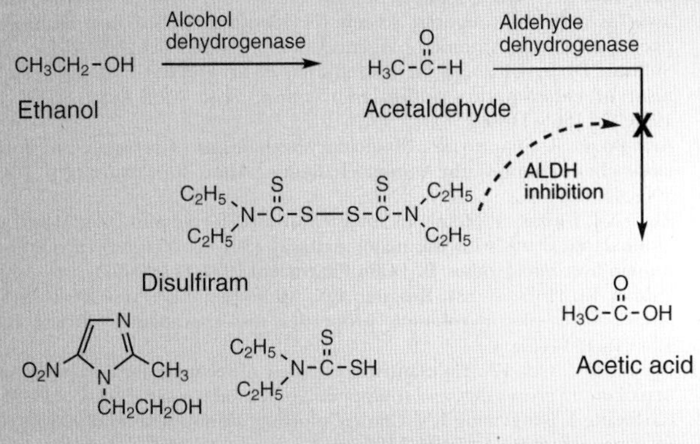

Metronidazole Diethyldithiocarbamate

The true incidence of disulfiram-like reactions during metronidazole treatment is difficult to estimate. Unfortunately, most reports citing this adverse effect arise from case reports, which may be confounded by patient comorbidities, polypharmacy, and/or use of other drugs of abuse. More recent literature has called the mechanism of this reaction (with metronidazole) into question. Certainly, metronidazole's lack of a disulfide moiety capable of engaging in a redox reaction with free sulfhydryl groups on biologically relevant proteins would argue against an identical mechanism of action. A relatively recent article confirms that metronidazole "neither inhibits ALDH of the liver nor increases blood acetaldehyde" (92). However, the slight inhibition of ADH by metronidazole may explain some of the alcohol intolerance symptoms observed when alcohol is consumed during therapy (nausea, dizziness, blurred vision). It was also demonstrated that the "disulfiram-like reaction" induced by metronidazole may be due to the synergistic activity it has with ethanol in elevating central serotonin levels, which has been termed "serotonergic duplication" by these authors (92).

Despite the lack of ALDH inhibiting action by metronidazole, most clinicians continue to counsel patients on the avoidance of alcohol (or alcohol-containing medications) during metronidazole treatment, as the unpleasant symptoms observed are real despite the difference in mechanism.

CASE STUDY

Victoria Roche and S. William Zito

DD is a 28-year-old woman who recently completed a PhD in Public Health. A person with a strong social conscience, she has been very troubled by the continuing suffering of the Haitian people more than 1 year after the devastating 2010 earthquake. She and her husband, who finished his PhD in civil engineering a month after DD defended her thesis, decided to spend the next year in Port-au-Prince using their professional expertise and commitment to global health to help in any way possible with the rebuilding.

Three months into their Haitian service immersion they found out that DD was pregnant, but she felt certain she could continue in her service mission until it was time to deliver. However, 2 weeks later, with the onset of the rainy season, she fell ill with what was ultimately diagnosed as "water-borne diarrhea" caused from exposure to *Giardia* parasites in standing water. In light of her early pregnancy, they have flown home to ensure that she receives the proper medical treatment and totally recovers before they return to Haiti to complete their mission. She is staying well-hydrated and is now about to be placed on an antiprotozoal agent to help eradicate the offending *Giardia lamblia* organism.

Because of her pregnancy, DD is taking no medications other than the vitamins and supplements recommended by her obstetrician. As the pharmacist consulting with her medical team, consider the structure of the three potential therapeutic choices below and make the best antiprotozoal drug product selection for this patient.

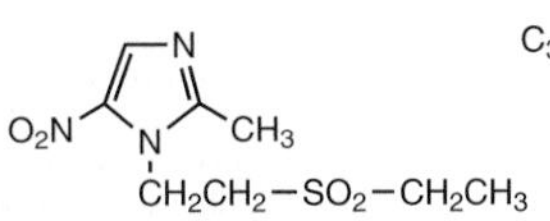

1

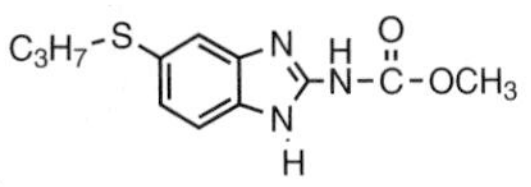

2

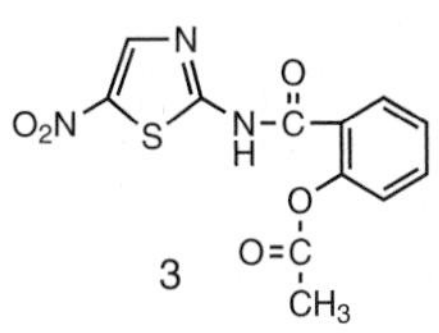

3

1. Conduct a thorough and mechanistic SAR analysis of the three therapeutic options in the case.
2. Apply the chemical understanding gained from the SAR analysis to this patient's specific needs to make a therapeutic recommendation.

References

1. El-Sayed NM, Myler PJ, Blandin G, et al. Comparative genomics of trypanosomatid parasitic protozoa. Science 2005;309:404–409.
2. El-Sayed NM, Myler PJ, Bartholoneu DS, et al. The genome sequence of *Trypanosoma cruzi*, etiologic agent of Chagas' disease. Science 2005;309:409–415.
3. Berriamn M, Ghedin E, Hertz-Fowler C, et al. The genome of the African trypanosome *Trypanosoma brucei*. Science 2005;309:416–422.
4. Barrett MP, Burchmore RJB, Stich A, et al. The trypanosomiases. Lancet 2003;362:1469–1480.
5. DoCampo R. Sensitivity of parasites to free radical damage by antiparasitic drugs. Chem Biol Interact 1990;73:1–27.
6. Lau AH, Lam NP, Piscitelli SC, et al. Clinical pharmacokinetics of metronidazole anti-infectives. Clin Pharmacokinet 1992;23:328–364.
7. Koch R, Beaulieu BB, Chrystal EJT, et al. Metronidazole metabolite in urine and its risk. Science 1981;211:399–400.
8. Drugs for parasitic infections. Med Lett 1998;40:1–12.
9. The choice of antibacterial drugs. Med Lett 1998;40:33–42.
10. Sisson G, Goodwin A, Raudonikiene A, et al. Enzyme associated with reductive activation and action of nitazoxanide, nitrofurans, and metronidazole in *Helicobacter pylori*. Antimicrob Agents Chemother 2002;46:2116–2123.
11. Stockis A, DeBruyn S, Gengler C, et al. Nitazoxanide pharmacokinetics and tolerability in man during 7 days dosing with 0.5 g and 1 g b.i.d. Int J Clin Pharmacol Ther 2002;40:221–227.
12. Nitazoxanide (Alinia)—a new antiprotozoal agent. Med Lett 2003;45:29–31.
13. Vohringer H-F, Arasteh K. Pharmacokinetic optimization in the treatment of *Pneumocystis carinii* pneumonia. Clin Pharmacokinet 1993;24:388–412.
14. Fishman JA. Treatment of infections due to *Pneumocystis carinii*. Antimicrob Agents Chemother 1998;42:1309–1314.
15. Fry M, Pudney M. Site of action of the antimalarial hydroxymaphthoquinoine, 2-[*trans*-4-(4′-chlorophenyl)cyclohexyl]-3-hydroxy-1,4-naphthoquinone (566C80). Biochem Pharmacol 1992;43:1545–1553.
16. Hughes WT, Gray VL, Gutteridge WE, et al. Efficacy of a hydroxynaphthoquinone, 566C80, in experimental *Pneumocystis carinii* pneumonitis. J Antimicrob Chemother 1990;34:225–228.
17. Allegra CJ, Kovacs JA, Drake JC, et al. Activity of antifolates against *Pneumocystis carinii* dihydrofolate reductase and identification of a potent new agent. J Exp Med 1987;165:926–931.
18. Koda RT, Dube' MP, Li WY, et al. Pharmacokinetics of trimetrexate and dapsone in AIDS patients with *Pneumocystis carinii* pneumonia. J Clin Pharmacol 1999;39:268–274.
19. Wang CC. Molecular mechanisms and therapeutic approaches to the treatment of African trypanosomiasis. Annu Rev Pharmacol Toxicol 1995;35:93–127.
20. Edwards KJ, Jenkins T, Neidle S. Crystal structure of a pentamidine–oligonucleotide complex: implications for DNA-binding properties. Biochemistry 1992;31:7104–7109.
21. Shapiro T, Englund PT. Selective cleavage of kinetoplast DNA minicircles promoted by antitrypanosomal drugs. Proc Natl Acad Sci U S A 1990;87:950–954.
22. Dykstra CC, Tidwell RR. Inhibition of topoisomerase from *Pneumocystis carinii* by aromatic dicationic molecules. J Protozool 1991;38:78S–81S.
23. Metcalf BW, Bey P, Danzin C, et al. Catalytic irreversible inhibition of mammalian ornithine decarboxylase (E.C. 4.1.1.17) by substrate and product analogues. J Am Chem Soc 1978;100:2551–2553.
24. Bacchi CJ, Nathan HC, Hutner SH, et al. Polyamine metabolism: a potential therapeutic target in trypanosomes. Science 1980;210:332–334.
25. Poulin R, Lu L, Ackermann B, et al. Mechanism of the irreversible inactivation of mouse ornithine decarboxylase by α-difluoromethylornithine. J Biol Chem 1992;267:150–158.
26. Bacchi CJ, Garofalo J, Ciminelli M, et al. Resistance to DL-α-difluoromethylornithine by clinical isolates of *Trypanosoma brucei rhodeniense*: role of S-adenosylmethionine. Biochem Pharmacol 1993;46:471–481.
27. Henderson GB, Ulrich P, Fairlamb AH, et al. "Subversive" substrates for the enzyme trypanothione disulfide reductase. Alternative approach to chemotherapy of Chagas' disease. Proc Natl Acad Sci U S A 1988;85:5374–5378.
28. Cana JD, Bollo S, Nunez-Vergara LJ, et al. *Trypanosoma cruzi*: effect and mode of action of nitroimidazole and nitrofuran derivatives. Biochem Pharmacol 2003;65:999–1006.
29. Fairlamb AH, Henderson GB, Cerami A. Trypanothione is the primary target for arsenical drugs against African trypanosomes. Proc Natl Acad Sci U S A 1989;86:2607–2611.
30. Berman JD. Chemotherapy for leishmaniasis: biochemical mechanisms, clinical efficacy, and future strategies. Rev Infect Dis 1988;10:560–586.
31. Cook GC. Leishmaniasis: some recent developments in chemotherapy. J Antimicrob Chemother 1993;31:327–330.
32. Singh S, Sivakumar R. Challenges and new discoveries in the treatment of leishmaniasis. J Infect Chemother 2004;10:307–331.
33. Griewank K, Gazeau C, Eichhorn A et al. Miltefosine efficiently eliminates *Leishmania major* amastigotes from infected murine dendritic cells without altering their immune functions. Antimicrob Agents Chemother 2010;54:652–659.
34. Ward SA. Mechanisms of chloroquine resistance in malarial chemotherapy. Trends Pharmacol Sci 1988;9:241–246.
35. Hempelmann E. Hemozoin biocrystallization in *Plasmodium falciparum* and the antimalarial activity of crystallization inhibitors. Parasitol Res 2007;100:671–676.
36. Kurosawa Y, Dorn A, Kitsuji-Shirane M, et al. Hematin polymerization assay as a high-throughput screen for identification of new antimalarial pharmacophores. Antimicrob Agents Chemother 2000;44:2638–2644.
37. Sullivan DJ Jr, Gluzman IY, Russell DG, et al. On the molecular mechanism of chloroquine's antimalarial action. Proc Natl Acad Sci U S A 1996;93:11865–11869.
38. Arav-Boger R, Shapiro TA. Molecular mechanisms of resistance in antimalarial chemotherapy: the unmet challenge. Annu Rev Pharmacol Toxicol 2005;45:565–585.
39. Zhao X-J, Ishizaki T. Metabolic interactions of selected antimalarial and non-antimalarial drugs with the major pathway (3-hydroxylation) of quinine in human liver microsomes. Br J Clin Pharmacol 1997;44:505–511.
40. Palmer KJ, Holliday SM, Brogden RN. Mefloquine: a review of its antimalarial activity, pharmacokinetic properties, and therapeutic efficacy. Drugs 1993;45:430–475.
41. Bryson HM, Goa KL. Halofantrine: a review of its antimalarial activity, pharmacokinetic properties, and therapeutic potential. Drugs 1992;43:236–258.
42. Karbwang J, Bangchang KN. Clinical pharmacokinetics of halofantrine. Clin Pharmacokinet 1994;27:104–119.
43. Augusto O, Schrieber J, Mason RP. Direct ESR detection of a free radical intermediate drug in the peroxidase-catalyzed oxidation of the antimalarial drug primaquine. Biochem Pharmacol 1988;37:2791–2797.
44. Mihaly GW, Ward SA, Edwards G, et al. Pharmacokinetics of primaquine in man: identification of the carboxylic acid derivative as a major plasma metabolite. Br J Clin Pharmacol 1984;17:441–446.
45. Ferone R, Burchall JJ, Hitchings GH. *Plasmodium berghei* dihydrofolate reductase isolation, properties, and inhibition by antifolates. Mol Pharmacol 1969;5:49–59.
46. Triglia T, Cowman AF. Primary structure and expression of the dihydropteroate synthetase gene of *Plasmodium falciparum*. Proc Natl Acad Sci U S A 1994;91:7149–7153.
47. Olliaro P. Mode of action and mechanisms of resistance for antimalarial drugs. Pharmacol Ther 2001;89:207–219.
48. Cumming JN, Ploypradith P, Posner GH. Antimalarial activity of artemisinin (Qinghaosu) and related trioxanes: mechanism(s) of action. Adv Pharmacol 1997;37:253–297.
49. Meshnick SR, Taylor TE, Kamchonwongpaisan S. Artemisinin and the antimalarial endoperoxides: from herbal remedy to targeted chemotherapy. Microbiol Rev 1996;60:301–315.
50. Posner GH, Cumming JN, Woo S-H, et al. Orally active antimalarial 3-substituted trioxanes: new synthetic methodology and biological evaluation. J Med Chem 1998;41:940–951.
51. Cumming JN, Wang D, Shapiro TA, et al. Design, synthesis, derivatization, and structure–activity relationships of simplified, tetracyclic, 1,2,4-trioxane alcohol analogues of the antimalarial artemisinin. J Med Chem 1998;41:952–964.
52. Eckstein-Ludwig, Webb RJ, van Goethem DK, et al. Artemisinins target the SERCA of *Plasmodium falciparum*. Nature 2003;424:957–961.
53. Hencken CP, Kalinda AS, D'Angelo JG. The anti-infective and anti-cancer properties of artemisinin and its derivatives. Ann Rev Med Chem 2009;44:359–378.
54. Rosenthal PJ. Antimalarial drug discovery: old and new approaches. J Exp Biol 2003;206:3735–3744.
55. Wiesner J, Ortmann R, Jomaa H, et al. New antimalarial drugs. Angew Chem Int Ed 2003;42:5274–5293.
56. de Silva N, Guyatt H, Bundy D. Anthelmintics: a comparative review of their clinical pharmacology. Drugs 1997;53:769–786.
57. Townsend LB, Wise DS. The synthesis and chemistry of certain anthelmintic benzimidazoles. Parasitol Today 1990;6:107–112.
58. Prichard RK. Mode of action of the anthelmintic thiabendazole in *Haemonchus contortus*. Nature 1970;228:684–685.
59. Friedman PA, Platzer EG. Interaction of anthelmintic benzimidazoles and benzimidazole derivatives with bovine brain tubulin. Biochim Biophys Acta 1978;544:605–614.
60. Lacey E. Mode of action of benzimidazoles. Parasitol Today 1990;6:112–115.
61. Braithwaite PA, Roberts MS, Allan RJ, et al. Clinical pharmacokinetics of high-dose mebendazole in patients treated for hydatid disease. Eur J Clin Pharmacol 1982;22:161–169.
62. Gottschall DW, Theodorides EJ, Wang R. The metabolism of benzimidazole anthelmintics. Parasitol Today 1990;6:115–124.
63. Marriner SE, Morris DL, Dickson B, et al. Pharmacokinetics of albendazole in man. Eur J Clin Pharmacol 1986;30:705–708.
64. Hawking F. Diethylcarbamazine and new compounds for the treatment of filariasis. Adv Pharmacol Chemother 1979;16:129–194.
65. Cesbron J-Y, Capron A, Vargaftig BB, et al. Platelets mediate the action of diethylcarbamazine on microfilariae. Nature 1987;325:533–536.
66. Florencio MS, Peixoto CA. The effect of diethylcarbamazine on the ultrastructure of microfilariae of *Wuchereria bancrofti*. Parasitology 2003;126:551–554.

67. Fujimaki Y, Ehara M, Kimura E, et al. Diethylcarbamazine, antifilarial drug, inhibits microtubule polymerization and disrupts preformed microtubules. Biochem Pharmacol 1990;39:851–856.
68. Maizels RM, Denham DA. Diethylcarbamazine (DEC): immunopharmacological interactions of an antifilarial drug. Parasitol 1992;105:S49–S60.
69. Mackenzie CD. Diethylcarbamazine: a review of its action in onchocerciasis, lymphatic filariasis, and inflammation. Trop Disease Bull 1985;82:R1–R37.
70. Goa KL, McTavish D, Clissold SP. Ivermectin: a review of its antifilarial activity, pharmacokinetic properties and clinical efficacy in onchocerciasis. Drugs 1991;42:640–658.
71. Ottesen EA, Campbell WC. Ivermectin in human medicine. J Antimicrob Chemother 1994;34:195–203.
72. Forrester SG, Beech RN, Prichard RK. Agonist enhancement of macrocyclic lactone activity at a glutamate-gated chloride channel subunit from *Haemonchus contortus*. Biochem Pharmacol 2004;67:1019–1024.
73. Wiest PM, Li Y, Olds GR, et al. Inhibition of phosphoinositide turnover by praziquantel in *Schistosoma mansoni*. J Parasitol 1992;78:753–755.
74. Xiao S-H, Catto BA, Webster LT Jr. Effects of praziquantel on different developmental stages of *Schistosoma mansoni* in vitro and in vivo. J Infect Dis 1985;151:1130–1137.
75. Fallon PG, Cooper RO, Probert AJ, et al. Immune-dependent chemotherapy of schistosomiasis. Parasitology 1992;105:S41–S48.
76. Utzinger J, Keiser J, Shuhua X, et al. Combination chemotherapy of schistosomiasis in laboratory studies and clinical trials. Antimicrob Agents Chemother 2003;47:1487–1495.
77. Cioli D, Pica-Mattoccia L, Archer S. Antischistosomal drugs: past, present … and future? Pharmacol Ther 1995;68:35–85.
78. Buhring KU, Diekmann HW, Muller H, et al. Metabolism of praziquantel in man. Eur J Drug Metab Pharmacokinet 1978;3:179–190.
79. Austin WC, Courtney WC, Danilewicz W, et al. Pyrantal tartrate, a new anthelmintic effective against infections of domestic animals. Nature 1966;212:1273–1274.
80. Narahashi T. Nerve membrane ionic channels as the primary target of pyrethroids. Neurotoxicology 1985;6:3–22.
81. Vijverberg HPM, de Weille JR. The interaction of pyrethroids with voltage-dependent Na channels. Neurotoxicology 1985;6:23–34.
82. Grammon DW, Sanders G. Pyrethroid–receptor interactions: stereospecific binding and effects on sodium channels in mouse brain preparations. Neurotoxicology 1985;6:35–46.
83. Lombet A, Mourre C, Lazdunski M. Interaction of insecticides of the pyrethroid family with specific binding sites on the voltage-dependent sodium channel from mammalian brain. Brain Res 1988;459:44–53.
84. Soderund DM. Metabolic consideration in pyrethroid design. Xenobiotica 1992;22:1185–1194.
85. Ruzo LO, Casida JE. Metabolism and toxicology of pyrethroids with dihalovinyl substituents. Environ Health Perspect 1977;21:285–292.
86. Taplin D, Meinkin TL, Joaquin BA, et al. Comparison of crotamiton 10% cream (Eurax) and permethrin 5% cream (Elimite) for the treatment of scabies in children. Pediatr Dermatol 1990;7:67–73.
87. Amer M, El-Ghariband I. Permethrin versus crotamiton and lindane in the treatment of scabies. Int J Dermatol 1992;31:357–358.
88. Stough D, Shellabarger S, Quiring J, et al. Efficacy and safety of spinosad and permethrin cream rinses for pediculosis capitis (head lice). Pediatrics 2009;124:e389–e395.
89. Spinosad: a new organically acceptable insecticide. Available at: www.jlgardencenter.com/uploads/handouts/Spinosad.pdf. Accessed March 13, 2011.
90. Millar NS, Denholm I. Nicotinic acetylcholine receptors: targets for commercially important insecticides. Invert Neurosci 2007;7:53–66.
91. Salgado VL, Sheets JJ, Watson GB. Studies on the mode of action of spinosad: the internal effective concentration and the concentration dependence of neural excitation. Pest Biochem Physiol 1998;60:103–110.
92. Karamanakos PN, Pappas P, Boumba VA, et al. Pharmaceutical agents known to produce disulfiram-like reaction: effects of hepatic ethanol metabolism and brain monoamines. Int J Toxicol 2007;26:423–432.

Suggested Readings

Freeman CD, Klutman EE, Lamp KC. Metronidazole: a therapeutic review and update. Drugs 1997;54:679–708.
Greenwood BM, Fidock DA, Kyle DE, et al. Malaria: progress, perils, and prospects for eradication. J Clin Invest 2008;118:1266–1276.
Maizels RM, Bundy DAP, Selkirk ME, et al. Immunological modulation and evasion by helminth parasites in human populations. Nature 1993;365: 797–805.
Wilson JD, Braunwald E, Isselbacher KJ, et al., eds. Harrison's Principles of Internal Medicine, 12th Ed. New York: McGraw-Hill, 1991:772.

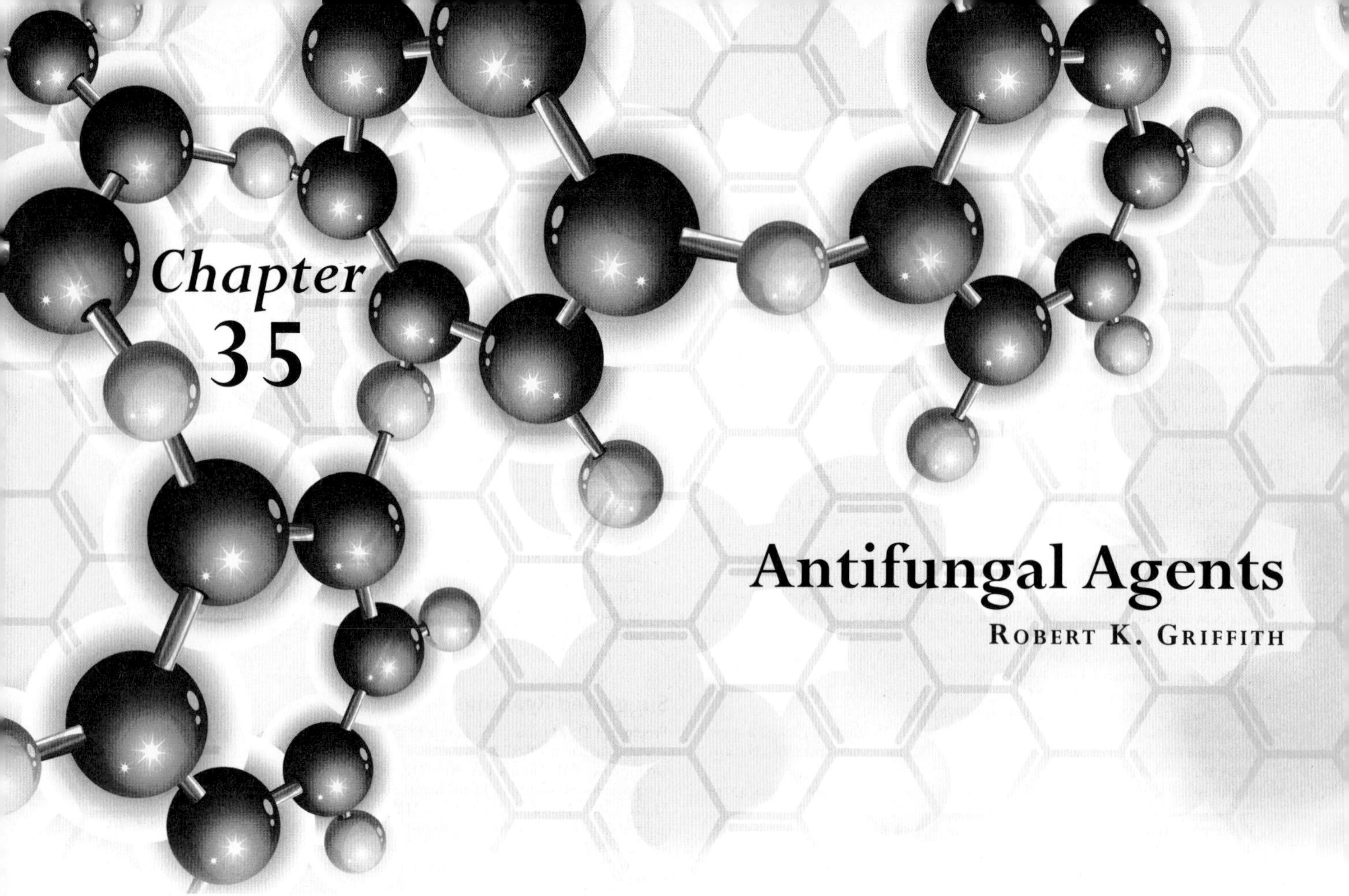

Chapter 35

Antifungal Agents

Robert K. Griffith

*Drugs Covered in This Chapter**

Polyenes
- Amphotericin B
- Natamycin
- Nystatin

Azoles
- Butoconazole
- Clotrimazole
- Econazole
- Miconazole
- Oxiconazole
- Sertaconaole
- Sulconazole
- Terconazole
- Tioconazole

Allylamines
- Butenafine
- Naftifine
- Terbinafine

Morpholines
- *Amorolfine*

Echinocandins
- Anidulafungin
- Caspofungin
- Micafungin

Miscellaneous agents
- Ciclopirox
- Flucytosine
- Griseofulvin
- Haloprogin
- Tolnaftate
- Undecylenic acid

Abbreviations

AUC, area under the curve
CNS, central nervous system
5-FU, 5-fluorouracil
IV, intravenous

Scenario

Douglas Slain, Pharm.D. BCPS

A 55 year old Caucasian female with a history of atrial fibrillation, rheumatoid arthritis, and diabetes mellitus is diagnosed with moderate pulmonary histoplasmosis. The patient is started on itraconazole in the hospital and sent home after a three day stay on itraconazole 200 mg orally twice a day for 8–10 weeks. Her other medications are metformin, prednisone, and digoxin. After about a week of her itraconazole therapy she started to feel very nauseated and tired. She called the pharmacist to see if this could be from the itraconazole. The patient's daughter also told the pharmacist that her mother's pulse rate was very low (50 BPM). The pharmacist recognized that this was more consistent with too much digoxin and referred her to her physician.

(The reader is directed to the clinical solution and chemical analysis of this case at the end of the chapter).

*Drugs listed include those available inside and outside of the United States; drugs available outside of the United States are shown in italics.

INTRODUCTION

Until recently, chemotherapy of fungal infections has lagged far behind chemotherapy of bacterial infections. This lack of progress has resulted, in part, because the most common fungal infections in humans have been relatively superficial infections of the skin and mucosal membranes, and potentially lethal deep-seated infections have been quite rare. Because most humans with a normally functioning immune system are able to ward off invading fungal pathogens with little difficulty, the demand for improvements in antifungal therapy has been small. Immunocompromised patients, however, are very susceptible to invasive fungal infections. The onset of the AIDS epidemic, combined with the increased use of powerful immunosuppressive drugs for organ transplants and cancer chemotherapy, has resulted in a greatly increased incidence of life-threatening fungal infections and a corresponding increase in demand for new agents to treat these infections. The number of effective antifungal agents available is quite small compared to those available to treat bacterial infections, but research in this area is quite active. Several new agents have been introduced in the last few years.

FUNGAL DISEASES

The fungal kingdom includes yeasts, molds, rusts, and mushrooms. Most fungi are saprophytic, which means that they live on dead organic matter in the soil or on decaying leaves or wood. A few of these fungi can cause opportunistic infections if they are introduced into a human through wounds or by inhalation. Some of these infections can be fatal. There are relatively few obligate animal parasites (i.e., microorganisms that can only live on mammalian hosts) among the fungi, although *Candida albicans* is commonly found as part of the normal flora of the gastrointestinal tract and vagina. The obligatory parasites are limited to dermatophytes that have evolved to live on/in the keratin-containing hair and skin of mammals, where they cause diseases such as ringworm and athletes foot. (Ringworm is not caused by a parasitic worm but, rather, is named for the ring-like appearance of this fungal infection of the skin.) A detailed description of fungal infections is beyond the scope of this book, but comprehensive treatises are available (1).

Most fungal infections are caused primarily by various yeasts and molds. Yeasts, such as the opportunistic pathogen *Candida albicans* and the baker's yeast *Saccharomyces cerevisiae*, typically grow as single oval cells and reproduce by budding. *C. albicans* and some other pathogenic yeasts also can grow in multicellular chains called hyphae. Infection sites may contain both yeast and hyphal forms of the microorganism. Molds, such as *Trichophyton rubrum*, one of the causative agents of ringworm, grow in clusters of hyphae called a mycelium. All fungi produce spores, which may be transported by direct contact or through the air. Although most topical fungal infections are readily treated, the incidence of life-threatening systemic fungal infections, including those caused by yeasts such as *C. albicans* and molds such as *Aspergillus fumigans* are increasing, and mortality remains high (2).

Dermatophytes

Dermatophytes are fungi causing infections of skin, hair, and nails (3). The dermatophytes obtain nutrients by attacking the cross-linked structural protein keratin, which other fungi cannot use as a food source. Dermatophytic infections, known as tinea, are caused by various species of three genera (*Trichophyton, Microsporum,* and *Epidermophyton*) and are named for the site of infection rather than for the causative organism. Tinea capitis is a fungal infection of the hair and scalp. Tinea pedis refers to infections of the feet, including athlete's foot, tinea manuum to fungal infection of the hands, tinea cruris to infection of the groin (jock itch), and tinea unguium to infection of the fingernails. Athlete's foot in particular may be an infection involving several different fungi, including yeasts. Tinea unguium, also known as onychomycosis, whether of the fingernails or toenails, can be particularly difficult to treat, because the fungi invade the nail itself. Appropriate drug therapy prevents the fungus from spreading to the newly formed nail. Penetration of drugs into previously existing nail is problematic, however, and with some drug regimens, the infection is not cured until an entirely new, fungus-free nail has grown in. Because this can take months, patient compliance with a lengthy drug regimen can be a problem.

Yeasts

The most common cause of yeast infections is *Candida albicans,* which is part of the normal flora in a significant portion of the population where it resides in the oropharynx, gastrointestinal tract, vagina, and surrounding skin (4). It is the principal cause of vaginal yeast infections and oral yeast infections (thrush). These commonly occur in mucosal tissue when the normal population of flora has been disturbed by treatment of a bacterial infection with an antibiotic or when growth conditions are changed by hormonal fluctuations, such as occur in pregnancy. *C. albicans* can cause infections of the skin and nails, although the latter are not common. In persons with healthy immune systems, *Candida* infections are limited to superficial infections of the skin and mucosa. In persons with impaired immune systems, however, *C. albicans* also may cause deep-seated systemic infections, which can be fatal. Several other infections with *Candida* species occur, including *C. tropicalis, C. krusei, C. parapsilosis,* and *C. glabrata* (also known as *Torulopsis glabrata*). These organisms are becoming more common and often do not respond to antifungal therapy as readily as *C. albicans.*

CLINICAL SIGNIFICANCE

Antifungal agents include diverse compounds with varied actions. A few key examples can highlight the importance of medicinal chemistry to clinical practice. Knowledge about the molecular structure of polyene antifungal agents, such as amphotericin B, is essential for understanding how they work. These agents are macrocyclic lactones with distinct hydrophilic and lipophilic regions. One of the putative mechanisms of polyene action involves the formation of pores in the fungal cell membrane. The lipophilic regions of the polyene molecules facilitate the binding to the cell membrane sterols. The hydrophilic portions of the molecule align to create a hydrophilic pore in the sterol-containing cell membrane. As a result, there is membrane depolarization and increased membrane permeability and, eventually, fungal cell death. The lipophilic regions of amphotericin B also contribute to its poor solubility in aqueous solutions.

The traditional intravenous formulation of amphotericin B includes a dispersing agent, deoxycholate, which facilitates formation of the required micellar dispersion when administered in a 5% dextrose in water solution. 5-Flucytosine (5-FC) is an analogue of the natural pyrimidine cytosine that is converted to 5-fluorouracil (5-FU) in susceptible fungi. Formation of 5-FU is essential to the antimycotic effect of 5-FC; 5-FU acts as a pyrimidine antimetabolite and is phosphorylated to the cytotoxic agent 5-fluorodeoxyuridine monophosphate. All of these facts are commonly emphasized in a medicinal chemistry sequence, and readers probably are aware that 5-FU is a chemotherapeutic agent that causes myelosuppression as its major toxicity. Therefore, it should not be surprising that the same side effect can be seen in patients receiving 5-FC. The newest antifungals, echinocandins, are macromolecular structures with high molecular weights (1,000 dalton), which can be visualized easily by looking at the chemical structure. Their relatively low volume of distribution in the body can be partially explained by their size. Clinically, these agents have not achieved high concentrations in the central nervous system and the vitreous chamber of the eye, two compartments that are subject to fungal invasion.

Douglas Slain, PharmD, BCPS
Associate Professor
College of Pharmacy
West Virginia University

Cryptococcus neoformans is a yeast commonly found in bird droppings, particularly pigeon droppings (5). When dust contaminated with spores is inhaled by persons with a competent immune system, the organism causes a minor, self-limiting, lung infection. Such infections frequently are mistaken for a cold, and medical treatment is not sought. In immunocompromised persons, however, the organism can be carried by the circulatory system from the lungs to many other organs of the body, including the central nervous system (CNS). Infection of the CNS is uniformly fatal unless treated.

Although most yeast infections are caused by various species of *Candida* or *Cryptococcus*, other yeasts also can cause infections in humans, including *Malassezia furfur*, *Trichosporon beigelii*, and *Blastoschizomyces capitatus* (6). These infections are relatively rare and are difficult to treat.

Thermally Dimorphic Fungi (Endemic Mycoses)

Thermally dimorphic fungi are saprophytes that grow in one form at room temperature and in a different form in a human host at 37°C (7). The most common infectious agents are *Blastomyces dermatitidis*, *Paracoccidioides brasiliensis*, *Coccidioides immitis*, and *Histoplasma capsulatum*, the causative agents of blastomycosis, paracoccidiomycosis, coccidiomycosis (valley fever), and histoplasmosis, respectively. All these organisms live in soil and cause disease through inhalation of contaminated dust. The resulting lung infections are often mild and self-limiting, but they may progress to a serious lung infection. The circulatory system may transport the organisms to other tissues, where the resulting systemic infection may be fatal. *B. dermatitidis* is endemic to south central United States and *P. brasiliensis* to Central and South America, where it is the most common cause of fungal pulmonary infections. *C. immitis* is endemic to the dry areas of the southwestern United States and northern Mexico. It is particularly prevalent in the San Joaquin Valley of California, hence the name valley fever. *H. capsulatum* is endemic to the Mississippi and Ohio River valleys of the United States, where nearly 90% of the population tests positive for exposure to the organism.

Molds

Various *Aspergillus* species are found worldwide and are virtually ubiquitous in the environment. The most common organisms causing disease are *A. fumigatus*, *A. niger*, and *A. flavus*. Several other *Aspergillus* species are known to cause infection, and some, such as *A. nidulans*, are becoming more common. *Aspergillus* spp. very rarely cause disease in persons with normal immune systems but are very dangerous to persons with suppressed immune systems. Because *Aspergillus* spores are everywhere, inhalation is the most common route of inoculation, but infection through wounds, burns, and implanted devices (e.g., catheters) also is possible. Nosocomial (hospital-derived) aspergillosis is a major source of infection in persons with leukemia and in those receiving organ or bone marrow transplants. Aspergillosis of the lungs may be contained, but systemic aspergillosis has a high mortality rate.

Zygomycosis (mucormycosis) is a term used to describe infections caused by the genera *Rhizopus*, *Mucor*, and *Absidia* of the fungal order Mucorales (8). As with several other opportunistic fungal pathogens, these soil microorganisms generally are harmless to those with a competent immune system but can cause rapidly developing, fatal infections in an immunosuppressed patient. These organisms can infect the sinus cavity, from which they spread rapidly to the CNS. Blood vessels also may be attacked and ruptured. Zygomycoses spread rapidly and are often fatal.

BIOCHEMICAL TARGETS FOR ANTIFUNGAL CHEMOTHERAPY

Antifungal chemotherapy depends on biochemical differences between fungi and mammals (9,10). Unlike bacteria, which are prokaryotes, both fungi and mammals are eukaryotes, and the biochemical differences between them are not as great as one might expect. At the cellular level, the greatest difference between fungal cells and mammalian cells is that fungal cells have both a cell membrane and an outer cell wall whereas mammalian cells have only a cell membrane. The fungal cell wall therefore is a logical target for a similar class of drugs, which would be expected to be potent antifungals yet have little human toxicity. Only recently, however, have a few potent inhibitors of fungal cell wall biosynthesis become available for clinical use (11). Other targets for antifungal agents include inhibitors of DNA biosynthesis, disruption of mitotic spindles, and general interference with intermediary metabolism. The difference between fungal and mammalian cells that is most widely exploited, however, is that the cell membranes of fungi and mammals contain different sterols. Sterols are important structural components of both fungal cell and mammalian cell membranes and are critical to the proper functioning of many cell membrane enzymes and ion-transport proteins. Mammalian cell membranes contain cholesterol as the sterol component, whereas fungal cell membranes contain ergosterol (12).

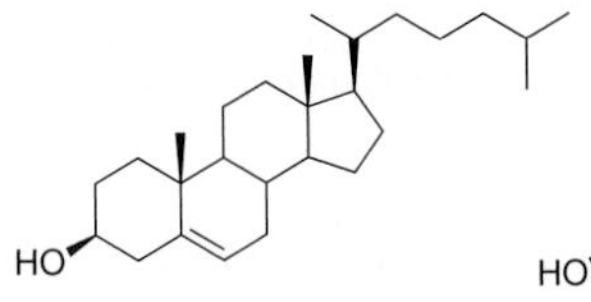

Cholesterol

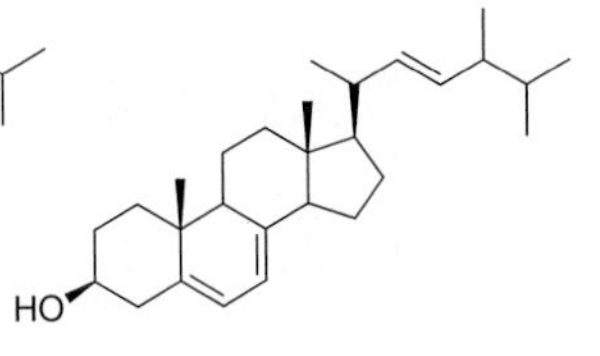

Ergosterol

Although the two sterols are quite similar, the side chains are slightly different, and when three-dimensional models are constructed, the ring system of ergosterol is slightly flatter because of the additional double bonds in the B ring. Nevertheless, with only a few exceptions, this difference in sterol components provides the biochemical basis of selective toxicity for most of the currently available antifungal drugs.

Polyene Membrane Disruptors: Amphotericin B, Nystatin, and Congeners

Before the mid-1950s, effective antifungal therapy was limited to topical applications of undecylenic acid derivatives, mixtures of benzoic acid and salicylic acid, and a few other agents of modest efficacy. No reliable treatments existed for the few cases of deep-seated systemic fungal infections that did occur. The discovery of the polyene antifungal agents, however, provided a breakthrough into both a new class of antifungal agents and the first drug to be effective against deep-seated fungal infections (13). The polyenes are macrocyclic lactones with distinct hydrophilic and lipophilic regions. The hydrophilic region contains several alcohols, a carboxylic acid, and usually, a sugar. The lipophilic region contains, in part, a chromophore of four to seven conjugated double bonds. The number of conjugated double bonds correlates directly with antifungal activity in vitro and, inversely, with the degree of toxicity to mammalian cells. That is, not only are the compounds with seven conjugated double bonds, such as amphotericin B, approximately 10-fold more fungitoxic, they are the only ones that may be used systemically (14).

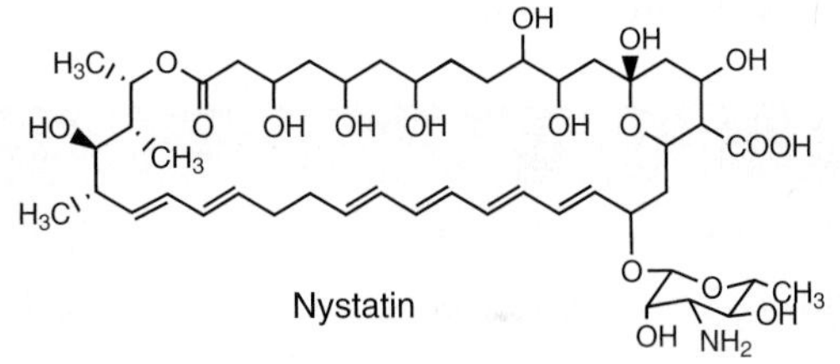
Nystatin

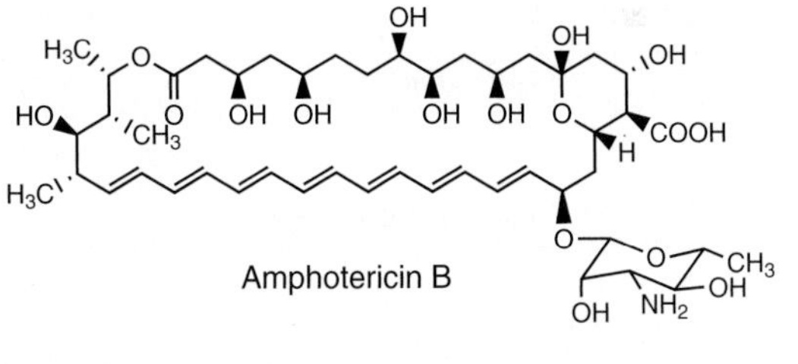
Amphotericin B

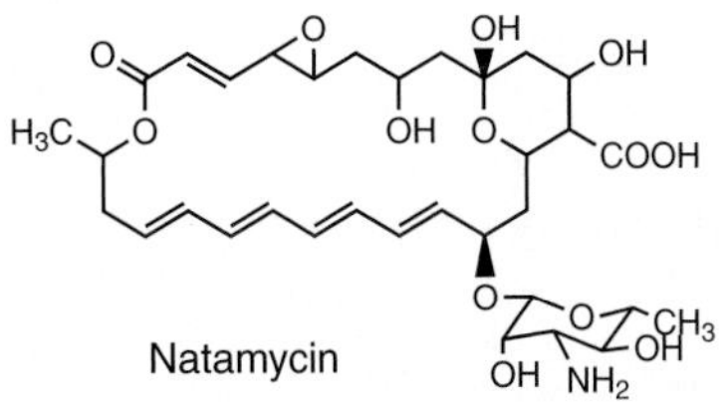
Natamycin

Mechanism of Action

The polyenes have an affinity for sterol-containing membranes, insert into the membranes, and disrupt membrane functions. The lipophilic polyene portion crosses the cell lipid bilayer forming a pore in the cell membrane. The membranes of cells treated with polyenes become leaky, and eventually, the cells die because of the loss of essential cell constituents, such as ions and small organic molecules (15). Polyenes have a demonstrably higher affinity for membranes containing ergosterol over cholesterol-containing membranes (16). This is the basis for their greater toxicity to fungal cells. Some evidence suggests that the mechanism of insertion differs between the types of cells. Polyene molecules may insert individually into ergosterol-containing membranes but require prior formation of polyene micelles before inserting into cholesterol-containing membranes.

Specific Drugs

NYSTATIN Nystatin, the first clinically useful polyene antifungal antibiotic, is a conjugated tetraene isolated from cultures of the bacterium *Streptomyces noursei* in 1951 (13). Nystatin is an effective topical antifungal against a wide variety of organisms and is available in a variety of creams and ointments. Nystatin is too toxic to be used systemically, but because very little drug is absorbed following oral administration, it may be administered by mouth to treat fungal infections of the mouth and gastrointestinal tract (Table 35.1). Although nystatin itself was not a breakthrough in systemic antifungal therapy, the search for other polyenes led to the discovery of a polyene that can be used systemically.

AMPHOTERICIN B Amphotericin B, which as a heptaene has low enough toxicity to mammalian cells to permit intravenous (IV) administration, was discovered in 1956 (13). Amphotericin B is nevertheless a very toxic drug and must be used with caution. Adverse effects include fever, shaking chills, hypotension, and severe kidney toxicity. Despite its toxicity, amphotericin B is considered to be the drug of choice for many systemic, life-threatening fungal infections. The drug cannot cross the blood–brain barrier and must be administered intrathecally for treatment of fungal infections of the CNS. Closely related heptaenes are candicidin, hamycin, and trichomycin.

The nephrotoxicity of amphotericin B has been a serious drawback to the use of this drug since its introduction. Recently, however, the toxicity of the drug has been decreased substantially by changes in formulation (Table 35.2). The polyenes are only sparingly soluble in water, and amphotericin B has long been formulated as a complex with deoxycholic acid for IV administration. More recently developed formulations of amphotericin B, such as liposomal encapsulation and lipid complexes, have dramatically decreased the toxicity of the drug to humans, which permits higher plasma levels to be employed (17). The mechanisms by which the new

TABLE 35.1 Topical Antifungals

Chemical Class	Generic Name	Trade Name	Dosage Form
Allylamine	Butenafine	Lotrimin Ultra	1% cream
		Mentax	
	Naftifine	Naftin	1% cream, gel
	Terbinafine	Lamisil	1% cream
		Lamisil DermGel	10 mg/g gel
	Tolnaftate (thiocarbamate)	Various	1% cream, solution
		Absorbine Athlete's Foot Cream	1% cream
		Genaspor	1% cream
		Tinactin	1% cream, solution, powder, spray powder, spray liquid
		Aftate	1% gel, spray powder, spray liquid
Imidazole	Butoconazole	Femstat-3	2% cream
		Gynazole 1	2% cream
	Clotrimazole	Cruex	1% cream
		Lotrimin AF	1% cream, lotion, solution
		Desenex	1% cream
	Econazole	Various	1% cream
		Spectazole	1% cream
	Sertaconazole	Ertaczo	2% cream
	Ketoconazole	Nizoral	2% cream, shampoo
	Miconazole	Micatin	2% cream, powder, spray powder, spray liquid

(Continued)

TABLE 35.1 Topical Antifungals (*Continued*)

Chemical Class	Generic Name	Trade Name	Dosage Form
		Monistat-Derm	2% cream
		Maximum Strength Desenex	2% cream
		Fungoid Creme	2% cream
		Lotrimin AF	2% cream, spray powder
		Zeasorb AF	2% cream
		Prescription Strength Desenex	2% spray liquid
		Funcoid Tincture	2% solution
	Oxiconazole	Oxistat	1% cream, lotion
	Sulconazole	Exelderm	1% cream, solution
	Tioconazole	Vagistat-1	6.5% oinment
Triazole	Terconazole	Terazol	Topical 0.4%–0.8% cream, suppository
Polyene	Nystatin	Mycostatin	100,000 U/g cream, ointment, powder
		Nilstat	100,000 U/g cream, ointment
		Nystex	100,000 U/g cream, ointment
	Natamycin	Alcon	5% ophthalmic solution
Miscellaneous	Ciclopirox	Loprox	0.77% cream, gel, suspension
			1% shampoo
		Penlac	8% nail lacquer
	Haloprogin	Halotex	1% cream, solution
	Undecylenic acid	Protectol Medicated	15% powder
		Caldesene	10% powder
		Cruex	10% powder
		Cruex Aerosol	19% powder
		Desenex	25% powder
		Phicon F	8% cream
		Various	2%–25% creams, powders, ointments

formulations decrease the toxicity are not entirely clear, but altered distribution is clearly a factor. Because the blood vessels at the site of infection are more permeable than those of normal tissue, the large suspended particles of the lipid formulations can penetrate the site of infection more readily than they can penetrate healthy tissue. The result is selective delivery of drug to the site of infection. Some evidence also indicates that the newer formulations transfer amphotericin B to ergosterol-containing fungal cells more efficiently than to cholesterol-containing mammalian cells (17).

Natamycin Natamycin, a tetraene, is available in the United States as a 5% suspension applied topically for the treatment of fungal infections of the eye (Table 35.1).

Ergosterol Biosynthesis Inhibitors

A schematic of fungal ergosterol biosynthesis starting from squalene is shown in Figure 35.1. The biosynthetic pathway has been simplified to emphasize steps important to the action of currently employed antifungal drugs (12). The last nonsteroidal precursor to both ergosterol and cholesterol is the hydrocarbon squalene. Squalene is converted to squalene epoxide by the enzyme squalene epoxidase. Squalene epoxide is then cyclized to lanosterol, the first steroid in the biosynthetic pathway. The steps involved in converting the side chain of lanosterol to the side chain of ergosterol, and the steps in removal of the geminal dimethyl groups on position 4, are not shown, because none of these reactions is targeted by clinically employed antifungal agents.

TABLE 35.2 Systemic Antifungal Agents

Chemical Class	Generic Name	Trade Name	Dosage Form
Allylamine	Terbinafine	Lamisil	250-mg tablets
Azole – imidazole	Ketoconazole	Various	200-mg tablets
		Nizoral	200-mg tablets
Azole – triazole	Fluconazole	Diflucan	50-, 100-, 150-, 200-mg tablets; 350-mg (10 mg/mL reconst.) powder for oral suspension; 100-, 200-mL (2 mg/mL) solution for injection
	Voriconazole	Vfend	50- and 200-mg tablets; 200-mg powder for injection; 45 g (40 mg/mL reconst.) powder for oral suspension
	Itraconazole	Various	100-mg capsules
		Sporanox	100-mg capsules; 10-mg/mL injection solution; oral solution 10 mg/mL
	Posaconazole	Noxafil	105-mL bottle, 40-mg/mL oral suspension
Echinocandins	Caspofungin	Cancidas	50- and 70-mg powder for injection
	Anidulafungin	Eraxis	50-mg powder for injection
	Micafungin	Mycamine	50-mg powder for injection
Polyene	Amphotericin B	Amphocin (desoxycholate)	50-mg powder for injection
		Fungizone (desoxycholate)	50-mg powder for injection
		Abelcet (lipid complex)	Suspension 100 mg/20 mL, single-use vials
		Amphotec (cholesteryl)	50 mg/20 mL and 100 mg/50 mL powder, single-use vials
		AmBisome (lipisomal)	Powder, single-use vials
Miscellaneous	Flucytosine	Ancobon	250- and 500-mg capsules
	Griseofulvin	Fulvicin, Grifulvin, Grisactin	250- and 500-mg microsize tablets; 125- to 330-mg ultramicrosize tablets

A key step in conversion of lanosterol to both cholesterol and ergosterol is removal of the 14α-methyl group. This reaction is carried out by a cytochrome P450 enzyme, 14α-demethylase, also known as CYP51 (18). The mechanism of this reaction involves three successive hydroxylations of the 14α-methyl group, converting it from a hydrocarbon through the alcohol, aldehyde, and carboxylic acid oxidation states (Fig. 35.2). The methyl group is eliminated as formic acid to afford a double bond between C-14 and C-15 of the D ring. This enzyme is the primary target of the azole antifungal agents discussed below.

Eventually, either before or after modification of the side chain, the Δ^{14} double bond is reduced by a Δ^{14}-reductase to form a *trans* ring juncture between the C and D rings. Several steps later, the double bond between C-8 and C-9 is isomerized to a Δ^{7} double bond by the enzyme Δ^{8},Δ^{7}-isomerase. Many of the steps are identical to those involved in mammalian cholesterol biosynthesis, and the basis for selective toxicity to fungal cells will be discussed under the specific agents.

Azoles—Imidazoles and Triazoles

Azole antifungal agents are the largest class of antimycotics available today, with more than 20 drugs on the market. Some are primarily used topically to treat superficial dermatophytic and yeast infections (Table 35.1), whereas others are administered orally for the treatment of systemic fungal infections (Table 35.2). The oral bioavailability of some azoles, in contrast to amphotericin B, combined with their generally broad spectrum of activity has led to their widespread use in treating a variety of serious infections. The characteristic chemical feature of azoles from which their name is derived is the presence of a five-membered aromatic ring containing either two or three nitrogen atoms. Imidazole rings have two nitrogens and triazoles three. In both cases, the azole ring is attached through N_1 to a side chain containing at least one aromatic ring. Imidazole-containing agents are shown in Figure 35.3 (for triazoles, see Fig. 35.6).

MECHANISM OF ACTION All the azoles act by inhibiting ergosterol biosynthesis through inhibition of the

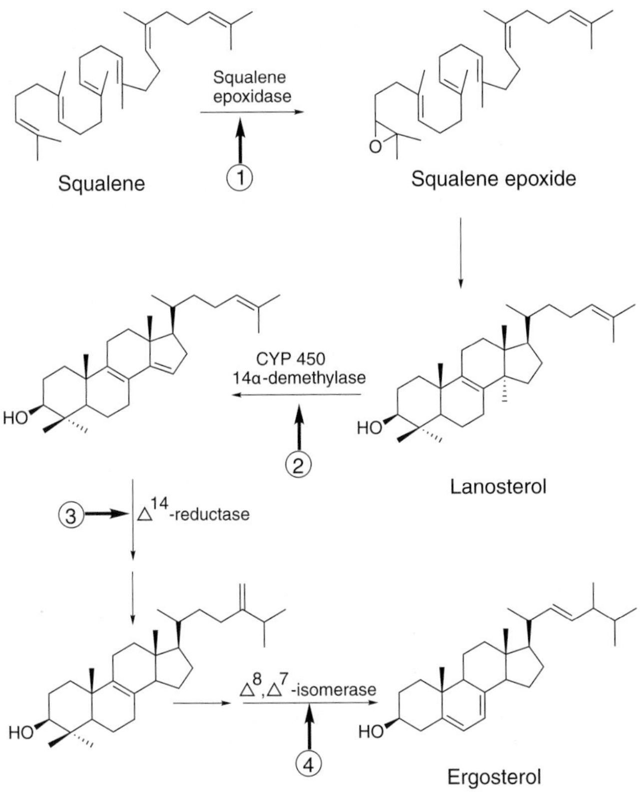

FIGURE 35.1 Ergosterol biosynthesis from squalene with key steps shown in this simplified figure. Enzymatic steps known to be the site of action of currently employed antifungal agents are indicated by a heavy black arrow and a number.

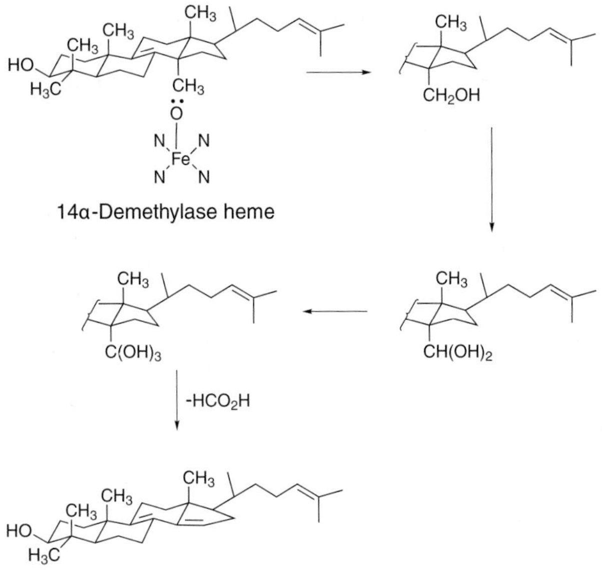

FIGURE 35.2 Demethylation of the 14α-methyl group from lanosterol carried out by the cytochrome P450 enzyme sterol 14α-demethylase, CYP51. The mechanism involves three successive heme-catalyzed insertions of activated oxygen into the three carbon–hydrogen bonds of the 14α-methyl group which raises the oxidation state of the methyl group to a carboxylic acid. The group is finally eliminated as formic acid to create a double bond between carbons 14 and 15.

14α-demethylase, CYP51, discussed earlier under ergosterol biosynthesis (Fig. 35.1, site 2). The basic N3 atom of the azole forms a bond with the heme iron of the CYP450 prosthetic group in the position normally occupied by the activated oxygen (Fig. 35.4). The remainder of the azole antifungal forms bonding interactions with the apoprotein in a manner that determines the relative selectivity of the drug for the fungal demethylase versus other CYP450 enzymes.

Inhibition of the 14α-demethylase results in accumulation in the fungal cell membrane of sterols still bearing a 14α-methyl group. These sterols do not have the exact shape and physical properties of the normal membrane sterol ergosterol. This results in permeability changes, leaky membranes, and malfunction of membrane-imbedded proteins. These effects taken together lead to fungal cell death. Because biosynthesis of the mammalian membrane sterol cholesterol also employs a CYP450 14α-demethylase, why do 14α-methyl sterols not accumulate in human cell membranes? The reason is in the relative strength of inhibition of the same enzyme from different species. For example, the median inhibitory concentration (IC_{50}) for ketoconazole against the enzyme from *Candida albicans* is approximately 10^{-8} mol/L versus approximately 10^{-6} mol/L for mammalian enzymes (19). This two orders of magnitude difference in strength of inhibition provides the therapeutic index with respect to this particular enzyme. As discussed later, however, many of the azoles are powerful inhibitors of other mammalian CYP450 enzymes.

The early azole antifungal drugs were all either extensively and rapidly degraded by first-pass metabolism or too toxic for systemic use. As a result, only those drugs with reduced or slow first-pass metabolism (ketoconazole, fluconazole, itraconazole, voriconazole, and posaconazole) are used systemically. The other azoles (clotrimazole, tioconazole, terconazole, butoconazole, econazole, oxiconazole, sulconazole, miconazole, and ketoconazole) are available in a variety of creams and ointments for topical treatments of dermatophytic infections and intravaginal use for vaginal yeast infections (Table 35.1).

Specific Drugs

Ketoconazole Ketoconazole (Fig. 35.3), an imidazole antifungal, was the first orally active antifungal azole to be discovered and, as a consequence, has been widely studied and employed for the treatment of systemic fungal infections, primarily candidiasis. Ketoconazole has little effect on *Aspergillus* or *Cryptococcus*. Ketoconazole is highly dependent on low stomach pH for absorption, and antacids or drugs that raise stomach pH will lower the bioavailability of ketoconazole. As with other azoles, it is extensively metabolized by microsomal enzymes (Fig. 35.5). All the metabolites are inactive. Evidence that CYP3A4 plays a significant role in metabolism of

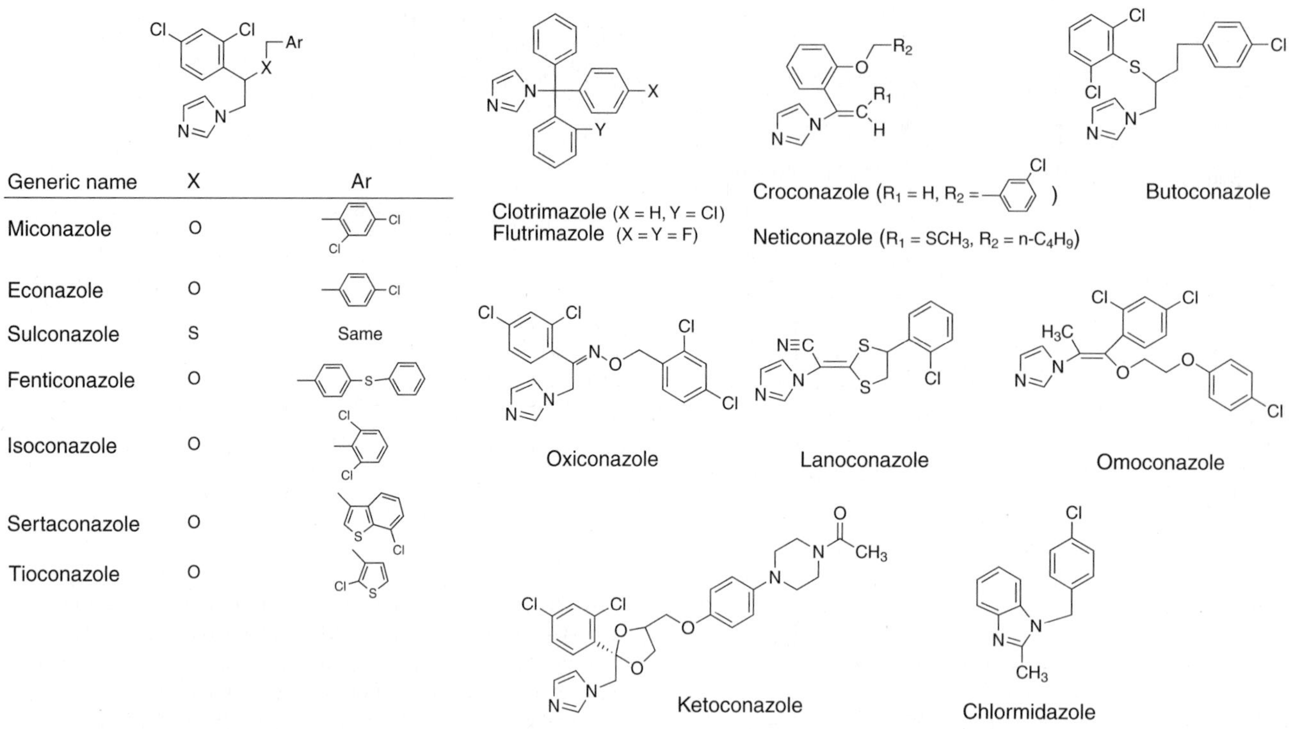

FIGURE 35.3 Imidazole antifungal agents.

ketoconazole is that coadministration of CYP3A4 inducers, such as phenytoin, carbamazepine, and rifampin, can cause as much as a 50% reduction in levels of ketoconazole (20). Ketoconazole also is a powerful inhibitor of human CYP3A4 and, as a consequence, has many serious interactions with other drugs. For example, coadministration of ketoconazole with the hypnotic triazolam results in a 22-fold increase in triazolam's area under the curve (AUC) and a sevenfold increase in half-life. CYP3A4 also is present in the gut and may contribute substantially to the metabolism of many drugs, such as the immunosuppressant agent cyclosporine, thus the potential for drug–drug interaction. Ketoconazole is a weak inhibitor of CYP2C9, which is the enzyme responsible for the metabolism of several narrow therapeutic index drugs, such as warfarin and phenytoin. As better systemic agents have become available, ketoconazole's clinical use has become limited to topical applications in a variety of dosage forms, including creams, lotions, suppositories, and shampoos.

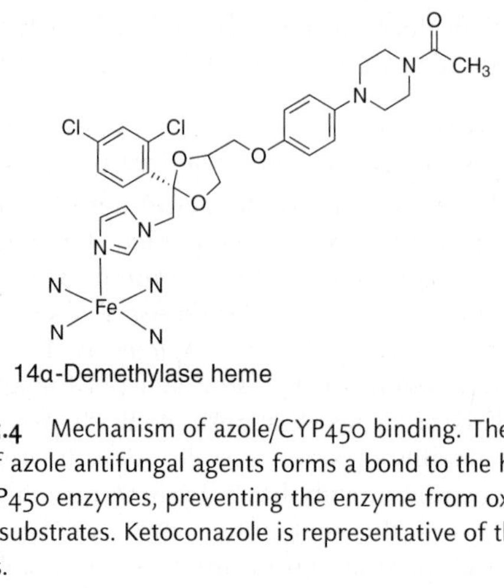

FIGURE 35.4 Mechanism of azole/CYP450 binding. The basic nitrogen of azole antifungal agents forms a bond to the heme iron of CYP450 enzymes, preventing the enzyme from oxidizing its normal substrates. Ketoconazole is representative of the azole antifungals.

Itraconazole Itraconazole was, along with fluconazole, one of the first triazoles introduced into clinical use (Fig. 35.6) (21). Itraconazole's oral bioavailability is variable and is influenced by food and stomach pH, a strongly acidic pH being required for good absorption. Like ketoconazole, itraconazole is extensively metabolized by CYP3A4 following oral administration, and levels are markedly reduced by coadministration of the CYP3A4-inducers phenytoin, carbamazepine, and rifampin (20). Additionally, like ketoconazole, itraconazole has been demonstrated to be a strong inhibitor of CYP3A4 (22). This interaction has proven to be of clinical significance because of the risk of developing rhabdomyolysis following lovastatin or simvastatin therapy with coadministration of itraconazole (23–25). Therefore, itraconazole is likely to have serious interactions with any other drug metabolized by CYP3A4. Again like ketoconazole, itraconazole appears to have little or no effect on CYP2C9-mediated metabolism of warfarin and phenytoin.

Terconazole Terconazole (Fig. 35.6) is a close analog of ketoconazole and itraconazole. It is approved only for the treatment of vaginal candidiasis and is not used systemically (Table 35.1) (26,27).

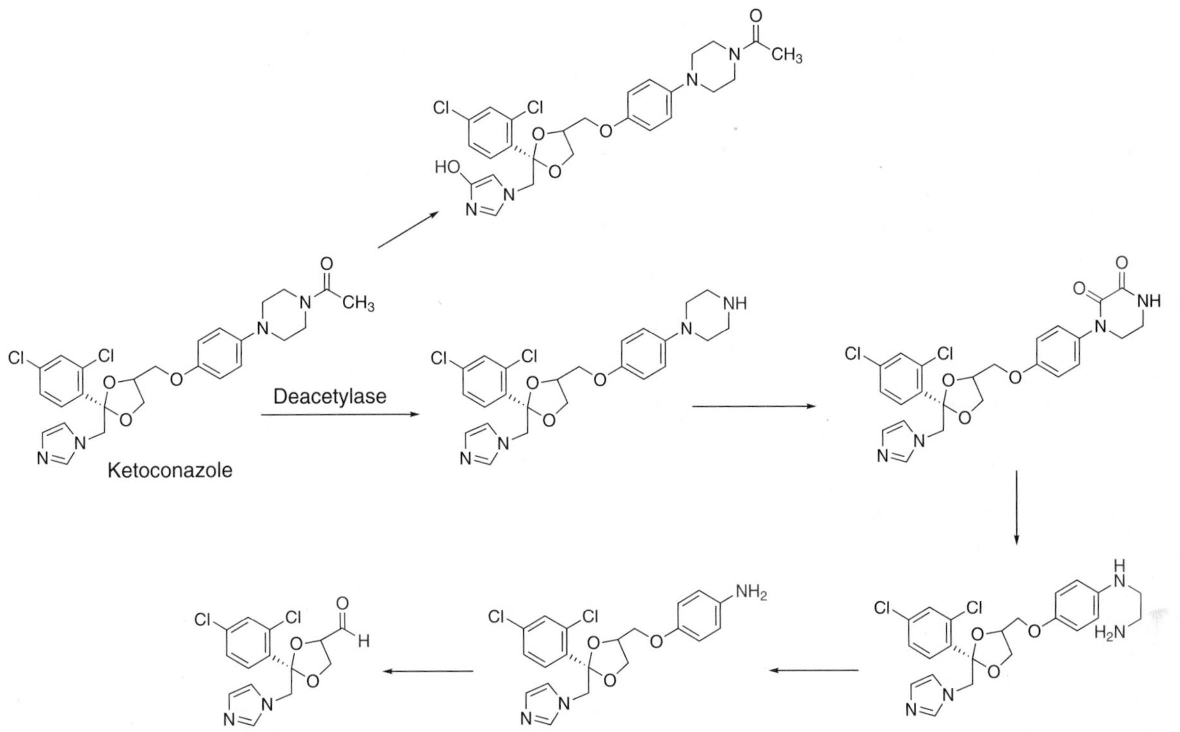

FIGURE 35.5 Extensive metabolism of ketoconazole involving hydrolysis of the *N*-acetyl by a deacetylase. The oxidation reactions are catalyzed by CYP3A4 and flavin-linked mixed-function oxidase. All metabolites are inactive.

FLUCONAZOLE Fluconazole (Fig. 35.6), which was introduced at the same time as itraconazole, differs from ketoconazole and itraconazole in that it is equally bioavailable when given orally or IV. Two major advantages of fluconazole over other antifungal agents are that it can cross the blood–brain barrier and has efficacy against *Cryptococcus neoformans* (28). Fluconazole also differs in that it is only a weak inhibitor of CYP3A4 but a strong inhibitor of CYP2C9 (29). For instance, fluconazole doubles the AUC of (*S*)-warfarin (the active enantiomer) and greatly prolongs the prothrombin time in patients receiving warfarin anticoagulant therapy (30). Because warfarin has such a narrow therapeutic index and excessive anticoagulation can be extremely harmful, this interaction is considered to be of major clinical significance. Fluconazole also decreases the metabolism of the CYP2C9 substrate phenytoin, an antiepileptic agent that also has a narrow therapeutic index (31). Depending on the dose of fluconazole, coadministration with phenytoin can result in a 75% to 150% increase in the phenytoin AUC, and numerous case reports have documented substantial adverse effects following this regimen. Fluconazole also will inhibit CYP3A4, although not to the same degree as ketoconazole and itraconazole. Fluconazole exhibits a dose-dependent inhibition of triazolam metabolism (a CYP3A4 reaction) causing as much as a fourfold increase in triazolam AUC.

Fluconazole has limited water solubility, and current IV formulations of only 2 mg/mL require high-volume infusions, which is a drawback for rapid administration in seriously ill patients. For this reason, a highly water-soluble fluconazole prodrug, fosfluconazole (Fig. 35.6), is being developed with a water solubility greater than 100 mg/mL (32). Fosfluconazole is a phosphate ester that is rapidly converted to fluconazole in vivo by alkaline phosphatases. This new prodrug allows much lower volume bolus injections to be administered, with over 90% of the prodrug rapidly converted to active fluconazole (33,34).

VORICONAZOLE Voriconazole (Fig. 35.6) is a fluconazole analog that was developed to overcome some of the limitations of fluconazole (35) and does, indeed, have a broader spectrum of activity than fluconazole, having activity against *Aspergillus* and fluconazole-resistant strains of *Candida* and *Cryptococcus* (36). Voriconazole is orally absorbed and penetrates the blood–brain barrier. Unfortunately, voriconazole is extensively metabolized CYP450 enzymes (Fig. 35.7) and is an inhibitor of CYP2C19, CYP2C9, and CYP3A4, leading to many drug interactions (37,38). Voriconazole exhibits nonlinear, saturable kinetics, and because CYP2C19 exhibits genetic polymorphisms, plasma levels can be higher in poor metabolizers versus extensive metabolizers (39,40).

POSACONAZOLE Posaconazole (Fig. 35.6), a recently introduced triazole, has a number of advantages over previous agents (41,42). Posaconazole has a wide spectrum of activity compared to other azoles, particularly against *Aspergillus* and other increasingly common nosocomial

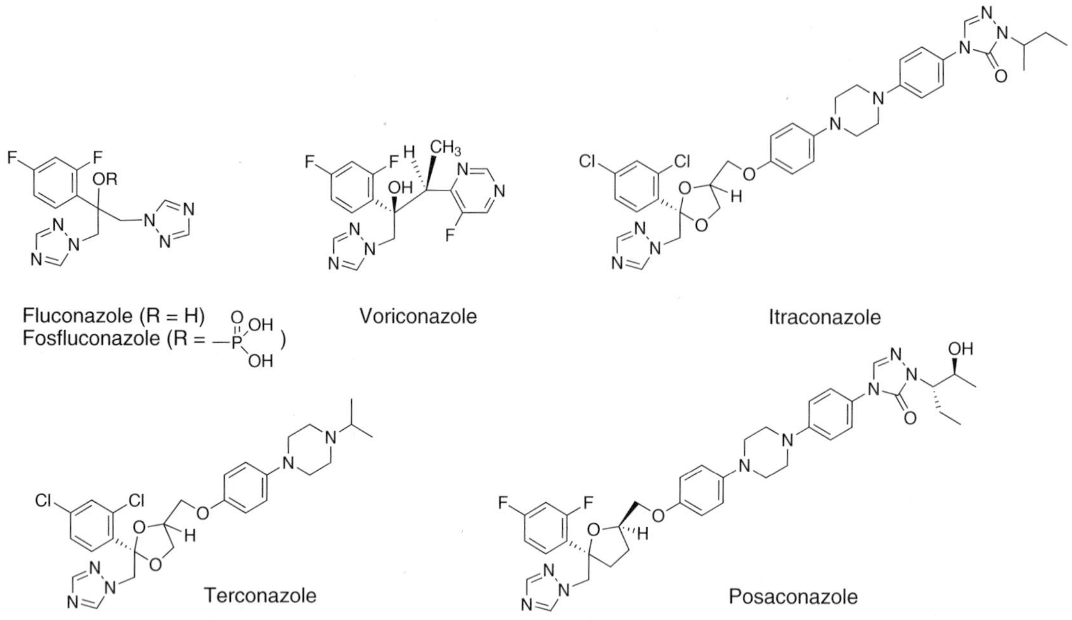

FIGURE 35.6 Triazole antifungal agents.

infections resistant to treatment by other antifungal drugs. *Aspergillus* resistance to azole antifungals has been attributed to the unique presence in *Aspergillus* of two distinct 14α-demethylases CYP51A and CYP51B (43). *Aspergillus* CYP51B is sensitive to fluconazole and itraconazole, but CYP51A remains functional, allowing the fungus to synthesize needed ergosterol. Posaconazole is active against both *Aspergillus* CYP51 enzymes accounting for its greater activity against the fungus compared to other azoles (44).

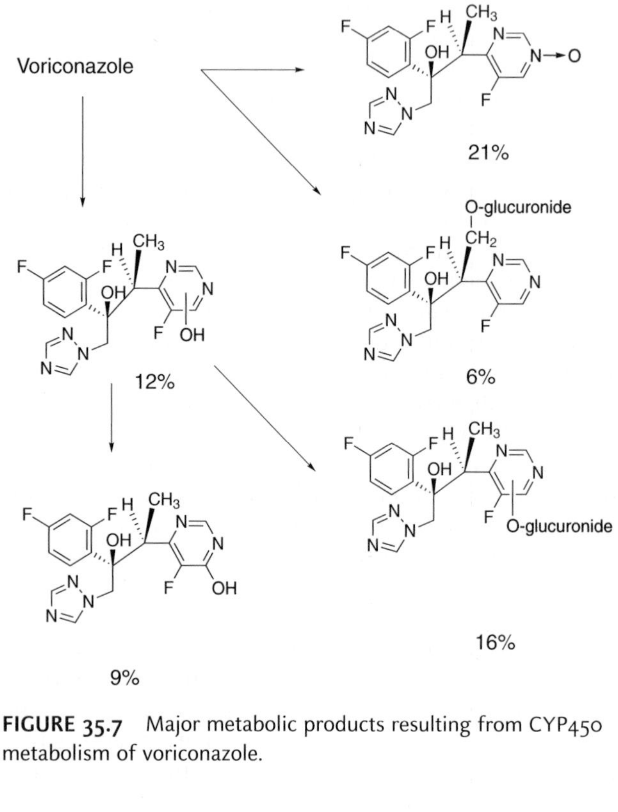

FIGURE 35.7 Major metabolic products resulting from CYP450 metabolism of voriconazole.

Posaconazole is metabolized primarily by phase 2 glucuronide conjugation and has little interaction with most oxidative CYP450 drug-metabolizing enzymes, but is an inhibitor of CYP3A4 (45,46). Posaconazole is structurally similar to itraconazole and saperconazole, but it contains a tetrahydrofuran ring in place of the dioxolan ring of those agents, which may account for some of its unique properties.

Azole Antifungals and P-Glycoprotein

In addition to being substrates and inhibitors of various cytochrome P450 enzymes, azole antifungals can also be inhibitors and/or substrates for the multidrug resistance enzyme P-glycoprotein. As discussed in Chapters 4 and 5, P-glycoprotein is an adenosine triphosphate–dependent pump that expels some drugs from blood circulation into the lumen of the small intestine and is also a component part of the blood–brain barrier. Therefore, P-glycoprotein is an important contributor to drug distribution and plasma levels and can be a major factor in drug–drug interactions. Fluconazole (47) and voriconazole (48) have little or no effect on P-glycoprotein, being neither substrates nor inhibitors. Itraconazole and ketoconazole bind tightly to P-glycoprotein and appear to be substrates for the transporter as well as strong inhibitors of its actions on other drugs (47). The most recently introduced azole, posaconazole, is also both a substrate and inhibitor of P-glycoprotein (49).

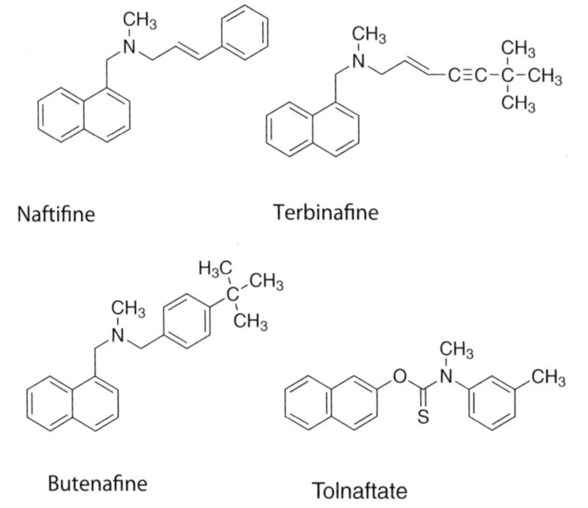

FIGURE 35.8 The squalene epoxidase inhibitors, allylamines. Naftifine was the first drug shown to act by inhibition of squalene epoxidase as was the much older thiocarbamate, tolnaftate.

Allylamines and Other Squalene Epoxidase Inhibitors

The group of agents generally known as allylamines (50) strictly includes only naftifine and terbinafine, but because butenafine and tolnaftate function by the same mechanism of action, they are included in this class and are shown in Figure 35.8. One can, of course, consider the benzyl group of butenafine to be bioisosteric with the allyl group of naftifine and terbinafine. Tolnaftate, a much older drug, is chemically a thiocarbamate but has the same mechanism of action as the allylamines. These drugs have a more limited spectrum of activity than the azoles and are effective only against dermatophytes. Therefore, they are employed in the treatment of fungal infections of the skin and nails (51).

Mechanism of Action All of the drugs in Figure 35.8 act through inhibition of the enzyme squalene epoxidase (Fig. 35.1, site 1). Inhibition of this enzyme has two effects, both of which appear to be involved in the fungitoxic mechanism of this class (52). First, inhibition of squalene epoxidase results in a decrease in total sterol content of the fungal cell membrane. This decrease alters the physicochemical properties of the membrane, resulting in malfunctions of membrane-imbedded transport proteins involved in nutrient transport and pH balance. Second, inhibition of squalene epoxidase results in a buildup within the fungal cell of the hydrocarbon squalene, which is itself toxic when present in abnormally high amounts. Mammals also employ the enzyme squalene epoxidase in the biosynthesis of cholesterol, but a desirable therapeutic index arises from the fact that the fungal squalene epoxidase enzyme is far more sensitive to the drugs than the corresponding mammalian enzyme. Terbinafine has a K_i of 0.03 μmol/L versus squalene epoxidase from *Candida albicans* but a K_i of only 77 μmol/L versus the same enzyme from rat liver—a 2,500-fold difference (53).

Specific Drugs

Naftifine Naftifine (Fig. 35.8) was the first allylamine to be discovered and marketed (50). Because of its extensive first-pass metabolism, naftifine is not used orally and is only available in topical preparations (Table 35.1). The widest use of naftifine is against various tinea infections of the skin.

Terbinafine Terbinafine (Fig. 35.8) is available in both topical and oral dosage forms (Tables 35.1 and 35.2) and is effective against a variety of dermatophytic infections when employed topically or systemically (53). A unique property of terbinafine is its effectiveness in the treatment of onychomycoses (nail infections) (54). Given orally, the highly lipophilic drug redistributes from the plasma into the nail bed and into the nail itself, where the infection resides (55,56), making terbinafine superior to other agents for treating this particular type of infection. Terbinafine is extensively metabolized by several CYP450 enzymes, including CYP1A2, CYP2C19, CYP2C9, CYP2C8, CYP3A4, and CYP2B6 (57). Because there are so many pathways for terbinafine metabolism, inhibition of any one has very little effect on overall clearance of the drug, although drugs that inhibit several CYP450 enzymes, such as cimetidine, can increase terbinafine plasma levels. Although not a substrate for the enzyme, terbinafine is a strong inhibitor of CYP2D6 and can have significant interactions with drugs that are metabolized by this enzyme, such as codeine and desipramine (29,58).

Butenafine and Tolnaftate Butenafine and tolnaftate, like naftifine (Fig. 35.8), are only available in topical preparation for the treatment of dermatophytic infections (Table 35.1). Tolnaftate has been marketed in a variety of nonprescription drug preparations for decades. Butenafine, discovered more recently, has a somewhat wider spectrum of activity than tolnaftate. For example, butenafine is active against superficial *Candida albicans* infections, which are not affected by tolnaftate (59).

Morpholines

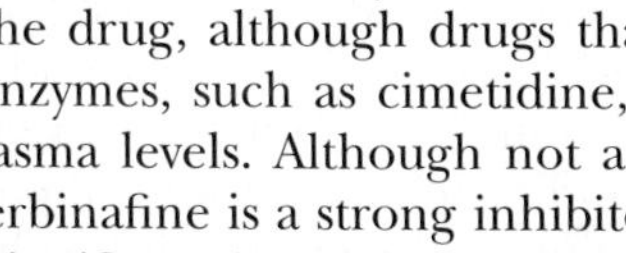

Amorolfine

Amorolfine is the only drug in this class that is employed clinically in the treatment of human fungal infections. Amorolfine is not currently available in the

United States, but it is marketed in Europe and Asia for the topical treatment of dermatophytic infections (60).

Morpholine antifungals inhibit ergosterol biosynthesis by acting on the enzymes Δ^{14}-reductase and Δ^8,Δ^7-isomerase (Fig. 35.1, sites 3 and 4) (61). Inhibition of these enzymes results in incorporation into fungal cell membranes of sterols retaining a Δ^{14} double bond, a Δ^8 double bond, or both. None of these will have the same overall shape and physicochemical properties as the preferred sterol, ergosterol. As with the antifungals already discussed, this results in membranes with altered properties and malfunctioning of membrane-embedded proteins.

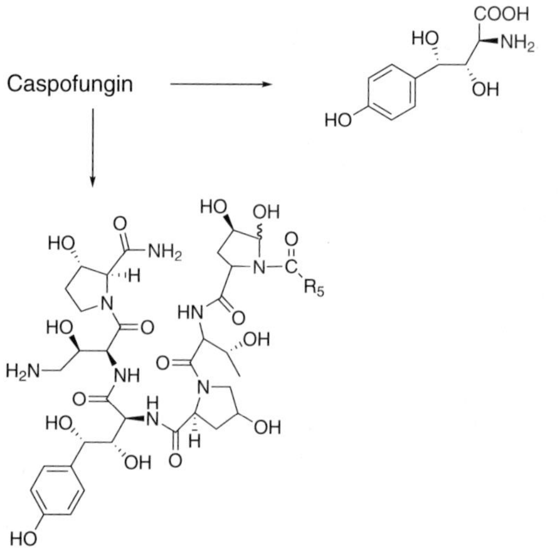

FIGURE 35.10 Metabolic products formed from caspofungin.

Inhibitors of Cell Wall Biosynthesis—Echinocandins

The most notable difference between fungal and mammalian cells is that fungi have a cell wall and mammals do not. Drugs interfering with cell wall biosynthesis would be expected to be relatively nontoxic to mammals. Such drugs have been the foundation of antibacterial therapy since the discovery of penicillin and the development of dozens of effective penicillins and cephalosporins. Only recently, however, have a few drugs affecting fungal cell wall biosynthesis become available. Echinocandins, a group of cyclic peptides with long lipophilic side chains and sometimes called lipopeptides, have been under investigation for a number of years (Fig. 35.9) (62). Echinocandins interfere with cell wall biosynthesis through inhibition of the enzyme β-1,3-glucan synthase. β-Glucan is an important polymer component of many fungal cell walls, and reduction in the glucan content severely weakens the cell wall, leading to rupture of the fungal cell.

Caspofungin, Anidulafungin, and Micafungin

Recently, three semisynthetic echinocandins have been approved for use in treating life-threatening systemic fungal infections (63). These are caspofungin, anidulafungin, and micafungin (Fig. 35.9). These drugs represent the first class of antifungal agents with a novel mechanism of action to be marketed in more than 35 years and are a very valuable contribution to therapy for systemic fungal infections. They are effective against a variety of *Candida* species that have proven to be resistant to other agents as well as effective against azole-resistant *Aspergillus*. Therefore, these drugs are truly life saving for those afflicted with these previously resistant fungi. Unfortunately, these echinocandins are not effective against *Cryptococcus neoformans*. None of these drugs is orally active, and all must be administered by IV infusion. Because of limited hepatic metabolism, drug–drug interactions are not a problem. Caspofungin is metabolized by hydrolysis in two portions of the hexapeptide ring (Fig. 35.10) (64), whereas anidulafungin does not appear to be actively metabolized but rather slowly degrades (65). Micafungin is metabolized by a sulfotransferase and by catechol-*O*-methyltransferase, but no significant drug interactions are known (66).

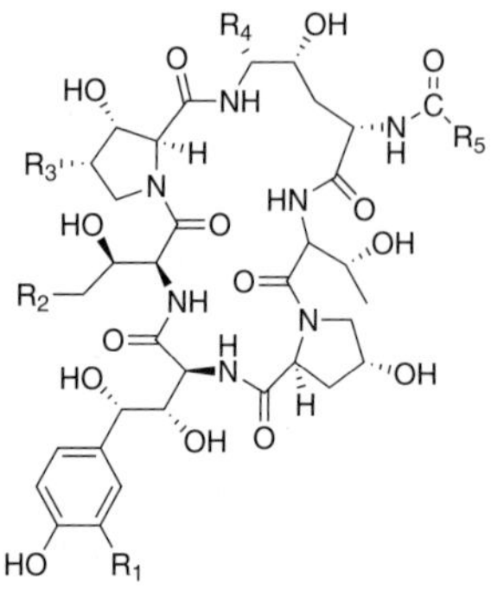

Drug	R_1	R_2	R_3	R_4	R_5
Caspofungin (Cancidas)	H	CH_2NH_2	H	$NHCH_2CH_2NH_2$	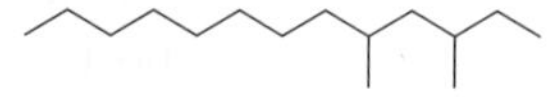
Anidulafungin (Eraxis)	H	H	CH_3	OH	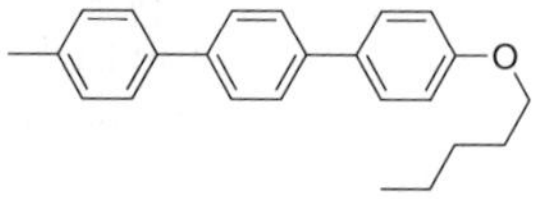
Micafungin (Mycamine)	OSO_3H	$CONH_2$	CH_3	OH	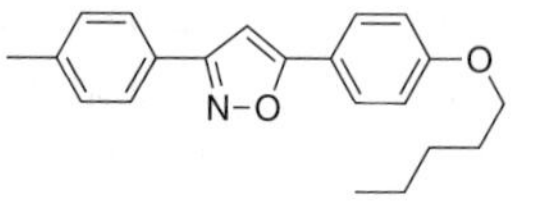

FIGURE 35.9 Echinocandins.

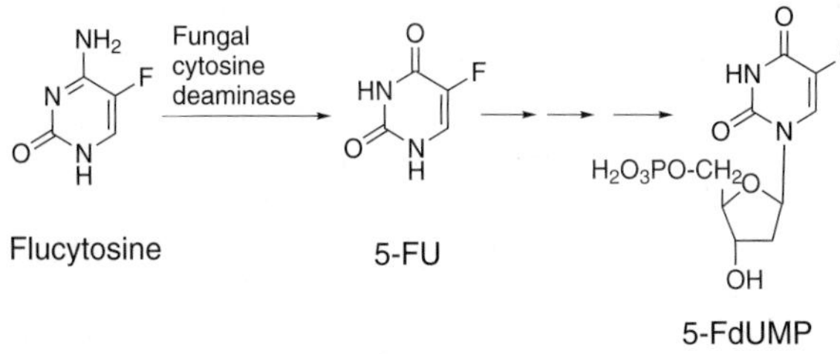

FIGURE 35.11 Flucytosine, a prodrug, is converted by fungal cytosine deaminase to 5-fluorouracil (5-FU). This reaction does not occur in mammalian cells. A further transformation of 5-FU to the actual cytotoxic agent 5-fluorodeoxyuridinemonophosphate (5-FdUMP) also occurs.

Drugs Acting Through Other Mechanisms

Flucytosine

Flucytosine is a powerful antifungal agent used in the treatment of serious systemic fungal infections, such as *Cryptococcus neoformans* and *Candida* spp. (Table 35.2). Flucytosine itself is not cytotoxic but, rather, is a prodrug that is taken up by fungi and metabolized to 5-fluorouracil (5-FU) by fungal cytidine deaminase (Fig. 35.11) (67). Then, 5-FU is converted to 5-fluorodeoxyuridine, which is a thymidylate synthase inhibitor that interferes with both protein and RNA biosynthesis. 5-Fluorouracil is cytotoxic and is employed in cancer chemotherapy (see Chapter 37). Human cells do not contain cytosine deaminase and, therefore, do not convert flucytosine to 5-FU. Some intestinal flora, however, do convert the drug to 5-FU, so human toxicity does result from this metabolism. Resistance rapidly develops to flucytosine when used alone, so it is almost always used in conjunction with amphotericin B. Use of flucytosine has declined since the discovery of fluconazole.

Griseofulvin

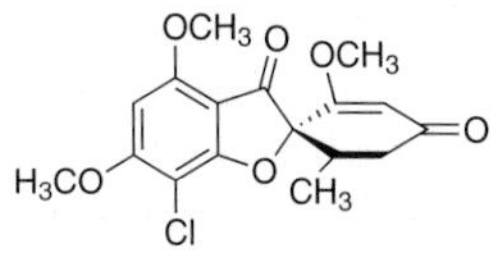

Griseofulvin

Griseofulvin is an antifungal antibiotic produced by an unusual strain of *Penicillium* (68). It is used orally to treat superficial fungal infections, primarily fingernail and toenail infections, but it does not penetrate skin or nails if used topically (Table 35.2). When given orally, however, plasma-borne griseofulvin becomes incorporated into keratin precursor cells and, ultimately, into keratin, which cannot then support fungal growth. The infection is cured when the diseased tissue is replaced by new, uninfected tissue, which can take months. The mechanism of action of griseofulvin is through binding to the protein tubulin, which interferes with the function of the mitotic spindle and, thereby, inhibits cell division. Griseofulvin also may interfere directly with DNA replication. Griseofulvin is gradually being replaced by newer agents (69).

Haloprogin

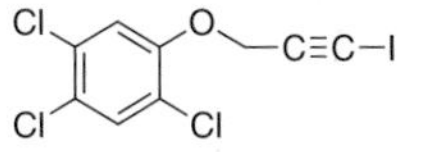

Haloprogin

Haloprogin is an iodinated acetylene active against dermatophytes (70). Haloprogin is only used for topical applications (Table 35.1). The mechanism of haloprogin is not clear, but it appears to lead to nonspecific metabolic disruption. It has been demonstrated to interfere with DNA biosynthesis and cell respiration.

Ciclopirox

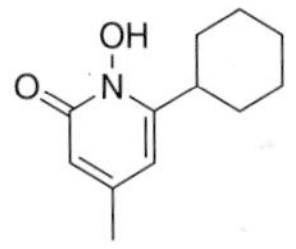

Ciclopirox

Ciclopirox is a hydroxylated pyridinone that is employed for superficial dermatophytic infections, principally onychomycosis. Ciclopirox has a unique mechanism of action through chelation of polyvalent cations, such as Fe^{3+}, which causes inhibition of a number of metal-dependent enzymes within the fungal cell. Although ciclopirox has been available for more than 30 years, a new formulation of an 8% lacquer has been recently introduced for treating nail infections (71).

Undecylenic Acid

$$H_2C{=}CH(CH_2)_8COOH$$

Undecylenic acid

Undecylenic acid is widely employed, frequently as the zinc salt, in over-the-counter preparations for topical treatment of infections by dermatophytes (Table 35.1) (72). Undecylenic acid is a fungistatic that acts through a nonspecific interaction with components in the fungal cell membrane.

SCENARIO: OUTCOME AND ANALYSIS

Outcome

Douglas Slain, PharmD, BCPS

The patient was told to go to the emergency room at the hospital. They measured her plasma digoxin concentration, which was found to be very elevated (3.3 ng/mL). The pharmacist at the emergency department found reports in the medical literature of interactions between itraconazole and digoxin. The team monitored and stabilized the patient. They decided to lower her digoxin dose by 50%. A week later, digoxin concentration was again tested and was within the desired range (1.9 ng/mL), and there were no signs of toxicity. The patient was able to remain on the reduced digoxin dose while finishing the course of itraconazole. Fluconazole does not have an interaction with digoxin, but it is not as effective for treating histoplasmosis.

Chemical Analysis

Victoria Roche, PhD, and S. William Zito, PhD

The interaction is due to the fact that itraconazole is a P-glycoprotein inhibitor. Digoxin is a substrate of P-glycoprotein. From a chemical standpoint, itraconazole and ketoconazole bind tightly to P-glycoprotein and serve as significant inhibitors and substrates. Structures that bind to P-glycoprotein are often lipophilic entities with molecular weights between 300 and 1,000. Conazole antifungal agents commonly have a structural pattern of three electron donor groups separated by 4.6 Angstroms, a motif known to be recognized by this efflux protein (73). Fluconazole does not appear to bind to P-glycoprotein. It is a much smaller structure than either itraconazole or ketoconazole, and it is significantly less lipophilic. As a result, it has been claimed to distribute ineffectively across membranes and experience difficulty reaching and interacting with the P-glycoprotein binding site (47). Therefore, a P-glycoprotein–mediated interaction with digoxin would not be expected from fluconazole.

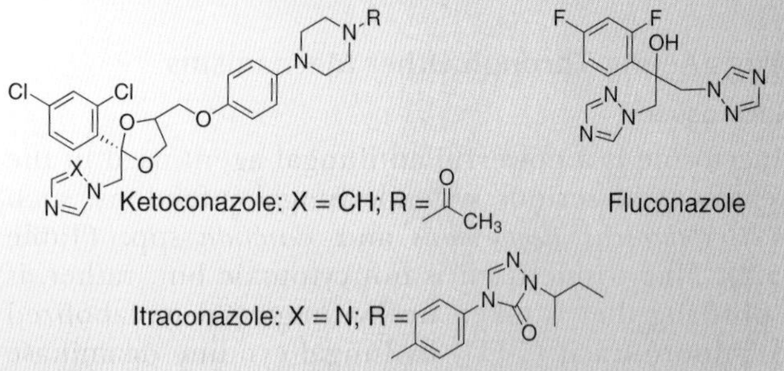

Agents that are CYP3A4 substrates and inhibitors are often P-glycoprotein substrates and inhibitors. Newer azoles like voriconazole and posaconazole appear to bind to P-glycoprotein but have not been as well studied.

CASE STUDY

Victoria Roche and S. William Zito

HN is a 64-year-old custodian at a brick plant located in the deep South. He is currently being treated for prostate cancer, and the antineoplastic drug he's on (docetaxel) has left him feeling weak and tired. He knows this drug is toxic to the bone marrow and leaves him vulnerable to infection. Despite feeling lethargic, he really needs the money (not to mention the company's insurance) and is currently cleaning six nights a week. When he's around people he wears a surgical mask to minimize his exposure to bacteria- and virus-laden environmental hazards. However, he works the night shift and is often alone, so he doesn't usually wear the mask while he's cleaning.

From a weather-related perspective, this was a horrible spring, with many devastating tornados and monsoon-like rainstorms pelting the region. A tornado-damaged roof allowed several areas of the large plant to flood, and the steamy late June heat that's now descended is close to intolerable. For the past several weeks HN had noticed a musty smell in several areas of the plant, and told his supervisor about a greenish-brown discoloration that was forming on some ceiling tiles and drywall in the more remote maintenance-related workrooms. He has been trying to clean the drywall but has not had much permanent success. Recently he began to experience new and disturbing symptoms, including shortness of breath, headaches, and nosebleeds. When he reported this to his oncologist, he was sent to an infectious disease specialist who diagnosed an invasive aspergillosis infection.

As the pharmacist working with the infectious disease team, you know that systemic mold infections are tough to treat, and HN's immunocompromised status is not helping matters (in fact, it contributed significantly to his fungal susceptibility). Taking into account that his anticancer drug (docetaxel) is inactivated exclusively by CYP3A4-mediated aliphatic hydroxylation and his pain medication (oxycodone) is activated by CYP2D6-mediated O-dealkylation, you consider the structure of the following antifungal candidates.

(continued)

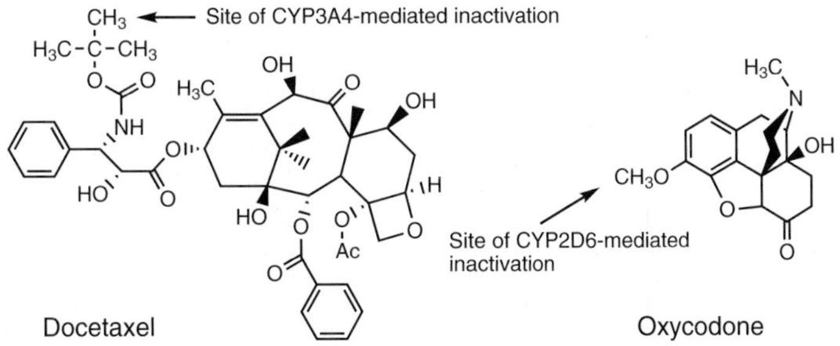

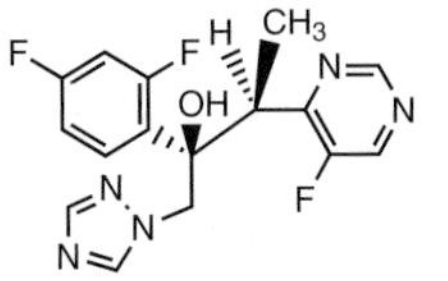

1

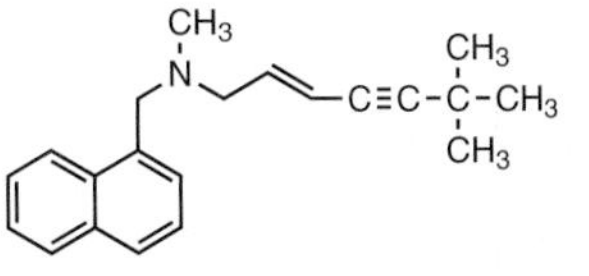

2

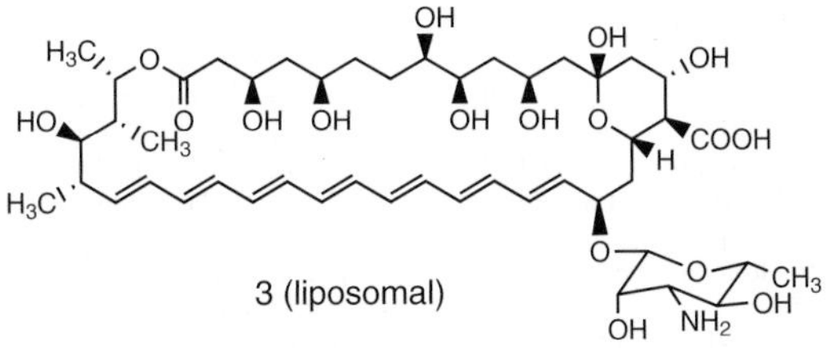

3 (liposomal)

1. Conduct a thorough and mechanistic SAR analysis of the three therapeutic options in the case.
2. Apply the chemical understanding gained from the SAR analysis to this patient's specific needs to make a therapeutic recommendation.

References

1. Anaissie EJ, McGinnis MR, Pfaller MA, eds. Clinical Mycology. New York: Churchill Livingstone, 2003.
2. Pfaller MA, Wenzel RP. The epidemiology of fungal infections. In: Anaissie EJ, McGinnis MR, Pfaller MA, eds. Clinical Mycology. New York: Churchill Livingstone, 2003:3–19.
3. Hiruma M, Yamaguchi H. Dermatophytes. In: Anaissie EJ, McGinnis MR, Pfaller MA, eds. Cinical Mycology. New York: Livingstone Churchill, 2003:370–379.
4. Digani MC, Solomkin JS, Anaissie EJ. Candida. In: Anaissie EJ, McGinnis MR, Pfaller MA, eds. Clinical Mycology. New York: Churchill Livingstone, 2003:195–239.
5. Viviani MA, Tortorano AM, Ajello L. Cryptococcus. In: Anaissie EJ, McGinnis MR, Pfaller MA, eds. Clinical Mycology. New York: Churchill Livingstone, 2003:240–259.
6. Maenza JR, Merz WG. Infections caused by non-candida non-cryptoccus yeasts. In: Anaissie EJ, McGinnis MR, Pfaller MA, eds. Clinical Mycology. New York: Churchill Livingstone, 2003:260–272.
7. Pera S, Patterson TF. Endemic mycoses. In: Anaissie EJ, McGinnis MR, Pfaller MA, eds. Clinical Mycology. New York: Churchill Livingstone, 2003:352–369.
8. Dromer F, McGinnis MR. Zygomycosis. In: Anaissie EJ, McGinnis MR, Pfaller MA, eds. Clinical Mycology. New York: Churchill Livingstone, 2003:297–308.
9. Fernandes PB, ed. New Approaches for Antifungal Drugs. Boston: Birkhauser, 1992.
10. Koller W, ed. Target Sites of Fungicide Action. Boca Raton, FL: CRC Press, 1992.
11. Zaas AK, Alexander BD. Echinocandins: role in antifungal therapy, 2005. Expert Opin Pharmacother 2005;6:1657–1668.
12. Koller W. Antifungal agents with target sites in sterol functions and biosynthesis. In: Koller W, ed. Target Sites of Fungicide Action. Boca Raton, FL: CRC Press, 1992:119–206.
13. Hamilton-Miller JM. Chemistry and biology of the polyene macrolide antibiotics. Bacteriol Rev 1973;37:166–196.
14. Kotler-Brajtburg J, Medoff G, Kobayashi GS, et al. Classification of polyene antibiotics according to chemical structure and biological effects. Antimicrob Agents Chemother 1979;15:716–722.
15. Bolard J. How do the polyene macrolide antibiotics affect the cellular membrane properties? Biochim Biophys Acta 1986;864:257–304.
16. Cotero BV, Rebolledo-Antunez S, Ortega-Blake I. On the role of sterol in the formation of the amphotericin B channel. Biochim Biophys Acta 1998;1375:43–51.
17. Wong-Beringer A, Jacobs RA, Guglielmo BJ. Lipid formulations of amphotericin B: clinical efficacy and toxicities. Clin Infect Dis 1998;27:603–618.
18. Lepesheva GI, Waterman MR. Sterol 14alpha-demethylase cytochrome P450 (CYP51), a P450 in all biological kingdoms. Biochim Biophys Acta 2007;1770:467–477.
19. Bossche HV, Janssen PA. Target sites of sterol biosynthesis inhibitors: secondary activities on cytochrome P-450 dependent reactions. In: Koller W, ed. Target Sites of Fungicide Action. Boca Raton, FL: CRC Press, 1992:227–254.
20. Tucker RM, Denning DW, Hanson LH, et al. Interaction of azoles with rifampin, phenytoin, and carbamazepine: in vitro and clinical observations. Clin Infect Dis 1992;14:165–174.
21. Warnock DW. Itraconazole and fluconazole: new drugs for deep fungal infection. J Antimicrob Chemother 1989;24:275–277.
22. Colburn DE, Giles FJ, Oladovich D, Smith JA. In vitro evaluation of cytochrome P450-mediated drug interactions between cytarabine, idarubicin, itraconazole and caspofungin. Hematology 2004;9:217–221.
23. Horn M. Coadministration of itraconazole with hypolipidemic agents may induce rhabdomyolysis in healthy individuals. Arch Dermatol 1996;132:1254.
24. Neuvonen PJ, Jalava KM. Itraconazole drastically increases plasma concentrations of lovastatin and lovastatin acid. Clin Pharmacol Ther 1996;60:54–61.
25. Vlahakos DV, Manginas A, Chilidou D, et al. Itraconazole-induced rhabdomyolysis and acute renal failure in a heart transplant recipient treated with simvastatin and cyclosporine. Transplantation 2002;73:1962–1964.
26. Doering PL, Santiago TM. Drugs for treatment of vulvovaginal candidiasis: comparative efficacy of agents and regimens. DICP 1990;24:1078–1083.
27. Van Cutsem J, Van Gerven F, Zaman R, et al. Terconazole: A new broad-spectrum antifungal. Chemotherapy 1983;29:322–331.
28. Bailey EM, Krakovsky DJ, Rybak MJ. The triazole antifungal agents: a review of itraconazole and fluconazole. Pharmacotherapy 1990;10:146–153.
29. Venkatakrishnan K, von Moltke LL, Greenblatt DJ. Effects of the antifungal agents on oxidative drug metabolism: clinical relevance. Clin Pharmacokinet 2000;38:111–180.

30. Kunze KL, Wienkers LC, Thummel KE, et al. Warfarin-fluconazole. I. Inhibition of the human cytochrome P450-dependent metabolism of warfarin by fluconazole: in vitro studies. Drug Metab Dispos 1996;24:414–421.
31. Niwa T, Shiraga T, Takagi A. Effect of antifungal drugs on cytochrome P450 (CYP) 2C9, CYP2C19, and CYP3A4 activities in human liver microsomes. Biol Pharm Bull 2005;28:1805–1808.
32. Sobue S, Sekiguchi K, Shimatani K, et al. Pharmacokinetics and safety of Fosfluconazole after single intravenous bolus injection in healthy male Japanese volunteers. J Clin Pharmacol 2004;44:284–292.
33. Sobue S, Tan K, Layton G, et al. Pharmacokinetics of fosfluconazole and fluconazole following multiple intravenous administration of fosfluconazole in healthy male volunteers. Br J Clin Pharmacol 2004;58:20–25.
34. Sobue S, Tan K, Shaw L, et al. Comparison of the pharmacokinetics of fosfluconazole and fluconazole after single intravenous administration of fosfluconazole in healthy Japanese and Caucasian volunteers. Eur J Clin Pharmacol 2004;60:247–253.
35. Sabo JA, Abdel-Rahman SM. Voriconazole: a new triazole antifungal. Ann Pharmacother 2000;34:1032–1043.
36. Herbrecht R, Denning DW, Patterson TF, et al. Voriconazole versus amphotericin B for primary therapy of invasive aspergillosis. N Engl J Med 2002;347:408–415.
37. Niwa T, Inoue-Yamamoto S, Shiraga T, et al. Effect of antifungal drugs on cytochrome P450 (CYP) 1A2, CYP2D6, and CYP2E1 activities in human liver microsomes. Biol Pharm Bull 2005;28:1813–1816.
38. Roffey SJ, Cole S, Comby P, et al. The disposition of voriconazole in mouse, rat, rabbit, guinea pig, dog, and human. Drug Metab Dispos 2003;31:731–741.
39. Cocchi S, Codeluppi M, Guaraldi G, et al. Invasive pulmonary and cerebral aspergillosis in a patient with Weil's disease. Scand J Infect Dis 2005;37:396–398.
40. Ghannoum MA, Kuhn DM. Voriconazole: better chances for patients with invasive mycoses. Eur J Med Res 2002;7:242–256.
41. Barchiesi F, Schimizzi AM, Caselli F, et al. Activity of the new antifungal triazole, posaconazole, against *Cryptococcus neoformans*. J Antimicrob Chemother 2001;48:769–773.
42. Torres HA, Hachem RY, Chemaly RF, et al. Posaconazole: a broad-spectrum triazole antifungal. Lancet Infect Dis 2005;5:775–785.
43. Mellado E, Diaz-Guerra TM, Cuenca-Estrella M, et al. Identification of two different 14-alpha sterol demethylase-related genes (cyp51A and cyp51B) in *Aspergillus fumigatus* and other *Aspergillus* species. J Clin Microbiol 2001;39:2431–2438.
44. Warrilow AG, Melo N, Martel CM, et al. Expression, purification, and characterization of *Aspergillus fumigatus* sterol 14-alpha demethylase (CYP51) isoenzymes A and B. Antimicrob Agents Chemother 2010;54:4225–4234.
45. Krieter P, Flannery B, Musick T, et al. Disposition of posaconazole following single-dose oral administration in healthy subjects. Antimicrob Agents Chemother 2004;48:3543–3551.
46. Wexler D, Courtney R, Richards W, et al. Effect of posaconazole on cytochrome P450 enzymes: a randomized, open-lable, two-way crossover study. Eur J Pharm Sci 2004;21:645–653.
47. Wang E, Lew K, Casciano CN, et al. Interaction of common azole antifungals with P-glycoprotein. Antimicrob Agents Chemother 2002;46:160–165.
48. Leveque D, Nivoix Y, Jehl F, et al. Clinical pharmacokinetics of voriconazole. Int J Antimicrob Agents 2006;27:274–284.
49. Sansome-Parsons A, Krishna G, Simon J, et al. Effects of age, gender, and race/ethnicity on the pharmacokinetics of posaconazole in healthy volunteers. Antimicrob Agents Chemother 2007;51:495–502.
50. Petranyi G, Ryder NS, Stutz A. Allylamine derivatives: new class of synthetic antifungal agents inhibiting fungal squalene epoxidase. Science 1984;224:1239–1241.
51. Gupta AK, Sauder DN, Shear NH. Antifungal agents: an overview. Part II. J Am Acad Dermatol 1994;30:911–933.
52. Georgopapadakou NH, Bertasso A. Effects of squalene epoxidase inhibitors on *Candida albicans*. Antimicrob Agents Chemother 1992;36:1779–1781.
53. Petranyi G, Stutz A, Ryder NS. Experimental antimycotic activity of naftifine and terbinafine. In: Fromtling RA, ed. Recent Trends in the Discovery, Development, and Evaluation of Antifungal Agents. Barcelona, Spain: Prous Science, 1987:441–459.
54. Gupta AK, Ryder JE, Chow M, et al. Dermatophytosis: the management of fungal infections. Skinmed 2005;4:305–310.
55. Zaias N. Management of onychomycosis with oral terbinafine. J Am Acad Dermatol 1990;4:810–812.
56. Finlay AY. Pharmacokinetics of terbinafine in the nail. Br J Dermatol 1992;126(Suppl 39):28–32.
57. Vickers AE, Sinclair JR, Zollinger M, et al. Multiple cytochrome P-450s involved in the metabolism of terbinafine suggest a limited potential for drug-drug interactions. Drug Metab Dispos 1999;27:1029–1038.
58. Abdel-Rahman SM, Marcucci K, Boge T, et al. Potent inhibition of cytochrome P-450 2D6-mediated dextromethorphan O-demethylation by terbinafine. Drug Metab Dispos 1999;27:770–775.
59. Odom RB. Update on topical therapy for superficial fungal infections: focus on butenafine. J Am Acad Dermatol 1997;36:S1–S2.
60. Zaug M, Bergstraesser M. Amorolfine in the treatment of onychomycoses and dermatomycoses (an overview). Clin Exp Dermatol 1992;17(Suppl 1):61–70.
61. Polak A. Preclinical data and mode of action of amorolfine. Dermatology 1992;184(Suppl 1):3–7.
62. Debono M, Gordee RS. Antibiotics that inhibit fungal cell wall development. Annu Rev Microbiol 1994;48:471–497.
63. Denning DW. Echinocandin antifungal drugs. Lancet 2003;362:1142–1151.
64. Balani SK, Xu X, Arison BH, et al. Metabolites of caspofungin acetate, a potent antifungal agent, in human plasma and urine. Drug Metab Dispos 2000;28:1274–1278.
65. Raasch RH. Anidulafungin: review of a new echinocandin antifungal agent. Expert Rev Anti Infect Ther 2004;2:499–508.
66. Hebert MF, Smith HE, Marbury TC, et al. Pharmacokinetics of micafungin in healthy volunteers, volunteers with moderate liver disease, and volunteers with renal dysfunction. J Clin Pharmacol 2005;45:1145–1152.
67. Revankar SG. Antifungal therapy. In: Anaissie EJ, McGinnis MR, Pfaller MA, eds. Clinical Mycology. New York: Churchill Livingstone, 2003:157–194.
68. Hunter PA, Darby GK, Russell NJ, eds. Fifty Years of Antimicrobials: Past Perspectives and Future Trends. Cambridge, UK: Cambridge University Press, 1995. Symposia of the Society for General Microbiology.
69. Cole GW, Stricklin G. A comparison of a new oral antifungal, terbinafine, with griseofulvin as therapy for tinea corporis. Arch Dermatol 1989;125:1537–1539.
70. Rezabek GH, Friedman AD. Superficial fungal infections of the skin. Diagnosis and current treatment recommendations. Drugs 1992;43:674–682.
71. Gupta AK, Fleckman P, Baran R. Ciclopirox nail lacquer topical solution 8% in the treatment of toenail onychomycosis. J Am Acad Dermatol 2000;43(4 Suppl):S70–S80.
72. Diehl KB. Topical antifungal agents: an update. Am Fam Physician 1996;54:1687–1692.
73. Seeling A. Eur J Biochem 1998; 251:262–261.

Chapter 36

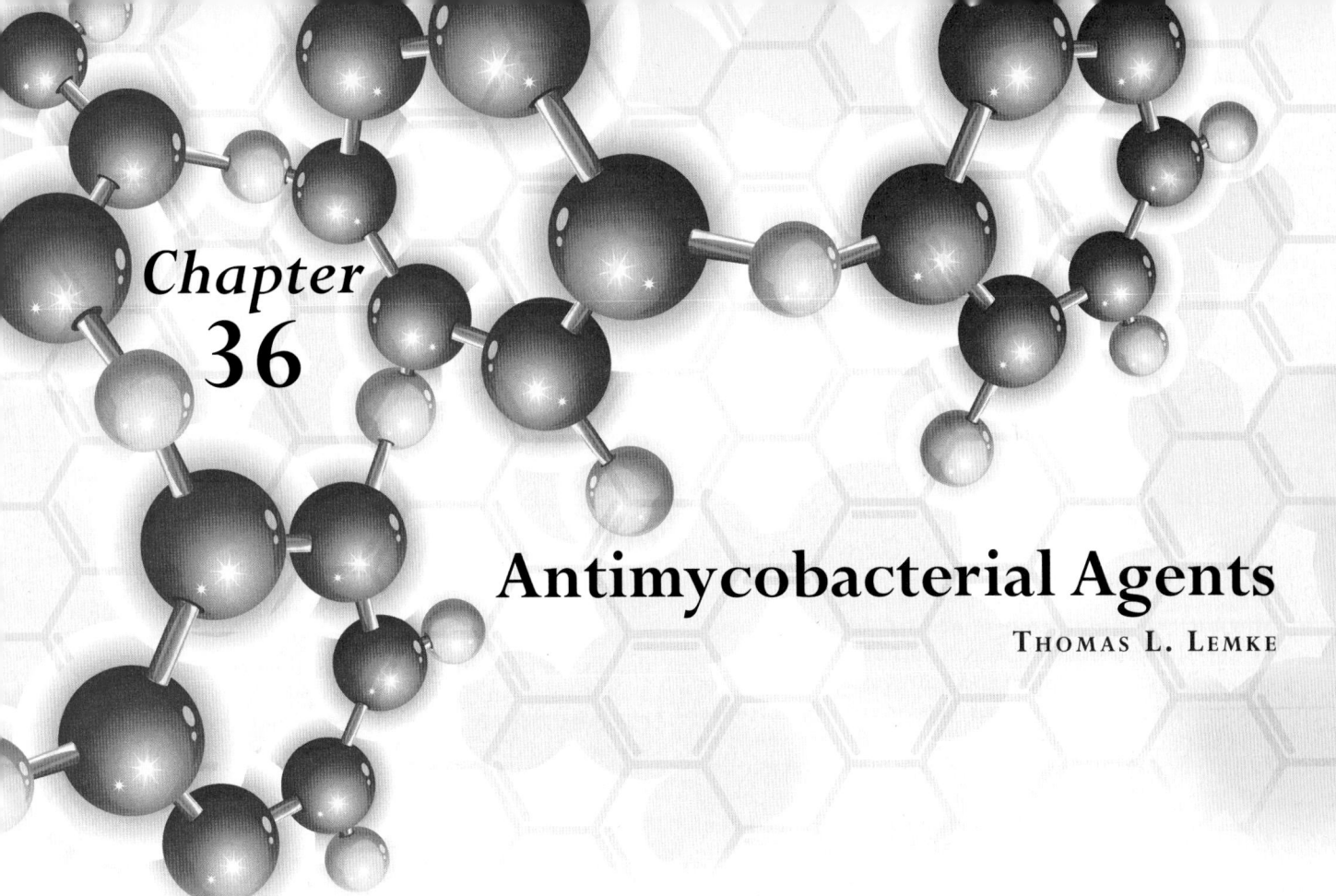

Antimycobacterial Agents

THOMAS L. LEMKE

Drugs Covered in This Chapter

ANTITUBERCULIN DRUGS
- Capreomycin
- Cycloserine
- Ethambutol
- Ethionamide
- Isoniazid
- Kanamycin
- Para-aminobenzoic acid
- Pyrazinamide
- Rifabutin
- Rifampin
- Rifapentine
- Streptomycin

MAC THERAPY
- Azithromycin
- Clarithromycin

LEPROSTATIC DRUGS
- Clofazimine
- Dapsone
- Rifampin
- Thalidomide

Abbreviations

AG, arabinogalactan
ATP, adenosine triphosphate
CDC, Centers for Disease Control and Prevention
CNS, central nervous system
DDRP, DNA-dependent RNA polymerase
DOTS, direct observed treatment, short-course
EMB, ethambutol
ENL, erythema nodosum leprosum
FDA, U.S. Food and Drug Administration
GI, gastrointestinal
G6PD, glucose-6-phosphate dehydrogenase
INH, isoniazid
LAM, lipoarabinomannan
MAC, *Mycobacterium avium–intracellulare* complex
MDR-TB, multidrug-resistant tuberculosis
PAS, *p*-aminosalicylic acid
RIF, rifampin
SAR, structure–activity relationship
STM, streptomycin
TB, tuberculosis
XTR-TB, extensively drug-resistant tuberculosis

SCENARIO

Elizabeth Coyle, PharmD

RG is a 48-year-old man who had a positive tuberculin skin test (PPD). One week ago he began taking isoniazid 300 mg daily for 9 months for the treatment of latent tuberculosis (TB). RG's medical history is unremarkable except for a right lower extremity deep vein thrombosis (DVT) 3 months ago, for which he is taking warfarin 5 mg daily. His anticoagulation has been fine with his International Normalization Ratio (INR) therapeutic at 2.5 when it was taken 2 weeks ago. However, over the last week he has noticed increased bruising, and his INR is now 5.5. He is taking no other medications, and his diet has stayed the same.

(The reader is directed to the clinical solution and chemical analysis of this case at the end of the chapter).

GENERAL CONSIDERATIONS

Mycobacteria are a genus of acid-fast bacilli belonging to the Mycobacteriaceae, which include the organisms responsible for tuberculosis and leprosy as well as a number of other, less common diseases. Characteristic of mycobacteria is that these organisms tend to be slow-growing and difficult to stain and, when they are stained with basic dye, can resist decolorization with acid alcohol. The staining characteristics relate to the abnormally high lipid content of the cell wall. In fact, the cell wall or cell envelope of the mycobacterium holds the secret to many of the characteristics of this genus of organisms. The cell envelope is unique in both structure and complexity. It has been suggested that the cell envelope is responsible for mycobacterium pathogenicity or virulence, multiple drug resistance, cell permeability, immunoreactivity, and inhibition of antigen responsiveness, as well as disease persistence and recrudescence. In addition, several of the successful chemotherapeutic agents are known to inhibit the cell envelope synthesis as their mechanism of action. It is no wonder that significant effort has been put forth to define the chemical structure of the mycobacterium cell envelope.

A series of papers were presented and reported in 1991 dealing with the topic of the structure and functions of the cell envelope of mycobacterium (1). As illustrated in Figure 36.1, the mycobacterial cell envelope contains, on the interior surface, a plasma membrane similar to that found in most bacteria. A conventional peptidoglycan layer affording the organism rigidity appears next. This layer is composed of alternating *N*-acetyl-D-glucosamines (Glu) linked to *N*-glycoyl-D-muramic acids (Mur) through 1–4 linkages that, in turn, is attached to the peptido chain of D-alanine (A), D-glutamine (G), meso-diaminopimelic acid (DP), and L-alanine (A). A novel disaccharide phosphodiester linker made up of *N*-acetyl-D-glucosamine and rhamnose connects the muramic acid to a polygalactan and polyarabinose chain. The latter polysaccharides are referred to as the arabinogalactan (AG) portion of the cell envelope. The manner in which the arabinosyl and galactosyl resides are arranged is still under investigation. It is known that the arabinosyl chains terminate in mycolic acid residues. (The mycolates will be discussed in more detail later in this chapter.) Noncovalently bound to the mycolates are a number of free nonpolar and polar lipids (the phthiocerol lipids and the glycopeptidolipids, respectively). Finally, spanning from the interior, embedded in the plasma membrane, to the exterior is the lipoarabinomannan (LAM) polymer. As indicated, this unit is composed of polyarabinose, polymannan, and various lipids attached through a phosphatidylinositol moiety (2,3).

SPECIFIC DISEASES

Leprosy (Hansen Disease)

Throughout the Bible, one finds reference to the condition of leprosy, such as that described in *Leviticus*: "[I]s there any flesh in the skin of which there is a burn by fire and the quick flesh of the burn becomes a bright spot, reddish white or white, ... and if the hair in the bright spot is turned white and it appears deeper than the skin, it is leprosy broken out in the burn." Associated with the disease was a belief that individuals suffering from this disease were unclean. Today, leprosy (Hansen disease) is recognized as a chronic granulomatous infection caused by *Mycobacterium leprae*. The disease can consist of lepromatous leprosy, tuberculoid leprosy, or a condition with characteristics between these two poles and referred to as borderline leprosy. The disease is more common in tropical countries but is not limited to warm climate regions. It is thought to afflict some 10 to 20 million individuals. Children appear to be the most susceptible population, but the signs and symptoms do not usually occur until much later in life. The incubation period is usually 3 to 5 years. The disease is contagious, but the infectiousness is quite low. Person-to-person contact appears to be the means by which the disease is spread, with entrance into the body occurring through the skin or the mucosa of the upper respiratory tract. Skin and peripheral nerves are the regions most susceptible to attack.

The first signs of the disease consist of hypopigmented or hyperpigmented macules. Anesthetic or paresthetic patches can be additionally experienced by the patient. Neural involvement in the extremities leads ultimately to muscle atrophy, resorption of small bones, and spontaneous amputation. When facial nerves are involved, corneal ulceration and blindness can occur. The identification of

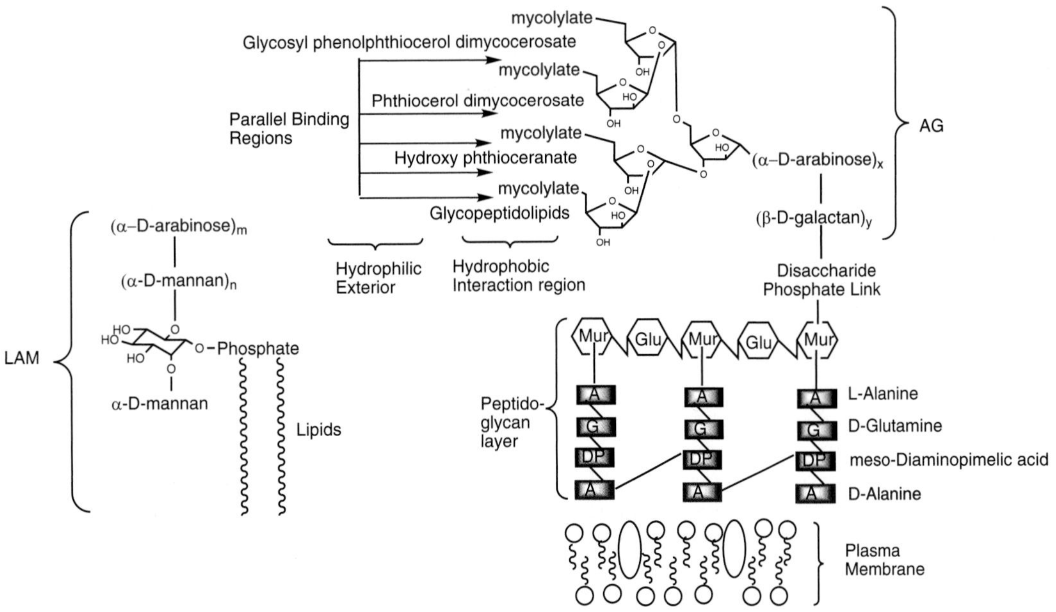

FIGURE 36.1 Diagramatic representation of the cell wall/cell envelope of mycobacterium with drug sites of action highlighted in *red*.

M. leprae in skin or blood samples is not always possible, but the detection of the antibody to the organism is an effective diagnostic test, especially for the lepromatous form of the disease.

Tuberculosis

Tuberculosis (TB) is a disease that has been known from the earliest recorded history. It is characterized as a chronic bacterial infection caused by *Mycobacterium tuberculosis*, an acid-fast, aerobic bacillus with the previously discussed, unusual cell wall. The cell wall has a high lipid content, resulting in a high degree of hydrophobicity and resistance to alcohol, acids, alkali, and some disinfectants. After staining with a dye, the *M. tuberculosis* cell wall cannot subsequently be decolorized with acid wash, thus the characteristic of being an acid-fast bacillus. It is estimated that today, one-third to one-half of the world population is infected with *M. tuberculosis*, leading to approximately 6% of all deaths worldwide (~2 million deaths) (4,5). TB is the leading worldwide cause of mortality resulting from an infectious bacterial

CLINICAL SIGNIFICANCE

Diseases caused by mycobacteria such as TB and MAC are of great concern to both healthcare workers and the public. Understanding the infectivity and pathophysiology of mycobacteria and the medicinal chemistry of the antimicrobials in the complex treatment of mycobacteria infections can help facilitate a clinician's pharmacotherapy decisions. Mycobacteria are very slow-growing organisms that grow both intracellularly and extracellularly. Because of their growth, the treatment of mycobacterial infections, especially TB, requires long-term treatment with a combination of agents to effectively eradicate the disease and prevent resistance. In addition, many of these agents are associated with significant side effects and drug interactions. A good understanding of the medicinal chemistry of antimycobacterial agents helps the clinician to determine the most effective and safe combination for an individual patient.

Continuing interest in the study of the medicinal chemistry of antimycobacterial agents is prudent in the development of newer and safer agents. Research efforts are continuously being made, looking at agents which have more rapid antimycobacterial activity as well as lower resistance and fewer side effects. The discovery of such agents would have a significant effect on increasing the eradication of this worldwide epidemic. Shorter-course therapies would lead to an increase in patient compliance and possible decrease in mycobacterial resistance. As newer and more effective therapies are developed, clinicians will need to stay informed about their pharmacokinetic and pharmacodynamic profiles so patients can receive the most optimal and effective treatment.

Elizabeth Coyle PharmD
Clinical Assistant Professor
Department of Clinical Sciences & Administration
University of Houston College of Pharmacy
Houston, Texas

agent. A steady decline in the reported cases of TB had been occurring in the United States from the 1950s until 1985. From 1985 until 1988, however, this decline leveled off, but beginning in 1989, an increase was noted. In 1991, the Centers for Disease Control and Prevention (CDC) reported 25,701 new cases of TB. Today, the press and professional publications announce the "epidemic" spread of TB. The resurgence has been linked to urban crowding, homelessness, immigration, drug abuse, the disappearance of preventive-medicine health clinics, crowded prisons, and the AIDS epidemic. "Most alarming is the emergence of multidrug-resistant TB" (MDR-TB) (6). Before 1984, only 10% of the organisms isolated from patients with TB were resistant to any drug. In 1984, 52% of the organisms were resistant to at least one drug, and 32% were resistant to more than one drug. MDR-TB can have a fatality rate as high as 50%. The World Health Organization estimates that as many as 5% of all TB cases are MDR-TB. MDR-TB is associated with resistance to the two most potent first-line anti-TB drugs (i.e., isoniazid and rifampicin). More patients are being diagnosed with extensively drug-resistant TB (XTR-TB), a condition in which the organism is resistant to either isoniazid or rifampicin, any fluoroquinolone, and at least one of the three second-line injectable drugs (i.e., capreomycin, kanamycin, and amikacin). As a result of MDR-TB and XTR-TB, isolates of *M. tuberculosis* should be tested for antimicrobial susceptibility. In fact, drug resistance is encountered in patients who have never been treated with any of the TB drugs.

M. tuberculosis is transmitted primarily via the respiratory route. The organism appears in water droplets expelled during coughing, sneezing, or talking. Either in the droplet form or as the desiccated airborne bacilli, the organism enters the respiratory tract. The infectiousness of an individual will depend on the extent of the disease, the number of organisms in the sputum, and the amount of coughing. Within 2 weeks of beginning therapy, the infected individual will usually no longer be infectious. TB is a disease that mainly affects the lungs (80% to 85% of the cases), but *M. tuberculosis* can spread through the bloodstream and the lymphatic system to the brain, bones, eyes, and skin (extrapulmonary TB). In pulmonary TB, the bacilli reach the alveoli and are ingested by pulmonary macrophages. Substances secreted by the macrophages stimulate surrounding fibroblasts to enclose the infection site, leading to formation of granulomas or tubercles. The infection, thus contained locally, can lie dormant, encapsulated in a fibrotic lesion, for years and then reappear later. Extrapulmonary TB is much more common in HIV-infected patients (40% to 75%).

Because of the effect of the AIDS virus on the immune system, all HIV-infected individuals should be screened for TB, and if infected, the patient should be treated for TB before an active infection develops. Patients with HIV infection and TB are 100-fold more likely to develop an active infection than noninfected patients. Individuals diagnosed with active TB should be counseled and tested for HIV because TB could have developed in conjunction with the weakened immune system seen in the patient with HIV infection. TB is the leading cause of death in patients who are HIV positive. Complicating treatment of HIV–TB coinfections is that drug interactions are quite common between the standard TB treatment regimens and antiretroviral drugs.

Mycobacterium Avium–Intracellulare Complex

Mycobacterium avium and *Mycobacterium intracellulare* are atypical acid-fast bacilli that are ubiquitous in the environment and considered usually to be nonpathogenic in healthy individuals. Unfortunately, in immunocompromised individuals, these and possibly other, unidentified mycobacteria cause severe, life-threatening infections. Disseminated *Mycobacterium avium–intracellulare* complex (MAC) is the most common bacterial opportunistic infection seen in patients with AIDS and the third most common opportunistic infection behind candidal esophagitis and primary *Pneumocystis jirovecii* pneumonia (PCP) reported in patients with AIDS. Between 1981 and 1987 and before the availability of effective antiretroviral medication, the incidence of MAC was reported as 5%. Today, approximately half of all patients with AIDS develop an infection caused by MAC. The lungs are the organs most commonly involved in patients without AIDS, but the infection can involve bone marrow, lymph nodes, liver, and blood in patients with AIDS. The CD4 T-lymphocyte count is used as a predictor for risk of disseminated MAC; a count of less than 50 cells/mm^3 in an HIV-infected person (adult or adolescent) is an indication of a potential infection and a recommendation for chemoprophylaxis. The MAC organisms grow within macrophages; therefore, the drug must be capable of penetration of the macrophage. Treatment of MAC, both prophylactically and for diagnosed infections, requires the use of multidrug therapy, and for disseminated MAC, this treatment is for the life of the patient.

GENERAL APPROACHES TO DRUG THERAPY

The mycobacteria have a number of characteristics in common, but it is important to recognize that the species vary widely in their susceptibility to the different drugs and that, in turn, this can relate to significant differences in the organisms. Some species, such as *M. tuberculosis,* are very slow-growing, with a doubling time of approximately 24 hours, whereas others, such as *Mycobacterium smegmatis,* double in 2 to 3 hours. The pathogenic mycobacterial organism can be divided into organism that are actively metabolizing and rapidly growing; semidormant bacilli, which exhibit spurts of metabolism; bacilli that exist at low pH and exhibit low metabolic activity; and dormant or persisters. The latter characteristic is the most problematic and responsible for treatment failures. Most current TB drugs are those that are effective against actively metabolizing and rapidly growing bacilli. Thus, successful chemotherapy calls for drugs with bactericidal action against all stages of the organisms—but especially against the persisters. The use of combination therapy over an extended period of time is one answer to successful treatment.

DRUG THERAPY FOR TUBERCULOSIS

Drug therapy for the treatment of TB has been greatly hampered by the development of MDR-TB (and more recently XDR-TB) and the lack of new classes of drugs. In fact, no new drugs have been developed in the last 45 years. The only change in the treatment of TB has been the strategy of using direct observed treatment, short-course (DOTS), with an emphasis on patient-centered care (7). Additionally, although the course of treatment has been reduced through the use of drug combinations to 6 months, patient compliance continues to be a serious problem, which in turn can be associated with the development of bacterial resistance.

First-Line Agents

Isoniazid (Isonicotinic Acid Hydrazide, Nydrazid, Laniazid)

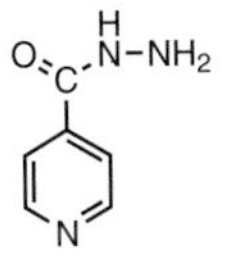

Isoniazid (INH) is a synthetic antibacterial agent with bactericidal action against *M. tuberculosis*. The drug was discovered in the 1950s as a beneficial agent effective against intracellular and extracellular bacilli, and it is generally considered to be the primary drug for treatment of *M. tuberculosis*. Its action is bactericidal against replicating organisms, but it appears to be only bacteriostatic at best against semidormant and dormant populations. After treatment with INH, *M. tuberculosis* loses its acid fastness, which can be interpreted as indicating that the drug interferes with cell wall development.

MECHANISM OF ACTION Although extensively investigated, the mechanism of action of INH has remained unknown until recently. New investigations into mechanisms of bacterial resistance have shed light on the molecular mechanism of action of INH (8). It is generally recognized that INH is a prodrug that is activated through an oxidation reaction catalyzed by an endogenous enzyme (9). This enzyme, katG, which exhibits catalase-peroxidase activity, converts INH to a reactive species capable of acylation of an enzyme system found exclusively in *M. tuberculosis*. Evidence in support of the activation of INH reveals that INH-resistant isolates have decreased catalase activity and that the loss of catalase activity is associated with the deletion of the catalase gene, *katG*. Furthermore, reintroduction of the gene into resistant organisms results in restored sensitivity of the organism to the drug. Reaction of INH with catalase-peroxidase results in formation of isonicotinaldehyde, isonicotinic acid, and isonicotinamide, which can be accounted for through the reactive intermediate isonicotinoyl radical or isonicotinic peroxide, as shown in Figure 36.2 (10). Evidence has been offered both for and against the reaction of catalase-peroxidase activated INH with a portion of the enzyme inhA, which is involved in the biosynthesis of the mycolic acids (Fig. 36.3) (11–13). The mycolic acids are important constituents of the mycobacterial cell wall in that they provide a permeability barrier to hydrophilic solutes. The enzyme inhA, produced under the control of the *inhA* gene, is an NADH-dependent, enoyl reductase protein thought to be involved in double-bond reduction during fatty acid elongation (Fig. 36.4). Isoniazid specifically inhibits long-chain fatty acid synthesis (>26 carbon atoms). It should be noted that the mycolic acids are α-branched lipids having a "short" arm of 20 to 24 carbons and a "long" arm of

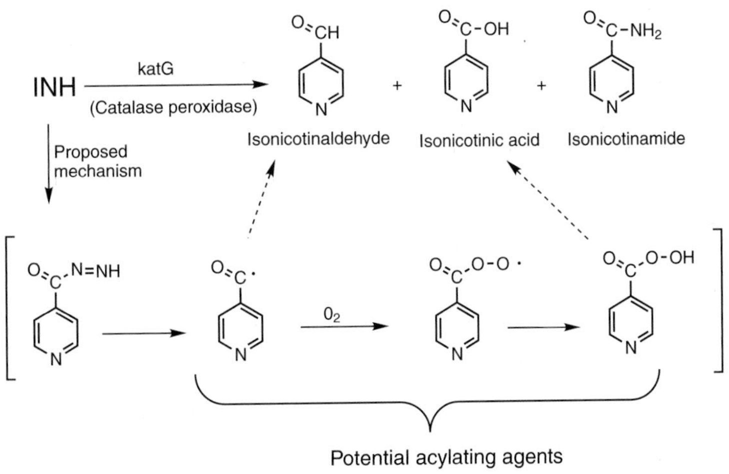

FIGURE 36.2 Reaction products formed from catalase-peroxidase reaction with isoniazid (INH).

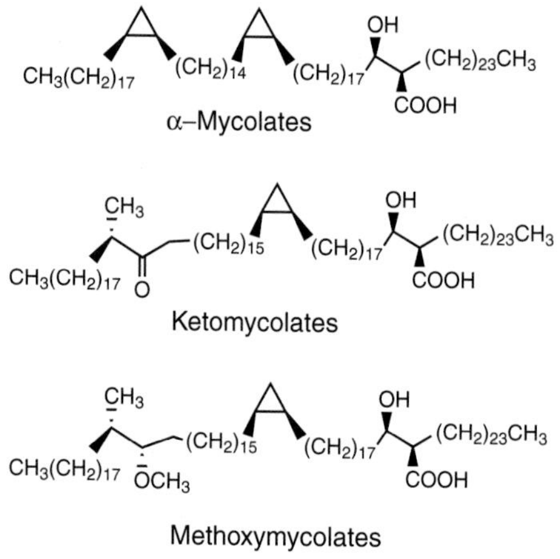

FIGURE 36.3 Mycolic acids.

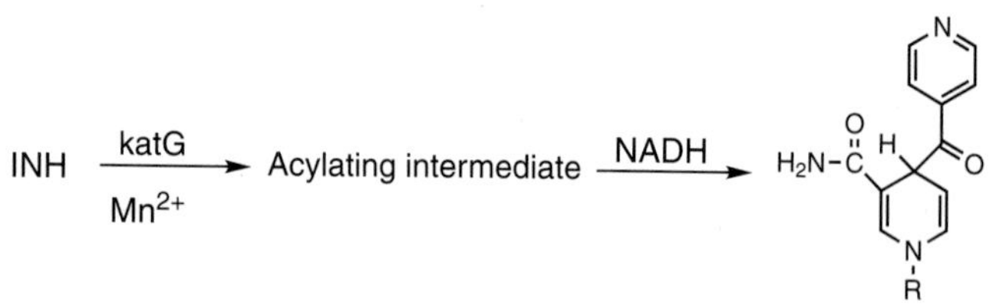

FIGURE 36.5 Acylation of NADH and NADH-dependent enoylacyl protein (inhA).

50 to 60 carbons. It has been proposed that INH is activated to an electrophilic species that acylates the four position of the NADH (Fig. 36.5). The acylated NADH is no longer capable of catalyzing the reduction of unsaturated fatty acids, which are essential for the synthesis of the mycolic acids (14–16).

The mechanism of resistance to INH appears to be a very complicated process, possibly involving mutations in multiple genes including *katG* and *inhA*. It is possible that different mutations result in different degrees of resistance. This seems to be especially true in MDR-TB. A high level of resistance is reported to occur through *katG* mutation, which leads to a Ser-315 to Thr-315 in katG catalase-peroxidase and prevents INH activation (17).

Structure–Activity Relationship An extensive series of derivatives of nicotinaldehyde, isonicotinaldehyde, and substituted isonicotinic acid hydrazides have been prepared and investigated for their tuberculostatic activity. Isoniazid hydrazones were found to possess activity, but these compounds were shown to be unstable in the gastrointestinal (GI) tract, releasing the active isonicotinic acid hydrazide (i.e., INH). Thus, it would appear that their activity resulted from the INH and not from the derivatives (18,19). Substitution of the hydrazine portion of INH with alkyl and aralkyl substituents resulted in a series of active and inactive derivatives (20–23).

Substitution on the *N*-2 position resulted in active compounds (R1 and/or R2 = alkyl; R3 = H), whereas any substitution of the *N*-1 hydrogen with alkyl groups destroyed the activity (R1 and R2 = H; R3 = alkyl). None of these changes produced compounds with activity superior to that of INH.

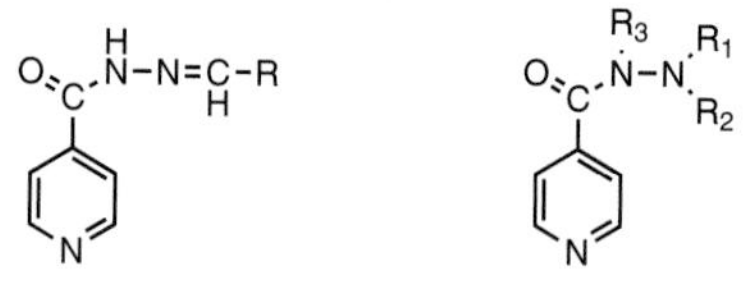

Isoniazid hydrazones Isonicotinic acid hydrazides

Metabolism Isoniazid is extensively metabolized to inactive metabolites (Fig. 36.6) (24,25). The major metabolite is *N*-acetylisoniazid. The enzyme responsible for acetylation, cytosolic *N*-acetyltransferase, is produced

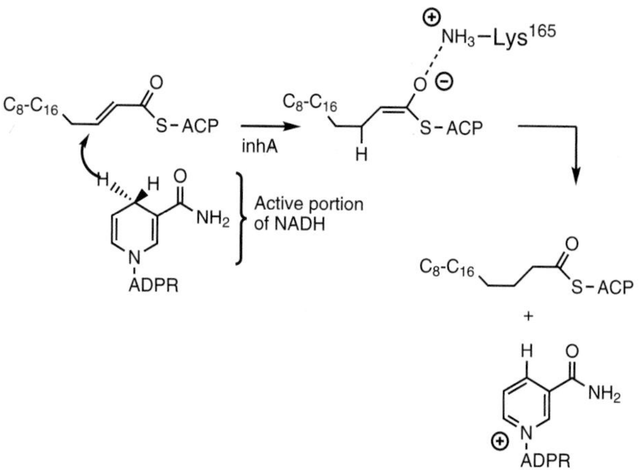

FIGURE 36.4 Enoylthioester. ACP, acyl carrier (protein) reduction catalyzed by NADH and inhA.

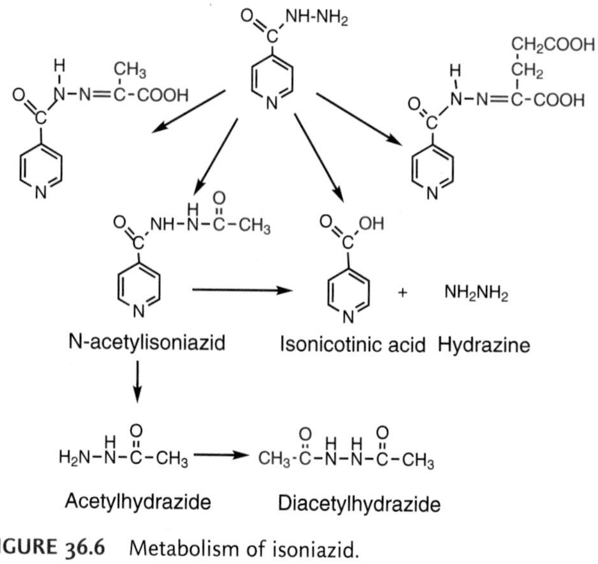

FIGURE 36.6 Metabolism of isoniazid.

under genetic control in an inherited autosomal fashion. Individuals who possess high concentrations of the enzyme are referred to as rapid acetylators, whereas those with low concentrations are slow acetylators. This can result in a need to adjust the dosage for fast acetylators. The *N*-acetyltransferase is located primarily in the liver and small intestine. Other metabolites include isonicotinic acid, which is found in the urine as a glycine conjugate, and hydrazine. Isonicotinic acid can also result from hydrolysis of *N*-acetylisoniazid, but in this case, the second product of hydrolysis is acetylhydrazine. Mono-*N*-acetylhydrazine is acetylated by *N*-acetyltransferase to the inactive *N*-diacetyl product. This reaction occurs more rapidly in rapid acetylators. The formation of *N*-acetylhydrazine is significant in that this compound has been associated with hepatotoxicity, which can occur during INH therapy. *N*-Acetylhydrazine has been postulated to serve as a substrate for microsomal P450, resulting in the formation of a reactive intermediate that is capable of acetylating liver proteins, in turn resulting in liver necrosis (26). It has been suggested that an *N*-hydroxylamine intermediate is formed that results in a reactive acetylating agent (Fig. 36.7). The acetyl radical/cation acylates liver protein (see Chapter 4).

Pharmacokinetics Isoniazid is readily absorbed following oral administration. Food and various antacids, especially aluminum-containing antacids, can interfere with or delay the absorption; therefore, it is recommended that the drug be taken on an empty stomach. The drug is well distributed to body tissues, including infected tissue. A long-standing concern about the use of INH during preventive therapy for latent TB has been the high incidence of hepatotoxicity. Recent studies have concluded that, excluding patients over 35 years of age, if relevant clinical monitoring is employed, the rate of hepatotoxicity is quite low (27). The risk of hepatotoxicity is associated with increasing age and, for unknown reasons, appears to be higher in women than in men.

Rifamycin Antibiotics

The rifamycins are members of the ansamycin class of natural products produced by *Streptomyces mediterranei*. This chemical class is characterized as molecules with an aliphatic chain forming a bridge between two nonadjacent positions of an aromatic moiety.

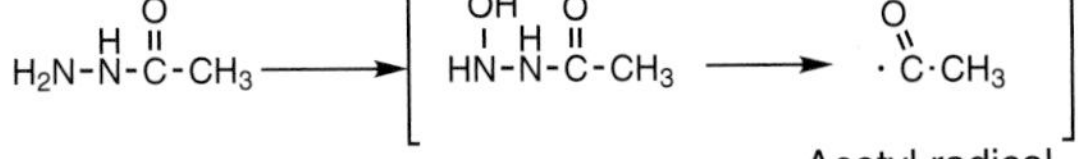

Acetylhydrazide

Acetyl radical

FIGURE 36.7 Acylating metabolite of isoniazid.

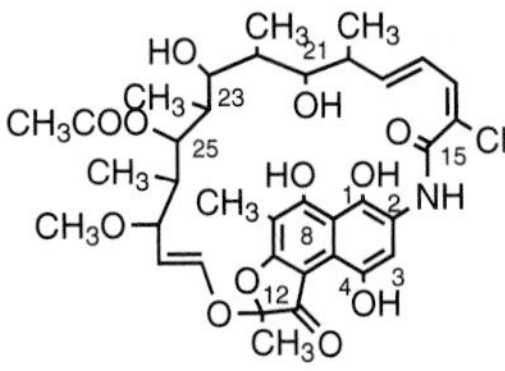

Rifamycin SV

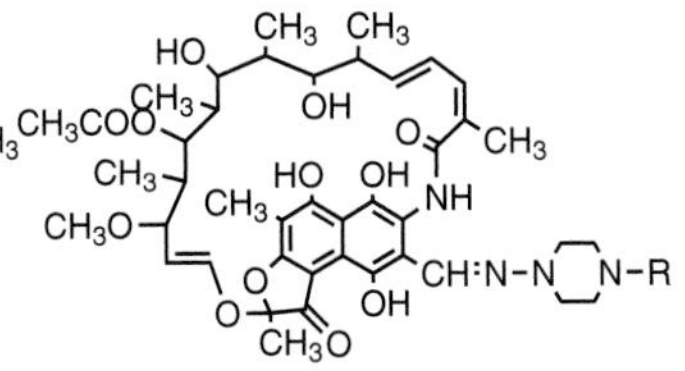

Rifampin R = CH_3

Rifapentine R = 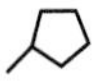

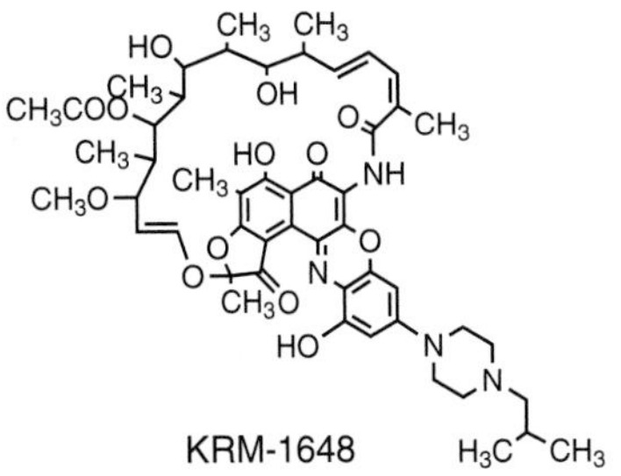

KRM-1648

While investigating the biologic activity of the naturally occurring rifamycins (B, O, and S), a spontaneous reaction gave the biologically active rifamycin SV, which was later isolated from natural sources. Rifamycin SV was the original rifamycin antibiotic chosen for clinical development (28). Semisynthetic derivatives are prepared via conversion of the natural rifamycins to 3-formylrifamycin, which is derivatized with various hydrazines to give products such as rifampin (RIF) and rifapentine. RIF and rifapentine have significant benefit over previously investigated rifamycins in that they are orally active, are highly effective against a variety of both gram-positive and gram-negative organisms, and have high clinical efficacy in the treatment of TB. The rifamycin antibiotics are active against both growing and slow-metabolizing, nongrowing bacilli.

Mechanism of Action The rifamycins inhibit bacterial DNA-dependent RNA polymerase (DDRP) by binding to the β-subunit of the enzyme and are highly active against rapidly dividing intracellular and extracellular bacilli. RIF is active against DDRP from both gram-positive and gram-negative bacteria, but because of poor penetration of the cell wall of gram-negative organisms by RIF, the drug has less value in infections caused by such organisms. Inhibition of DDRP leads to blocking the initiation of chain formation in RNA synthesis. It has been suggested that the naphthalene ring of the rifamycins π-π bonds to an aromatic amino acid ring in the DDRP protein (29). The DDRP is a metalloenzyme that contains two zinc atoms. It is further postulated that the oxygens at C-1 and C-8 of a rifamycin can chelate to a zinc atom, which increases the binding to DDRP, and finally, the oxygens at C-21 and C-23 form strong hydrogen bonds to the DDRP. The binding of the rifamycins to DDRP results in the inhibition of the RNA synthesis. Specifically, RIF has been shown to inhibit the elongation of full-length transcripts, but it has no effect on transcription initiation (8). Resistance develops when a mutation occurs in the gene responsible for the β-subunit of the RNA polymerase (*rpoB* gene), resulting in an inability of the antibiotic to readily bind to the RNA polymerase (30).

Structure–Activity Relationship A large number of derivatives of the naturally occurring rifamycins have been prepared (31). From these compounds, the following generalizations can be made concerning the structure–activity relationship (SAR): 1) Free –OH groups are required at C-1, C-8, C-21, and C-23; 2) these groups appear to lie in a plane and to be important binding groups for attachment to DDRP, as previously indicated; 3) acetylation of C-21 and/or C-23 produces inactive compounds; 4) reduction of the double bonds in the macro ring results in a progressive decrease in activity; and 5) opening of the macro ring also gives inactive compounds. These latter two changes greatly affect the conformational structure of the rifamycins, which in turn decreases binding to DDRP. Substitution at C-3 or C-4 results in compounds with varying degrees of antibacterial activity. The substitution at these positions appears to affect transport across the bacterial cell wall. A compound incorporating such substitution is the benzoxazinorifamycin KRM-1648, which is proceeding through clinical investigation. In vitro studies have shown rapid tissue sterilization and encouraging results concerning combination therapy for TB and, possibly, MAC.

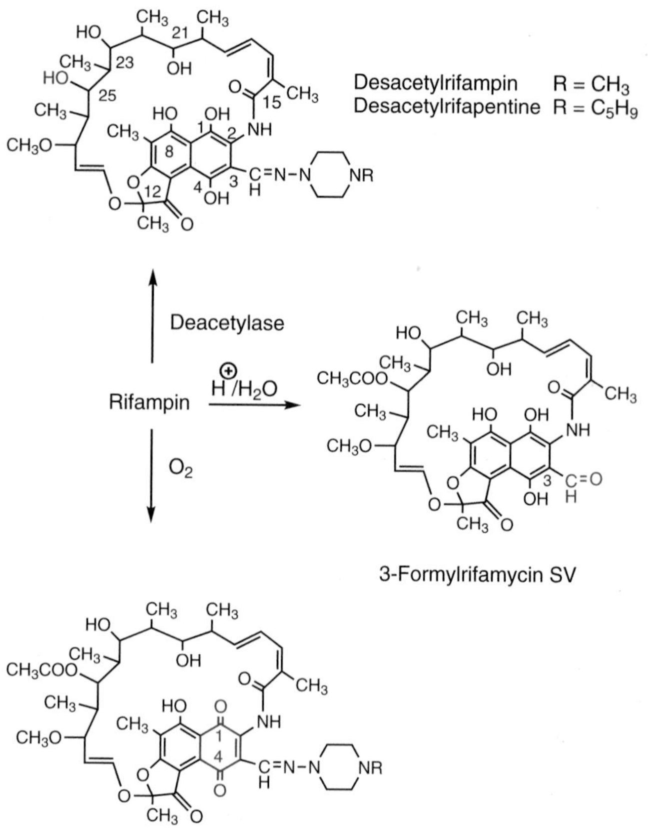

FIGURE 36.8 Metabolism and in vitro reactions of rifampin.

Metabolism RIF and rifapentine are readily absorbed from the intestine, although food in the tract can affect absorption. RIF's absorption can be reduced by food in the intestine; therefore, the drug should be taken on an empty stomach (25). Intestinal absorption of rifapentine has been reported to be enhanced when taken after a meal (32). Neither drug appears to interfere with the absorption of other antituberculin agents, but there are conflicting reports on whether INH affects absorption of RIF. The major metabolism of RIF and rifapentine is deacetylation, which occurs at the C-25 acetate (Fig. 36.8). The resulting products, desacetylrifampin and desacetylrifapentine, are still active antibacterial agents. The majority of both desacetyl products are found in the feces, but desacetylrifampin glucuronide can be found in the urine as well. 3-Formylrifamycin SV has been reported as a second metabolite after administration of both RIF and rifapentine. This product is thought to arise in the gut from an acid-catalyzed hydrolysis reaction. Formylrifamycin is reported to possess a broad spectrum of antibacterial activity (33).

Physicochemical Properties RIF and rifapentine are red-orange, crystalline compounds with zwitterionic properties. The presence of the phenolic groups results in acidic properties ($pK_a \sim 1.7$), whereas the piperazine moiety gives basic properties ($pK_a \sim 7.9$). These compounds are prone to acid hydrolysis, giving rise to 3-formylrifamycin SV, as indicated earlier. RIF and presumably rifapentine are prone to air oxidation of the *p*-phenolic groups in the naphthalene ring to give the *p*-quinone (C-1,4 quinone) (Fig. 36.8). RIF, rifapentine, and their metabolites are excreted in the urine, feces (biliary excretion), saliva, sweat, and tears. Because these agents have dye characteristics, one can note discoloration of the body fluids containing the drug. Notably, the tears can be discolored, and permanent staining of contact lenses can occur.

Therapeutic Application

Rifampin (Rifadin, Rimactane) With the introduction of RIF in 1967, the duration of combination therapy for the treatment of TB was significantly reduced (from 18 to 9 months). RIF is nearly always used in combination with one or more other antituberculin agents. The drug is potentially hepatotoxic and can produce GI disturbances, rash, and thrombocytopenic purpura. RIF is known to be a potent inducer of the hepatic CYP3A4 and can decrease the effectiveness of oral contraceptives, corticosteroids, warfarin, quinidine, methadone, zidovudine, clarithromycin, and the azole antifungal agents (see Chapter 4) (34). In addition, the rifamycins appear to increase the expression of P-glycoproteins, which increase the efflux of various drugs.

Because of the decreased effectiveness of protease inhibitors and nonnucleoside reverse transcriptase inhibitors used in the treatment of HIV, the CDC has recommended avoidance of RIF in treatment of HIV-infected patients presently on these HIV therapies.

Rifapentine (Priftin) Rifapentine is the first new agent introduced for the treatment of pulmonary TB in the last 25 years. The drug's major advantage over RIF is the fact that when used in combination therapy, rifapentine can be administered twice weekly during the "intense" phase of therapy, followed by once-a-week administration during the "continuous" phase. In contrast, RIF normally is administered daily during the "intense" phase, followed by twice-a-week dosing during the "continuous" phase. Because relapse and the emergence of resistant strains of bacteria are associated with poor patient compliance, reduced dosing is expected to increase compliance. Initial clinical studies actually showed that the relapse rates in patients treated with rifapentine (10%) were higher than those in patients treated with RIF (5%). It was found that poor compliance with the nonrifamycin antituberculin agents was responsible for the increased relapse (32).

Rifapentine is readily absorbed following oral administration and is highly bound to plasma protein (97.7% vs. 80% for RIF). Related to the higher plasma binding, rifapentine has a longer mean elimination half-life (13.2 hours in healthy male volunteers) in comparison with the half-life reported for RIF (~2 to 5 hours). Greater than 70% of either drug is excreted in the feces. Rifapentine is generally considered to be more active than RIF and can be used in patients with varying degrees of hepatic dysfunction without the need for dose adjustment (35). This drug, similar to what is seen with RIF, induces hepatic microsomal enzymes (CYP3A4 and CYP2C8/9) but appears to have less of an inducing effect on cytochrome P450 than RIF. Rifapentine has been reported to be teratogenic in rats and rabbits (32).

Pyrazinamide

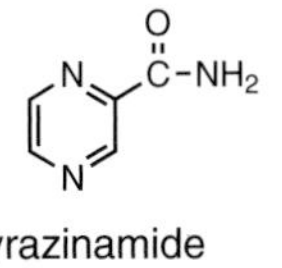

Pyrazinamide

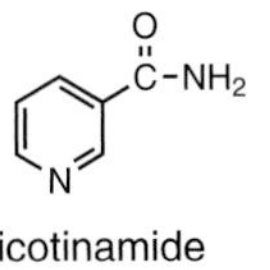

Nicotinamide

Pyrazinamide (pyrazinecarboxamide) was discovered while investigating analogs of nicotinamide. Pyrazinamide is a bioisostere of nicotinamide and possesses bactericidal action against *M. tuberculosis*. Pyrazinamide has become one of the more popular antituberculin agents despite the fact that resistance develops quickly. Combination therapy, however, has proven to be an effective means of reducing the rate of resistant strain development. The activity of pyrazinamide is pH dependent with good in vivo activity at pH 5.5, but the compound is nearly inactive at neutral pH.

Mechanism of Action The mechanism of action of pyrazinamide is unknown, but recent findings suggest that pyrazinamide can be active either totally or in part as a prodrug. Susceptible organisms produce pyrazinamidase, which is responsible for conversion of pyrazinamide to pyrazinoic acid intracellularly (8). Mutation in the pyrazinamidase gene (*pncA*) results in resistant strains of M. tuberculosis (37). Pyrazinoic acid has been shown to possess biologic activity at a pH 5.4 or lower, in contrast in vitro tests that show pyrazinoic acid is 8- to 16-fold less active than pyrazinamide (38). Pyrazinoic acid can lower the pH in the immediate surroundings of the M. tuberculosis to such an extent that the organism is unable to grow, but this physicochemical property appears to account for only some of the activity. The protonated pyrazinoic acid can also permeate the mycobacterial membrane to lower the pH of the cytoplasm. Recent evidence suggests that pyrazinoic acid decreases membrane potential in older, nonreplicating bacilli, thus decreasing membrane transport, and interferes with the energetics of the membrane (39).

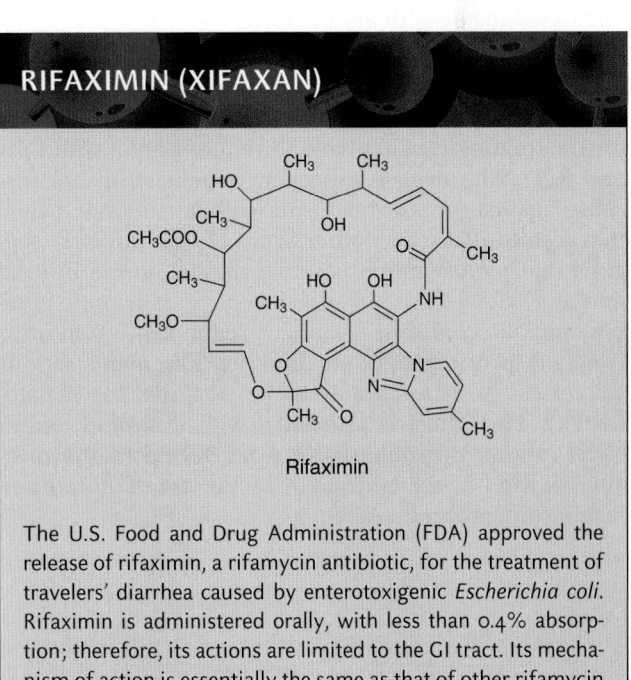

RIFAXIMIN (XIFAXAN)

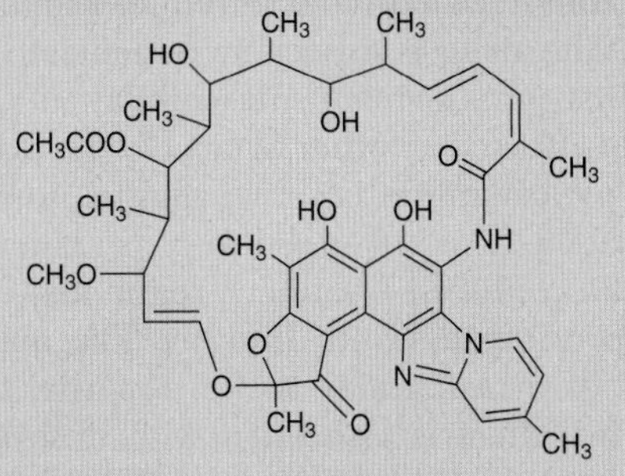

Rifaximin

The U.S. Food and Drug Administration (FDA) approved the release of rifaximin, a rifamycin antibiotic, for the treatment of travelers' diarrhea caused by enterotoxigenic *Escherichia coli*. Rifaximin is administered orally, with less than 0.4% absorption; therefore, its actions are limited to the GI tract. Its mechanism of action is essentially the same as that of other rifamycin antibiotics (36).

STRUCTURE–ACTIVITY RELATIONSHIP Previous structural modification of pyrazinamide has proven to be ineffective in developing analogs with increased biologic activity. Substitution on the pyrazine ring or use of alternate heterocyclic aromatic rings has given compounds with reduced activity (40). More recently, using quantitative SAR, a series of analogs have been prepared with improved biologic activity. The requirements for successful analogs include 1) provision for hydrophilicity to allow sufficient plasma concentrations such that the drug can be delivered to the site of infection, 2) lipophilicity to allow penetration into the mycobacterial cell, and 3) susceptibility to hydrolysis such that the prodrug is unaffected by the "extracellular" enzymes but is readily hydrolyzed at the site of action. Two compounds have been found that meet these criteria: *tert*-butyl 5-chloropyrazinamide and 2′-(2′-methyldecyl) 5-chloropyrazinamide (41).

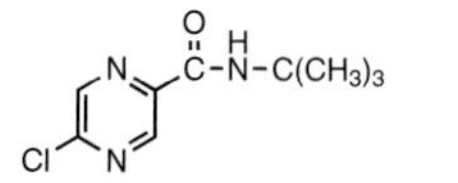

tert-butyl 5-chloropyrazinamide

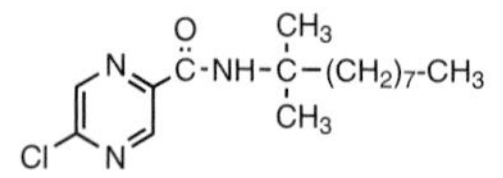

2'-(2'-methyldecyl) 5-chloropyrazinamide

METABOLISM Pyrazinamide is readily absorbed after oral administration, but little of the intact molecule is excreted unchanged (Fig. 36.9). The major metabolic route consists of hydrolysis by hepatic microsomal pyrazinamidase to pyrazinoic acid, which can then be oxidized by xanthine oxidase to 5-hydroxypyrazinoic acid. The latter compound can appear in the urine either free or as a conjugate with glycine (24).

THERAPEUTIC APPLICATION Pyrazinamide has gained acceptance as an essential component in combination therapy for the treatment of TB (component of Rifater with INH and RIF). The drug is especially beneficial in that it is active against semidormant intracellular tubercle bacilli that are not affected by other drugs (7,35). Evidence suggests that pyrazinamide is active against nonreplicating persister bacilli. The introduction of pyrazinamide combinations has reduced treatment regimens to 6 months from the previous 9-month therapy. The major serious side effect of pyrazinamide is the potential for hepatotoxicity. This effect is associated with dose and length of treatment. Pyrazinamide is not affected by the presence of food in the GI tract or by the use of aluminum-magnesium antacids (42).

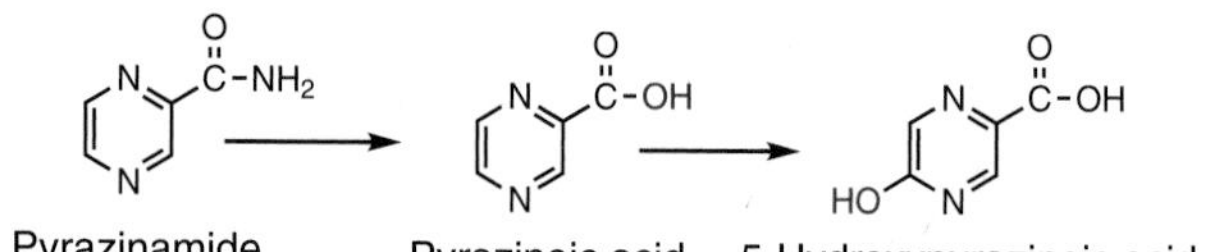

FIGURE 36.9 Metabolism of pyrazinamide.

Ethambutol (Myambutol)

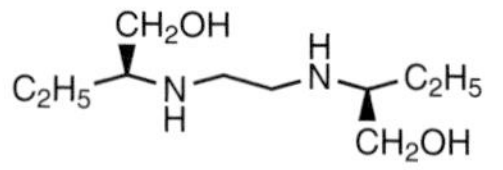

Ethambutol

Ethambutol (EMB), an ethylenediiminobutanol, is administered as its (+)-enantiomer, which is 200- to 500-fold more active than its (−)-enantiomer. The difference in activity between the two isomers suggests a specific receptor for its site of action. EMB is a water-soluble, bacteriostatic agent that is readily absorbed (75% to 80%) after oral administration.

MECHANISM OF ACTION The mechanism of action of EMB remains unknown, although mounting evidence suggests a specific site of action for EMB. It has been known for some time that EMB affects mycobacterial cell wall synthesis; however, the complicated nature of the mycobacterial cell wall has made pinpointing the site of action difficult. In addition to the peptidoglycan portion of the cell wall, the mycobacterium have a unique outer envelope consisting of arabinofuranose and galactose (AG), which is covalently attached to the peptidoglycan and an intercalated framework of LAM (Fig. 36.1). The AG portion of the cell wall is highly branched and contains distinct segments of galactan and distinct segments of arabinan. At various locations within the arabinan segments (terminal and penultimate), the mycolic acids are attached to the C-5′ position of arabinan (43,44). Initially, Takayama et al. (45) reported that EMB inhibited the synthesis of the AG portion of the cell wall. More recently, it has been reported that EMB inhibits the enzyme arabinosyl transferase. One action of arabinosyl transferase is to catalyze the polymerization of d-arabinofuranose, leading to AG (46,47). EMB mimics arabinan, resulting in a buildup of the arabinan precursor β-d-arabinofuranosyl-1-monophosphoryldecaprenol and, as a result, a block of the synthesis of both AG and LAM (Fig. 36.10) (48). The mechanism of resistance to EMB involves a gene overexpression of arabinosyl transferase, which is controlled by the *embAB* gene (49).

This mechanism of action also accounts for the synergism seen between EMB and intracellular drugs, such as RIF. Damage to the cell wall created by EMB improves the cell penetration of the intracellular drugs, resulting in increased biologic activity.

STRUCTURE–ACTIVITY RELATIONSHIP An extensive number of analogs of EMB have been prepared, but none has proven to be superior to EMB itself. Extension of the ethylene diamine chain, replacement of either nitrogen, increasing the size of the nitrogen substituents, and moving the location of the alcohol groups are all changes that drastically reduce or destroy biologic activity (Note: The drug candidate SQ109, which is in phase I/II of the

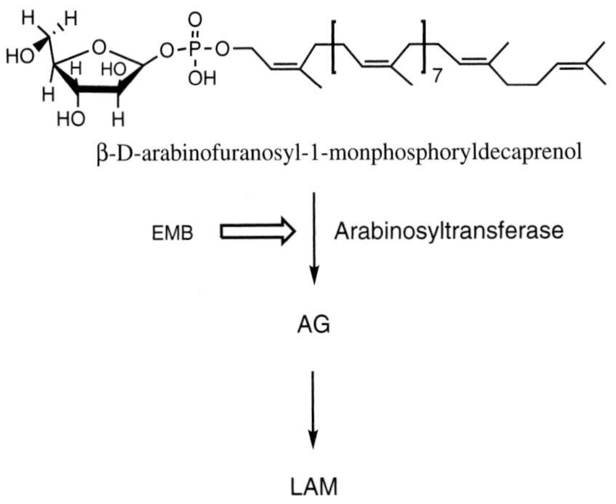

FIGURE 36.10 Site of action of ethambutol (EMB) in cell wall synthesis.

TB pipeline, is considered an analog of EMB; see the Antituberculin Drugs in the Pipeline box).

METABOLISM The majority of the administered EMB is excreted unchanged (73%), with no more than 15% appearing in the urine as either Metabolite A or Metabolite B (Fig. 36.11). Both metabolites are devoid of biologic activity.

Streptomycin

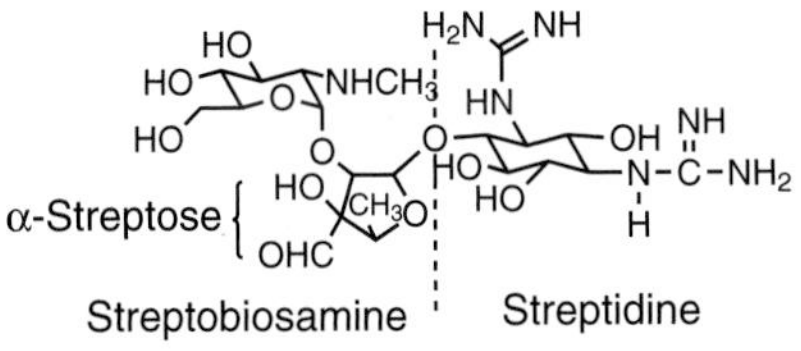

Streptomycin

Streptomycin (STM) was first isolated by Waksman and coworkers in 1944 and represented the first biologically active aminoglycoside. The material was isolated from a manure-containing soil sample and, ultimately, was shown to be produced by *Streptomyces griseus*. The structure was proposed and later confirmed by Kuehl et al. (50) in 1948. STM is water soluble, with basic properties. The compound is usually available as the trihydrochloride or sesquisulfate salt, both of which are quite soluble in water. The hydrophilic nature of STM results in very poor absorption from the GI tract. Orally administered STM is recovered intact from the feces, indicating that the lack of biologic activity results from poor absorption and not chemical degradation.

MECHANISM OF ACTION The mechanism of action of STM and the aminoglycosides in general has not been fully elucidated. It is known that the STM inhibits protein synthesis, but additional effects on misreading of an mRNA

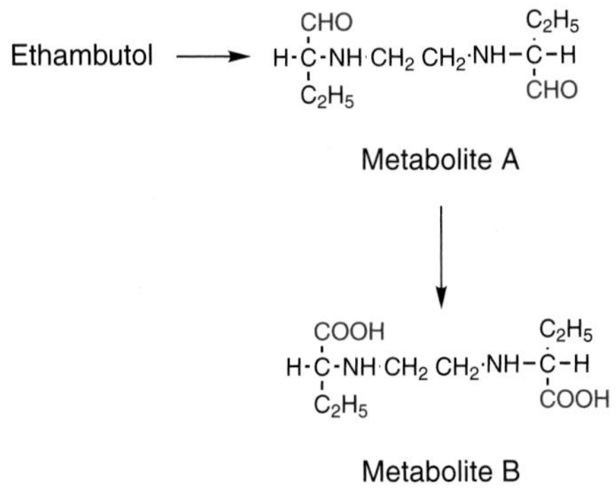

FIGURE 36.11 Metabolism of ethambutol.

template and membrane damage can contribute to the bactericidal action of STM. STM is able to diffuse across the outer membrane of *M. tuberculosis* and, ultimately, to penetrate the cytoplasmic membrane through an electron-dependent process. Through studies regarding the mechanism of drug resistance, it has been proposed that STM induces a misreading of the genetic code and, thus, inhibits translational initiation. In STM-resistant organisms, two changes have been discovered: First, S12 protein undergoes a change in which the lysine present at amino acids 43 and 88 in ribosomal protein S12 is replaced with arginine or threonine; and second, the pseudoknot conformation of 16S rRNA, which results from intramolecular base pairing between GCC bases in regions 524 to 526 of the rRNA to CGG bases in regions 505 to 507, is perturbed (51). It is thought that S12 protein stabilizes the pseudoknot, which is essential for 16S rRNA function. By some yet-to-be-defined mechanism, STM interferes with one or both of the normal actions of the 16S protein and 16S rRNA.

STRUCTURE–ACTIVITY RELATIONSHIP All of the aminoglycosides have very similar pharmacologic, pharmacodynamic, and toxic properties, but only STM and, to a lesser extent, kanamycin and possibly amikacin are used to treat TB. This is an indication for the narrow band of structurally allowed modifications giving rise to active analogs. Modification of the α-streptose portion of STM has been extensively studied. Reduction of the aldehyde to the alcohol results in a compound, dihydrostreptomycin, that has activity similar to STM but with a greater potential for producing delayed, severe deafness. Oxidation of the aldehyde to a carboxyl group or conversion to Schiff base derivatives (oxime, semicarbazone, or phenylhydrazone) results in inactive analogs. Oxidation of the methyl group in α-streptose to a methylene hydroxy gives an active analog that has no advantage over STM. Modification of the aminomethyl group in the glucosamine portion of the molecule by demethylation or by replacement with larger alkyl groups reduces activity; removal or modification of either guanidine in the streptidine nucleus also decreases activity.

Metabolism No human metabolites of STM have been isolated in the urine of patients who have been administered the drug, with approximately 50% to 60% of the dose being recovered unchanged in the urine (25). Metabolism appears to be insignificant on a large scale, but it is implicated as a major mechanism of resistance. One problem with STM that was recognized early was the development of resistant strains of *M. tuberculosis.* Combination drug therapy was partially successful in reducing this problem, but over time, resistance has greatly reduced the value of STM as a chemotherapeutic agent for treatment of TB. Various mechanisms can lead to the resistance seen in *M. tuberculosis.* Permeability barriers can result in STM not being transported through the cytoplasmic membrane, but the evidence appears to suggest that enzymatic inactivation of STM represents the major problem. The enzymes responsible for inactivation are adenyltransferase, which catalyzes adenylation of the C-3 hydroxyl group in the *N*-methylglucosamine moiety to give the *O*-3-adenylated metabolite, and phosphotransferase, which phosphorylates the same C-3 hydroxyl to give the *O*-3-phosphorylate metabolite (Fig. 36.12). This latter reaction appears to be the most significant clinically. The result of these chemical modifications is that the metabolites produced will not bind to ribosomes.

Second-Line Agents

A number of drugs, including ethionamide, *p*-aminosalicylic acid, cycloserine, capreomycin, kanamycin, and amikacin are considered to be second-line agents (it should be noted that some authorities classify STM as a second-line agent). These agents are active antibacterial agents, but they are usually less well tolerated or have a higher incidence of adverse effects. These agents are used in cases of resistance (MDR-TB), retreatment, or intolerance to the first-line drugs.

Ethionamide (Trecator-SC)

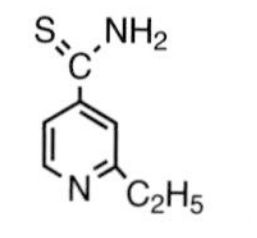

Ethionamide

The synthesis of analogs of isonicotinamide resulted in the discovery of ethionamide and a homolog in which the ethyl group is replaced with a propyl (prothionamide). Both compounds have proven to be bactericidal against *M. tuberculosis* and *Mycobacterium leprae.*

Mechanism of Action Evidence has been presented suggesting that the mechanism of action of ethionamide is similar to that of INH (see *Mechanism of Action* under *Isoniazid*) (11,15). Similar to INH, ethionamide is considered to be a prodrug that is converted via oxidation by catalase-peroxidase to an active acylating agent, ethionamide sulfoxide, which in turn inactivates the inhA enoyl reductase enzyme (Fig. 36.13). In the case of ethionamide, it has been proposed that the ethionamide sulfoxide acylates Cys-243 in inhA protein.

Metabolism Ethionamide is orally active but is not well tolerated in a single large dose (>500 mg). The GI irritation can be reduced by administration with meals. Additional side effects can include central nervous system (CNS) effects, hepatitis, and hypersensitivities. Less than 1% of the drug is excreted in the free form, with the remainder of the drug appearing as one of six metabolites. Among the metabolites are ethionamide sulfoxide, 2-ethylisonicotinamide, and the *N*-methylated-6-oxodihydropyridines (Compounds A, B, and C in Fig. 36.14) (52).

p-Aminosalicylic Acid

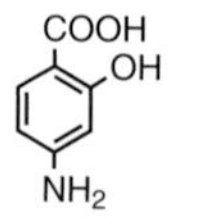

Para-aminosalicylic acid

Once a very popular component in TB therapy, *p*-aminosalicylic acid (PAS) is used as a second-line agent today. A combination of bacterial resistance and severe side effects has greatly reduced is value.

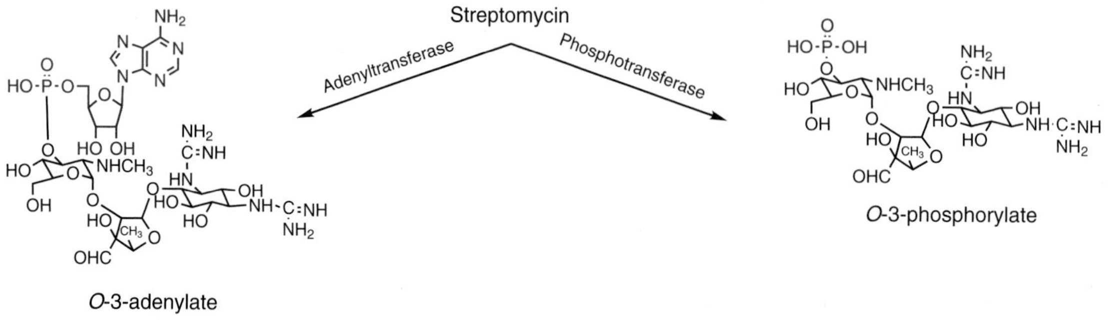

FIGURE 36.12 Metabolism of streptomycin (STM) as a mechanism of resistance.

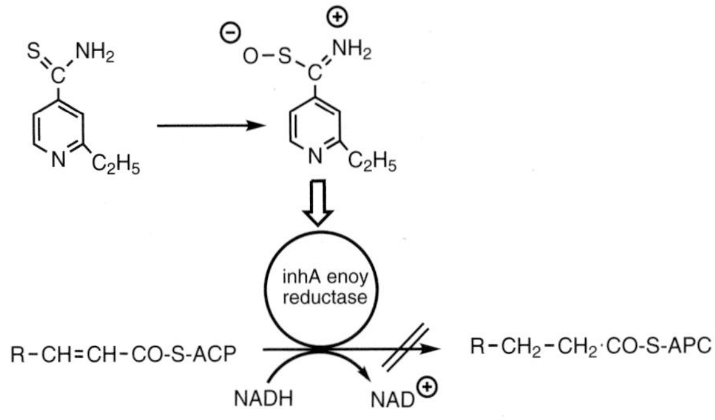

FIGURE 36.13 Mechanism of action of ethionamide.

As a bacteriostatic agent, PAS is used at a dose of up to 12 g/day, which causes considerable GI irritation. In addition, hypersensitivity reactions occur in 5% to 10% of the patients, with some of these reactions being life-threatening.

Mechanism of Action PAS is thought to act as an antimetabolite interfering with the incorporation of *p*-aminobenzoic acid into folic acid. When coadministered with INH, PAS is found to reduce the acetylation of INH, itself being the substrate for acetylation, thus increasing the plasma levels of INH. This action can be especially valuable in patients who are rapid acetylators.

Metabolism PAS is extensively metabolized by acetylation of the amino group and by conjugation with glucuronic acid and glycine at the carboxyl group. It is used primarily in cases of resistance, retreatment, and intolerance of other agents and is available from the CDC.

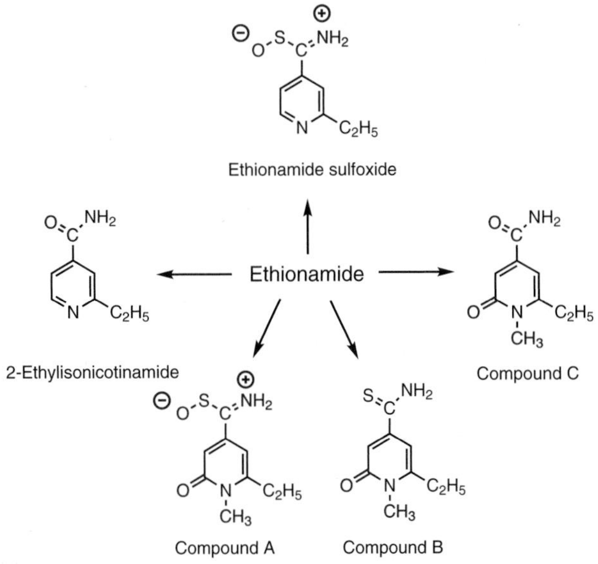

FIGURE 36.14 Metabolism of ethionamide.

Cycloserine (Seromycin)

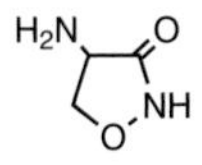

Cycloserine

Cycloserine is a natural product isolated from *Streptomyces orchidaceus* as the D-(+)-enantiomer.

Mechanism of Action D-Cycloserine is considered to be the active form of the drug, having its action associated with the ability to inhibit two key enzymes, D-alanine racemase and D-alanine ligase. D-Alanine is an important component of the peptidoglycan portion of the mycobacterial cell wall. Mycobacteria are capable of using naturally occurring L-alanine and converting the L-alanine to D-alanine via the enzyme D-alanine racemase. The resulting D-alanine is coupled with itself to form a D-alanine–D-alanine complex under the influence of D-alanine ligase, and this complex is incorporated into the peptidoglycan of the mycobacterial cell wall (Fig. 36.15). D-Cycloserine is a rigid analog of D-alanine; therefore, it competitively inhibits the binding of D-alanine to both of these enzymes and its incorporation into the peptidoglycan (Fig. 36.15) (53). Resistance is associated with an overexpression of D-alanine racemase.

Side Effects Cycloserine is readily absorbed after oral administration and is widely distributed, including the CNS. Unfortunately, D-cycloserine binds to neuronal *N*-methylasparate receptors and, in addition, affects synthesis and metabolism of γ-aminobutyric acid, leading to a complex series of CNS effects. As a second-line agent, cycloserine should only be used when retreatment is necessary or when the organism is resistant to other drugs. Cycloserine should not be used as a single drug; it must be used in combination.

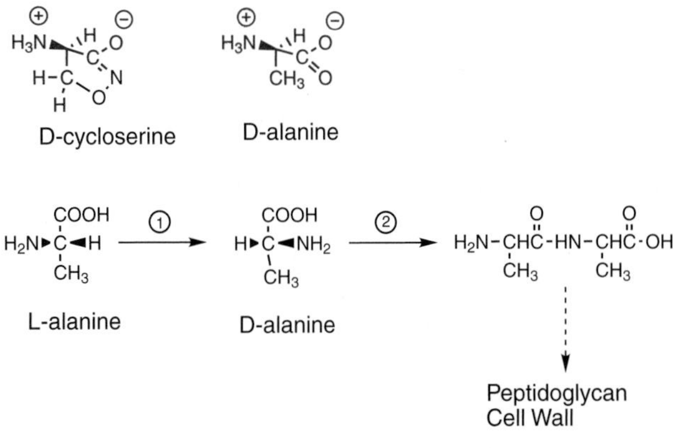

FIGURE 36.15 Sites of action of D-cycloserine: 1, D-alanine racemase; 2, D-alanine ligase.

Capreomycin (Capastat)

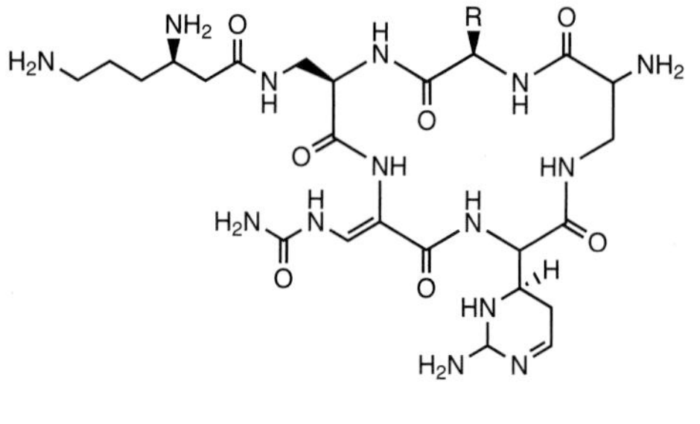

Capreomycin

Capreomycin is a mixture of four cyclic polypeptides, of which capreomycin Ia (R = OH) and Ib (R = H) make up 90% of the mixture. Capreomycin is produced by *Streptomyces capreolus* and is quite similar to the antibiotic viomycin. Little is known about its mechanism of action, but if the chemical and pharmacologic similarity to viomycin carries over to the mechanism of action, then one might expect something similar. Viomycin is a potent inhibitor of protein synthesis, particularly that which depends on mRNA at the 70S ribosome (54). Viomycin blocks chain elongation by binding to either or both the 50S or 30S ribosomal subunits. As a polypeptide, the drug must be administered parenterally, with the preferred route of administration being intramuscular. As a second-line bacteriostatic antituberculin drug, it is reserved for "resistant" infections and cases of treatment failure. The drug should not be given as a single agent; rather, it should be used in combination with EMB or INH. Reported toxicity of capreomycin includes renal and hepatic damage, hearing loss, and allergic reactions.

Kanamycin (Kanamycin A, R = OH; Kanamycin B, R = NH_2; Kantrex)

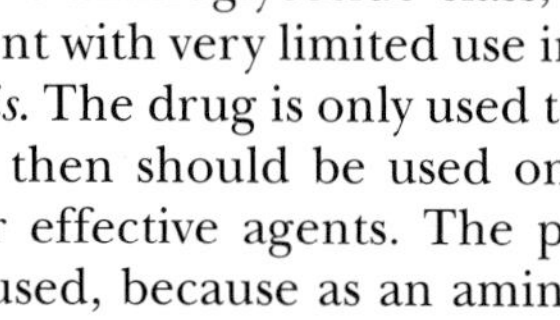

Kanamycin

A member of the aminoglycoside class, kanamycin is a second-line agent with very limited use in the treatment of *M. tuberculosis.* The drug is only used to treat resistant organisms and then should be used only in combination with other effective agents. The parenteral form of the drug is used, because as an aminoglycoside, the drug is poorly absorbed via the oral route. The narrow range of effectiveness and the severe toxicity, especially if the drug is administered over a long period of time, have limited is usefulness. (For additional information on kanamycin and aminoglycosides in general, see Chapter 33.)

Fluoroquinolones

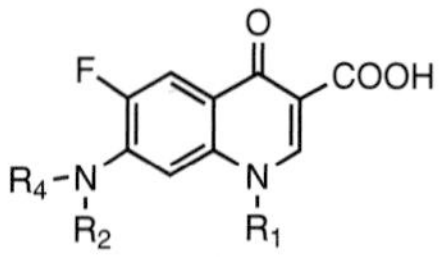

6-Fluoro- 4-quinolones

The fluoroquinolones are a broad-spectrum class of antibacterials that have been demonstrated to have activity against a wide range of gram-negative and gram-positive pathogens, including *M. tuberculosis, Mycobacterium kansasii, Mycobacterium xenopi, Mycobacterium fortuitum,* MAC, and *M. leprae.* The quinolones are attractive in that they are active at low concentrations, concentrate within macrophages, and have a low frequency of side effects.

Mechanism of Action The mechanism of action of the fluoroquinolones is reported in detail in Chapter 33 and basically involves binding to DNA gyrase–DNA complex (GyrA and GyrB), inhibiting bacterial DNA replication and transcription. As a result, these drugs exhibit bactericidal activity.

Structure–Activity Relationship The structural requirements for activity against mycobacterium and, specifically, for activity against the MAC have been explored (55,56). It is known that nonfluorinated quinolones are inactive against mycobacteria. In addition, it has been reported that certain fragments or substructures within the quinolones improve activity toward the MAC (biophores), whereas other fragments deactivate the quinolones (biophobes). The important structural features acting as biophores include: 1) a cyclopropyl ring at the *N*-1 position, 2) fluorine atoms at positions C-6 and C-8, and 3) a C-7 heterocyclic substituent. Excessive lipophilicity at *N*-1 can decrease activity (i.e., 2,4-difluorobenzene). The C-7 substituents with greatest activity against mycobacteria include the substituted piperazines and pyrrolidines (Fig. 36.16). Two biophobes have also been reported and are shown in Figure 36.17.

Several C-8 methoxy–substituted fluoroquinolones have been reported with superior activity over earlier quinolones (57,58). Moxifloxacin (Fig. 36.18) is reported to be active against *M. tuberculosis* when combined with INH.

Therapeutic Application Fluoroquinolone therapy for TB is predominantly used in patients infected with multidrug-resistant organisms. Resistance to the quinolones has been reported and appears to be associated with mutations in the *gyrA* and *gyrB* genes, leading to single-amino-acid substitution in the DNA

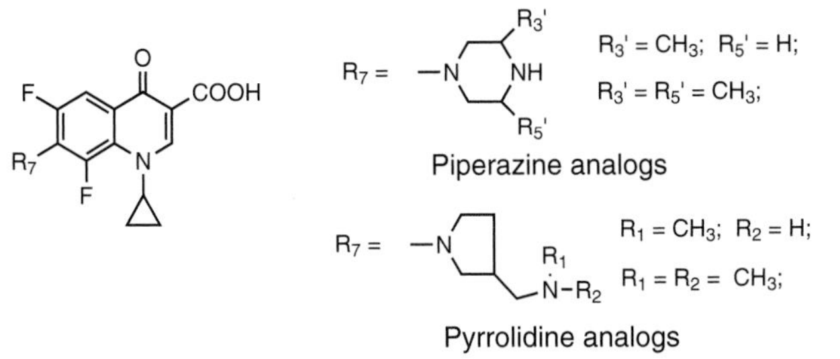

FIGURE 36.16 4-Quinolones demonstrating high activity against mycobacteria.

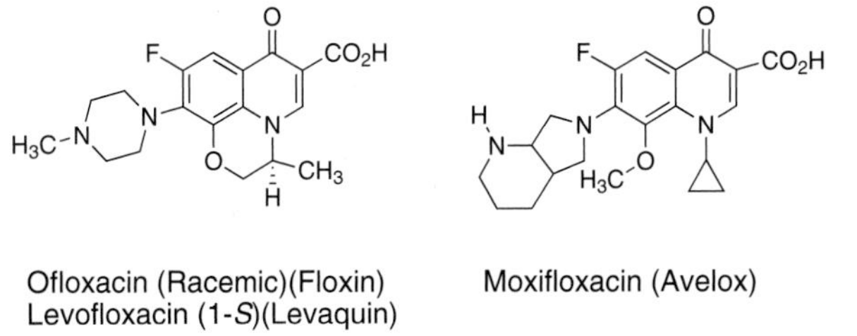

FIGURE 36.18 Fluoroquinolones active against *Mycobacterium tuberculosis*.

gyrase protein (8). As a result, use of the fluoroquinolones must be monitored in the treated patient population. The most active fluoroquinolones available for treatment of TB are ofloxacin, levofloxacin (the levo isomer of ofloxacin), and moxifloxacin (Fig. 36.18) (59).

Therapeutic Considerations for Treatment of Tuberculosis

Overview

Various stages of infectious organisms have been identified that can require special consideration for chemotherapy. The organism can be in a dormant stage, which is usually not affected by drugs. The continuously growing stage of the organism can find the bacteria either in an extracellular or an intracellular location. A stage of the organism, which is classified as the very slowly metabolizing bacteria, exists also in a relatively acidic environment. Finally, the organism can exhibit a stage in which it is dormant, followed by spurts of growth. As noted in the discussion of specific drugs, one stage or another can be more or less susceptible to a particular drug based on the above characteristics. It is also recognized that organisms from some geographic regions can show a low incidence of drug resistance, whereas those from other regions have a high incidence of drug resistance.

For patients with TB likely to be infected with organisms suspected of showing low rates of drug resistance, the American Thoracic Society currently recommends a minimum 26-week treatment period, consisting of an initial 2-month (8-week) phase, followed by a continuation phase of either 4 or 7 months. Four basic regimens are recommended for treatment of susceptible *M. tuberculosis* infections in adults. During the initial phase, three of the four regimens use a combination

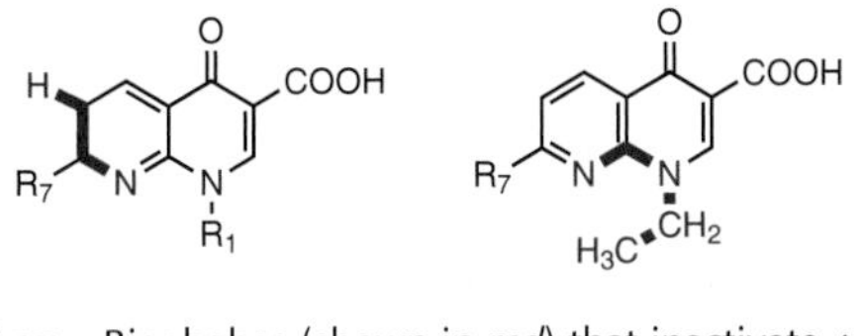

FIGURE 36.17 Biophobes (shown in *red*) that inactivate 4-quinolones toward mycobacteria.

of INH, RIF, pyrazinamide, and EMB, given either 7, 5, or 3 days per week. The fourth regimen uses INH, RIF, and EMB given 7 or 5 days per week (when drugs are administered DOTS, the drugs can be given less often). The four-drug regimen is administered based on the assumption that a proportion of the organisms are resistant to INH. For treatment of children when visual acuity cannot be tested, EMB is usually not recommended. Several options for drug treatment exist for the continuation phase of treatment (60). In a majority of cases, the continuation phase will last 4 months. Here again, if DOTS is used, the patient might only need to be treated two or three times weekly; without DOTS, the treatment is daily. The drug combination of INH and RIF is used during the continuation phase. Typical daily doses are 300 mg of INH, 600 mg of RIF, 2 g of pyrazinamide, and 1 g of EMB. The addition of pyrazinamide to the drug regimen results in a reduction of treatment time from 9 to 6 months. Individuals on any of these regimens are considered to be noninfectious after the first 2 weeks. This same group of drugs is recommended for patients with both TB and AIDS. The "cardinal rules" for all TB regimens are: 1) get drug susceptibility information as soon as possible; 2) always begin therapy with at least three drugs; 3) at all costs, avoid a regimen using only one effective drug; and 4) always add at least two drugs to a failing regimen (6,34,61). In addition, it is recommended that consideration be given to treating all patients with DOTS.

The only proven treatment for prophylaxis of TB (patients with a positive skin test or a high-risk factor) is INH used for 6 or 12 months. High-risk persons are considered to be adults and children with HIV infection, close contacts of infectious cases, and those with fibrotic lesions on chest radiographs. Adverse effects when using INH over a long treatment period can be a serious problem. Isoniazid can cause severe liver damage, and the drug should be removed if serum aminotransferase activity increases to three- to fivefold the normal level or the patient develops symptoms of hepatitis. Peripheral neuropathy can be seen with INH therapy. This condition can be prevented by coadministration of pyridoxine. Persons who are presumed to be infected with INH-resistant organisms should be treated with RIF rather than INH. Hepatitis, thrombocytopenia, and nephrotoxicity can be seen with RIF therapy. RIF is thought to potentiate the hepatitis caused by INH. GI upset and staining effects caused by RIF are of minor importance.

Although drug-susceptible TB has been successfully treated, the long period of treatment and low patient adherence have in part led to the development of drug-resistant TB, both MDR-TB and XDR-TB. In such situations, a new treatment paradigm has become necessary. For treatment of MDR-TB a five- to six-drug regimen is commonly used (Table 36.1) (62,63). The particular regimen should be based on drug susceptibility testing or previous treatment history. With duel mycobacterium resistance to INH and RIF, a combination of an aminoglycoside from group III drugs, a fluoroquinolone from group II drugs, along with EMB and pyrazinamide and ethionamide or prothionamide from groups I and IV, respectively, can be used at the doses indicated. If resistance to all group I drugs occurs, then *p*-aminosalicylic acid and cycloserine are added to the previous indicated drug list of an aminoglycoside, a fluoroquinolone, and ethionamide or prothionamide. The treatment should continue for up to 18 months after smear conversion to negativity as recommended by the World Health Organization.

DRUG THERAPY FOR MAC

Drug therapy for the treatment of MAC is complicated. It underwent significant changes in the early 1990s, but little has changed during the last 15 years. Recommendations for treatment are presently based on small and, in some cases, incomplete studies; more changes can be expected in the future. For the most up-to-date information, the reader is referred to the CDC's homepage (www.cdc.gov). The 1997 guidelines for prophylaxis of MAC advise that all adults and adolescents with HIV infection and a CD4 lymphocyte count of less than 50 cells/mL receive clarithromycin 500 mg twice a day or azithromycin 1,200 mg once a week. This recommendation is considered to be a standard of care (64–66). For treatment of MAC, it is recommended that a combination therapy be used that includes at least two drugs (either clarithromycin or azithromycin plus EMB

TABLE 36.1 Grouping of Drugs Used to Treat MDR-TB and XDR-TB

Drug Group	Drugs	Doses
I. First-line oral TB drugs	Isoniazid	5 mg/kg
	Rifampicin	10 mg/kg
	Ethambutol	15–25 mg/kg
	Pyrazinamide	30 mg/kg
II. Fluoroquinolones	Ofloxacin	15 mg/kg
	Levofloxacin	15 mg/kg
	Moxifloxacin	7.5–10 mg/kg
III. Injectable TB drugs	Streptomycin	15 mg/kg
	Kanamycin	15 mg/kg
	Amikacin	15 mg/kg
	Capreomycin	15 mg/kg
IV. Second-line TB drugs	Ethionamide/prothionamide	15 mg/kg
	Cycloserine/terizidone	15 mg/kg
	p-Aminosalicylic acid	150 mg/kg
V. Less effective drugs (efficacy uncertain)	Clofazimine	100 mg
	Amoxicillin/clavulanate	875/125 mg every 12 hours
	Linezolid	600 mg
	Imipenem	500–1,000 mg every 6 hours
	Clarithromycin	500 mg every 12 hours
	Thioacetazone	150 mg

for life). Other drugs that can be added to the combination consist of rifabutin, fluoroquinolones, and amikacin. It should be noted that INH and pyrazinamide are ineffective in the treatment of disseminated MAC.

Macrolides

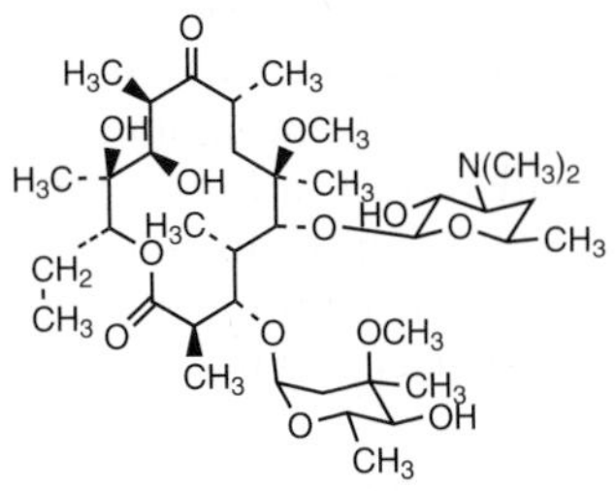

Clarithromycin

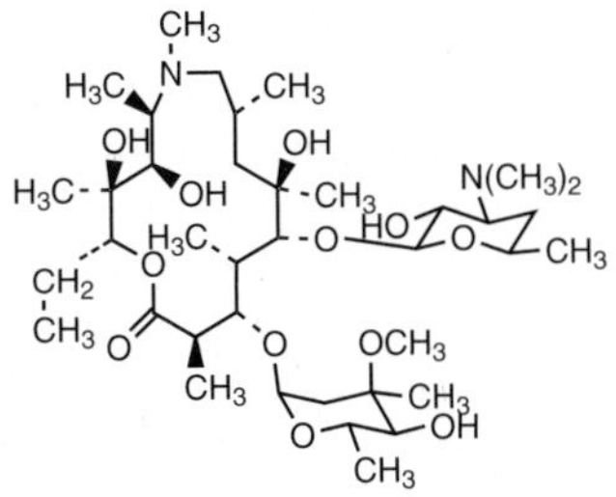

Azithromycin

Both clarithromycin and azithromycin are considered to be first-line agents for the prevention and treatment of MAC and have replaced rifabutin. Both macrolides are concentrated in macrophages (clarithromycin concentration is 17.3-fold higher in macrophage cells than in extracellular fluid) and appear to be equally effective, although clarithromycin has a lower minimum inhibitory concentration. Azithromycin has an intra-alveolar macrophage half-life of 195 hours, compared to a 4-hour half-life for clarithromycin. For prevention, the macrolides can be used as single agents, although there is a risk of resistant organisms forming and of a cross-resistance between clarithromycin and azithromycin. In one study, the combination of azithromycin and rifabutin proved to be more effective than either drug used alone. For the treatment of MAC, combination therapy is recommended.

Mechanism of Action

The macrolide antibiotics are bacteriostatic agents that inhibit protein synthesis by binding to the 50S ribosomal units. (For a more detailed discussion, see Chapter 33.)

Metabolism

Clarithromycin is metabolized in the liver to an active metabolite, 14-hydroxyclarithromycin, which is less active than the parent molecule. In addition, the drug is an inhibitor of CYP3A4, which could lead to increased concentrations of some drugs, such as rifabutin (see below). Azithromycin is primarily excreted unchanged in the gut, and at present, there is no evidence of CYP3A4 induction or inhibition.

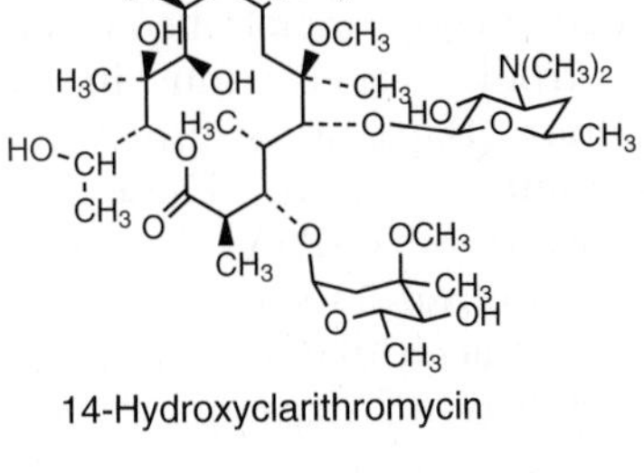

14-Hydroxyclarithromycin

Rifamycins

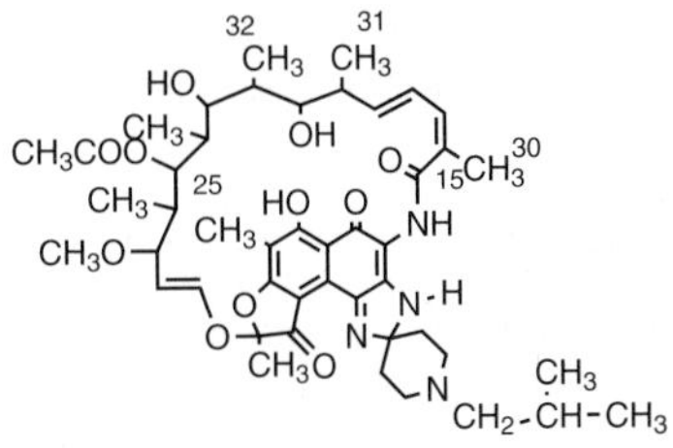

Rifabutin

Various rifamycin derivatives have been investigated or are under investigation for use in the prevention and treatment of MAC. Up until 1997, rifabutin (Mycobutin) was considered to be the drug of choice for prophylaxis of MAC-infected patients. Studies since 1995, however, have suggested that the macrolides are more effective (survival rates), present fewer side effects, and cause less drug interactions than rifabutin. Early treatment of MAC bacteremia consists of multidrug regimens, usually involving four or five drugs. Drug interactions and, in some studies, exceptionally high drug doses have given confusing results. It is generally agreed that rifabutin should be used in treatment when macrolides have failed or can be combined with azithromycin for prophylaxis or treatment when clarithromycin is unsuccessful.

Drug Interactions

The most significant drug interaction identified with rifabutin is associated with the fact that the drugs in this class are inducers of CYP3A4 and the CYP2C family. As a result, certain drugs that are substrates for these isoforms will show reduced activity. Rifabutin has been shown to reduce the area under the curve and the maximum concentration of clarithromycin and most HIV protease inhibitors. This action could lead to inactivity or resistance to these agents. In addition, because the HIV protease inhibitors are inhibitors of CYP3A4, a combination of rifabutin plus an HIV protease inhibitor is expected to increase the rifabutin area under the curve and maximum concentration, thus increasing the risk of rifabutin side effects. The most serious side effect of rifabutin is uveitis (inflammation of the iris). Under these conditions, appropriate changes in dosing are required. If combination therapy is desirable for the treatment of MAC, the combination of azithromycin and rifabutin is recommended, because no significant change in mean serum drug concentration is reported to occur with either agent when used in combination.

Drug Metabolism

The hepatic metabolism of rifabutin is complex, with as many as 20 metabolites having been reported. The structure of most of the metabolites remains unknown, but several have been identified, including 25-desacetylrifabutin, 25-desacetylrifabutin-*N*-oxide, 31-hydroxyrifabutin, 32-hydroxyrifabutin, and

32-hydroxy-25-desacetylrifabutin. The metabolites appear in the urine (50%) and in the feces (30%). Based on the activity of other rifamycins, it might be expected that one or more of the metabolites possess antimycobacterial activity.

Additional Drugs

Various other agents have been combined with the macrolides or RIF for the prophylaxis and treatment of MAC. As indicated earlier, the effectiveness of each component in multidrug treatment is not easily defined. The additional drugs used include EMB, ciprofloxacin, amikacin, and clofazimine. EMB and ciprofloxacin appear to have good activity against MAC, but clofazimine has shown unfavorable results. The FDA has advised against the use of clofazimine during initial therapy for MAC (65).

LEPROSY

Sulfones

The diaryl sulfones represent the major class of agents used to treat leprosy. The initial discovery of the sulfones came about as a result of studies directed at exploring the SAR of sulfonamides (Fig. 36.19). A variety of additional chemical modifications have produced several other active agents, but none has proved to be more beneficial than the original lead, 4,4′-diaminodiphenylsulfone. Dapsone was first introduced into the treatment of leprosy in 1943.

Dapsone

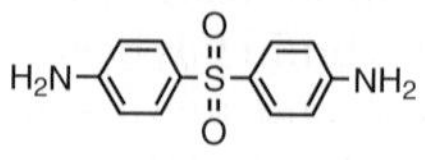

4,4'-Diaminodiphenylsulfone (Dapsone)

Dapsone, a diaminodiphenylsulfone, is a nearly water-insoluble agent that is very weakly basic ($pK_a \sim 1.0$). The lack of solubility can account, in part, for the occurrence of GI irritation. Despite the lack of solubility, the drug is efficiently absorbed from the GI tract. Although dapsone is bound to plasma protein (~70%), it is distributed throughout the body.

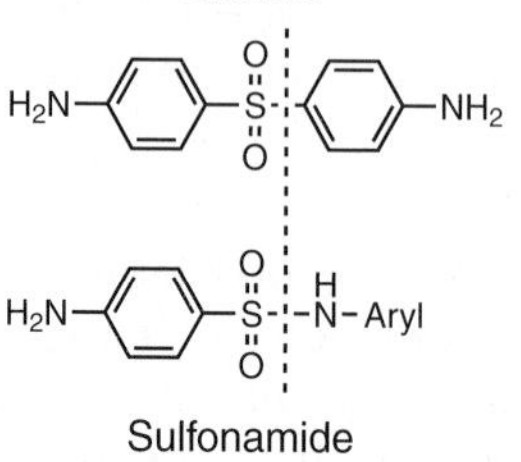

FIGURE 36.19 Structural comparison of sulfones versus sulfonamide.

Mechanism of Action Dapsone, a bacteriostatic agent, is thought to act in a manner similar to that of the sulfonamides—namely, through competitive inhibition of *p*-aminobenzoic acid incorporation into folic acid (see *Sulfonamides* in Chapter 33). Bacteria synthesize folic acid, but host cells do not. As a result, coadministration of dapsone and *p*-aminobenzoic acid will inactivate dapsone. Both dapsone and clofazimine have significant anti-inflammatory actions, which may or may not play a role in the antimicrobial action. The anti-inflammatory action can also be a beneficial side effect, offsetting the complication of erythema nodosum leprosum seen in some patients. The anti-inflammatory action can come about by inhibition of myeloperoxidase-catalyzed reactions (69).

Structure–Activity Relationship Several derivatives of dapsone have been prepared in an attempt to increase the activity. Isosteric replacement of one benzene ring resulted in the formation of thiazolsulfone. Although still active, it is less effective than dapsone. Substitution on the aromatic ring, to produce acetosulfone, reduced activity while increasing water solubility and decreasing GI irritation. A successful substitution consists of adding methanesulfinate to dapsone to give sulfoxone sodium. This water-soluble form of dapsone is hydrolyzed in vivo to produce dapsone. Sulfoxone sodium is used in individuals who are unable to tolerate dapsone because of GI irritation, but it must be used in a dose threefold that of dapsone because of inefficient metabolism to dapsone. The chemical modification of dapsone derivatives continues to be pursued with the intent of finding newer agents useful for the treatment of resistant strains of *Mycobacterium leprae* (70).

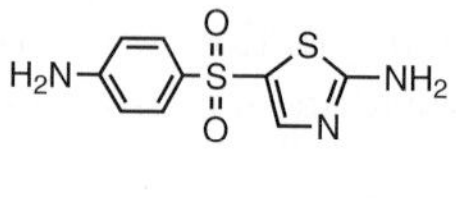

Thiazolsulfone

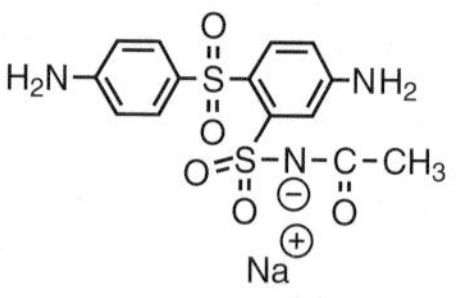

Acetosulfone

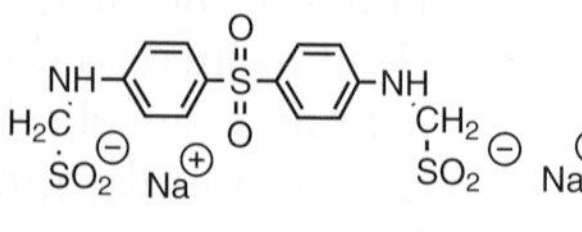

Sulfoxone sodium

Metabolism The major metabolic product of dapsone results from *N*-acetylation in the liver by *N*-acetyltransferase. Dapsone is also *N*-hydroxylated to the hydroxylamine derivative. These metabolic reactions are catalyzed by CYP3A4 isoforms. Neither of these compounds possesses significant leprostatic activity, although *N*-acetyldiaminodiphenylsulfone can be deacetylated back to dapsone. Products found in

ANTITUBERCULIN DRUGS IN THE PIPELINE

The need for new drugs to treat TB continues to mount, and as many as 10 compounds are presently moving through the clinical testing and approval process. Several of these drugs are already marketed for treatment of bacterial infections and include the fluoroquinolones (moxifloxacin and gatifloxacin), the oxazolidinone linezolid and a close analog, PNU-100480, and an analog of EMB (SQ109). Several new chemical entities offer hope in that they appear to act by unique mechanisms and include the nitroimidazoles PA-824 and OPC-67863. A drug candidate presently in phase II clinical studies is a diarylquinoline TMC207.

Oxazolidinones:

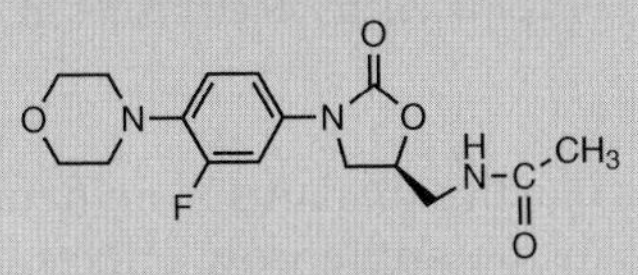

Linezolid

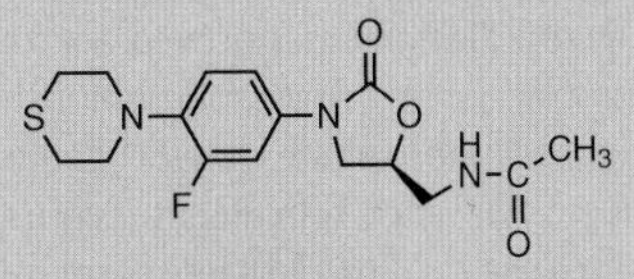

PNU-100480

Ethylene diamines:

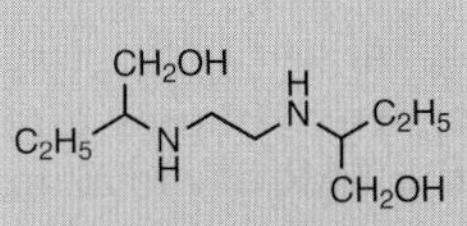

Ethambutol

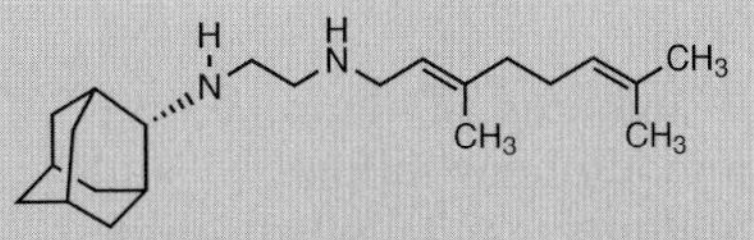

SQ109

Nitroimidazole:

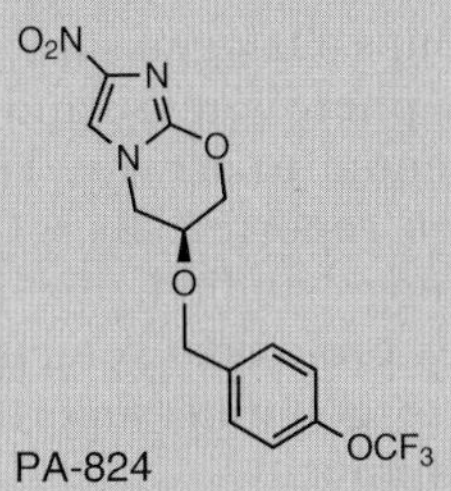

PA-824

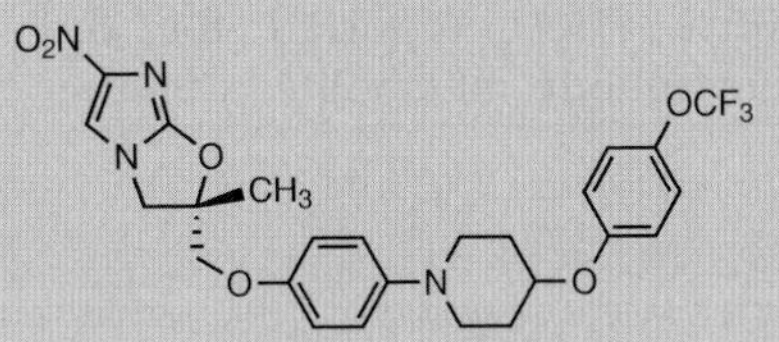

OPC-67863

Diarylquinoline (DARQ):

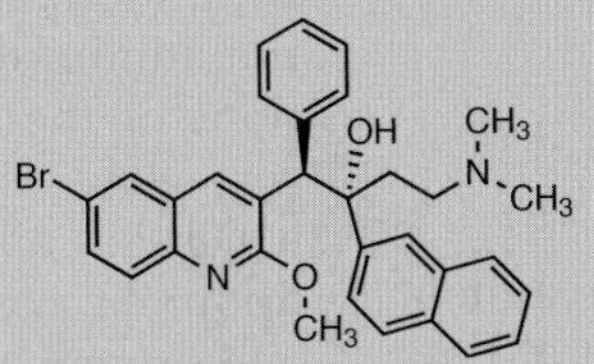

TMC207

Early studies with PNU-100480 are encouraging and show that it is more active than linezolid in treatment of TB. The chemical is in phase I investigation (62). SQ109 has been reported to have a mechanism different from that of EMB, possibly acting on the cell wall of the mycobacterium. The drug is presently in early phase II studies, but no recent information is available. The nitroimidazoles, PA-824 and OPC-67863, appear to be prodrugs and are reduced to the active drug, which in turn interferes with mycolic acid synthesis and thus cell wall synthesis. The two drugs are at various stages of early clinical investigation (63). The uniqueness of the nitroimidazoles is that they are active against both replicating and nonreplicating bacteria (67). Probably the most interesting compound is the diarylquinoline TMC207 due to its novel mechanism of action, which involves inhibition of F1Fo proton adenosine triphosphate (ATP) synthase and the enzyme involved in ATP synthesis (61,67). The drug is active against nonreplicating persisters. Recently it has been shown that the inhibitory action is selective against mycobacterium with only weak inhibitory activity against mammalian cells (68).

ADDITIONAL USES FOR DAPSONE

Dapsone has a variety of uses in addition to the treatment of leprosy. These include the treatment of dermatitis herpetiformis as well as an unlabeled use in the treatment of brown recluse spider bites, inflammatory bowel disorders, leishmaniasis, malaria prophylaxis, relapsing polychondritis, rheumatic and connective tissue disorders, and prophylaxis of *Pneumocystis jiroveci* pneumonia in HIV-infected patients and organ transplant patients. Recently, dapsone has been approved for the treatment of acne. Under the trade name of Aczone, the drug is available as a 5% gel. Glucose-6-phosphate dehydrogenase (G6PD) levels, blood hemoglobin, and reticulocyte counts should be followed in patients with G6PD deficiency anemia and predisposed to increased hemolytic effects.

the urine consist of small amounts of dapsone, the metabolites *N*-acetyldiaminodiphenylsulfone and *N*-hydroxydiaminodiphenylsulfone, and glucuronide and sulfates of each of these substances (Fig. 36.20).

Although the acetylated metabolites of dapsone are inactive, there is growing concern over the adverse hematologic effects of the hydroxylated metabolite. The specific adverse effect reported for the *N*-hydroxydiaminodiphenylsulfone metabolite is methemoglobinemia (71).

Clofazimine (Lamprene)

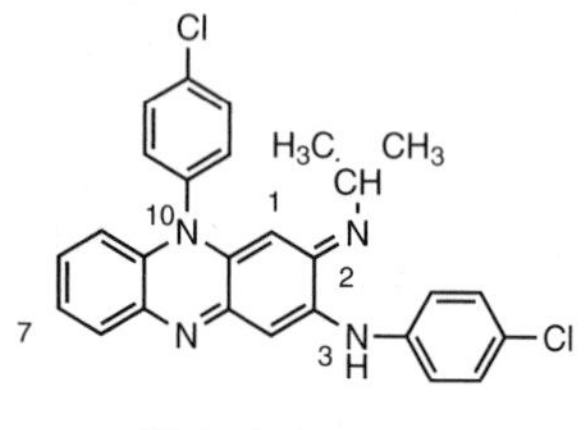

Clofazimine

Although classified as a secondary drug for the treatment of leprosy and commonly used as a component of multidrug therapy, clofazimine appears to be increasing in use. Clofazimine was first used to treat advanced leprosy unresponsive to dapsone or STM in 1966. The chemical, a phenazine derivative, is a water-insoluble dye (dark-red crystals) that leads to pigmentation of the skin. In addition, discoloration (pink, red, or brownish-black) of the feces, eyelid lining, sputum, sweat, tears, and urine is seen.

Mechanism of Action The mechanism of action remains unclear at the present time. The molecule possesses direct antimycobacterial and immunosuppressive properties. It has been shown that clofazimine increases prostaglandin synthesis and the generation of antimicrobial

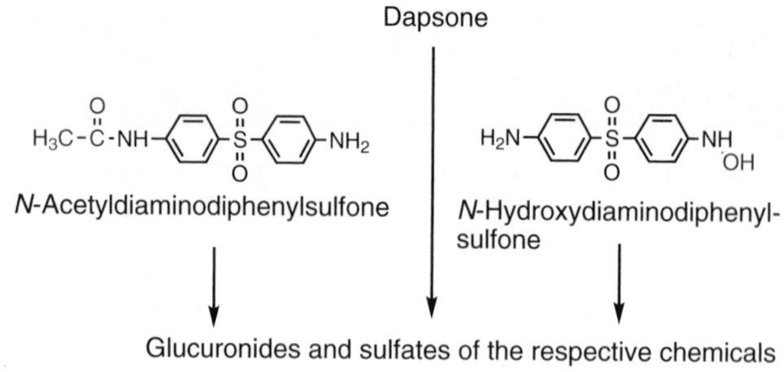

FIGURE 36.20 Metabolites of dapsone.

reactive oxidants from neutrophils, which can play a role in the antileprosy effects. The host cell defense can be stimulated by clofazimine, resulting in the generation of oxidants, such as the superoxide anion, which in turn could have a lethal effect on the organism (72,73).

Structure–Activity Relationship Several investigators have reported studies directed toward an understanding of the SAR of clofazimine (74–76). Substituents on the imino group at position 2, *p*-chloro substitution on the phenyls at C-3 and N-10, and substituents at position 7 have been investigated. The imino group at C-2 appears to be essential, with activity increased when the imino group is substituted with alkyl and cycloalkyl groups. Halogen substitution on the para position of the two phenyls at C-3 and N-10 enhance activity but are not essential to activity. The following order of activity has been reported: Br > Cl > CH_3 > EtO > H or F. In the analogs studied, the increased activity correlates well with pro-oxidative activities of the molecule (e.g., ability to generate superoxide anion) as well as increased lipophilicity.

Metabolism Various metabolites of clofazimine have been identified, but these account for less than 1% of the administered dose. The lack of higher concentrations of the metabolites can, in part, result from the very slow elimination of clofazimine from the body, which has an estimated half-life of 8.8 to 69 days. The lipophilic nature of clofazimine results in distribution and storage of the drug in fat tissue. There appears to be some discrepancy as to the structures of the metabolites (76,77). The most recent studies suggest the presence of two conjugates, with the possibility of intermediates (Fig. 36.21). Clofazimine is thought to undergo hydroxylic dehalogenation on the 3-chloroaniline, followed by sulfate conjugation and 4-hydroxylation, followed by glucuronic acid conjugation.

Rifampin (Rifadin, Rimactane)

RIF, an antituberculin drug, has already been discussed. Its actions against *Mycobacterium leprae* parallel those effects reported for *M. tuberculosis*. Today, RIF is considered to be an effective antileprosy agent when used in combination with the sulfones.

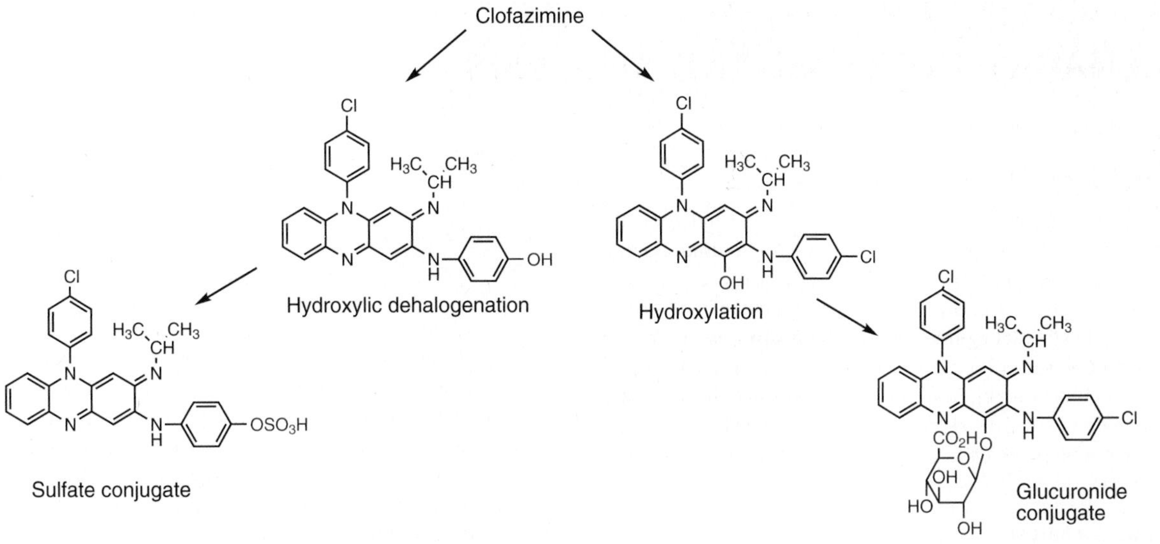

FIGURE 36.21 Human metabolic products of clofazimine.

Thalidomide (Thalomid)

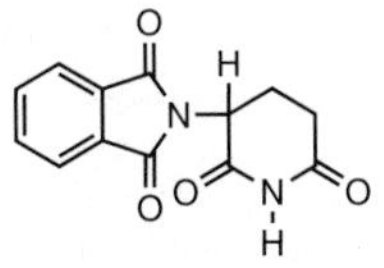

Thalidomide

The development of painful, tender, inflamed, subcutaneous nodules that can last a week or two but can reappear and last for long periods is seen in a number of diseases. In the case of leprosy, the condition is referred to as erythema nodosum leprosum (ENL). The condition appears to be a hypersensitivity reaction, and although it can appear in nontreated patients, it commonly is seen as a complication of the chemotherapy of leprosy. In addition to painful nodules, the patient can experience fever, malaise, wasting, vasculitis, and peripheral neuritis. This condition has been successfully treated with thalidomide. Recently, thalidomide has been approved by the FDA for treatment of ENL and is considered to be the drug of choice (78,79). The mechanism whereby thalidomide produces relief is thought to be associated with the drug's ability to control inflammatory cytokines. Specifically, thalidomide inhibits the synthesis and release of tumor necrosis factor-α, which is synthesized and released by blood mononuclear cells and appears in the serum during ENL; concentrations drop when the patient is treated with thalidomide. In addition to the treatment of ENL, thalidomide has been reported to exhibit beneficial effects in the treatment of aphthous ulcers in HIV-positive patients, Behcet disease, chronic graft-versus-host disease, rash caused by systemic or cutaneous lupus erythematosus, pyoderma gangrenosum, and multiple myeloma.

Thalidomide is a very potent teratogenic agent, with a history of an estimated 10,000 deformed infants born to mothers who used the drug during pregnancy. It can be used safely in postmenopausal women, but strict controls are required for women of childbearing age. Although no evidence suggests that men can transmit the drug during sex, the use of condoms by male patients will be required.

Therapeutic Considerations

Since its introduction into the chemotherapy of leprosy in 1947, dapsone has proved to be the single most effective agent. This drug was used as a monotherapeutic agent despite the recognition that resistant strains were beginning to emerge. Since 1977, monotherapy with dapsone is no longer recognized as an acceptable method for the treatment of leprosy. Today, combination chemotherapy is the method of choice. The combination consists of RIF (600 mg monthly), dapsone (100 mg daily), and clofazimine (300 mg monthly, with 50 mg daily added for patients with multibacillary leprosy, which is defined as five or more skin lesions). Therapy is usually continued for at least 2 years or as long as skin smears are positive. The patient is kept under supervision for 5 years following completion of chemotherapy. A similar treatment regimen is recommended for treatment of paucibacillary leprosy (defined as five or fewer skin lesions) except that treatment is continued for 6 months and the patient is kept under observation for an additional 2 years (80,81). It should be noted that the patient is noninfectious within 72 hours of starting treatment. Other combinations that have been reported include RIF plus ofloxacin and minocycline or ofloxacin plus minocycline. The new regimens allow a shortened treatment period and a reduced rate of relapse.

An important aspect of therapy for leprosy involves the treatment of peripheral nerve damage. This nerve damage can be treated with steroids, such as prednisolone. For severe cases, however, thalidomide is used.

SCENARIO: OUTCOME AND ANALYSIS

Outcome

Elizabeth Coyle, PharmD

After reviewing RG's medication list, it is realized that the increase in RG's INR is most likely due to a drug interaction between isoniazid and warfarin. Both drugs are metabolized through the liver, and isoniazid is a known inhibitor of many hepatically metabolized drugs. The pharmacist decides to decrease RG's warfarin dose to 2.5 mg daily, to recheck his INR in 2 days, and to continue to decrease the warfarin until RG's INR is again therapeutic at 2.5. The pharmacist will make sure to increase the warfarin dose once RG is finished taking 9 months of isoniazid.

Chemical Analysis

S. William Zito and Victoria Roche

Isoniazid is an aromatic hydrazide that that kills replicating *M. tuberculosis* organisms and halts the replication of dormant organisms. Its mechanism of action is to acylate NADH and an inhA enzyme that generates mycolic acids required for bacterial cell wall synthesis. The specific acylating intermediates are produced by the action of a catalase-peroxidase known as katG. The most important ones are the phenylacyl radical, phenylacylperoxy radical, and isonicotinic peroxide. The terminal nitrogen of isoniazid can be substituted with lipophilic alkyl groups without loss of activity, but the greatest potency is realized in the unsubstituted primary hydrazide. Isoniazid is metabolized via N-acetylation by an N-acetyltransferase to a metabolite that, in turn, generates an extremely hepatotoxic acetyl radical via a hydroxylamine intermediate. Patients who are slow acetylators express lower amounts of this transferase enzyme than those who are fast acetylators, and therefore they are less likely to experience hepatotoxicity from this agent. Oral absorption of this drug is good, but it is slowed by food and metal-containing antacids.

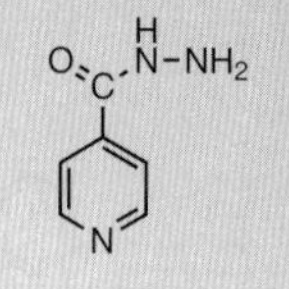

Isoniazid

Warfarin is a 3-aralkyl-4-hydroxycoumarin derivative. It was developed from structure activity relationship studies of the bishydroxycoumarin (dicoumarol) that was discovered to cause bleeding in cattle that ingested fermented sweet clover. Its anticoagulant activity derives from its ability to interfere with the cyclic interconversion of vitamin K and vitamin K 2,3-epoxide. Vitamin K is an essential cofactor necessary for the γ-carboxylation of the glutamic acid residues on the N-terminal of clotting factors II, VII, IX, and X. The 4-hydroxy substituent confers water solubility and the substituent at position 3 affects the pharmacokinetic parameters of onset, duration, and half-life. Warfarin is the only coumarin used in the United States. It is rapidly absorbed and highly protein bound.

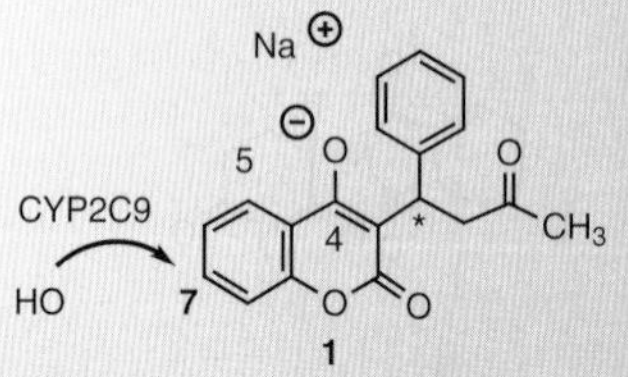

Warfarin sodium
(Coumadin)

Warfarin is metabolized by CYP2C9 to both 6- and 7-hydroxywarfarins, with the 7-hydroxy metabolite being the major oxidation product. When one thinks of warfarin drug-drug interactions, it is usually that, because warfarin is highly protein bound, other coadministered drugs will displace it and lead to higher blood levels and therefore enhanced anticoagulant activity. However, in this case it is more likely that the isoniazid is inhibiting the action of CYP2C9 on warfarin, leading to potentiation of its anticoagulant activity.

CASE STUDY

S. William Zito and Victoria Roche

LT is a 35-year-old female veterinary pathologist who was recently involved with the clinical and pathological evaluation of a dog that had presented with symptoms of a central nervous system disease. However, before a diagnosis could be made, the dog rapidly deteriorated and died. The postmortem examination revealed systemic mycobacteriosis, and *Mycobactrium tuberculosis* was identified by polymerase chain reaction amplification of DNA samples. Infection in companion animals is mainly acquired from close contact to a diseased human. LT, who performed the necropsy on the dog, tested positive for *M. tuberculosis*. Her accidental infection was most likely caused by inhalation of *M. tuberculosis*–containing aerosols created by using an electric saw to open the brain cavity.

LT presents to her physician with all the signs and symptoms of early infection (persistent cough, pain in the chest, fatigue, and loss of appetite). A thorough medical workup reveals that LT has hypertension, which is treated with extended-release diltiazem (120 mg/daily); no history of liver or kidney disease; and is taking oral contraceptives (BCs) that contain ethinyl estradiol and levonorgestrel. Her physician wants to treat LT with a four-drug regimen, and decides to use isoniazid, pyrazinamide, and ethambutal; however, he is undecided about which of the following antimycobacterial drugs to use as the fourth agent. What is your opinion?

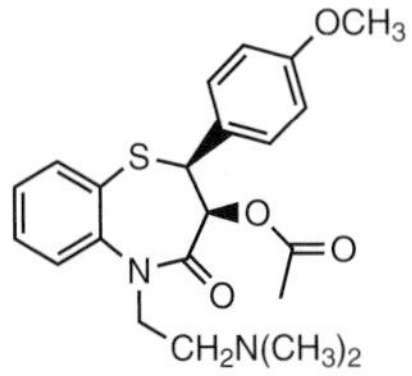

Diltiazem

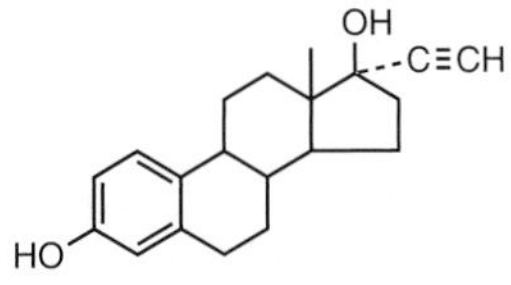

Ethinyl estradiol

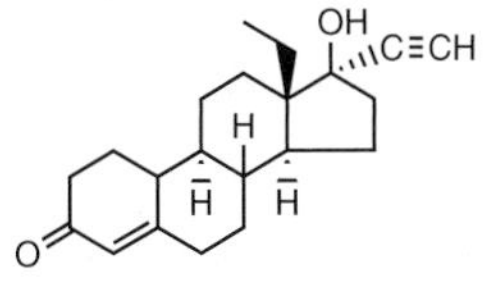

Levonorgestrel

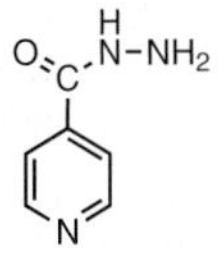

Isoniazid

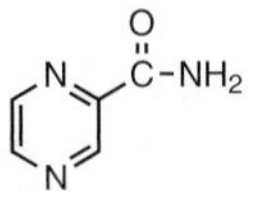

Pyrazinamide

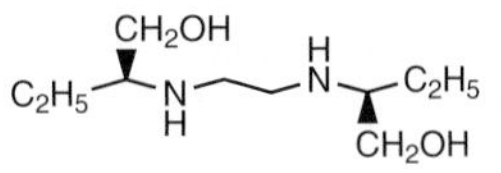

Ethambutol

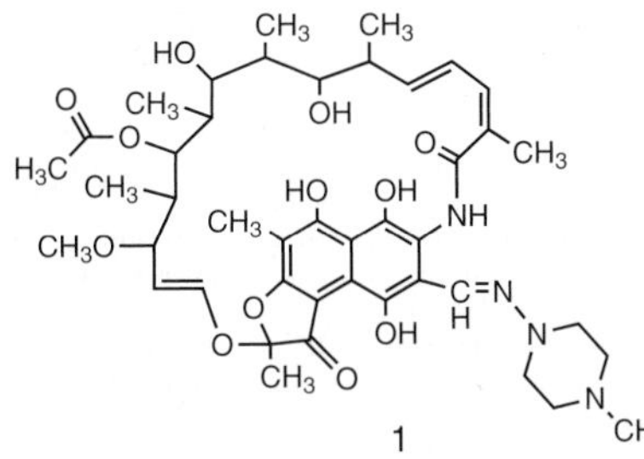

1

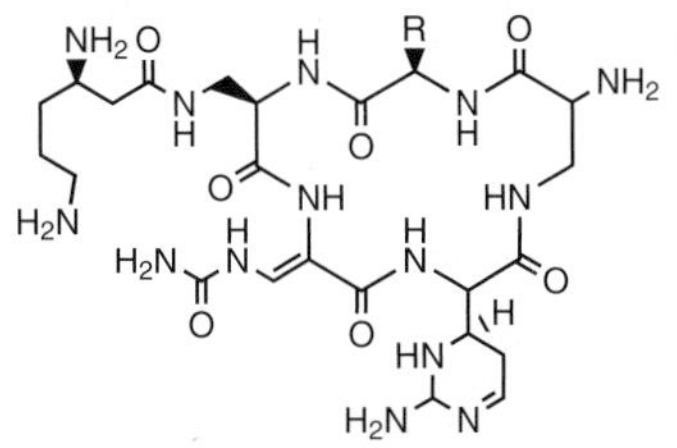

2

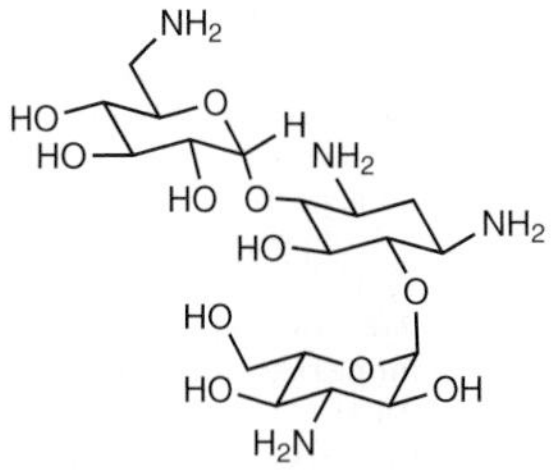

3

1. Conduct a thorough and mechanistic SAR analysis of the three therapeutic options in the case.
2. Apply the chemical understanding gained from the SAR analysis to this patient's specific needs to make a therapeutic recommendation.

References

1. Rastogi N. Structure and functions of the cell envelope in relation to mycobacterial virulence, pathogenicity and multiple drug resistance. 7th Form in microbiology. Res Microbiol 1991;142:419–481.
2. Minnikin DE. Chemical principles in the organization of lipid components in the mycobacterial cell envelope. Res Microbiol 1991;142:423–427.
3. McNeil MR, Brennan PJ. Structure, function and biogenesis of the cell envelope of mycobacteria in relation to bacterial physiology, pathogenesis and drug resistance. Some thoughts and possibilities arising from recent structural information. Res Microbiol 1991;142:451–463.
4. Marwick C. Do worldwide outbreaks mean tuberculosis again becomes 'captain of all these men of death'? JAMA 1992;267:1174–1175.
5. Daniel TM. Tuberculosis. In: Wilson JD, Braunwald E, Isselbacher KJ, et al., eds. Harrison's Principles of Internal Medicine, 12th Ed. New York: McGraw-Hill, 1991:637–645.
6. Taylor HG. The tuberculosis epidemic and the pharmacist's role. Am Pharm 1992;32:41–44.
7. Zhang Y. The magic bullets and tuberculosis drug targets. Annu Rev Pharmacol Toxicol 2005;45:529–564.
8. Blanchard JS. Molecular mechanisms of drug resistance in *Mycobacterium tuberculosis*. Annu Rev Biochem 1996;65:215–239.
9. Zhang Y, Heym B, Allen B, et al. The catalase-peroxidase gene and isoniazid resistance of *Mycobacterium tuberculosis*. Nature 1992;358:591–593.
10. Johnsson K, Schultz PG. Mechanistic studies of the oxidation of isoniazid by the catalase-peroxidase from *Mycobacterium tuberculosis*. J Am Chem Soc 1994;116:7425–7426.
11. Banerjee A, Dubnau E, Quemard A, et al. *inhA*, a gene encoding a target for isonaizid and ethionamide in *Mycobacterium tuberculosis*. Science 1994;263:227–230.
12. Mdluli K, Sherman DR, Hickey MJ, et al. Biochemical and genetic data suggest that inhA is not the primary target for activated isoniazid in *Mycobacterium tuberculosis*. J Infect Dis 1996;174:1085–1090.
13. Basso LA, Zheng R, Musser JM, et al. Mechanism of isoniazid resistance in *Mycobacterium tuberculosis*: enzymatic characterization of enoyl reductase mutants identified in isoniazid-resistant clinical isolates. J Infect Dis 1998;178:769–775.
14. Quemard A, Sacchettini JC, Dessen A, et al. Enzymatic characterization of the target for isoniazid in *Mycobacterium tuberculosis*. Biochemistry 1995;34:8235–8241.
15. Johnsson K, King DS, Schultz PG. Studies on the mechanism of action of isoniazid and ethimamide in the chemotherapy of tuberculosis. J Am Chem Soc 1995;117:5009–5010.
16. Rozwarski DA, Grant GA, Barton DHR, et al. Modification of the NADH of the isoniazid target (Inha) from *Mycobacterium tuberculosis*. Science 1998;279:98–102.
17. van Soolingen D, de Haas PEW, van Doorn HR, et al. Mutations at amino acid position 315 of the katG gene are associated with high-level resistance to isoniazid, other drug resistance and successful transmission of *Mycobacterium tuberculosis* in the Netherlands. J Infect Dis 2000;182:1788–1790.
18. Bavin EM, James B, Kay E, et al. Further observations on the antibacterial activity to *Mycobacterium tuberculosis* of a derivative of isoniazid, o-hydroxybenzalisonicotinylhydrazone (NUPASAL-213). J Pharm Pharmacol 1955;7:1032–1038.
19. Bavin EM, Drain DJ, Seiler M, et al. Some further studies on tuberculostatic compounds. J Pharm Pharmacol 1952;4:844–855.
20. Fox HH, Gibas JT. Synthetic tuberculostats. IV. Pyridine carboxylic acid hydrazides and benzoic acid hydrazides. J Org Chem 1952;17:1653–1660.
21. Fox HH, Gibas JT. Synthetic tuberculostats. VIII. Monoalkyl derivatives of isonicotinylhydrazine. J Org Chem 1953;18:994–1002.
22. Fox HH, Gibas JT. Synthetic tuberculostats. IX. Dialkyl derivatives of isonicotinylhydrazine. J Org Chem 1955;20:60–69.
23. Fox HH, Gibas JT. Synthetic tuberculostats. XI. Trialkyl and other derivatives of isonicotinylhydrazine. J Org Chem 1956;21:356–361.
24. Weber WW, Hein DW. Clinical pharmacokinetics of isoniazid. Clin Pharmacokinet 1979;4:401–422.
25. Holdiness MR. Clinical pharmacokinetics of the antituberculosis drugs. Clin Pharmacokinet 1984;9:511–544.
26. Timbrell JA, Mitchell JR, Snodgrass WR, et al. Isoniazid hepatotoxicity: the relationship between covalent binding and metabolism in vivo. J Pharmacol Exp Ther 1980;213:364–369.
27. Nolan CM, Goldberg SV, Buskin SE. Hepatotoxicity associated with isoniazid preventing therapy. JAMA 1999;281:1014–1018.
28. Lancini G. Ansamycins. In: Pape H, Rehm H-J, ed. Biotechnology: Microbial Products II, Vol 4. Deerfield Beach, FL: VCH, 1986.

29. Arora SK. Correlation of structure and activity in ansamycins: structure, conformation and interactions of antibiotic rifamycin S. J Med Chem 1985;28:1099–1102.
30. Levin ME, Hatfull GF. *Mycobacterium smegmatis* RNA polymerase: DNA supercoiling, action of rifampicin and mechanism of rifampicin resistance. Mol Microbiol 1993;8:277–285.
31. Lancini G, Zanchelli W. Structure–activity relationship in rifamycins. In: Perlman D, ed. Structure–Activity Relationship Among the Semisynthetic Antibiotics. New York: Academic Press, 1977.
32. Jarvis B, Lamb HM. Rifapentine. Drugs 1998;56:607–616.
33. Reith K, Keung A, Toren PC, et al. Disposition and metabolism of ^{14}C-rifapentine in healthy volunteers. Drug Met Dispos 1998;26:732–738.
34. Drugs for tuberculosis. The Medical Letter, 37, The Medical Letter, Inc., New Rochelle, NY, August 4, 1995:67–70.
35. Keung ACF, Eller MG, Weir SJ. Pharmacokinetics of rifapentine in patients with varying degrees of hepatic dysfunction. J Clin Pharmacol 1998;38:517–524.
36. Steffen R, Sack DA, Riopel L, et al. Therapy of travelers' diarrhea with rifaximin on various continents. Am J Gastroenterol 2003;98:1073–1078.
37. Scorpio A, Zhang Y. Mutations in *pncA*, a gene encoding pyrazinamidase/nicotinamidase, cause resistance to the antituberculous drug pyrazinamide in tubercle bacillus. Nat Med 1996;2:662–667.
38. Heifets LB, Flory MA, Lindholm-Levy PJ. Does pyrazinoic acid as an active moiety of pyrazinamide have specific activity against *Mycobacterium tuberculosis*? Antimicrob Agents Chemother 1989;33:1252–1254.
39. Zhang Y, Wade MM, Scorpio A, et al. Mode of action of pyrazinamide: disruption of mycobacterium tuberculosis membrane transport and energetics by pyrazinoic acid. Antimicrob Chemother 2003;52:790–795.
40. Kushner S, Dalalian H, Sanjurjo JL, et al. Experimental chemotherapy of tuberculosis. II. The synthesis of pyrazinamides and related compounds. J Am Chem Soc 1952;74:3617–3621.
41. Bergmann KE, Cynamon MH, Welch JT. Quantitative structure–activity relationships for the in vitro antimycobacterial activity of pyrazinoic acid esters. J Med Chem 1996;39:3394–3400.
42. Peloquin CA, Bulpitt AE, Jaresko GS, et al. Pharmacokinetics of pyrazinamide under fasting conditions, with food and with antacids. Pharmacotherapy 1998;18:1205–1211.
43. Daffe M, Brennan PJ, McNeil MR. Predominant structural features of the cell wall arabinogalactan of *Mycobacterium tuberculosis* as revealed through characterization of oligoglycosyl alditol fragments by gas chromatography/mass spectrometry and by ^{1}H and ^{13}C NMR analysis. J Biol Chem 1990;265:6734–6743.
44. Wolucka BA, McNeil MR, de Hoffmann E, et al. Recognition of the lipid intermediate for arabinogalactan/arabinomannan structure of cell wall of mycobacterium: biosynthesis and its relation to the mode of action of ethambutol in mycobacteria. J Biol Chem 1994;269:23328–23335.
45. Takayama K, Kilburn JO. Inhibition of synthesis of arabinogalactan by ethambutol in *Mycobacterium smegmatis*. Antimicrob Agents Chemother 1989;33:1493–1499.
46. Mikusova K, Slayden RAS, Besra GS, et al. Biogenesis of the mycobacterial cell wall and the site of action of ethambutol. Antimicrob Agents Chemother 1995;39:2484–2489.
47. Lee RE, Mikusova, Brennan PJ, et al. Synthesis of the mycobacterial arabinose donor beta-D-arabinofuranosyl-1-monophosphoryl decaprenol, development of a basic arabinosyl-transferase assay, and identification of ethambutol as an arabinosyl transferase inhibitor. J Am Chem Soc 1995;117:11829–11832.
48. Khoo K-H, Douglas E, Azadi P, et al. Truncated structural variants of lopoarabinomannan in ethambutol drug-resistant strains of *Mycobacterium smegmatis*. J Biol Chem 1996;271:28628–28690.
49. Belanger AE, Besra GS, Ford ME, et al. The *embAB* genes of *Mycobacterium avium* encode an arabinosyl transferase involved in cell wall arabinan biosynthesis that is the target for the antimycobacterial drug ethambutol. Proc Natl Acad Sci U S A 1996;93:11919–11924.
50. Kuehl FA, Peck RL, Hoffhine CE Jr, et al. Streptomyces antibiotics. XVIII. Structure of streptomycin. J Am Chem Soc 1945;70:2325–2329.
51. Finken M, Kirschner P, Meier A, et al. Molecular basis of streptomycin resistance in *Mycobacterium tuberculosis*: alterations of the ribosomal protein S12 gene and point mutations within a functional 16S ribosomal RNA pseudoknot. Mol Microbiol 1993;9:1239–1246.
52. Bieder A, Brunel P, Mazeau L. Identification de trois nouveaux metabolites de l'ethionamide: chromatographie, spectrophotometrie, polarographie. Ann Pharmaceut Francais 1966;24:493–500.
53. Caceres NE, Harris NB, Wellehan JF, et al. Overexpression of the D-alanine racemase gene confers resistance to D-cycloserine in *Mycobacterium smegmatis*. J Bacteriol 1997;179:5046–5055.
54. Gale EF, Cundliffe E, Reynolds PE, et al. The Molecular Basis of Antibiotic Action, 2nd Ed. London: Wiley & Sons, 1981.
55. Jacobs MR. Activity of quinolones against mycobacteria. Drugs 1995;49(Suppl 2):67–75.
56. Renau TE, Sanchez JP, Gage JW, et al. Structure–activity relationships of the quinolone antibacterials against mycobacteria: effect of structural changes at N-1 and C-7. J Med Chem 1996;39:729–735.
57. Miyazaki E, Miyazaki M, Chen JM, et al. Moxifloxacin (BAY-12-8039), a new 8-methoxyquinolone, is active in the mouse model of tuberculosis. Antimicrob Agents Chemother 1999;43:85–89.
58. Zhao BY, Pine R, Domagala J, et al. Fluoroquinolone action against clinical isolates of *Mycobacterium tuberculosis*: effects of a C-8 methoxy group on survival in liquid media and in human macrophages. Antimicrob Agents Chemother 1999;43:661–666.
59. Yew WW, Kwan SY, Ma WK, et al. In vitro activity of ofloxacin in *Mycobacterium tuberculosis* and its clinical efficacy in multiply resistant pulmonary tuberculosis. J Antimicrob Chemother 1990;26:227–236.
60. American Thoracic Society, Centers for Disease Control and Prevention, Infectious Disease Society of America. Treatment of tuberculosis. Am J Respir Crit Care Med 2003;167:604–661.
61. Reinke CM, Albrant DH. An old scourge: tuberculosis in the 1990s. US Pharmacist Hospital Edition 1991;16(October):37–72.
62. Nuermberger EL, Spigelman MK, Yew WW. Current development and future prospects in chemotherapy of tuberculosis. Respirology 2010;15:764–778.
63. Caminero JA, Sotgiu G, Zumla A, et al. Best drug treatment for multidrug-resistant and extensively drug-resistant tuberculosis. Lancet Infect Dis 2010;10:621–629.
64. Amsdenn GW, Peloquin CA, Berning SE. The role of advanced generation macrolides in the prophylaxis and treatment of *Mycobacterium avium* complex (MAC) infections. Drugs 1997;54:69–80.
65. Wright J. Current strategies for the prevention and treatment of disseminated *Mycobacterium avium* complex infection in patients with AIDS. Pharmacotherapy 1998;18:738–747.
66. Faris MA, Raasch RH, Hopfer RL, et al. Treatment and prophylaxis of disseminated *Mycobacterium avium* complex in HIV-infected individuals. Ann Pharmacother 1998;32:561–573.
67. Ma Z, Lienhardt C, McIlleron H, et al. Global tuberculosis drug development pipeline: the need and the reality. Lancet 2010;375:2100–2109.
68. Haagsma AC, Rooda A-I, Wagner MJ, et al. Selectivity of TMC207 towards mycobacterial ATP synthase compared with that towards the eukaryotic homologue. Antimicrob Agents Chemother 2009;53:1290–1292.
69. van Zyl JM, Basson K, Kriegler A, et al. Mechanisms by which clofazimine and dapsone inhibit the myeloperoxidase system. Biochem Pharmacol 1991;42:599–608.
70. Dhople AM. In vitro and in vivo activity of K-130, a dihyrofolate reductase inhibitor, against *Mycobacterium leprae*. Arzneim-Forsch Drug Res 1999;49:267–271.
71. Ward KE, McCarthy MW. Dapsone-induced methemoglobinemia. Ann Pharmacother 1998;32:549–552.
72. Savage JE, O'Sullivan JF, Zeis BM, et al. Investigation of the structural properties of dihydrophenazines which contribute to their pro-oxidative interaction with human phagocytes. J Antimicrob Chemother 1989;23:691–700.
73. Franzblau SG, White KE, O'Sullivan JF. Structure–activity relationships of tetramethylpiperdine-substituted phenazines against *Mycobacterium leprae* in vitro. Antimicrob Agents Chemother 1989;33:2004–2005.
74. Arutla S, Arra GS, Prabhakar CM, et al. Pro- and antioxidant effects of some antileprotic drugs in vitro and their influence on super oxide dismutase activity. Arzneim-Forsch Drug Res 1998;48:1024–1027.
75. O'Sullivan JF, Conalty ML, Morrison NE. Clofazimine analogues active against a clofazimine-resistant organism. J Med Chem 1988;31:567–572.
76. Kapoor VK. Clofazimine. In: Florey K, ed. Analytical Profiles of Drug Substances, Vol 18. San Diego: Academic Press, 1989.
77. Krishna DR, Mamidi RNVS, Hofmann U, et al. Characterization of clofazimine metabolites in humans by HPLC-electrospray mass spectrometry. Arzneim-Forsch Drug Res 1997;47:303–306.
78. Stirling D, Sherman M, Strauss S. Thalidomide: a surprising recovery. J Am Pharm Assoc 1997;37:306–313.
79. Thalidomide. The Medical Letter, 40, The Medical Letter, Inc., New Rochelle, NY, October 23, 1998:103–104.
80. Lambert HP, O'Grady FW. Antibiotic and Chemotherapy, 6th Ed. Edinburgh: Churchill Livingstone, 1992.
81. Lockwood DNJ, Kumar B. Treatment of leprosy. BMJ 2004;328:1447–1448.

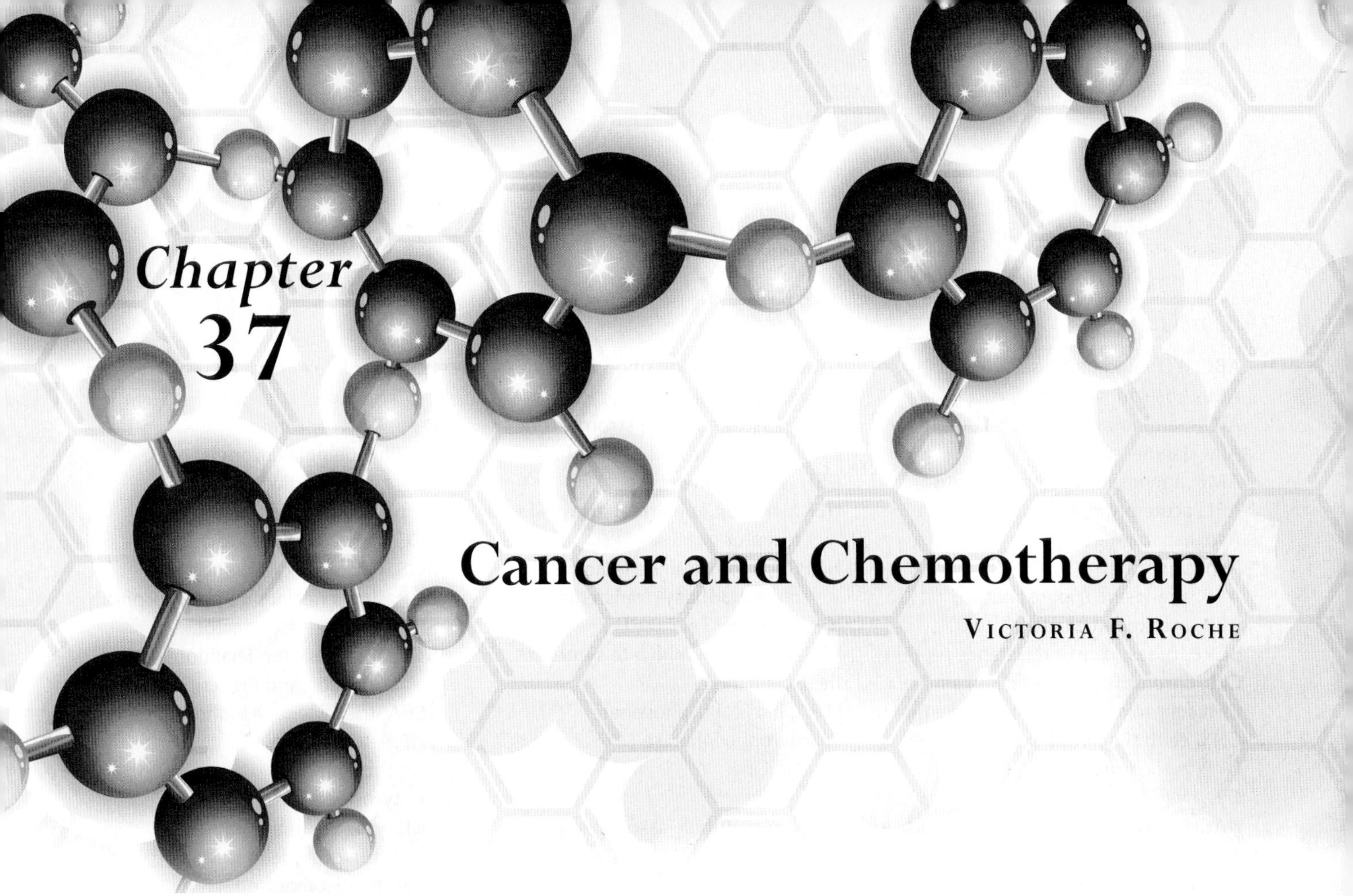

Chapter 37

Cancer and Chemotherapy

VICTORIA F. ROCHE

Drugs Covered in This Chapter

DNA CROSS-LINKING AGENTS

Miscellaneous DNA alkylating agents
- Altretamine
- Busulfan

Nitrogen mustards
- Bendamustine
- Chlorambucil
- Cyclophosphamide
- Ifosfamide
- Mechlorethamine
- Melphalan
- Thiotepa

Nitrosoureas
- Carmustine
- Lomustine
- Streptozocin

Organoplatinum complexes
- Carboplatin
- Cisplatin
- Oxaliplatin
- Picoplatin
- Satraplatin

Procarbazine and triazenes
- Dacarbazine
- Procarbazine
- Temozolomide

ANTIMETABOLITES

Antifolates
- Methotrexate
- Pemetrexed
- Pralatrexate

DNA methyltransferase inhibitors
- Azacitidine
- Decitabine
- Nelarabine

DNA polymerase inhibitors
- Cladribine
- Clofarabine
- Cytarabine
- Fludarabine
- Gemcitabine

Miscellaneous antimetabolites
- Hydroxyurea
- Pentostatin

Pyrimidine antagonists
- Capecitabine
- Floxuridine
- Fluorouracil

Purine antagonists
- Mercaptopurine
- Thioguanine

HISTONE DEACETYLASE INHIBITORS
- Romidepsin
- Vorinostat

IMMUNOMODULATORS
- Lenalidomide
- Thalidomide

MISCELLANEOUS ANTIBIOTICS
- Bleomycin
- Dactinomycin
- Mitomycin

MISCELLANEOUS ANTICANCER AGENTS
- Arsenic trioxide
- Bortezomib

MITOSIS INHIBITORS
- Cabazitaxel
- Docetaxel
- Estramustine
- Ixabepilone
- Paclitaxel
- Vinblastine
- Vincristine
- Vinorelbine

TOPOISOMERASE POISONS
- Daunorubicin
- Doxorubicin
- Epirubicin
- Etoposide
- Idarubicin
- Irinotecan
- Mitoxantrone
- Teniposide
- Topotecan
- Valrubicin

TYROSINE KINASE AND RELATED INHIBITORS
- Dasatinib
- Erlotinib
- Everolimus

- Gefitinib
- Imatinib
- Lapatinib
- Nilotinib
- Sorafenib
- Sunitinib
- Temsirolimus

Abbreviations

ABC, ATP-binding cassette
ABL, Abelson
AIC, 5-aminoimidazole-4-carboxamide
Ala, alanine
AMP, adenosine monophosphate
APL, acute promyelocytic leukemia
Asn, asparagine
Asp, aspartate
ATP, adenosine triphosphate
BCR, breakpoint cluster
BCRP, breast cancer resistance protein
CLL, chronic lymphocytic leukemia
CML, chronic myelogenous leukemia
CNS, central nervous system
CYP, cytochrome P450
Cys, cysteine
DACH, diaminocyclohexane
DHF, dihydrofolate
DHFR, dihydrofolate reductase
DPD, dihydropyrimidine dehydrogenase
dTMP, deoxythymidine monophosphate
dUMP, deoxyuridine monophosphate
EGCG, epigallocatechin-3-gallate
EGFR, epidermal growth factor receptor
FDA, U.S. Food and Drug Administration
FPGS, folyl polyglutamate synthase
GAR, glycine amide ribonucleotide
GI, gastrointestinal
GIST, gastrointestinal stromal tumors
GMP, guanosine monophosphate
GSH, glutathione
HER2, human epidermal growth factor receptor 2
HGPRT, hypoxanthine guanine phosphoribosyl transferase
His, histidine
hTS, human thymidylate synthase
Ile, isoleucine
ITPA, inositol triphosphate pyrophosphatase
Leu, leucine
Lys, lysine
MAP, microtubule-associated protein
MDR, multidrug resistance
Met, methionine
MMR, mismatch repair
MoAb, monoclonal antibody
MTIC, 3-methyl-(triazen-l-yl) imidazole-4-carboxamide
mTOR, mammalian target of rapamycin
NER, nucleotide-excision repair protein
NHL, non-Hodgkin lymphoma
PDGFR, platelet-derived growth factor receptor
P-gp, P-glycoprotein
Ph, Philadelphia chromosome
Phe, phenylalanine
Pt, platinum
RCC, renal cell carcinoma
ROS, reactive oxygen species
SNP, single nucleotide polymorphism
SPF, sun protection factor
STEPS, System for Thalidomide Education and Prescribing Safety
TEPA, triethylenephosphoramide
THF, tetrahydrofolate
Thr, threonine
TK, tyrosine kinase
TKI, tyrosine kinase inhibitor
TNM, tumor-node-metastasis
TopI, topoisomerase I
TopIIα, topoisomerase IIα
TPMT, thiopurine methyl transferase
Trp, tryptophan
Tyr, tyrosine
Val, valine
VEGFR, vascular endothelial growth factor receptor

SCENARIO

Kelly Nystrom, PharmD, BCOP

DT, a 37-year-old white man, was diagnosed with precursor B-cell acute lymphoblastic leukemia approximately 1 year ago. He was treated with a R-Hyper-CVAD program (cyclophosphamide, mesna, vincristine, doxorubicin and dexamethasone alternating with rituximab, high-dose methotrexate and cytarabine) and achieved a complete remission. He presented to the office 1 month ago with complaint of mild headaches (treated with ibuprofen 800 mg orally every 6 hours as needed) and left upper quadrant pain. A workup showed disease relapse and DL was admitted for cycle 2 of re-induction with a R-Hyper-CVAD program.

(The reader is directed to the clinical solution and chemical analysis of this case at the end of the chapter.)

INTRODUCTION

Healthy cells are under strict biochemical control for growth and differentiation. Cells divide and proliferate under the influence of various growth stimulators and are subject to arrested growth (senescence) and programmed cell death (apoptosis). In cancer, these regulatory processes have gone awry, and cells grow and divide uncontrollably, consuming energy and losing both structure and function due to an inability to adequately differentiate. To add insult to injury, rampant cell division is accompanied by disabled cell-death processes, leading first to cellular immortality and, eventually, to genetic instability. The causes of cancer are many and varied (e.g., chemical, environmental, viral, and mutagenic), but all ultimately lead to an aberration in the expression of proto-oncogenes, the products of which control normal cell life. When these genes mutate to become oncogenes in a sequential, multistep process, cancer results. Oncogenes (e.g., *myc* and *ras*) can either overexpress or underexpress regulatory biochemicals, resulting in preferential and accelerated cellular growth. Concomitantly, tumor suppressor genes (e.g., anti-oncogenes like *p53*, *p21*, p^{INK4A}, and *retinoblastoma*) can be inhibited (1).

Initially, tumors grow exponentially, taking a consistent amount of time for every doubling of the tumor cell population. In fact, the majority of a cancer cell's lifetime is spent before the tumor presents clinically. Initially, growth is very rapid (doubling time measured in days), but doubling time can slow to weeks or months as the tumor ages due to increasingly poor vascularization and the resulting decrease in access to blood and essential nutrients (2).

TABLE 37.1 · Oncogenic Origin of Selected Cancers

Cancer Type	Common Oncogenic or Tumor Suppressor Gene Origin
Chronic myelogenous leukemia	*bcr-abl* proto-oncogene translocation
Follicular lymphoma	*bcl-2* amplification, *myc* mutation
Sporadic thyroid cancer	*ret* mutation
Colorectal and gastric cancer	*APC* gene mutation
Familial breast and ovarian cancer	*BRCA1*, *BRCA2* mutation
Invasive ductal breast cancer	*HER2* amplification
Familial melanoma	$p16^{INK4A}$ mutation
Childhood neuroblastoma, small cell lung cancer	*N-myc* amplification
Leukemia, breast, colon, gastric, and lung cancer	*c-MYC* amplification
Renal cell cancer	*VHL* dysfunction

SELECTED DEFINITIONS

Oncogenes and Tumor Suppressor Genes

Oncogenes are regulators of cellular communication with the outside environment. They are derived through the mutation of proto-oncogenes, which are normal and ubiquitous genes involved in the regulation of homeostatic cellular functions. Mutations in proto-oncogenes can occur as spontaneous point mutations, inherited germline mutations, chromosomal rearrangements or through augmentation of gene expression. Regardless of the mutational mechanism, when the mutated oncogenes are stimulated by exposure to chemical, environmental, or viral carcinogens, they produce proteins that are either wrongly expressed within their normal cell or expressed in inappropriate tissues. In either case, cellular proliferation leading to cancer results (1,3).

Tumor suppressor genes are intended to keep oncogenes in check by halting uncontrolled cellular growth. In direct opposition to oncogenes, which induce cancer when stimulated or amplified, tumor suppressor genes promote cancer when inactivated or attenuated. Two of the most prevalent tumor suppressor genes involved in the generation of cancer are *p53* and *retinoblastoma*, or *Rb*. When either of these two suppressor genes loses function, the negative control on cellular proliferation is lifted and cells gain immortality (an essential quality of a cancer cell). The loss or disruption of function of the *p53* tumor suppressor gene is found in approximately half of human cancers and is a harbinger of a poor prognosis.

Oncogenes and tumor suppressor genes that have been linked to specific types of cancer are identified in Table 37.1 (1,3). Table 37.2 relates oncogenic markers of selected cancers to disease prognosis and treatment strategy (1).

Cell Cycle

When cells reproduce, they do so via a very specific game plan known as the cell cycle. Cell division (mitosis) kicks off the cycle, and after a period of 30 to 60 minutes, the cells go into either a resting phase (called G_0) or a presynthetic (gap) phase (called G_1), in which enzyme production occurs in preparation for de novo nucleic acid synthesis. Production of DNA then occurs in an S phase that can last up to 20 hours. The S phase is followed by a gap phase (G_2), in which RNA, critical proteins, and the mitotic spindle apparatus are generated for the next mitotic (M) phase (3,4).

This is important to our discussion since some anticancer agents are specific for a certain phase of the cell cycle. For example, antimetabolite antineoplastics damage cells in the S phase, whereas mitosis inhibitors pack their greatest cell-killing punch in the M phase. The administration of cell cycle phase-specific antineoplastics is carefully planned so that the drug encounters cancer cells at their most vulnerable moments. This often involves continuous infusion therapy or treatments spread over several days. Other antineoplastic agents are toxic to cells regardless of cycle phase (e.g., DNA alkylating agents and most antineoplastic antibiotics). These cell cycle phase-nonspecific agents can often be administered as a single bolus injection and/or at any time that is feasible for the provider and convenient for the patient.

In general, cancer cells undergoing rapid division are most vulnerable to the cytotoxic action of antineoplastic agents, and antineoplastic therapy holds its greatest promise for positive outcomes if initiated when the tumor is small but growing aggressively. Conversely, slow-growing tumors with a high percentage of cells remaining in the

CLINICAL SIGNIFICANCE

Chemotherapy has significantly changed the treatment of cancer since the first agents were studied in the 1940s. Understanding the chemical mechanism of action for traditional chemotherapy agents, including whether the agent is cell-cycle specific or cell-cycle nonspecific, is important so administration can be planned accordingly and co-administration of agents with similar toxicities can be avoided.

The disadvantage of traditional chemotherapy agents is the inability of the agent to recognize the difference between normal and cancer cells. So, although the agents may shrink or eliminate the tumor, the treatment is accompanied by many unwanted side effects. There are numerous examples where the chemical understanding of the chemotherapy agent is necessary. For example, when an anthracycline, such as doxorubicin, is given, free radicals are formed through an iron-dependent process that begins with the reduction of the anthracycline quinone ring to a hydroquinone. These free radicals can cause significant cardiac damage if left unmonitored. Dexrazoxane is a product that is predictably hydrolyzed to an electron-rich metabolite that binds to iron and prevents these toxic free radicals from being formed, thus reducing damage to the heart. Another example can be found when using cyclophosphamide or ifosfamide. The dissociation of aldophosphamide produces the active compound phophoramide mustard, but also produces acrolein, an electrophilic aldehyde, which can cause significant damage to the bladder by forming covalent bonds with cysteine residues of essential proteins. This bladder damage, or hemorrhagic cystitis, can be prevented with the use of mesna, a sulfhydryl-containing cysteine decoy that inactivates the effects of acrolein in the bladder. In addition, deficiencies found in individual patients can impact toxicities of certain chemotherapy agents.

Dihydropyrimidine dehydrogenase (DPD) is needed to deactivate both fluorouracil and capecitabine, which is a prodrug of fluorouracil. About 5% of the population has a deficiency of DPD, which results in accumulation of the drug and leads to severe toxicity if fluorouracil or capecitabine are administered. Recognizing the metabolic profile of these agents allows pharmacists to identify pharmacogenetically "at-risk" patients so that the safest dose of these highly toxic drugs can be administered.

Understanding the chemical basis for the toxicities seen with chemotherapy is imperative in managing or preventing them in clinical practice.

Kelly Nystrom, Pharm.D., BCOP
Associate Professor
Pharmacy Practice Department
School of Pharmacy and Health Professions
Creighton University

G_0 phase (e.g., non-small cell lung cancer) are often nonresponsive to cell cycle-specific chemotherapy (4). If the tumor is not detected until it is quite large, therapy can also be compromised by inefficient or substandard drug delivery due to poor tumor vascularization.

Metastasis

Metastasis refers to the process by which malignant cells leave the parent tumor, migrate to distant sites, and invade new tissue. The primary metastatic highways used by meandering cancer cells are the blood and lymph fluids. Sloughed cells must find a biologic environment with all of their essential growth factors in place before they can put down roots and evolve into a full-fledged metastatic tumor. Since many distinct and interdependent steps must be accomplished to establish metastatic disease, the process has been termed the "metastatic cascade" (5). Fortunately, there are many opportunities within the cascade for the body to mount a successful defense and destroy the potential invaders.

Cancer Staging

Clinicians need to have a common language through which to communicate about disease severity to make the best team-based decisions about the relative risks and benefits of treatment options. In the tumor-node-metastasis

TABLE 37.2 Oncogenic Markers and Therapeutic Strategies in Selected Cancers

Cancer Type	Oncogenic Marker	Prognosis/Responsiveness to Chemotherapy	Approach
Breast cancer	*HER2* amplification	Poor	Aggressive chemotherapy, targeted therapy
Acute myelogenous leukemia	t(8;21) or inv(16) translocation	Good	Standard chemotherapy
Acute lymphocytic leukemia	*bcr-abl* rearrangement	Poor	Bone marrow transplantation

(TNM) cancer staging classification, the severity of solid tumor neoplastic growth is characterized by the size of the tumor mass (T_1 to T_4), the extent of lymph node involvement (N_0 to N_3), and whether distant metastasis has occurred (M_0 or M_1). The larger the subscripted number in each of these parameters, the more advanced and/or disseminated the disease. Taken together, the TNM characteristics of a tumor can be translated into a comprehensive staging scale ranging from I (localized) to IV (metastatic). The intermediate disease severity stages indicate local (stage II) or regional (stage III) tissue invasion (3). Staging is an essential prerequisite for the prediction of prognosis and the identification of the most appropriate treatment plan and optimal dosing regimen (2).

Response Criteria

In this era of patient-centered, team-based care, it is equally beneficial to quantify a patient's clinical response to therapy in a manner that is consistent and universally understood by all health care providers. Five discrete anticancer therapy response categories have been defined, with criteria established for each (3). Whereas *cure* is obviously the most noble goal, it is very difficult to achieve in most types of cancer. A cure for all cancers except breast and melanoma equates to no evidence of disease for a minimum of 5 years. More commonly, the response category viewed as the pinnacle is *complete response,* in which the patient has no evidence of cancer for at least 1 month following the cessation of therapy, but where relapses are still possible. A *partial response* is claimed when tumor size has been reduced by 30% or more and there is no evidence of new lesions at the primary site or elsewhere for a minimum of 1 month. If this level of clinical improvement is not reached, yet the patient has experienced significant attenuation of symptoms and/or enhancement of quality of life, the response is termed *clinical benefit.* A less optimistic response category is *stable disease,* in which tumor size has either increased by less than 20% or decreased by less than 30%. Most dire is *progression,* a category that is characterized by tumor growth at the 20% or higher level and/or the formation of new lesions during therapy.

HISTORICAL BACKGROUND (6)

> "Those who have not been trained in chemistry or medicine, which after all is only applied chemistry, may not realize how difficult the problem of [cancer] treatment really is. It is almost, not quite, but almost as hard as finding some agent that will dissolve away the left ear, say, yet leave the right ear unharmed: so slight is the difference between the cancer cell and its normal ancestor."

Thus wrote noted cancer researcher and physician Dr. William H. Woglom in a monograph published by the American Association for the Advancement of Science in 1947 (7). Although somewhat predictive of what we now know to be true regarding the relationship between resident genes and oncogenes, Dr. Woglom's rather gloomy prognosis of our ability to meet cancer on its own ground and beat it was underpinned by centuries of unsuccessful attempts to treat neoplastic disease with toxic metals, including lead, arsenic, silver, zinc, antimony, mercury, and bismuth. However, the era of more promising chemotherapy was just on the horizon even as Woglom penned his words of therapeutic woe.

Among the first nonmetallic therapeutic agents to show benefit in the treatment of cancer was cortisone and, later, prednisone. In the 1940s, these glucocorticoids were shown to induce tumor regression in a laboratory cancer model (murine lymphosarcoma) and in acute leukemia. In the same decade, the retrospective recognition that World War I soldiers exposed to sulfur mustard gas, used as an agent of war, suffered from damaged lymphoid tissue and bone marrow led to the development of the cytotoxic nitrogen mustards for the treatment of lymphoma. Chemists then used their scientific understanding of mustard reactivity to design agents that were either "superpotent" and nonselective (e.g., highly toxic) or of lower reactivity so as to provide oral activity and less systemic toxicity.

The discovery in 1940 that *p*-aminobenzenesulfonamide was effective against streptococcal infections ushered in the era of antimetabolite chemotherapy. The development of antifolate antineoplastics, which were shown to be effective in combating childhood leukemias, got its start in the late 1940s. In the mid to late 1950s, on the heels of the success of antifolates, came the development of antimetabolites based on the structures of endogenous purine and pyrimidine bases. Perhaps the most exciting discovery in this regard was the recognition that a very simple analog of the endogenous pyrimidine uracil (5-fluorouracil) was a potent inhibitor of deoxythymidine monophosphate biosynthesis and that inhibiting the production of this essential nucleotide produced positive results in patients suffering from colon, stomach, pancreatic, and breast cancers. Antimetabolites that target DNA polymerase (e.g., cytarabine) were conceptualized and synthesized in the late 1950s and subsequently shown to be effective in acute myeloblastic leukemia.

The antibiotic antineoplastics came into clinical utility when the highly toxic actinomycin (discovered in the 1940s) was found to be effective in the treatment of human testicular cancer and uterine choriocarcinoma. Other natural anticancer antibiotics, such as bleomycin, subsequently were found to be active against various hematologic cancers and solid tumors (1960s), which led in more recent times to the development of semisynthetic analogs with both high potency and wider margins of safety. The antimitotic vinca alkaloids vincristine and vinblastine were shown to have activity against Hodgkin's disease and acute lymphoblastic leukemia around the same time that the antibiotic antineoplastics were being developed.

Cancer chemotherapy appears to have come full circle since the "metal-intense Renaissance," because some of the newer anticancer drugs to join the U.S. market are organometallic platinum (Pt) complexes. The activity of cisplatin (the first such complex to be commercially available) against lymphosarcoma and solid tumors of the head, neck, and reproductive organs was first noted in the early 1970s. The fortuitous discovery of organoplatinum complexes in the treatment of cancer is attributed to Dr. Barnett Rosenberg, who was studying the impact of electromagnetic radiation on bacterial cell growth using platinum electrodes. He followed up on the astute observation that the bacteria exposed to the electrodes experienced profound changes in cellular structure, which ultimately were attributed to the in situ generation of cisplatin. Both Pt(II) and Pt(IV) analogs of cisplatin, which offer high potency coupled with lower resistance potential and fewer use-limiting side effects (e.g., oto-, nephro-, and hematotoxicity), are currently on the market and in clinical trials. In addition to organometallics, the efficacy of sex hormones and hormone antagonists in fighting hormone-dependent cancers (e.g., estrogen receptor–positive breast cancer or prostate cancer) and the advent of therapeutic biologic response modifiers with direct antiproliferative effects (e.g., interferons) have added significantly to the therapeutic options available to providers and the cancer patients for whom they care.

The later 1990s saw the introduction of the tyrosine kinase inhibitors (TKIs) to the antineoplastic armamentarium. The recognition in 1960 that a mutant chromosome known as BCR-ABL (or the Philadelphia [Ph] chromosome) appeared consistently in the cells of patients with chronic myelogenous leukemia (CML) represented the first time a chromosomal aberration had been directly linked to a neoplastic disorder. The product of this abbreviated chromosome, the Bcr-Abl protein, is an unregulated tyrosine kinase that promotes cellular proliferation at the expense of apoptosis. Imatinib, the first rationally designed drug in the TKI class, was made available in 2001 and dramatically changed the treatment and clinical outcome of Ph-positive leukemias. Although imatinib selectively targets the Bcr-Abl protein, other inhibitors with selectivity for epidermal growth factor receptor (EGFR) and vascular endothelial growth factor receptor (VEGFR) kinases soon followed. These growth factor–selective TKIs show efficacy in the treatment of solid tumors of the lung, breast, pancreas, and kidney.

Despite the wide range of antineoplastic agents currently available, it has been estimated that approximately 40% of patients with cancer ultimately succumb to their disease (3). Novel therapies based on an in-depth understanding of the molecular mechanisms involved in the complex cascade of events we call cancer are urgently needed. Fortunately, molecular targets for focused chemotherapeutic interventions are being discovered with increasing regularity, opening the door for the scientifically grounded development of new drugs. The critical role of computer-based technology in facilitating the ability of chemists to conceptualize and visualize molecular interactions between potential drugs and putative receptor targets that lead to rational drug design and development, as well as in analyzing and managing the overwhelming amounts of data that are generated from these studies, cannot be overestimated. Likewise, the availability of viable tumor cell lines has facilitated a disease-specific orientation to the hunt for more effective therapies. Currently, there are tumor cell lines for lung, colon, breast, ovarian, brain, and kidney cancers, as well as for melanoma and leukemia (8).

Several monoclonal antibodies targeted to tumor cell antigens or proteins critical to cellular proliferation (e.g., human epidermal growth factor, vascular endothelial growth factor, tyrosine kinase, and proteasomes) have found their way to the U.S. market. In addition, several new targets for anticancer drug development currently are being actively explored by biomedical scientists (1,8). For example, cancer cells overexpress the enzyme telomerase, which inhibits the natural destruction of chromosomal telomeres (DNA caps), leading to unwanted cellular immortality. Telomerase inhibitors would be expected to reestablish cellular senescence and to halt uncontrolled cell division by maintaining the integrity of the telomeres and are being pursued as a new biochemical approach to disease attenuation or control (9). Other potential antineoplastic drug targets being seriously investigated are aberrant genes or enzymes unique to specific tumors and P-glycoprotein (P-gp), which is overexpressed in many cancers as a result of an amplified *mdr-1* gene and responsible for the rapid ejection of antineoplastic agents from target cells. Other multidrug resistance–associated proteins (the MRP family) involved in this devastating rebound of the cancer cell are also being investigated as potential sites of therapeutic intervention. The intense focus on resistance molecules such P-gp is warranted because patients whose tumors express this efflux-promoting protein respond poorly to chemotherapy and have a poor prognosis (2).

It is hoped that clinicians will one day be able to generate a genetic expression profile for each patient to help them assess the likelihood of response to all possible therapies and to guide pharmacotherapy selection. Pharmacogenomics-based predictors of therapeutic response to anticancer drugs currently being explored include single nucleotide polymorphisms (SNPs) and the multiplicity of genes and gene products within a single biochemical pathway (10). While there are multiple scientific, regulatory, and ethical barriers to overcome before the full power of pharmacogenomics can positively impact the care of every cancer patient, these issues are being actively addressed at the national level, giving hope that the age of individualized cancer chemotherapy may indeed be close at hand.

DISEASE STATE

Cancers can usually be classified as lymphatic, epithelial, nerve, or connective tissue related, and tumor nomenclature is based on tissue of origin as follows: carcinoma (epithelial origin), sarcoma (muscle or connective tissue origin), leukemia and lymphoma (lymphatic or hematologic origin), and glioma (neural origin). The risk of developing epithelial-derived cancers increases with age.

Incidence

In 2007, approximately 1.4 million people received a diagnosis of cancer, and approximately 560,000 died of the disease (3). The American Cancer Society estimates that over 1.5 million new cases of cancer will be diagnosed in 2010 (11). If the ratio of new diagnoses to deaths observed in 2007 holds steady, over 555,000 lives will be lost. The most commonly acquired cancers include those of the prostate, breast, lung, colon, and rectum. Lung cancer is the most fatal and will be responsible for approximately 157,000 U.S. deaths in 2010. These prominent cancers (prostate/breast, lung, and colorectal) occur with very similar frequency in men and women, and few gender-related differences in mortality have been noted (Table 37.3) (11). Some geographical differences in incidence have been observed, with lung cancer being more prevalent in rural southern U.S. states, and breast and colon cancer more commonly diagnosed in the "northeast corridor" of the United States (12).

TABLE 37.4 The American Cancer Society's Major Warning Signs of Cancer

Cancer Warning Signs in Adults	Cancer Warning Signs in Children
Change in bowel or bladder habits	Continued unexplained weight loss
A sore that does not heal	Frequent headaches, with vomiting
Unusual bleeding or discharge	Persistent pain in bones or joints
Thickening or lump in breast or elsewhere	Any unusual mass or swelling
Indigestion or difficulty in swallowing	Sudden eye or vision changes
Obvious change in a wart or mole	Recurrent or unexplained fever
Nagging cough or hoarseness	Excessive bruising or bleeding
	Noticeable paleness or loss of energy

Signs and Symptoms

The clinical manifestations of cancer can vary widely depending on type and stage of neoplastic disease. The American Cancer Society has been promulgating its list of the major warning signs of cancer for decades (Table 37.4) (3,13). Patients are well-served by being familiar with these early warning signs because cancer is most effectively treated when diagnosed before advanced disease develops. Recognizing that the first letters of each sign spell the word "caution" can help adults remember them. One readily recognized symptom of cancer is persistent weight loss (especially in children), and severe, unrelenting pain is a hallmark symptom of cancer in the later stages. Solid tumors can become palpable or observable masses when the cancer is advanced.

Biochemical Bases and Causes of Cancer

Currently, it is understood that cancer is caused by mutations in "resident" or normal genes rather than by the introduction of foreign genes into otherwise healthy systems (1,3). The single-gene theory of cancer (where a single mutation could result in neoplastic disease) has been abandoned in favor of the multiple mutation prerequisite, and complex gene pathways, interactions, and communications are now the focus of study in the understanding of malignant processes and their treatments. Once determined, the "mutational profile" of malignant cells may very well predict such parameters as disease severity, most promising therapeutic interventions, and clinical outcome.

The development of cancer occurs in four discrete steps or phases. In the **initiation** phase, exposure to a precipitating carcinogen prompts irreversible mutation in a number of different genes. The **promotion** phase is a time during which mutated cells arising from altered genes grow preferentially compared to normal cells. This preferential growth may result from continued exposure to the original carcinogen or from promotion by environmental "accelerants." This stage is reversible, so cancer sometimes can be avoided with appropriate changes in diet and lifestyle. The **transformation** phase is the 5- to 20-year progression of a mutated cell to a cancer cell. Cellular proliferation, clonal colony development, tissue invasion and destruction, and metastasis define the final **progression** phase of cancer development (3).

TABLE 37.3 Estimated 2010 U.S. Incidence and Mortality of Common Cancers

	Prostate/Breast		Lung and Bronchus		Colorectal	
	Men	Women	Men	Women	Men	Women
Incidence	217,730 (28%)	207,090 (28%)	116,750 (15%)	105,770 (14%)	72,090 (9%)	70,480 (10%)
Mortality	32,050 (11%)	39,840 (15%)	86,220 (29%)	71,080 (26%)	26,580 (9%)	24,790 (9%)

As previously mentioned, the genetic mutations leading to the diseases that we call cancer can be stimulated by a variety of chemical, environmental, and viral triggers. Both RNA retroviruses and DNA viruses have been implicated in human cancer causation (Table 37.5), although many more DNA than RNA viruses have oncogenic potential (14,15).

Individuals in certain occupations may be at enhanced risk for the development of some cancers due to unavoidable exposure to carcinogenic chemicals (12). Perhaps the best-known example of occupationally induced cancer involves exposure to asbestos, which has been conclusively linked with the development of lung, pleural, and peritoneal malignancies. Miners exposed to radon are also at a significantly enhanced risk for the development of lung cancer, as are individuals exposed through their work to soot, tars, hexavalent chromium, and nickel-containing compounds. The aromatic amines β-naphthylamine and 4-aminobiphenyl are known to induce bladder cancer, and exposure to the common organic solvent benzene has been linked to the development of leukemia.

Environmental carcinogens are all around us (Table 37.6) (12). Fortunately, individuals can do many things to protect themselves from exposure or from negative consequences of limited exposure. The chemicals deposited in the lungs from inhaling cigarette smoke are the primary cause of lung cancer in the United States, but smokers who quit decrease their risk for this often-fatal cancer by 67% or more after 10 smoke-free years (12). Nonsmokers can protect themselves from the cancer-promoting effects of secondhand smoke by removing themselves from smoke-filled environments. Smoking combined with alcohol has a synergistic effect in promoting the development of oral cancer. In addition to quitting smoking, abstaining from alcohol or drinking in moderation is a choice that individuals can make in an effort to decrease their overall risk of developing cancer. Other measures that patients can take to minimize the risk of cancer from environmental causes include protection from damaging ultraviolet rays through the use of high-SPF (sun protection factor) sunscreens and the consumption of foods that are low in fat but rich in carotenoids, vitamins A and C, folate, selenium, and/or fiber (12).

TABLE 37.6 Some Environmental Precipitants of Cancer

Environmental Cancer Precipitant	Cancer Type
Tobacco	Lung, oral, bladder, pancreatic, stomach, and renal cancer
Alcohol	Liver, rectal, and breast cancer
Tobacco plus alcohol	Oral cancers
Radon	Lung cancer
Halogenated compounds	Bladder cancer
Immunosuppressive agents	Lymphoma
Herbicides	Lymphoma
Ionizing or ultraviolet radiation	Leukemia, breast, thyroid, lung, and skin cancer

TABLE 37.5 RNA and DNA Viruses Associated with Cancer Development

Virus	Cancer
RNA Virus	
Human T-lymphotrophic virus	Adult T-cell leukemia
Hepatitis C	Hepatocellular carcinoma
DNA Virus	
Hepadnavirus	Hepatocellular carcinoma
Papillomavirus	Skin cancer, cervical cancer, anogenital cancer
Epstein-Barr virus	Burkett lymphoma, Hodgkin's disease, anaplastic nasopharyngeal carcinoma, gastric cancer
Herpes	Karposi sarcoma

GENERAL THERAPEUTIC APPROACHES

Cancer treatment can be comprised of surgery, radiation, antineoplastic chemotherapy, and/or therapy with biologic response modifiers, which stimulate the patient's own immunologic defense mechanisms. Surgery and radiation (ionizing, thermal, or photodynamic) are favored for isolated or localized cancers; chemotherapy and biologic response modifiers (with or without surgery and/or radiation) are reserved for disseminated or systemic cancers. Chemotherapy can also be used after surgery and/or radiation as an "insurance policy" against microscopic metastatic disease (adjuvant therapy) or before surgery to decrease the size of the mass to be removed (neoadjuvant therapy).

Unfortunately, cancer cells do not simply lie down in the face of chemotherapeutic intervention. Rather, these aggressive cells fight back in an attempt to retain their immortality. Some cancer cells acquire resistance to anticancer drugs by downregulating enzymes essential for drug transport or for the activation of antineoplastic prodrugs, or by upregulating enzymes involved in inactivating biotransformation. As noted previously, other mechanisms of biochemical retaliation include downregulation of target enzymes, altered drug uptake and efflux mechanisms (e.g., amplification of the gene that encodes for P-gp or the multidrug resistance–associated protein), inhibition of cellular repair proteins, and apoptosis inhibition (2–4).

Cancer Chemotherapy

The word *antineoplastic* means "against new growth." In general, the mechanism of cytotoxic action for all antineoplastic agents is interference with cellular synthesis or the function of RNA, DNA, and the proteins that sustain life. All antineoplastic agents are poisons because they are designed to kill cells. Currently available anticancer drugs are often highly and generally toxic, especially for cells with short half-lives. For example, nonspecific destruction of the rapidly dividing cells of the gastrointestinal (GI) tract leads to the severe nausea and vomiting associated with cancer chemotherapy, whereas alopecia and fatigue (as well as susceptibility to infection) are the result of the destruction of rapidly dividing cells in hair follicles and bone marrow, respectively. Factors such as the extent and severity of the disease, individual sensitivity to the antineoplastic mechanism employed by the drugs selected for use, the kinetics controlling drug transport, and cell cycle specificity all impact the chance for chemotherapeutic success (2).

Because cancer chemotherapy is most often given in several courses or "rounds," with an interval of several days or weeks in between to permit attenuation of side effects, three distinct aspects of drug dosing must be considered when determining the impact of antineoplastic therapy on overall patient welfare. First, the dose that ideally should be given per course has been identified for each commonly employed antineoplastic agent but can be altered significantly by individual patient health status (e.g., hepatic, renal, cardiovascular, hematopoietic, pulmonary, and/or other comorbidities), activity/performance status, genetic makeup, and the nature and anticipated severity of side effects. Each round of antineoplastic therapy kills a given percentage of cancer cells with each administration ("cell kill hypothesis"), and the percentage killed rises proportionally with the dose of drug. If chemotherapy can shrink tumors to 10^4 or fewer cells, normal host defense systems are usually capable of eradicating them (2,3). Therefore, the dose of drug that comes as close as possible to the recommended dose is the goal. Expect significant interpatient variation in response to the same chemotherapeutic regimen secondary to individual genetics, level of debilitation, extent of tissue invasion, critical organ system function (including bone marrow), and past exposure to chemotherapeutic agents.

As alluded to earlier, an ever-growing understanding of genetic polymorphism and its impact on the biosynthesis of target proteins and metabolizing enzymes is helping health care providers make wiser decisions about antineoplastic therapy and drug regimens. The length of the "drug-free" interval is the second important drug-dosing consideration because a shorter interval (or higher dose intensity—the "one-two punch") is associated with a more aggressive inhibition of tumor growth. Most often, patients cannot tolerate the debilitating side effects (e.g., myelosuppression) without a prolonged interval between rounds. The advent of genetically engineered biologic response modifiers, such as granulocyte colony-stimulating factor, which boosts the ability of bone marrow to produce neutrophils, has had a positive impact on optimizing dosing intensity/density.

Finally, many chemotherapeutic agents produce serious chronic or delayed toxicities that may be irreversible, particularly in heart, lung, and kidneys, which demands that the total cumulative dose be taken into account when designing the regimen. The ultimate balancing act is to give the patient as much antineoplastic drug as is normally recommended in the time frame most likely to kill the greatest percentage of cancer cells without inducing intolerable or life-threatening toxicity in healthy organs and tissues. Armed with the knowledge of the biochemical and/or molecular basis of toxicity, the pharmacist is in an excellent position to employ appropriate pharmacotherapeutic agents to attenuate unavoidable side effects.

One approach for minimizing unwanted toxicity is to employ a chemotherapeutic regimen of several drugs that act by distinct mechanisms and/or precipitate different side effects. Attacking the tumor with different therapeutic "guns" should target a larger variety of the mutant cells that comprise the tumor and permit a lower dose of each to be used compared to single-agent therapy. Minimizing side effect overlap provides a greater chance that the patient will be able to tolerate therapy and accommodate a shorter interval between courses.

It is essential that the oncology pharmacist be well versed in the pharmacotherapy-based management of severe pain, infection, and the nausea, vomiting, and fatigue associated with chemotherapy. The provision of contemporary and valid drug information to patients and families is essential, as is assistance in helping with the interpretation of information that patients and loved ones secure either through their health care providers or independently (e.g., from the Internet).

THERAPEUTIC CLASSES OF ANTICANCER DRUGS

DNA Cross-Linking Agents (Alkylators and Organometallics)

The primary target of DNA cross-linking agents is the actively dividing DNA molecule. The DNA cross-linkers are all extremely reactive electrophilic (δ^+) structures. When encountered, the nucleophilic groups on various DNA bases (particularly, but not exclusively, the N^7 of guanine) readily attack the electrophilic drug, resulting in irreversible alkylation or complexation of the DNA base.

Some DNA alkylating agents, such as the nitrogen mustards and nitrosoureas, are bifunctional, meaning that one molecule of the drug can bind two distinct DNA bases. Most commonly, the alkylated bases are on different DNA molecules, and interstrand DNA cross-linking through two guanine N^7 atoms results. The DNA alkylating antineoplastics are not cell cycle specific, but they are more toxic to cells in the late G_1 or S phases of the cycle.

This is the time when DNA is unwinding and exposing its nucleotides, increasing the chance that vulnerable DNA functional groups will encounter the electrophilic antineoplastic drug and launch the nucleophilic attack that leads to its own destruction. The DNA alkylators have a great capacity for inducing both mutagenesis and carcinogenesis; in other words, they can promote cancer in addition to treating it.

Organometallic antineoplastics (platinum coordination complexes) also cross-link DNA, and many do so by binding to adjacent guanine nucleotides, called diguanosine dinucleotides, on a single strand of DNA. This leads to intrastrand DNA cross-linking. The anionic phosphate group on a second strand of DNA stabilizes the drug–DNA complex and makes the damage to DNA replication irreversible. Some organometallic agents also damage DNA through interstrand cross-linking.

Nitrogen Mustards and Aziridine-Mediated Alkylators

Nitrogen mustards are bis(β-haloalkyl)amines. The term "bis" means two, and the "halo" (short for halogen) in the nomenclature is invariably chlorine. The two chlorine atoms dramatically decrease the basic strength of the amino nitrogen through a strong negative inductive effect. As a result, the unionized conjugate of these drugs predominates at physiologic pH. This is intentional because it is the unionized amine (with its lone pair of electrons) that allows the formation of the highly electrophilic aziridinium ion, which is the reactive DNA-destroying intermediate generated by all true mustards.

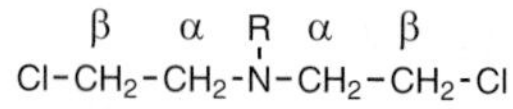

Bis-β-haloalkylamine

Mechanism of Action The mechanism of action of the nitrogen mustards (16) is depicted in Figure 37.1. In step 1, the lone pair of electrons on the unionized amino group conducts an intramolecular nucleophilic attack at the β-carbon of the mustard, displacing chloride anion and forming the highly electrophilic aziridinium ion intermediate, a quaternary amine. The carbon atoms of this strained cyclic structure are highly electrophilic due to the strong negative inductive effect of the positively charged nitrogen atom.

In step 2, a DNA nucleophile conducts an intermolecular nucleophilic attack, which breaks the aziridine ring and alkylates DNA. Although guanine is the preferred nucleic acid base involved in the alkylation reaction, adenine is also known to react. Of critical importance is the fact that the lone pair of electrons on the mustard nitrogen is regenerated when the aziridine ring cleaves.

Steps 3 and 4 are simply repetitions of steps 1 and 2, respectively, involving the second arm of the mustard and a second molecule of DNA. Ultimately, two molecules of DNA will be cross-linked through the carbon atoms of what was once the nitrogen mustard. Finally, hydrolytic depurination (step 5) cleaves the bound guanine residues from the DNA strand. This is an attempt to liberate the DNA from the mustard's covalent "stranglehold," but the DNA released from this mustard trap is damaged and unable to replicate. Cell death is the inevitable result. If

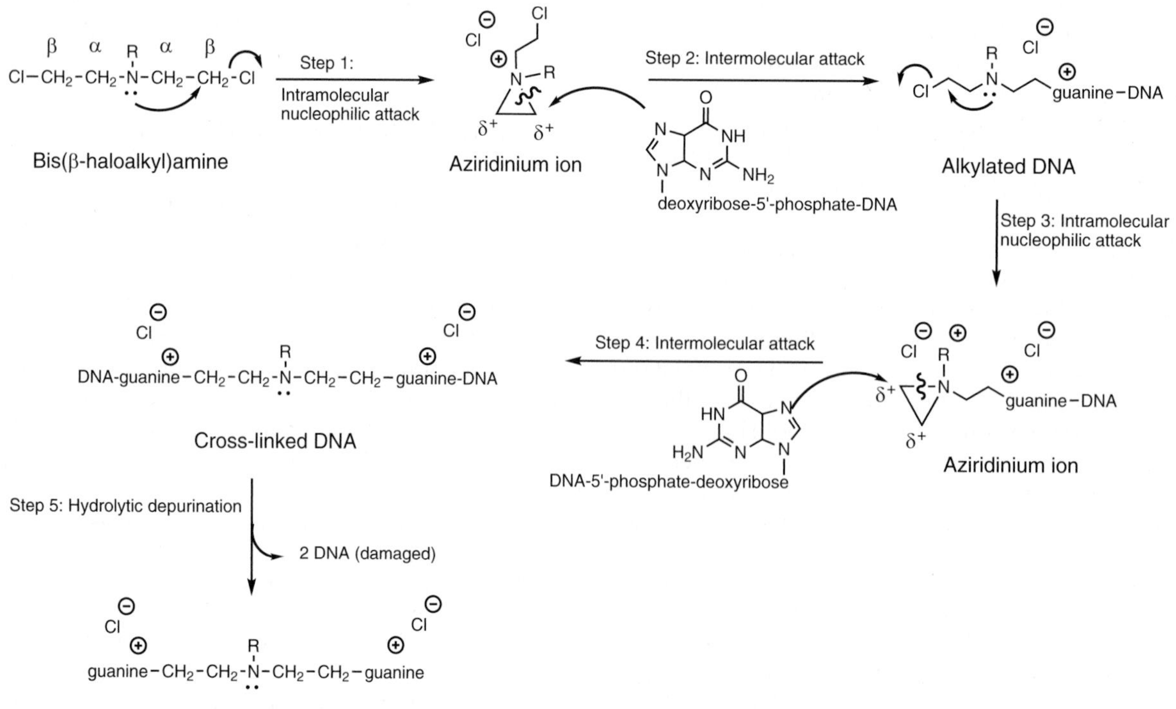

FIGURE 37.1 DNA destruction through nitrogen mustard–mediated alkylation.

this is happening in a tumor cell, the therapeutic goal has been accomplished. If it is happening in a healthy cell, particularly one with a short half-life, then the patient may experience side effects that can be use-limiting.

CHEMISTRY The structure of nitrogen mustards differs only in the nature of the third group (R) attached to the amino nitrogen. This group, which can be either aliphatic or aromatic, is the prime determinant of chemical reactivity, oral bioavailability, and the nature and extent of side effects.

An aliphatic nitrogen substituent (e.g., CH_3) will release electrons to the amine through σ bonds. This electronic enrichment enhances the nucleophilic character of the lone pair of electrons and increases the speed at which the δ^+ β-carbon of the mustard will be attacked. Whether in a tumor cell or a healthy cell, as soon as the aziridinium ion forms, it will react with unpaired DNA and/or other cell nucleophiles, such as electron-rich SH (mercapto or sulfhydryl), OH (hydroxyl), and NH (amino) groups of amino acids on enzymes or membrane-bound receptors. The body's water can also react with (and inactivate) the aziridinium ion. The intra- and intermolecular reactions designated as steps 1 through 4 in Figure 37.1 happen so rapidly that almost no chance exists for tissue or cell specificity, which means a greatly increased risk of serious side effects and use-limiting toxicity.

Conversely, an aromatic nitrogen substituent (e.g., phenyl) conjugated with the mustard nitrogen will stabilize the lone pair of electrons through resonance. Resonance delocalization significantly slows the rate of intramolecular nucleophilic attack, aziridinium ion formation, and DNA alkylation. Aromatic mustards have a reactivity sufficiently controlled to permit oral administration and attenuate the severity of side effects. The higher stability also provides the chance for enhanced tissue selectivity by giving the intact mustard time to reach malignant cells before generating the electrophilic aziridinium ion.

Nitrogen mustards can decompose in aqueous media through formation of the inactive dehalogenated diol shown in Figure 37.2. Both the mustard nitrogen (pathway a) and the oxygen of water (pathway b) can act as nucleophiles to advance this degradative process. The decomposition reactions can be inhibited if the nucleophilic character of these atoms is eliminated through protonation, so buffering solutions to a slightly acidic pH helps to enhance stability in aqueous solution.

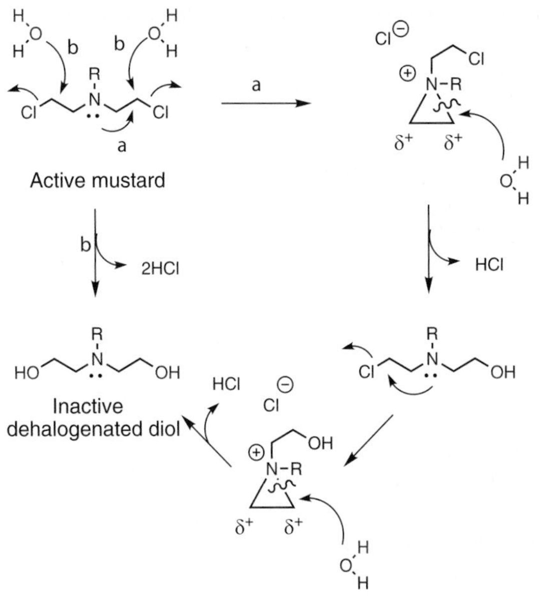

FIGURE 37.2 Aqueous decomposition of nitrogen mustards.

SPECIFIC DRUGS (FIG. 37.3)

Mechlorethamine Hydrochloride Mechlorethamine is the only aliphatic nitrogen mustard currently on the U.S. market. Its use is limited by extremely high reactivity, which leads to rapid and nonspecific alkylation of cellular nucleophiles and excessive toxicity. It is a severe vesicant, and if accidental skin contact occurs, the drug must be inactivated with 2% sodium thiosulfate ($Na_2S_2O_3$) solution. This reagent reacts with the mustard to create an inactive, highly ionized, and water-soluble thiosulfate ester that can be washed away (Fig. 37.4). The affected tissue should also be treated with an ice compress for 6 to 12 hours.

Mechlorethamine is marketed in hydrochloride salt form to provide water solubility for intravenous or intracavitary administration. The strong electron-withdrawing effect of the two chlorine atoms reduces the pK_a of mechlorethamine to 6.1, which gives a ratio of un-ionized to ionized drug forms of approximately 20:1 at pH 7.4. This agent is too reactive for oral administration and too toxic to use alone. In addition to severe nausea and vomiting, myelosuppression (lymphocytopenia and granulocytopenia), and alopecia, it can cause myelogenous leukemia with extended use due to its mutagenic/carcinogenic effects on bone marrow stem cells. Mechlorethamine is still used in regimens for cancers of the blood (e.g., Hodgkin's disease, chronic myelocytic leukemia, chronic lymphocytic leukemia); fortunately, safer and still highly potent antineoplastic agents are now available.

Melphalan This aromatic mustard, used primarily in the treatment of multiple myeloma, is able to stabilize the lone pair of electrons on the mustard nitrogen through resonance with the conjugated phenyl ring, slowing the formation of the reactive aziridinium ion. The L-isomer of the amino acid phenylalanine (L-Phe) was purposefully incorporated into this antineoplastic agent because naturally occurring L–amino acids are preferentially transported into cells by the action of specific amino acid carrier proteins. It was assumed that the L-Phe would act as a homing device and actively transport the toxic mustard inside the tumor cells, but some studies indicate that melphalan enters cells through facilitated diffusion rather than by active transport (17).

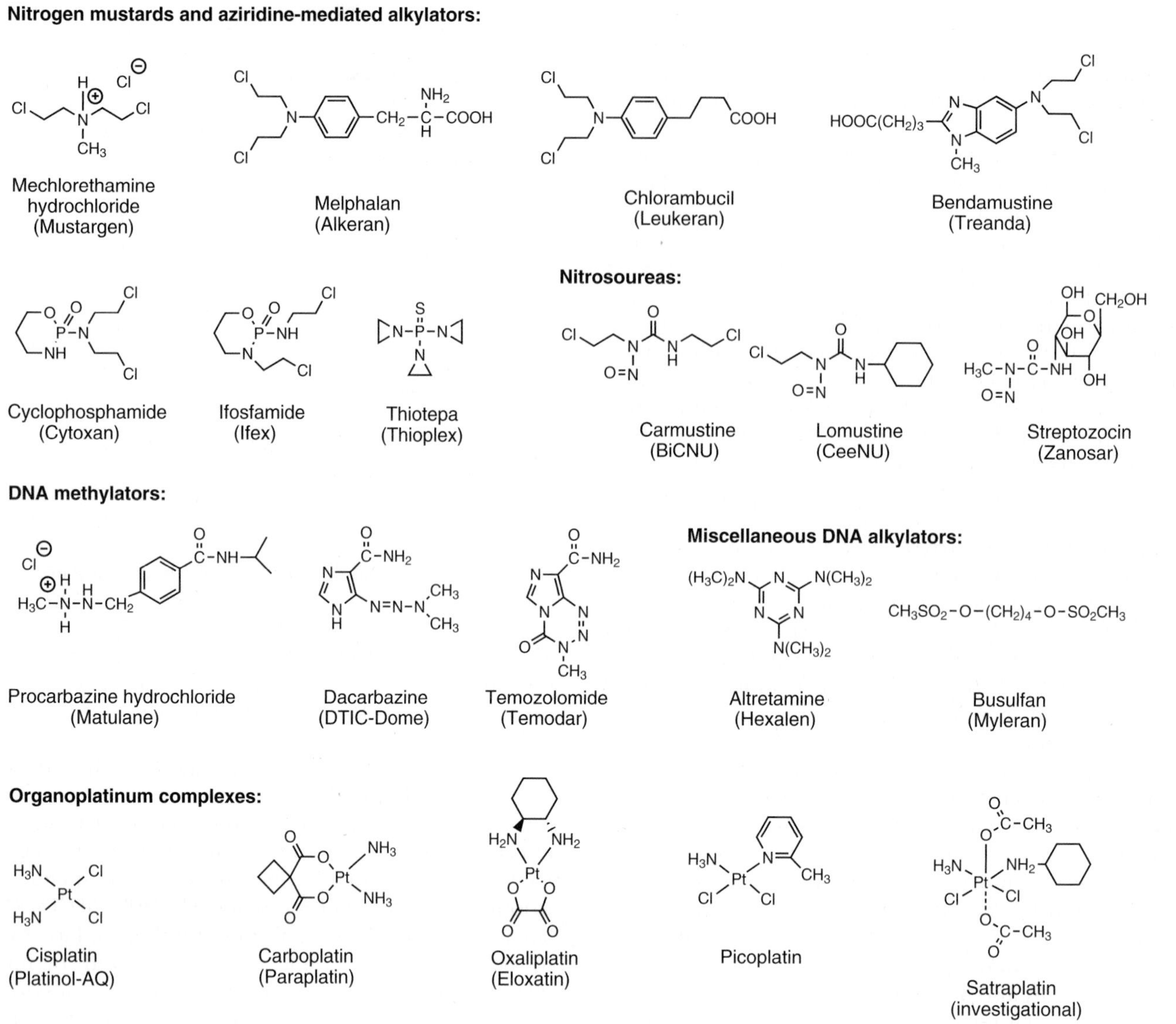

FIGURE 37.3 DNA cross-linking agents.

Because the lone pair of electrons of melphalan (and other aromatic mustards) is less reactive than the lone electron pair on aliphatic mustards, there is a greater opportunity for distribution to cancer cells and a decreased incidence of severe side effects. There is a lower incidence of nausea and vomiting compared to mechlorethamine, but patients still experience myelosuppression, which can be severe. This drug is also mutagenic and can induce leukemia.

Melphalan is orally active, but absorption can be erratic. Absorption is decreased with food, but dosing regimens do not demand an empty stomach. The hydrochloride salt is available for intravenous administration, but the risk of serious side effects is higher. Melphalan distributes into body water, so toxicity can be pronounced in dehydrated patients or in those with renal dysfunction. Dehydration can be corrected, but dosage adjustments should be considered in patients with renal disease.

Chlorambucil Like melphalan, chlorambucil has good oral bioavailability (which is decreased in the presence of food) and the potential to induce nonlymphocytic leukemia. This drug is active intact and also undergoes β-oxidation to provide an active phenylacetic acid mustard metabolite, which is responsible for some of the observed antineoplastic activity. It is used in the palliative treatment of chronic lymphocytic leukemia, malignant lymphoma, and Hodgkin disease.

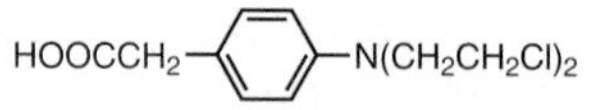

Phenylacetic acid mustard (an active chlorambucil metabolite)

Bendamustine Hydrochloride Bendamustine is an excellent chemical example of the adage "everything old is new again." First synthesized in 1963, serious interest in it as a

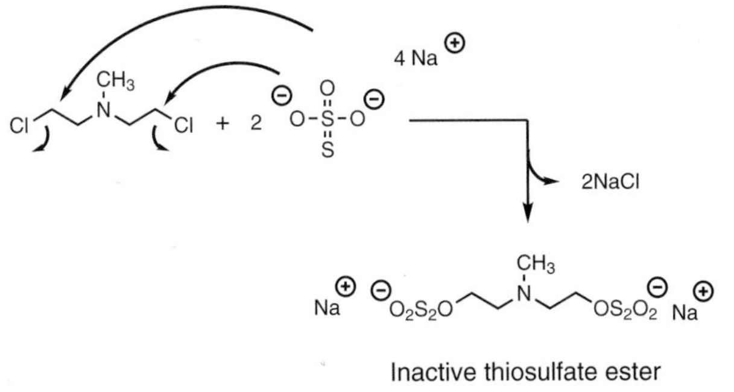

FIGURE 37.4 Mechlorethamine inactivation by sodium thiosulfate.

viable therapeutic agent surfaced only recently after several well-designed and appropriately executed clinical trials documented its value in the treatment of hematologic cancers, specifically chronic lymphocytic leukemia (CLL) and non-Hodgkin's lymphoma (NHL). Bendamustine is the *N*-methylbenzimidazole analog of chlorambucil, and the substitution of this purine-like aromatic ring was purposefully done to promote an antimetabolite mechanism along with DNA alkylation. DNA damage is more extensive and less repairable than that induced by other alkylating agents, and the drug is unique in its ability to stimulate *p21* and *p53*-induced apoptosis, S-phase cell cycle arrest, and "mitotic catastrophe" (18). The risk of acquired resistance and cross-resistance appears lower than with other DNA alkylators (19).

Unlike chlorambucil, bendamustine is given only intravenously on days 1 and 2 of a 21-day (NHL) or 28-day (CLL) cycle. It can be given alone or, in the case of slow-growing, refractory, and/or relapsed (indolent) lymphomas, in combination with other antineoplastic agents (e.g., the anticancer monoclonal antibody rituximab and/or the topoisomerase poison mitoxantrone). It undergoes minor CYP1A2-catalyzed *N*-demethylation and γ-hydroxylation. While active, these metabolites are clinically insignificant. There is currently no evidence of serious metabolism-based interactions or toxicities associated with bendamustine; however myelosuppression, hypersensitivity/anaphylaxis, and skin reactions have been noted with its use. Pretreatment with antihistamines and corticosteroids can help to minimize infusion reactions, a major cause of drug discontinuation.

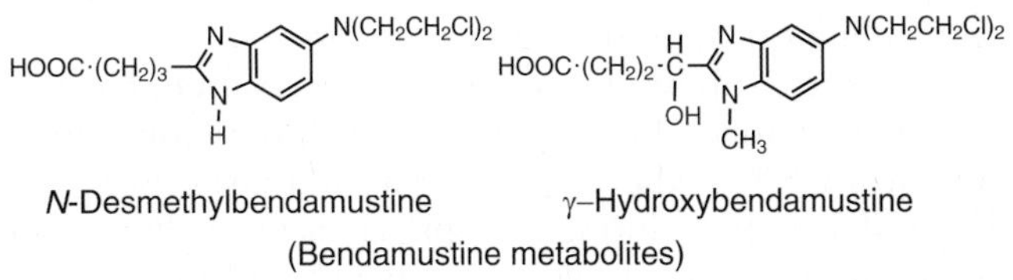

Cyclophosphamide Cyclophosphamide is a chiral prodrug antineoplastic agent requiring activation by metabolic and nonmetabolic processes (20) (Fig. 37.5). The initial metabolic step is mediated primarily by CYP2B6 (and, to a lesser extent, by CYP3A4 and CYP2C isoforms) and involves regioselective hydroxylation at C_4 of the oxazaphosphorine ring to generate a carbinolamine (20,21). This hydroxylation reaction must occur before the molecule will be transported into cells, and approximately 90% of an administered dose will be appropriately converted (20). CYP3A4 and CYP2B6 stereospecifically catalyze an inactivating *N*-dechloroethylation reaction on the *R* and *S* isomers, respectively, which yields highly nephrotoxic and neurotoxic chloroacetaldehyde (20,21). Chloroacetaldehyde toxicity is accompanied by glutathione depletion, indicating that, as expected, this

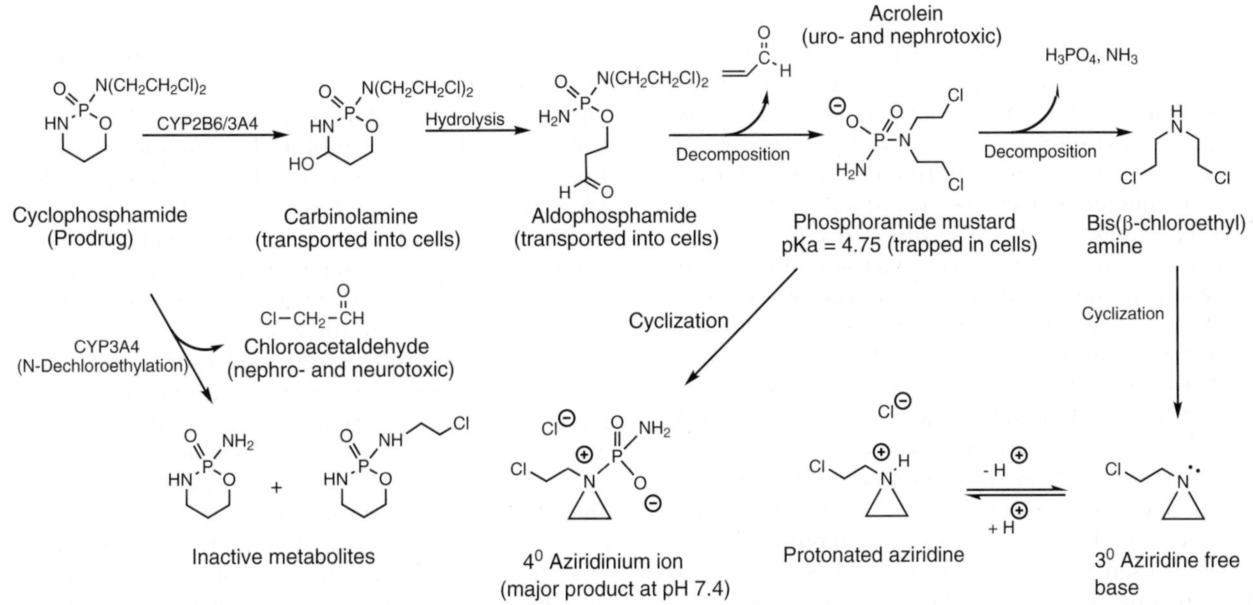

FIGURE 37.5 Cyclophosphamide metabolism.

electrophilic by-product alkylates cysteine (Cys) residues of critical cell proteins (22). Alkylation of lysine, adenosine, and cytidine residues is also possible.

The CYP-generated carbinolamine undergoes nonenzymatic hydrolysis to provide the aldophosphamide either in the bloodstream or inside cells. If this hydrolysis occurs extracellularly, the aldophosphamide is still able to penetrate cell membranes to reach the intracellular space. Once inside the cell, acrolein (a highly reactive α,β-unsaturated aldehyde) is cleaved via spontaneous β-elimination, generating phosphoramide mustard. With a pK_a of 4.75, the mustard will be persistently anionic at intracellular pH and trapped inside the cell.

The fate of phosphoramide mustard is varied. Most of it cyclizes to form the quaternary aziridinium ion, which alkylates DNA in the manner of all mustards. Some of it will decompose, losing phosphoric acid (H_3PO_4) and ammonia (NH_3) and leaving the naked bis(β-chloroethyl) amine mustard. This secondary amine cyclizes in a manner similar to the tertiary phosphoramide mustard, forming a tertiary aziridine (rather than a quaternary aziridinium) species. The free tertiary aziridine can protonate at intracellular pH to provide the cationic aziridine species, which is in equilibrium with the free base form. Some electrophilic character is lost, but the carbon atoms in both forms are still δ^+ enough to attract DNA nucleophiles, albeit less vigorously. The net result is DNA alkylation and cell death. Oxidation of oxazaphosphorine intermediates along the metabolic pathway by cytosolic alcohol or aldehyde dehydrogenase is inactivating (20).

The need for metabolic activation in the liver means lowered GI toxicity and less nonspecific toxicity for cyclophosphamide compared with other DNA alkylating agents, but cyclophosphamide is not without its toxic effects. Acrolein, generated during the formation of phosphoramide mustard, is a very electrophilic and highly reactive species, and it causes extensive damage to cells of the kidney and bladder. While acrolein can be produced in kidney via CYP3A4-mediated metabolism, it is predominantly generated in liver, where it readily conjugates with reduced glutathione (GSH) as expected (23, 24). However, when the acrolein-GSH or mercapturic acid conjugate is delivered to the bladder for excretion, the conjugate can cause direct toxicity or cleave to release electrophilic, reactive acrolein to the cells (23). Without additional GSH to re-scavenge liberated toxin, the acrolein will be attacked at its δ^+ terminal carbon by the nucleophilic SH of bladder cell Cys residues (Fig. 37.6). More complex biochemical events involving increased levels of preoxynitrite and subsequent lipid peroxidation also contribute to the observed urotoxicity (20). Physiologic results can include severe hemorrhage, sclerosis, and, on occasion (e.g., 5%), induction of bladder cancer. Acrolein also damages the nephron, particularly when used in high doses, in children, in patients with only one kidney, or when coadministered with other nephrotoxic agents (e.g., cisplatin). To minimize

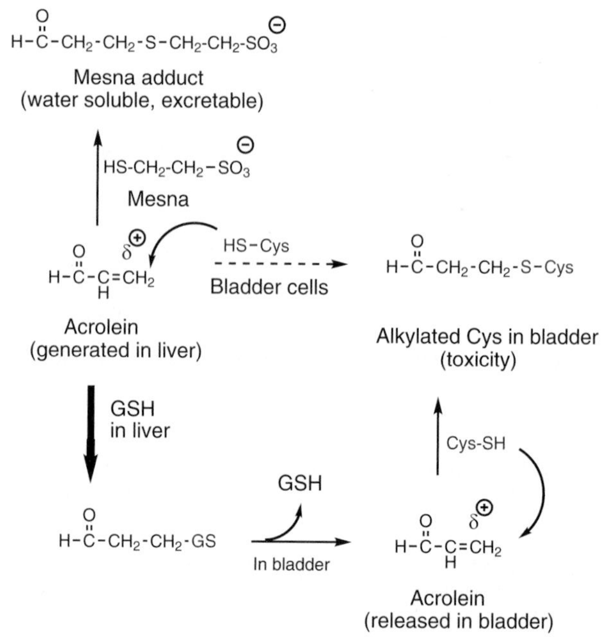

FIGURE 37.6 Sulfhydryl alkylation by acrolein.

the risk of bladder toxicity from acrolein, fluids should be forced and the bladder irrigated. Mesna (Mesnex) is available as adjuvant therapy in case of overt toxicity or as a prophylactic protectant. A sulfhydryl reagent, mesna is transported in the bloodstream as the inactive oxidized disulfide (dimesna) and selectively reduced to the reactive sulfhydryl in the proximal tubules (20). Once excreted into the bladder, the reactive SH group competes with Cys residues for the alkylating acrolein, as shown in Figure 37.6. Mesna concentrates in the bladder and will prevent damage to those cells. It does not concentrate to any appreciable extent in the nephron and, therefore, is not good protection against cyclophosphamide-induced nephrotoxicity.

As effective as mesna is for preventing acrolein-induced urotoxicity, it does little to spare the kidney and nerve cells from chloroacetaldehyde, the other toxic by-product of cyclophosphamide metabolism (25). Luckily, only approximately 10% of a standard dose of cyclophosphamide undergoes the dechloroethylation reaction, and most of the chloroacetaldehyde generated can be scavenged by GSH. However, since the competing hydroxylation reaction is saturable, this percentage can rise if higher doses are used (21).

Cyclophosphamide is most commonly used in combination with other antineoplastic agents to treat a wide range of neoplasms, including leukemias and malignant lymphomas, multiple myeloma, ovarian adenocarcinoma, and breast cancer. The drug is metabolized in the liver and eliminated via the kidney, with approximately 15% of a given dose being excreted unchanged. Doses should be reduced in patients with creatinine clearance levels less than 30 mL/min. Interestingly, hepatic dysfunction does not seem to alter the metabolism of this drug, but caution should be exercised in patients with inhibited CYP450 enzymes or with a combination of factors that could negatively impact drug activation/inactivation pathways. Significant stereochemistry-based variation in the metabolic, enzyme inhibition, excretion, and toxicity profiles of cyclophosphamide and related oxazaphosphorine antineoplastic agents have been described in the literature (20).

Ifosfamide This cyclophosphamide analog has the two arms of the mustard on different nitrogen atoms. Ifosfamide also requires metabolic activation (Fig. 37.7), but this time, it is the CYP3A4 isoform that converts the majority of the dose to the carbinolamine, with CYP2B6 taking on a minor supporting role (26). Because ifosfamide has a lower affinity for the hydroxylating CYP3A4 and CYP2B6 enzymes, presumably as a result of steric hindrance, bioactivation proceeds at a slower rate (27). Doses three- to fourfold higher than cyclophosphamide are required to achieve the same antineoplastic result.

Unlike cyclophosphamide, dechloroethylation is a significant metabolic pathway for ifosfamide, and up to 60% of a standard dose will undergo this toxicity-inducing biotransformation (20,28). CYP3A4/3A5 catalyzes approximately 70% of ifosfamide dechloroethylation, with CYP2B6 taking care of the remainder (21). So much chloroacetaldehyde is generated that the endogenous GSH

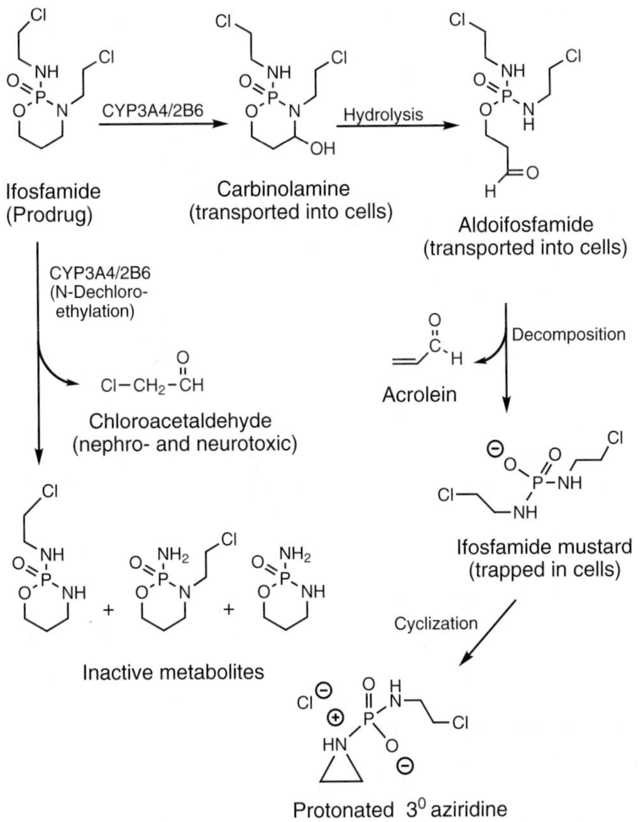

FIGURE 37.7 Ifosfamide metabolism.

decoy (available in limited quantities) just cannot keep up. The fact that this reaction can occur in the renal tubule, generating chloroacetaldehyde right in the nephron, contributes to a significantly higher nephrotoxicity that can result in glomerular and renal tubular failure (27). Neurotoxicity is most commonly central in origin (e.g., mental status dysfunction, seizures). Ultimately, both chloroalkyl groups are lost before the compound is excreted.

It bears repeating that there is a significantly higher risk of bladder toxicity and nephrotoxicity with ifosfamide than with cyclophosphamide. The higher risks of these toxicities result because significantly more chloroacetaldehyde is generated through CYP3A4- and CYP2B6-mediated dechloroethylation. Although this toxic by-product has been claimed to have some antitumor activity (20), the biotransformation can take place in the nephron, which generates chloroacetaldehyde right where it will do the most unwanted cellular damage. Ifosfamide is also more water soluble than cyclophosphamide and will concentrate in the renal system. In addition, higher doses must be administered to achieve the same degree of antineoplastic action, so more molecules of acrolein and chloroacetaldehyde will be produced.

Because acrolein is generated during the bioactivation of ifosfamide, the same precautions against hemorrhagic cystitis that were previously outlined for cyclophosphamide must be taken: hydrate well, irrigate thoroughly, and administer with mesna. As previously stated, mesna will not prevent chloroacetaldehyde-induced toxicity. GSH-based rescue agents such as *N*-acetylcysteine may have some benefit in attenuating ifosfamide-induced nephrotoxicity, but because they do not penetrate the blood–brain barrier, they would be of little value in neurotoxicity prophylaxis (20).

Ifosfamide is currently used as third-line therapy in testicular cancer, although it has also shown activity in a number of other solid tumors and hematologic cancers. Patients on ifosfamide (but not cyclophosphamide) commonly exhibit cerebral neuropathy attributed to the significantly higher levels of chloroacetaldehyde generated by this drug (20). In severe forms, CNS depression can progress to coma and death.

A new chiral oxazaphosphorine, trofosfamide, is currently undergoing clinical trials for the palliative care of solid tumor and NHL patients. Trofosfamide is rapidly dechloroethylated at the mustard and oxazaphosphorine nitrogen atoms to form ifosfamide (predominant) and cyclophosphamide, respectively (20).

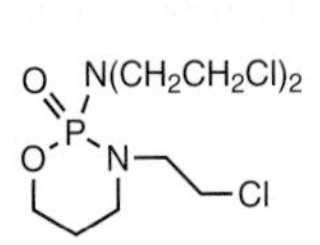

Trofosfamide

Thiotepa Thiotepa, a tertiary aziridine, is less reactive than quaternary aziridinium compounds and is classified as a weak alkylator. It is possible for the nitrogen atoms to protonate before reacting with DNA. However, the electron-withdrawing effect of the sulfur atom decreases the pK_a to approximately 6, which keeps the percentage ionized at pH 7.4 relatively low. Thiotepa undergoes oxidative desulfuration, forming an active cytotoxic metabolite known as TEPA (triethylenephosphoramide). Both thiotepa and TEPA have been proposed to alkylate DNA through the hydrolytic release of aziridine, a more easily protonated structure, which is, therefore, a more attractive target for DNA nucleophiles. In this mechanistic model, the parent drug and the TEPA metabolite serve as carriers to transport aziridine-releasing drug across tumor cell membranes. (Fig. 37.8). Thiotepa, but not TEPA, is capable of direct, regioselective DNA alkylation due to its slower rate of intracellular hydrolysis (29).

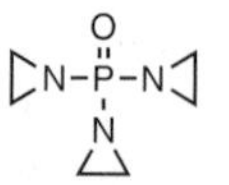

Triethylenephosphoramide
(an active thiotepa metabolite)

Thiotepa is most commonly employed in the treatment of ovarian and breast cancers, as well as papillary carcinoma of the bladder. Thiotepa and its TEPA metabolite readily enter the central nervous system (CNS) after systemic administration, leading to dizziness, blurred vision, and headaches. More critically, these agents are also severe myelosuppressants and can induce leukopenia, thrombocytopenia, and anemia. Patients treated with thiotepa are at high risk for infection and hemorrhage. Oral absorption is unreliable, so thiotepa is either given intravenously, or instilled intravesically in the treatment of bladder cancer. Even when administered locally in bladder cancer, high levels of this lipophilic drug reach the systemic circulation, resulting in bone marrow depression. Patients have died from myelosuppression after intravesically administered thiotepa. The drug also causes damage to the hepatic and renal systems. Dose and/or administration frequency should be increased slowly, even if the initial response to the drug is sluggish, or unacceptable toxicity may result.

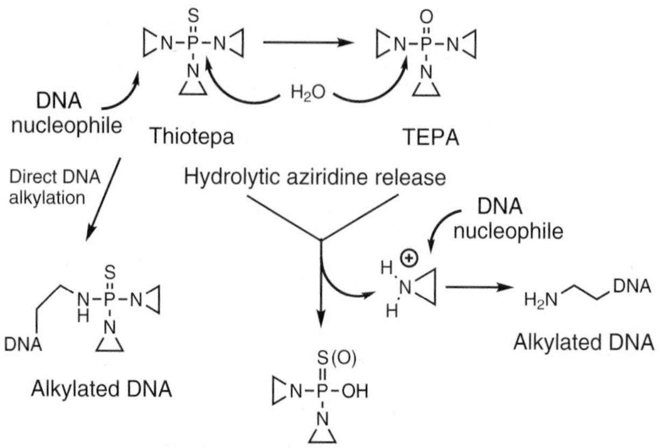

FIGURE 37.8 Mechanism of thiotepa DNA alkylation.

Nitrosoureas

MECHANISM OF ACTION The nitrosoureas are unstable structures that decompose readily in the aqueous environment of the cell. Nonenzymatic fragmentation is stimulated by the loss of proton from the urea moiety. Cyclization of the resultant anion to an unstable oxazolidine (pathway A) is followed by decomposition to vinyl diazotic acid and a substituted isocyanate, both of which release a gaseous fragment (nitrogen and carbon dioxide, respectively) to generate cytotoxic electrophiles (Fig. 37.9). Vinyl carbocation, acetaldehyde, and 2-chloroethylamine generated from the 2-chloroethylisocyanate moiety of carmustine are all capable of alkylating DNA in the standard manner (30). A second decomposition mechanism (pathway B)

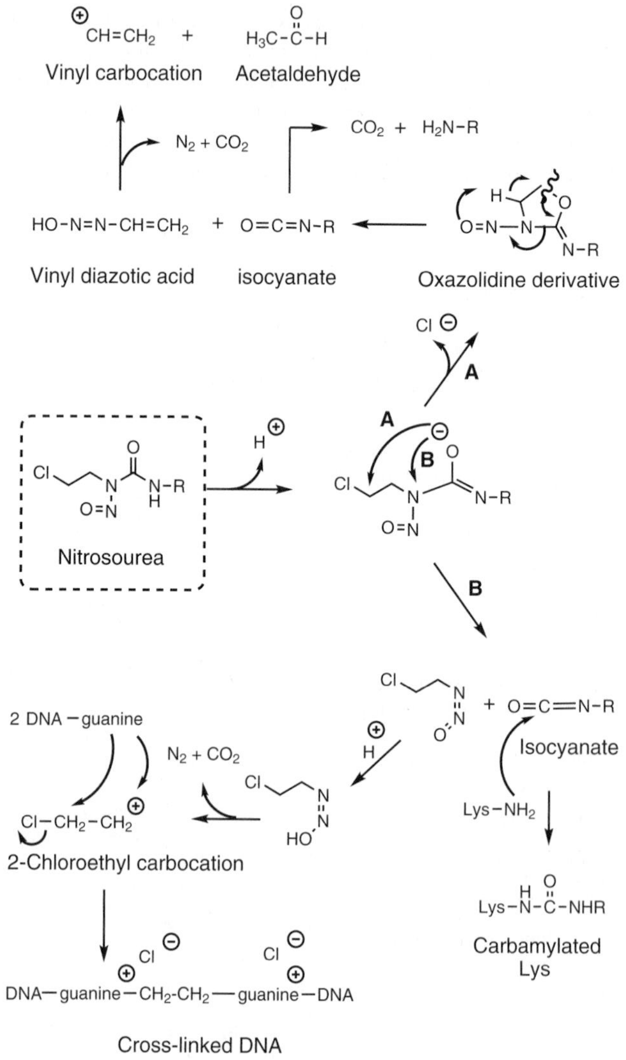

FIGURE 37.9 Nitrosourea decomposition to cytotoxic electrophiles.

ultimately produces an electrophilic 2-chloroethylcarbocation capable of DNA alkylation at guanine-N^7 and O^6, as well as an isocyanate that can carbamylate amino acid residues (e.g., lysine [Lys]).

Specific Drugs (Fig. 37.3)

Carmustine and Lomustine Carmustine and lomustine are both highly lipophilic chloroethylnitrosourea analogs marketed for use in brain tumors and Hodgkin's disease. Carmustine has also shown value in the treatment of NHL and multiple myeloma, and it is given intravenously or incorporated into biodegradable wafers that are implanted directly into the CNS after tumor resection. The high lipophilicity of carmustine precludes a totally aqueous intravenous formulation, and the drug is administered in 10% ethanol. Although carmustine degrades within 15 minutes of intravenous administration, lomustine is stable enough for oral use and is marketed in capsule form. Carmustine can also decompose in vitro if exposed to temperatures around 90°F. Pure carmustine is a low-melting solid, but the decomposed product is an oil and, therefore, readily detected. Vials of carmustine that appear oily should be discarded.

Both carmustine and lomustine can induce thrombocytopenia and leukopenia, leading to hemorrhage and massive infection. Acute (as well as potentially fatal delayed) pulmonary toxicity is also a risk. Pulmonary toxicity is dose-related, and individuals who received the drug in childhood or early adolescence are at higher risk for the delayed reaction. The grand mal seizures that are possible from the wafer formulation of carmustine appear to result from the wafer rather than from the nitrosourea. Resistance to carmustine involves upregulation of O^6-methylguanine-DNA methyltransferase with the subsequent repair of drug-induced DNA damage, and possibly sequestration by neuroprotective metallothionein proteins (31).

Streptozocin The glucopyranose moiety of streptozocin confers both islet cell specificity and high water solubility to this nitrosourea-based antineoplastic. As a result, it is used exclusively in metastatic islet cell carcinoma of the pancreas and is administered intravenously in D5W or normal saline. Lacking the 2-chloroethyl substituent of carmustine and lomustine, it is much less reactive as a DNA alkylating agent. Myelotoxicity, while not unknown, is relatively rare. However, cumulative, dose-related renal toxicity may be severe or fatal, and 67% of patients receiving this drug will exhibit some kidney-related pathology. Good hydration is essential to successful therapy, and kidney function should be monitored weekly.

Procarbazine and Triazines

Mechanism of Action Procarbazine and the triazenes dacarbazine and temozolomide act by different mechanisms, but they all exert an antineoplastic effect through the O^6-methylation of guanine nucleotides. O^6-Methylguanine pairs preferentially with thymine, and these "mispairs" prompt point mutations during subsequent DNA replication cycles and trigger cell destruction through the activation of the normal postreplication mismatch repair system. Patients who are able to repair this damage through the action of O^6-alkylguanine-DNA-alkyltransferase, which transfers the offending CH_3 group to a Cys residue on the alkyltransferase protein, will exhibit resistance to these agents, whereas those who underexpress this protein should respond well (32). Since the alkyltransferase is irreversibly inactivated in the DNA rescue process, enzyme depletion with subsequent loss of DNA repair capability is a significant risk.

Procarbazine metabolism involves CYP1A and CYP2B enzymes (33), and DNA alkylation operates through a free radical mechanism (Fig. 37.10). The major degradation pathway involves benzylic oxidation of azoprocarbazine, producing methylhydrazine that generates a methyl radical through an unstable diazene intermediate (34,35). In addition to O^6, the reactive methyl radical formed can

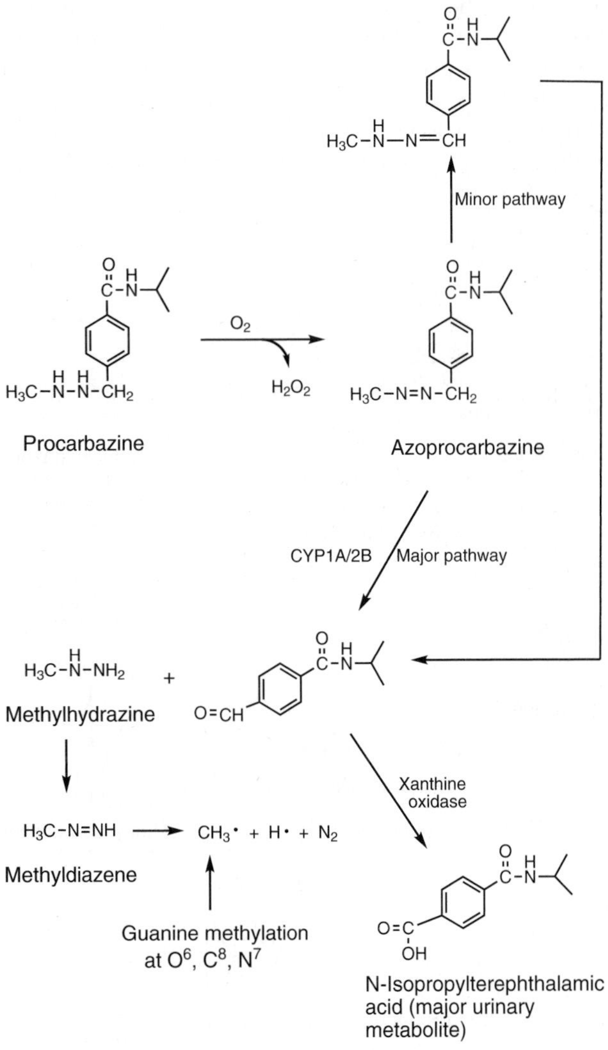

FIGURE 37.10 Procarbazine metabolism and mechanism of action.

alkylate the C^8 and N^7 positions of guanine. In contrast, the triazenes methylate DNA guanine via diazomethane and/or methyl carbocation generated in situ. Although temozolomide is converted to the diazomethane precursor 3-methyl-(triazen-l-yl)imidazole-4-carboxamide (MTIC) through nonenzymatic mechanisms, the conversion of dacarbazine to MTIC depends on the action of CYP1A1 and CYP1A2 enzymes, with a smaller contribution by CYP2E1 (Fig. 37.11) (33, 36). The O^6 and N^7 positions of guanine are the most vulnerable to triazene methylation.

Specific Drugs (Fig. 37.3)

Procarbazine Hydrochloride This methyl radical generator is used predominantly in the treatment of Hodgkin's disease. It is administered as part of a multidrug regimen that also includes a nitrogen mustard (mechlorethamine), a mitosis inhibitor (vincristine), and prednisone. It is administered as capsules and is well absorbed after oral administration. Procarbazine is extensively metabolized in the liver, and 70% of an administered dose is excreted in the urine as *N*-isopropylterephthalamic acid (Fig. 37.10). In addition to methylating DNA guanine residues, it is proposed to inhibit the de novo synthesis of proteins and nucleic acids. Procarbazine inhibits monoamine oxidase, leading to several significant and potentially fatal drug–drug and drug–food interactions. Facial flushing and other disulfiram-like symptoms are noted when alcohol is concomitantly consumed because the drug also inhibits enzymes involved in ethanol metabolism.

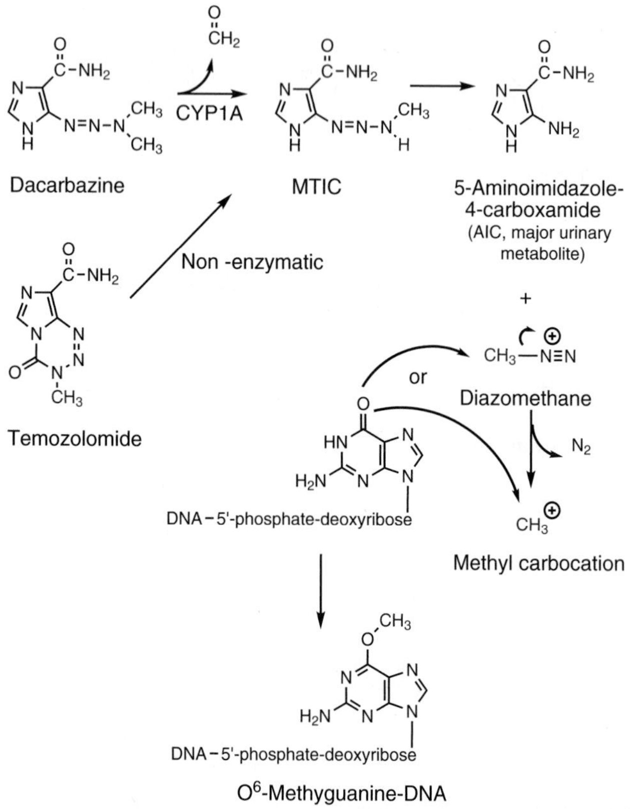

FIGURE 37.11 Metabolic activation of triazenes.

Dacarbazine This DNA methylating agent is administered intravenously as a single agent in the treatment of malignant melanoma and in combination with other agents in the treatment of metastatic melanoma. Approximately 40% of the drug is excreted unchanged, but both the 5-aminoimidazole-4-carboxamide (AIC, formed through the action of CYP1A enzymes) and the carboxylic acid (AIC hydrolysis product) are major urinary metabolites (Fig. 37.11). Leukopenia and thrombocytopenia are the most common side effects and can be fatal. Patients are also at risk for hepatotoxicity, including hepatocellular necrosis.

Temozolomide This imidazolotetrazine derivative is administered orally in capsule form for the treatment of glioblastoma multiforme or in patients with anaplastic astrocytoma who have not responded to procarbazine or the nitrosoureas. Oral absorption is rapid and complete. While CYP450 enzymes are not extensively involved in temozolomide metabolism, less than 6% of the drug is excreted unchanged in the urine. Women clear the drug less effectively than men and have a higher incidence of severe neutropenia and thrombocytopenia in the initial therapy cycle. Food decreases temozolomide absorption, and myelosuppression is the most significant adverse effect. Resistance involves drug-induced damage reversal by O^6-methylguanine-DNA methyltransferase, and some authors are advocating the design of inhibitors of this potential target for use in combination with temozolomide and other guanine O^6-methylating antineoplastics (37).

Miscellaneous DNA Alkylating Agents (Fig. 37.3)

Altretamine This unique hexamethylmelamine structure is believed to damage tumor cells through the production of the weakly alkylating species formaldehyde, a product of CYP450-mediated *N*-demethylation. Administered orally, altretamine is extensively metabolized on first pass, producing primarily mono- and didemethylated metabolites. Additional demethylation reactions occur in tumor cells, releasing formaldehyde in situ before the drug is excreted in the urine. The carbinolamine (methylol) intermediates of CYP450-mediated metabolism can also generate electrophilic iminium species that are capable of reacting covalently with DNA guanine and cytosine residues, as well as protein (Fig. 37.12). Iminium-mediated DNA cross-linking and DNA-protein interstrand cross-linking, mediated through both the iminium intermediate and formaldehyde, have been demonstrated (38,39), although the significance of DNA cross-linking on altretamine antitumor activity is uncertain. Resistance to altretamine has been shown to parallel resistance to formaldehyde-induced cytotoxicity (38). Its use currently is restricted to patients with ovarian cancer who have not responded to organoplatinum therapy. The toxicities

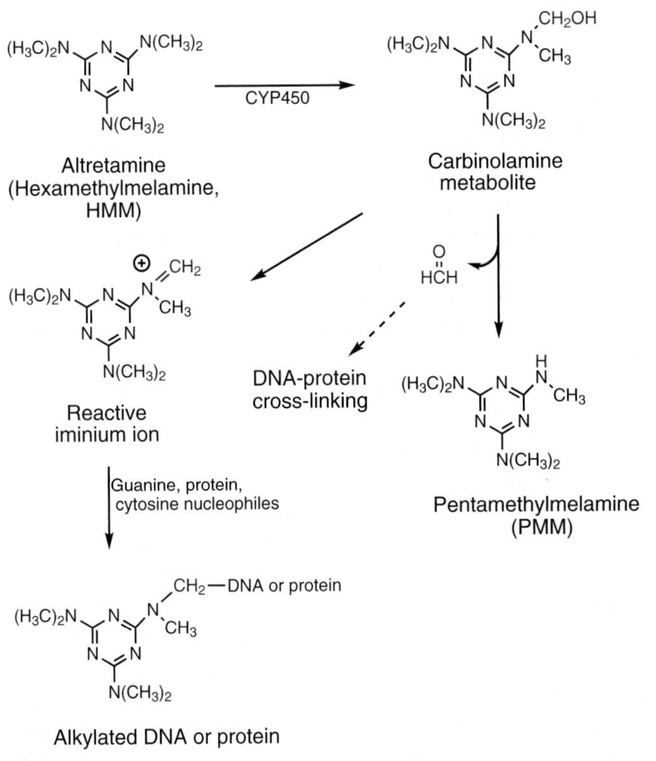

FIGURE 37.12 Altretamine metabolism and mechanism of action.

induced by altretamine are GI, neurologic, and hematologic in nature. An orally active liposomal formulation containing sodium deoxycholate has been investigated but is not currently commercially available (40).

BUSULFAN Chemically, busulfan is classified as an alkyl sulfonate. One or both of the methylsulfonate ester moieties can be displaced by the nucleophilic N^7 of guanine, leading to monoalkylated and cross-linked DNA as shown in Figure 37.13. The extent of alkyl sulfonate–mediated DNA interstrand cross-linking has been shown to vary with the length of the alkyl chain between sulfonate esters, with the tetramethylene-containing busulfan showing less interstrand cross-linking capability than hexamethylene, methylene, or octamethylene analogs (41). Intrastrand cross-linking also occurs, preferentially at 5′-GA-3′ but also at 5′-GG-3′ sequences (42). Alkylation of Cys sulfhydryl groups is yet another mechanism of cytotoxicity. Busulfan is used in the treatment of CML and can be administered either orally or by intravenous infusion. Serious bone marrow hypoplasia and myelosuppression are possible with this agent, and recovery from busulfan-induced pancytopenia can take up to 2 years.

Organoplatinum Complexes

MECHANISM OF ACTION Organoplatinum antineoplastic agents contain an electron-deficient metal atom that acts as a magnet for electron-rich DNA nucleophiles. Like nitrogen mustards, organoplatinum complexes are bifunctional and can accept electrons from two DNA nucleophiles. Intrastrand cross-links most frequently occur between adjacent guanine residues referred to as diguanosine dinucleotides (60% to 65%) or adjacent guanine and adenine residues (25% to 30%) (43). Interstrand cross-linking, which occurs much less frequently (1% to 3%), usually involves guanine and adenine bases (44).

CHEMISTRY All the currently marketed organoplatinum anticancer agents are Pt(II) complexes with square planar geometry, although an octahedral Pt(IV) complex currently is undergoing clinical trials. Platinum is inherently electron deficient, but the net charge on the organometallic complex is zero due to the contribution of electrons by two of the four ligands bound to the parent structure. Most commonly, the electron-donating ligand is chloride. Before reacting with DNA, the electron-donating ligands are displaced through nucleophilic attack by cellular

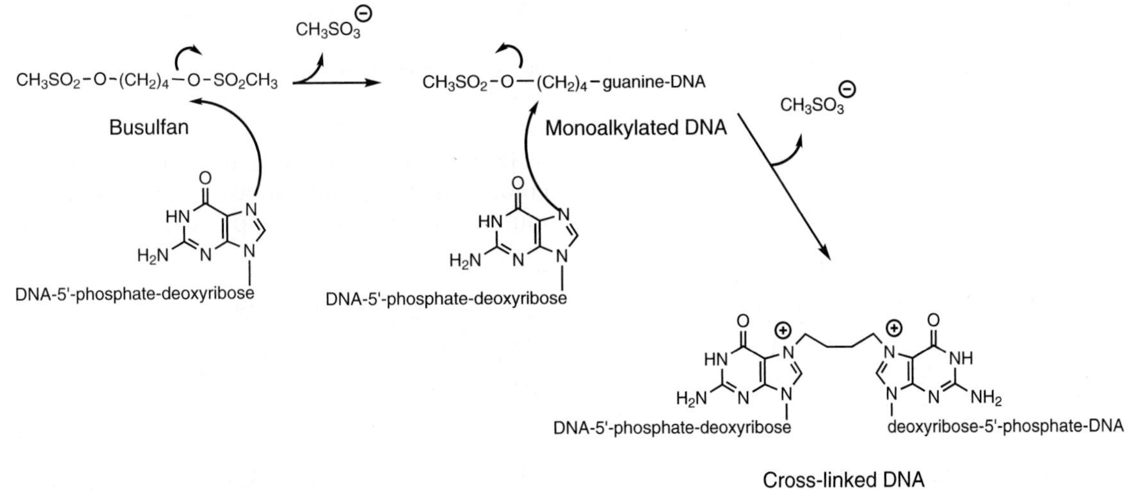

FIGURE 37.13 Busulfan-mediated DNA alkylation.

water. When the displaced ligands are chloride anions (e.g., cisplatin), the chloride-poor environment of the tumor cell facilitates the process, driving the generation of the active, cytotoxic hydrated forms (Fig. 37.14). Since the original ligands leave the metal with their electrons, the hydrated organoplatinum molecule has a net positive charge (45).

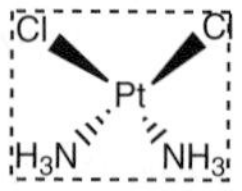

Cisplatin (square planar geometry)

The hydrated platinum analogs are readily attacked by DNA nucleophiles (e.g., the N^7 of adjacent guanine residues) due to the net positive charge that has been regained on the Pt atom (Fig. 37.14). The DNA bases become coordinated with the platinum, and in the cis configuration, DNA repair mechanisms are unable to permanently correct the damage. The net result is a major change in DNA conformation such that base pairs that normally engage in hydrogen bond formation are not permitted to interact. The two ammine ligands of the complex are bound irreversibly to the Pt atom through very strong coordinate covalent bonds. They cannot be displaced by DNA nucleophiles, but they do stabilize the cross-linked DNA–platinum complex by forming strong ion-dipole bonds with the anionic phosphate residues on DNA. The DNA distortion prompts a futile cycle of damage recognition and repair before giving up the ghost and succumbing to cell cycle arrest and apoptosis.

Specific Drugs (Fig. 37.3)

Cisplatin The simplest of the organometallic antineoplastic agents, cisplatin is used intravenously in the treatment of metastatic testicular and ovarian cancer and advanced bladder cancer. It is rapidly hydrated, resulting in a short plasma half-life of less than 30 minutes. It is eliminated predominantly via the kidney, but approximately 10% of a given dose undergoes biliary excretion. It is highly nephrotoxic and can cause significant damage to the renal tubules, especially in patients with preexisting kidney disease, with one kidney, or who are concurrently receiving other nephrotoxic drugs (e.g., cyclophosphamide or ifosfamide). Dosages should be reduced in any of these situations. Clearance decreases with chronic therapy, and toxicities can manifest at a later date.

To proactively protect against kidney damage, patients should be aggressively hydrated with chloride-containing solutions. Saline or mannitol diuretics can be administered to promote continuous excretion of the drug and its hydrated analogs. Sodium thiosulfate, which accumulates in the renal tubules, has also been used to neutralize active drug in the kidneys in an effort to avoid nephrotoxicity (Fig. 37.15). The reaction of sodium thiosulfate with cisplatin in the serum is much less significant because the drug does not concentrate there, and what is there is very strongly bound to serum proteins. The very strong protein binding explains why dialysis, even when prolonged, cannot rescue patients from cisplatin toxicity.

Cisplatin is a very severe emetogen, and vomiting almost always occurs unless antiemetic therapy is coadministered. Myelosuppression and ototoxicity that can lead to irreversible hearing loss can also occur with cisplatin use. A recent study has shown that, in medulloblastoma patients 3 to 21 years of age, bolus administration of the thiol-generating prodrug amifostine, both immediately before and again during cisplatin infusion, significantly decreased ototoxicity and the need for a hearing aid after therapy (46). Alkaline phosphatase, amifostine's activating enzyme, shows a higher activity in normal tissue compared to tumor tissue. This allows for higher levels of drug destruction in nontarget healthy cells and provides protection against unwanted toxicity without compromising cisplatin's antineoplastic action.

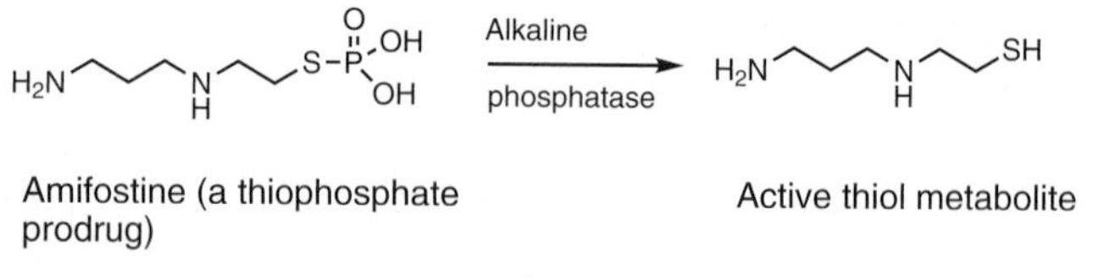

Resistance to cisplatin therapy can be intrinsic in colorectal, lung, and breast cancer, or acquired after multiple courses of therapy (e.g., in ovarian cancer).

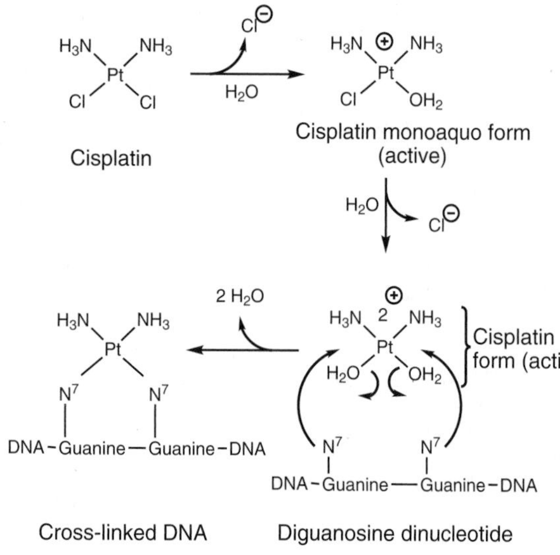

FIGURE 37.14 Cisplatin activation and DNA cross-linking.

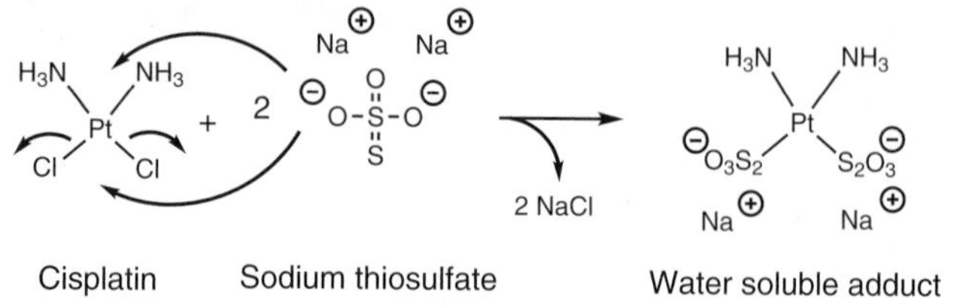

FIGURE 37.15 Cisplatin inactivation by sodium thiosulfate.

Resistance is mediated through several distinct mechanisms, including: 1) compromised carrier-mediated cellular transport via the copper transporting protein CTR1; 2) enhanced intracellular inactivation through drug trapping in vesicles; 3) drug inactivation through conjugation to Cys and/or methionine (Met)-containing GSH and metallothionein proteins; and 4) increased DNA repair and/or tolerance to cisplatin-induced DNA damage (47). Regarding the latter mechanism, cisplatin damage can be successfully repaired by nucleotide-excision repair proteins (NERs), which remove platinum-damaged segments from the DNA, and these proteins are often upregulated in cisplatin-resistant tumors. Cisplatin (and carboplatin)–DNA adducts are also recognized by mismatch repair proteins (MMRs). The downregulation of MMRs in cisplatin (and carboplatin)–treated cancer cells induces resistance through the loss of an apoptotic response that normally follows several ill-fated attempts to repair organoplatinum-induced damage. Testicular tumors are particularly responsive to cisplatin due to their inherent deficiency in DNA repair processes. Cellular efflux mediated by P-gp (a product of the *ABCB1* gene), a resistance mechanism common to natural product anticancer agents, is not believed to be a component of resistance to organometallics (47).

Cisplatin and the other organoplatinum anticancer agents react with aluminum and cannot be administered through aluminum-containing needles. The drug is photosensitive, is packaged in amber bottles, and must be protected from light.

Carboplatin Carboplatin, another square planar Pt(II) complex, forms the same cytotoxic hydrated intermediate as cisplatin but does so at a 10-fold slower rate, making it a 20- to 40-fold less potent chemotherapeutic agent (47). The ultimate damage done to cells as a result of carboplatin use approaches that of cisplatin, but the side effect profile is significantly milder. Suppression of platelets and white blood cells is the most significant toxic reaction, and nonhematologic toxicities (e.g., emesis, nephrotoxicity, and ototoxicity) are rare. The plasma half-life of carboplatin is 3 hours, and the drug is less extensively bound to serum proteins than cisplatin. Excretion is still predominantly renal, however, and doses must be reduced in patients with kidney disease.

Carboplatin is only approved for use in the treatment of advanced ovarian cancer, although clinical trials have shown that it may have a future in the treatment of hormone-refractory prostate cancer. Carboplatin can be used in combination with docetaxel (often considered the standard of care for prostate cancer) and estramustine (a less commonly used mitosis inhibitor). This drug has provided therapeutic benefit as a single agent in patients whose cancer has progressed after docetaxel therapy. Unlabeled uses for carboplatin include combination therapy in lung and head and neck cancers.

Oxaliplatin This Pt(II) complex loses oxalate dianion ($^{-}$OOC-COO^{-}) in vivo to form the mono- and dihydrated diaminocyclohexane (DACH) platinum analogs shown in Figure 37.16. The trans-(*R*,*R*)-DACH structure serves as the carrier for the cytotoxic hydrated platinum and extends into the major groove of DNA when the DNA–Pt complex forms (48). Hydrophobic DNA intrusion is believed to contribute to the cytotoxicity of this organometallic. Oxaliplatin engages primarily in intrastrand cross-linking with diguanosine dinucleotides, adjacent A-G nucleotides, and guanines that are separated by one nucleotide (G-X-G). Interstrand cross-linking, although less common, also occurs.

The adduct formed between oxaliplatin and DNA diguanosine dinucleotides is conformationally distinct from the adduct formed with cisplatin or carboplatin. Specifically, whereas the cisplatin diguanosine dinucleotide adduct bends the DNA by 60 to 80 degrees and presents a relatively wide minor groove, the oxaliplatin adduct produces a 31-degree bend with a comparatively narrow minor groove (49). This distinct oxaliplatin conformation is believed to result from the steric impact of the (*R*,*R*)-DACH carrier, which permits the *cis*-NH_3 moieties to hydrogen bond with a guanine-O^6, a bond that the inactive (*S*,*S*)-isomer cannot make (50). The conformation of the oxaliplatin-DNA adduct is much less likely to be recognized by MMR proteins, and the effectiveness of oxaliplatin in MMR-deficient cells is, at least in part, responsible for the lack of resistance that has plagued cisplatin and carboplatin (51,52). Oxaliplatin is also less dependent on CRT1 active transporting proteins for intracellular access and often retains activity in patients who are no longer responding to the first-generation organometallics. It is significantly less mutagenic, nephrotoxic, hematotoxic, and ototoxic than cisplatin. Excretion is via the kidney. Oxaliplatin decomposes in alkaline media and should not be coadministered with drugs that will increase the pH of the intravenous solution.

Oxaliplatin is used in the treatment of metastatic colon or rectal cancer, either alone or in combination with fluorouracil. Pulmonary fibrosis and peripheral sensory

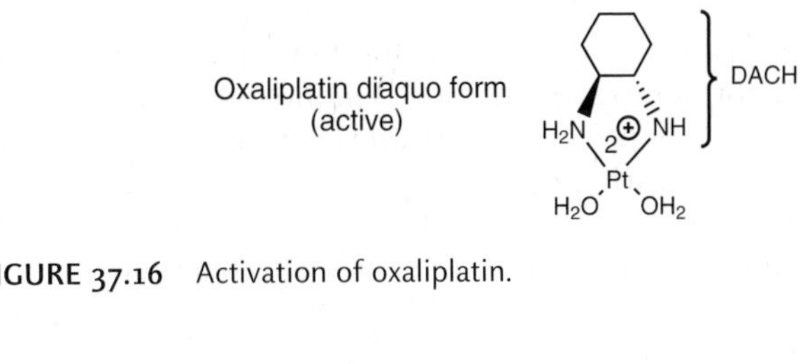

FIGURE 37.16 Activation of oxaliplatin.

neuropathies that can be life-threatening are known to occur. It has been proposed that the latter adverse effect is caused by oxalate-based chelation of intracellular Ca^{2+}, which inhibits voltage-gated sodium channels in sensory nerve cells (53). This hypothesis is supported by the observation that infusions of calcium or magnesium salts can significantly attenuate oxaliplatin-induced neuropathy without compromising therapeutic efficacy (54). In the future, exploitation of genetic differences in the expression of various repair proteins, growth factors, and metabolizing enzymes may allow the tailoring of oxaliplatin therapy based on an individual's pharmacogenetic profile (52).

Picoplatin Picoplatin is a Pt(II) organometallic currently designated as an orphan drug for the treatment of small cell lung cancer. It is also being investigated for use in platinum-sensitive ovarian cancer (in combination with paclitaxel), prostate cancer (in combination with docetaxel), and colorectal cancer (in combination with fluorouracil/leucovorin). The name of this antineoplastic is derived from the 2-methylpyridine (picoline) ring associated with the platinum atom. The intentional incorporation of bulk around the platinum decreases intracellular inactivation through attack by the sulfhydryl-containing glutathione peptide and metallothionein proteins, allowing continued efficacy in cisplatin-resistant tumors. This platin is active by the intravenous and oral routes. Like carboplatin, the drug is not nephro- or neurotoxic, but does induce myelosuppression that reverses upon drug discontinuation (47,55).

Satraplatin This asymmetrical organometallic agent is a Pt(IV) complex. As with the Pt(II) complexes, the platinum has no net charge in the parent drug since its original +4 charge has been "neutralized" by the donation of electrons from the chloride and acetate ligands. Unlike most marketed square-planar Pt(II) complexes, it is active by the oral route. Oral efficacy is enhanced by administering the drug on an empty stomach, using a 5 consecutive day regimen within a 28- to 35-day cycle. It is metabolized quickly in whole blood, producing up to six metabolites. The major metabolite is the desacetoxy analog. As with other organoplatinum complexes, the diaquo form is active.

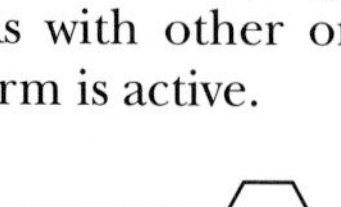

Desacetoxysatraplatin

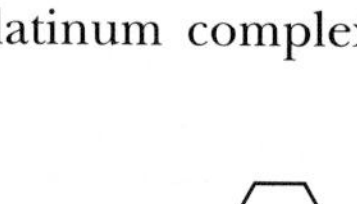

Diaquo satraplatin (active)

Satraplatin is currently in clinical trials as a second-line agent for the treatment of hormone-refractory prostate cancer. Trials pairing satraplatin with prednisolone have been particularly promising, with patients on the combination therapy showing a 40% reduction in progression compared to patients on the corticosteroid alone. Other trials in patients with small cell or non-small cell lung cancer are investigating the benefits of satraplatin as a single agent and satraplatin–paclitaxel combination therapy, respectively. Data analyzed to date suggest that satraplatin (administered as a single agent) is as effective as cisplatin or carboplatin in the treatment of small cell lung cancer and ovarian cancer. Satraplatin is also being paired with the pyrimidine antagonist capecitabine, the DNA polymerase inhibitor gemcitabine, or the mitosis inhibitor docetaxel in clinical trials in patients with advanced solid tumors.

Satraplatin retains activity in cisplatin-resistant cancers. Satraplatin-induced DNA damage is not recognized by MMR proteins, and its higher lipophilicity liberates it from dependence on CTR1 for cellular uptake. Resistance to satraplatin therapy can occur, but it is mediated through the intracellular sequestering of the drug in cytoprotective vesicles, a resistance pathway it shares with other organometallics. Its toxicity profile is mild, with dose-related, but noncumulative, myelosuppression (particularly neutropenia and thrombocytopenia), anemia, and diarrhea being the major use-limiting side effects (47,51,55,56).

Topoisomerase Poisons

Topoisomerases are enzymes that control the degree of DNA supercoiling and, in so doing, maintain proper DNA structure during replication and transcription to RNA (57). Topoisomerase IIα (TopIIα) cleaves double-stranded DNA during the replication phase via a transesterification reaction involving a topoisomerase tyrosine residue and a terminal 5′ phosphate but, through a reverse transesterification, repairs its own damage after replication is complete (58). Topoisomerase I (TopI) functions in essentially the same way, but cuts and religates a single DNA strand. Antineoplastic agents that function as topoisomerase poisons stimulate the DNA cleavage reaction but inhibit the DNA resealing activity of the enzymes, leaving the DNA irreversibly damaged and unable to replicate.

Three chemically distinct classes of anticancer agents can be classified as topoisomerase poisons: camptothecins, epipodophyllotoxins, and anthracyclines (discussed under antineoplastic antibiotics).

Camptothecins

MECHANISM OF ACTION Camptothecins are chiral, extensively conjugated, amine-containing pentacyclic lactones (Fig. 37.17). The biologic target of camptothecins is TopI, rather than the TopIIα enzyme that serves as the receptor for the epipodophyllotoxins and anthracyclines. However, as noted earlier, the mechanism of antineoplastic action of both enzyme inhibitors is stabilization of a cleavable ternary DNA–enzyme complex that does not permit the resealing of nicked DNA. Although the fragmented DNA is capable of resealing in the absence of drug, when DNA replication forks encounter the fragmented DNA, a double-stranded DNA break occurs, killing the cell.

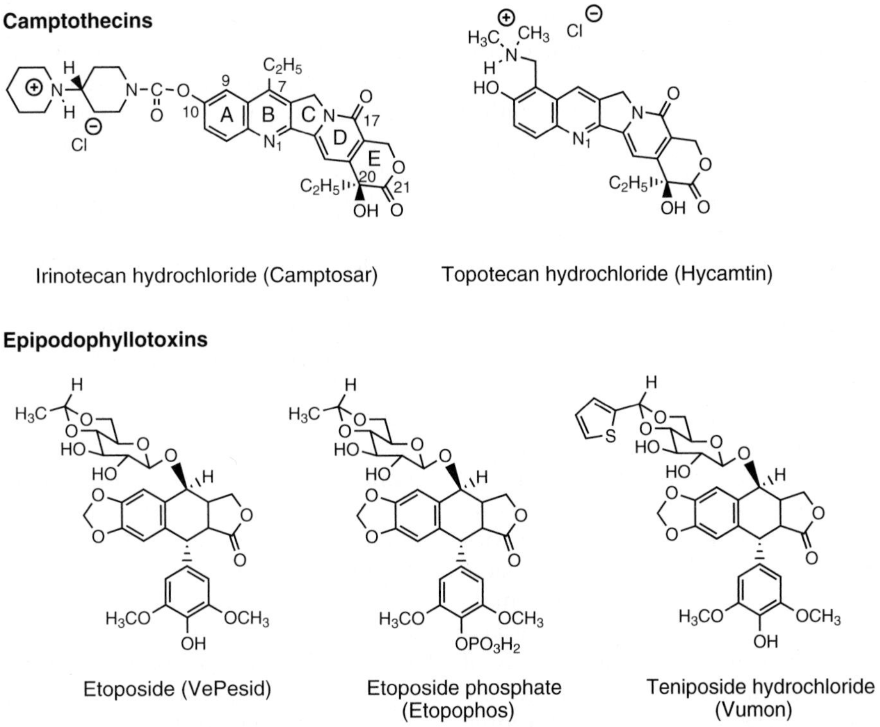

FIGURE 37.17 Camptothecins and epipodophyllotoxins: topoisomerase poisons.

The binding of camptothecins occurs in such a way as to stabilize a covalent DNA–topoisomerase bond at the point of single-strand breakage (tyrosine [Tyr] at 723 on the human enzyme) but sterically keep a TopI Lys532 residue from catalyzing the DNA religation reaction (59,60). The binding pocket, located within the DNA strand, is revealed only after the normal DNA nicking has occurred, explaining why these poisons preferentially bind to the enzyme–DNA complex rather than to unoccupied DNA or enzyme. The flat camptothecin ring system intercalates DNA at the site of cleavage, mimicking a DNA base pair (59). The crystal structures of human ternary complexes involving the parent alkaloid, camptothecin, and the semisynthetic analog, topotecan (Fig. 37.17), have been solved, and important drug–protein interacting entities are noted in Table 37.7 (59–61). The bulky substituents at C_7, C_9, and C_{10} of the marketed compounds, which project into the major groove of DNA, do not hinder binding.

Camptothecins are most toxic to cells undergoing active DNA replication and cell division (e.g., they are S-phase specific). Mechanisms of resistance are similar to those operational in many other classes of antineoplastic drugs and include downregulation or mutation of the target enzyme, downregulation of enzymes needed for drug activation, and cellular efflux. Breast cancer resistance protein and multidrug resistance (MDR)–associated proteins, such as MAP-2 and MAP-3, rather than P-gp, appear to mediate resistance to these agents (62,63).

Chemistry The parent camptothecin alkaloid, isolated from the bark of *Camptotheca acuminata* (the Chinese xi shu or "happy tree") (64), has antitumor activity, but its limited water solubility necessitates delivery as the sodium salt of the significantly less active hydrolyzed lactone. Lactonization of the hydroxy acid in acidic urine is significant, and elevated levels of active intact alkaloid in the kidney account for the hemorrhagic cystitis induced by this compound.

Camptothecin's quinoline ring system is unsubstituted, but currently marketed analogs have a basic side chain incorporated at either C_9 (topotecan) or C_{10} (irinotecan), allowing the formation of water-soluble salts of the intact semisynthetic alkaloid. At pH 7.4, the active lactone exists in equilibrium with the hydroxy acid hydrolysis product, with the direction dictated by the extent of binding to serum albumin. The preferential protein

TABLE 37.7 Topotecan–Topoisomerase I Interactions

Topotecan Functional Group	Topoisomerase I Residue
Pyridine N_1	Arg364
C_{10}-OH	Enzyme-associated water (H-bond)
C_{17}-pyridone carbonyl	Asn722
C_{20}-OH	Asp533 (H-bond)
C_{21}-lactone carbonyl	Tyr723-phosphate, Lys532

binding of the lactone, which occurs with irinotecan, shifts the equilibrium to favor the production of the more active lactone, thus enhancing potency.

Some authors have recently pondered whether camptothecins are making a clinical comeback (64). A quantitative study on camptothecin structure–property relationships has recently been published (65), as has a review summarizing the current literature describing outcomes in preliminary, preclinical, and clinical in vivo studies for camptothecins and various small and macromolecular analogs of the natural products (66).

Specific Drugs (Fig. 37.17)

Irinotecan Hydrochloride In combination with fluorouracil, this prodrug camptothecin analog is considered first-line therapy in the treatment of metastatic colorectal cancer. It has also shown efficacy in small cell and non–small cell lung cancers when used in combination with cisplatin. Given intravenously, the drug is slowly bioactivated in the liver through hydrolysis of the C_{10}-carbamate ester. The catalyzing enzyme is a saturable carboxylesterase known as irinotecan-converting enzyme. Levels of active metabolite, known as SN-38 (Fig. 37.18), are 50- to 100-fold lower than the parent drug, but preferential protein binding of the lactone (95%) permits significant plasma levels of the optimally active SN-38 compared to the hydroxy acid metabolite. SN-38 has a terminal half-life of 11.5 hours (compared with 5.0 to 9.6 hours for the prodrug parent) and is glucuronidated or sulfated at the C_{10} phenol before elimination. CYP3A4 also cleaves the terminal piperidine ring through oxidation at the α-carbons. This is followed by hydrolysis of the resultant amides, which produces inactive metabolites. Excretion of the parent drug and metabolites is renal (14% to 37%) and, to a lesser extent, biliary.

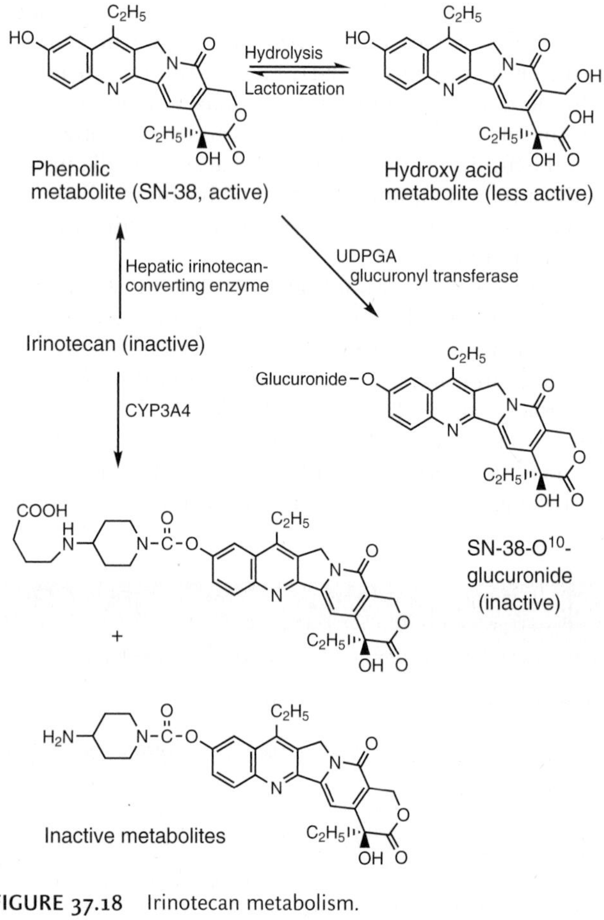

FIGURE 37.18 Irinotecan metabolism.

Delayed diarrhea induced by irinotecan is dose-limiting and potentially fatal, and vigorous loperamide therapy should be instituted at the first sign of symptoms. Acute diarrhea is attributed to the drug's ability to inhibit acetylcholinesterase and can be addressed through anticholinergic pretreatment. Pretreatment also helps patients to avoid "cholinergic syndrome," a collection of annoying side effects that include flushing, sweating, blurred vision, lacrimation, and less commonly, bradycardia. Camptothecins are also myelosuppressive, and leukoneutropenia can be severe, particularly in patients with elevated bilirubin levels. Extensive biotransformation also demands cautious use of irinotecan in patients with hepatic dysfunction. Prophylactic antiemetic therapy should be given at least 30 minutes before the administration of irinotecan to minimize the nausea and vomiting associated with this anticancer agent.

It is now recognized that patients, particularly those of Asian heritage, may be pharmacogenetically predisposed to life-threatening toxicity from camptothecin therapy. Variations in expression of gene(s) involved in the inactivating glucuronidation of irinotecan (specifically overexpression of the low activity UGT1A1*6 allele) are deemed responsible, and genotyping efforts are being made to more safely and effectively individualize therapy in "at-risk" individuals (67,68).

Topotecan Hydrochloride This active camptothecin analog is used by the intravenous route in the treatment of ovarian and small cell lung cancer that has not responded to first-line therapy. Myelosuppression, particularly neutropenia, is use-limiting and has precluded combination therapy with other bone marrow-suppressing drugs. Thrombocytopenia and anemia occur in approximately one-third of treated patients. Schedules that call for daily (for 5 days) administration can also result in serious mucositis and diarrhea.

Topotecan elimination is biphasic with a terminal half-life of 2.0 to 3.5 hours. Lactone hydrolysis is rapid, and binding to serum proteins is limited to between 25% and 40%. CYP3A4-mediated *N*-dealkylation to mono- and di-dealkylated metabolites occurs to a limited extent, and the *O*-glucuronides that form at multiple points along the metabolic path are excreted via the kidney (Fig. 37.19). Extensive renal clearance demands dosage adjustment in patients with kidney disease. A nanoliposomal formulation of topotecan with an enhanced cytotoxic and pharmacokinetic profile is currently in development (69).

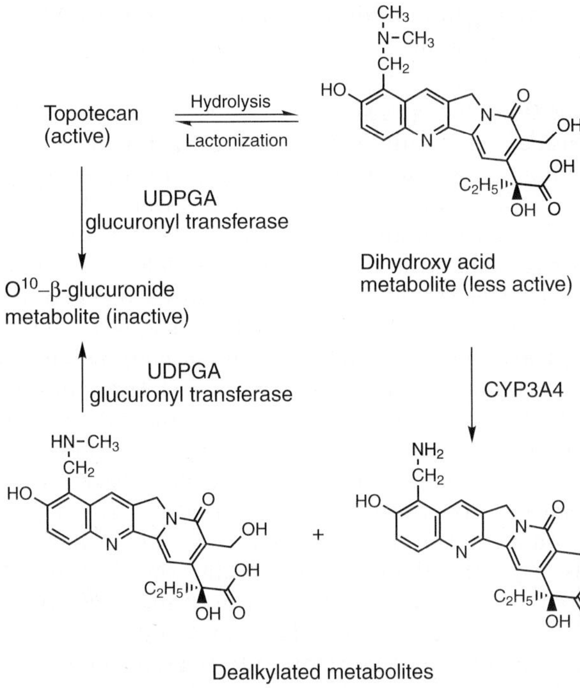

FIGURE 37.19 Topotecan metabolism.

Because both topotecan and irinotecan are metabolized by CYP3A4, the potential for drug–drug interactions must be evaluated. Reduced clearance was noted when azole antifungal agents and cyclosporine were coadministered with irinotecan, and accelerated clearance was observed when topotecan was coadministered with CYP3A4 inducers such as phenobarbital and phenytoin. Unlike irinotecan, at the time of this writing, there have been no published reports correlating the risk of topotecan toxicity to UGT1A1 polymorphism.

Epipodophyllotoxins

The epipodophyllotoxins (Fig. 37.17) are semisynthetic glycosidic derivatives of podophyllotoxin, the major component of the resinous podophyllin isolated from the dried roots of the American mandrake or mayapple plant (*Podophyllum peltatum*). Although these compounds are capable of binding to tubulin and inhibiting mitosis, their primary mechanism of antineoplastic action is TopIIα poisoning, a mechanism that they share with anthracyclines (see antineoplastic antibiotics). TopIIα has two distinct DNA-independent binding sites for the epipodophyllotoxins, one within the catalytic domain and a second within the *N*-terminal adenosine triphosphate (ATP)-binding domain (70). Once bound, the toxins stabilize the cleavable ternary drug–enzyme–DNA complex, stimulating DNA ligation but inhibiting resealing. The DNA-topoisomerase fragments accumulate in the cell, ultimately resulting in apoptosis. The RNA transcription processes are also disrupted by the interaction of epipodophyllotoxins with TopIIα (63). The epipodophyllotoxin binding site has recently been probed with a carbene-generating diazirine photoaffinity label (71), and a virtual library of 143 epipodophyllotoxin derivatives has been docked to a three-dimensional human TopIIα receptor model in order to identify key drug–enzyme interactions (Fig. 37.20) (72). This valuable information should serve as the starting point for the rational development of more potent and target-specific epipodophyllotoxins.

Epipodophyllotoxins are cell cycle specific and have their most devastating impact on cells in the S or early G_2 phase. For this reason, doses are divided and administered over several days. Resistance is multifaceted and involves downregulation of TopIIα, attenuation of enzymatic activity levels, development of novel DNA repair mechanisms, and P-gp–mediated cellular efflux.

CHEMISTRY Structurally, the two marketed epipodophyllotoxins, etoposide and teniposide, differ only in the nature of one β-D-glucopyranosyl substituent (methyl or thienyl, respectively). Both are highly water insoluble, but teniposide's higher lipophilicity facilitates cellular uptake and results in a 10-fold enhancement of potency (63). The need for solubility enhancers, such as polysorbate 80 (Tween, etoposide) or polyoxyethylated castor oil (Cremophor EL, teniposide), in intravenous formulations puts patients at risk for hypersensitivity reactions that can manifest as hypotension and thrombophlebitis. Epinephrine, antihistamines, and corticosteroids are often coadministered to minimize risk. A water-soluble phosphate ester analog of etoposide can be administered in standard aqueous vehicles, permitting higher doses than the oil-modified formulations would allow. The phosphate ester is rapidly cleaved to the free alcohol in the blood.

METABOLISM Epipodophyllotoxins are subject to metabolic transformation before renal and nonrenal elimination (Fig. 37.21). Etoposide is stable enough for oral administration, although a dose approximately twice that of the intravenous formulation must be administered. Teniposide is more extensively metabolized, presumably due to its enhanced ability to penetrate into hepatocytes, and no oral dosage form is marketed. Both

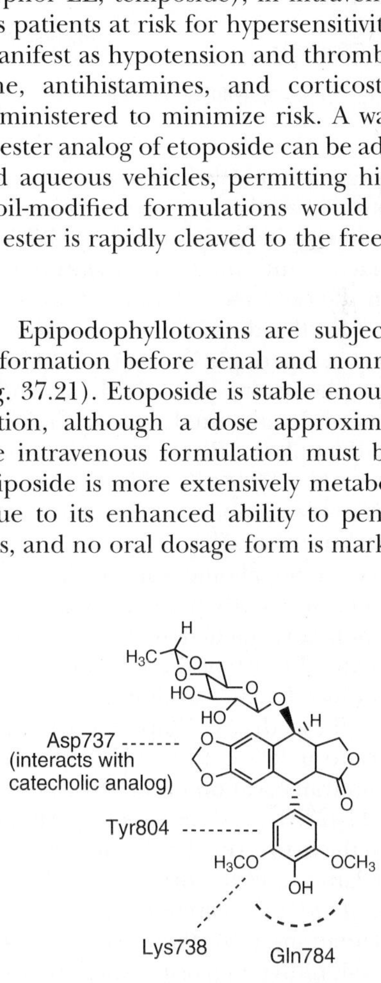

FIGURE 37.20 Proposed etoposide–TopIIα binding interactions.

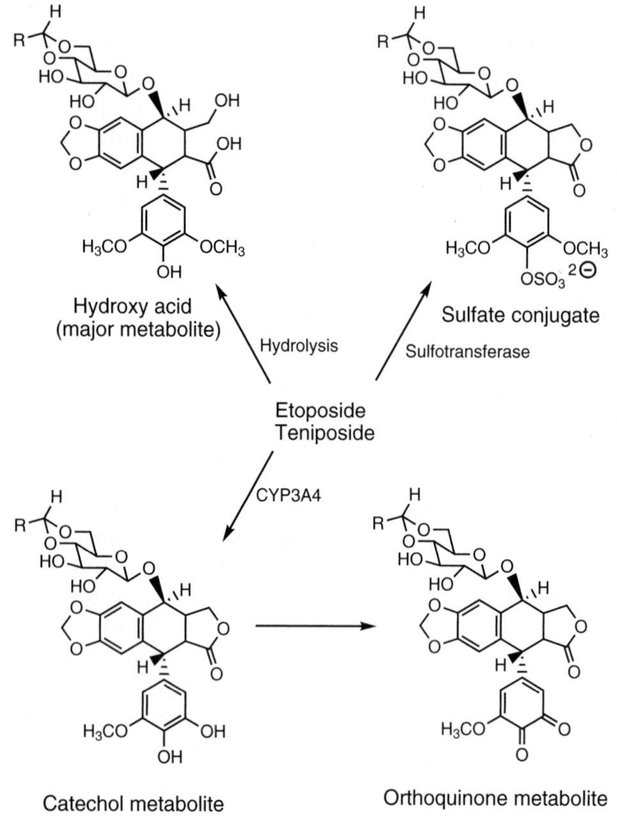

FIGURE 37.21 Epipodophyllotoxin metabolism.

drugs undergo lactone hydrolysis to generate the inactive hydroxy acid as the major metabolite, but the parent drugs can also be transformed by CYP3A4-catalyzed *O*-demethylation and phase 2 glucuronide or sulfate conjugation. Phase 2 metabolism accounts for between 5% and 22% of the dose. Clinically significant interactions between epipodophyllotoxins and CYP3A4 inducers, such as phenytoin, phenobarbital, and St. John's wort, have been documented, and coadministration can enhance antineoplastic drug clearance by as much as 77%. Conversely, CYP3A4 inhibitors, such as cyclosporine or macrolide antibiotics, can decrease clearance, leading to unwanted toxicity.

The catechol metabolite can oxidize to a reactive orthoquinone, and both have been proposed to promote topoisomerase-mediated DNA cleavage, potentially enhancing the risk of the translocations that result in therapy-induced acute myeloid leukemia in children treated with these drugs. Epipodophyllotoxin-induced leukemia occurs in 2% to 12% of patients and is believed to result from translocation of the *MLL* gene at chromosome band 11q23. The mean latency period of 2 years is shorter than the 5- to 7-year latency for leukemia induced by DNA alkylators, and the drug-induced cancer is often resistant to standard treatment (including bone marrow transplantation) (73). Other serious adverse effects include dose-limiting mucositis and myelosuppression, particularly leukopenia. Alopecia is common, and nausea and vomiting, most noticeable with the oral dosage form, are generally mild.

Specific Drugs (Fig. 37.17)

Etoposide Etoposide is used in the treatment of small cell lung cancer and in combination with other agents in refractory testicular cancer. Both intravenous and oral formulations are available. Oral bioavailability is concentration-dependent and runs approximately 50% for the 50-mg capsule. Little first-pass metabolism is noted with the gelatin capsule dosage form. The drug is more than 96% protein bound, undergoes biphasic elimination, and has a terminal half-life of 4 to 11 hours. Approximately 35% to 45% of a dose is eliminated via the kidneys, with less than 6% excreted in feces. The drug should be used with caution in patients with renal or liver disease. Specifically, doses should be decreased in patients with creatinine clearance of less than 50 mL/min or bilirubin levels of greater than 1.5 mg/dL, and the drug should not be used in patients with bilirubin levels of greater than 3.1 mg/dL. Organoplatinum anticancer agents (e.g., cisplatin) decrease etoposide clearance, especially in children. If used in combination, administration must be separated by at least 2 days.

Teniposide Teniposide is used in combination with other agents for the treatment of refractory childhood acute lymphoblastic leukemia. Compared to etoposide, it is more tightly protein bound (>99%), more extensively metabolized, more slowly cleared (terminal half-life, 5 to 40 hours), and less dependent on renal elimination (10% to 21%). Exposure to heparin can cause teniposide to precipitate, so lines must be thoroughly flushed before and after teniposide administration. The drug can also spontaneously precipitate, particularly if solutions are overagitated, and patients receiving 24-hour infusions should be monitored for blockage of access catheters. Teniposide and etoposide are Category D teratogens and, if at all possible, should not be used in women of childbearing age.

Antibiotics

The antibiotic antineoplastics (Fig. 37.22) are a broad category of natural or semisynthetic compounds that block DNA transcription by inhibiting enzymes critical to the DNA replication process and/or by nicking and/or inducing point mutations in the DNA strand. Antibiotic antineoplastics that interact directly with DNA first intercalate the double-stranded helix by inserting between the base pairs and forming strong noncovalent interactions with DNA bases. The highly stabilized complex deforms and uncoils the DNA, prohibiting proper replication. To bulldoze its way between the bonded DNA strands, a segment of the antibiotic must have the trigonal coplanar geometry guaranteed by aromaticity.

The antineoplastic anthracycline antibiotics function as TopIIα poisons. Another mechanism of cytotoxic

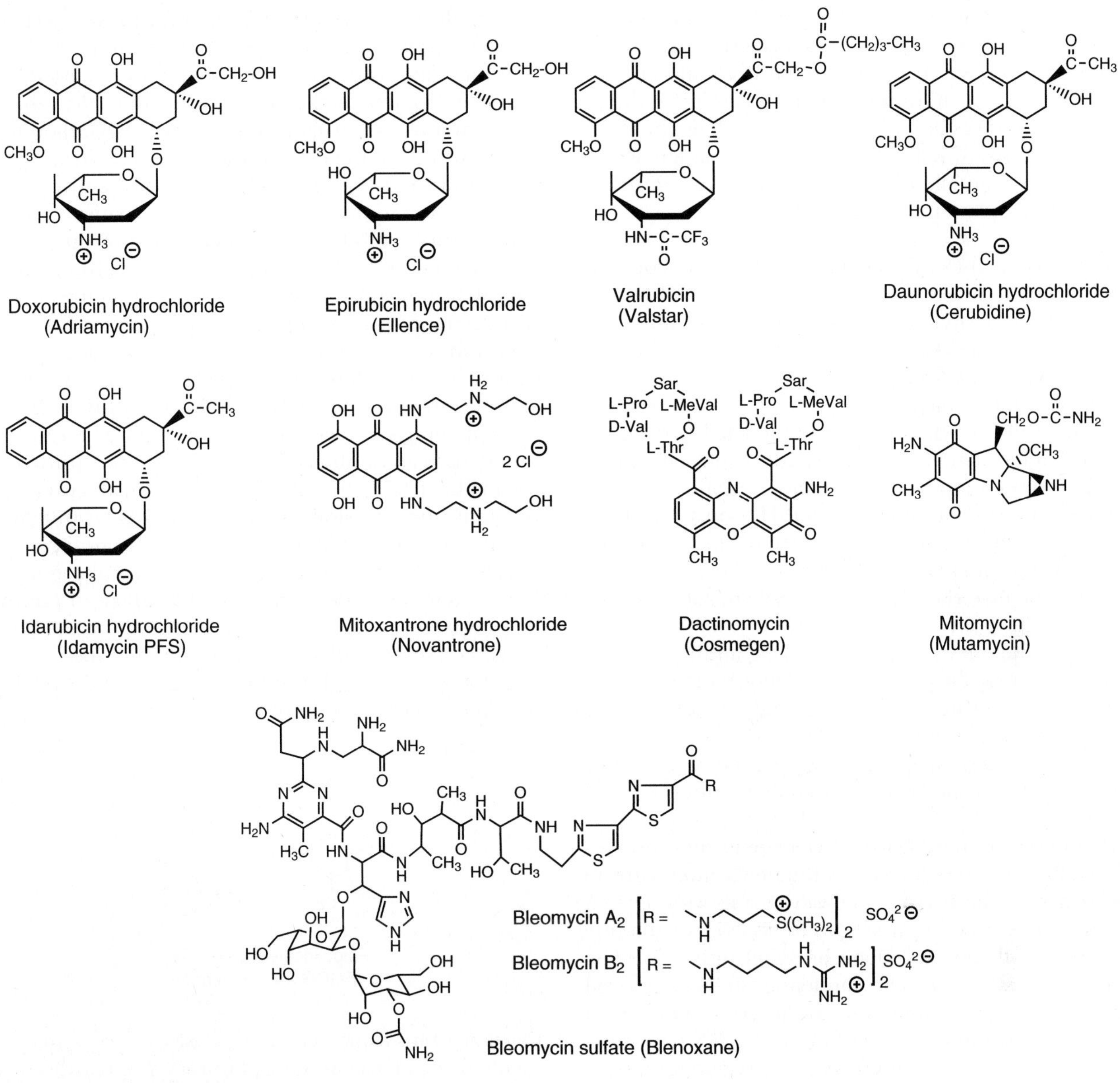

FIGURE 37.22 Anticancer antibiotics.

action, particularly for one antibiotic (bleomycin), is the generation of cytotoxic free radicals that cause single-strand breaks in DNA. Another antibiotic (mitomycin) is capable of alkylating DNA, a mechanism more commonly associated with the nitrogen mustard antineoplastics but that is predictable from the nucleophilic aziridine ring found within the structure of this anticancer agent.

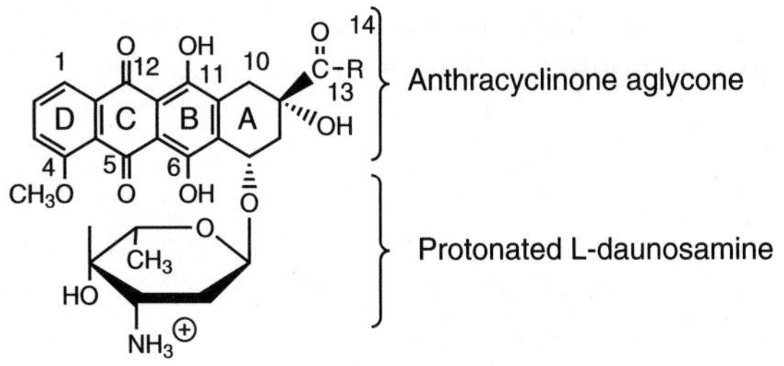

Anthracyclines and Anthracenediones

Anthracycline antineoplastic antibiotics are very closely related to the tetracycline antibacterials. Structurally, they are glycosides and contain a sugar portion (L-daunosamine) and a nonsugar organic portion. The nonsugar portion of glycosides is generically referred to as an aglycone. In anthracyclines, the aglycone moiety is specifically called anthracyclinone or anthroquinone.

MECHANISM OF ACTION Anthracycline-based antineoplastic agents act by poisoning TopIIα through the stabilization of the ternary drug–enzyme–DNA cleavable complex. Like the topoisomerase poisons discussed earlier, they allow DNA to be cut and covalently linked to the conserved topoisomerase Tyr residue but inhibit the resealing reaction. The flat, aromatic portion of the anthracyclinone ring system and the daunosamine sugar bind to DNA, whereas the anthracyclinone A ring is believed to bridge the gap between DNA and enzyme (57,74). Since a small number of anthracycline-induced DNA breaks can result in a high level of cell death, it has been hypothesized that the site of DNA cleavage, which contains an essential thymine-adenine (T-A) dinucleotide, is particularly lethal to the cell (75).

Chemistry DNA intercalation initiates the antineoplastic action of the anthracyclines (58). Rings B, C, and D slide between the two DNA strands, orienting the anthracyclinone moiety in a perpendicular fashion relative to the long axis of DNA and stabilizing the complex through π stacking and other affinity-enhancing interactions. A recent study in which doxorubicin was docked in a modeled DNA "post-cleavage" intercalation site proposed highly efficacious H-bonds between top Ser740 and the C_5 quinone oxygen (ring C), top Thr744 and the C_4-OCH_3 (ring D), and a DNA thymine base and the C_9-OH (ring A) (58). If present, a C_{14}-OH should H-bond with the carbonyl oxygen of a DNA thymine base (Fig. 37.23). Interestingly, although the C_4-OCH_3 helps hold drug to TopIIα enzyme, its removal increases antitumor activity by enhancing anthracyclinone planarity (thereby facilitating intercalation) and by directing the binding of the daunosamine sugar to stabilize the inhibitory ternary cleavable complex (76).

The daunosamine sugar is known to bind in the minor groove of DNA at the DNA-topoisomerase interface and subsequently orchestrate the DNA sequence specificity of the intercalation and overall DNA poisoning process (58,74). Binding roles for the protonated 3′-amino group have run the gamut from ion–ion paring with a DNA phosphate to covalently linking to the C_2-NH_2 of guanine via a formaldehyde methylene bridging unit (77). The aforementioned molecular modeling study suggested that the cationic daunosamine amino group binds with high affinity to the carbonyl oxygen of a DNA thymine base when in the naturally occurring α configuration. In the epimerized β configuration, there is an increased distance between these two moieties and an unfavorable steric interaction with other DNA residues. While the loss or epimerization of the daunosamine 3′-amino moiety decreases DNA binding, it does not destroy it. In fact, it has been stated that the antitumor activity of anthracyclines is related more to the proper positioning and stabilization of the drug within the "cleavable ternary complex" of drug–topoisomerase–DNA than to the actual affinity of the drug for the DNA (74,76).

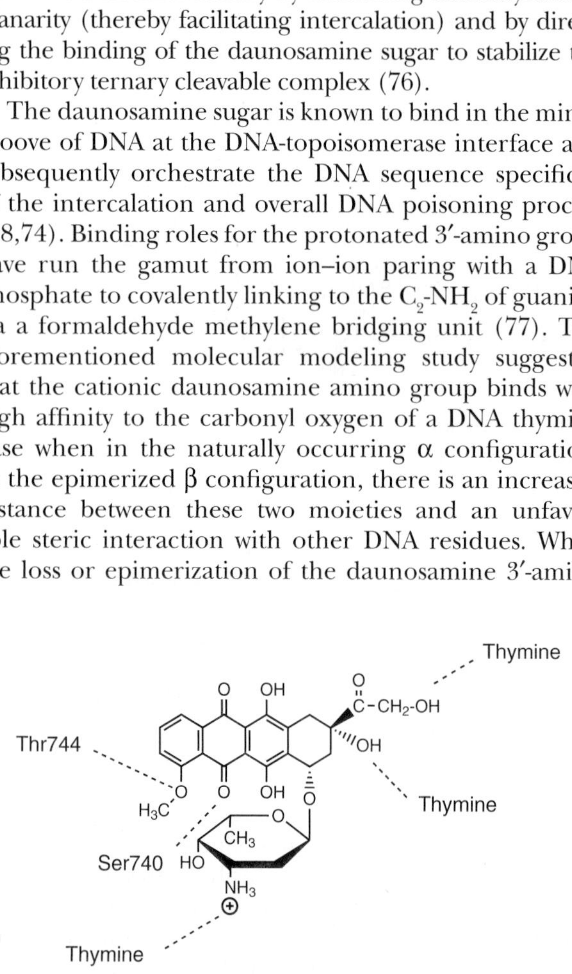

FIGURE 37.23 Proposed interaction between doxorubicin, DNA, and topoisomerase IIα.

Resistance to anthracycline chemotherapy can be intrinsic or acquired. The major mechanisms through which cancer cells fight back include compromised drug transport across cell membranes, active efflux via P-gp and MDR transporters, changes in tumor cell responsiveness to apoptotic triggers, alterations in TopIIα expression and activity, and augmented biochemical defenses against anthracycline-induced oxidative stress (78).

Interestingly, some authors have shown that the polyphenol epigallocatechin-3-gallate (EGCG, found in green tea) can inhibit cellular efflux of the anthracycline doxorubicin (79,80) and sensitize doxorubicin-treated/resistant human colon carcinoma cells (81). In addition to the scientific evidence supporting the positive doxorubicin–EGCG interaction, Sadzuka and colleagues (80) holistically state, "We think that the intake of a favorite beverage favors a positive mental attitude of the patient and increases the efficacy of the chemotherapeutic index, and that this efficacy is useful for improving the quality of life on cancer chemotherapy."

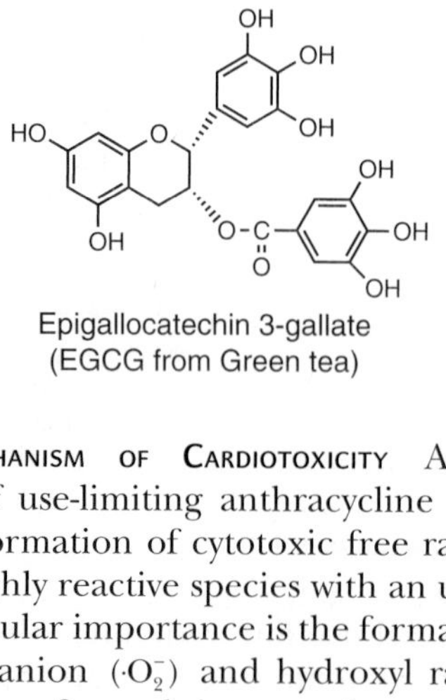

Epigallocatechin 3-gallate
(EGCG from Green tea)

Chemical Mechanism of Cardiotoxicity An important mechanism of use-limiting anthracycline cardiotoxicity involves the formation of cytotoxic free radicals. A free radical is a highly reactive species with an unpaired electron. Of particular importance is the formation of superoxide radical anion ($\cdot O_2^-$) and hydroxyl radical ($\cdot OH$), both of which are formed via a one-electron reduction of the anthracyclinone quinone (ring C) to hydroquinone by NADPH/CYP450 reductase. The mechanism by which these reactive oxygen species (ROS) are generated is shown in Figure 37.24.

When NADPH/CYP450 reductase reduces the quinone ring to a hydroquinone, superoxide radical anions ($\cdot O_2^-$) are generated. Superoxide radical anions react to generate hydrogen peroxide (H_2O_2), a reaction that requires protons and is catalyzed by the enzyme superoxide dismutase in a Cu^{2+}-mediated process. The fate of this hydrogen peroxide dictates the degree of cytotoxicity observed from the anthracycline.

In the presence of the enzyme catalase, hydrogen peroxide is rapidly converted to water and oxygen, which

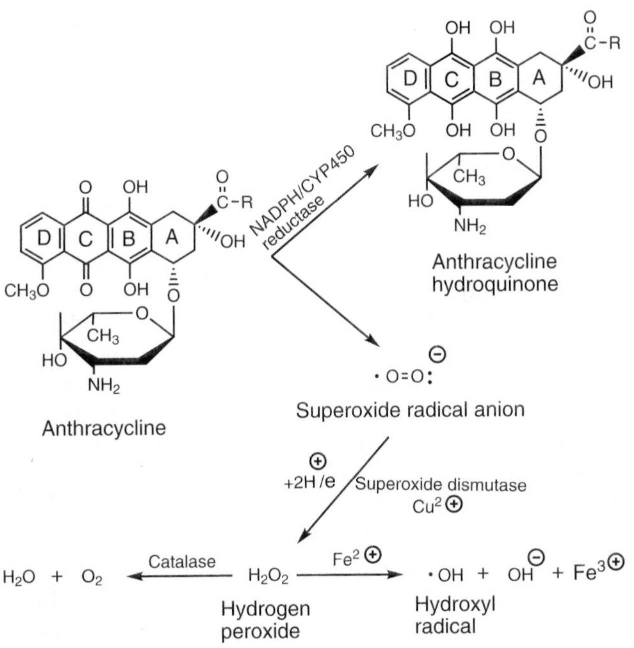

FIGURE 37.24 Anthracycline-mediated free radical formation.

obviously are harmless chemicals as far as the body is concerned. However, in the presence of ferrous ion (Fe^{2+}), hydrogen peroxide is converted into the highly toxic hydroxyl radical through a process called the Fenton reaction. Hydroxyl radicals promote single-strand breaks in DNA, which is therapeutically desirable to treat the uncontrolled growth of cancer cells. Anthracycline anticancer agents are also known to interfere with normal ferritin-iron mobilization, resulting in iron accumulation (82). The anthracyclines chelate strongly with di- and trivalent cations, including intracellular Fe^{2+}, so the generation of cytotoxic hydroxyl radicals after the initial NADPH/CYP450 reductase reduction is essentially guaranteed. Hydroxide anion and Fe^{3+} are also formed during the production of hydroxyl radicals. Anthracycline–iron complexes (particularly those involving Fe^{+3}) can also spontaneously generate ROS without the aid of enzymatic catalysis (83).

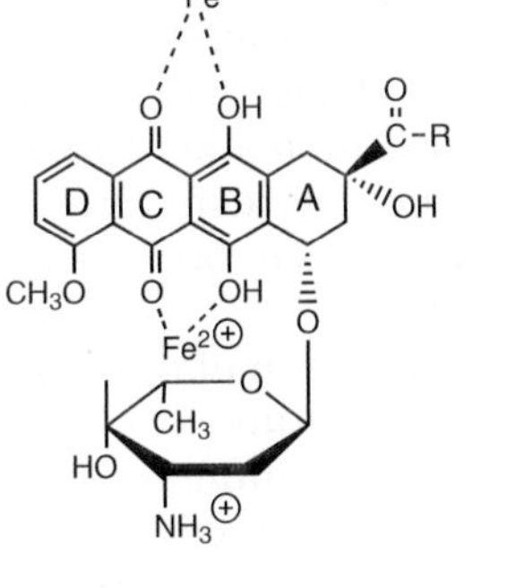

The generation of hydroxyl radicals inside the tumor cell could augment the antineoplastic effect of the anthracyclines, but such generation is uncommon at standard antineoplastic doses (75). These cytotoxic radicals are generated within the heart, however, and can lead to acute, albeit reversible, cardiotoxicity. Cardiac tissue is particularly vulnerable to free radical damage by the anthracyclines because it does not contain significant amounts of catalase and other relevant cytoprotective enzymes (84). When hydrogen peroxide forms in the myocardium, it has no choice but to go down the Fenton pathway. Cardiac toxicity is the major use-limiting side effect of anthracycline use, but coadministration of dexrazoxane (an antioxidant and iron chelator) has been shown to lower its incidence (85).

A role for nitric oxide metabolism, particularly nitric oxide synthase, in anthracycline-mediated cardiotoxicity has also been proposed (83,86). The reactive nitrogen species of greatest concern is peroxynitrite ($ONOO^-$), a strong oxidant that shows no selectivity in its destruction of life-sustaining macromolecules.

Although the rate of quinone metabolism influences the risk of acute anthracycline-induced cardiotoxicity, metabolism at C_{13} is believed to be responsible for the more life-threatening chronic cardiotoxicity that some patients experience. The C_{13}-carbonyl is reduced via a two-electron mechanism to a commonly less active (87,88) or inactive (83) secondary alcohol via cytosolic aldoketoreductase enzymes (Fig. 37.25), and the larger the R group, the slower this reaction and the longer the

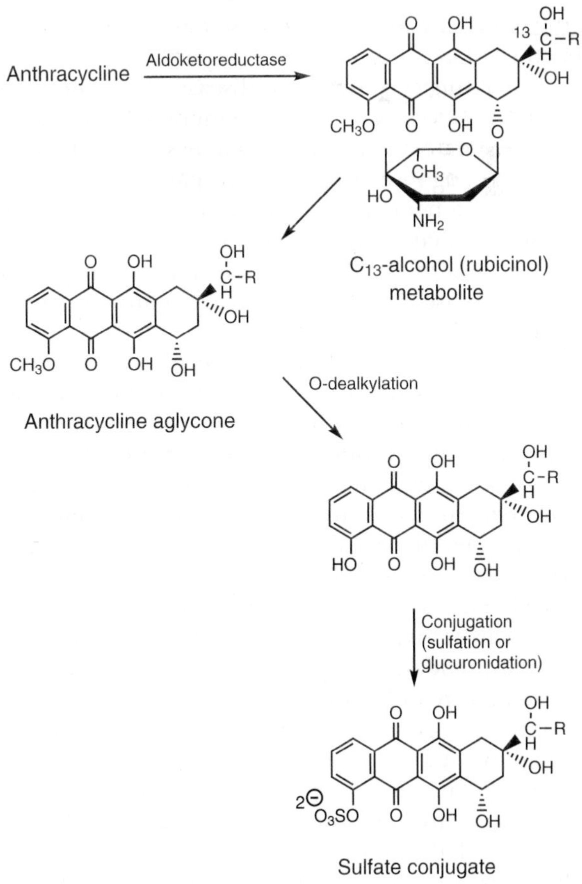

FIGURE 37.25 Anthracycline metabolism.

duration of antineoplastic action. The C_{13}-substituents found on most marketed anthracyclines include CH_3 (daunorubicin and idarubicin) and CH_2OH (doxorubicin and epirubicin). Before excretion, anthracyclines are further metabolized via hydrolytic or reductive deglycosidation to their 7-hydroxy or 7-deoxy aglycones, respectively, followed by *O*-dealkylation of the C_4 methoxy ether (if present) and conjugation with either glucuronic acid or sulfate. The aglycones may also have cardiotoxic properties (83).

The secondary alcohol ("rubicinol") metabolites formed by aldoketoreductase concentrate in cardiomyocytes and induce a prolonged inhibition of calcium loading, open a selective ion channel, inhibit Ca^{2+},Mg^{2+}-ATPase leading to increased cytosolic levels of Ca^{2+} in the sarcoplasmic reticulum, and inhibit Na^{+},K^{+}-ATPase action in the sarcolemma. Collectively, these cellular events can induce a chronic cardiomyopathy that presents as severe congestive heart failure involving systolic and diastolic dysfunction (82). As the rubicinol metabolites form a "long-lived reservoir" of cardiotoxic drug within the myocardium, chronic anthracycline-induced congestive heart failure can manifest without warning years after therapy, and it is often unresponsive to therapeutic intervention (83). It has been estimated that more than half of the patients diagnosed with chronic anthracycline-induced congestive heart failure will die within 2 years (83). Elevated risk has been related to age (both very young and very old), genetic polymorphisms impacting ROS production and/or anthracycline transport, underlying cardiovascular disease, high cumulative doses, and cyclophosphamide co-therapy. Females and blacks appear to be at risk for increased incidence or severity of drug-induced cardiomyopathy. Because toxicity is dose-dependent, patients with liver dysfunction who cannot adequately metabolize and clear anthracyclines are also at risk. Dosage adjustments in patients with liver disease must be made to avoid life-threatening toxicity.

Although the acute and chronic phases of anthracycline-induced cardiomyopathy appear metabolically distinct, a "unifying hypothesis" has recently been put forward to suggest that induction of ROS-mediated oxidative stress that characterizes acute cardiac toxicity may upregulate aldoketoreductase, thereby facilitating the development of rubicinol-induced chronic toxicity (83). As noted earlier, the pharmacotherapeutic approach currently used to attenuate anthracycline-induced cardiotoxicity is coadministration of dexrazoxane, an antioxidant and prodrug iron chelating agent. Dexrazoxane readily enters cells and is hydrolyzed to the active Fe^{2+} and Fe^{3+} chelating form (ADR-925). Although the affinity of ADR-925 for iron surpasses that of doxorubicin, iron-independent mechanisms for this cardioprotectant have also been proposed (83). This prodrug chelator can also be used to prevent serious tissue injury following accidental anthracycline extravasation (89).

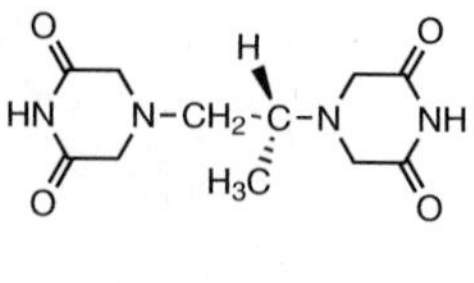

Dexrazoxane

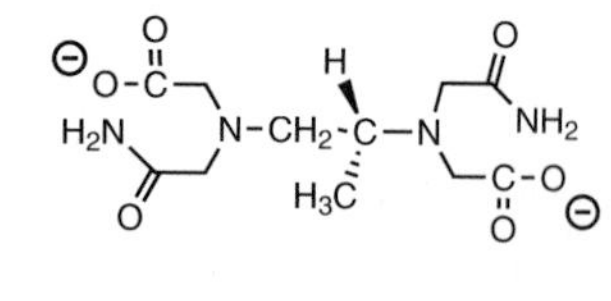

ADR-925

Other Toxicities In addition to cardiac toxicity, all anthracycline antineoplastics can cause severe myelosuppression (especially leukocytopenia) as well as moderate to severe nausea and vomiting, mucositis leading to hemorrhage and potentially fatal infection, and alopecia. Side effects are dose-dependent. Most of the anthracyclines are orally inactive and must be given by intravenous injection. They are highly necrotic to skin and, if extravasation occurs, can cause such severe blistering and ulceration that skin excision, followed by plastic surgery, may be indicated. The anthracyclines contain photosensitive phenolic groups that must be protected from light and air. The highly conjugated structure imparts a reddish-orange color to these compounds (implied in the name "rubicin"), which is maintained when these compounds are excreted in the urine. Patients should be warned that the reddish urine they will experience is not hemorrhagic but, rather, simply the result of the conjugated chemistry of this class of drugs.

The risk of serious or life-threatening adverse reactions can potentially outweigh the therapeutic benefits of anthracyclines in some patients, which has fueled the search for biomarkers that will predict tumor responsiveness to these powerful antineoplastic agents (90).

Specific Drugs (Fig. 37.22)

Doxorubicin Hydrochloride The C_{13} substituent of doxorubicin is hydroxymethyl, which retards the action of cytosolic aldoketoreductase and slows the conversion to the less active and chronically cardiotoxic doxorubicinol. This contributes to the longer duration of action compared to analogs that have CH_3 at this position (e.g., daunorubicin). Doxorubicin is highly lipophilic and concentrates in the liver, lymph nodes, muscle, bone marrow, fat, and skin. Elimination is triphasic, and the drug has a terminal half-life of 30 to 40 hours. The majority of an administered dose is excreted in the feces, approximately half of it unchanged (83). Doxorubicin is used either alone or in combination therapy to treat a wide range of neoplastic disorders, including hematologic cancers and solid tumors in breast, ovary, stomach, bladder, and thyroid gland.

A liposomal formulation of doxorubicin, marketed as Doxil, is used in the treatment of AIDS-related Kaposi sarcoma and organoplatinum-resistant ovarian cancer. Liposomes are taken up selectively into tumor cells, presumably due to their persistence in the bloodstream and enhanced permeability of tumor vascular membranes. In liposomal form, the drug is protected against enzymes that generate cardiotoxic free radicals and is less likely to concentrate in the heart (91). However, because this form of the drug can still induce potentially fatal congestive heart failure, all precautions outlined for the use of doxorubicin are employed when the liposomal formulation is used. The half-life of Doxil is extended to approximately 55 hours, and it is administered in doses ranging from 20 to 50 mg/m^2 every 3 to 4 weeks. The area under the curve of the liposomal formulation is approximately triple that of the free drug formulation. It is cleared more slowly than conventional doxorubicin and generates very little of the doxorubicinol metabolite. Significant side effects have occurred when the liposomal formulation is erroneously dispensed, so pharmacists must be vigilant when interpreting therapeutic orders.

Epirubicin Hydrochloride This stereoisomer of doxorubicin has the 4′-hydroxy group of the daunosamine sugar oriented in the unnatural β-position. However, this relatively modest structural change has a large impact on pharmacokinetic properties. Epirubicin is reduced to the C_{13} alcohol (epirubicinol) to a much lower (60%) extent than doxorubicin, and it is not highly susceptible to ROS-generating one-electron oxidation. The overall cardiotoxicity has been estimated at 30% lower than doxorubicin, but the margin of safety is mitigated somewhat by epirubicin's greater propensity to accumulate in myocardiocytes (83). The epirubicinol metabolite has an antitumor potency one-tenth that of the parent drug and does not contribute significantly to the therapeutic action. Both parent drug and metabolite readily undergo *O*-dealkylation/glucuronidation, resulting in a shortened terminal half-life compared to doxorubicin. Cleavage to the aglycone will occur prior to elimination (57,83). Although excretion is primarily biliary, dosage reduction in severe renal impairment, as well as in hepatic dysfunction, is warranted.

Epirubicin is indicated for use in breast cancer, and the starting dose is 100 to 120 mg/m^2 (compared to a starting dose of 60 to 75 mg/m^2 for doxorubicin). The side effects and precautions are as outlined previously for doxorubicin, although, as noted, there is a lower risk of serious myocardial toxicity or myelotoxicity.

Valrubicin Chemically, valrubicin differs from its doxorubicin parent by the addition of a C_{14}-valerate ester and a 3′-trifluoroacetamide moiety. The carbon-rich valerate is obviously lipophilic, and acylation of the daunosamine amino group makes the 3′-substituent nonionizable. Both of these structural changes promote a more rapid and extensive penetration into tumor cells.

Valrubicin currently has orphan drug status in the treatment of bacille Calmette-Guérin–refractory bladder cancer (the total patient population is ~1,000 individuals) and is used in patients for whom surgical intervention would result in high morbidity or death. It is administered directly into the bladder through a catheter (intravesically). The lipophilic drug is water insoluble, but it dissolves in an aqueous vehicle that includes polyethoxylated castor oil (Cremophor EL) and ethanol. The patient retains the drug in the bladder for 2 hours and then voids the solution in the normal fashion.

Valrubicin is an active antineoplastic as administered, although it does not function as a TopIIα poison. Rather, the intact drug inhibits the incorporation of nucleosides into DNA and RNA, which induces chromosomal damage and cell cycle arrest (92). Despite the fact that hydrolysis of the ester and trifluoroacetamide can be readily envisioned, it is excreted essentially unchanged. Less than 1% of an administered dose is absorbed systemically, so there is essentially no exposure to metabolizing enzymes. The reduced C_{13}-alcoholic metabolite does not form to any appreciable extent during the 2-hour treatment period. Therapy is considered to be almost exclusively local, and there is little risk for cardiac toxicity, bone marrow suppression, drug–drug interactions, or other side effects. Systemic exposure to the drug and its hydrolyzed (and cardiotoxic) metabolites *N*-trifluoroacetyldoxorubicin and *N*-trifluoroacetyldoxorubicinol would, of course, be greater in patients whose bladder wall integrity has been compromised by disease. These patients should not receive valrubicin. The most commonly reported adverse reactions to valrubicin are abdominal pain, urinary tract infection, hematuria, and dysuria. Some patients experience severe allergic reactions, most probably due to the Cremophor EL solubilizer that is notorious for inducing hypersensitivity reactions. Unlike other anthracyclines, valrubicin is not necrotic to skin.

Daunorubicin Hydrochloride The absence of the OH group at C_{14} in daunorubicin results in a faster conversion to the less active and chronically cardiotoxic C_{13}-ol metabolite (daunorubicinol) compared to hydroxymethyl-substituted anthracyclines like doxorubicin. The 18.5-hour terminal half-life of daunorubicin is approximately half that of doxorubicin, and the terminal half-life of the daunorubicinol metabolite is 26.7 hours. Excretion is approximately 40% biliary and 25% urinary. Daunorubicin is administered intravenously at a dose of 45 mg/m^2 for the treatment of lymphocytic and nonlymphocytic leukemia. The toxicity and side effect profile of this anthracycline is similar to that of doxorubicin, and all previously identified precautions apply.

The citrate salt of daunorubicin is marketed as a liposomal formulation, which promotes the use of this agent in solid tumors. Like Doxil (the liposomal formulation of doxorubicin), DaunoXome is indicated for use in AIDS-related Kaposi sarcoma and is administered intravenously at a dose of 40 mg/m^2 every 2 weeks. The pharmacokinetic profiles of Doxil and DaunoXome are similar.

Idarubicin Hydrochloride Idarubicin is the 4-desmethoxy analog of daunorubicin. The loss of the C_4-ether flattens the D ring, facilitating intercalation between DNA base pairs. In turn, this orients the daunosamine sugar in the minor groove in a way that better stabilizes the ternary complex between drug, DNA, and topoisomerase (76).

The loss of the 4-methoxy moiety also makes this compound more lipophilic than either doxorubicin or daunorubicin. This results in a better penetration into tumor cells and an enhanced antineoplastic potency. Increased rates of remission have been noted with the use of idarubicin compared to other anthracycline antineoplastic agents. Unlike its congeners, idarubicin shows significant oral bioavailability and is lipophilic enough to penetrate the blood–brain barrier. Currently, it is given only by the intravenous route and is not used in the treatment of brain cancer. Its primary indication is in acute myeloid leukemia, and it is administered in combination with other antileukemic drugs.

Idarubicin is reduced by aldoketoreductases to idarubicinol which, unlike other rubicinols, is as active an antitumor agent as the parent drug (88). Because there is no aromatic methoxy group, there is no *O*-dealkylation to the C_4-phenol. The major metabolite is free, unconjugated idarubicinol. The half-lives of idarubicin and idarubicinol are 22 and 45 hours, respectively. Idarubicin is administered intravenously at a dose of 10 to 12 mg/m^2/day for 3 to 4 days, and the idarubicinol metabolite can still be found in therapeutic concentrations in the blood 8 days after administration. Like other anthracyclines, excretion primarily is fecal, with a lesser dependence on renal elimination. Some authors have shown that idarubicin is transported into cardiac tissue via a saturable transporter and that the coadministration of methylxanthines (e.g., caffeine) can increase both myocardial drug concentrations and the risk of idarubicin-induced cardiotoxicity (93).

Mitoxantrone Hydrochloride Chemically, mitoxantrone is classified as an anthracenedione. The sugar moiety is missing, but the cationic side-chain amino nitrogens could bind to the anionic phosphate residue of the DNA backbone in the same fashion that the cationic L-daunosamine amino group of the true anthracyclines has been presumed to do. This molecule has the structural features needed to intercalate DNA and inhibit TopIIα, but the enhanced stability of the quinone ring (possibly through an increased potential for intramolecular hydrogen bonding) makes the ring highly resistant to NADPH/CYP450 reductase. This limits the formation of the highly toxic ROS. In addition, there is no active cardiotoxic metabolite to induce chronic toxicity by disrupting the movement of myocardial cations. The chance of cardiovascular toxicity from mitoxantrone is significantly decreased, although patients who have been previously treated with anthracycline antineoplastics may still be at risk. It is thought that any observed myocardial toxicity may be operating through mechanisms other than the generation of cytotoxic radicals.

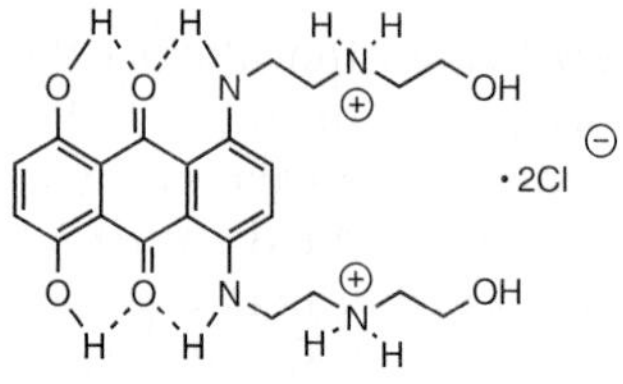

In addition, the risk of ulceration and necrosis on extravasation, as well as of non–marrow-related toxicities such as nausea, vomiting, mucositis, and alopecia, is significantly less than observed with true anthracyclines. There is a significant risk of bone marrow suppression, however. The risk of myelosuppression increases with dose, but it can be observed even when low doses are used.

Mitoxantrone excretion primarily is biliary. Both the unchanged drug and inactive metabolites resulting from *N*-dealkylation, deamination, and oxidation of the resultant aldehyde to the carboxylic acid are observed. Both arms of the structure can be metabolized, leading to mono- or dicarboxylic acid metabolites (Fig. 37.26), which are excreted as the glucuronide conjugate. The conjugated metabolites are an intense, dark blue in color and will result in blue-green excrement. The whites of the eyes and, in some cases, the skin may also take on a bluish cast.

Mitoxantrone is used in combination with other agents during the initial treatment of acute nonlymphocytic leukemia and hormone-refractory prostate cancer. Mitoxantrone also decreases the rate of relapse and disease progression in patients with multiple sclerosis (94). Although too toxic for use in patients with primary progressive disease, it is available for the treatment of chronic progressive, progressive relapsing, or deteriorating relapsing-remitting multiple sclerosis.

Miscellaneous Antibiotics (Fig. 37.22)

Dactinomycin Dactinomycin has two pentapeptide lactones attached to an aromatic (and, therefore, flat) actinocin (or phenoxazinone) structure. It is capable of intercalating DNA and binds preferably between guanine and cytosine residues on a single DNA strand. This interaction results in DNA elongation and distortion, commonly referred to as a point mutation. When sliding between adjacent DNA base pairs, the actinocin orients itself perpendicular to the main DNA axis, allowing the pentapeptide lactone units to bind to residues in the minor groove of DNA through hydrophobic and

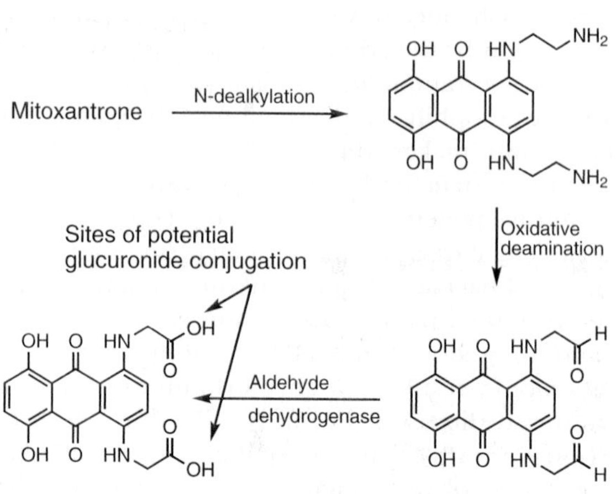

FIGURE 37.26 Mitoxantrone metabolism.

hydrogen bonds. An affinity-enhancing bond between the threonine carbonyl oxygen and a protonated C_2-amino group of guanine also forms. Other hydrogen, hydrophobic, and π-stacking interactions form between the lactone and DNA residues, particularly guanine and cytosine.

The binding of the actinocin and polypeptide lactone portions of dactinomycin to DNA is cooperative, meaning that the binding of one unit facilitates the binding of the other, most likely by promoting an optimal orientation. This significantly enhances drug-DNA affinity. The binding of dactinomycin to DNA, although noncovalent, is much stronger than that observed with the anthracyclines. Drug dissociation from DNA is slow, leading to a pseudoirreversible effect. Dactinomycin blocks gene transcription and translation processes, and RNA polymerase is inhibited, resulting in a decrease in de novo RNA (especially mRNA) and protein synthesis. A recent study has also documented the drug's ability to inhibit the polymerization of oligonucleotides containing the oncogenic c-Myc promoter G-quadruplex sequence through direct binding to this DNA segment (95).

The *p*-benzoquinoneimine segment of dactinomycin renders the molecule vulnerable to NADPH/CYP450 reductase. Free radicals can be generated, and additional single-strand DNA breaks can result. The loss of either aromatic methyl group results in a loss of activity. The reason for this profound impact on pharmacologic action and therapeutic utility is unknown.

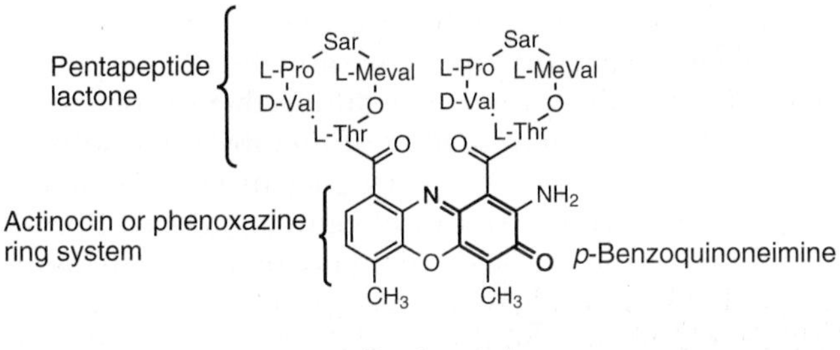

Dactinomycin

Dactinomycin is used for the treatment of various solid tumors and muscle-related cancers. It induces severe side effects, and nausea and vomiting can be use-limiting. Myelosuppression is also common and, most often, is the dose-limiting toxic effect. The drug is usually given by the intravenous route, but toxicity can be limited if the tumor can be perfused with drug (assuming minimal distribution into the general circulation). Dactinomycin is a severe blistering agent, and extravasation can cause irreversible and profound tissue damage. The side effects of radiation therapy are significantly exaggerated by the concurrent use of dactinomycin. The drug's 36-hour half-life is the result of a very high affinity for DNA, a large volume of distribution, and minimal metabolic breakdown. Dactinomycin is photosensitive and must be protected from light.

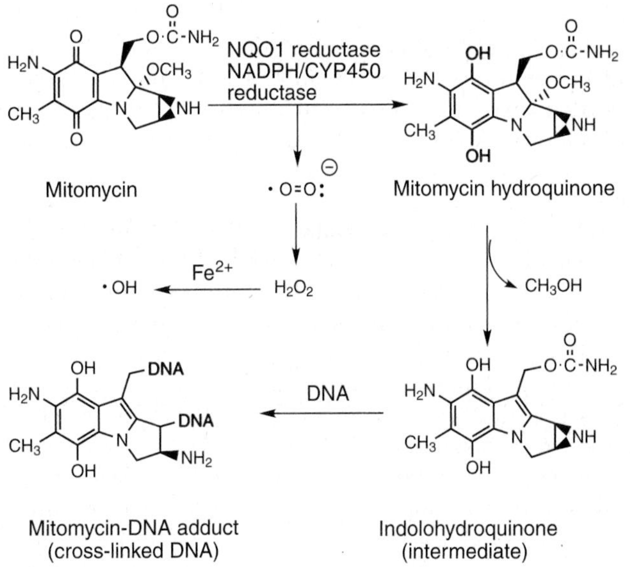

FIGURE 37.27 Mitomycin metabolism.

Mitomycin As shown in Figure 37.27, mitomycin is activated through a two-electron bioreductive process using NADPH/CYP450 reductase and/or NAD(P)H quinone oxidoreductase 1 (NQO1 reductase), an enzyme extensively expressed in many neoplastic cells (96–99). Through these enzymes, the quinone ring of mitomycin is readily reduced to the hydroquinone, generating superoxide radicals in the process that ultimately will be converted to cytotoxic hydroxyl radicals through the Fenton reaction. As previously discussed, hydroxyl radicals induce single-strand breaks in DNA. Formation of the hydroquinone is followed by aromatization to the indole ring through the loss of methanol. Both the electrophilic aziridine ring and the δ^+ methylene group adjacent to the carbamate ester are vulnerable to attack by DNA nucleophiles, such as the $2\text{-}NH_2$ group of guanine or the $4\text{-}NH_2$ group of cytosine, and can conceivably result in cross-linked DNA and cell death. The fact that mitomycin activating enzymes are predominantly cytosolic has brought into question the nuclear mechanisms long thought operational with this antibiotic. A recent report has provided evidence for 18S rRNA as the true therapeutically relevant target of mitomycin. Through the inhibition of cytosolic rRNA, mitomycin would induce cell death through "genome-wide translational silencing" (98).

Mitomycin is administered intravenously in the treatment of disseminated adenocarcinoma of the stomach or pancreas, and it has been used intravesically in superficial bladder cancer. Biotransformation pathways are saturable, and approximately 10% of an administered dose is eliminated unchanged via the kidneys. Myelosuppression is the major use-limiting side effect of this drug, which is slow to manifest but quite prolonged in duration. Severe skin necrosis can occur on extravasation, and potentially fatal pulmonary toxicities have been noted as well. Mitomycin can induce hemolytic uremia accompanied by irreversible renal dysfunction and thrombocytopenia, and the drug should not be administered to patients with serum creatinine levels greater than 1.7 mg/dL. Severe bronchospasm has also been noted in patients treated with vinca alkaloids who are also receiving (or who have previously received) mitomycin.

Bleomycin The commercially available bleomycin drug product is a mixture of naturally occurring glycopeptides, predominantly bleomycin A_2. Through DNA intercalation, the aromatic bithiazole ring system positions bleomycin for DNA destruction via cytotoxic free radicals. The disaccharide, polyamine, imidazole, and pyrimidine structures are very electron rich and readily chelate intracellular Fe^{2+}. Once chelated, Fe^{2+} is oxidized to Fe^{3+} with a concomitant reduction of bound oxygen. The ferric hydroperoxide bleomycin complex is considered the cytotoxic form (100). Through the direct abstraction of a hydrogen atom from 4′ of deoxyribose, a free radical is generated that subsequently decomposes to a highly electrophilic base propenal that inactivates essential cellular proteins via Cys alkylation (Fig. 37.28). Reduced GSH is proposed to serve a protective role by acting as propenal scavenger and, until depleted, saves cellular proteins from alkylation (101).

Bleomycin is a natural product isolated from *Streptomyces verticillus*. It is normally chelated with Cu^{2+}, which must be removed via catalytic reduction before marketing. This increases the cost of the drug, but it frees up the critical bleomycin functional groups for chelation with intracellular Fe^{2+}.

The action of bleomycin is terminated through the action of bleomycin hydrase, a cytosolic aminopeptidase that cleaves the terminal amide moiety to form the inactive carboxylate metabolite (Fig. 37.29). The metabolic replacement of the electron-withdrawing amide with an electron-donating carboxylate increases the pK_a of

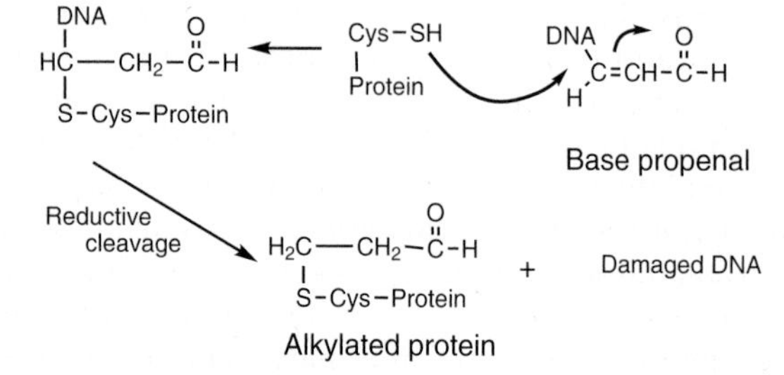

FIGURE 37.28 Mechanism of bleomycin-induced DNA cleavage.

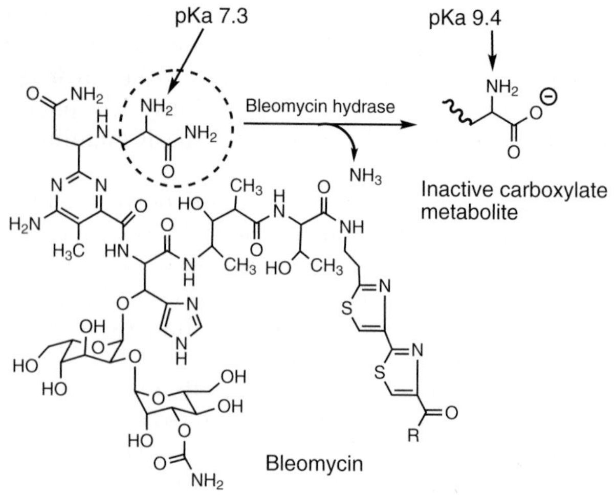

FIGURE 37.29 Bleomycin hydrase-mediated inactivation of bleomycin.

the α-amino group, which normally interacts with DNA in the un-ionized conjugate form. After hydrolysis, the ratio of ionized to un-ionized forms of this critical amine increases approximately 126-fold, destroying DNA affinity and leading to the loss of therapeutic action. Drug destruction via the bleomycin hydrase pathway is rapid, and tumors will be resistant to bleomycin if they contain high concentrations of the enzyme. Conversely, tumors that are poor in bleomycin hydrase (e.g., squamous cell carcinoma) respond well to this agent.

Bleomycin hydrase is found in all tissues except skin and lung. Approximately 10% of patients who are administered bleomycin will experience potentially fatal pulmonary fibrosis, which can occur during therapy or several months following termination of therapy, often without warning. The copper-complexing agent tetrathiomolybdate may reduce the risk of bleomycin-induced fibrosis by inhibiting the action of copper-dependent inflammatory cytokines (102). A recent report also supports the protective effect of inhibitors of the N-terminal catalytic site of angiotensin-converting enzyme (e.g., *N*-acetyl-Ser-Asp-Lys-Pro or AcSDKP) (103). Erythema and hypertrophic modifications in skin are also common side effects that manifest after 2 to 3 weeks of bleomycin therapy.

Bleomycin is used intravenously in the palliative treatment of squamous cell head and neck cancers, testicular and other genital carcinomas, Hodgkin's lymphoma, and NHL. It is excreted via the kidneys, and serum concentrations of active drug are increased in patients with renal disease. The elimination half-life can rise from 2 to 4 hours to more than 20 hours in renal failure, resulting in significant toxicity, especially pulmonary toxicity. Dosage adjustments are warranted. Unlike many antineoplastic agents, bleomycin does not suppress the bone marrow, and it is often given in combination with compounds that do so that the dose of all drugs can be optimized. Nausea and vomiting are also relatively mild, but approximately 1% of lymphoma patients who are treated with bleomycin will experience an immediate or delayed severe idiosyncratic reaction that mimics anaphylaxis.

Antimetabolites

MECHANISM OF ACTION The antineoplastic agents discussed thus far have all damaged existing DNA (or, less commonly, RNA) and inhibited its ability to replicate. The antimetabolites, on the other hand, most commonly stop the de novo synthesis of DNA by inhibiting the formation of the nucleotides that make up these life-sustaining polymers. We will see that the rate-limiting enzymes of nucleotide biosynthesis are often the primary targets for the antimetabolites since inhibition of these key enzymes is the most efficient way to shut down any biochemical reaction sequence. Antimetabolites are also capable of inhibiting other enzymes required in the biosynthesis of DNA, and many can arrest chain elongation by promoting the incorporation of false nucleotides into the growing DNA strand.

The antimetabolites serve as false substrates for critical nucleotide biosynthesis enzymes. These enzyme inhibitors are structurally "dolled up" to look like a super attractive version of the normal (endogenous) substrate. Speaking anthropomorphically, through a form of chemical entrapment, they entice the enzymes to choose them over the endogenous substrate and, once they do, the antimetabolites bind them irreversibly or pseudoirreversibly. If the building block nucleotides cannot be synthesized, then DNA synthesis (and tumor growth) is stopped dead in its tracks. If tumor growth is arrested, then metastasis slows, and the patient has a fighting chance for remission and/or cure.

Many antimetabolite antineoplastics are categorized by the class of nucleotide they inhibit. Purine antagonists inhibit the synthesis of the purine-based nucleotides adenosine monophosphate (AMP) and guanosine monophosphate (GMP), and the pyrimidine antagonists stop the production of the pyrimidine-based nucleotides, primarily deoxythymidine monophosphate (dTMP).

Pyrimidine Antagonists: dTMP Synthesis Inhibitors

DTMP BIOSYNTHESIS Looked at simply, dTMP is produced via C_5-methylation of deoxyuridine monophosphate (dUMP). The rate-limiting enzyme of the dTMP synthetic pathway is the sulfhydryl-containing thymidylate synthase, with 5,10-methylenetetrahydrofolate (5,10-methylene-THF) serving as the methyl-donating cofactor. All dTMP synthesis inhibitors will inhibit thymidylate synthase either directly or indirectly, and this will result in a "thymineless death" in actively dividing cells. Without dTMP and its deoxythymidine triphosphate metabolite, DNA will fragment, and the cell will die.

To understand how an antimetabolite inhibits a biochemical pathway, we must first understand completely how the pathway normally functions. A quick look at the dTMP synthesis pathway (Fig. 37.30) will confirm that our "simple methylation reaction" is comprised of several important steps, each of which is analyzed in turn below.

The synthase enzyme is very large and contains a deep pocket for the binding of both substrate and cofactor. It may be illuminating to think of this binding pocket like a big cooking pot. Once the "ingredients" are added (substrate and cofactor), the process of making the product (dTMP) can begin. The active site binding motifs for both substrate and cofactor are highly conserved among all thymidylate synthase enzymes, regardless of source (104). Whereas early studies on binding were conducted with bacteria-derived synthases, the human enzyme (human thymidylate synthase [hTS]) has now been crystallized and some binding residues identified (105,106).

As shown in Figure 37.31 (hTS sequence numbers are given where known), Asp226 forms essential hydrogen bonds with the dUMP pyrimidine 4-oxo and N_3-H moieties, whereas His196 forms a hydrogen bond with the pyrimidine 4-oxo moiety. The main-chain amide of Asp218 forms a hydrogen bond with the pyrimidine 2-oxo moiety. Four arginine residues (50, 175′, 176′, and 215) form electrostatic bonds with the anionic deoxyribose-5′-phosphate, and Tyr (H-donor) and histidine (His) (H-acceptor) residues form hydrogen bonds with the deoxyribose 3′-OH. As noted in the dTMP synthesis pathway (Fig. 37.30), Cys195 forms a transient covalent bond with pyrimidine C_6.

The glutamate tail of 5,10-methylene-THF cofactor binds to Phe80, Lys, and His residues of the synthase, whereas Leu221, Ile108, Phe80, and Phe225 interact with the *p*-aminobenzoic acid component of the folate. Asp218, Leu221, and Phe225 are known to interact with the pteridine portion of the cofactor (Fig. 37.31) (105–107).

The binding of both substrate and cofactor promotes a conformational change in the synthase protein and causes the N-terminal portion of the synthase to change its location, which covers the opening of the binding "pot" like a big lid. The conformational change positions the pteridine ring of the folate cofactor "face to face" with the dUMP substrate, permitting the ring stacking that properly orients all key functional groups for the reaction to come (106).

CHEMISTRY The C_6 position of the dUMP substrate is surrounded by electron-withdrawing nitrogen and oxygen atoms, leaving it highly electrophilic (δ^+) and ready to be attacked by the nucleophilic Cys195 of the synthase. The Cys sulfhydryl (SH) group launches an intermolecular nucleophilic attack, forming a new covalent bond between the sulfur and C_6 of the substrate (step 1). The bond that breaks in response to this attack is the 5,6-double bond of dUMP, which attacks the methylene group of the cofactor (step 2). With the release of the N_{10} nitrogen, the cofactor imidazolidine ring breaks (step 3). Taken together, steps 1 to 3 generate a ternary complex of enzyme, substrate, and cofactor (Fig. 37.30).

A series of reactions involving bond breaking and bond making are shown in Figure 37.30, leading to formation of dTMP, 7,8-dihydrofolate (7,8-DHF), and

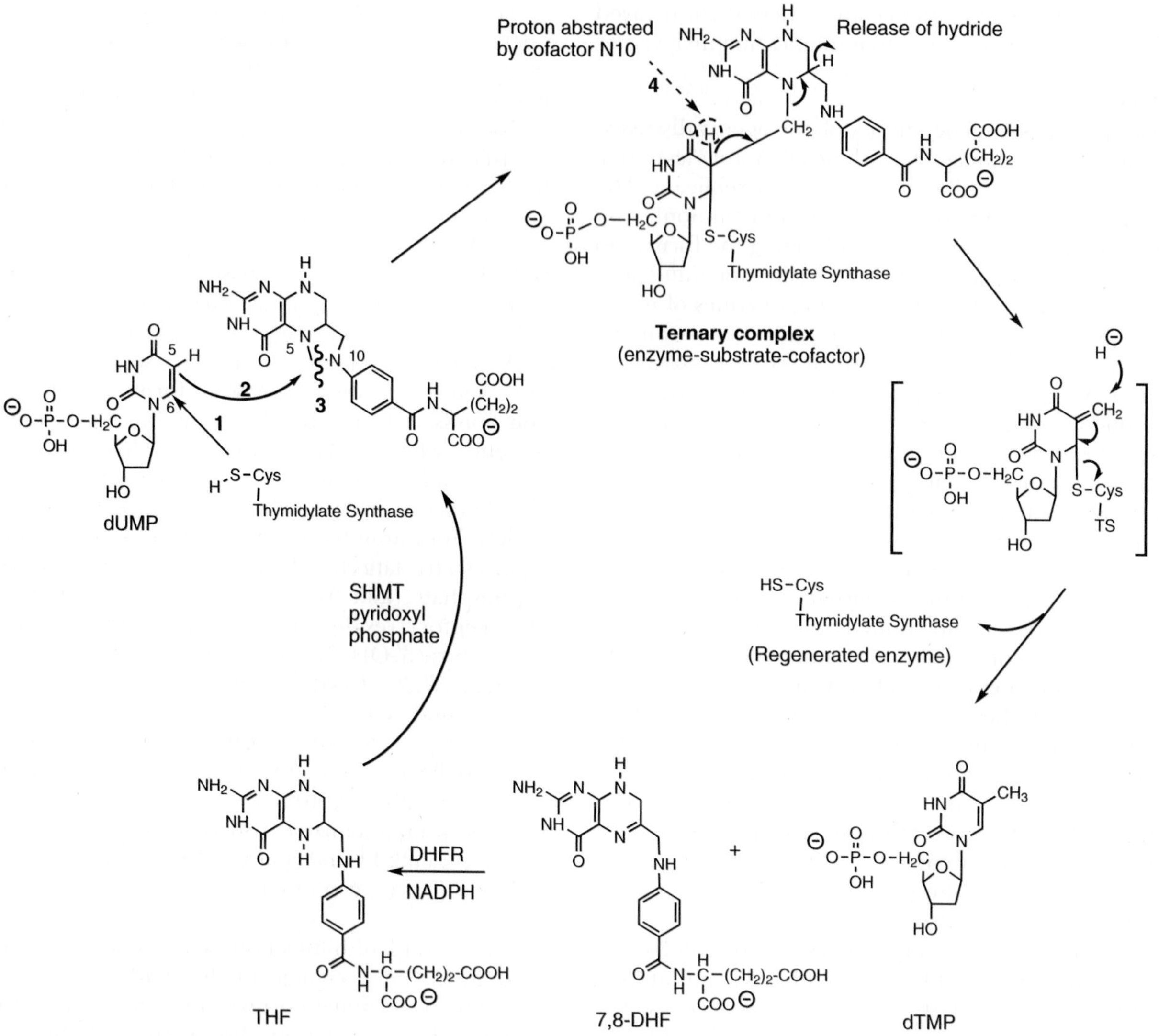

FIGURE 37.30 Synthesis of deoxythymidine monophosphate (dTMP).

regenerated thymidylate synthase. The C_5-H abstraction by N_{10} of the cofactor (step 4) is essential for synthesis of dTMP. To complete the biochemical cycle, 7,8-DHF must be reduced to tetrahydrofolate (THF) via dihydrofolate reductase (DHFR) using NADPH. Finally, THF is converted to 5,10-methylene-THF through the action of serine hydroxymethyltransferase and vitamin B_6.

With the enzyme and cofactor both regenerated and with plenty of dUMP stored in cellular pools, the cell is ready to synthesize another molecule of dTMP. This happens at a regular pace in healthy cells and at an uncontrolled rate in tumor cells.

Specific Drugs: Pyrimidine Analogs (Fig. 37.32)

Fluorouracil To bind to thymidylate synthase, this fluorinated pyrimidine prodrug must be converted to its deoxyribonucleotide form (Fig. 37.33). The active form of fluorouracil differs from the endogenous substrate only by the presence of the 5-fluoro group, which holds the key to the cell-killing action of this drug. The C_6 position of the false substrate is significantly more electrophilic than normal due to the strong electron-withdrawing effect of the C_5 fluorine. This greatly increases the rate of attack by Cys195, resulting in a very fast formation of a fluorinated ternary complex (Fig. 37.34). The small size of the fluorine atom assures no steric hindrance to the formation of this false complex.

The next step in the pathway required the abstraction of the C_5-H (as proton) by N_{10} of the cofactor, but this is no longer possible. Not only is the C_5-fluorine bond stable to cleavage, the fluorine atom and N_{10} would repel one another because they are both electron rich. The false ternary complex cannot break down, no product is formed, no cofactor is released, and most importantly, the rate-limiting enzyme (thymidylate synthase) is not regenerated. With thymidylate synthase directly and irreversibly inhibited, dTMP can no longer be synthesized and the cell will die.

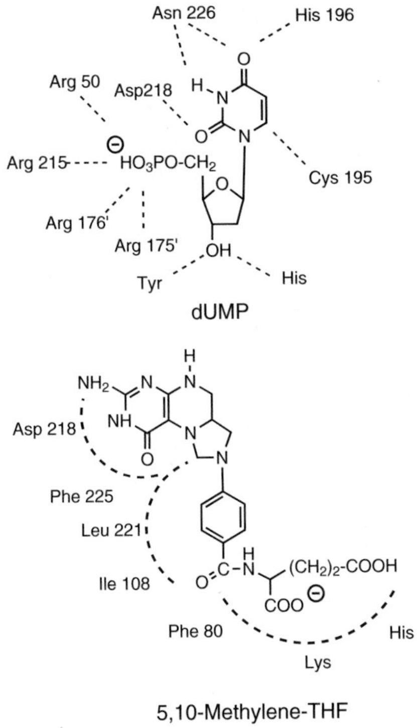

FIGURE 37.31 dUMP and 5,10-methylene-THF binding to thymidylate synthase.

Fluorouracil is administered intravenously in the palliative treatment of colorectal, breast, stomach, and pancreatic cancers. Patients are treated for 4 consecutive days, followed by treatment on odd-numbered days up to a maximum of 12 days. Fluorouracil is rapidly cleared from the bloodstream, and although up to 20% of a dose is excreted unchanged in the urine, most undergoes hepatic catabolism via a series of enzymes that includes the polymorphic dihydropyrimidine dehydrogenase (DPD) (Fig. 37.35). Patients who are genetically deficient in this enzyme (~5% of the population) will experience a more pronounced effect from this drug and are at significant risk for use-limiting or life-threatening toxicity unless doses are appropriately adjusted (108). It has been estimated that between 40% and 60% of patients who experience severe toxicity from fluorouracil are deficient in DPD (109). The incidence of DPD deficiency in African Americans is threefold higher than in Caucasians, and black women have a threefold higher incidence of DPD deficiency than black men (109). In patients with normal DPD activity, dosage adjustments are usually not required in hepatic or renal dysfunction. Major toxicities are related to bone marrow depression, stomatitis/esophagopharyngitis, and potential GI ulceration. Nausea and vomiting are common. Solutions of fluorouracil are light sensitive, but discolored products that have been properly stored and protected from light are still safe to use.

Floxuridine This deoxyribonucleoside prodrug is bioconverted via 2′-deoxyuridine kinase–mediated phosphorylation to the same active 5-fluoro-dUMP structure generated in the multistep biotransformation of fluorouracil (Fig. 37.33). It is given by intra-arterial infusion for the palliative treatment of GI adenocarcinoma that has metastasized to the liver and that cannot be managed surgically. Because floxuridine does not generate fluorouracil, its kinetic profile is not impacted by DPD pharmacogenetic status.

Capecitabine Although capecitabine is a carbamylated analog of cytidine, the drug actually is another 5-fluoro-dUMP prodrug (Fig. 37.36). Given orally, it is extensively metabolized to fluorouracil, which is then converted to the active fluorinated deoxyribonucleotide as previously described. Thymidine phosphorylase, an enzyme involved in this biotransformation, is much more active in tumors than in normal tissue, which improves the tumor-selective generation of fluorouracil. Levels of active drug in the tumor can be up to 3.5-fold higher than in surrounding tissue, leading to a lower incidence of side effects compared to fluorouracil therapy (110). Because capecitabine is biotransformed to fluorouracil, it follows the same catabolic and elimination pathways reported for fluorouracil (Figs. 37.33 and 37.35). Doses should be attenuated in moderate to severe renal impairment, and the caution relative to the augmented risk of toxicity in patients with dihydropyrimidine dehydrogenase deficiency applies.

Capecitabine is indicated for use as first-line therapy in patients with colorectal cancer. It is also used alone or in combination with docetaxel in patients with metastatic breast cancer who have experienced disease progression or recurrence after anthracycline therapy. Given twice daily in tablet form, the total daily dose is calculated based on patient body surface area and is taken 30 minutes after eating to avoid food-induced decreases in absorption. In addition to bone marrow suppression, nausea, and vomiting, the drug can induce severe diarrhea and a potentially disabling disorder termed "hand-and-foot syndrome" (palmar-plantar erythrodysesthesia).

Capecitabine inhibits CYP2C9 and, along with competition for serum protein binding sites, results in clinically significant drug–drug interactions with both warfarin and phenytoin. The interaction with warfarin can result in potentially fatal bleeding episodes, which can appear within days of combination therapy or be delayed up to 1 month after discontinuation of capecitabine therapy.

SPECIFIC DRUGS: ANTIFOLATES (FIG. 37.32)

Methotrexate Methotrexate is a folic acid antagonist structurally designed to compete successfully with 7,8-DHF for the DHFR enzyme. The direct inhibition of DHFR causes cellular levels of 7,8-DHF to build up, which in turn results in feedback (indirect) inhibition of thymidylate synthase. Methotrexate is also effective in inhibiting glycine amide ribonucleotide (GAR) transformylase

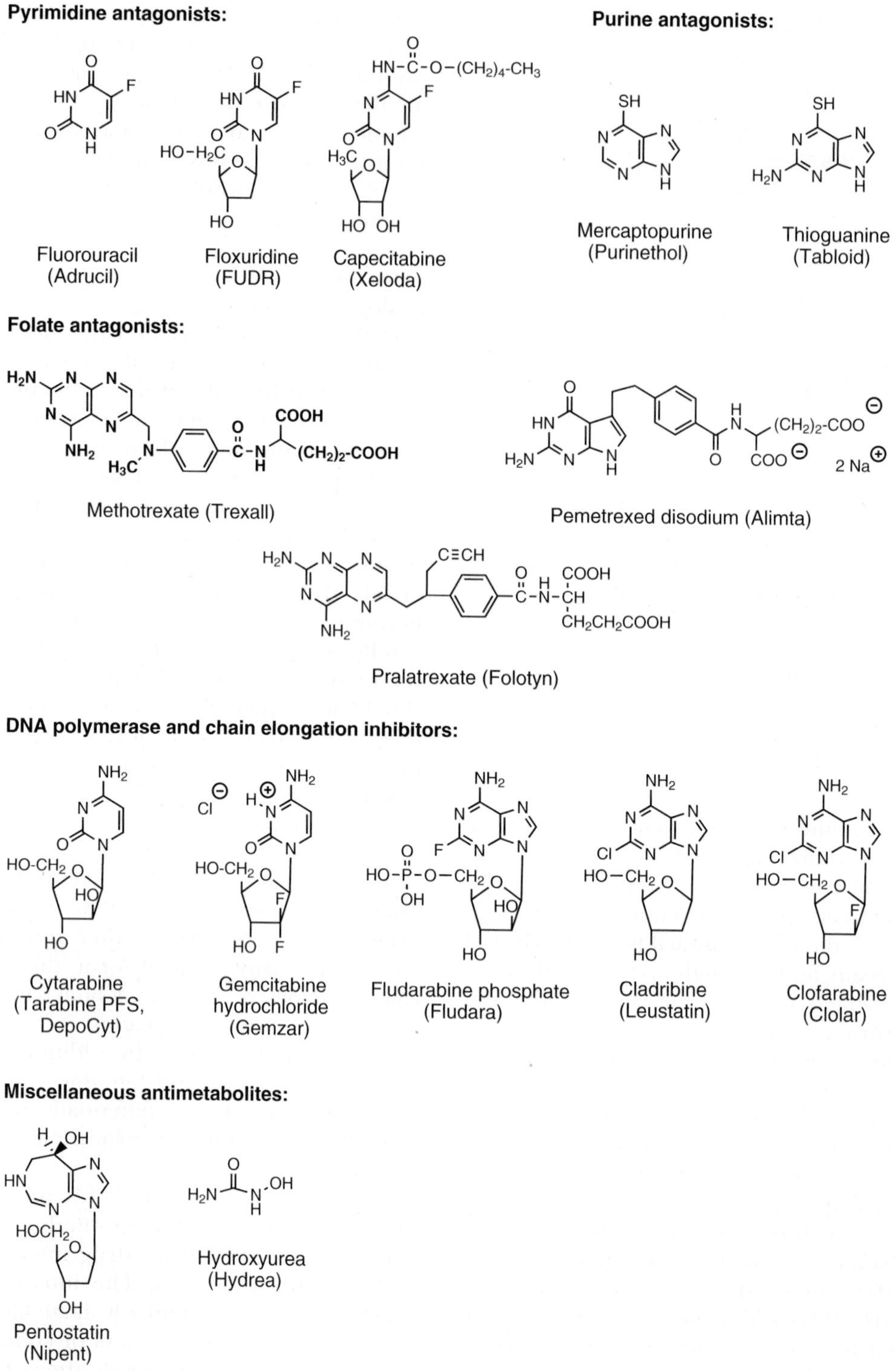

FIGURE 37.32 Antimetabolites.

(see Fig. 37.38), a key enzyme in the synthesis of purine nucleotides.

Methotrexate's C_4-NH_2 substituent, along with its lack of a 7,8-double bond, hold the key to its DHFR-inhibiting action. It has been proposed that the N_5 position of DHF is protonated by Glu30 of DHFR (111) and, in cationic form, binds to DHFR Asp27 through an electrostatic bond (Fig. 37.37). N_5 is the strongest base in the DHF structure, in part due to attenuating the impact of the C_4 carbonyl on electron density around N_1. Additional affinity-enhancing interactions between enzyme and substrate have also been identified (112,113), and once bound, the substrate's 5,6-double bond is positioned close to the NADPH cofactor so that the transfer of hydride can proceed.

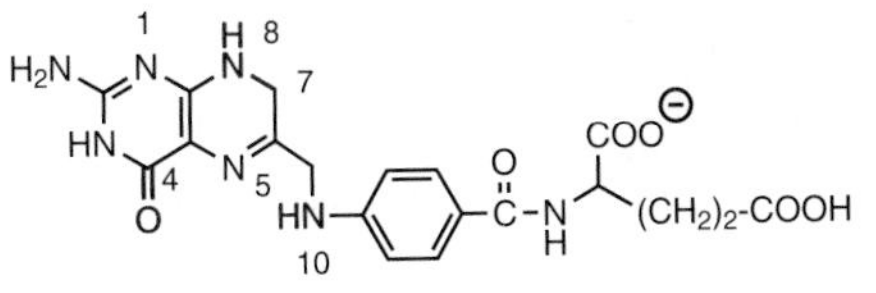

7,8-Dihydrofolate

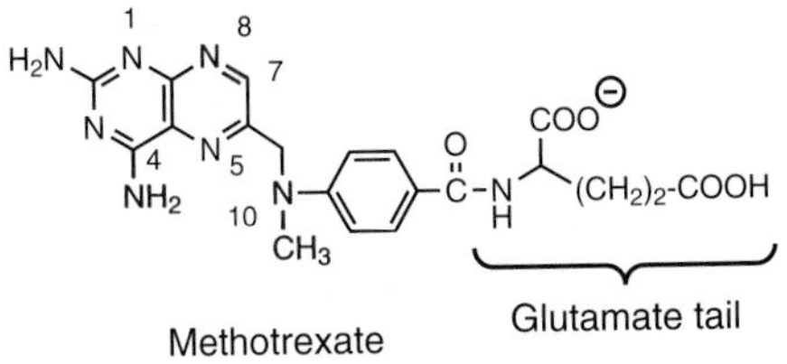

Methotrexate

In contrast, the C_4-NH_2 substituent of methotrexate enriches electron density at N_1 through π-electron donation, increasing its basic character between 10- and 1,000-fold and promoting protonation by Glu30 at the expense of N_5. Because N_1 and N_5 are across the pteridine ring from one another, the interaction of N_1 with the DHFR Asp27 will effectively stand the false substrate

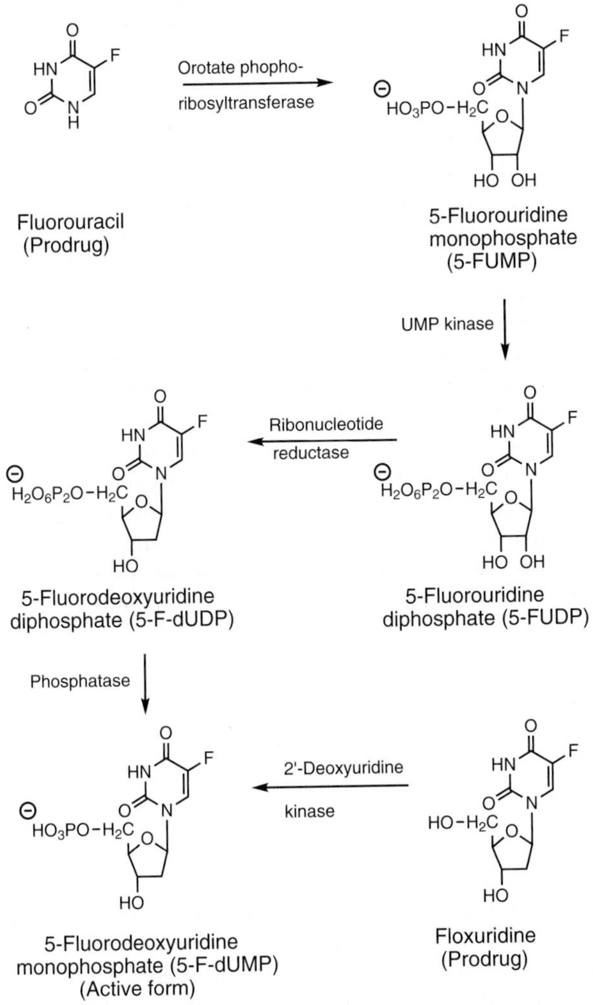

FIGURE 37.33 Activation of fluorouracil and floxuridine.

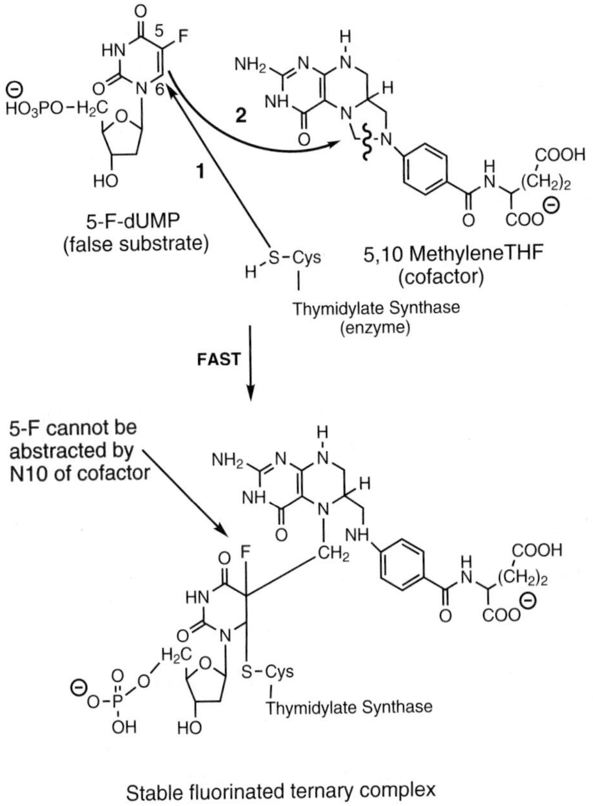

FIGURE 37.34 Mechanism of action of fluorouracil.

"on its head" relative to the orientation of 7,8-DHF (Fig. 37.37) (113,114). With the 5,6-double bond of methotrexate 180 degrees away from the bound NADPH cofactor and stabilized by the fully aromatic pteridine ring, the possibility for reduction is eliminated (113). The DHFR enzyme will be pseudoirreversibly bound to a molecule it cannot reduce, which ties up the DHFR enzyme and prevents the conversion of DHF to THF. In turn, this halts the synthesis of the 5,10-methylene-THF cofactor required for dTMP biosynthesis and causes feedback inhibition of the thymidylate synthase enzyme. The cell will die a "thymineless death."

Methotrexate is given orally in the treatment of breast, head and neck, and various lung cancers as well as in NHL. The sodium salt form is also marketed for intravenous, intramuscular, intra-arterial, or intrathecal injection. Oral absorption is dose-dependent and peaks at 80 mg/m^2 due to site saturation. The monoglutamate tail of methotrexate permits active transport into cells via a reduced folate carrier (RFC1), which predominates at serum concentration levels lower than 100 μmol/L. Methotrexate undergoes intracellular folyl polyglutamate synthase (FPGS)-catalyzed polyglutamation, which adds several anionic carboxylate groups to the molecule and traps the drug at the site of action. Polyglutamation is more efficient in tumor cells than in healthy cells, which promotes the selective toxicity of this drug. The polyglutamated drug will be hydrolyzed back

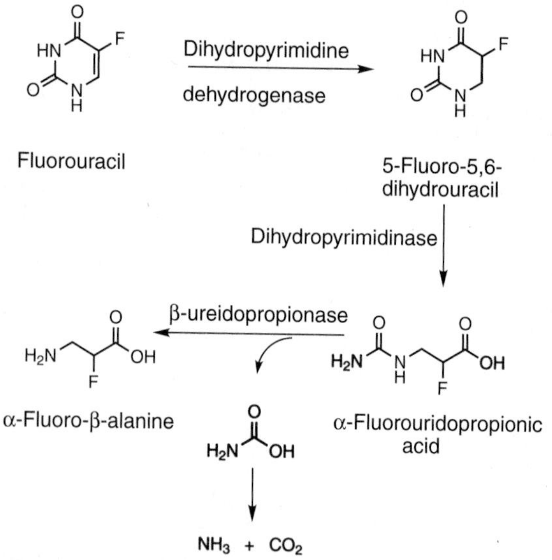

FIGURE 37.35 Fluorouracil metabolism.

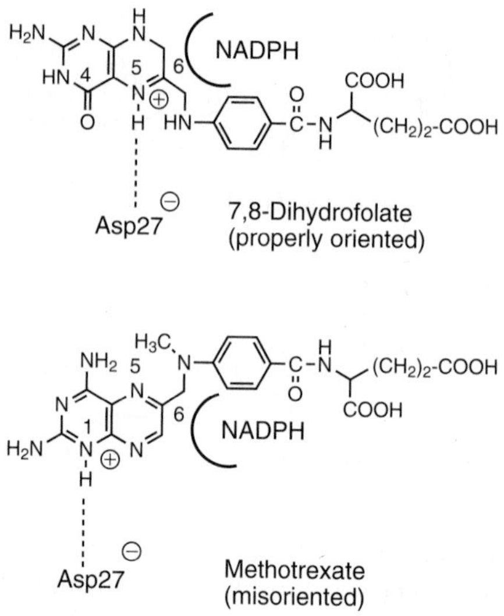

FIGURE 37.37 Misorientation of methotrexate at DHFR.

to the parent structure before renal elimination. Up to 90% of an administered dose of methotrexate is excreted unchanged in the urine within 24 hours.

Methotrexate toxicity occurs with high doses if "third space" fluids allow drug to accumulate in ascites and pleural effusions and/or when renal excretion is impaired by kidney disease. When used in high doses, methotrexate and its 7-hydroxymetabolite (which has a three- to fivefold lower water solubility) can precipitate in the renal tubule, causing damaging crystalluria. Methotrexate-induced lung disease is a particularly critical problem because it arises at any time and at any dose and can be fatal. Methotrexate use also precipitates severe GI side effects, including ulcerative stomatitis and hemorrhagic enteritis, leading to intestinal perforation. Potentially fatal skin reactions are a risk as well. As a Category X teratogen, this drug should not be given to women who are pregnant or planning to become pregnant.

If severe methotrexate toxicity occurs, reduced folate replacement therapy with 5-formyltetrahydrofolate (leucovorin) must be initiated as soon as possible. Leucovorin generates the folate cofactors needed by DHFR and GAR transformylase to ensure the continued synthesis of pyrimidine and purine nucleotides in healthy cells. "Leucovorin rescue" therapy is often given as prophylaxis after high-dose methotrexate therapy.

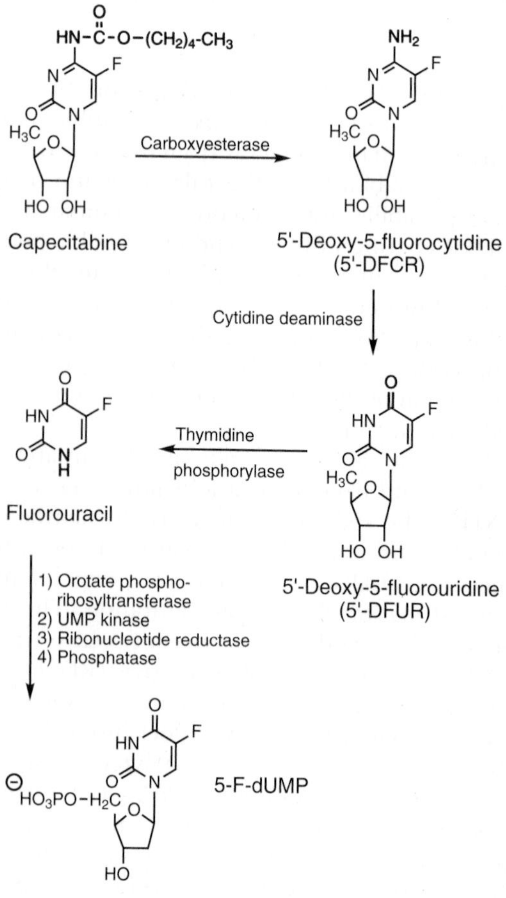

FIGURE 37.36 Capecitabine activation.

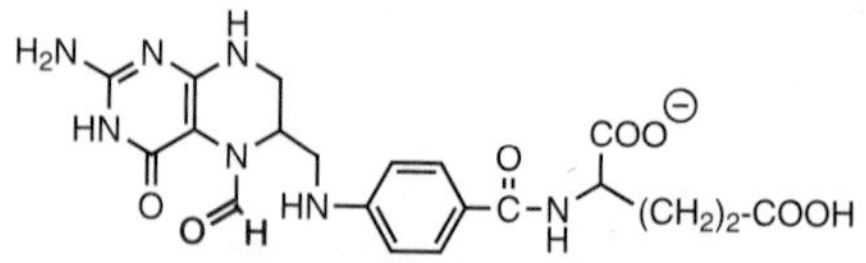

5-Formyltetrahydrofolate
(Leucovorin)

Cancer cells can become resistant to methotrexate over time. Acquired resistance mechanisms include increased DHFR expression, impaired transport, active cellular efflux, and/or attenuated intracellular polyglutamation.

Pemetrexed Disodium Pemetrexed is a novel multitarget antifolate administered by the intravenous route for the treatment of advanced or metastatic nonsquamous non-small cell lung cancer (115) and in combination with cisplatin in malignant pleural mesothelioma. Like methotrexate, it is actively transported into tumor cells via RFC1. Pemetrexed has a higher affinity for FPGS than methotrexate, so more polyglutamated drug is generated (and trapped) inside the cancer cell. Tetra- and pentaglutamates predominate. Both mono- and polyglutamated forms of pemetrexed are capable of inhibiting DHFR, and they do so with comparable activity (116,117). Unlike methotrexate, pemetrexed does not distribute centrally to any significant extent (117).

In addition to DHFR, polyglutamated pemetrexed (but not the monoglutamated parent) binds tightly to thymidylate synthase and GAR transformylase (116,118,119). Since intracellular polyglutamation of pemetrexed is so efficient, this drug realizes a significant portion of its potent anticancer activity through the inhibition of these two enzymes. In fact, thymidylate synthase is considered its primary target. Fortunately, the affinities of the polyglutamated forms of pemetrexed for this enzyme are higher than that of the monoglutamate parent form, so efficacy is not sacrificed for enhanced localization at the site of action. Pemetrexed is often used in combination with the organometallic cisplatin (116). A synergistic effect with gemcitabine (a DNA polymerase inhibitor) in the treatment of lung cancer patients has also been noted as long as gemcitabine is administered immediately prior to the antifolate (117).

Patients on pemetrexed must take folic acid (commonly 400 μg daily) and vitamin B_{12} (1 g on an established schedule) to reduce the risk of bone marrow suppression (neutropenia, thrombocytopenia, and anemia) and use-limiting GI side effects like mucositis and stomatitis. Pretreatment with corticosteroids can reduce the risk of drug-induced skin rash. Antiemetic therapy to proactively combat drug-induced nausea and vomiting is also warranted (117). Pemetrexed has a half-life of 3.5 hours and is excreted primarily unchanged via the kidneys.

Resistance to pemetrexed is mediated through a decrease in FPGS activity, enhanced hydrolysis of pemetrexed polyglutamates via γ-glutamyl hydrolase enzymes, and upregulation of the thymidylate synthase target. Significant cross-resistance has been noted between pemetrexed and other pyrimidine and folate antagonists (116,120). A recent study has shown that pharmacogenetic differences in ATP-binding cassette (ABC) C11 transporters may be an important predictor of sensitivity to pemetrexed chemotherapy (121). In the ABCC11 SNP 538G>A, the A/A variant (unlike the G/G or G/A) does not promote pemetrexed efflux from the cancer cell. ABCC11 genotype also impacts the nature of earwax, and it has been noted that East Asians (80% to 95% of whom express the A/A variant and have dry earwax) are particularly responsive to pemetrexed–cisplatin chemotherapy. Patients expressing the other ABCC11 variants would be at risk for pemetrexed resistance due to excessive drug efflux.

Pralatrexate The only structural difference between pralatrexate and methotrexate is in the area of N_{10}; pralatrexate is a 10-deaza analog where the carbon atom replacing N_{10} has been substituted with a triple bond-containing propargyl group. This structural alteration results in a significantly enhanced tumor cell uptake via RFC1 and FPGS-mediated polyglutamation compared to methotrexate and pemetrexed without compromising affinity for target enzymes (122,123). The rate of active transport of pralatrexate into tumor cells by RFC1 has been measured at approximately 12 to 14 times that of methotrexate, and a 10-fold higher FPGS polyglutamation efficacy has been estimated (124,125). This translates to more active drug inside the tumor cell for a longer period of time. Pralatrexate is excreted intact in the urine.

Unlike pemetrexed, which is also more extensively polyglutamated than methotrexate, pralatrexate's primary antineoplastic enzymatic target is DHFR. Although it interacts with and inhibits the isolated DHFR enzyme 2- to 3-fold less vigorously than methotrexate (K_i apparent = 26 and 45 nmol/L, respectively), the cellular influx and polyglutamation first-order rate constants (V_{max}/K_m) are 12- and 10-fold greater, respectively (126). Higher concentrations of active polyglutamated drug trapped within the cell provide a more potent DHFR inhibitory effect compared to methotrexate and a greater antitumor response than either methotrexate or pemetrexed (123,126).

Pralatrexate dosing is based on body surface area in order to standardize exposure to active drug. Some T-cell lymphoma patients treated with pralatrexate have achieved complete remission (124). In addition to T-cell lymphoma (127), pralatrexate might eventually find use in the treatment of non-small cell lung cancer and, in combination with the DNA polymerase inhibitor gemcitabine, in NHL. When used in combination with gemcitabine, the synergistic apoptotic effect is maximized when the antifolate is administered before the polymerase inhibitor (126). Pralatrexate is not effective against B-cell lymphoma (125). As with other antifolates, patients on pralatrexate should receive daily folic acid supplementation and vitamin B_{12} to reduce the risk of mucositis/stomatitis and bone marrow suppression. Whereas the latter adverse effect is viewed as a minor risk (126), mucositis has been termed the major dose-limiting adverse reaction, particularly in patients with high levels of methylmalonic acid (128). Unlike methotrexate, acquired resistance to pralatrexate is believed to be more highly dependent on a reduced expression of RFC1 than on an increased expression of DHFR (129).

Purine Antagonists: Amidophosphoribosyl Transferase Inhibitors

AMP AND GMP BIOSYNTHESIS Purine antagonists inhibit the de novo biosynthesis of AMP and GMP. The rate-limiting enzyme in the synthesis of these purine nucleotides is amidophosphoribosyl transferase (also known as phosphoribosylpyrophosphate amido transferase), which is a major target for one of the two thiol-containing purine anticancer antimetabolites on the U.S. market (mercaptopurine).

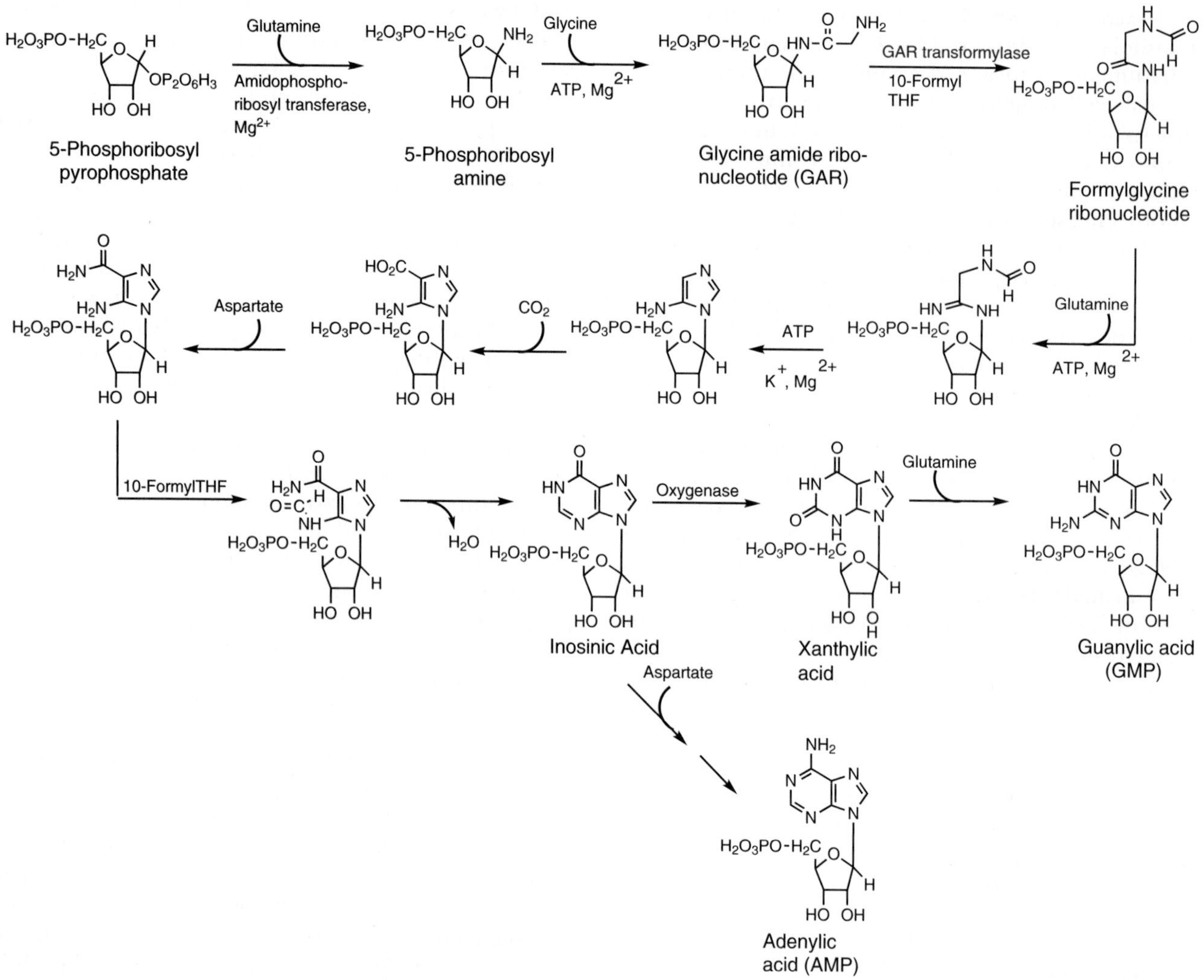

FIGURE 37.38 Biosynthesis of purine nucleotides.

The pathway outlining the synthesis of AMP and GMP is provided in Figure 37.38. It is important to recognize that the rate-limiting step is the first of the pathway; if that step is inhibited, no other step can proceed. Since the rate-limiting transferase enzyme works on a phosphorylated ribose substrate, no enzyme in the sequence will function without its presence. The formylation reaction catalyzed by GAR transformylase requires the methyl-donating 10-formyltetrahydrofolate and can be inhibited by the antifolates methotrexate and pemetrexed.

Chemistry The two currently marketed purine anticancer agents are both 6-thio analogs of the endogenous purine bases guanine and purine, also known as inosine (Fig. 37.32). They are prodrugs and must be converted to ribonucleotides by hypoxanthine guanine phosphoribosyl transferase (HGPRT) before they can exert their cytotoxic actions (Fig. 37.39). Mercaptopurine, acting through a methylated ribonucleotide metabolite, inhibits the target amidophosphoribosyl transferase enzyme, leading to the true antimetabolic effect of lowered AMP and GMP biosynthesis. A second mechanism of antineoplastic activity for mercaptopurine (and the predominant mechanism for thioguanine) involves the incorporation of di- and triphosphate deoxy- and ribonucleotides generated within the tumor cell into DNA and RNA, respectively (130). This illicit substitution inhibits further elongation of the strands and promotes apoptosis.

Thiopurines are metabolized by *S*-methylation via the polymorphic enzyme thiopurine methyl transferase (TPMT) with *S*-adenosylmethionine serving as cofactor. The methylated thiopurine bases cannot react with HGPRT and, therefore, cannot form the active false ribonucleotides. Drug manufacturers take this into account when establishing dosing regimens. The active false ribonucleotide 6-thioinosinic acid is also subject to extensive TPMT-catalyzed methylation. The *S*-methyl-6-thioinosinic acid metabolite is a potent inhibitor of the amidophosphoribosyl transferase enzyme and contributes to the cytotoxic action of the parent drug (Fig. 37.39). In contrast, little or no 6-methylthioguanylic acid is produced inside the cell (130,131).

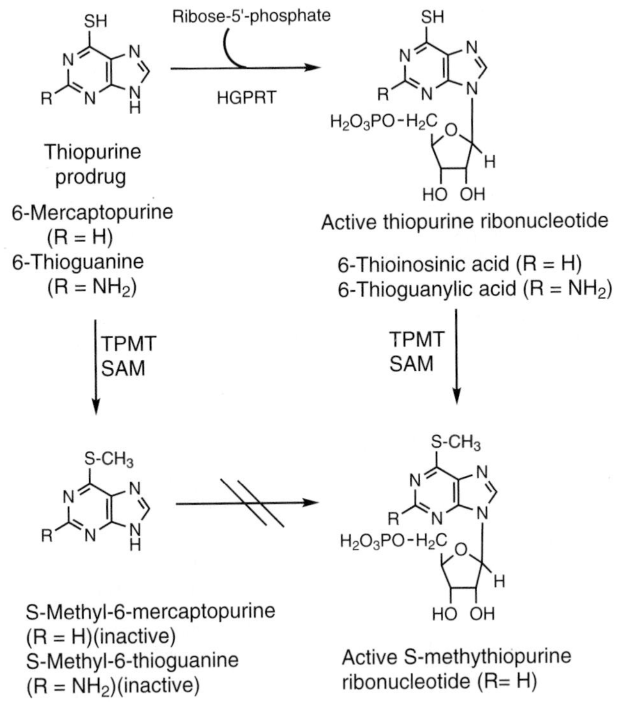

FIGURE 37.39 Thiopurine metabolism leading to activation and inactivation.

TPMT is polymorphic in humans, and some individuals do not express this protein to any significant extent (132). Patients who are poor TPMT metabolizers (e.g., 10% of Caucasians, but also evident in other races) will not experience the activity-attenuating metabolic effect and will generate more active ribonucleotide per dose than patients with normal or excessive levels of the enzyme. The TPMT genotype of patients should be assessed before initiating thiopurine therapy because poor metabolizers are at a high risk of life-threatening myelosuppression from elevated levels of false ribonucleotides, even when standard doses are administered (131). In addition, the accumulation of mutagenic thiopurine-based ribonucleotides puts these patients at higher risk for secondary malignancies (130). Thiopurines can still be used in poor TPMT metabolizers, but the dose should be decreased significantly (e.g., 10- to 15-fold) and white blood cell counts monitored vigilantly. Mercaptopurine appears to be more significantly impacted by TPMT genotype than thioguanine (133).

Genes that encode for inositol triphosphate pyrophosphatase (ITPA) are also known to impact the metabolic and toxicity profiles of mercaptopurines. Carriers of the rs41329251 ITPA allele appear to be at significantly higher risk for the development of mercaptopurine-induced febrile neutropenia even after TPMT genotype-based dosage adjustment (132,134).

Extensive TPMT metabolizers, who represent up to 90% of patients on thiopurine therapy, will form lower amounts of apoptotic 6-thiolated ribonucleotides. In the case of mercaptopurine, the molecules of ribonucleotide generated will be methylated very rapidly to the antimetabolic 6-methylthioinosinic acid, thus enhancing sensitivity to the drug (131). In contrast, extensive TPMT metabolizers show a decreased sensitivity to thioguanine because there is no compensatory increase in the formation of methylated ribonucleotide to offset the decreased production of 6-thioguanylic acid (130).

Xanthine oxidase competes with TPMT for mercaptopurine (but not for thioguanine) and converts it to inactive 6-thiouric acid, which is excreted in the urine (Fig. 37.40) (135). 6-Thioinosinic acid is also subject to metabolism via the xanthine oxidase pathway, ultimately forming the same inactive metabolite. Allopurinol, which inhibits xanthine oxidase and increases levels of active 6-thioinosinic acid, can be coadministered with mercaptopurine to increase its duration of action and antineoplastic potency. The dose of mercaptopurine can be cut approximately in half when coadministered with allopurinol. Coadministration of allopurinol with thioguanine is not warranted, since the impact of xanthine oxidase on its metabolic degradation is minor.

Specific Drugs (Fig. 37.32)

Mercaptopurine Mercaptopurine is used in the treatment of acute lymphatic and myelogenous leukemia. It is available in an oral dosage form, but absorption can be erratic and is reduced by the presence of food. The drug is extensively metabolized on first pass and excreted by the kidneys. Bone marrow suppression is the major use-limiting toxicity, although the drug can be hepatotoxic in high doses. Dosage adjustments should be considered in the face of renal or hepatic impairment. Since the major mechanism of action of mercaptopurine is inhibition of de novo purine nucleotide biosynthesis rather than apoptosis secondary to the incorporation of false nucleotides into DNA, there is a lower risk for mutagenesis and secondary malignancy compared to thioguanine (130).

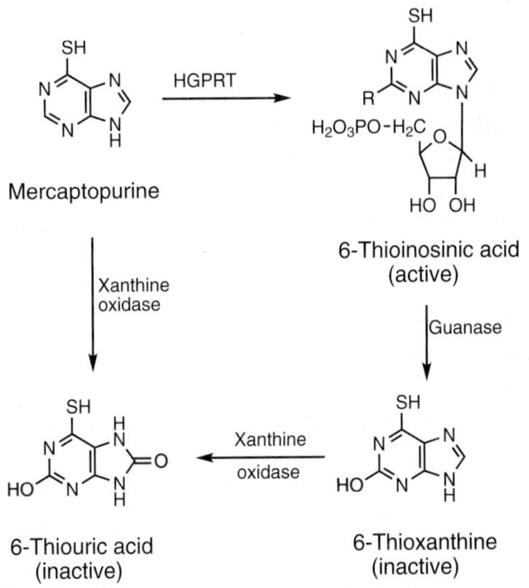

FIGURE 37.40 Xanthine oxidase inactivation of mercaptopurine and 6-thioinosinic acid.

Resistance to mercaptopurine (and thioguanine) therapy may have as much to do with attenuated active uptake via nucleoside transporters as with the more commonly cited deficiency in the activating HGPRT enzyme (136).

Thioguanine Thioguanine is administered orally in the treatment of nonlymphocytic leukemias. Like mercaptopurine, absorption is incomplete and variable, and the toxicity profiles are similar except where previously noted.

DNA Polymerase/DNA Chain Elongation Inhibitors

MECHANISM OF ACTION Five halogenated and/or ribose-modified DNA nucleoside analogs are marketed for the treatment of a wide variety of hematologic cancers and solid tumors (Fig. 37.32). These agents have complex and multifaceted mechanisms. All include inhibition of DNA polymerase and/or DNA chain elongation among their actions and all nucleosides must be converted to triphosphate nucleotides before activity is realized.

CHEMISTRY As nucleosides, the DNA polymerase inhibitors are actively taken up into cells via a selective nucleoside transporter protein, so tumors deficient in this transporter system will be resistant to these anticancer agents. Once inside the cell, specific kinases conduct the essential phosphorylation reactions. In active triphosphate form, they can be mistakenly incorporated into the growing DNA chain, thus arresting further elongation, and/or inhibit enzymes essential for DNA synthesis. All drugs in this group are administered intravenously, are excreted via the kidneys, and induce myelosuppression as their major use-limiting side effect. Resistance can involve aberrations in the expression of metabolizing enzymes as well as of transporting and efflux proteins. Some in vitro evidence points to the loss of functional nucleoside transporter proteins (specifically hENT1/SLC29A1) and deoxycytidine kinase enzymes as the primary causes of acquired resistance to DNA polymerase inhibitors (137).

As alluded to earlier, there is significant commonality in the enzymes involved in the activation and inactivation of these five antineoplastics, and the search is on for biomarkers that can reliably predict the degree of sensitivity to their therapeutic and potentially fatal toxic effects. Several polymorphic genes are under active investigation as candidates to assist practitioners in successfully individualizing antimetabolite chemotherapy (138).

SPECIFIC DRUGS (FIG. 37.32)

Cytarabine and Gemcitabine Both of these cytidine-based anticancer agents undergo initial phosphorylation by deoxycytidine kinase to the monophosphate with subsequent phosphorylations catalyzed by pyrimidine monophosphate and diphosphate kinases. Cytarabine, an arabinoside, is catabolized by cytidine and deoxycytidylate (deoxycytidine monophosphate) deaminases to inactive uracil analogs (Fig. 37.41). The significantly longer half-life of gemcitabine (19 hours) compared to conventional cytarabine (3.6 hours) is due to the inhibitory action of the difluorodeoxycytidine triphosphate

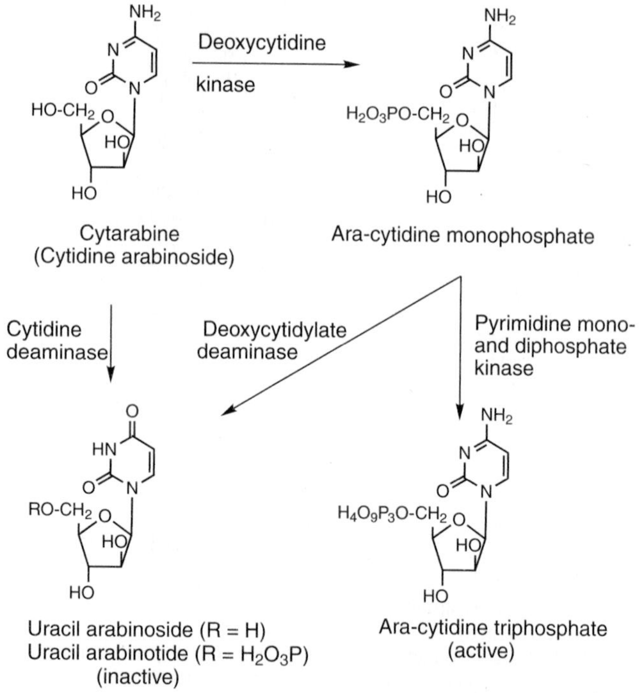

FIGURE 37.41 Cytarabine metabolism.

metabolite on the potentially degradative deoxycytidine monophosphate deaminase enzyme (110). Gemcitabine elimination is gender-dependent, with women having the greater risk for toxicity due to lower renal clearance. Gemcitabine is indicated in the treatment of breast, pancreatic, and non-small cell lung cancers. Cytarabine, which can be administered subcutaneously and intrathecally in additison to intravenously, is used in the treatment of various leukemias. A liposomal formulation of cytarabine is available for the treatment of lymphomatous meningitis.

Fludarabine, Cladribine, and Clofarabine Like their pyrimidine counterparts, these 3-halogenated adenosine-based nucleosides undergo conversion to the active triphosphate nucleotides after active transport into tumor cells. All are initially phosphorylated by deoxycytidine kinase, and cells with high levels of this enzyme should respond well to these agents. The C_2-halogen renders the molecules relatively resistant to the degradative action of adenosine deaminase, and a significant fraction of the dose is eliminated unchanged via the kidneys. Fludarabine, an arabinoside, is marketed as the monophosphate nucleotide to enhance water solubility for intravenous administration, but this group is cleaved rapidly in the bloodstream, allowing the free nucleoside to take advantage of the nucleoside-specific transporting proteins.

Cladribine is indicated in the treatment of hairy cell leukemia, whereas fludarabine phosphate is used in chronic lymphocytic leukemia. In addition to myelosuppression, fludarabine phosphate can induce hemolytic anemia, and severe CNS toxicity has been noted with high doses.

Clofarabine is used in acute lymphoblastic leukemia patients who are 21 years or less and who have failed with at least two previous regimens. In addition to inhibiting DNA chain elongation, this drug also inhibits ribonucleotide reductase and facilitates the release of proapoptotic proteins from mitochondria. The rapid attenuation of leukemia cells after administration of this agent can result in a condition known as tumor lysis syndrome, and respiratory and cardiac toxicities can occur secondary to cytokine release. Toxicity can progress to potentially fatal capillary leak syndrome and organ failure, and patients should receive intravenous fluids for the entire 5-day course of therapy to minimize risk of serious adverse events.

DNA Methyltransferase Inhibitors

Mechanism of Action In contrast to the DNA alkylating agents discussed earlier in this chapter, three nucleic acid–based chemotherapeutic agents, azacitidine, decitabine, and nelarabine (Fig. 37.42), block abnormal cellular proliferation by inhibiting DNA alkylation (specifically methylation) on genes responsible for differentiation and growth. The hypomethylation effect, mediated through the inhibition of DNA methyltransferase, can sometimes restore normal gene function while selectively killing cells that have stopped responding to the body's cellular proliferation control processes.

All of the marketed DNA methyltransferase inhibitors are nucleoside analogs that, once converted to triphosphate nucleotides, are mistakenly incorporated into DNA in lieu of their cytidine or guanine nucleotide counterparts. Interaction of the false nucleotide with methyltransferase results in an irreversible inhibition of the enzyme.

Chemistry All of these nucleoside analogs hydrolyze in aqueous solution and must be administered soon after the dose is constituted. Their vulnerability to deaminase enzymes explains their short elimination half-lives of less than or equal to 4 hours. Nelarabine will also be *O*-demethylated prior to DNA incorporation and can be further metabolized to guanine, xanthine, and uric acid. Anemia, neutropenia, and thrombocytopenia are among the most common side effects of this class of drugs.

Specific Drugs (Fig. 37.42)

Nelarabine Nelarabine is considered third-line treatment for T-cell acute lymphoblastic leukemia or lymphoma. The drug can induce severe and potentially irreversible neurologic symptoms including convulsions, severe central depression, and peripheral neuropathy that can mimic Guillain-Barré syndrome. These adverse effects are considered dose-limiting. As noted earlier, nelarabine can be metabolized to uric acid. Along with hydration and urine basification, the xanthine oxidase inhibitor allopurinol can be given prophylactically to minimize risk of nelarabine-induced hyperuricemia.

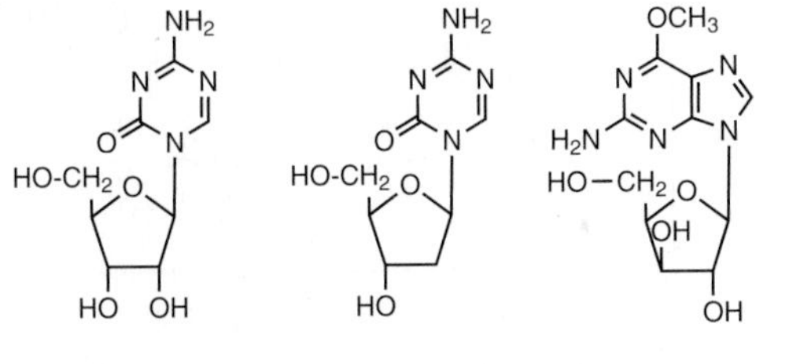

FIGURE 37.42 DNA methyltransferase inhibitors.

Azacitidine and Decitabine Azacitidine and decitabine are given intravenously (and, in the case of azacitidine, subcutaneously) for the treatment of myelodysplastic syndrome. Patients should be monitored for hematologic and renal toxicities while undergoing therapy with either agent, although renal toxicity is a more serious concern with azacitidine use. Both drugs are known to cause fetal harm, and patients should be actively counseled to take appropriate reproductive precautions.

Miscellaneous Antimetabolites (Fig. 37.32)

Pentostatin Pentostatin is a ring-expanded purine ribonucleoside that inhibits adenosine deaminase and is primarily used in the treatment of hairy cell leukemia. The elevated levels of deoxyadenosine triphosphate that result from inhibition of this degradative enzyme inhibit the action of ribonucleotide reductase (the enzyme that converts ribose diphosphate to deoxyribose diphosphate), thus halting DNA synthesis within the tumor cell. When used in chronic lymphocytic leukemia, some authors claim pentostatin offers a therapeutic efficacy comparable to fludarabine, but with a lower risk of toxicity (139).

Hydroxyurea Hydroxyurea, a drug with a 100-plus year history, blocks the synthesis of DNA by trapping a tyrosyl free radical species at the catalytic site of ribonucleotide reductase, thereby inhibiting the enzyme that converts ribonucleotide diphosphates into their corresponding deoxyribonucleotides. It is used orally for the treatment of melanoma, metastatic or inoperable ovarian cancer, resistant chronic myelocytic leukemia, and as an adjunct to radiation in the treatment of squamous cell carcinoma and cancer of the head and neck. Hydroxyurea increases the effectiveness of radiation therapy through its selective toxicity to cells in the radiation-resistant S phase and by stalling the cell cycle in the G_1 stage, in which radiation therapy does the greatest damage. It addition, hydroxyurea thwarts the normal damage-repair mechanisms of surviving cells. A review of its chemical, pharmacologic, metabolic, and therapeutic properties has recently been published (140).

Hydroxyurea has excellent oral bioavailability (80% to 100%), and serum levels peak within 2 hours of consuming the capsules. If a positive response is noted within 6 weeks, toxicities are mostly mild enough to permit long-term or indefinite therapy on either a daily or every-3-day basis. Leukopenia and, less commonly, thrombocytopenia and/or anemia are the most serious adverse effects. Excretion of the unchanged drug and the urea metabolite is via the kidneys. The carbon dioxide produced as a by-product of hydroxyurea metabolism is excreted in the expired air.

Mitosis Inhibitors

The mitotic process depends on the structural and functional viability of microtubules (polymeric heterodimers consisting of isotypes of α- and β-tubulin proteins). These distinct but nearly identical 50-kd proteins lie adjacent to one another within the tubule and roll up to form an open, pipe-like cylinder akin to a hollow peppermint candy stick. A γ-tubulin protein is found at the organizational center of the microtubule. The tubulin isotypes found in the microtubule are conserved throughout specific tissues within a given species and will impact the cell's sensitivity to mitosis inhibitors.

During cell division, tubulin undergoes intense, sporadic, and alternating periods of structural growth and erosion known as "dynamic instability." The proteins alternatively polymerize and depolymerize through guanosine triphosphate- and Ca^{2+}-dependent processes. Polymerization involves the addition of tubulin dimers to either end of the tubule, although the faster-growing (+) end is more commonly involved. Polymerization results in tubular elongation, whereas depolymerization results in the shortening of the structure. The frenetic alteration in structure, facilitated by microtubule-associated proteins (MAPs), ultimately allows the formation of the mitotic spindle and the attachment to chromosomes that are prerequisites to cell division. Inhibiting the essential hyperdynamic changes in microtubular structure results in mitotic arrest and apoptosis. Two general chemical classes of mitosis inhibitors have historically been marketed for the treatment of cancer: taxanes, and vinca alkaloids (141). They have been joined by the single agents estramustine, an estrogen-based nitrogen mustard–like carbamate originally thought to act via DNA alkylation, and the epothilone ixabepilone (Fig. 37.43).

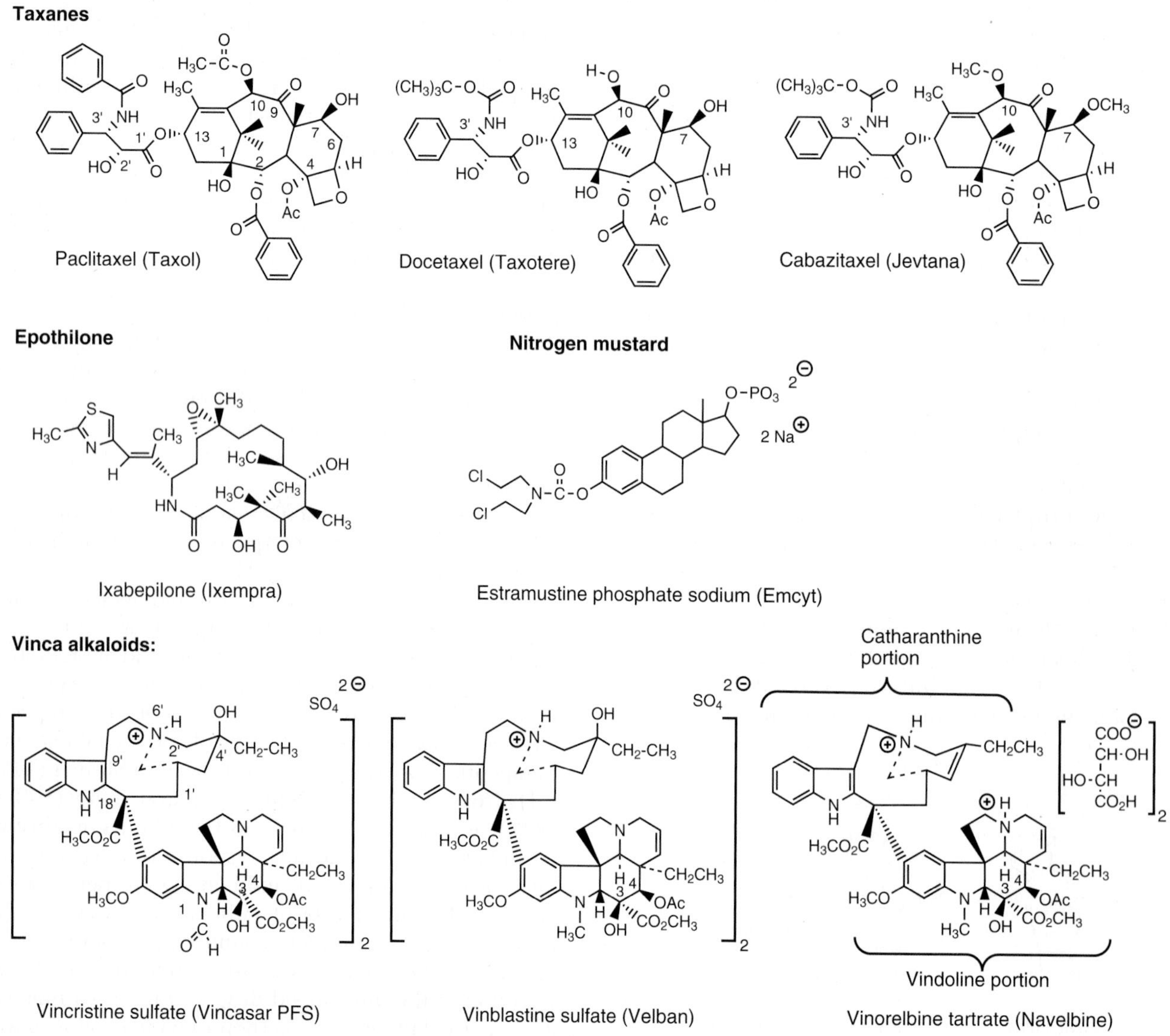

FIGURE 37.43 Mitosis inhibitors.

Taxanes

Mechanism of Action Anticancer taxanes initially were isolated from the bark of the Pacific yew (*Taxus brevifolia*) but are now produced semisynthetically from an inactive natural precursor (10-deactetylbaccatin III) found in the leaves of the European yew (*Taxus baccata*), a renewable resource. Taxanes bind to polymerized (elongated) β-tubulin at a specific hydrophobic receptor site comprised of the 31 N-terminal residues located deep within the tubular lumen (142). At standard therapeutic doses (which should lead to intracellular concentrations of 1 to 20 μM), taxane-tubulin binding promotes a stable tubulin conformation similar to that of the guanosine triphosphate-bound protein, which renders the microtubules resistant to depoly-merization and prone to polymerization (143). This promotes the elongation phase of microtubule dynamic instability at the expense of the shortening phase and inhibits the disassembly of the tubule into the mitotic spindle. In turn, this interrupts the normal process of cell division. At these concentrations, extensive polymerization causes the formation of large and dense aberrant structures known as asters, which contain stabilized microtubule bundles.

Taxanes are substrates for P-gp, and cellular efflux via this carrier protein is a major mechanism of taxane resistance. It has also been demonstrated that patients who express a mutant variety of the oncogene *p53* that causes the overexpression of MAP4, and subsequently promotes microtubular polymerization/elongation, show enhanced sensitivity to taxane chemotherapy and a resistance to vinca alkaloids (144).

Chemistry Chemically, diterpenoid taxanes consist of a 15-membered tricyclic taxane ring system (tricyclo[9.3.1.0]pentadecane) fused to an oxetane (D) ring and contain an esterified β-phenylisoserine side chain at C_{13}. As shown in Figure 37.43, the three marketed taxane antineoplastics differ in substitution pattern at C_{13} (benzamido or *t*-butoxycarboxamido), C_{10} (secondary alcohol, acetate ester, or methoxy ether), and/or C_7 (secondary alcohol or methoxy ether). The taxane ring system is often conceptualized as having "northern" and "southern" halves. The "southern" segment is critical to receptor binding, whereas the "northern" section ensures the proper conformation of essential functional groups, including the C_{13}-isoserine side chain [with its C_1-carbonyl, free C_2-(*R*)-OH and C_3-(*S*)-benzamido or *t*-butoxycarboxamido groups], the benzoyl and acetyl esters at C_2 and C_4, respectively, and the intact oxetane ring (145–147).

The key taxane–tubulin binding interactions are identified in Table 37.8 using paclitaxel as ligand (133,148,149). Paclitaxel interacts at the β-tubulin binding site in a folded ("T" or "butterfly") conformation that places C_2-benzoyl and the C_3-benzamido groups in close proximity (145,149). Their independent intermolecular engagement with a critical β-tubulin His residue perfectly positioned between them keeps them from interacting with one another. The oxetane ring of taxanes, although capable of enhancing receptor affinity through hydrogen bonding (146,148), is believed to serve a more critical role in properly orienting the C_4-acetyl moiety for interaction within its hydrophobic binding pocket (146). The C_1-OH also promotes conformational stability through intramolecular interaction with the carbonyl oxygen of the C_2 benzoyl moiety (145). The areas of the paclitaxel structure where steric influences are most critical to receptor binding have been identified (147).

Metabolism The taxanes are metabolized to significantly less cytotoxic metabolites by CYP450 enzymes (Fig. 37.44). In humans, CYP2C8 bioconverts paclitaxel to 6α-hydroxypaclitaxel, the major metabolite, which is 30-fold less active than the parent structure

TABLE 37.8 Paclitaxel–β-Tubulin Binding Interactions (142,145,146)

Paclitaxel Functional Group	β-Tubulin Binding Residues	Interaction
C_2-benzoyl phenyl	Leu217, Leu219, His229, Leu230	Hydrophobic
C_2-benzoyl carbonyl	Arg278	Hydrogen bond
$C_{3'}$-benzamido NH	Asp26	Hydrogen bond
$C_{3'}$-benzamido carbonyl	His229	Hydrogen bond
$C_{3'}$-phenyl	Ala233, Ser236, Phe272	Hydrophobic
C_4-acetyl	Leu217, Leu230, Phe272, Leu275	Hydrophobic
C_7-OH	Thr276 Ser277, Arg278	Hydrogen bond
C_{12}-CH_3	Leu217, Leu230, Phe272, Leu275	Hydrophobic
$C_{3'}$-OH	Arg369, Gly370 (NH)	Hydrogen bond
$C_{3'}$-carbonyl	Gly370 (NH)	Hydrogen bond
Oxetane oxygen	Thr276 (NH)	Hydrogen bond

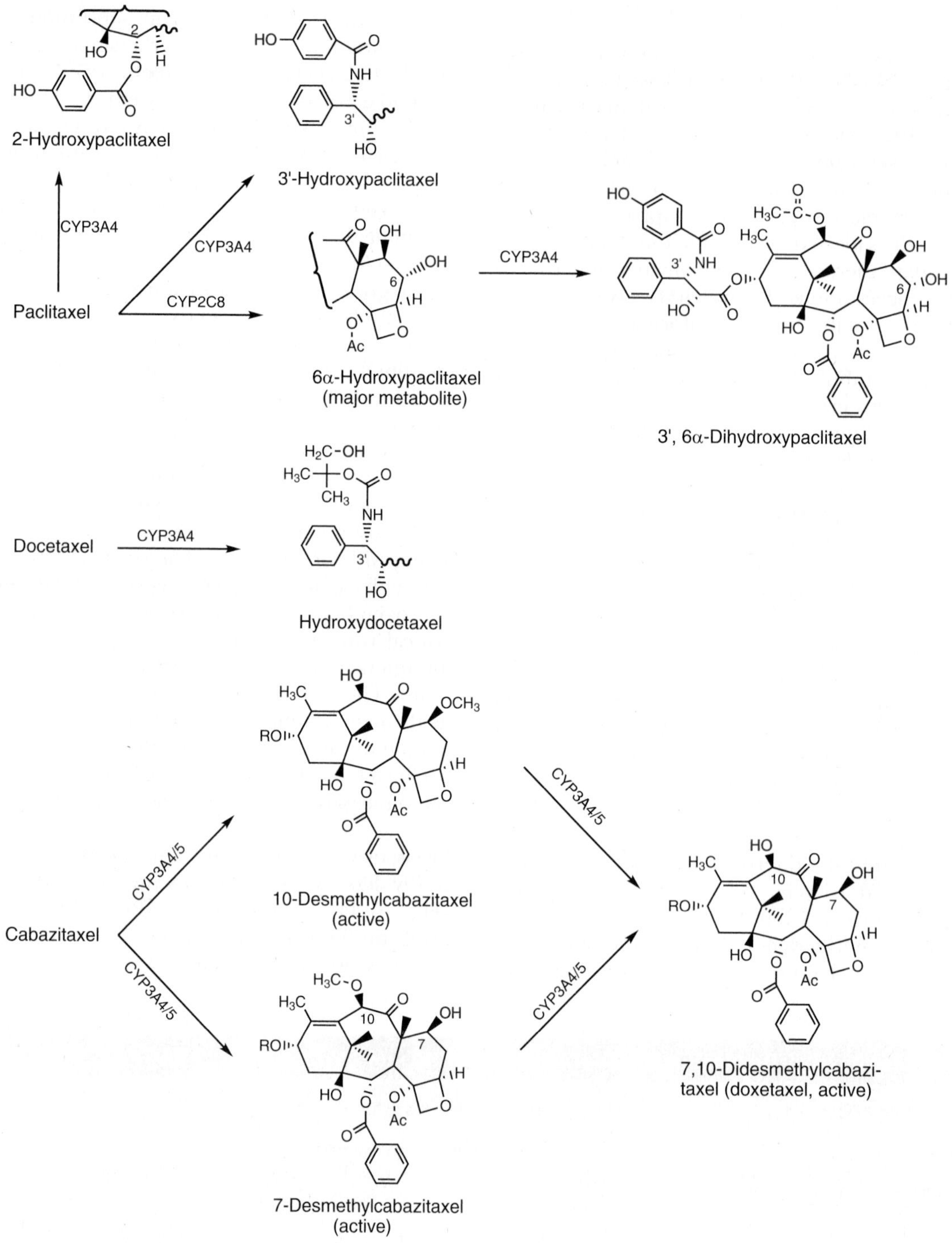

FIGURE 37.44 Metabolism of the taxane analogs.

(150–153). CYP3A4 mediates the formation of additional minor *p*-hydroxylated metabolites of the benzamido and benzoyl moieties at $C_{3'}$ and $C_{2'}$ respectively, and the 10-desacetyl metabolite has been documented in urine and plasma. Docetaxel is oxidized exclusively by CYP3A4/5, with CYP3A4 having a 10-fold higher affinity for the drug than CYP3A5. The major metabolite, known as hydroxydocetaxel, is the hydroxymethyl derivative of the 3′-*t*-butoxycarboxamide side chain (153). Hydroxydocetaxel is further oxidized and cyclized to isomeric oxazolidinediones before excretion. Cabazitaxel is metabolized predominantly (80% to 90%) by CYP3A4/5, with CYP2C8 taking on a minor biotransformation role. Three active metabolites (including docetaxel) result from *O*-demethylation at C_7 and/or C_{10}. The elimination of taxanes is predominantly biliary.

The metabolic patterns of these closely related structures are distinct, and it has been hypothesized that the C_{13} side chain plays a major role in positioning the compounds in the catalytic site of CYP450 enzymes. Specifically, the 3′-phenyl ring of paclitaxel has been proposed to properly orient C_6 for hydroxylation through π-stacking interactions with CYP2C8 active site residues while decreasing affinity for CYP3A4 binding groups. The hydrophobic character of the 10-acetoxy group, found in paclitaxel, enhances CYP450-mediated hydroxylation two- to fivefold by facilitating substrate binding or augmenting catalytic capability. Both isoforms are impacted by the presence of this ester, often to the same extent (153).

Epothilones

Chemistry Low water solubility is a significant drawback to the therapeutic utility of the taxanes. This is particularly true of paclitaxel, which has a more lipophilic acetate moiety at C_{10} compared to docetaxel's more polar hydroxyl group. Paclitaxel must be administered in a vehicle of 50% alcohol/50% polyoxyethylated caster oil (Cremophor EL), which can lead to an enhanced risk of hypersensitivity reactions (dyspnea, hypotension, angioedema, and urticaria) in patients not pretreated with H_1 and H_2 antagonists and dexamethasone (154). As noted previously, high P-gp–mediated cellular efflux of paclitaxel and docetaxel can result in drug resistance. To overcome these problems, epothilones, 16-membered macrolides structurally unrelated to the taxanes but with functional groups properly positioned to mimic critical tubulin-binding groups, are being actively investigated for use in a variety of solid tumor and hematologic cancers (Fig. 37.45). Epothilone B, one of the original structures investigated, binds with very high affinity to the taxane binding site on polymerized β-tubulin, and it acts through the same cytotoxic mechanism. In addition to enhanced water solubility and a lack of P-gp affinity, epothilone is more efficiently produced through fermentation with the myxobacterium *Sorangium cellulosum* and

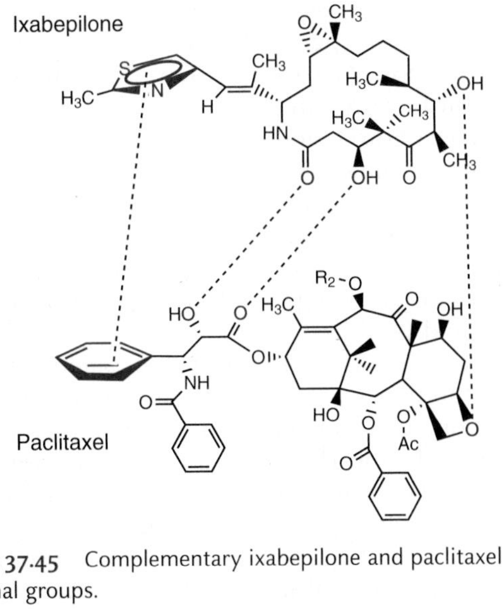

FIGURE 37.45 Complementary ixabepilone and paclitaxel functional groups.

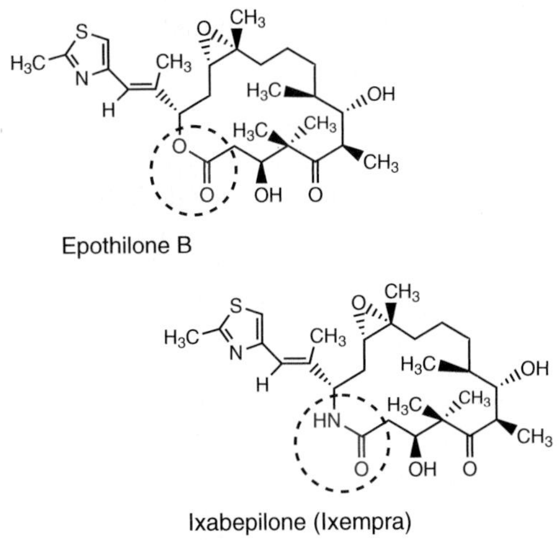

FIGURE 37.46 Epothilones.

has a higher antineoplastic potency (149,155,156). The lactam analog ixabepilone has a comparable anticancer activity with an even higher water solubility and better in vivo and in vitro stability (Fig. 37.46). The story of the discovery and subsequent development of this lactam as the lead compound in the search for a paclitaxel alternative makes for interesting reading (157).

Despite some conformational differences in ring system substituents between epothilones and taxanes, they are presumed to share a common or overlapping tubulin binding site, an assumption supported by the discovery of tubulin mutants that are resistant to both classes of antimitotics (158). Comparing crystal structures of tubulin-bound epothilone A (the 12-desmethyl derivative of epothilone B) and paclitaxel documents that the smaller macrolide fills only about half the binding site volume of the larger taxane ligand. The binding site is plastic, and residues adjust their side-chain conformations to accommodate either drug. Despite being surrounded by identical tubulin residues, the only common binding interaction involves a hydrogen bond between Arg282 and the 7-OH group of taxanes or epothilones.

Specific Drugs (Fig. 37.43)

Paclitaxel Paclitaxel, which is claimed to be "the best-selling anticancer drug in history" (145), is indicated for intravenous use in combination with cisplatin as first-line therapy for advanced ovarian and non-small cell lung cancer. It is also used alone or in combination with the fluorouracil prodrug capecitabine in anthracycline-resistant metastatic breast cancer. Paxclitaxel's ability to upregulate thymidine phosphorylase, one of capecitabine's activating enzymes, is the rationale behind the combination therapy (159). Solution (Taxol, Onxol) and albumin-bound (Abraxane) formulations are available and cannot be used interchangeably. Abraxane, which does not require the hypersensitivity-inducing Cremophor EL in its formulation, has also been used in various solid tumors of the GI and genitourinary tracts. Solution-based infusions usually are administered over 3 to 24 hours and can be passed through an in-line, 0.22-μm filter to reduce vehicle-related cloudiness. The albumin-bound form is given over 30 minutes and should be well mixed (but not filtered) to ensure complete suspension of the protein-drug particles. A paclitaxel receptor targeting peptide conjugate designed for selective drug delivery to the CNS is in clinical trials (142).

Besides hypersensitivity reactions common with the non–albumin-bound formulations, the major use-limiting adverse effect of paclitaxel is dose-dependent myelosuppression, particularly neutropenia, and first doses might need to be decreased in patients with hepatic dysfunction. Subsequent dose reductions, if any, should be tailored to individual response. The drug should not be given to patients who have baseline neutrophil counts below 1,500 cells/mm^3. The albumin-bound formulation is also associated with sensory neuropathy. As noted earlier, all patients receiving solution-based paclitaxel should be pretreated with antihistamines and a corticosteroid to minimize the risk of potentially fatal hypersensitivity reactions. Paclitaxel is a Category D teratogen and carries a high risk of fetal intrauterine mortality. Both male and female patients are advised not to attempt conception while on this drug. Due caution should be observed when coadministering paclitaxel with drugs that inhibit or compete for metabolizing enzymes, particularly CYP2C8 (e.g., 17α-ethinylestradiol and diazepam).

Docetaxel The indications for docetaxel as a rule mirror those of paclitaxel, although docetaxel is not used in ovarian cancer. It has greater water solubility than paclitaxel due to presence of the free C_{10}-OH group, and it is formulated with polysorbate 80 rather than with polyoxyethylated castor oil. Hypersensitivity reactions, while less likely, are still possible, and all patients should receive corticosteroid premedication. In addition to neutropenia and teratogenicity, this taxane can induce significant fluid retention, and 2-kg weight gains are not uncommon. Although rare, onycholysis has also been reported. Drug–drug interactions have been noted when docetaxel is coadministered with drugs that inhibit or compete for CYP3A4 enzymes (e.g., "azole" antifungals, erythromycin, and cyclosporine) (160).

Cabazitaxel Cabazitaxel is the 7,10-dimethoxy analog of docetaxel. Conversion of the two secondary alcohol groups to methoxy ethers dramatically lowers affinity for P-gp, resulting in sustained retention in tumor cells along with a higher blood–brain barrier penetration (161). Cabazitaxel has shown efficacy in docetaxel-resistant cell lines where resistance was due to P-gp overexpression. Although currently approved for use only in docetaxel-resistant metastatic prostate cancer, cabazitaxel has shown activity against a wide variety of human tumors including colon, lung, pancreas, squamous cell, head and neck, and metastatic breast cancers (161–163). Neutropenia is the most problematic dose-limiting reaction, although its incidence and severity are no worse than observed with other taxanes. Cabazitaxel does not promote the fluid retention commonly observed with docetaxel, but peripheral motor and/or sensory neuropathy can be persistent. Its relatively high incidence of diarrhea (~50%) may be explained by the accumulation of the drug in enterocytes, cells that constitutively express P-gp and, therefore, actively evict other taxanes. Despite the conversion of the two secondary alcohols to more lipophilic ethers, cabazitaxel's aqueous solubility is on a par with docetaxel's. Like docetaxel, it is formulated with polysorbate 80 rather than the more hypersensitivity-inducing Cremophor EL, although antihistamine/corticosteroid pretreatment is still recommended (160). It is administered by intravenous infusion in doses of 25 mg/m^2 every 3 weeks.

Ixabepilone The epothilone ixabepilone is used in combination with the thymidylate synthesis inhibitor capecitabine in anthracycline- and/or taxane-resistant advanced or metastatic breast cancer, or when these alternative drugs are contraindicated. Some phase II clinical trials have shown overall response rates to this agent as high as 57% in previously untreated breast cancer patients and up to 30% in patients who had been heavily pretreated (164). As noted previously, the lactam moiety provides stability to in vivo hydrolysis by carboxylesterases, but the drug is extensively metabolized by CYP3A4 to over 30 inactive metabolites prior to predominately fecal excretion. Drug–drug interactions with CYP3A4 substrates, inducers, or inhibitors have been reported, and dosage adjustments may be warranted if coadministration cannot be avoided. Like cabazitaxel, ixabepilone's serious use-limiting adverse reactions include peripheral neuropathy (67%) and neutropenia. Like paclitaxel, it requires Cremophor EL for solubilization, so hypersensitivity reactions are likely, and prophylactic premedication is required. The most common intravenous dosage regimen is 40 mg/m^2 administered over 3 hours every third week.

Vinca Alkaloids

MECHANISM OF ACTION Several alkaloids found naturally in *Catharanthus roseus* (periwinkle) have potent antimitotic activity. In opposition to the taxoids, vinca alkaloids halt cell division by inhibiting polymerization. They bind at the interface of two heterodimers within the inner tubular lumen at a single high-affinity site on β-tubulin in the vicinity of the guanosine triphosphate binding site on the (+) end of the tubules. Once bound, these alkaloids attenuate the uptake of the guanosine triphosphate essential to tubule elongation (165). Simultaneous binding to α- and β-tubulin results in protein cross-linking, which promotes a stabilized protofilament structure (166). Inhibition of microtubule elongation occurs at substoichiometric concentrations, at which alkaloid occupation of only 1% to 2% of the total number of high-affinity sites can result in up to a 50% inhibition of microtubule assembly (167,168). At high concentrations, when alkaloid binding to high-affinity sites becomes stoichiometric and lower-affinity binding sites on the tubule wall are also occupied, microtubular depolymerization is stimulated, leading to the exposure of additional alkaloidal binding sites and resulting in dramatic changes in microtubular conformation. Spiral aggregates, protofilaments, and highly structured crystals form, and the mitotic spindle ultimately disintegrates (143,159). The loss of the directing mitotic spindle promotes chromosome "clumping" in unnatural shapes (balls and stars), leading to cell death (154). Other nonmitotic toxicities related to the microtubule-disrupting action of the vinca alkaloids include inhibition of axonal transport and secretory processes and disturbances in platelet structure and function (167).

As noted earlier, the mutant *p53* oncogene is associated with resistance to vinca alkaloid–induced cytotoxicity due to its augmentation of MAP4-mediated microtubulin polymerization, which counteracts the depolymerizing mechanism of the alkaloids. In addition, the mutant oncogene gives a degree of immortality to stathmin, a cytosolic protein that must be inactivated for mitosis to begin. Finally, *p53* upregulates the MRP-1 efflux protein that ejects vinca alkaloids from cells. It has been suggested that *p53* phenotype could be harnessed to better predict a patient's anticipated susceptibility to various mitosis inhibitor antineoplastic therapy options (144).

Chemistry The specific chemical nature of the vinca binding site remains elusive due to difficulties encountered in binding assay development and implementation, as well as in data analysis. It is known that the active site is close to residue 339 and residue 390 on α- and β-tubulin, respectively (168). Of the three marketed vinca alkaloids (vincristine, vinblastine, and vinorelbine), vincristine binds most tightly, whereas vinblastine has the lowest affinity (167). Because vinca alkaloids enter cells by simple passive diffusion, unbound vinorelbine and vinblastine (being more lipophilic than vincristine) may be more extensively taken up into tissues. Vincristine, however, is cleared more slowly from the system and has the longest terminal half-life of the three agents, resulting in a more prolonged tumor cell exposure (143,167). Like the taxanes, tumor resistance to vinca alkaloids is mediated, in part, through P-gp.

The vinca alkaloids are complex structures composed of two polycyclic segments known as catharanthine (or velbanamine) and vindoline (Fig. 37.43), both of which are essential for high-affinity tubulin binding. The three commercially available anticancer alkaloids differ in the length of the alkyl chain bridging positions 6′ and 9′ of the catharanthine moiety (methylene or ethylene), in the substituents at position 4′ (olefin or tertiary alcohol), and in the N_1 vindoline indole nitrogen (methyl or formyl). Although subtle, these structural changes lead to significant differences in clinical spectrum, potency, and toxicity. For example, vincristine's relative lack of bone marrow toxicity at standard therapeutic doses makes it popular in combination therapy with more myelosuppressive anticancer agents, whereas vinblastine's relative lack of neurotoxicity permits its coadministration with cisplatin. It is known that acetylation of either hydroxyl group destroys antineoplastic activity and reduction of the vindoline olefinic linkage greatly attenuates antineoplastic action (154). The $C_{18'}$-methoxycarbonyl and the stereochemistry at positions 18′ and 2′ are also believed to be critical to activity (169).

Vinca alkaloids undergo O_4-deacetylation to yield metabolites equal to or more active than the parent drug. They are also subject to extensive CYP3A4/5-mediated metabolism before biliary excretion, although the structures of these metabolites are currently unknown (170–173).

Specific Drugs (Fig. 37.43)

Vincristine Sulfate It has been estimated that over half of U.S. children with cancer who receive chemotherapy will be given vincristine, as will more than 300,000 adult cancer patients per year (170). The drug is given by the intravenous bolus or continuous infusion routes in the treatment of acute leukemia and various Hodgkin's lymphomas and NHLs. Toxicity is often more pronounced by the latter route.

Elimination of vincristine is triphasic, with the first phase (5 minutes) representing rapid uptake into tissues and the last phase (85 hours) representing release back to the plasma from tubulin-containing cells. Since the drug is extensively metabolized by O_4-deacetylation and CYP3A5-catalyzed oxidation in the liver, patients with hepatic dysfunction are at an increased risk for toxicity, and dosage reductions should be considered. The most significant dose-limiting adverse effect is peripheral neuropathy, which is initially manifested as numbness and painful paresthesias in the extremities and progresses to muscular pain, severe weakness, and loss of coordination. Patients can also experience constipation secondary to intestinal neurotoxicity, which may require treatment with cathartics. African American patients, who commonly carry the CYP3A5*1 allele that expresses a catalytically active CYP3A5 enzyme, are at lower risk for severe and/or prolonged neurotoxicity than Caucasians, who carry less active/inactive alleles (170). Myelosuppression is not particularly problematic because it occurs at doses higher than those that can be tolerated. As previously noted, coadministration with mitomycin can induce acute or delayed pulmonary toxicity characterized by severe bronchospasm.

All vinca alkaloids are severe vesicants that can induce necrosis, cellulitis, and/or thrombophlebitis. Proper needle placement before administration should be assured to eliminate the risk of extravasation. Unlike the tissue damage caused by the vesicant action of nitrogen mustards and antibiotic antineoplastics, cold exacerbates tissue destruction. If extravasation occurs, apply heat for 1 hour 4 times a day for 3 to 5 days, coupled with local hyaluronidase injections. Vinca alkaloids are all Category D teratogens and are fatal if administered by the intrathecal route.

Vinblastine Sulfate In addition to the hematologic indications that it shares with vincristine, vinblastine has found utility in the treatment of advanced testicular carcinoma (often in combination with bleomycin), advanced mycosis fungoides, Kaposi sarcoma, and histiocytosis X. Leukopenia is the dose-limiting side effect, and dose reductions are warranted in patients with serum bilirubin levels greater than 3 mg/dL. The drug-related impact on erythrocyte and thrombocyte levels is usually insignificant. Like vincristine, it is administered as an intravenous bolus or infusion. The initial elimination half-life of 3.7 minutes is similar to vincristine, but the 24.8-hour terminal half-life is significantly shorter.

Vinorelbine Tartrate Vinorelbine is used alone or in combination with cisplatin for first-line treatment of non-small cell lung cancer. This semisynthetic alkaloid is unique in having oral bioavailability (167), but it is currently available only for intravenous injection. The initial phase elimination half-life is on a par with that observed for vincristine and vinblastine, and the terminal phase half-life is between 28 and 44 hours. Although dose-limiting granulocytopenia is the major adverse effect, potentially fatal interstitial pulmonary changes have been noted. Patients with symptoms of respiratory distress should be promptly evaluated. Biotransformations include deacetylation and *N*-oxidation. As with all vinca alkaloids, elimination is primarily hepatobiliary, and dosage reduction should be considered in patients with liver dysfunction.

Estramustine Phosphate Sodium Because this anticancer agent contains a carbamylated nitrogen mustard moiety, it was originally thought to function as a DNA alkylator; however, it is now known that its primary mechanism of antineoplastic action is inhibition of mitosis. Estramustine binds to MAP-4, prompting dissociation of this protein from the microtubule and promoting depolymerization and disassembly. It can also bind directly to α- and β-tubulin at a site distinct from the vinca alkaloid and taxane binding sites, although paclitaxel exerts a noncompetitive inhibition of estramustine binding to tubulin. A specific estramustine binding protein in prostate tissue is believed to facilitate its action in the treatment of metastatic carcinoma of the prostate. Estramustine has a low affinity for the β_m tubulin isotype, which is often overexpressed in estramustine-resistant prostatic neoplasms as one defense against this therapeutic intervention (159,174).

Estramustine's resonance-stabilized, mustard-like β-haloalkylamine carbamate structure uses an estradiol carrier to selectively deliver drug to steroid-dependent prostate tissue, and its use is limited to the palliative treatment of progressive prostate cancer. The ionized sodium phosphate ester makes the compound water soluble and able to distribute in the blood. The phosphate ester is readily cleaved during absorption to provide the active 17β-OH. The 3-carbamate group is also cleaved in vivo to generate estradiol (Fig. 37.47), which explains why this drug is not used to treat estrogen-dependent tumors (e.g., estrogen-dependent breast cancer). The liberated estradiol may also increase blood pressure and induce blood clots, leading to myocardial infarction. Fortunately, the myocardial infarctions are usually nonfatal, but the drug should be used with extreme caution in men who are predisposed to clotting disorders or who have a history of cerebral vascular disease or coronary artery disease. Hepatotoxicity is also associated with estramustine use.

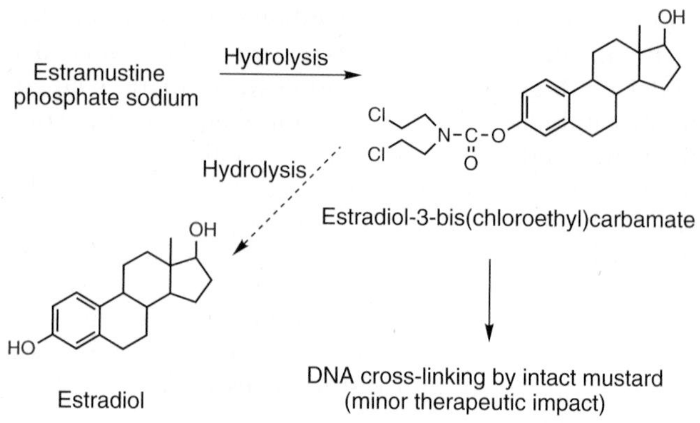

FIGURE 37.47 Estramustine metabolism.

Tyrosine Kinase and Related Inhibitors

Aberrations in the activity of protein tyrosine kinases (TKs) are associated with several neoplastic disorders, and it has been estimated that more that 80% of human oncogenes and proto-oncogenes direct the expression of these essential phosphorylating enzymes. When functioning normally, TKs regulate cell proliferation, differentiation, and survival. When functioning in a deregulated manner, they accelerate cell signaling cascades and cellular growth, induce tumors, augment antiapoptotic processes, and, in so doing, confer resistance to many chemotherapeutic drugs.

MECHANISM OF ACTION TKs are of two general types, receptor-associated and cellular (nonreceptor), both of which are ATP-dependent. The highly conserved ATP binding domain of the TKs serves as the receptor for antineoplastic TK inhibitors (TKIs, or tyrphostins). This hydrophobic domain, a depression or groove rich in isoleucine (Ile), leucine (Leu), alanine (Ala), and valine (Val) residues, is found in the "hinge region" that connects the amino terminal (N) and carboxy terminal (C) lobes of the catalytic unit. A minimum of five potential binding pockets surround this site, which may help explain the otherwise surprising degree of selectivity exhibited by many anticancer TKIs (175). Van der Waals, hydrophobic, hydrogen-bonding, and electrostatic interactions are all of prime importance in holding ATP and the TKIs to this enzymatic domain (175,176).

TKs that serve as targets for anticancer TKIs include EGFR, VEGFR, human epidermal growth factor receptor 2 (HER2), platelet-derived growth factor receptor (PDGFR), Bcr-Abl (a product of the translocated breakpoint cluster [BCR]-Abelson [ABL] gene known as the Philadelphia, or Ph, chromosome), and Src. Bcr-Abl and Src are nonreceptor kinases, whereas the remaining are receptor-associated enzymes. Type 1 inhibitors bind to the active conformation of the kinase, whereas type 2 TKIs inhibit the enzyme in its inactive conformation. Since the inactive conformation of TKs differs in structure to a greater degree than the active conformer, it has been proposed that type 2 inhibitors may have a better opportunity for selectivity (175,177). Promiscuous TKIs inhibit several kinase enzymes and are referred to as "multikinase inhibitors."

CYP3A4 is a common TKI-metabolizing isoform, and many TKIs inhibit a variety of cytochrome P450 (CYP) enzymes. Several TKIs are also substrates for, and inhibitors of, cellular efflux pumps like P-gp and breast cancer resistance protein (BCRP). All are excreted predominantly in the feces. The structures of the currently marketed TKIs are shown in Figure 37.48.

Bcr-Abl Inhibitors: Imatinib, Nilotinib, and Dasatinib

Chemistry Bcr-Abl inhibitors were the first TKIs to be introduced, and they literally changed the face of CML therapy. The aberrant Ph chromosome is viewed as the

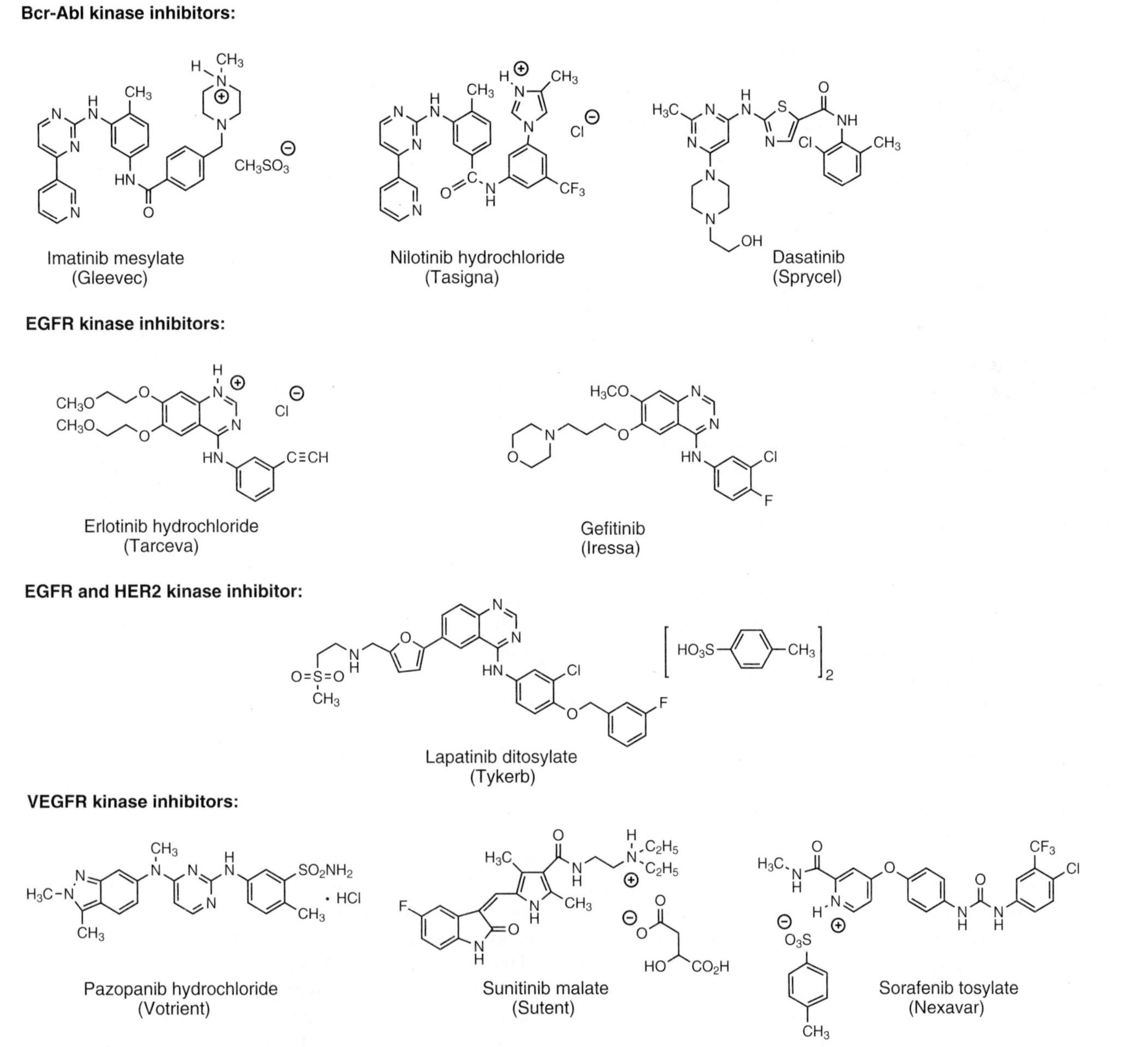

FIGURE 37.48 Tyrosine kinase inhibitors.

single cause of more than 90% of adult CML. The clinical availability of imatinib, discovered serendipitously in a search for new anti-inflammatory agents, allowed patients to realistically anticipate a 5-year survival, as opposed to the 2- to 3-year prognosis for patients with untreated disease. The drug has its greatest effect in the initial (chronic) phase of CML and is significantly less effective in the accelerated or highly fatal blastic phases.

As is the case with so many chemotherapeutic agents, acquired resistance has undermined the positive clinical outcomes this drug first promised. Resistance mechanisms are often associated with point mutations in the Abl (kinase) domain, in particular a threonine (Thr) to Ile mutation at position 315 (T315I). Residue 315 is known as the "gatekeeper" to the hydrophobic binding pocket, and the more significant bulk of the Ile residue blocks imatinib's access to this receptor through steric interference with the benzyl moiety (175,178). Alternate mechanisms of resistance are related to *BRC-ABL* gene amplification, P-gp overexpression, underexpression of an organic cation transporter-1 protein that helps imatinib (but not nilotinib) gain access to cells, and activation of Src kinases. Although nilotinib can show activity in some imatinib-resistant mutants, it cannot overcome the resistance induced by T315I. Twelve percent of all Bcr-Abl mutations are T315I, and CML patients carrying this mutation have a poor prognosis.

The Bcr-Abl inhibitors imatinib and nilotinib contain a 2-phenylaminopyrimidine pharmacophore. They are relatively large, extended structures that bind to both the ATP hinge region and to adjacent hydrophobic subdomains of the Bcr-Abl protein. As type 2 inhibitors, they bind to the inactive conformation of the kinase known as the "DFG-out state" (177). In this conformation, an enzymatic aspartate (Asp^{175}) (D)-Mg^{+2} interaction is broken, and a Phe residue is pushed out toward the aqueous environment, occluding the approach of ATP and generating a new binding area that attracts type 2 Bcr-Abl inhibitors. This conformation is also stabilized by an unphosphorylated Tyr^{393}, which orients toward the center of the enzyme and H-bonds with Asp^{363} (179).

The *o*-methyl substituent found on imatinib and nilotinib confers selectivity for the cytosolic Bcr-Abl protein in its inactive conformation, although the benzamide moiety permits some inhibition of PDGFR kinase. It is the PDGFR-related component of the activity profile that is believed responsible for the fluid retention induced by these two TKIs. These agents also contain a pyridyl substituent at C_4 of the pyrimidine ring, which enhances affinity through H-bonding with the amide NH of Met^{318} within the hinge region of the kinase (Fig. 37.49). The amide moiety, inverted in nilotinib compared to imatinib, forms H-bonds with Glu^{286} and Asp^{381} (180,181). Yet another H-bond is formed between gatekeeper Thr^{315} and the NH group connecting the pyrimidine and phenyl rings. Water solubility and the favorable oral bioavailability profiles of imatinib and nilotinib are conferred by the substituted piperazine and imidazole

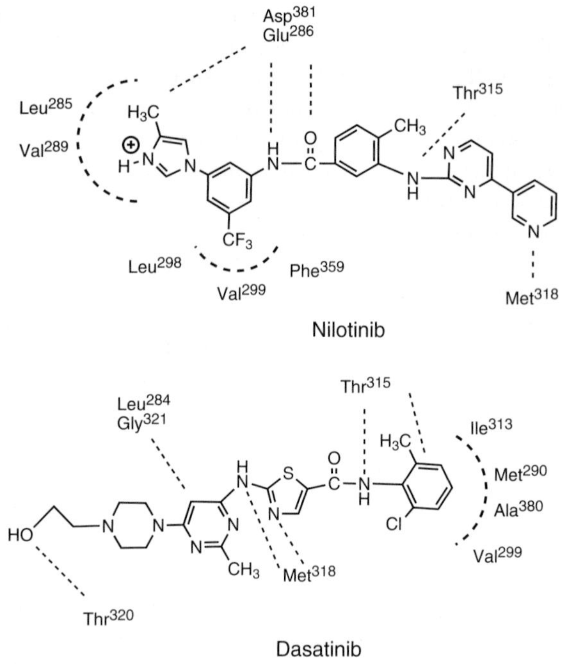

FIGURE 37.49 Binding interactions between tyrosine kinase and selected Bcr-Abl inhibitors.

rings, respectively. The lower pK_a of imidazole compared to piperazine explains why nilotinib is not a substrate for the organic cation transporter-1 protein that ferries imatinib into cells and contributes to imatinib resistance (182).

The trifluoromethyl moiety of nilotinib engages in unique affinity-enhancing hydrophobic interactions with Leu^{298}, Val^{299}, and Phe^{359}, which are, in part, responsible for nilotinib's 30- to 50-fold increase in TK-inhibiting potency compared to imatinib. The methylimidazole moiety also augments affinity through hydrophobic interactions with Leu^{285}, Glu^{286}, and Val^{289}, while leaving the basic nitrogen exposed to the aqueous environment (175,177–179).

In contrast to imatinib and nilotinib, dasatinib is a mixed type 1 and type 2 Bcr-Abl kinase inhibitor that also has significant affinity for cellular Src kinases. Although it contains a pyrimidine ring, this moiety does not bind in the hinge region as the pyrimidine rings of imatinib and nilotinib do. Rather, this binding honor goes to aminothiazole, and it is facilitated by a critical hydrogen bond between the thiazole nitrogen and the amide NH of Met^{318}. Met^{318}'s carbonyl oxygen also binds to the hydrogen of the amino group connecting the thiazole and pyrimidine rings. A third hydrogen bond between the drug's amide nitrogen and the hydroxyl of gatekeeper residue Thr^{315} ensures high affinity for the active (DFG-in) state of the kinase (178).

The 2-chloro-6-methylbenzamide segment of dasatinib binds deep within the hydrophobic pocket of the kinase in an area distinct from the ATP-binding site. Interactions between this aromatic moiety and Thr^{315}, Met^{290}, Val^{299},

Ile[313], and Ala[380] are known (183). Hydrophobic interactions with Leu[248] and Gly[321] also hold the pyrimidine ring to the kinase. As in imatinib, dasatinib's water solubility is assured through the hydroxyethyl-substituted piperazine ring, which is oriented toward the hinge region and is solvent-exposed. An H-bond between this moiety and the backbone carbonyl oxygen of Thr[320] is known to occur.

Dasatinib's ability to bind to the active kinase conformation has been attributed to the fact that it does not insert into the hydrophobic pocket containing Phe(F)[382], as the substituted benzyl moiety of imatinib does (175). Because it can bind to both the active and inactive conformations of Bcr-Abl kinase, dasatinib has a potency approximately 325 times that of imatinib, and it can be used in patients resistant to imatinib or nilotinib. Most mutations that confer resistance to imatinib occur in the P-loop of the kinase, an area not important to dasatinib binding (183). Dasatinib is effective against all imatinib-resistant mutants except T315I, retains activity in cells made resistant to imatinib via activation of Src kinases, and does not bind to P-gp.

EGFR and EGFR/HER2 Inhibitors: Erlotinib, Gefitinib, and Lapatinib

Chemistry EGFR and HER2 are closely related membrane-bound TKs. EGFR expression in solid tumors of the breast, lung, bladder, esophagus, and oral cavity has been clearly correlated with decreased life expectancy (184), and it is a consistent presence in almost all epithelial-derived cancers. Likewise, HER2 overexpression is a classic feature of treatment-resistant breast, ovarian, lung, and gastric cancers, and it endows tumors with what's been called an "antiapoptotic shield" (185). A unique Cys residue is located within the ATP-binding domain, and TKIs capable of irreversibly inactivating the protein through covalent bond formation with Cys[797] (e.g., neratinib) are now being investigated (175,176).

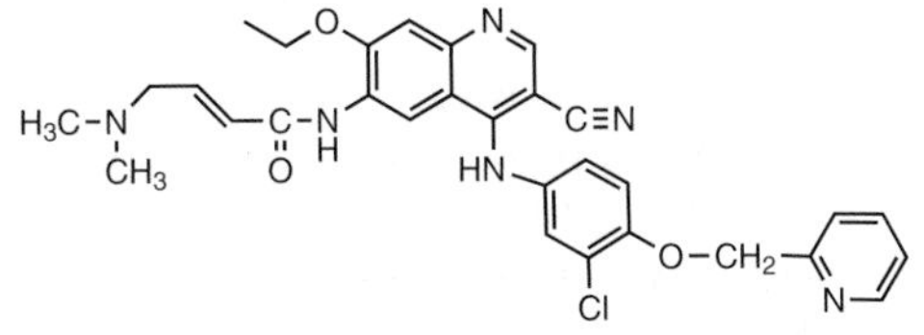

Neratinib (Irreversible tyrosine kinase inhibitor)

The currently marketed reversible EGFR TKIs all contain a 4-anilinoquinazoline pharmacophore with an oxygen-containing substituent at C_6. Ether-containing moieties of varying size are also permitted at C_7. An electron-withdrawing substituent at position 3′ of the aniline phenyl ring provides high selectivity for EGFR kinase as long as the 4′ position remains unsubstituted (erlotinib) or is modified with a very small substituent such as fluorine (gefitinib). Erlotinib and gefitinib are quintessential type 1 TKIs, with the *m*-substituted phenyl ring of the aniline moiety enhancing affinity through binding with back pocket residues of the active (open) enzyme. The H-bonds formed between the quinazoline nitrogen atoms and hinge residues Met[793] (N_1) and Thr[790] (N_3) are crucial to activity. The halogenated and acetylene-substituted phenyl rings of gefitinib and erlotinib, respectively, are maintained at a 42-degree angle relative to the quinazoline ring and, in this orientation, bind well in the hydrophobic pocket near Thr[790] as long as this gatekeeper residue remains small (175). A T790M mutation is believed responsible for acquired resistance to these highly selective TKIs (186,187). Unlike the acquired Bcr-Abl kinase resistance, which was steric in nature, an unfavorable TKI/ATP binding affinity ratio in the T790M mutant has been proposed to explain acquired resistance to EGFR TKIs (175).

Increasing the size of the 4′ substituent with groups like *m*-fluorobenzyloxy (lapatinib) restricts access to only the inactive conformation of EGFR (175) and broadens TK specificity to include HER2. The entire substituted aniline structural component of lapatinib binds within a lipophilic pocket of the HER2 kinase in its inactive (closed) conformation. The quinazoline ring of EGFR/HER2 inhibitors again affiliates with residues in the hinge region of the ATP-binding domain. Selectivity for the inactive conformation of its target kinases (which requires a conformational change to dislodge the inhibitor) may contribute to the very slow (300 minutes) enzyme dissociation half-life compared to erlotinib and gefitinib (30 minutes) (175).

Lapatinib's 2-furanyl substituent can be further substituted at position 5 with long, unbranched chains that extend out into the aqueous environment. The addition of a methylsulfone moiety to the chain terminus enhances water solubility. The ionizable morpholine ring of gefitinib serves a similar purpose. The water solubility of erlotinib is predictably low given the relative lack of polar functional groups in this area of the molecule.

VEGFR Inhibitors: Sunitinib, Sorafenib, and Pazopanib

Chemistry VEGF2 is a key enzymatic player in the generation of new blood vessels. Inhibition of this important TK starves tumors by inhibiting angiogenesis and keeping oxygen and essential nutrients from supporting their continued uncontrolled growth. This deprivation, coupled with the buildup of cellular waste materials, kills cells treated with TKIs that target this kinase. Augmenting the cytotoxic effect is the fact that VEGF inhibition decreases the permeability of tumor cell vasculature and eases intracellular delivery of chemotherapeutic agents (188).

The binding of sorafenib to VEGFR in its inactive conformation is believed to be similar to its interaction with its originally recognized kinase target B-RAF, a component of the RAS signal transduction network (175). Assuming so, the pyridine nitrogen in its un-ionized form and the nearby methylamide NH moiety H-bond with the amide group of Cys919 in the hinge region (NH and carbonyl oxygen, respectively). The trifluoromethylphenyl moiety binds in a hydrophobic pocket, possibly occupying the site normally reserved for Phe1047 in the "DFG-in" (active) conformation, and the urea moiety forms H-bonds with several residues, including the Asp1046 of the DFG trio.

Unlike sorafenib, a type 2 TKI, sunitinib can inhibit VEGFR in both its active and inactive conformations. The indolinone (or oxindole) moiety of sunitinib has been shown to confer high affinity for a hydrophobic pocket within the ATP-binding domain of kinases (189). However, the selectivity of VEGFR TKIs is low, since this kinase domain is replicated in many closely related enzymes, such as PDGFRα and c-kit, that are associated with GI stromal tumors (GISTs) (190). Broad activity against several kinases is expected, particularly from inhibitors that are retained exclusively within this conserved nucleotide-binding region and that avoid neighboring residues that permit differentiation of kinase affinity profiles (e.g., sunitinib). Sorafenib's pyridine ring interacts with amino acids in the kinase ATP-binding domain, whereas the urea component of the bisarylurea moiety augments affinity through H-bonding.

Geometric isomerism is important to the TKI activity of sunitinib, with the lower energy *Z* isomer being over 100 times as potent as the higher energy *E* isomer. Exposure to light will prompt a *Z* to *E* isomeric inversion, with a return to the lower energy *Z* state over time in the dark (191).

Sunitinib and sorafenib enter cells via passive diffusion as opposed to carrier-mediated transport (192). All currently marketed VEGFR TKIs are used in the treatment of renal cell carcinoma (RCC), a highly vascularized tumor (177).

Specific Drugs (Fig. 37.48)

Imatinib Mesylate Imatinib is indicated in Ph⁺ CML, acute lymphoblastic leukemia, GIST (a tumor expressing a c-kit kinase mutation), and myeloproliferative diseases. Available in 100- and 400-mg tablets, recommended doses in patients with adequate renal function run mostly between 400 and 600 mg daily. The drug should be taken with a large glass of water and with food to minimize GI distress.

Imatinib has a 98% mean oral bioavailability, and maximum serum concentrations are achieved within 4 hours. It is metabolized predominantly by CYP3A4-mediated *N*-dealkylation to an equally active desmethyl metabolite (191). Serum levels of imatinib will increase if coadministered with CYP3A4 inhibitors, and the drug should not be given with grapefruit juice. Conversely, the dose of imatinib should be increased by 50% if coadministration with potent CYP3A4 inducers (e.g., cyclosporine) is warranted. Imatinib is a competitive inhibitor of CYP3A4, CYP2C9, and CYP2D6, and care should be taken when substrates of these isozymes are coadministered. The parent drug and active desmethyl metabolite have elimination half-lives of 18 and 40 hours, respectively. Approximately 25% of a dose is excreted as the unchanged drug. Although well tolerated, common adverse effects include edema, diarrhea, nausea, and rash. Myocardial toxicity and hepatotoxicity, while potentially severe, are rare.

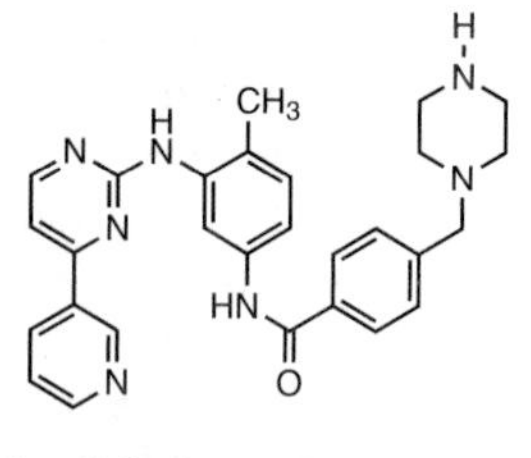

Imatinib desmethyl metabolite
(active)

Nilotinib Hydrochloride Nilotinib is indicated in newly diagnosed or imatinib-resistant Ph⁺ CML. It is supplied as 150- and 200-mg capsules, and twice-daily doses of 300 mg (new diagnosis) and 400 mg (resistant disease) are standard. The oral bioavailability of nilotinib is much lower than imatinib (30% vs. 98%, respectively). Taking the drug within 30 minutes of a high-fat meal increases oral bioavailability to 50% and the area under the curve by 82% (193), and this can result in an increased risk of serious toxicity. No food should be eaten 2 hours before or 1 hour after administration. Biotransformation is limited, with the major metabolite being a carboxylic acid arising from CYP3A4-mediated hydroxylation of an aromatic methyl group. No metabolites are active. Sixty-nine percent of a dose is excreted unchanged (191).

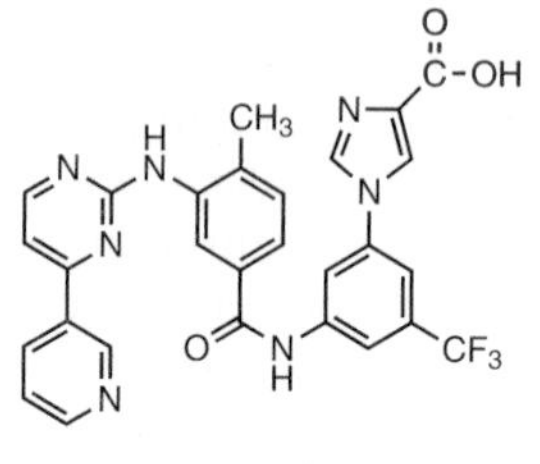

Nilotinib oxidized metabolite
(inactive)

Nilotinib is associated with life-threatening toxicities, including QT interval prolongation that can progress to torsades de pointes, sudden death, and myelosuppression. The risk of potentially fatal myocardial toxicity is elevated if the drug is taken with food or coadministered with potent CYP3A4 inhibitors. Nilotinib doses should be cut in half if CYP3A4 inhibitors must be coadministered and reduced in patients with hepatic impairment. Patients should also be counseled to avoid grapefruit juice and St. John's wort.

Dasatinib Dasatinib is available as 20-, 50-, 70-, and 100-mg tablets for use in Ph⁺ CML and acute lymphoblastic leukemia patients who are resistant or intolerant to other therapies, including imatinib. The starting dose is 140 mg once daily, and patients should be titrated up or down to the maximum dose tolerated. Doses higher than 180 mg daily are not recommended. Oral bioavailability is low due to poor absorption and rapid first-pass CYP3A4-mediated metabolism. Biotransformations include aromatic hydroxylation, benzylic hydroxylation, *N*-dealkylation, *N*-oxidation (at piperazine N_4), and oxidation of the hydroxyethyl moiety (Fig. 37.50).

FMO-3 and uridine diphosphate glucuronyl transferase also catalyze minor metabolic reactions (193). All five CYP3A4-generated metabolites retain activity, but represent only 5% of the parent area under the curve, so their clinical relevance is questionable. The *p*-hydroxylated metabolite can be oxidized to a potentially hepatotoxic quinoneimine (191). The mean elimination half-life of dasatinib is 3 to 5 hours, and 19% of a dose is excreted unchanged (191). Doses should be decreased (20 to 40 mg daily) or increased (as tolerated) if CYP3A4 inhibitors or inducers, respectively, must be coadministered. Like other drugs in this class, dasatinib also inhibits CYP3A4, and it should not be taken with grapefruit juice.

Dasatinib can be taken with or without food, and myelosuppression, peripheral edema, and GI distress are the most commonly encountered adverse effects. Unlike nilotinib, there is no black box warning related to prolongation of the QT interval, but the potential of dasatinib to exacerbate the toxicity of agents that do should not be ruled out.

Erlotinib Hydrochloride Erlotinib is used in the treatment of non-small cell lung cancer in patients whose disease has either stabilized after four rounds of organoplatinum therapy or progressed after completion of a non–TKI-based chemotherapeutic regimen. It is also used in combination with gemcitabine as first-line therapy in advanced or metastatic pancreatic cancer. Doses of 100 to 150 mg daily are common, and the product is marketed as 25-, 100-, and 150-mg tablets. Because administration with food significantly increases oral absorption from 60% to 100%, patients are instructed to take the drug 1 hour before or 2 hours after eating to minimize toxicity risks.

Extensive CYP3A4-mediated *O*-dealkylation of the terminal methoxy group of the C_6 side chain occurs, and some molecules of the primary alcohol are further oxidized by cytosolic enzymes to the carboxylic acid. CYP1A1 and CYP1A2 can also catalyze this reaction, and erlotinib's half-life and area under the curve are dramatically decreased in cigarette smokers (191). Coadministration of strong CYP3A4 inducers has the same effect. Conversely, erlotinib doses must be decreased in 50-mg increments if serious side effects occur with coadministration of CYP3A4 inhibitors. The potentially fatal hepatotoxicity that can be induced by this drug might be due, at least in part, to the formation of an electrophilic quinoneimine from a CYP3A4- and CYP1A1-generated phenolic metabolite (Fig. 37.51) (191).

In addition to hepatotoxicity, erlotinib can cause diarrhea and a maculopapular skin rash that has been positively correlated with therapeutic efficacy. The rash worsens when exposed to sunlight, so patients should be counseled to take appropriate precautions. Erlotinib is both a substrate and an inhibitor of P-gp and, like other TKIs, it inhibits CYP isoforms, specifically CYP3A4 and CYP3A5.

Gefitinib Gefitinib is used exclusively as a single agent in the treatment of organoplatinum- and docetaxel-refractory non-small cell lung cancer. One 250-mg tablet

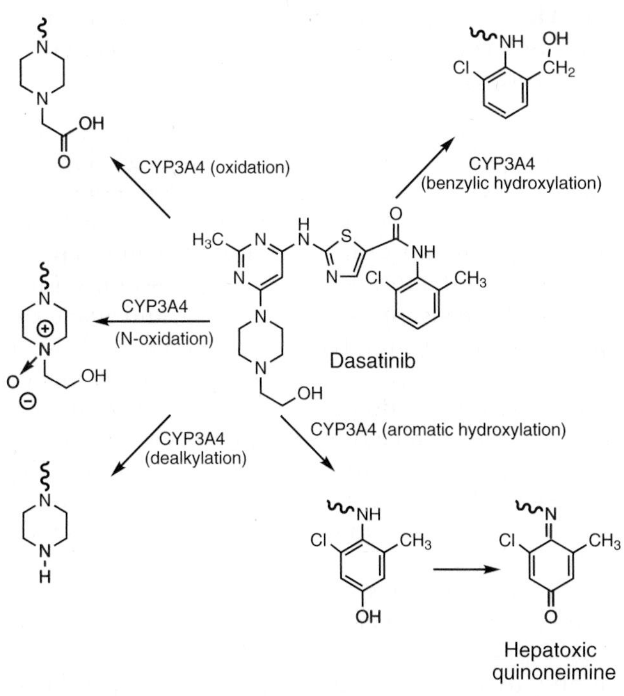

FIGURE 37.50 Dasatinib metabolism.

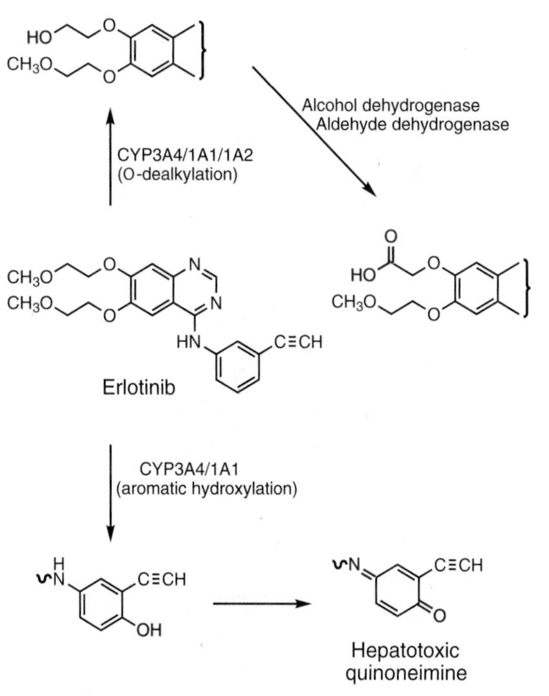

FIGURE 37.51 Erlotinib metabolism.

is administered daily without regard to meals. Higher doses induce more toxicity without additional therapeutic benefit.

CYP2D6, along with CYP3A4/3A5, catalyzes the dealkylation of the quinazoline 7-methoxy ether to a phenolic metabolite with equal in vitro EGFR-inhibiting action but limited therapeutic relevance due to polarity-induced difficulties in tumor cell penetration (193). Enzymatic cleavage and subsequent loss of the morpholine ring occur to a lesser extent, as do defluorination and subsequent *p*-hydroxylation of the aniline phenyl moiety. As noted with other TKIs, oxidation of the *p*-phenol to a reactive quinoneimine may occur in both liver (CYP3A4) and lung (CYP1A1) (Fig. 37.52). Smokers can generate up to 12 times more of this reactive metabolite than nonsmokers (191).

Like erlotinib, gefitinib induces rash (a consequence of its EGFR kinase specificity) and diarrhea. Between 40% and 50% of patients on the 250-mg daily dose will experience these two side effects. Infrequent but serious toxicities include potentially fatal interstitial lung disease (possibly related to quinoneimine formation), interstitial pneumonia, worsening pulmonary fibrosis, and corneal ulceration. The drug induces aberrant eyelash growth, which can induce eye pain.

Lapatinib Ditosylate This dual kinase inhibitor is used in combination with capecitabine as second-line therapy in the treatment of HER2-positive advanced or metastatic breast cancer. Patients receiving this drug should have previously received anthracycline, taxane, and trastuzumab therapy. Five 250-mg tablets are administered daily on an empty stomach. The drug is very expensive ($2,500 to $3,000 per month), and the fact that the area under the curve can be increased threefold by taking the drug with a high-fat meal has caused some to question whether this pharmacokinetic profile could be safely harnessed to lower costs without compromising clinical outcomes (191).

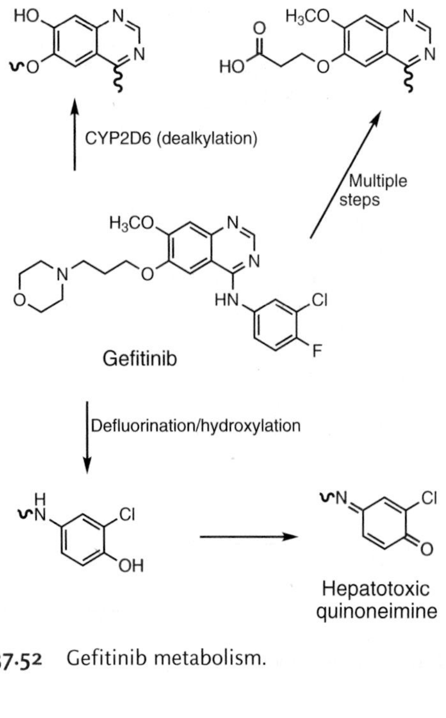

FIGURE 37.52 Gefitinib metabolism.

CYP3A4 is the major lapatinib-metabolizing enzyme and catalyzes the oxidative removal of the *m*-fluorobenzyl moiety. Doses are decreased to 500 mg daily when potent CYP3A4 inhibitors are coadministered, and titrated up to a maximum of 4,500 to 5,500 mg daily (as tolerated) when exposure to potent CYP3A4 inducers is required.

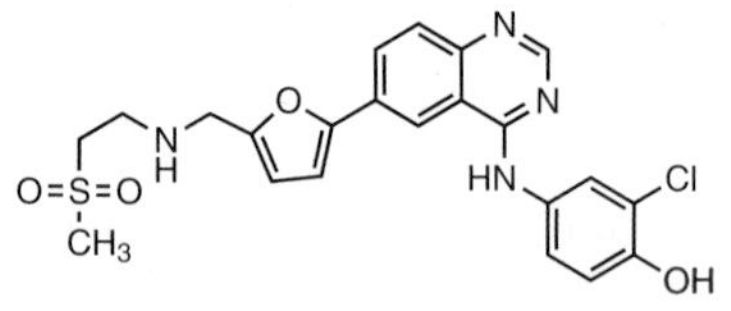

Lapatinib dealkylated metabolite

Severe diarrhea is the most common dose-limiting adverse reaction, but potentially fatal hepatotoxicity was the prompt for a black box toxicity warning for this agent. Given that the *o*-chlorinated phenolic metabolite generated by CYP3A4 could generate a quinoneimine as electrophilic and hepatotoxic as the one formed from gefitinib (Fig. 37.52), along with the high (1,250 mg) daily dose, the warning is not surprising. Other serious side effects are cardiovascular in nature and include decreased left ventricular ejection fraction and arrhythmia. The characteristic EGFR kinase-related rash is experienced by approximately 28% of patients taking this drug. Lapatinib's 24-hour half-life is along the lines of other TKIs. Like other drugs in this class, lapatinib inhibits CYP isoforms (CYP3A4 and CYP2C8), P-gp, and BCRP efflux proteins.

Sunitinib Malate Sunitinib is indicated in the treatment of advanced RCC and imatinib-resistant kit-positive GIST. Its introduction in 2006 more than doubled the rate of positive therapeutic outcomes previously achieved with interferon-α or interleukin-2 in RCC patients (40% vs. 2% to 20% response rates) (191). The drug is supplied as 12.5-, 25-, and 50-mg capsules and is administered daily on a 4 weeks on/2 weeks off regimen. Patients are usually started on 50 mg and then titrated up or down in 12.5-mg increments until an acceptable balance of benefit-to-toxicity is achieved. Absorption is independent of food, but could possibly be impacted by body mass index, which could partially explain the wide individual variability in bioavailability (193).

CYP3A4 deethylates sunitinib to an equally active secondary amine metabolite whose serum levels are approximately one-third of the parent drug (191). All precautions outlined for other CYP3A4-vulnerable kinase inhibitors should be taken.

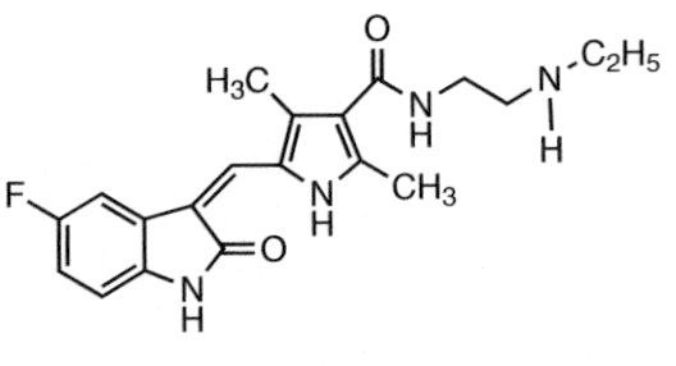

Sunitinib dealkylated metabolite (active)

Like many TKIs, sunitinib is a substrate for P-gp. The terminal half-life of sunitinib and its *N*-deethylated metabolite can extend up to 60 and 100 hours, respectively. The highly conjugated structure imparts a yellow color to the drug and its metabolites, which can be transferred to skin and body fluids. Patients often experience diarrhea, hand-foot syndrome (a consequence of drug leakage from palmar and plantar capillaries), and fatigue. More serious treatment-associated adverse events include potentially fatal hepatotoxicity, left ventricular dysfunction and arrhythmias, and elevated blood pressure. It has been estimated that almost one-fifth of patients on this drug discontinue it, with women and the elderly being at highest risk for adverse events (191).

Sorafenib Tosylate This TKI is indicated for the treatment of advanced RCC and unresectable hepatocellular carcinoma. For either indication, the dosing regimen is one 200-mg tablet twice daily on an empty stomach. Nonlinear kinetics manifest when doses of more than 400 mg/day are administered. Important to its use in hepatocellular carcinoma, doses are cut in half in patients with moderate hepatic impairment, and patients with severe hepatic impairment cannot usually take this drug. Interestingly, when hepatic dysfunction progresses to the very severe stage, 200-mg maximum daily doses are again tolerated (191). Slow tablet disintegration in the GI tract and enterohepatic circulation may contribute to interpatient variability in serum concentrations, and about half of an administered dose of drug will be lost to direct fecal elimination.

Between 9% and 16% of a dose of sorafenib is biotransformed by CYP3A4-mediated *N*-oxidation to an equally active metabolite, which subsequently undergoes glucuronic acid conjugation. Side effects are similar to those induced by sunitinib. Sorafenib is known to inhibit a number of CYP isoforms including CYP3A4, CYP2D6, CYP2B6, CYP2C19, and CYP2C8, but there appear to be no clinically significant interactions with substrates or modifiers of these enzymes (193,194).

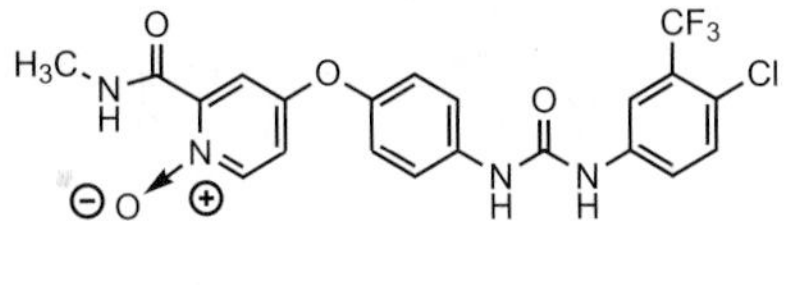

Sorafenib *N*-oxide metabolite (active)

Pazopanib Hydrochloride Like others in its class, pazopanib is indicated in RCC and administered at 800 mg once daily on an empty stomach. Nonlinear kinetics are observed when doses exceed this maximum. The drug is a substrate for CYP3A4 and P-gp, and it has a half-life of approximately 31 hours. Drug-induced hepatotoxicity can be severe, and patients with moderate hepatic dysfunction should not take more than 200 mg daily. Serious cardiovascular and GI toxicities have also been noted.

mTOR Inhibitors

MECHANISM OF ACTION Mammalian target of rapamycin (mTOR) is a serine/threonine kinase that is regulated through the action of phosphatidylinositol (175). When activated, it phosphorylates kinases that ultimately result in the de novo synthesis of proteins (including VEGF) that promote growth. The kinase domain of this 289-kd protein is in the C-terminal area, with the 100-residue macrolide-binding domain (known as FKBP12-FRB) located just to its N-terminal side. The two marketed mTOR inhibitors are O_{13} analogs of rapamycin, a bacterium isolated from soil (Fig. 37.53).

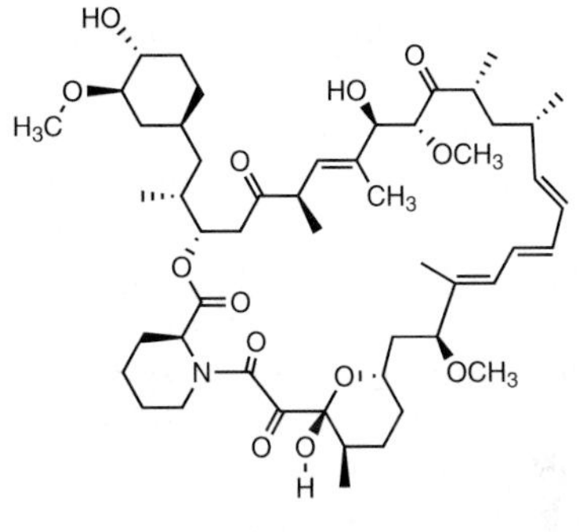

Rapamycin

CHEMISTRY Rapamycin binds tightly to FKBP12 and FBR and, by burrowing into the domain "gap" between these proteins, promotes an interaction that is not observed in the absence of the macrolide. This inhibits the ability of the kinase to function, albeit in a manner not yet understood. Van der Waals interactions with a number of Tyr, Phe, and tryptophan (Trp) residues in the FKBP12

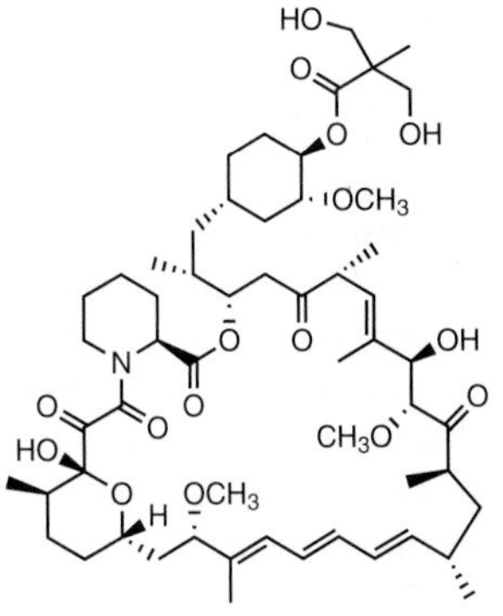

Temsirolimus (Torisel)

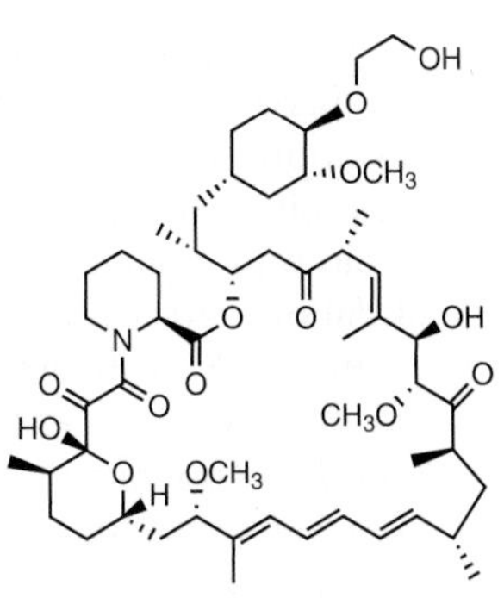

Everolimus (Afinitor)

FIGURE 37.53 mTOR inhibitors.

domain along with H-bonds with Asp and Tyr side chains promotes high-affinity binding between inhibitor and enzyme. Hydrophobic interactions between the carbon-rich macrolide and the kinase are known to occur and are the only interactions believed to form with the FBR domain (175). Rapamycin is 92% buried when bound to these two mTOR domains, and only O_{13} (the site of modification in the commercially available rapamycin-based inhibitors), C_{40}, and C_{41} (of the cyclohexane ring) contact the surrounding environment. The polar nature of the O_{13} ester and alcoholic substituents of temsirolimus and everolimus would promote solubility in these aqueous fluids.

Specific Drugs (Fig. 37.53)

Temsirolimus Temsirolimus is given as a 25-mg intravenous infusion once weekly to patients with advanced RCC. Patients receiving this agent should be pretreated with 25 to 50 mg of diphenhydramine (or a related antihistamine) 30 minutes prior to administration of the macrolide to minimize the risk of hypersensitivity reactions. In patients still responding positively after 6 months of therapy, the drug should be continued for an additional 6 months or for 2 months after complete remission, whichever occurs first. CYP3A4-mediated metabolism to rapamycin (an active metabolite) demands avoidance of inducers or inhibitors of this isoform if at all possible. If coadministration of these agents is essential, appropriate dosage adjustments should be made.

As an immunosuppressive agent, temsirolimus increases the risk of infection and delays wound healing. It also elevates blood glucose, cholesterol, and triglyceride levels. Potentially fatal adverse events associated with temsirolimus include interstitial lung disease, bowel perforation, renal failure, and cerebral hemorrhage.

Everolimus Everolimus is an orally active rapamycin analog that is supplied as 0.25-, 0.5-, 0.75-, 5-, and 10-mg tablets. Ten-milligram doses are administered once daily in the treatment of advanced RCC resistant to sunitinib or sorafenib, whereas the lower doses (<1 mg) are used to stop rejection of transplanted kidneys. In patients with moderate hepatic dysfunction, the antineoplastic dose is cut to 5 mg once daily.

Unlike temsirolimus, therapy can continue for as long as positive therapeutic outcomes are being achieved. However, like temsirolimus, CYP3A4-mediated metabolism requires appropriate dosage adjustments if strong inducers or inhibitors of this isoform must be coadministered. Major biotransformations involve monohydroxylation, *O*-dealkylation, and cleavage of the large lactone ring. None of these metabolites are active. Everolimus shares many of the same adverse effects as temsirolimus (immunosuppression, blood glucose elevation, and dyslipidemias) and can also induce angioedema and ulceration of the oral cavity.

Histone Deacetylase Inhibitors

Mechanism of Action Several structural prototypes can inhibit the deacetylation of Lys residues of the highly basic histone proteins involved in regulating gene transcription. Exposure to these inhibitors is associated with an increase in the antioncogene *p21*, induction of cell cycle arrest, and subsequent apoptosis (195). The fact that a wide variety of proteins can undergo acetylation helps explain the significant impact of this therapy on cellular homeostasis (196). These agents are currently used intravenously in the treatment of cutaneous T-cell lymphoma.

Specific Drugs (Fig. 37.54)

Romidepsin Romidepsin is a depsipeptide histone deacetylase inhibitor that induces a caspase-dependent apoptosis and retains efficacy in cells overexpressing the prosurvival protein Bcl-2 (197). It is a substrate for CYP3A4 and P-gp. Side effects are, as a rule, manageable, with fatigue, fever, and sepsis being the most commonly observed adverse reactions.

Myelosuppression and GI distress are rare. The belief that this agent induces QT interval prolongation has recently been challenged, although serum electrolytes, particularly potassium and magnesium, should be brought within normal range before instituting therapy with this agent (198).

Vorinostat This hydroxamic acid histone deacetylase inhibitor has an overlapping mechanism with romidepsin, but is not vulnerable to P-gp–mediated efflux and loses it caspase-dependent apoptotic action in cells that overexpress Bcl-2 (197). It is inactivated by direct glucuronic acid conjugation and/or hydrolysis at the hydroxamic acid end of the molecule and subsequent β-oxidation to 4-anilino-4-oxobutanoic acid (199). Side effects are classified as GI, constitutional (e.g., chills, fever), hematologic (thrombocytopenia, anemia), and taste-related. Pulmonary embolism is also a risk of vorinostat therapy.

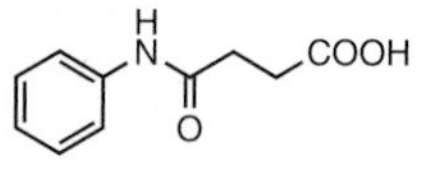

4-Anilino-4-oxobutanoic acid

Vorinostat is available only to patients who are enrolled in a manufacturer-sponsored program entitled Accessing Coverage Today. Patients must specify their pharmacy so

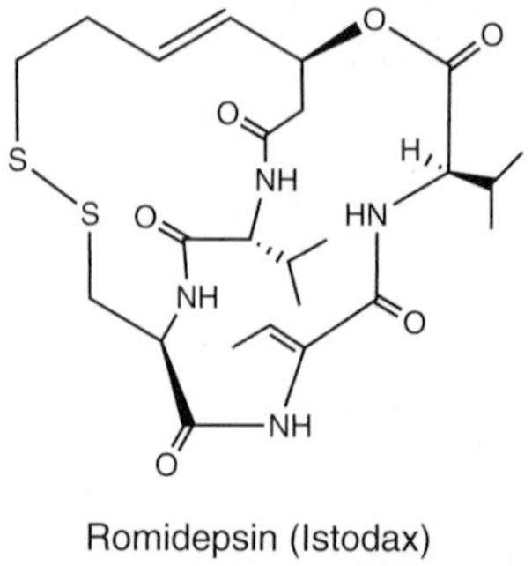

Romidepsin (Istodax)

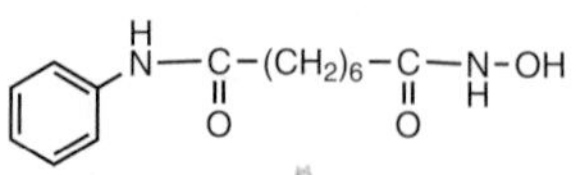

Vorinostat (Zolinza)

FIGURE 37.54 Histone deacetylase inhibitors.

that the medication can be provided for distribution by those specific pharmacists. Pharmacists dispensing this drug to approved patients do not require special certification or program enrollment (200).

Immunomodulators

Specific Drugs (Fig. 37.55)

Thalidomide Anyone of the "baby boomer" or World War II generation will recognize the name of the drug thalidomide because it induced perhaps the most well-known incident of drug-associated birth defects in recent history (201). Used in the late 1950s and early 1960s as an antiemetic and sedative in pregnant women, more than 10,000 European children were born with flipper-like arms and legs, a condition called phocomelia or "seal limb." Approximately half of those afflicted survived. Although it is known that the teratogenic and sedative actions of chiral thalidomide are mediated by different stereoisomers (202), the in vivo conversion of the therapeutic *R*-isomer to its cytotoxic *S*-enantiomer prohibited the use of this drug in women who were or could become pregnant. Although not licensed in the United States during these early years, the drug was banned by the U.S. Food and Drug Administration (FDA) until 1997 (203).

Despite this troubled beginning, the therapeutic potential of thalidomide, when used wisely and rationally, is significant (204). Its action as a tumor necrosis factor α inhibitor prompted the lifting of the FDA ban to allow its use in the treatment of leprosy. Its antiproliferative and proapoptotic actions have now allowed it to be approved for use in combination with dexamethasone in multiple myeloma (205,206). In addition to arresting uncontrolled cell growth, thalidomide denies multiple myeloma cells access to bone marrow stromal cells and various growth factors needed for tumor cell survival and augments circulating levels of natural killer cells, interleukin-2, and interferon-γ (202). The benefit of adding thalidomide to other chemotherapeutic regimens for multiple myeloma, and in treating other neoplastic disorders, is under active investigation (207).

Thalidomide is marketed as 50-, 100-, and 200-mg capsules. If tolerated, a 200-mg dose is administered at least 1 hour after the evening meal, preferably at bedtime. It undergoes spontaneous hydrolysis of the phthalimide and glutarimide moieties to generate 12 distinct hydrolysis products prior to renal elimination (208). Thalidomide has a minor vulnerability to stereoselective CYP2C19-catalyzed metabolism, and three metabolites have been identified (Fig. 37.56). However, the extent of formation shows significant individual variability, and the clinical significance of this potential metabolic pathway in vivo is highly questionable.

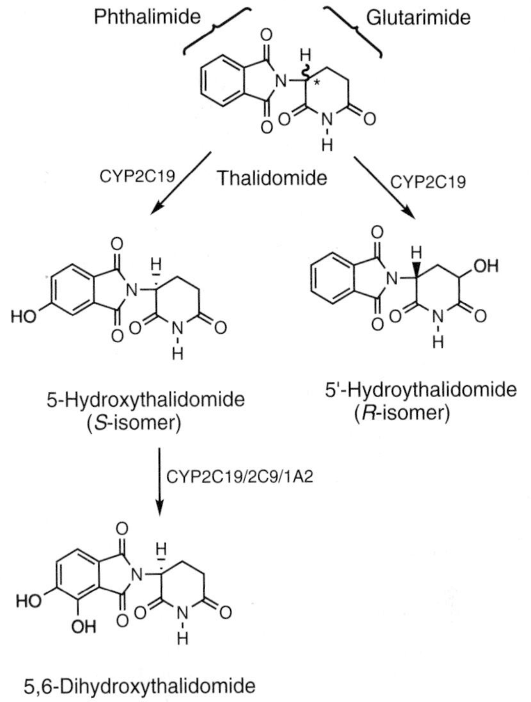

FIGURE 37.56 CYP2C19-mediated thalidomide metabolism.

Thalidomide can only be dispensed by pharmacists or other qualified providers who are registered with the System for Thalidomide Education and Prescribing Safety (STEPS) distribution program (209), and women of childbearing age may be given this drug only if no viable alternative exists, and then only with ongoing weekly (first therapeutic month) and monthly (thereafter) proof of nonpregnant status. Because the drug also finds its way into semen, male thalidomide patients capable of having sexual relations must agree to safety-promoting restrictions on reproductive activities. Use-limiting adverse effects include peripheral neuropathy that can be irreversible (most commonly with chronic use) and thromboembolic events (e.g., deep vein thrombosis, pulmonary emboli). The latter side effect is exacerbated by the coadministered dexamethasone. Other potentially problematic, but less serious, side effects include sedation, fatigue, and constipation (202).

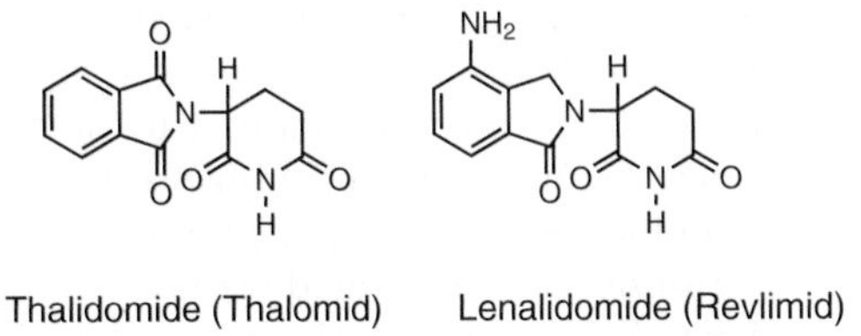

FIGURE 37.55 Thalidomide-based immunomodulators.

Lenalidomide Lenalidomide has a similar activity profile to its predecessor immunomodulator, thalidomide, but is effective at a little more than one-tenth of the dose (25 mg daily as opposed to 200 mg). The side effect profile is milder, although because the drug is also coadministered with dexamethasone, significant thromboembolic events can still occur. Neutropenia and thrombocytopenia can also be dose-limiting. The potential for serious dose-independent teratogenicity is the basis for restricted use in people of reproductive potential. Practitioners dispensing lenalidomide must be registered with RevAssist, a distribution program similar to STEPS (210).

Despite having retained the glutarimide moiety that was a prime target for nonenzymatic hydrolysis in thalidomide, approximately two-thirds of a dose of lenalidomide is excreted unchanged in the urine. The drug is not a substrate for or an inhibitor or inducer of CYP enzymes (211).

Miscellaneous Anticancer Agents

Specific Drugs

Arsenic Trioxide (Proapoptotic) As noted at the start of this chapter, the toxic effects of arsenic have been recognized for millennia (212). Arsenic trioxide (As_2O_3, known commercially as Trisenox) was originally introduced into Western medicine in the late 19th century for the treatment of leukemia and then fell out of favor as newer chemotherapeutic and radiation-based approaches to care became available. The drug experienced a pharmacotherapeutic renaissance in the late 20th century, and it is currently used intravenously to induce remission in patients with acute promyelocytic leukemia (APL). APL is characterized by the reciprocal translocation of chromosomes 15 and 17, resulting in the abnormal joining of the promyelocytic gene and retinoic acid receptor α (213). This, in turn, results in the generation of immature leukemia cells, differentiation arrest, and the induction of serious/fatal hemorrhagic and other coagulation-related disorders. Arsenic trioxide induces remission in APL patients through the destruction of the offending fusion protein, promotion of promyelocyte differentiation, and stimulation of apoptosis in malignant cells. One documented chemical apoptotic mechanism is inhibition of intracellular catalase and glutathione peroxidase, with the resultant accumulation of the free radical precursor H_2O_2. Another is the downregulation of the antiapoptotic protein Bcl-2 (212). Arsenic trioxide's indication specifies use after therapy with an anthracycline and a retinoid (e.g., tretinoin, *trans*-retinoic acid) has failed, but there is evidence to show its efficacy as first-line therapy in newly diagnosed or previously untreated patients (213). Although patient numbers were relatively small, complete remission rates ranging between 73% and 92% have been reported.

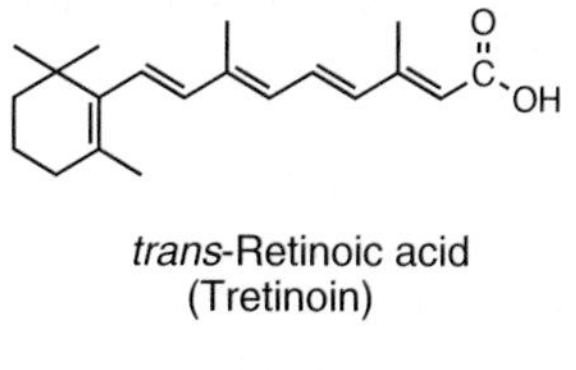

trans-Retinoic acid
(Tretinoin)

The pentavalent As(V) in the parent drug is reduced to the active trivalent As(III) by arsenate reductase. Prior to excretion, As(III) is methylated to mono- and dimethylarsonic acid. Although arsenic trioxide is usually well tolerated, the possibility of QT interval prolongation, torsades de pointes, and complete atrioventricular block demands an assessment of serum electrolytes (particularly magnesium and potassium) prior to the initiation of therapy. APL differentiation syndrome (also known as retinoic acid syndrome and characterized by pleural/pericardial/pulmonary infiltrates or effusions, dyspnea, weight gain, and fatigue) responds to corticosteroid intervention. Reversible hepatotoxicity has also been noted, and the strong emetogenic potential of As_2O_3 warrants coadministration of drugs to control nausea and vomiting.

Bortezomib (Proteasome Inhibitor) Facilitated by ubiquitin tagging, proteasomes selectively clear cells of cytoplasmic regulatory proteins by cleaving them into short peptides. Inhibition of this homeostatic process induces apoptosis, at least in part through the dysregulation of unfolded protein response gene expression (214) and the inhibition of the activation of antiapoptotic factor nuclear factor-κB by proteasome substrate IκBα (215). Bortezomib binds to the 20S proteasome (or "core particle") component of the 26S proteasome, a highly conserved protein that can cleave proteins essentially anywhere along the chain (216). The binding selectivity is quite high, as the estimated affinity ratio for this proteasome and the next most attractive target protein is over 1,500 (215). The crystal structure of the bortezomib-20S proteasome complex from yeast has been reported, and specific drug–proteasome interactions have been identified (217). The multiplicity of potential binding sites encompassing multiple 20S subunits confirms the complex nature of its activity and may pave the way for the development of more selective inhibitors with higher affinities and more desirable pharmacokinetic properties.

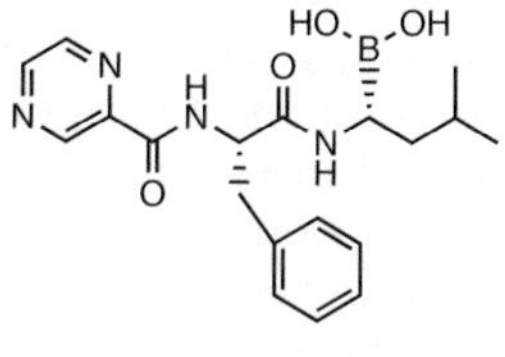

Bortezomib (Velcade)

Bortezomib is used intravenously in the treatment of multiple myeloma and mantle cell lymphoma. The boronic acid moiety is essential, as CYP-mediated deboronation yields a metabolite that does not inhibit the 26S proteasome. The drug is hydroxylated at various positions prior to excretion, and the CYP isoforms involved in the biotransformations include CYP3A4, CYP2C19, and CYP1A2. Like many other anticancer agents, the drug suppresses bone marrow, leading to neutropenia and thrombocytopenia, and can induce serious sensory (and less commonly motor) peripheral neuropathy. Neuropathy can often be managed with dose reduction, although drug discontinuation is required with grade 4 dysfunction (215). Cardiac and pulmonary complications have also been reported.

OTHER CHEMOTHERAPEUTIC APPROACHES

Hormone Therapy

Glucocorticoids (e.g., prednisone and methylprednisolone) are commonly administered with anticancer agents to suppress lymphocytic activity and to enhance the chance of success in the treatment of leukemias and lymphomas. In addition, some tumors, such as estrogen-dependent breast cancer, endometrial cancer, and metastatic cancer of the prostate, depend on the presence of sex hormones for viability. In these neoplastic diseases, the use of steroid receptor antagonists, synthesis inhibitors, or gonadotropin secretion inhibitors, either alone or in combination with other antineoplastic drugs, is a common approach to chemotherapeutic care. Antiestrogens (e.g., tamoxifen), antiandrogens (e.g., flutamide), progestins (e.g., megestrol acetate), aromatase nhibitors (e.g., exemestane), and luteinizing hormone-releasing hormone agonists (e.g., leuprolide acetate) are all available for use in managing hormone-dependent tumors and are often employed after surgery, radiation therapy, and/or other chemotherapy.

Enzyme Therapy

Exogenous asparagine (Asn) is essential to the survival of malignant lymphocytic leukemia cells, because these cells lack asparagine synthetase enzymes. L-Asparaginase (also known as L-asparagine amidohydrolase) or its derivatives can be added to the chemotherapeutic regimen of patients with leukemia to deplete serum Asn by hydrolysis to aspartate and ammonia. Being deprived of this avenue for Asn acquisition, tumor cells die from an inability to synthesize essential proteins. Normal cells, which contain asparagine synthetase, are able to synthesize this essential nutrient and can withstand therapy.

Monoclonal Antibodies

Seven human, humanized, or chimeric monoclonal antibodies (MoAbs), as well as three MoAbs conjugated with either a cytotoxic calicheamicin-based antibiotic or γ- and/or β-emitting radioisotopes, are also commercially available for the treatment of various neoplasms (Table 37.9) (218). The two murine MoAbs on the market (ibritumomab tiuxetan and tositumomab) have a momab ending in their names (mouse), as opposed to the humanized antibodies, which most commonly end in umab (human). Whether future marketed anticancer MoAbs will support this helpful hint to antibody origin remains to be seen.

MoAbs target tumor cell antigens, and in unconjugated form, the complex recruits endogenous immunomodulator and cell-destroying cytokines (e.g., natural killer cells, macrophages) to stop the advancement of the cancer. The protein components of conjugated MoAbs are homing devices designed to selectively deliver cell-killing chemicals attached to the antibody to tumor cells. It should be noted that some endogenous immunomodulator/biologic response modifying proteins (e.g., interleukin-2) are also available as drug products to treat selected solid and hematologic cancers.

The selected targeting of tumor cells over healthy cells (which do not express the target antigen to the extent malignant cells do) should promote a higher margin of safety for MoAbs when compared to administering toxins that can distribute as widely as their chemical properties allow. The engineering of humanized or chimeric MoAbs has significantly attenuated the risk of therapy-sabotaging immunologic responses to the murine-derived proteins found in the early agents. However, black box warnings for all MoAb anticancer agents except one (ofatumumab) caution against such potentially fatal events as infusion/hypersensitivity reactions, cytopenias, hemorrhage, hepatotoxicity, infection, tumor lysis syndrome, cardiomyopathy, and cardiopulmonary arrest.

The interested reader is directed to several reviews on the clinical use of anticancer MoAbs that have recently appeared in the literature (219–222).

TABLE 37.9 Anticancer MoAbs (217)

MoAb	Drug/Nuclide Conjugate?	Cellular Target	Cancer
Alemtuzumab	No	CD52	B-cell CLL
Bevacizumab	No	VEGF	Colorectal, lung
Cetuximab	No	EGFR	Colorectal, head and neck
Gemtuzumab ozogamicin	Calicheamicin	CD33	Acute myeloid leukemia
Ibritumomab tiuxetan (murine)	^{90}Y (β-emitting isotope)	CD20	NHL
Ofatumumab	No	CD20	CLL
Panitumumab	No	EGFR	Colorectal
Rituximab	No	CD20	NHL
Tositumomab (murine)	^{131}I (γ- and β-emitting isotope)	CD20	NHL
Trastuzumab	No	HER2	Breast

SCENARIO: OUTCOME AND ANALYSIS

Outcome

Kelly Nystrom, PharmD, BCOP

Despite maintaining urinary pH at or above 7.0, DT's 24-hour level of methotrexate (MTX) was reported at 3.57 μM, and leucovorin (prophylactic cells rescue from excessive MTX toxicity) was increased from 15 mg to 50 mg IV every 6 hours. The pharmacist reviewed DT's medications and, noting that he was taking ibuprofen around the clock for headache, discontinued that medication. Subsequently, DL's 48-hour level of MTX dropped to an acceptable 0.03 μM, and he was discharged.

Chemical Analysis

Victoria Roche and S. William Zito

The stronger of methotrexate's two glutamate COOH groups (α-COOH) would exist predominately in water-soluble anionic conjugate base form at DL's urinary pH (i/u = 1587/1 at pH 7.0). However, DL's chronic use of ibuprofen is compromising his renal function and allowing MTX to rise to toxic levels in the blood, necessitating additional rescue therapy with leucovorin.

Ibuprofen, an arylpropionic acid nonsteroidal anti-inflammatory drug (NSAID), inhibits COX-1 and COX-2 isoforms of cyclooxygenase that are responsible for the production of prostaglandin. COX-1 serves homeostatic functions in many tissues, including the kidney, and inhibition can result in a serious (e.g., up to 40%) decrease in glomerular filtration rate and potentially fatal renal insufficiency. Ibuprofen also inhibits proximal tubule transporter proteins (MRP2 and MRP4) used by MTX, resulting in a lower renal tubular efflux of MTX. COX-2 selective inhibitors (sulfonamide or sulfone-containing diarylheteroaromatic structures) do not alter MTX renal clearance kinetics, but COX-2 selective inhibitors are not used to treat headache.

MTX is approximately 50% bound to serum proteins; its 7-hydroxy metabolite is ~93% protein bound with a small volume of distribution. Ibuprofen's serum protein binding approaches 99%. All drugs are anionic in the bloodstream, contributing to their ability to compete for limited protein binding sites. Displacement of MTX and its cytotoxic 7-hydroxy metabolite from serum proteins secondary to ibuprofen co-therapy can result in abnormally high blood levels of free drug. Because ibuprofen also inhibits the urinary excretion of MTX, life-threatening toxicity results. The toxicity is addressed by increasing the dose of leucovorin ("rescue") and discontinuing use of the offending NSAID.

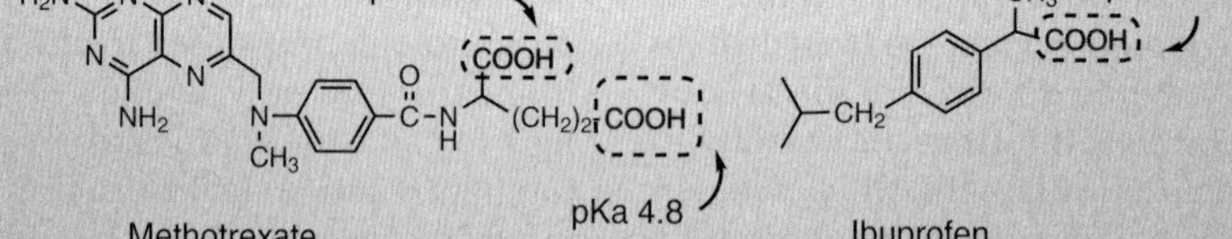

CASE STUDY

Victoria Roche and S. William Zito

KV is a 48-year-old firefighter who has been called into action over the past several years fighting wildfires in Arizona, Montana, Wyoming, and California. An increased incidence of testicular cancer has been noted among men in KV's line of work, and he received this difficult diagnosis a little more than a month ago. Fortunately his cancer is still in the early stages (stage IB).

KV's oncologist has elected the "BEP regimen," which combines bleomycin, etoposide, and cisplatin. He has been through one round of chemotherapy but is not responding as well as anticipated. KV's oncologist suspects intrinsic resistance to cisplatin. In addition, KV read on the internet about the possibility of hearing loss with this platinum coordination complex, and he has verbalized his fear that this permanent toxic effect could keep him from returning to work once he is (hopefully) in full remission. He also experienced hypersensitivity to the etoposide infusion, which, while initially managed with an infusion rate adjustment, corticosteroids, and antihistamines, progressed to the point where epinephrine was required to reverse bronchospasm.

The oncologist is consulting with you about appropriate next steps that could be taken to develop a chemotherapy regimen for KV that would give him the best chance for recovery with a high quality of life. A decision is made to change both the etoposide and the platinum complex in the regimen. Which of the structures in each pair of molecules below might be viable alternatives to accomplish the desired outcome? If you made any of these alterations in therapy, would you also recommend the coadministration of either compounds **A** or **B**?

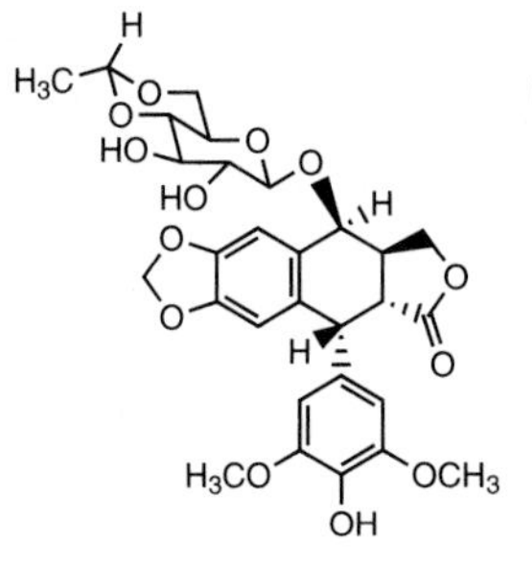

Etoposide

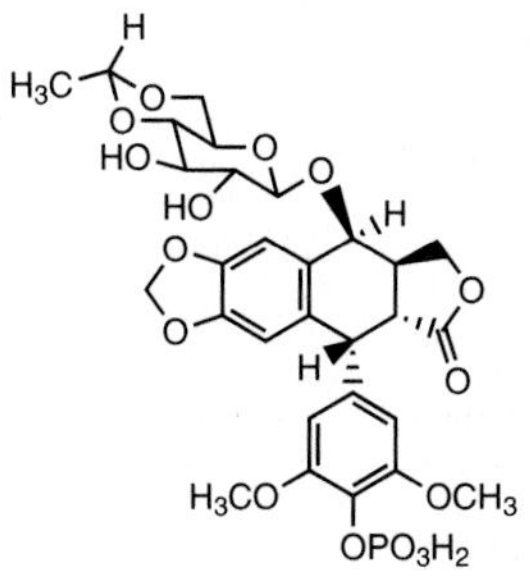

Etoposide alternative 1

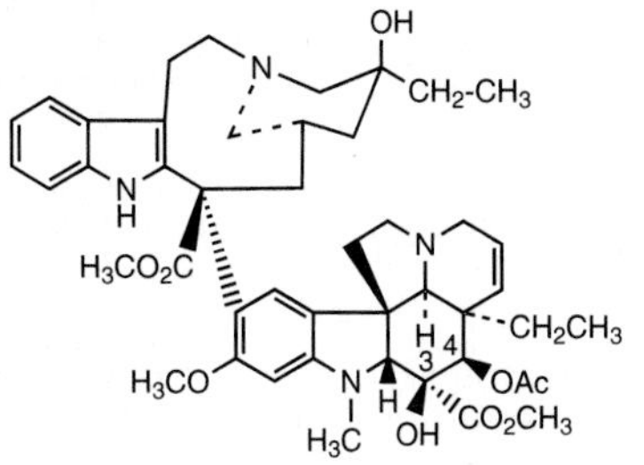

Etoposide alternative 2

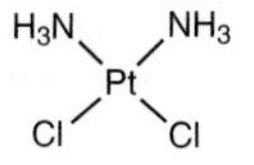

Cisplatin

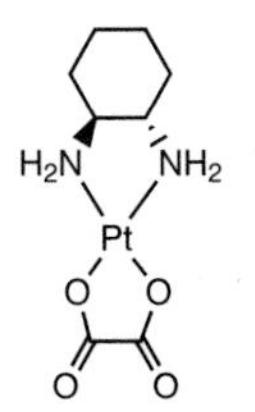

Cisplatin alternative 1

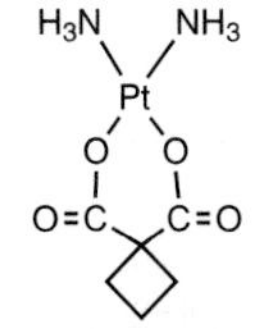

Cisplatin alternative 2

$MgSO_4$

A

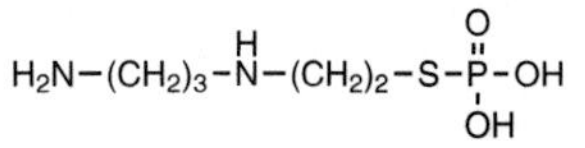

B

1. Conduct a thorough and mechanistic SAR analysis of the three therapeutic options in the case.
2. Apply the chemical understanding gained from the SAR analysis to this patient's specific needs to make a therapeutic recommendation.

References

1. Liu ET. Oncogenes and suppressor genes: genetic control of cancer. In: Goldman L, Ausiello D, eds. Cecil Textbook of Medicine, 22nd ed. Philadelphia: W.B. Saunders, 2004:1108–1116.
2. Bertino JR, Hait W. Principles of cancer therapy. In: Goldman L, Ausiello D, eds. Cecil Textbook of Medicine, 22nd ed. Philadelphia: W.B. Saunders, 2004:1137–1150.
3. Medina PJ, Fausel C. Cancer treatment and chemotherapy. In: DiPiro JT, Talbert RL, Yee GC, et al., eds. Pharmacotherapy: A Pathophysiologic Approach, 7th ed. New York: McGraw-Hill, 2008:2085–2119.
4. Chabner BA, Amrein PC, Drucker BJ, et al. Antineoplastic agents. In: Brunton LL, Lazo JS, Parker KL, eds. Goodman & Gilman's The Pharmacological Basis of Therapeutics, 11th ed. New York: McGraw Hill, 2005:1319–1321.
5. Minn AJ, Massague J. Invasion and metastases. In: DeVita VT Jr, Lawrence TS, Rosenberg SA, eds. Cancer: Principles and Practice of Oncology, 8th ed. Baltimore: Lippincott Williams & Wilkins, 2008:117–118.
6. Burchenal JH. The historical development of cancer chemotherapy. Semin Oncol 1977;4:135–146.
7. Woglom WH. General review of cancer therapy. In: Moulton FR, ed. Approaches to Tumor Chemotherapy. Washington, DC: AAAS, 1947:1.
8. Sznol M. Pharmacology of cancer chemotherapy: drug development. In: DeVita VT Jr, Lawrence TS, Rosenberg SA, eds. Cancer: Principles and Practice of Oncology, 8th ed. Baltimore: Lippincott Williams & Wilkins, 2008:385–392.
9. Wong K-K, Sharpless NE, Depinho RA. Telomeres, telomerase, and cell immortalization. In: DeVita VT Jr, Lawrence TS, Rosenberg SA, eds. Cancer: Principles and Practice of Oncology, 8th ed. Baltimore: Lippincott Williams & Wilkins, 2008:53–66.
10. El-Khoueiry A, Lenz HJ. Pharmacogenomics. In: DeVita VT Jr, Lawrence TS, Rosenberg SA, eds. Cancer: Principles and Practice of Oncology, 8th ed. Baltimore: Lippincott Williams & Wilkins, 2008:402–407.
11. American Cancer Society. Cancer facts and figures, 2010. http://www.cancer.org/acs/groups/content/@epidemiologysurveilance/documents/document/acspc-026238.pdf. Accessed December 2, 2010.
12. Blot WJ. Epidemiology of cancer. In: Goldman L, Ausiello D, eds. Cecil Textbook of Medicine, 22nd ed. Philadelphia: W.B. Saunders, 2004:1116–1120.
13. The signs of cancer. http://www.radoncgroup.com/signsofcancer.pdf. Accessed December 16, 2010.
14. Buchschacher GL Jr, Wong-Staal F. Etiology of cancer: viruses: RNA viruses. In: DeVita VT Jr, Lawrence TS, Rosenberg SA, eds. Cancer: Principles and Practice of Oncology, 8th ed. Baltimore: Lippincott Williams & Wilkins, 2008:169–177.
15. Howley PM, Ganem D, Kieff E. Etiology of cancer: viruses: DNA viruses. In: DeVita VT Jr, Lawrence TS, Rosenberg SA, eds. Cancer: Principles and Practice of Oncology, 8th ed. Baltimore: Lippincott Williams & Wilkins, 2008:177–189.
16. Ludeman SM. The chemistry of the metabolites of cyclophosphamide. Curr Pharm Des 1999;5:627–643.
17. Goldenberg GJ, Lee M, Lam HY, et al. Evidence for carrier-mediated transport of melphalan by L5178Y lymphoblasts in vitro. Cancer Res 1977;37:755–760.
18. Tageja N, Nagi J. Bendamustine: something old, something new. Cancer Chemother Pharmacol 2010;66:413–423.
19. Montillo M, Ricci F, Tedeschi A, et al. Bendamustine: new perspective for an old drug in lymphoproliferative disorders. Expert Rev Hematol 2010;3:131–148.
20. Giraud B, Herbert G, Deroussent A, et al. Oxazaphosphorines: new therapeutic strategies for an old class of drugs. Expert Opin Drug Metab Toxicol 2010;6:919–938.
21. Huang A, Roy P, Waxman DJ. Role of human liver microsomal CYP3A4 and CYP2B6 in catalyzing N-dechloroethylation of cyclophosphamide and ifosfamide. Biochem Pharmacol 2000;59:961–972.
22. Lind MJ, McGown AT, Hadfield JA, et al. The effect of ifosfamide and its metabolites on intracellular glutathione levels in vitro and in vivo. Biochem Pharmacol 1989;38:1835–1840.
23. Ramu K, Fraiser LH, Mamiya B, et al. Acrolein mercapturates: synthesis, characterization and assessment of their role in the bladder toxicity of cyclophosphamide. Chem Res Toxicol 1995;8:515–524.
24. Ramu K, Perry CS, Ahmed T, et al. Studies on the basis for the toxicity of acrolein mercapturates. Toxicol Appl Pharmacol 1996;140;487–498.
25. Springate JE. Ifosfamide metabolite chloroacetaldehyde causes renal dysfunction in vivo. J Appl Toxicol 1997;17:75–79.
26. Roy P, Yu LJ, Crespi CL, et al. Development of a substrate-activity based approach to identify the major human liver P-450 catalysts of cyclophosphamide and ifosfamide activation based on cDNA-expressed activities and liver microsomal P-450 profiles. Drug Metab Dispos 1999;27:655–666.
27. Woodland D, Ito S, Granvil CP, et al. Evidence of renal metabolism of ifosfamide to nephrotoxic metabolites. Life Sci 2000;68:109–117.
28. Storme T, Deroussent A, Mercier L, et al. New ifosfamide analogs designed for lower associated neurotoxicity and nephrotoxicity with modified alkylating kinetics leading to enhanced in vitro anticancer activity. J Pharmacol Exp Ther 2009;328:598–609.
29. Kheffache D, Ouameraldi O. Some physicochemical properties of the antitumor drug thiotepa and its metabolite tepa as obtained by density functional theory (DFT) calculations. J Mol Model 2010;16:1383–1390.
30. Eisenbrand G, Muller N, Denkel E, et al. DNA adducts and DNA damage by antineoplastic and carcinogenic N-nitroso compounds. J Cancer Res Clin Oncol 1986;112:196–204.
31. Bacolod MD, Fehdrau R, Johnson SP, et al. BCNU sequestration by metallothioneines may contribute to resistance in a medulloblastoma cell line. Cancer Chemother Pharmacol 2009;63:753–758.
32. Kyrtopoulos SA, Anderson LM, Chhabra SK, et al. DNA adducts and the mechanism of carcinogenesis and cytotoxicity of methylating agents of environmental and clinical significance. Cancer Detect Prev 1997;21:391–405.
33. Patterson LH, Murray GI. Tumour cytochrome P450 and drug activation. Curr Pharm Des 2002;8:1335–1347.

34. Moloney SJ, Wiebkin P, Cummings SW, et al. Metabolic activation of the terminal N-methyl group of N-isopropyl-alpha-(2-methylhydrazino)-p-toluamide hydrochloride (procarbazine). Carcinogenesis 1985;6:397–401.
35. Moloney SJ, Prough RA. Studies on the pathway of methane formation from procarbazine, a 2-methylbenzylhydrazine derivative, by rat liver microsomes. Arch Biochem Biophys 1983;221:577–584.
36. Yamagata S, Ohmori S, Suzuki N, et al. Metabolism of dacarbazine by rat liver microsomes: contribution of CYP1A enzymes to dacarbazine N-demethylation. Drug Metab Dispos 1998;26:379–382.
37. Cai W, Maldonado NV, Cui W, et al. Activity of irinotecan and temozolomide in the presence of O^6-methylguanine-DNA methyltransferase inhibition in neuroblastoma pre-clinical models. Br J Cancer 2010;103:1369–1379.
38. Coley HM, Brooks N, Phillips DH, et al. The role of N-(hydroxymethyl) melamines as antitumour agents: mechanism of action studies. Biochem Pharmacol 1995;9:1203–1212.
39. Ames MM. Hexamethylmelamine: pharmacology and mechanism of action. Can Treat Rev 1991;18(Suppl A):3–14.
40. Deng SJ, Wang S, Cao J, et al. Liposomes incorporating sodium deoxycholate for hexamethylmelamine (HMM) oral delivery: development, characterization, and in vivo evaluation. Drug Deliv 2010;17:164–170.
41. Ponti M, Souhami RL, Fox BW, et al. DNA interstrand crosslinking and sequence selectivity of dimethanesulphonates. Br J Cancer 1991;63:743–747.
42. Iwamoto T, Hiraku Y, Oikawa S, et al. DNA intrastrand cross-link at the 5'-GA-3' sequence formed by busulfan and its role in the cytotoxic effect. Cancer Sci 2004;95:454–458.
43. Teicher B. Newer cytotoxic agents: attacking cancer broadly. Clin Cancer Res 2008;24:1610–1617.
44. Chaney SG, Campbell SL, Bassett E, et al. Recognition and processing of cisplatin- and oxaliplatin-DNA adducts. Crit Rev Oncol Hematol 2005;53:3–11.
45. Raymond E, Faivre S, Woynarowski JM, et al. Oxaliplatin: mechanism of action and antineoplastic activity. Semin Oncol 1998;25(Suppl 5):4–12.
46. Fouladi M, Chintagumpala M, Ashley D, et al. Amifostine protects against cisplatin-induced ototoxicity in children with average risk medulloblastoma. J Clin Oncol 2008;26:3749–3755.
47. Kelland L. The resurgence of platinum-based cancer chemotherapy. Nat Rev 2007;7:573–584.
48. Mishima M, Samimi G, Kondo A, et al. The cellular pharmacology of oxaliplatin resistance. Eur J Cancer 2002;38:1405–1412.
49. Chaney SG, Campbell SL, Temple B, et al. Protein interactions with platinum-DNA adducts: from structure to function. J Inorg Biochem 2004;98:1551–1559.
50. Barnes KR, Lippard SJ. Cisplatin and related anticancer drugs: recent advances and insights. Met Ions Biol Syst 2004;42:143–177.
51. McKeage MJ. New-generation platinum drugs in the treatment of cisplatin-resistant cancers. Expert Opin Invest Drugs 2005;14:1033–1046.
52. Kweekel DM, Gelderblom H, Guchelaar H-J. Pharmacology of oxaliplatin and the use of pharmacogenomics to individualize therapy. Cancer Treat Rev 2005;31:90–105.
53. Grolleau F, Gamelin L, Boisdron-Celle M, et al. A possible explanation for a neurotoxic effect of the anticancer agent oxaliplatin on neuronal voltage-gated sodium channels. J Neurophysiol 2001;85:2293–2297.
54. Gamelin L, Boisdron-Celle M, Delva R, et al. Prevention of oxaliplatin-related neurotoxicity by calcium and magnesium infusions: a retrospective study of 161 patients receiving oxaliplatin combined with 5-fluorouracil and leucovorin for advanced colorectal cancer. Clin Cancer Res 2004;10:4055–4061.
55. Kelland L. Broadening the clinical use of platinum drug-based chemotherapy with new analogs: satraplatin and picoplatin. Expert Opin Invest Drugs 2007;16:1009–1021.
56. Choy H, Park C, Yao M. Current status and future prospects for satraplatin, an oral platinum analog. Clin Cancer Res 2008;14:1633–1638.
57. Pommier Y, Leo E, Zhang HL, et al. DNA topoisomerases and their poisoning by anticancer and antibacterial drugs. Chem Biol Rev 2010;17:421–433.
58. Dal Ben D, Palumbo M, Zagotto G, et al. DNA topoisomerase II structures and anthracycline activity: insights into ternary complex formation. Curr Pharm Des 2007;13:2766–2780.
59. Staker BL, Hjerrild K, Feese MD, et al. The mechanism of topoisomerase I poisoning by a camptothecin analog. Proc Natl Acad Sci 2002;99:15387–15392.
60. Giordano M, D'Annessa I, Coletta A, et al. Structural and dynamical effects induced by the anticancer drug topotecan on the human topoisomerase I-DNA complex. PLos One 2010;5:e10934.
61. Staker BL, Feese MD, Cushman M, et al. Structures of three classes of anticancer agents bound to the human topoisomerase I-DNA covalent complex. J Med Chem 2005;48:2336–2345.
62. Chabner BA, Ryan DP, Paz-Ares L, et al. Antineoplastic agents. In: Hardman JG, Limbird LE, eds. Goodman & Gilman's The Pharmacological Basis of Therapeutics, 10th ed. New York: McGraw Hill, 2001:1389–1459.
63. Takimoto CH. Topoisomerase interactive agents. In: DeVita VT Jr, Hellman S, Rosenberg SA, eds. Cancer: Principles and Practice of Oncology, 7th ed. Baltimore: Lippincott Williams & Wilkins, 2005:375–390.
64. Kirschbaum M. A comeback for camptothecins? Leuk Lymph 2009;50:1914–1915.
65. Xu C, Barchet TM, Mager DE. Quantitative structure-property relationships of camptothecins in humans. Cancer Chemother Pharmacol 2009;65:325–333.
66. Venditto VJ, Simanek EE. Cancer therapies using the camptothecins. A review of the in vivo literature. Mol Pharmacol 2010;7:307–349.
67. Shimoyama S. Pharmacogenetics of irinotecan. An ethnicity based prediction of irinotecan adverse effects. World J Gastrointest Surg 2010;2:14–21.
68. Onoue M, Terada T, Kobayashi M, et al. UGT1A1*6 polymorphism is most predictive of severe neutropenia induced by irinotecan in Japanese cancer patients. Int J Clin Oncol 2009;14:136–142.
69. Drummond DC, Noble CO, Guo Z, et al. Development of a highly stable and targetable nanoliposomal formulation of topotecan. J Control Release 2010;141:13–21.
70. Vilain N, Tsai-Pflugfelder M, Benoit A, et al. Modulation of drug sensitivity in yeast cells by the ATP-binding domain of human DNA topoisomerase IIalpha. Nucleic Acids Res 2003;31:5714–5722.
71. Chee GL, Yalowich JC, Bodner A, et al. A diazirine-based photoaffinity etoposide probe for labeling topoisomerase II. Bioorg Med Chem 2010;18:830–838.
72. Naik PK, Dubey A, Soni K, et al. The binding modes and binding affinities of epipodophyllotoxin derivatives with human topoisomerase IIα. J. Molec Graph Model 2010;29:546–564.
73. Felix CA. Secondary leukemias induced by topoisomerase-targeted drugs. Biochim Biophys Acta 1998;1400:233–255.
74. Binaschi M, Bigioni M, Cipollone A, et al. Anthracyclines: selected new developments. Curr Med Chem 2001;1:113–130.
75. Gerwirtz DA. A critical evaluation of the mechanisms of action proposed for the antitumor effects of the anthracycline antibiotics Adriamycin and daunorubicin. Biochem Pharmacol 1999;57:727–741.
76. Zunino F, Pratesi G, Perego P. Role of the sugar moiety in the pharmacological activity of anthracyclines: development of a novel series of disaccharide analogs. Biochem Pharmacol 2001;61:933–938.
77. Piestrzeniecwicz MK, Wilmanska D, Szemraj J, et al. Interactions of novel morpholine and hexamethylene derivatives of anthracycline antibiotics with DNA. Z Naturforsch 2004;59:739–748.
78. Chien AJ, Moasser MM. Cellular mechanisms of resistance against taxanes and anthracyclines in cancer: intrinsic and acquired. Semin Oncol 2008;35(Suppl 2):S1–S14.
79. Mei Y, Qian F, Wei M, et al. Reversal of cancer by green tea polyphenols. J Pharm Pharmacol 2004;56:1307–1314.
80. Sadzuka Y, Sugiyama T, Sonobe T. Efficacies of tea components on doxorubicin induced antitumor activity and reversal of multidrug resistance. Toxicol Lett 2000;114:155–162.
81. Stammler G, Volm M. Green tea catechins (EGCG and EGC) have modulating effects on the activity of doxorubicin in drug resistant cell lines. Anticancer Drugs 1997;8:265–268.
82. Kwok JC, Richardson DR. Examination of the mechanism(s) involved in doxorubicin-mediated iron accumulation in ferritin: studies using metabolic inhibitors, protein synthesis inhibitors and lysosomotropic agents. Mol Pharmacol 2004;65:181–195.
83. Mordente A, Meucci E, Silvestrini GE, et al. New developments in anthracycline-induced cardiotoxicity. Curr Med Chem 2009;16:1656–1672.
84. Lothstein L, Israel M, Sweatman TW. Anthracycline drug targeting: cytoplasmic versus nuclear-a fork in the road. Drug Res Updates 2001;4:169–177.
85. Swain SM, Vici P. The current and future role of dexrazoxane as a cardioprotectant in anthracycline treatment: expert panel review. J Cancer Res Clin Oncol 2004;130:1–7.
86. Fogli S, Nieri P, Breschi MC. The role of nitric oxide in anthracycline toxicity and prospects for pharmacologic prevention of cardiac damage. FASEB J 2004;18:664–675.
87. Kassner N, Huse K, Martin HJ, et al. Carbonyl reductase 1 is a predominant doxorubicin reductase in human liver. Drug Metab Dispos 2008;36:2113–2120.
88. Yamashita T, Fukushima T, Ueda T. Pharmacokinetic self-potentiation of idarubicin by induction of anthracycline carbonyl reducing enzymes. Leuk Lymph 2008;49:809–814.
89. Hasinoff BB. The use of dexrazoxane for the prevention of anthracycline extravasation injury. Expert Opin Invest Drugs 2008;17:217–223.
90. Moretti E, Oakman C, Di Leo A. Predicting anthracycline benefit: have we made any progress? Curr Opin Oncol 2009;21:507–515.
91. Waterhouse DN, Tardi PG, Mayer LD, et al. A comparison of liposomal formulations of doxorubicin with drug administered in free form: changing toxicity profiles. Drug Saf 2001;24:903–920.
92. Grossman HB, O'Donnell MA, Cookson MS, et al. Bacillus Calmette-Guerin failures and beyond: contemporary management of non-muscle invasive bladder cancer. Rev Urol 2008;10:281–289.
93. Kang W, Weiss M. Caffeine enhances the myocardial uptake of idarubicin but reverses its negative inotropic effect. Naunyn Schmiedelbergs Arch Pharmacol 2003;367:151–155.
94. Correale J, Rush C, Amengual A, et al. Mitoxantrone as rescue therapy in worsening relapsing-remitting MS patients receiving IFN-beta. J Neuroimmunol 2005;162:173–183.
95. Kang H-J, Park H-J. Novel molecular mechanism for actinomycin D activity as an oncogenic promoter G-quadruplex binder. Biochemistry 2009;48:7392–7398.
96. Basu S, Brown JE, Flannigan GM, et al. The immunohistochemical analysis of NAD(P)H:quinone oxidoreductase and NADPH cytochrome P450 reductase in human superficial bladder tumours: relationship between tumour enzymology and clinical outcome following intravesical mitomycin C therapy. Int J Cancer 2004;109:703–709.
97. Zappa F, Ward T, Pedrinis E, et al. NAD(P)H:quinone oxidoreductase 1 expression in kidney podocytes. J Histochem Cytochem 2003;51:297–302.

98. Snodgrass RG, Collier AC, Coon AE, et al. Mitomycin C inhibits ribosomal RNA: a novel cytotoxic mechanism for bioreductive drugs. J Biol Chem 2010;285:19068–19075.
99. Colucci MA, Moody CJ, Couch GD. Natural and synthetic quinones and their reduction by the quinone reductase enzyme NQO1: from synthetic organic chemistry to compounds with anticancer potential. Org Biomol Chem 2008;6:637–656.
100. Chow MS, Liu LV, Soloman EI. Further insights into the mechanism of the reaction of activated bleomycin with DNA. Proc Natl Acad Sci 2008;105:13241–13245.
101. Grollman AP, Takeshita M, Pillai KMR, et al. Origin and cytotoxic properties of base propenals derived from DNA. Cancer Res 1985;45:1127–1131.
102. Brewer GJ, Dick R, Ullenbruch MR, et al. Inhibition of key cytokines by tetrathiomolybdate in the bleomycin model of pulmonary fibrosis. J Inorg Biochem 2004;98:2160–2167.
103. Li P, Xiao HD, Xu J, et al. Angiotensin converting enzyme N-terminal inactivation alleviates bleomycin-induced lung injury. Am J Pathol 2010;177:1113–1121.
104. Guliana S, Polkinghorne I, Smith GA, et al. Macropodid herpesvirus 1 encodes genes for both thymidylate synthase and ICP34.5. Virus Genes 2002;24:207–213.
105. Schiffer CA, Clifton IJ, Davisson VJ, et al. Crystal structure of human thymidylate synthase: a structural mechanism for guiding substrates into the active site. Biochemistry 1995;34:16279–16287.
106. Jarmula A, Fraczyk T, Cieplak P, et al. Mechanism of influence of phosphorylation on serine 124 on a decrease of catalytic activity of human thymidylate synthase. Bioorg Med Chem 2010;18:3361–3370.
107. Kamb A, Finer-Moore J, Calvert AH, et al. Structural basis for recognition of polyglutamyl folates by thymidylate synthase. Biochemistry 1992;31:9883–9890.
108. Lee A, Ezzeldin H, Fourie J, et al. Dihydropyrimidine dehydrogenase deficiency: impact of pharmacogenetics on 5-fluorouracil therapy. Clin Adv Hematol Oncol 2004;2:527–532.
109. Mattison LK, Fourie J, Desmond RA, et al. Increased prevalence of dihydropyrimidine dehydrogenase deficiency in African-Americans compared to Caucasians. Cancer Ther Clin 2006;12:5491–5495.
110. Kummar S, Noronha V, Chu E. Antimetabolites. In: DeVita VT Jr, Hellman S, Rosenberg SA, eds. Cancer: Principles and Practice of Oncology, 7th ed. Baltimore: Lippincott Williams & Wilkins, 2005:365–374.
111. Dummins PL, Gready JE. Energetically most likely substrate and active-site protonation sites and pathways in the catalytic mechanism of dihydrofolate reductase. J Am Chem Soc 2001;123:3418–3428.
112. Cody V, Luft JR, Ciszak E, et al. Crystal structure determination at 2.3 angstrom of recombinant human dihydrofolate reductase ternary complex with NADPH and methotrexate-γ-tetrazole. Anticancer Drug Des 1992;7:483–491.
113. Cannon WR, Garrison BJ, Benkovic SJ. Consideration of the pH-dependent inhibition of dihydrofolate reductase by methotrexate. J Mol Biol 1997;271:656–668.
114. Meiering EM, Li H, Delcamp TJ, et al. Contributions of tryptophan 24 and glutamate 30 to binding long-lived water molecules in the ternary complex of human dihydrofolate reductase with methotrexate and NADPH studies by site directed mutagenesis and nuclear magnetic resonance spectroscopy. J Mol Biol 1995;241:309–325.
115. Fuld AD, Dragnev KH, Rigas JR. Pemetrexed in advanced non-small cell lung cancer. Expert Opin Pharmacother 2010;11:1387–1402.
116. Joerger M, Omlin A, Cerny T, et al. The role of pemetrexed in advanced non small-cell lung cancer: special focus on pharmacology and mechanism of action. Curr Drug Topics 2010;11:37–47.
117. Villela LR, Stanford BL, Shah SR. Pemetrexed, a novel antifolate therapeutic alternative for cancer chemotherapy. Pharmacotherapy 2006;26:641–654.
118. Mendelsohn LG, Shih C, Chen VJ, et al. Enzyme inhibition, polyglutamation and the effect of LY231514 (MTA) on purine biosynthesis. Semin Oncol 1999;26(Suppl 6):42–47.
119. Sayre PH, Finer-Moore JS, Fritz TA, et al. Multi-targeted antifolates aimed at avoiding drug resistance form covalent closed inhibitory complexes with human and Escherichia coli thymidylate synthases. J Mol Biol 2001;313:813–829.
120. Raymond E, Louvet C, Tournigand C, et al. Pemetrexed disodium combined with oxaliplatin, SN38, or 5-fluorouracil, based on the quantition of drug interactions in human HT29 colon cancer cells. Int J Oncol 2002;21:361–367.
121. Uemura T, Oguri T, Ozasa H, et al. ABCC11/MRP8 confers pemetrexed resistance in lung cancer. Cancer Sci 2010;101:2404–2410.
122. Sirotnak FM, Schmid GA, Samuels LL, et al. 10-Ethyl-10-deaza-aminopterin: strucrtural design and biochemical, pharmacologic, and antitumor properties. Natl Cancer Inst Monogr 1987;5:127–131.
123. Izbicka E, Diaz A, Streeper R, et al. Distinct mechanistic activity profile of pralatrexate in comparison to other antifolates in in vitro and in vivo models of human cancers. Cancer Chemother Pharmacol 2009;64:993–999.
124. O'Connor OA, Hamlin PA, Portlock C, et al. Pralatrexate, a novel class of antifol with high affinity for the reduced folate carrier-type 1, produces marked complete and durable remissions in a diversity of chemotherapy refractor cases of T-cell lymphoma. Br J Haematol 2007;139:425–428.
125. O'Connor OA. Pralatreate: an emerging new agent with activity in T-cell lymphoma. Curr Opin Oncol 2006;18:591–597.
126. Molina JR. Pralatrexate, a dihydrofolate reductase inhibitor for the potential treatment of several malignancies. IDrugs 2008;11:508–521.
127. Rueda A, Casanova M, Quero C, et al. Pralatrexate, a new hope for aggressive T-cell lymphoma? Clin Transl Oncol 2009;11:215–220.
128. Mould DR, Sweeney K, Duffull SB, et al. A population pharmacokinetic and pharmacodynamic evaluation of pralatrexate in patients with relapsed or refractory non-Hodgkin's or Hodgkin's lymphoma. Clin Pharmacol Ther 2008;86:190–196.
129. Serova M, Bieche I, Sablin MP, et al. Single agent and combination studies of pralatexate and molecular correlates of sensitivity. Br J Cancer 2011;104:272–280.
130. Coulthard SA, Hogarth LA, Little M, et al. The effect of thiopurine methyltransferase expression on sensitivity to thiopurine drugs. Mol Pharamcol 2002;62:102–109.
131. Cara CJ, Pena AS, Sans M, et al. Reviewing the mechanism of action of thiopurine drugs: towards a new paradigm in clinical practice. Med Sci Mont 2004;10:247–254.
132. Marsh S, Booven DJ. The increasing complexity of mercaptopurine pharmacogenomics. Clin Pharmacol Ther 2009;85:139–141.
133. Hartford C, Vasquez E, Schwab M, et al. Differential effects of targeted disruption of thiopurine methyltransferase on mercaptopurine and thioguanine pharmacodynamics. Cancer Res 2007;67:4965–4972.
134. Stocco G, Cheok MH, Crews KR, et al. Genetic polymorphism of inositol triphosphate pyrophosphatase is a determinant of mercaptopurine metabolism and toxicity during treatment for lymphoblastic leukemia. Clin Pharmacol Ther 2009;85:164–172.
135. Coulthard S, Hogarth L. The thiopurines: an update. Invest New Drugs 2005;23:523–532.
136. Fotoohi AK, Lindqvist M, Peterson C, et al. Impaired transport as a mechanism of resistance to thiopurines in human T-lymphoblastic leukemia cells. Nucleosides Nucleotides Nucleic Acids 2006;25:1039–1044.
137. Cai J, Damaraju VL, Grouix N, et al. Two distinct molecular mechanisms underlying cytarabine resistance in human leukemic cells. Cancer Res 2008;68:2349–2357.
138. Lamba JK. Genetic factors influencing cytarabine therapy. Pharmacogenomics 2009;10:1657–1674.
139. Lamanna N, Kay NE. Pentostatin treatment combinations in chronic lymphocytic leukemia. Clin Adv Hematol Oncol 2009;7:386–392.
140. Kovacic P. Hydroxyurea (therapeutics and mechanism): metabolism, carbamoyl nitroso, nitroxyl, radicals, cell signaling and clinical applications. Med Hypotheses 2011;76:24–31.
141. Chen S-H, Hong J. Novel tubulin-interacting agents: a tale of *Taxus brevifolia* and *Cantharanthus roseus*-based drug discovery. Drugs Future 2006;31:123–150.
142. Yue QX, Liu X, Guo DA. Microtubule-binding natural products for cancer therapy. Planta Med 2010;76:1037–1043.
143. Lee JJ, Harris LN. Antimicrotubule agents. In: DeVita VT Jr, Lawrence TS, Hellman, eds. Cancer: Principles and Practice of Oncology, 8th ed. Baltimore: Lippincott Williams & Wilkins, 2008:447–456.
144. Hait WN, Yang J-M. The individualization of cancer therapy: the unexpected role of p53. Transact Am Clin Climatol Assoc 2006;117:85–101.
145. Maccari L, Manetti F, Corelli, F, et al. 3D QSAR studies for the β-tubulin binding site of microtubule-stabilizing anticancer agents (MSAAs). A pseudoreceptor model for taxanes based on the experimental structure of tubulin. Il Farmaco 2003;58:659–668.
146. Gueritte F. General and recent aspects of the chemistry and structure-activity relationships of taxoids. Curr Pharm Des 2001;7:1229–1249.
147. Islam MN, Song Y, Iskander MN. Investigation of structural requirements of anticancer activity at the paclitaxel/tubulin binding site using CoMFA and CoMSIA. J Mol Graph Model 2003;21:263–272.
148. Manetti F, Forli S, Maccari L, et al. 3D QSAR studies of the interaction between β-tubulin and microtubule stabilizing antimitotic agents (MSAA). A combined pharmacophore generation and pseudoreceptor modeling approach applied to taxanes and epothilones. Il Farmaco 2003;58:357–361.
149. Manetti F, Maccari L, Corelli F, et al. 3D QSAR models of interactions between β-tubulin and microtubule stabilizing antimitotic agents (MSAA): a survey on taxanes and epothilones. Curr Topics Med Chem 2004;4:203–217.
150. Yang Y, Alcaraz AA, Snyder JP. The tubulin-bound conformation of paclitaxel: T-taxol vs. "PTX-NY." J Natl Prod 2009;72:422–429.
151. Vaclavikova R, Soucek P, Svobodova L, et al. Different in vitro metabolism of paclitaxel and docetaxel in humans, rats, pigs and minipigs. Drug Metab Dispos 2004;32:666–674.
152. Vaclavikova R, Horsky S, Simek P, et al. Paclitaxel metabolism in rat and human liver microsomes is inhibited by phenolic antioxidants. Naunyn-Schmiedelbergs Arch Pharmacol 2003;368:200–209.
153. Cresteil T, Monsarrat B, DuBois J, et al. Regioselective metabolism of taxoids by human CYP3A4 and 2C8: structure-activity relationship. Drug Metab Dispos 2002;39:438–445.
154. Chabner BA, Ryan DP, Paz-Ares L, et al. Antineoplastic agents. In: Hardman JG, Limbird LE, eds. Goodman & Gilman's The Pharmacological Basis of Therapeutics, 10th ed. New York: McGraw Hill, 2001:1389–1459.
155. Buey RM, Diaz JF, Andreu JM, et al. Interation of epothilone analogs with the paclitaxel binding site: relationship between binding affinity, microtubule stabilization, and cytotoxicity. Chem Biol 2004;11:225–236.
156. Altmann K-H. Epothilone B and its analogs: a new family of anticancer agents. Mini Rev Med Chem 2003;3:149–158.
157. Hunt JT. Discovery of ixabepilone. Mol Cancer Ther 2009;8:275–281.
158. Heinz DW, Schubert W-D, Hofle G. Much anticipated–the bioactive conformation of epothilone and its binding to tubulin. Angew Chem Int Ed 2005;44:1298–1301.

159. Hait WN, Rubin E, Goodin S. Tubulin-targeting agents. In: Giaconne G, Schilsky R, Sondel P, eds. Cancer Chemotherapy and Biological Response Modifiers. New York: Elsevier B.V., 2003:41–67.
160. Engles FK, Ten-Tije AJ, Baker SD, et al. Effect of cytochrome P450 3A4 inhibition on the pharmacokinetics of docetaxel. Clin Pharmacol Ther 2004;75:448–454.
161. Mita AC, Denis LJ, Rowinsky EK, et al. Phase I and pharmacokinetic study of XRP6258 (RPR 116258A), a novel taxane, administered as a 1-hour infusion every 3 weeks in patients with advanced solid tumors. Clin Cancer Res 2009;15:723–730.
162. Pivot X, Koralewski P, Hidalgo JL, et al. A multicenter phase II study of XRP2658 administered as a 1-hr i.v. infusion every 3 weeks in taxane-resistant metastatic breast cancer patients. Ann Oncol 2008;19:1547–1552.
163. Yoo GH, Kafri Z, Ensley JF, et al. XRP6258-induced gene expression patterns in head and neck cancer carcinomas. Laryngoscope 2010;120:1114–1119.
164. Donovan D, Vahdat LT. Epothilones: clinical update and future directions. Oncology 2008;22:408–416.
165. Pellegrini F, Budman DR. Review: tubulin function, actions of antitubulin drugs, and new drug development. Cancer Invest 2005;23:264–273.
166. Gigant B, Wang C, Ravelli RBG, et al. Structual basis for the regulation of tubulin by vinblastine. Nature 2005;435:519–522.
167. Beck WT, Cass CE, Houghton PJ. Microtubule-targeting anticancer drugs derived from plants and microbes: vinca alkaloids, taxanes and epothiolones. In: Bast RC Jr, Kufe DW, Pollock RE, et al., eds. Cancer Medicine, 5th ed. New York: BC Decker Inc., 2003:680–698.
168. Islam MN, Iskander MN. Microtubulin binding sites as target for developing anticancer agents. Mini Rev Med Chem 2004;4:1077–1104.
169. Himes RH. Interactions of the catharanthus (vinca) alkaloids with tubulin and microtubules. Pharmacol Ther 1991;51:257–267.
170. Egbelakin A, Ferguson MJ, MacGill EA. Increased risk of vincristine neurotoxicity associated with low CYP3A5 expression genotype in children with acute lymphoblastic leukemia. Pediatr Blood Cancer 2011;56:361–367.
171. Wu ML, Deng JF, Wu JC, et al. Severe bone marrow depression induced by the anticancer herb *Cantharanthus roseus*. J Toxicol Clin Toxicol 2005;43:667–671.
172. Beulz-Riche D, Grude P, Puozzo C, et al. Characterization of human cytochrome P450 isoenzymes involved in the metabolism of vinorelbine. Fundam Clin Pharmacol 2005;19:545–553.
173. Jakita J, Kuwabara T, Kobayashi H, et al. CYP3A4 is mainly responsible for the metabolism of a new vinca alkaloid, vinorelbine, in human liver microsomes. Drug Metab Dispos 2000;28:1121–1127.
174. Laing N, Dahllof B, Hartley-Asp B, et al. Interaction of estramustine with tubulin isotypes. Biochemistry 1997;36:871–878.
175. Johnson LN. Protein kinase inhibitors: contributions from structure to clinical compounds. Quart Rev Biophys 2009;42:1–40.
176. McInnes C, Fisher PM. Strategies for the design of potent and selective kinase inhibitors. Curr Pharm Des 2005;11:1845–1863.
177. Morphy R. Selectively nonselective kinase inhibition: striking the right balance. J Med Chem 2010;53:1413–1437.
178. Muller BA. Imatinib and its successors: how modern chemistry has changed drug development. Curr Pharm Des 2009;15:120–133.
179. Deininger MWN, Druker BJ. Specific targeted therapy of chronic myelogenous leukemia with imatinib. Pharmacol Rev 2003;55:401–422.
180. Weisberg E, Manley PW, Breitenstein W, et al. Characterization of AMN107, a selective inhibitor of native and mutant Bcr-Abl. Cancer Cell 2005;7:129–141.
181. Schenone S, Bruno O, Radi M, et al. New insights into small-molecule inhibitors of Bcr-Abl. Med Res Rev 2009;31:1–41.
182. Jarkowski A III, Sweeny RP. Nilotinib: a new tyrosine kinase inhibitor for the treatment of chronic myelogenous leukemia. Pharmacotherapy 2008;28:1374–1382.
183. Tokarski JS, Newitt JA, Chang CYJ, et al. The structure of dasatinib (BMS-354825) bound to activated Abl kinase domain elucidates its inhibitory activity against imatinib-resistant Abl mutants. Cancer Res 2006;66:5790–5797.
184. Fry DW, Kraker AJ, McMichael A, et al. A specific inhibitor of the epidermal growth factor receptor tyrosine kinase. Science 1994;265:1093–1095.
185. Levitzki A. Protein tyrosine kinase inhibitors as novel therapeutic agents. Pharmacol Ther 1999;82:231–239.
186. Michalczyk A, Kluter S, Rode HB, et al. Structural insights on how irreversible inhibitors can overcome drug resistance in EGFR. Bioorg Med Chem 2008;16:3482–3488.
187. Kettle JG, Ward RA. Toward the comprehensive systematic enumeration and synthesis of novel kinase inhibitors based on a 4-anilinoquinazoline binding mode. J Chem Inf Model 2010;50:525–533.
188. Erman M. Molecular mechanisms of signal transduction: epidermal growth factor receptor family, vascular endothelial growth factor family, kit, platelet-derived growth factor receptor, ras. J BUON 2007;12(Suppl 1):S83–S94.
189. Mohammadi M, McMahon G, Sun L, et al. Structures of the tyrosine kinase domain of fibroblast growth factor receptor in complex with inhibitors. Science 1997;276:955–960.
190. LoRusso PM, Ryan AJ, Boerner SA, et al. Small-molecule tyrosine kinase inhibitors. In: DeVita VT Jr, Lawrence TS, Rosenberg SA, eds. Cancer: Principles and Practice of Oncology, 8th ed. Baltimore: Lippincott Williams & Wilkins, 2008:457–468.
191. Duckett DR, Cameron MD. Metabolism considerations for kinase inhibitors in cancer treatment. Expert Opin 2010;6:1775–1193.
192. Chen HS, Franke R, Orwick S, et al. Interaction of the multikinase inhibitors sorafenib and sunitinib with solute carriers and ATP-binding cassette transporters. Clin Cancer Res 2009;15:6062–6069.
193. Van Erp NP, Gelderblom H, Guchelaar H-J. Clinical pharmacokinetics of tyrosine kinase inhibitors. Cancer Treat Rev 2009;35:692–706.
194. Grandinetti CA, Goldspiel BR. Sorafenib and sunitinib: novel targeted therapies for renal cell cancer. Pharmacotherapy 2007;27:1125–1144.
195. Vinodhkumar R, Song YS, Devaki T. Romidepsin (depsipeptide) induced cell cycle arrest, apoptosis and histone hyperacetylation in lung carcinoma cells (A549) are associated with increase in p21 and hypophosphorylated retinoblastoma protein expression. Biomed Pharmacother 2008;62:85–93.
196. Gore SD, Baylin SB, Herman JG. Histone deacetylase inhibitors and demethylating agents. In: DeVita VT Jr, Lawrence TS, Rosenberg SA, eds. Cancer: Principles and Practice of Oncology, 8th ed. Baltimore: Lippincott Williams & Wilkins, 2008:477–485.
197. Newbold A, Lindemann RK, Cluse LA, et al. Characterisation of the novel apoptotic and therapeutic activities of the histone deacetylase inhibitor romidepsin. Mol Cancer Ther 2008;7:1066–1079.
198. Whittaker SJ, Demierre M-F, Kim EJ, et al. Final results from a multicenter, international, pivotal study of romidepsin in refractory cutaneous T-cell lymphoma. J Clin Oncol 2010;28:4485–4491.
199. Du L, Musson DG, Wang AQ, Stability studies of vorinostat and its two metabolites in human plasma, serum, and urine. J Pharm Biomed Anal 2006;42:556–564.
200. Zolinza. http://www.zolinza.com/vorinostat/zolinza/consumer/about/act-program.jsp. Accessed January 9, 2011.
201. Lecutier MA. Phocomelia and internal defects due to thalidomide. Br Med J 1962;2:1147–1147.
202. Copur MS, Rose M, Gettinger SN. Miscellaneous chemotherapeutic agents. In: DeVita VT Jr, Lawrence TS, Rosenberg SA, eds. Cancer: Principles and Practice of Oncology, 8th ed. Baltimore: Lippincott Williams & Wilkins, 2008:490–495.
203. Rutter T. Thalidomide ban to be lifted in the US. Br Med J 1997;315:699.
204. Grover JK, Vats K. Thalidomide: from teratogen to antiangiogenic. Indian J Cancer 2001;38:22–32.
205. Von Lillenfeld TM, Hahn AC, Furkert K, et al. A systematic review of phase II trials of thalidomide/dexamethasone combination therapy in patients with relapsed or refractory multiple myeloma. Eur J Haematol 2008;81:247–252.
206. Cavello F, Boccadoro M, Palumbo A. Review of thalidomide in the treatment of newly diagnosed multiple myeloma. Ther Clin Risk Manag 2007;3:543–552.
207. Offidani M, Leoni P, Bringhen S, et al. Melphalan, prednisone, and thalidomide versus thalidomide, dexamethasone, and pegylated liposomal doxorubicin regimen in very elderly patients with multiple myeloma: a case match-study. Leuk Lymphoma 2010;51:1444–1449.
208. Lepper ER, Smith NF, Cox MC, et al. Thalidomide metabolism and hydrolysis: mechanisms and implications. Curr Drug Metab 2006;7:677–685.
209. Zeldis JB, Williams BA, Thomas SD, et al. Thalidomide S.T.E.P.S.: a comprehensive program for controlling and monitoring access to thalidomide. Clin Ther 1999;21:319–330.
210. Castaneda CP, Zeldis JB, Feeman J, et al. RevAssist: a comprehensive risk minimization program for preventing fetal exposure to lenalidomide. Drug Saf 2008;31:743–752.
211. Kumar G, Lau H, Laskin O. Lenalidomide: in vitro evaluation of the metabolism and assessment of cytochrome P450 inhibition and induction. Cancer Chemother Pharmacol 2009;63:1171–1175.
212. Bairey O, Vanichkin A, Shpilberg O. Arsenic-trioxide-induced apoptosis of chronic lymphocytic leukemia cells. Int J Lab Hematol 2010;32:e77–e85.
213. Leu L, Mohassel L. Arsenic trioxide as first line treatment for acute promyelocytic leukemia. Am J Health Syst Pharm 2009;66:1913–1918.
214. Dong H, Chen L, Chen X, et al. Dysregulation of unfolded protein response partially underlies proapoptotic activity of bortezomib in multiple myeloma cells. Leuk Lymphoma 2009;50:974–984.
215. Terpos E, Roussou M, Meletios-Athanassios D. Bortezomib in multiple myeloma. Expert Opin Drug Metab Toxicol 2008;4:639–654.
216. Molineaux CJ, Crews CM. Proteasome inhibitors. In: DeVita VT Jr, Lawrence TS, Rosenberg SA, eds. Cancer: Principles and Practice of Oncology, 8th ed. Baltimore: Lippincott Williams & Wilkins, 2008:486–490.
217. Groll M, Berkers CR, Ploegh HL, et al. Crystal structure of the boronic acid-based proteasome inhibitor bortezomib in complex with the yeast 20S proteasome. Structure 2006;14:451–456.
218. Robinson MK, Borghaci H, Adams GP, et al. Monoclonal antibodies. In: DeVita VT Jr, Lawrence TS, Rosenberg SA, eds. Cancer: Principles and Practice of Oncology, 8th ed. Baltimore: Lippincott Williams & Wilkins, 2008:537–548.
219. Tol J, Punt CJ. Monoclonal antibodies in the treatment of colorectal cancer: a review. Clin Ther 2010;32:437–453.
220. Oei AL, Sweep FC, Thomas CM, et al. The use of monoclonal antibodies for the treatment of epithelial ovarian cancer (review). Int J Oncol 2008;32:1145–1157.
221. Youssoufian H, Hicklin DJ, Rowinsky EK. Review: monoclonal antibodies to the vascular endothelial growth factor receptor-2 in cancer therapy. Clin Cancer Res 2007;13:5544s–5548s.
222. Alpaugh K, von Mehren M. Monoclonal antibodies in cancer treatment: a review of recent progress. BioDrugs 1999;12:209–236.

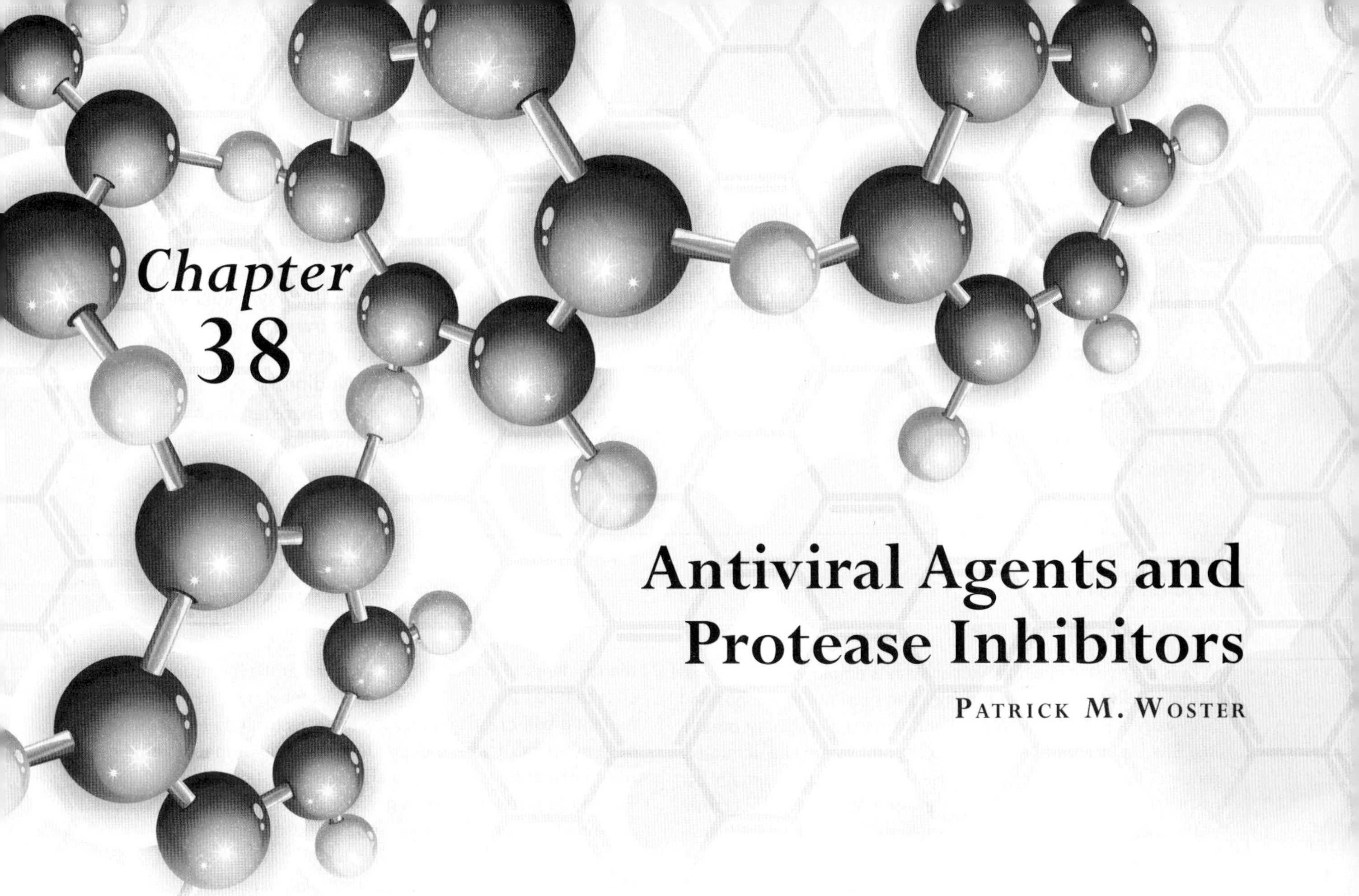

Chapter 38

Antiviral Agents and Protease Inhibitors

PATRICK M. WOSTER

*Drugs Covered in This Chapter**

ACYCLIC NUCLEOSIDE ANALOGUES
- Acyclovir
- Adefovir dipivoxil
- Cidofovir
- 6-Deoxyacyclovir
- Famciclovir
- Ganciclovir
- Valacyclovir

AGENTS AFFECTING THE RIBOSOME
- *Methisazone*

ANTIRETROVIRAL AGENTS: NUCLEOSIDE REVERSE TRANSCRIPTASE INHIBITORS
- Abacavir
- Didanosine
- Emtricitabine
- Lamivudine
- Stavudine
- Tenofovir disoproxil
- Zalcitabine
- Zidovudin

ANTIRETROVIRAL AGENTS: NONNUCLEOSIDE REVERSE TRANSCRIPTASE INHIBITORS
- Delavirdine
- Efavirenz
- Nevirapine

CONVENTIONAL NUCLEOSIDE ANALOGUES
- Cytarabine
- Idoxuridine
- Ribavirin
- Trifluorothymidine
- Vidarabine

FUSION INHIBITORS
- Enfuvirtide
- Maraviroc

HIV INTEGRASE INHIBITORS
- Raltegravir

HIV PROTEASE INHIBITORS
- Amprenavir
- Atazanavir
- Darunavir
- Fosamprenavir
- Indinavir
- Lopinavir
- Nelfinavir
- Ritonavir
- Saquinavir
- Tipranavir

INHIBITORS OF VIRAL ATTACHMENT, PENETRATION, OR EARLY REPLICATION
- Amantadine
- Interferon
- Rimantadine

NEURAMINIDASE INHIBITORS
- Oseltamivir
- Peramivir
- Zanamivir

NON NUCLEOSIDE ANALOGUES
- Boceprevir
- *Fomivirsen*†
- Foscarnet
- Telaprevir

Abbreviations

AIDS, acquired immunodeficiency syndrome
ara-HX, arabinosyl hypoxanthine
ARC, AIDS-related complex
AUC, area under plasma concentration–time curve
CCD, catalytic core domain
cDNA, complementary DNA
CMV, cytomegalovirus
CNS, central nervous system
CSF, cerebrospinal fluid
D4T, stavudine

* Drugs listed include those available inside and outside of the United States; drugs available outside of the United States are shown in italics.
† Fomivirsen has been withdrawn from the U.S. market.

DANA, 2-deoxy-2,3-dehydro-*N*-acetylneuraminic acid
ddI, didanosine
ddC, zalcitabine
DMSO, dimethylsulfoxide
EBV, Epstein-Barr virus
FDA, U.S. Food and Drug Administration
GI, gastrointestinal
HA, hemagglutinin
HAART, highly active antiretroviral therapy
HAV, hepatitis A virus
HBV, hepatitis B virus
HCV, hepatitis C virus
HEV, hepatitis E virus
HHV, human herpesvirus
HIV, human immunodeficiency virus
HPV, human papilloma virus
HSV, herpes simplex virus
HTLV-1, human T-cell leukemia virus 1
IC_{50}, half maximal inhibitory concentration
IV, intravenous
MHC, major histocompatibility complex
NA, neuraminidase
RNAi, RNA interference
RSV, respiratory syncytial virus
RT, reverse transcriptase
siRNA, short interfering RNAs
3TC, lamivudine
VZV, varicella-zoster virus
ZDV, zidovudine

SCENARIO

Douglas Slain, PharmD, BCPS

WM is a 37-year-old white woman who is employed as a nurses' aid in an elder care nursing home. She presents to the hospital with extreme flu-like symptoms and is having difficulty breathing. She is placed in the intensive care unit where she ultimately requires intubation and mechanical ventilation to maintain her respiratory function. WM is also given empiric broad-spectrum antibiotics in case of bacterial pneumonia. A rapid influenza test is positive. She needs anti-influenza therapy, but oral oseltamivir and inhaled zanamivir cannot be reliably delivered given her sedation, intubation, and mechanical ventilation. Many of the residents of her nursing home had an H1N1 strain of influenza that has the neuraminidase-resistant H274Y mutation. This mutation will drastically reduce the effectiveness of neuraminidase inhibitors that are dependent on C6 hydrophobic binding. Most circulating strains have also been resistant to rimantadine. Treatment options to consider are investigational intravenous zanamivir and investigational intravenous peramivir.

(The reader is directed to the clinical solution and chemical analysis of this case at the end of the chapter.)

INTRODUCTION

Viruses are the smallest of the human infectious agents and range in size from about 20 nm to about 300 nm in diameter (1,2). They contain one kind of nucleic acid, either RNA or DNA, as their entire genome, which codes for a variety of enzymes and other proteins used in replication and transmission of the organism. It can be argued that a virus does not qualify as a true life form, since it is nothing more than a nucleic acid strand with associated proteins, and it cannot move on its own power. However, when it attaches itself to a host cell, it internalizes itself and forces the host to make additional copies of the virus, demonstrating a clear reproductive plan. During replication, it uses host cellular biochemicals and processes and, thus in a sense, takes in "nutrients" in order to survive and multiply. In some cases, viruses respond to external conditions and escape the immune response by integrating into the host DNA, demonstrating the ability to respond to external stimuli. Although viruses are simple organisms, they are a significant causative agent for numerous human diseases and, as such, represent one of the major challenges in the area of drug discovery. Agents that are used clinically for a variety of viral diseases act by targeting processes that are specific to the virus, such as a unique viral enzyme or a necessary process such as transcription. However, to date, no drug has been discovered that is truly curative for viral infection. In addition, because viruses have the ability to undergo mutations, resistance to existing therapies can develop. The discovery of new antiviral agents is thus an important ongoing effort in medicinal chemistry.

VIRUS STRUCTURE AND CLASSIFICATION (1,2)

Numerous species of virus that infect bacteria, plants, and animals have been identified, and they exhibit a remarkable range of diversity. All viruses exist as obligate cellular parasites, and as such, they do not possess the complex biochemical machinery that is characteristic of higher organisms. However, they do have a defined macromolecular structure that is designed to protect them from the environment and facilitate their entry into cells. The basic subunit of a virus is its genome, which can be made up of either DNA or RNA. The nucleic acid portion of a virus can be single or double stranded, and may be present in linear or circular form. Viral genomic DNA or RNA is often associated with basic nucleoproteins and may be surrounded by a symmetrical protein known as a capsid. The capsid is made up of repeating structural units known as protomers, which themselves are made up of nonidentical protein subunits. The combination of the nucleic acid core and the capsid is termed the nucleocapsid, and in some cases, this comprises the entire virus. In other cases, the nucleocapsid structure is surrounded by a lipid-containing membrane that is derived during viral maturation, when the virus undergoes budding through the host cell membrane. The complete virus particle, with or without an envelope, is termed the virion. Viral architecture can be grouped into three types based on the arrangement of morphologic subunits, and each virus exhibits cubic (icosahedral) symmetry, helical symmetry, or has a complex structure. Icosahedral virions are symmetrical structures that contain 20 surfaces, each of which is an equilateral triangle. A sufficient number of capsid structural units must be employed in the icosahedron to make a capsid large enough to encapsulate the viral genome. Morphologic units called capsomeres are seen on the surface of icosahedral virus particles. These structures are clusters of polypeptides, but they do not necessarily correspond to the chemically defined structural units. Some viruses arrange their structural subunits into a standard helical formation. In viruses with helical symmetry, protein subunits systematically bind to the viral nucleic acid, ultimately forming a nucleocapsid helix. The filamentous nucleocapsid is then coiled inside a lipid-containing envelope. Unlike icosahedral virions, regular, periodic interaction between capsid protein and viral nucleic acid prevents the formation of "empty" helical particles. Finally, some virus particles, such as the large and complex poxviruses, do not exhibit cubic or helical symmetry, but instead form more complicated structures that can be spherical, brick-shaped, or ovoid. A subset of complex viruses is termed pleomorphic, in that they assume multiple complex morphologies. Advances in the visualization of viral capsid structure suggest that the assembly and processing of viral proteins could serve as a new target for antiviral drug development (3).

Viral taxonomy is complex, and viruses are classified according to a number of factors, including morphology, properties of the genome (i.e., DNA vs. RNA, single strand vs. double strand, linear vs. circular, sense vs. antisense), physicochemical properties, structure of associated proteins, replication strategy, and so on. Viruses are separated into major groups called families, with names that end in the suffix –viridae, and then into genera that end in –virus. Thus, pox viruses are in the family Poxviridae, and in the genus *Poxvirus*. A comparison of the genetic and structural features of viral families with members that can infect humans appears in Table 38.1.

CLINICAL SIGNIFICANCE

Antiviral agents include diverse compounds with varied actions. A thorough clinical understanding of most of these compounds is dependent on a basic appreciation of biochemistry and medicinal chemistry. Viruses are mainly composed of either RNA or DNA nucleic acid strands. As such, one of the most ideal targets for treating viral pathogens has been the inhibition of viral replication. Successful viral replication is dependent on enzyme-mediated transcription of viral RNA or DNA. A significant number of antiviral agents, including HIV nucleoside reverse transcriptase inhibitors, and a majority of antiherpes agents are designed to be "false" substrates of viral transcription enzymes. It is through competitive inhibition that these agents are able to fulfill their intended effect. Their chemical structures are similar to naturally occurring substrate nucleoside purines (adenosine and guanosine) and pyrimidines (thymidine and cytidine). However, as they are purposely modified in key positions with functional groups designed to foil polymerase enzymes, their incorporation will lead to termination of replication. While these nucleoside antiviral agents are often actively carried into cells via specific nucleoside transporting proteins, they typically require triphosphorylation to become active intracellularly. It is important to recognize that resistance to these antiviral medications can develop when genetic mutations alter the ability for viral enzymes to phosphorylate the drugs. Drugs like cidofovir and tenofovir are nucleotide analogs, which means they are already monophosphorylated. As a result, these agents can maintain activity against viruses that have developed resistance to other nucleoside agents through certain resistant mutations.

In clinical practice, HIV antiretroviral regimens usually require a pair of nucleoside reverse transcriptase inhibitors in the regimen. It is of paramount importance that combinations of "like" nucleosides analogs (e.g., two thymidine, two cytosine) are not used together as they have displayed antagonism and reduced viral load suppression. Nonnucleoside reverse transcriptase inhibitors are not structurally related to nucleic purines and pyrimidines; therefore, they do not act as substrates of the target enzyme.

Protease inhibitors, which are the most potent antiretroviral agents available, were the end result of coordinated chemical design and structure-based computational analysis of the protease enzyme. With identification of the protease crystalline structure and identification of active binding sites, scientists were able to create compounds that would fit the protease enzyme with strong affinity, and cause an inhibition of protease function. The clinical impact of these man-made drugs is regarded by many as the greatest single advance in the treatment of HIV infection.

Douglas Slain, PharmD, BCPS
Associate Professor
College of Pharmacy
West Virginia University
Morgantown, WV

TABLE 38.1 Characteristics of Virus Families Containing Members That Infect Humans

Family	Examples	Genome	Capsid Symmetry	Size (nm^{-1})	Envelope	Diseases
Parvoviridae	Parvovirus B19	ssDNA sense or antisense	Icosahedral	18–26	No	Erythema infectiosum (fifth disease); polyarthralgia arthritis; aplastic crisis, anemia
Papillomaviridae	Human papilloma (wart) virus; polyoma virus; SV 40	ds, circular DNA	Icosahedral	55	No	Warts; salivary gland infection; multifocal leukoencephalopathy; tumors (i.e., cervical)
Adenoviridae	Multiple types (40 adenoviruses and mastadenovirus)	dsDNA	Icosahedral	70–90	No	Infections of the eye and respiratory tract; tumors
Hepadnaviridae	Hepadnavirus, hepatitis B virus	dsDNA, circular, one ss region	Icosahedral	40–48	Yes	Hepatitis B; tumors
Herpesviridae	Herpes simplex I and II; varicella zoster; herpes zoster; cytomegalovirus; Epstein-Barr virus	dsDNA	Icosahedral	150–200	Yes	Eye, skin and genital infection; chickenpox; shingles; mononucleosis; tumors
Poxviridae	Variola; vaccinia	dsDNA	Complex	230–400	Complex	Smallpox; cowpox; chickenpox; tumors
Picornaviridae	Hepatitis A virus; poliovirus; enterovirus; rhinovirus, coxsackie virus A and B	ssRNA, sense	Icosahedral	28–30	No	Respiratory diseases; gastrointestinal diseases; polio; aseptic meningitis
Astroviridae	Astrovirus	ssRNA, sense	Icosahedral	28–30	No	Diarrhea in infants and immunocompromised patients
Caliciviridae	Norwalk virus	ssRNA, sense	Icosahedral	27–40	No	Epidemic gastroenteritis
Togaviridae	Rubella virus; alphavirus, arbovirus	ssRNA, sense	Icosahedral	50–70	Yes	Measles (rubella)
Flaviviridae	Hepatitis C virus; arbovirus; yellow fever virus; dengue virus; West Nile virus	ssRNA, sense	Complex	40–60	Yes	Hepatitis C; yellow fever; dengue fever; encephalitis; tumors
Coronaviridae	Coronavirus	ssRNA, sense	Complex	120–160	Yes	Colds; gastroenteritis in infants; SARS
Retroviridae	HIV I and II; lentivirus; human T-cell lymphotropic viruses	ssRNA as dimer	Complex	80–100	Yes	AIDS; AIDS-related complex; breast cancer; human T-cell leukemia; nasopharyngeal carcinoma
Arenaviridae	Arenavirus	ssRNA, antisense	Complex	50–300	Yes	Lassa fever; hemorrhagic fever; choriomeningitis
Orthomyxoviridae	Influenza virus A, B, C	ssRNA, antisense	Helical	80–120	Yes	Influenza
Bunyaviridae	Hantavirus	ssRNA, antisense	Helical	80–120	Yes	Hemorrhagic fever
Rhabdoviridae	Rhabdovirus; rabies virus; encephalitis virus	ssRNA, antisense	Helical	75–180	Yes	Rabies; encephalitis
Paramyxoviridae	Syncytial virus; parainfluenza virus	ssRNA, antisense	Helical	150–300	Yes	Mumps; measles (rubeola)
Filoviridae	Marburg virus; Ebola virus	ssRNA, antisense	Helical	80–800	Yes	Marburg viral fever; ebola hemorrhagic fever
Reoviridae	Reovirus; rotavirus; orbivirus	dsRNA in 10–12 pieces	Icosahedral	60–80	No	Mild respiratory and gastrointestinal infection; Colorado tick fever
Prion	Prion proteinaceous material	None	NA	NA	No	Bovine spongiform encephalopathy; Creu tzfeldt-Jakob disease

ds, double stranded; NA, not applicable; SARS, severe acute respiratory syndrome; ss, single stranded.

VIRAL REPLICATION, CELLULAR EFFECTS, AND PATHOGENESIS (2,4)

As mentioned earlier, all viruses exist as obligate intracellular parasites, and as such, they rely on the cellular machinery of the host for their growth, development, and replication. In order to synthesize the proteins needed for viral replication, the organism must be capable of producing usable mRNA in sufficient quantities to compete with host mRNA for protein synthesis. During viral replication, all of the macromolecules required by the virus are synthesized in a highly organized sequence. The replication cycle (Fig. 38.1) begins when the intact virion binds to a host cell through electrostatic adsorption to a specific "receptor" site. This process is known as the attachment phase. Attachment is most likely a fortuitous event resulting from structural complementarity between the exterior structure of the virion and a normal cell surface structure on the host cell. For example, HIV binds to the CD4 receptor on cells of the immune system, rhinoviruses bind ICAM-1, and Epstein-Barr virus recognizes the CD21 receptor on B cells. Recent studies suggest that some mammalian cells can develop proteins that restrict the binding of viral capsid structures, thus preventing entry into noninfected cells (5). When attachment has been achieved, the virion enters the penetration phase, the process by which it gains entry into the host cell. Penetration may occur by receptor-mediated endocytosis, fusion of the viral envelope with the cell membrane, or in some cases direct penetration of the membrane. Following penetration of the cell, viruses must be uncoated, resulting either in the naked nucleic acid or in the nucleocapsid form, which usually contains polymerase enzymes. After they have been uncoated, viruses are no longer infectious.

Once the virus has penetrated the cell and uncoated, it enters a segment of its life cycle known as the eclipse period, the length of which varies with the type of virus. It is during this time that the virus utilizes host resources to replicate and produce necessary viral proteins. Cells that can support viral reproduction are termed permissive, and as a result, the infection is known as productive, since it results in new viral particles. When new infectious viral particles are produced, host cellular metabolism may be completely directed to the production of viral products, resulting in destruction of the cell. In other cases, host cell metabolism is not dramatically altered, and the infected cell can survive. During viral reproduction, up to 100,000 new virions can be produced, and the replication cycle can vary from a few hours to more than 3 days. Some cells types, called nonpermissive, are unable to support the reproduction of an infective virion, resulting in an abortive infection. Abortive infections also occur when the virus itself is defective. Either situation can lead to a latent infection, where the viral genome may persist in a surviving host cell. As will be described below, such

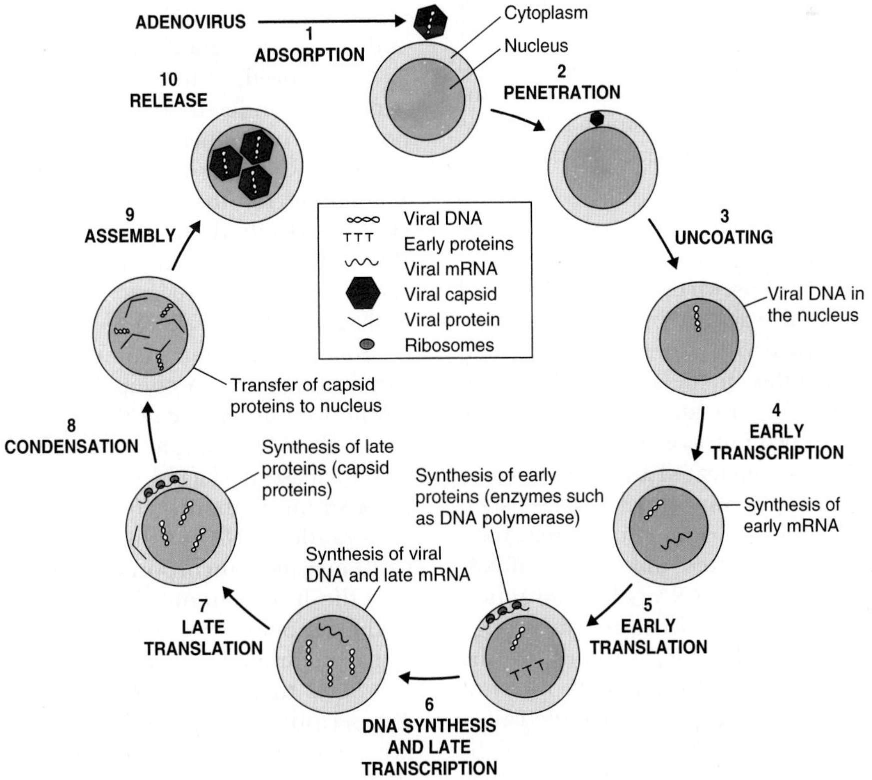

FIGURE 38.1 Steps involved in the viral life cycle. (Used with permission from Brooks GF, Butel JS, Morse SA, et al. Jawetz, Melnick and Adelberg's Medical Microbiology, 23rd Ed. New York: McGraw-Hill Companies, 2004.)

an infection can lead to the transformation of a cell from normal to malignant.

DNA Virus

The strategies used by various viruses to replicate vary widely, but all are characterized by the need to transcribe mRNA that is suitable for translation of viral proteins. There are several pathways leading to the required mRNA, after which the host enzymes and raw materials are used to make viral proteins. Early viral proteins used in replication are synthesized immediately after infection, while late proteins used to produce the complete virion structure are synthesized after viral nucleic acid synthesis. Most DNA viruses contain double-stranded DNA as their genome and thus can replicate using host cell machinery to produce mRNA directly. Papillomavirus, adenovirus, and herpesvirus are replicated in the host nucleus, and thus use transcriptional enzymes of the host (i.e., DNA-dependent RNA polymerase) to synthesize mRNA. This mRNA is then translated to form proteins needed by the virus, including enzymes (e.g., DNA-dependent DNA polymerase) used to produce progeny DNA copies. These progeny DNA strands are infectious. By contrast, poxviruses replicate in the cytoplasm using a mechanism that is not well understood, wherein the genome is initially transcribed by a viral enzyme in the virion core. Parvoviruses contain a single-stranded DNA genome, and must synthesize double-stranded DNA in the host nucleus prior to synthesis of mRNA and translation of proteins. This process may or may not require a helper virus such as herpes simplex. The hepatitis B viral genome, comprised of double-stranded DNA, contains numerous gaps that must be repaired using a DNA polymerase packaged in the virion before transcription to form mRNA.

RNA Virus

Compared to DNA viruses, those viruses with RNA-based genomes have evolved a wide variety of reproductive strategies. The single-stranded RNA viruses may be divided into three groups that differ in the method by which the RNA genome is utilized. In all three groups, the RNA genome must serve two functions: to be translated to form protein and to be replicated to form progeny RNA strands. The first group is comprised of viruses such as picornaviruses, flaviviruses, and togaviruses that have an RNA genome that can be used directly as mRNA. Viral RNA that can be used as mRNA is by convention termed (+) or sense-strand RNA. In most cases (e.g., picornaviruses), this sense-strand RNA binds to the host ribosome shortly after entering the cell, where it is read and used to produce a single polypeptide called the polyprotein. The polyprotein is then processed by autocatalysis and various proteolytic enzymes to produce the required viral proteins. In some cases (e.g., togaviruses), only a portion of the RNA genome is available to be translated by the host ribosome. Following the initial translation of the sense strand, it serves a second function, namely to serve as a template for the synthesis of a (–) or antisense strand via an RNA-dependent RNA polymerase. This antisense strand then can be used to produce additional sense-strand RNAs that are infectious and can also serve as mRNA. These progeny sense RNA strands are then packaged into an intact virion prior to transmission to another host cell.

The second group of single-stranded RNA viruses, including orthomyxoviruses, bunyaviruses, arenaviruses, paramyxoviruses, filoviruses, and rhabdoviruses, all contain an antisense RNA genome that can only be used for transcription of new RNA. All antisense RNA viruses contain an RNA transcriptase as part of their virion, because the host cell does not have this type of RNA-dependent RNA polymerase. In the first round of genome expression, a series of short sense-strand RNAs are made and then translated to form the required viral enzymes for replication. Ultimately, these enzymes are used to produce a full-length sense RNA strand, which is then used to make multiple copies of the antisense viral genome. The progeny antisense DNA strands by themselves are not infectious, because they have not yet been packaged with the required RNA transcriptase. When the progeny antisense RNA has been synthesized, it is packaged into an intact virion, in which form it becomes infectious prior to transmission to another cell.

The third group of RNA viruses is the retroviruses, in which single-stranded RNA exists as a dimer of a sense and antisense strand. The genomic RNA strands can be base-paired, although the structure of this complex is not well understood, or the strands can be hydrogen bonded to other macromolecules in the virion. Retroviral genomic RNA serves a single function, namely, to act as a template for the formation of double-stranded viral DNA. Host cells do not contain an enzyme that can form DNA from viral RNA, and thus the virion of a retrovirus must contain a reverse transcriptase (RT) enzyme, as well as various host tRNA molecules. Transcription of the genome begins when a complex of RT and tRNA binds to the viral genome. A complimentary DNA strand is then synthesized using one of the host tRNAs as a primer, and the original RNA strand is digested by RNAse H, and viral ribonuclease packaged in the virion. A complimentary DNA strand is then synthesized, and the resulting double-stranded DNA is translocated to the nucleus, where viral enzymes incorporate genome-length viral DNA into the host genome. In some cases, the viral portion of the genome can remain dormant for long periods, or it may be immediately used to make progeny viral RNA, a process that is catalyzed by host RNA polymerase II. Transcription produces both shortened segments that are used to make polyproteins and full length progeny RNA. The polyproteins are processed to form various viral proteins, while the full-length RNA is packaged into an infectious virion.

Virus Protein

In addition to replication of the viral genome, a number of other structures associated with the complete virion can also be made. A number of viral proteins may be synthesized that have important functions in the structure, transmission, and survival of the virus. These proteins can protect the genetic material in the virus from destruction by nucleases, participate in the attachment process, and provide structure and symmetry to the virion. In addition, in certain cases where the virus requires an enzymatic process for which there is no host enzyme, a virion may include enzymes such as RNA polymerases or an RT. Some viruses require a lipid envelope that contains transmembrane proteins specifically coded for by the virus and that envelops the genetic material during viral budding. Viral envelopes contain glycoproteins that are involved in cell recognition during attachment to the host cell. These glycoproteins often reflect the composition of glycoproteins in the host cell. They are a determinant of the antigenic nature of viruses, and thus facilitate recognition by the immune system of the host. However, depending on their composition, they can also help the virus elude neutralization by the immune system.

Cellular Egress

Viruses use one of two strategies for exiting infected cells. Nonenveloped viruses (picornaviruses, rheoviruses, etc.) complete their maturation by assembling into their corresponding virion within the cell nucleus or the cytoplasm. For example, picornaviruses assemble by clustering 60 copies of each of three viral proteins, called VP0, VP1, and VP3, into a structure called a procapsid. Viral RNA is then packaged into the procapsid, and proteolytic cleavage of VP0 produces two new viral proteins called VP2 and VP4. The resulting conformational change produces a stable and symmetrical structure that shields the genome from degradation by host nucleases. In most cases, destruction of the host cell is required when the virion exits. Enveloped viruses (all antisense RNA viruses, togaviruses, flaviviruses, coronaviruses, hepadnaviruses, herpesviruses, and retroviruses) contain proteins that carry signal sequences and markers that cause them to be inserted into the inner and outer surface of the host cell cytoplasmic membrane. Viral proteins on the outer surface are glycosylated using host enzymes and then displace host cell surface proteins and collect into patches. Viral nucleocapsids recognize proteins on the inner surface of the membrane, where they bind and are engulfed by the patch area of the membrane. The completed virion exits the cell by budding and release into the extracellular space. Viral egress can have a variety of effects on the host cell, ranging from destruction of the cell to minimal noncytolytic effects. Herpesviruses differ from other enveloped viruses in the manner in which they form their envelope. The nucleocapsid is formed in the nucleus, and final maturation of the virion occurs only on the inner surface of the host cell membrane, forming vesicles that are stored in between the inner and outer aspect of the cell membrane. Egress of the herpesvirus vesicle always occurs through destruction of the host cell.

Virus Pathogenesis

A complete discussion of viral pathogenesis is beyond the scope of this chapter. However, in general it may be considered that the symptoms of a viral infection arise from the response to viral replication and cell injury in the host. These responses range from asymptomatic or subclinical to severe clinical manifestations, and may be either local or systemic. Understanding the biochemical events that produce viral diseases can aid in the design of effective and specific therapies. Not surprisingly, viral pathogenesis occurs in distinct steps: 1) viral entry into the host and primary viral replication; 2) viral spread; 3) cellular injury and host immune response; 4) viral clearance or establishment of persistent infection; and 5) viral shedding. Most viruses enter the host through the respiratory or gastrointestinal tract, but may also penetrate the skin, urogenital tract, or conjunctiva. In a few cases, virus particles can enter through direct injection (e.g., HIV and hepatitis) or through insect bites (arboviruses). When a local infection occurs, the virus replicates near the site of entry, and the underlying tissue is not affected. However, some viruses are able to migrate to other sites, usually through the bloodstream or lymphatic system, to produce systemic infections. When infection occurs at a remote site, most viruses demonstrate tissue or organ preference (e.g., herpesvirus localizes in nerve ganglia, and the rabies virus migrates to the CNS). Localization of a virus in a particular tissue can be the result of cell receptor specificity or can arise because a virus may be activated by proteolytic enzymes in a specific cell type.

Clinical disease develops through a complex series of events when virus-infected cells are destroyed or their function is impaired, and some symptoms such as malaise and anorexia can result from host responses such as cytokine release. Disease-mediated damage may become chronic when cell types that do not regenerate (e.g., brain tissue) are involved. Ultimately, the host either succumbs to the infection; develops a chronic, latent, or subclinical infection; or completely recovers. In chronic infections, the virus can be continuously detected, at low levels, and either mild or no clinical symptoms may present. By contrast, latent infections are those in which the virus persists for extended periods of time in an inactive form or a location not exposed to the immune response. Intermittent flare-ups of clinical disease can occur, during which time infectious virus can be detected. Subclinical infections are those that give no overt sign of their presence. Humoral and cell-mediated immunity, interferon and other cytokines, and other host defense factors, depending on the type of virus, are common mediators of recovery, and begin to develop very soon after infection. Infiltration with mononuclear cells and lymphocytes is responsible for the inflammatory reaction in uncomplicated viral lesions. Virus-infected cells can be lysed by

T lymphocytes through recognition of viral polypeptides on the cell surface, and humoral immunity protects the host against reinfection by the same virus. Neutralizing antibodies that are directed against capsid proteins can prevent viral infection by disrupting viral attachment or uncoating. Interestingly, viruses have evolved a variety of survival tactics that serve to suppress or evade the host immune response. Because viruses are obligate intracellular parasites, a method of transmission from one host to another is required for survival of the species. Thus, during an active infection, shedding of the infectious virion into the environment is a required step in the life cycle of the virus and ensures transmission of the virus to new hosts. Shedding usually occurs at the same site where the infection was initiated and can occur at various stages of the disease course.

VIRAL DISEASES (6,7)

HIV

The human immunodeficiency virus (HIV-1) was first identified in 1979 and was found to be the cause of acquired immunodeficiency syndrome (AIDS) in 1981 (8). Since that time, AIDS had become a serious worldwide epidemic that continues to expand. The Joint United Nations Program on HIV/AIDS estimated that by the end of 2005, a total of 40.3 million people worldwide were living with HIV/AIDS, the majority having been infected by heterosexual contact. After four decades, the number of infected individuals has begun to drop slightly, and that number stands at 33.3 million in 2010. Only 5 million of these patients are receiving treatment for the disease. In 2005, more than 3.1 million people died of AIDS, and 4.9 million new cases of HIV were diagnosed, including more than 700,000 children (9). The number of new infections dropped to 2.9 million in 2009, and annual deaths decreased to 1.8 million (10). The incidence of the disease varies by location, with sub-Saharan Africa having the highest incidence of the disease. In the Third World, HIV infection is often comorbid with neglected tropical diseases (trypanosomiasis, leishmaniasis), malaria, and tuberculosis, causing a higher level of mortality (11). Because it is sexually transmitted, a high percentage of infected individuals are young adult workers, and as such, the disease has a significant economic impact in some regions. In addition, infected mother-to-fetus transmission occurs between 13% and 40% of the time. Although a variety of drugs have been developed for treating AIDS patients, none have proven successful in curing the disease. The basic difficulty experienced with this viral infection is the ability of virus to mutate, leading to rapid drug resistance.

The HIV-1 genome consists of two identical 9.2-kb single-stranded RNA molecules within the virion, each of which contains information for only nine genes. Following infection of the host cell, the persistent form of the HIV-1 genome is proviral double-stranded DNA. Mature HIV virions are spherical and consist of a lipid bilayer membrane surrounding a nucleocapsid that contains genomic RNA, a viral protease, RT, an integrase, and some other cellular factors. The HIV life cycle is depicted in Figure 38.2, and begins when the viral extracellular protein gp120 attaches to the CD4 receptor on T lymphocytes. Following attachment, the viral envelope and host cell membrane are fused, and the nucleocapsid is released into the cytoplasm. The nucleocapsid is uncoated, and the resulting RNA serves as a substrate for RT, producing a proviral double-stranded DNA that migrates to the nucleus and is incorporated into host DNA by integrase. This DNA is not expressed in resting

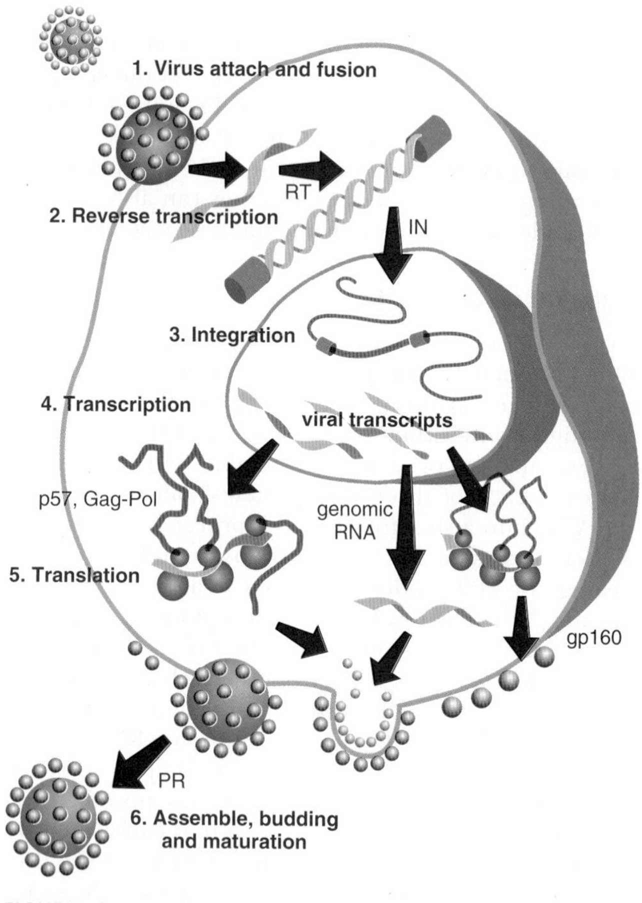

FIGURE 38.2 Replicative cycle of HIV. (1) The virus gp120 protein binds to CD4, resulting in fusion of the viral envelope and the cellular membrane and the release of viral nucleocapsid into the cytoplasm. (2) The nucleocapsid is uncoated, and viral RNA is reverse transcribed by reverse transcriptase (RT). (3) The resulting double-stranded proviral DNA migrates into the cell nucleus and is integrated into the cellular DNA by integrase (IN). (4) Proviral DNA is transcribed by the cellular RNA polymerase II. (5) The mRNAs are translated by the cellular polysomes. (6) Viral proteins and genomic RNA are transported to the cellular membrane and assemble. Immature virions are released. Polypeptide precursors are processed by the viral protease (PR) to produce mature viral particles. (Used with permission from Tyler KL, Fields BN. Fields Virology, 2nd Ed. New York: Raven Press, 1990:191–239.)

T lymphocytes, but when the cell is activated, proviral DNA is transcribed by host RNA polymerase II. The viral RNA and proteins are transported to the cell membrane, where they assemble, form a viral bud, and are released from the lymphocyte membrane. This produces an immature virion, and processing of the viral surface proteins by HIV protease then affords the mature, infectious virus.

About 50% of HIV infections are asymptomatic, whereas the other 50% produce flu-like symptoms within 4 weeks. During this initial phase, viral titers are very high and decline as specific antibodies are formed. The latent period is mediated by factors that are not well understood and can last several years. During this time, viral replication continues, and the level of CD4-positive T lymphocytes steadily declines. Eventually, the patient immune system becomes compromised, resulting in a variety of opportunistic infections. RT sometimes makes mistakes reading the viral RNA sequence, leading to mutations in the virus and changes in the structure of the surface proteins. Thus vaccines, which induce the production of antibodies that recognize and bind to very specific viral surface molecules, are unlikely to be effective in HIV therapy. As will be discussed below, other viral processes, such as reverse transcription and proteolytic processing, are viable targets for small-molecule therapy.

Kaposi sarcoma is a common complication of AIDS and has been shown to arise from a complex interaction between HIV and the human herpesvirus 8 (HHV-8). This disease presents as a reddish or purple lesion on various areas of the skin, and in advanced state may involve the lungs or gastrointestinal tract. HHV-8 does not work alone, but rather in combination with a patient's altered response to cytokines and the HIV-1 transactivating protein Tat, which promotes the growth of endothelial cells. HHV-8 can then encode interleukin-6 viral proteins, specific cytokines that stimulate cell growth in the skin. HHV-8 destroys the immune system further by directing a cell to remove the major histocompatibility complex (MHC-1) proteins that protect it from invasion. These proteins are then transferred to the interior of the cell and are destroyed, leaving the cell unguarded and vulnerable to pathogens that would normally be cleared by the immune system. It has recently been discovered that xCT, the 12-transmembrane light chain of the human cystine/glutamate exchange transporter system, serves as a receptor for internalization of HHV-8 (12).

Herpesvirus (2)

The herpesvirus family contains several of the most important human pathogens, which are responsible for causing a spectrum of common diseases. A common and significant feature of the herpesviruses is their ability to establish lifelong persistent infections in their hosts and to undergo periodic reactivation. Herpesviruses possess a large number of genes, and some of the resulting proteins are targets for antiviral chemotherapy. The herpesviruses that commonly infect humans include herpes simplex virus (HSV) types 1 and 2, varicella-zoster virus, cytomegalovirus, Epstein-Barr virus, human herpesviruses 6 (HHV-6) and 7 (HHV-7), and Kaposi sarcoma–associated herpesvirus HHV-8 (also known as KSHV). Herpesviruses are large viruses that have identical morphology and consist of a core of linear, double-stranded DNA surrounded by a protein coat that exhibits icosahedral symmetry and has 162 capsomeres. The genome is large and encodes at least 100 different proteins, including polypeptides involved in viral structure, the viral envelope, and enzymes involved in nucleic acid metabolism, DNA synthesis, and protein regulation. Oral cold sores and genital herpes infections are caused by HSV1 and HSV2, respectively. These viruses can establish a latent infection in the ganglia of nerves that supply the site of the primary infection, and the latent disease is reactivated by a number of stress factors. It is estimated that virtually 100% of adult humans are infected with HSV1, although many infections are subclinical and asymptomatic. The varicella virus is the cause of chickenpox, and the herpes zoster virus is responsible for shingles. Human cytomegalovirus rarely causes disease in healthy people, but when infection occurs in adulthood, it may cause an infectious mononucleosis-like illness. Primary infection with the Epstein-Barr virus is the cause of infectious mononucleosis, and this virus is thought to be a factor in the development of Burkitt lymphoma and other malignancies. HHV-6 is thought to cause roseola and mononucleosis, whereas HHV-7 is probably not involved in any human diseases. The role of HHV-8 in the pathogenesis of Kaposi sarcoma has been discussed earlier.

Hepatitis (2)

Viral hepatitis is a systemic disease, but primarily involves the liver. Hepatitis A virus (HAV) is responsible for infectious hepatitis, hepatitis B virus (HBV) is associated with serum hepatitis, and hepatitis C virus (HCV) is a common cause of posttransfusion hepatitis. Another viral agent, hepatitis E virus (HEV), causes an enterically transmitted form of hepatitis. On occasion, disease can arise from hepatic infection with yellow fever virus, cytomegalovirus, Epstein-Barr virus, herpes simplex virus, rubella virus, and the enteroviruses. Viral hepatitis usually involves acute inflammation of the liver, fever, nausea, vomiting, and jaundice, and all forms of hepatitis produce identical histopathologic lesions in the liver during acute disease. HAV is a member of the picornavirus family and carries a single-stranded RNA genome; only one strain of the virus exists. The onset of HAV hepatitis occurs within 24 hours, in contrast to the slower onset of clinical symptoms with HBV and HCV infection. Complete recovery occurs in most HAV cases, and chronic infection never occurs. HBV is classified as a hepadnavirus with a double-stranded circular DNA genome. The outcome of HBV infection ranges from complete recovery to progression to chronic hepatitis and, rarely, death. HBV establishes chronic infections, especially in infants; 80% to 95% of infants and young children infected with HBV become chronic carriers and are at high risk of developing hepatocellular carcinoma. In adults, 65% to 80% of infections are asymptomatic, and 90% to 95% of all patients recover completely. HCV is a positive-stranded RNA flavivirus and exists in at least six major genotypes. Most cases of posttransfusion hepatitis are caused by HCV, and these infections are usually subclinical with minor elevation of liver enzymes and a low incidence of jaundice. However, 70% to 90% of HCV patients develop chronic hepatitis, and many are at risk of progressing to chronic active hepatitis and cirrhosis decades later. HEV is transmitted enterically and occurs in epidemic form in developing countries, where water supplies are sometimes contaminated with feces. The disease is more severe in adults than in children, who are usually asymptomatic.

Influenza (2)

Respiratory illnesses commonly known as colds and flu account for more than half of all acute illnesses in the United States each year. Influenza viruses belong to the Orthomyxoviridae family and are a major source of morbidity and mortality caused by respiratory disease. Outbreaks of infection can occur in worldwide epidemics that have resulted in millions of deaths worldwide. Genetic mutations often cause antigenic changes in the structure of viral surface glycoproteins, making influenza viruses extremely difficult to control. Three immunologic types of influenza viruses are known and are termed influenza A, B, and C. Antigenic changes are very common in the type A group of influenza viruses, which are responsible for the majority of influenza epidemics. Influenza type B undergoes more infrequent antigenic changes and is less often the cause of an influenza epidemic, whereas influenza type C is antigenically stable and causes only mild illness in immunocompetent individuals. The viruses carry a single-stranded, negative-sense RNA genome that has eight segments in influenza A and B. Influenza C viruses contain only seven segments of RNA and lack a neuraminidase gene (see below). The complete virion in each type contains nine different structural proteins. A nucleoprotein associates with viral RNA to form a ribonucleoprotein structure that makes up the viral nucleocapsid. Three other large proteins are bound to the viral ribonuclear protein and are responsible for RNA transcription and replication. A matrix protein is also included in the virion that forms a shell underneath the viral lipid envelope and comprises about 40% of all viral protein.

The influenza virion structure also includes a lipid envelope derived from the host cell. This envelope contains two viral surface glycoproteins called hemagglutinin (HA) and neuraminidase (NA). Mutations cause antigenic changes in the structure of these two surface glycoproteins, and thus, they are the main determinants of antigenicity and host immunity. The ability of the virus to change the structure of HA on the virus surface is primarily responsible for the continual evolution of new strains, sometimes leading to subsequent influenza epidemics. NA is an enzyme that removes sialic acid from surface glycoproteins during viral maturation and is required to produce infectious particles and lower the viscosity of the mucin layer of the respiratory tract. Influenza virus spreads through airborne droplets or contact with contaminated hands or surfaces and has an incubation period that varies from 1 to 4 days. However, transmission of the virus begins to occur 24 hours prior to the onset of symptoms. Interferon is detectable in respiratory secretions at the onset of symptoms, and the host response to interferon contributes to recovery. Antibodies and other cell-mediated responses are seen 1 to 2 weeks after infection. It is well established that secondary infections from other viruses or bacteria can occur, and Reye syndrome, an acute encephalopathy occurring in children and adolescents, is a rare complication of influenza B, influenza A, and herpesvirus varicella-zoster infections. The chances of contracting Reye syndrome are increased when salicylates are used in children suffering from influenza and related respiratory diseases.

Tumor Viruses (2,13–17)

Viruses are etiologic factors in the development of several types of human tumors, most notably cervical cancer and liver cancer. At least 15% of all human tumors worldwide have a viral cause. Tumor viruses can be found in both the RNA and DNA virus kingdoms (18). The list of human viruses presently known to be involved in tumor development includes four DNA viruses (Epstein-Barr virus [EBV], certain papilloma viruses, HBV, and the Kaposi sarcoma herpesvirus HHV-8) and two RNA viruses, (human T-cell leukemia virus 1 [HTLV-1] and HCV). Nearly every case of cervical cancer is known to be caused by human papillomavirus (HPV), a fact that spurred the development of the HPV vaccines Gardasil and Cervarix (19). Tumor viruses alter cellular behavior through the use of a small amount of genetic information, using two general strategies. The tumor virus either introduces a new "transforming gene" into the cell (direct-acting), or the virus alters the expression of a preexisting cellular gene or genes (indirect-acting). In both cases, normal regulation of cellular growth processes is lost. Viruses alone cannot act as carcinogens, and other events are necessary to disable regulatory pathways and checkpoints in order to produce transformed, malignant cells. The processes used in the transformation of host cells by human tumor viruses are very diverse.

Cellular transformation may be defined as a stable, heritable change in the growth control of cells that results in tumor formation. Transformation from a normal to a neoplastic cell generally requires the retention of viral genes in the host cell. In the majority of cases, this is accomplished by the integration of certain viral genes into the host cell genome. Retroviruses incorporate their proviral DNA, formed through the action of reverse transcriptase, into host cell DNA. By contrast, DNA tumor viruses integrate a portion of the DNA of the viral genome into the host cell chromosome.

All RNA tumor viruses are members of the retrovirus family and belong to one of two classes (14,15,17). Class I RNA viruses are direct-transforming and carry an oncogene obtained through accidental incorporation from the host cell. No class I RNA viruses are known to produce tumors in humans. Class II or chronic RNA tumor viruses are weakly transforming and do not carry host cell–derived oncogenes. The two known cancer-causing retroviruses in humans act indirectly. They often act by inserting their proviral DNA into the immediate neighborhood of a host cellular oncogene. The human adult T-cell leukemia virus HTLV-1 acts in this manner, thus increasing the number of preneoplastic cells and facilitating secondary cellular changes leading to transformation.

DNA tumor virus strains exist among the papilloma-, polyoma-, adeno-, herpes-, hepadna-, and poxvirus groups (16). DNA tumor viruses encode viral oncoproteins that are important for viral replication, but also affect cellular growth control pathways. For example, inactivation of Rb and the p53 pathway by viral transforming proteins is a common strategy used by papillomaviruses and adenoviruses. As mentioned earlier, all DNA tumor viruses kill their host cell when the infectious virion is released to infect other cells. Thus, transformation and tumorigenicity are entirely dependent on a host cell interaction with the virus that does not involve viral spread to other cells, and cells transformed by DNA tumor viruses depend on the continued expression of the virally encoded oncogene.

Recent studies have revealed that the human tumor viruses EBV, HHV-8, HPV, HBV, HCV, and HTLV-1 express proteins that are targeted to the mitochondria (13). Because the mitochondria play a critical role in energy production, cell death, calcium homeostasis, and redox balance, these proteins have profound effects on host cell physiology. Further study of these proteins and their interactions with mitochondria will aid in the understanding of the mechanisms of viral replication and tumorigenesis and could reveal important new targets for antitumor therapy.

Prion Diseases (20–22)

Although they are not viruses, the infective proteins known as prions have sufficient similarities to viruses to warrant their discussion in this chapter. Prions are small proteins that have been shown to cause a variety of transmissible spongiform encephalopathies, which are rare neurodegenerative disorders typified by symptoms in the central nervous system (CNS) such as spongiform changes, neuronal loss, glial activation, and the accumulation of amyloid aggregates of an abnormally folded host protein. Human prion diseases include kuru, Creutzfeldt-Jakob disease (variant, sporadic, familial, and iatrogenic), Gerstmann-Sträussler-Scheinker syndrome, and fatal familial insomnia. The disease in cattle known as bovine spongiform encephalopathy and the related disease scrapie exhibit similar pathologic features. Following exposure, prions accumulate in lymphoid tissue such as the spleen, lymph nodes, and tonsils and in Peyer's patches (specialized lymphoid follicles located in the submucosa of the small intestine). This accumulation of the infectious agent is necessary for invasion of the CNS. In humans, the incubation period of the disease can vary between 18 months and 40 years. Prions appear to be variant, improperly folded versions of a normal cellular protein called PrP^c, a 30- to 35-kd protein with two sites for *N*-glycosylation that is anchored in the neuronal cell membrane. PrP^c protein contains three α-helices, a short β-pleated sheet region, and a long, unstructured portion that comprises half of the molecule. The variant, infectious form of the protein is known as PrP^{sc} and is produced autocatalytically from PrP^c. Prion diseases are always fatal, with no known cases of remission or recovery. The host shows no inflammatory response or immune response and no production of interferon, and there is no effect on host B-cell or T-cell function. At present, there are no effective agents to treat prion diseases.

VIRAL CHEMOTHERAPY

General Approaches (23,24)

The principles involved in the design of antiviral agents are similar to those used in the design of all chemotherapeutic agents. Drugs in this category are targeted to some process in the virus that is not present in the host cell. The earliest examples of antiviral agents did not achieve this goal, and these drugs were toxic at therapeutic levels or had a limited spectrum of activity. A variety of factors make the design of effective antiviral agents difficult, including their ability to undergo antigenic changes, the latent period during which there are no symptoms, and their reliance on host enzymes and other processes. This problem is compounded by the fact that host immunity is not well understood and that symptoms of viral infection may not appear until replication is complete and the viral genome has been incorporated into infected cells. Nonetheless, the continuing identification of new targets for antiviral agents provides new avenues for the discovery of small-molecule therapies. The following section includes information on currently marketed antiviral compounds that have been designed in eight general areas:

1. Agents that disrupt virus attachment to host cell receptors, penetration, or uncoating.
2. Agents that inhibit virus-associated enzymes such as DNA polymerases and others.
3. Agents that inhibit viral transcription.
4. Agents that inhibit viral translation.
5. Agents that interfere with viral regulatory proteins.
6. Agents that interfere with glycosylation, phosphorylation, sulfation, and so on.
7. Agents that interfere with the assembly of viral proteins.

8. Agents that prohibit the release of viruses from cell surface membranes.

The remainder of this chapter deals primarily with small-molecule antiviral agents that have been approved by the U.S. Food and Drug Administration (FDA) and are clinically effective in the treatment of viral infection. Immunizing biologic agents such as vaccines, as well as antineoplastic agents with antiviral activity, are not covered. Some compounds used primarily in the treatment of bacterial infections, such as rifampicin, bleomycin, doxorubicin, and actinomycin, also inhibit viral replication. However, these antibiotics do not affect the transcription or translation of viral mRNA and are only effective in high concentrations. Therefore, such antibiotics are not commonly used for viral infections. There is a continuing need for new antiviral agents, primarily because viral infections are not curable after the virus invades the host cell and begins to replicate. Vaccines are effective, but they are only able to prevent an infection, and only in cases where specific virus strains are involved. For example, immunization against influenza, which is a yearly routine in many parts of the world, can only provide immunity against specific strains that are represented in that preparation. New virulent strains may arise from nonhuman sources, such as the so-called swine flu or avian flu viruses, and currently available vaccines would have no effect against these new strains. With regard to small-molecule antiviral agents, the ideal drug would have broad-spectrum antiviral activity, completely inhibit viral replication, maintain efficacy against mutant viral strains, and reach the target organ without interfering with normal cellular processes or the immune system of the host.

ANTIVIRAL AGENTS (23,24)

Agents Inhibiting Virus Attachment, Penetration, and Early Viral Replication (Table 38.2)

Amantadine

Mechanism of Action Amantadine hydrochloride (1-adamantanamine hydrochloride) is a symmetrical tricyclic primary amine that inhibits penetration of RNA virus particles into the host cell (Fig. 38.3) (25). It also inhibits the early stages of viral replication by blocking the uncoating of the viral genome. Recent studies suggest that amantadine inhibits viral replication by blocking the influenza A virus M2 proton-selective ion channel.

Clinical Application Amantadine is clinically effective in preventing and treating all A strains of influenza, particularly A2 strains of Asian influenza virus and, to a lesser extent, German measles (rubella) or togavirus. It also shows in vitro activity against influenza B, parainfluenza (paramyxovirus), respiratory syncytial virus (RSV), and some RNA viruses (murine, Rous, and Esh sarcoma viruses). Many prototype influenza A viruses

TABLE 38.2 Antiviral Agents Interfering with Cellular Penetration and Early Replication

Generic Name	Trade Name	Spectrum of Activity	Dosage Form
Amantadine	Symmetrel	Influenza A	Cap (100 mg), syrup (50 mg/5 mL)
Rimantadine	Flumadine	Influenza A	Cap (100 mg)
Interferon α-2a	Roferon A Alferon Intron Wellferon	Chronic hepatitis, CMV, HSV, papillomavirus, rhinovirus, and others	Injectable (3, 5, 10, 18, 25, and 50 million units/mL)
Interferon α-2b	Interon A	Chronic hepatitis B and C, many other viruses	Injectable (3, 5, 10, 18, 25, and 50 million units/mL)
γ-Interferon	Actimmune	Chronic hepatitis B and C, many other viruses	Injectable (100 mcg/0.5 mL)
Tilorone	Amixin IC	Induces the production of interferons	Variable single doses given by injection
Zanamivir	Relenza	Influenza A and B	Inhaled powder (5 mg)
Oseltamivir	Tamiflu	Influenza A and B	Cap (75 mg)
Peramivir	Experimental	H1N1	600 mg daily by IV administration
Enfuvirtide	Fuzeon	HIV	Adult: 90 mg SQ BID Age 6–16: 2 mg/kg SQ BID
Maraviroc	Selzentry	HIV	300 mg orally twice daily

BID, twice a day; Cap, capsule; SQ, subcutaneous.

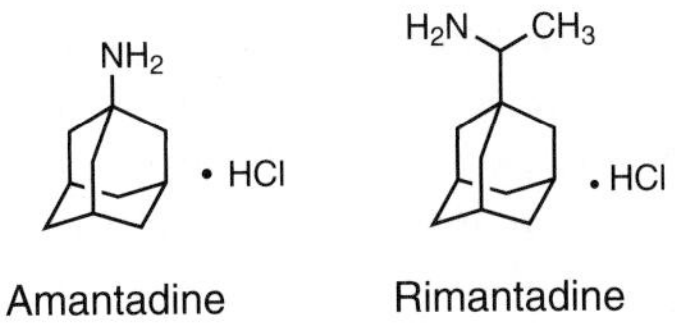

FIGURE 38.3 Agents that inhibit virus attachment, penetration, and early viral replication.

of different human subtypes (H1N1, Fort Dix, H2N2, Asian type, and H3N2, Hong Kong type) are also inhibited by amantadine hydrochloride in vitro and in animal model systems. If given within the first 48 hours of onset of symptoms, amantadine hydrochloride is effective in respiratory tract illness resulting from influenza A but not influenza B virus infection, adenoviruses, and RSV.

PHARMACOKINETICS Amantadine is well absorbed orally, and the usual dosage for oral administration is 100 mg twice daily. A 100-mg oral dose produces blood serum levels of 0.3 mg/mL within 1 to 8 hours. Maximum tissue concentration is reached in 48 hours when a 100-mg dose is given every 12 hours. In healthy adults receiving 25-, 100-, and 150-mg doses of the drug twice daily, steady-state trough plasma concentrations were 110, 302, and 588 mg/mL, respectively. Usually, no neurotoxicity is observed if the plasma level of amantadine is no more than 1.00 mg/mL. Amantadine crosses the blood–brain barrier and is distributed in saliva, nasal secretions, and breast milk (26). Approximately 90% of the drug is excreted unchanged by the kidney, primarily through glomerular filtration and tubular secretion, and there are no reports of metabolic products. Acidification of urine increases the rate of amantadine excretion. The half-life of the drug is 15 to 20 hours in patients with normal renal function.

SIDE EFFECTS Generally, the drug has low toxicity at therapeutic levels but may cause severe CNS symptoms such as nervousness, confusion, headache, drowsiness, insomnia, depression, and hallucinations. Gastrointestinal (GI) side effects include nausea, diarrhea, constipation, and anorexia. Convulsions and coma occur with high doses and in patients with cerebral arteriosclerosis and convulsive disorders. Chronic toxicity with amantadine is unexpected since few side effects have been experienced when the drug has been used for long-term therapy for Parkinson disease. Some serious reactions, however, include depression, orthostatic hypotension, psychosis, urinary retention, and congestive heart failure. Amantadine hydrochloride should be used with caution in patients who have a history of epilepsy, severe arteriosclerosis, liver diseases, and eczematoid dermatitis. Because amantadine does not appear to interfere with the immunogenicity of inactivated influenza A virus vaccine, patients may continue the use of amantadine for 1 week after influenza A vaccination. A virus resistant to amantadine has been obtained in cell culture and from animals, but these reports are not confirmed in humans.

Rimantadine

MECHANISM OF ACTION Rimantadine hydrochloride (α-methyl-1-adamantanemethylamine hydrochloride) is a synthetic adamantane derivative that is structurally and pharmacologically related to amantadine (Fig. 38.3) (27,28). It appears to be more effective than amantadine hydrochloride against influenza A virus with fewer CNS side effects. Rimantadine hydrochloride is thought to interfere with virus uncoating by inhibiting the release of specific proteins. It may act by inhibiting RT or the synthesis of virus-specific RNA but does not inhibit virus adsorption or penetration. It appears to produce a virustatic effect early in the virus replication. It is used widely in Russia and Europe.

CLINICAL APPLICATION Rimantadine hydrochloride has activity against most strains of influenza A including H1N1, H2N2, and H3N2 but has no activity against influenza B virus. It is used for prevention of infection caused by various human, animal, or avian strains of influenza A virus in adults and children. The side effects are nightmares, hallucinations, and vomiting. The most common side effects of rimantadine are associated with the CNS and GI tract.

PHARMACOKINETICS Rimantadine is metabolized in the liver, and about 90% is excreted in the urine within 24 hours. The major urinary metabolites are ring-hydroxylated derivatives, a small percentage of which are glucuronidated. The half-life of rimantadine in adults ranges from 24 to 36 hours. Over 90% of rimantadine doses are absorbed in 3 to 6 hours. Steady-state plasma concentrations range from 0.10 to 2.60 mg/mL at doses of 3 mg/kg/d in infants to 100 mg twice daily in the elderly. Nasal fluid concentrations of rimantadine at steady-state were 1.5 times higher than plasma concentration.

Interferon (29,30)

Isaacs and Lindenmann discovered interferon in 1957. When they infected cells with viruses, interference with the cellular effects of viral infection was observed. Interferon was subsequently isolated and found to protect the cells from further infection. When interferon was administered to other cells or animals, it displayed biologic properties such as inhibition of viral growth, cell multiplication, and immunomodulatory activities. The results led to the speculation that interferon may be a natural antiviral factor, possibly formed before antibody production, and may be involved in the normal mechanism of resistance displayed against viral infection. Some investigators relate interferon to the polypeptide hormones and suggest that interferon functions in cell-to-cell communication by transmitting specific messages. Recently, antitumor and anticancer properties of interferon have evoked worldwide interest in the possible use of this agent in therapy for viral diseases, cancer, and immunodeficiency disorders. Host cells in response to various inducers synthesize interferons.

Interferon Structure Interferon consists of a mixture of small proteins with molecular weights ranging from 20,000 to 160,000 daltons. They are glycoproteins that exhibit species-specific antiviral activity. Human interferons are classified into three types: alpha (α), beta (β), and gamma (γ) (31). The α-type is secreted by human leukocytes (white blood cells, non–T lymphocytes), and the β-type is secreted by human fibroblasts. Lymphoid cells (T lymphocytes), which either have been exposed to a presensitized antigen or have been stimulated to divide by mitogens, secrete α-interferon. γ-Interferon is also called "immune" interferon. Interferons are active in extremely low concentrations.

Mechanism of Action Although, interferons are mediators of immune response, different mechanisms for the antiviral action of interferon have been proposed. α-Interferon possesses broad-spectrum antiviral activity, and acts on virus-infected cells by binding to specific cell surface receptors. It inhibits the transcription and translation of mRNA into viral nucleic acid and protein. Studies in cell free systems have shown that the addition of adenosine triphosphate and double-stranded RNA to extracts of interferon-treated cells activates cellular RNA proteins and a cellular endonuclease. This activation causes the formation of translation inhibitory protein, which terminates production of viral enzyme, nucleic acid, and structural proteins (32). Interferon may also act by blocking synthesis of a cleaving enzyme required for viral release.

Clinical Application Interferon has been tested for use in chronic HBV infection, herpetic keratitis, herpes genitalis, herpes zoster, varicella-zoster, chronic hepatitis, influenza, and common cold infections. Other uses of interferon are in the treatment of cancers, such as breast cancer, lung carcinoma, and multiple myeloma. Interferon has had some success when used as a prophylactic agent for cytomegalovirus (CMV) infection in renal transplant recipients. The scarcity of interferon and the difficulty in purifying it have limited clinical trials. Supplies have been augmented by recombinant DNA technology, which allows cloning of the interferon gene (33), although the high cost still hinders clinical application. The FDA has approved recombinant interferon α-2a and α-2b and γ-interferon for the treatment of hairy cell leukemia (a rare form of cancer), AIDS-related Kaposi sarcoma, and genital warts (condyloma acuminatum). Subcutaneous injection of recombinant interferon α-2b has been approved for the treatment of chronic HCV. Some foreign countries have approved α-interferon for the treatment of cancers such as multiple myeloma (cancer of plasma cells), malignant melanoma (skin cancer), and Kaposi sarcoma (cancer associated with AIDS). Both β- and γ-interferons and interleukin-2 may be commercial drugs of the future for the treatment of cancers and viral infections, including genital warts and the common cold.

Pharmacokinetics The pharmacokinetics of interferon are not well understood. Maximum levels in blood after intramuscular injection were obtained in 5 to 8 hours. Interferon does not penetrate well into cerebrospinal fluid (CSF). Oral administration of interferon does not indicate a detectable serum level, and as such, oral administration is clinically ineffective. After intramuscular or subcutaneous injection, drug concentration in the plasma is dose related. Clinical use of interferon is limited to topical administration (nasal sprays) for prophylaxis and treatment of rhinovirus infections. Adverse reactions and toxicity include influenza-like syndrome of fever, chills, headache, myalgias, nausea, vomiting, diarrhea, bone marrow suppression, mental confusion, and behavioral changes. Intranasal administration produces mucosal friability, ulceration, and dryness. Two long-acting forms of interferon have recently become available. The addition of polyethylene glycol to the formulation of interferon α-2a and interferon α-2b affords an injectable form of each drug that has an extended half-life.

Because viruses were found to induce the release of interferon, efforts were made to induce the production or release of interferon in humans by the administration of chemical "inducers" (34). Various small molecules (substituted propanediamine) and large polymers (double-stranded polynucleotides) were used to induce interferons. Statolon, a natural double-stranded RNA produced in *Penicillium stoloniferum* culture, and a double-stranded complex of polyriboinosinic acid and polyribocytidylic acid (poly I:C) have been used as nonviral inducers for releasing preformed interferons. A modification of poly I:C stabilized with poly-L-lysine and carboxymethylcellulose (poly ICLC) has been used experimentally in humans. Clinically, it prevented coryza when used locally in the nose and conjunctival sacs. This substance was found to be a better interferon inducer than poly I:C. Another interferon inducer is Ampligen, a polynucleotide derivative of poly I:C with spaced uridines. It has anti-HIV activity in vitro and is an immunomodulator.

Other chemical inducers, such as pyran copolymers, tilorone, diethylaminoethyl dextran, and heparin, have also been used. Tilorone is an effective inducer of interferon in mice but is relatively ineffective in humans. Initial use of interferon and its inducers instilled intranasally after rhinovirus exposure was successful in the prevention of respiratory diseases.

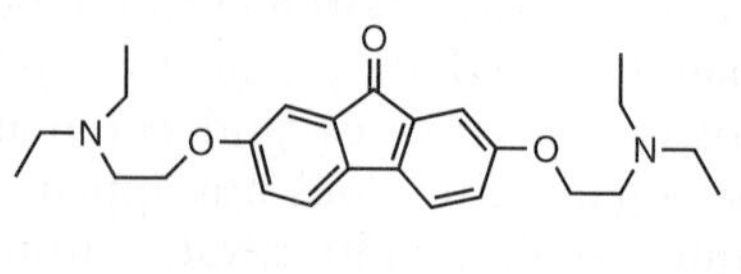

Tilorone

The clinical success of interferon and its inducers has not yet been established, although they may play a significant role in cell-mediated immunity to viral infections and cancer. Disadvantages of interferon use include unacceptable side effects, such as fever, headache, myalgias, leukopenia, nausea, vomiting, diarrhea, hypotension, alopecia, anorexia, and weight loss.

Neuraminidase Inhibitors (35)

Virus Activation

The role played by the surface glycoproteins HA, an enzyme important for viral binding to host cell receptors via a terminal sialic acid residue, and NA, an enzyme involved in various aspects of activation of influenza viruses, was discussed earlier. Freshly shed virus particles are coated with sialic acid residues. NA is found in both influenza A and B viruses and is thought to be involved in catalytically cleaving glycosidic bonds between terminal sialic acid residues and adjacent sugars on HA. The cleavage of sialic acid bonds facilitates the spread of viruses by enhancing adsorption to cell surface receptors, and thus increases the infective level of the virus. In the absence of sialic acid cleavage from HA, viral aggregation or inappropriate binding to HA will occur, interfering with the spread of the infection. NA also appears to play a role in preventing viral inactivation by respiratory mucus (Fig. 38.4).

Mechanism of Action

Since NA plays such an important role in the activation of newly formed viruses, it is not surprising that the development of NA inhibitors has become an important potential means of inhibiting the spread of viral infections. X-ray crystallography of NA has shown that while the amino acid sequence of NA from various viruses is considerably different, the sialic acid binding site is quite similar for type A and B influenza viruses. In addition, it is believed that the hydrolysis of sialic acid proceeds through an oxonium cation–stabilized carbonium ion as shown in Figure 38.4. Mimicking the transition state with novel carbocyclic derivatives of sialic acid has led to the development of transition state–based inhibitors (36). The first of these compounds, 2-deoxy-2,3-dehydro-*N*-acetylneuraminic acid (DANA; Fig. 38.5), was found to be an active neuraminidase inhibitor but lacked specificity for viral neuraminidase. Upon determination of the crystal structure of neuraminidase, more sophisticated measurements of the binding site for sialic acid led to the development of zanamivir and, later, oseltamivir.

Specific Drugs

Zanamivir Crystallographic studies of DANA bound to NA defined the receptor site to which the sialic acid portion of the virus binds. These studies suggested that substitution of the 4-hydroxy with an amino group or the larger guanidino group should increase binding of the inhibitor to NA. The 4-amino derivative was found to bind to a glutamic acid (Glu 119) in the receptor through a salt bridge, whereas the 4-guanidino derivative was able to form both a salt bridge to Glu 119 and a charge–charge interaction with a glutamic acid at position 227. The result of these substitutions was a dramatic increase in binding capacity of the 4-amino and 4-guanidino derivatives to NA, leading to effective competitive inhibition of the enzyme. The result has been the development of the 4-guanidino analog as zanamivir (Fig. 38.5), which has become an effective agent against influenza A and B virus.

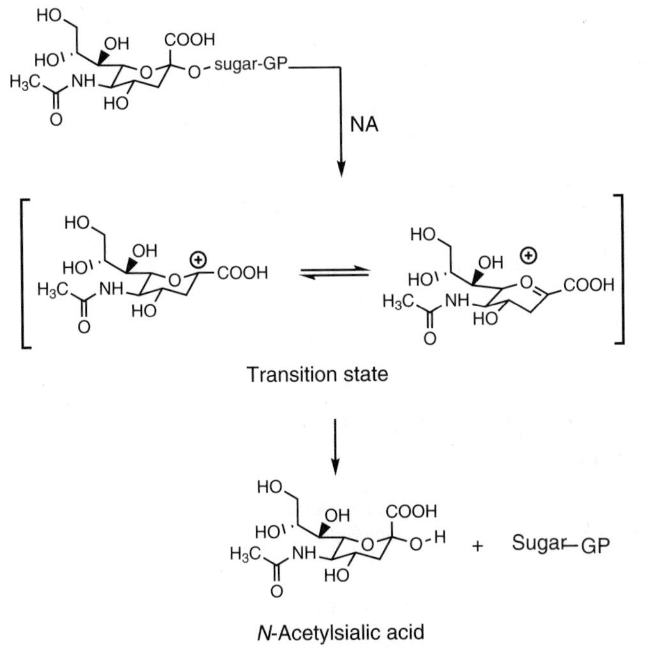

FIGURE 38.4 Neuraminidase-catalyzed removal of a sialic acid residue from a glycoprotein chain. GP, glycoprotein; NA, neuraminidase.

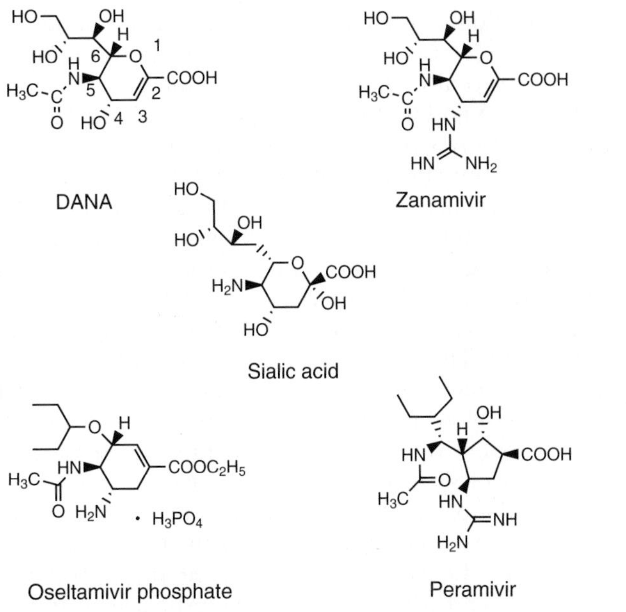

FIGURE 38.5 Neuraminidase inhibitors based on sialic acid.

Zanamivir is effective when administered via the nasal, intraperitoneal, and intravenous routes but is inactive when given orally (Table 38.2). Animal studies have shown 68% recovery of the drug in the urine following intraperitoneal administration, 43% urinary recovery following nasal administration, and only 3% urinary recovery following oral administration. Human data gave similar results to those obtained in animal models. Human efficacy studies with nasal drops or sprays demonstrated that the drug was effective when administered before exposure and after exposure to influenza A or B virus. When given before viral inoculation, the drug reduced viral shedding, infection, and symptoms. When administered beginning at either 26 or 32 hours after inoculation, there was a reduction in shedding, viral titer, and fever. Presently the drug is available as a dry powder for oral inhalation by adults and adolescents who have been symptomatic for no more than 2 days. Zanamivir is able to more rapidly resolve influenza symptoms and improve recovery (from 7 days with placebo to 4 days with treatment). Additional studies have suggested the prophylactic benefit of zanamivir when administered to family members after one member of the family developed flu-like symptoms. As a result, the manufacturer has submitted an application for the use of the drug for the prevention of influenza A and B.

Oseltamivir X-ray crystallographic studies further demonstrated that additional binding sites exist between NA and substrate involving the C-5 acetamido carbonyl of DANA and an arginine (Arg 152), the C-2 carboxyl and arginines as 118, 292, and 371, and the potential for hydrophobic binding to substituents at C-6 (with glutamic acid, alanine, arginine, and isoleucine). Structure–activity relationship studies showed that maximum binding occurred to NA when C-6 (based on DANA numbering) was substituted with the 3-pentyloxy side chain such as the one found in oseltamivir (Fig. 38.5). In addition, esterification with ethanol gave rise to a compound that is orally effective. Oseltamivir phosphate was approved as the first orally administered NA inhibitor used against influenza A and B (Table 38.2). The drug is indicated for the treatment of uncomplicated acute illness due to influenza infection. Recently, the manufacturer has submitted a request for approval of the drug for prevention of influenza A and B for use in adults, adolescents, and children 1 year of age and older. The drug is effective in treating influenza if administered within 2 days after onset of symptoms. The recommended dose is 75 mg twice daily for 5 days. The prophylactic dose is 75 mg taken once daily for 7 days. Oseltamivir is readily absorbed from the GI tract following oral administration. It is a prodrug that is extensively metabolized in the liver undergoing ester hydrolysis to the active carboxylic acid (Fig. 38.6). Two oxidative metabolites have also been isolated, with the major oxidation product being the ω-carboxylic acid (37). Side effects with oseltamivir are minor, consisting of nausea and vomiting that occur primarily in the first 2 days of therapy.

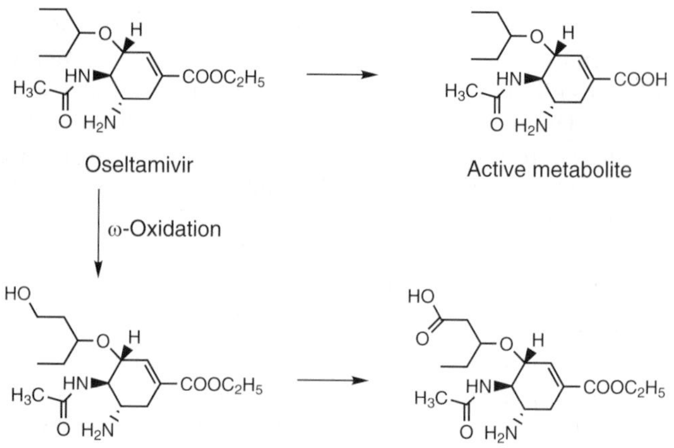

FIGURE 38.6 Metabolism of oseltamivir by hydrolysis and ω-oxidation.

Peramivir In 2009, the experimental NA inhibitor peramivir (Fig. 38.5, Table 38.2) received emergency FDA approval for use in treatment of certain hospitalized patients with known or suspected H1N1 influenza infections. This represents the first time in which an experimental drug in phase III clinical trials has received an emergency use approval. The drug is only available by electronic request from the U.S. Strategic National Stockpile. The use of peramivir is restricted to severe H1N1 influenza cases where other antiviral agents (including NA inhibitors) have failed (38). For example, a patient infected with an H1N1 strain of influenza that is resistant to oseltamivir and who is unable to inhale zanamivir would be a candidate for peramivir treatment. Peramivir is structurally distinct from oseltamivir and zanamivir in that it contains a cyclopentane ring structure that replaces the sialic acid core and because it does not contain a glycerol side chain, which is thought to reduce the oral bioavailability of oseltamivir and zanamivir. The structure of peramivir was proposed using the technique of structure-based design. In this approach, in silico docking of proposed NA inhibitors suggested that peramivir bound most efficiently to the four known binding pockets in the viral NA catalytic site. Peramivir is administered intravenously as a single dose (0.5 to 8 mg/kg) or as two daily doses (4 mg/kg). It has a serum half-life of 7.7 to 20 hours, and 90% of the drug is excreted unchanged in the urine. Because peramivir is still in phase III clinical trials, efficacy data have not yet been released.

Entry (Fusion) Inhibitors

Enfuvirtide (39,40)

N-acetyl-Tyr-Thr-Ser-Leu-Ile-His-Ser-Leu-Ile-Glu-Glu-Ser-Gln-Asp-Gln-Gln-Glu-Lys-Asp-Glu-Gln-Glu-Leu-Leu-Glu-Leu-Asp-Lys-Try-Ala-Ser-Leu-Try-Asp-Try-Phe-NH_2

Enfuvirtide

Entry inhibitors, also known as fusion inhibitors, are a new class of drugs for the treatment of HIV infection, and enfuvirtide is the first compound of this family to be approved for clinical use. Enfuvirtide is an oligopeptide consisting of 36 amino acids. It is a synthetic peptide that mimics an HR2 fragment of gp41, blocking the formation of a six-helix bundle structure that is critical in the fusion of the HIV-1 virion to a CD4-positive T lymphocyte. Specifically, it binds to the tryptophan-rich region of the gp41 protein. Enfuvirtide is used in combination with other antiretrovirals and works against a variety of HIV-1 variants, but it is not active against HIV-2. Resistance to enfuvirtide can develop when the virus produces changes in a 10–amino acid domain between residues 36 to 45 in the gp41 HIV surface glycoprotein. The drug is administered twice daily as a subcutaneous injection and has a complex absorption pattern. Enfuvirtide is highly bound to plasma protein (~92%) and is prone to proteolytic metabolism. Adverse reactions include pain, erythema, and pruritus at the site of injection and insomnia.

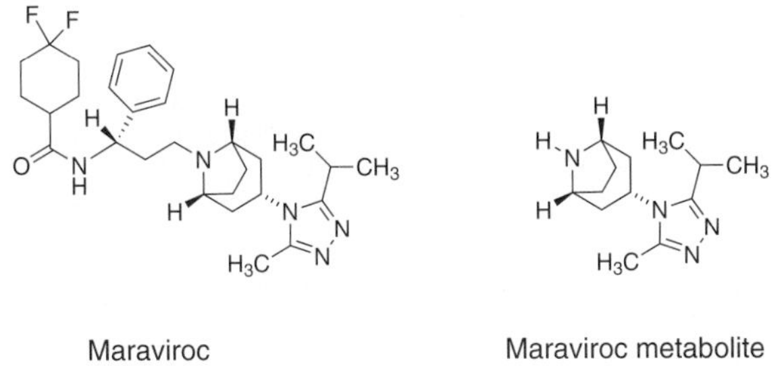

Maraviroc

CCR5 is a protein produced by humans that is a member of the chemokine coreceptor family and is located in the cell membrane of specific human cells (i.e., T cells, macrophages, dendritic cells, microglia). Although there are a number of natural substrates for this receptor protein, HIV can use this G protein–coupled receptor in part as a coreceptor for entry into its targeted cells. In addition, individuals who have a mutation in the *CCR5* gene (*CCR5*-δ32) have a deletion of a portion of the *CCR5* gene, which in turn leads to reduced or absent expression of *CCR5* in heterozygous or homozygous genotypes, respectively, with no apparent deleterious consequences. Individuals homozygous with respect to *CCR5*-δ32 have a high degree of resistance to HIV infection, whereas heterozygotes have a reduced rate of disease progression. As a result, CCR5 antagonists represent a promising new class of cell entry inhibitor drugs under development for the treatment of HIV-1 infection (fusion inhibitor). The CCR5 antagonist maraviroc has potent anti-HIV activity in vitro and is safe and well-tolerated at multiple doses up to 300 mg twice daily in healthy volunteers. Maraviroc was recently approved by the FDA (Selzentry; Pfizer). Maraviroc is an orally administered drug available as 150- and 300-mg film-coated tablets. The current FDA-approved dosage of maraviroc is 300 mg twice daily, and it must be used in combination with other antiretroviral medications. Maraviroc is actively absorbed following oral administration but has a low bioavailability (~23%) and is a substrate for P-glycoprotein, possibly accounting for the poor bioavailability. The drug is highly bound to plasma proteins (~76%) and is metabolized to inactive metabolites via CYP3A4. The major metabolite results from *N*-dealkylation.

Agents Interfering with Viral Nucleic Acid Replication (Table 38.3)

Acyclic Nucleoside Analogs (Fig. 38.7)

Acyclovir

Mechanism of Action Acyclovir is a synthetic analog of deoxyguanosine in which the carbohydrate moiety is acyclic (Fig. 38.7) (41). Because of this difference in structure as compared to other antiviral compounds (idoxuridine, vidarabine, and trifluridine, see below), acyclovir possesses a unique mechanism of antiviral activity. The mode of action of acyclovir consists of three consecutive mechanisms (42). The first of these mechanisms involves conversion of the drug to active acyclovir monophosphate within cells by viral thymidine kinase (Fig. 38.8). This phosphorylation reaction occurs faster within cells infected by herpesvirus than in normal cells because acyclovir is a poor substrate for the normal cell thymidine kinase. Acyclovir is further converted to di- and triphosphates by a normal cellular enzyme called guanosine monophosphate kinase. In the second mechanism, viral DNA polymerase is competitively inhibited by acyclovir triphosphate with a lower half maximal inhibitory concentration (IC_{50}) concentration than that for cellular DNA polymerase. Acyclovir triphosphate is incorporated into the viral DNA chain during DNA synthesis. Because acyclovir triphosphate lacks the 3'-hydroxyl group of a cyclic sugar, it terminates further elongation of the DNA chain. The third mechanism depends on preferential uptake of acyclovir by herpes-infected cells as compared to uninfected cells, resulting in a higher concentration of acyclovir triphosphate and leading to a high therapeutic index between herpes-infected cells to normal cells. Acyclovir is active against certain herpes virus infections. These viruses induce virus-specific thymidine kinase and DNA polymerase, which are inhibited by acyclovir. Thus, acyclovir significantly reduces DNA synthesis in virus-infected cells without significantly disturbing the active replication of uninfected cells.

Clinical Application Acyclovir has potent activity against several DNA viruses including HSV-1, the common cause of labial herpes (cold sore), and HSV-2, the common cause of genital herpes (Table 38.3) (43). Varicella-zoster virus (VZV) and some isolates of EBV are affected to a lesser extent by acyclovir. However, CMV is less sensitive to acyclovir, which has no activity against vaccinia virus, adenovirus, and parainfluenza infections. An ointment containing 5% acyclovir has been used in a regimen of five times a day for up to 14 days for the treatment of herpetic keratitis and primary and recurrent infections of herpes genitalis. Mild pain, transient burning, stinging, pruritus, rash, and vulvitis have been noted. The

TABLE 38.3 Antiviral Agents Interfering with Viral Nucleic Acid Replication

Generic Name	Common Name	Trade Name	Spectrum of Activity	Dosage Form (mg/unit)
Acyclic nucleoside analogs (Fig. 38.7)				
Acyclovir	Acyclo-G	Zovirax	HSV-1; HSV-2; VZV; EBV	5% Oint, Inj (5mg/ml), Cap (200), Tab (400, 800), Susp (200/5 mL)
Valacyclovir		Valtrex	HSV-1; VZV; CMV	Tab (500)
Cidofovir	HPMPC	Vistide	CMV; HSV-1; HSV-2; VZV; CMV; EBV	Inj (75/mL)
Famciclovir	FCV	Famvir	HSV; VZV; EBV; chronic HBV	Tab (125, 250, 500)
Ganciclovir	DHPG	Cytovene Vitrasert	CMV retinitis	Inj (50/mL), Cap (250, 500), Insert (4.5/insert)
Adefovir dipivoxil		Hepsera	Hepatitis B	Tab (10)
Conventional nucleoside analogs (Fig. 38.11)				
Idoxuridine	5-IUDR	Herplex Stoxil	HSV keratitis	0.1% Sol, 0.5% Oint
Ribavirin		Virazole	RSV; influenza A and B; HIV-1; parainfluenza	Aerosol (20/mL)
Trifluorothymidine	TFT, FT3	Viroptic	HSV-1	1% Sol
Vidarabine	Ara-A	Vira A	HSV-1; HSV-2	3% Oint (monohydrate)
Cytarabine	Ara-C	Cytosar	Herpes zoster	Inj (10, 20, 50, 100/mL)
Non-nucleoside analogs (Fig. 38.13)				
Boceprevir		Victrelis	HCV	Tab (200)
Fomivirsen			CMV retinitis	
Foscarnet	PFA	Foscavir	CMV retinitis; HSV	Inj (24/mL)
Telaprevir		Incivek	HCV	Tab (375)

CMV, cytomegalovirus; EBV, Epstein-Barr virus; HBV, hepatitis B virus; HSV, herpes simplex virus; VZV, varicella-zoster virus.

FDA has approved topical and intravenous (IV) acyclovir preparations for initial herpes genitalis and HSV-1 and HSV-2 infections in immunocompromised patients (44). In these individuals, early use of acyclovir shortens the duration of viral shedding and lesion pain. Oral doses of 200 mg of acyclovir, taken five times a day for 5 to 10 days, have not proven successful because of the low bioavailability of current preparations. Oral doses of 800 mg of the drug given five times daily for 7 to 10 days have been approved by the FDA for treatment of herpes zoster infection. This treatment shortens the duration of viral shedding in chickenpox and shingles. The IV injection of the drug (10 mg/kg three times daily for 10 to 12 days) has been approved for the treatment of herpes simplex encephalitis (45). Excessive and high doses of acyclovir have, however, caused viruses to develop resistance to the drug. This resistance results from reduction of virus-encoded thymidine kinase, which does not effectively activate the drug.

Pharmacokinetics Pharmacokinetic studies show that IV dose administration of acyclovir 2.5 mg/kg results in peak plasma concentrations of 3.4 to 6.8 mg/mL (46,47). The bioavailability of acyclovir is 15% to 30%, and it is metabolized to 9-carboxymethoxymethylguanine, which is inactive. Plasma protein binding averages 15%, and approximately 70% of acyclovir is excreted unchanged in the urine by both glomerular filtration and tubular secretion. The half-life of the drug is approximately 3 hours in patients with normal renal function. In an individual with renal diseases, the half-life of the drug is prolonged. Therefore, acyclovir dosage adjustment is necessary for patients with renal impairment. Acyclovir easily penetrates the lung, brain, muscle, spleen, uterus, vaginal mucosa, intestine, liver, and kidney.

VALACYCLOVIR Valacyclovir hydrochloride is an amino acid ester prodrug of acyclovir, which exhibits antiviral activity only after metabolism in the intestine or liver to

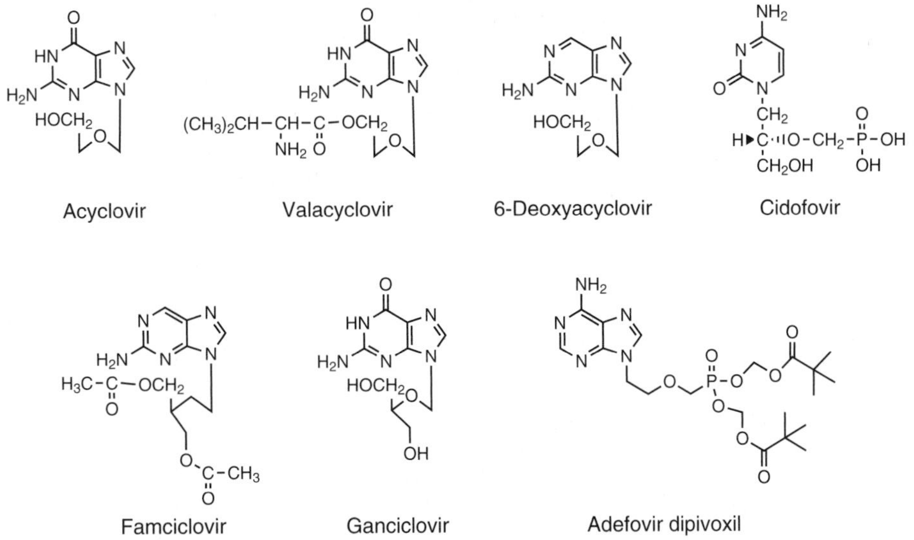

FIGURE 38.7 Agents that interfere with viral nucleic acid replication: acyclic nucleosides.

acyclovir followed by conversion to the triphosphate as shown in Figure 38.8 (48). Structurally, it differs from acyclovir by the presence of the amino acid valine attached to the 5′-hydroxyl group of the nucleoside. Valacyclovir's benefit comes from an increased GI absorption resulting in higher plasma concentrations of acyclovir, which is normally poorly absorbed from the GI tract. As with acyclovir, valacyclovir is active against HSV-1, VZV, and CMV because of its affinity for the viral form of the enzyme thymidine kinase. Oral valacyclovir is used for the treatment of acute, localized herpes zoster (shingles) in immunocompetent patients and may be given without meals. It is also used for the initial and recurrent episodes of genital herpes infections (Table 38.3). The adverse effects are similar to acyclovir and include nausea, headache, vomiting, constipation, and anorexia. The binding of valacyclovir to human plasma proteins ranges from 13.5% to 17.9%. The plasma elimination half-life of acyclovir is 2.5 to 3.3 hours. The bioavailability of valacyclovir hydrochloride is 54% compared to approximately 20% for oral acyclovir. It is as effective as acyclovir in decreasing the duration of pain associated with posttherapeutic neuralgia and episodes of genital lesion healing. The related analog 6-deoxyacyclovir (Fig. 38.8) is a prodrug form of acyclovir that is activated through metabolism by xanthine oxidase. This drug, which has improved solubility characteristics when compared to acyclovir, is used for the treatment of VZV infection.

Cidofovir

Mechanism of Action Cidofovir (1-[(*S*)-3-hydroxy-2-(phosphonomethoxy)propyl]cytosine) is a synthetic acyclic purine nucleotide analog of cytosine (Fig. 38.7) (49). It is a phosphorylated nucleotide that is additionally phosphorylated by host cell enzymes to its active intracellular metabolite, cidofovir diphosphate. This reaction occurs without initial virus-dependent phosphorylation by viral nucleoside kinases. It produces antiviral effects through interfering with DNA synthesis and inhibiting viral replication.

Clinical Application Cidofovir is active against herpes viruses including HSV-1 and HSV-2, VZV, CMV, and EBV. It is effective against acyclovir-resistant strains of HSV and ganciclovir-resistant strains of CMV. Cidofovir is a long-acting drug for the treatment of CMV retinitis in AIDS patients given as IV infusion or intravitreal injection. It is not a curative drug, and its benefit over foscarnet or ganciclovir is yet to be determined. The major adverse effect is nephrotoxicity, which appears to result in renal tubular damage. Concomitant administration of cidofovir with probenecid is contraindicated because of increased risk of nephrotoxicity. Topical cidofovir (0.2%) is as effective as trifluridine (1%) in reducing HSV-1 shedding and healing time in rabbits with dendritic keratitis. Cidofovir is administered IV, topically, and by ocular implant (Table 38.3). Peak plasma concentration of 3.1 to 23.6 mg/mL is achieved with doses of 1.0 to 10.0 mg/kg, respectively. The terminal plasma half-life is 2.6 hours, and 90% of the drug is excreted in the urine. It has a variable bioavailability (2% to 26%).

Famciclovir

Mechanism of Action Famciclovir is a synthetic purine nucleoside analog related to guanine (50,51). It is the diacetyl 6-deoxy ester of penciclovir, which is structurally related to ganciclovir. Its pharmacologic and microbiologic activities are similar to acyclovir. Famciclovir is a prodrug of penciclovir (Fig. 38.9), which is formed in vivo by hydrolysis of the acetyl groups and oxidation at the 6-position by mixed function oxidases. Penciclovir and its metabolite penciclovir triphosphate possess antiviral activity resulting from inhibition of viral DNA polymerase.

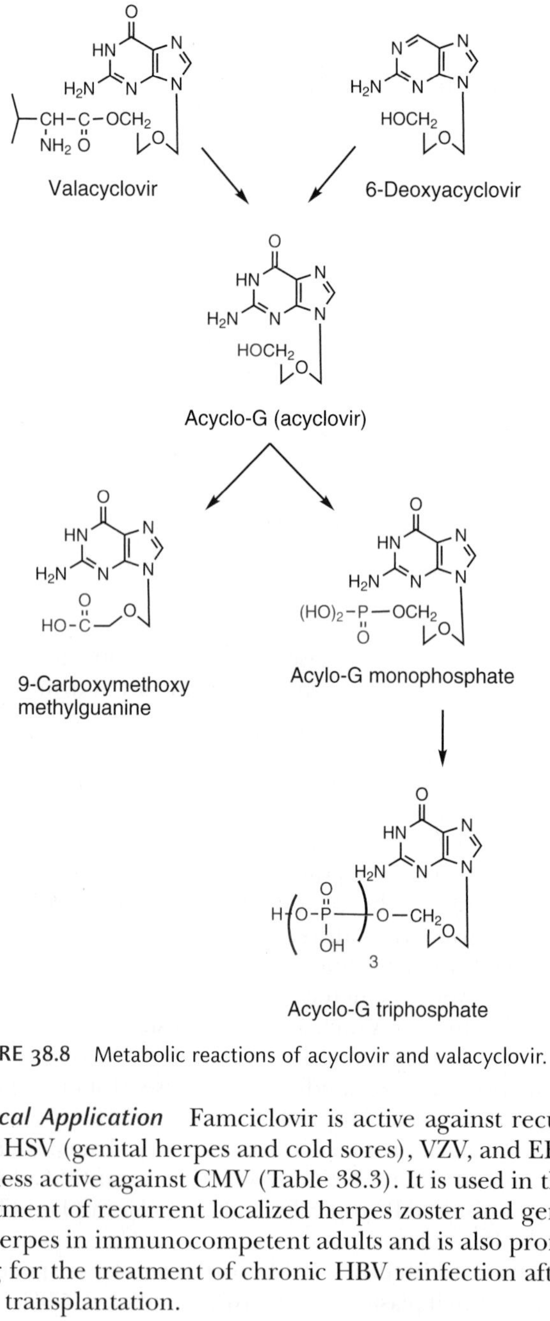

FIGURE 38.8 Metabolic reactions of acyclovir and valacyclovir.

Clinical Application Famciclovir is active against recurrent HSV (genital herpes and cold sores), VZV, and EBV but less active against CMV (Table 38.3). It is used in the treatment of recurrent localized herpes zoster and genital herpes in immunocompetent adults and is also promising for the treatment of chronic HBV reinfection after liver transplantation.

Pharmacokinetics Famciclovir can be given with or without food. The most common adverse effects are headache and GI disturbances. Concomitant use of famciclovir with probenecid results in increased plasma concentrations of penciclovir. The recommended dose of famciclovir is 500 mg every 8 hours for 7 days. The absolute bioavailability of famciclovir is 77%, and area under plasma concentration–time curve (AUC) is 86 mcg/mL. Famciclovir with digoxin increased plasma concentration of digoxin to 19% as compared to digoxin given alone.

Ganciclovir

Mechanism of Action Ganciclovir sodium is an acyclic deoxyguanosine analog of acyclovir (52). Its active form is ganciclovir triphosphate, which is an inhibitor of viral rather than cellular DNA polymerase. The phosphorylation of ganciclovir does not require a virus-specific thymidine kinase for its activity against CMV. The mechanism of action is similar to that of acyclovir; however, ganciclovir is more toxic to human cells than is acyclovir. Ganciclovir has greater activity than acyclovir against CMV and EBV infection in immunocompromised patients. It is also active against HSV infection and in some mutants resistant to acyclovir. In AIDS patients, ganciclovir stopped progressive hemorragic retinitis and symptomatic pneumonitis related to CMV infection.

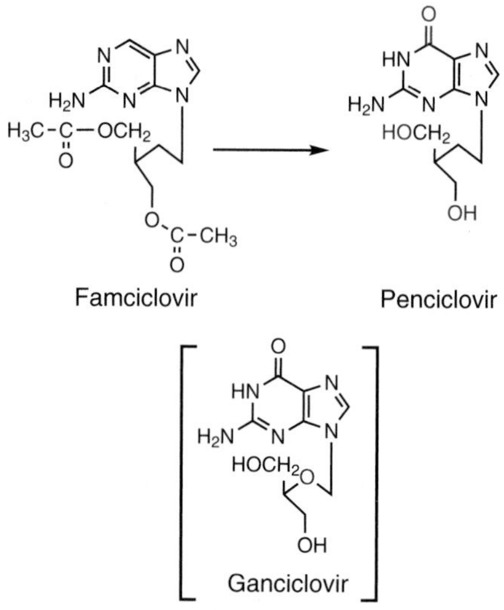

FIGURE 38.9 Metabolic activation of famciclovir.

Clinical Application Ganciclovir is absorbed and phosphorylated by infection-induced kinases of HSV and VZV infections. Common side effects are leukopenia, neutropenia, and thrombocytopenia. Ganciclovir with zidovudine causes severe hematologic toxicity. Ganciclovir is available only as an IV infusion because oral bioavailability is poor (Table 38.3). It is given in doses of 5 mg/kg twice daily for 14 to 21 days. When ganciclovir is given by IV administration, concentrations of the drug in the CSF and the brain vary from 25% to 70% of the plasma concentration. After minimal metabolism, ganciclovir is excreted in the urine. In adults with normal renal function, the serum half-life of the drug is approximately 3 hours. Ganciclovir has been approved by the FDA for the treatment of CMV retinitis in immunocompromised and AIDS patients.

Adefovir Dipivoxil (53)

Mechanism of Action Adefovir dipivoxil is an orally active prodrug indicated for the treatment of chronic HBV (Fig. 38.7). The drug is hydrolyzed by extracellular esterases to produce adefovir, which in turn is phosphorylated by adenylate kinase to adefovir phosphate, which inhibits HBV DNA polymerase. Incorporation of adefovir into viral DNA also leads to DNA chain termination.

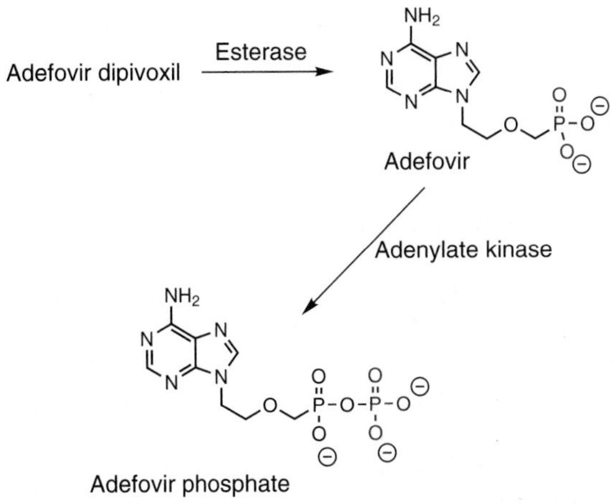

FIGURE 38.10 Activation of the prodrug adefovir dipivoxyl by esterase and adenylate kinase.

As shown in Figure 38.10, adefovir dipivoxil is activated in two steps involving an esterase that exposes a free phosphate group (adefovir), followed by addition of a second phosphate by adenylate kinase to form adefovir phosphate.

Pharmacokinetics Adefovir is poorly absorbed orally, but the bioavailability of adefovir dipivoxil reaches approximately 59%. The drug is absorbed to an equal extent with or without the presence of food, and it is excreted unchanged by the kidney. Adefovir dipivoxil joins interferon and lamivudine in the treatment of chronic HBV. It can be used singly or in combination with lamivudine. Early clinical studies indicate benefit of the use of adefovir dipivoxil to treat lamivudine-resistant HBV with a low level of resistant virus developing to monotherapy with adefovir dipivoxil.

Conventional Nucleoside Analogs (Fig. 38.11)

Idoxuridine

Mechanism of Action Idoxuridine is a nucleoside analog of thymidine containing a halogenated pyrimidine (54). It acts as an antiviral agent against DNA viruses by interfering with their replication based through competitive inhibition. Idoxuridine is first phosphorylated by the host cell virus-encoded enzyme thymidine kinase to an active triphosphate form. The phosphorylated drug inhibits cellular DNA polymerase to a lesser extent than HSV DNA polymerase, which is necessary for the synthesis of viral DNA. The triphosphate form of the drug is then incorporated during viral nucleic acid synthesis by a false pairing system that replaces thymidine. When transcription occurs, faulty viral proteins are formed, resulting in defective viral particles (55).

Clinical Application Idoxuridine is available as ophthalmic drops (0.1%) and ointment (0.5%) for the treatment of HSV keratoconjunctivitis (Table 38.3). Because of its poor solubility, the drug is ineffective in labial or genital HSV or for cutaneous herpes zoster infection. Idoxuridine in dimethylsulfoxide (DMSO), however, has been used in mucocutaneous HSV infection of the mouth and nose. Because DMSO facilitates drug absorption and also has some therapeutic effect, a 40% solution of idoxuridine in DMSO is more effective than idoxuridine used without this vehicle. Therefore, the FDA approved idoxuridine only for topical treatment of herpes simplex keratitis, and it is more effective in epithelial than in stromal infections. It is less effective for recurrent herpes keratitis, probably because of the development of drug-resistant virus strains.

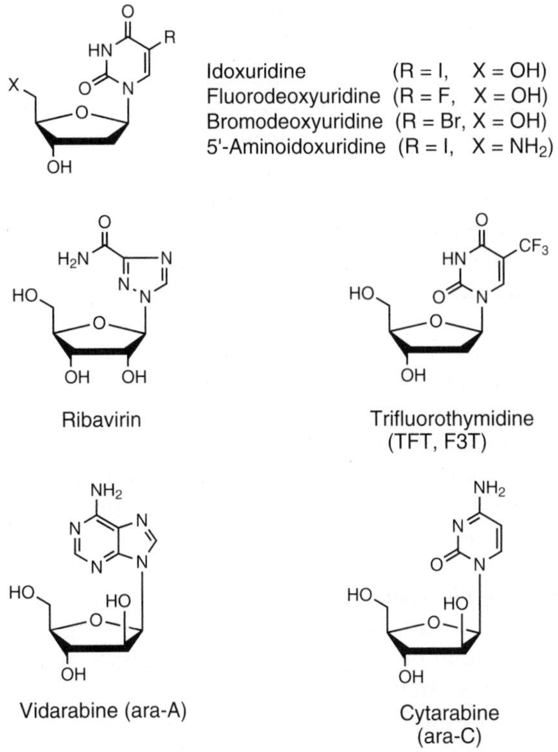

FIGURE 38.11 Agents that interfere with viral nucleic acid replication: conventional nucleosides.

Side Effects Adverse reactions of idoxuridine include such local reactions as pain, pruritus, edema, burning, and hypersensitivity. Systemic administration of idoxuridine by IV injection may be given in an emergency but leads to bone marrow toxicities such as leukopenia, thrombocytopenia, and anemia. It may also induce stomatitis, nausea, vomiting, abnormalities of liver functions, and alopecia. Idoxuridine has a plasma half-life of 30 minutes and is rapidly metabolized in the blood to idoxuracil and uracil.

Other halogenated uridine derivatives can also be used as antiviral agents (Fig. 38.11). Fluorodeoxyuridine has in vitro antiviral activity but is not used in clinical practice. Bromodeoxyuridine has been used in subacute sclerosing panencephalitis, a deadly virus-induced CNS disease. This agent appears to interfere with DNA synthesis in the same way as idoxuridine. The 5′-amino analog of idoxuridine (5-iodo-5′-amino-2,′5′-dideoxyuridine) is a better antiviral agent than idoxuridine and is less toxic. It is metabolized in herpesvirus-infected cells only by thymidine kinase to di- and triphosphoramidates. These metabolites inhibit HSV-specific late RNA transcription, causing reduction of less infective abnormal viral proteins. Although all of these analogs of idoxuridine have been studied for various clinical applications, none are presently marketed in the United States.

Ribavirin

Mechanism of Action Ribavirin, a guanosine analog, has broad-spectrum antiviral activity against both DNA and RNA viruses (Fig. 38.11) (56,57). It is phosphorylated by adenosine kinase to the triphosphate, resulting in inhibition of viral-specific RNA polymerase, disrupting messenger RNA and nucleic acid synthesis.

Clinical Application Ribavirin is highly active against influenza A and B and the parainfluenza group of viruses, genital herpes, herpes zoster, measles, and acute hepatitis types A, B, and C. Aerosolized ribavirin has been approved by the FDA for the treatment of lower respiratory tract infections (bronchiolitis and pneumonia) and serious RSV infections, but it can cause cardiopulmonary and immunologic disorders in children. Ribavirin inhibits in vitro replication of HIV-1; clinically, ribavirin was shown to delay the onset of full-blown AIDS in patients with early symptoms of HIV infection. Some viruses are less susceptible, for example, poliovirus, herpes viruses excluding varicella, vaccinia, mumps, reovirus, and rotavirus. A randomized double-blind study of aerosolized ribavirin treatment of infants with RSV infections indicated significant improvement in the severity of infection with a decrease in viral shedding (58).

Pharmacokinetics Oral or IV forms of ribavirin are useful in the prevention and treatment of Lassa fever. The oral bioavailability is approximately 45%, and serum half-life is 9 hours. Peak plasma level after 1 hour is 1 to 3 mg/mL. IV administration of the drug has higher peak plasma levels. Aerosol preparation delivery of drug (0.8 mg/kg/hour) produced drug levels in respiratory secretions of 50 to 200 mg/mL (Table 38.3). The clinical benefits of this agent have yet to be confirmed. Its few side effects are generally limited to GI disturbances, such as nausea, vomiting, and diarrhea. The drug is contraindicated in asthma patients because of deterioration of pulmonary function. Viral strains susceptible to ribavirin have not been found to develop drug resistance, as is the case with other antiviral agents, such as acyclovir, idoxuridine, and bromovinyldeoxyuridine.

Trifluorothymidine

Mechanism of Action Trifluorothymidine is a fluorinated pyridine nucleoside structurally related to idoxuridine (Fig. 38.11) (59). It has been approved by the FDA and is a potent, specific inhibitor of replication of HSV-1 in vitro. Its mechanism of action is similar to that of idoxuridine. Like other antiherpes drugs, it is first phosphorylated by thymidine kinase to mono-, di-, and triphosphate forms, which are then incorporated into viral DNA in place of thymidine to stop the formation of late virus mRNA and subsequent synthesis of the virion proteins.

Clinical Application Because of its greater solubility in water, it is active against HSV-1 and HSV-2. It is also useful in treating infections caused by human CMV and VZV infections. The advantage of use of this agent over idoxuridine is its high topical efficacy in the cure of primary keratoconjunctivitis and recurrent epithelial keratitis. It is also useful for difficult cases of herpetic iritis and established stromal keratitis.

Pharmacokinetics Trifluorothymidine is available as a 1% ophthalmic solution, which is effective in dendritic ulcers (Table 38.3). Generally, a 1% eye solution of trifluorothymidine is well tolerated. Cross-hypersensitivity and cross-toxicity between trifluorothymidine, idoxuridine, and vidarabine are rare. The most frequent side effects are temporary burning, stinging, localized edema, and bone marrow toxicity. It is less toxic but more expensive than idoxuridine. Trifluorothymidine, given intravenously, shows a plasma half-life of 18 minutes and is excreted in urine unchanged or as the inactive metabolite 5-carboxyuracil.

Vidarabine

Mechanism of Action Vidarabine is an adenosine nucleoside obtained from cultures of *Streptomyces antibioticus* (Fig. 38.11) (60). Cellular enzymes convert vidarabine to mono-, di-, and triphosphate derivatives that interfere with viral nucleic acid replication, specifically inhibiting the early steps in DNA synthesis. This agent was used originally as an antineoplastic drug. Its antiviral effect is, in some cases, superior to that of idoxuridine or cytarabine.

Clinical Application Vidarabine is used mainly in human HSV-1 and HSV-2 encephalitis, decreasing the mortality rate from 70% to 30%. Whitley et al. (61) reported that early vidarabine therapy is helpful in controlling complications of localized or disseminated herpes zoster in immunocompromised patients. Vidarabine is also useful in neonatal herpes labialis or genitalis, vaccinia virus, adenovirus, RNA viruses, papovavirus, CMV, and smallpox virus infections. Given the efficacy of vidarabine in certain viral infections, the FDA approved a 3% ointment for the treatment of herpes simplex keratoconjunctivitis and recurrent epithelial keratitis and a 2% IV injection for the treatment of herpes simplex encephalitis and herpes zoster infections (Table 38.3). A topical ophthalmic preparation of vidarabine is useful in herpes simplex keratitis but shows little promise in herpes simplex labialis or genitalis. The monophosphate esters of vidarabine are more water-soluble and can be used in smaller volumes and even intramuscularly. These esters are under clinical investigation for the treatment of HBV, systemic and cutaneous herpes simplex, and herpes zoster virus infections in immunocompromised patients.

Pharmacokinetics Vidarabine is deaminated rapidly by adenosine deaminase, which is present in serum and red blood cells. The enzyme converts vidarabine to its principal metabolite, arabinosyl hypoxanthine (ara-HX), which has weak antiviral activity (Fig. 38.12) (62). The half-life of vidarabine is approximately 1 hour, whereas ara-HX has a half-life of 3.5 hours. The drug is detected mostly in the kidney, liver, and spleen because 50% of it is recovered in the urine as ara-HX. Levels of vidarabine in CSF are 50% of those in the plasma. The most common side effects of vidarabine are GI disturbances such as anorexia, nausea, vomiting, and diarrhea. CNS side effects include tremors, dizziness, pain syndromes, and seizures. Bone marrow suppression is reported at higher doses. Because vidarabine is reported to be mutagenic, carcinogenic, and teratogenic in animal studies, its use in pregnant women is to be avoided. Allopurinol and theophylline may interfere with the metabolism of vidarabine at higher doses because of the xanthine oxidase metabolism of vidarabine. Therefore, this agent should be avoided or given with caution to patients receiving these medications concurrently. Also, adjustment of the dose is necessary in patients with renal insufficiency.

CYTARABINE

Mechanism of Action Cytarabine (1-β′-arabinofuranosylcytosine) is a pyrimidine nucleoside related to idoxuridine (Fig. 38.11) (63). It is used primarily as an anticancer rather than an antiviral agent (see Chapter 37). Cytarabine acts by blocking the utilization of deoxycytidine, thereby inhibiting the replication of viral DNA. The drug is first converted to mono-, di-, and triphosphates, which interfere with DNA synthesis by inhibiting both DNA polymerase and the reductase that promotes the conversion of cytidine diphosphate into its deoxy derivatives.

Clinical Application Cytarabine is used to treat Burkitt lymphoma and both myeloid and lymphatic leukemias. Its antiviral use is in the treatment of herpes zoster (shingles) infection. It is also used to treat herpetic keratitis and viral infections resistant to idoxuridine. The drug is usually used topically, but it has been given by IV injection to individuals with serious herpes infection (64). Cytarabine is deaminated rapidly in the body to an inactive compound, arabinosyluracil, which is excreted in the urine. The half-life of the drug in plasma is 3 to 5 hours. The toxic effects of cytarabine are chiefly on bone marrow, the GI tract, and the kidney. The drug is not given in the early months of pregnancy because of its teratogenic and carcinogenic effects in animals.

Nonnucleoside Analogs (Fig. 38.13)

FOMIVIRSEN SODIUM Fomivirsen was the first antisense oligonucleotide agent approved as an alternative medicine for patients with CMV retinitis for whom other agents did not work. Fomivirsen is a 21-mer phosphorothioate oligodeoxynucleotide (Fig. 38.13). Fomivirsen was used to treat CMV, which causes opportunistic retinitis in patients with AIDS. Such patients respond to fomivirsen but not to other treatment for CMV retinitis, which leads to blindness (65). It works by inhibiting synthesis of proteins responsible for the regulation of viral gene expression that is involved in infection of CMV retinitis. Fomivirsen has recently been withdrawn from the market by the drug manufacturer Novartis and is thus no longer available.

FOSCARNET SODIUM Foscarnet is a trisodium phosphoformate hexahydrate that inhibits DNA polymerase of herpes viruses including CMV and retroviral RT (Fig. 38.13) (66). It is not phosphorylated into an active form by viral host cell enzymes. Therefore, it has the advantage of not requiring an activation step before attacking the target viral enzyme. Foscarnet sodium was approved by the FDA

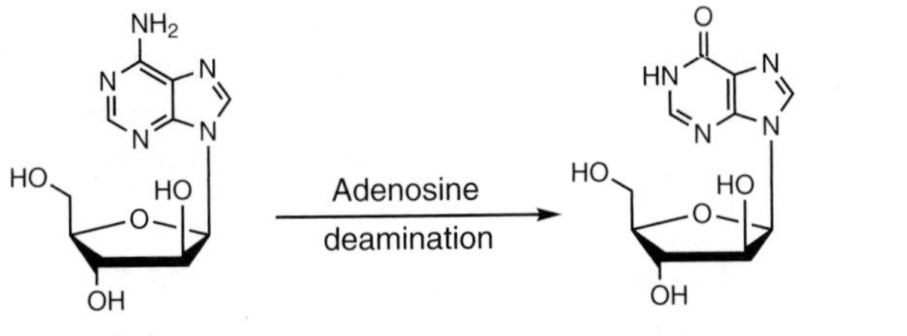

Vidarabine (ara-A)

Arabinofuranosylhypoxanthine (ara-HX)

FIGURE 38.12 Metabolism of vidarabine by adenosine deaminase.

5'-GCG TTT GCT CTT CTT CTT GCG-3'

Fomivirsen

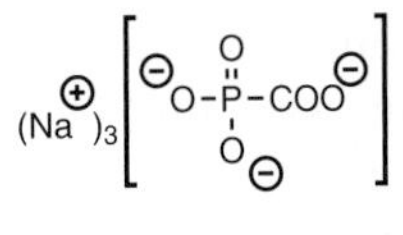

Foscarnet sodium

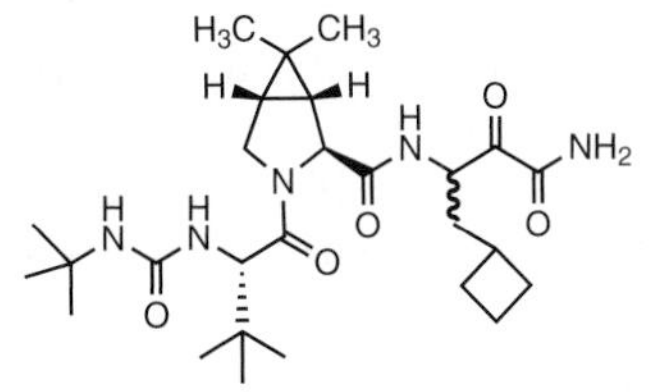

Boceprevir

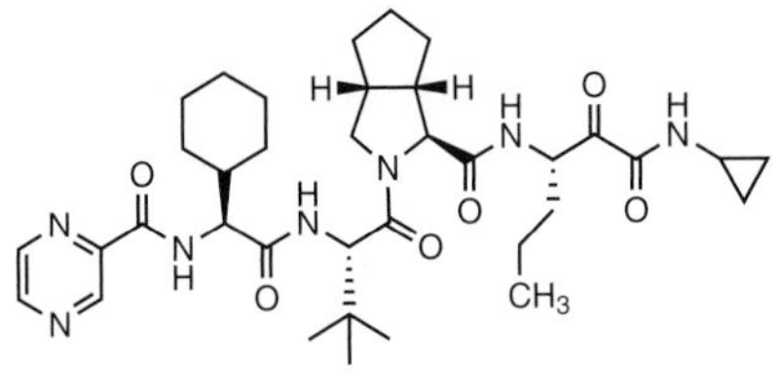

Telaprevir

FIGURE 38.13 Nonnucleoside inhibitors of viral replication.

for the treatment of CMV retinitis in AIDS patients. In combination with ganciclovir, the results have been promising, even in progressive disease with ganciclovir-resistant strains. Foscarnet sodium is also effective in the treatment of mucocutaneous diseases caused by acyclovir-resistant strains of HSV and VZV in AIDS patients. The drug is administered intravenously (60 mg/kg) three times a day for initial therapy and at a dose of 90 to 120 mg/kg daily for maintenance therapy (Table 38.3). The plasma-half life is 3 to 6 hours. Foscarnet sodium penetrates into the CSF and the eye. The drug is neurotoxic, and common adverse effects include phlebitis, anemia, nausea, vomiting, and seizures. Foscarnet sodium carries risk of severe hypocalcemia, especially with concurrent use of IV pentamidine. Foscarnet sodium used with zidovudine has an additive effect against CMV and acts synergistically against HIV.

Boceprevir and Telaprevir Boceprevir (SCH 503034, Victrelis) (67) and telaprevir (VX-950, Incivek) (68) represent significant advances in the treatment of HCV infection (Fig. 38.13) (Table 38.3). HCV is an enveloped, single-stranded sense RNA virus that encodes a polyprotein precursor of about 3,000 amino acids. The essential HCV enzyme NS3-4A protease is responsible for cleaving this HCV polyprotein at four sites to generate four peptides called NS4A, NS4B, NS5A, and NS5B. Boceprevir and telaprevir act as potent inhibitors of the HCV NS3-4A protease, and this inhibition prevents the processing of the HCV polyprotein and prevents the virus from replicating. Both compounds have recently been approved by the FDA and can be used in combination with pegylated interferon and ribavirin (69). For untreated HCV infection, telaprevir is administered for the first 12 weeks of therapy at 750 mg three times per day in combination with pegylated interferon α-2a 180 μg/week, and ribavirin 1.0 to 1.2 g/day according to body weight. After 12 weeks, telaprevir is discontinued, and pegylated interferon α-2a and ribavirin are continued until HCV RNA is undetectable in serum. Boceprevir must be administered using a different regimen. For untreated HCV infection, pegylated interferon α-2b and ribavirin are given alone for 4 weeks, and then boceprevir (800 mg three times a day) is given in combination with pegylated interferon α-2b (1.5 μg/kg/week) and ribavirin (0.8 to 1.4 g/day according to body weight) for 24 weeks. Total treatment duration is 28 weeks if patients test negative for HCV RNA but may need to be continued for an additional 20 weeks to clear the infection if HCV RNA is still detected after 28 weeks.

Agents Affecting Translation by the Ribosome

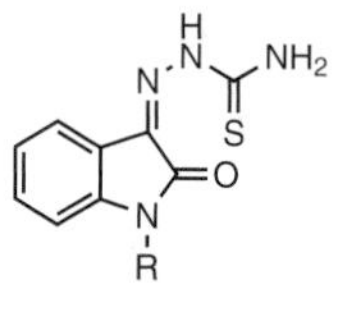

Methisazone (R = CH_3)

Methisazone (70)

Methisazone interferes with the translation of mRNA message at the ribosome, preventing the synthesis of protein synthesis. Ultimately, it produces a defect in protein incorporation into the virus. Although viral DNA increases and host cells are damaged, an infectious virus is not produced. Methisazone is active against poxviruses, including variola and vaccinia (71). Some RNA viruses, such as rhinoviruses, echoviruses, reoviruses, influenza, parainfluenza, and polioviruses are also inhibited. Therapeutically, methisazone is given in 1.5- to 3.0-g doses, twice daily by mouth. It has also been used as a prophylactic agent against smallpox. Historically, methisazone was one of the first antiviral compounds used in clinical practice. It is orally absorbed, with nausea and vomiting as the principal side effects. The drug is also used in vaccinia gangrenosa and disseminated vaccinia infections. This drug is not available in the United States, but it has been used in Europe for some time. Several analogs of methisazone (R = H, R = ethyl) possess activity against variola, neurovaccinia, smallpox in mice, Rous sarcoma virus, and vaccinia generalisata.

Antiretroviral (Anti-HIV) Agents Including Protease Inhibitors (72,73)

While there can be no permanent cure of AIDS without prevention or elimination of HIV infection, AIDS patients can prolong their life if the disease is diagnosed early and treatment is promptly initiated. Initial HIV treatment requires specific drugs that inhibit RT and HIV protease. In advanced HIV infection, AIDS is complicated by other organisms that proliferate in immunocompromised hosts, known as opportunistic infections. Such patients are treated symptomatically with a variety of drugs depending on the opportunistic infections (74–76). Anti-HIV agents have side effects, but patients can be managed by a careful monitoring of the drugs. Opportunistic diseases include infections by parasites, bacteria, fungi, and viruses. Neoplasms including Kaposi sarcoma and Burkitt lymphoma also commonly occur.

Anti-HIV agents are classified according to the mode of action. The drugs inhibiting RT interfere with replication of HIV and stop synthesis of infective viral particles. They are further classified into nucleoside and nonnucleoside RT inhibitors. The drugs inhibiting HIV protease inactivate RT activity and block release of viral particles from the infected cells. The chemistry, pharmacokinetics, side effects, toxicity, and drug interactions of RT inhibitors and protease inhibitors are discussed in the following sections.

Nucleoside Reverse Transcriptase Inhibitors (77,78)

The synthesis of viral DNA under the direction of RT requires availability of purines and pyrimidine nucleosides and nucleotides. Therefore, it is not surprising that a variety of chemical modifications of natural nucleosides have been investigated. Two such modifications have resulted in active drugs. Removal of the ribosyl 3′-hydroxyl group of the deoxynucleosides has given rise to dideoxy*adenosine* (didanosine is the prodrug for this derivative) (79,80), dideoxy*cytidine* (81–83), and didehydrodideoxy*thymidine* (84). Replacement of the 3′-deoxy with an azido group has given 3′-azido*thymidine* (85–88) and 3′-azido*uridine* (no longer used as a drug) (Fig. 38.14 and Table 38.4) (89). All of these drugs have similar mechanisms of action in that their incorporation into the viral DNA will ultimately lead to chain-terminating blockade due to the lack of a 3′-hydroxyl needed for the DNA propagation.

Zidovudine

Mechanism of Action Zidovudine (ZDV) is an analog of thymidine in which the azido group is substituted at the 3-carbon atom of the dideoxyribose moiety (Fig. 38.14). It is active against RNA tumor viruses (retroviruses) that are the causative agents of AIDS and T-cell leukemia. Retroviruses, by virtue of RT, direct the synthesis of a provirus (DNA copy of a viral RNA genome). Proviral DNA integrates into the normal cell DNA, leading to the HIV infection. ZDV is converted to 5′-mono-, di-, and triphosphates by the cellular thymidine kinase. These phosphates are then incorporated into proviral DNA, because RT uses ZDV-triphosphate as a substrate. This process prevents normal 5′,3′-phosphodiester bonding, resulting in termination of DNA chain elongation due to the presence of an azido group in ZDV. The multiplication of HIV is halted by selective inhibition of RT and thus viral DNA polymerase by ZDV-triphosphate at the required dose concentration. ZDV is a potent inhibitor of HIV-1 but also inhibits HIV-2 and EBV.

Clinical Application ZDV is used in AIDS and AIDS-related complex (ARC) to control opportunistic infections by raising absolute $CD4^+$ lymphocyte counts. ZDV was first synthesized by Horwitz (1964) (90), biologic activity was reported by Ostertag et al. (1974) (91), and in 1986, Yarchoan et al. (92) demonstrated application of ZDV in clinical trials of AIDS and related diseases. ZDV is recommended in the control of the disease in asymptomatic patients in whom absolute $CD4^+$ lymphocyte counts are less than $200/mm^3$. It prolongs the life of patients affected with *Pneumocystis jirovecii* pneumonia and improves the condition of patients with advanced ARC by reducing the severity and frequency of opportunistic infections. Substantial benefits are obtained when the drug is given after the $CD4^+$ cell counts fall below $500/mm^3$. Therefore, ZDV is used in early and advanced symptomatic treatment of AIDS or ARC patients. ZDV with other RT inhibitors or in combination with protease inhibitors is more beneficial when resistance to ZDV occurs.

HIV attacks susceptible cells and interacts mainly with $CD4^+$ cell surface proteins of helper T cells. As discussed earlier, the viral glycoprotein gp120 forms a complex with CD4 receptor on host cells and enters the cells by endocytosis. The sequence of events is shown in Figure 38.2. Ultimately, the immune system of the host is altered and AIDS symptoms appear. AIDS patients have symptoms such as high fever, weight loss, lymphadenopathy, chronic diarrhea, myalgias, fatigue, and night sweats. ZDV is given in such conditions. However, the drug is toxic to the bone marrow and causes macrocytic anemia, neutropenia, and granulocytopenia. Other adverse reactions include headache, insomnia, nausea, vomiting, seizures, myalgias, and confusion.

Pharmacokinetics ZDV is available in 100-mg capsules for oral administration. For asymptomatic adults, the initial recommended dosage is 1,200 mg daily (200 mg every 4 hours) reducing to 600 mg daily (100 mg every 4 hours) for patients with advanced disease (Table 38.4).

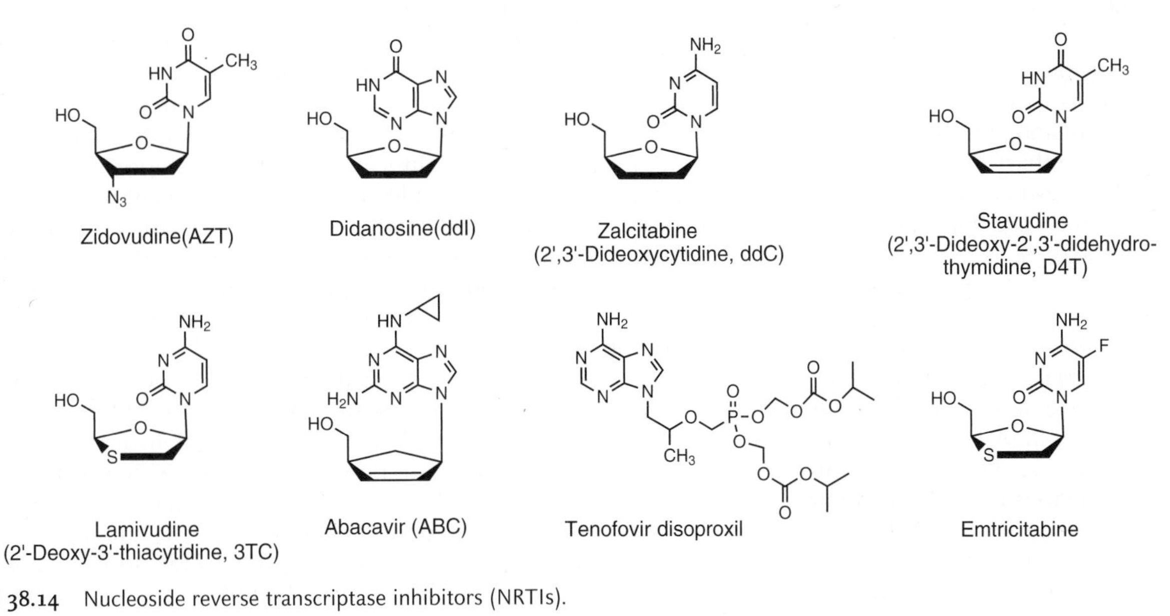

FIGURE 38.14 Nucleoside reverse transcriptase inhibitors (NRTIs).

TABLE 38.4 HIV Reverse Transcriptase Inhibitors

Generic Name	Common Name	Trade Name	Dosage Form (mg/unit)
Nucleoside reverse transcriptase inhibitors			
Zidovudine	AZT ZDV	Retrovir	Tab (300), Cap (100), Syrup (50/5 mL), Inj (10/mL)
Didanosine	ddI	Videx	Tab (25, 50, 100, 150, 200)
Dideoxyadenosine	ddA		Powder for oral Sol (100, 167, 250)
Zalcitabine	ddC	Hivid	Tab (0.375)
Stavudine	D4T	Zerit	Cap (15, 20, 30, 40) Powder for oral Sol (1/mL)
Lamivudine	3TC	Epivir Epivir HBV	Tab (150), Sol (10/mL) Tab (100), Sol (5/mL)
Abacavir	ABC	Ziagen	Tab (300), Sol (20/mL)
Tenofovir disoproxil		Viread	Tab (300)
Emtricitabine		Emtriva	Cap (200)
Nonnucleoside reverse transcriptase inhibitors			
Nevirapine		Viramune	Tab (200)
Delavirdine		Rescriptor	Tab (100)
Efavirenz		Sustiva	Cap (50, 100, 200)

Cap, capsule; Inj, injection; Sol, solution; Tab, tablet.

The maintenance dose is 600 mg daily in symptomatic patients. ZDV is sensitive to heat and light because of its azide group and should be stored in colored bottles at 15° to 25°C. ZDV is well absorbed through the GI tract. It concentrates in the body tissues and fluids, including CSF. The bioavailability of the drug was found to be approximately 65%. Its half-life is approximately 1 hour. IV doses of 2.5 mg/kg or oral doses of 5 mg/kg yielded peak plasma concentrations of 5 mmol/L. Plasma protein binding was approximately 30%. Most of the drug is converted to its inactive glucuronide metabolite and is excreted unchanged through urine. ZDV also crosses the blood–brain barrier. Pentamidine, dapsone, amphotericin B, flucytosine, and doxorubicin may increase the toxic effects of ZDV. Probenecid prolongs the plasma half-life of the drug.

Didanosine

Mechanism of Action Didanosine (ddI) is a purine dideoxynucleoside analog of inosine. Chemically, it is 2′,3′-dideoxyinosine and differs from inosine by having hydrogen atoms in place of 2′- and 3′-hydroxyl groups on the ribose ring (Fig. 38.14). ddI is a prodrug that is bioactivated by metabolism to dideoxyadenosine triphosphate. Dideoxyadenosine triphosphate is a competitive inhibitor of viral RT and is incorporated into the developing viral DNA in place of deoxyladenosine triphosphate. As such this agent causes chain termination due to the absence of a 3′-hydroxyl group. ddI inhibits HIV RT and exerts a virustatic effect on the retroviruses. Combined with ZDV, antiretroviral activity of ddI is increased.

Pharmacokinetics ddI has a plasma half-life of 1.5 hours and is given in 200-mg dose twice daily. Oral bioavailability of the drug is approximately 25% at doses of 7 mg/kg or less. It significantly decreases p24 antigen levels and increases $CD4^+$ cell counts. In some cases, viral resistance to ddI has been known to occur after treatment for 1 year. It is given in advanced HIV infection, ZDV intolerance, or significant clinical/immunologic deterioration. The major side effects of ddI are painful peripheral neuropathy and pancreatitis. Some of the minor side effects include abdominal pain, nausea, and vomiting. The use of products, such as pentamidine, sulfonamides, and cimetidine should be avoided with ddI.

ZALCITABINE Zalcitabine (ddC) is a useful alternate to ZDV and is a synthetic pyrimidine nucleoside analog. It differs from 2′-deoxycytidine in that the 3′-hydroxyl group of the 2′-deoxyribose moiety is replaced with a hydrogen atom (Fig. 38.14). It is given in combination with ZDV when $CD4^+$ cell counts fall below 300 cells/mm^3. Monotherapy with ddC was more active than ZDV. Its oral bioavailability is 87%, and plasma half-life is approximately 1 hour.

It has side effects such as stomatitis, rash, fever, malaise, arthritis, and arthralgia. In low doses (0.005 mg/kg every 4 hours), ddC produced sustained decrease in p24 antigen level and increase in CD4+ cell counts. The CSF fluid/plasma ratio of ddC is 0.2.

After oral administration, bioavailability of ddC was less than 80%, which was further reduced with food. The mean maximum plasma concentration of the drug was also reduced from 25.2 to 15.5 ng/mL when the drug was taken with food. Dideoxyuridine is the major metabolite in urine and feces. The drug demonstrated penetration through blood–brain barrier. The major toxicity of ddC is peripheral neuropathy, in which case it should be discontinued. Pancreatitis occurs in some cases when given alone or in combination with ZDV.

STAVUDINE Stavudine (D4T) is a pyrimidine nucleoside analog that has significant activity against HIV-1 after intracellular conversion of the drug to a D4T-triphosphate. It differs in structure from thymidine by the replacement of the 3′-hydroxyl group with a hydrogen atom and a double bond in the 2′ and 3′ positions on the deoxyribose ring (Fig. 38.14). It decreased p24 antigen and raised CD4+ cell counts. D4T is beneficial for patients in whom CD4+ cell counts do not decrease below 300 cells/mm^3 with ZDV and ddI. It was shown to be more effective than ZDV or ddC in delaying the progression of HIV infection. It is recommended for patients with advanced HIV infection.

Pharmacokinetics D4T is rapidly absorbed, and absolute bioavailability in adults is 85% at an oral dose of 4 mg/kg. A peak plasma concentration in a dose-dependent manner occurs within an hour. It can be taken with food. The apparent volume of distribution after oral dose is 66 L. The plasma half-life of D4T is approximately 1.5 hours, and the intracellular half-life of D4T-triphosphate is 3.5 hours. It is less toxic to bone marrow but causes peripheral neuropathic toxicity. The side effects include pain, tingling, and numbness in the hands and feet.

LAMIVUDINE Lamivudine (3TC) is an analog of ddC in which 3′-methylene group is replaced with a sulfur (S) atom in the ribose ring (Fig. 38.14) (93). It exerts virustatic effect against retroviruses by competitively inhibiting HIV RT after intracellular conversion of the drug to its active 5′-3TC-triphosphate form. It is usually given with other antiretroviral agents, such as ZDV or D4T. 3TC in a 600 mg/day dose reduced HIV cells by 75%, and in combination with ZDV, the reduction in viral load was 94%. 3TC is rapidly absorbed through the GI tract. Its bioavailability is approximately 86% after oral administration of 2 mg/kg twice daily; peak serum 3TC concentration was approximately 2 mg/mL. 3TC binding to human plasma was approximately 36%. In vivo, it is converted to *trans* sulfoxide metabolite, and a majority of the drug is eliminated unchanged in urine. The FDA approved 3TC in combination with ZDV for the treatment of disease progression caused by HIV infection. The combinations of 3TC with ddI, ddC, or D4T also are used for advanced HIV infection. Such combinations have the ability to delay resistance to ZDV and restore ZDV sensitivity in AIDS patients. Recently, oral therapy in lower doses of 3TC (Table 38.4) has been approved by the FDA for treatment of chronic HBV. Peripheral neuropathy and GI disturbances are the major side effects of 3TC. The minor side effects are nausea, vomiting, and diarrhea.

ABACAVIR SULFATE Abacavir was approved in 1998 as a nucleoside reverse transcriptase inhibitor to be used in combination with other drugs for the treatment of HIV and AIDS. The drug is extensively metabolized via stepwise phosphorylation to 5′-mono-, di-, and triphosphate. Abacavir is well absorb (>75%) and penetrates the CNS and can be taken without regard to meals. The drug does not show any clinically significant drug–drug interactions but has been reported to produce life-threatening hypersensitivity reactions. The major use of abacavir appears to be in combination with other nucleoside reverse transcriptase inhibitors. A fixed combination product has recently been approved by the FDA under the trade name of Trizivir and consists of 300 mg of abacavir, 150 mg of 3TC, and 300 mg of ZDV. The combination has been shown to be superior to other combinations in reducing viral load as well as showing improvement in CD4+ cell count. The most common adverse effects reported with abacavir include headache, nausea, vomiting, malaise, and diarrhea.

TENOFOVIR DISOPROXIL (94)

Mechanism of Action Tenofovir is a prodrug with a bioavailability of 25%, which is improved in the presence of food (35%). The drug is approved for the treatment of HIV infections in adult patients. Tenofovir diphosphate is an HIV reverse transcriptase inhibitor. The drug is hydrolyzed via plasma esterase to tenofovir, which is then phosphorylated to the active tenofovir diphosphate, as shown in Figure 38.15. The diphosphate competes with

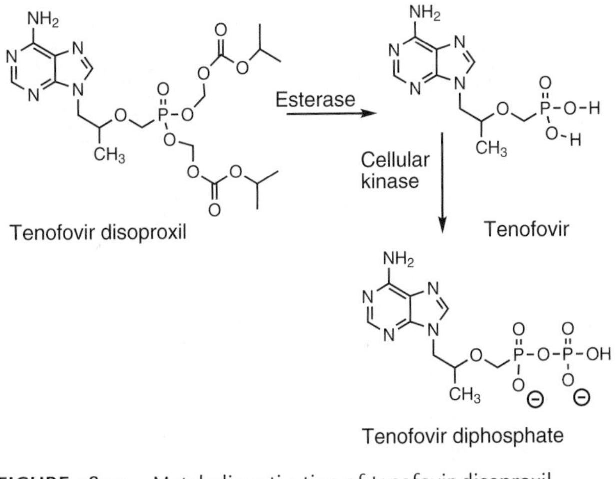

FIGURE 38.15 Metabolic activation of tenofovir disoproxil.

deoxyadenosine triphosphate for incorporation into viral DNA, and when incorporated, tenofovir diphosphate results in premature termination of DNA growth and inhibition of DNA polymerase. Tenofovir disoproxil is indicated for treatment-experienced patients with HIV-1. The drug appears to also be effective in treatment-naive patients, but initial approval is for treatment-experienced patients. The drug is administered as one tablet once daily (300 mg). It is recommended that the drug be combined with other reverse transcriptase inhibitors or HIV protease inhibitors, which results in additive or synergistic activity. At present, two fixed combinations exist that contain tenofovir: tenofovir disoproxil fumarate plus emtricitabine (Truvada) and a fixed triple combination of tenofovir, emtricitabine, and efavirenz (Atripla). Other fixed-dose products may be approved in the future for treatment of HIV.

Emtricitabine (95) Emtricitabine is an orally active nucleoside RT inhibitor (Fig. 38.14). It is metabolized in vivo to the 5′-triphosphate, which in turn competes with the normal substrate (deoxycytidine-5′-triphosphate) for incorporation into DNA. In addition, incorporation of emtricitabine into viral DNA inhibits further chain elongation, resulting in chain termination. The drug is administered orally once daily. The (−)-enantiomer is the most active form of the drug, although the (+)-isomer is also active. Emtricitabine is not bound to plasma protein, and approximately 86% is excreted unchanged in the urine. The only metabolites identified consist of the 3′-sulfoxide and the 2′-*O*-glucuronide. Emtricitabine is reported to be more active than 3TC with a low level of resistance developing when used in combination therapy with efavirenz and ddI. As indicated earlier, the drug is also available in fix-dosed combinations with tenofovir.

Nonnucleoside Reverse Transcriptase Inhibitors

The FDA has recently approved several nonnucleosides that inhibit RT activity (Fig. 38.16 and Table 38.4). They are used with nucleoside drugs to obtain synergistic activity in decreasing the viral load and increasing $CD4^+$ cell count. These drugs are primarily designed and synthesized by protein structure-based drug design methodologies. Their use as monotherapy may be limited because of rapid onset of resistance and hypersensitivity reactions. However, interaction of nonnucleoside drugs with other protease inhibitors, such as saquinavir, indinavir, and ritonavir, is being investigated. In addition, interaction of these drugs with clarithromycin, ketoconazole, rifabutin, and rifampin is under study.

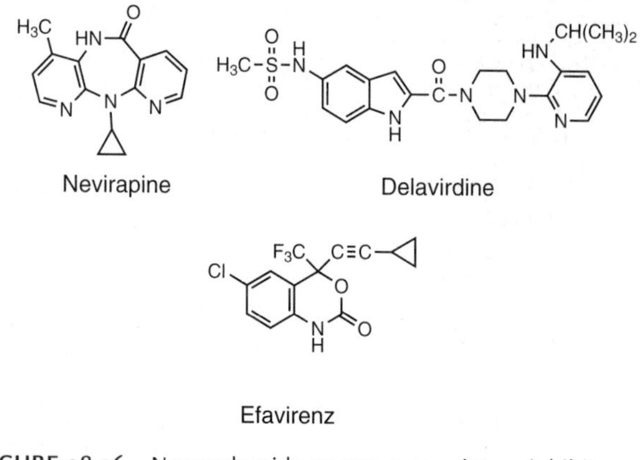

FIGURE 38.16 Nonnucleoside reverse transcriptase inhibitors (NNRTI).

Nevirapine

Mechanism of Action Nevirapine and its analogs exhibit antiretroviral effects against AZT-resistant HIV strains (96). Nevirapine in combination with ZDV and ddI produced approximately 18% higher $CD4^+$ cell counts and a decrease in viral load compared with ZDV and ddI. Nevirapine is recommended with nucleosides for HIV-1–infected patients who have experienced clinical or immunologic deterioration. The significant side effects of nevirapine are liver dysfunction and skin rashes. Nevirapine is a dipyridodiazepinone derivative, which binds directly to RT. Thus, it blocks RNA- and DNA-dependent polymerase activities by causing a disruption of the RT catalytic site. HIV-2 RT and human DNA polymerases are not inhibited by nevirapine. The 50% inhibitory concentration ranged from 10 to 100 nmol/L against HIV-1.

Pharmacokinetics Nevirapine is rapidly absorbed after oral administration, and its bioavailability is approximately 95%. Peak plasma nevirapine concentrations of 2 ± 0.4 mg/mL (7.5 mmol/L) are obtained in 4 hours after a single 200-mg dose (Table 38.4). Following multiple doses, nevirapine concentrations appear to increase linearly in the dose range of 200 to 400 mg/day. Nevirapine is about 60% bound to plasma proteins in the plasma concentration range of 1 to 10 mg/mL. It readily crossed the placenta and was found in breast milk. Nevirapine is metabolized as glucuronide conjugates of hydroxylated metabolites, which are excreted in urine. In vivo, ketoconazole did not produce any significant inhibitory effect on nevirapine metabolism. The plasma concentrations of nevirapine were elevated or reduced in patients receiving cimetidine or rifabutin, respectively.

Delavirdine Delavirdine, a bisheteroarylpiperazine derivative, is a potent nonnucleoside RT inhibitor with activity specific for HIV-1 (97). The FDA has approved this drug in combination with other anti-HIV agents (Table 38.4). In phase I/II trials, it demonstrated sustained improvements in $CD4^+$ cell counts, p24 antigen levels, and RNA viral load. Promising results were obtained when the drug was used in two- or three-drug combination with nucleoside drugs. Combination of delavirdine with ddI, ddC, or ZDV demonstrated additive or synergistic effect. However, delavirdine with ZDV was more beneficial in early HIV infection. Combinations of nevirapine and delavirdine have an antagonistic effect on HIV-1 RT inhibition. Delavirdine directly inhibits RT and DNA-directed DNA polymerase activities of HIV-1 after the formation of the enzyme–substrate complexes, thereby causing chain termination effects.

Pharmacokinetics Delavirdine is rapidly absorbed by oral administration, and peak plasma concentration is obtained in 1 hour. The single-dose bioavailability of delavirdine tablets relative to oral solution was approximate 85%. The 50% inhibitory concentration for delavirdine against RT activity was 6.0 nmol/L. Delavirdine is extensively bound to plasma protein (~98%). Delavirdine is metabolized to its inactive *N*-desisopropyl metabolite in liver, and the pharmacokinetics is nonlinear. This reaction is catalyzed by CYP3A4, and delavirdine appears to be an inhibitor of this enzyme, increasing the risk for drug–drug interactions with other drugs that are substrates for this cytochrome isoform. Skin rashes are the major side effect of delavirdine therapy. Cross-resistance between delavirdine and protease inhibitors, such as indinavir, nelfinavir, ritonavir, and saquinavir, is unlikely because they act at different target enzymes.

EFAVIRENZ Efavirenz is a new nonnucleoside RT inhibitor that was approved by the FDA (Table 38.4) as a potent inhibitor of wild-type and resistant mutant HIV-1, which is inhibited up to 95% with efavirenz concentrations of 1.5 mmol/L (98). In combination with indinavir, a mean reduction in HIV-RNA of 1.68 log and an increase in $CD4^+$ cell counts of 96 cells/mm^3 were reported. Coadministration of efavirenz with indinavir reduced indinavir concentration (AUC) by approximately 35%.

Pharmacokinetics Efavirenz is administered once a day and can be used as a substitute for indinavir in combination therapy with standard drugs, such as ZDV and 3TC (also as a fixed combination of tenofovir, emtricitabine, and efavirenz [Atripla]). Because it is given once a day, this cuts down the number of pills that an AIDS patient has to swallow. In the current cocktail therapy of AIDS patients, efavirenz is a good option for reducing the many side effects of cocktail therapy. It is administered to both adults and children and may be less expensive than indinavir. The side effects of efavirenz include dizziness, insomnia, impaired concentration, abnormal dreams, and drowsiness. The most common adverse effect is a skin rash. Other side effects are diarrhea, headache, and dizziness. Efavirenz is recommended to be taken at bedtime with or without food. Avoiding driving or operating machinery and intake of high-fat meals are recommended. It should always be taken in combination with at least one other anti-HIV agent. Efavirenz is contraindicated with midazolam, triazolam, or ergot derivatives.

TABLE 38.5 HIV Protease Inhibitors

Generic Name	Trade Name	Dosage Form (mg/unit)
Saquinavir	Invirase	Cap (200)
	Fortovase	Cap (200)
Ritonavir	Norvir	Cap (200)
Indinavir	Crixivan	Cap (200, 400)
Nelfinavir	Viracept	Tab (250), Powder (50/g)
Amprenavir	Agenerase	Cap (50, 150) Sol (15/mL)
Lopinavir/ritonavir	Kaletra	Cap (133.3/33.3) Sol (80/20 per mL)
Atazanavir	Reyataz	Cap (150, 200)
Fosamprenavir	Lexiva	Tab (700)
Tipranavir	Aptivus	Cap (250)
Darunavir	Prezista	Tab (75, 150, 300, 400 or 600)

Cap, capsule; Sol, solution; Tab, tablet.

HIV Protease Inhibitors (Table 38.5) (99)

Mechanism of Action

The HIV genome contains various structural genes, such as the *gag* and *gag-pol* genes, that are translated into precursor polyproteins that form immature viral particles. These precursor protein molecules are processed (cleaved) by an essential viral pol-encoded aspartic proteinase, HIV protease, to form the desired structural proteins of the mature viral particle that are necessary for virus replication and survival. For example, the structural proteins p7, p9, p17, and p24, which play important roles in infectivity of HIV, are products of the *pol* gene. HIV protease also activates RT and plays an important role in the release of infectious viral particles. Thus, an area of considerable interest has been the development of drugs that act as inhibitors of HIV protease. Such inhibitors act on HIV protease and prevent posttranslational processing and budding of immature viral particles from the infected cells. This group of drugs represents a major breakthrough in treatment of HIV when used in combination with RT inhibitors, and their development is one of the most significant advances in medicinal chemistry.

Functional HIV protease exists as a dimer in which each monomer contains one of two conserved aspartate residues at the active site. There are several HIV protease cleavage sites on the protein precursors, but the enzyme prefers to perform the hydrolysis of the peptide bond on the amino terminal side of a proline (100). As shown in Figure 38.17, the amino acid R groups flanking the scissile bond are designated P1, P2, and so on, on the amino terminus, and P1′, P2′, and so on, on the carboxyl terminus of the cleavage site (Fig. 38.17A). The corresponding pockets on the enzyme that are responsible for binding

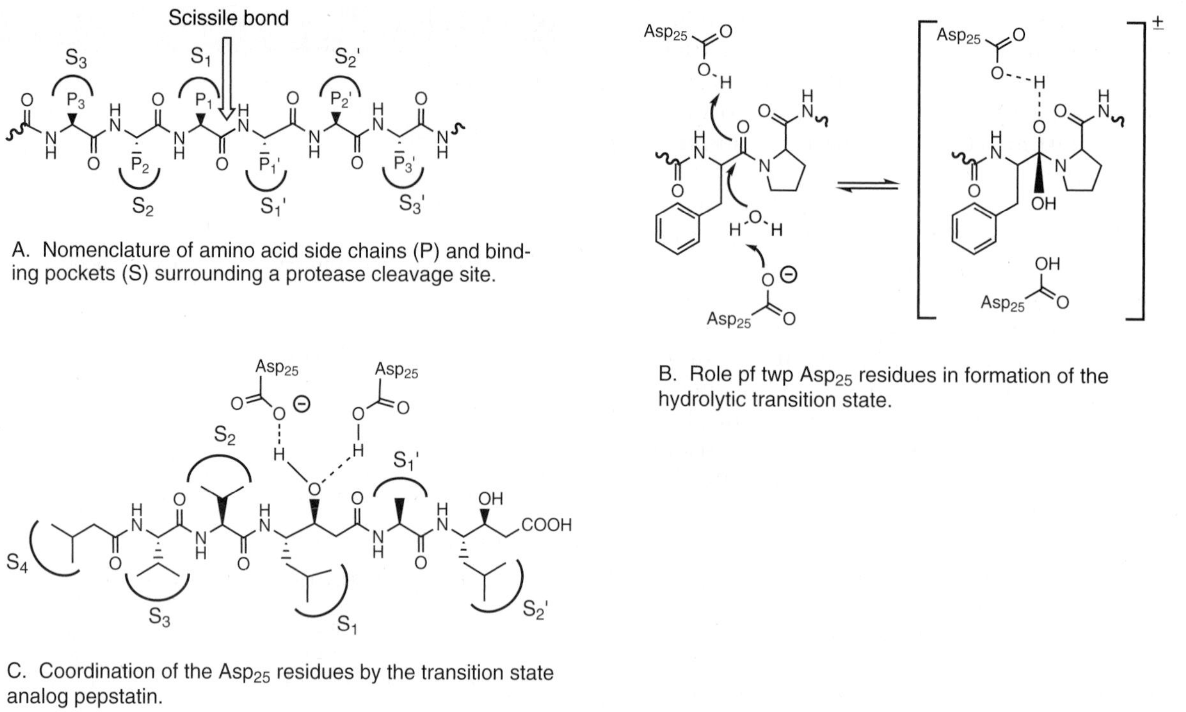

A. Nomenclature of amino acid side chains (P) and binding pockets (S) surrounding a protease cleavage site.

B. Role pf twp Asp_{25} residues in formation of the hydrolytic transition state.

C. Coordination of the Asp_{25} residues by the transition state analog pepstatin.

FIGURE 38.17 Principles of the design of transition-state analog inhibitors of HIV protease.

the P groups are termed S1, S2, S1′, S2′, and so on. In the active site, a pair of aspartates (the Asp25 on each of the two subunits of the protein) work together to complete the reaction (Fig. 38.17B). One coordinates the water that performs the hydrolysis, while the other coordinates the carboxyl group on the P1′ amino acid. Rationally designed drugs that inhibit HIV protease are designed as transition-state mimics that align at the active site of HIV-1 protease, as defined by three-dimensional crystallographic analysis of the protein structure. Figure 38.17C shows the aspartic protease inhibitor pepstatin bound in the HIV protease active site. Pepstatin is an inhibitor of all aspartic proteases, but can be used to illustrate the mechanism by which transition-state analogs inhibit HIV protease (101). Pepstatin contains an unnatural amino acid core known as statine (Fig. 38.18), and the hydroxyl-bearing sp3 carbon of this core mimics the tetrahedral transition state that occurs during hydrolysis of the peptide bond. Other transition-state cores have been used in the design of highly potent aspartic protease inhibitors, including the hydroxyethylene and hydroxyethylamine cores (Fig. 38.18). The crystal structures of several HIV protease inhibitors bound to wild-type and mutant HIV proteases have been solved by x-ray crystallography. The structure of the HIV protease inhibitor lopinavir bound to wild-type HIV protease is depicted in Figure 38.19. Note that the hydroxyl group of the transition-state core is hydrogen bonded to the two Asp25 carboxylate moieties at a distance of about 3 Å. A number of oligopeptide-like analogs have been synthesized that differentially inhibit viral and mammalian aspartic proteases, and the most useful of these are selective for the viral enzyme HIV-1 protease. Structurally, these agents are either peptidomimetic or nonpeptide compounds. Their effectiveness is related to their ability to inhibit the processing of the gag-pol precursor polyprotein to p24, p55, and p160. Consequently, the infectivity of HIV-1 is diminished. Although, some compounds exhibit in vitro and in vivo antiviral activities, optimization of their pharmacokinetic and pharmacodynamic properties has presented major problems. In view of the great demand for successful anti-AIDS drugs, the FDA has approved the protease inhibitors described in the following sections using the accelerated approval process. The structures of currently marketed HIV protease inhibitors are shown inn Figure 38.20.

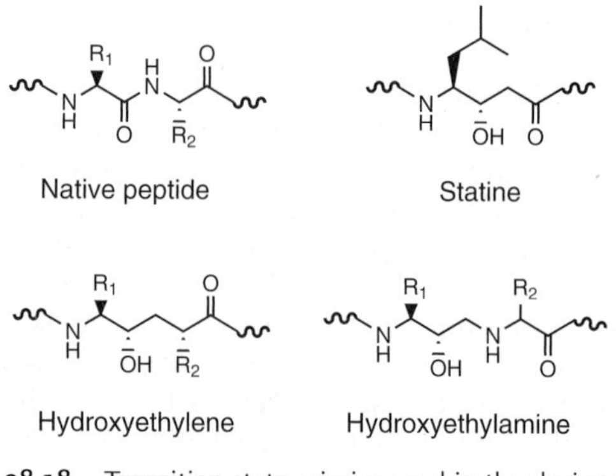

FIGURE 38.18 Transition-state mimics used in the design of HIV protease inhibitors.

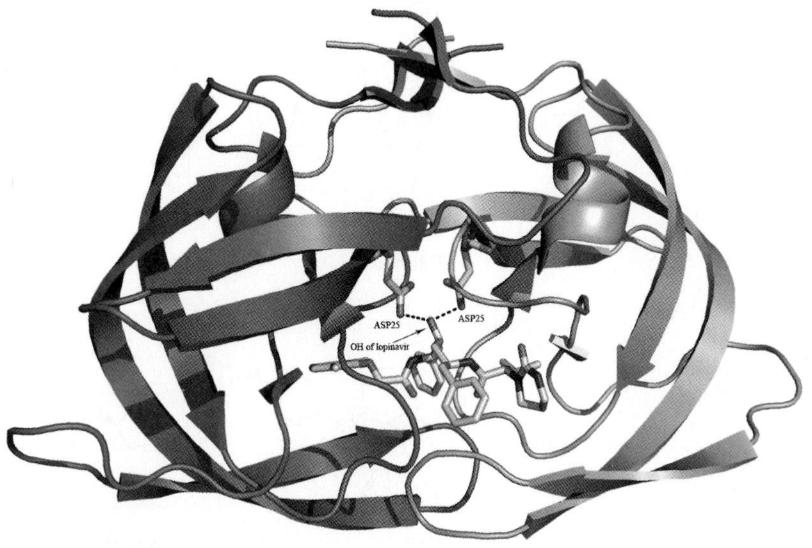

FIGURE 38.19 Model of the HIV protease inhibitor lopinavir bound to wild-type HIV protease.

Potential Drug Interactions

Protease inhibitors have a high potential for drug interactions, stemming from the fact that they are substrates for and inhibitors of the CYP3A4 enzyme system. As a result, concurrent use of protease inhibitors with other drugs metabolized by CYP3A4 may be contraindicated, and in some cases, the resulting drug interactions can be life-threatening. The most potent CYP450 inhibitor in this class is ritonavir (used to advantage in combination with lopinavir and other HIV protease inhibitors), followed by indinavir, nelfinavir, and amprenavir (moderate inhibitors) and saquinavir (the least potent inhibitor). Drug interactions have been reported with bepridil, dihydroergotamine, and a number of benzodiazepines. Marked increases in the activity of amiodarone, lidocaine (systemic), quinidine, the tricyclic antidepressants, and warfarin might be expected (102). Other interactions have been reported with rifampin, rifabutin, phenobarbital, phenytoin, dexamethasone, or carbamazepine. Because the protease inhibitors are themselves metabolized by CYP450, their action may be altered by other agents that induce or inhibit this system. In the case of rifabutin, which inhibits CYP3A4 in the gut, relative bioavailability of the protease inhibitors is increased, and the dose of the protease inhibitor may need to be decreased.

HIV Protease Inhibitors that are Used Clinically (Fig. 38.20)

SAQUINAVIR MESYLATE

Clinical Application Saquinavir was the first protease inhibitor approved by the FDA in December 1995 (103,104). It is a carboxamide derivative used in the treatment of advanced HIV infection in selected patients. Saquinavir is used concomitantly in either ZDV-untreated patients or ddC-treated patients previously treated with prolonged ZDV therapy. Although combined therapy did not slow progression of disease, $CD4^+$ cell counts were increased in patients infected with HIV in the United States and European countries. Triple therapy with saquinavir, ZDV, and ddC has been more effective than double therapy with saquinavir plus ZDV or ddC. Thus, combination therapy slowed disease progression and mortality.

The IC_{50} concentration of saquinavir in both acutely and chronically infected cells was 1 to 30 nmol/L. In combination with ZDV, ddC, or ddI, the activity of saquinavir was increased without increased cytotoxicity. The resistance of HIV isolates to saquinavir was observed due to substitution mutations in the HIV protease at amino acid positions 48 (glycine to valine) and 90 (leucine to methionine).

Pharmacokinetics The bioavailability of saquinavir in a single 600-mg dose following a high-fat meal was shown to be about 4%. Approximately 30% of a 600-mg dose of saquinavir reached the liver, where it showed first-pass metabolism. The metabolites, various mono- and dihydroxylated compounds of which the major metabolites are the monohydroxylated products shown in Figure 38.21, are not active. Approximately, 88% and 19% of a 600-mg oral dose was found in the feces and urine, respectively. The volume of distribution after IV administration of a 12-mg dose of saquinavir was 700 L. The drug is 98% bound to plasma proteins, and a very low concentration of saquinavir was found in CSF. The steady-state AUC was 2.5 times higher than that observed after a single dose of 600 mg in HIV-infected patients after a meal as compared to multiple dosing. Saquinavir has a plasma half-life of approximately 1.8 hours. Although saquinavir hard-gel capsule in combination with other antiretroviral drugs reduced the risk of disease progression or death, it has limited bioavailability. To overcome this limitation, the FDA has approved saquinavir soft-gel capsules. Saquinavir is well tolerated in combination with ZDV and/or ddC

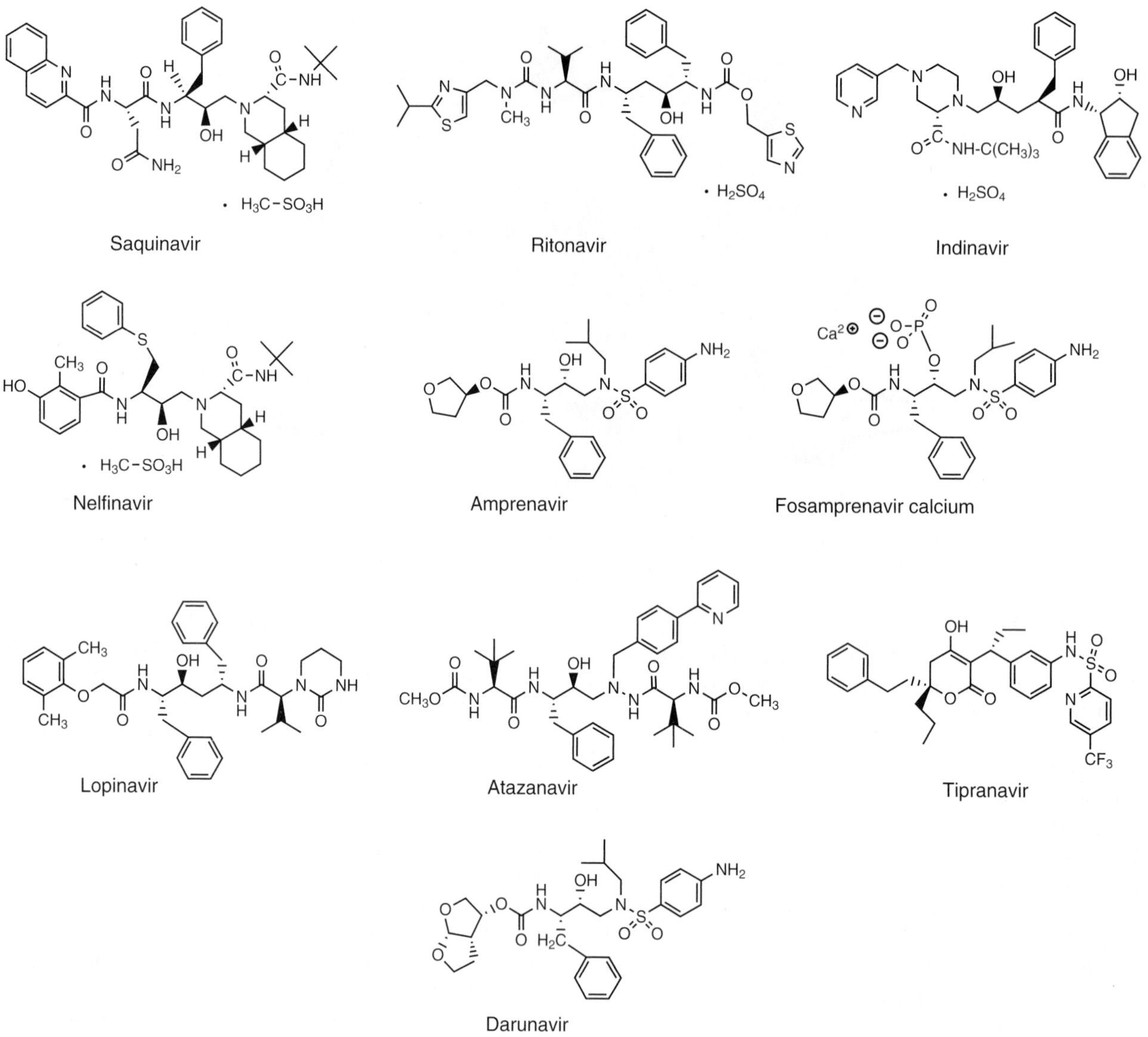

FIGURE 38.20 Structures of HIV protease inhibitors that are used clinically.

and has few side effects, but GI disturbances were common adverse effects. Saquinavir has a few mild side effects, such as headache, rhinitis, nausea, and diarrhea.

Ritonavir Ritonavir is another HIV protease inhibitor that was approved by the FDA in March 1996 (Fig. 38.20) (105). Ritonavir is a peptidomimetic inhibitor of both the HIV-1 and HIV-2 proteases. A 50% reduction in viral replication was obtained at a 3.8 to 153 nmol/L concentration of ritonavir.

Pharmacokinetics After a 600-mg dose of an oral solution, peak concentrations of ritonavir were obtained in approximately 2 or 4 hours under fasting or nonfasting conditions, respectively. Under nonfasting conditions, peak ritonavir concentrations decreased 23%, and the extent of absorption decreased 7% relative to fasting conditions. In two separate studies, the capsule and oral solution indicated AUC values of 129.5 ± 47.1 and 129.0 ± 39.3 mg/hour/mL, respectively, when a 600-mg dose was given under nonfasting conditions. Five ritonavir metabolites have been isolated from human urine and feces. The isopropylthiazole oxidation product was the major active metabolite (M2) (Fig. 38.22).

As with saquinavir, ritonavir is metabolized by CYP3A4 and is an inhibitor of the CYP450 system. Ritonavir is contraindicated with several compounds, such as clarithromycin, desipramine, ethinyl estradiol, rifabutin, sulfamethoxazole, and trimethoprim because of increased concentrations of these drugs in the plasma due to inhibited oxidative metabolism. Ritonavir alone or in combination with 3TC, ZDV, saquinavir, or ddC increased $CD4^+$ cell counts and decreased HIV RNA particle levels. Cross-resistance between ritonavir and RT inhibitors is unlikely because of the different mode of action and enzyme involved. Common adverse reactions, such as nausea,

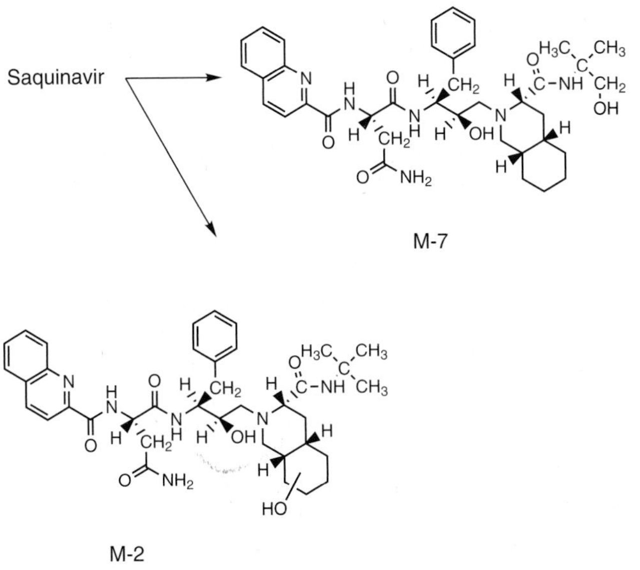

FIGURE 38.21 Major metabolic products from saquinavir.

diarrhea, vomiting, anorexia, abdominal pain, and neurologic disturbances, were reported with the use of ritonavir alone or in combination with other nucleoside analogs. Ritonavir is used for the treatment of advanced HIV infection including opportunistic infections. In combination with nucleoside drugs, ritonavir reduced the risk of mortality and clinical progression.

INDINAVIR SULFATE Indinavir, a pentanoic acid amide derivative, was approved by the FDA in March 1996 (Fig. 38.20) (106). The 95% inhibitory concentration against laboratory-adapted HIV variants, primary clinical isolates and clinical resistant virus to indinavir analogs, is 25 to 100 nmol/L in drug combination studies with ZDV and ddI. However, HIV has shown ritonavir resistance in some patients. This resistance is due to mutation of the virus that is correlated with the expression of amino acid substitutions in the viral protease. Cross-resistance to indinavir is observed with other protease inhibitors but not with the RT inhibitor. For this reason, indinavir is beneficial with ZDV and other nucleoside drugs.

Pharmacokinetics Indinavir is rapidly absorbed in fasting patients, and plasma peak concentration is observed in about 1 hour. At a dose of 800 mg every 8 hours, peak plasma concentration is approximately 300 nmol/L. The drug is approximately 60% bound to human plasma proteins. Indinavir is metabolized via oxidation and glucuronide conjugation. These metabolites were recovered in feces and urine, with about 20% of the drug excreted in the urine. The half-life of indinavir is approximately 1.8 hours. Because of indinavir's metabolism, a number of drug interactions are possible. Indinavir interacts with rifabutin or ketoconazole, leading to increased or decreased indinavir concentration, respectively, in the blood plasma. Administration of drug combinations of indinavir with antiviral nucleoside analogs, cimetidine, quinidine, trimethoprim–sulfamethoxazole, fluconazole, or isoniazid resulted in an increased activity of indinavir. Indinavir is contraindicated in patients taking triazolam or midazolam because inhibition of metabolism of these drugs may result in prolonged sedation, nephrolithiasis, asymptomatic hyperbilirubinemia, and GI problems (anorexia, constipation, dyspepsia, and gastritis). The usual oral dose for indinavir alone or in combination with other antiviral agents is one 800-mg capsule every 8 hours. The drug is well absorbed if given on an empty stomach or 1 hour before or 2 hours after a light meal with water. The dose is reduced to 600 mg every 8 hours if given concurrently with ketoconazole. Indinavir activity is increased when combined with RT inhibitors.

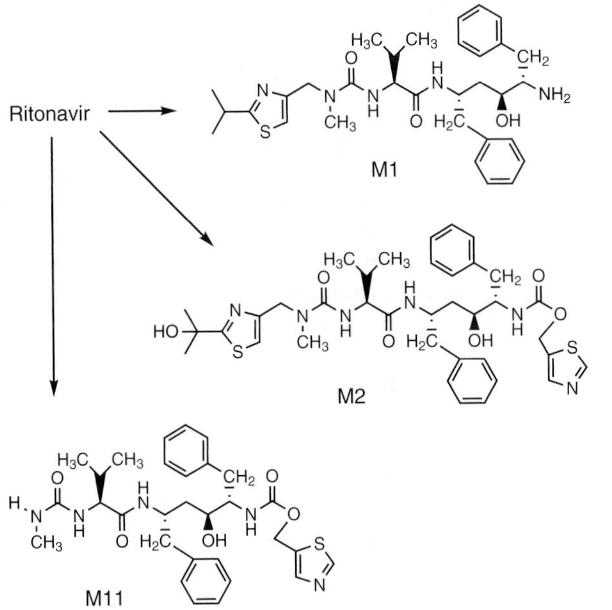

FIGURE 38.22 Major metabolic products from CYP3A4 metabolism of ritonavir.

NELFINAVIR MESYLATE Nelfinavir is a peptidomimetic drug that is effective in HIV-1 and HIV-2 wild-type and ZDV-resistant strains (Fig. 38.20). ED_{50} concentrations range from 9 to 60 nmol/L (95% effective dose was 0.04 mg/mL) (107). After IV administration, the elimination half-life of nelfinavir was about 1 hour. In combination with D4T, nelfinavir reduced HIV viral load by about 98% after 4 weeks. It is well tolerated when used with azole antifungals (ketoconazole, fluconazole, or itraconazole) or macrolide antibiotics (erythromycin, clarithromycin, or azithromycin). However, it causes diarrhea and other side effects common to nonnucleoside drugs. Following oral administration, nelfinavir peak levels in plasma ranged from 0.34 mg/mL (10 mg/kg in the dog) to 1.7 mg/mL (50 mg/kg in the rat). Nelfinavir was slowly absorbed, and bioavailability was 47% in the dog. The drug appeared to be metabolized in the liver, and the major excretory route was in feces.

Amprenavir Amprenavir is the fifth in a series of protease inhibitors to be approved for marketing in the United States. While structurally unique from the previous agents, its pharmacologic profile does not appear to differ significantly from the previously marketed agents. Early studies suggest that a different resistance profile may exist and that the drug may be effective against some resistant strains of HIV. Side effects appear to be more common than with other protease inhibitors and include nausea, vomiting, paresthesia, depression, and rash. Because amprenavir is a sulfonamide, there is some concern for cross-sensitivity with antibacterial sulfonamides. Although this has not been reported, care should be taken if sensitivity to trimethoprim–sulfamethoxazole, used in *Pneumocystis jirovecii* pneumonia, is reported.

Pharmacokinetics Amprenavir is rapidly absorbed following oral administration and may be taken with or without food. High-fat meals decrease the absorption of the drug and therefore should be avoided. The product is available in capsule and liquid form. The recommended adult and adolescent dose of 1,200 mg twice daily requires the patient to take eight capsules (150 mg) twice daily. The liquid preparation is recommended for children between 4 and 12 years of age or for patients 13 to 16 years of age who weigh less than 50 kg. The dose is 22.5 mg/kg twice daily or 17 mg/kg three times a day. Since this preparation contains the excipient propylene glycol, it is not recommended for children less than 4 years of age and certain other individuals who are unable to metabolize this alcohol.

Fosamprenavir Calcium (108) Fosamprenavir has been approved for the treatment of HIV in adults when used in combination with other anti-HIV drugs. It is a prodrug that, upon hydrolysis by serum phosphatases, gives rise to amprenavir, which as indicated earlier is a peptidomimetic transition-state inhibitor that targets HIV-1 protease and reduces viral replication and, thus, infectiousness of HIV-1. It is commonly administered in combination with RT inhibitors to produce excellent efficacy in AIDS patients. The drug is administered as two 700-mg tablets twice daily or, in combination with ritonavir, can be given as two 700-mg tablets once daily or one 700-mg tablet twice daily. Fosamprenavir is a slow-release version of amprenavir and, as a result, decreases the pills required for the patient and lowers the "pill burden" in AIDS patients.

Lopinavir/Ritonavir Recently, the FDA has approved the release of lopinavir/ritonavir combination in patients who have not responded to other regimens for treatment of HIV. The product is available in a soft gelatin capsule containing 133.3 mg of lopinavir and 33.3 mg of ritonavir, as well as oral solutions containing 80 mg/mL of lopinavir and 20 mg/mL of ritonavir. The small amount of ritonavir is not expected to have antiretroviral activity, but rather the ritonavir is meant to increase the plasma concentrations of lopinavir by inhibiting lopinavir's metabolism by CYP3A4. These drugs, in combination with other antiretroviral agents, have been approved for use in adults and patients between the ages of 6 months and 12 years. This is the first protease inhibitor to be indicated for the very young.

Atazanavir Calcium (109) Atazanavir is an antiretroviral agent approved for use in combination with other antiretroviral agents for the treatment of HIV infections (Fig. 38.20). It targets HIV-1 protease and reduces viral replication and thus virulence of HIV-1. Similar to saquinavir, ritonavir, indinavir, nelfinavir, amprenavir, and lopinavir, the drug is used in combination with RT inhibitors to produce excellent efficacy in AIDS patients. Atazanavir is dosed orally once daily, thus reducing "pill burden," and seems to have a minimum impact on lipid parameters, but does increase total bilirubin. The drug is well absorbed when administered orally with food (bioavailability ~68%). The drug is highly bound to plasma protein (86%) and is metabolized by CYP3A isoenzyme. Atazanavir is a moderate inhibitor of CYP3A, and potential drug–drug interactions are possible with CYP3A inhibitors and inducers.

Tipranavir Tipranavir is a recently approved, nonpeptidic inhibitor of HIV protease (Fig. 38.20) (110). It is indicated for patients who have developed resistance to other antiretroviral drugs, including other HIV protease inhibitors. Although it is very potent, it also exhibits more severe side effects than other HIV protease inhibitors, including intracranial hemorrhage, hepatitis, and diabetes mellitus. It is dosed at 500 mg twice daily in combination with 200 mg of ritonavir to suppress metabolism by cytochrome P450 (111). There is evidence that tipranavir induces its own metabolism, but using twice-daily coadministration of tipranavir and ritonavir at varying doses, tipranavir levels were 24- to 70-fold higher than levels achieved with administration of tipranavir alone.

Darunavir Darunavir is a second-generation HIV protease inhibitor that can be used in treatment-naive and treatment-experienced adult and pediatric patients (Fig. 38.20) (112). It was designed to bind tightly and specifically to HIV protease and thereby overcome the problems associated with first-generation drugs, including toxicity, high dose, expensive manufacture, and susceptibility to resistance. Like other HIV protease inhibitors, darunavir is metabolized by cytochrome P450, and thus, the drug is dosed at 800 mg once daily in combination with 100 mg of ritonavir (113).

HIV Integrase Inhibitors

Raltegravir

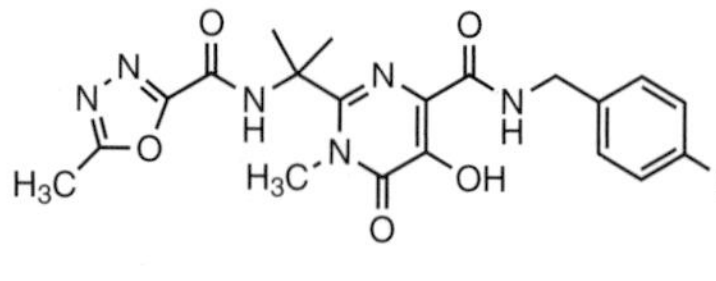

Mechanism of Action Raltegravir (Isentress) is the first (and thus far only) FDA-approved treatment for HIV that acts by inhibition of HIV integrase (114). A second HIV integrase inhibitor, elvitegravir, is currently in phase III clinical trials. Like HIV protease, HIV integrase is essential for replication of the HIV virus and, as such, has become a validated target for drug discovery. Each HIV particle contains 40 to 100 integrase molecules the role of which is to facilitate the insertion of viral complementary DNA (cDNA) into the host cell genome. Following host cell infection, the viral RNA is converted to cDNA via the action of RT. The preparation of cDNA for insertion requires integrase-mediated trimming of the 3′-ends of the viral DNA (3′-processing). The 3′-processing occurs within the cytoplasm, and the processed cDNA plus integrase complex, which also contains viral and cellular protein, is referred to as the preintegration complex. This complex is transported into the nucleus of the host cell where integration into the host DNA occurs through the catalytic action of integrase. The 3′-OH of the cDNA is joined to the 5′-phosphate of the host chromosome with both ends of the cDNA being joined to the host DNA. This very complex integration of cDNA into the host genome involves numerous viral and host proteins. Integrase itself is a 32-kd protein with three structural domains: 1) amino-terminal domain; 2) catalytic core domain (CCD); and 3) carboxy-terminal domain. All three domains are essential for integration, whereas only the CCD is required for the reverse reaction referred to as disintegration. The amino-terminal domain binds zinc, while the CCD binds manganese (Mn^{2+}) and magnesium (Mg^{2+}). It has been proposed that raltegravir acts by inhibiting cDNA integration via chelation to the divalent cations in the CCD at the interface the integrase-donor-acceptor complex (Fig. 38.23).

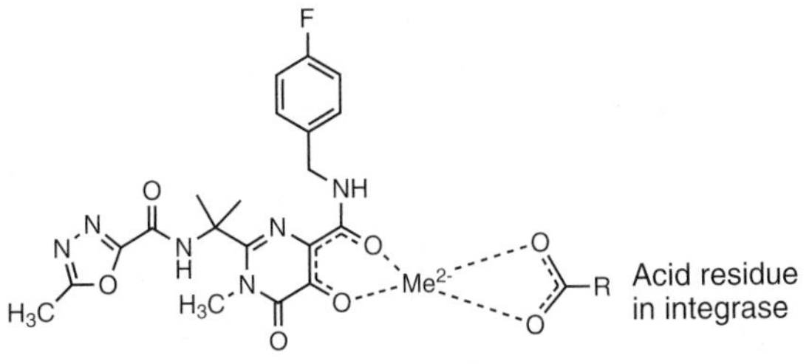

Raltegravir

FIGURE 38.23 Chelation complex between raltegravir and integrase.

Pharmacokinetics Raltegravir is readily absorbed following oral administration. The drug is highly bound to plasma protein (~83%). Food does not appear to affect the rate of absorption. The major route of metabolism is glucuronidation mediated by uridine diphosphate-glucuronosyl-transferase.

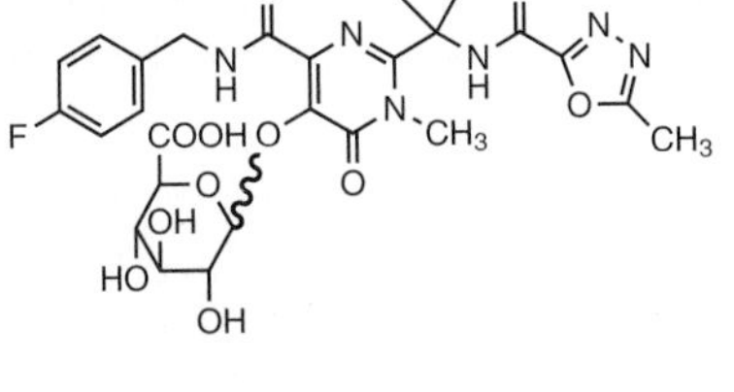

Approximately 51% of the drug is recovered in the feces unchanged, and 32% is recovered in the urine where 23% is the glucuronide. Glucuronidation inhibitors have the potential for drug–drug interactions, although there was no clinically significant effect when administered with atazanavir. Raltegravir is recommend for use in combination therapy and in patients who have demonstrated resistance to previous regimens.

Raltegravir was approved in 2008 for use in individuals whose infection has proven resistant to highly active antiretroviral therapy drugs (see next section), and in 2009, the FDA expanded approval for use in all patients. It is taken twice daily, and doses of 200, 400, and 600 mg have been used.

Combination Drug Therapy (115,116)

When several antiretroviral drugs, typically three or four, are taken in combination for the treatment of HIV, the approach is known as highly active antiretroviral therapy (HAART). Multiple HAART therapies have been undertaken, and the National Institutes of Health recommends that all infected patients should be treated in this manner (114). The synergistic antiviral effects of rimantadine with ribavirin and tiazofurin against influenza B virus and ganciclovir with foscarnet against HSV-1 and HSV-2 are noteworthy. The synergistic action of either trifluorothymidine or acyclovir with leukocyte interferon has been used in the topical treatment of human herpetic keratitis. During the past decade, research into combination antiretroviral therapy for AIDS patients has made remarkable progress. ZDV, the first approved drug for HIV-infected patients, produced bone marrow toxicity. To overcome toxic effects, combinations of ZDV with foscarnet, ddC, or ddI have been used. Such combination therapy indicated improved efficacy and decreased side effects as compared to either drug used alone. The combination of ZDV with α-interferon has been used to treat patients with AIDS-related Kaposi sarcoma. This combination drug therapy delayed emergence of ZDV-resistant HIV strains.

A combination of granulocyte-macrophage colony-stimulating factor with ZDV and α-interferon has been successful in managing treatment-related cytopenia in HIV-infected patients. The advantages of combination therapy include therapeutic antiviral effect, decreased toxicity, and low incidence of drug-resistant infection. In recent years, emergence of drug resistance has been demonstrated in patients receiving single antiviral agent therapy. Resistance to amantadine, acyclovir, ribavirin, ganciclovir, ZDV, and other antiviral agents is noteworthy.

Combined antiretroviral drug therapy serves different purposes. It prolongs the life of AIDS patients, removes drug resistance, and/or reduces toxicity of drugs. With these objectives, successful combinations of ZDV have been reported with ddC, ddI, 3TC, or D4T. Recently, combinations of nucleosides drugs (ZDV, ddC, ddI, 3TC) are used with protease inhibitors (saquinavir, indinavir, ritonavir) for delaying HIV infection. Combined nucleoside drugs are known to delay progression of HIV infection.

Antiretroviral therapy includes nucleosides or non-nucleoside RT inhibitors and protease inhibitors. These drugs inhibit HIV replication at different stages of viral infection. Nucleoside and nonnucleoside drugs inhibit RT by preventing RNA formation or viral protein synthesis. Nonnucleoside drugs inhibit RT by inactivating the catalytic site of the enzyme. Protease inhibitors act after HIV provirus has integrated into the human genome. These drugs inhibit protease, which is an enzyme responsible for cleaving viral precursor polypeptides into effective virions. Thus, protease inhibitors combined with RT inhibitors act by a synergistic mechanism to interrupt HIV replication.

Two-drug combinations, such as ZDV plus ddI or ddC, 3TC plus ZDV, and D4T plus ddI, have been successful in raising $CD4^+$ cell counts and decreasing HIV RNA viral load. Triple-drug therapy consisting of ZDV, 3TC, and a protease inhibitor (indinavir, ritonavir, nelfinavir) has been more effective than two-drug therapy consisting of two nonnucleoside analog combinations. In addition, fewer opportunistic infections were noted when patients took the three-drug combination. ZDV can also be combined with immunomodulators to increase immunologic response in AIDS patients. ZDV has been combined with α-interferon to obtain synergistic activity of the drug. An ideal approach of combined antiretroviral drug therapy would be drugs acting at different stages of HIV cell replication.

Investigational Antiviral Agents: Short Interfering RNA (117)

The field of directed RNA interference (RNAi) has rapidly developed into a highly promising approach for specifically interrupting gene function in order to alleviate disease pathology. This technique was first described in 1998, and the inventors of this technology, Andrew Fire and Craig C. Mello, were awarded a Nobel Prize in 2006 for their work with RNAi. RNAi is a natural mechanism for silencing gene expression that has been conserved through evolution in eukaryotes ranging from plants to humans. In this process, double-stranded duplexes 21 to 25 nucleotides in length are created from a parent double-stranded RNA molecule by an enzyme known as dicer. These short interfering RNAs (siRNA) bind to specific mRNAs that feature a complimentary sequence to form an RNA-induced silencing complex, and thereby block the expression of predetermined specific proteins at the posttranscriptional level. This binding also appears to direct the cell to cleave target mRNA/siRNA complexes. Many research groups are attempting to develop RNAi therapies that induce the degradation of target mRNA involved in inherited or acquired disorders. This technology is especially well suited to treating viral infections, and numerous examples now illustrate that a wide range of viruses can be inhibited with RNAi, both in vitro and in vivo. Antiviral RNAi therapies can be tailored to the biochemical characteristics of each pathogen and can be made more specific through choice of delivery vehicle, route of administration, selection of gene targets, and regulation of RNAi induction. As mentioned earlier, successful antiviral therapeutics possess the ability to discriminate virus from host. However, because viruses rely extensively on host cell machinery for many functions and activities involved in viral replication, they offer a very limited number of therapeutic targets. Because RNAi specifically targets a short stretch of viral nucleic acids rather than a viral protein, even a small viral genome can provide a large number of potential targets.

Researchers are continuing to look for suitable siRNA treatments for viral infections such as HBV, HCV, and HIV. Despite extensive research, the development of an siRNA-based therapy for viral infection faces significant barriers including poor siRNA stability, inefficient cellular uptake, widespread biodistribution, activation of immune response, and occurrence of nonspecific (i.e., off-target) effects (118). The most notable of these barriers is the delivery of intact siRNA molecules to the interior of virus-infected cells. A number of approaches have been tried, including bioconjugation of siRNA with lipids, incorporation into nanoparticles, and in situ biosynthesis of siRNAs. Although this strategy for antiviral development shows great promise, a reliable siRNA-based therapy for viral infection will likely not be realized in the near future.

SCENARIO: OUTCOME AND ANALYSIS

Outcome

Douglas Slain, PharmD, BCPS

WM was started on the investigational zanamivir intravenous formulation. After about 5 days of therapy, the patient became clinically stable and was able to come off of mechanical ventilation. She ultimately recovered. Resistance testing did show that she had an H1N1 strain that had the H274Y mutation.

Chemical Analysis

Victoria Roche and S. William Zito

These three antiviral molecules all take advantage of the research conducted to map the binding site of the influenza virus activating enzyme neuraminidase. Neuraminidase facilitates the spread of shed viruses by cleaving sialic acid (*N*-acetylneuraminic acid) from the saccharide-coated viral particles, which promotes their receptor-mediated absorption into unaffected cells.

SCENARIO: OUTCOME AND ANALYSIS *(Continued)*

The potentially cationic amino (oseltamivir) and guanidine (zanamivir and peramivir) moieties bind to one or more anionic glutamate residues on the neuraminidase enzyme. Neuraminidase is rich in Arg residues, and the acetamido carbonyl oxygen atom found on all three antiviral agents forms an ion-dipole bond with cationic Arg152. Several Arg residues also interact with the anionic carboxylate moieties of zanamivir and peramivir. Presumably, the nonionizable ester of oseltamivir is able to form an ion-dipole bond with this cationic collection of residues.

The major affinity difference among these neuraminidase inhibitors relates to their ability to interact with a hydrophobic area of the neuraminidase that is known to bind with the 3-pentyloxy side chain found at position 6 of oseltamivir and related inhibitors. Peramivir has a lipophilic 3-pentyl moiety that extends from the carbon atom connecting the acetamido moiety to the cyclopentane ring. This lipophilic group presumably interacts hydrophobically with the neuraminidase enzyme in a manner similar to 3-pentyloxy group of oseltamivir.

Since WM was infected with a strain of H1N1 that is resistant to drugs that interact hydrophobically with neuraminidase, the selection of an inhibitor without this capability was justified. Zanamivir has an oxygen-rich trihydroxypropyl (glycerol) moiety at position 6, which significantly detracts from its lipophilic character and, therefore, its ability to bind within the hydrophobic cavity of neuraminidase. As a neuraminidase inhibitor that is not dependent on hydrophobic bonding, it would stand the best chance of helping this patient successfully overcome her H274Y-mutated influenza infection.

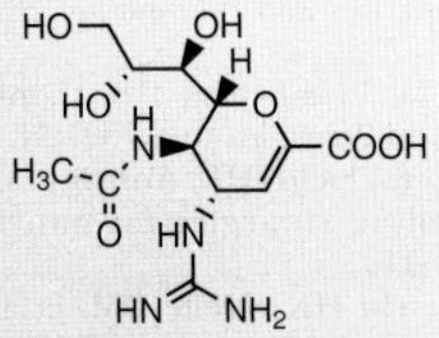

Zanamivir

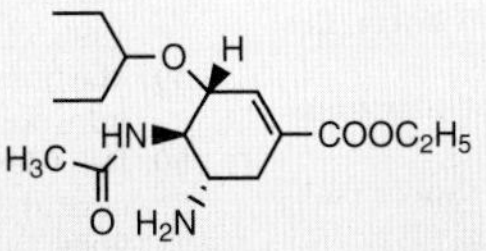

Oseltamivir

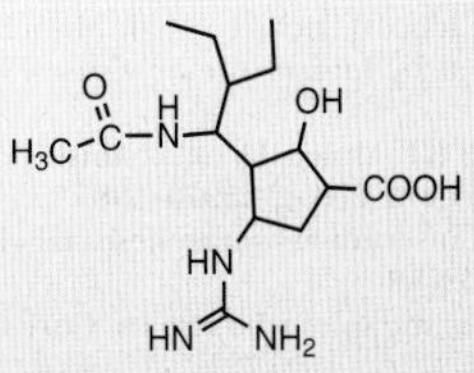

Peramivir

CASE STUDY

Victoria Roche and S. William Zito

LP is a 29-year-old man from a disadvantaged background who recently found new hope for his future through his affiliation with Homeboy Industries, an LA-based organization founded by Fr. Greg Boyle that assists former gang members in redirecting their lives through job training, education, and holistic support (www.homeboy-industries.org). Though he is regularly urged to return to the streets by his former "friends," LP is now seeing the potential for a better life and is trying to stick it out despite his apprehension. Through frequent unprotected sexual activity, LP contracted genital herpes several years ago and routinely had been given oral acyclovir (when available) and some acyclovir ointment by physicians working pro bono at a downtown free clinic. In the past, LP was minimally compliant with his regimen, and he has admitted to both overusing the topical preparation and stopping oral therapy prematurely. Now this drug is no longer effective in managing his outbreaks, and partial resistance to this therapy is presumed. He has presented to the clinic with painful genital lesions, most likely exacerbated by the stress he is currently undergoing as he tries to turn his life around.

As a new pharmacist donating your professional services to the patients of this clinic, you are speaking with LP about his disease state. This young man is now involved in a serious relationship, and he says he is committed to taking his medication as directed and practicing safe sex. Though your choice of therapies is limited to what's been donated to the clinic, three options (drawn below) present themselves. Although none may be truly optimal, which would be your first choice to help this patient through his latest HSV-2 outbreak?

1. Conduct a thorough and mechanistic SAR analysis of the three therapeutic options in the case.
2. Apply the chemical understanding gained from the SAR analysis to this patient's specific needs to make a therapeutic recommendation.

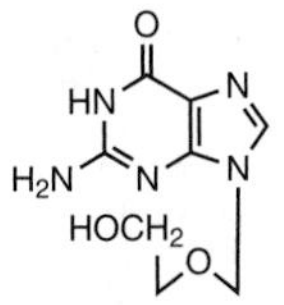

Acyclovir

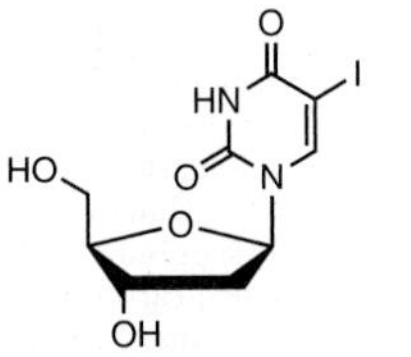

1

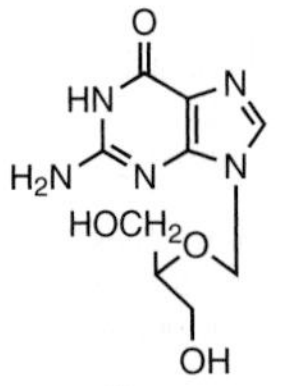

2

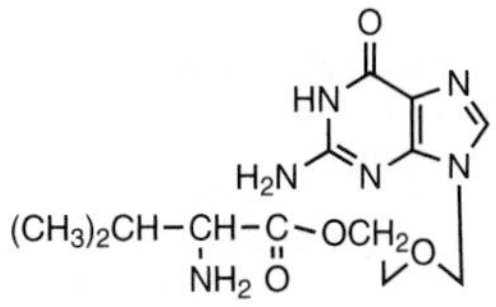

3

References

1. Baron S. Medical Microbiology, 3rd Ed. New York: Churchill Livingstone, 1991:555–652.
2. Brooks GF, Butel JS, Morse SA, et al. Jawetz, Melnick and Adelberg's Medical Microbiology, 23rd Ed. New York: McGraw-Hill Companies, 2004.
3. Pornillos O, Ganser-Pornillos BK, Yeager M. Atomic-level modelling of the HIV capsid. Nature 2011;469:424–427.
4. Tyler KL, Fields BN. Fields Virology, 2nd Ed. New York: Raven Press, 1990:191–239.
5. Ganser-Pornillos BK, Chandrasekaran V, Pornillos O, et al. Hexagonal assembly of a restricting TRIM5alpha protein. Proc Natl Acad Sci U S A 2011;108:534–539.
6. Gallo RC. History of the discoveries of the first human retroviruses: HTLV-1 and HTLV-2. Oncogene 2005;24:5926–5930.
7. Sierra S, Kupfer B, Kaiser R. Basics of the virology of HIV-1 and its replication. J Clin Virol 2005;34:233.
8. Gallo RC, Montagnier L. The discovery of HIV as the cause of AIDS. N Engl J Med 2003;349:2283–2285.
9. World Health Organization. Joint United Nations Programme on HIV/AIDS (UNAIDS): AIDS epidemic update 2005. Available at: http://www.who.int/hiv/epiupdates/en/index.html.
10. UNAIDS. UNAIDS report on the global aids epidemic 2010. Available at: http://www.unaids.org/globalreport/Global_report.htm.
11. Hotez PJ, Molyneux DH, Fenwick A, et al. Incorporating a rapid-impact package for neglected tropical diseases with programs for HIV/AIDS, tuberculosis, and malaria. PLoS Med 2006;3:e102.
12. Kaleeba JAR, Berger EA. Kaposi's sarcoma-associated herpesvirus fusion-entry receptor: cystine transporter xCT. Science 2006;311:1921–1924.
13. D'Agostino DM, Bernardi P, ChiecoBianchi L, et al. Mitochondria as functional targets of proteins coded by human tumor viruses. Adv Cancer Res 2005;94:87–142.
14. Grassmann R, Aboud M, Jeang KT. Molecular mechanisms of cellular transformation by HTLV-1 tax. Oncogene 2005;24:5976–5985.
15. Mikkers H, Berns A. Retroviral insertional mutagenesis: tagging cancer pathways. Adv Cancer Res 2003;88:53–99.
16. O'Shea CC. DNA tumor viruses: the spies who lyse us. Curr Opin Genet Dev 2005;15:18–26.
17. Robinson HL. Retroviruses and cancer. Rev Infect Dis 1982;4:1015–1025.
18. Klein G. Perspectives in studies of human tumor viruses. Front Biosci 2002;7:d268–d274.
19. Saslow D, Castle PE, Cox JT, et al. American Cancer Society Guideline for human papillomavirus (HPV) vaccine use to prevent cervical cancer and its precursors. CA Cancer J Clin 2007;57:7–28.
20. Johnson RT. Prion diseases. Lancet Neurol 2005;4:635–642.
21. Mabbott NA, MacPherson GG. Prions and their lethal journey to the brain. Nat Rev Microbiol 2006;4:201–211.
22. Weissmann C. Birth of a prion: spontaneous generation revisited. Cell 2005;122:165–168.
23. Mandell GL. Principles and Practice of Infectious Diseases New York: Churchill Livingstone, 1995.
24. Mills J, Corey L. Antiviral Chemotherapy: New Directions for Clinical Application and Research, Vol. 3. Englewood Cliffs, NJ: PTR Prentice Hall, 1993.
25. Burlington DB, Meiklejohn G, Mostow SR. Anti-influenza A virus activity of amantadine hydrochloride and rimantadine hydrochloride in ferret tracheal ciliated epithelium. Antimicrob Agents Chemother 1982;21:794–799.
26. Hayden FG. Combinations of antiviral agents for treatment of influenza virus infections. J Antimicrob Chemother 1986;18(Suppl B):177–183.
27. Wingfield WL, Pollack D, Grunert RR. Therapeutic efficacy of amantadine HCl and rimantadine HCl in naturally occurring influenza A2 respiratory illness in man. N Engl J Med 1969;281:579–584.
28. Wintermeyer SM, Nahata MC. Rimantadine: a clinical perspective. Ann Pharmacother 1995;29:299–310.
29. Francis ML, Meltzer MS, Gendelman HE. Interferons in the persistence, pathogenesis, and treatment of HIV infection. AIDS Res Hum Retroviruses 1992;8:199–207.
30. Hayden FG. Clinical Aspects of Interferons. Boston: Kluwer Academic Publishers, 1988.
31. Streuli M, Nagata S, Weissmann C. At least three human type alpha interferons: structure of alpha 2. Science 1980;209:1343–1347.
32. Baglioni C, Maroney PA. Mechanisms of action of human interferons. Induction of 2′5′-oligo(A) polymerase. J Biol Chem 1980;255:8390–8393.
33. Taniguchi T, Guarente L, Roberts TM, et al. Expression of the human fibroblast interferon gene in Escherichia coli. Proc Natl Acad Sci U S A 1980;77:5230–5233.
34. Pollard RB. Interferons and interferon inducers: development of clinical usefulness and therapeutic promise. Drugs 1982;23:37–55.
35. Calfee DP, Hayden FG. New approaches to influenza chemotherapy. Neuraminidase inhibitors. Drugs 1998;56:537–553.
36. Kim CU, Lew W, Williams MA, et al. Influenza neuraminidase inhibitors possessing a novel hydrophobic interaction in the enzyme active site: design, synthesis, and structural analysis of carbocyclic sialic acid analogues with potent anti-influenza activity. J Am Chem Soc 1997;119:681–690.
37. Sweeny DJ, Lynch G, Bidgood AM, et al. Metabolism of the influenza neuraminidase inhibitor prodrug oseltamivir in the rat. Drug Metab Dispos 2000;28:737–741.
38. Mancuso CE, Gabay MP, Steinke LM, et al. Peramivir: an intravenous neuraminidase inhibitor for the treatment of 2009 H1N1 influenza. Ann Pharmacother 2010;44:1240–1249.
39. Lalezari JP, Henry K, O'Hearn M, et al. Enfuvirtide, an HIV-1 fusion inhibitor, for drug-resistant HIV infection in North and South America. N Engl J Med 2003;348:2175–2185.
40. Poveda E, Briz V, Soriano V. Enfuvirtide, the first fusion inhibitor to treat HIV infection. AIDS Rev 2005;7:139–147.
41. Field HJ. A perspective on resistance to acyclovir in herpes simplex virus. J Antimicrob Chemother 1983;12(Suppl B):129–135.
42. Elion GB, Furman PA, Fyfe JA, et al. Selectivity of action of an antiherpetic agent, 9-(2-hydroxyethoxymethyl) guanine. Proc Natl Acad Sci U S A 1977;74:5716–5720.
43. Whitley RJ, Alford CA. Antiviral agents: clinical status report. Hosp Pract (Off Ed) 1981;16:109–121.
44. Mitchell CD, Bean B, Gentry SR, et al. Acyclovir therapy for mucocutaneous herpes simplex infections in immunocompromised patients. Lancet 1981;1:1389–1392
45. Whitley RJ, Alford CA, Hirsch MS, et al. Vidarabine versus acyclovir therapy in herpes simplex encephalitis. N Engl J Med 1986;314:144–149.
46. Brigden D, Bye A, Fowle AS, et al. Human pharmacokinetics of acyclovir (an antiviral agent) following rapid intravenous injection. J Antimicrob Chemother 1981;7:399–404.
47. de Miranda P, Whitley RJ, Blum MR, et al. Acyclovir kinetics after intravenous infusion. Clin Pharmacol Ther 1979;26:718–728.
48. Perry CM, Faulds D. Valaciclovir. A review of its antiviral activity, pharmacokinetic properties and therapeutic efficacy in herpesvirus infections. Drugs 1996;52:754–772.
49. Martinez CM, Luks-Golger DB. Cidofovir use in acyclovir-resistant herpes infection. Ann Pharmacother 1997;31:1519–1521.
50. De Clercq E, Field HJ. Antiviral prodrugs: the development of successful prodrug strategies for antiviral chemotherapy. Br J Pharmacol 2006;147:1–11.
51. Schacker T, Hu HL, Koelle DM, et al. Famciclovir for the suppression of symptomatic and asymptomatic herpes simplex virus reactivation in HIV-infected persons. A double-blind, placebo-controlled trial. Ann Intern Med 1998;128:21–28.
52. Fletcher CV, Balfour HH Jr. Evaluation of ganciclovir for cytomegalovirus disease. DICP 1989;23:5–12.
53. Dando T, Plosker G. Adefovir dipivoxil: a review of its use in chronic hepatitis B. Drugs 2003;63:2215–2234.
54. Whitley RJ. The past as prelude to the future: history, status, and future of antiviral drugs. Ann Pharmacother 1996;30:967–971.
55. Farah A. Handbook of Experimental Biology, Vol 38/2. Berlin: Springer, 1975.
56. Hall CB, McBride JT. Vapors, viruses, and views. Ribavirin and respiratory syncytial virus. Am J Dis Child 1986;140:331–332.
57. Sidwell RW, Huffman JH, Khare GP, et al. Broad-spectrum antiviral activity of virazole: 1-beta-D-ribofuranosyl-1,2,4-triazole-3-carboxamide. Science 1972;177:705–706.
58. Fox CF, Robinson WS. Virus Research. New York: Academic Press, 1973.
59. Power WJ, Benedict-Smith A, Hillery M, et al. Randomised double-blind trial of bromovinyldeoxyuridine (BVDU) and trifluorothymidine (TFT) in dendritic corneal ulceration. Br J Ophthalmol 1991;75:649–651.
60. Whitley RJ, Soong SJ, Dolin R, et al. Adenine arabinoside therapy of biopsy-proved herpes simplex encephalitis. National Institute of Allergy and Infectious Diseases collaborative antiviral study. N Engl J Med 1977;297:289–294.
61. Whitley RJ, Soong SJ, Dolin R, et al. Early vidarabine therapy to control the complications of herpes zoster in immunosuppressed patients. N Engl J Med 1982;307:971–975.
62. Chao DL, Kimball AP. Deamination of arabinosyladenine by adenosine deaminase and inhibition by arabinosyl-6-mercaptopurine. Cancer Res 1972;32:1721–1724.
63. Ward RL, Stevens JG. Effect of cytosine arabinoside on viral-specific protein synthesis in cells infected with herpes simplex virus. J Virol 1975;15:71–80.
64. Nutter RL, Rapp F. The effect of cytosine arabinoside on virus production in various cells infected with herpes simplex virus types 1 and 2. Cancer Res 1973;33:166–170.
65. Field AK. Viral targets for antisense oligonucleotides: a mini review. Antiviral Res 1998;37:67–81.
66. Chrisp P, Clissold SP. Foscarnet. A review of its antiviral activity, pharmacokinetic properties and therapeutic use in immunocompromised patients with cytomegalovirus retinitis. Drugs 1991;41:104–129.
67. Venkatraman S, Bogen SL, Arasappan A, et al. Discovery of (1R,5S)-N-[3-amino-1-(cyclobutylmethyl)-2,3-dioxopropyl]- 3-[2(S)-[[[(1,1-dimethylethyl)amino] carbonyl]amino]-3,3-dimethyl-1-oxobuty 1]- 6,6-dimethyl-3-azabicyclo[3.1.0] hexan-2(S)-carboxamide (SCH 503034), a selective, potent, orally bioavailable hepatitis C virus NS3 protease inhibitor: a potential therapeutic agent for the treatment of hepatitis C infection. J Med Chem 2006;49:6074–6086.

68. Lin K, Perni RB, Kwong AD, et al. VX-950, a novel hepatitis C virus (HCV) NS3-4A protease inhibitor, exhibits potent antiviral activities in HCv replicon cells. Antimicrob Agents Chemother 2006;50:1813–1822.
69. Pawlotsky JM. The results of phase III clinical trial with telaprevir and boceprevir presented at the Liver Meeting 2010: a new standard of care for hepatitis c virus genotype 1 infection, but with issues still pending. Gastroenterology 2011;140:746–754.
70. Blair E, Darby G. Antiviral Therapy. New York: BIOS Scientific Publishers, 1998.
71. do Valle LA, de Melo PR, de Gomes LF, et al. Methisazone in prevention of variola minor among contacts. Lancet 1965;2:976–978.
72. Mohan P, Baba M. Anti-AIDS Drug Development: Challenges, Strategies and Prospects. Chur, Switzerland: Harwood Academic, 1995.
73. Sethi ML. Current concepts in HIV/AIDS pharmacotherapy. Consultant Pharmacists: 1998;13:1224–1245.
74. Berger TG. Treatment of bacterial, fungal, and parasitic infections in the HIV-infected host. Semin Dermatol 1993;12:296–300.
75. Goa KL, Barradell LB. Fluconazole. An update of its pharmacodynamic and pharmacokinetic properties and therapeutic use in major superficial and systemic mycoses in immunocompromised patients. Drugs 1995;50:658–690.
76. Sattler FR, Feinberg J. New developments in the treatment of Pneumocystis carinii pneumonia. Chest 1992;101:451–457.
77. Mitsuya H. Anti-HIV Nucleosides: Past, Present and Future. New York: Chapman and Hall, 1997.
78. Gorbach SL, Barlett JG, Blacklow NR. Infectious Diseases. Philadelphia: W.B. Saunders Co., 1998.
79. MacDonald L, Kazanjian P. Antiretroviral therapy in HIV-infection: an update. Formulary 1996;31:780–804.
80. Faulds D, Brogden RN. Didanosine. A review of its antiviral activity, pharmacokinetic properties and therapeutic potential in human immunodeficiency virus infection. Drugs 1992;44:94–116.
81. Beach JW. Chemotherapeutic agents for human immunodeficiency virus infection: mechanism of action, pharmacokinetics, metabolism, and adverse reactions. Clin Ther 1998;20:2–25.
82. Lipsky JJ. Zalcitabine and didanosine. Lancet 1993;341:30–32.
83. Shelton MJ, O'Donnell AM, Morse GD. Zalcitabine. Ann Pharmacother 1993;27:480–489.
84. Neuzil KM. Pharmacologic therapy for human immunodeficiency virus infection: a review. Am J Med Sci 1994;307:368–373.
85. Fischl MA, Richman DD, Grieco MH, et al. The efficacy of azidothymidine (AZT) in the treatment of patients with AIDS and AIDS-related complex. A double-blind, placebo-controlled trial. N Engl J Med 1987;317:185–191.
86. Fischl MA, Richman DD, Hansen N, et al. The safety and efficacy of zidovudine (AZT) in the treatment of subjects with mildly symptomatic human immunodeficiency virus type 1 (HIV) infection. A double-blind, placebo-controlled trial. The AIDS Clinical Trials Group. Ann Intern Med 1990;112:727–737.
87. Nasr M, Litterst C, McGowan J. Computer-assisted structure-activity correlations of dideoxynucleoside analogs as potential anti-HIV drugs. Antiviral Res 1990;14:125–148.
88. Sethi ML. Zidovudine, Vol. 20. San Diego: Academic Press, 1991.
89. Hoth DF Jr, Myers MW, Stein DS. Current status of HIV therapy: I. Antiretroviral agents. Hosp Pract (Off Ed) 1992;27:145–156.
90. Horwitz JP, Chua J, Noel M, et al. Nucleosides. Iv. 1-(2-deoxy-beta-D-lyxofuranosyl)-5-iodouracil. J Med Chem 1964;7:385–386.
91. Ostertag W, Roesler G, Krieg CJ, et al. Induction of endogenous virus and of thymidine kinase by bromodeoxyuridine in cell cultures transformed by Friend virus. Proc Natl Acad Sci U S A 1974;71:4980–4985.
92. Yarchoan R, Klecker RW, Weinhold KJ, et al. Administration of 3′-azido-3′-deoxythymidine, an inhibitor of HTLV-III/LAV replication, to patients with AIDS or AIDS-related complex. Lancet 1986;1:575–580.
93. Perry CM, Faulds D. Lamivudine. A review of its antiviral activity, pharmacokinetic properties and therapeutic efficacy in the management of HIV infection. Drugs 1997;53:657–680.
94. Barditch-Crovo P, Deeks SG, Collier A, et al. Phase I/II trial of the pharmacokinetics, safety, and antiretroviral activity of tenofovir disoproxil fumarate in human immunodeficiency virus-infected adults. Antimicrob Agents Chemother 2001;45:2733–2739.
95. Bang LM, Scott LJ. Emtricitabine: an antiretroviral agent for HIV infection. Drugs 2003;63:2413–2424.
96. Tan B, Ratner L. The use of new antiretroviral therapy in combination with chemotherapy. Curr Opin Oncol 1997;9:455–464.
97. Freimuth WW. Delavirdine mesylate, a potent non-nucleoside HIV-1 reverse transcriptase inhibitor. Adv Exp Med Biol 1996;394:279–289.
98. Graul AI, Rabesseda X, Castaner J. Efavirenz. Drugs Future 1998;23:133–141.
99. Deeks SG, Volberding PA. HIV-1 protease inhibitors. AIDS Clin Rev 1997;145–185.
100. Bihani S, Das A, Prashar V, et al. X-ray structure of HIV-1 protease in situ product complex. Proteins 2009;74:594–602.
101. Rich DH, Sun ET. Mechanism of inhibition of pepsin by pepstatin. Effect of inhibitor structure on dissociation constant and time-dependent inhibition. Biochem Pharmacol 1980;29:2205–2212.
102. Josephson F. Drug-drug interactions in the treatment of HIV infection: focus on pharmacokinetic enhancement through CYP3A inhibition. J Intern Med 2010;268:530–539.
103. Hoetelmans RM, Meenhorst PL, Mulder JW, et al. Clinical pharmacology of HIV protease inhibitors: focus on saquinavir, indinavir, and ritonavir. Pharm World Sci 1997;19:159–175.
104. Perry CM, Noble S. Saquinavir soft-gel capsule formulation. A review of its use in patients with HIV infection. Drugs 1998;55:461–486.
105. Markowitz M, Saag M, Powderly WG, et al. A preliminary study of ritonavir, an inhibitor of HIV-1 protease, to treat HIV-1 infection. N Engl J Med 1995;333:1534–1539.
106. Deeks SG, Smith M, Holodniy M, et al. HIV-1 protease inhibitors. A review for clinicians. JAMA 1997;277:145–153.
107. Perry CM, Benfield P. Nelfinavir. Drugs 1997;54:81–87; discussion 88.
108. Falcoz C, Jenkins JM, Bye C, et al. Pharmacokinetics of GW433908, a prodrug of amprenavir, in healthy male volunteers. J Clin Pharmacol 2002;42:887–898.
109. Colonno RJ, Thiry A, Limoli K, et al. Activities of atazanavir (BMS-232632) against a large panel of human immunodeficiency virus type 1 clinical isolates resistant to one or more approved protease inhibitors. Antimicrob Agents Chemother 2003;47:1324–1333.
110. Courter JD, Teevan CJ, Li MH, et al. Role of tipranavir in treatment of patients with multidrug-resistant HIV. Ther Clin Risk Manag 2010;6:431–441.
111. Hughes CA, Robinson L, Tseng A, et al. New antiretroviral drugs: a review of the efficacy, safety, pharmacokinetics, and resistance profile of tipranavir, darunavir, etravirine, rilpivirine, maraviroc, and raltegravir. Expert Opin Pharmacother 2009;10:2445–2466.
112. Boyd MA, Hill AM. Clinical management of treatment-experienced, HIV/AIDS patients in the combination antiretroviral therapy era. Pharmacoeconomics 2010;28(Suppl 1):17–34.
113. McCoy C. Darunavir: a nonpeptidic antiretroviral protease inhibitor. Clin Ther 2007;29:1559–1576.
114. Al-Mawsawi LQ, Neamati N. Allosteric inhibitor development targeting HIV-1 integrase. Chem Med Chem 2011;6:228–241.
115. Fischl MA, Stanley K, Collier AC, et al. Combination and monotherapy with zidovudine and zalcitabine in patients with advanced HIV disease. The NIAID AIDS Clinical Trials Group. Ann Intern Med 1995;122:24–32.
116. Havlir DV, Lange JM. New antiretrovirals and new combinations. AIDS 1998;12(Suppl A):S165–S174.
117. Leonard JN, Schaffer DV. Antiviral RNAi therapy: emerging approaches for hitting a moving target. Gene Ther 2006;13:532–540.
118. Chen Y, Cheng G, Mahato RI. RNAi for treating hepatitis B viral infection. Pharm Res 2008;25:72–86.

Suggested Readings

Bamford DH, Burnett RM, Stuart DI. Evolution of viral structure. Theoret Population Biol 2002;61:461–470.

Brooks GF, Butel JS, Morse SA, et al. Jawetz, Melnick and Adelberg's Medical Microbiology, 23rd Ed. New York: McGraw-Hill Companies, 2004:Chapters 29–44.

De Clercq E. Antiviral drug discovery and development: where chemistry meets with biomedicine. Antiviral Res 2005;67:56–75.

De Clercq E. Antiviral drugs in current clinical use. J Clin Virol 2004;30:115–133.

De Clercq E. Antivirals and antiviral strategies. Nat Rev Microbiol 2004;2:704–720.

De Clercq E. Recent highlights in the development of new antiviral drugs. Curr Opin Microbiol 2005;8:552–560.

De Clercq E, Field HJ. Antiviral prodrugs: the development of successful prodrug strategies for antiviral chemotherapy. Br J Pharmacol 2006;147:1–11.

Fung SK, Lok AS. Drug insight: nucleoside and nucleotide analog inhibitors for hepatitis B. Nat Clin Pract Gastroenterol Hepatol 2004;1:90–97.

Grassmann R, Aboud M, Jeang KT. Molecular mechanisms of cellular transformation by HTLV-1 Tax. Oncogene 2005;24:5976–5985.

Mabbott NA, MacPherson GG. Prions and their lethal journey to the brain. Nat Rev Microbiol 2006;4:201–211.

Moscona A. Neuraminidase inhibitors for influenza. N Engl J Med 2005;353:1363–1373.

O'Shea CC. DNA tumor viruses: the spies who lyse us. Curr Opin Genet Dev 2005;15:18–26.

Robinson HL. Retroviruses and cancer. Rev Infect Dis 1982;4:1015–1025.

Sierra S, Kupfer B, Kaiser R. Basics of the virology of HIV-1 and its replication. J Clin Virol 2005;34:233–244.

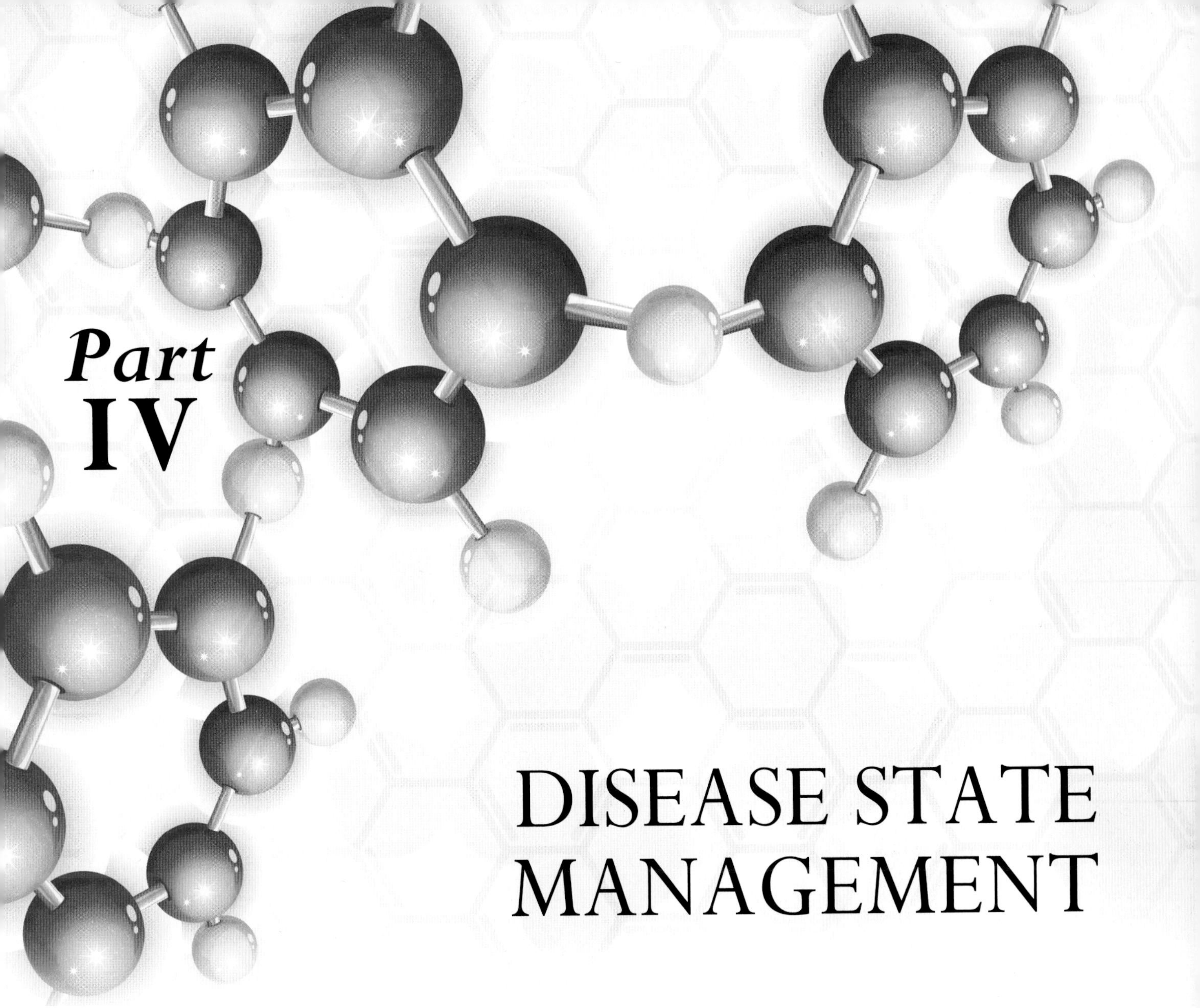

Part IV

DISEASE STATE MANAGEMENT

Chapter 39

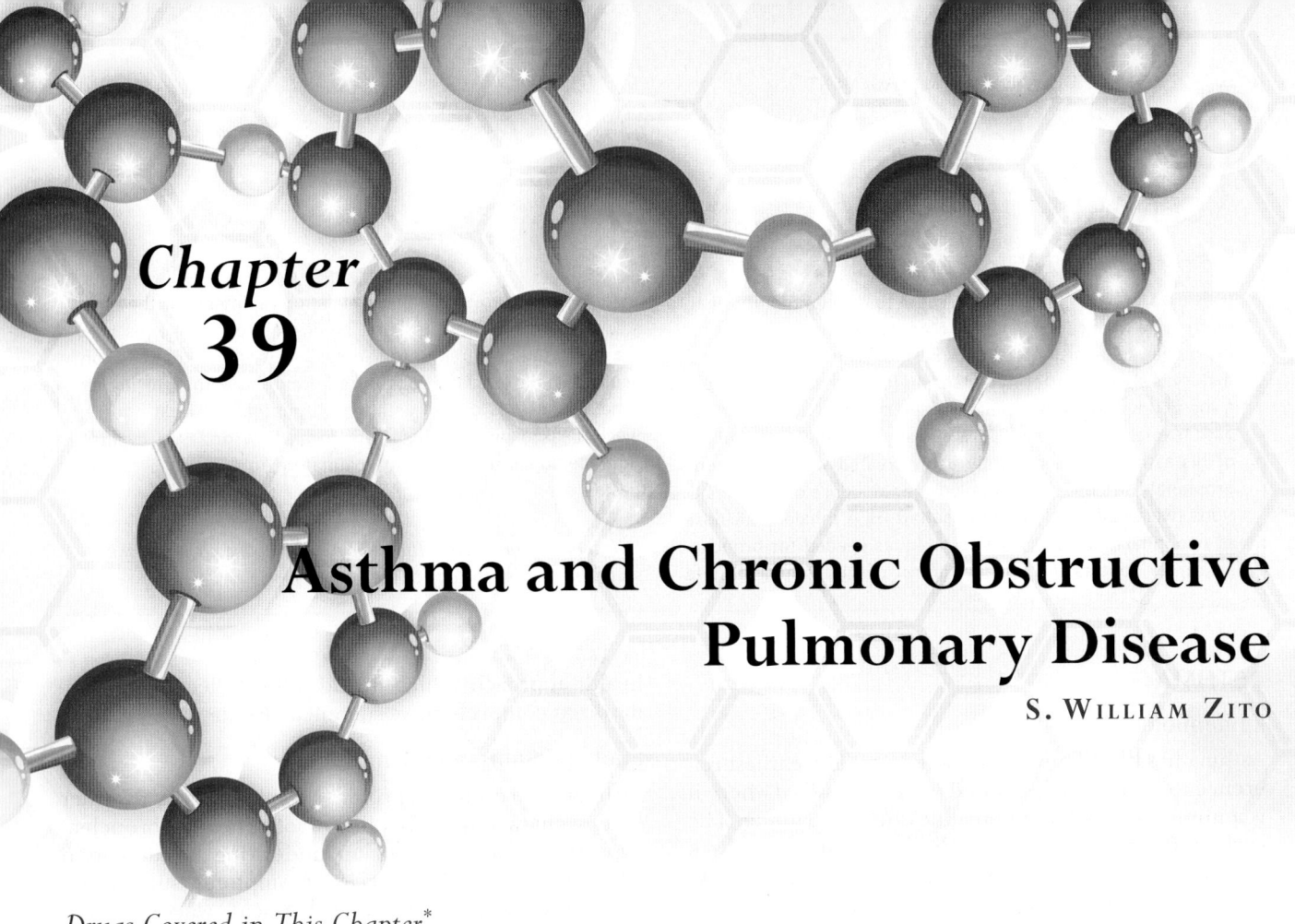

Asthma and Chronic Obstructive Pulmonary Disease

S. WILLIAM ZITO

Drugs Covered in This Chapter*

ADRENOCORTICOIDS
- Beclomethasone dipropionate
- Budesonide
- *Ciclesonide*
- Flunisolide
- Fluticasone propionate
- Hydrocortisone
- Methylprednisolone
- Mometasone furoate
- Prednisolone
- Triamcinolone acetonide

β_2-ADRENERGIC AGONISTS
- Albuterol
- Bitolterol mesylate
- Epinephrine (Adrenalin)
- *Fenoterol hydrobromide*
- Formoterol fumarate (arformoterol)
- Isoetharine hydrochloride
- Metaproterenol sulfate
- Salmeterol xinafoate
- Terbutaline sulfate

ANTIMUSCARINICS
- *Aclidinium bromide*
- Ipratropium hydrobromide
- Tiotropium bromide

LEUKOTRIENE MODIFIERS
- Montelukast
- Zafirlukast
- Zileuton

MAST CELL DEGRANULATION INHIBITORS
- Cromolyn sodium (*sodium cromoglycate*)
- Nedocromil sodium

METHYLXANTHINES
- Dyphylline
- Theophylline

MONOCLONAL ANTI-IGE ANTIBODY
- Omalizumab

PHOSPHODIESTERASE INHIBITORS
- Roflumilast

Abbreviations

AMP, adenosine monophosphate
ATT, α_1-antitrypsin
cAMP, cyclic adenosine monophosphate
cGMP, cyclic guanosine monophosphate
COMT, catechol *O*-methyl transferase
COPD, chronic obstructive pulmonary disease
CRF, corticotrophin-releasing factor
cysLT, cysteinyl leukotriene
EPI, epinephrine
FcεRI, high-affinity Fc immunoglobulin E receptor
FDA, U.S. Food and Drug Administration
FEV_1, forced expiratory volume in 1 second
FLAP, 5-lipoxygenase–activating protein
FVC, forced vital capacity
GI, gastrointestinal
GOLD, Global Initiative for Chronic Lung Disease
HDAC2, histone deacetylase 2
HPA, hypothalamus-pituitary-adrenal
HRE, hormone response element
Ig, immunoglobulin
IL, interleukin
IV, intravenous
L-DOPA, L-dihydroxyphenylalanine
MAO, monoamine oxidase
MIH, macrophage migration inhibitory factor
NE, norepinephrine
NIH, National Institutes of Health
PDE, phosphodiesterase
PEF, peak expiratory flow
SRS-A, slow-reacting substance of anaphylaxis
TSLP, thymic stromal lymphopoietin

*Drugs listed include those available inside and outside of the United States; drugs available outside of the United States are shown in italics.

SCENARIO

Joseph V. Etzel, PharmD

JP is a 42-year old man who presents to his community pharmacy for a Medication Therapy Management consultation for his moderate-persistent asthma. Besides asthma, JP's medical history is significant for hypertension (controlled with ramipril 5 mg PO daily) and perennial allergic rhinitis (well controlled with fexofenadine 60 mg PO twice daily). For the management of his asthma, JP is currently being treated with fluticasone propionate 110 mcg inhalation powder at a dose of two inhalations twice daily and albuterol sulfate HFA inhaler at a dose of two inhalations every 4 to 6 hours as needed for bronchospasm. JP reports inadequate control of his asthma despite being adherent to the above medication regimens for the past several months. He states that he is required to use his albuterol inhalation three to four times per week for the relief of acute asthma exacerbations. In addition, he admits to nighttime awakenings due to asthmatic symptoms at least once a week. Peak expiratory flow rate (peak flow or FEV_1) evaluations demonstrate values approximately 70% of his personal best.

(The reader is directed to the clinical solution and chemical analysis of this case at the end of the chapter).

ASTHMA

Epidemiology

Asthma has been known since antiquity. The earliest reference to asthma can be found in Homer's *Iliad* where it is a noun used to denote breathlessness or panting. The earliest use of the term as a medical condition dates back to Ancient Greece, in Hippocrates' *Corpus Hippocraticum*, and the best clinical description of asthma from antiquity was offered by the physician Aretaeus of Cappadocia who practiced in the first century AD (1).

Over the period of 1980 to 1999, asthma prevalence increased in the United States. However, since then, asthma prevalence has stopped increasing, and in addition, asthma-related mortality and hospitalizations have decreased, which perhaps is an indication of improved disease state management (2,3). According to U.S. population data gathered by the National Health Interview Survey, the lifetime estimate of the number of people who were ever diagnosed with asthma is 34 million, or 11.5% of the population. The current percentages for asthma prevalence as of 2007 are 9.1% for children less than 18 years old and 7.3% for adults over age 18 years. Boys have a higher incidence of asthma than girls (9.7% vs. 8.5%); however, this reverses in adulthood, when females show a higher prevalence compared to males (9% vs. 5.4%) (4). In a recent study, over a 1-year period (2004–2005), 15% of all children in the study population (>4 million) age less than 17 years were dispensed an asthma-related medication (5). Race/ethnicity plays a significant role in the prevalence of asthma. Blacks have the highest prevalence, followed by whites and Hispanics (10.2% vs. 7.6% vs. 6.8%, respectively) (4). If asthma is not controlled, it can result in death. Over a 3-year period (2001–2003), 4,210 asthma-related deaths occurred, of which over 50% occurred in persons older than age 65. These prevalence, morbidity, and mortality data demonstrate the significant public health burden of asthma in the United States and why the Centers for Disease Control and Prevention (CDC) have established an asthma public health approach, which includes the collection of standardized comprehensive surveillance data (3).

Etiology, Signs, and Symptoms

Asthma is a common chronic, complex, airway disorder that is characterized by airflow obstruction, bronchial hyperresponsiveness, and an underlying inflammation that leads to variable degrees of symptoms, such as difficulty breathing (paroxysmal dyspnea), wheezing, and cough (6). The National Institutes of Health (NIH) Expert Panel Report 3, "Guidelines for the Diagnosis and Management of Asthma," simply defines asthma as a chronic inflammatory response of the airways (6,7).

The most common form of asthma is allergic asthma (atopic or extrinsic asthma), and it is associated with environmental allergens, such as plant pollens, house dust mites (*Dermatophagoides farinae*), domestic pet dander, molds, and foods. The less common form, intrinsic asthma, has no known allergic cause and usually occurs in adults older than 35 years. Intrinsic asthma may result from an autonomic dysfunction characterized by excess cholinergic and/or tachykinin activity, but this hypothesis has never been proven (8). Aside from environmental allergens, an asthmatic attack may be precipitated by respiratory infection, strenuous physical exercise, polyps, drugs (e.g., aspirin and β-adrenergic antagonists), and environmental pollutants, primarily cigarette smoke. Strong emotional stress and breathing cold dry air can also precipitate an asthmatic onset (9).

Why has there been a marked increase in asthma in affluent industrialized countries? To answer this question, recent thought has focused on the "hygiene hypothesis," which implicates an imbalance of TH_1 and TH_2 lymphocytes as a major cause of the increased prevalence of asthma (10). The TH_1 lymphocytes are the type of $CD4^+$ T lymphocyte associated with defense against bacterial infection, whereas the TH_2 type predominates in allergic inflammation. The hypothesis claims that because bacterial infections have significantly decreased in industrialized nations, there is an imbalance, in

CLINICAL SIGNIFICANCE

The therapeutic approach to the management of asthma and chronic obstructive pulmonary disease (COPD) has changed dramatically over the past several decades. Treatment guidelines have evolved based on a better understanding of these disease states as well as on the development of newer and more efficacious treatment modalities through the application of structure-activity relationships (SARs) of chemical lead compounds. Although both disease states are characterized by pulmonary obstruction and chronic inflammation, the nature of such pulmonary abnormalities differ between the two conditions. Traditional therapy had focused on the symptomatic relief of airflow obstruction through the use of bronchodilators, such as adrenergic agonists and anticholinergics. Today, however, evidence-based consensus guidelines for the treatment of asthma emphasize interventions to manage the underlying inflammation of this condition and minimize disease progression. Likewise, the goal of managing COPD is to use agents to achieve and maintain clinical control by preserving airway patency.

The current therapeutic approach to managing these diseases includes the use of rapidly acting drugs to relieve acute symptoms as well as the use of maintenance medications either to minimize inflammation or control long-term symptoms, thereby limiting the need for symptomatic relief. Short-acting adrenergic agonists are those most commonly used to manage acute exacerbations of these disease states. Though effective, older agents, such as epinephrine and isoproterenol, were limited in their pharmacokinetic profile as well as in their lack of pulmonary selectivity. Modifying the chemical structure of these compounds, however, has resulted in the development of agents with significant clinical advantages in terms of duration of action and adverse effects profiles. Similarly, the application of SAR principles to the development of anti-inflammatory agents, such as corticosteroids, leukotriene modifers, and mast-cell stabilizers, has lead to the availability of superior long-term controlling agents in terms of potency, pharmacokinetic profile, and safety.

When treating patients with asthma and COPD, clinicians should be mindful of the SARs of those agents being employed. The application of these principles should be used to determine the most appropriate drug therapy in light of patient-specific needs and desired outcomes. In addition, clinicians can look forward to the availability of newer and more clinically appropriate agents for the management of asthma and COPD as our understanding of these conditions evolve and as advances in medicinal chemistry and biotechnology result in the development of increasingly selective drug entities and improved receptor targeting modalities.

Joseph V. Etzel, Pharm.D.
Assistant Dean of Student Affairs
Associate Clinical Professor of Pharmacy
College of Pharmacy & Allied Health Professions
St. John's University
Jamaica, New York

susceptible children, in favor of the TH$_2$-type lymphocytes, and this imbalance therefore favors allergic asthma (11). However, it is an oversimplification to claim that asthma inflammation is simply an overproduction of TH$_2$-type lymphocytes. Recent studies have discovered that a number of other T-helper cell subtypes are also involved in allergic inflammation, including TH$_9$, TH$_{17}$, TH$_{25}$, and TH$_3$ cells, and that regulatory T cells also contribute to asthma pathogenesis (12).

Asthma frequently occurs in families, and studies have shown that this results, at least in part, from mutually shared genes (13,14). Asthma is a complex disorder and lacks a mendelian genetic pattern, so it is difficult to study. To date, however, genetic research indicates that what is inherited is the susceptibility to develop asthma. It is clear that genes alone are not responsible for the development of asthma, because environmental factors also play a major role. Numerous genes on various chromosomes have been linked to asthma. Table 39.1 shows several gene products that may influence the development of asthma (13–19). In reality, however, there is little correlation between gene expression and clinical symptoms. The one exception to this is the low-expression allele of macrophage migration inhibitory factor (MIF), which has been shown to have a strong association with patients who have mild asthma (20). Drug development of MIF inhibitors might lead to future treatments for asthma as well as other inflammatory diseases (21).

Pathogenesis of Asthma

For a long time, asthmatic symptoms were thought to be the result of airway smooth muscle abnormalities, resulting in episodic bronchoconstriction. Today, however, it is clear that the constriction of bronchial smooth muscle is only one of many effects of chronic airway inflammation. Evidence of inflammation appears very soon after the onset of symptoms; therefore, treatment algorithms for asthma now emphasize quick relief of the bronchoconstriction and the amelioration of the underlying inflammation (22).

Inflammation in asthma is characterized by mucous plugging, epithelial shedding, basement membrane thickening, inflammatory cell infiltration, and smooth muscle hypertrophy and hyperplasia. An acute extrinsic asthmatic attack begins when allergens interact with lung epithelia, which causes the release of cytokines (thymic stromal lymphopoietin [TSLP], interleukin

TABLE 39.1 Putative Asthma-Associated Gene Products

Gene Products
β_2-Adrenergic receptor
Interleukin-4, -5, -9, and -13
Interleukin-4 receptor α (Il-4Rα)
β Chain of the high-affinity immunoglobulin E receptor (FcεRIβ)
Tumor necrosis factor α (TNFα)
Major histochemical complex (MHC)
T-cell receptor a/δ complex
ADAM33 (a disintegrin and metalloproteinase)
Dipeptidyl peptidase 10
PHD finer protein 11
Prostanoid DP1 receptor
Macrophage migration inhibitory factor (MIF)

[IL]-33, and IL-25). TSLP mediates migration and maturation of dendritic cells and production of IL-4 from competent T-helper cells (T_{FH}), leading to the activation of B cells to produce immunoglobulin (Ig) E antibody, which in turn binds to high-affinity Fc IgE receptors (FCεRI) on the mast cells. Activation of mast cells occurs when an antigen cross-links with IgEs on their surface. This IgE complex triggers mast cell degranulation, leading to the rapid release of inflammatory mediators, such as histamine, prostaglandins, leukotrienes, and cytokines (including tumor necrosis factor-α and ILs). The initial attack generally resolves within an hour; however, a second phase begins 4 to 6 hours after exposure and can last up to 24 hours. This late phase is the result of recruitment of additional inflammatory cells, primarily eosinophils, by the release of cytokines (IL-4, IL-13, IL-5, IL-9, and IL-3) from macrophages and TH_2-type lymphocytes in the lower lung (Fig. 39.1) (23,24).

Clinical Evaluation

Most patients with asthma are asymptomatic between acute exacerbations. The onset of symptoms can be sudden or gradual and frequently occurs during the night or early in the morning. Acute symptoms include shortness of breath, wheezing or whistling at the end of exhalation, cough, and chest tightness. Patients with chronic and poorly controlled asthma develop barrel chest and diminished diaphragm movement, both of which are evidence of chronic pulmonary hyperinflation.

Acute asthmatic attacks may be mild, moderate, or severe depending on the degree of airway obstruction. The determination of the degree of airflow obstruction is accomplished by pulmonary function testing. The most common pulmonary function test uses spirometry, which measures the rate at which the lung changes volume during forced breathing maneuvers. The most important spirometric measure is the forced vital capacity (FVC). This requires the patient to exhale as rapidly and as completely as possible after a maximal inhalation. Normal lungs generally can empty their volume in 6 seconds or less. When airflow is obstructed, however, the expiratory time may increase by as much as fivefold. In practice, the forced expiratory volume in 1 second (FEV_1) is measured and compared to the FVC and then recorded as the ratio of FEV_1 to FVC (FEV_1/FVC) (Fig. 39.2) (measurement is done by means of a spirometer). Healthy persons normally can expel at least 75% of their FVC in the first second. Decreases in the FEV_1/FVC ratio indicate obstruction, and a decrease below 40% indicates severe asthma (22,23).

A more convenient way to measure airway obstruction is to determine the peak expiratory flow (PEF) rate. The PEF rate correlates well with the FEV_1; can be determined using inexpensive, handheld, peak flow meters; and is easily and simply measured at home. The PEF rate is the maximal rate of flow that is produced through forced expiration. Peak flow meters come with a chart that lists predicted PEF rates based on the patient's age, gender, and height. The patient or clinician can then compare the determined PEF rate with the predicted PEF rate and make an evaluation regarding the severity of an asthmatic attack. The PEF rate or the FEV_1/FVC ratio, along with the frequency of daytime and nighttime symptoms, forms the basis for the classification of the severity of an asthmatic attack. Table 39.2 shows the severity classification of asthma established by the NIH Expert Panel Report 3, "Guidelines for the Diagnosis and Management of Asthma" (6).

GENERAL THERAPEUTIC APPROACHES TO THE TREATMENT AND MANAGEMENT OF ASTHMA

Asthma symptoms are caused by bronchoconstriction and inflammation, and approaches to treatment are directed at both of these physiologic problems. Therefore, drugs that affect adrenergic/cholinergic bronchial smooth muscle tone and drugs that inhibit the inflammatory process are used to treat and control asthma symptoms. In the normal lung, bronchiole smooth muscle tone results from the balance between the bronchoconstrictive effects of the cholinergic system and the bronchodilating effects of the adrenergic system on the smooth muscles of the bronchioles. Pharmacologic treatment of asthmatic bronchoconstriction consists of either increasing adrenergic tone with an adrenergic agonist or inhibiting cholinergic tone with an anticholinergic agent.

The inflammatory effects seen in asthma are the result of the release of physiologically active chemicals from a variety of inflammatory cells. Pharmacologic treatment, therefore, uses anti-inflammatory drugs

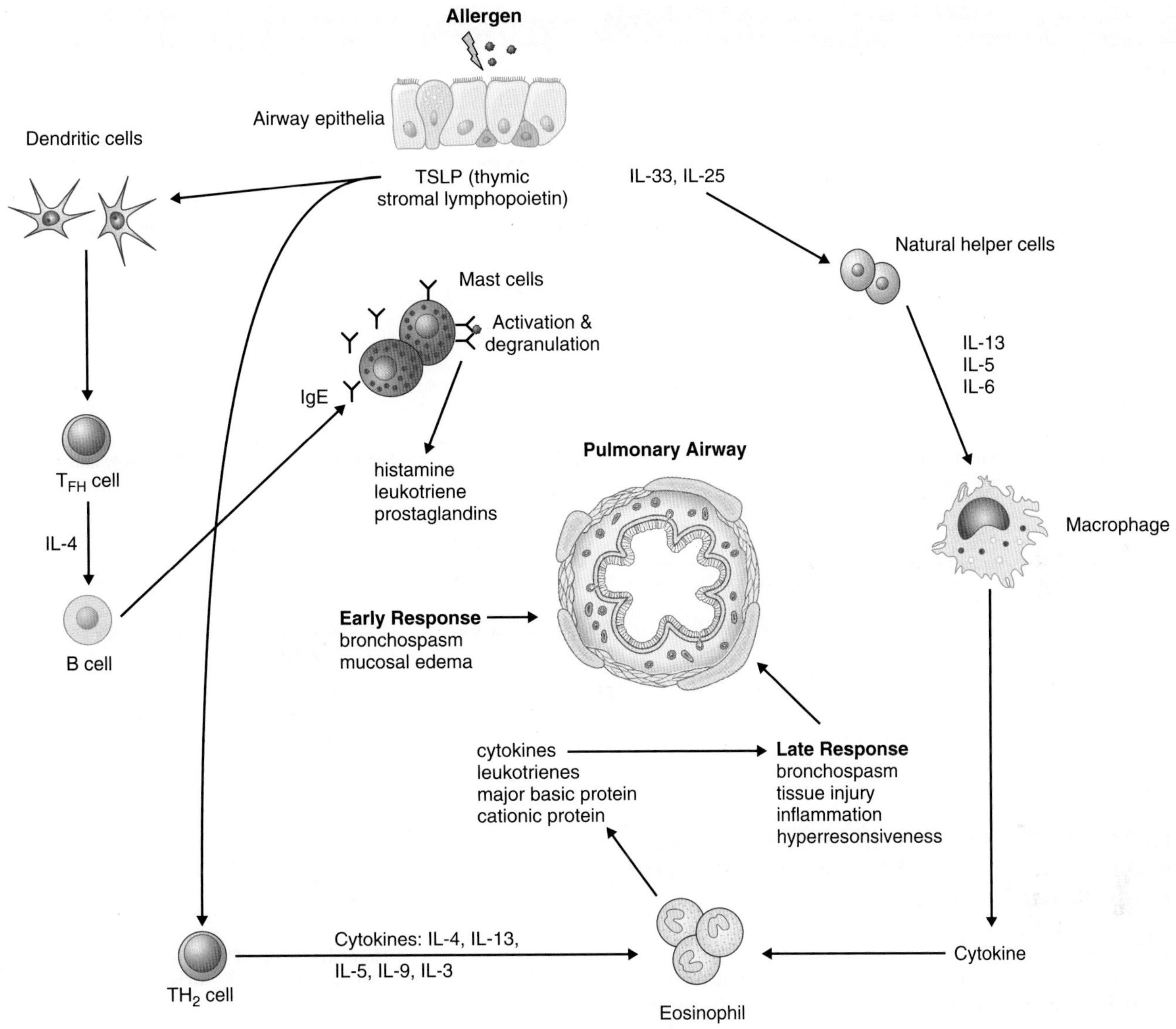

FIGURE 39.1 Pictorial summary of asthma pathogenesis.

(corticosteroids), mast cell stabilizers, leukotriene modifiers, and IgE monoclonal antibodies. Figure 39.3 depicts the overall approach to the pharmacologic treatment of asthma.

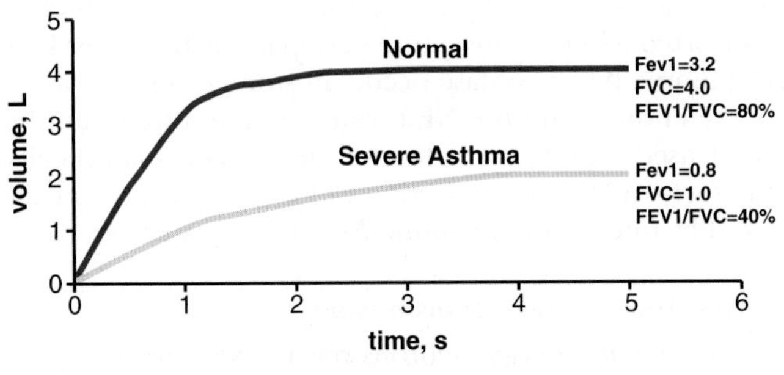

FIGURE 39.2 Spirometric comparison of normal and severe asthma. FEV_1, forced expiratory volume in 1 second; FVC, forced vital capacity.

Therapeutic management of asthma requires the use of quick-acting drugs to relieve an acute attack as well as drugs that control symptoms over the long-term. The current approach to asthma management uses a stepwise approach (6). The quick-reliever medication is almost always an inhaled short-acting β_2-adrenergic agonist, whereas controller drugs are inhaled corticosteroids, long-acting β_2-agonists, leukotriene modifiers, cromolyn sodium, and/or methylxanthines. The dose, route of administration, and number of controller drugs depend on the severity of the patient's disease. Recently, the U.S. Food and Drug Administration (FDA) has recommended that long-acting β_2-agonists should never be used alone in the treatment of asthma in children or adults based on analyses of studies showing an increased risk of severe worsening of asthma symptoms, leading to hospitalizations and even death in some patients (25). Table 39.3 shows the stepwise approach to asthma management based on disease severity.

TABLE 39.2 Classification of Asthma Severity (6)

Components of Severity		Intermittent Step 1		Persistent	
			Mild Step 2	Moderate Step 3	Severe Step 4 or 5
	Symptoms	≤ 2 days/week	>2 days/week but not daily	Daily	Throughout the day
Impairment	Nighttime awakenings	≤ 2x/month	3-4x/month	>1x/week but not nightly	Often 7x/week
Normal FEV_1/FCV:	Rescue inhaler use	≤ 2 days/week	> 2 days/week but not daily and not > 1x on any day	Daily	Several times per day
8-19 yr 85%					
20-39 yr 80%					
40-59 yr 75%	Interference with normal activity	None	Minor limitation	Some limitation	Extremely limited
60-80 yr 70%					
	Lung function	Normal FEV_1 between exacerbation			
		FEV_1 >80% predicted	FEV_1 >80% predicted	FEV_1 >60% but <80% predicted	FEV_1 <60% predicted
		FEV_1/FVC normal	FEV_1/FVC normal	FEV_1/FVC reduced 5%	FEV_1/FVC reduced >5%

FEV1, forced expiratory volume in 1 second; FVC, forced vital capacity

THERAPEUTIC CLASSES OF DRUGS USED TO TREAT ASTHMA AND CHRONIC OBSTRUCTIVE PULMONARY DISEASE

β_2-Adrenergic Agonists

What structural features make a drug an adrenergic agonist? What features make it a selective β_2-agonist? The answers to these questions lie in the structural relationship of a drug to that of norepinephrine (NE), the physiologic neurotransmitter of the sympathetic branch of the autonomic nervous system. Drugs that act on postsynaptic sympathetic receptors in the same way as NE are called sympathomimetics or, more commonly, adrenergic agonists. The related natural agonist epinephrine (EPI; adrenalin) is the predominant adrenergic hormone produced in the chromaffin cells of the adrenal medulla. EPI interacts just like NE at all adrenergic receptors.

Chemistry and Biochemistry of Norepinephrine and Epinephrine

Chemically, NE is classified as a catecholamine. A catechol is a 1,2-dihydroxybenzene, and NE is a β-hydroxyethylaminodihydroxybenzene. EPI is the *N*-methyl derivative of NE, and they both have acidic and basic functional groups. Physiologically, however, they behave as a base, being more than 90% protonated at pH 7.4 ($pK_a = 9.6$) and functioning as an ionized acid.

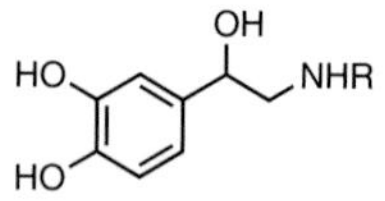

Norepinephrine R = H
Epinephrine R = CH_3

NE is biosynthesized in the neurons of both the central nervous system and the autonomic nervous system, whereas EPI is formed in the chromaffin cells of the adrenal medulla. Both NE and EPI are derived from L-tyrosine by a series of enzyme-catalyzed reactions (Fig. 39.4 depicts the overall pathway). L-Tyrosine hydroxylase hydroxylates the meta position of L-tyrosine, producing L-dihydroxyphenylalanine (L-DOPA), and is the rate-limiting step. The L-DOPA is then decarboxylated by L-aromatic amino acid decarboxylase to form dopamine, which is converted to NE by the action of dopamine β-hydroxylase. Dopamine β-hydroxylase occurs in storage vesicles of the nerve ending, and the NE formed is stored there until it is released into the synaptic cleft. In the chromaffin cells, the formed NE is converted to EPI by *N*-methylation catalyzed by phenylethanolamine *N*-methyltransferase.

Termination of Neurotransmission

Stimulated adrenergic neurons release NE into the synaptic cleft, which then binds reversibly with receptors to produce a characteristic adrenergic response. Termination

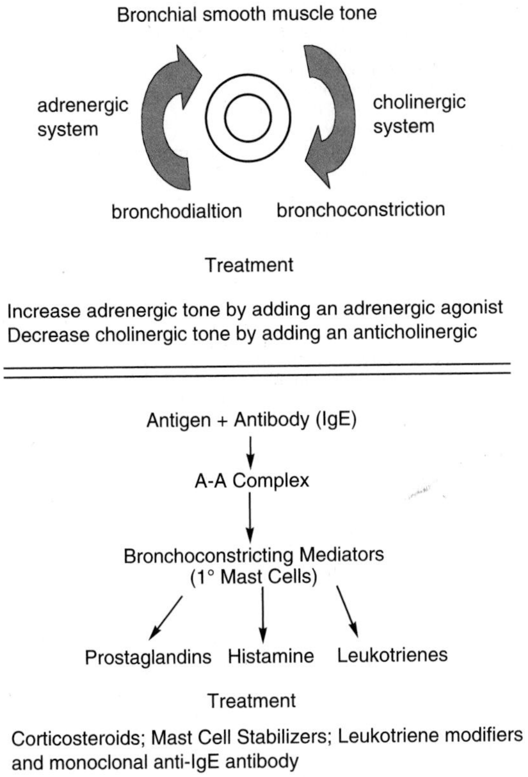

FIGURE 39.3 Overview of pharmacologic treatment for asthma.

of the adrenergic response occurs primarily by reuptake (uptake-1) into the presynaptic neuron; however, diffusion away from the receptors and extracellular metabolism also occur to a limited extent. The NE that is taken back up into the presynaptic neuron is either used again as a neurotransmitter or is metabolized by mitochondrial monoamine oxidase (MAO). The extraneuronal NE that diffuses away from the neurons is either metabolized by catechol *O*-methyl transferase (COMT) in situ or reaches the circulatory system and is metabolized by COMT and MAO in various tissues, most importantly the liver, gastrointestinal (GI) tract, and the lungs. Figure 39.5 depicts the possible metabolic pathways for both NE and EPI. It is important to note that agonists that are resistant to MAO and/or COMT have greater oral availability and longer duration of action.

Adrenergic Receptors

The adrenergic receptors have long been pharmacologically classified as α or β based on their interaction with NE, EPI, and the adrenergic prototype, isoproterenol (26).

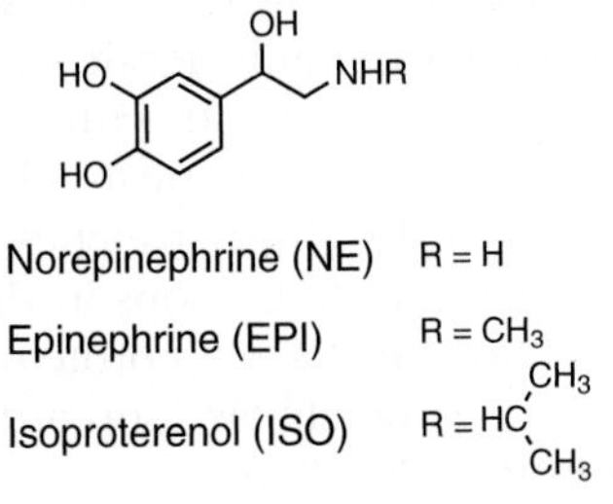

TABLE 39.3 Stepwise Medication Management of Asthma

All Asthma Patients: Short-acting inhaled β_2-agonist as needed for acute exacerbations (SABA)

Severity Classification	Long-term Control
Step 1: Intermittent Asthma Persistent Asthma	*Preferred*: SABA PRN
Step 2: Mild	*Preferred:* Low-dose Inhaled corticosteroid (ICS) *Alternative:* Cromolyn, Nedocromil, Leukotriene receptor antagonist (LTRA) or theophylline
Step 3: Moderate	*Preferred:* Low-dose ICS + long-acting β_2-agonist (LABA) or medium-dose ICS *Alternative:* Low-dose ICS + either LTRA, Theophylline or Zileutin
Step 4: Severe	*Preferred:* Medium-dose ICS + LABA *Alternative:* Medium-dose ICS + either LTRA, Theophylline or Zileutin
Step 5: Severe	*Preferred:* High-dose ICS + LABA and *Consider:* Omalizumab for patients who have allergies
Step 6: Severe	*Preferred:* High-dose ICS + LABA + oral corticosteroid and *Consider:* Omalizumab for patients who have allergies

NE and EPI are nonselective and interact with all adrenergic receptors, but isoproterenol selectively interacts only with the β-receptors. The adrenergic receptors have been further divided into three groups, α_1, α_2, and β, each of

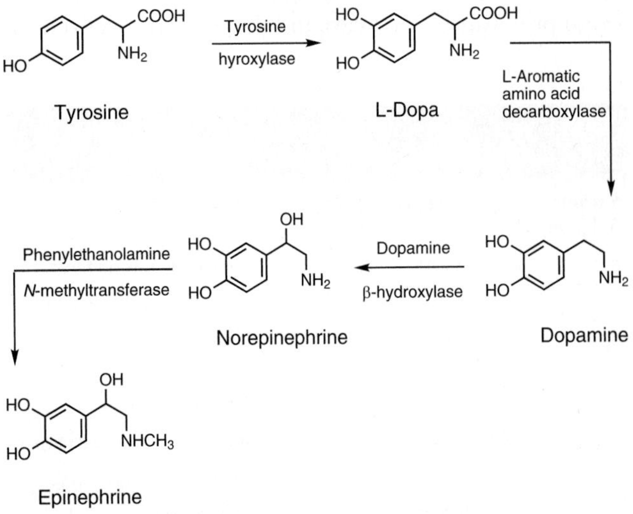

FIGURE 39.4 The biosynthesis of norepinephrine and epinephrine from tyrosine.

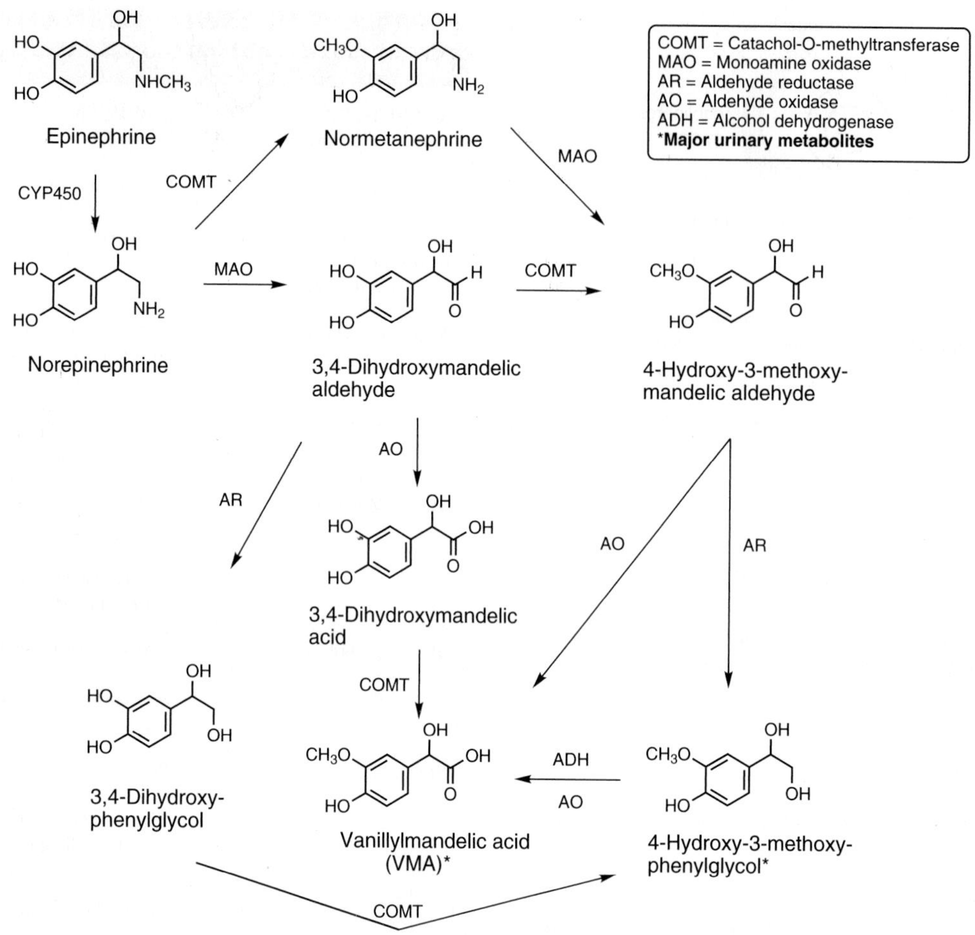

FIGURE 39.5 Metabolic pathways for norepinephrine and epinephrine.

which has been further divided into three receptor subtypes based on their organ distribution and physiologic activities (27). Therefore, there are now a total of nine adrenergic receptor subtypes, but the most important in relation to the treatment of asthma and chronic obstructive pulmonary disease (COPD) are the β_1 and β_2 subtypes that are found primarily in the heart and the lung, respectively. As may be deduced from Table 39.4, adrenergic agonists that are selective for the β_2 subtype will cause bronchial dilation and might be expected to relieve the bronchospasm of an asthmatic attack. Nonselective β-agonists, however, will have stimulatory cardiac effects and, therefore, would have limited use in cardiac patients with asthma.

TABLE 39.4 Physiologic Response in Relationship to β-Receptor Subtype and Organ Site

Receptor Subtype	Organ Location	Response
β_1	Heart	Increased rate and force
		Increase conduction velocity
β_2	Bronchiole smooth muscle	Dilation
	Intestine	Decreased motility
	Liver	Increased gluconeogenesis
		Increased glycogenolysis
	Uterus	Contraction
	Lungs	Bronchial dilation

Adrenergic Receptor Structure and Agonist Interactions

The adrenergic receptors are members of the guanine nucleotide binding regulatory protein–coupled receptor family more commonly referred to as G protein–coupled receptors. They affect biologic activity by releasing secondary messenger molecules inside the cell after they bind an extracellular agonist. This process usually is referred to as signal transduction and is common to hormone and neurotransmitter receptors found in the muscarinic, serotonergic, dopaminergic, and adrenergic systems. All the G protein–coupled receptors are structurally similar, being comprised of seven transmembrane α-helix bundles. The helices are connected by short stretches of hydrophilic residues, which form multiple loops in the intracellular and extracellular domains. The G proteins generally are bound to the third intracellular loop and imbedded in the inner membrane (Fig. 39.6).

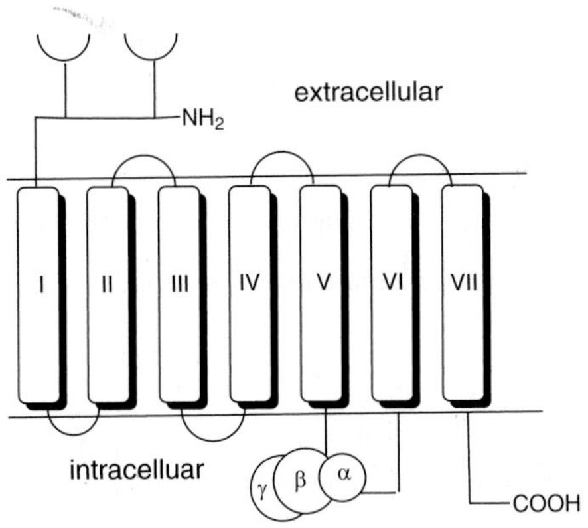

FIGURE 39.6 Representations of the G protein–coupled receptor.

All the β-adrenergic receptors are coupled to adenylate cyclase via specific G stimulatory proteins (Gs). When agonist binds to the β-adrenergic receptors, the α-subunit migrates through the membrane and stimulates adenylate cyclase to form cyclic adenosine monophosphate (cAMP) from adenosine triphosphate. Once formed in the cell, cAMP activates protein kinase A, which catalyzes the phosphorylation of numerous proteins, thereby regulating their activity and leading to characteristic cellular responses. The intracellular enzyme phosphodiesterase (PDE) hydrolyzes cAMP to form adenosine monophosphate (AMP) and terminates its action (Fig. 39.7).

A great deal of research has been done to identify the binding residues of the adrenergic receptors. Molecular modeling methods have been used to construct three-dimensional models for agonist complexes with the β-adrenergic receptors. The picture that has emerged is that NE binds ionically via its protonated amine to Asp-113 in helix 3 and hydrogen bonds to both hydroxyls of the catechol ring with Ser-204 and Ser-207 in helix 5. That binding limits configurational and rotational freedoms, which allows reinforcing van der Waals interactions between the aromatic ring with residues Phe-290 in helix 6 and Val-114 in helix 3. The *N*-alkyl substituents are believed to fit into a pocket formed between aliphatic residues in helix 6 and helix 7. Stereochemistry also plays an important role in receptor binding. The β-carbon in NE/EPI is chiral and can be either *R* or *S* in configuration. Endogenous NE/EPI exists in the *R* configuration so that the β-hydroxyl is oriented toward the receptor Asn-293 (28,29) (Fig. 39.8).

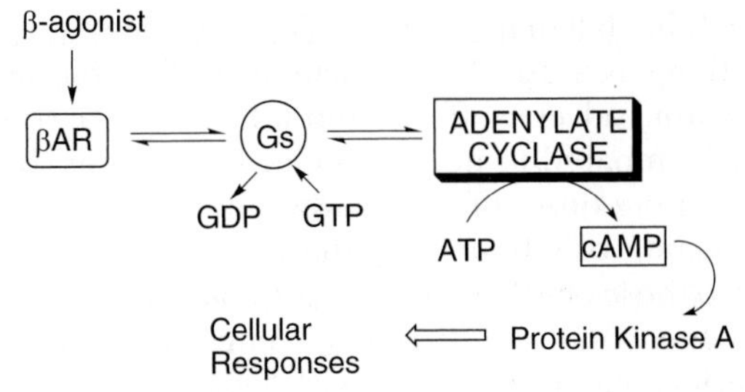

FIGURE 39.7 β-Adrenergic receptor G protein coupling to adenylate cyclase.

Adrenergic Agonist Structure–Activity Relationships

The fundamental pharmacophore for all adrenergic agonists is a substituted β-phenylethylamine (Table 39.5). The nature and number of substituents on the pharmacophore influences whether an analog will be direct-acting or indirect-acting or have a mixture of direct and indirect action. In addition, the nature and number of substituents also influences the specificity for the β-receptor subtypes. Direct-acting adrenergic agonists bind the β-adrenergic receptors just like NE/EPI, producing a sympathetic response. Indirect-acting agonists cause their effect by a number of mechanisms. They can stimulate the release of NE from the presynaptic terminal, inhibit the reuptake of released NE, or inhibit the metabolic degradation of NE by neuronal MAO (i.e., MAO inhibitors). Mixed-acting agonists work as their name implies (i.e., they have both direct and indirect abilities). Table 39.5 shows the relationship between substituents and the mechanisms of action by adrenergic agonists.

Relationship of Structure to α- or β-Receptor Selectivity

The substituents on the amino group (R_1) determine α- or β-receptor selectivity. As was noted earlier, when the *N*-substituent was changed from hydrogen (NE) to methyl (EPI) to isopropyl, the receptor affinity went from nonselective for NE/EPI to β-selective for isopropyl. Therefore, one can say that the larger the bulk of the *N*-substituent, the greater the selectivity for the β-receptor. As a matter of fact, if R_1 is *t*-butyl or aralkyl, there is complete loss of α-receptor affinity, and the β-receptor affinity shows preference for the β_2-receptor. It must be said that receptor selectivity is dose related, and when the dose is high enough, all selectivity can be lost.

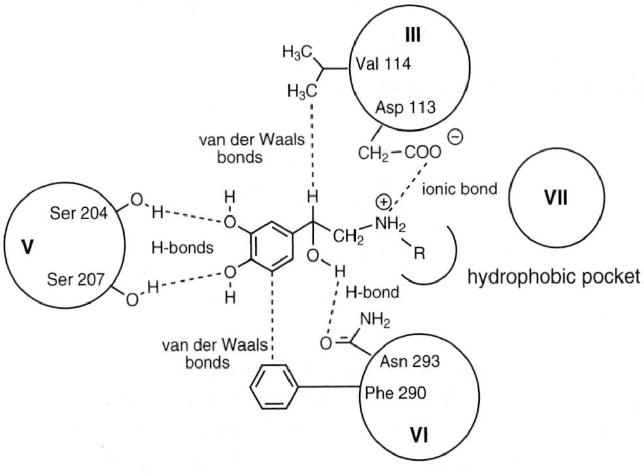

FIGURE 39.8 Ligand binding to key residues in the adrenergic receptor.

TABLE 39.5 Relationship of Substituents to Adrenergic Agonist Mechanism of Action

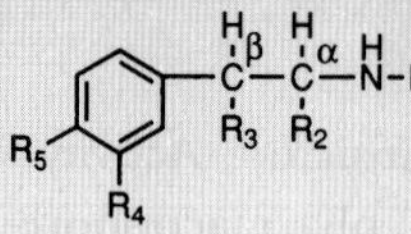

Action	R_3	R_4	R_5
Direct[a]	OH	OH	OH
or	OH	OH	H
Indirect[b]	H	H	H
or	H	H	OH
Mixed[c]	H	OH	OH
or	OH	H	OH

[a]β-OH (R_3) necessary for direct action, optimal if in the R-configuration; *m*-OH (R_4) also necessary for direct action; *p*-OH (R_5) can be an H or OH, however catechol optimal.
[b]Without the catechol OHs (R_4 and R_5) or β-OH (R_3) there is little affinity for the β-receptor; *p*-OH does not contribute to β-receptor binding affinity.
[c]β-OH (R_3) or *m*-OH (R_4) contribute to direct action.

Substituents on the α-carbon (R_2) other than hydrogen will show an increased duration of action, because they make the compound resistant to metabolism by MAO. In addition, if the substituent is ethyl, there is selectivity for the β_2-receptor, which is enhanced by a bulky *N*-substituent. Interestingly, α-methyl substitution shows a slight β-receptor enhancement and only for the *S*-configuration.

For an adrenergic agonist to demonstrate significant β_2-receptor selectivity, there needs to be, in addition to the bulky *N*-substituent, an appropriately substituted phenyl ring. The currently marketed adrenergic agonists contain a resorcinol ring, a salicyl alcohol moiety, or an *m*-formamide group (Fig. 39.9). In addition, these ring configurations are resistant to COMT metabolism and will increase the duration of action.

Specific Adrenergic Drugs Used to Treat Asthma

For a more detailed discussion of the chemistry of adrenergic agents, see Chapter 10.

Epinephrine (Adrenalin)

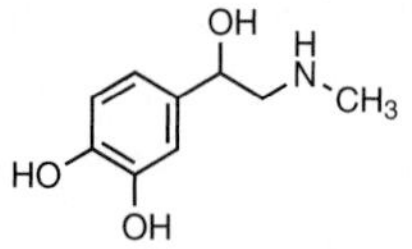

Epinephrine (Epi Pen)

The combination of the catechol nucleus, the β-hydroxyl group, and the *N*-methyl give EPI a direct action and a strong affinity for all adrenergic receptors. Epinephrine and all other catechols are chemically susceptible to oxygen and other oxidizing agents, especially in the presence of bases and light, quickly decomposing to inactive quinones. Therefore, all catechol drugs are stabilized with antioxidants and dispensed in air-tight amber containers.

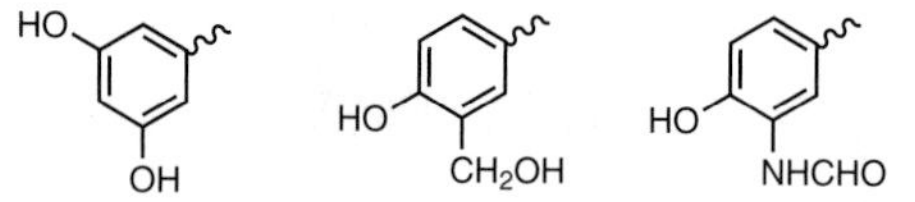

Resorcinol   Salicyl alcohol   *N*-formamide

FIGURE 39.9 Ring configurations that contribute to β_2-receptor selectivity.

Epinephrine is ultimately metabolized by COMT and MAO to 3-methoxy-4-hydroxymandelic acid (vanillylmandelic acid), which is excreted as the sulfate or glucuronide in the urine (Fig. 39.5). Only a very small amount is excreted unchanged.

Epinephrine usually is administered slowly by intravenous (IV) injection to relieve acute asthmatic attacks not controlled by other treatments. IV injection produces an immediate response. Use of EPI with drugs that enhance cardiac arrhythmias (digitalis or quinidine) is not recommended. Tricyclic antidepressants and MAO inhibitors will potentiate the effects of EPI on the heart. Epinephrine should be used with caution in individuals suffering from hyperthyroidism, cardiovascular disease, hypertension, or diabetes. Adverse effects include palpitations, tachycardia, sweating, nausea and vomiting, respiratory difficulty, dizziness, tremor, apprehension, and anxiety.

Isoetharine Hydrochloride

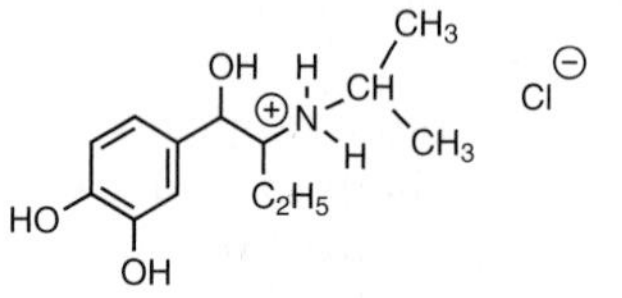

Isoetharine hydrochloride

The α-ethyl group confers β_2-selectivity, and the β-hydroxyl group and catechol nucleus makes it a direct-acting drug. It is susceptible to COMT metabolism; however, the α-ethyl group inhibits MAO. Therefore, one would expect some oral activity.

Isoetharine is dispensed as a solution only for inhalation administration to treat reversible bronchospasm of asthma. It has fallen into relative disuse, because with high doses, there is a significant incidence of cardiovascular (β_1-receptor) adverse effects, and it has a low β_2-receptor potency compared to newer β_2-selective agonists. It has a 2- to 4-minute onset of action when inhaled and a duration of action of 3 hours. Isoetharine has adverse effects similar to those of EPI, including palpitations, tachycardia, nausea and vomiting, dizziness, tremor, and headache. Isoetharine may cause decreased levels of theophylline when coadministered. Cardiovascular effects are a concern when isoetharine is taken with other asthma drugs.

Metaproterenol Sulfate

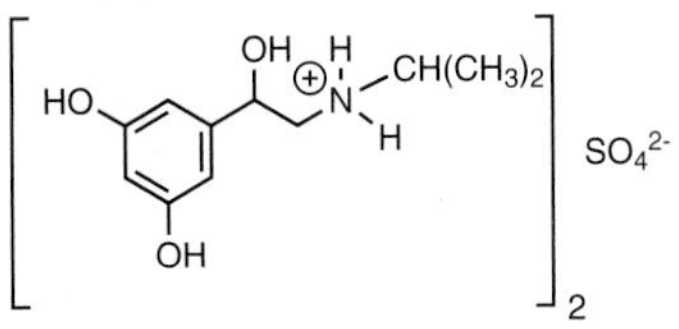

Metaproterenol sulfate
(Alupent, Metaprel)

Metaproterenol is a direct-acting resorcinol analog of isoproterenol. The *N*-isopropyl is β-directing, and the combination with the resorcinol ring system enhances the selectivity for the β_2-receptors. It is the least potent of the β_2-selective agonists, however, most likely because of the poor β_2-selectivity of the isopropyl group. It has good oral bioavailability being resistant to COMT and only slowly metabolized by MAO. When administered orally, it has an onset of approximately 30 minutes with a 4-hour duration. Inhaled metaproterenol can have an onset as rapidly as 5 minutes; however, it can be as long as 30 minutes in susceptible individuals. Metaproterenol is available in tablet, syrup, and inhalation dosage forms and is recommended for bronchial asthma attacks and treatment of acute asthmatic attacks in children 6 years of age and older (5% solution for inhalation only). Metaproterenol has the same adverse effect profile as other adrenergic agonists, but with a decreased incidence of arrhythmias.

Terbutaline Sulfate

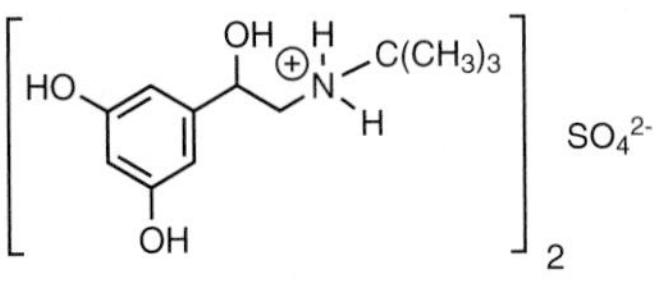

Terbutaline sulfate
(Brethine, Brethaire)

Terbutaline is the *N-t*-butyl analog of metaproterenol and, as such, would be expected to have a more potent β_2-selectivity. When compared to metaproterenol, terbutaline has a threefold greater potency at the β_2-receptor. Like metaproterenol, it is resistant to COMT and slowly metabolized by MAO, and thus has good oral bioavailability, with similar onset and duration. Terbutaline is available as tablets and solutions for injection and inhalation. Adverse effects are similar to other direct-acting β_2-selective agonists, but with a greater incidence of palpitations.

Bitolterol Mesylate

Bitolterol is a prodrug that releases colterol on activation by esterases in the lung (Fig. 39.10). Colterol is a direct-acting agonist, and the *N-t*-butyl group makes it β_2-selective with a binding potency equivalent to that of isoetharine and terbutaline. The ester form is lipophilic, which helps to keep it local in the lung and resistant to COMT, which tends to increase its duration of action.

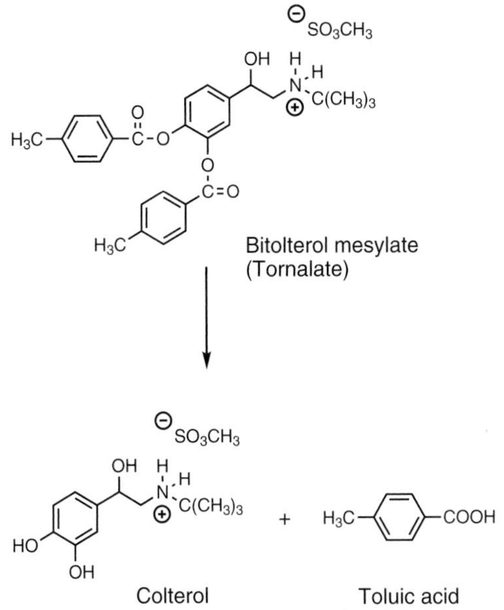

FIGURE 39.10 Esterase hydrolysis of bitolterol.

Onset begins 2 to 4 minutes after administration, and the effect can last as long as 8 hours. It has an adverse effect profile similar to that of other β_2-selective agonists, with less drowsiness and restlessness compared to other direct-acting agonists.

Albuterol

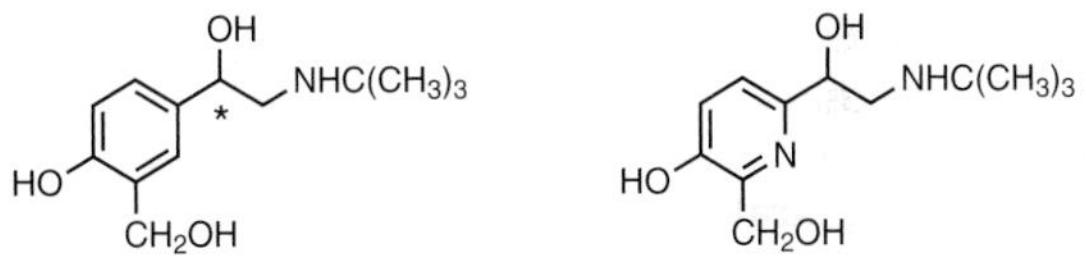

dl-Albuterol (Proventil, Ventolin)
Levalbuterol (Xopenex)

Pirbuterol (Maxair)

Albuterol has the *N-t*-butyl and a salicyl alcohol phenyl ring, which gives it optimal β_2-selectivity. It is resistant to COMT and slowly metabolized by MAO, thus having good oral bioavailability. Its onset by inhalation is within 5 minutes, with a duration of action between 4 and 8 hours. It currently is the drug of choice for relief of the acute bronchospasm of an asthmatic attack. Levalbuterol is the *R*-(−)-isomer of albuterol and is available only in solution to be administered via nebulizer. Because it is the active isomer, the dose is fourfold less than that of albuterol. Pirbuterol is the pyridine isostere of albuterol. It has pharmacokinetics similar to albuterol but is half as potent at the β_2-receptor. Pirbuterol is only available as an inhaler, whereas albuterol comes in tablet, syrup, solution, and aerosol formulations. Adverse effects of pirbuterol are nervousness, tremor, and headache, which are less than the profile for albuterol, which adds nausea, vomiting, dizziness, hypertension, insomnia, tachycardia, and palpitations.

Salmeterol Xinafoate

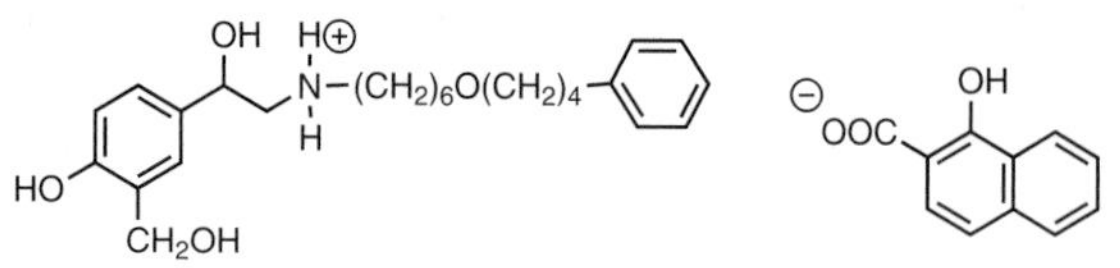

Salmeterol xinafoate
(Serevent diskus)

Salmeterol has an *N*-phenylbutoxyhexyl substituent in combination with a β-hydroxyl group and a salicyl phenyl ring for optimal direct-acting β_2-receptor selectivity and potency. Salmeterol has the greatest receptor affinity of all the adrenergic agonists. It is resistant to both MAO and COMT and that, together with its increased lipophilicity, gives salmeterol a long duration of action. It is postulated that the phenylbutoxyhexyl *N*-substituent binds outside of the receptor site and keeps the active pharmacophore moiety in position for prolonged stimulations. It is available only as a powder for inhalation, with a 20-minute onset of action, which lasts for 12 hours. It is used as a controller for the long-term treatment of asthma and is not recommended for quick relief of an acute attack. It also is available in combination with the steroid fluticasone propionate (Advair Diskus). There was a small but significant increase in asthma-related deaths among patients receiving salmeterol during a large clinical trial, and as a result, the FDA has recommended that it not be used as monotherapy for asthma in either children or adults. Subgroup analyses suggested that the risk may be greater in black patients compared with Caucasian patients (25,30).

Formoterol Fumarate

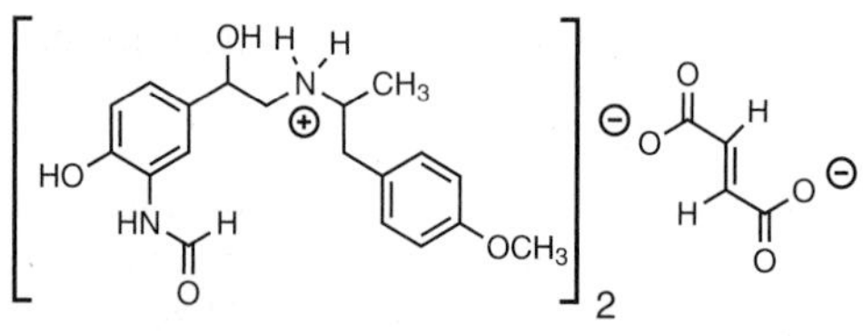

Formoterol fumarate (Foradil aerosolizer)
Arformoterol (*R,R*-Formoterol [Brovana])

Formoterol has a β-directing *N*-isopropyl-*p*-methoxyphenyl group and a unique *m*-formamide and *p*-hydroxyphenyl ring, which provides selectivity for β_2-receptors. It is resistant to MAO and COMT, making it a long-acting agonist. The most prominent metabolic pathway involves direct glucuronidation at the phenolic hydroxyl group (31). *O*-Demethylation followed by conjugation at the phenolic 2′-hydroxyl group also occurs and appears to involve four cytochrome P450 isozymes (CYP2D6, CYP2C19, CYP2C9, and CYP2A6).

Formoterol has a more rapid onset as compared to salmeterol while maintaining the same long duration of action. This is believed to result from formoterol's greater water solubility, allowing it to get to receptor sites faster, whereas its moderate lipophilicity keeps it in the lungs longer. It is indicated for the long-term maintenance treatment of asthma and for patients with symptoms of nocturnal asthma who require regular treatment with inhaled, short-acting, β_2-agonists. It is not indicated for patients whose asthma can be managed by occasional use of inhaled, short-acting, β_2-agonists. Formoterol is available only as a powder in a capsule for administration via the aerosolizer. Patients should be cautioned not to take the capsules orally and to keep them in a safe place to avoid accidental oral administration.

Formoterol has two asymmetric centers and, therefore, can exist in four possible enantiomers. The *R,R*-enantiomer is active and reported to be 1,000 times more active than the *S,S*-enantiomer and twice as potent as racemic formoterol. It is available under the name arformoterol (Brovana), undergoes the same metabolism, and is only indicated for the treatment of COPD.

Fenoterol Hydrobromide

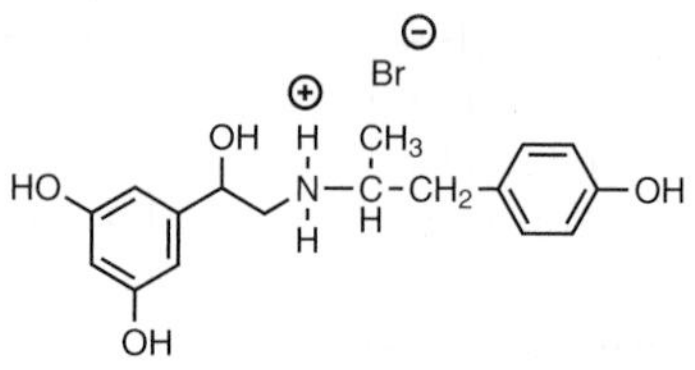

Fenoterol hydrobromide
(Berotec)

Fenoterol is an investigational drug in the United States that has been in use in Europe since 1970. It is the *p*-hydroxyphenyl derivative of metaproterenol, and the combination of the resorcinol ring and the bulky *p*-hydroxyphenyl isopropyl group on the nitrogen gives fenoterol significant β_2-receptor selectivity. It has approximately half the affinity for the β_2-receptor as compared to albuterol. The resorcinol ring is resistant to COMT metabolism, and the bulky nitrogen substituent greatly retards MOA metabolism as well giving fenoterol a reasonable oral bioavailability with pharmacokinetics similar to albuterol (i.e., rapid onset and a 4- to 6-hour duration of action after oral inhalation).

Antimuscarinics

Acetylcholine is the endogenous neurotransmitter of the parasympathetic nervous system. The parasympathetic nerve fibers are found in both the autonomic and central nervous systems. These fibers are classified into those that are stimulated by muscarine and those that are stimulated by nicotine. Nicotine, an alkaloid from *Nicotiana tabacum*, stimulates preganglionic fibers in both the parasympathetic and sympathetic systems as well as the somatic motor fibers of the skeletal system. Muscarine, an alkaloid from the poisonous mushroom *Amanita muscaria*, stimulates postganglionic parasympathetic fibers

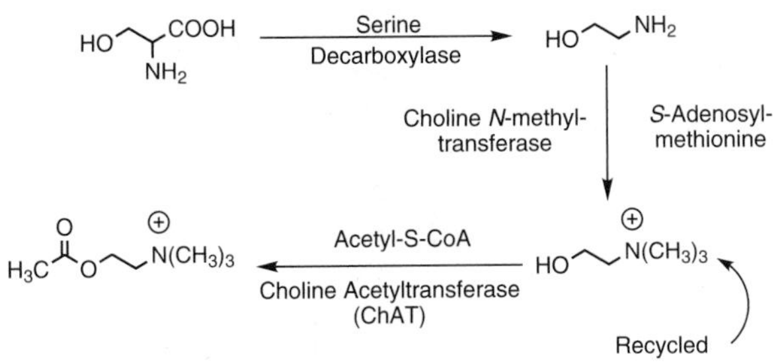

FIGURE 39.11 Biosynthesis of acetylcholine.

with receptors found on autonomic effector cells. The central nervous system has fibers that contain both nicotinic and muscarinic receptors. In this chapter, we are most interested in the drugs that block the muscarinic fibers (antimuscarinics), because blocking them results in cardiovascular, mydriatic, antispasmodic, antisecretory, and bronchodilatory effects.

Biochemistry and Metabolism of Acetylcholine

Acetylcholine is the ester formed between acetylcoenzyme A and choline by the action of choline acetyltransferase in the presynaptic cholinergic neurons. Most of the choline used to biosynthesize acetylcholine comes via uptake from the synaptic space, where it is produced from the hydrolysis of acetylcholine by acetylcholinesterase, a serine hydroxylase. Additionally, some choline is biosynthesized in the presynaptic neurons from serine (Fig. 39.11). Once formed, acetylcholine is stored in vesicles from which it is released on stimulation.

The duration of action of acetylcholine is very short, because it is rapidly hydrolyzed by the acetylcholinesterase present in the synaptic space. This hydrolysis is a straightforward splitting of the acetylcholine into acetic acid and choline; however, the way this happens is very interesting and begins by the proper binding of acetylcholine in the catalytic pocket. Binding of the cationic *N*-end to tyrosine, glutamate, and tryptophan via a combination of π-cation and electrostatic forces places the acyl head of acetylcholine in the correct position for attack by the serine hydroxyl group (Fig. 39.12).

Once properly bound, the hydrolysis actually involves two hydrolytic steps. The first step is the hydrolysis of acetylcholine by nucleophilic attack at the carbonyl carbon by the serine hydroxyl group, which liberates choline and leaves the enzyme acetylated. A triad formed between glutamine, histidine, and the serine at the catalytic site activates the serine for the nucleophilic attack. The second step is the hydrolysis of the acetylated enzyme by water to regenerate the free enzyme. The water is activated by hydrogen-bonding to the histidine residue, which increases the nucleophilic character of the oxygen of water. The activated water attacks the electrophilic carbonyl carbon of the acetyl group to generate acetate and regenerate the free hydroxyl group of serine (Fig. 39.13) (32).

Muscarinic Receptor Structure and Agonist/Antagonist Interactions

The muscarinic receptors are considered to be part of the superfamily of G protein–coupled receptors. They consist of seven transmembrane helices and are linked to their G protein through interaction with the second and third intracellular loops (33). There are five subtypes of receptor, designated M_{1-5}, and the odd-numbered receptors (M_1, M_3, and M_5) are coupled to the G_q/G_{11} class. This class of receptors activates intracellular phospholipase C to hydrolyze phosphatidylinositol 4,5-diphosphate to diacylglycerol and inositol triphosphate as intracellular messengers. The even-numbered receptors (M_2 and M_4) are coupled to the G_i/G_o class, which mediates the inhibition of adenylate cyclase (Fig. 39.14).

Table 39.6 lists the physiologic action of the M_3 receptors. Because the M_3 receptors cause bronchiole constriction, they counterbalance the bronchiole dilation of the β_2-adrenergic receptors in the lung, resulting in maintenance of bronchiole tone. This forms the basis for the therapeutic use of inhaled antimuscarinics, because they block cholinergic bronchiole constriction and allow adrenergic bronchiole dilation to help overcome the pulmonary constriction associated with an asthmatic attack.

Affinity labeling and mutagenic studies have established that acetylcholine binds to its receptor in a narrow region of the circular arrangement of the seven transmembrane helices approximately 10 to 15 angstroms away from the membrane surface. The cationic nitrogen of acetylcholine binds to the anionic carboxylate of an Asp located in helix 3 (34). As depicted in Figure 39.15, the ionic interaction is

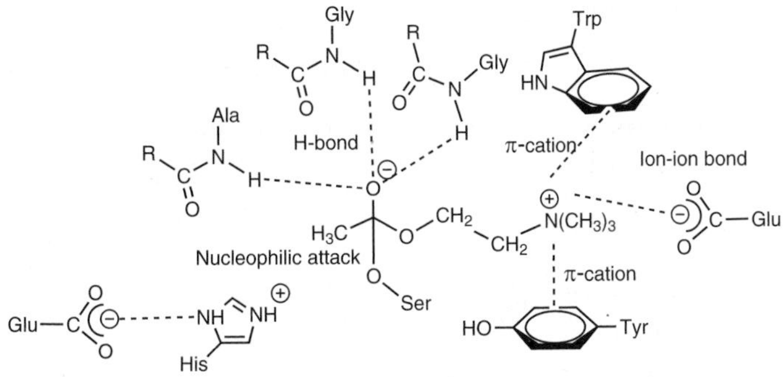

FIGURE 39.12 Binding of acetylcholine in the catalytic site of acetylcholinesterase.

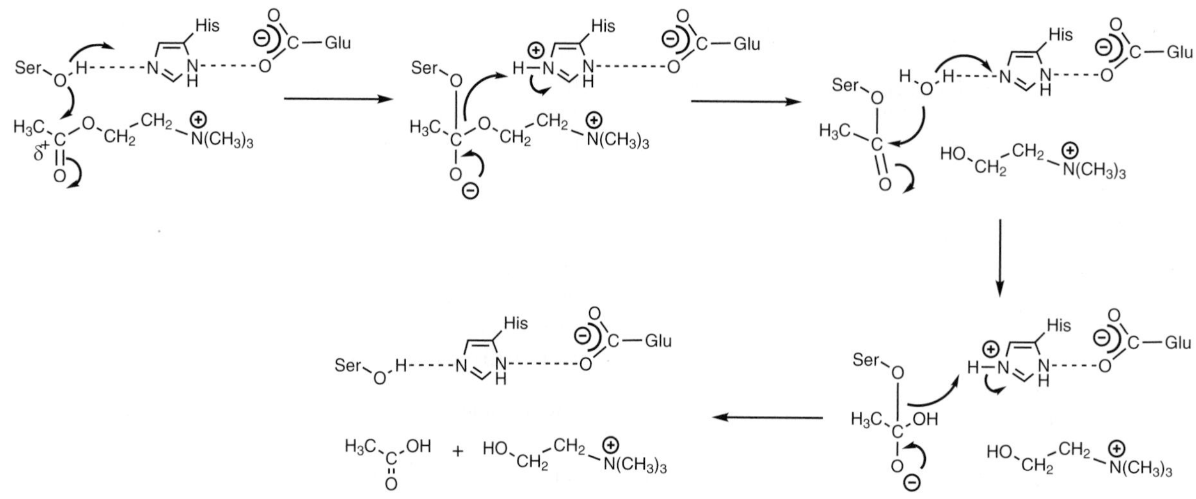

FIGURE 39.13 The role of the triad formed between glutamine, histidine, and serine in the hydrolysis of acetylcholine by acetylcholinesterase.

stabilized by hydrogen-bonding with a Tyr in helix 5 and a Thr in helix 5. It is postulated that muscarinic antagonists (see *Structure–Activity Relationships of Antimuscarinic Agents* below) bind to the Asp and contain hydrophobic substituents that bind to a hydrophobic pocket in the receptor, which does not allow the change in conformation needed to transfer the agonist signal to the coupled G protein (35).

Structure–Activity Relationships of Antimuscarinic Agents

The structural pharmacophore for all antimuscarinic drugs is an acetylcholine analog in which the acetyl methyl group is substituted with at least one phenyl ring. This pharmacophore generally is classified as an amino alcohol ester. The ester function can be replaced with different moieties to produce different classes of antimuscarinic drugs. When the ester function is replaced by an ether function, the amino alcohol ether class is produced. When the ester function is replaced by a saturated carbon, the amino alcohols are obtained when R_1 is a hydroxyl group, and the amino amides are obtained when R_1 is an amido group (Fig. 39.16).

The classic chemical prototype for the antimuscarinics is atropine, an alkaloid from *Atropa belladonna*. Buried within its structure is the amino alcohol ester pharmacophore, where R_1 is a hydroxymethyl group, R_2 is hydrogen, and the nitrogen is part of a bicyclic ring system called tropine (Fig. 39.17).

Although atropine does not have a quaternary nitrogen, the nitrogen is protonated at physiologic pH;

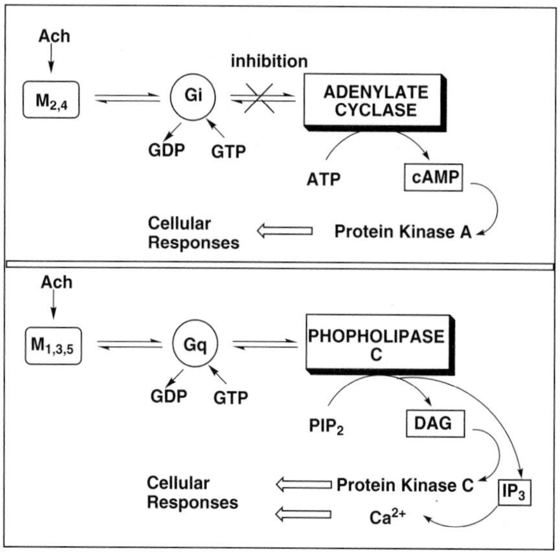

FIGURE 39.14 Comparison of the role of G protein in odd- and even-numbered muscarinic receptors.

TABLE 39.6 Physiologic Action Associated with the M3 Muscarinic Receptors

Organ	M_3-Receptor Effect
Eye	
Iris circular muscle	Contracts
Ciliary muscle	Contracts
Heart	
Sinoatrial node	Decelerates
Atrial contractility	Decelerates
Bronchiole smooth muscle	Contracts
Gastrointestinal tract	
Smooth muscle	Contracts
Secretions	Increases
Sphincters	Relaxes

From Katzung B. Introduction to autonomic pharmacology. In: Katzung B, ed. Basic and Clinical Pharmacology. 8th Ed. New York: Lange Medical Books/McGraw-Hill, 2001:75–191; with permission.

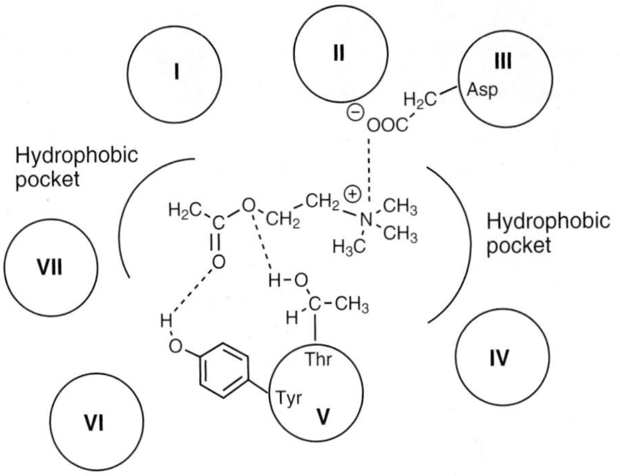

FIGURE 39.15 Acetylcholine binding to residues in the muscarinic receptor.

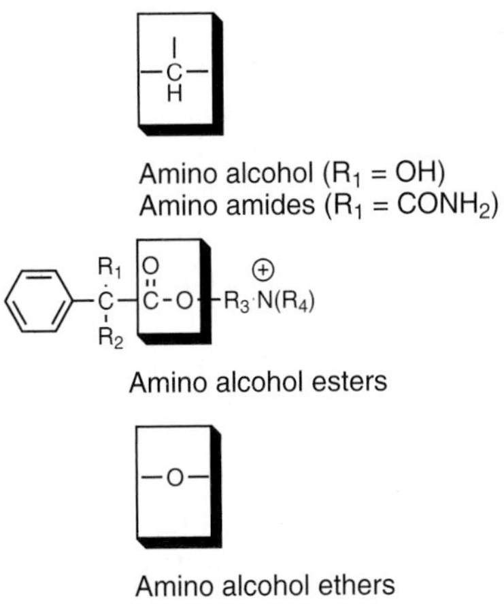

FIGURE 39.16 The pharmacophore for all classes of antimuscarinic agents.

therefore, it can bind to the anionic Asp residue in the muscarinic receptor. The nitrogen is not absolutely necessary for activity and can be replaced with a carbon atom. This leads to a substantial loss of binding affinity, however, and there are no marketed drugs with this configuration. The nitrogen can be substituted with alkyl groups, and methyl is the optimal size. When the nitrogen is made quaternary, the molecule loses its oral availability but leads to compounds that can be administered effectively by inhalation. The asterisks in atropine (Fig. 39.17) refer to chiral carbons. When stereochemistry is present in the amino alcohol moiety (tropine), there is little difference between the activities of the *R*- and *S*-configurations. When stereochemistry is found in the acid moiety, however, the *R* configuration is approximately 100-fold more active than the *S*-isomer. This indicates the importance of the binding role for the phenyl ring in causing the uncoupling of the G protein, which leads to receptor inhibition.

Specific Antimuscarinic Drugs Used to Treat Asthma

For a more detailed discussion of the chemistry of cholinergic agents see Chapter 9.

Ipratropium Hydrobromide

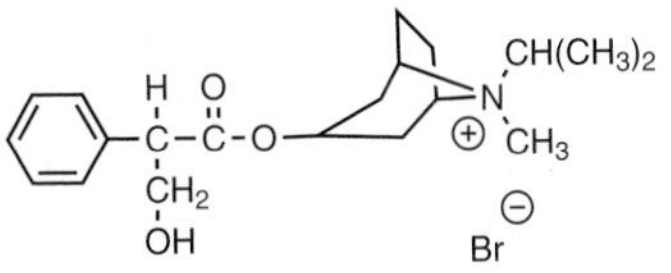

Ipratropium hydrobromide
(Atrovent)

Ipratropium is the *N*-isopropyl analog of atropine. Its quaternary cationic nature makes it highly hydrophilic and poorly absorbed from the lungs after inhalation via solution or aerosol. Much of an inhaled dose is swallowed. There is no significant absorption, however, and the bronchodilation effect can be considered to be a local, site-specific effect. Ipratropium is indicated primarily for the relief of bronchospasms associated with COPD and has seen little application for the treatment of asthma. It also is administered by nasal spray for the relief of rhinorrhea associated with the common cold and perennial rhinitis. Inhaled ipratropium has a 15-minute onset of action and a rather short duration of action (<4 hours); therefore, it is dosed four times a day. Other drugs, including adrenergic agonists, methylxanthines, steroids, and cromolyn sodium, can be coadministered with ipratropium without adverse drug reactions. The little ipratropium that reaches the circulation is minimally protein bound and is partially metabolized to by esterase to inactive products. Most adverse effects from ipratropium are common to antimuscarinics and include blurred vision, dry mouth, tachycardia, urinary difficulty, and headache. Patients should be careful not to spray ipratropium into their eyes, because its dilation effects can precipitate or exacerbate narrow-angle glaucoma.

Tiotropium Bromide

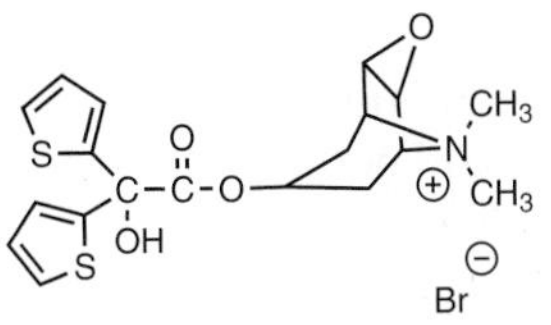

Tiotropium bromide
(Spiriva)

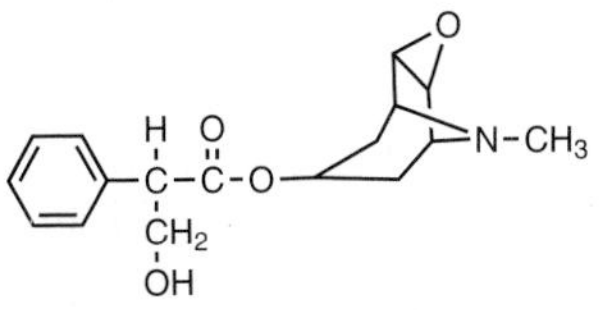

Scopolamine

Tiotropium is the dithienyl derivative of *N*-methyl scopolamine, a quaternary analog of naturally occurring scopolamine in *Atropa belladonna*. It is indicated primarily for

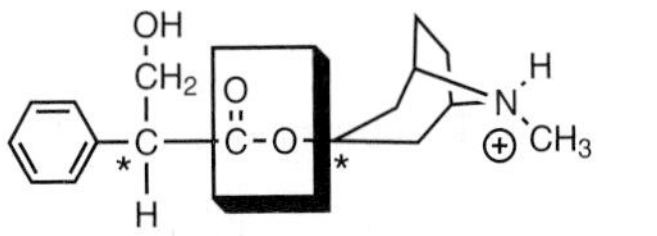

FIGURE 39.17 Atropine is an example of the amino alcohol ester class of antimuscarinic agents.

the relief of bronchospasms associated with COPD and can be considered to be a site-specific, local medication to the lung. Tiotropium is administered as a dry powder via inhalation using a HandiHaler, in which is placed the drug, contained in a green capsule. Patients should be cautioned not to be confused and take the medication orally. Systemic distribution following oral inhalation is minimal, essentially because of its hydrophilic character. If swallowed, only approximately 14% of the dose is eliminated in the urine, with the remainder being found in the feces. Inhaled tiotropium has a 30-minute onset of action but a much longer duration of action than ipratropium (24 hours vs. <4 hours, respectively). Tiotropium is metabolized by both CYP3A4 and CYP2D6, followed by glutathione conjugation to a variety of metabolites. Only a very small amount is nonenzymatically hydrolyzed to inactive products. Tiotropium has an adverse reaction profile similar to that of ipratropium, with dry mouth being the most common adverse effect; however, blurred vision, tachycardia, urinary difficulty, headache precipitation, and exacerbation of narrow-angle glaucoma have been reported.

ACLIDINIUM BROMIDE: ANTIMUSCARINIC DRUG IN THE PIPELINE

Aclidinium bromide is new antimuscarinic drug currently in phase III clinical trials. It is recommended for the inhalation treatment of COPD. Structurally, aclidinium bromide is related to tiotropium bromide in that it is a dithienyl derivative where the *N*-methyl scopolamine moiety is replaced by an *N*-phenoxypropyl-1-aza bicyclo [2,2,2]octane. This change results in a molecule with kinetic selectivity for the M_3 versus the M_2 muscarinic receptors. Aclidinium bromide is reported to be a long-acting bronchodilator with a fast onset of action. Aclidinium bromide undergoes rapid hydrolysis of its ester bond in human plasma to its constituent acid and alcohol derivatives with a half-life of 2.4 minutes in humans. In comparison, more than 70% of tiotropium bromide remains intact in plasma after 60 minutes. The acid and alcohol metabolites do not contribute to the bronchodilator activity of aclidinium bromide, and the short half-life combined with the lack of antimuscarinic activity of its hydrolysis products suggest that aclidinium may have reduced antimuscarinic side effects. Although the major metabolites of aclidinium bromide are the ester hydrolysis products, it also undergoes, to a minor extent, oxidative metabolism, yielding mono-oxygenated phenyl and the loss of one of the thienyl rings mediated by CYP3A4 and CYP2D6 isoforms. In a small clinical trial in patients with moderate to severe COPD, aclidinium bromide demonstrated significant elevation in FEV_1 from baseline, producing sustained bronchodilation over 24 hours, and no side effects were related to the treatment protocol (36–38).

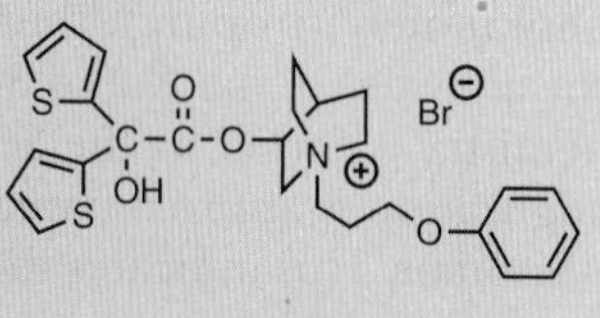

Aclidinium bromide (Almirall)

Methylxanthines

The methylxanthines naturally occur in coffee (*Coffea arabica*), cacao (*Theobroma cacao*), and tea (*Camellia sinensis*) (39). The major methylxanthines are caffeine, theophylline, and theobromine, and they differ by the position and number of methyl groups on their xanthine ring system (Fig. 39.18).

The most common source of these xanthines is in the beverages coffee, tea, and cocoa, which are universally consumed mainly for their stimulant properties. A cup of coffee or tea contains between 60 and 85 mg of caffeine, and a cup of cocoa can have as much as 250 mg of theobromine. Caffeine frequently is added to cola drinks and to over-the-counter analgesics and stimulants. Theophylline is used for its bronchodilating effects in the treatment of asthma. Its importance has declined greatly since the development of the inhaled β_2-adrenergic agonists and inhaled steroids and because it has a narrow therapeutic window, which requires close patient monitoring and periodic blood level determination to avoid serious side effects.

Theophylline Mechanism of Action and Metabolism

Despite a great deal of investigation, just how theophylline causes bronchodilation is not clearly understood. Inhibition of the enzyme PDE, which is responsible for the hydrolysis of cAMP and cyclic guanosine monophosphate (cGMP), generally is put forth as the mechanism of action; however, theophylline also is an adenosine antagonist and has been implicated in stimulation of the release of catecholamines. It has been clearly shown that theophylline does inhibit PDEs in vitro, and x-ray crystallographic studies have identified the binding residues that interact with the methylxanthines (Fig. 39.19).

Theophylline binds to a subpocket of the active site and appears to be sandwiched between a phenylalanine and a valine via hydrophobic bonds. Its binding affinity is reinforced by hydrogen-bonding between a tyrosine and N-7 and a glutamine and O-6 of the xanthine ring system. There are more than 11 families of PDEs, and studies have shown that theophylline binds in a similar manner to both the PDE4 and PDE5 family isoforms (40).

Chemically, theophylline is 1,3-dimethylxanthine and contains both an acidic and a basic nitrogen (N-7 and N-9, respectively). Physiologically, it behaves as an acid (pK_a = 8.6), and its poor aqueous solubility

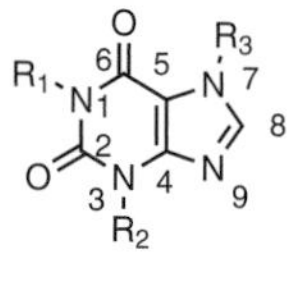

	R_1	R_2	R_3
Caffeine	CH_3	CH_3	CH_3
Theophylline	CH_3	CH_3	H
Theobromine	H	CH_3	CH_3

FIGURE 39.18 Structural differences between the methylxanthines.

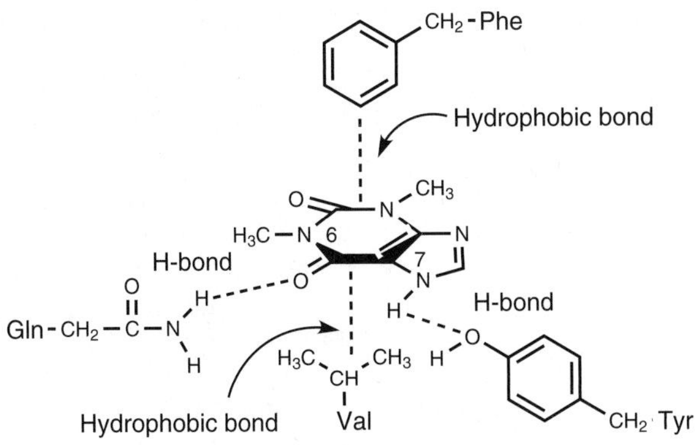

FIGURE 39.19 Methylxanthine binding interactions in the catalytic pocket of phosphodiesterase.

can be enhanced by salt formation with organic bases. Theophylline is metabolized by a combination of C-8 oxidation and *N*-demethylation to yield methyluric acid metabolites (Fig. 39.20). The major urinary metabolite is 1,3-dimethyl uric acid, which is the product of the action of xanthine oxidase. Because none of the metabolites is uric acid itself, theophylline can be safely given to patients who suffer from gout.

Methylxanthine Drugs Used to Treat Asthma

Theophylline

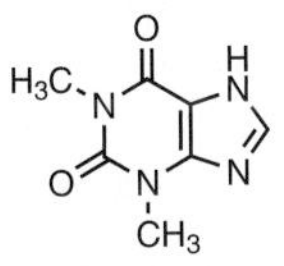

Theophylline
(Elixophylline, Bronkodyl,
various others)

The primary indication for theophylline is as a controller medication for the treatment of bronchospasm of asthma and COPD. In addition to bronchodilation

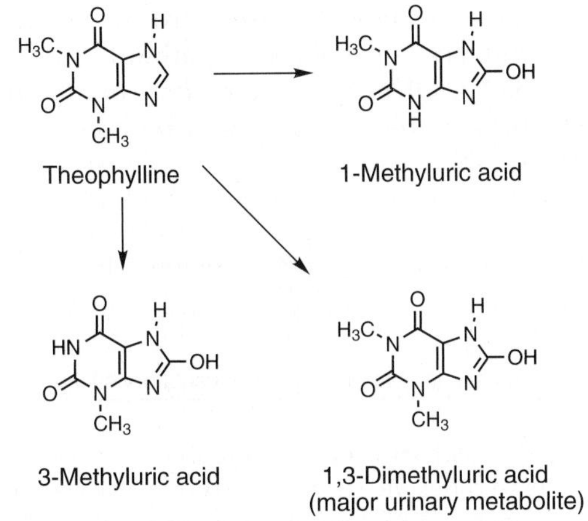

FIGURE 39.20 Metabolism of theophylline.

effects, theophylline dilates pulmonary blood vessels, acts centrally to stimulate respiration, acts as a diuretic, increases gastric acid secretion, and inhibits uterine contractions. Dosing requires the determination of plasma levels, with 10 to 20 μg/mL associated with the least incidence of side effects. Overdose of theophylline can result in a quick onset of ventricular arrhythmias, convulsions, or even death without any previous warning. Many drugs increase the plasma concentration of theophylline, including quinolone and macrolide antibiotics, nonselective β-blockers, ephedrine, calcium channel blockers, cimetidine, and oral contraceptives. Theophylline is available in tablet, capsule, liquid, and parenteral dosage preparations. There also are combination products with guaifenesin and ephedrine available as tablet and liquid dosage forms. There are two products that are theophylline salts. Aminophylline is theophylline ethylenediamine, which contains 70% theophylline and is available in tablets, liquid, parenteral, and suppository dosage forms. Oxytriphylline is the choline salt of theophylline, and it contains 64% theophylline in tablets and liquid dosage forms. Care must be taken to correctly calculate the equivalent dose when switching a patient from theophylline to one of its salts.

Dyphylline (Dihydroxypropyl Theophylline)

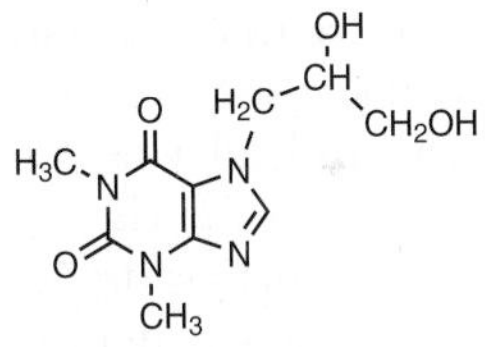

Dyphylline

Dyphylline is the N-7 dihydroxypropyl derivative of theophylline and is not a theophylline salt. Dyphylline does not get metabolized to theophylline in vivo, and even though it contains 70% theophylline by molecular weight ratio, the equivalent amount to theophylline is not known. Dosing must be accomplished independently by monitoring dyphylline blood levels. Dyphylline has a diminished bronchodilator effect compared to theophylline, but it may have lower and less serious side effects. Dosage forms available are an elixir and tablets.

Adrenocorticoids Used to Treat Asthma and COPD

Steroids are a large class of tetracyclic terpene compounds that are widely distributed in plants and animals. Many synthetic analogs have been made to take advantages of their various pharmacologic activities. There are four major classes of steroids: the adrenocorticoids, the sex hormones, the bile acids, and the vitamins. The adrenocorticoids are formed in the adrenal cortex and are subdivided into the glucocorticoids and mineralocorticoids. The glucocorticoids are so named because they affect glucose homeostasis, but they also have significant anti-inflammatory activity. The mineralocorticoids affect sodium and water retention. The reproductive organs, in both the male and female, produce steroid hormones, which are responsible for the differentiation of the sex characteristics and the development of muscle and hair. The bile acids are derived from cholesterol and are an essential aid to the action of lipase in the digestion of fats, and vitamin D and its derivatives are associated with calcium homeostasis. We will limit our discussion to the glucocorticoids, because their anti-inflammatory activity makes them useful for the treatment of asthma and COPD. Of note, because the major role of the glucocorticoids is to provide the body with levels of glucose that are compatible with life, they should be used with caution in patients with diabetes. Similarly, because the major role of the mineralocorticoids is to maintain blood volume and regulate electrolyte balance, their use in patients with hypertension should be monitored carefully. (For more detail regarding the adrenal corticosteroids, see Chapter 28.)

Steroid Nomenclature

The basic structure of a steroid is a tetracyclic cyclopentanoperhydrophenanthrene, referred to as the steroid nucleus, as depicted in Figure 39.21. The addition of methyl groups at C-10 and C-13 and of an ethyl group at C-17 to the steroid nucleus gives a 21-carbon base structure called pregnane. All glucocorticoids are substituted pregnanes. Rings A, B, and C are in the chair conformation, and all ring junctions are *trans*, giving the glucocorticoids a rigid backbone with α and β faces. The glucocorticoids bind to their receptor via the β face. All glucocorticoids have at least one double bond in ring A and hydroxyl groups at C-11, C-17, and C-21 as well as 3- and 20-keto groups. For example, hydrocortisone is Δ^4- 11β,17α,21-trihydroxy-3,20-pregnenedione. A more complete discussion of steroid nomenclature and stereochemistry has been published elsewhere (41).

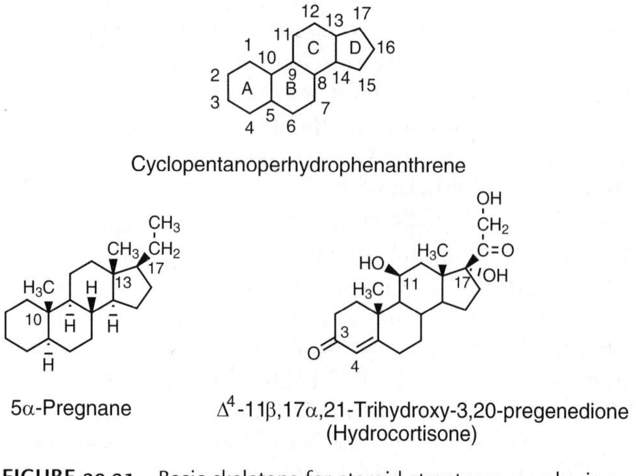

FIGURE 39.21 Basic skeletons for steroid structures, numbering, and nomenclature.

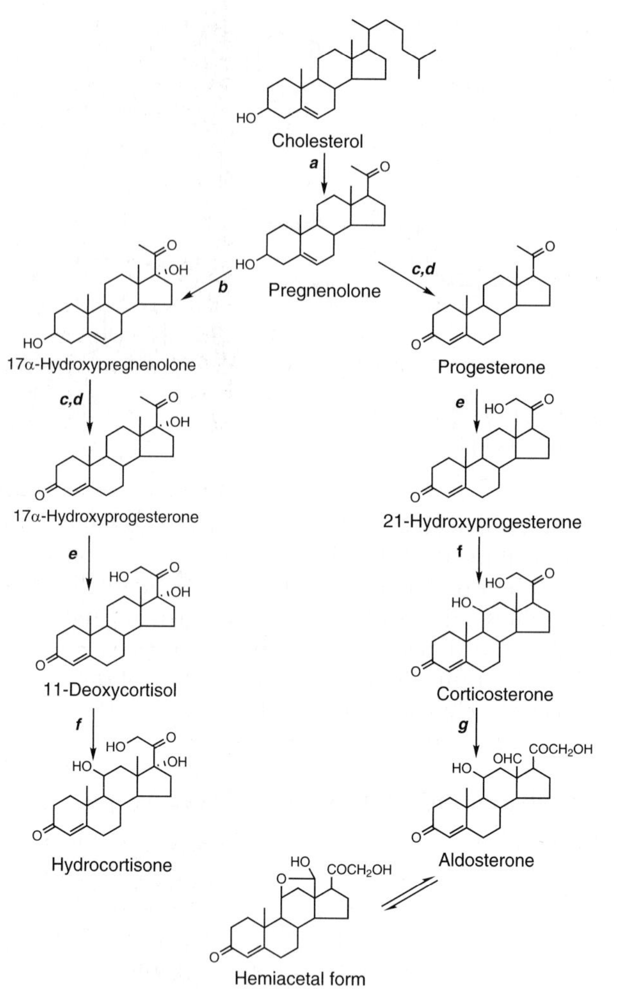

FIGURE 39.22 Biosynthesis of the adrenocorticoids from cholesterol. The enzymes involved are (*a*) side chain cleavage, (*b*) 17α-hydroxylase, (*c*) 5-ene-3β-hydroxy-steroid dehydrogenase, (*d*) 3-oxosteroid-4,5-isomerase, (*e*) 21-hydroxylase, (*f*) 11β-hydroxylase, and (*g*) 18-hydroxylate.

Steroid Biosynthesis and Secretion

Steroids are biosynthesized from cholesterol. Cholesterol is obtained through our diet (~0.3 g/day), but the majority is biosynthesized from acetate in the liver (~1 g/day). The complete pathway can be seen in Figure 39.22. Of note is the central branching role played by pregnenolone, leading to both classes of the adrenocorticoids.

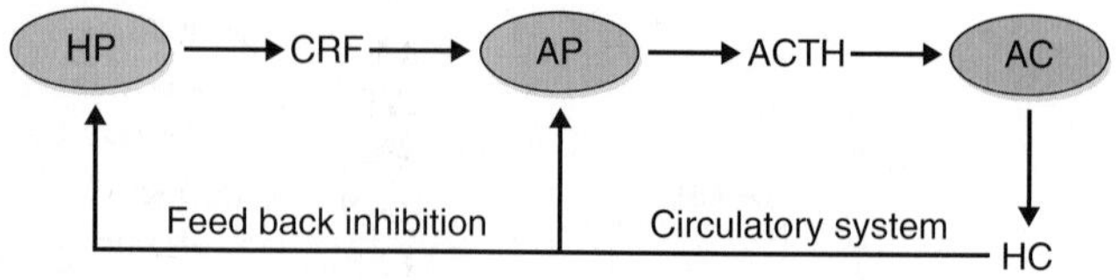

FIGURE 39.23 Mechanism of adrenocorticoid secretion and control. AC, adrenal cortex; ACTH, adrenocorticotrophic hormone; AP, anterior pituitary; CRF, corticotrophin-releasing factor; HC, hydrocortisone; HP, hypothalamus.

Once formed, the adrenocorticoids are secreted into the circulatory system, and circulating levels are maintained via a feedback mechanism (Fig. 39.23). When circulating levels are low, the hypothalamus secretes corticotrophin-releasing factor (CRF). In turn, CRF stimulates the anterior pituitary to secrete adrenocorticotrophic hormone, which stimulates the adrenal cortex to synthesize and secrete the adrenocorticoids (mainly hydrocortisone and aldosterone). When circulating levels of the adrenocorticoids are sufficiently high, they feedback-inhibit CRF secretion from the hypothalamus and adrenocorticotrophic hormone release from the anterior pituitary gland. It should be noted that chronic use of steroids inhibits the adrenal cortex from producing glucocorticoids. This is known as hypothalamus-pituitary-adrenal (HPA) suppression. If steroid therapy is stopped abruptly, the lack of endogenous glucocorticoids can be life-threatening. A slow and gradual withdrawal from exogenous steroid therapy is always warranted to allow the HPA axis to recover.

Steroid Pharmacologic Action

The major pharmacologic activities of the glucocorticoids are anti-inflammation, inhibition of cytokines, and inhibition of mast cell release of autocoids. The anti-inflammatory activity of the glucocorticoids is derived from their ability to affect protein synthesis. Specifically, they stimulate the synthesis of lipocortin, a protein that inhibits phospholipase A_2, which is an enzyme that catalyzes the breakdown of membranes to release arachidonic acid, the first step in the arachidonic acid cascade that results in the production of inflammatory prostaglandins and leukotrienes (Figs. 39.24 and 39.25). Therefore, inhibition of phospholipase A_2 ultimately results in the reduction of the inflammatory prostaglandins and leukotrienes.

A second anti-inflammatory mechanism of glucocorticoids involves inhibition of IL-1. IL-1 stimulates the proliferation of T and B lymphocytes that are responsible for the production of the cytokines and antibodies, which in turn are important in the inflammatory and immune responses to antigens. The glucocorticoids, by their ability to inhibit IL-1, cause a decrease in T and B lymphocytes, leading to immunosuppression, and therefore must be used with caution in patients with infection. A third action of glucocorticoids is to inhibit the synthesis and release of histamine and other autocoids from mast cells. These pharmacologic activities make the glucocorticoids especially useful for treating the inflammatory processes associated with asthma and COPD.

Steroid Mechanism of Action

How do glucocorticoids and other adrenocorticoids affect the levels of proteins and other biologically important compounds? The short answer is that these steroids bind to their receptor in the cytoplasm and that the glucocorticoid–receptor complex travels into the nucleus, where it binds to DNA and affects gene transcription, which increases and, sometimes, decreases the production of important biologically active compounds. The detail of just how the glucocorticoids accomplish this is quite interesting and is depicted in Fig. 39.26.

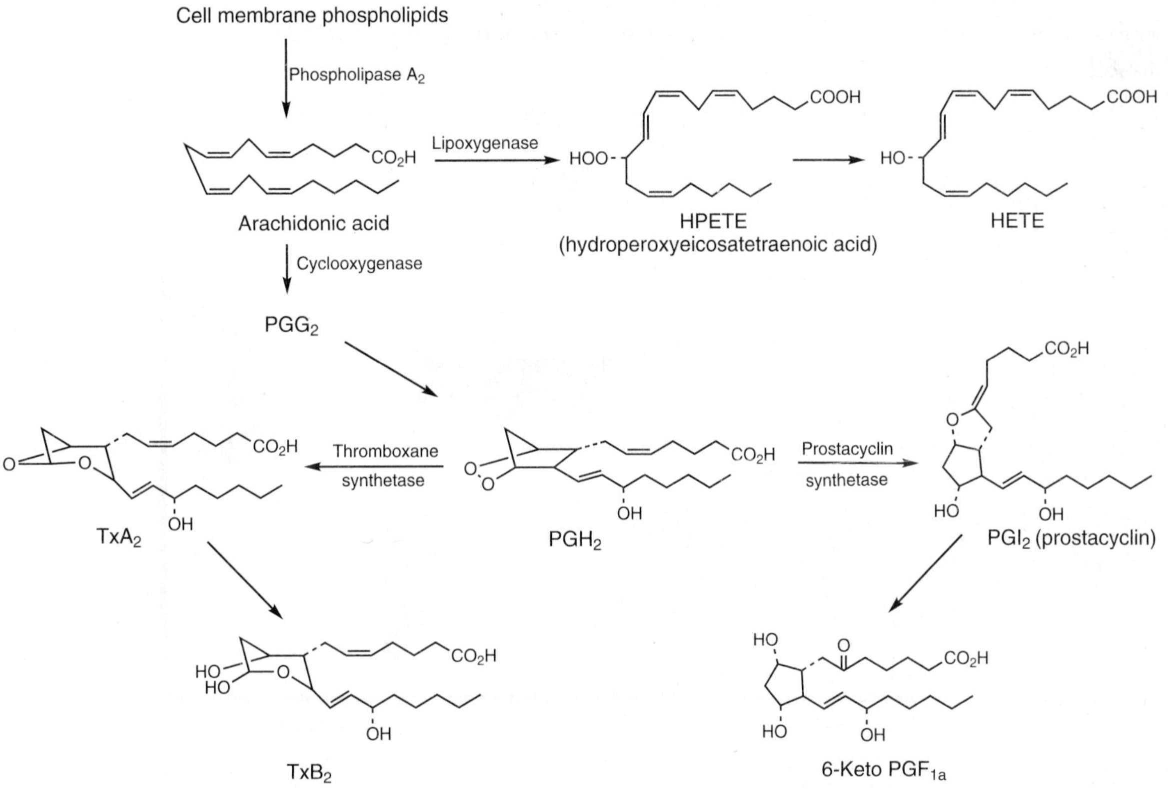

FIGURE 39.24 Biosynthesis of thromboxanes, prostacyclin, and prostaglandins.

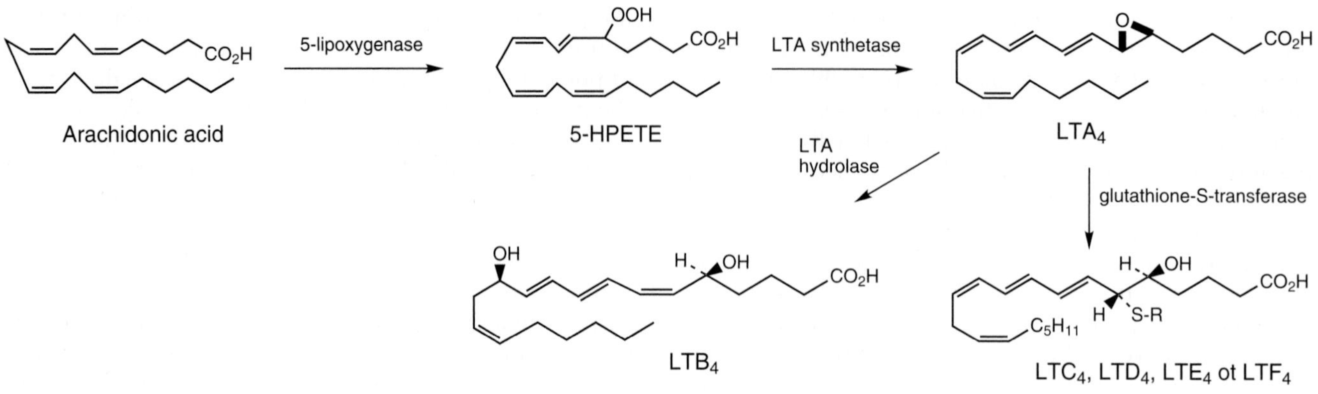

FIGURE 39.25 Biosynthesis of leukotrienes.

Circulating glucocorticoids enter the target cell by simple diffusion, because they are relatively lipophilic. The glucocorticoid receptor occurs inside the cell in combination with a heat shock protein. The glucocorticoid receptor has three distinct regions: the amino terminal for maximum activity, a middle region for binding to DNA, and the carboxy terminal, where the glucocorticoids bind. When the glucocorticoid binds to its receptor, the heat shock protein is released, with a conformational change in the steroid–receptor complex. The glucocorticoid–receptor complex then translocates into the nucleus of the cell, where it binds to specific sequences of DNA called hormone response elements (HREs), which are located in the promoter areas of hormone-responsive genes. The DNA binding region of the glucocorticoid receptor contains eight cysteine amino acid residues that coordinate two zinc ions that form peptide loops called zinc fingers. When the zinc finger domains bind to the HRE of DNA, it dimerizes the glucocorticoid–receptor complex, placing each subunit in adjacent binding grooves. In most cases, binding causes gene transcription and protein synthesis; however, in some instances, binding will block transcription (42). A more precise understanding of just how the glucocorticoids inhibit the expression of inflammatory proteins has only recently become understood. In the inflammatory cells, such as macrophages, inflammatory protein genes are activated by the acetylation of core histones, which are entwined in DNA. This acetylation opens the chromatin structure allowing gene transcription and synthesis of inflammatory proteins. Glucocorticoids recruit histone deacetylase 2 (HDAC2) to actively transcribing genes, which reverses this process and switches off inflammatory gene transcription (43).

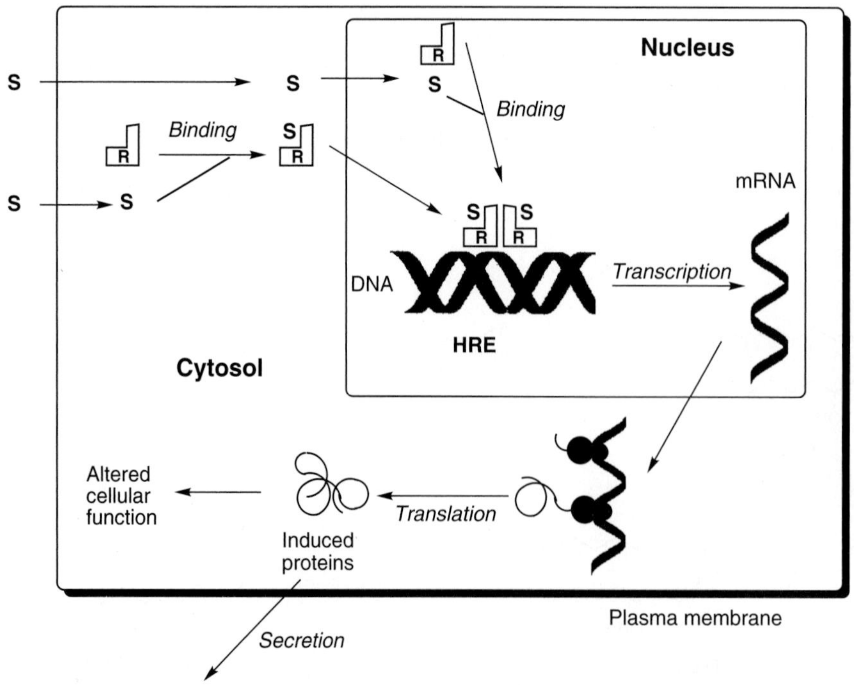

FIGURE 39.26 Mechanism of steroid hormone action. S, steroid; R, receptor.

Receptor Structure and Glucocorticoid Binding

The glucocorticoid receptor is a member of the nuclear receptor superfamily, which includes the receptors for the steroid hormones, retinoids, peroxisomal activators, vitamin D, and thyroid hormones. The steroid receptor is a soluble protein found in the cytosol of the cell. The binding domain of all the steroid receptors consists of 11 α-helices and 4 β-strands. X-ray crystallographic structural analysis, however, has revealed a unique binding pocket for the glucocorticoid receptor, which makes it distinct from the estrogen receptor, androgen receptor, and mineralocorticoid receptor. When a glucocorticoid binds to the receptor, it is completely enclosed within a pocket formed by helices 3, 4, 5, 6, 7, and 10 and β-strands 1 and 2. The strong binding affinity for the glucocorticoids is a result of the hydrophobic and hydrophilic interactions with amino acid residues in the ligand binding domain. Nearly every atom of the glucocorticoid contacts one or more amino acid residues. The most significant contacts are the hydrogen-bonding between every hydrophilic group on the glucocorticoid structure (Fig. 39.27). The carbonyl group on ring A forms hydrogen bonds with both Arg-611 and the amide of Gln-570. The hydroxyls at C-11 and C-21 hydrogen bond with the side chain of Asn-564. The C-17 hydroxyl group hydrogen bonds with Gln-642, and the C-20 carbonyl group bonds with Thr-739. Glucocorticoid binding to the ligand binding domain releases the heat shock protein and stabilizes the receptor in an active form capable of dimerization subsequent to HRE site binding (44,45).

Glucocorticoid Structure–Activity Relationships

There are essential structural features that are necessary for glucocorticoid activity. The natural glucocorticoids also interact with the mineralocorticoid receptor and, therefore, will have salt-retaining properties. A large number of synthetic analogs have been prepared to decrease the mineralocorticoid effects in favor of increasing the glucocorticoid (anti-inflammatory) effect of the steroids. In addition, many derivatives are prepared to enhance pharmacokinetic parameters, most notably the synthesis of lipophilic and hydrophilic esters.

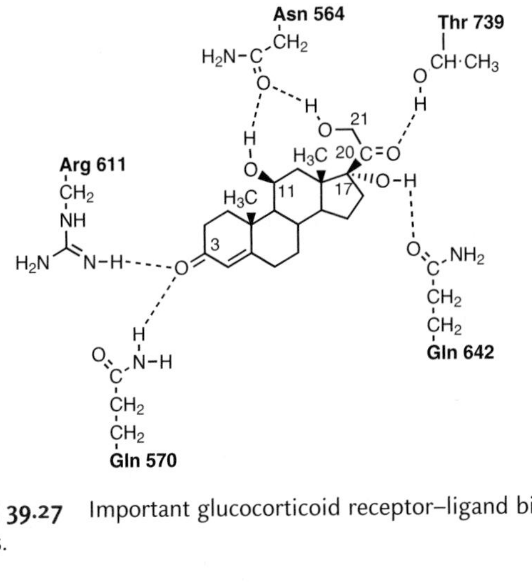

FIGURE 39.27 Important glucocorticoid receptor–ligand binding residues.

Functional groups that are essential for both mineralocorticoid and glucocorticoid activity include the pregnane skeleton with an all-*trans* backbone, the ring A-en-one system (Δ^4-3-one ring A), and the 17β-ketol side chain (C-20-keto-C-21-hydroxy). The C-21 hydroxyl group must be free for both mineralocorticoid and glucocorticoid activity. An exception to this rule are the C-21 chloro and C-20 fluoromethyl thio ester ($-SCH_2F$) derivatives that retain anti-inflammatory activity when applied topically or by inhalation. Glucocorticoids that are used for their anti-inflammatory effects and that have both glucocorticoid and mineralocorticoid activity are hydrocortisone, cortisone, prednisone, and prednisolone.

Many derivatives of the fundamental glucocorticoid skeleton have been synthesized with the intention of enhancing anti-inflammatory activity and decreasing the salt-retaining properties of the glucocorticoids when administered in therapeutic doses. Figure 39.28 depicts those positions where substituents will affect anti-inflammatory and/or mineralocorticoid activity. The triangles indicate those positions where substitutions will increase the anti-inflammatory activity, the open circles indicate those positions where substituents will increase both anti-inflammatory and mineralocorticoid properties, the closed circle is the position where substituents will decrease the mineralocorticoid activity, and the open box is where specific substituents can either increase anti-inflammatory activity or decrease mineralocorticoid properties depending on the specific substituent. Therefore, the anti-inflammatory activity will be greatly increased by flattening ring A by adding a double bond at C-1 (Δ^1) and also by adding a hydroxyl group at C-11. A 17α-hydroxy increases both activities, as does 9α-fluoro or 9α-chloro. Mineralocorticoid activity is substantially eliminated by 16α- or 16β-methyl groups, a 16α-hydroxyl group, or a 16α,17α-acetonide. A C-6α-methyl group only slightly enhances the anti-inflammatory activity, whereas a C-6α-fluoro has twice as much anti-inflammatory effect. Both substituents, in combination with a C-16 substituent, will greatly decrease the mineralocorticoid effects.

Therefore, synthetic compounds can be prepared with marked glucocorticoid activity and little if any significant mineralocorticoid activity. These include triamcinolone, methylprednisolone, fluticasone, beclomethasone, budesonide, mometasone, and ciclesonide.

Glucocorticoid Metabolism

If one or more of the essential functional groups on the glucocorticoid skeleton are modified by metabolism, glucocorticoid activity will be lost. There are three major metabolic reactions that will eliminate glucocorticoid activity. They are ring A reductions, C-17 oxidation, and C-11 keto-enol isomerization. Reduction of the ring A 3-keto to a 3α-hydroxy by 3α-hydroxysteroid dehydrogenase and the reduction of the 4,5-double bond by

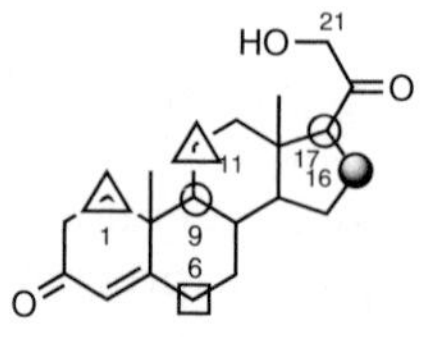

Both anti-inflammatory and mineralcorticoid activity increased (open circle)	Anti-inflammatory activity increased (triangle and square)	Mineralocorticoid activity decreased (closed circle and square)
17α-OH	1-dehydro	6α-CH_3
9α-F	6α-F	16α-& 16β-CH_3
9α-Cl	11β-OH	16α,17α-acetonide
21-OH		16α-OH

FIGURE 39.28 Glucocorticoid structure–activity relationship.

5β-reductase to produce the A/B *cis*-fused ring give rise to inactive metabolites (Fig. 39.29). Oxidation of the C-17 side chain to produce a 17-keto steroid requires both the C-17 hydroxyl group and a free C-21 hydroxyl group. Esterification of one or both will inhibit this metabolism and prolong the duration of action. The rapid in vivo equilibrium that exists between cortisone (11-keto) and hydrocortisone (11-β-hydroxy) is catalyzed by 11β-hydroxysteroid dehydrogenase and produces the keto form that is inactive but also the hydroxy form that is highly glucocorticoid enhancing and found on all glucocorticoids. Figure 39.29 summarizes the metabolism of hydrocortisone.

Synthetic Steroid Esters

The glucocorticoids are lipophilic despite having at least three hydroxyl groups. The hydroxyl groups can be esterified with an appropriate acid that will either enhance or decrease that lipophilicity. The C-21 hydroxyl group is the most accessible and, therefore, is the easiest to esterify. The C-17 hydroxyl group also is easily esterified, but because it is slightly hindered by the C-17 side chain, it will react more slowly. The C-11 hydroxyl group is highly hindered by the C-10 and C-13 methyl groups and will not react with acids to form esters. In addition, esterification has an effect on both receptor affinity and glucocorticoid metabolism. Because the C-21 must be free to hydrogen bond to the Arg-564 in the glucocorticoid receptor, C-21 esters are prodrugs requiring hydrolysis to become active. Also, the C-17 hydroxyl group needs to be free to be metabolically oxidized; therefore, esterification of the C-17 hydroxyl group inhibits oxidation to the C-17 keto group, thus prolonging duration of action. Duration

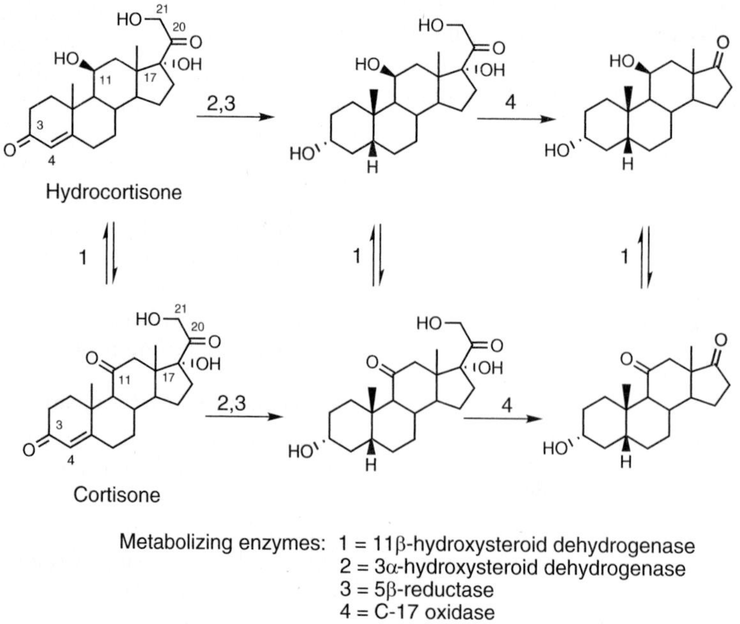

Metabolizing enzymes: 1 = 11β-hydroxysteroid dehydrogenase
2 = 3α-hydroxysteroid dehydrogenase
3 = 5β-reductase
4 = C-17 oxidase

FIGURE 39.29 Metabolic pathways for hydrocortisone.

also is prolonged because of the fact that the lipophilic glucocorticoid esters do not concentrate in the urine (i.e., they undergo tubular reabsorption after glomerular filtration).

The lipophilicity of a glucocorticoid can be enhanced by esterification with lipophilic acids. Doing so results in a number of effects, including increasing the logP, which provides local activity with less systemic absorption and decreased side effects. The fact that C-21 lipophilic esters are prodrugs means that they have a longer duration of action. They also have a slower onset, because the lipophilic esters generally are bulky and retard hydrolytic enzymes.

These lipophilic prodrugs can be administered orally to treat a variety of conditions, by inhalation to treat asthma and COPD, and topically to treat various types of dermatitis. When administered orally, their longer duration of action means that they can be given less frequently, which often results in better compliance. When administered topically, C-21 lipophilic ester prodrugs are activated by hydrolysis by skin esterases (46,47), which slows their systemic absorption. Systemically absorbed glucocorticoids are further metabolized in the liver as depicted in Figure 39.29. Figure 39.30 shows the structures of the most common C-21 lipophilic esters found on commercially available glucocorticoids.

Diesters and ketals provide a further enhancement of logP (i.e., increased lipophilicity) and an increased duration of action because they are slow to metabolize. It should be noted that diesters and hexacatonides (Fig. 39.31) are prodrugs, whereas plain ketals are not (i.e., they already have a free C-21 hydroxyl group). Diesters are formed at C-21 and at either the C-17 or, if present, the C-16 hydroxyl groups. The diesters are prodrugs; however, the esters at C-17 or C-16 are active intact. The most common diesters are either the diacetate or dipropionate.

A ketal is a cyclic derivative formed between hydroxyl groups on adjacent carbons and a carbonyl carbon of a ketone. The most common ketal found in glucocorticoids is called an acetonide and is the condensation product formed between the C-16 and C-17 hydroxyl groups and the carbonyl carbon of acetone (CH_3COCH_3)

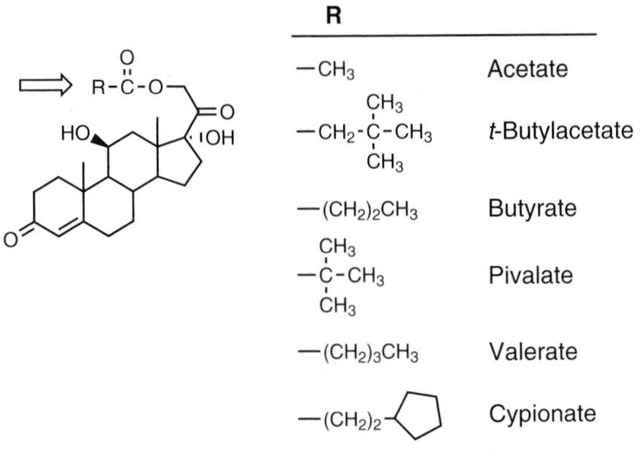

FIGURE 39.30 Common lipophilic esters of glucocorticoids.

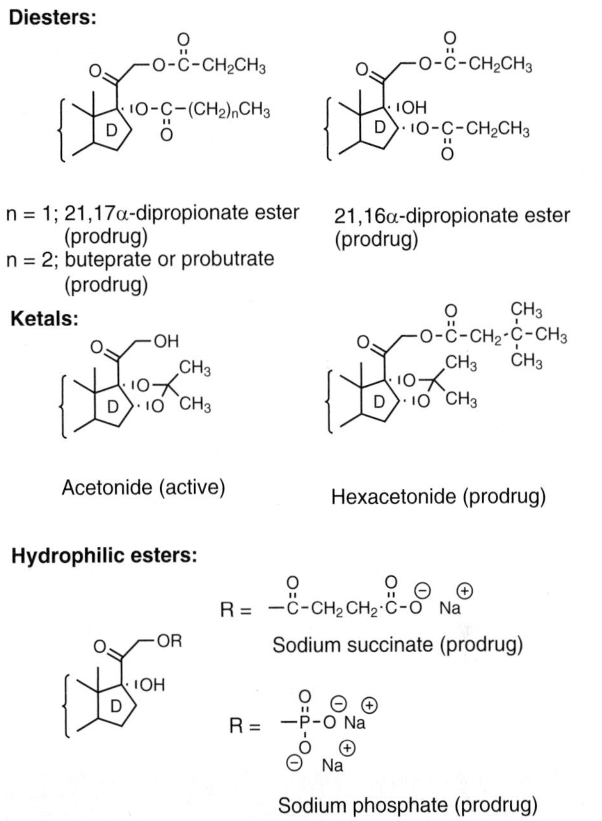

FIGURE 39.31 Examples of glucocorticoid lipophilic diesters and ketals and hydrophilic esters.

(Fig. 39.31). If the acetonide is found along with a C-21-*t*-butylacetate ester, it is named a hexacetonide; the "hex" refers to the total number of carbons found in the butylacetate group. The hexacetonides are prodrugs and must hydrolyze to become active. The buteprate (i.e., probutate) is a diester consisting of a propionate at C-21 and a butyrate at C-17 (Fig. 39.31). It also is a prodrug, and the C-21 ester must be hydrolyzed to yield the active form.

Esterification also can be used to increase the hydrophilicity of the glucocorticoids, making them water-soluble prodrugs. The synthetic approach here is to use either a dicarboxylic acid or phosphoric acid to condense with the C-21 hydoxyl group (Fig. 39.31). This places an ionizable group (a carboxylate or phosphate) on the prodrug, yielding water-soluble esters. These derivatives are used to prepare aqueous injectable products that can be administered intramuscularly or IV.

Hydrophilic glucocorticoid prodrugs have a rapid onset, because they are readily hydrolyzed by plasma esterases. In contrast to the lipophilic prodrugs, their water solubility allows them to be easily excreted through the kidney, resulting in a shorter duration of action. Hydrophilic prodrugs have more systemic side effects because of their wide distribution that comes from their high solubility in the blood. Along with their ability to be injected IV, this property makes them useful in asthmatic emergencies (i.e., status asthmaticus) during which the patient is unable to take oral medication. Table 39.7 summarizes glucocorticoid prodrug derivatives.

Glucocorticoid Drugs Used to Treat Asthma

Systemic Glucocorticoids

Hydrocortisone

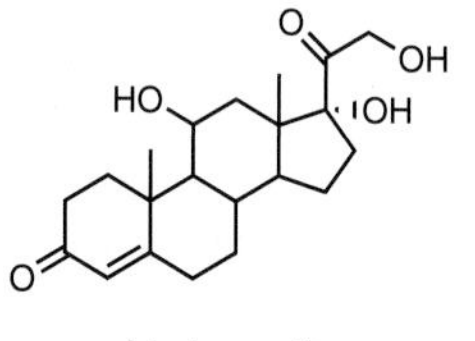

Hydrocortisone
(Cortisol)

Δ^4-11β,17α,21-trihydroxy-3,20-pregnenedione

Hydrocortisone is endogenous, and it has both glucocorticoid and mineralocorticoid activity. It is the fundamental structure by which the glucocorticoid and mineralocorticoid activities of all other corticosteroids are judged. Functional groups that are essential for both mineralocorticoid and glucocorticoid activity include the pregnane skeleton with an all-*trans* backbone, the ring A-en-one system (Δ^4-3-one ring A), and the 17β-ketol side chain (C-20-keto-C-21-hydroxy). The glucocorticoid activity is enhanced by the C-11 and C-17 hydroxyl groups. Hydrocortisone can be used to treat severe asthmatic attacks that do not respond to conventional treatment. It is available as various ester forms (Table 39.7).

TABLE 39.7 Glucocorticoid Prodrug Derivatives

Drug	Trade Name	Site of Ester	Route of Administration
Hydrocortisone derivatives			
Hydrocortisone phosphate		C-21	IM, IV, SC
Sodium succinate	A-Hydrocort Sulucortef	C-21	IM, IV
Cypionate	Cortef	C-21	PO
Acetate	Cortaid	C-21	Topical
Butyrate	Locoid	C-21	Topical
Buteprate	Pandel	C-21	Topical
Valerate	Westcort	C-21	Topical
Prednisolone derivatives			
Phosphate	Hydeltrasol	C-21	IV, IM
Acetate	Key-Pred	C-21	Topical
Di-*t*-butylacetate (tebutate)	Prednisol TBA	C-17, 21	Topical
Methylprednisolone derivatives			
Sodium succinate	Solu-medrol	C-21	IV, IM
	A-Methapred		
Acetate	Depo-Medrol		
	Depoject	C-21	IM

IM, intramuscular; IV, intravenous; PO, oral; SC, subcutaneous.

Prednisolone

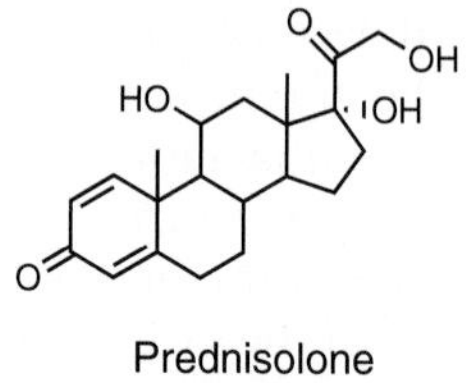

Prednisolone
(Delta-Cortef)

$\Delta^{1,4}$-11β,17α,21-trihydroxy-pregnadiene-3,20-dione

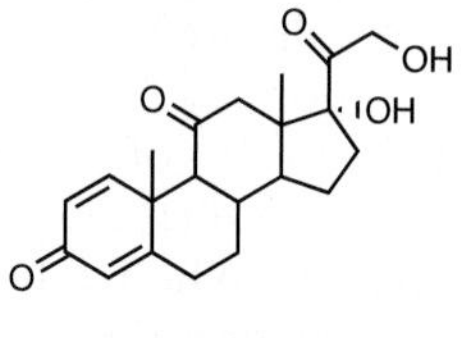

Prednisone
(Deltasone, Meticortin)

$\Delta^{1,4}$-17α,21-dihydroxy-pregnadiene-3,11,20-trione

Prednisolone is hydrocortisone to which has been added a Δ^1 double bond. This places two double bonds in ring A, which flattens it and increases glucocorticoid action at the expense of mineralocorticoid activity. Prednisolone has fourfold the glucocorticoid activity of hydrocortisone while having approximately half its mineralocorticoid activity. In addition, prednisolone has an increased duration of action compared to hydrocortisone, because the extra double bond in ring A retards its metabolic reduction.

Prednisolone can be used to treat severe asthmatic attacks that do not respond to conventional treatment, and it is available as the free alcohol for oral administration. The C-21 sodium phosphate (Hydeltrasol) ester is available for parenteral use. Various ester prodrugs are available, as listed in Table 39.7. A prodrug of prednisolone is prednisone. It is the 11-keto analog of prednisolone and must be converted in vivo to the active 11β-hydroxy compound, which is necessary to hydrogen bond to Asn-564 in the glucocorticoid receptor. Prednisone should not be used in patients with hepatic dysfunction, because their ability to reduce the 11-keto group with 11β-hydroxysteroid dehydrogenase to the active metabolite may be impaired.

Methylprednisolone

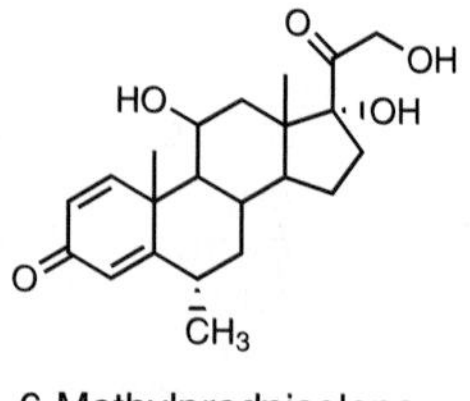

6-Methylprednisolone
(Medrol)

$\Delta^{1,4}$-6α-methyl-11α,17α,21-trihydroxy-pregnadiene-3,20-dione

Adding a 6α-methyl group to prednisolone increases the glucocorticoid activity and effectively abolishes mineralocorticoid action. It has fivefold the glucocorticoid activity of hydrocortisone (prednisolone has fourfold the glucocorticoid activity) and none of its mineralocorticoid properties. It is used almost exclusively as a systemic product and is available as the free alcohol for oral administration and as various esters (Table 39.7).

Side Effects

Systemic administration of glucocorticoids can result in a large number of adverse effects on prolonged use. As already stated, there is the severe risk of HPA axis suppression, requiring the slow tapering off of the dose. In addition, glucocorticoids have cardiovascular effects (thromboembolism, hypertension, and arrhythmias), central nervous system effects (convulsions and steroid psychosis), dermatologic effects (impaired wound healing and hair growth), endocrine effects (amenorrhea, postmenstrual bleeding, and suppression of growth in children), electrolyte disturbances (sodium and fluid retention, hypertension, and metabolic alkalosis), GI effects (pancreatitis, increased appetite, and peptic ulcer), musculoskeletal effects (muscle weakness, steroid myopathy, and osteoporosis), and ophthalmic effects (cataracts, increased intraocular pressure, and glaucoma).

Glucocorticoids for Inhalation

Beclomethasone Dipropionate

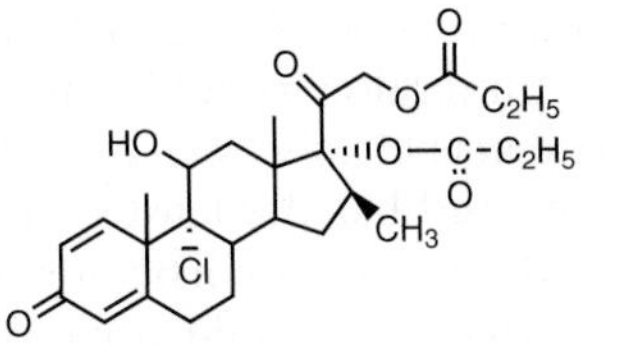

Beclomethasone dipropionate
(QVAR, Vanceril)

9α-Chloro-16β-methyl-11β,17α,21-trihydroxypregna-1,4-diene-3,20-dione 17,21-dipropionate

Beclomethasone dipropionate is a lipophilic prodrug that, when inhaled, shows a systemic bioavailability of approximately 20% of the administered dose. The 16β-methyl group decreases mineralocorticoid activity, and the 9α-chloro group increases both the glucocorticoid and mineralocorticoid activity, resulting in potent anti-inflammatory activity with little or no salt-retaining effects. The main adverse effects are headache, sinusitis, and pain. Beclomethasone dipropionate is metabolized to the more active 17α-monopropionate derivative during absorption from the lungs and then further metabolized to the free alcohol in the liver. The dipropionate also is metabolized to the inactive 21-monopropionate in the liver. Beclomethasone dipropionate and its metabolites are mainly excreted in the feces, with less than 10% excreted in the urine.

Budesonide

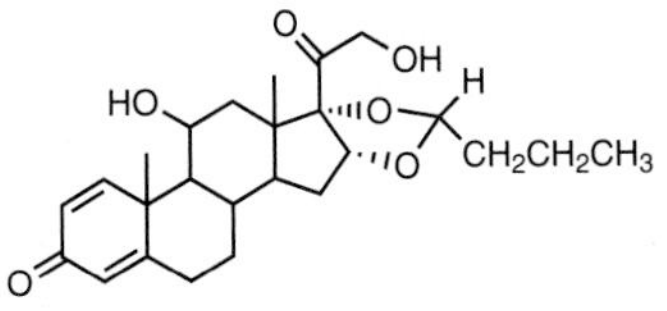

Budesonide
(Pulmacort tubuhaler, Respules)

16α,17–[(*R,S*-butylidenebis(oxy)]-11β,21-dihydroxypregna-1,4-diene-3,20-dione

Budesonide is an acetal formed between the 16α,17α-dihydroxyl groups and butanal. It is a nonhalogenated glucocorticoid with a 16,17-acetal that decreases the mineralocorticoid activity. In receptor affinity studies, the *R*-epimer was twofold more active than the *S*-epimer. Because the C-21 hydroxy is free, budesonide is not a prodrug and is active as administered. Only 34% of the metered dose of inhaled budesonide reaches the lung. Systemically absorbed budesonide is highly protein bound and metabolized to 16α-hydroxyprednisolone and 6β-hydroxybudesonide in the liver. Both metabolites have less than 1% of the glucocorticoid activity of the parent compound. Inhaled budesonide is excreted mainly as metabolites via both the feces (15%) and the urine (32%). Budesonide is available as a powder delivered through an aerosol or as a suspension for inhalation.

Ciclesonide

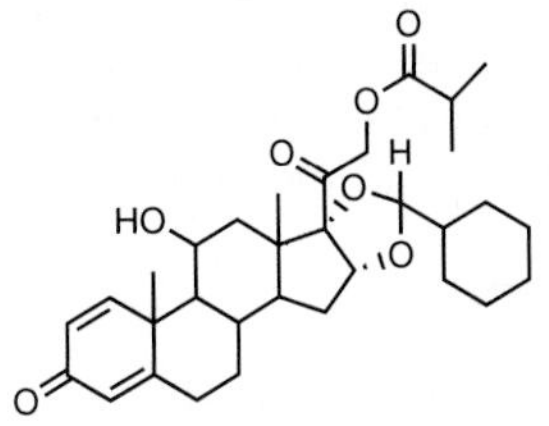

Ciclesonide (Alvesco, Omnaris)

16α,17-[(*R*-cyclohexylmethene]bis(oxy)]-11β-hydroxy-21-(2-methyl-1-oxopropoxy)-[regma-1,4-diene-3,20-dione

Ciclesonide is a glucocorticoid with an acetal formed at positions 16 and 17 with cyclohexylcarboxaldehyde. Acetals at this position decrease mineralocorticoid activity. In addition, ciclesonide has a Δ^1 double bond that retards ring A reduction, promoting a longer duration of action, and also flattens ring A, which increases glucocorticoid action at the expense of mineralocorticoid activity. Ciclesonide is a prodrug that is converted to its active form desisobutyryl-ciclesonide via esterases in the lung. It is reported to have a relative potency equivalent to fluticasone, mometasone, budesonide, and beclomethasone dipropionate. Lung deposition on inhalation is 52%, and the oral bioavailability is less than 1%, presumably due to low GI absorption and high first-pass metabolism. Des-ciclesonide is metabolized in the liver to additional metabolites mainly by CYP3A4 and to a lesser extent CYP2D6. Ciclesonide is available in a hydrofluoroalkane propellant metered-dose formulation for inhalation. Ciclesonide is also used for the treatment of hay fever in the form of a nasal spray under the trade name of Omnaris.

Flunisolide

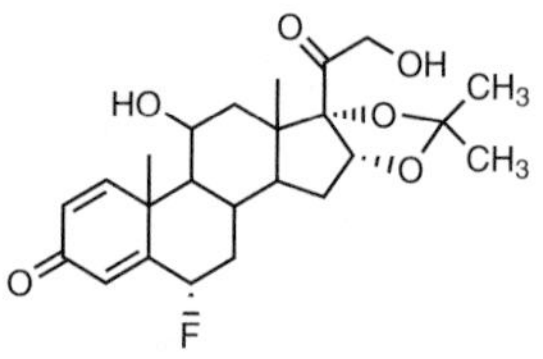

Flunisolide
(Aerobid)

6α–Fluoro-11β,21-dihydroxy-16α,17-[(1-methyl-ethylidene)bis(oxy)]pregna-1,4-diene-3,20-dione

Flunisolide is an acetone ketal (acetonide) with a 6α-fluoro group and a free C-21 hydroxyl group. The acetonide decreases mineralocorticoid activity, and the 6α-fluoro group increases glucocorticoid activity. It is not a prodrug, because it has the free hydroxyl group at C-21. Flunisolide has approximately 20% of the receptor affinity as budesonide, and approximately 40% of the inhaled dose is systemically bioavailable. Flunisolide is quickly metabolized by CYP3A4 to the 6β-hydroxy metabolite, which has less than 1% of the activity of the parent compound. This, along with the rapid elimination of both flunisolide and its metabolite as glucuronides, greatly limits any systemic adverse effects. Flunisolide is available as a microcrystalline powder aerosol.

Fluticasone Propionate

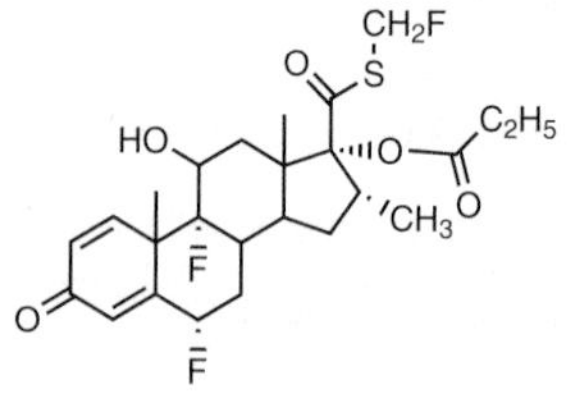

Fluticasone propionate (Flovent, Flonase)

6α,9α-Difluoro-S-fluoromethyl-11β-hydroxy-16α-methyl-3-oxo-17α-propionyloxyandrosta-1, 4-diene-17α-carbothioate

Fluticasone propionate has a unique C-20 thioflouromethyl group, and that, in combination with the 17α-propionate ester, gives it 36-fold the glucocorticoid receptor affinity as compared to beclomethasone dipropionate and twofold the affinity as compared to budesonide. The 9α-flouro group increases both glucocorticoid and mineralocorticoid activities, and the 6α-flouro group enhances only the glucocorticoid action. Studies have determined that the effectiveness of inhaled fluticasone propionate results from a local rather than a systemic effect. Interestingly, less than 1% of the swallowed dose is bioavailable, in contrast to the fact that the majority of the inhaled dose is systemically available and highly protein bound. Fluticasone propionate is not a prodrug and is extensively metabolized by the liver. The only detectable metabolite is the 17β-carboxylic acid derived from CYP3A4 oxidation. This metabolite has a 2,000-fold less affinity for the glucocorticoid receptor than the parent drug. Elimination is through both the feces and the urine, with the relative amounts determined by the route of administration. Fluticasone propionate is available in aerosol and powder inhalation formulations.

Mometasone Furoate

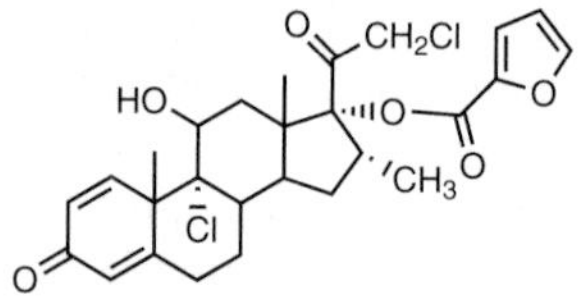

Mometasone furoate (Asmanex Twisthaler)

9α,21-dichloro-17α–[(2-furanylcarbonyl)oxy]-11β-hydroxy-16α-methylpregna-1,4-diene-3,20-dione

Mometasone furoate has a number of unique functional groups that confer enhanced glucocorticoid activity as well as pharmacokinetic advantages. The combination of the C-21 chloro and the furoic acid ester at C-17 results in the highest glucocorticoid receptor affinity of any topical corticosteroid. The 16α-methyl decreases the mineralocorticoid effects, and the 9α-chloro group increases both glucocorticoid and mineralocorticoid activities. Inhaled mometasone furoate acts locally as an anti-inflammatory treatment for asthma and has the least systemic bioavailability of all the inhaled glucocorticoids (<1%). It is extensively metabolized, with 6β-hydroxymometasone and 21-hydroxymometasone being found among the metabolites. Inhaled mometasone furoate is mainly excreted in the feces (~74%) as metabolites and only minimally excreted in the urine (~8%). It has a relatively long half-life in the lung and is administered once daily, usually in the evening.

Triamcinolone Acetonide

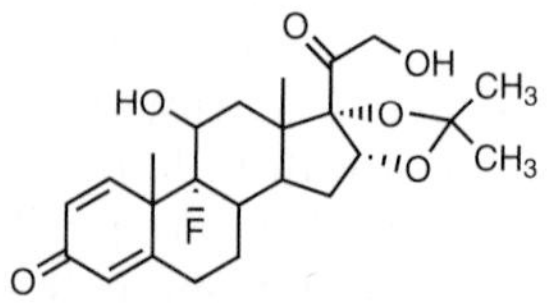

Triamcinolone acetonide (Azmacort)

9α–Fluoro-11β,17α,21-trihydroxypregna-1,4-diene-3,20-dione-16α,17-acetonide

Triamcinolone acetonide has the acetonide function, which greatly decreases its mineralocorticoid activity.

The 9α-flouro group increases both the glucocorticoid and the mineralocorticoid activities. Triamcinolone acetonide has a receptor affinity that is 10-fold that of beclomethasone dipropionate but 6-fold less than that of mometasone furoate. After oral inhalation, as much as 25% of triamcinolone acetonide can be detected systemically; a good proportion of that is assumed to be from swallowing and absorbed from the GI tract unchanged. It is metabolized in the liver to a number of metabolites, including 6β-hydroxytriamcinolone acetonide and the C-21 carboxy-6β-hydroxytriamcinolone acetonide, both of which are readily excreted via the kidneys. The acetonide remains intact during metabolic reactions and, therefore, is highly resistant to hydrolytic cleavage. Triamcinolone acetonide is excreted mainly as metabolites in the urine (40%) and in the feces (60%), with less than 1% being excreted unchanged.

Mast Cell Degranulation Inhibitors

The discovery that a Middle Eastern herb, *Ammi visnaga* (Khella, Bishop's weed), had mild bronchodilation effects led to the isolation of a benzopyrone (a chromone), khellin. Khellin had only weak bronchodilator effects, so synthetic analogs were prepared in an attempt to enhance the bronchodilation. All analogs were less active; however, it was noted by Dr. Roger Altounyans, who was experimenting on himself with these analogs, that one of them, if inhaled before an asthmatic attack, gave excellent protection against the attack's severity (48). The active compound was identified as a bischromone and named cromolyn sodium in the United States and sodium cromoglycate in Europe (Fig. 39.32).

This class of mast cell degranulation inhibitors prevents the release of histamine, leukotrienes, prostaglandins, and other inflammatory autocoids by interaction with the sensitized mast cell before antigenic challenge and does not inhibit the binding of IgE to the mast cell or the antigen to IgE. The exact mechanism of action is still not completely understood; however, it is clear that inhibition of the role of calcium in the degranulation process is involved. A number of membrane and cellular proteins that bind cromolyn sodium are known to regulate intracellular calcium levels and include basophilic membrane protein, nucleoside diphosphate kinase, calgranulins B and C, and annexins I through V (49,50). Mast cell degranulation inhibitors also are used topically in the eye to treat allergic reactions; in addition to cromolyn sodium, they include nedocromil sodium, lodoxamide tromethamine, and pemirolast potassium. (For additional details about this class of compounds, see Chapter 32.)

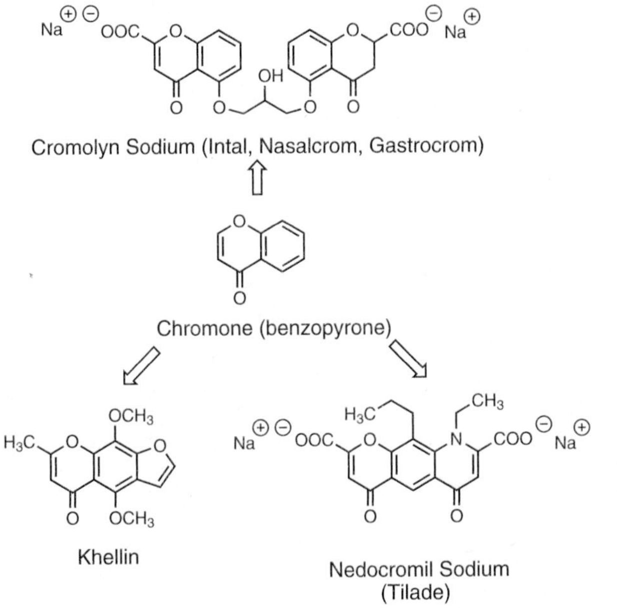

FIGURE 39.32 Structures of several chromosome mast cell stabilizers.

Mast Cell Stabilizers Used to Treat Asthma

Cromolyn Sodium

Cromolyn sodium is a bischromone that contains the fundamental benzopyrone moiety of khellin (Fig. 39.32). The two chromone rings are necessary for activity and must be coplanar, with a linking chain of no longer than six carbons. If one changes the linking chain to positions 8 and 8′, coplanarity cannot be maintained, and the compound loses all activity. Cromolyn sodium is poorly absorbed from the lungs (~8%), insignificantly from the eye (~0.07%), and by approximately 1% from the GI tract. What little that finds its way into systemic circulation is eliminated intact in the urine and the bile. For the treatment of asthma, cromolyn sodium is available as a solution for both intranasal and inhalation administration. There also is an oral concentrate (100 mg/5 mL), which is administered as a 200-mg dose given four times a day.

Nedocromil Sodium

Nedocromil sodium was developed by changing the furan ring of khellin to a piperidinone ring (Fig. 39.32). In vitro, nedocromil sodium inhibits the release of inflammatory response mediators from a variety of cells, including neutrophils, mast cells, macrophages, and platelets. Inhaled nedocromil sodium is poorly absorbed into the systemic circulation, with approximately 3% of an inhaled dose excreted in the urine during the first 6 hours after administration. Only 2% of orally dosed nedocromil sodium is bioavailable, 89% of which is protein bound. When administered IV, nedocromil sodium is not metabolized and is excreted unchanged in the bile and the urine. Nedocromil sodium is available in aerosol canisters for oral inhalation via a mouthpiece.

Leukotriene Modifiers

It has been known for more than 40 years that a substance called SRS-A (slow-reacting substance of anaphylaxis) produced a slowly developing, long-lasting contraction of isolated guinea pig ileum and that this same substance was associated with the pathophysiology of asthma.

Subsequently, it was determined that SRS-A actually was a mixture of triene-containing lipids, designated as cysteine-leukotrienes: LTC_4, LTD_4, and LTE_4. Determination of the chemical structure of these biologically active compounds led to the development of biosynthesis inhibitors as well as receptor antagonists that are useful in the treatment of asthma (51).

Biosynthesis of Leukotrienes

The leukotrienes occur in a variety of inflammatory cells that are abundant in asthma, including eosinophils, mast cells, and macrophages. They are derived from arachidonic acid via a branch of the common pathway to the prostacyclins and thromboxanes. Arachidonic acid itself is produced by the action of phospholipase A_2 on cell walls. Unlike the prostacyclins and thromboxanes, excess arachidonic acid does not activate the pathway. Instead, the first step in the conversion of arachidonic acid to produce the leukotrienes is controlled by an activating protein, 5-lipoxygenase–activating protein (FLAP), which regulates the interaction of 5-lipoxygenase with its substrate. Figure 39.33 depicts the biosynthetic pathway and shows that 5-lipoxygenase oxidizes arachidonic acid to the unstable peroxide intermediate, 5-hydroperoxyeicosatetraenoic acid, which is quickly dehydrated to LTA_4, which in turn is further metabolized by LTA_4 hydrolase to LTB_4 and by LTA_4 synthase to the glutathione adduct, LTC_4. Cleavage of γ-glutamic acid by γ-glutamyl transpeptidase converts LTC_4 to LTD_4, which in turn is converted to LTE_4 by the removal of glycine under the action of dipeptidase. The three leukotrienes produced from LTA_4 have strong bronchoconstrictive activity: LTD_4 is the most potent bronchoconstrictor, with the fastest onset of action; however, LTB_4 has no bronchoconstrictive activity but is a potent neutrophil chemotactic agent.

Leukotriene Receptors

The cysteinyl leukotriene (cysLT) receptors are of the rhodopsin family of the G protein–coupled receptor family. As such, they consist of seven transmembrane-spanning helices that activate intracellular signaling pathways in response to their endogenous ligands (LTC_4, LTD_4, and LTE_4). Studies have identified two distinct cysLT receptors, and molecular biologists have cloned the human genes for both the $cysLT_1$ receptor and the $cysLT_2$ receptor (52). Pharmacology studies distinguished between the two cysLT receptors by evaluating their interaction with known antagonists, showing that the $cysLT_1$ receptor is competitively inhibited from binding LTD_4, whereas the $cysLT_2$ receptor was not. In addition, there is a slight difference in ligand-binding affinities between the two receptors. The $cysLT_1$ receptors have an affinity profile of $LTD_4 > LTC_4 = LTE_4$, whereas the $cysLT_2$ receptors show an affinity profile of $LTC_4 = LTD_4 > LTE_4$. Both receptor types occur in the lungs and spleen. The $cysLT_1$ receptor is found only in the placenta and small intestines, whereas the $cysLT_2$ receptor occurs only in the heart, lymph nodes, and brain. The incomplete overlap of tissue distribution along with their distinct ligand-binding

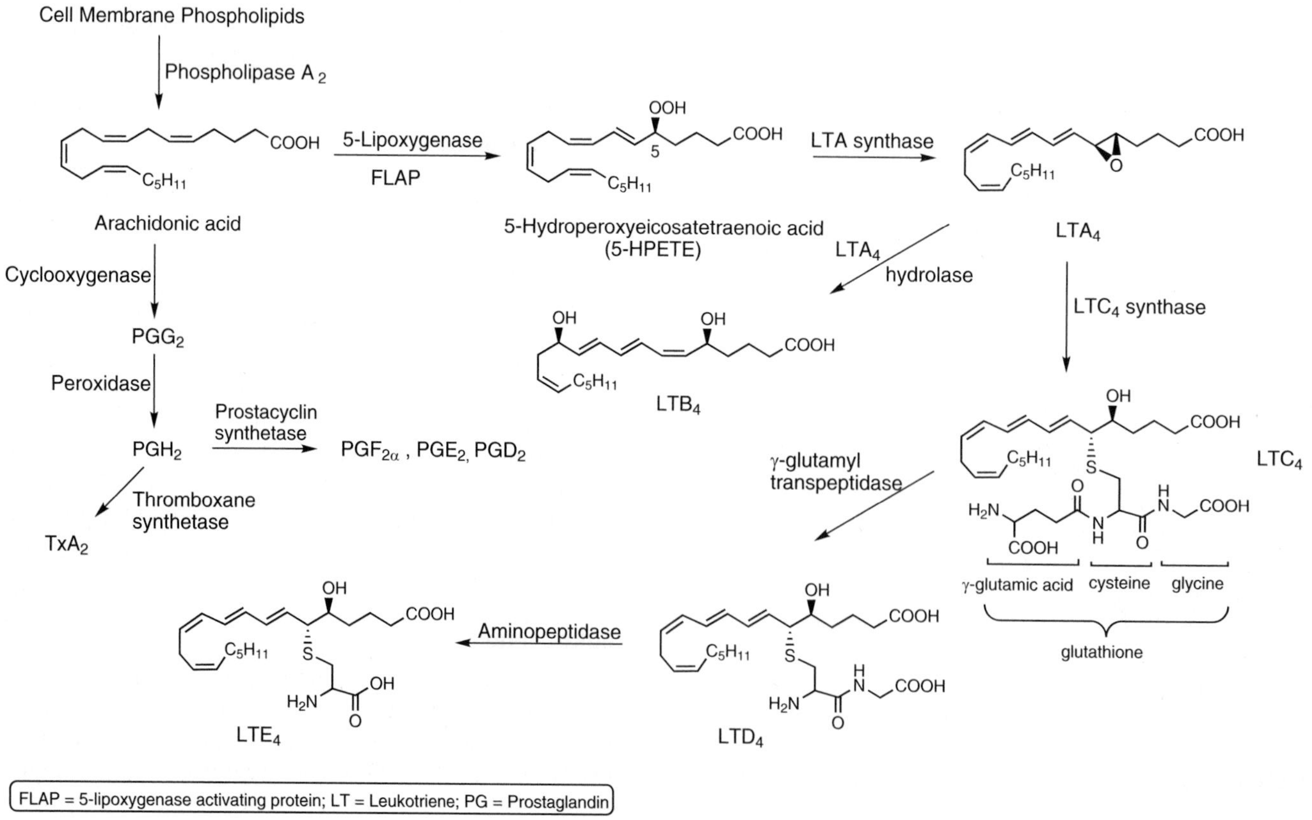

FIGURE 39.33 Biochemical pathways leading to the leukotrienes.

properties suggests the $cysLT_1$ receptors and the $cysLT_2$ receptors might serve different functions in vivo (53), and because the $cysLT_1$ receptors are inhibited by selective antagonists, they have importance in the treatment of leukotriene-related bronchoconstriction in asthma.

Leukotriene Modifier Drugs

Two approaches to the development of leukotriene modifiers have been taken. The first approach was to block their biosynthesis by looking for compounds that inhibit one or more of the enzymes involved in the biochemical pathway. The second approach was to identify antagonists with selective affinity for the $cysLT_1$ receptors.

Leukotriene Biosynthesis Inhibitors

The search for orally active 5-lipoxygenase inhibitors has resulted in only a few classes of compounds that are effective in animals and humans with the *N*-hydroxyureas, yielding a useful product (54). The 5-lipoxygenase inhibitors block the production of LTB_4 as well as LTC_4, LTD_4, and LTE_4, thereby decreasing both the bronchoconstrictive and chemotactic effects of the leukotrienes.

ZILEUTON

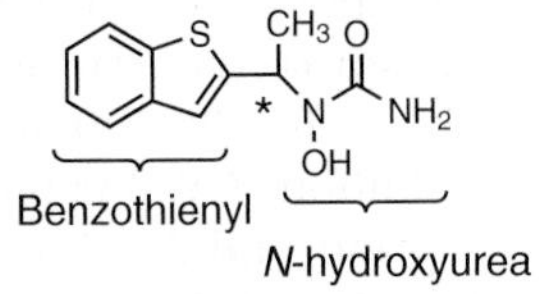

Zileuton (Zyflo)

Zileuton is the first *N*-hydroxyurea 5-lipoxygenase inhibitor to be marketed. It is the ethylbenzothienyl derivative of *N*-hydroxyurea and occurs as the racemic mixture of *R*-(+)- and *S*-(−)-enantiomers, both of which are pharmacologically active. The *N*-hydroxyl group is essential for inhibitory activity, with the benzothienyl group contributing to its overall lipophilicity. Zileuton is rapidly absorbed orally and is 93% protein bound in the plasma. Metabolism occurs in the liver, with the inactive *O*-glucuronide being the major metabolite, along with less than 0.5% inactive *N*-dehydroxylated and unchanged zileuton. The glucuronidation is stereoselective, with the *S*-isomer being metabolized and eliminated more quickly (55). Greater than 90% of an oral dose is bioavailable, and 95% is excreted as metabolites in the urine, with a half-life of 2.5 hours, thus requiring four-times-a-day dosing. Zileuton increases the plasma levels of propranolol, theophylline, and warfarin, and dosing of these drugs should be reduced and the serum levels monitored carefully in patients taking both drugs. The most serious side effect of zileuton is elevation of liver enzymes; if symptoms of liver dysfunction (e.g., nausea, fatigue, pruritus, jaundice, or flu-like symptoms) occur, the drug should be discontinued.

Leukotriene Receptor Antagonists

The search for leukotriene receptor antagonists began without the aid of ligand–receptor binding data and took the form of three approaches. These included the design of leukotriene structural analogs and quinoline analogs and the random screening of compounds. The combination of these efforts led to a simple structure–activity relationship: The lipophilic tetraene tail of LTD_4 can be mimicked by a variety of more stable aromatic rings, the thioether of the glycinylcysteinyl dipeptide can be replaced by an alkyl carboxylic acid, and the C_1 carboxylate of LTD_4 needs to be retained. Additional research focusing on the three-dimensional requirements for antagonist binding to the cysLT receptors further clarified that the pharmacophore needs to consist of an acidic or negative ionizable functional group, a hydrogen-bond acceptor function, and three hydrophobic regions (56). Based on this background, synthetic efforts resulted in the development of montelukast and zafirlukast as $cysLT_1$ receptor antagonists. Figure 39.34 demonstrates how both these antagonists fit the pharmacophore model.

MONTELUKAST

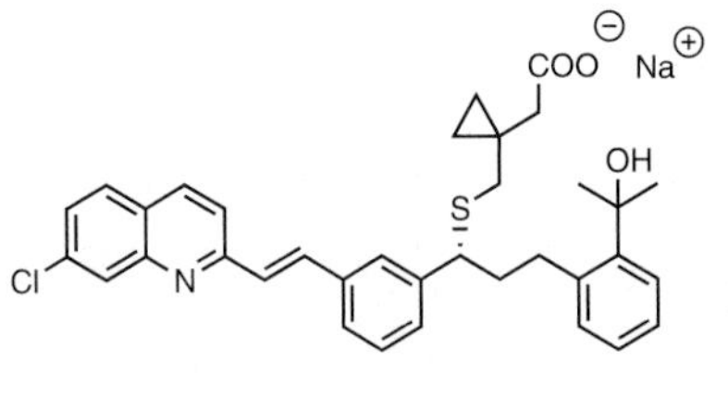

Montelukast (Singulair)

Montelukast was developed from other weakly antagonistic quinoline derivatives. A number of changes can be made to the structure without the loss of activity. These include changing the double bond between the two aromatic rings to an ether linkage, reducing the quinoline ring, changing the chlorine to a fluorine, and/or exchanging the sulfur for an amide group. Montelukast is a high-affinity, selective antagonist of the $cysLT_1$ receptor. It is rapidly absorbed orally, with a bioavailability of 64%. Montelukast is 99% bound to plasma proteins and is metabolized extensively in the liver by CYP3A4 and CYP2C9 to oxidated products. CYP3A4 oxidizes the sulfur and the C-21 benzylic carbon, whereas CYP2C9 is selectively responsible for the methyl hydroxylation. Figure 39.35 shows the primary metabolic pathway for montelukast in humans (57). More than 86% of an oral dose is eliminated as metabolites through the bile. Montelukast did not demonstrate any significant adverse effects greater than placebo in clinical trials; however, because it is metabolized by the cytochrome P450 enzymes, its plasma levels should be monitored when coadministered with cytochrome P450–inducing drugs, such as phenobarbital, rifampin, and phenytoin. Montelukast is available in tablet, chewable tablet, and granules for administration mixed with food.

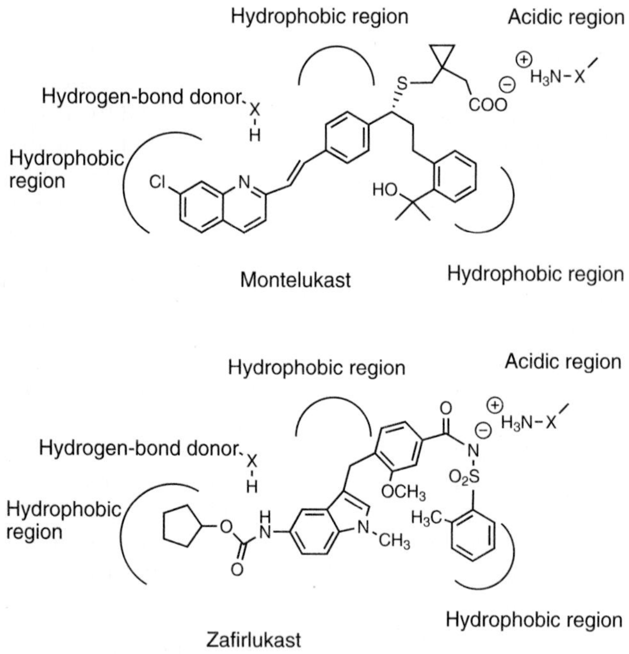

FIGURE 39.34 Interaction of montelukast and zafirlukast with cysteinyl leukotriene (cysLT) receptor model.

Zafirlukast

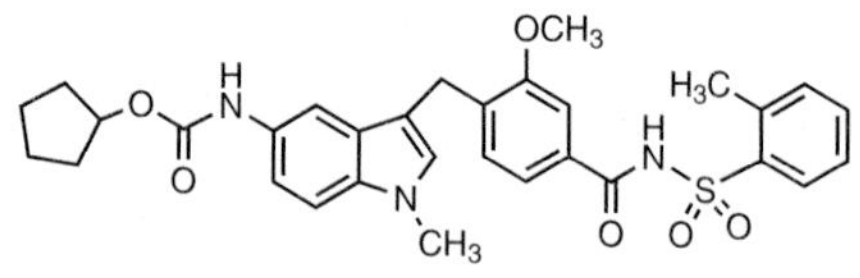

Zafirlukast (Accolate)

Zafirlukast is an indole derivative with a sulfonamide group that fulfills the need for an ionizable moiety on the pharmacophore. A large number of analogs have been prepared; however, they all resulted in a decrease in antagonist activity. Zafirlukast, like montelukast, is a selective antagonist for the $cysLT_1$ receptor and antagonizes the bronchoconstrictive effects of all leukotrienes (LTC_4, LTD_4, and LTE_4). Zafirlukast is well absorbed orally; however, food will decrease its absorption by as much as 40%. Zafirlukast is primarily metabolized in the liver by CYP2C9 and CYP3A4 to hydroxylated metabolites (58). Zafirlukast also has been shown to undergo carbamate hydrolysis, followed by *N*-acetylation. Additionally, zafirlukast is known to produce an idiosyncratic hepatotoxicity in susceptible patients. This appears to result from the formation of an electrophilic α,β-unsaturated iminium intermediate evidenced by the formation of a glutathione adduct on the methylene carbon bridging the indole ring to the methoxybenzene moiety of the molecule (59).

Figure 39.36 summarizes the metabolism of zafirlukast. More than 90% of its metabolites are excreted in the feces, with the remaining found in the urine. Zafirlukast inhibits CYP3A4 and CYP2C9 in concentrations equivalent to clinical plasma levels and, therefore, should be used with caution in patients taking drugs metabolized by these enzymes. Specifically, coadministration with warfarin results in a significant increase in prothrombin time. Other drugs metabolized by CYP2C9 are phenytoin and carbamazepine. In addition, CYP3A4-metabolized drugs are cyclosporine, cisapride, and the dihydropyridine class of calcium channel blockers. Of particular interest is the fact that aspirin increases the plasma levels of zafirlukast, and theophylline decreases the plasma levels of zafirlukast.

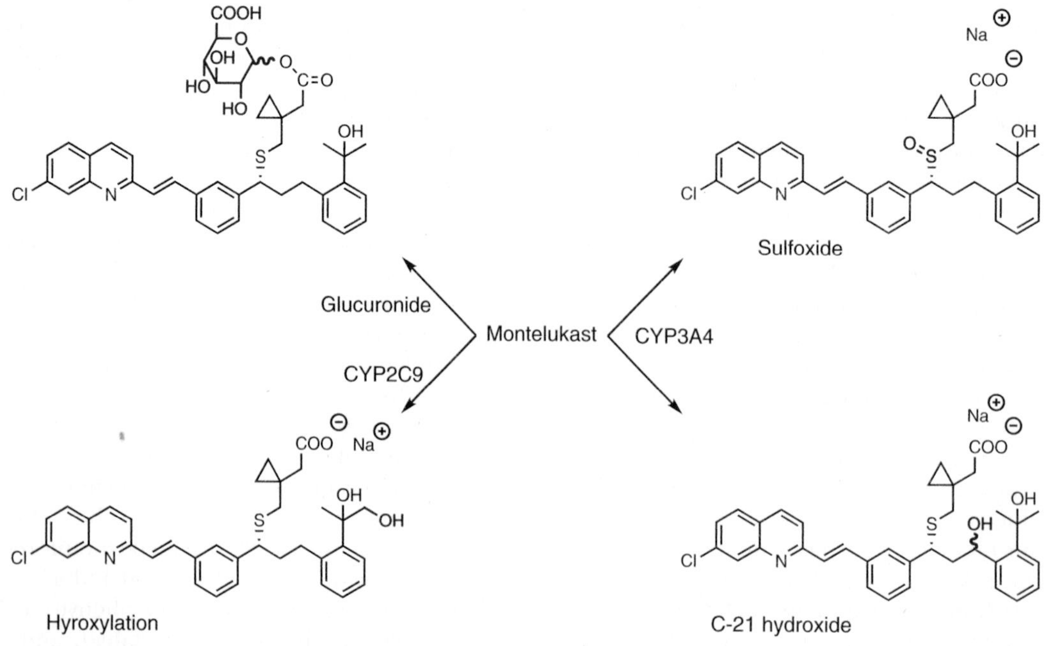

FIGURE 39.35 Metabolism of montelukast.

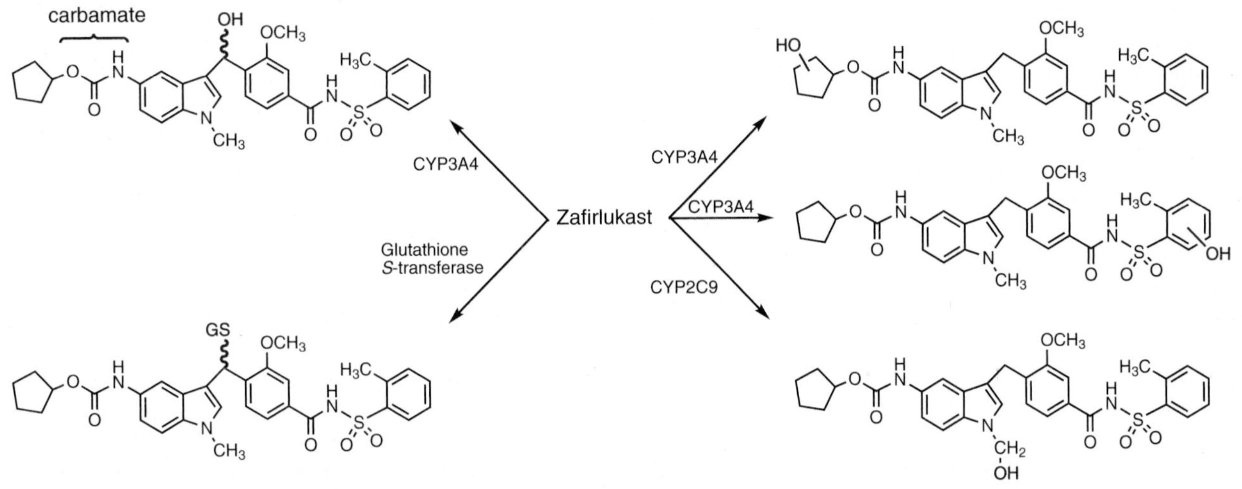

FIGURE 39.36 Metabolism of zafirlukast to oxidative products and a glutathione adduct.

Care should be taken when coadministering with erythromycin, because this decreases the bioavailability of zafirlukast. Zafirlukast is only available in tablet formulations.

Monoclonal Anti-IgE Antibody

The pathophysiology of allergic asthma, as already discussed, ultimately results in the production of allergen-specific IgE by activated B lymphocytes. The IgE binds to high-affinity (FcεRI) receptors on mast cells. The site where IgE binds to the receptor is located on the Fc fragment area of the C-ε-3 region, hence the acronym FcεRI (Fig. 39.37A). Subsequent allergen exposure causes cross-linking of bound IgE molecules, which triggers degranulation of these cells, resulting in the release of asthma mediators. Monoclonal anti-IgE antibody development is designed to moderate the role of IgE in activating mast cells, thereby decreasing the severity of allergic asthmatic attacks, and may also have beneficial effects in treating seasonal allergic rhinitis.

Omalizumab Development and Pharmacology

Omalizumab is a monoclonal antibody developed through somatic cell hybridization techniques and was identified as a murine anti-human IgE antibody, originally called MAE11 (60). It is designed to interact with the site that binds to FcεRI on mast cells. Additional amino acid sequences have been incorporated into the antibody so that a humanized product resulted that only differs by 5% nonhuman amino acid residues.

In vitro, omalizumab has been shown to complex with free IgE, forming trimers consisting of a 2:1 complex of IgE to omalizumab or a 1:2 complex of IgE to omalizumab. In addition, larger complexes also are formed, consisting of a 3:3 ratio of each (Fig. 39.37B). Omalizumab does not bind to IgE already bound to mast cells and, therefore, does not cause the degranulation that might be expected from such interaction. Thus, omalizumab effectively neutralizes free IgE and, aside from the obvious decrease of available IgE, also causes the down-regulation of FcεRI receptors on the mast cell surface, resulting in a decrease of IgE bound to the mast cell.

Omalizumab (Xolaire)

The clinical role for omalizumab is in the treatment of allergic asthma. It is approved for the treatment of adults and adolescents 12 years of age and older whose symptoms

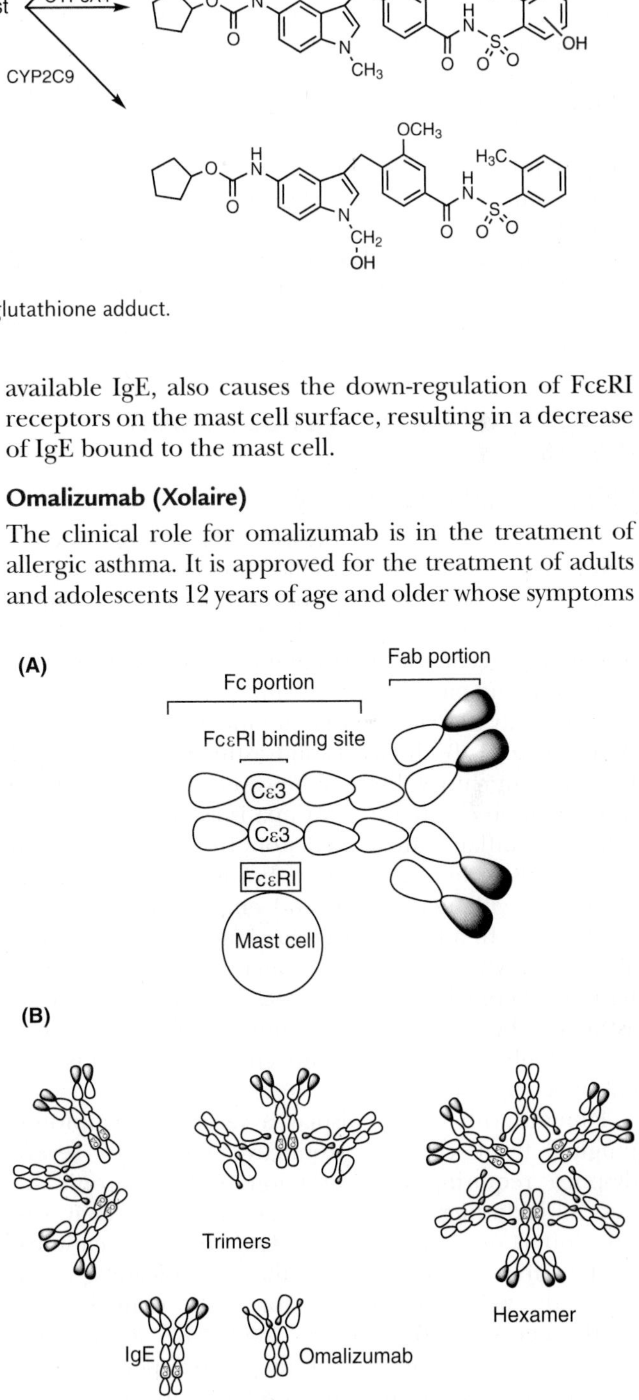

FIGURE 39.37 (A) Graphic representation of IgE binding to the FcεRI on a mast cell. (B) Graphic representation of immune complexes formed between omalizumab. Hexamers predominate when components are in a 1:1 ratio, and the trimers predominate when one of the components is in excess.

are not controlled with inhaled glucocorticoids and who have a positive skin test for airborne allergens. The bioavailability after subcutaneous administration is 62%, with slow absorption resulting in peak serum levels in 7 to 8 days from a single dose. Steady-state plasma concentration is reached in 14 to 29 days with multiple dosing regimens. The elimination of omalizumab is not clearly understood; however, studies have determined that intact IgE is excreted via the bile and that omalizumab:IgE complexes are cleared faster than uncomplexed omalizumab and slower than free IgE. This means that over time, total IgE concentrations (free and complexed IgE) increase, because the complex is cleared more slowly. The metabolism of omalizumab is not known, and the clearance of the complex is similar to the liver elimination of another immunoglobulin, IgG. The reticuloendothelial system degrades IgG, and it is believed that the same process occurs for the omalizumab:IgE complex. Omalizumab is available as a lyophilized powder for injection in single-use, 5-mL vials.

CHRONIC OBSTRUCTIVE PULMONARY DISEASE

Definition and Epidemiology

COPD is characterized by persistent breathing difficulty that is not completely reversible and is progressive over time. It usually is the result of an abnormal inflammatory response to airborne toxic chemicals. Thus, COPD is a general term and most commonly refers to chronic bronchitis and emphysema. Asthma is considered to be a disease entity unto itself and is not included in the definition of COPD. Both COPD and asthma are considered to be inflammatory diseases; however, the nature of the inflammation is different. Asthma is associated with the release of inflammatory mediators from mast cells and eosinophils, whereas chronic bronchitis is primarily associated with neutrophils and emphysema with alveoli damage. In addition, asthma is more often than not allergenic, whereas chronic bronchitis and emphysema have no allergic component. Finally, it is uncommon for asthma to be associated with smoking, whereas there is a very high incidence of both chronic bronchitis and emphysema in smokers.

Patients with COPD display a variety of symptoms, ranging from chronic productive cough to severe dyspnea requiring hospitalization. Other chronic illnesses, including cardiac, endocrine, and renal disease, often occur along with COPD in many patients. In the United States, COPD is the fourth leading cause of death, being responsible for more than 100,000 deaths per year (61). During 2000–2005, COPD was the underlying cause of death for 718,077 persons aged 25 years or older in the United States, with the mortality rate for women being almost twice that of men (11% vs. 5%) (62). It has been estimated that between 16 and 24 million people in the United States have COPD and that those with chronic bronchitis outnumber those with emphysema. Rates of COPD-related death among women have tripled over the last 30 years, and this is being attributed to their increase in smoking. COPD is recognized as a global health problem, and in 2001, the NIH and the World Health Organization developed the Global Initiative for Chronic Lung Disease (GOLD) guidelines, which present only evidence-based recommendations for the treatment of COPD (63,64).

Pathogenesis

The single most important risk factor for the development of COPD is smoking. It is estimated that 85% of COPD cases are attributable to cigarette smoking. Not all people who smoke, however, develop the disease, which means other factors are involved. It seems that genetics, environmental pollutants, and infection along with bronchial hyperreactivity all play an important role.

Cigarette smoke attracts inflammatory cells into the lungs and stimulates the release of the proteolytic enzyme elastase. Elastase breaks down elastin, which is a needed structural component of lung tissue. Normally, the lung is protected from elastase by an inhibitor, α_1-antitrypsin (ATT). Cigarette smoke, however, causes an abnormal amount of elastase to be produced that ATT cannot counter, leading to lung damage. Smokers with an inherited deficiency of ATT have a greatly increased risk of developing emphysema, especially at an early age. Patients with COPD show an accelerated decline in lung function (50 to 90 mL FEV_1/year) as compared to nonsmokers (20 to 30 mL/year) (see earlier discussion of FEV_1 under *General Therapeutic Approaches to the Treatment and Management of Asthma*). Patients with COPD who stop smoking slow down the progression of the disease. Unfortunately, however, they do not improve, because the symptoms are an indication of irreparable lung tissue damage.

The role of other risk factors for developing COPD is not clear. Air pollution and occupational exposure to gases and particulates from the incomplete combustion of coal, diesel, and gasoline are related to the development of cough and sputum, but development of COPD seems to occur only in susceptible individuals. Passive cigarette smoke comes from the burning end of the cigarette and actually is higher in toxic substances compared with exhaled smoke. It has been established that respiratory infections as well as cough and sputum production are more common in children who live in households where one or both parents smoke. Chinese and Afro-Caribbean races have a reduced incidence of COPD, whereas COPD in American blacks is on the rise (61,62).

Permanent destructive enlargement of the air spaces distal to the terminal bronchioles without obvious fibrosis is the pathologic characteristic of emphysema. On the other hand, chronic bronchitis is characterized by hypersecretion of mucus, most of which is produced by the trachea and first branches of the bronchi. The smaller bronchi and terminal bronchioles, however, are the site of the increased airway resistance in chronic bronchitis. In the early stages of chronic bronchitis, the mucus and inflammation contribute to "smoker's cough," with little effect on airway obstruction. As inflammation continues, cell wall edema and the production of large amounts of mucus contribute to airway narrowing and the difficulty in breathing associated with COPD. Even though bronchospasm may seem to be involved in COPD, there is little related pathogenesis. Chronic obstructive pulmonary disease is a disease of the small airways and their adjacent alveoli. In chronic bronchitis, there are structural changes in the small airways as a result of persistent inflammatory irritation, which leads to airway narrowing. Emphysema on the other hand is the result of loss of lung elastic recoil because of inflammation and alveolar wall destruction. Both diseases often occur together, with one predominate over the other. An important clinical manifestation between chronic bronchitis and emphysema is that there is significant hypoxia and carbon dioxide retention with chronic bronchitis, which does not happen with emphysema. Because of this, emphysema patients are referred to as "pink puffers," whereas patients with chronic bronchitis are called "blue bloaters" (63).

Pharmacotherapy

All the medications used to treat COPD have already been covered in the previous section on asthma. The GOLD guidelines base their treatment protocols on a classification of disease severity divided into five stages (63–65). Stages 0 and I are defined as "at risk" (0) and mild COPD (I). In stage 0, the patient has normal lung function, with chronic cough and sputum production. Treatment at this stage is to counsel the patient to reduce risks and, especially, to stop smoking. In stage I, there is minor airway limitation, characterized as FEV_1/FVC <70% but FEV_1 ≥80% of the predicted value. Stage I treatment is to use a short-acting bronchodilator, usually as needed, but regular use is effective in patients with concurrent asthma. The most frequently used short-acting bronchodilator is the β_2-agonist albuterol, although pirbuterol and the anticholinergic ipratropium can be just as effective, but with a slightly longer onset of action. The patient also should take precautions to avoid bacterial or viral infections by receiving vaccinations against influenza and pneumococcal pneumonia.

Stage II COPD is a moderate disease condition in which the patient demonstrates shortness of breath on exertion and spirometry reveals FEV_1/FVC <70% and FEV_1 between 50% and 80% of the predicted value. Stage II drug treatment requires the addition of a long-acting bronchodilator along with the short-acting bronchodilator. Salmeterol and formoterol are long-acting β_2-agonists, and tiotropium is the long-acting anticholinergic most often used. Alternatively, the addition of ipratropium along with the short-acting β_2-agonist also can be effective at this stage. Extended-release theophylline is an option for patients who do not receive adequate relief of symptoms or who cannot tolerate other bronchodilators.

Stage III is a severe form of COPD, with FEV_1/FVC <70% and FEV_1 between 30% and 50% of the predicted value. The patient experiences increasing dyspnea that affects his or her ability to perform routine tasks (i.e., climbing stairs). A course of oral glucocorticoids (i.e., prednisone) may be used to control a severe attack. The role of inhaled glucocorticoids is not clearly established, and no evidence suggests that an inhaled glucocorticoid has any advantage in patients who can maintain their FEV_1 with bronchodilators. However, the combination of an inhaled glucocorticoid with a long-acting β_2-agonist has been shown to be more effective than either drug class alone in reducing exacerbations and improving lung function. The combination formulation of fluticasone propionate and salmeterol dosage (250 μg/50 μg) is approved for twice-daily administration.

Stage IV is the most severe form of COPD, with airflow restriction of FEV_1/FVC <70% and FEV_1 <30% of the predicted value along with chronic respiratory failure. At this stage, the patient is experiencing debilitating exacerbations that are not controlled by medication and requires daily oxygen for respiratory failure. Surgery also is an option, but it is not without serious risks. Surgical options include bullectomy (removal of large blebs in the lungs), lung transplant (uncommon), and lung volume reduction surgery (removal of lung sections affected by emphysema).

Patients with emphysema that is associated with ATT deficiencies can receive weekly IV infusions of ATT to maintain acceptable antiprotease activity that can minimize their disease progression. The three approved ATT products are Aralast, Prolastin, and Zemaira. Because these protein products are derived from human plasma, there is the risk of transmission of viral infection and Creutzfeldt-Jakob disease.

New Drug Classes for Treatment of Asthma and COPD

Phosphodiesterase Inhibitors

A number of important therapeutic agents owe their pharmacologic action to their ability to inhibit the enzyme PDE. In the treatment of asthma, theophylline, at least in part, relaxes bronchospasm by relaxing bronchiole smooth muscles; amrinone and milrinone are ionotropic agents that relax vasculature, causing vasodilation; sildenafil and vardenafil relax smooth muscle of the vasculature in the penis; dipyramidole inhibits platelet aggregation; and the alkaloid papaverine relieves smooth and cardiac muscle spasms through its ability to inhibit PDE. These pharmacologic effects are the result of inhibiting the ability of PDE to break down cAMP and cGMP and prolong their action as secondary messengers within a variety of cell types throughout the body. The PDE inhibitors also are implicated in an anti-inflammatory role by increasing cAMP and cGMP levels in cell types associated with the release of inflammatory chemicals from T and B cells, monocytes, neutrophils, and eosinophils. This last discovery is the impetus to develop new PDE inhibitors to treat asthma (eosinophils) and COPD (neutrophils).

New Phosphodiesterase Inhibitors Progress in the development of PDE inhibitors to treat COPD and asthma awaited the basic pharmacologic research that identified the specific PDE isoforms associated with inflammatory cells so that selective inhibitors could be designed and synthesized (66). There are 11 families of PDEs, with PDE4 being associated with inflammatory processes. Specifically, three PDE4 subtypes (PDE4A, PDE4B, and PDE4D) are found in inflammatory cells (with PDE4B being predominant). Therefore, recent efforts in this area have been directed toward the development and synthesis of selective PDE4 inhibitors. Two PDE4 inhibitors are being investigated for their possible use in treating asthma and COPD. In the United States, cilomilast is being investigated for the treatment of COPD, and in Europe, roflumilast is being investigated for the treatment of both asthma and COPD. Progress of these and other PDE4 inhibitors toward marketing has been slow because of lack of clinical efficacy and dose-limiting side effects (nausea, diarrhea, and headache). The primary problem is the low therapeutic ratio of these compounds because the tolerated dose is either subtherapeutic or at the very bottom of the effective dose–response curve (67,68).

Cilomilast

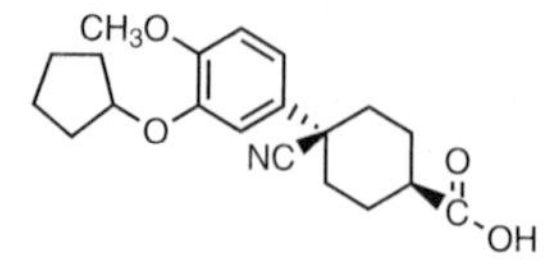

Cilomilast (Ariflo)

Cilomilast contains the dialkoxyphenyl ring characteristic of selective PDE4 inhibitors. The ether oxygens hydrogen bond to a glutamine in the binding pocket, and the cyclopentyl ring adds additional hydrophobic interactions. The oxygen atoms of the carboxyl group form hydrogen bonds with water that is coordinated with Mg^{2+} located in the distal end of the binding pocket. Orally administered cilomilast is 96% bioavailable. Food does not interfere with the overall absorption; however, food does slow down the rate. Cilomilast is 99% bound to albumin in the plasma and is metabolized in the liver by CYP2C8. The metabolism is extensive and results in oxidation, carboxyl group glucuronidation, and dealkylation of the cyclopentyl group, followed by glucuronidation or sulfation. A major difficulty with cilomilast is that in therapeutic doses, patients during clinical trials have experienced significant diarrhea and nausea. These effects appear to be significant enough to keep cilomilast off the market. These side effects, theoretically, result from its inhibition of the PDE4D receptor subtype.

Roflumilast (Daliresp)

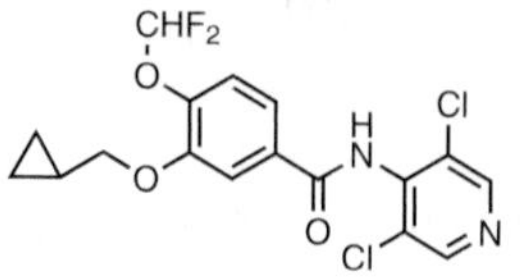

Roflumilast (Daxas)

The PDE4 receptor binding of roflumilast is similar to that of cilomilast. The dialkylphenyl oxygens hydrogen bond to a glutamine deep inside the binding pocket. The diflouromethoxy group and the cyclopropyl group contribute hydrophobic bonds; however, the cyclopentyl group on cilomilast makes far more interactions compared with the cyclopropyl group. The water molecule coordinated to the Mg^{2+} hydrogen bonds to the dichloropyridyl group just like the carboxylic acid oxygens in cilomilast. These structural differences make roflumilast a more potent inhibitor than cilomilast toward PDE4B (69). Roflumilast is well absorbed on oral administration and has a half-life of 10 hours. Roflumilast is metabolized in the liver to its *N*-oxide derivative, which also is a PDE4 inhibitor, and it has a plasma half-life of 20 hours. Roflumilast's preclinical pharmacology continues to be understood, which enables it to be an effective oral treatment for COPD with an acceptable tolerability profile (70). Roflumilast was approved for treatment of COPD associated with chronic bronchitis in the European Union in 2010 and in the U.S. in 2011.

Anticytokine Therapies

Because glucocorticoids are not effective in suppressing or controlling inflammation symptoms in asthmatics and those suffering from COPD, there continues to be a need to develop new approaches to novel therapeutic treatments. Most of these approaches are focused on the inhibition of the chemokines and cytokines associated with the inflammatory process.

The following is a brief overview, because a detailed discussion of each of these novel approaches is beyond the scope of this chapter. Anti-eosinophil attack includes targeting cytokines (anti–IL-4, -13, and -5), their receptors (βc), and the chemokine receptor (CRR3). Anti–IL-4 and anti–IL-13 therapies have been shown to be effective in allergen challenge tests. TPA ASM-8 (a mixture of two antisense oligonucleotides), which is a CCR3/βc antagonist, also has been shown to be effective. Evaluation of both of these approaches is in very early stages, and much longer studies are needed. Anti–IL-5 had no effect on allergen challenge, which indicates that targeting just one cytokine may not be the best approach to the development of new therapies. Anti–tumor necrosis factor-α therapies have shown some clinical efficacy, but there is a lingering concern about serious side effects, such as infection and malignancy. Therefore, it is likely that inhaled glucocorticoid and β_2-agonist treatments for both asthma and COPD are to be the standard of treatment for now and in the near future (71).

SCENARIO: OUTCOME AND ANALYSIS

Outcome

Joseph V. Etzel, PharmD

The goal of asthma treatment is to achieve and maintain clinical control of symptoms and minimize the occurrence of symptoms. After reviewing JP's case, the pharmacist concludes that JP's disease state is not well controlled, as suggested by his frequent exacerbations requiring short-acting β_2-agonist use, occasional nighttime awakenings, and diminished FEV_1 values. After confirming the patient's medication adherence, appropriate inhalation techniques, and environmental control, the pharmacist recommends a step up in therapy to achieve better management of JP's asthma. Because JP's asthma is inadequately controlled with a medium-dose inhaled corticosteroid, the pharmacist recommends the addition of a long-acting β_2-agonist (LABA), such as salmeterol 50 mcg inhalation twice daily. This recommendation is based on comparative studies that demonstrate significantly greater improvements in asthma control when an LABA is added to medium-dose inhaled corticosteroid therapy compared with other adjunctive therapies. Although salmeterol is available as a single entity product, the pharmacist recommends a twice-daily combination dry-powder inhalation product containing both fluticasone (250 mcg) and salmeterol (50 mcg) to improve patient adherence. Once therapy is adjusted, the patient should be re-evaluated in 2 to 6 weeks to ensure adequate response. Although comorbid disease states, such as allergic rhinitis, may exacerbate asthma, this patient's allergies appear to be well controlled and no intervention seems to be necessary.

Chemical Analysis

S. William Zito and Victoria Roche

It is recommended in this case to add an LABA to JP's asthma treatment. The fundamental pharmacophore for all adrenergic agonists is a substituted β-phenylethylamine.

The number and nature of substituents on the pharmacophore influences the specificity for the β-receptor subtypes. The substituents on the amino group (R_1) determines α- or β-receptor selectivity: the larger the bulk of the N-substituent, the greater the selectivity for the β-receptor. If R_1 is *t*-butyl or aralkyl, there is complete loss of α-receptor affinity, and the β-receptor affinity shows preference for the β_2-receptor. It must be said that receptor selectivity is dose related, and when the dose is high enough, all selectivity can be lost. Substituents other than hydrogen on the α-carbon (R_2) will show an increased duration of action because they make the compound resistant to metabolism by MAO. For an adrenergic agonist to demonstrate significant β_2-receptor selectivity there needs to be an appropriately substituted phenyl ring. The currently marketed adrenergic agonists contain a resorcinol ring, a salicyl alcohol moiety, or an m-formamide group. In addition, these ring configurations confer resistant to COMT metabolism and will increase their duration of action. So, as can be seen in the structure of salmeterol, there are two moieties that contribute to its β_2-agonist activity as well as its duration of action: (1) the phenylbutoxyhexyl N-substituent, which confers β_2-selectivity, and (2) the salicyl alcohol ring, which both reinforces β_2-selectivity and increases duration of action due to inhibition of COMT metabolism.

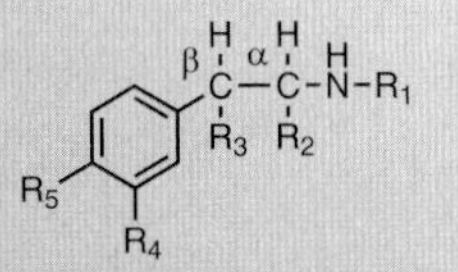

Adrenergic agonist pharmacophore

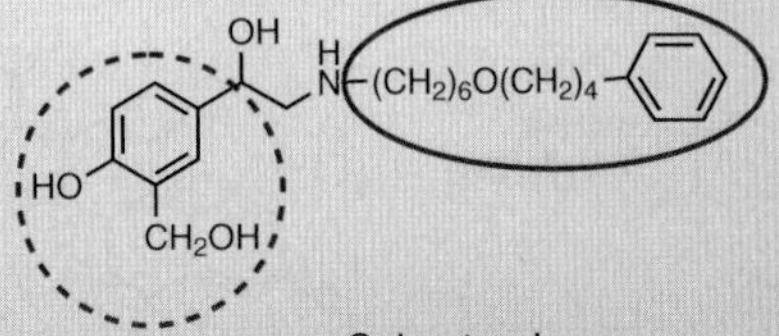

Salmeterol

CASE STUDY

S. William Zito and Victoria Roche

TJ is a 65-year-old woman who presents to the emergency department with difficulty breathing because of uncontrollable wheezing and tightness of the chest, which was brought on as a consequence of a weekend camping and fishing trip. TJ has a long history of severe persistent asthma and does not regularly monitor peak flow levels at home. TJ's asthma is treated with fluticasone proprionate (2 puffs BID), zafirlukast (20 mg BID), and albuterol (2 puffs BID; four times a day PRN).

TJ says that the albuterol usually controls her acute attacks but it did not work this morning, leaving her feeling as if she could not breath at all. On the way to the emergency department she was treated with two albuterol nebs (2.5 mg each) and 0.5 mg SQ epinephrine. In the emergency department, TJ demonstrated a peak flow of 175 L/min (baseline of last office visit was 480 L/min). The attending physician administered supplemental oxygen by nasal cannula to achieve an O_2 saturation of ≥95% and continued the albuterol at 2.5 mg every 1 hour as needed. In addition, the attending physician wants to add an oral corticosteroid to achieve a response to therapy above 60% of baseline peak expiratory flow sustained for at least 60 minutes. Evaluate the three structures for use in this case.

1. Conduct a thorough and mechanistic SAR analysis of the three therapeutic options in the case.
2. Apply the chemical understanding gained from the SAR analysis to this patient's specific needs to make a therapeutic recommendation.

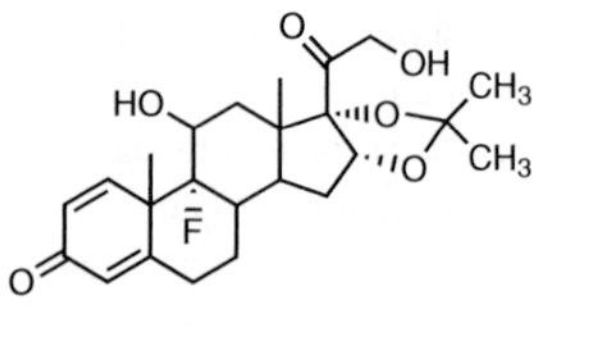

Triamcinolone acetonide

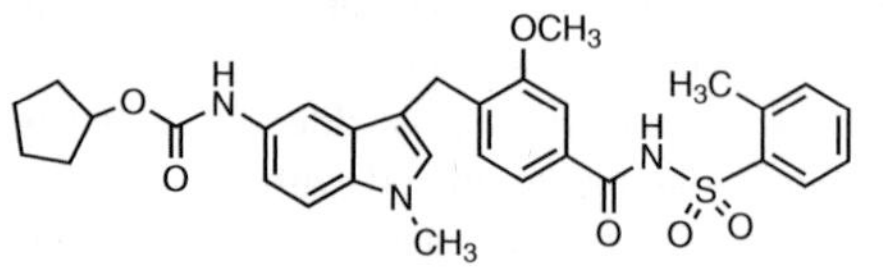

Zafirlukast

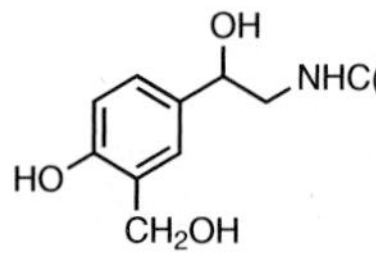

Albuterol

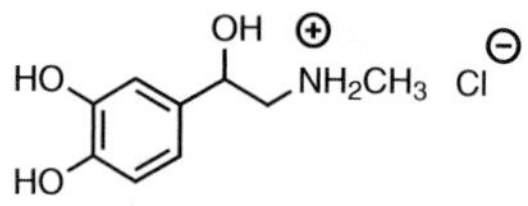

Epinephrine

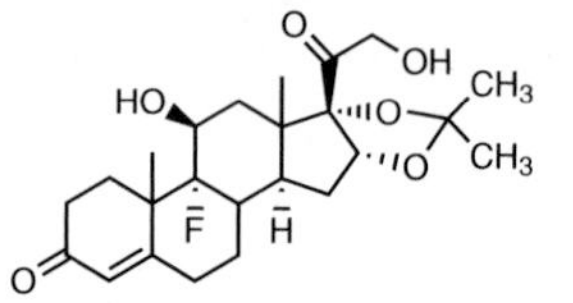

1

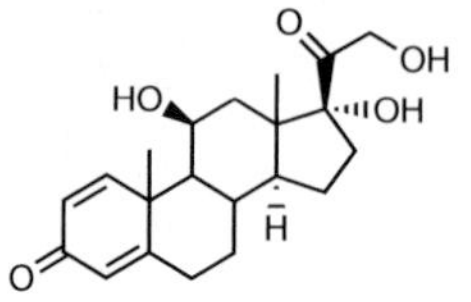

2

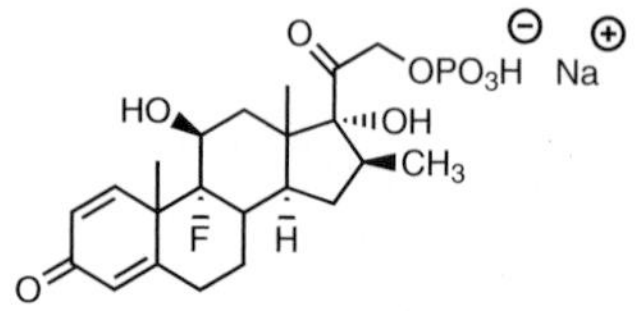

3

References

1. Marketos S, Ballas CN. Bronchial asthma in the medical literature of Greek antiquity. J Asthma 1982;19:263–269.
2. Mannino D, Homa DM, Akinbami LJ, et al. Surveillance for asthma: United States, 1980–1999. Morbid Mortal Wkly Rep 2002;51(SS-1):1-14.
3. Moorman J, Rudd RA, Johnson CA, et al. Surveillance for asthma: United States, 1908-2004. Morbid Mortal Wkly Rep 2007;56(SS-8):1–15.
4. Sondik E, Madans JH, Gentleman JF. Summary health statistics for U.S. adults: National Health Interview Survey, 2008. 2010; Available from: Available at: http://www.cdc.gov/asthma/asthmadata.htm.
5. Korelitz J, Zito JM, Gavin NI, et al. Asthma-related medication use among children in the United States. Ann Allerg Asthma Immunol 2008;100:222–229.
6. Busse WW. Expert Panel Report 3 (EPR-3): guidelines for the diagnosis and management of asthma–summary report 2007. J Allerg Clin Immunol 2007;120(Suppl 1):S94–S138.
7. Busse WW. National Heart, Lung, and Blood Institute, National Asthma Education and Prevention Program, Expert Panel Report 3: guidelines for the diagnosis and management of asthma. Full Report 2007. Available at: http://www.nhlbi.nih.gov/guidelines/asthma/asthgdln.htm.
8. Elias J, Lee CG, Zheng T, et al. New insights into the pathogenesis of asthma. J Clin Invest 2003;111:291–297.
9. Centers for Disease Control and Prevention. Important asthma triggers. 2010. Available at: http://www.cdc.gov/asthma/triggers.
10. Weiss ST. Eat dirt: the hygiene hypothesis and allergic diseases. N Engl J Med 2002;347:930–931.
11. Bach J-F. The Effect of Infections on susceptibility to autoimmune and allergic diseases. N Engl J Med 2002;347:911–920.
12. Vock C, Hauber H, Wegmann M. The other T helper cells in asthma pathogenesis. J Allerg 2010;519298:1-14.
13. Cookson W. The alliance of genes and environment in asthma and allergy. Nature 1999;402(Suppl 6760):B5–B11.
14. Ober C. Perspectives on the past decade of asthma genetics. J Allerg Clin Immunol 2005;116:274–278.
15. Sandford AJ, Pare PD. The genetics of asthma. The important questions. Am J Respir Crit Care Med 2000;161:S202–S206.
16. Tattersfield A, Knox AJ, Britton JR, et al. Asthma. Lancet 2002;360:1313–1322.
17. Bochner B, Busse WW. Allergy and asthma. J Allerg Clin Immunol 2005;115:953–959.
18. Lilly CM. Diversity of asthma: evolving concepts of pathophysiology and lessons from genetics. J Allerg Clin Immunol 2005;115:S526–S531.
19. Moffatt MF, Gut IG, Demenais F, et al. A large-scale, consortium-based genomewide association study of asthma. N Eng J Med 2010;363:1211–1221.

20. Mizue Y, Ghani S, Lang L, et al. Role for macrophage migration inhibitory factor in asthma. Proc Natl Acad Sci U S A 2005;102:14410–14415.
21. Hare AA, Leng L, Gandavadi S, et al. Optimization of N-benzyl-benzoxazol-2-ones as receptor antagonists of macrophage migration inhibitory factor (MIF). Bioorg Med Chem Lett 2010;20:5811–5814.
22. Peters J, Levine SM. Introduction to pulmonary function testing. In: DiPiro JT, Talbert RL, Yee GC, et al., eds. Pharmacotherapy: A Pathophysiologic Approach. Stamford, CT: McGraw-Hill, 2002:463–473.
23. Welsh D, Thomas DA. Obstructive lung disease. In: Ali J, Levitzky MG, eds. Pulmonary Pathophysiology. New York: Lange Medical Books/McGraw-Hill, 2005:85–91.
24. Locksley RM. Asthma and allergic inflammation. Cell 2010;140:777–783.
25. U.S. Food and Drug Administration. Drug safety communication: new safety requirements for long-acting inhaled asthma medications called long-acting beta-agonists (LABAs). 2010; Available at: http://www.fda.gov/Drugs/DrugSafety/PostmarketDrugSafetyInformationforPatientsandProviders/ucm200776.htm.
26. Ahlquist RP. A study of the adrenotropic receptors. Am J Physiol 1948;153:586–600.
27. Philipp M, Hein L. Adrenergic receptor knockout mice: distinct functions of 9 receptor subtypes. Pharmacol Ther 2004;101:65–74.
28. Bikker JA, Trumpp-Kallmeyer S, Humblet C. G-protein coupled receptors: models, mutagenesis, and drug design. J Med Chem 1998;41:2911–2927.
29. Furse KE, Lybrand TP. Three-dimensional models for β-adrenergic receptor complexes with agonists and antagonists. J Med Chem 2003;46:4450–4462.
30. Nelson HS, Weiss ST, Bleecker ER, et al. The Salmeterol Multicenter Asthma Research Trial. Chest 2006;129:15–26.
31. Zhang M, Fawcett JP, Kennedy JM, et al. Stereoselective glucuronidation of formoterol by human liver microsomes. Br J Clin Pharmacol 2000;49:152–157.
32. Kua J, Zhang Y, Eslami AC, et al. Studying the roles of W86, E202, and Y337 in binding of acetylcholine to acetylcholinesterase using a combined molecular dynamics and multiple docking approach. Protein Sci 2003;12:2675–2684.
33. Kostenis E, Zeng FY, Wess J. Structure-function analysis of muscarinic acetylcholine receptors. J Physiol Paris 1998;92:265–268.
34. Katzung B. Introduction to autonomic pharmacology. In: Katzung B, ed. Basic and Clinical Pharmacology. New York: Lang Medical Books/McGraw-Hill, 2001:75–191.
35. Wess J, Blin N, Mutschler E, et al. Muscarinic acetylcholine receptors: structural basis of ligand binding and G protein coupling. Life Sci 1995;56:915–922.
36. Joos G, Schelfhout VJ, Pauwels RA, et al. Bronchodilatory effects of aclidinium bromide, a long-acting muscarinic antagonist, in COPD patients. Respir Med 2010;104:865–872.
37. Albertí J, Sentellas S, Salvà M. In vitro liver metabolism of aclidinium bromide in preclinical animal species and humans: identification of the human enzymes involved in its oxidative metabolism. Biochem Pharmacol 2011;81:761–776.
38. Sentellas S, Ramos I, Albertí J, et al. Aclidinium bromide, a new, long-acting, inhaled muscarinic antagonist: in vitro plasma inactivation and pharmacological activity of its main metabolites. Eur J Pharm Sci 2010;39:283–290.
39. Robbers J, Speedie MK, Tyler VE. Pharmacognosy and Pharmacobiotechnology. Baltimore: Williams and Wilkins, 1996.
40. Huai Q, Liu Y, Francis SH, et al. Crystal structures of phosphodiesterases 4 and 5 in complex with inhibitor 3-isobutyl-1-methylxanthine suggest a conformation determinant of inhibitor selectivity. J Biol Chem 2004;279:13095–13101.
41. IUPAC-IUB Joint Commission on Biochemical Nomenclature (JCBN). The nomenclature of steroids. Eur J Biochem 1989;186:429–458.
42. Luisi BF, Xu W, Otwinowski Z, et al. Crystallographic analysis of the interaction of the glucocorticoid receptor with DNA. Nature 1991;352:497–505.
43. Bhavsar P, Ahmad T, Adcock IM. The role of histone deacetylases in asthma and allergic diseases. J Allerg Clin Immunol 2008;121:580–584.
44. Bledsoe RK, Montana V, Stanley T, et al. Crystal structure of the glucocorticoid receptor ligand binding domain reveals a novel mode of receptor dimerization and coactivator recognition. Cell 2002;110:93–105.
45. Hammer S, Spika I, Sippl W, et al. Glucocorticoid receptor interactions with glucocorticoids: evaluation by molecular modeling and functional analysis of glucocorticoid receptor mutants. Steroids 2003;68:329–339.
46. Jewell C, Prusakiewicz JJ, Ackermann C, et al. The distribution of esterases in the skin of the minipig. Toxicol Lett 2007;173:118–123.
47. Thompson R, Whittaker VP. The esterases of skin. Biochem J 1944;38:295–299.
48. Howell J. Roger Altounyan and the discovery of cromolyn (sodium cromoglycate). J Allerg Clin Immunol 2005;115:882–885.
49. Hemmerich S, Yarden Y, Pecht I. A cromoglycate binding protein from rat mast cells of a leukemia line is a nucleoside diphosphate kinase. Biochemistry 1992;31:4574–4579.
50. Oyama Y, Shishibori T, Yamashita K, et al. Two distinct anti-allergic drugs, amlexanox and cromolyn, bind to the same kinds of calcium binding proteins, except calmodulin, in bovine lung extract. Biochem Biophys Res Commun 1997;240:341–347.
51. Samuelsson B, Dahlén SE, Lindgren JA, et al. Leukotrienes and lipoxins: structures, biosynthesis, and biological effects. Science 1987;237:1171–1176.
52. Capra V. Molecular and functional aspects of human cysteinyl leukotriene receptors. Pharmacol Res 2004;50:1–11.
53. Kanaoka Y, Boyce JA. Cysteinyl leukotrienes and their receptors: cellular distribution and function in immune and inflammatory responses. J Immunol 2004;173:1503–1510.
54. Brooks CDW, Summers JB. Modulators of leukotriene biosynthesis and receptor activation. J Med Chem 1996;39:2629–2654.
55. Sweeny DJ, Nellans HN. Stereoselective glucuronidation of zileuton isomers by human hepatic microsomes. Drug Metab Dispos 1995;23:149–153.
56. Palomer A, Pascual J, Cabré F, et al. Derivation of pharmacophore and CoMFA models for leukotriene D4 receptor antagonists of the quinolinyl(bridged) aryl series. J Med Chem 2000;43:392–400.
57. Chiba M, Xu X, Nishime J, et al. Hepatic microsomal metabolism of montelukast, a potent leukotriene D4 receptor antagonist, in humans. Drug Metab Dispos 1997;25:1022–1031.
58. Savidge RD, Bui K, Birmingham B, et al. Metabolism and excretion of zafirlukast in dogs, rats, and mice. Drug Metab Dispos 1998;26:1069–1076.
59. Kassahun K, Skordos K, McIntosh I, et al. Zafirlukast metabolism by cytochrome P450 3A4 produces an electrophilic α,β-unsaturated iminium species that results in the selective mechanism-based inactivation of the enzyme. Chem Res Toxicol 2005;18:1427–1437.
60. Buhl R. Anti-IgE antibodies for the treatment of asthma. Curr Opin Pulm Med 2005;11:27–34.
61. Mannino D, Homa DM, Akinbami LJ, et al. Chronic obstructive pulmonary disease surveillance—United States, 1971-2000. Morbid Mortal Wkly Rep Surv Summ 2002;51(SS-6):1–18.
62. Brown D, Croft JB, Greenlund KJ, et al. Deaths from chronic obstructive pulmonary disease: United States, 2000–2005. Morbid Mortal Wkly Rep 2008;57:1229–1232.
63. Pauwels RA, Buist A, Claverley P, et al. Global strategy for the diagnosis, management, and prevention of chronic obstructive pulmonary disease. NHLBI/WHO Global Initiative for Chronic Obstructive Lung Disease (GOLD) Workshop Summary. Am J Respir Crit Care Med 2001;163:1256–1276.
64. Global strategy for diagnosis, management, and prevention of COPD–updated 2009. Available at: http://www.goldcopd.com/GuidelinesResources.asp?l1=2&l2=0.
65. Konzem S, Stratton MA. Chronic obstructive lung disease. In: DiPiro JT, Talbert RL, Yee GC, et al., eds. Pharmacotherapy: A Pathophysiologic Approach. Stamford, CT: McGraw-Hill, 2002.
66. Lipworth BJ. Phosphodiesterase-4 inhibitors for asthma and chronic obstructive pulmonary disease. Lancet 2005;365:167–175.
67. Spina D. PDE4 Inhibitors: current status. Br J Pharmacol 2008;155:308–315.
68. Giembycz M. Can the anti-inflammatory potential of PDE4 inhibitors be realized: guarded optimism or wishful thinking? Br J Pharmacol 2008;155:288–290.
69. Card GL, England B, Suzuki Y, et al. Structural basis for the activity of drugs that inhibit phosphodiesterases. Structure 2004;12:2233–2247.
70. Hatzelmann A, Morcillo EJ, Lungarella G, et al. The preclinical pharmacology of roflumilast: a selective, oral phosphodiesterase 4 inhibitor in development for chronic obstructive pulmonary disease. Pulm Pharmacol Ther 2010;23:235–256.
71. Bhowmick B, Singh D. Novel anti-inflammatory treatments for asthma. Exp Rev Respir Med 2008;2:617–629.

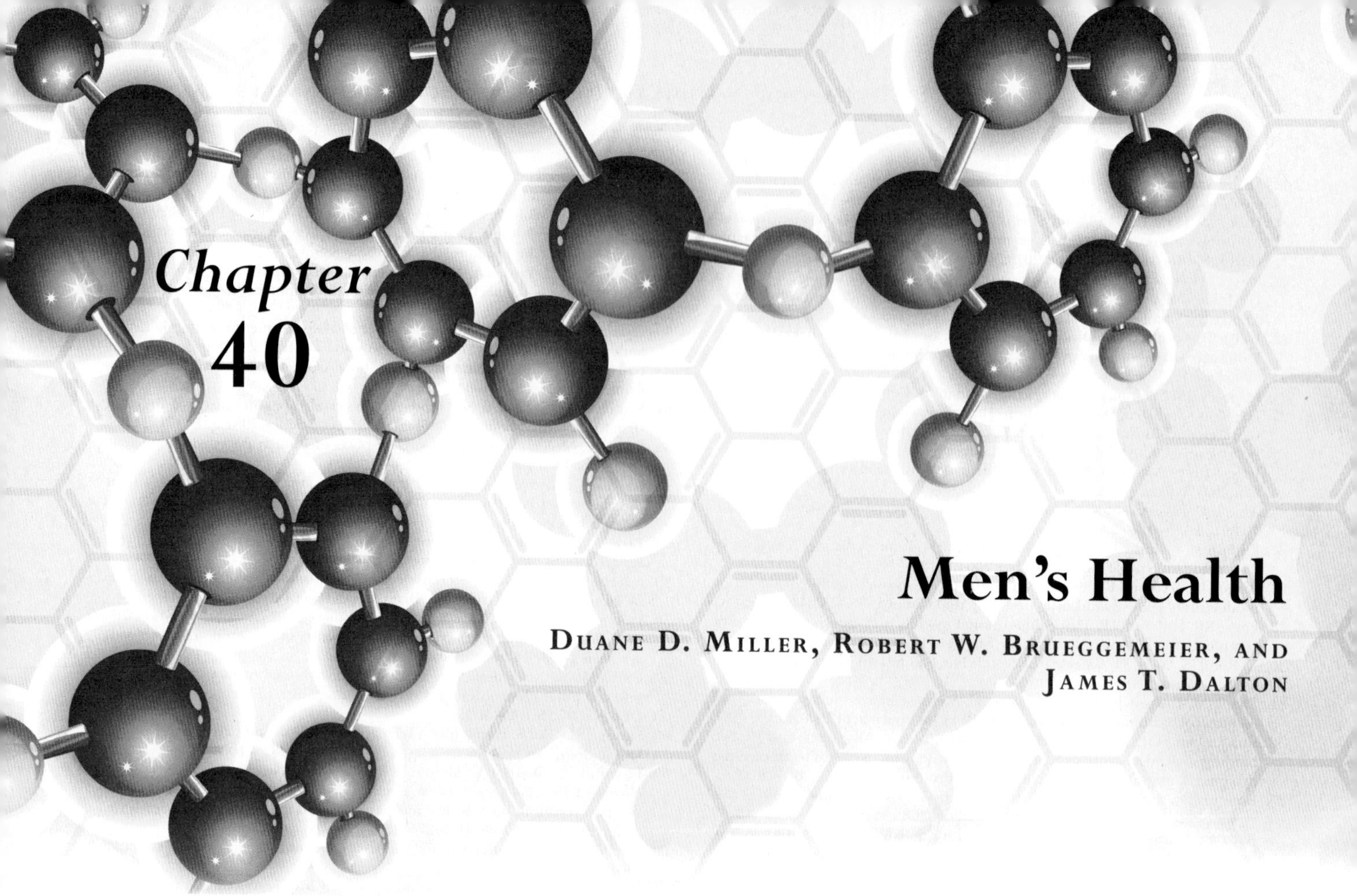

Chapter 40

Men's Health

Duane D. Miller, Robert W. Brueggemeier, and James T. Dalton

Drugs Covered in This Chapter*

Anabolic agents
- Nandrolone
- Oxandrolone
- Oxymetholone
- Stanozolol
- *Testolactone*

Chemotherapy and immunotherapy
- Docetaxel
- Sipuleucel-T

Drugs for the treatment of benign prostatic hyperplasia

α_1-Adrenergic antagonists
- Alfuzosin
- Doxazosin
- Silodosin
- Tamsulosin
- Terazosin

5α-Reductase inhibitors
- Dutasteride
- Finasteride

Drugs for treatment of erectile dysfunction

Phosphodiesterase-5 inhibitors
- Sildenafil
- Tadalafil
- Vardenafil

Miscellaneous drugs
- Prostaglandin E1
- Papaverine
- Phentolamine

Testosterone products
- Fluoxymesterone
- Methyltestosterone
- Testosterone
- Testosterone esters

Therapies for prostate cancer

Luteinizing hormone–releasing hormone agonists
- Goserelin
- Leuprolide

Luteinizing hormone–releasing hormone antagonist
- Degarelix

Antiandrogens
- Bicalutamide
- Flutamide
- Nilutamide

Abbreviations

AR, androgen receptor
ARE, androgen response element
AUA, American Urological Association
BPH, benign prostatic hyperplasia
cAMP, cyclic adenosine monophosphate
cGMP, cyclic guanosine monophosphate
DBD, DNA binding domain
DHEA, dehydroepiandrosterone
DHT, dihydrotestosterone
ED, erectile dysfunction
FSH, follicle-stimulating hormone
IC_{50}, median inhibitory concentrations
IM, intramuscular
LBD, ligand binding domain
LH, luteinizing hormone
LHRH, luteinizing hormone–releasing hormone
NCI, National Cancer Institute
NO, nitric oxide
PAP, prostatic acid phosphatase
PDE, phosphodiesterase
PGE_1, prostaglandin E_1
PSA, prostate-specific antigen
SARM, selective androgen receptor modulator
SHBG, sex hormone binding globulin
TRT, testosterone replacement therapy

*Drugs listed include those available inside and outside the United States; drugs available outside of the United States are shown in italics.

SCENARIO

Autumn Stewart, PharmD

NP is 68-year-old African American man presenting to his community pharmacy with a new prescription for itraconazole 200 mg QD for 12 weeks for onychomycosis. The patient had the following prescriptions refilled 1 week earlier: dutasteride 0.5 mg QD, doxazosin 4 mg HS, and amlodipine 10 mg QD. While conducting a prospective drug review of the patient's medications, the pharmacist identifies a potential drug interaction between itraconazole and dutasteride. After consultation with the physician, the patient is counseled to monitor for adverse effects and report any new symptoms immediately.

(The reader is directed to the clinical solution and chemical analysis of this case at the end of the chapter).

INTRODUCTION

This chapter focuses on the physiology, pharmacology, metabolism, and structure–activity relationships for therapeutic and emerging classes of drugs that are used almost exclusively in men. Major differences in endocrine hormones and the anatomy and physiology of the reproductive system and genitourinary tract between males and females make men uniquely susceptible to a variety of disorders, including aging-related androgen insufficiency (hypogonadism and andropause), prostate and testicular cancer, benign prostatic hyperplasia (BPH), and erectile dysfunction (ED). The majority of these disorders and their treatments are associated with the male sex hormones (i.e., androgens), their pharmacologic target (i.e., the androgen receptor [AR]), and the tissues that rely on the androgens.

Prostate problems are common in older men, particularly those age 50 years and older. A man may have prostate problems for a number of reasons, including an infection of the prostate (prostatitis), a noncancerous enlargement of the prostate (BPH), or prostate cancer, the second most common cancer in men. BPH is the most common disease of the prostate, occurring in 50% to 60% of men in their 60s and up to 80% to 90% of men over the age of 70 years (1). Risk of prostate cancer also increases with age; approximately 70% of all cases of the disease are diagnosed in men age 65 years and older. Prostate problems often are discovered by men themselves. The signs of prostate problems include frequent urge to urinate, blood in the urine, painful or burning urination, difficulty urinating, or inability to urinate.

Aging-related androgen insufficiency (male hypogonadism) is a physiologic condition characterized by the inability of the testes to produce sufficient testosterone to maintain sexual function, muscle strength, bone mineral density, and fertility (spermatogenesis). One in five men older than 50 years will exhibit symptoms of this condition. Symptoms of aging-related androgen insufficiency may include lethargy or decreased energy, decreased libido or interest in sex, ED (with loss of erections), muscle weakness and aches, inability to sleep, hot flashes, night sweats, depression, infertility, thinning of bones or bone loss, and cardiovascular disease. By the time that men are between the ages of 40 and 55 years, some may experience a phenomenon similar to the female menopause called andropause. Whether andropause is more common than hypogonadism in the aging male is a matter for debate. The decline in testosterone occurs very gradually in men over several decades and may be accompanied by loss of bone mass (osteoporosis), loss of muscle mass and strength (sarcopenia), and changes in fat distribution, cholesterol levels, spermatogenesis, sexual performance, quality of life, and impotence (i.e., ED). Studies show that a decline in testosterone actually can put men at risk for other health problems, such as heart disease, metabolic syndrome, and weak bones. Psychological stress, alcohol abuse, injuries or surgery, medications, obesity and infections, tobacco, and drugs, such as decongestants, antihypertensives, tranquilizers, statins, or antiseizure agents, can contribute to the onset of these conditions. There is no way of predicting who will experience the symptoms of androgen insufficiency that are of sufficient severity to seek medical help; neither is it predictable at what age the symptoms of aging-related androgen insufficiency will occur in a particular individual. Each man's symptoms also may be different. Because all this happens at a time of life when many men begin to question their values, accomplishments, and direction in life, it often is difficult to realize that the changes occurring are related to more than just external conditions. Now that men are living longer, there is heightened interest in aging-related androgen insufficiency, its risks for other health problems, and its treatment.

Testicular cancer is the most common form of cancer among males age 15 to 44 years and is approximately four times more common in white men than in African American men. After motor vehicle accidents and suicide, cancer is the leading cause of death in this age group, followed by homicide, heart disease, and HIV. Testicular cancer is known as "young man's cancer." Early detection is the key to survival. Testicular cancer is androgen-dependent, with a very fast onset, because the tumors can be very aggressive. When the cancer is confined to the testicles, there often is no pain, but by the time pain develops, it often is a sign that the cancer has already spread. Survival rates increase significantly if treatment has begun before the cancer has a chance to metastasize. Testicular cancer is most often discovered

CLINICAL SIGNIFICANCE

The therapeutics of men's health is currently experiencing significant changes that will impact the pharmacist's role in providing care to this population. The use of treatments for male andropause is becoming more popular as men seek medical advice for the treatment of erectile dysfunction (ED) and other associated symptoms. Though androgen replacement therapy is becoming more common, it has not replaced the phosphodiesterase (PDE5) inhibitors' role as the drug of choice for the treatment of ED. Both Viagra (sildenafil) and Cialis (tadalafil) were among the Top 200 Drugs dispensed in 2009. There are advantages and disadvantages to each of these PDE5 inhibitors. Some can be taken with food whereas others cannot. Some have optimal durations of action, and others durations of action are much shorter. However, all have been known to have adverse effects and drug interactions in common. Some of these adverse effects can be rather severe, and the drug interactions with nitrates can be fatal.

The development of newer, more effective, and less deleterious agents is essential for the treatment of ED. Agents that are more selective for PDE5 and avoid other PDEs are critical to this endeavor. By studying the structure–activity relationships between the PDEs and the inhibitors, this can be achieved. Minor changes to the side chains or functional groups of the currently available PDE inhibitors can potentially eliminate the adverse effects and drug interactions that limit the use of these agents. As new agents become available, clinicians continually compare and contrast them to the ones that are currently available in an effort to improve patient care. This is an ongoing, joint effort by chemists and clinicians alike to optimize patient care, either indirectly or directly, by continually making adjustments to either chemical structures or therapeutic treatment plans for the patient.

Autumn Stewart, PharmD
Assistant Professor of Pharmacy Practice
Duquesne University
School of Pharmacy
Pittsburgh, Pennsylvania

by self-examination. Therefore, all men should conduct testicular self-examinations at least monthly and, preferably, every time they shower for any changes or lumps and see a doctor immediately if any changes are noted. The diagnosis is noninvasive and involves using ultrasound to look at the density, size, and shape of the testicles and other masses in the scrotum.

Men who experience any of these symptoms associated with the prostate, aging-related androgen insufficiency, and testicular cancer should see a doctor to find out the cause of the problem and to talk about possible treatment.

Testosterone and its metabolite, dihydrotestosterone (DHT), are the primary endogenous androgens and play crucial physiologic roles in establishing and maintaining the male phenotype (2). Their actions are essential for the differentiation and growth of male reproductive organs, initiation and regulation of spermatogenesis, and control of male sexual behavior. In addition, androgens are important for the development of male characteristics in certain extragenital structures, such as muscle, bone, hair, larynx, skin, lipid tissue, and kidney (3). In females, the precise physiologic roles of androgens are not completely understood, but the aging-related decline in circulating androgen levels has been linked to symptoms such as decreased libido and sexuality, lack of vigor, diminished well-being, and loss of bone mineral density in postmenopausal women (4–6).

THE SEX HORMONES

The sex steroid hormones are steroid molecules that are necessary for reproduction in females and males and that affect the development of secondary sex characteristics in both sexes. The sex steroids are comprised of three classes: estrogens, progestins, and androgens (Fig. 40.1). The two principal classes of female sex steroid hormones are estrogens and progestins (for further discussion, see Chapter 41). Chemically, the naturally occurring estrogens are C-18 steroids and have in common a planar unsaturated A ring with a 3-phenolic group that distinguish them from the other sex steroid hormones. The most potent endogenous estrogen is estradiol (Fig. 40.1). The naturally occurring progestins are C-21 steroids and have in common a 3-keto-4-ene structure in the A ring and a ketone at the C-21 position. The most potent endogenous progestin is progesterone (Fig. 40.1). The principal class of the male sex steroid hormone is the androgens. The naturally occurring androgens are C-19 steroids and have in common oxygen atoms (as either hydroxyl or ketone groups) at both the

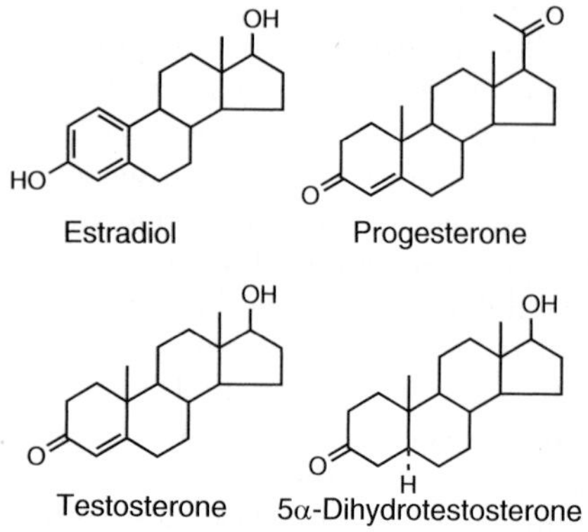

FIGURE 40.1 The sex hormones.

C-3 and C-17 positions. Testosterone is a potent androgen that is found in the blood at higher concentrations than other androgens (Fig. 40.1), whereas DHT (Fig. 40.1) is a more potent metabolite of testosterone that is formed in certain androgen target tissues including the prostate and scalp. All three classes of endogenous steroids are present in both males and females. The production and circulating plasma levels of estrogens and progestins are higher in females, however, and the production and circulating plasma levels of androgens are higher in males.

DISCOVERY OF ANDROGENS

One of the earliest and most unusual experiments with testicular extracts was carried out in 1889 by the French physiologist Charles Brown-Séquard. He administered such an extract to himself and reported that he felt an increased vigor and capacity for work (7). In 1911, Pézard showed that extracts of testicular tissue increase comb growth in capons (8). Early attempts to isolate pure male hormones from the testes failed, because only small amounts are present in this tissue.

The earliest report of an isolated androgen was presented by Butenandt (9) in 1931. He isolated 15 mg of crystalline androsterone from 15,000 L of human male urine. A second crystalline compound, dehydroepiandrosterone, which has weak androgenic activity, was isolated by Butenandt and Dannenberg (10) in 1934. During the following year, testosterone was isolated from bull testes by David et al. (11). This hormone was shown to be 6 to 10 times more active than androsterone.

Shortly after testosterone was isolated, Butenandt and Hanisch (12) reported its synthesis. In that same year, extracts of urine from males were shown to cause nitrogen retention (a measure of protein anabolism) as well as the expected androgenic effects (13). Many steroids with androgenic activity have subsequently been synthesized. Steroid hormones may have many potent effects on various tissues, and slight chemical alterations of androgenic steroids may increase some of these effects without altering others.

Testosterone was the first androgen to be used clinically for its anabolic activity. New sources of the hormone were needed, however, because only 270 mg could be isolated from a ton of bull testes (14). Commercially, testosterone is prepared from various steroids, including sarsasapogenin, diosgenin, and certain androgens found in stallion urine. Because of its androgenic action, testosterone is limited in its use in humans as an anabolic steroid. Many steroids were synthesized in an attempt to separate the androgenic and the anabolic actions. Because testosterone had to be given parenterally, it also was desirable to find orally active agents.

In the United States, most of the androgens and anabolic steroid products are subject to control by the U.S. Federal Control Substances Act as amended by the Anabolic Steroid Control Act of 1990 as Schedule III drugs.

ANDROGEN PHYSIOLOGY

The overall physiologic effects of endogenous androgens are contributed by testosterone and its active metabolites, DHT and estradiol. Testosterone and DHT execute their actions predominantly through the AR, which belongs to the nuclear receptor superfamily and functions as a ligand-dependent transcription factor. Circulating testosterone is essential for the differentiation and growth of male accessory reproductive organs (e.g., prostate and seminal vesicles), control of male sexual behavior, and the development and maintenance of male secondary characteristics that involve muscle, bone, larynx, and hair. Healthy young adult men produce approximately 3 to 10 mg of testosterone per day, with circulating plasma levels ranging from approximately 500 to 1,000 ng/dL in eugonadal (normal) men. Circulating testosterone and estradiol participate in the feedback regulation of androgen production by the hypothalamus- pituitary-testis axis, as shown in Figure 40.2. Testosterone, luteinizing hormone (LH), and LH-releasing hormone (LHRH; also known as gonadotropin-releasing hormone) constitute the elements of a negative feedback control mechanism, whereby testosterone controls its own release. Low circulating testosterone levels increase the hypothalamic secretion of LHRH, which leads to increased production of LH and, consequently, increased testosterone production by the Leydig cells. More than 95% of circulating testosterone is synthesized and secreted by the Leydig cells in the testes. High testosterone levels, on the other hand, inhibit LHRH release, thus suppressing both LH secretion and testosterone secretion. The LHRH is released from the hypothalamus in short, intermittent pulses every 2 hours and at greater magnitude in the morning, which in turn stimulates the pulsatile secretion of LH and follicle-stimulating hormone (FSH) from the pituitary. FSH stimulates the Sertoli cells controlling spermatogenesis and development of the testis. Thus, testosterone

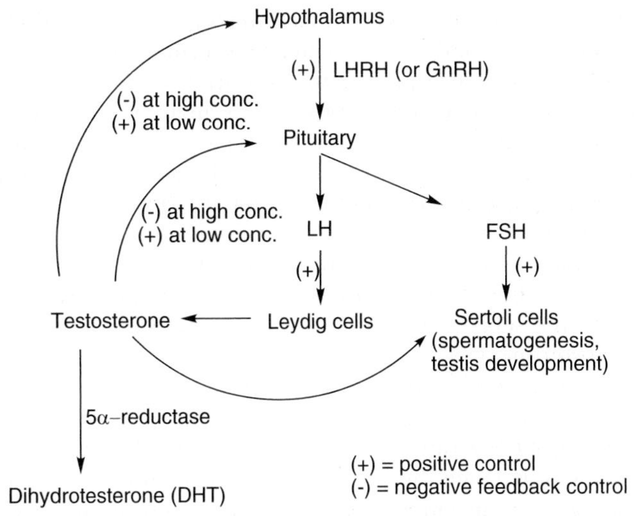

FIGURE 40.2 Hypothalamus-pituitary-testicular axis. (+), positive control; (–), negative feedback control.

secretion likewise is pulsatile and diurnal, with the highest concentration occurring at approximately 8:00 AM and the lowest at approximately 8:00 PM. In older men, especially those older than 60 years, the body does not produce enough testosterone that is needed to do all the intended work, and the testosterone levels remain relatively constant, without the morning pulses observed in young adult men. Average plasma testosterone concentrations in older men peak in the morning, with daily ranges of approximately 300 to 550 ng/dL by 70 years of age. The diurnal cycling is blunted as men age (15). In women, testosterone levels range from 15 to 100 ng/dL. Starting at approximately 40 years of age, testosterone levels drop by approximately 10% every decade in men. In the normal functioning of the male hormonal system, 97% to 98% of plasma testosterone is bound to sex hormone binding globulin (SHBG), essentially making it unavailable to the body's tissues due to the high binding affinity of testosterone for SHBG. The remaining 2% to 3% is known as "bioavailable" or free testosterone. Serum concentrations of SHBG increase with age in men, resulting in a corresponding decrease in free testosterone as men age. Free testosterone levels in serum are positively correlated with muscle strength and bone mineral density in elderly men, but negatively correlated with fat mass (16).

In the testis, FSH directly interacts with FSH receptors expressed in Sertoli cells and stimulates spermatogenesis, whereas LH indirectly stimulates spermatogenesis through testosterone synthesized by Leydig cells. Testosterone and its aromatized metabolite (estradiol) negatively regulate circulating levels of testosterone in the hypothalamus and pituitary. Activin and inhibin produced by Sertoli cells stimulate or inhibit, respectively, the secretion of FSH from the pituitary (17). High concentrations of intratesticular testosterone are essential for the initiation and maintenance of spermatogenesis, as evidenced by the infertility of hypogonadal men. Results from both animal models and humans, however, support the idea that both FSH and testosterone are required to achieve quantitative and qualitative spermatogenesis.

Androgens also are needed for the development of secondary sex characteristics. The male voice deepens because of thickening of the laryngeal mucosa and lengthening of the vocal cords. In both men and women, they play a role first in stimulating the growth of hair on the face, arms, legs, and pubic areas and later in the recession of the male hairline. The fructose content of human semen and both the size and the secretory capacity of the sebaceous glands also depend on the levels of testosterone.

Testosterone causes nitrogen retention by increasing the rate of protein synthesis and muscle mass while decreasing the rate of protein catabolism. The positive nitrogen balance therefore results from both decreased catabolism and increased anabolism of proteins that are used in male sex accessory apparatus and muscle. The actions of androgen in the reproductive tissues, including prostate, seminal vesicle, testis, and accessory structures, are known as the androgenic effects, whereas the nitrogen-retaining effects of androgen in muscle and bone are known as the anabolic effects. Although the precise mechanism of androgen action on muscle remains unknown, the common hypothesis is that androgens promote muscle protein synthesis. Evidence supports the idea that testosterone supplementation increases muscle protein synthesis in elderly men (18) and young hypogonadal men (19). Also, androgen-induced increases in muscle mass appear to arise from muscle fiber hypertrophy rather than hyperplasia (i.e., cellular enlargement rather than cellular proliferation) (20).

The thickness and linear growth of bones are stimulated and, later, limited by testosterone because of closure of the epiphyses. Androgens affect bone mineral density by changing overall osteoblast (bone-forming cell) activity and osteoclast (bone-resorbing cell) activity, resulting from changes in the total number of each cell type and individual cell functional capacity (21,22). Androgens seem to have the ability to decelerate the bone remodeling cycle and tilt the focal balance of that cycle toward bone formation. The loss of androgens is thought to increase the rate of bone remodeling by removing the restraining effects on osteoblastogenesis and osteoclastogenesis.

ANDROGEN BIOSYNTHESIS

The major pathways for the biosynthesis of the sex steroid hormones are summarized in Figure 40.3. Cholesterol is stored in endocrine tissues and is converted to androgen, estrogen, or progesterone when the tissue is stimulated by a gonadotropic hormone. Androgens (male sex hormones) primarily are synthesized from cholesterol in the testes, whereas estrogens are biosynthesized chiefly in the ovary in mature, premenopausal women and adipose tissue in men. This is not surprising, because androgens are intermediates in the biosynthesis of estrogens. In the liver, androgens are formed from C-21 steroids. During pregnancy, the placenta is the main source of estrogen biosynthesis, and pathways for production change (23,24). Small amounts of these hormones also are synthesized by the adrenal cortex, the hypothalamus, and the anterior pituitary in both sexes. The major source of estrogens in both postmenopausal women and men is adipose tissue (25).

LH binds to its receptor on the surface of the Leydig cells to initiate testosterone biosynthesis. As in other endocrine cells, the binding of gonadotropin activates the G_s signal transduction pathway, increasing intracellular cyclic adenosine monophosphate (cAMP) levels via activation of adenylate cyclase. One of the processes influenced by elevated cAMP levels is the activation of cholesterol esterase, which cleaves cholesterol esters and liberates free cholesterol. The free cholesterol is then converted in mitochondria to pregnenolone via the side-chain cleavage reaction (Fig. 40.3).

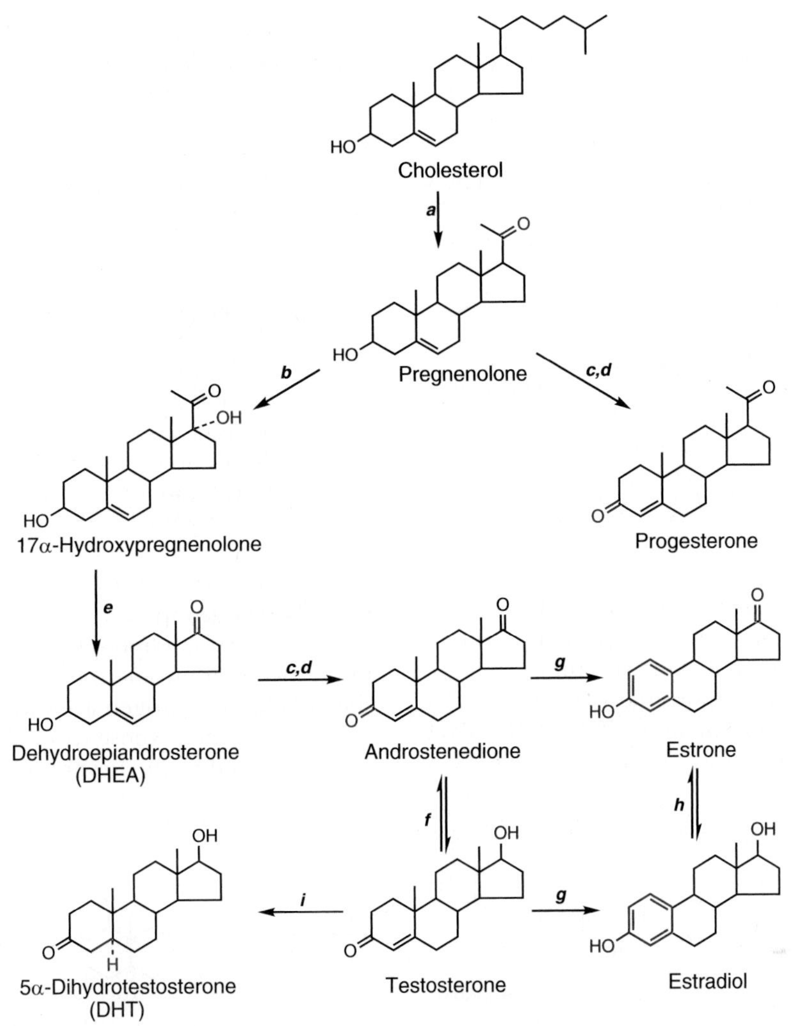

FIGURE 40.3 Biosynthesis of androgens and other sex steroid hormones. The enzymes involved in this biosynthesis are (*a*) side-chain cleavage, (*b*) 17α-hydroxylase, (*c*) 5-ene-3β-hydroxysteroid dehydrogenase, (*d*) 3-oxosteroid-4,5-isomerase, (*e*) 17,20-lyase, (*f*) 17β-hydroxysteroid dehydrogenase, (*g*) aromatase, (*h*) estradiol dehydrogenase, and (*i*) 5α-reductase.

Pregnenolone is converted by 17α-hydroxylase to 17α-hydroxypregnenolone and then to dehydroepiandrosterone (DHEA; a C-19 steroid) via 17,20-lyase, which involves cleavage of the C-17 to C-20 carbon–carbon bond and loss of the 17β-acetyl side chain (26). The 17α-hydroxylase is found in the endoplasmic reticulum membrane and is comprised of the CYP17A protein and the ubiquitous NADPH-P450 reductase. CYP17A is expressed by the *CYP17* gene found on chromosome 10 in humans. Alternatively, progesterone can be formed from pregnenolone via the action of 5-ene-3β-hydroxysteroid dehydrogenase and 3-oxosteroid-4,5-isomerase. These same enzymes are responsible for the conversion of DHEA to the 17-ketosteroidal androgen, androstenedione (Fig. 40.3).

Testosterone is formed by reduction of the 17-ketone of androstenedione by 17β-hydroxysteroid dehydrogenase type 5, also known as aldo-ketoreductase 1C3, or AKR1C3 (27,28). Testosterone and androstenedione are metabolically interconvertible (Fig. 40.3). Loss of the C-19 angular methyl group and aromatization of the A ring of testosterone or androstenedione is catalyzed by the microsomal cytochrome P450 enzyme complex, called aromatase, and results in the C-18 steroids—namely, 17β-estradiol or estrone, respectively—as shown in Figure 40.4. 17β-Estradiol and estrone are also metabolically interconvertible, catalyzed by estradiol dehydrogenase. Research interests in the aromatization reaction continue to expand from basic endocrinology and reproductive biology studies to aromatase inhibition for the treatment of estrogen-dependent cancers, as illustrated in several conferences and reviews (29–32). Androstenedione is the preferred substrate for aromatization, and three molecules of NADPH and three molecules of oxygen are necessary for conversion of one molecule of androgen to estrogen (33).

The most potent endogenous androgen is the 5α-reduced steroid, DHT, which is biosynthesized by two 5α-reductase isoforms, type 1 and type 2. Type 1 5α-reductase is expressed predominantly in sebaceous

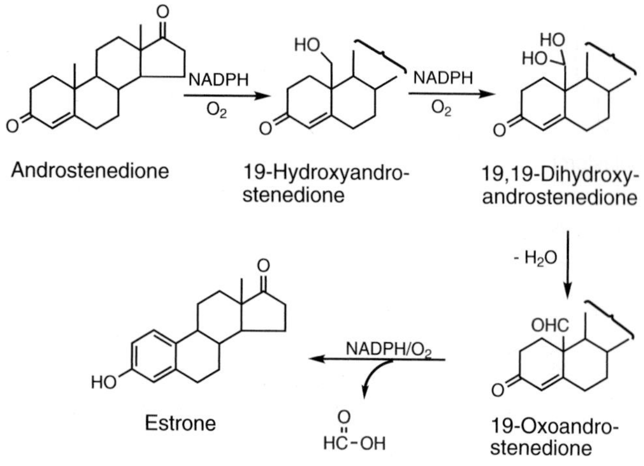

FIGURE 40.4 Aromatase mechanism.

glands of the skin, scalp, and liver and is responsible for approximately one-third of the circulating DHT. Type 2 5α-reductase is found primarily in prostate, seminal vesicles, epididymides, genital skin (scrotum), hair follicles, and liver, and it is responsible for two-thirds of the circulating DHT. Approximately 6% to 8% of testosterone is converted to DHT. 5α-Reductase has been found in both the microsomal fraction and the nuclear membrane of homogenized target tissues, and it catalyzes an irreversible reduction reaction, which requires NADPH as a cofactor, that provides the α-hydrogen at C-5 (34,35). Conversion to DHT amplifies the action of testosterone by three to five times because of the greater binding affinity of DHT as compared to testosterone for the ARs (36).

ANDROGEN METABOLISM

Testosterone can be metabolized in either its target tissues or the liver (37–39), as shown in Figure 40.5. In androgen target tissues, testosterone can be converted to physiologically active metabolites. In the prostate gland, skin, and liver (40), testosterone is reduced to DHT by 5α-reductase (types 1 and 2) (41). On the other hand, a small amount of testosterone (0.3%) also can be converted to estradiol by aromatase through cleavage of the C-19 methyl group and aromatization of ring A, which mainly occurs in adipose tissue. This process also occurs in the ovaries of women. In men, approximately 80% of the circulating estrogen arises from aromatization of testosterone in the adipose tissue (42), with the other 20% being secreted by the Leydig cells in the testes (43).

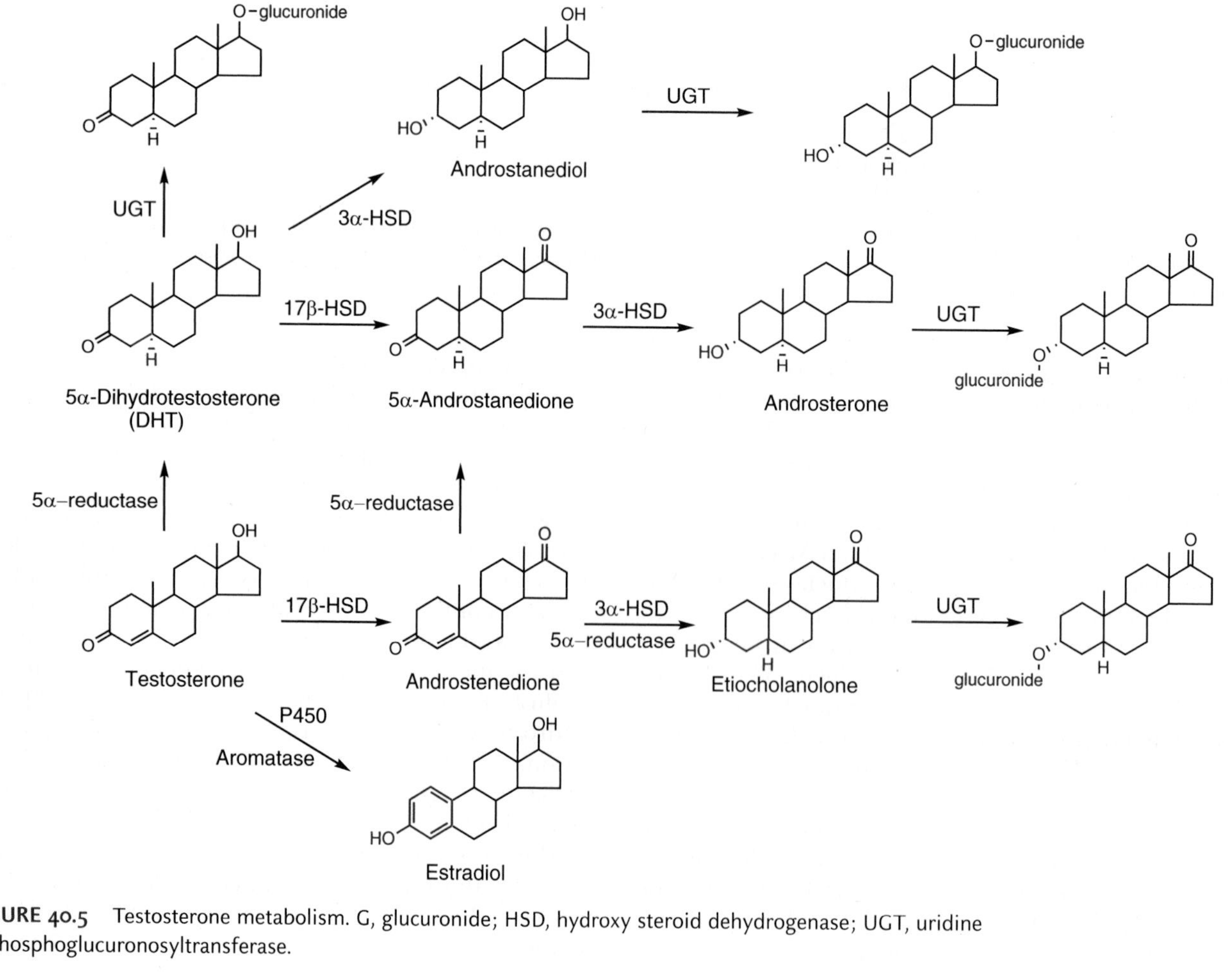

FIGURE 40.5 Testosterone metabolism. G, glucuronide; HSD, hydroxy steroid dehydrogenase; UGT, uridine diphosphoglucuronosyltransferase.

Both 5α-reduction and aromatization are irreversible processes. In addition to these pathways, testosterone also can be further inactivated in the liver through reduction and oxidation, followed by glucuronidation and renal excretion. It can be metabolized to androstenedione through oxidation of the 17β-OH group and to androstenedione with 5α-reduction of ring A. Androstenedione can be further converted to androsterone after 3-keto group reduction. Alternatively, androstenedione also can be converted to etiocholanolone through 5β- and 3-keto reduction. Similarly, DHT can be converted to androstenedione, androsterone, and androstenediol (44).

After the administration of radiolabeled testosterone, approximately 90% of the radioactivity is found in the urine, and 6% is recovered in the feces through enterohepatic circulation (45). Major urinary metabolites include androsterone and its 5α-diastereoisomer etiocholanolone, both of which are inactive metabolites. They are excreted mainly as glucuronide conjugates or, to a lesser extent, as sulfate conjugates (46). The reduction of testosterone to its *cis* A/B ring juncture (5β) conformation, etiocholanolone, explains its complete loss of activity, because the *cis* A/B ring no longer has affinity for the AR, as shown in Figure 40.6. Most of the other metabolites mentioned earlier undergo extensive glucuronidation of the 3α- or 17β-OH groups as well, either in the target tissues or in the liver (46) and are further excreted in the urine. Therefore, following oral administration, the plasma testosterone half-life is less than 30 minutes because of extensive hepatic metabolism. Approximately 90% of an oral dose of testosterone undergoes first-pass metabolism before it reaches the systemic circulation. A number of minor metabolites of testosterone also have been isolated from urine and identified as 5α-androstanes and 5β-androstanes with a 3α-hydroxyl function. Most 17-ketosteroids isolated from the urine result from catabolism of the adrenocorticoids rather than from metabolism of androgens.

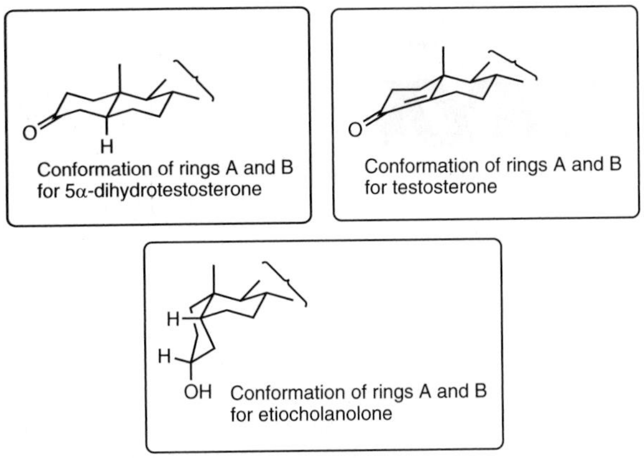

FIGURE 40.6 Conformations of dihydrotestosterone (DHT), testosterone (T), and etiocholanolone A and B rings.

MECHANISMS OF ANDROGEN ACTION

Testosterone, DHT, and other androgens execute their actions predominantly through the AR. The AR is mainly expressed in androgen target tissues, such as the prostate, skeletal muscle, liver, and central nervous system, with the highest expression level being observed in the prostate, adrenal gland, and epididymis (47). Testosterone is thought to be largely responsible for initiation of AR action in muscle, bone, brain, and bone marrow, whereas DHT plays a major role in genitalia, prostate, skin, and hair follicles due to their higher expression of 5α-reductase enzymes. The AR is a member of the steroid and nuclear receptor superfamily, which is composed of more than 100 members and continues to grow. Among this large family of proteins, only five vertebrate steroid receptors (estrogen, progesterone, androgen, glucocorticoid, and mineralocorticoid receptors) are known. Like other steroid receptors, AR is a soluble protein that functions as an intracellular transcriptional factor. The AR function is regulated by the binding of androgens, which initiates sequential conformational changes of the receptor that affect receptor–protein interaction and receptor–DNA interactions (48).

The AR gene is more than 90 kb long and codes for a protein of 919 amino acids that has three major functional domains, as illustrated in Figure 40.7. The N-terminal domain, which serves a modulatory function, is encoded by exon 1 (1,586 bp). The DNA binding domain (DBD) is encoded by exons 2 and 3 (152 and 117 bp, respectively). The ligand binding domain (LBD) is encoded by five exons, which vary from 131 to 288 bp in size. There also is a small hinge region between the DBD and LBD. Two transactivation functions have been identified. The N-terminal activation function (AF1) is not conserved in sequence and is ligand-independent (constitutively active), whereas the C-terminal activation function (AF2) is conserved in sequence and functions in a ligand-dependent manner (49). A nuclear localization signal spans the region between the DBD and the hinge region.

Similar to the other steroid receptors, unbound AR is mainly located in the cytoplasm and associated with a complex of heat shock proteins through interactions with LBD (50). On agonist binding (51), AR goes through a series of conformational changes: The heat shock proteins dissociate from AR, and the transformed AR undergoes dimerization, phosphorylation, and translocation to the nucleus, which is mediated by the nuclear localization signal, as shown in Figure 40.8. Translocated receptor then binds to androgen-response elements (AREs) in DNA, which are characterized by a six-nucleotide half-site consensus sequence 5′-TGTTCT-3′ spaced by three random nucleotides and are located in the promoter or enhancer region of AR gene targets. Recruitment of other transcription coregulators (including coactivators and corepressors) and transcriptional machinery further ensures the transactivation of AR-regulated gene expression. All these complicated processes are initiated by the ligand-induced conformational changes in the LBD.

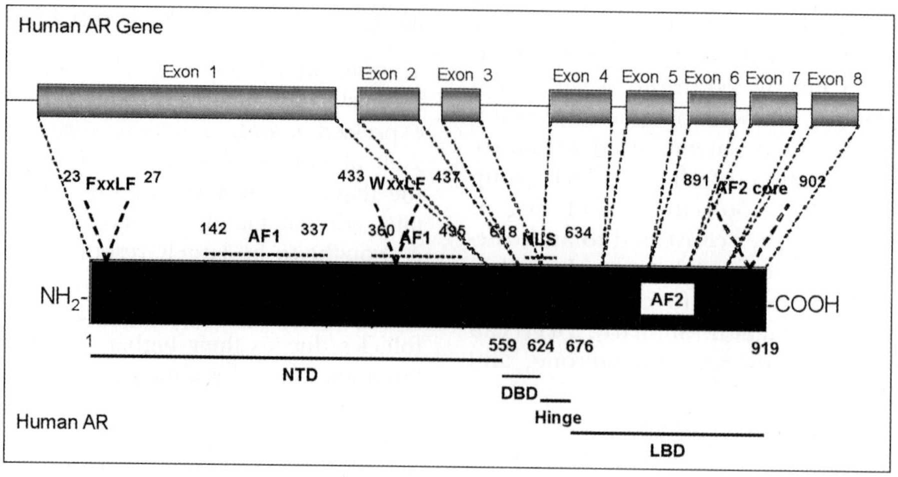

FIGURE 40.7 Structural domains of the androgen receptor gene and protein.

Ligand-induced AR conformational changes provide the structural basis for the recruitment of cofactor proteins and transcriptional machinery, which also is required for the assembly of AR-mediated transcription complexes (52), as shown in Figure 40.8. The formation of an activation complex is known to involve AR, coactivators, and RNA polymerase II recruitment to both the enhancer and promoter, whereas the formation of a repression complex involves factors bound only at the promoter and not at the enhancer. Because the formation of a functional AF2 region provides a structural basis for ligand-induced protein–protein interaction, ligand-specific recruitment of coregulators might be crucial for the agonist or antagonist activity of AR ligands.

Binding of DNA also is required for AR-regulated gene expression, which is known as the classic genomic function of AR. The ARE half-site sequence can be arranged either as inverted repeats or as direct repeats (52,53), and AR recognizes and binds to the ARE site through two zinc fingers located in the DBD. Like other steroid receptors, ligand-bound AR forms homodimers and appears to form "head-to-head" dimers (54) even when it is bound to the direct repeats of ARE. Selective recognition of specific ARE sequences could be regulated by ligand binding (55) and/or the presence of other transcriptional factors, which bind to their own DNA binding sites as well (combinatorial regulation) (56).

Besides the genomic pathway, the nongenomic pathway of AR also has been reported in oocytes (57), skeletal muscle cells (58), osteoblasts (59,60), and prostate cancer cells (61,62). As compared to the genomic pathway, the nongenomic actions of steroid receptors are

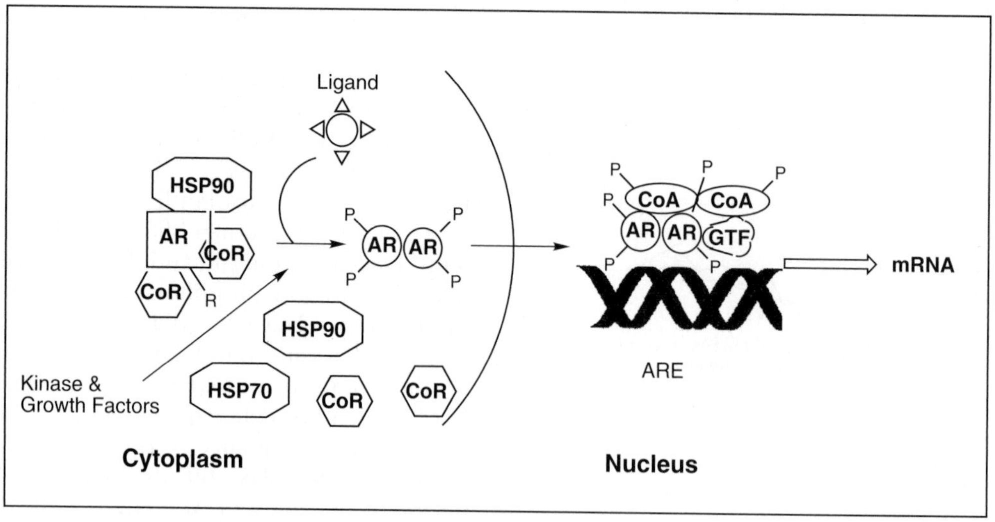

FIGURE 40.8 Mechanism of androgen action. The androgen receptor (AR) is maintained in an inactive complex by heat shock protein (HSP) 70, HSP90, and corepressors (CoR). On ligand binding, it homodimerizes and enters the nucleus. The receptor is basally phosphorylated (P) in the absence of hormone, and hormone binding increases the phosphorylation status of the receptor. The AR binds to the androgen response element (ARE) on the promoter of androgen responsive genes, leading to the recruitment of coactivators (CoA) and general transcription factors (GTF), leading to gene transcription.

characterized by the rapidity of the action, which varies from seconds to an hour or so, and by interaction with plasma membrane–associated signaling pathways (63). Nevertheless, the structural basis for nongenomic action is direct interactions between AR and cytosolic proteins from different signaling pathways, which could be closely related to the ligand-induced conformational change of the LBD or, indirectly, the N-terminal domain. Functionally, the nongenomic action of androgen involves either rapid activation of kinase-signaling cascades or modulation of intracellular calcium levels, which could be related to stimulation of gap junction communication, neuronal plasticity, and aortic relaxation (64). Separation of the genomic and nongenomic functions of steroid receptors using specific ligands also was proposed as a new strategy to achieve tissue selectivity (63,65).

DRUGS USED IN THE TREATMENT OF AGING-RELATED ANDROGEN INSUFFICIENCIES

Male Hypogonadism

Male hypogonadism (testosterone deficiency) is the inability of the testes to produce sufficient testosterone to maintain sexual function, muscle strength, bone mineral density, and fertility (spermatogenesis). In men, there is a gradual decline of approximately 1% per year in the production of testosterone beginning around 40 years of age. For most men, testosterone levels naturally decline with advancing age but still remain within the physiologic range throughout their lifetimes, causing no significant problems. Approximately 20% of men older than age 60 years and 30% to 40% of men older than 80 years have plasma testosterone levels indicative of hypogonadism (<280 to 300 ng/dL). Male hypogonadism is most commonly primary hypogonadism (testicular failure to produce testosterone for various reasons), secondary hypogonadism (hypothalamic-pituitary failure to stimulate testicles to produce testosterone), or a combination of both.

Testosterone and structurally related steroidal androgens have been used for decades to treat male hypogonadism, Klinefelter syndrome (a chromosomal abnormality resulting in testicular dysfunction), anemia secondary to chronic renal failure, aplastic anemia, protein wasting diseases associated with cancer, burns, traumas, AIDS, short stature, breast cancer (as an antiestrogen), and hereditary angioedema. However, these agents have been demoted to the therapy of final resort for anemia and cancer because of serious hepatotoxicity and the recent development of more effective therapies (e.g., erythropoietin, aromatase inhibitors, and taxanes). Although severe hypogonadism is uncommon, aging-related androgen insufficiency is much more frequent. Low endogenous testosterone concentrations are associated with sarcopenia and frailty arising from decreased fat-free mass, lessened muscle strength, and reduced bone mineral density (osteoporosis). Low testosterone concentrations also are associated with decreased sexual libido and ED. More than 30 million men older than 40 years in the United States are estimated to suffer from ED. Although androgens are not essential for erection (66), transdermal and intramuscular (IM) testosterone replacement therapy often is employed in hypogonadal men with ED (67). Furthermore, selective phosphodiesterase (PDE5) inhibitors that increase penile blood flow are considered to be the treatment of choice for men with ED. Hormone replacement therapy with testosterone in aging men also improves body composition, bone and cartilage metabolism, and memory and cognition, and it even decreases cardiovascular risk (68).

Low testosterone concentrations frequently are seen in patients with ED, aging, type 2 diabetes, HIV/AIDS, osteoporosis, depression, obesity, alcohol abuse, anabolic steroid abuse, chronic inflammatory disease, cancer, and glucocorticoid use.

Andropause

Andropause was first described in the medical literature in the 1940s, but the ability to diagnose it is relatively new. The idea that men, as well as women, might be subject to sex hormone fluctuations in later life has been a topic of debate among endocrinologists and men's health professionals (69). Andropause affects men between the ages of 40 and 55 years, but unlike women, men do not have a clear-cut signpost, such as the cessation of menstruation, to mark this transition. Men's "transition" may be much more gradual and expand over many decades, and men will very likely experience andropausal symptoms including ED, loss of muscle mass, irritability, generalized fatigue, and even problems with memory and cognition. A decline in testosterone levels will occur in virtually all men, and there is no way of predicting who will experience andropausal symptoms of sufficient severity to seek medical help. It is estimated that 30% of men in their 50s, and up to 50% of men older than 65 years, will have testosterone levels low enough to cause noticeable symptoms. Once andropause is discovered, the process of replacing the missing testosterone is either by injection, locally applied hormone gel, transdermal patch, or implanted pellets.

Testosterone Replacement Therapy

The acceptance of testosterone replacement therapy (TRT) has been hampered by the lack of orally active preparations with good efficacy and, particularly, a safe profile (70). Progress has been limited over the last three decades in developing synthetic molecules that could separate the desirable physiologic functions normally regulated by endogenous androgens from the undesirable or dose-limiting side effects. The abuse of synthetic anabolic steroids by athletes and body builders has contributed to the general perception of certain undesirable side effects, such as aggressive behavior, liver toxicity, acne, or impotency.

Current formulations for TRT largely are restricted to injectable formulations of testosterone esters, transdermal delivery formulations (scrotal or nonscrotal patches or gel), or buccal testosterone. Marketed injectable forms of testosterone esters (e.g., testosterone enanthate, propionate, or cypionate) produce undesirable fluctuations in testosterone blood levels, with supraphysiologic concentrations early and subphysiologic levels toward the end of the period before the next injection. These fluctuations provide an unsatisfactory benefits profile and, in some cases, undesired side effects. Skin patches provide a better blood level profile of testosterone, but skin irritation and daily application limit the usefulness and acceptability of this form of therapy. Topical gels (AndroGel and Testim) are widely used for TRT, but must be cautiously used in homes with children due to the risk of virilization. Oral preparations such as fluoxymesterone and 17α-methyltestosterone are only sparingly used because of concerns about liver toxicity linked to the 17α-alkyl group and because of somewhat lower efficacy (70). Thus, these oral androgens are generally considered to be obsolete and do not represent a viable form of therapy.

Benefits and Risks of Testosterone Replacement Therapy

Multiple large-scale and long-term clinical trials of TRT have been conducted in aging men to evaluate the risk–benefit ratio of TRT, but no agreement exists regarding the benefits and risks of TRT (Table 40.1) [for review, see Hijazi and Cunningham (69) and Rhoben and Morgentaler (70)]. The potential benefits of TRT include increase in bone mineral density and improvement in muscle mass and strength, cognitive function, mood, and sexual function. The potential risks of TRT, however, including those in the cardiovascular system, blood (e.g., hematocrit and hemoglobin levels), and prostate, are routinely experienced. An emerging class of drugs known as selective androgen receptor modulators (SARMs) may soon transform the therapeutic landscape of androgen use by selectively stimulating anabolic targets and avoiding steroid-related side effects. Because of the long-term effects of TRT in otherwise healthy men remain unclear, guidelines published by The Endocrine Society recommend a general policy that TRT not be offered to older men with low serum testosterone levels and that TRT only be used in men with clinically significant symptoms of androgen deficiency and serum total testosterone concentrations approaching 200 ng/dL (71).

Clearly, TRT is beneficial for hypogonadal men with androgen insufficiency to restore sexual function and muscle strength, to prevent bone loss, and to protect against heart disease (atherosclerosis) (70). Increasing testosterone levels with TRT, however, may pose problems by stimulating the growth of the prostate. Long-term TRT could cause prostate gland enlargement, which might exacerbate BPH or fuel the growth of prostate cancer that is already present and could cause breast enlargement in men (gynecomastia). This is especially

TABLE 40.1 Testosterone Replacement Therapy

Benefits	Risks
Improved sexual performance and desire	Stimulated growth of preexisting prostate cancer
More energy and improved quality of life	Greater chance for benign prostatic hyperplasia
More energy and sense of well-being	Increased hemoglobin levels to above the physiologic range
Increased bone mineral density Improved muscle mass strength	Problems with voiding; symptoms includes poor urine flow and hesitancy before urinating
Improved (lower) low-density lipoprotein profile	Increased potential for liver damage from oral preparations Sleep apnea (stopping of breathing during sleep)
Decreased irritability and depression	Breast tenderness and swelling (gynecomastia)
Improved cognitive function	Testicular shrinkage (testicular atrophy)
Increased hemoglobin levels to the physiologic range	Infertility (decreased spermatogenesis) Skin reaction from patches or gel
Thickened body hair and skin	Pain, soreness, or bruising from injection Increased fluid retention Increased skin problems (acne, oily skin) Increased body hair

worrisome because of the high prevalence of BPH in older men and the possibility that many men may have prostate cancer that is undiagnosed. In fact, men with a palpable prostate nodule, a prostate-specific antigen level greater than 4 ng/mL, or severe lower urinary tract symptoms associated with BPH are usually advised to avoid TRT.

In elderly men, testosterone effects on muscle mass and strength have not been consistent or impressive, possibly because of the low dosages used in clinical trials. The high correlation between the dose (and plasma concentration) and the anabolic actions of androgen in muscle suggests that androgen administration of higher doses in elderly men may significantly increase muscle mass and strength, but high doses might increase the adverse effects and the aromatization of testosterone to estrogen (72).

Types of Testosterone Replacement Therapy

Several types of TRT exist. Choosing a specific therapy depends on the patient's preference of a particular delivery system, the side effects, and the cost. Types include injection, transdermal, buccal mucosal, and oral (Table 40.2).

Injection Orally administered testosterone is ineffective in the treatment of male androgen insufficiency syndromes due to extensive presystemic first-pass metabolism. IM injections bypass the problems of first-pass metabolism. IM injections are depot formulations of testosterone esters that undergo differing rates of in vivo ester hydrolysis to release free testosterone over an extended period of time. Typically, the depot esters are administered IM into a large muscle once every 2 to 4 weeks depending on the depot ester used (Table 40.2). They are safe, effective, and the least expensive androgen preparations available. The major disadvantage with the IM route for the depot esters is that testosterone plasma concentrations exhibit a saw-toothed pattern, with supraphysiologic levels within 2 to 4 days following the IM injection and subphysiologic levels before the next injection. A more satisfactory physiologic replacement therapy without the fluctuations in free testosterone plasma levels would be to administer a lower IM dose (i.e., 100 mg) on a weekly or biweekly schedule. Because IM injection of testosterone or its esters causes local irritation, the rate of absorption may be erratic.

Esters of testosterone available for IM administration include the 17β-propionate, 17β-enanthate, and the cypionate (17β-cyclopentylpropionate) (Fig. 40.9). Testosterone enanthate and cypionate are commonly used and demonstrate comparable pharmacokinetics. Testosterone enanthate is formed by esterification of the 17β-hydroxy group of testosterone with heptanoic acid, while testosterone cypionate is formed with cyclopentanepropionic acid. Sterile solutions of these esters are available in a suitable vegetable oil, such as cottonseed oil. Unlike oral testosterone, with a half-life of 10 to 100 minutes, IM testosterone administration avoids first-pass metabolism and exhibits a longer duration due to the slow hydrolysis and release of testosterone from the depot injection site. Generally, the concentration of SHBG in plasma determines the distribution of testosterone between free and bound forms. The bulky cypionate and enanthate esters of testosterone have a duration of action of up to 2 to 4 weeks, whereas the shorter propionate ester has a shorter duration of action of 1 to 2 weeks. Doses may be adjusted by aiming for midphysiologic (400 to 600 ng/dL) testosterone values after 1 week or at the low end (300 to 400 ng/dL) just before the next injection is due.

Implant Subcutaneous implantation of testosterone pellets (Testopel) is much less flexible for dose adjustment as compared to transdermal, oral, or IM injection. Fat-soluble pellets containing 75 mg of testosterone can be implanted subcutaneously on the anterior abdominal wall or buttocks to deliver testosterone over a 3- to 4-month period. The longer duration of action of the pellets is accompanied by a larger dose requirement as compared to weekly or biweekly IM injections. In general, two 75-mg pellets provide an equivalent dose of testosterone over 3 months to weekly 25-mg IM injections of testosterone propionate. Approximately one-third of the material from the pellet is absorbed in the first month, one fourth in the second month, and one sixth in the third month. Adequate effects from the pellets can occasionally continue for as long as 6 months.

Transdermal Transdermal TRT systems are, perhaps, the most commonly used systems for delivering testosterone to bypass the rapid first-pass metabolism associated with oral testosterone. Clinical studies have shown that these formulations are effective forms of testosterone replacement, with peak response within 3 to 6 months. Use of the transdermal formulation should be discontinued if the desired response is not reached within this time period. Skin irritation is more common with the transdermal formulations, with more than 50% experiencing some form of skin irritation at some point during the treatment. Pretreatment with corticosteroid creams (not with the ointment) has been shown to reduce the severity and incidence of skin irritation without significantly affecting testosterone absorption from the formulation. With the transdermal formulations, testosterone levels were maintained within physiologic values, and a beneficial effect was observed on general mood and sexual functioning. A plasma concentration in the midphysiologic range (400 to 600 ng/dL) is the goal.

Matrix-Type Transdermal Systems This type of patch (scrotal patch; Testoderm) must be applied to dry, clean (shaven) scrotal skin, which is 5 to 30 times more permeable to testosterone than other skin sites, every 24 hours to produce an adequate testosterone plasma concentration.

TABLE 40.2 Testosterone Products and Properties[a]

Product	Trade Name	Onset of Peak Response	Duration of Action	Time to Peak Conc.	Time to Steady-State Conc.	Dose (mg)	Oral Frequency of Dosing	Bioavailability (%)	Elimination Half-life
Methyltestosterone	Android	—	24 hours	2 hours	—	10–50	Daily	70	3 hours
	Testred								
	Virilon								
	Oreton Methyl								
Fluoxymesterone	Halotestin	—	24 hours	—	—	5–40	Daily	80	9 hours
	Android-F								
Testosterone undecanoate	Andriol	6 hours	10 hours	~6 hours	—	40–120	Daily	<10	3 hours
Testosterone propionate	Testex	6–24 hours	1–2 weeks	3–36 hours	—	10–50	Two or three times per week	—	—
Testosterone cypionate	Andronate Depotestosterone Depotest	6–24 hours	2–4 weeks	24 hours	—	50–400	2–4 weeks	—	8 days
Testosterone enanthate	Andro-LA	6–24 hours	2–4 weeks	24 hours	—	50–400	2–4 weeks	—	8 days
	Andryl								
	Delatestryl								
	Delatest								
	Everone								
	Testamone								
	Testrin-PA								
Testosterone pellets	Testopel	1–2 months	3–6 months	1 month	1–2 weeks	150–450	3–6 months	—	—
Trandermal patches	Androderm	3–6 months	24 hours	2–4 hours	2–3 days	2–5	24 hours	—	10–100 minutes
	Testoderm TTS								
	Testoderm								
Transdermal gels	AndroGel	3–6 months	5 days	4 (2–6) hours	2–3 days	50–100	24 hours	—	10–100 minutes
	Testim								
Buccal mucosal	Striant	—	24 hours	5 (0.5–12) hours	2–3 days	30	Every 12 hours	—	6 hours

[a]Thompson Healthcare, Inc. Micromedex Healthcare Series. Available at: http://www.Thompsonhc.com.

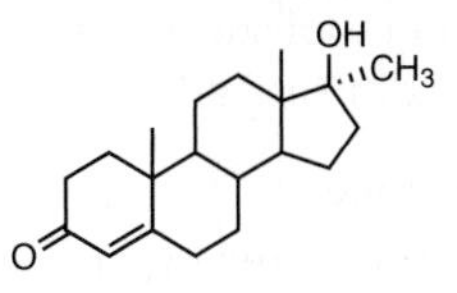

17α-Methyltestosterone

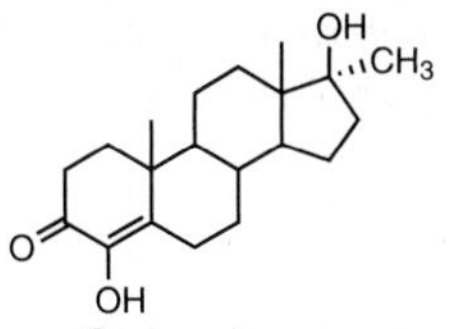

Oxymesterone

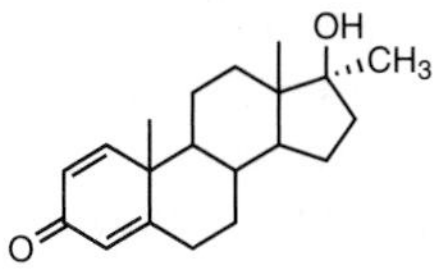

Methandrostenolone

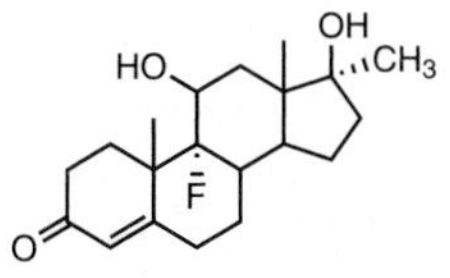

Fluoxymesterone

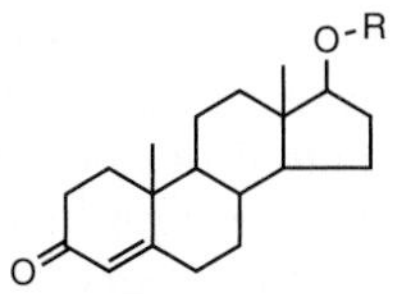

Testosterone 17β-propionate: R = CH_3CH_2CO
Testosterone 17β-enanthanate: R = $CH_3(CH_2)_5CO$
Testosterone 17β-undecanoate: R = $CH_3(CH_2)_9CO$
Testosterone 17β-cyclopentylpropionate

R = 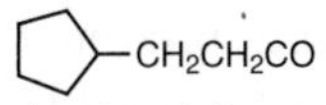

(cypionate)

FIGURE 40.9 Testosterone esters and synthetic testosterone derivatives.

The matrix system is described as a "drug-in-adhesive film," in which the drug is located on the adhesive layer of the film; thus, it is thinner and less bulky than the reservoir system. The advantage of the matrix system is that it produces supraphysiologic levels of DHT because of the high 5α-reductase enzyme activity of the scrotal tissue. The patches have an occlusive backing that prevents sex partners from coming in contact with the active drug. A matrix transdermal system will not produce adequate plasma testosterone concentrations if applied to nonscrotal skin. Plasma testosterone concentrations are reached in approximately 2 to 4 hours. Although testosterone is absorbed throughout a 24-hour period, concentrations do not simulate the circadian rhythm of endogenous testosterone in normal (eugonadal) males. Within 24 hours after application of the matrix system, plasma testosterone concentration gradually falls to 60% to 80% of the peak plasma concentration, and when the system is removed, testosterone plasma concentration declines to baseline within 2 hours. Inadequate scrotal size and adherence problems are limitations. Skin irritation does occur in those with sensitive scrotal skins.

Reservoir-Type Transdermal Systems The reservoir-type patch (nonscrotal patch; Androderm, Testoderm TTS) is not applied to scrotal skin but, rather, to the abdomen, back, thighs, or upper arms every 24 hours (see Table 40.2 for dosage strength). This type of patch is membrane-controlled for the drug to diffuse continuously over 24 hours from the reservoir into the skin. Thus, this type of patch is thicker than the matrix (scrotal) patch. The patches have an occlusive backing that prevents sex partners from coming in contact with the active drug. The site of the application is rotated at 7-day intervals between applications to lessen skin reactions at the same application site. The advantage of the reservoir transdermal system is that it achieves normal testosterone circadian rhythm as seen in younger men, peaking in the morning and decreasing throughout the rest of the day. The reservoir-type patch, when applied to nonscrotal skin, produced physiologic DHT and estradiol plasma concentrations. Steady-state plasma concentrations of testosterone, which are approximately 10 times baseline values, are reached in about 6 hours (range, 4 to 10 hours depending on application patch location), which then fall to 60% to 80% of the peak plasma concentration within 24 hours after application of the transdermal system. Thus, physiologic plasma testosterone concentrations are maintained over 24 hours with this type of patch. Drug accumulation does not occur with repeated applications. When the system is removed, testosterone plasma concentrations decline to baseline within 2 hours. A usual dose for the reservoir-type transdermal results in the systemic absorption of 2 to 10 mg daily in hypogonadal men.

Gel Testosterone gel (AndroGel, Testim) is a 1% testosterone hydroalcoholic gel that provides continuous transdermal delivery of testosterone for 24 hours once the gel is rubbed into the skin on the lower abdomen, upper arm, or shoulder. It should not be applied to scrotal tissue (Table 40.2). Because there is a continuous release of testosterone over 24 hours, the normal circadian rhythm is not observed. As the gel dries, approximately 10% of the testosterone is absorbed through the skin. Gel application of TRT appears to cause fewer skin reactions than occur with the patches. Men should avoid showering or bathing for several hours after an application to ensure adequate absorption. A potential side effect of the gel is the possibility of transferring the medication to a partner; skin-to-skin contact should be avoided either until the gel is completely dry or by covering the area after an application. Skin-to-skin contact with children is of particular concern and is included as a "black box" warning for these products. Following the application of 5 g of gel, which will deliver 50 mg of testosterone, the mean peak testosterone concentrations are reached in approximately 2 hours, which are about two to three times baseline values. For optimum results, the gel is best applied in the evening to allow maximum concentration to occur early in the morning hours. Doses of the gel may be adjusted by aiming for midphysiologic (400 to 600 ng/dL) testosterone values after 1 week. When the gel treatment is discontinued, plasma testosterone levels remain in the physiologic range for 24 to 48 hours, then return to their pretreatment levels within 5 days following the last application. An increase in plasma testosterone can be observed within 30 minutes of application. Plasma concentrations approximate the steady-state level by the end of the first 24 hours and are at steady-state by the second or third day of dosing.

Buccal Mucosal Striant is a gel-like substance that adheres to the gumline, which softens to deliver physiologic amounts of testosterone to the systemic circulation, thereby producing circulating testosterone concentrations in hypogonadal males that approximate physiologic levels seen in healthy young men (400 to 700 ng/dL). One buccal system (30 mg) is applied to the gum region twice daily, morning and evening, approximately 12 hours apart. Because there is a continuous release of testosterone over 24 hours, the normal circadian rhythm is not observed. Peak plasma testosterone concentrations are reached within 10 to 12 hours and are stable within a few days of the buccal preparation. The buccal preparation is difficult for patients to get used to, because the side effects may include gum irritation or pain, bitter taste, and headache. A study found that this form of TRT delivers a steadier dose of testosterone throughout the day without significant adverse effects, comparable to the gel.

ORAL Orally administered testosterone is ineffective in the treatment of male androgen deficiency syndromes because of extensive presystemic first-pass metabolism, primarily to inactive 17-ketosteroid, etiocholanolone and androsterone, and androstenediol metabolites in the gastrointestinal mucosa during absorption and in the liver (Fig. 40.5). Oral administration results in supraphysiologic elevations of testosterone and undesirable variability of plasma concentrations. The plasma half-life of testosterone is less than 30 minutes. Generally, the amount of SHBG in plasma determines the distribution of testosterone between free and bound forms. Approximately 90% of a dose of testosterone is metabolized, and its metabolites are excreted in the urine primarily as glucuronide conjugates, with approximately 6% of a dose being excreted in the feces as unmetabolized testosterone. Comparative dosage ranges for testosterone and its synthetic preparations are shown in Table 40.2. Taking testosterone orally (Android, Testred), in the form of methyltestosterone, is not recommended for long-term replacement. Oral testosterone may cause an unfavorable cholesterol profile and increase the risk of blood clots and heart and liver problems.

The androgenic activity of lipophilic long-chain ester testosterone 17β-undecanoate (Android Testocaps are not approved for use in the United States) (Fig. 40.9) has been attributed to formation of testosterone via systemic ester hydrolysis of lymphatically transported testosterone undecanoate (73). Its oral bioavailability was approximately 3%. Lymphatically transported testosterone undecanoate accounted for between 90% and 100% of the systemically available ester, and 83% to 85% of the systemically available testosterone resulted from systemic hydrolysis of lymphatically transported testosterone undecanoate. These data demonstrate that intestinal lymphatic transport of testosterone undecanoate produces increased systemic exposure of testosterone by avoiding the extensive first-pass hepatic metabolism responsible for the inactivation of testosterone after oral administration.

Synthetic Derivatives of Testosterone

Some of the early studies with androgens included structural modifications of the naturally occurring hormones to avoid first-pass metabolism. Blocking the metabolism of the 17β-hydroxy group with substituents in the 17α-position resulted in androgens with an increased bioavailability and duration of action when given orally. The synthetic androgens include methyltestosterone and fluoxymesterone (Fig. 40.9). The long-term use of oral androgens has been associated with liver cancer.

17α-METHYLTESTOSTERONE The synthesis of 17α-methyltestosterone made available a compound that was orally active (74) in daily doses between 10 and 50 mg (Android, Testred), which is equivalent to a 400-mg oral dose of testosterone. The presence of a 17α alkyl group reduces susceptibility to hepatic oxidative metabolism, thereby increasing oral bioavailability (~70%) by slowing metabolism. Following oral administration, methyltestosterone is well absorbed from the gastrointestinal tract, with a half-life of approximately 3 hours. This drug has the androgenic and anabolic activities of testosterone. Although orally active, it is more effective when administered sublingually. The alkylated oral androgens are seldom used due to their potential hepatotoxicity.

FLUOXYMESTERONE By substituting a 9α-fluoro group onto an analog of 17α-methyltestosterone, fluoxymesterone has 20 times the anabolic and 10 times the androgenic activity of 17α-methyltestosterone (Fig. 40.9) (74). It has a bioavailability of approximately 80% and a mean half-life of 9 hours, and less than 5% of the drug is excreted unchanged. Daily doses of 5 to 20 mg (Androxy) are generally used for TRT, but, like methyltestosterone, concerns related to the potential hepatotoxicity of alkylated androgens have limited the clinical use of this drug. Fluoxymesterone is also associated with sodium and water retention, which could lead to edema.

Structure–Activity Relationships of Steroidal Androgens

Until the discovery of nonsteroidal androgens (discussed later), it was believed that a substance must contain a steroid skeleton to have androgenic activity (75). Oxygen functional groups normally occurring at positions 3 and 17 of the steroid ring system are not essential, because the basic nucleus, 5α-androstane, has androgenic activity (Fig. 40.1). This appears to be the minimal structural requirement for hormonal activity of steroids. For derivatives of etiocholane, in which the hydrogen is in the 5β-position, thereby affording a *cis* A/B ring juncture, no active androgens and anabolic agents are known (75). Generally, ring expansion (to form homo derivatives by inserting a methylene group into one of the rings in the steroid nucleus) or ring contraction (by removing a methylene group) significantly reduces or destroys the androgenic and anabolic activities.

Introduction of a 3-ketone function or a 3α-OH group enhances androgenic activity. A hydroxyl group in the 17α-position of androstane contributes no androgenic or anabolic activity; no known substituent can approach the effectiveness of a 17β-OH group. Evidence indicates that the longer-acting esters of the 17β-OH compounds are hydrolyzed in vivo to the free alcohol, which is the active species. The 17β-oxygen atom is important for attachment to the receptor site, while 17α-alkyl groups are important for preventing metabolic changes at this position (74). Such 17α-substituents render the compounds orally active.

Increasing the length of the alkyl side chain at the 17α-position, however, resulted in decreased activity, and the incorporation of other substituents, such as the 17α-ethynyl group, produced compounds with useful progestational activity (progestins) (see Chapter 41), such as ethisterone. Attaching an isoxazole ring to ethisterone produced danazol (Danatrol, Danocrine), which exhibited potent antigonadotropic properties, weak androgen and anabolic properties, and no estrogen or progestin activity.

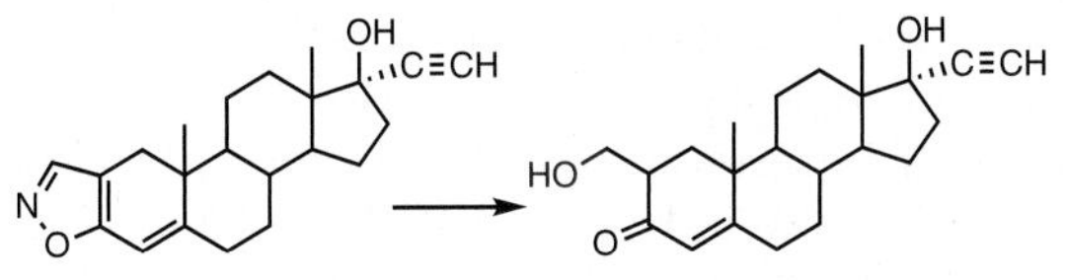

Danazol

2-Hydroxymethylethisterone (Danazol metabolite)

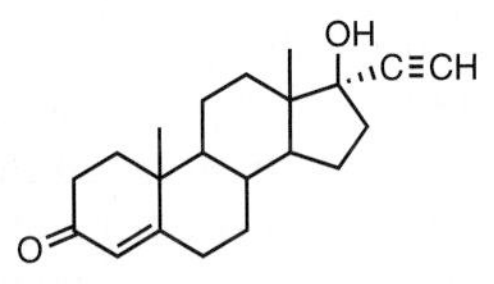

Ethisterone

As a gonadotropin inhibitor, danazol suppresses the surge of LH and FSH from the pituitary, thus suppressing ovarian steroidogenesis. For this reason, it is used in the treatment of endometriosis. Previous treatment of endometriosis had been surgical or medical, with progestins or a combination of estrogen and progestin. Danazol is metabolized by CYP3A4 to its inactive metabolite, 2-hydroxymethylethisterone.

Several modifications of 17α-methyltestosterone lead to potent, orally active anabolic agents. Two hydroxylated analogs include oxymesterone (Fig. 40.9) and oxymetholone (Fig. 40.10). These drugs have at least three times the anabolic and half the androgenic activity of testosterone (74).

Halogen substitution produces compounds with decreased activity except when inserted into positions 4 or 9 (e.g., fluoxymesterone). Replacement of a carbon atom in position 2 by oxygen has produced the only clinically successful heterocyclic steroid (oxandrolone) among a number of azasteroids and oxasteroids. Some of the 2-oxasteroids are potent anabolic agents.

Introduction of a sp^2 hybridized carbon atom into the A ring (methenolone, testolactone, Fig. 40.10) renders the ring more planar, and in turn, this may be responsible for greater anabolic activity. The 19-norsteroids (nandrolone) are of interest, because these agents seem to produce a more favorable ratio of anabolic to androgenic activity. Vida (74) has extensively reviewed the replacement of various hydrogens on the androgen steroid skeleton by other functional groups. It appears that certain substitutions at positions 1, 2, 7, 17, and 18 may result in compounds with favorable activities that will be of clinical importance.

Adverse Effects Testosterone replacement therapy can have undesirable side effects depending on the type of delivery system used. The adverse effects from oral testosterone include stomach upset, headache, acne, increased hair growth on the face or body, jaundice (liver toxicity), anxiety, change in sex drive, sleeplessness,

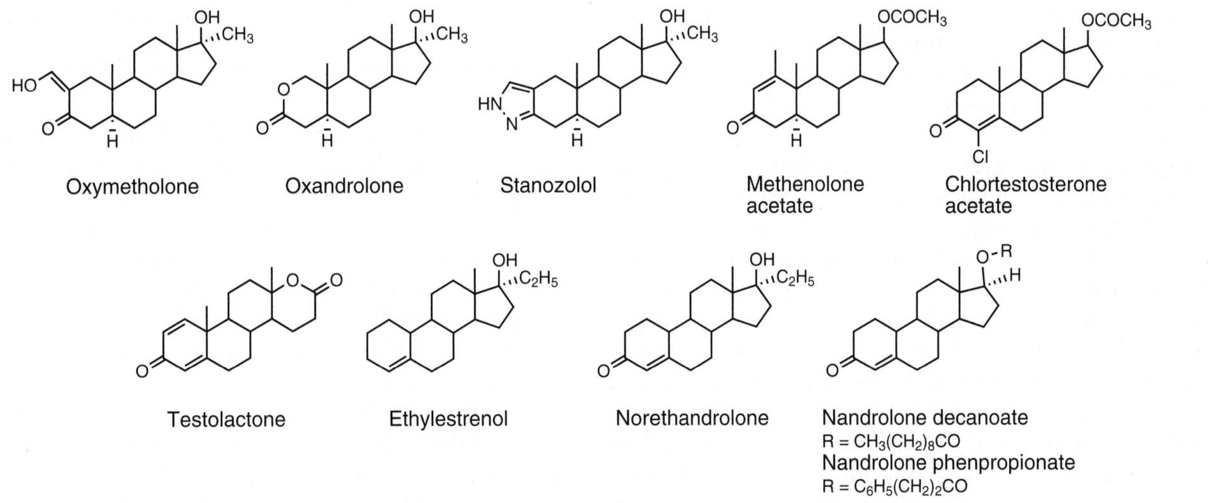

FIGURE 40.10 Anabolic steroids.

increased urination, depression, enlargement of breasts, and increased frequency and duration of erections (70–72). Breast enlargement can develop because testosterone can be converted to estradiol via aromatase. Other adverse effects include water retention, liver toxicity, cardiovascular disease, sleep apnea, and prostate enlargement. These risks are relatively uncommon when the dosage is closely monitored to maintain physiologic plasma testosterone concentrations. Testosterone replacement therapy is contraindicated in men with carcinoma of the breast or with known or suspected BPH or carcinoma of the prostate. Therefore, pretreatment screening for any prostate dysfunction is mandatory before starting TRT.

Anabolic Agents

Because complete dissociation of anabolic and androgenic effects is not possible, many of the actions of anabolic steroids are similar to those of androgens. Comparative dosage ranges for the anabolic steroids are shown in Table 40.2.

Selenium dioxide dehydrogenation of 17α-methyltestosterone yields the 1,4-diene analog, methandrostenolone, which has several-fold the anabolic activity of the starting material. It has low androgenic activity but, apparently, can produce mammogenic effects in men. These effects are thought to result from estrogenic metabolites.

The 17α-alkylated anabolic steroids in clinical use are oxandrolone (Anavar, Oxandrin), oxymetholone (Anadrol-50), stanozolol (Winstrol), nandrolone decanoate (Deca-Durabolin, Hybolin), and nandrolone phenpropionate, as shown in Figure 40.10.

A 2-oxasteroid analog of 17α-methyltestosterone is oxandrolone, which contains a lactone in the A ring (oxygen bio-isostere of ring A) and, therefore, is susceptible to in vivo hydrolysis. It has three times the anabolic activity of 17α-methyltestosterone but exhibits slight androgenic activity (76). A pyrazole heterocyclic compound used for its anabolic effects is stanozolol (76).

The anabolic steroid oxymetholone (Anadrol) was used primarily to stimulate production of erythropoietin in the treatment of anemias resulting from bone marrow failure before the advent of erythropoietin, but is seldom used today due to its association with hepatitis and liver tumors.

Testolactone (Teslac), a 18-oxasteroid, is a D-homo-oxoandrostandienedione analog, with ring D being a six-membered lactone ring. Although testolactone possesses some anabolic activity with weak androgenic effects, it was used primarily in the treatment of breast cancer as a noncompetitive irreversible inhibitor of aromatase to suppress the formation of estrogens that would stimulate the growth of breast tissue (77). It is primarily excreted in the urine unchanged, but it is metabolized in the liver by partial reduction of the 4-ene double bond in ring A to the 5β-metabolite (*cis* A/B ring juncture). Testolactone was discontinued in 2008 and is no longer available for clinical use.

Alkylation in the 1, 2, 7, and 18 positions of the androstane molecule generally increases anabolic activity (74). One of these derivatives, methenolone acetate, is an example of a potent anabolic agent that does not have an alkyl substituent at the 17α-position. A halogenated anabolic agent used in about the same dosage is chlortestosterone acetate (Fig. 40.10).

Androgens, having no methyl group in position 10 of the steroid nucleus, are an important class of anabolic agents often referred to as the 19-norandrogens, as shown in Figure 40.10. The removal of the 19-CH_3 group of the androgen results in reduction of its androgenic properties but retention of its anabolic, tissue-building properties. These steroids can be synthesized by the Birch reduction of the aromatic A ring of a 3-methoxy estrogen to a 2,5(10)-estradiene. Cleavage of the enol ether with HCl results in the 19-nortestosterone derivative. In animal assays, 19-nortestosterone has about the same anabolic activity as the propionate ester of testosterone, but its androgenic activity is much lower. Because 19-nortestosterone showed some separation of anabolic and androgenic activities, related analogs were synthesized and biologically investigated. Two of the more potent members of the series are norethandrolone and ethylestrenol and are shown in Figure 40.10. Norethandrolone has a better ratio of anabolic to androgenic activity than either 19-nortestosterone or 17α-methyl-19-nortestosterone (78). Both androgenic and progestational side effects have been observed with this agent. Ethylestrenol is more potent than norethandrolone as an anabolic agent and is used in a dosage of 4 mg per day orally.

Nandrolone phenpropionate and nandrolone decanoate are esters of 19-nortestosterone, as shown in Figure 41.10. When administered IM, slow in vivo hydrolysis of the ester occurs, releasing free 19-nortestosterone over a prolonged period. Nandrolone decanoate is the longer-acting ester intended for deep IM injection, preferably into the gluteal muscle, in the treatment of anemia associated with renal insufficiency. Nandrolone phenpropionate has a shorter duration of action than the decanoate and is used in the treatment of metastatic breast cancer in women.

Abuse of Steroidal Anabolic Agents to Enhance Athletic Performance

Performance-enhancing substances are now a point of major interest for athletes, government, and news media. These substances are having a major impact on sports and the public in general. It appears that we are headed for much greater antidoping efforts in sports. A great deal of interest has recently been shown in "designer" anabolic steroids for their high-muscle-building effects, as shown in Figure 40.11. Tetrahydrogestrinone and desoxymethyltestosterone (Fig. 40.11) brought a great deal of interest to the performance-enhancing area, because their use was very difficult to detect (79,80). Tetrahydrogestrinone is thought to have been derived from gestrinone, a substance that has been used for the treatment of a variety of gynecologic disorders. Tetrahydrogestrinone also

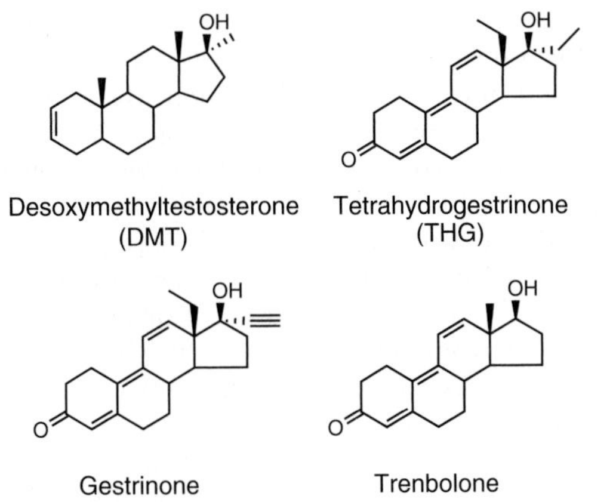

FIGURE 40.11 Illegal anabolic agents.

is related to trenbolone, which has been used by body builders and by ranchers to build up cattle before marketing. Before tetrahydrogestrinone, both gestrinone and trenbolone had been on the banned anabolic steroid list of the International Olympic Committee. Tetrahydrogestrinone was very difficult to trace, however, because it was unstable under the normal conditions of testing for anabolic steroids. Once a suitable assay was developed, it was possible to go back and test samples of athletes around the world, and several were found to have taken tetrahydrogestrinone.

Nonsteroidal Androgens

Selective Androgen Receptor Modulators (SARMs)

The successful marketing and clinical application of selective estrogen receptor modulators (see Chapter 41) raised the possibility of developing selective ligands for other members of the nuclear receptor superfamily. The concept of SARMs (81–83) recently emerged—namely, a compound that is an antagonist or weak agonist in the prostate but agonist in the bone and muscle and is orally available with low hepatotoxicity. For an ideal SARM, the antagonist or weak agonist activity in the prostate will reduce concern for the potential to stimulate nascent or undetected prostate cancer, whereas the strong agonist activity in the muscle and bone can be used to treat muscle-wasting conditions, hypogonadism, and/or aging-related frailty. Currently, research on SARMs is in its early stages—namely, preclinical discovery and the early phase of clinical development. Late-stage clinical trials planned in the next 3 to 5 years, however, should reveal the true promise of this exciting new therapeutic class of drugs.

The SARM pharmacophores can be classified into four categories: *N*-arylpropionamide (83), bicyclic hydantoin (84), tricyclic quinolines (85), and tetrahydroquinoline (86) analogs, as shown in Figure 40.12. These nonsteroidal AR ligands are not substrates for aromatase or 5α-reductase but exhibit affinity as full AR agonists in anabolic organs (e.g., muscle and bone) or as partial AR agonists in androgenic tissues (e.g., prostate and seminal vesicles).

STRUCTURE–ACTIVITY RELATIONSHIPS FOR THE *N*-ARYLPROPIONAMIDES

The majority of published preclinical research has focused on a series of *N*-arylpropionamide analogs as AR agonists or partial agonists, using the key structural elements of bicalutamide, an androgen antagonist (83,87).

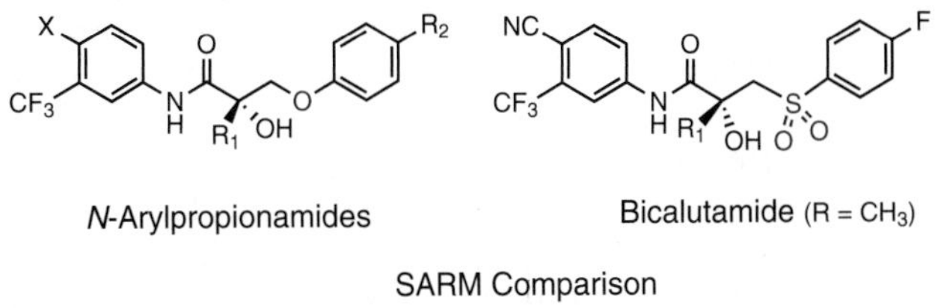

A series of chiral bicalutamide analogs, which bear electron-withdrawing groups (either a cyano or a nitro group at the 4-position and a trifluoromethyl group at the 3-position) in ring A, with a fluoro or acetylamino substituents at the para position in ring B (R_2) demonstrated high in vitro AR binding affinity and in vivo androgenicity and anabolic activity in rats (88,89). The *R*-isomer analogs, which have a trifluoromethyl group instead of a methyl group at the R_2 position, exhibited higher AR binding affinity and more potent activity than their corresponding *S*-isomers (90). The sulfide analogs (replacement of ether oxygen with sulfur) exhibited greater AR binding affinity, except that hepatic oxidation of the sulfur linkage led to rapid in vivo inactivation and reduced efficacy. Partial androgen agonist activity was observed when position 3 of ring A was substituted with a trifluoromethyl group (91). Replacing the aromatic ring A with a heterocyclic ring derivative failed to retain AR binding affinity, which probably arose from steric hinderance on binding with the AR; however, a heterocyclic B ring retained AR binding affinity. Small size electron-withdrawing moieties at R_2, such as fluoro, chloro, nitro, or cyano groups, are optimum. Because aromatic nitro groups are associated with hepatotoxicity, the nitro group was replaced with a nonreducible electron-withdrawing group (i.e., a cyano group), which gave the most potent and efficacious *N*-arylpropionamide SARM with favorable pharmacokinetic properties. As evidenced from

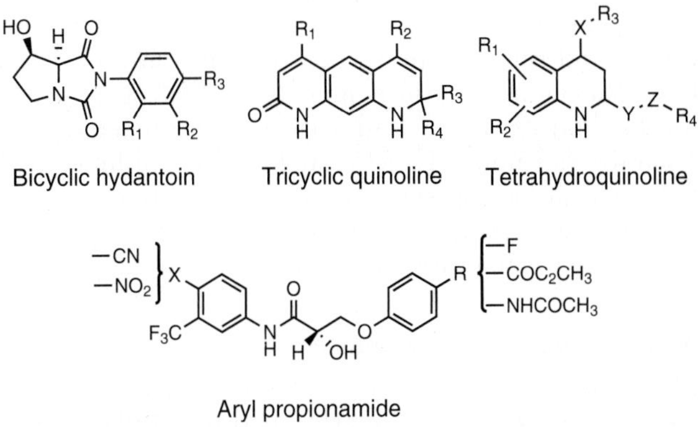

FIGURE 40.12 Selective androgen receptor modulators.

structure–activity relationship studies, minor differences in ligand structure can lead to either agonist or antagonist activity. Full or partial agonist binding to AR is influenced by stereoisomeric conformation as well as by steric and electronic effects of the substituents. Molecular modeling of *N*-arylpropionamide AR ligands was used in conjunction with pharmacology, pharmacodynamics, pharmacokinetics, and metabolism to examine and optimize structural properties.

Results from in vitro and in vivo animal studies suggest that the therapeutic promise of SARMs as treatment for muscle wasting, osteoporosis, hormonal male contraception, BPH, or other conditions associated with aging or androgen deficiency—without unwanted side effects associated with testosterone—may be soon realized (92). The AR specificity and lack of steroidal-related side effects clearly distinguish these drugs from their steroidal predecessors and open the door for expanded clinical use of androgens. As the molecular mechanisms of action of SARMs on target tissues become more fully understood, the discovery of novel SARMs and expansion into broader therapeutic applications will be more feasible. Currently, research concerning SARMs is in preclinical discovery and the early phase of clinical development with the expectations that SARMs, with the beneficial pharmacologic activity of androgens without the unwanted side effects, will provide individual patients who have various androgen-dependent disorders with a significantly improved quality of life.

TREATMENT OF PROSTATIC DISEASES

Diseases of the prostate represent some of the greatest threats to men's health. Incidence rates for BPH escalate rapidly with age, from approximately 50% of men at age 50 years to approximately 90% at age 90 years in the United States. Drugs that inhibit the metabolism of testosterone to DHT (i.e., 5α-reductase inhibitors) (93) or block urethral constriction (α_1-adrenergic receptor antagonists) (94) are used as front-line treatment for urinary obstruction associated with BPH. Surgery is also commonly performed as treatment for early-stage prostate cancer (i.e., prostatectomy) and transurethral resection of the prostate, making these some of the most common surgeries performed on men.

Prostate cancer is the most common noncutaneous cancer and remains the second leading cause of death from cancer in American men (95). Androgen receptor antagonists (i.e., antiandrogens) and gonadotropin-releasing hormone (LHRH) analogs are routinely used for medical management of patients with early-stage prostate cancer, whereas patients with advanced prostate cancer are treated with anticancer chemotherapy.

Benign Prostatic Hyperplasia

BPH is the noncancerous proliferation of the prostate gland. The major problem associated with BPH is lower urinary tract symptoms. Approximately 80% of men will develop BPH within their lifetime. Although the cause of BPH is not well understood, it occurs mainly in older men, and it does not develop in men whose testes were removed before puberty. As men age, the concentration of free testosterone in the blood decreases due to increases in SHBG, while the concentrations of estradiol increase due to aromatization in adipose tissue. Animal studies have suggested that BPH may result from the increased concentration of estradiol or DHT within the gland, which promotes cell growth (96). Men who do not produce DHT do not develop BPH (97).

The symptoms of BPH stem from obstruction of the urethra by an enlarged prostate and the gradual loss of bladder function, which results in incomplete emptying of the bladder. The symptoms of BPH vary, but the most common symptoms involve changes or problems with urination. The typical symptoms of BPH are obstructive (e.g., poor urine stream, dribbling, and large residual urine volume) and irritative (e.g., hesitancy, increased frequency of urination, and nocturia), which can significantly compromise the quality of life for men. The enlarging prostate increases the adrenergic tone of the prostate in patients with BPH, which results in further tightening of the urethra. When partial obstruction is present, urinary retention also can be brought on by alcohol, cold temperatures, a long period of immobility, or the ingestion of over-the-counter cold or allergy medicines that contain a sympathomimetic decongestant drug or anticholinergics.

Severe BPH can cause serious problems over time, including urinary retention and strain on the bladder, which can lead to urinary tract infections, bladder or kidney damage, bladder stones, and incontinence.

Before and during adulthood, DHT plays a critical role in determining prostate size, and multiple lines of evidence suggest the importance of DHT in the development of BPH (98,99). For instance, BPH does not develop in males with certain type 2 5α-reductase mutations or in males with very low levels of androgen because of prepubertal castration or hypopituitarism-related hypogonadism. Moreover, clinical treatment of BPH either by chemical or surgical castration or by type 2 5α-reductase inhibitor (e.g., finasteride or dutasteride) induces apoptosis of epithelial cells, which in turn significantly decreases the volume of the prostate (99). Recently, the role of age-dependent changes in the intraprostatic hormonal environment in the development of BPH was evaluated (93). Despite the aging-related decrease in testosterone and intraprostatic DHT production, an increased estradiol/DHT ratio was observed in the aging human prostate, which can be relevant to the development of BPH. Furthermore, estradiol is capable of inducing precancerous lesions and prostate cancer in aging dogs (100). Therefore, TRT in older men raises concern regarding acceleration of BPH and/or prostate cancer.

Surgical procedures often are used to reduce a large prostate mass, but there are early pharmacologic treatments for BPH including α_1-adrenergic blockers, 5α-reductase inhibitors, and phytotherapy.

The α_1-adrenergic antagonists treat the increased adrenergic tone of the sympathetic nervous system by relaxing the muscles at the neck of the bladder and in the prostate, thereby reducing the pressure on the urethra and increasing the flow of urine (94). They do not cure BPH but, rather, help to alleviate some of the symptoms. Approximately 60% of men find that symptoms improve significantly within the first 2 to 3 weeks of treatment with an α_1-antagonist. Alfuzosin, tamsulosin, and silodosin are used exclusively as first-line α_1-adrenergic antagonists for the treatment of BPH, while doxazosin and terazosin have also been used to treat high blood pressure. Prazosin, another α_1-antagonist, is not indicated for the treatment of BPH. Tamsulosin, alfuzosin, and silodosin are uroseletive α_1-adrenergic antagonists developed specifically to treat BPH.

The 5α-reductase inhibitors work by suppressing the production of intraprostatic DHT, thereby reducing the size of the prostate (93). Finasteride and dutasteride are the most commonly used drugs for this purpose. Unlike α_1-antagonists, 5α-reductase inhibitors are able to reverse BPH to some extent and so may delay the need for surgery. Several months of treatment may be needed before the benefit is noticed.

α_1-Adrenergic Antagonists

Mechanism of Action α_1-Adrenoceptors are widely distributed in the human body and play important physiologic roles (see Chapter 10). Of the three α_1-adrenoceptor subtypes (α_{1A}, α_{1B}, and α_{1D}), α_{1A}-adrenoceptors, expressed in prostate and urethral tissue, and α_{1D}-adrenoceptors, expressed mainly in the detrusor muscle of the bladder and the sacral region of the spinal cord, have been shown mediate smooth muscle contraction and antagonists provide relief from the symptoms of BPH. The vast majority of α-adrenoceptors expressed in the prostate are of the α_{1A} (70%) and α_{1D} subtypes (27%). α_{1B}-Adrenoceptor is known to be important in the regulation of blood pressure (101). The predominant expression of the α_{1A}-adrenoceptor subtype in the prostatic and urethral smooth muscle cells led to the design of drugs with uroselectivity for this receptor subtype. Thus, alfuzosin (an aminoquinazoline), tamsulosin (an *N*-substituted, catecholamine-related sulfonamide), and silodosin (a substituted indole carboxamide) were designed for the treatment of BPH (Fig. 40.13) (99). Doxazosin and terazosin, along with prazosin, originally were used as antihypertensives but also were found to be effective for the treatment of BPH based on their common mechanism of action. Comparisons of the affinities (K_i, nmol/L) of the α_{1A}-adrenoceptor antagonists (Table 40.3) did not show substantial differences for the quinazoline α_{1A}-antagonists (alfuzosin, doxazosin, and terazosin) but some uroselectivity for tamsulosin and silodosin (94,102,103). In vivo studies showed that those α_{1A}-adrenoceptor antagonists without in vitro adrenoceptor subtype selectivity, such as alfuzosin and doxazosin, showed uroselectivity (terazosin was not uroselective), whereas tamsulosin, which exhibited in vitro selectivity for the α_{1A}-adrenoceptor, did not show the expected in vivo uroselectivity (104). Silodosin, the most recent addition to this class of drugs, showed both in vitro and in vivo uroselectivity. However, these differences between in vitro and in vivo studies suggest that these drugs modify urethral pressures in a manner that is not directly correlated with their selectivity for the cloned α_{1A}-adrenoceptor subtypes. It is apparent that the existing α_{1A}-adrenoceptor antagonists have different in vivo pharmacologic profiles that are not yet predictable from their receptor based on the current state of knowledge regarding the α_{1A}-adrenoceptor classification (104).

Thus, tamsulosin, alfuzosin, and silodosin are first-line drugs for the treatment of BPH and have no utility in treating hypertension, because they have fewer cardiovascular effects than terazosin and doxazosin. Some of the basic physicochemical and pharmacokinetic properties of the α_1-antagonists are summarized in Table 40.3. Improvements in urine flow occur 4 to 8 hours after the first dose and in BPH symptoms within 1 week.

Adverse Reactions In patients with BPH, the most common adverse effects for α_1-adrenergic antagonists are

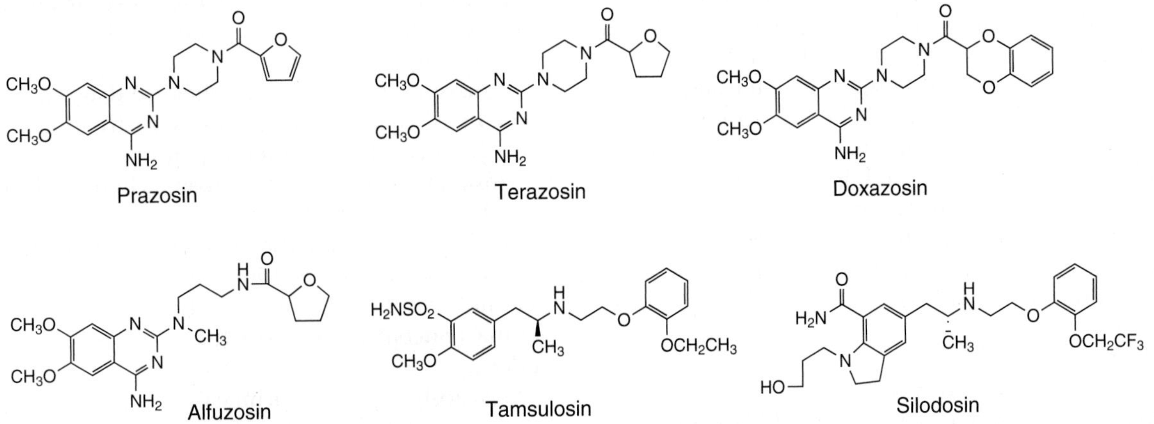

FIGURE 40.13 α_1-Adrenergic antagonists for treatment of benign prostatic hyperplasia.

TABLE 40.3 Some Properties and Pharmacokinetics of the α-Adrenergic Antagonists

Drug	Alfuzosin	Doxazosin	Silodosin	Tamsulosin	Terazosin
Trade name	Uroxatral	Cardura	Rapaflo	Flomax	Hytrin
cLogP[a]	−1.0 ± 0.4	0.7 ± 0.4	2.97	2.2 ± 0.4	−1.0 ± 0.4
logD[a] (pH 7)	−1.3	−0.5	0.5	−0.5	−1.0
Oral bioavailability (%)	65	65 (62–69)	32	<50 with food	90
				>90 fasted	
Onset of action (weeks)[b]	<2	1–2	<1	1	2
Duration of action (hours)	>48	18–36	24	>24	>18
Protein binding (%)	82–90	98	97	94	95
Time to peak concentration (hours)	1–2	2–5	2-3	4–5	1
Volume of distribution (L/kg)	2.5–3.2	1.0–3.4	50	18	25–30
Elimination half-life (hours)	3–10	18–22	13	9–13	9–12
				14–15 elderly	
Cytochrome isoforms	3A4	3A4	3A4	3A4, 2D6	—
Excretion (%)	69 feces	63–65 feces	33 urine	21 feces	55–65 feces
	24–30 urine (metabolites)	~20 urine ~10 unchanged	55 feces glucuronides	76 urine 10 unchanged	30 urine 10–20 unchanged
K_i (nmol/L) for α_{1A}	2.4	2.7	1.0	0.5	2.5

[a]Chemical Abstracts, American Chemical Society, calculated using Advanced Chemistry Development (ACD/Labs) Software V8.14 for Solaris (1994–2006 ACD/Labs).
[b]Time for improvement in urine flow observed.

related to abnormal ejaculation and orthostatic hypotension, with vasodilation, dizziness, headache, and tachycardia also occurring in some patients during the first 2 weeks of treatment (105). Therefore, a dose titration usually is required, especially in patients taking doxazosin and terazosin or older than 60 years. These cardiovascular side effects are attributed to a nonselective blockade of α_1-adrenoceptors present in vascular smooth muscle in addition to the required blockade of α_1-adrenoceptors in prostate. No first-dose effect and fewer vasodilatory adverse events have been reported with silodosin and the sustained-release formulations of other drugs, which occur more frequently with the immediate-release formulation. At higher doses, orthostatic hypotension occurs more frequently. The first-dose phenomenon of orthostatic hypotension and syncope has been reported occasionally in elderly patients and in those concurrently receiving calcium antagonists, diuretics, and β-blockers. Concomitant use of the α_1-adrenoceptor antagonists with PDE5 inhibitors (used commonly for ED in older men) is associated with a higher risk for dizziness and symptomatic hypotension

Classes of α_1-Adrenergic Antagonists.

Quinazolines Prazosin was the first selective quinazoline α_1-blocker to be discovered in the late 1960s as an antihypertensive. Alfuzosin, doxazosin, and terazosin are structurally similar (a 4-amino-6,7-dimethoxyquinazoline ring system) but differ in the attached side chain as a piperazine ring or open-chain analog as shown in Figure 40.13. The other structural differences are the acyl groups attached to the second nitrogen of the piperazine or the aminopropyl chain. The differences in these groups afford dramatic differences in some of the pharmacokinetic properties for these agents (see Table 40.3). Perhaps most significant are the long half-lives and durations of action for these drugs that permit once-a-day dosing and, generally, lead to increased patient compliance.

Alfuzosin is a first-line uroselective drug for the treatment of BPH, but with no utility in treating hypertension, because it has fewer cardiovascular effects than terazosin and doxazosin. Alfuzosin is hepatically metabolized by 7-*O*-demethylation and *N*-dealkylation, primarily by CYP3A4, to inactive metabolites. In patients with moderate or severe hepatic insufficiency, a reduction in clearance resulted in a three to four times increase in its plasma concentrations, which may require a reduction in dose.

Doxazosin is primarily metabolized by 7-*O*-demethylation, hydroxylation of the benzodioxan ring, and oxidation of the piperazine ring to inactive metabolites. In patients with renal insufficiency, the elimination half-life was not significantly different from healthy volunteers.

Terazosin is similarly metabolized via 7-*O*-demethylation and *N*-dealkylation to four metabolites: 6- and 7-*O*-demethyl terazosin, the piperazine derivative of terazosin, and the diamine metabolite of the piperazine compound.

Catecholamine-Sulfonamide Tamsulosin exhibits uroselectivity and is a first-line drug for the treatment of BPH, with no utility for treating hypertension, because of its fewer cardiovascular effects. Tamsulosin is *O*-deethylated by CYP3A4 to phenolic metabolites that are conjugated to glucuronide or sulfate before renal excretion and by *O*-demethylation and 3′-hydroxylation to catechol metabolites that also are conjugated with glucuronide and sulfate.

Indole Carboxamide Silodosin is the most uroselective of the α_1-adrenoceptor antagonists, demonstrating 160- and 50-fold higher affinity for binding to α_{1A}- as compared to α_{1B}- and α_{1D}-adrenoceptors, respectively (103). Silodosin undergoes extensive metabolism through glucuronidation, alcohol and aldehyde dehydrogenase, and CYP3A4. The glucuronide conjugate (formed via direct glucuronidation of the alcohol) of silodosin is active, has a longer half-life (24 hours) than the parent drug, and achieves a plasma exposure (area under the curve) four times higher than that of silodosin.

5α-Reductase Inhibitors

The development of BPH requires a combination of intraprostatic DHT and the aging process. Although not elevated in BPH, levels of DHT in the prostate remain at a physiologic levels with aging despite a decrease in plasma testosterone. Adult males with genetically inherited, type 2 5α-reductase deficiency also have decreased DHT levels. These 5α-reductase–deficient males have a small prostate gland throughout life and do not develop BPH. Except for the associated urogenital defects that are present at birth, no other clinical abnormalities related to 5α-reductase deficiency have been observed in these individuals.

Mechanism of Action Inhibitors of DHT biosynthesis can result in a decrease in both circulating and target-tissue (prostate and skin) DHT concentrations, thus blocking its androgenic action in these tissues. The critical enzyme targeted for DHT inhibition is 5α-reductase, which converts testosterone to DHT. The first agent to demonstrate 5α-reductase inhibition was a progestin analog, medrogesterone (106) (Fig. 40.14). Two azasteroid-17-amide derivatives of medrogesterone have been developed as potent irreversible inhibitors of 5α-reductase and approved for the treatment of BPH: finasteride, a selective inhibitor of type 2 5α-reductase (107,108), and dutasteride, a nonselective inhibitor of type 1 and type 2 5α-reductase (109) (Fig. 40.14). Thus, the inhibition of type 2 5α-reductase suppresses the metabolism of testosterone to DHT, resulting in significant decreases in plasma and intraprostatic DHT concentrations (108–110).

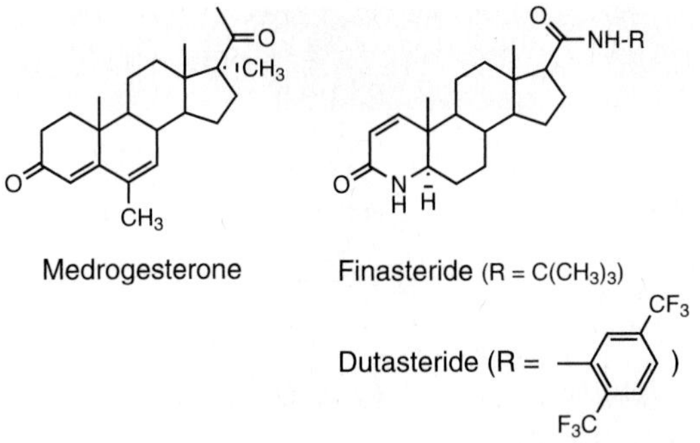

FIGURE 40.14 5α-Reductase inhibitors for the treatment of benign prostatic hyperplasia.

Finasteride and dutasteride are both mechanism-based inhibitors of type 1 and type 2 5α-reductase isoenzymes that inactivate 5α-reductase by an apparent irreversible modification of 5α-reductase (111,112). The inhibition constants (median inhibitory concentrations [IC_{50}]) in Table 40.4 suggest that finasteride is 30 times more selective for type 2 5α-reductase, whereas dutasteride appears to be approximately 2 times more potent as an inhibitor of type 2 5α-reductase than as an inhibitor of type 1 5α-reductase. The reduction of finasteride to dihydrofinasteride proceeds through an enzyme-bound, NADP-dihydrofinasteride adduct (see Chapter 8) (111). The mechanism-based inhibition explains the exceptional potency and specificity of finasteride and dutasteride in the treatment of BPH. This concept of mechanism-based inhibition may have application to the development of other inhibitors of pyridine nucleotide–linked enzymes.

Drug Interactions Because finasteride and dutasteride are metabolized primarily by CYP3A4, the CYP3A4 inhibitors, such as ritonavir, ketoconazole, verapamil, diltiazem, cimetidine, and ciprofloxacin, may increase these drugs' blood levels and, possibly, cause drug–drug interactions. Clinical drug interaction studies have shown no pharmacokinetic or pharmacodynamic interactions between dutasteride and tamsulosin or terazosin, warfarin, digoxin, and cholestyramine.

Finasteride The selective inhibition of the type 2 5α-reductase isozyme by finasteride produces a rapid reduction in plasma DHT concentration, reaching 65% suppression within 24 hours of administering a 1-mg oral tablet (113). At steady-state, finasteride suppresses DHT levels by approximately 70% in plasma and by as much as 85% to 90% in the prostate. The remaining DHT in the prostate likely is the result of type 1 5α-reductase. The mean circulating levels of testosterone and estradiol

TABLE 40.4 Some Properties and Pharmacokinetics of the 5α-Reductases

Drugs	Finasteride	Dutasteride
Trade name	Proscar	Avodart
cLogP[a]	3.2 ± 0.4	5.6 ± 0.6
logD[a] (pH 7)	3.2	5.6
Oral bioavailability (%)	65 (26–170)	60 (40–94)
Onset of action (hours)	<24	—
Duration of action (hours)	—	>5 weeks
Protein binding (%)	90	99
Time to peak concentration (hours)	—	2–3
Volume of distribution (L/kg)	76 (44–96)	300–500
Elimination half-life (hours)	5–6 (18–60 years)	5 weeks
	>8 (60+ years)	
Cytochrome isoforms	3A4	3A4
Active metabolites	None	6-*p*-OH
Excretion (%)	57 feces and 40 urine as metabolites	40 feces metabolites
		5 unmetabolized urine
IC_{50} (nmol/L)	313 Type 1	3.9 Type 1
	11 Type 2	1.8 Type 2

[a]Chemical Abstracts, American Chemical Society, calculated using Advanced Chemistry Development (ACD/Labs) Software V8.14 for Solaris (1994–2006ACD/Labs).

remained within their physiologic concentration range. Long-term therapy with finasteride can reduce clinically significant end points of BPH, such as acute urinary retention or surgery. Finasteride is most effective in men with large prostates. Finasteride has no affinity for the AR and no androgenic, antiandrogenic, estrogenic, antiestrogenic, or progestational effects.

Pharmacokinetics The mean oral bioavailability of finasteride is 65%, as shown in Table 40.4, and is not affected by food (113). Approximately 90% of circulating finasteride is bound to plasma proteins. Finasteride has been found to cross the blood–brain barrier, but levels in semen were undetectable (<0.2 ng/mL). Finasteride is extensively metabolized in the liver, primarily via CYP3A4 to two major metabolites: monohydroxylation of the *t*-butyl side chain, which is further metabolized via an aldehyde intermediate to the second metabolite, a monocarboxylic acid (Fig. 40.15). The metabolites show approximately 20% the inhibition of finasteride for 5α-reductase. The mean terminal half-life is approximately 5 to 6 hours in men between 18 and 60 years of age and 8 hours in men older than 70 years of age. Following an oral dose of finasteride, approximately 40% of the dose was excreted in the urine as metabolites and approximately 57% in the feces. Even though the elimination rate of finasteride is decreased in the elderly, no dosage adjustment is necessary. No dosage adjustment is necessary in patients with renal insufficiency. A decrease in the urinary excretion of metabolites was observed in patients with renal impairment, but this was compensated for by an increase in fecal excretion of metabolites. Caution should be used during administration to patients with liver function abnormalities, because finasteride is metabolized extensively in the liver. Finasteride can be absorbed through the skin. As such, tablets, especially broken ones, should not be handled by women who are pregnant or could become pregnant due to a risk of fetal exposure.

DUTASTERIDE Similar to finasteride, dutasteride is a competitive and mechanism-based inhibitor not only of type 2 but also of type 1 5α-reductase isoenzymes, with which stable enzyme-NADP adduct complexes are formed, inhibiting the conversion of testosterone to DHT (112). The suppression of both type 1 and type 2 isoforms results in greater and more consistent reduction of plasma DHT than that observed for finasteride (114–116). The more effective dual inhibition of type 1 and type 2 5α-reductase isoforms lowers circulating DHT to a greater extent than with finasteride and shows advantages in treating BPH and other disease states (e.g., prostate cancer) that are DHT-dependent.

The maximum effect of 0.5-mg daily doses of dutasteride on the suppression of DHT is dose-dependent and is observed within 1 to 2 weeks. After 2 weeks of 0.5-mg daily dosing, median plasma DHT concentrations were reduced by 90%, and after 1 year, the median decrease in plasma DHT was 94% (115,116). The median increase in plasma testosterone was 19% but remained within the physiologic range. The drug also reduced serum prostatic-specific antigen (PSA) by approximately 50% at 6 months and total prostate volume by 25% at 2 years. Dutasteride produced improvements in quality of life and peak urinary flow rate and reduction of acute urinary retention without the need for surgery. The main side effects are ED, decreased libido, gynecomastia, and ejaculation disorders. Long-term use (>4 years), however, did not reveal increased onset of sexual side effects. A combination product (Jalyn) containing dutasteride (0.5 mg) and tamsulosin (0.4 mg) was approved by the U.S. Food and Drug Administration in 2010 based on clinical studies showing that the combination was more effective than either monotherapy as assessed by prostate symptom score and maximal urine flow rates. The decreased adrenergic tone associated with tamsulosin and long-term reduction in prostate size (obstruction) associated with dutasteride provide rapid and sustained symptomatic relief for men with BPH.

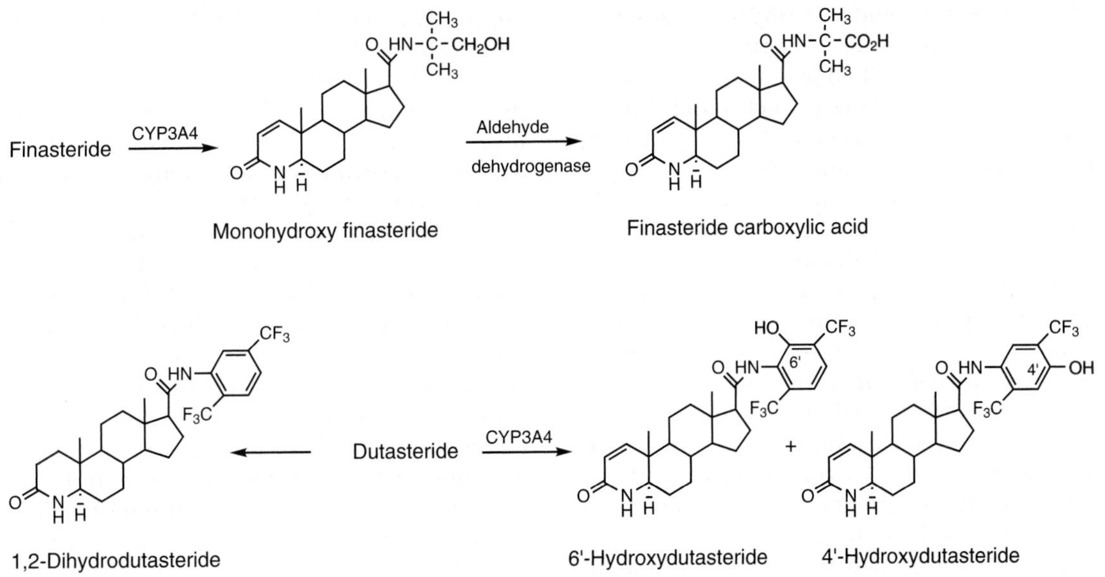

FIGURE 40.15 Metabolites of finasteride and dutasteride.

Pharmacokinetics Following oral administration, peak plasma concentrations of dutasteride occur in approximately 2 to 3 hours, with a bioavailability of approximately 60% (Table 40.4), and no meaningful reduction in absorption occurs with food (113,114). Dutasteride is highly bound to plasma proteins 99%. The concentrations of dutasteride in semen averaged approximately 3 ng/mL, with no significant effects on DHT plasma levels of sex partners. Dutasteride is extensively metabolized in humans by CYP3A4 to three major metabolites: 4′-hydroxydutasteride and 1,2-dihydrodutasteride, which are less potent than parent drug, and 6′-hydroxydutasteride, which is comparable to the parent drug as an inhibitor of both type 1 and type 2 5α-reductases (Fig. 40.15). Dutasteride and its metabolites are excreted mainly (40%) in feces as dutasteride-related metabolites. The terminal elimination half-life of dutasteride is approximately 5 weeks. Because of its long half-life, plasma concentrations remain detectable for up to 4 to 6 months after discontinuation of treatment. No dose adjustment is necessary in elderly patients, even though its half-life increased with age from approximately 170 hours in men between age 20 and 49 years to 300 hours in men older than age 70 years (113,116). No adjustment in dosage is necessary for patients with renal impairment. Like finasteride, dutasteride can be absorbed through the skin. As such, dutasteride capsules should not be handled by women who are pregnant or could become pregnant.

Phytotherapy

A number of plant extracts are popularly used to alleviate BPH, although formal evidence that they are effective is often scanty (117). Extracts of the saw palmetto berry (*Serenoa repens*) are widely used for the treatment of BPH, often as an alternative to pharmaceutical agents. In a national survey conducted in 2002, 1.1% of the adult male population in the United States, or approximately 2.5 million males, reported using saw palmetto. The herb is widely used in Europe, where half of the German urologists prefer prescribing plant-based extracts rather than synthetic drugs. The most common nonstandardized preparation used is either the hexane-extract (Permixon) or the ethanol or carbon dioxide extraction of the dried ripe fruit from the American dwarf saw palmetto plant (*S. repens*), which is rich in fatty acids and plant sterols. The plant sterols appear to be the primary active constituents. The U.S. Pharmacopeia states that the liposterolic extract product should contain 70% to 95% fatty acids and 0.2% to 0.5% sterols. Other substances in the extracts include polyprenic compounds and flavonoids. The usual therapeutic dose of the extracts is 320 mg daily.

Serenoa repens had been popular in the United States during the 19th century as a treatment for a variety of urogenital disorders and had been mentioned as a treatment for prostate problems as early as 1899. Research into the effects of *S. repens* in many European countries appeared to confirm a positive action on BPH. The mechanism of action for the saw palmetto is not clearly established, but the sterols may have, as one mechanism of action, the inhibition of 5α-reductase and a decrease in DHT production. Therapeutic results should be expected in 6 to 8 weeks, but clinical efficacy is observed with BPH for 6 months or longer. The liposterolic extract is largely devoid of the side effects noted for prescription BPH drugs.

Although most previous randomized trials of saw palmetto have reported small improvements in the symptoms of BPH or in urinary flow rates, these studies were limited by the small numbers of subjects enrolled, their short duration, failure to use standardized products, their failure to use standard outcome measures, and the lack of information from participants concerning how effectively the placebo was blinded. Using widely accepted outcome measures from the American Urological Association (AUA) and a matched placebo capsule, a randomized, 1-year, double-blind saw palmetto trial (funded by the National Institutes of Health National Institute on Complementary and Alternative Medicine) was performed to determine the efficacy of saw palmetto for the treatment of BPH (118). A total of 225 men age 50 years and older with documented disease received 160 mg of a standardized saw palmetto extract twice a day or a matching-placebo capsule. Over the course of a year, the men made eight office visits and were evaluated for assessment of AUA standardized changes, which included maximal urine flow, postvoid residual urine volume, prostate size, and other health-related outcomes. In contrast to most previous studies, this study reported no significant benefit of saw palmetto on urinary symptoms in terms of objective measures of BPH over a 1-year period.

Despite the differences between these studies, the weight of evidence suggests that saw palmetto may induce mild to moderate improvements in urinary symptoms and flow measures.

Other Western herbs that have been investigated for the treatment of BPH include pumpkin seeds (*Cucurbita pepo*), nettle root (*Urtica dioica* or *Urtica urens*), bee pollen (particularly that from the rye plant), African potato (tubers of *Hypoxis rooperi*), and the African tree *Pygeum africanum*, also known as *Prunus africanum*. In most cases, but particularly with pumpkin seeds and African potato, the main active components are sterols, such as β-sitosterol, which also has been used for BPH. Triterpenoids in *Pygeum* sp. also have been proposed to be active components, potentially having the action of reducing prostate swelling. Among the Chinese herbs recommended for BPH, the iridoid glycosides may be the active components from plantago seed, catalpol from rehmannia, and morroniside from cornus (an ingredient in the rehmannia formulas). Iridoids have not been found in the Western herbal therapies for BPH and represent a potential new area for future investigation. Iridoids are the recognized active constituents of the Western herb chaste tree berry (*Vitex agnus costus*), which has been shown to reduce prolactin levels in women; elevated prolactin may be a risk factor for prostate enlargement in men. Triterpenoids found in vaccaria and alisma (an ingredient in rehmannia formulas) could contribute to their therapeutic effects in a manner similar to that suggested for pygeum.

Prostatic Cancer

Prostate cancer is the second leading cause of cancer death and the most commonly diagnosed cancer in American men (95). Prostate cancer is more common in African American males, in whom it tends to be more aggressive and progressive, leading to advanced disease. The incidence of prostate cancer increases with age. Traditional treatments for localized prostate cancer include watchful waiting, surgery (radical prostatectomy), and external-beam radiation, whereas surgical and pharmacologic approaches to induce androgen deprivation are used for advanced prostate cancer.

Huggins and Hodges won the 1966 Nobel Prize for describing the relationship between testosterone and prostate cancer, having shown that marked reductions in serum testosterone by castration or estrogen treatment caused metastatic prostate cancer to regress in 1941 (119). Androgen deprivation therapy has remained an important component in the treatment of prostate cancer since then. Testicular surgery (bilateral orchiectomy) to prevent testosterone production was once the most common treatment for advanced prostate cancer and is still used today. Although this surgery is not a cure, it delays the advance of the disease. Numerous refinements in therapy have occurred since this time, including androgen deprivation therapy with diethylstilbestrol (seldom used now), gonadotropin-releasing hormone agonists and antagonists, antiandrogens, and chemotherapy for advanced cases. Chemotherapy is used in the most advanced stages of the disease when the cancer is no longer responding to hormonal treatment.

Because prostate cancer typically grows slowly and causes no symptoms, digital rectal examination and the serum PSA test are most often used to screen for prostate cancer. The PSA test is also used to evaluate and manage other prostate problems, most notably BPH. However, the PSA screening test cannot tell the difference between prostate cancer and other prostate problems. PSA is a protein made by prostate tissue and prostate cancer cells. Men with prostate cancer often have elevated PSA levels, because the cancer cells make excessive amounts of this protein under the control of testosterone.

Radical prostatectomy (surgical removal of the prostate gland) is an effective treatment for cancer that remains localized to the prostate gland. However, prostate cancer may have already invaded the surrounding tissues (e.g., pelvic lymph nodes) at the time of surgery. Months, even years, may pass before this latent prostate cancer produces sufficient PSA to be detected by modern assays. When detected, increasing levels of PSA are referred to as biochemical recurrence and signal the re-emergence of the disease and the progression to advanced prostate cancer, with a median survival of approximately 10 to 15 years (120). Advanced prostate cancer in its earliest stages is thought to be dependent on androgens (i.e., testosterone and DHT) for growth. As such, androgen deprivation therapy, either by surgical castration or pharmacologic suppression of LH, is used as first-line treatment for advanced prostate cancer.

Luteinizing Hormone–Releasing Hormone Therapy

The goal of LHRH therapy for advanced prostate cancer is to suppress the production of testosterone in the testis by shutting down the production of LH by the pituitary. Both LHRH agonists and LHRH antagonists are used. The LHRH agonists (Fig. 40.16), such as leuprolide acetate (Lupron Depot and Eligard) and goserelin acetate (Zoladex), when administered in a continuous,

H-5 oxoPro-His-Trp-Ser-Tyr-D-Leu—Leu-Arg—Pro-NH-C_2H_5

Leuprolide

H-5 oxoPro·His—Trp-Ser-Tyr-D-Ser(t-Bu)-Leu-Arg-Pro-N(H)-N(H)-C(=O)-NH_2

Goserelin

[Note: H-5 oxoPro = pGlu (PyroGlu)]

FIGURE 40.16 Nonsteroidal antiandrogens.

nonpulsatile manner, suppress serum testosterone levels to a similar extent as surgical castration (i.e., <50 ng/dL). The LHRH agonists bind with higher affinity to the LHRH receptor than does the endogenous hormone, causing desensitization of the LHRH receptor complex on the gonadotroph cells in the anterior pituitary gland (121). After a brief surge, pituitary biosynthesis and secretion of LH stops, serum LH levels fall, and testicular production of testosterone ceases (see the hypothalamus-pituitary-testis axis in Fig. 40.2). A surge in serum testosterone levels accompanies the surge in pituitary LH production within the first 3 to 7 days of initiation of therapy and can exacerbate symptoms (serum PSA levels or bone pain) in some men. Castration (i.e., serum testosterone levels <50 ng/dL) is generally achieved with 2 weeks after administration of the first dose. A variety of depot formulations for intramuscular administration of leuprolide and goserelin are available, with durations of action ranging from 1 to 4 months.

Degarelix (Firmagon) is the only LHRH antagonist approved for use in the treatment of advanced prostate cancer. It competes reversibly with the endogenous LHRH for receptor binding on the pituitary gonadotroph cells and directly inhibits LH production.

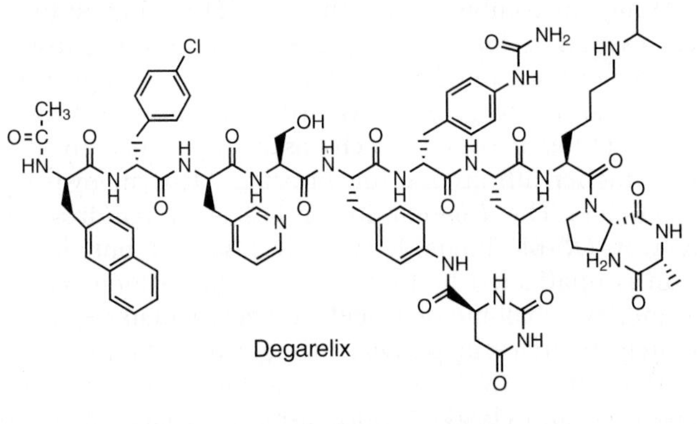

Degarelix

Because degarelix acts as an antagonist, there is no surge in pituitary LH or testicular androgen production as is observed with the LHRH agonists. As such, approximately 96% of men achieve castration levels of serum testosterone within 3 days of receiving their first dose (240 mg as two subcutaneous injections of 120 mg) of degarelix. Lower doses of degarelix (80 mg) are administered every 28 days thereafter to maintain castration.

Androgen deprivation therapy with LHRH significantly reduces serum testosterone levels, thereby depriving prostate cancer cells of their primary signal for growth (i.e., testosterone) and alleviating or easing the symptoms associated with advanced prostate cancer. However, LHRH agonists and antagonists are not cures for prostate cancer. They are considered as palliative care. The most common side effects associated with LHRH therapy are hot flashes, but osteoporosis (due to androgen and estrogen deprivation), impotence, loss of libido, and changes in serum lipids may also occur. Long-term use of LHRH therapy is associated with osteoporosis, decreased cognitive abilities, fatigue, and vascular stiffness. Symptoms may worsen over the first few weeks of treatment. Periodic monitoring of PSA and plasma testosterone levels is recommended. Tumor flare reactions may occur transiently but can be prevented by antiandrogens or by short-term estrogens at low dose for several weeks.

Antiandrogens (Androgen Antagonists)

Treatment for advanced prostate cancer also involves the use of hormone-blocking drugs called antiandrogens. The goal of antiandrogen therapy is to block the actions of testosterone and DHT on ARs. Antiandrogens, however, are not a cure for prostate cancer. Nonsteroidal antiandrogens (Fig. 40.17), such as flutamide, nilutamide, and bicalutamide, are referred

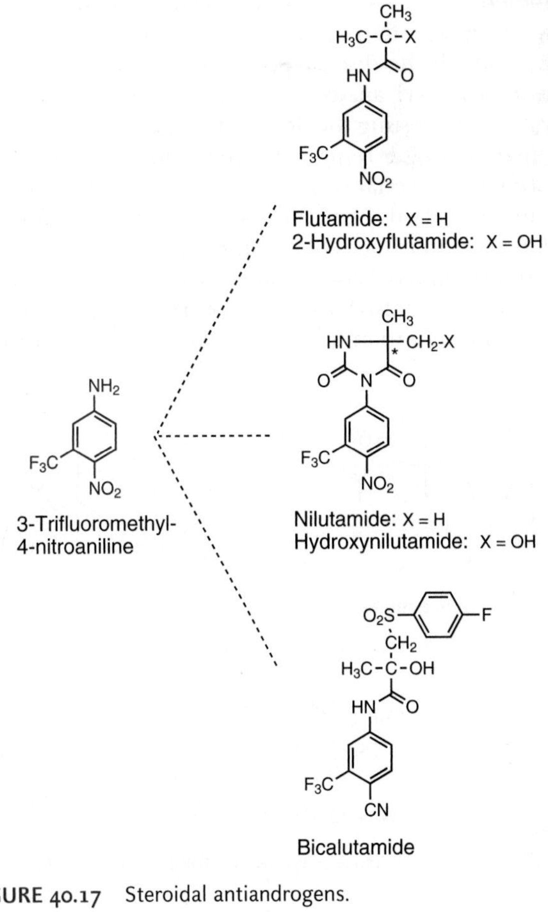

FIGURE 40.17 Steroidal antiandrogens.

to as pure antiandrogens, because they bind exclusively to AR and, thus, are devoid of antigonadotropic, antiestrogenic, and progestational effects (122). These agents have advantages over steroidal antiandrogens, such as megestrol acetate or cyproterone acetate (Fig. 40.18), in terms of specificity, selectivity, and pharmacokinetic properties.

Antiandrogens block the binding of DHT at the AR and block or diminish the effectiveness of androgens in androgen-sensitive tissues. Such compounds have shown potential therapeutic use in the treatment of acne, virilization in women, and hyperplasia and neoplasia of the prostate (123). Several steroidal and nonsteroidal agents have demonstrated antiandrogenic activity. Cyproterone acetate suppresses gonadotropin release and binds with high affinity to the AR (124,125). Oxandrolone also acts by competing for the receptor binding sites (126). A novel AR antagonist, WIN 49,596, has been described (127) that contains a fused pyrazole ring at carbons 2 and 3 of the steroid nucleus. A potent nonsteroidal antiandrogen, flutamide, has been shown to compete with DHT for the AR (128). Its hydroxylated metabolite is a more powerful antiandrogen in vivo, and it has a higher affinity for the receptor than the parent compound (129).

Antiandrogens are useful for the treatment of advanced prostate cancer during its early stages. Although approved as monotherapy for the treatment of advanced prostate cancer in Europe, antiandrogens are only indicated for combined use with an LHRH analog in the United States. Prostate cancer often advances to a "castration-resistant" state, in which the disease progresses in the presence of continued LHRH analog therapy or even after surgical castration, suggesting the development of prostate cancer cells that no longer require androgen for their growth or the ability of adrenal or intratumoral androgens to support tumor growth. Antiandrogens are most commonly used in the latter stages of the disease in order to achieve total androgen blockade. Instances of antiandrogen withdrawal syndrome also have been reported after prolonged treatment with antiandrogens. Antiandrogen withdrawal syndrome is commonly observed clinically and is defined in terms of the tumor regression or symptomatic relief observed on cessation of antiandrogen therapy. The AR mutations that result in receptor promiscuity and the ability of these antiandrogens to exhibit agonist activity may account, at least in part, for this phenomenon. For example, hydroxyflutamide and bicalutamide act as AR agonists in AR mutants with an alanine residue at position 877 or leucine residue at position 741 (as opposed to threonine or tryptophan residues, respectively, which are present at these positions in the wild-type AR) (130,131).

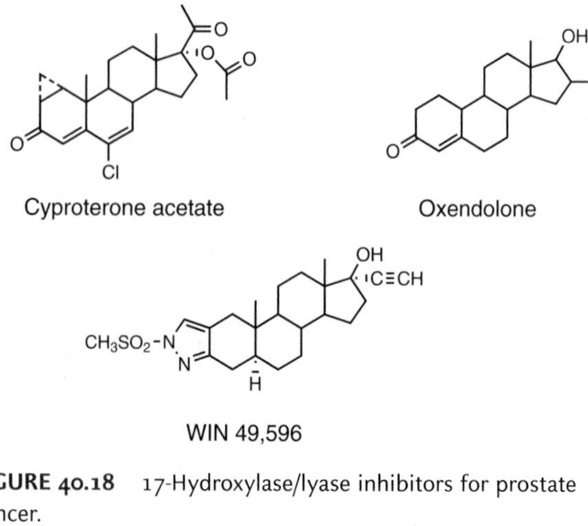

FIGURE 40.18 17-Hydroxylase/lyase inhibitors for prostate cancer.

The search for nonsteroidal antiandrogens led to the development of the substituted toluidides, flutamide and bicalutamide, and nilutamide, a hydantoin that is structurally related to the toluidides (Fig. 40.17). These compounds are pure antiandrogens and compete with DHT for the human prostate AR. They are used in combination with other drugs in the treatment of advanced prostate cancer. Although these compounds possess no intrinsic hormonal activity, their antiandrogenic mechanism of action is via competitive blockade of ARs for DHT in the hormone-sensitive tumor cells of the prostate (132). As a result of this antagonism, androgen-dependent DNA and protein synthesis is inhibited, causing arrest or regression of the prostatic tumor. Because these nonsteroidal antiandrogens are metabolized extensively in the liver, they should be used with caution in patients who have liver function abnormalities.

Specific Drugs

Bicalutamide Bicalutamide is a nonsteroidal pure antiandrogen given at a dosage of 150 mg once daily as monotherapy for the treatment of early (localized or locally advanced) nonmetastatic prostate cancer in Europe (133). It also can be used at a lower dosage (50 mg) in combination with a LHRH analog or surgical castration for the treatment of advanced prostate cancer in the United States. Bicalutamide is a racemate, and its antiandrogenic activity resides almost exclusively in the (*R*)-enantiomer, which has an approximately fourfold higher affinity for the prostate AR than hydroxyflutamide. The (*S*)-enantiomer has no antiandrogenic activity. (*R*)-Bicalutamide is slowly absorbed, but absorption is unaffected by food (134). It has a long plasma elimination half-life of 1 week and accumulates approximately 10 times in plasma during daily administration (Table 40.5). (*S*)-Bicalutamide is much more rapidly absorbed and cleared from plasma. At steady-state, the plasma levels of (*R*)-bicalutamide are 100 times higher than those of (*S*)-bicalutamide. Although mild to moderate hepatic impairment does not affect its pharmacokinetics, evidence suggests slower elimination of (*R*)-bicalutamide in subjects with severe hepatic impairment (134). Bicalutamide metabolites are excreted almost equally in urine and feces, with little or no unchanged drug excreted in urine. Unmetabolized drug predominates in the plasma. Following oral administration, the racemate displays stereoselective oxidative metabolism

TABLE 40.5 Some Properties and Pharmacokinetics of the Antiandrogens

Drugs	Bicalutamide	Flutamide	Nilutamide
Trade name	Casodex	Eulexin	Nilandron
cLogP[a]	4.9 ± 0.7	3.7 ± 0.4	3.3 ± 0.6
logD (pH 7)	4.9	3.7	3.3
Oral bioavailability (%)	80–90	—	—
Onset of action (weeks)[b]	8–12	2–4	1–2
Duration of action	8 days	3 months to 2.5 years	1–3 months
Protein binding (%)	96	94–96	80–84
Time to peak concentration (hours)	31	2–3	1–4
Elimination half-life (hours)	~6	8 (10 active metabolite)	40–60
	10 elderly	60–120 met	
Cytochrome isoforms	3A4	1A2	Flavin monooxygenase, CYP2C
Active metabolites	None	2-hydroxy	Yes
Excretion (%)	43 feces	<10 feces	<10 feces
	34 urine/glucunomide	~28 urine	62 urine
	metabolites	<10 unchanged	<2 unchanged

[a]Chemical Abstracts, American Chemical Society, calculated using Advanced Chemistry Development (ACD/Labs) Software V8.14 for Solaris (1994–2006 ACD/Labs).
[b]Time for significant improvement in prostate-specific antigen or other biomarkers.

of its (*R*)-enantiomer, with an elimination half-life of approximately 6 days. (*R*)-Bicalutamide is cleared almost exclusively by CYP3A4-mediated metabolism, but glucuronidation is the predominant metabolic route for (*S*)-bicalutamide. No evidence indicates CYP3A4 induction in humans.

Flutamide After oral administration (usual dose is 250 mg every 8 hours), flutamide is completely absorbed from the gastrointestinal tract and undergoes extensive first-pass metabolism by CYP1A2 to its major metabolite, 2-hydroxyflutamide, and its hydrolysis product, 3-trifluoromethyl-4-nitroaniline (Fig. 40.17) (129). 2-Hydroxyflutamide is a more powerful antiandrogen in vivo, with higher affinity for the receptor than that of flutamide (135). 2-Hydroxyflutamide has an elimination half-life of approximately 8 hours. These studies show the principal role of CYP1A2 in the metabolism of flutamide to 2-hydroxyflutamide, with minor contribution from CYP3A4. 2-Hydroxyflutamide inhibits the metabolism of flutamide and both 2- and 4-hydroxylation of estradiol. Flutamide is a pure antagonist, whereas 2-hydroxyflutamide is a more potent AR antagonist but also can activate the androgenic receptor at higher concentrations (135). These findings raise the possibility that increased conversion of flutamide to 2-hydroxyflutamide or accumulation of 2-hydroxyflutamide in cells may contribute to the anomalous responses to flutamide that are observed in some advanced prostate cancers. Rare reports of liver failure have been associated with flutamide, mandating regular monitoring of liver function tests in men taking flutamide therapy.

Nilutamide Nilutamide is a nitroaromatic antiandrogen used for the treatment of metastatic prostate carcinoma in men (124). It is a competitive antagonist of the AR. Nilutamide is a nitroaromatic hydantoin analog of flutamide, as shown in Figure 40.17, that is completely absorbed after oral administration, with a mean elimination half-life of approximately 50 hours (Table 40.5) (136). Daily oral doses of nilutamide range from 150 to 300 mg per day. One of the methyl groups attached to the hydantoin ring is stereoselectively hydroxylated to a chiral metabolite, which subsequently is oxidized to its carboxylic acid metabolite. Less than 2% of nilutamide is excreted unchanged in the urine. In vitro, the nitro group of nilutamide was reduced to the amine and hydroxylamine moieties by nitric oxide (NO) synthases, a flavin monooxygenase system (137). The therapeutic effects of nilutamide are overshadowed, however, by the occurrence of several adverse reactions mediated by toxic mechanisms, which are poorly investigated. The reduction of nilutamide is catalyzed by NO synthases via formation of a nitro anion free radical or via its reduction to its hydroxylamino derivative, which could explain some of the toxic effects of this drug (138). NO synthases also are involved in the formation of reactive NO and oxygen species and in the interactions with some xenobiotic compounds.

Chemotherapy and Immunotherapy

Because of the long time course for progression of prostate cancer, many men with advanced prostate cancer will die from other diseases (e.g., cardiovascular) and not from their cancer. However, advanced prostate cancer invariably progresses to a castration-resistant state, necessitating the need for increasingly harsh treatment to reduce androgen production or stop the growth of the cancer. Therapy with an LHRH agonist or antagonist alone is followed by combination therapy with an antiandrogen, which is ultimately followed by cancer chemotherapy or immunotherapy for those who are no longer responsive to any of the available hormonal therapies.

Docetaxel (Taxotere) is the only chemotherapeutic agent specifically approved for use in men with advanced prostate cancer (see Chapter 37). Infusions of 75 mg/m^2 of docetaxel over 1 hour once every 3 weeks in combination with 5 mg of prednisone daily was shown to increase survival to 18.9 months, or approximately 2 months longer as compared to treatment with mitoxantrone and prednisone (139).

Sipuleucel-T (Provenge) (a therapeutic cancer vaccine) was approved for the treatment of asymptomatic or minimally symptomatic metastatic castrate-resistant (hormone-refractory) prostate cancer in 2010. Sipuleucel-T is an autologous cellular immunotherapy. Although the precise mechanism of action is unknown, sipuleucel-T is designed to induce an immune response targeted against prostatic acid phosphatase (PAP), an antigen expressed in most prostate cancers. Three doses are usually administered at approximately 2-week intervals, with each dose containing a minimum of 50 million autologous $CD54^+$ cells activated with PAP–granulocyte-macrophage colony-stimulating factor. Patients must be given oral acetaminophen and an antihistamine, such as diphenhydramine, approximately 30 minutes prior to administration due to the high (~70%) prevalence of acute infusion reactions. Clinical trials with sipuleucel-T demonstrated a 4-month improvement in survival as compared to placebo (140).

Inhibitors of Androgen Biosynthesis

Extragonadal (e.g., adrenal or intratumoral) androgen sources may sustain prostate tumor growth despite a castrate environment in men with castration-resistant prostate cancer. A variety of experimental approaches to better reduce androgen biosynthesis have been evaluated and are in clinical development.

17α-HYDROXYLASE/17,20-LYASE INHIBITORS 17α-Hydroxylase/17,20-lyase is the key enzyme that converts pregnenolone to DHEA and, subsequently, to testosterone (Fig. 40.3). Because testosterone has androgenic activity, inhibition of its biosynthesis would be useful in treating androgen-dependent diseases, such as prostate cancer (141). Inhibitors of 17α-hydroxylase/17,20-lyase inhibitors could prevent androgen biosynthesis in the testes, adrenals, or tumor and may provide effective treatment of patients with advanced prostate cancer. Because this is an early step in steroid biosynthesis, inhibition of this enzyme efficiently may reduce androgen biosynthesis, but lead to an accumulation of serum mineralocorticoids.

The antifungal agent ketoconazole (Fig. 40.19) is an effective inhibitor of 17α-hydroxylase (IC_{50} = 76 nmol/L), which has demonstrated the promise of 17α-hydroxylase inhibitors for the treatment of metastatic prostate cancer patients (142). The nonsteroidal imidazole agent R 75251 (Liarozole) (Fig. 40.19) (143) is under development as a potentially more selective inhibitor of 17α-hydroxylase/17,20-lyase. The steroidal compounds MDL 27,302 (144), abiraterone (CB7598), and Sa40 (145) (Fig. 40.19) were designed as mechanism-based inhibitors of 17α-hydroxylase/17,20-lyase. For MDL 27,302, inhibition is specific to the cyclopropylamino compound, because the isopropylamino- or the cyclobutylamino-analogs were not inhibitory. Enzymatic specificity of MDL 27,302 of 17α-hydroxylase/17,20-lyase was demonstrated by its failure to inhibit steroid 21-hydroxylase and the cholesterol side-chain cleavage enzyme (CYP450scc). Both the 17α-hydroxylase and 17/20-lyase activities of human testicular microsomes were inhibited by MDL 27,302. Abiraterone and Sa40 are heterocyclic analogs of MDL 27,302 and potent irreversible inhibitors of 17α-hydroxylase (IC_{50} = 4 and 24 nmol/L, respectively) (145). Inhibition studies show that the 16,17-double bond is necessary for irreversible binding of these 17-pyridyl and 17-pyrimidyl steroids to 17α-hydroxylase. Oxidation to an epoxide probably is not involved, however, because the epoxide was a weak inhibitor (IC_{50} = 260 nmol/L). Recently completed clinical studies showed that abiraterone reduced serum PSA levels in men with advanced prostate cancer who had failed ketoconazole therapy. Substantial declines in serum androgen levels

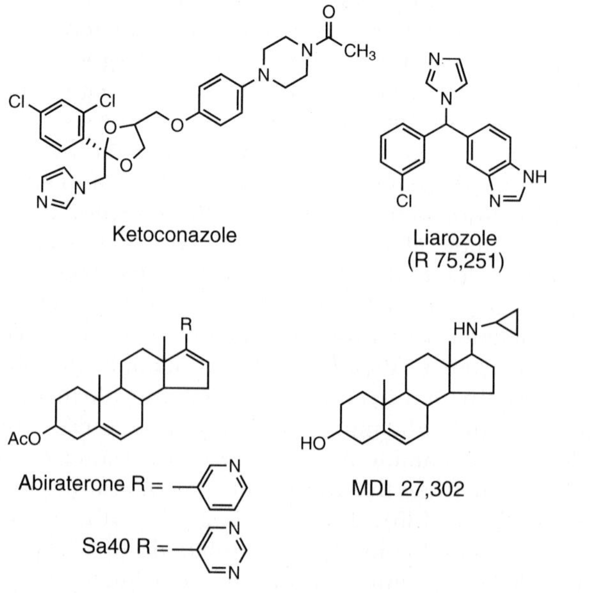

FIGURE 40.19 Luteinizing hormone–releasing hormone (LHRH) agonists used for the treatment of prostate cancer.

and increases in serum mineralocorticoids were seen at all doses (146).

5α-Reductase Inhibitors The association between lifetime exposure to testosterone and DHT and the risk of developing prostate cancer suggests that chemoprevention with specific inhibitors of key enzymes associated with androgen biosynthesis may be possible (138). Two key enzymes considered for inhibition are 5α-reductase, which inhibits the formation of DHT, and 17α-hydroxylase/17,20-lyase, which inhibits testosterone biosynthesis (Fig. 40.3).

The 5α-reductase inhibitors have been discussed previously (see *Benign Prostatic Hyperplasia*). The results of the Prostate Cancer Prevention Trial (147) for finasteride showed a 25% relative risk reduction in prostate cancer in men aged 55 years or older, albeit at an increased risk of invasive tumors (148). The risk of invasive tumors may outweigh the benefit of these agents. The 5α-reductase inhibitors have not been proven to be effective as chemoprevention against clinically significant prostate cancer. Similar results were recently reported with dutasteride (149).

Bone-Protecting Treatments

The most common site for the spread of prostate cancer is bone. Most symptoms of advanced prostate cancer are caused by the presence of disease in the bone. These symptoms can be mitigated with a drug called zoledronic acid (Zometa), a bisphosphonic acid administered by intravenous infusion that inhibits osteoclastic bone resorption, which can slow the spread of disease, reducing the development of bone pain and inhibiting bone fractures.

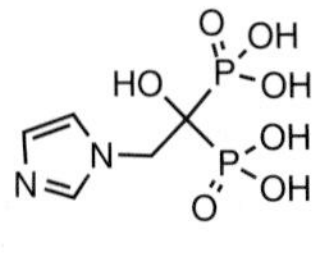

Zoledronic acid

Zoledronic acid is most commonly given to patients whose cancer is no longer responding to hormones, but it also may be given to prevent the bone thinning and weakening that result from hormonal treatments.

Treatment of Prostatitis

Prostatitis is a broad term used to identify inflammation of the prostate gland associated with lower urinary tract symptoms in men (150). Prostatitis rarely occurs in males younger than 30 years; however, it is a common problem in older males, being described as acute bacterial prostatitis, chronic bacterial prostatitis, or nonbacterial prostatitis. Because antimicrobial drug penetration generally is poor into the prostate gland, with poor efficacy of the antimicrobial agents and long duration of treatment; a 30% to 40% failure rate occurs with common treatment modalities. Three major factors determine the diffusion and concentration of antimicrobial agents in prostatic fluid and tissue: the lipid solubility of the antimicrobial agent, its dissociation constant (pK_a), and the percentage of plasma protein binding. The physiologic pH of human prostatic fluid is 6.5 to 6.7, but it increases in chronic prostatitis, ranging from 7.0 to 8.3 (151). A greater concentration of antimicrobial agents in the prostatic fluid occurs in the presence of a pH gradient across the membrane separating plasma from prostatic fluid. Of the available antimicrobial agents, β-lactam drugs have a low pK_a and poor lipid solubility and, thus, penetrate poorly into prostatic fluid, except for some cephalosporins. Good to excellent penetration into prostatic fluid and tissue has been demonstrated with many antimicrobial agents, including tobramycin, tetracyclines, macrolides, fluoroquinolones, sulfonamides, and nitrofurantoin. The diagnosis and therapy of prostatitis remains a challenge. Because prostatitis usually requires prolonged therapy, patients must understand the importance of compliance, and physicians should screen for drug interactions that may decrease compliance and efficacy.

Acute bacterial prostatitis is the least common of the prostate infections and, usually, is accompanied by a urinary tract infection with positive cultures. The symptoms include sudden onset of fever, chills, and low back pain, as well as complaints of urinary obstruction (e.g., dysuria, nocturia, urgency, frequency, and burning) and urinary irritation (e.g., hesitancy, straining, dribbling, weak stream, and incomplete emptying). The most commonly prescribed antimicrobials for acute bacterial prostatitis are trimethoprim–sulfamethoxazole, doxycycline, and the fluoroquinolones, ciprofloxacin, ofloxacin, and norfloxacin (see Chapter 33). The concentrations of these antimicrobial agents in the prostatic fluid are two to three times that in plasma, thus achieving adequate concentrations in prostatic tissues to eradicate the most common causative pathogens. The recommended duration of treatment for acute bacterial prostatitis is 4 to 6 weeks. A short-course therapy is not recommended because of the risk of relapse or progression to chronic bacterial prostatitis.

Chronic bacterial prostatitis occurs when acute bacterial prostatitis has been inadequately treated because of pathogen resistance, relapse, or short-course therapy or because of blocked drainage of secretions from the prostate. Most men with chronic prostatitis will have had a previous bout of acute prostatitis. The most common clinical feature of chronic prostatitis is recurrent urinary tract infections and the symptoms and complaints of acute bacterial prostatitis. Fluoroquinolones, trimethoprim–sulfamethoxazole, doxycycline, and nitrofurantoin are used in the management of chronic prostatitis. Chronic prostatitis warrants at least 10 to 12 weeks of therapy. Poor clinical outcomes, however, have been observed because of poor diffusion of antimicrobials into the prostate.

Nonbacterial prostatitis is the most common type of prostatitis. It occurs more frequently than bacterial prostatitis, with the same signs and symptoms as bacterial prostatitis except that prostatic fluid cultures are negative for presence of bacteria. Inflammation is evident on prostate gland examination. Treatment includes minocycline, doxycycline, or erythromycin. Treatment duration is approximately 2 to 4 weeks.

DRUGS USED FOR ERECTILE DYSFUNCTION

Phosphodiesterase Inhibitors

The currently available first- and second-generation oral PDE5 inhibitors, sildenafil, tadalafil, and vardenafil, have emerged as the first-line treatment for ED because of patient convenience, safety, and clinical efficacy and have markedly improved the quality of life in men with ED of various etiologies. As defined by the National Institutes of Health Consensus Development Panel on Impotence in 1993, ED is the inability to achieve or maintain an erection sufficient for satisfactory sexual performance. It is estimated that 10 to 30 million men in the United States, and more than 100 million men worldwide, experience some form of ED. This condition is strongly associated with age, and according to the community-based Massachusetts Male Aging Study, the prevalence of ED in men between 40 and 70 years of age is 52%. The general classification of ED includes psychogenic ED (e.g., depression, psychological stress, relationship problems, and performance anxiety), organic ED (e.g., diabetes, hypertension, spinal cord injuries, and some medications), and mixed psychogenic and organic ED.

Treatment options for men with ED have changed significantly over the past three decades and have progressed from psychosexual therapy and penile prostheses (1970s) through revascularization, vacuum constriction devices, and intracavernosal injection therapy (1980s) to transurethral and oral drug delivery (1990s). The introduction of the first PDE5 inhibitor, sildenafil citrate (Viagra), in 1998 revolutionized the treatment of men with ED of a broad-spectrum of etiologies and acknowledged the need for pharmacologic agents in the treatment of ED (152). With the recognition of the prevalence of ED by the public and the effectiveness of agents like sildenafil, there was an increased effort in the search for new agents with fewer side effects that led to the development of the second-generation PDE5 inhibitors, vardenafil and tadalafil, which have since been introduced into the world market at differing potencies and pharmacokinetics.

Mechanism of Action

The physiologic mechanism to achieve penile erection is mediated via an NO/cyclic guanosine monophosphate (cGMP) pathway. During sexual stimulation, parasympathetic neurons and vascular endothelial cells release NO, which activates soluble guanylate cyclase, thereby increasing the level of cGMP in the corpus cavernosum and relaxation (vasodilation) of vascular smooth muscle. PDE5 is a cGMP-specific hydrolyzing enzyme and is present at high concentrations in the smooth muscle of the penile corpus cavernosum (153,154). One of the more effective methods for elevating cGMP levels in this tissue is to use PDE5 inhibitors. Other PDE isoenzymes also found in the human cavernous smooth muscle include PDE3 (cGMP-inhibited PDE) and PDE4 (cAMP-specific PDE). Thus, inhibitors of PDE, especially PDE5, have been shown to be an effective means for treating ED by enhancing and maintaining erections during sexual stimulation through sustaining sufficient cellular levels of cGMP in both the corpus cavernosum and the blood vessels supplying it. The increased vasodilation of the corporeal sinusoids allows more blood flow into the penis, thereby enhancing an erection.

Structure–Activity Relationships

The chemical similarities and distinct differences between sildenafil, vardenafil, and tadalafil regarding their selectivity for the inhibition of PDE5 and other PDE isoforms and their pharmacokinetic disparities largely affect the efficacy profile of these compounds. The obvious difference for the three drugs is the heterocyclic ring systems used to mimic the purine ring of cGMP. Although the heterocyclic ring systems and the *N*-substituent (ethyl vs. methyl) attached to the piperazine side chain (Fig. 40.20) are the only two structural

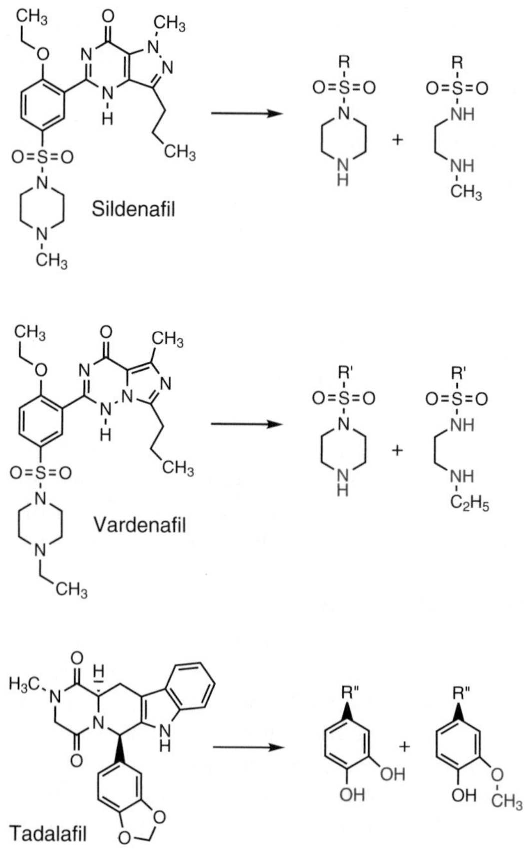

FIGURE 40.20 Phosphodiesterase 5 inhibitors for erectile dysfunction and their primary metabolites.

differences between sildenafil and vardenafil, these differences do not explain why vardenafil has a more than 20 times greater potency than sildenafil for inhibiting PDE5. A structure–activity relationship analysis for the difference in potency between sildenafil and vardenafil revealed that the methyl/ethyl group on the piperazine moiety plays very little role in the potency difference for inhibiting PDE5, whereas the differences in the heterocyclic ring systems play a critical role in higher potency for vardenafil (155).

A comparison of the in vitro inhibition values (IC_{50}) reveals that vardenafil is approximately 10 times more selective as an inhibitor of PDE5 than sildenafil and tadalafil (Table 40.6) (155). Furthermore, vardenafil also was approximately four times more selective than sildenafil for the inhibition of PDE1 and PDE6, as shown by its IC_{50} selectivity ratios: a PDE5/PDE1 ratio of 257 for vardenafil and 60 for sildenafil, and a PDE5/PDE6 ratio of 16 for vardenafil and 7.4 for sildenafil (Table 40.6). The low PDE5/PDE6 selectivity ratio suggests that at therapeutic doses, sildenafil is only approximately 10 times as potent for PDE5 as for PDE6, which is a retinal enzyme found in the photoreceptors of the human retina. This lower PDE5/PDE6 selectivity ratio toward PDE6 for sildenafil indicates it is more likely to inhibit PDE6, which is presumed to be the cause for color vision abnormalities observed with high doses or plasma levels of sildenafil.

Pharmacokinetics

Sildenafil, vardenafil, and tadalafil have only limited oral bioavailability because of extensive presystemic metabolism in the intestine and hepatic first-pass metabolism via the CYP3A isoform family (Table 40.6) (156). The three drugs are rapidly absorbed after oral administration and reach peak plasma concentrations within 30 to 60 minutes. Rapid absorption and lipophilicity are considered to be a prerequisite for their rapid onset of efficacy and sexual satisfaction. Sildenafil and vardenafil are both rapidly absorbed, but with a significant difference in their mean bioavailability of approximately 15% for vardenafil and 40% for sildenafil. The administration of a high-fat meal had no significant effect on the rate and extent of absorption of tadalafil but did decrease the

TABLE 40.6 Some Properties and Pharmacokinetics of the Phosphodiesterase 5 Inhibitors

Drugs	Sildenafil	Vardenafil	Tadalafil
Trade Name	Viagra	Levitra	Cialis
cLogP[a]	2.3 ± 0.7	3.0 ± 0.7	1.4 ± 0.8
logD (pH 7)	2.2	3.0	1.4
Oral bioavailability (%)	38–40	15 (8–25)	~36
Onset of action (hours)	<0.5	<1	0.5–1
Duration of action (hours)	<4	<1	<36
Protein binding (%)	96	94	94
Time to peak concentration (hours)	0.5–2	0.5–3	0.5–6
Volume of distribution (L/kg)	105	208	63
Peak plasma concentration (nmol/L)	1–2	0.03	0.84
Elimination half-life (hours)	3–5	4–5	18
Cytochrome isoforms	3A4 (major)	3A4 (major)	3A4 (primary)
	2C9 (minor)	2C9 (minor)	
Active metabolites	*N*-desmethyl	*N*-desethyl	None
Excretion (%)	~80 feces/met	>90 feces/met	~60 feces/met
	~13 urine/met	<10 urine/met	~35 urine/met
PDE5 IC_{50} (nmol/L)	3.9 (3–7)	0.16 (0.09–0.7)	1.8 (0.9–5)
PDE5/PDE6 IC_{50}	7.4	16	85
PDE5/PDE1 IC_{50}	60	257	—

[a]Chemical Abstracts, American Chemical Society, calculated using Advanced Chemistry Development (ACD/Labs) Software V8.14 for Solaris (1994–2006 ACD/Labs).
IC_{50}, median inhibitory concentration; met, metabolite; PDE, phosphodiesterase.

rate of absorption for sildenafil and vardenafil, which is consistent with their calculated lipophilicity (Table 40.6). It remains unclear whether food has any effect on their absorption and therapeutic efficacy. They are all highly protein bound, with free plasma concentration fractions of only 4% to 6%. Although the bioavailability for tadalafil has not been reported, pharmacokinetic studies and its long duration of action suggest that it is predominately metabolized by hepatic CYP3A4 to catechol metabolites, with minimal presystemic metabolism.

The major route of elimination for the three PDE5 inhibitors is hepatic metabolism, with renal excretion of unmetabolized drug accounting for 1% or less of the elimination pathways (Fig. 40.20) (156). CYP3A is the major drug-metabolizing enzymes for the three PDE5 inhibitors. CYP2C9, CYP2C19, and CYP2D6, however, also contribute to the metabolism of sildenafil, and CYP2C9 contributes to the metabolism of vardenafil. Both sildenafil and vardenafil have active metabolites that reach plasma concentrations high enough to contribute to the overall efficacy and safety profile of their parent-drug molecules. Grapefruit juice increases the bioavailability of sildenafil and vardenafil as well as delays their absorption. The pharmacokinetics of sildenafil and vardenafil may become less predictable in patients who also drink grapefruit juice. Although patients usually will not be endangered by concomitant use of grapefruit juice, it seems advisable to avoid this combination, which can cause systemic vasodilatation.

The larger differences in their volumes of distribution, together with the substantial differences in their systemic clearance, result in distinct differences in their elimination half-lives: 3 to 5 hours for sildenafil and vardenafil, compared with approximately 18 hours for tadalafil.

Hepatic CYP3A and CYP2C activity has been described as being age-dependent, with reduced activity being exhibited in elderly compared to young individuals. This decrease in metabolic activity is reflected by a corresponding increase in plasma concentrations of all three PDE5 inhibitors, warranting dose reductions for sildenafil and vardenafil in elderly patients. Similarly, ethnicity-dependent differences in the pharmacokinetics of all three PDE5 inhibitors may be expected based on known ethnic differences in CYP3A4/5 activity. Gender differences in pharmacokinetics have not been described for any of the three PDE5 inhibitors, which seems to be in agreement with the literature. Severe renal impairment resulted in an increase in plasma concentrations for all the drugs, and this warrants dose reductions for sildenafil and tadalafil in the affected patient population.

Drug Interactions

None of the three PDE5 inhibitors have been identified as CYP inhibitors, including CYP3A or CYP2C substrates. Because metabolism via CYP3A is the major elimination pathway for all three drugs (sildenafil, vardenafil, and tadalafil), all inducers and inhibitors of CYP3A activity have the potential to interfere with the elimination of these drugs. This interaction potential has been verified clinically for inducers of CYP3A activity only for rifampicin and tadalafil (156). The strong inhibitors of CYP3A4 (ritonavir, indinavir, saquinavir, erythromycin, and ketoconazole) increased the plasma levels for sildenafil, vardenafil, and tadalafil. Grapefruit juice, a selective inhibitor of CYP3A intestinal metabolism, also increased the plasma concentrations of sildenafil and vardenafil but not of tadalafil. Ritonavir, as an inhibitor of CYP3A4 and CYP2C9, increased the plasma levels for vardenafil by 50 to 300 times, most likely as a consequence of the simultaneous inhibition of both CYP3A4 and CYP2C9, the major metabolism pathways for vardenafil. The effect of ritonavir on sildenafil was much less pronounced (11 times), because other compensatory CYP-mediated metabolism pathways were still available. Ritonavir increased the plasma levels for tadalafil (CYP3A4) by approximately three times.

Adverse Effects

A number of side effects have been reported with these drugs, including nausea, indigestion, cutaneous flushing, headache, and retinal effects, including a bluish haze and increased light sensitivity. It has been suggested that some of these side effects result from the inhibition of other PDEs, including the isoform PDE6 (156,157). The search is on for even more selective ED agents to see if additional side effects can be eliminated. If one is taking α-adrenergic blockers for high blood pressure, one should consult a physician before using the agents together (156). Other vasodilators associated with regulating the intracellular levels of cGMP, such as nitroglycerin, should not be used in combination with the PDE5 inhibitors.

Therapeutic Effects

The first line of treatment of ED is PDE5 inhibition, because the three drugs can be given orally. If the PDE5 inhibitors are not effective, then the cause may be low libido, and men should have their testosterone blood levels checked (in some instances, TRT may help to resolve ED). Other alternative drugs currently available for the treatment of ED include prostaglandin E_1, which is given by injection at the base of the penis or by suppository into the tip of the penis, as well as the α_1-adrenergic blocker and the nonselective PDE inhibitor papaverine. Apomorphine is a dopamine agonist that can be used for treating ED but, in humans, has the undesirable emetic side effect. Some selective dopamine D_4 agents are now being investigated for treatment of ED. Vacuum devices and penile implants are also available.

Specific Drugs for Erectile Dysfunction

Sildenafil In 1998, sildenafil was the first selective PDE inhibitor to be approved and found to be effective in treating ED (152). Sildenafil has approximately one-tenth the selectivity for PDE5 as for PDE6, which is found in the photoreceptors of the human retina. In vitro metabolism studies for sildenafil have shown that the primary metabolite, *N*-desmethylsildenafil, and the minor metabolite, oxidative opening of the piperazine ring, are mediated by CYP3A4, CYP2C9, CYP2C19, and CYP2D6 (Fig. 40.20). The estimated relative contributions to clearance were 79% for CYP3A4, 20% for CYP2C9, and less than 2% for CYP2C19 and CYP2D6. These results demonstrate that CYP3A4 is the primary cytochrome mediating *N*-demethylation and that drugs inhibiting CYP3A4 likely impair sildenafil biotransformation and clearance. The pharmacokinetics of radiolabeled sildenafil were consistent with rapid absorption, first-pass metabolism, and primarily fecal elimination of *N*-demethylated metabolites. The absorption of sildenafil following oral administration was rapid (~92%), whereas the oral bioavailability was approximately 38% as a result of first-pass metabolism.

Vardenafil Vardenafil was the second agent to be marketed and had the advantage that its onset time was not reduced by taking the medication on a full stomach (Table 40.6) (156,158). It is 30 times more potent as an inhibitor of PDE5 (mean IC_{50} = 3.9 nmol/L) than sildenafil and 10 times more potent than tadalafil, with a greater selectivity (>1,000 times) for human PDE5 than for human PDE2, PDE3, and PDE4 and moderate selectivity (>80 times) for PDE1 (155,159) (Table 40.6). Vardenafil specifically inhibited the hydrolysis of cGMP by PDE5, with an IC_{50} of 0.7 nmol/L (sildenafil, 6.6 nmol/L). The IC_{50} of vardenafil for PDE1 was 180 nmol/L, for PDE6 11 nmol/L, and for PDE2, PDE3, and PDE4 more than 1,000 nmol/L.

Tadalafil Tadalafil was the latest agent to be released and can be taken on a full stomach without slowing the onset (Table 40.6) (156). It has a much longer duration of action, lasting up to 48 hours, compared with sildenafil and vardenafil, which last for approximately 4 hours. The longer half-life of tadalafil results in a lengthened period of responsiveness as compared to sildenafil and vardenafil. This longer therapeutic window requires fewer time constraints for the effectiveness of tadalafil and has been interpreted as being advantageous through providing the option for more spontaneous sexual activity. Because of its long half-life, however, tadalafil has been detected in plasma even 5 days after oral administration. This suggests the possibility of accumulation if taken regularly and in short intervals, which may result in an increased risk of side effects with the excessive use of this PDE5 inhibitor. The 3,4-methylenedioxy substitution on the phenyl ring was significant for increasing its potency as a PDE5 inhibitor. Optimization of the chain on the piperazinedione ring resulted in no significant change in IC_{50}. Tadalafil is a highly potent PDE5 inhibitor (IC_{50} = 5 nmol/L), with high selectivity for PDE5 versus PDE1 through PDE4 (160). The PDE5/PDE6 selectivity ratio is 85.

Prostaglandin E_1 Prostaglandin E_1 (PGE_1; Alprostadil) is approved for the intracavernosal (Caverject, Edex) or intraurethral suppository (Muse) treatment of ED. A three-drug combination of PGE_1, papaverine, and phentolamine sometimes is used as an intracavernosal injection to achieve a synergistic action. ED that is medication-induced or caused by endocrine problems, such as hypogonadism or hyper- or hypothyroidism, should be evaluated and appropriately treated before PGE_1 treatment is considered. PGE_1 is produced endogenously to relax vascular smooth muscle and cause vasodilation by activating the adenylate cyclase/cAMP pathway. Recent studies show that cAMP is important in the PGE_1 relaxation of penile erectile tissue and vasodilation of penile resistance arteries (161). Moreover, agents that stimulate the release of cAMP also cross-activate the NO/cGMP cascade.

When administered by intracavernosal injection or as an intraurethral suppository, PGE_1 acts locally to relax the smooth muscle of the corpora cavernosa and the cavernosal arteries. Swelling, elongation, and rigidity of the penis result when arterial blood rapidly flows into the corpus cavernosum to expand the lacunar spaces. The entrapped blood reduces the venous blood outflow as sinusoids compress against the tunica albuginea. Adding papaverine and phentolamine to the PGE_1 regimen synergistically increases arterial blood flow via separate mechanisms. Papaverine relaxes the sinusoid and the smooth muscle of the helicine arteries, whereas phentolamine relaxes arterial smooth muscle and blocks both of the α-adrenergic receptors that inhibit an erection. PGE_1 is rapidly metabolized within the urethra, prostate, and corpus cavernosum to 7α-hydroxy-5,11-diketotetranorprosta-1,16-dioic acid and 5α,7α-dihydroxy-11-ketotetranor-prostane-1,16-dioic acid (162). The major route of excretion of PGE_1 metabolites is via the kidney. Its elimination half-life is 5 to 10 minutes. If any alprostadil is systemically absorbed, it is metabolized by a single pass through the lungs. The onset of action is within 10 minutes, and the time to peak effect is less than 20 minutes. The duration of action is 1 to 3 hours for the intracavernosal injection and 30 to 60 minutes for the intraurethral suppository.

Papaverine (Intracavernosal) Papaverine is used, sometimes in combination with phentolamine, by intracavernosal injection to facilitate erections in men with ED. In general, papaverine is most useful in patients with organic ED (neurogenic and, to a lesser extent, vascular). It is less useful in patients with ED resulting from endocrine problems (hypogonadism or hyper- or hypothyroidism) or medications. When administered by intracavernosal injection, papaverine, a weak and nonspecific PDE inhibitor, is thought to cause relaxation of the cavernous smooth muscles and vasodilation of the penile arteries by inhibition of PDE (163). These effects result in increased arterial blood flow into the corpus cavernosa and in swelling and elongation of the penis. Venous outflow also is reduced, possibly as a result of increased venous resistance. Adding phentolamine and PGE_1 to the papaverine regimen synergistically increases arterial blood flow via their separate mechanisms. Papaverine is slowly released into the venous circulation with minimal systemic effects. The time to peak effect usually is within 10 minutes, and the duration of action is 1 to 6 hours with concurrent administration with phentolamine.

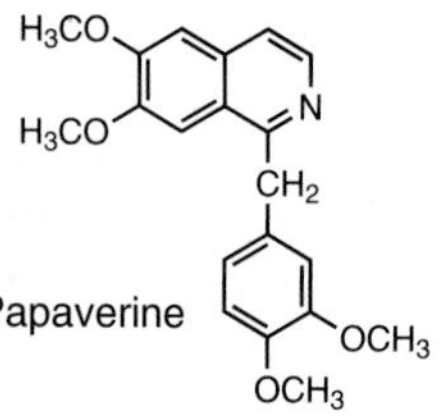

Papaverine

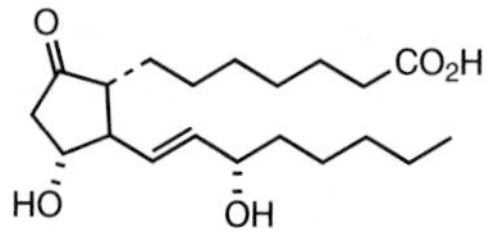

PGE_1

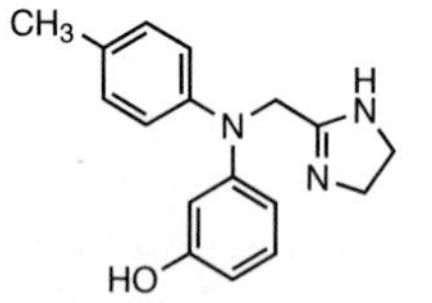

Phentolamine

Phentolamine (Intracavernosal; Rogitine)

Phentolamine is used in combination with papaverine, by intracavernosal injection, to facilitate erections in men with impotence (see *Papaverine* above). Its mechanism of action is as an α-adrenergic antagonist (see Chapter 10) of both α_1- and α_2-receptors, causing vasodilation and reduction in peripheral resistance. When administered by intracavernosal injection, it is thought to cause relaxation of the cavernous smooth muscles and vasodilation of the penile arteries. This results in increased arterial blood flow into the corpus cavernosa as well as swelling and elongation of the penis. Venous outflow also is reduced, possibly as a result of increased venous resistance. Phentolamine is slowly released into venous circulation with minimal, if any, systemic effects. Time to peak effect is within 10 minutes, and duration of action when used with papaverine is 1 to 6 hours.

TESTICULAR CANCER

Testicular cancer develops in the testicles and, according to the National Cancer Institute (NCI), accounts only for approximately 1% of all cancers in men. Compared with prostate cancer, testicular cancer is relatively rare. It is most common among males between 15 and 40 years of age and is approximately fourfold more common in white men than in black men.

Nearly all testicular tumors originate from germ cells, the specialized sperm-forming cells within the testicles. These tumors fall into one of two types, seminomas or nonseminomas (164). Seminomas account for approximately 40% of all testicular cancer and are made up of immature germ cells. Seminomas are slow-growing and tend to stay localized in the testicle for long periods. Nonseminomas arise from more mature, specialized germ cells and tend to be more aggressive than seminomas. According to the American Cancer Society, 60% to 70% of patients with nonseminomas have cancer that has spread to the lymph nodes. α-Fetoprotein is a tumor-associated marker in blood for testicular cancer. Its measurement can help to show how well the chemotherapeutic drugs are working. Because seminomas are slow-growing, they tend to stay localized and usually are diagnosed at stage I (confined to testicle) or stage II (spread to lymph nodes). Treatment might be a combination of testicle removal, radiation, or chemotherapy. Most nonseminomas are not diagnosed at stage I. Advanced testicular cancer (stage III, metastasized to other tissues) seminomas, as well as stage II and stage III nonseminomas, usually are treated with multidrug chemotherapy. The majority of cases are stage I when first identified; stage III cases are relatively rare.

Chemotherapy is the standard treatment, with or without radiation, when the cancer has spread to other parts of the body. The drugs approved to treat testicular cancer include ifosfamide, etoposide, vinblastine, bleomycin, and cisplatin (Chapter 37). Cisplatin usually is given in combination with bleomycin and etoposide or other chemotherapy drugs following surgery or radiation therapy. Testicular cancer has one of the highest cure rates of all cancers, essentially 100% at stage I. Approximately 90% of men with advanced testicular cancer can be cured, according to the NCI. Because testicular cancer is curable when detected early, the NCI recommends regular monthly testicular self-examination after a hot shower, when the scrotum is looser, feeling for lumps or enlargement.

MALE OSTEOPOROSIS

Osteoporosis is a common condition in men that usually develops after the age of 70 years and affects approximately 2 million men in the United States (165). Osteoporosis occurs less frequently in men because of greater skeletal bone mass during growth (i.e., greater bone size). Approximately 20% to 25% of all hip fractures occur in men, however, and the age-adjusted prevalence of vertebral deformities appears to be similar in men and in women. Currently, bisphosphonates (alendronate and risedronate) (see Chapter 30) are the therapy of choice for increasing bone mineral density to decrease the risk of fracture in the treatment of male osteoporosis, and a short course of parathyroid hormone (1-34; teriparatide) may be indicated for men with very low bone mineral density or for those in whom bisphosphonate therapy is unsuccessful. Antiandrogen therapy for the treatment of prostate cancer, hypogonadism, and diabetes are some of the risk factors for osteoporosis and fracture. Vitamin D and calcium have been shown to help improve bone mineral density. Testosterone replacement therapy is controversial except in men who clearly have hypogonadism and low levels of testosterone; in those men, treatment with testosterone appears to increase bone density.

SCENARIO: OUTCOME AND ANALYSIS

Outcome

Autumn Stewart, PharmD

NP presents 2 weeks later complaining of sexual dysfunction. Symptoms related to benign prostatic hypertrophy remain controlled and the nail infection appears to be improving. The patient's physician is consulted and a change is made from dutasteride to finasteride 5.0 mg QD. The patient follows up 2 weeks later and reports that adverse effects related to sexual function have resolved and no new problems have arisen.

Chemical Analysis

S. William Zito and Victoria Roche

NP has experienced sexual dysfunction after being treated with itraconazole for onychomycosis due to a drug-drug interaction with dutasteride, used here to treat benign prostatic hypertrophy. Itraconazole is an inhibitor of CYP3A4, and because dutasteride is metabolized by CYP3A4, inhibiting its metabolism leads to increased plasma levels and sexual dysfunction (SD). The sexual dysfunction side effect of dutasteride is most likely associated with the progestin activity of this analog. Dutasteride is a selective inhibitor of both type 1 and type 2 isoforms of 5 α-reductase, which blocks conversion of testosterone to dihydrotestosterone (DHT). DHT is an androgen primarily responsible for the growth and enlargement of the prostate gland. Switching NP to finasteride results in moderating the sexual dysfunction side effects, presumably because of a much lower incidence of SD (4.7% vs. 1.8%).

Dutasteride is a 4-azasteroid progestin analog related to medrogesterone (6-methyl-6-dehydro-17-methylprogesterone). Specifically it is a 17β-bis(trifluoromethyl) azaandrostene-carboxamide. Its mechanism of action involves binding to the NADPH cofactor of 5 α-reductase and forming a complex that is slowly released from the enzyme resulting in essentially irreversible inhibition. The key reaction is between the Δ-1 double bond of dutasteride and NADPH.

Finasteride also is a 4-azasteroid progestin analog related to medrogesterone. It differs from dutasteride only in being a 17β-1,1-dimethylethyl carboxamide. Though dutasteride inhibits both isoforms of 5 α-reductase, finasteride inhibits only the type II isozyme, which is primarily found in the prostate, seminal vesicles, epididymides, and hair follicles, as well as the liver. The type I isozyme is responsible for one third of the circulating DHT, whereas type II isozyme is responsible for two thirds. Finasteride has the same mechanism of action as dutasteride but a lower incidence of sexual dysfunction side effects.

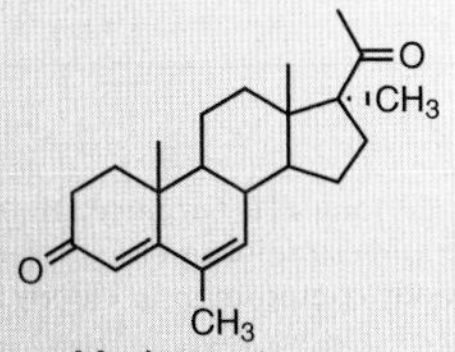

Medrogesterone

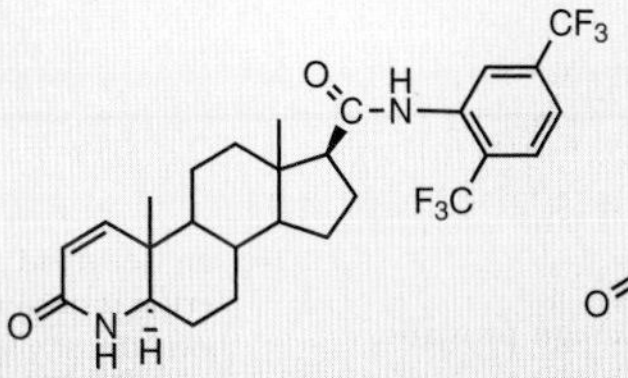

Dutasteride

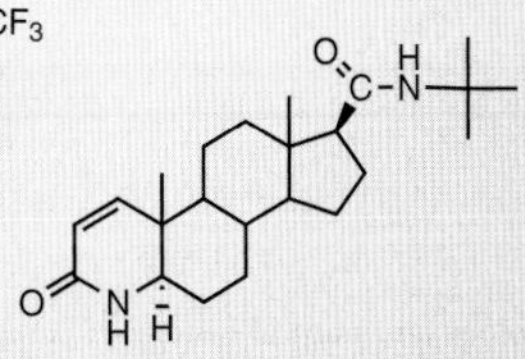

Finasteride

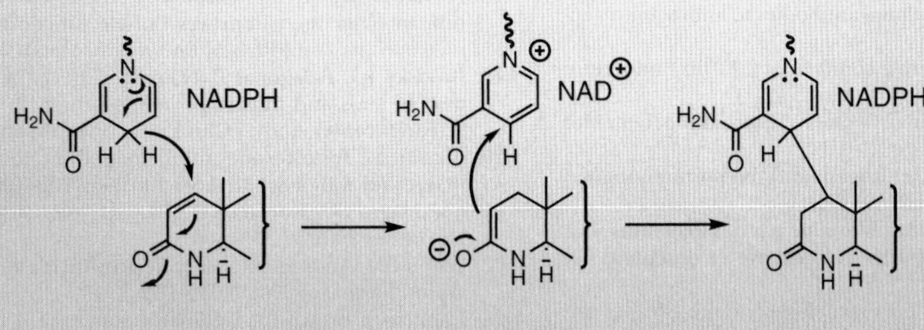

Dutasteride Dutasteride Dutasteride-NADPH Complex

CASE STUDY

S. William Zito and Victoria Roche

BJ is a 62-year-old man. He has had chronic stable angina (CSA) for the past 3 years, which is under control with isosorbide mononitrate CR (60 mg daily). BJ reports that although he carries around sublingual nitroglycerine for acute attacks, he hasn't ever had to use it. His medical history includes type 2 diabetes mellitus since he was 45 years old, which he controls with diet and metformin (850 mg/day). He appears today at your ambulatory care clinic to speak to his primary care physician. He explains that he feels great and has become active again. He now plays tennis three times a week and swims most mornings at the local pool with his wife. He is really enjoying life but has not had an erection for the last 12 months and wants to continue to have a healthy sexual relationship with his wife. Physical examination shows a blood pressure of 125/80 mm Hg and his electrocardiogram is normal. Laboratory tests show the following values: fasting blood glucose, 90 mg/dL; glycosylated hemoglobin, 6.0%; creatinine, 1.1 mg/dL; total cholesterol, 160; LDL, 120; HDL, 45; and triglycerides, 119 mg/dL. BJ was examined by his physician, who measured the blood flow through his penis using an echo Doppler. It was found to be below the normal range. In addition, a biothesiometry study was conducted to see if there was any nerve deterioration due to his diabetes, and the results were negative. Evaluate the following three drug choices for use in this case.

1. Conduct a thorough and mechanistic SAR analysis of the three therapeutic options in the case.
2. Apply the chemical understanding gained from the SAR analysis to this patient's specific needs to make a therapeutic recommendation.

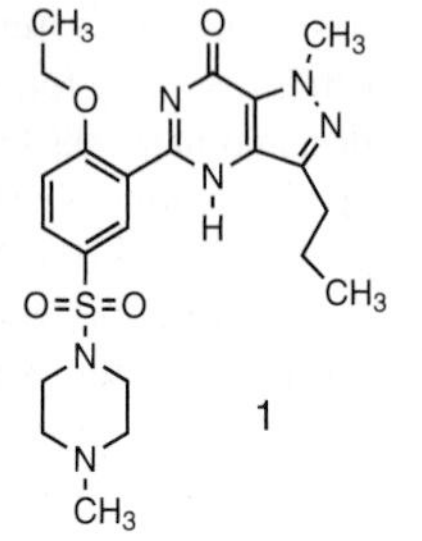
1

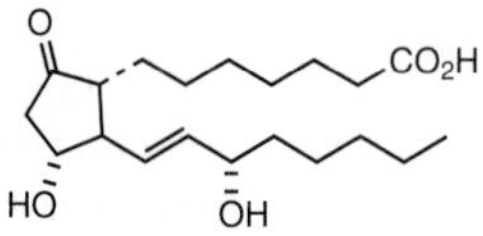
2

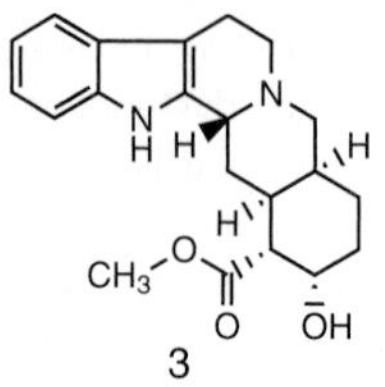
3

References

1. Bushman W. Etiology, epidemiology and natural history of benign prostatic hyperplasia. Urol Clin North Am 2009;36:403–415.
2. Mooradian AD, Morley JE, Korenman SG. Biological actions of androgens. Endocr Rev 1987;8:1–28.
3. Takeda H, Chodak G, Mutchnik S, et al. Immunohistochemical localization of androgen receptors with mono- and polyclonal antibodies to androgen receptor. J Endocrinol 1990;126:17–25.
4. Davis S. Androgen replacement in women: a commentary. J Clin Endocrinol Metab 1999;84:1886–1891.
5. Davis SR. The therapeutic use of androgens in women. J Steroid Biochem Mol Biol 1999;69:177–184.
6. Davis SR, Burger HG. Clinical review 82: androgens and the postmenopausal woman. J Clin Endocrinol Metab 1996;81:2759–2763.
7. Brown-Sequard CE. Des effects produits chez Phomme par des injections sous cutanées d'un liquide retire des testicules frais de cobaye et de chien. CR Seanc Soc Biol 1889;1:420–430.
8. Pezard A. Sur la determination des caractéres sexuels secondaire chez les gallinacés. C R H Acad Sci 1911;153:1027–1034.
9. Butenandt A. Chemical investigation of the sex hormones. Angew Chem 1931;44:905–908.
10. Butenandt AH, Dannenberg H. Androsterone, a crystalline male sex hormone. III. Isolation of a new physiologically inert sterol derivative from male urine, its relationship to dehydroandrosterone and androsterone. Z Physiol Chem 1934;229:192–208.
11. David K, Dingemanse E, Freud J, et al. Crystalline male hormone from testes (testosterone), more active than androsterone prepared from urine or cholesterol. Z Physiol Chem 1935:281–282.
12. Butenandt A, Hanisch G. Testosterone. Transformation of dehydroandrosterone into androstenediol and testosterone; a way to the preparation of testosterone from cholestrol. Chem Ber 1935;68B:1859–1862.
13. Kochakian CD, Murlin JR. Effect of male hormone on the protein and energy metabolism of castrate dogs. J Nutr 1935;10:437–459.
14. Kock FC. The chemistry and biology of the male sex hormones. Bull N Y Acad Med 1938;14:655–680.
15. Bremner WJ, Vitiello MV, Prinz N. Loss of circadian rhythmicity in blood testosterone levels with aging in normal men. J Clin Endocrinol Metab 1983;56:1278–1281.
16. van den Beld AW, de Jong FH, Grobbee DE, et al. Measures of bioavailable serum testosterone and estradiol and their relationships with muscle strength, bone density and body composition in elderly men. J Clin Endocrinol Metab 2000;85:3276–3282.
17. Vale W, Wiater E, Gray P, et al. Activins and inhibins and their signaling. Ann N Y Acad Sci 2004;1038:142–147.
18. Ferrando AA, Sheffield-Moore M, Yeckel CW, et al. Testosterone administration to older men improves muscle function: molecular and physiological mechanisms. Am J Physiol Endocrinol Metab 2002;282:E601–E607.
19. Brodsky IG, Balagopal P, Nair KS. Effects of testosterone replacement on muscle mass and muscle protein synthesis in hypogonadal men—a clinical research center study. J Clin Endocrinol Metab 1996;81:3469–3475.
20. Bhasin S. Testosterone supplementation for aging-associated sarcopenia. J Gerontol A Biol Sci Med Sci 2003;58:1002–1008.
21. Manolagas SC, Kousteni S, Jilka RL. Sex steroids and bone. Recent Prog Horm Res 2002;57:385–409.
22. Wiren KM. Androgens and bone growth: it's location, location, location. Curr Opin Pharmacol 2005;5:626–632.
23. Fishman J, Brown JB, Hellman Leon, et al. Estrogen metabolism in normal and pregnant women. J Biol Chem 1962;237:1489–1494.
24. Gurpide E, Angers M, Vande Wiele RL, et al. Determination of secretory rates of estrogens in pregnant and nonpregnant women from the specific activities of urinary metabolites. J Clin Endocrinol Metab 1962;22:935–945.
25. Simpson ER, Merrill JC, Hollub AJ, et al. Regulation of estrogen biosynthesis by human adipose cells. Endocr Rev 1989;10:136–148.
26. Nakajin S, Hall PF. Microsomal cytochrome P-450 from neonatal pig testis. Purification and properties of a C-21 steroid side-chain cleavage system (17α-hydroxylase-C17,20-lyase). J Biol Chem 1981;256:3871–3876.
27. Baulieu EE, Wallace W, Lieberman S. The conversion in vitro of Δ^5-androstene-3β,17β-diol-17α-H3 to testosterone-17α-H3 by human adrenal and placental tissue. J Biol Chem 1963;238:1316–1319.
28. Rosner JM, Horita S, Forsham PH. Androstenediol, a probable intermediate in the in vitro conversion of dehydroepiandrosterone to testosterone by the rabbit testis. Endocrinology 1964;75:299–303.
29. Brodie A. Aromatase inhibitors: introduction and perspective. J Enzyme Inhib 1990;42:75–77.
30. Brueggemeier RW, Hackett JC, Diaz-Cruz ES. Aromatase inhibitors in the treatment of breast cancer. Endocr Rev 2005;26:331–345.

31. Miller WR, Anderson TJ, Evans DB, et al. An integrated view of aromatase and its inhibition. J Steroid Biochem Mol Biol 2003;86:413–421.
32. Osborne CK, Schiff R. Aromatase inhibitors: future directions. J Steroid Biochem Mol Biol 2005;95:183–187.
33. Thompson EA Jr, Siiteri PK. The involvement of human placental microsomal cytochrome P-450 in aromatization. J Biol Chem 1974;249:5373–5378.
34. Bruchovsky N, Wilson JD. The conversion of testosterone to 5-α-androstan-17-β-ol-3-one by rat prostate in vivo and in vitro. J Biol Chem 1968;243:2012–2021.
35. Ofner P. Effects and metabolism of hormones in normal and neoplastic prostate tissue. Vitam Horm 1968;26:237–291.
36. Liao S, Liang T, Fang S, et al. Steroid structure and androgenic activity. Specificities involved in the receptor binding and nuclear retention of various androgens. J Biol Chem 1973;248:6154–6162.
37. Brueggemeir R. Male sex hormones, analogues, and antagonists. In: Burger A, Abraham DJ, eds. Burger's Medicinal Chemistry and Drug Discovery, 6th Ed. Hoboken, NJ: Wiley, 2003.
38. Dorfman RI, Ungar F. Metabolism of Steroid Hormones. 2nd Ed. Academic Press: New York, 1965:716.
39. Thigpen AE, Silver RI, Guileyardo JM, et al. Tissue distribution and ontogeny of steroid 5α-reductase isozyme expression. J Clin Invest 1993;92:903–910.
40. Russel DW, Berman DM, Bryant JT, et al. The molecular genetics of steroid 5α-reductases. Recent Prog Horm Res 1994;49:275–284.
41. Johansen KL. Testosterone metabolism and replacement therapy in patients with end-stage renal disease. Semin Dial 2004;17:202–208.
42. Vermeulen A, Kaufman JM, Goemaere S, et al. Estradiol in elderly men. Aging Male 2002;5:98–102.
43. Fotherby K, James F, Atkinson L, et al. Studies in the aromatization of a synthetic progestin. J Endocrinol 1972;52:v–vi.
44. Belanger A, Pelletier G, Labrie F, et al. Inactivation of androgens by UDP-glucuronosyltransferase enzymes in humans. Trends Endocrinol Metab 2003;14:473–479.
45. Taylor W, Scratcherd T. Steroid metabolism in the rabbit. Biliary and urinary excretion of metabolites of [4-14-C] testosterone. Biochem J 1967;104:250–253.
46. Dorfman RI, Hamilton JB. Urinary excretion of androgenic substances after intramuscular and oral administration of testosterone propionate to humans. J Clin Invest 1939;18:67–71.
47. Gao W, Bohl CE, Dalton JT. Chemistry and structural biology of androgen receptor. Chem Rev 2005;105:3352–3370.
48. Chawnshang C. Androgens and androgen receptor: mechanisms, functions, and clinical applications. Boston: Kluwer Academic Publishers, 2002.
49. Freedman LP. Molecular Biology of Steroid and Nuclear Hormone Receptors. Progress in Gene Expression. Boston: Birkhauser, 1998.
50. Pratt WB, Toft DO. Steroid receptor interactions with heat shock protein and immunophilin chaperones. Endocr Rev 1997;18:306–360.
51. Shang Y, Myers M, Brown M. Formation of the androgen receptor transcription complex. Mol Cell 2002;9:601–610.
52. Claessens F, Verrijdt G, Schoenmakers E, et al. Selective DNA binding by the androgen receptor as a mechanism for hormone-specific gene regulation. J Steroid Biochem Mol Biol 2001;76:23–30.
53. Haelens A, Verrijdt G, Callewaert L, et al. DNA recognition by the androgen receptor: evidence for an alternative DNA-dependent dimerization, and an active role of sequences flanking the response element on transactivation. Biochem J 2003;369(Pt 1):141–151.
54. Shaffer PL, Jivan Arif, Dollins DE, et al. Structural basis of androgen receptor binding to selective androgen response elements. Proc Natl Acad Sci U S A 2004;101:4758–4763.
55. Hsiao PW, Thin TH, Lin DL, et al. Differential regulation of testosterone vs. 5α-dihydrotestosterone by selective androgen response elements. Mol Cell Biochem 2000;206:169–175.
56. Remenyi A, Scholer HR, Wilmanns M. Combinatorial control of gene expression. Nat Struct Mol Biol 2004;11:812–815.
57. Lutz LB, Jamnongjit M, Yang WH, et al. Selective modulation of genomic and nongenomic androgen responses by androgen receptor ligands. Mol Endocrinol 2003;17:1106– 1116.
58. Estrada M, Espinosa A, Mueller M, et al. Testosterone stimulates intracellular calcium release and mitogen-activated protein kinases via a G protein–coupled receptor in skeletal muscle cells. Endocrinology 2003;144:3586–3597.
59. Kousteni S, Bellido T, Plotkin LI, et al. Nongenotropic, sex-nonspecific signaling through the estrogen or androgen receptors: dissociation from transcriptional activity. Cell 2001;104:719–730.
60. Zagar Y, Chaumaz G, Lieberherr M. Signaling cross-talk from Gβ4 subunit to Elk-1 in the rapid action of androgens. J Biol Chem 2004;279:2403–2413.
61. Kampa M, Papakonstanti EA, Hatzoglou A, et al. The human prostate cancer cell line LNCaP bears functional membrane testosterone receptors that increase PSA secretion and modify actin cytoskeleton. FASEB J 2002;16:1429–1431.
62. Unni E, Sun S, Nan B, et al. Changes in androgen receptor nongenotropic signaling correlate with transition of LNCaP cells to androgen independence. Cancer Res 2004;64:7156–7168.
63. Norman AW, Mizwicki MY, Norman DP. Steroid-hormone rapid actions, membrane receptors, and a conformational ensemble model. Nat Rev Drug Discov 2004;3:27–41.
64. Simoncini T, Genazzani AR. Nongenomic actions of sex steroid hormones. Eur J Endocrinol 2003;148:281–292.
65. Kousteni S, Chen J-R, Bellido T, et al. Reversal of bone loss in mice by nongenotropic signaling of sex steroids. Science 2002;298:843–846.
66. Bancroft J, Wu FC. Changes in erectile responsiveness during androgen replacement therapy. Arch Sex Behav 1983;12:59–66.
67. Arver S, Dobs AS, Meikle AW, et al. Improvement of sexual function in testosterone deficient men treated for 1 year with a permeation enhanced testosterone transdermal system. J Urol 1996;155:1604–1608.
68. Oettel M. Testosterone metabolism, dose–response relationships, and receptor polymorphisms: selected pharmacological/toxicological considerations on benefits versus risks of testosterone therapy in men. Aging Male 2003;6:230–256.
69. Hijazi RA, Cunningham GR. Andropause: is androgen replacement therapy indicated for the aging male? Annu Rev Med 2005;56:117–137.
70. Rhoben EL, Morgentaler A. Risks of testosterone replacement therapy and recommendations for monitoring. N Engl J Med 2004;350:482–492.
71. Testosterone therapy in adult men with androgen deficiency syndromes: an Endocrine Society clinical practice guideline. J Clin Endocrinol Metab 2010;95:2536–2559.
72. Basaria S, Coviello AD, Travison TG, et al. Adverse events associated with testosterone administration. N Engl J Med 2010;363:109–122.
73. Shackleford DM, Faassen WA, Houwing N, et al. Contribution of lymphatically transported testosterone undecanoate to the systemic exposure of testosterone after oral administration of two andriol formulations in conscious lymph duct–cannulated dogs. J Pharmacol Exp Ther 2003;306:925–933.
74. Vida JA. Androgens and Anabolic Agents: Chemistry and Pharmacology. New York: Academic Press, 1969.
75. Segaloff A, Gabbard RB. 5α-Androstane—an androgenic hydrocarbon. Endocrinology 1960;67:887–889.
76. Arnold A, Potts GO, Beyler AL. The ratio of anabolic to androgenic activity of (7,17) 17-dimethyltestosterone, oxymesterone, mestanolone, and fluoxymesterone. J Endocrinol 1963;28:87–92.
77. Cocconi G. First generation aromatase inhibitors–aminoglutethimide and testololactone. Breast Cancer Res Treat 1994;30:57–80.
78. Kicman AT. Pharmacology of anabolic steroids. Br J Pharmacol 2008;154:502–521.
79. Catlin DH, Sekera MH, Ahrens BD, et al. Tetrahydrogestrinone: discovery, synthesis, and detection in urine. Rapid Commun Mass Spectrom 2004;18:1245–1249.
80. Jasuja R, Catlin DH, Miller A, et al. Tetrahydrogestrinone is an androgenic steroid that stimulates androgen receptor-mediated, myogenic differentiation in C3H10T1/2 multipotent mesenchymal cells and promotes muscle accretion in orchidectomized male rats. Endocrinology 2005;146:4472–4478.
81. Zhi L, Martinborough E. Selective androgen receptor modulators (SARMs). Ann Rep Med Chem 2001;36:169–180.
82. Negro-Vilar A. Selective androgen receptor modulators (SARMs): a novel approach to androgen therapy for the new millennium. J Clin Endocrinol Metab 1999;84:3459–3462.
83. Dalton JT, Mukherjee A, Zhu Z, et al. Discovery of nonsteroidal androgens. Biochem Biophys Res Commun 1998;244:1–4.
84. Balog A, Salvati ME, Weifang S, et al. The synthesis and evaluation of [2.2.1]-bicycloazahydantoins as androgen receptor antagonists Bioorg Med Chem Lett 2004;14:6107–6111.
85. Higuchi RI, Edwards JP, Caferro TR, et al. 4-Alkyl- and 3,4-dialkyl-1,2,3,4-tetrahydro-8-pyridono[5,6-g]quinolines: potent, nonsteroidal androgen receptor agonists. Bioorg Med Chem Lett 1999;9:1335–1340.
86. Zhi L, Tegley CM, Marschke KB, et al. Switching androgen receptor antagonists to agonists by modifying C-ring substituents on piperidino[3,2-g]quinolinone. Bioorg Med Chem Lett 1999;9:1009–1012.
87. Tucker H, Crook JW, Chesterson GJ. Nonsteroidal antiandrogens. Synthesis and structure–activity relationships of 3-substituted derivatives of 2-hydroxypropionanilides. J Med Chem 1998;31:954–959.
88. Yin D, He Y, Perera MA, et al. Key structural features of nonsteroidal ligands for binding and activation of the androgen receptor. Mol Pharmacol 2003;63:211–223.
89. He Y, Yin D, Perera M, et al. Novel nonsteroidal ligands with high binding affinity and potent functional activity for the androgen receptor. Eur J Med Chem 2002;37:619–634.
90. Kirkovsky L, Mukherjee A, Yin D, et al. Chiral nonsteroidal affinity ligands for the androgen receptor. 1. Bicalutamide analogues bearing electrophilic groups in the B aromatic ring. J Med Chem 2000;43:581–590.
91. Bohl CE, Gao W, Miller DD, et al. Structural basis for antagonism and resistance of bicalutamide in prostate cancer. Proc Natl Acad Sci U S A 2005;102:6201–6206.
92. Mohler ML, Bohl CE, Jones A, et al. Nonsteroidal selective androgen receptor modulators (SARMs): dissociating the anabolic and androgenic activities of the androgen receptor for therapeutic benefit. J Med Chem 2009;52:3597–3617.
93. Tarter TH, Vaughan ED Jr. Inhibitors of 5α-reductase in the treatment of benign prostatic hyperplasia. Curr Pharm Des 2006;12:775–783.
94. Martin DJ. Preclinical pharmacology of α1-adrenoceptor antagonists. Eur Urol 1999;36(Suppl 1):35–41.
95. American Cancer Society. Cancer Facts and Figures 2010. Atlanta, GA: American Cancer Society, 2010.

96. Shibata Y, Ito K, Suzuki K. Changes in the endocrine environment of the human prostate transition zone with aging: simultaneous quantitative analysis of prostatic sex steroids and comparison with human prostatic histological composition. Prostate 2000;42:45–55.
97. Lee M, Sharifi R. Benign prostatic hyperplasia: diagnosis and treatment guideline. Ann Pharmacother 1997;31:481–486.
98. Tan SY, Antonipillai I, Murphy BE. Inhibition of testosterone metabolism in the human prostate. J Clin Endocrinol Metab 1974;39:936–941.
99. Andriole G, Bruchovsky N, Chung LW, et al. Dihydrotestosterone and the prostate: the scientific rationale for 5α-reductase inhibitors in the treatment of benign prostatic hyperplasia. J Urol 2004;172:1399–1403.
100. Liang T, Cascieri MA, Cheung AH, et al. Species differences in prostatic steroid 5α-reductases of rat, dog, and human. Endocrinology 1985;117:571–579.
101. Cavalli A, Lattion AL, Hummler E, et al. Decreased blood pressure in mice deficient of the alpha 1b-adrenergic receptor. Proc Natl Acad Sci USA 1997;94:11589–11594.
102. Amadesi S, Varani K, Spisani L, et al. Comparison of prazosin, terazosin, and tamsulosin: functional and binding studies in isolated prostatic and vascular human tissues. Prostate 2001;47:231–238.
103. Tatemichi S, Tomiyama Y, Maruyama I, et al. Uroselectivity in male dogs of silodosin (KMD-3213), a novel drug for the obstructive component of benign prostatic hyperplasia. Neurourol Urodyn 2006;25:792–799.
104. Foglar R, Shibata K, Horie K, et al. Use of recombinant α_1-adrenoceptors to characterize subtype selectivity of drugs for the treatment of prostatic hypertrophy. Eur J Pharmacol 1995;288:201–207.
105. Michel MC. The forefront for novel therapeutic agents based on the pathophysiology of lower urinary tract dysfunction: alpha-blockers in the treatment of male voiding dysfunction–how do they work and why do they differ in tolerability? J Pharmacol Sci 2010;112:151–157.
106. Peterson CM. Progestogens, progesterone antagonists, progesterone, and androgens: synthesis, classification, and uses. Clin Obstet Gynecol 1995;38:813–820.
107. Rasmusson GH, Reynolds GF, Steinberg NG, et al. Azasteroids: structure–activity relationships for inhibition of 5α-reductase and of androgen receptor binding. J Med Chem 1986;29:2298.
108. McConnell JD, Wilson JD, George FW, et al. Finasteride, an inhibitor of 5α-reductase, suppresses prostatic dihydrotestosterone in men with benign prostatic hyperplasia. J Clin Endocrinol Metab 1992;74:505–508.
109. Djavan R, Milani S, Fong YK. Dutasteride: a novel dual inhibitor of 5α-reductase for benign prostatic hyperplasia. Expert Opin Pharmacother 2005;6:311–317.
110. Vermeulen A, Giagulli VA, De Schepper P, et al. Hormonal effects of an orally active 4-azasteroid inhibitor of 5α-reductase in humans. Prostate 1989;14:45–53.
111. Bull G, Garcia-Calvo M, Andersson, S, et al. Mechanism-based inhibition of human steroid 5α-reductase by finasteride: enzyme-catalyzed formation of NADP-dihydrofinasteride, a potent bisubstrate analogue inhibitor. J Am Chem Soc 1996;118:2359–2365.
112. Darren SJ, Lee FW, Simpson ND, et al. Pharmacokinetic parameters and mechanisms of inhibition of rat type 1 and 2 steroid 5α-reductases: determinants for different in vivo activities of GI198745 and finasteride in the rat. Biochem Pharmacol 2001;62:933–942.
113. Steiner JF. Clinical pharmacokinetics and pharmacodynamics of finasteride. Clin Pharmacokinet 1996;30:16–27.
114. Frye SV. Discovery and clinical development of dutasteride, a potent dual 5α-reductase inhibitor. Curr Top Med Chem 2006;6:405–421.
115. Dolder CR. Dutasteride: a dual 5α-reductase inhibitor for the treatment of symptomatic benign prostatic hyperplasia. Ann Pharmacother 2006;40:658–665.
116. Roehrborn CG, Boyle P, Nickel JC, et al. Efficacy and safety of a dual inhibitor of 5α-reductase types 1 and 2 (dutasteride) in men with benign prostatic hyperplasia. Urology 2002;60:434–441.
117. Buck AC. Is there a scientific basis for the therapeutic effects of *Serenoa repens* in benign prostatic hyperplasia? Mechanisms of action. J Urol 2004;172:1792–1799.
118. Bent S, Kane C, Shinohara K, et al. Saw palmetto for benign prostatic hyperplasia. N Engl J Med 2006;354:557–566.
119. Huggins C, Hodges CV. Studies on prostatic cancer, I: the effect of castration, of estrogen and of androgen injection on serum phosphatases in metastatic carcinoma of the prostate. Cancer Res 1941;1:293–297.
120. Roberts WB, Han M. Clinical significance and treatment of biochemical recurrence after definitive therapy for localized prostate cancer. Surg Oncol 2009;18:268–274.
121. Oesterling JE. LHRH agonists. A nonsurgical treatment for benign prostatic hyperplasia. J Androl 1991;12:381–388.
122. Neumann F, Topert M. Pharmacology of antiandrogens. J Steroid Biochem 1986;25:885–895
123. Martini L, Motta M. Androgens and Antiandrogens. New York: Raven Press, 1977:77–89.
124. Neri RO. Antiandrogens. Adv Sex Horm Res 1976;2:233–262.
125. Yoshioka K, et al. Studies on antiandrogenic agents. Synthesis of 16β-ethyl-19-nortestosterone. Chem Pharm Bull (Tokyo) 1975;23:3203–3207.
126. Wakeling AE, Furr B, Glen T, et al. Receptor binding and biological activity of steroidal and nonsteroidal antiandrogens. J Steroid Biochem 1981;15:355–359.
127. Snyder BW, Winneker RC, Batzold FH. Endocrine profile of Win 49596 in the rat: a novel androgen receptor antagonist. J Steroid Biochem 1989;33:1127–1132.
128. Liao S, Howell DK, Chang TN. Action of a nonsteroidal antiandrogen, flutamide, on the receptor binding and nuclear retention of 5α-dihydrotestosterone in rat ventral prostate. Endocrinology 1974;94:1205–1209.
129. Shet MS, Mcphaul M, Fisher CW, et al. Metabolism of the antiandrogenic drug (flutamide) by human CYP1A2. Drug Metab Dispos 1997;25:1298–1303.
130. Suzuki H, Akakura K, Komiya A, et al. Codon 877 mutation in the androgen receptor gene in advanced prostate cancer: relation to antiandrogen withdrawal syndrome. Prostate 1996;29:153–158.
131. Hara T, Miyazaki J, Araki H, et al. Novel mutations of androgen receptor: a possible mechanism of bicalutamide withdrawal syndrome. Cancer Res 2003;63:149–153.
132. Fang S, Liao S. Antagonistic action of antiandrogens on the formation of a specific dihydrotestosterone-receptor protein complex in rat ventral prostate. Mol Pharmacol 1969;5:428–431.
133. Furr BJ, Tucker H. The preclinical development of bicalutamide: pharmacodynamics and mechanism of action. Urology 1996;47(Suppl 1A):13–25.
134. Cockshott ID. Bicalutamide: clinical pharmacokinetics and metabolism. Clin Pharmacokinet 2004;43:855–878.
135. Marugo M, Bernasconi D, Miglietta L, et al. Effects of dihydrotestosterone and hydroxyflutamide on androgen receptors in cultured human breast cancer cells (EVSA-T). J Steroid Biochem Mol Biol 1992;42:547–554.
136. Creaven PJ, Pendyala L, Tremblay D. Urology. Pharmacokinetics and metabolism of nilutamide. 1991;37(2 Suppl):13–19.
137. Ask K, Decologne N, Ginies C, et al. Metabolism of nilutamide in rat lung. Biochem Pharmacol 2006;71:377–385.
138. Ask K, Dijols S, Giroud C, et al. Reduction of nilutamide by NO synthases: implications for the adverse effects of this nitroaromatic antiandrogen drug. Chem Res Toxicol 2003;16:1547–1554.
139. Tannock IF, de Wit R, Berry WR, et al. Docetaxel plus prednisone or mitoxantrone plus prednisone for advanced prostate cancer. N Engl J Med 2004;351:1502–1512.
140. Kantoff PW, Higano CS, Shore ND, et al. Sipuleucel-T immunotherapy for castration-resistant prostate cancer. N Engl J Med 2010;363:411–422.
141. Van Wauwe J, Janssen PA. Is there a case for P-450 inhibitors in cancer treatment? J Med Chem 1989;32:2231–2239.
142. Barrie SE, Potter GA, Goddard PM, et al. Pharmacology of novel steroidal inhibitors of cytochrome P45017α (17β-hydroxylase/C17-20 lyase). J Steroid Biochem Mol Biol 1994;50:267–273.
143. Angelastro MR, Laughlin ME, Schatzman GL, et al. 17β-(Cyclopropylamino)-androst-5-en-3β-ol, a selective mechanism-based inhibitor of cytochrome P450(17α) (steroid 17α-hydroxylase/C17-20 lyase). Biochem Biophys Res Commun 1989;162:1571.
144. Haidar S, Ehmer PB, Barassin S, et al. Effects of novel 17α-hydroxylase/C17,20-lyase (P450 17, CYP 17) inhibitors on androgen biosynthesis in vitro and in vivo. J Steroid Biochem Mol Biol 2003;84:555–562.
145. Oottamasathien S, Crawford ED. Recent advances in hormonal therapy for advanced prostate cancer. Oncology 2003;17:1047–1052.
146. Ryan CJ, Smith MR, Fong L, et al. Phase I clinical trial of the CYP17 inhibitor abiraterone acetate demonstrating clinical activity in patients with castration-resistant prostate cancer who received prior ketoconazole therapy. J Clin Oncol 2010;28:1481–1488.
147. National Cancer Institute. The prostate cancer prevention trial. Available at: http://www.cancer.gov/pcpt.
148. Thompson IM, Goodman PJ, Tangen CM, et al. The influence of finasteride on the development of prostate cancer. N Engl J Med 2003;349:215–224.
149. Andriole GL, Bostwick DG, Brawley OW, et al. Effect of dutasteride on the risk of prostate cancer. N Engl J Med. 2010;362:1192–1202.
150. Stevermer JJ, Easley SK. Treatment of prostatitis. Am Fam Physician 2000;61:3015–3022.
151. Charalabopoulos K, Karachalios G, Baltogiannis D, et al. Penetration of antimicrobial agents into the prostate. Chemotherapy 2003;49:269–279.
152. Boolell M, Allen MJ, Ballard SA, et al. Sildenafil: an orally active type 5 cyclic GMP-specific phosphodiesterase inhibitor for the treatment of penile erectile dysfunction. Int J Impot Res 1996;8:47–52.
153. Setter SM, Iltz JL, Fincham JE, et al. Phosphodiesterase-5 inhibitors for erectile dysfunction. Ann Pharmacother 2005;39:1286–1295.
154. Pissarnitski D. Phosphodiesterase-5 (PDE5) inhibitors for the treatment of male erectile disorder: attaining selectivity versus PDE6. Med Res Rev 2006;26:369–395.
155. Saenz de Tejada I, Angulo J, Cuevas P, et al. The phosphodiesterase inhibitory selectivity and the in vitro and in vivo potency of the new PDE5 inhibitor vardenafil. Int J Impot Res 2001;13:282–290.
156. Gupta M, Kovar A, Meibohm B. The clinical pharmacokinetics of phosphodiesterase-5 inhibitors for erectile dysfunction. J Clin Pharmacol 2005;45:987–1003.

157. Kloner RA. Cardiovascular effects of the three phosphodiesterase-5 inhibitors approved for the treatment of erectile dysfunction. Circulation 2004;110:3149–3155.
158. Porst H, Rosen R, Padma-Nathan H, et al. The efficacy and tolerability of vardenafil, a new, oral, selective phosphodiesterase type 5 inhibitor, in patients with erectile dysfunction: the first at-home clinical trial. Int J Impot Res 2001;13:192–199.
159. Corbin JD, Beasley A, Blount MA, et al. Vardenafil: structural basis for higher potency over sildenafil in inhibiting cGMP-specific phosphodiesterase-5 (PDE5). Neurochem Int 2004;45:859–863.
160. Kuan J, Brock G. Selective phosphodiesterase type 5 inhibition using tadalafil for the treatment of erectile dysfunction. Expert Opin Invest Drugs 2002;11:1605–1613.
161. Beckman TJ, Abu-Lebdeh HS, Mynderse LA. Evaluation and medical management of erectile dysfunction. Mayo Clin Proc 2006;81:385–390.
162. McDonald-Gibson WJ, McDonald-Gibson RG, Greaves MW. Prostaglandin E_1 metabolism by human plasma. Prostaglandins 1972;2:251–263.
163. Bechara A, Casabe A, Cheliz G, et al. Comparative study of papaverine plus phentolamine versus prostaglandin E_1 in erectile dysfunction. J Urol 1997;157:2132–2134.
164. McGlynn KA, Devesa SS, Sigurdson AJ, et al. Trends in the incidence of testicular germ cell tumors in the United States. Cancer 2003;97:63–70.
165. Kamel HK. Male osteoporosis: new trends in diagnosis and therapy. Drugs Aging 2005;22:741–748.

Suggested Readings

Gao W, Dalton JT. Androgen receptor. In: Bunce CM, Campbell MJ, eds. Nuclear Receptors, Current Concepts and Future Challenges. New York: Springer, 2010:143–182.

McKenna NJ, O'Malley BW. SnapShot: nuclear receptors I. Cell 2010;142:822–822.

McKenna NJ, O'Malley BW. SnapShot: nuclear receptors II. Cell 2010;142:986.

Mohler ML, Bohl CE, Narayanan R, et al. Nonsteroidal tissue-selective androgen receptor modulators. In: Ottow E, Weinmann H, eds. Nuclear Receptors as Drug Targets. Berlin: Wiley-VCH, 2008:249–304.

Nieschlag E, Behre HM. Testosterone: Action, Deficiency, Substitution, 3rd Ed. Cambridge, UK: Cambridge University Press, 2004.

Nuclear Receptor Signalling Atlas. Available at: Availawww.nursa.org.

Proteau PL. Steroids and therapeutically related compounds. In: Block JH, Beale JM Jr, eds. Wilson and Gisvold's Textbook of Organic Medicinal and Pharmaceutical Chemistry, 11th Ed. Baltimore: Lippincott Williams & Wilkins, 2004:767–817.

Snyder PJ. Androgens. In: Brunton L, Lazo J, Parker K, eds. Goodman & Gilman's The Pharmacological Basis of Therapeutics, 11th Ed. New York: McGraw-Hill, 2006:1573–1586

Stanisić V, Lonard DM, O'Malley BW. Modulation of steroid hormone receptor activity. Prog Brain Res 2010;181:153–176.

Xie W, ed. Nuclear Receptors in Drug Metabolism. Hoboken, NH: Wiley & Sons, 2009.

Zeelen FJ. Medicinal Chemistry of Steroids. Amsterdam: Elsevier, 1990.

Chapter 41

Women's Health

ROBIN M. ZAVOD

Drugs Covered in This Chapter*

AROMATASE INHIBITORS
- Anastrozole
- Exemestane
- Letrozole

FULVESTRANT

INFERTILITY DRUGS
- Clomiphene citrate
- Follicle-stimulating hormone
- Gonadotropin-releasing hormone
- Lutropin alfa

PROGESTERONE RECEPTOR ANTAGONISTS
- Mifepristone
- Ulipristal acetate

PROGESTINS
- Desogestrel
- Dienogest
- Drospirenone
- *Elcometrine*
- Etonogestrel
- *Gestodene*
- Medroxyprogesterone acetate
- Megestrol acetate
- Nomegestrol acetate
- Norethindrone
- Norgestimate
- Norgestrel/Levonorgestrel
- *Trimegestone*

SELECTIVE ESTROGEN RECEPTOR MODULATORS
- Tamoxifen
- Toremifene

STEROIDAL ESTROGENS
- Conjugated estrogens
- Estradiol
- Ethinyl estradiol
- Mestranol

Abbreviations

cAMP, cyclic adenosine monophosphate
CEE, conjugated equine estrogen
CoA, coactivator
CYP, cytochrome P450
DES, diethylstilbestrol
DHEA, dehydroepiandrosterone
EE, ethinyl estradiol
ER, estrogen receptor
ERE, estrogen response element
ERT, estrogen replacement therapy
FDA, U.S. Food and Drug Administration
FSH, follicle-stimulating hormone
GI, gastrointestinal
GnRH, gonadotropin-releasing hormone
hCG, human chorionic gonadotropin
hCG-H, hyperglycosylated human chorionic gonadotropin
HDL, high-density lipoprotein
HPO, hypothalamic-pituitary-ovary
HRT, hormone replacement therapy
HSDD, hypoactive sexual desire disorder
5-HT, serotonin
IUD, intrauterine device
IUI, intrauterine insemination
IVF, in vitro fertilization
LDL, low-density lipoprotein
LH, luteinizing hormone
OC, oral contraceptive
OHSS, ovarian hyperstimulation syndrome
SERM, selective estrogen receptor modulator
SHBG, sex hormone binding globulin
SSRI, selective serotonin reuptake inhibitor
VTE, venous thromboembolism
WHI, Women's Health Initiative

*Drugs listed include those available inside and outside of the United States; drugs available outside of the United States are shown in italics.

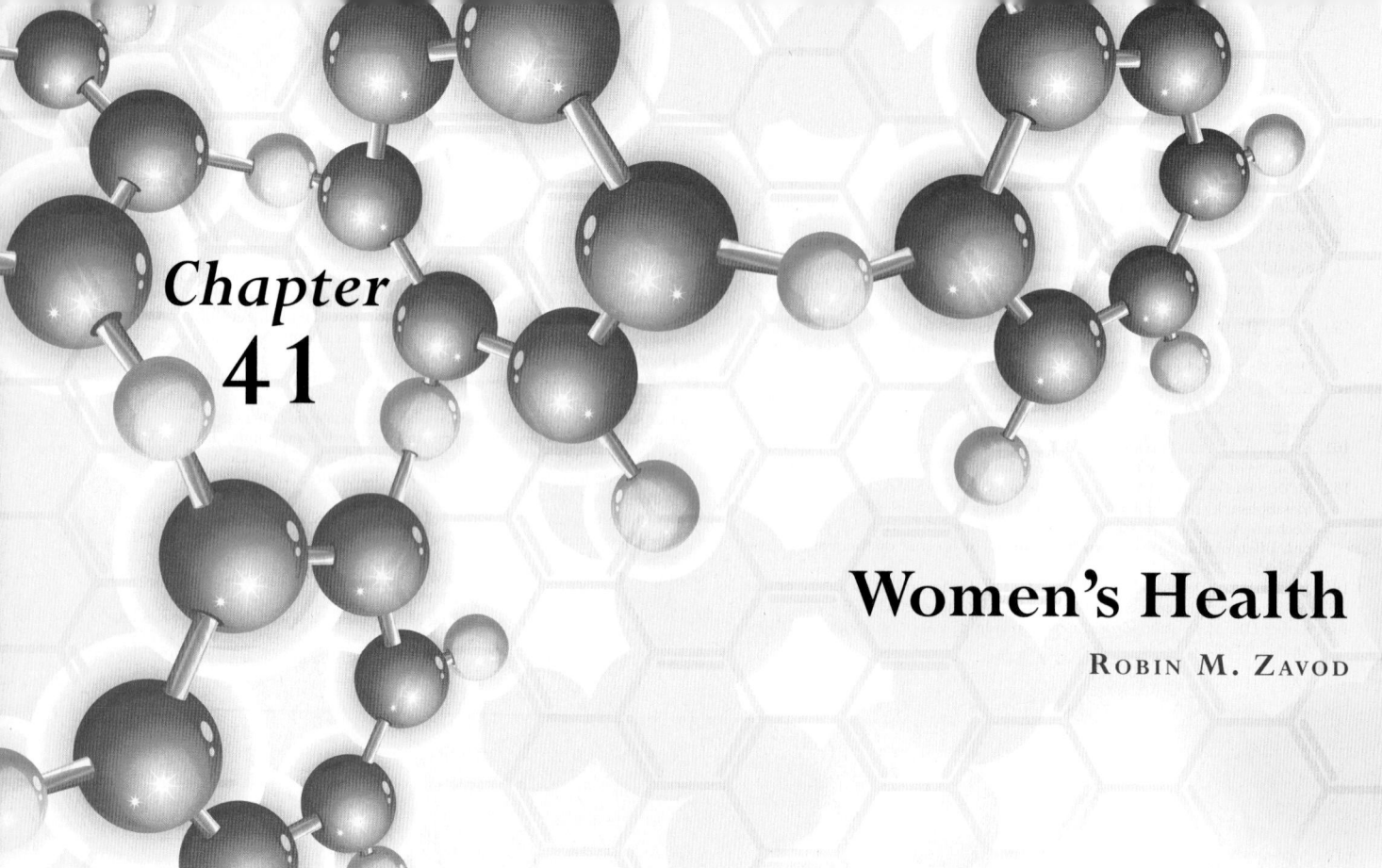

SCENARIO

Nancy Ordonez, PharmD

CC is a 20-year-old college student who comes to the family medicine clinic for her annual physical and gynecologic exam. She wants to discuss options for contraception. She is currently taking a combined oral contraceptive (COC) containing ethinyl estradiol 0.03 mg/levonorgesterel 0.15 mg, which she has been taking for 6 months. She is a very busy computer science major and handles a heavy academic load in addition to being a member of the winning college softball team. She is a runner and works part-time at the school's recreation center as a swimming instructor. She admits that she has not been very diligent in taking her COC on a regular basis due to her busy schedule, and she would like to have a more long-term contraceptive agent. She is taking no other medications except a multivitamin once daily. She has no significant medical history and is negative for tobacco use. Her pregnancy test in the clinic is negative.

(The reader is directed to the clinical solution and chemical analysis of this case at the end of the chapter).

INTRODUCTION

The sex hormones are specific steroids necessary for reproduction and for the development of secondary sex characteristics in both sexes. The sex steroids are comprised of three classes: estrogens, progestins, and androgens. In this chapter, the two principal classes of female sex hormones, estrogens and progestins, will be discussed. The naturally occurring estrogens are C_{18} steroids and contain an aromatic A ring with a hydroxyl group at the 3 position. The most potent endogenous estrogen is estradiol. The naturally occurring progestins are C_{21} steroids and contain a 3-keto-4-ene structure in the A ring and a ketone at the C_{21} position. The most potent endogenous progestin is progesterone. The class of steroids that contains the male sex hormones is the androgen class. The naturally occurring androgens are C_{19} steroids and contain either a hydroxyl or ketone functional group at both the C_3 and C_{17} positions. The primary androgen found in the blood is testosterone, with the active metabolite 5α-dihydrotestosterone formed in certain target tissues. All three classes of endogenous steroids are present in both sexes, but the production and circulating plasma levels of estrogens and progestins are substantially higher in females.

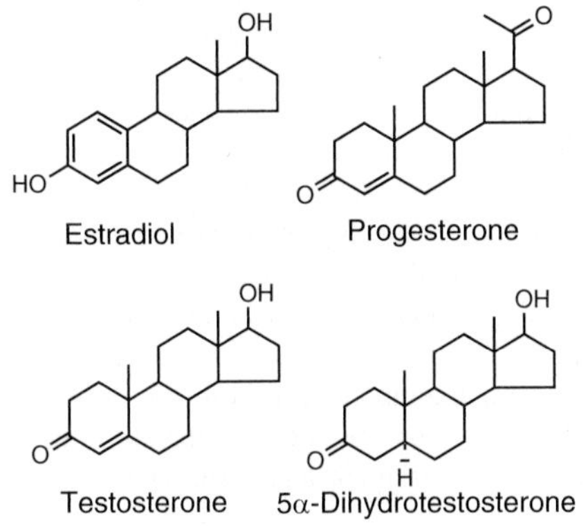

SEX HORMONES: REPRODUCTIVE CYCLE

The female reproductive cycle is controlled by an integrated system involving the hypothalamus, anterior pituitary gland, ovary, and reproductive tract (Fig. 41.1). The hypothalamus exerts its action on the pituitary gland via the hormone signal gonadotropin-releasing hormone (GnRH). This hormone is released by the hypothalamus in a pulsatile fashion and stimulates the release of the gonadotropins, follicle-stimulating hormone (FSH), and luteinizing hormone (LH) from the anterior pituitary.

The two main gonadotropins, FSH and LH, regulate production of the sex hormones estrogen and progesterone. As the name implies, FSH promotes the initial development and growth of immature ovarian follicles, and as these follicles mature, they secrete estradiol. During the follicular phase, when estrogen levels are elevated, the endometrium undergoes proliferation as a direct result of estrogenic stimulation. As estradiol levels increase, the production of FSH decreases via feedback inhibition, and LH release is stimulated. The level of LH rises to a sharp peak (LH surge) at the midpoint of the menstrual cycle. This serves to cause the dominant follicle to rupture and release its egg (ovulation). The luteal phase follows ovulation and ends at menses. During this phase, the endometrium shows secretory activity, and cell proliferation declines. Once ovulation has occurred, LH induces luteinization of the tissue that remains from the ruptured follicle, which leads to formation of the corpus luteum. The corpus luteum is responsible for the biosynthesis and

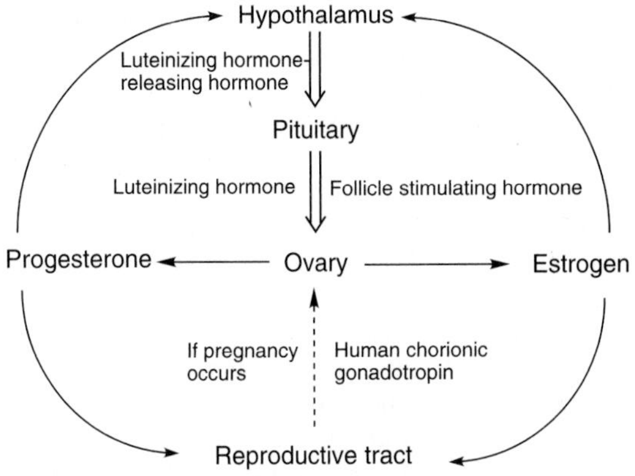

FIGURE 41.1 Hypothalamic, ovarian, and reproductive tract interrelationships.

secretion of progesterone during the luteal phase of the menstrual cycle. This phase occurs when endometrial preparation for pregnancy occurs, as well as during the early weeks of a pregnancy.

If the egg remains unfertilized, the corpus luteum degrades, and the levels of progesterone and estrogen decline. This leads to sloughing off of the endometrial lining, known as menstruation. At this point in the menstrual cycle, estrogen and progesterone levels are low, and hormonal feedback to the hypothalamus ceases. Without the influence of these hormonal signals, the hypothalamus releases additional GnRH, and the cycle begins again. A single menstrual cycle starts with the onset of menses (day 1) and ends with the start of the next menstrual period. This interval varies from 20 to 35 days, with an average length of 28 days. The major events of the ovarian cycle are summarized in Figure 41.2.

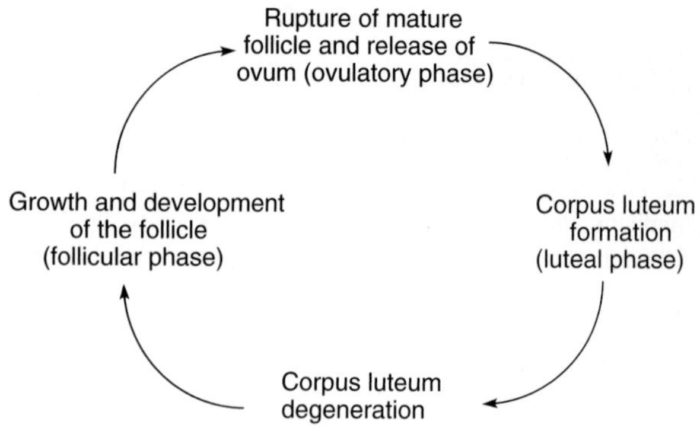

FIGURE 41.2 Ovarian cycle.

If the egg is fertilized successfully, then the menstrual cycle is interrupted because of the release of a gonadotropin synthesized in the placenta, human chorionic gonadotropin (hCG). The role of this glycoprotein is to maintain the corpus luteum. Fourteen days after egg fertilization, the level of urinary hCG reaches a concentration that can be detected by a home pregnancy test. Levels of this gonadotropin peak around the seventh week of pregnancy and then decrease to a level that is maintained throughout pregnancy.

For the first 9 weeks of pregnancy, the corpus luteum produces an adequate level of estrogen and progesterone to maintain the pregnancy. After this period, the placenta assumes these responsibilities. Both estrogen and progesterone levels increase during pregnancy, finally reaching their maximal concentrations a few days before labor and delivery.

Over the course of a woman's lifetime, her hormonal status and ability to reproduce vary considerably. Sexual maturation and the onset of the reproductive period are correlated with the start of cyclic menstrual bleeding. This typically occurs between the ages of 8 and 17 years (average age, 11 years). Later in life, reproductive capacity begins to wane, and women gradually lose ovarian function, which causes intermittent maturation of follicles and, therefore, irregular production of the corpus luteum. This is referred to as perimenopause. Eventually, cessation of menses occurs, resulting in menopause and the loss of reproductive capacity. This typically occurs between the ages of 45 and 55 years. Throughout a woman's reproductive life cycle, various types of hormone therapy play key roles in regulating this hormone cycle.

CLINICAL SIGNIFICANCE

Women's health issues encompass a variety of disease states and range from contraception to infertility, menopause, osteoporosis, and oncology. Pharmacologic agents treating these disease states are numerous and their uses are wide-ranging. Recent developments of drugs dealing with women's health issues not only have focused on producing better oral contraceptives but have expanded to designing drugs for the treatment of osteoporosis, infertility, and breast cancer. With so many medications from which to choose, the clinician must be knowledgeable about the drug's pharmacodynamic, pharmacokinetic, and medicinal chemistry properties to optimize therapy. For example, with so many oral contraceptives (OCs) on the market, the clinician must apply his or her knowledge about the drug to tailor the therapy. For patients with acne, OCs with low androgenic characteristics would be appropriate. Postpartum mothers who are breastfeeding and want to start taking OCs will need to use a product containing progestin only. In addition to OCs, drugs used to treat infertility must be customized to fit the patient's clinical picture. A variety of medications are used to treat infertility, ranging from clomiphene citrate, an antiestrogen, to products containing follicle-stimulating hormone.

Advancements in the treatment of bone disorders and cancer in women have resulted from the increased knowledge of estrogen receptors and the development of selective estrogen receptor modulators (SERMs). Modifications in the structure–activity relationships of SERMs produce drugs with favorable side effect profiles that are effective for osteoporosis and breast cancer. Many ongoing research investigations continue to develop drugs for treating the assortment of health care issues faced by women. An essential component in both the development and the clinical applications of these drugs is the utilization of knowledge regarding the drugs' medicinal chemistry properties.

Nancy Ordonez, PharmD
Clinical Assistant Professor
University of Houston
College of Pharmacy
Houston, Texas

HOME PREGNANCY TESTS

With the increased availability of a variety of home diagnostic tests, the sale of home pregnancy, ovulation, and fertility tests alone was a $227 million dollar business in 2009. Home pregnancy tests have been used since 1976, with approximately 26 devices currently available in the United States. These tests claim that they can be used on the first day of a missed menstrual period (or, for certain devices, even earlier) with more than 99% diagnostic accuracy for pregnancy. Despite these claims, accurate results are obtained only a fraction of the time (Table 41.1) (1).

Home pregnancy tests are qualitative tests and simply detect the presence of the α and β subunits of hCG in a small sample of urine collected early in the day (Table 41.2) (2,3). Their detection limits range from 6.3 to 50 IU/L, and all are calibrated using regular hCG. A positive response indicates that the anti-hCG monoclonal or polyclonal antibodies found within the tests have successfully bound to a specific site along hCG. A second antibody linked to an enzyme that reacts with this anti-hCG complex causes a color change (3). What is not clear is if it is the regular hCG or the hyperglycosylated hCG (hCG-H) that is the source for the immunoreactivity observed during the weeks immediately following implantation. Compelling evidence suggests that hCG-H may be the principle source of hCG immunoreactivity, yet the detection limits for this glycoprotein are poorer than those reported for regular hCG. Only 6 of 15 home pregnancy tests evaluated were equally capable of detecting hCG-H and regular hCG (2).

False-positive results can stem from a recent birth, miscarriage, or the use of menotropins or hCG injections in women experiencing infertility, in whom hCG levels may still be elevated (4). Although unlikely because of the use of monoclonal antibody technology, there also may be false-positive results from pharmacologic sources, including methadone, promethazine, or chlordiazepoxide (3). False-negative results generally are a consequence of errors in using the device or in handling the urine sample.

This chapter will focus primarily on hormonal therapies for the treatment and/or management of contraception, endometriosis, infertility, menopause, and breast cancer.

STEROID HORMONES

Estrogens

Three endogenous estrogens are present in women. Estradiol, the most potent of the three, represents 10% to 20% of the circulating estrogen. Estrone is 10-fold less potent than estradiol and accounts for 60% to 80% of the circulating estrogen. The remaining 10% to 20% is in the form of estriol, a very weak estrogen. Estrone was the first estrogen to be isolated in crystalline form from the urine of pregnant women. The two other C_{18} estrogen steroids, 17β-estradiol and estriol, were isolated and characterized later.

TABLE 41.1 Clinical Sensitivity Evaluation of Home Pregnancy Tests (1)

Name of Device	Confidence in Positive Results (%)	Clinical Sensitivity (%)
EPT	45	16
Clear Blue Easy Earliest Results	100	80
First Response Early Result	100	>95
Fact Plus Select	24	<16
Accu-Clear	22	<16

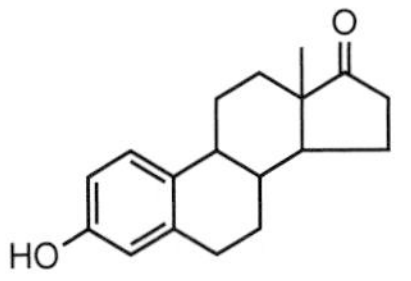

Estrone

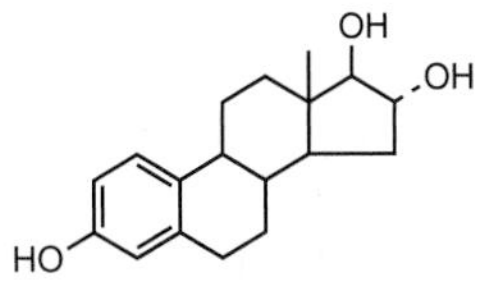

Estriol

Biosynthesis

Estrogens are biosynthesized in the maturing dominant follicle and in the corpus luteum in premenopausal women. During pregnancy, the placenta becomes the primary location of estrogen biosynthesis (5,6). Approximately 50% of estrone production occurs in the ovaries. The remaining estrone is biosynthesized from estradiol, as well as from the conversion of estrone sulfate to estrone in the adrenal gland and the aromatization of androstenedione. In contrast to premenopausal women, in whom the natural estrone-to-estradiol ratio is 1:2, postmenopausal women have an estrone-to-estradiol ratio of 2:1, which reflects the loss of ovarian function.

In endocrine tissues, cholesterol is the steroid that is stored and converted to estrogen, progesterone, or androgen when the tissue is stimulated by a gonadotropic hormone. The major pathways for the biosynthesis of sex steroid hormones are summarized in Figure 41.3. In the ovary, FSH acts on the preovulatory follicle to stimulate the biosynthesis of estrogens. The thecal cells of the preovulatory follicle convert cholesterol into androgens, whereas the granulosa cells convert androgens to estrogens.

Cleavage of the side chain of cholesterol produces pregnenolone (step a in Fig. 41.3), which can then be transformed into progesterone or, via several biosynthetic steps, to the aromatic A ring containing structures such as those found in estrogens (7). Pregnenolone is converted by 17α-hydroxylase to 17α-hydroxypregnenolone (step b), which then proceeds on to the intermediate dehydroepiandrosterone (DHEA) via the 17,20-lyase reaction (step e) (8). DHEA is converted by 5-ene-3β-hydroxysteroid dehydrogenase and 3-oxosteroid-4,5-isomerase to the 17-ketosteroid, androstenedione (steps c and d), which is interconvertible with testosterone via

TABLE 41.2 Evaluation of Home Pregnancy Tests with Regular Human Chorionic Gonadotropin (hCG) and Hyperglycosylated hCG (H-hCG) Standards (2)

Name of Device	Regular hCG (IU/L)				H-hCG (IU/L)				hCG Limit (IU/L)
	6.3	13	25	50	6.3	13	25	50	
EPT	–	–	+	++	–	+	+	++	40
Clear Blue Easy	+	+	++	++	–	–	+	+	50
First Response Early Result	–	+	+	++	–	–	+	++	~50
Fact Plus Select	–	–	+	+	–	–	+	+	100
Answer	–	–	+	++	–	–	±	+	100

–, negative result observed; ±, exceptionally faint positive result observed; +, clear positive result observed; ++, strongly positive result observed.

17β-hydroxysteroid dehydrogenase (step f). The final step in the biosynthesis is the conversion of the C_{19} androgens to the C_{18} estrogens via the loss of the C_{19} angular methyl group and aromatization of ring A to form 17β-estradiol or estrone (step g) catalyzed by aromatase. The interconversion of 17β-estradiol and estrone is catalyzed by estradiol dehydrogenase (step h), a member of the 17β-hydroxysteroid dehydrogenase family.

Metabolism

Metabolism of the estrogens to their water-soluble glucuronide and sulfate conjugates occurs mainly in the liver. Creation of an estrogen reservoir occurs as a result of enterohepatic recycling, a process by which estrogens undergo desulfation followed by resulfation.

Approximately 50% of an exogenous dose of 17β-estradiol undergoes hepatic first-pass metabolism to

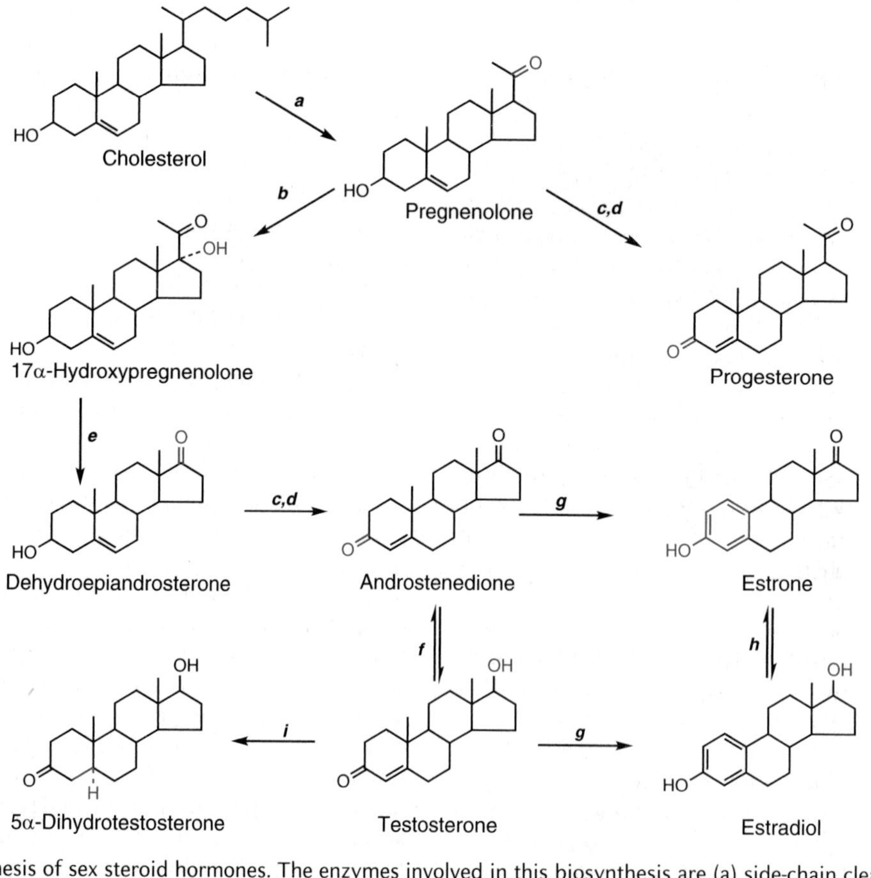

FIGURE 41.3 Biosynthesis of sex steroid hormones. The enzymes involved in this biosynthesis are (a) side-chain cleavage, (b) 17α-hydroxylase, (c) 5-ene-3β-hydroxysteroid dehydrogenase, (d) 3-oxosteroid-4,5-isomerase, (e) 17,20-lyase, (f) 17β-hydroxysteroid dehydrogenase, (g) aromatase, (h) estradiol dehydrogenase, and (i) 5α-reductase.

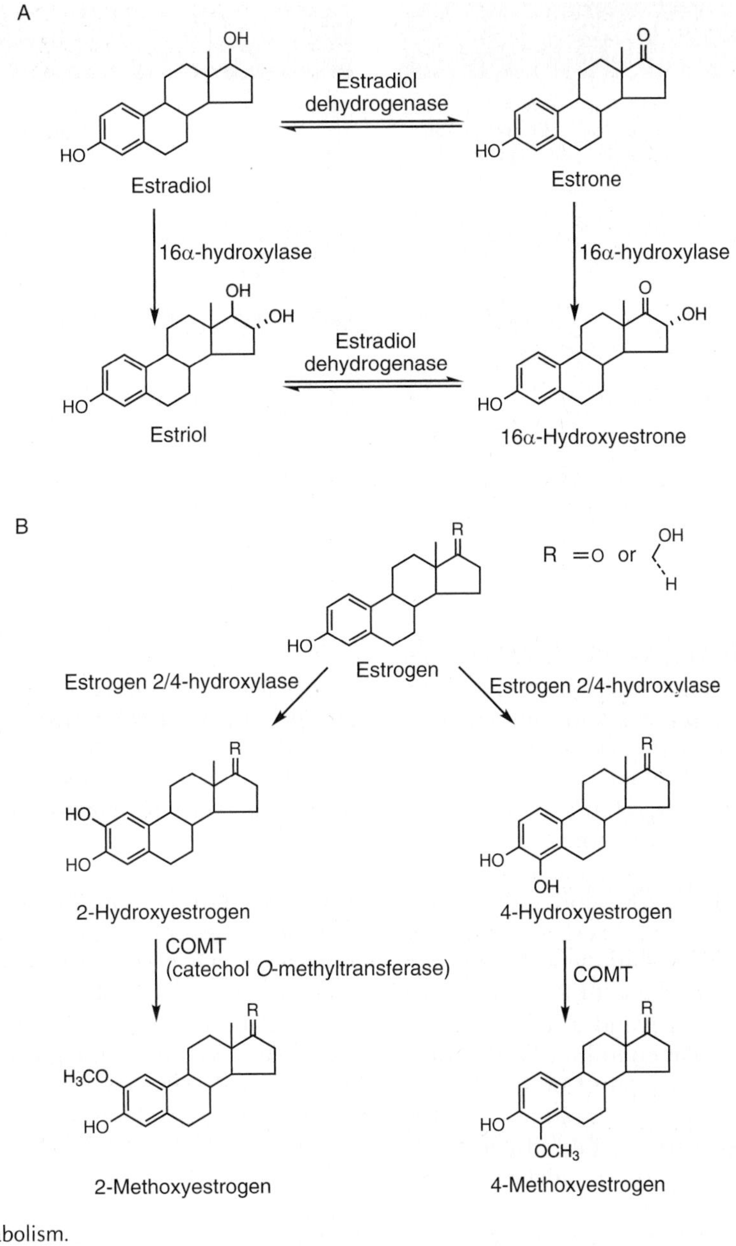

FIGURE 41.4 Estrogen metabolism.

metabolites that are readily excreted via the kidney, and the remaining 50% is found in bile fluid (9). Much of the material found in bile subsequently enters the intestine, where it is reabsorbed and returned to the liver. Only 10% of an administered dose is found in the feces (5). Both 17β-estradiol and estrone are converted by 16α-hydroxylase to yield estriol (Fig. 41.4A), which is found in the urine as the glucuronide conjugate.

Estrogens are metabolized by estrogen 2/4-hydroxylase (CYP3A4) at positions ortho to the 3-phenolic group to form the 2-hydroxyestrogens and the 4-hydroxyestrogens (Fig. 41.4B). The resulting catechol estrogens bind to estrogen receptors (ERs) and produce weak to moderate estrogenic effects. These metabolites are unstable in vivo, however, and are rapidly converted to their 2-methoxy and 4-methoxyestrogen metabolites as well as to their glucuronide, sulfate, and glutathione conjugates. These metabolites are found in comparatively large amounts in the urine (9,10).

Estradiol is 37% bound to sex hormone binding globulin (SHBG) and 61% bound to albumin, leaving only 2% free in circulation (Table 41.3) (11,12). The affinity of estrone and of the sulfated esters of estrone and estradiol for SHBG is less than that that of estradiol; however, they are more tightly bound to albumin than estradiol is. These proteins are vital to the transport, distribution, and metabolic clearance rate of estrogens (13). In addition, estradiol is capable of inducing the synthesis of SHBG.

TABLE 41.3 Estrogenic Affinity for Binding Proteins and Metabolic Clearance Rate (11,12)

Estrogen	RBA to SHBG	% Bound to SHBG	% Bound to Albumin	Metabolic Clearance Rate (L/day/m²)
17β Estradiol	50	37	61	580
Estrone	12	16	80	1050
Estriol	0.3	1	91	1100
Estrone sulfate	0	0	99	80
Equilin sulfate	0			175

RBA, relative binding affinity (testosterone, 100%); SHBG, sex hormone-binding globulin.

TABLE 41.4 Relative Binding Affinities of Endogenous and Exogenous Estrogens (14)

Estrogen	ERα Binding Affinity	ERβ Binding Affinity
17β Estradiol	100	100
Estrone	60	37
Estrone sulfate	<1	<1
Estriol	14	21
Coumestrol	94	185
Genistein	5	36
Tamoxifen	7	6
Clomiphene	25	12
Diethylstilbestrol	468	295

ER, estrogen receptor.

Mechanism of Estrogenic Action

MOLECULAR INTERACTIONS Estradiol plays a key role in several physiologic processes, including development of secondary sex characteristics during puberty and stimulation of the mammary glands during pregnancy, and has thermoregulatory capacity. Estradiol facilitates these processes via its biologic target, the ER, of which there are two subtypes (ERα and ERβ). The two receptors differ in size: ERα is composed of 595 amino acids, and ERβ is composed of 485 amino acids. The expression and distribution of these subtypes is inconsistent between the various tissues and organs, which may explain the wide response that is observed (11). The predominant ER in the female reproductive tract and mammary glands is ERα, whereas ERβ is found primarily in vascular endothelial cells, bone, and male prostate tissues. Expression of both ERα and ERβ can be regulated hormonally via estradiol. Estradiol has similar affinities for both ERα and ERβ (Table 41.4), which is not the case for certain nonsteroidal estrogenic compounds and antiestrogens (14).

Within each target cell are two receptor locations, one within the nucleus, where a genomic mechanism predominates, and a second within the cell membrane, where a nongenomic mechanism prevails. Unlike the nuclear receptors, the cell membrane receptors are coupled to G proteins that are linked to a cascade of intracellular signals. Nuclear ERα and ERβ are virtually identical in their DNA binding sites but are only approximately 60% homologous in the C-terminal ligand binding domain (11,13).

When estradiol binds either ERα or ERβ, the receptor protein is phosphorylated and undergoes a conformational change to produce either homo- or heterodimers (ERα/ERα, ERβ/ERβ, or ERα/ERβ) (15). The dimeric ER complex then migrates from the cytosol to the cell nucleus, where it teams up with specific estrogen response elements (EREs) found within an adaptor protein, typically a promoter, which aids in binding of the complex to estrogen activated genes (11,13). This complex also enlists a coactivator (CoA) complex to this promoter, which regulates DNA transcription (Fig. 41.5). Because the ER can interact with other nuclear receptors as well as with transcription factors, it is not easy to tease out all the factors that control estrogen-mediated biologic responses.

PHYSIOLOGIC EFFECTS One of the principal actions of the estrogens is to promote the development of female secondary sex characteristics. These feminizing attributes include hair growth, skin softening, breast growth, and accumulation of fat in the thighs, hips, and buttocks. Estrogen also stimulates the growth and development of the female reproductive tract, including the uterine oviduct, cervix, and vagina.

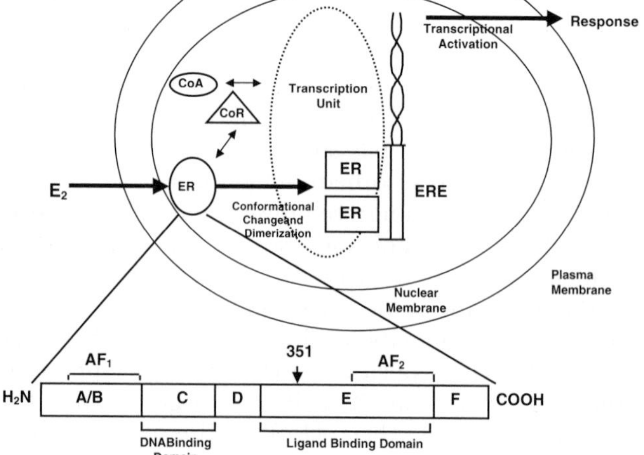

FIGURE 41.5 A subcellular model of estradiol (E_2) action in a target tissue. The abbreviations used are as described in the text.

Estrogens play a significant role in breast tissue as well. Considerable research has focused on understanding breast cancer and the factors that influence its growth. Estrogens serve as "fuel" for hormone-dependent mammary carcinoma and cause proliferation of breast cells. They also stimulate gene expression and, therefore, the production of several proteins, including intracellular proteins important for breast cell function and growth, as well as proteins that influence tumor growth and metastasis. Some of these intracellular proteins include the enzymes needed for DNA synthesis, such as DNA polymerase, thymidine kinase, thymidylate synthetase, and dihydrofolate reductase (16,17).

TABLE 41.5 Potencies of Orally Administered Estrogens (12,13)

Type of Estrogen	FSH Suppression	Serum SHBG Suppression
Piperazine estrone sulfate	1.1	1
Micronized estradiol	1.3	1
Conjugated estrogens	1.4	3.2
Ethinyl estradiol	80–200	614

FSH, follicle-stimulating hormone; SHBG, sex hormone-binding globulin

Steroidal Estrogens

Estradiol Estradiol is the most potent endogenous estrogen, exhibiting high affinity for the ER and high potency when administered parenterally. When administered orally, estradiol is promptly conjugated in the intestine and oxidatively metabolized by the liver, resulting in its low oral bioavailability and therapeutic effectiveness.

Ethinyl Estradiol and Mestranol One method to increase the oral bioavailability of estradiol is to prevent metabolic oxidation of the estradiol C_{17} hydroxyl group to the corresponding ketone (estrone). This is readily accomplished via alkylation of the C_{17} position with a chemically inert alkyne group (e.g., ethinyl estradiol [EE]) (Fig. 41.6). This synthetic analog is several hundred–fold more potent than estradiol, with doses in the microgram rather than the milligram range (Table 41.5) (18). Following oral administration, EE is rapidly and almost completely absorbed, with an oral bioavailability of approximately 40% and an elimination half-life of 26 hours (Table 41.6). EE undergoes extensive first-pass metabolism to its 3-*O*-glucuronide and 3-*O*-sulfate metabolites and, via aromatic hydroxylation, to 2–hydroxyethinylestradiol and its *O*-methyl metabolites. EE undergoes extensive enterohepatic recycling. The bacteria in the gastrointestinal (GI) tract hydrolyze the glucuronide and sulfate conjugates, thereby permitting reabsorption of EE. It is for this reason that a number of antibacterial agents have an adverse effect on oral contraceptive (OC) efficacy.

Another semisynthetic estrogen, mestranol, is the 3-*O*-methyl ether of EE (Fig. 41.6). Mestranol is a prodrug and, following oral administration, is rapidly metabolized to EE via hepatic oxidative *O*-demethylation. Mestranol and EE are used primarily in OC combination formulations (19).

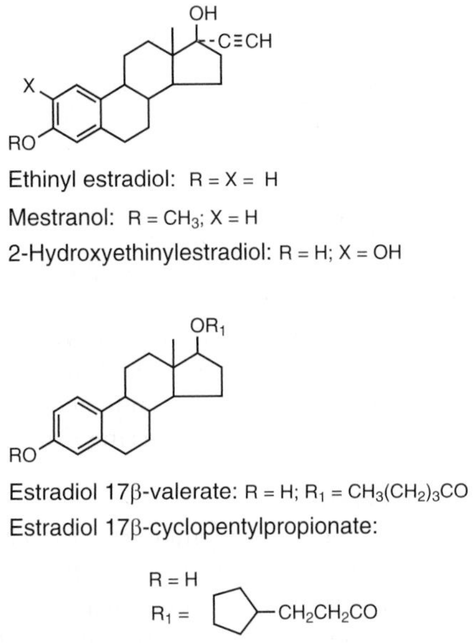

FIGURE 41.6 17α-Ethynyl estrogens and estradiol esters.

Esters of Estradiol To deliver estrogens with a longer duration of action, 17β-estradiol must be derivatized into an ester prodrug. In contrast to the ethinyl derivatives delivered orally, these estrogen analogs usually are administered intramuscularly. Slow hydrolysis of the ester releases free estradiol over a prolonged period of time. The therapeutically useful esters of estradiol include 17β-valerate and 17β-cyclopentylpropionate (cypionate) (Fig. 41.6). Estradiol cypionate (Depo-Estradiol) is available as a sterile solution of the drug in oil (e.g., cottonseed oil), with a duration of action of 14 to 28 days. Estradiol valerate (Delestrogen) is available as a sterile solution in a vegetable oil (e.g., sesame oil or castor oil), with a duration of action of 14 to 21 days. Estradiol valerate is also the estrogenic component of a newly approved combination OC (Natazia). After oral administration, estradiol valerate undergoes metabolic activation during absorption through GI mucosa and first pass through the liver via CYP3A pathways to 17β-estradiol (20).

Conjugated Estrogens Pregnant mares produce two unique estrogenic compounds, equilenin and equilin, that are excreted in the urine as sodium sulfate conjugates. These conjugated metabolites also are used as estrogen preparations (Fig. 41.7). Conjugated Estrogens USP is a mixture of the sodium salts of the sulfate esters of estradiol derived from equine urine or prepared synthetically from estrone and equilin. These preparations (Premarin) are composed of a mixture of sodium

TABLE 41.6 Pharmacokinetic Properties for Some Estrogenic and Progestinal Agents[a]

Drug	Protein[b] Binding	Oral Bioavailability	Biotransformation	Elimination Half-life (hrs)	Time to Peak Conc. (hrs)	Peak Serum Conc.(ng/mL)	Elimination (%)
Estradiol	50–80%	Poor	Hepatic first pass metabolism	20 minutes		0.1–0.2	Renal: 90[d]
Ethynyl estradiol	98%	40%		26 (6–20)	1–2	33	
Progesterone							
Oral 200 mg micronized	>90%	<10%	Hepatic first pass metabolism	<5 minutes	2–4	24.3	Renal: 50–60[d]
IM 45 mg			Hepatic	10 weeks	28	39.1	Fecal: 10
IM 90 mg				19.6	9.2	53.8	
Vaginal gel 45 mg				34.8	6.8	14.9	
Medroxyprogesterone acetate: Oral 10 mg	>90%	High	Hepatic	30	2–4	19–35	Renal: 15–22[d]
IM 150 mg/mL every 3 months			No first-pass hepatic metabolism	50 days	3 weeks	1–7	Fecal: 45–80
Megestrol acetate							
Oral 160 mg	>90	ND	Hepatic	38 (13–104)	2–3	200	Renal: 66[d]
Oral 600 mg					2–3	753	Fecal: 20
Norgestrel	>90%	60%	Hepatic	20	24	ND	Renal: 45[d] Fecal: 32
Levonorgestrel 3/12/60 months implants 216 mg loading dose[d]	>90	60	No first-pass Hepatic metabolism	16 (8–30)	24	1,6 first week, then 0.26–0.4	Renal: 45[d] Fecal: 32
Desogestrel (Desogen) (as 3-keto-desogestrel)	>90	76	First pass to 3-ketodesogestrel active metabolite	12–58	1–2	2–6	Renal: 43[d] Fecal: 50
Norethindrone	>80	65	Hepatic first pass metabolism	8 (5–14)	0.5–4.0	5–10	Renal: 50[d] Fecal: 20–40
Norethindrone acetate	>80	65	Hepatic first pass metabolism	8 (5–14)	0.5–4.0	5–10	Renal: 50[d] Fecal: 20–40
Norgestimate as (desacetylnorgestimate)	>50–60 >90	60	First pass to desacetylnorgestimate	37	1–2	0.5–0.7	Renal: 47[d] Fecal: 37

[a]USP Drug Information 2000.
[b]Sex hormone binding globulin (SHBG) synthesis is stimulated by estrogens and inhibited by androgens: levels are twice as high in women as in men.
[c]Progesterone binds strongly to cortisol binding globulin (CBG; 17.7%) and SHBG (0.6%) and weakly to albumin (79.3%). Absorption is the rate-limiting step for the elimination half-life of Levonorgestrel: free, 1.1–1.7%; SHBG, 92–62%; and albumin, 37.56%; but suppresses SHBG by 33%. Norethindrone: free, 3.5%; SHBG, 35.5%; and albumin, 61%. Medroxyprogesterone does not bind SHBG. 3-Keto-desgestrel, 64%; albumin, 32%. Norgestimate >90% protein bound.
[d]A mean dose of 35 µg levonorgestrel is released daily.
ND, no data available.

estrone sulfate (52.5% to 61.5%) and sodium equilin sulfate (22.5% to 30.5%) as well as several lesser metabolites (e.g., 17α- and 17β-dihydroequilenin or 17α- and 17β-estradiol) as sodium sulfate conjugates. Esterified Estrogens USP (Menest) is a blend of estrone sodium sulfate (75% to 85%) and sodium equilin sulfate (6% to 15%) (Fig. 41.7).

Synthetic conjugated estrogens A (Cenestin) contains a mixture of 9 of the 10 known synthetic conjugated estrogenic substances present in Conjugated Estrogens USP. This includes a mixture of the sodium salts of estrogen sulfates, including estrone sulfate and sodium equilin sulfate. Synthetic conjugated estrogens B (Enjuvia) contains the same set of synthetic estrogens as Cenestin, as well as sodium $\Delta^{8,9}$-dehydroestrone sulfate.

Another sulfate conjugate that is orally effective is estropipate (piperazine estrone sulfate; Ortho-Est) (Fig. 41.7). This derivative has the same actions and utility as the conjugated, naturally occurring estrogens.

Nonsteroidal Estrogens

Stilbene Derivatives The steroid nucleus is not required for estrogenic action. Several derivatives of stilbene (diphenylethylene) that were used therapeutically demonstrate potent estrogenic activity. Diethylstilbestrol (DES), prepared in 1939, was one of these stilbenes (Fig. 41.8).

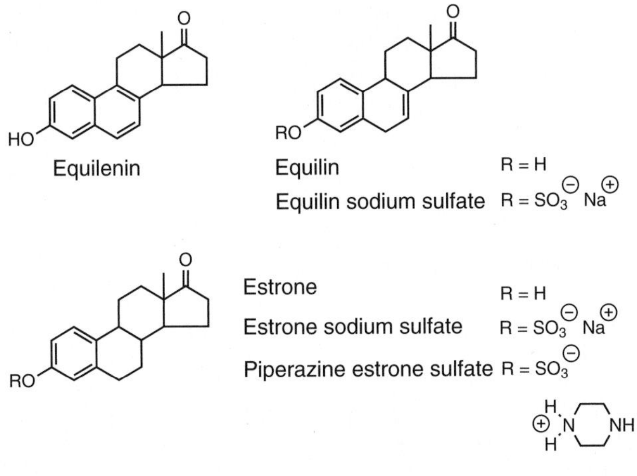

FIGURE 41.7 Conjugated and esterified estrogens.

A *trans* stilbene, DES has 10-fold the estrogenic potency of its *cis* isomer, largely because the *trans* isomer more closely resembles estradiol (21). Unfortunately, when DES was administered to relieve pregnancy-related symptoms, it was correlated with abnormal growth in the offspring. Studies are now suggesting that women exposed to DES prenatally have a higher incidence of breast cancer after age 40 (22). It has been hypothesized that the catechol metabolites of estradiol and DES are oxidized to the corresponding *O*-quinones. A quinone-DNA reaction leads to depurination that generates mutations that may represent a critical step in the initiation of cancer (Fig. 41.9) (23).

Structure–Activity Relationships

As a result of numerous studies, there is an extensive body of knowledge regarding structure–activity relationships for estrogens (24–27). The aromatic A ring and the C_3 hydroxyl group are structural features essential for estrogenic activity. The 17β-hydroxyl, the distance between the C_3 and C_{17} hydroxyl groups, and the presence of planar hydrophobic scaffolding also are important structural contributors and help to optimize estrogenic activity. Ideally, the distance between the oxygen atoms of the C_3 and C_{17} hydroxyl groups should range from 10.3 to 12.1 Å.

Substitution of the estrogen steroid nucleus can significantly modify estrogenic activity. Functionality at the C_1 position greatly reduces activity, and only small groups can be accommodated at the 2 and 4 positions. Addition of hydroxyl groups at positions 6, 7, and 11 reduces activity. Removal of the oxygen function from position 3 or 17 or epimerization of the 17β-hydroxyl group of estradiol to the α-configuration results in estrogenic analogs that are less active (28). The equine estrogens contain one or two additional double bonds in the steroidal B ring (equilin and equilenin, respectively) (Fig. 41.7). The presence of this unsaturation substantially boosts the estrogenic potency of these estrogens. Substituents at the 11β position are tolerated; for example, 11β-methoxy or 11β-ethyl has significantly greater affinity for the ER as compared to estradiol.

Certain modifications at the 17α and 16 positions can lead to enhanced activity. For example, the 17α-ethynyl or 17α-vinyl groups provide the greatest activity, whereas highly polar substituents at this position are poorly tolerated. At the 16 position, moderate size and polarity are tolerated. Enlargement of the D ring (i.e., D-homoestradiol) greatly reduces estrogenic activity.

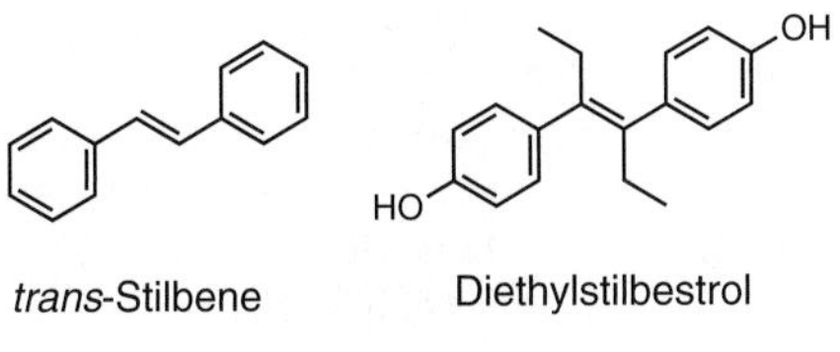

FIGURE 41.8 Nonsteroidal estrogens.

Pharmacokinetics

The bioavailability observed varies with the route of estrogen administration. When administered subcutaneously, the order of bioavailability of the three naturally occurring steroids is estradiol > estrone > estriol. When administered orally, this order changes to estriol > estradiol > estrone (29). Although all three of these estrogens demonstrate at least minimal bioavailability when administered orally, chemical modifications have led to estrogen analogs with improved oral activity. For example, EE is a more effective oral estrogen because of its resistance to metabolism in the GI tract and in the liver. Other types of highly active, orally bioavailable estrogen analogs include those with a labile ether [e.g., 3-(2-tetrahydropyranyl) and 17β-(2-tetrahydropyranyl) estradiol] (30). These drugs proved to be 12- and 15-fold as active, respectively, as estradiol.

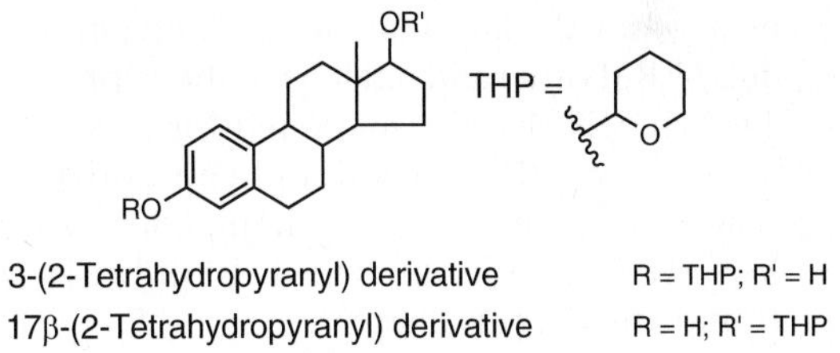

Estrogen Antagonists

Agents that antagonize the actions of estrogen are of particular interest for their contraceptive utility and for the treatment of estrogen-dependent breast cancer. There are three classes of agents that either interfere with estrogen activation of its receptor (e.g., impeded estrogens or triphenylethylene antiestrogens) or limit estrogen biosynthesis (e.g., aromatase inhibitors).

IMPEDED ESTROGENS The impeded estrogens (e.g., estriol) interact with the ER in target tissues but dissociate from the receptor too rapidly to produce a significant estrogenic effect. If, however, the impeded estrogens are present in a high enough local concentration, they will compete with or impede estradiol access to its receptor site, thereby reducing the effect of estradiol on the cell (5,31).

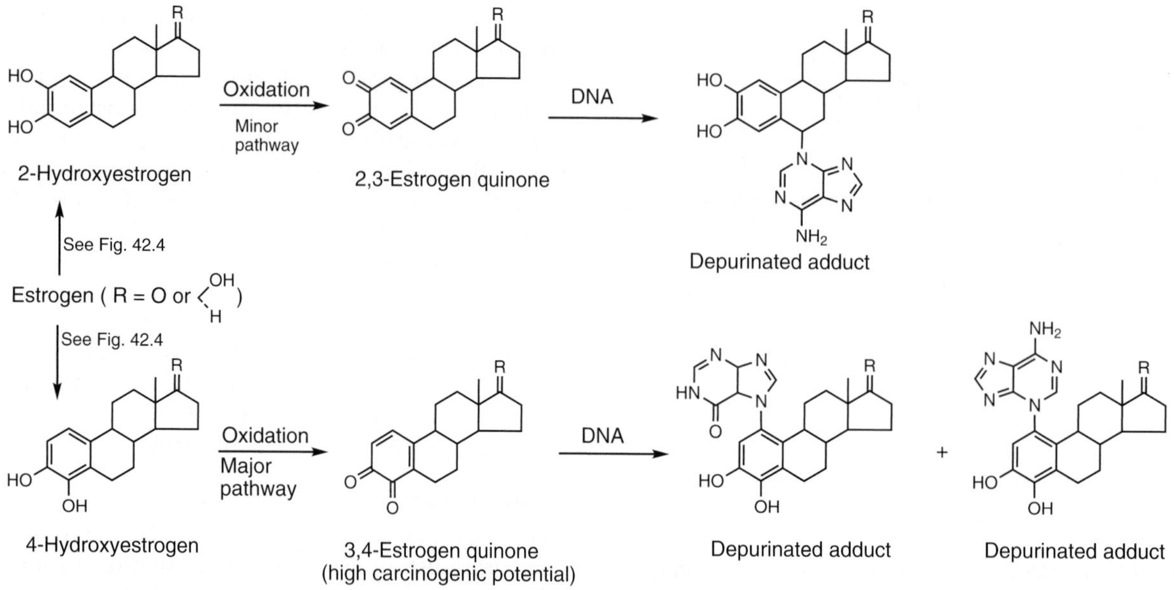

FIGURE 41.9 Metabolic pathways involving estrogens leading to DNA damage through depurination.

ANTIESTROGENS—TRIPHENYLETHYLENE ANALOGS The triphenylethylene antiestrogens (Fig. 41.10) are structurally related to the stilbene family of estrogens and exhibit high affinity for the ER. They prevent translocation of the estrogen–receptor complex into the nucleus of target cells and interfere with the binding of the receptor–hormone complex to the acceptor site of the chromatin (32,33).

Advances in the molecular pharmacology of estrogen and ERs have led to the development of selective estrogen receptor modulators (SERMs). These agents exhibit tissue-specific estrogen agonist or antagonist activity (34). The 3,4-dihydronaphthalene- and benzothiophene-containing SERMs are rigid analogs of the triphenylethylenes. The first SERM to be marketed for the treatment of osteoporosis was the benzothiophene raloxifene, an estrogen agonist at the bone (see Chapter 30). Discussion about the SERMs used in the treatment of breast cancer can be found later in this chapter.

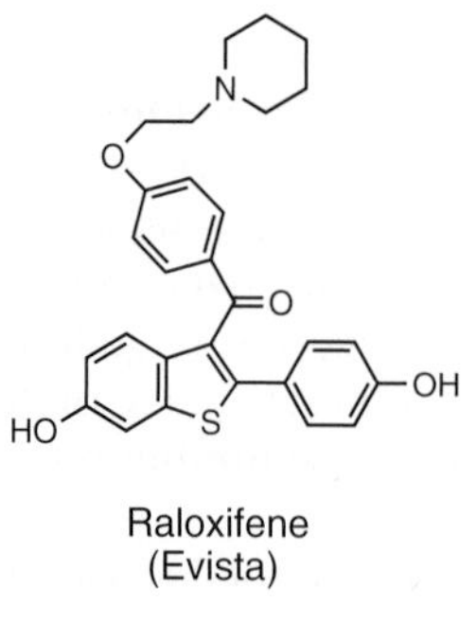

Raloxifene
(Evista)

AROMATASE INHIBITORS

Androstenedione Derivatives Inhibitors of aromatase block the conversion of androgens to estrogens and, therefore, have the therapeutic potential to control reproductive functions and aid in the treatment of estrogen-dependent cancers, such as breast cancer. These steroidal agents compete with androstenedione for the active site of the aromatase enzyme. The structure–activity relationships for steroidal aromatase inhibitors indicate that the best agents are substrate analogs, with only small structural changes to the A ring and at C_{19} permitted (Fig. 41.11). Analogs that contain aryl functionalities at the 7α position have enhanced affinity for the enzyme. In addition, 4-hydroxy-androstenedione, several androst-1,4-diene-3,17-diones, and 10β-propynylestr-4-ene-3,17-dione act as enzyme-activated irreversible

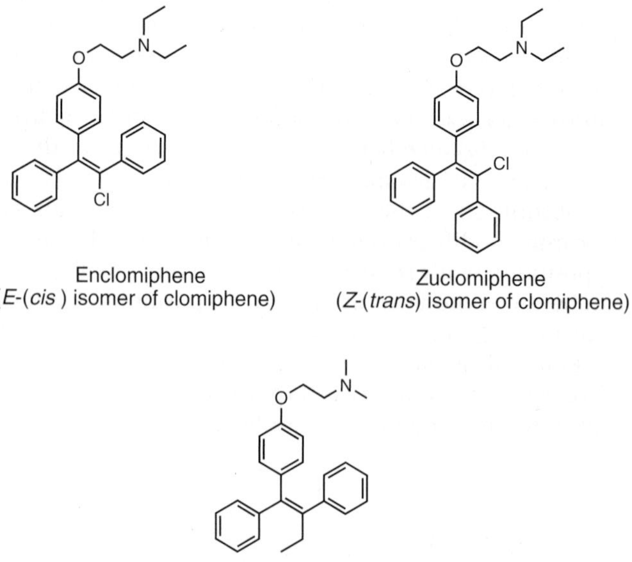

Enclomiphene
(*E*-(*cis*) isomer of clomiphene)

Zuclomiphene
(*Z*-(*trans*) isomer of clomiphene)

Tamoxifen
(*Z*-diastereomer)

FIGURE 41.10 Antiestrogens—triphenylethylene analogs.

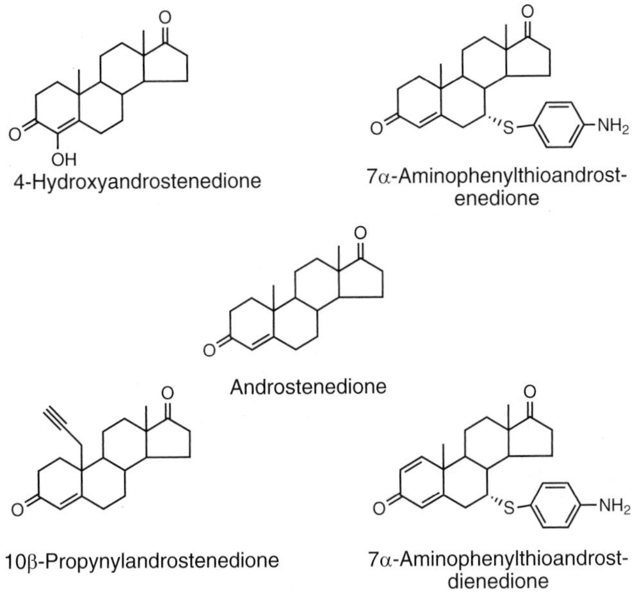

FIGURE 41.11 Androstenedione aromatase inhibitors.

inhibitors (suicide substrates) in vitro. Additional information about the use of aromatase inhibitors in the treatment of breast cancer can be found later in this chapter.

Triazole Derivatives Triazole-based aromatase inhibitors were developed based on the aromatase inhibitor aminoglutethimide (35,36) and include anastrozole (37) and letrozole (38) (Fig. 41.12). The triazoles inhibit aromatase as a result of the N-4 nitrogen of the triazole ring interaction with the heme iron atom of this CYP19 enzyme complex. Anastrozole and letrozole are competitive inhibitors of aromatase and selectively inhibit the conversion of testosterone to estrogens in all tissues and, thereby, reduce serum concentrations of circulating estrone, estradiol, and estrone sulfate. Because estrogen acts as a growth factor for hormone-dependent breast cancer cells, reduction of serum and tumor concentrations of estrogen inhibits tumor growth and delays disease progression. Ovarian production of estrogen declines in postmenopausal women, so the conversion of androstenedione and testosterone to estrone and estradiol in peripheral tissues becomes the primary source of estrogen. The structure–activity relationships of these inhibitors have

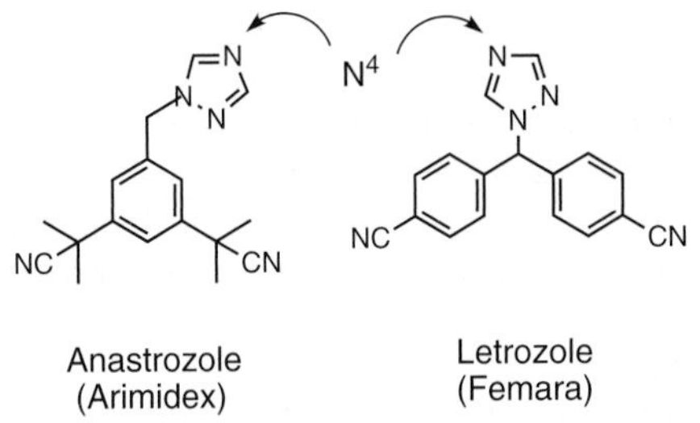

FIGURE 41.12 Triazole aromatase inhibitors.

been reviewed elsewhere (39–41). Additional information about the triazole derivatives as it relates to the treatment of breast cancer can be found later in this chapter.

Clinical Applications

Estrogens are used in the treatment of a wide variety of menstrual-related disturbances, including the management of menopausal symptoms (e.g., vulvar and vaginal atrophy); female hypoestrogenism resulting from hypogonadism, castration, or primary ovarian failure; and amenorrhea, dysmenorrhea, and oligomenorrhea. They also are effective in the management of ovarian development failure, acne, and senile vaginitis. After childbirth, estrogens have been used to suppress lactation in women who elect not to participate in breastfeeding. More detailed discussions about the clinical application of estrogens in the treatment of several disease states can be found later in this chapter.

Administration of estrogens may promote sodium retention and, as a result, cause retention of water and, possibly, edema. This effect, however, is less pronounced than that observed with the glucocorticoids. More detailed information regarding the pharmacology and toxicology of estrogens can be found in published reviews (5,24,42).

Progestins

Fraenkel (43) first observed in 1903 that removal of the corpus luteum shortly after conception resulted in pregnancy termination. In 1929, Corner and Allen (44) developed an assay method for progestogenic activity, and by 1934, the hormone progesterone had been isolated by several research groups (29).

Biosynthesis

Progesterone biosynthesis is initiated when LH, secreted from the anterior pituitary, binds to the target cell surface LH receptor. Activation of the LH receptor results in an increase of intracellular cyclic adenosine monophosphate (cAMP) levels via activation of a G protein and adenylate cyclase. In the presence of elevated concentrations of cAMP, cholesterol esterase activation occurs. This enzyme catalyzes the cleavage of cholesterol esters to free cholesterol, which is then converted in mitochondria to pregnenolone as described previously. The formation of progesterone from pregnenolone is catalyzed by 5-ene-3β-hydroxysteroid dehydrogenase and 3-oxosteroid-4,5-isomerase (steps c and d in Fig. 41.3).

Progesterone is secreted primarily from the ovaries (30 mg/day), particularly by the corpus luteum in reproductive-age women and by the placenta during pregnancy. Compared with the ovaries, the adrenal gland produces only a small fraction of progesterone (1 mg/day).

Metabolism

Progesterone is rapidly metabolized by the liver, regardless of the route of administration, and has a half-life of 5 to 10 minutes (Fig. 41.13). Progesterone is mainly excreted renally as the glucuronide and sulfate conjugates

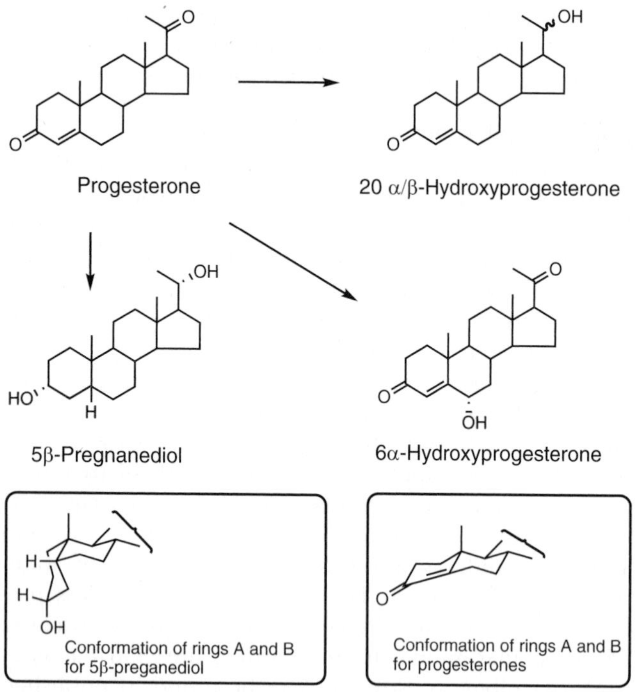

FIGURE 41.13 Metabolism of progesterone.

of 5β-pregnanediol. The glucuronide metabolite serves as an index of the corpus luteum activity, and a premature drop in its level may be a warning of possible miscarriage.

Other routes of metabolism include 6α-hydroxylation and reduction of the 20-ketone. These metabolites have no significant progestogenic activity. The formation of 5β-pregnanediol from progesterone is characterized by reduction of the 4,5-double bond to create a *cis* A/B ring juncture and reduction of the 3-ketone to a 3α-hydroxy group.

In the serum, progesterone is bound to either cortisol binding globulin or albumin, with only a small fraction being freely available. The metabolic clearance rate for progesterone is 2,100 to 2,500 L/day, for which protein binding has no role.

Mechanism of Progestin Action—Molecular Interactions

The progesterone receptor is a ligand-activated transcription factor and a member of the nuclear receptor superfamily. All nuclear receptors have three conserved functional domains, including the DNA binding domain, the N-terminal domain, and the C-terminal ligand binding domain (42). Very little is known about the structure of the N-terminal domain. The DNA binding domain contains two asymmetric zinc fingers with four cysteine residues coordinated to each zinc atom. Between the zinc fingers is an α helix, which has specific interactions with the DNA. The ligand binding domain is composed of 12 α helices and four β sheets that ultimately form a hydrophobic cavity in which the receptor agonist binds (45). When progesterone binds to its receptor, a conformational change in the receptor occurs, transforming it into an active transcriptional factor. Phosphorylation of the receptor occurs at this point, but it is unclear what biochemical role that plays. The receptor then undergoes dimerization to form PR-A and PR-B, which are not structurally identical. These isoforms have similar activities related to steroid hormone and DNA binding, but their functional activities are unique. The dimer interacts with specific nuclear DNA sequences (hormone response elements) within progesterone-responsive genes. The receptor agonist–receptor dimer complex combines with coactivators that link the complex to gene transcription (46). The rate of gene transcription is then either increased or decreased. Once gene transcription is initiated, proteins are biosynthesized, and physiologic effects are observed in target cells and organs.

Physiologic Effects

The primary physiologic site of action of progesterone is the uterus. It acts on both the endometrium (inner mucous lining) and the myometrium (muscle mass) of the uterus. The effect of progesterone on the endometrium, already primed by estrogens, is to induce the secretory phase of the menstrual cycle. During this phase, the endometrial glands grow and secrete large amounts of carbohydrates that can be used by the fertilized ovum as an energy source. The primary function of progesterone with respect to the myometrium is to stop spontaneous rhythmic contractions of the uterus.

Progesterone often is referred to as the "hormone of pregnancy." For the first trimester, the corpus luteum serves as the primary source of progesterone, at which point the developing placenta takes over as the major source of progesterone and estrogen. The high level of progesterone that is produced during pregnancy sends a signal to the hypothalamus via the negative feedback system to prevent release of the FSH and LH necessary for the development of new ova.

In general, the nonreproductive effects of progesterone are fairly insignificant. Progesterone is able to antagonize the actions of aldosterone, and as a result, there is an increase in sodium excretion. When sodium levels drop, aldosterone secretion is stimulated, and sodium is retained (47). It has been suggested that the temperature-raising effect of progesterone may be the result of a reduction in perspiration. This effect is not unique to progesterone, because other steroids in the pregnane and androstane series have a similar effect (48).

Ovarian biosynthesis and secretion of progesterone is controlled by the release of LH from the anterior pituitary during ovulation. The LH induces progesterone secretion from the corpus luteum during the second half of the menstrual cycle. If conception does not occur, the corpus luteum degenerates, and progesterone production decreases. As progesterone levels drop, endometrial sloughing occurs—otherwise known as menstruation.

Side Effects

Characteristic progestin-related side effects include nausea and vomiting, drowsiness, and breakthrough and irregular bleeding. With prolonged therapy, a greater incidence of these effects may occur, along with edema and weight gain, breast pain, decreased libido, and masculinization of the female fetus.

Structure–Activity Relationships

Progestin activity is restricted to those molecules with a steroid nucleus. The synthetic progestins generally can be divided into two steroidal classes: the androstanes (including the 19-norandrostanes), and the pregnanes (including the 19-norpregnanes) (46–51). In the androstane series, a 17α-substituent, such as ethynyl, methyl, ethyl, and variations of these, provides oral bioavailability.

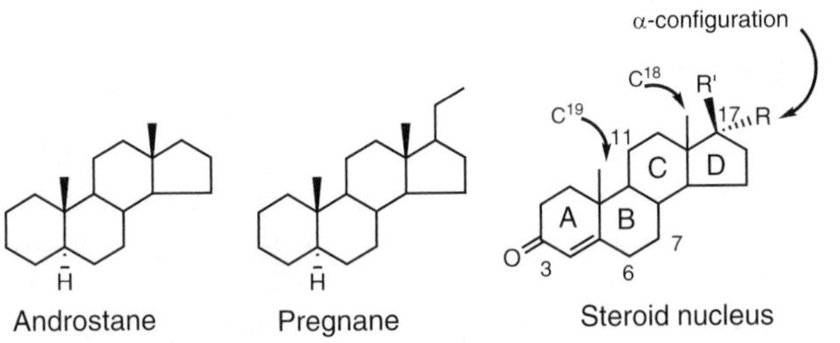

Ethisterone (17β-hydroxy-17α-ethynyl progesterone) (Fig. 41.14), the first androstane found to be effective, has only about one-third the activity of progesterone when delivered subcutaneously, but is 15-fold more active than progesterone when administered orally. Closely related to testosterone, this progestin has significant androgenic activity. Removal of the CH_3 group at position 19 leads to norethindrone (norethisterone; 19-norandrostane) (Fig. 41.14), which has 5- to 10-fold more progestin activity. The activity of norethindrone is increased further by the addition of a chlorine substituent at position 21 (blocks metabolic hydroxylation) or by the addition of a methyl group at carbon 18 (norgestrel) (Fig. 41.14). Ethynodiol diacetate, another 19-norandrostane, is an extremely potent oral progestin. It is more active when administered orally than parenterally and, when combined with an estrogen, is effective as an OC.

Further unsaturation of the B or C ring of androstane derivatives usually enhances progestin activity. Introduction of a halogen or methyl substituent in the 6α or 7α positions generally increases hormonal activity. Acetylation of the 17β-OH of norethindrone increases the duration of action of the drug. Removal of the 3-keto function of norethindrone allows retention of potent progestin activity without androgenic effects.

Activity of the pregnanes and 19-norpregnanes is enhanced by unsaturation at C_6 and C_7 and by substitution of a methyl group or a halogen at C_6. This activity

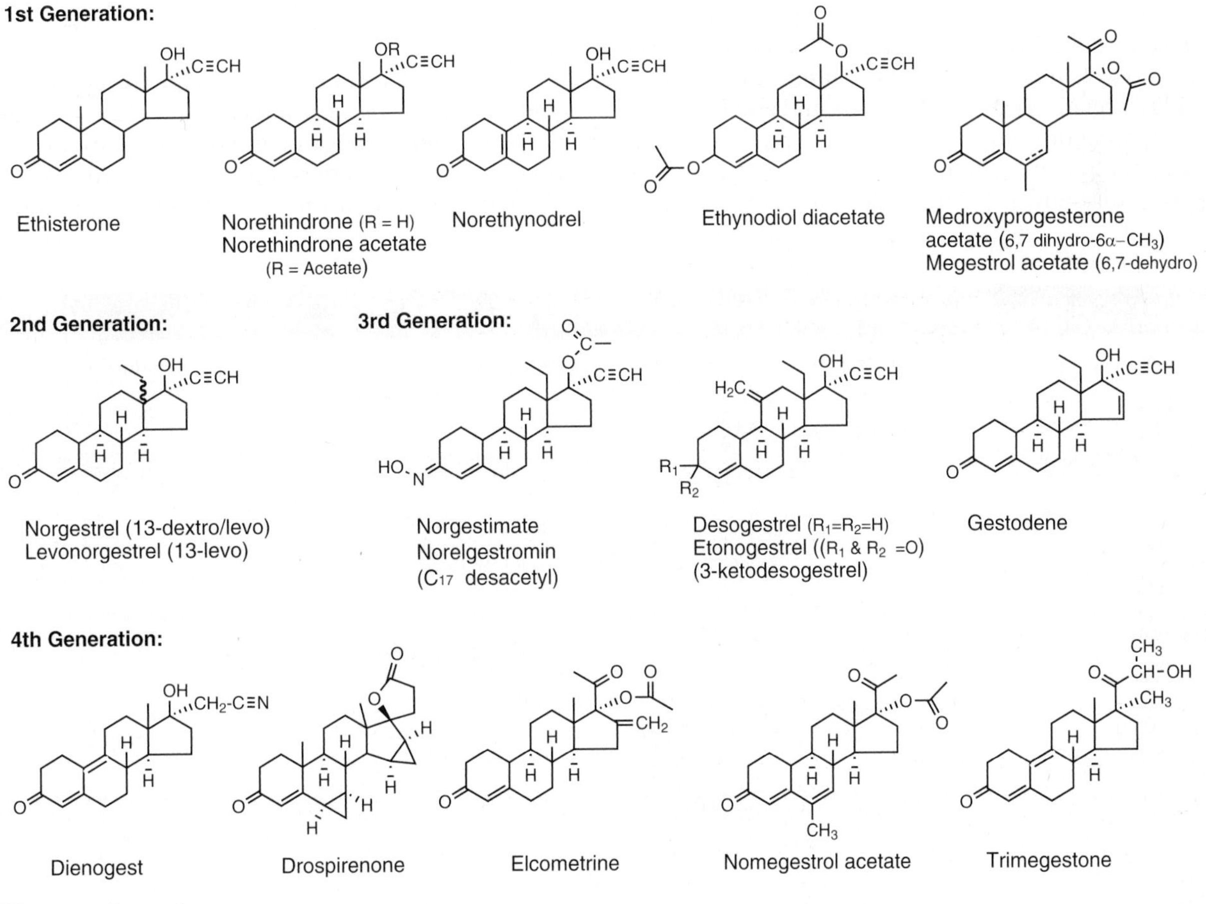

FIGURE 41.14 Progestins.

may be further increased by introducing a CH_3 group at C_{11}. These substitutions prevent metabolic reduction of the two carbonyl groups and metabolic oxidation at C_6. Substitution of a fluoro group at C_{21} prevents metabolic hydroxylation and enhances oral effectiveness.

Because glucocorticoid receptor activity is not desirable yet is innate to those derivatives that bind with high affinity to the progesterone receptor, structural alterations have been investigated to pare out this biologic activity. Small B-ring substituents serve to decrease glucocorticoid action, as do substituents at the C_{17} position.

Synthetic Progestins

Early generations of the progestins were used primarily for contraceptive purposes, so antigonadotropic activity was considered to be desirable. Unfortunately, many of these agents were plagued by androgenic activity and the corresponding adverse effects (Table 41.7) (11). Development of newer progestins is now focused on analogs with improved progesterone receptor selectivity (Table 41.8) and little or no effect on the androgen, estrogen, or glucocorticoid receptors (43). From a structural perspective, these synthetic progestins contain either a pregnane or androstane steroid nucleus.

Not only can the progestins be classified by type of steroid ring system, they also can be organized by generation. The first-generation agents include the pregnanes (medroxyprogesterone acetate, megestrol acetate, 17α-acetoxy progesterone) (Fig. 41.14), the androstanes (ethisterone, dimethisterone), and the 19-norandrostanes (norethynodrel, norethindrone, norethindrone acetate, ethynodiol acetate) (Fig. 41.14). Norgestrel and levonorgestrel (19-norandrostanes) are two of the predominant agents in the second generation (Fig. 41.14). The levonorgestrel derivatives (19-norandrostanes) desogestrel, gestodene, and norgestimate compose the third generation (Fig. 41.14), and the newer, fourth generation includes nomegestrol acetate (19-norpregnane) and trimegestone (pregnane) (Fig. 41.14). In addition, there is one nonethynylated 19-norandrostane, dienogest, and one spironolactone derivative, drospirenone, to round out the fourth generation (43). The antiandrogenic activity associated with several fourth-generation agents (e.g., trimegestone, drospirenone, and dienogest) makes this group of progestins unique (Table 41.7) (11). Trimegestone and elcometrine are the most potent progestins, with the third-generation levonorgestrel and etonogestrel (3-ketodesogestrel) being slightly less potent (Table 41.8).

Progesterone and Its Derivatives

Progesterone has a significant role in priming the uterine endometrium for implantation of a potential blastocyst. It also is involved in formation of the placenta postimplantation, the development of mammary glands, and by preventing contraction of the uterine musculature, pregnancy maintenance. Progesterone also has inhibitory roles, including ovulation prevention via an antigonadotropic effect and inhibition of the conversion of testosterone to dihydrotestosterone, an active metabolite, by virtue of its ability to be a substrate for 5α-reductase (46). Interestingly, progesterone reduces nuclear ER levels and induces 17-hydroxysteroid dehydrogenase, the enzyme that catalyzes the conversion of estradiol to the less potent estrone (52,53).

There are some limitations as to how progesterone can be administered, because it has relatively low bioavailability when administered orally. The pharmacokinetics for progesterone and its derivatives are listed in Table 41.6. To achieve consistent therapeutic benefit, progesterone

TABLE 41.7 Hormonal Activities of Representative Progestins (11)

Progestogen	Antiestrogenic	Androgenic	Antiandrogenic	Glucocorticoid	Antimineralocorticoid
Progesterone	++	–	+	++	++
Medroxyprogesterone acetate	++	+	–	++	–
Norethisterone (1)	++	++	–	–	–
Levonorgestrel (2)	++	++	–	–	–
Etonogestrel (3)	++	++	–	+	–
Norgestimate (3)	++	++	–	?	?
Drospirenone (4)	++	–	++	–	++
Elcometrine (4)	++	–	–	–	?
Nomegestrol acetate (4)	++	–	++	–	–
Trimegestone (4)	++	–	+	–	+
Dienogest (4)	++	–	++	–	–

The numbers in parentheses indicate the generation of progestogen. ++, effective; +, weekly effective; –, not effective; ?, unknown.

TABLE 41.8 Steroid Receptor Binding Affinities (11,43)

Progestogen	Progesterone	Androgen	Glucocorticoid	Mineralocorticoid
Progesterone	50	0	10	100
Medroxyprogesterone acetate (1)	115	5	29	160
Norethisterone (1)	75	15	0	0
Levonorgestrel (2)	150	45	1	75
Etonogestrel (3)	150	20	14	0
Norgestimate (3)	15	0	1	0
Gestodene (3)	90	85	27	290
Drospirenone (4)	35	65	6	230
Elcometrine (4)	136	0	38	?
Nomegestrol acetate (4)	125	42	6	0
Trimegestone (4)	330	1	9	120
Dienogest (4)	5	10	1	0

The numbers in parentheses indicate the generation of progestogen.

must be administered either by injection or intravaginally. Progesterone may need to be administered over a relatively long period of time to maintain a pregnancy, so it is important to note that neither of the two routes just mentioned is without significant adverse effects. As a result, development of orally active derivatives has been a significant priority.

MEDROXYPROGESTERONE ACETATE The initial structural modifications made to progesterone led to only weakly active or inactive analogs. For example, 17α-acetoxyprogesterone had limited activity when administered orally (54). Further structural modification of 17α-acetoxyprogesterone was aimed at limiting metabolic hydroxylation at C_6. This was accomplished by the addition of a C_6 substituent, and the resulting analog displayed improved biologic activity (51).

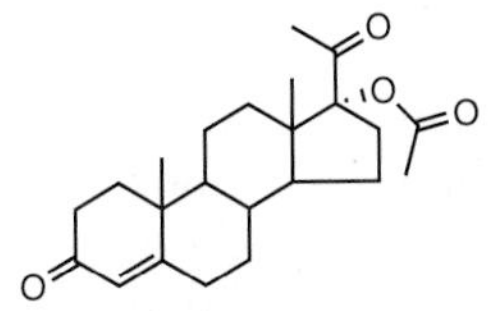

17α-Acetoxyprogesterone

Among the first of these substituted 17α-acetoxyprogesterone analogs to be used therapeutically was medroxyprogesterone acetate, a 6α-methyl progesterone analog (Fig. 41.14) (55). This analog is 25-fold more active than ethisterone. Following oral administration, medroxyprogesterone acetate is completely and rapidly deacetylated by first-pass metabolism to medroxyprogesterone. Medroxyprogesterone is extensively metabolized via pathways similar to those for progesterone, except for 6α-hydroxylation. Most medroxyprogesterone acetate metabolites are excreted in the urine, primarily as glucuronide conjugates. Plasma protein binding for medroxyprogesterone is approximately 86%, primarily to serum albumin, with no binding to SHBG.

MEGESTROL ACETATE (MEGACE) Progestin activity is further enhanced when a double bond is introduced between positions 6 and 7, as is found in megestrol acetate (Fig. 41.14). Megestrol is used primarily in the treatment of breast and endometrial carcinomas and in postmenopausal women with advanced hormone-dependent carcinoma. Less than 10% of an oral dose undergoes metabolism. Several major metabolites appear in the urine (e.g., 2-hydroxy and 6-hydroxymethyl megestrol and their glucuronide conjugates).

Synthetic Progestins

ETHISTERONE AND ITS ANALOGS Ethisterone (Fig. 41.14), a 17α-ethynyl derivative of testosterone, is one of the first synthetic progestins to be used therapeutically. In 1937, this agent was synthesized from male sex hormones (androstanes) in an attempt to find an orally active androgen (56). Ethisterone later proved to be an effective oral progestin and became useful in the treatment of menstrual dysfunctions (52). Several molecular modifications of ethisterone have improved progestogenic action, including introduction of methyl groups in the $C_{6\alpha}$ and C_{21} positions (42).

A second breakthrough was made in 1944, when Ehrenstein (57) discovered that the C_{19} methyl group is not necessary for progestogenic activity. In fact, this work showed that loss of the C_{19} methyl results in analogs with activity equal to or greater than that of parenterally administered progesterone. In 1953, Djerassi et al. (58) synthesized 19-norprogesterone. This drug differed from the natural hormone only in replacement of the C_{19} angular methyl group with a hydrogen atom. When administered parenterally, this analog was eightfold more active than progesterone and, at the time, was the most potent progestin known. While these drugs were important compounds in the development of the progestins, none are used singly or in combination today.

Norethindrone/Norethisterone and Norethynodrel Research on 19-norsteroids as potential progestins culminated in the synthesis of two potent, orally active progestins, norethindrone and norethynodrel (Fig. 41.14) (49). These two substances were among the first 19-norsteroids to be used clinically for progesterone-related disorders. When combined with estrogens, such as EE or mestranol, these agents were effective contraceptives. Because the progestogenic action of norethynodrel is approximately one-tenth that of norethindrone, it is no longer used in OC formulations. Although norethindrone is a weak androgen, it does not exhibit any glucocorticoid or antimineralocorticoid activity (Table 41.7).

After oral administration, norethindrone acetate is completely and rapidly deacetylated by hepatic and intestinal first-pass metabolism to norethindrone, with an oral bioavailability of approximately 64%. Subsequent metabolism of norethindrone includes reduction of the Δ^4 double bond to both the 5α- and 5β-dihydronorethindrone products as well as reduction of the ketone. The pharmacokinetics for norethindrone acetate are indistinguishable from those of orally administered norethindrone. Roughly 36% of norethindrone is bound to SHBG, and 61% is bound to albumin (11).

Norethindrone acetate also can be administered transdermally along with estradiol when formulated as a patch. This combination of hormones can be used as part of either a continuous or a cyclic hormone replacement regimen.

Norgestrel and Levonorgestrel Norgestrel is formulated as a racemic mixture despite the fact that only its levo isomer, levonorgestrel, is pharmacologically active (Fig. 41.14). Levonorgestrel exhibits some androgenic activity but no glucocorticoid or antimineralocorticoid action. Levonorgestrel can be administered orally, transdermally (combined with estradiol and formulated as a 7-day patch), and for prolonged, continuous use, via an intrauterine device (IUD). The oral bioavailability of levonorgestrel is approximately 95% (11). From a protein binding perspective, 48% of an oral dose is bound to SHBG, and 50% is bound to albumin. Levonorgestrel undergoes metabolic reduction of its ketone and is hydroxylated.

Norgestimate and Desogestrel Norgestimate (Fig. 41.14) is considered to be a pro-progestin (prodrug), because it rapidly undergoes a two-step metabolic transformation to form two active products, norelgestromine (levonorgestrel 3-oxime) and levonorgestrel (Fig. 41.14). Deacetylation occurs in the intestine and liver, whereas conversion of the 3-oxime to the corresponding ketone occurs primarily in the liver. Unlike the other progestins mentioned, norgestimate and its metabolites are not bound to SHBG.

Norgestimate exhibits high selectivity for the progesterone receptor and low androgenic activity as a result of a large drug-induced increase in the production of SHBG. As a component of both mono- and triphasic OC formulations, this progestin exhibits fewer androgenic side effects, including less of a detrimental effect on the patient's lipid profile and lack of significant weight gain (58). Rates of breakthrough bleeding were lower with a triphasic regimen including norgestimate compared to a monophasic regimen containing norethindrone acetate. Norgestimate is metabolized to norelgestromine, the primary active metabolite and the active progestin found in the contraceptive patch (Ortho Evra).

Desogestrel also is a prodrug and is rapidly metabolized in the intestinal mucosa and via first pass through the liver to its active metabolite, etonogestrel (3-ketodesogestrel) (Fig. 41.14). Following oral administration, the relative bioavailability for desogestrel is approximately 84%. Desogestrel also exhibits high selectivity for the progesterone receptor and low androgenic activity, and it does not diminish the beneficial effects of estrogen on the lipid profile. The rates of breakthrough bleeding are low with the monophasic desogestrel/EE formulation, which has improved therapy discontinuation percentages. Unfortunately, there is evidence that suggests that there is a twofold increase in the risk of venous thromboembolism with desogestrel-containing preparations (59).

Gestodene Unlike the other members of the third generation of progestins, gestodene is not a prodrug (Fig. 41.14). It exhibits nearly 100% oral bioavailability and excellent receptor binding affinity for the progesterone receptor. Because the SHBG level is considered to be a surrogate marker for venous thromboembolism (VTE) risk, it is important to note that an increase in SHBG levels is evident both in monophasic combination OC preparations (200% to 300% increase) and in triphasic preparations (150% increase) that contain gestodene (60). Both the monophasic and triphasic preparations also cause an increase in triglyceride and total cholesterol levels, although the increase is smaller in magnitude than those associated with desogestrel and norgestimate. An increase in high-density lipoprotein (HDL) levels was not observed (61). The effectiveness of a gestodene/EE sustained-release, matrix-type transdermal patch (weekly administration) is currently under investigation. Products containing gestodene are available in Europe, but not the United States.

Dienogest, Drospirenone, Elcometrine, Nomegestrol Acetate, and Trimegestone Classified as a testosterone-like, norethindrone-related progestin, dienogest is structurally unique in that it contains an estrane skeleton, a C_{17} cyanomethyl group that replaces the C_{17} ethynyl group, and Δ^9 unsaturation (Fig. 41.14). An effective OC preparation results when dienogest is combined with EE or estradiol valerate (Fig. 41.6). The OC preparation of dienogest/estradiol valerate is the first to be used in a four-phase dosage regimen (Natazia). The pharmacologic profile for this progestin includes antiandrogenic action similar to drospirenone (see below) without the risk of hyperkalemia. Correction of menopausal symptoms results when dienogest is combined with estradiol valerate. Limited evidence suggests that this combination has a positive impact on cognition, which is in direct opposition to the Women's Health Initiative (WHI) study data regarding the combination of medroxyprogesterone acetate and conjugated estrogens. Dienogest bioavailability is approximately 90%, and it is metabolized extensively by the CYP3A4 pathway. Coadministration of inhibitors or inducers of CYP3A4 will alter plasma concentrations of dienogest and, as a result, cause deviation from therapeutic efficacy.

Derived from spironolactone, drospirenone (Fig. 41.14) is the only progestin with antimineralocorticoid activity. Its affinity for the mineralocorticoid receptor is fivefold greater than that of aldosterone. Drospirenone has progestogenic action, but only 10% that of levonorgestrel. Drospirenone also has antiandrogenic action because it blocks testosterone from binding to androgenic receptors; however, it does not exhibit estrogenic or glucocorticoid receptor activity.

This androstane-based progestin has several distinctive functional groups: two cyclopropyl groups, one that includes C_6 and C_7 and the other C_{15} and C_{16}, and a C_{17} lactone. When combined with EE, drospirenone is effective in a monophasic OC (Table 41.9). In addition, drospirenone plus estradiol (Angeliq) is used in the treatment of various menopausal symptoms. The unique antimineralocorticoid activity of drospirenone effectively negates the side effects related to angiotensinogen production (causing an increase in sodium and water retention) associated with EE. Remarkably, within the first several cycles, women actually lost weight when using this combination of hormones (46). Regrettably, this benefit was lost, and statistically significant weight gain occurred as the number of cycles approached 13 (59). Drospirenone can cause potassium retention, and therefore, hyperkalemia is a possibility in patients concurrently taking other potassium-sparing drugs including nonsteroidal anti-inflammatory drugs, diuretics, angiotensin-converting enzyme inhibitors, and/or potassium chloride.

Elcometrine (Fig. 41.14) is a member of the 19-norprogesterone class of progestins. When administered subcutaneously (implant), intravaginally (vaginal ring), or transdermally, elcometrine is an exceptionally potent progestin. It is 100-fold more potent when administered subcutaneously than when delivered orally. Its oral bioavailability is only 10%, with a half-life of just 1 to 2 hours because of rapid metabolism (11). The C_{16} methylene functionality substantially increases its affinity for the progesterone receptor. Elcometrine does not bind to the androgenic receptor and, therefore, does not possess either androgenic or antiandrogenic activity (11). Unfortunately, like medroxyprogesterone acetate, elcometrine has affinity for the glucocorticoid receptor, although adverse effects were noted only at exceptionally high doses. Because of its antiestrogenic action, elcometrine also can be administered transdermally along with estradiol as a treatment for menopausal symptoms (46). From a protein binding perspective, elcometrine does not bind to SHBG but, rather, to albumin (11). This progestin is not available in the United States but is marketed in several Spanish-speaking countries.

Nomegestrol acetate (Fig. 41.14) is structurally similar to megestrol acetate but lacks the angular C_{19} methyl group. It has substantially better selectivity for the progesterone receptor and higher potency than medroxyprogesterone acetate. Nomegestrol acetate has potent antigonadotropic action and, therefore, is an appropriate progestin to use in an OC preparation. It exhibits no glucocorticoid, antimineralocorticoid, or androgenic activity; however, it does demonstrate significant antiandrogenic action (11). This progestin is bound primarily to albumin. Like desogestrel, it does not diminish the beneficial effects of estrogen on the lipid profile (11).

Trimegestone, the most potent of the 19-norprogesterones, contains an unusual C_{21} hydroxyl group (Fig. 41.14). It has very high affinity for the progesterone receptor but only weak affinity for the mineralocorticoid receptor. Trimegestone displays no glucocorticoid, androgenic, or antiandrogenic action. This progestin undergoes metabolic hydroxylation to produce metabolites with substantial progestogenic action. Either alone or in combination with estradiol, trimegestone has shown favorable results regarding bone loss and bone turnover (46). Given with estradiol, this hormone replacement therapy (HRT) combination is effective in the treatment of postmenopausal symptoms regardless of whether it is administered continuously or as part of cyclic therapy. Like desogestrel and nomegestrol acetate, this progestin does not diminish the beneficial effects of estrogen on the lipid profile (11). Although available outside of the United States, this progestin is not presently marketed in the United States.

CHLORMADINONE ACETATE

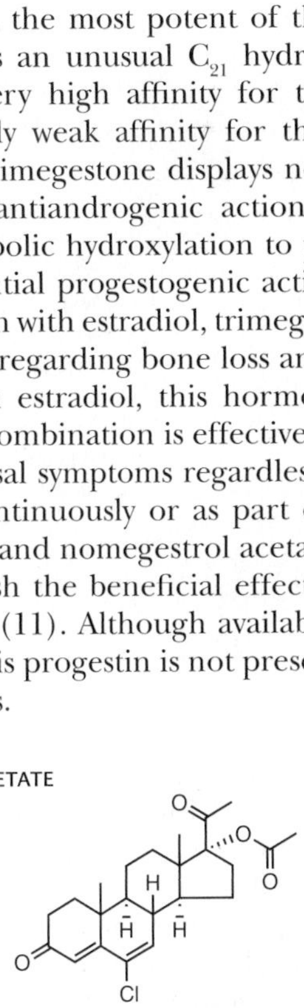

Chlormadinone acetate was first synthesized in 1961 and is a progestin with a pharmacologic profile that

TABLE 41.9 Components of a Representative Set of Oral Contraceptives (74)

Type of Contraceptive	Trade Name	Estrogen	Progestin
Monophasic combination oral contraceptives	Lybrel (continuous)	EE (20 mcg)	Levonorgestrel (0.09 mg)
	Aviane	EE (20 mcg)	Levonorgestrel (0.1 mg)
	Loestrin-21	EE (20 mcg)	Norethindrone acetate (1 mg)
	YAZ	EE (20 mcg)	Drospirenone (3 mg)
	Yasmin	EE (30 mcg)	Drospirenone (3 mg)
	Loestrin-21	EE (30 mcg)	Norethindrone acetate (1.5 mg)
	Lo/Ovral	EE (30 mcg)	Norgestrel (0.3 mg)
	Desogen	EE (30 mcg)	Desogestrel (0.15 mg)
	Ortho-Cept	EE (30 mcg)	Desogestrel (0.15 mg)
	Levora	EE (30 mcg)	Levonorgestrel (0.15 mg)
	Nordette-28	EE (30 mcg)	Levonorgestrel (0.15 mg)
	Jolessa (3 months)	EE (30 mcg)	Levonorgestrel (0.15 mg)
	Seasonale (3 months)	EE (30 mcg)	Levonorgestrel (0.15 mg)
	Necon 1/35	EE (35 mcg)	Norethindrone (1 mg)
	Modicon	EE (35 mcg)	Norethindrone (0.5 mg)
	Femcon Fe (chewable)	EE (35 mcg)	Norethindrone (0.4 mg) + 7 ferrous fumarate tabs
	Balziva	EE (35 mcg)	Norethindrone (0.4 mg)
	Ortho-Cyclen	EE (35 mcg)	Norgestimate (0.25 mg)
	Zovia 1/35E	EE (35 mcg)	Ethynodiol diacetate (1 mg)
	Ovcon-50	EE (50 mcg)	Norethindrone (1 mg)
	Zovia 1/50E	EE (50 mcg)	Ethynodiol diacetate (1 mg)
	Ovral	EE (50 mcg)	Norgestrel (0.5 mg)
	Ortho-Novum 1/50	Mestranol (50 mcg)	Norethindrone (1 mg)
	Beyaz	EE 20 mcg	Drospirenone (3 mg) + 0.0451 mg levomefolate calcium
	Safyral	EE 30 mcg	Drospirenone (3 mg) + 451 mcg levomefolate calcium
Biphasic combination oral contraceptives	Mircette	EE (20 mcg) days 1–21	Desogestrel (0.15 mg)
	Ortho-Novum 10/11	EE (10 mcg) days 24–28	Desogestrel (0.0 mg)
	LoSeasonique (3 months)	EE (35 mcg)	Norethindrone (0.5 mg)
	Seasonique (3 months)	EE (35 mcg)	Norethindrone (1 mg)
	LO Loestrin Fe	EE (20 mcg)	Levonorgestrel (0.1 mg)
		EE (10 mcg)	Levonorgestrel (0.0 mg)
		EE (30 mcg)	Levonorgestrel (0.15 mg)
		EE (10 mcg)	Levonorgestrel (0.0 mg)
		EE (10 mcg)	Norethindrone (1 mg)
		EE (10 mcg)	Norethindrone (0 mg)
Triphasic combination oral contraceptives	Tri-Legest	EE (20/30/35 mcg)	Norethindrone acetate (1 mg)
	Cyclessa	EE (25 mcg)	Desogestrel (0.1/0.125/0.15 mg)
	Ortho TriCyclen Lo	EE (25 mcg)	Norgestimate (0.18/0.215/0.25 mg)
	Trivora	EE (30/40/30 mcg)	Levonorgestrel (0.05/0.075/0.125 mg)
	Ortho TriCyclen	EE (35 mcg)	Norgestimate (0.18/0.215/0.25 mg)
	Ortho Novum 7/7/7	EE (35 mcg)	Norethindrone (0.5/0.75/1 mg)
	Ananelle	EE (35 mcg)	Norethindrone (0.5/1/0.5 mg)
4-Phasic combination oral contraceptive	Natazia	Estradiol valerate (30/20/20/10 mcg)	Dienogest (0/2/3/0 mg)
Progestin-only agents	Ortho Micronor		Norethindrone (0.35 mg)

EE, ethinyl estradiol.

includes a high affinity for the progesterone receptor, antiestrogenic action, and moderate antiandrogenic activity (62). Unlike progesterone, chlormadinone acetate acts as a weak glucocorticoid agonist, is a competitive inhibitor of 5α-reductase, and has no antimineralocorticoid activity. Chlormadinone acetate effectively suppresses gonadotropin secretion, thereby preventing follicular growth and maturation. The mechanisms associated with its contraceptive efficacy are similar to other progestins. It is five times more potent than norethindrone. Combined with EE (Belara; not U.S. Food and Drug Administration [FDA] approved), it is an effective OC with a good side effect profile, including excellent resolution of mild to moderate acne. The thromboembolic risk associated with this progestin is not significant. Like elcometrine and nomegestrol, chlormadinone acetate is bound to albumin.

17α-Hydroxyprogesterone Caproate (Gestiva)

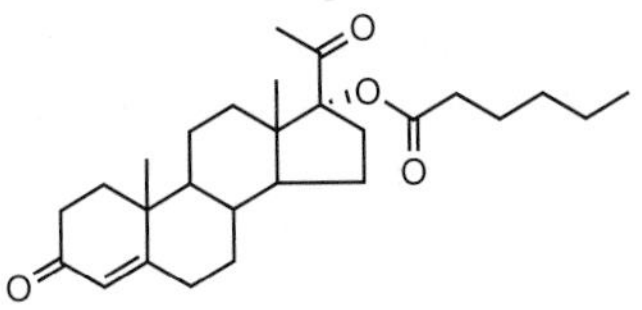

17α-Hydroxyprogesterone caproate

Originally marketed (Delalutin) nearly 50 years ago to prevent impending miscarriages, 17α-hydroxyprogesterone caproate was removed from the market in 2000 when its efficacy was called into question. 17α-Hydroxyprogesterone caproate, a synthetic injectable progesterone, was approved by the FDA in 2011 to reduce the risk of preterm delivery in women who have already experienced a preterm birth. It has not been shown to be effective in women carrying multiple fetuses. Injections begin between 16 and 21 weeks and are associated with pain, swelling, or itching at the injection site, hives, nausea, and diarrhea. Follow-up studies of the children born to women who used this drug indicate that developmental milestones were achieved at 2.5 and 5 years of age (63). A number of other pharmacologic agents are currently available for the prevention of preterm delivery including agents that can alter intracellular messengers (e.g., β-adrenergic receptor agonists, nitric oxide donors, magnesium sulfate and calcium channel blockers) and agents that modulate myometrial stimulants (e.g., inhibitors of prostaglandin synthesis and oxytocin antagonists) (64).

17α-Hydroxyprogesterone caproate binds extensively to albumin and SHBG. From a metabolic perspective, it undergoes reduction, hydroxylation, and conjugation reactions, including becoming glucuronidated, sulfated, and acetylated. It induces several cytochrome P450 (CYP) isozymes including CYP1A2, CYP2A6, and CYP2B6 (65).

Progestin Antagonists

An antiprogestin is a substance that competes with progesterone for its receptor and, ultimately, prevents progesterone from binding to and activating its receptor. Because progesterone is integral to the continuation of an early pregnancy, it is expected that antiprogestins will interfere with pregnancy maintenance. In 1982, the first antiprogestin, mifepristone (RU 486), was reported (66).

Mifepristone (Mifeprex) Mifepristone was shown to interrupt early stages of implantation and pregnancy in humans (Fig. 41.15) (67). After oral administration, mifepristone is rapidly absorbed, with a peak plasma concentration in approximately 90 minutes, an oral bioavailability of approximately 70%, and a terminal elimination half-life of 18 hours. It is 98% protein bound, primarily to albumin and α_1-acid glycoprotein. Mifepristone is metabolized primarily via CYP3A4 pathways involving mono- and di-oxidative *N*-demethylation and terminal hydroxylation of the 17-propynyl chain. The fact that approximately 83% of the drug is recovered in the feces and 9% in the urine suggests a biliary route of elimination. Mifepristone also demonstrates antiglucocorticoid activity (68).

Additional antiprogestin analogs, such as onapristone (ZK 98,299), exhibit less antiglucocorticoid activity (69). These antiprogestins also have demonstrated therapeutic potential for the treatment of hormone-dependent breast cancer (70). Telapristone acetate (Proellex) is in early clinical trial for the treatment of symptomatic uterine fibroids and amenorrhea.

Ulipristal Acetate (ellaOne) Ulipristal acetate (FDA approved in 2010) is a synthetic progestin used similarly to levonorgestrel in the prevention of pregnancy following unprotected intercourse or suspected contraceptive failure (Fig. 41.15). It is not intended for routine use as a contraceptive.

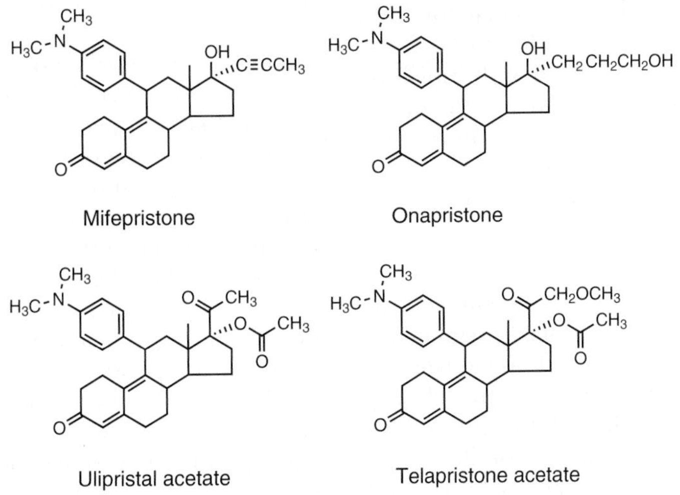

FIGURE 41.15 Progesterone antagonists.

The mechanism by which ulipristal acetate exerts its effect is dependent on when it is administered during the menstrual cycle. As a selective progesterone receptor modulator, it can delay or inhibit ovulation (progesterone agonist action) or alter the endometrium to prevent uterine implantation (progesterone antagonist action). If used within 120 hours of unprotected intercourse, ulipristal acetate reduces the pregnancy rate when compared to the rate in the absence of emergency contraception (71). Ulipristal acetate has very high affinity for the progesterone receptors, and it may reduce the effectiveness of hormonal contraceptive methods. Once administered as emergency contraception, it is recommended that a barrier method of contraception should be used for the remainder of that menstrual cycle.

Adverse events reported during clinical trials do not differ significantly from those found with other progestins and include headache (18%), abdominal pain (12%), and nausea (12%). Subsequent menses may occur later or earlier by a few days following use of ulipristal acetate (71).

Ulipristal acetate is metabolized to mono- and di-*N*-demethylated metabolites via CYP3A4, with the mono-*N*-demethylated metabolite retaining pharmacologic activity. Coadministration of inducers of CYP3A4 (e.g., carbamazepine, St. John's wort) will likely reduce the effectiveness of ulipristal acetate, and coadministration of inhibitors of CYP3A4 will cause an increase in therapeutic action (71).

Selective progesterone receptor modulators that are continuously administered have been evaluated as effective estrogen-free contraception and as treatment for the heavy and irregular menstrual bleeding associated with fibroids. Weekly oral administration and intrauterine and vaginal routes are under investigation (72,73).

THERAPEUTIC APPLICATIONS

A woman's reproductive life cycle spans nearly four decades. During this time, her hormonal status and ability to reproduce vary considerably. The need for hormonal intervention during this time period varies from person to person and, typically, requires highly individualized medication regimens. The remainder of this chapter will focus on hormonal and selected nonhormonal therapies for the management of contraception, endometriosis, infertility, menopause, and breast cancer.

Contraceptive Methods

Despite the availability of a wide variety of contraceptive methods and technologies, nearly half of all pregnancies in the United States are unplanned, and one-fourth are terminated. You might expect that cost, adverse effects, and inconvenience would be some of the hurdles to achieving contraceptive efficacy, but one of the greatest barriers is ineffective patient education (74). Despite ease of use, nearly 50% of those patients who have chosen an OC regimen discontinue their therapy within a year (75). If information regarding potential side effects, dosing requirements, and how the therapy is able to prevent pregnancy is provided in an accessible fashion, however, there may be many fewer patients who discontinue their contraceptive therapy (74,76,77).

Behavioral and Barrier Methods

Behavioral methods, such as natural family planning, fertility awareness, coitus interruptus, and lactation infertility, typically result in the highest pregnancy rates of all of the contraceptive methods. To be effective, these methods require disciplined effort on the part of the patient and her partner and somewhat detailed patient training. Barrier methods, such as male and female condoms (FC2 approved by FDA in 2009; FC1 approved by FDA in 1993), diaphragms, Today Sponge (including nonoxynol-9 spermicide; FDA approved in 2005), and cervical caps, still require a very conscientious and often preplanned effort on the part of the patient as well as fairly detailed patient training. Unplanned pregnancy rates with these barrier methods are approximately 12% to 15%.

Pharmacologic contraception, including OCs, patches, vaginal rings, IUDs, and injectable medications, provides substantially lower pregnancy rates with diligent use, relatively limited patient effort, and patient education that is focused largely on adverse effects.

Combination Oral Contraceptives

Available since the early 1960s, most OC pills contain both an estrogen and a progestin component. The estrogen component, either EE or mestranol, suppresses FSH release and, therefore, prevents the formation of a dominant follicle during the follicular phase of the menstrual cycle. The dominant follicle is responsible for producing estradiol, which sends a negative feedback signal to the hypothalamus to prevent the secretion of additional gonadotropins and, therefore, prevent maturation of additional follicles. The estrogen component also is responsible for maintaining the stability of the endometrial lining (78). The progestin component, of which there are many available, suppresses the LH surge and, therefore, blocks ovulation.

In the more than 45-year evolution of OCs, the estrogen dose has dropped to one-sixth and the progestin dose to one-tenth of the original levels. This makes the newer OC agents substantially safer but also prone to causing adverse effects, such as irregular and breakthrough bleeding. In addition to these dosage changes, the progestin components have become progressively more selective in their binding to the progesterone receptor, thereby limiting the androgenic side effects that were characteristic of the older progestins (59).

There are three generations of OCs that are classified based on the progestin component and the pharmacologic profile. The first-generation OCs contain either norethisterone or norethindrone acetate along with 35 to 50 mcg of EE. Their pharmacologic profile includes high affinity for the progesterone receptor, strong antigonadotropic action, and intermediate affinity for androgen receptors (79). Second-generation OCs contain levonorgestrel (along with 20 to 50 mcg EE) and have an even higher affinity for both the progesterone and androgen receptors than the first-generation agents (79). The third-generation OCs contain desogestrel, gestodene (available in Europe), or norgestimate (along with 15 to 30 mcg of EE) and have some affinity for the androgen receptor, which results in fewer androgenic side effects. This generation was supposed to have less metabolic side effects. The fourth generation of OCs contain chlormadinone acetate (not available in the United States), drospirenone, or cyproterone acetate (along with 20 to 30 mcg of EE) (79).

OC agents are either monophasic or multiphasic in their hormone composition (Table 41.9). The multiphasic formulations more closely mimic the natural changes in both hormone concentrations that occur throughout the menstrual cycle. Most of the OC formulations are administered for 21 days, followed by 7 drug-free days to allow monthly withdrawal bleeding. Extended-cycle products (Seasonale and Seasonique) have efficacies similar to that of the standard 28-day regimen (Table 41.9) and allow the patient to experience only 7 drug-free days every 3 months. Another nonstandard combination OC consists of EE plus a progestin for 21 days, followed by 2 hormone-free days and then 5 days of EE (Mircette and Kariva) (Table 41.9) (76). A continuous regimen of low-dose EE and levonorgestrel (Lybrel) that completely eliminates the menstrual cycle is also available (80).

Another monophasic low-dose formulation (YAZ) (Table 41.9), comprised of estradiol and drospirenone, has the added benefit of diuretic action. The dosing regimen for this OC is comprised of 24 days of drug therapy, followed by drug-free days to allow for withdrawal bleeding. The 3-mg drospirenone component of this preparation is equivalent to 25 mg of spironolactone in terms of diuretic potential. Because of the diuretic action of drospirenone, the drug has the potential to cause hyperkalemia. Diminished fluid-related weight gain is an obvious advantage to this OC formulation, but caution is advised in patients with renal or adrenal insufficiency, with hepatic dysfunction, or who are receiving chronic pharmacotherapy that may increase serum potassium levels (e.g., angiotensin-converting enzyme inhibitors and potassium-sparing diuretics). This product joins a previous OC formulation that contains drospirenone (Yasmin) (Table 41.9). It should be noted that intracyclic bleeding (spotting) is more prevalent with EE doses of less than 30 mcg, as is the case with these OCs. Studies have shown that the incidence of this adverse effect was greatest during the first cycle of OC use and diminished to very low incidence within three cycles (81).

In an attempt to reduce the risk of neural tube defects in pregnancies that occur during use or shortly after discontinuation of OCs, there are two formulations available that contain levomefolate calcium.

Although the adverse effects of OC therapy include an increased risk of stroke, acute myocardial infarction, and VTE disease, the incidence of cardiovascular disease in this patient population (age, <35 years) is already low (76). In women older than 35 years, the natural incidence of cardiovascular disease increases, so these adverse effects become more important to consider. The risk of VTE in patients who use a third-generation OC (ethinyl estradiol + desogestrel or norgestimate) is about twice that of patients who use a second-generation OC (ethinyl estradiol + levonorgestrel) and five times greater than in nonusers (82). The risk of VTE is greatest in the first 3 months of OC use. From a metabolic perspective, the primary adverse effect of the estrogen component is an increase in hepatic production of proteins, including those that enhance venous and arterial thromboembolism (83). In addition, the progestin component has an adverse effect on the lipid profile, including an elevation of serum triglyceride and a decrease in HDL levels. Generally speaking, the estrogen component of a combination OC balances out this negative impact on a patient's lipid profile. The degree to which the lipid profile is altered is dependent not only on the amount of hormone delivered, but also on the route of administration (84). It has been suggested that cholesterol levels change over the course of a given menstrual cycle (~20% change), with cholesterol levels being highest during the first half of the cycle. As the level of estrogen increases over time, the level of HDL cholesterol increases to the highest point at ovulation, whereas the levels of low-density lipoprotein (LDL) cholesterol and triglycerides drop over the same interval (85). Neoplastic effects are associated with OCs as well, such as an increased risk of cervical cancer and a decreased risk of colorectal, endometrial, and ovarian cancers that persists long after the discontinuation of therapy. Women taking OCs who require thyroid hormone replacement may require a dosage adjustment of thyroid hormone because use of OCs may cause an increase in serum concentrations of thyroid-binding globulin (20). See Table 41.10 for preferred contraceptive methods with coexisting disease states (86).

Contraceptive effectiveness certainly relies on patient adherence and consistent timing of the daily dose; however, there are other factors that can contribute to poor efficacy. Low serum EE levels have been associated with elevated body weight (87). Studies that evaluated the therapeutic efficacy of OCs in obese women yielded conflicting results. Vomiting and diarrhea for longer than 24 hours, as well as any chronic malabsorption condition, can cause a decrease in the absorption of both OC components and, therefore, a significant enough decrease in effectiveness to warrant the use of an additional form of contraception. Drug efficacy may also be reduced in the presence of one or more drugs that induce liver enzymes (e.g., carbamazepine, phenytoin, topiramate, barbiturates) or that can alter the enterohepatic recycling of the hormones (e.g., certain antibiotics).

TABLE 41.10 Contraception Considerations with Coexisting Medical Conditions (86)

Medical Condition	Concern	Preferred Contraceptive Method
Bariatric surgery	Reduced absorption	Nonoral contraceptive (malabsorptive surgery); all okay (sleeve or banding surgery)
Breast cancer	Increased risk, worsening, or recurrence	All okay (+ family history); copper IUD (current or past history)
Breast feeding	Estrogen may reduce milk production	Progestin only
Diabetes	Impaired glucose control and carbohydrate metabolism	Copper IUD (no vascular disease); progestin only or copper IUD (with vascular complications)
Epilepsy	Induction of metabolic enzymes	Avoid estrogen-containing preparations (lamotrigine); depot medroxyprogesterone and IUDs (carbamazepine, phenytoin, barbiturates, topiramate)
Hypercoagulable conditions	Increased coagulation and risk of thromboembolism	All okay (+ family history); copper IUD or progestin only (personal history of DVT or PE + no anticoagulant therapy); avoid estrogen-containing preparations (personal history of DVT or PE + anticoagulant therapy)
Headache/ migraine	Increased risk of stroke	All okay (nonmigraine headaches); copper IUD or progestin only (migraine without aura); copper IUD (migraine with aura); continuous or extended combined OCs (menstrual migraine)
Hyperlipidemia	Increase in triglyceride levels (estrogen) and LDL levels (progestin)	Copper IUD; other types of contraceptive forms may be acceptable depending on type of dyslipidemia
Hypertension	Increase in blood pressure and increase in cardiovascular events	No estrogen-containing types (controlled blood pressure); copper IUD or progestin only (uncontrolled/elevated blood pressure)
Obesity	Increased risk of VTE	All okay except contraceptive patch (BMI <40)
Systemic lupus erythematosus	Increased risk of ischemic heart disease, stroke, and VTE.	Copper IUD only (+ or unknown antiphospholipid antibody test)

BMI, body mass index; DVT, deep vein thrombosis; IUD, intrauterine device; LDL, low-density lipoprotein; OC, oral contraceptive; PE, pulmonary embolism; VTE, venous thromboembolism.

Progestin-Only Oral Contraceptives

A few contraceptive formulations only contain progestins (Table 41.9). Their contraceptive effects are accomplished via several mechanisms. From a hormonal perspective, progestins are able to suppress ovulation by preventing mid–menstrual cycle LH and FSH peaks via negative feedback inhibition. They also thicken cervical mucus to prevent entry of sperm into the endometrial cavity as well as transform the endometrium into an unsuitable environment for embryo implantation. Although the progestins suppress ovulation, they only do so 60% of the time, which generally is not sufficient for young women. The progestin-only OCs are an appropriate choice, however, for older women in whom fertility is diminished, for patients with contraindications to exogenous estrogen (e.g., smoking or high blood pressure), or for a lactating patient who is already experiencing prolactin-induced ovulation suppression (74). Unlike the combination oral agents, timing of administration is critical, because the effect of the progestin on the cervical mucus lasts for only 27 hours. If there is more than a 3-hour delay in the time of administration from the previous day, that dose is considered to be "missed," and additional contraceptive methods are recommended.

The first progestin-only "mini-pills" contained either norethindrone or norgestrel. Their adverse effect profile is limited, because there is no estrogen component to increase the risk of VTE or other cardiovascular related risks. Agents that induce metabolic enzymes (e.g., primidone, carbamazepine, topiramate, rifampin, ritonavir, St. John's wort) may decrease the efficacy of the minipills by reducing the circulating levels of hormone (88). Antibiotics do not alter the enterohepatic recycling of progestins as they do with estrogens.

Transdermal Contraceptive Patch

Despite the ease of administration of the OCs, poor patient adherence rates have fueled the development of several long-acting contraceptive formulations (Table 41.11). The contraceptive patch, containing a combination of norelgestromin and EE, is applied to the upper arm, lower abdomen, upper torso, or buttocks once per week on the same day of the week for 3 weeks, followed by a patch-free week to allow for withdrawal bleeding (89). After several weeks of therapy (several patches applied), the mean and steady-state serum concentrations were in the range needed for contraceptive efficacy (90). Despite the absence of first-pass metabolism with this route of administration, the EE component undergoes hydroxylation and is conjugated to the corresponding glucuronide and sulfate derivatives. Contraceptive efficacy is compromised with coadministration of various metabolic enzyme inducers. If more than 48 hours elapse between patch removal and administration, it is recommended to start a new 4-week cycle with the newly administered patch, and an additional

TABLE 41.11 Contraceptive Methods Using Nonoral Routes of Administration

Trade Name	Estrogen	Progestin	Route of Administration
Ortho Evra	EE (0.75 mg)	Norelgestromin (6 mg)	Transdermal patch
NuvaRing	EE (0.015 mg daily)	Etonogestrel (0.12 mg daily)	Vaginal ring
Lunelle[a]	Estradiol cypionate (5 mg)	Medroxyprogesterone acetate (25 mg)	IM
Depo-Provera		Medroxyprogesterone acetate (150 mg/mL)	IM (400–1,000 mg weekly)
Norplant II		Levonorgestrel (36 mg/rod)	2 Subdermal rods (3 years)
Jadelle[a]		Levonorgestrel (75 mg/rod)	2 Subdermal rods (5 years)
Implanon		Etonogestrel (68 mg/rod)	1 Subdermal rod (3 years)
Mirena		Levonorgestrel (52 mg)	IUD (5 years)

[a]Not available in the United States.
EE, ethinyl estradiol; IM, intramuscular; IUD, intrauterine device.

method of contraception should be used for 1 week (91). The patch provides equivalent efficacy to the OCs; however, it may not be as effective for women who weigh more than 90 kg (92). The adverse effects associated with the patch are headache, nausea, breast and abdominal pain, and application site irritation.

The revised Ortho Evra labels include statements that the patch can cause blood clots that could lead to a pulmonary embolism were based on the results of studies that show that this formulation exposes users to 60% more estrogen than OC users (containing 35 mcg EE) and that patients 15 to 44 years of age are at an increased risk for pulmonary embolism. Patients using this contraception formulation were twice as likely to develop blood clots and therefore at much greater risk for developing a VTE (93).

A transparent transdermal patch containing EE (0.9 mg) and gestodene (1.9 mg) is currently under investigation, as is a patch containing EE and levonorgestrel.

Contraceptive Vaginal Ring

The vaginal ring (NuvaRing), another long-acting contraceptive, continually delivers a low dose of etonogestrel and EE directly into the vagina (Table 41.11). The ring is inserted into the vagina by the patient and remains in place for 3 weeks. Again, 1 drug-free week allows appropriate withdrawal bleeding. Unscheduled removal of the ring is allowed, but the ring must be reinserted within 3 hours to ensure continued therapeutic efficacy (77). This formulation has comparable efficacy with the OCs yet provides continuous hormone delivery, thereby minimizing the side effects caused by the pulsatile delivery associated with oral dosing regimens (77,94). This formulation is not without adverse effects, including decreased libido, nausea, vaginitis, and breast tenderness.

A vaginal ring with a longer duration of action (1 year) is in phase II clinical trials. The active agents in this delivery system are nestorone and EE.

Contraceptive Injectables

An intramuscular formulation that contains an aqueous suspension of medroxyprogesterone acetate and estradiol cypionate is available but is not currently marketed in the United States (Table 41.11). The 28- to 33-day dosing interval provides excellent contraceptive effectiveness. There are several advantages to this contraceptive method, including scheduled withdrawal bleeding and a quick return to a fertile state on discontinuation of therapy. The adverse effects are similar to those seen with other combination OC formulations, including headache, weight gain, decreased libido, and breast tenderness (77).

Progestin-Only Injectables and Implants

The issue regarding timing of administration all but disappears when a progestin injection is administered every 3 months. In this formulation, medroxyprogesterone acetate is an aqueous microcrystalline suspension (Table 41.11). The mechanisms by which this progestin accomplishes contraceptive efficacy are the same as those discussed previously for other progestins. Despite the ease of use, the continuation rate after a year of injections is less than 30%, largely because of the adverse effects, including irregular and heavy bleeding, amenorrhea, and infertility that lasts for 9 to 21 months after the last injection (74). Improved patient education concerning the potential side effects may be a simple solution to discontinuation of therapy.

Several subdermal implants are available that provide contraceptive efficacy for 1 to 5 years depending on the formulation (Table 41.11). These implants consist of progestins contained within individual rods that are surgically implanted into the inner side of the upper nondominant arm. As indicated in Table 41.11, varying durations of action can be expected depending on the number of rods implanted. Implanon (etonogestrel) is available in the United States. This formulation is subject to the same adverse effects as other progestin-only formulations. Age-appropriate fertility returns within 1 week of removal.

Intrauterine Devices

There are two forms of IUDs: one that releases the progestin levonorgestrel (Table 41.10), and one that is copper-coated. Both devices are T-shaped and must be inserted into the uterus by a physician. These devices mechanically irritate the endometrium and create an inflammatory environment that is toxic to sperm and ova and is not conducive to embryo implantation (74). The copper coating further enhances this inflammatory response. The copper-based IUD can be used continuously for 10 years, whereas the progestin-containing device is only approved for 5 years of use (95). Although generally well tolerated, ectopic pregnancy and infection (related to device insertion or to the device itself) are two serious potential complications. Discontinuation of use often is a result of breakthrough and/or heavy withdrawal bleeding.

Emergency Contraception

Emergency contraception is defined as any method that prevents pregnancy after intercourse. This type of therapy is available in either combination (Yuzpe method) or single-agent formulations. The progestin-only formulations contain either levonorgestrel (two 0.75-mg tablets = Plan B; one 1.5-mg tablet = Plan B One Step) or ulipristal acetate (Ella) (Fig. 41.15). The combination regimens (multiple tablets of 21/7 or 24/4 regimens) include EE and levonorgestrel (Table 41.12) (96). Typically, these agents are administered as one dose within 72 hours of intercourse, with another dose taken 12 hours later. Nausea and vomiting are common side effects. If the patient is hormone adverse, then insertion of a copper IUD within 5 days of ovulation (the earliest estimated date) will prevent implantation (97).

Mifepristone (Mifeprex) is a 19-nortestosterone–based antiprogestogen that competes with the endogenous agonist for the progesterone receptor (see previous discussion). If administered within 5 days of unprotected intercourse, it also will prevent pregnancy. Despite the presence of the bulky 11β-diethylamino phenyl group, mifepristone has higher receptor affinity for the progesterone receptor than the natural agonist. It is not completely understood how mifepristone inactivates the progesterone receptor. Of note is that mifepristone and progesterone do not interact similarly with the ligand binding domain, such that in the presence of mifepristone, the conformational change that occurs in this domain is unique from that produced by the natural agonist (45).

TABLE 41.12 Representative Choices for Emergency Contraception (96)

Trade Name	Ethinyl Estradiol Content	Levonorgestrel	Pills per Dose; No. of Doses
Plan B	None	0.75 mg	1 tablet; 2
Ogestrel	0.50 mcg	0.25 mg	2 tablets; 2
Cryselle	0.15 mcg	0.30 mg	4 tablets; 2
Seasonale	0.15 mcg	0.30 mg	4 tablets; 2
Aviane	0.20 mcg	0.10 mg	5 tablets; 2

Endometriosis

Endometriosis, a condition present in 1 of 10 menstruating women, is characterized by implantation of endometrial tissue outside the uterus, typically within the pelvic region (98,99). During a normal menstrual cycle, hormonal signals cause the endometrial tissues to thicken in anticipation of embryo implantation. If a pregnancy does not occur, then these tissues are shed, resulting in monthly menses. When endometrial tissues implant outside the uterus, they respond identically to those within the uterus, such that when hormones fall in response to a nonpregnant state, these tissues are shed—yet have no natural exit. This tissue may form cysts, which in turn may form scar tissue and/or adhesions. Typically, the presence of one or more of these elicits significant pain and discomfort, especially during menstruation. Because the resulting scars and/or adhesions can cause infertility, treatment should be sought if the patient wishes to have children (98).

The cause of endometriosis is not completely understood. Sampson's hypothesis in 1927 suggests that menstrual fluids flow back (retrograde) through the fallopian tubes, where the endometrial cells can then implant and grow. Another theory proposes that the bloodstream is responsible for transporting the endometrial cells to regions outside the uterus. A third hypothesis is that endometriosis is a genetically acquired disease and that environmental factors trigger disease initiation (98,99). One of the hypotheses currently gaining some strength involves the immune system. Abnormal B- and T-cell function is evident in endometrial lesions, as are abnormal levels of cytokines, growth factors, and interleukins (100). Regardless of the biochemical cause, the growth of these endometrial lesions is controlled by both estrogen and progesterone (101), which means that hormonal intervention is likely to be effective in the treatment of this condition.

Pharmacologic Management

Treatment of endometriosis largely depends on the severity of the symptoms experienced by the patient. Characteristic symptoms experienced by patients include dysmenorrhea, pelvic and lower abdominal pain, and dyspareunia (101). The American Association of Reproductive Medicine has a four-tiered system to describe the severity of the endometriotic disease, ranging from stage I (mild) to stage IV (severe) (100).

Pharmacologic management looks to achieve two primary goals: pain management and prevention/delay of disease progression. Nonsteroidal anti-inflammatory drugs (e.g., ibuprofen) that inhibit prostaglandin biosynthesis may be sufficient to ease menstrual pain, but this pain may not be adequately managed even at the maximum dose. Endometriotic pain is directly related to the fluctuating levels of endogenous hormones. Clear evidence indicates that endometriosis-related symptoms improve substantially during pregnancy and after menopause. Because OCs chemically produce a "pregnant" state, one might expect this type of hormone therapy to be a viable treatment option.

Combination Oral Contraceptives There are a number of hormone-based pharmacologic options for the treatment of endometriosis. If a woman wishes to achieve complete cessation of endometriosis-related pain, a 3- to 4-month regimen using a combination OC is recommended. This forces the body into a chemically "pregnant" state, such that hormone fluctuations and ovulation cease. As a result, menstrual flow decreases, and the size of the endometrial implants diminish. No evidence suggests that one OC combination is more efficacious than another (100). After 3 to 4 months of continuous OC therapy, 1 drug-free week is required to allow withdrawal bleeding to occur. If daily administration is difficult for the patient to manage, then selection of one of several delivery systems that allow less frequent dosing (e.g., transdermal patch or vaginal ring) is appropriate. Cyclic dosing is more appropriate if the patient does not experience symptoms continually throughout the menstrual cycle. Adverse effects include nausea, headache, and breakthrough bleeding.

Gonadotropin-Releasing Hormone Agonists The GnRH agonists leuprolide (Lupron), goserelin (Zoladex), triptorelin (Trelstar Depot), and nafarelin (Synarel) downregulate the hypothalamic-pituitary GnRH receptors, thereby limiting the secretion of FSH and LH and causing suppression of ovarian function (Fig. 41.16) (98,100). This creates an estrogen-deficient environment that prevents menstruation and reduces the size of wayward endometrial implants. These agents have enjoyed success in the treatment of endometriosis (85% to 100% success with 6 months of therapy), but they come with a price. The GnRH agonists generate a state of artificial menopause, which can cause classical vasomotor symptoms, urogenital atrophy, and insomnia. Bone mineral density suffers substantially after prolonged use, so the duration of this type of therapy is limited to 6 months (102). One way to extend the duration of therapy is to coadminister agents that address these side effects. Suggested "add-back" therapies include a progestin alone (e.g., norethindrone), a progestin and a bisphosphonate (e.g., etidronate), or a progestin and an estrogen (e.g., conjugated equine

1 2 3 4 5 6 7 8 9 10
pyroGlu–His–Trp–Ser–Tyr–Gly–Leu–Arg–Pro–Gly-NH_2

GnRh

pyroGlu–His–Trp–Ser–Tyr–D-Leu—Leu-Arg—Pro-NH-C_2H_5

Leuprolide

pyroGlu–His–Trp-Ser–Tyr-D-Ser(t-Bu)–Leu-Arg-Pro–NH–NH–C(=O)–NH_2

Goserelin

pyroGlu–His–Trp–Ser–Tyr–D-NaL—Leu–Arg–Pro–Gly-NH_2

Nafarelin (D-NaL = 3-(2-naphthyl)-D-alanyl)

FIGURE 41.16 Structure of GnRH and its analogs.

estrogen [CEE]). The amount of estrogen that is added back is enough to counteract the side effects of the GnRH agonists but insufficient to cause endometrial tissue growth (100). A serious limitation to multidrug therapy is the considerable cost associated with these agents as compared to the OCs or progestin injectables.

It should be noted that the same mechanism by which these agents are effective in the treatment of endometriosis is also applicable to the treatment of fibroids. Leuprolide acetate effectively shrinks the fibroid size by decreasing the supply of hormones that "feed" fibroids.

Gonadotropin-Releasing Hormone Antagonists Non–peptide-based GnRH antagonists offer several significant advantages over the injectable GnRH agonists in the treatment of endometriosis. Mechanistically, these agents provide rapid hormone suppression without the characteristic hormone flare. Because they are non–peptide based, they are easily formulated for oral delivery. Elagolix, an orally active nonpeptide GnRH antagonist, is in phase II clinical trial for the treatment of endometriosis. In clinical trials, it produced statistically significant reductions in dysmenorrhea, nonmenstrual pelvic pain, and dyspareunia—all of which are symptoms of endometriosis. An important advantage of an orally available agent is the ability to modulate estrogen levels to maximize pain relief while minimizing bone loss.

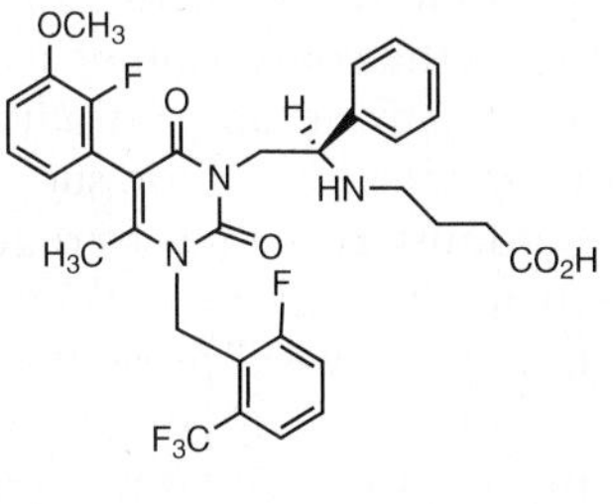

Elagolix

Androgenic Agents Danazol, a synthetic analog of 17α-ethinyl testosterone, induces amenorrhea, anovulation, and endometrial atrophy via suppression of the hypothalamic-pituitary-ovary (HPO) axis (98,100).

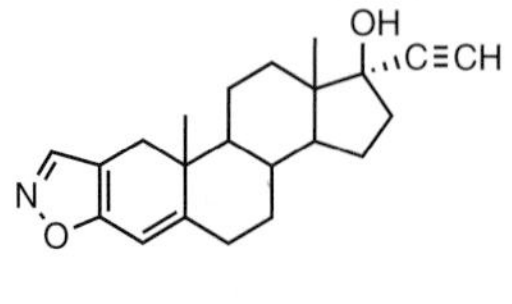

Danazol
(Danocrine)

This causes an estrogen-deficient state, but it also causes an increase in androgen production. Danazol generally is not well tolerated because of its androgenic and anabolic side effects, including acne, decreased breast size, facial hair, weight gain, and oily skin (98,99). This type of therapy is not a viable option for women with liver disease or hyperlipidemia. Because danazol is teratogenic, it is recommended that effective contraception be used during treatment (98,100). Gestrinone, a 19-nortestosterone, has androgenic activity, antiestrogen activity, and antiprogesterone action (Fig. 41.14). Administered twice weekly, gestrinone decreases the secretion of LH and FSH via interaction with receptors within the HPO axis. The side effect profile includes weight gain, acne, seborrhea, and hirsutism.

Progestins Medroxyprogesterone acetate (Fig. 41.14), administered by injection (Depo-Provera), orally (Provera), or via IUD, effectively suppresses the HPO axis, induces anovulation, and reduces serum estrogen levels (103). This prevents menstruation and endometrial implant growth. As a result, endometriosis-related pain is minimized in approximately 90% of the patients. Levonorgestrel intrauterine system (Mirena) has also been found to be effective in managing endometriosis. Drug therapy selection should reflect the fact that pharmacologic therapy is likely to be required on a chronic basis. The progestins are fairly well tolerated and relatively inexpensive, but they are not without adverse effects, including nausea, breakthrough bleeding, weight gain, mood swings, and depression.

Aromatase Inhibitors Normal endometrial tissues are devoid of aromatase activity. In patients with endometriosis, evidence suggests that high levels of aromatase are present in endometrial implants. Aromatase is the enzyme that catalyzes the conversion of androstenedione and testosterone to estrone and estradiol, respectively (Fig. 41.3). If an aromatase inhibitor, such as anastrozole (Fig. 41.12), is administered, then estrogen production will be decreased in the endometrial implants. A local state of estrogen deficiency will prevent growth of these implants (104). Unfortunately, one outcome of prolonged aromatase therapy is the development of osteoporosis. As a result, an OC typically is coadministered to provide baseline estrogen concentrations to limit the risk of osteoporosis.

Selective Estrogen Receptor Modulators To be effective in the treatment of endometriosis without therapy-limiting side effects, a SERM must behave as an estrogen antagonist at the endometrium and as an agonist at the bone. An investigational agent, TZE-5323, has antiestrogenic action by virtue of its ability to inhibit binding of estrogen to ERα and ERβ and then limit subsequent transcriptional activation (105). This agent may prove to be beneficial in the treatment of endometriosis.

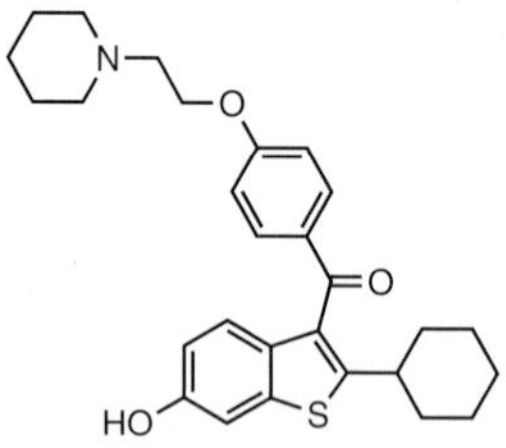

TZE-5323

Progesterone Receptor Modulators
Like the SERMs, the selective progesterone receptor modulators bind to the progesterone receptors and act as either an agonist or antagonist depending on the absence or presence of progesterone and the tissue that is being targeted. In the absence of progesterone, these agents demonstrate progestin activity. In the presence of progesterone, they exhibit antiprogestin activity in some target tissues, particularly the endometrium (101). Several investigational agents, including asoprisnil, have suppressed the growth of endometrial implants while estrogen concentrations remained at similar levels to those found during the follicular phase of the menstrual cycle (106). Recently, phase III clinical trials with asoprisnil were halted due to endometrial changes found in patients.

Surgical Intervention Laparoscopic surgical intervention to remove the endometrial implants is recommended for those patients who do not wish to use pharmacologic methods because of their immediate interest in having children. It should be noted that as many as 20% of patients do not respond to surgical intervention. This results, in part, from a failure to identify and excise all of the errant endometrial tissues (100). Adjunct therapy is not routinely used, because study data fail to consistently show efficacy (107).

Hypoactive Sexual Desire Disorder

Low libido for long periods of time is the hallmark of hypoactive sexual desire disorder (HSDD). This affects 9% to 26% of women depending on age and menopausal status. Both hormonal and nonhormonal solutions are under investigation to treat this female sexual problem.

Though originally designed and evaluated as an antidepressant, flibanserin's side effect profile included enhanced libido. Phase III clinical trial data suggested that patients derived meaningful benefit from treatment with flibanserin. Side effects included dizziness, nausea, and fatigue. In June 2010, the FDA failed to approve flibanserin for the treatment of HSDD based on lack of efficacy. A transdermal testosterone gel (LibiGel) is also in phase III clinical trials for the treatment of HSDD in menopausal women. Once-daily topical application of a pea-sized dose on the upper arm followed by rapid absorption into the skin delivers testosterone evenly to the bloodstream over time.

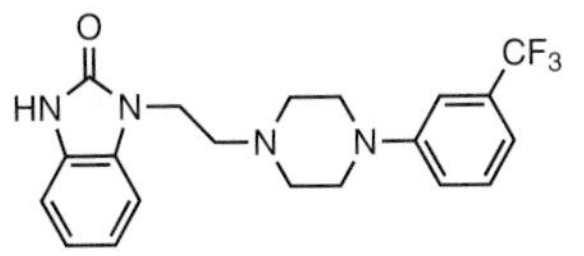

Flibanserin

Menorrhagia

Heavy menstrual bleeding (menorrhagia) is a condition reported by 3 million U.S. women annually. It is characterized by normal intervals of menstruation with an excessive volume (>80 mL) of blood loss per cycle. Tranexamic acid (Lysteda) was approved by the FDA in 2009 for the treatment of menorrhagia. As an orally available lysine receptor antagonist, tranexamic acid acts as an antifibrinolytic by preventing the activation of plasminogen to plasmin. Plasmin is the serine protease that is responsible for the degradation of fibrin.

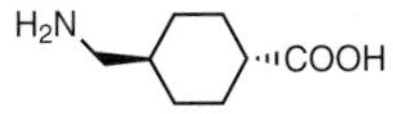

Tranexamic acid

Infertility

Infertility is not a disease state of the "individual" but, rather, often is considered to be a disease state of the "couple." Defined as the inability to conceive a pregnancy after 12 months of unprotected intercourse, infertility affects 10% to 13% of couples. Identification of the cause of infertility requires thorough medical histories as well as several diagnostic tests (Table 41.13) (108,109). The causes of infertility include ovulatory disorders as well as situations in which tubal factors, uterine factors, cervical factors, and/or immunologic and thrombophilic factors play a substantial role (Table 41.14) (110).

In 2010, one in seven babies were born to women at least 35 years of age, an interesting statistic that highlights the recent trend to delay having children. With this delay comes an age-related reduction in fertility and the need to employ one or more pharmacologic therapies to achieve a live birth. As of 2006, there had been more than 3 million babies born as a result of in vitro fertilization (IVF), with nearly one in three embryo-transfer cycles

TABLE 41.13 Infertility Medical Evaluation (88,89)

Male	Female
Fertility in other relationships	Previous pregnancies, fertility in other relationships; onset of menstrual cycle
Medication use	Medication use, including contraceptive use
Alcohol or recreational drug use, cigarette smoking	Alcohol or recreational drug use, cigarette smoking
Environmental exposure (e.g., sauna, hot tub), chemotherapy or radiation exposure	Environmental exposure (e.g., DES), chemotherapy or radiation exposure
Sexual dysfunction/frequency of intercourse	Frequency of intercourse
Semen analysis	Ovulation documentation
	Screening tests: pap smear, cervical cultures, mammogram, infectious disease screening
	Day 3 FSH levels (>10 mIU/mL = low rate of pregnancy)
	Thyroid panel, including TSH levels
	Fasting Prolactin levels
	Clomiphene citrate challenge test + FSH and estradiol levels (assess ovarian reserve)
	Hysterosalpingogram (assess tubal patency, shape of intrauterine cavity)
	Laparoscopy (assess endometriosis or if adhesions are present)
	Hysteroscopy (assess interuterine lesions or abnormalities)

DES, diethylstilbestrol: FSH, follicle-stimulating hormone; TSH, thyroid-stimulating hormone.

TABLE 41.14 Infertility Classification and Causes (90)

Ovulatory Disorders	Characteristics	Therapeutic Regimen
WHO Class I Hypogonadotropic, hypogonadal anovulation	Low or low normal FSH, low estradiol due to decreased Gn-RH or pituitary not responding to Gn-RH	Weight gain, reduce exercise, pulsatile Gn-RH
WHO Class II Normogonadotropic, normoestrogenic anovulation	Normal gonadotropins and estrogens, FSH secretion during follicular stage is subnormal, includes women with PCOS	Weight loss, clomiphene with or without metformin, aromatase inhibitors
WHO Class III Hypergonadotropic, hypoestrogenic anovulation	Premature ovarian failure, ovarian resistance	
Hyperprolactinemic anovulation	Elevated levels of prolactin inhibits gonadotropin and therefore estrogen secretion	Dopamine agonists (bromocriptine)
Tubal Factor Infertility		Hysterosalpinogram, IVF, tubal reconstruction, laparoscopic surgery (endometriosis)
Uterine Factor Infertility		Leiomyoma, polyp removal
Cervical Factor Infertility		IUI, IVF
Immunologic and Thrombophilic Factor Infertility		Low dose aspirin and heparin, anticoagulation therapy
Unexplained Infertility		Clomiphene with or without IUI, gonadotropins with IUI, ART

ART, assisted reproduction technology; FSH, follicle-stimulating hormone; nGnRH, gonadotropin-releasing hormone; IUI, intrauterine insemination; IVF, invitro fertilization; PCOS, polycystic ovarian syndrome, WHO, World Health Organization.

resulting in a live birth (111). Many infertility treatment options and protocols are available, most of which are highly individualized (Table 41.15) (109).

Intrauterine Insemination and In Vitro Fertilization

Intrauterine insemination (IUI) involves induction of ovulation, followed by transfer of motile sperm directly into the uterine cavity. This type of procedure is indicated if erectile dysfunction or male infertility (low motility, low count, and/or poor morphology) has been identified, if the cervical environment (e.g., presence of antisperm antibodies) is not conducive for effective sperm motility and/or sustenance, and if there are any physiologic dysfunctions (112).

IVF involves hyperstimulation of the ovaries to produce multiple mature follicles. Once the follicles reach 18 to 21 mm in diameter, hCG is administered, and within 34 to 36 hours, all the mature follicles are aspirated and their eggs removed. Depending on the couple, fertilization of the oocyte by the sperm may or may not require assistance. The resulting fertilized oocytes or embryos are then sustained and monitored for 3 to 5 days. Embryo characterization is performed daily to identify the most advanced embryos of good quality for subsequent transfer into the uterine cavity. Preimplantation genetic diagnosis can be performed with a single cell biopsied from each embryo that reaches the six- to eight-cell stage by day 3. The genetic tests performed (on all chromosomes) will help the physician and patient to identify those embryos with normal genetic makeup (including sex determination). Despite these advanced technologies and regardless of the age group, the pregnancy rate does not exceed 50%, and the risk for multiple births is substantially higher than that observed in the general population.

Clomiphene Citrate (Clomid)

Clomiphene citrate is by far the most frequently prescribed agent to stimulate ovulation. It is administered orally as a mixture of two geometric isomers. The *Z* (*cis*, zuclomiphene)-diastereomer displays estrogenic activity, and the *E* (*trans*, enclomiphene)-diastereomer exhibits antiestrogenic activity (Fig. 41.10). Its ability to stimulate ovulation stems from its action at the hypothalamic ERs, where it serves to block these receptors and interfere with natural feedback inhibition. When an estrogen deficiency is perceived by the hypothalamus, it responds by secreting GnRH. This peptide hormone signals the pituitary to release the gonadotropins FSH and LH. Elevated FSH levels promote follicular development, which in turn causes the maturing follicles to secrete estradiol. Clomiphene is administered orally (50 or 100 mg) for 5 consecutive days, typically on days 5 to 9 of the menstrual cycle. Approximately 7 days after the last clomiphene tablet is taken, the hypothalamus finally is able to detect that estradiol levels are elevated, and it then signals the pituitary to secrete LH. This surge in LH causes the dominant

TABLE 41.15 Representative Infertility Treatment Options (89)

Treatment Option	Patient Characteristics	Pharmacological Therapy
Intrauterine insemination	Mild endometriosis Unexplained infertility Mild male factors	Clomiphene citrate (days 5–9), monitor LH levels
Ovulation induction	Ovulatory disorder PCOS Hyperprolactinemia Hypothalamic amenorrhea Premature ovarian failure	Progestin challenge test; gonadotropin therapy (hMG and/or FSH)
In vitro fertilization (with or without donor oocytes)	Tubal factor Severe endometriosis Unexplained infertility	Ovarian hyperstimulation, hCG
Therapeutic donor insemination	Women without partners Severe male factor	Sperm donor

FSH, follicle-stimulating hormone; hCG, human chorionic gonadotropin; hMG, human menopausal gonadotropin; LH, luteinizing hormone; PCOS, polycystic ovarian syndrome.

follicle to rupture and release an egg, a process known as ovulation.

The clomiphene citrate challenge test is a diagnostic tool used to evaluate ovarian reserve in women older than 35 years of age. The protocol involves measurement of FSH and estradiol levels on day 3 of the cycle, followed by administration of 100 mg of clomiphene citrate on days 5 to 9 and measurement of FSH and estradiol on day 10 of the cycle. Elevated estrogen levels on day 3 are a good predictor of a poor pregnancy prognosis. Any FSH measurement that is high (>10 mIU/mL), even if other levels measured within the same cycle are within the normal range, is interpreted to mean a significantly limited reproductive potential because of poor ovarian reserve (108,113). The adverse effects associated with clomiphene include thickening of the cervical mucus, which creates a substantial barrier for motile sperm. A postcoital test can be performed to determine if this, in fact, represents an insurmountable hurdle. If so, an IUI is warranted to bypass this cervical challenge. Another adverse effect is endometrial thinning, which is not conducive to embryo implantation; if this is the case, additional pharmacologic therapies are recommended to thicken the endometrial lining. Other adverse effects include hot flashes and mood swings (114).

Women with low estrogen levels or hypothalamic disorders that result in irregular or absent ovulation are not candidates for clomiphene therapy. There is a 10% chance of having twins and a slightly higher risk of miscarriage in women stimulated with clomiphene (114). Clomiphene-based ovulatory stimulation should only be considered for a maximum of six cycles.

Clomiphene is readily absorbed from the GI tract following oral administration, with a half-life of approximately 5 days. It is metabolized in the liver, and its metabolites are excreted principally in the feces via enterohepatic recirculation.

Human Chorionic Gonadotropin (Pregnyl)

Human chorionic gonadotropin mimics LH both in structure and in function. It is produced by the placenta during pregnancy and is isolated from the urine of pregnant women. In the protocols for IUI or IVF, exogenous hCG must be administered to stimulate a scheduled ovulation. Between 36 and 72 hours after intramuscular administration, the dominant follicle ruptures and releases its egg. At that point, the scheduled IUI or IVF occurs. The hCG can be given in combination with clomiphene citrate to enhance ovulation (114). (For an in-depth discussion of hCG, see Chapter 6.)

Choriogonadotropin Alfa (Ovidrel [r-hCG])

The biologic activities of r-hCG are identical to those of placental and human pregnancy (urine) u-hCG. From a structural perspective, this glycoprotein has an α chain that is identical to hCG, LH, and FSH with some variation in the branching and extent of sialyation of the oligosaccharides (115). The structure and glycosylation pattern of the β chain is similar to u-hCG.

Human Menopausal Gonadotropin (Repronex, Menopur)

Human menopausal gonadotropin (menotropins) is composed of equal parts FSH and LH and is derived from the urine of menopausal women. This type of therapy is used after clomiphene-based therapy has failed or if a patient does not produce sufficient levels of FSH or LH and experiences amenorrhea. These hormones directly stimulate the ovaries to develop multiple follicles per reproductive cycle (114).

Human menopausal gonadotropin has a substantial role in several IVF protocols. It typically is administered via injection (75 or 150 U) starting on day 2 or 3 of the menstrual cycle and is administered continuously (7 to 12 days) until shortly before the patient is ready to undergo follicle retrieval. The size and number of maturing follicles, as well as the patient's estrogen level, are closely monitored to maximize the number of follicles retrieved and to minimize the risk of ovarian hyperstimulation syndrome (OHSS) (114). Adverse effects include injection site reactions and inflammation as well as the possibility of developing OHSS. Menopur, another formulation of menotropins that also contains equal parts FHS and LH, has been shown to cause fewer injection site reactions.

Follicle-Stimulating Hormone (Bravelle, Follistim, Gonal-F)

Two types of products are available that contain FSH. Bravelle contains FSH isolated from the urine of menopausal women and does not contain significant amounts of LH. Follistim and Gonal-F are products that contain only purified synthetic (recombinant) FSH. The recombinant products are more effective at stimulating the development of multiple follicles (111,112). All three agents are administered as subcutaneous injections. Administration of exogenous FSH circumvents the influence of both the hypothalamus and the pituitary on the ovaries and causes direct stimulation of ovarian follicle growth. Women who fail to achieve pregnancy with clomiphene assistance or who are diagnosed with polycystic ovarian syndrome are candidates for this type of therapy (114). (For additional discussion of FSH, see Chapters 6.)

Dopamine Agonists—Bromocriptine and Cabergoline

The hormone prolactin is responsible for stimulating the production of breast milk in mothers of newborns as well as for inducing lactation infertility. In this situation, FSH and LH secretion is inhibited; therefore, ovulation is prevented. In other populations of women, elevated levels of prolactin can result from the presence of an adenoma or a benign pituitary tumor or because the pituitary cells that produce prolactin are hyperactive. This hyperactivity may have a pharmacologic genesis (e.g., antipsychotics, tranquilizers, painkillers, or alcohol) or a pathophysiologic origin (e.g., kidney or thyroid disease). Both bromocriptine and cabergoline suppress prolactin production. Bromocriptine is available as a tablet or capsule and is administered one to four times daily. It also is available as an intravaginal formulation. Cabergoline tablets are administered one to two times weekly. Once the prolactin levels drop to normal levels, the patient should experience improved fertility. If pregnancy is not achieved despite normal prolactin levels, then addition of clomiphene or gonadotropins is warranted (114).

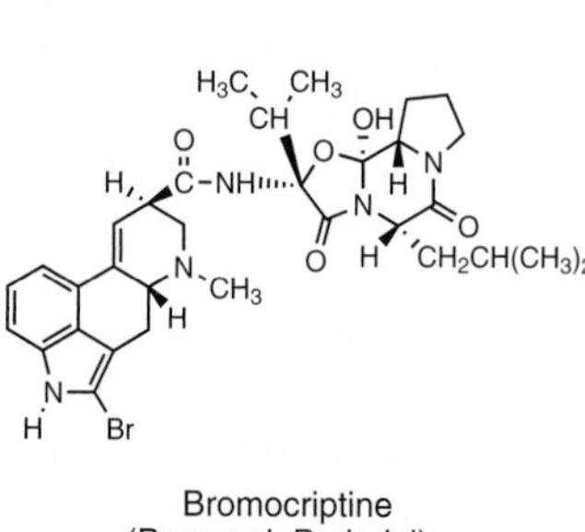

Bromocriptine
(Pergonal, Parlodel)

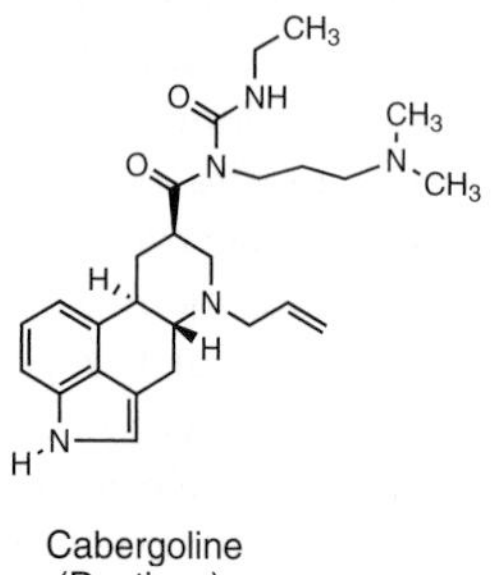

Cabergoline
(Dostinex)

Gonadotropin-Releasing Hormone

GnRH is secreted from the hypothalamus in a pulsatile fashion once roughly every 90 minutes. It is rapidly degraded by pituitary endopeptidases and has a circulatory half-life of 2 to 4 minutes. Degradation occurs primarily at the Gly^6 residue (Fig. 41.16). Synthetic efforts to improve peptide stability have resulted in several successful GnRH agonists that contain hydrophobic D-amino acids replacing Gly^6 (see below) (116).

When GnRH binds to and activates its pituitary cell surface receptor, it sends a signal for the pituitary to biosynthesize and secrete FSH and LH. This receptor is part of the family of G protein–coupled receptors and is composed of seven-transmembrane domains. Eventually, the receptor hormone complex is internalized, the ligand degraded, and the receptor partially recycled (116).

If a patient is unable to produce sufficient quantities of GnRH, then replacement therapy is available. To mimic normal secretion patterns, this hormone is delivered by infusion every 90 minutes via an external pump worn by the patient (114).

Gonadotropin-Releasing Hormone Agonists and Antagonists

Typically, GnRH agonists are administered continuously and not in normal physiologic pulses. As a result of constant stimulation of the GnRH receptors, an initial hyperstimulation of the pituitary occurs, causing a surge in FSH and LH secretion, which is quickly followed by complete cessation of their release. Ultimately, this causes the production of estrogen and progesterone to stop, which prevents ovulation from occurring. In patients who do not have a regular ovulatory cycle, these medications are used to squelch all internal influence over ovulation. Once internal hormonal signaling has been silenced, human menopausal gonadotropin can be administered, permitting the physician exquisite control over the levels of pituitary hormones. With exogenous FSH and LH now present, follicle development is stimulated, and oocyte retrieval for IVF is possible. When used continuously, GnRH agonists stifle the natural LH surge associated with ovulation, so hCG must be administered 34 to 36 hours before oocyte retrieval to launch ovulation.

Several GnRH agonists are available, including leuprolide acetate (Lupron) and goserelin acetate (Zoladex), which are injectable agents, and nafarelin acetate (Synarel), which is administered via nasal spray (Fig. 41.16). GnRH is rapidly degraded by peptidases (half-life = 2 to 4 minutes) between amino acids 5 and 6, 6 and 7, and 9 and 10. These analogs of GnRH have altered amino acids at these positions in order to improve analog stability. (Discussion about structure–activity relationships can be found in Chapter 6.)

Two GnRH antagonists, ganirelix acetate (Antagon) and cetrorelix acetate (Cetrotide), are administered by intramuscular injection (114). The primary advantage of the GnRH antagonists over the agonists is that they interact with and effectively block the GnRH receptor without causing an initial surge of FSH and LH. The primary role of both the antagonists and agonists is to prevent a premature LH surge.

In an IVF cycle, the GnRH antagonist is not administered until the dominant follicle reaches 14 mm in diameter, which is nearly a week after gonadotropin therapy is initiated. The GnRH antagonists suffer from low solubility and the tendency to form gels in aqueous solutions (116). Ganirelix acetate has a short half-life and must be administered daily until hCG is administered, whereas cetrorelix has a longer half-life and can be administered once every 3 to 4 days (112). (Discussion about structure–activity relationships can be found in Chapter 6.)

Women whose ovulatory cycle has been managed by gonadotropin therapy have a 25% risk of multiple pregnancies. Some evidence suggests a lower pregnancy rate in patients using protocols that include a GnRH antagonist (116,117). Adverse effects include injection site pain and inflammation, abdominal bloating, mood swings, and menopausal symptoms, including hot flashes and vaginal dryness. The likelihood of developing OHSS is fairly small in protocols that include GnRH agonists or antagonists. In these regimens, the physician has control over the hCG injection necessary to trigger ovulation and can delay—or even withhold—this injection if estrogen levels are too high, a factor that predisposes the patient to develop OHSS (114). It should be noted that GnRH downregulation caused by these agents may have an adverse effect on oocyte quality, which has a negative impact on an IVF cycle (111).

As part of an assisted reproductive technology protocol, the use of both a GnRH agonist or antagonist and exogenous gonadotropins provides significant benefits, including enhanced stimulation of follicular development, improved oocyte quality, and LH surge suppression, all of which lead to fewer cycle cancellations and improved reproductive capability (111).

Lutropin Alfa (Luveris)

Lutropin alfa is the first recombinant human form of LH approved by the FDA. This agent serves as LH replacement therapy for women who are hypogonadotropic and hypogonadal with a substantial deficiency in LH (<1.2 IU/L). Lutropin alfa typically is used in combination with follitropin alfa to induce follicular growth and development. Both of these agents are administered subcutaneously.

The half-life of lutropin alfa is approximately 10 hours. Treatment should not exceed 14 days unless follicular development is clearly evident. Adverse effects include headache, breast and abdominal pain, and nausea. Lutropin alfa can contribute to the development of OHSS and should not be used in women with primary ovarian failure or uncontrolled thyroid or adrenal dysfunction or who are pregnant.

Progesterone (Endometrin)

Since natural progesterone levels can be compromised by IVF, progesterone supplementation is recommended to provide luteal phase support. Formulated as a vaginal insert, micronized progesterone is administered to support embryo implantation and early pregnancy as a component of assisted reproductive technology treatment. Drug administration begins at the time of oocyte retrieval and continues two to three times per day for the following 10 weeks or until menses occur, indicating cycle failure. Higher progesterone serum concentrations were achieved more quickly with this formulation as compared to progesterone 8% gel (Crinone).

Menopause

Physiologically, menopause is described as the loss of ovarian follicle function, followed by the cessation of menses. Before menopause, the body typically is engaged in a 2- to 4-year preamble, complete with the signs and symptoms of menopause (e.g., hot flashes and night sweats). This stage is termed perimenopause and is characterized by a gradual decline in the secretion of estrogen and progesterone. When the ovary no longer prepares follicles for ovulation and the resulting corpus luteum is not formed, a dramatic decrease in the production of estrogen and progesterone occurs, along with the resulting physiologic changes, including bone loss, urogenital atrophy, and perhaps, incontinence, vasomotor symptoms, enhanced risk of cardiovascular disease, sexual dysfunction including decreased libido, and reduced skin elasticity (118). Many, if not most, of these changes have a negative effect on the quality of life for women during what is considered to be an exceptionally productive time in their lives. Identification of pharmacologic and nonpharmacologic methods to alleviate these symptoms is essential to improving quality of life during this turbulent hormonal phase at the end of a woman's reproductive lifetime.

History

As early as 1899, the Merck Manual listed several treatments for menopausal symptoms, including the drug Ovarin, which was composed of desiccated and pulverized cow ovaries flavored with vanilla. In 1932, this formulation was largely replaced by products that contained components isolated from the urine of pregnant women. By the late 1930s, these human-derived products were supplanted by Premarin, which contained components isolated from the urine of pregnant mares (119). Other formulations that take advantage of other routes of administration have been available for quite some time as well; for example, in 1928, the first estrogen patch was developed by Searle.

By the 1960s and 1970s, the first studies regarding serious adverse effects associated with estrogen therapy were reported, including severe hypertensive episodes and increased thromboembolic events. In 1978, the FDA mandated that a comprehensive warning be distributed with all estrogen products, including OCs. This document listed the approved indications and fully described the potential risks of using an estrogen-containing formulation. Despite these warnings, the use of estrogen-containing products actually increased as a result of the

FDA notice that stated that these agents were effective for the prevention of osteoporosis (119).

Hormone Replacement Therapy

Until mid-2002, HRT continued to be considered as first-line therapy for the pharmacologic management of menopausal symptoms and for health preventive purposes in postmenopausal women. At that point, the results from the WHI study and, eventually, the WHI Memory Study (120) were released and clearly identified that although HRT (combination of 0.625 mg/day of CEE and 2.5 mg/day of medroxyprogesterone acetate) reduced the incidence of colorectal and endometrial cancers as well as hip fracture, it also increased the incidence of heart attacks, stroke, and breast cancer and increased global cognitive impairment (121). Ultimately, the FDA mandated that safety warnings appear on the package labels for both combination and estrogen-only products to warn women about these risks.

Medical management of menopause largely revolves around treatment of the symptoms caused by estrogen deficiency. Without regular maturation of ovarian eggs, follicles are not consistently formed and, therefore, do not consistently secrete the same levels of estrogen as found in premenopausal women. In postmenopausal women, the primary source of endogenous estrogen (albeit a fraction of that found in premenopausal women) comes from the transformation of androstenedione into estrone. Because the release of FSH and LH by the pituitary gland is governed by estrogen concentrations via negative feedback inhibition, it is no surprise that menopausal women have FSH levels 10- to 15-fold higher and LH levels 4- to 5-fold higher than those found in premenopausal women (53). In addition, low estrogen levels prevent launch of the normal LH surge that is key to follicular rupture, followed by formation of the corpus luteum. Because the corpus luteum is responsible for the secretion of progesterone, it is, again, no surprise that the levels of this hormone also are out of balance during menopause (122). The vasomotor symptoms associated with menopause represent some of the most disturbing and, potentially, embarrassing menopause-related effects experienced by women. Since the early 1940s, estrogen replacement therapy (ERT) with CEE has been indicated for the treatment of these symptoms as well as for the treatment of urogenital atrophy and vaginal dryness. For patients with an intact uterus, progesterone was administered along with the estrogen to prevent endometrial hyperplasia and endometrial cancer. This type of combination therapy is referred to as HRT. Nearly 90% of menopausal patients experience symptom relief after initiation of either ERT or HRT (Table 41.16) (123,124). Each patient requires individual dose titration to maximize menopausal symptom relief and to minimize side effects (e.g., breast tenderness, weight gain, and vaginal bleeding). Because of the WHI findings, HRT is considered as safe to administer if used short term and if dose reduction occurs after 2 to 3 years of treatment.

Despite the WHI findings, estrogen remains the gold standard in relief of menopausal symptoms. Recently, pharmaceutical manufacturers have concentrated on the development of alternate dosage forms that deliver the minimum dose of estrogen to minimize adverse effects, to maximize therapeutic benefit, and to maintain a more normal ratio of estrone to estradiol. These formulations include several different types of transdermal products, vaginal rings, and vaginal creams. The estrogens found in these products include estradiol, EE (synthetic), piperazine estrone sulfate, and conjugated estrogens. Unfortunately, these estrogens do not have identical potencies. Conjugated equine estrogens, esterified estrogens, and estrone sodium sulfate at 0.625 mg are equivalent to 1 mg of micronized estrogen, 0.75 mcg of piperazine estrone sulfate, 5 to 10 mcg of EE, or 0.50 mcg of transdermal estrogen.

Although estradiol is the most potent endogenous estrogen, it has poor oral bioavailability. Oral administration of estrogen in a conjugated (e.g., estradiol valerate) or micronized (Estrace) form enhances absorption by the GI mucosa; however, when administered via this route, estradiol undergoes extensive hepatic metabolism (CYP3A4) to the corresponding ketone (estrone) (Fig. 41.3), which is much less potent. Only 10% of an oral dose of estradiol reaches the circulation (53). Estrone then undergoes sulfate conjugation to an inactive product. In effect, estrone sulfate represents a stable reservoir of circulating estradiol (12,13). Piperazine estrone sulfate (estropipate) also is quickly converted to estrone sulfate when administered orally. In premenopausal women, the physiologic ratio of estradiol to estrone is 2:1, but after oral administration of estradiol, this ratio shifts substantially in favor of higher circulating estrone levels.

One mechanism to increase the oral bioavailability of estradiol is to prevent metabolic oxidation of the estradiol C_{17} hydroxyl group to the corresponding ketone. This is readily accomplished via alkylation of the C_{17} position with a chemically inert alkyne group (e.g., EE, Fig. 41.6). This synthetic analog is several hundred-fold more potent than estradiol, with doses in the microgram rather than the milligram range.

Conjugated equine estrogen, isolated from the urine of pregnant mares, currently is the most popular form of ERT. In addition to the ring B saturated hormones already discussed (45% estrone sulfate), CEE also contains equilin estrogens that have an unsaturated B ring, including equilin sulfate (25%) and 17α-dihydroequilin (15%). Comparison between human and equine-derived estrogens yields nearly equivalent binding properties between equilin and estrone as well as similar metabolic fates (12). Another method to keep the ratio of estrone to estradiol more equivalent is to use formulations that deliver estrogen via routes that are not subject to first-pass metabolism (e.g., transdermal, intravaginal, and intranasal). In addition, these routes permit ratios of estradiol to estrone similar to those found in premenopausal women (53). Transdermal formulations (Table 41.16) permit utilization of a lower drug dose and provide continuous systemic availability.

TABLE 41.16 Hormone Replacement Therapy for Treatment of Menopausal Vasomotor Symptoms (117,123,124)

Dosage Form	Trade Name	Estrogen	Progesterone
Tablets: estrogen only			
	Femtrace	Estradiol acetate	
	Premarin	Conjugated estrogens	
	Cenestin	Conjugated estrogens (plant derived)	
	Menest, Estratab	Esterified estrogen	
	Estrace	Micronized 17β-estradiol	
	Ortho-Est, Ogen	Estropipate	
	Enjuva[a]	Conjugated estrogens	
		$\Delta^{8,9}$-dehydroestrone sulfate	
Tablets: estrogen/progestin combination			
	Angeliq	Estradiol	Drospirenone
	Prempro	Conjugated estrogens	Medroxyprogesterone acetate (daily)
	Premphase	Conjugated estrogens	Medroxyprogesterone acetate (cyclic)
	FemHRT	Ethinyl estradiol	Norethindrone acetate
	Activella	Estradiol	Norethindrone acetate
	Prefest	Estradiol	Norgestimate
Transdermal or percutaneous			
• Transdermal spray (solution)	Evamist	Estradiol	
• Transdermal emulsion	Estrasorb	Estradiol	
• Transdermal gel	Estrogel	Estradiol	
	Divigel	Estradiol	
	Elestrin	Estradiol	
• Patch (estrogen)	Alora (biweekly)	Estradiol	
	Climera (weekly)	Estradiol	
	Estraderm (biweekly)	Estradiol	
	Menostar (weekly)	Estradiol	
	Vivelle dot (biweekly)	Estradiol	
• Patch (combo)	Climera Pro	Estradiol	Levonorgestrel
	Combipatch	Estradiol	Norethindrone acetate
Capsules	Prometrium		Micronized progesterone
Intravaginal delivery			
• Tablets	Vagifem	Estradiol	
• Cream	Estrace Vaginal	Estradiol	
	Premarin Vaginal	Conjugated estrogens	
	SCE-A Vaginal Cream	Synthetic conjugated estrogens A	
• Ring	Ogen Vaginal	Estradiol	
	Estring	Estradiol acetate	
	Femring	Estradiol acetate	
Intramuscular injection	Delestrogen	Estradiol valerate	
	Depo-Estradiol	Estradiol cypionate	

Intravaginal administration of micronized estradiol tablets (Table 41.16) represents another avenue for effective estradiol absorption without concern about first-pass metabolism (12). Originally approved as a 25-mcg tablet, Vagifem (10 mcg estradiol) was approved in 2009 by the FDA as a low-dose formulation for the treatment of vaginal atrophy. Unfortunately, vaginal creams containing estradiol only achieve 25% of the absorption expected for a similar oral dose. As a result, this formulation is best used for the treatment of urogenital atrophy. A sustained-release depot formulation of estradiol is available in the form of a vaginal ring (Femring, Estring) (Table 41.16). This type of formulation elutes estradiol or estradiol acetate over a 90-day period, thereby limiting the effort required by the patient. Estring delivers 7.5 mcg of estradiol per day and is indicated for the treatment of urogenital atrophy. Available in two strengths, Femring releases the equivalent of 50 or 100 mcg of estradiol per day via estradiol acetate, which subsequently is hydrolyzed to estradiol after release. This ring is indicated for the treatment of several urogenital symptoms associated with postmenopausal atrophy as well as for the treatment of vasomotor symptoms as a result of delivery of sufficient systemic estrogen. Two vaginal creams have been approved by the FDA for the treatment of vulvar and vaginal atrophy due to menopause. Synthetic Conjugated Estrogens-A (plant derived) is to be administered as 1 g once daily (0.625 mg/g cream) for 1 week followed by 1 g twice weekly. Conjugated estrogens (Premarin) are administered as a cyclic regimen with delivery of 0.5 to 2 g of cream daily for 21 days and then off for 7 days. Premarin vaginal cream (0.5g), administered twice weekly or using the cyclic regimen, has also been approved for the treatment of moderate to severe dyspareunia (painful sexual intercourse).

Although easy to use, percutaneous preparations (topical emulsion) (Table 41.16) suffer from inconsistent absorption. The FDA has approved several transdermal estradiol gels (Divigel, Elestrin, EstroGel) for the treatment of moderate to severe hot flashes. Divigel, sold in individual-use packets (0.50 mg estradiol), is a quick-drying gel that is applied daily to a 5 × 7 inch area on the thigh. Elestrin is supplied as a metered-dose applicator that delivers 0.87 g of gel per actuation (0.52 mg estradiol). The gel is applied directly to the upper arm and dries within 1 to 2 minutes (125). EstroGel is also delivered in a metered-dose applicator with 1.25 g of gel supplied per actuation (0.75 mg estradiol). It is recommended that Estrogel be applied in a thin layer from shoulder to wrist (~750 cm^2 area). Divigel and Elestrin are the lowest dose transdermal gels approved for the relief of hot flashes.

Evamist (estradiol), approved by the FDA in 2007, is a metered-dose transdermal spray that is to be applied to the inside of the forearm. Each spray (90 μL) delivers 1.53 mg of estradiol. Dosage adjustments can be easily made by increasing or decreasing the number of sprays applied daily. The FDA has warned that children and pets should not be exposed to those areas of the skin that have been treated, as premature puberty in girls and gynecomastia in boys developed in children of adult patients several weeks to months after initiation of Evamist therapy.

In addition to those identified by the WHI study, the adverse effects of ERT include nausea, headache, breast tenderness, and heavy withdrawal bleeding. Transdermal delivery minimizes headache and nausea, and use of a low-dose oral regimen lessens breast tenderness (5).

Micronized progesterone (Table 41.16) in combination with oral CEE provides valuable therapeutic benefit in the treatment of menopausal symptoms without the risk of endometrial hyperplasia. Unless micronized, progesterone is poorly absorbed when administered orally (12). Intravaginal administration of a controlled-release progesterone gel (Table 41.16) results in excellent absorption and more consistent serum levels than orally administered micronized progesterone. Systemic absorption is limited when progesterone is delivered by this route. Intramuscular administration of a progesterone in oil formulation produces the highest serum concentrations but is least likely to be tolerated by patients. The adverse effects associated with the use of oral progestins include irritability, depression, weight gain, and headache. These can be minimized if other routes of administration are used (e.g., IUD).

To minimize patient effort and to maximize patient adherence, a number of estrogen/progesterone combination products are commercially available (Table 41.17). Four types of combination regimens are available (oral and transdermal), including both continuous and cyclic therapeutic options. Cyclic regimens require a minimum of 12 to 14 days of progestin administration to prevent endometrial hyperplasia.

Used in perimenopause, administration of a synthetic progestin supplements the waning progesterone produced in the luteal phase of the menstrual cycle. This helps to prevent endometrial hyperplasia and to ensure

TABLE 41.17 Combination Therapies for the Treatment of Menopausal Symptoms (50)

Type of Therapy	Effect of Therapy	Regimen
Oral continuous-cyclic (sequential)	Scheduled withdrawal bleeding	CEE (1-14) + [CEE + MPA] (15-28)
Transdermal continuous-cyclic (sequential)	Scheduled withdrawal bleeding	17β-Estradiol + norethindrone acetate
Oral continuous-combined	Prevents monthly bleeding; unpredictable breakthrough bleeding likely to occur for first 6–12 months	CEE + MPA, 17β-estradiol + norethindrone acetate, ethynyl estradiol + norethindrone acetate
Transdermal continuous-combined	Prevents monthly bleeding	17β-estradiol + norethindrone acetate
Continuous long cycle (cyclic withdrawal)	Reduced monthly bleeding	Estrogen administered daily, progestin given six times/year for 12–14 days
Intermittent-combined (Continuous pulse)	Prevents monthly bleeding	3 days of estrogen alone, followed by 3 days estrogen and progestin combo, repeat continuously

CEE, conjugated equine estrogen; MPA, medroxyprogesterone acetate.

regular menses despite the irregularity of the menstrual cycle.

A unique investigational SERM RAD1901 is able to cross the blood–brain barrier and activate centrally located estrogen receptors (126). It retains ER agonist action at the bone and antagonist action in uterine and breast tissues. It is in phase II clinical trials for the treatment of menopausal hot flashes.

With such concern and confusion surrounding the use of either ERT or HRT for the treatment of menopausal symptoms and postmenopausal health benefits, women have turned to other natural or nonhormonal pharmacologic sources of relief (Table 41.18) (127,128). There are three groups of phytoestrogens that are found in over-the-counter supplements: the coumestans, lignans, and isoflavones (129). "Hormonal herbs," such as soy, black cohosh, and red clover, are purported to contain some or all of the phytoestrogens genistein, daidzein, and coumestrol (Fig. 41.17), which possess at least weak estrogenic activity (Table 41.19) (127–130) but structurally are nonsteroidal. The isoflavones genistein and daidzein are metabolized to other compounds including equol, which exerts estrogenic action. Other sources of nonsteroidal phytoestrogens, such as resveratrol from the skin of wine grapes (e.g., *Vitis vinifera*), currently are under investigation for their purported estrogenic effects (131). Small studies have indicated that the phytoestrogens may have additional beneficial effects on lipid profile and bone density (53).

MF-101 (Menerba) is an ERβ-selective agonist in phase II clinical trials for the treatment of the vasomotor symptoms associated with menopause. It does not stimulate the endometrium or breast tissue and therefore is unlikely to increase the risk of either uterine or breast cancer and thus may be a safer alternative to HRT. MF-101 is derived from 22 herbs used in traditional Chinese medicine for

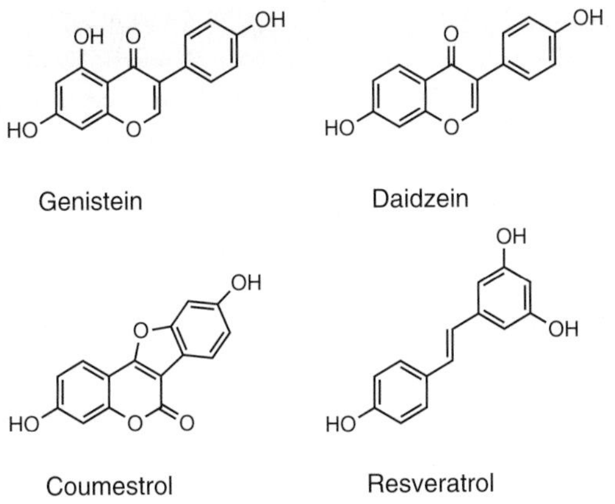

FIGURE 41.17 Naturally occurring phytoestrogens

the treatment of menopause. The active isolates include liquiritigenin and chalcone (126,132).

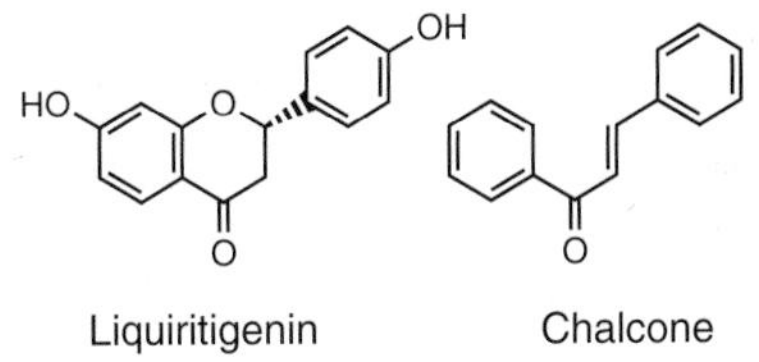

Several of the newer antidepressants, specifically those that modulate serotonergic neurotransmission, have become more prominent in the treatment of menopausal symptoms (Table 41.18). Some even consider this as first-line treatment when hormone therapy is contraindicated. Venlafaxine, a dual serotonin and norepinephrine reuptake inhibitor, has been found to decrease the frequency and substantially reduce the intensity of vasomotor symptoms and to improve problems of fatigue and sleep difficulty in more than 50% of the participants in clinical trials (127,133,134). With a 75-mg/day dose of venlafaxine, patients obtained relief from hot flashes within 1 to 2 weeks of treatment initiation. In comparison, fluoxetine and sertraline, which are selective serotonin reuptake inhibitors (SSRIs), only modestly improve the frequency and intensity of vasomotor symptoms. The effectiveness and onset of action of paroxetine, another SSRI, mirror those of venlafaxine. A low-dose paroxetine mesylate formulation (Mesafem) is in phase II clinical trials. A deuterated analog of paroxetine (CTP-347) demonstrates less CYP2D6 inhibition, thereby alleviating the drug interactions characteristic of paroxetine (126). Interestingly, the SSRI citalopram not only is similarly effective as paroxetine but also is effective in patients in whom vasomotor symptoms did not resolve with venlafaxine treatment. Desvenlafaxine has been shown to decrease the frequency of moderate to severe hot flashes by 65% and also significantly reduced the severity of hot flashes (135). Mirtazapine is an α_2-receptor antagonist and a serotonergic ($5\text{-}HT_2$) antagonist. The role of serotonin in modulation of the thermoregulatory processes is only starting to become clear. There is evidence that indicates that activation of central $5\text{-}HT_2$

TABLE 41.18 Nonhormone Replacement Remedies for Vasomotor Symptoms of Menopause (103,104)

Serotonin Based	Adrenergic Based	GABA Based	Herbals
Venlafaxine (SNRI)	Clonidine	Gabapentin	Soy
Paroxetine (SSRI)	Mirtazepine		Black cohosh
Fluoxetine (SSRI)			Garden sage
Citalopram (SSRI)			Dong quai
Sertraline (SSRI)			Kava
Mirtazepine			Valerian
			Red clover
			Flaxseed

GABA, γ-aminobutyric acid; SNRI, serotonin and norepinephrine reuptake inhibitor; SSRI, selective serotonin uptake inhibitor

TABLE 41.19 Herbal Products with Purported Utility in Postmenopausal Women (103–105)

Herb	Purported Use	Potential Problems
Soy (beans) *Glycine max*	Contains phytoestrogens—varied evidence for success in treatment of hot flashes	No concurrent treatment with tamoxifen
Black cohosh (root) *Actacea racemosa*	Contains phytoestrogens—purported use for hot flashes, additional studies needed	Possible liver issues
Sage (leaves, flowers) *Salvia officinalis*	Reduces night sweats and hot flashes	Kidney damage (large amounts)
Kava *Piper methysticum*	Reduces anxiety—no evidence for use in hot flashes	Liver damage
Red clover (leaf) *Trifolium pretense*	Contains phytoestrogens—not clinically significant reduction in hot flashes	Interaction with warfarin that can cause bleeding issues
Dong quai (root) *Angelica sinensis*	Not effective in treating hot flashes	Interaction with warfarin that can cause bleeding issues
Valerian (root) *Valeriana officinalis*	Treats hot flashes and insomnia	Morning drowsiness
Ginseng (root) *Panax ginseng*	May help with quality of life issues (mood, sleep) but does not help with hot flashes	
Flaxseed	No significant evidence that it helps hot flashes	Alters activity of antiplatelet and anticoagulant drugs

receptors results in hyperthermia; therefore, administration of a 5-HT_2 receptor antagonist should alleviate the thermoregulatory dysfunction associated with estrogen deficiency (127). Interestingly, an endogenous estrogen deficiency causes a reduction in the expression of central 5-HT_2 receptors, which is reversible on administration of an exogenous source of estrogen.

There is limited evidence that gabapentin (including an unapproved extended-release formulation Serada) and clonidine are effective in reducing the frequency of hot flashes (45% to 49% decrease) (133). There is also tentative evidence that gabapentin improves sleep quality in menopausal women. Although not indicated for the treatment of vasomotor symptoms associated with menopause, pregabalin (Lyrica) has also demonstrated the ability to decrease the frequency and severity of hot flashes.

There are nonpharmacologic avenues to consider when trying to limit the rise in body temperature, including avoidance of caffeine, alcohol, spicy foods, anxiety, and physical contact. Maintaining a good diet and exercise program is also thought to be beneficial because obesity and a sedentary lifestyle have been related to hot flashes (129).

Hormone-Dependent Breast Cancer

Background and Introduction

In the United States, the lifetime risk of developing breast cancer is one in eight, with the greatest incidence in women older than 60 years of age (136). It is the second leading cause of death from cancer in women (lung cancer is number one). An evaluation of 51 studies that represented 52,000 women with breast cancer showed a 15% increase in the risk of breast cancer in patients who had taken a combination of estrogen and progestin for less than 5 years. As treatment duration increased, this risk was amplified (137). In the HRT arm of the WHI study, the risk of breast cancer increased, yet in the ERT arm, there was no change in this risk (138). It should be noted that this increase in risk occurred 3 years after initiation of the study. To make matters worse, the breast cancers found in women of the HRT arm were likely to be more advanced than those found in women of the placebo arm of the study. Both arms of the WHI study were terminated prematurely, because the health risks incurred outweighed the benefits. No increased incidence of breast cancer was found in the ERT arm. The incidence of stroke did increase, however, and there was no benefit as it related to coronary heart disease (139).

According to the WHI study, there was no increased risk of endometrial cancer in patients taking HRT. If unopposed estrogen is administered to a patient with an intact uterus, then a significant increase in the risk of uterine cancer occurs within 2 years of treatment initiation (149). As the dose and duration of treatment increase, this risk grows.

Estrogen deficiency has been correlated with the development of colorectal cancer, the third most commonly diagnosed cancer. When estrogen levels are low, expression of the ER diminishes. Colorectal cells without ER expression are ripe to become cancerous. If estrogen levels are boosted by HRT, then ER expression should improve correspondingly, thereby reducing the number of colorectal cells primed to become malignant. The WHI study clearly shows a substantial decrease (37%) in the occurrence of colorectal cancer in patients treated with HRT.

MENOPAUSE AND LIBIDO

Despite what you might gather from promotional ads on the television and radio, sexual dysfunction in women occurs much more frequently than in men. Regardless of age (18 to 59 years), the prevalence of a lack of interest in sex among U.S. women is approximately 30% (140). This loss of sexual desire, a general feeling of lethargy or loss of energy, and reduced muscle strength can be attributed largely to an androgen deficiency. Urogenital atrophy and a decrease in vaginal lubrication in postmenopausal women also are potential reasons for a woman to experience an arousal disorder. These symptoms are directly linked to an estrogen deficiency. Administration of an exogenous androgen, typically testosterone, eases some of these symptoms, but it is unclear if this is a result of androgen receptor activation or of conversion into estradiol. Testosterone can be administered via several routes, including intramuscularly, subcutaneously (implants), or transdermally (patches). Estrogen replacement therapy effectively manages vasomotor symptoms as well as urogenital atrophy and dryness and diminishes some of the psychological symptoms, but it has virtually no effect on the waning libido experienced by many menopausal women. A method to address both sets of symptoms is to administer an oral estrogen/androgen combination (Estratest [methyltestosterone + esterified estrogen]) daily (53). With this type of regimen, it is imperative that the testosterone dose only generates physiologic serum testosterone levels so as to maximize therapeutic benefit and minimize undesirable side effects, including virilization and fluid retention (141).

Nonhormonal strategies also are available to treat female sexual arousal disorder. A transdermal formulation of alprostadil, used to treat male erectile dysfunction, has been shown to improve the arousal success rate. Applied 15 minutes before intercourse, this cream can cause local irritation, which is reversible on cleansing (142).

Molecular Mechanism of Action of the SERMs

The precise mechanism of SERM action is not well understood, but clearly, the ER is a primary target, as a signal transduction pathway, to modulate drug action in different tissues. Different concentrations of ER are present in breast cancers, which can be explained by heterogeneity in the tumor cell population. The more cells in the tumor that contain ERs, the higher the overall ER content, and the more likely the tumor will respond to antiestrogen therapy. Approximately 60% of ER-positive (receptor-rich) tumors are responsive to any form of additive or ablative endocrine therapy, whereas only 10% of ER-negative (receptor-poor) tumors respond to endocrine therapy (150). The current standard of care is to determine the ER status of the tumor in all patients with breast cancer.

The ER is divided into six regions (A–F, as shown in Fig. 41.5) (151). The DNA-binding domain (region C) is essential for the interaction of the ER with an ERE (152). The ligand-binding domain (region E) is the site of estradiol binding and the site of competitive binding by antiestrogens. The activating function (AF-1 and AF-2) regions are the areas of the ER that interact with coactivator molecules to form an effective transcription unit at an estrogen-responsive gene (153).

Crystallization of the ligand-binding domain (region E) of the ER with estradiol, DES, and raloxifene (154) as well as 4-hydroxytamoxifen (128) has provided an important insight regarding the conformational changes that occur with agonist or antagonist ER complexes. Figure 41.18 illustrates the crystal structure of the estradiol and raloxifene receptor complexes. The most important difference is the position of helix 12, which is essential for the correct binding of coactivators to form a transcription complex at an estrogen-responsive gene. Estradiol causes helix 12 to seal the ligand inside the hydrophobic pocket of the ligand-binding domain. It is hypothesized that this conformation allows coactivator binding. By contrast, raloxifene prevents helix 12 from sealing the hydrophobic pocket, and gene transcription is prevented (because coactivators cannot bind) (154). A similar

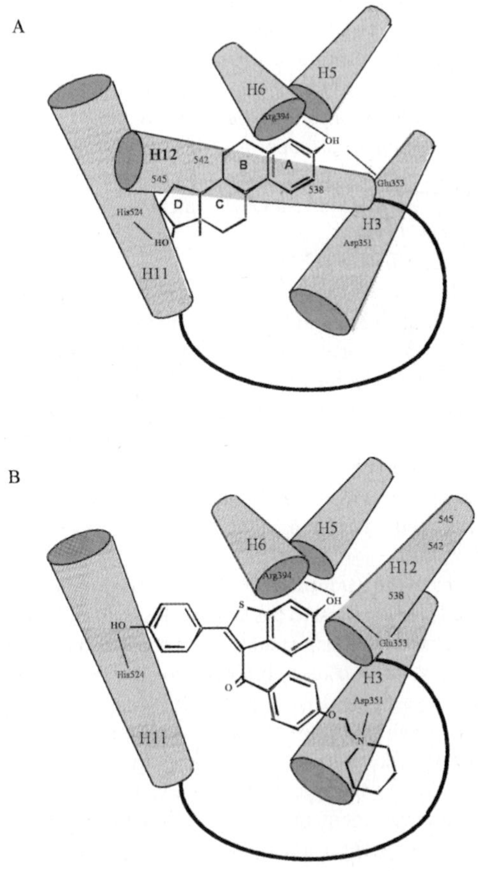

FIGURE 41.18 Comparison of the binding of estradiol (A) and raloxifene (B) in the ligand binding domain of the human estrogen receptor (ER). The key event in estrogen action is the repositioning of helix 12 (H12) to seal the steroid into the hydrophilic pocket so that coactivators can bind at the key amino acids indicated on H12. This cannot happen in the raloxifene–ER complex.

MENOPAUSE AND OSTEOPOROSIS

Osteoporosis causes 1.5 million fractures annually, including hip and spine fractures that increase both morbidity and mortality. In women older than 50 years, one in six will experience a hip fracture, and only 40% of patients older than 55 years with a hip fracture actually recover their mobility (143). (A comprehensive review of pharmacologic therapies available for the treatment and prevention of osteoporosis can be found in Chapter 30).

The estrogen deficiency associated with menopause has a detrimental effect on bone composition and quality. Before 65 years of age, postmenopausal women lose 3% to 5% of their bone mass on an annual basis. After this point, bone loss occurs at a rate of 0.5% to 1.0% annually. This results, in part, from an increase in circulating cytokines (e.g., tumor necrosis factor α, interleukin-1, and interleukin-6) when estrogen levels are low. These cytokines stimulate differentiation and proliferation of osteoclasts, the cells that normally degrade bone. The WHI study shows a positive correlation between HRT and a substantial decrease in fractures (24%). Currently, HRT (0.625 mg of CEE with 2.5 mg of medroxyprogesterone acetate) is recommended for the prevention, but not the treatment, of osteoporosis. This type of therapy should be initiated shortly after menopause and continued for at least 7 years (122). A lower dose of estrogen (0.3 mg) along with a progestin also may afford ample prevention. Despite the well-documented benefits of HRT in the prevention of osteoporosis, this should not be the primary therapeutic indication. In addition, no estrogen- or progestin-containing products have an FDA indication for the treatment of osteoporosis (119).

Studies that evaluate the benefit of combination OCs on bone mineral density have produced mixed results. Nearly one-third of these studies indicate no benefit, but the rest show a beneficial effect, including a 25% reduction of hip fractures in postmenopausal women (144). In patients using a combination OC containing at least 50 mcg of the estrogen component, this reduction in the risk of hip fracture improved to 44% (66). In general, the maximal benefits on bone mineral density are observed when the patients are older, have taken OCs for 5 or more years, and have used an OC preparation containing at least 50 mcg of estradiol.

Climara Pro (transdermal patch with estradiol [0.045 mg/day] and levonorgestrel [0.015 mg/day]) is indicated for the treatment of the vasomotor symptoms related to menopause. This formulation has also been approved for the prevention of postmenopausal osteoporosis.

Tamoxifen and raloxifene are SERMs and represent effective nonsteroidal therapy for the treatment of breast cancer and bone loss, respectively. The SERMs are a unique drug class in that a single agent may act as a receptor agonist in select tissues but a receptor antagonist in other tissues. In theory, it might be possible to protect a woman from osteoporosis and to reduce her risk for endometrial, breast, and colorectal cancers without worsening menopausal vasomotor symptoms with one drug. To date, no SERM can meet all these goals simultaneously. Raloxifene, a second-generation SERM, is an estrogenic agonist at the bone and is very effective for preventing osteoporosis without negative endometrial consequences or increasing the risk of breast cancer (see Chapter 30) (53). It is classified as an antiresorptive agent and has been approved by the FDA for both the treatment and prevention of osteoporosis. It also has a beneficial role in reducing the risk of cardiovascular events in postmenopausal women because of its antiatherogenic effects (reduces LDL levels) as well as in decreasing the risk of breast cancer (145). Unlike the bisphosphonates, which decrease both hip and vertebral fractures by 30% to 50%, raloxifene reduces only vertebral fractures by the same percentage. Raloxifene only has an effect on skeletal sites composed of cancellous bone. Unfortunately, raloxifene causes or worsens vasomotor symptoms in approximately 25% of patients, which represents a limitation to its use. In addition, raloxifene causes a threefold increase in the risk for VTE, which makes it contraindicated in women with a history of thrombosis. Following oral administration, raloxifene undergoes rapid first-pass metabolism to form its glucuronide conjugates and, thus, has oral bioavailability (~2%).

Because raloxifene only reduces the risk of vertebral fracture, there is a need to identify agents that are effective at multiple skeletal sites with minimal side effects. The novel SERM HMR-3339 improves bone mineral density in adult ovariectomized rats at a variety of skeletal sites (e.g., lumbar spine, tibia, and femur), including those sites composed of cortical bone (145,146). An additional benefit afforded by HMR-3339 is a reduction in total cholesterol (10% to 15%) and LDL (10% to 24%). This antiatherogenic activity, coupled with promising reductions in fracture risk across multiple skeletal sites, makes HMR-3339 a very exciting drug candidate for the treatment of multiple postmenopausal conditions.

HMR-3339

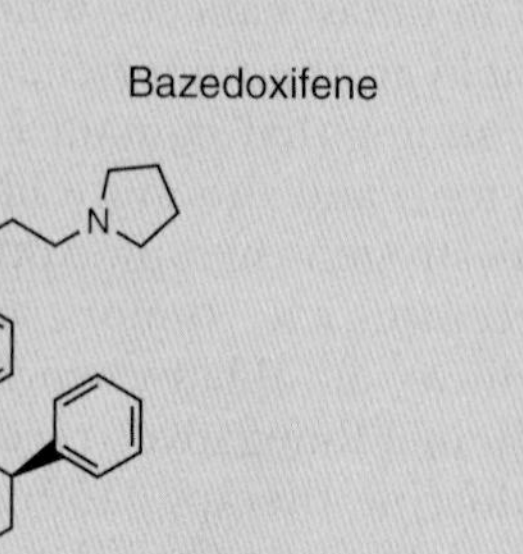

Bazedoxifene

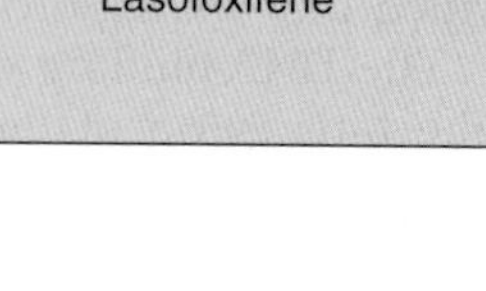

Lasofoxifene

(Continued)

MENOPAUSE AND OSTEOPOROSIS (Continued)

Bazedoxifene

Bazedoxifene is an indole-based third-generation SERM currently in phase III clinical trials for the prevention of postmenopausal osteoporosis. Similar to raloxifene, it is an ER antagonist in both breast and uterine tissues and an ER agonist on bone and the cardiovascular system. Bazedoxifene has been shown to reduce the risk of new vertebral fractures and reduce the risk of nonvertebral fracture in those at higher risk for fracture by 50% (147). Coadministration with conjugated estrogens has been shown effective in the management of menopausal symptoms.

Lasofoxifene

Lasofoxifene is a naphthalene-based third-generation SERM currently in phase III clinical trials for the prevention of postmenopausal osteoporosis. Similar to raloxifene, it is an ER antagonist in both breast and uterine tissues and an ER agonist on bone and the cardiovascular system. Lasofoxifene has been shown to reduce the risk of both vertebral and nonvertebral fractures. Increases in BMD in the femoral neck (2.9%), lumbar spine (3.1%), and hip (2.7%) have been reported (147).

Additional SERMs are presently undergoing clinical evaluation for treatment of osteoporosis and menopause-related vaginal atrophy (see Chapter 30).

Ibandronate sodium (Boniva) is one example of the bisphosphonate class of antiresorptive agents and is effective in the treatment and prevention of postmenopausal osteoporosis (see Chapter 30) (148).

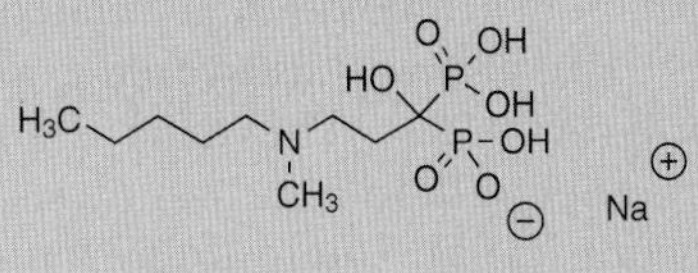

Ibandronate sodium

It was first approved as a tablet (2.5 mg) to be administered daily and later approved as the first once-monthly formulation (150 mg) for the treatment and prevention of osteoporosis (148). In January 2006, the FDA approved an intravenous formulation of ibandronate sodium (3 mg) to be administered every 3 months for the treatment of osteoporosis. This type of formulation benefits patients who have difficulty swallowing oral dosage forms or are unable to remain upright for 30 to 60 minutes. The injectable formulation generated a larger increase in lumbar spine bone mineral density compared to the oral formulations. Bone mineral density in the hip, femoral neck, and trochanter was improved as well. Adverse events associated with the injectable formulation included arthralgia, back and abdominal pain, and hypertension. There is a risk of renal toxicity that is inversely related to the rate of administration of this formulation. Caution is advised in patients who have renal impairment or who are receiving other pharmacologic therapy that may negatively affect renal function (145).

model is proposed for the 4-hydroxytamoxifen ER complex, but it is clear from studies in vitro that the raloxifene– and 4-hydroxytamoxifen–receptor complexes have different efficacies (155,156).

The antiestrogenic and some of the estrogen-like actions of SERMs can be explained by the different conformations of the ERα complexes attracting novel coactivators or corepressors (Fig. 41.5) to modulate estrogen action at different sites. In this model, the receptor would be the same at each site, yet the coactivators and corepressors would be distributed differently at different targets (157).

Alternatively, ERα could be modulated by different concentrations of ERβ at different sites. It has been suggested that ERβ could enhance estrogen-like gene activation through a protein–protein interaction at AP-1 (*fos* and *jun*) sites (158). At present, it is not entirely clear how SERM action is modulated at each target. Indeed, more than one mechanism may occur.

Selective Estrogen Receptor Modulators

Lerner et al. (159) described the first nonsteroidal antiestrogen, ethamoxytriphetol (MER25) (Fig. 41.19). This compound is an antiestrogen, with no other hormonal or antihormonal action. Although MER25 behaved as a "morning after" pill in laboratory animals (160), clinical trials associated with other reproductive and gynecologic applications showed that the drug had low potency and

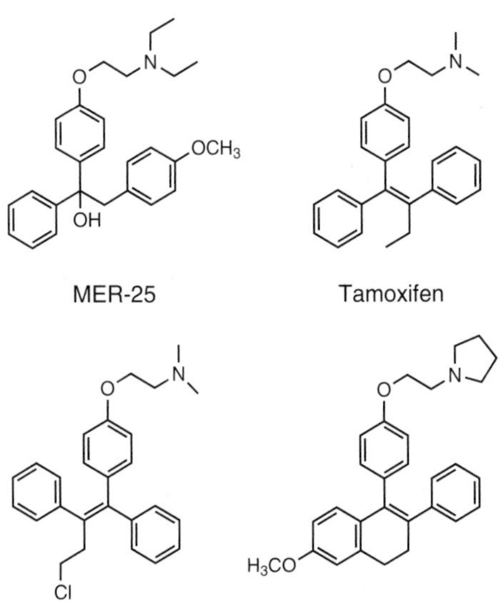

FIGURE 41.19 Nonsteroidal antiestrogens.

that the dose required caused central nervous system toxicity (161). In the search for more potent antiestrogens, clomiphene also was identified as an effective postcoital contraceptive in laboratory animals (Fig. 41.9) (162). Clinical trials in humans, however, demonstrated that clomiphene induces ovulation (163) and does not prevent implantation. Tamoxifen, a related triphenylethylene (Fig. 41.10), also was discovered as part of a fertility-control program (164). This drug is administered as the *Z*-diastereomer and, in some countries, is used for ovulation induction (165). Interestingly tamoxifen, clomiphene, and a rigid analog of tamoxifen, nafoxidine (Fig. 41.19), all inhibit the binding of [^{3}H]estradiol to ER; therefore, it was logical to test their efficacy as breast cancer treatments. Clomiphene and nafoxidine were not pursued after initial testing as a result of concerns about toxic side effects (166). Although a very low incidence of side effects is associated with tamoxifen, vasomotor symptoms often are evident and negatively affect patient quality of life (167–169). During the past 30 years, tamoxifen has become the endocrine treatment of choice for all stages of breast cancer and the first agent to reduce the incidence of breast cancer in high-risk pre- and postmenopausal women (170–172). Tamoxifen has now replaced endocrine ablative surgery in both pre- and postmenopausal patients with advanced breast cancer.

TAMOXIFEN (NOLVADEX) Tamoxifen (Fig. 41.19) is a SERM that is used as an antiestrogen in the treatment of estrogen-dependent breast cancer following primary treatment (chemotherapy and/or surgery). Therapy is limited to 5 years, because no additional benefit has been identified for treatment regimens of longer duration. Tamoxifen demonstrates only weak estrogenic effects at several sites, including the endometrium and bone, and on the lipid profile (169). Tamoxifen undergoes rapid oxidative *N*-demethylation to its major metabolite, *N*-demethyltamoxifen, via CYP3A4 and to its minor metabolite, 4-hydroxytamoxifen, via CYP2D6 (Fig. 41.20). Evidence suggests that 4-hydroxytamoxifen is the active metabolite of tamoxifen (173,174), with a higher binding affinity than the parent drug for the ER (173). Circulating levels of the demethylated metabolite at steady-state are up to twice the level of the parent drug, because the elimination half-life of *N*-demethyl tamoxifen is 14 days, compared with 7 days for tamoxifen (175). The aminoethyl ether side chain of the triphenylethylene antiestrogens is critical for the antiestrogenic activity of these agents.

Tamoxifen is rapidly absorbed from the GI tract with 100% bioavailability. It undergoes minimal first-pass metabolism and is highly protein bound, primarily to albumin. Tamoxifen's terminal elimination half-life is 5 to 7 days, which is indicative of enterohepatic recycling, elevated protein binding, and metabolic autoinhibition (169). For patients receiving concurrent anticoagulation therapy, a dosage reduction of the anticoagulant may be warranted.

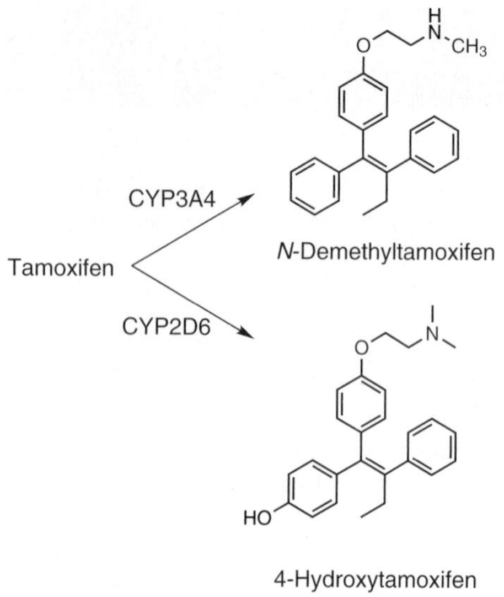

FIGURE 41.20 Metabolism of tamoxifen.

Agents that strongly inhibit CYP2D6 (e.g., paroxetine, fluoxetine, bupropion, duloxetine, thioridazine, quinidine, ticlopidine, terfenadine, cinacalcet) should be avoided in patients taking tamoxifen because these agents will prevent the metabolism of tamoxifen to its active metabolite (endoxifen). CYP2D6 genotyping will help to identify if a patient will respond to tamoxifen treatment.

After 5 years of tamoxifen therapy, a significant number of patients experience a relapse, primarily because of tamoxifen resistance. What is observed clinically is that the weak estrogenic effects of tamoxifen begin to predominate and effectively "feed" the hormone-dependent tumor.

TOREMIFENE (FARESTON) Toremifene is structurally and pharmacologically related to tamoxifen. It differs structurally from tamoxifen because of halogenation (chlorination) of the ethyl side chain, which reduces its antiestrogenic potency (Fig. 41.19). Toremifene demonstrates beneficial effects on the bone and cardiovascular system and increases HDL levels (169).

Toremifene is rapidly absorbed from the GI tract, with 100% bioavailability. It undergoes minimal first-pass metabolism and is highly protein bound, primarily to albumin. Toremifene, like tamoxifen, undergoes rapid oxidative *N*-demethylation, catalyzed by CYP3A4, to its active metabolite, *N*-demethyltoremifene. It also undergoes deamination-hydroxylation to ospemifene (Fig. 41.21) (169). Because toremifene is extensively metabolized in the liver, it should be used cautiously in patients with hepatic impairment. The terminal elimination half-life for toremifene is 5 to 6 days, which again is indicative of enterohepatic recycling and high protein binding (167).

Ospemifene (Ophena) is another SERM that is in phase III clinical trials for the treatment of postmenopausal

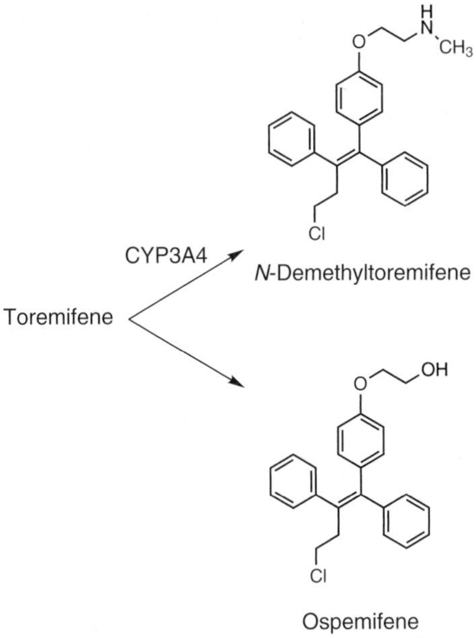

FIGURE 41.21 Metabolism of toremifene.

osteoporosis and postmenopausal vaginal syndrome (which includes vaginal atrophy, dryness, irritation, and dyspareunia) (176). As a metabolite of toremifene, it also is under evaluation as an effective treatment for breast cancer. In addition to its beneficial effects on the bone, ospemifene lowers LDL levels, improves the symptoms of vaginal dryness, and does not induce hot flashes.

Raloxifene Hydrochloride (Evista)

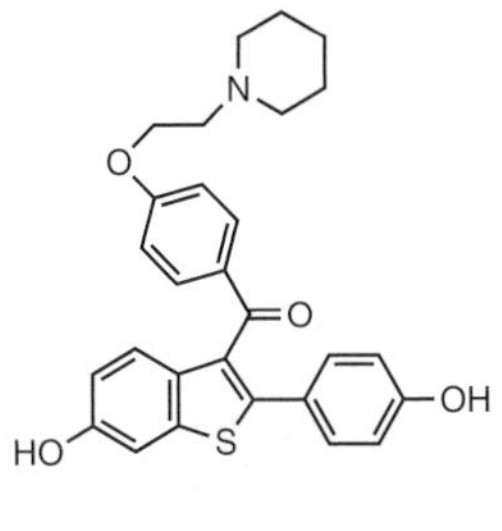

Originally indicated for the prevention and treatment of osteoporosis in postmenopausal women, raloxifene hydrochloride was approved by the FDA in 2007 to reduce the risk of invasive breast cancer in postmenopausal women with osteoporosis and postmenopausal women at high risk for invasive breast cancer (177). Raloxifene hydrochloride is a benzothiophene derivative and acts as ER antagonist in the breast and uterus while maintaining agonist action at the bone. See Chapter 30 for additional information.

Pure Antiestrogens

Despite the fact that 30% to 40% of patients with advanced breast cancer respond to tamoxifen therapy, this response only lasts for 12 to 18 months. Tamoxifen resistance is caused, in part, by its intrinsic agonist activity at the ER. In addition, tamoxifen only inhibits the AF-2 activation pathway but does not play a role in AF-1 pathway inhibition. Pure antiestrogens do not possess any estrogenic activity in any species or target tissue and, therefore, offer an additional avenue of treatment when resistance to tamoxifen occurs. In addition, because they are devoid of estrogenic action, these agents cannot be classified as SERMs.

Fulvestrant (Faslodex)

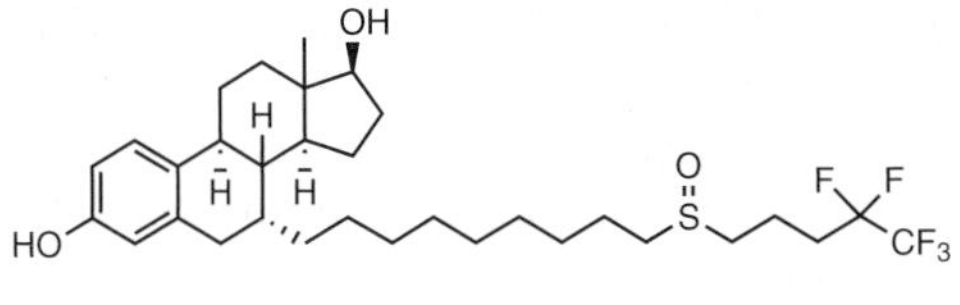

Fulvestrant

Fulvestrant is effective in preventing the growth of tamoxifen-resistant breast cancers (178) both in the laboratory (179,180) and in clinical trials. It is indicated following antiestrogen therapy for the treatment of ER-positive metastatic breast cancer that has continued to progress (181). Fulvestrant is an estradiol analog with a hydrophobic side chain in the 7α position. Oral bioavailability is poor despite metabolic protection on the end of the hydrophobic side chain. The rationale for this stems from the fact that fulvestrant is virtually insoluble. As a result, it is administered by intramuscular injection once a month. Metabolism of fulvestrant to both active and less active metabolites is similar to that observed with the endogenous steroids (181). Side effects appear to be minimal and include several GI symptoms, headache, and hot flashes. There is no clinical evidence of uterine stimulation or laboratory evidence of stimulation of endometrial carcinoma models (182). Fulvestrant should not be administered to women who are pregnant, who are taking anticoagulants, or who have thrombocytopenia.

Acolbifene

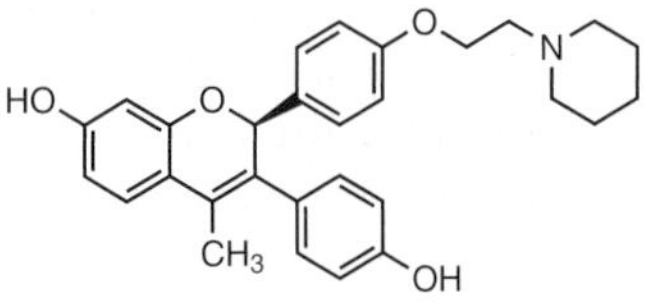

Acolbifene

Acolbifene is a nonsteroidal antiestrogen that is presently in phase II clinical studies (183). This fourth-generation antiestrogen is 200-fold more potent than tamoxifen in breast and uterine cancer cells and is effective in patients for whom tamoxifen therapy has failed. The mechanistic rationale for the effectiveness of acolbifene in tamoxifen-resistant tumors is based on the fact that it inhibits both the AF-1 and AF-2 activation pathways and does not possess any intrinsic estrogenic action. Acolbifene enjoys a 60% breast cancer cure rate (184). Structurally, acolbifene resembles raloxifene, with a benzopyran ring substituted for the benzothiophene ring. An additional benefit observed with acolbifene is its protective effect on bone loss. Adverse effects include nausea and vomiting.

Aromatase Inhibitors

Aromatase inhibitors are considered to be first-line therapy in postmenopausal women with metastatic, hormone receptor–positive breast cancer who do not tolerate tamoxifen. Aromatase is a viable target for drug action in the treatment of breast cancer, because it is the enzyme that catalyzes the conversion of androstenedione and testosterone to estrone and estradiol, respectively (Fig. 41.3, g and h). Inhibition of this enzyme limits estrogen production and effectively starves the hormone-dependent tumor. Studies do not clearly indicate that aromatase inhibitors are better first-line agents than tamoxifen and have not clearly identified a portion of this patient population that is more likely to benefit from this class of agents. It is recommended that postmenopausal women who have completed a 5-year regimen of tamoxifen for the treatment of early-stage, hormone receptor–positive breast cancer consider extending their treatment with an aromatase inhibitor. It has not yet been definitively established what the optimum duration of treatment should be or whether an aromatase inhibitor should supplant or be sequenced after tamoxifen therapy. The aromatase inhibitors are associated with a lower risk of endometrial cancer and thromboembolic events but with higher rates of fractures and myalgia as compared to tamoxifen.

LETROZOLE (FEMARA) Letrozole (Fig. 41.12) is a nonsteroidal aromatase inhibitor that was approved for the treatment of postmenopausal women with hormone receptor–positive or hormone receptor–unknown, locally advanced or metastatic breast cancer. By binding to the heme group of aromatase, letrozole inhibits the aromatase and causes a reduction in plasma estrogen levels. Inhibition of aromatase by letrozole is competitive and highly specific, with no effect on enzymes that are responsible for the production of glucocorticosteroids and mineralocorticosteroids (185).

This agent is significantly more effective than tamoxifen in treating hormone-dependent cancer. Letrozole reduces the rate of tumor progression for 9.4 months compared with 6 months for tamoxifen. Because tamoxifen therapy is limited to only 5 years, patients with breast cancer are left vulnerable to the return of their cancer. There is a 2% to 4% chance each year that the cancer might return. Taking letrozole after this 5-year period decreases the risk of the cancer returning by half. Letrozole also is used in patients who were treated for early forms of breast cancer to prevent disease from recurring. In clinical trials, it was shown that this type of preventive treatment cut the recurrence risk in half.

Letrozole is administered orally (2.5 mg daily) and is rapidly absorbed from the GI tract. Absorption is not affected by food. It is slowly metabolized (CYP3A4 and CYP2A6) to an inactive agent that is subsequently glucuronidated and eliminated renally. Letrozole strongly inhibits CYP2A6 and moderately inhibits CYP2C19. Its metabolism is induced by tamoxifen (169). Letrozole may increase the risk of osteoporosis and can cause hot flashes and night sweats. An increased incidence of hypercholesterolemia also has been documented.

For those women who are looking to cryopreserve oocytes or embryos prior to initiating chemotherapy for the treatment of breast cancer, letrozole can serve as an ovarian stimulant without increasing their estrogen and gonadotropin exposure. However, there are concerns that letrozole can cause birth defects and miscarriage if used off-label as a fertility drug.

ANASTROZOLE (ARIMIDEX) Anastrozole (Fig. 41.12) is a potent and highly selective, nonsteroidal aromatase inhibitor used in the treatment of advanced breast cancer that is hormone responsive. It is considered to be second-line therapy (after tamoxifen) in the treatment of postmenopausal breast cancer. Anastrozole, a benzyltriazole derivative, competes with the natural substrate for binding to the active site of the aromatase. The mechanism of enzyme inhibition resides in the coordination of the triazole ring with the heme iron atom of the aromatase enzyme complex (186,187). This coordination ultimately prevents aromatization of androgens into estrogens and, therefore, deprives the tumor of estrogen. This effect is reversible. In the presence of anastrozole, estradiol levels are reduced to undetectable levels, with no adverse effects on levels of any other hormone, including cortisol and aldosterone.

Anastrozole is well absorbed orally, with biliary elimination as its primary route (85%) and an elimination half-life of approximately 50 hours (186). Approximately 60% of an oral dose is metabolized in the liver by oxidative *N*-dealkylation, hydroxylation, and glucuronidation to inactive triazole metabolites.

EXEMESTANE (AROMASIN)

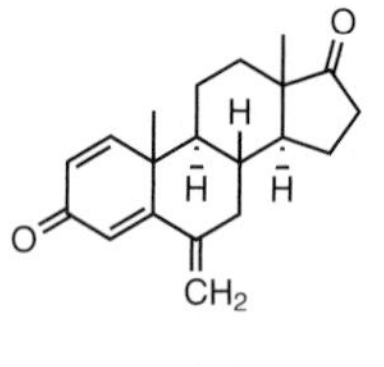

Exemestane is a steroid-based, irreversible aromatase inhibitor that is approved for the treatment of estrogen-dependent tumors and postmenopausal breast cancer. It also has been approved overseas as adjuvant therapy after 2 to 3 years of adjuvant tamoxifen treatment of ER-positive, invasive early breast cancer. The structure of exemestane is related to androstenedione. It is important to consider the woman's menstrual status when using this agent, because the synthesis of ovarian aromatase is part of a negative feedback loop such that decreased levels of circulating estrogen will promote increased biosynthesis of aromatase. As a result, exemestane should not be administered to premenopausal women or those who are pregnant. Exemestane binds irreversibly to aromatase and, therefore, is classified as a suicide inhibitor. Because this agent has high binding affinity and specificity for aromatase, it is able to suppress the activity of this enzyme by 97.7% (anastrozole, 92% to 96%; letrozole, 98%) (188).

Exemestane is administered orally (25 mg daily); however, only 50% of a given dose is absorbed. Absorption is improved if the medication is taken following a high-fat meal. Approximately 90% of a dose is bound to plasma proteins. Exemestane undergoes extensive metabolism by CYP3A4, and dosage adjustments may be necessary if given concomitantly with a CYP3A4 inducer (188). Adverse reactions reported in patients with early breast cancer include hot flashes, arthralgia, and fatigue, whereas hot flashes and nausea were the primary adverse reactions noted in patients with advanced breast cancer.

SUMMARY

Throughout a woman's reproductive life cycle, there are a number of disease states or life circumstances that can be successfully managed with one or more hormone-related therapeutic strategies. Not only is it important to select an appropriate therapeutic regimen for each individual, but it is also essential to determine which route of administration and, therefore, which formulation is the most therapeutically advantageous. A number of formulations are available for several single and multicomponent products, and maximizing patient compliance should be considered when recommending a particular product. There are no products devoid of adverse effects, so it is important that these be explained to the patient to minimize discontinuation of the recommended therapy.

The alarming results generated by the WHI studies have fueled the development of new estrogen-containing products designed to deliver lower doses of estrogen to minimize systemic exposure and decrease the risk of cardiovascular disease and development of cancer. In addition, a number of alternative therapies are under investigation for the treatment of menopausal symptoms. Agents that modulate serotonergic neurotransmission seem to be especially promising, because many of these therapies are already known commercial entities.

Pharmacologic management of breast cancer continues to make progress with advanced characterization techniques and the use of aromatase inhibitors and SERMs. Future generations of SERMs will need to be completely devoid of estrogenic activity to prevent the development of resistance, as is occurring with tamoxifen.

SCENARIO: OUTCOME AND ANALYSIS

Outcome

Nancy Ordonez, PharmD

CC was offered several options for contraception:

1. Depo-medroxyprogesterone is an injectable progestin-only contraceptive administered every 12 weeks.
2. Transdermal patch containing ethinyl estradiol 0.75 mg and norelgestromin 6 mg. The patch is applied to the abdomen, buttock, upper arm or upper torso and is changed on a weekly basis.
3. Vaginal contraceptive ring contains etonogestrel 0.12 mg/day and ethinyl estradiol 0.015 mg/day and is inserted vaginally for duration of 3 weeks.

She chose to use the vaginal contraceptive ring due to the longer duration of contraception and, with her job as a swimming instructor, she was afraid that the patch may become detached.

Chemical Analysis

Victoria F. Roche and S. William Zito

The vaginal contraceptive ring selected by CC and her provider is a combination product containing the estrogen ethinyl estradiol and the progestin etonogestrel. Both drugs have the 17α-ethinyl moiety that promotes female hormonal action, protects the essential 17β-OH group from inactivating oxidation to a 17-keto steroid, and promotes oral bioavailability.

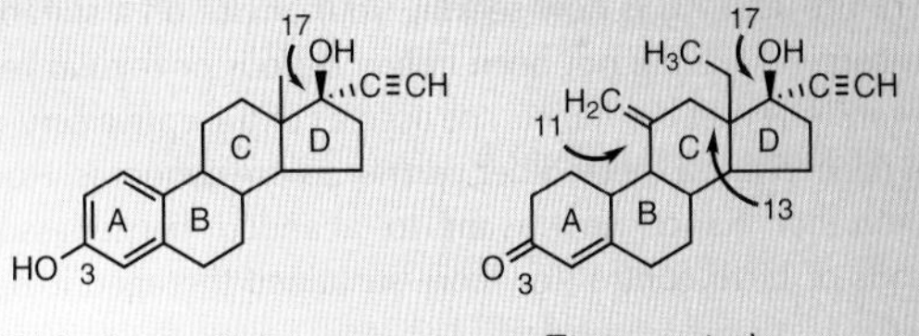

Ethinyl estradiol Etonogestrel

The aromatic ring is unique to estrogenic steroids and is a defining and essential structural feature of the pharmacological class. The phenolic OH group is also essential and forms a critical hydrogen bond with estrogen receptor Arg and Glu residues. The 17β-OH forms its own essential hydrogen bond with an estrogen receptor His residue. The remainder of the steroid hydrocarbon skeleton has been proposed to serve as a molecular scaffold to keep these two essential H-bonding hydroxyl groups separated by the appropriate distance for optimal estrogen receptor binding. The estrogenic component of a combination oral contraceptive acts by halting the secretion of follicle-stimulating hormone and other pregnancy-supporting gonadotropins.

The antiovulatory action of the C_{18} progestin etonogestrel depends on the 17α-ethinyl group; without it, a significant amount of androgenic activity might be observed. In addition, the C_{13}-ethyl group enhances progestational activity over the methyl substituent found on endogenous and most synthetic female sex

SCENARIO: OUTCOME AND ANALYSIS *(Continued)*

steroids. The unique exocyclic 11-methylene moiety adds unsaturation to ring C, another structural modification that promotes antiovulatory action in C_{18} steroids. The Δ^4-3-one A ring is found in all C_{21} and most C_{18} progestational steroids, and it has a higher receptor affinity than any other A-ring structural pattern. The 3-keto group is known to serve a H-bonding role and interacts with progesterone receptor Gln and Arg residues. Once bound to the progesterone receptor, etonogestrel prevents pregnancy by inhibiting ovulation and promoting changes in cervical and endometrial environments that are hostile to fertilization and implantation.

The use of the NuvaRing contraceptive vaginal ring would allow CC to avoid both injections and worry about the loss of a patch formulation because of sweat or chlorinated water. Because she has been noncompliant with oral medications, she could "set it and forget it" for 3 weeks, which should decrease the risk of accidental conception. The continuous release of an appropriate dose of contraceptive steroids should also result in fewer adverse effects than are commonly observed with orally administered contraceptive agents. This was a wise therapeutic choice for this patient.

CASE STUDY

Victoria Roche and S. William Zito

AG is 40-year-old New York advertising executive who has spent her adult life advancing her career in the high-pressure world of designer fashion. She lives life in the fast lane, and she purposefully chose a single life to give herself the freedom to do what she needed to do when she needed to do it, including traveling to exotic spots around the globe to promote her clients' work. Despite her best intentions, AG fell in love with a noted photographer who contracts with her agency, and they will be married next month. Though committed to making their marriage work, neither plans to give up their career. They have agreed that children are not in their future, and AG is now seeking your advice on a suitable oral contraceptive. Having not been in any serious or regular relationships until she met her fiancé, she used a contraceptive cervical cap when needed and expected her partner to use condoms. However, she and her fiancé now want to abandon barrier-associated methods of birth control for more sustained therapeutic options.

AG is a smoker whose moderately elevated blood pressure is kept under control with amlodipine besylate (Norvasc). Both of her parents are alive and doing well, but there is cardiovascular disease in her family history, and she lost her maternal grandfather to an acute myocardial infarction when he was in his early 60s. AG is known to be a rapid 2C9 metabolizer.

After reviewing AG's medical history, you consider the structures of the following steroid-based options before deciding which should be used, either alone or in combination.

1. Conduct a thorough and mechanistic SAR analysis of the three therapeutic options in the case.
2. Apply the chemical understanding gained from the SAR analysis to this patient's specific needs to make a therapeutic recommendation.

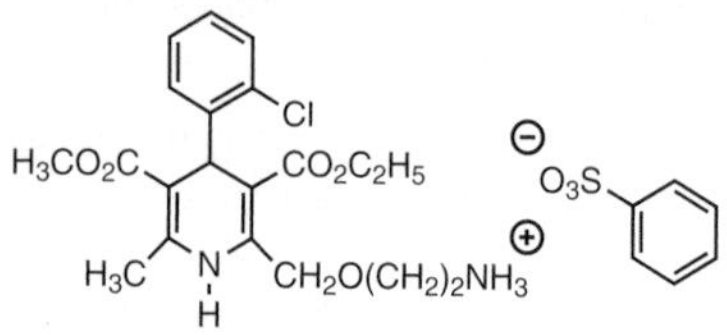

Amlodipine

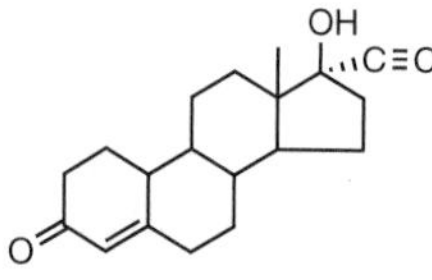

1

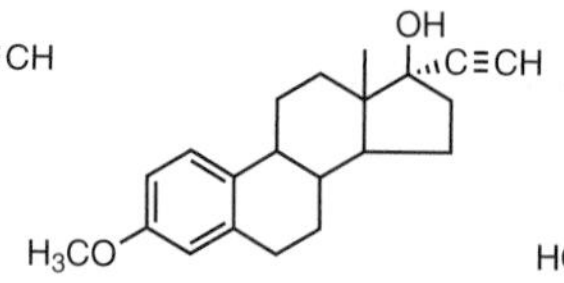

2

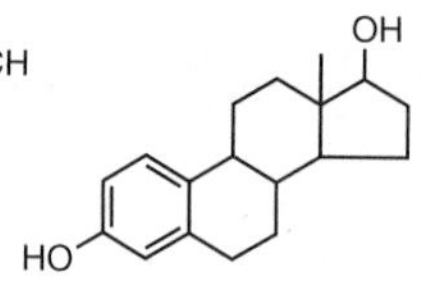

3

References

1. Cole LA, Sutton-Riley JM, Khanlian SA, et al. Sensitivity of over-the-counter pregnancy tests: comparison of utility and marketing messages. J Am Pharm Assoc 2005;45:608–615.
2. Butler SA, Khanlian SA, Cole LA. Detection of early pregnancy forms of human chorionic gonadotropin by home pregnancy test devices. Clin Chem 2001;47:2131–2136.
3. Hulisz DT, Urbanski CM. Home pregnancy testing kits. US Pharmacist 2002;21:22–32.
4. Eichner SF, Timpe EM. Urinary-based ovulation and pregnancy: point-of-care testing. Ann Pharmacother 2004;38:325–331.
5. Williams C, Stancel GM. Estrogens and progestins. In: Hardman JG, Limbard LE, Moliwoff PB, eds. Goodman and Gilman's The Pharmacological Basis of Therapeutics, 9th Ed. New York: Pergamon Press, 1996:1411–1440.
6. Gurpide E, Anger H, Vande Wicke RL, et al. Determination of secretory rates of estrogens in pregnant and nonpregnant women from the specific activities of urinary metabolites. J Clin Endocrinol Metab 1962;22:935–945.
7. O'Malley BW, Means AR. Receptors for Reproductive Hormones. New York: Plenum Press, 1974.
8. Najakin S, Hall PF. Microsomal cytochrome P-450 from neonatal pig testis. Purification and properties of a C_{21} steroid side-chain cleavage system (17α-hydroxylase-C17,20 lyase). J Biol Chem 1981;256:3871–3876.
9. Brown JB. Determination and significance of the natural estrogens. Adv Clin Chem 1960;3:157–233.
10. Diczfalusy E, Lauritzen C. Oestrogen bein Menschen. Berlin: Springer, 1961.
11. Kuhl H. Pharmacology of estrogens and progestins: influence of different routes of administration. Climacteric 2005;8(Suppl 1):3–63.
12. Grow DR. Metabolism of endogenous and exogenous reproductive hormones. Obstet Gynecol Clin North Am 2002;29:425–436.

13. Ansbacher R. The pharmacokinetics and efficacy of different estrogens are not equivalent. Am J Obstet Gynecol 2001;184:255–263.
14. Kuiper GGJM, Carlsson B, Grandien K, et al. Comparison of the ligand binding specificity and transcript tissue distribution of estrogen receptors α and β. Endocrinology 1997;138:863–870.
15. Ray S, Rastogi R, Kumar A. Current status of estrogen receptors. Prog Drug Res 2002;59:201–232.
16. Aitken SC, Lippman ME. Hormonal regulation of.de novo pyrimidine synthesis and utilization in human breast cancer cells in tissue culture. Cancer Res 1983;43:4284–4290.
17. Aitken SC, Lippman ME. Effect of estrogens and antiestrogens on growth-regulatory enzymes in human breast cancer cells in tissue culture. Cancer Res 1985;45:1611–1620.
18. Inhoffen HH, Hohlweg W. Neue per os-wirksame weibliche keimdrüsen-hormon-derivate: 17-aethynyl-oestradiol und pregnen-in-on-3-ol-17. Naturwissenschaften 1938;26:96–100.
19. Colton LB, Nysted CN, Riegel B, et al. 17-Alkyl-19-nortestosterones. J Am Chem Soc 1957;79:1123–1127.
20. Hussar D. New therapeutic agents marketed in the first half of 2010. Pharmacy Today 2010;16:53–63.
21. Solmssen UV. Synthetic estrogens and the relation between their structure and their activity. Chem Rev 1945;37:481–598.
22. Saeed M, Rogan E, Cavalieri EL. Mechanism of metabolic activation and DNA adduct formation by the human carcinogen diethylstilbestrol: the defining link to natural estrogens. Int J Cancer 2009;124:1276–1284.
23. Cavalieri EL, Chakravarti D, Guttenplan J, et al. Catechol estrogen quinines as initiators of breast and other human cancers: implications for biomarkers of susceptibility and cancer prevention. Biochim Biophys Acta Rev Cancer 2006;1766:63–78.
24. Bentley PJ. Endocrine Pharmacology. Cambridge, UK: Cambridge University Press, 1980.
25. Anstead GM, Carlson KE, Katzenellenbogen JA. The estradiol pharmacophore: ligand structure–estrogen receptor binding affinity relationships and a model for the receptor binding site. Steroids 1997;62:268–303.
26. Brzozowski AM, Pike ACW, Dauter Z, et al. The crystallization of the ligand-binding domain (LBD) of the estrogen receptor (ER) with 17β-estradiol and raloxifene. Nature 1997;389:753–758.
27. Shiau AK, Barstad D, Loria PM, et al. The structural basis of estrogen receptor/coactivator recognition and the antagonism of this interaction by tamoxifen. Cell 1998;95:927–937.
28. Baran JS. Synthesis of 11β-hydroxyestrone and related 16- and 17-hydroxyestratrienes. J Med Chem 1967;10:1188–1190.
29. Fieser LF, Fieser M. Steroids. New York: Reinhold, 1959:421.
30. Cross AD, Denot E, Carpio H, et al. Steroids CCLXX. Biologically-active labile ethers. II. A new group of potent orally active estrogens. Steroids 1965;4:423–432.
31. Funder JW, Feldman D, Highheel E, et al. Molecular modifications of antialdosterone compounds: effects on affinity of spirolactones for renal aldosterone receptors. Biochem Pharmacol 1974;23:1493–1501.
32. Katzenellenbogen BS, Ferguson ER. Antiestrogen action in the uterus: biological ineffectiveness of nuclear bound estradiol after antiestrogen. Endocrinology 1975;97:1–12.
33. Clark JH, Peck EJ Jr, Anderson JN, et al. Estrogen receptors and antagonism of steroid hormone action. Nature 1974;251:442–448.
34. Jordan VC. Selective estrogen receptor modulators. In: Williams DA, Lemke T, eds. Foye's Principles of Medicinal Chemistry, 5th Ed. Baltimore: Lippincott Williams & Wilkins, 2002:1059–1069.
35. Salhanick HA. Basic studies on aminoglutethimide. Cancer Res 1982;42(Suppl 8):3315S–3321S.
36. Bhatnagar AS, Hausler A, Schieweck K, et al. Novel aromatase inhibitors. J Steroid Biochem Mol Biol 1990;37:363–367.
37. Buzdar AU, Jonat W, Howell A, et al. ARIMIDEX: a potent and selective aromatase inhibitor for the treatment of advanced breast cancer. J Steroid Biochem Mol Biol 1997;61:145–150.
38. Bhatnagar AS, Hausler A, Schieweck K, et al. Highly selective inhibition of estrogen biosynthesis by CGS 20267, a new nonsteroidal aromatase inhibitor. J Steroid Biochem Mol Biol 1990;37:1021–1027.
39. Brueggemeier RW. Biochemical and molecular aspects of aromatase. J Enzyme Inhib 1990;4:101–111.
40. Johnston JO, Metcalf BW. In: Sunkara P, ed. Novel Approaches to Cancer Chemotherapy. New York: Academic Press, 1984:307–358.
41. Banting L, Nicholls PJ, Shaw MA, et al. Recent developments in aromatase inhibition as a potential treatment for estrogen-dependent breast cancer. Prog Med Chem 1989;26:253–298.
42. Rucnitz PC. Female sex hormones and analogs. In: Wolff ME, ed. Burger's Medicinal Chemistry, Vol. 4, 5th Ed. New York: Wiley, 1997:553–588.
43. Fraenkel L. Arch Gynaek 1903;68:438.
44. Corner GW, Allen WM. Physiology of the corpus luteum. Am J Physiol 1929;88:326–339.
45. Leonhardt SA, Edwards DP. Mechanism of action of progesterone antagonists. Exp Biol Med 2002;227:969–980.
46. Sitruk-Ware R. New progestogens: a review of their effects in perimenopausal and postmenopausal women. Drugs Aging 2004;21:865–883.
47. Fotherby K. The biochemistry of progesterone. Vitam Horm 1964;22:153–204.
48. Salhanick HA, ed. Metabolic Effects of Gonadal Hormones and Contraceptive Steroids. New York: Plenum Press, 1969:668.
49. Lednicer D, ed. Contraception: The Chemical Control of Fertility. New York: Marcel Dekker, 1969.
50. Heftmann E. Steroid Biochemistry. New York: Academic Press, 1970:140.
51. Klopper A. Developments in steroidal hormonal contraception. Br Med Bull 1970;26:39–44.
52. Klimstra PD. Progestational agents. Am J Pharm Educ 1970;34:630–647.
53. Kalantaridou SN, Davis SR, Calis KA. Hormone therapy in women. In: DiPiro JT, Talbert RL, Yee GC, et al., eds. Pharmacotherapy: A Pathophysiologic Approach, 6th Ed. New York: McGraw-Hill, 2005.
54. Davis ME, Wied GL. 17α-Hydroxyprogesterone caproate: a new substance with prolonged progestational activity: a comparison with chemically pure progesterone. J Clin Endocrinol Metab 1955;15:923–930.
55. Babcock JC. 6α-Methyl-17α-hydroxyprogesterone 17-acylates: a new class of potent progestins. J Am Chem Soc 1958;80:2904–2905.
56. Ruzicka L, Hofmann K. Sexual hormone XXIV. Über die anlagerung von acetylen an die 17-ständige ketogruppe bei trans-androsteron und Δ^5-trans-dehydro-androsteron. Helv Chim Acta 1937;20:1280–1282.
57. Ehrenstein M. Investigations on steroids. VIII. Lower homologues of hormones of the pregnane series: 10-nor-11-desoxycorticosterone acetate and 10-norprogesterone. J Org Chem 1944;9:435–456.
58. Djerassi C, et al. Steroids. XLVIII. 19-Norprogesterone, a potent progestational hormone. J Am Chem Soc 1953;75:4440–4442.
59. Kaunitz AM. Enhancing oral contraceptive success: the potential for new formulations. Am J Obstet Gynecol 2004;190:S23–S29.
60. Sitruk-Ware R. Pharmacological profile of progestins. Maturitas 2004;47:277–283.
61. Teichmann A. Metabolic profile of six oral contraceptives containing norgestimate, gestodene, and desogestrel. Int J Fertil Menopausal Stud 1995;40(Suppl 2):98–104.
62. Bouchard P. Chlormadinone acetate (CMA) in oral contraception. A new opportunity. Fertil Contracept 2005;10(Suppl 1):7–11.
63. Kotz D. Drug aims to reduce risk of premature labor. Globe Newspaper Company. Available at: http://www.boston.com/community/moms/articles/2011/02/04/fda_approves_first_drug_to_halt_premature_labor/. Accessed November 19, 2011.
64. Simhan HN, Caritis SN. Prevention of preterm delivery. N Engl J Med 2007;357:477–487.
65. Ther-Rx Corporation. Makena, 2011. Available at: http://www.makena.com/media/PDFs/full-pi.pdf. Accessed November 19, 2011.
66. Philibert D, Deraedt R. RU 38486: a new lead for steroidal antihormones. 64th Annual Meeting of the Endocrine Society, San Francisco, CA, June 1982, Abstract No. 668.
67. Baulieu EE. Contragestion and other clinical applications of RU 486, an antiprogesterone at the receptor. Science 1989;245:1351–1357.
68. Agarwal MK, Hainque B, Moustaid N, et al. Glucocorticoid antagonists. FEBS Lett 1987;217:221–226.
69. Elger W, Beier S, Chwalisz K, et al. Studies on the mechanisms of action of progesterone antagonists. J Steroid Biochem Mol Biol 1986;25:835–845.
70. Horwitz KB. The molecular biology of RU486. Is there a role for antiprogestins in the treatment of breast cancer? Endocr Rev 1992;13:142–163.
71. Hussar D. New therapeutic agents marketed in the second half of 2010. Pharmacy Today 2011;17:69–80.
72. Heikinheimo O, Vani S, Carpen O, et al. Intrauterine release of progesterone antagonist ZK230211 is feasible and results in novel endometrial effects: a pilot study. Hum Reprod 2007;22:2515–2522.
73. Sitruk-Ware R. Vaginal delivery of contraceptives. Expert Opin Drug Delivery 2005;2:729–736.
74. Himmerick KA. Enhancing contraception: a comprehensive review. JAAPA 2005;7:26–33.
75. Mishell DR Jr. State of the art in hormonal contraception: an overview. Am J Obstet Gynecol 2004;190:S1–S4.
76. Edwards LA. An update on oral contraceptive options. Formulary 2004;39:104–121.
77. Forinash AB, Evans SL. New hormonal contraceptives: a comprehensive review of the literature. Pharmacotherapy 2003;23:1573–1591.
78. Dickerson LM, Bucci KK. Contraception. In: DiPiro JT, Talbert RL, Yee GC, et al., eds. Pharmacotherapy: A Pathophysiologic Approach, 6th Ed. New York: McGraw-Hill, 2005.
79. Ouzounian S, Verstraete L, Chabbert-Buffet N. Third generation oral contraceptives: future implications of current use. Expert Rev Obstet Gynecol 2008;3:189–201.
80. Shrader SP, Dickerson LM. Extended- and continuous cycle oral contraceptives. Pharmacotherapy 2008;28:1033–1040.
81. Cibula D, Karck U, Weidenhammer HG, et al. Efficacy and safety of a low-dose 21-day combined oral contraceptive containing ethynyl estradiol 20 μg and drospirenone 3 mg. Clin Drug Investig 2006;26:143–150.
82. Vandenbroucke JP, Helmerhorst FM, Bloemenkamp KW, et al. Third generation oral contraceptive and deep venous thrombosis: from epidemiologic controversy to new insight in coagulation. Am J Obstet Gynecol 1997;177:887–891.

83. Mishell DR Jr. The pharmacologic and metabolic effects of oral contraceptives. Int J Fertil 1989;34(Suppl):21–26.
84. Shufelt CL, Bairey Merz CN. Contraceptive hormone use and cardiovascular disease. J Am Coll Cardiol 2009;53:221–231.
85. Mann D. Menstrual cycle affects cholesterol levels. WebMD Health News. Available at: http://women.webmd.com/news/20100812/menstrual-cycle-affects-cholesterol-levels. Accessed November 19, 2011.
86. Contraception for women with chronic medical conditions. Pharmacist's Letter/Prescriber's Letter 2011;27:270306.
87. Trussell J, Schwartz EB, Guthrie K. Obesity and oral contraceptive failure. Contraception 2009;79:334–338.
88. Erkkola R, Landren B-M. Role of progestins in contraception. Acta Obstet Gynecol Scand 2005;84:207–216.
89. Milanes-Skopp R, Nelson AL. Transdermal contraceptive patches: current status and future potential. Expert Rev Clin Pharmacol 2009;2:601–607.
90. Goa KL, Warner GT, Easthope SE. Transdermal ethynyl estradiol/norelgestromin: a review of its use in hormonal contraception. Treat Endocrinol 2003;2:191–206.
91. Hitchens K. Birth control now comes in a patch for women. Drug Topics 2002;19.
92. Zieman M, Guillebaud J, et al. Contraceptive efficacy and cycle control with the Ortho Evra/Evra transdermal system: the analysis of pooled data. Fertil Steril 2002;77(Suppl 2):S13–S18.
93. Ortho Evra (norelgestromin/ethinyl estradiol transdermal system) package insert. Raritan, NJ: Ortho-McNeil-Janssen Pharmaceuticals, Inc., March 2008.
94. Bjarnadottir RI, Tuppurainen M, Killick SR. Comparison of cycle control with a combined contraceptive vaginal ring and oral levonorgestrel/ethynyl estradiol. Am J Obstet Gynecol 2002;186:389–395.
95. Sivin I, Stern J. Health during prolonged use of levonorgestrel 20 micrograms/d and the copper TCu 380Ag intrauterine contraceptive devices: a multicenter study: International Committee for Contraception Research (ICCR). Fertil Steril 1994;61:70–77.
96. Downing D, Kasperowicz M, Rowe EL. Emergency Contraception: The Pivotal Role of the Pharmacist, American Pharmacists Association Special Report, a Continuing Education Program for Pharmacists, 2007, 1-20. Available at: http://www.pharmacist.com/AM/Template.cfm?Section=APhA_Special_Reports.
97. Glasier A. Emergency postcoital contraception. N Engl J Med 1997;337:1058–1064.
98. Crosignani P, Olive D, Berqqvist A, et al. Advances in the management of endometriosis: an update for clinicians. Hum Reprod Update 2006;12:179–189.
99. Saljoughian M. Understanding endometriosis and its treatment. US Pharmacist 2005;HS5–HS8.
100. Sturpe DA, Patel AD. Endometriosis. In: DiPiro JT, Talbert RL, Yee GC, et al., eds. Pharmacotherapy: A Pathophysiologic Approach, 6th Ed. New York: McGraw-Hill, 2005.
101. Garcia-Velasco JA, Quea G. Medical treatment of endometriosis. Minerva Ginecol 2005;57:249–255.
102. Valle RF, Sciarra JJ. Endometriosis: treatment strategies. Ann NY Acad Sci 2003;997:229–239.
103. Luciano AA, Turksoy RN, Carleo J. Evaluation of oral medroxyprogesterone acetate in the treatment of endometriosis. Obstet Gynecol 1988;72:323–327.
104. Bulun SE, Fang Z, Imir G, et al. Aromatase and endometriosis. Semin Reprod Med 2004;22:45–50.
105. Saito T, Yoshizawa M, Yamaguchi Y, et al. Effects of the novel orally active antiestrogen TZE-5323 on experimental endometriosis. Arzneimittelforschung 2003;53:507–514.
106. DeManno D, Elger W, Garg R, et al. Asoprisnil (J867): a selective progesterone receptor modulator for gynecological therapy. Steroids 2003;68:1019–1032.
107. Olive DL, Pritts EA. The treatment of endometriosis: a review of the evidence. Ann NY Acad Sci 2002;955:360–372.
108. Pal L, Santoro N. Age-related decline in fertility. Endocrinol Metab Clin North Am 2003;32:669–688.
109. Gharib S, Chapin MD, Rein MS, et al. Infertility: A Guide to Evaluation, Treatment and Counseling. Boston: Brigham and Women's Hospital Mary Horrigan Connors Center for Women's Health, 2003:1–10.
110. Kuohung W, Barbieri RL. Overview of treatment of female infertility. Available at: http://www.uptodate.com/contents/overview-of-treatment-of-female-infertility?selectedTitle=3%7E70&type=A. Accessed November 19, 2011.
111. Arslan M, Bocca S, Mirkin S, et al. Controlled ovarian hyperstimulation protocols for in vitro fertilization: two decades of experience after the birth of Elizabeth Carr. Fertil Steril 2005;84:555–569.
112. Hugues J-N. Ovarian stimulation for assisted reproductive technologies. Available at: http://whqlibdoc.who.int/hq/2002/9241590300.pdf. Accessed November 19, 2011.
113. Scott RT, Leonardi MR. A prospective evaluation of clomiphene citrate challenge test screening of the general infertility population. Obstet Gynecol 1993;82:539–544.
114. American Society for Reproductive Medicine: Ovulation Drugs: A Guide for Patients. Birmingham, AL: American Society for Reproductive Medicine, 2000:1–19.
115. Ovidrel (choriogonadotropin alfa) injection, solution [EMD Serono, Inc.]. Available at: http://dailymed.nlm.nih.gov/dailymed/drugInfo.cfm?id=19008. Accessed November 19, 2011.
116. Schultze-Mosgau A, Griesinger G, Altgassen C, et al. New developments in the use of peptide gonadotropin-releasing hormone antagonists versus agonists. Expert Opin Investig Drugs 2005;14:1085–1097.
117. Al Inany H, Aboulghar M. GnRH antagonist in assisted reproduction: a Cochrane review. Hum Reprod 2002;17:874–885.
118. Utian WH. Psychosocial and socioeconomic burden of vasomotor symptoms in menopause: a comprehensive review. Health Qual Life Outcomes 2005;3:47–56.
119. Stefanick ML. Estrogens and progestins: background and history, trends in use, and guidelines and regimens approved by the U.S. Food and Drug Administration. Am J Med 2005;118:64S–73S.
120. Shumaker SA, Legault C, Rapp SR, et al. Estrogen plus the incidence of dementia and mild cognitive impairment in postmenopausal women: The Women's Health Initiative Memory Study: a randomized, controlled study. JAMA 2003;289:2651–2662.
121. Shumaker SA, Legault C, Kuller L, et al. Conjugated equine estrogens and incidence of probable dementia and mild cognitive impairment in postmenopausal women: Women's Health Initiative Memory Study. JAMA 2004;291:2947–2968, 3005–3007.
122. Smoot LC. Hormone replacement therapy: where do we stand now? Drug Topics 2004;84–93.
123. Estrogen Monograph: Facts and Comparisons, Version 4.1. Available at: http://online.factsandcomparisons.com. Accessed April 7, 2011.
124. Estrogens and Progestins Combined Monograph: Facts and Comparisons, Version 4.1. Available at: http://online.factsandcomparisons.com. Accessed November 19, 2011.
125. Sites CK. Bioidentical hormones for menopausal therapy. Womens Health 2008;4:163–171.
126. Rovner SL. Hot flashes: still a mystery. Chem Engineering News 2009;87:33–35.
127. Perez DG, Loprinzi CL. Newer antidepressants and other nonhormonal agents for the treatment of hot flashes. Compr Ther 2005;31:224–236.
128. Bhatti WH, Gaich CL, Menke GL. Natural hormone replacement therapy. US Pharmacist 2004;41–54.
129. Kelley KW, Carroll DG. Evaluating the evidence for over-the-counter alternatives for relief of hot flashes in menopausal women. Pharmacy Today 2010;16:59–68.
130. National Institutes of Health State-of-the-Science. Conference statement: management of menopause-related symptoms. Ann Intern Med 2005;142:1003–1013.
131. Gehm BD, McAndrews JM, Chien PY, et al. Resveratrol, a polyphenolic compound found in grapes and wine, is an agonist for the estrogen receptor. Proc Natl Acad Sci USA 1997;94:14138–14143.
132. Stovall DW, Pinkerton JV. MF-101, an estrogen receptor beta agonist for the treatment of vasomotor symptoms in peri- and postmenopausal women. Curr Opin Investig Drugs 2009;10:365–371.
133. Carroll DG, Kelley KW. Use of antidepressants for management of hot flashes. Pharmacotherapy 2009;29:1357–1374.
134. Sulli M, See S, Kanmaz T. Nonhormonal therapy for hot flashes. US Pharmacist 2003;28:41–54.
135. Muse K, Kirby L, Constantine G, et al. Desvenlafaxine succinate (DVS) results in a sustained reduction in number of moderate-to-severe hot flushes (HFs) [abstract]. Fertil Steril 2007;88(Suppl 1):S246.
136. Swanson GM. Breast cancer risk estimation: a translational statistic for communication to the public. J Natl Cancer Inst 1993;85:848–849.
137. Collaborative Group on Hormonal Factors in Breast Cancer. Breast cancer and hormone replacement therapy: collaborative reanalysis of data from epidemiological studies of 52,705 women with breast cancer and 108,411 women without breast cancer. Lancet 1997;350:1047–1059.
138. Stefanick ML, Anderson GL, Margolis KL, et al. Effects of conjugated equine estrogens on breast cancer and mammography screening in postmenopausal women with hysterectomy. JAMA 2006;295:1647–1657.
139. Women's Health Initiative Steering Committee. Effect of conjugated equine estrogen in postmenopausal women with hysterectomy. JAMA 2004;291:1701–1712.
140. Warnock JK. Female hypoactive sexual desire disorder: epidemiology, diagnosis, and treatment. CNS Drugs 2002;16:745–753.
141. Arlt W. Androgen therapy in women. Eur J Endocrinol 2006;154:1–11.
142. Palkhivala A. Alprostadil cream may be effective against female sexual arousal disorder. ASRM 2005 Annual Meeting: Abstract O-322. Presented October 19, 2005.
143. Greenblatt D. Treatment of postmenopausal osteoporosis. Pharmacotherapy 2005;25:574–584.
144. Michaelsson K, Baron JA, Farahmand BY, et al. Oral contraceptive use and risk of hip fracture: a case-control study. Lancet 1999;353:1481–1484.
145. Vogelvang TE, Mijatovic V, Kenemans P, et al. HMR 3339, a novel selective estrogen receptor modulator, reduces total cholesterol, low-density lipoprotein cholesterol, and homocysteine in healthy postmenopausal women. Fertil Steril 2004;82:1540–1549.

146. Ammann P, Bourrin S, Brunner F, et al. A new selective estrogen receptor modulator HMR-3339 fully corrects bone alterations induced by ovariectomy in adult rats. Bone 2004;35:153–161.
147. Silverman S. New selective estrogen receptor modulators (SERMs) in development. Curr Osteporos Rep 2010;8:151–153.
148. Bisphosphonate Monograph, Facts and Comparisons 4.1. Available at: http://online.factsandcomparisons.com. Accessed November 19, 2011.
149. Casper RF. Estrogen with interrupted progestin HRT: a review of experimental and clinical studies. Maturitas 2000;34:97–108.
150. McGuire WL, Carbone PP, Volliner EP. Estrogen Receptors in Human Breast Cancer. New York: Raven Press, 1975.
151. Kumar V, Green S, Stack G, et al. Functional domains of the human estrogen receptor. Cell 1987;51:941–951.
152. Green S, Chambon P. Estradiol induction of a glucocorticoid-responsive gene by a chimeric receptor. Nature 1987;325:75–78.
153. Kraus WL, McInerney EM, Katzenellenbogen BS. Ligand-dependent, transcriptionally productive association of the amino- and carboxyl-terminal regions of a steroid hormone nuclear receptor. Proc Natl Acad Sci USA 1995;92:12314–12318.
154. Brzozowski AM, Pike AC, Dauter Z, et al. Molecular basis of agonism and antagonism in the estrogen receptor. Nature 1997;389:753–758.
155. Shiau AK, Barstad D, Loria PM, et al. The structural basis of estrogen receptor/coactivator recognition and the antagonism of this interaction by tamoxifen. Cell 1998;95:927–937.
156. Jordan VC. Antiestrogenic action of raloxifene and tamoxifen: today and tomorrow. J Natl Cancer Inst 1998;90:967–971.
157. Wijayaratne AL, Nagel SC, Paige LA, et al. Comparative analyses of mechanistic differences among antiestrogens. Endocrinology 1999;140:5828–5840.
158. Paech K, Webb P, Kuiper GG, et al. Differential ligand activation of estrogen receptors ER-α and ER-β at AP1 sites. Science 1997;277:1508–1510.
159. Lerner LJ, Holthaus JF, Thompson CR. A nonsteroidal estrogen antagonist 1-(p-2-diethylaminoethoxyphenyl)-1-phenyl-2-p-methoxyphenylethanol. Endocrinology 1958;63:295–318.
160. Segal JS, Nelson WO. An orally active compound with antifertility effects in rats. Proc Soc Exp Biol Med 1958;98:431–436.
161. Lerner LJ. The first nonsteroidal antiestrogen–MER 25. In: Nonsteroidal Antiestrogens: Molecular Pharmacology and Antitumor Activity. Sydney, Australia: Sydney Academic Press, 1981:1–6.
162. Holtkamp DE, Greslin SC, Root CA, et al. Gonadotropin inhibiting and antifecundity effects of chloramiphene. Proc Soc Exp Biol Med 1960;105:197–201.
163. Greenblatt R, Roy S, Mahesh V. The induction of ovulation. Am J Obstet Gynecol 1962;84:900–912.
164. Harper MJ, Walpole AL. A new derivative of triphenylethylene: effect on implantation and mode of action in rats. J Reprod Fertil 1967;13:101–119.
165. Furr BJ, Jordan VC. The pharmacology and clinical uses of tamoxifen. Pharmacol Ther 1984;25:127–205.
166. Legha SS, Carter SK. Antiestrogens in the treatment of breast cancer. Cancer Treat Rev 1976;3:205–216.
167. Cole MP, Jones CT, Todd ID. A new antiestrogenic agent in late breast cancer. An early clinical appraisal of ICI42474. Br J Cancer 1971;25:270–275.
168. Ward HW. Antiestrogen therapy for breast cancer: a trial of tamoxifen at two dose levels. Br Med J 1973;1:13–14.
169. Morella KC, Wurz GT, DeGregorio MW. Pharmacokinetics of selective estrogen receptor modulators. Clin Pharmacokinet 2003;42:361–372.
170. Lerner LJ, Jordan VC. Development of antiestrogens and their use in breast cancer: Eighth Cain Memorial Award Lecture. Cancer Res 1990;50:4177–4189.
171. Osborne CK. Tamoxifen in the treatment of breast cancer. N Engl J Med 1998;339:1609–1618.
172. Fisher B, Costantino JP, Wickerham DL, et al. Tamoxifen for prevention of breast cancer: report of the National Surgical Adjuvant Breast and Bowel Project P-1 Study. J Natl Cancer Inst 1998;90:1371–1388.
173. Jordan VC, Collins MM, Rowsby L, et al. A monohydroxylated metabolite of tamoxifen with potent antiestrogenic activity. J Endocrinol 1977;75:305–316.
174. Jordan VC, Murphy CS. Endocrine pharmacology of antiestrogens as antitumor agents. Endocr Rev 1990;11:578–610.
175. Jordan VC. Biochemical pharmacology of antiestrogen action. Pharmacol Rev 1984;36:245–276.
176. Gennari L. Ospemifene hormos. Current Opin Invest Drugs 2004;5:448–455.
177. Thomsen A, Kolesar JM. Chemoprevention of Breast Cancer. Am J Health Syst Pharm 2008;65:2221–2228.
178. Howell A, DeFriend DJ, Robertson JF, et al. Pharmacokinetics, pharmacological, and antitumor effects of the specific antiestrogen ICI 182780 in women with advanced breast cancer. Br J Cancer 1996;74:300–308.
179. Wakeling AE, Dukes M, Bowler J. A potent specific pure antiestrogen with clinical potential. Cancer Res 1991;51:3867–3873.
180. Osborne CK, Coronado-Heinsohn EB, Hilsenbeck SG, et al. Comparison of the effects of a pure steroidal antiestrogen with those of tamoxifen in a model of human breast cancer. J Natl Cancer Inst 1995;87:742–750.
181. Faslodex (fulvestrant injection), prescribing information. London, UK: AstraZeneca Pharmaceuticals, 2004.
182. O'Regan RM, Cisneros A, England GM, et al. Effects of the antiestrogens tamoxifen, toremifene, and ICI 182,780 on endometrial cancer growth. J Natl Cancer Inst 1998;90:1552–1558.
183. Simard J, Sanchez R, Poirier D, et al. Blockade of the stimulatory effect of estrogens, OH-tamoxifen, OH-toremifene, droloxifene, and raloxifene on alkaline phosphatase activity by the antiestrogen EM-800 in human endometrial adenocarcinoma Ishikawa cells. Cancer Res 1997;57:3494–3497.
184. Labrie F, Champagne P, Labrie C, et al. Activity and safety of the antiestrogen EM-800, the orally active precursor of acolbifene, in tamoxifen-resistant breast cancer. J Clin Oncol 2004;22:864–871.
185. Femara (letrazole tablets), prescribing information. Basel, Switzerland: Novartis, 2001.
186. Higa GM, Al-Khouri N. Anastrozole: a selective aromatase inhibitor for the treatment of breast cancer. Am J Health Syst Pharm 1998;55:445–452.
187. Higa GM. Altering the estrogenic milieu of breast cancer with a focus on the new aromatase inhibitors. Pharmacotherapy 2000;20:280–291.
188. Higa GM. Exemestane: treatment of breast cancer with selective inactivation of aromatase. Am J Health Syst Pharm 2002;59:2194–2201.

Chapter 42

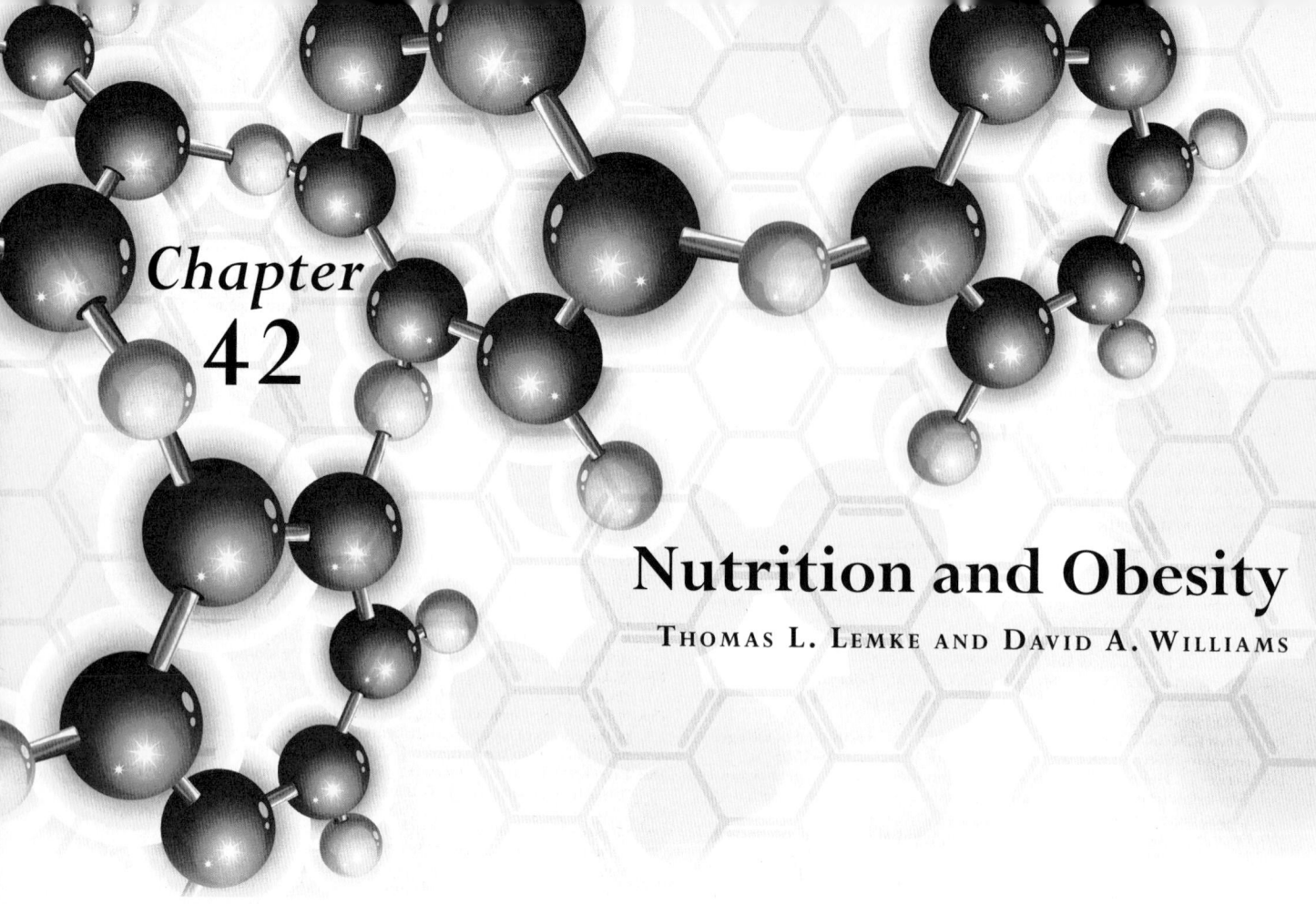

Nutrition and Obesity

THOMAS L. LEMKE AND DAVID A. WILLIAMS

*Nutrients/Drugs Covered in This Chapter**

DRUGS

- Amphetamine
- Benzphetamine
- Diethylpropion
- Ephedrine
- Fenfluramine
- Mazindol
- Olestra
- Orlistat
- Phendimetrazine
- Phenmetrazine
- Phentermine
- Phenylpropanolamine
- Pseudoephedrine
- Sibutramine

MACRONUTRIENTS

- Acesulfame-K
- Aspartame
- *Cyclamate*
- Fatty acids
  - Saturated
  - Unsaturated (polyunsaturated)
- Fiber
- Glycogen
- Neotame
- Rebaudioside A
- Saccharin
- Starch
- Sucralose
- Xylitol

MICRONUTRIENTS

- Sodium chloride
- Tocopherols
- Vitamin A
  - Carotenes
  - Lutein
  - Retinol
- Vitamin C (ascorbic acid)
- Vitamin D
- Vitamin E
- Vitamin K

Abbreviations

ATP, adenosine triphosphate
BMI, body mass index
BMR, basal metabolic rate
CHD, coronary heart disease
CNS, central nervous system
CoA, coenzyme A
DIT, diet-induced thermogenesis
DRI, Dietary Reference Intake
DSHEA, Dietary Supplement Health and Education Act
DV, daily value
EEA, energy of expenditure of activity
FDA, U.S. Food and Drug Administration
GI, gastrointestinal
GRAS, generally recognized as safe
HDL, high-density lipoprotein
LDL, low-density lipoprotein
NLEA, Nutrition Labeling and Educational Act
PKU, phenylketonuria
PUFA, polyunsaturated fatty acids
RAE, retinol activity equivalent
RDA, Recommended Dietary Allowance
RDI, Recommended Daily Intakes
ROS, reactive oxygen species
RS, resistant starch
SSRI, selective serotonin reuptake inhibitor
TEE, total energy expenditure
TFA, *trans* fatty acid

*Nutrients/Drugs listed include those available inside and outside of the United States; the nutrient shown in italics is no longer available in the United States.

SCENARIO

Beverly Lukawski, PharmD, and Jennifer Campbell, PharmD

JL, a 25-year-old Hispanic woman, presented to the emergency room after experiencing syncope during her morning workout and subsequent tightness in her chest. JL is 5′6″ and 115 kg. The patient has a past medical history of migraines and currently treats them using over-the-counter aspirin with caffeine. The patient states that she also takes an oral contraceptive and recently initiated a weight-loss dietary supplement called Kwik Loss (ingredients: bitter orange, caffeine, and vitamins B_6, B_{12}, and C) to help her lose weight for an upcoming wedding. The patient presents with a blood pressure of 141/82 mm Hg and a heart rate of 75 beats/min. All other vital signs are within normal limits.

(The reader is directed to the clinical solution and chemical analysis of this case at the end of the chapter.)

INTRODUCTION

Every living cell in the human body and the cells of other living organisms require essential ingredients to survive. These essential ingredients are chemical substances, both organic and inorganic, that are not generally produced in the body, or if they are, they are not produced in sufficient quantities to meet the cellular or body needs. These chemical substances are commonly referred to as nutrients, and the utilization of these substances for normal body development and growth is called nutrition. Poor nutrition can result from both insufficient quantities of nutrients and overconsumption of nutrients. Examples of diseases associated with low levels of nutrients are blindness (vitamin A deficiency), osteoporosis (vitamin D, calcium, and phosphate deficiencies), scurvy (vitamin C deficiency), and kwashiorkor (protein deficiency). Excessive intake of nutrients can lead to obesity, which in turn has been associated with cardiovascular diseases, osteoarthritis, sleep apnea, respiratory problems, and type 2 diabetes, to mention only a few. Nutritional balance will always be critical to overall body health and will be emphasized throughout this chapter. Complicating the science of nutrition is the fact that nutrition is affected by age, sex, experience, religion, lifestyle, culture, economics, and a wide variety of other factors. From our standpoint, nutrition is essential for body growth and maintenance and will be presented in this context.

NUTRIENT CLASSIFICATION

The nutrients essential to man and animals can be classified as macronutrients or micronutrients. Those chemicals that must be taken in large quantities are referred to as macronutrients, whereas those that are required in small quantities are referred to as micronutrients. The macronutrients consist of carbohydrates, fats, proteins, and water, whereas the micronutrients consist of vitamins and minerals. The quantities of macro- and micronutrients change with age. From conception until the mid-teens, the body undergoes considerable growth, and the quantities of nutrients required for good health will be high. From the teens throughout much of the remainder of life, nutrients are expected to maintain the structure of the body. In the elderly, the demand for some nutrients may actually decrease, although this may be more associated with reduced physical activity. During much of our adult life (20 years of age and older), nutrition serves the role of maintaining the body by replacing essential chemicals lost due to normal turnover and supplying energy for running the body. The energy supplied to the body is primarily met through the macronutrients and, more specifically, by carbohydrates and fats. Body composition and weight will generally be relatively stable in an individual with good health, but depending on the eating habits and physical activity, serious medical issues may arise. This chapter is intended to address the issues of energy needs, nutritional sources of energy and balance, the disease state of obesity, and the types of chemicals that can be substituted for high-caloric nutrients. The simplistic view of excessive body weight or the medical condition of obesity occurs when the intake of macronutrients exceeds the energy needs of the body and nutrients are put into storage. Carbohydrates are stored in the form of glycogen; amino acids, the absorbable form of protein, are stored in the form of protein; and fats are stored as fats or lipids (Fig. 42.1).

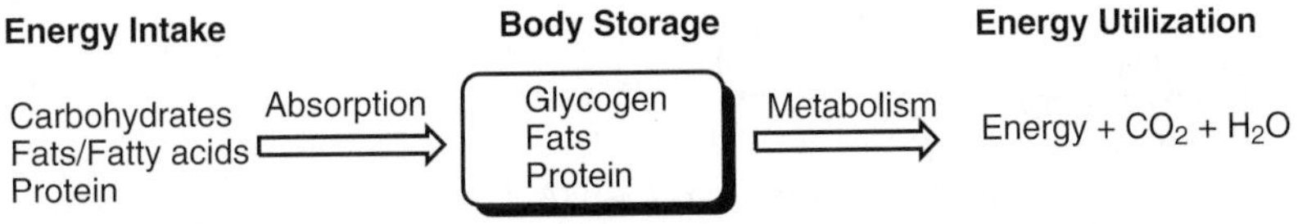

FIGURE 42.1 Diagrammatic representation of macronutrient absorption, storage, and utilization needed to run the body.

CLINICAL SIGNIFICANCE

Obesity, defined by a body mass index (BMI) of >30 kg/m², is a current public health crisis in the United States. In 2009, Colorado was the only state to have less than a 20% prevalence of obesity, whereas in nine states, 30% or more of residents had a BMI of >30 kg/m². Although diet and exercise are promoted as the first-line approach to weight loss for the majority of people, many are not successful in these attempts. As a result, they turn to prescription or over-the-counter medications or dietary supplements to aid in their weight loss. In 2005, more than $1.6 billion was spent on dietary supplements for weight loss.

While the chemical relationship to therapeutic action of previously available prescription drugs is well known, the same cannot be said for the ingredients in dietary supplements. Products touted as "metabolism boosters" once contained the ingredient ephedra, a source of ephedrine alkaloids, with these nonphenolic phenethylamines showing an affinity for presynaptic norepinephrine reuptake sites. In 2004, ephedra was removed from the market due to safety concerns; a postmarketing meta-analysis detailed more than 16,000 adverse drug events attributed to ephedra-containing ingredients, ranging from liver disease and seizure to myocardial infarction and stroke (1). After the removal of ephedra, "ephedra-free" products were soon on the shelves of pharmacies and supplement stores. Many of these products had replaced ephedra with bitter orange (*Citrus aurantium*). Bitter orange contains both octopamine and its metabolite synephrine, compounds structurally related to ephedrine. While the full chemical composition of bitter orange products is under debate, synephrine's stimulant properties are supported by numerous case studies detailing cardiovascular incidents, including angina, syncope, and myocardial infarction, that occurred in people taking ephedra-free dietary supplements (2). Applying well-known adrenergic agonist structure–activity relationships to the synephrine molecule would have allowed health providers to accurately predict many of these effects.

As the market for these products grows, so do the number of products aimed at overweight and obese patients. It is vital that pharmacists understand the chemistry of the ingredients in dietary supplements used for weight loss, the mechanisms of action this chemistry predicts, and the physiologic impact these products may have. This knowledge will enable pharmacists to identify potential drug–herb interactions and potential adverse drug reactions and will help pharmacists adequately counsel patients who rely on their expertise to help understand when to use or avoid these products.

Beverly Lukawski, PharmD, and Jennifer Campbell, PharmD
Department of Pharmacy Practice
Creighton University, School of Pharmacy
Omaha, Nebraska

BODY ENERGY NEEDS

The energy needed to meet body demands is derived from ingested organic macronutrients. Specifically, carbohydrates, fats, and proteins serve as potential sources of energy, and the oxidative breaking of carbon–carbon and carbon–hydrogen bonds converts this potential energy into the body's energy carrier adenosine triphosphate (ATP) (Fig. 42.2). ATP in turn is used to carry out biochemical processes in the body such as muscle contraction for external work, vascular and heart contraction for blood flow, active transport of molecules and ions, biosynthesis of macromolecules, and a whole host of other cellular functions. The conversion of foods to energy (food energy) is not a very efficient process, and as a result, nearly half of the potential energy of the macronutrients is lost in the form of heat. The unit of measure of potential energy is that of the calorie (Cal or kcal) and is defined as the amount of energy required to heat 1 kg of water 1°C from 15°C to 16°C. Note, that the terminology *Cal* (spelled with an uppercase "C") replaces the older unit terminology *cal* (spelled with a lowercase "c"), which is 1/1,000 of a kcal. Nutritional labels report caloric content of foods in the form of calories (Cal). One may also see energy reported in joules or kilojoules (kJ) where 1 kcal equals 4.184 kJ, a standard set by the International System of Units. The hydrolysis of ATP, a phosphoric acid anhydride, releases approximately 12 kcal/mol and results from the exothermic hydrolysis of an anhydride bond and the resulting stabilization of the phosphate anion through resonance stabilization (Fig. 42.3).

The measure of potential energy present in any particular foodstuff can be determined experimentally by complete combustion of a particular foodstuff within an instrument called a calorimeter. The calorimeter consists of a combustion chamber submerged in a water bath. The foodstuff is combusted within the chamber, and the

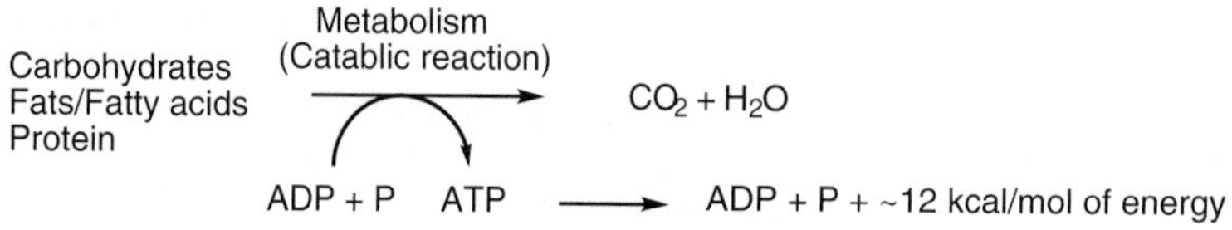

FIGURE 42.2 Conversion of foodstuff to ATP, the body energy currency.

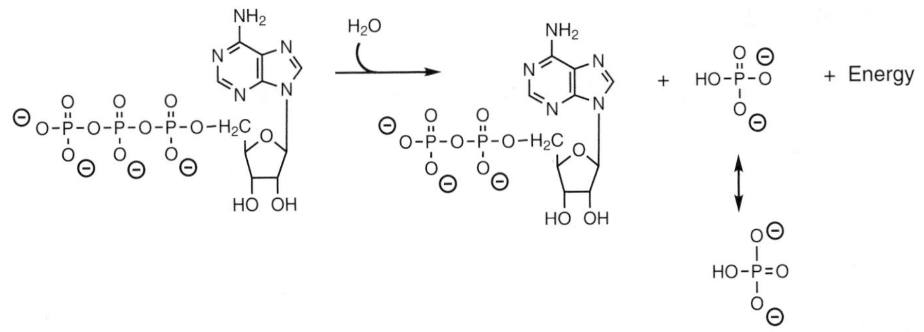

FIGURE 42.3 Energy release reaction involving ATP hydrolysis to adenosine diphosphate (ADP) plus phosphate.

rise in water temperature is measured, which in turn indicates the energy released during combustion. On average, carbohydrates release 4.1 kcal/g, proteins release 4.2 kcal/g, and fats release 9.3 kcal/g of energy (Fig. 42.4). Several attributes can be noted by viewing the chemical structures of the macronutrients. Complete combustion of the carbon atoms in these molecules gives rise to carbon dioxide and water. Nitrogen within the structure of proteins is not oxidized and is not a source of energy. The carbons in carbohydrates are already in a partially oxidized form (C-OH), as are several of the carbons in a protein (C-NH, C=O), whereas a fatty acid has a large number of carbon–carbon and carbon–hydrogen bonds that are available for metabolism. Thus by simple observation of the chemical structures of the macronutrients, one can see that fatty acids would be expected to have a significantly larger potential for generating energy.

Ideally, the amount of energy being generated from the macronutrients should equal the amount of energy needed to run and maintain the body. Actually there are two sources of macronutrient calories; those arising from the external foods that are eaten are called exogenous calories, and those calories that are found stored in the body are called endogenous calories (Fig. 42.5). In an attempt to quantify the number of calories expended on a daily basis, various calculations and formulas have been developed. In most cases, these calculations have either been too complicated to be of practical value or

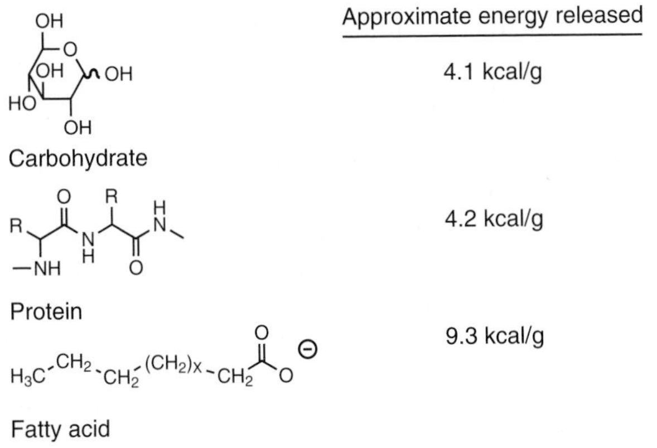

FIGURE 42.4 Potential energy derived from various foodstuffs.

are only a rough approximation of actual caloric consumption. One simplistic approximate measure of calories needed to maintain the body at a resting state (i.e., energy needed for cellular metabolism plus energy for blood circulation and respiration) is the basal metabolic rate (BMR). Combining the BMR with the energy expenditure of activity (EEA), also known as the total energy expenditure (TEE), and the diet-induced thermogenesis (DIT) can give an estimate of daily energy needs, which if combined with an estimate of calories consumed will help the individual determine their balance between calorie intake and calorie expenditure. BMR calculations can be done with the formula shown in Equation 42.1. As indicated, the BMR is dependent on the gender of the individual and the individual's weight, height, and age.

42.1

$$\begin{aligned}&\text{BMR (in Cal/day for women)}\\&\quad = 655 + (9.6 \times W) + (1.8 \times H) - (4.7 \times A)\\&\text{BMR (in Cal/day for men)}\\&\quad = 66 + (13.7 \times W) + (5 \times H) - (6.8 \times A)\end{aligned}$$

where W = weight in kilograms of the individual (1 kg = 2.2 lb), H = height in centimeters of the individual (1 in = 2.54 cm), and A = age of the individual.

A generalization can be made for lifestyle activities; for a sedentary lifestyle, the EEA is between 400 and 800 Cal/day; for a moderately active lifestyle, the EEA would be 1,200 to 1,800 Cal/day; and for an individual involved in heavy labor, the EEA would be 1,800 to 4,500 Cal/day. An energy expenditure calculator can be found at www.healthcalc.com/diet/energy-expenditure-advanced. Table 42.1 lists a number of physical activities along with an approximation of the calorie expenditure. A third component of the calculation of daily caloric needs is DIT. The DIT is defined as the energy expenditure above basal fasting levels divided by the energy content of the food ingested over a 24-hour period and is expressed as a percentage (3). The DIT is different for each nutrient, but normally, the DIT for a mixed diet is in the range of 10% of the total amount of energy ingested. The DIT is associated with the energy required for nutrient absorption, steps involved in metabolism, and storage of the absorbed nutrients. Ideally, the sum of the BMR, EEA, and DIT should equal the dietary daily intake so as to protect against weight gain or weight loss.

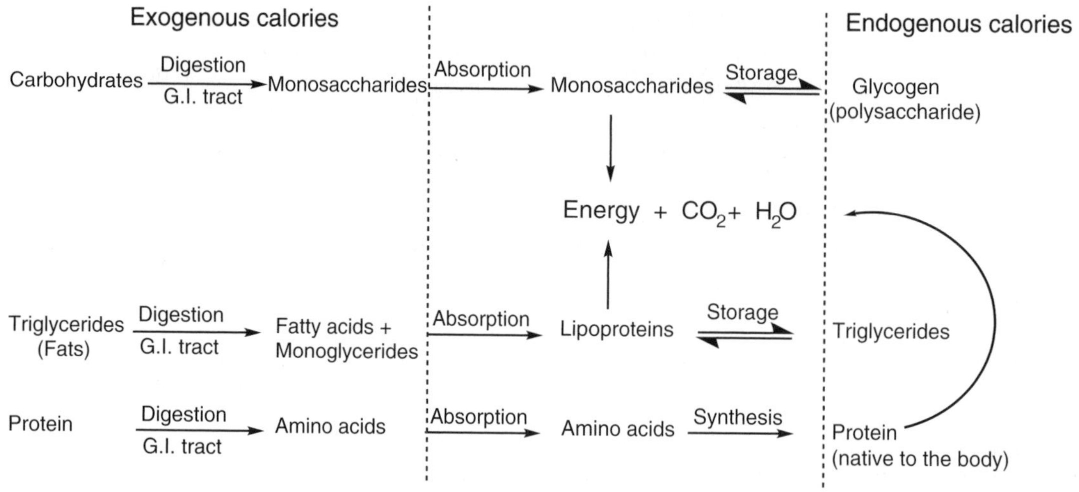

FIGURE 42.5 Digestion, absorption, and storage of macromolecules and conversion to energy.

OVERWEIGHT AND OBESITY

Worldwide, overweight and obesity have become major health issues, and nowhere can this be seen more dramatically than in the United States. In a report issued by Ogden et al. (4) in 2006, it was estimated that obesity in U.S. adults (age 20 and older) has doubled between the years of 1980 and 2002 to 32.2%, whereas overweight in children age 6 to 19 years has tripled to 17.2% (5). Today, obesity is considered to be a chronic disease, which is directly or indirectly related to the other diseases, including coronary heart disease, hypertension, stroke, and type 2 diabetes, and various other conditions, including an increase in death rates. It has been reported that even among overweight individuals, the risk of death for middle-age men and women increases by 20% to 40% compared with people who maintain a desirable weight (6). Some have suggested that obesity should be considered an epidemic. The significance of overweight and obesity in children can only be expected to create serious problems as they grow into maturity and for public health issues in the future. In 1995, the National Health and Nutrition Examination Survey estimated that 97 million Americans, or 37% of the population, were overweight or obese, whereas the Cleveland Clinic report in 2010 estimated that 66% of the U.S. population was considered overweight or obese (7). By definition, obesity is defined as excessive body fat, whereas overweight is defined as excessive body weight composed of bone, muscle, fat, and water. It is generally agreed that men with more than 25% body fat and women with more than 30% body fat are obese. There are various methods for measuring body fat both directly and indirectly. Underwater weighing, also known as hydrodensitometry, and dual-energy x-ray absorptiometry can give direct measures of body fat content, but these methods tend to be expensive. More commonly used are the BMI calculation and waist circumference measurement, which give a good, but indirect estimate of total body fat. The BMI is a simple calculation useful for adults and is shown in Equation 42.2.

TABLE 42.1 Energy Expended During Typical Exercises[a]

Activity	Calories Used per Hour
Bicycling (6 mph)	240
Bicycling (12 mph)	410
Jogging (7 mph)	920
Running in place	650
Jumping rope	720
Swimming (50 yd/min)	500
Walking (2 mph)	240
Walking (3 mph)	320
Walking (4.5 mph)	440

[a]For a more detailed list of activities, see Appendix B in McArdle WD, Katch FI, Katch VL. Sports and Exercise Nutrition, 3rd Ed. Baltimore: Lippincott Williams & Wilkins, 2009.

42.2
$$\text{BMI} = \text{Weight(kg)} / \text{Height(m)}^2$$
$$\text{BMI} = \text{Weight(lb)} / \text{Height(in)}^2 \times 703$$

Individuals with a BMI of <25 are considered normal, individuals with a BMI of 25 to 29.9 are classified as overweight, and individuals with a BMI ≥30 are said to be obese. With a BMI ≥40, the person is considered morbidly obese. It should be noted that there are individual who have a normal amount of body fat, but because of a high muscular content may have an "obese" BMI; this may be seen in athletes, especially football players. The elderly may actually have an underestimate of body fat based on BMI calculations because of the loss of muscle mass. However, in general, the BMI gives a good estimate of total body fat. The relationship of BMI to potential

TABLE 42.2 Relationship of BMI to Health Risk		
BMI Category	**Health Risk**	**Risk Adjusted to Comorbidity**
<25	Minimal	Low
25 to <27	Low	Moderate
27 to <30	Moderate	High
30 to <35	High	Very high
35 to <40	Very high	Extremely high

health risks is shown in Table 42.2. The presence of excessive abdominal fat can also be used as an indicator of health risk, and this is done through the measuring of waist circumference. The waist circumference gives a good measure of abdominal fat mass. The circumference is measured as a horizontal plane at the iliac crest (Fig. 42.6). A high-risk waist circumference is >40 inches in a man and >35 inches in a woman.

A commonly asked question is: To what extent are overweight and obesity related to genetics and environment? Current research appears to point to environment as a major contributor to overweight and obesity. A combination of increased calorie consumption and reduced physical activity over a long enough period of time leads to excessive body weight. As reported by Putnam et al. (8), between 1985 and 2000, the average consumption of calories increased by 12%, or approximately 300 calories/day. It was estimated that of this 300-calorie increase, fats and sugars accounted for 24% and 23%, respectively. An increase in 300 calories/day without a compensatory increase in physical activity could lead to a weight gain of 22 lbs. It was further reported that in 2000, an increase in fat intake occurred, while protein and carbohydrate intake remained unchanged. In another study, it was reported that between 1977 and 1996, food portions increased both inside and outside the home, resulting in increases in calories of salty snacks (93 kcal), soft drinks (49 kcal), hamburgers (97 kcal), French fries (68 kcal), and Mexican dishes (133 kcal) (9). An increase of 10 kcal/day could lead to an increase in body weight by 1 lb per year. All of this suggests that an imbalance between calorie consumption and physical activity may contribute to the increase in body weight that now threatens the U.S. population.

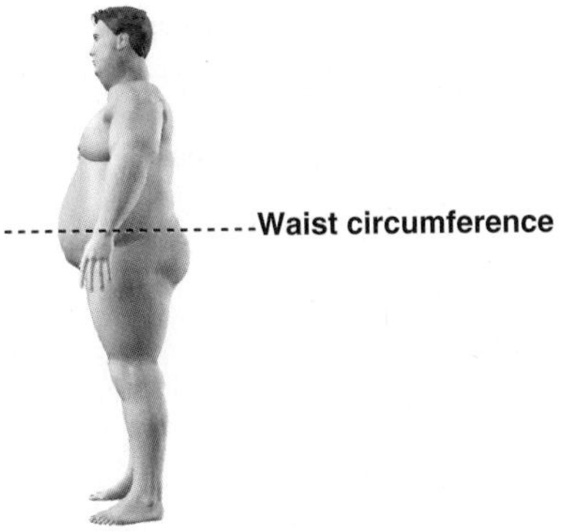

FIGURE 42.6 Measurement of waist circumference at iliac crest.

Food Labels

Food labels are meant to help individuals manage their caloric and nutrient intake, and thus, it is important to understand the terminology used on food labels. Figure 42.7 illustrates an example of a typical food label. The label will indicate a "normal" serving size and the number of calories obtained from this size serving. Following

Nutrition Facts

Serving size	3/4 c (28 g)
Servings per container	14
Amount per serving	
Calories	110
Calories from fat	9
	% Daily Value*
Total Fat 1 g	2%
Saturated fat 0 g	0%
Trans fat 0 g	0%
Cholesterol 0 mg	0%
Sodium 250 mg	10%
Total Carbohydrate 23 g	8%
Dietary fiber 1.5 g	6%
Sugars 10 g	
Protein 3 g	
Vitamin A	25%
Vitamin C	25%
Calcium	2%
Iron	25%

*Percent Daily Values are based on a 2000 calorie diet. Your daily values may be higher or lower depending on your calorie needs.

	Calories	2000	2500
Total fat	Less than	65 g	80 g
Sat Fat	Less than	20 g	25 g
Cholesterol	Less than	300 mg	300 mg
Sodium	Less than	2400 mg	2400 mg
Total Carbohydrate		300 g	375 g
Fiber		25 g	30 g

Calories per gram:

Fat	9
Carbohydrates	4
Protein	4

INGREDIENTS: Corn, whole wheat, sugar, rolled oats, brown sugar, rice, partially hydrogenated vegetable oir (sunflower and/or canola oil), wheat flour, salt, malted barley flour, corn syrup, whey (from milk), malted corn and barley syrup, honey, artificial flavor, annatto etract (color), BHT added to packaging material to preserve product freshness.
VITAMINS AND MINERALS: Reduced iron, niacinamide, vitamin B6, Vitamin A palmitate zinc oxide (source of zinc), riboflavin (vitamin B2), thiamin mononitrate (vitamin B1), folic acid, vitamin B12, vitamin D.

EXCHANGE: 1-1/2 starch, exchange calculations based on *Exchange Lists for Meal Planning* ©1995, American Diabetes Association, Inc. and The American Dietetic

FIGURE 42.7 Typical food label.

this, the actual content of total fats (including cholesterol), carbohydrates, and protein, as well as the micronutrients, which include minerals (sodium, calcium, and iron) and vitamins (vitamins A and C), is shown. The recommended calorie intake for individuals over the age of 4 years is presently set at 2,000 calories, which serves as the basis for listing the percentage of daily value (DV) for nutrients, which is also shown on the typical label. It should be noted that the U.S. Food and Drug Administration (FDA) has the authority to manage food labels and derives this authority from the Federal Food Drug & Cosmetic Act of 1938, the updated Nutrition Labeling and Educational Act of 1990 (NLEA), and the Dietary Supplement Health and Education Act of 1994 (DSHEA). The DVs are actually based on the highest Recommended Dietary Allowance (RDA) for the age or gender groups listed for RDAs and therefore would be a high-end recommendation. The RDAs are given in gram or milligram quantities, representing the average daily nutrient intake level required to meet the daily needs of an individual for good health, whereas the DV values are a percentage of the total daily requirements. These numbers are reviewed and updated by the Food and Nutrition Board of the Institute of Medicine, in partnership with Health Canada. RDAs, also referred to as the Recommended Daily Intakes (RDIs), have become part of a broader dietary guidelines known as the Dietary Reference Intake (DRI), which is revised and updated continually and serves as the basis for determination of the % DV. Based on the most up-to-date scientific findings, the RDI may be greater than, lesser than, or equal to the older RDA numbers. Presently, the RDI is 300 g for total carbohydrates, 65 g for fats, and 50 g for protein (Table 42.3). The intent of these numbers and percentages is to help the consumer judge the nutritional value of a particular food by seeing the actual nutrient content in a serving of the food and the percentage of that nutrient toward reaching a 2,000-calorie daily intake for a cross-section of American/Canadian consumers. A further interpretation of the RDA information is that a DV of 20% or greater is considered a "high" quantity of the nutrient, whereas a DV of 5% or less is considered a "low" nutrient quantity. The expectation is that a consumer seeing a "high" DV (e.g., sodium in Fig. 42.7) might wish to choose a product with a lower value and vice versa for foods with a "low" DV (e.g., fiber in Fig. 42.7). It should be noted that carbohydrate and protein do not have a DV percent list, which is because there is no consensus on the quantitative intake of these two nutrients. However because both carbohydrates and proteins are important and essential nutrients in the diet, their RDAs/RDIs are listed to help consumers manage their intake. Nutrients present in less than 500 mg/serving may be listed as 0.0 g, and therefore may be present, but need not be listed. Finally, it was not until 2003 that *trans* fatty acids were required to be reported.

MACRONUTRIENTS

To address the issue of overweight and obesity from the standpoint of overconsumption of calories, one must first identify the sources of calories within our food. The macronutrients (carbohydrates, fats, and proteins) are the source of calories in our diet (Figs. 42.1 through 42.5). In fact, carbohydrates and fats are the usual organic nutrients from which the majority of our nutrients arise.

TABLE 42.3 Dietary Recommendations for Various Nutrients

		Micronutrients			
Macronutrients	RDI	Vitamins	RDI	Minerals	RDI
Carbohydrates	300 g	A	5,000 IU	Sodium	2.3 g
Fiber	25 g	D	400 IU	Potassium	4.7 g
Total fat	65 g	E	30 IU	Calcium	1.0 g
Saturated fat	20 g	K	80 mcg	Iron	18 mg
Protein	50 g	C	60 mg	Phosphorus	1.0 g
		Thiamin	1.2 mg	Iodine	150 mcg
		Riboflavin	1.7 mg	Magnesium	400 mg
		Niacin	20 mg	Zinc	15 mg
		B_6	2 mg	Selenium	70 mcg
		Folate	20 mg	Copper	2 mg
		B_{12}	400 mcg	Manganese	2 mg
		Biotin	300 mcg	Chromium	120 mcg
		Pantothenic acid	10 mg	Chloride	3.4 g

Carbohydrates

Carbohydrates are compounds composed of carbon, hydrogen, and oxygen and consist of simple monosaccharides such as glucose, galactose, and fructose; disaccharides such as sucrose (table sugar), maltose, and lactose (milk sugar); and polysaccharides such as starch, glycogen, and cellulose (Fig. 42.8). The absorbable form of a carbohydrate is the monosaccharide; disaccharides and polysaccharides must first be hydrolyzed in the gastrointestinal (GI) tract before absorption.

Monosaccharide Absorption

Absorption of the very hydrophilic monosaccharides requires facilitated absorption/transport, both from the intestine and from body fluids into the cytoplasm of cells. Two families of membrane proteins involved in monosaccharide transport are the glucose transporter proteins (GLUT1 to GLUT5) and the Na^+-glucose cotransporters (SGLT1 to SGLT3). The GLUTs are 12 membrane–spanning proteins of approximately 500 amino acids found in red blood cells, the blood–brain barrier, liver cells, fat cells, and brush borders of the intestine. The role of these GLUT transporters is to facilitate the absorption of glucose and fructose. The SGLTs are 12 membrane–spanning proteins that are unrelated to the GLUTs, which exhibit high affinity for glucose following binding to sodium ion (Chapter 5). The SGLT1 is primarily expressed in the small intestine, whereas SGLT2 is expressed in the kidney, where they increase the absorption of glucose from the gut and reabsorb glucose from the kidney tubules, respectively. SGLTs also show affinity for galactose transport. Because monosaccharides account for the major source of energy to human cells, the role of GLUTs and SGLTs is quite important.

Disaccharide Metabolism

Disaccharides require hydrolysis to monosaccharides; for example, sucrose is hydrolyzed to glucose and fructose prior to absorption. Various enzymes present in the brush border of the intestine are involved in the hydrolytic process (i.e., sucrase-isomaltase, lactase-phlorizin hydrolase, maltase-glucoamylase, and trehalase).

Starch Metabolism

Starch is a polysaccharide of glucose that exists as a straight chain polymer called amylose with three or more glucose monomers linked via α-1,4-linkages and amylopectin, a highly branched polymer consisting of α-1,4-linkages together with α-1,6-linkages similar to what is seen in glycogen (Fig. 42.8). Amylose exists in a helix configuration. Starch is a major constituent of plants with various ratios of amylose to amylopectin (for example, potato is 20% amylose and 80% amylopectin; rice is 18.5% amylose and 81.5% amylopectin). The hydrolytic metabolism of starch begins in the oral cavity where α-amylase, which attacks the α-1,4-linkages, is secreted by the salivary glands and later by α-amylase secreted by the pancreas in the duodenum. Glucoamylase in the small intestine is also involved

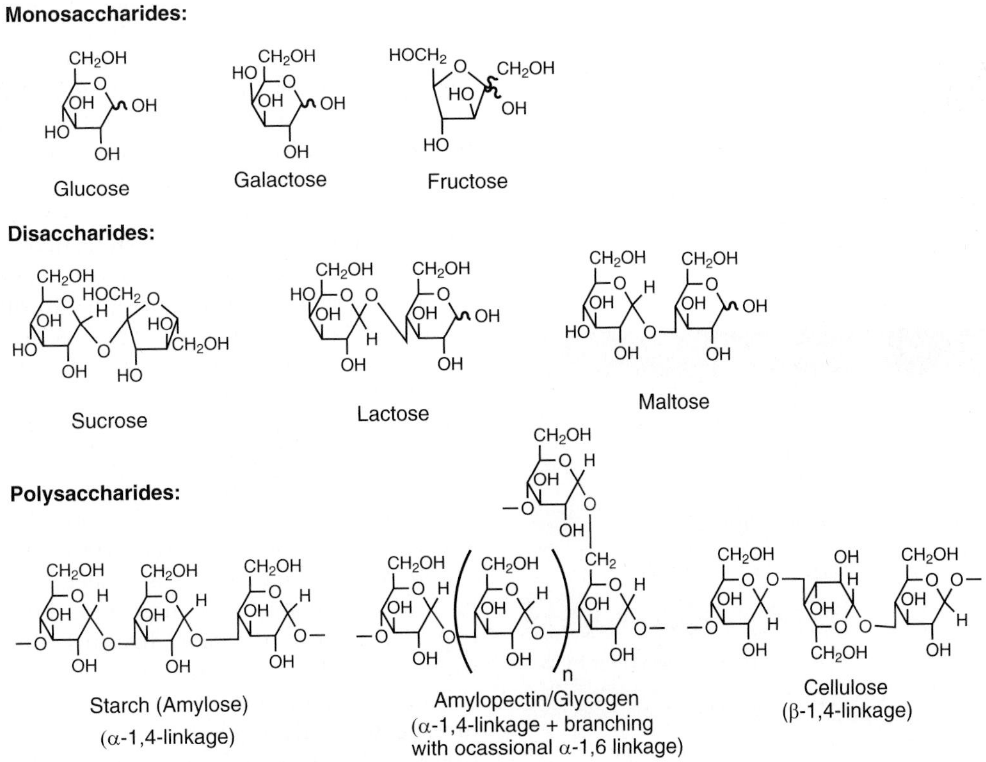

FIGURE 42.8 Structures of common carbohydrates.

in starch hydrolysis. The result of the amylase metabolism is that maltose and maltotriose (a three α-1,4 glucose unit molecule) are formed, at which point final hydrolysis occurs via the previously mentioned brush border disaccharidases, leading to formation of absorbable glucose.

Glycogen Synthesis and Metabolism

Glycogen is the human storage form for glucose, with storage occurring in the liver and muscle tissue. Once glucose is absorbed and phosphorylated to glucose-1-phosphate, it is then incorporated into glycogen through the action of glycogen synthase and glycogen branching enzyme. The structure of glycogen is similar to starch, with both α-1,4-links and α-1,6-links (Fig. 42.8). The process of glycogen formation differs from glycogen degradation. Glycogen hydrolysis occurs when the body requires energy, which involves a process of phosphorylation, transferase, and a debranching enzyme, leading to the release of glucose into the bloodstream.

Cellulose

Cellulose is a major polysaccharide found in plants (Fig. 42.8). It is a linear polymer of glucose but differs from starch by the fact that the linkage between the glucose monomeric units has the β-1,4-linkage, which increases the stability of the polymer through internal hydrogen bonding to produce a strong linear configuration. This configuration prevents hydrolytic metabolism by human enzymes that are specific for α-1,4-linkages. The β-1,4-linkage can be hydrolyzed by cellulase found in some bacteria, protozoa, and fungi and in bovine animals.

Fiber

Fiber or, more specifically, dietary fiber is made up of nondigestible oligosaccharides usually of plant origin, such as the polysaccharides cellulose and pectin (polysaccharide containing 1,4-α-D-galactosyluronic acid monomeric units), or complex material found in wood and cell walls of plants such as lignin (Table 42.4). There is no FDA definition of what a dietary fiber actually is. Fibers may be further classified as soluble fibers (water soluble) such as pectin or insoluble fibers such as cellulose, hemicellulose, and lignin.

TABLE 42.4 Classes of Dietary Fibers

Oligosaccharides	Source
Cellulose	Bran, legumes, peas, vegetables, cabbage, seeds, and apple skin
Hemicellulose	Bran and whole grains
Polyfructose	Oligofructans and insulin
Gums	Oatmeal, barley, and legumes
Pectin	Apples, strawberries, and citrus fruits
Resistant starches	Ripe bananas and potatoes
Nonsaccharide lignin	Root vegetables, wheat, fruits, strawberries

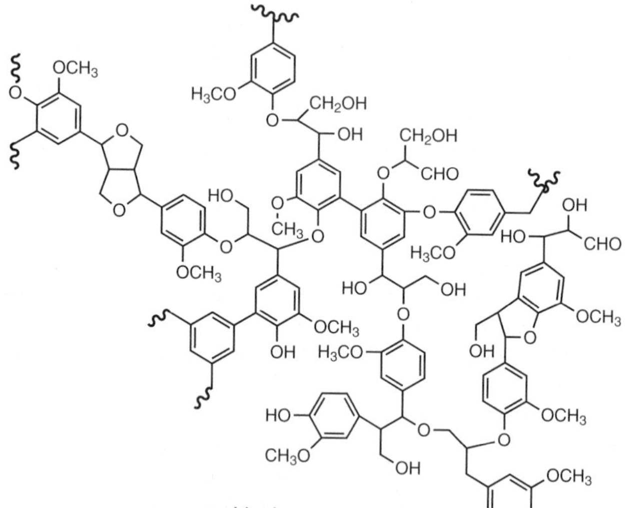

Lignin

As the name would imply, soluble fibers absorb and dissolve in water forming gels that are prone to fermentation by bacteria that are located in the colon, generating short-chain fatty acids, such as butyric acid, through the benefit of epithelial cells in the colon. Insoluble fibers create bulk, which is suggested to be beneficial via increased stomach transit time and a reduction of intestinal transit time. This is thought to decrease the urge to eat and cause a reduction in the ability for chemical absorption to occur from the intestine. Although evidence supporting the health benefits of dietary fibers is suggestive at best, there is general agreement that fiber in the diet can lower the incidence of obesity (creates a feeling of satiety) (10), reduce insulin resistance and the risk of type 2 diabetes, reduce the risk of heart disease (decrease cholesterol absorption from the intestine), and reduce the risk of colon cancer (decrease absorption of potential carcinogens from the gut). Insoluble fibers also act as bulk laxatives. The average American diet contains 12 to 15 g of fiber compared to 40 to 150 g of fiber in the diets of Africans and Indians. Recommendations for fiber content in the diet are presently 38 g/day for men under the age of 50, 30 g/day for men over the age of 50, 25 g/day for women under the age of 50, and 20 g/ day for women over the age of 50. Recently, food manufacturers have been studying starches referred to as resistant starch (RS). Resistant starch is expected to resist digestion by amylase and amylopectinase and, therefore, would be expected to have the same health benefits claimed for the dietary fibers. Various classes of RS, some of which are natural while others are manufactured, are being investigated (informally classified as RS1 through RS5). Changes in crystalline structure of the RS, increases in branching and cross-linking within the starch, and starch–lipid complexes cause the starch to become more resistant to hydrolysis (11).

Although nondigestible fibers have little or no caloric value, the soluble fiber that is fermented in the colon can be a source of energy and is given a caloric value of 4 kcal/g.

Properties of Sugars

Sugar is defined as a sweet-tasting crystalline carbohydrate, and in most cases, when one refers to sugar, the person is referring to sucrose (table sugar), although glucose, galactose, lactose, and fructose are sugars having similar properties. Normally, carbohydrates make up 40% to 70% of the human daily caloric intake, and the majority of the carbohydrates come in the form of starch, but sizable quantities of sucrose and lactose are also commonly found in the diet. It is estimated that the average American adult consumes 64 lb of sucrose/year, while children may consume as much as 140 lb/year. Approximately one-third of sugar is ingested from the table sugar bowl, and two-thirds is found in commercially processed food, mostly as high-fructose corn syrup. The consumption of sugar has both a physiologic and a psychological basis. The perception of sweetness is detected by G protein–coupled receptors located in the taste buds on the tongue. Sweetness is one of the five basic tastes that the human body has evolved to detect, and humans crave sweet materials as a way of supplying the body with sufficient energy to meet the daily needs. However, children have been taught to crave sweet foods since sweets are commonly used to bribe children. As a result, we crave sweet foods, namely carbohydrates, in excess to what is actually needed for good health. Excessive intake of sucrose or high-fructose corn syrup is directly related to the development of tooth caries and indirectly related to the development of overweight and obesity, which in turn is related to the onset of type 2 diabetes. Although it might be assumed that a good approach to the health issues associated with excessive consumption of carbohydrates, sugars in particular, would be to reduce the intake of these macronutrients, there seems to be an ingrained pattern that replacement is more acceptable than restraint. Thus, because of the mounting concern regarding overweight and obesity and the need to reduce calorie intake and yet the desire to meet the craving for sweet substances, nonnutritive sweeteners have gained universal acceptance.

Nonnutritive Sweeteners

Saccharin (Sweet'N Low)

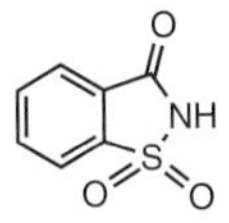

Saccharin

The history of saccharin began with its synthesis in 1878, and over the past 130 plus years, this food additive has been part of the human food scene. Saccharin's history has included a period when it was ban from the market as an adulterant only to be returned as a sugar substitute. It has had limited use directed toward diabetics, carried a warning as a possible carcinogen, and is now openly available for consumer use and a common ingredient in a host of food products. Saccharin's colorful history has recently been presented in a book titled *Empty Pleasures: The Story of Artificial Sweeteners from Saccharin to Splenda* (12).

The properties of saccharin include a sweetness 300-fold that of sucrose with zero calories (Table 42.5). Saccharin does have a bitter aftertaste, a fact that makes saccharin less than the ideal nonnutritive sweetener, and instability to prolonged heating, thus limiting its use to nonbaked products. The bitter aftertaste has been masked by the addition of other sweeteners. The biggest health-related problem associated with saccharin was a scare resulting from the development of bladder cancer in male rats reported in 1977 and titled the "Canadian Rat Study." This study resulted in the banning of saccharin by the FDA, but the passage of the Saccharin Study and Labeling Act in 1977 by the U.S. Congress allowed saccharin to remain on the market with the required label that saccharin-containing products were potentially carcinogenic. (*This product contains saccharin, which has been determined to cause cancer in laboratory animals.*) Saccharin-containing products retained this label until December

TABLE 42.5 Comparison of the Sweetness of Nutritive and Nonnutritive Sweeteners

	Sweetness	Calories per 100 g
Nutritive sweetener		
Sucrose	100%	All mono- and disaccharides ~370
Glucose	60%–70%	
Fructose	110%–180%	
Maltose	33%–50%	
Galactose	15%–40%	
Xylitol	100%	~192
Nonnutritive sweetener		
Saccharin	300x sucrose	0
Sodium cyclamate	30x sucrose	0
Aspartame	200x sucrose	~0.05
Neotame	7,000x sucrose	0
Acesulfame-K	200x sucrose	0
Sucralose	600x sucrose	0
Rebaudioside A	200x sucrose	0

2000 when the warning label was removed following presentation of evidence that male rats are unique in that a combination of high bladder pH, high calcium phosphate concentrations, and a specific protein that favors crystal formation occurs in the presence of saccharin. The formation of microcrystals in the bladder of male rats causes damage to the bladder wall, which over an extended period of time led to tumor formation. These conditions do not exist in humans, and therefore, a threat of saccharin-induced tumors is not possible (13).

Cyclamate (Sucaryl)

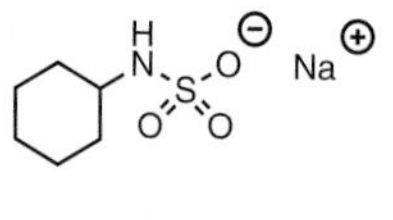

Cyclamates were first synthesized in 1937 and reached the U.S. market in the 1950s. This artificial sweetener has several advantages over saccharin in that it does not possess a bitter aftertaste and is stable to heat. The compound is 30 to 50 times sweeter than sucrose with zero caloric value (Table 42.5). During the 1960s, the cyclamates became very popular as nonnutritive sweeteners when directly added to foods, used in baked products, and added to soft drinks and canned fruits. In 1958, cyclamate was added to the generally recognized as safe (GRAS) list, but in 1969, the chemical was banned by the FDA for use in the United States due to what was reported to be the development of bladder cancer in rats possibly due to metabolism of cyclamate to cyclohexylamine. While studies to repeat these results were claimed by the manufacturer to be irreproducible, the chemical has never returned to the U.S. market, although the chemical is still sold in many countries throughout the world.

Aspartame (Equal, NutraSweet) and Neotame

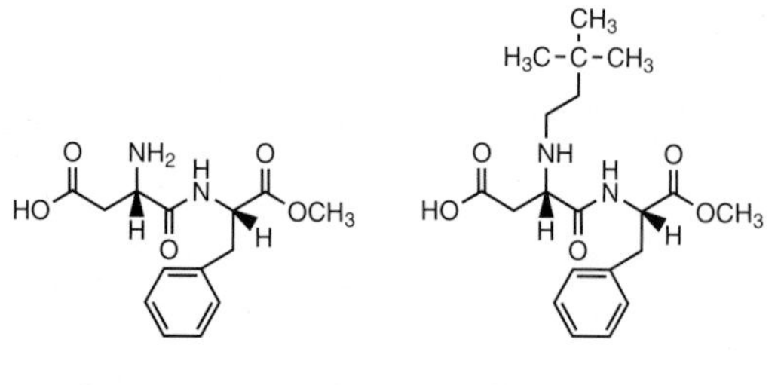

In 1965, a chemist working at G.D. Searle & Company discovered that a compound composed of the methyl ester of the dipeptide of two natural amino acids, L-phenylalanine and L-aspartic acid, had an outstanding sweet taste. This dipeptide was later named aspartame. Coming at a time when both saccharin and cyclamate were facing intense scrutiny as synthetic, nonnutritive sweeteners, aspartame was seen as a potentially significant breakthrough in the nonnutritive sweetener market. The properties of aspartame included a sweetness 200-fold sucrose with no bitter aftertaste. A single serving of aspartame, equivalent to an equally sweet 180-calorie serving of sucrose, contains only 0.1 calories (Table 42.5). While still not stable to prolonged heating, aspartame's other major attraction was the fact that it was composed of L-phenylalanine and L-aspartic acid, two naturally occurring amino acids. At a time when the consumer was (and still is) concerned about synthetic, unnatural chemicals, aspartame offered a marketing windfall. Present in the form of a dipeptide methyl ester, aspartame was first approved for marketing in 1974, but concerns about tumors, brain damage, and testing procedures delayed its introduction to the market until July 1981. By 1985, aspartame was consumed to the extent of 800 million pounds/year, and 2 years later, it was estimated that aspartame appeared in more than 1,200 products.

Aspartame, being a dipeptide, is prone to hydrolytic metabolism, either in the intestine or mucus membrane of the intestinal lining, to produce phenylalanine, aspartic acid, and methanol (Fig. 42.9). This metabolism in turn raised the question of the safety of the products formed. Methanol, or wood alcohol, is a potential toxin when absorbed into the bloodstream, where it can be converted into formaldehyde and then to formic acid, which could potentially lead to systemic metabolic acidosis and blindness (14). It was found that the quantity

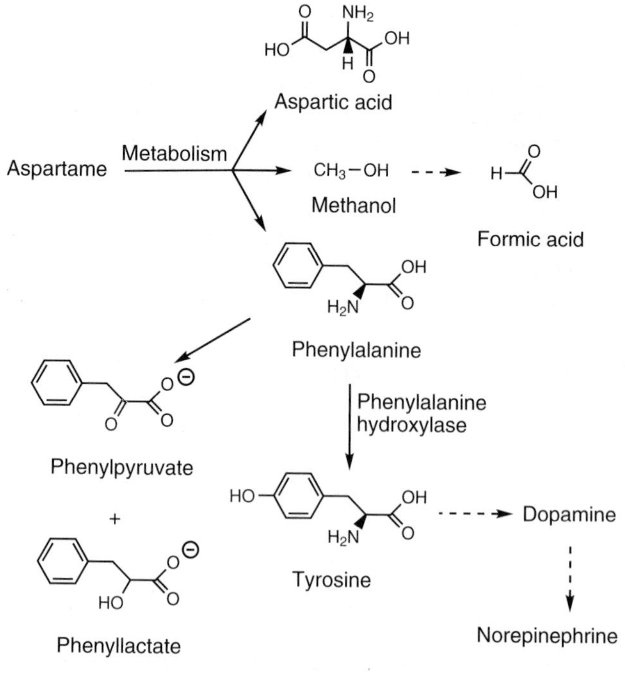

FIGURE 42.9 Metabolism of aspartame and its metabolites.

of formic acid detected in the urine (studies could not detect formic acid in the blood after aspartame administration) following large doses of aspartame generated less formic acid from the aspartame than that found after consuming some fruit juices.

The second concern for aspartame is the effect of phenylalanine on individuals who suffer from phenylketonuria (PKU). PKU is a genetic condition in which children are born with a deficiency of phenylalanine hydroxylase, an enzyme that converts phenylalanine into tyrosine. A lack of this enzyme leads to higher than normal levels of phenylalanine in the blood, which leads to formation of catabolic products such as phenylpyruvate and phenyllactate. These products can result in a reduced level of tyrosine and possibly the neurotransmitters formed from tyrosine (norepinephrine, and dopamine). If not diagnosed within a few days of birth, PKU can lead to central nervous system (CNS) damage and mental retardation. The exact cause of the mental retardation is not known, but it is assumed that one or all of the abnormal conditions cited above may have a role in PKU. Although phenylalanine is still essential in PKU patients, a diet with low phenylalanine levels is important in the prevention of the serious outcomes of excessive phenylalanine in PKU patients. As a result, the consumption of aspartame by women during pregnancy who might give birth to a PKU infant and administering aspartame-containing foods to a child diagnosed with PKU have raised concerns. Studies demonstrated that abusive doses of aspartame (200 mg/kg in an adult or 100 mg/kg in a child) or successive doses of aspartame (three 10 mg/kg doses in a child) did not lead to phenylalanine levels equal to or above those approved for adults or children with PKU (14). These studies suggested that aspartame-containing foods and beverages are unlikely to have adverse effects on patients with PKU, although there is no reason for infants with or without PKU to be using nonnutritive sweeteners. Aspartame-containing foods contain a warning indicating its presence and its potential for harm in patients with PKU.

In 2002, an analog of aspartame, neotame was approved for marketing in the United States. This compound differs from aspartame by the addition of a dimethylbutyl substituent on the nitrogen of aspartic acid. The result of this substitution is that sweetness is 30-fold greater than aspartame and from 7,000- to 13,000-fold greater than sucrose. Metabolism of neotame results in formation of methanol, but significantly less phenylalanine and *N*-dimethylbutylaspartic acid. The nitrogen substitution also decreases the hydrolysis of the dipeptide, and only 20% to 30% of the neotame is absorbed, presumably as the individual amino acids (15). Since the sweetness of neotame is so much higher than aspartame, a much lower dose would be required to meet the desired sweetness of a neotame-containing food. As a result, it is estimated that the amount of methanol absorbed after an appropriate dose of neotame is approximately 1.3 mg/L, whereas the methanol content from some juices is calculated to be approximately 140 mg/L. The amount of phenylalanine produced from neotame is estimated to be 2.6 mg/day in an adult and 1.5 mg/day in a child, whereas the restricted diet content of phenylalanine for a child with PKU is set at 0.4 to 0.6 g/day, and the average adult consumes 2.5 to 10 g/day of phenylalanine. The amount of phenylalanine obtained from a dose of neotame would have a negligible effect on a patient with PKU. Presently, there do not appear to be any food products that contain neotame.

Acesulfame-K (Sunette)

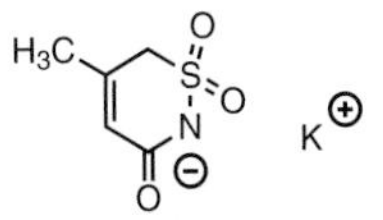

Acesulfame

Discovered in 1967, acesulfame-K is a nonnutritive sweetener that is approximately 200 times sweeter than sucrose and heat stable and therefore can be used in cooking and baking (Table 42.5). The compound is not metabolized and shows structural similarity to saccharin. Acesulfame-K is commonly used in combination with other sweeteners due to its bitter aftertaste, a property it has in common with saccharin (both chemicals affect the same bitter receptor) (16). The chemical was approved for use in the United States in 1988 in dry food, and by 2003, it was approved as a general purpose sweetener, allowing for its added use in carbonated and noncarbonated beverages.

Sucralose (Splenda)

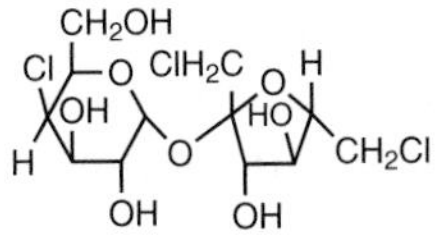

Sucralose

Sucralose is a synthetic derivative of sucrose in which three hydroxyl groups have been replaced with chlorine atoms. As a result, the compound is not metabolized by the body but retains the sweet taste of sucrose, and in fact, the sweetness is increased by approximate 600-fold. The chloride substitution, in addition to preventing the metabolism of Sucralose, increases stability of the chemical to heat. Sucralose can be used in baking and cooking (15). In 1999, sucralose was approved as a general purpose sweetener in the United States. Its general purpose use is indicative of its safety as judged by the FDA.

Rebaudioside A (Truvia, Rebiana, or Reb-A)

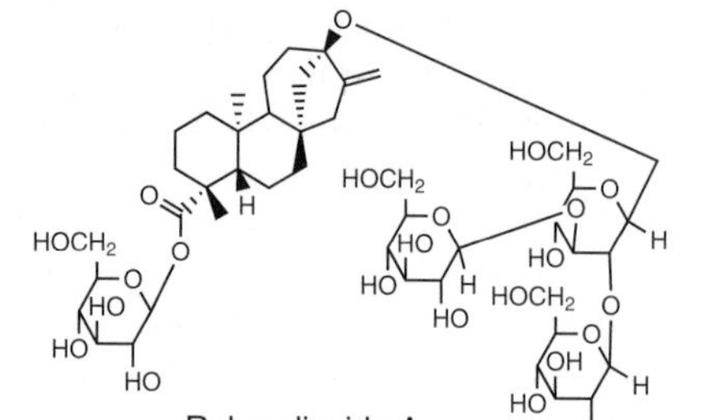

Rebaudioside A

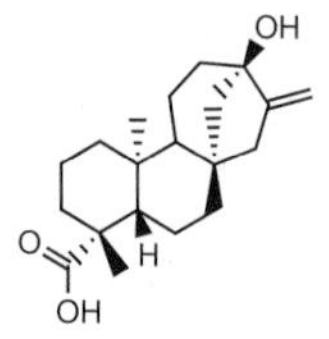

Steviol

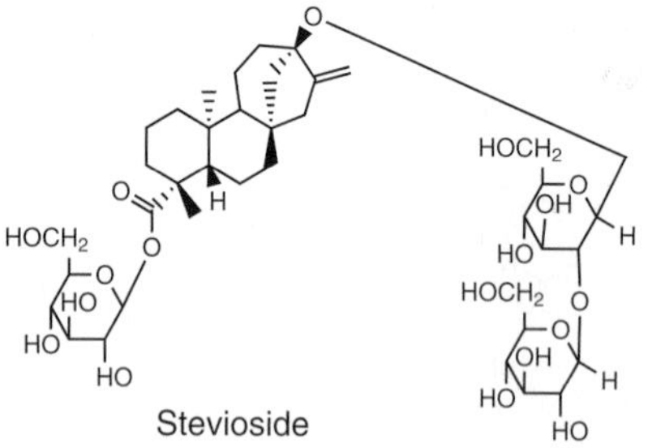

Stevioside

For many centuries, the leaves of the stevia plant (*Stevia rebausiana* Bertoni) have been used for their sweet taste (15,17), but not until the last decade has commercial interest in this plant resulted in a marketed product derived from the stevia plant. Two major glycosides possess much of the sweet taste; these are stevioside and rebaudioside A, which has been developed and introduced onto the market as a nonnutritive sweetener. Rebaudioside A, known by the trade name Rebiana or Reb-A, is a diterpene glycoside that possesses a sweetness approximately 200-fold greater than sucrose (Table 42.5) and has zero calories. As a glycoside, it is prone to acid-catalyzed hydrolysis. At low pHs, stevioside can undergo hydrolysis by intestinal bacterial flora, leading to the formation of steviol, the aglycone component of the rebiosides. Human metabolic studies on stevioside have shown that only trace amounts of stevioside can be detected in blood and no steviol is detected. Because steviol has been shown to exhibit positive genetic toxicology as well as the ability to induce chromosome breakage in bacteria, stevioside, stevia extracts, and, to some extent, rebaudioside A have been studied in depth for their safety (17,18). These studies have concluded that stevioside and rebaudioside A are not genotoxic or carcinogenic in vitro or in vivo and that the only cell-damaging effects of steviol occurred in in vitro studies at excessive concentrations.

In 2008, the FDA approved inclusion of rebaudioside A in the GRAS list as well as its use in foods and beverages as a nonnutritive sweetener. Prior to these approvals, rebaudioside A was available in the United States as a dietary supplement. In the single-component product Truvia, erythritol (a four-carbon polyhydroxy sugar alcohol) is added as a sweetener to mask the aftertaste of licorice, which appears to be associated with rebaudioside A. Erythritol itself has a caloric content of 0.2 kcal/g.

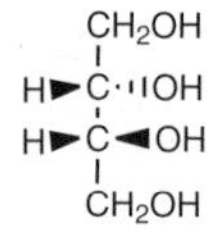

Erythritol

Xylitol

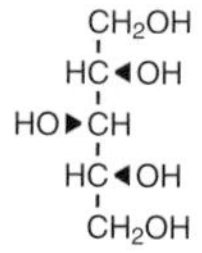

Xylitol

Xylitol is a polyol (a five-carbon polyhydroxy sugar alcohol) with structural similarity to glucose and erythritol. It has been used since the 1960s as a sugar substitute with a sweetness comparable to sucrose but with 40% fewer calories (Table 42.5). Xylitol is commonly found in chewing gums because it does not promote the development of dental caries or plaque formation and yet satisfies the need for sweetness. This property is due to the fact that the polyols are not metabolized to organic acids in the oral cavity. Xylitol can be added to the gum, and the gum can still be labeled as sugar "free" (15). Unfortunately, if consumed in large quantities, xylitol can have a laxative effect due to its poor absorption and water osmotic effect. Xylitol can be consumed by diabetics and will not affect blood sugar levels. Xylitol is found commonly in fruits such as raspberries and plums and can be prepared from the hydrogenation of xylose, which is found in corncobs and wood pulp.

Fats and Fatty Acids

Chemistry of Fats and Fatty Acids

By definition, a fat is a neutral molecule composed of three fatty acids attached to the alcohol glycerol, thus referred to as triglycerides, and represents a storage and transport form for fatty acids.

Glycerin

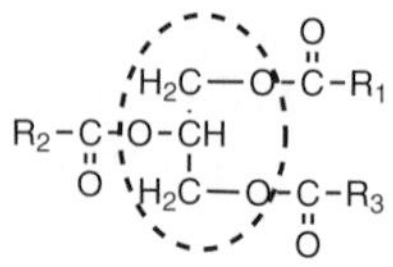

Triglyceride
(Fat)

Fatty acids themselves play multiple biologic roles, including the following: They are components of the cell wall, usually in the form of phospholipids, glycolipids, and fatty acid acetylated proteins; a high-energy source of calories; and hormone and intracellular messengers.

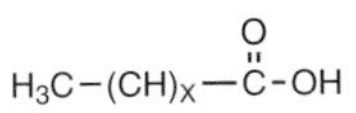

x	Common name	Official name
10	Lauric acid	*n*-Dodecanoic acid
12	Myristic acid	*n*-Tetradecanoic acid
14	Palmitic acid	*n*-Hexadecanoic acid
16	Stearic acid	*n*-Octadecanoic acid
18	Arachidic acid	*n*-Eicosanoic acid
20	Behenic acid	*n*-Docosanoic acid
22	Lignoceric acid	*n*-Tetracosanoic acid

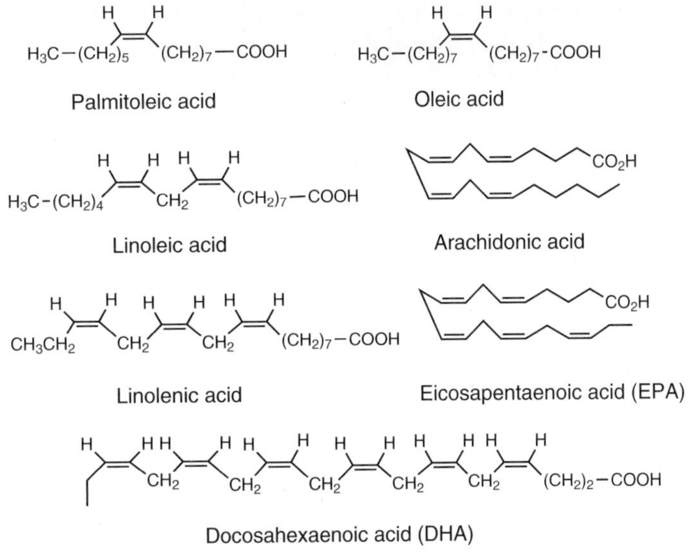

FIGURE 42.10 Structures of unsaturated, monounsaturated, and polyunsaturated fatty acids.

The fatty acids are classified based on the presence or absence of double bonds. The natural fatty acids with no double bonds are referred to as saturated fatty acids; they are totally saturated with hydrogen. The naturally occurring saturated fatty acids contain 12 to 24 carbon atoms (Fig. 42.10) and have an even number of carbon atoms, which results from the fact that they are biosynthesized from the two-carbon acetate unit. A second group of fatty acids is the monounsaturated fatty acids, consisting of palmitoleic acid (9*Z*-hexadecenoic acid) and oleic acid (9*Z*-octadecenoic acid). These acids have a single double bond, and it should be noted that the stereochemistry of these and other naturally occurring unsaturated fatty acids contain the *cis* or *Z* configuration. A third class of fatty acids are the polyunsaturated fatty acids (PUFA) and consist of linoleic and linolenic acid (9*Z*,12*Z*-octadecadienoic acid and 9*Z*,12*Z*,15*Z*-octadecatrienoic acid, respectively). Additional fatty acids of nutritional significance are arachidonic acid (C20:4 *cis* double bonds), eicosapentaenoic acid (EPA) (C20:5 *cis* double bonds), and docosahexaenoic acid (C22 with 6 *cis* double bonds), which are shown in Figure 42.10. A commonly used nomenclature refers to fatty acids with a double bond three carbons from the end of the fatty acid chain as the ω-3 fatty acids. Linolenic acid, eicosapentaenoic acid, and docosahexaenoic acid constitute the ω-3 fatty acids.

Physical-Chemical Properties

A distinguishing physical-chemical property of the various classes of fatty acids is that as the degree of unsaturation increases, the melting point decreases. The saturated fatty acids tend to be low-melting solids, whereas the unsaturated fatty acids and PUFAs are liquids (Table 42.6). The saturated fatty acids tend to be found in higher concentrations in animal fats, whereas the unsaturated and polyunsaturated fatty acids are found in high concentrations in vegetable oils (Table 42.7). It is interesting that as the consumer demand moves away from saturated fats and toward unsaturated fats that seed manufacturers are turning to genetically modified plant seeds to product plants that produce increased levels of monounsaturated fatty acids and reduced levels of saturated and polyunsaturated fatty acids (19).

TABLE 42.6 Melting Points of Saturated and Unsaturated Fatty Acids

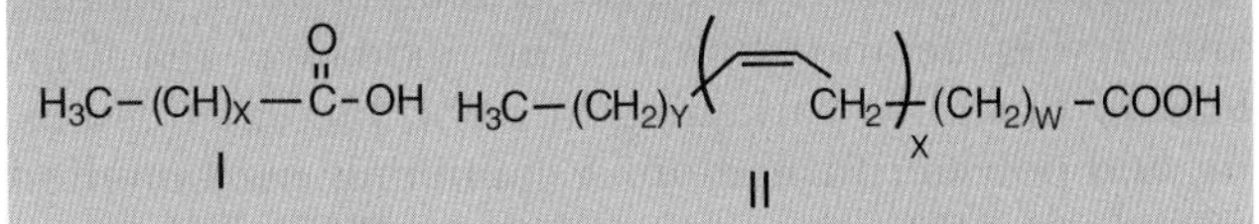

Common name	x			mp (°C)
Saturated (I)				
Lauric acid	10			44
Myristic acid	12			58
Palmitic acid	14			63
Stearic acid	16			70
Unsaturated (II)	w	x	y	
Palmitoleic acid	6	1	5	−1
Oleic acid	6	1	7	4
Linoleic acid	6	2	4	−5
Linolenic acid	6	3	1	−12
Arachidonic acid	2	5	1	−49.5

TABLE 42.7 Approximate Percentage of Fatty Acids in Various Food

Food	Saturated Fatty Acids (%)	Monounsaturated Fatty Acids (%)	Polyunsaturated Fatty Acids (%)
Butter fat	60	36	4
Pork fat	59	39	2
Beef	53	44	2
Chicken fat	39	44	21
Margarines[a]	20	40	40
Salmon oil	24	39	36
Corn oil	15	31	53
Soybean oil	14	24	53
Olive oil	14	75	11
Sunflower	10	22	66
Canola	7	61	22

[a]Fatty acid content shows considerable variations between percentage of saturated fatty acids (palmitic acid and stearic acid), monounsaturated fatty acid (oleic acid), and polyunsaturated fatty acid (linoleic acid) as well as *cis/trans* ratio in various brand name margarines.
Nazir DJ, Moorecroft BJ, Mishkel MA. Fatty acid composition of margarines. Am J Clin Nutr 1976;29:331–339.

In part, this relates to a second physical-chemical property of the fatty acids. The fats containing saturated fatty acids generally have a more stable shelf-life and are stable at elevated temperatures to air oxidation. The PUFAs within the fat are susceptible to oxidation reactions, especially at elevated temperature (baking and frying temperatures). The oxidative reactions lead to rancidity, darkening in color, increased viscosity, and polymer formation. A commonly used method of reducing the concentration of the PUFA is through partial hydrogenation (leading to the hydrogenated oils). Catalytic hydrogenation involves a reversible addition of hydrogen and catalyst to the double bond followed by the irreversible addition of a second hydrogen to the initial double bond (Fig. 42.11). The reversibility of the initial step in the hydrogenation leads to loss of the hydrogen from the saturated carbon and formation of both the initial alkene and a new alkene with the more stable *trans* or *E* stereochemistry and, thus, formation of a *trans* fatty acid (TFA) impurity. The quantity of TFAs formed by catalytic hydrogenation can be reduced by changes in the conditions used for the hydrogenation process (20). The 2006 report of a Canadian study, "Transforming the Food Supply: Report of the Trans Fat Task Force," submitted to the Minister of Health reports that of the fats present in food, the TFA levels may be as high as 24% to 33% for bakery products, 20% to 40% for margarines, and as high as 40% for snack foods, nachos, and nachos cheese sauces (21). The concern is that TFA consumption increases the levels of low-density lipoprotein (LDL) cholesterol, reduces the level of high-density lipoprotein (HDL) cholesterol, and increases the ratio of total cholesterol to HDL cholesterol, which are measures that are associated with increased risk of coronary heart disease (CHD) (22). Other endogenous changes have been associated with TFA consumption including changes in triglyceride levels, promotion of inflammatory reactions, and endothelial dysfunction. Generally, *trans* fats composed of one or more TFAs attached to the glycerin backbone are not normally present in natural foods with the exception of small amounts in meats coming from cows, sheep, and other ruminants in which bacteria within the stomach of ruminants produce the TFAs. It is estimated that this accounts for approximately 0.5% of the total caloric intake. But commercially deep-fried foods, bakery products, packaged snack foods, margarines, and crackers prepared with *trans* fat–containing oils may increase the amount of *trans* fats in our diet, leading to 2% to 3% of the total caloric intake being TFAs. Thus, considerable concern has been generated in the press, health professionals, and the public about the long-term effects of *trans* fats. This has led to changes in the manufacture of cooking

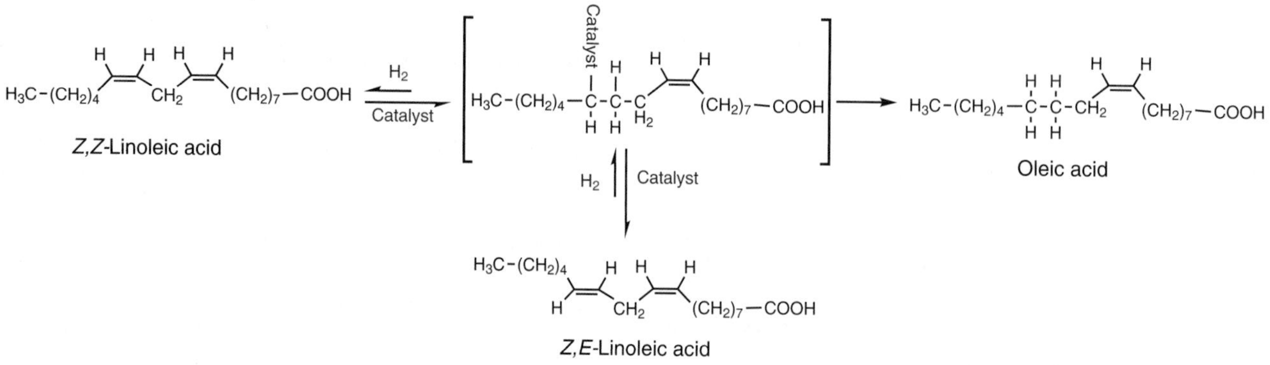

FIGURE 42.11 Catalytic hydrogenation of a polyunsaturated fatty acid to a monounsaturated fatty acid.

oils and the use of oils containing *trans* fats, including in some cases, legislation outlawing the use of *trans* fat–containing oils. It has been suggested that a 2% increase in energy intake from TFAs could result in a 23% increase in the incidence of CHD (20). Over the past several years, the presence of TFAs in food products has declined as indicated by the labeling of foods as having zero *trans* fats, although such a label does not guarantee zero grams per serving. The FDA allows a report of zero grams per serving if the food contains <500 mg/serving of *trans* fats.

Fat and Fatty Acid Absorption

The major nutritional value of fats comes from the fatty acids, which upon metabolism are a high-density source of energy. In order for this to occur, the fat must be absorbed, transported via the bloodstream either to the cells in tissue where the energy is needed or to storage sites in adipose cells for future energy needs, and finally moved into a cell's mitochondria for metabolism, with the release of energy in the form of ATP units. This process is complicated by the fact that fats themselves cannot be transported across cell membranes due to their low hydrophilicity. Rather, a sequence of hydrolysis and ester formation occurs at various stages in the absorption-transport-storage-utilization process.

Consumed fats travel to the small intestine where they are emulsified with the aid of bile acids and are then hydrolyzed through the action of pancreatic lipase. The resulting fatty acids and glycerol can now be absorbed into the intestinal mucosa. At this point, the fat is reformed and, in the presence of apoproteins and cholesterol, is converted to chylomicrons (large lipoprotein particles consisting of 85% to 92% triglycerides), which are capable of entering the bloodstream for transport to storage sites in adipocytes or muscle cells for utilization as an energy source. Once again, for transport into adipocytes or muscle cells, the fat must be hydrolyzed by lipases, absorbed across the cell membrane, and re-esterified to the triglycerol fat for storage in adipocytes or metabolized in the mitochondria of the muscle cell (myocytes) (23).

Mobilization of fats from adipocytes is a G protein–innervated process involving β-adrenergic receptors and various hormones including glucagon, epinephrine, and β-corticotropin. Release of fatty acids from the adipocytes into the bloodstream allows for the transport to myocytes with the aid of blood albumin and ultimately passive absorption into the myocytes. It should be noted that insulin can inhibit the release of fatty acids from adipocytes by inhibition of adenylcyclase. Once again, transport into the mitochondria from the cytoplasm requires esterification to a fatty acyl-coenzyme A (CoA), transport across the outer mitochondria membrane, transesterification to fatty acylcarnitine, transport across the inner mitochondria, and transesterification back to fatty acyl-CoA, which can now be metabolized in the Krebs cycle to carbon dioxide, water, and release of ATP.

Nutritional Properties

It is estimated that 35% to 40% of the caloric intake in the United States comes in the form of fat, with greater than 90% of the fat being in the form of triglycerides (free fatty acids, cholesterol, and phospholipids represent the remaining amount of fat in the diet). This amounts to approximately 100 to 150 g/day of triglycerides. The RDI for fat is 65 g/day consisting of 20 g/day of saturated fats and 300 mg of cholesterol. This is based on a 2,000-calorie diet for an adult. Obviously the typical diet of 100 to 150 g/day of fat will lead to an excessive caloric intake of this macronutrient and an associated potential for overweight and obesity.

Fats have an essential role in the health of the body. In addition to being a major source of body energy (80% to 90%), fatty acids are an endogenous source of cholesterol via acetyl-CoA units. Cholesterol is the precursor to hormones of the body (bile salts, vitamin D, sex hormones, and adrenocortical hormones). Phospholipids and unsaturated fatty acids are components of the cell membrane, and subcutaneous fats give the body thermal insulation. However, excessive quantities of fats are associated with significant human disease.

Health Issues

As already indicated, fats and fatty acids as a source of calories are associated with overweight and obesity, but this is true of any calorie source because a calorie is a calorie irrespective of whether it comes from fats, carbohydrates, or proteins. There are particular disease states in which evidence points to dietary fats as a major contributor to the condition. CHD, which includes ischemic heart disease, myocardial infarction, and angina pectoris, is a condition in which fats and cholesterol have a significant role (Chapter 25). Countries that have diets low in saturated fats and cholesterol have a low incidence of ischemic heart disease, whereas Western industrialized countries with high dietary fat intake show significant increases in heart disease. A strong link exists between high blood lipid levels (e.g., LDL) and atherosclerosis, which in turn is tied to CHD. A reversible relationship also exists between CHD and the lowering of blood lipid levels. Thus, a goal is to reduce total fat calories to less than 35% of caloric intake.

Epidemiologic studies suggest that colorectal cancer is correlated with high calorie intake, diets rich in meat protein, and elevated dietary fats and oils. Metabolic processes in the GI tract and low fiber in the diet have been suggested as possible mechanisms.

It is generally agreed that a relationship exists between fats and insulin resistance, leading to type 2 diabetes, and diets consisting of low fat content and high carbohydrate content are commonly recommended. Obesity is certainly considered a predisposing factor to type 2 diabetes, but other than fats being a significant source of calories, the relationship between diabetes and fats is tenuous. Animal studies support the relationship of saturated fats and decreased insulin sensitivity, but whether these studies can be carried over to humans is debatable. Because of the complexity of diets, human variability, and the lack of long-term studies, it is difficult to associate fats with type 2 diabetes, although evidence points to beneficial effects of low saturated fats, low *trans* fats, and high PUFA combined with high-fiber diets in reducing the risk of type 2 diabetes (24).

Fats and Fatty Acid Substitution

As with carbohydrates, replacement of fats and fatty acids with nonfats or reduced-fat calories is desirable. Other than reducing the proportion of fats in the diet, the options for fat substitutes are far less than the choices available with sugar substitutes.

Skimmed Milk Skimmed milk is a dairy product in which nearly all of the butterfat is removed, whereas whole milk contains approximately 3.5 g of a mixture of fats in 100 g of fluid. The fatty acid content of whole milk consists of saturated fatty acids (palmitic acid [31%], myristic acid [12%], and stearic acid [11%]) and unsaturated fatty acids (oleic acid [24%], palmitoleic acid [4%], and linoleic acid [3%]). Various other milk products are available such as reduced-fat (2% fat) and low-fat milk (~1% fat). Because of the low-fat content of skimmed milk, the caloric content of 100 g of skimmed milk is approximately 34 calories compared with 64 calories in 100 g of whole milk. Ice cream prepared from cow's milk contains from 10% to 19% fat, a varying content of cholesterol (~97 mg/100 g of ice cream), and a caloric content of approximately 274 calories. In contrast, frozen yogurt made from skimmed milk has very little fat, but may have significant calorie content due to added sucrose.

Olestra (Olean)

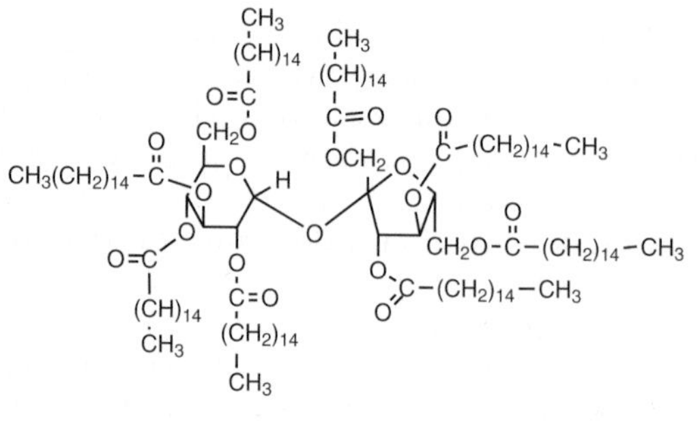

Olestra

Olestra is composed of a sucrose nucleus with all of the alcohol groups substituted with stearic acid. As a result of the bulky substituents, the compound is not readily hydrolyzed to the fatty acids and sucrose; thus, olestra is advertized as a "fat-free" material. The properties of olestra include a high boiling point with stability to baking and cooking and a taste and feel similar to fat. As a result, olestra is used as a frying oil to prepare potato chips. Americans purchased more than 1.6 billion pounds of potato chips, pretzels, and microwave popcorn in 1999 (25). Olestra-prepared chips have 0 g of fat and 70 calories, whereas an equivalent quantity of normally prepared chips has 10 g of fat and 160 calories. The lower metabolism is associated with poor absorption of the olestra, and as a highly fatty material, it has the potential for dissolving the fat-soluble vitamins (vitamins A, D, E, and K), increasing the potential for hypovitaminosis of these vitamins. Most significantly, olestra causes cramping and loose stools, which have seriously affected the sales of olestra-containing products. To offset the potential for fat-soluble vitamin deficiencies, olestra-containing foods commonly are fortified with small amounts of the fat-soluble vitamins.

Various nondigestible fibers from oats have been developed that can be used in foods as fat replacements products, but these appear to have low commercial value at the present time.

Protein

The third major macronutrient is protein. As indicated earlier, proteins are essential to the body as a source of amino acids. Proteins, as a polymer of amino acids, are not absorbed as such but must be metabolized by peptidases in the GI tract to the monomeric amino acids and di- and tripeptides, which can then be absorbed from the GI tract via active transport. Protein makes up 12% to 14% of our normal diet. The body's energy needs are met primarily by fat (~15 kg in the body), whereas carbohydrates in the form of glycogen give rise to immediate energy needs, but its presence in the body is quite small (~0.2 kg). Protein, in the form of muscle mass, accounts for approximately 6 kg of body weight and is a source of potential energy via metabolism to amino acids, which are converted into glucose through the biochemical process called gluconeogenesis. In general, proteins are used for body structure (muscle), hormones, and enzymes and as a source of nitrogen for the synthesis of key chemical components such as purine for RNA and DNA synthesis; only as a last resort will the body use protein as a source of energy.

Twenty amino acids are essential to the human body and are normally obtained from the proteins in the diet. Once absorbed, these essential amino acids can be used for protein synthesis through the action of DNA and RNA (see Chapter 6). The actual RDAs for individual amino acids are not known, and it is not possible to accurately determine the RDAs for protein that have varying quantities of individual amino acids. It is generally accepted that males have an RDA of 45 to 63 g of protein/day, whereas females have an RDA of 44 to 50 g/day. These numbers are greatly affected by pregnancy and lactation in women (RDA may increase by as much as 50%), but can also be affected in both men and women by chronic stress, where the level of protein requirement will increase.

PHARMACOTHERAPY OF OVERWEIGHT AND OBESITY

Overweight and obesity are complex chronic conditions for which successful treatment is not easily attained. Although the cause of obesity and overweight can be easily defined as resulting from a chronic intake of calories in excess to what the body needs, the involvement of social, behavioral, cultural, physiologic, metabolic, and genetic factors makes treatment extremely difficult. Dieting and physical activity can normally produce a loss of weight, but the long-term maintenance of the desired body weight is extremely difficult. Health hazards are associated with both excessive body weight and weight cycling, which commonly occurs through the loss and regaining of weight. A comprehensive study of the issues and treatment of overweight and obesity was reported in 1997 by the National Heart, Lung, and Blood Institute Obesity Education Initiative titled "Clinical Guidelines on the Identification, Evaluation, and Treatment of Overweight and Obesity in Adults" in which drug therapy was addressed as being one of several methods that can be helpful to long-term treatment (26). Presently, only one agent is available on the U.S. market, whereas other drugs are at various stages of development.

Orlistat (Alli, Xenical)

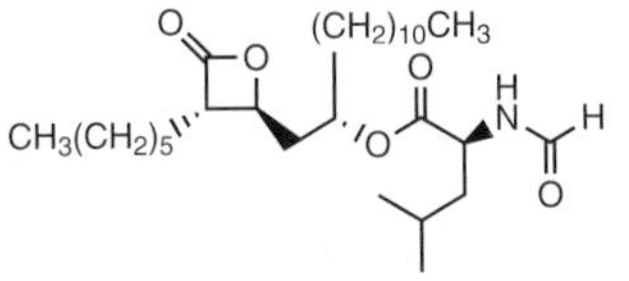

Orlistat, tetrahydrolipstatin, is a semisynthetic derivative of the natural product lipstatin produced by *Streptomyces toxytricini*. The compound acts as an irreversible inhibitor of pancreatic lipase and several other lipases and, as such, prevents the normal metabolic breakdown of fats, leading to reduced absorption of fatty acids from the GI tract (27,28). Fecal fat loss increases by as much as 30% after treatment with orlistat, thus indicating that reduced activity of intestinal lipases increases the loss of undigested fats. Studies with porcine pancreatic lipase show that acylation of serine 152 is responsible for this inhibition of lipase activity (28) (Fig. 42.12), suggesting a similar mechanism for orlistat in human intestine. Orlistat itself is not absorbed to any appreciable extent and is lost from the body via the GI tract. In addition, drug interaction studies indicate that orlistat may interfere with the absorption of a wide spectrum of drugs, such as cyclosporin, some diabetes medications, levothyroxine and warfarin, and with the fat-soluble vitamins with the exception of vitamin E (29).

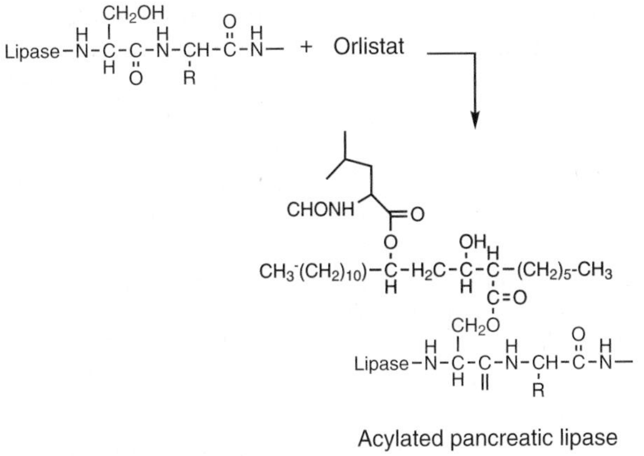

FIGURE 42.12 Irreversible acylation of a serine in pancreatic lipase by orlistat.

As might be expected, the most common adverse events were associated with the lack of absorption of fats and consisted of oily stools, spotting bowel movements, stomach pain, and flatulence. These events occurred in approximately 5% of the patients receiving orlistat at 30 to 360 mg/day. Additionally, it was noted that while on orlistat, obese patients showed a decrease in LDL and total cholesterol levels and that HbA_{1c} levels decreased in patients with type 2 diabetes.

Orlistat is available in a nonprescription product (Alli, 60 mg taken with each fat-containing meal up to 3 doses/day) and a prescription product (Xenical, 120 mg taken with each fat-containing meal up to 3 doses/day). Orlistat is used as an adjunct to diet and exercise and can be used for long-term therapy.

ANOREXIANTS AS PHARMACOLOGIC AGENTS IN THE MANAGEMENT OF OBESITY

The anorexiants constitute the starting place of pharmacologic therapy for obesity. Other terms for these agents include *anorectics* or *anorexigenics*, *antiobesity agents*, and *appetite suppressants*. These drugs are used as adjuncts in weight reduction programs under physician supervision for morbidly obese patients (BMI >30 kg/m^2) who are on a caloric reduction diet, exercise program, and behavioral therapy program, who may need to reduce weight over months or years. Appetite is clearly a very important instinct to promote survival (30). Arguably any drug that would abolish appetite may carry a high mortality risk and may be unsuitable for clinical use. Because the human body uses various neurochemicals and hormones to protect its stores of fat (a reaction probably useful to our ancestors when food was scarce), a "silver bullet," or a way to completely circumvent this natural habit of protecting excess food stores, has not yet been found. As a result, anorexiants/antiobesity drugs are not a practical long-term solution for people who are overweight. Appetite suppressants should not be used in place of proper diet.

For best results, these drugs must be used along with a medically approved diet and exercise program.

The anorectic drugs currently available can be divided into sympathomimetic amines (adrenergic agents) and serotonergic agents. The anorexiants shown in Figure 42.13 are structurally and pharmacologically related to the amphetamines (phenylisopropylamines) (see also Chapter 10). Although, anorexiants are primarily intended to suppress the appetite, most of the drugs in this class appear to be CNS stimulants, with a potential for abuse or addiction (31). Therefore, the antiobesity drugs are classified as schedule I, II, III, IV, and V as determined by the Controlled Substances Act of 1971 (Fig. 42.13). For example, schedule I drugs have a very high potential for abuse and addiction but no legitimate medical use, whereas schedule V drugs have the lowest potential for abuse and addiction and a legitimate medical use.

The anorexiants are associated with abuse and addiction because they are chemically and pharmacologically related to amphetamine. The dependence associated with these agents may be psychological and/or physiologic and is usually associated with long-term therapy or abuse. If the patient continues to lose weight and does not develop side effects or dependence, therapy may be continued past 12 weeks. If the patient does not continue to lose weight, then the dosage should not be increased, and the agent should be discontinued. Total length of therapy with the anorexiant agents should not exceed 6 months.

Sympathomimetic Amines

Sympathomimetic amines are drugs that act by releasing norepinephrine from storage vesicles in the adrenergic neuron and by blocking norepinephrine reuptake from the synapse (see Chapter 10). These drugs also act as reuptake inhibitors of dopamine, which is believed to be linked with their abuse and addiction potential. Although the mechanism of action of the sympathomimetic amines in the treatment of obesity is not fully known, this class of compounds has no primary effect on the appetite brain center; rather, its appetite-suppressant action appears to be secondary to CNS stimulation. These drugs are FDA approved for short-term use and include phentermine (Ionamin), diethylpropion (Tenuate), mazindol (Sanorex), benzphetamine (Didrex), and phendimetrazine (Bontril) (Fig. 42.13). Sympathomimetic appetite suppressants are used in the short-term treatment of obesity, usually for no more than 12 weeks. Their appetite-reducing effect tends to decrease after a few weeks of treatment. As a result, the sympathomimetic amines are useful only during the first few weeks of a weight-loss program. These drugs should not be taken with other appetite suppressants due to the possibility of serious side effects. The sympathomimetic amines may cause withdrawal reactions, especially if they have been used regularly for a long time or in high doses. In such cases, withdrawal symptoms (such as depression and severe fatigue) may occur if these medications are suddenly stopped.

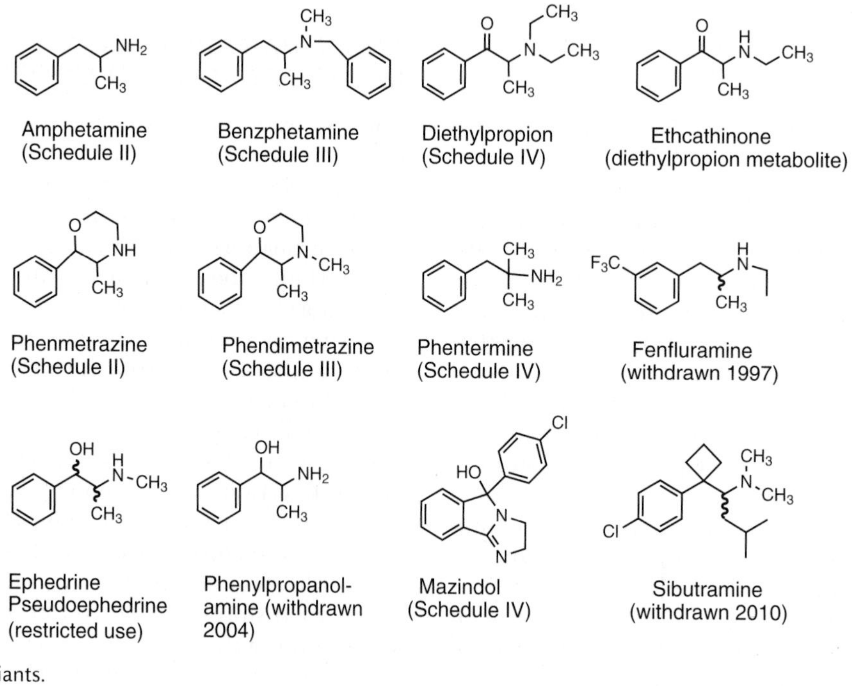

FIGURE 42.13 Anorexiants.

Amphetamine

Amphetamine is the prototypical anorexiant and a psychostimulant drug of the phenylisopropylamine family that produces increased wakefulness and decreased fatigue and appetite (Fig. 42.13). The drug has also been used recreationally and as a performance enhancer. Amphetamine is ranked as the most addictive and most harmful of the appetite suppressants (32). Amphetamine is a chiral compound, and its racemate can be divided into levo- and dextroamphetamine. Dextroamphetamine was used for treatment of obesity. Other derivatives of amphetamine used as recreational drugs are described in Chapter 19.

Amphetamine was first synthesized in 1887 as a synthetic substitute for ephedrine. No pharmacologic use was found for amphetamine until 1933 when the pharmaceutical company Smith, Kline and French began selling the volatile base form of the drug as a nasal inhaler under the trade name Benzedrine as a nasal decongestant. Shortly after marketing Benzedrine inhaler, the psychostimulant properties of amphetamine were discovered; these included a sense of well-being and a feeling of exhilaration, lessened fatigue in work, and loss of appetite. During World War II, amphetamine was extensively used to combat fatigue and increase alertness in soldiers, especially fighter and bomber crews. After decades of reported abuse, the FDA banned Benzedrine inhalers and limited amphetamine to prescription use in 1965, but nonmedical use remained common. Amphetamine became a schedule II drug under the Controlled Substances Act in 1971. An analog of amphetamine is methamphetamine; the *N*-methyl analog was also synthesized as an ephedrine derivative in 1920, but by 1941, it became a controlled substance because of abuse and was eventually banned.

Amphetamine became popular for weight loss during the late 1930s. The appetite-suppressant action for amphetamine appears to be secondary to CNS stimulation, along with other beneficial effects such as increased alertness. Use of amphetamine increased over the subsequent decades, culminating in the "rainbow pill" regimen. This was a combination of multiple pills, all thought to help with weight loss, taken throughout the day. Typical regimens included stimulants such as amphetamine, thyroxine, diuretics, digitalis, laxatives, and often a barbiturate to suppress the side effects of the stimulants. As a result of deaths attributed to diet pills and the gradual implementation of greater restrictions on diet pills, in 1979, the FDA banned the use of amphetamine in diet pills.

Benzphetamine

Benzphetamine (Didrex) is the *N*-benzyl analog of methamphetamine FDA approved in 1960 (Fig. 42.13). Because it is closely related to amphetamine, its anorexiant and pharmacologic properties appear to be similar to amphetamine. It is used as a short-term adjunct in management of morbid obesity. Benzphetamine is primarily *N*-demethylated to *N*-benzylamphetamine and to the minor metabolites methamphetamine, amphetamine, and their hydroxylated metabolites (33). Because benzphetamine is poorly metabolized to methamphetamine and amphetamine in the liver regardless of route of administration, benzphetamine is classified as schedule III appetite suppressant because it still has the potential for abuse and addiction, but much less so than amphetamine. Benzphetamine should not be given to patients who have a history of drug abuse.

Diethylpropion

Diethylpropion (Tenuate) was developed in 1958 as an anorexiant alternative to amphetamine and phenmetrazine without the psychostimulant side effects and abuse potential and does not affect blood pressure (Fig. 42.13). The appetite-suppressant effect of diethylpropion is due to its *N*-monodeethylation to ethocathinone (34). It is used along with a medically approved, reduced-calorie diet, exercise, and behavior change program to help one lose weight. Like the other sympathomimetic appetite suppressants, taking this medication late in the day may cause trouble sleeping (insomnia). This drug is classified as schedule IV, and therefore, abuse and addiction are low but possible with this medication. Increasing the dose or frequency of use is contraindicated, as is using diethylpropion beyond the normal prescribing time.

Phenmetrazine and Phendimetrazine

PHENMETRAZINE Phenmetrazine (Preludin) is a stimulant drug of the morpholine chemical class that was previously used as an appetite suppressant but has since been withdrawn from the U.S. and world market due to its great potential for abuse and addiction. It has been replaced by its *N*-methyl analog phendimetrazine, which functions as a prodrug to phenmetrazine (Fig. 42.13). Phenmetrazine was first patented in Germany in 1952 by Boehringer-Ingelheim as an anorectic drug without the side effects of amphetamine. The drug is a cyclized analog of ephedrine. It was introduced into clinical use in 1954 and withdrawn from the market in 1965. Phenmetrazine has a high potential for abuse and addiction and therefore is classified as schedule II. In a study of the effectiveness on weight loss between phenmetrazine and dextroamphetamine, phenmetrazine was found to be slightly more effective (35). Phenmetrazine causes the release of norepinephrine and dopamine but not of serotonin and inhibits the reuptake of norepinephrine and dopamine. Phenmetrazine was used recreationally in the United States during the 1960s and the early 1970s.

PHENDIMETRAZINE Phendimetrazine (Bontril) is also a stimulant drug of the morpholine chemical class approved as an appetite suppressant. Phendimetrazine is the *N*-methyl analog of phenmetrazine with anorexigenic action resulting from a combination of its own lesser activity plus that resulting from *N*-demethylation to phenmetrazine (Fig. 42.13). Thus, phendimetrazine functions as a prodrug to phenmetrazine; approximately 30% of an oral dose is converted into phenmetrazine. Because of its slow conversion to phenmetrazine, phendimetrazine is a less abusable version of phenmetrazine and is classified as schedule III. In addition, approximately 30% of the administered dose of phendimetrazine is excreted unchanged, and 25% is excreted as inactive *N*-oxide.

Phentermine

Phentermine (Ionamin) is structurally similar to amphetamine and is currently used as a single weight-loss agent to decrease appetite (Fig. 42.13). Phentermine received approval from the FDA in 1959 as an appetite-suppressing drug and became available in the early 1970s. Phentermine is a contraction of phenyl-tertiary-butylamine and is related to amphetamine. Phentermine is approved as an appetite suppressant to help reduce weight in obese patients when used short term (<12 weeks) and combined with exercise, diet, and behavioral modification. Phentermine has fewer psychostimulant effects and less abuse and addiction potential than amphetamine and therefore is classified as schedule IV appetite suppressant (36). Its side effects are consistent with its norepinephrine-releasing properties, but the incidence and magnitude of these effects are less than with amphetamine. After short-term use, tolerance begins and can be followed by rebound weight gain. However, phentermine was not a popular appetite suppressant drug until 1992 when Weintraub reported that combining phentermine with fenfluramine (Pondimin) (serotonergic appetite suppressant) caused a 10% weight loss, which was maintained for over 2 years (37). Thus, Fen-Phen rapidly became the most commonly prescribed diet medication. Dexfenfluramine (Redux) was developed in the mid-1990s as an alternative to fenfluramine with less side effects and received regulatory approval in 1996. However, after 24 cases of heart valve disease in Fen-Phen users were reported, fenfluramine and dexfenfluramine were voluntarily taken off the market at the request of the FDA (38). Studies later proved that the abnormal valve findings were due to the serotonergic effect of fenfluramine or dexfenfluramine on the heart valve. The FDA did not ask manufacturers to remove phentermine from the market.

Ephedrine and Pseudoephedrine

A number of over-the-counter dietary supplements and Internet products (Herbal Fen-Phen, PhenTrim, Phen-Cal, Xenadrine) contain ephedrine, which is derived from the ephedra herb, ma huang. Ephedra is one of a group of plants that are a source of ephedrine alkaloids, including ephedrine and pseudoephedrine (Fig. 42.13) (see Chapter 10). Ephedrine can cause a number of side effects, including rapid heartbeat, high blood pressure, psychosis, heart attacks, and seizures. Pseudoephedrine, a related stereoisomer of ephedrine, is commonly found in many antihistamines and cold medicines, has similar effects, and is sometimes used by dieters. Pseudoephedrine has also been used for its CNS stimulant properties. The structural similarity of pseudoephedrine to the amphetamines has made the drug a sought-after chemical precursor in the illicit manufacture of methamphetamine. As a result, the U.S. Congress recognized that pseudoephedrine is used in the illegal manufacture of methamphetamine, and passed the Combat Methamphetamine Epidemic Act of 2005, restricting the sale of pseudoephedrine-containing products (i.e., Sudafed), as well as to all over the counter products containing ephedrine, pseudoephedrine, and phenylpropanolamine. Other countries also restrict the sale of pseudoephedrine. In 2004, the FDA prohibited the sale of any dietary supplement containing ephedra/ephedrine in the United States due to an unreasonable risk to those who use it. Ephedra has become an increasingly popular ingredient in dietary supplements promoted for weight loss and boosting athletic performance or energy. The FDA reports little evidence supporting ephedra's effectiveness in promoting anything but modest, short-term weight loss without any clear health benefit. In addition, ephedra raises blood pressure and puts additional stress on the circulatory system, and these actions have been linked to heart attack and stroke. In 2006, the FDA declared all dietary supplements containing ephedrine alkaloids to be adulterated, and therefore illegal for marketing in the U. S. However, ephedrine is still legal for other medical uses, and purchase is restricted from state to state. However, the safety of dietary supplements containing ephedrine alkaloids and pseudoephedrine is closely regulated by the FDA, for these hazards.

Phenylpropanolamine

Phenylpropanolamine (Dexatrim), a sympathomimetic drug and a synthetic derivative of ephedrine, was available as an over-the-counter appetite suppressant and decongestant in cold medicines (Nyquil). Individuals who took 25 to 75 mg of phenylpropanolamine experienced some weight loss (Fig. 42.13). Common adverse effects included nervousness, insomnia, dizziness, palpitations, and headaches, but not a clinically significant increase in blood pressure. In 2005, the FDA removed phenylpropanolamine from over-the-counter sale due to a proposed increased risk of stroke in younger women and because of its potential use in amphetamine manufacture; it is controlled by the Combat Methamphetamine Epidemic Act of 2005. Canada withdrew phenylpropanolamine in 2001 for the same reasons. The drug is still available in Europe by prescription and over the counter.

Mazindol

Mazindol (Sanorex) differs from the prototypical amphetamine analogs by being a fused tricyclic imidazo-isoindole compound (Fig. 42.13). However, mazindol exhibits pharmacologic effects similar to those of amphetamine. Like other sympathomimetic appetite suppressants, mazindol is thought to act as a reuptake inhibitor of norepinephrine and dopamine, which stimulates the CNS and increases heart rate and blood pressure. Similar to amphetamine, patients report a decrease in appetite and an increase in energy, but mazindol has a low potential for abuse and addiction. Thus, mazindol is classified as a schedule IV appetite suppressant. As with other schedule

IV appetite suppressants, this drug is used in the short-term treatment (<12 weeks) of obesity, in combination with a weight-loss program based on caloric restriction, exercise, and behavior modification in patients with a BMI of 30 kg/m^2 or in patients with a BMI of 27 kg/m^2 in the presence of risk factors such as hypertension, diabetes, or hyperlipidemia. Its appetite-suppressing effect tends to decrease after a few weeks of treatment. Because of this effect, mazindol is useful only during the first few weeks of a weight-loss program.

Serotonergic Agents

To circumvent the feedback mechanisms that prevent most monotherapies from producing sustained large amounts of weight loss, it has been hypothesized that combinations of drugs may be more effective by targeting multiple pathways and possibly inhibiting feedback pathways that work to cause a plateau in weight loss. This was evidenced by the early success of combining phentermine and fenfluramine or dexfenfluramine, popularly referred to Fen-Phen or Redux, in producing significant weight loss. However, as previously described, Fen-Phen was removed from the market due to safety fears regarding a potential link to heart valve damage and primary pulmonary hypertension. The damage was found to be a result of activity of fenfluramine and dexfenfluramine at the 5-HT$_{2B}$ serotonin receptor in heart valves.

Fenfluramine

Fenfluramine (Pondimin) was part of the Fen-Phen antiobesity medication controversy as previously described. Fenfluramine was introduced on the U.S. market in 1973 as an appetite suppressant but was not very popular until combined with phentermine. It exists as the racemic mixture of two enantiomers: dextrofenfluramine and levofenfluramine (Fig. 42.13). The drug and its metabolite, norfenfluramine, cause the release of serotonin from vesicular storage sites and inhibit serotonin transporter reuptake of serotonin from the synaptic cleft, thus acting on the hypothalamus to decrease satiety. The end result is a feeling of fullness and loss of appetite. The neurotransmitter serotonin regulates mood, appetite, and other functions. Selective serotonin reuptake inhibitors (SSRIs) also suppress appetite (39) (see Chapter 18).

One mechanism to explain valvular abnormality involves heart valve serotonin receptors, which are thought to help regulate growth. Because fenfluramine and its active metabolite norfenfluramine stimulate 5-HT$_{2B}$ serotonin receptors, this may have caused the damage by stimulation of these receptors, leading to inappropriate valve cell division (38). Fenfluramine is no longer marketed worldwide.

Sibutramine

Sibutramine (Meridia) is an adrenergic/serotonergic agent approved by the FDA in 1997 for use in the management of obesity, including weight loss and maintenance of weight loss, and should be used in conjunction with a reduced-calorie diet (Fig. 42.13). The drug was recommended for obese patients with an initial BMI of greater than 30 kg/m^2. Sibutramine and its metabolite inhibit norepinephrine and serotonin reuptake, suppressing appetite similar to SSRIs. Sibutramine may also stimulate thermogenesis by activating the β3 system in brown adipose tissue. Initially tested for its antidepressant activity, sibutramine was found to cause modest weight loss. However, weight was regained even in subjects taking high-dose sibutramine.

Since its approval in 1997, sibutramine has exhibited an increased risk of nonfatal but serious cardiovascular events in patients with a known or high risk for cardiovascular disease (40). As a result of safety concerns, minimal efficacy as an appetite suppressant, and increased risk of adverse cardiovascular events, in 2010, Abbot Laboratories withdrew sibutramine from the U.S. and European markets under pressure from the FDA and European Medicines Agency (41).

Counterfeit weight-loss products have been on the increase, prompting the FDA in 2008 and 2009 to issue safety alerts to consumers naming more than 60 different products marketed as "dietary supplements" for weight loss that illegally contain undisclosed amounts of sibutramine, sometimes containing as much as twice the dosage of the prescription drug. The safety alerts underscore the risks associated with unregulated "herbal supplements" in unsuspecting persons. This concern is especially relevant to those with underlying medical conditions incompatible with undeclared pharmaceutical adulterants (42).

The drug rimonabant was approved as an antiobesity drug in Europe that acted centrally through antagonism of cannabinoid receptors resulting in a reduced appetite. Concerns about psychiatric effects lead Sanofi-Aventis to remove the drug from FDA consideration as an antiobesity agent in 2008 and 2009.

Over-the-Counter Drugs and Herbal Remedies

People must be cautious when using any weight-loss medications, including over-the counter diet pills and herbal or so-called natural remedies. The following are examples of some products being sold for weight loss.

The Internet is a source of large numbers of products that are advertised as aids to promote weight loss. Many of these products consist of mixtures of natural products that also contain unlisted anorexiants such as ephedrine, propanolamine, or sibutramine, which the manufacturers claim will burn fats and create significant weight loss. None of these products have been approved by the FDA and are sold based on testimonials with some literature references suggesting effects on fat metabolism but, in most cases, without any documented clinical support. An example of such a product is LipoFuze, which the manufacturer states is a combination of "six patented and four clinically tested fat burning ingredients." The list of ingredients includes evodiamine, raspberry ketone, fucoxanthin, *Coleus foskohlii* extract, guggulsterones,

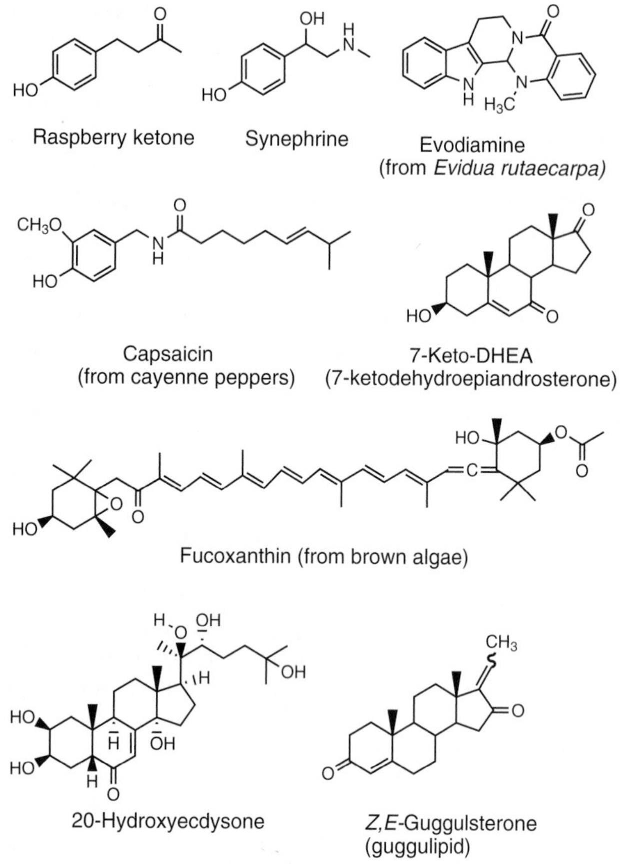

FIGURE 42.14 Partial list of ingredients in LipoFuze.

black pepper extract, green tea, capsaicin, synephrine hydrochloride, 7-oxo DHEA, cinnamon, phenylethylamine, ginger, and 20-hydroxyecdysone (Fig. 42.14). Classified as dietary supplements, the products are not tightly controlled by the FDA, and thus it is up to the consumer to be aware of their effectiveness and safety.

MICRONUTRIENTS

Vitamins

Vitamins are organic chemicals found in microorganisms, plants, and animals, but not man, that are essential to man and higher animals for the maintenance of growth, physiologic function, metabolism, and reproduction. The role of vitamins in the body is to act as catalysts for the biochemical reactions of the body, and although they are not consumed in these reactions, vitamins do have a normal turn over and elimination and therefore must be continuously resupplied to the body. The reader is referred to a biochemistry textbook for a discussion of the molecular mechanisms involving vitamins, as well as earlier chapters in this text (see Chapter 26 for vitamin K and Chapter 30 for vitamin D). The RDIs for the vitamins are given in Table 42.3. It is not our intention to review all of the vitamins in depth, but rather to describe nutritional properties of a select few vitamins.

The vitamins are divided into fat-soluble and water-soluble vitamins based on their physical-chemical properties. The fat-soluble vitamins include vitamins A, D, E, and K, whereas all of the remaining vitamins are considered water soluble (the B complex vitamins: thiamine [vitamin B_1], riboflavin [vitamin B_2], niacin [vitamin B_3], pantothenic acid [vitamin B_5], pyridoxal/pyridoxine [vitamin B_6], cobalamin [vitamin B_{12}], folic acid, and biotin; and vitamin C). Diseases associated with the vitamins most commonly occur due to deficiencies of the vitamins (hypovitaminosis) (Table 42.8), but can also occur due to excessive quantities of a vitamin (hypervitaminosis). Because of the lack of water solubility, the fat-soluble vitamins can build up in the body and therefore are commonly associated with hypervitaminosis, but the water-soluble vitamins can also cause hypervitaminosis. Vitamin deficiencies can be classified as either primary hypovitaminosis or secondary hypovitaminosis. Primary hypovitaminosis is the result of inadequate diet because of a lack of foods containing the vitamins or an inadequate diet due to poor use of foods. The latter may occur if the individual is dieting and not consuming a balanced diet or possibly because of food faddism where a variety of foods are not being used. Secondary hypovitaminosis may be the result of poor health or chronic disease states. Examples might be hyperthyroidism, chronic diarrhea, liver disease, or diseases of the GI tract. There are times in the life of an individual when demands for vitamins increase, such as during pregnancy and lactation in the female when the RDIs for all nutrients increase. Unless an increase in vitamin consumption occurs, the female will suffer hypovitaminosis. The use of drugs can also result in hypovitaminosis. An alcoholic may experience both primary and secondary deficiencies. While consuming alcohol, an alcoholic may not be eating a balanced diet and thus is at risk for a primary deficiency. Alcohol also damages both the intestinal lining and the liver, and nutrients cannot be absorbed through the damaged mucosal membrane or properly used by a damaged liver.

Vitamin A (Retinol, Retinal, Carotenes)

Vitamin A and its precursors, the carotenes, are fat soluble and found in high concentrations in liver and fish oils, yellow and green leafy vegetables, eggs, and whole-milk products. β-Carotene is also found in high levels in carrots and is highly lipophilic and readily absorbed. The carotenes, α- and β-carotene, are oxidatively converted into all-*trans*-retinal, which in turn can be converted into all-*trans*-retinol (Fig. 42.15), and thus the carotenes can be considered provitamin A's. *Trans*-retinol is generally considered the active form of vitamin A, whereas β-carotene has approximately half the activity of retinol, with α-carotene being a far less efficient source of vitamin A activity. Retinol is commonly found as a lipid-soluble ester with either palmitic acid or acetic acid. The carotinoids, a combination of

TABLE 42.8 Vitamins, Outward Disease(s), and Common Sources and Roles

Vitamin	Specific Disease(s)	Source	Role
Fat soluble			
Vitamin A	Xerophthalmia Nyctalopia	Yellow and green leafy vegetables, carrots, yellow fruits, fish oils, milk, fats and egg yolk, apricots, peaches, and sweet potatoes	Necessary for normal eye function, integrity of the epithelium, synthesis of adrenocortical steroids
Vitamin D	Rickets Osteomalacia	Egg yolks, dairy products, fish, and UV light	Calcium absorption and bone formation
Vitamin E	Spinocerebellar ataxia Skeletal myopathy	Cereals, nuts, unsaturated oils, leafy green and yellow vegetables, milk, muscle meats, and butter	Health of sensory neurons leading to peripheral neuropathy if absent
Vitamin K	Pigmented retinopathy Hypoprothrombinemia	Synthesized in the intestinal tract by bacteria and found in leafy green vegetables	Involved in the blood-clotting process
Water soluble			
Vitamin C (ascorbic acid)	Scurvy	Citrus fruits, cabbage, peppers, berries, melons, and salad greens	Prevents scurvy, necessary for proper bone and teeth formation
Vitamin B_1 (thiamine)	Beriberi Wernicke encephalopathy	Yeast, beans, brown rice, lean pork, whole-wheat bread, liver, and outer layers of seeds of plants or unrefined cereal grains	Prevents beriberi (leg edema, paralysis, muscle atrophy)
Vitamin B_2 (riboflavin)	Anemias	Liver, kidney, milk, yeast, heart, anaerobic fermenting bacteria, and many vegetables	Deficiency leads to lip lesions, seborrheic dermatitis
Vitamin B_3 (niacin)	Pellagra	Liver, kidney, lean meat, soybeans, wheat germ, broccoli, and avocados	Prevents pellagra (dermatitis, diarrhea, dementia)
Vitamin B_5 (pantothenic acid)	Rare, no specific disease	Muscle meats, outer layer of whole grains, broccoli, and avocados	Deficiencies are rare, but may appear as numbness, paresthesia, and muscle cramps
Vitamin B_6 (pyridoxal)	Homocystinuria	Wheat germ, milk, yeast, liver	Prevents dermatitis sicca in adults and convulsions in infants, essential to biochemical reactions
Vitamin B_{12} (cobalamin)	Pernicious anemia	Liver, kidney, muscle meats	Prevents pernicious anemia
Folic acid	Megaloblastic anemia NTDs	Leafy vegetables, beans, peas, liver, kidney, baker's yeast, grains, various nuts, and sunflower seeds	Important for prevention of NTDs, necessary to DNA and RNA synthesis and other biochemical reactions
Biotin	Rare, no specific disease	Tomatoes, kidney, egg yolk, peanuts, chocolates, yeast, and liver	Deficiency causes myodermatitis, lassitude, gastrointestinal symptoms, and hyperesthesias, including muscle pain

NTD, neural tube defect; UV, ultraviolet.

all sources of vitamin A, have used various measures to define their biologic activity. Since 2001, the retinol activity equivalent (RAE) has been used, which defines 1 mcg of RAE as equal to 1 mcg of all-*trans*-retinol and equal to 2 mcg of β-carotene, which is equal to 12 mcg of food-based β-carotene and 24 mcg of other food-based all-*trans* provitamin A carotenoids. Presently, the recommendation is that men should receive a dose of 900 mcg daily, whereas women should receive 700 mcg/day. Of course, the female dose should be increased during pregnancy and lactation (770 and 1,300 mcg, respectively) (43).

Physiologic Action of Vitamin A

Vision One commonly thinks of vitamin A and its role in vision. A simplistic outline of the process of vision is shown in Figure 42.16. To initiate the process, *trans*-retinol is isomerized to 11-*cis*-retinol, which in turn is oxidized to 11-*cis*-retinal, the aldehyde that forms a Schiff base with the protein opsin to form rhodopsin, which is the functional

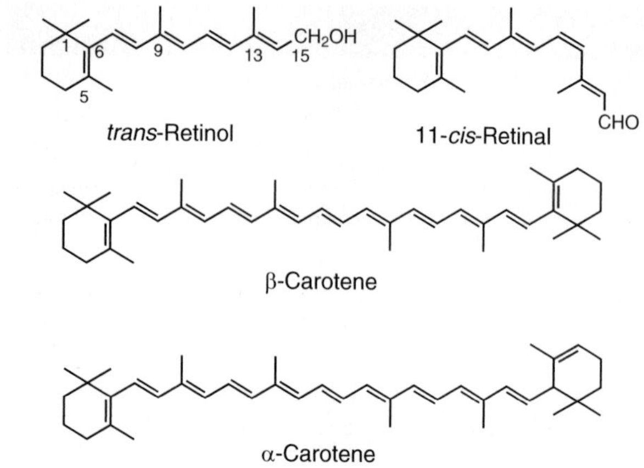

FIGURE 42.15 Naturally occurring carotenoids.

form of vitamin A. The absorption of a photon of light by the rhodopsin results in sodium conductance at a G protein–coupled receptor, leading to signaling in the visual center in the cortex via the optic nerve and release of opsin and *trans*-retinal, which is recycled through conversion back to *trans*-retinol. A deficiency of vitamin A (i.e., hypovitaminosis A) in the rods of the retina will initially lead to night blindness, nyctalopia, which is a reversible condition. Vitamin A deficiency in a child has much more severe consequences and is a leading cause of blindness (xerophthalmia) in many third-world nations.

Other Effects of Vitamin A Animal studies suggest additional roles for vitamin A in the development of epithelial tissue, mucus-producing tissue, reproduction, and bone growth. Whether these activities relate to human conditions is not known, and the evidence appears to point to retinoic acid as being important for these actions. Carotenoids have also been suggested to function as antioxidants and therefore have been proposed as valuable agents in the prevention of heart disease and cancer. The data supporting this notion are weak at best. A specific carotenoid, lutein, as well as β-carotene in combination with vitamin E, vitamin C, and zinc have been claimed to show benefit in the treatment of age-related macular degeneration.

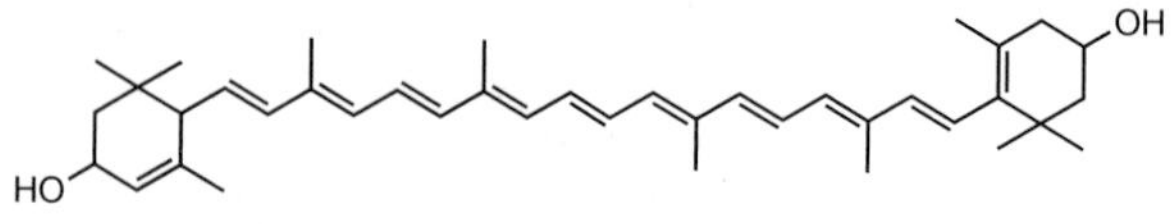

Lutein

Once again, the scientific evidence supporting these claims is weak.

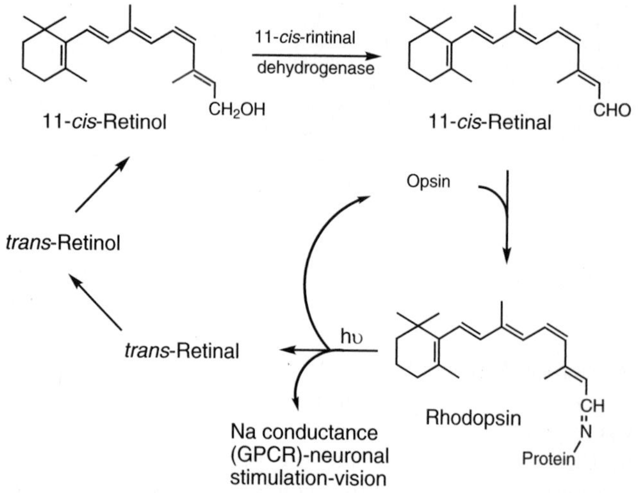

FIGURE 42.16 Role of vitamin A leading to visual signaling in the cortex.

Absorption The absorbable form of vitamin A is usually considered to be retinol. When vitamin A is administered as a retinol ester, hydrolysis is required in the intestine to release the free alcohol. If the source of vitamin A is β-carotene, oxidative cleavage is required to produce two molecules of retinal, which in turn are reduced to all-*trans*-retinol. Studies have shown that β-carotene can be absorbed as such, but quite inefficiently. Oxidative cleavage of β-carotene does not always occur symmetrically, in which case the yield of vitamin A is less than two molecules per molecule of β-carotene. Approximately 70% to 90% of absorption of vitamin A occurs from the small intestine, with much of the vitamin A being transported to the liver for storage.

Hypervitaminosis A Lay press publications claiming unsubstantiated benefits from vitamin A have resulted in consumers ingesting vitamin A in doses beyond normal daily requirements (doses as high as 25,000 IU or 7,500 mcg). Because of the lipid nature of vitamin A, large quantities can be retained and stored in the body, leading to hypervitaminosis A. The signs and symptoms of hypervitaminosis A include headache, fatigue, insomnia, cracked bleeding lips, cirrhosis-like damage of the liver, birth defects, and yellow skin coloration. Adverse events associated with vitamin A will not normally be seen unless the vitamin is consumed in large quantities over an extended period of time, and these effects are reversible upon discontinuance of the vitamin. The upper safe limit for vitamin A consumption is considered to be 3,000 mcg. The relationship between vitamin A and birth defects appears to be primarily associated with the intake of 13-*cis*-retinoic acid (Accutane), which is a known teratogen if consumed during the first trimester of pregnancy. There does not appear to be evidence that retinol, retinal, or β-carotene are sources of retinoic acid or 13-*cis*-retinoic acid, but cautious intake of vitamin A should be advised.

Vitamin D (Sunshine Vitamin, Calcitriol, Calciferols)

Vitamin D is an interesting fat-soluble vitamin because the vitamin can be synthesized in the body via a series of reactions including an ultraviolet-stimulated ring cleavage (ultraviolet B radiation) and hydroxylation reactions that occur in the liver and kidney (Fig. 42.17). Since the vitamin can be and is synthesized in the body, it should be considered a hormone rather than a vitamin. However, the absence of sufficient sunlight will lead to vitamin D–associated diseases, and therefore, additional quantities of vitamin D (actually its precursors) are required, and thus the vitamin nature of the calcitriol. Because the amount of sunlight that an individual receives can vary considerably, the actual daily needs for an individual can also vary considerably, and the recommended intake for vitamin D cannot be accurately defined. It is generally accepted that 5 mcg (200 IU) is sufficient for those under the age of 50 years, with increased quantities for those between 51 and 70 years (400 IU) and those over 71 years (600 IU). However, clinicians are recommending up to 2,000 mcg/day, especially for individuals living in the northern latitudes. A scan of the Internet shows that the consumer can purchase vitamin D_3 (cholecalciferol) in doses as high as 5,000 IU/dose.

Physiologic Action of Vitamin D The major role of vitamin D is to regulate the serum levels of ionic calcium and phosphate, which in turn affects bone ossification and neuromuscular function. 7-Dehydrocholesterol is found in most tissues, but that which is in the epidermis can be cleaved (between the C9 and C10 position) by the energy of absorbed ultraviolet light that is unfiltered by window glass. Following isomerization, vitamin D_3 is formed and circulates in the blood (Fig. 42.17). In the liver, vitamin D_3 is hydroxylated to 25-hydroxycholecalciferol, the primary circulating form of vitamin D. Final activation of vitamin D occurs in the kidney where hydroxylation occurs at the 1-postion to give the active 1,25-dihydroxycholecalciferol (calcitriol). Calcitriol is transported through the serum into the target tissue of the intestine and bone where it governs the transcription of mRNA, leading to synthesis of proteins, which increase the absorption of calcium from the gut or resorption of calcium from the bones in conjunction with parathyroid hormone (see Chapter 30). The termination of the action of calcitriol occurs through further hydroxylation, leading to any of a number of tri- and tetrahydroxycholecalciferols (24-hydroxylation is shown in Fig. 42.17).

Hypovitaminosis D, resulting from insufficient vitamin D serum levels, leads to poor absorption of calcium and phosphate from the intestine, which can result in mobilization of calcium from bones (resorption) in order to meet serum needs for the ion. In an infant, this can lead to rickets, whereas in an adult, osteomalacia will result. To prevent these conditions, it has become common practice to fortify milk and other food products with vitamin D as well as to recommend that women who breastfeed their infant should supplement their diet with vitamin D. There are indications that the vitamin D content of breast milk from many lactating women may

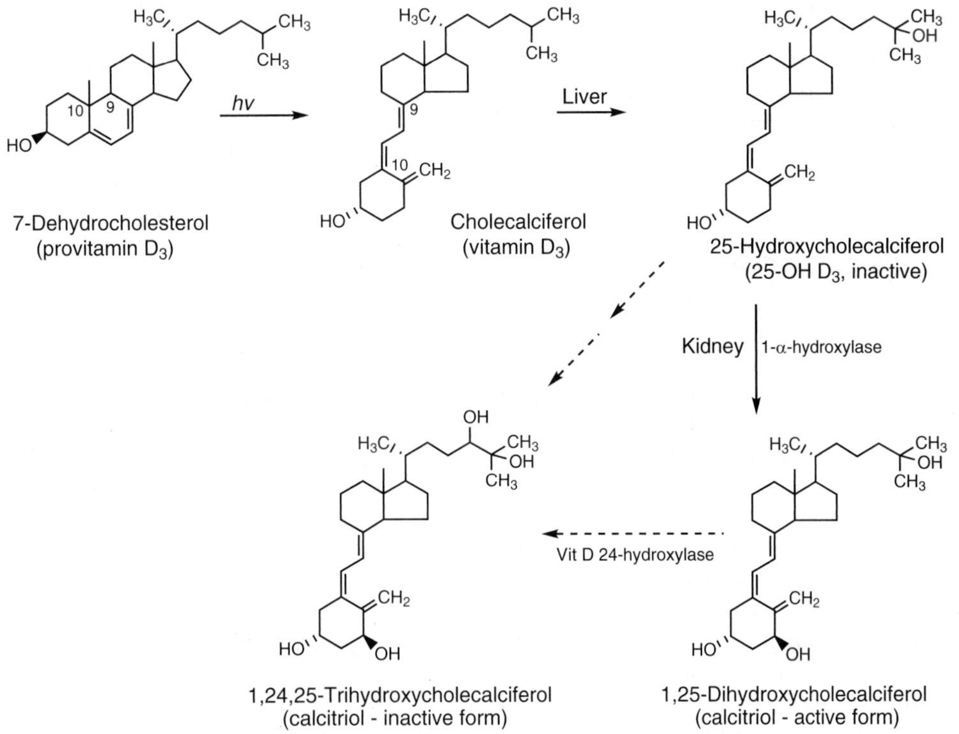

FIGURE 42.17 Bioactivation and inactivation of vitamin D.

be low in vitamin D. Hypovitaminosis D is common in the elderly due to the inability of the aged skin to form vitamin D_3 and because window glass filters out the beneficial ultraviolet light wavelengths. Hypovitaminosis D has also been found to be a factor in individuals with autoimmune diseases, such as diabetes, multiple sclerosis, irritable bowel syndrome, and rheumatoid arthritis, but the significance of the deficiency in these diseases has not been determined.

Hypervitaminosis D, resulting from consumption of high doses of vitamin D supplements, appears to be far less of a problem than earlier literature suggested, although doses of 10,000 IU/day or greater are considered problematic. High serum calcium levels increase the likelihood for precipitation of calcium salts in soft tissue such as kidney and heart. This could lead to a decrease in renal function and kidney stones, although the more common symptoms of hypervitaminosis D include constipation, bone pains and stiffness, and confusion. Treatment of hypervitaminosis D consists of removal of the source of vitamin D and reduction in exposure to the sun along with hydration and diuresis.

Vitamin E (Tocopherols)

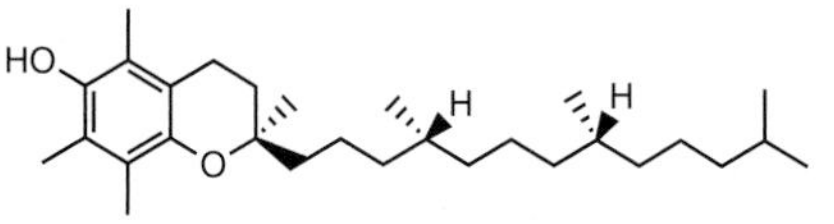

α-Tocopherol

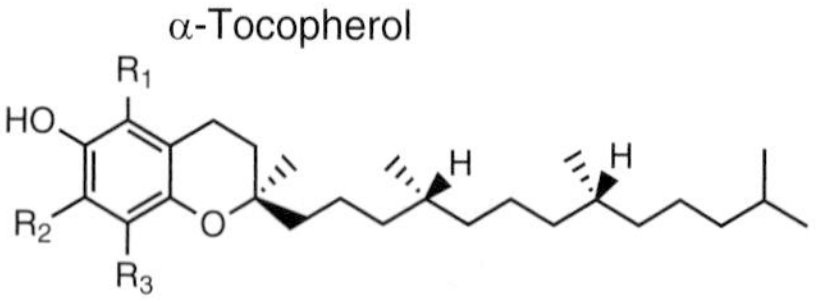

β-Tocopherol (R_2 = H, R_1 = R_3 = CH_3)
γ-Tocopherol (R_1 = H, R_2 = R_3 = CH_3)
δ-Tocopherol (R_1 = R_2 = H, R_3 = CH_3)

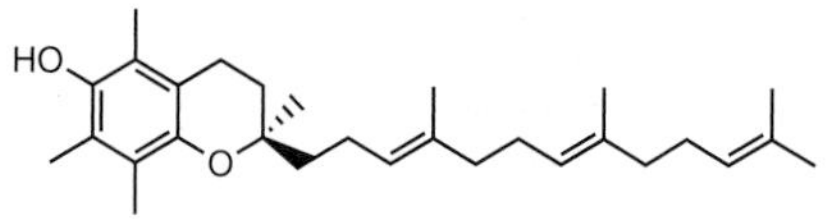

α-Tocotrienol

Vitamin E consists of a group of fat-soluble compounds composed of α-, β-, γ-, δ-tocopherol and α-, β-, γ-, δ-tocotrienol. α-Tocopherol and γ-tocopherol represent the two major tocopherols, whereas the tocotrienols are normally found in low concentrations in nature and are the unsaturated analogs of the respective tocopherols. Since the tocopherols have three chiral centers, a total of eight stereoisomers are possible for each of the tocopherols. The tocotrienols have only a single asymmetric center, resulting in two isomers for each of these products. Both the tocopherols and tocotrienols make up what is normally called vitamin E. The interest in vitamin E arose from studies of infertile male rats, which were shown to be deficient in a substance with vitamin E biologic activity. The substance was isolated and given the name of tocopherol, which is derived from the Greek words meaning "bring forth childbirth." Vitamin E is known as the antisterility vitamin, although there is no known correlation between low levels of vitamin E in male humans and infertility. The commercially available vitamin E may be a single isomer of one of the tocopherols or a mixture of tocopherols, although it is generally considered that α-tocopherol or *R,R,R*-α-tocopherol is the more active form of vitamin E. The tocotrienols may also be present in commercial vitamin E, but far less is known about the effects of these materials. The tocopherols may come in the form of an ester of the primary alcohol with the acetate ester being a common form of the vitamin. The quantization of vitamin E is based on a direct analytical measure or an indirect biologic rat assay method.

Physiologic Action of Vitamin E The search for a human function for vitamin E has not been an easy task. Vitamin E is ubiquitous in nature, and therefore, human deficiency in this vitamin is uncommon. The source of vitamin E include cereals, nuts, unsaturated oils, leafy green and yellow vegetables, milk, muscle meats, and butter (Table 42.8), although the distribution of the tocopherols and tocotrienols in nature is not uniform. Tocopherols are found in oils, seeds, leaves, and other green part of higher plants, whereas tocotrienols are limited to bran and germ fractions of certain seeds and cereals. In either case, nearly every diet will have a source of vitamin E. A reference to generic vitamin E would usually include products containing both tocopherols and tocotrienols. The difficulty of identifying a role for vitamin E has been that the lay press contains numerous articles claiming favorable actions for vitamin E, including improving wound healing without scarring, slowing down the ageing process, protecting against various cancers, preventing heart disease, and improving the performance of athletes. Many of these claims are not substantiated by scientific studies, although a common thread linking these claims is that vitamin E has the chemical property of being a fat-soluble antioxidant. Located in cell membranes, vitamin E could act by virtue of its high reactivity toward reactive oxygen species (ROS), thus protecting cellular components from oxidation (antioxidant). A diagram representing the action of an antioxidant such as vitamin E is shown in Figure 42.18. The tocopherols are thought to protect PUFA from ROS-catalyzed reactions that result in lipid

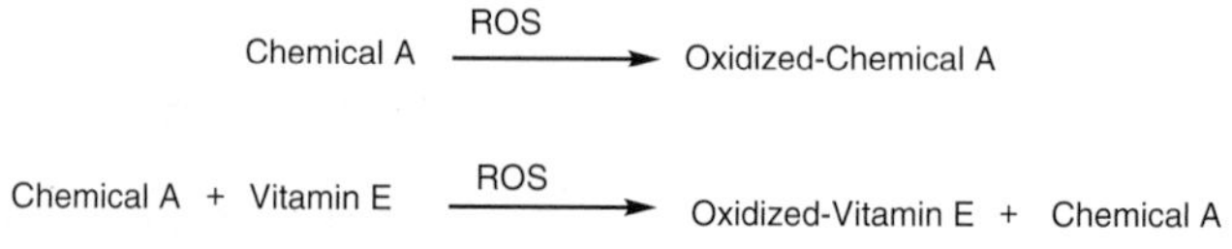

FIGURE 42.18 Vitamin E acting as an antioxidant to protect Chemical A.

peroxide radicals, which through a series of chain reactions damage PUFA.

Mechanism of Antioxidant Activity Vitamin E and especially α-tocopherol are substituted nicely to preferentially scavenge a lipid peroxyl radical. The mechanism and products of this reaction are shown in Figure 42.19. ROS can readily oxidize PUFA via abstraction of a hydrogen from the fatty acid, leaving behind a dienyl radical (44). This dienyl radical combines with oxygen to give a mixture of *cis/trans* lipid peroxyl radicals, which if left unchecked will lead to severe cellular damage through a series of hydrogen abstraction chain reactions with biomolecules (i.e., PUFA, DNA, RNA, etc.). In the presence of vitamin E, the lipid free radical abstracts a hydrogen from the phenolic group of α-tocopherol to produce a relatively stable tocopherol radical, thus effectively chain-breaking the auto-oxidation of the PUFA. α-Tocopherol is very efficient in acting as an antioxidant by virtue of the stability of the α-tocopherol radical, which results from the chemical substituents attached to the chroman ring system. Stabilization of the α-tocopherol radical is increased by the electron-donating *ortho* methyl groups, with only α-tocopherol having methyls in both *ortho* positions. Additionally, resonance stabilization by the *para* oxygen in the chroman ring improved the stability of the α-tocopherol radical (45,46).

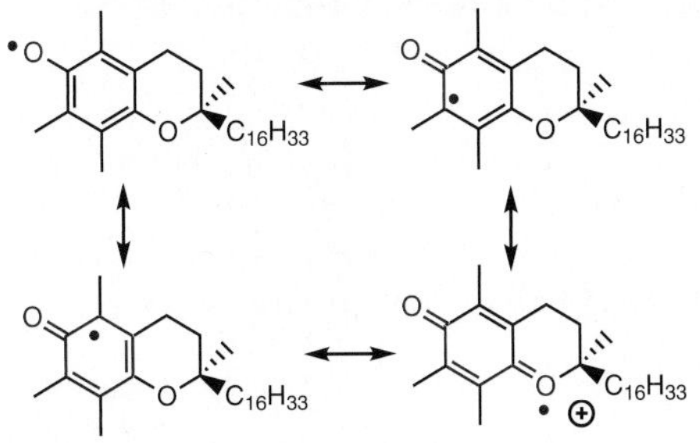

Resonance stabilization of α-tocopherol radical

The quenching of the α-tocopherol radical leads to formation of α-tocopherolquinone and the epoxytoxopherones (Fig. 42.19).

Absorption and Metabolism The absorption of vitamin E, both the tocopherols and the tocotrienols, occurs readily provided that two conditions are met. First, if vitamin E is administered as an ester, the ester must initially be hydrolyzed. This is easily done by esterases present in the intestine. Second, absorption is dependent on the presence of bile acids in the GI tract. Bile acids favor micelle

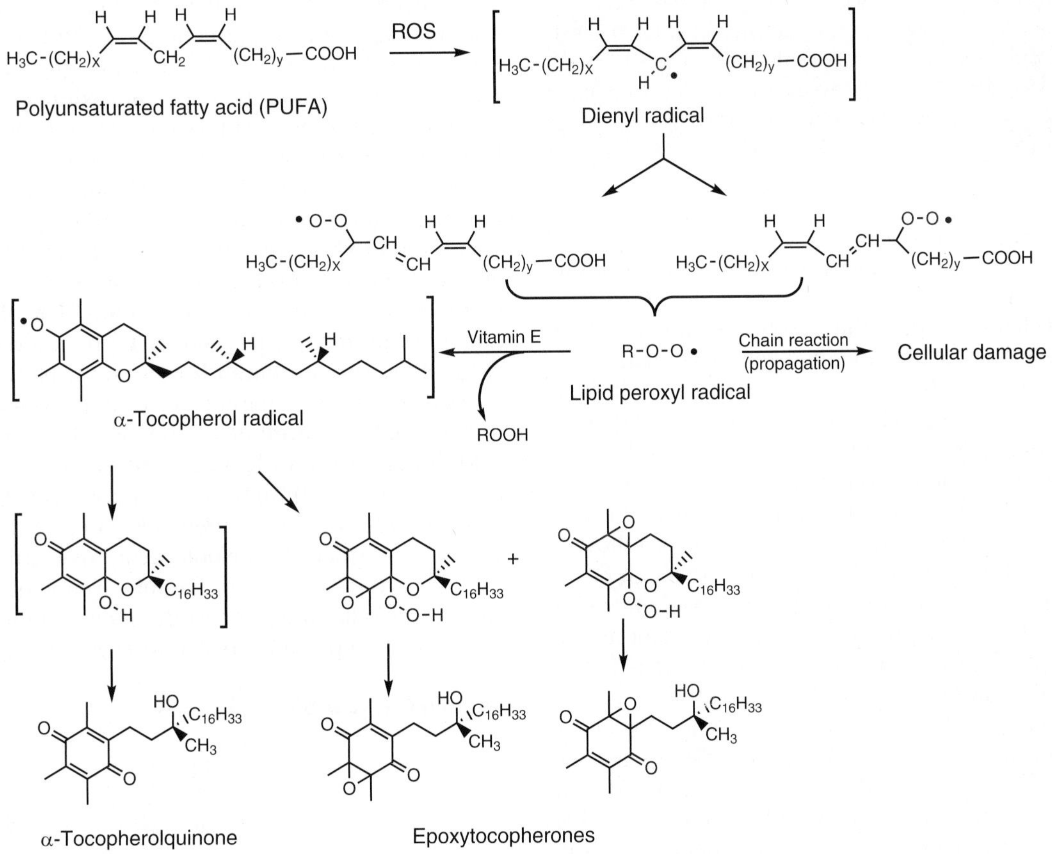

FIGURE 42.19 The action of vitamin E in decreasing cellular damage via reaction with PUFA free radicals.

REACTIVE OXYGEN SPECIES

A variety of chemicals found in the human body possess the chemical property of being an ROS. These include molecular oxygen, superoxide, hydrogen peroxide, and the hydroxy radical. A characteristic of an ROS is that it is highly reactive due to the presence of or ability to produce a single unshared valance shell electron, which is known as a free radical.

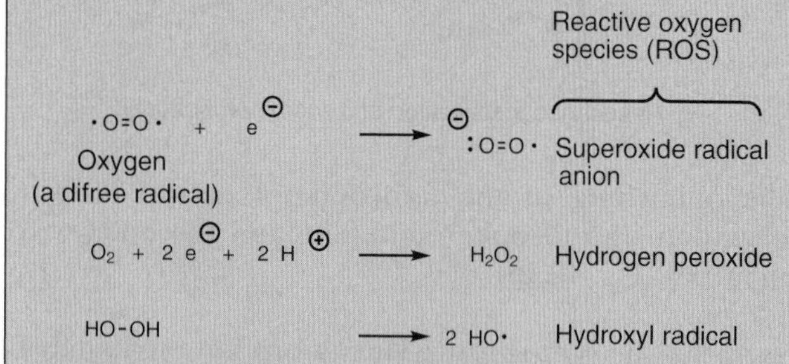

Free radicals such as molecular oxygen, superoxide radical anion, or hydroxy radical are very reactive and can attack cellular components leading to oxidation by abstracting an electron from the cellular component. DNA, RNA, protein, and PUFA are all prone to oxidative reactions catalyzed by the ROS. Generally, the body has sufficient enzymes, such as catalase, superoxide dismutase, and ubiquinone (coenzyme Q_{10}), along with natural antioxidants such as glutathione, vitamin E, vitamin C, vitamin A, and carotenes, to protect the cells against damage from ROS. Under oxidative stress, cellular damage may occur, and some theories suggest that chronic damage to key components of the cell may account for various cancers, cardiovascular disease, and even the ageing process.

formation, which is essential for absorption of these fat-soluble materials.

A general characteristic of the fat-soluble vitamins is their high lipophilicity and the potential for hypervitaminosis to occur; however in the case of vitamin E, hypervitaminosis is quite uncommon. This may be due to the fact that both the tocopherols and the tocotrienols are oxidized to more water-soluble chemicals that can be readily excreted from the body. The common metabolism consists of ω-oxidation of the lipophilic side chain of vitamin E followed by progressive shortening of the side chain through β-oxidation and the elimination of acetic and propionic acids (Fig. 42.20). The final products of these oxidations are the hydroxychromans as shown in Figure 42.20 (47–49). The ω-oxidation and apparently the β-oxidations are catalyzed by CYP4F2, and these series of reactions also occur with the tocotrienols, although the rates of these reactions and the amount of each of the metabolites may differ. It should be noted that whether the side chain of the vitamin E is saturated or unsaturated similar metabolic products are formed (how or when the alkene is reduced is not presently known). Thus, the plasma level of the particular vitamin E derivative may differ depending on the tocopherols or tocotrienols that are administered, which in turn may affect the antioxidant benefit of vitamin E.

Vitamin K (Menadiones)

Vitamin K, the fourth of the fat-soluble vitamins, derives its name from the German word *koagulation* and is similar to vitamin E in that there is no single chemical entity that possesses the biologic activity attributed to vitamin K. The major activity associated with vitamin K is catalyzing a posttranslation carboxylation of several proteins that are involved in blood coagulation (see Chapter 26). The basic nucleus of all vitamin K compounds is the 2-methyl-1,4-naphthoquinone to which various chain lengths of the 5-carbon isoprenoid unit are attached at the 3-position (Fig. 42.21). Green plants produce phylloquinone or vitamin K_1, which represents a major dietary source of the vitamin. Bacteria, some of which live in the intestine, produce various chain length methaquinones, where n varies from 4 to 9, that are abbreviated MK-n, and these compounds are referred to as vitamin K_2. Animals, including man, but not bacteria, can synthesize MK-4 from phylloquinone as well as from menadione, which is a synthetic form of vitamin K.

Sources and Properties of Vitamin K As previously indicated, vitamin K is found in leafy green vegetables such as collards, spinach, and salad greens, which have the highest concentrations (300 to 400 mcg/100 g), and from fats and oils such as soybean and canola oil (50,51). The RDA is rather low, being 1 mcg/kg body weight/day, while the DRI varies considerably from approximately 2 mcg/day for infants to 90 to 120 mcg/day for females and males between the ages of 19 and 70 years. One might expect that vitamin K deficiencies would be uncommon since various foods and intestinal bacterial flora are sources of this vitamin, and although this is generally true, the bioavailability of phylloquinone is in the range of 15% to 20%, and turnover of the vitamin occurs rapidly. The absorption of dietary vitamin K occurs via the lymphatic system, whereas the metabolism of vitamin K is not well characterized.

As discussed in Chapter 26, vitamin K is essential for the normal functioning of the blood clotting cascade. Additionally, vitamin K is thought to have a role in bone mineralization, although the exact role remains unclear.

Vitamin K toxicity has often been cited, and in fact, menadione is considered to be potentially toxic, a toxicity associated with interference with the functioning of glutathione. However, phylloquinone and the menaquinones have not been shown to produce toxic effects even at high doses.

Vitamin C (Ascorbic Acid)

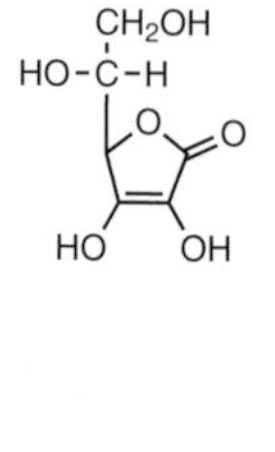

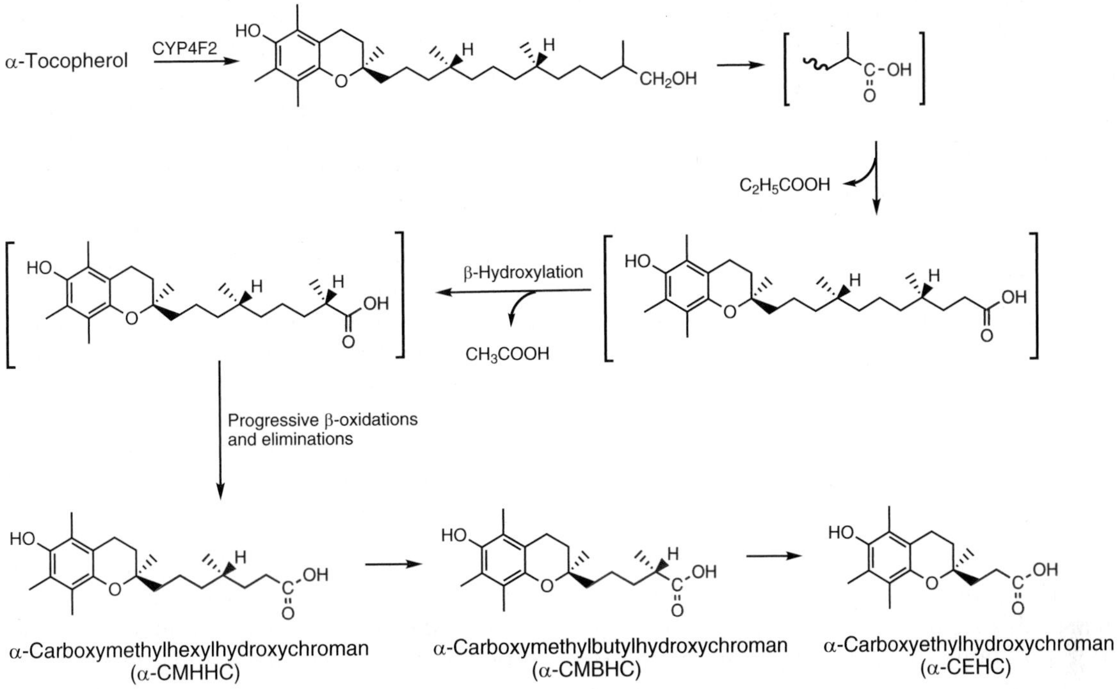

FIGURE 42.20 Metabolism of α-tocopherol.

Vitamin C, or ascorbic acid, is a water-soluble vitamin. The deficiency of vitamin C, known as scurvy, has a long history dating back to 3000 BC. Scurvy is a condition characterized by subcutaneous hemorrhage due to blood vessel rupture, commonly seen in the gingival, skin, and GI mucosa. With severe scurvy, loss of teeth, bone damage, internal bleeding, and infections occur, ultimately leading to death. Although the condition was described in the literature, it was not until the 1800s that its relationship to a chemical present in fruit juices became well known. It was another 100 years before Albert Szent-Gyorgyi identified and named the chemical in fruit juices that could prevent scurvy as ascorbic acid. Vitamin C is synthesized in plants from glucose and fructose, and most mammals can also synthesize this substance with the exception of humans, nonhuman primates, including guinea pigs, and several other animal species. Water-soluble vitamin C is often considered to be a vitamin that is not stored in the body and thus excessive levels will not build up in the body. Neither of these ideas is entirely correct. Vitamin C is stored in quantities sufficient to prevent scurvy for approximately 30 to 40 days, whereas large doses of vitamin C do have the potential for adverse effects (see below).

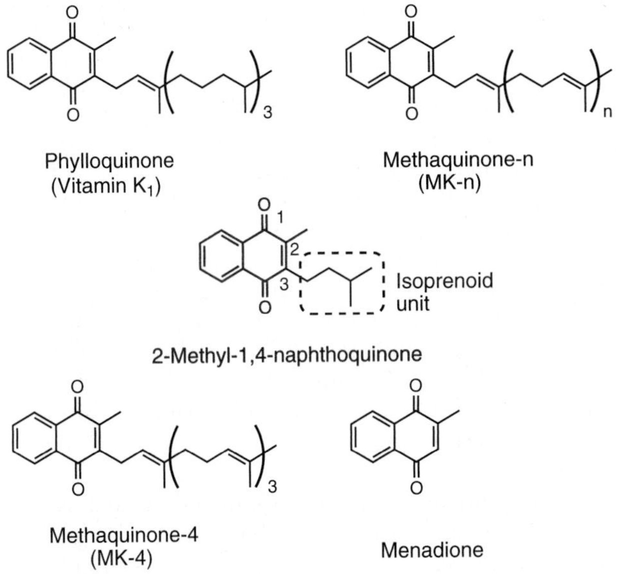

FIGURE 42.21 Structures of various vitamin K analogs.

Biologic Action Vitamin C is a water-soluble antioxidant by virtue of its ability to give up two electrons and in the process become oxidized (Fig. 42.22). The driving force for this activity resides in the fact that the ascorbyl free radical is stable and, with the loss of the second electron, ascorbic acid becomes dehydroascorbic acid, which following hydration is recycled back to ascorbic acid by reduction via glutathione. The relationship between the antioxidant property of vitamin C and scurvy is not known with certainty, but it is known that vitamin C is a cofactor in the hydroxylation of the amino acids proline and lysine, which are essential components of collagen. The hydroxylated amino acids have a role in stabilizing the helix structure of collagen,

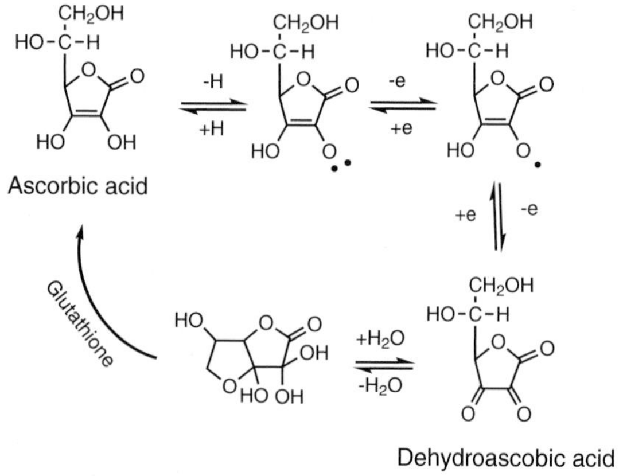

FIGURE 42.22 Antioxidant property of ascorbic acid.

and therefore, deficiency of vitamin C may impair the proper function of collagen. Collagen is part of the structural make up of connective tissue; thus vitamin C deficiency leads to gum deterioration and bleeding, adverse effects on bone integrity leading to teeth loss, and skin discoloration.

The antioxidant property of vitamin C has led to many suggestions as to additional biologic activity for vitamin C, which includes benefits in prevention of cardiovascular diseases. The anthrogenic properties of LDL are thought to relate to the oxidation of LDL to a peroxy radical, which then plaques onto the walls of blood vessels. Vitamin C may inhibit the initial oxidation. Increased consumption of vitamin C has been reported to correspond to a reduction in ischemic heart disease and a reduction in hypertension. Increased plasma levels of vitamin C, associated with increased consumption of fruits and vegetables (common sources of vitamin C), have been linked with a decrease in various cancers including oral cavity, esophagus, stomach, colon, and lung cancers. Suppression of ROS or radical intermediates serves as the basis for these claims. Doses in the gram quantity are often recommended for these actions, but clinical data are normally absent or complicated by other factors such as the benefits derived from simply increasing the intake of fruits and vegetables in the diet. Linus Pauling championed the concept that vitamin C was beneficial in treating some terminally ill cancer patients and could prevent or promote the recovery from the common cold. Data did not support the use of doses of up to 10 g/day for terminally ill cancer patients. As to the benefit of vitamin C in treatment of the common cold, it is felt that vitamin C will not prevent the common cold but may hasten the recovery from the cold. There is some evidence showing that vitamin C may increase the body's production of interferons, which in turn possess antiviral activity, thus supporting the claim for benefit in the common cold and potentially the treatment of viral-associated cancers.

Hypervitaminosis C The RDA for vitamin C is in the range of 60 to 75 mg/day, with higher amounts recommended for women during pregnancy and lactation and for smokers. Vitamin C–containing products are available with daily doses in the range of the RDAs all the way up to products that contain 1,000 mg per tablet or capsule. With such potent products available to the consumer, it is not uncommon for the patient to be consuming excessive quantities of vitamin C. High doses of vitamin C have been associated with increased oxalate excretion, with the potential for oxalate-based kidney stones, and will lower urine pH, affecting drug excretion. High doses, in the range of 3 g/day, may cause diarrhea and bloating, while even normal doses of vitamin C increase iron absorption, which in some individuals may cause health issues. Vitamin C prevents intestinal oxidation of ferrous ion to ferric ion, which is poorly absorbed from the GI tract.

Although vitamin C is an essential component in our diet, its role in good health and the biochemistry of the body is still not clear, and additional benefits can be expected to be elucidated in the future.

Sodium Chloride (Table Salt, NaCl)

The human body is composed of both organic and inorganic compounds. The inorganic nutrients generally are considered under the title of micronutrients and, just as with the organic micronutrients, are too numerous to cover in this chapter. The essential minerals include calcium, chromium, copper, iodine, iron, magnesium, manganese, molybdenum, phosphorus, selenium, and zinc, along with the essential electrolytes of sodium, potassium, and chloride. This discussion will be limited to sodium and chloride ions.

Dietary Role Sodium ion, most commonly consumed in the form of sodium chloride, is essential for various roles in the body. What is not known is just how much sodium chloride represents the minimum amount needed for good health. It is estimated that Americans consume approximately 10 to 12 g/day, which qualifies it as the second most common food additive (~15 lb/year). There is no RDA set for sodium chloride, although it is thought that an intake of less than 1,000 mg/day would meet the needs for a normal adult. The adequate intake and upper limit for sodium chloride are given as approximately 3.8 and 9.1 g/day, respectively, which would result in 1.5 to 3.6 g/day of sodium and 2.3 to 5.5 g/day of chloride (39.6% of sodium chloride is sodium and 60.4% of sodium chloride is chloride). The 2005 dietary guideline for sodium chloride consumption was established at 5.8 g/day (~1 teaspoon), or 2.3 g/day of sodium.

The human appetite for sodium chloride has both a physiologic and an educated basis. Taste receptors in the oral cavity can detect a salty taste presumably as a means of encouraging and assuring the intake of sodium chloride. But the human also has an educated appetite for salt. Commercially processed food commonly has added sodium, usually in the form of sodium chloride, as a preservative but also to improve the taste. It is estimated that as much as 65% to 85% of the daily consumed sodium chloride is present as "hidden salt" in processed food. In the case of baby food, sodium chloride may be added to meet the need to satisfy the parent who tastes the food rather than to meet a nutritional need of the child. As a result, the child grows up with a conditioned belief that a specific food must have a certain degree of saltiness, whether natural or "man enhanced." Many adults salt their food prior to tasting it because again they have a belief that the food must meet an expected level of saltiness.

The concern about sodium intake is not a new concern as indicated by the White House Conference on Food, Nutrition, and Health, which issued a report in which the role of sodium in hypertension was emphasized. Since this report, additional reports and studies have appeared, all of which suggest that Americans need to reduce their intake of sodium in the form of sodium chloride and that high sodium intake is associated with elevated blood pressure, heart disease, stroke, congestive heart failure, and renal disease. In the 1980s, the FDA made an attempt to sensitize the public to this growing public health issue, which at best resulted in a public awareness of sodium intake from processed foods and resulted in some manufacturers producing low-salt products, but in general attempts to actually reduce salt intake have failed. These efforts by the FDA were directed primarily at consumer education, and it was estimated that only about 30% of the consumers actually attempted to reduce sodium intake. In 2009, the Institute of Medicine Committee on Strategies to Reduce Sodium Intake convened and issued their report in 2010 (52). This comprehensive report indicates that although dietary sources of sodium are plentiful, a major contributor to sodium intake is processed and restaurant foods, whereas sodium added to food from the salt shaker amounts to only 5% of the sodium consumed. The report reached the conclusion that standards for sodium intake need to be set by the FDA and that a progressive decrease in sodium content of processed food and restaurant food needs to occur but that this reduction needs to be done in a way acceptable to the consumer. It is also noted that sodium does appear in the GRAS list, giving the FDA authority to set standards, but that these standards need to be done within the confines of GRAS and that sodium should not be removed from GRAS. A total of five recommendations were made (39), and basically the GRAS status of salt needs to be changed over time and in cooperation with the food industry. Throughout the changes in sodium content in foods, efforts need to be made to educate the public to the need for lowering sodium intake so as to lead to successful behavioral changes in the taste expectations of the public.

DIETARY SUPPLEMENTS

Two legislative acts that were passed by Congress in the 1990s have impacted nutrition in the United States. These are the NLEA of 1990 and the DSHEA of 1994. The NLEA allows companies, through petition to the FDA, to label their product with health claims linking food or food components to a reduced risk of a specific disease. The petitioning company is responsible for presenting evidence to support its claims. Among the claims that have appeared since this legislation went into effect are the following:

- Low sodium and a reduced risk of hypertension
- Calcium for the treatment of osteoporosis
- Fiber containing grains and a reduction in the risk of cancer
- Fruits, vegetables, and grains and the prevention of coronary heart disease
- Folic acid and the prevention of neural tube defects
- Soy protein and the prevention of coronary heart disease
- Whole-grain foods and the prevention of specific cancers
- Dietary lipids as the cause of cancer
- Dietary sugar alcohols and protection of dental caries
- Soluble fibers and the prevention of heart disease

The second act, DSHEA, allows companies to introduce dietary supplements without FDA approval provided "there is a history of use or other evidence to establishing safety." This legislation allows "structure-function" claims but not health claims without supportive evidence. The manufacturer must show safety of ingredients. A dietary supplement is a product that contains dietary ingredients, is taken by mouth, and is intended to supplement one's diet. Such products include vitamins, minerals, herbs, enzymes, amino acids, and metabolites.

As a result of these acts, various classes of nutrients have appeared on the market including nutraceuticals, functional foods, and the official use of foods titled as "organic foods." Nutraceuticals are defined as dietary supplements, foods, or medical foods that possess health benefits and that are safe for human consumption in such quantities and such frequency as required to realize beneficial properties. A functional food is a product that is conveyed in a conventional food format and has health benefits. Through these acts, various natural products have appeared as dietary supplements including *S*-adenosylmethionine (SAM-e), plant stanols, soy protein in "milk" products, and a number of herbal products being sold as dietary supplements.

SCENARIO: OUTCOME AND ANALYSIS

Outcome

Beverly Lukawski, PharmD, and Jennifer Campbell, PharmD

JL was diagnosed with exercise-induced syncope. After noting no previous medical or family history of cardiac conditions, the pharmacist recommended that she stop taking Kwik Loss and discussed the benefits a low-calorie, high-fiber diet and exercise.

Chemical Analysis

Victoria Roche and S. William Zito

Bitter orange contains an ephedrine-like alkaloid known as ρ-synephrine. Unlike ephedrine, ρ-synephrine has a phenolic OH group located *para* to the ethanolamine side chain, which prevents its entry into the CNS. Because it cannot reach α-adrenoceptors in the brain, it cannot stimulate them to induce an anorexic effect. It also cannot act indirectly to increase central levels of the endogenous α-receptor agonist norepinephrine. Therefore, this compound would have no value in a product designed to induce weight loss.

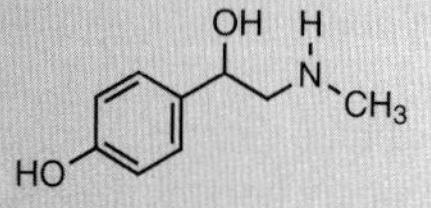

ρ-Synephrine

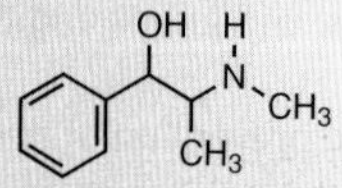

Ephedrine

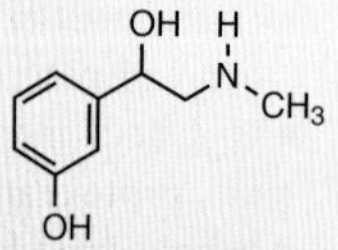

m-Synephrine

However, ρ-synephrine does have all the structural features required for direct stimulation of β-adrenergic receptors in the periphery. These features include a potentially cationic amine (ion–ion anchoring to Asp), benzylic OH (H donor in a hydrogen bond to Asn), and an N-CH_3 substituent (hydrophobic interaction with several residues within a spacious β-receptor lipophilic cleft). Although it is missing the catechol nucleus found on the most potent direct-acting adrenoceptor stimulators, the ρ-hydroxyl group is known to be most important for high β-receptor affinity. Stimulation of the β_1 receptors of the heart can induce tachycardia and an increased force of myocardial contraction. The enhanced cardiac output can elevate blood pressure, albeit not as significantly as α-receptor stimulation. It is the β_1-receptor stimulation of ρ-synephrine that is likely responsible for JL's rapid heart rate and (perhaps with some weak, residual α-receptor stimulation) her moderate, and hopefully transient, hypertension.

In contrast, a *m*-phenol selectively directs phenylethanolamines to α-adrenoceptors. *m*-Synephrine is commercially available as phenylephrine (Neo-Synephrine). Its vasoconstrictive properties make it useful as a nasal decongestant when administered locally (nasal spray) or orally, and it restores blood pressure in hypotensive crises when administered intravenously. *m*-Synephrine is not found naturally in bitter orange.

The other phenolic alkaloids associated with bitter orange are octopamine and *N*-methyltyramine. While extracts of bitter orange contain *N*-methyltyramine concentrations that are approximately 6% of ρ-synephrine's, the neutraceutical dosage form has concentrations of octopamine and *N*-methyltyramine that are 0.8% and 3.1% of the ρ-synephrine concentration, respectively (53). It is clear from their structures that both octopamine and *N*-methyltyramine would have activities similar to those exhibited by ρ-synephrine, and to the extent they are present, they would have contributed to JL's clinical presentation.

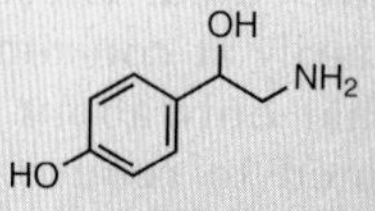

Octopamine

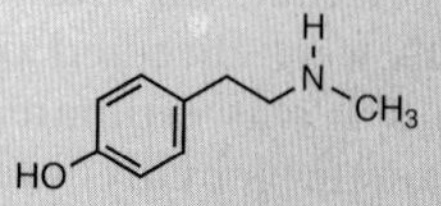

N-Methyltyramine

CASE STUDY

Victoria Roche and S. William Zito

BW is a 58-year-old woman who has been approximately 30 pounds overweight for as long as you, her neighborhood pharmacist, have known her. She sees you regularly because you are a Certified Diabetes Educator and BW, a type 2 diabetic, is taking a glipizide/metformin combination product in an attempt to stay off insulin for as long as possible. She does pretty well on this therapy, although she occasionally experiences drug-induced loose stools.

BW has always had good intentions of losing weight and following your wise counsel for modifying her diet and increasing her level of physical activity. She even bought a membership to the local gym. However, she is self conscious about being seen in exercise wear and always finds excuses to not go. In addition, she has an affinity for salty snacks (especially Kettle chips) that she knows are really bad for her, but she says she cannot help eating them when she feels hungry. Unfortunately, she generally enjoys a sugared soda when munching on those chips.

Today you are offering BW your condolences on the death of her father, who recently died from an aggressive form of colon cancer. Knowing the genetic implications of this cancer (and many others), BW says she is now more determined than ever to regain and maintain good health and to reach her target weight by exercising and eating right. She asks your advice about a natural way to "jump start" her weight loss initiative so she can achieve some initial success in the first few months of her new lifestyle. Specifically, she asks about snack foods that contain olestra, switching to diet soda (which contains aspartame), or taking Metamucil fiber supplement, which contains a hemicelluloses comprised of β-1,4-xylose units substituted with arabinose and additional xylose sugars. Which of those would you recommend to help BW on her way to a sustainably healthy lifestyle?

1. Conduct a thorough and mechanistic SAR analysis of the three therapeutic options in the case.
2. Apply the chemical understanding gained from the SAR analysis to this patient's specific needs to make a therapeutic recommendation.

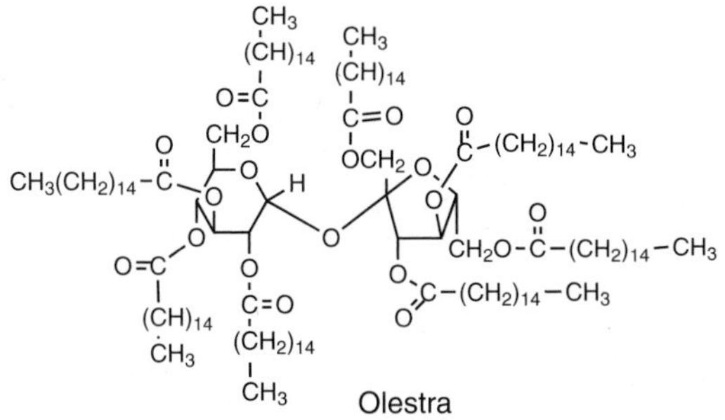

Olestra

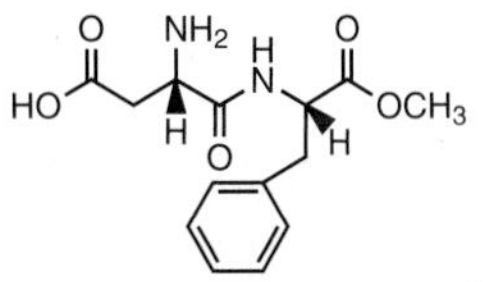

Aspartame

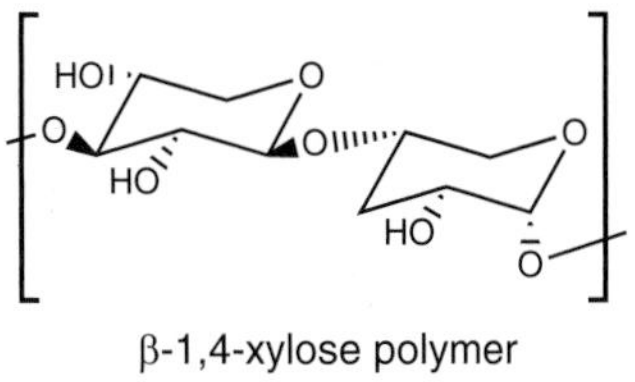

β-1,4-xylose polymer

References

1. Marinac JSM, Buchinger CL, Godfrey LA, et al. Herbal knowledge and dietary supplements: a survey of use, attitudes, and knowledge among older adults. J Am Osteopath Assoc 2007;107:13–23.
2. Bitter Orange. Natural Medicines Comprehensive Database. Available at: http://naturaldatabase.therapeuticresearch.com/home.aspx?cs=SCHOOLNOPL&s=ND. Accessed May 17, 2011.
3. Westerterp KR. Diet induced thermogenesis. Nutr Metab 2004;1:1-5.
4. Ogden CL, Carroll MD, Curtin LR, et al. Prevalence of overweight and obesity in the United States, 1999–2004. JAMA 2006;295:1549–5155.
5. National Heart, Lung, and Blood Institute Obesity Education Initiative. Clinical guidelines on the identification, evaluation, and treatment of overweight and obesity in adults. Bethesda, MD: National Institutes of Health, 1998. NIH Publication No. 98-4083.
6. Adams KF, Schatzkin A, Harris TB, et al. Overweight, obesity, and mortality in a large prospective cohort of persons 50 to 71 years old. N Engl J Med 2006;355:763–778.
7. Cleveland Clinic. Understanding adult obesity. Available at: http://my.clevelandclinic.org/disorders/obesity/hic_understanding_adult_obesity.aspx Accessed January 2011.
8. Putnam J, Allshouse J, Kantor LS. U.S. per capita food supply trends: more calories, refined carbohydrates, and fats. Food Rev 2002;25:2–15.
9. Nielsen SJ, Popkin BM. Patterns and trends in food portion sizes, 1977–1998. JAMA 2003;289:450–453.
10. Howarth NC, Saltzmen E, Roberts SB. Dietary fiber and weight regulation. Nutr Rev 2001;59:129–139.
11. Kemsley J. New fibers for foods. Chem Eng News 2010:38–40.
12. DeLaPena C. Empty Pleasures: The Story of Artificial Sweeteners from Saccharin to Splenda. Chapel Hill, NC: The University of North Carolina Press, 2010.
13. Whysmer J, Williams GM. Saccharin mechanistic data and risk assessment: urine composition, enhanced cell proliferation, and tumor promotion. Pharmacol Ther 1996;71:225–252.
14. Stegink L. The aspartame story: a model for the clinical testing of a food additive. Am J Clin Nutr 1987;46:204–215.
15. Kroger M, Meister K, Kava R. Low-calorie sweeteners and other sugar substitutes: a review of the safety issues. Compr Rev Food Sci Food Safety 2006;5:35–47.
16. Kuhn C, Bufe B, Winnig M, et al. Bitter taste receptors for saccharin and acesulfame-K. J Neurosci 2004;24:10260–10265.

17. Brusick DJ. A critical review of the genetic toxicity of steviol and steviol glycosides. Food Chem Toxicol 2008;46:S83–S91.
18. Pezzuto JM, Compadre CM, Swanson SM, et al. Metabolically-activated steviol, the aglycone of stevioside, is mutagenic. Proc Natl Acad Sci U S A 1985;82:2478–2482.
19. Jacoby M. Sowing the seeds of oil customization. Chem Eng News 2010:52–55.
20. Eller FJ, List GR, Teel JA, et al. Preparation of spread oils meeting U.S. Food and Drug Administration labeling requirements for trans fatty acids via pressure-controlled hydrogenation. J Agric Food Chem 2005;53:5982–5984.
21. Health Canada. Transforming the food supply: Report of the Trans Fat Task Force submitted to the Minister of Health. Available at: http://www.hc-sc.gc.ca/fn-an/nutrition/gras-trans-fats/tf-ge/tf-gt_rep-rap_e.html. Accessed February 2011.
22. Mozaffarian D, Katan MB, Ascherio A, et al. Trans fatty acids and cardiovascular disease. N Engl J Med 2006;354:1601–1613.
23. Wiley. Tutorial on fatty acid metabolism. Available at: http://www.wiley.com/college/pratt/0471393878/student/animations/fatty_acid/index.html.
24. Hu FB, van Dam RM, Liu S. Diet and risk of type II diabetes: the role of types of fat and carbohydrates. Diabetologia 2001;44:805–817.
25. Allshouse J, Frazao B, Turpening J. Are Americans turning away from lower fat salty snacks? Food Rev 2002;25:37–43.
26. National Heart, Lung, and Blood Institute Obesity Education Initiative. Clinical guidelines on the identification, evaluation, and treatment of overweight and obesity in adults. Bethesda, MD: National Institutes of Health, 1998. NIH Publication No. 98-4083.
27. Hadvary P, Lengsfeld H, Wolfer H. Inhibition of pancreatic lipase in vitro by the covalent inhibitor tetrahydrolipstatin. Biochem J 1988;256:357–361.
28. Hadvary P, Sidler W, Meister W, et al. The lipase inhibitor tetrahydrolipstatin binds covalently to the putative active site serine of pancreatic lipase. J Biol Chem 1991;266:2021–2027.
29. McNeely W, Benfield P. Orlistat. Drugs 1998;56:241–249.
30. Centers for Disease Control and Prevention. The Practical Guide: Identification, Evaluation and Treatment of Overweight and Obesity in Adults. Druid Hills, GA: Centers for Disease Control and Prevention, 2000.
31. WebMD. Diet pills and prescription weight loss drugs: how they work. Available at: http://www.webmd.com/diet/guide/weight-loss-prescription-weight-loss-medicine. Accessed June 8, 2011.
32. Nutt D, King LA, Saulsbury W, et al. Development of a rational scale to assess the harm of drugs of potential misuse. Lancet 2007;369:1047–1053.
33. Inoue T, Suzuki S. The metabolism of 1-phenyl-2-(N-methyl-N-benzylamino) propane (benzphetamine) and 1-phenyl-2-(N-methyl-N-furfurylamino)propane (furfenorex) in man. Xenobiotica 1986;16:691–698.
34. Rothman RB, Baumann MH. Therapeutic potential of monoamine transporter substrates. Curr Top Med Chem 2006;6:1845–1859.
35. Phenmetrazine hydrochloride. JAMA 1957;163:357.
36. The American Society of Health-System Pharmacists. Phentermine. Available at: http://www.drugs.com/monograph/phentermine.html. Accessed June 8, 2011.
37. Weintraub M, Sundaresan PR, Schuster B, et al. Long-term weight control study. I-IV. An open-label study of dose adjustment of fenfluramine and phentermine. Clin Pharmacol Ther 1992;51:595–633.
38. Connolly HM, Crary JL, McGoon MD, et al. Valvular heart disease associated with fenfluramine-phentermine. N Engl J Med 1997;337:581–588.
39. Wong DT, Fuller RW. Serotonergic mechanisms in feeding. Int J Obes 1987;11(Suppl 3):125–133.
40. Torp-Pedersen C, Caterson I, Coutinho W, et al. Cardiovascular responses to weight management and sibutramine in high-risk subjects: an analysis from the SCOUT trial. Eur Heart J 2007;28:2915–2923.
41. James WP, Caterson ID, Coutinho W, et al. Effect of sibutramine on cardiovascular outcomes in overweight and obese subjects. N Engl J Med 2010;363:905–917.
42. U.S. Food and Drug Administration Center for Drug Evaluation and Research. Consumer directed questions and answers about FDA's initiative against contaminated weight loss products. Available at: http://www.fda.gov/Drugs/ResourcesForYou/Consumers/QuestionsAnswers/ucm136187.htm. Accessed June 8, 2011.
43. Ross AC. Vitamin A and carotenoids. In: Shils ME, Shike M, Ross AC, et al., eds. Modern Nutrition in Health and Disease, 10th Ed. Philadelphia: Lippincott Williams & Wilkins, 2006.
44. Porter NA, Caldwell SE, Mills KA. Mechanisms of free radical oxidation of unsaturated lipids. Lipids 1995;30:277–290.
45. Kamal-Eldin A, Appelqvist L. The chemistry and antioxidant properties of tocopherols and tocotrienols. Lipids 1996;31:671–701.
46. Liebler DC, Burr JA. Antioxidant stoichiometry and the oxidative fate of vitamin E in peroxyl radical. Lipids 1995;30:789–793.
47. Sontag TJ, Parker RS. Cytochrome P450 omega-hydroxylase pathway of tocopherol catabolism novel mechanism of regulation of vitamin E status. J Biol Chem 2002;277:25290–25296.
48. Birringer M, Pfluger P, Kluth D, et al. Identities and differences in the metabolism of tocotrienols and tocopherols in HepG2 cells. J Nutr 2002;132:3113–3118.
49. Lodgea JK, Ridlingtonb J, Leonarda S, et al. Tocotrienols are metabolized to carboxyethyl-hydroxychroman derivatives and excreted in human urine. Lipids 2001;36:43–48.
50. Suttie JW. Vitamin K. In: Shils ME, Shike M, Ross AC, et al., eds. Modern Nutrition in Health and Disease, 10th Ed. Philadelphia: Lippincott Williams & Wilkins, 2006.
51. Booth SL, Suttie JW. Dietary intake and adequacy of vitamin K. J Nutr 1998;128:785–788.
52. Henney JE, Taylor CL, Boon CS, eds. Strategies to Reduce Sodium Intake in the United States. Institute of Medicine (US) Committee on Strategies to Reduce Sodium Intake. Washington, DC: National Academies Press, 2010.
53. Nelson BC, Putzbach K, Sharpless KE, et al. Mass spectrometric determination of the predominant adrenergic protoalkaloids in bitter orange (*Citrus aurantium*). J Agric Food Chem 2007;55:9769–9775.

APPENDIX A. pK_a and CLogP Values for Some Drugs and pK_a Values for Miscellaneous Organic Acids and Bases

DAVID A. WILLIAMS

TABLE A.1 pK_a Values for Some Drugs and Miscellaneous Organic Acids and Bases

Drugs	pK_a Values		ClogP*	Drugs	pK_a Values		ClogP*
	HA	HB^+			HA	HB^+	
Acebutolol		9.2	1.77	Amoxapine		7.6	1.89
Acenocoumarol	4.7		3.24	Amoxicillin	2.4	9.6	−1.99
Acetaminophen	9.7		0.8	Amphetamine		10.0	1.76
Acetanilide		0.5	1.14	Amphotericin B	5.5	10.0	2.30
Acetazolamide	7.4, 9.1		−0.26	Ampicillin	2.5	7.2	−1.28
α-Acetylmethadol		8.6	3.03	Amprenavir	1.76, 11.54		2.68
Acetysalicylic acid	3.5		1.19	Anileridine		3.7, 7.5	2.96
Acyclovir	9.3	2.3	−1.47	Antazoline		2.5, 10.1	3.58
Adriamycin		8.2	0.10	Antipyrine		1.5	0.28
Ajmaline		8.2	1.81	Apomorphine	8.9	7.0	1.70
Albuterol	10.3	9.3	0.69	Apraclonidine		9.22	0.87
Alclofenac	4.3		2.48	Aprobarbital	8.0		1.28
Alfentanil		6.5	2.16	Ariprazole		7.6[c]	3.76
Alfuzosin		8.13	1.26	Ascorbic acid	4.2, 11.6		−1.64
Allobarbital	7.8		0.94	Atomoxetine		9.23	3.36
Allopurinol	9.4		−0.14	Atenolol		9.6	0.33
Alphaprodine		8.7	2.49	Atropine		9.8	1.83
Alprenolol		9.7	2.89	Azatadine		9.3	2.69
Altretamine		10.3	2.52	Azathioprine	8.0		0.02
Amantadine		9.0	2.44	Azlocillin	2.8		0.83
Amiloride		8.7	0.93	Aztrenam	0.7, 2.9	3.9	0.49
Aminoacrine		10.0	2.74	Bacampicillin		6.8	3.52
p-Aminobenzoic acid	4.9	2.5	0.78	Baclofen	5.4	9.5	−0.96
Aminocaproic acid	4.4	10.8	−2.70	Barbital	7.9		0.70
Aminopterin	5.5		−0.9	Bendroflumethiazide	8.5		1.95
Aminopyrine		5.0	0.8	Benzocaine		2.5	1.86
p-Aminosalicylic acid	3.6	1.8	1.24	Benzphetamine		6.6	3.84
Aminothiadiazole		3.2	0.38	Benzquinamide		5.9	0.46
Amiodarone		6.6	7.81	Benztropine		10.0	4.03
Amitriptyline		9.4	4.41	Betaprodine		8.7	2.49
Amlodipine		8.7	3.01	Bethanidine		10.6	1.73
Amobarbital	7.8		1.58	Bitolterol			4.16

(Continued)

TABLE A.1 pK_a Values for Some Drugs and Miscellaneous Organic Acids and Bases (*Continued*)

Drugs	pK_a Values		ClogP*	Drugs	pK_a Values		ClogP*
	HA	HB+			HA	HB+	
Brimonidine		7.78	1.20	Cephacetrile			−1.60
Bosentan	5.46		4.36	Cephalexin[b]	3.2		0.35
Bromazepam	11.0	2.9	1.69	L-Cephaloglycin	4.6	7.1	−0.38
Bromocriptine[a]	15	6.6	–	Cephaloridine	3.4		−2.10
Bromodiphenhydramine		4.9	4.03	Cephalothin	2.5		−0.41
Brompheniramine		3.6, 9.8	3.24	Cephapirin			−0.41
Brucine		8.2, 2.5	1.41	Cephradine			0.48
Bufuralol		8.9	3.54	Cetirizine	2.9	8.3	1.62
Bumetanide	5.2, 10.0		2.88	Cevimeline		8.5	2.44
Bunolol		9.3	1.96	Chloral hydrate	10.0		0.99
Bupivacaine		8.1	3.31	Chlorambucil	5.8		2.61
Buprenorphine		8.42	2.83	Chlorcyclizine		2.1, 8.2	3.24
Bupropion		7.0	2.32	Chlordiazepoxide		4.8	2.49
Butabarbital	7.9		1.67	Chlorhexidine		10.8	4.57
Butacaine		9.0	4.62	Chloroquin		8.1, 9.9	4.41
Butaclamol		7.2	3.81	Chlorothiazide	6.8, 9.5		−0.24
Butamben		5.4	2.85	Chlorpheniramine		9.0	2.97
Butorphanol		8.6	3.54	Chlorphentermine		9.6	2.78
Butylated hydroxytoluene	7.5		5.17	Chlorpromazine		9.3	5.35
Butylparaben	8.5		3.57	Chlorpropamide	4.9		2.30
Caffeine	>14.0	0.6	−0.63	Chlorprothixene		8.8, 7.6	5.31
Camptothecin		10.8	0.95	Chlortetracycline[c]	3.3, 7.4	9.3	1.32
Captopril	3.7, 9.8		1.99	Chlorthalidone	9.4	1	0.70
Carbenicillin	2.7		1.13	Chlorzoxazone	8.3		2.25/1.82 lactam
Carbenoxolone	6.7, 7.1		6.63	Cimetidine		6.8	0.56
Carbidopa	7.8		−1.75	Cinchonine		4.3, 8.4	3.69
Carbinoxamine		8.1	2.69	Ciprofloxacin	6.0	8.8	1.63
Carisoprodol		4.2	2.10	Citalopram		9.59	3.47
Carpindolol		8.8	2.93	Clindamycin		7.5	1.75
Carvedilol		7.8	4.11	Clofibrate	3.5		3.88
Carteolol		9.74	1.34	Clonazepam	10.5	1.5	2.41
Cefaclor	1.5	7.2	0.14	Clonidine		8.3	1.52
Cefamandole	2.7		0.25	Clopenthixol		6.7, 7.6	3.91
Cefazolin	2.1		−0.70	Clopidogrel		4.55	2.50
Cefoperazone	2.6		−1.11	Clotrimazole		4.7	4.92
Cefotaxime	3.4		−0.51	Cloxacillin	2.8		2.83
Cefoxitin	2.2		−0.02	Clozapine		3.7, 7.4	3.94
Ceftazidime	1.8, 2.7	4.1	−2.50	Cocaine		8.7	2.28
Ceftizoxime	2.7	2.1	−0.65	Codeine		8.2	1.39
Ceftriaxone	3.2, 4.1	3.2	−0.54	Colchicine		1.9	1.07
Cefuroxime			0.26	Cromolyn	1.1, 1.9		2.00
Celecoxib	11.2		2.59	Cyclacillin	2.7	7.5	1.21

TABLE A.1 pK_a Values for Some Drugs and Miscellaneous Organic Acids and Bases (*Continued*)

Drugs	pK_a Values HA	pK_a Values HB+	ClogP*	Drugs	pK_a Values HA	pK_a Values HB+	ClogP*
Cyclamate	1.9		1.03	Diethazine		9.1	5.55
Cyclazocine		9.4	3.52	Diethylcarbamazepine		7.7	1.66
Cyclizine		8.0, 2.5	2.47	Diflunisal	3.0		3.65
Cyclobarbital	8.6		1.50	Dihydroergocriptine		6.9	6.37
Cyclobenzaprine		8.5	6.19	Dihydroergocristine		6.9	6.55
Cyclopentamine		11.5	2.46	Dihydroergotamine		6.9	5.69
Cyclopentolate		7.9	0.99	Dihydrostreptomycin		7.8	−1.49
Cycloserine		4.5, 7.4	−2.99	Dilevalol		9.5	3.09
Cyclothiazide[c]	9.1, 10.5		1.73	Diltiazem		7.7	4.73
Cyproheptadine		8.9	4.92	Dimethadione	6.1		0.77
Cytarabine		4.3	−2.17	Dimethisoquin		6.3	4.04
Dacarbazine		4.4	−0.24	Dinoprost[e]	4.9		2.59
Dantrolene	7.5		1.07	Dinoprostone	4.6		2.97
Dapsone		1.3, 2.5	0.99	Diperodon		8.4	4.65
Darifenicin		9.20	3.78	Diphenhydramine		9.1	3.27
Daunorubicin		8.4	0.54	Diphenoxin			3.97
Debrisoquin		11.9	0.75	Diphenoxylate		7.1	4.51
Dehydrocholic acid	5.12		1.89	Diphenylpyraline		8.9	3.43
Demeclocycline	3.3, 7.2	9.4	0.94	Dipipanone		8.5	5.10
Demoxepam		4.5, 10.6	0.73	Dipyridamole		6.4	3.35
Deprenyl		7.4	2.68	Disopyramide	10.2	8.4	2.33
Deserpidine[d]		6.7	4.95	Donepezil		9.1	3.91
Desipramine		10.4	3.97	Dobutamine		9.5	2.53
Desloratadine		4.2, 9.7	3.50	Dopamine	10.6	8.9	0.05
Desvenlafaxine				Dozazosin		6.93	2.85
Dextroamphetamine		9.9	1.76	Doxepin		9.0	3.85
Dextrobrompheniramine		9.3	3.24	Doxorubicin		8.2, 10.2	0.24
Dextrochlorpheniramine		9.2	2.97	Doxycycline	3.4, 7.7	9.5	1.78
Dextrofenfluramine		9.1	3.55	Doxylamine		4.4, 9.2	2.34
Dextroindoprofen	4.6		2.82	Droperidol		7.6	3.10
Dextromethorphan		8.3	3.89	Duloxetine		9.34	4.81
Dextromoramide		7.0	2.53	Emetine		8.2, 7.4	3.82
Diacetylmorphine (heroin)		7.8	1.58	Enalapril	3.0	5.5	3.25
Diatrizoic acid	3.4		0.49	Enalaprilat	2.3, 3.4	8.0	3.63
Diazepam		3.4	2.82	Entacapone	4.5, 10.72		3.02
Diazoxide	8.5		1.09	Ephedrine		9.6	1.43
Dibenzepin		8.3	3.26	Epinephrine	8.9	10.0	−0.54
Dibucaine		8.9	4.40	Ergometrine		7.3	2.48
Dichlorphenamide	7.4, 8.6		0.34	Ergonovine		6.8	2.48
Diclofenac	4.5		4.55	Ergotamine		6.4	7.37
Dicloxacillin	2.8		3.10	Erythromycin		8.8	2.48
Dicoumarol	4.4, 8.0		2.05	Esmolol		9.5	1.92
Dicyclomine		9.0	4.64	Estrone[f]	10.8		3.62

(*Continued*)

TABLE A.1 pK_a Values for Some Drugs and Miscellaneous Organic Acids and Bases (*Continued*)

Drugs	pK_a Values		ClogP*	Drugs	pK_a Values		ClogP*
	HA	HB+			HA	HB+	
Ethacrynic acid	3.50		2.84	Guanethidine		8.3, 11.9	1.10
Ethambutol		6.3, 9.5	−0.29	Guanabenz		8.1	2.66
Ethoheptazine		8.5	2.41	Guanoxan		12.3	0.83
Ethopropazine		9.6	4.77	Haloperidol		8.3	3.76
Ethosuximide	9.5		0.25	Hexobarbital	8.2		1.46
Ethyl biscoumacetate	7.5		1.61	Hexylcaine		9.1	3.65
Ethylmorphine		8.2	1.90	Hexylresorcinol	9.5		3.77
Ethylnorepinephrine		8.4	−0.40	Homatropine		9.7	1.30
Etidocaine		7.9	3.57	Hycanthone		3.4	3.81
Etomidate		4.2	3.05	Hydralazine		0.5, 7.1	1.00
Eugenol	9.8		2.40	Hydrochlorothiazide	7.0, 9.2		−0.02
Fenclofenac	4.5		4.59	Hydrocodone		8.9	2.57
Fenfluramine		9.1	3.55	Hydrocortisone	–		1.76
Fenoterol	10.0	8.6	1.33	Hydroflumethiazide	8.9, 10.7		−0.07
Fenoprofen	4.5		3.72	Hydromorphone		8.2	2.13
Fentanyl		8.4	3.68	Hydroxyamphetamine		9.3	1.14
fesoterodine		9.28	5.08	Hydroxyzine		2.0, 7.1	2.32
Fexofenadine	4.25	9.53	3.73	Hyoscyamine		9.7	1.79
Finasteride		12.4	3.83	Ibuprofen	5.2		3.50
Flurbiprofen	4.3		3.66	Imipramine		9.5	4.35
Flucloxacillin	2.7		2.89	Indacaterol			3.88
Flufenamic acid	3.9		5.22	Indapamide	8.8		1.96
Flumizole	10.7		4.26	Indomethacin	4.5		4.25
Flunitrazepam		1.8	2.13	Indoprofen	5.8		2.82
Fluoxetine		8.7	3.93	Indoramin		7.7	2.87
Flupenthixol		7.8	3.67	Iocetamic acid[g]	4.1 or 4.3		4.57
Fluphenazine enanthate		3.5, 8.2	7.29	Iodipamide	3.5		5.10
Fluphenazine		3.9, 8.1	3.92	Iodoquinol	8.0		4.10
Flurazepam	8.2	1.9	4.84	Iopanoic acid	4.8		4.65
Flutamide	13.12		3.52	Iprindole	8.2		5.02
Formoterol	7.9	9.2	2.03	Iproniazid		8.1	0.41
Furosemide	3.9		2.30	Ipronidazole		2.7	0.96
Fusidic acid	5.4		5.76	Irbesartan	4.9		5.25
Fluvoxamine		9.39	3.71	Isocarboxazid		10.4	1.63
Gabapentin	3.7	10.7	1.08	Isoniazid		2.0, 3.5, 10.8	−0.77
Galantamine		8.2	−0.05	Isoproterenol	10.1, 12.1	8.6	0.32
Gentamicin[b]		8.2	−3.55	Isoxsuprine	9.8	8.0	2.80
Glibenclamide	5.3		3.08	Kanamycin		7.2	–
Glipizide	5.9		1.88	Ketamine		7.5	3.01
Glutethimide	9.2		1.75	Ketobemidone		8.7	0.80
Glyburide	5.3		3.08	Ketoconazole		2.9, 6.5	404
Glycyclamine		5.5	2.81	Ketoprofen[h]	4.8		2.91
Guanfacine		7.1	1.33	Labetalol	8.7	7.4	2.72

TABLE A.1 pK_a Values for Some Drugs and Miscellaneous Organic Acids and Bases (*Continued*)

Drugs	pK_a Values		ClogP*	Drugs	pK_a Values		ClogP*
	HA	HB^+			HA	HB^+	
Lansoprazole		3.9	2.58	Methenamine		4.8	−0.17
Leucovorin	3.1, 8.1, 10.4		−1.43	Methicillin	3.0		1.02
Levallorphan	4.5	6.9	3.85	Methohexital	8.3		2.01
Levobunolol		9.2	1.96	Methotrexate	3.8, 4.8	5.6	−0.45
Levodopa	2.3, 9.7, 13.4	8.7	−1.15	Methotrimeprazine		9.2	4.94
Levonordefrin	9.8	8.6	−0.91	Methoxamine		9.2	0.61
Levorphanol		9.2	3.26, 3.26	Methoxyphenamine		10.1	2.12
Lidocaine		7.8	2.20	Methyclothiazide	9.4		1.42
Lincomycin		7.5	0.72	Methyl nicotinate		3.1	0.79
Liothyronine	8.4		3.91	Methyl paraben	8.4		1.88
Lisinopril	1.7, 3.3, 11.1	7.0	3.47	Methyl salicylate	9.9		2.52
Loperamide		8.6	4.15	Methyldopa	2.3, 10.4, 12.6	9.2	−0.74
Loratadine		5.0, 9.8	3.90	Methylergonovine		6.6	2.99
Lorazepam	11.5	1.3	2.35	Methylphenidate		8.8	2.31
Losartan	4.9, 4.7		3.46	Methylthiouracil	8.2		0.14
Loxapine		6.6	2.41	Methyprylon	12.0		0.65
Lysergide		7.5	2.71	Methysergide		6.62	1.81
Maprotiline		10.2	4.36	Metoclopramide		0.6, 9.3	2.16
Mazindol		8.6	2.36	Metolazone	9.7		3.16
Mecamylamine		11.2	2.98	Metopon		8.1	2.41
Meclizine		3.1, 6.2	5.28	Metoprolol		9.88	1.63
Meclofenamic acid	4.0		5.44	Metronidazole		2.6	−0.14
Medazepam		6.2	3.89	Metyrosine	2.7, 10.1		00.01
Mefenamic acid	4.2		4.83	Mexiletine		9.1	2.12
Memantine		10.8	3.0	Mezlocillin	2.7		0.33
Mepazine		9.3	5.04	Miconazole		6.7	4.97
Meperidine		8.7	2.19	Midazolam		6.2	3.80
Mephentermine		10.4	2.61	Minocycline	2.8, 5.0, 7.8	9.5	2.12
Mephobarbital	7.7		1.23	Minoxidil		4.6	1.62
Mepindolol		8.9	2.30	Mitomycin		10.9	−0.30
Mepivacaine		7.7	1.78	Molindone		6.9	−1.32
Mercaptopurine	7.8	11.0	−0.04	Montelukast	5.7		5.81
Mesalamine	2.7	5.8	0.74	Morphine	9.9	8.0	0.87
Metaproterenol	11.8	8.8	0.28	Morpholine		8.33	−0.79
Metaraminol		8.6	0.25	Moxalactam	2.5, 7.7, 10.2		−2.56
Methacycline	3.5, 7.6	9.5	1.35	Nabilone[b]	13.5		7.25
Methadone		8.3	3.93	Nadolol		9.67	0.56
Methamphetamine		10.0	2.20	Nafcillin	2.7		2.60
Methapyrilene		3.7, 8.9	2.78	Nalbuphine	10.0	8.7	1.21
Methaqualone		2.5	2.50	Nalidixic acid	6.0		0.03
Metharbital	8.2		1.50	Nalorphine		7.8	1.59
Methazolamide	7.3		0.13	Naloxone		7.9	1.78
Methdilazine		7.5	4.64	Naltrexone		8.13	2.05

(*Continued*)

TABLE A.1 pK_a Values for Some Drugs and Miscellaneous Organic Acids and Bases (*Continued*)

Drugs	pK_a Values		ClogP[*]	Drugs	pK_a Values		ClogP[*]
	HA	HB^+			HA	HB^+	
Naphazoline		10.9	2.99	Pentazocine	10.0	8.5	4.15
Naproxen	4.2		2.88	Pentobarbital	8.1		2.18
Nebivolol		7.1	4.08	Pentoxiphylline		0.3	0.29, 0.29
Nelfinavir	7.53	9.58	7.28	Pergolide		7.8[b]	3.90
Niacin/nicotinic acid	2.0	4.8	0.22	Perphenazine		3.7, 7.8	3.94
Nicotinamide		0.5, 3.4	−0.37	Perhexilene			6.46
Nicotine		3.1, 8.0	0.57	Phenacetin		2.2	1.66
Nikethamide		3.5	0.92	Phencyclidine		8.5	4.25
Nitrazepam	10.8	3.2	2.35	Phendimetrazine		7.6	1.64
Nitrofurantoin	7.1		−0.47	Phenethicillin	2.8		2.29
Norcodeine		5.7	0.52	Phenindamine		8.3	3.81
Nordefrin	9.8	8.5	−0.91	Phenindione	4.1		3.13
Norepinephrine	9.8, 12.0	8.6	−1.26	Pheniramine		4.2, 9.3	2.20
Norfenephrine		8.7	−0.60	Phenmetrazine		8.5	1.74
Normorphine		9.8	0.00	Phenobarbital	7.4		0.53
Nortriptyline		9.7	3.97	Phenolphthalein	9.7		1.91
Noscapine		6.2	2.38	Phenothiazine		2.5	4.15
Novobiocin	4.3, 9.1		3.74	Phenoxybenzamine		4.4	3.69
Nystatin[i]	8.9	5.1	2.46	Phentermine		10.1	2.20
Octopamine	9.5	8.9	−0.59	Phentolamine		7.7	4.08
Olanzapine		5.0, 7.4	3.08	Phenylbutazone	4.5		3.38
Omeprazole		4.0	2.36	Phenylephrine	10.1	8.8	0.12
Ondansetron		7.7	1.55	Phenylpropanolamine		9.4	0.36
Orphenadrine		8.4	3.33	Phenylsalicylate	2.98, 8.80[c]		2.75
Oxacillin	2.7		2.55	Phenyltoloxamine		9.1	3.46
Oxazepam	11.6	1.8	2.22	Phenyramidol		5.9	2.32
Oxprenolol		9.5	2.15	Phenytoin	8.3		2.47
Oxybutynin		7.0	5.05	Physostigmine		2.0, 8.2	1.27
Oxycodone		8.9	1.59	Pilocarpine		1.6, 7.1	−0.24
Oxymorphone	9.3	8.5	1.15	Pimozide		7.3, 8.6	5.76
Oxyphenbutazone	4.7		3.28	Pindolol		8.8	1.68
Oxypurinol	7.7		0.18	Piperazine		5.6, 9.8	−1.50
Oxytetracycline[c]	3.3, 7.3	9.1	0.48	Pipradrol		9.7	3.61
Pamaquine		1.3, 3.5, 10.0	4.38	Pirbuterol		3.0, 7.0, 10.3	0.04
Papaverine		6.4	2.95	Piroxicam	4.6		0.59
Pantoprazole	8.19	3.8	1.48	Pivampicillin		7.0	3.88
Pargyline		6.9	1.68	Polythiazide	9.8		2.05
Pemoline		10.5	0.42	Practolol		9.5	0.59
Penbutolol[c]		9.3	4.02	Pramipexole		10.8	2.35
Penicillamine	1.8, 10.5	7.9	0.85	Pramoxine		6.2	2.59
Penicillin G	2.8		1.92	Prasugrel		5.4	4.31
Penicillin V	2.7		1.94	Prazepam		2.9	3.70
Pentamidine		11.4	2.85	Prazosin		6.5	2.14

TABLE A.1 pK_a Values for Some Drugs and Miscellaneous Organic Acids and Bases (*Continued*)

Drugs	pK_a Values		ClogP*	Drugs	pK_a Values		ClogP*
	HA	HB^+			HA	HB^+	
Pregabalin	4.2	10.6	1.09	Serotonin	9.8	4.9, 9.1	0.54
Prenalterol	10.0	9.5	1.27	Sertraline		9.5	5.08
Prilocaine		7.9	2.03	Silodosin			2.52
Probenecid	3.4		2.51	Solifenacin		6.44	3.70
Procainamide		9.2	1.32	Sotalol	8.5	9.8	0.24
Procaine		8.8	2.26	Spiperone		8.3, 9.1	3.25
Procarbazine		6.8	0.06	Streptozocin		1.3	−1.23
Prochlorperazine		3.7, 8.1	4.65	Strychnine		2.3, 8.0	1.93
Promazine		9.4	4.69	Sufentanil		8.0	3.95
Promethazine		9.1	4.89	Sulfacetamide	5.4	1.8	−0.96
Proparacaine		3.2	3.46	Sulfadiazine	6.5	2.0	0.12
Propoxycaine		8.6	2.70	Sulfaguanidine	12.1	2.8	−1.22
Propoxyphene		6.3	4.10	Sulfamerazine	7.1	2.3	0.11
Propranolol		9.5	2.90	Sulfamethazine	7.4	2.4	0.30
Propylhexedrine		10.4	2.98	Sulfamethoxazole	5.6		0.66
Propylthiouracil	7.8		1.15	Sulfasalazine	2.4, 9.7, 11.8		3.05
Pseudoephedrine		9.5	1.43	Sulfathiazole	7.1	2.4	0.05
Pyrathiazine		8.9	4.15	Sulfinpyrazone	2.8		1.89
Pyrazinamide		0.5	−0.17	Sulfisoxazole	5.0		1.01
Pyridoxine	8.96	5.0	−0.83	Sulindac	4.5		2.55
Pyrilamine		4.0, 8.9	2.67	Sulpiride		9.1	0.78
Pyrimethamine		7.3	2.75	Sulthiame	10.0		0.56
Pyrrobutamine		8.8	4.57	p-Synephrine	10.2	9.3	0.13
Quinacrine		8.2, 10.2	5.59	Talbutal	7.8		1.79
Quinidine		4.2, 7.9	2.82	Tamsulosin	10.23	8.37	2.14
Quinine		4.2, 8.5	2.82	Tamoxifen		8.9	5.13
Ranitidine		2.3, 8.2	−0.07	Tapentadol		9.34	3.02
Resperidone	3.11	8.24	3.04	Terazosin		7.1	0.80
Reserpine		6.6	3.65	Temazepam		1.6	2.19
Rifampin	1.7	7.9	2.05	Terbutaline	10.1, 11.2	8.8	0.70
Rimoterol	10.3	8.7	0.74	Tetracaine		8.4	3.75
Ritodrine		9.0	2.04	Tetracycline	3.3, 7.7	9.7	0.62
Rivastigmine		8.85	2.05	Tetrahydrocannabinol (THC)		10.6	6.84
Rolitetracycline	7.4		1.66	Tetrahydrozoline		10.5	2.85
Ropinirole		9.5	2.49	Theobromine	10.1	0.1	−1.06
Rotoxamine		8.1	2.69	Theophylline	8.6	3.5	−0.02
Saccharin	1.6		0.91	Thiazbendazole		4.7	2.47
Salicylamide	8.2		1.35	Thiamylal	7.5		2.81
Salicylic acid	3.0, 13.4		2.01	Thioguanine	8.2		−0.28
Salmeterol	9.26	9.99	3.71	Thiopental	7.5		2.63
Salsalate	3.5, 9.8		3.29	Thiopropazate		3.2, 7.2	4.76
Scopolamine		7.6	0.69	Thioridazine		9.5	5.90
Secobarbital	7.9, 12.6		2.30	Thiothixene		7.7, 7.9	3.72

(*Continued*)

TABLE A.1 pK_a Values for Some Drugs and Miscellaneous Organic Acids and Bases (*Continued*)

Drugs	pK_a Values		ClogP*	Drugs	pK_a Values		ClogP*
	HA	HB+			HA	HB+	
Thiouracil	7.5		0.85	Vidarabine		3.5, 12.5	−1.23
Thonzylamine		2.2, 9.0	1.86	Vigabatrin	4.02	9.72	−0.30
l-Thyroxine	2.2, 6.7	10.1	4.72	Viloxazine		8.1	1.24
tiagabine	3.3	9.4	4.03	Vinblastine		5.4, 7.4	5.92
Ticarcillin	2.6, 3.4		1.24	Vincristinej		5.0, 7.4	5.75
Ticrynafen	2.7		3.05	Vindesine		6.0, 7.7	4.94
Timolol		8.8	1.28	Voriconazole	2.72, 11.54		1.21
Timoprazole		3.1, 8.8	1.22	Warfarin	5.1		3.13
Tiotidine		6.8	0.35	Xylometazoline		10.2	4.59
Tobramycin		6.7, 8.3, 9.9	−4.22	Zimeldine		3.8, 8.74	3.07
Tocainide		7.5	0.81	Zonisamide		10.2	0.72
Tolamolol		7.9	2.03	Miscellaneous organic acids and bases			
Tolazamide	3.1	5.7	1.54	Acetic acid	4.8		
Tolazoline		10.3	1.80	Allylamine			
Tolbutamide	5.4		2.36	6-Aminopenicillanic acid	2.3		
tolcapone	10.63		2.12	Ammonia		9.3	
Tolmetin	3.5		2.68	Aniline		4.63	
Toloteridine		9.87	5.23	Benzoic acid	4.2		
Topiramate	8.67		2.16	Benzyl alcohol	18.0		
Tramadol		9.41	2.32	Benzylamine		9.33	
Tramazoline		10.7	2.78	Butyric acid	4.8		
Tranylcypromine		8.2	1.47	Carbonic acid	6.4, 10.4		
Trazodone		6.7	2.76	Citric acid	3.1, 4.8, 5.4		
Triamterene		6.2	1.16	Diethanolamine		8.9	
Trichlormethiazide	8.6		0.13	Diethylamine		11.09	
Trifluoperazine		3.9, 8.1	4.62	Dimethylamine		10.73	
Triflupromazine		9.2	5.16	Ethanol	15.6		
Trimeprazine		9.0	5.04	Ethanolamine		9.5	
Trimethobenzamide		8.3	1.26	Ethylamine		10.7	
Trimethoprim		6.6	0.91	Ethylenediamine		7.56, 10.71	
Trimipramine		8.0	4.71	Fumaric acid	3.0, 4.4		
Tripelennamine		4.2, 8.7	2.78	Gluconic acid	3.6		
Triprolidine		6.5	3.25	Glucuronic acid	3.2		
Troleandomycin		6.6	3.46	Guanidine		13.6	
Tropicamide		5.3	0.64	Imidazole		7.0, 14.9	
Tuaminoheptane		10.5	2.43	Isopropylamine		10.63	
Tubocurarine		8.1, 9.1	0.77	Lactic acid	3.9		
Tyramine	10.9	9.3	0.78	Maleic acid	1.9		
Valdenafil	6.13, 2.02	9.11	3.64	Mandelic acid	3.4		
Valproic acid	4.8		2.58	Methylamine		10.66	
Valsartan	6.0		4.02	Monochloroacetic acid	2.9		
Venlafaxine		9.4	2.47	N-propylamine		10.6	
Verapamil		8.9	4.02	Nitromethane	11.0		

TABLE A.1 pK_a Values for Some Drugs and Miscellaneous Organic Acids and Bases (*Continued*)

Drugs	pK_a Values		ClogP*	Drugs	pK_a Values		ClogP*
	HA	HB^+			HA	HB^+	
Phenol	9.9			Trichloroacetic acid	0.9		
Phthalic acid	2.9			Triethanolamine		7.8	
Resorcinol	9.2, 11.3			Triethylamine		10.75	
Sorbic acid	4.8			Trimethylamine		9.8	
Succinimide	9.6			Tropic acid	4.1		
Tartaric acid	3.0, 4.4			Tropine		10.8	
p-Toluidine		5.3		Uric acid	5.4		

*ClogP values calculated on basis of unionized molecules. Calculate Log $D_{pH\,7.4}$ to determine distribution/partition coefficient at pH 7.4. ClogP cacluated with ACD/Log P 12v., Advanced Chemical Development, Toronto, Canada, 2010.
[a]Determined in methyl cellosolve/water (8:2 w/w mixture).
[b]Determined in 66% dimehylformamide.
[c]Determined in 25% to 30% ethanol.
[d]Determined in 40% methanol.
[e]Prostaglandin $F_{2\alpha}$.
[f]Spectrophotometric determination.
[g]The p*K*a values of the four optical isomers are 4.1 for two isomers and 4.25 for two isomers.
[h]Determined in methanol/water (3:1 mixture).
[i]Determined in dimethylformamide/water (1:1 mixture).
[j]Determined in 33% dimehylformamide.

General References for pK_a and ClogP Values

Albert A, Serjeant EP. The Determination of Ionization Constants of Acids and Bases: A Laboratory Manual, 3rd ed. New York: Chapman and Hall, 1984.

Florey K, ed. Analytical Profiles of Drugs Substances. New York: Academic Press, 1978.

Hansch C, Leo AJ. Substituent Constants for Correlation Analysis in Chemistry and Biology. New York: Wiley, 1979.

Hansch C, Sammes PG, Taylor JB, eds. Comprehensive Medicinal Chemistry, vol 6. Oxford: Pergamon Press, 1990.

O'Neil A, Heckelman PE, Koch CB, et al. The Merck Index, 14th ed. Rahway, NJ: Merck and Co, 2006.

Perrin DD, Dempsey B, Serjeant EP. p*K*a Prediction for Organic Acids and Bases. New York: Chapman and Hall, 1981.

Serjeant EP, Dempsey B. Ionization Constants of Organic Acids in Aqueous Solution. IUPAC Chemical Data Series No. 23. Oxford, UK: Pergamon Press, 1979.

Sinko P. Martin's Physical Pharmacy and Pharmaceutical Sciences, 5th ed. Baltimore: Lippincott Williams & Wilkins, 2005.

APPENDIX B. pH Values for Tissue Fluids

David A. Williams

TABLE B.1 pH Values for Tissue Fluids

Fluid	pH
Aqueous humor	7.2
Blood, arterial	7.4
Blood, venous	7.4
Blood, maternal umbilical	7.3
Cerebrospinal fluid	7.4
Colon[a]	
Fasting	5–8
Fed	5–8
Duodenum[a]	
Fasting	4.4–6.6
Fed	5.2–6.2
Feces[b]	7.1 (4.6–8.8)
Ileum[a]	
Fasting	6.8–8.6
Fed	6.8–8.0
Intestine, microsurface	5.3
Lacrimal fluid (tears)	7.4
Milk, breast	7.0
Muscle, skeletal[c]	6.0
Nasal secretions	6.0
Prostatic fluid	6.5
Saliva	6.4
Semen	7.2
Stomach[a]	
Fasting	1.4–2.1
Fed	3–7
Sweat	5.4
Urine	5.8 (5.5–7.0)
Vaginal secretions, premenopause	4.5
Vaginal secretions, postmenopause	7.0

[a]Dressman JB, Amidon GL, Reppas C, et al. Dissolution testing as a prognostic tool for oral drug absorption. Pharm Res 1998;15:11–22.
[b]Value for normal, soft, formed stools. Hard stools tend to be more alkaline, whereas watery, unformed stools are acidic.
[c]Studies conducted intracellularly on the rat.

Drug Index

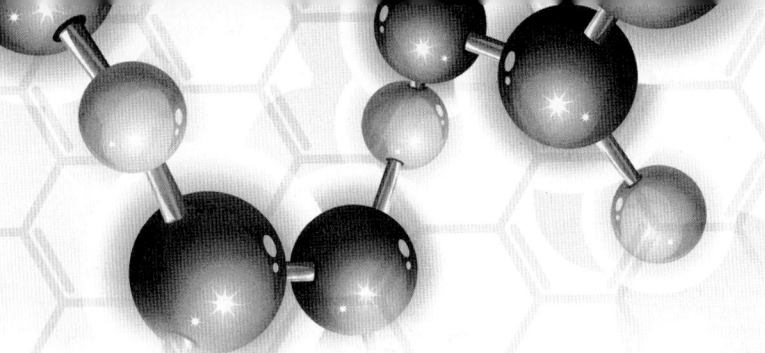

Page numbers followed by "f" indicate illustrations and chemical structures those followed by "t" indicate to tables. Drugs are listed under the generic name.

Subject Index

Note: Page numbers followed by "f" indicate illustrations and chemical structures; those followed by "t" indicate to tables. Drugs are listed under the generic name.

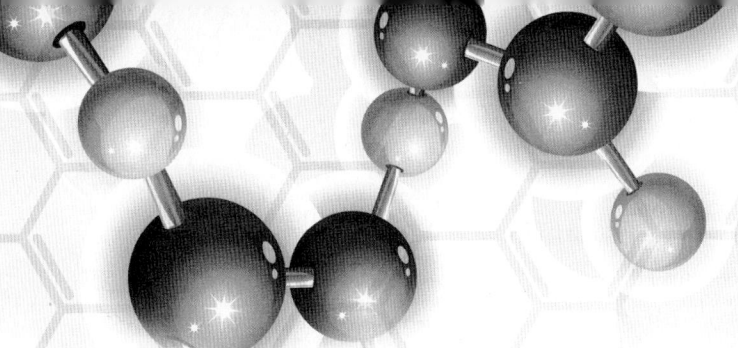

D